The 5-Minute Clinical Consult 2025

2025

33rd EDITION

The 5-Minute Clinical Consult 2025

33rd Edition

Editor-in-Chief

Frank J. Domino, MD
Professor and Director of Predoctoral Education
Department of Family Medicine and Community Health
UMass Chan Medical School
Worcester, Massachusetts

Associate Editors

Robert A. Baldor, MD, FAAFP
Professor and Founding Chair
Department of Family Medicine
UMass Chan Medical School-Baystate
Springfield, Massachusetts
Designated Institutional Official
Baystate Franklin Medical Center
Greenfield, Massachusetts

Kathleen A. Barry, MD
Associate Professor
UMass Chan Medical School
Department of Family Medicine and Community Health
Hahnemann Family Health Center
Worcester, Massachusetts

Jeremy Golding, MD, FAAFP
Professor of Family Medicine and Obstetrics & Gynecology
UMass Chan Medical School
Department of Family Medicine and Community Health
University of Massachusetts Memorial Health Care
Hahnemann Family Health Center
Worcester, Massachusetts

Mark B. Stephens, MD, MS, FAAFP
Associate Dean for Medical Education
Professor of Family and Community Medicine
Professor of Humanities
Penn State College of Medicine
University Park, Pennsylvania

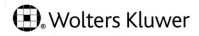 Wolters Kluwer

Philadelphia · Baltimore · New York · London
Buenos Aires · Hong Kong · Sydney · Tokyo

5MinuteConsult™

Director, Medical Practice: Brian Brown
Associate Director of Medicine Content Development: Anne Malcolm
Acquisitions Editor: Joe Cho
Development Editor: Cindy Yoo
Editorial Assistant: Kristen Kardoley
Marketing Manager: Kirsten Watrud
Production Project Manager: Bridgett Dougherty
Manager, Graphic Arts & Design: Stephen Druding
Manufacturing Coordinator: Lisa Bowling
Prepress Vendor: Absolute Service, Inc.

33rd edition

9 8 7 6 5 4 3 2 1

Printed in Mexico

Library of Congress Cataloging-in-Publication Data available from the Publisher upon request.
ISBN-13: 978-1-9752-3472-0

shop.lww.com

QUADM0324

This edition is dedicated to Lauren Evelyn Clark.

MARK B. STEPHENS, MD, MS, FAAFP

PREFACE

"...to know that one life has breathed easier because you lived. This is to have succeeded."

This is the last line of poem attributed to Ralph Waldo Emerson. I share it with my fourth-year med students every year. And added it to this book a few years back.

Very few professions offer this opportunity to help someone "breathe easier," both literally and metaphorically. We have challenging and amazing professions. To know more about someone than their spouse; sometimes even more than they know about themselves and the opportunity to help them live physically, mentally, and emotionally better is a huge task and our "superpower."

Yet, in the hectic minutes of our busy days, we may not be aware of or mindful of all that we have and all that we do.

Anthropologist Jane Goodall reminds us:

"You cannot get through a single day without having an impact on the world around you. What you do makes a difference, and you have to decide what kind of difference you want to make."

Making the decision to have this impact, to make one person's world, and the entire world, a better place comes at great personal cost and sacrifice (I know). The fulfillment of helping someone breathe easier is your gift. And maybe your payment.

Thank you.

Welcome to the 2025 edition of *The 5-Minute Clinical Consult*. Your clinical practice is full of challenges and unanswered questions. Your use of this amazing tool will provide you with the answers needed to help your patients live to their fullest.

The 5-Minute Clinical Consult is here to assist in fulfilling our role as health care providers. In each patient interaction, in addition to bringing your clinical expertise, remember how your patients view you—as their advocate, someone who prioritizes their well-being unlike anyone else.

Our editorial team has collaborated with hundreds of authors so that you may deliver your patients the best care. Each topic provides you with quick answers you can trust, where and when you need them most, either in print or online.

This highly organized content online provides you with the following:
- Differential diagnosis support from our expanded collection of algorithms
- Current evidence-based designations highlighted in each topic covering 500+ commonly encountered diseases in print, with an additional 1,000 online adult and pediatric diseases and conditions topics:
- FREE point-of-care CME and CE: 1/2-hour credit for every digital search
- A to Z drug database from Facts & Comparisons
- Laboratory test interpretation from *Wallach's Interpretation of Diagnostic Tests*
- More than 3,000 patient handouts in English and Spanish
- ICD-10 codes; additionally, SNOMED codes are available online.

Our Web site delivers quick answers to your questions. It is an ideal resource for patient care. Integrating *The 5-Minute Clinical Consult* content into your workflow is easy and fast, and our patient education handouts can assist in helping you meet meaningful use compliance.

The site provides an easy-to-use interface, allowing smooth maneuverability between topics, algorithms, images, videos, and patient education materials as well as more than 1,000 online-only topics.

Evidence-based health care is the integration of the best medical information with the values of the patient and your skill as a clinician. We have updated our evidence-based medicine (EBM) content so you can focus on how to best apply it in your practice.

The algorithm section includes both diagnostic and treatment algorithms. This easy-to-use graphic method helps you evaluate an abnormal finding and prioritize treatment. They are also excellent teaching tools, so share them with the learners in your office.

This book and Web site are a source to solve problems and to help evaluate, diagnose, and treat patients' concerns. Use your knowledge, expressed through your words and actions, to address their anxiety.

The 33rd edition means I have had the great fortune to help grow and support this content for half of its life. I am honored to play this role and hope to keep doing so for some years to come. I thank you, the reader, and the team at Wolters Kluwer for your support.

The 5-Minute Clinical Consult editorial team values your observations, so please share your thoughts, suggestions, and constructive criticism through our Web site's contact form.

FRANK J. DOMINO, MD

EVIDENCE-BASED MEDICINE

WHAT IS EVIDENCE-BASED MEDICINE?

We used to treat every otitis media with antibiotics. These recommendations came about because we applied logical reasoning to observational studies. If bacteria cause an acute otitis media, then antibiotics should help it resolve sooner, with less morbidity. Yet, when rigorously studied (via a systematic review), we found little benefit to this intervention.

The underlying premise of EBM is the evaluation of medical interventions and the literature that supports those interventions in a systematic fashion. EBM hopes to encourage treatments proven to be effective and safe. And when insufficient data exist, it hopes to inform you on how to safely proceed.

EBM uses end points of real patient outcomes, morbidity, mortality, and risk. It focuses less on intermediate outcomes (bone density) and more on patient conditions (hip fractures).

Implementing EBM requires three components: the best medical evidence, the skill and experience of the provider, and the values of the patients. Should this patient be screened for prostate cancer? It depends on what is known about the test, on what you know of its benefits and harms, your ability to communicate that information, and that patient's informed choice.

This book hopes to address the first EBM component, providing you access to the best information in a quick format. Although not every test or treatment has this level of detail, many of the included interventions here use systematic review literature support.

The language of medical statistics is useful in interpreting the concepts of EBM. Below is a list of these terms, with examples to help take the confusion and mystery out of their use.

> **Prevalence:** proportion of people in a population who have a disease (in the United States, 0.3% [3 in 1,000] people >50 years old have colon cancer)
> **Incidence:** how many *new* cases of a disease occur in a population during an interval of time; for example, "The estimated incidence of colon cancer in the United States is 104,000 in 2005."
> **Sensitivity:** percentage of people with disease who test positive; for mammography, the sensitivity is 71–96%.
> **Specificity:** percentage of people without disease who test negative; for mammography, the specificity is 94–97%.

Suppose you saw ML, a 53-year-old woman, for a health maintenance visit, ordered a screening mammogram, and the report demonstrates an irregular area of microcalcifications. She is waiting in your office to receive her test results; what can you tell her?

Sensitivity and specificity refer to people who are known to have disease (sensitivity) or those who are known not to have disease (specificity). But what you have is an abnormal test result. To better explain this result to ML, you need the positive predictive value.

> **Positive predictive value (PPV):** percentage of positive test results that are truly positive; the PPV for a woman aged 50 to 59 years is approximately 22%. That is to say that only 22% of abnormal screening mammograms in this group truly identified cancer. The other 78% are false positives.

You can tell ML only 1 out of 5 abnormal mammograms correctly identifies cancer; the other four are false positives, but the only way to know which mammogram is correct is to do further testing.

> **The corollary of the PPV is the negative predictive value (NPV),** which is the percentage of negative test results that are truly negative.

The PPV and NPV tests are population dependent, whereas the sensitivity and specificity are characteristics of the test and have little to do with the patient in front of you. So when you receive an abnormal lab result, especially a screening test such as mammography, understand their limits based on their PPV and NPV.

Treatment information is a little different. In discerning the statistics of randomized controlled trials of interventions, first consider an example. The Scandinavian Simvastatin Survival Study (4S) (*Lancet.* 1994;344[8934]:1383–1389) found using simvastatin in patients at high risk for heart disease for 5 years resulted in death for 8% of simvastatin patients versus 12% of those on placebo; this results in a relative risk of 0.70, a relative risk reduction of 33%, and a number needed to treat of 25.

There are two ways of considering the benefits of an intervention with respect to a given outcome. The absolute risk reduction is the difference in the percentage of people with the condition before and after the intervention. Thus, if the incidence of myocardial infarction (MI) was 12% for the placebo group and 8% for the simvastatin group, the absolute risk reduction is 4% (12% − 8% = 4%).

The relative risk reduction reflects the improvement in the outcome as a percentage of the original rate and is commonly used to exaggerate the benefit of an intervention. Thus, if the risk of MI were reduced by simvastatin from 12% to 8%, then the relative risk reduction would be 33% (4% / 12% = 33%); 33% sounds better than 4%, but the 4% is the absolute risk reduction and reflects the true outcome.

Absolute risk reduction is usually a better measure of clinical significance of an intervention. For instance, in one study, the treatment of mild hypertension has been shown to have relative risk reduction of 40% over 5 years (40% fewer strokes in the treated group). However, the absolute risk reduction was only 1.3%. Because mild hypertension is not strongly associated with strokes, aggressive treatment of mild hypertension yields only a small clinical benefit. Don't confuse relative risk reduction with relative risk.

> **Absolute (or attributable) risk (AR):** the percentage of people in the placebo or intervention group who reach an end point; in the 4S, the absolute risk of death was 8%.

Relative risk (RR): the risk of disease of those treated or exposed to some intervention (i.e., simvastatin) divided by those in the placebo group or who were untreated

- If RR is <1.0, it reduces risk—the smaller the number, the greater the risk reduction.
- If RR is >1.0, it increases risk—the greater the number, the greater the risk increase.

Hazard ratio: the probability of an event in a treatment group versus the probability of events in a control group at a given time (can be calculated at any time in the study; often applied to observational data); like RR, if HR is statistically <1.0, it reduces risk; if >1.0, increases risk.

Relative risk reduction (RRR): the relative decrease in risk of an end point compared to the percentage of that end point in the placebo group

If you are still confused, just remember that the RRR is an overestimation of the actual effect.

Number needed to treat (NNT): This is the number of people who need to be treated by an intervention to prevent one adverse outcome. A "good" NNT can be a large number (100) if risk of serious outcome is great. If the risk of an outcome is not that dangerous, then lower (25) NNTs are preferred.

The NNT should be compared to a similar statistic, the number needed to harm (NNH). This is the number of people who have to be given treatment before one excess side effect or harm occurs. When the NNT is compared to the NNH, you and the patient can judge whether the benefit of the intervention is great enough to outweigh the risk of harm.

EVIDENCED-BASED GRADING

To help you interpret diagnostic and treatment recommendations within *The 5-Minute Clinical Consult*, we have graded the best information within the text and highlighted this content.

An "A" grade means the reference is from the highest quality resource, such as a systematic review. A systematic review is a summary of the medical literature on a given topic that uses strict, explicit methods to perform a thorough search of the literature and then provides a critical appraisal of individual studies, concluding in a recommendation. The most prestigious collection of systematic reviews is from the Cochrane Collaboration (www.cochrane.org).

A "B" grade means the data referenced comes from high-quality randomized controlled trials performed to minimize bias in their outcome. Bias is anything that interferes with the truth; in the medical literature, it is often unintentional, but it is much more common than we appreciate. In short, always assume some degree of bias exist in any research endeavor.

A "C" grade implies the reference used does not meet the A or B requirements; they are often treatments recommended by consensus groups (such as the American Cancer Society). In some cases, they may be the standards of care. But implicit in a group's recommendation is the bias of the author or the group that supports the reference.

BIAS

Bias is anything that interferes with the truth. There are many types of bias that should be considered by the publishers of medical information. Below describes a number of bias types that often affect our care without us knowing it is present.

Publication bias occurs when research is not published. The motivation to publish information that "didn't work" is low. It is estimated up to 40% of all medical research never gets published. When you read of an effective intervention, wonder if other studies did not show benefit and went unpublished.

Comparator bias occurs when research compares an intervention to not the standard of care. Knowing a new treatment is more effective than placebo for treating a condition is not helpful if you typically use a drug or procedure. Why not study comparing the new to the standard of care? Sometimes, the new treatment is no better than the current standard. And if a study was done to see if the new is better than the old and not published, you have an example of publication bias.

Selection bias involves choosing study populations that might be different than the average patient or just reporting a just subset of study participants from a study. Either will result in the data being skewed because it can only be applied to small subset of people.

Attrition bias and the concept of intention to treat. Attrition bias is when researchers address how a study deals with participants who do not adhere to the research protocol or drop out completely. Intention to treat analysis hopes to diminish attrition bias by statistically considering the nonadhering or dropped out patients as unsuccessfully benefiting from the intervention.

Commercial (funder) bias involves who paid for the research being done, and do they have a vested interest in the outcome. If the developer of a new drug does a large study, or a researcher has a personal financial interest in seeing a study succeed, they may consciously or unconsciously alter what is reported. The data may be accurate, but until this is studied by less vested interests, it is difficult to accept the conclusions.

A systematic review gathers all the literature on a topic, say using antibiotics to treat otitis media, and combines the data to determine if the sum of all the trials tells a different story than any single trial. The large number of participants in this type of research results in a much more statistically (and clinically) significant conclusion than any single paper.

A meta-analysis is a quantitative systematic review and demonstrates its outcomes in the form of a forest plot. The interpretation of a forest plot is to look for the diamond on the bottom. If it is totally to LEFT of the vertical line, it means risk of an outcome was reduced by the intervention. If it is fully to the RIGHT, then risk of that outcome was increased. And if the diamond touches the vertical line, it means there was no statistical influence of the intervention on the outcome.

We hope this brief introduction to EBM has been informative, clear, and helpful. If any of the information above seems unclear, or if you have a question, please contact us via the 5MinuteConsult Web site.

ACKNOWLEDGMENTS

This is the 33rd edition of *The 5-Minute Clinical Consult*, a comprehensive point-of-care tool to assist in the care of patients. From beginning to end, one cannot find a more current and easy-to-use collection of clinically useful content.

Developing and maintaining a book and Web site of this magnitude requires an equally broad effort from its supporting team. I wish to thank the dedication and tireless efforts of many: Rebecca Schmidt, product lead, medical education and medical practice; Cindy Yoo, development editor; Joe Cho, acquisitions editor; and Lisa McAllister, vice president, medical practice.

This 2025 edition is the direct result of the dedication and insights of our associate editors. I wish to thank Drs. Robert A. Baldor, Jeremy Golding, Mark B. Stephens, and Kathleen A. Barry for their hard work and overwhelming commitment to *The 5-Minute Clinical Consult*.

I wish to especially thank my wife, Sylvia, and my daughter, Molly, who have given greatly for this book.

The challenge of completing a book covering this broad spectrum of medicine requires insights and skills far beyond my own. Many thanks to my mentors, Bob Baldor and Mark Quirk, who have been an enormous support—always there to encourage, reassure, and impart wisdom.

Many in the academic and health care worlds are due thanks for support, insight, and friendship:

M. Diane McKee, Michele Pugnaire, Karen Rayla, Maryanne Adams, Erica White, Phil Fournier, Erik Garcia, Jeff Stovall, Jim Comes, Leah Honor, J. Herb Stevenson, Michael Kidd, Zainab Nawab, Sanjiv and Amita Chopra, Vasilios (Bill) Chrisostomidis, James (Jay) Broadhurst, Christina Kim, Madhavi Medipally, the staff of Shrewsbury Family Medicine, Ben Babbitt, Joyce Paquette, Priscila Velez, Brittany McLean, Michelle Leboeuf, Chad Ren, Joseph Frappier, my amazing colleagues Mark Powicki, Steve Messineo, Jill Terrien, Susan Feeney, Mariyan Montaque, Jillian Joseph, Jim Nairus, Kayla Chalmers, Danielle Ferreira, Rick Watson, and Sara Floros, and the faculty and students of the University of Massachusetts Medical School.

Medicine is a challenge I have fortunately not had to meet alone. Thanks to my parents, Frank and Angela (Jean); my brother, John, and his family, Marylou, Cate, and Jane; Frank, Mary Anne, Diane, and David Christian; the Diana and Hymie Lipschitz family; and the Bob and Ruth Pabreza family; they are responsible for who I am and my success in life.

I am blessed with the best of friends; without them, I would not be a physician. Thanks to Bob Bacic; Ron Jautz; Richard Onorato; John Horcher; Auguste Turnier; Bob Smith; Paul Saivetz; Bob and Nancy Gallinaro; Drew and Jill Grimes; Louay Toma; Laurie, Alan, Daniel, Jenny, and Matt Bugos; Alan Ehrlich; Andy Jennings; Bill Demianiuk; John and Kathleen Polanowicz; Phil and Carol Pettine; Mark and Linda Shelton; Steve Bennett; Vicki Triolo; and Bob and Laurie Jenal, Mike Rousse, Cliff Sterns, and Conor Wallace.

—FRANK J. DOMINO, MD

CONTRIBUTING AUTHORS

Hanadi Abou Dargham, MD
Associate Program Director
Department of Family Medicine
St. Joseph's Medical Center
Stockton, California

Laith Abushanab, MD
Emergency Medicine Resident
Department of Emergency Department
Rutgers Robert Wood Johnson Medical School
New Brunswick, New Jersey

Adel M. Abuzeid, MBBS
Associate Professor, Surgery
Augusta University Medical Center
Augusta, Georgia

Ryan Accomazzo, MD, MPH
Concord, North Carolina

Cyrus Adams-Mardi, MD, MS
The George Washington University School of Medicine and Health Sciences
Washington, District of Columbia

Ronald N. Adler, MD, FAAFP
Associate Professor
Department of Family Medicine and Community Health
University of Massachusetts Medical School
Worcester, Massachusetts

Adwoa A. Adu, MD
Family Medicine Core Faculty
Department of Family Medicine
University of South Carolina
Greenville, South Carolina

Faraz Ahmad, MD, MPH†
Assistant Clinical Professor
Department of Family and Community Medicine
Ohio State University
Columbus, Ohio

Hiba Ahmad, PharmD, BCOP†
Clinical Oncology Pharmacist
University of Colorado
Aurora, Colorado

Yasir Ahmed, MD
Cornea, Cataract, and Refractive Surgeon
Eye Center of Texas
Houston, Texas

Stephanie Algenio-Anciro, MD
Resident Physician
Department of Family Medicine
David Grant Medical Center
Travis Air Force Base, California

Fozia Akhtar Ali, MD, FAAFP
Diplomat of American Board of Obesity Medicine
Associate Professor
Family and Community Medicine Department
UT Health San Antonio
San Antonio, Texas

Nabeel Ali, MD
Associate Program Director
Department of Family Medicine
Baptist Memorial Medical Education
Southaven, Mississippi

Aya Allam, MD
Department of Family Medicine
Creighton University
Omaha, Nebraska

Richard W. Allinson, MD
Associate Professor
Department of Ophthalmology
Texas A&M Health Science Center
Bryan, Texas
Senior Staff Physician
Baylor Scott & White Clinic
Waco, Texas

Alqasem Alsaqri, MD
Resident Physician
Department of Family Medicine
Advocate Christ Medical Center Family Medicine Program
Oak Lawn, Illinois

Bremmy L. Alsbrooks, DO, MPH
Resident Physician
Department of Graduate Medical Education
HCA Medical City Arlington
Arlington, Texas

Maureen Alvarado, DO
Assistant Professor/Clinical
Department of Family and Community Medicine
UT Health San Antonio
San Antonio, Texas

Christoffer Amdahl, MD
Resident Physician
Department of Family Medicine
HCA Medical City Arlington
Arlington, Texas

Khorshid Amirkhosravi, MD
UT Health
San Antonio, Texas

Alyssa Anderson, MD
Assistant Professor
Department of Family and Community Medicine
Penn State College of Medicine
Hershey, Pennsylvania

Garland E. Anderson II, MD
Associate Clinical Professor
Department of Rural Family Medicine
Louisiana State University Health Sciences Center New Orleans
New Orleans, Louisiana

Justin Ryan Andrada, DO
Resident Physician
Department of Family Medicine
St. Joseph Hospital Chicago
Chicago, Illinois

Rose Katherine Appel, DO
Associate Program Director
Department of Graduate Medical Education
AdventHealth East Orlando
Orlando, Florida

Camille A. Archer, MD
Director of Child & Adolescent Outpatient Psychiatry
Department of Child & Adolescent Psychiatry
Brookdale Hospital Medical Center, One Brooklyn Health
Brooklyn, New York

Ann M. Aring, MD, FAAFP
Associate Program Director
Department of Family Medicine Residency
OhioHealth Riverside Methodist Hospital
Columbus, Ohio

Alaina Aristide, MD
Resident Physician
Lawrence Family Medicine Residency
Lawrence, Massachusetts

Michael A. Armstrong, MD
Resident Physician
Department of Family Medicine
HCA Medical City Arlington
Arlington, Texas

James J. Arnold, DO, FACOFP†
Director of Medical Education
96th Medical Group/Eglin Hospital
Eglin Air Force Base, Florida

Michael J. Arnold, MD†
Assistant Professor
Department of Family Medicine
Uniformed Services University of the Health
    Sciences
Bethesda, Maryland

Chris Artner, MD
Resident
Department of Internal Medicine Residency
    Program
University of Louisville
Louisville, Kentucky

Ashley Asensio, DO
Resident Physician
Department of Emergency Medicine
Rutgers Robert Wood Johnson Medical School
New Brunswick, New Jersey

Maximos Attia, MD, FAAFP
Associate Professor
Department of Family Medicine
Guthrie
Sayre, Pennsylvania

Justin Atwood, MD
Prisma Health
Columbia, South Carolina

Frantz Aubry, MD
Clinical Fellow
Department of Psychiatry
One Brookdale Health
Brooklyn, New York

Sandra S. Augusto, MD, MPH
Education Director
Barre, Worcester Family Residency Program
Assistant Professor, UMass Chan Medical
    School
Full Spectrum Family Medicine with OB Faculty,
    BFHC
Department of Family Medicine and Community
    Health
UMass Memorial Hospital
Worcester, Massachusetts

Sudeep K. Aulakh, MD, FACP, FRCPC
Director, Ambulatory Education
UMass Chan Medical School-Baystate
Springfield, Massachusetts

Ben Ayotte, MD
Clinical Assistant Professor, Division of Hospital
    Medicine
Department of Internal Medicine
Michigan Medicine, University of Michigan
Ann Arbor, Michigan

Sanaa Ayyoub, MD
Endocrinologist
Dartmouth-Hitchcock Medical Center
Manchester, New Hampshire

**Sultan Mahmood Babar, MD, CAQSM,
    FAAFP**
Consultant Physician
Department of Emergency Medicine
King Faisal Specialist Hospital & Research
    Centre
Riyadh, Kingdom of Saudi Arabia

Franklyn C. Babb, MD, FAAFP
Professor
Department of Family and Community Medicine
Texas Tech University Health Sciences Center
    School of Medicine
Lubbock, Texas

Melissa E. Badowski, PharmD, MPH
Clinical Associate Professor
Department of Pharmacy Practice
University of Illinois at Chicago College of
    Pharmacy
Chicago, Illinois

Andrew Baird, MD
PGY-3 Family Medicine Resident
HCA Healthcare/Mercer University School of
    Medicine
Grand Strand Medical Center
Family Medicine Residency Program
Myrtle Beach, South Carolina

Frederic Baker Mills IV, MD, MS
Orthopaedic Surgery Resident
Department of Orthopaedic Surgery
Duke University Health System
Durham, North Carolina

Robert A. Baldor, MD, FAAFP
Professor and Founding Chair
Department of Family Medicine
UMass Chan Medical School-Baystate
Springfield, Massachusetts
Designated Institutional Official
Baystate Franklin Medical Center
Greenfield, Massachusetts

Kenneth A. Ballou, MD
Associate Professor of Clinical Medicine
Department of Family Medicine
University of California at Riverside School of
    Medicine
Riverside, California

Laurel Banach, MD
Department of Family Medicine
UMass Memorial Medical Center
Worcester, Massachusetts

Tara Baney, MS, CRNP
Nurse Practitioner
Department of Family and Community Medicine
Penn State Health
State College, Pennsylvania

Zeina M. Bani Hani, MBBS
The George Washington University
Washington, District of Columbia

Sophia R. Barber, DO
PGY-1
Department of Family Medicine
AHN Forbes Family Medicine Residency
Monroeville, Pennsylvania

Elise Joyce Barney, DO
Clinical Assistant Professor
Department of Internal Medicine
University of Arizona College of Medicine
Phoenix, Arizona

John P. Barrett, MD, MPH, MS†
COL, MC, USA
Adjunct Associate Professor
Deputy Director
Uniformed Services University
War Related Illness and Injury Study Center
Washington DC VA Medical Center
Washington, District of Columbia

Kathleen A. Barry, MD
Associate Professor
UMass Chan Medical School
Department of Family Medicine and Community
    Health
Hahnemann Family Health Center
Worcester, Massachusetts

Tricia Bautista, MD
Resident Physician
Family Medicine Residency Program
Adventist Health Hanford
Hanford, California

Orly Bell, MD, MPH
Resident Physician
Department of Family Medicine
University of California Los Angeles
Los Angeles, California

Paul P. Belliveau, PharmD
Professor of Pharmacy Practice
Department of Pharmacy Practice
Massachusetts College of Pharmacy and Health
    Sciences
Worcester, Massachusetts

Brandis Belt, MD, MPH
Assistant Residency Director
Department of Family Medicine
Robert Wood Johnson University Hospital
    Somerset
Somerville, New Jersey

Brock A. Benedict, DO
US Army
Family Physician
Womack Army Community Hospital
Fort Liberty, North Carolina

Ambreka Benons, MD
Psychiatry Resident
Brooklyn, New York

Ivan Berezowski, MD
Resident Physician
Department of General Internal Medicine
The George Washington University Hospital
Washington, District of Columbia

Jasmine S. Beria, DO, MPH
Assistant Professor
Department of Medicine
NYU Langone Hospital Long Island
Mineola, New York

Bryan G. Beutel, MD
Assistant Professor
Kansas City University College of Medicine
Kansas City, Missouri

Rajarshi Bhadra, MD
Clinical Fellow
Department of Nephrology
University of Massachusetts Medical School
Worcester, Massachusetts

Prarthna V. Bhardwaj, MBBS
Fellow, Department of Hematology Oncology
UMass Chan Medical School-Baystate
Springfield, Massachusetts

Siddhi Bhivandkar, MD
Department of Psychiatry
St. Elizabeth's Medical Center
Boston University
Boston, Massachusetts

Ghazaleh Bigdeli, MD, FCCP
Pulmonary Rehab Associates
Youngstown, Ohio

Wendy S. Biggs, MD
Professor, Family Medicine
Central Michigan University College of
    Medicine
Saginaw, Michigan

Dmitry Bisk, MD
Associate Director
HonorHealth Scottsdale Osborn Family
    Medicine Residency Program
HonorHealth
Scottsdale, Arizona

Haley Bodette, MD
Resident Physician
Department of Family Medicine
ProHealth Waukesha Memorial Hospital
Waukesha, Wisconsin

Frances J. Boly, DO
Department of Infectious Diseases
Advocate Christ Medical Center
Oak Lawn, Illinois

Curtis W. Bone, MD, MHS
Assistant Professor
Department of Family and Community Medicine
Penn State Health Milton S. Hershey Medical
    Center
Hershey, Pennsylvania

Marie L. Borum, MD, EdD, MPH[†]
Professor of Medicine
Director of the Division of Gastroenterology
    and Liver Diseases
Department of Medicine
George Washington University School of
    Medicine and Health Care Sciences
Washington, District of Columbia

Katherine E. Bouchard, DO
Department of Family Medicine
Methodist Charlton Medical Center
Dallas, Texas

Melissa Boucher, DO, MPH
Chief Resident, Ascension St. Joseph Family
    Medicine Residency
Department of Family Medicine
Ascension St. Joseph Hospital
Chicago, Illinois

William McCormick Bowen, MD
Program Director
UNM Santa Fe Family Medicine Residency
Santa Fe, New Mexico

Greg Bowlin, MD
Assistant Professor
Primary Care Sports Medicine
Texas A&M College of Medicine
College Station, Texas

William B. Bradley, MD
Florida State University College of Medicine
Tallahassee, Florida

Makenna Brezitski, MD, Med
Resident Physician
Department of Family & Community Medicine
Penn State Health Milton S. Hershey Medical
    Center
Hershey, Pennsylvania

**Katy (Ekaterina) Brodski-Quigley, MD,
    EdM**
Physician, Urgent Care
Waltham, Massachusetts

David T. Broome, MD
Assistant Professor
Department of Internal Medicine
Division of Metabolism, Endocrinology, and
    Diabetes
University of Michigan
Ann Arbor, Michigan

Kathryn M. Brown, MD, MS
Assistant Professor
Department of Family Medicine and Community
    Health
University of Minnesota
Minneapolis, Minnesota

Phillip Charles Brown, MD
Assistant Clinical Professor
UCLA Family Medical Department
Los Angeles, California

Daniella Davida Brutman, MD
Physician
Department of Family Medicine
AMITA Health Saint Joseph Hospital Chicago
Chicago, Illinois

Liz Buck, MD
Department of Family Medicine
University of Washington
Seattle, Washington

Bonnie A. Buechel, MD, MS
Resident Physician
Department of Family and Community Medicine
Penn State Health Milton S. Hershey Medical
    Center
Hershey, Pennsylvania

Han Q. Bui, MD, MPH[†]
Chief Medical Officer
International SoS
Houston, Texas

Dylan Buller, MD
Resident
Department of Urology
UConn Health
Farmington, Connecticut

Chelsea Leigh Bunce, DO
New Brunswick, New Jersey

Kyle Burke, DO
Department of Family and Community Medicine
Penn State Health Milton S. Hershey Medical
    Center
Hershey, Pennsylvania

Liam P. Burke, MD
Assistant Professor
Department of Family Medicine and Community
    Health
University of Massachusetts Medical School
Worcester, Massachusetts

Harold J. Bursztajn, MD
Associate Professor of Psychiatry, Part-Time
Department of Psychiatry
Beth Israel Deaconess Medical Center
Harvard Medical School
Boston, Massachusetts

Jared Caballes, MD
Resident Physician
Department of Family Medicine
Kaweah Health Medical Center
Visalia, California

Jennifer W. Caceres, MD
Associate Professor of Medicine
Department of Medicine
Schmidt College of Medicine at Florida Atlantic
    University
Boca Raton, Florida

David C. Cadena Jr., MD†
Assistant Professor
Department of Family and Community Medicine
University of Texas Health Science Center at
    San Antonio
San Antonio, Texas

Kristen R. Canady, MD, PhD
Department of Family and Community Medicine
University of Texas Health Science Center at
    San Antonio
San Antonio, Texas

Justin Paul Canakis, DO
Resident Doctor
Department of Internal Medicine
George Washington University
Washington, District of Columbia

Etny Raul Candelario, MD, MS
Department of Family and Community Medicine
University of Texas Health Science Center
San Antonio, Texas

**Dana G. Carroll, PharmD, BCPS, CDCES,
    BCGP**
Clinical Professor
Department of Pharmacy Practice
Auburn University Harrison School of Pharmacy
Tuscaloosa, Alabama

Samantha Carroll, MD
Hospitalist
Department of Pediatrics
AdventHealth for Children
Orlando, Florida

Elizabeth H. Carver, DNP, FNP-BC, CNE
Nurse Practitioner
Occupational Health and Wellness
Duke University
Durham, North Carolina

Robert J. Casey, MD
Affiliate Assistant Professor
Clerkship Director, Pediatrics
Department of Women's and Children's Health
Charles E. Schmidt College of Medicine
Florida Atlantic University
Boca Raton, Florida

Casandra Cashman, MD, FAAFP
Assistant Director
Community East Family Medicine Residency
    Program
Indianapolis, Indiana

Michelle Caster, MD
Assistant Professor
Department of Family Medicine
University Hospitals
Cleveland, Ohio

Jennifer E. Cavin, MD
Assistant Professor
Department of Family Medicine
Dell Medical School, The University of Texas at
    Austin
Austin, Texas

William E. Cayley Jr., MD, Mdiv
Adjunct Clinical Professor
University of Wisconsin School of Medicine and
    Public Health
Prevea Family Medicine Residency
Eau Claire, Wisconsin

Jan Cerny, MD, PhD†
Associate Professor of Medicine
Department of Medicine
Division of Hematology/Oncology
University of Massachusetts Medical School
Worcester, Massachusetts

Morgan Lee Chambers, MD, MEd
PGY2
Department of Family and Community Medicine
Penn State Health Milton S. Hershey Medical
    Center
Hershey, Pennsylvania

Ronald G. Chambers Jr., MD, FAAFP†
Program Director
Department of Family Medicine
Dignity Health
Sacramento, California

Christine Chan, MD
Faculty
Hawai'i Island Family Medicine Residency
Hilo Medical Center
Hilo, Hawaii

Sangili Chandran, MD
Director, Primary Care Sports Medicine
Advocate Christ Medical Center
Oak Lawn, Illinois
Associate Professor
Department of Family Medicine
Chicago Medical School
Roslind Franklin University of Medicine and
    Science
Chicago, Illinois

Clifford M. Chang, MD
Resident Physician
Department of Emergency Medicine
Inspira Vineland Medical Center
Vineland, New Jersey

Felix B. Chang, MD, DABMA, ABIHM, ABIM
Director, Inpatient Service
University of Massachusetts Fitchburg Family
    Medicine Residency Program
Hospitalist, Family Medicine University of
    Massachusetts Medical School
Worcester, Massachusetts
Hospitalist
Department of Hospital Medicine
University of Massachusetts Memorial Medical
    Group
Leominster, Massachusetts

Jennifer G. Chang, MD†
LtCol, USAF, MC
Department of Family Medicine Residency
96th Medical Group
Eglin Air Force Base, Florida

Juliana Chang, MD
Rheumatology Fellow
University of California, Irvine
Irvine, California

Jason Chao, MD, MS
Professor
Department of Family Medicine and Community
    Health
Case Western Reserve University and University
    Hospitals Cleveland Medical Center
Cleveland, Ohio

Kathya M. Chartre, MD
Department of Family Medicine
AMITA Health Saint Joseph Hospital
Chicago, Illinois

Parul Chaudhri, DO
Assistant Professor, Director of Osteopathic
    Education
Department of Family Medicine
University of Toledo
Toledo, Ohio

Summer Chavez, DO, MPH, MPM
Clinical Assistant Professor
Department of Health Systems and Population
    Health Sciences
University of Houston
Houston, Texas

Janet Chen, DO
AdventHealth
Orlando, Florida

Jeffrey Chen, MD
Clinical Instructor
Department of Internal Medicine
University of Texas at Houston, McGovern
    Medical School
Houston, Texas

Rensa Chen, DO
Resident Physician
Department of Family and Community Medicine
Penn State Health Milton S. Hershey Medical
    Center
Hershey, Pennsylvania

Teresa M. Chirayil, MD[†]
Resident Physician, Family Medicine
Advocate Christ Family Medicine Residency
Oak Lawn, Illinois

Luke Thomas Chmielecki, MD
Clinical Instructor
Department of Internal Medicine
Boston Medical Center
Boston, Massachusetts

Ratnesh Chopra, MD
Assistant Professor of Medicine
University of Massachusetts Medical School
Worcester, Massachusetts

Efstathia Choros, MD, CPA
Emergency Medicine Physician
Department of Emergency Medicine
University of Massachusetts Memorial
    Healthcare
Worcester, Massachusetts

Megan Ann Christopher, MD, MPH
Resident Physician
Department of Family Medicine
Dell Medical School, The University of Texas at
    Austin
Austin, Texas

Justin Chu, MD
Internal Medicine & Pediatrics
University of Louisville School of Medicine
Louisville, Kentucky

Vivian Nnenna Chukwuma, MD
Resident
Department of Internal Medicine
Advocate Christ Medical Center
Oak Lawn, Illinois

S. Lindsey Clarke, MD, FAAFP[†]
Medical University of South Carolina Area
    Health Education Consortium Professor
    (Greenwood/Family Medicine)
Director of Resident Education and Associate
    Program Director
Self Regional Healthcare
Greenwood, South Carolina

Karl T. Clebak, MD, MHA, FAAFP[†]
Associate Professor, Program Director
Department of Family and Community Medicine
Penn State Health Milton S. Hershey Medical
    Center
Hershey, Pennsylvania

Gregorio Climaco, MD
PGY-2 Family Medicine Resident
SouthWestern Illinois Family Medicine Resident
St. Elizabeth's Hospital
O'Fallon, Illinois

Cerrone A. Cohen, MD
Assistant Professor
Duke Psychiatry and Behavioral Sciences
Duke Family Medicine and Community Health
Duke University
Durham, North Carolina

Timothy J. Coker, MD, FAAFP[†]
United States Air Force Academy
Air Force Academy, Colorado

Erik Colegrove, MD
Department of Family Medicine
Central Michigan University
Mount Pleasant, Michigan

Irene Coletsos, MD
Community Psychiatrist
Department of Behavioral Health
VinFen, Department of Mental Health
Quincy, Massachusetts

Jennifer R. Collins, PharmD
Clinical Pharmacy Specialist - Ambulatory Care
Community Health Network
Indianapolis, Indiana

Christina Conrad, DO
Department of Pediatric Emergency Medicine
Phoenix Children's Hospital
Phoenix, Arizona

Sabina M. Constantine, DO
Clinical Assistant Professor
NYU Long Island School of Medicine
NYU Langone Hospital—Long Island
Mineola, New York

Stephanie L. Conway-Allen, PharmD, RPh
Associate Professor
Department of Pharmacy Practice
Massachusetts College of Pharmacy and Health
    Sciences University
Worcester, Massachusetts

Tonya M. Cook, PharmD
Faculty, Clinical Pharmacist
Department of Family Medicine Residency
St. Mary's Medical Center Family Medicine
    Residency
Grand Junction, Colorado

Corey J. Costanzo, DO, MPH, MS
Assistant Professor
Department of Family Medicine
UMass Chan School of Medicine
Worcester, Massachusetts

Samantha Cotler, DO, MBA
Family Medicine Residency
AdventHealth East Orlando
Orlando, Florida

Benjamin Cottrell, DO
Resident Physician
AdventHealth East Orlando
Orlando, Florida

Caroline E. Cox, MD
Division of Surgery
Spartanburg Regional Medical Center
Spartanburg, South Carolina

Julie A. Creech, DO[†]
Family Medicine Physician, Sports Medicine
Physician, Primary Care Sports Medicine Fellow
United States Air Force
O'Fallen, Illinois

Jason Cross, PharmD, BCPS, BCACP
Associate Professor of Pharmacy Practice
Massachusetts College of Pharmacy and Health
    Sciences University
Worcester, Massachusetts

Hongyi Cui, MD, PhD
Associate Professor of Surgery, Associate
    Director, Acute Care Surgery
Department of Surgery
University of Massachusetts Memorial Medical
    Center
Worcester, Massachusetts

Shani H. Cunningham, DO, MEd, FAAP
Assistant Professor
AdventHealth for Children
Orlando, Florida

Madeleine Cutrone, MD
Resident Physician
Department of Family Medicine
Novant Health Family Medicine Residency
    Program
Huntersville, North Carolina

Tina D'Amato, DO
Attending Family Physician
Charlotte Family Medicine
Charlotte, Vermont

Darnel Viray Dabu, MD, MPH, FAAFP
Faculty
Department of Family Medicine
Lakeside Medical Center
Belle Glade, Florida

Pawan Daga, MD
Resident
Department of Internal Medicine
University of Louisville
Louisville, Kentucky

Heather Ann Dalton, MD, FAAFP†
Hospice and Palliative Medicine Fellow
Department of Internal Medicine
UT Southwestern Medical Center
Dallas, Texas

Paul E. Daniel Jr., MD
Hospitalist
UMass Memorial Healthcare
Division of Hospital Medicine
Worcester, Massachusetts

Akhil Das, MD, FACS
Professor
Department of Urology
Thomas Jefferson University
Philadelphia, Pennsylvania

Amanda Kimberley Davis, MD, MBBS
Department of Family Medicine
Tallahassee Memorial Health Care FMRP
Tallahassee, Florida

Michelle A. Davis, DO
Resident Physician
Family and Community Medicine
University of Texas Health Science Center
San Antonio, Texas

Ana De Diego, MD
Resident Physician
Department of Internal Medicine
University of Miami at Holy Cross
Miami, Florida

Niyomi De Silva, MD
Associate Program Director
Department of Family Medicine
HCA Medical City Arlington
Arlington, Texas

Iain W. Decker, DO
Resident Physician
Department of Ophthalmology
Kettering Health Network Grandview Medical
    Center
Dayton, Ohio

Henry Del Rosario, MD
Assistant Professor
Department of Family Medicine and Community
    Health
University of Massachusetts Memorial Medical
    School
Worcester, Massachusetts

Emilee J. Delbridge, PhD, LMFT
Assistant Professor of Clinical Family Medicine
Department of Family Medicine
Indiana University
Indianapolis, Indiana

**Konstantinos E. Deligiannidis, MD, MPH,
    FAAFP**
Assistant Professor
Department of Family Medicine
Donald and Barbara Zucker School of Medicine
    at Hofstra/Northwell
Hempstead, New York

Malhar Desai, DO, MS, BA
Resident
Robert Wood Johnson - Emergency Department
Rutgers Robert Wood Johnson Medical School
New Brunswick, New Jersey

Michael DiGaetano, MD
Resident Physician
Department of Emergency Medicine
Rutgers Robert Wood Johnson University
    Hospital
New Brunswick, New Jersey

Sherilyn DeStefano, MD
Assistant Professor
Department of Family Medicine
Oregon Health and Science University
Portland, Oregon

Hillary Kieran Deveaux, MBBS
Resident
Department of Internal Medicine
Advocate Christ Medical Center
Oak Lawn, Illinois

Bradley Devrieze, MD
Assistant Professor
Department of Internal Medicine
Creighton University School of Medicine
Omaha, Nebraska

Gabriel J. Diaz, CRNP-BC, MS
Nurse Practitioner
Department of Gastroenterology
The George Washington University
Washington, District of Columbia

Amanda M. DiSabato, DO
Resident Physician
Department of Family Medicine
OhioHealth Riverside Methodist Hospital
Family Medicine Residency Program
Columbus, Ohio

Lena Dung Doan, DO
Resident Physician
Department of Family Medicine
Texas A&M Health Science Family Medicine
    Residency Program
Bryan, Texas

Loreal Dolar, DO
Resident Physician
Orlando, Florida

Frank J. Domino, MD
Professor and Director of Predoctoral Education
Department of Family Medicine and Community
    Health
UMass Chan Medical School
Worcester, Massachusetts

Andrea B. Dotson, MD, MSPH
Assistant Professor
Department of Family Medicine and Community
    Health
Durham, North Carolina

Ian P. Downin, MD, MHA
Resident Physician
Department of Family and Community Medicine
Penn State Health Milton S. Hershey Medical
    Center
Hershey, Pennsylvania

Joanna Drowos, DO, MPH, MBA
Associate Dean for Faculty Affairs
Associate Professor of Family Medicine
Charles E. Schmidt College of Medicine
Florida Atlantic University
Boca Raton, Florida

Milap Dubal, MD, MPH
Assistant Professor
Department of Family and Community Medicine
Penn State Health
Fishburn, Pennsylvania

Michelle E. Duffelmeyer, MD
Director of Didactic Education
College of Health Science
Westfield State University
Westfield, Massachusetts

Carla Dugas, DO
Core Faculty, Attending Physician
Department of Emergency Medicine
Inspira Medical Center
Vineland, New Jersey

Maurice Duggins, MD, FAAFP
Faculty
Clinical Associate Professor
Department of Family and Community Medicine
Ascension Via Christi Family Medicine
　Residency
Kansas University School of Medicine–Wichita
Wichita, Kansas

Ashten Duncan, MD, MPH, CPH
Resident Physician, PGY-3
Family and Community Medicine
University of New Mexico—Santa Fe Family
　Medicine Residency
Santa Fe, New Mexico

Muhammad I. Durrani, DO, MS†
Assistant Research Director, Core Faculty
Department of Emergency Medicine
Inspira Medical Center
Vineland, New Jersey

Sudeshna Dutta, MD
Resident
Department of Family Medicine
Creighton University
Omaha, Nebraska

Farzad Effan, MBBS
Resident
Department of Family Medicine
Creighton University
Omaha, Nebraska

Stephany Giraldo Eierle, DO, MPH
UMass Memorial Chan Medical School
Worcester, Massachusetts

William G. Elder, PhD
Professor and Chair
Department of Behavioral and Social Sciences
University of Houston
Houston, Texas

Pamela Ellsworth, MD
Professor of Urology
University of Central Florida
Orlando, Florida

John F. Emerson, MD
Associate Professor
Department of Family Medicine
Prisma Health
Greenville, South Carolina

Deborah R. Erlich, MD, MmedEd, FAAFP
Associate Professor
Department of Family Medicine
Family Medicine Clerkship Director
Tufts University School of Medicine
Boston, Massachusetts

Justin T. Ertle, MD
Assistant Professor
Department of Internal Medicine
Medical College of Georgia at Augusta
　University
Augusta, Georgia

Emily J. Eshleman, DO, MS
Resident Physician
Department of Family Medicine
University of Massachusetts Medical School
Worcester, Massachusetts

Tyler R. Evans, DO
Assistant Professor
Department of Family and Community Medicine
University of Texas Southwestern Medical
　Center
Dallas, Texas

Vanessa Joyce M. Evardone, MD, BSMT
Fellow
Department of Geriatric Medicine
Florida Atlantic University (FAU)—West Palm
　Beach VA Medical Center
Boca Raton, Florida

Idil D. Ezhuthachan, MD, MS
Assistant Professor
Department of Pediatrics
Children's Healthcare of Atlanta
Assistant Professor
Department of Pediatrics
Emory University
Atlanta, Georgia

Pang-Yen Fan, MD
Professor of Medicine
Division of Renal Medicine
University of Massachusetts Medical School
Worcester, Massachusetts

Jennifer Fantasia, MD
Assistant Professor
Department of Urology
University of Massachusetts Medical School
Worcester, Massachusetts

N. Max Farenwald, DO
Virginia Tech Carillon Clinic
Roanoke, Virginia

Rhonda A. Faulkner, PhD†
Director of Behavioral Medicine
Department of Family Medicine
AMITA Health Saint Joseph Hospital Chicago
University of Illinois College of Medicine Master
　Affiliate
Chicago, Illinois

Jeffrey P. Feden, MD, FACEP
Associate Professor, Clinician Educator
Department of Emergency Medicine
The Warren Alpert Medical School of Brown
　University
Providence, Rhode Island

A. Susan Feeney, MS, DNP, FNP-BC
Assistant Professor
Director of Family and Adult-Gerontology NP
　Programs
Tan Chingfen Graduate School of Nursing
UMass Chan Medical School
Worcester, Massachusetts

Neil Feldman, DPM†
Central Massachusetts Podiatry, PC
Worcester, Massachusetts

Nolan P. Feola, MD†
Capt., Eglin Air Force Base Family Medicine
　Residency
Eglin Air Force Base
Shalimar, Florida

Gregory John Ferenchak, MD
Faculty Physician
Department of Family Medicine
Allegheny Health Network, Forbes Family
　Medicine Residency
Monroeville, Pennsylvania

Ulysses Fernandez-Miro, DO†
Department of Family Medicine
Air Force/Saint Louis University
O'Fallon, Illinois

Allison H. Ferris, MD
Associate Professor of Medicine
Chair of Department of Medicine
Program Director of Internal Medicine
　Residency
Florida Atlantic University Schmidt College of
　Medicine
Boca Raton, Florida

Anna Sophia Fields, MD
Memorial Family Medicine Residency
Houston, Texas

Matthew J. Filippo, DO
Associate Professor, Teaching/Clinical
　Psychiatrist
Department of Psychiatry
Advocate Lutheran General Hospital
Park Ridge, Illinois

Theodore B. Flaum, DO
Associate Professor
Department of Osteopathic Manipulative
　Medicine
NYIT College of Osteopathic Medicine
Old Westbury, New York

Kyle J. Fletke, MD
Assistant Professor
Department of Family and Community Medicine
University of Maryland School of Medicine
Baltimore, Maryland

Suzanne Florczyk, PharmD
Clinical Pharmacist
Novant Health
Cornelius, North Carolina

Jane Marie Forbes, MD
Assistant Professor
Department of Family Medicine
University of Virginia
Charlottesville, Virginia

Jennifer G. Foster, MD, MBA, FACP
Associate Professor of Medicine
Charles E. Schmidt College of Medicine
Florida Atlantic University
Boca Raton, Florida

Zoe Foster, MD, FAAFP
Program Director
Department of Family and Preventive Medicine
Prisma Health
University of South Carolina
Columbia, South Carolina

Robert L. Frachtman, MD, FACG
Clinical Assistant Professor of Internal Medicine
Department of Internal Medicine/
   Gastroenterology
Dell Medical School, The University of Texas at
   Austin
Austin, Texas

Alex T. Fredrickson, MD
St. John's Family Medicine Residency
St. Paul, Minnesota

Bruce Palmer Freshley Jr., MD
Fellow, Primary Care Sports Medicine
Department of Family and Community Medicine
Medical College of Georgia at Augusta
   University
Augusta, Georgia

Minjin Fromm, MD
Assistant Professor
Department of Orthopedics and Physical
   Rehabilitation
University of Massachusetts Medical School
Worcester, Massachusetts

Calli M. Fry, DO
Resident
Department of Family Medicine
Texas A&M Family Medicine Residency
Bryan, Texas

Mmaserame Gaefele, MD
Resident Physician, Family Medicine
UMass Chan Medical School-Baystate Health
Greenfield, Massachusetts

Rishi Gaiha, MD
Medical Director, Pain Management
Advocate Illinois Masonic Medical Center
Chicago, Illinois

Steven W. Gale, MD
Family Medicine Physician
Prevea Health
Green Bay, Wisconsin

Moises Gallegos, MD, MPH
Clinical Assistant Professor
Department of Emergency Medicine
Stanford University School of Medicine
Stanford, California

Pooja Gandhi, DO
PGY-2
University of Louisville Internal Medicine
   Residency
Louisville, Kentucky

Mark A. Gardon, DO, MS
Resident Physician
Department of Internal Medicine
University of Louisville
Louisville, Kentucky

Taylor Gaudard, MD, IBCLC
Assistant Professor
Department of Family Medicine
Central Michigan University College of
   Medicine
Saginaw, Michigan

Hermione Gaw, MD
Resident Physician
Department of Family Medicine Residency
Dignity Health Sacramento
Sacramento, California

Breanna Gawrys, DO
Associate Professor
Department of Family Medicine
Uniformed Services University
Bethesda, Maryland

Tamara L. Gayle, MD, Med
Department of Pediatric Hospital Medicine
Children's National Medical Center
Washington, District of Columbia

Kamini Geer, MD, MPH
Women's Health Fellowship Director
AdventHealth Winter Park
Winter Park, Florida

Joanne E. Genewick, DO, FAIHM
Assistant Professor of Family Medicine
Mayo Clinic Family Medicine Residency–
   Mankato
Mayo Clinic Health System
Mankato, Minnesota

Michelle A. Georgia, DO
Resident Physician
Department of Pediatrics
University of Massachusetts
Worcester, Massachusetts

Corinne Gibbons, MD, MPH
Family Physician
Greater Lawrence Family Health Center
Lawrence, Massachusetts

Lawrence M. Gibbs, MD, MSEd
Program Director
HCA Healthcare KC/Lees Summit Family—
   Medical Center Program
Lee's Summit, Missouri

Daniel V. Girzadas Jr., MD
Department of Emergency Medicine
University of Illinois
Chicago, Illinois
Department of Emergency Medicine
Advocate Christ Medical Center
Oak Lawn, Illinois

Lawrence Go, MD
Resident
Department of Family and Community Medicine
Penn State Health
State College, Pennsylvania

Krystyna Guinevere Golden, MD[†]
Resident Physician
Eglin Family Medicine Residency
Eglin Air Force Base Hospital
Eglin Air Force Base, Florida

Jeremy Golding, MD, FAAFP
Professor of Family Medicine and Obstetrics &
   Gynecology
UMass Chan Medical School
Department of Family Medicine and Community
   Health
University of Massachusetts Memorial Health
   Care
Hahnemann Family Health Center
Worcester, Massachusetts

Frances L. Gonzalez Gonzalez, MD[†]
Family Medicine Resident Physician
AdventHealth
Winter Park, Florida

Lislie Lisete Gonzalez Veitia, MD
Geriatric Fellow
Department of Medical Education
Florida Atlantic University
Boca Raton, Florida

Hansaa Gopalakrishnan, MD
Resident Physician
Department of Family Medicine
HCA Houston Healthcare West/University of
    Houston
Houston, Texas

Emily Ann Gorman, DO
Assistant Program Director
Department of Family Medicine
OhioHealth Riverside Family Medicine
Columbus, Ohio

Kristina Gracey, MD, MPH
Assistant Professor
Department of Family Medicine and Community
    Health
University of Massachusetts
Worcester, Massachusetts

Michael Gray, MD
Springfield Hospital
Springfield, Vermont

Whitney Green, MD
Resident Physician
Department of Family Medicine
UTHSC–St. Francis
Memphis, Tennessee

Ramanpreet Grewal, MD
Family Medicine
Galesburg Cottage Hospital
Galesburg, Illinois

Hunter Grey, OD
Physician
Department of Ophthalmology/Optometry
Baylor Scott & White Medical Center
Waco, Texas

Simon B. Griesbach, MD†
Assistant Director
Department of Family Medicine
Waukesha Family Medicine Residency at
    ProHealth Care
Waukesha, Wisconsin
Clinical Adjunct Assistant Professor
Department of Family Medicine and Community
    Health
Madison, Wisconsin
Assistant Clinical Professor
Department of Family and Community Medicine
Medical College of Wisconsin
Milwaukee, Wisconsin

Lauren A. Griffin, DO
Resident
Department of Family Medicine
Novant Health
Cornelius, North Carolina

Andrew Grimes, MD
Affiliate Clinical Faculty
Department of Perioperative Medicine
Dell Medical School, The University of Texas at
    Austin
Austin, Texas

Neena R. Gupta, MD†
Associate Professor
Department of Pediatric Nephrology
UMass Memorial Medical Center
Worcester, Massachusetts

Sonia Gupta, MD
Resident
Department of Internal Medicine
Creighton University
Omaha, Nebraska

Emmeline Ha, MD
Health Policy Research Fellow
George Washington University
Washington, District of Columbia

Michael Haddadin, MD
Fellow
Department of Hematology
Oncology University of Massachusetts
Worcester, Massachusetts

Reem Hadi, MD
Board-Certified Family Physician
Forward Health
San Antonio, Texas

Matthew A. Halfar, MD
Assistant Professor
Department of Family and Community Medicine
Creighton University
Omaha, Nebraska

Thomas J. Hansen, MD†
System Vice President Chief Academic Officer
Department of Academic Affairs
Advocate Aurora Health
Downers Grove, Illinois

Allison Hargreaves, MD
Assistant Professor of Family Medicine and
    Community Health
UMass Chan Medical School
Worcester, Massachusetts

Chelsea Harris, MD
Faculty
Department of Family Medicine
Lawrence Family Medicine Residency
Lawrence, Massachusetts

Alyssa Jeanne Vest Hart, DO, FAAFP
Program Director, St. Joseph Family Medicine
    Residency
Chicago, Illinois

Chandra Hartman, MD, FAAFP
Program Director
Greenfield Family Medicine Residency
UMass Chan Medical School-Baystate Health
Greenfield, Massachusetts

Fern R. Hauck, MD, MS, FAAFP
Professor
Spencer P. Bass, MD, Twenty-First Century
    Professor of Family Medicine
Professor of Public Health Sciences
Director of Research and Faculty Development
University of Virginia School of Medicine
Charlottesville, Virginia

Kelsey R. Henry, MD
Chief Resident
Department of Family Medicine
Ascension St. Vincent's
Jacksonville, Florida

Luke T. Hentrich, PharmD
PGY-2 Pharmacotherapy Resident
The University of Tennessee Health Science
    Center
College of Pharmacy
Knoxville, Tennessee

Tony Cha Her, MD
Assistant Professor and Director of Anatomical
    Programs
Surgery Department
Charles E. Schmidt College of Medicine
Florida Atlantic University
Boca Raton, Florida

Emily N. Hernandez, DO
Resident Physician
Department of Family Medicine
Advocate Christ Medical Center
Oak Lawn, Illinois

Katelyn Hernandez, DO
Resident Physician
Department of Pediatrics
AdventHealth for Children
Orlando, Florida

**Pablo I. Hernandez Itriago, MD, MHCM,
    FAAFP**
Chief Medical Officer
Edward M. Kennedy Community Health Center
Assistant Professor
Department of Family Medicine and Community
    Health
UMass Chan Medical School
Worcester, Massachusetts

Christopher R. Heron, MD, BS
Associate Professor
Department of Family and Community Medicine
Penn State Health Milton S. Hershey Medical
    Center
Hershey, Pennsylvania

Lisa Hertz, MD
Department of Gastroenterology
Long Beach Memorial Medical Center
Long Beach, California

Zachary H. Hicks, DO
Family Medicine Resident
Family Medicine Residency Clinic
Travis Air Force Base
Fairfield, California

Jordan Patrick Hilgefort, MD
Assistant Professor
Department of Family and Geriatric Medicine
University of Louisville School of Medicine
Louisville, Kentucky

Joseph Daniel Hogue, MD, MBA
Program Director, Family Medicine Residency at
    Baptist Desoto
Baptist Memorial Medical Education
Memphis, Tennessee

Allison Holley, MD
Assistant Professor of Family Medicine
Florida Atlantic University College of Medicine
Boca Raton, Florida

Stanton C. Honig, MD†
Clinical Professor of Urology
Department of Urology
Yale University School of Medicine
New Haven, Connecticut

**Steven A. House, MD, FAAFP, FAAHPM,
    HMDC**
Professor, Program Director
Department of Family and Geriatric Medicine
University of Louisville/Glasgow
Glasgow, Kentucky

Jordan Howard-Young, MD
Assistant Professor of Family Medicine and
    Community Health
Assistant Professor of Psychiatry
UMass Chan Medical School
Worcester, Massachusetts

Vincent Huang, MD
Resident Physician
Department of Internal Medicine
Pennsylvania Hospital
Philadelphia, Pennsylvania

Dennis E. Hughes, DO, FACEP
Attending Physician
CoxHealth
Springfield, Missouri

Pamela R. Hughes, MD†
Military Program Director
Department of Family Medicine
St. Louis University Southwest Illinois Family
    Medicine Residency
O'Fallon, Illinois

Lauren A. Hutka, DO
Resident Physician
Obstetrics and Gynecology, Aultman Hospital
Canton, Ohio

Daniel Idahosa, MD, BS
Resident Physician
Department of Emergency Medicine
Robert Wood Johnson University Hospital
New Brunswick, New Jersey

Adora Ilochonwu, MD
Resident Physician
Department of Family Medicine
Advocate Christ Medical Center
Oak Lawn, Illinois

Adedapo Iluyomade, MD, MBA
Clinical Faculty
Division of Cardiology
University of Miami Hospital and Clinics
Miami, Florida

Oleg Isakov, MD
Clinical Assistant Professor
SUNY Downstate School of Medicine
Brooklyn, New York

Bashyam Iyengar, MD, MPH
Faculty, Family Medicine
Ascension St. Vincent
Jacksonville, Florida

Vasudha Jain, MD
Core Faculty
Department of Family Medicine
Tidelands Health
Myrtle Beach, South Carolina

Nikhil Jaiswal, MD
Texas A&M University
College Station, Texas

Pooja Mira Jayaprakash, MD
Adjunct Assistant Clinical Professor
Department of Community Health and Family
    Medicine
University of Florida
Gainesville, Florida

Zaiba Jetpuri, DO, MBA, FAAFP
Associate Professor
Department of Family and Community Medicine
UT Southwestern Medical Center
Dallas, Texas

Dongsheng Jiang, MD, MSc
Associate Professor
Penn State University
State College, Pennsylvania

James F. Jiang, MD
Department of Urology
UC Irvine Urology
Orange, California

Joanna Jiang, MD
Medical Resident
Ohio State University
Columbus, Ohio

Nasheena Jiwa, MD
Physician/Fellow
Department of Pulmonary and Critical Care
University of Connecticut Health Center
Farmington, Connecticut

Brett Johnson, MD
Program Director, Family Medicine
Methodist Health System
Dallas, Texas

Erin Johnson, MD
UMass Chan Medical School
Worcester, Massachusetts

Katherine G. W. Johnson, MD
Assistant Professor
Department of Family Medicine
Self Regional Healthcare
Greenwood, South Carolina

Lars J. Johnson, MD
Clinical Instructor
Department of Internal Medicine
University of Michigan
Ann Arbor, Michigan

Tyler Johnson, DO
Surgical Resident
Department of General Surgery
Spartanburg Regional Medical Center
Spartanburg, South Carolina

Julie Johnston, MD, FAAFP
Faculty Physician
Lawrence Family Medicine Residency
Lawrence, Massachusetts

Melody A. Jordahl-Iafrato, MD, FAAFP
Assistant Program Director
Community Hospital East Family Medicine
    Residency
Department of Family Medicine
Community Hospital
East Indianapolis, Indiana

Jillian K. Joseph, MPAS, PA-C
Instructor
Department of Family Medicine and Community
    Health
UMass Memorial Health
Worcester, Massachusetts

Nisarg Joshi, MD, BS
Junior Attending, Vitreoretinal Surgery Fellow
Department of Ophthalmology
University of South Florida
Tampa, Florida

Patrick Wakefield Joyner, MD, MS[†]
Assistant Professor
Department of Orthopedic Surgery
ORTHOCOLLIER
Naples, Florida

Tya-Mae Y. Julien, MD
Gastroenterologist, Independent Contractor
North Texas Bioethics Network
UT Southwestern Medical Center
Dallas, Texas

Khadija Kabani, DO, FAAFP
Associate Program Director
Department of Family Medicine
Methodist Health System
Dallas, Texas

Hamid Kadiwala, MD
Neurologist/Epileptologist
Fort Worth Epilepsy Clinic
Fort Worth, Texas

Afsha Rais Kaisani, MD
Core Faculty
Medical City Arlington Family Medicine
    Residency Program - HCA Medical City
    Healthcare UNT-TCU Graduate Medical
    Education Consortium
Arlington, Texas

Mwangi Kamau, MD
University of Massachusetts Medical School
Worcester, Massachusetts

Donna Kaminski, DO, MPH, FAAFP
Assistant Director
Somerset Family Medicine Residency Program
Rutgers Health Robert Wood Johnson University
    Hospital
Somerville, New Jersey

Lovella Kanu, MD, FAAFP, Dipl. ABOM
Assistant Program Director
Advocate Family Medicine Residency Program
Oak Lawn, Illinois

Rahul Kapur, MD
Assistant Professor
Department of Family Medicine and Community
    Health
University of Minnesota
Minneapolis, Minnesota

Nioti R. Karim, MD
Core Faculty
Department of Family Medicine
University of Houston
Houston, Texas

Chelsea Karson, MD
Resident Physician
Department of Psychiatry
Advocate Lutheran General Hospital
Park Ridge, Illinois

Clara M. Keegan, MD
Associate Professor
Department of Family Medicine
The Robert Larner, M.D. College of Medicine at
    The University of Vermont
Burlington, Vermont

Priscilla L. Kha, DO, MPH[†]
Resident Physician
Family and Community Medicine
University of Texas at Southwestern Medical
    Center
Dallas, Texas

Mohamad Khalil, MD
Department of Family and Community Medicine
Creighton University
Omaha, Nebraska

Anila Khaliq, MD
Faculty
Department of Family Medicine
Touro College of Osteopathic Medicine
Middletown, New York

Hiba A. Khan, DO
Oak Lawn, Illinois

Catherine Khoo, MD, FAAFP
Adjunct Clinical Assistant Professor of Family
    Medicine (Voluntary) at the Keck School of
    Medicine
Family Medicine Residency Program
California Hospital Medical Center
Los Angeles, California

Alexander J. Kiener, MD
Post-Doctoral Clinical Fellow
Department of Cardiology
Baylor College of Medicine/Texas Children's
    Hospital
Houston, Texas

Barbara M. Kiersz Mueller, DO
Family and Osteopathic Medicine Physician
Austin Regional Clinic—Far West
Austin, Texas

Caleb Weiss Kiesow, MD, BS
Resident
Department of Family Medicine
SLU/SWIL USAF Family Medicine Residency
O'Fallon, Illinois

Catherine Kim, MD
Resident Physician
Department of Family Medicine
HCA Medical City Arlington
Arlington, Texas

Michael J. Kim, MD, FAAFP
Assistant Professor
Department of Family Medicine
Uniformed Services University of the Health
    Sciences
Bethesda, Maryland

Walter M. Kim, MD, PhD
Lecturer
Department of Medicine
Harvard Medical School
Associate Physician
Division of Gastroenterology, Hepatology and
    Endoscopy
Brigham and Women's Hospital
Chief
Department of Gastroenterology
Lemuel Shattuck Hospital
Boston, Massachusetts

Brian J. Kimbrell, MD, FACS
Assistant Professor of Surgery
University of Florida
Trauma Medical Director
Medical Director of Critical Care Medicine
Blake Medical Center
Bradenton, Florida

Thomas Kingsley, MD, MPH, MS
Assistant Professor of Medicine and Biomedical
    Informatics
Department of Medicine and Epidemiology
Mayo Clinic
Rochester, Minnesota

Marni Klessman Gleiber, MD
Assistant Professor of Physical Medicine and
    Rehabilitation
Director of Ethics, Professionalism &
    Professional Identity Thread
Charles E. Schmidt College of Medicine
Florida Atlantic University
Boca Raton, Florida

Laura K. Klug, PharmD
Associate Professor
Department of Pharmacy Practice and Family
    and Community Medicine
Creighton University
Omaha, Nebraska

Arturas Klugas, MD, FAAFP
Assistant Professor
Department of Family Medicine
MSU/Alma Family Medicine Residency
Alma, Michigan

Egle Klugiene, MD
Faculty Physician
Department of Family Medicine
MidMichigan Medical Center
Gratiot, Michigan

Jennifer Koch, MD
Professor
Department of Medicine
University of Louisville
Louisville, Kentucky

Sharon L. Koehler, DO, FACS†
Assistant Professor, Breast Surgery
Department of Clinical Specialties
New York Institute of Technology College of
    Osteopathic Medicine
Old Westbury, New York

Sumira A. Koirala, MD, FAAFP
Faculty, Associate Professor of Family and
    Community Medicine
St. Elizabeth Boardman Family Medicine
    Residency
Bon Secours Mercy Health
Boardman, Ohio

Ashley Koontz Sturts, DO
Assistant Professor
Department of Family and Community Medicine
Penn State Health Milton S. Hershey Medical
    Center
Hershey, Pennsylvania

Scott E. Kopec, MD, FCCP
Program Director, Internal Medicine Residency
Department of Pulmonary, Allergy, and Critical
    Care Medicine
UMass Chan Medical School
Worcester, Massachusetts

Matthew J. Kor, MD
Family Medicine Physician
Department of Family Medicine
Dignity Health
San Andreas, California

Lukas D. Kost, MD
Resident
Department of Family Medicine
United Health Services
Binghamton, New York

Nora Elizabeth Kratz, MD
Resident Physician
Department of Family Medicine and Community
    Medicine
University of New Mexico
Albuquerque, New Mexico

Pankaj Ksheersagar, MD
Department of Family Medicine and Community
    Health
University of Massachusetts
Worcester, Massachusetts

Mukti Kulkarni, MD, MPH
Assistant Professor
Family Medicine and Community Health
UMass Chan Medical School
Worcester, Massachusetts

Shalini Kumar, MD
Family Medicine Resident, PGY-2
Department of Family Medicine
Advocate Christ Medical Center
Oak Lawn, Illinois

Daniel B. Kurtz, PhD, BS†
Professor Emeritus
Department of Biology
Utica College
Utica, New York

Melinda Kwan, DO, MPH
Urgent Care Physician
Department of Urgent Care
Southwest Medical Associates
Las Vegas, Nevada

Makayla Lagerman, MD
Resident Physician
Department of Family and Community Medicine
Penn State Health Milton S. Hershey Medical
    Center
Hershey, Pennsylvania

**Jason Edward Lambrecht, MD, FHM, FACP,
    PharmD†**
Assistant Professor
Critical Care Fellow
Department of Internal Medicine
Creighton University
Omaha, Nebraska

Anne Campbell Larkin, MD
Associate Professor
Department of Surgery
UMass Chan Medical School
Worcester, Massachusetts

Shane L. Larson, MD†
Assistant Professor of Family Medicine
Uniformed Services University of the Health
    Sciences
Womack Army Medical Center
Fort Bragg, North Carolina

Justin P. Lavin Jr., MD, FACOG
Professor and Chairman Emeritus
Department of Obstetrics and Gynecology
Cleveland Clinic Akron General
Akron, Ohio

Kelley V. Lawrence, MD, IBCLC
Assistant Campus Director
Department of UNC School of Medicine
    Charlotte Campus
Novant Health
Charlotte, North Carolina

Justin D. Leavitt, MD
Resident Physician
Department of General Surgery
Novant New Hanover Regional Medical Center
Wilmington, North Carolina

Bianca Lee, DO, MS
Department of Internal Medicine
Nassau University Medical Center
East Meadow, New York

Daniel T. Lee, MD, MA
Clinical Professor
Department of Family Medicine
University of California, Los Angeles
Los Angeles, California

David L. Lee, MD
Assistant Professor
Department of Family and Community Medicine
Penn State Health Milton S. Hershey Medical
    Center
Hershey, Pennsylvania

Hobart Lee, MD, FAAFP
Associate Professor
Department of Family Medicine
Loma Linda University School of Medicine
Loma Linda, California

Junseo Bernard Lee, MD
Resident
Department of Internal Medicine
George Washington University
Washington, District of Columbia

F. Stuart Leeds, MD, MS
Associate Professor
Department of Family Medicine
Wright State University Boonshoft School of
    Medicine
Dayton, Ohio

Brett Lehner, MD
UMass Memorial Medical Center
Worcester, Massachusetts

Angelia Leipelt, BA, IBCLC, ICCE, CLE
Lactation Consultant
Dignity Health Methodist Hospital of
    Sacramento
Sacramento, California

Mollie R. Lerner, DO, MS
Resident
Department of Family Medicine
Novant Health
Cornelius, North Carolina

Nikki A. Levin, MD, PhD
Associate Professor
Department of Dermatology
University of Massachusetts Medical School
Worcester, Massachusetts

Gary I. Levine, MD
Associate Professor
Department of Family Medicine
Brody School of Medicine
East Carolina University
Greenville, North Carolina

Briana Lindberg, MD, CAQSM
Associate Program Director
Department of Family Medicine
Womack Army Medical Center Family Medicine
    Residency Program
Fort Bragg, North Carolina

Stephen W. Line, DO, CAQSM
Associate Program Director
Primary Care Sports Medicine Fellowship
Clinical Assistant Professor
Department of Primary Care and Rural Health
Texas A&M University
College Station, Texas

Evan R. Locke, MD
Resident Physician
Department of Family Medicine
David Grant Medical Center
Travis Air Force Base, California

Daud Lodin, MD, MPH
Surgical Resident
Department of Surgery
Charles E. Schmidt College of Medicine
Florida Atlantic University
Boca Raton, Florida

Jacquelynn P. Luker, MD
Assistant Professor
Department of Family, Internal, and Rural
    Medicine
The University of Alabama
Tuscaloosa, Alabama

Nica E. Lurtsema, MD, MPH
Department of Family and Community Medicine
Texas Tech University Health Sciences Center
    School of Medicine
Lubbock, Texas

Ryan D. Lurtsema, MD
Assistant Professor
Sports Medicine, Family and Community
    Medicine
Texas Tech University Health Sciences Center
Lubbock, Texas

Eileen Ly, MD
Family Medicine Resident
Travis Family Medicine Residency Program
Fairfield, California

Ann M. Lynch, PharmD, RPh, AE-C
Professor
Department of Pharmacy Practice
Massachusetts College of Pharmacy and Health
    Sciences University
Worcester, Massachusetts

**Jonathan Edward MacClements, MD,
    FAAFP**
Professor
Department of Medical Education and
    Population Health
Dell Medical School, The University of Texas at
    Austin
Austin, Texas

Nathan J. Macedo, MD, MPH
Assistant Professor
Department of Family Medicine
UMass Chan Medical School-Baystate
Springfield, Massachusetts

Theodore E. Macnow, MD
Assistant Professor of Pediatrics
Department of Pediatric Emergency
UMass Memorial Children's Medical Center
Worcester, Massachusetts

Michael J. Maddaleni, MD
Department of Family Medicine/Sports Medicine
University of Massachusetts Medical School
Worcester, Massachusetts

Manju Mahajan, MD, FAAFP
Faculty
Department of Family Medicine and Community
    Health
Hahnemann Family Health Center
UMass Chan Medical School
Worcester, Massachusetts

Shayan Mahapatra, MBBS, MD
Internal Medicine Resident
Cleveland Clinic Florida
Weston, Florida

Deepali Maheshwari, DO, MPH[†]
Fellow
Department of Obstetrics and Gynecology
University of Massachusetts Medical School
Worcester, Massachusetts

Daniel John Majarwitz, MD
Resident Physician
Department of Internal Medicine/Psychiatry
East Carolina University
Greenville, North Carolina

Shivani Malhotra, MD, FAAFP
Associate Professor & Regional Chair
Department of Family Medicine
UAB Family Medicine Program
Huntsville, Alabama

Samir Malkani, MD, MRCP–UK
Professor
Department of Medicine
University of Massachusetts Medical School
Worcester, Massachusetts

Boyd S. Malphrus, BA, MPAS
Physician Assistant
Duke Employee Occupational Health and
    Wellness
Duke University Medical Center
Durham, North Carolina

Michael Mamone, MD
St. Georges University School of Medicine
True Blue, Grenada

Lee A. Mancini, MD, CSCS*D, CSN
Associate Professor
Department of Family Medicine and Community
    Health
Chief, Division of Sports and Exercise Medicine
Director, Primary Care Sports and Exercise
    Medicine Fellowship
University of Massachusetts
Worcester, Massachusetts

Eric J. Mao, MD
Assistant Professor
Department of Medicine
Division of Gastroenterology and Hepatology
University of California, Davis
Sacramento, California

Laura Marsh, MD, CAQSM
Program Director
Sports Medicine Fellowship
Clinical Assistant Professor
Department of Primary Care and Rural
    Medicine
Texas A&M University
College Station, Texas

Wendy K. Marsh, MD, MSc
Associate Professor
Department of Psychiatry
University of Massachusetts Medical School
Worcester, Massachusetts

Bethany P. Marshall, PharmD
Faculty
Prisma Sumter Family Medicine Residency
Prisma Health
Sumter, South Carolina

Nicholas R. Martin, MD
Resident
Department of Family Medicine and Community
    Health
University of Massachusetts Medical School
Worcester, Massachusetts

Stephen A. Martin, MD, EdM
Associate Professor
Department of Family Medicine and Community
    Health
University of Massachusetts Medical School
Worcester, Massachusetts

William Edwin Martin, MD, MBA, MPH
Medical Director
Mediprise
Houston, Texas

Lisa C. Martinez, MD
Associate Professor
Department of Medicine
Florida Atlantic University
Boca Raton, Florida

Marni L. Martinez, APRN
Clinical Nurse Specialist
Austin Gastroenterology
Austin, Texas

George W. Matar, MD
Resident Physician
Department of Family and Community Health
University Hospital Cleveland Medical Center
Cleveland, Ohio

Donnah Mathews, MD, FACP
Assistant Professor
Department of Internal Medicine
Alpert School of Medicine at Brown University
Providence, Rhode Island

Daniel R. Matta, MD
Family Medicine Residency Faculty
Department of Family Medicine
Tallahassee Memorial Hospital Family Medicine
Residency Program
Tallahassee, Florida

Douglas M. Maurer, DO, MPH, FAAFP[†]
Director Medical Education
Department of Family Medicine
Madigan Army Medical Center
Tacoma, Washington

George Maxted, MD
Associate Clinical Professor
Department of Family Medicine
Tufts University School of Medicine
Boston, Massachusetts

Jeremy Maxwell, MBBS
PGY-2 Resident
Department of Family Medicine
Tallahassee Memorial Healthcare
Tallahassee, Florida

Beth K. Mazyck, MD
Associate Professor
Department of Family Medicine and Community
Health
University of Massachusetts Medical School
Worcester, Massachusetts

Andrew McBride, MD
Family Medicine Liaison
Department of Family Medicine
University of Colorado
Aurora, Colorado
Department of Family Medicine and Sports
Medicine
Boulder Community Health
Boulder, Colorado

Adam McConnell, MD
Faculty
SSM Family Medicine Residency
Oklahoma City, Oklahoma

Lindsay McCormack, MD
Department of Dermatology
University of Massachusetts Medical School
Worcester, Massachusetts

Oregon J. McDiarmid, MD
Resident Physician
GME – Family Medicine
Medical City Arlington
Arlington, Texas

Susan McDiarmid, EdD, MS, PA-C
Assistant Program Director
Physician Assistant Program
Westfield State University
Westfield, Massachusetts

Michelle Moran McDonough, MD
Co-Chief Resident
Department of Family Medicine Residency
Program
Mayo Clinic—Mankato
Mankato, Minnesota

Paul McFarlane, MBBS
Resident Physician
Department of Family Medicine Residency
Program
Tallahassee Memorial Healthcare
Tallahassee, Florida

Marc McKenna, MD, CAQSM
Program Director
Chestnut Hill Family Medicine Residency
Philadelphia, Pennsylvania

Donna Marie McMahon, DO, FAAP
Associate Professor, Associate Dean Student
Affairs
Department of Clinical Specialties, Pediatrics
NYIT College of Osteopathic Medicine
Old Westbury, New York

Brock McMillen, MD, FFAFP
Assistant Professor of Clinical Family Medicine
Indiana University School of Medicine
Indianapolis, Indiana

Susan Medalie, DO
Core Faculty, FM/OB—Lehigh Valley Health
Network
Schuylkill Rural Residency
Pottsville, Pennsylvania

Christopher Medrano, MD
Department of Family Medicine
Saint Joseph Hospital
Chicago, Illinois

Jennifer A. Meeks, DO
Assistant Director
Department of Family Medicine
AdventHealth
Orlando, Florida

Randi Cheree Melton, DO
Assistant Professor
Department of Family Medicine
Tuscaloosa Family Medicine Residency Program
Tuscaloosa, Alabama

Donna I. Meltzer, MD
Clinical Associate Professor
Department of Family, Population & Preventive
Medicine
Stony Brook Medicine
Stony Brook, New York

Adam Mendonca, MD[†]
Family Medicine
Resident Physician
Family and Community Medicine
Baylor College of Medicine
Houston, Texas

Chelsea Mendonca, MD[†]
Assistant Professor
Department of Family and Community Medicine
Baylor College of Medicine
Houston, Texas

Caleb J. Mentzer, DO
Assistant Professor
Department of Surgery
Division of Trauma, Critical Care, & Acute Care
Surgery
Spartanburg Regional Medical Center
Spartanburg, South Carolina

Marcelle Meseeha, MD
Assistant Professor
Department of Internal Medicine Guthrie
Sayre, Pennsylvania

Eric Robert Messner, PhD, FNP-BC
Associate Medical Director
Department of Family and Community Medicine
Inpatient Service
Assistant Professor
Department of Family and Community Medicine
Penn State Health Milton S. Hershey Medical
Center
Hershey, Pennsylvania

Katherine Metropulos, DO
Resident Physician
Department of Family Medicine
Advocate Christ Medical Center Family
    Medicine Program
Oak Lawn, Illinois

Sloan F. Miler, MD
Department of Medicine
Lemuel Shattuck Hospital
Jamaica Plain, Massachusetts

Jan Estes Miller, MD
Associate Program Director
SSM Health St Anthony Family Medicine
    Residency
Oklahoma City, Oklahoma

Paul G. Millner, MD
Assistant Professor
Department of Internal Medicine
Creighton University
Omaha, Nebraska

Tasaduq Hussain Mir, MD, FAAFP
Faculty
Department of Family Medicine
Medical City Arlington
Arlington, Texas

Shabia Mohammed, DO
Resident Physician
Department of Family Medicine
Advocate Christ Medical Center
Oak Lawn, Illinois

Hammad Mohsin, MD
Assistant Professor
Department of Psychiatry
Mather at Northwell Health
Port Jefferson, New York

Saadia Mohsin, MD
Physician
Capital Health
Pennington, New Jersey

**Katherine Montag Schafer, PharmD,
    BCACP**
Assistant Professor
Department of Family Medicine and Community
    Health
University of Minnesota
Minneapolis, Minnesota

Nicholas Moore, MD, FAAFP, CAQSM
Medical Director
Motor City Orthopedics & Sports Medicine
Associate Director
Providence Sports Medicine Fellowship Program
Assistant Professor
Michigan State University College of Human
    Medicine
Novi, Michigan

Elias Moreno, DO
Tallahassee Memorial Healthcare
Tallahassee, Florida

Jared Morphew, MD
Assistant Professor
Department of Family and Community Medicine
UT Southwestern Medical Center
Dallas, Texas

Daniel Scott Morrison, MD
Associate Professor
Department of Emergency Medicine
Rutgers Robert Wood Johnson Medical School
New Brunswick, New Jersey

Christopher Morrow, PA-C†
United States Army

Rachel Kristina Moyer, MD
Resident Physician
Department of Family Medicine
David Grant Medical Center
Fairfield, California

David Mullen, MD
Assistant Professor of Clinical Family Medicine
Department of Family Medicine
Indiana University School of Medicine
Indianapolis, Indiana

Sahil Mullick, MD
Associate Program Director, Director of
    Inpatient Service, Assistant Clinical Professor,
    Hospitalist, Core Faculty
Department of Family and Community Medicine
Creighton University School of Medicine
Omaha, Nebraska

Carolyn Murphy, MD
Assistant Professor
Department of Palliative Care
University of Massachusetts
Worcester, Massachusetts

Rachel C. Murphy, DO
Spartanburg Regional Medical Center
Spartanburg, South Carolina

Mark T. Nadeau, MD, MBA†
Professor and Program Director
Department of Family and Community Medicine
University of Texas Health Science Center at
    San Antonio
San Antonio, Texas

Sabari Nair, DO
Resident Physician
Department of Family Medicine
Lakeside Medical Center
Belle Glade, Florida

Munima Nasir, MD
Associate Professor
Department of Family and Community Medicine
Penn State Health Milton S. Hershey Medical
    Center
Hershey, Pennsylvania

Ned Francis Nasr, MD, FASA
Vice Chair for Education, Department of
    Anesthesiology
Program Director, Anesthesiology Residency
    Program
Advocate Illinois Masonic Medical Center
Chicago, Illinois

Kristen Nayak, MD
Clinical Assistant Professor
Department of Medicine
Division of Primary Care and Population Health
Stanford University School of Medicine
Stanford, California

Katharine L. Neff, DO
United States Air Force
Tucson, Arizona

Michelle Nelson, MD
Core Faculty
Department of Family Medicine
MidMichigan Medical Center—Gratiot
Alma, Michigan

Vicki R. Nelson, MD, PhD
Associate Professor
Department of Family Medicine
Prisma Health-Upstate
University of South Carolina School of Medicine
    Greenville
Greenville, South Carolina

David Neuberger, MD
Assistant Professor
Department of Family and Geriatric Medicine
University of Louisville
Louisville, Kentucky

Sandra N. New, DNP
Retired
Knoxville, Tennessee

Annemarie Newark, MD
Physician
Department of Obstetrics and Gynecology
Cleveland Clinic Akron General
Akron, Ohio

Jacob Thomas Newman, DO
Resident Physician
Department of Internal Medicine
The George Washington University Hospital
Washington, District of Columbia

Roland W. Newman II, DO
Assistant Professor
Associate Program Director—Family and
    Community Medicine Residency Program
Department of Family and Community Medicine
Penn State Health Milton S. Hershey Medical
    Center
Hershey, Pennsylvania

Melinda W. Ng, MD
Resident Physician
Department of Family Medicine
David Grant Medical Center
Fairfield, California

Elizabeth T. Nguyen, MD
Department of Texas A&M Athletics
Department of Primary Care and Rural
    Medicine
Texas A&M University
College Station, Texas

Huong N. Nguyen, DO, MS
Resident Physician
Department of Family and Community Medicine
Penn State Health Milton S. Hershey Medical
    Center
Hershey, Pennsylvania

Nancy V. Nguyen, DO
Core Faculty, Methodist Hospital FMRP
Chair Family Medicine
Dignity Health Methodist Hospital of
    Sacramento
Sacramento, California

Tam T. Nguyen, MD
Washington Township Medical Group
Union City, California

Tu Dan Nguyen, MD, CAQSM
Director of Sports Medicine
Department of Family Medicine
Memorial Family Medicine Residency Program
Sugar Land, Texas

Sarah E. Nickolich, MD
Assistant Professor
Department of Family and Community Medicine
Penn State Health
Hershey, Pennsylvania

Frederick W. Nielson, MD†
MAJ, USAF, MC
Department of Family Medicine
US Air Force
Eielson Air Force Base, Alaska

Matthew Nodelman, MD
Assistant Medical Director
Associate Program Director
Department of Family Medicine
Prisma Health/University of South Carolina
    School of Medicine—Columbia
Columbia, South Carolina

Benjamin Nolasco, MD, MHS
Resident Physician
Valley Stream Health System
Las Vegas, Nevada

Victoria Allon Nutting, DO, MS
Resident Physician
Department of Family Medicine Residency
Texas A&M University
College Station, Texas

Davis M. O'Brien, MD
Resident Physician
Department of Surgery
Medical College of Georgia
Augusta, Georgia

Smriti Ohri, MD
Assistant Professor
Department of Family Medicine
University of Connecticut
Hartford, Connecticut

Alicia Leandra Olowu, DO
Core Faculty
Department of Family Medicine
Garnet Health Medical Center
Middletown, New York

Opeoluwa Olukorede, MD
Resident
Department of Family Medicine and Community
    Health
UMass Chan Medical School
Worcester, Massachusetts

Adedamola Ayo Omole, MD
Adventist Health Hanford
Hanford, California

Daniela Rangel Orozco, MD, MHP, MS
Associate Program Director
Department of Family Medicine
Kaweah Health
Visalia, California

Seniha Ozudogru, MD
Assistant Professor
Department of Neurology
University of Pennsylvania
Philadelphia, Pennsylvania

Kelly Pagidas, MD
Professor, Texas Christian University
Fort Worth, Texas

Chris Para, MD
Resident
Department of Internal Medicine
Advocate Christ Medical Center
Oak Lawn, Illinois

Jon S. Parham, DO, MPH, FAAFP
Associate Professor
Department of Family Medicine
University of Tennessee Graduate School of
    Medicine
Knoxville, Tennessee

Nisha J. Parikh, MD, MPH
Emergency Medicine Resident
Department of Emergency Medicine
Rutgers Robert Wood Johnson Medical School
New Brunswick, New Jersey

Doyun Park, MD
Attending Physician
Department of Hematology
Baystate
Springfield, Massachusetts

Morgan J. Parker, DO
PGY-1 Resident
Department of Family Medicine
Novant Health
Cornelius, North Carolina

Naomi Parrella, MD, FAAFP, Dipl. ABOM
Associate Professor and Medical Director
Department of Family Medicine
Department of Surgery
Rush University Medical Center
Chicago, Illinois

Elyas Parsa, DO
Program Director
Department of Family Medicine
San Joaquin General Hospital
French Camp, California

Michael T. Partin, MD
Assistant Professor
Department of Family and Community Medicine
Penn State Health Milton S. Hershey Medical
    Center
Hershey, Pennsylvania

Bindusri Paruchuri, MD
Assistant Professor
Department of Family Medicine
University of Tennessee Health Science Center
Nashville Family Medicine Residency Program
Murfreesboro, Tennessee

Ankit Patel, MD
Resident Physician
Department of Internal Medicine
George Washington University
Washington, District of Columbia

Avignat S. Patel, MD
Senior Physician
Department of Pulmonary Critical Care
    Medicine
Lahey Hospital and Medical Center
Burlington, Massachusetts
Assistant Professor
Department of Medicine
Tufts University School of Medicine
Boston, Massachusetts

Birju B. Patel, MD, FACP†
Adjunct Assistant Professor of Medicine
Emory University School of Medicine
Atlanta, Georgia

Damini Patel, DO
Attending
Department of Family Medicine
Advocate Christ Medical Center
Oak Lawn, Illinois

Jay Patel, DO
Resident
Department of Family Medicine
Dell Medical School, The University of Texas at
    Austin
Austin, Texas

Nihal K. Patel, MD
Assistant Clinical Professor
Department of Medicine
University of Connecticut School of Medicine
Harford, Connecticut

Mahesh C. Patel, MD
Professor
Department of Internal Medicine-Infectious
    Diseases
University of Illinois at Chicago
Chicago, Illinois

Jyothi R. Patri, MD, MHA, FAAFP, HMDC
Program Director
Adventist Health Hanford Family Medicine
    Residency Program
Adventist Health Hanford Central Valley
    Network
Hanford, California

Jared M. Patton, MD, MS†
Senior Medical Officer
Camp Kinser Branch Medical Clinic
United States Navy
Okinawa, Japan

Amrutha Pavle, MD
Assistant Professor
Department of Family and Community Medicine
UT Southwestern Medical Center
Dallas, Texas

Amena Payami, DO
Family Medicine Resident Physician
AdventHealth East Orlando
Orlando, Florida

William Pearce, MD
Harvard Medical School
Boston, Massachusetts

Rade N. Pejic, MD
Associate Professor
Department of Family Medicine
Tulane University School of Medicine
New Orleans, Louisiana

Tristan M. Pennella, DO
Family Medicine Resident
Mayo Clinic Health System Mankato
Mankato, Minnesota

Daniel Perez, MD
Faculty
Department of Family Medicine
Lakeside Medical Center
Belle Glade, Florida

Juan Perez, DO
Assistant Professor
Department of Family Medicine
Penn State University
State College, Pennsylvania

Mayra A. Perez, DO
Clinical Assistant Professor
Department of Family and Community Medicine
UT Health San Antonio
San Antonio, Texas

Christine S. Persaud, MD, MBA
Assistant Professor, Program Director–Sports
    Medicine Fellowship
Department of Orthopedic Surgery &
    Rehabilitation Medicine
SUNY Downstate Health Sciences University
Brooklyn, New York

Parvathi Perumareddi, DO
Associate Professor
Charles E. Schmidt College of Medicine
Florida Atlantic University
Boca Raton, Florida

Casey Petronella, DO
Resident Physician, Family Medicine
Garnet Health Medical Center
Middletown, New York

Kelsey E. Phelps, MD†
Assistant Professor of Family Medicine
Louisiana State University Rural Family
    Medicine Residency
Bogalusa Louisiana State University
Bogalusa, Louisiana

Shawn Phillips, MD
Associate Professor
Department of Family and Community Medicine
    and Orthopedics and Rehabilitation
Penn State College of Medicine
Hershey, Pennsylvania

Grant Pierre, MD, CAQSM
Faculty UMass Sports Medicine Fellowship
Department of Family Medicine
University of Massachusetts
Worcester, Massachusetts

Sreelakshmi Surendran Pillai, MD
Resident
Department of Family medicine
Creighton University Medical Center
Omaha, Nebraska

Jared Piotrowski, MD
Lead Hospitalist
Associate Program Director Internal Medicine
    Residency
Department of Hospital Medicine
Cleveland Clinic Florida
Weston, Florida

Karly Pippitt, MD
Assistant Dean, Community Faculty
Department of Family and Preventive Medicine
University of Utah School of Medicine
Salt Lake City, Utah

William Andrew Pleasant, MD
Assistant Professor
Department of Emergency Medicine
Rutgers Robert Wood Johnson Medical School
New Brunswick, New Jersey

Meghan Plunkett, MD
96 MDG
Eglin Air Force Base, Florida

Ryan S. Poland, MD
Resident Physician
Department of Family and Community Medicine
Ohio State University Wexner Medical Center
Columbus, Ohio

Yevgeniy Popov, DO, MPH
Fellow
Department of Rheumatology
University of Massachusetts Medical School
Worcester, Massachusetts

Matthew E. Posen, DO
Resident Physician
Department of Internal Medicine
Advocate Christ Medical Center
Oak Lawn, Illinois

Donna R. Potts, MD
Faculty
Department of Family Medicine
Ascension St. Vincent's
Jacksonville, Florida

Stacy E. Potts, MD, Med
Professor
Executive Vice Chair of Education
Department of Family Medicine and Community
    Health
UMass Chan Medical School
Worcester, Massachusetts

James E. Powers, DO, FACEP, FAAEM
Professor of Emergency Medicine
Campbell University School of Osteopathic
    Medicine
Lillington, North Carolina

Sourabh Prabhakar, MD
Department of Cardiology
ProMedica Toledo Hospital
Toledo, Ohio

Meenu Prasad, DO
Resident Physician
Family Medicine
Garnet Health Medical Center
Middletown, New York

Priya Prasher, MBBS
Pediatric Emergency Medicine Fellow
Department of Emergency Medicine
Phoenix Children's Hospital
Phoenix, Arizona

Bethany Price, DO
Residency Faculty
Department of Family Medicine
Saint Mary's Family Medicine Residency
Grand Junction, Colorado

Bliss Puthenpurayil, MD
Department of Family Medicine
University of Texas Southwestern
Dallas, Texas

Natasha J. Pyzocha, DO, FAWM, FAAFP
Medical Director
98point6
Seattle, Washington

Jana Wei Qiao, MD
Resident Physician
Department of Family Medicine
Penn State Health Milton S. Hershey Medical
    Center
Hershey, Pennsylvania

Juan Qiu, MD, PhD
Professor
Department of Family and Community Medicine
Pennsylvania State University College of
    Medicine
State College, Pennsylvania

**Christine A. Quartuccio-Carran, DO,
    FAAFP**
Associate Program Director
Valley Health System Family Medicine
    Residency Program
Las Vegas, Nevada

Alexandria Quinere, DO, MBS[†]
Resident Physician, Family Medicine
Garnet Health Medical Center
Middletown, New York

Jeffrey D. Quinlan, MD, FAAFP[†]
Professor, Chair, and DEO
Department of Family Medicine
Roy J. and Lucille A. Carver College of Medicine,
    University of Iowa
Iowa City, Iowa

Sana W. Qureshi, DO
Department of Family Medicine
Medical City Arlington
Arlington, Texas

Alexander Sasha Rackman, MD
Assistant Professor
Department of Medicine
Florida Atlantic University
Boca Raton, Florida

Naureen Bashir Rafiq, MD, FAAFP
Associate Professor and Core faculty
Department of Family Medicine
Creighton University School of Medicine
Omaha, Nebraska

Kalyanakrishnan Ramakrishnan, MD
Professor
Department of Family and Preventive Medicine
University of Oklahoma Health Sciences Center
Oklahoma City, Oklahoma

Jason R. Ramos, MD, FAAFP
Family Medicine Program Director
Family Physician
Department of Family Medicine
Honor Community Health
Pontiac, Michigan

Melinda M. Rathkopf, MD, MBA
Allergist/Immunologist, Associate Professor of
    Pediatrics
Division of Allergy/Immunology, Children's
    Healthcare of Atlanta
Emory University School of Medicine
Atlanta, Georgia

Raye Reeder, MD, MPH
Assistant Professor
Department of Family and Community Medicine
OU School of Community Medicine
Tulsa, Oklahoma

Robyn Lee Reese, DO
Resident Physician
Department of Family Medicine
Mayo Clinic
Jacksonville, Florida

Jameson Reich, DO
David Grant Medical Center
Fairfield, California

Brittany M. Reid, MBBS
Resident Physician
Department of Family Medicine and Community
    Health
UMass Chan Medical School
Worcester, Massachusetts

Kimberly Resnick, MD
Director of Gynecologic Oncology
MetroHealth Medical Center
Cleveland, Ohio

Morgan Adams Rhodes, PharmD
Associate Professor
Department of Family and Preventive Medicine
University of South Carolina/Prisma Health
Columbia, South Carolina

Andrew J. Richardson, MD
Department of Family Medicine
Baylor Scott & White Health
College Station, Texas

Michael Richardson, MD
Clinical Assistant Professor
Family Medicine
Tufts University School of Medicine
Boston, Massachusetts

**Jacob Ringenberg, MD, CAQSM, MUSC,
    AHEC**
Assistant Professor
Self Regional Hospital
Greenwood, South Carolina

Bryce Ringwald, MD
Family Medicine Resident
OhioHealth Riverside Methodist Hospital
Columbus, Ohio

Michele Roberts, MD, PhD
Paxton, Massachusetts

Cecile T. Robes, DO
Associate Professor
Department of Family Medicine
Novant Health Family Medicine Residency
Cornelius, North Carolina

Sean C. Robinson, MD, CAQSM
Assistant Professor
Department of Family Medicine and Sports
    Medicine
Oregon Health & Science University
Portland, Oregon

Sylvia M. Robinson, MD
Physician
Department of Pediatrics
Rush University Medical Center
Chicago, Illinois

Chelsea E. Robitaille, MS, PA-C
Professor
Physician Assistant Program
Westfield State University
Westfield, Massachusetts

Leigh A. Romero, MD, CAQSM
Assistant Professor
Department of Population Health—Family
    Medicine
Dell Medical School, The University of Texas at
    Austin
Austin, Texas

Jennifer M. Romeu, MD, MSM
Associate Program Director
Family Medicine Residency Program
Central Michigan University College of
    Medicine
Saginaw, Michigan

Scott Rosen, MD
Assistant Professor
Department of Internal Medicine
Baptist Memorial Medical Education
Southaven, Mississippi

Laura Ross, MD
Hospitalist
Novant Health Huntersville Medical Center
Huntersville, North Carolina

Stacy P. Rubin, MD
Assistant Professor
Department of Internal Medicine
Charles E. Schmidt College of Medicine
Florida Atlantic University
Boca Raton, Florida

Emerald Russell-Nathan, MD
PGY-2 Pediatric Resident
AdventHealth for Children
Orlando, Florida

**Anup Sabharwal, MD, MBA, FACE, FASPC,
    FNLA**
Professor
Department of Endocrinology, Diabetes, and
    Metabolism
Florida International University
Miami Beach, Florida

Omar B. Saeed, DO, MPH
Resident Physician
Department of Ophthalmology
Kettering Health Dayton
Dayton, Ohio

Artika Saharan, MD
New Brunswick, New Jersey

Kristen EB Said, MD, MPH
Assistant Professor
Department of Family Medicine and Community
    Health
Duke University
Durham, North Carolina

Amulya Sajja, MD
Resident Physician
Department of Family Medicine
HCA Medical City Arlington
Arlington, Texas

Lewjain Sakr, MD
Department of Internal Medicine
Cleveland Clinic Florida
Weston, Florida

Akanksha Samal, DO
Department of Family Medicine
AdventHealth East Orlando
Orlando, Florida

Kyle M. Samyn, DO, MS
Resident Physician
Department of Family Medicine
Oakland Primary Care
Warren, Michigan

Vicente T. San Martin, MD
Medical Director
Department of Endocrinology
Macromedica Dominicana
Santo Domingo, Dominican Republic

Sagar Saoji, MD
Resident
Department of Family Medicine
Lakeside Medical Center
Belle Glade, Florida

Arindam Sarkar, MD
Assistant Professor
Department of Family and Community Medicine
Baylor College of Medicine
Houston, Texas

Katelyn D. Sarkar, PA-C
Physical Medicine & Rehabilitation
UTHealth Houston
Houston, Texas

Luay Sarsam, MD
Department of Cardiovascular Disease
Arnot Ogden Medical Center
Elmira, New York

Durr-e-Shahwaar Sayed, DO
Attending Physician
Department of Family Medicine
Inspira Medical Group
Woodbury, New Jersey

Payam Sazegar, MD†
Kaiser Permanente San Diego Family Medicine
    Residency
San Diego, California

Natasha E. Scaria, MD
Resident
Department of Family Medicine
Advocate Christ Medical Center
Oak Lawn, Illinois

Christina Scartozzi, DO
Assistant Professor
Department of Family and Community Medicine
Penn State Health St. Joseph Medical Center
Reading, Pennsylvania

Reid Evan Schalet, DO, BA
Resident Physician
Department of Gastroenterology
George Washington University Hospital
Washington, District of Columbia

Samuel A. Schueler, MD
The George Washington University School of
    Medicine and Health Sciences
Washington, District of Columbia

Jennifer Schwartz, MD†
Newton Wellesley Hospital
Newton, Massachusetts

Ingrid U. Scott, MD, MPH†
Jack and Nancy Turner Professor of
    Ophthalmology
Professor of Public Health Sciences
Penn State College of Medicine
Hershey, Pennsylvania

Kasey M. Scott, MD
Chief Resident
Department of Internal Medicine
University of Louisville Hospital
Louisville, Kentucky

Stephanie Mayle Scott, DO
Department of Internal Medicine
Prisma Health Midlands
Columbia, South Carolina

Timothy A. Scully, DO
Chief Resident
Department of Internal Medicine
Augusta University Medical Center
Augusta, Georgia

Daniel Scura, DO
Sports Medicine Fellow
Department of Orthopedics
Downstate Medical Center
Brooklyn, New York

David P. Sealy, MD, CAQSM, FAAFP, FAMSSM
Professor
Department of Family Medicine/Sports Medicine
Medical University of South Carolina
Area Health Education Consortium Greenwood
Self Regional Healthcare, Primary Care Sports Medicine Fellowship
Greenwood, South Carolina

LaRae L. Seemann, MD
Department of Family Medicine
Mayo Clinic
Jacksonville, Florida

Jarrett Keller Sell, MD, FAAFP, AAHIVS
Associate Professor
Department of Family and Community Medicine
Penn State Health Milton S. Hershey Medical Center
Hershey, Pennsylvania

Nicolas Semenchuk, MD, MS
PGY-2
Department of Emergency Medicine
Advocate Christ Medical Center
Oak Lawn, Illinois

Anthony Shadiack, DO, CAQSM
Associate Program Director, Family Medicine
HCA Healthcare/Mercer University School of Medicine
Grand Strand Medical Center
Myrtle Beach, South Carolina

Chirag N. Shah, MD
Associate Professor
Department of Emergency Medicine
Rutgers Robert Wood Johnson Medical School
New Brunswick, New Jersey

Nehal R. Shah, MD†
Associate Professor of Medicine
VCU Health System
Richmond, Virginia

Samir A. Shah, MD, FACG, FASGE, AGAF
Clinical Professor of Medicine
Department of Medicine/Gastroenterology
Alpert Medical School of Brown University
Chief of Gastroenterology
Department of Gastroenterology
The Miriam Hospital
Providence, Rhode Island

Ammar Shahid, MD†
Department of Sports Medicine
Tower Health and Drexel University
Philadelphia, Pennsylvania

Rahim Shareef, DO
Resident Physician, Family Medicine
Advocate Christ Family Medicine Residency
Oak Lawn, Illinois

Raksha Sharma, MD
Department of Internal Medicine
Florida Atlantic University
Boca Raton, Florida

Denise Sharon, MD, PhD, FAASM†
Independent Contractor
PVHMC Adult and Children Sleep Disorders Center
Pomona Valley Hospital and Medical Center
Claremont, California

Tyler D. Sharpe, MD
Associate Professor
Department of Internal Medicine
University of Louisville
Louisville, Kentucky

Zahra Sardar Sheikh, MD, MPH, CMD
Assistant Professor of Medicine
Department of Geriatric Medicine
University of Massachusetts
Worcester, Massachusetts

Leslie Shelton, DO
Department of Family Medicine
Honor Health
Scottsdale, Arizona

Victoria Shepard, MD
Assistant Professor
Dell Medical School Family Medicine Residency
Austin, Texas

Chelsea M. Shine, DO
Resident
Department of Family Medicine
Methodist Charlton Family Medicine Center
Dallas, Texas

Irfan H. Siddiqui, MD
Attending Physician, Faculty
Department of Internal Medicine
Advocate Christ Medical Center
Oak Lawn, Illinois

Karlynn Sievers, MD
Associate Program Director
Department of Family Medicine
St. Mary's Family Medicine Residency Program
Grand Junction, Colorado

Matthew A. Silva, PharmD, RPh, BCPS
Professor
Department of Pharmacy Practice
Massachusetts College of Pharmacy and Health Sciences
Worcester, Massachusetts

Lauren Simms, MD
Urogynecology Fellow
Department of Urogynecology
University of Massachusetts Medical School
Worcester, Massachusetts

Madhavi Singh, MD†
Assistant Professor
Department of Family and Community Medicine
Penn State College of Medicine
Hershey, Pennsylvania

Navpreet K. Singh, MD
Department of Family Medicine and Sleep Medicine
Temple University
Philadelphia, Pennsylvania

Nelly Singh, DO
Family Medicine Resident Physician
Garnet Health Medical Center
Middletown, New York

Sareena Singh, MD, FACOG
Assistant Professor
Department of Obstetrics and Gynecology, Gynecologic Oncology
Northeast Ohio Medical University
Rootstown, Ohio

Antoine Sioufi, MD
Resident
Department of Family Medicine
Creighton University
Omaha, Nebraska

Brian G. Skotko, MD, MPP
Emma Campbell Endowed Chair on Down Syndrome
Department of Pediatrics
Massachusetts General Hospital
Associate Professor
Department of Pediatrics
Harvard Medical School
Boston, Massachusetts

Jeremy W. Smith, MD
Resident Physician
Department of Family Medicine
Medical City Arlington
Arlington, Texas

Joan Elizabeth Smith, DNP
Nurse Practitioner
Division of Gastroenterology and Liver Diseases
Medical Faculty Associates
George Washington University
Washington, District of Columbia

Melissa L. Smith, MD, MS, FAAFP
Lee's Summit Family Medicine
Lee's Summit, Missouri

Nicholas Smith, MD
Family Medicine Resident
Department of Family Medicine
Tallahassee Memorial Hospital Family Medicine
Residency Program
Tallahassee, Florida

Christian Soeharsono, MD
Medical Resident
Department of Pediatrics
AdventHealth
Orlando, Florida

Mina Soliman, MD
Department of Family Medicine
Creighton University
Omaha, Nebraska

**D'Ann Wilson Somerall, FAANP, FNP-BC,
DNP, CRNP, MAEd**
Nurse Practitioner
Adjunct Assistant Professor
University of Alabama at Birmingham School
of Nursing
Birmingham, Alabama

William E. Somerall Jr., MD, MAEd
Associate Professor
Department of School of Nursing
University of Alabama at Birmingham
Birmingham, Alabama

Nicole D. Somes, MD
Resident Physician
Department of Family Medicine
UMass Chan School of Medicine
Worcester, Massachusetts

Kento Sonoda, MD
Assistant Professor
Department of Family and Community Medicine
Saint Louis University
St. Louis, Missouri

Chantal Soobhanath, MD
Resident Physician
Department of Pediatrics
AdventHealth for Children
Orlando, Florida

Mikayla L. Spangler, PharmD
Associate Professor
Department of Pharmacy Practice and Family
Medicine
Creighton University
Omaha, Nebraska

Dana Sprute, MD, MPH, FAAFP
Associate Professor, Division of Family Medicine
Department of Population Health
Dell Medical School, The University of Texas at
Austin
Austin, Texas

Brianna Stadsvold, MD
Resident
Department of Surgery
Medical College of Georgia at Augusta
University
Augusta, Georgia

Ross C. Stanton, MD, JD, MPH
Resident Physician
Department of Family and Community Medicine
Saint Louis University (Southwest Illinois) Family
Medicine Residency Program
O'Fallon, Illinois

Diana V. Steau, MD
Department of Family Medicine
Creighton University
Omaha, Nebraska

Daniel J. Stein, MD, MPH
Instructor/Associate Physician
Harvard Medical School
Department of Internal Medicine
(Gastroenterology)
Brigham and Women's Hospital
Boston, Massachusetts

Keith L. Stelter, MD
Assistant Professor
Department of Family Medicine
Mayo Clinic
Rochester, Minnesota

Mark B. Stephens, MD, MS, FAAFP
Associate Dean for Medical Education
Professor of Family and Community Medicine
Professor of Humanities
Penn State College of Medicine
University Park, Pennsylvania

Frederick C. Stone Jr., MD, MPH[†]
Clinical Assistant
Professor of Family Medicine
University of South Carolina—Columbia
Columbia, South Carolina

Sibley Strader, MD
Department of Family Medicine and Community
Health
University Hospitals Cleveland Medical Center
Cleveland, Ohio

Adam Strosberg, DNP, ARNP-BC
Visiting Professor
Chamberlain University
Fort Lauderdale, Florida

Mary E. Stuckey, MD
Resident Physician, PGY-2
Department of Emergency Medicine
Rutgers Robert Wood Johnson Medical School
New Brunswick, New Jersey

Moez K. Sumar, MD, BSc
Anesthesiology Resident
Department of Anesthesiology
Advocate Illinois Masonic Medical Center
Chicago, Illinois

Jennifer E. Svarverud, DO[†]
Family Medicine Resident
Nellis Family Medicine Residency
Nellis Air Force Base, Nevada

Sasha Svendsen, MD
Child Abuse Pediatrician
UMass Memorial Children's Assistant Professor
of Pediatrics
UMass Chan Medical School
Worcester, Massachusetts

Neha Syed, DO, BS
Resident Physician
Department of Internal Medicine
Advocate Christ Medical Center Internal
Medicine Residency Program
Oak Lawn, Illinois

Nergess T. Taheri, DO, MSBI
Assistant Program Director
Department of Family Medicine/GME
Lakeside Medical Center
Belle Glade, Florida

Shelby Takeshita, MD
Department of Family Medicine Residency
David Grant Medical Center
Travis Air Force Base, California

Yuki Takeuchi, MD
Resident, Family Medicine
University of Rochester Medical Center
Rochester, New York

Irene J. Tan, MD, FACR[†]
Clinical Professor of Medicine
Department of Medicine
Sidney Kimmel Medical College
Thomas Jefferson University
Department of Medicine, Division of
Rheumatology
Einstein Medical Center Philadelphia
Philadelphia, Pennsylvania

Asma Tariq, MD
Core Faculty
Department of Family Medicine
Kaweah Health
Visalia, California

Madeline Taskier, MD
Research Instructor—Health Policy Fellow
Department of Family Medicine
George Washington University School of
Medicine and Health Sciences
Washington, District of Columbia

Yutthapong Temtanakitpaisan, MD, FACC, FSCAI
Interventional Cardiologist
Department of Cardiology
Bangkok Hospital Khon Kaen
Muang, Khon Kaen, Thailand

Clare W. Teng, MD
Researcher
Department of Ophthalmology
University of Pennsylvania
Philadelphia, Pennsylvania

Jason Teng, MD[†]
Attending Physician
Emergency Department
Virginia Hospital Center
Arlington, Virginia

Janki Thakkar, MD
Resident Physician
Department of Psychiatry
Advocate Lutheran General Hospital
Park Ridge, Illinois

Rebecca Thal, NP-C, AAHIVS
Nurse Practitioner
Family Health Center of Worcester
Worcester, Massachusetts

Kelly S. Thao, MD
Resident
Department of Family Medicine
St. John's Family Medicine
St. Paul, Minnesota

Erin Thomas, MD, BS
Medical Resident
Department of Internal Medicine
University of Massachusetts Medical School
Worcester, Massachusetts

Sarah Marie Tiggelaar, MD, CLC, FAAFP
Assistant Professor of Family Medicine
Maternal Child Health Fellowship Director
Department of Family Medicine
University of Rochester
Rochester, New York

Kliment Todosov, MD
PGY-2 Resident
Department of Family Medicine
Garnet Health Medical Center
Middletown, New York

Anna Marie Tran, DO
Resident Physician, Family Medicine
Ascension St. Vincent's Hospital
Jacksonville, Florida

Thomas Triantafillou, MD
Assistant Professor
Department of Medicine
Advocate Christ Medical Center
Oak Lawn, Illinois

Alec L. Tributino, DO
Resident
Department of Family Medicine
University of Massachusetts
Worcester, Massachusetts

Zoltan Trizna, MD, PhD
Director
Dermatology and Dermatological Surgery
Austin, Texas

Meiline Troeung, DO[†]
Resident
Family and Community Medicine
University of Texas Southwestern
Dallas, Texas

Elizabeth J. Trout, MD, MLS
Assistant Program Director
Novant Health Family Medicine Residency Program
Cornelius, North Carolina

Edison Tsui, MD
Department of Hematology and Oncology
Baystate Medical Center
Springfield, Massachusetts

Jonathan Tsui, MD
Resident Physician
Department of Ophthalmology
Geisinger Eye Institute
Danville, Pennsylvania

Terrence Tsui, DO
Primary Care Sports Medicine Fellow
Department of Orthopedics
Bayhealth Medical Center
Dover, Delaware

Priscilla Tu, DO, FAAFP, FAOASM, FACOFP, FAAMA
Associate Program Director, Virginia Tech Carilion Family Medicine Residency
Associate Professor, Virginia Tech Carilion
Roanoke, Virginia

Nouf O. Turki, MD
Department of Gastroenterology and Hepatology
George Washington University Hospital
Washington, District of Columbia

Alethea Y. Turner, DO, FAAFP
Associate Director
Department of Family Medicine Residency Program
HonorHealth
Scottsdale, Arizona

Rod J. Turner Jr., MD, CAQSM, MS
Assistant Professor
Department of Family Medicine
UTHealth Houston
Houston, Texas

Sahel Uddin, DO
Resident
Department of Family and Community Medicine
Penn State Health Milton S. Hershey Medical Center
Hershey, Pennsylvania

Victoria Udezi, MD, MPH, FAAFP[†]
Assistant Professor
Department of Family Medicine
UT Southwestern Medical Center
Dallas, Texas

Ulunma Natalie Umesi, MD, MBA
Resident Physician
Brooklyn, New York

Lyncean Ung, DO
Nassau University Medical Center
East Meadow, New York

Kaitlin Unser, DO
New York Institute of Technology
Old Westbury, New York

Haris Vakil, MD
Resident
Department of Family Medicine
UTMB
Galveston, Texas

Santiago O. Valdes, MD, FAAP
Associate Professor
Department of Pediatric Cardiology
Baylor College of Medicine/Texas Children's Hospital
Houston, Texas

Marvin Valencia, DO
Primary Care Sports Medicine Fellow
Department of Population Health
Dell Medical School, The University of Texas at Austin
Austin, Texas

Emily Valentin-Mendez, MD
Resident Physician
Department of Family Medicine
Novant Health Family Medicine Residency
Cornelius, North Carolina

Christine M. Van Horn, MD, MS
Resident Physician
Department of Urology
University of Massachusetts Medical School
Worcester, Massachusetts

Alexander Vavra, DO[†]
Captain
Department of Medical Corps
United States Air Force
Scott Air Force Base, Illinois

Kathleen M. Vazzana, DO, MSc
Pediatric Rheumatologist
Department of Pediatric Rheumatology
Arnold Palmer Hospital for Children
Orlando, Florida

Benjamin J. Velky, MD
Faculty Physician
Department of Family Medicine
Montgomery Center for Family Medicine
Greenwood, South Carolina

Ashley L. Vertente, MD, MBA
Resident Physician, PGY-3
Saint Francis Hospital
Wilmington, Delaware

Brian P. Vickery, MD
Associate Professor of Pediatrics
Emory University School of Medicine
Children's Healthcare of Atlanta
Atlanta, Georgia

Astrud S. A. Villareal, MD, FAAFP†
Assistant Professor
Department of Family and Community Medicine
University of Texas Southwestern Medical
   Center
Dallas, Texas

Tamanna Vir, DO
Department of Family Medicine
Medical City Arlington
Arlington, Texas

Dana M. Vlachos, DO
Faculty Attending
Department of Family Medicine Residency
Advocate Christ Medical Center
Oak Lawn, Illinois

Jenney Vongprathoum, MD
Resident
Department of Family Medicine
Dell Medical School, The University of Texas at
   Austin
Austin, Texas

Yongkasem Vorasettakarnkij, MD, MSc†
Assistant Professor
Department of Medicine
Chulalongkorn University
Cardiac Center
King Chulalongkorn Memorial Hospital
Thai Red Cross Society
Bangkok, Thailand

Stephanie Vaux Voyles, MD
Faculty Physician
Department of Family Medicine Residency
St. Mary's Medical Center
Grand Junction, Colorado

Joseph R. Wagner, MD
Chair, Department of Urology
Chair, Robotic Surgery Council
Hartford HealthCare
Hartford, Connecticut

Mako Wakabayashi, MD
Department of Family Medicine
Oregon Health and Science University
Portland, Oregon

Trent Walradt, MD
Fellow
Department of Gastroenterology, Hepatology,
   and Endoscopy
Brigham and Women's Hospital
Boston, Massachusetts

Anne Walsh, MMSc, PA-C, DFAAPA
Clinical Associate Professor
Department of PA Studies
Chapman University
Irvine, California

Thandi Walters, MD
Department of Family Medicine
Tallahassee Memorial Hospital
Tallahassee, Florida

Kellie Wang, PharmD
Pharmacist
Department of Pharmacy
Sarasota Memorial Hospital
Sarasota, Florida

Samuel C. Wang, MD
Program Director
Memorial Family Medicine Residency Program
Houston, Texas

Daniel L. Warden, MD
Primary Care Sports Medicine Fellow
Department of Sports Medicine
Ascension Providence
Novi, Michigan

Waiz Wasey, MD
Assistant Professor Family Medicine, Sleep
   Medicine
Department of Family Medicine
Southern Illinois University
Springfield, Illinois

Leigh Weatherly, DO
Family Medicine, PGY-1
UMass Chan Medical School
Worcester, Massachusetts

Grant Wei, MD, FACEP
Associate Professor and Program Director
Department of Emergency Medicine
Rutgers Robert Wood Johnson Medical School
New Brunswick, New Jersey

Jill T. Wei Doherty, MD
Department of Family Medicine
Santa Monica Family Physicians
Santa Monica, California

Lisa Weiss, MD, Med, FAAFP
Associate Professor
Bon Secours Mercy Health
Boardman, Ohio

Maggie C. Wertz, MD†
Faculty Physician
Eglin Family Medicine Residency
Eglin Air Force Base, Florida

Todd A. Wical, DO†
Squadron Flight Surgeon
Department of Primary Care
Blanchfield Army Community Hospital
Fort Campbell, Kentucky

Joseph P. Wiedemer, MD, FAAFP
Associate Professor
Department of Family and Community Medicine
Penn State Health
State College, Pennsylvania

Sarah Wiggill, MD
Assistant Professor of Family Medicine
Department of Medicine
Charles E. Schmidt College of Medicine
Florida Atlantic University
Boca Raton, Florida

Susanne Wild, MD
Clinical Associate Professor
Department of Family Medicine
Family Medicine Residency
University of Arizona College of Medicine—
   Phoenix
Phoenix, Arizona

Alec M. Wilhelmi, MD
Resident Physician
Department of Family Medicine and Population
   Health
Dell Medical School, The University of Texas at
   Austin
Austin, Texas

Faren H. Williams, MD, MS†
Clinical Professor
Department of Orthopedics and Physical
   Rehabilitation
University of Massachusetts Medical School
Worcester, Massachusetts

Katherine Williams, MD
Attending Physician
Department of Family Medicine
Summa Health Medical Group
Rootstown, Ohio

Norton Winer, MD[†]
Assistant Clinical Professor of Neurology
Department of Neurology
University Hospitals Cleveland
Cleveland, Ohio

Fawn J. Winkelman, DO
Department of Osteopathic Family Medicine
Nova Southeastern University College of
    Osteopathic
Owner/Physician, Elite Medicine and Aesthetic
    Institute
Fort Lauderdale, Florida

Jay Winner, MD, FAAFP
Family Physician and Director Stress Reduction
    Program
Department of Family Medicine
Sansum Clinic
Santa Barbara, California

Christopher M. Wise, MD
Professor of Internal Medicine
Department of Internal Medicine/
    Rheumatology, Allergy, and Immunology
Virginia Commonwealth University Health
    System
Richmond, Virginia

Jeffrey Wisinski, DO
Assistant Professor
Department of Family Medicine/Sports Medicine
Prisma Health
Columbia, South Carolina

Anita Wong, MD
Assistant Clinical Professor
Department of Family Medicine
University of California, Los Angeles
Los Angeles, California

William W. Wong, DO
Assistant Professor of Medicine
Department of Pulmonary and Critical Care
    Medicine
UMass Chan Medical School
Worcester, Massachusetts

Frances Yung-tao Wu, MD
Clinical Assistant Professor
Department of Family Medicine
Rutgers Robert Wood Johnson Medical School
New Brunswick, New Jersey
Assistant Director
Department of Family Medicine Residency
Robert Wood Johnson University Hospital
    Somerset
Somerville, New Jersey

Velyn Wu, MD, MACM
Assistant Clinical Professor
Department of Community Health and Family
    Medicine
University of Florida College of Medicine
Gainesville, Florida

Sujitha Yadlapati, MD
HCA Corpus Christi Medical Center—Bay Area
Dermatology Residency Program
McAllen, Texas

Pratiksha Yalakkishettar, MD[†]
Preventive Medicine Fellow and Family
    Physician
Family Medicine and Community Health
UMass Chan Medical School
Worcester, Massachusetts

Johnny J. Yang, MD, MS
Saba University School of Medicine
Devens, Massachusetts

Michael Y. Yang, MD, CAQSM[†]
Section Chief of Sports Medicine
Mercy Orthopedics and Sports Medicine
Mercy Catholic Medical Center
Darby, Pennsylvania

Margaret Yip, DO
Resident Physician
Orlando, Florida

Emily A. Yocom, DO
Department of Family Medicine
Travis Air Force Base
Fairfield, California

Dinesh Yogaratnam, PharmD, BCPS,
    BCCCP
Associate Professor
Massachusetts College of Pharmacy and Health
    Sciences University
Worcester, Massachusetts

James R. Yon, MD
Department of Trauma and Acute Care Surgery
New Hanover Regional Medical Center
Wilmington, North Carolina

Jocelyn C. Young, DO, MSc
Clinical Assistant Professor
Department of Family Medicine
SUNY Upstate Medical University
Assistant Clinical Professor
Department of Family Medicine
United Health Services/Wilson Family Medicine
    Residency Program
Faculty Physician
Department of Family Medicine
United Health Services Hospitals
Johnson City, New York

Faraz Yousefian, DO
Department of Internal Medicine
Texas Institute for Graduate Medical Education
    and Research
San Antonio, Texas

Nida Zahra, MD, FAAFP
Associate Professor
Department of Family and Community Medicine
UT Southwestern Medical Center
Dallas, Texas

Touqir Zahra, MD, FACP
Assistant Professor
Department of Internal Medicine
Florida Atlantic University
Boca Raton, Florida

Rochelle Zak, MD
Associate Professor
Department of Medicine/Sleep Disorders Center
University of California at San Francisco
San Francisco, California

Batoul Zalkout, DO
Resident Physician, Family Medicine
Advocate Christ
Oak Lawn, Illinois

Anna K. Zheng, MD
OB Lead
Department of Family Medicine
Edward M. Kennedy Community Health Center
Assistant Professor
Department of Family Medicine and Community
    Health
University of Massachusetts Medical Center
Worcester, Massachusetts

Svitlana Zhukivska, MD
Associate Professor
Department of Family Medicine
University of Toledo
Toledo, Ohio

Erika Zimmons, DO, MS
Assistant Professor
Department of Family Medicine and Community
    Health
University of Massachusetts Medical School
Worcester, Massachusetts

[†]The views expressed are those of the authors
and do not reflect the official policy of the
Department of the Army, Department of
the Navy, Department of the Air Force, the
Department of Defense, or the United States
Government.

CONTENTS

Topics

Diagnosis and Treatment: An Algorithmic Approach

This section contains flowcharts (or algorithms) to help the reader in the diagnosis of clinical signs and symptoms and treatment of a variety of clinical problems. They are organized by the presenting sign, symptom, or diagnosis.

These algorithms were designed to be used as a quick reference and adjunct to the reader's clinical knowledge and impression. They are not an exhaustive review of the management of a problem, nor are they meant to be a complete list of diseases.

ABDOMINAL PAIN, CHRONIC

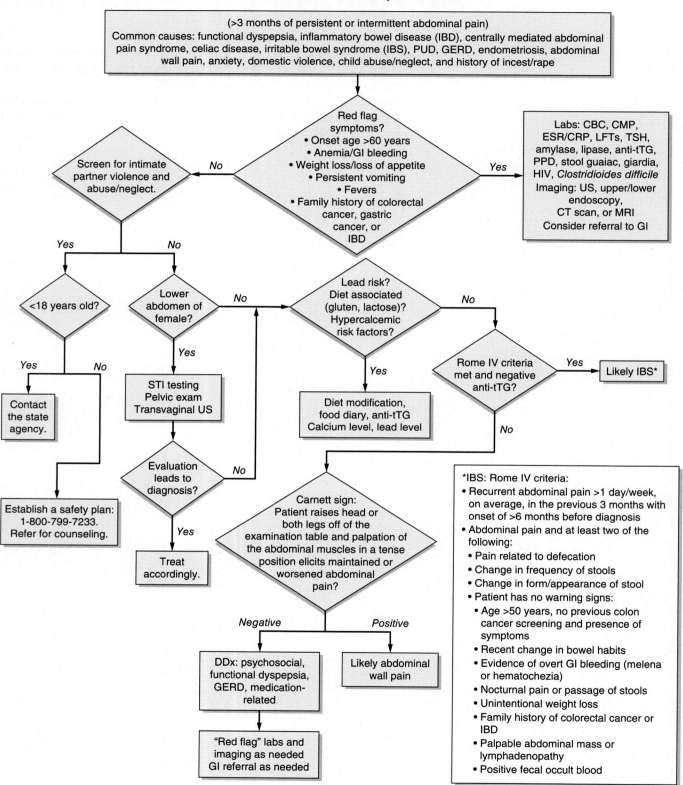

(>3 months of persistent or intermittent abdominal pain)
Common causes: functional dyspepsia, inflammatory bowel disease (IBD), centrally mediated abdominal pain syndrome, celiac disease, irritable bowel syndrome (IBS), PUD, GERD, endometriosis, abdominal wall pain, anxiety, domestic violence, child abuse/neglect, and history of incest/rape

Red flag symptoms?
• Onset age >60 years
• Anemia/GI bleeding
• Weight loss/loss of appetite
• Persistent vomiting
• Fevers
• Family history of colorectal cancer, gastric cancer, or IBD

Screen for intimate partner violence and abuse/neglect. — *No*

Yes → Labs: CBC, CMP, ESR/CRP, LFTs, TSH, amylase, lipase, anti-tTG, PPD, stool guaiac, giardia, HIV, *Clostridioides difficile* Imaging: US, upper/lower endoscopy, CT scan, or MRI Consider referral to GI

Yes / *No*

<18 years old?

Lower abdomen of female? — *No*

Lead risk? Diet associated (gluten, lactose)? Hypercalcemic risk factors? — *No*

Rome IV criteria met and negative anti-tTG? — *Yes* → **Likely IBS***

Yes / *No*

Contact the state agency.

STI testing Pelvic exam Transvaginal US

Yes

Diet modification, food diary, anti-tTG Calcium level, lead level

No

Establish a safety plan: 1-800-799-7233. Refer for counseling.

Evaluation leads to diagnosis? — *No*

Yes

Treat accordingly.

Carnett sign: Patient raises head or both legs off of the examination table and palpation of the abdominal muscles in a tense position elicits maintained or worsened abdominal pain?

Negative / *Positive*

DDx: psychosocial, functional dyspepsia, GERD, medication-related

Likely abdominal wall pain

"Red flag" labs and imaging as needed GI referral as needed

*IBS: Rome IV criteria:
• Recurrent abdominal pain >1 day/week, on average, in the previous 3 months with onset of >6 months before diagnosis
• Abdominal pain and at least two of the following:
• Pain related to defecation
• Change in frequency of stools
• Change in form/appearance of stool
• Patient has no warning signs:
  • Age >50 years, no previous colon cancer screening and presence of symptoms
  • Recent change in bowel habits
  • Evidence of overt GI bleeding (melena or hematochezia)
  • Nocturnal pain or passage of stools
  • Unintentional weight loss
  • Family history of colorectal cancer or IBD
  • Palpable abdominal mass or lymphadenopathy
  • Positive fecal occult blood

Kamini Geer, MD, MPH and Frances L. Gonzalez Gonzalez, MD

Sabo CM, Grad S, Dumitrascu DL. Chronic abdominal pain in general practice. *Dig Dis*. 2021;39(6):606–614.

ABDOMINAL PAIN, LOWER

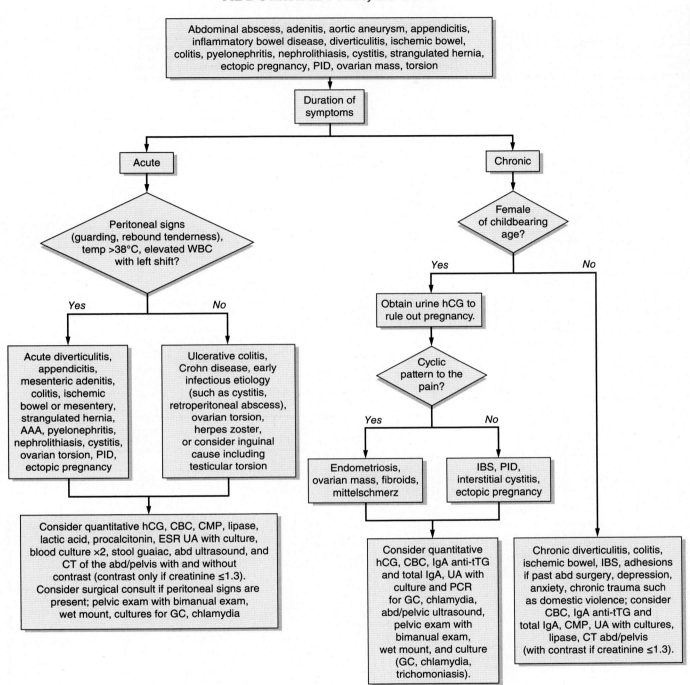

Kenneth A. Ballou, MD

Cullison KM, Franck N. Clinical decision rules in the evaluation and management of adult gastrointestinal emergencies. *Emerg Med Clin North Am.* 2021;39(4):719–732.

ABDOMINAL PAIN, UPPER

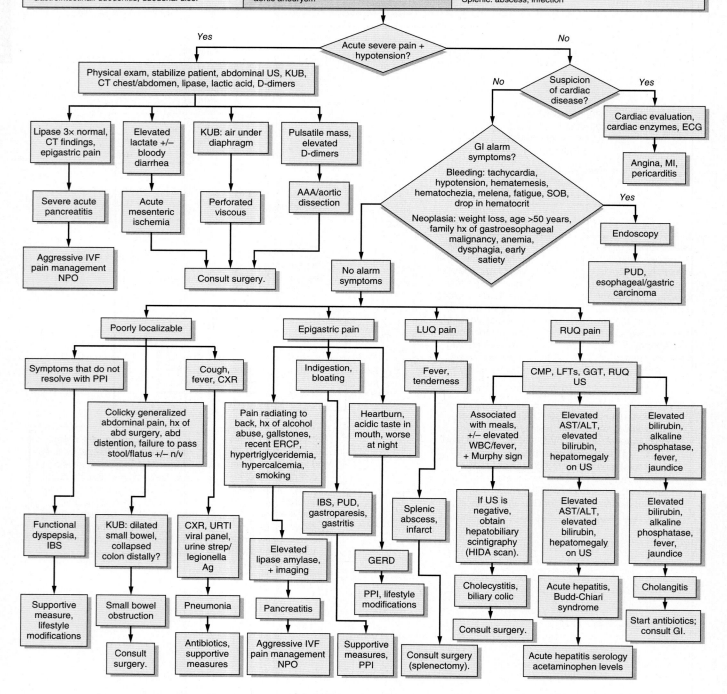

Right upper quadrant abdominal differential diagnosis:
- Biliary: cholecystitis, cholelithiasis, cholangitis
- Cardiac: myocardial infarction, pericarditis, angina
- Hepatic: abscess, hepatitis, mass
- Bowel: colitis, diverticulitis, appendicitis
- Pulmonary: pneumonia, pulmonary emboli, pleurisy
- Renal: nephrolithiasis, pyelonephritis
- Pancreas: mass, pancreatitis
- Gastrointestinal: duodenitis, duodenal ulcer

Epigastric abdominal differential diagnosis:
- Biliary: cholecystitis, cholelithiasis, cholangitis
- Cardiac: myocardial infarction, pericarditis, angina
- Gastric: esophagitis, gastritis, GERD, functional dyspepsia, gastric or duodenal ulcer disease/perforation
- Bowel: irritable bowel syndrome
- Pancreatic: mass, pancreatitis
- Vascular: aortic dissection, mesenteric ischemic, aortic aneurysm

Left upper quadrant abdominal differential diagnosis:
- Cardiac: myocardial infarction, pericarditis, angina
- Gastric: esophagitis, gastritis, GERD, functional dyspepsia, gastric or duodenal ulcer disease/perforation
- Pancreatic: mass, pancreatitis
- Renal: nephrolithiasis, pyelonephritis
- Pulmonary: pneumonia, emboli
- Vascular: aortic dissection, mesenteric ischemic, aortic aneurysm
- Splenic: abscess, infection

Acute severe pain + hypotension?

Yes → Physical exam, stabilize patient, abdominal US, KUB, CT chest/abdomen, lipase, lactic acid, D-dimers

- Lipase 3× normal, CT findings, epigastric pain → Severe acute pancreatitis → Aggressive IVF pain management NPO
- Elevated lactate +/– bloody diarrhea → Acute mesenteric ischemia → Consult surgery.
- KUB: air under diaphragm → Perforated viscous → Consult surgery.
- Pulsatile mass, elevated D-dimers → AAA/aortic dissection → Consult surgery.

No → **Suspicion of cardiac disease?**

Yes → Cardiac evaluation, cardiac enzymes, ECG → Angina, MI, pericarditis

No → **GI alarm symptoms?**

Bleeding: tachycardia, hypotension, hematemesis, hematochezia, melena, fatigue, SOB, drop in hematocrit

Neoplasia: weight loss, age >50 years, family hx of gastroesophageal malignancy, anemia, dysphagia, early satiety

Yes → Endoscopy → PUD, esophageal/gastric carcinoma

No alarm symptoms →

Poorly localizable
- Symptoms that do not resolve with PPI
  - Functional dyspepsia, IBS → Supportive measure, lifestyle modifications
- Colicky generalized abdominal pain, hx of abd surgery, abd distention, failure to pass stool/flatus +/– n/v
  - KUB: dilated small bowel, collapsed colon distally? → Small bowel obstruction → Consult surgery.
- Cough, fever, CXR
  - CXR, URTI viral panel, urine strep/legionella Ag → Pneumonia → Antibiotics, supportive measures

Epigastric pain
- Indigestion, bloating
  - Pain radiating to back, hx of alcohol abuse, gallstones, recent ERCP, hypertriglyceridemia, hypercalcemia, smoking
    - Elevated lipase amylase, + imaging → Pancreatitis → Aggressive IVF pain management NPO
  - IBS, PUD, gastroparesis, gastritis → Supportive measures, PPI
- Heartburn, acidic taste in mouth, worse at night → GERD → PPI, lifestyle modifications

LUQ pain
- Fever, tenderness → Splenic abscess, infarct → Consult surgery (splenectomy).

RUQ pain
- CMP, LFTs, GGT, RUQ US
  - Associated with meals, +/– elevated WBC/fever, + Murphy sign → If US is negative, obtain hepatobiliary scintigraphy (HIDA scan). → Cholecystitis, biliary colic → Consult surgery.
  - Elevated AST/ALT, elevated bilirubin, hepatomegaly on US → Elevated AST/ALT, elevated bilirubin, hepatomegaly on US → Acute hepatitis, Budd-Chiari syndrome → Acute hepatitis serology acetaminophen levels
  - Elevated bilirubin, alkaline phosphatase, fever, jaundice → Elevated bilirubin, alkaline phosphatase, fever, jaundice → Cholangitis → Start antibiotics; consult GI.

Brock McMillen, MD, FFAFP, Emilee J. Delbridge, PhD, LMFT, and David Mullen, MD

Yew KS, George MK, Allred HB. Acute abdominal pain in adults: evaluation and diagnosis. *Am Fam Physician.* 2023;107(6):585–596.

ACETAMINOPHEN POISONING, TREATMENT

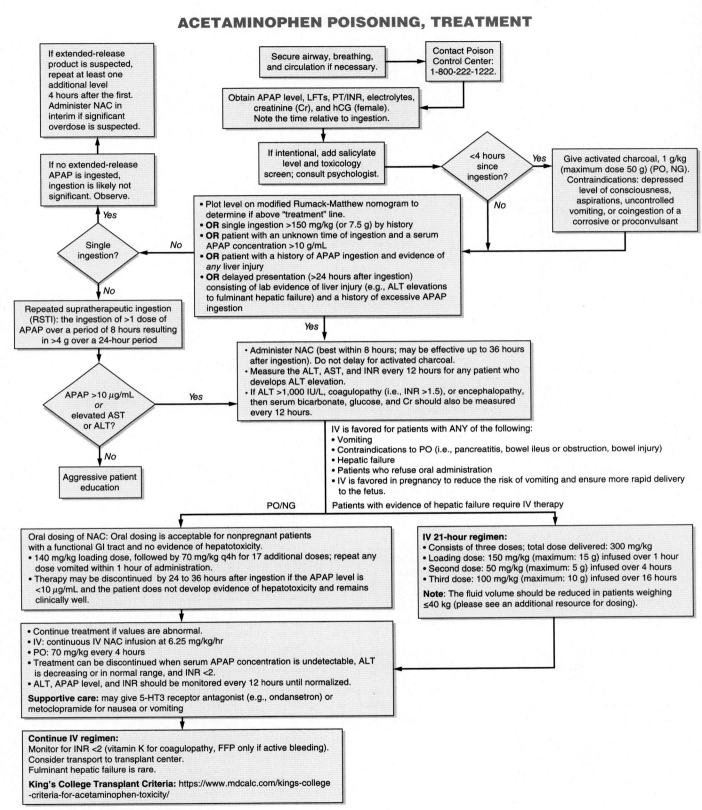

If extended-release product is suspected, repeat at least one additional level 4 hours after the first. Administer NAC in interim if significant overdose is suspected.

If no extended-release APAP is ingested, ingestion is likely not significant. Observe.

Single ingestion? — Yes

Single ingestion? — No

Repeated supratherapeutic ingestion (RSTI): the ingestion of >1 dose of APAP over a period of 8 hours resulting in >4 g over a 24-hour period

APAP >10 μg/mL or elevated AST or ALT? — Yes / No

Aggressive patient education

Secure airway, breathing, and circulation if necessary.

Contact Poison Control Center: 1-800-222-1222.

Obtain APAP level, LFTs, PT/INR, electrolytes, creatinine (Cr), and hCG (female). Note the time relative to ingestion.

If intentional, add salicylate level and toxicology screen; consult psychologist.

<4 hours since ingestion? — Yes / No

Give activated charcoal, 1 g/kg (maximum dose 50 g) (PO, NG). Contraindications: depressed level of consciousness, aspirations, uncontrolled vomiting, or coingestion of a corrosive or proconvulsant

- Plot level on modified Rumack-Matthew nomogram to determine if above "treatment" line.
- **OR** single ingestion >150 mg/kg (or 7.5 g) by history
- **OR** patient with an unknown time of ingestion and a serum APAP concentration >10 g/mL
- **OR** patient with a history of APAP ingestion and evidence of *any* liver injury
- **OR** delayed presentation (>24 hours after ingestion) consisting of lab evidence of liver injury (e.g., ALT elevations to fulminant hepatic failure) and a history of excessive APAP ingestion

— Yes

- Administer NAC (best within 8 hours; may be effective up to 36 hours after ingestion). Do not delay for activated charcoal.
- Measure the ALT, AST, and INR every 12 hours for any patient who develops ALT elevation.
- If ALT >1,000 IU/L, coagulopathy (i.e., INR >1.5), or encephalopathy, then serum bicarbonate, glucose, and Cr should also be measured every 12 hours.

IV is favored for patients with ANY of the following:
- Vomiting
- Contraindications to PO (i.e., pancreatitis, bowel ileus or obstruction, bowel injury)
- Hepatic failure
- Patients who refuse oral administration
- IV is favored in pregnancy to reduce the risk of vomiting and ensure more rapid delivery to the fetus.

PO/NG — Patients with evidence of hepatic failure require IV therapy

Oral dosing of NAC: Oral dosing is acceptable for nonpregnant patients with a functional GI tract and no evidence of hepatotoxicity.
- 140 mg/kg loading dose, followed by 70 mg/kg q4h for 17 additional doses; repeat any dose vomited within 1 hour of administration.
- Therapy may be discontinued by 24 to 36 hours after ingestion if the APAP level is <10 μg/mL and the patient does not develop evidence of hepatotoxicity and remains clinically well.

IV 21-hour regimen:
- Consists of three doses; total dose delivered: 300 mg/kg
- Loading dose: 150 mg/kg (maximum: 15 g) infused over 1 hour
- Second dose: 50 mg/kg (maximum: 5 g) infused over 4 hours
- Third dose: 100 mg/kg (maximum: 10 g) infused over 16 hours

Note: The fluid volume should be reduced in patients weighing ≤40 kg (please see an additional resource for dosing).

- Continue treatment if values are abnormal.
- IV: continuous IV NAC infusion at 6.25 mg/kg/hr
- PO: 70 mg/kg every 4 hours
- Treatment can be discontinued when serum APAP concentration is undetectable, ALT is decreasing or in normal range, and INR <2.
- ALT, APAP level, and INR should be monitored every 12 hours until normalized.

Supportive care: may give 5-HT3 receptor antagonist (e.g., ondansetron) or metoclopramide for nausea or vomiting

Continue IV regimen:
Monitor for INR <2 (vitamin K for coagulopathy, FFP only if active bleeding).
Consider transport to transplant center.
Fulminant hepatic failure is rare.

King's College Transplant Criteria: https://www.mdcalc.com/kings-college-criteria-for-acetaminophen-toxicity/

APAP, acetaminophen; NAC, *N*-acetylcysteine.

Pankaj Ksheersagar, MD

Dart RC, Mullins ME, Matoushek T, et al. Management of acetaminophen poisoning in the US and Canada: a consensus statement. *JAMA Netw Open.* 2023;6(8):e2327739. doi:10.1001/jamanetworkopen.2023.27739.

ACIDOSIS

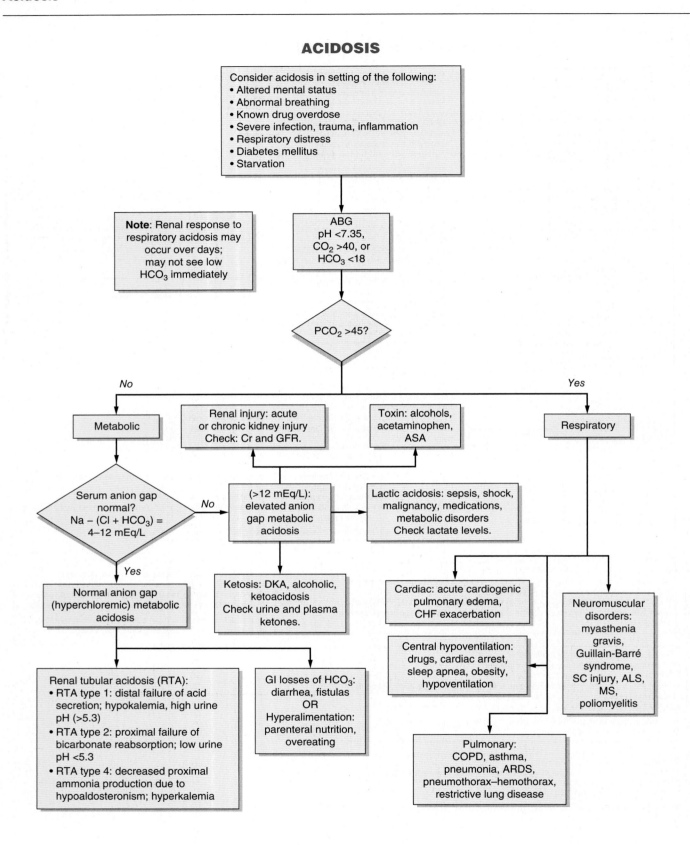

Consider acidosis in setting of the following:
- Altered mental status
- Abnormal breathing
- Known drug overdose
- Severe infection, trauma, inflammation
- Respiratory distress
- Diabetes mellitus
- Starvation

Note: Renal response to respiratory acidosis may occur over days; may not see low HCO_3 immediately

ABG
pH <7.35,
CO_2 >40, or
HCO_3 <18

PCO_2 >45?

No   *Yes*

Metabolic

Renal injury: acute or chronic kidney injury
Check: Cr and GFR.

Toxin: alcohols, acetaminophen, ASA

Respiratory

Serum anion gap normal?
$Na - (Cl + HCO_3) = 4-12$ mEq/L

No

(>12 mEq/L): elevated anion gap metabolic acidosis

Lactic acidosis: sepsis, shock, malignancy, medications, metabolic disorders
Check lactate levels.

Yes

Normal anion gap (hyperchloremic) metabolic acidosis

Ketosis: DKA, alcoholic, ketoacidosis
Check urine and plasma ketones.

Cardiac: acute cardiogenic pulmonary edema, CHF exacerbation

Neuromuscular disorders: myasthenia gravis, Guillain-Barré syndrome, SC injury, ALS, MS, poliomyelitis

Central hypoventilation: drugs, cardiac arrest, sleep apnea, obesity, hypoventilation

Renal tubular acidosis (RTA):
- RTA type 1: distal failure of acid secretion; hypokalemia, high urine pH (>5.3)
- RTA type 2: proximal failure of bicarbonate reabsorption; low urine pH <5.3
- RTA type 4: decreased proximal ammonia production due to hypoaldosteronism; hyperkalemia

GI losses of HCO_3: diarrhea, fistulas
OR
Hyperalimentation: parenteral nutrition, overeating

Pulmonary: COPD, asthma, pneumonia, ARDS, pneumothorax–hemothorax, restrictive lung disease

Shivani Malhotra, MD, FAAFP

Kraut JA, Madias NE. Serum anion gap: its uses and limitations in clinical medicine. *Clin J Am Soc Nephrol.* 2007;2(1):162–174.

ACNE

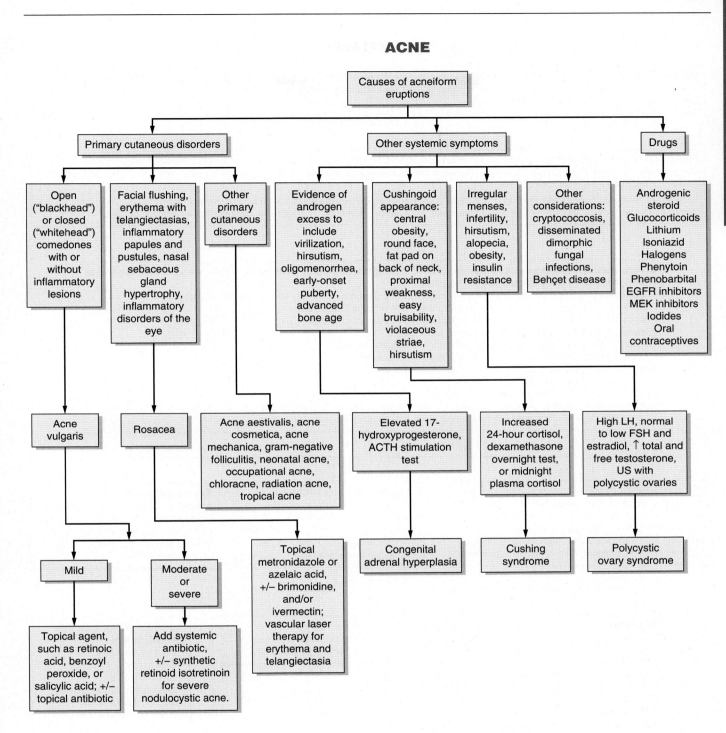

Christine A. Quartuccio-Carran, DO, FAAFP and Benjamin Nolasco, MD, MHS

Ogé LK, Broussard A, Marshall MD. Acne vulgaris: diagnosis and treatment. *Am Fam Physician*. 2019;100(8):475–484.

ALCOHOL WITHDRAWAL, TREATMENT

History: duration and quantity of alcohol intake for 2 weeks prior to presentation, time since last drink, previous episodes of alcohol withdrawal, concurrent substance use, preexisting medical and psychiatric conditions, prior detoxification admissions, prior seizure activity, living situation, social supports, stressors, triggers

Physical: VS (fever, tachycardia, tachypnea, hypertension), **CIWA** (see below), MSE (arousal, orientation, hallucinations), HEENT (diaphoresis, scleral icterus), CV (arrhythmias), evaluate s/sx of liver failure (ascites, varices, caput medusae, asterixis, palmar erythema), neuro (nystagmus, tremor, seizure activity)

Include assessment of conditions likely to *complicate*, *exacerbate*, or *precipitate* alcohol withdrawal: anxiety, arrhythmias, CHF, CAD, dehydration, depression, GI bleeding, history of traumatic experience, infections, liver disease, pancreatitis, neurologic deficits.

Clinical Institute Withdrawal Assessment (CIWA) of Alcohol Scale (For patients in the ICU who cannot respond to questions, the MINDS protocol should be used.)
- Nausea and vomiting 0–7 (0, none; 4, intermittent; 7, constant nausea; frequent dry heaves/vomiting)
- Tremor 0–7 (0, none; 4, moderate; 7, severe; even with arms not extended)
- Paroxysmal sweats 0–7 (0, none; 4, beads of sweat; 7, drenching sweats)
- Anxiety 0–7 (0, none; 4, moderate; 7, acute panic state)
- Agitation 0–7 (0, none; 4, moderately restless; 7, constantly thrashing about or pacing)
- Tactile disturbances 0–7 (0, none; 1–3, for pruritus or paresthesias; 4–7, for hallucinations)
- Auditory disturbances 0–7 (0, none; 1–3, for increased sensitivity; 4–7, for hallucinations)
- Visual disturbances 0–7 (0, none; 1–3, for increased sensitivity; 4–7, for hallucinations)
- Headache 0–7 (0, no headache; 4, moderate; 7, extremely severe)
- Orientation 0–4 (0, fully oriented; 1, cannot do serial additions or is uncertain about date; 2, disoriented to date but within 2 calendar days; 3, disoriented to date by >2 days; 4, disoriented to place or person)

Mild withdrawal—CIWA 0–7 onset 5–8 hours after cessation or significant decrease in consumption: anxiety, restlessness, agitation, mild nausea, decreased appetite, sleep disturbance, facial sweating, mild tremulousness, fluctuating tachycardia and hypertension, possible mild cognitive impairment

Moderate withdrawal—CIWA 8–14 onset 24–48 hours after cessation: marked restlessness and agitation, moderate tremulousness with constant eye movement, diaphoresis, nausea, vomiting, anorexia, diarrhea

Severe withdrawal/delirium tremens—CIWA 15–30 onset 48–96 hours after alcohol cessation: marked tremulousness, fever, drenching sweats, severe hypertension and tachycardia, delirium

Good candidate for outpatient therapy:
- Not pregnant
- No comorbid illnesses requiring hospitalization
- No history of seizures
- Not a suicide risk
- Low risk of delirium tremens
- No history of unsuccessful outpatient detoxification
- Good access to follow-up medical care
- Tolerating oral medication
- Adequate social support available

Outpatient therapy contraindicated: pregnant, history of seizures or withdrawal seizures, chronic or acute comorbid illness requiring inpatient observation, lack of ability to follow-up

High risk of delirium tremens:
- Age >30 years
- Heavy drinking >8 years
- Drinking >100 g ethanol per day (>8 drinks per day)
- Random BAC >200 mg/dL
- Elevated MCV
- Cirrhosis

Admit to inpatient detoxification program:
- Replete thiamine IV as below before giving glucose and/or fluids containing dextrose to prevent Wernicke encephalopathy.
- VS q4h
- CIWA q4h
- Institute seizure precautions.
- IV fluids

Admit to ICU for inpatient detoxification:
- VS q15min
- CIWA q1h
- NPO, IV fluids
- Lateral decubitus position, restrain if necessary
- Glucose, sodium, potassium, phosphate, and magnesium replacement as needed

Treat as outpatient:
- Thiamine 100 mg once daily for 5 days
- Folic acid 1 g once daily for 5 days
- Evaluate daily until symptoms decrease.
- Assess blood pressure, heart rate, and CIWA-Ar score at each follow-up visit.
- Perform alcohol breath analysis randomly.
- Facilitate entry into a long-term outpatient therapy program (Alcoholics Anonymous).
- **If patient misses an appointment or resumes drinking, refer to addiction specialist or inpatient treatment facility.**
- Evaluate daily until symptoms decrease—usually for about 5 days. Face to face preferred but can alternate with telemedicine visits if necessary.
- Discuss any additional postwithdrawal treatment options through primary care or a specialized alcohol treatment program.

Labs:
- Toxicology screen/EtOH level to assess need for and timing of withdrawal regimen
- CBC, electrolytes, phosphate, magnesium; vitamin B_{12} and folate to be repleted regardless of blood levels
- Amylase/lipase if suspected pancreatitis
- PT, PTT if suspected liver failure
- LFTs, GGT
- UPT if premenopausal

Imaging:
- Head CT if history of trauma, mental status changes greater than expected, or focal neurologic changes
- Consider addition of EEG if focal neurologic signs or prolonged postictal state seizure.
- Consider addition of ECG if there is a history of cardiac problems.

Medications:
- Diazepam 5–20 mg IV q10min until calm and then q1h to maintain light somnolence for duration of delirium

If severe liver disease, severe asthma or respiratory failure, elderly, debilitated, or low serum albumin:
- Lorazepam 1–4 mg IV q10min until calm and then q1h to maintain light somnolence for duration of delirium

Example outpatient regimen:
Fixed diazepam schedule
Day 1: 10 mg q6h
Day 2: 10 mg q8h
Day 3: 10 mg q12h
Day 4/5: 10 mg at bedtime

Symptom-triggered diazepam schedule:
Give dose if CIWA >8.
Day 1: 10 mg q4h PRN
Day 2: 10 mg q6h PRN
Day 3: 10 mg q6h PRN
Days 4/5: 10 mg twice a day PRN
Pt with transaminitis, LFT >3 times normal USE lorazepam (Ativan) in tapering doses over 5 days; may start with 2 mg q4h PRN

Fixed chlordiazepoxide (Librium) schedule:
Day 1: 50 mg PO q6h
Day 2: 25 mg q6h
Day 3: 25 mg q6h
Avoid in renal disease, liver disease, or elderly.

If benzodiazepines are contraindicated or if preference is to start with non-benzodiazepine agent, gabapentin is an alternative.

Immediate release: oral: initial: 300 mg/q6h on day 1, then 300 mg/q8h on day 2, then 300 mg/q12h on day 3, then 300 mg at night on day 4.
In addition to scheduled doses, provide one additional PRN 300 mg dose per day for breakthrough withdrawal symptoms.

Discharge planning:
- CIWA scores <8–10 for 24 hours
- Begin 1:1 or group therapy.
- Discharge to treatment center, day program, home.
- Facilitate entry into Alcoholics Anonymous.
- Evaluate for outpatient treatment with benzodiazepine.
- Nutrition/social work consultation
- Close follow-up with primary care physician

Medications:
Nutritional replacement
- Thiamine 100 mg IV/IM or PO once daily for 5 days
- Folic acid 1 g PO once daily for 5 days

Sympatholytic adjunctive therapy (no effect on prevention of withdrawal seizure and should be used with benzodiazepine therapy)
- Atenolol 50–100 mg once daily
- Clonidine 0.2 mg 3 times daily

For hallucinations associated with withdrawal:
- Haloperidol 2–5 mg IM/PO q1–4h max 5 mg/day
- Use only in conjunction with benzodiazepines and with extreme caution because haloperidol may lower seizure threshold.
- Frequent reassurance, re-orientation to time and place, and nursing care are recommended nonpharmacologic interventions.

Supportive care
- Frequent reorientation to time and place may be needed for patient.
- Decrease stimulation.
- Encourage PO fluid intake of noncaffeinated beverages.

Medications:
Long-acting benzodiazepines (diazepam or chlordiazepoxide) provide lower chance of recurrent withdrawal or seizures. Symptom-triggered regimen is preferred over fixed dose regimen. If patient is at greater risk of complications, can consider front-loading approach (CIWA score of 19 or greater)

Symptom triggered (Assess using CIWA q1h. Once moderate symptoms are controlled, can reduce assessment to q4–6h)
- Diazepam 10–20 mg (until CIWA-Ar <10)
  OR
- Chlordiazepoxide 50–100 (until CIWA-Ar <10)

Front loading
- Diazepam 10 mg PO q1h until CIWA-Ar <10

Fixed schedule
- Diazepam 20 mg PO q2–3h for three doses
  OR
- Chlordiazepoxide, 50 mg q6h for four doses, then 25 mg q6h for eight doses

Short-acting benzodiazepines (lorazepam) may have lower risk when there is concern about prolonged sedation, for example, h/o liver disease, LFT >3 times normal limit, elderly patients, or those with severe hepatic insufficiency.
- Lorazepam 1–2 mg PO q2–4h until CIWA <8

Astrud S. A. Villareal, MD, FAAFP, Priscilla L. Kha, DO, MPH, and Victoria Udezi, MD, MPH, FAAFP

The ASAM clinical practice guideline on alcohol withdrawal management. *J Addict Med.* 2020;14(3S Suppl 1):1–72. *Erratum in: J Addict Med.* 2020;14(5):e280.

ALKALINE PHOSPHATASE ELEVATION

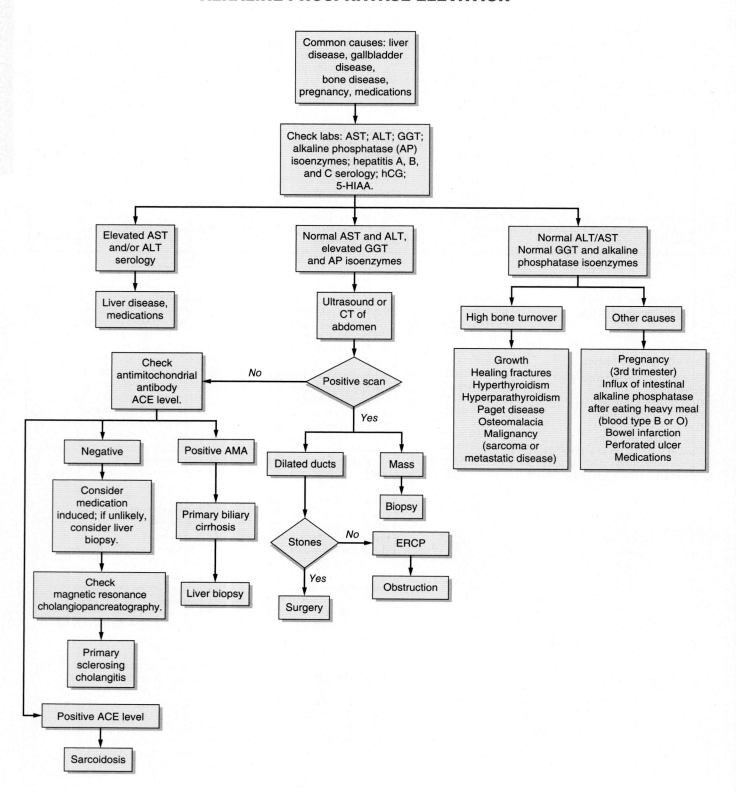

Reem Hadi, MD and Fozia Akhtar Ali, MD, FAAFP

Siddique A, Kowdley KV. Approach to a patient with elevated serum alkaline phosphatase. *Clin Liver Dis*. 2012;16(2):199–229.

AMENORRHEA, SECONDARY

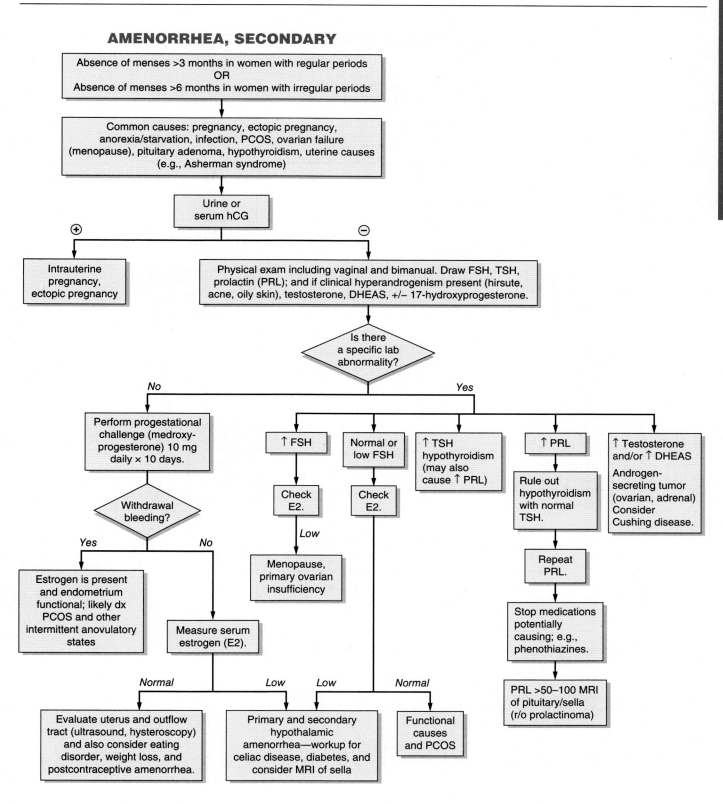

Jeremy Golding, MD, FAAFP

Klein DA, Paradise SL, Reeder RM. Amenorrhea: a systematic approach to diagnosis and management. *Am Fam Physician*. 2019;100(1):39–48.

ANEMIA

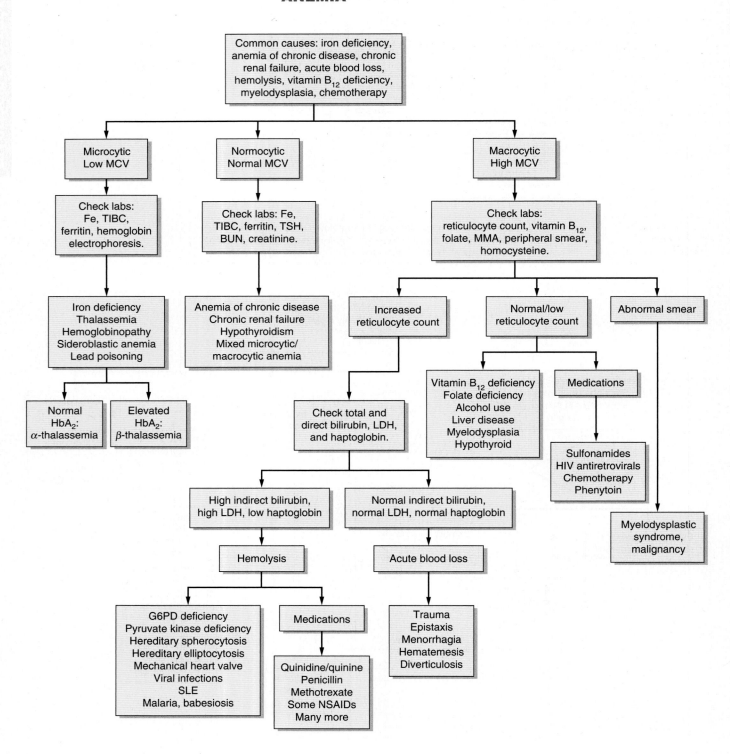

Brittany M. Reid, MBBS and Sandra S. Augusto, MD, MPH

Lanier JB, Park JJ, Callahan RC. Anemia in older adults. *Am Fam Physician*. 2018;98(7):437–442.

AST ELEVATION

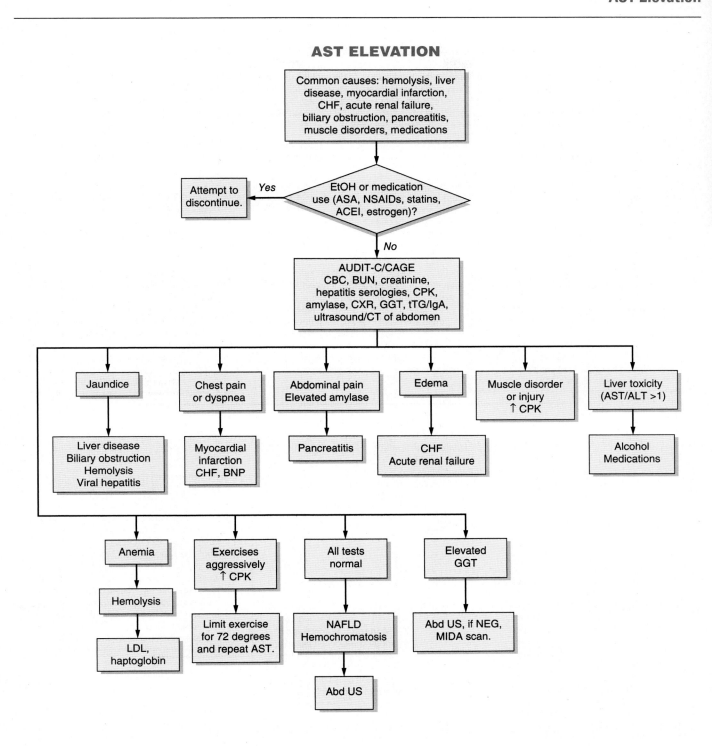

Common causes: hemolysis, liver disease, myocardial infarction, CHF, acute renal failure, biliary obstruction, pancreatitis, muscle disorders, medications

EtOH or medication use (ASA, NSAIDs, statins, ACEI, estrogen)?

Yes → Attempt to discontinue.

No →

AUDIT-C/CAGE
CBC, BUN, creatinine, hepatitis serologies, CPK, amylase, CXR, GGT, tTG/IgA, ultrasound/CT of abdomen

Jaundice
→ Liver disease
Biliary obstruction
Hemolysis
Viral hepatitis

Chest pain or dyspnea
→ Myocardial infarction
CHF, BNP

**Abdominal pain
Elevated amylase**
→ Pancreatitis

Edema
→ CHF
Acute renal failure

**Muscle disorder or injury
↑ CPK**

**Liver toxicity
(AST/ALT >1)**
→ Alcohol
Medications

Anemia
→ Hemolysis
→ LDL, haptoglobin

**Exercises aggressively
↑ CPK**
→ Limit exercise for 72 degrees and repeat AST.

All tests normal
→ NAFLD
Hemochromatosis
→ Abd US

Elevated GGT
→ Abd US, if NEG, MIDA scan.

Bryce Ringwald, MD and Emily Ann Gorman, DO

Giboney PT. Mildly elevated liver transaminase levels in the asymptomatic patient. *Am Fam Physician*. 2005;71(6):1105–1110.

ASTHMA EXACERBATION, PEDIATRIC ACUTE

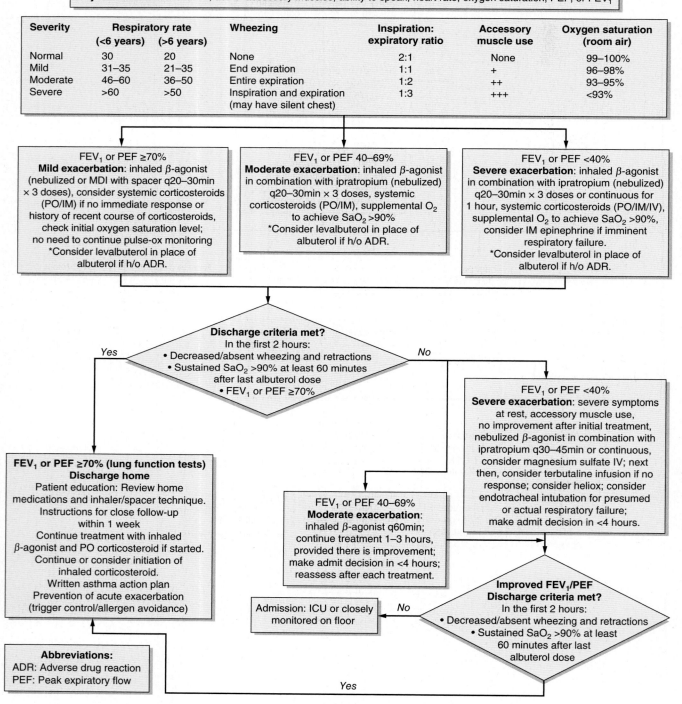

Initial evaluation: brief history of present illness, physical exam
Asthma history: emergency department visits, hospital and ICU admissions, home medications, frequency of oral steroid use, history of intubation, rapidly progressive episodes, food allergies, smoking history
Physical exam: auscultation, use of accessory muscles, ability to speak, heart rate, oxygen saturation, PEF, or FEV_1

Severity	Respiratory rate (<6 years)	Respiratory rate (>6 years)	Wheezing	Inspiration: expiratory ratio	Accessory muscle use	Oxygen saturation (room air)
Normal	30	20	None	2:1	None	99–100%
Mild	31–35	21–35	End expiration	1:1	+	96–98%
Moderate	46–60	36–50	Entire expiration	1:2	++	93–95%
Severe	>60	>50	Inspiration and expiration (may have silent chest)	1:3	+++	<93%

FEV_1 or PEF ≥70%
Mild exacerbation: inhaled β-agonist (nebulized or MDI with spacer q20–30min × 3 doses), consider systemic corticosteroids (PO/IM) if no immediate response or history of recent course of corticosteroids, check initial oxygen saturation level; no need to continue pulse-ox monitoring
*Consider levalbuterol in place of albuterol if h/o ADR.

FEV_1 or PEF 40–69%
Moderate exacerbation: inhaled β-agonist in combination with ipratropium (nebulized) q20–30min × 3 doses, systemic corticosteroids (PO/IM), supplemental O_2 to achieve SaO_2 >90%
*Consider levalbuterol in place of albuterol if h/o ADR.

FEV_1 or PEF <40%
Severe exacerbation: inhaled β-agonist in combination with ipratropium (nebulized) q20–30min × 3 doses or continuous for 1 hour, systemic corticosteroids (PO/IM/IV), supplemental O_2 to achieve SaO_2 >90%, consider IM epinephrine if imminent respiratory failure.
*Consider levalbuterol in place of albuterol if h/o ADR.

Discharge criteria met?
In the first 2 hours:
• Decreased/absent wheezing and retractions
• Sustained SaO_2 >90% at least 60 minutes after last albuterol dose
• FEV_1 or PEF ≥70%

Yes / No

FEV_1 or PEF <40%
Severe exacerbation: severe symptoms at rest, accessory muscle use, no improvement after initial treatment, nebulized β-agonist in combination with ipratropium q30–45min or continuous, consider magnesium sulfate IV; next then, consider terbutaline infusion if no response; consider heliox; consider endotracheal intubation for presumed or actual respiratory failure; make admit decision in <4 hours.

FEV_1 or PEF ≥70% (lung function tests)
Discharge home
Patient education: Review home medications and inhaler/spacer technique.
Instructions for close follow-up within 1 week
Continue treatment with inhaled β-agonist and PO corticosteroid if started.
Continue or consider initiation of inhaled corticosteroid.
Written asthma action plan
Prevention of acute exacerbation (trigger control/allergen avoidance)

FEV_1 or PEF 40–69%
Moderate exacerbation:
inhaled β-agonist q60min; continue treatment 1–3 hours, provided there is improvement; make admit decision in <4 hours; reassess after each treatment.

Admission: ICU or closely monitored on floor

No

Improved FEV_1/PEF Discharge criteria met?
In the first 2 hours:
• Decreased/absent wheezing and retractions
• Sustained SaO_2 >90% at least 60 minutes after last albuterol dose

Yes

Abbreviations:
ADR: Adverse drug reaction
PEF: Peak expiratory flow

Jan Estes Miller, MD and Adam McConnell, MD

Cloutier MM, Baptist AP, Blake KV, et al; for Expert Panel Working Group of the National Heart, Lung, and Blood Institute (NHLBI); National Asthma Education and Prevention Program Coordinating Committee (NAEPPCC). 2020 Focused updates to the asthma management guidelines: a report from the National Asthma Education and Prevention Program Coordinating Committee Expert Panel Working Group. *J Allergy Clin Immunol.* 2020;146(6):1217–1270.

Asthma Treatment and Maintenance, Adults and Adolescents ≥12 Years

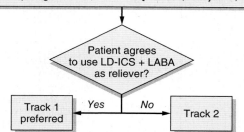

Confirm diagnosis
- History/PE
- Spirometry w/ reversibility
- Symptom frequency
- Modifiable risk factors
- Comorbidities (allergic rhinitis, inhalants [tobacco, marijuana, vaping, etc.])

Patient agrees to use LD-ICS + LABA as reliever?

Yes → Track 1 preferred
No → Track 2

Treatment approach
- Use of spacer for all MDIs (β-agonist, ICS) to improve delivery, decrease side effects

Assess, Adjust, Review
- Once good asthma control has been achieved for 2–3 months, consider stepping down therapy.
- Before stepping up, confirm symptoms are due to asthma and review/address common issues (inhaler technique, adherence, allergen exposure, etc.).

Track 1: Patient agrees to use LD-ICS + LABA as reliever (preferred).
Track 2: Patient prefers to use SABA as reliever and ICS as controller.

Symptoms	Step 1 Sx <2 times a month	Step 2 >2 times a month/ <4–5 times a week	Step 3 Daily symptoms/ waking ≥1/week	Step 4 Uncontrolled/ acute exacerbation	Step 5 Persistent symptoms/ exacerbations despite optimized step 4 treatments
Track 1	Preferred: As needed LD-ICS + formoterol	Preferred: As needed LD-ICS + formoterol	Preferred: LD-ICS + formoterol (MART)	Preferred: MD-ICS + formoterol (MART)	Preferred: Add on LAMA, HD-ICS, phenotype assessment Consider: Anti-IgE therapy (omalizumab) Anti-IL-5 therapy Anti-IL-4 antibody (dupilumab) Anti-TSLP (tezepelumab)
Track 2	Alternative: LD-ICS when SABA is used	Alternative: Daily LD-ICS and as needed SABA	Alternative: Daily LD-ICS + LABA	Alternative: Daily MD-ICS + LABA or HD-ICS + LABA	Alternative: Add on LAMA, HD-ICS, phenotype assessment; Consider: Anti-IgE therapy (omalizumab) Anti-IL-5 therapy Anti-IL-4 antibody (dupilumab) Anti-TSLP (tezepelumab)
		Other options: Daily LTRA	Other options: MD-ICS or HDM SLIT HDM SLIT	Other options: Add LAMA or Daily LTRA or HD-ICS	Other options: Add azithromycin or LD-OCS.

Adults and adolescents Inhaled corticosteroid	Total daily ICS dose (μg)		
	Low	Medium	High
BDP (pMDI, HFA)	200–500	>500–1,000	>1,000
BDP (DPI or pMDI, extrafine particle, HFA)	100–200	>200–400	>400
Budesonide (DPI or pMDI, HFA)	200–400	>400–800	>800
Ciclesonide (pMDI, extrafine particle, HFA)	80–160	>160–320	>320
Fluticasone furoate (DPI)	100		200
Fluticasone propionate (DPI)	100–250	>250–500	>500
Fluticasone propionate (pMDI, HFA)	100–250	>250–500	>500
Mometasone furoate (DPI)	Depends on DPI device		
Mometasone furoate (pMDI, HFA)	200–400		400

BDP: beclomethasone dipropionate
pMDI: pressurized MDI
HFA: hydrofluoroalkane
DPI: dry powder inhaler
LD: low dose
MD: medium dose
HD: high dose
LD-OCS: low-dose oral corticosteroids
ICS: inhaled corticosteroids
SABA: short-acting β-agonist

LABA: long-acting β-agonist
MART: maintenance and reliever therapy
LAMA: long-acting muscarinic antagonist
LTRA: leukotriene receptor antagonist
HDM SLIT: house dust mite sublingual immunotherapy

Frank J. Domino, MD, Shayan Mahapatra, MBBS, MD, and Jared Piotrowski, MD

Global Initiative for Asthma. Global strategy for asthma management and prevention, 2022. https://www.ginasthma.org. Accessed December 2, 2023.

Asthma Treatment and Maintenance, Children Ages 5 Years and Younger

Confirm diagnosis
– History/PE
– Symptom frequency
– Modifiable risk factors
– Comorbidities (allergic rhinitis, exposures [tobacco, marijuana, vaping, etc.])

Treatment approach
– Use of spacer for all MDIs (β-agonist, ICS) to improve delivery, decrease side effects
Assess, Adjust, Review
– Once good asthma control has been achieved for 2–3 months, consider stepping down therapy.
– Before stepping up, confirm symptoms are due to asthma and review/address common issues (inhaler technique, adherence, allergen exposure, etc.).

Track 1: Patient agrees to use ICS as controller (preferred).

Track 2: Patient prefers to use SABA as reliever and ICS as controller.

Symptoms	Step 1 Infrequent viral URI wheezing Few interval symptoms	Step 2 Wheezing requiring SABA ≥3 times a year	Step 3 Asthma diagnosis and not well controlled on LD-ICS; review alternative diagnosis and exposure risks.	Step 4 Asthma not controlled on double-dose ICS; review alternative diagnosis and exposure risks.
Preferred	Preferred: SABA as needed	Preferred: Daily LD-ICS + SABA as needed	Preferred: Double LD-ICS SABA as needed	Preferred: Refer to pediatric pulmonary.
Controller options (lacks evidence)	Consider LD-OCS at onset of viral illness.	Daily LTRA; consider LD-OCS at onset of viral illness.	LD-ICS + LTRA; consider refer to pediatric pulmonary.	Add LTRA or increase ICS frequency.

Children 6–11 years Inhaled corticosteroid	Total daily ICS dose (μg)		
	Low	Medium	High
BDP (pMDI, HFA)	100–200	>200–400	>400
BDP (pMDI, extrafine particle, HFA)	50–100	>100–200	>200
Budesonide (DPI)	100–200	>200–400	>400
Budesonide (nebules)	250–500	>500–1,000	>1,000
Ciclesonide (pMDI, extrafine particle, HFA)	80	>80–160	>160
Fluticasone furoate (DPI)	50		–
Fluticasone propionate (DPI)	50–100	>100–200	>200
Fluticasone propionate (pMDI, HFA)	50–100	>100–200	>200
Mometasone furoate (pMDI, HFA)	100		200

BDP: beclomethasone dipropionate
pMDI: pressurized MDI
HFA: hydrofluoroalkane
DPI: dry powder inhaler
LD: low dose
LD-OCS: low-dose oral corticosteroids

ICS: inhaled corticosteroids
SABA: short-acting β-agonist
LTRA: leukotriene receptor antagonist

Frank J. Domino, MD

Global Initiative for Asthma. Global strategy for asthma management and prevention, 2022. https://www.ginasthma.org. Accessed December 2, 2023.

Asthma Treatment and Maintenance, Children Ages 6–11

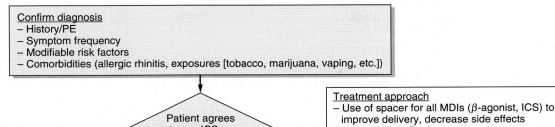

Confirm diagnosis
– History/PE
– Symptom frequency
– Modifiable risk factors
– Comorbidities (allergic rhinitis, exposures [tobacco, marijuana, vaping, etc.])

Patient agrees to use ICS as controller?

Yes — Track 1 preferred
No — Track 2

Treatment approach
– Use of spacer for all MDIs (β-agonist, ICS) to improve delivery, decrease side effects
Assess, Adjust, Review
– Once good asthma control has been achieved for 2–3 months, consider stepping down therapy.
– Before stepping up, confirm symptoms are due to asthma and review/address common issues (inhaler technique, adherence, allergen exposure, etc.).

Track 1: Patient agrees to use ICS as controller (preferred).

Track 2: Patient prefers to use SABA as reliever and ICS as controller.

Symptoms	Step 1 Sx <1 a month	Step 2 2 times a month but <1 a week	Step 3 Daily symptoms or waking ≥1 a week	Step 4 Symptoms most days Waking ≥1 week Low lung function	Step 5 Persistent symptoms/ exacerbations despite optimized step 4 treatments
Track 1	Preferred: LD-ICS when SABA is used	Preferred: LD-ICS	Preferred: LD-ICS + formoterol (MART) or MD-ICS or very LD-ICS + formoterol	Preferred: MD-ICS + formoterol (MART) or LD-ICS + formoterol (MART) Refer to pediatric pulmonary	Preferred: HD-ICS, phenotype assessment; Consider: Anti-IgE therapy (omalizumab) Anti-IL-5 therapy Anti-IL-4 antibody (dupilumab)
Track 2 (lacks efficacy evidence)	Alternative: LD-ICS + SABA as needed	Alternative: Daily LTRA or LD-ICS when SABA is used	Alternative: Daily LD-ICS + LTRA; SABA or LD-ICS + formoterol as reliever	Alternative: Add tiotropium or LTRA; SABA or LD-ICS + formoterol as reliever	Alternative: As last resort, add on LD-OCS but consider side effects.

Children 6–11 years Inhaled corticosteroid	Total daily ICS dose (μg) Low	Medium	High
BDP (pMDI, HFA)	100–200	>200–400	>400
BDP (pMDI, extrafine particle, HFA)	50–100	>100–200	>200
Budesonide (DPI)	100–200	>200–400	>400
Budesonide (nebules)	250–500	>500–1,000	>1,000
Ciclesonide (pMDI, extrafine particle, HFA)	80	>80–160	>160
Fluticasone furoate (DPI)	50		–
Fluticasone propionate (DPI)	50–100	>100–200	>200
Fluticasone propionate (pMDI, HFA)	50–100	>100–200	>200
Mometasone furoate (pMDI, HFA)	100		200

BDP: beclomethasone dipropionate
pMDI: pressurized MDI
HFA: hydrofluoroalkane
DPI: dry powder inhaler
LD: low dose
MD: medium dose
HD: high dose
LD-OCS: low-dose oral corticosteroids

ICS: inhaled corticosteroids
SABA: short-acting β-agonist
MART: maintenance and reliever therapy
LTRA: leukotriene receptor antagonist

Frank J. Domino, MD

Global Initiative for Asthma. Global strategy for asthma management and prevention, 2022. https://www.ginasthma.org. Accessed December 2, 2023.

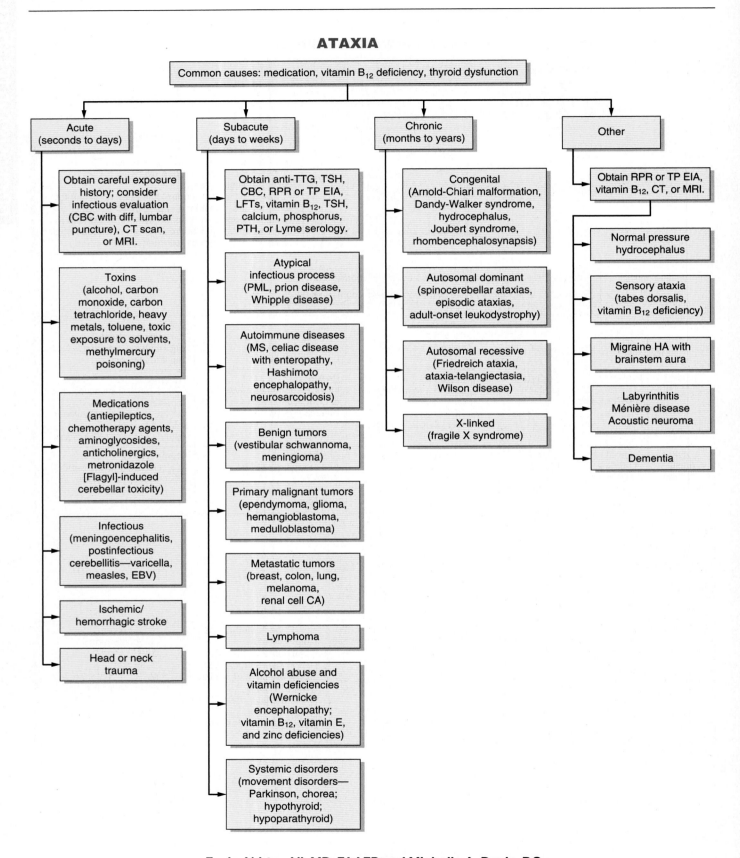

Fozia Akhtar Ali, MD, FAAFP and Michelle A. Davis, DO

Brunberg JA; for Expert Panel on Neurologic Imaging. Ataxia. *AJNR Am J Neuroradiol.* 2008;29(7):1420–1422.

AZOTEMIA AND UREMIA

Azotemia is the elevation of blood urea nitrogen (BUN). It can be divided into prerenal, intrinsic renal, and postrenal azotemia based on the cause. This is important because treatments differ. Azotemia is called uremia if signs and symptoms, for example, nausea, vomiting, severe metabolic acidosis, hyperkalemia, and fluid overload, among others, develop. Uremia is mostly due to the accumulation of BUN and other toxins or waste products normally filtered by the kidney, and it may progress to seizures, coma, and death if left untreated. Dialysis is often the treatment of choice for severe uremia.

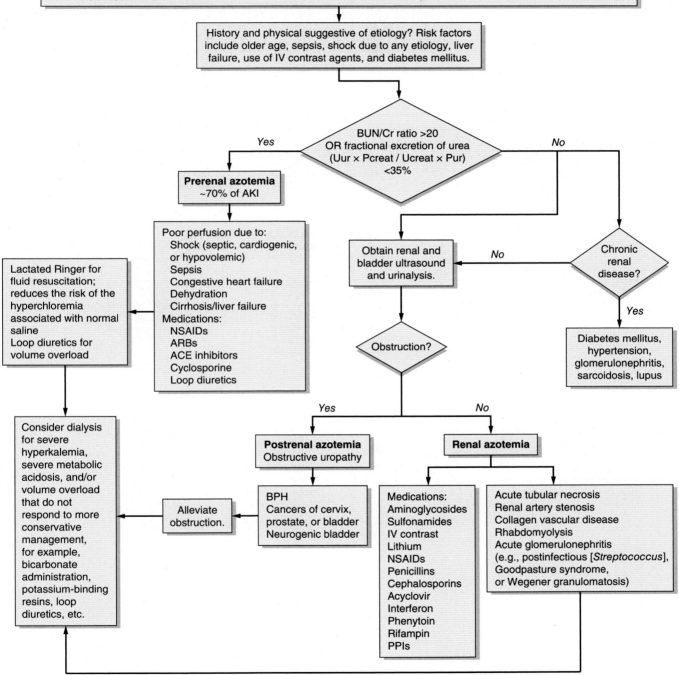

History and physical suggestive of etiology? Risk factors include older age, sepsis, shock due to any etiology, liver failure, use of IV contrast agents, and diabetes mellitus.

BUN/Cr ratio >20 OR fractional excretion of urea (Uur × Pcreat / Ucreat × Pur) <35%

Yes — **Prerenal azotemia** ~70% of AKI

Poor perfusion due to:
Shock (septic, cardiogenic, or hypovolemic)
Sepsis
Congestive heart failure
Dehydration
Cirrhosis/liver failure
Medications:
NSAIDs
ARBs
ACE inhibitors
Cyclosporine
Loop diuretics

Lactated Ringer for fluid resuscitation; reduces the risk of the hyperchloremia associated with normal saline
Loop diuretics for volume overload

No — Chronic renal disease?

No — Obtain renal and bladder ultrasound and urinalysis.

Yes — Diabetes mellitus, hypertension, glomerulonephritis, sarcoidosis, lupus

Obstruction?

Yes — **Postrenal azotemia** Obstructive uropathy

No — **Renal azotemia**

BPH
Cancers of cervix, prostate, or bladder
Neurogenic bladder

Alleviate obstruction.

Medications:
Aminoglycosides
Sulfonamides
IV contrast
Lithium
NSAIDs
Penicillins
Cephalosporins
Acyclovir
Interferon
Phenytoin
Rifampin
PPIs

Acute tubular necrosis
Renal artery stenosis
Collagen vascular disease
Rhabdomyolysis
Acute glomerulonephritis
(e.g., postinfectious [*Streptococcus*],
Goodpasture syndrome,
or Wegener granulomatosis)

Consider dialysis for severe hyperkalemia, severe metabolic acidosis, and/or volume overload that do not respond to more conservative management, for example, bicarbonate administration, potassium-binding resins, loop diuretics, etc.

Steven A. House, MD, FAAFP, FAAHPM, HMDC

Mercado MG, Smith DK, Guard EL. Acute kidney injury: diagnosis and management. *Am Fam Physician*. 2019;100(11):687–694.

CARDIAC ARRHYTHMIAS

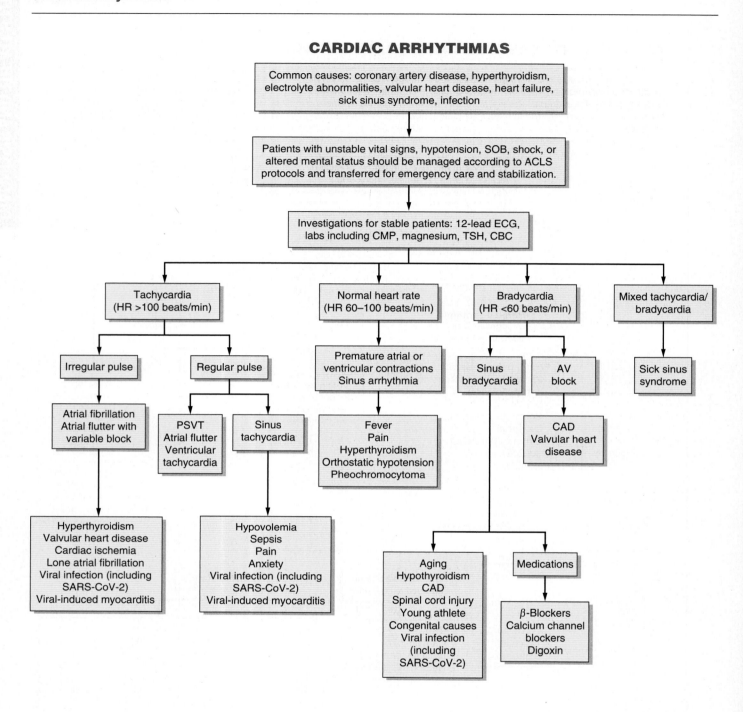

Common causes: coronary artery disease, hyperthyroidism, electrolyte abnormalities, valvular heart disease, heart failure, sick sinus syndrome, infection

Patients with unstable vital signs, hypotension, SOB, shock, or altered mental status should be managed according to ACLS protocols and transferred for emergency care and stabilization.

Investigations for stable patients: 12-lead ECG, labs including CMP, magnesium, TSH, CBC

Tachycardia (HR >100 beats/min)

Normal heart rate (HR 60–100 beats/min)

Bradycardia (HR <60 beats/min)

Mixed tachycardia/ bradycardia

Irregular pulse

Regular pulse

Premature atrial or ventricular contractions Sinus arrhythmia

Sinus bradycardia

AV block

Sick sinus syndrome

Atrial fibrillation Atrial flutter with variable block

PSVT Atrial flutter Ventricular tachycardia

Sinus tachycardia

Fever Pain Hyperthyroidism Orthostatic hypotension Pheochromocytoma

CAD Valvular heart disease

Hyperthyroidism Valvular heart disease Cardiac ischemia Lone atrial fibrillation Viral infection (including SARS-CoV-2) Viral-induced myocarditis

Hypovolemia Sepsis Pain Anxiety Viral infection (including SARS-CoV-2) Viral-induced myocarditis

Aging Hypothyroidism CAD Spinal cord injury Young athlete Congenital causes Viral infection (including SARS-CoV-2)

Medications

β-Blockers Calcium channel blockers Digoxin

William E. Cayley Jr., MD, Mdiv

Byrnes TJ, Costantini O. Tachyarrhythmias and bradyarrhythmias: differential diagnosis and initial management in the primary care office. *Med Clin North Am.* 2017;101(3):495–506.

CERVICAL HYPEREXTENSION INJURY

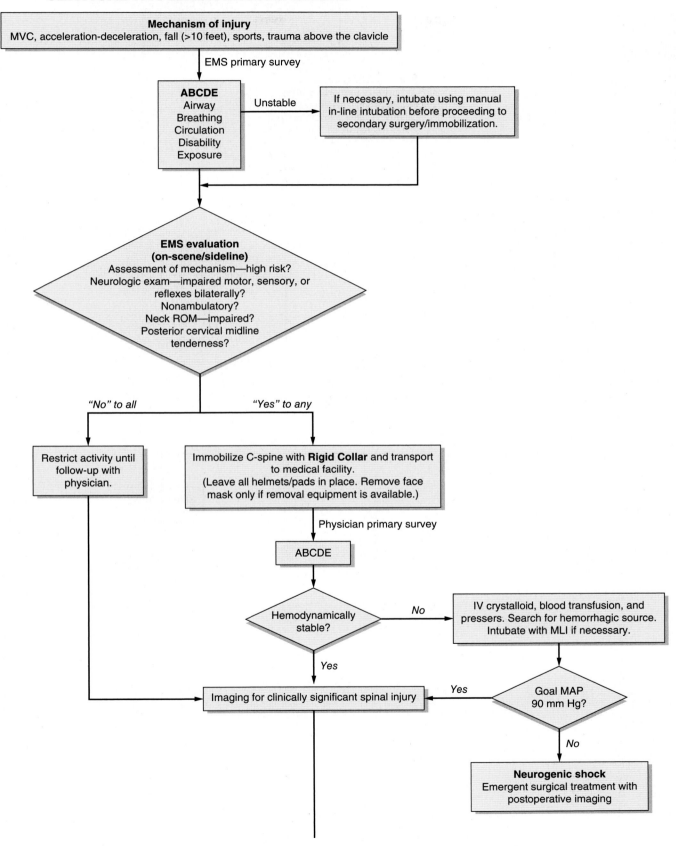

Mechanism of injury
MVC, acceleration-deceleration, fall (>10 feet), sports, trauma above the clavicle

EMS primary survey

ABCDE
Airway
Breathing
Circulation
Disability
Exposure

Unstable → If necessary, intubate using manual in-line intubation before proceeding to secondary surgery/immobilization.

EMS evaluation (on-scene/sideline)
Assessment of mechanism—high risk?
Neurologic exam—impaired motor, sensory, or reflexes bilaterally?
Nonambulatory?
Neck ROM—impaired?
Posterior cervical midline tenderness?

"No" to all

"Yes" to any

Restrict activity until follow-up with physician.

Immobilize C-spine with **Rigid Collar** and transport to medical facility.
(Leave all helmets/pads in place. Remove face mask only if removal equipment is available.)

Physician primary survey

ABCDE

Hemodynamically stable?

No → IV crystalloid, blood transfusion, and pressers. Search for hemorrhagic source. Intubate with MLI if necessary.

Yes

Goal MAP 90 mm Hg?

Yes → Imaging for clinically significant spinal injury

No

Neurogenic shock
Emergent surgical treatment with postoperative imaging

A-21

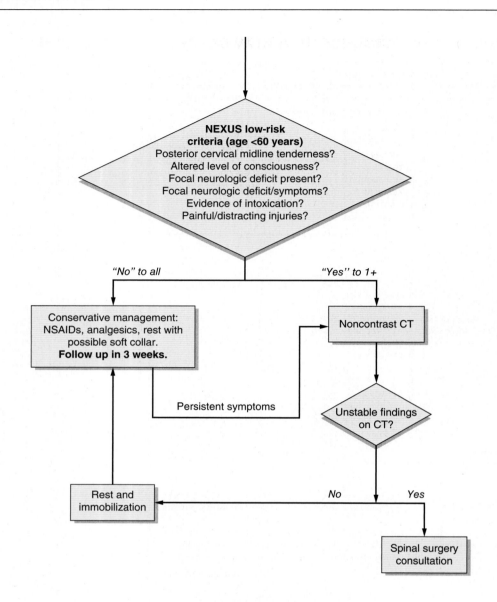

NEXUS low-risk
criteria (age <60 years)
Posterior cervical midline tenderness?
Altered level of consciousness?
Focal neurologic deficit present?
Focal neurologic deficit/symptoms?
Evidence of intoxication?
Painful/distracting injuries?

"No" to all

"Yes" to 1+

Conservative management:
NSAIDs, analgesics, rest with
possible soft collar.
Follow up in 3 weeks.

Noncontrast CT

Persistent symptoms

Unstable findings
on CT?

Rest and
immobilization

No

Yes

Spinal surgery
consultation

Ashley L. Vertente, MD, MBA and Michael Y. Yang, MD, CAQSM

Schleicher P, Pingel A, Kandziora F. Safe management of acute cervical spine injuries. *EFORT Open Rev.* 2018;3(5):347–357.

CHEST PAIN/ACUTE CORONARY SYNDROME

Common DDx: STEMI, NSTEMI/unstable angina, PE, aortic dissection, PTX, pericarditis, Boerhaave syndrome, anxiety, costochondritis, GI-related, domestic violence

↓

ECG

STEMI criteria
Any of the following
- 1 mm ST elevation in any two contiguous leads except V_2 and V_3
  - In women: 1.5 mm elevation in V_2 or V_3
  - In men aged <40 years: 2.5 mm elevation in V_2 or V_3
  - In men aged ≥40 years: 2 mm in V_2 or V_3

STEMI equivalents
- de Winter T waves
- ST depression in V_2 and V_3 and concerning posterior ECG
- LBBB or paced rhythm with Sgarbossa criteria*
- Hyperacute T waves

*Sgarbossa Criteria:
- Concordant ST-Elevation of ≥1 mm = 5 points
- Concordant ST-depression of ≥1 mm in V_1–V_3 = 3 points
- Discordant ST-elevation of >5 mm = 2 points
Score of ≥3 has a 90% specificity for myocardial infarction; not sensitive

STEMI criteria or STEMI equivalent → *Alert cardiology*

162–325 mg ASA
O_2 if SpO_2 <90%
SL NTG q5min × 3 PRN for pain
(avoid in inferior STEMI)
Load with dual antiplatelet agent
- Clopidogrel 300 mg
~OR~
- Ticagrelor 180 mg
~OR~
- Prasugrel 60 mg
Heparin bolus
Avoid morphine if possible
(may interfere with antiplatelet agent).
Troponin, CXR

No STEMI criteria or STEMI equivalent

ASA 162–325 mg, serial troponin, serial ECG if continuing chest pain, CXR

↓

Serial troponin positive?

Yes:
- Admit
- Heparin bolus
- ASA daily
- Consider nitrates, clopidogrel, β-blocker, ACEi, and statin.

No: Risk stratify for CAD
- High risk
- Medium risk
- Low risk

High risk / Medium risk Positive stress test → Cardiology evaluation for consideration of cardiac catheterization

Medium risk → **Stress test**
- Positive → Cardiology evaluation for consideration of cardiac catheterization
- Negative → Discharge home with PCP follow-up.

Low risk → Discharge home with PCP follow-up.

Review DDx: anxiety, GERD, PE, biliary dysfunction, MSK pain, domestic violence.

PCI available within 120 minutes?

Yes: PCI

No: Administer thrombolytic within 30 minutes if unable to PCI within 120 minutes.

Successful treatment?
- **No:** Consider CABG.
- **Yes:** Medical therapy

Medical therapy
- ASA 81 mg
- Clopidogrel 75 mg/day
- High-intensity statin
- β-blocker unless CHF or shock
- Cardiac rehabilitation
- ACE inhibitor for patients with reduced EF
- Consider aldosterone antagonist if EF <40%.

Jason Teng, MD and Moises Gallegos, MD, MPH

Kontos MC, de Lemos JA, Deitelzweig SB, et al. 2022 ACC expert consensus decision pathway on the evaluation and disposition of acute chest pain in the emergency department: a report of the American College of Cardiology Solution Set Oversight Committee. *J Am Coll Cardiol.* 2022;(20):1925–1960. doi:10.1016/j.jacc.2022.08.750.

CHILD ABUSE: NONACCIDENTAL TRAUMA

When should you consider NAT in young children?

Skin Injury	**Age <6 months** • Any bruise or oral injury **Age 6 months–4 years** • Unexplained bruises in noncruising children • Bruises on the trunk, ear, neck, jaw line, cheek • Patterned bruising • Subconjunctival hemorrhage • Frenular tears
Burns	**Any age** • Unexplained burns • Burns in the shape of a heated object • Immersion burns • Burns on both the perineum and lower extremities
Fractures	**Age <6 months** • Any fracture **Age 6–11 months** • Linear parietal skull fractures without history • Any nonlinear parietal skull fracture • Any fracture of the ribs, femur, or humerus • Nonskull fractures in nonambulatory children • Any other fracture without history **Age 12–23 months** • Any rib or femur fracture • Nonsupracondylar humerus fracture • Any other fracture without history **Age 24 months–4 years** • Any rib fracture • Any other fracture without history
Intracranial	**Age <12 months** • Any subdural hemorrhage or hygroma **Age 12 months–4 years** • Acute subdural hematoma without history of high energy trauma (e.g., MVC, long-distance fall)
Visceral	**Age <12 months** • Any visceral injury **Age 12 months–4 years** • Unexplained traumatic visceral injury • Trauma to pancreas • Proximal hollow viscus injury

When should you consider NAT in older children?

• When a child makes a disclosure
• When there is no or inconsistent history to explain an injury
• When a prepubertal child displays sexualized behaviors
• When a prepubertal child has genital injury or infection
• Any pregnancy in a child <16 years old

Medical History

• If possible, interview the child separate from their guardian.
• Ask open-ended questions that do not introduce concepts of intentional injury or inappropriate behavior.
• When a child makes a disclosure, listen attentively, believe them, and thank them for telling you.

1. Obtain a focused injury history, especially a clear timeline.
2. PMH, that is, prior traumas, injuries, surgeries, hospitalizations
3. Family bleeding, bruising, bone, metabolic, or genetic history
4. Developmental and behavioral history
5. Social history, including living situation, other children in household, substance use, psychosocial stressors

Physical Examination

1. General assessment (alertness, demeanor, growth, evidence of neglect like severe caries, neglected wound care, etc.)
2. Skin exam, noting bruises, lacerations, burns, bites, etc.
3. Complete neurologic exam.
4. Consider secure photographs or sketches of physical signs.
5. If suspecting sexual violence, a specialized provider like a SANE nurse should perform the genital exam, if available.

Diagnostic Testing for Suspected NAT

1. Skeletal survey for those <24 months old
2. Head CT or MRI if <6 months or concerned for head trauma
3. Consider basic lab evaluation: AST/ALT, urine toxicology
4. If bruising: CBC, PT, aPTT, von Willebrand, factor VIII + IX
5. If fractures: Ca, Mg, phos, alk phos, PTH, vitamin D
6. If focal neuro findings or IC bleeding: Consult ophthalmology.

Management of Suspected NAT

1. Consult social work and child protection team.
2. Refer to child protection agencies when appropriate.
3. Document as objectively as possible.
4. Refer for mental health support early.

Cultural and Social Considerations

• Take the time to look into practices that differ from your own with a sense of curiosity and cultural humility, recognizing that parenting practices differ between cultures.
• NAT should never be the only thing on your differential.

• In many states, medical providers are mandated reporters when NAT is suspected, but we also have a responsibility to obtain a complete and accurate history to inform our degree of suspicion.
• The professional opinion of a medical provider is taken very seriously by child protective agencies and can have significant impact on the agencies' determinations.
• Although the investigation of cases of suspected NAT is intended to protect children, many forms of agency involvement, particularly family separation, are inherently trauma inducing.

• Recognize that structural racism and other forms of oppression drive disparities in which families are suspected, referred, investigated, surveilled, and separated.
• Despite NAT being less likely to occur in families of color when controlling for other risk factors, children of color and Latinx children are overrepresented in child protective agencies, whereas cases of NAT among white, non-Latinx children are potentially missed.
• These structures of oppression, and the long history of medicine's involvement in their creation and perpetuation, create an understandable level of mistrust in some families.
• This mistrust can result in guarded responses, declining to volunteer information, or skepticism of medical recommendations, all of which may be misinterpreted by medical providers as suspicious.

Jordan Howard-Young, MD and Stephany Giraldo Eierle, DO, MPH

Child Welfare Information Gateway. *Child Welfare Practice to Address Racial Disproportionality and Disparity.* Washington, DC: Children's Bureau; 2021. https://www.childwelfare.gov/pubPDFs/racial_disproportionality.pdf. Accessed December 7, 2022.

CHRONIC JOINT PAIN AND STIFFNESS

Common causes: osteoarthritis, rheumatoid arthritis, septic arthritis, gout, pseudogout, fibromyalgia → Joint pain lasting >6 weeks

Yes | *No*

No systemic s/sx
Morning stiffness <1 hour ← <2,000 WBCs

Warm, swollen joints
Morning stiffness >1 hour
± Systemic s/sx

Worse w/ weight-bearing ± Swelling

Diffuse arthralgia, myalgia

Check ESR, Lyme serology, joint aspiration for cell count, cultures, crystals.

Osteoarthritis

Fibromyalgia

Acetaminophen, NSAIDs, topical NSAIDs

Graduated exercise program
Pregabalin
Amitriptyline
Duloxetine

>3,000–50,000 WBCs
>50% PMNs

Variable cell counts
Negative culture
Symmetric joint involvement

>50,000 WBCs
>75% PMNs

Low-impact exercise, PT
Staging with MRI
Complementary therapies

Crystals present

↑ESR
No crystals
Negative culture

Viral

Septic arthritis

Urate, negative birefringence

Calcium phosphate dihydrate
Positive birefringence

Check autoimmune markers, systemic symptoms.

Check for hep B, hep C, HIV, parvovirus B19, or other suspected viruses.

Emergent empirical IV Abx.
Consult orthopedics for irrigation, biopsy.
Narrow Abx to clinical response, microbiology sensitivities.

Gout

Pseudogout

NSAIDs
colchicine, steroids

NSAIDs
intra-articular steroid

Joint treatment is largely supportive.

↑RF, anti-CCP

Malar rash
Oral ulcers
↑ANA,
anti-dsDNA,
anti-Smith Ab

Asymmetric joints affected
Involvement of SI joint, spine
Negative RF

Bilateral shoulder and hip involvement

Xerophthalmia
Xerostomia

IBD

Rheumatoid arthritis

Polymyalgia rheumatica

Sjögren syndrome

IBD arthritis

NSAIDs
Methotrexate
Biologics

SLE

Spondyloarthropathy

Oral steroids

Hydroxy-chloroquine
Steroids
Methotrexate

Immunomodulators
Anticytokines

NSAIDs, hydroxychloroquine

HLA-B27

Urethritis
Conjunctivitis

Scaly rash
Dactylitis

Ankylosing spondylitis

Reactive arthritis

Psoriatic arthritis

NSAIDs
PT

Treat primary etiology.
NSAIDs
Sulfasalazine

NSAIDs
Methotrexate
Biologics

Tristan M. Pennella, DO and Joanne E. Genewick, DO, FAIHM

Foster ZJ, Day AL, Miller J. Polyarticular joint pain in adults: evaluation and differential diagnosis. *Am Fam Physician*. 2023;107(1):42–51.

CHRONIC OBSTRUCTIVE PULMONARY DISEASE (COPD), DIAGNOSIS AND TREATMENT

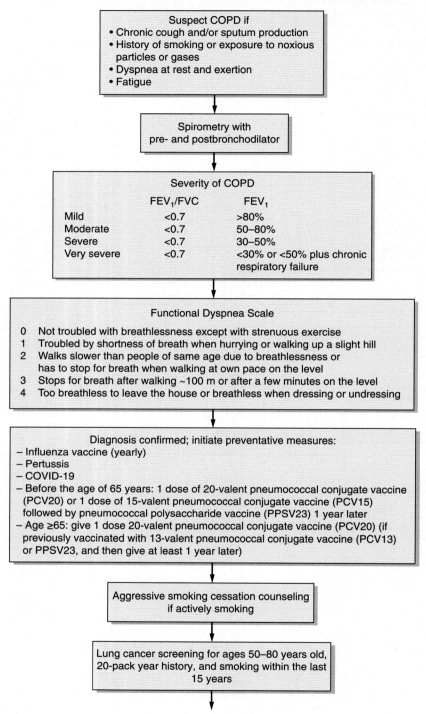

Suspect COPD if
- Chronic cough and/or sputum production
- History of smoking or exposure to noxious particles or gases
- Dyspnea at rest and exertion
- Fatigue

Spirometry with pre- and postbronchodilator

Severity of COPD

	FEV$_1$/FVC	FEV$_1$
Mild	<0.7	>80%
Moderate	<0.7	50–80%
Severe	<0.7	30–50%
Very severe	<0.7	<30% or <50% plus chronic respiratory failure

Functional Dyspnea Scale

0 Not troubled with breathlessness except with strenuous exercise
1 Troubled by shortness of breath when hurrying or walking up a slight hill
2 Walks slower than people of same age due to breathlessness or has to stop for breath when walking at own pace on the level
3 Stops for breath after walking ~100 m or after a few minutes on the level
4 Too breathless to leave the house or breathless when dressing or undressing

Diagnosis confirmed; initiate preventative measures:
– Influenza vaccine (yearly)
– Pertussis
– COVID-19
– Before the age of 65 years: 1 dose of 20-valent pneumococcal conjugate vaccine (PCV20) or 1 dose of 15-valent pneumococcal conjugate vaccine (PCV15) followed by pneumococcal polysaccharide vaccine (PPSV23) 1 year later
– Age ≥65: give 1 dose 20-valent pneumococcal conjugate vaccine (PCV20) (if previously vaccinated with 13-valent pneumococcal conjugate vaccine (PCV13) or PPSV23, and then give at least 1 year later)

Aggressive smoking cessation counseling if actively smoking

Lung cancer screening for ages 50–80 years old, 20-pack year history, and smoking within the last 15 years

Group **A**/mild COPD

– FDS = 0 or 1
– 0–1 exacerbations annually (not leading to hospitalization)

Treatment:
– Short-acting β-agonist or anticholinergic PRN

Group **B**/moderate COPD

– FDS ≥2
– 0–1 exacerbations annually (not leading to hospitalization)

Treatment:
– Long-acting β-agonist plus long-acting anticholinergic combination inhaler
– Short-acting β-agonist or anticholinergic PRN

Group **E**/severe COPD

– FDS ≥2
– 0–1 exacerbations annually (not leading to hospitalization)
– ≥2 exacerbations annually or ≥1 exacerbation leading to hospitalization

Treatment:
– Long-acting β-agonist plus long-acting anticholinergic combination inhaler or inhaled corticosteroids plus long-acting β-agonist plus long-acting anticholinergic combination inhaler, if eosinophils are ≥100
– Short-acting β-agonist or anticholinergic PRN
– Pulmonary rehabilitation
– Assess for supplemental oxygen
– Consider surgical options and/or add a phosphodiesterase-1 inhibitor.
– Consider azithromycin 3 times a week to daily in patients with frequent exacerbations.

William W. Wong, DO and Scott E. Kopec, MD, FCCP

Global Initiative for Chronic Obstructive Lung Disease. 2022 Global strategy for prevention, diagnosis and management of COPD. https://goldcopd.org/2022-gold-reports/. Accessed September 19, 2023.

CIRRHOSIS

Common causes: alcoholic liver disease, chronic hepatitis B and C, α_1-antitrypsin deficiency, nonalcoholic steatohepatitis, hemochromatosis, medications, primary biliary cirrhosis, primary sclerosing cholangitis, autoimmune hepatitis, Wilson disease

↓

Check liver function tests: HCV Ab, HBsAg, HBsAb, Fe, TIBC, ferritin, CBC w/ diff, antimitochondrial antibodies (AMAs), US or CT of liver antinuclear and smooth muscle antibodies, serum α_1-antitrypsin, serum ceruloplasmin.

↓

History of alcohol or hepatotoxic medication exposure?

Yes ────────────────── **No**

Yes:

Alcoholic hepatitis

Medications
↓
Methotrexate
Amiodarone
INH
Valproic acid
Many others

No:

+ Viral studies
↓
Hepatitis B
Hepatitis C

− Viral studies

Elevated Fe/TIBC and increased ferritin
↓
Hemochromatosis

Normal Fe studies
↓
Order AMA, anti-smooth muscle antibody (ASMA), ANA, liver–kidney microsomal type 1 antibody (LKM-1).
↓
No autoimmune findings

Elevated ASMA, LKM-1, and CRP
↓
Autoimmune hepatitis / Total serum immunoglobulin G elevated

Elevated AMA
↓
Primary biliary cirrhosis

Decreased α_1-antitrypsin levels
↓
α_1-Antitrypsin deficiency

History of inflammatory bowel disease
↓
Primary sclerosing cholangitis

Fatty infiltration on liver imaging
↓
Nonalcoholic steatohepatitis

Kayser-Fleischer rings
↓
Wilson disease

Chelsea Mendonca, MD and Adam Mendonca, MD

Smith A, Baumgartner K, Bositis C. Cirrhosis: diagnosis and management. *Am Fam Physician*. 2019;100(12):759–770.

CONCUSSION, SIDELINE EVALUATION
Stable, No C-Spine Injury

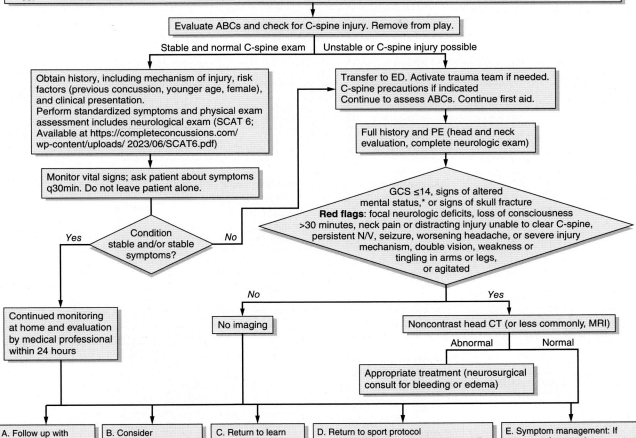

Concussion: traumatic event AND change in neurologic function OR one of the following signs/symptoms: **somatic** (HA, nausea/vomiting [N/V], dizziness, vertigo, visual problems, sensitivity to light or sound, numbness/tingling), **cognitive** (LOC, memory problems, feeling "foggy," slower reaction times, confusion), **emotional/behavioral** (i.e., irritability, sadness), **sleep** (i.e., drowsiness)

Evaluate ABCs and check for C-spine injury. Remove from play.

Stable and normal C-spine exam — Unstable or C-spine injury possible

Obtain history, including mechanism of injury, risk factors (previous concussion, younger age, female), and clinical presentation.
Perform standardized symptoms and physical exam assessment includes neurological exam (SCAT 6; Available at https://completeconcussions.com/wp-content/uploads/ 2023/06/SCAT6.pdf)

Transfer to ED. Activate trauma team if needed. C-spine precautions if indicated
Continue to assess ABCs. Continue first aid.

Full history and PE (head and neck evaluation, complete neurologic exam)

Monitor vital signs; ask patient about symptoms q30min. Do not leave patient alone.

GCS ≤14, signs of altered mental status,* or signs of skull fracture **Red flags**: focal neurologic deficits, loss of consciousness >30 minutes, neck pain or distracting injury unable to clear C-spine, persistent N/V, seizure, worsening headache, or severe injury mechanism, double vision, weakness or tingling in arms or legs, or agitated

Yes — Condition stable and/or stable symptoms? — **No**

Continued monitoring at home and evaluation by medical professional within 24 hours

No — No imaging

Yes — Noncontrast head CT (or less commonly, MRI)

Abnormal — Normal

Appropriate treatment (neurosurgical consult for bleeding or edema)

A. Follow up with medical professional in the next 24 hours.
- History and PE (including complete neurologic exam and symptom checklist)
- Patient should undergo physical and cognitive rest while symptoms persist.
- If at neurologic baseline, review return to play protocol and return to learn protocol.
- If not at neurologic baseline, consider ED evaluation or neuroimaging, close follow-up, and symptomatic treatment.

B. Consider neuropsych testing (paper-and-pencil, ImPACT, CogState, HeadMinder, ANAM, etc.).
- The ideal timing, frequency, and type of neuropsych testing have not been determined.
- Most concussions can be managed appropriately without the use of neuropsych testing.
- Neuropsych testing may be most helpful for high-risk athletes, those with prior concussions, and those who may downplay symptoms in an effort to return to play sooner.

C. Return to learn protocol
- Daily activities that do not result in more than mild exacerbation of symptoms related to current concussion (5–15 minutes and increase gradually)
- School activities: homework, reading, or other cognitive activities
- Return to school part-time: gradual introduction of school work (i.e., partial school day with greater access to breaks)
- Return to school full-time

D. Return to sport protocol
- Stage 1: symptom-limited activity; daily activities that do not exacerbate symptoms (walking)
  - Goal: gradual reintroduction
- Stage 2A: aerobic exercise (light): 55% max HR
- Stage 2B: aerobic exercise (moderate): 70% max HR (stationary cycling)
  - Goal: increase HR
- Stage 3: individual sport-specific exercise
  - Goal: additional movement, change of direction
- Stages 4–6 should begin after the resolution of any symptoms, abnormalities and cognitive function and any other clinical findings related to the current caution.
- Stage 4: noncontact training drills
  - Goal: resume usual intensity of exercise, coordination, and increased thinking
- Stage 5: full contact practice
  - Goal: restore confidence and assess functional skills
- Stage 6: return to sport
  - Goal: normal game play

E. Symptom management: If concussive symptoms (typically HA, sleep, cognitive, and mood disturbances) are persistent and interfering with function, consider symptomatic treatment.
- In the acute setting, ASA and NSAIDs should be used with caution due to increased risk of intracranial bleeding. Acetaminophen and physical modalities are OK.
- If HA persists for a few days, consider typical abortive treatment. There is no established role for pharmacotherapy in the acute treatment of concussion-induced sleep, cognitive, or mood disturbances.
- If symptoms persist beyond 4 weeks, consider referral to specialist (neurology, sports medicine, etc.). Multidisciplinary approach is often needed.

*Signs of altered mental status: agitation, somnolence, repetitive questioning, or slow response to verbal communication.

Anthony Shadiack, DO, CAQSM and Andrew Baird, MD

Patricios JS, Schneider KJ, Dvorak J, et al. Consensus statement on concussion in sport: the 6th International Conference on Concussion in Sport–Amsterdam, October 2022. *Br J Sports Med.* 2023;57(11):695–711. doi:10.1136/bjsports-2023-106898.

CONGESTIVE HEART FAILURE: DIFFERENTIAL DIAGNOSIS

Common causes: CAD, MI, valvular disease, arrhythmia, idiopathic cardiomyopathy, pulmonary HTN, renal disease, medication nonadherence

Diagnosis made clinically

History: exercise intolerance, dyspnea on exertion or at rest, cough, orthopnea, paroxysmal nocturnal dyspnea, chest discomfort, fatigue, weight gain

Exam: elevated jugular venous pressure, rales, S_3/S_4 gallop, hepatojugular reflux, increased abdominal distention, pallor, lower extremity edema

Testing: chest x-ray, ECG, troponin, echo, BNP, BMP, LFTs, TSH, UA, uric acid

Diagnosis of (C)HF: Framingham Diagnostic Criteria
Requires 2 major criteria or 1 major and 2 minor criteria

Major criteria
- Acute pulmonary edema
- Cardiomegaly
- Hepatojugular reflux
- Elevated jugular venous pressure
- Paroxysmal nocturnal dyspnea
- Rales
- S_3

Minor criteria
- Ankle edema
- Dyspnea on exertion
- Hepatomegaly
- Nocturnal cough
- Pleural effusion
- Tachycardia to >120 beats/min

97% and 89% sensitive for systolic and diastolic heart failure (HF), respectively

BNP <80

BNP 80–500

Indeterminate. Consider (C)HF AND alternative diagnoses:
- COPD
- Asthma
- Lung disease
- Pulmonary embolus

LVEF <40% (HFrEF, systolic HF)

EF 40–50% (HFmrEF)

LVEF >50% (HFpEF, diastolic HF)

BNP >500

Likely (C)HF

(C)HF essentially ruled out

Ischemic
- History of CAD/MI
- Positive stress test
- CAD on cardiac catheterization
- Troponin elevation

Cardiac catheterization unless contraindicated

Evaluate for causes of (C)HF.
- Ischemic: CAD/MI
- Nonischemic: HTN, idiopathic CM, valvular disease, HOCM, arrhythmia, myocarditis/pericarditis, collagen vascular disease
- Due to volume: medication noncompliance, renal failure

Nonischemic cardiomyopathy

Idiopathic cardiomyopathy

Others: HTN, thyrotoxicosis, alcoholism, chemotherapy induced, cocaine, autoimmune, collagen vascular disease, infiltrative (amyloid, hemochromatosis), obstructive sleep apnea

Tachycardia mediated (atrial fibrillation/flutter, SVT, frequent PVCs)

Valvular disease cardiomyopathy

Viral mediated (coxsackievirus, adenovirus, HIV, EBV)

Abbreviations:
HFpEF, heart failure with preserved ejection fraction; HFmrEF, heart failure with midrange ejection fraction; HFrEF, heart failure with reduced ejection fraction

Jeremy Golding, MD, FAAFP

King M, Kingery J, Casey B. Diagnosis and evaluation of heart failure. *Am Fam Physician.* 2012;85(12):1161–1168.

CONSTIPATION, DIAGNOSIS AND TREATMENT (ADULT)

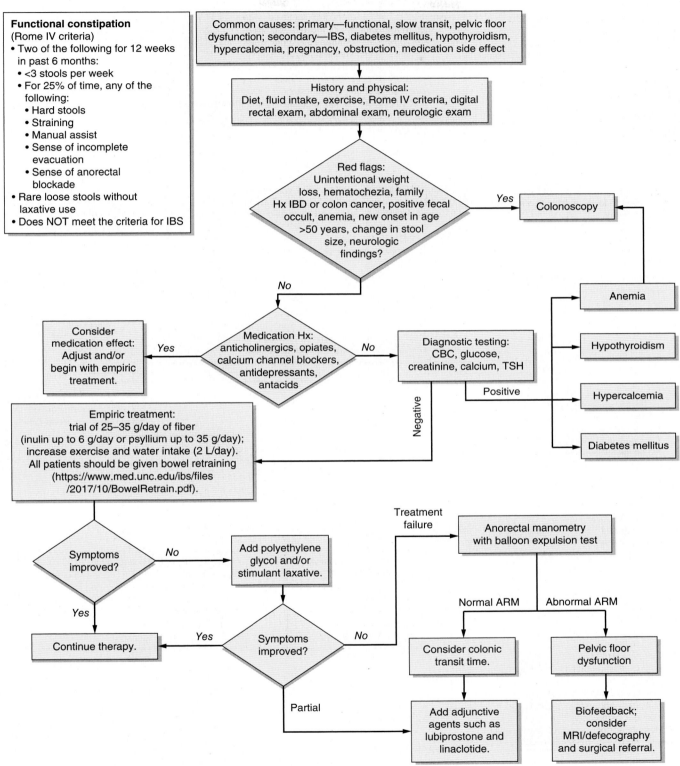

Functional constipation
(Rome IV criteria)
- Two of the following for 12 weeks in past 6 months:
  - <3 stools per week
  - For 25% of time, any of the following:
    - Hard stools
    - Straining
    - Manual assist
    - Sense of incomplete evacuation
    - Sense of anorectal blockade
- Rare loose stools without laxative use
- Does NOT meet the criteria for IBS

Common causes: primary—functional, slow transit, pelvic floor dysfunction; secondary—IBS, diabetes mellitus, hypothyroidism, hypercalcemia, pregnancy, obstruction, medication side effect

History and physical: Diet, fluid intake, exercise, Rome IV criteria, digital rectal exam, abdominal exam, neurologic exam

Red flags: Unintentional weight loss, hematochezia, family Hx IBD or colon cancer, positive fecal occult, anemia, new onset in age >50 years, change in stool size, neurologic findings? — **Yes** → Colonoscopy

No

Medication Hx: anticholinergics, opiates, calcium channel blockers, antidepressants, antacids — **Yes** → Consider medication effect: Adjust and/or begin with empiric treatment.

No → Diagnostic testing: CBC, glucose, creatinine, calcium, TSH

Positive → Anemia / Hypothyroidism / Hypercalcemia / Diabetes mellitus

Negative

Empiric treatment: trial of 25–35 g/day of fiber (inulin up to 6 g/day or psyllium up to 35 g/day); increase exercise and water intake (2 L/day). All patients should be given bowel retraining (https://www.med.unc.edu/ibs/files/2017/10/BowelRetrain.pdf).

Symptoms improved? — **No** → Add polyethylene glycol and/or stimulant laxative.

Yes → Continue therapy.

Symptoms improved? — **Yes** → Continue therapy. / **Partial** → Add adjunctive agents such as lubiprostone and linaclotide. / **No** →

Treatment failure → Anorectal manometry with balloon expulsion test

Normal ARM → Consider colonic transit time. → Add adjunctive agents such as lubiprostone and linaclotide.

Abnormal ARM → Pelvic floor dysfunction → Biofeedback; consider MRI/defecography and surgical referral.

Daniel J. Stein, MD, MPH

Lacy BE, Mearin F, Chang L, et al. Bowel disorders. *Gastroenterology*. 2016;150(6):1393.e5–1407.e5.

CONSTIPATION, TREATMENT (PEDIATRIC)

*Red flags:
No meconium passed >48 hours in a term newborn
Constipation <1 month of age
Family history of Hirschsprung disease
Ribbon stools
Blood in the stools in the absence of anal fissures
Failure to thrive
Fever
Bilious vomiting
Severe abdominal distension
Abnormal thyroid gland
Abnormal position of the anus
Perianal fistula
Absent anal or cremasteric reflex
Decreased lower extremity strength/tone/reflex
Sacral dimple
Tuft of hair on spine
Gluteal cleft deviation
Anal scars
Extreme fear during anal inspection

Rome Criteria
Rome IV infants and children aged <4 years
○ ≥1 month with two or more of following:
• ≤2 bowel movements (BMs) per week
• History of excessive stool retention
• History of painful or hard BMs
• History of large-diameter stools
• Presence of large fecal mass in rectum
○ If child is toilet trained, **criteria** include the following:
• ≥1 episode per week of incontinence
• History of large stools that may block toilet
○ Potential accompanying symptoms
• Irritability, decreased appetite, early satiety which resolve immediately after passing of a large stool

Rome IV diagnostic children and adolescents aged 4–18 years (developmental age ≥4 years)
○ ≥1 month with two or more of following, at least once a week:
• ≤2 BMs per week
• ≥1 episode per week of incontinence after toilet training
• History of retentive behavior or excessive volitional stool retention
• History of painful or hard BMs
• Presence of large fecal mass in rectum
• History of large stools that may block toilet
○ After appropriate evaluation, symptoms cannot be attributed to another medical condition.

Careful history and physical exam; digital rectal exam is not required for diagnosis.

Are red flags present?

Yes

Obtain based on symptoms: CBC, TSH, calcium, glucose, creatinine, tissue transglutaminase (tTG), and endomysium antibody (EMA).

Differential diagnosis:
Celiac disease
Hypothyroidism
Hypercalcemia
Hypokalemia
Diabetes mellitus
Drugs/toxins—opiates, anticholinergics, antidepressants, chemotherapy, heavy metals
Vitamin D intoxication
Botulism
Cystic fibrosis
Hirschsprung disease
Anal achalasia
Colonic inertia
Anal malformations
Pelvic mass
Spinal cord abnormalities
Abnormal abdominal musculature
Pseudoobstruction
Multiple endocrine neoplasia type 2B

No

Functional constipation

Fecal impaction?

Yes

First line: polyethylene glycol (PEG) 3350 1.0–1.5 g/kg/day PO (as effective as enemas)

Second line: enemas daily for 3–6 days

No

Initial therapy: PEG 0.4 g/kg/day PO
Maintenance therapy: PEG 0.2–0.8 g/kg/day PO titrated to response; continue for 2 months until symptoms resolved for 1 month and then D/C gradually.

PEG is superior to lactulose.

Education: recognition of withholding behaviors; use of behavioral interventions: regular toileting routines, diaries, reward systems
Dietary/lifestyle recommendations:
– Normal fiber, fluid intake, physical activity
– No defined role for prebiotic or probiotic

Refer for specialty evaluation.

A. Susan Feeney, MS, DNP, FNP-BC

Tabbers MM, DiLorenzo C, Berger MY, et al; for European Society for Pediatric Gastroenterology, Hepatology, and Nutrition, North American Society for Pediatric Gastroenterology. Evaluation and treatment of functional constipation in infants and children: evidence-based recommendations from ESPGHAN and NASPGHAN. *J Pediatr Gastroenterol Nutr.* 2014;58(2):258–274.

CONTRACEPTION

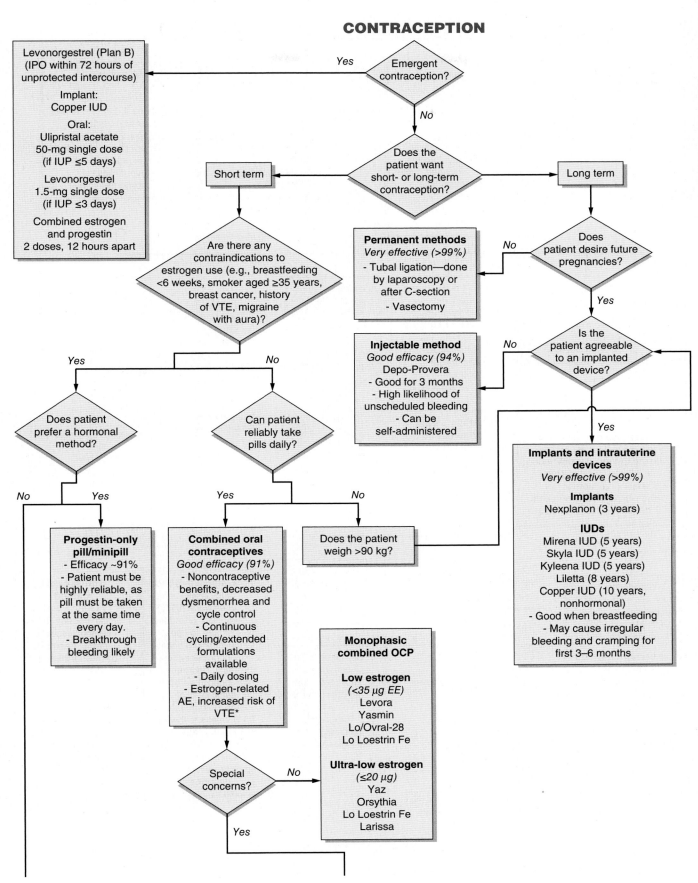

Levonorgestrel (Plan B) (IPO within 72 hours of unprotected intercourse)

Implant: Copper IUD

Oral: Ulipristal acetate 50-mg single dose (if IUP ≤5 days)

Levonorgestrel 1.5-mg single dose (if IUP ≤3 days)

Combined estrogen and progestin 2 doses, 12 hours apart

Emergent contraception? — Yes → (box above); No ↓

Does the patient want short- or long-term contraception? — Short term / Long term

Are there any contraindications to estrogen use (e.g., breastfeeding <6 weeks, smoker aged ≥35 years, breast cancer, history of VTE, migraine with aura)? — Yes / No

Permanent methods
Very effective (>99%)
- Tubal ligation—done by laparoscopy or after C-section
- Vasectomy

Does patient desire future pregnancies? — No → Permanent methods; Yes ↓

Injectable method
Good efficacy (94%)
Depo-Provera
- Good for 3 months
- High likelihood of unscheduled bleeding
- Can be self-administered

Is the patient agreeable to an implanted device? — No → Injectable method; Yes ↓

Does patient prefer a hormonal method? — No / Yes

Can patient reliably take pills daily? — Yes / No

Implants and intrauterine devices
Very effective (>99%)

Implants
Nexplanon (3 years)

IUDs
Mirena IUD (5 years)
Skyla IUD (5 years)
Kyleena IUD (5 years)
Liletta (8 years)
Copper IUD (10 years, nonhormonal)
- Good when breastfeeding
- May cause irregular bleeding and cramping for first 3–6 months

Progestin-only pill/minipill
- Efficacy ~91%
- Patient must be highly reliable, as pill must be taken at the same time every day.
- Breakthrough bleeding likely

Combined oral contraceptives
Good efficacy (91%)
- Noncontraceptive benefits, decreased dysmenorrhea and cycle control
- Continuous cycling/extended formulations available
- Daily dosing
- Estrogen-related AE, increased risk of VTE*

Does the patient weigh >90 kg?

Monophasic combined OCP

Low estrogen
(<35 µg EE)
Levora
Yasmin
Lo/Ovral-28
Lo Loestrin Fe

Ultra-low estrogen
(≤20 µg)
Yaz
Orsythia
Lo Loestrin Fe
Larissa

Special concerns? — No → Monophasic combined OCP; Yes ↓

Contraception

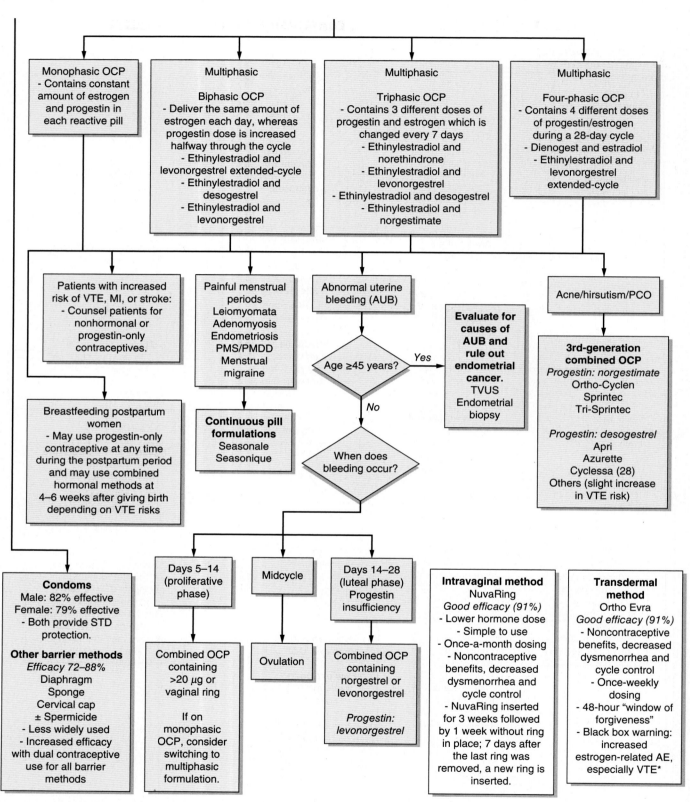

Monophasic OCP
- Contains constant amount of estrogen and progestin in each reactive pill

Multiphasic

Biphasic OCP
- Deliver the same amount of estrogen each day, whereas progestin dose is increased halfway through the cycle
- Ethinylestradiol and levonorgestrel extended-cycle
- Ethinylestradiol and desogestrel
- Ethinylestradiol and levonorgestrel

Multiphasic

Triphasic OCP
- Contains 3 different doses of progestin and estrogen which is changed every 7 days
- Ethinylestradiol and norethindrone
- Ethinylestradiol and levonorgestrel
- Ethinylestradiol and desogestrel
- Ethinylestradiol and norgestimate

Multiphasic

Four-phasic OCP
- Contains 4 different doses of progestin/estrogen during a 28-day cycle
- Dienogest and estradiol
- Ethinylestradiol and levonorgestrel extended-cycle

Patients with increased risk of VTE, MI, or stroke:
- Counsel patients for nonhormonal or progestin-only contraceptives.

Painful menstrual periods
Leiomyomata
Adenomyosis
Endometriosis
PMS/PMDD
Menstrual migraine

Abnormal uterine bleeding (AUB)

Evaluate for causes of AUB and rule out endometrial cancer.
TVUS
Endometrial biopsy

Acne/hirsutism/PCO

Age ≥45 years? *Yes* →

No

Continuous pill formulations
Seasonale
Seasonique

When does bleeding occur?

3rd-generation combined OCP
Progestin: norgestimate
Ortho-Cyclen
Sprintec
Tri-Sprintec

Progestin: desogestrel
Apri
Azurette
Cyclessa (28)
Others (slight increase in VTE risk)

Breastfeeding postpartum women
- May use progestin-only contraceptive at any time during the postpartum period and may use combined hormonal methods at 4–6 weeks after giving birth depending on VTE risks

Condoms
Male: 82% effective
Female: 79% effective
- Both provide STD protection.

Other barrier methods
Efficacy 72–88%
Diaphragm
Sponge
Cervical cap
± Spermicide
- Less widely used
- Increased efficacy with dual contraceptive use for all barrier methods

Days 5–14 (proliferative phase)

Midcycle

Days 14–28 (luteal phase)
Progestin insufficiency

Intravaginal method
NuvaRing
Good efficacy (91%)
- Lower hormone dose
- Simple to use
- Once-a-month dosing
- Noncontraceptive benefits, decreased dysmenorrhea and cycle control
- NuvaRing inserted for 3 weeks followed by 1 week without ring in place; 7 days after the last ring was removed, a new ring is inserted.

Transdermal method
Ortho Evra
Good efficacy (91%)
- Noncontraceptive benefits, decreased dysmenorrhea and cycle control
- Once-weekly dosing
- 48-hour "window of forgiveness"
- Black box warning: increased estrogen-related AE, especially VTE*

Combined OCP containing >20 μg or vaginal ring

If on monophasic OCP, consider switching to multiphasic formulation.

Ovulation

Combined OCP containing norgestrel or levonorgestrel

Progestin: levonorgestrel

*Consult CDC MEC guidelines for contraindications to use.

Susan Medalie, DO

Madden T, Secura GM, Nease RF, et al. The role of contraceptive attributes in women's contraceptive decision making. *Am J Obstet Gynecol.* 2015;213(1):46.e1–46.e6.

DEEP VENOUS THROMBOSIS, DIAGNOSIS AND TREATMENT

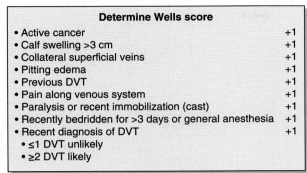

Determine Wells score

- Active cancer   +1
- Calf swelling >3 cm   +1
- Collateral superficial veins   +1
- Pitting edema   +1
- Previous DVT   +1
- Pain along venous system   +1
- Paralysis or recent immobilization (cast)   +1
- Recently bedridden for >3 days or general anesthesia   +1
- Recent diagnosis of DVT   +1
  - ≤1 DVT unlikely
  - ≥2 DVT likely

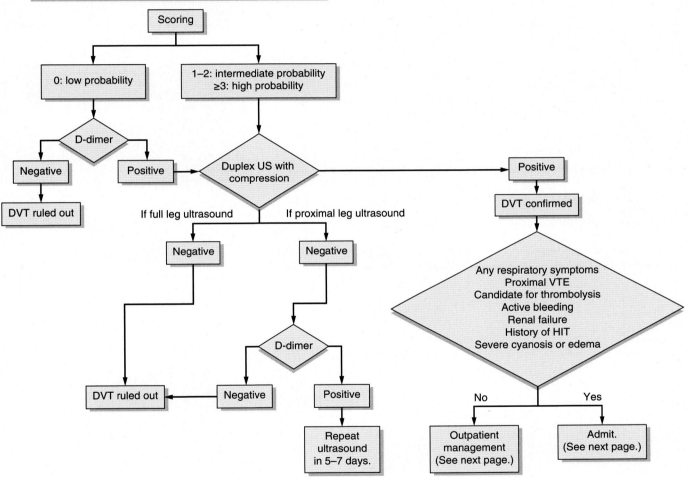

Treatment

```
          Outpatient                                    Inpatient
          management                                   management
                                                       indications
```

Therapy options:

Low-molecular-weight heparin (LMWH), unfractionated heparin (UF), or fondaparinux with warfarin bridging

- Treatment with LMWH, UFH, or fondaparinux is recommended for at least 5 days AND until INR ≥2 for 2 consecutive days.
  ○ Enoxaparin 1 mg/kg SC BID OR
  ○ UFH preferred in patients with renal impairment
- Start warfarin on same days as LMWH, UFH, and fondaparinux.
  ○ Goal INR 2–3
  ○ Continue for 3–6 months after first DVT.
  ○ Warfarin is contraindicated in pregnancy.

LMWH, UF, or fondaparinux followed by dabigatran
- Dabigatran 150 mg BID after 7–10 days of LMWH and continue for at least 6 months
- Adjust dose for CrCl <50 mL/min.
- Do not use in CrCl <15 mL/min.

Direct oral anticoagulants (rivaroxaban or apixaban) does not need bridge.

- Rivaroxaban
  ○ 15 mg BID with food for 21 days followed by 20 mg daily for at least 3 months
  ○ Avoid in patients with CrCl < 30 mL/min.

- Apixaban
  ○ 10 mg BID for 7 days followed by 5 mg BID for at least 3 months

- Massive DVT
- Symptomatic PE
- High-risk bleeding with anticoagulation therapy
- Comorbid condition
- Phlegmasia cerulea dolens
- History of HIT

- IV UFH : 80 U/kg bolus or to a max 5,000 units → continuous infusion with initial dose 18 U/kg/hr → titrate to goal PTT 60–85 seconds ~OR~
- UFH 250 U/kg SC BID ~OR~
- Enoxaparin 1.5 kg/mg SC daily ~OR~
- Fondaparinux 5–10 mg SC daily depending on weight

Jason Teng, MD and Moises Gallegos, MD, MPH

Lim W, Le Gal G, Bates SM, et al. American Society of Hematology 2018 guidelines for management of venous thromboembolism: diagnosis of venous thromboembolism. *Blood Adv.* 2018;2(22):3226–3256.

DEHYDRATION, PEDIATRIC

Causes of dehydration in pediatric patients include gastrointestinal losses (vomiting, diarrhea), losses from skin (sweat, fever, burns), and urinary loses (glycosuria, diuretics).

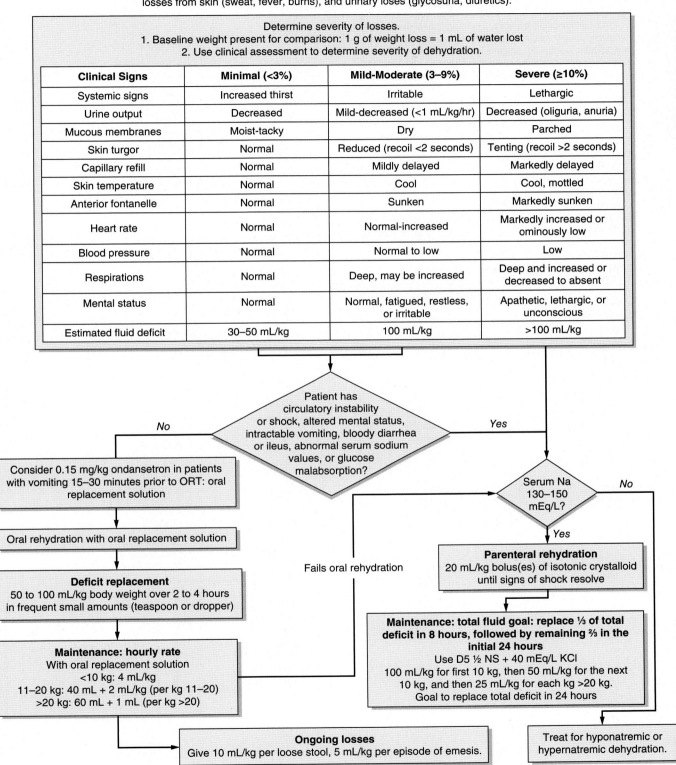

Determine severity of losses.
1. Baseline weight present for comparison: 1 g of weight loss = 1 mL of water lost
2. Use clinical assessment to determine severity of dehydration.

Clinical Signs	Minimal (<3%)	Mild-Moderate (3–9%)	Severe (≥10%)
Systemic signs	Increased thirst	Irritable	Lethargic
Urine output	Decreased	Mild-decreased (<1 mL/kg/hr)	Decreased (oliguria, anuria)
Mucous membranes	Moist-tacky	Dry	Parched
Skin turgor	Normal	Reduced (recoil <2 seconds)	Tenting (recoil >2 seconds)
Capillary refill	Normal	Mildly delayed	Markedly delayed
Skin temperature	Normal	Cool	Cool, mottled
Anterior fontanelle	Normal	Sunken	Markedly sunken
Heart rate	Normal	Normal-increased	Markedly increased or ominously low
Blood pressure	Normal	Normal to low	Low
Respirations	Normal	Deep, may be increased	Deep and increased or decreased to absent
Mental status	Normal	Normal, fatigued, restless, or irritable	Apathetic, lethargic, or unconscious
Estimated fluid deficit	30–50 mL/kg	100 mL/kg	>100 mL/kg

Patient has circulatory instability or shock, altered mental status, intractable vomiting, bloody diarrhea or ileus, abnormal serum sodium values, or glucose malabsorption?

No → Consider 0.15 mg/kg ondansetron in patients with vomiting 15–30 minutes prior to ORT: oral replacement solution

Yes → Serum Na 130–150 mEq/L?

Oral rehydration with oral replacement solution

Deficit replacement
50 to 100 mL/kg body weight over 2 to 4 hours in frequent small amounts (teaspoon or dropper)

Maintenance: hourly rate
With oral replacement solution
<10 kg: 4 mL/kg
11–20 kg: 40 mL + 2 mL/kg (per kg 11–20)
>20 kg: 60 mL + 1 mL (per kg >20)

Fails oral rehydration

Serum Na 130–150 mEq/L? — *No*

Yes →

Parenteral rehydration
20 mL/kg bolus(es) of isotonic crystalloid until signs of shock resolve

Maintenance: total fluid goal: replace ⅓ of total deficit in 8 hours, followed by remaining ⅔ in the initial 24 hours
Use D5 ½ NS + 40 mEq/L KCl
100 mL/kg for first 10 kg, then 50 mL/kg for the next 10 kg, and then 25 mL/kg for each kg >20 kg.
Goal to replace total deficit in 24 hours

Ongoing losses
Give 10 mL/kg per loose stool, 5 mL/kg per episode of emesis.

Treat for hyponatremic or hypernatremic dehydration.

Bindusri Paruchuri, MD and Sarah Marie Tiggelaar, MD, CLC, FAAFP

Santillanes G, Rose E. Evaluation and management of dehydration in children. *Emerg Med Clin North Am*. 2018;36(2):259–273. doi:10.1016/j.emc.2017.12.004.

DELIRIUM

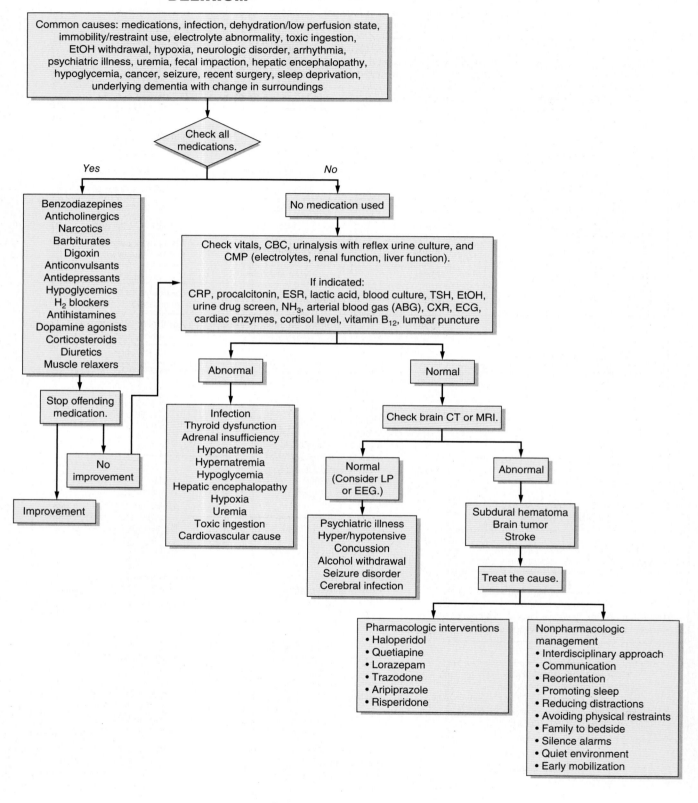

Common causes: medications, infection, dehydration/low perfusion state, immobility/restraint use, electrolyte abnormality, toxic ingestion, EtOH withdrawal, hypoxia, neurologic disorder, arrhythmia, psychiatric illness, uremia, fecal impaction, hepatic encephalopathy, hypoglycemia, cancer, seizure, recent surgery, sleep deprivation, underlying dementia with change in surroundings

Check all medications.

Yes

Benzodiazepines
Anticholinergics
Narcotics
Barbiturates
Digoxin
Anticonvulsants
Antidepressants
Hypoglycemics
H_2 blockers
Antihistamines
Dopamine agonists
Corticosteroids
Diuretics
Muscle relaxers

Stop offending medication.

No improvement

Improvement

No

No medication used

Check vitals, CBC, urinalysis with reflex urine culture, and CMP (electrolytes, renal function, liver function).

If indicated:
CRP, procalcitonin, ESR, lactic acid, blood culture, TSH, EtOH, urine drug screen, NH_3, arterial blood gas (ABG), CXR, ECG, cardiac enzymes, cortisol level, vitamin B_{12}, lumbar puncture

Abnormal

Infection
Thyroid dysfunction
Adrenal insufficiency
Hyponatremia
Hypernatremia
Hypoglycemia
Hepatic encephalopathy
Hypoxia
Uremia
Toxic ingestion
Cardiovascular cause

Normal

Check brain CT or MRI.

Normal
(Consider LP or EEG.)

Psychiatric illness
Hyper/hypotensive
Concussion
Alcohol withdrawal
Seizure disorder
Cerebral infection

Abnormal

Subdural hematoma
Brain tumor
Stroke

Treat the cause.

Pharmacologic interventions
• Haloperidol
• Quetiapine
• Lorazepam
• Trazodone
• Aripiprazole
• Risperidone

Nonpharmacologic management
• Interdisciplinary approach
• Communication
• Reorientation
• Promoting sleep
• Reducing distractions
• Avoiding physical restraints
• Family to bedside
• Silence alarms
• Quiet environment
• Early mobilization

Corey J. Costanzo, DO, MPH, MS

Thom RP, Levy-Carrick NC, Bui M, et al. Delirium. *Am J Psychiatry*. 2019;176(10):785–793.

DEMENTIA

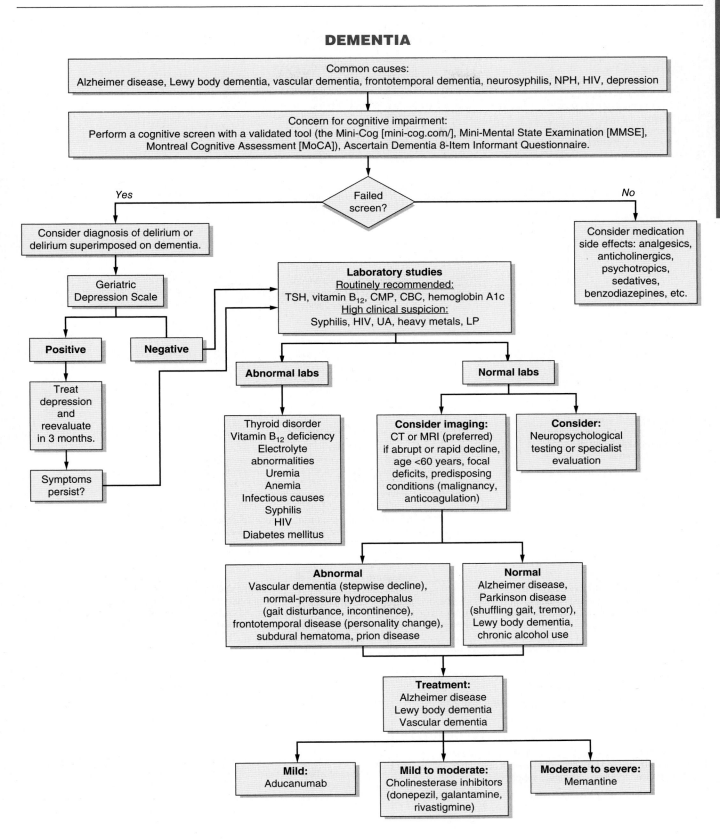

Common causes:
Alzheimer disease, Lewy body dementia, vascular dementia, frontotemporal dementia, neurosyphilis, NPH, HIV, depression

Concern for cognitive impairment:
Perform a cognitive screen with a validated tool (the Mini-Cog [mini-cog.com/], Mini-Mental State Examination [MMSE], Montreal Cognitive Assessment [MoCA]), Ascertain Dementia 8-Item Informant Questionnaire.

Failed screen?

Yes

No

Consider diagnosis of delirium or delirium superimposed on dementia.

Consider medication side effects: analgesics, anticholinergics, psychotropics, sedatives, benzodiazepines, etc.

Geriatric Depression Scale

Laboratory studies
Routinely recommended:
TSH, vitamin B_{12}, CMP, CBC, hemoglobin A1c
High clinical suspicion:
Syphilis, HIV, UA, heavy metals, LP

Positive

Negative

Treat depression and reevaluate in 3 months.

Abnormal labs

Normal labs

Symptoms persist?

Thyroid disorder
Vitamin B_{12} deficiency
Electrolyte abnormalities
Uremia
Anemia
Infectious causes
Syphilis
HIV
Diabetes mellitus

Consider imaging:
CT or MRI (preferred) if abrupt or rapid decline, age <60 years, focal deficits, predisposing conditions (malignancy, anticoagulation)

Consider:
Neuropsychological testing or specialist evaluation

Abnormal
Vascular dementia (stepwise decline), normal-pressure hydrocephalus (gait disturbance, incontinence), frontotemporal disease (personality change), subdural hematoma, prion disease

Normal
Alzheimer disease, Parkinson disease (shuffling gait, tremor), Lewy body dementia, chronic alcohol use

Treatment:
Alzheimer disease
Lewy body dementia
Vascular dementia

Mild:
Aducanumab

Mild to moderate:
Cholinesterase inhibitors (donepezil, galantamine, rivastigmine)

Moderate to severe:
Memantine

Adam Mendonca, MD and Chelsea Mendonca, MD

Falk N, Cole A, Meredith TJ. Evaluation of suspected dementia. *Am Fam Physician*. 2018;97(6):398–405.

DEPRESSIVE EPISODE, MAJOR

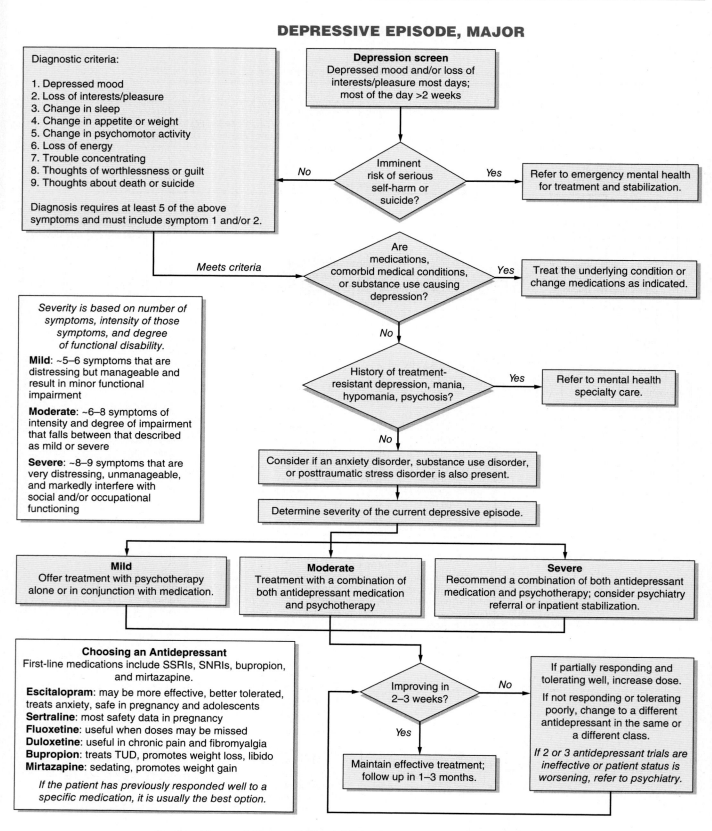

Diagnostic criteria:

1. Depressed mood
2. Loss of interests/pleasure
3. Change in sleep
4. Change in appetite or weight
5. Change in psychomotor activity
6. Loss of energy
7. Trouble concentrating
8. Thoughts of worthlessness or guilt
9. Thoughts about death or suicide

Diagnosis requires at least 5 of the above symptoms and must include symptom 1 and/or 2.

Depression screen
Depressed mood and/or loss of interests/pleasure most days; most of the day >2 weeks

Imminent risk of serious self-harm or suicide? — No / Yes

Yes → Refer to emergency mental health for treatment and stabilization.

Meets criteria

Are medications, comorbid medical conditions, or substance use causing depression? — Yes → Treat the underlying condition or change medications as indicated.

No

History of treatment-resistant depression, mania, hypomania, psychosis? — Yes → Refer to mental health specialty care.

No

Consider if an anxiety disorder, substance use disorder, or posttraumatic stress disorder is also present.

Determine severity of the current depressive episode.

Severity is based on number of symptoms, intensity of those symptoms, and degree of functional disability.

Mild: ~5–6 symptoms that are distressing but manageable and result in minor functional impairment

Moderate: ~6–8 symptoms of intensity and degree of impairment that falls between that described as mild or severe

Severe: ~8–9 symptoms that are very distressing, unmanageable, and markedly interfere with social and/or occupational functioning

Mild
Offer treatment with psychotherapy alone or in conjunction with medication.

Moderate
Treatment with a combination of both antidepressant medication and psychotherapy

Severe
Recommend a combination of both antidepressant medication and psychotherapy; consider psychiatry referral or inpatient stabilization.

Choosing an Antidepressant
First-line medications include SSRIs, SNRIs, bupropion, and mirtazapine.

Escitalopram: may be more effective, better tolerated, treats anxiety, safe in pregnancy and adolescents
Sertraline: most safety data in pregnancy
Fluoxetine: useful when doses may be missed
Duloxetine: useful in chronic pain and fibromyalgia
Bupropion: treats TUD, promotes weight loss, libido
Mirtazapine: sedating, promotes weight gain

If the patient has previously responded well to a specific medication, it is usually the best option.

Improving in 2–3 weeks? — No / Yes

No → If partially responding and tolerating well, increase dose.

If not responding or tolerating poorly, change to a different antidepressant in the same or a different class.

If 2 or 3 antidepressant trials are ineffective or patient status is worsening, refer to psychiatry.

Yes → Maintain effective treatment; follow up in 1–3 months.

Jordan Howard-Young, MD and Stephany Giraldo Eierle, DO, MPH

U.S. Department of Veterans Affairs, U.S. Department of Defense. *VA/DoD Clinical Practice Guideline for Management of Major Depressive Disorder.* Washington, DC: U.S. Department of Veterans Affairs, U.S. Department of Defense; 2016.

DIABETIC KETOACIDOSIS (DKA), TREATMENT

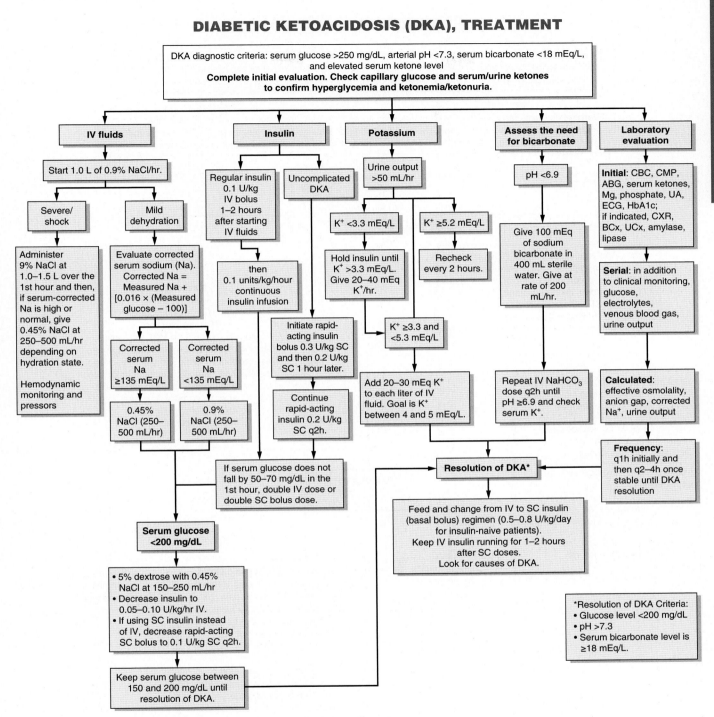

DKA diagnostic criteria: serum glucose >250 mg/dL, arterial pH <7.3, serum bicarbonate <18 mEq/L, and elevated serum ketone level
Complete initial evaluation. Check capillary glucose and serum/urine ketones to confirm hyperglycemia and ketonemia/ketonuria.

IV fluids

Start 1.0 L of 0.9% NaCl/hr.

Severe/shock

Administer 9% NaCl at 1.0–1.5 L over the 1st hour and then, if serum-corrected Na is high or normal, give 0.45% NaCl at 250–500 mL/hr depending on hydration state.

Hemodynamic monitoring and pressors

Mild dehydration

Evaluate corrected serum sodium (Na). Corrected Na = Measured Na + [0.016 × (Measured glucose − 100)]

Corrected serum Na ≥135 mEq/L

0.45% NaCl (250–500 mL/hr)

Corrected serum Na <135 mEq/L

0.9% NaCl (250–500 mL/hr)

Serum glucose <200 mg/dL

- 5% dextrose with 0.45% NaCl at 150–250 mL/hr
- Decrease insulin to 0.05–0.10 U/kg/hr IV.
- If using SC insulin instead of IV, decrease rapid-acting SC bolus to 0.1 U/kg SC q2h.

Keep serum glucose between 150 and 200 mg/dL until resolution of DKA.

Insulin

Regular insulin 0.1 U/kg IV bolus 1–2 hours after starting IV fluids

Uncomplicated DKA

then 0.1 units/kg/hour continuous insulin infusion

Initiate rapid-acting insulin bolus 0.3 U/kg SC and then 0.2 U/kg SC 1 hour later.

Continue rapid-acting insulin 0.2 U/kg SC q2h.

If serum glucose does not fall by 50–70 mg/dL in the 1st hour, double IV dose or double SC bolus dose.

Potassium

Urine output >50 mL/hr

K⁺ <3.3 mEq/L

Hold insulin until K⁺ >3.3 mEq/L. Give 20–40 mEq K⁺/hr.

K⁺ ≥5.2 mEq/L

Recheck every 2 hours.

K⁺ ≥3.3 and <5.3 mEq/L

Add 20–30 mEq K⁺ to each liter of IV fluid. Goal is K⁺ between 4 and 5 mEq/L.

Assess the need for bicarbonate

pH <6.9

Give 100 mEq of sodium bicarbonate in 400 mL sterile water. Give at rate of 200 mL/hr.

Repeat IV NaHCO₃ dose q2h until pH ≥6.9 and check serum K⁺.

Resolution of DKA*

Feed and change from IV to SC insulin (basal bolus) regimen (0.5–0.8 U/kg/day for insulin-naive patients). Keep IV insulin running for 1–2 hours after SC doses. Look for causes of DKA.

Laboratory evaluation

Initial: CBC, CMP, ABG, serum ketones, Mg, phosphate, UA, ECG, HbA1c; if indicated, CXR, BCx, UCx, amylase, lipase

Serial: in addition to clinical monitoring, glucose, electrolytes, venous blood gas, urine output

Calculated: effective osmolality, anion gap, corrected Na⁺, urine output

Frequency: q1h initially and then q2–4h once stable until DKA resolution

*Resolution of DKA Criteria:
- Glucose level <200 mg/dL
- pH >7.3
- Serum bicarbonate level is ≥18 mEq/L.

Astrud S. A. Villareal, MD, FAAFP, Meiline Troeung, DO, and Tyler R. Evans, DO

Westerberg DP. Diabetic ketoacidosis: evaluation and treatment. *Am Fam Physician*. 2013;87(5):337–346.

DIARRHEA, CHRONIC

Common causes: infectious (bacterial, viral, parasitic), inflammatory bowel disease (IBD), irritable bowel syndrome (IBS), medications, endocrine diarrhea (tumors, systemic), malignancy, radiation, food additives, malabsorption syndromes (celiac disease, pancreatic insufficiency, bile acid malabsorption [BAM])

History: characteristics of stool, associated symptoms, iatrogenic risk factors (medications, radiotherapy), antibiotics, recent hospitalization, medical and surgical history, dietary history (carbohydrates, sugar, alcohol, coffee, fatty food), recent travel, family history, sexual history, immunosuppression

Alarm signs? GI bleeding, fever, significant weight loss?

Yes

No

Labs: stool studies (multiplex PCR, culture, *Clostridium difficile*, ova + parasites, fat, electrolytes, calprotectin, blood), blood tests (TSH, glucose, celiac serology [TTG IgA], HIV Ab, GI peptide assays, C4/FGF19), hydrogen breath test

Abnormal

Normal

No

Medication induced? Acid-reducing agents (PPIs, H_2 blockers), antacids (containing Mg), antibiotics, β-blockers, NSAIDs, colchicine, digoxin, SSRIs, metformin, olmesartan, mycophenolate mofetil, herbal medications, vitamin and mineral supplements, antineoplastic agents, sorbitol, fructose abuse, chronic laxative abuse

Yes

Stool positive for ova and parasites, *C. difficile* toxin, pathogenic bacteria, or PCR → infectious diarrhea

Positive fecal blood, leukocytes, calprotectin → inflammatory diarrhea → colonoscopy

Positive celiac serology → upper endoscopy

Positive fecal fat → See "Malabsorption Syndrome" algorithm.

Positive hydrogen breath test → small intestinal bacterial overgrowth

Colonoscopy

Abnormal exam and/or biopsies

Normal

IBD, malignancy, ischemic colitis, infectious colitis, microscopic colitis

Evaluate for IBS/Rome criteria: Symptom onset for at least 6 months Recurrent abdominal pain, on average, at least 1 day/week in the last 3 months, associated with two or more of the following criteria:

- Related to defecation
- Associated with a change in frequency of stool
- Associated with a change in form (appearance) of stool

Consider alternative medications.

If no improvement with IBS treatment and limited FODMAP diet trial, consider empiric trial of bile acid sequestrants to determine if BAM is present.

Jennifer M. Romeu, MD, MSM

Schiller LR. Evaluation of chronic diarrhea and irritable bowel syndrome with diarrhea in adults in the era of precision medicine. *Am J Gastroenterol.* 2018;113(5):660–669.

DIZZINESS

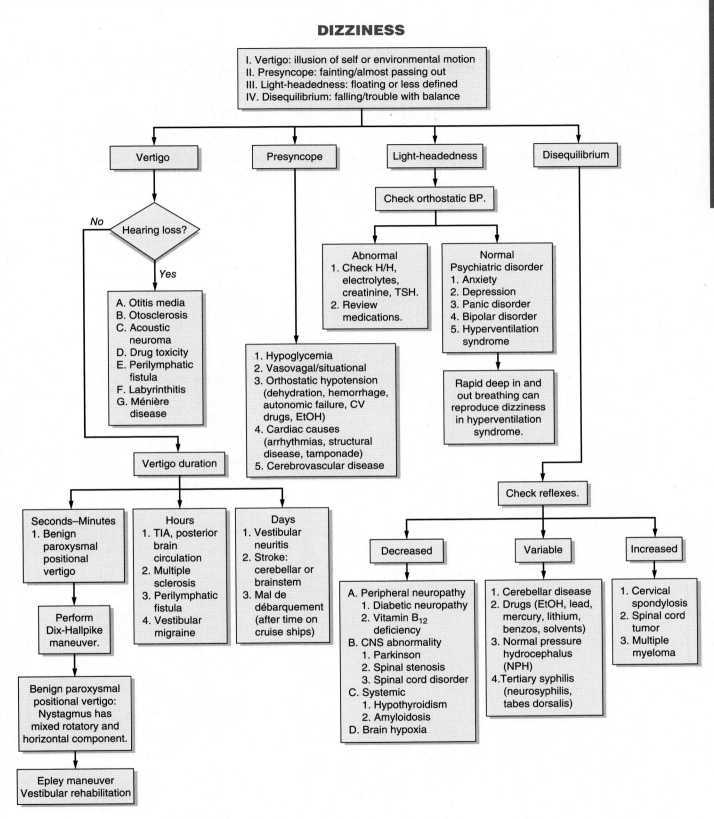

I. Vertigo: illusion of self or environmental motion
II. Presyncope: fainting/almost passing out
III. Light-headedness: floating or less defined
IV. Disequilibrium: falling/trouble with balance

Vertigo

Hearing loss? — *No*

Yes

A. Otitis media
B. Otosclerosis
C. Acoustic neuroma
D. Drug toxicity
E. Perilymphatic fistula
F. Labyrinthitis
G. Ménière disease

Vertigo duration

Seconds–Minutes
1. Benign paroxysmal positional vertigo

Perform Dix-Hallpike maneuver.

Benign paroxysmal positional vertigo: Nystagmus has mixed rotatory and horizontal component.

Epley maneuver Vestibular rehabilitation

Hours
1. TIA, posterior brain circulation
2. Multiple sclerosis
3. Perilymphatic fistula
4. Vestibular migraine

Days
1. Vestibular neuritis
2. Stroke: cerebellar or brainstem
3. Mal de débarquement (after time on cruise ships)

Presyncope

1. Hypoglycemia
2. Vasovagal/situational
3. Orthostatic hypotension (dehydration, hemorrhage, autonomic failure, CV drugs, EtOH)
4. Cardiac causes (arrhythmias, structural disease, tamponade)
5. Cerebrovascular disease

Light-headedness

Check orthostatic BP.

Abnormal
1. Check H/H, electrolytes, creatinine, TSH.
2. Review medications.

Normal
Psychiatric disorder
1. Anxiety
2. Depression
3. Panic disorder
4. Bipolar disorder
5. Hyperventilation syndrome

Rapid deep in and out breathing can reproduce dizziness in hyperventilation syndrome.

Disequilibrium

Check reflexes.

Decreased

A. Peripheral neuropathy
   1. Diabetic neuropathy
   2. Vitamin B_{12} deficiency
B. CNS abnormality
   1. Parkinson
   2. Spinal stenosis
   3. Spinal cord disorder
C. Systemic
   1. Hypothyroidism
   2. Amyloidosis
D. Brain hypoxia

Variable

1. Cerebellar disease
2. Drugs (EtOH, lead, mercury, lithium, benzos, solvents)
3. Normal pressure hydrocephalus (NPH)
4. Tertiary syphilis (neurosyphilis, tabes dorsalis)

Increased

1. Cervical spondylosis
2. Spinal cord tumor
3. Multiple myeloma

Jennifer G. Foster, MD, MBA, FACP

Stern SC, Cifu AS, Altkorn D, eds. *Symptom to Diagnosis: An Evidence-Based Guide*. 3rd ed. New York, NY: McGraw-Hill; 2014.

DYSPEPSIA

Dyspepsia: predominant symptom of epigastric pain for at least 1 month, associated with other symptoms, such as nausea, vomiting, or heartburn; common causes: GERD, peptic ulcer (<10%), gastroesophageal cancer (<1%), gastroparesis, functional dyspepsia (>70%)

Functional dyspepsia: dyspepsia with normal endoscopy. Main forms of functional dyspepsia: epigastric pain syndrome (intermittent pain/burning in epigastrium at least weekly) and postprandial distress syndrome (at least several episodes weekly of bothersome fullness after meals or early satiety). The two syndromes may both be present in the same patient.

Alarm features of dyspepsia: areas where gastric cancer is common (e.g., Southeast Asia), overt GI bleeding, progressive dysphagia and odynophagia, persistent vomiting, unintentional weight loss, family history upper GI cancer, palpable abdominal mass or lymphadenopathy, unexplained iron deficiency anemia

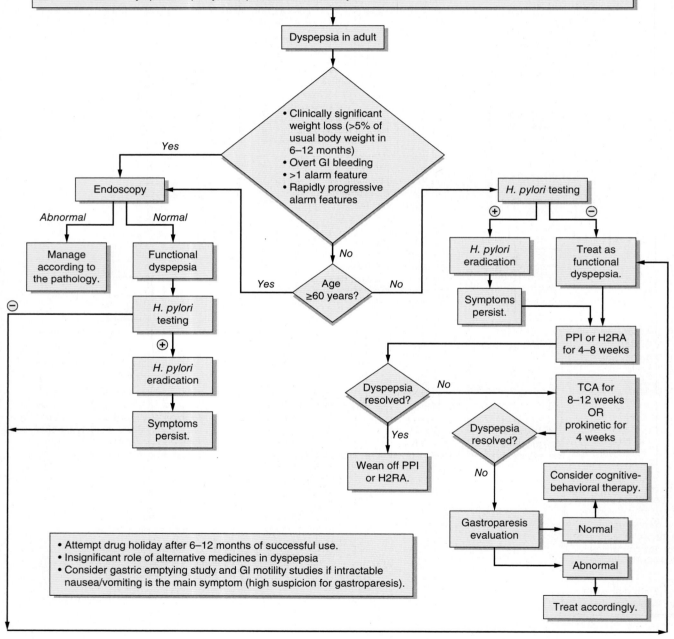

Adwoa A. Adu, MD

Moayyedi P, Lacy BE, Andrews CN, et al. ACG and CAG clinical guideline: management of dyspepsia. *Am J Gastroenterol*. 2017;112(7):988–1013.

DYSPHAGIA

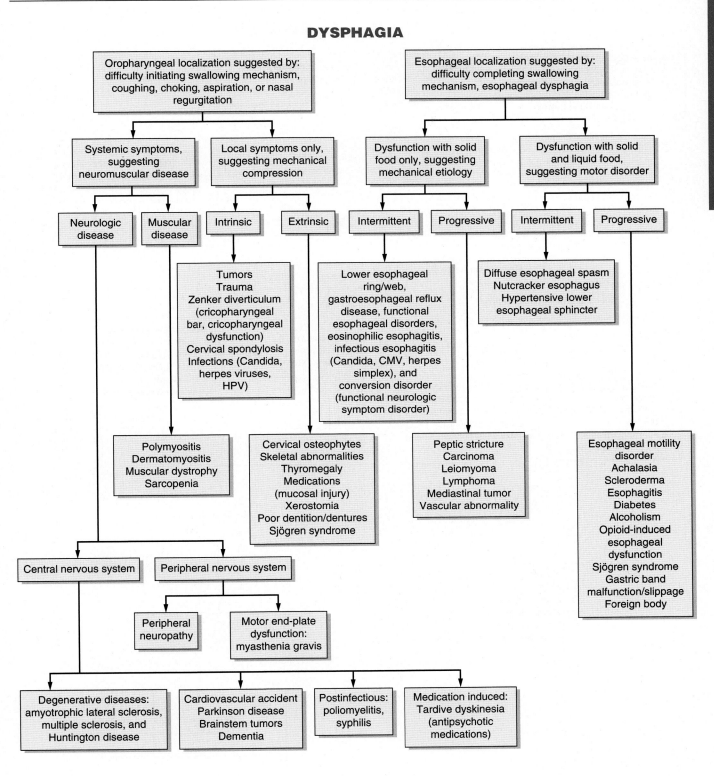

Oropharyngeal localization suggested by: difficulty initiating swallowing mechanism, coughing, choking, aspiration, or nasal regurgitation

Esophageal localization suggested by: difficulty completing swallowing mechanism, esophageal dysphagia

- **Systemic symptoms, suggesting neuromuscular disease**
  - Neurologic disease
  - Muscular disease
- **Local symptoms only, suggesting mechanical compression**
  - Intrinsic
  - Extrinsic
- **Dysfunction with solid food only, suggesting mechanical etiology**
  - Intermittent
  - Progressive
- **Dysfunction with solid and liquid food, suggesting motor disorder**
  - Intermittent
  - Progressive

Intrinsic: Tumors, Trauma, Zenker diverticulum (cricopharyngeal bar, cricopharyngeal dysfunction), Cervical spondylosis, Infections (Candida, herpes viruses, HPV)

Intermittent (solid): Lower esophageal ring/web, gastroesophageal reflux disease, functional esophageal disorders, eosinophilic esophagitis, infectious esophagitis (Candida, CMV, herpes simplex), and conversion disorder (functional neurologic symptom disorder)

Intermittent (motor): Diffuse esophageal spasm, Nutcracker esophagus, Hypertensive lower esophageal sphincter

Muscular disease: Polymyositis, Dermatomyositis, Muscular dystrophy, Sarcopenia

Extrinsic: Cervical osteophytes, Skeletal abnormalities, Thyromegaly, Medications (mucosal injury), Xerostomia, Poor dentition/dentures, Sjögren syndrome

Progressive (solid): Peptic stricture, Carcinoma, Leiomyoma, Lymphoma, Mediastinal tumor, Vascular abnormality

Progressive (motor): Esophageal motility disorder, Achalasia, Scleroderma, Esophagitis, Diabetes, Alcoholism, Opioid-induced esophageal dysfunction, Sjögren syndrome, Gastric band malfunction/slippage, Foreign body

Neurologic disease:
- Central nervous system
- Peripheral nervous system
  - Peripheral neuropathy
  - Motor end-plate dysfunction: myasthenia gravis

Degenerative diseases: amyotrophic lateral sclerosis, multiple sclerosis, and Huntington disease

Cardiovascular accident, Parkinson disease, Brainstem tumors, Dementia

Postinfectious: poliomyelitis, syphilis

Medication induced: Tardive dyskinesia (antipsychotic medications)

Joanna Drowos, DO, MPH, MBA and Sarah Wiggill, MD

Wilkinson JM, Codipilly DC, Wilfahrt RP. Dysphagia: evaluation and collaborative management. *Am Fam Physician*. 2021;103(2):97–106.

ERYTHROCYTOSIS

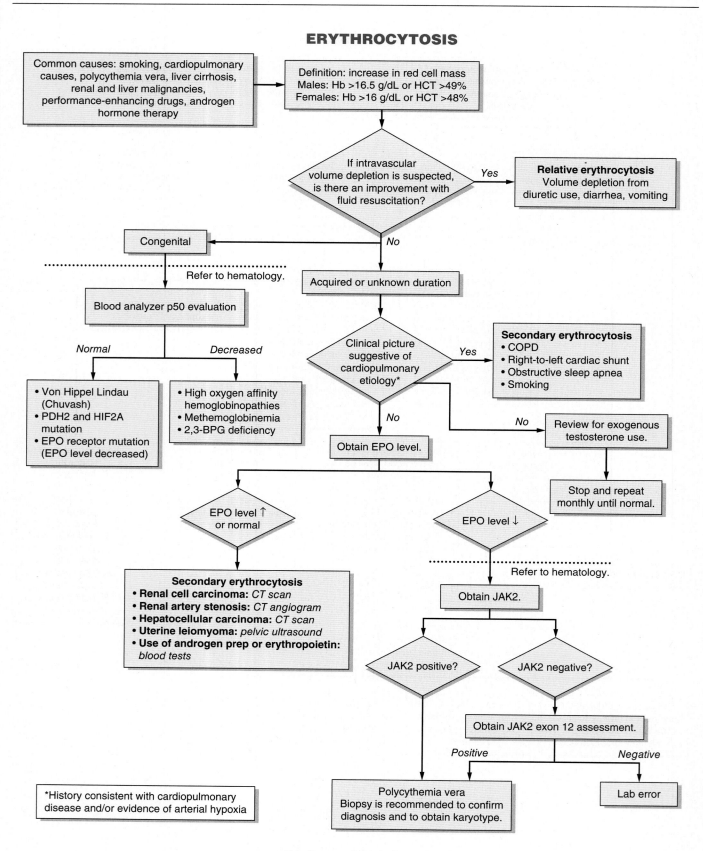

Common causes: smoking, cardiopulmonary causes, polycythemia vera, liver cirrhosis, renal and liver malignancies, performance-enhancing drugs, androgen hormone therapy

Definition: increase in red cell mass
Males: Hb >16.5 g/dL or HCT >49%
Females: Hb >16 g/dL or HCT >48%

If intravascular volume depletion is suspected, is there an improvement with fluid resuscitation?

Yes → **Relative erythrocytosis**
Volume depletion from diuretic use, diarrhea, vomiting

No

Congenital

Refer to hematology.

Acquired or unknown duration

Blood analyzer p50 evaluation

Normal / *Decreased*

• Von Hippel Lindau (Chuvash)
• PDH2 and HIF2A mutation
• EPO receptor mutation (EPO level decreased)

• High oxygen affinity hemoglobinopathies
• Methemoglobinemia
• 2,3-BPG deficiency

Clinical picture suggestive of cardiopulmonary etiology*

Yes → **Secondary erythrocytosis**
• COPD
• Right-to-left cardiac shunt
• Obstructive sleep apnea
• Smoking

No

No → Review for exogenous testosterone use.

Obtain EPO level.

Stop and repeat monthly until normal.

EPO level ↑ or normal

EPO level ↓

Secondary erythrocytosis
• **Renal cell carcinoma:** *CT scan*
• **Renal artery stenosis:** *CT angiogram*
• **Hepatocellular carcinoma:** *CT scan*
• **Uterine leiomyoma:** *pelvic ultrasound*
• **Use of androgen prep or erythropoietin:** *blood tests*

Refer to hematology.

Obtain JAK2.

JAK2 positive?

JAK2 negative?

Obtain JAK2 exon 12 assessment.

Positive / *Negative*

Polycythemia vera
Biopsy is recommended to confirm diagnosis and to obtain karyotype.

Lab error

*History consistent with cardiopulmonary disease and/or evidence of arterial hypoxia

Frank J. Domino, MD

Tefferi A, Barbui T. Polycythemia vera and essential thrombocythemia: 2021 update on diagnosis, risk-stratification and management. *Am J Hematol.* 2020;95(12):1599–1613.

FATIGUE

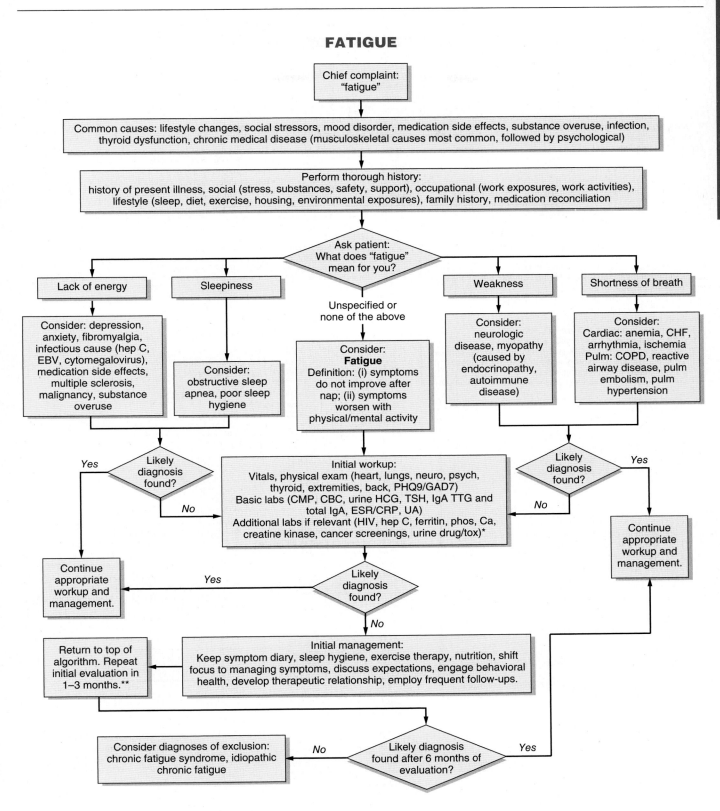

Chief complaint: "fatigue"

Common causes: lifestyle changes, social stressors, mood disorder, medication side effects, substance overuse, infection, thyroid dysfunction, chronic medical disease (musculoskeletal causes most common, followed by psychological)

Perform thorough history: history of present illness, social (stress, substances, safety, support), occupational (work exposures, work activities), lifestyle (sleep, diet, exercise, housing, environmental exposures), family history, medication reconciliation

Ask patient: What does "fatigue" mean for you?

Lack of energy
Consider: depression, anxiety, fibromyalgia, infectious cause (hep C, EBV, cytomegalovirus), medication side effects, multiple sclerosis, malignancy, substance overuse

Sleepiness
Consider: obstructive sleep apnea, poor sleep hygiene

Unspecified or none of the above
Consider: **Fatigue** Definition: (i) symptoms do not improve after nap; (ii) symptoms worsen with physical/mental activity

Weakness
Consider: neurologic disease, myopathy (caused by endocrinopathy, autoimmune disease)

Shortness of breath
Consider: Cardiac: anemia, CHF, arrhythmia, ischemia Pulm: COPD, reactive airway disease, pulm embolism, pulm hypertension

Likely diagnosis found? — Yes / No

Likely diagnosis found? — Yes / No

Initial workup: Vitals, physical exam (heart, lungs, neuro, psych, thyroid, extremities, back, PHQ9/GAD7) Basic labs (CMP, CBC, urine HCG, TSH, IgA TTG and total IgA, ESR/CRP, UA) Additional labs if relevant (HIV, hep C, ferritin, phos, Ca, creatine kinase, cancer screenings, urine drug/tox)*

Continue appropriate workup and management.

Continue appropriate workup and management.

Likely diagnosis found? — Yes / No

Continue appropriate workup and management.

Initial management: Keep symptom diary, sleep hygiene, exercise therapy, nutrition, shift focus to managing symptoms, discuss expectations, engage behavioral health, develop therapeutic relationship, employ frequent follow-ups.

Return to top of algorithm. Repeat initial evaluation in 1–3 months.**

Consider diagnoses of exclusion: chronic fatigue syndrome, idiopathic chronic fatigue

Likely diagnosis found after 6 months of evaluation? — No / Yes

Stacy E. Potts, MD, Med

Wright J, O'Connor KM. Fatigue. *Med Clin North Am*. 2014;98(3):597–608.

FEVER IN FIRST 60 DAYS OF LIFE

Algorithm for:
• Well-appearing
• Full term (≤37 weeks)
• Previously healthy
• No focal source of infection

Ill-appearing or altered mental status? Initiate sepsis care with antibiotics listed in "Empiric Treatment" below.

**HSV Risk Factors
• Ill-appearing, seizures, abnormal neurologic exam
• Maternal primary HSV or active lesions with vaginal delivery
• Vesicular rash, mucous membrane lesions
• Hepatosplenomegaly or ALT >40
• Household contact with active HSV lesions

Rectal temperature ≥38°C or 100.4°F

Age <28 days?

Yes

1. Admit.
   C-reactive protein (CRP) and/or procalcitonin (PCT), if available
2. CBC w/ diff, ALT, AST, UA, blood culture, straight catheterization urine culture
   If <21 days, obtain LP; if ≥22 days and reassuring CBC/inflammatory markers (IM), may consider watching patient off of antibiotics
3. LP CSF: Gram stain, protein, glucose, culture CSF HSV and enterovirus PCR
4. Stool analysis and PCR if diarrhea
5. Respiratory viral panel (including COVID-19)
6. CXR if respiratory distress, hypoxia, crackles
7. HSV testing (CSF HSV PCR, serum HSV PCR, skin/eye/mouth swab PCR) if age <21 days or age >21 days and elevated transaminases or CSF pleocytosis

Empiric treatment

Ampicillin (IM/IV)
<7 days and <2 kg: 50 mg/kg q12h
<7 days and >2 kg: 50 mg/kg q8h
≥7 days and <2 kg: 50 mg/kg q8h
≥7 days and >2 kg: 50 mg/kg q6h
and
Gentamicin
<8 days: 2.5 mg/kg IV/IM q12h
8–90 days: 2.5 mg/kg IV/IM q8h

If concern for CNS disease, add cefotaxime (IM/IV)
≤7 days: <2 kg: 50 mg/kg q12h; >2 kg: 50 mg/kg q12h
>7 days: <1.2 kg: 50 mg/kg q12h; 1.2–2.0 kg: 50 mg/kg q8h; >2 kg: 50 mg/kg q6h

If <21 days, initiate empiric acyclovir therapy 20 mg/kg q8h if infant has **HSV risk factors.

If >21 days, add acyclovir if mucocutaneous vesicles, elevated transaminases, seizures, or CSF pleocytosis.

Add acyclovir 20 mg/kg q8h if mucocutaneous vesicles, elevated transaminases, seizures, or CSF pleocytosis.

Add vancomycin 15 mg/kg q8h if MRSA is suspected.

No

1. CBC w/ diff, UA, blood culture, straight catheterization urine culture
2. Respiratory viral panel (including COVID-19)
3. Stool analysis and culture if diarrhea
4. Consider HSV testing if risk criteria** are met in infants <42 days.
5. CXR if respiratory distress, hypoxia, crackles

Low-Risk Criteria

• WBC 5–15,000/μL
• Absolute band count ≤1,500/μL
• IMs: PCT ≤0.5 ng/dL and/or CRP <20 mg/dL
• UA <10 WBC/HPF and no bacteria
• Stool <5 WBC/HPF
• Stool culture
• Nontoxic appearance
• No focus of infection (i.e., bone, skin)
• Reliable PCP follow-up

Yes

Outpatient management if patient able to be reevaluated in 24 hours
1. Consider empiric therapy with daily follow-up: *only* if LP done; ceftriaxone IV/IM 50–100 mg/kg/day
2. Await blood and urine cultures.

No

Admission recommended
1. Perform LP CSF: Gram stain, protein, glucose, culture.
2. Initiate empiric therapy: ceftriaxone IV/IM 50–100 mg/kg/day.
3. Await blood and urine cultures.
4. If MRSA is suspected, or ill-appearance, add vancomycin.
5. If mucocutaneous vesicles, seizures, or CSF pleocytosis, add acyclovir 20 mg/kg q8h.

Cultures at 24 hours?

Negative

Febrile?

No → Observe.

Yes → Febrile but low risk:
Clinical reexamination + repeat follow-up within 24 hours
Consider repeat ceftriaxone on case-specific basis.

Positive → Immediately reevaluate patient. LP recommended (if not already performed) and/or admission for IV antibiotics

Chandra Hartman, MD, FAAFP

Pantell RH, Roberts KB, Adams WG, et al; for Subcommittee on Febrile Infants. Evaluation and management of well-appearing febrile infants 8 to 60 days old. *Pediatrics.* 2021;148(2):e2021052228.

FEVER OF UNKNOWN ORIGIN

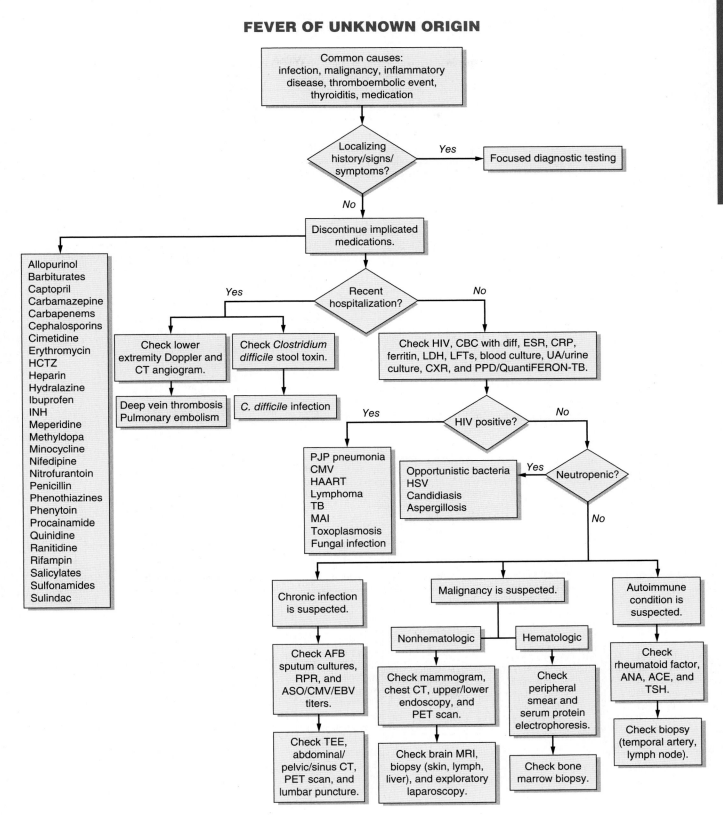

Common causes:
infection, malignancy, inflammatory disease, thromboembolic event, thyroiditis, medication

Localizing history/signs/symptoms? → *Yes* → Focused diagnostic testing

No

Discontinue implicated medications.

Allopurinol
Barbiturates
Captopril
Carbamazepine
Carbapenems
Cephalosporins
Cimetidine
Erythromycin
HCTZ
Heparin
Hydralazine
Ibuprofen
INH
Meperidine
Methyldopa
Minocycline
Nifedipine
Nitrofurantoin
Penicillin
Phenothiazines
Phenytoin
Procainamide
Quinidine
Ranitidine
Rifampin
Salicylates
Sulfonamides
Sulindac

Recent hospitalization?

Yes

Check lower extremity Doppler and CT angiogram.

Deep vein thrombosis
Pulmonary embolism

Check *Clostridium difficile* stool toxin.

C. difficile infection

No

Check HIV, CBC with diff, ESR, CRP, ferritin, LDH, LFTs, blood culture, UA/urine culture, CXR, and PPD/QuantiFERON-TB.

HIV positive?

Yes

PJP pneumonia
CMV
HAART
Lymphoma
TB
MAI
Toxoplasmosis
Fungal infection

Opportunistic bacteria
HSV
Candidiasis
Aspergillosis

Yes ← Neutropenic? ← *No*

No

Chronic infection is suspected.

Check AFB sputum cultures, RPR, and ASO/CMV/EBV titers.

Check TEE, abdominal/pelvic/sinus CT, PET scan, and lumbar puncture.

Malignancy is suspected.

Nonhematologic

Check mammogram, chest CT, upper/lower endoscopy, and PET scan.

Check brain MRI, biopsy (skin, lymph, liver), and exploratory laparoscopy.

Hematologic

Check peripheral smear and serum protein electrophoresis.

Check bone marrow biopsy.

Autoimmune condition is suspected.

Check rheumatoid factor, ANA, ACE, and TSH.

Check biopsy (temporal artery, lymph node).

Pankaj Ksheersagar, MD

Hersch EC, Oh RC. Prolonged febrile illness and fever of unknown origin in adults. *Am Fam Physician*. 2014;90(2):91–96.

GAIT DISTURBANCE

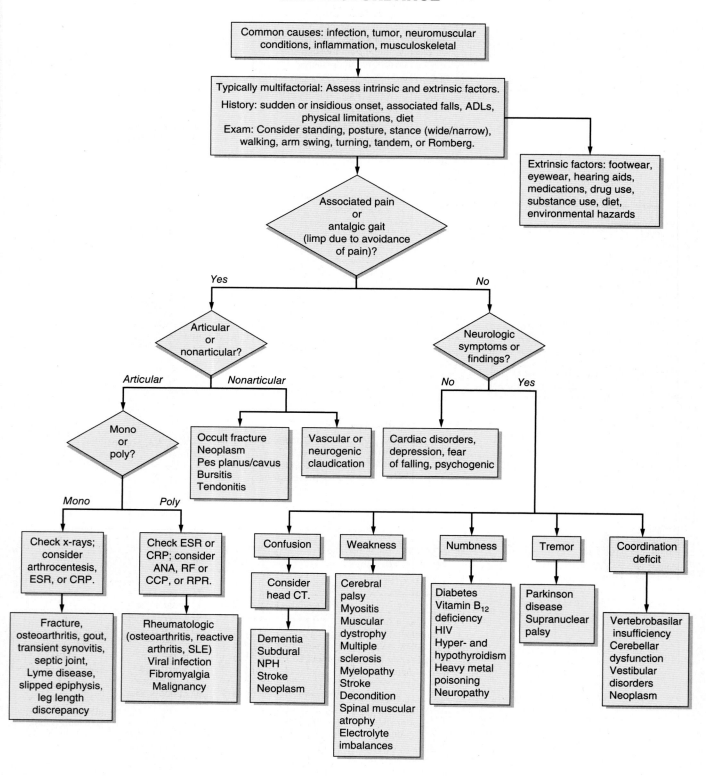

Common causes: infection, tumor, neuromuscular conditions, inflammation, musculoskeletal

Typically multifactorial: Assess intrinsic and extrinsic factors.
History: sudden or insidious onset, associated falls, ADLs, physical limitations, diet
Exam: Consider standing, posture, stance (wide/narrow), walking, arm swing, turning, tandem, or Romberg.

Extrinsic factors: footwear, eyewear, hearing aids, medications, drug use, substance use, diet, environmental hazards

Associated pain or antalgic gait (limp due to avoidance of pain)?

Yes → **Articular or nonarticular?**

No → **Neurologic symptoms or findings?**

Articular → **Mono or poly?**

Nonarticular → Occult fracture, Neoplasm, Pes planus/cavus, Bursitis, Tendonitis | Vascular or neurogenic claudication

No → Cardiac disorders, depression, fear of falling, psychogenic

Mono → Check x-rays; consider arthrocentesis, ESR, or CRP. → Fracture, osteoarthritis, gout, transient synovitis, septic joint, Lyme disease, slipped epiphysis, leg length discrepancy

Poly → Check ESR or CRP; consider ANA, RF or CCP, or RPR. → Rheumatologic (osteoarthritis, reactive arthritis, SLE), Viral infection, Fibromyalgia, Malignancy

Yes (Neurologic) →

Confusion → Consider head CT. → Dementia, Subdural, NPH, Stroke, Neoplasm

Weakness → Cerebral palsy, Myositis, Muscular dystrophy, Multiple sclerosis, Myelopathy, Stroke, Decondition, Spinal muscular atrophy, Electrolyte imbalances

Numbness → Diabetes, Vitamin B_{12} deficiency, HIV, Hyper- and hypothyroidism, Heavy metal poisoning, Neuropathy

Tremor → Parkinson disease, Supranuclear palsy

Coordination deficit → Vertebrobasilar insufficiency, Cerebellar dysfunction, Vestibular disorders, Neoplasm

Frank J. Domino, MD

Attaullah AHM, De Jesus O. *Gait Disturbances*. Treasure Island, FL: StatPearls Publishing; 2022. https://www.ncbi.nlm.nih.gov/books/NBK560610/. Accessed January 11, 2023.

GASTROESOPHAGEAL REFLUX DISEASE (GERD), DIAGNOSIS AND TREATMENT

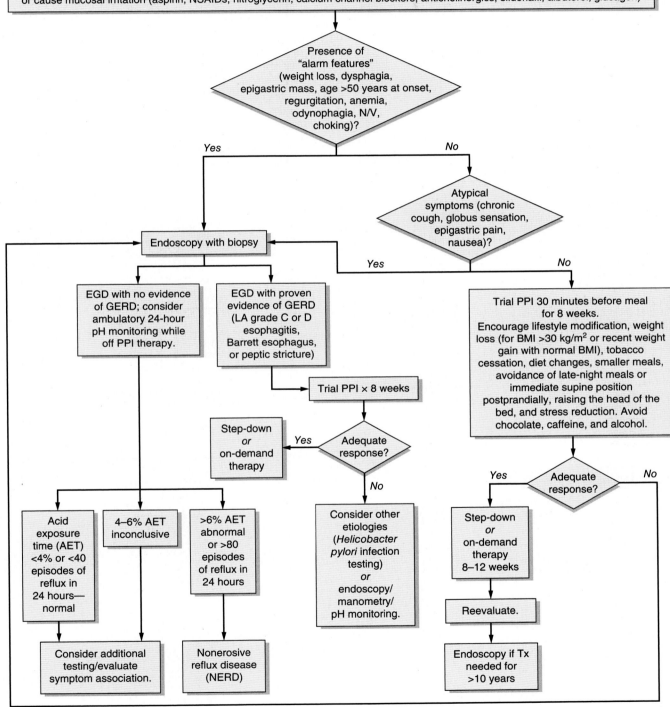

Mmaserame Gaefele, MD and Nathan J. Macedo, MD, MPH

Kellerman R, Kintanar T. Gastroesophageal reflux disease. *Prim Care*. 2017;44(4):561–573. doi:10.1016/j.pop.2017.07.001.

GENITAL ULCERS

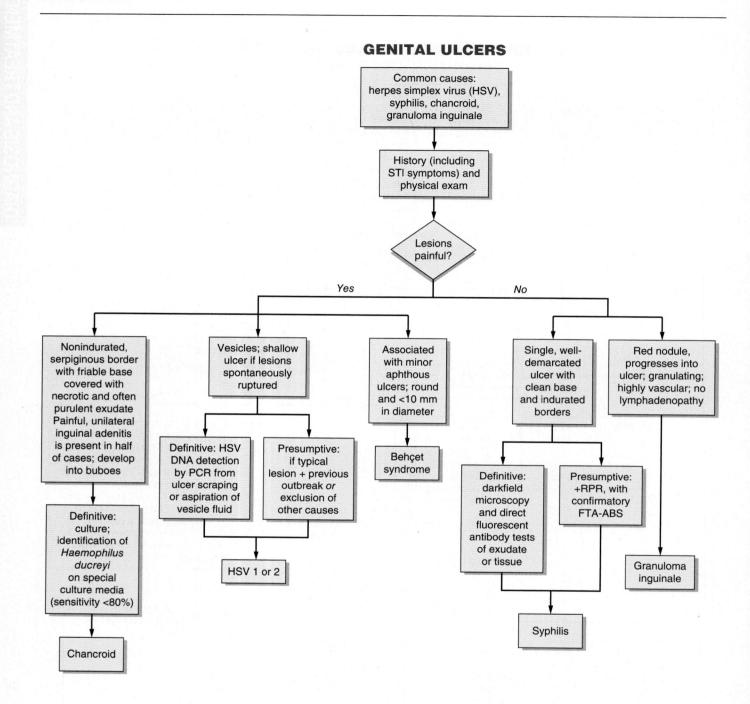

Common causes: herpes simplex virus (HSV), syphilis, chancroid, granuloma inguinale

↓

History (including STI symptoms) and physical exam

↓

Lesions painful?

Yes

- Nonindurated, serpiginous border with friable base covered with necrotic and often purulent exudate Painful, unilateral inguinal adenitis is present in half of cases; develop into buboes
  - **Definitive:** culture; identification of *Haemophilus ducreyi* on special culture media (sensitivity <80%)
    - **Chancroid**

- Vesicles; shallow ulcer if lesions spontaneously ruptured
  - **Definitive:** HSV DNA detection by PCR from ulcer scraping or aspiration of vesicle fluid
  - **Presumptive:** if typical lesion + previous outbreak *or* exclusion of other causes
    - **HSV 1 or 2**

- Associated with minor aphthous ulcers; round and <10 mm in diameter
  - **Behçet syndrome**

No

- Single, well-demarcated ulcer with clean base and indurated borders
  - **Definitive:** darkfield microscopy and direct fluorescent antibody tests of exudate or tissue
  - **Presumptive:** +RPR, with confirmatory FTA-ABS
    - **Syphilis**

- Red nodule, progresses into ulcer; granulating; highly vascular; no lymphadenopathy
  - **Granuloma inguinale**

Madeline Taskier, MD

Roett MA. Genital ulcers: differential diagnosis and management. *Am Fam Physician.* 2020;101(6):355–361.

GRANULOCYTOSIS (LEUKOCYTOSIS)

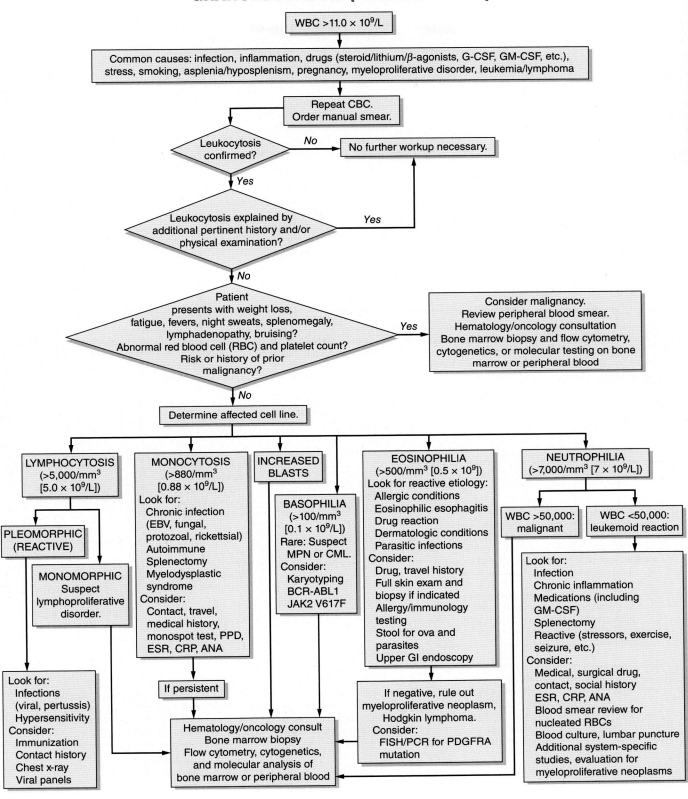

WBC >11.0 × 10⁹/L

Common causes: infection, inflammation, drugs (steroid/lithium/β-agonists, G-CSF, GM-CSF, etc.), stress, smoking, asplenia/hyposplenism, pregnancy, myeloproliferative disorder, leukemia/lymphoma

Repeat CBC.
Order manual smear.

Leukocytosis confirmed? — No → No further workup necessary.

Yes

Leukocytosis explained by additional pertinent history and/or physical examination? — Yes →

No

Patient presents with weight loss, fatigue, fevers, night sweats, splenomegaly, lymphadenopathy, bruising? Abnormal red blood cell (RBC) and platelet count? Risk or history of prior malignancy? — Yes → Consider malignancy. Review peripheral blood smear. Hematology/oncology consultation Bone marrow biopsy and flow cytometry, cytogenetics, or molecular testing on bone marrow or peripheral blood

No

Determine affected cell line.

LYMPHOCYTOSIS (>5,000/mm³ [5.0 × 10⁹/L])

PLEOMORPHIC (REACTIVE)

MONOMORPHIC Suspect lymphoproliferative disorder.

Look for:
Infections (viral, pertussis)
Hypersensitivity
Consider:
Immunization
Contact history
Chest x-ray
Viral panels

MONOCYTOSIS (>880/mm³ [0.88 × 10⁹/L])
Look for:
Chronic infection (EBV, fungal, protozoal, rickettsial)
Autoimmune
Splenectomy
Myelodysplastic syndrome
Consider:
Contact, travel, medical history, monospot test, PPD, ESR, CRP, ANA

If persistent

INCREASED BLASTS

BASOPHILIA (>100/mm³ [0.1 × 10⁹/L])
Rare: Suspect MPN or CML.
Consider:
Karyotyping
BCR-ABL1
JAK2 V617F

EOSINOPHILIA (>500/mm³ [0.5 × 10⁹])
Look for reactive etiology:
Allergic conditions
Eosinophilic esophagitis
Drug reaction
Dermatologic conditions
Parasitic infections
Consider:
Drug, travel history
Full skin exam and biopsy if indicated
Allergy/immunology testing
Stool for ova and parasites
Upper GI endoscopy

If negative, rule out myeloproliferative neoplasm, Hodgkin lymphoma.
Consider:
FISH/PCR for PDGFRA mutation

NEUTROPHILIA (>7,000/mm³ [7 × 10⁹/L])

WBC >50,000: malignant

WBC <50,000: leukemoid reaction

Look for:
Infection
Chronic inflammation
Medications (including GM-CSF)
Splenectomy
Reactive (stressors, exercise, seizure, etc.)
Consider:
Medical, surgical drug, contact, social history
ESR, CRP, ANA
Blood smear review for nucleated RBCs
Blood culture, lumbar puncture
Additional system-specific studies, evaluation for myeloproliferative neoplasms

Hematology/oncology consult
Bone marrow biopsy
Flow cytometry, cytogenetics, and molecular analysis of bone marrow or peripheral blood

Edison Tsui, MD

George TI. Malignant or benign leukocytosis. *Hematology Am Soc Hematol Educ Program.* 2012;2012:475–484.

HEADACHE, CHRONIC

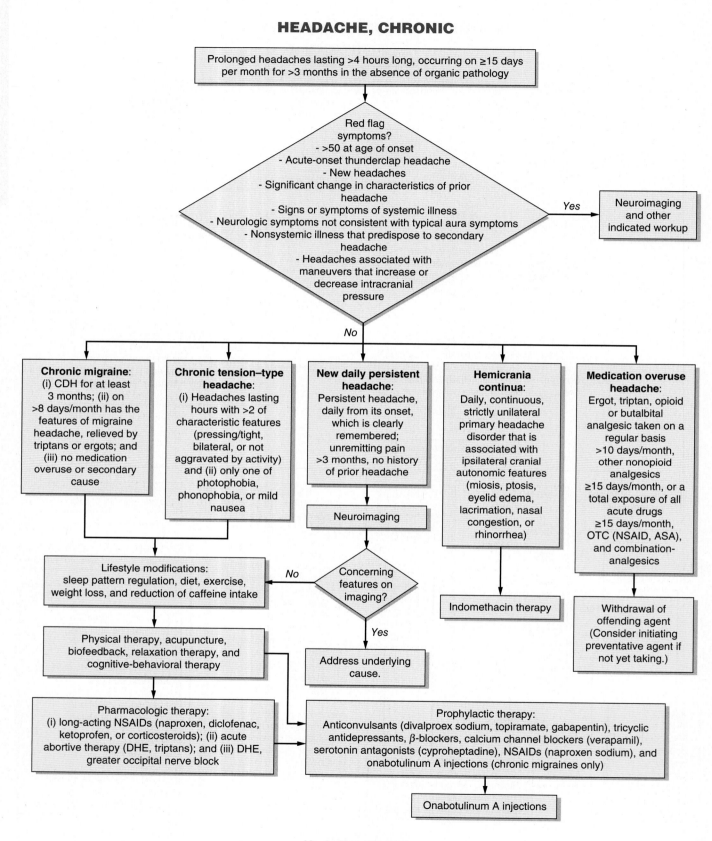

Karly Pippitt, MD

Dodick D, Dilli E. *Chronic Daily Headache*. Mt. Royal, NJ: American Headache Society; 2018. https://americanheadachesociety.org/wp-content/uploads/2018/05/David_Dodick_and_Esma_Dilli_-_Chronic_Daily_Headache.pdf. Accessed December 12, 2022.

HEART MURMUR

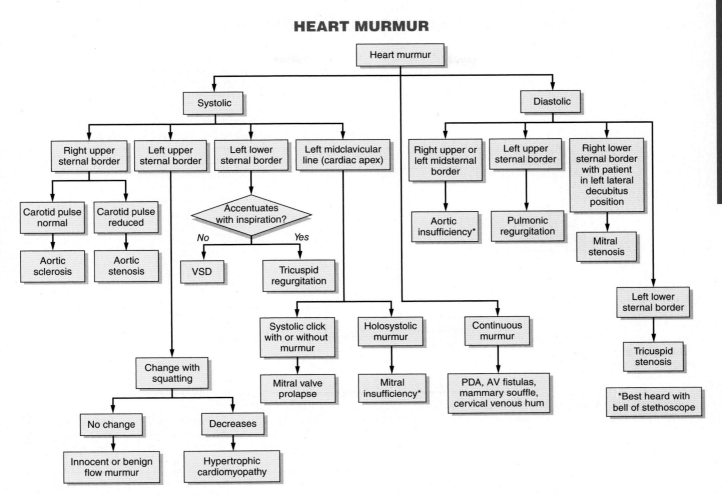

Navpreet K. Singh, MD

Bonow RO, Carabello BA, Chatterjee K, et al; for 2006 Writing Committee Members and American College of Cardiology/American Heart Association Task Force. 2008 Focused update incorporated into the ACC/AHA 2006 guidelines for the management of patients with valvular heart disease: a report of the American College of Cardiology/American Heart Association Task Force on Practice Guidelines (writing committee to revise the 1998 guidelines for the management of patients with valvular heart disease): endorsed by the Society of Cardiovascular Anesthesiologists, Society for Cardiovascular Angiography and Interventions, and Society of Thoracic Surgeons. *Circulation*. 2008;118(15):e523–e661.

HEMATEMESIS (BLEEDING, UPPER GASTROINTESTINAL)

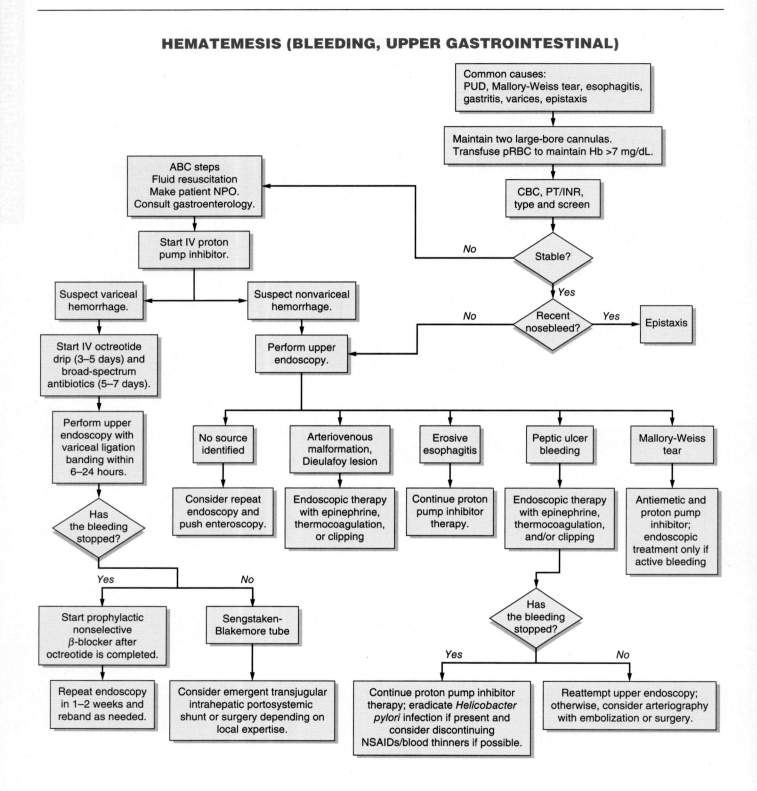

Manju Mahajan, MD, FAAFP

Kamboj AK, Hoversten P, Leggett CL. Upper gastrointestinal bleeding: etiologies and management. *Mayo Clin Proc.* 2019;94(4):697–703.

HEMATURIA

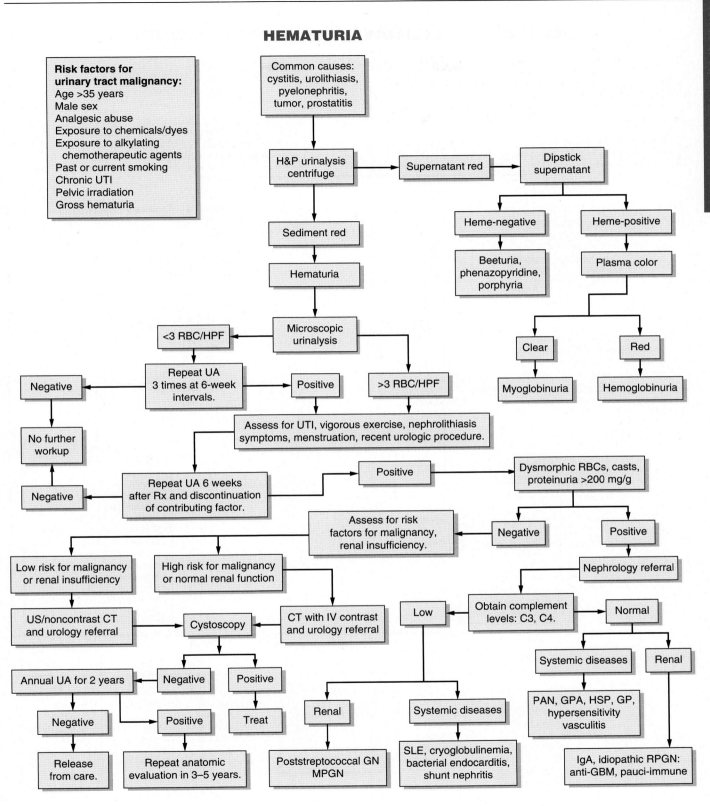

Risk factors for urinary tract malignancy:
Age >35 years
Male sex
Analgesic abuse
Exposure to chemicals/dyes
Exposure to alkylating chemotherapeutic agents
Past or current smoking
Chronic UTI
Pelvic irradiation
Gross hematuria

Common causes: cystitis, urolithiasis, pyelonephritis, tumor, prostatitis

H&P urinalysis centrifuge → Supernatant red → Dipstick supernatant

Dipstick supernatant → Heme-negative → Beeturia, phenazopyridine, porphyria

Dipstick supernatant → Heme-positive → Plasma color

Plasma color → Clear → Myoglobinuria

Plasma color → Red → Hemoglobinuria

Sediment red → Hematuria → Microscopic urinalysis

Microscopic urinalysis → <3 RBC/HPF → Repeat UA 3 times at 6-week intervals.

Repeat UA 3 times at 6-week intervals → Negative → No further workup

Repeat UA 3 times at 6-week intervals → Positive

Microscopic urinalysis → >3 RBC/HPF

Assess for UTI, vigorous exercise, nephrolithiasis symptoms, menstruation, recent urologic procedure.

Repeat UA 6 weeks after Rx and discontinuation of contributing factor.

Repeat UA 6 weeks after Rx... → Negative → No further workup

Repeat UA 6 weeks after Rx... → Positive → Dysmorphic RBCs, casts, proteinuria >200 mg/g

Dysmorphic RBCs, casts, proteinuria >200 mg/g → Negative → Assess for risk factors for malignancy, renal insufficiency.

Dysmorphic RBCs, casts, proteinuria >200 mg/g → Positive → Nephrology referral

Assess for risk factors for malignancy, renal insufficiency → Low risk for malignancy or renal insufficiency

Assess for risk factors for malignancy, renal insufficiency → High risk for malignancy or normal renal function

Low risk for malignancy or renal insufficiency → US/noncontrast CT and urology referral

High risk for malignancy or normal renal function → CT with IV contrast and urology referral

US/noncontrast CT and urology referral → Cystoscopy
CT with IV contrast and urology referral → Cystoscopy

Cystoscopy → Negative → Annual UA for 2 years

Cystoscopy → Positive → Treat

Annual UA for 2 years → Negative → Release from care.

Annual UA for 2 years → Positive → Repeat anatomic evaluation in 3–5 years.

Nephrology referral → Obtain complement levels: C3, C4.

Obtain complement levels: C3, C4 → Low

Obtain complement levels: C3, C4 → Normal

Low → Renal → Poststreptococcal GN MPGN

Low → Systemic diseases → SLE, cryoglobulinemia, bacterial endocarditis, shunt nephritis

Normal → Systemic diseases → PAN, GPA, HSP, GP, hypersensitivity vasculitis

Normal → Renal → IgA, idiopathic RPGN: anti-GBM, pauci-immune

Michael T. Partin, MD and Karl T. Clebak, MD, MHA, FAAFP

Ingelfinger JR. Hematuria in adults. *N Engl J Med.* 2021;385(2):153–163.

HEPATOMEGALY

Common causes: liver disease, obesity (nonalcoholic fatty liver disease and steatohepatitis), neoplasms, infection, vascular disease, fat/glycogen storage disorders, biliary disease, toxins, and metabolic disturbances

History: Evaluate for heart failure, obesity, alcohol use, drug abuse, infections, genetic diseases, recent exposures, medications, and travel.

Physical exam: inspection, look for jaundice, auscultation, palpation, percussion, and estimation of liver and spleen size

Initial labs:
- ALT/AST, GGT
- Total bilirubin (indirect/direct)
- Alkaline phosphatase
- Hepatitis serologies
- HIV

Normal

Imaging: CT, ultrasound

Abnormal

Normal

Reevaluate in 6 months.

Persistent hepatomegaly

Liver biopsy

Normal

Liver is normal; reevaluate in 1 year.

Abnormal

Cholestatic injury: predominant elevation of bilirubin and alkaline phosphatase

- Primary sclerosing cholangitis
- Primary biliary cholangitis
- Malignancy
- Biliary obstruction

Abnormal

Hepatocellular injury: predominant elevation of ALT and AST

Viral hepatitis

Malignancy

Consider the following diagnoses:
- Cirrhosis
- α_1-Antitrypsin deficiency
- Chronic hepatitis
- Wilson disease
- Hemochromatosis
- Glycogen and fat storage disease (pediatric patients)
- Extramedullary hematopoiesis
- Malignancy
- Biliary obstruction
- Nonalcoholic fatty liver disease

Medications/toxins:
- Acetaminophen
- Statins
- Idiosyncratic drug reactions
- Mushroom poisoning

Other:
- Autoimmune hepatitis
- Wilson disease
- α_1-Antitrypsin deficiency
- Hemochromatosis
- Nonalcoholic fatty liver disease
- Alcoholic hepatitis

Vascular congestion:
- Hepatic congestion secondary to heart failure
- Budd-Chiari syndrome
- IVC obstruction

Uniformly enlarged

Liver biopsy +/– FibroSURE

Vascular

Vascular congestion:
- Heart failure
- Budd-Chiari syndrome
- IVC obstruction

Cyst
- *Entamoeba histolytica*
- Polycystic liver disease
- Benign cysts

Abscess

Pyogenic liver abscesses usually develop following peritonitis or direct spread of biliary infection.

Mass
- Primary liver tumor (benign or malignant)
- Metastatic liver disease
- Granulomatous liver disease (TB, sarcoidosis, etc.)

Liver biopsy

Cirrhotic

Cirrhosis:
- Hepatitis
- Alcohol liver disease
- Nonalcoholic fatty liver disease

Manju Mahajan, MD, FAAFP

Kwo PY, Cohen SM, Lim JK. ACG clinical guideline: evaluation of abnormal liver chemistries. *Am J Gastroenterol*. 2017;112(1):18–35.

HYPERBILIRUBINEMIA AND JAUNDICE

Jaundice: a yellow discoloration of the skin, sclera and mucous membranes by bilirubin, a bile pigment formed by the breakdown of heme ring; detected when the serum bilirubin level >3 mg/dL

Bilirubin: a product of hemoglobin breakdown in the spleen; heme is converted to unconjugated bilirubin, bound to albumin, and transported to the liver where it is then conjugated.

Common causes of hyperbilirubinemia: Gilbert syndrome, hemolysis, hepatitis, and choledocholithiasis

History and physical: alcohol and drug use, fever, prodromal viral symptoms, weight loss, asterixis, mental status, bruising, spider angiomas, palmar erythema, gynecomastia, hepatomegaly, splenomegaly, right upper quadrant tenderness, ascites

Evaluation: CBC w/ diff; LFTs: AST, ALT, serum alkaline phosphatase (AP), albumin, protein, total bilirubin (TB), and direct bilirubin (DB); prothrombin and/or international normalized ratio (INR), haptoglobin, gamma-glutamyltransferase, LDH; viral and autoimmune hepatitis serologies; amylase, lipase; hCG; US, CT, or MRI

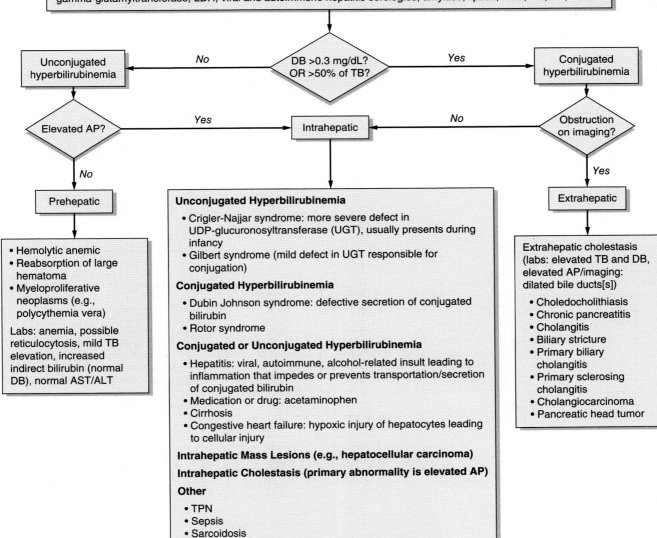

DB >0.3 mg/dL? OR >50% of TB?

No → **Unconjugated hyperbilirubinemia** → **Elevated AP?**
- Yes → **Intrahepatic**
- No → **Prehepatic**

Yes → **Conjugated hyperbilirubinemia** → **Obstruction on imaging?**
- No → **Intrahepatic**
- Yes → **Extrahepatic**

Prehepatic
- Hemolytic anemic
- Reabsorption of large hematoma
- Myeloproliferative neoplasms (e.g., polycythemia vera)

Labs: anemia, possible reticulocytosis, mild TB elevation, increased indirect bilirubin (normal DB), normal AST/ALT

Unconjugated Hyperbilirubinemia
- Crigler-Najjar syndrome: more severe defect in UDP-glucuronosyltransferase (UGT), usually presents during infancy
- Gilbert syndrome (mild defect in UGT responsible for conjugation)

Conjugated Hyperbilirubinemia
- Dubin Johnson syndrome: defective secretion of conjugated bilirubin
- Rotor syndrome

Conjugated or Unconjugated Hyperbilirubinemia
- Hepatitis: viral, autoimmune, alcohol-related insult leading to inflammation that impedes or prevents transportation/secretion of conjugated bilirubin
- Medication or drug: acetaminophen
- Cirrhosis
- Congestive heart failure: hypoxic injury of hepatocytes leading to cellular injury

Intrahepatic Mass Lesions (e.g., hepatocellular carcinoma)

Intrahepatic Cholestasis (primary abnormality is elevated AP)

Other
- TPN
- Sepsis
- Sarcoidosis

Extrahepatic

Extrahepatic cholestasis (labs: elevated TB and DB, elevated AP/imaging: dilated bile ducts[s])
- Choledocholithiasis
- Chronic pancreatitis
- Cholangitis
- Biliary stricture
- Primary biliary cholangitis
- Primary sclerosing cholangitis
- Cholangiocarcinoma
- Pancreatic head tumor

Catherine Khoo, MD, FAAFP

Fargo MV, Grogan SP, Saguil A. Evaluation of jaundice in adults. *Am Fam Physician.* 2017;95(3):164–168.

HYPERCALCEMIA

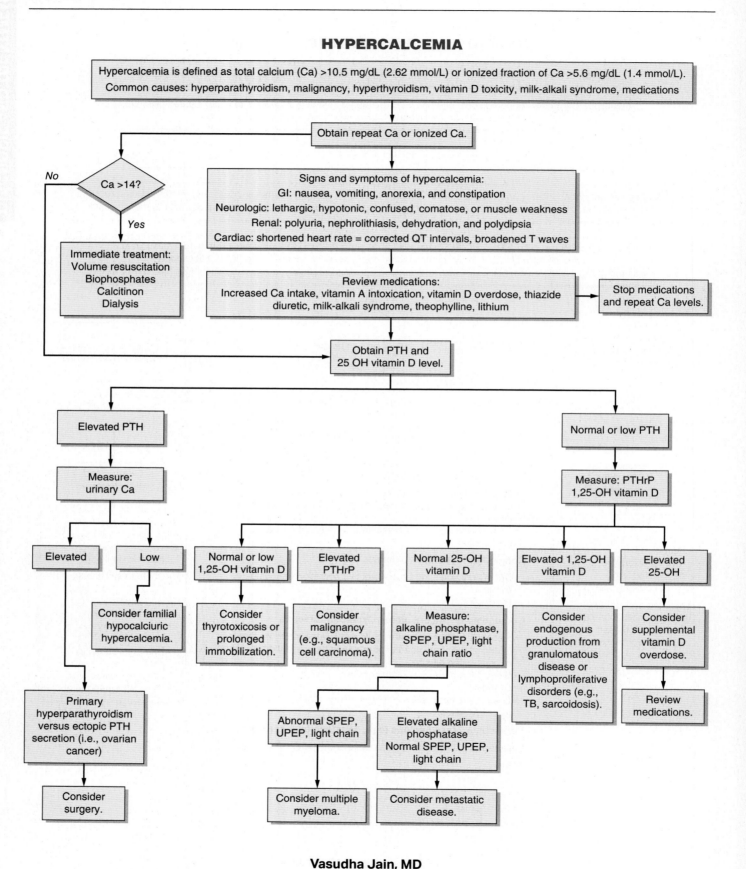

Hypercalcemia is defined as total calcium (Ca) >10.5 mg/dL (2.62 mmol/L) or ionized fraction of Ca >5.6 mg/dL (1.4 mmol/L).
Common causes: hyperparathyroidism, malignancy, hyperthyroidism, vitamin D toxicity, milk-alkali syndrome, medications

Obtain repeat Ca or ionized Ca.

Ca >14?

No

Yes

Immediate treatment:
Volume resuscitation
Biophosphates
Calcitinon
Dialysis

Signs and symptoms of hypercalcemia:
GI: nausea, vomiting, anorexia, and constipation
Neurologic: lethargic, hypotonic, confused, comatose, or muscle weakness
Renal: polyuria, nephrolithiasis, dehydration, and polydipsia
Cardiac: shortened heart rate = corrected QT intervals, broadened T waves

Review medications:
Increased Ca intake, vitamin A intoxication, vitamin D overdose, thiazide diuretic, milk-alkali syndrome, theophylline, lithium

Stop medications and repeat Ca levels.

Obtain PTH and 25 OH vitamin D level.

Elevated PTH

Normal or low PTH

Measure: urinary Ca

Measure: PTHrP 1,25-OH vitamin D

Elevated

Low

Normal or low 1,25-OH vitamin D

Elevated PTHrP

Normal 25-OH vitamin D

Elevated 1,25-OH vitamin D

Elevated 25-OH

Consider familial hypocalciuric hypercalcemia.

Consider thyrotoxicosis or prolonged immobilization.

Consider malignancy (e.g., squamous cell carcinoma).

Measure: alkaline phosphatase, SPEP, UPEP, light chain ratio

Consider endogenous production from granulomatous disease or lymphoproliferative disorders (e.g., TB, sarcoidosis).

Consider supplemental vitamin D overdose.

Primary hyperparathyroidism versus ectopic PTH secretion (i.e., ovarian cancer)

Review medications.

Abnormal SPEP, UPEP, light chain

Elevated alkaline phosphatase Normal SPEP, UPEP, light chain

Consider surgery.

Consider multiple myeloma.

Consider metastatic disease.

Vasudha Jain, MD

Renaghan AD, Rosner MH. Hypercalcemia: etiology and management. *Nephrol Dial Transplant.* 2018;33(4):549–551.

HYPERKALEMIA

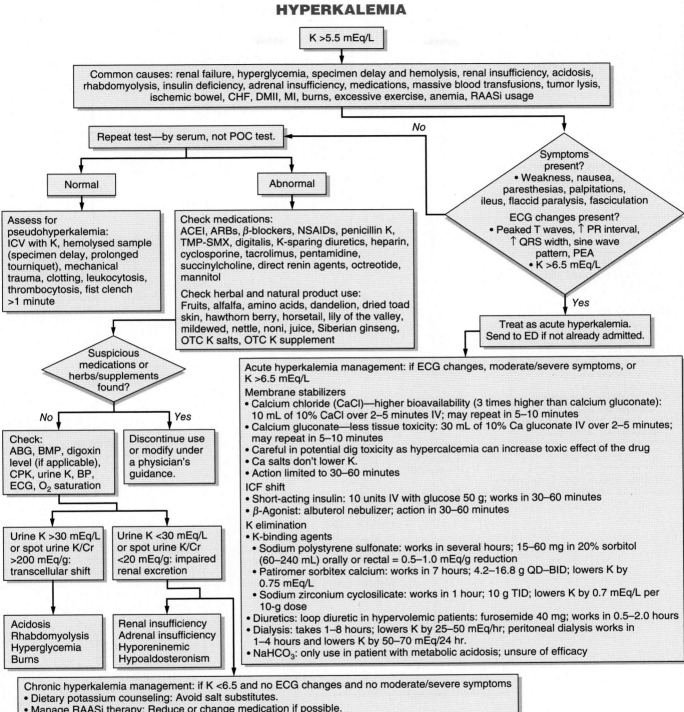

K >5.5 mEq/L

Common causes: renal failure, hyperglycemia, specimen delay and hemolysis, renal insufficiency, acidosis, rhabdomyolysis, insulin deficiency, adrenal insufficiency, medications, massive blood transfusions, tumor lysis, ischemic bowel, CHF, DMII, MI, burns, excessive exercise, anemia, RAASi usage

Repeat test—by serum, not POC test.

No

Symptoms present?
• Weakness, nausea, paresthesias, palpitations, ileus, flaccid paralysis, fasciculation

ECG changes present?
• Peaked T waves, ↑ PR interval, ↑ QRS width, sine wave pattern, PEA
• K >6.5 mEq/L

Yes

Treat as acute hyperkalemia. Send to ED if not already admitted.

Normal

Abnormal

Assess for pseudohyperkalemia: ICV with K, hemolysed sample (specimen delay, prolonged tourniquet), mechanical trauma, clotting, leukocytosis, thrombocytosis, fist clench >1 minute

Check medications: ACEI, ARBs, β-blockers, NSAIDs, penicillin K, TMP-SMX, digitalis, K-sparing diuretics, heparin, cyclosporine, tacrolimus, pentamidine, succinylcholine, direct renin agents, octreotide, mannitol

Check herbal and natural product use: Fruits, alfalfa, amino acids, dandelion, dried toad skin, hawthorn berry, horsetail, lily of the valley, mildewed, nettle, noni, juice, Siberian ginseng, OTC K salts, OTC K supplement

Suspicious medications or herbs/supplements found?

No

Yes

Check: ABG, BMP, digoxin level (if applicable), CPK, urine K, BP, ECG, O_2 saturation

Discontinue use or modify under a physician's guidance.

Acute hyperkalemia management: if ECG changes, moderate/severe symptoms, or K >6.5 mEq/L

Membrane stabilizers
• Calcium chloride (CaCl)—higher bioavailability (3 times higher than calcium gluconate): 10 mL of 10% CaCl over 2–5 minutes IV; may repeat in 5–10 minutes
• Calcium gluconate—less tissue toxicity: 30 mL of 10% Ca gluconate IV over 2–5 minutes; may repeat in 5–10 minutes
• Careful in potential dig toxicity as hypercalcemia can increase toxic effect of the drug
• Ca salts don't lower K.
• Action limited to 30–60 minutes

ICF shift
• Short-acting insulin: 10 units IV with glucose 50 g; works in 30–60 minutes
• β-Agonist: albuterol nebulizer; action in 30–60 minutes

K elimination
• K-binding agents
 • Sodium polystyrene sulfonate: works in several hours; 15–60 mg in 20% sorbitol (60–240 mL) orally or rectal = 0.5–1.0 mEq/g reduction
 • Patiromer sorbitex calcium: works in 7 hours; 4.2–16.8 g QD–BID; lowers K by 0.75 mEq/L
 • Sodium zirconium cyclosilicate: works in 1 hour; 10 g TID; lowers K by 0.7 mEq/L per 10-g dose
• Diuretics: loop diuretic in hypervolemic patients: furosemide 40 mg; works in 0.5–2.0 hours
• Dialysis: takes 1–8 hours; lowers K by 25–50 mEq/hr; peritoneal dialysis works in 1–4 hours and lowers K by 50–70 mEq/24 hr.
• $NaHCO_3$: only use in patient with metabolic acidosis; unsure of efficacy

Urine K >30 mEq/L or spot urine K/Cr >200 mEq/g: transcellular shift

Urine K <30 mEq/L or spot urine K/Cr <20 mEq/g: impaired renal excretion

Acidosis Rhabdomyolysis Hyperglycemia Burns

Renal insufficiency Adrenal insufficiency Hyporeninemic Hypoaldosteronism

Chronic hyperkalemia management: if K <6.5 and no ECG changes and no moderate/severe symptoms
• Dietary potassium counseling: Avoid salt substitutes.
• Manage RAASi therapy: Reduce or change medication if possible.
• Diuretic therapy
• Oral $NaHCO_3$ (if appropriate)
• Fludrocortisone: can increase fluid retention, HTN, vascular injury
• Consider potassium binders—see acute management (elimination section).
• Monitor potassium 2 times per year.
• Review medications, herbs, and supplements.
• Multidisciplinary approach: patient education, physician education, dietitian, pharmacist

Manju Mahajan, MD, FAAFP and Michael Richardson, MD

Palmer BF, Carrero JJ, Clegg DJ, et al. Clinical management of hyperkalemia. *Mayo Clin Proc*. 2021;96(3):744–762.

HYPERLIPIDEMIA

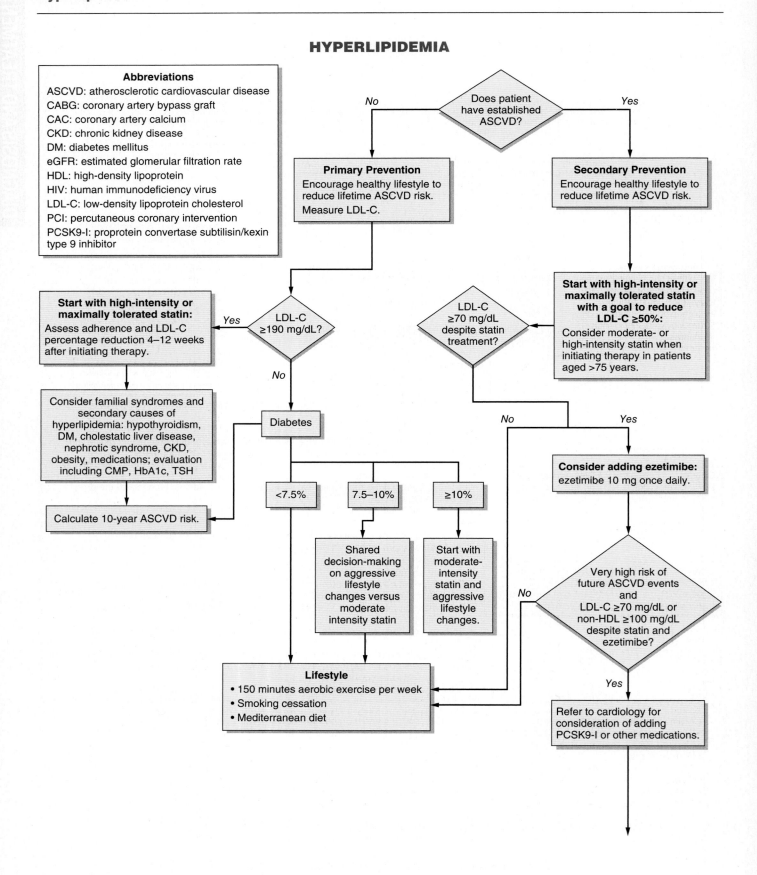

Abbreviations
ASCVD: atherosclerotic cardiovascular disease
CABG: coronary artery bypass graft
CAC: coronary artery calcium
CKD: chronic kidney disease
DM: diabetes mellitus
eGFR: estimated glomerular filtration rate
HDL: high-density lipoprotein
HIV: human immunodeficiency virus
LDL-C: low-density lipoprotein cholesterol
PCI: percutaneous coronary intervention
PCSK9-I: proprotein convertase subtilisin/kexin type 9 inhibitor

Does patient have established ASCVD?

No

Primary Prevention
Encourage healthy lifestyle to reduce lifetime ASCVD risk.
Measure LDL-C.

Yes

Secondary Prevention
Encourage healthy lifestyle to reduce lifetime ASCVD risk.

Start with high-intensity or maximally tolerated statin:
Assess adherence and LDL-C percentage reduction 4–12 weeks after initiating therapy.

Yes

LDL-C ≥190 mg/dL?

No

LDL-C ≥70 mg/dL despite statin treatment?

Start with high-intensity or maximally tolerated statin with a goal to reduce LDL-C ≥50%:
Consider moderate- or high-intensity statin when initiating therapy in patients aged >75 years.

Consider familial syndromes and secondary causes of hyperlipidemia: hypothyroidism, DM, cholestatic liver disease, nephrotic syndrome, CKD, obesity, medications; evaluation including CMP, HbA1c, TSH

Diabetes

No

Yes

Calculate 10-year ASCVD risk.

<7.5%

7.5–10%

≥10%

Consider adding ezetimibe:
ezetimibe 10 mg once daily.

Shared decision-making on aggressive lifestyle changes versus moderate intensity statin

Start with moderate-intensity statin and aggressive lifestyle changes.

Very high risk of future ASCVD events and LDL-C ≥70 mg/dL or non-HDL ≥100 mg/dL despite statin and ezetimibe?

No

Lifestyle
• 150 minutes aerobic exercise per week
• Smoking cessation
• Mediterranean diet

Yes

Refer to cardiology for consideration of adding PCSK9-I or other medications.

LDL-C reduction	≥50%	30–49%
Atorvastatin	40–80 mg/day	10–20 mg/day
Rosuvastatin	20–40 mg/day	5–10 mg/day
Simvastatin		20–40 mg/day
Pravastatin		40–80 mg/day
Lovastatin		40–80 mg/day
Fluvastatin		40 mg BID
Fluvastatin XL		80 mg/day
Pitavastatin		1–4 mg/day

Reassess 4–12 weeks after the start of treatment or after a change in medication dose:
Assess for medication and lifestyle adherence.
Measure LDL-C and determine percent reduction from baseline.
Reassess every 12 months.

**Cardiovascular Risk Assessment
(10-year, Revised Pooled Cohort Equations 2018)**
Available at
https://www.merckmanuals.com/medical-calculators/cvriskrevised2018-en.htm

**Jason Cross, PharmD, BCPS, BCACP, Dinesh Yogaratnam, PharmD, BCPS, BCCCP, and
Sudeep K. Aulakh, MD, FACP, FRCPC**

Grundy SM, Stone NJ, Bailey AL, et al. 2018 AHA/ACC/AACVPR/AAPA/ABC/ACPM/ADA/AGS/APhA/ASPC/NLA/PCNA guideline on the management of blood cholesterol: executive summary: a report of the American College of Cardiology/American Heart Association Task Force on Clinical Practice Guidelines. *J Am Coll Cardiol*. 2019;73(24):3168–3209.

HYPERNATREMIA

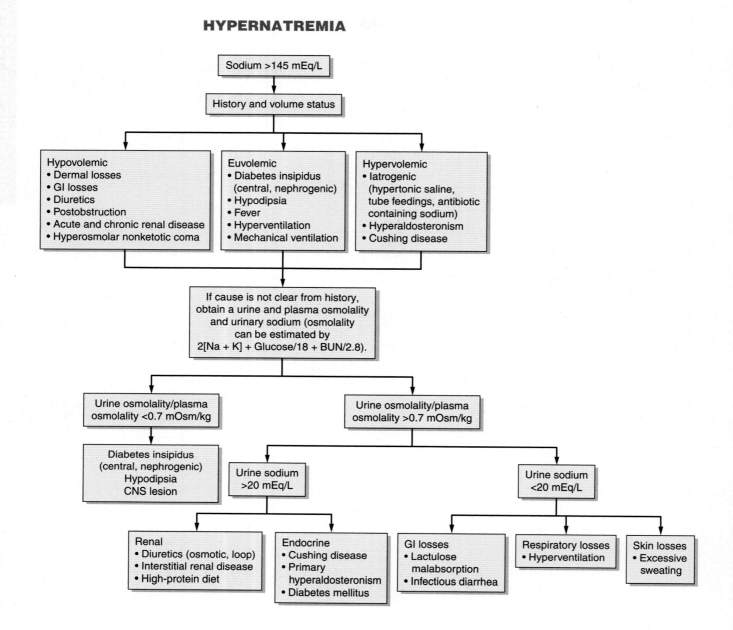

Timothy J. Coker, MD, FAAFP

Braun MM, Barstow CH, Pyzocha NJ. Diagnosis and management of sodium disorders: hyponatremia and hypernatremia. *Am Fam Physician*. 2015;91(5):299–307.

HYPERTRIGLYCERIDEMIA

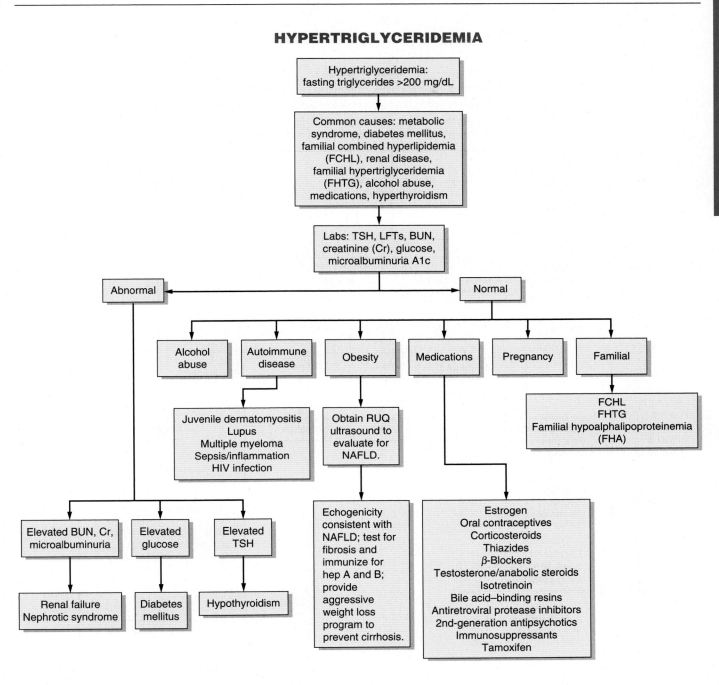

Steven W. Gale, MD and Timothy J. Coker, MD, FAAFP

Berglund L, Brunzell JD, Goldberg AC, et al; for Endocrine Society. Evaluation and treatment of hypertriglyceridemia: an Endocrine Society clinical practice guideline. *J Clin Endocrinol Metab*. 2012;97(9):2969–2989.

HYPOALBUMINEMIA

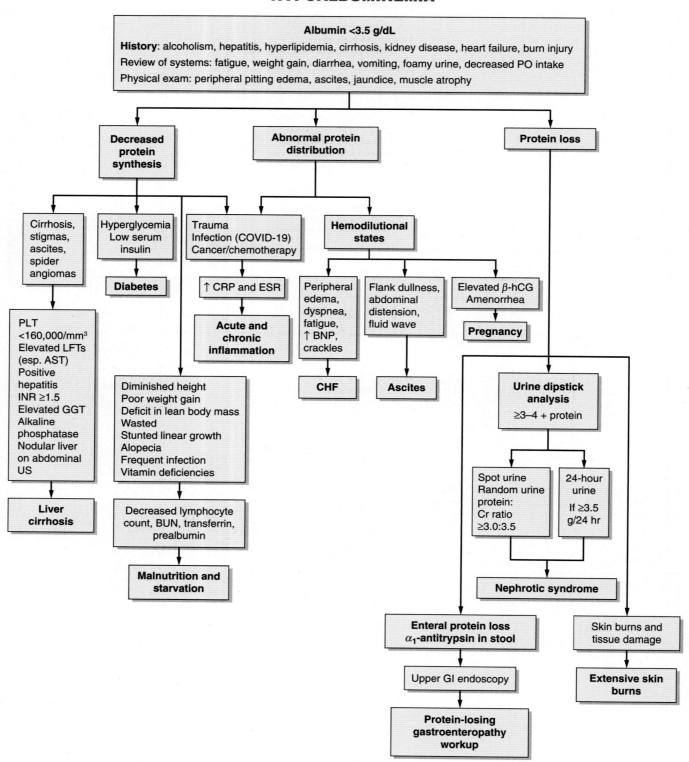

Albumin <3.5 g/dL

History: alcoholism, hepatitis, hyperlipidemia, cirrhosis, kidney disease, heart failure, burn injury
Review of systems: fatigue, weight gain, diarrhea, vomiting, foamy urine, decreased PO intake
Physical exam: peripheral pitting edema, ascites, jaundice, muscle atrophy

Decreased protein synthesis

Abnormal protein distribution

Protein loss

Cirrhosis, stigmas, ascites, spider angiomas

Hyperglycemia Low serum insulin

Diabetes

Trauma Infection (COVID-19) Cancer/chemotherapy

Hemodilutional states

PLT <160,000/mm³ Elevated LFTs (esp. AST) Positive hepatitis INR ≥1.5 Elevated GGT Alkaline phosphatase Nodular liver on abdominal US

↑ CRP and ESR

Acute and chronic inflammation

Peripheral edema, dyspnea, fatigue, ↑ BNP, crackles

Flank dullness, abdominal distension, fluid wave

Elevated β-hCG Amenorrhea

Pregnancy

Liver cirrhosis

Diminished height Poor weight gain Deficit in lean body mass Wasted Stunted linear growth Alopecia Frequent infection Vitamin deficiencies

CHF

Ascites

Urine dipstick analysis

≥3–4 + protein

Decreased lymphocyte count, BUN, transferrin, prealbumin

Spot urine Random urine protein: Cr ratio ≥3.0:3.5

24-hour urine

If ≥3.5 g/24 hr

Malnutrition and starvation

Nephrotic syndrome

Enteral protein loss α_1-antitrypsin in stool

Skin burns and tissue damage

Upper GI endoscopy

Extensive skin burns

Protein-losing gastroenteropathy workup

Anna Marie Tran, DO and Bashyam Iyengar, MD, MPH

Soeters PB, Wolfe RR, Shenkin A. Hypoalbuminemia: pathogenesis and clinical significance. *J Parenter Enteral Nutr.* 2019;43(2):181–193. doi:10.1002/jpen.1451.

HYPOCALCEMIA

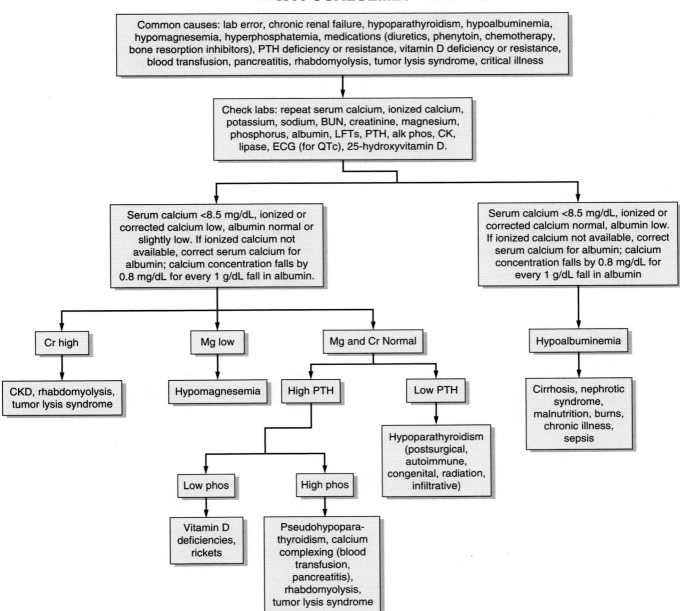

Parvathi Perumareddi, DO

Pepe J, Colangelo L, Biamonte F, et al. Diagnosis and management of hypocalcemia. *Endocrine.* 2020;69(3):485–495.

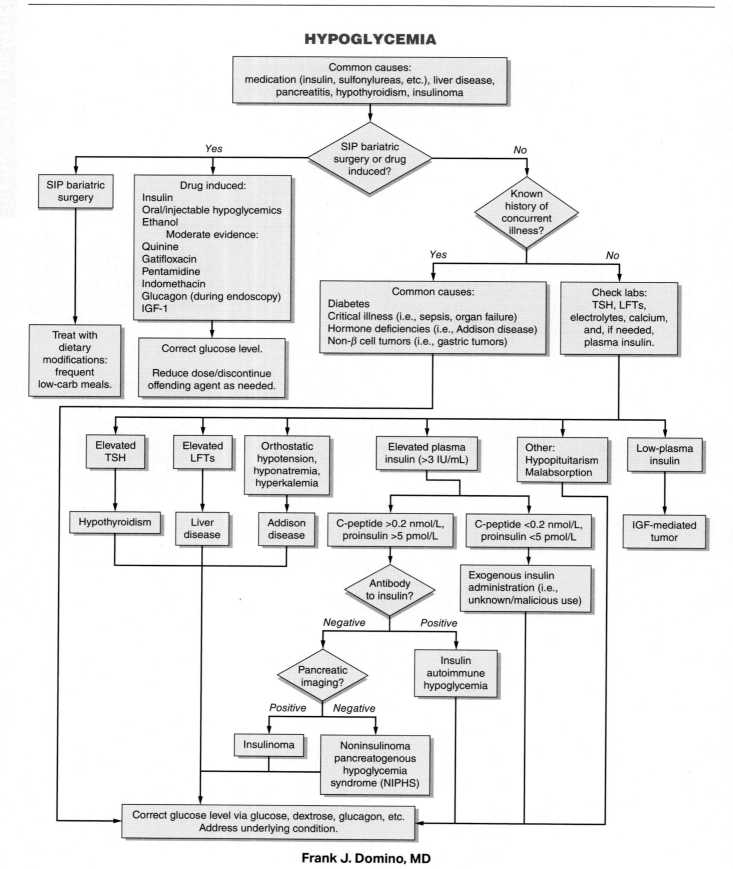

HYPOGLYCEMIA

Common causes:
medication (insulin, sulfonylureas, etc.), liver disease, pancreatitis, hypothyroidism, insulinoma

SIP bariatric surgery or drug induced?

Yes → *No*

SIP bariatric surgery

Drug induced:
Insulin
Oral/injectable hypoglycemics
Ethanol
    Moderate evidence:
Quinine
Gatifloxacin
Pentamidine
Indomethacin
Glucagon (during endoscopy)
IGF-1

Known history of concurrent illness?

Yes → *No*

Common causes:
Diabetes
Critical illness (i.e., sepsis, organ failure)
Hormone deficiencies (i.e., Addison disease)
Non-β cell tumors (i.e., gastric tumors)

Check labs:
TSH, LFTs, electrolytes, calcium, and, if needed, plasma insulin.

Treat with dietary modifications: frequent low-carb meals.

Correct glucose level.
Reduce dose/discontinue offending agent as needed.

Elevated TSH

Elevated LFTs

Orthostatic hypotension, hyponatremia, hyperkalemia

Elevated plasma insulin (>3 IU/mL)

Other: Hypopituitarism Malabsorption

Low-plasma insulin

Hypothyroidism

Liver disease

Addison disease

C-peptide >0.2 nmol/L, proinsulin >5 pmol/L

C-peptide <0.2 nmol/L, proinsulin <5 pmol/L

IGF-mediated tumor

Antibody to insulin?

Negative → *Positive*

Exogenous insulin administration (i.e., unknown/malicious use)

Pancreatic imaging?

Positive → *Negative*

Insulin autoimmune hypoglycemia

Insulinoma

Noninsulinoma pancreatogenous hypoglycemia syndrome (NIPHS)

Correct glucose level via glucose, dextrose, glucagon, etc. Address underlying condition.

Frank J. Domino, MD

Kandaswamy L, Raghavan R, Pappachan JM. Spontaneous hypoglycemia: diagnostic evaluation and management. *Endocrine.* 2016;53(1):47–57.

HYPOKALEMIA

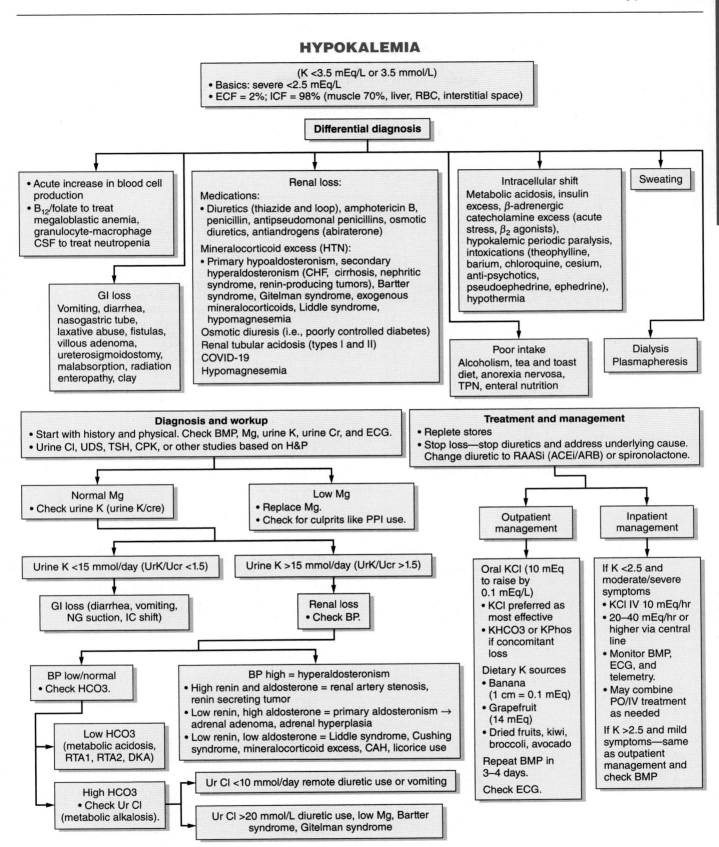

(K <3.5 mEq/L or 3.5 mmol/L)
- Basics: severe <2.5 mEq/L
- ECF = 2%; ICF = 98% (muscle 70%, liver, RBC, interstitial space)

Differential diagnosis

- Acute increase in blood cell production
- B₁₂/folate to treat megaloblastic anemia, granulocyte-macrophage CSF to treat neutropenia

GI loss
Vomiting, diarrhea, nasogastric tube, laxative abuse, fistulas, villous adenoma, ureterosigmoidostomy, malabsorption, radiation enteropathy, clay

Renal loss:
Medications:
- Diuretics (thiazide and loop), amphotericin B, penicillin, antipseudomonal penicillins, osmotic diuretics, antiandrogens (abiraterone)

Mineralocorticoid excess (HTN):
- Primary hypoaldosteronism, secondary hyperaldosteronism (CHF, cirrhosis, nephritic syndrome, renin-producing tumors), Bartter syndrome, Gitelman syndrome, exogenous mineralocorticoids, Liddle syndrome, hypomagnesemia

Osmotic diuresis (i.e., poorly controlled diabetes)
Renal tubular acidosis (types I and II)
COVID-19
Hypomagnesemia

Intracellular shift
Metabolic acidosis, insulin excess, β-adrenergic catecholamine excess (acute stress, β₂ agonists), hypokalemic periodic paralysis, intoxications (theophylline, barium, chloroquine, cesium, anti-psychotics, pseudoephedrine, ephedrine), hypothermia

Sweating

Poor intake
Alcoholism, tea and toast diet, anorexia nervosa, TPN, enteral nutrition

Dialysis
Plasmapheresis

Diagnosis and workup
- Start with history and physical. Check BMP, Mg, urine K, urine Cr, and ECG.
- Urine Cl, UDS, TSH, CPK, or other studies based on H&P

Treatment and management
- Replete stores
- Stop loss—stop diuretics and address underlying cause. Change diuretic to RAASi (ACEi/ARB) or spironolactone.

Normal Mg
- Check urine K (urine K/cre)

Low Mg
- Replace Mg.
- Check for culprits like PPI use.

Outpatient management

Inpatient management

Urine K <15 mmol/day (UrK/Ucr <1.5)

Urine K >15 mmol/day (UrK/Ucr >1.5)

GI loss (diarrhea, vomiting, NG suction, IC shift)

Renal loss
- Check BP.

Oral KCl (10 mEq to raise by 0.1 mEq/L)
- KCl preferred as most effective
- KHCO3 or KPhos if concomitant loss

Dietary K sources
- Banana (1 cm = 0.1 mEq)
- Grapefruit (14 mEq)
- Dried fruits, kiwi, broccoli, avocado

Repeat BMP in 3–4 days.

Check ECG.

If K <2.5 and moderate/severe symptoms
- KCl IV 10 mEq/hr
- 20–40 mEq/hr or higher via central line
- Monitor BMP, ECG, and telemetry.
- May combine PO/IV treatment as needed

If K >2.5 and mild symptoms—same as outpatient management and check BMP

BP low/normal
- Check HCO3.

BP high = hyperaldosteronism
- High renin and aldosterone = renal artery stenosis, renin secreting tumor
- Low renin, high aldosterone = primary aldosteronism → adrenal adenoma, adrenal hyperplasia
- Low renin, low aldosterone = Liddle syndrome, Cushing syndrome, mineralocorticoid excess, CAH, licorice use

Low HCO3 (metabolic acidosis, RTA1, RTA2, DKA)

High HCO3
- Check Ur Cl (metabolic alkalosis).

Ur Cl <10 mmol/day remote diuretic use or vomiting

Ur Cl >20 mmol/L diuretic use, low Mg, Bartter syndrome, Gitelman syndrome

Lisa Weiss, MD, Med, FAAFP and Sumira A. Koirala, MD, FAAFP

Kardalas E, Paschou SA, Anagnostis P, et al. Hypokalemia: a clinical update. *Endocr Connect.* 2018;7(4):R135–R146.

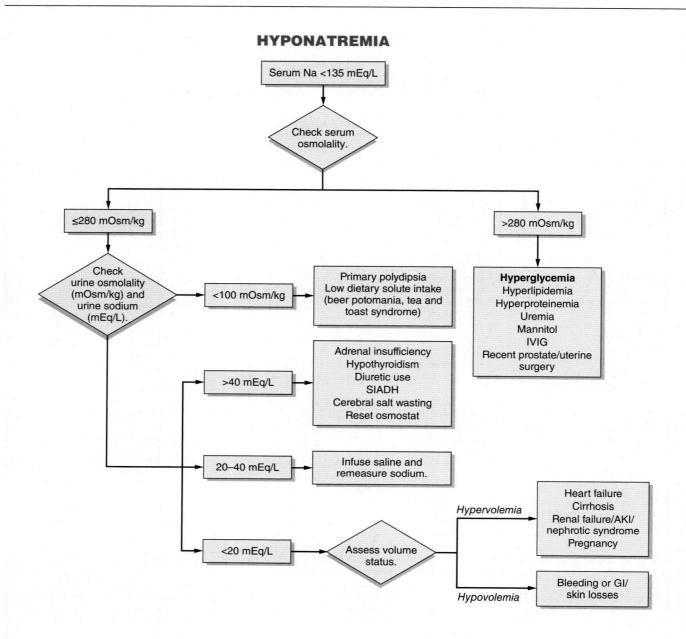

HYPONATREMIA

Serum Na <135 mEq/L

Check serum osmolality.

≤280 mOsm/kg

>280 mOsm/kg

Check urine osmolality (mOsm/kg) and urine sodium (mEq/L).

<100 mOsm/kg

Primary polydipsia
Low dietary solute intake (beer potomania, tea and toast syndrome)

>40 mEq/L

Adrenal insufficiency
Hypothyroidism
Diuretic use
SIADH
Cerebral salt wasting
Reset osmostat

20–40 mEq/L

Infuse saline and remeasure sodium.

<20 mEq/L

Assess volume status.

Hypervolemia

Heart failure
Cirrhosis
Renal failure/AKI/ nephrotic syndrome
Pregnancy

Hypovolemia

Bleeding or GI/ skin losses

Hyperglycemia
Hyperlipidemia
Hyperproteinemia
Uremia
Mannitol
IVIG
Recent prostate/uterine surgery

Chelsea Harris, MD and Corinne Gibbons, MD, MPH

Verbalis JG, Goldsmith SR, Greenberg A, et al. Diagnosis, evaluation, and treatment of hyponatremia: expert panel recommendations. *Am J Med*. 2013;126(10 Suppl 1):S1–S42.

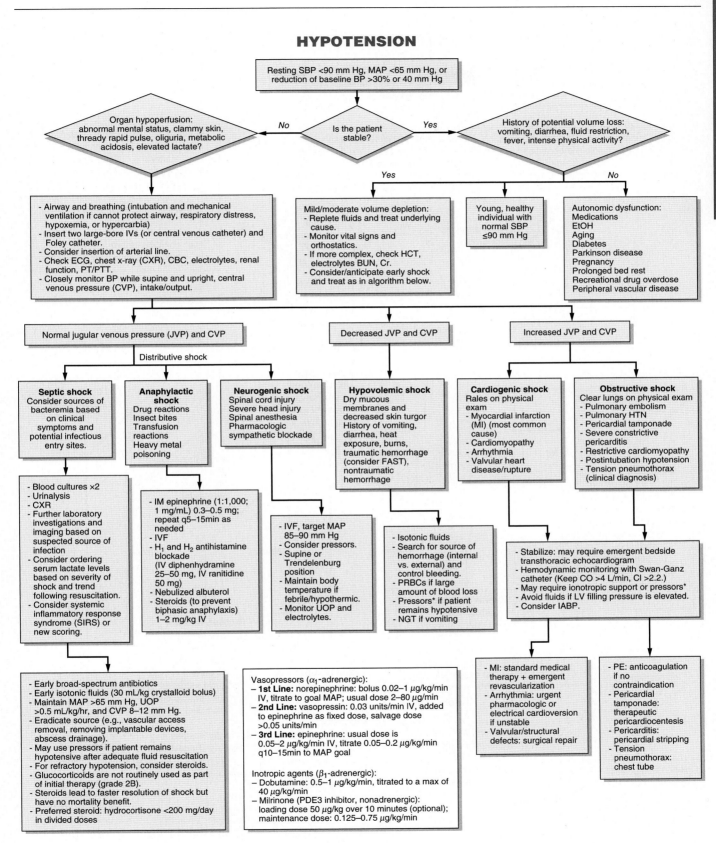

Frank J. Domino, MD

Thompson K, Venkatesh B, Finfer S. Sepsis and septic shock: current approaches to management. *Intern Med J.* 2019;49(2):160–170.

INFERTILITY

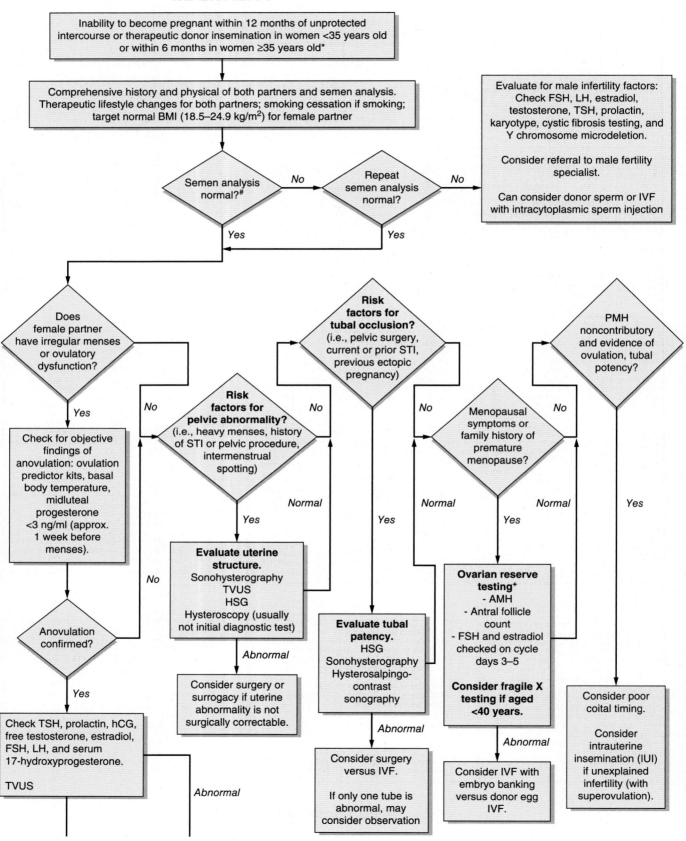

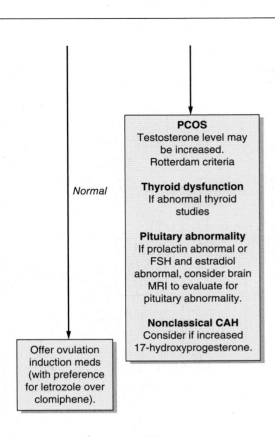

Normal

PCOS
Testosterone level may
be increased.
Rotterdam criteria

Thyroid dysfunction
If abnormal thyroid
studies

Pituitary abnormality
If prolactin abnormal or
FSH and estradiol
abnormal, consider brain
MRI to evaluate for
pituitary abnormality.

Nonclassical CAH
Consider if increased
17-hydroxyprogesterone.

Offer ovulation
induction meds
(with preference
for letrozole over
clomiphene).

*Common causes of infertility
- Male factor (40–50%)
- Diminished ovarian reserve
(premature menopause or
advanced age)
- Tubal or uterine abnormality
- Ovulatory dysfunction (PCOS,
thyroid abnormality, obesity/low
BMI, eating disorder,
hyperprolactinemia)
- Unknown (30%)

**\+Lab values consistent with
reduced ovarian reserve**
AMH <1 ng/mL
Antral follicle count <5–7
FSH >10 IU/L
Elevated estradiol (normal is
<60–80 pg/mL)
History of poor response to IVF
stimulation (<4 oocytes at egg
retrieval)

**\#Lower limit cutoffs for normal
semen analysis from WHO**
Ejaculate volume 1.5 mL
pH ≥7.2.
Sperm concentration at least
15×10^6/mL
Minimum total sperm
39×10^6/ejaculate
Total motility 40%
No sperm agglutination

TVUS: transvaginal ultrasound
HSG: hysterosalpingogram
AMH: Anti-müllerian hormone
CAH: congenital adrenal hyperplasia

Julie Johnston, MD, FAAFP and Alaina Aristide, MD

Practice Committee of the American Society for Reproductive Medicine. Fertility evaluation of infertile women: a committee opinion. *Fertil Steril*. 2021;116(5):1255–1265.

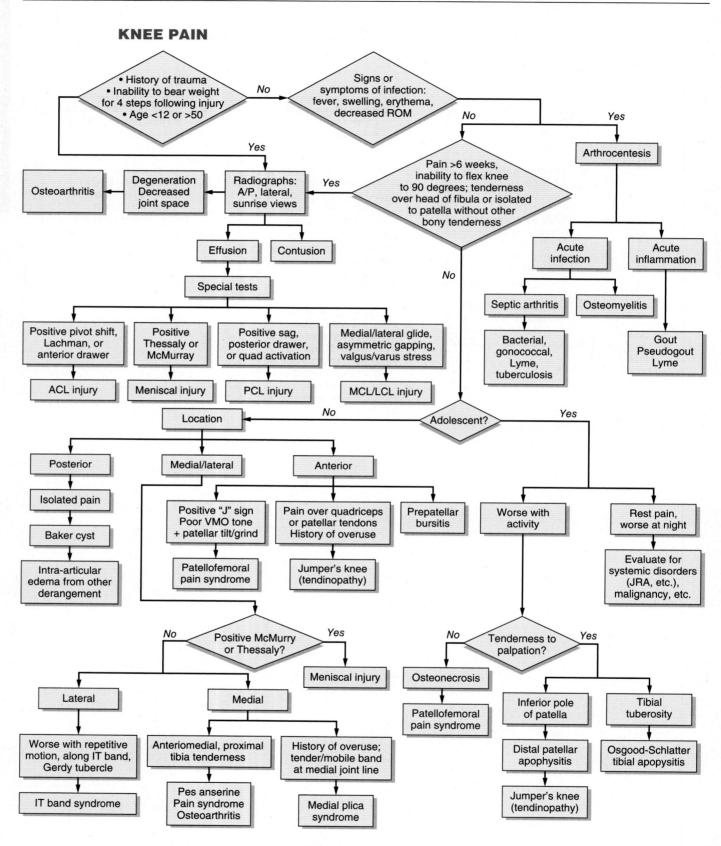

KNEE PAIN

KNEE PAIN

- History of trauma
- Inability to bear weight for 4 steps following injury
- Age <12 or >50

No → Signs or symptoms of infection: fever, swelling, erythema, decreased ROM

Yes →

Yes → Radiographs: A/P, lateral, sunrise views

Osteoarthritis ← Degeneration Decreased joint space ← Radiographs: A/P, lateral, sunrise views

No → Pain >6 weeks, inability to flex knee to 90 degrees; tenderness over head of fibula or isolated to patella without other bony tenderness

Yes → Arthrocentesis

Effusion | Contusion

Acute infection | Acute inflammation

Special tests

Septic arthritis | Osteomyelitis

Gout Pseudogout Lyme

Bacterial, gonococcal, Lyme, tuberculosis

Positive pivot shift, Lachman, or anterior drawer → ACL injury

Positive Thessaly or McMurray → Meniscal injury

Positive sag, posterior drawer, or quad activation → PCL injury

Medial/lateral glide, asymmetric gapping, valgus/varus stress → MCL/LCL injury

Location ← *No* ← Adolescent? → *Yes*

Posterior → Isolated pain → Baker cyst → Intra-articular edema from other derangement

Medial/lateral

Anterior

Positive "J" sign Poor VMO tone + patellar tilt/grind → Patellofemoral pain syndrome

Pain over quadriceps or patellar tendons History of overuse → Jumper's knee (tendinopathy)

Prepatellar bursitis

Worse with activity

Rest pain, worse at night → Evaluate for systemic disorders (JRA, etc.), malignancy, etc.

No ← Positive McMurry or Thessaly? → *Yes* → Meniscal injury

No ← Tenderness to palpation? → *Yes*

Lateral | Medial

Osteonecrosis → Patellofemoral pain syndrome

Inferior pole of patella | Tibial tuberosity

Worse with repetitive motion, along IT band, Gerdy tubercle → IT band syndrome

Anteriomedial, proximal tibia tenderness → Pes anserine Pain syndrome Osteoarthritis

History of overuse; tender/mobile band at medial joint line → Medial plica syndrome

Distal patellar apophysitis → Jumper's knee (tendinopathy)

Osgood-Schlatter tibial apopysitis

Tu Dan Nguyen, MD, CAQSM and Rod J. Turner Jr., MD, CAQSM, MS

Bunt CW, Jonas CE, Chang JG. Knee pain in adults and adolescents: the initial evaluation. *Am Fam Physician*. 2018;98(9):576–585.

LACTATE DEHYDROGENASE ELEVATION

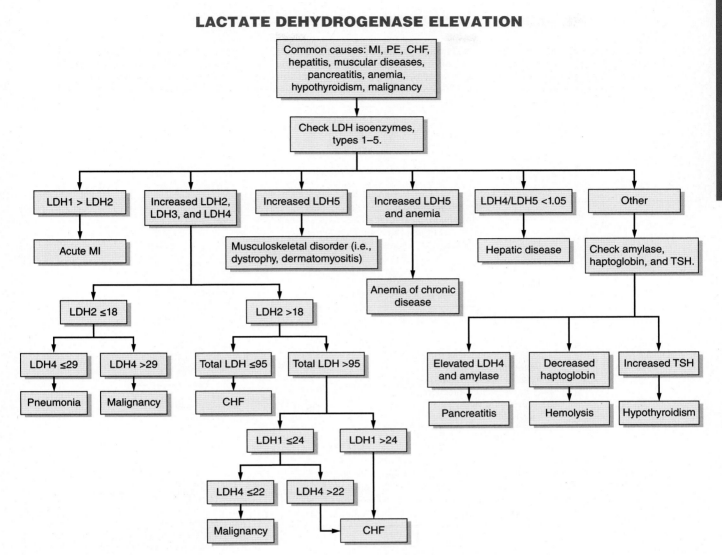

Frank J. Domino, MD

Lossos IS, Breuer R, Intrator O, et al. Differential diagnosis of pleural effusion by lactate dehydrogenase isoenzyme analysis. *Chest*. 1997;111(3):648–651.

LOW BACK PAIN, CHRONIC

Common causes: radiculitis, SI joint dysfunction, somatic dysfunction, structural skeletal deformities, trauma, trochanteric bursitis, piriformis syndrome, osteoporosis, osteoarthritis, pars interarticularis fracture, ankylosing spondylitis, spinal stenosis, compression fracture, epidural abscess, osteomyelitis, malignancy, postherpetic neuralgia, abdominal aortic aneurysm

Pain >3 months

Symptoms of cauda equina syndrome or malignancy? Abnormal gait, bowel/bladder incontinence, acute urinary retention, bilateral sciatica, saddle anesthesia, progressive neurologic symptoms, constitutional symptoms, history of malignancy, pain worse when supine?

Yes → Urgent MRI or CT and neurosurgery referral

No

Concern for infection? Fever, recent invasive spinal procedure, IV drug abuse, recent infection, overlying skin infection?

No → Concern for fracture? History of trauma, osteoporosis, chronic steroid use?

Yes ↓ (infection)

Urgent MRI or CT and laboratory evaluation: Consider CBC with diff, CRP/ESR, CMP, urinalysis, UDS, blood cultures, and TB testing.

Yes → Plain x-rays

No → No need for imaging

Neurosurgery or orthopedic spine referral

Negative / **Positive** / **Positive**

Negative →

Nonpharmacotherapy: patient education, structured exercise, multidisciplinary rehab, weight loss, yoga, tai chi, acupuncture, massage, osteopathic spinal manipulation therapy, progressive relaxation, motor control exercise, cognitive-behavioral therapy, stress management

Pharmacotherapy: topical or oral NSAIDs, antidepressants (i.e., duloxetine), anticonvulsants (i.e., topiramate), skeletal muscle relaxants* (i.e., tizanidine, cyclobenzaprine), Botox, tramadol,* other opioids,* injection therapy (i.e., corticosteroids, anesthetics, and other drugs administered at epidural sites, facet joints, or local sites)

Attempt to identify comorbid psychological problems and treatment barriers to improve long-term benefit.

*Use with caution

Nonpharmacotherapy: patient education, structured exercise, multidisciplinary rehab, weight loss, yoga, tai chi, acupuncture, massage, osteopathic spinal manipulation therapy, progressive relaxation, motor control exercise, cognitive-behavioral therapy, stress management

Pharmacotherapy: topical or oral NSAIDs, antidepressants (i.e., duloxetine), anticonvulsants (i.e., topiramate), skeletal muscle relaxants* (i.e., tizanidine, cyclobenzaprine), Botox, tramadol,* other opioids,* injection therapy (i.e., corticosteroids, anesthetics, and other drugs administered at epidural sites, facet joints, or local sites)

Attempt to identify comorbid psychological problems and treatment barriers to improve long-term benefit.

*Use with caution

No improvement: Consider surgical, psychiatry, or pain management referral.

N. Max Farenwald, DO and Priscilla Tu, DO, FAAFP, FAOASM, FACOFP, FAAMA

Will JS, Bury DC, Miller JA. Mechanical low back pain. *Am Fam Physician*. 2018;98(7):421–428.

LYMPHADENOPATHY

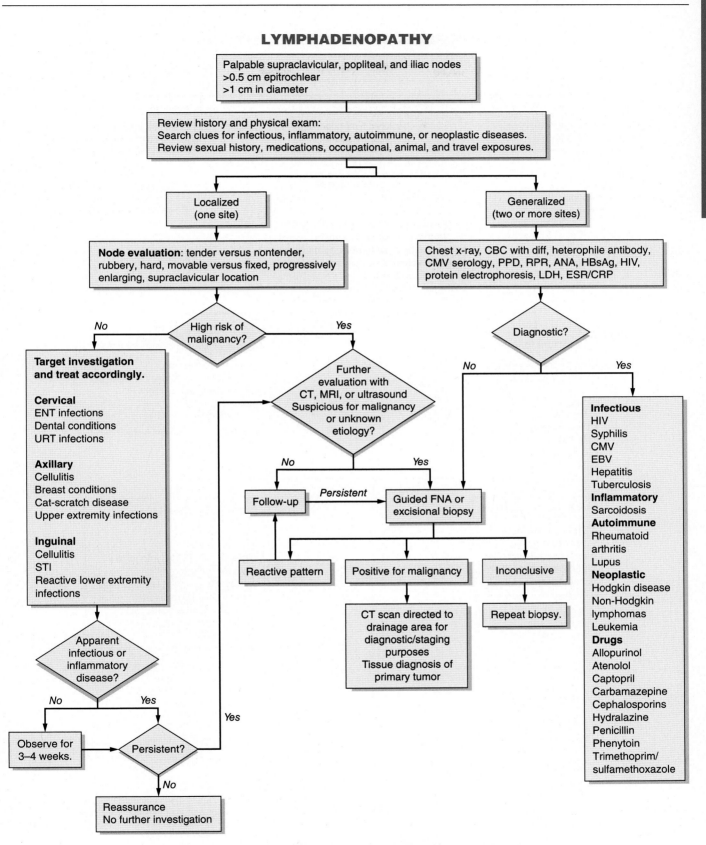

Palpable supraclavicular, popliteal, and iliac nodes
>0.5 cm epitrochlear
>1 cm in diameter

Review history and physical exam:
Search clues for infectious, inflammatory, autoimmune, or neoplastic diseases.
Review sexual history, medications, occupational, animal, and travel exposures.

Localized (one site)

Generalized (two or more sites)

Node evaluation: tender versus nontender, rubbery, hard, movable versus fixed, progressively enlarging, supraclavicular location

Chest x-ray, CBC with diff, heterophile antibody, CMV serology, PPD, RPR, ANA, HBsAg, HIV, protein electrophoresis, LDH, ESR/CRP

High risk of malignancy?

Diagnostic?

No

Yes

No

Yes

Target investigation and treat accordingly.

Cervical
ENT infections
Dental conditions
URT infections

Axillary
Cellulitis
Breast conditions
Cat-scratch disease
Upper extremity infections

Inguinal
Cellulitis
STI
Reactive lower extremity infections

Further evaluation with CT, MRI, or ultrasound Suspicious for malignancy or unknown etiology?

No

Yes

Follow-up

Persistent

Guided FNA or excisional biopsy

Reactive pattern

Positive for malignancy

Inconclusive

CT scan directed to drainage area for diagnostic/staging purposes
Tissue diagnosis of primary tumor

Repeat biopsy.

Infectious
HIV
Syphilis
CMV
EBV
Hepatitis
Tuberculosis
Inflammatory
Sarcoidosis
Autoimmune
Rheumatoid arthritis
Lupus
Neoplastic
Hodgkin disease
Non-Hodgkin lymphomas
Leukemia
Drugs
Allopurinol
Atenolol
Captopril
Carbamazepine
Cephalosporins
Hydralazine
Penicillin
Phenytoin
Trimethoprim/sulfamethoxazole

Apparent infectious or inflammatory disease?

No

Yes

Yes

Observe for 3–4 weeks.

Persistent?

No

Reassurance
No further investigation

Katy (Ekaterina) Brodski-Quigley, MD, EdM

Gaddey HL, Riegel AM. Unexplained lymphadenopathy: evaluation and differential diagnosis. *Am Fam Physician*. 2016;94(11):896–903.

LYMPHOPENIA OR LYMPHOCYTOPENIA

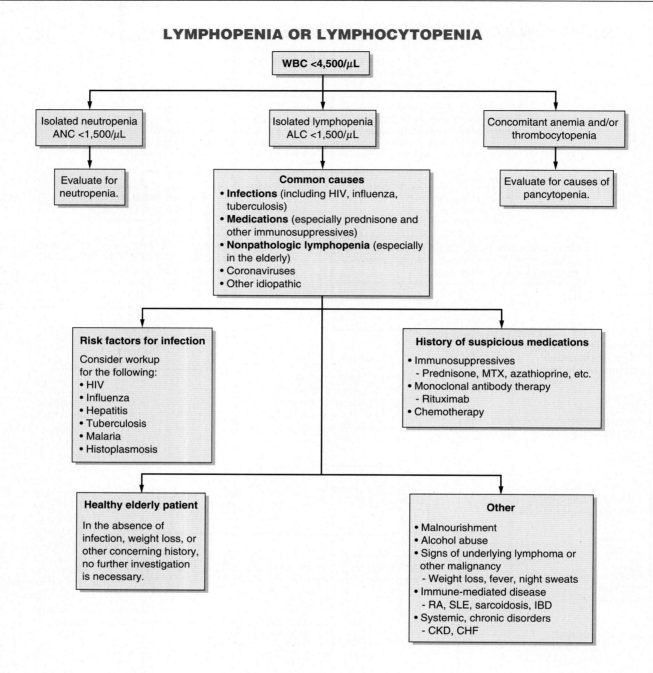

WBC <4,500/μL

Isolated neutropenia
ANC <1,500/μL

↓

Evaluate for neutropenia.

Isolated lymphopenia
ALC <1,500/μL

Concomitant anemia and/or thrombocytopenia

↓

Evaluate for causes of pancytopenia.

Common causes
- **Infections** (including HIV, influenza, tuberculosis)
- **Medications** (especially prednisone and other immunosuppressives)
- **Nonpathologic lymphopenia** (especially in the elderly)
- Coronaviruses
- Other idiopathic

Risk factors for infection

Consider workup for the following:
- HIV
- Influenza
- Hepatitis
- Tuberculosis
- Malaria
- Histoplasmosis

History of suspicious medications
- Immunosuppressives
  - Prednisone, MTX, azathioprine, etc.
- Monoclonal antibody therapy
  - Rituximab
- Chemotherapy

Healthy elderly patient

In the absence of infection, weight loss, or other concerning history, no further investigation is necessary.

Other
- Malnourishment
- Alcohol abuse
- Signs of underlying lymphoma or other malignancy
  - Weight loss, fever, night sweats
- Immune-mediated disease
  - RA, SLE, sarcoidosis, IBD
- Systemic, chronic disorders
  - CKD, CHF

Jillian K. Joseph, MPAS, PA-C and Allison Hargreaves, MD

Warny M, Helby J, Nordestgaard BG, et al. Lymphopenia and risk of infection and infection-related death in 98,344 individuals from a prospective Danish population-based study. *PLoS Med.* 2018;15(11):e1002685. doi:10.1371/journal.pmed.1002685.

MENOPAUSE, EVALUATION AND MANAGEMENT PART I

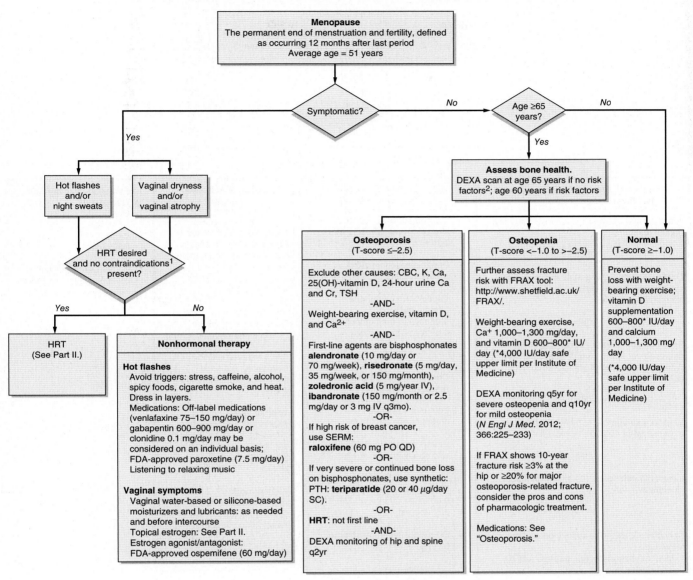

Menopause
The permanent end of menstruation and fertility, defined as occurring 12 months after last period
Average age = 51 years

Symptomatic?

No → **Age ≥65 years?** → No

Yes ↓

Hot flashes and/or night sweats

Vaginal dryness and/or vaginal atrophy

HRT desired and no contraindications[1] present?

Yes / No

HRT
(See Part II.)

Nonhormonal therapy

Hot flashes
Avoid triggers: stress, caffeine, alcohol, spicy foods, cigarette smoke, and heat.
Dress in layers.
Medications: Off-label medications (venlafaxine 75–150 mg/day) or gabapentin 600–900 mg/day or clonidine 0.1 mg/day may be considered on an individual basis; FDA-approved paroxetine (7.5 mg/day)
Listening to relaxing music

Vaginal symptoms
Vaginal water-based or silicone-based moisturizers and lubricants: as needed and before intercourse
Topical estrogen: See Part II.
Estrogen agonist/antagonist: FDA-approved ospemifene (60 mg/day)

Age ≥65 years? — Yes ↓

Assess bone health.
DEXA scan at age 65 years if no risk factors[2]; age 60 years if risk factors

Osteoporosis
(T-score ≤−2.5)

Exclude other causes: CBC, K, Ca, 25(OH)-vitamin D, 24-hour urine Ca and Cr, TSH
-AND-
Weight-bearing exercise, vitamin D, and Ca^{2+}
-AND-
First-line agents are bisphosphonates **alendronate** (10 mg/day or 70 mg/week), **risedronate** (5 mg/day, 35 mg/week, or 150 mg/month), **zoledronic acid** (5 mg/year IV), **ibandronate** (150 mg/month or 2.5 mg/day or 3 mg IV q3mo).
-OR-
If high risk of breast cancer, use SERM:
raloxifene (60 mg PO QD)
-OR-
If very severe or continued bone loss on bisphosphonates, use synthetic: PTH: **teriparatide** (20 or 40 μg/day SC).
-OR-
HRT: not first line
-AND-
DEXA monitoring of hip and spine q2yr

Osteopenia
(T-score <−1.0 to >−2.5)

Further assess fracture risk with FRAX tool: http://www.shetfield.ac.uk/FRAX/.

Weight-bearing exercise, Ca^+ 1,000–1,300 mg/day, and vitamin D 600–800* IU/day (*4,000 IU/day safe upper limit per Institute of Medicine)

DEXA monitoring q5yr for severe osteopenia and q10yr for mild osteopenia (*N Engl J Med.* 2012; 366:225–233)

If FRAX shows 10-year fracture risk ≥3% at the hip or ≥20% for major osteoporosis-related fracture, consider the pros and cons of pharmacologic treatment.

Medications: See "Osteoporosis."

Normal
(T-score ≥−1.0)

Prevent bone loss with weight-bearing exercise; vitamin D supplementation 600–800* IU/day and calcium 1,000–1,300 mg/day

(*4,000 IU/day safe upper limit per Institute of Medicine)

PART II

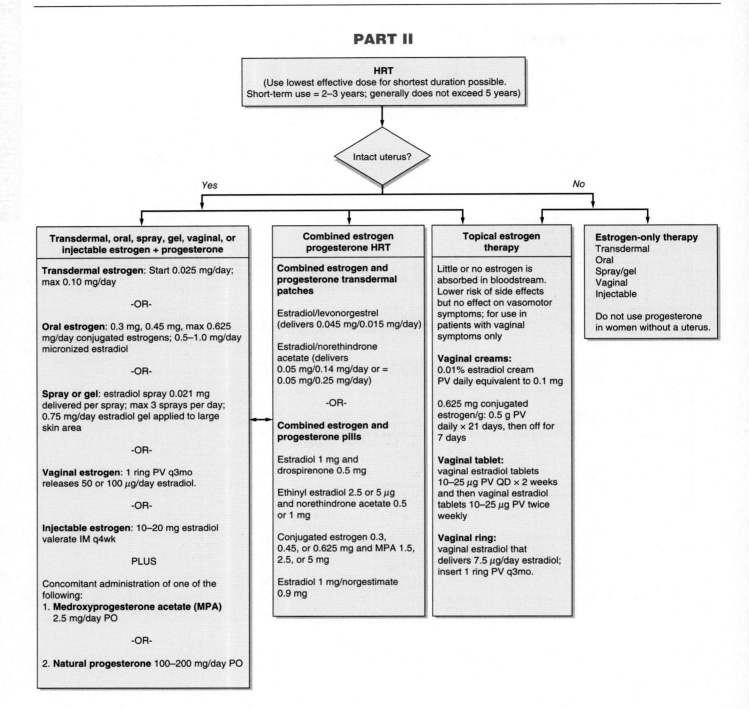

HRT
(Use lowest effective dose for shortest duration possible.
Short-term use = 2–3 years; generally does not exceed 5 years)

Intact uterus?

Yes — No

Transdermal, oral, spray, gel, vaginal, or injectable estrogen + progesterone

Transdermal estrogen: Start 0.025 mg/day; max 0.10 mg/day

-OR-

Oral estrogen: 0.3 mg, 0.45 mg, max 0.625 mg/day conjugated estrogens; 0.5–1.0 mg/day micronized estradiol

-OR-

Spray or gel: estradiol spray 0.021 mg delivered per spray; max 3 sprays per day; 0.75 mg/day estradiol gel applied to large skin area

-OR-

Vaginal estrogen: 1 ring PV q3mo releases 50 or 100 µg/day estradiol.

-OR-

Injectable estrogen: 10–20 mg estradiol valerate IM q4wk

PLUS

Concomitant administration of one of the following:
1. **Medroxyprogesterone acetate (MPA)** 2.5 mg/day PO

-OR-

2. **Natural progesterone** 100–200 mg/day PO

Combined estrogen progesterone HRT

Combined estrogen and progesterone transdermal patches

Estradiol/levonorgestrel (delivers 0.045 mg/0.015 mg/day)

Estradiol/norethindrone acetate (delivers 0.05 mg/0.14 mg/day or = 0.05 mg/0.25 mg/day)

-OR-

Combined estrogen and progesterone pills

Estradiol 1 mg and drospirenone 0.5 mg

Ethinyl estradiol 2.5 or 5 µg and norethindrone acetate 0.5 or 1 mg

Conjugated estrogen 0.3, 0.45, or 0.625 mg and MPA 1.5, 2.5, or 5 mg

Estradiol 1 mg/norgestimate 0.9 mg

Topical estrogen therapy

Little or no estrogen is absorbed in bloodstream. Lower risk of side effects but no effect on vasomotor symptoms; for use in patients with vaginal symptoms only

Vaginal creams:
0.01% estradiol cream PV daily equivalent to 0.1 mg

0.625 mg conjugated estrogen/g: 0.5 g PV daily × 21 days, then off for 7 days

Vaginal tablet:
vaginal estradiol tablets 10–25 µg PV QD × 2 weeks and then vaginal estradiol tablets 10–25 µg PV twice weekly

Vaginal ring:
vaginal estradiol that delivers 7.5 µg/day estradiol; insert 1 ring PV q3mo.

Estrogen-only therapy
Transdermal
Oral
Spray/gel
Vaginal
Injectable

Do not use progesterone in women without a uterus.

Kelly Pagidas, MD

Practice Bulletin No. 141: management of menopausal symptoms: correction. *Obstet Gynecol.* 2018;131(3):604.

MIGRAINE, TREATMENT

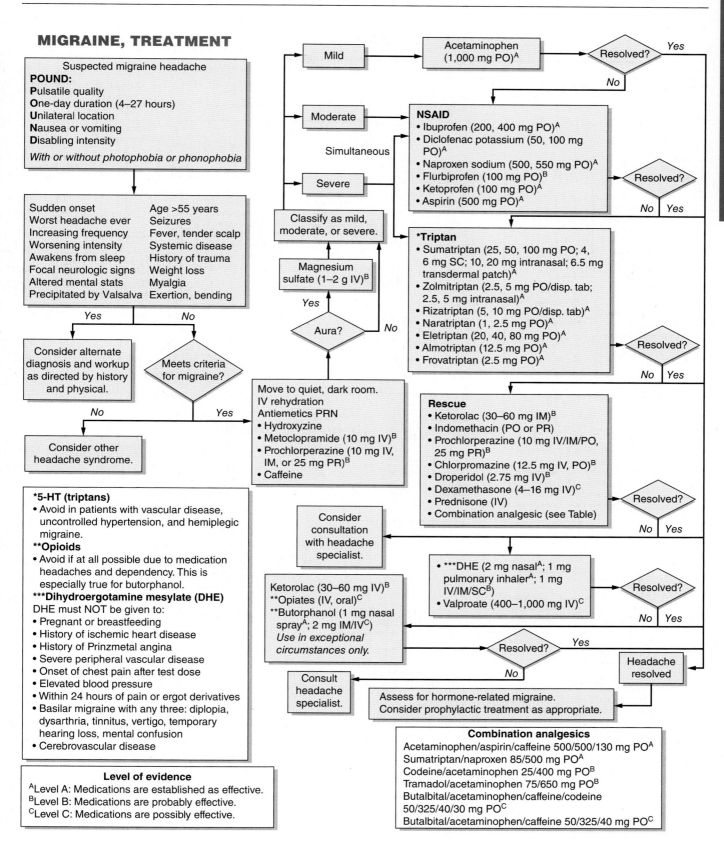

Suspected migraine headache
POUND:
Pulsatile quality
One-day duration (4–27 hours)
Unilateral location
Nausea or vomiting
Disabling intensity

With or without photophobia or phonophobia

Sudden onset
Worst headache ever
Increasing frequency
Worsening intensity
Awakens from sleep
Focal neurologic signs
Altered mental stats
Precipitated by Valsalva

Age >55 years
Seizures
Fever, tender scalp
Systemic disease
History of trauma
Weight loss
Myalgia
Exertion, bending

Yes → Consider alternate diagnosis and workup as directed by history and physical.

No → Meets criteria for migraine?

No → Consider other headache syndrome.

Yes → Move to quiet, dark room.
IV rehydration
Antiemetics PRN
• Hydroxyzine
• Metoclopramide (10 mg IV)[B]
• Prochlorperazine (10 mg IV, IM, or 25 mg PR)[B]
• Caffeine

Mild → Acetaminophen (1,000 mg PO)[A] → Resolved? Yes / No

Classify as mild, moderate, or severe.

Moderate / **Severe** (Simultaneous)

Magnesium sulfate (1–2 g IV)[B] → Aura? Yes / No

NSAID
• Ibuprofen (200, 400 mg PO)[A]
• Diclofenac potassium (50, 100 mg PO)[A]
• Naproxen sodium (500, 550 mg PO)[A]
• Flurbiprofen (100 mg PO)[B]
• Ketoprofen (100 mg PO)[A]
• Aspirin (500 mg PO)[A]
→ Resolved? No / Yes

*Triptan
• Sumatriptan (25, 50, 100 mg PO; 4, 6 mg SC; 10, 20 mg intranasal; 6.5 mg transdermal patch)[A]
• Zolmitriptan (2.5, 5 mg PO/disp. tab; 2.5, 5 mg intranasal)[A]
• Rizatriptan (5, 10 mg PO/disp. tab)[A]
• Naratriptan (1, 2.5 mg PO)[A]
• Eletriptan (20, 40, 80 mg PO)[A]
• Almotriptan (12.5 mg PO)[A]
• Frovatriptan (2.5 mg PO)[A]
→ Resolved? No / Yes

Rescue
• Ketorolac (30–60 mg IM)[B]
• Indomethacin (PO or PR)
• Prochlorperazine (10 mg IV/IM/PO, 25 mg PR)[B]
• Chlorpromazine (12.5 mg IV, PO)[B]
• Droperidol (2.75 mg IV)[B]
• Dexamethasone (4–16 mg IV)[C]
• Prednisone (IV)
• Combination analgesic (see Table)
→ Resolved? No / Yes

Consider consultation with headache specialist.

Ketorolac (30–60 mg IV)[B]
**Opiates (IV, oral)[C]
**Butorphanol (1 mg nasal spray[A]; 2 mg IM/IV[C])
Use in exceptional circumstances only.

• ***DHE (2 mg nasal[A]; 1 mg pulmonary inhaler[A]; 1 mg IV/IM/SC[B])
• Valproate (400–1,000 mg IV)[C]
→ Resolved? No / Yes

Resolved? Yes / No

Headache resolved

Consult headache specialist.

Assess for hormone-related migraine.
Consider prophylactic treatment as appropriate.

*5-HT (triptans)
• Avoid in patients with vascular disease, uncontrolled hypertension, and hemiplegic migraine.

**Opioids
• Avoid if at all possible due to medication headaches and dependency. This is especially true for butorphanol.

***Dihydroergotamine mesylate (DHE)
DHE must NOT be given to:
• Pregnant or breastfeeding
• History of ischemic heart disease
• History of Prinzmetal angina
• Severe peripheral vascular disease
• Onset of chest pain after test dose
• Elevated blood pressure
• Within 24 hours of pain or ergot derivatives
• Basilar migraine with any three: diplopia, dysarthria, tinnitus, vertigo, temporary hearing loss, mental confusion
• Cerebrovascular disease

Level of evidence
[A]Level A: Medications are established as effective.
[B]Level B: Medications are probably effective.
[C]Level C: Medications are possibly effective.

Combination analgesics
Acetaminophen/aspirin/caffeine 500/500/130 mg PO[A]
Sumatriptan/naproxen 85/500 mg PO[A]
Codeine/acetaminophen 25/400 mg PO[B]
Tramadol/acetaminophen 75/650 mg PO[B]
Butalbital/acetaminophen/caffeine/codeine 50/325/40/30 mg PO[C]
Butalbital/acetaminophen/caffeine 50/325/40 mg PO[C]

Katy (Ekaterina) Brodski-Quigley, MD, EdM

Marmura MJ, Silberstein SD, Schwedt TJ. The acute treatment of migraine in adults: the American Headache Society evidence assessment of migraine pharmacotherapies. *Headache.* 2015;55(1):3–20.

NAIL ABNORMALITIES

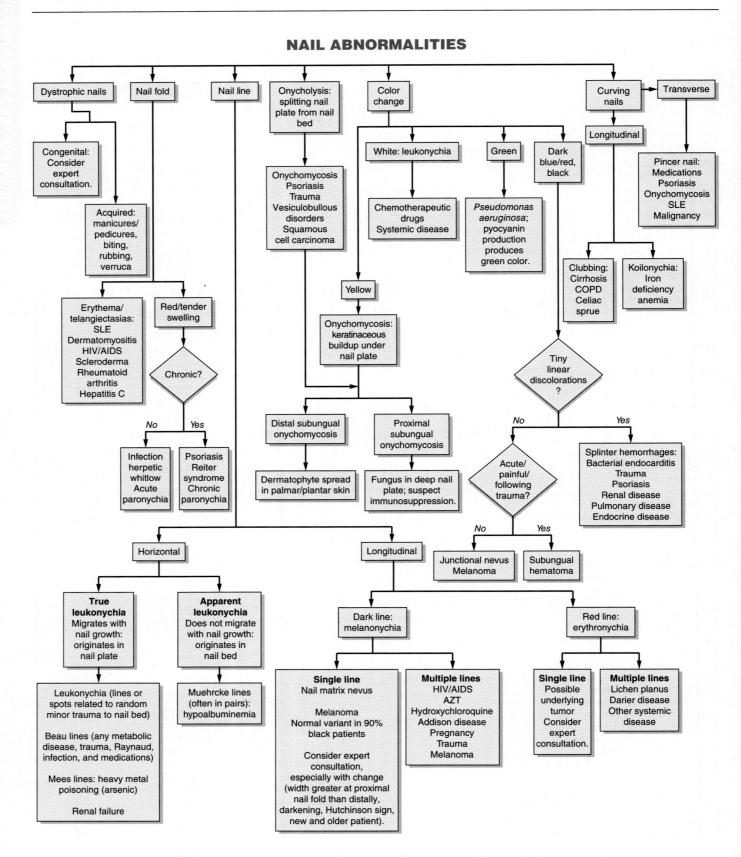

Natasha J. Pyzocha, DO, FAWM, FAAFP and Douglas M. Maurer, DO, MPH, FAAFP

Tully AS, Trayes KP, Studdiford JS. Evaluation of nail abnormalities. *Am Fam Physician*. 2012;85(8):779–787.

NEUTROPENIA

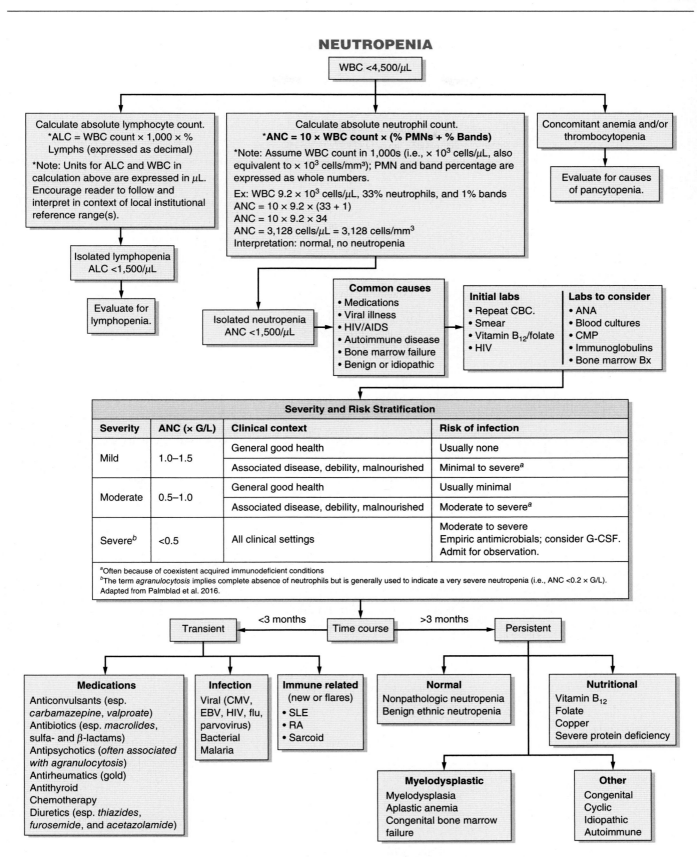

Ben Ayotte, MD, Lars J. Johnson, MD, and Thomas Kingsley, MD, MPH, MS

Palmblad J, Nilsson CC, Höglund P, et al. How we diagnose and treat neutropenia in adults. *Expert Rev Hematol*. 2016;9(5):479–487.

PAIN, CHRONIC, DIAGNOSIS

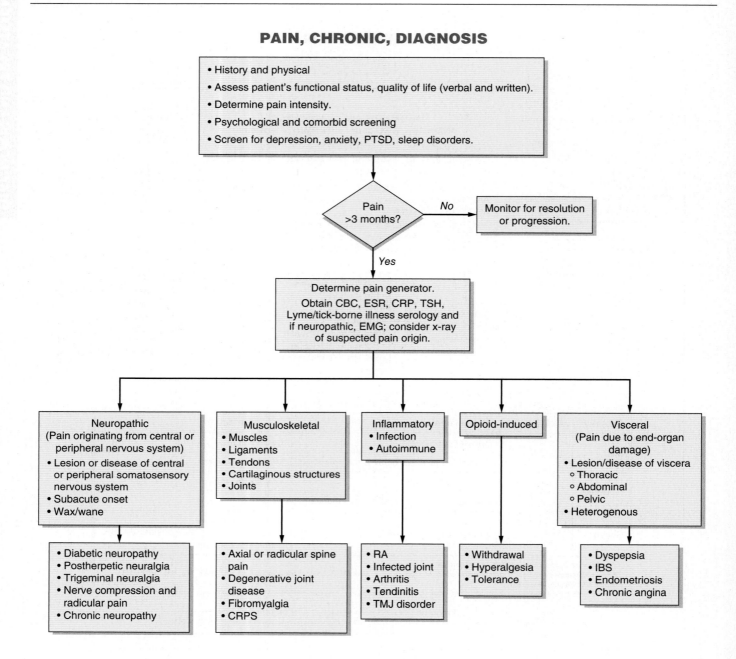

- History and physical
- Assess patient's functional status, quality of life (verbal and written).
- Determine pain intensity.
- Psychological and comorbid screening
- Screen for depression, anxiety, PTSD, sleep disorders.

Pain >3 months?

No → Monitor for resolution or progression.

Yes

Determine pain generator.
Obtain CBC, ESR, CRP, TSH, Lyme/tick-borne illness serology and if neuropathic, EMG; consider x-ray of suspected pain origin.

Neuropathic
(Pain originating from central or peripheral nervous system)
- Lesion or disease of central or peripheral somatosensory nervous system
- Subacute onset
- Wax/wane

Musculoskeletal
- Muscles
- Ligaments
- Tendons
- Cartilaginous structures
- Joints

Inflammatory
- Infection
- Autoimmune

Opioid-induced

Visceral
(Pain due to end-organ damage)
- Lesion/disease of viscera
  ○ Thoracic
  ○ Abdominal
  ○ Pelvic
- Heterogenous

- Diabetic neuropathy
- Postherpetic neuralgia
- Trigeminal neuralgia
- Nerve compression and radicular pain
- Chronic neuropathy

- Axial or radicular spine pain
- Degenerative joint disease
- Fibromyalgia
- CRPS

- RA
- Infected joint
- Arthritis
- Tendinitis
- TMJ disorder

- Withdrawal
- Hyperalgesia
- Tolerance

- Dyspepsia
- IBS
- Endometriosis
- Chronic angina

Bruce Palmer Freshley Jr., MD

Hooten M, Thorson D, Bianco J, et al. *Pain: Assessment, Non-Opioid Treatment Approaches and Opioid Management*. Bloomington, MN: Institute for Clinical Systems Improvement; 2017.

PALPABLE BREAST MASS

Obtain a detailed history and perform a clinical breast exam (CBE).

Order breast imaging:
- If <30 years old (yo), order a directed sonogram.
  - *If <30 yo and high clinical suspicion for malignancy or mass not visualized on ultrasound, also order a diagnostic mammogram.*
- If ≥30 yo, order a directed sonogram and diagnostic mammogram.

BI-RADS 1 or 3   BI-RADS 4 or 5   BI-RADS 2

Is clinical suspicion high or low?

Benign finding (i.e., cyst, lipoma, lymph node)

Low   *High*

Monitor

- If <30 yo, w/ CBE and/or sonogram every 6–12 months for 1–2 years
- If ≥30 yo, w/ CBE and sonogram/mammogram every 6 months for 1–2 years
- *CBE ideally performed on days 10–12 of menstrual cycle*

- Core needle biopsy by radiologist or surgeon
- If needle biopsy is not possible, refer to surgeon.

No

Is lesion unchanged?

Yes

Resume routine screening.

Adwoa A. Adu, MD

Salzman B, Collins E, Hersh L. Common breast problems. *Am Fam Physician*. 2019;99(8):505–514.

PALPITATIONS, ADULT

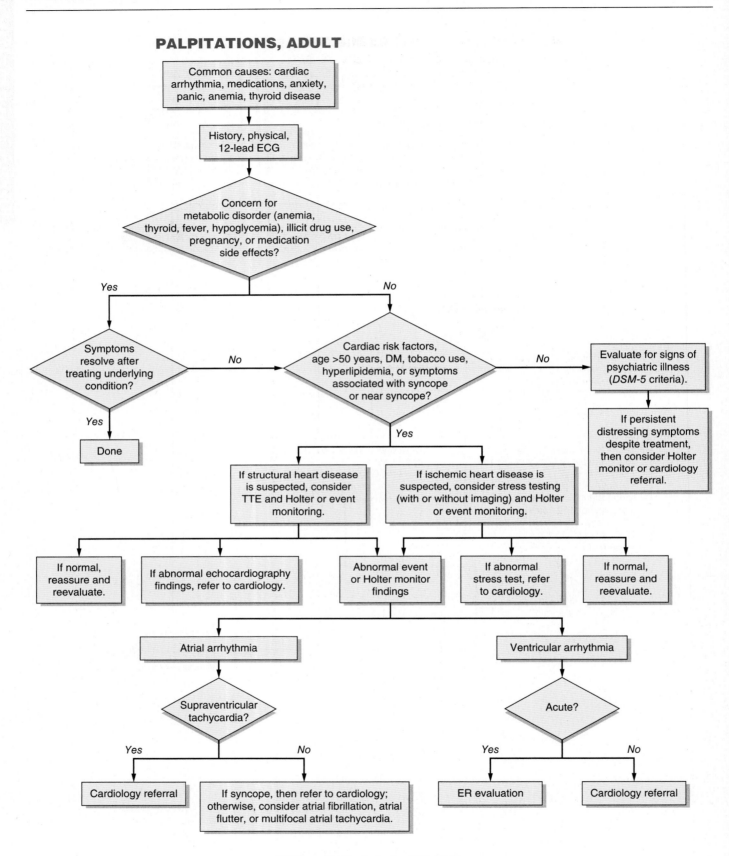

William E. Cayley Jr., MD, Mdiv

Wexler RK, Pleister A, Raman SV. Palpitations: evaluation in the primary care setting. *Am Fam Physician*. 2017;96(12):784–789.

DIAGNOSIS AND TREATMENT

PAP, NORMAL AND ABNORMAL IN NONPREGNANT WOMEN AGES 25 YEARS AND OLDER

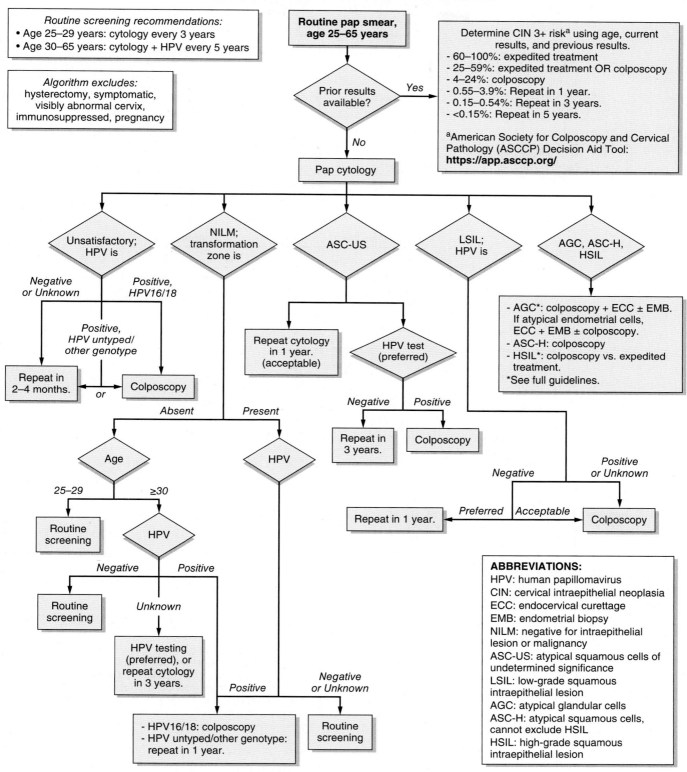

Emmeline Ha, MD and Kristen Nayak, MD

Perkins RB, Guido RS, Castle PE, et al; for 2019 ASCCP Risk-Based Management Consensus Guidelines Committee. 2019 ASCCP Risk-Based Management Consensus Guidelines for abnormal cervical cancer screening tests and cancer precursors. *J Low Genit Tract Dis.* 2020;24(2):102–131.

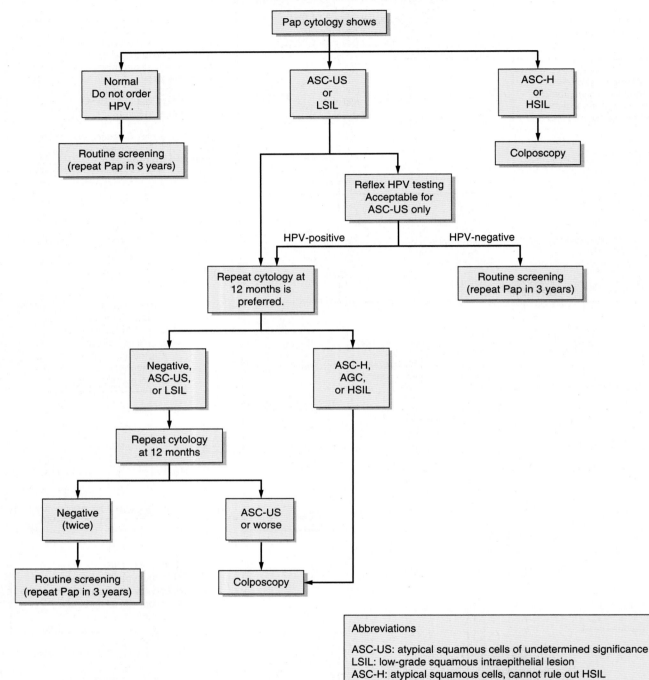

PAP, NORMAL AND ABNORMAL IN WOMEN AGES 21–24 YEARS

Pap cytology shows

- Normal — Do not order HPV. → Routine screening (repeat Pap in 3 years)
- ASC-US or LSIL → Reflex HPV testing Acceptable for ASC-US only
  - HPV-positive → Repeat cytology at 12 months is preferred.
    - Negative, ASC-US, or LSIL → Repeat cytology at 12 months
      - Negative (twice) → Routine screening (repeat Pap in 3 years)
      - ASC-US or worse → Colposcopy
    - ASC-H, AGC, or HSIL → Colposcopy
  - HPV-negative → Routine screening (repeat Pap in 3 years)
- ASC-H or HSIL → Colposcopy

Abbreviations

ASC-US: atypical squamous cells of undetermined significance
LSIL: low-grade squamous intraepithelial lesion
ASC-H: atypical squamous cells, cannot rule out HSIL
HSIL: high-grade squamous intraepithelial lesion
HPV: human papillomavirus
AGC: atypical glandular cells

Pratiksha Yalakkishettar, MD and Manju Mahajan, MD, FAAFP

Perkins RB, Guido RS, Castle PE, et al. 2019 ASCCP risk-based management guidelines for abnormal cervical cancer screening tests and cancer precursors. *J Low Genit Tract Dis*. 2020;24(2):102–131.

PARKINSON DISEASE, TREATMENT

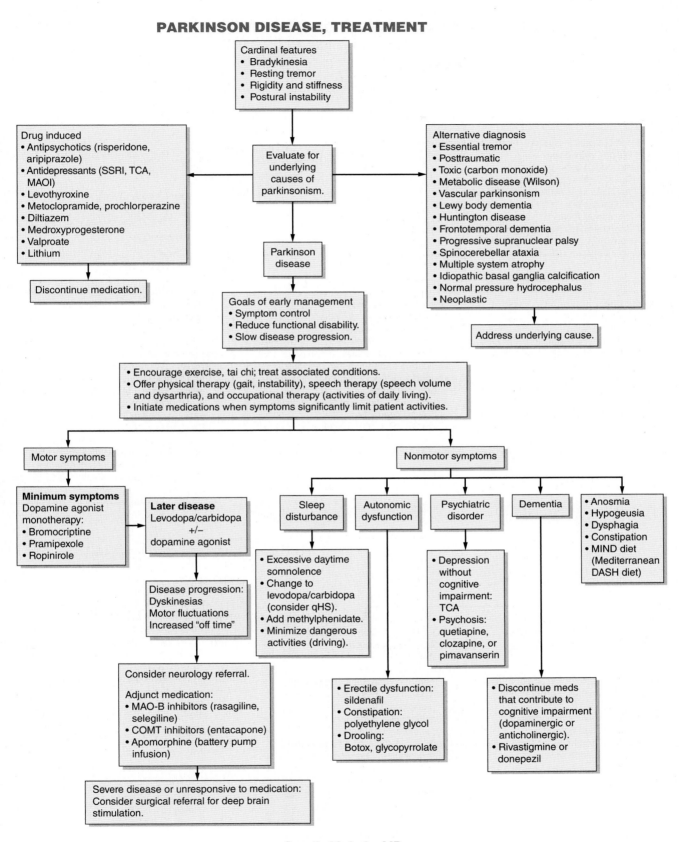

Cardinal features
- Bradykinesia
- Resting tremor
- Rigidity and stiffness
- Postural instability

Drug induced
- Antipsychotics (risperidone, aripiprazole)
- Antidepressants (SSRI, TCA, MAOI)
- Levothyroxine
- Metoclopramide, prochlorperazine
- Diltiazem
- Medroxyprogesterone
- Valproate
- Lithium

Evaluate for underlying causes of parkinsonism.

Alternative diagnosis
- Essential tremor
- Posttraumatic
- Toxic (carbon monoxide)
- Metabolic disease (Wilson)
- Vascular parkinsonism
- Lewy body dementia
- Huntington disease
- Frontotemporal dementia
- Progressive supranuclear palsy
- Spinocerebellar ataxia
- Multiple system atrophy
- Idiopathic basal ganglia calcification
- Normal pressure hydrocephalus
- Neoplastic

Discontinue medication.

Parkinson disease

Goals of early management
- Symptom control
- Reduce functional disability.
- Slow disease progression.

Address underlying cause.

- Encourage exercise, tai chi; treat associated conditions.
- Offer physical therapy (gait, instability), speech therapy (speech volume and dysarthria), and occupational therapy (activities of daily living).
- Initiate medications when symptoms significantly limit patient activities.

Motor symptoms

Nonmotor symptoms

Minimum symptoms
Dopamine agonist monotherapy:
- Bromocriptine
- Pramipexole
- Ropinirole

Later disease
Levodopa/carbidopa
+/–
dopamine agonist

Sleep disturbance

Autonomic dysfunction

Psychiatric disorder

Dementia

- Anosmia
- Hypogeusia
- Dysphagia
- Constipation
- MIND diet (Mediterranean DASH diet)

Disease progression:
Dyskinesias
Motor fluctuations
Increased "off time"

- Excessive daytime somnolence
- Change to levodopa/carbidopa (consider qHS).
- Add methylphenidate.
- Minimize dangerous activities (driving).

- Depression without cognitive impairment: TCA
- Psychosis: quetiapine, clozapine, or pimavanserin

Consider neurology referral.

Adjunct medication:
- MAO-B inhibitors (rasagiline, selegiline)
- COMT inhibitors (entacapone)
- Apomorphine (battery pump infusion)

- Erectile dysfunction: sildenafil
- Constipation: polyethylene glycol
- Drooling: Botox, glycopyrrolate

- Discontinue meds that contribute to cognitive impairment (dopaminergic or anticholinergic).
- Rivastigmine or donepezil

Severe disease or unresponsive to medication: Consider surgical referral for deep brain stimulation.

Saadia Mohsin, MD

Connolly BS, Lang AE. Pharmacological treatment of Parkinson disease: a review. *JAMA*. 2014;311(16):1670–1683.

PEDIATRIC EXANTHEMS, DIAGNOSTIC

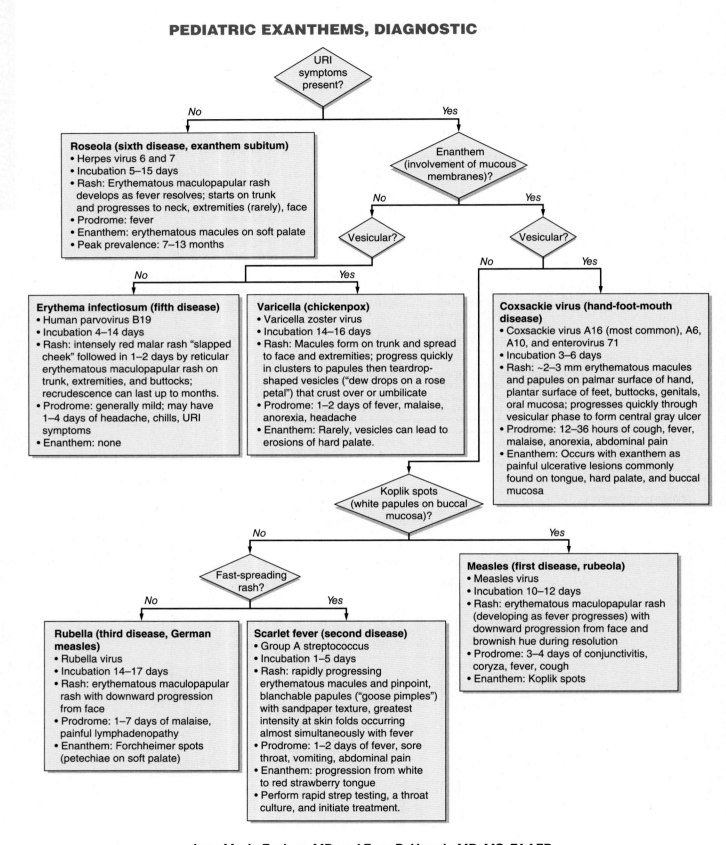

URI symptoms present?

No → **Roseola (sixth disease, exanthem subitum)**
- Herpes virus 6 and 7
- Incubation 5–15 days
- Rash: Erythematous maculopapular rash develops as fever resolves; starts on trunk and progresses to neck, extremities (rarely), face
- Prodrome: fever
- Enanthem: erythematous macules on soft palate
- Peak prevalence: 7–13 months

Yes → **Enanthem (involvement of mucous membranes)?**

No → **Vesicular?**

Yes → **Vesicular?**

Vesicular? No → **Erythema infectiosum (fifth disease)**
- Human parvovirus B19
- Incubation 4–14 days
- Rash: intensely red malar rash "slapped cheek" followed in 1–2 days by reticular erythematous maculopapular rash on trunk, extremities, and buttocks; recrudescence can last up to months.
- Prodrome: generally mild; may have 1–4 days of headache, chills, URI symptoms
- Enanthem: none

Vesicular? Yes → **Varicella (chickenpox)**
- Varicella zoster virus
- Incubation 14–16 days
- Rash: Macules form on trunk and spread to face and extremities; progress quickly in clusters to papules then teardrop-shaped vesicles ("dew drops on a rose petal") that crust over or umbilicate
- Prodrome: 1–2 days of fever, malaise, anorexia, headache
- Enanthem: Rarely, vesicles can lead to erosions of hard palate.

Vesicular? Yes → **Coxsackie virus (hand-foot-mouth disease)**
- Coxsackie virus A16 (most common), A6, A10, and enterovirus 71
- Incubation 3–6 days
- Rash: ~2–3 mm erythematous macules and papules on palmar surface of hand, plantar surface of feet, buttocks, genitals, oral mucosa; progresses quickly through vesicular phase to form central gray ulcer
- Prodrome: 12–36 hours of cough, fever, malaise, anorexia, abdominal pain
- Enanthem: Occurs with exanthem as painful ulcerative lesions commonly found on tongue, hard palate, and buccal mucosa

Koplik spots (white papules on buccal mucosa)?

No → **Fast-spreading rash?**

Yes → **Measles (first disease, rubeola)**
- Measles virus
- Incubation 10–12 days
- Rash: erythematous maculopapular rash (developing as fever progresses) with downward progression from face and brownish hue during resolution
- Prodrome: 3–4 days of conjunctivitis, coryza, fever, cough
- Enanthem: Koplik spots

Fast-spreading rash? No → **Rubella (third disease, German measles)**
- Rubella virus
- Incubation 14–17 days
- Rash: erythematous maculopapular rash with downward progression from face
- Prodrome: 1–7 days of malaise, painful lymphadenopathy
- Enanthem: Forchheimer spots (petechiae on soft palate)

Fast-spreading rash? Yes → **Scarlet fever (second disease)**
- Group A streptococcus
- Incubation 1–5 days
- Rash: rapidly progressing erythematous macules and pinpoint, blanchable papules ("goose pimples") with sandpaper texture, greatest intensity at skin folds occurring almost simultaneously with fever
- Prodrome: 1–2 days of fever, sore throat, vomiting, abdominal pain
- Enanthem: progression from white to red strawberry tongue
- Perform rapid strep testing, a throat culture, and initiate treatment.

Jane Marie Forbes, MD and Fern R. Hauck, MD, MS, FAAFP

Dyer JA. Childhood viral exanthems. *Pediatr Ann*. 2007;36(1):21–29.

PELVIC PAIN

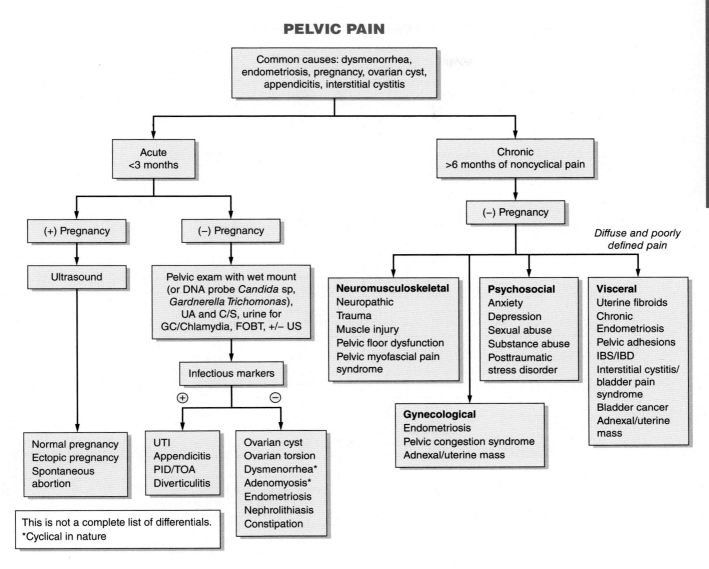

Common causes: dysmenorrhea, endometriosis, pregnancy, ovarian cyst, appendicitis, interstitial cystitis

Acute
<3 months

Chronic
>6 months of noncyclical pain

(+) Pregnancy

(−) Pregnancy

Ultrasound

Pelvic exam with wet mount (or DNA probe *Candida* sp, *Gardnerella Trichomonas*), UA and C/S, urine for GC/Chlamydia, FOBT, +/− US

(−) Pregnancy

Diffuse and poorly defined pain

Infectious markers

⊕   ⊖

Neuromusculoskeletal
Neuropathic
Trauma
Muscle injury
Pelvic floor dysfunction
Pelvic myofascial pain syndrome

Psychosocial
Anxiety
Depression
Sexual abuse
Substance abuse
Posttraumatic stress disorder

Visceral
Uterine fibroids
Chronic Endometriosis
Pelvic adhesions
IBS/IBD
Interstitial cystitis/bladder pain syndrome
Bladder cancer
Adnexal/uterine mass

Normal pregnancy
Ectopic pregnancy
Spontaneous abortion

UTI
Appendicitis
PID/TOA
Diverticulitis

Ovarian cyst
Ovarian torsion
Dysmenorrhea*
Adenomyosis*
Endometriosis
Nephrolithiasis
Constipation

Gynecological
Endometriosis
Pelvic congestion syndrome
Adnexal/uterine mass

This is not a complete list of differentials.
*Cyclical in nature

Wendy S. Biggs, MD and Taylor Gaudard, MD, IBCLC

Learman LA, McHugh KW; for American College of Obstetricians and Gynecologists' Committee on Practice Bulletins—Gynecology. ACOG Practice Bulletin Number 218: chronic pelvic pain. *Obstet Gynecol.* 2020;135(3):e98–e109.

POISON EXPOSURE AND TREATMENT
POISON EXPOSURE

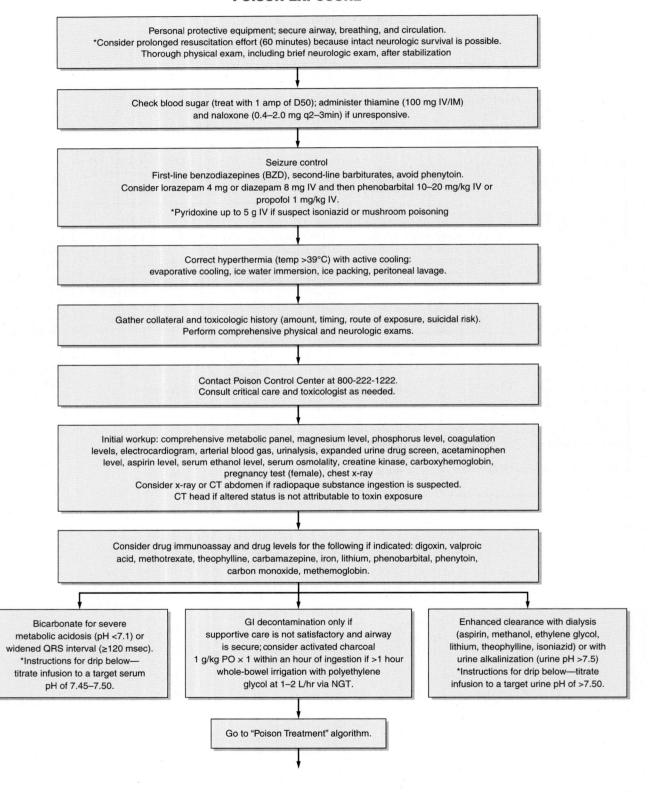

Personal protective equipment; secure airway, breathing, and circulation.
*Consider prolonged resuscitation effort (60 minutes) because intact neurologic survival is possible.
Thorough physical exam, including brief neurologic exam, after stabilization

Check blood sugar (treat with 1 amp of D50); administer thiamine (100 mg IV/IM)
and naloxone (0.4–2.0 mg q2–3min) if unresponsive.

Seizure control
First-line benzodiazepines (BZD), second-line barbiturates, avoid phenytoin.
Consider lorazepam 4 mg or diazepam 8 mg IV and then phenobarbital 10–20 mg/kg IV or
propofol 1 mg/kg IV.
*Pyridoxine up to 5 g IV if suspect isoniazid or mushroom poisoning

Correct hyperthermia (temp >39°C) with active cooling:
evaporative cooling, ice water immersion, ice packing, peritoneal lavage.

Gather collateral and toxicologic history (amount, timing, route of exposure, suicidal risk).
Perform comprehensive physical and neurologic exams.

Contact Poison Control Center at 800-222-1222.
Consult critical care and toxicologist as needed.

Initial workup: comprehensive metabolic panel, magnesium level, phosphorus level, coagulation
levels, electrocardiogram, arterial blood gas, urinalysis, expanded urine drug screen, acetaminophen
level, aspirin level, serum ethanol level, serum osmolality, creatine kinase, carboxyhemoglobin,
pregnancy test (female), chest x-ray
Consider x-ray or CT abdomen if radiopaque substance ingestion is suspected.
CT head if altered status is not attributable to toxin exposure

Consider drug immunoassay and drug levels for the following if indicated: digoxin, valproic
acid, methotrexate, theophylline, carbamazepine, iron, lithium, phenobarbital, phenytoin,
carbon monoxide, methemoglobin.

Bicarbonate for severe
metabolic acidosis (pH <7.1) or
widened QRS interval (≥120 msec).
*Instructions for drip below—
titrate infusion to a target serum
pH of 7.45–7.50.

GI decontamination only if
supportive care is not satisfactory and airway
is secure; consider activated charcoal
1 g/kg PO × 1 within an hour of ingestion if >1 hour
whole-bowel irrigation with polyethylene
glycol at 1–2 L/hr via NGT.

Enhanced clearance with dialysis
(aspirin, methanol, ethylene glycol,
lithium, theophylline, isoniazid) or with
urine alkalinization (urine pH >7.5)
*Instructions for drip below—titrate
infusion to a target urine pH of >7.50.

Go to "Poison Treatment" algorithm.

POISON TREATMENT

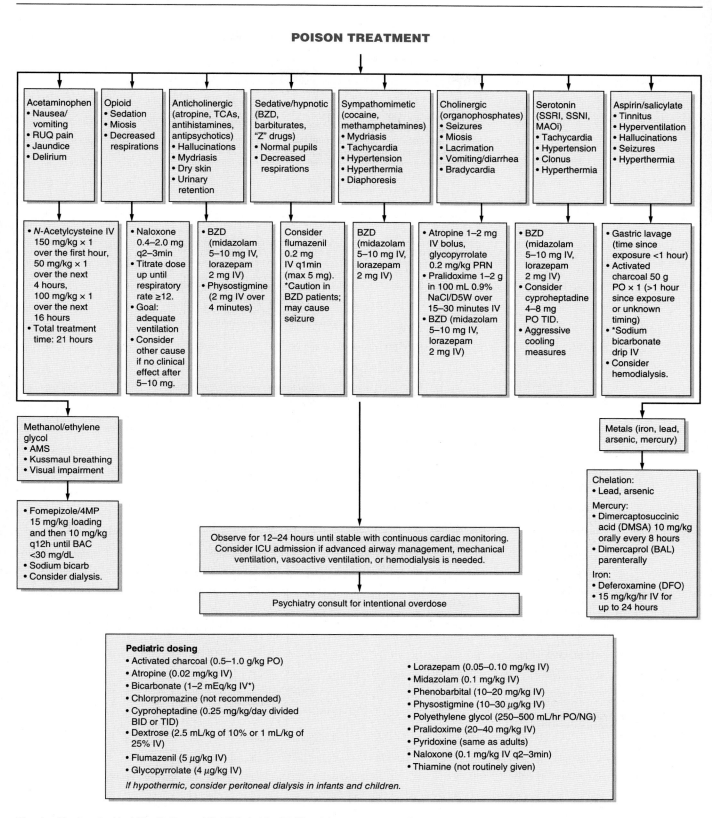

Acetaminophen
- Nausea/vomiting
- RUQ pain
- Jaundice
- Delirium

Opioid
- Sedation
- Miosis
- Decreased respirations

Anticholinergic (atropine, TCAs, antihistamines, antipsychotics)
- Hallucinations
- Mydriasis
- Dry skin
- Urinary retention

Sedative/hypnotic (BZD, barbiturates, "Z" drugs)
- Normal pupils
- Decreased respirations

Sympathomimetic (cocaine, methamphetamines)
- Mydriasis
- Tachycardia
- Hypertension
- Hyperthermia
- Diaphoresis

Cholinergic (organophosphates)
- Seizures
- Miosis
- Lacrimation
- Vomiting/diarrhea
- Bradycardia

Serotonin (SSRI, SSNI, MAOi)
- Tachycardia
- Hypertension
- Clonus
- Hyperthermia

Aspirin/salicylate
- Tinnitus
- Hyperventilation
- Hallucinations
- Seizures
- Hyperthermia

- *N*-Acetylcysteine IV 150 mg/kg × 1 over the first hour, 50 mg/kg × 1 over the next 4 hours, 100 mg/kg × 1 over the next 16 hours
- Total treatment time: 21 hours

- Naloxone 0.4–2.0 mg q2–3min
- Titrate dose up until respiratory rate ≥12.
- Goal: adequate ventilation
- Consider other cause if no clinical effect after 5–10 mg.

- BZD (midazolam 5–10 mg IV, lorazepam 2 mg IV)
- Physostigmine (2 mg IV over 4 minutes)

- Consider flumazenil 0.2 mg IV q1min (max 5 mg). *Caution in BZD patients; may cause seizure

- BZD (midazolam 5–10 mg IV, lorazepam 2 mg IV)

- Atropine 1–2 mg IV bolus, glycopyrrolate 0.2 mg/kg PRN
- Pralidoxime 1–2 g in 100 mL 0.9% NaCl/D5W over 15–30 minutes IV
- BZD (midazolam 5–10 mg IV, lorazepam 2 mg IV)

- BZD (midazolam 5–10 mg IV, lorazepam 2 mg IV)
- Consider cyproheptadine 4–8 mg PO TID.
- Aggressive cooling measures

- Gastric lavage (time since exposure <1 hour)
- Activated charcoal 50 g PO × 1 (>1 hour since exposure or unknown timing)
- *Sodium bicarbonate drip IV
- Consider hemodialysis.

Methanol/ethylene glycol
- AMS
- Kussmaul breathing
- Visual impairment

- Fomepizole/4MP 15 mg/kg loading and then 10 mg/kg q12h until BAC <30 mg/dL
- Sodium bicarb
- Consider dialysis.

Metals (iron, lead, arsenic, mercury)

Chelation:
- Lead, arsenic

Mercury:
- Dimercaptosuccinic acid (DMSA) 10 mg/kg orally every 8 hours
- Dimercaprol (BAL) parenterally

Iron:
- Deferoxamine (DFO)
- 15 mg/kg/hr IV for up to 24 hours

Observe for 12–24 hours until stable with continuous cardiac monitoring. Consider ICU admission if advanced airway management, mechanical ventilation, vasoactive ventilation, or hemodialysis is needed.

Psychiatry consult for intentional overdose

Pediatric dosing
- Activated charcoal (0.5–1.0 g/kg PO)
- Atropine (0.02 mg/kg IV)
- Bicarbonate (1–2 mEq/kg IV*)
- Chlorpromazine (not recommended)
- Cyproheptadine (0.25 mg/kg/day divided BID or TID)
- Dextrose (2.5 mL/kg of 10% or 1 mL/kg of 25% IV)
- Flumazenil (5 µg/kg IV)
- Glycopyrrolate (4 µg/kg IV)

- Lorazepam (0.05–0.10 mg/kg IV)
- Midazolam (0.1 mg/kg IV)
- Phenobarbital (10–20 mg/kg IV)
- Physostigmine (10–30 µg/kg IV)
- Polyethylene glycol (250–500 mL/hr PO/NG)
- Pralidoxime (20–40 mg/kg IV)
- Pyridoxine (same as adults)
- Naloxone (0.1 mg/kg IV q2–3min)
- Thiamine (not routinely given)

If hypothermic, consider peritoneal dialysis in infants and children.

*To mix a bicarbonate drip: 150 mEq (3 amps) $NaHCO_3$ in 1 L of D5W and then start at a rate of 150–200 mL/hr.

Erin Johnson, MD and Frank J. Domino, MD

Ornillo C, Harbord N. Fundaments of toxicology—approach to the poisoned patient. *Adv Chronic Kidney Dis.* 2020;27(1):5–10.

PRECOCIOUS PUBERTY

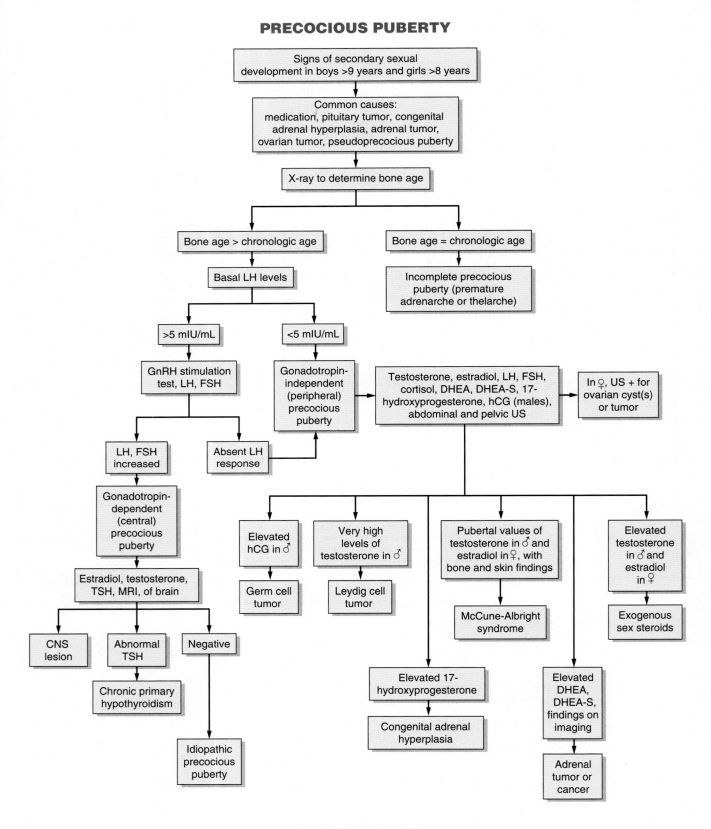

Frank J. Domino, MD

Berberoğlu M. Precocious puberty and normal variant puberty: definition, etiology, diagnosis and current management. *J Clin Res Pediatr Endocrinol.* 2009;1(4):164–174.

PREOPERATIVE EVALUATION OF NONCARDIAC SURGICAL PATIENT

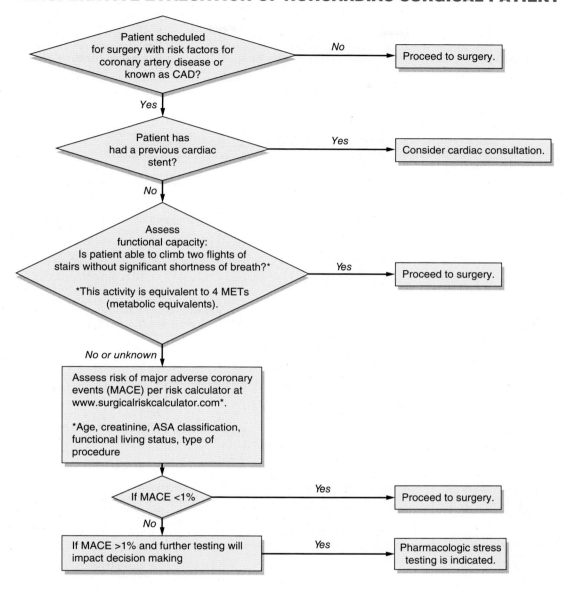

Andrew Grimes, MD

Smilowitz NR, Berger JS. Perioperative cardiovascular risk assessment and management for noncardiac surgery: a review. *JAMA*. 2020;324(3):279–290.

PROTEINURIA

Defined as >150 mg/24 hr urine
Common causes and reasons to screen: hypertension, diabetes, glomerular disease, cardiovascular disease, congestive heart disease, multiple myeloma, nephrotic syndrome, fever, urinary tract infection, orthostatic hypertension, lupus. Perform history and physical.

If at any point in the workup there is high clinical suspicion for disease, if the patient is symptomatic, GFR <30, or if renal disease is discovered, then consult nephrology.

Underlying cause of proteinuria identified through history and physical exam? — *Yes* → Treat underlying cause.

No

Obtain urinalysis.

Normal GFR range for healthy adults: greater than 90 mL/min/1.73 m^2

Semiquantitative urinalysis ranges (albumin)
Negative: 0 mg/dL
Trace: 15–30 mg/dL
1+: 30–100 mg/dL
2+: 100–300 mg/dL
3+: 300–1,000 mg/dL
4+: >1,000 mg/dL

Albuminuria and GFR are independent risk factors for the progression of chronic kidney disease.

Trace to 2+.

2+ or greater

Obtain repeat urinalysis in 1–2 weeks.

2+ or greater →

Obtain serum creatinine to determine GFR and urine albumin creatinine ratio (ACR) or instead evaluate with 24-hour urine.

ACR >30 mg/g + reduced GFR or ACR >300 mg/g or 24-hour urine > 2 g

<2+

ACR <300 mg/g without decreased GFR or 24-hour urine <2 g

Transient (Consider fever, heavy physical activity, UTI, CHF, urologic hemorrhage, orthostatic proteinuria.)
Reassurance and f/u as needed

Evaluate for orthostatic proteinuria with first morning void and random void. If normal first morning void and elevated random sample, diagnose orthostatic proteinuria.

Obtain renal ultrasound and UPEP. Consult nephrology.

If UPEP is abnormal, consult heme/onc; may be concern for multiple myeloma

Continue to monitor blood pressure, urinalysis, and renal function yearly.

Consider additional labs and evaluate for the following as clinically indicated:
• ANA (lupus)
• Antistreptolysin O titer (streptococcal glomerulonephritis)
• C3/C4 (glomerulonephritis)
• ESR (rule out inflammation/infection)
• Fasting glucose (diabetes)
• H/H (will be low in chronic renal failure)
• HIV, VDRL, hepatitis serologies
• Serum albumin and lipid levels (Consider nephrotic syndrome.)
• Serum electrolytes
• Serum urate (Elevation can cause tubulointerstitial disease.)
• Chest radiograph (systemic disease such as sarcoidosis, etc.)

Ulysses Fernandez-Miro, DO and Pamela R. Hughes, MD

Waheed S. Evaluation of proteinuria. https://bestpractice.bmj.com/topics/en-us/875. Updated February 25, 2022. Accessed October 12, 2022.

PULMONARY EMBOLISM, DIAGNOSIS

Assess Pulmonary Embolism Rule Out Criteria (PERC).
If any of the following are true, then the patient is considered PERC-positive;
1. Patient is >49 years.
2. Patient's pulse >99 beats/min
3. Patient's pulse oximetry reading <95% on room air
4. Patient with hemoptysis
5. Patient taking exogenous estrogen
6. Patient had a previous VTE diagnosis.
7. Patient had surgery or trauma, which required intubation or hospitalization in the last 4 weeks.
8. Patient has unilateral leg swelling of the calves.

*Age-adjusted D-dimer (for patients >50 years) Threshold = age × 10 ng/mL; D-dimer < age-adjusted cutoff is negative result; D-dimer > age-adjusted cutoff is positive result.

Assess mortality risk.
Simplified Pulmonary Embolism Severity Index (sPESI)

>80 years old	1
Cancer	1
Congestive heart failure	1
Heart rate >110 beats/min	1
Systolic blood pressure <100 mm Hg	1
O$_2$ saturation <90	1

0 points = can consider early discharge or outpatient treatment
≥1 point(s) = consider inpatient treatment

Clinical signs/symptoms of pulmonary embolism (PE)

Clinically stable? — **No** → Stabilize and consider empiric anticoagulation. TTE to evaluate RV strain or dysfunction

Yes

Clinical pretest probability score?

Stabilize and consider empiric anticoagulation. TTE to evaluate RV strain or dysfunction → PE confirmed → Thrombolysis, surgery, or catheter embolectomy if hypotensive

→ PE ruled out → Consider alternative diagnosis.

PERC score? ← <2   2–6   >6

Wells PE rule (pretest probability):

Variable	Points
Signs/symptoms of DVT	3
Alternative diagnosis less likely than PE	3
Pulse >100 beats/min	1.5
Immobility/surgery in prior 4 weeks	1.5
History of VTE	1.5
Active cancer	1
Hemoptysis	1

Negative   Positive

*Highly sensitive D-dimer?

Consider alternative diagnosis. ← Negative   Positive

Spiral CT angiography → Inconclusive results or unable to perform CT (i.e., renal failure or contrast allergy)

Positive

PE confirmed

V/Q scan

High probability of PE | Inconclusive (low to intermediate probability) | Low probability and low CPTP | Normal V/Q scan

Treat with anticoagulation and consider thrombolysis if becomes unstable.

Consider alternative imaging: serial lower extremity venous ultrasound, pulmonary angiography, MRA, or V/Q SPECT.

Consider alternative diagnosis.

sPESI score? → See "Pulmonary Embolism, Treatment" algorithm.

Lawrence M. Gibbs, MD, MSEd and Melissa L. Smith, MD, MS, FAAFP

Konstantinides SV, Meyer G, Becattini C, et al. 2019 ESC guidelines for the diagnosis and management of acute pulmonary embolism developed in collaboration with the European Respiratory Society (ERS). *Eur Heart J*. 2020;41(4):543–603.

PULMONARY EMBOLISM, TREATMENT

Probability of pulmonary embolism above treatment threshold

Anticoagulation contraindicated?
- Yes → **IVC filter**
- No ↓

- Consider oral anticoagulant. Apixaban or rivaroxaban do not need parenteral bridging, whereas dabigatran and edoxaban require 5–10 days of parental therapy.
- Alternatively, consider fondaparinux or argatroban (caution use of argatroban in liver disease) and vitamin K antagonist (warfarin) with at least 5 days of concomitant therapy. When used in combination, goal INR prior to discontinuation of the parenteral product is as follows: INR >2 (fondaparinux) or >4 (argatroban) × 24 hours. Of note, argatroban falsely elevates the INR, which can be misleading when given in combination with vitamin K antagonist. Once the INR is >4, discontinue the argatroban and recheck the INR in 4–6 hours with a goal INR 2–3.
- Prior to using vitamin K antagonist (warfarin) for new-onset heparin-induced thrombocytopenia, be sure platelets are >150,000.

For all patients, assess for treatment at home versus in hospital; for example, Pulmonary Embolism Severity Index (PESI):
- If very low or low risk: Consider outpatient management.
- If intermediate, high, or very high risk: Consider inpatient management.

Massive pulmonary embolism?
- SBP <90 mm Hg for 15 minutes
- Fall in SBP >40 mm Hg for 15 minutes
- Requiring vasopressors
- Persistent bradycardia
- Cardiac arrest

Yes → / No ↓

Thrombolysis contraindicated?
- Prior intracranial bleed
- Ischemic stroke <3 months
- Suspected aortic dissection
- Active bleeding diathesis
- Recent brain or spinal surgery
- Closed head or facial trauma

- No ↓ / Yes →

Benefits of thrombolysis may outweigh risks IF: hemodynamic instability, worsening oxygenation, severe RV, or major myocardial necrosis. Thrombolysis indicated?
- Yes →
- No ↓

- Interventional Radiology or surgical embolectomy, per local expertise
- ECMO

Thrombolysis using tPA (can be given systemically or catheter directed based on bleeding risk)

History of heparin-induced thrombocytopenia?
- Yes →
- No ↓

Clinical improvement?
- Yes →
- No →

Begin:
- Oral anticoagulant therapy: Apixaban or rivaroxaban do not need parenteral bridging, whereas dabigatran and edoxaban require 5–10 days of parenteral therapy.

  OR

- Therapeutic dose low-molecular-weight heparin (LMWH)

  OR

- Heparin infusion to therapeutic aPTT or therapeutic LMWH and warfarin, discontinuing LMWH when INR >2 for at least 24 hours and minimum 5 days of concomitant therapy; goal INR 2–3

Emmeline Ha, MD and Jason Teng, MD

Kearon C, Akl EA, Ornelas J, et al. Antithrombotic therapy for VTE disease: CHEST guideline and expert panel report. *Chest.* 2016;149(2):315–352. doi:10.1016/j.chest.2015.11.026.

RASH

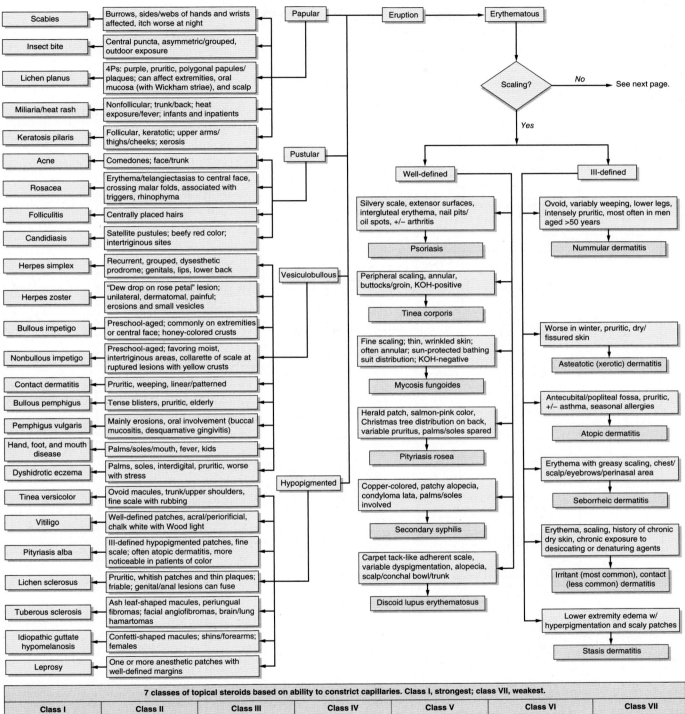

7 classes of topical steroids based on ability to constrict capillaries. Class I, strongest; class VII, weakest.						
Class I	**Class II**	**Class III**	**Class IV**	**Class V**	**Class VI**	**Class VII**
Clobetasol propionate ointment, cream, 0.05% (Temovate)	Fluocinonide ointment, cream, gel, 0.05% (Lidex)	Triamcinolone acetonide ointment, 0.1% (Aristocort A)	Triamcinolone acetonide cream, 0.1% (Kenalog)	Fluocinolone acetonide cream, 0.025% (Synalar)	Desonide cream, 0.05% (DesOwen)	Hydrocortisone, 0.5%, 1%, 2.5% (Hytone)
Betamethasone dipropionate ointment, cream, 0.05% (Diprolene, Diprosone)	Amcinonide ointment, 0.1% (Cyclocort)	Betamethasone valerate ointment, 0.01% (Valisone)	Mometasone furoate cream, 0.1% (Elocon)	Fluticasone propionate cream, 0.05% (Cutivate)	Prednicarbate 0.1% cream (Dermatop)	
Halobetasol propionate ointment, cream, 0.05% (Ultravate)	Desoximetasone ointment, cream, 0.25%; gel, 0.05% (Topicort)	Fluticasone propionate ointment, 0.05% (Cutivate)	Hydrocortisone valerate ointment, 0.2% (Westcort)	Hydrocortisone valerate cream, 0.2% (Westcort)	Alclometasone dipropionate ointment, cream, 0.05% (Aclovate)	

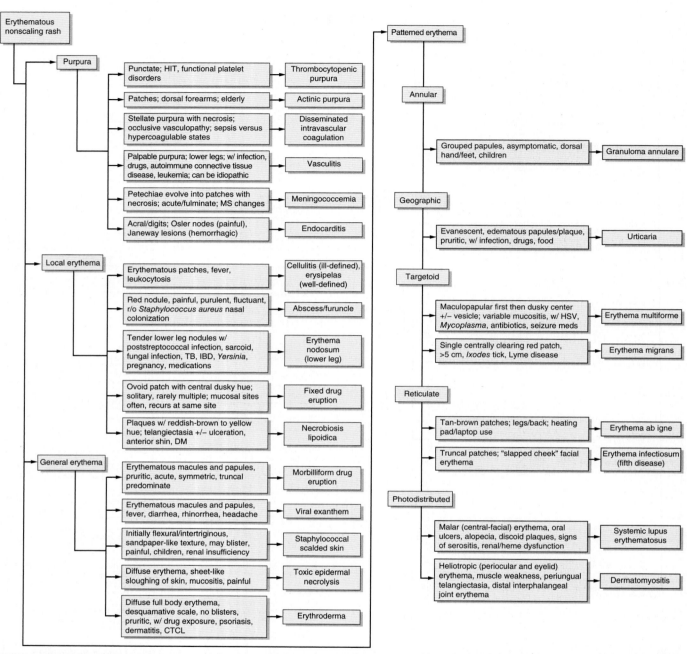

Erythematous nonscaling rash		

Purpura
- Punctate; HIT, functional platelet disorders → Thrombocytopenic purpura
- Patches; dorsal forearms; elderly → Actinic purpura
- Stellate purpura with necrosis; occlusive vasculopathy; sepsis versus hypercoagulable states → Disseminated intravascular coagulation
- Palpable purpura; lower legs; w/ infection, drugs, autoimmune connective tissue disease, leukemia; can be idiopathic → Vasculitis
- Petechiae evolve into patches with necrosis; acute/fulminate; MS changes → Meningococcemia
- Acral/digits; Osler nodes (painful), Janeway lesions (hemorrhagic) → Endocarditis

Local erythema
- Erythematous patches, fever, leukocytosis → Cellulitis (ill-defined), erysipelas (well-defined)
- Red nodule, painful, purulent, fluctuant, r/o *Staphylococcus aureus* nasal colonization → Abscess/furuncle
- Tender lower leg nodules w/ poststreptococcal infection, sarcoid, fungal infection, TB, IBD, *Yersinia*, pregnancy, medications → Erythema nodosum (lower leg)
- Ovoid patch with central dusky hue; solitary, rarely multiple; mucosal sites often, recurs at same site → Fixed drug eruption
- Plaques w/ reddish-brown to yellow hue; telangiectasia +/− ulceration, anterior shin, DM → Necrobiosis lipoidica

General erythema
- Erythematous macules and papules, pruritic, acute, symmetric, truncal predominate → Morbilliform drug eruption
- Erythematous macules and papules, fever, diarrhea, rhinorrhea, headache → Viral exanthem
- Initially flexural/intertriginous, sandpaper-like texture, may blister, painful, children, renal insufficiency → Staphylococcal scalded skin
- Diffuse erythema, sheet-like sloughing of skin, mucositis, painful → Toxic epidermal necrolysis
- Diffuse full body erythema, desquamative scale, no blisters, pruritic, w/ drug exposure, psoriasis, dermatitis, CTCL → Erythroderma

Patterned erythema

Annular
- Grouped papules, asymptomatic, dorsal hand/feet, children → Granuloma annulare

Geographic
- Evanescent, edematous papules/plaque, pruritic, w/ infection, drugs, food → Urticaria

Targetoid
- Maculopapular first then dusky center +/− vesicle; variable mucositis, w/ HSV, *Mycoplasma*, antibiotics, seizure meds → Erythema multiforme
- Single centrally clearing red patch, >5 cm, *Ixodes* tick, Lyme disease → Erythema migrans

Reticulate
- Tan-brown patches; legs/back; heating pad/laptop use → Erythema ab igne
- Truncal patches; "slapped cheek" facial erythema → Erythema infectiosum (fifth disease)

Photodistributed
- Malar (central-facial) erythema, oral ulcers, alopecia, discoid plaques, signs of serositis, renal/heme dysfunction → Systemic lupus erythematosus
- Heliotropic (periocular and eyelid) erythema, muscle weakness, periungual telangiectasia, distal interphalangeal joint erythema → Dermatomyositis

7 classes of topical steroids based on ability to constrict capillaries. Class I, strongest; class VII, weakest.						
Class I	**Class II**	**Class III**	**Class IV**	**Class V**	**Class VI**	**Class VII**
Clobetasol propionate ointment, cream, 0.05% (Temovate)	Fluocinonide ointment, cream, gel 0.05% (Lidex)	Triamcinolone acetonide ointment, 0.1% (Aristocort A)	Triamcinolone acetonide cream, 0.1% (Kenalog)	Fluocinolone acetonide cream, 0.025% (Synalar)	Desonide cream, 0.05% (DesOwen)	
Betamethasone dipropionate ointment, cream, 0.05% (Diprolene, Diprosone)	Amcinonide ointment, 0.1% (Cyclocort)	Betamethasone valerate ointment, 0.01% (Valisone)	Mometasone furoate cream, 0.1% (Elocon)	Fluticasone propionate cream, 0.05% (Cutivate)	Prednicarbate 0.1% cream (Dermatop)	Hydrocortisone, 0.5%, 1%, 2.5% (Hytone)
Halobetasol propionate ointment, cream, 0.05% (Ultravate)	Desoximetasone ointment, cream, 0.25%; gel, 0.05% (Topicort)	Fluticasone propionate ointment, 0.05% (Cutivate)	Hydrocortisone valerate ointment, 0.2% (Westcort)	Hydrocortisone valerate cream, 0.2% (Westcort)	Alclometasone dipropionate ointment, cream, 0.05% (Aclovate)	

Jennifer G. Foster, MD, MBA, FACP, Lisa C. Martinez, MD, and Allison H. Ferris, MD

Ely JW, Stone MS. The generalized rash: part I. Differential diagnosis. *Am Fam Physician*. 2010;81(6):726–734;
Ely JW, Stone MS. The generalized rash: part II. Diagnostic approach. *Am Fam Physician*. 2010;81(6):735–739.

RECTAL BLEEDING AND HEMATOCHEZIA

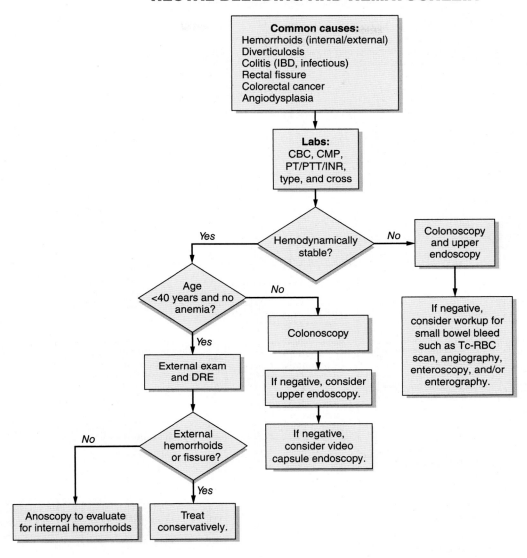

Common causes:
Hemorrhoids (internal/external)
Diverticulosis
Colitis (IBD, infectious)
Rectal fissure
Colorectal cancer
Angiodysplasia

Labs:
CBC, CMP,
PT/PTT/INR,
type, and cross

Hemodynamically stable?

Yes — Age <40 years and no anemia?

No — Colonoscopy and upper endoscopy

If negative, consider workup for small bowel bleed such as Tc-RBC scan, angiography, enteroscopy, and/or enterography.

No — Colonoscopy

If negative, consider upper endoscopy.

If negative, consider video capsule endoscopy.

Yes — External exam and DRE

External hemorrhoids or fissure?

No — Anoscopy to evaluate for internal hemorrhoids

Yes — Treat conservatively.

Allison Holley, MD

Almadi MA, Barkun AN. Patient presentation, risk stratification, and initial management in acute lower gastrointestinal bleeding. *Gastrointest Endosc Clin N Am.* 2018;28(3):363–377.

RED EYE

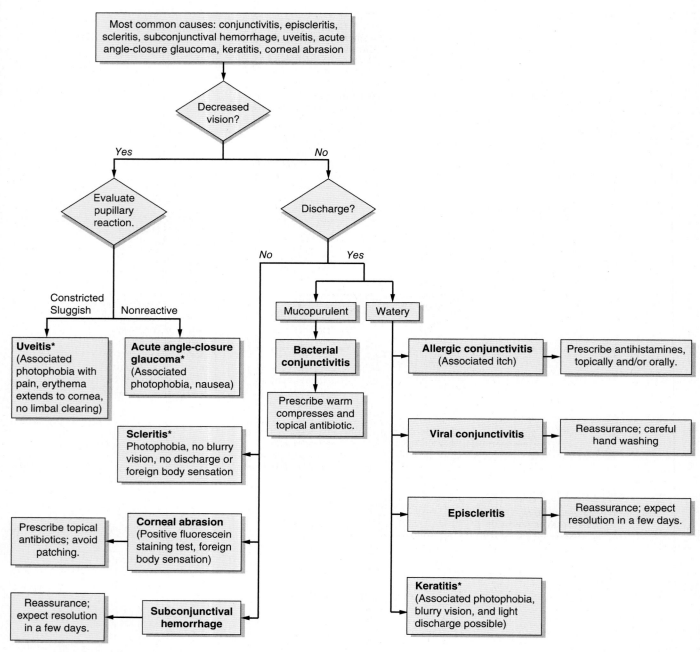

Most common causes: conjunctivitis, episcleritis, scleritis, subconjunctival hemorrhage, uveitis, acute angle-closure glaucoma, keratitis, corneal abrasion

Decreased vision?

Yes — Evaluate pupillary reaction.

No — Discharge?

Constricted Sluggish →

Uveitis* (Associated photophobia with pain, erythema extends to cornea, no limbal clearing)

Nonreactive →

Acute angle-closure glaucoma* (Associated photophobia, nausea)

Scleritis* Photophobia, no blurry vision, no discharge or foreign body sensation

Corneal abrasion (Positive fluorescein staining test, foreign body sensation)

Prescribe topical antibiotics; avoid patching.

Subconjunctival hemorrhage

Reassurance; expect resolution in a few days.

Discharge?

No

Yes

Mucopurulent → **Bacterial conjunctivitis** → Prescribe warm compresses and topical antibiotic.

Watery →

Allergic conjunctivitis (Associated itch) → Prescribe antihistamines, topically and/or orally.

Viral conjunctivitis → Reassurance; careful hand washing

Episcleritis → Reassurance; expect resolution in a few days.

Keratitis* (Associated photophobia, blurry vision, and light discharge possible)

*****Urgent ophthalmology consultation.**

Robert A. Baldor, MD, FAAFP

Cronau H, Kankanala RR, Mauger T. Diagnosis and management of red eye in primary care. *Am Fam Physician*. 2010;81(2):137–144.

SALICYLATE POISONING, ACUTE, TREATMENT

Assess airway, breathing, and circulation (ABC).
Provide appropriate ABC management. Avoid intubation unless patient is unable to protect airway. Intubation may increase acidosis and result in cardiovascular collapse.

Early toxicity: tachypnea, hyperpnea, nausea, vomiting, tinnitus, vertigo
Late toxicity: hyperthermia, hypotension, altered mental status

Does the patient exhibit signs of severe toxicity (altered mental status/coma, seizure, pulmonary edema, or need for endotracheal intubation and mechanical ventilation)?

No → **History and physical**
Obtain careful history of ingestion (time, reported ingestion, coingestants, etc.) and perform thorough physical exam for hemodynamic instability, alterations in respiratory pattern, and changes in mental status.

Yes → **Initiate emergent hemodialysis.**
Begin volume resuscitation and alkalinization using 150 mEq (3 amps) NaHCO$_3$ + 40 mEq KCl in 1 L D5W unless prohibited by cerebral/pulmonary edema. Administer 25 g (1 amp) D50 for altered mental status. Do not delay treatment for diagnostic studies.

Is the patient asymptomatic, stable, and known to have ingested <150 mg/kg?

Note: Volume resuscitation and alkalinization are the mainstays of therapy and should be given to all symptomatic patients unless pulmonary or cerebral edema is present. Respiratory alkalosis (pH >7.5) is NOT a contraindication to therapy. Do not delay for charcoal or diagnostic studies.

No → **Initial treatment**
1. Early volume resuscitation with isotonic saline or LR at rate of 10–20 mL/kg body wt for first 2 hours then adjust to maintain UOP of 1.0–1.5 mL/kg/hr.
2. Urinary alkalinization using 150 mEq (3 amps) NaHCO$_3$ + 40 mEq KCl mixed in 1 L D5W, infused at 2–3 mL/kg/hr
3. Administer first-dose activated charcoal at 1 g/kg (max 50 g) ONLY if patient is alert, cooperative, has bowel sounds on exam, and can tolerate. Consider additional doses of 50 g q4h for 2 more doses if patient continues to meet the aforementioned criteria.

Yes → **Evaluation/observation**
Obtain first salicylate level, noting time since ingestion occurred.

ASA detectable?

No → Recheck if within 2 hours of presentation. Discharge after 6 hours observation if patient remains asymptomatic and levels are nondetectable.

Yes → Recheck levels q2h until persistently within therapeutic range, trending down, or nondetectable. Routinely reassess for changes in clinical status and initiate treatment if indicated.

Obtain diagnostic studies.
Labs: salicylate level (note time since ingestion), ABG/VBG, basic electrolytes, BUN, creatinine, LFTs, coags, lactate, UA. Obtain tox screen if polysubstance overdose suspected.
Imaging: chest radiograph (to evaluate for pulmonary edema). Consider head CT for altered mental status to evaluate for cerebral edema or alternative causes of mental status changes.

Presence of salicylate level >90 mg/dL, arterial pH <7.3, pulmonary or cerebral edema, renal failure, or has patient deteriorated?

No → **Maintenance therapy and evaluation**
1. Continue bicarbonate infusion to maintain urine output of 1–2 mL/kg/hr.
2. Measure urine pH hourly and titrate infusion to goal pH of 7.5–8.0.
3. Measure serum K hourly and replete if <4.5 mEq/L.
4. Measure ABG or VBG hourly and decrease rate of bicarbonate drip if serum pH exceeds 7.6.
5. Measure serum salicylate level q2h until salicylate level begins to decline and acid–base status is normal.

Yes → Initiate hemodialysis.

Disposition
Treatment should be continued with frequent clinical assessment for improvement. Treatment and testing may be stopped ONLY when patient is asymptomatic, acid–base status is stable, AND salicylate level has fallen into therapeutic range (10–30 mg/dL).

Parvathi Perumareddi, DO

Juurlink DN, Gosselin S, Kielstein JT, et al; for EXTRIP Workgroup. Extracorporeal treatment for salicylate poisoning: systematic review and recommendations from the EXTRIP Workgroup. *Ann Emerg Med*. 2015;66(2):165–181.

SEIZURE, NEW ONSET

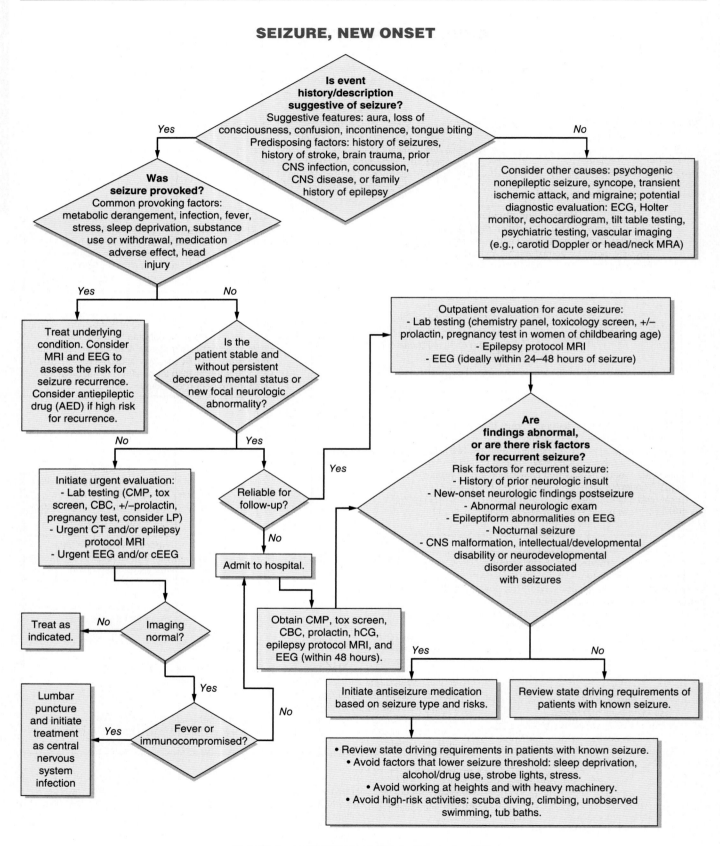

Is event history/description suggestive of seizure?
Suggestive features: aura, loss of consciousness, confusion, incontinence, tongue biting
Predisposing factors: history of seizures, history of stroke, brain trauma, prior CNS infection, concussion, CNS disease, or family history of epilepsy

Yes

No

Was seizure provoked?
Common provoking factors: metabolic derangement, infection, fever, stress, sleep deprivation, substance use or withdrawal, medication adverse effect, head injury

Consider other causes: psychogenic nonepileptic seizure, syncope, transient ischemic attack, and migraine; potential diagnostic evaluation: ECG, Holter monitor, echocardiogram, tilt table testing, psychiatric testing, vascular imaging (e.g., carotid Doppler or head/neck MRA)

Yes

No

Treat underlying condition. Consider MRI and EEG to assess the risk for seizure recurrence. Consider antiepileptic drug (AED) if high risk for recurrence.

Is the patient stable and without persistent decreased mental status or new focal neurologic abnormality?

Outpatient evaluation for acute seizure:
- Lab testing (chemistry panel, toxicology screen, +/–prolactin, pregnancy test in women of childbearing age)
- Epilepsy protocol MRI
- EEG (ideally within 24–48 hours of seizure)

No

Yes

Are findings abnormal, or are there risk factors for recurrent seizure?
Risk factors for recurrent seizure:
- History of prior neurologic insult
- New-onset neurologic findings postseizure
- Abnormal neurologic exam
- Epileptiform abnormalities on EEG
- Nocturnal seizure
- CNS malformation, intellectual/developmental disability or neurodevelopmental disorder associated with seizures

Initiate urgent evaluation:
- Lab testing (CMP, tox screen, CBC, +/–prolactin, pregnancy test, consider LP)
- Urgent CT and/or epilepsy protocol MRI
- Urgent EEG and/or cEEG

Reliable for follow-up?

Yes

No

Admit to hospital.

Treat as indicated.

No

Imaging normal?

Yes

Obtain CMP, tox screen, CBC, prolactin, hCG, epilepsy protocol MRI, and EEG (within 48 hours).

Yes

No

Initiate antiseizure medication based on seizure type and risks.

Review state driving requirements of patients with known seizure.

Lumbar puncture and initiate treatment as central nervous system infection

Yes

Fever or immunocompromised?

No

• Review state driving requirements in patients with known seizure.
• Avoid factors that lower seizure threshold: sleep deprivation, alcohol/drug use, strobe lights, stress.
• Avoid working at heights and with heavy machinery.
• Avoid high-risk activities: scuba diving, climbing, unobserved swimming, tub baths.

Yuki Takeuchi, MD and Kento Sonoda, MD

Gavvala JR, Schuele SU. New-onset seizure in adults and adolescents: a review. *JAMA*. 2016;316(24):2657–2668.

SHOULDER PAIN, TREATMENT

Analgesics, NSAIDs, ice, activity modification

Positive apprehension testing—GH instability

OA → PT → IACS → Surgical evaluation if refractory

Anterior dislocation → X-ray if first time and available → Reduce if negative fracture.

Myofascial or TrP → PT → Dry needling TrP injection OMT Massage Myofascial release Acupuncture

Humerus Clavicle Scapula Fracture → Pain management Fracture management

Pain and limitation with both active and passive ROM—adhesive capsulitis

Refer to PT. Consider IA CS injection.

Symptoms may last 1–3 years to resolve.

If not improving, consider:
– Repeat GH CS injection
– Distention
– Manipulation under anesthesia
– Surgical release
– ESWT

Acromioclavicular

Pain, limited ROM, and x-ray findings of degeneration and joint space narrowing-OA → PT → ICAS, consider PRP

Sprain/ separation → Immobilization for comfort

I, II, III → 2–3 days
III → 4–6 weeks → Conservative treatment

IV–VI → Surgical repair

Surgical evaluation if refractory

Pain with empty can, Hawkins and/or Neer's testing—impingement syndrome

PT CS OMT acupuncture → Surgery evaluation after 3 months if refractory

Rotator cuff

Tendinopathy → PT Consider PRP in first 3 months. Acupuncture TENS → SA or SD bursitis; CS → Surgical evaluation if refractory

Labral tear → PT

Tear → Partial, Complete → Consider early surgery if young and acute. → PT, NSAIDs, SA CS, DPT, PRP → Surgical consult if:
– Not improving
– Disabling

Abbreviations:
NSAIDs, nonsteroidal anti-inflammatory drugs; TrP, trigger point; GH, glenohumeral; PT, physical therapy plus home exercise plan; OA, osteoarthritis; IA, intra-articular; CS, corticosteroid; OMT, osteopathic manipulative therapy; SA, subacromial; SD, subdeltoid; DPT, dextrose prolotherapy; PRP, platelet-rich plasma; TENS, transcutaneous electrical nerve stimulation; ESWT, extracorporeal shock wave therapy

Vicki R. Nelson, MD, PhD

Greenberg DL. Evaluation and treatment of shoulder pain. *Med Clin North Am.* 2014;98(3):487–504.

SICKLE CELL ANEMIA, ACUTE, EVALUATION AND MANAGEMENT

This algorithm is meant to assist clinicians in the workup and management of common complications of sickle cell disease. It should not replace a physician's clinical judgment or be considered a standardized protocol for all patients.

Known Sickle Cell Patient (Part I of II)

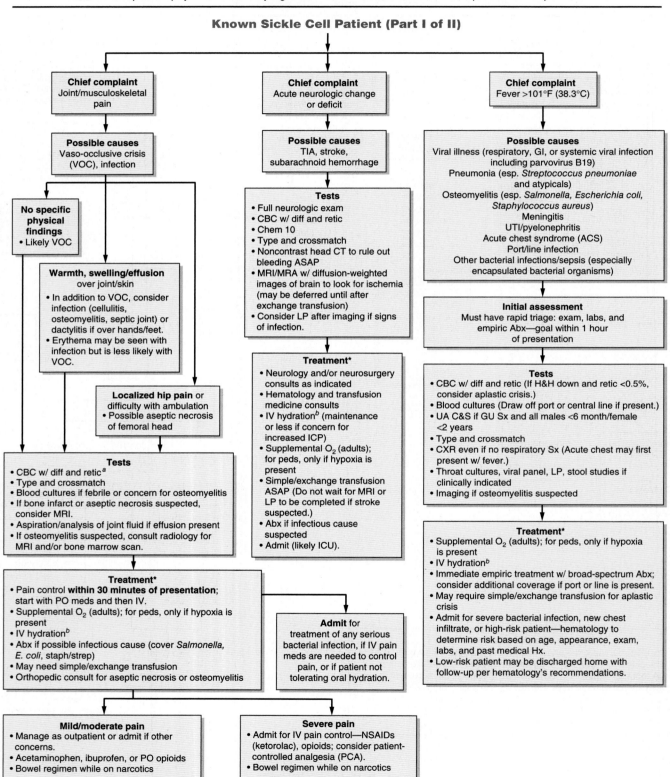

Chief complaint
Joint/musculoskeletal pain

Possible causes
Vaso-occlusive crisis (VOC), infection

No specific physical findings
• Likely VOC

Warmth, swelling/effusion
over joint/skin
• In addition to VOC, consider infection (cellulitis, osteomyelitis, septic joint) or dactylitis if over hands/feet.
• Erythema may be seen with infection but is less likely with VOC.

Localized hip pain or difficulty with ambulation
• Possible aseptic necrosis of femoral head

Tests
• CBC w/ diff and retic[a]
• Type and crossmatch
• Blood cultures if febrile or concern for osteomyelitis
• If bone infarct or aseptic necrosis suspected, consider MRI.
• Aspiration/analysis of joint fluid if effusion present
• If osteomyelitis suspected, consult radiology for MRI and/or bone marrow scan.

Treatment*
• Pain control **within 30 minutes of presentation**; start with PO meds and then IV.
• Supplemental O_2 (adults); for peds, only if hypoxia is present
• IV hydration[b]
• Abx if possible infectious cause (cover *Salmonella, E. coli,* staph/strep)
• May need simple/exchange transfusion
• Orthopedic consult for aseptic necrosis or osteomyelitis

Mild/moderate pain
• Manage as outpatient or admit if other concerns.
• Acetaminophen, ibuprofen, or PO opioids
• Bowel regimen while on narcotics

Severe pain
• Admit for IV pain control—NSAIDs (ketorolac), opioids; consider patient-controlled analgesia (PCA).
• Bowel regimen while on narcotics

Chief complaint
Acute neurologic change or deficit

Possible causes
TIA, stroke, subarachnoid hemorrhage

Tests
• Full neurologic exam
• CBC w/ diff and retic
• Chem 10
• Type and crossmatch
• Noncontrast head CT to rule out bleeding ASAP
• MRI/MRA w/ diffusion-weighted images of brain to look for ischemia (may be deferred until after exchange transfusion)
• Consider LP after imaging if signs of infection.

Treatment*
• Neurology and/or neurosurgery consults as indicated
• Hematology and transfusion medicine consults
• IV hydration[b] (maintenance or less if concern for increased ICP)
• Supplemental O_2 (adults); for peds, only if hypoxia is present
• Simple/exchange transfusion ASAP (Do not wait for MRI or LP to be completed if stroke suspected.)
• Abx if infectious cause suspected
• Admit (likely ICU).

Admit for treatment of any serious bacterial infection, if IV pain meds are needed to control pain, or if patient not tolerating oral hydration.

Chief complaint
Fever >101°F (38.3°C)

Possible causes
Viral illness (respiratory, GI, or systemic viral infection including parvovirus B19)
Pneumonia (esp. *Streptococcus pneumoniae* and atypicals)
Osteomyelitis (esp. *Salmonella, Escherichia coli, Staphylococcus aureus*)
Meningitis
UTI/pyelonephritis
Acute chest syndrome (ACS)
Port/line infection
Other bacterial infections/sepsis (especially encapsulated bacterial organisms)

Initial assessment
Must have rapid triage: exam, labs, and empiric Abx—goal within 1 hour of presentation

Tests
• CBC w/ diff and retic (If H&H down and retic <0.5%, consider aplastic crisis.)
• Blood cultures (Draw off port or central line if present.)
• UA C&S if GU Sx and all males <6 month/female <2 years
• Type and crossmatch
• CXR even if no respiratory Sx (Acute chest may first present w/ fever.)
• Throat cultures, viral panel, LP, stool studies if clinically indicated
• Imaging if osteomyelitis suspected

Treatment*
• Supplemental O_2 (adults); for peds, only if hypoxia is present
• IV hydration[b]
• Immediate empiric treatment w/ broad-spectrum Abx; consider additional coverage if port or line is present.
• May require simple/exchange transfusion for aplastic crisis
• Admit for severe bacterial infection, new chest infiltrate, or high-risk patient—hematology to determine risk based on age, appearance, exam, labs, and past medical Hx.
• Low-risk patient may be discharged home with follow-up per hematology's recommendations.

Known Sickle Cell Patient (Part II of II)

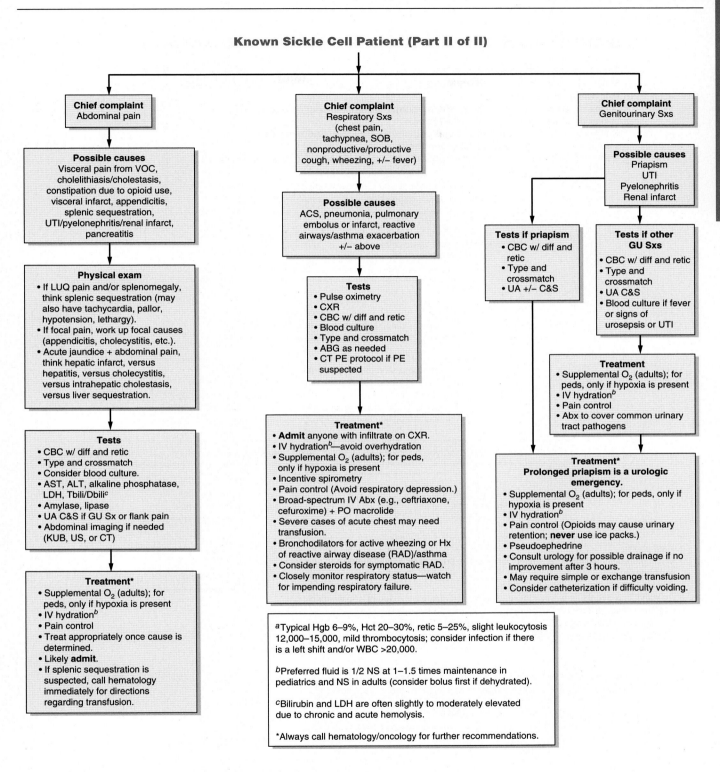

Chief complaint
Abdominal pain

Possible causes
Visceral pain from VOC, cholelithiasis/cholestasis, constipation due to opioid use, visceral infarct, appendicitis, splenic sequestration, UTI/pyelonephritis/renal infarct, pancreatitis

Physical exam
- If LUQ pain and/or splenomegaly, think splenic sequestration (may also have tachycardia, pallor, hypotension, lethargy).
- If focal pain, work up focal causes (appendicitis, cholecystitis, etc.).
- Acute jaundice + abdominal pain, think hepatic infarct, versus hepatitis, versus cholecystitis, versus intrahepatic cholestasis, versus liver sequestration.

Tests
- CBC w/ diff and retic
- Type and crossmatch
- Consider blood culture.
- AST, ALT, alkaline phosphatase, LDH, Tbili/Dbili[c]
- Amylase, lipase
- UA C&S if GU Sx or flank pain
- Abdominal imaging if needed (KUB, US, or CT)

Treatment*
- Supplemental O_2 (adults); for peds, only if hypoxia is present
- IV hydration[b]
- Pain control
- Treat appropriately once cause is determined.
- Likely **admit**.
- If splenic sequestration is suspected, call hematology immediately for directions regarding transfusion.

Chief complaint
Respiratory Sxs (chest pain, tachypnea, SOB, nonproductive/productive cough, wheezing, +/– fever)

Possible causes
ACS, pneumonia, pulmonary embolus or infarct, reactive airways/asthma exacerbation +/– above

Tests
- Pulse oximetry
- CXR
- CBC w/ diff and retic
- Blood culture
- Type and crossmatch
- ABG as needed
- CT PE protocol if PE suspected

Treatment*
- **Admit** anyone with infiltrate on CXR.
- IV hydration[b]—avoid overhydration
- Supplemental O_2 (adults); for peds, only if hypoxia is present
- Incentive spirometry
- Pain control (Avoid respiratory depression.)
- Broad-spectrum IV Abx (e.g., ceftriaxone, cefuroxime) + PO macrolide
- Severe cases of acute chest may need transfusion.
- Bronchodilators for active wheezing or Hx of reactive airway disease (RAD)/asthma
- Consider steroids for symptomatic RAD.
- Closely monitor respiratory status—watch for impending respiratory failure.

Chief complaint
Genitourinary Sxs

Possible causes
Priapism
UTI
Pyelonephritis
Renal infarct

Tests if priapism
- CBC w/ diff and retic
- Type and crossmatch
- UA +/– C&S

Tests if other GU Sxs
- CBC w/ diff and retic
- Type and crossmatch
- UA C&S
- Blood culture if fever or signs of urosepsis or UTI

Treatment
- Supplemental O_2 (adults); for peds, only if hypoxia is present
- IV hydration[b]
- Pain control
- Abx to cover common urinary tract pathogens

Treatment*
Prolonged priapism is a urologic emergency.
- Supplemental O_2 (adults); for peds, only if hypoxia is present
- IV hydration[b]
- Pain control (Opioids may cause urinary retention; **never** use ice packs.)
- Pseudoephedrine
- Consult urology for possible drainage if no improvement after 3 hours.
- May require simple or exchange transfusion
- Consider catheterization if difficulty voiding.

[a]Typical Hgb 6–9%, Hct 20–30%, retic 5–25%, slight leukocytosis 12,000–15,000, mild thrombocytosis; consider infection if there is a left shift and/or WBC >20,000.

[b]Preferred fluid is 1/2 NS at 1–1.5 times maintenance in pediatrics and NS in adults (consider bolus first if dehydrated).

[c]Bilirubin and LDH are often slightly to moderately elevated due to chronic and acute hemolysis.

*Always call hematology/oncology for further recommendations.

Paul E. Daniel Jr., MD and Efstathia Choros, MD, CPA

National Heart, Lung, and Blood Institute. Evidence-based management of sickle cell disease: expert panel report, 2014. https://www.nhlbi.nih.gov/health-topics/evidence-based-management-sickle-cell-disease. Published September 2014. Accessed January 31, 2021.

SUICIDE, EVALUATING RISK FOR

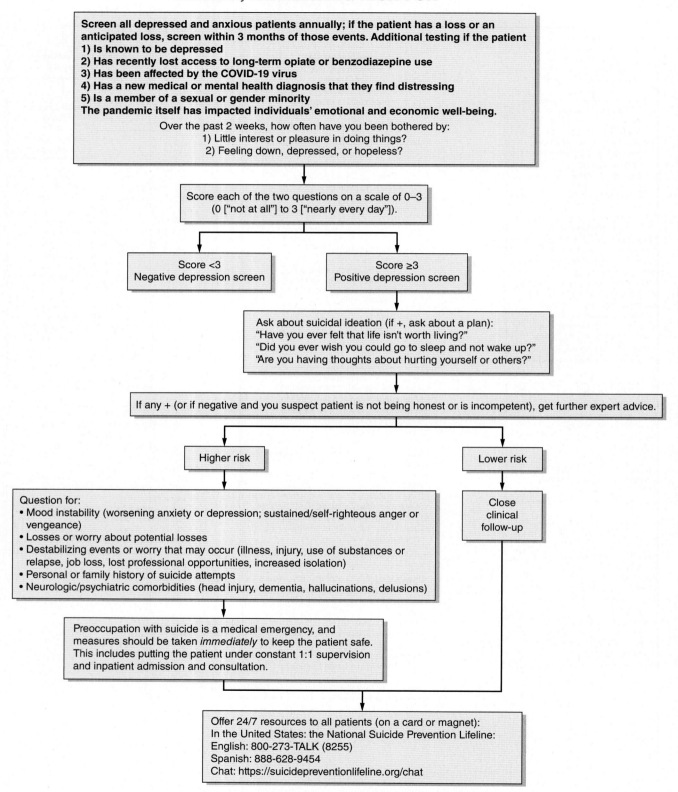

Screen all depressed and anxious patients annually; if the patient has a loss or an anticipated loss, screen within 3 months of those events. Additional testing if the patient
1) Is known to be depressed
2) Has recently lost access to long-term opiate or benzodiazepine use
3) Has been affected by the COVID-19 virus
4) Has a new medical or mental health diagnosis that they find distressing
5) Is a member of a sexual or gender minority
The pandemic itself has impacted individuals' emotional and economic well-being.

Over the past 2 weeks, how often have you been bothered by:
1) Little interest or pleasure in doing things?
2) Feeling down, depressed, or hopeless?

Score each of the two questions on a scale of 0–3
(0 ["not at all"] to 3 ["nearly every day"]).

Score <3
Negative depression screen

Score ≥3
Positive depression screen

Ask about suicidal ideation (if +, ask about a plan):
"Have you ever felt that life isn't worth living?"
"Did you ever wish you could go to sleep and not wake up?"
"Are you having thoughts about hurting yourself or others?"

If any + (or if negative and you suspect patient is not being honest or is incompetent), get further expert advice.

Higher risk

Lower risk

Question for:
• Mood instability (worsening anxiety or depression; sustained/self-righteous anger or vengeance)
• Losses or worry about potential losses
• Destabilizing events or worry that may occur (illness, injury, use of substances or relapse, job loss, lost professional opportunities, increased isolation)
• Personal or family history of suicide attempts
• Neurologic/psychiatric comorbidities (head injury, dementia, hallucinations, delusions)

Close
clinical
follow-up

Preoccupation with suicide is a medical emergency, and measures should be taken *immediately* to keep the patient safe. This includes putting the patient under constant 1:1 supervision and inpatient admission and consultation.

Offer 24/7 resources to all patients (on a card or magnet):
In the United States: the National Suicide Prevention Lifeline:
English: 800-273-TALK (8255)
Spanish: 888-628-9454
Chat: https://suicidepreventionlifeline.org/chat

Irene Coletsos, MD and Harold J. Bursztajn, MD

Posner K, Oquendo MA, Gould M, et al. Columbia Classification Algorithm of Suicide Assessment (C-CASA): classification of suicidal events in the FDA's pediatric suicidal risk analysis of antidepressants. *Am J Psychiatry.* 2007;164(7):1035–1043.

SYNCOPE

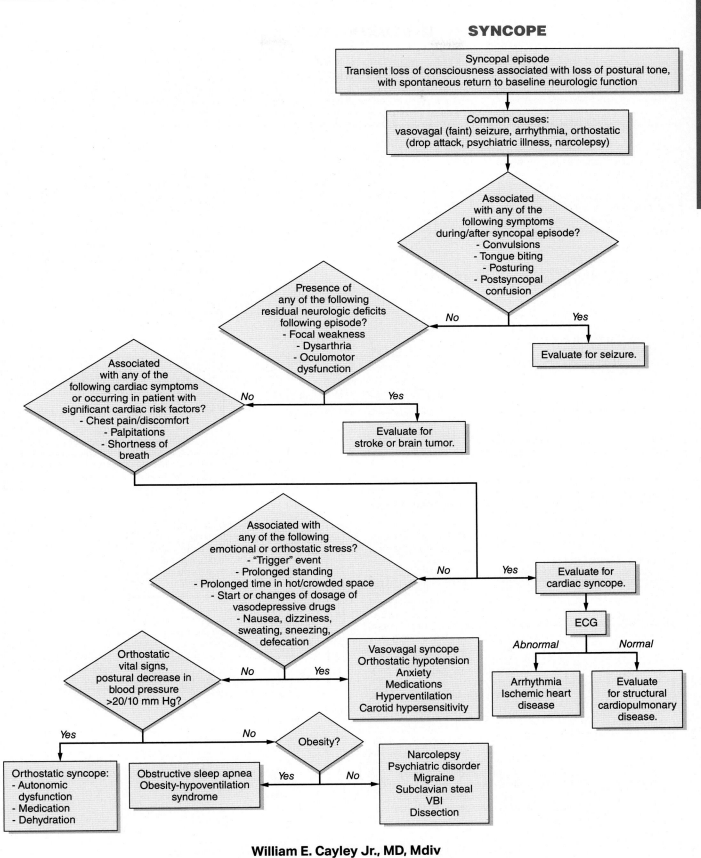

William E. Cayley Jr., MD, Mdiv

Runser LA, Gauer RL, Houser A. Syncope: evaluation and differential diagnosis. *Am Fam Physician*. 2017;95(5):303–312.

THROMBOCYTOPENIA

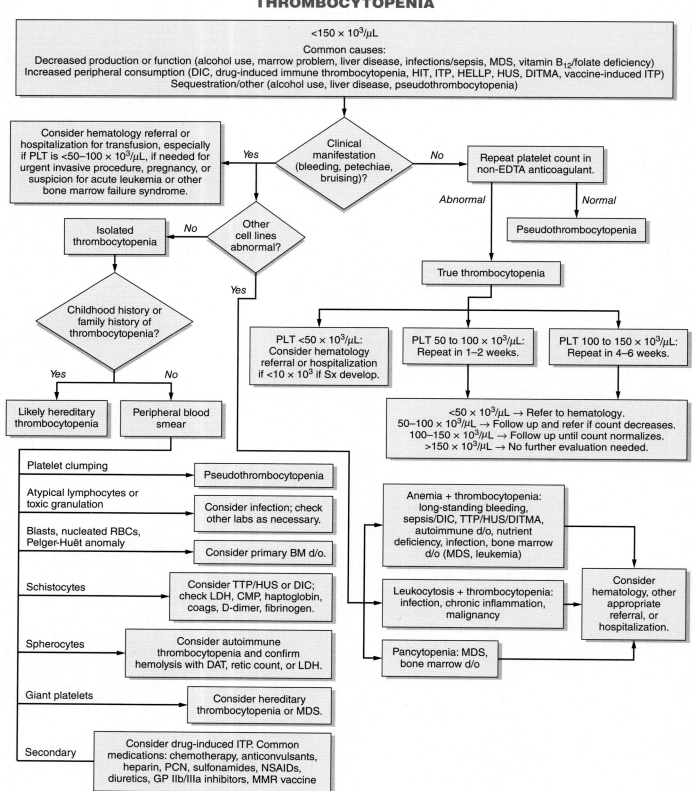

$<150 \times 10^3/\mu L$
Common causes:
Decreased production or function (alcohol use, marrow problem, liver disease, infections/sepsis, MDS, vitamin B_{12}/folate deficiency)
Increased peripheral consumption (DIC, drug-induced immune thrombocytopenia, HIT, ITP, HELLP, HUS, DITMA, vaccine-induced ITP)
Sequestration/other (alcohol use, liver disease, pseudothrombocytopenia)

Clinical manifestation (bleeding, petechiae, bruising)?

Yes → Consider hematology referral or hospitalization for transfusion, especially if PLT is $<50–100 \times 10^3/\mu L$, if needed for urgent invasive procedure, pregnancy, or suspicion for acute leukemia or other bone marrow failure syndrome.

No → Repeat platelet count in non-EDTA anticoagulant.
- *Normal* → Pseudothrombocytopenia
- *Abnormal* → True thrombocytopenia

Other cell lines abnormal?

No → Isolated thrombocytopenia → Childhood history or family history of thrombocytopenia?
- **Yes** → Likely hereditary thrombocytopenia
- **No** → Peripheral blood smear

True thrombocytopenia:
- PLT $<50 \times 10^3/\mu L$: Consider hematology referral or hospitalization if $<10 \times 10^3$ if Sx develop.
- PLT 50 to $100 \times 10^3/\mu L$: Repeat in 1–2 weeks.
- PLT 100 to $150 \times 10^3/\mu L$: Repeat in 4–6 weeks.

$<50 \times 10^3/\mu L \rightarrow$ Refer to hematology.
$50–100 \times 10^3/\mu L \rightarrow$ Follow up and refer if count decreases.
$100–150 \times 10^3/\mu L \rightarrow$ Follow up until count normalizes.
$>150 \times 10^3/\mu L \rightarrow$ No further evaluation needed.

Peripheral blood smear:
- Platelet clumping → Pseudothrombocytopenia
- Atypical lymphocytes or toxic granulation → Consider infection; check other labs as necessary.
- Blasts, nucleated RBCs, Pelger-Huët anomaly → Consider primary BM d/o.
- Schistocytes → Consider TTP/HUS or DIC; check LDH, CMP, haptoglobin, coags, D-dimer, fibrinogen.
- Spherocytes → Consider autoimmune thrombocytopenia and confirm hemolysis with DAT, retic count, or LDH.
- Giant platelets → Consider hereditary thrombocytopenia or MDS.
- Secondary → Consider drug-induced ITP. Common medications: chemotherapy, anticonvulsants, heparin, PCN, sulfonamides, NSAIDs, diuretics, GP IIb/IIIa inhibitors, MMR vaccine

Other cell lines abnormal? Yes:
- Anemia + thrombocytopenia: long-standing bleeding, sepsis/DIC, TTP/HUS/DITMA, autoimmune d/o, nutrient deficiency, infection, bone marrow d/o (MDS, leukemia)
- Leukocytosis + thrombocytopenia: infection, chronic inflammation, malignancy
- Pancytopenia: MDS, bone marrow d/o

→ Consider hematology, other appropriate referral, or hospitalization.

Jillian K. Joseph, MPAS, PA-C and Allison Hargreaves, MD

Gauer RL, Whitaker DJ. Thrombocytopenia: evaluation and management. *Am Fam Physician*. 2022;106(3):288–298.

TINNITUS

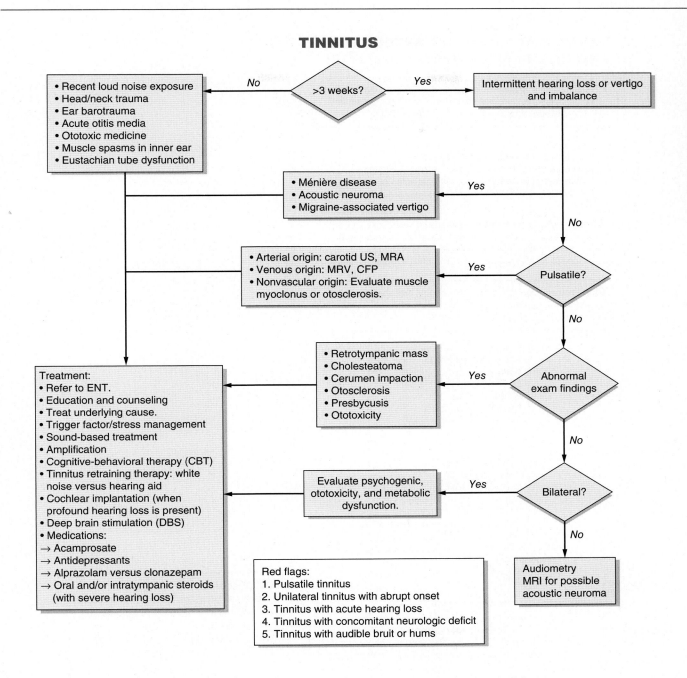

Recent loud noise exposure / Head/neck trauma / Ear barotrauma / Acute otitis media / Ototoxic medicine / Muscle spasms in inner ear / Eustachian tube dysfunction

>3 weeks?
- No → (left box)
- Yes → Intermittent hearing loss or vertigo and imbalance

Intermittent hearing loss or vertigo and imbalance
- Yes → Ménière disease / Acoustic neuroma / Migraine-associated vertigo
- No → Pulsatile?

Pulsatile?
- Yes → Arterial origin: carotid US, MRA / Venous origin: MRV, CFP / Nonvascular origin: Evaluate muscle myoclonus or otosclerosis.
- No → Abnormal exam findings

Abnormal exam findings
- Yes → Retrotympanic mass / Cholesteatoma / Cerumen impaction / Otosclerosis / Presbycusis / Ototoxicity
- No → Bilateral?

Bilateral?
- Yes → Evaluate psychogenic, ototoxicity, and metabolic dysfunction.
- No → Audiometry / MRI for possible acoustic neuroma

Treatment:
- Refer to ENT.
- Education and counseling
- Treat underlying cause.
- Trigger factor/stress management
- Sound-based treatment
- Amplification
- Cognitive-behavioral therapy (CBT)
- Tinnitus retraining therapy: white noise versus hearing aid
- Cochlear implantation (when profound hearing loss is present)
- Deep brain stimulation (DBS)
- Medications:
  → Acamprosate
  → Antidepressants
  → Alprazolam versus clonazepam
  → Oral and/or intratympanic steroids (with severe hearing loss)

Red flags:
1. Pulsatile tinnitus
2. Unilateral tinnitus with abrupt onset
3. Tinnitus with acute hearing loss
4. Tinnitus with concomitant neurologic deficit
5. Tinnitus with audible bruit or hums

Dongsheng Jiang, MD, MSc and Juan Qiu, MD, PhD

Henton A, Tzounopoulos T. What's the buzz? The neuroscience and the treatment of tinnitus. *Physiol Rev.* 2021;101(4):1609–1632.

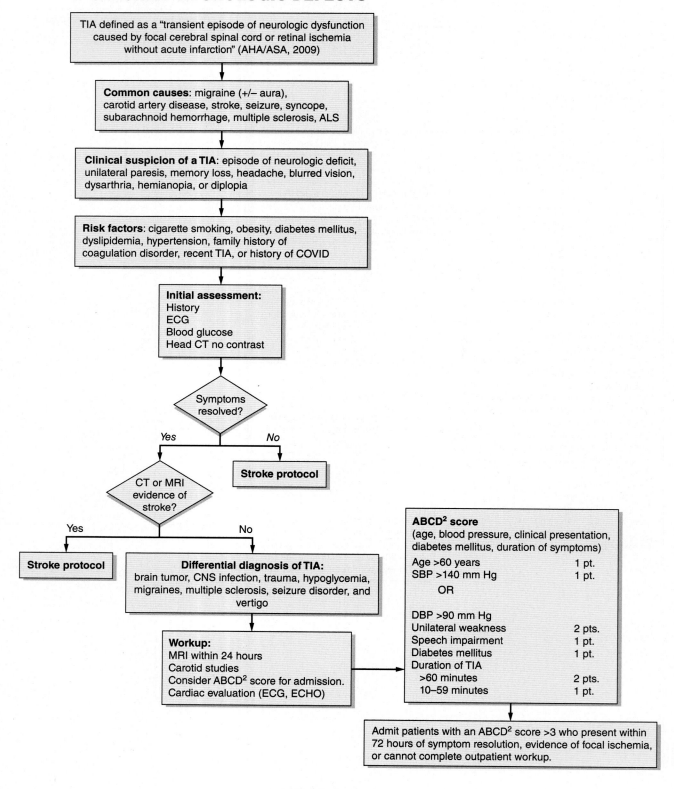

TRANSIENT ISCHEMIC ATTACK AND TRANSIENT NEUROLOGIC DEFECTS

TIA defined as a "transient episode of neurologic dysfunction caused by focal cerebral spinal cord or retinal ischemia without acute infarction" (AHA/ASA, 2009)

Common causes: migraine (+/– aura), carotid artery disease, stroke, seizure, syncope, subarachnoid hemorrhage, multiple sclerosis, ALS

Clinical suspicion of a TIA: episode of neurologic deficit, unilateral paresis, memory loss, headache, blurred vision, dysarthria, hemianopia, or diplopia

Risk factors: cigarette smoking, obesity, diabetes mellitus, dyslipidemia, hypertension, family history of coagulation disorder, recent TIA, or history of COVID

Initial assessment:
History
ECG
Blood glucose
Head CT no contrast

Symptoms resolved?

Yes — No

Stroke protocol

CT or MRI evidence of stroke?

Yes — No

Stroke protocol

Differential diagnosis of TIA:
brain tumor, CNS infection, trauma, hypoglycemia, migraines, multiple sclerosis, seizure disorder, and vertigo

Workup:
MRI within 24 hours
Carotid studies
Consider ABCD^2 score for admission.
Cardiac evaluation (ECG, ECHO)

ABCD^2 score
(age, blood pressure, clinical presentation, diabetes mellitus, duration of symptoms)

Age >60 years	1 pt.
SBP >140 mm Hg	1 pt.
OR	
DBP >90 mm Hg	
Unilateral weakness	2 pts.
Speech impairment	1 pt.
Diabetes mellitus	1 pt.
Duration of TIA	
>60 minutes	2 pts.
10–59 minutes	1 pt.

Admit patients with an ABCD^2 score >3 who present within 72 hours of symptom resolution, evidence of focal ischemia, or cannot complete outpatient workup.

Saadia Mohsin, MD

Simmons BB, Cirignano B, Gadegbeku AB. Transient ischemic attack: part I. Diagnosis and evaluation. *Am Fam Physician*. 2012;86(6):521–526.

TREMOR

Common causes: essential tremor, physiologic tremor, Parkinson disease, parkinsonian syndrome, medications, alcoholism, drug withdrawal, fragile X, metal toxicity, metabolic disturbances

If Taking:
- Anticonvulsants (valproic acid, lamotrigine, carbamazepine)
- Antidepressants (SSRIs/TCAs)
- Antipsychotics (Haldol/2nd gen)
- β-Agonists
- Cancer medications (vincristine, cisplatin, methotrexate)
- Cardiac medications (amiodarone, atorvastatin, verapamil)
- Corticosteroids
- Drugs/toxins (nicotine, alcohol, cocaine)
- Hypoglycemic agents
- Immunosuppressants (cyclosporine, glatiramer)
- Metoclopramide
- Mood stabilizers (lithium)
- Stimulants (caffeine, amphetamines, epinephrine, methylphenidate, pseudoephedrine)
- Thyroid hormones

No → Check TSH, CMP, RPR, vitamin B$_{12}$, ammonia, and magnesium.

Yes → Trial discontinuation should be attempted if clinically possible and check serum drug level if indicated.

Abnormal → Treat accordingly.

Normal

Resting tremor (tremor with limb supported against gravity)

Bradykinesia, rigidity, postural instability

- Parkinson disease
- Parkinsonian syndrome
- Severe essential tremor

Trial of β-blocker (in the case of severe essential tremor); trial of dopaminergic agents otherwise

Postural tremor (tremor with limb maintained against gravity)

- Alcohol withdrawal
- Panic disorder
- Anxiety
- Benzodiazepine withdrawal
- Essential tremor
- Handwriting tremor
- Peripheral neuropathy

For peripheral neuropathy, trial of gabapentin
For essential tremor, trial of β-blocker with or without anticonvulsants

Isometric tremor (tremor with muscle contraction against stationary object)

Kinetic tremor (tremor with voluntary movement)

Large extremity movement → Simple kinetic tremor

Tremor with visually guided limb movement → Intention tremor, cerebellar lesion (CVA, MS, tumor)

Obtain MRI or CT.

Psychogenic tremor (tremor relieved by distraction)

Stress reduction/ mental health counseling

Marni Klessman Gleiber, MD

van de Wardt J, van der Stouwe AMM, Dirkx M, et al. Systematic clinical approach for diagnosing upper limb tremor. *J Neurol Neurosurg Psychiatry.* 2020;91(8):822–830.

TYPE 2 DIABETES, TREATMENT

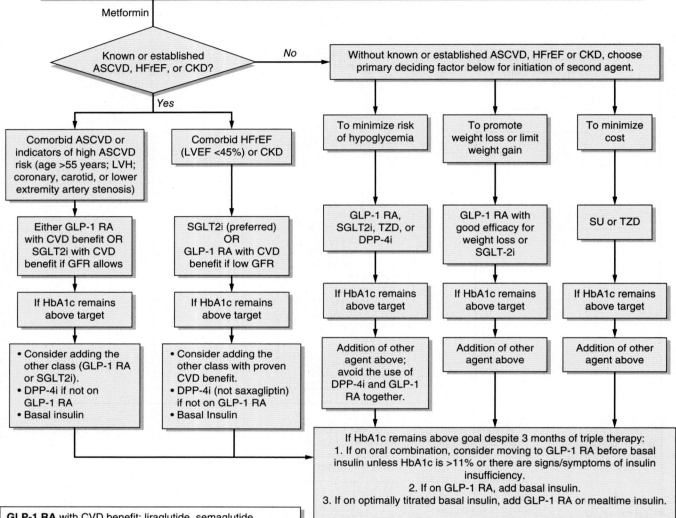

First-line therapy, comprehensive lifestyle changes (including weight management and physical activity)
If HbA1c remains above goal, proceed below.
If initial HbA1c ≥8.5% or 1.5% above HbA1c target, can consider initiation of dual therapy (metformin + second agent)
If initial HbA1c ≥10%, BG >300 mg/dL, or symptoms of hyperglycemia, can consider basal insulin therapy

Metformin

Known or established ASCVD, HFrEF, or CKD? — No → Without known or established ASCVD, HFrEF or CKD, choose primary deciding factor below for initiation of second agent.

Yes

Comorbid ASCVD or indicators of high ASCVD risk (age >55 years; LVH; coronary, carotid, or lower extremity artery stenosis)

Comorbid HFrEF (LVEF <45%) or CKD

To minimize risk of hypoglycemia

To promote weight loss or limit weight gain

To minimize cost

Either GLP-1 RA with CVD benefit OR SGLT2i with CVD benefit if GFR allows

SGLT2i (preferred) OR GLP-1 RA with CVD benefit if low GFR

GLP-1 RA, SGLT2i, TZD, or DPP-4i

GLP-1 RA with good efficacy for weight loss or SGLT-2i

SU or TZD

If HbA1c remains above target

If HbA1c remains above target

If HbA1c remains above target

If HbA1c remains above target

If HbA1c remains above target

- Consider adding the other class (GLP-1 RA or SGLT2i).
- DPP-4i if not on GLP-1 RA
- Basal insulin

- Consider adding the other class with proven CVD benefit.
- DPP-4i (not saxagliptin) if not on GLP-1 RA
- Basal Insulin

Addition of other agent above; avoid the use of DPP-4i and GLP-1 RA together.

Addition of other agent above

Addition of other agent above

If HbA1c remains above goal despite 3 months of triple therapy:
1. If on oral combination, consider moving to GLP-1 RA before basal insulin unless HbA1c is >11% or there are signs/symptoms of insulin insufficiency.
2. If on GLP-1 RA, add basal insulin.
3. If on optimally titrated basal insulin, add GLP-1 RA or mealtime insulin.

Metformin therapy should be maintained, if indicated, whereas other oral agents may be discontinued on an individual basis to avoid unnecessarily complex or costly regimens, side effects, and hypoglycemia.

GLP-1 RA with CVD benefit: liraglutide, semaglutide, dulaglutide; with greatest weight loss benefit: semaglutide, liraglutide, and dulaglutide
SGLT2i with CVD benefit: empagliflozin, canagliflozin, and dapagliflozin; requires renal dose adjustment
DPP-4i: linagliptin, saxagliptin, or sitagliptin; saxagliptin associated with increased risk of heart failure admissions
TZD: pioglitazone
SU: glimepiride, glyburide, or glipizide
Basal (long-acting) insulin: insulin glargine, insulin detemir, and insulin degludec. Start at 10 U or 0.1–0.2 U/kg/day SQ.

Glycemic Goals
- An HbA1c goal for newly diagnosed, nonpregnant adults with no comorbidities is <7%.
- If older age, multiple comorbidities, limited life expectancy, or high risk for hypoglycemia, higher HbA1c goals (such as <8%) may be appropriate.

Christine Chan, MD

Li J, Albajrami O, Zhuo M, et al. Decision algorithm for prescribing SGLT2 inhibitors and GLP-1 receptor agonists for diabetic kidney disease. *Clin J Am Soc Nephrol.* 2020;15(11):1678–1688.

VAGINAL BLEEDING, ABNORMAL

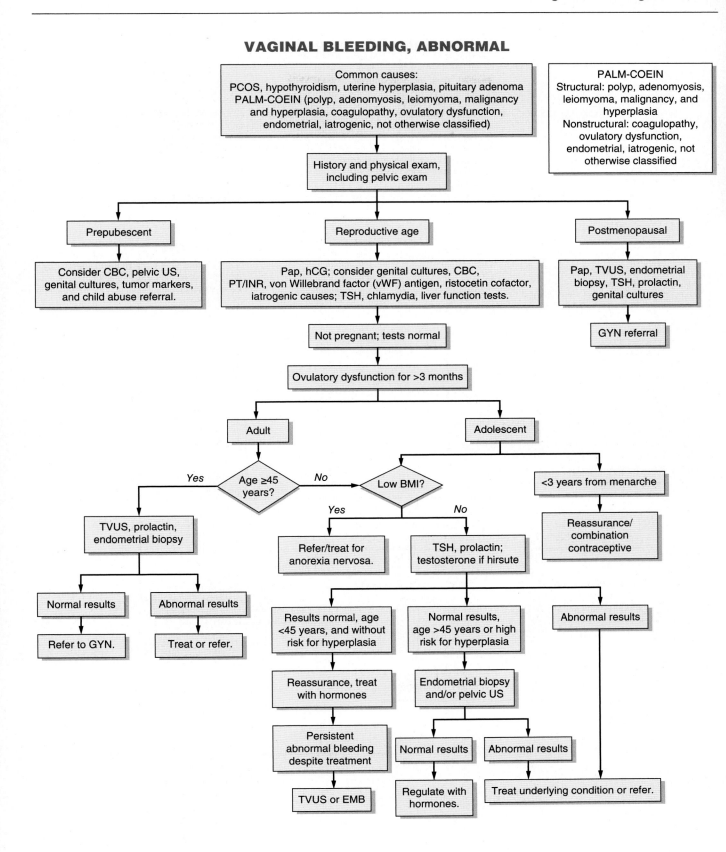

Common causes:
PCOS, hypothyroidism, uterine hyperplasia, pituitary adenoma
PALM-COEIN (polyp, adenomyosis, leiomyoma, malignancy
and hyperplasia, coagulopathy, ovulatory dysfunction,
endometrial, iatrogenic, not otherwise classified)

PALM-COEIN
Structural: polyp, adenomyosis, leiomyoma, malignancy, and hyperplasia
Nonstructural: coagulopathy, ovulatory dysfunction, endometrial, iatrogenic, not otherwise classified

History and physical exam, including pelvic exam

Prepubescent
Consider CBC, pelvic US, genital cultures, tumor markers, and child abuse referral.

Reproductive age
Pap, hCG; consider genital cultures, CBC, PT/INR, von Willebrand factor (vWF) antigen, ristocetin cofactor, iatrogenic causes; TSH, chlamydia, liver function tests.

Postmenopausal
Pap, TVUS, endometrial biopsy, TSH, prolactin, genital cultures

GYN referral

Not pregnant; tests normal

Ovulatory dysfunction for >3 months

Adult

Adolescent

Age ≥45 years? — Yes → TVUS, prolactin, endometrial biopsy

Age ≥45 years? — No → Low BMI?

Low BMI? — Yes → Refer/treat for anorexia nervosa.

Low BMI? — No → TSH, prolactin; testosterone if hirsute

<3 years from menarche → Reassurance/combination contraceptive

TVUS, prolactin, endometrial biopsy:
- Normal results → Refer to GYN.
- Abnormal results → Treat or refer.

Results normal, age <45 years, and without risk for hyperplasia → Reassurance, treat with hormones → Persistent abnormal bleeding despite treatment → TVUS or EMB

Normal results, age >45 years or high risk for hyperplasia → Endometrial biopsy and/or pelvic US:
- Normal results → Regulate with hormones.
- Abnormal results → Treat underlying condition or refer.

Abnormal results → Treat underlying condition or refer.

Frank J. Domino, MD

Wouk N, Helton M. Abnormal uterine bleeding in premenopausal women. *Am Fam Physician.* 2019;99(7):435–443.

VITAMIN D DEFICIENCY

Risk factors/common causes:

- Age >65 years
- Insufficient sunlight exposure (homebound, veiled)
- Renal disease
- Liver disease
- Depression
- Dark skin
- Insufficient dietary intake

- Obesity (BMI >30 kg/m^2)
- Immigrants to colder climates
- Chronic use of glucocorticoids
- Periosteal bone pain (e.g., sternum, tibia)
- GI malabsorption (celiac, cystic fibrosis, inflammatory bowel disease, exocrine pancreatic insufficiency, short bowel syndrome)

- Pregnancy
- Medications: anticonvulsants, antiretroviral, and glucocorticoids
- Gastrectomy or extensive bowel surgery
- Wearing clothing that covers a large portion of the body

Significant risk factors?

— No → Low suspicion for vitamin D deficiency

↓ Yes

Requirements:
<1 year old: 400 IU/day
>1 year old: 600 IU/day
To reach levels >30 ng/mL, may require 1,000 IU/day
Obese children: 2–3 times more vitamin D for their age group
Maintenance dose:
0–6 months old: 1,000–2,000 IU/day
6 months–1 year old: 1,500–2,000 IU/day
1–3 years old: 2,500–3,000 IU/day
4–8 years old: 3,000 IU/day
>8 years old: 2,000 IU/day
Vitamin D deficiency:
0–1 year old: 2,000 IU/day for 6 weeks or 50,000 IU weekly for 6 weeks followed by maintenance 400–1,000 IU/day
1–18 years old: 2,000 IU/day for 6 weeks or 50,000 IU weekly for 6 weeks followed by maintenance 600–1,000 IU/day

Yes ← **Age <18 years?** → No → **Lab:** serum 25-hydroxyvitamin D concentration

Level <20 ng/mL (vitamin D deficiency)

Level 20–29 ng/mL (vitamin D insufficiency)

Level ≥30 ng/mL normal

Treatment: Start 50,000 IU vitamin D$_2$ once a week for 8–12 weeks and then begin 2,000–3,000 IU vitamin D per day.

Treatment: 2,000–4,000 IU vitamin D per day

Maintenance: Supplement with 600–2,000 IU of vitamin D per day.

After 6 months, consider repeating serum 25-hydroxyvitamin D level.

Recheck serum 25-hydroxyvitamin D concentration.

Level <20 ng/mL? — No →

↓ Yes

Consult endocrinology if no malabsorptive disease.

Parvathi Perumareddi, DO

Holick MF, Binkley NC, Bischoff-Ferrari HA, et al; for Endocrine Society. Evaluation, treatment, and prevention of vitamin D deficiency: an Endocrine Society clinical practice guideline. *J Clin Endocrinol Metab.* 2011;96(7):1911–1930.

WEIGHT LOSS, UNINTENTIONAL

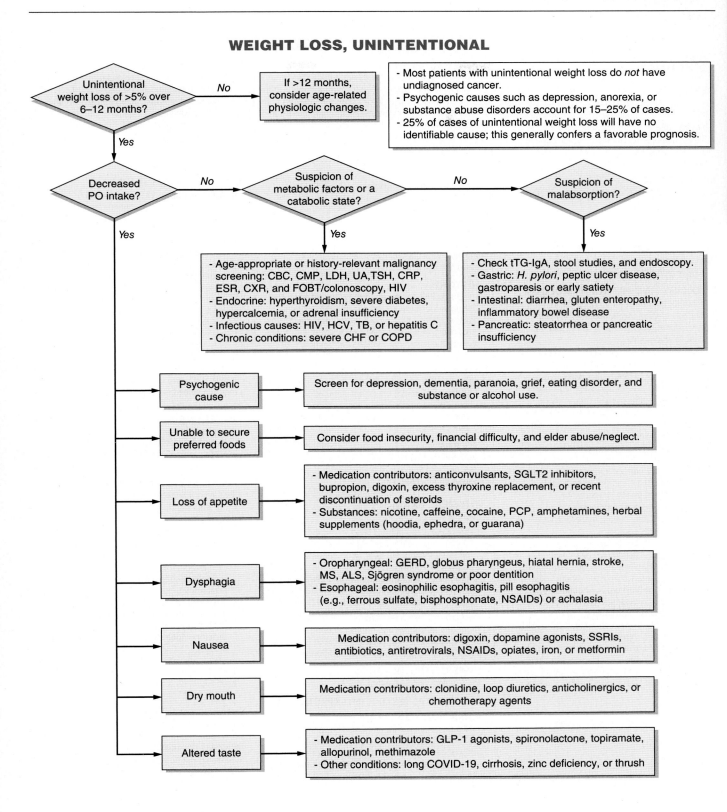

Arindam Sarkar, MD and Katelyn D. Sarkar, PA-C

Gaddey HL, Holder KK. Unintentional weight loss in older adults. *Am Fam Physician*. 2021;104(1):34–40.

ABNORMAL (DYSFUNCTIONAL) UTERINE BLEEDING

Jeremy Golding, MD, FAAFP • Zachary H. Hicks, DO

 BASICS

DESCRIPTION

- Abnormal uterine bleeding (AUB) is uterine bleeding that is irregular in quantity, frequency, or duration.
- May be acute or chronic (occurring >6 months)
- The International Federation of Gynecology and Obstetrics (FIGO) now uses AUB rather than dysfunctional uterine bleeding (DUB).

EPIDEMIOLOGY

Adolescent and perimenopausal women are affected most often.

Incidence

5% of reproductive-aged women will see a doctor in any given year for AUB.

Prevalence

3–30% of reproductive-aged women have AUB.

ETIOLOGY AND PATHOPHYSIOLOGY

- Anovulation accounts for 90% of AUB.
- Adolescent AUB is usually due to an immature hypothalamic-pituitary-ovarian (HPO) axis that leads to anovulatory cycles.
- The mnemonic PALM-COEIN (1) was developed to describe AUB in reproductive aged women.
- PALM (structural causes): polyp, adenomyosis, leiomyoma, and malignancy and/or hyperplasia
- COEIN (nonstructural causes): coagulopathy, ovulatory disorders, endometrial, iatrogenic, and not yet classified
- Coagulopathy
  - 20% of patients with heavy menstrual bleeding have a bleeding disorder.
  - Two most common coagulopathies involved: von Willebrand disease and thrombocytopenia
- Diseases causing ovulatory dysfunction
  - Hyperparathyroidism, hypothyroidism, adrenal disorders, pituitary disease (prolactinoma), PCOS, eating disorders
- Medications (iatrogenic causes)
  - Anticoagulants, steroids, tamoxifen (estrogen receptor antagonists), hormonal contraception, copper IUD, antipsychotic medications (mostly first generation), postmenopausal hormone replacement therapy, antiemetics (metoclopramide and domperidone specifically)
- Other causes of AUB not defined in PALM-COEIN: ectopic pregnancy, threatened or incomplete abortion or hydatidiform mole, upper genital tract infections, advanced or fulminant liver disease, chronic renal disease, nutritional deficiencies, inflammatory bowel disease, excessive weight gain, increased exercise

Genetics

Unclear but can include inherited disorders of hemostasis

RISK FACTORS

- Unopposed estrogen therapy (no. 1 risk factor for endometrial cancer)
- Increasing age, typically >40 years old; obesity; PCOS; diabetes mellitus; nulliparity; early menarche or late menopause (>55 years of age); chronic anovulation or infertility; history of breast cancer or endometrial hyperplasia; tamoxifen use; family history: gynecologic, breast, or colon cancer; thyroid disease

GENERAL PREVENTION

No direct preventive measure for AUB

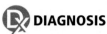 **DIAGNOSIS**

The most valuable in diagnosis and determining etiology is history.

HISTORY

- Menstrual history: onset, severity (quantified by pad/tampon use, presence and size of clots), timing of bleeding (unpredictable or episodic) over the last 6 months; also assess menopausal status.
- Association with other factors (e.g., coitus, contraception, weight loss/gain)
- Gynecologic history: gravidity and parity, STI history, previous Pap smear results
- Review of systems (Exclude symptoms of pregnancy, bleeding disorders, stress, exercise, recent weight change, visual changes, headaches, and galactorrhea.)

ALERT

Postmenopausal bleeding is any bleeding that occurs >1 year after the last menstrual period; cancer must always be ruled out (1)[C].

PHYSICAL EXAM

Evaluate for:

- Body mass index, pallor, vital signs, visual field defects (may suggest a pituitary lesion), vaginal discharge, hirsutism or acne, goiter, galactorrhea, purpura, ecchymosis
- Pelvic exam: uterine irregularities and Tanner stage, foreign bodies; rule out rectal or urinary tract bleeding; include Pap smear and tests for STIs (2)[C].

Pediatric Considerations

Premenarchal children with vaginal bleeding should be evaluated for foreign bodies, physical/sexual abuse, possible infections, and signs of precocious puberty.

DIFFERENTIAL DIAGNOSIS

See "Etiology and Pathophysiology."

DIAGNOSTIC TESTS & INTERPRETATION

Initial Tests (lab, imaging)

- All patients: urine hCG and CBC: For acute heavy/hemorrhagic bleeding, a type and crossmatch should be obtained.
- If coagulopathy is suspected, prothrombin time (PT), activated partial thromboplastin time (aPTT), and fibrinogen level; if abnormal, get von Willebrand factor, ristocetin cofactor assay, and factor VIII.

- Consider other tests based on differential diagnosis:
  - Suspected hormonal abnormalities: TSH, prolactin level, follicle-stimulating hormone (FSH)
  - Concern for infection: STI screening, KOH prep, vaginitis panel
  - Possible congenital adrenal hyperplasia: 17-Hydroxyprogesterone
  - Possible PCOS: testosterone and/or dehydroepiandrosterone sulfate (DHEA-S) if PCOS is suspected
- TVUS in postmenopausal AUB
  - American College of Obstetricians and Gynecologists (ACOG) continues to recommend endometrial sampling for postmenopausal women with AUB but states that a thin, homogeneous endometrial thickness (ET) <4 mm does not require endometrial sampling unless bleeding is persistent or recurrent, whereas ET >4 mm should prompt further evaluation (based on ACOG 2018 guidelines) (3)[C]. Sampling of thin endometrium is often unsatisfactory for histologic evaluation.
  - Incidentally found endometrial measurement >4 mm without associated bleeding in postmenopausal women should not trigger evaluation; however, assessment based on individual risk factors is appropriate.
- TVUS, sonohysterography, and hysteroscopy may be similarly effective in detection of intrauterine pathology in premenopausal women with AUB.

Follow-Up Tests & Special Considerations

It is appropriate to initiate medical therapy in females <35 years of age if low risk of uterine anatomic/histologic abnormality or adenomyosis prior to performing an endometrial biopsy (EMB)

Diagnostic Procedures/Other

- Pap smear to screen for cervical cancer if age >21 years (2)[C]
- EMB
  - Women aged >45 years with AUB to rule out cancer or premalignancy
  - Postmenopausal women with ET ≥4 mm
  - Women aged 18 to 45 years with AUB, a history of unopposed estrogen, and failed medical management
  - Women of any age without risk factors if they have abnormal findings following imaging (2)
  - Perform on or after day 18 of cycle, if known; secretory endometrium confirms that ovulation occurred.
- Hysteroscopy with targeted biopsy if suspected intrauterine lesion with negative EMB; NPV for endometrial cancer with negative hysteroscopy at any age is 99.5%.

Test Interpretation

Pap smear could reveal carcinoma or inflammation indicative of cervicitis. Most EMBs show proliferative or dyssynchronous endometrium (suggesting anovulation) but can show simple or complex hyperplasia without atypia, hyperplasia with atypia, or endometrial adenocarcinoma.

TREATMENT

GENERAL MEASURES

NSAIDs (naproxen sodium 500 mg BID, mefenamic acid 500 mg TID, ibuprofen 600 to 1,200 mg/day)

- Decreases amount of blood loss and pain compared with placebo
- "Surgical" approaches (including LNG-IUD) generally superior to medical approaches for long-term control (4)[A]

MEDICATION

First Line

- Acute, emergent, nonovulatory bleeding
  - Conjugated equine estrogen (Premarin): 25 mg IV q4h (max of 6 doses) stops bleeding within 8 hours in 72% of individuals, or 2.5 mg Premarin PO q6h should control bleeding in 12 to 24 hours (2)[A].
  - Tranexamic acid (TXA) 1.3 g PO or 10 mg/kg IV (max of 600 mg/dose) TID
  - Intrauterine tamponade by filling 26F foley bulb with 30 mL saline
  - D&C if no response after 2 to 4 doses of Premarin or sooner if bleeding >1 pad per hour
  - Change to oral contraceptive pill (OCP) or progestin for cycle regulation
- Acute, nonemergent, nonovulatory bleeding:
  - Monophasic combined OCPs with 35 μg of estrogen TID for 7 days shown to stop bleeding in 88% of women
  - Medroxyprogesterone acetate 20 mg PO TID for 7 days shown to stop bleeding in 76% of women in 3 days
- Nonacute, nonovulatory bleeding
  - Levonorgestrel IUD (Mirena) is the most effective (71–95% decrease in blood loss) form of progesterone delivery and not inferior to surgical management (4)[A].
  - Progestins: medroxyprogesterone acetate (Provera) 10 mg/day for 5 to 10 days each month; daily progesterone for 21 days per cycle results in significantly less blood loss (5)[A]; medroxyprogesterone acetate (Depo-Provera) 150 mg q12wk
  - OCPs: 20 to 35 μg daily estrogen plus progesterone (Consider especially for anovulatory females <18 years old who are not yet sexually active.)
  - TXA 1.0 to 1.5 g by mouth three times a day; avoid in patients with hypercoagulable states.
- Do not use estrogen if contraindications exist (suspicion for endometrial hyperplasia or carcinoma, history of DVT, migraine with aura, or smoking in women >35 years of age [relative contraindication]).
- Precautions
  - Failed medical treatment requires further workup and consideration of surgical management.
  - Consider DVT prophylaxis when treating with high-dose estrogens (2)[C].

Second Line

- Gonadotropin-releasing hormone (GnRH) agonists: leuprolide (varying doses and duration of action)
- GnRH antagonists (elagolix 300 mg BID): FDA approved for heavy menstrual bleeding due to uterine fibroids in premenopausal women combined with add-back therapy (1 mg estradiol/0.5 mg norethindrone acetate once a day)
- Danazol (200 to 400 mg/day for a maximum of 9 months) is more effective than NSAIDs but is limited by androgenic side effects and cost; now replaced by GnRH agonists
- Metformin or clomifene (Clomid) alone or in combination in women with PCOS who desire ovulation and pregnancy

ISSUES FOR REFERRAL

If an obvious cause for vaginal bleeding is not found in a pediatric patient, refer to a pediatric endocrinologist or pediatric/adolescent gynecology.

ADDITIONAL THERAPIES

- Antiemetics if treating with high-dose estrogen or progesterone (2)[C]
- Iron supplementation if anemia (usually iron deficiency) is identified

SURGERY/OTHER PROCEDURES

- Hysterectomy in cases of endometrial cancer, if medical therapy fails, or if other uterine pathology is found
- Endometrial ablation, less expensive than hysterectomy and associated with high patient satisfaction; this is a permanent procedure and should be avoided in patients who desire continued fertility.
- Uterine artery embolization if bleeding is refractory to medications or confirmed fibroids

ADMISSION, INPATIENT, AND NURSING CONSIDERATIONS

- Significant hemorrhage causing acute anemia with signs of hemodynamic instability; with acute bleeding, replace volume with crystalloid and blood, as necessary.
- Pad counts and clot size can be helpful to determine and monitor amount of bleeding.
- Discharge criteria: hemodynamic stability and control of vaginal bleeding

 ONGOING CARE

FOLLOW-UP RECOMMENDATIONS

Once stable from acute management, recommend follow-up evaluation in 4 to 6 months for further evaluation.

Patient Monitoring

Women treated with estrogen or OCPs should keep a menstrual diary to document bleeding patterns and their relation to therapy.

DIET

No restrictions, although a 5% reduction in weight can induce ovulation in anovulation caused by PCOS

PATIENT EDUCATION

https://www.acog.org/Patients

PROGNOSIS

- Varies with pathophysiologic process
- Most anovulatory cycles can be treated with medical therapy and do not require surgical intervention.

COMPLICATIONS

Iron deficiency anemia, mood disorders

REFERENCES

1. Wouk N, Helton M. Abnormal uterine bleeding in premenopausal women. *Am Fam Physician.* 2019;99(7):435–443.
2. Committee on Practice Bulletins—Gynecology. Practice Bulletin No. 128: diagnosis of abnormal uterine bleeding in reproductive-aged women. *Obstet Gynecol.* 2012;120(1):197–206.
3. Khafaga A, Goldstein SR. Abnormal uterine bleeding. *Obstet Gynecol Clin North Am.* 2019;46(4):595–605.
4. Marjoribanks J, Lethaby A, Farquhar C. Surgery versus medical therapy for heavy menstrual bleeding. *Cochrane Database Syst Rev.* 2016;2016(1):CD003855.
5. Lethaby A, Irvine G, Cameron I. Cyclical progestogens for heavy menstrual bleeding. *Cochrane Database Syst Rev.* 2008;(1):CD001016.

 SEE ALSO

- Dysmenorrhea; Menorrhagia (Heavy Menstrual Bleeding)
- Algorithm: Abnormal Uterine Bleeding

CODES

ICD10

- N93.9 Abnormal uterine and vaginal bleeding, unspecified
- N93.8 Other specified abnormal uterine and vaginal bleeding

CLINICAL PEARLS

- AUB is irregular uterine bleeding that occurs in the absence of pregnancy or pathology, making it a diagnosis of exclusion.
- Anovulation accounts for 90% of AUB.
- EMB should be performed in
  - Women aged >45 years with AUB
  - Women aged 18 to 45 years with AUB and a history of unopposed estrogen and failed medical management

ABNORMAL PAP AND CERVICAL DYSPLASIA

Anna K. Zheng, MD • Henry Del Rosario, MD

BASICS

DESCRIPTION
- Cervical dysplasia: premalignant cervical disease that is also called cervical intraepithelial neoplasia (CIN); precancerous epithelial changes in the transformation zone of the uterine cervix almost always associated with human papillomavirus (HPV) infections
- CIN encompasses a range of histologic diagnoses.
  - CIN I: mild dysplasia; low-grade lesion; cellular changes are limited to the lower 1/3 of the squamous epithelium.
  - CIN II: moderate dysplasia; high-grade lesion; cellular changes are limited to the lower 2/3 of the squamous epithelium.
  - CIN III or carcinoma in situ: severe dysplasia; high-grade lesion; cellular changes involve the full thickness of the squamous epithelium.
- System(s) affected: reproductive

Pediatric Considerations
Only 0.1% of cervical cancers occur before age 20 years. Screening any individual with a cervix age <21 years (regardless of sexual debut and history) does not reduce cervical cancer incidence and mortality compared with beginning screening at age 21 years.

Geriatric Considerations
- Any individual with a cervix and age >65 years who has had adequate prior screening and no history of CIN II+ in the last 20 years should not be screened for cervical cancer. Adequate prior screening is defined as three consecutive negative cytology-only results or two consecutive negative HPV testing alone or negative cytology "cotesting" with negative HPV results within 10 years before cessation of screening (with the most recent test within the last 5 years).
- Routine screening should continue for at least 25 years at 3-year intervals with HPV testing or cotesting after spontaneous regression or appropriate management of a high-grade precancerous lesion, even if this extends screening past the age 65 years (1)[C].

Pregnancy Considerations
- Squamous intraepithelial lesions can progress during pregnancy but often regress postpartum.
- Colposcopy only to exclude the presence of invasive cancer in high-risk individuals
- Unless cancer is identified or suspected, treatment of CIN is contraindicated during pregnancy.

EPIDEMIOLOGY
Cervical cancer is the fourth most common type of cancer in women worldwide. In the United States, cervical cancer has dropped to 20th place in causes of cancer deaths in 2021. Incidence of CIN III peaks between ages 25 and 29 years; invasive disease peaks 15 years later. Cervical cancer most commonly occurs in those aged 35 to 44 years. More than 15% of cervical cancer cases occur in those >65 years of age (occurs in those who did not get regular screening).

Incidence
In 2021, it was projected that there would be 14,480 new cases of cervical cancer diagnosed and 4,290 women will die from the disease. The incidence of cervical cancer in the United States has decreased by >50% in the past 40 years because of widespread cervical cancer screening tests.

Prevalence
Multiple studies in populations around the world have found that prevalence of high-grade dysplasia has fallen significantly in HPV-immunized populations.

ETIOLOGY AND PATHOPHYSIOLOGY
HPV is so common that most sexually active men and women will get at least one type of HPV at some point in their lives.
- High-risk HPV types: 16, 18, 31, 33, 35, 45, 52, and 58 are common oncogenic virus types for cervical cancer. HPV types 16 and 18 are associated with ~70% of all cervical cancers.
- Most HPV infections are transient, becoming undetectable within 1 to 2 years. Persistent infections are what place women at significant risk for developing precancerous lesions. Compared to younger women, women age >30 years are less likely to clear a new HPV infection.
- Low-risk types: HPV viral types 6, 11, 42, 43, and 44 are considered common low-risk types and may cause genital warts. HPV types 6 and 11 (cause 90% of benign anogenital warts) can lead to low-grade squamous intraepithelial lesion (LSIL) and CIN I.

RISK FACTORS
- HIV infection and other immunosuppressive conditions
- In utero exposure to diethylstilbestrol
- Cigarette smoking
- Multiple sexual partners
- Some correlation with low socioeconomic status, high parity, oral contraceptive use, and poor nutrition

GENERAL PREVENTION
Immunization: Immunization decreases high-risk HPV infections and CIN2/3 cervical pathology for at least 5 to 7 years but has not yet been shown to decrease cervical cancer. It is likely that prevention of invasive cancer will be demonstrated within a few years. Ideally, HPV immunization of girls, boys, and any individual with a cervix should be initiated prior to first intercourse. Per the Advisory Committee on Immunization Practices (ACIP), offer HPV vaccine to adolescents 11 to 12 years of age and can start vaccination as early as 9 years old. Gardasil 9: The U.S. FDA approved in October 2018 for use in females and males aged 9 to 26 years and via shared clinical decision for ages 27 to 45 years; 88% effective preventing dysplasia due to HPV types 16 and 18 (75% of cervical cancer), types 6 and 11 (anogenital warts), and protection against five additional HPV types, which cause approximately 25% of CIN II+ lesions
- Vaccine schedule: If the first vaccine dose was given before the 15th birthday, only 2 doses are required to complete the series, 6 to 12 months apart; if vaccine began on or after the 15th birthday: 3 doses at 0, 2, and 6 months
- Immunocompromising conditions: 3 doses needed

- Safe sex practices: condom use. Advise smoking cessation.
- Screening
  - Pap smear has been the main screening test for cervical cellular pathology, with or without cotesting for HPV.
  - Screening recommendations by age and source (see algorithm "Pap, Normal and Abnormal in Nonpregnant Women Ages 25 Years and Older" and separate algorithm "Pap, Normal and Abnormal in Women Ages 21–24 Years"). <21 years: Do not screen (USPSTF/ASCCP/ASCP/ACOG) (2)[A].
  - Frequency of screening recommendation: USPSTF/ASCCP/ASCP/ACOG generally agree by age and screen.
    - 21 to 29 years: Screen with cytology every 3 years. For patients aged ≥25 years, screen every 5 years with primary HPV testing using an assay method explicitly approved for primary HPV testing (preferred) or every 3 years with cytology (acceptable) (1).
    - 30 to 65 years: Screen with either primary HPV testing or cotesting every 5 years (1)[C]. Cytology every 3 years, if cotesting or HPV-only testing is not available, is also acceptable (1),(2).
    - >65 years (who have had adequate prior screening and are not high risk): Do not screen (2)[A].
  - The 2020 ACS recommendations differ from previous guidelines by screening at a later age of 25 years and preferring the HPV test alone (3) if available; ages 21 to 24 years: no screening.
- Special circumstances: patients after hysterectomy with removal of the cervix and with no history of CIN II+: Do not screen (2)[A]. Patients with history of CIN II+ or status treatment should continue screening until at least 25 years following their diagnosis of CIN II+ (1)[C].
- HIV-positive patients: Screen individuals every 3 years in those who have had three consecutive normal annual Pap tests and every 3 years cotesting in ages ≥30 years.

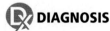
DIAGNOSIS

HISTORY
Usually asymptomatic until there is invasive disease

PHYSICAL EXAM
Pelvic exam occasionally reveals external HPV lesions. Examine for exophytic or ulcerative cervical lesions, with or without bleeding.

DIFFERENTIAL DIAGNOSIS
Acute or chronic cervicitis; cervical glandular hyperplasia; uterine malignancy

DIAGNOSTIC TESTS & INTERPRETATION
- Current evidence indicates no clinically important differences between conventional cytology and liquid-based cytology in detecting cervical cancer precursors. Conventional Pap smear involves a cervical sample plated on a microscope slide with fixative. ThinPrep is a liquid-based collection and thin-layer preparation.

- To ensure an adequate sample of both the ecto- and endocervix, use a cytobrush and an extended tip spatula.
- The sensitivity and specificity of using HPV and cytology testing together (cotesting) for dysplasia is near 100% and 92.5%, respectively. Cotesting leads to earlier diagnosis of CIN III+ and cancer than does cytology alone. Testing for high-risk HPV using an assay specifically approved for primary screening without cytology is preferred for individuals with a cervix aged ≥25 years, particularly for poorly screened or unscreened populations. Per updated 2019 ASCCP guidelines, cytology screening alone is also acceptable when HPV or cotesting is not feasible. Per 2020 ACS, HPV testing alone is preferred due to comparable sensitivity to HPV/Pap cotesting and being more efficient in effort and cost.
- Cytology report component: specimen type (conventional Pap smear or liquid based), adequacy (presence of endocervical cells), and categorization (negative for intraepithelial lesion or malignancy or epithelial cell abnormality; i.e., squamous/glandular)
- Bethesda 2014 system (cytologic grading) epithelial cell abnormalities
  - Squamous cell: atypical squamous cells (ASC) (of undetermined significance [ASC-US], cannot exclude high-grade squamous intraepithelial lesion or HSIL [ASC-H]). HPV, mild dysplasia, CIN I. Moderate/severe dysplasia CIS, CIN II, and CIN III
  - Glandular cell: atypical glandular cells (AGCs) favor neoplasia, not otherwise specified; AGCs: favor neoplasia. AIS (adenocarcinoma in situ), adenocarcinoma

Diagnostic Procedures/Other

Clinical action depend on immediate risk of CIN 3+ for cases aged ≥25 years (1)[C]. Algorithms from 2012 ASCCP guidelines differ for women aged 21 to 24 years, provided below (4)[C].

- ASC-US: (<25 years of age)
  - Option 1: HPV testing (preferred)
    - If HPV positive, proceed to clinical action depending on immediate CIN 3+ risk (1),(4)[C].
    - If HPV negative, repeat cotesting at 3 years (4)[C].
  - Option 2: Repeat cytology at 1 year (acceptable) (4)[C].
    - If repeat cytology ASC or greater, proceed to colposcopy or other clinical action if immediate CIN 3+ risk is known.
    - If repeat cytology is negative, proceed to routine screening.
- ASC-H (<25 years of age): colposcopy required
- LSIL: (<25 years of age)
  - LSIL with negative HPV test: Repeat cotesting at 1 year (preferred).
    - If cotesting is negative, repeat cotesting in 3 years.
    - If cotesting is positive, proceed to colposcopy or repeat cotesting in 1 year.
  - LSIL with no HPV test or positive HPV test: Proceed to colposcopy.
  - LSIL in pregnancy: colposcopy preferred, but it is acceptable to defer colposcopy to postpartum (4)[B].
- HSIL/CIN2 or 3+/AGCs/Atypical endometrial cells (≥21 years): likely colposcopy but clinical action ultimately depends on immediate CIN 3+ risk (1)[C]

- Age ≥25 years/special populations/rarely screened/status posttreatment/history of CIN 2, CIN 3, AIS or invasive cancer: clinical action only when immediate CIN 3+ risk is ≥4% with stress on shared decision-making; can proceed to treatment if immediate CIN 3+ risk is >60% and bypass colposcopy biopsy (1)

Test Interpretation

Atypical squamous or columnar cells, coarse nuclear material, increased nuclear diameter, koilocytosis (HPV hallmark)

TREATMENT

ASCCP smart-phone application includes 2019 guidelines: Evidence-based management phone application includes algorithms to guide Pap smear and post-colposcopic diagnostics and therapeutics are available online at https://www.asccp.org/mobile-app and https://www.asccp.org/management-guidelines (1),(4).

GENERAL MEASURES

Office evaluation and observation; promote smoking cessation; promote safe sex practices; promote immunization.

MEDICATION

Infective/reactive Pap smear: Treat organism/condition found on Pap smear results. Condyloma acuminatum treatment options: See chapter "Condylomata Acuminata."

SURGERY/OTHER PROCEDURES

- Expedited treatment that bypasses colposcopy biopsy is recommended for nonpregnant patients aged ≥25 years with immediate CIN 3+ risk of >60% and is acceptable for immediate CIN 3+ risk between 25% and 60% while stressing the importance of shared decision-making (1).
- Observation is preferred to treatment for CIN I (1). Colposcopy can be deferred for certain patients, and repeat HPV testing or cotesting in 1 year is recommended if immediate CIN 3+ risk is low risk (<4%).
- Excisional treatment is preferred to ablative treatment for histologic HSIL (CIN 2 or CIN 3). For AIS, excision is recommended (1).
- If cervical malignancy, see "Cervical Malignancy."

ONGOING CARE

FOLLOW-UP RECOMMENDATIONS

After treatment (excision or ablation) of HSIL, CIN II or III, or AIS and initial posttreatment management, women should reenter screening with HPV testing or cotesting at 3-year intervals for at least 25 years (1).

PATIENT EDUCATION

HPV vaccination, smoking cessation, protected intercourse, regular screening with Pap smear per guidelines

PROGNOSIS

- Progression of CIN to invasive cervical cancer is slow, and the likelihood of regression is high: Up to 43% of CIN II and 32% of CIN III lesions may regress. CIN III has a 30% probability of becoming invasive cancer over a 30-year period, although only about 1% if treated.

- CIN III becomes invasive: Lesions discovered early are amenable to treatment with excellent results and few recurrences.
- The 5-year survival rate for cervical cancer patients is 66.3%. The 5-year relative survival rate for patients diagnosed with localized disease is 91.9%.

COMPLICATIONS

Aggressive cervical surgery may be associated with cervical stenosis, cervical incompetence (leading to preterm labor), and scarring affecting cervical dilation in labor.

REFERENCES

1. Perkins RB, Guido RS, Castle PE, et al. 2019 ASCCP risk-based management consensus guidelines for abnormal cervical cancer screening tests and cancer precursors. *J Low Genit Tract Dis*. 2020;24(2):102–131.
2. Curry SJ, Krist AH, Owens DK, et al. Screening for cervical cancer: US Preventive Services Task Force recommendation statement. *JAMA*. 2018;320(7):674–686.
3. Fontham ETH, Wolf AMD, Church TR, et al. Cervical cancer screening for individuals at average risk: 2020 guideline update from the American Cancer Society. *CA Cancer J Clin*. 2020;70(5):321–346.
4. Massad LS, Einstein MH, Huh WK, et al. 2012 Updated consensus guidelines for the management of abnormal cervical cancer screening tests and cancer precursors. *J Low Genit Tract Dis*. 2013;17(5 Suppl 1):S1–S27.

ADDITIONAL READING

American Society for Colposcopy and Cervical Pathology. ASCCP diagnostic and management guidelines. https://www.asccp.org/management-guidelines. Accessed December 3, 2022.

 SEE ALSO

- Cervical Malignancy; Condylomata Acuminata; Trichomoniasis; Vulvovaginitis, Prepubescent
- Algorithms: Pap, Normal and Abnormal in Nonpregnant Women Ages 25 Years and Older; Pap, Normal and Abnormal in Women Ages 21–24 Years

 CODES

ICD10

- R87.619 Unspecified abnormal cytological findings in specimens from cervix uteri
- N87.9 Dysplasia of cervix uteri, unspecified
- N87.1 Moderate cervical dysplasia

CLINICAL PEARLS

- Vaccine should be offered prior to onset of any sexual activity for maximum effectiveness.
- Know and adhere to recognized screening guidelines to avoid the harms of over screening.
- Optimal screening strategy is in evolution. HPV-only screening is now preferred due to test being more sensitive than cytology alone (1), but the approved assay is not yet widely available in 2021.

ACETAMINOPHEN POISONING

Janet Chen, DO • Jennifer A. Meeks, DO

 BASICS

DESCRIPTION

- A disorder characterized by hepatic necrosis following large acetaminophen ingestions. Clinical manifestations of acetaminophen toxicity vary with time since ingestion and are generally classified into four stages.
- Single, large ingestions of acetaminophen account for a majority of poisonings. Toxicity can also occur with ingestions of lesser amounts in individuals who regularly abuse alcohol, are chronically malnourished, or take medications impacting hepatic metabolism. Ingestions greater than 12 g in adults and greater than 250 mg/kg in children are likely to cause toxicity.

EPIDEMIOLOGY

- Two-thirds of hospitalizations due to acetaminophen toxicity are due to intentional ingestion. Most (80%) are adults and 70% are women. 50% of poison control calls related to acetaminophen are related to unintentional ingestions in children under 5.
- Second leading factor associated with liver transplantation worldwide
- More than 50,000 emergency department visits, >2,500 hospitalizations, and nearly 500 deaths annually in the United States are associated with acetaminophen ingestion.

ETIOLOGY AND PATHOPHYSIOLOGY

Pharmacokinetics

- With oral therapeutic ingestion, acetaminophen is entirely absorbed from the duodenum and reaches peak serum concentrations of 10 to 20 μg/mL after up to 2 hours. This peak may be delayed with toxic ingestions.
- Therapeutic adult doses of acetaminophen are 325 to 1,000 mg q4–6h to a maximum dose of 4 g/day. Therapeutic pediatric doses are 10 to 15 mg/kg q4–6h, not to exceed 5 doses in 24 hours or 75 g/kg/day.
- The elimination half-life of acetaminophen ranges from 2 to 4 hours but may be delayed in extended-release formulation.

Pathophysiology

Ingestion of supratherapeutic doses of acetaminophen or subtherapeutic ingestions in individuals with compromised liver function can cause acetaminophen poisoning and result in hepatocellular damage. The liver metabolizes 96% of ingested acetaminophen and 2–4% is excreted in urine. Therapeutic doses break down into 90–95% benign metabolites and 5–10% of the toxic metabolite, N-acetyl-p-benzoquinone imine (NAPQI). NAPQI is rapidly conjugated with hepatic stores of glutathione to form a nontoxic metabolite to be excreted in the urine. Toxic ingestions of acetaminophen saturate the glucuronidation and sulfation pathways, depleting glutathione stores and result in accumulations of NAPQI that cause hepatocellular damage.

RISK FACTORS

Concurrent poisoning with other substances can impact the hepatic metabolism; psychiatric illness or history of suicide attempts; regular ingestion of large amounts of alcohol; chronic malnutrition and possible risk related to previous weight loss surgery

GENERAL PREVENTION

- Poison Control: 800-222-1222 for consultations and management guidance
- FDA labeling guidance: http://www.fda.gov/Drugs/GuidanceComplianceRegulatoryInformation/Guidances/default.htm

Geriatric Considerations

There is an increased risk of hepatic damage in elderly patients due to decreased hepatic metabolism and coingestion of other hepatotoxic medications. Keep dose of acetaminophen ≤3,000 mg/day in seniors and in patients with liver disease and/or alcohol abuse disorders.

Pediatric Considerations

Hepatic damage after ingestion of toxic acetaminophen doses can be less severe in young children, potentially because they have more stores of glutathione.

Pregnancy Considerations

There is an increased incidence of spontaneous abortion in pregnant patients with acetaminophen poisoning, especially with overdose at an early gestational age. Abortion incidence and possible fetal death is increased if N-acetylcysteine (NAC) treatment is delayed. IV NAC is generally preferred in pregnancy due to greater bioavailability.

 DIAGNOSIS

Signs and symptoms of poisoning develop over the first 24 hours following large ingestions. Symptoms may develop gradually in those with a history of long-term ingestion near supratherapeutic doses. Presentation of symptoms varies, and it is divided into four stages:

- Stage 1—first 24 hours after ingestion
  - Patient may be asymptomatic in first 8 hours following ingestion. Symptoms may include nausea, emesis, anorexia, and diaphoresis. Laboratory results are usually unremarkable at this time.
- Stage 2—days 2 to 3 following ingestion
  - Typically less nausea, vomiting, diaphoresis, and malaise than in stage 1. Right upper quadrant pain and hepatomegaly may become evident. Elevated aminotransferases are usually seen.
- Stage 3—days 3 to 4 following ingestion
  - Stage 1 symptoms such as nausea, vomiting, and malaise reappear. Severe poisonings may result in jaundice, confusion, somnolence, and coma. Marked liver enzyme elevations which usually peak at this point; prolonged prothrombin time (PT)/international normalized ratio (INR); typically negative acetaminophen levels. Multiorgan failure and death most commonly occur in this stage.
- Stage 4—days 5+ after ingestion
  - Possible recovery stage in patients with resolving stage 3 symptoms. Recovery may be prolonged, but is typically complete and without long-term sequelae. Laboratory abnormalities typically resolve. Fulminant hepatic failure occurs in <1% of adults and is very rare in children <6 years of age.

HISTORY

Primary questions should focus on what was ingested (extended release, hydrocodone-acetaminophen, co-ingestants, etc.), how much was ingested, and time of ingestion. Was the ingestion intentional or accidental? Also ask regarding current or history of alcohol abuse, hepatitis, and previous surgeries.

PHYSICAL EXAM

Physical exam findings will likely vary depending on stage of toxicity. In general, a full physical examination is warranted with vitals assessment.

- Assess individual's general appearance for somnolence, fatigue, pallor, diaphoresis, and signs of dehydration.
- Look for signs of hepatotoxicity: hepatomegaly and right upper quadrant pain.

DIFFERENTIAL DIAGNOSIS

- Consider presence of co-ingestants, especially alcohol, opiates, and aspirin.
- Other ingested toxins that produce severe acute hepatic injury, including the mushroom *Amanita phalloides* and products containing yellow phosphorus or carbon tetrachloride. Consider other causes of hepatitis: alcoholic, viral, ischemic.

DIAGNOSTIC TESTS & INTERPRETATION

Initial Tests (lab, imaging)

- Draw plasma acetaminophen levels on all patients ≥4 hours after ingestion (levels peak at 4 hours). Draw additional levels at 6 and 8 hours if extended-release form was ingested. Poison Control may help guide the frequency of exams, vitals, or any other ancillary testing that may be warranted.
  - If a sustained-released product has been ingested, obtain two serum acetaminophen levels 4 to 6 hours apart. Treat if either level is above the possible toxicity line.
  - For chronic toxicity or patients who present 24 hours post-ingestion, treat based on clinical effects, LFTs, and the acetaminophen level.
- Liver function tests: alanine transaminase (ALT), aspartate transaminase (AST), PT/INR, bilirubin, lactate dehydrogenase (LDH)
  - With severe poisonings, PT/INR rise in parallel with LFT changes. With toxic ingestions, AST, ALT, and bilirubin levels begin to rise in stage 2 and peak in stage 3. Improvement in ALT with therapy is an encouraging clinical sign.
- Additional labs: electrolytes, glucose, BUN, creatinine, urinalysis, urine drug screen (UDS), serum alcohol, and salicylate
  - Screen for coingestants with the above labs and consider searching for other medications/substances depending on the clinical history. Obtain a pregnancy screen in females (urine or serum) as it can influence management.
  - Consider an arterial blood gas (ABG): anion gap metabolic acidosis due to accumulation of 5-oxoproline may rarely be seen.
- Imaging: No specific imaging is required.

Follow-Up Tests & Special Considerations

During recovery, liver tests should normalize and complete restoration of liver function without long-term sequelae is expected.

Diagnostic Procedures/Other

Advanced imaging of the liver and/or kidney with ultrasound or CT should be considered when acute hepatitis or kidney injury is present to rule out alternative causes. Otherwise, imaging is not required and any abnormal findings, if present, may be nonspecific.

 TREATMENT

- Immediately contact a local Poison Control center for recommendations. Call (800) 222-1222 in the United States.
- NAC is a benign prodrug that provides cysteine as a substrate to detoxify acetaminophen metabolites and replenish glutathione stores in the liver. NAC administration may reduce mortality from 5% to 0.7%.
- The Rumack-Matthew nomogram:
  - A plot used to determine if acetaminophen levels are high enough to warrant treatment with NAC during acute toxic ingestions. The nomogram is not intended for sustained-release products or chronic ingestions.
  - Give NAC when acetaminophen plasma levels measured ≥4 hours after ingestion are at the "treatment line" or higher on the Rumack-Matthew nomogram.
  - Treatment line acetaminophen plasma levels on the nomogram correspond to >150 μg/mL (993 μmol/L), >75 μg/mL (497 μmol/L), and >37 μg/mL (244 μmol/L) at 4, 8, and 12 hours after ingestion, respectively.
- Initiate NAC (Mucomyst) within 8 hours of ingestion whenever possible; single-dose activated charcoal (1 g/kg PO) may be effective if given within 1 to 4 hours of ingestion. *Never* delay oral NAC for activated charcoal.
- Ipecac and gastric lavage are no longer recommended for routine use at home or in health care facilities (1).

MEDICATION

First Line

- Empirically start NAC within 8 hours even while awaiting lab results. It may be effective up to ≥36 hours after ingestion.
  - NAC may be given PO or IV, depending on situation and availability. IV NAC has been shown to decrease the length of hospitalization compared to PO NAC (1).
  - A two-bag regimen should be used to administer a total of 300 mg/kg IV NAC (Acetadote, Cetylev) over a 20-hour period to reduce adverse effects of NAC administration. Begin with a 200 mg/kg IV dose over 4 hours followed by a 100 mg/kg IV dose over 16 hours.
  - Use an oral loading dose of 140 mg/kg and then 70 mg/kg q4h for 17 additional doses (72-hour regimen).

- NAC precautions:
  - PO NAC may cause significant nausea and vomiting due to its sulfur content and is often poorly tolerated; consider a nasogastric tube.
  - IV NAC (Acetadote) may cause anaphylactoid reactions, (3–6%) including rash, bronchospasm, pruritus, angioedema, tachycardia, or hypotension (higher rates seen in asthmatics and those with atopy). Reactions usually occur with the loading dose. To prevent this, slow or temporarily stop the infusion; may concurrently treat with antihistamines.
  - Nausea can be treated with metoclopramide, 1 to 2 mg/kg IV, or ondansetron, 0.15 mg/kg IV.
  - NAC failure rates range from 3% to 7% (1).
- Give single-dose activated charcoal within 1 to 4 hours of ingestion (especially in cases of co-ingestants). Do not delay NAC administration for use of activated charcoal.

Second Line

In massive ingestions (levels >1,000 mg/L, severe acidosis, coma/hypotension) or when severe renal failure is present, hemodialysis may improve survival (1).

ISSUES FOR REFERRAL

- Behavioral health evaluation for intentional ingestions
- Child abuse reporting if neglect led to overdose

ADMISSION, INPATIENT, AND NURSING CONSIDERATIONS

- Consider hospitalization for toxic ingestions with vital instability and/or laboratory abnormalities. Consider transfer to a psychiatric facility for intentional ingestions when medically stable.
- IV fluids are generally provided for hydration purposes.

 ONGOING CARE

FOLLOW-UP RECOMMENDATIONS

- Evaluate all patients at an accredited health care facility. Evaluate patients with evidence of organ failure, increased LFTs, or coagulopathy for emergency liver transplant (ELT) at a transplant center.
- Restrict activity if hepatic damage is significant. Outpatient management is adequate for nontoxic accidental ingestions.

DIET

No special diet, except with severe hepatic damage

PATIENT EDUCATION

Counsel patients to avoid acetaminophen (Tylenol, others) or other forms of acetaminophen, particularly if using combination product(s) containing acetaminophen. Educate parents/caregivers during well-child visits regarding appropriate OTC dosing and medication storage. Provide anticipatory guidance for caregivers, family, and cohabitants of potentially suicidal patients. Educate patients on long-term acetaminophen therapy.

PROGNOSIS

- Complete recovery with early therapy is possible and more likely in stage 4 of toxicity.
- 10% of adult patients with severe liver complications develop necrosis, hepatic encephalopathy, or require transplant.
- Hepatic failure is rare in children <6 years of age.

COMPLICATIONS

Recovery after acute poisoning is complete and sequelae are rare.

REFERENCE

1. Chiew AL, Gluud C, Brok J, et al. Interventions for paracetamol (acetaminophen) overdose. *Cochrane Database Syst Rev*. 2018;(2):CD003328.

ADDITIONAL READING

Dart RC, Mullins ME, Matoushek T, et al. Management of acetaminophen poisoning in the US and Canada: a consensus statement. *JAMA Netw Open*. 2023;6(8):e2327739.

CODES

ICD10

- T39.1X4A Poisoning by 4-Aminophenol derivatives, undetermined, init
- K71.10 Toxic liver disease with hepatic necrosis, without coma
- T39.1X1A Poisoning by 4-Aminophenol derivatives, accidental, init

CLINICAL PEARLS

- Immediately call and notify the local Poison Control Center for management recommendations (800) 222-1222 (United States).
- Give NAC when plasma acetaminophen concentrations (measured ≥4 hours after ingestion) are in the "possible risk" or higher levels. This corresponds to acetaminophen levels >150 μg/mL (993 μmol/L), >75 μg/mL (497 μmol/L), and >37 μg/mL (265 μmol/L) at 4, 8, and 12 hours after ingestion, respectively.
- Start NAC within 8 hours of ingestion for best chance of hepatic protection. Empirically give NAC in patients presenting near 8 hours while waiting for labs. A two-bag IV dosing regimen over 20 hours is preferred.
- All patients with acetaminophen liver injury (even after 8 hours) should receive NAC.
- If using oral NAC, dilute with a palatable beverage. Serve in a cup with lid and straw.
- For extended-release acetaminophen, follow plasma levels at 4, 6, and 8 hours after ingestion. Start NAC if any level is elevated.

ACNE ROSACEA
Shane L. Larson, MD

 BASICS

DESCRIPTION
- Rosacea is a chronic condition characterized by recurrent episodes of facial flushing, erythema (due to dilatation of small blood vessels in the face), papules, pustules, and telangiectasia (due to increased reactivity of capillaries) in a symmetric, central facial distribution; sometimes associated with ocular symptoms (ocular rosacea)
- Four subtypes:
  - Erythematotelangiectatic rosacea (ETR)
  - Papulopustular rosacea (PPR)
  - Phymatous rosacea
  - Ocular rosacea
- System(s) affected: skin/exocrine
- Synonym(s): rosacea

Geriatric Considerations
- Chronic inflammatory dermatosis with middle-age onset
- Effects of aging might increase the side effects associated with oral isotretinoin used for treatment (at present, data are insufficient due to lack of clinical studies in elderly patients aged ≥65 years).

EPIDEMIOLOGY
Prevalence
- Predominant age of onset: 30 to 50 years
- Predominant sex: female > male. However, males are at greater risk for progression to later stages.
- More common in Fitzpatrick skin types I and II

ETIOLOGY AND PATHOPHYSIOLOGY
- No proven cause
- Possibilities include the following:
  - Thyroid and sex hormone disturbance
  - Alcohol, coffee, tea, spiced food overindulgence (unproven)
  - Demodex follicular parasite (suspected)
  - Exposure to cold, heat
  - Emotional stress
  - Dysfunction of the GI tract (possible association with *Helicobacter pylori*)

Genetics
- People of Northern European and Celtic background commonly afflicted
- Associated with three human leukocyte antigen (HLA) alleles: HLA-DRB1, HLA-DQB1, and HLA-DQA1 (MHC class II)

RISK FACTORS
- Exposure to spicy foods, hot drinks
- Environmental factors: sun, wind, cold, heat

GENERAL PREVENTION
No preventive measures known

COMMONLY ASSOCIATED CONDITIONS
- Seborrheic dermatitis of scalp and eyelids
- Keratitis with photophobia, lacrimation, visual disturbance
- Corneal lesions
- Blepharitis
- Uveitis

 DIAGNOSIS

HISTORY
- Usually have a history of episodic flushing with increases in skin temperature in response to heat stimulus in mouth (hot liquids), spicy foods, alcohol, sun exposure
- Acne may have preceded onset of rosacea by years; nevertheless, rosacea usually arises de novo without preceding history of acne or seborrhea.
- Excessive facial warmth and redness are the predominant presenting complaints. Itching is generally absent.

PHYSICAL EXAM
- Rosacea has four subtypes:
  - The rosacea diathesis: episodic erythema, "flushing and blushing"
  - ETR: persistent erythema with telangiectases
  - PPR: persistent erythema, telangiectases, papules, pustules
  - Phymatous: persistent deep erythema, dense telangiectases, papules, pustules, nodules; rarely persistent "solid" edema of the central part of the face (phymatous)
- Progression from one subtype to another is hypothetical.
- Facial erythema, particularly on cheeks, nose, and chin. At times, entire face may be involved.
- Inflammatory papules are prominent; pustules and telangiectasia may be present.
- Comedones are absent (unlike acne vulgaris).
- Women usually have lesions on the chin and cheeks, whereas the nose is commonly involved in men.
- Ocular findings (mild dryness and irritation with blepharitis, conjunctival injection, burning, stinging, tearing, eyelid inflammation, swelling, and redness) are present in 50% of patients.

DIFFERENTIAL DIAGNOSIS
- Drug eruptions (iodides and bromides)
- Granulomas of the skin
- Cutaneous lupus erythematosus
- Carcinoid syndrome
- Acne vulgaris
- Seborrheic dermatitis
- Steroid rosacea (abuse)
- Systemic lupus erythematosus
- Lupus pernio (sarcoidosis)

DIAGNOSTIC TESTS & INTERPRETATION
- Diagnosis is based on physical exam findings.
- A recent change in classification has been proposed based on the phenotype that reflects the clinical presentation and to better focus treatment options, which are targeted to address the main clinical presentation (1).

Test Interpretation
Histology of affected skin may reveal:
- Inflammation around hypertrophied sebaceous glands, producing papules, pustules, and cysts
- Absence of comedones and blocked ducts
- Vascular dilatation and dermal lymphocytic infiltrate
- Granulomatous inflammation

 TREATMENT

GENERAL MEASURES
- Proper skin care and photoprotection are important components of management plan (1)[B]. Use of mild, nondrying soap is recommended; local skin irritants should be avoided.
- Avoidance of triggers
- Reassurance that rosacea is completely unrelated to poor hygiene
- Treat psychological stress if present.
- Topical steroids should not be used because they may aggravate rosacea.
- Avoid oil-based cosmetics:
  - Others are acceptable and may help women tolerate symptoms.
- Electrodesiccation or chemical sclerosis of permanently dilated blood vessels
- Possible evolving laser therapy
- Support physical fitness.

MEDICATION
First Line
- Topical metronidazole preparations once (1% formulation) or twice (0.75% formulations) daily for 7 to 12 weeks was significantly more effective than placebo in patients with moderate to severe rosacea. A rosacea treatment system (cleanser, metronidazole 0.75% gel, hydrating complexion corrector, and sunscreen SPF 30) may offer superior efficacy and tolerability to metronidazole (2)[A].

- Azelaic acid (Finacea) is very effective as initial therapy; azelaic acid topical alone is effective for maintenance (3)[A].
- Topical ivermectin 1% cream (2)[A]
  - Recently found to be more effective than metronidazole for treatment of PPR
- Topical brimonidine tartrate 0.5% gel is effective in reducing erythema associated with ETR (4)[A].
  - α_2-Adrenergic receptor agonist; potent vasoconstrictor
- Oxymetazoline 1% cream, an α_{1A}-adrenergic receptor agonist recently approved for the treatment of persistent erythema associated with rosacea in adults (5)[B]
- Doxycycline 40-mg dose is at least as effective as 100-mg dose and has a correspondingly lower risk of adverse effects but is much more expensive (6)[A].
- Precautions: Tetracyclines may cause photosensitivity; sunscreen is recommended.
- Significant possible interactions:
  - Tetracyclines: Avoid concurrent administration with antacids, dairy products, or iron.
  - Broad-spectrum antibiotics: may reduce the effectiveness of oral contraceptives; however, this finding has only been confirmed with rifampin; consider adding barrier method.

Second Line
- Topical erythromycin
- Topical timolol maleate 0.5%
- Topical clindamycin (lotion preferred)
  - Can be used in combination with benzoyl peroxide; commercial topical combinations are available.
- Possible use of calcineurin inhibitors (tacrolimus 0.1%; pimecrolimus 1%). Pimecrolimus 1% is effective to treat mild to moderate inflammatory rosacea.
- Permethrin 5% cream; similar efficacy compared to metronidazole for severe cases, oral isotretinoin at 0.3 mg/kg for a minimum of 3 months

Pediatric Considerations
Tetracyclines: not for use in children <8 years

Pregnancy Considerations
- Tetracyclines: not for use during pregnancy
- Isotretinoin: teratogenic; not for use during pregnancy or in women of reproductive age who are not using reliable contraception; requires registration with iPLEDGE program

ADDITIONAL THERAPIES
Cyclosporine 0.05% ophthalmic emulsion may be more effective than artificial tears for ocular rosacea.

SURGERY/OTHER PROCEDURES
Laser treatment is an option for progressive telangiectasias or rhinophyma.

- Pulsed dye laser (585 nm or 595 nm) is effective in treating telangiectases and erythema.
- CO_2 fractional ablative laser can be used to treat rhinophyma.

 ONGOING CARE

FOLLOW-UP RECOMMENDATIONS
Outpatient treatment

Patient Monitoring
- Occasional and as needed
- Close follow-up and laboratory assessment for patients using isotretinoin per prescribing instructions and iPLEDGE program guidance
- Consider ophthalmology evaluation in patients with ocular symptoms.

DIET
Avoid alcohol and hot drinks of any type.

PROGNOSIS
- Slowly progressive
- Subsides spontaneously (sometimes)

COMPLICATIONS
- Rhinophyma (dilated follicles and thickened bulbous skin on nose), especially in men
- Conjunctivitis
- Blepharitis
- Keratitis
- Visual deterioration

REFERENCES

1. Schaller M, Almeida LMC, Bewley A, et al. Rosacea treatment update: recommendations from the global ROSacea COnsensus (ROSCO) panel. *Br J Dermatol*. 2017;176(2):465–471.
2. van Zuuren EJ, Fedorowicz Z, Carter B, et al. Interventions for rosacea. *Cochrane Database Syst Rev*. 2015;2015(4):CD003262.
3. van Zuuren EJ, Fedorowicz Z, Tan J, et al. Interventions for rosacea based on the phenotype approach: an updated systematic review including GRADE assessments. *Br J Dermatol*. 2019;181(1):65–79.
4. Fowler J Jr, Jackson M, Moore A, et al. Efficacy and safety of once-daily topical brimonidine tartrate gel 0.5% for the treatment of moderate to severe facial erythema of rosacea: results of two randomized, double-blind, and vehicle-controlled pivotal studies. *J Drugs Dermatol*. 2013;12(6):650–656.
5. Oxymetazoline cream (Rhofade) for rosacea. *Med Lett Drugs Ther*. 2017;59(1521):84–86.
6. Del Rosso JQ, Webster GF, Jackson M, et al. Two randomized phase III clinical trials evaluating anti-inflammatory dose doxycycline (40-mg doxycycline, USP capsules) administered once daily for treatment of rosacea. *J Am Acad Dermatol*. 2007;56(5):791–802.

ADDITIONAL READING

- Al Mokadem SM, Ibrahim ASM, El Sayed AM. Efficacy of topical timolol 0.5% in the treatment of acne and rosacea: a multicentric study. *J Clin Aesthet Dermatol*. 2020;13(3):22–27.
- Liu RH, Smith MK, Basta SA, et al. Azelaic acid in the treatment of papulopustular rosacea: a systematic review of randomized controlled trials. *Arch Dermatol*. 2006;142(8):1047–1052.
- Mikkelsen CS, Holmgren HR, Kjellman P, et al. Rosacea: a clinical review. *Dermatol Reports*. 2016;8(1):6387.
- van Zuuren EJ, Arents BWM, van der Linden MMD, et al. Rosacea: new concepts in classification and treatment. *Am J Clin Dermatol*. 2021;22(4):457–465.

 SEE ALSO

- Acne Vulgaris; Blepharitis; Dermatitis, Seborrheic; Lupus Erythematosus, Discoid; Uveitis
- Algorithm: Acne

 CODES

ICD10
- L71.9 Rosacea, unspecified
- L71.8 Other rosacea

CLINICAL PEARLS
- Rosacea usually arises de novo without any preceding history of acne or seborrhea.
- Rosacea may cause chronic eye symptoms, including blepharitis.
- Avoid alcohol, sun exposure, and hot drinks.
- Medication treatment resembles that of acne vulgaris, with oral and topical antibiotics.

ACNE VULGARIS

Gary I. Levine, MD

BASICS

DESCRIPTION
Acne vulgaris is a disorder of the pilosebaceous units, and a chronic inflammatory dermatosis notable for open/closed comedones, papules, pustules, and/or nodules.

Geriatric Considerations
Favre-Racouchot syndrome: comedones on face/head due to sun exposure

Pregnancy Considerations
- May result in a flare or remission of acne
- Typically improves in first trimester, may worsen in third trimester
- Can use topical benzoyl peroxide (BP), azelaic acid, erythromycin, or clindamycin; salicylic acid, oral erythromycin, azithromycin, cephalexin, or amoxicillin
- Avoid topical tretinoin, trifarotene, and adapalene—may cause retinoid embryopathy; class C
- Contraindicated: isotretinoin (Category X), tazarotene, tetracycline, doxycycline, minocycline, sarecycline

Pediatric Considerations
- Neonatal acne (neonatal cephalic pustulosis)—newborn to 8 weeks; lesions limited to face; usually self-limited, Rx topical ketoconazole 2% cream
- Infantile acne—6 weeks to 1 year; lesions on face, neck, back, chest; topical/systemic Rx
- Early to middle childhood acne—1 to 7 years; rare; consider hyperandrogenism.
- Preadolescent acne—7 to 12 years; common, 47% of children, usually due to adrenal awakening, comedonal lesions
- Do not use tetracyclines in those <8 years old; other therapies similar to adolescent

EPIDEMIOLOGY
- Predominant age: early to late puberty, may persist in 20–40% into 4th decade
- Male > female (teen), female > male (adult)

Prevalence
- 80–95% of adolescents affected; 8% of adults aged 25 to 34 years; 3% at aged 35 to 44 years
- African Americans 37%, Hispanic 32%, Caucasians 24%

ETIOLOGY AND PATHOPHYSIOLOGY
- Androgens (testosterone and dehydroepiandrosterone sulfate [DHEA-S]) stimulate sebum production/qualitative sebum changes and proliferation of keratinocytes in follicles. Keratin plug obstructs follicle os, causing sebum accumulation and follicular distention.
- *Cutibacterium acnes* phylotype IA1, an anaerobe, colonizes and proliferates within a biofilm in the plugged follicle. *C. acnes* promote proinflammatory mediators/cytokines (IL-1), causing inflammation of follicle/dermis.

Genetics
Familial association in 50%

RISK FACTORS
- Increased endogenous androgenic effect
- Oily cosmetics, cocoa butter, polyvinyl chloride, chlorinated hydrocarbons, cutting oil
- Occluding skin surface (e.g., sports equipment such as helmets and shoulder pads), cell phones, hands against the skin, or pandemic masks ("maskne"—subset of acne mechanica)
- Numerous drugs, including androgenic steroids (e.g., steroid abuse, some birth control pills), lithium, phenytoin
- Endocrine disorders: PCOS, Cushing syndrome, congenital adrenal hyperplasia, androgen-secreting tumors, acromegaly
- Psychological stress
- High-glycemic load, possibly high-dairy diets (skim milk), and whey protein supplements may exacerbate acne.
- Severe acne may worsen with smoking.

GENERAL PREVENTION
Avoidance of risk factors

COMMONLY ASSOCIATED CONDITIONS
- Acne conglobata, hidradenitis suppurativa
- Pomade acne—hair oils
- SAPHO syndrome (synovitis, acne, pustulosis, hyperostosis, and osteitis)
- Pyogenic arthritis, pyoderma gangrenosum, and acne (PAPA) and seborrhea, acne, hirsutism, and alopecia (SAHA)
- Dark-skinned patients: 50% keloidal scarring and 50% acne hyperpigmented macules

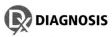

DIAGNOSIS

HISTORY
Ask about duration, relation to menses, medications, cleansing products, stress, smoking, exposures, diet, and family history.

PHYSICAL EXAM
- Closed comedones (whiteheads), open comedones (blackheads)
- Nodules or papules, pustules, cysts
- Scars: ice pick, rolling, boxcar, atrophic macules, hypertrophic, depressed, sinus tracts
- Consistent grading is useful; no specific universal grading system is recommended.
- Grading system (American Academy of Dermatology, 1990)
  – Mild: few papules/pustules; no nodules
  – Moderate: some papules/pustules; few nodules
  – Severe: many papules/pustules/nodules
  – Very severe: acne conglobata, acne fulminans, acne inversa
- Most common areas affected are face, chest, back, and upper arms (greatest concentration of sebaceous glands).
- Adult female—facial lesion distribution not limited to mandibular and perioral lesion location, similar to adolescents

DIFFERENTIAL DIAGNOSIS
Folliculitis: gram-negative, gram-positive, and pityrosporum; acne (rosacea, cosmetica, steroid induced); perioral dermatitis; pseudofolliculitis barbae; drug eruption; keratosis pilaris; sarcoidosis; seborrheic dermatitis; lupus erythematosus

DIAGNOSTIC TESTS & INTERPRETATION
Initial Tests (lab, imaging)
Only indicated if additional signs of androgen excess; if so, test for free and total testosterone and DHEA-S, and consider LH and FSH (PCOS).

TREATMENT

- Comedonal (grade 1): keratolytic agent
- Mild inflammatory acne (grade 2): BP +/− topical retinoid or BP +/− topical antibiotic +/− topical retinoid
- Moderate inflammatory acne (grade 3): Add time-limited systemic antibiotic to grade 2 regimen.
- Severe inflammatory acne (grade 4): as in grade 3, or isotretinoin
- Topical retinoid plus a topical antimicrobial agent (such as BP) is first-line treatment for more than mild disease (1)[A].
- Topical retinoid + antibiotic (topical or PO) is better than either alone for mild/moderate.
- Topical retinoids are first-line agents for maintenance therapy (1)[A]. Avoid long-term antibiotics for maintenance.
- Avoid oral or topical antibiotics as monotherapy. Use with topical BP +/− topical retinoid.
- Recommended vehicle type
  – Dry or sensitive skin: cream, lotion, or ointment
  – Oily skin, humid weather: gel, solution, wash
  – Hair-bearing areas: lotion, hydrogel, or foam
- Apply topical agents to entire affected area, not just visible lesions.
- Mild soap daily to control oiliness; avoid abrasives.
- Avoid drying agents; use gentle cleanser/non-comedogenic moisturizer to decrease irritation with keratolytic agents.

MEDICATION

ALERT
Most prescribed branded topical medications are very expensive.

- Keratolytic agents (α-hydroxy acids, salicylic acid, topical retinoids, azelaic acid) (Side effects include dryness, erythema, and scaling; start with lower strength or alternate day Rx; increase as tolerated.)
- Tretinoin (Retin-A, Retin-A Micro, Avita, Atralin, Altreno), 1st generation, varying strengths and formulations: wash skin; let skin dry for 30 minutes before application to reduce irritation. Apply pea-sized dose at bedtime. Retin-A Micro, Atralin, and Avita are less irritating and stable with BP; may cause an initial flare of lesions; may be eased by every other day application for the first 2 to 4 weeks
  – Avoid in pregnant and lactating women.
  – Cost varies based on formulation—$50 to $150 per tube for generic.
- Adapalene (Differin): 0.1%, apply topically HS, 3rd generation
  – Effective; less irritation than tretinoin or tazarotene (1)[A]
  – May be combined with BP (Epiduo) 0.1 or 0.3%/2.5%—very effective in skin of color
  – 0.1% gel is available over-the-counter (OTC); *much less* expensive than other Rx retinoids ($10 to $15)

- Tazarotene (Tazorac): Apply at bedtime; 3rd generation; most effective and most irritating; teratogenic, $400 per tube
- Trifarotene (Aklief): 0.005% cream, apply in PM, 4th-generation retinoid, greater selectivity, safer, $600
- Azelaic acid (Azelex): 20% topical cream BID, Finevin 15% gel
  - Keratinolytic, antibacterial, anti-inflammatory; reduces postinflammatory hyperpigmentation in dark-skinned individuals
  - Side effects: erythema, dryness, scaling, hypopigmentation
  - Effective in postadolescent acne; safe in pregnancy-risk category B
  - 20% Rx >$400 per tube, OTC 10% and 15% formulations cost $10 to $40 per tube.
- Salicylic acid: 0.5–2%, less effective and less irritating than tretinoin; α-Hydroxy acids, can use with BP and OTC medications
- Topical BP: generates oxygen free radicals, no resistance in *C. acnes*
  - 2.5% as effective as stronger preparations (5% and 10%); gel penetrates better into follicles.
  - When used with tretinoin, apply BP in morning/tretinoin at night (tretinoin is photolabile).
  - Microencapsulated BP 3% and tretinoin 0.1% (Twyneo) are now FDA-approved (expensive).
  - Side effects: concentration dependent irritation; may bleach clothes; photosensitivity
- Topical antibiotics (other than BP): Do not use as monotherapy due to antibiotic resistance.
  - Erythromycin 2%, clindamycin 1%, minocycline 4% topical foam (Amzeeq), metronidazole gel or cream: once daily
  - BP–erythromycin (Benzamycin): especially effective with azelaic acid
  - BP–clindamycin (BenzaClin, DUAC, Clindoxyl)
  - Tretinoin 0.025% clindamycin 1.2% gel (Veltin); apply HS.
  - BP–salicylic acid (Cleanse & Treat, Inova): similar in effectiveness to BP–clindamycin
  - Sodium sulfacetamide (Sulfacet-R, Novacet, Klaron): useful in acne with seborrheic dermatitis or rosacea
  - Dapsone (Aczone) 5% or 7.5% gel: useful in adult females with inflammatory acne; may cause yellow/orange skin discoloration when mixed with BP; very rare methemoglobinemia; glucose 6 phosphate deficiency, expensive—$350 per tube
- Oral antibiotics: use for shortest possible period, generally 6 to 12 weeks of therapy, limit to 3 months, max of 6 months if necessary; use when acne is more severe, trunk involvement, unresponsive to topical agents, or at greater risk for scarring; do not use as monotherapy.
  - Tetracycline: 500 to 1,000 mg/day divided BID; high dose initially, taper in 6 months, less effective than doxycycline or minocycline, take fasting or without dairy; side effects: photosensitivity, esophagitis
  - Minocycline: 100 to 200 mg/day, divided daily—BID; side effects include photosensitivity, urticaria, gray-blue skin, vertigo, autoimmune hepatitis, lupus; extended release preparation better tolerated

- Doxycycline: 20 to 200 mg/day, divided daily—BID; photosensitivity
- Erythromycin: 500 to 1,000 mg/day; divided BID–QID; decreasing effectiveness due to *C. acnes* resistance
- Trimethoprim-sulfamethoxazole (Bactrim DS, Septra DS): QD or BID
- Azithromycin (Zithromax): 500 mg 3 days/week × 1 month and then 250 mg every other day × 2 months
- Amoxicillin: 1,000 to 1,500 mg/day
- Oral retinoids
  - Isotretinoin: 0.5 to 1 mg/kg/day divided BID to maximum of 2 mg/kg/day divided BID for very severe disease; 60–90% cure rate; usually given for 12 to 20 weeks; maximum cumulative dose = 120 to 150 mg/kg; 20% of patients relapse and require retreatment, 0.25 to 0.40 mg/kg/day in moderately severe acne
    ○ Side effects: teratogenic, pancreatitis, excessive drying of skin, hypertriglyceridemia, hepatitis, blood dyscrasias, hyperostosis, premature epiphyseal closure, night blindness, erythema multiforme, Stevens-Johnson syndrome, possible suicidal ideation, psychosis
    ○ Avoid tetracyclines or vitamin A during isotretinoin.
    ○ Monitor for pregnancy, psychiatric/mood changes, CBC, lipids, glucose, and LFTs at baseline and every month.
    ○ Patient and provider must register with iPLEDGE program (https://www.ipledgeprogram.com), two forms of effective contraception required
  - Isotretinoin micronized (Absorica LD): 0.4 to 0.8 mg/kg/day BID × 15 to 20 weeks, may have fewer side effects, $1,100 per month
- Medications for women only
  - FDA-approved oral contraceptives (in order of possible effectiveness)
    ○ Drospirenone/ethinyl estradiol (Yaz), or drospirenone/ethinyl estradiol/levomefolate (Beyaz) > norgestimate/ethinyl estradiol > norethindrone acetate/ethinyl estradiol
    ○ Most combined contraceptives are also effective; may take 3 to 6 months
- Spironolactone (Aldactone); 25 to 200 mg/day; antiandrogen; reduces sebum production, not FDA-approved for acne Rx
- Other agent: clascoterone topical (Winlevi): 1% cream, antiandrogen, can use in both sexes; no systemic side effects; expensive, $500 to $675

ISSUES FOR REFERRAL
Management of acne scars

ADDITIONAL THERAPIES
- Acne hyperpigmented macules: topical hydroquinone (1.5–10%), azelaic acid (20%) topically, topical retinoids, corticosteroids: low dose, dapsone 5% gel (Aczone): sunscreen
- Light-based treatment—ultraviolet A/ultraviolet B (UVA/UVB); blue or blue/red light; pulse dye, infrared laser; photodynamic therapy with 5-aminolevulinic acid has best evidence.

SURGERY/OTHER PROCEDURES
- Comedo extraction after incising the layer of epithelium over closed comedo
- Inject large cystic lesions with 0.05 to 0.30 mL triamcinolone (Kenalog 2 to 5 mg/mL); 30-gauge needle, inject through pore, slightly distend cyst, can cause local atrophy.
- Acne scar treatment: retinoids, steroid injections, cryosurgery, electrodesiccation, micro-/dermabrasion, chemical peels, laser resurfacing, pulsed dye laser, microneedling, fillers, punch elevation

COMPLEMENTARY & ALTERNATIVE MEDICINE
Evidence suggests that tea tree oil, some plant extracts, and green tea extract may be useful.

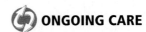 ONGOING CARE

FOLLOW-UP RECOMMENDATIONS
Limit use of oral antibiotics to 3 months; taper topical antibiotic as lesions resolve (2).

DIET
High-glycemic index foods, milk chocolate, and skim milk may worsen acne; paleo diet and high omega-3 fatty acid foods are helpful.

PATIENT EDUCATION
Lesions may worsen initially; improvement is typically seen after a minimum of 4 weeks of treatment.

PROGNOSIS
Gradual improvement over time (usually within 8 to 12 weeks after beginning therapy)

COMPLICATIONS
- Acne conglobata: severe confluent inflammatory acne with systemic symptoms; facial scarring, psychological distress, including anxiety, depression, and suicidal ideation
- Postinflammatory hyperpigmentation, keloids, scars—more common in skin of color

REFERENCES
1. Kolli SS, Pecone D, Pona A, et al. Topical retinoids in acne vulgaris: a systematic review. *Am J Clin Dermatol*. 2019;20(3):345–365.
2. Marson JW, Baldwin HE. An overview of acne therapy, part 1: topical therapy, oral antibiotics, laser and light therapy, and dietary interventions. *Dermatol Clin*. 2019;37(2):183–193.

 SEE ALSO

- Acne Rosacea
- Algorithm: Acne

 CODES

ICD10
L70.0 Acne vulgaris

CLINICAL PEARLS
Decrease topical frequency to every day or to every other day to lessen irritation.

ACUTE CORONARY SYNDROMES: NSTE-ACS (UNSTABLE ANGINA AND NSTEMI)

Asma Tariq, MD • Jared Caballes, MD • Daniela Rangel Orozco, MD, MHP, MS

BASICS

DESCRIPTION

- Unstable angina (UA) and non–ST-segment elevation myocardial infarction (NSTEMI) are acute coronary syndromes without ST-segment elevation (NSTE-ACS) that are differentiated from one another based on the myocardial necrosis/damage (no elevation in cardiac biomarkers in UA) that is present in NSTEMI.
- UA and NSTEMI are difficult to distinguish initially because elevation in troponin levels may not be detectable until several hours after presentation. Initial management for both syndromes is similar.
- Patient history alone is not sufficient to make a diagnosis of ACS, and the clinical dilemma of distinguishing between cardiac and noncardiac chest pain involves a combination of patient history, ECG, and cardiac biomarkers.

EPIDEMIOLOGY

Incidence
- The estimated annual incidence of new and recurrent MI is 605,000 and 200,000, respectively.
- In the United States, the average age at first MI is 65.6 years for males and 72.0 years for females, and males outnumber females at a 3:2 ratio.

ETIOLOGY AND PATHOPHYSIOLOGY

- NSTE-ACS is due to a sudden decrease in myocardial blood flow, resulting in an imbalance between myocardial oxygen consumption and demand. This can be due to acute plaque rupture or plaque erosion and leads to a partially occluding thrombus in the coronary artery, rather than a total or complete occlusion as seen in STEMI.
- Other mechanisms of NSTE-ACS include:
  - Prinzmetal angina or coronary vasospasm induced by tobacco use, hyperventilation, magnesium deficiency, cocaine, or methamphetamines.
  - Increased myocardial oxygen demand resulting in supply-demand mismatch (type 2 NSTEMI) due to underlying causes such as pulmonary embolism, sepsis, shock, and arrhythmias/tachycardia
  - Coronary microvascular dysfunction or endothelial dysfunction without epicardial coronary obstruction
  - Less commonly: coronary arterial aneurysm, spontaneous coronary artery dissection, and thromboembolism

Genetics
Genetic polymorphisms of MMP-3 5A/6A and ACE I/D along with conventional ischemic heart disease risk factors can increase the risk of occurrence of STEMI, while having no influence on the pathogenesis of NSTEMI or UA.

RISK FACTORS

- Traditional/classic: age, male sex, prior MI, hypertension (HTN), tobacco use, diabetes mellitus (DM), dyslipidemia, and family history of premature CAD (defined as age of onset prior to 55 years in males and 65 years in females)
- Novel/emerging risk factors: sedentary lifestyle, overweight/obesity (metabolic syndrome), inflammation (psoriasis, rheumatoid arthritis), cigarette smoking, psychosocial factors (anxiety/depression/ stress), chronic kidney disease (CKD), obstructive sleep apnea, environmental pollutants

GENERAL PREVENTION

Smoking cessation, normal body mass index, stress management, regular physical activity, glycemic control for patients with diabetes and blood pressure (BP) control in patients with HTN, risk-based statins, aspirin in those with documented CAD

DIAGNOSIS

HISTORY

- Chest heaviness/tightness lasting $\geq$10 minutes; with or without exertion; typically retrosternal and can radiate to the neck, jaw, interscapular area, upper extremities, or epigastrium; pain is typically described as a pressure, tightness, heaviness, squeezing, or fullness.
- Associated symptoms of palpitations, dyspnea, nausea/vomiting, diaphoresis, light-headedness, syncope, or dysphoria can occur.
- Atypical symptoms: stabbing or pleuritic pain, epigastric/abdominal pain, indigestion or isolated dyspnea; more common in those aged >75 years, in women, or in those with diabetes, renal insufficiency, and dementia; may present without chest pain and with symptoms of dyspnea, diaphoresis, and extreme fatigue which represent "anginal equivalents"

PHYSICAL EXAM

- Tachycardia or bradycardia, HTN or hypotension, widened pulse pressure, tachypnea, fever, poor dental hygiene
- Dysrhythmia, jugular venous distention (JVD), new murmur (third and fourth heart sounds), rub or gallop, diminished peripheral pulses, carotid bruits
- Tachypnea, $\uparrow$ work of breathing, crackles
- Pain reproducible with movement or palpation is unlikely to be cardiac.
- Cool skin, pallor, diaphoresis, signs of dyslipidemia (xanthomas, xanthelasma)

DIFFERENTIAL DIAGNOSIS

- Cardiac: aortic dissection, myocarditis, pericarditis, pericardial effusion/cardiac tamponade, heart failure with preserved and reduced ejection fraction, hypertensive emergency, stress cardiomyopathy (takotsubo), dysrhythmia, and mitral valve disease

- Pulmonary: pulmonary embolism, pneumothorax, pneumonia, pleuritis, bronchitis, pneumonitis, and pleuritis
- Psychiatric: panic attacks, anxiety
- Musculoskeletal: costochondritis, rib fracture
- Gastroenterology: gastroesophageal reflux disease, esophageal spasm, esophagitis, esophageal rupture or perforation, hiatal hernia, penetrating or perforating peptic ulcer, biliary or pancreatic pain

DIAGNOSTIC TESTS & INTERPRETATION

Initial Tests (lab, imaging)
- 12-lead ECG: should be obtained within 10 minutes of presentation; applies to both UA and NSTEMI
- CBC, BMP (to evaluate for electrolyte abnormalities), and serum troponin biomarkers (negative by definition in UA), which can be elevated within the first 2 to 3 hours since the onset of chest pain
- Chest x-ray, computed tomography with contrast (to exclude other etiologies if applicable), and transthoracic echocardiography are recommended.

Follow-Up Tests & Special Considerations
Fasting lipid profile, preferably within 24 hours, activated partial thromboplastin time (aPTT), TSH, HbA1c, and urine drug screen (in selected patients)

Diagnostic Procedures/Other
- For low- to intermediate-risk patients with resolution of symptoms and nondiagnostic ECG with negative biomarkers, consider noninvasive cardiac testing with standard exercise treadmill test, exercise stress echocardiography, or myocardial perfusion imaging using single-photon emission computed tomography.
- Alternatively, coronary computed tomography angiography can be performed as well in the same population at low to intermediate risk.

Test Interpretation
- ECG results in the setting of NSTE-ACS:
  - New ST-segment depression $\geq$0.5 mm in two or more contiguous leads and/or T-wave inversions $\geq$1 mm in two or more contiguous leads
  - ST depression and/or tall R wave in V_1/V_2 with upright T waves may indicate transmural STEMI of posterior wall. ECG with posterior leads (V_7–V_9) should be performed.
  - If initial ECG is nondiagnostic but symptoms persist with suspicion for ACS, perform serial ECGs at 15- to 30-minute intervals.
- Troponin concentration rises within 3 to 6 hours after onset of ischemic symptoms but can be delayed up to 8 to 12 hours (troponin T is not specific in patients with renal dysfunction).
  - NSTEMI can be diagnosed by initial concentration of >52 ng/L or a change in level from initial reading after 2 hours >10 ng/L.
  - In patients with symptoms suggestive of ACS, negative troponin at 6 hours can almost effectively rule out infarct in most patients (1).

- CK-MB has been shown to have better specificity than troponin in post-PCI MI. Troponin elevation will resolve in 3 to 10 days, CK-MB will return to normal within 3 to 4 days (1).
- Repeat biomarkers 8 to 12 hours from onset of symptoms to check if troponin levels have peaked. The expected rise and fall of troponin level in the setting of MI is an important diagnostic factor that can distinguish an MI from alternative causes of elevated troponin (1).

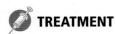 TREATMENT

GENERAL MEASURES

- Initial ABCDs; assess clinical stability (adequate oxygenation) and determine the next step.
- Risk stratify (TIMI or GRACE score) to select invasive approach (coronary angiography within 24 hours of admission) versus ischemia-guided therapy; urgent invasive management is required for very high-risk patients, such as those with hemodynamic instability, cardiogenic shock, recurrent or ongoing chest pain refractory to medical therapy, or life-threatening arrhythmias or cardiac arrest.
- TIMI risk score includes age >65 years, ≥3 CAD risk factors, known CAD with >50% stenosis, aspirin use within the last 7 days, severe angina in the preceding 24 hours, elevated cardiac markers, and ST deviation >0.5 mm. Low risk is a score of 0 to 2, intermediate risk with a score of 3 to 4, and high risk with a score of 5 to 7.
- GRACE risk score calculation uses eight parameters to predict death and MI in the hospital and at 6 months, which include age, heart rate, systolic BP, creatinine, Killip classification for heart failure, cardiac arrest, ST-segment deviation, and elevated cardiac enzymes.
- Bed/chair rest with continuous ECG monitoring, maintaining O_2 saturation >90%, and tight BP control; discontinue NSAIDs if possible. Support smoking cessation. Correct electrolyte abnormalities with potassium goal around 4 mEq/L and magnesium at 2 mg/dL.

MEDICATION
First Line
- Antiplatelet therapy: dual antiplatelet therapy for all patients with NSTE-ACS
- Aspirin, nonenteric coated, initial dose of 162 to 325 mg chewed or crushed; maintenance dose of 75 to 100 mg/day indefinitely, which can reduce the risk of death, MI, and stroke
- P2Y12 inhibitors should be given at the time of diagnosis unless invasive approach is planned in a high-bleeding risk patient:
  – Ticagrelor, loading dose of 180 mg PO, followed by 90 mg PO twice daily; avoid in patients with 2nd- and 3rd-degree heart block; can cause dyspnea in some patients; contraindicated in patients with severe liver dysfunction *or*
  – Prasugrel 60 mg PO, followed by maintenance dose of 10 mg PO daily; often reserved for post-PCI patients treated with coronary stents; contraindicated in patients aged ≥75 years or those with history of CVA/TIA *or*
  – Clopidogrel, loading dose of 300 to 600 mg PO, followed by maintenance dose of 75 mg PO daily; use with caution with thrombocytopenia and CKD (adding clopidogrel to aspirin may reduce the combined outcome of mortality).

- Nitroglycerin sublingual 0.4 mg every 5 minutes for total of 3 doses and then assess need for IV nitroglycerin based on blood pressure and pain relief. Nitroglycerin-induced hypotension may be attenuated with right ventricular infarction.
- Morphine sulfate (initial dose of 2 to 4 mg), with increments of 2 to 8 mg, can be repeated at 5- to 15-minute intervals for relief of severe, persistent chest pain.
- Oral β-blocker therapy should be initiated within 24 hours in patients without signs of heart failure, cardiogenic shock, or other contraindications to β-blockade (2nd- or 3rd-degree heart block without a pacemaker or active asthma).
  – In patients with concomitant ACS, stabilized heart failure, and reduced systolic function (LVEF <40%), the recommended β-blockers are metoprolol succinate, carvedilol, and bisoprolol.
- Lipid-lowering therapy: Initiate or continue high-intensity statin therapy (preferred due to nonlipid benefit on vascular function) with atorvastatin 80 mg/day or rosuvastatin 20 to 40 mg/day regardless of the patient's baseline LDL level. Ezetimibe and PCSK9 inhibitors (evolocumab, alirocumab) can be considered in statin-intolerant patients/complementary therapy.
- ACE inhibitor (ACEi) should be started and continued indefinitely in all patients with LVEF <40% and in those with diabetes or HTN, and it can lead to improved 30-day mortality in patients after an acute STEMI.
- Aldosterone antagonist (spironolactone or eplerenone) is recommended in NSTEMI for patients without significant renal dysfunction or hyperkalemia who are on a therapeutic dose of ACEi/ARB and β-blocker and have LVEF ≤40%, DM, or heart failure.
- Antithrombotic therapy: Initiate anticoagulant (unfractionated heparin, enoxaparin, bivalirudin or fondaparinux) therapy as soon as possible after presentation. For patients undergoing invasive management (PCI), stop at the end of procedure. For patients being treated with conservative approach, continue for a minimum of 48 hours. Unfractionated or low-molecular-weight heparin plus aspirin may reduce death or MI at 1 week, but longer-term benefits are unclear at this time. Warfarin has not been shown to be beneficial and can increase the risk of major bleeding.

Second Line
Nondihydropyridine calcium channel blockers (CCB) (verapamil or diltiazem) are used to reduce myocardial oxygen demand when β-blockers are contraindicated if left ventricular ejection fraction is normal. Long-acting CCBs are recommended in treatment of patients with epicardial or microvascular coronary artery spasm. Avoid in patients with heart block.

ISSUES FOR REFERRAL
- Cardiology consultation is indicated for NSTE-ACS.
- Referral to exercise-based cardiac rehabilitation program prior to hospital discharge is associated with decreased morbidity and mortality.

SURGERY/OTHER PROCEDURES
Some patients often undergo exercise stress testing a few weeks or more after hospital discharge as part of a cardiac rehabilitation program for activity counseling.

 ONGOING CARE

FOLLOW-UP RECOMMENDATIONS
- Patients with low-risk suspected ACS who have normal serial ECGs and cardiac troponin levels may have a treadmill ECG, stress myocardial perfusion imaging, or stress echocardiography within 72 hours after discharge.
- With LVEF <40%, repeat LVEF 1 to 3 months postdischarge.

DIET
- 1/3 of deaths caused by cardiovascular disease (CVD) can be prevented through healthy lifestyle choices including diet and physical activity.
- The Mediterranean diet is associated with reduced CVD mortality, whereas DASH diet is associated with reduced risk of CAD.
- There is an association with increased sodium intake and CVD risk, but reducing dietary sodium has not been shown to reduce CVD risk.

PATIENT EDUCATION
- May resume exercise and sexual activity within 2 weeks in asymptomatic patients after outpatient reevaluation
- Exercise recommendations for adults include at least 150 minutes of moderate-intensity aerobic activity per week and are associated with reduced CVD risk.

PROGNOSIS
- 50% of patients with UA progress to myocardial infarction within 30 days if left untreated.
- Between 9% and 19% of those with ACS die in the first 6 months after initial diagnosis, with about 1/2 of these deaths occurring within the first 30 days.

REFERENCE
1. Amsterdam EA, Wenger NK, Brindis RG, et al. 2014 AHA/ACC guidelines for the management of patient with non–ST-elevation acute coronary syndrome: a report of the American College of Cardiology/American Heart Association Task Force on Practice Guidelines. *J Am Coll Cardiol*. 2014;64(24):e139–e228.

 CODES

ICD10
- I24.9 Acute ischemic heart disease, unspecified
- I20.0 Unstable angina
- I21.4 Non-ST elevation (NSTEMI) myocardial infarction

CLINICAL PEARLS
- NSTEMI is diagnosed in patients who present with symptoms consistent with ACS and elevated troponin levels but without EKG changes suggestive of STEMI.
- UA can present similarly to NSTEMI but without evidence of myocardial necrosis in the form of elevated troponin levels, and initial management for both is the same.

ACUTE CORONARY SYNDROMES: STEMI

Yutthapong Temtanakitpaisan, MD, FACC, FSCAI

BASICS

DESCRIPTION
Acute myocardial infarction (AMI) is the rapid development of myocardial necrosis resulting from a sustained and complete absence of blood flow to a portion of the myocardium. ST-segment elevation myocardial infarction (STEMI) occurs when coronary blood flow ceases, usually following complete atherothrombotic occlusion of a large coronary artery, resulting in transmural ischemia. This is accompanied by release of serum cardiac biomarkers and ST-segment elevation on an electrocardiogram (ECG).

EPIDEMIOLOGY
Incidence
There are >650,000 cases of AMI reported annually in the United States. Early revascularization and AMI management has improved mortality, with a 30-day survival of 95%.

Prevalence
Atherosclerotic heart disease is the leading cause of morbidity and mortality in the United States. ~7.5 million people in the United States are affected by AMI. Prevalence increases with age and is higher in men (5.5%) compared to women (2.9%).

ETIOLOGY AND PATHOPHYSIOLOGY
- Atherosclerotic coronary artery disease (CAD): Atherosclerotic lesions can be fibrotic, calcified, or lipid laden. Thin-capped atheromas are more likely to rupture, causing atherothrombotic occlusion.
- Nonatherosclerotic causes:
  - Embolism from either infective vegetations, or thrombi originating within the right atrium across the foramen ovale ("paradoxical"), from the left atrium or from within the left ventricle
  - Spontaneous coronary artery dissection: prevalent in fibromuscular dysplasia (FMD) and in young women
  - Mechanical or iatrogenic obstruction: chest trauma, dissection of the aorta and/or coronary arteries
  - Coronary artery spasm from increased vasomotor tone; anginal variant
  - Arteritis and other etiologies: hematologic causes (disseminated intravascular coagulation [DIC], severe anemia), aortic stenosis, cocaine, IV drug use, severe burns, prolonged hypotension

RISK FACTORS
Advancing age, hypertension, tobacco use, diabetes mellitus, dyslipidemia, family history of premature onset of CAD, sedentary lifestyle

GENERAL PREVENTION
Smoking cessation/abstinence; healthy diet; weight loss/control; regular physical activity and exercise; control of hypertension, hyperlipidemia, and diabetes mellitus

COMMONLY ASSOCIATED CONDITIONS
Abdominal aortic aneurysm, cerebrovascular disease, atherosclerotic peripheral vascular disease

DIAGNOSIS

HISTORY
- Symptoms:
  - Classically, sudden onset of chest heaviness/tightness, with or without exertion, lasting minutes to hours
  - Pain/discomfort radiating to neck, jaw, interscapular area, upper extremities, and/or epigastrium
  - Patients with inferior MI may present primarily with abdominal discomfort
- Previous history of myocardial ischemia (stable or unstable angina, AMI, coronary bypass surgery, or percutaneous coronary intervention [PCI])
- Assess risk factors for CAD, history of bleeding, noncardiac surgery, and family history of premature CAD.
- Medications: Ask if there is a recent use of phosphodiesterase type 5 inhibitors (if recent use, avoid concomitant nitrates).
- Tobacco, alcohol, and/or drug abuse (especially cocaine)

PHYSICAL EXAM
- General: restlessness, agitation, hypothermia, fever
- Neurologic: dizziness, syncope, fatigue, disorientation (especially in the elderly)
- Cardiovascular (CV): dysrhythmia, hypotension, widened pulse pressure, S3 and S4, jugular venous distention (JVD)
- Respiratory: dyspnea, tachypnea, crackles, rales
- GI: abdominal pain, nausea, vomiting, hiccups
- Skin: cool skin, pallor, diaphoresis

Geriatric and Gender Considerations
- Elderly patients may have an atypical presentation, including silent or unrecognized MI. They may often present with syncope, weakness, shortness of breath, unexplained nausea, epigastric pain, altered mental status, or delirium.
- Women or patients with diabetes mellitus may present with typical and/or "atypical" symptoms such as fatigue, dyspnea, and malaise.

DIFFERENTIAL DIAGNOSIS
Unstable angina, aortic dissection, pulmonary embolism (PE), perforating gastric ulcer, pericarditis, dysrhythmias, gastroesophageal reflux disease (GERD), esophageal spasm, biliary/pancreatic pain, hyperventilation syndrome, anxiety/panic

DIAGNOSTIC TESTS & INTERPRETATION
Initial Tests (lab, imaging)
- 12-lead ECG:
  - ≥1 mm ST elevation in a regional pattern, involving at least two contiguous leads, with or without abnormal Q waves
  - STEMI of posterior wall: ST depression ± tall R waves in V_1–V_2
  - Absence of Q waves represents partial or transient occlusion or early infarction.
  - Consider right-sided and posterior chest leads if inferior MI pattern (examine V_3R, V_4R, V_7–V_9).
  - In the setting of ventricular pacing or a prior left bundle branch block (LBBB), the Sgarbossa criteria or BARCELONA algorithm (1) may be helpful.

- 2-Dimensional transthoracic echocardiography is useful in evaluating regional wall motion in MI, left ventricular function, mechanical complications, and mural thrombus.
- Once diagnosis is suspected, emergent coronary angiography with PCI is preferred.

Follow-Up Tests & Special Considerations
Serum biomarkers
- Troponin I and T (cTnI, cTnT) rise 3 to 6 hours after onset of ischemic symptoms.
- Elevations in cTnI persist for 7 to 10 days, whereas cTnT elevations persist for 10 to 14 days after MI.
- High-sensitivity troponin is highly sensitive and provides faster recognition of AMI.
- Myoglobin fraction of creatine kinase-MB (CK-MB) adds little diagnostic value in assessment of possible AMI to troponin testing.

Pregnancy Considerations
Pregnant patients presenting with STEMI will need discussion of risks and benefits of invasive coronary angiography with radiation exposure to fetus. Management should otherwise be the same as in nonpregnant patients.

Diagnostic Procedures/Other
- Portable chest x-ray; transthoracic echocardiography; chest computed tomography angiography (CTA) scan may occasionally be of value acutely in equivocal presentations to evaluate for alternative diagnoses (aortic dissection, PE, ventricular aneurysm).
- Coronary angiography is the definitive test.

ALERT
Patients with chronic kidney disease need special attention to amount of contrast media used.

TREATMENT

GENERAL MEASURES
Following emergent revascularization, admit the patient to the coronary care unit (CCU) or a telemetry unit with continuous ECG monitoring and bed rest and use:
- Antiarrhythmics as needed for unstable dysrhythmia
- Dual antiplatelet therapy (DAPT) with continuation of aspirin 81 mg/day with clopidogrel 75 mg/day or prasugrel 10 mg/day or ticagrelor 90 mg twice daily

MEDICATION
Medication recommendations are based on the 2013 American College of Cardiology (ACC)/American Heart Association (AHA) guideline (2)[C] and 2017 European Society of Cardiology (ESC) guideline (3)[C].

First Line
- Supplemental oxygen 2 to 4 L/min for patients with oxygen saturation <90% or respiratory distress
- Nitroglycerin (NTG) sublingual 0.4 mg q5min for a total of 3 doses, followed by NTG IV if ongoing pain and/or hypertension and/or management of pulmonary congestion if no contraindications exist such as systolic <90 mm Hg or >30 mm Hg below baseline, right ventricle (RV) infarct, use of sildenafil or vardenafil within 24 hours or within 48 hours of tadalafil

- Morphine sulfate 4 to 8 mg IV with 2 to 8 mg IV repeated at 5- to 15-minute intervals to relieve pain, anxiety, or pulmonary congestion
- Antiplatelet agents:
  – Aspirin (ASA), non–enteric-coated, initial dose of 162 to 325 mg chewed
  – A loading dose of a P2Y12 inhibitor is recommended for patients with STEMI for whom PCI is planned. Prasugrel or ticagrelor is preferred.
    ◦ Prasugrel 60 mg loading dose; prasugrel is contraindicated in patients with previous stroke/transient ischemic attack. Do not recommend in patients aged >75 years or in patients with low body weight (<60 kg).
    ◦ Ticagrelor 180 mg loading dose; ticagrelor may cause transient dyspnea.
    ◦ Clopidogrel 600 mg loading dose should be given if neither prasugrel nor ticagrelor is available.
    ◦ Cangrelor may be considered in patients not pretreated with oral P2Y12 receptor inhibitors at the time of PCI or in those who are unable to take oral agents.
    ◦ Standard recommendation for duration of DAPT is 6 to 12 months after PCI, depending on bleeding and ischemia risks.
- Anticoagulation therapy:
  – Unfractionated heparin (UFH) 70- to 100-U/kg IV bolus *or*
  – Enoxaparin 0.5-mg/kg IV bolus *or*
  – Bivalirudin 0.75-mg/kg IV bolus and then 1.75-mg/kg/hr infusion for up to 4 hours after procedure
- PCI versus fibrinolysis: The goal is to keep total ischemic time within 120 minutes. Door to needle time should be within 30 minutes or door to balloon time within 90 minutes.
  – Coronary reperfusion therapy
    ◦ Primary PCI (balloon angioplasty, coronary stents) in the following:
      ▪ Symptom onset of ≤12 hours
      ▪ Symptom onset of ≤12 hours and contraindication to fibrinolytic therapy irrespective of time delay
      ▪ Cardiogenic shock or acute severe heart failure (HF) irrespective of time delay from onset of MI
      ▪ Evidence of ongoing ischemia 12 to 24 hours after symptom onset
  – Procedural considerations: Radial access is recommended over femoral access. PCI of infarct-related artery (IRA) is indicated.
  – Fibrinolysis
    ◦ If presenting to a hospital without PCI capability and cannot be transferred to a PCI-capable facility to undergo PCI within 120 minutes of first medical contact
    ◦ If no contraindications, administer within 12 to 24 hours of symptom onset, if there is evidence of ongoing ischemia.
      ▪ Alteplase (tPA): 15-mg IV bolus, followed by 0.75 mg/kg (up to 50 mg) IV over 30 minutes and then 0.5 mg/kg (up to 35 mg) over 60 minutes; maximum of 100 mg over 90 minutes
      ▪ Reteplase (rPA): 10 units IV bolus; give second bolus 30 minutes apart.
      ▪ Tenecteplase (TNK-tPA): 30- to 50-mg (based on weight) IV bolus; recommend reducing to half dose in patients ≥75 years of age.

  ◦ Adjunctive antiplatelet therapy with fibrinolysis
    ▪ Aspirin: 162- to 325-mg loading dose followed by 81 mg/day indefinitely
    ▪ Clopidogrel (300-mg loading dose for patients <75 years of age, 75-mg dose for patients >75 years of age); clopidogrel 75 mg/day should be continued for at least 14 days and up to 1 year.
  ◦ Adjunctive anticoagulation therapy with fibrinolysis: Use anticoagulants (UFH, enoxaparin, or fondaparinux) as ancillary therapy to reperfusion therapy for a minimum of 48 hours and preferably duration of admission (up to 8 days) or until revascularization, if performed.
- Glycoprotein IIb/IIIa receptor antagonists at the time of primary PCI in selected patients if there is no reflow or thrombotic complications (abciximab, eptifibatide, or tirofiban)
- ACE inhibitors should be initiated orally within 24 hours of STEMI in patients with anterior infarction, HF, diabetes, or ejection fraction (EF) ≤0.40 unless contraindicated.
- High-intensity statin therapy should be started as early as possible.
- Mineralocorticoid receptor antagonist (spironolactone, eplerenone) is recommended in patients with EF <40% and HF or diabetes, who are already receiving an ACE inhibitor and a β-blocker (BB), if there is no renal failure or hyperkalemia.

Second Line
Long-acting nondihydropyridine calcium channel blocker (CCB) when BB is ineffective or contraindicated and EF is normal; do not use immediate-release nifedipine.

ISSUES FOR REFERRAL
Transfer high-risk patients who receive fibrinolytic therapy as primary reperfusion therapy at a non–PCI-capable facility to a PCI-capable facility as soon as possible.

SURGERY/OTHER PROCEDURES
Urgent coronary artery bypass graft (CABG) surgery is indicated in patients with STEMI and coronary anatomy not amenable to PCI who have ongoing or recurrent ischemia, cardiogenic shock, severe HF, or other high-risk features.

ADMISSION, INPATIENT, AND NURSING CONSIDERATIONS
All STEMI patients should be admitted to a CCU or an intensive cardiac care unit for evaluation and treatment.

ONGOING CARE

FOLLOW-UP RECOMMENDATIONS
STEMI patients should follow up with a cardiologist 1 to 2 weeks postdischarge, every 3 months for the 1st year and then yearly. Emphasize medication adherence and encourage smoking cessation. Strongly consider referral to an exercise-based cardiac rehabilitation program.

DIET
Low-fat/healthy-fat diet: reduced intake of saturated fats (to <7% of total calories), eliminate *trans*-fatty acids (to <1% of total calories); Mediterranean diet is healthy.

PATIENT EDUCATION
May resume sexual activity ≥1 weeks after uncomplicated MI or 6 to 8 weeks after CABG; smoking cessation and low-fat diet

COMPLICATIONS
- Advanced age, diabetes, delayed or unsuccessful revascularization, reduced left ventricular systolic function, and evidence of congestive HF are all associated with worse prognosis.
- HF, myocardial wall rupture, left ventricular aneurysm, pericarditis, dysrhythmias, acute mitral regurgitation, and depression (common)

REFERENCES
1. Di Marco A, Rodriguez M, Cinca J, et al. New electrocardiographic algorithm for the diagnosis of acute myocardial infarction in patients with left bundle branch block. *J Am Heart Assoc.* 2020;9(14):e015573.
2. O'Gara PT, Kushner FG, Ascheim DD, et al. 2013 ACCF/AHA guideline for the management of ST-elevation myocardial infarction. *J Am Coll Cardiol.* 2013;61(4):e78–e140.
3. Ibanez B, James S, Agewall S, et al; for ESC Scientific Document Group. 2017 ESC guidelines for the management of acute myocardial infarction in patients presenting with ST-segment elevation: The Task Force for the management of acute myocardial infarction in patients presenting with ST-segment elevation of the European Society of Cardiology (ESC). *Eur Heart J.* 2018;39(2):119–177.

 CODES

ICD10
- I24.9 Acute ischemic heart disease, unspecified
- I21.3 ST elevation (STEMI) myocardial infarction of unspecified site
- I25.10 Athscl heart disease of native coronary artery w/o ang pctrs

CLINICAL PEARLS
Early revascularization with PCI within 90 minutes of presentation at a PCI-capable hospital or within 120 minutes if transfer to a PCI-capable hospital is required. Fibrinolytic therapy should be initiated within 30 minutes if presenting to a hospital without PCI capability and if the patient cannot be transferred to a PCI-capable facility to undergo PCI within 120 minutes of first medical contact.

ACUTE KIDNEY INJURY

Michelle Nelson, MD • Arturas Klugas, MD, FAAFP

BASICS

DESCRIPTION
- An abrupt loss of kidney function, acute kidney injury (AKI) defined as (1):
  - Increase in serum creatinine (SCr) of ≥0.3 mg/dL within 48 hours
  - ≥50% increase in baseline SCr within 7 days
  - Urine output of <0.5 mL/kg/hr for 6 hours
- Staging is based on SCr or urine output:

Stage	Increase in Baseline Creatinine	Increase in Creatinine	Urine Output
1	1.5 times	≥0.3 mg/dL	<0.5 mL/kg/hr for 6–12 hours
2	2.0–2.9 times	N/A	<0.5 mL/kg/hr for ≥12 hours
3	3.0 times	≥4.0 mg/dL	<0.3 mL/kg/hr for ≥24 hours

- The result is retention of nitrogenous waste, electrolyte, acid–base, and volume abnormalities (1).

EPIDEMIOLOGY
Incidence
- 5% of hospital and 30% of ICU admissions have AKI. 25% of patients develop AKI while hospitalized; 50% of these cases are iatrogenic.
- Developing AKI as an inpatient is associated with >4-fold increased risk of death (2).

ETIOLOGY AND PATHOPHYSIOLOGY
Three categories: prerenal, intrarenal, and postrenal
- Prerenal (reduced renal perfusion, typically reversible):
  - Decreased renal perfusion (often due to hypovolemia) leads to a decrease in glomerular filtration rate (GFR)
  - Caused by hypotension, volume depletion (GI losses, excessive sweating, diuretics, hemorrhage); renal artery stenosis/embolism; burns; heart/liver failure; if decreased perfusion is prolonged or severe, can progress to ischemic acute tubular necrosis (ATN)
- Intrarenal (intrinsic kidney injury, often from prolonged or severe renal hypoperfusion)
  - ATN—from prolonged prerenal azotemia, radiographic contrast material, aminoglycosides, nonsteroidal anti-inflammatory drugs (NSAIDs), or other nephrotoxic substances
  - Glomerulonephritis (GN)
  - Acute interstitial nephritis (AIN; drug induced), arteriolar insults, vasculitis, accelerated hypertension, cholesterol embolization (following an intra-arterial procedure), intrarenal deposition/sludging (uric acid nephropathy and multiple myeloma [Bence Jones proteins])
- Postrenal (obstruction of the collecting system)
  - Extrinsic compression (e.g., benign prostatic hypertrophy [BPH], carcinoma, pregnancy); intrinsic obstruction (e.g., calculus, tumor, clot, stricture, sloughed papillae); decreased function (e.g., neurogenic bladder), leading to obstruction of the urinary collection system

Genetics
No known genetic pattern

RISK FACTORS
- Chronic kidney disease (CKD); comorbid conditions (e.g., diabetes mellitus, hypertension, heart failure, liver failure); advanced age; radiocontrast material exposure (intravascular), female gender, African American
- Medications that impair autoregulation of GFR (NSAIDs, angiotensin-converting enzyme inhibitors [ACEIs], angiotensin II receptor blockers [ARBs], cyclosporine/tacrolimus)
- Nephrotoxic medications (e.g., aminoglycoside antibiotics, platinum-based chemotherapy); hypovolemia (e.g., diuretics, hemorrhage, GI losses); sepsis, surgery, rhabdomyolysis, burns; solitary kidney (risk in nephrolithiasis); BPH; malignancy (e.g., multiple myeloma)

GENERAL PREVENTION
- Maintain adequate renal perfusion with isotonic fluids, vasopressor support if necessary.
- Avoid nephrotoxic agents.

COMMONLY ASSOCIATED CONDITIONS
Hyperkalemia, hyperphosphatemia, hypercalcemia, hyperuricemia, hydronephrosis, BPH, nephrolithiasis, congestive heart failure (CHF), uremic pericarditis, cirrhosis, CKD, malignant hypertension, vasculitis, drug reactions, sepsis, severe trauma, burns, transfusion reactions, recent chemotherapy, rhabdomyolysis, internal bleeding, dehydration

DIAGNOSIS

AKI is usually asymptomatic until the patient has experienced severe loss of function. Oliguria can be present, but it is neither specific nor sensitive.

HISTORY
- Thorough medication history; changes in oral intake, urine output, and body weight
- Prerenal: thirst, orthostatic symptoms, vomiting, diarrhea, bleeding
- Intrarenal: nephrotoxic medications, radiocontrast material, other toxins
- Postrenal: colicky flank pain that radiates to the groin suggests ureteric obstruction such as a stone; nocturia, frequency, and hesitancy suggest prostatic disease; suprapubic and flank pain are usually secondary to distension of the bladder and collecting system; anticholinergic drugs inhibit bladder emptying.
- Uremic symptoms: lethargy, altered mental status, nausea, vomiting, anorexia, metallic taste

PHYSICAL EXAM
- Uremic signs: altered mental status, seizures, myoclonus, pericardial friction rub, peripheral neuropathies
- Prerenal signs: tachycardia, decreased jugular venous pressure (JVP), orthostatic hypotension, dry mucous membranes, decreased skin turgor; comorbid stigmata of sepsis, liver disease, or heart failure
- Intrinsic renal signs: pruritic rash, livedo reticularis, subcutaneous nodules, ischemic digits despite good pulses
- Postrenal signs: suprapubic distension, flank pain, enlarged prostate

DIAGNOSTIC TESTS & INTERPRETATION
Initial Tests (lab, imaging)
- Compare to baseline renal function (creatinine [Cr] and GFR) (1)[A]
- Urinalysis: dipstick for blood and protein; microscopy for cells, casts, and crystals (1)[A]
- Sterile pyuria (especially WBC casts) suggests AIN; triad of fever, rash, and eosinophilia present in 10% of cases
- Proteinuria, hematuria, and edema, often with nephritic urine sediment (RBCs and RBC casts), suggest GN or vasculitis.
- Casts: transparent hyaline casts—prerenal etiology; pigmented granular/muddy brown casts—ATN; WBC casts—AIN; RBC casts—GN
- Urine eosinophils: ≥1% eosinophils suggest AIN (poor sensitivity)
- Urine electrolytes in an oliguric state
  - $FE_{Na} = [(\text{urinary Na} \times \text{serum Cr})/(\text{serum Na} \times \text{urinary Cr})]$
  - FE_{Na} <1% suggests prerenal etiology and >2% indicates intrinsic cause
  - If on diuretics, use FE_{urea} instead of FE_{Na}. FE_{urea} (percent) = $[(\text{serum Cr} \times \text{urine urea})/(\text{serum urea} \times \text{urinary Cr})] \times 100$; FE_{urea} <35% suggests prerenal etiology and >50% suggests intrinsic disease
- CBC, BUN, serum Cr, electrolytes (including Ca/Mg/P); consider arterial or venous blood gas (ABG/VBG)
- Common lab abnormalities in AKI
  - Increased: potassium, phosphate, magnesium, uric acid
  - Decreased: hemoglobin, calcium
- Calculate creatinine clearance (CrCl) to ensure appropriate medication dosing
- Imaging:
  - Renal ultrasound (US): first line; excludes postrenal causes; identifies kidney size, nephrolithiasis
  - Doppler-flow renal US: evaluates for renal artery stenosis/thrombosis
  - Abdominal x-ray (kidney, ureter, bladder [KUB]): identifies calcification, renal calculi, kidney size
- Novel biomarkers such as urinary IL-18, neutrophil gelatinase-associated lipocalin (NGAL), kidney injury molecule-1 (KIM-1), plasma cystatin C, TIMP-2, and *IGFBP7* under investigation (3)

Follow-Up Tests & Special Considerations
- Consider CK (rhabdomyolysis) and immunologic testing (if GN or vasculitis suspected).
- Advanced imaging if initial tests unrevealing
  - Prerenal: US as effective as CT for obstruction; noncontrast helical CT: most sensitive test for nephrolithiasis
  - Radionuclide renal scan: evaluates renal perfusion, function (GFR), and presence of obstructive uropathy and extravasation. MRI: acute tubulointerstitial nephritis with increased T2-weighted signal.
  - Avoid gadolinium contrast in at-risk patients (those with diabetes mellitus and GFR <45 mL/min/1.73 m², or those without diabetes and GFR <30 mL/min/1.73 m²). If necessary, use intravenous fluids before and after contrast administration.

Diagnostic Procedures/Other
Cystoscopy with retrograde pyelogram evaluates for bladder tumor, hydronephrosis, obstruction, and upper tract abnormalities without risk of contrast nephropathy.

Test Interpretation
Kidney biopsy: last resort if patient does not respond to therapy or if diagnosis remains unclear; most useful to evaluate intrinsic AKI of unclear cause (AIN, GN, vasculitis, or renal transplant rejection)

 TREATMENT

Fluid resuscitation is the mainstay of treatment of AKI, both in prerenal and in some forms of intrinsic kidney injury. In severe cases of kidney injury, renal replacement therapy (RRT) may be required. The most important aspect of treating AKI is determining the underlying cause.

GENERAL MEASURES
- Identify and correct prerenal and postrenal causes; stop nephrotoxic drugs and renally dose others. Strictly monitor intake/output and daily weight; optimize cardiac output to maintain renal perfusion. Optimize nutrition and treat any infections. Remove obstruction by placing a Foley catheter, suprapubic catheter, or nephrostomy tube as clinically indicated.
- Indications for RRT: volume overload, severe hyperkalemia, or metabolic acidosis refractory to medical management; advanced uremic complications (pericarditis, encephalopathy, bleeding diathesis); pulmonary edema

MEDICATION
First Line
- Find and treat the underlying cause. Correct electrolyte imbalances—particularly hyperkalemia.
  – If patient is oliguric and not volume overloaded, a monitored fluid challenge may help.
- Furosemide is ineffective in preventing and treating AKI but can (judiciously) be used to manage volume overload and/or hyperkalemia. Furosemide stress test may predict the likelihood of progressive AKI, need for RRT, and mortality.
- Fenoldopam, a dopamine agonist, has been equivocal in decreasing risk of RRT and mortality in AKI; not currently recommended (1)[C].
- Hyperkalemia with ECG changes: Give IV calcium gluconate, isotonic sodium bicarbonate (only if acidemic, and avoid use of hypertonic "amps" of $NaHCO_3$), glucose with insulin, and/or high-dose nebulized albuterol (to drive K^+ into cells); Kayexalate and/or furosemide (to increase K^+ excretion); hemodialysis if severe/refractory.
- Fluid restriction may be required for oliguric patients to prevent worsening hyponatremia.
- Effective strategies for AKI prevention: isotonic IVF, once-daily dosing of aminoglycosides; use of lipid formulations of amphotericin B, use of iso-osmolar nonionic contrast media.
- Risk of contrast-induced AKI is reduced by avoidance of hypovolemia:
  – Inpatients: Isotonic saline 1 mL/kg/hr 6–12 hours preprocedure, during the procedure and 6–12 hours postprocedure.
  – Outpatients: Isotonic saline 3 mL/kg/hr × 1 hour preprocedure, 1 to 1.5 mL/kg/hour × 4–6 hours during and after the procedure for a total of 6 ml/kg

Second Line
- Tamsulosin or other selective α-blockers for bladder outlet obstruction secondary to BPH.
- Dihydropyridine calcium channel blockers may have a protective effect in posttransplant ATN.

ISSUES FOR REFERRAL
- Consider nephrology consultation for potential initiation of RRT; persistent and prolonged anuria or oliguria and/or refractory elevation in BUN and/or Cr despite appropriate fluid and/or electrolyte replacement, and/or underlying structural or functional renal disease (e.g., glomerulonephropathies, SLE nephritis, cryoglobulinemia), and/or renal transplant patients.
- Consider urology consult for obstructive nephropathy.

SURGERY/OTHER PROCEDURES
- Relieve obstruction by retrograde ureteral catheters/percutaneous nephrostomy.
- Hemodialysis catheter placement

COMPLEMENTARY & ALTERNATIVE MEDICINE
Many herbal and dietary supplements are potentially nephrotoxic (aristolochic acid, ochratoxin A, Djenkol bean, impila [*Callilepis laureola*]), orellanine, cat's claw, Chinese yew (*Taxus celebica*), morning cypress (*Cupressus funebris* [Endl]), St. John's wort.

ADMISSION, INPATIENT, AND NURSING CONSIDERATIONS
- Treat life-threatening complications: hyperkalemia, metabolic acidosis, volume overload, and advanced uremia
- Monitor strict intake and output through fluid balance and daily weights.
- Consider urinary catheter placement to quantify urine output, weighing risks of catheter-associated urinary tract infection (CAUTI). Remove as soon as possible. Stabilize renal function and ensure treatment plan prior to discharge; dialysis if necessary.

 ONGOING CARE

FOLLOW-UP RECOMMENDATIONS
Nephrology follow-up if persistent renal impairment and/or proteinuria

DIET
- Total caloric intake of 20 to 30 kcal/kg/day (1)
- Restrict Na^+ to 2 g/day (unless hypovolemic); consider K^+ restriction (2 to 3 g/day) if hyperkalemic. If hyperphosphatemic, consider use of phosphate binders, although no evidence of benefit in AKI. Avoid magnesium- and aluminum-containing compounds.

PATIENT EDUCATION
- Keep well-hydrated. Avoid nephrotoxic drugs, such as NSAIDs and aminoglycosides.
- Acute Kidney Injury (AKI). National Kidney Foundation: https://www.kidney.org/atoz/content/AcuteKidneyInjury

PROGNOSIS
- In cases of prerenal and postrenal AKI, short duration of AKI correlates with good rates of recovery.
- Among patients who require RRT for AKI, recovery more likely with higher baseline GFR, AKI from ATN due to sepsis or surgery; recovery less likely with preexisting heart failure.

COMPLICATIONS
Death, sepsis, infection, CKD, seizures, paralysis, peripheral edema, CHF, arrhythmias, uremic pericarditis, bleeding, hypotension, anemia, hyperkalemia, uremia

REFERENCES
1. Kidney Disease: Improving Global Outcomes (KDIGO) Acute Kidney Injury Work Group. KDIGO Clinical Practice Guideline for Acute Kidney Injury. *Kidney Inter.* 2012;(Suppl 2):1–138.
2. Gonsalez SR, Cortês AL, Costa da Silva R, et al. Acute kidney injury overview: from basic findings to new prevention and therapy strategies. *Pharmacol Ther.* 2019;200:1–12.
3. Gameiro J, Fonseca JA, Outerelo C, et al. Acute kidney injury: from diagnosis to prevention and treatment strategies. *J Clin Med.* 2020;9(6):1704.

 SEE ALSO

- Chronic Kidney Disease; Glomerulonephritis, Acute; Hepatorenal Syndrome; Hyperkalemia; Prostatic Hyperplasia, Benign (BPH); Renal Insufficiency; Reye Syndrome; Rhabdomyolysis; Sepsis
- Algorithm: Anuria or Oliguria

CODES

ICD10
- N17.0 Acute kidney failure with tubular necrosis
- N17.1 Acute kidney failure with acute cortical necrosis
- N17.8 Other acute kidney failure

CLINICAL PEARLS
- Three categories of AKI:
  – Prerenal: decreased renal perfusion (often from hypovolemia) leading to a decrease in GFR; reversible
  – Intrarenal: intrinsic kidney damage; ATN most common due to ischemic/nephrotoxic injury
  – Postrenal: extrinsic/intrinsic obstruction of the urinary collection system
- Indications for emergent hemodialysis: severe hyperkalemia, metabolic acidosis, or volume overload refractory to conservative therapy; uremic pericarditis, encephalopathy, or neuropathy; and selected alcohol and drug intoxications
- Management of ATN is supportive; no specific treatments are proven to effectively hasten recovery.
- Fluid management remains a mainstay of treatment in prerenal and intrinsic kidney injury.

ADHESIVE CAPSULITIS (FROZEN SHOULDER)

Sultan Mahmood Babar, MD, CAQSM, FAAFP

 BASICS

DESCRIPTION

- Adhesive capsulitis (AC) or frozen shoulder:
  - Presents as progressive painful restriction in range of movement of the glenohumeral (GH) joint
  - Course usually involves diminishment of pain but can have residual pain and limits of active and passive range of motion (ROM)
- Subtypes:
  - Primary AC:
    - Idiopathic
    - Usually associated with diabetes mellitus (DM)
    - Typically resolves in 9 to 24 months
  - Secondary AC:
    - Typically due to prolonged immobilization
    - Most commonly due to a complication of rotator cuff impingement syndrome (rotator cuff tendonitis) that remains incompletely treated
    - Sometimes called "shoulder-hand-syndrome," which is a complex regional pain syndrome (CRPS) or reflex sympathetic dystrophy (RDS), if it is characterized by shoulder pain, diffuse swelling, and decreased ROM
- Clinical course:
  - Phase 1 (2 to 9 months): painful phase; pain is constant; diagnosis may be difficult if restricted movement is not present in early disease.
  - Phase 2 (4 to 12 months): stiffening or freezing phase; movement becomes restricted, especially with external rotation.
  - Phase 3 (12 to 42 months): resolution or thawing phase; gradual return to normal shoulder mobility

EPIDEMIOLOGY

Incidence
- 2.4/1,000 people per year
- Female:male ratio (1.4:1)

Prevalence
2–5% in the general population, 10–20% among diabetes (1)

ETIOLOGY AND PATHOPHYSIOLOGY
Underlying fundamental processes:
- Idiopathic
- Inflammation: Mast cells, T cells, B cells, and macrophages have been identified histologically, suggesting an inflammatory process. Studies confirm presence of elevated inflammatory cytokines such as IL-1, IL-6, TNF-α, COX-1, and COX-2 (1).
- Elevated markers for neoangiogenesis (CD34) and neoinnervation (GAP43, PGP9.5, NGFRp75) have been associated with AC which helps explain the acute painful phase. Additionally, one study showed that overexpression of TGF-β led to the development of AC in rats (1).
- Scarring: Fibroblasts and myofibroblasts have been identified histologically. Capsular contracture reduces the joint volume to 3 to 4 mL compared to the normal 10 to 15 mL. Intercellular adhesion molecule-1 (ICAM-1) facilitates leukocyte endothelial transmigration. It is elevated in both AC and DM.

- This scarring primarily effects the rotator interval (coracohumeral ligament (CHL), biceps tendon, and GH capsule). A contracted CHL is an essential finding in AC (1).
- Contracture of the GH capsule from loss of synovial layer, capsular adhesions, and loss of capsular volume are seen in AC.

RISK FACTORS
- Shoulder immobilization; often due to impingement syndrome (most significant risk factor)
- Increasing age
- Female gender
- Diabetes
- Thyroid disease
- Atherosclerotic cardiovascular disease (ASCVD): cerebrovascular accident (CVA)/myocardial infarction (MI)/hyperlipidemia
- Antiretroviral medication use
- Parkinson disease
- Trauma/surgery
- Prior history of AC in contralateral shoulder

GENERAL PREVENTION
- Active lifestyle, while avoiding shoulder injury
- Control of diabetes, atherosclerotic disease, thyroid, and autoimmune conditions

COMMONLY ASSOCIATED CONDITIONS
DM, autoimmune disorders, Parkinson disease, highly active antiretroviral therapy (HAART) use, CVA/MI, cervical disc disease, thyroid disorders

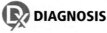 DIAGNOSIS

HISTORY
- Identify possible risk factors.
- Progressive and worsening stiffness of the GH joint
- Majority will have diffuse shoulder pain, especially at the beginning of the disease.
- On the late phase of the disease, stiffness becomes predominant.
- Rule out other pain invoking conditions such as fractures, osteoarthritis (OA), subacromial pathologies such as bursitis and rotator cuff tendinopathy, cervical radiculopathy, and GH arthrosis (1).

PHYSICAL EXAM
- Limitation in both active and passive ROM due to true mechanical restriction
- Capsular pattern of ROM restriction is demonstrated, with external rotation most affected, followed by abduction and then flexion.
- Pain with rotator cuff impingement tests
- Inability to reach overhead or back pocket
- Scapular substitution frequently accompanies active shoulder movement
- Loss of arm swing with gait

DIFFERENTIAL DIAGNOSIS
- Rotator cuff strain/tear/impingement syndrome
- GH or acromioclavicular joint OA
- Cervical strain/radiculopathy/OA

- Subacromial bursitis
- Parsonage-Turner syndrome: brachial plexus inflammation secondary to a trigger, such as an infection, trauma, or autoimmune condition
- Myofascial pain syndrome
- Calcific tendonitis
- Fracture
- Shoulder subluxation/dislocation
- Bony neoplasm/metastasis

DIAGNOSTIC TESTS & INTERPRETATION
AC is a clinical diagnosis that can further be guided by labs and images if needed. No single lab or imaging alone can make the diagnosis.

Initial Tests (lab, imaging)
- No labs are required for idiopathic AC. If other risk factor for a particular associated condition are present, then blood tests can be used to check for these conditions. This includes diabetes, thyroid disease, a stroke, autoimmune diseases, and, in rare cases, Parkinson disease.
  - For example, thyroid-stimulating hormone, hemoglobin A1C, erythrocyte sedimentation rate, C-reactive protein.
- Imaging
  - Plain radiographs of the affected shoulder (posteroanterior, external rotation, axillary, and supraspinatus outlet views)
    - Preferred initial tests
    - In most cases, will be negative
    - Used primarily to rule out other pathologies such as GH, OA, fractures, dislocation, or tumors
  - Magnetic resonance imaging (MRI)
    - Not indicated unless there is a concomitant pathology in the shoulder or neurologic deficit
    - May show thickening of the joint capsule and the CHL along with edema and increased joint fluid
    - Rotator interval/axillary joint capsule enhancement and inferior GH and/or CHL hyperintensity are the most diagnostic signs with sensitivity and specificity >80% (2).
  - Ultrasound (US)
    - Indications similar to those for MRI
    - Selection depends on individual cases and clinician's preference.
    - Can also reveal thickening of the CHL and soft tissues of the joint capsule and increased joint fluid
    - Doppler US can show increased vascularity around the intra-articular (IA) portion of the biceps tendon and CHL.

Follow-Up Tests & Special Considerations
- Shared decision-making regarding treatment
- Pain referral for CRPS

Diagnostic Procedures/Other
Injection test can be helpful in differentiating AC from subacromial pathologies such as rotator cuff tendinopathy (which should improve with injection of local anesthetics, in contrast to AC). This should only be done if the diagnosis is still uncertain after a thorough history and physical.

TREATMENT

- In most cases, self-limited
- Physical therapy with exercises within the limits of pain
- Manage patient expectations; resolution often takes 18 months of medication and rehabilitation.
- Treat any underlying medical conditions associated with AC such as DM and thyroid disorders.

MEDICATION

- Medication can be used to provide symptomatic relief.
- Acetaminophen or nonsteroidal anti-inflammatory drugs (NSAIDs) are first line of treatment.
- Glucocorticoid injections:
  - Single IA corticosteroid injections and multisite injections showed great statistical and clinical outcomes for pain when used in the beginning of the disease. IA corticosteroid injections in patients with frozen shoulder for <1 year duration showed greater benefits compared to other interventions and such benefits were shown to last as long as 6 months.
  - A course of physical therapy after an injection, for 4 to 6 weeks, with or without IA corticosteroid appeared to be associated with short-term benefits of improving pain and ROM.
  - Injection may be diluted with a local anesthetic such as lidocaine. Triamcinolone 20 to 40 mg or methylprednisolone 20 to 40 mg can be used.
  - Hydrodilation with normal saline combined with IA corticosteroid injection may expedite ROM recovery compared to corticosteroid injection alone (1).
- Although a short course of oral glucocorticoid can temporarily provide pain relief and improved mobility, the benefits were not greater than a few weeks. Studies have shown that IA corticosteroid injections are more effective than oral steroid treatment (1).

First Line

Conservative treatment
- Home exercises using climbing the wall.
  - Climbing the wall: Face a wall and place the hand from the affected shoulder flat on the surface of the wall; use the fingers to "climb" the wall; pause 30 seconds every few inches. Repeat the exercise after turning the torso 90 degrees to wall (abduction).
- Can also be used along with NSAIDs or glucocorticoid injections
- Oral steroids are usually not recommended.

Second Line

If there is no improvement in 6 to 8 weeks of conservative treatment, then more invasive treatment may be indicated.
- Hydrodilatation:
  - Injection of 10 to 20 mL of saline or 1% Lidocaine along with glucocorticoid
- Physical therapy should be continued.

ISSUES FOR REFERRAL

Surgical referral can be considered if symptoms have been present for >1 year and patients fail to make progress with appropriate management for 3 months.

ADDITIONAL THERAPIES

- Exercise and physical therapy:
  - Gentle ROM exercises should be offered to every patient.
  - Exercises should be performed daily and as tolerated. A structured plan should be given to the patient.
  - Physical therapy has been found to be beneficial especially in phases 2 and 3 of AC. Best data supports its use in conjunction with other treatment such as corticosteroid injections.
- Laser has been suggested as a possible treatment, particularly for pain relief; not enough evidence for support
- Suprascapular nerve block can provide temporary pain relief and may be a therapeutic option for AC refractory to IA corticosteroid injections; however, there is a lack of high-quality evidence for support (1).
- Other therapies that have been studied include whole-body cryotherapy and IA injection of botulinum toxin type A, both of which have demonstrated to improve pain and ROM but with limited evidence (1).

SURGERY/OTHER PROCEDURES

- Should be reserved for patients who do not respond to conservative measures for at least 1 year or is not showing any improvement conservatively.
- Some of the most common procedures include manipulation under anesthesia (MUA), arthroscopic capsular release (ARC), distension arthrogram, among others. One study comparing ARC, MUA, and physiotherapy showed that although all three treatments led to substantial improvements in pain and function, none of the treatments were clinically superior to another.

ONGOING CARE

FOLLOW-UP RECOMMENDATIONS

- After establishing a diagnosis, assess the need for pain control and start the patient on NSAIDs, in combination with a gentle exercise program with guidance with physical therapy.
- Follow up in 3 to 4 weeks: if no significant improvement, may consider IA corticosteroid injections
- Physical therapy should be concurrently used because it can hasten the rate of recovery and increase ROM.
- For secondary AC, consider evaluation and management of underlying condition.
- If no improvement, consider surgical intervention.

PATIENT EDUCATION

- Patient education is important; explain prognosis and ensure compliance with treatment.
- Climbing the wall: Face a wall and place the hand from the affected shoulder flat on the surface of the wall; use the fingers to "climb" the wall; pause 30 seconds every few inches. Repeat the exercise after turning the torso 90 degrees to wall (abduction).
- In case of secondary AC, address the importance of treating underlying causes.

PROGNOSIS

- Recovery is dependent on onset of treatment, symptoms, and comorbidities in patient.
- Variable duration, lasting 1 to 3 years without intervention
- Patients with idiopathic frozen shoulder have a good rate of recovery.

REFERENCES

1. Le HV, Lee SJ, Nazarian A, et al. Adhesive capsulitis of the shoulder: review of pathophysiology and current clinical treatments. *Shoulder Elbow*. 2017;9(2):75–84.
2. Suh CH, Yun SJ, Jin W, et al. Systematic review and meta-analysis of magnetic resonance imaging features for diagnosis of adhesive capsulitis of the shoulder. *Eur Radiol*. 2019;29(2):566–577.

CODES

ICD10
- M75.00 Adhesive capsulitis of unspecified shoulder
- M75.01 Adhesive capsulitis of right shoulder
- M75.02 Adhesive capsulitis of left shoulder

CLINICAL PEARLS

- Frozen shoulder or AC is generally a self-limiting global restriction in ROM of the shoulder joint. Up to 15% will have disability long-term.
- Natural course consists of a painful phase, freezing phase, and thawing phase. It occurs mostly in older women; total prevalence is 3–5% of the general population and roughly 10–20% of the diabetic population.
- An active and passive ROM restriction will be present; most common is the inability to externally rotate the shoulder. Other signs include pain on provocation of subacromial space and inability to reach overhead or for back pocket.
- Plain x-rays are the preferred initial imaging modality. MRI and US are done only if there is concomitant pathology or neurologic deficit.
- Treatment includes pain control and physical therapy; can progress to glucocorticoid therapy with a consideration for surgery
- Resolution of symptoms can take up to 24 months.
- Given the prevalence in patients who are middle-aged, it is also referred to the "50-year-old shoulder."

ADVANCE CARE PLANNING

Heather Ann Dalton, MD, FAAFP

BASICS

DESCRIPTION

- Advance care planning (ACP) allows patients to have a voice in the decisions that affect their care if they lose the ability to do so for themselves.
- There are several methods of addressing a patient's priorities in their care:
  - Advance directives, including living wills (LWs) and heath care durable powers of attorney (DPOA), also known as a medical power of attorney (MPOA)
  - Physician/medical orders for life-sustaining treatment (POLST/MOLST) and directives to physicians
  - Facilitated conversations with family and significant others
- ACP is an important aspect of patient-centered care as the population ages and individuals lose decision-making capacity, when new chronic medical conditions are diagnosed, or in the setting of severe acute illnesses like COVID-19.
- ACP helps to interpret patient's wishes in the context of individual illness circumstances, negotiate conflicts in decisions, and allow patients to determine what is in their best interest based on personal values.
- Definitions
  - Advance directives (1): written instructions to guide decision-making in the event a patient is unable to provide informed consent
    - LWs and MPOAs usually only take effect if the patient has been determined to lack capacity to decide care for himself or herself; otherwise, patient preference takes precedence (even if contradictory to an LW).
    - If done appropriately, these help patients avoid languishing in poor quality of life states or receiving unwanted care which can be associated with complex ethical dilemmas.
  - LW: a patient's explicit written instructions of his or her wishes regarding medical care
    - Each state has specific legal requirements. Certain states do not recognize LWs but have other "medical directive" forms. LWs and medical directives can take effect immediately (e.g., when a patient is diagnosed with a terminal illness) or when a patient can no longer make decisions for himself or herself.
    - LWs have direct treatment instructions.
    - Challenges of LWs include lack of standardization, narrow scope, and limited updating on changes in disease trajectory.
    - LWs do not expire, and they can be revised.
    - The LW is NOT a medical directive; so, it cannot prevent life-sustaining treatment in an emergent situation (as a POLST/MOLST can [see next]).

- MPOA: a written document designating a surrogate decision maker in the event a patient cannot speak for himself or herself
  - A health care proxy (HCP)/MPOA speaks on behalf of the patient to make decisions aligned as closely as possible to the patient's health care wishes. Ideally, this is someone the patient knows and trusts. It is also helpful if this individual has had discussions with the patient about his or her values and desires.
  - Different states have varying rules regarding precedence if there is a conflict between an LW provision and an HCP decision. When there is conflict, engage with palliative care, ethics, and legal.
  - If a patient has had goals of care discussions with friends or family but does not have a legally named HCP, those discussions can still help inform the decision-making process and elicit patient values.
  - POLST/MOLST: a medical directive which, unlike an LW, directs point of care decision-making by EMS/first responders
    - Designed to minimize confusion in emergent situations, these are adjunctive documents to LWs and MPOAs that provide clear instruction regarding resuscitation, intubation, and other life-sustaining treatments.
    - They are portable and follow a patient across different care settings. Given their simplicity, a POLST/MOLST is more likely to be followed than an LW, which can be difficult to locate.
    - Although EMS/first responders may be concerned about the legal implications of withholding life-sustaining treatment, POLST forms provide legal protection if patient wishes are followed.
- There are no authoritative guidelines for when to initiate discussions about ACP; age 65 years may be an appropriate time. Additionally, patient values and wishes should be discussed following a new diagnosis of a serious illness or a significant change in disease trajectory. Each conversation must be individualized.
- ACP should be completed while patients are able to make decisions about their future care. Every effort should be made to initiate discussions and complete required forms prior to incapacitating health changes.
- Nursing home residents and patients with dementia often do not have capacity to complete legal documents related to LW and MPOA.

Pediatric Considerations

For children with serious acute or terminal illness, it is a difficult (but important) part of treatment.

- Provider fears about increasing parental distress when discussing ACP are unfounded.
- ACP may unburden parents from difficult decisions and is associated with increased positive emotions, understanding of the patient's illness, and provider's rapport.

TREATMENT

- Suggested discussion points:
  - For all adult patients:
    - Assess willingness to engage in ACP. Do not force patients if they are not ready to have this potentially emotionally challenging conversation.
    - Ask patients to identify who they would like to make decisions for them if they were unable to do so.
    - Encourage patients to inform trusted family or friends about new diagnoses or changes in health.
    - Discuss what values are most important to patients.
    - Document decisions concisely and clearly.
  - For any patient with a chronic, serious, or terminal illness:
    - Discuss the natural course of disease progression, including time course and end-of-life expectations.
    - For example:
      - Chronic obstructive lung disease: exacerbations, decreased ability to perform activities of daily living, supplemental oxygen, mechanical ventilation
      - Malignancy: possibility of chronic pain, inability to swallow/poor appetite necessitating alternative feeding options, ascites and therapeutic procedures, treatment side effects
  - For older patients:
    - Consider routine discussions of ACP around age 65 years. It is crucial to speak with patients while they still have decision-making capacity. Discussions should be repeated regularly, especially if clinical course deteriorates, to ensure patient preferences have not changed.
    - Provide online resources for completing LWs.
    - Refer patients to legal or notary services for advance directive/MPOA, as applicable.
    - Complete POLST/MOLST forms in clinic, if applicable in your state.

– For any change in clinical status (including frequent ER visits or hospitalizations):
  ○ Changes in functional status should prompt a discussion about prognosis and future wishes. Hospitalizations are important milestones to discuss recovery or decline.
  ○ Consider palliative care services.
  ○ Consider support services to prevent caregiver burnout.
- At the end of life, if it is the patient's desire, it is important to engage hospice services in a timely manner.
  – ACP discussions are often complicated by social, familial, cultural, spiritual, and medical factors. It is important to be sensitive to each patient's individual context.
  – Do not force the conversation if a patient is resistant or unprepared to discuss ACP.
    ○ Motivational interviewing can be used to gauge interest and readiness to discuss ACP.
    ○ Addressing implications for friends and family who may be burdened with decision-making may help promote ACP conversations.
  – The first time ACP is brought up often serves as an introduction to the topic and an opportunity for the patient to consider options. Subsequent visits can address specific scenarios and choices.
  – Avoid medical jargon (i.e., CPR, mechanical ventilation, parenteral nutrition, etc.) when addressing options. Patients may not understand the severity or implications of advanced life-saving interventions. It may be more effective to describe how a particular intervention may affect the patient and what the resulting quality of life may look like.

ONGOING CARE

Reimbursement: The Centers for Medicare & Medicaid Services reimburses physicians for ACP discussions.
- Current CPT codes are 99497 for the first 16 to 45 minutes of discussion and completion of forms and 99498 as an add-on for a total of 46 to 75 minutes (2).
- There are no limits to the number of times ACP can be reported in a given period of time.
- An advance directive does not have to be completed in order to bill for services.
- No specific diagnosis is required for the ACP codes (3).

FOLLOW-UP RECOMMENDATIONS
Patient Monitoring
- There are no specific guidelines for how often an LW or DPOA discussion should be revisited after completion.
- When there is a new diagnosis or a significant change in clinical status, have the patient consider how it would affect his or her ACP decision-making.
- Have patients display POLST/MOLST forms prominently for ease of visibility to EMS, such as on their refrigerator.

PATIENT EDUCATION
- See references for links: The National Hospice and Palliative Care Organization, National Institute on Aging, Aging with Dignity, National Healthcare Decisions Day, and the American Bar Association have resources to help patients.
- Online platforms such as Prepare for your Care and MyDirectives allow patients to specify their wishes electronically.
- DeathWise is a nonprofit organization with worksheets that patients can use for the health, financial, care of body, and service components of ACP.

COMPLICATIONS
- Often LWs, MPOAs, and POLST/MOLSTs are completed, but physicians do not have access to them. Electronic health records are a convenient place to store documents, but they may be difficult to retrieve.
  – Any ACP form should be a part of the medical record with open access (if possible) to facilitate appropriate decision-making.
- Emergency rooms are vulnerable to uncertainty about what interventions patients want if they cannot communicate for themselves and guiding documents are often not readily available. POLST forms can help avoid confusion.
- There is often misunderstanding on the part of both doctors and patients regarding do-not-resuscitate (DNR) and do-not-intubate (DNI) orders.
  – DNR/DNI orders can be reversed and should be re-addressed as the patient's clinical status changes.
  – DNR/DNI in a person with a chronic progressive illness does not necessarily mean DNR/DNI for an acute reversible process.

REFERENCES

1. American Association of Retired Persons. Advance directive forms by state. http://www.aarp.org/home-family/caregiving/free-printable-advance-directives/. Accessed August 4, 2023.
2. Centers for Medicare & Medicaid Services. Medicare Learning Network: advance care planning. https://www.cms.gov/outreach-education/medicare-learning-network-mln/mlnproducts/downloads/advancecareplanning.pdf. Accessed August 4, 2023.
3. Bosisio F, Barazzetti G. Advanced care planning: promoting autonomy in caring for people with dementia. *Am J Bioeth*. 2020;20(8):93–95.

ADDITIONAL READING

- Aging with Dignity. Five wishes. https://www.aging-withdignity.org/. Accessed September 15, 2022.
- American Bar Association. Tool kit for health care advance planning. https://www.americanbar.org/groups/law_aging/resources/health_care_decision_making/consumer_s_toolkit_for_health_care_advance_planning.html. Accessed September 15, 2022.
- Heyland DK. Engaging seriously ill older patients in advance care planning. https://psnet.ahrq.gov/webmm/case/404/engaging-seriously-ill-older-patients-in-advance-care-planning. Accessed September 15, 2022.
- MyDirectives: https://www.mydirectives.com/
- National Healthcare Decisions Day: https://theconversationproject.org/nhdd/
- National Hospice and Palliative Care Organization. CaringInfo: http://www.caringinfo.org/
- Prepare for your Care: https://prepareforyourcare.org/en/welcome

 CODES

ICD10
- Z71.89 Other specified counseling
- Z51.5 Encounter for palliative care
- Z66 Do not resuscitate

CLINICAL PEARLS
- ACP is an important and underused element of compassionate and comprehensive patient-centered care.
- The primary barriers to discussing advanced directives from the patient's perspective include lack of knowledge, fear of burdening the family, and a desire for physicians to initiate the discussion.
- The primary barriers to discussing advanced directives from the physician's perspective include discomfort with the topic and lack of time to fully address the topic.
- Fewer unwanted interventions occur in emergency room and inpatient settings when ACP is actively reviewed and patient's wishes are documented and conveyed appropriately.

AIR TRAVEL EMERGENCIES
Theodore E. Macnow, MD • Michelle A. Georgia, DO

BASICS

DESCRIPTION
Physicians commonly help with in-flight medical events (IME). Many IMEs fall outside a practitioner's normal scope of practice. The aircraft environment is cramped with limited medical resources. Despite these obstacles, health care workers should be prepared to render assistance in these situations.

EPIDEMIOLOGY
Incidence
- 2.9 million passengers travel daily worldwide. In the United States, 1.7 million individuals travel by plane every day.
- Airlines estimate an IME occurs on 1 in 40 flights or in 1 per 7,500 to 40,000 passengers. Most are minors, and 65–70% are handled by the flight crew (1),(2).
- The likelihood of encountering an IME is increasing because of larger aircraft, longer flights, and an aging population.
- The most common IMEs involve syncope/near syncope (32.7%), gastrointestinal (14.8%), respiratory (10.1%), and cardiovascular symptoms (7%) (2).
- In otherwise healthy passengers, vasovagal syncope represents up to 90% of IMEs.
- 5% of passengers suffer from a chronic illness and account for 2/3 of IMEs.
- 15% of ground-based physician calls are for pediatric passengers.
- 3% of IMEs are fatal.

ETIOLOGY AND PATHOPHYSIOLOGY
Hypobaric hypoxia: Atmospheric pressure of oxygen drops from 160 mm Hg at sea level to 120 mm Hg at cruising altitude in a pressurized cabin. In healthy people, the arterial oxygen tension drops from 100 to 60 mm Hg with associated mean inflight oxygen saturations of 93% (range: 85 to 98).

> **ALERT**
> Passengers with chronic obstructive pulmonary disease (COPD) or other pulmonary disorders have a lower baseline PaO$_2$, so any drop in oxygen tension may occur on the steep part of the hemoglobin dissociation curve and may result in more significant hypoxemia. Passengers with unstable angina or heart failure may not be able to compensate for hypoxia.

- Gas expansion: Gases expand about 30% in flight. This can lead to a pneumothorax, wound dehiscence or perforation from bowel gas expansion, sinus pressure, and tympanic membrane rupture in children with ear infections.
- Venous thromboembolism: There is an increased risk of deep vein thromboses (DVTs) on longer flights and in passengers with underlying medical conditions because of prolonged sitting, hypoxic conditions, and dehydration.
- Stress: Travelling is mentally and physically stressful, which may lead to psychiatric emergencies or acute coronary syndrome (ACS).
- Insomnia: Passengers have disrupted circadian rhythms, which may trigger seizures and contribute to medication nonadherence.
- Turbulence: Motion sickness is common and traumatic injury can result from falling luggage.

- Medication nonadherence: Forgotten or checked medications may lead to glycemic control problems, seizures, blood pressure instability, and inaccessible as needed medications.
- Decreased access to food and drink: Vasovagal syncope may result from dehydration. Diabetics may suffer hypoglycemia.
- Low air humidity: Cabin air is <20% relative humidity, which contributes to dehydration, epistaxis, and asthma or COPD exacerbations.
- Viral infections: Parainfluenza and influenza are the most common viruses communicated by proximity. The cabin air is filtered and not infectious.

> **ALERT**
> Transmission of SARS-CoV-2 virus can occur on air travel. Like other viruses, the risk is mostly from proximity to infected passengers rather than cabin air flow. The risk may be mitigated by mask-wearing.

RISK FACTORS
- Recent surgery: Passengers are at risk for wound dehiscence, bowel perforation, and compartment syndrome from gas expansion.
- COPD, asthma, CHF, or coronary artery disease: Passengers may suffer from hypoxemia and may not be able to compensate appropriately.
- Recent cast placement: Passengers are at risk for compartment syndrome due to tissue edema.
- Hypercoagulability: Passengers with inherited or acquired hypercoagulable conditions, pregnancy, certain medications, heart disease, or recent surgery are at increased risk for DVTs.
- Recent scuba diving: Passengers are at risk for decompression syndromes.
- Long flights: The effects of hypoxia are cumulative and time dependent.

GENERAL PREVENTION
General guidelines:
- Travelers should discuss medication timing with their doctor and bring necessary medications and equipment onboard.
- Supplemental inflight oxygen is required for patients with a baseline PaO$_2$ <70 mm Hg or who are unable to walk a flight of stairs or 150 feet without having shortness of breath or experiencing angina (3)[C].

Pregnancy Considerations
Women are generally safe to fly until 36 weeks' gestation.

Pediatric Considerations
- Travelers with children should bring liquid formulations of medication in allowed quantities on the plane. Children with asthma should have a rescue inhaler with spacer and facemask.
- Specific guidelines:
  – Avoid flying 10 to 14 days after surgery (varies by type of surgery).
  – Casts may need to be bivalved if applied 24 to 48 hours before a flight.
  – Avoid scuba diving 24 hours before flying.
  – DVT prevention (3)[C]:
    ○ Adequately hydrate.
    ○ Stand, stretch, and exercise the legs in flight.
    ○ Passengers with risk factors may need compression stockings, aspirin, or anticoagulation.

DIAGNOSIS

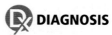

HISTORY
- Symptoms vary based on emergency; if the patient is alert, gather as much history as possible.
- Ask about past medical and surgical history, medications and compliance, and allergies.
- Inquire about illicit drug or alcohol use.
- Document findings and recommendations and save a secure copy for your records.

PHYSICAL EXAM
- Wear all available PPE. Protective gear is available on board.
- May need to obtain blood pressure by palpitation due to noise
- Assess vital signs, general appearance, and mental status. Look for signs of dehydration including skin perfusion.
- If stethoscope available, auscultate as best as possible.

> **ALERT**
> Assess for tension pneumothorax by listening for decreased lung sounds and contralateral tracheal deviation. A tension pneumothorax requires needle decompression.

DIFFERENTIAL DIAGNOSIS
- **Syncope or near-syncope:** vasovagal syncope, dehydration, hypoglycemia, intoxication, medication reaction or toxicity, ACS, arrhythmia, cerebrovascular accident, pulmonary thrombosis/air embolism, and hypoxia
- **Chest pain:** ACS, pulmonary embolism, pneumothorax, bronchospasm, aortic dissection, gastroesophageal reflux, musculoskeletal etiology, and anxiety
- **Shortness of breath:** COPD or asthma exacerbation, pneumonia, pulmonary thrombosis/air embolism, toxic exposure
- **Stroke-like symptoms:** cerebrovascular accident, transient ischemic attack, hypoglycemia, seizure, syncope, intracranial mass, and complex migraine
- **Seizure:** seizure, syncope, hypoglycemia, eclampsia, cardiac arrest
- **Gastrointestinal illness:** motion sickness, food-borne illness, gastritis, enteritis, gastroesophageal reflux, pancreatitis, medication or substance withdrawal
- **Obstetric emergency:** preterm labor, miscarriage, eclampsia, placenta previa
- **Allergic reaction:** urticaria, anaphylaxis, dermatitis
- **Cardiac arrest:** arrhythmia, pulmonary embolism, respiratory arrest, ACS, intoxication, syncope
- **Altered mental status:** use or withdrawal from drugs or alcohol (consider GI absorption from smuggling), hypoglycemia, panic attack, DKA, hypoxia, psychiatric emergency

DIAGNOSTIC TESTS & INTERPRETATION
The automated external defibrillator (AED) can be used as a cardiac monitor.

TREATMENT

GENERAL MEASURES
- **First aid and CPR:** If there is no pulse or not breathing, start CPR, BLS, ALS, and PALS as appropriate. Airline crew members are trained in first aid and CPR.
- **Ask for help:** Ask the flight crew and other passengers for equipment, medications, expertise, and lifting assistance.
- **Oxygen:** All flights have oxygen at 2 to 5 L per minute by facemask. This oxygen delivery at cruising altitude mimics conditions at sea level. Oxygen should be applied in all cases of respiratory distress, chest pain, seizures, and altered mental status.
- **Ground-based physician support:** Many airlines contract with companies that offer inflight medical advice, interpreter services, recommendations for diversion, and sometimes telemedicine technology.
- **Request to fly at lower attitude:** Flying <22,500 feet with cabin pressurization mimics sea level oxygen pressure. Flying lower uses more fuel and is slower; so, it may not be optimal to reach a hospital quickly.
- **Request a diversion:** The pilot can request an expedited landing, medical services on arrival, or a closer destination. Medical emergencies that involve resuscitation, persistent abnormal vital signs, chest pain, stroke symptoms, respiratory distress, unconsciousness, obstetrics, or psychiatric emergencies should be considered for diversion.

Table 1. FAA-Mandated Contents of Emergency Medical Kit

Equipment	Oropharyngeal airways (3 sizes)
	Cardiopulmonary resuscitation mask
	Manual resuscitation devices, 3 masks
	Adhesive tape, 1-inch
	Alcohol sponges
	IV administration set
	Needles
	Protective gloves
	Sphygmomanometer
	Stethoscope
	Tape scissors
	Tourniquet
	Instructions on kit use
Medications	Analgesic, nonnarcotic
	Antihistamine, 50 mg, injectable
	Antihistamine tablets, 25 mg
	Aspirin tablets, 325 mg
	Atropine, 0.5 mg, 5 mL
	Bronchodilator, inhaled (i.e., albuterol)
	Dextrose, 50%/50 mL, injectable
	Epinephrine 1:1,000, 1 mL, injectable
	Epinephrine 1:10,000, 2 mL, injectable
	Lidocaine, 5 mL, 20 mg/mL, injectable
	Nitroglycerine tablets
	Saline solution (minimum 500 cc)

MEDICATION
- All U.S. commercial aircraft have an emergency medical kit (EMK) as well as basic first aid kits on the aircraft. The contents vary among countries, airlines, and aircraft. Many airlines have adopted a more extensive EMK.
- The minimal contents in the EMK required by the Federal Aviation Administration are described in Table 1.
- Depending on the airline, local policies, and country of operation, nurse practitioners and physicians assistants may be able to open and use the EMK.
- All aircraft are equipped with an AED.

ALERT
Not usually found in the EMK are glucometers, intubation equipment, ACLS drugs, narcotics, insulin, or antibiotics. In a 2019 survey, only 35% of EMKs contain naloxone. Ask other passengers for needed medications or equipment.

Pediatric Considerations
The most common cause of airplane diversion in the pediatric population was secondary to seizures. Most EMKs do not contain anticonvulsant medications although the Aerospace Medical Association recommends the inclusion of them in EMKs. EMKs do not include liquid or suppository medications. Consider crushing tablets or asking other passengers for medication or equipment. A toilet paper roll or cut soda bottle can be taped to an albuterol pump to make a spacer.

ADDITIONAL THERAPIES
- **Cardiac Arrest:** CPR; early defibrillation; epinephrine 1:10,000 q3–5min (adults: 1 mg IV, pediatric: 0.01 mg/kg IV); lidocaine or atropine when indicated; recommend diversion.
- **ACS:** oxygen by facemask, aspirin 325 mg PO, nitroglycerin (0.4 mg sublingually q5–10min if systolic blood pressure > 100 mm Hg); apply AED; recommend diversion.
- **Asthma/COPD exacerbation:** oxygen, albuterol 2.5 mg inhaled (repeat as needed), steroid (if available), epinephrine 1:1,000 (autoinjector: adult: 0.3 mg, pediatric [<25 kg]: 0.15 mg IM; ampule: adult 0.3 mg, pediatric 0.01 mg/kg) if significant respiratory distress; consider diversion.
- **Allergic reaction:** diphenhydramine (PO or IV, adult: 25 to 50 mg, pediatric: 1 mg/kg); if anaphylaxis, epinephrine 1:1,000, (autoinjector: adult: 0.3 mg, pediatric [<25 kg]: 0.15 mg IM; ampule: adult: 0.3 mg, pediatric: 0.01 mg/kg); NS (IV, adults: 1 L, pediatric: 20 cc/kg); steroid (if available); divert if anaphylaxis.
- **Vasovagal syncope:** Elevate the legs. If alert and oriented, offer oral liquids. Consider IV fluid bolus. Consider hypoglycemia and offer oral glucose. Monitor blood pressure. Consider diversion if the patient remains symptomatic or has persistent abnormal vital signs.
- **Gastrointestinal:** Oral antiemetic and antacid may be available from the EMK or other passengers. If there is an abdominal pain, consider diversion.

- **Tension pneumothorax:** Needle thoracostomy is preferred over 2nd intercostal space midclavicular line.
- **Psychiatric emergency:** Consider intoxication, hypo-/hyperglycemia, and hypoxia. Attempt verbal de-escalation. The airline protocol should be used for physical restraint. Ask the patient and other passengers if they have oral anxiolytics. Monitor the patient for signs of respiratory distress or ACS if restrained. Consider diversion.
- **Opioid ingestion:** Rescue breathing as needed; naloxone if available in EMK or from other passengers 0.4 to 0.8 mg IV or 2 mg intranasal or IM

ONGOING CARE

PROGNOSIS
- The Aviation Medical Assistance Act of 1998 covers any person with a medical license who is qualified to provide medical care in the United States who act to the best they can within their training and do not demonstrate gross negligence or willful misconduct. This includes physicians, nurses, physician assistants, paramedics, and emergency medical technicians. No physician has been successfully sued in the United States for volunteering care in an IME.
- When overhead paged for assistance, health care workers responded 76% of the time, physicians in 48% of cases and 60% of IMEs improve with help from a health care provider.

REFERENCES
1. Hu JS, Smith JK. In-flight medical emergencies. *Am Fam Physician*. 2021;103(9):547–552.
2. Martin-Gill C, Doyle TJ, Yealy DM. In-flight medical emergencies: a review. *JAMA*. 2018;320(24):2580–2590.
3. Aerospace Medical Association Medical Guidelines Task Force. Medical guidelines for airline travel, 2nd ed. *Aviat Space Environ Med*. 2003;74(Suppl 5):A1–A19.

SEE ALSO
AirRx: smartphone app with information on protocols, diagnoses, and treatments for managing IMEs

CLINICAL PEARLS
- Medical emergencies on airplanes are common. Most are minor.
- Equipment and drugs on board airplanes can be extensive but vary widely.
- All flights are equipped with AEDs and oxygen.
- Many airlines partner with ground-based physician support.
- Utilize passengers as a resource for help, information, and supplies

ALCOHOL USE DISORDER (AUD)

Eric Robert Messner, PhD, FNP-BC • Curtis W. Bone, MD, MHS

 BASICS

DESCRIPTION

- Any pattern of alcohol use causing significant physical, mental, or social dysfunction; key features are tolerance, withdrawal, and persistent use despite problems.
- The severity of AUD exists on a spectrum but is classified as mild, moderate, or severe based on the number of clinical criteria that are met. Manifestation of 2 to 3 of the *DSM-5* criteria for substance use disorders is considered mild disease, 4 to 5 is classified as moderate, and ≥6 is severe AUD.
- *DSM-5* criteria for AUD
  - Tolerance or withdrawal
  - Loss of control over the amount of alcohol used
  - Alcohol cravings or unable to cut down or quit using alcohol
  - Alcohol use during hazardous situations or continued alcohol use that leads to hazardous situations
  - A large amount of time is spent using or recovering from alcohol.
  - Continued alcohol use despite known physical or psychological consequences (i.e., hypertension, hyperlipidemia, cirrhosis, depression, anxiety)
  - Continued use of alcohol despite a negative impact on relationships or failure to meet obligations at work or school
  - Social or occupational activities that were once important to the person are abandoned.
- National Institute on Alcohol Abuse and Alcoholism (NIAAA) criteria for low-risk alcohol use
  - Low-risk alcohol use: NIAAA criteria for low-risk drinking is no more than 14 drinks a week or >4 drinks per occasion. For women, low-risk drinking involves no more than 7 drinks a week or 3 drinks per occasion. Alcohol use that exceeds these levels does not always result in AUD but can still be problematic for an individual.
  - The safest level of use is considered no use because even low-level use is associated with reduction in grey matter and cognitive impairment.
  - Binge drinking: drinking that brings blood alcohol levels to 0.08 g/dL; this is usually 4 drinks for women and 5 drinks for men in 2 hours.
- Measuring alcohol use
  - A standard drink includes 14 g (0.6 fluid oz) of pure alcohol. This includes:
    - 12 oz of beer that are 5% alcohol
    - 5 oz of wine that are 12% alcohol
    - 1.5 oz of distilled spirits that are 40% alcohol

Geriatric Considerations
- Multiple drug interactions
- Signs and symptoms of AUD may be different or attributed to a chronic medical problem or dementia.
- Accelerated aging from frequent alcohol use together with increased consumption in middle-age and older adults increases risk of cognitive decline and dementia.

Pediatric Considerations
- Children of alcoholics are at increased risk; 2.5% of adolescents have AUD; 13.4% of youth aged 12 to 20 years report binge drinking in the past month; negative effect on maturation and normal brain development
- Early-onset drinkers (those who start drinking before age 21 years) are 4 times more likely to develop a problem than those who begin after age 21 years.

EPIDEMIOLOGY
Predominant age is 18 to 25 years, but all ages are affected; male > female (3:1)
- Young drinkers through college age commonly engage in heavy to binge drinking (4 drinks for women and 5 drinks for men in 2 hours) to extreme binge drinking (>15 drinks in one session) on weekends.
- New data reflects increased drinking in middle-age to older adults and binge drinking, especially in women, increasing risk of cognitive decline and dementia.
- In the United States, recent increases in AUD come from a dramatic rise in alcohol use in women (84%) as compared to men (35%).

Prevalence
- 27% of Americans aged ≥18 years reported binge drinking in the past month; 7% reported heavy alcohol use in the past month; 15 million adults (6%) aged >18 years has AUD.
- Excess drinking cost $249 billion in 2010 in the United States, and kills 88,000 Americans per year: approximately 1 in 10 working-age adults
- In the United States, harmful alcohol use is the third leading cause of preventable death and has become a major public health crisis.

ETIOLOGY AND PATHOPHYSIOLOGY
- Multifactorial: genetic, environment, psychosocial
- Alcohol is a CNS depressant, facilitating γ-aminobutyric acid (GABA) inhibition and blocking *N*-methyl-D-aspartate receptors.

Genetics
50–60% of risk is genetic.

RISK FACTORS
- Family history; depression; anxiety disorders; bipolar disorder; eating disorders
- Tobacco and/or other substance abuse
- Male gender; lower socioeconomic status; unemployment; poor self-esteem
- Posttraumatic stress disorder; antisocial personality disorder; criminal behavior

GENERAL PREVENTION
- Counsel patients with family history and risk factors.
- USPSTF recommended in 2018 to screen adults for alcohol use and provide brief counseling to those with risky drinking habits.
- Screening and brief intervention (SBI)

COMMONLY ASSOCIATED CONDITIONS
- Cardiomyopathy; atrial fibrillation; hypertension
- Peptic ulcer disease; cirrhosis; fatty liver; cholelithiasis; hepatitis; pancreatitis
- Diabetes mellitus; malnutrition; upper GI malignancies
- Peripheral neuropathy, seizures
- Abuse and violence
- Behavioral disorders (depression, bipolar, schizophrenia): >50% of patients have a comorbid substance abuse problem.

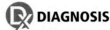 DIAGNOSIS

Use *DSM-5* criteria listed previously.

HISTORY
- Thorough behavioral history
- Anxiety, depression, insomnia, psychological and social dysfunction, marital, or relationship problems, domestic violence
- Complaints about alcohol-related behavior; frequent trauma, MVAs, ED visits

PHYSICAL EXAM
- General: fever, diaphoresis, agitation
- Cardiovascular: hypertension, dilated cardiomyopathy, tachycardia, arrhythmias
- Respiratory: aspiration pneumonia
- GI: stigmata of chronic liver disease, peptic ulcer disease, pancreatitis, esophageal malignancies, esophageal varices
- Musculoskeletal: poorly healed fractures, myopathy, osteopenia, osteoporosis, bone marrow suppression
- Neurologic: tremors, cognitive deficits (e.g., memory impairment), peripheral neuropathy, Wernicke-Korsakoff syndrome (from severe acute deficiency of thiamine: Korsakoff psychosis is a chronic neurologic sequela of Wernicke encephalopathy); Wernicke encephalopathy has the traditional triad of ophthalmoplegia, ataxia, and confusion.
- Dermatologic: burns (e.g., cigarettes), bruises, poor hygiene, palmar erythema, spider telangiectasias

DIFFERENTIAL DIAGNOSIS
- Other substance use disorders
- Depression, dementia; cerebellar ataxia; cerebrovascular accident (CVA); benign essential tremor; seizure disorder
- Hypoglycemia; diabetic ketoacidosis; viral hepatitis

DIAGNOSTIC TESTS & INTERPRETATION
Screening
- CAGE questionnaire: (**C**ut down, **A**nnoyed, **G**uilty, and **E**ye opener): >2 "yes" answers is 74–89% sensitive and 79–95% specific for AUD; less sensitive for white women, college students, elderly; not an appropriate tool for less severe forms of alcohol abuse
- Single question for unhealthy use: "How many times in the last year have you had X or more drinks in 1 day?" (X = 5 for men, 4 for women); 81.8% sensitive, 79% specific for AUDs
- Alcohol Use Disorders Identification Test (AUDIT): 10 items, if score is >4: 70–92% sensitive, better in populations with low incidence of alcoholism: https://www.nams.sg/helpseekers/alcohol/self-assessment-tool/Pages/default.aspx

- AUDIT-C is a three-item screening tool. Scores >4 for men and 3 for women are concerning for alcohol misuse.
  - Q#1: How often did you have a drink containing alcohol in the past year?
  - Q#2: How many drinks containing alcohol did you have on a typical day when you were drinking in the past year?
  - Q#3: How often did you have six or more drinks on one occasion in the past year?

Initial Tests (lab, imaging)
- CBC; liver function tests (LFTs); electrolytes; BUN/creatinine; lipid panel; PT/INR; thiamine; folate; hepatitis A, B, and C serology
- Amylase, lipase (if GI symptoms present)
- Serum levels increased in chronic abuse:
  - AST/ALT ratio >2.0; γ-glutamyl transferase (GGT); carbohydrate-deficient transferrin; uric acid
  - Elevated mean corpuscular volume (MCV); ↑ prothrombin time; triglycerides and cholesterol (total)
- Often decreased: serum protein, albumin; thiamine, folate
- CT scan or MRI of brain: cortical atrophy, lesions in thalamic nucleus, and basal forebrain
- Abdominal ultrasound (US): ascites, periportal fibrosis, fatty infiltration, inflammation
- Calculate MELD score.

Follow-Up Tests & Special Considerations
Abdominal US every 6 months to screen for hepatocellular carcinoma (HCC) among individuals with cirrhosis

TREATMENT

For management of acute withdrawal, see "Alcohol Withdrawal."

GENERAL MEASURES
- Brief interventions and counseling by clinicians have proven effective for problem drinking.
- Treat comorbid problems (sleep, anxiety, etc.), but use extreme caution in prescribing medications with cross tolerance to alcohol (benzodiazepines).
- Group programs and/or 12-step programs help patients accept treatment and develop insight (i.e., Alcoholics Anonymous groups).

MEDICATION
First Line
- Long-term treatment of AUD is initiated after resolution of acute withdrawal:
  - FDA approved
    - Naltrexone: 50 mg/day PO or 380 mg IM once every 4 weeks; most evidence-based FDA-approved medication for AUD; opiate antagonist reduces craving and likelihood of relapse and decreases number of heavy drinking days among people with AUD (IM route may enhance compliance and efficacy); will precipitate withdrawal if patient is on opioids

- Acamprosate (Campral): 666 mg PO TID after withdrawal completed; consider if contraindication to naltrexone; reduces relapse risk; if helpful, use for 1 year; caution if creatinine clearance is low
- Disulfiram: 250 to 500 mg/day PO; FDA approved but not considered first line given unproven efficacy and severe risks; may provide psychological deterrent; most effective if used with close supervision; extreme caution with use given potential for severe emesis in population at risk of esophageal varices; severe reactions may involve myocardial infarction, upper GI bleed, seizure, and death.
- Supplements for all
  - Thiamine: 100 mg/day (first dose IV prior to glucose to avoid Wernicke encephalopathy)
  - Folic acid: 1 mg/day
  - Multivitamin: daily
- Contraindications
  - Naltrexone: caution during pregnancy, acute hepatitis, hepatic failure
  - Acamprosate: caution if GFR <30

ALERT
Treat acute symptoms if in alcohol withdrawal; give thiamine 100 mg/day with first dose prior to glucose.

Second Line
Non–FDA-approved medications for long-term treatment of AUD (Initiate after resolution of acute withdrawal.)

- Topiramate (Topamax): 25 to 300 mg/day PO or divided BID; may enhance abstinence (off-label FDA use)
- Baclofen: initial dose of 5 mg TID; initial dose may be titrated to 10 mg TID with max dose of 60 mg/day in 3 divided doses; well tolerated in patients with cirrhosis; doses >60 mg/day provide no identifiable benefit.
- Selective serotonin reuptake inhibitors may be beneficial if comorbid depression exists.
- Varenicline may provide benefit to patients with AUD who also smoke.

ISSUES FOR REFERRAL
Addiction specialist, 12-step or long-term program, behavioral health professional

ADDITIONAL THERAPIES
Cognitive behavioral therapy, motivational interviewing, contingency management

 # ONGOING CARE

FOLLOW-UP RECOMMENDATIONS
Weekly follow up at the outset is often ideal with progressive spacing to 4-week follow up as condition stabilizes.

Patient Monitoring
- Outpatient detoxification: daily visits (not recommended for patients with heavy alcohol abuse)
- Early outpatient rehabilitation: weekly visits; detoxification alone is not sufficient.

PATIENT EDUCATION
- Substance Abuse and Mental Health Services Administration: (800) 662-HELP or https://www.samhsa.gov/find-help
- Alcoholics Anonymous: https://www.aa.org/
- Secular Organizations for Sobriety: https://www.sossobriety.org/

PROGNOSIS
- Chronic relapsing disease; mortality rate more than twice in general population, death 10 to 15 years earlier
- Abstinence benefits: survival, mental health, family, employment
- 12-step programs, cognitive behavior, and motivational therapies are often effective during 1st year following treatment.

ADDITIONAL READING
- Nadkarni A, Massazza A, Guda R, et al. Common strategies in empirically supported psychological interventions for alcohol use disorders: a meta-review. *Drug Alcohol Rev.* 2023;42(1):94–104.
- National Institute on Alcohol Abuse and Alcoholism. Helping patients who drink too much: a clinician's guide. https://www.niaaa.nih.gov/health-professionals-communities. Accessed October 12, 2023.
- National Institute on Alcohol Abuse and Alcoholism. Rethinking drinking: alcohol and your health. https://www.rethinkingdrinking.niaaa.nih.gov. Accessed October 12, 2023.
- Tucker JA, Chandler SD, Witkiewitz K. Epidemiology of recovery from alcohol use disorder. *Alcohol Res.* 2020;40(3):2.

CODES

ICD10
- F10.10 Alcohol abuse, uncomplicated
- F10.20 Alcohol dependence, uncomplicated
- F10.239 Alcohol dependence with withdrawal, unspecified

CLINICAL PEARLS
- CAGE questionnaire: >2 "yes" answers is 74–89% sensitive and 79–95% specific for AUD; less sensitive for white women, college students, elderly; not an appropriate tool for less severe forms of alcohol abuse
- Single question for unhealthy use screening: "How many times in the last year have you had X or more drinks in 1 day?" (X = 5 for men, 4 for women); 81.8% sensitive, 79% specific for AUDs
- NIAAA criteria for "at-risk" drinking: men >14 drinks a week or >4 per occasion; women: >7 drinks a week or >3 per occasion

ALCOHOL WITHDRAWAL

Ulunma Natalie Umesi, MD, MBA • Oleg Isakov, MD • Ambreka Benons, MD

BASICS

DESCRIPTION
Alcohol withdrawal syndrome (AWS) is a spectrum of symptoms resulting from abrupt cessation or reduction in alcohol intake, after a period of prolonged use. It ranges from minor symptoms, such as tremors and insomnia, to major complications, such as seizures and delirium tremors. Symptoms generally start within a few hours of the last drink and peak at 24 to 48 hours.

EPIDEMIOLOGY
Incidence
- In 2019, 14.5 million Americans met the diagnostic criteria for alcohol use disorder (AUD). Approximately 50% of those with AUD have experienced AWS in their lifetime.
- 32% of emergency room visits are alcohol related.

ETIOLOGY AND PATHOPHYSIOLOGY
- Consumption of alcohol stimulates γ-aminobutyric acid (GABA), resulting in decreased excitability with chronic ingestion; this repeated stimulation downregulates GABA inhibitory effects.
- Concurrently, alcohol ingestion inhibits glutamate on the central nervous system (CNS), with chronic alcohol use upregulation of excitatory *N*-methyl-D-aspartate glutamate receptors.
- When alcohol is abruptly stopped, the joint effect of a downregulated inhibitory system (GABA modulated) and upregulated excitatory system (glutamate modulated) results in brain hyperexcitability no longer suppressed by alcohol; clinically seen as AWS.

RISK FACTORS
- Long duration of heavy alcohol consumption
- Prior history of alcohol withdrawal episodes
- Elevated blood pressure on presentation, comorbid medical conditions, or surgical illness
- Physiological dependence on benzodiazepines (BZDs) or barbiturates

Geriatric Considerations
Elderly with AUD are more susceptible to withdrawal.

Pregnancy Considerations
Inpatient hospitalization for acute alcohol withdrawal management is recommended in pregnancy.

GENERAL PREVENTION
- The U.S. Preventive Services Task Force recommends universal screening all adults.
- The single screening question, "How many times in the past year have you had 5 or more (men) 4 or more (women) drinks in one day?" is the most sensitive and specific question for detecting unhealthy alcohol use.
- Brief, standard assessment screening tools include CAGE, AUDIT, or AUDIT-C to detect unhealthy alcohol use.

COMMONLY ASSOCIATED CONDITIONS
- General: weight loss and poor nutrition
- Renal: electrolyte abnormalities (hyponatremia, hypokalemia, hypomagnesemia, hypophosphatemia)
- GI: hepatitis, cirrhosis, esophageal varices, GI bleed, pancreatitis

- Heme: thrombocytopenia, macrocytic anemia
- Cardiovascular: hypertension, atrial fibrillation
- CNS: seizures, hallucinations, memory deficits, atrophy, Wernicke-Korsakoff syndrome
- Peripheral neuropathy
- Pulmonary: aspiration pneumonitis; increased risk of anaerobic infections
- Psychiatric: depression, posttraumatic stress disorder, bipolar disease, polysubstance use disorder
- Reproductive: sexual dysfunction and amenorrhea

DIAGNOSIS

- *Diagnostic and Statistical Manual of Mental Disorders*, 5th edition diagnostic criteria for AWS:
  – Two (or more) of the following present within a few hours after the cessation or reduction of heavy and prolonged alcohol ingestion:
    ○ Autonomic hyperactivity
    ○ Hand tremor
    ○ Insomnia
    ○ Psychomotor agitation
    ○ Anxiety
    ○ Nausea or vomiting
    ○ Generalized seizures
    ○ Transient visual, auditory, or tactile hallucinations or illusions
  – Signs or symptoms cause significant impairment in social, occupation or occupation areas.
  – Signs and symptoms are not secondary to an underlying medical or mental condition.
- Clinical manifestations
  – AWS can be divided into three cluster of symptoms.
  – Autonomic hyperactivity: onset a few hours of cessation and peak 24 to 48 hours
  – Neural excitation: Alcohol withdrawal–associated seizures are often brief and typically occur 12 to 48 hours after the last drink.
  – Alcohol withdrawal delirium: onset of 48 to 72 hours after cessation

HISTORY
- Duration and quantity of alcohol intake, time since last drink
- Prior symptoms of alcohol withdrawal or history of prior admissions for AUD
- Concurrent substance use
- Preexisting medical and psychiatric conditions, prior seizure activity
- Social history: living situation, social support, stressors, and triggers

PHYSICAL EXAM
Assess for conditions that are exacerbated by AWS.
- Cardiovascular: arrhythmias, heart failure, coronary artery disease
- GI: GI bleed, liver disease, pancreatitis
- Neuro: oculomotor dysfunction, gait ataxia, neuropathy
- Psych: orientation, memory (may be complicated by hepatic encephalopathy)
- General: hand tremor (6 to 8 cycles per second), infections

DIFFERENTIAL DIAGNOSIS
- Cocaine and amphetamines intoxication
- Opioid, marijuana, and other sedating substances withdrawal
- Anticholinergic drug toxicity
- Neuroleptic malignant syndrome
- Sepsis, CNS infection, or hemorrhage
- Mania, psychosis, anxiety, or panic disorder
- Thyroid crisis

DIAGNOSTIC TESTS & INTERPRETATION
Initial Tests (lab, imaging)
- Blood alcohol level, urine drug screen
- Complete blood count; comprehensive metabolic panel
- Lipase; amylase, GGT
- Head CT if change in mental status during withdrawal
- If first seizure, full neurologic workup, including EEG, brain imaging, and lumbar puncture

Follow-Up Tests & Special Considerations
- For patients reporting abnormal pain, elevate amylase or lipase; consider abdominal ultrasound or CT.
- Electrocardiogram is suggested for patients aged >50 years or for patients with history of cardiac problems.

Test Interpretation
Rate of metabolism of alcohol varies but is generally 10 to 15 mg/dL/hr; patients with prolonged alcohol use metabolize at a faster rate of 20 to 30 mg/dL/hr. Using these calculations can approximate when withdrawal symptoms may increase.
- Blood alcohol concentration (BAC): <100 grams of alcohol per 100 mL of blood (<100 mg%) loss of coordination and mood changes
- BAC: 100 to 199 neurologic impairment, slower reaction time or ataxia
- BAC: 200 to 299 obvious intoxication is present, unless person has marked tolerance.
- BAC: >300 can be associated with slurred speech, amnesia, coma, and death.

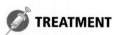

TREATMENT

GENERAL MEASURES
- Goals of therapy:
  – Provide a safe humane withdrawal from the drug(s) of dependence while protecting the individual's dignity.
  – Prepare for ongoing treatment of dependency.
- The Clinical Institute Withdrawal Assessment of Alcohol Scale, revised (CIWA-Ar) is useful for deciding medication dosing and frequency for AWS. Severity of symptoms are rated on a scale from 0 to 7, with 0 being without symptoms and 7 being the maximum score (except orientation and clouding of sensorium, scale 0 to 4) (1).
  – Nausea and vomiting
  – Tactile disturbances
  – Tremor
  – Auditory disturbances

– Paroxysmal sweats
– Visual disturbances
– Anxiety
– Headache or fullness in head
– Agitation
– Orientation and clouding of sensorium
- The maximum CIWA-Ar score achievable is 67.
  – Mild withdrawal: score ≤8: likely resolve without medication
  – Moderate withdrawal: 8 to 14: often require management with medication
  – Severe withdrawal: ≥15 are associated with the highest risk of seizures and development of DTs.
- Frequent reevaluation with CIWA-Ar score is crucial.

MEDICATION

First Line

- BZD monotherapy remains the treatment of choice for CIWA scores >10, based on the following considerations (1):
  – Agents with rapid onset control agitation more quickly (e.g., IV diazepam).
  – Long-acting BZDs (diazepam, chlordiazepoxide) are more effective at preventing breakthrough seizures and contribute to reduction in breakthrough or rebound symptoms.
  – Short-acting BZDs (lorazepam, oxazepam) are preferable when prolonged sedation is a concern (e.g., elderly patients or other serious concomitant medical illness) and preferable with severe hepatic impairment.
- Use symptom-triggered or fixed-schedule regimens.
  – Symptom-triggered regimens are preferred and associated with lower BZD amounts and reduce hospitalization length of stay.
  – Fixed-schedule regimens are appropriate if nursing staff do not have training for symptom-triggered regimens, in patient with severe coronary artery disease, or if history of past withdrawal seizures.
- Symptom-triggered regimen: Administer one of the following medications every 4 to 6 hours, with added doses PRN when CIWA-Ar ≥8. Assess the need for further medications 1 hour after each dose.
  – Chlordiazepoxide: 50 to 100 mg PO
  – Diazepam: 10 to 20 mg PO
  – Oxazepam: 30 to 60 mg PO
  – Lorazepam: 2 to 4 mg PO
- Fixed-schedule regimen: Administer one of the following medications every 6 hours:
  – Chlordiazepoxide: 50 mg PO for 4 doses and then 25 mg PO for 8 doses
  – Diazepam: 10 mg PO for 4 doses and then 5 mg PO for 8 doses
  – Lorazepam: 2 mg PO for 4 doses and then 1 mg PO for 8 doses
  – Important to monitor closely and provide additional BZDs if CIWA-Ar ≥8
- Folic acid: 1 mg/day
- Thiamine: 50 to 100 mg/day
  – Do not administer IV glucose before giving thiamine because this may precipitate Wernicke encephalopathy and Korsakoff psychosis.
- Correct electrolyte abnormalities/imbalance as they occur.

Second Line

- Gabapentin: reduces alcohol consumption, cravings, and may be effective for mild withdrawal
- β-Blockers (e.g., atenolol or propranolol) and α_2-agonists (e.g., clonidine) help to control hypertension and tachycardia but do not prevent severe symptoms such as DT or seizures; not used as monotherapy
- Carbamazepine: associated with reduced seizures and effective at mild withdrawal; should not be used as a monotherapy
- An antipsychotic (haloperidol) can be used for significant agitation and alcoholic hallucinosis but requires close observation because of lower seizure threshold.

ADDITIONAL THERAPIES

Peripheral neuropathy and cerebellar dysfunction merit physical therapy evaluation.

ADMISSION, INPATIENT, AND NURSING CONSIDERATIONS

Criteria for inpatient admission:

- CIWA-Ar score >15 or severe withdrawal
- Presence of ataxia, nystagmus, confusion
- Severe nausea or vomiting that prevents ingestion of medications
- Poor ability to follow up or no reliable social support
- Pregnancy
- History of seizure disorder, withdrawal seizures, or DTs
- Concurrent psychiatric illness, associated medical or surgical illness that requires treatment

 ONGOING CARE

FOLLOW-UP RECOMMENDATIONS

- Managing alcohol withdrawal is only a first step toward treating patient's underlying AUD; discharge arrangements should include outpatient substance use counseling, peer support groups, and/or residential treatment facility (2).
- Prescribe medication-assisted treatment:
  – Acamprosate (666 mg PO TID): glutamate and GABA modulator indicated to reduce cravings
  – Naltrexone (50 mg/day PO; 380 mg IM every 4 weeks): opiate receptor antagonist, reduce craving; initiate therapy after patient is opioid free for at least 7 days.
  – Disulfiram (250 mg/day PO): creates adverse reaction to alcohol by interfering with aldehyde dehydrogenase, blocking alcohol metabolism, leading to an accumulation of acetaldehyde

Patient Monitoring

Frequent follow-up to monitor for relapse

PATIENT EDUCATION

- Alcoholics Anonymous: https://www.aa.org/
- SMART Recovery (Self-Management and Recovery Training): https://www.smartrecovery.org/ (not spiritually based)
- National Institute on Alcohol Abuse and Alcoholism: https://www.niaaa.nih.gov/health-professionals-communities
- FamilyDoctor.Org: alcohol withdrawal syndrome (Spanish resources available)

PROGNOSIS

Mortality from severe withdrawal (DTs) is 1–5%.

REFERENCES

1. Rastegar DA, Fingerhood MI. *The American Society of Addiction Medicine Handbook of Addiction Medicine*. 2nd ed. New York, NY: Oxford University Press; 2020.
2. Tiglao SM, Meisenheimer ES, Oh RC. Alcohol withdrawal syndrome: outpatient management. *Am Fam Physician*. 2021;104(3):253–262.

 SEE ALSO

Substance Use Disorders

CODES

ICD10

- F10.239 Alcohol dependence with withdrawal, unspecified
- F10.230 Alcohol dependence with withdrawal, uncomplicated
- F10.231 Alcohol dependence with withdrawal delirium

CLINICAL PEARLS

- Any BZD dose should be patient specific, sufficient to achieve and maintain a "light somnolence" (e.g., sleeping but easily arousable) and should be tapered off carefully to prevent BZD withdrawal.
- Administer thiamine before patient receives glucose, so to not precipitate Wernicke encephalopathy.
- Avoid administering diazepam and lorazepam intramuscularly because of erratic absorption.
- Managing AWS is the first step toward treating AUD. Ensure patient has outpatient follow-up to continue treatment.

ALOPECIA

Melinda W. Ng, MD • Breanna Gawrys, DO

BASICS

Absence of hair from areas where it normally grows

DESCRIPTION
- Phases of the hair follicle cycle
  - Anagen phase (growth phase): 90% scalp hair follicles, lasts 2 to 6 years
  - Catagen phase (transition phase): regression of follicle, <1% follicles, lasts 3 weeks
  - Telogen phase (resting phase): club hair ready for shedding, lasts 2 to 3 months
- Scarring (cicatricial) alopecia
  - Inflammatory disorders leading to permanent follicle destruction and hair loss
  - Includes lymphocytic, neutrophilic, and mixed cicatricial alopecia
- Nonscarring (noncicatricial) alopecia
  - Mild or no inflammation, no destruction of follicle
  - Includes focal (alopecia areata [AA], traction alopecia), patterned (androgenic alopecia, female pattern hair loss), or diffuse hair loss (telogen effluvium, anagen effluvium)
- Structural hair disorders: Brittle hair from abnormal hair formation/external insult

EPIDEMIOLOGY
Prevalence
- Androgenic alopecia:
  - In males, 30% Caucasian by 30 years of age, 50% by 50 years of age, and 80% by 70 years of age
  - In females, 70% of women >65 years of age
- AA: 1/1,000 with lifetime risk 1–2%; men and women are affected equally.
- Scarring alopecia: rare, 3–7% of all hair disorder patients

ETIOLOGY AND PATHOPHYSIOLOGY
- Scarring (cicatricial) alopecia
  - Inflammatory disorders leading to permanent destruction of the follicle
  - Slick smooth scalp without follicles evident
  - Three subtypes based on inflammation: lymphocytic, neutrophilic, and mixed
  - Primary scarring includes discoid lupus, lichen planopilaris, frontal fibrosing alopecia, central centrifugal cicatricial alopecia, acne keloidalis nuchae, folliculitis decalvans, dissecting cellulitis of scalp, primary fibrosing, among others
  - Secondary scarring from infection, neoplasm, radiation, surgery, and other physical trauma, including tinea capitis
  - Central centrifugal cicatricial alopecia is the most common form of scarring hair loss in African American women; etiology unknown but possibly from hair care practices
- Nonscarring (noncicatricial) alopecia
  - Focal hair loss
    - AA: patchy hair loss, usually autoimmune, T cell–mediated inflammation resulting in premature transition to catagen and then telogen phases
      - May progress to alopecia totalis (entire scalp) or alopecia universalis (loss of all hair)
      - Nail disease frequently seen (10–20% of patients with AA)
      - High psychiatric comorbidity
    - Alopecia syphilitica: "moth-eaten" appearance, secondary syphilis

- Pressure-induced alopecia: hair loss from long periods of pressure on one area of scalp
- Temporal triangular alopecia: congenital patch of hair loss in temporal area
- Traction alopecia: due to physical stressor of tight braids, ponytails, hair weaves
- Patterned hair loss
  - Androgenic alopecia: hair transitions from terminal to vellus hairs
  - Male pattern hair loss: thinning in bitemporal or vertex areas (Hamilton-Norwood Scale, stages I to VII); results from increased androgen receptors, and increased 5-α reductase leads to increased testosterone conversion in follicle to dihydrotestosterone (DHT); this leads to decreased follicle size and vellus hair
  - Female pattern hair loss: thinning on frontal and vertex areas; unclear etiology, possible association with polycystic ovarian syndrome, adrenal hyperplasia, and pituitary hyperplasia
- Trichotillomania: intentional pulling of hair from scalp; presents various patterns
- Diffuse
  - Telogen effluvium: sudden shift of many follicles from anagen to telogen phase, resulting in decreased hair density but not bald areas
    - May follow major stressors, including childbirth, injury, illness; occurs 2 to 3 months after event
    - Can be chronic with ongoing illness (SLE, renal failure, IBS, HIV, thyroid/pituitary dysfunction)
    - Adding or changing medications (oral contraceptives, anticoagulants, anticonvulsants, SSRIs, retinoids, β-blockers, ACE inhibitors, colchicine, cholesterol-lowering medications, etc.)
    - Malnutrition from malabsorption, eating disorders; poor diet can contribute.
  - Anagen effluvium
    - Interruption of the anagen phase without transition to telogen phase; days to weeks after inciting event
    - Chemotherapy is the most common trigger. Radiation, anticancer drugs, and severe protein-calorie malnutrition can also trigger.
- Inherited and acquired structural hair disorders
  - Multiple inherited hair disorders including Menkes disease, monilethrix, and so forth; these result in the formation of abnormal hairs that are weakened.
  - May also result from chemical or heat damaging from hair processing treatments

Genetics
Family history of early patterned hair loss is common in androgenic alopecia, also in AA.

RISK FACTORS
- Genetic predisposition
- Chronic illness including autoimmune disease, infections, cancer
- Physiologic stress including pregnancy and childbirth
- Poor nutrition
- Medication, chemotherapy, radiation
- Hair chemical treatments, braids, weaves/extensions

GENERAL PREVENTION
Minimize risk factors if possible.

COMMONLY ASSOCIATED CONDITIONS
- See "Etiology and Pathophysiology."
- Vitiligo—4.1% patients with AA, may be the result of similar autoimmune pathways

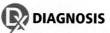

DIAGNOSIS

The diagnosis is clinical, made by history and examination.

HISTORY
- Description of hair loss problem: rate of loss, duration, distribution, degree of hair loss, hair care practices, and hair breakage versus hair shedding
- Associated symptoms: pruritus, pain, or burning
- Hair-care practices: use of prolonged heat, coloring, bleaching, chemical relaxers, and hairstyling (braids and ponytails)
- Medications
- Medical illness: recent illness/surgeries, pregnancy, thyroid disorder, iron deficiency, poisoning/exposures
- Psychological stress
- Dietary history and weight changes
- Family history of hair loss or autoimmune disorders

PHYSICAL EXAM
- Pattern of hair loss
  - Generalized, patterned, focal
  - Assess hair density, vellus versus terminal hairs, and broken hair.
- Scalp scaling, inflammation, papules, pustules
- Presence of follicular ostia to determine class of alopecia
- Hair pull test
  - Pinch 25 to 50 hairs between thumb and forefinger and exert slow, gentle traction while sliding fingers up.
    - Normal: 1 to 2 dislodge
    - Abnormal: ≥6 hairs dislodged
    - Broken hairs (structural disorder)
    - Broken-off hair at the borders patch that are easily removable (in AA)
- Hair loss at other sites, nail disorders, skin changes
- Clinical signs of thyroid disease, lupus, or other diseases
- Clinical signs of virilization: acne, hirsutism, acanthosis nigricans, truncal obesity

DIFFERENTIAL DIAGNOSIS
Search for type of alopecia and then for reversible causes.

DIAGNOSTIC TESTS & INTERPRETATION
Initial Tests (lab, imaging)
- No testing may be indicated depending on clinical appearance.
- For diffuse nonscarring alopecia, consider TSH, serum iron and ferritin, and CBC. Depending on clinical history and exam, consider LFT, BMP, zinc, RPR, ANA, and prolactin.
- If suspected hyperandrogenic state in female-pattern hair loss, consider free and/or total testosterone level and dehydroepiandrosterone sulfate.

Follow-Up Tests & Special Considerations
Consider visualization under dermatoscope; will see exclamation point hairs for AA

Diagnostic Procedures/Other
- Light hair-pull test: Pull on 25 to 50 hairs; ≥6 hairs dislodged is consistent with shedding (effluvium, AA).
- Direct microscopic exam of the hair shaft
  - Anagen hairs: elongated, distorted bulb with root sheath attached
  - Telogen hairs: rounded bulb, no root sheath
  - Exclamation point hairs: club-shaped root with thinner proximal shaft (AA)
  - Broken and distorted hairs may be associated with multiple hair dystrophies.
- Biopsy: scarring (cicatricial) alopecia or if diagnosis remains unknown
  - Recommend two 4-mm punch biopsies.
  - In scarring alopecia, take the biopsy at the edge of inflammation.
    - Lymphocytic inflammation with perifollicular fibrosis
  - In nonscarring alopecia, take the biopsy at an area with thinning hair but not complete hair loss.
    - Androgenic alopecia: ratio of terminal: vellus hair follicle <2:1, variable size of hair shafts, follicular miniaturization
    - Telogen effluvium: increased ratio of catagen: telogen, no change in number of hair follicles, no miniaturization of follicle
    - AA: increased ratio of catagen: telogen, no change in number of hair follicles, follicular miniaturization
- Ultraviolet light fluorescence and potassium hydroxide prep (to rule out tinea capitis)

 TREATMENT

GENERAL MEASURES
- Consider potential harms and benefits to the patient prior to treatment. Many will gain an improved quality of life.
- Treat underlying medical causes (e.g., thyroid disorder, syphilis).
- Traction alopecia: Change hair care practices; education.
- Trichotillomania: often requires psychological intervention to induce behavior change

MEDICATION
AA: Extent of hair loss and the patient are the most important factors influencing the approach to treatment. Spontaneous remission rates from 8% for extensive disease (>50% scalp involvement) to 68% (<25% scalp involvement) (1)
- <10 years old: topical 0.1% mometasone cream +/− topical 5% minoxidil foam/solution BID (1)[A]
- ≥10 years old:
  - <50% scalp involvement: topical corticosteroids +/− intralesional corticosteroids +/− topical 5% minoxidil (1)[C]
    - 0.05% clobetasol propionate foam
    - Triamcinolone acetonide 2.5 mg/mL
      - For scalp, inject 0.1 mL into deep dermal layer at 1.0 cm intervals with 1.5-inch, 30-G needle every 4 to 6 weeks; max of 40 mg per session
      - Adverse effects: itching, burning, acne, skin atrophy

- >50% scalp involvement; in addition to above treatments:
  - Topical immunotherapy: diphenylcyclopropenone (DPCP) or 3% squaric acid dibutyl ester (SADBE) (1)[C]
    - 2% DPCP for initial sensitization and then 0.001% DPCP applied with increased concentration weekly until patient develops desire effect; must be applied by physician or nurse weekly
    - Avoid topical immunotherapy in pregnant women due to teratogenic effects. Other side effects include severe eczema and cervical and occipital lymphadenopathy, among others.
  - JAK inhibitor +/− intralesional corticosteroid (2)[C]
    - Baricitinib 2 mg once daily; increase to 4 mg once daily if the response is not adequate after 3 months of treatment. Reduce back to 2 mg once daily once adequate response is achieved. If no response in 6 months, discontinue drug.
    - Must have baseline times prior to initiation: CBC, LFTs, lipid panel, viral hepatitis panel, latent TB, renal insufficiency, pregnancy
- **Androgenic alopecia**: Treatment must be continued indefinitely; can use in combination
- Minoxidil (Rogaine) (3)[A]: topical 2% solution 1 mL BID or 5% foam daily for women; topical 5% 1 mL BID solution or foam for men; adverse effects: skin irritation, hypertrichosis of face/hands, tachycardia; Category C in pregnancy
- Finasteride (Propecia) (3)[A]: oral 1 mg daily for men and women (off-label)
  - Adverse effects: loss of libido, gynecomastia, depression; caution in liver disease
  - Absolutely no use or contact during pregnancy, Category X, contraception required in female use
- Spironolactone (Aldactone) (3)[A]: 100 to 200 mg/day (off-label); adverse effects: dose-dependent, hyperkalemia, menstrual irregularity, fatigue; Category D in pregnancy
- Combination: Finasteride + minoxidil has superior efficacy to monotherapy.

SURGERY/OTHER PROCEDURES
- Wigs, hairpieces, extensions, scarfs, hats
- Surgical: graft transplantation, flap transplantation, or excision of the scarred area; used primarily in scarring alopecia
- Platelet-rich plasma: has been shown to restore dormant hair follicles and stimulate new hair growth

COMPLEMENTARY & ALTERNATIVE MEDICINE
- Many herbal medications are available; no clear evidence at this time
- Volumizing shampoos can help remaining hair look fuller.

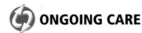 **ONGOING CARE**

DIET
If nutritional deficit is noted, supplementation may be necessary.

PATIENT EDUCATION
National Alopecia Areata Foundation: https://www.naaf.org/

PROGNOSIS
- *Cicatricial alopecia*: hair follicles permanently damaged; prognosis depends on type of alopecia and available treatments
- *AA*: often regrows within 1 year even without treatment; recurrence is common. 10% have severe, chronic form; poor prognosis is more likely with long duration, extensive hair loss, autoimmune disease, nail involvement, and young age.
- *Traction alopecia*: excellent prognosis with behavior modification
- *Androgenic alopecia*: Prognosis depends on response to treatment.
- *Telogen effluvium*: maximum shedding 3 months after the inciting event and recovery following correction of the cause; usually subsides in 3 to 6 months but takes 12 to 18 months for cosmetically significant regrowth; rarely, permanent hair loss, usually with long-term illness

REFERENCES
1. Strazzulla LC, Wang EHC, Avila L, et al. Alopecia areata: an appraisal of new treatment approaches and overview of current therapies. *J Am Acad Dermatol*. 2018;78(1):15–24.
2. King B, Ohyama M, Kwon O, et al; for BRAVE-AA Investigators. Two phase 3 trials of baricitinib for alopecia areata. *N Engl J Med*. 2022;386 (18):1687–1699.
3. Kanti V, Messenger A, Dobos G, et al. Evidence-based (S3) guideline for the treatment of androgenetic alopecia in women and in men— short version. *J Eur Acad Dermatol Venereol*. 2018;32(1):11–22.

 SEE ALSO

- Hyperthyroidism; Lichen Planus; Lupus Erythematosus, Systemic (SLE); Polycystic Ovarian Syndrome (PCOS); Syphilis; Tinea (Capitis, Corporis, Cruris)
- Algorithm: Alopecia

CODES

ICD10
- L65.9 Nonscarring hair loss, unspecified
- L64.9 Androgenic alopecia, unspecified
- L63.9 Alopecia areata, unspecified

CLINICAL PEARLS
- History and physical are necessary in determining type of alopecia for appropriate treatment.
- Treatment of underlying medical condition or removal of triggering medication will often resolve hair loss.
- Educating the patient about the nature of the condition and expectations is the key to care.
- Alopecia can affect the psychological condition of the patient, and it may be necessary to address this in any type of hair loss.

ALTITUDE ILLNESS

Andrew McBride, MD

BASICS

DESCRIPTION
- A spectrum of cerebral and pulmonary syndromes ranging from mild discomfort to fatal illness that occur on ascent to higher altitudes as a direct result of inadequate acclimatization
- Categories of altitude: high, 1,500 to 3,500 m; very high, 3,500 to 5,500 m; and extreme, 5,500 to 8,850 m (1).
- Altitude illness can affect anyone, including experienced and fit individuals. For most, it is an unpleasant (self-limited) syndrome that does not require medical intervention (2).
- Acute mountain sickness (AMS): symptoms associated with a physiologic response to a hypobaric, hypoxic environment; onset usually occurs within 6 to 12 hours after ascending >2,500 m. Neurologic symptoms predominate, ranging from mild/moderate headache and malaise to severe impairment.
- High-altitude pulmonary edema (HAPE): noncardiogenic pulmonary edema; typically after ≥2 days at altitudes >3,000 m, rare between 2,500 and 3,000 m
- High-altitude cerebral edema (HACE): a potentially fatal neurologic syndrome considered to be the end stage of AMS; onset after at least 2 days at altitudes >4,000 m
- System(s) affected: nervous/pulmonary
- Synonym(s): mountain sickness

Geriatric Considerations
- Risk does not increase with age.
- Age alone should not preclude travel to high altitude; allow extra time to acclimate.
- Worsening of preexisting medical problems referred to as altitude-exacerbated conditions

Pediatric Considerations
- Altitude illness seems to have the same incidence in children as in adults; diagnosis may be delayed in younger children.
- Any child who experiences behavioral symptoms after recent ascent should be presumed to have an altitude-related illness.

Pregnancy Considerations
- The risk during pregnancy is unknown.
- No evidence suggests that exposure to high altitudes (1,500 to 3,500 m) poses a risk to a normal pregnancy.

EPIDEMIOLOGY
Most epidemiologic studies are limited to relatively homogeneous male populations.

Incidence
- Incidence and severity increase with altitude and rate of ascent.
- AMS effects >25% of people who ascend to 3,500 m (11,500 ft) and >50% of those who ascend above 6,000 m (19,700 ft)
- HACE: in general population at 2,500 m (8,202 ft) is <0.01%, but increases to 1–2% in trekkers, climbers, and soldiers near a 4,000-m altitude
- HAPE: 0.01–0.1% in the general population at 2,500 m (8,202 ft) to 2–6% in trekkers and mountaineers at 4,000 m (13,123 ft)

ETIOLOGY AND PATHOPHYSIOLOGY
- Hypobaric hypoxia and hypoxemia are the pathophysiologic precursors to altitude illness.
- The conditions of AMS and HACE represent a pathophysiologic continuum (1).
- Symptoms of AMS may be the result of cerebral swelling, either through vasodilatation induced by hypoxia or through cerebral edema.
- Other mechanisms include impaired cerebral autoregulation, release of vasogenic mediators, and alteration of the blood–brain barrier.
- HAPE is a noncardiogenic pulmonary edema characterized by exaggerated pulmonary hypertension leading to vascular leakage through overperfusion, stress failure, or both.

Genetics
Genetic factors involved in predisposition to developing AMS are poorly understood.

RISK FACTORS
- Individuals with a prior history of AMS, HACE, or HAPE
- Failure to properly acclimatize at a lower altitude
- Ascent rate (sleeping elevation) >500 m/day (3)
- Trips to extreme altitude
- Increased duration at high altitude
- Higher altitude during sleep cycle
- Cardiac congenital abnormalities
- Younger age (<50 years) (1)

GENERAL PREVENTION
- The Richalet hypoxia sensitivity test (indicated for those who have never been at a high altitude and who face a journey to a high altitude without the possibility of acclimatization) helps predict altitude illness (positive predictive value of 79%) (1).
- General guidelines
  - Preacclimatization (exposure of hypoxia prior to ascent) protects against altitude illness.
  - Staged ascent (spending 6 to 7 days) at 2,200 to 3,000 m can also prevent altitude illness (3).
  - Ascending no >500 m/day.
  - Lower sleeping elevation: "Climb high and sleep low" for anyone going >3,500 m.
  - Avoid heavy exertion for the first 1 to 3 days at altitude.
  - Avoid respiratory depressants (alcohol and sedatives).
  - Preascent physical conditioning is not preventive.
- Pharmacologic prophylaxis
  - Acetazolamide, dexamethasone, and ibuprofen (see "Treatment")
  - For prevention of HAPE only (if at risk):
    - Consider nifedipine, dexamethasone, and tadalafil (see "Treatment").

DIAGNOSIS

HISTORY
- AMS:
  - Symptoms include headache, anorexia, irritability, marked fatigue, nausea, vomiting, dizziness, light-headedness, dyspnea with exertion, or insomnia.
  - Often, these symptoms resolve spontaneously after 18 to 36 hours without requiring descent (1).
  - Severity has been studied using the Lake Louise Questionnaire, which ranks four symptoms from 0 (none) to 3 (severe).
    - Headache, gastrointestinal symptoms, fatigue and/or weakness, and dizziness/light-headedness
    - AMS is considered diagnostic with a headache score of at least 1 point and a total score of at least 3 points.
    - Mild: 3 to 5 points; moderate: 6 to 9 points; severe: 10 to 12 points
    - Recommend calculating the score after 6 hours at altitude (to exclude travel and acute hypoxia symptoms) (1).
- HAPE symptoms: reduced exercise tolerance, exertional dyspnea, and cough followed by dyspnea at rest, cyanosis, and productive cough that may contain pink frothy sputum (3); begins within 1 to 3 days of reaching a new altitude, rarely occurring after 4 days; diagnose using the Lake Louise Questionnaire (1):
  - At least two of these symptoms: dyspnea, cough, asthenia, reduced physical performance, chest tightness, or congestion *plus*
  - At least two of these symptoms: crackles, whistles, tachypnea, or tachycardia
- HACE symptoms: altered mental status (irrational behavior, lethargy, obtundation, coma)
  - In less than 1% of cases, AMS can develop into HACE (1).

PHYSICAL EXAM
- HAPE
  - Lung crackles, whistles, or wheezing
  - Central cyanosis
  - Tachycardia
  - Tachypnea
- HACE
  - Abnormal mental status exam (behavioral change, lethargy, obtundation, coma)
  - Truncal ataxia
  - Papilledema, retinal hemorrhage, cranial nerve palsies
  - Focal neurologic deficits (rare)

DIFFERENTIAL DIAGNOSIS
- AMS/HACE
  - Dehydration
  - Ingestion of toxins, drugs, or alcohol
  - Subarachnoid hemorrhage, CNS mass, cerebrovascular accident
  - Migraine headache
  - Carbon monoxide exposure
  - CNS infection
  - Acute psychosis
- HAPE
  - Pneumonia, cardiogenic pulmonary edema
  - Spontaneous pneumothorax, pulmonary embolism
  - Asthma, bronchitis
  - Myocardial infarction
  - Hyperventilation syndrome
- Onset of symptoms >3 days at a given altitude, the absence of headache, or the lack of rapid response to oxygen or descent suggests an alternative diagnosis.

DIAGNOSTIC TESTS & INTERPRETATION
Initial Tests (lab, imaging)
- AMS: Laboratory studies are nonspecific and rarely required for diagnosis.
- HAPE: severe hypoxemia demonstrated with oximetry or blood gas analysis
  – Chest radiographs usually show patchy infiltrates. Clear lung fields suggest an alternate diagnosis.
- ECG may show sinus tachycardia or right-sided heart strain (2).

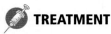 TREATMENT

GENERAL MEASURES
- Individuals without previous altitude exposure should adhere to acclimatization guidelines.
- Stop ascent, acclimatize at the same altitude, and/or descend if symptoms do not abate over 24 hours. Definitive treatment is to descend to a lower altitude. Dramatic improvement accompanies even modest reductions in altitude.
- Oxygen helps relieve symptoms. Give continuously by cannula or mask, and titrate to SaO$_2$ >90% (2).
- AMS and HACE
  – Acetazolamide reduces mild to moderate symptoms of AMS (see "Medication").
  – Dexamethasone may also be effective in treating moderate AMS (see "Medication").
- HACE
  – Acetazolamide may be used as prophylaxis (see "Medication").
  – Dexamethasone (see "Medication")
  – Immediate descent (3)[A]
  – Supplemental oxygen (highest flow available; maintain SaO$_2$ >90%) (3)[A]
  – Portable hyperbaric therapy if available and unable to descend (3)[B]
- HAPE
  – Supplemental oxygen (highest flow available; maintain SaO$_2$ >90%) (3)[A]
  – Minimize exertion and keep the patient warm.
  – Immediate descent or evacuation to a lower altitude (3)[A].
  – Portable hyperbaric therapy (2 to 15 psi using Gamow bag or Chamberlite) is an effective and practical alternative when descent is not possible (3)[C].
  – Nifedipine (see "Medication")

MEDICATION
First Line
- Oxygen: 2 to 15 L/min to maintain SaO$_2$ >90% until symptoms improve
- Acetazolamide: If patient has a history of problems at altitude and/or plans to ascend >500 m/day >2,500 m, consider therapy for primary prevention. Avoid in patients with a sulfonamide allergy.
  – Primary prevention of AMS: Adult dosing of 125 mg PO BID starting 24 hours before ascent and continued for 2 to 4 days at a stable altitude (3)[A]; pediatric dosing of 2.5 mg/kg (maximum of 125 mg) q12h (3)[C].
  – Treatment of AMS: 250 mg PO BID until symptoms resolve; pediatric dose: 2.5 mg/kg q12h (3)[C]

- Dexamethasone: may significantly reduce the incidence and severity of AMS. Adverse side effects are rare.
  – Prevention of AMS: 2 mg PO q6h or 4 mg PO q12h starting 1 day before ascent and discontinued cautiously after 2 days at maximum altitude; do not use for pediatric prevention (3)[A].
  – Prevention of HAPE: 8 mg PO q12h (3)[C]
  – Treatment of AMS: 4 mg PO/IV/IM q6h; pediatric dose: 0.15 mg/kg dose q6h (3)[B]
  – Treatment of HACE: 8 mg PO/IV/IM initially and then 4 mg q6h; pediatric dose: 0.15 mg/kg dose q6h (3)[B]
- Nifedipine (reduces pulmonary arterial pressure) (2)
  – Prevention of HAPE: 30 mg extended-release PO BID starting 1 day prior to ascent and continued for 2 days at maximum altitude (3)[B]
  – Treatment of HAPE: 30 mg extended-release PO q12h (likely unnecessary if oxygen is available) (3)[C]
- Tadalafil: Consider for the prevention of HAPE (2).
  – Prevention HAPE: 10 mg PO BID 1 day prior to ascent in HAPE-susceptible individual (3)[C]
  – Can be used for treatment of HAPE when descent is impossible or delayed, access to supplemental oxygen or portable hyperbaric therapy is impossible, and nifedipine is unavailable (3)[C]
- Adjunct therapy
  – Salmeterol
    ○ Possible treatment of HAPE (not well studied): 125 μg inhaled BID starting 1 day before ascent and continued for 2 days at maximum altitude
    ○ Not recommended for HAPE prevention (3)[B]
  – NSAIDs:
    ○ Aspirin: 325 mg PO q4h for a total of 3 doses
    ○ Ibuprofen: 600 mg PO q8h 3 times daily for 1 to 2 days for prophylaxis (3)[B]; can also be used to treat headache at high altitude
  – Antiemetics
    ○ Prochlorperazine: 10 mg PO/IM q6–8h
    ○ Promethazine: 25 to 50 mg PO/IM/PR q6h
- Other trialed therapies
  – Ginkgo biloba, inhaled budesonide, and acetaminophen should not be used for AMS prevention (3)[C]. Acetaminophen may be used to treat headache at high altitude.
  – Remote ischemic preconditioning (RIPC), as well as supplementation of antioxidants, dietary nitrites, leukotriene receptor blockers, phosphodiesterase inhibitors, salicylic acid, spironolactone, sumatriptan, or iron lack quality evidence supporting their use (3).
  – Coca-containing products have been used in the Andes but have not been well studied (3).
  – Furosemide: not recommended for prophylaxis; should not be used for treatment in HAPE (3)[C]

ADMISSION, INPATIENT, AND NURSING CONSIDERATIONS
Outpatient treatment for mild cases

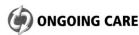 ONGOING CARE

FOLLOW-UP RECOMMENDATIONS
Patient Monitoring
- For mild cases, no follow-up is needed.
- For more severe cases, follow closely until symptoms subside.

PATIENT EDUCATION
Counsel patients about the risks of high-altitude travel and how to recognize symptoms of high-altitude illness.

PROGNOSIS
Most cases of mild to moderate AMS are self-limiting and do not require medical intervention. Patients may resume ascent once the symptoms subside. HAPE and HACE respond well to descent, evacuation, and/or pharmacologic treatment if identified early.

COMPLICATIONS
High-altitude retinal hemorrhage can cause visual changes but is usually asymptomatic.

REFERENCES
1. Savioli G, Ceresa IF, Gori G, et al. Pathophysiology and therapy of high-altitude sickness: practical approach in emergency and critical care. *J Clin Med*. 2022;11(14):3937.
2. Burtscher M, Hefti U, Hefti JP. High-altitude illnesses: old stories and new insights into the pathophysiology, treatment and prevention. *Sports Med Health Sci*. 2021;3(2):59–69.
3. Luks AM, Auerbach PS, Freer L, et al. Wilderness Medical Society clinical practice guidelines for the prevention and treatment of acute altitude illness: 2019 update. *Wilderness Environ Med*. 2019;30(4S):S3–S18.

ADDITIONAL READING
Ucrós S, Aparicio C, Castro-Rodriguez JA, et al. High altitude pulmonary edema in children: a systematic review. *Pediatr Pulmonol*. 2023;58(4):1059–1067.

 CODES

ICD10
- T70.20XA Unspecified effects of high altitude, initial encounter
- T70.20XD Unspecified effects of high altitude, subsequent encounter
- T70.20XS Unspecified effects of high altitude, sequela

CLINICAL PEARLS
- Slow ascent and timely descent are important to prevent and treat high-altitude illnesses.
- Lack of symptom resolution with appropriate descent suggests an alternative diagnosis.
- High-flow oxygen, followed by oxygen titrated to maintain SaO$_2$ >90%, is the first-line treatment for all patients with more than mild altitude illness.

ALZHEIMER DISEASE

John P. Barrett, MD, MPH, MS

BASICS

DESCRIPTION
- Alzheimer disease (AD) is a progressive, irreversible, degenerative neurologic disease that results in neuron death.
- AD represents 60–80% of dementia.
- AD is the sixth leading cause of death in the United States.
- People aged ≥65 years with new AD live 4 to 8 years on average.
- AD is underdiagnosed (~50%), and >50% with AD unaware of diagnosis
- Economic burden in 2023: ~$245 billion, projected $1.1 trillion by 2050 (1)
- Dementia should be distinguished from:
  - Age-related cognitive decline: lifelong changes in mental ability and memory; part of normal aging
  - Mild cognitive impairment (MCI): greater impairment than cognitive decline
    ○ MCI: People are generally able to live independently from a cognitive perspective.
    ○ MCI: affects 17–22% of those aged ≥65 years, with 32–38% developing dementia ≤5 years (1)
- AD diagnostic classification:
  - Preclinical AD: no cognitive symptoms, AD biomarkers present
  - MCI due to AD: very mild impairment
  - Dementia due to AD:
    ○ Mild: impairment in some activities
    ○ Moderate: impairment in many activities
    ○ Severe: impairment in most activities
- System(s) affected: nervous
- Synonym(s): presenile dementia; senile dementia of the Alzheimer type

EPIDEMIOLOGY
- Predominant age: >65 years
- Incidence: females = males
- Prevalence: females > males

Incidence
New cases of AD in the United States: 484,000/year
- 65 to 75 years: 2 new cases per 1,000 people
- 75 to 84 years: 11 new cases per 1,000 people
- ≥85 years: 37 new cases per 1,000 people

Prevalence
~6.7 million in the United States; ~50 million worldwide (1)
- 13.8 million in the United States by 2050
- 1 in 9 of those aged ≥65 years have AD dementia.
- 33.3% of those aged ≥85 years have AD dementia.
- ~200,000 in United States with early-onset AD (age <65 years)

ETIOLOGY AND PATHOPHYSIOLOGY
- Progressive, irreversible disease, worsening cognitive impairment
- β-Amyloid plaques outside of neurons and τ protein tangles inside of neurons, resulting in loss of connections and neuron death.
- Age, genetics, systemic diseases, and lifestyle behaviors may influence AD progression.

Genetics
- Autosomal dominant: <5% of AD, usually early onset (age <65 years)
- Familial inheritance AD (nonautosomal dominant): 15–25% of AD

RISK FACTORS
- Nonmodifiable risk factors: (1),(2),(3)
  - Age, gender (due to longer lifespan in women)
  - Family history, genetic mutations
  - APOE-e4 gene variant: e4 heterozygous 2- to 3-fold risk; e4 homozygous 8-fold risk
  - Racial and ethnic differences in AD exist.
- Cardiovascular disease–related risk factors:
  - Hypertension (HTN) (especially in midlife years); hyperlipidemia
  - Obesity, diabetes, and impaired glucose processing
  - Tobacco use, unhealthy diet, lack of physical activity
  - Cerebrovascular (stroke) risks and injury
- Other potentially modifiable risk factors:
  - Fewer years of formal education (<8th grade)
  - Lack of continuous brain activity—learning
  - Traumatic brain injuries: repetitive mild and moderate/severe
  - Lack of social engagement
  - Late-life depression
  - Poor quality and inadequate sleep
  - Hearing and vision deficits
  - High alcohol consumption
  - Environmental factors (e.g., air pollution)

GENERAL PREVENTION
- Cognitive decline and impairment are top concerns of people aged ≥50 years.
- HTN management, increased physical activity, and cognitive training may delay/prevent cognitive decline, MCI, and AD (3)[B].
- NSAIDs, estrogen, and vitamin E do not delay AD onset; insufficient evidence for statins and proton pump inhibitors (3)[B]
- Healthy lifestyles may prevent or delay AD (3)[B].
- Treat psychiatric conditions and avert delirium during hospitalizations.

COMMONLY ASSOCIATED CONDITIONS
- Down syndrome
- Depression

DIAGNOSIS

- "Welcome to Medicare" preventive visit and Medicare Annual Wellness Visit both require assessment of cognitive function.
- Diagnosis of dementia requires exclusion of delirium. Delineating specific dementia type requires a thorough H&P, cognitive and other diagnostic tests.
  - 2000 *DSM-IV-TR* criteria: progressive impairment in two or more areas of memory, executive function, attention, language, or visuospatial skills and significant interference in ability to function in work, home, or social interactions
  - 2013 *DSM-5* uses term "neurocognitive disorder" instead of dementia; impairment in one or more cognitive areas sufficient to disrupt independent living: complex attention, executive function, learning and memory, language, perceptual motor, social cognition

HISTORY
- Include informant: family member, caregiver, or friend
- Alzheimer's Association 10 signs:
  - Memory loss that disrupts daily life
  - Difficulty completing familiar tasks
  - Challenges in planning and problem-solving
  - New problems with words in speaking or writing
  - Trouble with visual images or spatial relationships
  - Changes in mood or personality
  - Misplacing things, losing ability to retrace steps
  - Decreased or poor judgment
  - Withdrawal from work or social activities
  - Confusion with time and place

PHYSICAL EXAM
- Exam to rule out other causes of dementia or delirium
- Noncognitive portions of physical exam often normal for age except in severe AD (2),(3)
- Neuro: speech, language, vision, hearing, gait, balance, reflexes, muscle strength and tone, tremor, abnormal movements (akathisia, bradykinesia/dyskinesia)
- Late stage: skin lesions, nutrition-hydration status
- Brief cognitive testing, such as: Mini-Cog, Montreal Cognitive Assessment (MoCA), Mini-Mental State Examination (MMSE)
- Assess depression: Patient Health Questionnaire-9, Geriatric Depression Scale (GDS).
- Functional assessment: instrumental activities of daily living (IADLs), Functional Activities Questionnaire (FAQ)

DIFFERENTIAL DIAGNOSIS
- Other dementias (most common):
  - Vascular (large and microvessel, mixed); mixed type (with AD)
  - Frontotemporal lobar degeneration; dementia with Lewy bodies
  - Parkinson disease; normal pressure hydrocephalus
  - Creutzfeldt-Jakob disease; Huntington disease; Wernicke-Korsakoff syndrome
- Metabolic: hyper-hypothyroid, vitamin-nutrient deficiency, uremia/renal, hepatic, hyponatremia
- Autoimmune: vasculitis, end-stage multiple sclerosis
- Infectious: HIV, syphilis, Lyme disease, varicella-zoster virus, prion
- Depression; brain tumor: primary or metastatic; subdural hematoma (usually acute presentation)
- Medications, drug-alcohol reactions/addiction

DIAGNOSTIC TESTS & INTERPRETATION
Neuropsychological testing for atypical symptoms, young age, unclear presentation, or need to determine independent decision making

Initial Tests (lab, imaging)
- To help rule out other causes of dementia (1),(2)
  - Complete blood count with differential; homocysteine level
  - Chemistry panel; thyroid function, syphilis testing, lipid panel, vitamin B_{12}
  - Special considerations: ESR, HIV, folate, C-reactive protein, HbA1c
- Imaging (biomarkers): Different professional standards exist; may help determine cause of dementia
  - Consider MRI (preferred) or computed tomography (CT) scan if MRI contraindicated.
    - Initial AD evaluation; recent or rapid decline, age <65 years, history of stroke, atypical presentation, concern for cancer, high bleeding risk
  - Single photon emission CT (SPECT) and positron emission tomography (PET): rarely indicated; *insufficient evidence to use alone*

Follow-Up Tests & Special Considerations
- Consider genetic testing with concern for autosomal dominant and familial AD.
- Cerebrospinal fluid biomarker testing not currently indicated

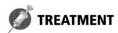 TREATMENT

GENERAL MEASURES
- Optimize treatment of risk factors and associated comorbid conditions (e.g., hearing).
- Advance care planning before individual loses ability for independent decisions
- Assess caregiver support and burnout.

ALERT
American Geriatrics Society recommends "Don't prescribe cholinesterase inhibitors (ChEIs) for dementia without periodic assessment for perceived cognitive benefits and adverse gastrointestinal effects" in its Choosing Wisely statement.

MEDICATION
First Line
- Acetylcholinesterase inhibitors (2)[A]
  - Best in mild to moderate disease; *may* be effective in Lewy body dementia
  - ChEIs equally effective; GI and other side effects, such as bradycardia/syncope
  - When used for at least 6 months, may provide mild benefit in cognition and behavior
  - Try different ChEI if no benefit.
  - Donepezil (Aricept): Start at 5 mg/day PO; may increase to 10 mg/day after 1 month and may increase to 23 mg/day after 3 months if needed
  - Orally disintegrating tablets; generic available
  - Caution with digoxin or β-blockers (Donepezil may prolong PR interval.)
  - Rivastigmine (Exelon): Start at 1.5 mg PO BID, increase by 1.5 mg BID q2wk; maintenance 6 to 12 mg/day total
  - Capsule, solution, or patch (reduced side effects)
  - Galantamine (Razadyne): Start at 4 mg BID for 4 weeks, increase by 4 mg BID every month; goal of 16 to 24 mg/day dose
  - Tablets, solution, extended-release (ER) capsule, and transdermal formulations

- Vitamin E —2,000 IU/day, mixed data, side effects exist (2)[B]
- Memantine, an *N*-methyl-D-aspartate (NMDA) receptor antagonist for moderate to severe AD
  - Monotherapy or in combination with acetylcholinesterase inhibitors (2)[A]
  - Memantine immediate release: 5 mg/day; titrate up to 10 mg BID, adding 5 mg/day qwk PRN.
  - Memantine ER: 7 mg/day up to 28 mg/day, adding 7 mg/day qwk PRN
- Aducanumab (Aduhelm): monoclonal antibody therapy targeting β-amyloid; limited benefit with side-effect concerns; recommend against routine use; aducanumab evaluation by physicians who specialize in AD (1)[C]
- Neuropsychiatric symptoms: assessment for delirium and reversible causes (sleep, hearing, environment); for moderate to severe symptoms—consider second-line care.

Second Line
- For moderate to severe depression: selective serotonin reuptake inhibitors (SSRIs) preferred
- Insomnia: Medications have little efficacy for sleep in AD (2)[A],(3)[A].
  - Avoid antihistamines in elderly.
  - Caution and use lowest dose possible: risperidone, trazodone, sleep aid (e.g., zolpidem)
- Moderate agitation, anxiety/restlessness: may consider low-dose risperidone or SSRIs (citalopram) (2)[B]
- Cautious use of low dose risperidone for severe psychosis
- Precautions
  - Avoid anticholinergic drugs when possible.
  - Benzodiazepines may produce paradoxical excitation or daytime drowsiness.
  - Triazolam (Halcion) can produce confusion, memory loss, and psychotic behavior.
  - Donepezil: caution with anticholinergics, sick sinus syndrome, and history of peptic ulcers

ISSUES FOR REFERRAL
Consider geriatric psychiatry referral for AD patients with behavioral symptoms requiring psychotropic medications.

ADDITIONAL THERAPIES
- Exercise to reduce restlessness; cognitive stimulation therapy
- Consider occupational, music, aroma, and pet therapy.

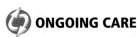 ONGOING CARE

FOLLOW-UP RECOMMENDATIONS
Patient Monitoring
- Medication reconciliation each visit, including OTCs
- Recommend: healthy lifestyle: exercise, nutrition, sleep, being social, and cognitive activity-stimulation
- Inform about unproven products advertised to improve brain health: some medications, nutritional supplements, and brain games.
- Frequently assess medication side effects and effectiveness (ChEIs/memantine).

- Late AD may require skilled care placement.
- Advance care planning is Medicare reimbursable.
- National Highway Traffic Safety Administration's safe driving assessment: https://www.nhtsa.gov/older-drivers/driving-safely-while-aging-gracefully

DIET
Consider trial of ketogenic diet; may improve cognition

PATIENT EDUCATION
- Alzheimer's Association: https://www.alz.org/
- Early advance care planning, such as advanced directives, financial planning, caregiver support

PROGNOSIS
Average survival from diagnosis is ages 4 to 8 years, and initial diagnosis is often delayed.

COMPLICATIONS
- Hostility, agitation, wandering, falls, "sundowning," depression, suicide
- Infections, inadequate nutrition/hydration, drug toxicity

REFERENCES
1. Alzheimer's Association. 2023 Alzheimer's disease facts and figures. *Alzheimers Dement*. 2023;19(4):1598–1695.
2. Atri A. The Alzheimer's disease clinical spectrum: diagnosis and management. *Med Clin North Am*. 2019;103(2):263–293.
3. Livingston G, Huntley J, Sommerlad A, et al. Dementia prevention, intervention, and care: 2020 report of the Lancet Commission. *Lancet*. 2020;396(10248):413–446.

ADDITIONAL READING
The Gerontological Society of America. *The GSA KAER Toolkit for Primary Care Teams*. Washington, DC: The Gerontological Society of America; 2020. https://www.geron.org/publications/kaer-toolkit. Accessed October 2, 2023.

 SEE ALSO

Delirium; Depression; Hypothyroidism, Adult; Substance Use Disorders

 CODES

ICD10
- G30 Alzheimer's disease
- G30.1 Alzheimer's disease with late onset
- G30.9 Alzheimer's disease, unspecified

CLINICAL PEARLS
- AD is very common, >33.3% in those aged >85 years, and greatly underdiagnosed.
- Imaging not needed for diagnosis for typical AD
- Early diagnosis allows advance care planning (e.g., advanced directives) and caregiver support.
- Atypical antipsychotic medications increase mortality.

AMENORRHEA

Michelle E. Duffelmeyer, MD • Susan McDiarmid, EdD, MS, PA-C

BASICS

DESCRIPTION
- Primary amenorrhea
  - No menses by age 13 years with absence of secondary sexual characteristics OR
  - No menses by age 15 years with normal secondary characteristics
- Secondary amenorrhea: cessation of menses for 3 months if previously normal menstrual cycles or 6 months if a history of irregular cycles
- System(s) affected: endocrine/metabolic; reproductive

Pregnancy Considerations
Pregnancy is by far the most common cause of secondary amenorrhea.

EPIDEMIOLOGY
Prevalence
- Primary amenorrhea: <1% of female population
- Secondary amenorrhea: 3–4% of female population
- No evidence for race and ethnicity affecting prevalence

ETIOLOGY AND PATHOPHYSIOLOGY
Absence of menses that can be temporary, intermittent, or permanent due to dysfunction of the hypothalamus, pituitary, uterus, ovaries, or vagina
- Primary amenorrhea
  - Gonadal dysgenesis (e.g., Turner syndrome [45,X]) or failure (e.g., autoimmune, idiopathic)
  - Anatomic abnormalities (e.g., müllerian agenesis, imperforate hymen, transverse vaginal septum)
  - Hypothalamic-pituitary abnormalities
    ○ Functional hypothalamic amenorrhea (abnormal GnRH secretion, stress, exercise, anorexia nervosa)
    ○ Physiological delay of puberty
    ○ Central lesions (tumors, hypophysitis, granulomas)
    ○ Pituitary dysfunction (hyperprolactinemia, abnormal follicle-stimulating hormone [FSH], luteinizing hormone [LH], or GnRH)
    ○ Thyroid dysfunction
  - Polycystic ovarian syndrome (PCOS)
  - Androgen insensitivity syndrome
  - Congenital adrenal hyperplasia
- Secondary amenorrhea
  - Pregnancy
  - Hypothalamic dysfunction (reduced GnRH secretion)
    ○ Functional hypothalamic amenorrhea (stress, anorexia nervosa, and/or excessive exercise)
    ○ Hypothalamic tumors
    ○ Severe systemic illness (e.g., diabetes mellitus type 1 or celiac disease)
  - Pituitary disease (e.g., hyperprolactinemia, Sheehan syndrome, Cushing syndrome)
  - Thyroid disease
  - PCOS
  - Ovarian disorders (e.g., primary ovarian insufficiency [due to chemotherapy, radiation, fragile X syndrome] or ovarian tumors)
  - Anatomic abnormalities (e.g., intrauterine adhesions [Asherman syndrome])
- Pathophysiology varies, depending on etiology.

Genetics
May occur with Turner syndrome or testicular feminization

RISK FACTORS
- Obesity
- Excessive exercise (commonly associated "female athlete triad")
- Eating disorders
- Malnutrition
- Stress (emotional or illness-induced)
- Family history of amenorrhea or early menopause
- Treatment with antipsychotic medications

GENERAL PREVENTION
Maintenance of proper body mass index (BMI) and healthy lifestyle with respect to food and exercise

COMMONLY ASSOCIATED CONDITIONS
- Primary ovarian insufficiency may be associated with autoimmune abnormalities (autoimmune thyroiditis, type 1 diabetes).
- PCOS is associated with insulin resistance and obesity.
- Decreased exposure to estrogen may increase risk for osteopenia or osteoporosis.

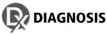

DIAGNOSIS

HISTORY
- Review of systems, including weight change, symptoms of pregnancy or menopause, virilizing changes, cyclic pelvic pain, galactorrhea, headaches, vision changes, fatigue, palpitations, polyuria/polydipsia
- Growth and pubertal development history, including age of breast development, pubertal growth spurt, and adrenarche (early sexual maturation)
- History of chronic illness, trauma, surgery, medications (including contraceptives), prior chemotherapy or radiation
- Obstetrical history
- Psychiatric history
- Social history, including diet and exercise history, drug abuse, sexual history, and stress
- Family history of delayed or absent puberty

PHYSICAL EXAM
- General appearance
- Vital signs, height, weight, growth percentile and BMI, hypotension, bradycardia, hypothermia (anorexia nervosa)
- HEENT exam: evidence of dental erosions, trauma to palate (bulimia), visual field defect, funduscopic changes, cranial nerve findings (prolactinoma), webbed neck (Turner syndrome), thyromegaly
- Skin exam: evidence of androgen excess (acne, hirsutism), acanthosis nigricans (PCOS), fine downy hair on body (anorexia nervosa), striae, vitiligo, easy bruisability
- Breast exam: state of development, evidence of galactorrhea (prolactinoma), shield chest (Turner syndrome)
- Pelvic exam: presence or absence of pubic hair (if sparse: androgen insensitivity or deficiency); clitoromegaly (androgen excess); distention or bulging of external vagina (imperforate hymen); thin, pale vaginal mucosa without rugae (estrogen deficiency and ovarian failure); presence of

cervical mucus (evidence for estrogen production); blind vaginal pouch (müllerian agenesis, androgen insensitivity syndrome); ovarian enlargement (tumors, PCOS)

DIAGNOSTIC TESTS & INTERPRETATION
Initial Tests (lab, imaging)
- Primary amenorrhea
  - Serum human chorionic gonadotropin (hCG), prolactin (PRL), thyroid-stimulating hormone (TSH), and FSH
  - If no or minor breast development:
    ○ Low FSH suggests primary hypothalamic-pituitary etiology or constitutional delay of puberty.
    ○ High FSH suggests gonadal failure, and karyotype analysis should be performed.
  - If normal breast development:
    ○ If low FSH, evaluate for anatomic abnormalities. If uterus is absent or abnormal, perform karyotype analysis, testosterone level, and dehydroepiandrosterone sulfate (DHEA-S).
- Secondary amenorrhea
  - Serum hCG, PRL, TSH, and FSH
    ○ PRL >50 ng/mL: suggests empty sella syndrome or pituitary adenoma; however, levels can transiently increase with stress. Repeat level and if elevated, perform MRI for evaluation.
    ○ PRL elevated but <50 ng/mL: Repeat fasting in the morning and before exercise.
    ○ If FSH high: Consider primary ovarian insufficiency or natural menopause.
  - To determine endogenous estrogen production, perform a progestin challenge (see "Treatment"): if withdrawal bleed, likely chronic anovulation (most commonly PCOS). If no withdrawal bleed, perform estrogen and progestin challenge (see "Treatment"):
    ○ If no bleed: Consider outflow tract obstruction or hypoestrogenism.
    ○ If bleed occurs: Check FSH/LH: elevated in premature ovarian failure; decreased in pituitary tumors, eating disorders, chronic illness
- If there is evidence for hyperandrogenism, measure total testosterone, DHEA-S, and 17-OH progesterone levels. Initiate evaluation for androgen-secreting tumor if testosterone >200 ng/dL.
- Imaging is not generally indicated as a first approach.
- US may show ovarian cysts (PCOS), presence or absence of uterus, and endometrial thickness (consider MRI if unable to tolerate US probe).

Follow-Up Tests & Special Considerations
- Women aged <30 years with ovarian failure (see below) should have karyotype analysis and be investigated for premutations of *FMR1* gene (fragile X syndrome) and for adrenal antibodies.
- If there is an absence of uterus or there is a foreshortened vagina, karyotype analysis should also be performed.
- Laparoscopy: diagnosis of streak ovaries (Turner syndrome) or polycystic ovaries
- Hysterosalpingogram: Rule out Asherman syndrome and other etiologies of outflow obstruction.

Diagnostic Procedures/Other
- If constitutional delay is suspected, obtain bone age.
- If hypothalamic amenorrhea from functional suppression is suspected, consider dual energy x-ray absorptiometry (DEXA) scan to assess bone loss (1).

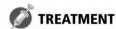

TREATMENT

GENERAL MEASURES
Identify and correct underlying pathology if possible.

MEDICATION
- Progesterone challenge and replacement: medroxyprogesterone (Provera): 10 mg/day for 10 days will result in withdrawal bleed within 7 days of last dose if hypothalamic–pituitary–gonadal axis is intact (i.e., amenorrhea is a consequence of anovulation and lack of progesterone), although experts disagree (2).
- Estrogen replacement: Cycling with a combination oral contraceptive (containing 35 or 50 μg of estrogen) or conjugated estrogen (Premarin) 0.625 mg for 25 days with progesterone added as above for the last 10 days will result in a withdrawal bleed if the uterus and lower genital tract are normal (hypothalamic-pituitary axis pathologic).
- Use of hormonal therapies will not correct the underlying problem. Other drugs might be required to treat specific conditions (e.g., dopamine agonist cabergoline or bromocriptine for hyperprolactinemia).
- Use of hormonal replacement therapy is not recommended for long-term management of amenorrhea in older women.
  - May be safe for symptom management in young women. Give to maintain secondary sex characteristics and to prevent osteoporosis in adolescents and young women (3)[A].
- Combination estrogen/progesterone contraceptives (oral contraceptive pills [OCPs], patch, ring) replace estrogen and prevent pregnancy.
  - Have a positive effect on bone mineral density in oligo-/amenorrheic women but not in functional hypothalamic amenorrhea (4)[A].
  - Can decrease hirsutism in PCOS
- Calcium supplementation: 1,500 mg/day if cause is hypoestrogenism
- Because PCOS is related to insulin resistance, metformin is used to correct metabolic abnormalities, improve ovulation, and restore normal menstrual patterns. Of note, treatment with metformin has shown an increase in clinical pregnancy rates but not in live birth rates (5)[A].
- Contraindications to estrogen administration
  - Pregnancy, thromboembolic disease, previous myocardial infarction or cerebrovascular accident, estrogen-dependent malignancy, severe hepatic impairment or disease
- Precautions
  - Patients with amenorrhea who desire pregnancy should not be given hormone replacement therapy but should receive treatment for infertility based on the specific cause.

ISSUES FOR REFERRAL
Many causes of amenorrhea require referral to specialists in OB/GYN, endocrine, surgery, and/or psychiatry.

SURGERY/OTHER PROCEDURES
- Hymenectomy for primary amenorrhea if due to imperforate hymen
- Lysis of adhesions in Asherman syndrome is often effective in restoring regular menses and fertility.
- If karyotype is XY, gonads must be removed due to increased risk of tumors.
- Patients with congenital short vagina can undergo surgery to create a functioning vagina.
- Treatment of prolactinomas may include surgical resection.

ONGOING CARE

FOLLOW-UP RECOMMENDATIONS
If excessive exercise is suspected, activity level should be reduced by 25–50%.

Patient Monitoring
- Depends on the cause and treatment chosen
- If hormonal replacement is used, discontinue after 6 months to assess spontaneous resumption of menses.

DIET
- Correct overweight or underweight by dietary management and behavior modification.
- If PCOS is the etiology, a weight-loss diet will help restore ovulation.

PATIENT EDUCATION
- Educate on the circumstances and complications of her condition and its underlying etiology.
- Specific educational resources are helpful.
- Discuss the expected duration of amenorrhea (temporary or permanent), its effect on fertility, and the long-term sequelae of untreated amenorrhea (e.g., osteoporosis, vaginal dryness).
- Appropriate contraceptive advice should be given because fertility returns before menses.
- Additional support may be needed if amenorrhea is associated with a reduction in, or loss of, fertility.

PROGNOSIS
Reflects the underlying cause. In functional hypothalamic amenorrhea, one study demonstrated 83% reversal rate in the presence of an obvious contributing factor.

COMPLICATIONS
- Estrogen-deficiency symptoms (e.g., hot flashes, vaginal dryness) and osteoporosis in prolonged hypoestrogenic amenorrhea
- Increased risk of endometrial cancer in patients whose amenorrhea is secondary to anovulation with estrogen excess (obesity, PCOS)
- Premature ovarian failure may increase cardiovascular risk.

REFERENCES
1. Gordon CM. Clinical practice. Functional hypothalamic amenorrhea. *N Engl J Med*. 2010;363(4):365–371.
2. Klein DA, Poth MA. Amenorrhea: an approach to diagnosis and management. *Am Fam Physician*. 2013;87(11):781–788.
3. Marjoribanks J, Farquhar C, Roberts H, et al. Long term hormone therapy for perimenopausal and postmenopausal women. *Cochrane Database Syst Rev*. 2012;(7):CD004143.
4. Liu SL, Lebrun CM. Effect of oral contraceptives and hormone replacement therapy on bone mineral density in premenopausal and perimenopausal women: a systematic review. *Br J Sports Med*. 2006;40(1):11–24.
5. Tang T, Lord JM, Norman RJ, et al. Insulin-sensitising drugs (metformin, rosiglitazone, pioglitazone, D-chiro-inositol) for women with polycystic ovary syndrome, oligo amenorrhoea and subfertility. *Cochrane Database Syst Rev*. 2012;(5):CD003053.

ADDITIONAL READING
- Practice Committee of American Society for Reproductive Medicine. Current evaluation of amenorrhea. *Fertil Steril*. 2008;90(Suppl 5):S219–S225.
- Santoro N. Update in hyper- and hypogonadotropic amenorrhea. *J Clin Endocrinol Metab*. 2011;96(11): 3281–3288.

 SEE ALSO

- Hyperthyroidism; Hypothyroidism, Adult; Osteoporosis and Osteopenia
- Algorithms: Amenorrhea, Primary (Absence of Menarche by Age 16 Years); Amenorrhea, Secondary; Delayed Puberty

CODES

ICD10
- N91.1 Secondary amenorrhea
- N91.2 Amenorrhea, unspecified
- N91.0 Primary amenorrhea

CLINICAL PEARLS
- First, evaluate whether amenorrhea is primary or secondary and exclude pregnancy. TSH and PRL are usual first blood tests.
- Progestin challenge may cause withdrawal bleed in women with intact hypothalamic–pituitary–gonadal axis.

ANAL FISSURE

Anne Walsh, MMSc, PA-C, DFAAPA • Lisa Hertz, MD

 BASICS

DESCRIPTION

Anal fissure (fissure in ano): longitudinal tear in the lining of the anal canal distal to the dentate line, most commonly at the posterior midline; characterized by a knifelike tearing sensation on defecation, often associated with bright red blood per rectum; this common benign anorectal condition is often confused with hemorrhoids; may be acute or chronic (>4 to 8 weeks in duration) and may be associated with the presence of hypertrophic papilla and sentinel pile (skin tag)

EPIDEMIOLOGY

- Affects all ages; common in infants 6 to 24 months; uncommon in older children: suspect abuse or trauma; elderly less common due to lower resting pressure in the anal canal
- Sex: male = female; women more likely to get anterior midline fissures (25%) versus men (8%)

Incidence

Exact incidence is unknown (1), as patients often treat with home remedies and do not seek medical care. However, one cohort study found the average lifetime risk in the United States to be 7.8%, equal to that of appendectomy (2).

Prevalence

- 80% of infants, usually self-limited
- 10–20% of adults, most of whom do not seek medical advice

ALERT

Secondary fissures:

- Lateral fissure: Rule out infectious disease.
- Atypical fissure: Rule out Crohn disease.

ETIOLOGY AND PATHOPHYSIOLOGY

High-resting pressure within the anal canal (usually as a result of constipation/straining) coupled with decreased perfusion of the posterior canal leads to ischemia of the anoderm, resulting in splitting of the anal mucosa during defecation and spasm of the exposed internal sphincter.

Genetics

None known

RISK FACTORS

- Constipation (25% of patients)
- Diarrhea (6% of patients)
- Passage of hard or large-caliber stool
- Low fiber diet
- High-resting pressure of internal anal sphincter (prolonged sitting, obesity)
- Trauma (sexual activity or abuse, foreign body, childbirth, mountain biking)
- Prior anal surgery with scarring/stenosis
- Inflammatory bowel disease (IBD) (Crohn disease)
- Infection (chlamydia, syphilis, herpes, tuberculosis)

GENERAL PREVENTION

All measures to prevent constipation; avoid straining and prolonged sitting on toilet.

COMMONLY ASSOCIATED CONDITIONS

Posterior midline location: constipation, irritable bowel syndrome (IBS); other/multiple locations: Crohn disease, tuberculosis, leukemia, and HIV

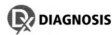 DIAGNOSIS

HISTORY

- Severe, sharp rectal pain, often with and following defecation but can be continuous; bright red blood on the stool or when wiping
- Occasionally, anal pruritus or perianal irritation

PHYSICAL EXAM

- Gentle spreading of the buttocks with close inspection of the anal verge will reveal a tender, smooth-edged tear in the anodermal tissue, typically posterior to midline, occasionally anterior to midline, and rarely eccentric to midline. Digital rectal exam and anoscopy are painful and can be deferred if inspection confirms the diagnosis.
- Minimal edema, erythema, or bleeding may be seen.
- Chronic fissures may demonstrate rolled edges, exposed muscle fibers, hypertrophic papillae at proximal end, and a sentinel pile (tag) at distal end.

DIFFERENTIAL DIAGNOSIS

- Thrombosed external hemorrhoid: swollen, painful mass at anal verge
- Perirectal abscess: tender, warm erythematous induration or fluctuance
- Perianal fistula: abnormal communication between rectum and perianal epithelium with feculent or purulent drainage
- Pruritus ani: shallow excoriations and erythema rather than true fissure

DIAGNOSTIC TESTS & INTERPRETATION

Diagnostic Procedures/Other

- Avoid anoscopy/sigmoidoscopy initially, unless necessary for differential diagnoses or chronic fissures.
- Due to pain, some patients may require exam under anesthesia in order to confirm the diagnosis.

 TREATMENT

The goal of treatment is to avoid repeated tearing of the anal mucosa with resultant spasm of the internal anal sphincter by decreasing the patient's high sphincter tone and addressing its underlying cause.

GENERAL MEASURES

- Wash the area gently with warm water, consume a high-fiber diet, increase fluid intake, add daily fiber supplement, avoid constipation, and maintain healthy weight.
- Medical therapy for chronic fissures is usually initiated in a stepwise manner when needed: topical nitrates, topical calcium channel blockers, botulinum toxin injections

MEDICATION

First Line

Acute fissures—50% will heal spontaneously with supportive measures (1)[C].

- Stool softeners (docusate) orally daily
- Osmotic laxatives (polyethylene glycol) orally daily as needed
- Fiber supplements (psyllium, methylcellulose, inulin) orally daily and increase fluid intake
- Topical analgesics (2% lidocaine gel or 3% cream) 2 to 3 times daily for pain control
- Topical lubricants/emollients (Balneol lotion, glycerin ointment, petroleum jelly) for comfort with defecation
- Topical hydrocortisone 1% cream short term for inflammation/pruritus
- Sitz baths (plain, warm-hot water soak of perineum for 10 to 20 minutes) 2 to 3 times daily after bowel movements

Second Line

Chronic fissures—will not heal without treatment, due to persistent internal sphincter spasm and ischemia:

- Chemical sphincterotomy—first-line treatment
  - Topical nitroglycerin 0.2–0.4% ointment applied BID; nitroglycerin (Rectiv) 0.4% ointment is available commercially: marginally but significantly better than placebo in healing (48.6% vs. 37%); late recurrence common (50%); reduces resting anal pressure through the release of nitric oxide and vasodilation; headache, hypotension, and dizziness are major side effects (20–30%).
  - Topical calcium channel blockers (nifedipine 0.2–0.3% gel, diltiazem 2% ointment), applied 2 to 4 times per day, relax the internal sphincter, thereby reducing the resting anal pressure; no better than nitrates for healing but fewer side effects (1)[C]; oral calcium channel blockers confer lower healing rates, more side effects, and equal rates of recurrence.
  - Botulinum toxin (Botox) 4 mL (20 units) injected into the internal sphincter muscle: no better than topical nitrates for healing but fewer side effects; inhibits the release of acetylcholine from nerve endings to inhibit muscle spasm (3)[C]

ISSUES FOR REFERRAL

- Persistent symptoms despite medical therapy, which is usually tried for 90 to 120 days prior to colorectal surgery referral. Select patients with chronic fissures may be referred directly for surgical therapy due to proven superior healing rates (1)[C].
- Late recurrence, which is common (50%) particularly if the underlying issue remains untreated (constipation, IBS)
- Secondary fissures (suspected infectious or IBD)

ADDITIONAL THERAPIES

Anococcygeal support (modified toilet seat) may offer an advantage in chronic fissures to avoid surgery.

SURGERY/OTHER PROCEDURES

- Surgery typically reserved for failure of medical therapy
- Lateral internal sphincterotomy (LIS) involves division of the internal sphincter muscle and is the surgical procedure of choice (95% healing rate) (1)[C].
  - Risk for fecal or flatus incontinence: up to 47% short term, up to 15% long term
  - Open and closed techniques have similar results and are equally acceptable (1)[C].
  - May be repeated for recurrent fissures with similar outcomes (1)[C]
  - Not typically performed on women of childbearing potential due to increased risk of fecal incontinence with or without subsequent obstetrical injury (1)
- A cutaneous flap to LIS in patients without anal hypertonia; less incontinence but lower healing rates (1)[C]
- Botulinum toxin injections also first-line treatment; less effective (60–80% healing) than surgery but fewer complications (3)[C]
  - Risk for fecal or flatus incontinence: 18% short term
  - May be repeated as needed with same efficacy; lower doses as effective as higher doses with lower rates of complications including incontinence and recurrence (4)[A]
  - Higher doses combined with fissurectomy may be as effective as surgical sphincterotomy.
- Controlled pneumatic balloon dilation may be used by gastroenterologists if surgical referral is not available; should not be used first line as benefits are not well documented; uncontrolled manual dilation is no longer recommended.

COMPLEMENTARY & ALTERNATIVE MEDICINE

Alternative therapies (hibiscus and other herbal extracts, clove and coconut oil, essential oils, homeopathic and ayurvedic medications, anal self-massage) need further study before they can be recommended as first-line treatment.

 ONGOING CARE

DIET

High fiber (>25 g/day; augment with daily fiber supplements); increase fluid intake; decrease caffeine.

PATIENT EDUCATION

- Avoid prolonged sitting or straining during bowel movements; drink plenty of fluids; avoid constipation; lose weight if obese.
- Avoid use of triple antibiotic ointment and long-term use of steroid creams to the anal area.
- Use a finger cot or glove when applying nitroglycerin ointment, and apply the first dose before bedtime to minimize side effects.
- Topical medications should be applied directly to anal verge; no need to insert rectally

PROGNOSIS

Most acute fissures heal within 6 weeks with conservative therapy. Medical therapy is less likely to be successful for chronic anal fissures (40% failure rate) but should remain as first-line treatment.

COMPLICATIONS

- Chronic fissure is a complication of nonhealing acute fissure.
- Recurrence is a common complication especially when underlying cause is not addressed.
- Abscess and fistula formation are less common complications.
- Fecal and flatus incontinence is primarily associated with surgery (5–47% postop), which may become permanent (up to 8% long term, primarily to flatus).

REFERENCES

1. Stewart DB Sr, Gaertner W, Glasgow S, et al. Clinical practice guideline for the management of anal fissures. *Dis Colon Rectum*. 2017;60(1):7–14.
2. Salati SA. Anal fissure—an extensive update. *Pol Przegl Chir*. 2021;93(4):46–56.
3. Wald A, Bharucha AE, Cosman BC, et al. ACG clinical guideline: management of benign anorectal disorders. *Am J Gastroenterol*. 2014;109(8):1141–1157.
4. Lin JX, Krishna S, Su'a B, et al. Optimal dosing of botulinum toxin for treatment of chronic anal fissure: a systematic review and meta-analysis. *Dis Colon Rectum*. 2016;59(9):886–894.

ADDITIONAL READING

- Fargo MV, Latimer KM. Evaluation and management of common anorectal conditions. *Am Fam Physician*. 2012;85(6):624–630.
- Sugerman DT. JAMA patient page. Anal fissure. *JAMA*. 2014;311(11):1171.

 CODES

ICD10

- K60.2 Anal fissure, unspecified
- K60.0 Acute anal fissure
- K60.1 Chronic anal fissure

CLINICAL PEARLS

- Avoid anoscopy or sigmoidoscopy initially, unless necessary for differential diagnoses (e.g., secondary fissures).
- Best chance to prevent recurrence is to treat the underlying cause (e.g., chronic constipation).
- No medical therapy approaches the cure with decreased recurrence rate of surgery for chronic fissure.

ANEMIA, CHRONIC DISEASE

Stephanie Algenio-Anciro, MD • Breanna Gawrys, DO

BASICS

DESCRIPTION
- Otherwise known as anemia of chronic inflammation
- During chronic systemic infection, inflammation, or malignancy, the production of proinflammatory mediators causes inhibition of erythropoiesis as well as the imbalance in iron homeostasis (1).
- A normocytic, normochromic, hypoproliferative anemia and classically has low serum iron levels, decreased total iron-binding capacity (TIBC), and elevated ferritin levels (1)
- Anemia is typically mild to moderate with hemoglobin (Hgb) rarely <8 g/dL.

EPIDEMIOLOGY
Prevalence
Anemia of chronic disease (ACD) is the second most common anemia after iron-deficiency anemia (IDA). Worldwide, estimates suggest up to 40% of all anemias can be considered from ACD or with ACD as a contributing factor, affecting >1 billion individuals.

ETIOLOGY AND PATHOPHYSIOLOGY
- Production of red blood cells is decreased as a result of functional iron deficiency.
- Three major pathways are involved as a result of proinflammatory cytokines: iron restriction, inflammatory suppression of erythropoietin (EPO), and decreased erythrocyte survival (2).
- Iron overload and the proinflammatory cytokines IL-1, IL-6, and BMP6 increase the production of the iron-regulating hormone hepcidin (1).
  - Hepcidin binds to ferroportin causing internalization and degradation, preventing efflux of iron from stores in macrophages and hepatocytes.
  - Hepcidin decreases iron absorption by duodenal enterocytes.
  - Newer studies show hepcidin may directly block iron export and limit erythropoiesis (2).
- EPO production and the response to EPO by erythroid bone marrow is suppressed by proinflammatory cytokines such as IL-1, TNF-α, and IFN-γ (1).
- Inflammatory cytokines may also cause erythrophagocytosis and oxidative damage, reducing RBC survival.
- It is unclear if the severity of anemia corresponds to the severity of disease.

RISK FACTORS
Hepatic disease, renal disease, infections, autoimmune causes (see "Commonly Associated Conditions")

GENERAL PREVENTION
Prevention of ACD involves timely identification and treatment of the underlying condition.

COMMONLY ASSOCIATED CONDITIONS
- Chronic inflammatory diseases
  - Rheumatoid arthritis (RA), systemic lupus erythematosus (SLE), sarcoidosis, temporal arteritis, inflammatory bowel disease (IBD)
- Cancer and hematologic malignancies

- Hepatic disease or failure
- Congestive heart failure or coronary artery disease
- Chronic kidney disease (CKD)
- Chronic obstructive lung disease
- Acute or chronic infections
  - Viral
    - HIV, HCV
  - Bacterial
    - Abscess, subacute bacterial endocarditis, tuberculosis, osteomyelitis
  - Fungal
  - Parasitic
- Malignancies
- Cytokine dysregulation (anemia of aging)
- Hypometabolic states
  - Protein malnutrition, thyroid disease, panhypopituitarism, diabetes mellitus, Addison disease

DIAGNOSIS

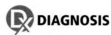

HISTORY
- ACD is often discovered incidentally on routine CBC with differential.
- ACD presents with the underlying causative infectious, inflammatory, or malignant process without any source of occult bleeding; often, patients will have mild and vague anemia symptoms, such as fatigue, light-headedness, and palpitations (1).
- Those with a cardiovascular condition may experience symptoms of angina, shortness of breath, and reduced exercise capacity with even a moderately low Hgb level (10 to 11 g/dL).

DIFFERENTIAL DIAGNOSIS
- IDA
- Anemia of CKD
- Drug-induced marrow suppression or hemolysis
- Endocrine disorders
- Thalassemia
- Sideroblastic anemia
- Dilutional anemia

DIAGNOSTIC TESTS & INTERPRETATION
Initial Tests (lab, imaging)
- Hgb (1)
  - Typically, <13 g/dL in males or <12 g/dL in females
  - An Hgb of <8 g/dL suggests a concurrent secondary cause for the anemia and warrants additional workup.
- MCV
  - Usually normal (80 to 100 fL), but microcytosis (<80 fL) may be present with concurrent iron deficiency or long-standing disease
- RBC morphology
  - Normocytic and normochromic
- Serum ferritin
  - Nonspecific acute phase reactant
  - Normal or slightly elevated (usually >100 μg/L) (2)
  - Serum ferritin levels <30 μg/L suggest coexisting iron deficiency.

- Serum iron levels
  - Low due to increased retention and decreased release from stores (<50)
- TIBC
  - Extremely low (<300)
- Absolute reticulocyte count
  - Inappropriately low (reticulocyte index, 20,000 to 25,000/mL) due to reduced erythropoiesis
- Serum B$_{12}$ and folate
  - Diminished due to decreased absorption or lacking in diet

	IDA	ACD	IDA + ACD
Iron	Low	Low	Low
Reticulocyte count	Low	Low	Low
Transferrin, TIBC	High	Low	Normal/high
Transferrin saturation	Low	Normal	Low
Ferritin	Low	Normal/high	Normal
sTfR* index	High	Low/normal	High
Hepcidin	Low	High	Normal
EPO	High	Normal/high	High
Inflammatory markers	Normal	High	High

*Soluble Transferrin Receptor

Diagnostic Procedures/Other
- Traditional gold standard: anemia, hypoferremia, and low TSAT combined with bone marrow biopsy with Prussian blue stainable iron (1)
  - Staining is qualitative and may not be accurate.
- Reticulocyte Hgb concentration <28 pg
- Measuring the hepcidin level via enzyme-linked immunosorbent assay can help differentiate IDA from ACD (3).
- Soluble transferrin receptor (sTfR) and the sTfR/log ferritin index
  - Ratio reflects erythropoiesis within bone marrow and differentiates among ACD, IDA, and ACD + IDA.
    - However, sTfR alone may have greater clinical value than the sTfR index because unlike ferritin, transferrin is not affected by chronic disease/inflammation.
      - Elevated sTfR indicates IDA, whereas normal values are more consistent with ACD.
- Functional test: supplemental iron increase H/H in IDA and little effect on ACD
- Although a known cause of anemia may be present, iron, B$_{12}$, and folate deficiencies should be ruled out.

TREATMENT

GENERAL MEASURES

- Primary management should focus on the underlying cause of ACD (1).
  - Treatment of the primary disease will generally restore Hgb back to baseline.
- In cases where primary treatment is not possible (e.g., terminal cancer, end-stage renal disease), additional treatment can be considered.
  - The two main forms of treatment are erythropoietin-stimulating agents (ESAs) and transfusions.
  - ACD is frequently responsive to ESAs (epoetin-α, darbepoetin) in pharmacologic doses.
  - Replete iron to maximize ESA effectiveness.
  - Transfusion should only be initiated in severe anemia or acute symptoms.
- Currently, no target Hgb exists, but treatment to Hgb >13 g/dL is associated with adverse outcomes (1).
- Coexisting B$_{12}$ or folate deficiency should be considered and corrected in severe cases of anemia.
  - Reduced dietary intake of nutrients is common among patients who are chronically ill.
  - Patients who regularly undergo hemodialysis will often lose these during treatment.

MEDICATION

- ESAs
  - Specifically approved for CKD, but there is evidence that they may also have applications in RA, IBD, HIV, and certain cancers (do not use in breast, cervical, head and neck, lymphoid, and non–small cell lung cancers); do not administer to patients with active malignancy not receiving curative therapy.
  - Indication for ESA therapy is an Hgb <10 g/dL.
  - ESAs have not been shown to improve symptoms or outcomes in mild anemia of CHF.
- Epoetin-α (1)
  - Indications
    - Hgb <10 g/dL
    - Fatigue or exertional intolerance
    - CKD (eGFR <60 mL/min)
    - Anemia due to IBD, RA, hepatitis C
    - Chemotherapy in patients with specific malignancies (palliative therapy)
  - Dosing and schedule
    - Lowest effective dose to maintain an Hgb level generally between 10 and 12 g/dL (1)
    - CKD associated: Start 50 to 100 U/kg SC/IV 3 times per week.
  - Patients with cancer who are undergoing chemotherapy: 150 U/kg SC 3 times per week or 40,000 U once a week
  - Adverse effects:
    - Increased risk of cardiovascular complications, mortality, and thromboembolism
    - Pure red cell aplasia (decrease in Hgb, low reticulocyte count, normal WBC and platelets)
    - Risk of tumor progression in certain cancer patients
- Darbepoetin-α
  - Long-acting, molecularly modified EPO preparation with a half-life 3 to 4 times longer than recombinant human EPO, reducing the frequency of injections to weekly or biweekly

  - Dosing and schedule
    - Administer SC/IV q1–2wk; hold if Hgb >12 g/dL; IV route is preferred in hemodialysis patients.
  - Adverse effects
    - Similar to EPO
- Epoetin-α or darbepoetin-α dose adjustments
  - Follow FDA-approved labeling.
  - Treatment beyond 6 to 8 weeks without appropriate rise of Hgb (>1 to 2 g/dL) is not recommended.

First Line

The best treatment for ACD is to address the underlying disease. Either epoetin-α or darbepoetin-α may be used as first-line treatment.

ADDITIONAL THERAPIES

- Iron supplementation (PO or IV)
  - Indicated in combined ACD and IDA
  - Forms
    - Oral: ferrous sulfate; poorly tolerated (GI side effects); incomplete absorption (due to hepcidin)
    - Intravenous: ferric gluconate, iron sucrose, iron dextran (potential allergic and anaphylactoid reactions), ferumoxytol
  - Adverse effects: may stimulate hepcidin production and exacerbate iron restriction
  - Benefits: relatively safe, inexpensive, may decrease ESA requirements (DRIVE study)
- Transfusions
  - 1 to 2 U packed red blood cells (1)
  - Indications
    - Life-threatening/severe anemia: A "restrictive threshold" of Hgb 7 to 8 g/dL to guide transfusion in asymptomatic patients should be used.
    - Patients with underlying cardiac or pulmonary disease, active ACS, elderly patients, or patients with acute bleeding or hemorrhagic shock may require transfusion at Hgb of higher threshold (>10 g/dL).
    - Symptomatic anemia (chest pain, SOB, reduced exercise capacity) and/or ECG changes
    - Lack of response to medical therapy
  - Possible adverse effects: infection (HIV, hepatitis), volume overload, transfusion reaction
  - Specific benefits: rapid correction of anemia
  - When an infection occurs during EPO therapy, it is best to cease EPO therapy and rely on transfusion therapy instead until the infection is properly treated.
- Future directions (1)
  - Hepcidin-antagonizing strategies
  - Anti-BMP, anti-IL-6 antibodies
  - Ferroportin stabilizers
  - Vitamin D (lowers hepcidin)
  - Heparin (impairs hepcidin transcription)

ONGOING CARE

FOLLOW-UP RECOMMENDATIONS

Patient Monitoring

- Hgb should not be increased >12 g/dL because normalization of Hgb has been associated with higher mortality.
- Baseline and periodic monitoring of transferrin saturation and ferritin levels every 3 months may be of value.

DIET

Many chronic conditions associated with ACD are impacted by diet. A well-balanced diet rich in fruits, vegetables, and legumes, including iron-rich foods, may be beneficial in treatment.

PATIENT EDUCATION

Patients receiving medical therapy should be advised about the following possible risks:

- Mortality, cardiovascular complications, thromboembolism, progression of cancer

COMPLICATIONS

- Adverse effects of ACD:
  - Mortality; cardiovascular complications; symptoms affecting daily life
- Adverse effects of ESAs:
  - Heightened risk of mortality and/or cardiovascular complications in CKD patients
  - Heightened risk of mortality and/or tumor progression in cancer patients
  - Elevated risk of thromboembolism

REFERENCES

1. Gangat N, Wolanskyj AP. Anemia of chronic disease. *Semin Hematol*. 2013;50(3):232–238.
2. Weiss G, Ganz T, Goodnough LT. Anemia of inflammation. *Blood*. 2019;133(1):40–50.
3. Karlsson T. Evaluation of a competitive hepcidin ELISA assay in the differential diagnosis of iron deficiency anaemia with concurrent inflammation and anaemia of inflammation in elderly patients. *J Inflamm (Lond)*. 2017;14:21.

ADDITIONAL READING

Besarab A, Bolton WK, Browne JK, et al. The effects of normal as compared with low hematocrit values in patients with cardiac disease who are receiving hemodialysis and epoetin. *N Engl J Med*. 1998;339(9):584–590.

SEE ALSO

Anemia, Iron Deficiency

CODES

ICD10

- D63.1 Anemia in chronic kidney disease
- D63.8 Anemia in other chronic diseases classified elsewhere

CLINICAL PEARLS

- ACD is the second most common anemia seen clinically.
- One of the most common diagnostic problems is making the distinction between ACD, IDA, and combined ACD + IDA.
  - Iron level is usually nondiagnostic.
  - Use markers such as transferrin/TIBC, TSAT, sTfR, sTfR index, hepcidin, and ferritin to distinguish.
- Hgb should be kept in low to normal range; do not replete beyond 12 g/dL.

ANEMIA, IRON DEFICIENCY
Deborah R. Erlich, MD, MmedEd, FAAFP

 BASICS

DESCRIPTION
- Low serum iron associated with low hemoglobin (Hgb) or microcytic, hypochromic red blood cells (RBCs)
- Because normal Hgb varies with age and sex, anemia is defined as Hgb level 2 standard deviations below normal for age and sex (1).
- Onset acute (rapid blood loss) or chronic (slow blood loss, deficient iron intake, or poor absorption)
- Both low Hgb per RBC and fewer RBC in total lead to blood oxygen deficiency, which can have serious systemic consequences
- System(s) affected: hematologic, lymphatic, immunologic, cardiac, and gastrointestinal (GI) systems

Geriatric Considerations
- Iron deficiency anemia (IDA) is associated with increased hospitalization, morbidity, and mortality in older adults.
- Older patients with suspected IDA should undergo endoscopy to evaluate for occult GI malignancy.

Pediatric Considerations
- Risks for IDA in children include low birth weight, history of prematurity, lead exposure, low-income status, immigrant status, and drinking cow's milk before 12 months of age.
- The U.S. Preventive Services Task Force (USPSTF) did not find sufficient evidence for screening low-risk infants; the Centers for Disease Control (CDC) recommends screening high-risk infants at 6 to 12 months of age, and the American Academy of Pediatrics (AAP) recommends universal screening at 12 months (1).
- Should screening be done, include both Hgb and ferritin.

Pregnancy Considerations
- The USPSTF did not find sufficient evidence for screening pregnant women for IDA; the CDC recommends screening women for anemia at the first prenatal visit and giving low-dose iron to all pregnant women, whereas the American College of Obstetricians and Gynecologists (ACOG) recommends screening all pregnant women for IDA and treating those with IDA.
- Iron supplements are recommended during pregnancy to improve maternal hematologic indexes, although significant clinical outcomes have not been proven (2)[A].

EPIDEMIOLOGY
- Iron deficiency is the most common nutritional deficiency in the world, and IDA is the most common cause of anemia (50%).
- Predominant age: all ages but especially toddlers and menstruating and pregnant women
- Predominant sex: female
- Common in developing and developed countries

Incidence
- Adults: men 2%, women 15–20% annually
- Infants and toddlers: 3–5% annually
- Pregnant patients: may be as high as 20% (1)

Prevalence
2 billion people worldwide
- Infants and children aged <12 years: 4–7%
- Men: 2–5%
- Menstruating women: 30%

ETIOLOGY AND PATHOPHYSIOLOGY
Depletion of iron stores leads to decrease in both reticulocyte count and production of Hgb. Causes:
- Blood loss (menses, GI bleeding, trauma)
- Poor iron intake
- Poor iron absorption (e.g., atrophic gastritis, postgastrectomy, celiac disease)
- Increased demand for iron (e.g., infancy, adolescence, pregnancy, breastfeeding)

RISK FACTORS
- Premenopausal woman
- Frequent blood donor
- Pregnancy/lactation, young maternal age
- Strict vegan diet
- Use of NSAIDs
- Hospitalized with frequent blood draws
- Living in or visiting countries with endemic hookworm infection

GENERAL PREVENTION
- Consider screening asymptomatic pregnant women and high-risk children at 1 year of age (guidelines vary) (1)[C].
- Supplementation in asymptomatic children aged 6 to 12 months if at risk for IDA (e.g., malnutrition, abuse) (1),(2)
- Iron- and vitamin C–rich diet for menstruating women
- Iron 30 mg/day for asymptomatic pregnant women (2)

COMMONLY ASSOCIATED CONDITIONS
- GI tract malignancy, peptic ulcer disease (PUD), *Helicobacter pylori* infection, irritable bowel disease
- Hookworm or other parasitic infestations
- Hyper metrorrhagia
- Pregnancy
- Obesity treated with gastric bypass surgery
- Malnutrition
- Medications such as NSAIDs or antacids

ⅅℝ DIAGNOSIS

HISTORY
Asymptomatic in most cases; symptoms may occur in severe anemia:
- Weakness, fatigue, malaise, headaches, and/or inability to concentrate
- Exertional dyspnea
- Angina with coronary artery disease
- Melena
- Pica (ice chewing)

PHYSICAL EXAM
- Pallor (skin, conjunctivae, sublingual)
- Tachycardia, tachypnea
- Cool extremities
- Brittle nails/hair
- Signs of heart failure

DIFFERENTIAL DIAGNOSIS
- GI bleeding (e.g., gastritis, PUD, carcinoma, varices, celiac disease)
- Chronic intravascular hemolysis (e.g., paroxysmal nocturnal hemoglobinuria, malfunctioning prosthetic valve)
- Defective iron usage (e.g., thalassemia trait, sideroblastosis, G6PD deficiency)
- Defective iron reutilization (e.g., infection, inflammation, cancer, hypothyroid, chronic diseases)
- Hypoproliferation (e.g., decreased erythropoietin from hypothyroidism, renal failure)
- Other anemias such as anemia of chronic disease, thalassemia, lead poisoning

DIAGNOSTIC TESTS & INTERPRETATION
Initial Tests (lab, imaging)
- Obtain: Hgb, HCT, ferritin, serum iron, total iron binding capacity (TIBC)
- Hgb (to define anemia):
  - <13 g in men and <12 g in women
  - Hgb 2 standard deviations below normal for age and sex (1)
  - Patients with comorbidities (e.g., chronic hypoxemia, smokers, high altitudes) may be anemic at higher Hgb levels.
- Mean corpuscular volume (MCV): <80 Fl
  - MCV may be low normal in mild anemia or hidden by large cells (reticulocytes, macrocytes).
- Ferritin is most sensitive and specific for diagnosing iron deficiency as cause of anemia:
  - <15 μg/L diagnoses IDA (<30 μg/L likely) (1).
  - >100 μg/L rules out iron deficiency.
- Iron studies:
  - Decreased: ferritin, serum iron, transferrin saturation (TF = [serum iron] $\times$ 100 / TIBC)
  - Increased: TIBC, transferrin
- Red cell distribution width (RDW) increases with a mixed population of cells (e.g., mixed IDA and vitamin B_{12} deficiency).
- CBC with differential, peripheral smear, reticulocyte count, and index
  - Peripheral smear usually shows hypochromia and microcytosis but may be normal, and reticulocyte production index is low (1).
- When comorbidity is suspected:
  - Consider testing for G6PD deficiency.
  - Evaluate for thalassemia.
    - Very low MCV <80, elevated Hgb A2 or Hgb F, family history, and especially high or high normal RBC count
    - Microcytosis with ovalocytosis and unresponsive to iron suggests the thalassemia trait.
- Celiac disease: IgA antiendomysial antibodies (IgA anti-EmA) and/or IgA antitissue transglutaminase (IgA anti-TTG)
- TSH for hypothyroidism
- An empiric trial of iron at 3 mg/kg/day may help diagnose decreased iron stores in children; reticulocytes become elevated in 7 to 10 days or Hgb increases >1 g/dL weekly, indicating iron deficiency.

- Drugs that may alter lab results:
  - Iron supplements or multivitamin–mineral preparations that contain iron
- Disorders that may alter lab results:
  - Elevated ferritin: acute inflammation, liver disease, Hodgkin disease, acute leukemia, solid tumors, fever, renal dialysis
  - Elevated Hgb: smoking, chronic hypoxemia, high altitude

Diagnostic Procedures/Other
- Stool guaiac (low sensitivity, so if negative, consider further evaluation)
- Stool for ova and parasites if at risk
- Colonoscopy and endoscopy to evaluate for bleeding sites and colorectal and gastric carcinoma for:
  - Premenopausal women with negative GYN workup and/or lack of response to iron
  - Men and postmenopausal women (1)[C]
- Bone marrow aspiration rarely performed

 TREATMENT

GENERAL MEASURES
- Search for underlying cause and correct it.
- Avoid transfusions, except in rare cases.

MEDICATION
- Elemental iron 100 to 200 mg/day for adults (whether pregnant or not) (2)
- Elemental iron 3 to 6 mg/kg/day for children
- Ferrous sulfate 325 mg TID, ferrous gluconate 300 mg 1 to 3 tablets BID–TID or ferrous fumarate 324 mg 1 tablet BID on an empty stomach 1 hour before meals (1)[C]
- Concomitant vitamin C enhances absorption.
- Medications that reduce gastric acid secretion, such as proton pump inhibitors and H_2 antagonists, reduce iron absorption (1).
- Special oral iron formulations (e.g., enteric-coated iron) are expensive and reduce symptoms only to the degree that they reduce the delivery of iron.
- IV iron is indicated for patients who cannot tolerate oral replacement (e.g., pregnant people or patients with GI disorders) or for those who insufficiently respond to oral replacement. Other indications for IV iron: Hgb <6 g/dL, bariatric surgery status, heavy uterine bleeding, malabsorption, inflammatory bowel disease, ongoing/severe losses.
- Outside of the United States, IV iron is becoming first line ahead of oral iron for its superiority in efficacy and toxicity.
- IV iron formulations available in the United States:
  - Low-molecular-weight iron dextran 1,000 mg over 1 hour
  - Ferumoxytol 510 mg over 3 minutes
  - Ferric carboxymaltose 750 mg over 15 minutes
- Liquid iron preparations (used for children) can also be used in adults when tablets are not absorbed or well tolerated.

- Formula to determine elemental iron needed: elemental iron (mg) = dose (mL) = 0.0442 (desired Hgb [g/dL] − current Hgb [g/dL]) × lean body weight (LBW in kg) + (0.26 × LBW)
  - For males: LBW = 50 kg + 2.3 kg for each inch of height >5 feet
  - For females: LBW = 45.5 kg + 2.3 kg for each inch of height >5 feet
  - Normal Hgb (males and females)
    - >15 kg (33 lb) . . . 14.8 g/dL
    - <15 kg (33 lb) . . . 12 g/dL
- Relative contraindications for oral iron: tetracycline, allopurinol, antacids, penicillamine, fluoroquinolones, vitamin E
- Precautions
  - Iron may cause dark stools and constipation. Consider a stool softener.
  - Iron overdose is highly toxic; absorption is limited to 1 to 2 mg daily; keep tablets and liquids out of reach of children.
- Blood transfusion for severe acute blood loss or severely symptomatic patients (e.g., demand ischemia due to anemia). Hgb threshold varies by risk factors and clinical scenario. Pregnant women with Hgb <6 should be transfused (1)[C].

ISSUES FOR REFERRAL
- Men and postmenopausal women with IDA (Test for colon cancer.)
- Pregnant women with Hgb level <9 g/dL
- Nonpregnant adults with Hgb <6 g/dL
- Failure to respond to a 4- to 6-week trial of oral iron

 ONGOING CARE

FOLLOW-UP RECOMMENDATIONS
Patient Monitoring
- Monitor patients every 3 months after Hgb normalizes for a year and then yearly (1)[C].
- Hgb increases 1 g/dL every 3 to 4 weeks.
- Iron stores may take up to 4 weeks to correct after Hgb normalizes.

DIET
- Iron-rich foods include red meat, poultry, fish, and eggs (all heme iron sources, best absorbed); and lentils, beans, dark green vegetables, raisins, tofu, and iron-fortified breads/cereals (non-heme iron sources, less well absorbed).
- Foods and beverages containing ascorbic acid (vitamin C) enhance iron absorption when taken simultaneously, such as citrus, tomatoes, dark green leafy vegetables, and berries.
- Avoid milk or dairy products within 2 hours of iron tablet ingestion.
- Limit milk to 16 oz/day (adults).
- Limit tea, coffee, and caffeinated beverages.
- Increase fluid and dietary fiber to decrease likelihood of constipation.
- Limit foods with high levels of chemicals (phytates and polyphenols).

PATIENT EDUCATION
- https://familydoctor.org/condition/anemia/
- https://patient.info/pdf/4392.pdf

PROGNOSIS
- IDA can be resolved with iron therapy if the underlying cause is treated.
- Treat coexisting subclinical hypothyroidism. Failure to treat hypothyroidism results in poor response to iron therapy.

COMPLICATIONS
- Ischemic events or heart failure, especially in elderly
- Poor growth, failure to thrive, motor and cognitive developmental delay in children

REFERENCES

1. Short MW, Domagalski JE. Iron deficiency anemia: evaluation and management. *Am Fam Physician*. 2013;87(2):98–104.
2. McDonagh M, Cantor A, Bougatsos C, et al. *Routine Iron Supplementation and Screening for Iron Deficiency Anemia in Pregnant Women: A Systematic Review to Update the U.S. Preventive Services Task Force Recommendation. Evidence Syntheses No. 123*. Rockville, MD: Agency for Healthcare Research and Quality; 2015.

ADDITIONAL READING

National Institutes of Health Office of Dietary Supplements. Iron: fact sheet for health professionals. https://ods.od.nih.gov/factsheets/Iron -HealthProfessional/. Accessed September 21, 2022.

SEE ALSO

Algorithm: Anemia

CODES

ICD10
- D50.9 Iron deficiency anemia, unspecified
- D50 Iron deficiency anemia
- O99.01 Anemia complicating pregnancy

CLINICAL PEARLS
- IDA due to poor dietary iron intake is the most common anemia.
- Blood loss and reduced iron stores due to poor utilization or malabsorption are risk factors for IDA.
- Premenopausal women and children are at the greatest risk for IDA.

ANEMIA, SICKLE CELL

Joseph P. Wiedemer, MD, FAAFP • Dongsheng Jiang, MD, MSc

BASICS

DESCRIPTION
- Hereditary, hemoglobinopathy marked by chronic hemolytic anemia, acute episodes of painful crises, and increased susceptibility to infections
- The heterozygous condition (Hb AS), sickle cell trait, is usually asymptomatic without anemia.
- Synonym(s): sickle cell disease (SCD); HbSS disease

Pediatric Considerations
- Sequestration crises and hand–foot syndrome are seen typically in infants/young children.
- Strokes occur mainly in childhood.
- Adolescence/young adulthood:
  - Frequency of complications and organ/tissue damage increases with age.
  - Psychological complications: body image, interrupted schooling, restriction of activities; stigma of disease; low self-esteem

Pregnancy Considerations
- Complicated, especially during 3rd trimester and delivery
  - Fetal mortality: 35–40%; fetal survival is >90% if the fetus reaches the 3rd trimester.
  - High prevalence of small for gestational age (SGA) babies
  - 6 times higher maternal mortality compared to control
- Increased risk of thrombosis, preterm delivery, pain, toxemia, infection, pulmonary infarction, and phlebitis
- Partial exchange transfusion in 3rd trimester may reduce maternal morbidity and fetal mortality but is controversial.
- Chronic transfusions have been effective in diminishing pain episodes in pregnant women. However, this method should be used with caution due to risk of alloimmunization.

EPIDEMIOLOGY
Prevalence
- ~100,000 Americans have sickle cell anemia (SCA), and ~3 million people in the United States have sickle cell trait.
- The condition affects mainly people of African descent. Hispanic, Middle Eastern, Asian Indian, and Mediterranean ancestry may also be affected.

ETIOLOGY AND PATHOPHYSIOLOGY
- Hemoglobin S (HbS) results from the substitution of the amino acid valine for glutamic acid at the sixth position of the β-globin chain. Hydrophobic valine residues interact with other hydrophobic residues, contributing to HbS polymerization.
- HbS polymerization occurs in the RBC with increased concentrations of HbS and in deoxygenated states, resulting in RBC sickling.
- Sickle RBCs exhibit increased adhesion, are inflexible, and have decreased ability to maneuver through small vessels leading to increased blood viscosity, stasis, and vasoocclusion of small arterioles and capillaries, resulting in ischemia.

- Chronic anemia; crises:
  - Vaso-occlusive crisis: tissue ischemia and necrosis; progressive organ failure/tissue damage from repeated episodes
  - Hand–foot syndrome: Vessel occlusion/ischemia affects small blood vessels in hands or feet.
  - Aplastic crisis: suppression of RBC production by severe infection (e.g., parvovirus and other viral infections)
  - Suppression of RBC production
  - Hyperhemolytic crisis: accelerated hemolysis with reticulocytosis; increased RBC fragility/shortened lifespan
  - Sequestration crisis: splenic sequestration of blood (only in young children as spleen is later lost to autoinfarction)
- Susceptibility to infection: impaired/absent splenic function leading to decreased ability to clear infection; defect in alternate pathway of complement activation
- Increased red cell destruction causes decreased hemoglobin levels and results in anemia and fatigue.

Genetics
- Autosomal recessive; homozygous condition, HbSS; heterozygous condition, HbAS
- The heterozygote condition can also be combined with other hemoglobinopathies: Sickle cell hemoglobin C (HbSC) disease and $S\beta$ + thalassemia are clinically similar to the heterozygous condition, whereas $S\beta$ thalassemia is clinically similar to the homozygous condition.

RISK FACTORS
- Vaso-occlusive crisis ("painful crisis"): hypoxia, dehydration, high altitudes, stress, fever, infection, acidosis, cold, anesthesia, strenuous physical exercise, alcohol, smoking
- Aplastic crisis (suppression of RBC production): severe infections, human parvovirus B19 infection, folic acid deficiency
- Hyperhemolytic crisis (accelerated hemolysis with reticulocytosis): acute bacterial infections, exposure to oxidant

GENERAL PREVENTION
- Prevention of crises
  - Avoid hypoxia, dehydration, cold, infection, fever, acidosis, and anesthesia.
  - Prompt management of fever, infections, pain
  - Avoid alcohol and smoking. Avoid high-altitude areas.
- Minimizing trauma: Aseptic technique is imperative.

DIAGNOSIS

HISTORY
- Often asymptomatic in early months of life due to presence of fetal hemoglobin
- In those >6 months of age, the earliest symptoms: irritability and painful swelling of the hands and feet (hand–foot syndrome); pneumococcal sepsis or meningitis, severe anemia and acute splenic enlargement (splenic sequestration), acute chest syndrome, pallor, jaundice, or splenomegaly

- Manifestations in older children include anemia, severe or recurrent musculoskeletal or abdominal pain, aplastic crisis, acute chest syndrome, splenomegaly or splenic sequestration, and cholelithiasis.
- Painful crises in bones, joints, abdomen, back, and viscera account for 90% of all hospital admissions.
- Acute chest syndrome: tachycardia, fever, bilateral infiltrates caused by pulmonary infarctions

DIAGNOSTIC TESTS & INTERPRETATION
Initial Tests (lab, imaging)
- Screening test: Sickledex test/hemoglobin electrophoresis (diagnostic test of choice); SCA (FS pattern)
  - 80–100% HbS, variable amounts of HbF, and no HbA1
  - Sickle cell trait (FS pattern): 30–45% HbS, 50–70% HbA1, minimal HbF
- Hemoglobin ~5 to 10 g/dL; RBC indices: mean corpuscular volume (MCV) normal to increased; mean corpuscular hemoglobin concentration (MCHC) increased; reticulocytes 3–15%
- Leukocytosis; bands in absence of infection, platelets elevated; peripheral smear: sickled RBCs, nucleated RBCs, Howell-Jolly bodies
- Serum bilirubin mildly elevated (2 to 4 mg/dL); ferritin very elevated in patients with multiple previous transfusions; serum lactate dehydrogenase (LDH) elevated, fecal/urinary urobilinogen high
- Haptoglobin absent or very low
- Urine analysis: hemoglobinuria, hematuria (sickle cell trait may have painless hematuria), increased albuminuria (Monitor for progressive kidney disease.)
- Imaging depends on clinical circumstances.
  - Bone scan to rule out osteomyelitis
  - CT/MRI to rule out CVA; high index of suspicion required for any acute neurologic symptoms other than mild headache
  - Chest x-ray: may show enlarged heart; diffuse alveolar infiltrates in acute chest syndrome
  - Transcranial Doppler: Start at age 2 years; repeat yearly. Transcranial Doppler ultrasound identifies children aged 2 to 16 years at higher risk of stroke; may be normal in clinically silent strokes
  - ECG to detect pulmonary hypertension and echocardiogram every other year from age ≥15 years

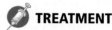

TREATMENT

GENERAL MEASURES
- Painful crises: hydration, analgesics; oxygen regardless of whether the patient is hypoxic
- Retinal evaluation starting at school age to detect proliferative sickle retinopathy
- Occupational therapy, cognitive and behavioral therapies, support groups
- All standard childhood vaccinations should be administered accordingly.
- Special immunizations
  - Influenza vaccine yearly
  - Conjugated pneumococcal vaccine (PCV13) at ages 2, 4, and 6 months; booster at ages 12 to 15 months

– Patients <5 years of age with incomplete vaccination history should receive catch-up doses accordingly.
– Adults 19 to 64 years of age: Pneumococcal 20-valent conjugate vaccine (Prevnar 20) is recommended.

- Meningococcal vaccine:
  – 6 weeks old: Hib-MenCY at ages 2, 4, 6, and 12 months
  – 9 months old: 2 doses of MCV4 separated by 3 months
  – ≥2 years of age: 2 doses of MCV4-D-CRM separated by 2 months; boosters recommended every 5 years

MEDICATION

First Line

- Four FDA approved medications for SCD treatment (1),(2):
  – Hydroxyurea: decrease in painful events including acute chest syndrome; age ≥9 months; dose: initial: 20 mg/kg daily; maintenance: 20 to 35 mg/kg; maximum dose: 2,500 mg daily
  – L-glutamine: reduction in vaso-occlusive episodes (VOE) and hospitalization; age ≥5 years; dose: weight <30 kg: 5 g BID; 30 to 65 kg: 10 g BID; >65 kg: 15 kg BID
  – Crizanlizumab: reduction in VOE; age ≥16 years; loading: 5 mg/kg IV every 2 weeks for 2 doses; maintenance: 5 mg/kg IV every 4 weeks
  – Voxelotor: increase in hemoglobin; age ≥4 years; dose: <40 kg: 600 to 900 mg once daily; ≥40 kg: 1,500 mg once daily
- Prophylactic penicillins indicated in infants and children starting at 2 months: A dose of 125 mg BID is recommended for children aged <3 years. A dose of 250 mg BID is recommended for children aged 3 to 5 years. Amoxicillin 20 mg/kg/day is an alternative to penicillin. Penicillin can be discontinued at age 5 years unless the patient has had a splenectomy or invasive pneumococcal infection.
- Supplemental oxygen
- Painful crises (mild, outpatient)—nonopioid analgesics (ibuprofen)
- Painful crises (severe, hospitalized)—parenteral opioids (e.g., morphine on fixed schedule); patient-controlled analgesia (PCA) pump may be useful. Patients given strong opioids in the acute care setting should be safely monitored.
- Acute chest syndrome: Patients may deteriorate quickly; monitor patients with vaso-occlusive crisis with incentive spirometry. Treat with aggressive management with oxygen, analgesics, antibiotics, and simple or exchange transfusion.
- Empiric antibiotics to cover *Mycoplasma pneumoniae* and *Chlamydia pneumoniae* (cephalosporins or azithromycin); if osteomyelitis, cover for *Staphylococcus aureus* and *Salmonella* (e.g., ciprofloxacin).
- Precautions: Avoid high-dose estrogen oral contraceptives; consider medroxyprogesterone (Depo-Provera). G-CSF use is contraindicated as it may lead to VOE and multiorgan failure.

Second Line

Folic acid: 0 to 6 months old: 0.1 mg/day; 6 to 12 months old: 0.25 mg/day; 1 to 2 years of age: 0.5 mg/day; >2 years of age: 1 mg/day

ADDITIONAL THERAPIES

- Transfusion: It increases oxygen-carrying capacity and improves blood flow in severe anemia.
  – It is the main treatment during an acute episode and is helpful in splenic sequestration, aplastic crisis, stroke, acute chest syndrome, multiple organ failure, priapism, etc. (3)
  – Prophylactic transfusions for primary or secondary stroke prevention in children
  – Preoperative transfusions have been shown to reduce the risk of perioperative complications with goal Hgb >10 g/dL.
- Chelation with oral deferasirox if the patient is multiply transfused (after age 2 years).
- Red cell exchange is indicated to minimize the level of HbS (<30%) as well as prevent iron overload.

SURGERY/OTHER PROCEDURES

- Hematopoietic stem cell transplant (HSCT): curative
- Endothelin-1 has therapeutic potential for prevention of renal and pulmonary complications of SCD.
- Oral therapy with L-glutamine
- Monoclonal antibodies that bind P-selectin

ADMISSION, INPATIENT, AND NURSING CONSIDERATIONS

Admission criteria/initial stabilization: severe pain, suspected infection or sepsis, evidence of acute chest syndrome

 ONGOING CARE

FOLLOW-UP RECOMMENDATIONS

Patient Monitoring

- Treat infections early. Any ≥101°F (38.3°C) requires immediate medical attention.
- Monitor for hepatitis C and hemosiderosis in patients who receive chronic transfusions.
- Periodic eye evaluations: starting at age 10 years for proliferative sickle retinopathy; rescreen 1- to 2-year intervals.
- Biannual examination for hepatic, renal, and pulmonary dysfunction
- Neuroimaging screening for risk of stroke: transcranial Doppler beginning at age 2 years and continuing up to age 16 years
- Baseline pulmonary evaluation at each visit to assess for wheezing, shortness of breath, or cough (indicators of disease severity and pulmonary hypertension); echocardiography for symptomatic patients; right heart catheterization for diagnosis
- Screening for albuminuria should be performed annually starting at age 10 years, with introduction of ACE/ARB therapy for management of confirmed albuminuria.
- SCD may be considered a provoking factor for VTE, but decisions on anticoagulation duration and prophylaxis should be a shared decision-making process.

DIET

- Avoid alcohol (leads to dehydration); maintain hydration.
- Multivitamin without iron is recommended; vitamin D deficiency and decreased bone marrow density in SCD patients

PROGNOSIS

- Anemia occurs in infancy; sickle cell crises at 1 to 2 years of age; some children die in their 1st year.
- In adulthood, fewer crises but more complications; median age of death is 42 years for men and 48 years for women.

COMPLICATIONS

- Alloimmunization, bone infarct and osteomyelitis, aseptic necrosis of femoral head
- Cerebral strokes (peak age 6 to 7 years), impaired mental development, even without history of stroke
- Cholelithiasis/abnormal liver function
- Chronic leg ulcers, poor wound healing
- Impotence, priapism, hematuria/hyposthenuria, renal complications (proteinuria)
- Retinopathy, splenic infarction (by age 10 years)
- Acute chest syndrome (infection/infarction) leading to chronic pulmonary disease
- Infections (pneumonia, osteomyelitis, meningitis, pyelonephritis); sepsis (leading cause of morbidity and mortality)
- Hemosiderosis (secondary to multiple transfusions)
- Risk of opioid tolerance and substance abuse in chronic, uncontrolled patients

REFERENCES

1. Kavanagh PL, Fasipe TA, Wun T. Sickle cell disease: a review. *JAMA*. 2022;328(1):57–68.
2. Brandow AM, Liem RI. Advances in the diagnosis and treatment of sickle cell disease. *J Hematol Oncol*. 2022;15(1):20.
3. Parikh T, Goti A, Yashi K, et al. Pediatric sickle cell disease and stroke: a literature review. *Cureus*. 2023;15(1):e34003.

 SEE ALSO

Algorithm: Anemia

CODES

ICD10

- D57.212 Sickle-cell/Hb-C disease with splenic sequestration
- D57.211 Sickle-cell/Hb-C disease with acute chest syndrome
- D57.21 Sickle-cell/Hb-C disease with crisis

CLINICAL PEARLS

- Use 1/2 NS because NS may theoretically increase the risk of sickling.
- Painful crises in bones, joints, abdomen, back, and viscera account for 90% of all hospital admissions. Management of pain should follow individualized pain plans or hospital protocol for SCD crises without discrimination.

ANEURYSM OF THE ABDOMINAL AORTA

Jeffrey Chen, MD

 BASICS

DESCRIPTION

- There are two types of aneurysm: true and false. A true aneurysm involves all three vessel wall layers. False aneurysms or pseudoaneurysms occur when the intimal and medial layers are disrupted and the dilated segment is surrounded by the adventitia only. Ruptures are usually higher with false aneurysms due to poor support of the aneurysmal wall.
- Abdominal aortic aneurysm (AAA) is the most common true arterial aneurysm. False aneurysms of the abdominal aorta are usually due to trauma or infection.
- The average diameter of the infrarenal aorta is 2 cm; an aortic diameter of ≥3 cm is considered aneurysmal.
- In men, AAA diameters are predictive of clinical events. In women, aneurysms are still defined as >3 cm, but the aortic scaling index (ASI; diameter [cm] / body surface area [m^2]) is more predictive of clinical events.
- System(s) affected: cardiovascular; neurologic; heme/lymphatic/immunologic
- Synonym(s): aortic aneurysms; AAA

Geriatric Considerations
Incidence of AAA, risk of rupture, and operative morbidity and mortality all rise with age.

Pediatric Considerations
Rare in children; may be associated with umbilical artery catheters, connective tissue diseases, arteritides, or congenital abnormalities

EPIDEMIOLOGY

- Estimated prevalence of AAA in developed countries is 2–8%. Age-related increase is seen more with men than women.
- Ultrasound studies show that 4–8% of older men have an occult AAA.
- 90% of all AAA >4 cm are related to atherosclerotic disease, with the vast majority located infrarenally.
- Predominant sex: male > female

Incidence
- Roughly 15,000 deaths per year and the 15th leading cause of death in the United States
- 0.4–0.67% in Western populations or 2.5 to 6.5 aneurysms per 1,000 patient-years
- If stratified into years, the incidence of AAA is increased in the older populations. For example, the incidence increases from 55 to 298 per 100,000 patient-years if comparing men aged 65 to 74 years versus men >85 years of age.

Prevalence
- The prevalence of AAA-associated mortality has decreased by 50% since the 1990s, likely due to the decline in cigarette smoking, increased screening for AAA detection, and early interventions.
- With the increasing life expectancy in developed countries, the prevalence of AAA is expected to increase, but the decreased prevalence of smoking will have the opposite effect.

ETIOLOGY AND PATHOPHYSIOLOGY

- AAAs are caused by degradations of abnormal production of elastin and collagen, the structural components of the aortic wall.
- There are many causes of aortic aneurysms: inflammation, degenerative disorders, vasculitis, infections, and trauma. However, the vast majority of AAA are caused by inflammation with atherosclerosis as the inciting factor.
- Although most aortic aneurysms are caused by inflammatory or degenerative destruction of elastin and collagen, infections, trauma, and connective tissue disorders can also degrade elastin and collagen, leading to similar presentations.
- The natural course of an AAA is progressive expansion, based on multiple factors, the most important being ongoing smoking.

Genetics
- Familial AAAs have a variable polygenetic inheritance pattern.
- Monogenetic inheritance patterns such as: Marfan syndrome (fibrillin-1 defect), Ehlers-Danlos syndrome (type IV collagen defect), or Loeys-Dietz syndrome are more commonly associated with thoracoabdominal aortic aneurysms.

RISK FACTORS
Older age, male sex, Caucasian race, family history, smoking, hypertension (HTN), hyperlipidemia, atherosclerosis, peripheral aneurysms, obesity

GENERAL PREVENTION
- Address cardiovascular disease risk factors.
- Follow screening guidelines: U.S. screening for detection of AAA in male patients, aged 65 to 75 years, who have ever smoked.

COMMONLY ASSOCIATED CONDITIONS
- HTN, myocardial infarction (MI), heart failure, carotid artery atherosclerosis, lower extremity peripheral arterial disease, tobacco abuse
- Screening for thoracic aneurysm should also be considered.
- 20% of patients with AAA have concurrent thoracic aneurysm (1).

DIAGNOSIS

- Asymptomatic AAA (majority)
  - USPSTF recommends a one-time screen for an AAA by abdominal ultrasonography for men aged 65 to 75 years with a smoking history (2)[A].
  - Selective screening for AAAs in nonsmoker men aged 65 to 75 years can be offered based on personal or family history and patient's preferences (2)[A].
  - Women with a first-degree relative with an AAA can be offered screening via abdominal ultrasonography (1)[C].

ALERT
- Symptomatic: The triad of shock, pulsatile mass, and abdominal pain always suggest rupture of AAA, and immediate surgical evaluation is recommended (1)[A].
  - Hemodynamically stable patients (shock is absent as the rupture is contained) may undergo a CT abdomen with IV contrast for evaluation of an AAA.
  - Unstable patients (rupture is uncontained) undergo a focused bedside ultrasound and surgical repair if AAA is present.

- Unusual presentations:
  - Primary aortoenteric fistula: erosion/rupture of AAA into duodenum
  - Aortocaval fistula: erosion/rupture of AAA into vena cava or left renal vein: 3–6%

HISTORY
- Abdominal, back, or flank pain
- AAA risk factors, hypotension if presenting in an emergency situation
- Found on routine screening if presenting in an outpatient setting

PHYSICAL EXAM
- Pulsatile supraumbilical mass
- Encroachment by aneurysm
  - Vertebral body erosion, gastric outlet obstruction, ureteral obstruction
  - Lower extremity ischemia secondary to embolization of mural thrombus
- Rupture leads to tachycardia, hypotension, evidence of shock and anemia, and possible flank contusion (Grey Turner sign).

DIFFERENTIAL DIAGNOSIS
- Other abdominal masses
- Other causes of abdominal or back pain (e.g., peptic ulcer disease, renal colic, diverticulitis, appendicitis, incarcerated hernia, bowel obstruction, GI hemorrhage, arthritis, metastatic disease, MI)

DIAGNOSTIC TESTS & INTERPRETATION

Initial Tests (lab, imaging)
- If rupturing AAA is considered: complete blood chemistry (chemistries, PT/INR, PTT, type and cross), ECG
- Ultrasound: simplest and least expensive diagnostic procedure with a high sensitivity (94–100%) and specificity (98–100%); test of choice for an asymptomatic AAA (1)[A]
- Surveillance of asymptomatic aneurysm
  - 2.6 to 2.9 cm: Screen at 10-year intervals.
  - 3 to 3.9 cm: Screen at 3-year intervals.
  - 4 to 4.9 cm: Screen at 12-month intervals.
  - 5 to 5.4 cm: Screen every 6 months.
- CT scans are preferred preoperative study (caution with IV contrast in renal failure) if a symptomatic AAA is suspected.
- MRI/MRA can visualize AAA but is often not possible in emergent situations.
- Abdominal x-rays can be diagnostic if calcifications exist; not a diagnostic tool of choice

Follow-Up Tests & Special Considerations
- Evaluation for coronary artery disease is appropriate prior to elective AAA repair, including stress test, echocardiography, and ECG if appropriate.
- If AAA was discovered at any location, then full assessment of entire aorta, including thoracic aorta and aortic valve, is recommended (1)[C].

Diagnostic Procedures/Other

ALERT
Use clinical judgment: Patients with known AAA having abdominal or back pain symptoms may be rupturing despite a negative CT scan.

TREATMENT

GENERAL MEASURES
- Treat atherosclerotic risk factors: HTN, dyslipidemia, diabetes mellitus, and smoking (2)[A].
- Smoking was associated with a 0.35 mm/year AAA growth, twice as fast as AAA growth in nonsmokers, and is the most important AAA outcome predictor (1).
- Emergent treatment in unstable or symptomatic patients requires immediate vascular surgery consultation, adequate IV access and resuscitation, type and cross for multiple units, and rapid bedside ultrasound (1).
- Less acute prevention of AAA rupture is elective repair and risk factor modification.

MEDICATION
- β-Blockers, aspirin, and statins theoretically reduce the rate of growth of AAAs by decreasing shear wall stress, inflammation, and prevention of an intraluminal mural thrombus. However, there are conflicting RCT and meta-analysis trials. Because concomitant atherosclerosis is often a precipitating factor in AAAs, their use is recommended for reduced mortality in patients with coronary artery disease or its equivalents (3)[A].
- The use of ACE inhibitors has shown to be inconclusive with regard to growth of AAA; however, studies do indicate a decreased rate of AAA rupture (3)[A].
- Doxycycline and roxithromycin, theorized to decreased wall inflammation, have not been shown to have any effect on AAA (4).

SURGERY/OTHER PROCEDURES
Current recommendations are the following:
- Elective
  - 5.5-cm diameter is threshold for repair in "average" patient (1)[C].
  - Younger, low-risk patients with long-life expectancy may prefer early repair.
  - Saccular aneurysms should be considered for elective repair (1)[C].
  - Women or AAA with high risk of rupture: Consider elective repair at 4.5 to 5 cm.
    - Consider delayed repair in high-risk patients.
    - 5% perioperative mortality for open elective repair (1)
- High risk of rupture
  - Expansion >0.5 cm/year; poorly controlled HTN; smoking/severe COPD
- High-risk patients for elective repair
  - Risk factors for open repair include age >75 years, COPD, chronic kidney disease with Cr >1.75, and suprarenal clamp site.
  - The leading cause of early mortality after AAA repair is coronary artery disease, with open AAA repair being much higher risk than endovascular AAA repair (1)[C].
- The RCT IMPROVE trial showed a similar 30-day mortality for patients with ruptured AAA who underwent endovascular repair versus open repair (35.4% vs. 37.4%); 1-year follow-up all-cause mortality between the two groups (41.1% vs. 45.1%) (4)[A]

- Perioperative morbidity rates are lower for EVAR, suggesting that an EVAR is preferable in patients with a ruptured AAA with poor prognostic factors for an open repair, such as SBP <80 mm Hg, age >80 years, Cr >1.3 on admission, ischemic heart disease, female sex, and hemoglobin <9.0 on admission (2),(4)[A].
- Contraindications for AAA endovascular repair are an aortic neck >32 mm and a ruptured AAA with aortic neck length <7 mm. In these patients, an open AAA repair is performed due to anatomic constrictions.

ADMISSION, INPATIENT, AND NURSING CONSIDERATIONS
Risk of abdominal compartment syndrome after repair, 4–12%; usually associated with large fluid resuscitation

 ONGOING CARE

FOLLOW-UP RECOMMENDATIONS
Patient Monitoring
- May do a CT scan 5 years after an open repair for possible late aortic dilatation or pseudoaneurysm (2)[C]
- Follow-up imaging should be tailored to patient. Once renal function stabilizes postoperatively, a CT can be performed to evaluate the endograft (2)[C].
- Aggressive risk factor modification always recommended postoperatively (2)[A].

DIET
Low-fat, low-salt, and low-caffeine diet; optimize nutrition prior to elective repair.

PATIENT EDUCATION
Smoking cessation, aerobic exercise, and aggressive control of atherosclerotic risk factors such as HTN

PROGNOSIS
- Naturally progressive disorder, expands at an average rate of 0.3 to 0.4 cm/year; a fast expansion is considered >0.6 cm/year and should be evaluated for operative management.
- Possibility of rupture increases with an aneurysm diameter of >5.5 cm or a fast rate of expansion (>0.5 cm over a 6-month period), continued cigarette use, female sex, recent surgery, uncontrolled HTN, and aneurysm couture.

COMPLICATIONS
- Emergent AAA repair and elective AAA repair have similar complications, with a higher incidence in emergent AAA repair.
- Complications include MI, respiratory failure, and acute kidney injury in the early period.
- Late complications such as aortic graft infection, aortoenteric fistula, and graft occlusion have similar rates between emergent and elective repair.
- Ischemic bowel and abdominal compartment syndrome are complications usually after a ruptured open AAA repair given the massive blood loss, increased operative time, and magnitude of fluid resuscitation.

REFERENCES
1. Chaikof EL, Dalman RL, Eskandari MK, et al. The Society for Vascular Surgery practice guidelines on the care of patients with an abdominal aortic aneurysm. *J Vasc Surg*. 2018;67(1):2–77.e2.
2. LeFevre ML; for U.S. Preventive Services Task Force. Screening for abdominal aortic aneurysm: U.S. Preventive Services Task Force recommendation statement. *Ann Intern Med*. 2014;161(4):281–290.
3. Guessous I, Periard D, Lorenzetti D, et al. The efficacy of pharmacotherapy for decreasing the expansion rate of abdominal aortic aneurysms: a systematic review and meta-analysis. *PLoS One*. 2008;3(3):e1895.
4. Braithwaite B, Cheshire NJ, Greenhalgh RM, et al; for IMPROVE Trial Investigators. Endovascular strategy or open repair for ruptured abdominal aortic aneurysm: one-year outcomes from the IMPROVE randomized trial. *Eur Heart J*. 2015;36(31):2061–2069.

ADDITIONAL READING
Aggarwal S, Qamar A, Sharma V, et al. Abdominal aortic aneurysm: a comprehensive review. *Exp Clin Cardiol*. 2011;16(1):11–15.

 SEE ALSO

Aortic Dissection; Arteritis, Temporal; Ehlers-Danlos Syndrome; Marfan Syndrome; Polyarteritis Nodosa; Turner Syndrome

 CODES

ICD10
- I71.4 Abdominal aortic aneurysm, without rupture
- I71.3 Abdominal aortic aneurysm, ruptured

CLINICAL PEARLS
- Men with a smoking history aged 65 to 75 years should undergo a one-time screening abdominal ultrasound to evaluate for an AAA. Men and women with a first-degree relative with an AAA should be considered for a screening with abdominal ultrasound.
- Larger AAAs should be screened more often, with elective repair with AAA >5.5 cm or an expansion of >0.5 cm every 6 months.
- Patients with a ruptured AAA present in shock, with abdominal pain and a pulsatile mass. A bedside ultrasound should be done quickly to evaluate for an AAA, or an emergent CT scan can be performed if the patient is hemodynamically stable.
- AAAs are treated either openly or endovascularly as an elective or emergent procedure. 30-day and 1-year mortality between the two methods remain the same; however, there is an increased mortality with an emergent AAA repair.
- Patients require aggressive risk factor modification, especially smoking cessation.

ANGIOEDEMA

Kathryn M. Brown, MD, MS • Katherine Montag Schafer, PharmD, BCACP

 BASICS

Angioedema (AE) is acute, localized swelling of skin, mucosa, and submucosa caused by extravasation of fluid into the affected tissues (1).

DESCRIPTION
- AE commonly occurs as a part of the presentation of urticaria, but when it presents without wheals, it should be diagnosed as a distinct disease (1).
- AE develops in minutes to hours and resolves in hours to days but can be life-threatening if the upper airway is involved.
- Two major classifications of AE exist, both with unique subtypes (1):
  - Acquired AE (AAE): involves all cases that are not considered to be hereditary AE (HAE)
    ○ Idiopathic histaminergic (IH-AAE): no cause identified, response to antihistamine treatment
    ○ Idiopathic non-histaminergic (InH-AAE): no cause identified, no response to antihistamine treatment
    ○ Angiotensin-converting enzyme-inhibitor (ACEI)-related AAE (ACEI-AAE)
    ○ C1-inhibitor (C1-INH) deficiency-related AAE (C1-INH-AAE)
  - HAE: mediated by changes in the genes that regulate the compliment cascade, also known as bradykinin-mediated AE
    ○ C1-INH-HAE: caused by C1-INH deficiency
    ○ FXII-HAE: Patients have a normal C1-INH but a FXII mutation.
    ○ U-HAE: Patients have a normal C1-INH, unknown cause.
- Synonym(s): angioneurotic edema; Quincke edema

EPIDEMIOLOGY
- Predominant age of onset
  - AAE (1):
    ○ IH-AAE, InH-AAE, ACEI-AAE: any age
    ○ C1-INH-AAE: age >40 years
  - HAE: infancy to 2nd decade of life
- Predominant gender: male = female, except FXII-HAE which predominantly affects females

Prevalence
- AAE:
  - IH-AAE: most common form of AE
  - ACEI-AAE: 0.1–2.2% of patients receiving ACEI (1)
    ○ The incidence of AE related to ACEI use in black individuals is as high as four times that of whites. Note: Race is now recognized as a social, not biological, construct and decisions about initiation of ACEI should not be influenced by self-identified race.
  - C1-INH-AAE: 1:500,000 (1)
- HAE
  - C1-INH-HAE: 1:10,000 to 100,000 (1)
  - C1-INH accounts for 85% of cases of HAE (2)

ETIOLOGY AND PATHOPHYSIOLOGY
- AAE:
  - IH-AAE: due to release of vasoactive substances
  - ACEI-AAE: thought to be due to elevated plasma levels of bradykinin
  - C1-INH-AAE: nongenetic changes to C1-INH function, can be due to autoantibodies
    ○ Can be associated with other lymphoproliferative conditions like systemic lupus erythematosus

- HAE:
  - Attacks are triggered by prolonged mechanical pressure, cold, heat, trauma, emotional stress, menses, illness, and inflammation.
  - C1-INH-HAE
    ○ Type I: decreased production of C1-INH
    ○ Type II: normal or high levels of C1-INH; however, is dysfunctional
  - FXII-HAE
    ○ normal C1-INH with presence of mutation in coagulation FXII gene
    ○ Formerly type III HAE
    ○ Symptoms, often estrogen-dependent, are induced with estrogen administration (hormone replacement therapy or oral contraceptives [OCPs]) or with pregnancy
  - U-HAE
    ○ Normal C1-INH, without presence of FXII gene mutation

Genetics
- HAE types I and II are autosomal dominant, whereas HAE with normal C1-INH is dominant X-linked.
- Spontaneous genetic mutations responsible for 25% of HAE cases

RISK FACTORS
- Consuming medications and foods that can cause allergic reactions
- Positive family history

GENERAL PREVENTION
- Avoid known triggers.
- Do not use ACEI in type I or II HAE.

COMMONLY ASSOCIATED CONDITIONS
- Quincke disease (AE of the uvula)
- Urticaria

 DIAGNOSIS

- AAE:
  - Lack of positive family history of AE
  - Assess for:
    ○ Exposure to common allergens: foods (shellfish, nuts, eggs, milk, wheat soy), latex, insect bites/stings, medication (antibiotics, aspirin, narcotics, NSAIDs, and OCPs)
      ▪ Allergy can be confirmed with positive skin prick test
    ○ Exposure to ACEI
    ○ Exposure to physical stimuli (cold or vibration)
  - If ACEI, allergy, or other causes have been ruled out, then deemed IH-AAE
    ○ If AE recurs despite prophylactic antihistamine use, then deemed InH-AAE
- HAE:
  - Positive family history of AE in second-degree relative
  - C1-INH-HAE, FXII-HAE, and U-HAE require laboratory confirmation.

HISTORY
- Acute, typically asymmetric, swelling with onset in minutes to hours
- In comparison with urticaria, AE presents without wheals, typically is nonpruritic, but can cause a painful, burning sensation.

- Recent exposure to food allergens or medications
- Identify potential triggers such as environmental exposure or trauma.
- Family history of AE
- Recent infection, history of autoimmune disease, or malignancy

PHYSICAL EXAM
- Vitals: Symptoms of hypotension, tachycardia, and tachypnea indicate systemic involvement and increased severity.
- Tense, nonpitting skin swelling that is skin colored or slightly erythematous
- Commonly affects the mucus membranes of the face including periorbital, lips, tongue, or larynx but can involve any part of the body
- Evaluate for involvement of oropharynx or symptoms such as stridor.
- GI tract involvement is more common in forms of HAE and may manifest as intermittent, unexplained abdominal pain.

ALERT
- Increased risk for early intubation and tracheostomy with involvement of the anterior tongue, base of the tongue or larynx, stridor within 4 hours of onset of symptoms, and drooling.
- Patients with HAE are at higher risk for intubation, tracheostomy, and death, although these complications can occur with any subtype.

DIFFERENTIAL DIAGNOSIS
Urticaria; anaphylaxis; contact dermatitis; food/drug allergy; erysipelas; connective tissue disease: systemic lupus erythematosus, dermatomyositis; lymphedema; insect bite reaction; diffuse subcutaneous infiltrative process

DIAGNOSTIC TESTS & INTERPRETATION
Initial Tests (lab, imaging)
- Initial diagnosis should be based on history and clinical assessment alone.
- Laboratory testing includes CBC, ESR, complement testing (C4, C1-INH, C1-INH function), allergy testing, and screening for paraproteinemia (SPEP, UPEP).
- Complement testing assists in distinguishing between various types of AE; this assessment should be done in collaboration with an allergy specialist:
  - Low serum C4 is a sensitive but nonspecific screening test for hereditary and acquired C1-INH deficiency.
  - If C4 is normal, determine C1-INH level and function and recheck C4 during an acute attack.
  - If C4 level and C1-INH level and function are still normal, consider other causes and/or require genetic assessment (i.e., FXII gene).
  - If C4 level, C1-INH level, and C1-INH function are low, these indicate C1-INH-HAE type I.
  - C1-INH-HAE type II is characterized by low C4 and low C1-INH function, but C1-INH level can be normal or elevated.
- For recurrent AE with urticaria, complement levels should be obtained in addition to allergy testing for potential triggers.
- Abdominal radiographs and CT scan can demonstrate GI AE or ileus.

- C1-INH deficiency may occur in association with internal malignancy. In rare cases, AE can be a para-neoplastic disease. Imaging (CT scan, radiography, etc.) would be done as part of a neoplastic workup for patients with AAE.

Follow-Up Tests & Special Considerations
If C4 and C1q antigen are low (as in AAE), neoplastic and autoimmune workup is warranted. CBC, a peripheral smear, protein electrophoresis, immunophenotyping of lymphocytes, and imaging studies are often undertaken to rule out hematologic malignancies or cancer.

 TREATMENT

GENERAL MEASURES
- Intubation if airway is threatened
- Eliminate suspected trigger.
- Volume replacement is essential for patients who are unstable or refractory to initial therapy.

MEDICATION
First Line
- If AE presenting with signs of anaphylaxis (hypotension, respiratory compromise): epinephrine 1:1,000; 0.1 mg/kg (maximum 0.3 mg for children, 0.5 mg for adults) intramuscularly q5–15min
- If cause of AE is unknown, use first-line therapy:
  – Epinephrine, if airway involvement
  – H_1 antagonist (IV diphenhydramine, adult: 25 to 50 mg, children: 1 mg/kg, maximum 50 mg). In older adults, side effects can include delirium, urinary retention, constipation, and increased ocular pressure.
  – H_2 antagonists (IV ranitidine, adult: 50 mg, children: 1 mg/kg, maximum 50 mg)
  – Corticosteroids (IV hydrocortisone, adult: 200 mg, children: maximum 100 mg; or IV methylprednisolone, adult: 50 to 100 mg, children: 1 mg/kg, maximum 50 mg)
- AAE
  – IH-AAE (1)
    ○ Acute treatment: first-line therapy, as above
    ○ Prevention: second-generation antihistamines (cetirizine, fexofenadine, loratadine, etc.), administered daily; may need to escalate to higher than standard doses, up to four times labeled dosing, before considering treatment failure or alternative diagnosis, that is, InH-AAE (1)
  – InH-AAE
    ○ Acute treatment: Antihistamines are ineffective; corticosteroids, epinephrine, if upper airway involvement
    ○ Prevention: Consider tranexamic acid: adult up to 3 g/day or specialty referral for immunosuppressive agents (1).

  – ACEI-AAE
    ○ Acute treatment:
      ▪ Remove causative agent.
      ▪ May be ineffective: first-line therapy, as above
      ▪ Off label: bradykinin receptor antagonist (icatibant), C1-INH replacement (Berinert, Ruconest), kallikrein inhibitor (ecallantide)
    ○ Prevention: Remove causative agent; angiotensin receptor blockers (ARBs) are an appropriate substitute as they have a low incidence of cross-reactivity.
  – C1-INH-AAE
    ○ Acute treatment:
      ▪ Off label: bradykinin receptor antagonist (icatibant), C1-INH replacement (Berinert, Ruconest), kallikrein inhibitor (ecallantide)
      ▪ H1/H2 antagonists, corticosteroids, and epinephrine are ineffective and not recommended.
      ▪ Associated improvement through treatment of underlying disease
    ○ Prevention: possible remission through treatment of underlying disease
- HAE
  – C1-INH-HAE
    ○ Berinert (human C1 esterase inhibitor) 20 IU/kg IV (2)
    ○ Ruconest (recombinant C1 esterase inhibitor) 50 IU/kg IV or 4,200 IU IV if 85kg or age ≥13 years or older (2)
  – FXII-HAE/U-HAE:
    ○ Patients with U-HAE/HXII-HAE do not respond to corticosteroids and antihistamine.
    ○ Treatment choice should be driven by allergy/immunology specialist and may include C1-INH agents, icatibant, ecallantide, progesterone, danazol, and tranexamic acid (1).
    ○ Prevention: In women, symptoms may be provoked by hormone therapy or pregnancy. Avoidance of these conditions may prevent clinical attacks (1).

Second Line
HAE acute treatment: FFP can be considered if first-line treatments unavailable; however, can potentially worsen attack, so caution is required.

ISSUES FOR REFERRAL
Patients presenting with first episode of AE with a positive family history or recurrent AE will benefit from management from allergy/immunology specialist.

ADMISSION, INPATIENT, AND NURSING CONSIDERATIONS
Need for admission is based on severity of airway involvement. Ishoo criteria can be used for risk stratification. All patients with respiratory distress or in need of airway support will benefit from treatment in an intensive care unit.

 ONGOING CARE

PATIENT EDUCATION
Educate on avoidance of identified triggers, types of treatment, when to seek emergency care, and wearing medical alert bracelet.

PROGNOSIS
- AE symptoms often resolve in hours to 2 to 4 days. If airway is compromised, AE can be life-threatening.
- Patients with HAE have an average of 20 attacks per year; each may last 3 to 5 days. Prophylaxis can decrease the frequency of events and number of missed days of school or work.

REFERENCES
1. Cicardi M, Aberer W, Banerji A, et al. Classification, diagnosis, and approach to treatment for angioedema: consensus report from the Hereditary Angioedema International Working Group. *Allergy.* 2014;69(5):602–616.
2. Patel G, Pongracic JA. Hereditary and acquired angioedema. *Allergy Asthma Proc.* 2019;40(6):441–445.

 SEE ALSO

Anaphylaxis; Urticaria

 CODES

ICD10
- T78.3XXA Angioneurotic edema, initial encounter
- D84.1 Defects in the complement system

CLINICAL PEARLS
- AE is an acute, localized swelling of skin, mucosa, and submucosa caused by extravasation of fluid into the affected tissues.
- If AE occurs in the presence of wheals, the patients should be diagnosed with urticaria and not AE.
- Onset is in minutes to hours and often resolves in hours to days, but it can be life-threatening if the upper airway is involved.
- There are two major classifications of AE: AAE and HAE.
- Any recurrent AE requires referral for specialist management.
- ARBs are an appropriate substitute for patients with ACEI-AAE because they have a low incidence of cross-reactivity.

ANKLE FRACTURES

Jeffrey P. Feden, MD, FACEP

BASICS

- Bones: tibia, fibula, talus
- Mortise joint: tibial plafond, fibula above (forming medial and lateral malleolus) and talus below
- Ligaments: syndesmotic, lateral collateral, and medial collateral (deltoid) ligaments

DESCRIPTION
- Two common classification systems help describe most fractures (but do not always predict fracture stability).
  - Danis-Weber: based on level of the fibular fracture in relationship to the tibiotalar joint
    - Type A (30%): below ankle joint; usually stable
    - Type B (63%): at the level of the ankle joint; may be stable or unstable
    - Type C (7%): above ankle joint; usually unstable
  - Lauge-Hansen (LH): based on foot position and direction of applied force relative to the tibia
    - Supination-adduction (SA)
    - Supination-external rotation (SER): most common (40–75% of fractures)
    - Pronation-abduction (PA)
    - Pronation-external rotation (PER)
- Stability-based classification
  - Stable
    - Isolated lateral malleolar fractures (Weber A/B) without talar shift and with negative stress test
    - Isolated nondisplaced medial malleolar fractures
  - Unstable
    - Bi- or trimalleolar fractures
    - High fibular fractures (Weber C) or lateral malleolar fracture with medial injury and positive stress test
    - Lateral malleolar fracture with talar shift/tilt (bimalleolar equivalent)
    - Displaced medial malleolar fractures
- Pilon fracture: tibial plafond fracture due to axial loading (unstable)
- Maisonneuve fracture: fracture of proximal 1/3 of fibula associated with ankle fracture or ligament disruption (unstable); high risk of peroneal nerve injury

Pediatric Considerations
- Ankle fractures are more common than sprains in children compared to adults because ligaments are stronger than physis.
- Talar dome fracture: osteochondral fracture of talar dome; suspect in child with nonhealing ankle "sprain" or recurrent effusions
- Tillaux fracture: isolated Salter-Harris III of distal tibia with growth plate involvement
- Triplane fracture: Salter-Harris IV with fracture lines oriented in multiple planes: 2-, 3-, and 4-part variants

EPIDEMIOLOGY
- Ankle fractures are responsible for 9% of all adult and 5% of all pediatric fractures.
- Peak incidence: females 45 to 64 years; males 8 to 15 years (average is 46 years)

Incidence
107 to 184 per 100,000 people per year

ETIOLOGY AND PATHOPHYSIOLOGY
- Most common: falls (38%), inversion injury (32%), sports related (10%)
- Plantar flexion (joint less stable in this position)
- Axial loading: tibial plafond or pilon fracture

RISK FACTORS
- Age, fall, fracture history, polypharmacy, intoxication
- Obesity, sedentary lifestyle
- Sports, physical activity
- History of smoking or diabetes
- Alcohol or slippery surfaces

GENERAL PREVENTION
- Nonslip, flat, protective shoes
- Fall precautions in elderly

COMMONLY ASSOCIATED CONDITIONS
- Most ankle fractures are isolated injuries, but 5% have associated fractures, usually in ipsilateral lower limb.
- Ligamentous or cartilage injury (sprains)
- Tibiotalar or subtalar dislocation
- Other axial loading or shearing injuries (i.e., vertebral compression or pelvic fractures)

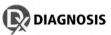

DIAGNOSIS

HISTORY
- Location of pain, timing, and mechanism of injury (key historical element is exact mechanism)
- Weight-bearing status after injury
- History of ankle injury or surgery
- Tetanus status
- Assess for safety and fall risk (especially in elderly)

PHYSICAL EXAM
- Examine skin integrity (open vs. closed fracture).
- Assess point of maximal tenderness.
- Palpate joints above and below, especially noting tenderness at the proximal fibula.
- Assess neurovascular status and ability to bear weight.
- Consider associated injuries.
- Assess ankle stability: anterior drawer test for the anterior talofibular ligament (ATFL), talar tilt test for lateral and medial ligaments, squeeze test and external rotation stress test for the tibiofibular syndesmosis

DIFFERENTIAL DIAGNOSIS
- Ankle sprain, including syndesmotic ("high ankle") sprain
- Other fractures: talus, 5th metatarsal, calcaneus
- Achilles tendon injury

DIAGNOSTIC TESTS & INTERPRETATION
- Plain radiographs: first line for suspected fractures based on pretest probability (Ottawa Ankle Rules [OAR])
- OAR: Overall sensitivity of 98% in adults increases to 99.6% if applied within the first 48 hours after trauma (1)[A].

- OAR—obtain films in patients aged 18 to 55 years if:
  - Tenderness at the posterior edge of distal 6 cm of tibia or tip of the medial malleolus, *or*
  - Tenderness at the posterior edge or distal 6 cm of fibula or tip of the lateral malleolus, *or*
  - Inability to bear weight both immediately and in the ED for four steps, *or*
  - Tenderness at navicular or 5th metatarsal (Ottawa Foot Rules)
- If initial x-ray is normal, but severe symptoms persist past 48 to 72 hours, obtain repeat x-rays.
- In children >1 year old, OAR sensitivity is 98.5%.
- OAR not valid for intoxicated patients, those with multiple injuries, or sensory deficits (neuropathy)
- Three standard views
  - Anteroposterior (AP)
  - Lateral: talar dome/distal tibia incongruity indicates instability.
  - Mortise (15- to 25-degree internal rotation view): symmetry of mortise; space between the medial malleolus and talus (i.e., medial clear space) should be ≤4 mm.
  - Additional stress view may demonstrate instability (e.g., increased medial clear space with manual external rotation).

Pediatric Considerations
- Consider tenderness over distal fibula with normal films as Salter-Harris I.
- Stress views are unnecessary in children and may cause physeal damage.
- Salter-Harris V often missed and diagnosed with leg-length discrepancy or angular deformity after Salter-Harris I; rare, 1% of fractures

Follow-Up Tests & Special Considerations
- CT recommended for operative planning in trimalleolar, Tillaux, triplane, pilon fractures, or fractures with intra-articular involvement
- CT may be considered for radiographically occult talus fracture if clinical suspicion warrants.
- MRI not routinely indicated; does not increase sensitivity for detecting complex ankle fractures
  - MRI useful for chronic instability, osteochondral lesions, occult fractures, and unexpected stiffness in children

Diagnostic Procedures/Other
- Ultrasound for soft tissue injury associated with displaced fractures
- Bone scan or MRI for stress fracture

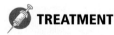

TREATMENT

GENERAL MEASURES
- Immobilize in temporary cast/splint and protect with crutches/non–weight-bearing.
  - 1 to 2 weeks to allow decreased swelling, if not open or irreducible fracture
- Ice and elevate the extremity; pain due to swelling is best controlled with elevation.
  - Compression stockings offer no benefit for swelling.

- Closed ankle fractures—must determine stability
  - Stable = nonoperative management
  - Unstable = surgery
  - Lateral shift of talus ≥2 mm or displacement of either malleolus by 2 to 3 mm = surgery
  - In adults with displaced fractures: insufficient evidence if surgery or nonoperative management produces superior long-term outcomes (2)[A]
- Stable syndesmosis injury = nonoperative
- Fracture dislocations: urgent reduction
  - Do not wait for imaging if neurovascular compromise, obvious deformity, or skin tenting.
  - Flex hip and knee 90 degrees for easier reduction.
  - Postreduction: neurovascular exam and x-rays

MEDICATION
First Line
- NSAIDs and/or acetaminophen for pain
- Initial IM pain injection (i.e., ketorolac, ≥50 kg adult: 60 mg or 30 mg q6h, max 120 mg daily; children 2 to 16 years old, <50 kg or age of ≥65 years: 1 mg/kg, 30 mg, or 15 mg q6h, max 60 mg daily)
- For suspected open fractures: tetanus booster, broad-spectrum cephalosporin and aminoglycoside within 3 hours postinjury
- Intra-articular or hematoma block

ISSUES FOR REFERRAL
- Consultation for neurovascular compromise, tenting of skin or open fracture, displaced or unstable fracture, compartment syndrome
- All other fractures: Follow up within 1 week and if remain non–weight-bearing. Consult orthopedics if uncomfortable with routine fracture management.

ADDITIONAL THERAPIES
- Nonoperative = cast immobilization
  - No difference in type of immobilization (Air-Stirrup ankle brace, cast, orthosis)
  - Initially, non–weight-bearing with crutches and then advance to 50% with crutches; full weight-bearing after 6 weeks postinjury
  - If removable cast, gentle range of motion exercises at 4 weeks
- Open ankle fractures (2%)
  - Remove gross debris/contamination in ED.
  - Duration of optimal antibiotic therapy controversial
  - Surgical emergency; best if repaired within 24 hours

SURGERY/OTHER PROCEDURES
- Surgical options
  - Open reduction and internal fixation (ORIF); preferred in athletes and unstable fractures
  - External fixation may be preferred in extreme tissue injury or comminuted fractures; may have more malunion compared to ORIF but no difference in wound complications
- Timing of surgery
  - Immediately if neurovascular compromise, open fracture, unsuccessful reduction, tissue necrosis
  - Otherwise, delay >5 days postinjury because inflammation can affect wound healing.
- Length of recovery is usually 6 to 8 weeks.

Pediatric Considerations
- Salter-Harris I and II = nonoperative
  - Distal tibia: long leg cast for 4 to 6 weeks and then short leg cast for 2 to 3 weeks
  - Distal fibula: posterior splint or ankle brace 3 to 4 weeks, weight-bearing; if displaced, then short leg cast 4 to 6 weeks, non–weight-bearing
  - Limit reduction attempts because of potential injury to growth plate.
  - Reduction not recommended if presenting ≥1 week postinjury
  - Intra-articular displacement of ≥2 mm in child with >2 years growth remaining = ORIF
- Salter-Harris III and IV:
  - Distal tibia: if >2 mm displacement = ORIF
  - Distal fibula: rare, usually stable after tibial reduction
  - Tillaux and triplane fractures: ORIF if displaced ≥2 mm

Geriatric Considerations
- Higher surgical risk due to age/comorbidities
- Osteoporosis increases risk of implant/fixation failure (2)[A].
- Risks from surgery/anesthesia: wound healing problems, pulmonary embolism, mortality, amputation, reoperation

ADMISSION, INPATIENT, AND NURSING CONSIDERATIONS
- Admit if:
  - Emergency surgery required
  - Patient nonadherent, lacks social support, unable to maintain non–weight-bearing status, or has significant associated injuries
  - Concerning mechanism of injury (i.e., syncope, myocardial infarction, head injury)
- Nursing: non–weight-bearing; maintain splint/cast; apply ice; keep leg elevated; pain control; assist ADLs.
- Discharge criteria:
  - Ambulates with walker or crutches
  - Medical workup (if needed) completed
  - Orthopedic follow-up arranged

ONGOING CARE

FOLLOW-UP RECOMMENDATIONS
Patient Monitoring
- Orthopedic follow-up: serial x-rays
  - In children, sclerotic lines on x-ray (Parker-Harris growth arrest lines) indicate growth disturbance.
- Immobilize for 4 to 6 weeks and then progressive activity, weight-bearing, with removable splint or boot.
- Physical therapy referral: no difference in outcomes between stretching, manual therapy, exercise program

PATIENT EDUCATION
- Ice and elevate for 2 to 3 weeks; use crutches/cane as instructed; splint/cast care (avoid getting wet, etc.)
- Notify physician if swelling increases, paresthesias, pain, or change in color of extremity.

PROGNOSIS
- Good results can be achieved without surgery if fracture is stable.
  - Most return to activity within 3 to 4 months.
- Most athletes return to preinjury activity levels.
- Increasing age, *not* injury severity, is associated with worsening mobility after fracture.

COMPLICATIONS
- Displaced fracture or instability
- Delayed union, malunion, or nonunion (0.9–1.9%)
- Postsurgical wound problems: loss of fixation, further surgery, amputation
- Deep venous thrombosis
- Complex regional pain syndrome, extensor retinaculum syndrome in children
- Infection (osteomyelitis)
- Posttraumatic arthritis, degenerative joint disease, growth arrest in children

REFERENCES
1. Polzer H, Kanz KG, Prall WC, et al. Diagnosis and treatment of acute ankle injuries: development of an evidence-based algorithm. *Orthop Rev (Pavia)*. 2012;4(1):e5.
2. Donken CCMA, Al-Khateeb H, Verhofstad MHJ, et al. Surgical versus conservative interventions for treating ankle fractures in adults. *Cochrane Database Syst Rev*. 2012;(8):CD008470.

CODES

ICD10
- S82.899A Oth fracture of unsp lower leg, init for clos fx
- S82.899B Oth fracture of unsp lower leg, init for opn fx type I/2
- S82.56XA Nondisp fx of medial malleolus of unsp tibia, init

CLINICAL PEARLS
- OAR are nearly 100% sensitive in determining the need for x-rays.
- Assess neurovascular status, ability to bear weight, and associated injuries.
- Assess joint above/below to avoid overlooking extent of injury (i.e., Maisonneuve fracture).
- Consider possibility of radiographically occult fracture (e.g., talus fracture).
- Normal x-rays with point tenderness suggest Salter-Harris type I fractures in children.
- Assessment of fracture stability (using classification systems) often dictates conservative versus operative management.

ANKYLOSING SPONDYLITIS

Elizabeth T. Nguyen, MD

BASICS

DESCRIPTION
- Ankylosing spondylitis (AS) is an axial inflammatory spondyloarthropathy (axSpA) characterized by chronic low back pain (>3 months duration) and evidence of sacroiliitis (sclerosis, erosions, and changes in joint width) on plain radiography.
  - Terminology of "axSpA" comprises whole spectrum of patients with radiographic evidence of sacroiliitis (AS) or nonradiographic axSpA (nr-axSpA)
  - Both AS and nr-axSpA are largely similar in disease presentation and treatment received.
- Systems affected: musculoskeletal; ophthalmic; cardiovascular; neurologic; pulmonary; gastrointestinal
- Synonyms: Marie–Strümpell disease; "bamboo spine"

EPIDEMIOLOGY
- Peak onset typically before age of 30 years; rarely occurs after age 45 years
- Male > female (approximately 2:1) for AS
  - Studies vary with effect of gender on AS.
  - Peripheral disease
    - Higher prevalence of anterior uveitis in men versus higher prevalence of peripheral arthritis and psoriasis in women
  - Men with family history of AS at higher risk
- Approximately 1 in 200 people affected by AS and >1 in 100 by axSpA (axial spondyloarthritis)

Incidence
Affects 0.1–0.5% of the population

Prevalence
Prevalence of axSpA among adults in the USA varies from 0.9% to 1.4%.

ETIOLOGY AND PATHOPHYSIOLOGY
- Autoinflammation at sites of bacterial exposure (e.g., intestines) or mechanical stress in genetically susceptible individuals
- Inflammation at the insertion of tendons, ligaments, and fasciae to bone (enthesopathy) causes erosion, remodeling, and new bone formation.

Genetics
- 85–95% of patients with AS are *HLA-B27*–positive (1)[C].
- Other genetic associations include endoplasmic reticulum aminopeptidase 1 (*ERAP1*) and interleukin-23 receptor (*IL23R*).

RISK FACTORS
- Positive family history
  - Concordance rates of 63% for HLA-B27–positive monozygotic twins and 27% for dizygotic twins
- Gut microbiome theory
  - 57–70% of patients with AS had asymptomatic intestinal inflammation in terminal ileum.
- Current smoking (not history of smoking)

COMMONLY ASSOCIATED CONDITIONS
- Peripheral arthritis
- Enthesopathy: Achilles tendonitis, plantar fasciitis (prevalence of 35–60%)
- Uveitis (prevalence of 6–30%)
- Psoriasis(prevalence of 10%)
- Dactylitis "sausage digit"
- Inflammatory bowel disease (IBD) (prevalence of 4–6%)

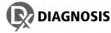

DIAGNOSIS

HISTORY
- Inflammatory back pain
  - Insidious onset typically at age <45 years; duration >3 months; insidious onset; nighttime awakenings secondary to back pain; pain and stiffness increase at rest and improve with activity.
- Alternating buttock/hip pain and constitutional symptoms (fatigue, poor sleep, weight loss, low-grade fever) are common and may appear before radiographic evidence of the disease.
- Other symptoms associated with enthesopathy (Achilles tendon pain, plantar fascia pain), dactylitis (sausage digits), iritis (unilateral pain, red eye, photophobia, vision changes/blurring)

PHYSICAL EXAM
- Sacroiliac (SI) joint tenderness, loss of lumbar lordosis, and cervical spine rotation
  - Low sensitivity and specificity for physical examination of sacroiliitis
- Diminished range of motion in the lumbar spine in all three planes of motion
- Tenderness of tendon insertional sites—Achilles, plantar fascia
- Peripheral oligoarthritis/dactylitis seen mostly with peripheral SpA
- Extra-articular manifestations: uveitis, psoriasis, IBD

DIFFERENTIAL DIAGNOSIS
- Mechanical low back pain
- Other inflammatory arthritis
- Osteoarthritis or erosive osteochondritis of the axial spine
- Infectious arthritis or discitis, unilateral sacroiliitis
- Vertebral compression fracture
- Fibromyalgia—tender points can mimic enthesitis findings

DIAGNOSTIC TESTS & INTERPRETATION
- ESR and C-reactive protein (CRP) may be mildly elevated or normal; if high, correlates with disease activity and prognosis
- HLA-B27 testing
- SI joints:
  - Can do a single, anteroposterior view. Oblique view may also provide useful information but require slightly higher radiation levels.
  - Radiographic interpretation can vary in results for interpretation of sacroiliitis and can be challenging.
- If pelvic radiographic negative or equivocal, consider pelvic MRI to evaluate for active inflammation.
- Spine: lateral view preferred
  - Can help rule out other causes of back pain
- In adults with AS of unclear activity while on a biologic, conditionally recommendations are to obtain a spinal or pelvis MRI to assess activity. No recommendation to obtain spinal or pelvis MRI to confirm inactivity of adults with stable AS (2)

Initial Tests (lab, imaging)
Diagnosis is based off of the Assessment of SpondyloArthritis international Society (ASAS) criteria.
- 2009 ASAS classification:
  - If a patient has low back pain for at least 3 months and is <45 years old and there is concern for AS based off of history and physical, obtain an anterior-posterior x-ray of the SI joints.
    - If sacroiliitis suspected on imaging plus at least 1 or more SpA feature *or*
    - HLA-B-27–positive plus at least 2 or more SpA features (as below):
      - SpA features include arthritis, colitis, Crohn disease, dactylitis, elevated CRP, enthesitis, family history of SpA, good response to nonsteroidal anti-inflammatory drugs (NSAIDs), positive HLA-B27, inflammatory back pain, psoriasis, or uveitis
- 1984 modified New York criteria for AS—must fulfill radiologic criteria and at least one or more clinical criteria
  - Clinical criteria
    - Low back pain and stiffness >3 months that improves with exercises and not relieved by rest
    - Limitation of motion of lumbar spine in flexion and extension
    - Limitation of chest expansion relative to normal values correlated for age and sex
  - Radiological criteria
    - Sacroiliitis at least grade 2 bilaterally or grade 3–4 unilaterally
  - If patients have negative radiographic imaging and negative HLA-B27 but two to three SpA features, can consider MRI of SI joint

Follow-Up Tests & Special Considerations
- Routine monitoring of radiographic changes with serial spine radiographs is not recommended (2)
- If significant change in course of disease occurs, causes other than inflammation, such as spinal fracture, should be considered and appropriate evaluation should be performed (3).

TREATMENT

GENERAL MEASURES
- Symptom control, maintaining spinal flexibility and normal posture, reducing functional limitations, maintaining work ability, and decreasing disease complications are primary treatment goals.
- Aggressive physical therapy is the most important nonpharmacologic management (3)[A].

MEDICATION
First Line
- NSAIDs are first-line pharmacologic agent for pain and stiffness in AS.
  - Naproxen, up to 500 mg BID; celecoxib, up to 200 mg BID; ibuprofen, up to 800 mg TID
  - In adults with stable AS, when continuous use is not needed to control symptoms, conditionally recommend per American College of Rheumatology (ACR) on-demand treatment with NSAIDs (3)[A].

- Precautions
  - Consider CVD, GI, and renal risks of NSAIDs. Use with caution in patients with a bleeding diathesis or on anticoagulants.
- Injection of intra-articular corticosteroids into SI joints and prostheses can provide transient relief, but systemic corticosteroids are not recommended.
  - Consider with patients with mainly peripheral symptoms (i.e., isolated sacroiliitis or enthesitis) who have had limited response to NSAIDs

Second Line
- Biologic agents: tumor necrosis factor inhibitors (TNFi), interleukin-17 inhibitors (IL-17i), and Janus kinase inhibitors (JAKi)
  - TNFi: infliximab, etanercept, adalimumab, certolizumab, golimumab
  - IL-17i: secukinumab, ixekizumab
  - JAKi: tofacitinib
- Recommended for active disease after lack of response to at least two different NSAIDs over 2–4 weeks and primarily axial disease (vs. mainly peripheral symptoms).
- In adults with active AS despite treatment with NSAIDs, recommend treatment with TNFi first, and then treatment with secukinumab (IL-17i) or ixekizumab (IL-17i) over sulfasalazine, methotrexate, or tofacitinib (JAKi) (2).
  - If history of recurrent uveitis or active IBD: can use TNFi monoclonal antibody
  - If history of significant psoriasis: IL-17i preferred
- Precautions with TNFi
  - TNFi increase the risk of serious bacterial, mycobacterial, fungal, opportunistic, malignancies, and viral infections. Screen for tuberculosis and hepatitis B.
  - Immunizations (especially live vaccines) should be updated before initiating anti-TNFs; live vaccines are contraindicated once patients receive anti-TNFs.
- Disease-modifying antirheumatic drugs (DMARDs), such as methotrexate and sulfasalazine, are ineffective for axial disease; sulfasalazine may be effective for peripheral arthritis; this class may be considered in patients with contraindications to TNF agents (2)[C].
- Recommendations for tapering if in remission or switching choices differ currently between ACR and ASAS-EULAR.

ISSUES FOR REFERRAL
- Coordinate care with a rheumatologist for diagnosis, monitoring, and management (anti-TNF therapy).
- Management of extra-articular manifestations and other systemic conditions may require referral to appropriate specialty.

SURGERY/OTHER PROCEDURES
- Evaluate for C-spine ankylosis/instability before intubation in patients with AS undergoing surgery.
- Consider total hip arthroplasty in patients with refractory pain or disability and radiographic evidence of structural damage, independent of age.
- Spinal corrective osteotomy can be considered in patients with severe disabling deformity, although less evidence for this and recommendations differ (i.e., between ACR and ASAS-EULAR).

 ## ONGOING CARE

FOLLOW-UP RECOMMENDATIONS
Patient Monitoring
- Monitor posture and range of motion with 6- to 12-month visits; increase frequency if higher disease activity.
- Bath Ankylosing Spondylitis Disease Activity Index (BASDAI) or Ankylosing Spondylitis Disease Activity Score (ASDAS) can be used to measure disease activity.
- Fall prevention/evaluation
- Regular-interval monitoring of CRP or ESR
- Screening for osteopenia/osteoporosis with dual energy x-ray absorptiometry scan

PATIENT EDUCATION
- Maintain physical activity and posture. Avoid trauma/contact sports.
- Swimming, water aerobics, tai chi, and walking are excellent activities.
- Arthritis Foundation: http://www.arthritis.org
- Spondylitis Association of America: http://www.spondylitis.org

PROGNOSIS
Extent and rapidity of progression of condition are highly variable.

COMPLICATIONS
- MSK/spine: osteoporosis, spinal fusion causing kyphosis, c-spine fracture or subluxation, cauda equina syndrome (rare)
- Pulmonary: restrictive lung disease, upper lobe fibrosis (rare)
- Cardiac: conduction defects at atrioventricular (AV) node, aortic insufficiency, aortitis, pericarditis (extremely rare)
- Eye: uveitis, cataracts
- Renal: IgA nephropathy, amyloidosis (<1%)
- GI: microscopic, subclinical ileal, and colonic mucosal ulcerations in up to 50% of patients, mostly asymptomatic

REFERENCES
1. Hwang MC, Ridley L, Reveille JD. Ankylosing spondylitis risk factors: a systematic literature review. *Clin Rheumatol*. 2021;40(8):3079–3093.
2. Ward MM, Deodhar A, Gensler LS, et al. 2019 Update of the American College of Rheumatology/Spondylitis Association of America/Spondyloarthritis Research and Treatment Network Recommendations for the Treatment of Ankylosing Spondylitis and Nonradiographic Axial Spondyloarthritis. *Arthritis Rheumatol*. 2019;71(10):1599–1613.
3. Ramiro S, Nikiphorou E, Sepriano A, et al. ASAS-EULAR recommendations for the management of axial spondyloarthritis: 2022 update. *Ann Rheum Dis*. 2023;82(1):19–34.

ADDITIONAL READING
- Adams K, Bombardier C, van der Heijde DM. Safety of pain therapy during pregnancy and lactation in patients with inflammatory arthritis: a systematic literature review. *J Rheumatol Suppl*. 2012;90: 59–61.
- Gensler L, Inman R, Deodhar A. The "knowns" and "unknowns" of biologic therapy in ankylosing spondylitis. *Am J Med Sci*. 2012;343(5):360–363.
- Mease PJ. Fibromyalgia, a missed comorbidity in spondyloarthritis: prevalence and impact on assessment and treatment. *Curr Opin Rheumatol*. 2017;29(4):304–310.
- Sieper J. Treatment challenges in axial spondylarthritis and future directions. *Curr Rheumatol Rep*. 2013;15(9):356.
- Sieper J, Rudwaleit M, Baraliakos X, et al. The Assessment of Spondyloarthritis International Society (ASAS) handbook: a guide to assess spondyloarthritis. *Ann Rheum Dis*. 2009; 68(Suppl 2):ii1–ii44.
- Walsh JA, Magrey M. Clinical manifestations and diagnosis of axial spondyloarthritis. *J Clin Rheumatol*. 2021;27(8):e547–e560.

 ## SEE ALSO

Arthritis, Psoriatic; Arthritis, Rheumatoid (RA); Crohn Disease; Reactive Arthritis (Reiter Syndrome); Ulcerative Colitis

 ## CODES

ICD10
- M45.0 Ankylosing spondylitis of multiple sites in spine
- M45.6 Ankylosing spondylitis lumbar region
- M45.7 Ankylosing spondylitis of lumbosacral region

CLINICAL PEARLS
- Diagnosis of AS is suggested by a history of inflammatory back pain, restricted spinal motion, radiographic evidence of sacroiliitis, and response to NSAIDs.
- HLA-B27 testing supports the diagnosis if clinical features are not definitive.
- MRI is more sensitive at detecting SI joint inflammation than plain radiography.
- Physical therapy is important in helping to maintain posture and mobility.
- NSAIDs and TNFi are the mainstays of pharmacologic treatment of AS.

ANOREXIA NERVOSA

Jennifer E. Cavin, MD

BASICS

DESCRIPTION

- An eating disorder characterized by the restriction of food intake leading to significantly low weight with intense fear of weight gain and distorted perception of body weight and shape
- *Diagnostic and Statistical Manual of Mental Disorders*, 5th edition (*DSM-5*) divides anorexia into two types:
  - Restricting type: characterized by restricting intake of calories or extreme amounts of exercise without binge-eating and purging behaviors within the last 3 months
  - Binge-eating/purging type: regular engagement in binge intake or purging behaviors within the past 3 months
- System(s) affected: nervous, cardiovascular, endocrine, metabolic, pulmonary, gastrointestinal, reproductive, ophthalmic, taste, and dermatologic
- Severity of anorexia nervosa (AN) is based on BMI; severe is <15 kg/m².

EPIDEMIOLOGY
Prevalence
- Estimated lifetime prevalence among U.S. adults of 0.5%
- Median age of onset age: 17 years
- Predominant sex: female > male (10:1 to 20:1 female-to-male ratio)

ETIOLOGY AND PATHOPHYSIOLOGY
- Complex relationships among genetic, biologic, environmental, psychological, and social factors that result in the development of this disorder
- Serotonin, norepinephrine, and dopamine neuronal systems are implicated.

Genetics
- Aggregates in families—11-fold risk among female relatives of a proband with the disorder
- Evidence of high concordance rates in monozygotic than in dizygotic twins
- GWAS study showing 8 loci exceeding genome wide significance on chromosomes 1, 3, 10, and 11.

RISK FACTORS
- Body dissatisfaction, negative self-evaluation
- Perfectionism, high parental demands, academic pressure, severe life stressors
- History of sexual or physical abuse or parental maltreatment
- Participation in sports or activities that emphasize leanness: ballet, figure skating, gymnastics, cheerleading
- Type 1 diabetes mellitus
- Family history of substance abuse, affective disorders, or eating disorders

GENERAL PREVENTION
Prevention programs for adolescents and young women ≥15 years can reduce risk factors and future onset of eating disorders.
- Encourage realistic and healthy weight management strategies and attitudes.
- Promote self-esteem; reduce focus on thin as ideal.
- Decrease co-occurring anxiety/depressive symptoms and improve stress management.

COMMONLY ASSOCIATED CONDITIONS
- Suicide, mood and anxiety disorders
- Substance use disorder
- Cluster C personality disorder

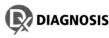DIAGNOSIS

DSM-5 diagnosis of AN requires these three criteria:
- Restriction of energy intake that leads to a low body weight
- Intense fear of weight gain or becoming obese, or continuous behavior that prevents weight gain, despite being considered underweight
- Distorted perception of body weight, body shape, and undue influence of weight on self-worth or denial of the medical seriousness of low body weight

HISTORY
- Onset may be insidious or stress related.
- Patient unlikely to self-identify problem
- Restriction of required energy intake, leading to significantly low body weight
- Fear of weight gain and/or distorted body image and preoccupation with body size (even of certain body parts and weight control)
- Elaborate food preparation and eating rituals.
- Other possible signs and symptoms:
  - Extensive exercise
  - Amenorrhea
  - Weakness, fatigue, cognitive impairment
  - Cold intolerance
  - Constipation, bloating, early satiety
  - Growth arrest, delayed puberty
  - Fractures
- Screening recommended by the USPSTF (SCOFF) (1)
  - Do you make yourself Sick because you feel uncomfortably full? (Yes is abnormal.)
  - Do you worry you have lost Control over how much you eat? (Yes is abnormal.)
  - Have you recently lost more than One stone (14 pounds or 6.35 kg) in a 3-month period? (Yes is abnormal.)
  - Do you believe yourself to be Fat when others say you are too thin? (Yes is abnormal.)
  - Would you say that Food dominates your life? (Yes is abnormal.)

PHYSICAL EXAM
- May be normal
- Abnormal vital signs: hypothermia, bradycardia, orthostatic hypotension
- Body weight <85% of expected (may wear extra clothes or hide heavy objects to increase weight on scale)
- Cardiac: dysrhythmias, midsystolic click from mitral valve prolapse
- Skin/extremities: dry skin; lanugo hair on extremities, face, and trunk; hair loss; peripheral edema
- Neurologic and abdominal exams: to rule out other causes of weight loss and vomiting
- Gynecologic: amenorrhea

DIFFERENTIAL DIAGNOSIS
- Hyperthyroidism, adrenal insufficiency
- IBS, malabsorption
- Immunodeficiency, chronic infections
- Uncontrolled diabetes
- Bulimia, body dysmorphic disorder, restrictive eating disorder not otherwise specified
- Depressive, anxiety, or conversion disorders

DIAGNOSTIC TESTS & INTERPRETATION
Initial Tests (lab, imaging)
- Vitals: hypotension, bradycardia, hypothermia
- UA: low specific gravity, ketone, low urine creatinine excretion
- CBC: anemia, leukopenia, thrombocytopenia
- Low-serum LH, FSH; low-serum testosterone in men
- Thyroid function tests: low thyroid-stimulating hormone with normal T_3/T_4
- LFT: abnormal liver enzymes
- Chem 7: altered BUN, creatinine clearance; electrolyte disturbances including hyponatremia, hypokalemia
- Hypoglycemia, hypercholesterolemia, hypercortisolemia, hypophosphatemia, hypomagnesemia
- Low vitamin D and hypocalcemia
- 12-Lead EKG to assess for prolonged QT interval
- If underweight for >6 months: DEXA scan to assess for diminished bone density

Follow-Up Tests & Special Considerations
Weighting is an anxiety-provoking test but an important marker to assess progress. Ask staff to be nonjudgmental. Try to weight patients in a gown, as many intend to exaggerate their weight by hiding heavy objects or wearing baggy clothes.

Test Interpretation
- Osteoporosis/osteopenia, pathologic fractures
- Sick euthyroid syndrome, dehydration

TREATMENT

GENERAL MEASURES
- OP treatment: for patients who are not medically unstable, are highly motivated, and able to control eating and exercising behaviors
  - Interdisciplinary team (primary care physician, mental health provider, dietitian)
  - Average weekly weight gain goal: 0.5 to 1.0 kg, with stepwise increase in calories
  - CBT
  - Focus on health, not on weight gain alone.
  - Build trust and a treatment alliance.
  - Involve the patient in establishing diet and exercise goals.
  - Help the patient to recognize feelings that lead to disordered eating.
  - In chronic cases, goal may be to achieve a safe weight rather than a healthy weight.

- Inpatient treatment if medically unstable, or with comorbid psychiatric issues, or unable to control eating and exercise behaviors
  - If possible, admit to a specialized eating disorders unit.
  - Monitor vital signs, electrolytes, cardiac function, edema, and weight.
  - Assess risk for refeeding syndrome—potentially fatal shift in fluid and electrolyte balance with restoration of nutrition characterized by hypophosphatemia, hypokalemia, seizures, CHF, rhabdomyolysis, peripheral edema
  - Initial supervised meals may be necessary.
  - Stepwise increase in activity
  - Tube feeding or TPN is used only as a last resort.
- CBT has demonstrated effectiveness as a means of improving treatment adherence and minimizing dropout among patients with AN (2)[A].

MEDICATION

First Line
- No medications are available that effectively treat patients with AN, but pharmacotherapy may be used as an adjuvant to CBTs (3)[A].
- If medications are used, start with low doses due to increased risk for adverse effects.
- SSRIs may:
  - Help to prevent relapse after weight gain.
  - Treat comorbid depression or OCD.
  - Use of atypical antipsychotics is being studied with mixed findings to date. Olanzapine is potentially beneficial as an adjuvant treatment of underweight individuals in the inpatient settings.
- Attend to black box warnings.
- Bupropion should be avoided because it is associated with a higher incidence of seizures.

Second Line
- Management of osteopenia:
  - Primary treatment is weight gain.
  - Elemental calcium 1,200 to 1,500 mg/day plus vitamin D 800 IU/day
  - No indication for bisphosphonates in AN
  - Weak evidence for use of hormone-replacement therapy
- Psyllium to prevent constipation

ISSUES FOR REFERRAL
Patients with AN benefit from an interdisciplinary team

ADMISSION, INPATIENT, AND NURSING CONSIDERATIONS
- Suggested physiologic values to admit: heart rate <40 beats/min, BP <90/60 mm Hg, symptomatic hypoglycemia, temperature <97°F (36.1°C), dehydration, other cardiovascular abnormalities, weight <75% of expected, rapid weight loss, lack of improvement while in OP therapy
- Suggested psychological indications: poor motivation/insight, lack of cooperation with OP treatment, inability to eat, need for nasogastric feeding, suicidal intent or plan, severe coexisting psychiatric disease, problematic family environment
- Suggested lab indications: potassium <3 mmol/L, prolonged QTC (>0.499 ms), urine specific gravity >1.03 or <1.01

Pediatric Considerations
- Children often present with nausea, abdominal pain, fullness, and inability to swallow.
- Additional indications for hospitalization: heart rate <50 beats/min, orthostatic BP, hypokalemia or hypophosphatemia, rapid weight loss even if weight not <75% below normal

Geriatric Considerations
- Late-onset AN (>50 years of age) may be a long-term disease or triggered by death of loved one, marital discord, divorce, or depression.
- Always consider other organic causes of weight loss.

ONGOING CARE

FOLLOW-UP RECOMMENDATIONS
- Family and individual therapy is extremely important for long-term outcomes.
- Emphasize importance of moderate activity for health.

Patient Monitoring
- Level of exercise activity
- Weigh weekly until stable, then monthly.
- Depression, suicidal ideation

DIET
Dietary consultation and nutritional education programs

PATIENT EDUCATION
- http://www.mayoclinic.org/diseases-conditions/anorexia/home/ovc-20179508
- National Alliance on Mental Illness: http://www.nami.org/Learn-More/Mental-Health-Conditions/Eating-Disorders

PROGNOSIS
- Prognosis: ~50% recover, 30% improve, 20% are chronically ill
- Mortality: 5–18% (annual mortality rate of 5 per 1,000 person-years)

ALERT
High risk of suicide (approximately 1 in 5 individuals with AN who died had committed suicide) (4)[A]

COMPLICATIONS
- Refeeding syndrome
- Cardiac arrhythmia, cardiac arrest, cardiomyopathy, congestive heart failure
- Delayed gastric emptying, necrotizing colitis
- Seizures, Wernicke encephalopathy, peripheral neuropathy, cognitive deficits
- Osteopenia, osteoporosis

Pregnancy Considerations
- Behaviors may persist, decrease, or recur during pregnancy and the postpartum interval.
- Increased risk for preterm labor, operative delivery, and infants with low birth weight; anemia, genitourinary infections, and labor induction should be managed as high risk.

REFERENCES

1. Hill LS, Reid F, Morgan JF, et al. SCOFF, the development of an eating disorder screening questionnaire. *Int J Eat Disord*. 2010;43(4):344–351.
2. Galsworthy-Francis L, Allan S. Cognitive behavioural therapy for anorexia nervosa: a systematic review. *Clin Psychol Rev*. 2014;34(1):54–72.
3. Claudino AM, Hay P, Lima MS, et al. Antidepressants for anorexia nervosa. *Cochrane Database Syst Rev*. 2006;(1):CD004365.
4. Arcelus J, Mitchell AJ, Wales J, et al. Mortality rates in patients with anorexia nervosa and other eating disorders. A meta-analysis of 36 studies. *Arch Gen Psychiatry*. 2011;68(7):724–731.

ADDITIONAL READING

American Psychiatric Association. *Practice Guideline for the Treatment of Patients with Eating Disorders*. 3rd ed. Arlington, VA: American Psychiatric Association; 2006.

SEE ALSO

- Amenorrhea; Bulimia Nervosa; Osteoporosis and Osteopenia
- Algorithm: Weight Loss, Unintentional

CODES

ICD10
- F50.01 Anorexia nervosa, restricting type
- F50.02 Anorexia nervosa, binge eating/purging type
- F50.00 Anorexia nervosa, unspecified

CLINICAL PEARLS

- "Are you satisfied with your eating patterns?" or "Do you worry that you have lost control over how you eat?" may help to screen those with an eating problem.
- Assess for suicide risk.
- Studies have shown that patients with AN will not accept medications unless combined with psychotherapy.
- To care for a patient with AN, an interdisciplinary team that includes a medical provider, a dietitian, and a behavioral health professional is the most accepted approach.

ANTIPHOSPHOLIPID ANTIBODY SYNDROME

Juliana Chang, MD

 BASICS

DESCRIPTION

Antiphospholipid antibody syndrome (APS) is a systemic autoantibody-mediated thrombophilic disorder characterized by recurrent arterial or venous thrombosis and/or recurrent fetal loss in the presence of persistent antiphospholipid antibodies (APAs) as evidenced by lupus anticoagulant (LAC), anticardiolipin antibodies (aCL), and/or anti–β_2 glycoprotein-I (GPI) antibody. The APAs enhance clot formation by interacting with phospholipid-binding plasma proteins. The resulting APS can cause morbidity and mortality in both pregnant and nonpregnant individuals:

- Types of APS (based on clinical presentation)
  - Primary: no underlying condition evident
  - Secondary: most commonly associated with autoimmune diseases like systemic lupus erythematosus (SLE); transient APAs have been linked to certain infections, drugs, and malignancies.
  - Catastrophic APS (CAPS) a.k.a. Asherson syndrome (<1%)
    - Most severe form of disease; characterized by thrombotic microangiopathy and associated with multiorgan failure that develops at the same time
    - High mortality if treatment is delayed

Pregnancy Considerations
- Complications include maternal venous thromboembolism, stroke, fetal demise, preeclampsia and placental insufficiency, fetal growth retardation, miscarriage, and preterm birth.
- Low-dose aspirin and low-molecular-weight heparin (LMWH) or unfractionated heparin are the drugs of choice in pregnancy.
- Prophylactic-dose heparin is recommended in the postpartum period (unless patient is on therapeutic anticoagulation) given high risk of thrombosis. With adequate treatment, >70% of patients with APS deliver viable infants.

EPIDEMIOLOGY
- The prevalence of APAs increases with age but is not necessarily associated with a higher risk of thrombosis.
- For APS, female > male

Incidence
- Incidence of APS is around 5 new cases per 100,000 persons per year.
- In patients with positive APAs without prior risk of thrombosis, the annual incident risk of thrombosis is 0–3.8%. This risk is increased to 5.3% in those with triple positivity. 10–15% of recurrent abortions are attributable to APS.

Prevalence
Prevalence around 40 to 50 cases per 100,000 persons per year; APAs are present in 1–5% of the general population and in ~40% of those with SLE. A higher prevalence of 10–15% is seen in those with venous thromboembolism, fetal loss, and stroke.

ETIOLOGY AND PATHOPHYSIOLOGY
- Anti–β_2-GP1 antibodies play a central role in the pathogenesis of APS. The procoagulant effect is mediated by various possible mechanisms:
  - Endothelial effects: inhibition of prostacyclin production and loss of annexin V cellular shield
  - Platelet activation resulting in adhesion and aggregation

- Interference of innate anticoagulant pathways (such as inhibition of protein C)
  - Complement activation
- Pregnancy-related complications are also a result of autoantibody-mediated effects:
  - Interference with expression of trophoblastic adhesion molecules resulting in abnormal placentation and placental thrombosis
- Proposed mechanisms: excess production of natural antibodies, molecular mimicry due to infections, exposure of phospholipid antigens during platelet activation, cardiolipin peroxidation, and genetic predisposition
- A "second hit" by environmental factors is often required to manifest APS.

Genetics
Most cases of APS are acquired.

RISK FACTORS
- Age >55 years in males, >65 years in females
- Cardiovascular risk factors (hypertension [HTN], hyperlipidemia, diabetes, obesity, smoking, combined oral contraceptive use)
- Underlying autoimmune disease (SLE, rheumatoid arthritis, collagen vascular disease, Sjögren syndrome, idiopathic thrombocytopenic purpura, Behçet syndrome)
- Positive APAs
- Surgery, immobilization, pregnancy

GENERAL PREVENTION
Risk factor modification: control HTN and diabetes; smoking cessation; avoidance of oral estrogen contraceptives in high-risk patients; start thromboprophylaxis in established cases; preconception assessment

COMMONLY ASSOCIATED CONDITIONS
- Autoimmune diseases: SLE (most common), scleroderma, Sjögren syndrome, dermatomyositis, and rheumatoid arthritis
- SLE is the most common autoimmune disease associated with APS.
- Malignancy
- Infections: viral, bacterial, parasitic, and rickettsial
- Certain drugs associated with APA production without increased risk of thrombosis: phenothiazines, hydralazine, procainamide, and phenytoin
- Hemolysis, elevated liver enzymes, and low platelet count in association with pregnancy (HELLP) syndrome
- Sneddon syndrome (APS variant syndrome with livedo reticularis, HTN, and stroke)

DIAGNOSIS

Sapporo criteria (also called Sydney criteria), revised 2006:
- At least one of the following clinical criteria:
  - Vascular thrombosis
    - ≥1 clinical episodes of arterial, venous, or small vessel thrombosis, occurring within any tissue or organ and confirmed by unequivocal imaging studies or histopathology without associated inflammation in the vessel wall
    - Superficial venous thrombosis does not meet the criteria for APS.

- Complications of pregnancy (any one of the following):
  - ≥3 consecutive spontaneous abortions before the 10th week of pregnancy, unexplained by maternal/paternal chromosomal abnormalities or maternal anatomic/hormonal causes
  - ≥1 unexplained deaths of morphologically normal fetuses (documented by ultrasonography or by direct examination) at ≥10th week of gestation
  - ≥1 premature births of morphologically normal newborn babies at ≤34th week of pregnancy due to severe preeclampsia, eclampsia, or placental insufficiency
- *And* the presence of at least one of three laboratory findings (confirmed on ≥2 occasions at least 12 weeks apart):
  - LAC detected in blood
  - Anticardiolipin IgG and/or IgM antibodies present at moderate or high levels in the blood (>40 GPL or MPL or >99th percentile) via a standardized ELISA
  - Anti–β_2-GP1 IgG and/or IgM antibodies in blood at a titer >99th percentile by standardized ELISA

HISTORY
- History of venous thromboembolism or arterial thrombosis (stroke, MI)
- History of recurrent fetal loss or other obstetric complications (one miscarriage >10 weeks or one or more premature births before the 34th week of gestation due to preeclampsia, eclampsia, or placenta insufficiency of >3 unexplained consecutive abortions before the 10th week of gestation with maternal anatomic or hormonal abnormalities)
- Bleeding from thrombocytopenia if severe or acquired factor II deficiency
- Personal or family history of autoimmune disease

PHYSICAL EXAM
- Signs of venous thrombosis in extremities
- Skin manifestations, including a vasculitic rash in the form of palpable purpura or livedo reticularis, superficial thrombophlebitis, or lower extremity ulcers
- Livedo reticularis
- Cardiac murmurs
- Focal neurologic or cognitive deficits

DIFFERENTIAL DIAGNOSIS
- Thrombophilic conditions
  - Inherited: deficiency of protein C, protein S, antithrombin III; mutation of factor V Leiden, prothrombin gene mutation
  - Acquired: neoplastic and myeloproliferative disorders, hyperviscosity syndromes, nephrotic syndrome
- Embolic disease secondary to atrial fibrillation, LV dysfunction, endocarditis, cholesterol emboli
- Disseminated intravascular coagulation
- Paroxysmal nocturnal hemoglobinuria
- Heparin-induced thrombocytopenia
- Behçet syndrome
- CAPS: hemolytic-uremic syndrome, TTP, or malignant HTN

DIAGNOSTIC TESTS & INTERPRETATION

- LAC assay and IgG and IGM aCL by ELISA and anti–β_2-GP1 IgG and IgM antibodies are diagnostic tests of choice.
- The LAC assay combines at least two out of three screening tests (prolongation of aPTT, dilute Russell viper venom time [dRVVT], and kaolin clotting) with two confirmatory tests.
- A weakly positive LAC result should be considered clinically important (1).
- Anti–β_2-GP1 antibodies are important in the pathogenesis of thrombosis. A positive LAC assay recognizes antibodies against β_2-GP1 and prothrombin.

Initial Tests (lab, imaging)
- CBC, PT/INR, aPTT, LAC, aCL, anti–β_2-GP1 antibodies
- Prevalence of APAs in SLE ranges from 11% to 87%; hence, it is important to screen for SLE.
- Imaging is based on clinical picture, suspected sites of thrombosis, and organ involvement.

Follow-Up Tests & Special Considerations
- The results of LAC are difficult to interpret in patients treated with warfarin. Unfractionated heparin or LMWH and fondaparinux do not affect the LAC assay.
- Repeat testing at 12 weeks for persistence of APA.

Diagnostic Procedures/Other
Biopsy of the affected organ system may be necessary to distinguish from vasculitis.

Test Interpretation
Usual finding is thrombosis and minimal vascular or perivascular inflammation:

- Acute changes: capillary congestion and noninflammatory fibrin thrombi
- Chronic changes: ischemic hypoperfusion, atrophy, and fibrosis

 TREATMENT

MEDICATION

First Line
- Primary thromboprophylaxis is controversial in patients with APS and no clinical symptoms. A 2018 Cochrane review involving nine studies and 1,044 randomized participants failed to show conclusive benefit of aspirin in patients without a thrombotic event. Low-dose aspirin or heparin is indicated only in patients with a high risk of thrombosis because the overall risk of thrombosis is <4%.
- Secondary thromboprophylaxis: All symptomatic, nonpregnant patients with APS need indefinite anticoagulation. The target INR depends on the severity and type of thrombosis:
  – Venous thrombosis (first episode): warfarin with target INR of 2 to 3
  – Arterial thrombosis or recurrent venous thrombosis despite anticoagulation: warfarin with target INR of 3 to 4
  – LMWH and fondaparinux are alternatives.

- Direct oral anticoagulants (DOACs) such as rivaroxaban, apixaban, and dabigatran; all have been approved for treatment of DVT/PE; however, studies in APS are lacking; a prospective randomized trial in 2016 of warfarin versus rivaroxaban in patients with thrombotic APS showed increase in endogenous thrombin potential in patients who switched to rivaroxaban. The 15th International Congress on Antiphospholipid Antibodies Task Force published in 2017 concluded that there is an insufficient evidence to recommend DOACs in APS. DOACs may be alternatives to warfarin in patients intolerant to warfarin. A 3-year, open-label, randomized noninferiority trial in 2019 did not show noninferiority of rivaroxaban to dose-adjusted VKAs for thrombotic APS and moreover showed a non-statistically significant near doubling of the risk for recurrent thrombosis.
  – Rituximab may be an option in severe cases, possibly in those with thrombotic microangiopathy.
- Danaparoid, fondaparinux, and argatroban can be considered in heparin-induced thrombocytopenia.
- Statins can decrease proinflammatory and pro-thrombotic state in APS but are not recommended in the absence of hyperlipidemia.
- Hydroxychloroquine can be added in recalcitrant APS.
- Eculizumab may be useful in refractory cases.
- Vitamin D deficiency/insufficiency should be corrected in all APA-positive patients.
- Low-dose aspirin is superior to low-dose aspirin with low-dose warfarin due to decreased bleeding risk with no differences in number of thrombosis.
- CAPS: Anticoagulants and high-dose steroids may suffice in less severe cases. Aggressive treatment with either IVIG or plasma exchange is often required in severe cases. These measures have improved survival up to 66%.
- Treatment in pregnancy:
  – Patients with APS and no prior thrombotic events may be offered low-dose aspirin during pregnancy; treatment decisions should be individualized though.
  – For women with no prior history of thrombosis and ≥2 early miscarriages, treat with either 81 mg aspirin alone or in combination with unfractionated heparin (5,000 to 10,000 U SC q12h) or LMWH (prophylactic dose). In those with a previous late pregnancy loss (>10 weeks' gestation) or preterm (<34 weeks) delivery due to severe preeclampsia, a combination of aspirin and heparin is recommended.
  – Preconception assessment and treatment with low-dose aspirin, vitamin D, and folate should be offered in selected patients.
  – In those with a history of thrombosis, low-dose aspirin plus either therapeutic low-dose heparin (dosed every 8 to 12 hours to maintain mid-interval aPTT or factor Xa levels) or LMWH (therapeutic dose)
  – Refractory cases: Up to 30% of patients have recurrent pregnancy loss despite the use of aspirin and heparin. There is no role for warfarin due to risk of teratogenicity. Such cases are best managed in consultation with a maternal–fetal medicine specialist.

 ONGOING CARE

DIET
Patients on warfarin should limit foods rich in vitamin K (kale, spinach, sprouts, greens).

PATIENT EDUCATION
- Compliance with warfarin therapy to keep INR at goal
- Awareness of drug and diet interactions with warfarin
- Avoid oral hormonal contraceptives.

PROGNOSIS
- Pulmonary HTN, neurologic involvement, myocardial ischemia, nephropathy, gangrene of extremities, and CAPS are associated with a worse prognosis.
- 30% risk of recurrent thrombosis in the absence of adequate anticoagulation

COMPLICATIONS
- Pregnancy complications and pulmonary HTN are associated with higher morbidity and mortality.
- Thrombotic complications are the common cause of death.

REFERENCE

1. Bertolaccini ML, Amengual O, Andreoli L, et al. 14th International Congress on Antiphospholipid Antibodies Task Force. Report on antiphospholipid syndrome laboratory diagnostics and trends. *Autoimmun Rev*. 2014;13(9):917–930.

CODES

ICD10
- D68.61 Antiphospholipid syndrome
- D68.69 Other thrombophilia
- D68.62 Lupus anticoagulant syndrome

CLINICAL PEARLS

- APS is a multisystem autoimmune disorder with recurrent arterial/venous thrombosis and fetal loss and positive APAs.
- Both clinical and laboratory criteria are required for diagnosis. The latter must be confirmed on two separate occasions at least 12 weeks apart.
- APS requires lifelong anticoagulation.

ANXIETY (GENERALIZED ANXIETY DISORDER)

Rhonda A. Faulkner, PhD • Daniella Davida Brutman, MD

 BASICS

DESCRIPTION
- Persistent, excessive, and difficult-to-control worry associated with significant symptoms of motor tension, autonomic hyperactivity, and/or disturbances of sleep or concentration
- System(s) affected: nervous (increased sympathetic tone and catecholamine release), cardiac (tachycardia), pulmonary (dyspnea), and GI (nausea, irregular bowels)

EPIDEMIOLOGY
Prevalence
- Lifetime prevalence in United States: 5.1–11.9%
- Onset at any age but typically during adulthood; median age of onset in the United States is 31 years.
- Female > male (2:1)

ETIOLOGY AND PATHOPHYSIOLOGY
- May be mediated by abnormalities of neurotransmitter systems (serotonin, norepinephrine, γ-aminobutyric acid [GABA])
- Associated with altered regional brain function (increased activity in the amygdala and prefrontal cortex)

Genetics
A serotonin transporter gene (5HT1A) may contribute to GAD.

RISK FACTORS
- Adverse life events (illness, poverty, etc.)
- Family history
- Comorbid psychiatric disorders (1)

GENERAL PREVENTION
- Physical activity and cardiorespiratory fitness are associated with decreased generalized anxiety.
- Cognitive-behavioral therapy (CBT) and parental intervention in children with early anxiety may protect against GAD (1).

COMMONLY ASSOCIATED CONDITIONS
- Major depressive disorder (>60%), dysthymia, bipolar disorder, schizophrenia
- Alcohol/drug abuse; cigarette smoking
- Panic disorder, agoraphobia, phobia, social anxiety disorder, anorexia nervosa, PTSD, ADHD
- Somatoform and pain disorders

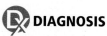 **DIAGNOSIS**

HISTORY
Diagnosis is primarily through history. Pathologic anxiety must be distinguished from normal anxiety reactions.
- *DSM-5* criteria are as follows:
  - Symptoms of excessive anxiety and worry occur more often than not for at least 6 months.
  - Difficult to control the worry.
  - At least three additional criteria for diagnosis of GAD in adults; only one in children
    ○ Restlessness or feeling keyed up or on edge
    ○ Easily fatigued

○ Difficulty concentrating or mind going blank
○ Irritability
○ Muscle tension
○ Sleep disturbances (difficulty falling or staying asleep)
- Persistent worry must cause significant distress or impairment in social, occupational, or other areas of functioning.
- Focus of anxiety and worry is not consistent with or limited to the occurrence of other types of psychiatric disorders and is not directly related to PTSD.
- Symptoms are not the result of a substance, another medical condition, or other *DSM-5* diagnosis.

PHYSICAL EXAM
No specific physical findings in GAD; patients may exhibit irritability, bitten nails, tremor, or clammy hands.

DIFFERENTIAL DIAGNOSIS
- Cardiovascular: ischemic heart disease, mitral valve prolapse, cardiomyopathies, arrhythmias, congestive heart failure
- Respiratory: asthma, chronic obstructive pulmonary disease, pulmonary embolism
- CNS: stroke, seizures, dementia, migraine, vestibular dysfunction, neoplasms
- Metabolic and hormonal: hyper- or hypothyroidism, pheochromocytoma, adrenal insufficiency, Cushing syndrome, hypokalemia, hypoglycemia, hyperparathyroidism
- Drug-induced anxiety: alcohol, sympathomimetics (cocaine, amphetamine, caffeine), corticosteroids, herbals (ginseng)
- Withdrawal: alcohol, sedative-hypnotics
- Psychiatric: panic disorder, OCD, PTSD, social phobia, adjustment disorder, and somatization disorder

DIAGNOSTIC TESTS & INTERPRETATION
Initial Tests (lab, imaging)
- Lab tests are normal. Initial tests may include thyroid-stimulating hormone, CBC, BMP, urine drug screen, and ECG.
- GAD-2: two-question self-reporting scale (22% positive predictive value [PPV]/78% negative predictive value [NPV])
- PHQ-4 provides a very brief screen for both anxiety and depression (1).

Diagnostic Procedures/Other
Psychological testing
- GAD-7: provides more detailed information for treatment (29% PPV/71% NPV); also may be indicative of panic disorder (GAD-7: 29% PPV/71% NPV)
- Hamilton Anxiety Scale (HAM-A), Anxiety Disorders Interview Schedule (ADIS-IV)
- Children: ADIS-IV Parent and Child Version, Multidimensional Anxiety Scale for Children (MASC), Screen for Child Anxiety Related Emotional Disorders (SCARED)

 TREATMENT

GENERAL MEASURES
- Assess for suicidality.
- Identify and treat coexisting substance abuse and other psychiatric conditions.
- Delayed treatment may result in poorer outcomes compared with treatment within 1 year of symptom onset.
- Remission may not occur until 4 to 6 months of treatment. Treat for ≥12 months.
- Psychotherapeutic approaches
  - Psychological treatments are effective in treating GAD: number needed to treat (NNT) = 2 (2)[A].
  - CBT: most well-studied psychological treatment; may improve comorbid conditions; treatment of choice (1)[A]
  - Psychodynamic psychotherapy: patient discovering and verbalizing unconscious conflicts (1)[C]

MEDICATION
First Line
- SSRIs and SNRIs have demonstrated efficacy, are well-tolerated, do not cause abuse/dependence, and treat comorbid depression. Data to compare between agents are limited (3)[A].
- Medication selection based on side-effect profile, drug–drug interactions, and/or patient treatment history/preference.
- For SSRIs/SNRIs, start at lowest available dose, uptitrate every 2 to 4 weeks, use highest tolerated FDA-approved dose for at least 4 to 6 weeks before deeming ineffective or switching to a different SSRI/SNRI. Taper gradually to discontinue.
- Switching between medications without adequate dose or duration of therapy can lead to ineffective treatment.
- Common side effects of SSRIs: nausea, diarrhea, insomnia, agitation or sedation, drug interactions, weight gain, and sexual side effects (decreased libido, delayed orgasm)
- Common side effects of SNRIs: nausea, dizziness, insomnia, sedation, constipation, sweating, and blood pressure elevation
- SSRI: escitalopram (Lexapro): initially 10 mg/day; may titrate to a max of 20 mg/day (4)[A]
- SNRIs:
  - Duloxetine (Cymbalta): initially 30 mg/day; may titrate by 30 mg/day qwk to a max of 120 mg/day; doses >60 mg/day rarely more effective (4)[A]
  - Venlafaxine XR (Effexor XR): initially 37.5 to 75.0 mg; may titrate up by 75 mg every 4 days to a max of 225 mg/day (4)[A]
- Pregabalin (Lyrica): decreases anxiety scores and reduces relapse at 75 to 300 mg BID; less sexual dysfunction and sleep disruption than SSRIs; taper to discontinue; rapid onset of action (off-label) (4)[A]

Second Line

- Sertraline (Zoloft): initially 25 mg/day; may titrate by 25 to 50 mg/day qwk to a max of 200 mg/day (4)[B]
- Azapirones: buspirone (BuSpar): less dependence risk; 15 mg/day divided BID–TID initially; max of 60 mg/day divided BID–TID (4)[B]
- Fluoxetine (Prozac): 10 to 20 mg/day; may titrate up to 60 mg/day (off-label) (4)[B]
- Mirtazapine (Remeron): 15 mg nightly; titrate in increments of 15 mg qwk; max dose of 45 mg daily; use as monotherapy or adjunct to SSRI; most common side effect is drowsiness (off-label) (4)[B].
- Paroxetine (Paxil): initially 10 to 20 mg/day; may titrate by 10 mg/day qwk to a max of 50 mg/day (no added benefit >20 mg/day); efficacious but poorly tolerated (4)[A]
- Quetiapine (Seroquel): optimal dose 150 mg/day; efficacious but less well tolerated than SSRIs; consider as augmentation (4)[A].
- Citalopram (Celexa) likely has efficacy for GAD but does not have FDA indication.
- Benzodiazepines: efficacious in the short term, less effective in the long term, risk for dependence/abuse (3),(4)[A]
  - Clonazepam (Klonopin): 0.25 mg BID; may increase to 4 mg/day divided BID
  - Diazepam (Valium): 2 to 5 mg BID–QID; may increase to max of 40 mg/day
  - Lorazepam (Ativan): 0.5 mg BID–TID; may increase to 6 mg/day divided TID
  - Alprazolam (Xanax): 0.25 mg TID; may increase to 4 mg/day
- Hydroxyzine (Vistaril, Atarax): CNS depressant, antihistamine, anticholinergic; decreased risk of dependence: usual dose: 50 to 100 mg PO QID; limit use in the elderly (2)[B].

Geriatric Considerations

- Avoid TCAs and long-acting benzodiazepines.
- Pregabalin may cause dizziness and somnolence.

Pediatric Considerations

- CBT is the first-line treatment for mild to moderate GAD.
- CBT with SSRI is the first-line treatment for severe GAD.
- Black box warning (SSRIs): Antidepressants increase the risk of suicidal thinking and behavior in children, adolescents, and young adults.
- SSRIs and SNRIs have all been shown to be effective, with SSRIs as the first-line choice.
- Anxiety and ADHD often co-occur. Treat the more debilitating first and consider using nonstimulating medications.

Pregnancy Considerations

- Buspirone: Category B, secreted in breast milk; inadequate studies to assess risk
- Benzodiazepines: Category D, may cause lethargy and weight loss in nursing infants; avoid breastfeeding if the mother is taking chronically or in high doses. The use shortly before delivery is associated with floppy infant syndrome.
  - Prenatal exposure to diazepam increases absolute risk of oral cleft by 0.01% (5).

- SSRIs: If possible, taper and discontinue. After 20 weeks' gestation, there is an increased risk of pulmonary hypertension; mild transient neonatal syndrome of CNS; and motor, respiratory, and GI signs. Studies regarding risk of autism show mixed results. Most are Category C, except for:
  - Paroxetine: Category D; conflicting evidence regarding risk of congenital cardiac defects and other congenital anomalies in 1st trimester; fetal echocardiography should be performed in mothers with 1st trimester exposure.
  - Hydroxyzine: Category C; case reports of neonatal withdrawal

ALERT

- Benzodiazepines: age >65 years, respiratory disease/sleep apnea, contraindicated with narrow-angle glaucoma, precaution with open-angle glaucoma; sudden discontinuation increases seizure risk. Long-term use has potential for tolerance and dependence; use with caution in patients with history of substance abuse.
- Buspirone: hepatic and/or renal dysfunction; mono-amine oxidase inhibitor (MAOI) treatment
- SSRIs: Use caution in those with comorbid bipolar disorder; may increase risk of serotonin syndrome, especially in combination with other serotonergic drugs

COMPLEMENTARY & ALTERNATIVE MEDICINE

- Probable benefit but more study needed for acupuncture, yoga, massage, tai chi, and aromatherapy (6)[B]
- Mindfulness-based stress reduction is noninferior to escitalopram in treating anxiety (3)
- Kava: some evidence for benefit in mild to moderate anxiety, but concern regarding potential hepatotoxicity (6)[B]
- Strong evidence to support regular physical activity (6)[A]
- Possible benefit from repetitive transcranial magnetic stimulation for pharmacotherapy treatment refractory patients
- Cannabidiol may have a beneficial role in the treatment of anxiety-related disorders and COVID-19 disease-related anxiety; more longitudinal studies are needed.
- Psilocybin with behavioral intervention may have a substantial additive benefit.

ONGOING CARE

FOLLOW-UP RECOMMENDATIONS

Patient Monitoring

- Follow up within 2 to 4 weeks from starting new medications.
- Medications should be continued past the initial period of response, and recommend continued treatment for 12 months.
- Monitor mental status on benzodiazepines and avoid drug dependence or abrupt discontinuation.
- Monitor all patients for suicidal ideation, especially those on SSRIs and SNRIs.
- Clinical follow-up with patient every 6 months is recommended.

DIET

Limit caffeine; avoid alcohol and nicotine.

PATIENT EDUCATION

- Regular exercise may be beneficial.
- Psychoeducation regarding normal versus pathologic anxiety and the physiology of anxiety can be helpful.

PROGNOSIS

Probability of recovery is 40–60%, but comorbid psychiatric disorders and poor relationships with family make relapse more likely.

REFERENCES

1. Patel G, Fancher TL. In the clinic. Generalized anxiety disorder. *Ann Intern Med.* 2013;159(11):ITC6-1–ITC6-12.
2. Cuijpers P, Sijbrandij M, Koole S, et al. Psychological treatment of generalized anxiety disorder: a meta-analysis. *Clin Psychol Rev.* 2014;34(2):130–140.
3. Huh J, Goebert D, Takeshita J, et al. Treatment of generalized anxiety disorder: a comprehensive review of the literature for psychopharmacologic alternatives to newer antidepressants and benzodiazepines. *Prim Care Companion CNS Disord.* 2011;13(2):PCC.08r00709.
4. Slee A, Nazareth I, Bondaronek P, et al. Pharmacological treatments for generalised anxiety disorder: a systemic review and network meta-analysis. *Lancet.* 2019;393(10173):768–777.
5. Armstrong C. ACOG guidelines on psychiatric medication use during pregnancy and lactation. American Family Physician. https://www.aafp.org/pubs/afp/issues/2008/0915/p772.html. Accessed October 3, 2023.
6. Sarris J, Moylan S, Camfield DA, et al. Complementary medicine, exercise, meditation, diet, and lifestyle modification for anxiety disorders: a review of current evidence. *Evid Based Complement Alternat Med.* 2012;2012:809653.

 SEE ALSO

Algorithms: Anxiety; Depressive Episode, Major

 CODES

ICD10

F41.1 Generalized anxiety disorder

CLINICAL PEARLS

- Psychiatric comorbidities, especially depression, are common with GAD; patients are at increased risk for suicidality.
- CBT and SSRIs/SNRIs are the treatments of choice.
- Start medication at low doses, with careful titration to therapeutic dosing, to minimize side effects and maximize efficacy.
- Benzodiazepines may be used initially but should be tapered and withdrawn if possible.

AORTIC VALVULAR STENOSIS

Grant Wei, MD, FACEP • Nisha J. Parikh, MD, MPH • Chirag N. Shah, MD

BASICS

DESCRIPTION
- Aortic stenosis (AS) is a narrowing of the aortic valve area (AVA) from leaflet fibrosis or calcification, leading to obstruction of the left ventricular (LV) outflow tract.
- AS has a long asymptomatic latency period.
- Development of severe obstruction, syncope, angina, and symptoms of congestive heart failure (CHF) have high mortality without surgical intervention.

EPIDEMIOLOGY
- AS is the most common acquired valve disease leading to operative intervention in Europe and North America (1).
- Cause by age at presentation: <30 years, congenital; 30 to 65 years, congenital or rheumatic fever (RF); >65 years, degenerative calcification of aortic valve

Prevalence
- Affects 1% of population 65 to 74 years old, 2% of 75 to 84 years old, 4% of >84 years old
- Bicuspid aortic valve present in 1–2% of population predisposes to AS at an earlier age.
- Progressive aortic leaflet thickening and calcification results in LV outflow obstruction. Obstruction causes increased afterload and decreased cardiac output.

ETIOLOGY AND PATHOPHYSIOLOGY
- An increase in LV systolic pressure is required to preserve cardiac output leading to concentric LV hypertrophy (LVH). This preserves ejection fraction but adversely affects heart functioning. LVH impairs coronary blood flow during diastole by compression of coronary arteries and reduced capillary ingrowth into hypertrophied muscle.
  - LVH results in diastolic dysfunction by reducing ventricular compliance. Diastolic dysfunction necessitates stronger left atrial (LA) contraction to augment preload and maintain stroke volume. Loss of LA contraction by atrial fibrillation can induce acute deterioration.
- Diastolic dysfunction may persist after AS interventions due to the presence of interstitial fibrosis.
- Degenerative calcific changes to aortic valve (2)
  - AS has an initiation phase caused by endothelial dysfunction and lipid deposition, followed by an inflammatory response, fibrosis, and calcification (3).
- Congenital: unicuspid valve, bicuspid valve, tricuspid valve with fusion of commissures, hypoplastic annulus
- RF: chronic scarring with fusion of commissures

Genetics
Bicuspid aortic valves display genetic variants involving mutations in NOTCH1 and GATA1 genes, which involve accelerated calcification in AS (3).

RISK FACTORS
- Congenital unicommissural valve or bicuspid valve
- RF
  - Prevalence of chronic rheumatic valvular disease has declined significantly in the United States. Most cases are associated with mitral valve disease.
- Degenerative calcific changes
  - Most common cause of acquired AS in the United States. Risk factors include hypercholesteremia, hypertension, cigarette smoking, male gender, age, diabetes mellitus, and arterial hypertension

GENERAL PREVENTION
Optimal management of hypertension, cardiac comorbid conditions, and smoking cessation; angiotensin-converting enzyme (ACE) and ARB inhibitors decrease LV fibrosis.

COMMONLY ASSOCIATED CONDITIONS
- Coronary artery disease (CAD) (50% of patients); hypertension (40% of patients)
- Aortic insufficiency (common in calcified bicuspid valves and rheumatic disease)
- Mitral valve disease: 95% of patients with AS from RF also have mitral valve disease.
- LV dysfunction and CHF
- Acquired von Willebrand disease: Impaired platelet function and decreased von Willebrand factor results in bleeding (ecchymosis and epistaxis) in 20% of AS patients. Severity of coagulopathy is directly related to severity of AS.
- Gastrointestinal arteriovenous malformations (AVMs)
- Cerebral or systemic embolic events due to calcium emboli

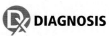

DIAGNOSIS

HISTORY
- Primary symptoms: angina, syncope, and heart failure; angina is the most frequent symptom. Syncope is often exertional. Heart failure symptoms include fatigue, exertional dyspnea, orthopnea, paroxysmal nocturnal dyspnea, and shortness of breath.
- Palpitations
- Neurologic events (transient ischemic attack or cerebrovascular accident) secondary to embolization
- Geriatric patients may have subtle symptoms such as fatigue and exertional dyspnea.
- Note: Symptoms do not always correlate with valve area (severity of AS) but most commonly occur when AVA is <1 cm², jet velocity is >4 m/s, or the mean transvalvular gradient is ≥40 mm Hg.

PHYSICAL EXAM
- Auscultation
  - Harsh, systolic crescendo–decrescendo murmur is best heard at 2nd right sternal border and radiates into the carotid arteries. Peak of murmur correlates with severity of stenosis; later peaking murmur suggests greater severity.
  - High-pitched blowing diastolic murmur suggests associated aortic insufficiency.
  - Paradoxically split S_2 or absent A_2. Note: Normally split S_2 reliably excludes severe AS.
  - S_4 due to stiffening of the left ventricle
- Other associated signs include *pulsus parvus et tardus*: decreased and delayed carotid upstroke, LV heave, and findings of CHF: pulmonary and/or lower extremity edema

DIFFERENTIAL DIAGNOSIS
- Mitral regurgitation: High-frequency, pansystolic murmur, best heard at the apex, often radiates to the axilla.
- Hypertrophic obstructive cardiomyopathy: also systolic crescendo–decrescendo murmur but best heard at left sternal border and may radiate into axilla; murmur intensity increases by changing from squatting to standing and/or by Valsalva maneuver.

- Discrete fixed subaortic stenosis: 50–65% has associated cardiac deformity (patent ductus arteriosus [PDA], ventricular septal defect [VSD], aortic coarctation).
- Aortic supravalvular stenosis: Williams syndrome, homozygous familial hypercholesterolemia

DIAGNOSTIC TESTS & INTERPRETATION
Initial Tests (lab, imaging)
- Chest x-ray (CXR)
  - May be normal in compensated, isolated valvular AS; boot-shaped heart reflective of concentric hypertrophy; poststenotic dilatation of ascending aorta and calcification of aortic valve (seen on PA/Lateral CXR)
- ECG: often normal ECG (ECG is nondiagnostic), or may show LVH, LA enlargement, and nonspecific ST- and T-wave abnormalities
- Echo indications
  - Initial workup
    - ○ Transthoracic echocardiogram (TTE): primary test in the diagnosis and evaluation of AS (1); assesses valve anatomy; severity of disease; LV wall thickness, size, and function; and pulmonary artery pressure
  - Based on AS severity, asymptomatic patients should have repeated TTE.
    - ○ Mild: every 3 to 5 years, moderate: 1 to 2 years, and severe: 6 to 12 months
- Echo findings
  - Aortic valve thickening, calcification; decreased aortic valve excursion; reduced AVA; transvalvular gradient across aortic valve; LVH and diastolic dysfunction; LV ejection fraction altered; wall-motion abnormalities suggesting CAD; evaluate for concomitant aortic insufficiency or mitral valve disease.
- AS severity based on echo values (2)[B]
  - Stage A (at risk): bicuspid aortic valve, sclerosis, or other congenital abnormality; mean pressure gradient: 0 mm Hg; jet velocity <2 m/s
  - Stage B (progressive): bicuspid or trileaflet valve
    - ○ Mild: mean pressure gradient: <20 mm Hg; jet velocity 2.0 to 2.9 m/s
    - ○ Moderate: mean pressure gradient: 20 to 40 mm Hg; jet velocity 3.0 to 3.9 m/s
  - Stage C (asymptomatic severe AS):
    - ○ C1 (without LV dysfunction): AVA ≤1 cm² or AVAi ≤0.6 cm²/m²; mean pressure gradient: 40 to 60 mm Hg; jet velocity ≥4 to 5 m/s
    - ○ C2 (with LV dysfunction): AVA ≤1 cm² or AVAi ≤0.6 cm²/m²; mean pressure gradient: ≥40 mm Hg; jet velocity ≥4 m/s
  - Stage D (symptomatic severe AS):
    - ○ D1 (high gradient): AVA ≤1 cm²; mean pressure gradient: >40 mm Hg; jet velocity >4 m/s
    - ○ D2 (low flow/low gradient with reduced EF <50%): AVA ≤1 cm²; mean pressure gradient: <40 mm Hg; jet velocity <4 m/s
    - ○ D3 (low gradient, normal EF ≥50% or paradoxical low-flow severe AS): AVA ≤1 cm²; AVAi ≤0.6 cm²/m²; stroke volume index <35 mL/m²; mean pressure gradient: <40 mm Hg; jet velocity <4 m/s

Diagnostic Procedures/Other

- Exercise stress testing
  - Asymptomatic patients with severe AS: helpful to uncover subtle symptoms or changes, abnormal BP (increase <20 mm Hg), and ECG changes (ST depressions). 1/3 of patients develop symptoms with exercise testing; *Stop* testing at this point.
  - Symptomatic patients: *Do not* perform exercise stress testing because it may induce hypotension or ventricular tachycardia.
  - CHF patients: Dobutamine stress echocardiography is reasonable to evaluate patients with low-flow/low-gradient AS and LV dysfunction.
- Cardiac catheterization
  - Perform prior to aortic valve replacement (AVR) in patients with suspected CAD; determines need for coronary artery bypass graft (CABG); if unambiguous diagnosis of AS, perform only coronary angiography.
  - Measures transvalvular flow and transvalvular pressure gradient, which facilitates calculation of effective valve area
- CT calcium scoring
  - Patient with low-flow, low-gradient AS with preserved AF
  - Calcium score >1,200 AU for women and >2,000 AU for men help predict severity AS and clinical outcomes.

Test Interpretation

- Aortic valve: nodular calcification on valve cusps (initially at bases), cusp rigidity, cusp thickening, and fibrosis
- LVH, myocardial interstitial fibrosis
- 50% incidence of concomitant CAD

 TREATMENT

MEDICATION

- No effective medical therapy for severe or symptomatic AS
- Currently, more research into the pro-inflammatory cytokines, clotting factors, and proteins involved in promoting calcification in AS are potential novel targets for medications.
  - PCSK9 inhibitors, simvastatin/ezetimib combination, and medications lowering lipoprotein A are promising therapeutics to prevent mild AS from worsening.
- Prevention: currently no recommended medical therapy; statins have been thought to slow progression if initiated during mild disease. However, this has not been supported by large, randomized controlled trials.
- Antibiotic prophylaxis against recurrent RF is indicated for patients with rheumatic AS (penicillin G 1,200,000 U IM q4wk; duration varies with age and history of carditis).
- Antibiotic prophylaxis is no longer indicated for prevention of infective endocarditis.
- Comorbidities: hypertension: ACE inhibitors, start with low dose and increase cautiously. Be cautious of vasodilators, which may cause hypotension.

SURGERY/OTHER PROCEDURES

- AVR is recommended for most symptomatic patients with evidence of significant AS on echocardiography.
  - If the AVA is >1.5 cm² and the mean pressure gradient is <15 mm Hg, there is no benefit from AVR.
- Transcatheter AVR (TAVR) versus surgical AVR has shown no difference in all-cause mortality in 1 year in severe, asymptomatic AS in ages ≥70 years with moderately increased operative risk.
- Indications for AVR surgery (2)[B]:
  - Symptomatic and severe high-gradient AS by history or exercise testing when surgical risk is low or intermediate
  - Asymptomatic, severe AS, and LVEF <50%
  - Severe AS (stage C or D) when undergoing other cardiac surgery
- AVR surgery is reasonable in patients who are (2)[B]:
  - Asymptomatic with severe AS (C1) with jet velocity ≥5 m/s and low surgical risk, decreased exercise tolerance, or have an exercise fall in blood pressure
  - Symptomatic stage D2 with low-dose dobutamine stress with jet velocity ≥4 m/s or mean pressure gradient ≥40 mm Hg with AVA ≤1 cm² at any dobutamine dose
  - Symptomatic stage D3 with LVEF >50% if clinical and hemodynamic data support valve obstruction as the likely cause of symptoms
  - Stage B patients who are undergoing other cardiac surgery, or asymptomatic stage C1 with rapid disease progression and low surgical risk
- TAVR offers a less invasive option for some patients (1)[C].
  - For those who are at high surgical risk and considered inoperable, TAVR has been shown to be superior to medical therapy.
  - For those who are at high surgical risk, TAVR has demonstrated noninferiority to surgical AVR.
  - For those who are at low or intermediate surgical risk, TAVR now a reasonable alternative to surgical AVR
  - Valve-in-valve TAVR can be considered in high-risk patients with failed surgically implanted bioprosthetic valves.
- Percutaneous balloon valvuloplasty may have role in palliation or as a bridge to valve replacement in hemodynamically unstable or high-risk patients but is not recommended as an alternative to valve replacement.

 ONGOING CARE

FOLLOW-UP RECOMMENDATIONS

Report symptoms referable to AS (angina, syncope). Asymptomatic patients: yearly history and physical; serial ECHO: yearly for severe AS, every 1 to 2 years for moderate AS, every 3 to 5 years for mild AS

PATIENT EDUCATION

Physical activity limitations

- Asymptomatic mild AS: no restrictions; asymptomatic moderate to severe AS: Avoid strenuous exercise. Consider exercise stress test prior to starting exercise program.

PROGNOSIS

- Although survival in asymptomatic patients is comparable to that in age- and sex-matched control patients, it decreases rapidly after symptoms appear.
- 25% mortality per year in symptomatic patients who do not undergo valve replacement; average survival is 2 to 3 years without AVR surgery; median survival in symptomatic AS: heart failure: 2 years; syncope: 3 years; angina: 5 years
- Perisurgical mortality: AVR surgery has 4% mortality rate; AVR + CABG has 6.8% mortality rate; adverse postoperative prognostic factors: age, heart failure New York Heart Association (NYHA) class III/IV, cerebrovascular disease, renal dysfunction, CAD

REFERENCES

1. Baumgartner H, Falk V, Bax JJ, et al; for ESC Scientific Document Group. 2017 ESC/EACTS guidelines for the management of valvular heart disease. *Eur Heart J.* 2017;38(36):2739–2791.
2. Nishimura RA, Otto CM, Bonow RO, et al. 2017 AHA/ACC focused update of the 2014 AHA/ACC guideline for the management of patients with valvular heart disease: a report of the American College of Cardiology/American Heart Association Task Force on Clinical Practice Guidelines. *Circulation.* 2017;135(25):e1159–e1195.
3. Goody PR, Hosen MR, Christmann D, et al. Aortic valve stenosis: from basic mechanisms to novel therapeutic targets. *Arterioscler Thromb Vasc Biol.* 2020;40(4):885–900.

CODES

ICD10

- I35.0 Nonrheumatic aortic (valve) stenosis
- I06.0 Rheumatic aortic stenosis
- Q23.0 Congenital stenosis of aortic valve

CLINICAL PEARLS

- AS is diagnosed on physical exam by a systolic crescendo–decrescendo murmur and delayed/diminished pulses.
- Symptomatic AS most commonly presents as angina, syncope, and heart failure.
- Symptomatic AS has a very poor prognosis unless treated with surgical intervention.

APPENDICITIS, ACUTE

Grant Wei, MD, FACEP • Mary E. Stuckey, MD • Chirag N. Shah, MD

BASICS

DESCRIPTION
- Acute inflammation of the appendix
- Simple or uncomplicated appendicitis occurs when there is no clinical or radiologic sign of perforation. Complicated or perforated appendicitis is defined by a palpable mass and phlegmon, perforation, or abscess on imaging.
- Arising from the base of the cecum in right lower quadrant (RLQ), the appendix can be anterior, posterior, medial, or lateral to the cecum as well as in the pelvis; vascular supply provided by appendicular artery, a branch of the ileocolic artery; nerve supply derived from the superior mesenteric plexus
- Most common cause of acute surgical abdomen

EPIDEMIOLOGY
- Predominant age: 10 to 30 years; rare in infancy; although uncommon, it can be more challenging to diagnose in elderly.
- Predominant sex: slight male predominance
  – Ages 10 to 30 years: male > female (3:2)
  – Age >30 years: male = female

Incidence
- 1 case per 1,000 people per year
- Lifetime incidence of 1 in every 15 people (7%)

Pregnancy Considerations
- Most common extrauterine surgical emergency
- Incidence similar in pregnancy
- Higher rate of perforation; more likely to present with peritonitis

ETIOLOGY AND PATHOPHYSIOLOGY
Obstruction of the appendiceal lumen is thought to lead to distention, ischemia, and bacterial overgrowth. Without intervention, appendicitis can lead to perforation and subsequent abscess formation or generalized peritonitis. Causes of obstruction are as follows:
- Fecaliths (most common)
- Lymphoid tissue hyperplasia (in children)
- Vegetables, fruit seeds, and other foreign bodies
- Intestinal worms (ascarids)
- Strictures, fibrosis, neoplasms

Genetics
First-degree relative with history of appendicitis increases risk; no direct genetic link found.

RISK FACTORS
Adolescent males, familial tendency, intra-abdominal tumors

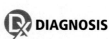

DIAGNOSIS

- Diagnosis relies on history and physical examination with supporting laboratory studies and imaging.
- Modified Alvarado Scoring System (MASS): The use of MASS in the diagnosis of acute appendicitis improves diagnostic accuracy and reduces negative appendectomy and complication rates (1)[B].
  – Pain migrating to RLQ (1 point)
  – Nausea/vomiting (1 point)
  – Anorexia (1 point)
  – RLQ tenderness (2 points)
  – Rebound tenderness (1 point)
  – Elevated temperature (1 point)

  – Leukocytosis (2 points)
  – Left shift (1 point)
  – A MASS score >7 suggests appendicitis without the need for further imaging.
  – A MASS score of 4 to 6 requires a CT scan for diagnosis of appendicitis. A cutoff point of 6 for the MASS score yields higher sensitivity but is also associated with a higher negative appendectomy rate (normal appendix).
  – A MASS score of ≤3 does not warrant a CT scan as appendicitis is seen as less likely.
  – Supplement MASS in female patients with additional investigations (e.g., abdominal ultrasound or laparoscopy).
- Pediatric Appendicitis Score—helps predict the likelihood of acute appendicitis (diagnosis is still clinical)

HISTORY
- Classic history is vague periumbilical pain, followed by anorexia, nausea, and vomiting. Over the next 4 to 48 hours, pain migrates to the RLQ.
- Only 50% of patients present with a classic history.
- Pain before vomiting (~100% sensitive), abdominal pain (~100%), pain migration (50%)
- Anorexia (~100%), nausea (90%), vomiting (75%), obstipation
- Atypical symptoms and pain suggest a retrocecal or pelvic appendix.

PHYSICAL EXAM
- Fever; temperature >100.4°F (may be absent); tachycardia
- RLQ tenderness; maximal tenderness at McBurney point (1/3 the distance from the anterior superior iliac spine to the umbilicus)
- Voluntary and involuntary guarding
- Rovsing sign: RLQ pain with palpation of left lower quadrant
- Psoas sign: pain with right thigh extension (retrocecal appendix)
- Obturator sign: pain with internal rotation of flexed right thigh (pelvic appendix); local and suprapubic pain on rectal exam (pelvic appendix)
- Pelvic and rectal exams are helpful to assess other causes of lower abdominal pain (e.g., pelvic inflammatory disease, prostatitis).
- Serial exams can be useful in indeterminate cases.

DIFFERENTIAL DIAGNOSIS
- GI
  – Gastroenteritis, inflammatory bowel disease
  – Diverticulitis, ileitis
  – Cholecystitis, pancreatitis
  – Intussusception, volvulus
- Gynecologic
  – Pelvic inflammatory disease, ectopic pregnancy
  – Ovarian cyst, ovarian torsion, tubo-ovarian abscess
  – Endometriosis
  – Ruptured graafian follicle
- Urologic
  – Testicular torsion, epididymitis
  – Kidney stones, prostatitis, cystitis, pyelonephritis
- Systemic
  – Diabetic ketoacidosis
  – Henoch-Schönlein purpura
  – Sickle cell crisis
  – Porphyria

- Other
  – Acute mesenteric lymphadenitis
  – No organic pathologic condition
  – Hernias
  – Psoas abscess
  – Rectus sheath hematoma
  – Epiploic appendagitis
  – Pneumonia (basilar)

Pediatric Considerations
- Decreased diagnostic accuracy of history and physical exam
- Higher fever; more vomiting and diarrhea

Pregnancy Considerations
- Appendicitis is more difficult to diagnose in pregnancy.
- Normal inflammatory response is suppressed.
- Appendix displaced out of pelvis by gravid uterus

Geriatric Considerations
Decreased diagnostic accuracy, more likely to be an atypical presentation

DIAGNOSTIC TESTS & INTERPRETATION

Initial Tests (lab, imaging)
- Leukocytosis: WBC >10,000/mm³ (70%)
- Polymorphonuclear predominance—"left shift" (>90%)
- Urinalysis: hematuria, pyuria (30%)
- Human chorionic gonadotropin (hCG) (If positive, rule out ectopic pregnancy.)
- C-reactive protein: nonspecific inflammatory marker; when paired with an elevated WBC, increases predictive value for appendicitis
- Drugs may alter lab results: antibiotics, steroids.
- Imaging if the diagnosis is not clear; helps to detect complications (abscess, perforation)
- Plain films: minimal utility, nonspecific findings, may visualize fecalith
- CT with contrast: sensitivity 91–98%; specificity 95–99%; imaging modality of choice; consider radiation dose, particularly in young patients.
- Ultrasound: alternative in pregnancy, children, and women with suspected gynecologic pathology; sensitivity and specificity vary with skill of the ultrasonographer; increasing use in adult populations, with positive predictive value approaching 100% in some studies; can rule in appendicitis but cannot reliably exclude the diagnosis; an effective strategy is to start with ultrasound and, if negative, obtain a CT scan if suspicion warrants.
- MRI: increasing use in pregnant patients; may help in patients with contrast allergies and renal failure; limitations include cost, availability, and time required to complete the study.
- Radioisotope-labeled WBC scans: may be used in patients with indeterminate CT scans and suspected appendicitis as an alternative to observation or surgery; limitations include availability and time required to complete the study.

Diagnostic Procedures/Other
- Exploratory laparotomy/laparoscopy
- Acceptable appendectomy rates vary based on age and gender and may be higher for females of childbearing age than males.

Test Interpretation
- Acute appendiceal inflammation, local vascular congestion, obstruction
- Gangrene, perforation with abscess (15–30%)
- Fecalith

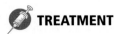 **TREATMENT**

GENERAL MEASURES
- Surgery (appendectomy) has been the standard of care for acute, uncomplicated appendicitis. Evidence suggests nonoperative management with antibiotics may be noninferior to appendectomy after 30 days but carries a 29% rate of recurrence with need for appendectomy within 90 days. Surgical treatment of uncomplicated appendicitis has a higher complication-free success rate (82.3%) than that of antibiotic treatment alone (67.2%) in both adult and pediatric patients.
- Generally, surgery is indicated for complicated or perforated appendicitis with abscess formation. For larger drainable abscesses, percutaneous drainage and antibiotics are recommended.

MEDICATION
First Line
- Uncomplicated acute appendicitis: perioperative dose of antibiotic: single dose of cefoxitin or ampicillin/sulbactam (Unasyn) or cefazolin plus metronidazole
- Nonoperative antibiotic of choice: IV ertapenem for 2 days followed by 5 days PO levofloxacin and metronidazole (2)[B]
- Gangrenous or perforating appendicitis
  - Broadened antibiotic coverage for aerobic and anaerobic enteric pathogens
  - Piperacillin and tazobactam (Zosyn) or ticarcillin and clavulanate (Timentin) or a 3rd-generation cephalosporin plus metronidazole are initial options.
  - Adjust dosage and choice of antibiotic based on intraoperative cultures.
  - Continue antibiotics for at least 7 days postoperatively or until patient becomes afebrile with normal WBC count.

Second Line
- Uncomplicated acute appendicitis: clindamycin plus one of the following: ciprofloxacin, levofloxacin, gentamicin, or aztreonam
- In the case of acute appendicitis complicated by abscess formation or phlegmon in pediatric patients, some studies show initial conservative management with antibiotics alone to carry fewer risks and complications than emergent appendectomy.
- Gangrenous or perforated appendicitis: ciprofloxacin or levofloxacin plus metronidazole or monotherapy with a carbapenem (imipenem and cilastatin, meropenem, ertapenem)

ISSUES FOR REFERRAL
All cases of appendicitis require emergent surgical consultation.

ADDITIONAL THERAPIES
A newer option for the treatment of acute appendicitis is currently being studied—endoscopic retrograde appendicitis therapy (ERAT). Studies thus far indicate high technical and clinical success rates (>99%), with very low rates of complication (0.19%) and a much lower recurrence rate (6.01%) than treatment with antibiotics only.

SURGERY/OTHER PROCEDURES
- The American College of Surgeons, Society for Surgery of the Alimentary Tract, and others recommend surgery as the treatment of choice.
- Antibiotic treatment might be used as an alternative in specific patients or if surgery is contraindicated.
- Nonoperative management with antibiotics with up to a reported 39% recurrence rate at 5 years for uncomplicated acute appendicitis

ADMISSION, INPATIENT, AND NURSING CONSIDERATIONS
- Admit all patients with appendicitis.
- Fluid resuscitation with normal saline (NS) or lactated Ringer (LR) solution
- Correct fluid and electrolyte deficits.
- Discharge when tolerating oral intake, return of bowel function, afebrile, normal WBC.

 ONGOING CARE

FOLLOW-UP RECOMMENDATIONS
- Return to work in 1 to 2 weeks is typical, following most cases of uncomplicated appendicitis.
- Restrict activity for 4 to 6 weeks after surgery: no heavy lifting (>10 lb) or strenuous physical activity.
- If managed nonoperatively and patient is >40 years of age, consider colonoscopy to rule out malignancy.

PATIENT EDUCATION
Postoperative warning signs:
- Anorexia, nausea, vomiting
- Abdominal pain, fever, chills
- Signs/symptoms of wound infection

PROGNOSIS
- Generally uncomplicated course in young adults with unruptured appendicitis
- Extremes of age and appendiceal rupture increase morbidity and mortality.
- Morbidity rates
  - Nonperforated appendicitis: 3%
  - Perforated appendicitis: 47%
- Mortality rates
  - Unruptured appendicitis: 0.1%
  - Ruptured appendicitis: 3%
  - Patients >60 years of age make up 50% of total deaths from appendicitis.
  - Older patients with ruptured appendix: 15%

Pediatric Considerations
- Rupture earlier
- Rupture rate: 15–60%

Pregnancy Considerations
- Rupture rate: 40%
- Fetal mortality rate: 2–8.5%

Geriatric Considerations
Rupture rate: 67–90%

COMPLICATIONS
- Intestinal fistulas
- Intestinal obstruction, paralytic ileus, incisional hernia
- Liver abscess (rare), pyelophlebitis
- Stump appendicitis: recurrence of appendicitis at appendiceal stump after appendectomy

REFERENCES
1. Abdella Bahta NN, Zeinert P, Rosenberg J, et al. The Alvarado score is the most impactful diagnostic tool for appendicitis: a bibliometric analysis. *J Surg Res*. 2023;291:557–566.
2. Sippola S, Haijanen J, Grönroos J, et al. Effect of oral moxifloxacin vs intravenous ertapenem plus oral levofloxacin for treatment of uncomplicated acute appendicitis: the APPAC II randomized clinical trial. *JAMA*. 2021;325(4):353–362.

 SEE ALSO

Algorithm: Abdominal Rigidity

CODES

ICD10
- K35.80 Unspecified acute appendicitis
- K35.2 Acute appendicitis with generalized peritonitis
- K35.3 Acute appendicitis with localized peritonitis

CLINICAL PEARLS
- Anorexia with periumbilical pain localizing to RLQ is the classic history for acute appendicitis.
- Diagnosis is more challenging in children, pregnant patients, and the elderly due to varying symptoms and signs.
- In equivocal cases, CT scan is the diagnostic test of choice. Ultrasound and MRI are alternatives.
- Acute appendicitis is the most common surgical emergency during pregnancy.

APPROACH TO TRAVEL MEDICINE COUNSELING

Benjamin Cottrell, DO • Rose Katherine Appel, DO

 BASICS

DESCRIPTION
Pretravel consultations help determine potential health hazards, allow the opportunity to discuss risks, and maximize prevention.

EPIDEMIOLOGY

Incidence
In 2022, >900 million international arrivals were recorded across the globe. In the United States, ~22 million international visitors arrived in 2021, whereas ~10 million Americans visited foreign countries around the world (figures been impacted by COVID-19). As more and more people begin to travel again, illness and injury will be increasingly common.

RISK FACTORS
Risks vary by destination, length of the trip, planned activities, age, and health status of the traveler.
- Traveler details
  - Past medical history (age, gender, medical conditions, allergies, medications)
    ○ Flying is contraindicated within 3 weeks of a myocardial infarction and within 10 days of thoracic or abdominal surgery. Consider nasal spray before air travel if there is preexisting eustachian tube dysfunction (1).
  - Special conditions (pregnancy, breastfeeding, disability or handicap, immunocompromised state, older age)
    ○ Flying is often discouraged after the 36th week of pregnancy.
  - Immunization history
  - Prior travel experience (previous malaria prophylaxis, experience with altitude, illnesses related to prior travel)
- Trip details
  - Itinerary (countries/specific regions, rural or urban; side trips); timing (length, season, time until departure); reason for travel; special activities (disaster relief, medical care, high altitude or climbing, diving, cruise ship, rafting, cycling, extreme sports)

GENERAL PREVENTION
- Routine vaccinations
  - *Haemophilus influenzae* type b; hepatitis B—for last minute travelers, can offer accelerated vaccine schedule for hepatitis A and hepatitis B with Twinrix or accelerated schedule for hepatitis B alone with Heplisav-B
  - Influenza
  - Measles, mumps, rubella—more common in countries without routine childhood immunization, including Europe
  - Meningococcal—outbreaks common in sub-Saharan Africa especially during the dry season (December through June); Saudi Arabia requires the quadrivalent vaccine for Hajj pilgrims. Hajj visas require vaccine to be administered ≥10 days and ≤3 years (≤5 years for conjugate vaccine) before arriving in Saudi Arabia (2).
  - Pneumococcal
  - Polio—wild poliovirus type 1 circulates currently in Afghanistan and Pakistan (2).
  - Rotavirus—common in developing countries; does not usually cause travelers' diarrhea in adults, so vaccination is only recommended for children
  - Tetanus, diphtheria, pertussis
  - Varicella—more common in countries without routine childhood immunization
  - Zoster—stress may trigger reactivation.
  - Human papillomavirus (HPV)—sexual activity during travel may lead to HPV infection.
- Travel-specific vaccinations (destination dependent)
  - Hepatitis A
  - Japanese encephalitis—most of Asia and parts of Western Pacific; 2-dose series given 28 days apart but may be given as early as 7 days; it must be given at least 1 week prior to travel.
  - Rabies—if immunoglobulin would be difficult to obtain, consider vaccination to simplify postexposure prophylaxis.
  - Tick-borne encephalitis (not available in the United States) is endemic in European and Asian countries.
  - Typhoid—highest risk in India, Pakistan, and Bangladesh; do not give live oral vaccine to pregnant women, immunocompromised patients, or if antibiotics are taken in the previous 72 hours (2). Oral vaccination is available for ages ≥6 years, and injectable vaccination options are available for ages ≥2 years. Oral vaccination is given at least 1 week prior to travel via four capsules taken every other day. Infectible vaccination is given at least 2 weeks prior to travel as a single dose.
  - Yellow fever—highest risk in sub-Saharan Africa and the Amazon regions of South America; vaccination is not considered valid until 10 days after administration (2); approved for ages ≥9 months as a single dose which provides lifelong protection for most people
- Malaria prophylaxis
  - Based on destination, types of planned activities, and patient preferences; CDC has up-to-date recommendations.
  - Chloroquine-sensitive malaria (2),(3)
    ○ Chloroquine—begin 1 to 2 weeks prior to travel, continue 4 weeks after leaving malaria-endemic area; may increase QTc interval (particularly if given with other QTc-prolonging drugs); adult dose: 300-mg base (500-mg salt) orally once weekly; pediatric dose: 5 mg/kg base (8.3 mg/kg salt) orally once weekly (up to 300-mg base per dose)
    ○ Hydroxychloroquine—begin 1 to 2 weeks prior to travel, continue for 4 weeks after leaving malaria-endemic area; dosed weekly; adult dose: 310-mg base (400-mg salt) orally once weekly; pediatric dose: 5 mg/kg base (6.5 mg/kg salt) orally once weekly (up to 310 mg base per dose)
  - Chloroquine-resistant malaria (2),(3)
    ○ Atovaquone/proguanil—begin 1 to 2 days before travel and continue for 1 week after leaving malaria-endemic area; adult dose: 250 mg/100 mg atovaquone/proguanil PO daily; pediatric dose: Tablets contain 62.5 mg/25 mg atovaquone/proguanil hydrochloride; 5 to 10 kg: 1/2 pediatric tablet daily; 10 to 20 kg: 1 pediatric tablet daily; 20 to 30 kg: 2 pediatric tablets daily; 30 to 40 kg: 3 pediatric tablets daily; >40 kg: 1 adult tablet daily
    ○ Doxycycline—begin 1 to 2 days before travel and continue for 4 weeks after leaving malaria-endemic area; adult dose: 100 mg orally daily; pediatric dose: ≥8 years old 2.2 mg/kg up to adult dose of 100 mg daily
    ○ Mefloquine—begin 1 to 2 weeks before travel and continue for 4 weeks after leaving malaria-endemic area; has a number of drug interactions; not recommended for people with cardiac conduction abnormalities (especially ventricular arrhythmias), major psychiatric disorders, or seizures; adult dose: 228-mg base (250-mg salt) orally once weekly; pediatric dose: ≤9 kg: 4.6 mg/kg base (5 mg/kg salt) orally once weekly; 10 to 19 kg: 1/4 tablet once weekly; 20 to 30 kg: 1/2 tablet once weekly; 31 to 45 kg: 3/4 tablet once weekly; >45 kg: 1 tablet once weekly
- Protection against mosquitoes and ticks
  - Avoid areas of known outbreaks of communicable disease. Refer to the CDC travelers' health Web site for updates.
  - Avoid peak exposure times and places. Mosquitoes may bite at any time of the day. Peak biting activity for vectors of some diseases (such as dengue, Zika, and chikungunya) is during daylight hours. Peak biting activity for vectors of other diseases (such as malaria, West Nile, and Japanese encephalitis) are most active in twilight periods (dawn and dusk) or after dark.
  - Wear appropriate clothing: Minimize exposed skin. Check for ticks. Use bed nets.
  - Insecticides and repellants—reapply regularly.
    ○ DEET, picaridin, oil of lemon eucalyptus, IR3535, 2-Undecanone
- Zika virus
  - Transmitted via mosquito bite (*Aedes* species) or via sexual intercourse; vaccinations are not currently available, but use preventative techniques such as mosquito repellants or wearing long clothing to avoid mosquito bites.
  - Most infections are asymptomatic. Pregnant women should avoid travel to any area with risk of Zika virus transmission. Women planning for pregnancy should consider waiting 2 months after returning from Zika-endemic area prior to conceiving.
- SARS-coronavirus-2
  - CDC recommends receiving COVID-19 primary series and boosters as recommended by traveler age group.
  - Check travel restrictions, testing, vaccination, and mask requirements of each destination before you travel.
  - Consider delaying or cancelling planned trips if case numbers are high in originating location or destination.
  - Do not travel if you have any symptoms. Avoid contact with anyone who is sick. Consider wearing masks in congested areas, especially indoor public transportation. Consider getting tested for COVID-19 ≤3 days prior to your departure and 3 to 5 days after your arrival back home. Bring extra supplies, such as masks and hand sanitizer. Respect physical distancing recommendations by staying at least 6 feet apart from others. Wash your hands often or use hand sanitizer (with at least 60% alcohol).

- Mpox
  - Since April 2022, there has been a recent rise in mpox cases; transmitted via contaminated fomites, skin lesions, or body fluids from an infected person; symptoms include flulike symptoms followed by a rash (vesiculopustular) and may have umbilication. CDC recommends vaccination prior to travel if travelers fall into high-risk populations, including the immunocompromised. Postexposure prophylaxis (PEP) is also available for those who have been exposed to mpox. Decrease risk of infection by avoiding congregate areas, practicing safe sex, and avoiding contact with those infected with mpox.
- Traveler's diarrhea
  - Symptoms range from mild abdominal cramping and urgent loose stools to severe abdominal pain, fever, vomiting, and bloody diarrhea; differs from food poisoning in which preformed toxins are ingested in food; nausea and vomiting may both be present although usually resolve within 12 hours; approximately 80–90% bacterial, 5–8% viral, 10% protozoal (1)
  - High-risk areas include Asia, Middle East, Africa, Mexico, and Central and South America (2).
  - Intermediate-risk areas include countries in Eastern Europe, South Africa, and some Caribbean islands (2).
  - Strategies to minimize diarrhea (2)
    - Wash hands or use sanitizer prior to eating. Avoid raw or undercooked meat, fish or shellfish, salads, uncooked vegetables, unpasteurized fruit juices, or unpasteurized milk or milk products. Avoid unpeeled raw fruit. Peel it yourself if possible. Tap water may be unsafe for drinking, making ice, preparing food, washing dishes, or brushing teeth; use sealed bottled water if possible.
  - For high-risk patients—bismuth subsalicylate reduces incidence of travelers' diarrhea by 50%; 2 oz of liquid or two chewable tablets QID (not recommended for children aged <3 years or pregnant women); note darkening of stool as a side effect (2).
  - Treatment based on severity of disease (2)
    - Mild—diarrhea is tolerable, not distressing, and does not interfere with activities; does not require antibiotics
    - Moderate—diarrhea is distressing and interferes with planned activities. Antibiotics such as fluoroquinolones, azithromycin, or rifaximin; loperamide can be used as a monotherapy.
    - Severe—incapacitating diarrhea; azithromycin is the preferred agent, although fluoroquinolones and rifaximin can also be used.
  - Antibiotic options for travelers' diarrhea treatment
    - Azithromycin—1,000 mg one-time dose; if symptoms are not resolved in 24 hours, then continue daily dosing for 3 days. Alternate dosing is 500 mg daily for 3 days.
    - Ciprofloxacin—750 mg one-time dose; if symptoms are not resolved in 24 hours, then continue daily dosing for 3 days. Alternate dosing is 500 mg BID × 3 days.
    - Rifaximin—200 mg TID × 3 days

- Adjunct medications
  - Loperamide—4 mg initially followed by 2 mg after each loose stool (max of 16 mg/day); pediatric dose: not recommended for children aged <6 years; 6 to 8 years old—2 mg initial dose, followed by 1 mg after each loose stool (max of 4 mg/day); 9 to 11 years old—2 mg after initial dose, followed by 1 mg after each loose stool (max of 6 mg/day); ≥12 years old: Refer to adult dosing.
  - Diphenoxylate: 5 mg (2 tablets) TID or QID until control is achieved (max of 20 mg/day); pediatric dose: not recommended for children aged <2 years; 0.3 to 0.4 mg/kg/day in 4 divided doses
- Altitude illness
  - More likely at an altitude of 8,000 feet (2,500 m) or higher, although can occur at lower altitudes; children and adults are equally susceptible. Factors that increase risk are elevation at destination, rate of ascent, and exertion (2).
  - Acute mountain sickness (AMS)—most common; typically presents with headache starting 2 to 12 hours after arrival; other symptoms include fatigue, loss of appetite, nausea, and vomiting; usually resolves within 24 to 48 hours of acclimatization (2)
  - High-altitude cerebral edema (HACE)—severe progression of AMS; rare, although most often associated with high-altitude pulmonary edema (HAPE); lethargy, drowsiness, confusion, ataxia; requires immediate descent (2)
  - HAPE—Symptoms include shortness of breath, weakness, and cough; requires supplemental oxygen and immediate descent.
  - Preventive measures
    - Ascend gradually. Avoid alcohol.
  - Preventive medications:
    - Recommended for those at high risk for AMS
    - Acetazolamide—AMS/HACE prevention dose: 125 mg BID (250 mg BID if >100 kg); pediatric dose: 2.5 mg/kg q12h; AMS treatment dose: 250 mg BID; pediatric dose: 2.5 mg/kg q12h; used as an adjunct to dexamethasone (2)
    - Dexamethasone—usually reserved for treatment; prevention dose: 2 mg q6h or 4 mg q12h; should not be used for prophylaxis in pediatric patients; AMS treatment dose: 4 mg q6h PO, IV, or IM; HACE treatment dose: 8 mg once and then 4 mg q6H PO, IV, or IM; pediatric dose: 0.15 mg/kg/dose q6h up to 4 mg (2)
    - Nifedipine—for prevention and treatment of HAPE; dose: 30 mg SR q12h (2)
    - Tadalafil—for prevention of HAPE only; dose: 10 mg BID (2)
    - Sildenafil—for HAPE prevention; dose: 50 mg q8h (2)
- Jet lag
  - Before travel, adjust sleep cycle (and possibly meal times) 1 to 2 hours earlier or later (depending on direction of travel) for several days prior to departure. Drink plenty of water to remain hydrated. Optimize sunlight exposure to destination. Sedative hypnotics (nonbenzodiazepine), such as zolpidem, can be useful. If using benzodiazepines, use short-acting agents, such as temazepam.
- Motion sickness
  - High risk individuals include children aged 2 to 12 years; patients who are pregnant, menstruating, or on hormones; patients who get migraines; and patients who are using certain medications.

- Prevention strategies include avoiding known triggers and using strategic positioning (front of car, over wing of aircraft).
  - Treatment
    - Dimenhydrinate: pediatric dose: 1.0 to 1.5 mg/kg 1 hour before travel and every 6 hours during the trip
    - Diphenhydramine: pediatric dose: 0.5 to 1 mg/kg/dose up to 25 mg 1 hour before travel and every 6 hours during the trip
    - Scopolamine: transdermal patch to hairless area behind ear at least 4 hours prior to exposure and every 3 days as needed; should not be used in children
- Environmental hazards
  - Avoid walking barefoot (parasites can enter skin). Avoid swimming in freshwater where there is a risk for schistosomiasis or leptospirosis. Use sunscreen.
  - If scuba diving, avoid flying or altitude exposure >2,000 feet (2); ≥12 hours after surfacing from nondecompression dive; ≥18 hours after repetitive dives or multiple days of diving; 24 to 28 hours after a dive that required decompression stops
- Other considerations
  - Consider travel insurance, including coverage for evacuation.
  - Carry medications on carry-on or personal luggage.

REFERENCES

1. Potin M, Carron PN, Genton B. Injuries and medical emergencies among international travelers. *J Travel Med.* 2023;taad088.
2. Brunette GW, Nemhauser JB, Kozarsky PE, et al. *CDC Yellow Book 2020: Health Information for International Travel.* New York, NY: Oxford University Press; 2019.
3. Murray HW. The pretravel consultation: recent updates. *Am J Med.* 2020;133(8):916–923.e2.

ADDITIONAL READING

Centers for Disease Control and Prevention. Travelers' health. https://www.cdc.gov/travel. Accessed November 1, 2023.

 CODES

ICD10
- Z71.9 Counseling, unspecified
- Z71.89 Other specified counseling

CLINICAL PEARLS

- The COVID-19 pandemic has drastically altered the landscape of domestic and international travel.
- The CDC Travelers' Health Web site is a useful point-of-care tool for destination-specific travel advice (https://wwwnc.cdc.gov/travel/).
- To allow adequate time for vaccine response and delivery of necessary pretravel medications, patients should seek advice several weeks prior to anticipated travel.

ARTERITIS, TEMPORAL

Irfan H. Siddiqui, MD • Neha Syed, DO, BS

BASICS

DESCRIPTION
- Also known as giant cell arteritis (GCA), Horton disease, and cranial arteritis
- Temporal arteritis is a chronic inflammatory disease involving large- and medium-sized arteries, most commonly cranial arteries originating from aortic arch. Inflammation of the aorta is observed in 50% of cases.
- New headache is a common presenting symptom and occurs in more than 2/3 of patients. Other symptoms include jaw claudication, vision loss, fatigue, fever, weight loss, symptoms of polymyalgia rheumatica (PMR), and aortic arch syndrome (decreased or absent peripheral pulses, discrepancies of blood pressure, arterial bruits). Onset of symptoms is usually subacute; however, acute presentations can also occur.
- Considered medical emergency due to risk of irreversible vision loss if not treated due to arteritic anterior ischemic optic neuropathy, central or branch artery occlusion, posterior ischemic optic neuropathy, or rarely cerebral ischemia

EPIDEMIOLOGY
- Most common form of systemic vasculitis affecting persons ≥50 years old
- 80% of cases occur at ages 70 to 80 years.
- Women are affected approximately 3 times more than men in persons of Northern European descent.
- Most common vasculitis in individuals of Northern European descent

Incidence
- Incidence varies by ethnicity; in the United States, approximately 1% in women and 0.5% in men
- Prevalence in Northern Europeans is 2 per 1,000 persons.
- Peaks in patients 70 to 80 years old, >80% of patients

ETIOLOGY AND PATHOPHYSIOLOGY
- The exact etiology of GCA remains unknown, although current theory suggests that advanced age, ethnicity, and specific genetic predisposition lead to a maladaptive response to endothelial injury, intimal hyperplasia, and ultimately vascular stenosis.
- GCA is a chronic, systemic vasculitis primarily affecting the elastic lamina of medium- and large-sized arteries. Histopathology of affected arteries is marked by transmural inflammation of the intima, media, and adventitia, as well as patchy infiltration by lymphocytes, macrophages, and multinucleated giant cells. Mural hyperplasia can result in arterial luminal narrowing, resulting in subsequent distal ischemia.
- Current theory regarding the etiology of GCA is that a maladaptive response to endothelial injury leads to an inappropriate activation of T-cell–mediated immunity via immature antigen-presenting cells. The subsequent release of cytokines within the arterial vessel wall can attract macrophages and multinucleated giant cells, which form granulomatous infiltrates and give diseased vessels their characteristic histology. This also leads to an oligoclonal expansion of T-cells directed against antigens in or near the elastic lamina. Ultimately, this cascade results in vessel wall damage, intimal hyperplasia, and eventual stenotic occlusion.

- In recent years, GCA and PMR have increasingly been considered to be closely related conditions.
- Varicella zoster virus has been proposed as possible immune trigger for GCA; however, this has not been substantiated, and adjunctive treatment with antivirals remains controversial.

Genetics
The gene for *HLA-DRB1*04* has been identified as a risk factor for GCA, and polymorphisms of *ICAM-1* and *PTPN-22* have also been implicated.

RISK FACTORS
- Increasing age (>70 years) is the greatest risk factor.
- Females
- Genetic predisposition—occasional family clustering has been reported.
- Environmental factors influence susceptibility.
- History of smoking
- Early menopause (<43 years) and lower BMI at menopause in women 50 to 69 years old

COMMONLY ASSOCIATED CONDITIONS
Population studies have shown 40–60% of patients diagnosed with GCA also have PMR symptoms, and 16–21% of patients with PMR have GCA.

DIAGNOSIS

HISTORY
- Most common presenting symptom is headache (2/3 of patients).
- Constitutional symptoms (fever, fatigue, weight loss)
- Any visual disturbances (amaurosis fugax, diplopia)
- Vision loss (20% of patients); unilateral is most common, often proceeds to bilateral if untreated
- Jaw claudication (Presence of symptom significantly increases likelihood of a positive biopsy.)
- Scalp tenderness or sensitivity
- Claudication of upper extremities or tongue
- Symptoms of PMR (shoulder and hip girdle pain and stiffness)
- Distal extremity swelling/edema
- Upper respiratory symptoms

PHYSICAL EXAM
- Temporal artery abnormalities (beading, prominence, tenderness)
- Typically, appear "ill"
- Decreased peripheral pulses in the presence of large vessel diseases
- Funduscopic exam shows pale and edema of the optic disc, scattered cotton wool patches, and small hemorrhages.
- Unlike other forms of vasculitis, GCA rarely involves the skin, kidneys, and lungs.
- Supraclavicular, axillary, and supraorbital bruits

DIFFERENTIAL DIAGNOSIS
- Migraines
- Herpes zoster
- Other vasculitis (Takayasu arteritis, Wegner, PAN)
- Other rheumatologic condition (RA, PMR, MCTD)

DIAGNOSTIC TESTS & INTERPRETATION
- American College of Rheumatology 1990 classification criteria are as follows:
  - Age >50 years
  - New localized headache
  - Temporal artery abnormality (tenderness to palpation, decreased or absent pulses)
  - ESR >50 mm/hr
  - Abnormal temporal artery biopsy showing vasculitis with predominance of mononuclear cell infiltration or granulomatous inflammation
- Three or more of the American College of Rheumatology criteria demonstrate a sensitivity of 94.5% and a specificity of 91.2%.

Initial Tests (lab, imaging)
- ESR >50 mm/hr (86% sensitivity), although non-specific (27%); infrequently, may be normal
- C-reactive protein (CRP) >2.45 mg/dL is a more sensitive marker of inflammation (97% sensitivity) and is associated with increased odds of a positive biopsy result.
- A normal ESR and/or CRP renders the diagnosis of GCA unlikely.
- Acute-phase reactants (fibrinogen, interleukin-6) are frequently elevated but very nonspecific and reserved for diagnostically difficult cases.
- Mild anemia: very nonspecific but may be associated with a lower rate of ischemic complications
- Color Doppler US of the temporal artery may identify vascular occlusion, stenosis, or edema ("halo sign"); it is low cost and noninvasive but also very operator dependent and does not significantly improve on the clinical exam. It may aid in the diagnosis of larger vessel involvement.
- Atherosclerotic disease with carotid intima-media thickness >0.9 mm may mimic halo sign.
- MRI and MRA may be beneficial in diagnosis (78% sensitive, 90% specific) if performed within 5 days of steroids.
- Positron emission tomography (PET), like MRI/MRA and color Doppler, may be useful in diagnostically difficult cases to quantify the inflammatory burden and early in the course of disease, as the metabolic changes occur prior to structural vascular damage, but it also lacks studies to support its use.

Follow-Up Tests & Special Considerations
- Development of aortic aneurysms (late and potentially serious complication of GCA) can lead to aortic dissection.
- Due to the risk of irreversible vision loss, treatment with high-dose steroids should be started on strong clinical suspicion of GCA, prior to the temporal biopsy being done.

Diagnostic Procedures/Other
- Gold standard diagnostic study: histopathologic examination of the temporal artery biopsy specimen (Do not delay starting medication if suspicion as pathology remains up to 14 days after starting steroids.)
- The temporal artery is chosen because of its accessibility in the systemic disease; alternatively, facial artery or other cranial arteries may be used.
- Length of biopsy specimen should be at least 7 to 10 mm to avoid false-negative results because skip lesions may occur.

- Diagnostic yield of biopsy may be increased if procedure is coupled with imaging (high-resolution MRI or color Doppler US).
- Bilateral temporal artery biopsy should not be performed, unless the initial histopathology is negative and the suspicion for GCA remains high.
- May be negative in up to 42% of patients with GCA, especially in a large-vessel disease, and a negative biopsy alone should not dictate treatment
- Biopsy results are not affected by prior glucocorticoids; so, treatment should not be delayed.

Test Interpretation
- Inflammation of the arterial wall, with fragmentation and disruption of the internal elastic lamina
- Multinucleated giant cells are found in <50% of cases and are not specific for the disease.
- GCA occurs in three histologic patterns: classic, atypical, and healed.

TREATMENT

MEDICATION
First Line
Glucocorticoids:

- The typical dose of prednisone is between 60 and 80 mg/day (or 1 mg/kg/day), and the dose may be titrated up to relieve symptoms. Steroids should not be in the form of alternate day therapy because this is more likely to lead to a relapse of vasculitis (1)[A].
- IV steroids indicated if vision loss has been noted, otherwise PO steroids are equally effective (1)[C]
- Given risk of irreversible vision loss, immediate steroid therapy should be initiated prior to confirmation by biopsy.
- The initial dose of steroids is continued for 2 to 4 weeks and slowly tapered over 9 to 12 months. Tapering may require ≥2 years (1)[A]. Assess for relapse during taper by monitoring symptoms, ESR, and CRP.
- Tocilizumab (an IL-6 receptor antagonist) 162 mg SQ weekly or biweekly in addition to prednisone may be superior to prednisone alone, although it does carry a black box warning regarding increased risk of opportunistic infections.
- It has been suggested that low-dose aspirin might be effective for patients with GCA.

Second Line
- Methotrexate as an adjunct to glucocorticoid therapy may have a modest effect in decreasing the relapse rate of GCA.
- Cyclophosphamide have shown some benefit in patients who have not adequately responded to glucocorticoids.
- Azathioprine and abatacept can also be used as adjuncts to glucocorticoids.
- Therapies directed at TNF as adjunct to steroids have not shown significant benefit (1)[B].

ONGOING CARE

FOLLOW-UP RECOMMENDATIONS
Sun avoidance and protection of the head and the face from photodamage may eventually prove to be important preventive measures for GCA.

Patient Monitoring
- GCA is typically self-limited and lasts several months or years.
- Overall, GCA does not seem to decrease longevity. Nevertheless, it may lead to serious complications such as visual loss, which occurs in about 15–20% of patients.
- Another complication of GCA is the development of aortic aneurysms, usually affecting the ascending aorta. Yearly, chest x-rays may be useful to identify this problem.
- About 50% of the patients with GCA will eventually develop PMR (stiffness of shoulder and hip girdle).
- Low-dose aspirin should be given as indicated by atherosclerosis guidelines.

DIET
Calcium and vitamin D supplementation should be administered for osteoporosis prevention associated with prolonged corticosteroid therapy.

PATIENT EDUCATION
- Consequences of discontinuing steroids abruptly (adrenal insufficiency, disease relapse)
- Risks of long-term steroid use (infection, hyperglycemia, weight gain, impaired wound healing, osteoporosis, hypertension)
- Possibility of relapse and importance of reporting new headaches and vision changes to provider immediately

PROGNOSIS
- Variable duration of disease, from 1 year to chronic course
- Life expectancy is not affected by the disease unless severe aortitis is present.
- Once vision loss has occurred, it is unlikely to be recovered, but treatment resolves the other symptoms and prevents future vision loss and stroke.
- In most patients, glucocorticoid therapy can eventually be discontinued without complications. In patients with chronic disease, however, prednisone may need to be continued for years.
- Disease relapse is possible.

COMPLICATIONS
- Vision loss with delayed diagnosis
- Glucocorticoid-related toxicity

REFERENCE
1. Borchers AT, Gershwin ME. Giant cell arteritis: a review of classification, pathophysiology, geoepidemiology and treatment. *Autoimmun Rev.* 2012;11(6–7):A544–A554.

ADDITIONAL READING
De Miguel E, Beltran LM, Monjo I, et al. Atherosclerosis as a potential pitfall in the diagnosis of giant cell arteritis. *Rheumatology (Oxford).* 2018;57(2):318–321.

SEE ALSO

Depression; Fibromyalgia; Headache, Cluster; Headache, Tension; Polymyalgia Rheumatica; Polymyositis/Dermatomyositis

CODES

ICD10
- M31.6 Other giant cell arteritis
- M31.5 Giant cell arteritis with polymyalgia rheumatica

CLINICAL PEARLS
- Due to the risk of irreversible vision loss, treatment with high-dose steroids (prednisone 60 mg/day) should be started immediately in patients suspected of GCA.
- Temporal artery biopsy is the gold standard for diagnosis. Temporal artery biopsy is not likely to be affected by a few weeks of treatment.
- Treatment consists of a very slow steroid taper. Bone protection therapy and low-dose aspirin should be considered.
- Normal ESR level = value of age / 2 for men and age + 10 / 2 for women
- Patients on corticosteroids should be placed on therapy to minimize osteoporosis, unless there are contraindications.

ARTHRITIS, JUVENILE IDIOPATHIC

Donna Marie McMahon, DO, FAAP • Kathleen M. Vazzana, DO, MSc

BASICS

DESCRIPTION
- Juvenile idiopathic arthritis (JIA) is the most common chronic pediatric rheumatologic disease.
- JIA can be associated with significant disability:
  - Age of onset: <16 years of age
  - Common symptoms: joint swelling, restricted range of motion, warmth, redness, pain
  - ≥6 weeks of symptoms prior to diagnosis
- Seven (International League of Associations for Rheumatology [ILAR]) subtypes determined by clinical characteristics in first 6 months of illness (1):
  - Systemic: 10%; preceded by febrile onset of ≥2 weeks with rash, serositis, hepatosplenomegaly, or lymphadenopathy (1)
  - Polyarticular rheumatoid factor (RF) positive: 2–7%; ≥5 joints involvement (1); large and small joints; RF positive on two tests ≥3 months apart (2)
  - Polyarticular RF negative: 10–30%; ≥5 (large and small) joints involved (1); RF negative (2)
  - Oligoarticular: 30–60%; involvement of 1 to 4 joints; risk for chronic uveitis in antinuclear antibodies (ANA) positive females (1) and axial skeletal involvement in older boys (2); types: (i) persistent (40%): knee, ankle, elbow; (ii) extended type (20%): >4 joints after first 6 months
  - Psoriatic arthritis: 5%; arthritis with psoriasis or arthritis with >2 of the following: dactylitis, nail changes (pitting), psoriasis in first-degree relative (1)
  - Enthesitis-related arthritis: 1–11%; arthritis and enthesitis or one of them plus at least two of the following: sacroiliac or lumbosacral pain, Reiter syndrome or acute anterior uveitis in first-degree relative, acute symptomatic anterior uveitis, human leukocyte antigen (HLA)-B27 positive, history of ankylosing spondylitis, sacroiliitis with inflammatory bowel disease, onset of arthritis in male >6 years old (1)[C]
  - Undifferentiated arthritis (11–21%): presents with overlapping symptoms in ≥2 categories above or arthritis that does not fulfill above categories (2)
- Systems affected: musculoskeletal, hematologic, lymphatic, immunologic, dermatologic, ophthalmologic, gastrointestinal
- Synonyms: juvenile chronic arthritis; juvenile arthritis; juvenile rheumatoid arthritis (JRA); Still disease (2)

EPIDEMIOLOGY
54% of cases occur in children aged 0 to 5 years.

Incidence
2 to 20/100,000 children aged <16 years in developed nations

Prevalence
16 to 150/100,000 children aged <16 years in developed nations (1)

ETIOLOGY AND PATHOPHYSIOLOGY
- Humoral and cellular immunodysregulation; T lymphocytes play a key role.
- Genetic predisposition; IL2RA/CD25 and VTCN1 implicated as genetic loci
- Environmental triggers, possibly infectious
  - Rubella or parvovirus B19
  - Heat shock proteins
- Immunoglobulin or complement deficiency

RISK FACTORS
Female gender 3:1

COMMONLY ASSOCIATED CONDITIONS
Other autoimmune disorders, chronic anterior uveitis (iridocyclitis), nutritional impairment, growth issues

DIAGNOSIS

Clinical criteria: age of onset <16 years and >6 weeks duration of objective arthritis (swelling or restricted range of motion of a joint with heat, pain, or synovial tenderness and no other form of childhood arthritis) in ≥1 joints

HISTORY
- Arthralgias, fever, fatigue, malaise, myalgias, weight loss, morning stiffness, rash
- Limp if lower extremity involvement
- Arthritis for ≥6 weeks

PHYSICAL EXAM
- Arthritis: swelling, effusion, loss of musculoskeletal landmarks, limited range of motion, tenderness, pain with motion, warmth
- Rash, rheumatoid nodules (uncommon), lymphadenopathy, hepato- or splenomegaly, enthesitis, dactylitis (mainly in psoriatic type)

DIFFERENTIAL DIAGNOSIS
- Legg-Calvé-Perthes disease, toxic synovitis, growing pains
- Septic arthritis, osteomyelitis, viral infection, mycoplasmal infection, Lyme disease/Lyme arthritis
- Reactive arthritis: postinfectious, rheumatic fever, Reiter syndrome
- Inflammatory bowel disease
- Hemoglobinopathies, hemarthrosis, rickets
- Leukemia (particularly acute lymphocytic leukemia), bone tumors (osteoid osteoma), neuroblastoma
- Vasculitis, immunoglobulin A vasculitis, Kawasaki disease
- Systemic lupus erythematosus, dermatomyositis, mixed connective tissue disease, sarcoidosis, systemic sclerosis, collagen disorders
- Farber disease
- Accidental or nonaccidental trauma

DIAGNOSTIC TESTS & INTERPRETATION

Initial Tests (lab, imaging)
- CBC: leukocyte count is normal or elevated (systemic); lymphopenia, reactive thrombocytosis, anemia; liver function test (LFT; hepatic involvement) and renal function studies (prior to therapy with nephrotoxic drugs)
- Joint-fluid aspiration/analysis to exclude infection
- ESR and C-reactive protein typically elevated; C-reactive protein often disproportionately high
- Myeloid-related proteins (MRP 8/14) associated with flares
- ANA-positive patients have increased risk of uveitis; ANA positive in up to 70% with oligoarticular JIA
- RF positive: 2–10% (usually polyarticular); poor prognosis
- HLA-B27 positive: enthesitis-related arthritis
- Diagnostic radiography, MRI, ultrasound, and CT; no one modality has superior diagnostic value
- Radiograph of affected joint(s): *early* radiographic changes: soft tissue swelling, periosteal reaction, juxta-articular demineralization; *later* changes: joint space loss, articular surface erosions, subchondral cyst formation, sclerosis, joint fusion
- If orthopnea, obtain ECG to rule out pericarditis.
- Radionuclide scans: for infection/malignancy
- CT is best for bony abnormalities; MRI can assess synovial hypertrophy and cartilage degeneration; MRI more sensitive to monitor disease activity and clinical responsiveness to treatment in peripheral joints

Follow-Up Tests & Special Considerations
Use pediatric (not adult) controls when interpreting results of dual energy x-ray absorptiometry.

Diagnostic Procedures/Other
- Ultrasound: Assess for effusions.
- Synovial biopsy: if synovial fluid cannot be aspirated or if infection is suspected in spite of negative synovial fluid culture

Test Interpretation
Synovial biopsy → synovial cell hyperplasia, hyperemia, infiltration of small lymphocytes and mononuclear cells (rarely done)

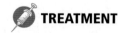 TREATMENT

GENERAL MEASURES
- The goal is to control active disease, minimize extra-articular manifestations, and achieve clinical remission.
- All patients require regular (every 3 to 4 months for oligoarticular JIA and in ANA-positive patients) ophthalmic exams to uncover asymptomatic eye disease, particularly for the first 3 years following diagnosis.
- Moist heat or electric blanket for morning stiffness
- Splints for contractures
- Aerobic exercise: weight-bearing or aquatic therapy to improve functional capacity

MEDICATION

First Line

- ≤4 joints
  - NSAIDs (ibuprofen, naproxen, celecoxib): adequate in ~50%; symptoms often improve within days; full efficacy 2 to 3 months
    - Precautions: may worsen bleeding diatheses; use caution in renal insufficiency and hypovolemic states; take with food.
    - Significant drug interactions: may lower serum levels of anticonvulsants and blunt the effect of loop diuretics; NSAIDs may increase serum methotrexate levels.
  - Intra-articular long-acting corticosteroids: immediately effective; improve synovitis, joint damage, contractures, prevent leg length discrepancy
    - Indication: patients with oligoarthritis who fail a 2-month NSAID trial or with poor prognosis (2)
- ≥5 joints
  - If high disease activity or a failed 1 to 2 months NSAID trial → methotrexate

Second Line

- 30–40% of patients require addition of disease-modifying antirheumatic drugs (DMARDs): methotrexate, sulfasalazine, leflunomide, and tumor necrosis factor (TNF) antagonists (etanercept, infliximab, adalimumab); newer biologic therapies, including IL-1 and IL-6 receptor antagonists, are currently under investigation.
- Methotrexate: 10 mg/m^2/week PO or SC
- Sulfasalazine: oligoarticular and HLA-B27 spondylarthritis
- Etanercept: 0.8 mg/kg (max of 50 mg/dose) given SC q1wk or 0.4 mg/kg SC twice a week (max of 25 mg/dose)
- Infliximab: 5 mg/kg q6–8wk
- Adalimumab: if weight 15 kg to <30 kg, 20 mg SC q2wk; if weight ≥30 kg, 40 mg SC q2wk
- Rituximab: for polyarticular RF positive who have failed two TNF-α inhibitors
- Tocilizumab: for RF-pJIA who have failed two TNF-α inhibitors
- Begin treatment with TNF-α inhibitors in children with a history of arthritis in ≤4 joints and significant active arthritis despite treatment with methotrexate or arthritis in ≥5 joints and any active arthritis following an adequate trial of methotrexate.
- Anakinra: IL-1 receptor antagonist; begin treatment with anakinra in children with systemic arthritis and active fever whose treatment requires a second medication, in addition to systemic glucocorticoids.

ISSUES FOR REFERRAL

- Consult pediatric rheumatologist for assistance with management of JIA.
- Orthopedics as needed for articular complications

- Ophthalmology to evaluate for uveitis and continued screening
- Physical therapy to maintain range of motion, improve muscle strength, and prevent deformities
- Occupational therapy to maintain and improve appropriate age-related functional activities
- Behavioral health if difficulty coping with disease

SURGERY/OTHER PROCEDURES

- Total hip and/or knee replacement for severe disease
- Soft tissue release if splinting/traction unsuccessful
- Correct limb length or angular deformities.
- Synovectomy is rarely performed.

ADMISSION, INPATIENT, AND NURSING CONSIDERATIONS

- Hospitalize if:
  - Patient unable to ambulate
  - Signs/symptoms of pericarditis
  - Persistent fever or diagnostic confusion to facilitate evaluation and workup
  - Need for surgery
- Discharge when fever and serositis resolved

 ONGOING CARE

FOLLOW-UP RECOMMENDATIONS

Patient Monitoring

Determined by medication and disease activity

- NSAIDs: periodic CBC, urinalysis, LFTs, renal function tests
- Aspirin and/or other salicylates: transaminase and salicylate levels weekly for 1 month and then every 3 to 4 months
- Methotrexate: monthly LFTs, CBC, BUN, creatinine

PATIENT EDUCATION

- Psychosocial needs; school issues; behavioral strategies for dealing with pain and noncompliance; available health care resources; support groups
- American College of Rheumatology: https://www.rheumatology.org/I-Am-A/Patient-Caregiver

PROGNOSIS

- 50–60% of patients will ultimately achieve remission.
- Functional ability depends on adequacy of therapy (disease control, maintaining muscle and joint function).
- Poor prognosis: patients with active disease at 6 months; polyarticular disease; extended pauciarticular disease course; female gender; RF positive; ANA positive; persistent morning stiffness; rapid appearance of erosions; hip involvement

COMPLICATIONS

- Blindness, band keratopathy, glaucoma, short stature, micrognathia if temporomandibular joint involvement, debilitating joint disease, disseminated intravascular coagulation, hemolytic anemia
- NSAIDs: peptic ulcer, GI hemorrhage, CNS reactions, renal disease, leukopenia
- DMARDs: bone marrow suppression, hepatitis, renal disease, dermatitis, mouth ulcers, retinal toxicity (antimalarials; rare)
- TNF antagonists: higher risk of infection
- Osteoporosis, avascular necrosis
- Methotrexate: Folate supplementation decreases hepatic/GI symptoms; may reduce stomatitis
- Macrophage activation syndrome: decreased blood cell precursors secondary to histiocyte degradation of marrow

REFERENCES

1. Giancane G, Alongi A, Ravelli A. Update on the pathogenesis and treatment of juvenile idiopathic arthritis. *Curr Opin Rheumatol.* 2017;29(5): 523–529.
2. Saad N, Onel K. Overview of juvenile idiopathic arthritis. *Open Orthop J.* 2020;14:101–109.

ADDITIONAL READING

Ringold S, Angeles-Han ST, Beukelman T, et al. 2019 American College of Rheumatology/Arthritis Foundation guideline for the treatment of juvenile idiopathic arthritis: therapeutic approaches for non-systemic polyarthritis, sacroiliitis, and enthesitis. *Arthritis Rheumatol.* 2019;71(6):846–863.

 CODES

ICD10

- M08.90 Juvenile arthritis, unspecified, unspecified site
- M08.80 Other juvenile arthritis, unspecified site
- M08.00 Unsp juvenile rheumatoid arthritis of unspecified site

CLINICAL PEARLS

- JIA is the most common form of arthritis in children.
- Consider JIA in any child presenting with a limp.
- High-titer RF correlates with disease severity; prognosis worse if positive RF titers
- DMARDs improve JIA-associated symptoms.
- NSAIDs are typically first-line choice of medication.

ARTHRITIS, PSORIATIC

Nikki A. Levin, MD, PhD • Lindsay McCormack, MD

 BASICS

A chronic, destructive, seronegative arthropathy in patients with long-standing psoriasis

DESCRIPTION
- Psoriatic arthritis (PsA) is a seronegative spondylo-arthropathy characterized by inflammatory arthritis and enthesitis.
- Five patterns of arthritis in PsA:
  – Asymmetric oligoarthritis: <5 joints
  – Distal interphalangeal (DIP) joint predominant: osteoarthritis-like, associated with nail psoriasis
  – Symmetric polyarthritis: may be indistinguishable from rheumatoid arthritis (RA)—typically milder
  – Spondyloarthritis: asymmetric and discontinuous, unlike ankylosing spondylitis (AS)
  – Arthritis mutilans: destructive, resorptive arthritis; produces "opera-glass" or "telescoping" digit
- Psoriasis may be limited in extent.
  – Course of arthritis and extent of psoriasis do not correlate.
  – Other extra-articular features, such as iritis, are less common.
  – Damaging joint disease may occur in 40–60%. Characteristic radiologic changes include "pencil-in-cup" deformity and periostitis.
- Rheumatoid factor (RF) and anti–cyclic citrullinated peptide (anti-CCP) antibody are usually negative. HLA-B27 may be positive.

EPIDEMIOLOGY
- Peak onset age: 30 to 50 years
- Predominant gender: female = male
- Polyarthritis is more common in women.
- Spondylitis in up to 25%, more common in males
- Psoriasis precedes arthritis in most patients by an average of 12 years. Arthritis preceding psoriasis occurs in up to 15% of patients, usually children. Arthritis and psoriasis may present simultaneously.
- Psoriasis occurs in 2–3% of the U.S. population; 6–42% will develop PsA (1).

Prevalence
Prevalence: 1 to 2/1,000 population (1)

ETIOLOGY AND PATHOPHYSIOLOGY
- CD4+/CD8+ T cells; tumor necrosis factor α (TNF-α); interleukin 1 (IL-1), IL-6, IL-8, IL-10, IL-17 and IL-23; and matrix metalloproteases present in synovial fluid
- Osteoclast precursor cell upregulation
- Unknown. Probably multifactorial: immunologic, genetic, environmental factors

Genetics
- 30–40% concordance in identical twins
- HLA-B27 in 15–50% with PsA (spondylitis pattern) versus 90% in AS
- Other HLA associations in PsA: HLA-B7, HLA-B38, HLA-B39, HLA-Cw6

RISK FACTORS
- Psoriasis
- Family history of PsA
- Obesity

GENERAL PREVENTION
No known prevention strategies; unknown whether early treatment of psoriasis prevents onset of PsA

COMMONLY ASSOCIATED CONDITIONS
Psoriasis

 DIAGNOSIS

- A history of inflammatory arthritis, dactylitis, or enthesitis in patients with existing psoriasis helps establish the diagnosis. It can be difficult to differentiate PsA from other inflammatory arthropathies.
- Use Classification of PsA (CASPAR) criteria (91% sensitivity; 99% specificity) to screen patients for PsA. Inflammatory articular disease (joint, spine, or entheseal) with ≥3 points from the following five categories:
  – Evidence of current psoriasis, a personal or family history of psoriasis (2 points)
  – Typical psoriatic nail dystrophy, including ony-cholysis, pitting, and hyperkeratosis (1 point)
  – Negative RF (ELISA preferred) (1 point)
  – Current or prior history of dactylitis (1 point)
  – Radiologic evidence of new bone formation (excluding osteophyte formation) on plain radiographs of the hand or foot (1 point)

HISTORY
History and physical exam help establish the diagnosis of PsA.
- (Generally) long-standing history of psoriasis
- Morning stiffness of hands, feet, or low back for >30 minutes
- Pain of involved joints
- Swelling or redness of peripheral joints
- Low back or buttock pain
- Ankle or heel pain
- Dactylitis or uniform swelling of an entire digit

PHYSICAL EXAM
- Affected peripheral joints may have overlying erythema, warmth, and swelling.
  – Synovitis
  – Dactylitis
  – Swelling of tendons (e.g., Achilles tendon) and tenderness at insertion sites (e.g., calcaneus)
  – Limited range of motion of axial skeleton
  – Pain with stress of the sacroiliac joint
- Well-demarcated pink-to-red erythematous plaques with a white silvery scale; common locations include scalp, ears, trunk, buttocks, gluteal cleft, elbows and forearms, knees and legs, and palms and soles.
- Nails may be dystrophic with pits, oil spots, crumbling, leukonychia, and red lunulae.

DIFFERENTIAL DIAGNOSIS
- Reactive arthritis
- Psoriasis and RA
- Psoriasis and osteoarthritis
- Psoriasis and polyarticular gout
- Psoriasis and AS

DIAGNOSTIC TESTS & INTERPRETATION
Initial Tests (lab, imaging)
- Serum RF (usually negative)
- Anti-CCP (usually negative)
- Antinuclear antibodies (usually negative)
- Acute-phase reactants (ESR and C-reactive protein) may be elevated.
- HLA-B27 is noted in 50–70% with axial disease and <15% with peripheral disease.
- Baseline radiographs of affected joints
- Plain radiographs may aid diagnosis, assess joint damage, disease progression, and response to therapy.
- Juxta-articular new bone formation (periostitis) and marginal joint erosions that progress centrally ("pencil-in-cup" erosions) are characteristic radio-graphic features.
- In patients with psoriasis, detection of enthesitis on ultrasound may be associated with higher risk of PsA.

Follow-Up Tests & Special Considerations
Follow-up radiographs; interval based on severity

Diagnostic Procedures/Other
Diagnosis is typically clinical.

Test Interpretation
Biopsy of skin or synovium is not usually required.

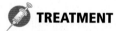 **TREATMENT**

GENERAL MEASURES
Physical therapy and/or occupational therapy benefit all stages of disease.
- Treatment algorithms for PsA are based on severity of joint symptoms, extent of structural damage, and severity of psoriasis. Patients with moderate to severe arthritis should be started on disease-modifying antirheumatic drugs (DMARDs) to reduce or prevent joint damage and preserve joint integrity and function.
- In addition to pharmacotherapy, patients should be educated on lifestyle modifications such as smoking cessation, diet, weight reduction, joint protection, physical activity, exercise, work participation, and stress coping mechanisms (2),(3).

MEDICATION
First Line
- NSAIDs to control symptoms of mild disease. Intermittent intra-articular glucocorticoid injections may help.
- There are no systematic trials of NSAIDs for PsA. Dose NSAID to suppress mild inflammation. NSAID selection is based on patient preference and dosing convenience. Sample NSAIDs include ibuprofen 400 to 800 mg PO TID–QID, naproxen 250 to 500 mg PO BID–TID, diclofenac 100 to 150 mg QD, indomethacin 100 to 150 mg QD.
- Monotherapy is as effective as combination therapy (≥2 drugs from the following: analgesics, NSAIDs, opioids, opioid-like drugs, and neuromodulators [antidepressants, anticonvulsants, and muscle relaxants]).

Second Line

- Recommended DMARDs include sulfasalazine, leflunomide, methotrexate. There is no evidence to support the use of combination DMARD therapy.
- Initial dosing regimens for DMARDs: sulfasalazine (2 to 3 g/day PO divided in BID dosing), leflunomide (loading dose of 100 mg/day PO for 3 days and then 20 mg/day PO), methotrexate (1 test dose of 2.5 to 5.0 mg PO to assess for significant bone marrow suppression and then 15 to 25 mg once weekly), azathioprine (0.5 mg/kg/day, with a max dose of 2.5 mg/kg/day if no signs of cytopenia at lower doses)
- Avoid systemic corticosteroids if possible (may help in short term for severe flares while initiating a biologic agent).
- Biologic therapies, particularly anti–TNF-α agents, are indicated for patients who do not respond to at least one standard DMARD or in patients with poor prognosis, even if they have not failed a standard DMARD (3).
- Dosing regimens for anti–TNF-α agents:
  – Adalimumab 40 mg SC q2wk
  – Certolizumab pegol 200 mg every 2 week; for maintenance dosing or 400 mg every 4 weeks
  – Etanercept 50 mg SC weekly
  – Golimumab 50 mg SC monthly
  – Infliximab 5 mg/kg at 0, 2, and 6 weeks, q8wk afterward
- Anti–IL-17 agents include the following:
  – Ixekizumab 80 mg q4wk
  – Secukinumab 150 mg weekly from 0 to 4 weeks and then monthly
  – Brodalumab 210 mg SC × 1 weekly from 0 to 2 and then q2wk (4)
- Anti–IL-12/IL-23 agents include the following:
  – Ustekinumab is currently dosed at 45 or 90 mg (depending on weight) at 0, 4, and 12 weeks and then q12wk thereafter.
- IL-23 selective inhibitor include the following:
  – Risankizumab 150 mg SC × 1 on week 0, 4, and then q12wk
  – Guselkumab 100 mg SC × 1 at 0 and 4 weeks and then q8wk
- PDE4 inhibitors include the following:
  – Apremilast 30 mg PO BID
- JAK 1, JAK 2, and JAK 3 inhibitors include the following:
  – Tofacitinib citrate dosed at 5 mg PO BID immediate release or 11 mg once daily extended release (1)
  – Upadacitinib dosed at 15 mg PO QD
- Selective T-cell costimulation blocker:
  – Abatacept dosed at 125 mg once weekly SC or according to body weight. Following the initial IV infusion (using the weight-based dosing), repeat IV infusion (using the same weight-based dosing) q2wk and q4wk after the initial infusion, and q4wk thereafter (1).

- Above medications are FDA-approved for PsA.
- Do not use anti-TNF agents in the setting of active infection (including TB and hepatitis B). Do not use anti-TNF agents with concurrent live vaccinations, with New York Heart Association classes III to IV congestive heart failure, with malignancy, or in patients with a history of demyelinating disease.
- Do not use biologic therapies in patients with active infection, with concurrent live vaccinations, or with history of malignancy.
- Do not use JAK inhibitors in patients with active infection or malignancy or those with risk factors for cardiovascular and thromboembolic disease.

Pregnancy Considerations

- Avoid teratogenic medications (e.g., methotrexate, leflunomide) during pregnancy.
- Adalimumab, etanercept, golimumab, infliximab, ustekinumab, and certolizumab pegol, secukinumab, are currently listed as Category B medications. Apremilast, abatacept, tofacitinib citrate, ixekizumab, and guselkumab are listed as pregnancy Category C medication. Upadacitinib is pregnancy Category D medication.

ISSUES FOR REFERRAL

- Rheumatology
- Dermatology

SURGERY/OTHER PROCEDURES

Joint fusion or replacement for advanced destruction

ONGOING CARE

FOLLOW-UP RECOMMENDATIONS

Epidemiologic data suggest a relationship between psoriasis, metabolic syndrome, type 2 diabetes, Crohn disease, myocardial infarction, and stroke. Control of weight, blood pressure, lipids, and glucose is recommended (2).

PATIENT EDUCATION

- National Psoriasis Foundation: https://www.psoriasis.org/about-psoriatic-arthritis/
- Arthritis Foundation: http://www.arthritis.org/about-arthritis/types/psoriatic-arthritis/
- American College of Rheumatology: https://www.rheumatology.org

PROGNOSIS

- Course is typically insidious with chronic joint disease and recurring/remitting skin disease.
- Prognosis is more favorable than for RA (except for patients who develop arthritis mutilans).

COMPLICATIONS

- Disability
- Psychosocial impact of PsA: anxiety and depression

REFERENCES

1. Ritchlin CT, Colbert RA, Gladman DD. Psoriatic arthritis. *N Engl J Med*. 2017;376(10):957–970.
2. Ruta S, Jaldin Cespedes R, Cuellar L, et al. Psoriatic arthritis: differential features at the time of clinical presentation in a large cohort of patients with polyarthralgia. *Eur J Rheumatol*. 2023;10(1):12–17.
3. Gwinnutt JM, Wieczorek M, Balanescu A, et al. 2021 EULAR recommendations regarding lifestyle behaviours and work participation to prevent progression of rheumatic and musculoskeletal diseases. *Ann Rheum Dis*. 2023;82(1):48–56.
4. Singh JA, Guyatt F, Ogdie A, et al. Special article: 2018 American College of Rheumatology/National Psoriasis Foundation guideline for the treatment of psoriatic arthritis. *Arthritis Rheumatol*. 2019;71(1):5–32.

ADDITIONAL READING

- Norden A, Oulee A, Ivanic M, et al. The use of ultrasound to detect enthesitis as a potential guide for intervention in patients with psoriasis at risk of psoriatic arthritis: a systematic review. *Int J Dermatol*. 2023;62(8):973–979.
- Ruyssen-Witrand A, Perry R, Watkins C, et al. Efficacy and safety of biologics in psoriatic arthritis: a systematic literature review and network meta-analysis. *RMD Open*. 2020;6(1):e001117.

CODES

ICD10

- L40.50 Arthropathic psoriasis, unspecified
- L40.51 Distal interphalangeal psoriatic arthropathy
- L40.53 Psoriatic spondylitis

CLINICAL PEARLS

- One in four patients with psoriasis develops PsA.
- The severity of psoriasis correlates with the likelihood of developing arthritis, not the severity of arthritis.
- Commonly overlooked locations of psoriasis include scalp, ears, umbilicus, and gluteal cleft.
- Osteoarthritis and polyarticular gout may mimic or coexist with PsA.
- The polyarticular pattern of PsA mimics RA. The presence of both enthesitis and psoriasis helps differentiate PsA from RA.
- Therapies for PsA are rapidly expanding and include NSAIDs; DMARDs; immunosuppressants, biologics, and JAKi.

ARTHRITIS, RHEUMATOID (RA)
Sonia Gupta, MD

 BASICS

DESCRIPTION
Rheumatoid arthritis (RA) is a symmetric inflammatory disease primarily causing synovial inflammation and leading to the destruction of bone and cartilage.

EPIDEMIOLOGY
Incidence
Annual incidence: The United States is approximately 40 per 100,000 persons.

Prevalence
- Prevalence: 0.24% of the general population worldwide; in the United States, the prevalence is between 0.5% and 1.0%.
- Female:male, 2:1
- The lifetime risk of developing RA: 3.6% in women and 1.7% in men

ETIOLOGY AND PATHOPHYSIOLOGY
RA is a chronic inflammatory disease. The end result is damage to cartilage and bone, potentially leading to significant disability. Multiple cytokines have been identified in the pathophysiology of RA. These include tumor necrosis factor (TNF)-α, interleukin (IL)-1, IL-6, and IL-17. Macrophages and osteoclast activation are also involved in the disease process, ultimately leading to bony erosion and degradation.

Genetics
Estimated heritability 40%, >100 risk loci, HLA-DRB1 (the strongest genetic predisposition)

RISK FACTORS
Family history, genetic predisposition, middle-aged, female, lower socioeconomic status, cigarette smoking, infection, environmental, chronic inflammatory mucosal conditions

GENERAL PREVENTION
Smoking cessation, a well-balanced diet, achieving a healthy weight, regular physical activity, good dental hygiene

COMMONLY ASSOCIATED CONDITIONS
- Interstitial lung disease
- Pyoderma gangrenosum

 DIAGNOSIS

Early diagnosis is essential to maximize therapeutic effectiveness, to minimize disease progression, and to maximize quality of life.

HISTORY
- Join pain is the primary symptom. It is insidious in onset, often symmetrically involving small (peripheral) joints.
- Morning stiffness (≥1 hour) is common.
- Improvement of pain and stiffness with activity, low-grade fever, and weight loss are other historical features.
- Joint deformity is a longer term sequela.

PHYSICAL EXAM
- Symmetric swelling and tenderness of metacarpophalangeal (MCP), proximal interphalangeal (PIP), metatarsophalangeal (MTP), and spare distal interphalangeal (DIP) joints
- Ulnar deviation, boutonnière deformity, MCP joint subluxation, radial deviation at the wrist, hammer-toe deformity, extensor tendon rupture
- Subcutaneous nodules
- Extra-articular manifestations: keratoconjunctivitis, episcleritis, scleritis, rales, crackles, pericardial friction, rubs, splinter hemorrhage, palpable purpura, skin ulceration, nail fold infarcts, sensory and/or motor deficit, osteoporosis
- Cervical spine instability

DIFFERENTIAL DIAGNOSIS
Systemic lupus erythematosus, osteoarthritis, viral hepatitis, tophaceous gout, calcium pyrophosphate dihydrate deposition (CPPD), arthropathy, gout, polymyalgia rheumatica (PMR), postinfectious reactive arthritis, Lyme arthritis

DIAGNOSTIC TESTS & INTERPRETATION
- Diagnostic criteria
  - American College of Rheumatology criteria (1)
    - At least one joint with clinical synovitis that cannot be explained by another condition
    - A score of ≥6 classifies as RA Joint involvement
      - 1 large joint (0 point), 2 to 10 large joints (1 point), 1 to 3 small joints (2 points), 4 to 10 small joints (3 points), >10 joints (5 points)
    - Serology
      - Negative RF or low-positive anticyclic citrullinated peptide (anti-CCP) antibodies (0 point)

- Low-positive RF or low-positive anti-CCP antibodies (2 points)
- High-positive RF or high-positive anti-CCP antibodies (3 points)
  - Acute phase reactants
    - Normal CRP or ESR (0 point)
    - Abnormal CRP or ESR (1 point)
  - Duration of symptoms
    - <6 weeks (0 point)
    - ≥6 weeks (1 point)
- Anemia of chronic disease, mild thrombocytosis, elevated ESR, and CRP
- Serology: elevated rheumatoid factor and anti-CCP antibodies
- X-ray: joint space narrowing, juxta-articular osteopenia, marginal erosions
- Ultrasound can assess synovial thickening/erosions.
- MRI of hands and wrists (erosions, pannus, synovitis)

Initial Tests (lab, imaging)
- Imaging
- CT findings in RA—RA-associated lung disease: usual interstitial pneumonia pattern, nonspecific interstitial pneumonia pattern
- RA pleural effusion: typically exudative; elevated LDH, low pH <7.3, and glucose <60 mg/dL

Follow-Up Tests & Special Considerations
Laboratory monitoring for DMARD: CBC, liver transaminases, serum creatinine, albumin

Diagnostic Procedures/Other
- Joint aspiration to exclude crystal arthropathy and septic arthritis
- Synovial fluid analysis in RA: yellowish-white, turbid, white blood cell increased (3,500 to 50,000 cells/mm), protein: ~4.2 g/dL (42 g/L), serum-synovial glucose difference >30 mg/dL

Test Interpretation
- Anti-CCP antibodies are present in 60–70% of patients with RA but are 90–98% specific for RA. They are often present years before clinical arthritis. It correlates with erosive disease.
- Rheumatoid factor is positive in 50% of patients at the time of diagnosis and an additional 20–35% becomes positive in 6 months.
- Imaging: x-ray to follow the progression and identify the destruction of the disease; MRI of hands and wrists (erosions, pannus, synovitis) and ultrasound can assess synovial thickening/erosions.

TREATMENT

Treat-to-target approach is strongly recommended over usual care for patients who have not been previously treated with DMARDS (both traditional and biologics).

GENERAL MEASURES
Smoking cessation, well-balanced diet, regular physical activity, good dental hygiene

MEDICATION
- Conventional synthetic disease-modifying antirheumatic drugs (csDMARDs) are recommended as first line: Hydroxychloroquine, leflunomide, methotrexate (MTX), and sulfasalazine are the most common—MTX is the most used first-line RA drug worldwide and is generally preferred as the first-line DMARD. 7.5 mg/week is a typical starting dose for MTX.
- TNF-α inhibitors: etanercept, infliximab, adalimumab, certolizumab, and golimumab have the longest safety data and are the initial choice for biologic agents. Etanercept is an engineered biologic combination of the TNF-α receptor extracellular domain with IgG Fc. A common dose is 50 mg SC per week.
- IL inhibitors (anakinra, rilonacept, canakinumab, tocilizumab, ustekinumab) suppress IL-1, IL-6, IL-12, and IL-23.
- Abatacept suppresses CTLA-4.
- Rituximab is an anti-CD20 antibody.
- JAK inhibitors include tofacitinib, baricitinib, and upadacitinib.
- Treatment recommendations
  - In DMARD-naive patients in moderate to high activity, MTX monotherapy is preferred over other treatments.
  - The addition of other agents is conditionally recommended over triple therapy for patients taking a maximally tolerated dose of MTX who are not at the target.
  - Continuation of DMARDS at their current dose is conditionally recommended over a dose reduction.
  - If the disease flares in a patient on traditional DMARD, TNF inhibitor, or non-TNF biologics therapy, a short-term glucocorticoid can be added at the lowest possible dose and for the shortest possible duration.

- Before starting medication
  - Screening for hepatitis B and hepatitis C infection
  - Quant TB test
  - Baseline ophthalmologic examination for patients receiving hydroxychloroquine use

First Line
csDMARDs

Second Line
Biologics synthetic disease-modifying antirheumatic drugs (adalimumab, certolizumab, etanercept, golimumab, infliximab), T cell costimulatory agents (abatacept), IL-6 receptor inhibitors (tocilizumab, sarilumab), anti-CD20 antibody (rituximab), targeted synthetic disease-modifying antirheumatic drugs, JAK inhibitors (tofacitinib, baricitinib, upadacitinib)

ISSUES FOR REFERRAL
- Rheumatology for management of biologics
- Pulmonology: interstitial lung disease
- Ophthalmology: scleritis, episcleritis, screening patients on hydroxychloroquine (Plaquenil)

SURGERY/OTHER PROCEDURES
Synovectomy, tendon alignment, arthrodesis

COMPLEMENTARY & ALTERNATIVE MEDICINE
Psychosocial interventions, physical and occupational therapies

ADMISSION, INPATIENT, AND NURSING CONSIDERATIONS
For serious infection, diverticulitis, and gastrointestinal perforation

ONGOING CARE

FOLLOW-UP RECOMMENDATIONS
Patient Monitoring
Drug toxicity monitoring regularly, monitoring for extra-articular manifestation

DIET
Avoid fatty foods and eat lots of fruits and vegetables.

PATIENT EDUCATION
Smoking cessation; avoid alcohol and pregnancy while on MTX.

PROGNOSIS
Poor prognosis with an autoantibody and longer disease duration, HLA, erosive disease

COMPLICATIONS
Joint deformities, malignancies (lymphoma, lung cancer, skin cancer), pulmonary disease, infection, cardiovascular diseases

REFERENCE
1. Aletaha D, Neogi T, Silman AJ, et al. 2010 Rheumatoid arthritis classification criteria: an American College of Rheumatology/European League Against Rheumatism collaborative initiative. *Arthritis Rheum*. 2010;62(9):2569–2581.

ADDITIONAL READING
- Cush JJ. Rheumatoid arthritis: early diagnosis and treatment. *Med Clin North Am*. 2021;105(2): 355–365.
- Sánchez-Flórez JC, Seija-Butnaru D, Valero EG, et al. Pain management strategies in rheumatoid arthritis: a narrative review. *J Pain Palliat Care Pharmacother*. 2021;35(4):291–299.

CODES

ICD10
- M06.9 Rheumatoid arthritis, unspecified
- M05.60 Rheu arthritis of unsp site w involv of organs and systems
- M05.30 Rheumatoid heart disease w rheumatoid arthritis of unsp site

CLINICAL PEARLS
- Early treatment with DMARDs is essential; treat-to-target approach
- MTX is the first-line treatment for active disease.
- Biologic agents continue to rapidly evolve and are a critical element of the ongoing treatment of RA. Selection of specific agents is dependent on individual patient characteristics and is best done with rheumatologic support.

ARTHRITIS, SEPTIC

Shane L. Larson, MD • Briana Lindberg, MD, CAQSM

 BASICS

DESCRIPTION
- Infection due to bacterial invasion of the joint space
- Systems affected: musculoskeletal
- Synonyms: suppurative arthritis; infections arthritis; pyarthrosis; pyogenic arthritis; bacterial arthritis

EPIDEMIOLOGY
Gender differences:
- Gonococcal: female > male
- Nongonococcal: male > female

Incidence
- May occur at any age, bimodal incidence with peaks in childhood and age ≥55 years
- 40 to 60 cases per 100,000 population/year overall (1)
- 70 cases per 100,000 population/year in immuno-compromised and patients with prosthetic joints
- Disseminated gonococcal infection is 3 cases per 100,000 population/year.

Prevalence
- 27% of patients presenting with monoarticular arthritis have nongonococcal septic arthritis (1).
- Given rising prevalence of prosthetic joints, infected hardware is now most common form of septic arthritis (~2–10% of all joint recipients)

ETIOLOGY AND PATHOPHYSIOLOGY
- Multiple pathogens
- Nongonococcal: *Staphylococcus aureus* (most common in adults)
  – MRSA risk increased in elderly, intravenous drug users (IVDU), postsurgical
  – *Streptococcus* spp. (second most common in adults)
  – Gram-negative rods (GNR): IVDU, trauma, extremes of age, immunosuppressed
- *Neisseria gonorrhoeae* (most common in young, sexually active adults)
- Polymicrobial infections: *Pantoea agglomerans*, Nocardia asteroides; typically occur after penetrating trauma such as bite wounds or organic foreign body penetration
- Other: rickettsial (e.g., Lyme), fungal, mycobacterial
- Risk by specific age:
  – <1 month: *S. aureus*, group B streptococcus (GBS), GNR
  – 1 month to 4 years: *S. aureus*, *Streptococcus pneumoniae*, *Neisseria meningitidis*
  – 16 to 40 years: *N. meningitidis*, *S. aureus*
  – >40 years: *S. aureus*
- Patients with native joint infection are at increased risk for infection of prosthesis (of same joint should it require replacement).
- Specific high-risk groups:
  – Rheumatoid arthritis (RA): *S. aureus*
  – IVDU: *S. aureus*, GNR, opportunistic pathogens
  – Neonates: GBS
  – Immunocompromised: gram-negative bacilli, fungi
  – Trauma patients with open injuries: mixed flora
- Pathogenesis:
  – Hematogenous spread (most common)
  – Direct inoculation by microorganisms secondary to trauma or iatrogenesis (e.g., joint surgery)
  – Adjacent spread (e.g., osteomyelitis)

- Pathophysiology:
  – Microorganisms initially enter through synovial membrane and spread to the synovial fluid.
  – Resulting inflammatory response releases cytokines and destructive proteases leading to systemic symptoms and joint damage.

RISK FACTORS
- Age >80 years
- Low socioeconomic status, alcoholism
- Cellulitis and skin ulcers
- Violation of joint capsule
  – Prior orthopedic surgery
  – Intraarticular injection
  – Trauma
- History of previous joint disease
  – Inflammatory arthritis (RA: 10-fold increased risk)
  – Osteoarthritis
  – Crystal arthritides
- Systemic illness: diabetes mellitus, liver disease, HIV, malignancy, end-stage renal disease/hemodialysis, immunosuppression, sickle cell anemia
- Risks for hematogenous spread: IVDU, severe sepsis/systemic infection

GENERAL PREVENTION
- Prompt treatment of skin and soft tissue infections
- Control risk factors.
- Immunizations (*S. pneumoniae*, *N. meningitidis*)

COMMONLY ASSOCIATED CONDITIONS
Preexisting joint conditions, previous joint trauma or surgery, prosthetic joint

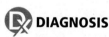 **DIAGNOSIS**

HISTORY
- Typically presents with a combination of joint pain, swelling, warmth, and decreased range of motion
- Nongonococcal arthritis: mostly monoarticular (80%)
  – Typically large joints: knee (50%), hip (20%), shoulder (8%), ankle (7%)
  – Most patients report fever.
  – IV drug users may develop infection in axial joints (e.g., sternoclavicular joint).
  – Prosthetic joints may be minimally symptomatic and present with draining sinus over joint.
  – Patients on chronic immunosuppressive drugs and those receiving articular corticosteroid injections may have atypical presentations (absent fever or joint pain).
- Pediatric considerations:
  – Infants may avoid moving limb (often mistaken for neurologic problem).
  – Hip pain may commonly refer to knee and/or thigh.
- Gonococcal arthritis
  – Bacteremic phase: migratory polyarthritis, teno-synovitis, high fever, chills, pustules (dermatitis–arthritis syndrome)
  – Localized phase: less symptomatic—often mono-articular, low-grade fever
- Approximately 22% of all patients with culture-proven septic arthritis had no associated risk factors or underlying joint disease.

PHYSICAL EXAM
- Physical exam has poor sensitive and specificity for septic arthritis; however, common findings include:
  – Fever
  – Limited range of motion
  – Joint effusion and tenderness
  – Erythema and warmth over affected joint
  – Pain with passive range of motion
- Hip and shoulder involvement may reveal severe pain with range of motion and less obvious swelling.
- Infants with septic hip arthritis maintain the joint in flexion and external rotation as position of comfort.
- Purpura associated with disseminated gonococcal infection

DIFFERENTIAL DIAGNOSIS
- Crystal arthritis: gout, pseudogout, calcium oxalate, cholesterol
- Infectious arthritis: fungi, spirochetes, rheumatic fever, HIV, viral
- Inflammatory arthritis: RA, spondyloarthropathy, systemic lupus erythematosus, sarcoidosis
- Osteoarthritis
- Trauma: meniscal tear, fracture, hemarthrosis
- Other: bursitis, cellulitis, tendinitis

DIAGNOSTIC TESTS & INTERPRETATION
Initial Tests (lab, imaging)
- Synovial fluid analysis is the gold standard of diagnosis.
  – Obtain prior to antibiotic therapy when possible.
  – Include Gram stain, culture, cell count/differential, and crystal analysis.
  – Use blood culture bottles to increase yield.
  – Gram stain (sensitivity 29–65%); culture (positive in 80%) (1)
  – >50,000 WBCs/HPF with >90% polymorpho-nuclear leukocytes is suggestive.
    ○ Synovial WBC (sWBC) *count alone is insufficient to rule in or rule out septic arthritis* (1).
    ○ Likelihood of septic arthritis increases as sWBC rises >100,000/HPF (1).
  – Analysis of synovial fluid leukocyte esterase is associated with a high negative predictive value (NPV) (2).
  – Crystals (e.g., urate or calcium pyrophosphate) *do not exclude concurrent infectious arthritis*.
  – Prosthetic joint: WBC count is unreliable; a lower number of sWBCs may indicate infection.
- Serum tests:
  – WBC count alone is neither sensitive nor specific.
  – ESR > 15 mm/hr has sensitivity up to 94% but poor specificity (3).
  – CRP > 20 mg/L has sensitivity of 92% (3).
  – Synovial lactate is a potential biomarker to rule out septic arthritis when <250 U/L; however, more study is needed (1).
  – Blood cultures positive in ~50% of cases
- Other tests:
  – Disseminated gonococcus: culture blood, cervix, urine, urethra, pharynx in addition to joint fluid
  – Suspect Lyme arthritis: PCR and serum titers for *Borrelia* IgM and IgG indicate exposure.

- Pediatrics: No single lab test distinguishes septic arthritis from transient synovitis.
  - The combination of fever, non–weight-bearing, and elevated ESR/CRP is suspicious; obtain synovial fluid for analysis when possible.
- Imaging:
  - Can help identify effusion but does not further differentiate causes of arthritis
  - Plain films
    - Nondiagnostic for septic arthritis; useful for trauma, soft tissue swelling, osteoarthritis, or osteopenia
    - May show nonspecific inflammatory arthritic changes (i.e., erosions, joint destruction, or joint space loss)
  - Ultrasound
    - Useful for guiding arthrocentesis
    - Recommended for aspiration of deep joints such as the hip
  - MRI
    - Highly sensitive for effusion, may help differentiate between transient synovitis and septic arthritis in children
  - Other imaging
    - CT is not routinely indicated.
    - Bone scans are not performed unless there is concurrent suspicion for osteomyelitis.

Diagnostic Procedures/Other
Arthrocentesis in all suspected cases (prior to starting antibiotics): Avoid contaminated tissue (e.g., overlying cellulitis) when performing arthrocentesis.

Test Interpretation
Synovial biopsy shows polymorphonuclear leukocytes and (possibly) the causative organism.

 TREATMENT

GENERAL MEASURES
- Admit for parenteral antibiotics and monitoring
  - Begin antibiotics immediately after arthrocentesis.
- Drainage of purulent material is *required* if:
  - Pediatric: Surgical drainage and irrigation is recommended if there is a hip involvement due to high risk of avascular necrosis.
  - Prosthetic Joint: antibiotics and consult with orthopedics for consideration of revision arthroplasty, resection arthroplasty, or débridement
- Antibiotic therapy for a total of 4 to 6 weeks in most cases
  - Native joint infections require at least 2 weeks; prosthetics longer
  - Each case should be evaluated individually and contextually, consulting infectious disease specialists when appropriate.
  - Exception: gonococcal arthritis; treated for 2 to 3 weeks
- Intra-articular antibiotics are not typically recommended or used.

MEDICATION
First Line
- Initial antibiotic choice is guided by Gram stain or most likely organism based on age, clinical history, and risk factors (1)[C].
- Nongonococcal (1)[C],(2)[C]:
  - Gram-positive cocci: Vancomycin 15 to 20 mg/kg 2 to 3 times daily or linezolid 600 mg twice daily
  - Gram-negative bacilli:
    - Cefepime 2 g twice daily or ceftriaxone 2 g daily or ceftazidime 2 g 3 times daily or cefotaxime 2 g 3 times daily
    - For cephalosporin allergy: Consider treatment with ciprofloxacin 400 mg 3 times daily.
  - Negative Gram stain: Vancomycin 15 to 20 mg/kg 2 to 3 times daily plus 3rd-generation cephalosporin until cultures and susceptibilities return
  - Duration of therapy: typically 2 weeks of IV and additional 2 to 4 weeks PO while monitoring therapeutic response closely
- Gonococcal:
  - Ceftriaxone 1 g IV/IM daily for 7 to 14 days
    - Continue at least 24 to 48 hours after symptom resolution.
    - May require concurrent drainage of affected joint
    - Concomitant treatment for *Chlamydia* (doxycycline 100 mg twice daily or azithromycin 1 g once)
- Other considerations:
  - Narrow antibiotic therapy based on culture results.
  - Consider *Salmonella* in pediatric patients with history of sickle cell disease.
    - 3rd-generation cephalosporins in this instance
  - Lyme arthritis: doxycycline 100 mg PO twice daily or amoxicillin 500 mg PO 3 times daily for 28 days if no neurologic involvement, otherwise ceftriaxone 2 g IV daily

ISSUES FOR REFERRAL
- Infectious disease specialist consult for IVDU and immunosuppressed patients
- Orthopedic consultation for prosthetic joint infections (1)[C]

SURGERY/OTHER PROCEDURES
- Consider drainage in all cases—particularly shoulder, hip, and prosthetic joints (1)[C].
- Other treatment options include repeat needle aspiration, arthroscopy, or arthrotomy.

ADMISSION, INPATIENT, AND NURSING CONSIDERATIONS
Mean duration of hospitalization is 12 days.

 ONGOING CARE

FOLLOW-UP RECOMMENDATIONS
Patient Monitoring
- Can monitor synovial fluid to verify decreasing WBC and sterile fluid after initial treatment
- If no improvement in 24 hours, reevaluate and consider arthroscopy.
- Follow up at 1 week and 1 month after stopping antibiotics to exclude relapse.

PROGNOSIS
- Early treatment improves functional outcome.
- Delayed recognition/treatment is associated with higher morbidity and mortality.
- Elderly, concurrent RA, *S. aureus* infections, and infection of hip and shoulder also increase risk of poor outcome.

COMPLICATIONS
- Mortality rates between 3% and 25% (1)
- Limited joint range of motion, ankylosis, osteomyelitis, postinfectious synovitis
- Secondary osteoarthritis; flail, fused, or dislocated joint; sepsis, septic necrosis
- Sinus formation
- Osteomyelitis, postinfectious synovitis
- Limb length discrepancy (primarily in cases prior to skeletal maturity)

REFERENCES
1. Long B, Koyfman A, Gottlieb M. Evaluation and management of septic arthritis and its mimics in the emergency department. *West J Emerg Med*. 2019;20(2):331–341.
2. Dey M, Al-Attar M, Peruffo L, et al. Assessment and diagnosis of the acute hot joint: a systematic review and meta-analysis. *Rheumatology (Oxford)*. 2022;62(5):1740–1756.
3. Aggarwal P, Mahapatra S, Avasthi S, et al. Role of serum and synovial procalcitonin in differentiating septic from non-septic arthritis—a prospective study. *J Clin Orthop Trauma*. 2022;31:101948.

CODES

ICD10
- M00.079 Staphylococcal arthritis, unspecified ankle and foot
- M00.829 Arthritis due to other bacteria, unspecified elbow
- M00.011 Staphylococcal arthritis, right shoulder

CLINICAL PEARLS
- Arthrocentesis and synovial fluid analysis are mandatory in cases of suspected septic arthritis.
- Gram stain has variable sensitivity in septic arthritis. sWBC count is generally >50,000/HPV but is unreliable as a sole diagnostic feature and should be interpreted in context.
- Early IV antibiotics and (if necessary) drainage of infected joints are critical to successful management.
- Crystalline disease may coexist with septic arthritis.
- Initial antibiotic therapy is guided by arthrocentesis results (Gram stain), age, and patient-specific risk factors.

ARTHROPOD BITES AND STINGS

James E. Powers, DO, FACEP, FAAEM

BASICS

DESCRIPTION

- Arthropods are the largest division of the animal kingdom. Two classes, insects and arachnids, have the greatest impact on human health. Arthropods affect humans by inoculating venom, microorganisms, or irritative substances through a bite or sting; by invading tissue, or by contact allergy to their skin, hairs, or secretions.
- Transmission of infectious microorganisms during feeding is of the greatest concern.
- Sequelae of bites, stings, or contact include:
  - Local redness with itch, pain, and swelling: common, usually immediate and transient; large local reactions that increase over 24 to 48 hours; systemic reactions with anaphylaxis, neurotoxicity, organ damage, or other systemic toxin effects; tissue necrosis or secondary infection

EPIDEMIOLOGY

Incidence
Arthropod bites and stings account for up to 1 million emergency department visits annually in the United States.

Prevalence
Widespread, with regional and seasonal variations

ETIOLOGY AND PATHOPHYSIOLOGY

- Arthropods: four medically important classes
  - Insects: *Hymenoptera* (bees, wasps, hornets, fire ants), mosquitoes, bed bugs, flies, lice, fleas, beetles, caterpillars, and moths
  - Arachnids: spiders, scorpions, mites, and ticks
  - Chilopods: centipedes
  - Diplopods: millipedes
- Four general categories of pathophysiologic effects: toxic, allergic, infectious, and traumatic
  - Toxic effects of venom: local (tissue inflammation or destruction) versus systemic (neurotoxic or organ damage)
  - Allergic: Antigens in saliva or venom may cause local inflammation. Exaggerated immune responses may result in anaphylaxis or serum sickness.
  - Trauma: Mechanical injury from biting or stinging causes pain, swelling, and portal of entry for bacteria and secondary infection. Retention of arthropod parts can cause a granulomatous reaction.
  - Infection: Arthropods transmit bacterial, viral, and protozoal diseases.

Genetics
Family history of atopy may be a factor in the development of more severe allergic reactions.

RISK FACTORS
Previous sensitization; although most arthropod contact is inadvertent, certain activities, occupations, and travel exposures increase risk; greater risk for adverse outcomes in young, elderly, immunocompromised, and those with chronic or poorly controlled cardiac or respiratory disease; increased risk of anaphylaxis, especially to *Hymenoptera* stings, in patients with mastocytosis

GENERAL PREVENTION

- Avoid common arthropod habitats.
- Insect repellents (not effective for bees, spiders, scorpions, caterpillars, bed bugs, fleas, ants)
  - N,N-diethyl-meta-toluamide (DEET)
    - Most studied repellent; broadest spectrum of activity against biting arthropods (1)[A]
    - Concentrations of 20–35% offer approximately 5 hours of protection (1)[A]. Safe for children >2 months of age and pregnant and lactating women (1)[A]
  - Picaridin (also known as icaridin)
    - 20% spray comparable to 20% DEET for mosquito and tick protection
  - p-Menthane-3,8-diol (PMD; lemon eucalyptus extract)
    - 30% concentrations give 4 to 5 hours of protection against mosquitoes and ticks. Not for use on children <3 years old
  - There are many other products but lack evidence regarding efficacy, duration of action, and safety.
- Barrier methods: clothing, bed nets. Use of light-colored pants, long-sleeved shirts, and hats may reduce arthropod impact. Permethrin: synthetic insecticide derived from chrysanthemum plant. Do not apply directly to skin. Permethrin-impregnated clothing provides good protection against arthropods. Mosquito nets: advised for all travelers to disease-endemic areas at risk from biting arthropods. Permethrin-treated nets may offer additional protection.
- Risk of tick-borne diseases may be decreased by removal of ticks within 24 hours of attachment.

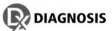 DIAGNOSIS

HISTORY

- Sudden onset of pain or itching with visualization of arthropod
- Many cases unknown to patient or asymptomatic initially (bed bugs, lice, scabies, ticks). Consider in patients presenting with localized erythema, urticaria, wheals, papules, pruritus, or bullae
- May identify insect by its habitat or by remnants brought by the patient. History of prior exposure useful but not always available or reliable. Travel, occupational, social, and recreational history may identify risk factors for arthropod exposure.

PHYSICAL EXAM

- If stinger is present, remove by flicking or scraping away from skin.
- Anaphylaxis is a clinical diagnosis. Signs and symptoms include:
  - Erythema, flushing, urticaria, angioedema: Caution—skin involvement absent in up to 20% of cases. Itching/edema of lips, tongue, uvula; drooling; respiratory distress, wheeze, repetitive cough, stridor, dysphonia
  - Hypotension, dysrhythmia, syncope, confusion, chest pain

- If no evidence of anaphylaxis, the exam focuses on the sting or bite itself. Common findings include local erythema, swelling, wheals, urticaria, papules, or bullae; excoriations from scratching may be present
- Thorough exam to look for arthropod infestation (lice, scabies) or attached ticks. Body lice usually found in seams of clothing; skin scraping to identify scabies. Signs of secondary bacterial infection after 24 to 48 hours: increasing erythema, pain, fever, lymphangitis, or abscess

DIFFERENTIAL DIAGNOSIS

- Urticaria and localized dermatologic reactions:
  - Contact dermatitis, drug eruption, mastocytosis, bullous diseases, dermatitis herpetiformis, tinea, eczema, vasculitis, pityriasis, erythema multiforme, viral exanthem, cellulitis, abscess, impetigo, folliculitis, erysipelas, necrotizing fasciitis
- Anaphylactic-type reactions
  - Cardiac, hemorrhagic, or septic shock; myocardial infarction; acute respiratory failure, asthma; angioedema, urticarial vasculitis; flushing syndromes (catecholamines, vasoactive peptides); syncope; scombroid

DIAGNOSTIC TESTS & INTERPRETATION

Initial Tests (lab, imaging)
Seldom needed; basic lab parameters are usually normal.

Follow-Up Tests & Special Considerations

- Severe envenomations may affect organ function and require monitoring of lab values (CBC, comprehensive metabolic panel, prothrombin time/international normalized ratio).
- Potential arthropod-borne diseases:
  - Ticks: Lyme disease, Rocky Mountain spotted fever, relapsing fever, anaplasmosis, babesiosis, tularemia; ehrlichiosis, Powassan virus disease; Heartland virus (HRTV); Bourbon virus. Noninfectious complications of tick bites include tick paralysis and α-Gal sensitization resulting in meat allergy.
  - Flies: tularemia, leishmaniasis, African trypanosomiasis, bartonellosis, loiasis, anthrax
  - Fleas: plague, tularemia, murine typhus
  - Chigger mites: scrub typhus (Asia-Pacific regions)
  - Body lice: epidemic typhus, relapsing fever
  - Kissing bugs: Chagas disease
  - Mosquitoes: malaria, yellow fever, dengue fever, West Nile virus, chikungunya, Zika virus, lymphatic filariasis, Rift Valley fever virus; Japanese, Eastern equine, and St. Louis encephalitis
- Patients with anaphylaxis or significant systemic symptoms should be referred to an allergist for formal testing (1)[A].

Diagnostic Procedures/Other
Skin and immunologic tests available to identify specific allergens; baseline serum tryptase levels for follow-up of anaphylaxis

TREATMENT

Most treatments are based on consensus recommendations, clinical experience, or retrospective studies.

ALERT
- Anaphylaxis is potentially life-threatening. Most deaths occur within 30 to 60 minutes.
- Give epinephrine as soon as diagnosis of anaphylaxis is suspected. Delay associated with increased morbidity and mortality (2)[A].
- Antihistamines and steroids do not replace epinephrine and are never the initial therapy in anaphylaxis (2)[A].

GENERAL MEASURES
Routine management of arthropod bites and stings is directed at relieving itching, pain, and swelling; includes local wound care, ice compress, topical corticosteroids, systemic antihistamines, and analgesics.

MEDICATION
First Line
- For arthropod bites/stings with anaphylaxis (2)[C]
  - Epinephrine: most important: IM injection in midanterolateral thigh
    ○ IM dose: epinephrine 1:1,000 (1 mg/mL): adult: 0.3 to 0.5 mg per dose; pediatric: 0.01 mg/kg to a maximum dose of 0.3 mg per dose; can repeat every 5 to 15 minutes
  - High flow oxygen up to 100%, as needed
  - Establish 1 to 2 large-bore IV lines. Normal saline bolus 20 to 30 mL/kg; repeat as needed
  - Antihistamines: H_1 and H_2 antagonists are poorly effective in treating cardiovascular and respiratory impacts of anaphylaxis; may have adjunctive role after treatment with epinephrine
  - Corticosteroids: 2012 Cochrane review showed no benefit in acute anaphylaxis. No clear benefit in reducing risk for biphasic reactions.
  - Prednisone, methylprednisolone still frequently used
- Arthropod bites/stings without anaphylaxis
  - Routine wound care, wash with soap and water; antibiotics only if an infection
  - Tetanus booster, as indicated
  - Oral antihistamines may be helpful in controlling itch/hives. Commonly utilized H_1 and H_2 antagonists include:
    ○ Diphenhydramine adults: 25 to 50 mg PO every 4 to 6 hours; pediatrics: 1 to 1.5 mg/kg PO (max of 25 to 50 mg/dose) every 6 to 8 hours; daily maximum dose of 300 mg for adults and 5 mg/kg (to max of 300 mg) for pediatrics
    ○ Cetirizine adults: 5 to 10 mg PO daily; pediatrics: 6 to 23 months—2.5 mg PO daily; 2 to 5 years—5 mg PO daily; ≥6 years—5 to 10 mg PO daily
    ○ H_2 antagonists: famotidine adults: 10 to 20 mg PO 1 to 2 times daily as needed; children and adolescents: 0.5 mg/kg/dose PO 1 to 2 times daily (maximum dose is 40 mg PO twice per day). H_2 antagonists are not FDA-approved for the treatment of hives or pruritus.
  - Oral steroids: Consider short course for severe pruritus or local reactions.
    ○ Prednisone or prednisolone: adults: 5 to 60 mg/day PO; infants, children, adolescents: 1 to 2 mg/kg/day in 1 to 4 divided doses (maximum of 60 mg/day)

- Consider topical steroid cream or ointment for 3 to 5 days.
  ○ OTC 1% hydrocortisone; may consider higher potency such as triamcinolone 0.1%, fluocinolone 0.025%
- Other specific therapies:
  ○ Scorpion stings: Treat excess catecholamine release (nitroprusside, prazosin, β-blockers). Atropine for hypersalivation. One FDA-approved scorpion antivenom in the United States. Consider in patients with severe symptoms and in consultation with a toxicologist (1)[B].
  ○ Black widow bites: Treat muscle spasms with benzodiazepines and opioid analgesics. Antivenom is available but only administered for severe symptoms and in consultation with a toxicologist (1)[B].
  ○ Consult Poison Control hotline for questions regarding any envenomation management: 1-800-222-1222.
- Fire ants: characteristically cause sterile pustules; leave intact—do not open or drain.
- Brown recluse spider: local wound care, tetanus prophylaxis as indicated, pain control, supportive treatment; surgical consult if débridement or scar revision needed (1)[C]
- Ticks: early removal to reduce risk of disease transmission
- Pediculosis: head, pubic, and body lice
  ○ First line: permethrin 1% topical lotion (3)[A]; alternatives: pyrethrins; ivermectin PO shown to be effective but not FDA-approved for pediculosis. Repeat treatment in 7 to 10 days.
  ○ Body lice usually treated successfully by bathing and laundering clothing and linens in hot water (3)[A].
- Sarcoptes scabiei—scabies
  ○ Permethrin 5% cream is treatment of choice: Apply to entire body. Wash off after 8 to 14 hours. Repeat in 1 week (3)[A].
  ○ Ivermectin: 200 μg/kg PO once; repeat in 2 weeks shown to be effective but not FDA-approved for scabies.

ISSUES FOR REFERRAL
Patients with anaphylaxis or significant systemic symptoms should be referred to an allergist for formal testing (1)[A].

SURGERY/OTHER PROCEDURES
Débridement and delayed skin grafting may be required for severe brown recluse spider and other bites.

COMPLEMENTARY & ALTERNATIVE MEDICINE
- Ice, cool compresses. Calamine lotion commonly used, but no clear benefit.
- A paste of 3 tsp of baking soda and 1 tsp water may help salve bites.

ADMISSION, INPATIENT, AND NURSING CONSIDERATIONS
Admission required for anaphylaxis, vascular instability, neuromuscular events, pain, GI symptoms, renal damage/failure

 ONGOING CARE

FOLLOW-UP RECOMMENDATIONS
Venom immunotherapy is the cornerstone of treatment for *Hymenoptera* stings; 80–98% effective so patients with anaphylaxis should be referred to allergist for testing.

Patient Monitoring
Monitor for delayed effects, including infectious diseases from arthropod bites. Serum sickness reactions, vasculitis (rare)

PATIENT EDUCATION
Provide instruction on symptomatic care, arthropod avoidance, and infection and vector-borne disease surveillance. For patients with anaphylaxis, provide action plan and instructions on the use of epinephrine (2)[C].

PROGNOSIS
- Excellent for local reactions and mild systemic symptoms
- In anaphylaxis, immediate treatment with epinephrine significantly reduces morbidity and mortality.

COMPLICATIONS
- Anaphylaxis
- Secondary bacterial infection; arthropod-associated infectious diseases; scarring; psychological effects, phobias

REFERENCES
1. Herness J, Snyder MJ, Newman RS. Arthropod bites and stings. *Am Fam Physician*. 2022;106(2): 137–147.
2. Cardona V, Ansotegui IJ, Ebisawa M, et al. World Allergy Organization anaphylaxis guidance 2020. *World Allergy Organ J*. 2020;13(10):100472.
3. Kamath S, Kenner-Bell B. Infestations, bites, and insect repellents. *Pediatr Ann*. 2020;49(3): e124–e131.

 CODES

ICD10
- T63.481A Toxic effect of venom of arthropod, accidental, init
- T63.301A Toxic effect of unsp spider venom, accidental, init
- T63.484A Toxic effect of venom of oth arthropod, undetermined, init

CLINICAL PEARLS
- Urgent administration of epinephrine is the key to successful treatment of anaphylaxis.
- Local treatment and symptom management are sufficient in most insect bites and stings.
- Tick-borne illness is on the rise in the United States.

ASCITES

Tasaduq Hussain Mir, MD, FAAFP • Afsha Rais Kaisani, MD • Jeremy W. Smith, MD

 BASICS

DESCRIPTION
- Ascites is the pathologic accumulation of fluid in the peritoneal cavity and the most common complication of cirrhosis (1).
- It may occur in conditions that cause generalized edema like nephrotic syndrome, heart failure, and malignancy.
- Amount of fluid accumulation:
  - Grade 1: mild ascites—only detected by ultrasound (US); responsive ascites
  - Grade 2: moderate ascites—moderate symmetric distension of abdomen; recurrent ascites
  - Grade 3: large or gross ascites—marked distension of the abdomen; refractory ascites (RA)
    - Ascitic fluid that recurs after paracentesis or cannot be prevented by treatment
- Men generally have no fluid in peritoneal cavity; women may have up to 20 mL depending on menstrual phase.

EPIDEMIOLOGY
- Children: most commonly associated with nephrotic syndrome and malignancy
- Adults: cirrhosis (81%), cancer (10%), heart failure (3%), tuberculosis (TB) 2%, other (6%)
- 50% of patients with decompensated cirrhosis develop ascites.

Incidence
Approximately 50–60% of cirrhotic patients develop ascites within 10 years (2). The presence of ascites in cirrhotic patients is a poor prognostic indicator with mortality of about 44% in 5 years (1).

Prevalence
10% of patients with cirrhosis have ascites.

ETIOLOGY AND PATHOPHYSIOLOGY
- Portal hypertension versus nonportal hypertension
  - Cannot reliably establish/confirm etiology without paracentesis
  - Serum-ascites albumin gradient (SAAG): (serum albumin level: ascites albumin level) helps to differentiate
- High portal pressure (SAAG ≥1.1 g/dL)—reflects portal hypertension
  - Cirrhosis, hepatitis (alcoholic, viral, autoimmune, medications), acute liver failure, liver malignancy (primary or metastatic), heart failure or constrictive pericarditis, Budd-Chiari syndrome, and portal vein thrombosis
- Normal portal pressure (SAAG <1.1 g/dL)—excludes portal hypertension
  - Peritoneal carcinomatosis, TB, severe hypoalbuminemia (nephrotic syndrome; severe enteropathy with protein loss), Meigs syndrome (ovarian cancer), lymphatic leak (chylous ascites), pancreatitis, inflammatory (vasculitis, lupus serositis, sarcoidosis), other infections (parasitic, fungal), hemoperitoneum (trauma or ectopic pregnancy)
- Pathogenesis of ascites in the setting of portal hypertension (cirrhotic ascites): backward transmission of increased pressure to the visceral capillary bed with subsequent dilation and shift of fluid to the peritoneal cavity
  - This decreases intravascular volume and leads to hypotension. Systemic hypovolemia triggers renin-angiotensin–aldosterone system.

RISK FACTORS
- Cirrhosis—hepatitis B and C; alcohol abuse
- Congestive heart failure (CHF); advanced kidney disease; malignancy
- TB

GENERAL PREVENTION
Lifestyle—appropriate diet; physical activity; safe sexual practices; avoid alcohol misuse and hepatotoxic medications.

COMMONLY ASSOCIATED CONDITIONS
Nephrotic syndrome, liver cancer, heart failure

 DIAGNOSIS

History, physical examination, and diagnostic abdominal paracentesis are key to diagnosis.

HISTORY
- Address risk factors (e.g., EtOH use, TB exposure, prior malignancies, sexual partners, transfusion history, metabolic syndrome, increased risk of nonalcoholic steatohepatitis progressing to cirrhosis, previous history of cardiac illness).
- Assess for symptoms of underlying disease (chest pain, dyspnea, orthopnea, peripheral edema, asterixis, weight loss, night sweats, chronic cough).
- Assess for complications (fever/abdominal pain might indicate spontaneous bacterial peritonitis [SBP], progressive dyspnea due to increased abdominal girth).
- Progressive abdominal distention may be painful.

PHYSICAL EXAM
- Abdominal distention with flank/shifting dullness is the most sensitive (83%) and specific (56%) exam finding; requires >1,500 mL of fluid to detect
- Signs of right sided heart failure: peripheral edema (penile/scrotal, pedal), increased jugular venous pressure
- Stigmata of chronic liver cirrhosis (palmar erythema, spider angiomata, dilated abdominal wall collateral veins)
- Other signs of advanced liver disease: jaundice, muscle wasting, gynecomastia, leukonychia, asterixis
- Signs of underlying malignancy: cachexia; supraclavicular (Virchow) node suggests upper abdominal malignancy.

DIFFERENTIAL DIAGNOSIS
Obesity; large ovarian tumors; bowel obstruction; massive splenomegaly

DIAGNOSTIC TESTS & INTERPRETATION
Diagnostic abdominal paracentesis is the most cost-effective method.

Initial Tests (lab, imaging)
- US (can detect small volumes of ascitic fluid ~100 mL)
- Diagnostic paracentesis to rule out infection with clinically new-onset ascites or new abdominal pain in patient with ascites

- Ascitic fluid should be sent for analysis for cell count, protein, Gram stain, and culture (2)[C].
  - Cell count and differential: Polymorphonuclear (PMN) leukocytes ≥250 cells/mm³ is diagnostic of SBP.
  - Albumin to calculate SAAG (obtained by subtracting ascitic fluid albumin from serum albumin obtained on the SAME day):
    - <1.1 g/dL indicates a low portal pressure exudative process (i.e., inflammatory, biliary/pancreatic, carcinomatosis, TB).
    - ≥1.1 g/dL indicates portal hypertensive/transudative process (cirrhosis, CHF, constrictive pericarditis, thrombosis).
    - Other tests (based on clinical scenario to rule out etiologies other than cirrhosis) (2)[C]
- Abdominal US can confirm ascites; highly sensitive, cost-effective, involves no radiation
- Portal Doppler US can detect thrombosis or cirrhosis.
- CT scan for intra-abdominal pathology (malignancy)
- MRI preferred for evaluation of liver disease or confirmation of portal vein thrombosis

Follow-Up Tests & Special Considerations
- All patients with cirrhosis should be evaluated for hepatocellular carcinoma with US every 6 months
- Complete metabolic panel (CMP), Complete blood count (CBC), PT/INR should be checked every 6 months to calculate Child-Pugh and Model for End-Stage Liver Disease (MELD) scores.

Diagnostic Procedures/Other
Laparoscopy: if imaging and paracentesis are nondiagnostic
- Allows for direct visualization and biopsy of peritoneum, liver, and intra-abdominal lymph nodes
- Preferred for evaluating suspected peritoneal TB or malignancies

Test Interpretation
Cytology may reveal malignant cells: adenocarcinoma (ovary, breast, GI tract) or primary peritoneal carcinoma (most commonly associated with ascites).

 TREATMENT

For all patients, first-line treatment consists of:
- Daily weight
- Restrict dietary sodium to ≤2 g/day if the cause is due to portal hypertension (high SAAG).
- Water restriction (1.0 to 1.5 L/day) only necessary if evidence of hyponatremia (serum sodium <120 to 125 mEq/L)
- Avoid alcohol and ensure adequate nutrition if liver disease.
- Baclofen may be used to reduce alcohol craving/consumption in EtOH cirrhosis.

GENERAL MEASURES
Oral antibiotic prophylaxis against SBP should be initiated in patients with a history of SBP or ascitic fluid protein <1.5 g/dL (15 g/dL) and advanced liver disease (Child-Pugh score ≥9 or bilirubin ≥3 mg/dL) or kidney disease (serum creatinine ≥1.2 mg/dL, serum sodium ≤130 per mmol/L).

MEDICATION

ALERT
- Aggressive diuresis can induce acute kidney injury (AKI), encephalopathy, and hyponatremia. Monitor

creatinine and electrolytes closely. Serum creatinine >2 mg/dL or serum sodium <120 mmol/L warrants withdrawal of diuretics.
- Avoid nonsteroidal anti-inflammatory drugs (NSAIDs) (can exacerbate oliguria/azotemia).
- Angiotensin-converting enzyme (ACE) inhibitors and angiotensin receptor blockers (ARBs) may be harmful due to an increased risk of hypotension and renal failure. Avoid in RA.
- Consider discontinuing β-blockers in patients with RA, SBP, worsening hypotension (systolic blood pressure <90 mm Hg), AKI, hyponatremia <130 mEq/L, or azotemia.

First Line
- Sodium restriction and diuretics are the mainstay of treatment for patients with elevated portal pressures; other causes (e.g., carcinomatosis) are less likely to respond to medical therapy.
  - Spironolactone 100 to 400 mg/day PO; typical initial dose is 100 to 200 mg in AM.
  - Furosemide 40 to 160 mg/day PO; typical initial dose is 40 mg in AM.
  - Most common and preferred regimen is spironolactone and furosemide together, maintaining a 100:40 ratio, for maximum efficacy and potassium homeostasis.
- Diuretic-intractable/RA (10% of patients—50% mortality in 6 months) defined as:
  - Persistent or worsening ascites despite maximum doses of spironolactone (400 mg/day) and furosemide (160 mg/day) for at least 1 week
  - Recurrence of grade 2 or 3 ascites within 4 weeks of achieving minimal ascites
  - Diuretic induced complications like hepatic encephalopathy, hyponatremia to <125 mEq/L, renal impairment with creatinine rise of ≥100% to >2
- Treatment:
  - Routine dietary sodium restriction compliance using 24-hour urine sodium excretion.
  - Discontinue diuretics if urinary sodium excretion with diuretics is <30 mmol/day.
  - Therapeutic paracentesis or serial large-volume paracentesis (LVP) (See "Surgery/Other Procedures.")
  - IV furosemide reduces eGFR dramatically in ascitic patients and is better avoided.

Second Line
- Midodrine 7.5 mg TID can be used for RA or hypotensive patients and may improve survival (2)[B]. Titrate to blood pressure response.
- Alternatives to spironolactone: amiloride up to 40 mg/day; triamterene up to 200 mg/day in divided doses (2)[C]
- Alternatives to furosemide: torsemide up to 100 mg/day; bumetanide up to 4 mg/day (2)[C]
- Vaptans: FDA recommended avoiding use in chronic liver disease due to potential for inducing serious liver injury (3)[A].

ISSUES FOR REFERRAL
Liver transplant is the definitive treatment for portal hypertension. Consider referral for transplant in patients with decompensated liver disease, whether ascites is present/controlled (2)[B]. Patients with cirrhosis and MELD score of ≥15 should be referred for liver transplant.

SURGERY/OTHER PROCEDURES
- Therapeutic paracentesis
  - Initial therapy if tense ascites is present (2)[C]; serial (generally every 2 weeks) paracenteses can be used as second line after diuretics in patients with elevated portal pressures. Continue diuretics at 50% of the previous dose if transitioning to serial paracentesis in patients failing diuretic monotherapy.
  - Replace albumin when removing >5 L of ascites: 5.5 to 8.0 g albumin for each liter removed.
- Transjugular intrahepatic portosystemic shunt (TIPS): for patients with elevated portal pressures with RA
- Automated low flow ascites pump drains ascitic fluid from peritoneal cavity to urinary bladder for elimination. Mainly used in patients with contraindication to TIPS placement or liver transplant.
- Cell free and concentrated ascites reinfusion: used for management of malignant ascites. Protein collected from filtration and concentration of ascitic fluid is reinfused intravenously.
- Peritoneovenous shunt (LeVeen or Denver shunt): drains ascites directly into the inferior vena cava and reserved for patients with RA who are not candidates for TIPS or liver transplant and can't tolerate repeat paracentesis (2)[C]
- Indwelling catheters with external drainage: most useful in malignant ascites as a palliative measure
- Avoid percutaneous endoscopic gastrostomy (PEG) tube placement in patients with ascites due to high postprocedure mortality rate (2)[B].

ADMISSION, INPATIENT, AND NURSING CONSIDERATIONS
Admit patient in hospital who have cirrhosis and present with new abdominal pain, fever, and hypotension.

 ONGOING CARE

FOLLOW-UP RECOMMENDATIONS
Patient Monitoring
CMP, CBC, PT/INR should be checked every 6 months to calculate Child-Pugh and MELD scores

DIET
Low sodium diet (<2 g/day)

PROGNOSIS
Prognosis varies depending on underlying cause. Ascites in itself is rarely life threatening but can signify life-threatening underlying disease (e.g., cancer, end-stage liver disease).

COMPLICATIONS
- SBP: ascitic fluid PMN leukocyte count ≥250 cells/mm³ or positive culture
- Hepatorenal syndrome
  - Type 1—rapid acute worsening of renal function evolving in the setting of a known precipitating factor
  - Type 2—slowly progressive in the setting of RA
- Cellulitis: common in obese patients with brawny edema; treat with diuretics and antibiotics (2)[B].

REFERENCES
1. Chiejina M, Kudaravalli P, Samant H. Ascites. In: StatPearls [Internet]. Treasure Island, FL: StatPearls Publishing; 2022. https://www.ncbi.nlm.nih.gov/books/NBK470482. Accessed August 5, 2023.
2. Gallo A, Dedionigi C, Civitelli C, et al. Optimal management of cirrhotic ascites: a review for internal medicine physicians. *J Transl Int Med*. 2020;8(4):220–236.
3. Kockerling D, Nathwani R, Forlano R, et al. Current and future pharmacological therapies for managing cirrhosis and its complications. *World J Gastroenterol*. 2019;25(8):888–908.

ADDITIONAL READING
- Biggins SW, Angeli P, Garcia-Tsao G, et al. Diagnosis, evaluation, and management of ascites, spontaneous bacterial peritonitis and hepatorenal syndrome: 2021 practice guidance by the American Association for the Study of Liver Diseases. *Hepatology*. 2021;74(2):1014–1048.
- Garbuzenko DV, Arefyev NO. Current approaches to the management of patients with cirrhotic ascites. *World J Gastroenterol*. 2019;25(28):3738–3752.

 SEE ALSO

- Cirrhosis of the Liver; Hepatorenal Syndrome
- Algorithms: Congestive Heart Failure: Differential Diagnosis; Nephrotic Syndrome

CODES

ICD10
- R18.8 Other ascites
- R18.0 Malignant ascites
- K70.31 Alcoholic cirrhosis of liver with ascites

CLINICAL PEARLS
- Cirrhosis is the most common cause of ascites.
- Patients with new-onset ascites or hospitalized patients with ascites should undergo diagnostic paracentesis.
- First-line treatment: moderate sodium restriction and diuretics
- Second-line treatment: serial paracentesis or TIPS
- Avoid NSAIDs, ACE inhibitors, ARBs, and nonselective β-blockers in patients with ascites.
- Most common cause of "diuretic-intractable ascites" is the inability to adhere to dietary sodium restriction.

ASTHMA
Stacy E. Potts, MD, Med

BASICS

DESCRIPTION
- A heterogeneous disease characterized as chronic inflammation of the airway
- Common triggers: exercise, allergen-irritant exposure, change in weather, laughter, or viral respiratory infections
- Patient may experience symptoms-free periods alternating with sporadic flare-up (exacerbations).
- Most common asthma phenotypes:
  - Allergic asthma: usually present since childhood and has strong family history of allergic diseases
  - Nonallergic asthma
  - Late-onset asthma: more common in females
  - Asthma with fixed airflow limitation: due to airway remodeling
  - Asthma with obesity
- Asthma severity is assessed retrospectively from treatment required to control symptoms.
  - Mild asthma: well controlled with step 1 or 2 treatment (i.e., with as-needed ICS-formoterol alone or with low-intensity maintenance controller treatment)
  - Moderate asthma: well controlled with step 3 or 4 treatment (i.e., low- or medium-dose ICS-LABA)
  - Severe asthma: remains "uncontrolled" with optimized treatment with high-dose ICS-LABA or that requires high-dose ICS-LABA to prevent it from becoming "uncontrolled"

EPIDEMIOLOGY
Incidence
Traffic-related air pollution may be attributable to 13% of global asthma incidence.

Prevalence
Asthma affects 262 million individuals worldwide.
- 455,000 deaths worldwide reported in 2019 (1)
- African Americans are 3 times more likely to die from asthma.
- Asthma affects about 10% of children aged 5 to 18 years in the United States.
- Asthma prevalence is greater in boys than girls; however, in adults, women are more affected.
- Obesity is associated with increased prevalence and incidence of asthma.
- Rate of asthma deaths: largest among those aged ≥65 years

ETIOLOGY AND PATHOPHYSIOLOGY
Airway hyperreaction begins with inflammatory cell infiltration and degranulation, subbasement fibrosis, mucus hypersecretion, epithelial injury, significant smooth muscle hypertrophy and hyperreactivity, angiogenesis that then leads to intermittent airflow obstruction due to reversible bronchospasm.

Genetics
Genetic association with increased interleukin (IL) or IgE production and airway hyperresponsiveness leading to asthma

RISK FACTORS
- Host factors: genetic predisposition, sex, obesity, preterm or small for gestational age (SGA)
- Environmental: viral infections, animal and airborne allergens, tobacco smoke exposure, e-cigarette use, pollution, stress

- Aspirin or NSAIDs hypersensitivity
- Persons with food allergies and asthma are at increased risk for fatal anaphylaxis from those foods.

COMMONLY ASSOCIATED CONDITIONS
- Atopy: eczema, allergic conjunctivitis, allergic rhinitis
- Obesity (associated with higher asthma rates)
- Gastroesophageal reflux disease (GERD)
- Obstructive sleep apnea (OSA)

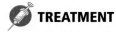

DIAGNOSIS

HISTORY
History of variable respiratory symptoms:
- More than one symptom such as wheeze, SOB, cough, chest tightness
- Symptoms worse at night, vary in time and intensity, worse with common triggers

PHYSICAL EXAM
- May be normal
- Focus on
  - Use of accessory muscles
  - Rhinitis, nasal polyps, swollen nasal turbinates
  - Expiratory wheezing, prolonged expiratory phase. Note: Wheezing may be absent in severe exacerbation due to severely reduced airflow.
  - Skin: eczema

DIFFERENTIAL DIAGNOSIS
- In children
  - Upper airway diseases (allergic rhinitis or sinusitis)
  - Large airway obstruction (foreign body aspiration, vocal cord dysfunction, vascular ring or laryngeal web, laryngotracheomalacia, enlarged lymph nodes, or tumor)
  - Small airway obstruction (viral bronchiolitis, cystic fibrosis, bronchopulmonary dysplasia, heart disease, primary ciliary dyskinesia, bronchiectasis)
  - Other causes (recurrent cough, chronic upper airway cough syndrome, aspiration/GERD)
- In adults: Chronic obstructive pulmonary disease, bronchiectasis, heart failure, pulmonary embolism, tumor, pulmonary infiltration with eosinophilia, Churg-Strauss syndrome, medication-induced cough (ACE inhibitors), vocal cord dysfunction

DIAGNOSTIC TESTS & INTERPRETATION
Initial Tests (lab, imaging)
- Blood tests are not required but may find eosinophilia or elevated serum IgE levels (allergic asthma).
- Documented variable expiratory airflow limitation:
  - Spirometry with methacholine challenge: Normal test does not rule out asthma; measures the FVC and the FEV_1; a reduced predicted ratio of FEV_1/FVC with reversibility (increase of 200 mL and 12% of FEV_1/FVC from baseline) after using a short-acting bronchodilator (SABA)
  - Excessive variability in twice daily peak expiratory flow (PEF) in 2 weeks (daily PEF variability >10%)
  - Bronchial challenge test: used mainly in adults, positive when there is a fall in FEV_1 >20% with methacholine or histamine; or >15% with hypertonic saline or mannitol challenge
  - Exercise challenge test: fall in FEV_1 >10% and 200 mL from baseline
  - Significant increase in lung function after 4 weeks of anti-inflammatory treatment
- Chest x-ray is used to exclude alternative diagnoses.

Follow-Up Tests & Special Considerations
- Asthma action plan: Patients monitor their own symptoms and/or peak flow measurements. Reassess action plan every 3 to 6 months.
- Assess asthma symptoms control with simple screening tools, such as consensus-based Global Initiative for Asthma (GINA) symptom control tool or Primary Care Asthma Control Screening Tool (PACS). Use the review, assess, adjust method of ongoing management.

Diagnostic Procedures/Other
- Allergy skin testing is not useful for diagnosis of asthma but may be to evaluate atopic triggers.
- Measurement of fractional concentration of exhaled nitric oxide (FeNO) suggests eosinophilic airway inflammation.

TREATMENT

GENERAL MEASURES
- Focus on symptom control and prevention of exacerbations.
- Use of holding chambers ("spacers") with inhaled agents improves clinical outcomes.
- Written asthma self-management action plan
- Encourage physical activity, weight loss, smoking cessation, avoidance of irritants, emotional stress.
- Avoidance of occupational exposure
- Annual influenza vaccine; pneumococcal vaccine is recommended for high-risk patients.
- Patients at risk for anaphylaxis carry epinephrine (EpiPen).
- Controller medications: used for regular maintenance, reduce airway inflammation, control symptoms, and reduce risk of exacerbations:
  - Inhaled corticosteroids (ICS)
  - Long-acting β-agonist (LABA) (formoterol, salmeterol)
- The ICS can be delivered by regular daily treatment or, in mild well-controlled asthma, by as-needed low-dose ICS-formoterol.

ALERT
- Treatment of asthma with SABAs alone is no longer recommended by the GINA Guidelines for adults and adolescents.
  - ICS therapy is essential to reduce risk of death and severe exacerbations.
- Reliever (rescue medication) provided to all patients for as-needed relief of breakthrough symptoms
  - SABA–albuterol/levalbuterol
- Add-on therapies for patients with severe asthma, when patients persist with symptoms despite optimized treatment with high-dose controller medications (ICS + LABA)

Pediatric Considerations
- Tiotropium is not indicated in children aged <12 years.
- Reliever for all management steps in children aged 6 to 11 years is as-needed SABA.
- School-based programs including asthma self-management reduce emergency department visits, hospitalizations, and days of reduced activity.

Pregnancy Considerations

- Do not use bronchial provocation test nor step down controller treatment until after delivery.
- Asthma symptoms tend to worsen in 1/3 of patients, 1/3 improves, and 1/3 remains unchanged.
- Exacerbations are common in 2nd trimester.
- Poorly controlled asthma results in low birth weight, increased prematurity, and perinatal mortality.
- All short-acting agents (SABA) are pregnancy Category C as well as ICS.
- Cessation of ICS during pregnancy is a significant risk factor for exacerbation.
- Leukotriene receptor antagonists (LTRA), montelukast, and zafirlukast are Category B but are not studied extensively in pregnancy.

Geriatric Considerations

Underdiagnosed due to comorbidities

MEDICATION

First Line

- Stepwise approach for asthma treatment for adolescents (age >12 years) and adults:
  - Step 1: symptom driven treatment: symptom driven as-needed low dose ICS-formoterol; alternative: low-dose ICS whenever SABA taken
  - Step 2: maintenance treatment: low-dose controller + as-needed reliever: daily low-dose ICS + as-needed SABA; controller alternative: LTRA or dust mite control/sublingual immunotherapy (if allergic asthma)
  - Step 3: one or two controllers + as-needed reliever: first (adults/adolescents): low-dose ICS-LABA; controller alternatives: medium-dose ICS or low-dose ICS with LTRA; preferred reliever: as-needed low-dose ICS/formoterol as both controller + reliever for those on maintenance therapy; first (ages 6 to 11 years) and second alternative (adults/adolescents): medium-dose ICS + SABA; third: low-dose ICS + LTRA
  - Step 4: two or more controllers + as-needed reliever: first (adults/adolescents): medium-dose ICS-LABA as controller; controller alternatives: high-dose ICS, add-on tiotropium, or LTRA; consider house dust mite SLIT for sensitized patient with normal spirometry and allergic rhinitis; preferred reliever: low-dose ICS-formoterol for those prescribed bud-form/BDP-form maintenance and reliever therapy, otherwise SABA reliever when on other ICS-LABA
  - Step 5: high-dose ICS-LABA, referral for phenotype assessment and consider add-on therapy (i.e., LAMA, anti-IgE, anti-IL5/5R, anti-IL4, tiotropium) or add low-dose OCS while considering risks versus benefits
- Combination therapy with a LABA + ICS resulted in fewer asthma exacerbations than treatment with ICS alone.
- COVID-19 special considerations
  - Patients with asthma should continue taking their prescribed asthma medications, particularly ICS-containing medication and oral corticosteroids if prescribed.
  - COVID-19 vaccination is recommended for people with asthma.

ISSUES FOR REFERRAL

- Specialized testing (e.g., bronchoprovocation)
- Specialized treatments (e.g., immunotherapy)
- Poorly controlled asthma, frequent exacerbation, or multiple emergency department visits
- Occupational asthma due to legal implications

ADDITIONAL THERAPIES

- Exercise-induced bronchoconstriction (EIB): SABA prior exercise (2) or LTRA/chromones
- Allergen immunotherapy when clear relationship between symptoms and exposure
- Management of acute exacerbation of asthma
  - Outpatient:
    - Mild: speak in full sentence, HR <120 beats/min, oxygen saturation 90–95%, and peak flow >50% of predicted can be managed as outpatient in clinic; should start SABA with ICS or formoterol/ICS and prednisolone; if symptoms resolve within 1 hour, could be discharged home with close follow-up
    - Severe symptoms: not able to speak in full sentence, HR >120 beats/min, oxygen saturation <90%, peak flow <50% predicted, drowsy, confused, or silent chest; transfer to inpatient facility.
  - Treatment for severe:
    - Oxygen: to maintain saturation 93–95%
    - SABA: within 1 hour of arrival; initially, around the clock followed by on demand
    - Systemic steroids: Oral is as effective as IV; 50 mg prednisolone (morning dose) or 200 mg hydrocortisone divided in doses; duration should be 5 to 7 days.
    - Epinephrine: only when asthma is associated with angioedema or anaphylaxis
    - Avoid sedative.
    - Vital signs, pulse oximetry, response and duration of response to SABA, a lung function such as PEF or FEV_1
    - Asthma education
  - Discharge criteria: minimal or absent asthma symptoms; hypoxia has resolved; FEV_1 or PEF ≥70% predicted or personal best; bronchodilator response sustained ≥60 minutes

ADMISSION, INPATIENT, AND NURSING CONSIDERATIONS

Admitted patients should continue, or commence, ICS-containing therapy.

 ## ONGOING CARE

Smoking cessation if indicated

FOLLOW-UP RECOMMENDATIONS

- Identify triggers and control exposures.
- Consider stepping down treatment once symptoms are controlled for 3 months.

PATIENT EDUCATION

- American Academy of Allergy, Asthma & Immunology: 1-800-822-2762 or https://www.aaaai.org/
- Asthma and Allergy Foundation of America: 1-800-727-8462 or https://www.aafa.org/

PROGNOSIS

Prognosis is good for male patients, nonsmokers, and children with mild disease.

COMPLICATIONS

- Atelectasis, pneumonia, medication-specific side effects/adverse effects/interactions
- Respiratory failure; death: ~50% of asthma deaths occur in the elderly (aged >65 years).

REFERENCES

1. GBD 2019 Diseases and Injuries Collaborators. Global burden of 369 diseases and injuries in 204 countries and territories, 1990–2019: a systematic analysis for the Global Burden of Disease Study 2019. *Lancet*. 2020;396(10258):1204–1222.
2. Global Initiative for Asthma. 2023 GINA main report: global strategy for asthma management and prevention. https://ginasthma.org/2023-gina-main-report/. Accessed November 3, 2023.

ADDITIONAL READING

Cloutier MM, Baptist AP, Blake KV, et al; for Expert Panel Working Group of the National Heart, Lung, and Blood Institute; National Asthma Education and Prevention Program Coordinating Committee. 2020 Focused updates to the asthma management guidelines: a report from the National Asthma Education and Prevention Program Coordinating Committee Expert Panel Working Group. *J Allergy Clin Immunol*. 2020;146(6):1217–1270.

CODES

ICD10

- J45.20 Mild intermittent asthma, uncomplicated
- J45.52 Severe persistent asthma with status asthmaticus
- J45.51 Severe persistent asthma with (acute) exacerbation

CLINICAL PEARLS

- SABA plus ICS or formoterol/ICS is the most effective rescue therapy for acute asthma symptoms.
- Holding chambers should be used by all.
- ICSs are the preferred long-term control therapy for patients of all ages.

ATELECTASIS

Chris Artner, MD • Jennifer Koch, MD

BASICS

DESCRIPTION
- Atelectasis is defined as the incomplete expansion of lung tissue due to collapse or closure.
- Broadly categorized as:
  - Obstructive: due to airway blockage
  - Nonobstructive: multiple etiologies including loss of contact between the parietal and visceral pleurae, replacement of lung tissue by scarring or infiltrative disease, surfactant dysfunction, and parenchymal compression
- Often asymptomatic; symptoms depend on the rate of collapse, the amount of lung involved, and whether the patient has underlying lung disease and/or comorbidities.
- Reduced respiratory gas exchange can cause hypoxemia.

EPIDEMIOLOGY
- Mean age is 60 years, but all ages are susceptible.
- Male = female; no racial or socioeconomic predilection
- Frequently occurs in patients on mechanical ventilation
- Increased risk in postoperative patients and patients with lung or chest wall injury

Incidence
Postoperative atelectasis, especially after major cardiovascular or gastrointestinal (GI) procedures; can be seen in up to 90% of patients

Prevalence
Rounded atelectasis can be seen in up to 65–70% of asbestos workers.

ETIOLOGY AND PATHOPHYSIOLOGY
- Obstructive (resorptive) atelectasis is caused by intrinsic airway blockage and is the most common variety. It can be caused by luminal blockage (i.e., foreign body, mucus plug, asthma, cystic fibrosis, trauma, mass lesion) or airway wall abnormality (i.e., congenital malformation, emphysema).
  - Distal to the obstruction, alveolar air is rapidly reabsorbed into the deoxygenated venous system, causing complete collapse of the alveolar tissue.
  - The patency and function of the collateral ventilatory systems in each lobe (pores of Kohn, canals of Lambert, and fenestrations of Boren) depends on multiple patient factors including age, underlying lung disease, and fraction of inspired oxygen (FiO_2).
  - In patients with emphysema, the fenestra of Boren become enlarged, which acts as a compensatory mechanism and can lead to a delay in atelectasis despite an obstructing lesion or mass.
- Nonobstructive atelectasis
  - Passive atelectasis (i.e., during a pleural effusion, pneumothorax, or large emphysematous bulla) is due to pleural membrane separation of the visceral and parietal layers.
  - Compression atelectasis occurs with space-occupying lesions, cardiomegaly, abscess, or significant lymphadenopathy. The increased chest wall pressure compresses the alveoli.

- Adhesive atelectasis occurs in the setting of acute respiratory distress syndrome (ARDS), radiation, smoke inhalation, posttraumatic lung contusion, or uremia. The underlying surfactant dysfunction causes increased surface tension and alveoli collapse.
  - Cicatrization atelectasis is common in granulomatous disease (i.e., sarcoidosis, TB), toxic or radiation exposure, and drug-induced fibrosis (i.e., amiodarone, cyclophosphamide). The scarring and fibrosis reduce lung expansion.
  - Replacement atelectasis: occurs when a tumor fills alveoli of a lobe causing complete lobar collapse
- Rounded atelectasis is a distinct form of atelectasis seen in patients with asbestos exposure.
- Muscular weakness: due to anesthesia side effect, or in neuromuscular diseases with respiratory muscle involvement

Pediatric Considerations
Children are at a higher risk of developing atelectasis due to their less developed collateral ventilation and compensatory mechanisms.

RISK FACTORS
- Critical care, surgery, and prolonged immobilization
- General anesthesia (including long-acting muscle relaxants, postoperative epidural anesthesia)
- Positive fluid balance
- Massive blood transfusion (≥4 units)
- Nasogastric tube placement
- Hypothermia
- Mechanical ventilation with high tidal volume (Vt >10 mL/kg) and plateau pressure (>30 cm H_2O)
- Patient risk factors for postoperative atelectasis:
  - Age >60 years and <6 years
  - Chronic obstructive pulmonary disease (COPD), obstructive sleep apnea, congestive heart failure (CHF), pulmonary hypertension
  - Alcohol abuse, smoking
  - Poor cough effort
  - Albumin <3.5 g/dL, hemoglobin <10 g/dL
  - BMI >27 kg/m² (weak evidence)
  - ASA class II + functional dependence in activities of daily living (ADLs)

GENERAL PREVENTION
- Early mobilization, deep breathing exercises, coughing, and frequent changes in body position
- Preoperative physical therapy lowered rates of atelectasis, pneumonia, and length of stay (LOS) in patients undergoing elective cardiac surgery (1)[A].
- Mechanical ventilation settings with high Vt (Vt >10 mL/kg) and plateau pressures (>30 cm H_2O) and without positive end-expiratory pressure (PEEP) are associated with postoperative pulmonary complications (i.e., pneumonia, respiratory failure) (2):
  - Minimize ventilator-induced injury by employing low Vt and plateau pressures at sufficient PEEP (3)[C].
  - Ensure lower FiO_2 during anesthetic induction and intraoperatively to prevent nitrogen washout (2)[A].

COMMONLY ASSOCIATED CONDITIONS
- Obstructive lung diseases (COPD and asthma)
- Trauma
- ARDS, neonatal RDS, pulmonary edema, pulmonary embolism, pneumonia, pleural effusion, pneumothorax
- Respiratory syncytial virus (RSV), bronchiolitis
- Bronchial stenosis, pulmonic valve disease, and pulmonary hypertension
- Neuromuscular disorders (muscular dystrophy, spinal muscular atrophy, spinal cord injury, and Guillain-Barré syndrome) and cystic fibrosis

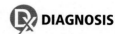

DIAGNOSIS

HISTORY
- Frequently asymptomatic
- Tachypnea and sudden-onset dyspnea
- Nonproductive cough
- Pleuritic pain on affected side
- History of smoking; COPD; pulmonary insufficiency; exposure to radiation, asbestos, or other air pollutants

PHYSICAL EXAM
- Signs of hypoxia or cyanosis
- Tracheal or precordial impulse displacement toward the affected side; dullness to percussion
- Bronchial breathing in patent airway
- Wheezing or absent breath sounds in occluded airway
- Diminished chest expansion

DIFFERENTIAL DIAGNOSIS
- Pneumonia
- Pleural effusion
- Neoplasm

DIAGNOSTIC TESTS & INTERPRETATION
Initial Tests (lab, imaging)
- CBC and respiratory Gram stain, culture, and viral panel if infection suspected
- ABG: Despite hypoxemia, $PaCO_2$ level is usually normal or low.
- Chest x-ray (CXR): PA and lateral

Follow-Up Tests & Special Considerations
- Chest CT or MRI may be indicated to visualize airway and mediastinal structures and identify cause of atelectasis in unclear cases.
- Chest ultrasound may differentiate atelectasis versus pleural effusion or consolidation.
- Pulmonary function tests (PFTs) can help identify obstructive or restrictive disease and decreased respiratory muscle pressures.
- Hypoalbuminemia (albumin <3.5 g/L) is a powerful marker of increased risk for postoperative pulmonary complications, including atelectasis.

Diagnostic Procedures/Other
Flexible fiber-optic bronchoscopy can be considered in unexplained or refractory cases.

TREATMENT

GENERAL MEASURES
- Identify and treat the underlying etiology.
- Pain control to facilitate deeper breathing
- Lie on the unaffected side, encourage frequent coughing, deep breathing exercises, and early mobility.
- PEEP for prevention following surgery or general anesthesia (2)[A]
- Regular use of incentive spirometer (3)[A]
- Mechanical ventilation with PEEP in severe respiratory distress or hypoxemia
- Continuous positive airway pressure (CPAP) may be beneficial in patients with hypoxemia in the setting of few secretions (3)[A].
- Patients with post operative atelectasis and significant secretions should be suctioned frequently and undergo chest physiotherapy.

MEDICATION
First Line
Pharmacotherapy should address underlying etiology:
- Effective analgesia to permit deep inspiration and coughing
- Antibiotics for infection
- Chemotherapy or radiation for malignancy
- Bronchodilators and corticosteroids for asthma
- Mucolytics can be considered to promote airway clearance.

Pediatric Considerations
- Dornase alfa may be effective clearing mucinous secretions in refractory mucous plugging in children (used in cystic fibrosis).
- Chest physiotherapy (i.e., percussion, drainage, deep insufflation, and saline lavage) is the most commonly used therapy in the inpatient setting.
- Other physically stimulating modalities (mechanical insufflation-exsufflation, intrapulmonary percussive ventilation, intermittent positive pressure breathing) may have utility in patients with neuromuscular disease and cystic fibrosis to enhance mucus clearance.
- Applying continuous distending pressure has shown some benefit in the treatment of preterm infants with RDS and has the potential to reduce lung damage particularly if used early.
- In obstructive atelectasis, bronchoscopy remains controversial. However, in the presence of a mucus plug or cast, bronchoscopy may be beneficial.

Second Line
Fiber-optic bronchoscopy to improve airway clearance has been efficacious in several studies; however, there is a debate regarding its efficacy in the treatment of atelectasis. It may be beneficial in those with unsuccessful attempts or contraindications to chest physiotherapy (i.e., chest wall trauma).

SURGERY/OTHER PROCEDURES
Appropriate surgical resection for underlying disease (i.e., tumor, severe lymphadenopathy)

ALERT
The association between postoperative atelectasis and fever is likely coincidental rather than causal.

ADMISSION, INPATIENT, AND NURSING CONSIDERATIONS
Ensure adequate oxygenation (may start with 100% FiO_2 then taper) and humidification. Note: If obstructive atelectasis is suspected, then judiciously increase FiO_2 to prevent nitrogen washout, which can hasten atelectasis.

 ONGOING CARE

FOLLOW-UP RECOMMENDATIONS
Patient Monitoring
- Frequency/adequacy of monitoring will vary by underlying cause and concurrent comorbidities.
- For uncomplicated cases of atelectasis, outpatient monitoring may be appropriate.

PATIENT EDUCATION
Maximize mobility as tolerated and encourage frequent coughing and deep breathing exercises. Seek further treatment or return to ED for worsening symptoms or shortness of breath.

PROGNOSIS
- Postoperative atelectasis usually spontaneous resolves within 24 hours but can persist for days.
- Resolution of lobar atelectasis due to endobronchial obstruction depends on treatment of underlying disease or malignancy.

COMPLICATIONS
- Pneumonia or other pulmonary infections
- Acute atelectasis: hypoxemia, respiratory failure, post obstructive drowning of the lung
- Chronic atelectasis: bronchiectasis, pleural effusion, empyema

REFERENCES
1. Hulzebos EHJ, Smit Y, Helders PPJM, et al. Preoperative physical therapy for elective cardiac surgery patients. *Cochrane Database Syst Rev.* 2012;11(11):CD010118.
2. Lagier D, Zeng C, Fernandez-Bustamante A, et al. Perioperative pulmonary atelectasis: part II. Clinical implications. *Anesthesiology.* 2022;136(1):206–236.
3. Marret E, Cinotti R, Berard L, et al.; and the PPV Study Group. Protective ventilation during anaesthesia reduces major postoperative complications after lung cancer surgery: a double-blind randomised controlled trial. *Eur J Anaesthesiol.* 2018;35(10):727–735.

ADDITIONAL READING
- Brower RG. Consequences of bed rest. *Crit Care Med.* 2009;37(Suppl 10):S422–S428.
- Guimarães MM, El Dib R, Smith AF, et al. Incentive spirometry for prevention of postoperative pulmonary complications in upper abdominal surgery. *Cochrane Database Syst Rev.* 2009;(3):CD006058.
- Mavros MN, Velmahos GC, Falagas ME. Atelectasis as a cause of postoperative fever: where is the clinical evidence? *Chest.* 2011;140(2):418–424.
- Tusman G, Böhm SH, Warner DO, et al. Atelectasis and perioperative pulmonary complications in high-risk patients. *Curr Opin Anaesthesiol.* 2012;25(1):1–10.
- Wu KH, Lin CF, Huang CJ, et al. Rigid ventilation bronchoscopy under general anesthesia for treatment of pediatric pulmonary atelectasis caused by pneumonia: a review of 33 cases. *Int Surg.* 2006;91(5):291–294.

 CODES

ICD10
- P28.10 Unspecified atelectasis of newborn
- J98.11 Atelectasis
- P28.19 Other atelectasis of newborn

CLINICAL PEARLS
- Low serum albumin (<3.5 g/L) is a strong predictor of postoperative pulmonary complications, including atelectasis.
- Anesthesia-induced atelectasis occurs in almost all anesthetized patients but can be reduced by employing PEEP intraoperatively or when reversing anesthesia.
- Early mobilization, coughing, deep breathing exercises, and treating the underlying cause are the mainstays of therapy.
- Bronchogenic carcinoma can present as atelectasis and must be excluded in all patients aged >35 years.
- No strong clinical evidence supports atelectasis as an early cause of postoperative fever.

ATRIAL FIBRILLATION AND ATRIAL FLUTTER

Bianca Lee, DO, MS • Lyncean Ung, DO

 BASICS

This topic covers both atrial fibrillation (AFib) and atrial flutter (AFlut).

DESCRIPTION

- AFib: paroxysmal or continuous supraventricular tachyarrhythmia characterized by rapid, uncoordinated atrial electrical activity and an irregularly irregular ventricular response; in most patients, the ventricular rate is rapid because the atrioventricular (AV) node is bombarded with very frequent atrial electrical impulses (400 to 600 beats/min).
- AFlut: paroxysmal or continuous supraventricular tachyarrhythmia with rapid but organized atrial electrical activity; the atrial rate is typically between 250 and 350 beats/min and is often manifested as "saw-tooth" flutter (F) waves on the ECG, particularly in the inferior leads and V_1. AFlut commonly occurs with 2:1 or 3:1 AV block, so the ventricular response may be regular and typically at a rate of 150 beats/min.
- AFib and AFlut are related arrhythmias, sometimes seen in the same patient. Distinguishing the two is important because there may be implications for management.
- Clinical classifications:
  – Paroxysmal: self-terminating episodes, usually <7 days
  – Persistent: sustained >7 days, usually requiring pharmacologic or electrical cardioversion to restore sinus rhythm
  – Permanent: Sinus rhythm cannot be restored or maintained.
  – Nonvalvular AFib: absence of moderate-to-severe mitral stenosis or a mechanical heart valve
- Lone AFib occurs in patients aged <60 years (with possible genetic predisposition) who have no clinical or echocardiographic evidence of cardiovascular disease, including hypertension (HTN).

EPIDEMIOLOGY
- Incidence/prevalence increases significantly with age.
- Young patients with AFib, particularly lone AFib, are most commonly males.

Incidence
- AFib: from <0.1%/year <40 years to >1.5%/year >80 years
- Lifetime risk: 25% for those aged ≥40 years
- AFlut is less common.

Prevalence
- Estimated at 0.4–1% in general population, with 2.7 million patients in America
- Increases with age, up to 8% in those ≥80 years

ETIOLOGY AND PATHOPHYSIOLOGY
- Cardiac: HTN, acute coronary syndrome (ACS), congestive heart failure (CHF), valvular heart disease, cardiomyopathy, pericarditis, and infiltrative heart disease
- Pulmonary: pulmonary embolism (PE), chronic obstructive pulmonary disease (COPD), obstructive sleep apnea, pneumonia
- Ingestion: ethanol, caffeine, nicotine
- Endocrine: hyperthyroidism, diabetes mellitus (DM)

- Obesity
- Postoperative: cardiac, pulmonary, or esophageal
- Idiopathic: lone AFib
- Iatrogenic: amiodarone
- Patients with paroxysmal episodes are usually associated with premature atrial beats and/or bursts of tachycardia, originating in pulmonary vein ostia or other sites.
- Many patients with AFib are thought to have some degree of atrial fibrosis or scarring.
- Autonomic (vagal and sympathetic) tone may play a role in triggering the arrhythmia.
- The presence of AFib is associated with electrical and structural remodeling processes that promote arrhythmia maintenance in the atria, termed "AFib begets AFib."

Genetics
Familial forms are rare but do exist. There are ongoing efforts to identify the genetic underpinnings of such cases.

RISK FACTORS
Age, HTN, and obesity are the most important risk factors for both AFib and AFlut.

GENERAL PREVENTION
Adequate control of HTN may prevent development of AFib due to hypertensive heart disease and is the most significant modifiable risk factor for AFib. Weight reduction may decrease the risk of AFib in obese patients. Ethanol consumption may trigger AFib.

COMMONLY ASSOCIATED CONDITIONS
HTN, stroke, and other cardiac diseases

 DIAGNOSIS

HISTORY
Symptoms vary from none to mild (palpitations, light-headedness, fatigue, poor exercise capacity) to severe (angina, dyspnea, syncope).

PHYSICAL EXAM
- AFib: irregularly irregular heart rate and pulse, pulse deficit
- AFlut: similar to AFib but may have regular pulse

DIFFERENTIAL DIAGNOSIS
- Multifocal atrial tachycardia
- Sinus tachycardia with frequent atrial premature beats
- Paroxysmal supraventricular tachycardia (Wolff-Parkinson-White [WPW] syndrome, atrioventricular nodal reentry tachycardia [AVNRT])

DIAGNOSTIC TESTS & INTERPRETATION
- Screening with ECG to detect asymptomatic cases of AFib has not been shown to detect more cases than screening focused on pulse palpation (1)[A]. Many "smartwatches" can detect dysrhythmia consistent with AFib.
- AFib: The ECG is diagnostic, with findings of low-amplitude fibrillatory waves without discrete P waves and an irregularly irregular pattern of QRS complexes. There is often tachycardia in the absence of heart rate–controlling medications (2).

- AFlut: The ECG is diagnostic. Saw-tooth F waves are the classic sign, generally best seen in the inferior leads, although ventricular rate may need to be slowed to see the waves. QRS complexes may be regular or irregular; there is usually tachycardia (2).
- Ambulatory rhythm monitoring (e.g., telemetry, Holter monitoring, event recorders) is helpful in confirming suspected paroxysmal AFib or AFlut and monitoring for recurrence (2).

Initial Tests (lab, imaging)
Thyroid-stimulating hormone, electrolytes, complete blood count, complete metabolic panel, 2D transthoracic echocardiogram, prothrombin time/international normalized ratio (INR) (if anticoagulation is contemplated); digoxin level (if appropriate)

Follow-Up Tests & Special Considerations
- Occasional Holter monitoring and/or exercise stress testing to assess for adequacy of rate and/or rhythm control
- Chest x-ray (CXR) for cardiopulmonary disease
- ECG for signs of cardiac hypertrophy, ischemia, and/or other arrhythmias
- Transesophageal echocardiogram to detect left atrial appendage thrombus if cardioversion is planned
- Sleep study may be useful if sleep apnea is suspected.

Test Interpretation
Evaluate for presence of atrial dilatation and fibrosis, atrial thrombus (especially in atrial appendage), valvular heart disease, cardiomyopathy.

 TREATMENT

- Two primary issues in the management of AFib and/or AFlut: decisions on heart rate control (control ventricular rate while allowing AFib to continue) or rhythm control (terminate AFib and restore normal sinus rhythm) and decision to anticoagulate or not
- Anticoagulation therapy to prevent thromboembolism (primarily stroke) reduces risk of stroke by about 2/3. Several calculators exist for estimating yearly risk of thromboembolic event (ATRIA, CHA_2DS_2VASc). If risk is sufficiently low, or risk of bleeding is high (HAS-BLED tool may assist in evaluation), no anticoagulation may be indicated. Clinical judgment and patient preference remain important.

MEDICATION
- American Heart Association/American College of Cardiology anticoagulation guidelines (the same for AFib and AFlut) (3)[C]:
  – CHA_2DS_2VASc scoring (**C**HF [1 point], **H**TN [1 point], **A**ge ≥75 years [2 points], **D**M [1 point], prior **S**troke or transient ischemic attack [TIA] or thromboembolism [2 points], **V**ascular disease [1 point], **A**ge 65 to 74 years [1 point], female **S**ex **c**ategory [1 point]); CHA_2DS_2VASc is the recommended stroke risk assessment for patients with nonvalvular AFib (3)[C].
    ○ In patients with nonvalvular AFib and a CHA_2DS_2VASc score of 0 in males or 1 in females, anticoagulant therapy may be omitted (3)[C].

- In patients with nonvalvular AFib and a CHA_2DS_2VASc score of 1 in males and 2 in females (with one non–sex-related risk factor), oral anticoagulant therapy may be considered (3)[C].
- In patients with nonvalvular AFib with any high-risk factors for stroke (prior TIA/cerebrovascular accident [CVA]/thromboembolism) or a CHA_2DS_2VASc score ≥2 in men or ≥3 in women should receive oral anticoagulants unless contraindicated (3)[C].

– Direct-acting oral anticoagulant (DOAC)/non–vitamin K oral anticoagulant (NOAC) agents are recommended over warfarin for most patients with nonvalvular AFib who should receive anticoagulant therapy (3)[C]. Oral anticoagulants include warfarin (3)[C] with maintenance of an INR of 2.0 to 3.0, dabigatran (Pradaxa), rivaroxaban (Xarelto), apixaban (Eliquis), or edoxaban (Savaysa) (3)[C]. Patients with valvular AFib should be treated with warfarin to maintain an INR of 2.0 to 3.0 or 2.5 to 3.5 dependent on the type and location of the prosthesis (2)[B].

– The selection of an anticoagulant should be individualized; consider the risks of each agent, cost, patient's preference, and tolerability.

ALERT

Renal and hepatic functions should be evaluated prior to initiation of direct thrombin or factor Xa inhibitors (3)[C]. Limited information is available about safety in patients on renal dialysis. Additional dosing considerations of age ≥80 years or weight ≤60 kg are recommended with apixaban (3)[C]. Dosing of such agents may need individualized adjustment. Specific reversal agents for life-threatening bleeding or urgent procedure are available:

- Idarucizumab (Praxbind) for dabigatran (3)[C]
- Coagulation factor Xa (recombinant), inactivated-zhzo (Andexxa) for apixaban and rivaroxaban (3)[C]
- In addition to anticoagulation, initial rate control must be achieved followed by a decision regarding long-term strategy: rate-control alone or rhythm control. Four classes of medications are available to achieve ventricular rate control: β-blockers (i.e., metoprolol), nondihydropyridine calcium channel blockers (i.e., verapamil, diltiazem), digoxin, and amiodarone. Optimal target for ventricular rate has not been firmly established, but there is an evidence that aggressive control of the ventricular rate (<80 beats/min) offers no benefit beyond more modest rate control (i.e., resting heart rate <110 beats/min) (2)[C].
- Patients in whom rate control cannot be achieved or who continue to have persistent symptoms despite reasonable heart rate control may require attempts at restoration of sinus rhythm.
- Restoration of sinus rhythm using electrical or pharmacologic cardioversion may significantly reduce the symptom burden of AFib or AFlut in many patients and may also be useful for controlling ventricular rate.
- Randomized clinical trials (AFFIRM and RACE) comparing the outcomes of rate versus rhythm control found no difference in morbidity, mortality, and stroke rates in patients assigned to one therapy or the other (2).

ISSUES FOR REFERRAL

Management of AFib or AFlut refractory to standard medical therapy (i.e., unable to achieve adequate rate control with medication or development of significant bradycardia with treatment) may require the use of more aggressive treatments.

SURGERY/OTHER PROCEDURES

- Electrophysiologic study and ablation may be considered for patients with either AFib or AFlut. In the case of AFlut, ablation is a procedure viewed as a first-line therapy. Ablation of AFib may be reasonable in symptomatic patients with heart failure with reduced ejection fraction (HFrEF) to lower mortality and reduce hospitalization (3)[C].
- Cardiac surgery (e.g., the maze procedure, occlusion of the left atrial appendage) may be considered in patients planning to undergo cardiac surgery for other reasons.
- Percutaneous left atrial appendage (LAA) occlusion with WATCHMAN device may be considered in those at increased risk of stroke and systemic embolism with contraindications to long-term anticoagulation (3)[C].

COMPLEMENTARY & ALTERNATIVE MEDICINE

The use of herbal remedies, dietary supplements, and vitamins should be thoroughly assessed to avoid medication interactions.

ADMISSION, INPATIENT, AND NURSING CONSIDERATIONS

- Patients with significant symptoms, RVR, AFib/AFlut triggered by an acute process (e.g., ACS, CHF, PE), or in whom antiarrhythmic therapy is being started likely require admission to the hospital for a period of stabilization.
- Acute therapy for symptomatic patients with AFib or AFlut:
  – IV β-blockers or nondihydropyridine calcium channel blockers (e.g., diltiazem, verapamil) for control of ventricular rate in patients without preexcitation (3)[C] (caution if wide QRS complex)
  – IV amiodarone or digoxin may be considered in patients with severe left ventricular dysfunction or hemodynamic instability (3)[C].
- Urgent direct-current cardioversion is recommended in patients with hemodynamic instability or inadequate rate control (3)[C].
- Consider the initiation of anticoagulation therapy.

 ## ONGOING CARE

Consider elective expert consultation.

FOLLOW-UP RECOMMENDATIONS

Patient Monitoring

- Adequate anticoagulation levels with warfarin should be determined weekly during initiation and at least monthly when stable (3)[C].
- If NOACs are employed, hepatic and renal functions should be reevaluated at least annually (3)[C].

DIET

Patients on warfarin should attempt to consume a stable amount of vitamin K.

PATIENT EDUCATION

For overweight and obese patients, weight loss combined with risk factor modification have demonstrated beneficial effects on controlling AFib (3)[C].

PROGNOSIS

AFib and AFlut may increase morbidity and mortality, but the overall prognosis is a function of underlying heart disease and adherence with therapy.

COMPLICATIONS

- Embolic stroke
- Peripheral arterial embolization
- Bleeding with anticoagulation
- Tachycardia-induced cardiomyopathy with prolonged periods of inadequate rate control

REFERENCES

1. Jonas DE, Kahwati LC, Yun JDY, et al. Screening for atrial fibrillation with electrocardiography: evidence report and systematic review for the US Preventive Services Task Force. *JAMA*. 2018;320(5):485–498.
2. January CT, Wann LS, Alpert JS, et al. 2014 AHA/ACC/HRS guideline for the management of patients with atrial fibrillation: executive summary: a report of the American College of Cardiology/American Heart Association Task Force on Practice Guidelines and the Heart Rhythm Society. *Circulation*. 2014;130(23):2071–2104.
3. January CT, Wann LS, Calkins H, et al. 2019 AHA/ACC/HRS focused update of the 2014 AHA/ACC/HRS guideline for the management of patients with atrial fibrillation: a report of the American College of Cardiology/American Heart Association Task Force on Clinical Practice Guidelines and the Heart Rhythm Society in collaboration with the Society of Thoracic Surgeons. *Circulation*. 2019;140(2):e125–e151.

CODES

ICD10

- I48.91 Unspecified atrial fibrillation
- I48.92 Unspecified atrial flutter
- I48.0 Paroxysmal atrial fibrillation

CLINICAL PEARLS

Reevaluation of the need for and choice of anticoagulation therapy at periodic intervals is recommended to reassess stroke and bleeding risks.

ATRIAL SEPTAL DEFECT

Jeremy Golding, MD, FAAFP

 BASICS

DESCRIPTION

- Atrial septal defect (ASD) is a congenital defect of the interatrial septum characterized by absent or insufficient tissue. Patent foramen ovale (PFO) is not considered an ASD, because no septal tissue is missing.
- Types classified by location and abnormal embryogenesis (1)
  - 75%: ostium secundum defect, located in the midseptum
  - 15–20%: ostium primum defect, located in the inferior septum, associated with cleft mitral valve and failure of endocardial cushion development
  - 5–10%: sinus venosus defect, located in the superior-posterior septum near the orifice of the superior vena cava, associated with partial defect in right upper pulmonary venous return
  - <1%: coronary sinus defect, absence of the entire common wall between the coronary sinus and the left atrium
- Hemodynamic effects
  - Left-to-right shunting in late ventricular systole and early diastole
  - Degree depends on size of the defect and relative pressures of the two ventricles.
  - Causes excessive blood flow through the right-sided circulation, ultimately leading to reactive pulmonary hypertension and heart failure
- Systems affected: cardiovascular; pulmonary

Pediatric Considerations

- Most cases of ASD are detected and corrected in the pediatric population.
- The smaller the defect and the younger the child, the greater the chance of spontaneous closure.

EPIDEMIOLOGY

Incidence

- Predominant age: present from birth, may be diagnosed at any age
- Female to male ratio 2–4:1
- No race predilection
- 1/1,500 live births
- Ostium secundum alone accounts for >90% of all congenital heart lesions in the adult population (2).

Prevalence

ASDs account for 13% of congenital heart disorders.

ETIOLOGY AND PATHOPHYSIOLOGY

- The flow across ASD is usually left-to-right because of higher left-sided pressures:
  - Minimal right-to-left shunting in early ventricular systole, especially during inspiration
  - Increased right-sided pressure/pulmonary arterial hypertension can cause reversal of shunt flow (Eisenmenger syndrome) with resulting cyanosis and clubbing.
- Symptoms typically occur due to right ventricular and pulmonary vascular volume overload and right-sided heart failure.

Genetics

- Majority of cases are spontaneous, although rare familial cases exist.
- 25% prevalence in Down syndrome
- 5% with chromosomal abnormalities

RISK FACTORS

- Family history, other congenital heart defects
- Maternal age >35 years
- Gestational exposures: thalidomide, alcohol, tobacco, elevated blood glucose

COMMONLY ASSOCIATED CONDITIONS

- 70% ASDs are isolated but may occur as a component of other complex cardiac structural defects, including anomalous pulmonary venous return.
- May be associated with rare underlying genetic syndromes, including Holt-Oram (ASD present in 66%), Ellis-van Creveld, VACTERL syndrome, Down syndrome, or Noonan syndrome

 DIAGNOSIS

HISTORY

- Most ASDs are small, asymptomatic in throughout childhood, and only found as an incidental cardiac murmur on routine physical examination.
- Infants with large ASDs may present with right-sided heart failure (more advanced, only 10% at diagnosis), tachypnea, recurrent respiratory infections, or failure to thrive.
- Uncorrected defects usually become symptomatic by 40 years of age and may present with palpitations (most frequently), exercise intolerance, dyspnea, syncope, peripheral edema, cyanosis, or fatigue.
- Children and young adults are rarely symptomatic but may present with exercise intolerance or atrial arrhythmias.

PHYSICAL EXAM

- Children and young adults are mostly asymptomatic, although they can rarely exhibit cyanosis and hyperdynamic precordium.
- Signs vary according to extent of shunting.
- Cardiac palpation
  - Hyperdynamic precordium over the right ventricle
  - Palpable pulmonary artery pulse at the left upper sternal border
- Cardiac auscultation
  - *Fixed, widely split S₂ (key physical finding)*
  - May also have
    - ○ Systolic ejection murmur (pulmonic flow murmur)
    - ○ Low-pitched diastolic rumble (tricuspid flow murmur)
    - ○ Diastolic murmur (pulmonic regurgitation)
    - ○ Systolic murmur (mitral regurgitation)
    - ○ Fourth heart sound in the setting of right-sided heart failure
- Signs of Eisenmenger syndrome:
  - Cyanosis and clubbing
  - Jugular venous distention and edema

DIFFERENTIAL DIAGNOSIS

- Other congenital heart disease
- Right bundle branch block (for widely split S₂)

DIAGNOSTIC TESTS & INTERPRETATION

Initial Tests (lab, imaging)

- Best initial test is transthoracic echocardiogram (TTE) with Doppler imaging of the entire atrial septum: sensitive for secundum (89%), primum (100%), and sinus venosus (44%) defects.
- If TTE is nondiagnostic or shows evidence of right ventricular overload, progression to transesophageal echocardiography (TEE) is warranted.
- Oximetry at rest and with activity: Cyanosis or SpO₂ <90% may suggest Eisenmenger syndrome (right-to-left shunting). In certain subsets of patients, these signs may only appear with activity (3).
- ECG is not typically diagnostic but may show various signs of right- or left-sided heart strain, inverted P wave in lead III (in sinus venosus), or leftward axis (ostium primum or sinus venosus).

Follow-Up Tests & Special Considerations

- Bubble contrast enhancement may be helpful.
- TEE may be required to define ASD morphology and to locate the pulmonary veins; often used prior to percutaneous closure. TEE has excellent sensitivity and specificity.

Diagnostic Procedures/Other

- Echocardiography is first line as noted above.
- Cardiac catheterization: used to characterize ASDs and concomitant heart disease and to assess presence of pulmonary vascular resistance or hypertension (particularly if considering surgery); this procedure is not indicated in young patients unless part of a planned closure, evaluating another disease simultaneously, or other visualization methods are insufficient (3).
- Cardiac magnetic resonance: noninvasive follow-up to echocardiography, used to evaluate sinus venosus defects/pulmonary veins, shunt fraction, and right ventricular function (3)
- Exercise testing: may be used to document change over time
- Chest x-ray: may be used to identify right ventricular or pulmonary artery enlargement
- Cardiac CT: may further define ASD but with significant radiation exposure

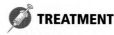 **TREATMENT**

GENERAL MEASURES

- 75% of small secundum ASDs (<8 mm) will close spontaneously by 18 months of age; however, close follow-up is warranted.
- Surgical closure is usually required for primum and sinus venosus defects.

MEDICATION

First Line

- Treatment of secondary cardiac or pulmonary vascular disease
  - Atrial fibrillation/supraventricular tachycardia (SVT) with anticoagulation and cardioversion/sinus rhythm or rate-control
  - Heart failure with diuretics, oxygen, digoxin, etc.
  - Remodeling therapy with prostaglandins, endothelin blockers, and PDE-5 inhibitors for patients with severe pulmonary arterial hypertension (3)
- Consider pulmonary vasodilator therapy for adults with progressive/severe pulmonary vascular disease.

Second Line

- Antibiotic prophylaxis is NOT recommended for unrepaired/isolated ASDs or as prophylaxis against infective endocarditis during dental procedures.
- To prevent thrombus formation after device deployment, aspirin alone or a combination of aspirin and clopidogrel 75 mg for at least 6 months is recommended.

SURGERY/OTHER PROCEDURES

- The majority of small secundum defects, <6 mm, close spontaneously by 2 years of age. Closure is generally indicated in children with defects >8 mm, defects of any size in children aged >5 years with related symptoms
- Closure for secundum defects is not recommended in asymptomatic patients before 2 years of age given the possibility of spontaneous closure. It is also contraindicated in patients with irreversible, severe pulmonary hypertension without continued shunting.
- In adults, secundum closure via percutaneous transcatheter device or surgery to reduce subsequent morbidity and mortality indicated in patients with right heart enlargement with or without symptoms, pulmonary systemic flow ratio of 2:1 (or >1.5:1 and <21 years old per the AHA), or symptoms including documented orthodeoxia/platypnea or paradoxical embolism. Treatment with a closure device does not significantly affect aortic/mitral valve function.
- Surgical repair is standard for a sinus venosus, coronary sinus, or primum ASD.
- Percutaneous closure with a closure device is considered the treatment of choice of secundum ASD in adults (3),(4). It is safe and effective with satisfactory long-term clinical follow-up. In addition, the use of closure device does not significantly affect aortic or mitral valve function (4).
- Maze procedure may be considered before or after closure for patients with intermittent or chronic atrial tachyarrhythmias.

ONGOING CARE

FOLLOW-UP RECOMMENDATIONS

- Outpatient cardiologist visits: every 3 months to 5 years depending on physiologic stage of the defect (3)
- ECG: every 1 to 5 years depending on physiologic stage of the defect
- TTE: every 1 to 5 years depending on physiologic stage of the defect
- Exercise stress test: every 6 to 24 months for advanced disease

Patient Monitoring

- In otherwise asymptomatic healthy children, follow up until defect has closed or become negligible in size.
- ASDs repaired in adulthood may require periodic long-term follow-up.
- ASDs repaired in childhood generally do not have late complications.
- Pregnancy is well tolerated in cases with repaired/small unrepaired ASDs but is not recommended in cases of unrepaired ASD/Eisenmenger syndrome due to increased risk of maternal and fetal mortality.
- Recommend consultation in patients with unrepaired ASDs prior to scuba diving or high-altitude travel.

PATIENT EDUCATION

For patient education materials on this topic, consult the American Heart Association or Mayo Clinic ASD webpages.

PROGNOSIS

- ASD closure in asymptomatic, minimally symptomatic, and symptomatic adults reduces morbidity especially if performed before 25 years of age (2),(3).
- ASD repair deferred until after adolescence may not decrease long-term risk of future atrial arrhythmias.
- In one study, prognosis after ASD closure saw a >20% reduction in pulmonary resistance by pretreatment with PAH therapies and pulmonary remodeling treatments (3).
- Unoperated ASDs: up to 25% mortality by 27 years, up to 90% mortality by 60 years, increased rates of atrial arrhythmias, reduced functional capacity, greater degrees of pulmonary arterial hypertension (2),(3)

COMPLICATIONS

- Unrepaired: congestive heart failure, stroke, atrial arrhythmias, increased infection risk (pulmonary, cerebral abscess, infective endocarditis); rarer complications include pulmonary arterial hypertension/Eisenmenger syndrome, and paradoxical embolism (3).
- Surgically repaired: late-onset arrhythmias 10 to 20 years after surgery (5%), perioperative atrial tachyarrhythmias (10–13% of patients), increased risk of arrhythmia-associated embolic events (2)
- Device closure: device embolization (1%), cardiac perforation, thrombus formation, endocarditis, supraventricular arrhythmias, and device erosions

REFERENCES

1. Bradley EA, Zaidi AN. Atrial septal defect. *Cardiol Clin*. 2020;38(3):317–324.
2. Oster M, Bhatt AB, Zaragoza-Macias E, et al. Interventional therapy versus medical therapy for secundum atrial septal defect: a systematic review (Part 2) for the 2018 AHA/ACC Guideline for the Management of Adults With Congenital Heart Disease: a report of the American College of Cardiology/American Heart Association Task Force on Clinical Practice Guidelines. *J Am Coll Cardiol*. 2019;73(12):1579–1595.
3. Stout KK, Daniels CJ, Aboulhosn JA, et al. 2018 AHA/ACC guideline for the management of adults with congenital heart disease: executive summary: a report of the American College of Cardiology/American Heart Association Task Force on Clinical Practice Guidelines. *J Am Coll Cardiol*. 2019;73(12):1494–1563.
4. Scacciatella P, Marra S, Pullara A, et al. Percutaneous closure of atrial septal defect in adults: very long-term clinical outcome and effects on aortic and mitral valve function. *J Invasive Cardiol*. 2015;27(1):65–69.

SEE ALSO

Aortic Valvular Stenosis; Coarctation of the Aorta; Patent Ductus Arteriosus; Pulmonary Valve Stenosis; Tetralogy of Fallot; Ventricular Septal Defect

CODES

ICD10

- Q21.2 Atrioventricular septal defect
- Q21.1 Atrial septal defect
- I23.1 Atrial septal defect as current complication following acute myocardial infarction

CLINICAL PEARLS

- ASD is often missed due to subtle clinical presentation.
- Ideally, hemodynamically significant ASDs should be closed in early childhood, although some benefit from closure is present in older patients.
- Many ASDs can be treated by catheter-directed percutaneous closure rather than open-heart surgery.
- Routine endocarditis prophylaxis is not recommended for unrepaired ASDs.
- Generally, symptomatic and hemodynamically significant ASDs are repaired; optimal management of asymptomatic small ASDs is unclear.
- PFOs, unlike large ASDs, are very common and generally require no treatment in asymptomatic individuals.

ATTENTION DEFICIT/HYPERACTIVITY DISORDER, ADULT

Ulunma Natalie Umesi, MD, MBA • Camille A. Archer, MD • Ambreka Benons, MD

 BASICS

- Adult attention deficit hyperactivity disorder (adult ADHD) is a pattern of behaviors that include inattention and/or hyperactivity or impulsivity. It is present in multiple settings that impair social, academic, or work performance.
- Complications of adult ADHD include employment, financial, and interpersonal difficulties, as well as increased risk for driving accidents and suicide.
- Adult ADHD typically begins in childhood and 30–60% will continue to meet criteria as adults.

DESCRIPTION
- Symptoms include difficulty concentrating, impulsivity, and hyperactivity/overactivity. Impairment in executive functioning and emotional dysregulation are common features.
- The three main types of ADHD are (i) hyperactivity-impulsivity predominant, (ii) inattentive predominant, and (iii) combined. The combined type is the most common, followed by the inattentive and hyperactive types.

EPIDEMIOLOGY
Prevalence
ADHD affects approximately 4.4–5.2% of adults between 18 and 44 years of age (1). ADHD is more common in men than women, who are less likely to be referred for assessment and more likely to be undiagnosed or misdiagnosed.

ETIOLOGY AND PATHOPHYSIOLOGY
Genetics
- ADHD appears to have a genetic component, with heritability of approximately 0.8, suggesting that genetic factors would account for about 65% of phenotypic variance.
- First-degree relatives of persons with ADHD reported to have 4 to 5 times greater risk than general population.

RISK FACTORS
- The risk of ADHD is increased among offsprings of mothers who smoked or had obesity and diabetes during pregnancy. Risk is also increased in those who had lead exposure in childhood. It is unknown whether these associations are causal.
- Premature birth; very low birth weight; and extreme neglect, abuse, or social deprivation also increase the risk as do certain infections during pregnancy, at birth, and in early childhood.
- Other factors associated with increased risk for ADHD include neurodevelopmental disorders including autism spectrum disorder and learning disabilities.

COMMONLY ASSOCIATED CONDITIONS
- Substance use and substance abuse disorders
- Mood and anxiety disorders
- Intellectual disabilities
- Obsessive-compulsive disorder (OCD)
- Tic disorders
- Delayed sleep-wake phase disorder

 DIAGNOSIS

- Diagnosis is made from patient's history and detailing patient's current level of functioning in at least two different settings (e.g., work and home).
- It is important to gather history of patient's childhood and school performance.

HISTORY
- Commonly reported symptoms of ADHD include poor concentration, disorganization, failure to complete projects, poor performance at work, and difficulty controlling temper.
- *DSM-5* criteria include (1):
  - At least five symptoms of inattention or hyperactivity/impulsivity
  - Several symptoms must be present before the age of 12 years (if not diagnosed in childhood, this is established by a historical assessment of childhood symptoms).
  - Symptoms must be present in two or more settings (home, work, etc.).
  - There must be clear evidence that symptoms interfere with or reduce quality of social, academic, or work functioning.
  - Symptoms must be present for >6 months.
- History of medication or substances that have side effects that impact attentiveness and mimic ADHD symptoms
- History of thyroid disorders, head injury or trauma, liver disease, seizure disorders
- Ask about cardiovascular disease and neurodevelopmental disorders including autism spectrum disorder, tic disorders, and learning disabilities.
- Ask about family history of ADHD and other psychiatric and neurologic problems.

PHYSICAL EXAM
- Physical exam is the key to rule out other medical conditions.
- Focus on thyroid and neurologic examinations; look for findings suggestive of substance abuse.
- Record BP and baseline weight; monitor if starting medical treatment.

DIFFERENTIAL DIAGNOSIS
Hearing impairment, hyperthyroid/hypothyroid, sleep deprivation, sleep apnea, phenylketonuria, OCD, lead toxicity, substance abuse (2)

DIAGNOSTIC TESTS & INTERPRETATION
- Adult ADHD screening tools:
  - Retrospective scales include the Childhood Symptom Scale and the Wender Utah Rating Scale
  - Current symptom scales include the Adult ADHD Rating Scale IV, Adult Self-Report Scale Symptom Checklist, and the Conners Adult Rating Scale (1). These scales can take 5 to 20 minutes to complete.
- Provider/patient screening checklist
  - https://add.org/wp-content/uploads/2015/03/adhd-questionnaire-ASRS111.pdf
  - https://nyulangone.org/files/psych_adhd_screener_0.pdf

Initial Tests (lab, imaging)
- Thyroid-stimulating hormone (TSH)
- ECG with concerns for cardiac disease in patient or family history
- Urine toxicology screen to rule out concomitant substance abuse disorder

Follow-Up Tests & Special Considerations
- Liver function test monitoring
- Consider polysomnography in patients with sleep disorder symptoms to rule out sleep apnea.
- A history of childhood behaviors is helpful, but adult patients often don't accurately recall childhood symptomology.
- Inquire about family history of ADHD, family and personal substance abuse, and tic disorders to facilitate formulation of an accurate diagnosis and recognition of high-risk behaviors.
- Caution against stimulant use in pregnancy because of high risk of low fetal birth weight and preterm birth. Risks and benefits of treatment must be discussed in detail with patient and preferably with his or her partner (3)[B].
- Caution against use of stimulants in adult patients with cardiac history.

ALERT
Mood disorders, generalized anxiety disorders, and substance abuse can also coexist with adult ADHD; treating both the ADHD and comorbid conditions will improve the patient's prognosis.

TREATMENT
- Most of the research and medication trials have been performed in children.
- There is an increasing evidence that medications used in children are also effective in adults (2)[A].

ALERT
Because stimulant medication may induce dependency, substance abuse, and diversion, it is recommended to do pill counts, screen urine for drugs, monitor behavior, and query prescription databases. Misuse of amphetamines may cause sudden death and serious cardiovascular adverse events.

GENERAL MEASURES
When substance abuse is not present, stimulants are first-line treatment for ADHD and highly efficacious. Patients may require trials of different dosages, formulations, and medications before an optimal response in symptoms and functions is achieved. Nonstimulants are useful when there is abuse potential, comorbid conditions, or poor response to stimulants.

MEDICATION
- Titrate slowly to effective dose to avoid side effects.
- Stimulants are more effective than antidepressants or nonstimulants, but up to 30% discontinue medications because of side effects.

- Stimulants can be grouped into those related to methylphenidate and those related to amphetamine. Both groups include both short- and long-acting preparations. Recent evidence suggests that adherence and persistence rates improve in those using long-acting agents (1).
- Antidepressants studied for ADHD include bupropion, which has been shown to have a medium effect compared with stimulants (2)[A].

First Line

D and D-L stimulant classes:

- Stimulants: methylphenidate (Concerta, Ritalin), dexmethylphenidate (Focalin), dextroamphetamine/amphetamine (Adderall), dextroamphetamine (Dexedrine), lisdexamfetamine (Vyvanse)
  - Methylphenidate preparations are available in short-acting, intermediate-acting, long-acting, and patch formulations.
  - Methylphenidate hydrochloride extended-release (Ritalin LA) may be used for patients who are naive to stimulants. It can be started at 20 mg/day and dose titrated by 10 mg increments weekly to symptoms response; max of 60 mg/day
  - Methylphenidate extended-release (Concerta) is another option in adults up to 65 years of age; starting dose of 18 mg/day; adjust in increments of 18 mg/weekly until symptoms improve; max of 72 mg/day
  - Dextroamphetamine is commonly used (half-life of 4 to 6 hours) with an initial dose of 5 mg BID; titrate up by 5 mg/week to a maximum of 20 mg BID.
  - Dextroamphetamine/amphetamine (Adderall) is a 75%/25% mix that also comes in an extended-release form. Initial dosing can be started at 5 mg BID for short acting or 20 mg/day for long acting and increased by 5 mg/week for short acting and 10 mg/week for long acting to a maximum of 60 mg total daily.
  - Lisdexamfetamine (Vyvanse) is an extended-release stimulant that is a prodrug requiring metabolization to active component, dextroamphetamine.
  - Common side effects of stimulants include hypertension (HTN), tachycardia, insomnia, weight loss, stomach upset, increased anxiety/irritability, or worsening of tics (2)[A].
- Nonstimulants:
  - Atomoxetine (Strattera) has been shown effective in adults with ADHD when compared to placebo (4)[B]. It may be given as a single dose or split dose and has low abuse potential. Onset of effect may take up to 4 weeks. Atomoxetine may be particularly useful when anxiety, mood, or tics co-occur with ADHD. There are rare cases of liver damage associated with these medications. Monitor for increased suicidal thinking.
  - Antidepressants: best used for those at high risk or with history of substance abuse disorder. Bupropion (Wellbutrin) is effective in adults with ADHD symptoms, especially if comorbid depression (3)[A].
  - Tricyclic antidepressants (desipramine and nortriptyline) have also shown to be effective in ADHD (1).

- α_2-Agonists (guanfacine, clonidine) have been found to be effective in children and adolescents; however, they have not been studied extensively in adults (5)[C]. These may be used with comorbid tics and/or disruptive behavior disorders.
  - Combining stimulants with a nonstimulant medication such as atomoxetine, guanfacine, or clonidine has shown positive effects among patients who are resistant to stimulants alone.

ISSUES FOR REFERRAL

Consider referral to obstetrician experienced in high-risk pregnancies when treating pregnant women with ADHD.

ADDITIONAL THERAPIES

- Cognitive-behavioral therapy (CBT) can be useful in conjunction with medication to help patient modify and cope with symptoms. CBT helps reduce impairments resulting from executive dysfunction (EDF) that is not optimally ameliorated with medication (1).
- Among adults with ADHD and EDFs, addition of memantine as an adjunct to extended release methylphenidate was associated with improved executive functioning, supporting the need for further research.

COMPLEMENTARY & ALTERNATIVE MEDICINE

- Mixed evidence that fatty acid supplementation in addition to medication may be beneficial (6)
- Eliminating artificial food coloration only shows a mild benefit in decreasing symptoms (7).
- Behavioral therapy
  - Providing rewards can motivate desired behaviors in this population.
  - Classroom performance shows significant improvement in schools emphasizing learning, minimizing punishment, and increasing a positive learning environment (8).

 ## ONGOING CARE

Transfer from pediatric to adult care must be closely coordinated to avoid hiatus in treatment.

FOLLOW-UP RECOMMENDATIONS

- Close follow-up of medication as dose is titrated to monitor for side effects.
- Repeat screening checklists to quantify benefits.
- Reinforce behavioral change (e.g., self-initiated through CBT), which is the essential goal of long-term management.

DIET

Limit caffeine intake while in prescribed stimulant medication.

PATIENT EDUCATION

Support groups (e.g., https://www.chadd.org/, https://www.add.org/)

COMPLICATIONS

Comorbid psychiatric conditions such as MDD, anxiety disorders, OCD, and tic disorders

REFERENCES

1. Young JL, Goodman DW. Adult attention-deficit/hyperactivity disorder diagnosis, management, and treatment in the DSM-5 era. *Prim Care Companion CNS Disord*. 2016;18(6).
2. Castells X, Ramos-Quiroga JA, Bosch R, et al. Amphetamines for attention deficit hyperactivity disorder (ADHD) in adults. *Cochrane Database Syst Rev*. 2011;(6):CD007813.
3. Verbeeck W, Tuinier S, Bekkering GE. Antidepressants in the treatment of adult attention-deficit hyperactivity disorder: a systematic review. *Adv Ther*. 2009;26(2):170–184.
4. Asherson P, Bushe C, Saylor K, et al. Efficacy of atomoxetine in adults with attention deficit hyperactivity disorder: an integrated analysis of the complete database of multicenter placebo-controlled trials. *J Psychopharmacol*. 2014;28(9):837–846.
5. Hirota T, Schwartz S, Correll CU. Alpha-2 agonists for attention-deficit/hyperactivity disorder in youth: a systematic review and meta-analysis of monotherapy and add-on trials to stimulant therapy. *J Am Acad Child Adolesc Psychiatry*. 2014;53(2):153–173.
6. Millichap JG, Yee MM. The diet factor in attention-deficit/hyperactivity disorder. *Pediatrics*. 2012;129(2):330–337.
7. Sonuga-Barke EJS, Brandeis D, Cortese S, et al; for European ADHD Guidelines Group. Nonpharmacological interventions for ADHD: systematic review and meta-analyses of randomized controlled trials of dietary and psychological treatments. *Am J Psychiatry*. 2013;170(3):275–289.
8. Feldman HM, Reiff MI. Clinical practice: attention deficit-hyperactivity disorder in children and adolescents. *N Eng J Med*. 2014;370(9):838–846.

ADDITIONAL READING

American Psychiatric Association. *Diagnostic and Statistical Manual of Mental Disorders*. 5th ed. Arlington, VA: American Psychiatric Association; 2013.

CODES

ICD10

- F90.9 Attention-deficit hyperactivity disorder, unspecified type
- F90.1 Attn-defct hyperactivity disorder, predom hyperactive type
- F90.0 Attn-defct hyperactivity disorder, predom inattentive type

CLINICAL PEARLS

- Adult ADHD results in inattention, easy distractibility, hyperactivity, and impulsive behavior; it is associated with low self-esteem, problematic interpersonal relationships, and difficulty meeting academic and job expectations.
- Psychotropic medications plus cognitive behavioral treatments are the cornerstone of management.
- Substance abuse is a common comorbidity; recommend use of nonstimulant medication in those at high risk.

ATTENTION DEFICIT/HYPERACTIVITY DISORDER, PEDIATRIC

Katherine Williams, MD

 BASICS

DESCRIPTION

- Attention deficit hyperactivity disorder (ADHD) is a neurodevelopmental disorder that manifests in early childhood characterized by distractibility, impulsivity, hyperactivity, and/or inattention.
- Three subsets: predominantly hyperactivity (ADHD-H), predominantly inattentive (ADHD-I), or combined (ADHD-C)
- System(s) affected: nervous

EPIDEMIOLOGY

- Predominant age: onset <12 years; lasts into adolescence and adulthood
- Predominant sex: assigned male at birth > assigned female at birth (2:1); ADHD-I is more common in patients assigned female at birth.

Prevalence
9–15% of children aged 4 to 17 years

ETIOLOGY AND PATHOPHYSIOLOGY
Not definitive—suggested pathogenesis includes imbalance of catecholamine metabolism and structural brain differences. Environmental influences are controversial.

RISK FACTORS

- Family history (genetic component)
- Medical causes (affecting brain development)—including prenatal tobacco exposure and prematurity

COMMONLY ASSOCIATED CONDITIONS

- Mood disorders—depression, anxiety
- Behavior disorders—oppositional defiant disorder, conduct disorder
- Autism spectrum disorder
- Physiologic disorders—sleep disorders, tics
- Learning disabilities, developmental coordination syndrome, language disorder
- Substance use disorders

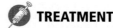 **DIAGNOSIS**

- American Academy of Pediatrics (AAP) guidelines recommend *DSM-5-TR* criteria to establish diagnosis.
- *DSM-5-TR* (1) criteria for children aged <17 years: ≥6 inattention criteria and/or ≥6 hyperactivity/impulsivity criteria; symptoms must occur often, be present before age of 12 years, for >6 months, be noticed in ≥2 settings (e.g., home, school), reduced quality of social or scholastic functioning, be excessive for development level of child, and are not better explained by or occur with another mental disorder (e.g., depression, anxiety, or personality disorder).
- Inattention
  - Careless mistakes in tasks; difficulty sustaining attention or in organizing
  - Does not seem to listen
  - Does not follow through or finish tasks
  - Avoids tasks that require sustained mental effort
  - Loses things
  - Forgetful in daily activities
  - Distracted by external stimuli
  - Forgetful

- Hyperactivity/impulsivity
  - Fidgets
  - Difficulty remaining seated
  - Runs/climbs excessively or inappropriately; difficulty playing quietly
  - Acts as if "driven by a motor" or seeming to always be "on the go"
  - Talks excessively
  - Blurts out answers before question is complete
  - Has difficulty waiting turn
  - Interrupts others
- Children undergoing extreme stress (divorce, illness, homelessness, abuse) may demonstrate ADHD behaviors secondary to stress.
- If diagnostic behaviors are noted in only one setting, explore the stressors in that setting.
- The diagnostic behaviors are more noticeable in tasks that require concentration or boredom tolerance.

HISTORY

- Birth and development history
- Psychosocial evaluation of home environment
- School performance and school absences
- Psychiatric history or history of comorbid disorder(s)
- Cardiac history

PHYSICAL EXAM

- Baseline weight, heart rate, blood pressure for future monitoring
- Note any soft neurologic signs, such as tics, clumsiness, and mixed handedness.
- Assess hearing and vision.

DIFFERENTIAL DIAGNOSIS

- Activity level appropriate for age
- Dysfunctional family situation or abuse
- Learning disability (e.g., dyslexia)
- Hearing/vision/language disorder
- Autism spectrum disorders
- Oppositional/defiant disorder or conduct disorder
- Seizure disorder
- Neurodevelopmental syndromes (e.g., fragile X)
- Lead poisoning
- Sequelae of central nervous system infection/trauma
- Medication effect
- Any of the comorbid conditions above

DIAGNOSTIC TESTS & INTERPRETATION

- Behavior rating scales completed by parents, caregivers, and teachers prior to initiation of therapy and then repeated after therapy (Vanderbilt ADHD Forms)
- National Institute for Children's Health Quality. Caring for children with ADHD: a resource toolkit for clinicians. https://www.nichq.org/resource/caring-children-adhd-resource-toolkit-clinicians
- Testing for learning disability: request from school

Initial Tests (lab, imaging)
Rarely needed; consider lead.

Diagnostic Procedures/Other
ECG prior to stating stimulant medication if positive family history of premature CV disease

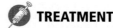 **TREATMENT**

GENERAL MEASURES

- Always develop a behavioral health plan with parents and school.
- Identify treatment goals based on behaviors which are most harmful to the child's development.
- Coordinate school and home behavioral plan.
- Children aged 4 to 5 years should begin with behavioral interventions
- Children aged 6 to 17 years begin with behavioral interventions and consider medication if behavioral goals are not being met over time.
- Behavioral counseling can be beneficial for both parents and child, including parent training, academic training, and social training.
- Behavioral modifications should involve repeated positive reinforcement with limiting negative comments, reward systems, environmental changes at both home and school (time out, quiet time), etc.

MEDICATION

- Stimulant medications are often considered first line as they have the highest efficacy, but they also carry greater risks.
- Atomoxetine may be used as first line, especially if there is a risk of diversion in the home, growth concerns (poor weight gain, sleep issues, etc.), or if parents wish to try nonstimulant medication.
- Stimulant choice should be based on cost, formulary, convenience, and duration. A second type of stimulant should be tried if the first treatment fails.

First Line
Stimulant:

- Methylphenidate
  - Short acting
    - Ritalin, Methylin: onset within 30 minutes; duration of 3 to 5 hours
  - Intermediate acting
    - Metadate ER: onset within 20 to 60 minutes and lasts for 8 hours
  - Long acting
    - Methylphenidate CD: combination of immediate release and delayed release for duration over 8 to 12 hours (bimodal)
    - Cotempla XR ODT: combination of immediate release and extended release for duration up to 12 hours
    - Quillivant XR: combination of immediate release and extended release for duration up to 12 hours
    - Quillichew ER: continuous release over 6 to 8 hours for duration up to 13 hours
    - Ritalin LA: combination of immediate release and delayed release for duration over 8 to 12 hours
    - Concerta/Relexxii: combination of immediate release and continuous release for duration over 10 to 12 hours
    - Aptensio XR: combination of immediate release and controlled release for duration of 12 hours
    - Adhansia XR: combination of immediate release and controlled release for duration of 16 hours

○ Jornay PM: night-time dosing where <5% of drug available within the first 10 hours of administration with a peak concentration at 14 hours and steady decline after
○ Daytrana transdermal patch: onset 2 hours after application for duration of 9 to 12 hours

- Dexmethylphenidate
  – Focalin: duration 5 to 6 hours
  – Focalin XR: combination of immediate release and delayed release over 10 to 12 hours
- Serdexmethylphenidate-dexmethylphenidate
  – Azstarys: 70% prodrug delayed and 30% immediate release drug; onset within 1 hour and duration of 13 hours
- Amphetamine
  – Immediate release
    ○ Evekeo/Evekeo ODT: onset within 20 to 60 minutes for duration of 4 to 6 hours
  – Extended release
    ○ Dyanavel XR: combination of immediate and extended release for duration of 13 hours (liquid + tab)
    ○ Adzenys XR-ODT: combination of immediate release and extended release; duration over 10 to 12 hours
- Dextroamphetamine
  – Immediate release
    ○ Dexedrine, ProCentra: onset within 20 to 60 minutes for duration of 4 to 6 hours
  – Extended release
    ○ Dextroamphetamine SR: combination of immediate release and continuous release; duration over 8 to 12 hours
    ○ Xelstrym patch: onset 2 hours after application for duration of 9 to 12 hours
- Dextroamphetamine/amphetamine mixed salts
  – Short acting
    ○ Adderall: onset within 20 to 60 minutes for duration of 4 to 6 hours
  – Long acting
    ○ Adderall XR: combination of immediate and continuous release for duration of 10 to 12 hours
    ○ Mydayis: combination of immediate and two different delayed-release beads; duration up to 16 hours
- Lisdexamfetamine
  – Vyvanse: prodrug converted to dextroamphetamine with effect over 10 hours

- Common adverse effects:
  – Anorexia, insomnia, growth delay, GI effects, CV effects, and headache
  – Rare: priapism, psychosis, tics, suicidal thinking
- Significant possible interactions: may increase levels of anticonvulsants, SSRIs, tricyclics, and warfarin
- High-caffeine energy drinks, albuterol inhalers, and decongestants may increase side effects.
- The FDA reports permanent skin discoloration with Daytrana patches.

Second Line
Nonstimulant:
- SNRI
  – Atomoxetine (Strattera): effects last at least 10 to 12 hours but must be taken daily without drug holidays
  – Viloxazine (Qelbree): lasts throughout the day, must be taken daily without drug holidays
- α_2-Agonist
  – Modest efficacy, high side effects; consider consultation before use.
    ○ Clonidine XR (Kapvay): duration of at least 10 to 12 hours
    ○ Guanfacine XR (Intuniv): duration of at least 10 to 12 hours

ISSUES FOR REFERRAL
Refer for children if there are additional mental health issues, developmental issues, or poor response to treatment.

COMPLEMENTARY & ALTERNATIVE MEDICINE
Parents of children with ADHD use herbals and complementary treatments frequently (20–60%) but very limited evidence to support any intervention, including video game therapies and trigeminal nerve stimulation.

ONGOING CARE

FOLLOW-UP RECOMMENDATIONS
Patient Monitoring
- Office visits to monitor side effects and efficacy: End points are improved grades, rating scales, family interactions, and peer interactions.
- Monitor growth (especially weight), HR, and BP.

PATIENT EDUCATION
- Excellent reference: http://www.parentsmedguide.org
- Teachers reference: ADDitude toolkit for parents and teachers

PROGNOSIS
- Relative deficits in academic and social functioning may persist into late adolescence/adulthood.
- Encourage career choices that allow autonomy and mobility.

COMPLICATIONS
Primarily from untreated ADHD:
- Increased failing in school, parental abuse, social isolation, poor self-esteem, risk of substance abuse, automobile accidents, and injuries

REFERENCE
1. American Psychiatric Association. *Diagnostic and Statistical Manual of Mental Disorders: DSM-5-TR.* 5th ed. Text rev. American Psychiatric Association Publishing; 2022.

ADDITIONAL READING
- Felt BT, Biermann B, Christner JG, et al. Diagnosis and management of ADHD in children. *Am Fam Physician.* 2014;90(7):456–464.
- National Institute for Children's Health Quality. Caring for children with ADHD: a resource toolkit for clinicians. https://www.nichq.org/resource/caring-children-adhd-resource-toolkit-clinicians. Published 2002. Accessed September 16, 2023.

 CODES

ICD10
- F90.2 Attention-deficit hyperactivity disorder, combined type
- F90.0 Attention-deficit hyperactivity disorder, predominantly inattentive type
- F90 Attention-deficit hyperactivity disorders

CLINICAL PEARLS
- Identify treatment goals before initiating any intervention and make treatment plan based on these goals.
- Behavioral therapy for child and parents and coordination with teachers and behavioral specialists in schools
- AAP recommends behavioral interventions for ages 4 to 5 years and behavioral interventions plus stimulant medications as first-line treatment for ages 6 to 17 years.
- Multiple medications—stimulants first line; titrate to patient response with close monitoring of response and side effects.

ATYPICAL MOLE (DYSPLASTIC NEVUS) SYNDROME

Sahil Mullick, MD • Farzad Effan, MBBS

 BASICS

Atypical mole syndrome (AMS), also known as dysplastic nevi syndrome (DNS), B-K mole syndrome, Clark nevi syndrome, or familial atypical multiple mole melanoma (FAMMM) syndrome, is a condition characterized by a large number of pigmented nevi with architectural disorder, which arise sporadically or by inheritance and are associated with an increased risk of melanoma.

DESCRIPTION

There is no consensus on criteria for AMS.

- Elevated total body nevi count, including clinically atypical nevi, is usually >50 and often >100.
  - Larger number in hereditary AMS versus sporadic atypical nevi (as few as <10)
- Increased risk of melanoma
  - Up to 90% occurrence by age 80 years in certain high-risk individuals
  - Earlier onset than in sporadic melanoma
  - More arise de novo than from an existing nevus
  - Higher risk for appearance at unusual sites (e.g., scalp, eyes, and sun-protected areas)
- Median age of diagnosis for melanoma in AMS is 10 to 20 years earlier than the general population, with documented cases of melanoma as early as in the 2nd and 3rd decades of life.

EPIDEMIOLOGY

Incidence
Uncertain due to phenotype variability, limited data

Prevalence
Affects between 2% and 8% of fair-skinned adults as well as those with high exposure to ultraviolet radiation

ETIOLOGY AND PATHOPHYSIOLOGY

- Cyclin-dependent kinase inhibitor 2A (*CDKN2A*) mutations have been observed in familial DNS and multiple melanomas. The *CDKN2A* gene on 9p21 encodes for the proteins p16 and p14. p16 binds to CDK4/6 and is a negative cell-cycle regulator via inhibition of the CDK-cyclin D interaction needed for cell cycle progression from G1 to S. p14 functions by stabilizing the tumor-suppressor protein p53 in the G1 phase of the cell cycle.
- Familial cases of germline *CDKN2A* mutations are transmitted in an autosomal dominant fashion.
- No clear somatic mutation patterns in sporadic cases

Genetics
CDKN2A gene mutation is observed in 25–40% of hereditary cases, with autosomal dominant inheritance but variable expressivity and incomplete penetrance.

RISK FACTORS
Family history of melanoma or multiple nevi, sun exposure, neonatal blue-light phototherapy, history of painful sunburns

GENERAL PREVENTION
- Primary prevention with sun avoidance, sun protection
- Secondary prevention of melanoma with routine skin exams, biopsy of suspect lesions, and environmental risk mitigation as above

COMMONLY ASSOCIATED CONDITIONS
- Malignant melanoma, including ocular melanoma
- Ocular nevi
- Pancreatic cancer in *CDKN2A* mutation

 DIAGNOSIS

AMS is a clinical diagnosis with various classifications schemes proposed. Although not widely accepted, diagnostic criteria, as defined by the NIH, require the three features of (i) malignant melanoma in ≥1 first- or second-degree relatives; (ii) numerous melanocytic nevi (frequently >50), some of which are clinically atypical; and (iii) nevi that have certain histologic features (1).

HISTORY
- Changing lesions: bleeding, scaling, size, texture, nonhealing, hyper- or hypopigmentation
- Large number of nevi
- Congenital nevi
- Sun exposure
- Prior skin biopsies
- Prior melanoma
- Immunosuppression (e.g., AIDS, chemotherapy, pancreatic cancer)
- First- or second-degree relatives with:
  - AMS
  - Melanoma
  - Pancreatic cancer

PHYSICAL EXAM
- Full-body skin exams, with photography to track new and changing nevi
- Goal to distinguish melanoma from atypical mole (AM)
- ABCDE mnemonic for skin lesions concerning for melanoma: Asymmetry, Border irregularity, Color variegation, Diameter >6 mm, and Evolving lesion
  - AM is often defined as ≥5 mm and at least two other features.
  - Melanoma typically has several characteristics of ABCDEs, with increased specificity for melanoma if lesion diameter is >6 mm.
- "Ugly duckling sign" (2)[B]:
  - Melanoma screening strategy for increasing accuracy of diagnosis of melanoma by identifying malignant nevi straying from the predominant nevus pattern when numerous atypical nevi are present
- Most common features of AM on dermoscopy include (3):
  - Reticular pattern most common
  - Uniform pigmentation most common followed by multifocal hypo- or hyperpigmentation
  - Homogenous brown globules
  - Pigmentation with central heterogeneity and abrupt termination
- Dermatoscopic features more suggestive of melanoma include (4):
  - Depigmented areas
  - Whitish veil
  - Homogenous areas distributed irregularly, in multiple areas, or >25% of total lesion
  - ≥4 colors

DIFFERENTIAL DIAGNOSIS
- Common nevus: acquired or congenital
- Melanoma
- Seborrheic keratosis
- Dermatofibroma
- Lentigo
- Pigmented actinic keratosis
- Pigmented basal cell carcinoma
- Blue rubber bleb nevus syndrome

DIAGNOSTIC TESTS & INTERPRETATION
Diagnosis is first suspected with history and physical exam and then confirmed by biopsy and histopathology.

Initial Tests (lab, imaging)
- Dermoscopy can be used for a more detailed exam of nevus to aid in distinguishing between benign and malignant lesions as well as for further classification to any of the 11 subtypes; however, the degree of success is dependent on the skill of the examiner.
- Reflectance confocal microscopy (RCM) may provide more specificity than dermoscopy in distinguishing AM from melanoma.
- When the total nevus count is high and following each nevus is impractical, total body photography may aid in the evaluation of evolving nevi as well as in documenting new nevi.

Follow-Up Tests & Special Considerations
Genetic testing is available for *CDKN2A* mutations, but it is not recommended outside of research studies because results cannot be adequately used for management or surveillance.

Diagnostic Procedures/Other
- Biopsy is recommended for any lesion where melanoma cannot be excluded or in the presence of clinically concerning features (e.g., recent growth) (5)[B].
- Biopsy entails full-thickness biopsy of the entire lesion with a narrow 1- to 3-mm margin of normal skin down to fat for adequate depth assessment (6)[C].
  - Excisional biopsy, elliptical or punch excision, provides the most accurate diagnosis and should be performed when possible.
  - Scoop shave biopsy can also be used, but care must be taken to not transect the lesion.
- Reexcision of mild to moderately dysplastic nevi with positive margins may not change pathologic diagnosis or outcomes (studies inconclusive) (7)[A], but for severely dysplastic nevi, consider reexcision, with surgical margins of 2 to 5 mm (8)[C].
- Genetic testing can help diagnosis in ambiguous situations, but studies are limited (9)[C].

Test Interpretation
"Dysplastic nevus" is a term more accurately reserved as a histologic diagnosis. Features may include melanocyte proliferation in the dermoepidermal junction extending through at least three rete ridges in a specific pattern, fusing of rete ridges, dermal fibrosis, neovascularization, and interstitial lymphocytic inflammation (8).

TREATMENT

MEDICATION
No medications have been shown to treat AMS (8)[C].

ISSUES FOR REFERRAL
- Routine skin exams for those patients at high risk for melanoma
- Ophthalmologic exams for ocular nevi/melanoma screening/papilledema
- Oncology or specialized genetics study group involvement if strong family predisposition to pancreatic cancer

ADDITIONAL THERAPIES
- Topical chemo- and immunotherapies have been unsuccessfully attempted to treat AMS (8)[C].
- Laser treatment should be avoided because it is both unsafe and ineffective for melanocytic nevi (8)[C].

SURGERY/OTHER PROCEDURES
Surgical excision of all atypical nevi is not recommended because most melanomas in AMS appear de novo on healthy skin and therefore has low clinical value and is not cost-effective. Excision of all atypical nevi also leads to both poor cosmetic outcomes and a false sense of security. Lesions suspicious for melanoma should be biopsied or removed surgically.

 ONGOING CARE

FOLLOW-UP RECOMMENDATIONS
Close follow-up with a dermatologist or other physician experienced with assessment of atypical nevi:
- Total body skin exam (including nails, scalp, genital area, and oral mucosa) every 6 months initially, starting at puberty; may be reduced to annually once nevi are stable
- Total body photography at baseline and intervals to track new and changing nevi
- Dermoscopic evaluation of suspicious lesions
- Excision of suspicious lesions
- Ocular exam for those with familial AMS

Patient Monitoring
Monthly self-exams of skin

PATIENT EDUCATION
For young adults with fair skin, counsel to minimize exposure to ultraviolet radiation to reduce risk of skin cancer (USPSTF grade B).
- Fair skin: light eye, hair, or skin color, freckles
- Educate on sun avoidance, proper application of sunscreen, use of protective clothing (e.g., hats), avoidance of tanning booths and sunburns.
- Teach "ABCDE" mnemonic + "ugly duckling sign" to assess nevi and identify potential melanomas.
- Provide instruction on skin self-exam techniques.

- A sample listing of patient-centric review sources on this topic are as follows:
  - Verywell Health (https://www.verywellhealth.com/the-abcdes-of-skin-cancer-514388)
  - Skin Cancer Foundation (https://www.skincancer.org/risk-factors/atypical-moles/)
  - Melanoma Research Foundation (https://melanoma.org/melanoma-education/what-melanoma-looks-like/)

PROGNOSIS
- Most AMs either regress or do not change.
- Multiple classification schemes have been developed over the years to delineate risk of melanoma in patients with AMS. Individuals with a family history of melanoma are at greatest risk. The Rigel classification system can be applied in the clinical setting. Points are assigned based on incidence of melanoma, with 1 point given for a personal history with melanoma and 2 points for each family member with melanoma (modified nuclear family consisting of first-degree relatives plus grandparents and uncles/aunts) and stratified as follows:
  - Score = 0, Rigel group 0, 6% 25-year accumulated risk for melanoma
  - Score = 1, Rigel group 1, 10% risk
  - Score = 2, Rigel group 2, 15% risk
  - Score ≥3, Rigel group 3, 50% risk
- The *CDKN2A* mutation has also been associated with a 60–90% risk of melanoma by age 80 years and a 17% risk for pancreatic cancer by age 75 years. In patients with melanoma, presence of the *CDKN2A* mutation may not worsen overall survival rates (10).

COMPLICATIONS
- Malignant melanoma
- Poor cosmetic outcomes from biopsy

REFERENCES
1. Goldsmith LA, Askin FB, Chang AE, et al. Diagnosis and treatment of early melanoma: NIH consensus development panel on early melanoma. *JAMA*. 1992;268(10):1314–1319.
2. Gaudy-Marqueste C, Wazaefi Y, Bruneu Y, et al. Ugly duckling sign as a major factor of efficiency in melanoma detection. *JAMA Dermatol*. 2017;153(4):279–284.
3. Hofmann-Wellenhof R, Blum A, Wolf IH, et al. Dermoscopic classification of atypical melanocytic nevi (Clark nevi). *Arch Dermatol*. 2001;137(12):1575–1580.
4. Salopek TG, Kopf AW, Stefanato CM, et al. Differentiation of atypical moles (dysplastic nevi) from early melanomas by dermoscopy. *Dermatol Clin*. 2001;19(2):337–345.
5. Wiedemeyer K, Hartschuh W, Brenn T. Dysplastic nevi: morphology and molecular and the controversies in-between. *Surg Pathol Clin*. 2021;14(2):341–357.
6. Strazzula L, Vedak P, Hoang MP, et al. The utility of re-excising mildly and moderately dysplastic nevi: a retrospective analysis. *J Am Acad Dermatol*. 2014;71(6):1071–1076.
7. Vuong KT, Walker J, Powell HB, et al. Surgical re-excision vs. observation for histologically dysplastic naevi: a systematic review of associated clinical outcomes. *Br J Dermatol*. 2018;179(3):590–598.
8. Duffy K, Grossman D. The dysplastic nevus: from historical perspective to management in the modern era: part I. Historical, histologic, and clinical aspects. *J Am Acad Dermatol*. 2012;67(1):1.e1–1.e18.
9. Helm TN, Helm MF, Helm KF. Melanoma arising in a persistent nevus: melanoma where "pseudomelanoma" is expected. *JAAD Case Rep*. 2021;12:5–7.
10. Dalmasso B, Pastorino L, Ciccarese G, et al. CDKN2A germline mutations are not associated with poor survival in an Italian cohort of melanoma patients. *J Am Acad Dermatol*. 2019;80(5):1263–1271.

ADDITIONAL READING
- Fleming NH, Shaub AR, Bailey E, et al. Outcomes of surgical re-excision versus observation of severely dysplastic nevi: a single-institution, retrospective cohort study. *J Am Acad Dermatol*. 2020;82(1):238–240.
- Perkins A, Duffy RL. Atypical moles: diagnosis and management. *Am Fam Physician*. 2015;91(11):762–767.
- Terushkin V, Ng E, Stein JA, et al. A prospective study evaluating the utility of a 2-mm biopsy margin for complete removal of histologically atypical (dysplastic) nevi. *J Am Acad Dermatol*. 2017;77(6):1096–1099.

 CODES

ICD10
- D22.9 Melanocytic nevi, unspecified
- D22.4 Melanocytic nevi of scalp and neck
- D22.30 Melanocytic nevi of unspecified part of face

CLINICAL PEARLS
- In describing nevi, "atypical" is a clinical term, whereas "dysplastic" is a histologic term.
- AMS is a risk factor for melanoma, although most atypical moles/dysplastic nevi are not precursors to melanoma. Melanoma in AMS tends to arise from healthy skin despite a large number of atypical nevi.
- ~20% of individuals with familial AMS will develop pancreatic cancer by age 75 years.
- Patients with AMS tend to produce neoplasms in unusual sites such as the scalp, eyes, and sun-protected areas (e.g., gluteal folds).

AUTISM SPECTRUM DISORDERS

Afsha Rais Kaisani, MD • Tasaduq Hussain Mir, MD, FAAFP • Catherine Kim, MD

BASICS

DESCRIPTION
- Group of neurodevelopmental disorders of early childhood characterized by (i) persistent deficits in social communication and interaction and (ii) restricted, repetitive patterns of behavior, interests, or activities
- *Diagnostic and Statistical Manual of Mental Disorders, 5th edition*: umbrella term autism spectrum disorder (ASD), which encompasses a group of pervasive developmental disorders with designations for varying severities and associated symptoms
- ASD combines former diagnoses, including autistic disorder, childhood disintegrative disorder, Asperger disorder, pervasive developmental disorder not otherwise specified (PDD-NOS), early infantile autism, childhood autism, Kanner autism, high-functioning autism, and atypical autism, many of which are still used by ICD-10 coding.
- Although symptoms must be present in early development period, they may not be apparent until social demands exceed capacity.
- Symptoms must cause functional impairment. Severity levels:
  – Level 1: requiring support—noticeable impairment
  – Level 2: requiring substantial support—marked deficits
  – Level 3: requiring very substantial support—severe impairments interfering with functionality
- Specifiers for associated symptoms include with catatonia; intellectual impairment; language impairment; known medical or genetic condition; and neurodevelopmental, mental, or behavioral disorders.
- Important to distinguish ASD from symptoms that could be better explained by intellectual disability or global developmental delay

EPIDEMIOLOGY
Onset in early childhood; predominant sex: male > female (approximately 4:1 ratio)

Pediatric Considerations
Symptom onset can often be seen in children <3 years of age but may not become apparent until social demands exceed capacity.

Prevalence
- Estimated prevalence has increased from approximately 1.1% in 2008 to 2.3% in 2018 among children aged 8 years in the United States (1).
- Higher prevalence contributed to changes in diagnostic criteria, increased awareness, improved ascertainment, and access to care (1).
- Higher percentage of ASD is observed in black, Hispanic, and Asian and Pacific Islander children than in white children, which may reflect improvements in identification among these groups (1).

ETIOLOGY AND PATHOPHYSIOLOGY
- No single cause has been identified. Variety of genetic and environmental factors have been associated with ASD but none with absolute specificity for ASD development (1).
- Epidemiologic evidence does not support association between immunizations and ASD.

Genetics
- Genetic concordance: A 2009 Swedish population-based cohort study of 2 million subjects showed a cumulative risk of 59% for monozygotic twins.

- The American College of Medical Genetics and Genomics practice guidelines list the risk of siblings of children diagnosed with ASD without an identifiable cause to be 7% if the affected child is female, 4% if the affected child is male, and >30% if there are two or more affected children.

RISK FACTORS
- Male sex, advanced paternal age, family history, very low birth weight
- Perinatal insults including toxic exposures, teratogens, prenatal infections, use of selective serotonin reuptake inhibitors (SSRI) or valproate during pregnancy

GENERAL PREVENTION
- Screening for early intervention is associated with improved prognosis, yet median age of diagnosis in the United States is >4 years.
- Routine screening for ASD with a validated tool is recommended at 18- and 24-month well-child visits to assist with early detection.
- Screening is indicated after 24 months if parents or clinician have concerns about ASD as less severe presentations may pass earlier routine screening.
- Children with false positives for ASD frequently have some form of developmental disorder and benefit from early intervention.
- Screening difficult due to variability of signs and symptoms of ASD and lack of unanimous consensus of social developmental milestones, thus leading to delayed diagnosis

COMMONLY ASSOCIATED CONDITIONS
- Intellectual disability (seizure in severe cases)
- Attention deficit hyperactivity disorder (ADHD), anxiety, depression, or obsessive behavior
- Motor impairments including hypotonia, apraxia, toe walking, or gross motor delays
- Phenylketonuria (PKU), tuberous sclerosis, fragile X syndrome, Angelman syndrome, Rett syndrome, CHARGE syndrome, Joubert syndrome, Smith-Lemli-Opitz syndrome, Timothy syndrome, and fetal alcohol syndrome (rare)
- Sleep issues: insomnia, circadian rhythm sleep–wake disorder, sleep-related movement disorder
- Change in bowel habits, abdominal pain

DIAGNOSIS

Based on developmental history and behavior.

HISTORY
Listen to parents' concerns and test early for suspicion of a neurodevelopmental disorder.
- Impairment in social-emotional reciprocity: failure of normal back-and-forth conversations; reduced sharing of interests, emotions, or affect; failure to initiate or respond to social interaction
- Deficits in nonverbal communication: abnormal eye contact or body language; deficits in understanding and use of gestures; lack of facial expression and nonverbal communication
- Deficits in developing, maintaining, and understanding relationships:
  – Difficulties adjusting behavior to suit various social contexts; difficulties in sharing imaginative play or in making friends; absence of interest and developing peer relationships
- Repetitive and stereotyped behavior patterns
  – Stereotyped or repetitive motor movements, use of objects, or speech

  – Insistence on sameness, ritualized patterns of behavior with intolerance to change
  – Highly restricted, fixated interests that are abnormal in intensity or focus
  – Hyper- or hyporeactivity to sensory input or unusual interest in sensory aspects of the environment
- Prenatal, neonatal, and developmental history; seizure disorder
- Family history of autism, genetic disorders, learning disabilities, psychiatric illness, or neurologic disorders

PHYSICAL EXAM
- Measurement of growth parameters: height, weight, head circumference (Macrocephaly is present in 25% of ASD.)
- Vision, hearing, speech/language, and communication assessments
- Developmental and sensorimotor testing
- Complete neurologic exam
- Examination for dysmorphic features consistent with genetic disorders
- Wood lamp skin exam to rule out skin manifestations of neurocutaneous disorders
- Red flags: early symptoms of ASD
  – By 9 months—does not respond to name or show facial expressions of emotions
  – By 12 months—does not play interactive games
  – By 18 months—does not point at objects

DIFFERENTIAL DIAGNOSIS
- Behavioral disorder: anxiety, obsessive-compulsive, reactive attachment
- Developmental disorders: elective mutism, Rett syndrome, language disorder, hearing impairment, intellectual disability/global developmental delay, social communication disorder, ADHD
- Others: fetal alcohol disorder, tic disorder, fragile X syndrome, acquired epileptic aphasia

DIAGNOSTIC TESTS & INTERPRETATION
- The American Academy of Pediatrics (AAP) recommends developmental and behavioral screening for all children during well-child visits at 9, 18, and 30 months.
- Recommendation for ASD screening at 18 and 24 months
- The Modified Checklist for Autism in Toddlers (M-CHAT): commonly used test to screen for ASD in children aged 12 to 30 months; additional information needed for children aged <12 months (M-CHAT) (2)[B].
- The Modified Checklist for Autism in Toddlers Revised with Follow-up (M-CHAT-R/F): improved PPV, lower false-positive rate in children aged 16 to 30 months, especially those with cultural barriers (M-CHAT-R/F) (2)[B]; children with M-CHAT-R/F total score >2 are considered at risk and require follow-up.
- Infant-Toddler Checklist (parent questionnaire): identifies language delay in low-risk patients between 6 and 24 months; useful in identifying infant siblings of children with ASD at increased risk for ASD (2)[B]
- Screening Tool for Autism in Toddlers & Young Children (STAT) shows promising evidence as level 2 screening to detect 2-year-olds with autism with other developmental disorders (2)[B].
- Autism Diagnostic Interview-Revised (ADI-R) is a semi-structured interview with the parent(s), whereas the Autism Diagnostic Observation Schedule, 2nd Edition (ADOS-2) is a semi-structured direct observation of a child's behavior with sensitivity of 80% and 91%, respectively, and specificity of 72% and 76%, respectively (1).

- ASD screening tools for older children: Autism Spectrum Quotient-Child and Childhood Autism Spectrum Test (ages 4 to 11 years), Autism Spectrum Screening Questionnaire (ages 6 to 17 years), the Developmental Behaviour Checklist (ages 4 to 18 years with intellectual disabilities), and Asperger Syndrome Diagnostic Scale (higher-functioning children aged 5 to 18 years)

Initial Tests (lab, imaging)
- Chromosomal microarray (CMA), DNA analysis (fragile X), and whole exome sequencing
- Complete blood count, thyroid-stimulating hormone, creatine kinase, and PKU screening; consider lead testing.
- Metabolic testing if signs of lethargy, limited endurance, hypotonia, recurrent vomiting and dehydration, developmental regression, or specific food intolerance
- TORCH (toxoplasmosis, others [syphilis, varicella-zoster, parvovirus B19], rubella, cytomegalovirus, HIV, and herpes) infection workup if microcephaly present
- MRI if focal neurologic symptoms

Follow-Up Tests & Special Considerations
- Children with ASD have the same general health care needs as other children and should receive the same preventative care.
- Follow-up appointments and testing recommended as indicated for comorbidities.
- Consider additional hearing tests with audiometry and brainstem auditory evoked response (BAER) or consultation to audiology.
- Speech and language evaluation
- Evaluation by multidisciplinary team: psychiatrist, genetic counselor, neurologist, psychologist, other autism specialists
- Monitoring of intellectual level

Diagnostic Procedures/Other
Electroencephalogram, if displaying signs or symptoms suggestive of epilepsy or specific developmental disorders associated with abnormal encephalographic findings (1)

 ## TREATMENT

The goal of therapy is to improve function and well-being (1).

GENERAL MEASURES
Two categories of evidence-based interventions exist: comprehensive treatment model (CTM) and focused interventions (1),(2).

- CTMs are replicable, intense, and specifically designed programs that address a broad range of symptoms and specific skill(s) or symptom(s). Services are provided through individual instruction or class settings, include parents, and may involve technology-assisted interventions. Some examples of CTMs include early intensive behavioral intervention with applied behavior analysis, focused on learning and reinforcing acceptable behaviors: Treatment and Education of Autistic and Related Communication-Handicapped Children (TEACCH) and the Early Start Denver Model (ESDM).
  - Treatment addresses social communication, language, play skills, and maladaptive behavior to improve cognitive, language, and adaptive skills.

- Focused intervention practices: designed to address a single or limited range of skills, such as increasing social communication or learning a specific task and generally arranged to be delivered over a short period of time
  - Cognitive-behavioral therapy: shown to reduce anxiety in older children with ASD with average to above-average IQ

MEDICATION
First Line
- FDA-approved psychotropic medications for irritability, aggression, and emotional dysregulation in individuals with ASD:
  - Risperidone: age >5 years—0.25 mg/day in <20 kg; 0.5 mg/day in >20 kg with effective dose range of 0.5 to 3.0 mg/day PO divided doses
  - Aripiprazole: ages 6 to 17 years; PO; initial dose of 2 mg daily for 2 days, increase up to 5 mg daily/week; max of 15 mg/day
- Stimulants (such as methylphenidate, atomoxetine, and guanfacine extended-release): efficacious in treating concomitant symptoms of ADHD; magnitude of response is less than in typically developing children, and adverse effects are frequent.
- SSRIs: limited evidence for ASD; shown to help in reducing ritualistic behavior, improve mood and language skills; initial choice for anxiety and depressive mood
- Melatonin used for patients with concomitant sleep disorders; shown mixed efficacy

ISSUES FOR REFERRAL
Refer early for evaluation of behavior and language, genetic counseling, and audiology; refer to geneticist if ASD associated with genetic syndrome based on family history and subsequent medical surveillance. Consider referrals to psychiatry, ophthalmology, otolaryngology, neurology, and nutrition. Refer family members to support groups.

COMPLEMENTARY & ALTERNATIVE MEDICINE
- Medications such as secretin, intravenous immunoglobulin, and vitamins and minerals: have no benefit; may carry risks
- Music, massage, therapeutic horseback riding, and other pet therapies merit further review.

 ## ONGOING CARE

Planning for transition to adulthood should begin around 12 to 14 years of age, with adaptation for developmental abilities.

FOLLOW-UP RECOMMENDATIONS
Patient Monitoring
- Constant monitoring by caregivers; evaluation every 6 to 12 months by physician for symptom and medical management
- Intellectual and language testing every 2 years in childhood
- Siblings of children with ASD should be monitored for symptoms of ASD.

DIET
Insufficient evidence for recommendations of any certain dietary modifications for ASD; gluten- and casein-free diets without benefit across several randomized clinical trials

PROGNOSIS
- Prognosis influenced by IQ, early intervention, strength of early language skills, and psychiatric comorbidities
- General expected course is for a lifelong need for supervised structured care; some patients will develop gainful employment, independent living, and social relationships.

COMPLICATIONS
Increased risk for physical and sexual abuse; with pica, increased risk of lead poisoning; gastrointestinal issues

REFERENCES
1. Hirota T, King BH. Autism spectrum disorder: a review. *JAMA*. 2023;329(2):157–168.
2. Hyman SL, Levy SE, Myers SM, et al. Identification, evaluation, and management of children with autism spectrum disorder. *Pediatrics*. 2020;145(1):e20193447.

ADDITIONAL READING
Sanchack KE, Thomas CA. Autism spectrum disorder: primary care principles. *Am Fam Physician*. 2016;94(12):972–979.

 SEE ALSO

Algorithm: Intellectual Disability

CODES

ICD10
- F84.5 Asperger's syndrome
- F84 Pervasive developmental disorders
- F84.2 Rett's syndrome

CLINICAL PEARLS
AAP ALARM mnemonic:
- **A**SD is prevalent (screen all children between 18 and 24 months).
- **L**isten to parents when they feel something is wrong.
- **A**ct early: Screen children with delayed language and social developmental milestones.
- **R**efer to multidisciplinary teams.
- **M**onitor support for patient and families.

BABESIOSIS

Frederick W. Nielson, MD

 BASICS

DESCRIPTION
- Rare tick-borne hemolytic disease caused by intraerythrocytic protozoan parasites of the genus *Babesia*
- Infrequently reported outside the United States
  - Internationally, sporadic cases have been reported from France, Italy, the United Kingdom, Ireland, the former Soviet Union, and Mexico. China, Italy, and Turkey have also reported cases.
  - In the United States, infections have been reported in many states. Transmission has primarily occurred in the Northeast and upper Midwest, especially in parts of New England, New York, Pennsylvania, New Jersey, Wisconsin, and Minnesota. Asymptomatic infection is common in these areas.
- Incubation period varies from 5 to 33 days:
  - Most patients do not recall specific tick exposure.
  - After transfusion of infected blood, the incubation period can be up to 9 weeks.
- System(s) affected: cardiovascular, gastrointestinal, hemic/lymphatic/immunologic, musculoskeletal, nervous, pulmonary, renal/urologic

Pediatric Considerations
Transplacental and perinatal transmission is rare. Atovaquone has been used safely in children who weigh >5 kg.

Pregnancy/Lactation Considerations
Safety data on use of atovaquone in pregnant women are limited. However, there are limited safety data available to suggest administration of quinine plus clindamycin during pregnancy may be safe. For this reason, this drug combination rather than atovaquone plus azithromycin is generally recommended for treatment of symptomatic babesiosis during pregnancy.

Geriatric Considerations
Morbidity and mortality are higher in elderly populations, especially with those who have comorbidities.

EPIDEMIOLOGY
- Babesiosis affects patients of all ages. Most patients present in their 40s or 50s.
- Coinfection with other tick-borne illness (anaplasmosis, ehrlichiosis, Lyme disease) is common.

Incidence
- Cases reported by the CDC hover around 2,000 per year (data last reported in 2020): https://www.cdc.gov/parasites/babesiosis/data-statistics/index.html.
- In patients at high risk for tick-borne diseases, seroconversion data show antibodies to *Babesia microti* in 7 of 671 individuals (1%).

Prevalence
Prevalence is difficult to estimate due to lack of surveillance and asymptomatic infections.

ETIOLOGY AND PATHOPHYSIOLOGY
- *B. microti* (in the United States) and *Babesia divergens* and *Babesia bovis* (in Europe) cause most human infections. *B. divergens* and a new strain *Babesia duncani* appear to be more virulent. Other species identified in case reports. All share morphologic, antigenic, and genetic characteristics.
- Ixodid (hard-bodied) ticks, particularly *Ixodes dammini* (*Ixodes scapularis*: deer tick) and *Ixodes ricinus*, are the primary vectors.
- The white-footed deer mouse is the primary reservoir.
- Infection is passed to humans through the saliva of a nymphal-stage tick during a blood meal. Sporozoites introduced at the time of the bite enter red blood cells and form merozoites through binary fission (classic morphology on blood smear). Humans are a dead-end host for *B. microti*.

RISK FACTORS
Those residing in endemic areas are at elevated risk for contracting babesiosis. Complications from the disease are highest in those with asplenia, who are immunocompromised or elderly.

GENERAL PREVENTION
- Avoid endemic regions during the peak transmission months of May to September.
- Appropriate insect repellent is advised during outdoor activities, especially in wooded or grassy areas.
  - 10–35% N,N-diethyl-meta-toluamide (DEET) provides adequate skin protection.
  - Acaricides, such as permethrin, provide impregnated clothing with even further protection.
- Daily skin checks to ensure early removal of ticks is essential.

COMMONLY ASSOCIATED CONDITIONS
- Coinfection with *Borrelia burgdorferi* and *B. microti* in endemic areas has been reported and rates may be as high as ~27%.
- Coinfection with *Ehrlichia* is not uncommon.

DIAGNOSIS

HISTORY
- Travel history to endemic regions as well as exposure history are helpful.
- The tick must remain attached for at least 24 hours before the transmission of *B. microti* occurs.
- Severe disease is more common in patients with comorbidities (immunosuppression, chronic disease), so maintaining a proper index of suspicion after exposure history may prompt workup and treatment.
- The disease presentation is similar to malaria (1): fever (68–89%), fatigue (78–79%), chills (39–68%), sweats (41–56%), headache (32–75%), myalgia (32–37%), anorexia (24–25%), cough (17–23%), arthralgias (17–32%), and nausea (9–22%). Other symptoms include abdominal pain, vomiting, diarrhea, and emotional lability.

PHYSICAL EXAM
- High fever (up to 40°C [104°F])
- Hemodynamic instability (shock in extremely ill)
- Hepatomegaly and splenomegaly (mild if noted)
- Rash (Uncommon; if rash is present, consider concurrent Lyme disease.)
- CNS involvement includes headache, photophobia, neck and back stiffness, altered sensorium, and emotional lability.
- Jaundice and dark urine may develop later in course of illness.

DIFFERENTIAL DIAGNOSIS
- Bacterial sepsis
- Hepatitis
- Lyme disease; ehrlichiosis; Rocky Mountain spotted fever
- Leishmaniasis
- Malaria
- HIV; EBV
- HELLP syndrome (in pregnancy)

DIAGNOSTIC TESTS & INTERPRETATION
Initial Tests (lab, imaging)
- Diagnosis requires a high index of clinical suspicion. Nonspecific laboratory clues include evidence of mild to severe hemolytic anemia, normal to slightly depressed leukocyte count, elevated LDH or transaminase level, elevated BUN and creatinine, proteinuria and hemoglobinuria.
- Definitive diagnosis is made by blood smear.
  - Wright- or Giemsa-stained peripheral blood smear demonstrates intraerythrocytic parasites (2)[B].
  - Dividing "cross-like" tetrads of merozoites (Maltese cross) are pathognomonic (2).
  - Serial blood smears may be required (low parasite load early in the illness) (2).
  - Can be confused with *Plasmodium falciparum* on peripheral smear
- If blood smears are negative but suspicion remains, IgM serologies through indirect immunofluorescent antibody testing (IFAT) for *B. microti* antigen:
  - Positive titer results vary by lab. Titers of >1:64 or a 4-fold increase from baseline are consistent with *B. microti* infection. Titers may be >1:1,024 in acute infection (2)[B]. Titers often elevated 8 to 12 months and can persist for years.
  - In New England, seroprevalence is 0.5–16%.
- Detection of *B. microti* by polymerase chain reaction (PCR) is more sensitive and equally specific in acute cases. PCR can also be used to monitor disease progression (2)[B]. Newer real-time PCR tests have a sensitivity and specificity approaching 100%.
- If lab tests are inconclusive and infection is strongly suspected, inoculation of laboratory animals with patient blood can reveal *B. microti* organisms in the blood of the animal within 2 to 4 weeks (2).

Follow-Up Tests & Special Considerations
Monitoring intraerythrocytic parasitemia helps guide treatment.

TREATMENT

GENERAL MEASURES
- In areas endemic for Lyme disease and ehrlichiosis, doxycycline 100 mg BID PO empirically treats coinfection until serologic testing is complete.
- Drug resistance has emerged in severely immunocompromised patients (2).
- Consider treating asymptomatic patients if parasitemia persists for >3 months; otherwise, do not treat in absence of symptoms.

MEDICATION
First Line
- Mild to moderate infection with *B. microti*:
  - 7 to 10 days of atovaquone 750 mg PO (with a fatty meal) BID *plus*
  - Azithromycin 500 mg/day PO BID on day 1, followed by 250 mg/day.
- Pediatrics: atovaquone 20 mg/kg (max of 750 mg) BID and azithromycin 10 mg/kg (max of 500 mg) on day 1 and then 5 mg/kg (max of 250 mg) (3)[C]
- For severe *B. microti* infection, the same dosing is recommended but azithromycin can be given IV.
- Alternative treatment option includes oral quinine 650 mg TID or QID plus IV clindamycin 300 to 600 mg QID for 7 to 10 days.
  - Pediatrics: clindamycin 7 to 10 mg/kg (max of 600 mg) TID or QID and quinine 8 mg/kg (max of 650 mg) TID
- Persistent or relapsing babesiosis: Treat for 6 weeks, including 2 weeks after Babesia is no longer detected on blood smear.

Second Line
- Combination of quinine sulfate 650 mg PO TID and clindamycin 600 mg PO TID or 1.2 g parenterally BID for 7 to 10 days is the most commonly used treatment; pediatric: quinine 8 mg/kg (max of 650 mg) q6–8h for 7 to 10 days and clindamycin 7 to 10 mg/kg (max of 600 mg) PO q6–8h for 7 to 10 days; some experts prefer this regimen for severe infections (3)[C].
- Other drugs including tetracycline, primaquine, sulfadiazine (Microsulfon), and sulfadoxine/pyrimethamine (Fansidar) have been evaluated. Results vary. Pentamidine (Pentam) is moderately effective in diminishing symptoms and decreasing parasitemia.

ALERT
Clindamycin can lead to *Clostridium difficile*–associated diarrhea.

ISSUES FOR REFERRAL
Consultation with hematology and infectious disease for exchange transfusion may be considered in severe disease (blood parasitemia >10%, massive hemolysis, and asplenia) (2)[C].

ADMISSION, INPATIENT, AND NURSING CONSIDERATIONS
Targeted organ damage due to disease by prompt inpatient management; select patients with severe babesiosis and organ compromise may be considered for exchange transfusion.

ONGOING CARE

FOLLOW-UP RECOMMENDATIONS
- If left untreated, silent babesiosis may persist for months or years (2).
- Alkaline phosphatase levels >125 U/L, WBC counts >5 × 10^9/L, history of cardiac abnormality, history of splenectomy, presence of heart murmur, and parasitemia of ≥4% are associated with disease severity.

Patient Monitoring
The need for monitoring depends on disease severity. In cases of severe infection, hematocrit and parasitemia levels can be followed until clinical improvement is evident and parasitemia is <5%. For mild to moderate disease, anticipate clinical improvement within 48 hours and complete resolution within 3 months.

COMPLICATIONS
- Many remain asymptomatic.
- Complications in hospitalized patients: CHF (12%), DIC (18%), ARDS (21%), renal failure (6%), coma/lethargy (9%), death (9%)
- Other reported complications include neutropenia and myocardial infarction.
- In asplenic patients, warm autoimmune hemolytic anemia has been reported.

REFERENCES
1. Waked R, Krause PJ. Human babesiosis. *Infect Dis Clin North Am*. 2022;36(3):655–670.
2. Vannier E, Krause PJ. Human babesiosis. *N Engl J Med*. 2012;366(25):2397–2407.
3. Krause PJ, Auwaerter PG, Bannuru RR, et al. Clinical practice guidelines by the Infectious Diseases Society of America (IDSA): 2020 guideline on the diagnosis and management of babesiosis. *Clin Infect Dis*. 2021;72(2):e49–e64.

ADDITIONAL READING
Centers for Disease Control and Prevention. Resources for health professionals. https://www.cdc.gov/parasites/babesiosis/health_professionals/index.html. Accessed October 13, 2023.

CODES
ICD10
B60.0 Babesiosis

CLINICAL PEARLS
- Ticks must remain in place for 24 hours to transmit infection. Encourage daily "tick checks" if people are exposed in high-risk areas.
- Most patients do not recall tick exposure, and incubation can last up to a month.
- If left untreated, silent babesial infection may persist for months or years.
- First-line treatment for mild or moderate disease is atovaquone plus azithromycin.
- Patients with mild-to-moderate disease should show clinical improvement within 48 hours after starting therapy. Symptoms should fully resolve in 3 months.
- Coinfection with *B. burgdorferi* and *Ehrlichia* species is common in endemic areas. In areas endemic for Lyme disease and ehrlichiosis, consider adding doxycycline until serologic testing is completed.

BACK PAIN, LOW

Ashley Koontz Sturts, DO • Makayla Lagerman, MD • Makenna Brezitski, MD, Med

BASICS

DESCRIPTION

- Low back pain (LBP) is a common chief complaint presenting to primary care and acute care settings.
  - 2.5 million were diagnosed with LBP in the United States between 2008 and 2015 (1).
  - Annual expenditure in the United States on LBP care >$100 billion dollars (1)
- Defined as a pain between the costal margins and the inferior gluteal folds (2)
- Suggested classification is by duration (2):
  - Acute: Most cases resolve in 4 to 6 weeks.
  - Recurrent: repetitive occurrence of symptoms in a year
  - Chronic: at least 3 months in duration
- LBP has significant implications on work-life balance.
  - LBP is the leading cause of loss of productivity worldwide (1).
  - LBP is the leading cause of years lived with disability across 126 countries (1).
- It is necessary to rule out "red" flag symptoms indicating the need for immediate intervention.
- System(s) affected: musculoskeletal, neurologic
- Synonym(s): lumbago, lumbar sprain/strain, low back syndrome

EPIDEMIOLOGY

Incidence
Annually, 7% in the United States (1)

Prevalence
Prevalence increases with age (2):
- 1–6% in children 7 to 10 years old
- 18% in adolescents
- 28–42% in ages 40 to 69 years (peak prevalence by age)

ETIOLOGY AND PATHOPHYSIOLOGY
Recent subcategorization by primary type of pain (1):
- Mechanical, including facet arthropathy, myofascial pain, sacroiliac joint dysfunction
- Inflammatory, including spondyloarthropathies
- Neuropathic/radicular (16–55% of chronic LBP)—classical symptoms radiating down legs in dermatomes (1)
  - Herniated disc is a common cause.
  - Spinal stenosis results from age-related degeneration.
  - Less common causes to consider: metastatic disease, herpes zoster
- Nociplastic—amplified pain from central nervous system (1)

RISK FACTORS
- Age
- High-risk activity (lifting, sudden twisting, bending)
- Obesity
- Sedentary lifestyle
- Physically strenuous work
- Psychosocial factors—anxiety, depression, stress
- Poor flexibility
- Smoking

GENERAL PREVENTION
There is no strong existing evidence for prevention; however, routine physical activity has been shown to be beneficial.

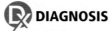

DIAGNOSIS

HISTORY
- Onset of pain (sudden or gradual)
- Inciting event, injury, or trauma
- Frequency of pain (episodic or constant with or without fluctuation)
- Characterization and location of pain:
  - Facet pain commonly radiates to sacroiliac joint/PSIS region.
  - Sacroiliac pain often refers to the thigh and can radiate below the knee.
  - Irritation, impingement, or compression of lumbar nerve roots often results in leg pain rather than back pain.
  - Pain from the L1–L3 nerve roots radiates to the hip and/or thigh; pain from the L4–S1 nerve roots radiates below the knee.
- Red flags (1)
  - Patient history: cancer, trauma, advanced age, weight loss, immunodeficiency, osteoporosis
  - Medications: IV drug use, corticosteroid use
  - Symptoms: fever, pain at night/at rest, saddle anesthesia, bowel/bladder dysfunction, gait abnormality, night sweats

Pediatric Considerations
A patient <4 years old with LBP should raise suspicion of abuse or a nonmechanical cause; consider malignancy, inflammatory, and infectious processes.

PHYSICAL EXAM
- Follow the "IPASS" system: inspection, palpation, active/passive range of motion, strength, special tests
  - Observe posture, gait, positioning, and muscle atrophy.
  - Evaluate for point tenderness at midline spinous processes and paraspinal muscle.
  - Lumbar spine range of motion evaluation— flexion, extension, rotation, sidebending
- Completely evaluate reflexes, strength, pulses, and sensation.
  - Slump test:
    - Have patient sit on table and slump shoulders forward.
    - Then have patient touch chin to chest and attempt to have them extend one leg at a time.
    - Symptom reproduction radiating down dermatomal distribution of lower extremities is consistent with lumbar radiculopathy, such as from a disk herniation.
  - Straight leg test:
    - With the patient supine, passively raise the patient's leg straight to at least 60 degrees keeping the knee straight and ankle dorsiflexed.
    - Pain, especially radiating down the leg, may also imply lumbar radiculopathy, such as from a disk herniation.
  - Stork test:
    - Have patient stand on one leg with opposite hip held in flexion.
    - Extend back.
    - Pain in lumbosacral area is a positive test— consider spondylolisthesis versus facet OA.
  - Evaluate for saddle anesthesia; anal wink reflex if concern for cauda equina syndrome exists
- Consider special testing of the hips for differentiation from sacroiliac-related back pain (e.g., FABER, FADIR).
- Evaluate mental and emotional well-being

DIFFERENTIAL DIAGNOSIS
- Intrinsic spine: fracture, disc herniation, stenosis, muscle strain, spondylolysis/spondylolisthesis/spondylosis (3)
- Systemic: infectious, inflammatory, malignancy, connective tissue disorder (3)
- Referred: abdominal aortic aneurysm, herpes zoster, other pelvic and retroperitoneal diagnoses (3)

DIAGNOSTIC TESTS & INTERPRETATION
Initial Tests (lab, imaging)
- Initial diagnosis is typically made clinically via history and physical exam.
- Imaging is NOT recommended in initial presentation, unless red flag symptoms are present.

Follow-Up Tests & Special Considerations
- MRI is recommended for chronic LBP or if surgical/procedural intervention is considered (2).
- X-ray can be considered if there is a concern for fracture, spondylolysis, or spondylolisthesis
- Blood work can be considered if inflammatory, infectious, or rheumatologic conditions are a concern.

Diagnostic Procedures/Other
Emergent neurosurgical consult for acute neurologic deficits or suspected cauda equina syndrome

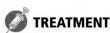 TREATMENT

GENERAL MEASURES
- Multidisciplinary biopsychosocial approach is encouraged.
- First-line management: activity modification, early return to routine duties, physical therapy

MEDICATION
First Line
NSAIDs may be considered if contraindications to therapy do not exist (2).

Second Line
- Opioids—rarely needed; use very low dose and shortest possible duration; educate on misuse.
- TCAs/SSRIs/SNRIs—assist with neuropathic symptoms and associated mental health concerns
- Gabapentinoids—assist with chronic neuropathic symptoms

ISSUES FOR REFERRAL
- If not responding to initial measures, can consider (2):
  – Osteopathic manipulative therapy, massage therapy, chiropractics
  – Psychological evaluation and treatment
  – TENS unit
- Referral to PM&R for epidural corticosteroid injection or radiofrequency denervation if radicular symptoms are present (2)
- Failure of conservative measures or presentation of alarm symptoms warrants referral to neurosurgery or orthopedics.

ADDITIONAL THERAPIES
There is no strong evidence to support bracing, therapeutic ultrasound, traction, or insoles (2).

COMPLEMENTARY & ALTERNATIVE MEDICINE
- Osteopathic manipulation has been found to be effective for nonspecific LBP and for chronic back pain.
- There is no strong evidence to support the use of acupuncture, dry needling, or meditation (2).

 ONGOING CARE

FOLLOW-UP RECOMMENDATIONS
- Initial follow up is recommended in 2 to 4 weeks for acute flare.
- Longer interval follow up of 6 to 12 weeks may be beneficial for chronic LBP.

REFERENCES
1. Knezevic NN, Candido KD, Vlaeyen JWS, et al. Low back pain. *Lancet*. 2021;398(10294):78–92.
2. Bailly F, Trouvin AP, Bercier S, et al. Clinical guidelines and care pathway for management of low back pain with or without radicular pain. *Joint Bone Spine*. 2021;88(6):105227.
3. Casazza BA. Diagnosis and treatment of acute low back pain. *Am Fam Physician*. 2012;85(4):343–350.

ADDITIONAL READING
- Almeida MO, Garcia AN, Menezes Costa LC, et al. The McKenzie method for (sub)acute non-specific low back pain. *Cochrane Database Syst Rev*. 2023;4(4):CD009711.
- Andronis L, Kinghorn P, Qiao S, et al. Cost-effectiveness of non-invasive and non-pharmacological interventions for low back pain: a systematic literature review. *Appl Health Econ Health Policy*. 2017;15(2):173–201.
- Phillips SF, Butts JF, Silvis M. Low back pain in youth: recognizing red flags. *J Fam Pract*. 2020;69(8):E1–E8.

 SEE ALSO

Algorithm: Low Back Pain, Acute

 CODES

ICD10
- M54.5 Low back pain
- G89.29 Other chronic pain
- M53.3 Sacrococcygeal disorders, not elsewhere classified

CLINICAL PEARLS
- LBP is a common cause for health care expenditure, disability, and loss of productivity worldwide.
- If no alarm symptoms are present, imaging is not beneficial in initial workup.
- Conservative management can be effective with physical therapy, activity modification, and NSAIDs.
- Referral for surgical evaluation is necessary if alarm symptoms develop.

BACTERIURIA, ASYMPTOMATIC

Johnny J. Yang, MD, MS • Bindusri Paruchuri, MD

BASICS

DESCRIPTION

Asymptomatic bacteriuria (ASB) is specific bacterial growth of $\geq 10^5$ CFU/mL in one and two consecutive midstream urine samples for men and women, respectively >18 years. This definition applies to individuals with no clinical symptoms.

EPIDEMIOLOGY

Incidence
- Premenopausal females: 1–6%
- Pregnancy: 2–10%
- Older females and males: 4–19%
  - ~22% of women >90 years old (1)
- Institutionalized older population: 15–50%

Prevalence
- Variable; increases with age, female gender, sexual activity, neurogenic bladder, and presence of genito-urinary (GU) abnormalities
- Pregnancy: 2–10%
- Short- and long-term indwelling catheter 9–23% and 100%, respectively
- Long-term care residents in women 25–50% and men 15–40%

ETIOLOGY AND PATHOPHYSIOLOGY
- Pathophysiology: Most cases are secondary to the ascension of bacteria from the urethra to bladder.
- Microbiology is similar to that of other urinary tract infections (UTI), with bacteria originating from the periurethral area, vagina, or gut.
- Organisms are less virulent in ASB than those causing UTI.
- The most common organism is *Escherichia coli*. Other common organisms are *Klebsiella pneumoniae*, *Enterobacter*, *Proteus mirabilis*, *Staphylococcus aureus*, group B *Streptococcus* (GBS), and *Enterococcus*.

Genetics
Genetic variations that reduce toll-like receptor-4 (*TLR4*) function have been associated with ASB by lowering innate immune response and delaying bacterial clearance.

RISK FACTORS
- Pregnancy
- Older age
- Female gender
- Sexual activity, use of diaphragm with spermicide
- GU abnormalities: neurogenic bladder, urinary retention, urinary catheter use (indwelling, intermittent, or condom catheter), or pathologic urinary fistulas

- Institutionalized elderly population
- Diabetes mellitus
- Immunocompromised status
- Spinal cord injuries or functional impairment
- Hemodialysis

COMMONLY ASSOCIATED CONDITIONS
Depends on the risk factors

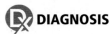

DIAGNOSIS

HISTORY
- Asymptomatic
- Lack of symptoms attributable to UTI such as fever, acute dysuria (<1 week), new or worsening urinary urgency/frequency/incontinence, or acute gross hematuria

PHYSICAL EXAM
- Afebrile
- No suprapubic and costovertebral angle tenderness

DIFFERENTIAL DIAGNOSIS
- UTI
- Uncomplicated cystitis
- Contaminated urine specimen

DIAGNOSTIC TESTS & INTERPRETATION

Initial Tests (lab, imaging)
- Urinalysis (UA):
  - The presence of pyuria, leukocyte esterase, and nitrite in ASB is common.
- Urine culture (clean catch)
- Screening urine culture in asymptomatic patients is indicated in only two conditions:
  - Pregnancy: screening between 12 and 16 weeks' gestation or at first prenatal visit if later
  - Prior to transurethral resection of prostate (TURP) or any urologic interventions when mucosal bleeding is anticipated
- Screening for ASB in men and nonpregnant women is not recommended.

Follow-Up Tests & Special Considerations
- Noncontaminated urine specimen should be used for urine culture.
- In pregnancy, periodic screening urine culture should be done after ASB treatment but not required in GBS bacteriuria (2).

Test Interpretation
- Patient with significant bacteriuria with or without pyuria and without symptoms referable to UTI should be diagnosed as ASB per Infectious Diseases Society of America.
  - Significant bacteriuria is defined based on type of urine specimen, sex, and the amount of bacteria.
  - By midstream, clean catch specimen
    - Male: >100,000 CFU/mL of single bacteria species
    - Female: the same criteria as male but needs two positive consecutive specimens
      - In pregnancy, if >10,000 CFU/mL of GBS, treatment is indicated (Grade B)
    - By catheterized specimen male and female: >100 CFU/mL of one bacterial species; required one-time collection only
- The presence of pyuria or leukocyte esterase is common but not a marker of infection.
- Positive nitrite is an indicator of the presence of bacteriuria but cannot differentiate UTI from ASB or poor collection technique.

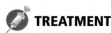

TREATMENT

GENERAL MEASURES

ALERT
- Antibiotic treatment of ASB is indicated in only two conditions:
  - Pregnancy
    - Rationale: Treatment prevents up to 70% of pregnant women from developing acute pyelonephritis, which reduces the risk of low birth weight and preterm delivery that are perinatal complications.
  - Prior to TURP
    - Rationale: Antibiotic treatment can effectively prevent postprocedure bacteremia and sepsis.
- Treatment of ASB in other conditions (nonpregnant women, diabetic women, indwelling catheter, patients with spinal cord injury, or the elderly living in the community) does not provide any known clinical benefit, does not reduce the risk of symptomatic infection, nor improve morbidity or mortality. It increases health care cost, adverse drug side effects, development of resistant organisms, and reinfection rate.
- Recommendation against screening all nonrenal solid organ transplant or after 1 month following renal transplant; inadequate evidence to guide management in nonurologic procedure (3)[A]

MEDICATION

- Pregnancy
  - Intrapartum antibiotic prophylaxis with IV penicillin or clindamycin (penicillin allergy) is recommended for women with GBS bacteriuria occurring at any stage of pregnancy and of any colony count to prevent GBS disease in the newborn.
  - No consensus on choice of antibiotics and duration of treatment in pregnancy; however, the cure rate is higher for the 4- to 7-day treatment than 1-day treatment.
  - Choice of antibiotics should be guided by bacterial pathogen, local resistance rate, adverse effects, and comorbidities of patients.
  - Common oral antibiotics (FDA pregnancy category B) that have been used
    - Nitrofurantoin 100 mg BID for 5 days (low level of resistance may cause hemolysis in glucose-6-phosphate dehydrogenase deficiency)
    - Amoxicillin/clavulanate 500/125 mg BID for 5 to 7 days
    - Cefuroxime 250 mg BID for 5 days
    - Cephalexin 500 mg BID for 5 days
    - Fosfomycin 3 g for 1 single dose (not effective when glomerular filtration rate is <30 mL/min, may be used in highly resistant bacteria such as methicillin-resistant *S. aureus* [MRSA], vancomycin-resistant enterococci [VRE], and extended-spectrum β-lactamase [ESBL]-producing organism and/or bacteria).
  - Avoid trimethoprim in 1st trimester and near term. Avoid sulfa after 32 weeks' gestation. This is due to a theoretical risk of kernicterus. However, this may be used if other options are unavailable or contraindicated.
  - Contraindicated: fluoroquinolones (FDA pregnancy category C), tetracyclines (FDA pregnancy category D)
- Prior to invasive urologic interventions
  - Initiate antibiotic the night before or immediately before the procedure.
  - Antibiotic should be continued until the indwelling catheter is removed postprocedure.

ONGOING CARE

FOLLOW-UP RECOMMENDATIONS

No consensus on rescreening frequency of ASB in pregnancy. Per American College of Gynecology (ACOG) guidelines, follow-up urine culture, after treatment, is recommended. Although more data is needed to determine the effectiveness of this recommendation.

Patient Monitoring

Development of any signs/symptoms of UTI should warrant antibiotic treatment.

DIET

Daily cranberry juice or cranberry capsules twice daily may reduce the frequency of ASB during pregnancy, but it has not been confirmed in large study.

PATIENT EDUCATION

Patient should seek medical attention when UTI symptoms develop.

COMPLICATIONS

- Late pregnancy pyelonephritis occurs in 20–35% of women with untreated bacteriuria (20- to 30-fold higher than women with negative initial screening urine cultures or in whom bacteriuria was treated). Pyelonephritis is associated with premature delivery and worse fetal outcomes (infant with GBS infections, low-birth-weight infant). Antimicrobial treatment will decrease the risk of subsequent pyelonephritis from 20–35% to 1–4% and the risk of having a low-birth-weight baby from 15% to 5%.
- If bacteriuria remains untreated in patients who undergo traumatic urologic procedures, up to 60% develop bacteremia after the procedure, and 5–10% progress to severe sepsis/septic shock.

REFERENCES

1. Owens DK, Davidson KW, Krist AH, et al; for US Preventive Services Task Force. Screening for asymptomatic bacteriuria in adults: US Preventive Services Task Force recommendation statement. *JAMA*. 2019;322(12):1188–1194.
2. Zolotor AJ, Carlough MC. Update on prenatal care. *Am Fam Physician*. 2014;89(3):199–208.
3. Nicolle LE, Gupta K, Bradley SF, et al. Clinical practice guideline for the management of asymptomatic bacteriuria: 2019 update by the Infectious Diseases Society of America. *Clin Infect Dis*. 2019;68(10):e83–e110.

CODES

ICD10

- N39.0 Urinary tract infection, site not specified
- B96.20 Unsp Escherichia coli as the cause of diseases classd elswhr
- B96.1 Klebsiella pneumoniae as the cause of diseases classd elswhr

CLINICAL PEARLS

- ASB is a common and benign disorder for which treatment is not indicated in most patients.
- The presence of pyuria, leukocyte esterase, and nitrite is common in ASB and not an indication for antimicrobial treatment.
- Antibiotic treatment is indicated for ASB in pregnancy, patients who require TURP, or any urologic interventions with mucosal bleeding.
- Treatment of ASB in other conditions does not decrease the frequency of UTI or improve outcome.
- Overtreatment of ASB may result in negative consequences such as antimicrobial resistance, adverse drug reaction, and unnecessary cost.

BALANITIS, PHIMOSIS, AND PARAPHIMOSIS
Margaret Yip, DO

 BASICS

DESCRIPTION
- Balanitis:
  - Balanitis is an inflammation of the glans penis.
  - Posthitis is an inflammation of the foreskin or prepuce.
  - Balanoposthitis is inflammation of both the glans penis and the foreskin.
  - Balanitis xerotica obliterans (BXO) is lichen sclerosus of the glans penis (uncommon).
- Phimosis and paraphimosis:
  - Phimosis: when the foreskin is too tight to retract back to expose glans penis; can be physiologic (normal) or pathologic
  - Paraphimosis: a urological emergency where the foreskin is retracted over the glans penis and cannot return to normal position which can lead to strangulation, vascular compromise, and even necrosis
- System(s) affected: renal/urologic; reproductive; skin/exocrine

ALERT
- Recurrent infections and irritations (for example condom catheter) can lead to pathologic phimosis.
- Inappropriate forced reduction of a physiologic foreskin can lead to chronic scarring and pathologic phimosis.
- Paraphimosis is a pediatric emergency; if left untreated, can lead to necrosis and autoamputation

EPIDEMIOLOGY
- Balanitis: predominant age: adult; predominant gender: male only
- Phimosis/paraphimosis: predominant age: infancy and adolescence; unusual in adults; risk returns in geriatrics; predominant sex: male only

Incidence
Balanitis: will affect 3–11% of males

Prevalence
Phimosis: in the United States: 8% of boys aged 6 years and 1% of men >16 years of age

ETIOLOGY AND PATHOPHYSIOLOGY
- Balanitis:
  - Allergic reaction (condom latex, contraceptive jelly, soaps)
  - Infections (*Candida albicans*, *Borrelia vincentii*, streptococci, *Trichomonas*, HPV)
  - Fixed-drug eruption (sulfa, tetracycline)
  - Plasma cell infiltration (Zoon balanitis)
  - Autodigestion by activated pancreatic transplant exocrine enzymes

- Phimosis:
  - Physiologic: present at birth; resolves spontaneously during the first 2 to 3 years of life through nocturnal erections, which slowly dilate the phimotic ring
  - Acquired: recurrent inflammation, trauma, or infections of the foreskin
- Paraphimosis:
  - Often iatrogenically or inadvertently induced by the foreskin not being pulled back over the glans after voiding, cleaning, cystoscopy, or catheter insertion

Geriatric Considerations
Condom catheters can predispose to balanitis.

Pediatric Considerations
Oral antibiotics predispose male infants to *Candida balanitis*. Most phimosis referrals seen in pediatric urology clinics are normal physiologically phimotic foreskins (1). Inappropriate care of physiologic phimosis can lead to acquired phimosis by repeated forced reduction of the foreskin. Uncircumcised penises require no special care and with normal hygiene, most foreskins will become retractile over time.

RISK FACTORS
- Balanitis:
  - Presence of foreskin
  - Morbid obesity
  - Poor hygiene
  - Diabetes; probably most common
  - Nursing home environment
  - Condom catheters
  - Chemical irritants
  - Edematous conditions: CHF, nephrosis
- Phimosis:
  - Poor hygiene
  - Diabetes by repeated balanitis
  - Frequent diaper rash in infants
  - Recurrent posthitis
- Paraphimosis:
  - Presence of foreskin
  - Inexperienced health care provider (leaving foreskin retracted after catheter placement)
  - Poor education about care of the foreskin

GENERAL PREVENTION
- Balanitis:
  - Proper hygiene and avoidance of allergens
  - Circumcision
- Phimosis/paraphimosis:
  - If the patient is uncircumcised, appropriate hygiene and care of the foreskin are necessary to prevent phimosis and paraphimosis.

DIAGNOSIS

HISTORY
- Balanitis:
  - Pain
  - Drainage
  - Dysuria
  - Odor
  - Ballooning of foreskin with voiding
  - Redness
- Phimosis:
  - Painful erections
  - Recurrent balanitis
  - Foreskin balloons when voiding
  - Inability to retract foreskin at appropriate age
- Paraphimosis:
  - Uncircumcised
  - Pain
  - Drainage
  - Voiding difficulty

PHYSICAL EXAM
- Balanitis:
  - Erythema
  - Tenderness
  - Edema
  - Discharge
  - Ulceration
  - Plaque
- Phimosis:
  - Foreskin will not retract.
  - Secondary balanitis
  - Physiologic phimosis—preputial orifice appears normal and healthy.
  - Pathologic phimosis—preputial orifice has fine white fibrous ring of scar.
- Paraphimosis:
  - Edema of prepuce and glans
  - Drainage
  - Ulceration

DIFFERENTIAL DIAGNOSIS
- Balanitis:
  - Leukoplakia
  - Lichen planus
  - Psoriasis
  - Reactive arthritis (formerly known as Reiter syndrome)
  - Lichen sclerosus et atrophicus
  - Erythroplasia of Queyrat
  - BXO: atrophic changes at end of foreskin; can form band that prevents retraction
- Phimosis/paraphimosis:
  - Penile lymphedema, which can be related to insect bites, trauma, or allergic reactions
  - Penile tourniquet syndrome: foreign body around penis, most commonly hair
  - Anasarca

DIAGNOSTIC TESTS & INTERPRETATION

Initial Tests (lab, imaging)
- Microbiology culture
- Wet mount
- Serology for syphilis
- Serum glucose; ESR (if concerns about reactive arthritis)
- STI testing
- HIV testing
- Gram stain

Diagnostic Procedures/Other
Biopsy, if persistent

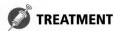 **TREATMENT**

GENERAL MEASURES
- Consider circumcision for recurrent balanitis and paraphimosis.
- Warm compresses or sitz baths
- Local hygiene

MEDICATION
- Balanitis:
  - Allergic/irritant:
    ○ Hydrocortisone 1% BID
  - Antifungal:
    ○ Clotrimazole (Lotrimin) 1% BID
    ○ Nystatin (Mycostatin) BID–QID
    ○ Fluconazole: 150 mg PO single dose
  - Antibacterial:
    ○ Bacitracin QID
    ○ Neomycin–polymyxin B–bacitracin (Neosporin) QID
    ○ If cellulitis, cephalosporin or sulfa drug PO or parenteral:
      ■ Dermatitis: topical steroids QID
      ■ Zoon balanitis: topical steroids QID
- Phimosis:
  - 0.05% fluticasone propionate daily for 4 to 8 weeks with gradual traction placed on foreskin
  - 1% pimecrolimus BID for 4 to 6 weeks; not for use in children aged <2 years
- Paraphimosis:
  - Manual reduction, if possible (should be done with the patient sedated); place the middle and index fingers of both hands on the engorged skin proximal to the glans. Place both thumbs on glans and, with gentle pressure, push on the glans and pull on the foreskin to attempt reduction. If unsuccessful, a dorsal slit will be necessary, with eventual circumcision after the edema resolves.

- Osmotic agents: granulated sugar placed on edematous tissue for several hours to reduce edema
- Puncture technique: Multiple punctures of foreskin with a 21-gauge needle will allow edematous fluid to escape and thus allow reduction.
- Dorsal slit; done by surgeon or urologist
- BXO:
  - 0.05% betamethasone BID
  - 0.1% tacrolimus BID

ISSUES FOR REFERRAL
Recurrent infections or development of meatal stenosis

SURGERY/OTHER PROCEDURES
- Balanitis and phimosis: Consider circumcision as preventive measure.
- For paraphimosis:
  - Represents a true surgical emergency to avoid necrosis of glans
  - Dorsal slit with delayed circumcision, if reduction is not possible
  - Operative exploration if the possibility of penile tourniquet syndrome cannot be eliminated; hair removal cream can be applied if a hair is thought to be the cause of the tourniquet.

ADMISSION, INPATIENT, AND NURSING CONSIDERATIONS
- Admission criteria/initial stabilization
  - Uncontrolled diabetes
  - Sepsis
- Appropriate hygiene if condom catheters are used
- Discharge on resolution of problem

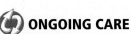 **ONGOING CARE**

FOLLOW-UP RECOMMENDATIONS
Patient Monitoring
Balanitis:
- Every 1 to 2 weeks until etiology has been established
- Persistent balanitis may require biopsy to rule out malignancy or BXO.
- Evaluation for resolution of phimosis

DIET
Weight reduction, if obese

PATIENT EDUCATION
- Need for appropriate hygiene
- Appropriate foreskin care
- Avoidance of known allergens such as soaps
- No sexual activity for 2 to 3 weeks after circumcision

PROGNOSIS
Should resolve with appropriate treatment

COMPLICATIONS
- Meatal stenosis
- Premalignant changes from chronic irritation
- UTIs
- Acquired phimosis
- Unreducible paraphimosis can lead to gangrene.
- Posthitis (inflammation of the prepuce)

REFERENCE
1. McGregor TB, Pike JG, Leonard MP. Pathologic and physiologic phimosis: approach to the phimotic foreskin. *Can Fam Physician*. 2007;53(3):445–448.

 SEE ALSO

Reactive Arthritis (Reiter Syndrome)

 CODES

ICD10
- N48.1 Balanitis
- N47.1 Phimosis
- N48.0 Leukoplakia of penis

CLINICAL PEARLS
- Balanitis is an inflammation of the glans penis. Posthitis is an inflammation of the foreskin. BXO is lichen sclerosus of the glans penis.
- With recurrent infections and a plaque, a biopsy should be done to rule out BXO or malignancy.
- If there is a true phimosis that interferes with appropriate hygiene, treat the phimosis with steroids or circumcision.

BARRETT ESOPHAGUS

Daniel J. Stein, MD, MPH • Trent Walradt, MD

BASICS

DESCRIPTION
- Metaplasia of the distal esophageal mucosa from native stratified squamous epithelium to abnormal columnar (intestinalized) epithelium; likely a consequence of chronic GERD
- Predisposes to the development of adenocarcinoma of the esophagus

EPIDEMIOLOGY
- Predominant age of >50 years, more common in men; estimated to be present in 1–2% of adult population
- Very rare in pediatric population

Incidence
- 10–15% of patients undergoing endoscopy for evaluation of reflux symptoms
- Incidence of esophageal adenocarcinoma (EAC) is rising in the United States (1); since 1970.
- Attributed to changes in smoking and obesity rather than reclassification or overdiagnosis
- Annual incidence of adenocarcinoma in all Barrett patients estimated at 0.5% per year

Prevalence
Potentially as many 1.5 to 2 million U.S. adults

ETIOLOGY AND PATHOPHYSIOLOGY
- Chronic gastric reflux injures the esophageal mucosa, triggering columnar metaplasia. Refluxed bile acids likely induce differentiation in gastroesophageal junction (GEJ) cells.
- Columnar cells in the esophagus have higher malignant potential than squamous cells. Activation of *CDX2* gene and overexpression of HER2/neu (ERBB2) oncogene promotes carcinogenesis.
- Elevated levels of COX-2 are associated with Barrett esophagus (BE).
- Classic progression: normal epithelium → esophagitis/reflux exposure → metaplasia (BE) → dysplasia (low → high-grade) → adenocarcinoma

Genetics
Familial predisposition to GERD and BE with multiple genetic markers have been identified.

RISK FACTORS
- Chronic reflux (>5 years); hiatal hernia
- Age >50 years; male gender
- Incidence in white males is much higher than white women and black men.
- Smoking history; intra-abdominal obesity
- Family history—at least one first-degree relative with BE or EAC

GENERAL PREVENTION
Weight loss, smoking cessation, robust intake of fruits and vegetables, and moderate wine consumption may decrease risk of BE and lower progression to esophageal cancer.

COMMONLY ASSOCIATED CONDITIONS
GERD, obesity, hiatal hernia

DIAGNOSIS

HISTORY
- Assess underlying risk factors.
- Common GERD symptoms: heartburn, regurgitation
- Atypical symptoms include chest pain, odynophagia, chronic cough, water brash, globus sensation, laryngitis, or wheezing.
- Symptoms suggestive of complicated GERD or cancer include weight loss, anorexia, dysphagia, odynophagia, hematemesis, or melena.

ALERT
BE is not by itself symptomatic; up to 50% of EAC and BE patients do not report GERD.

PHYSICAL EXAM
- No physical exam findings are specific for BE.
- Findings generally similar to GERD

DIFFERENTIAL DIAGNOSIS
Erosive esophagitis; uncomplicated GERD; hiatal hernia

DIAGNOSTIC TESTS & INTERPRETATION
Endoscopy with multiple biopsies demonstrating intestinal metaplasia extending ≥1 cm proximal to the GEJ is required to diagnose BE.

- Gastric cardia–type epithelium on pathology does not have clear malignant significance and may reflect sampling error.
- Specialized intestinal metaplasia at the GEJ: unclear significance; cancer risk difficult to assess with varying definitions of GEJ landmarks

ALERT
- Endoscopic screening is controversial. Consider one-time screening for patients with chronic GERD (>5 years) and/or frequent GERD symptoms with two or more risk factors: age >50 years, white ethnicity, central obesity, smoking history, family history of BE or EAC (ACG), or patients with multiple risk factors (2)[B].
- Screening for BE in the general population with GERD is *not* routinely recommended (2)[C].

Initial Tests (lab, imaging)
None
- *Helicobacter pylori* testing is *not* indicated.
- No current biomarkers are effective for diagnosis; some under investigation for risk stratification

Diagnostic Procedures/Other
- Endoscopy: Visualization of epithelial change with biopsy confirmation is standard.
- Classify disease extent: long segment (≥3 cm) versus short segment (<3 cm).

- Systematic endoscopic biopsies confirm diagnosis:
  - Seattle protocol: four-quadrant biopsies at regular intervals with biopsies of visible mucosal irregularities; more time-consuming but higher diagnostic yield than random biopsies
  - Capsule endoscopy has lower sensitivity than conventional endoscopy.
  - Chromoendoscopy (dye or virtual) should be used in addition to white light endoscopy.
- Swallowable capsule sponge devices combined with biomarkers are an alternative to endoscopy for screening.

Test Interpretation
- Specialized intestinal metaplasia (also called specialized columnar epithelium) is diagnostic of BE.
- Diagnosis of dysplasia (and grade) should be confirmed by two gastrointestinal pathologists before treatment. Benign BE is established by a single pathologist report.
- Cardia-type columnar epithelium may predispose to malignancy (unclear risk).
- If screening endoscopy reveals erosive esophagitis, repeat after 8 to 12 weeks of proton pump inhibitor (PPI) therapy to exclude underlying BE; defer biopsies until healing occurs (2)[C].

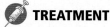

TREATMENT

MEDICATION
- The goal of medical therapy is to control GERD and to reduce esophagitis.
- Neither suppression of gastric acid production via high-dose PPIs nor reduction in esophageal acid exposure via antireflux surgery induces regression of BE. These therapies may, however, decrease progression/cancer risk.

First Line
- Patients with BE should be treated with a daily PPI. Patients should remain on lifetime therapy. If GERD symptoms were initially present, increase PPI until symptoms are controlled.
- Dose PPIs 30 to 60 minutes before a meal (ideally, the first meal of the day).

ALERT
Titrate PPI therapy to symptoms; routine pH monitoring is *not* recommended.

ISSUES FOR REFERRAL
- Most patients with low-grade dysplasia (except those who do not desire intervention) and all those with high-grade dysplasia or intramucosal carcinoma should be referred for endoscopic eradication of their BE.
- Refer patients who are considering esophagectomy (rare) to a high-volume institution.

ADDITIONAL THERAPIES

- Aspirin combined with high dose twice daily PPI may reduce progression to dysplasia (not yet routinely recommended).
  - COX-2 selective inhibitor celecoxib use not shown to affect progression of Barrett dysplasia to adenocarcinoma
  - Consider low-dose aspirin in patients with BE and risk factors for cardiovascular disease.
- Statins, alone or in combination with aspirin or NSAIDs, may be effective in chemoprevention.
- No dysplasia: No other therapy is generally indicated; continue regular surveillance (3)[C].
- Treatment of dysplasia:
  - Low-grade dysplasia: Refer for endoscopic therapy (usually radiofrequency ablation or cryotherapy) (3)[C].
  - High-grade dysplasia: Refer for endoscopic mucosal resection and/or endoscopic therapy to prevent progression to adenocarcinoma (3)[C].
  - Intramucosal carcinoma: endoscopic resection if possible, followed by ablation of remaining BE, with surgery as a backup
  - More advanced carcinoma: Refer to oncology and surgery to discuss resection.
  - Indeterminate grade dysplasia should have a re-evaluation with biopsies on increased PPI dosage.
  - Endoscopic eradication is successful in >90% of patients but often requires multiple sessions and can be associated with complications (3). Patients with prior ablation need ongoing surveillance for recurrence.

ALERT
Endoscopic eradication is not recommended for most BE without dysplasia

SURGERY/OTHER PROCEDURES

ALERT
- Antireflux surgery does not appear to decrease risk of esophageal cancer.
- Esophagectomy is definitive but should only be considered after failure of minimally invasive endoscopic eradication therapy for high-grade dysplasia. Morbidity and mortality are higher than with endoscopic treatment.

COMPLEMENTARY & ALTERNATIVE MEDICINE
Multivitamin, vitamin C, or vitamin E once a day may reduce progression to EAC in patients with BE.

Geriatric Considerations
Surveillance or no treatment in patients who are poor operative candidates; discontinue surveillance in patients who are not candidates for treatment.

 ONGOING CARE

FOLLOW-UP RECOMMENDATIONS
- Surveillance is recommended in high-risk patients with histologically confirmed BE.
- Surveillance intervals depend on grade of dysplasia.
- Patients diagnosed with BE on initial exam do not require endoscopy in 1 year (2)[C].
- No dysplasia: Survey every 3 to 5 years.
  - Discontinue surveillance if life expectancy is ≤5 years.
- Low-grade dysplasia not planning for ablation: Survey every 6 to 12 months (2),(3)[C].
  - Routine surveillance if patients have confirmed absence of low-grade dysplasia after two consecutive endoscopies
- Low-grade dysplasia with eradication therapy: Survey at 1 year and then every 2 years.
- Indefinite for dysplasia: Repeat after 3 to 6 months of increased acid suppression, and if unchanged, survey every 12 months.
- High-grade dysplasia without eradication therapy: Survey every 3 months; with eradication therapy: Survey at 3, 6, and 12 months and then annually.

ALERT
- Adherence to recommended surveillance protocols may improve rates of dysplasia and cancer detection.
- Continue surveillance even if the patient has had endoscopic ablation therapy, antireflux surgery, or esophagectomy.

DIET
Avoid foods that trigger reflux: caffeine, alcohol, chocolate, peppermint, carbonated drinks, garlic, onions, spicy foods, fatty foods, citrus, and tomato-based products.

PATIENT EDUCATION
- Lifestyle modifications: smoking cessation and weight loss; avoid supine position after meals; avoid tight-fitting clothes; elevate the head of bed.
- No evidence that treating GERD reverses BE or necessarily prevents esophageal cancer

PROGNOSIS
Annual incidence of esophageal cancer in patients with BE is estimated 0.12–0.6% per year:
- Low-grade dysplasia: may be transient; cancer risk 0.7–0.8% per year (3)
- High-grade dysplasia: cancer risk 5–9% per year (2),(3)
- Promising areas for research include the use of biomarkers for risk stratification, chemoprevention of neoplastic progression, advanced imaging, capsule endoscopy for screening, and the use of vitamins and antioxidants for prevention and treatment.

COMPLICATIONS
Same as GERD: stricture, bleeding, ulceration

REFERENCES

1. Muthusamy VR, Wani S, Gyawali CP, et al; for CGIT Barrett's Esophagus Consensus Conference Participants. AGA clinical practice update on new technology and innovation for surveillance and screening in Barrett's esophagus: expert review. *Clin Gastroenterol Hepatol*. 2022;20(12): 2696–2706.e1.
2. Bryce C, Bucaj M, Gazda R. Barrett esophagus: rapid evidence review. *Am Fam Physician*. 2022;106(4):383–387.
3. Qumseya B, Sultan S, Bain P, et al; for ASGE Standards of Practice Committee Chair. ASGE guideline on screening and surveillance of Barrett's esophagus. *Gastrointest Endosc*. 2019;90(3): 335–359.e2.

ADDITIONAL READING

- Cotton CC, Eluri S, Shaheen NJ. Management of dysplastic Barrett's esophagus and early esophageal adenocarcinoma. *Gastroenterol Clin North Am*. 2022;51(3):485–500.
- Sarem M, Martínez Cerezo FJ, Salvia Favieres ML, et al. Low-grade dysplasia in Barrett's esophagus: a problematic diagnosis. *Gastroenterol Hepatol*. 2023;46(8):637–644.

 CODES

ICD10
- K22.70 Barrett's esophagus without dysplasia
- K22.719 Barrett's esophagus with dysplasia, unspecified
- K22.710 Barrett's esophagus with low grade dysplasia

CLINICAL PEARLS

- Patients with BE and no dysplasia can be managed with endoscopic surveillance. Patients with low-grade dysplasia may be managed with either endoscopic surveillance or endoscopic eradication. Patients with BE and high-grade dysplasia can be managed with endoscopic eradication
- The highest incidence of BE is in white males >50 years of age.
- Esophagectomy is generally limited to patients with invasive carcinoma or those failing to respond to endoscopic therapy.

BASAL CELL CARCINOMA

Karl T. Clebak, MD, MHA, FAAFP • Jana Wei Qiao, MD

BASICS

DESCRIPTION
Basal cell carcinoma (BCC) is the most common type of skin cancer, originating from the basal cell layer of the skin appendages.
- Rarely metastasizes but is locally invasive and capable of local tissue destruction and disfigurement

EPIDEMIOLOGY
Most common cancer in Europe, Australia, and the United States; the most common type of skin cancer

Incidence
- Over 2 million new cases each year in the United States; 2.5 times more common than squamous cell carcinoma (SCC)
- White individuals have a 1 in 5 chance of developing BCC during their lifetime.
- Most common skin cancer in Asian and Hispanic individuals; second most common skin cancer in African American/black individuals (1)
- Predominant age: generally >60 years
- Predominant sex: male > female (2:1 ratio)

ETIOLOGY AND PATHOPHYSIOLOGY
UV radiation induces inflammation and cyclooxygenase activation in the skin.

Genetics
Several genetic conditions increase the risk of developing BCC:
- Albinism (recessive alleles)
- Xeroderma pigmentosum (autosomal recessive)
- Bazex-Dupré-Christol syndrome (rare, X-linked dominant)
- Nevoid BCC syndrome/Gorlin syndrome (rare, autosomal dominant)
- Cytochrome P450 CYP2D6 and glutathione S-transferase detoxifying enzyme gene mutations (especially in truncal BCC, marked by clusters of BCCs and a younger age of onset)
- Mutations in the tumor suppressor gene patched, or activated mutations in smoothened, resulting in upregulation of hedgehog pathway signaling

RISK FACTORS
- Chronic sun exposure (UV radiation); increased susceptibility in the following phenotypes:
  – Light complexion: skin type I (burns, but does not tan) and skin type II (usually burns, sometimes tans)
  – Red or blond hair
  – Blue or green eyes
- Tendency to sunburn
- Male sex, although increasing risk in women due to lifestyle changes, such as tanning beds
- Previous history of nonmelanoma skin cancer
- Family history of skin cancer
- Chronic immunosuppression: transplant recipients (5 to 10 times higher incidence), patients with HIV (2 times higher incidence), or lymphomas
- Arsenic exposure
- Immunosuppression
- UV radiation and/or use of tanning devices
- Xeroderma pigmentosum

GENERAL PREVENTION
- Use broad-spectrum sunscreens of at least SPF 30 daily at least 15 minutes before outdoor activity. Reapply every 2 hours, or immediately after swimming or sweating.
- Avoid overexposure to the sun. Avoid tanning beds.
- The USPSTF concludes that the current evidence is insufficient to assess the balance of benefits and harms of visual skin examination by a clinician to screen for skin cancer in adults. The American Cancer Society recommends cancer-related checkups every 3 years in patients aged 20 to 39 years old and yearly in patients aged ≥40 years.

COMMONLY ASSOCIATED CONDITIONS
- Cosmetic disfigurement (head and neck most often affected)
- Loss of vision with orbital involvement
- Loss of nerve function due to perineural spread or extensive and deep invasion
- Ulcerating neoplasms are prone to infections.

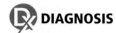

DIAGNOSIS

HISTORY
- Exposure to risk factors, family history of skin cancer
- History of a growing, ulcerating, or bleeding skin lesion often in a sun-exposed area

PHYSICAL EXAM
- 80% on face and neck, 20% on trunk and lower limbs
- Nodular: most common (50–80%); presents as pinkish, pearly papule, plaque, or nodule, often with telangiectatic vessels, ulceration, and a rolled periphery, usually on the head or neck
- Pigmented: presents as a translucent papule with "floating pigment"; more commonly seen in darker skin types; may give a blue, brown, or black appearance and be confused with melanoma (2)
- Superficial: 10–30%; light red, scaly plaque resembling eczema or psoriasis but with thin, rolled borders and central clearing, usually on trunk or extremities; least invasive of BCC subtypes (2)
- Morpheaform (sclerosing): 5–10%; resembles scar-like waxy plaque with poorly defined borders, occasionally with ulceration; most common on head or neck (2)

DIFFERENTIAL DIAGNOSIS
- SCC
- Sebaceous hyperplasia
- Epidermal inclusion cyst
- Intradermal nevi (pigmented and nonpigmented)
- Molluscum contagiosum
- Actinic keratosis
- Nummular dermatitis
- Psoriasis
- Melanoma (pigmented lesions)
- Atypical fibroxanthoma
- Fibrous papule
- Keratoacanthoma

DIAGNOSTIC TESTS & INTERPRETATION

Initial Tests (lab, imaging)
- Biopsy is necessary to confirm the diagnosis.
- Dermoscopy may improve diagnostic accuracy of BCCs.

Diagnostic Procedures/Other
- Clinical diagnosis and histologic subtype are confirmed through skin biopsy and pathologic examination.
- Shave biopsy is typically sufficient and used for nodular lesions. For flat lesions, punch biopsy or a shave biopsy with a scoop technique allows for the assessment of depth of tumor and perineural invasion. Excisional biopsy is rarely used.

Test Interpretation
- Nodular BCC
  – Extending from the epidermis are nodular aggregates of basaloid cells.
  – Tumor cells are uniform; rarely have mitotic figures; large, oval, hyperchromatic nuclei with little cytoplasm, surrounded by a peripheral palisade
  – Increased mucin in dermal stroma
- Superficial BCC
  – Appear as buds of basaloid cells attached to undersurface of epidermis
  – Peripheral palisading
- Morpheaform BCC
  – Thin cords and strands of basaloid cells; embedded in dense, fibrous, scar-like stroma
  – Less peripheral palisading and retraction, greater subclinical involvement
- Infiltrating BCC
  – Like morpheaform BCC but no scar-like stroma and thicker, spiky, irregular strands
  – Less peripheral palisading and retraction, greater subclinical involvement
- Micronodular BCC
  – Small, nodular aggregates of tumor cells
  – Less retraction artifact and higher subclinical involvement than nodular BCC

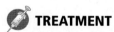

TREATMENT

GENERAL MEASURES
- Low risk BCC: curettage and electrodesiccation (C&E), standard excision, radiation therapy
- High risk BCC: standard excision, Mohs surgery, radiation therapy

MEDICATION
- May be especially useful in those who cannot tolerate surgical procedures, who refuse to have surgery, and who have low-risk superficial and/or nodular BCC
  – 5-Fluorouracil (5-FU) cream inhibits thymidylate synthetase, interrupting DNA synthesis for superficial lesions in low-risk areas; primary treatment only; 5% applied BID for 3 to 10 weeks
  – Imiquimod (Aldara) cream approved for treatment of low-risk superficial BCC; daily dosing for 6 to 12 weeks; 80% clearance rate (3)[A]

- Emerging therapies:
  - Vismodegib, a sonic hedgehog pathway inhibitor; for patients with advanced BCC failing other options; also beneficial for multiple BCC and BCC nevus syndrome
  - Intralesional injection: Efficacy for small (<1 cm) nodular and superficial BCCs varies from 67% to 94% based on the type of agent used (3)[C]; ingenol mebutate: from the plant *Euphorbia peplus*; in one trial, 63% of lesions, significant histologic cure rates were seen 85 days after treatment.
  - Laser therapy: Evidence for monotherapy is currently lacking in randomized controlled trials, but anecdotal evidence supports treatment for superficial BCC; one retrospective study with superpulsed carbon dioxide therapy for superficial and nodular BCC showed no recurrence in 3-year follow-up (3)[B].

First Line
Typically, surgical excision (See "Surgery/Other Procedures.")

ADDITIONAL THERAPIES
- Radiation therapy
  - Useful for patients, typically older (>60 years), who cannot not undergo surgery and for unresectable tumors
  - Used following surgery as adjuvant therapy, particularly if margins of tumor were not cleared
  - Cure rate is ~90%.
  - Recurrence rates are 4–16%.
- Photodynamic Therapy (PDT)
  - PDT uses photosensitizing agents (injected or topical) which becomes accumulated in the target cells.
  - Methyl aminolevulinate and 5-aminolevulinic acid, photosensitizers, are activated by specific wavelengths of light that destroy local tissue.
  - Currently approved in Canada, Europe, Australia, and New Zealand; off-label treatment for BCC in the United States

SURGERY/OTHER PROCEDURES
- Surgical excision is first-line treatment; specific treatment selection varies with extent and location of lesion as well as tumor border demarcation.
- High-risk areas
  - Inner canthus, nasolabial sulcus, philtrum, preauricular area, retroauricular sulcus, lip, temple, "mask areas" of the face
- C&E
  - If nodular lesion <1 cm, in low-risk area, not deeply invasive
  - Avoid in the hair-bearing areas due to risk of the tumor extending down follicular structures.
  - 5-year cure rate of 91–97%; recurrence as high as 27% for high-risk lesions (3)
  - Pathology sample sent at time of C&E to ensure absence of high-risk pathology
- Excision with postoperative margin assessment
  - Treatment of choice for low-risk lesions <2 cm in diameter
  - The goal is 4-mm margin.
  - 5-year cure rate of 98%

- Cryosurgery
  - Reserved for nodular and superficial BCC, not indicated for tumors with depth exceeding 3 mm
  - Contraindicated in hair-bearing areas and over the lower extremities (3)
  - Typically used for tumors with low risk of recurrence
  - Mean recurrence rates range from 0% to 39% across different studies.
- Mohs surgery
  - Surgical procedure where thin layers of the tumor are progressively removed and examined to determine tumor boarder, allowing only cancer-free tissue to remain
  - Preferred microsurgically controlled surgical treatment for lesions in high-risk areas, recurrent lesions, and lesions exhibiting an aggressive growth pattern
  - 5-year recurrence rates up to 10.1% in primary BCC, 17.4% in recurrent BCC
  - Requires referral to appropriately trained dermatologic surgeon

COMPLEMENTARY & ALTERNATIVE MEDICINE
Nicotinamide 500 mg BID lowers incidence of nonmelanoma skin cancers; β-carotene has not been shown effective.

ADMISSION, INPATIENT, AND NURSING CONSIDERATIONS
Outpatient, unless extensive lesion

ONGOING CARE

FOLLOW-UP RECOMMENDATIONS
- Seek shade, especially between 10 AM and 4 PM.
- Closer attention to prolonged duration around water, sand, and snow, which are UV-reflecting surfaces that can increase risk of skin damage
- Oral retinoids may prevent the development of new BCCs in patients with Gorlin syndrome, renal transplant recipients, and patients with severe actinic damage.

Patient Monitoring
- Every 6 to 12 months for the first 2 to 5 years and then annually for life; if no recurrence within the first 2 years, decreased frequency of monitoring can be considered.
- Increased risk of other skin cancers
- Recurrence:
  - Local: Follow NCCN 2022 guidelines for primary treatment.
  - Regional: surgery and/or radiation therapy
  - Metastatic: multidisciplinary tumor board consultation

PATIENT EDUCATION
- Monthly skin self-exam
- Educate patients concerning adequate vitamin D intake. Use broad-spectrum UVA/UVB sunscreen with SPF 15 or higher.
- Keep newborns out of the sun. Apply sunscreen to babies ≥6 months.

PROGNOSIS
- Proper treatment yields 90–95% cure.
- Most recurrences happen within 5 years. BCCs that develop in the head or neck area have a higher risk of recurring.
- Development of new BCCs: Many patients (30–50%) will develop a new lesion within 5 years.
- Cure rates with 5-FU, imiquimod, phototherapy, or cryotherapy may be 10% lower than surgical modalities.

COMPLICATIONS
- Recurrence rates >5 years postoperatively are up to 56% in primary BCC, 14% in recurrent BCC; long-term follow-up in high-risk tumors is indicated.
- Usually, recurrences will appear within 5 years.
- Metastasis: rare (<0.1%) but metastatic disease usually fatal within 8 months
  - Head and neck location, depth, and tumor diameter >4 cm are risk factors for metastasis and death.

REFERENCES
1. Hogue L, Harvey VM. Basal cell carcinoma, squamous cell carcinoma, and cutaneous melanoma in skin of color patients. *Dermatol Clin*. 2019;37(4):519–526.
2. Cameron MC, Lee E, Hibler BP, et al. Basal cell carcinoma: epidemiology; pathophysiology; clinical and histological subtypes; and disease associations. *J Am Acad Dermatol*. 2019;80(2):303–317.
3. Cameron MC, Lee E, Hibler BP, et al. Basal cell carcinoma: contemporary approaches to diagnosis, treatment, and prevention. *J Am Acad Dermatol*. 2019;80(2):321–339.

ADDITIONAL READING

Dzubow L, Goldberg LH, Lebwohl M, et al. *Basal Cell Carcinoma Prevention Guidelines*. New York, NY: The Skin Cancer Foundation; 2021. http://www.skincancer.org/skin-cancer-information/basal-cell-carcinoma/bcc-prevention-guidelines. Accessed October 13, 2021.

CODES

ICD10
- C44.711 Basal cell carcinoma of skin of unspecified lower limb, including hip
- C44.51 Basal cell carcinoma of skin of trunk
- C44.61 Basal cell carcinoma of skin of upper limb, including shoulder

CLINICAL PEARLS
- BCC is the most common cancer and skin malignancy, originating from the basal cell layer of the skin appendages.
- Chronic sun exposure and fair skin type increase risk with 80% on face and neck.
- Nodular type most common; telangiectasia seen at the borders

BED BUGS

Fawn J. Winkelman, DO • Adam Strosberg, DNP, ARNP-BC

 BASICS

DESCRIPTION
- Nocturnal obligate blood parasites residing in furniture and bedding
- 5 to 7 mm oval, reddish brown, flat, wingless morphology
- Microscopic evidence suggests a mature bed bug *Cimex lectularius* is approximately the size of an apple seed (1).

EPIDEMIOLOGY
Incidence
- Bed bug infestations are increasing in incidence and becoming more difficult to treat (2).
- Resurgence due to changes in pesticide, increased travel, use of secondhand furniture, and high turn-over rates of hotel guests

Prevalence
- Infestations have increased by 10–30% across the United States (1) in public places (schools, hospitals, hotels/motels, aircraft) over the past decade.
- The global population of bed bugs (*C. lectularius* and *Cimex hemipterus*, family Cimicidae) has undergone a significant resurgence since the late 1990s. This is likely due to an increase in global travel, trade, and the number of insecticide-resistant bed bugs. The global bed bug population is increasing annually.
- There are over 75 species of Insecta: Hemiptera: Cimicidae ("bed bugs") with the two genera and species implicated in human infestations being *C. lectularius* and *C. hemipterus* (1).
- *C. lectularius* lives in urban environments and *C. hemipterus* lives in tropical climates.

ETIOLOGY AND PATHOPHYSIOLOGY
- Insect family Cimicidae
- Three species bite humans: *C. lectularius, C. hemipterus,* and *Leptocimex boueti.*
- Most prevalent species is *C. lectularius.*

- Found in tropical and temperate climates
- Hide in crevices of mattresses, box springs, headboards, and baseboards
- Infestations occur in hotels/motels, hospitals, cinemas, vehicles, aircraft, and homes.
- Unlike other infestations, bed bug infestations are not associated with alterations in personal hygiene.
- Reactions range from an absent or minimal response to the typical pruritic, erythematous maculopapular rash. Less commonly, there is an urticarial or anaphylactoid response.
- Skin reactions are due to host immunologic response to parasite salivary proteins.
- Urticarial reactions are mediated via immunoglobulin (Ig) G antibody response to salivary proteins.
- Bullous reactions caused by an IgE-mediated hypersensitivity to nitrophorin in bug saliva
- Bugs are attracted to body warmth and exhaled carbon dioxide.
- Bites do not transmit other known pathogens.

RISK FACTORS
- Immunocompromise
- High hotel turnover
- Secondhand furniture in home

GENERAL PREVENTION
- Traps typically use carbon dioxide and heat to attract and trap bugs but can be cost prohibitive.
- Vector control: Vacuum regularly; reduce clutter; seal cracks in walls; inspect luggage and clothing.
- Launder all bedding and clothing in >130°F (50°C) for 2 hours or place in 20°F (−5°C) or cooler environment for at least 5 days.
- If present in the home, eradicate using professional extermination services. Some pest control companies use canines to detect live bed bugs and eggs based on pheromones from the bed bugs.

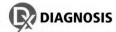 **DIAGNOSIS**

HISTORY
- Recent travel
- Bed bug sighting; blood specks on sheets
- New skin lesions in the morning
- Intense pruritus, pain, or burning

PHYSICAL EXAM
- Characteristic lesions are erythematous pruritic papules in an irregular linear pattern (1).
- Found on body surfaces exposed during sleeping such as face, neck, arms, legs, and shoulders
- May appear hours to days after being bitten
- Patients are usually asymptomatic but may present with papular urticaria, diffuse urticaria, bullous lesions, and/or anaphylactoid symptoms.

DIFFERENTIAL DIAGNOSIS
- Urticaria; insect or spider bite; scabies
- Dermatitis herpetiformis

DIAGNOSTIC TESTS & INTERPRETATION
Initial Tests (lab, imaging)
- Skin scraping with mineral oil preparation
- Skin biopsy

Test Interpretation
- Skin scraping is negative with mineral oil, which helps to exclude scabies.
- Skin biopsy shows nonspecific perivascular eosinophilic infiltrate consistent with arthropod bite reaction.

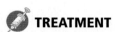 **TREATMENT**

GENERAL MEASURES
- Treatment should address three areas: treatment of the skin, eradication of the infestation, and assessment for potential behavioral health consequences (1).
- Most patients present for the treatment of skin irritation and lesions.
- Disease is self-limited and resolves within 1 to 2 weeks.
- Treat symptomatically.

MEDICATION

First Line

- Oral antihistamines (i.e., diphenhydramine, hydroxyzine)
- Topical antipruritics (i.e., pramoxine/calamine ointment or doxepin cream)
- Topical low-potency to mid-potency corticosteroids for 2 weeks (i.e., hydrocortisone, triamcinolone)
- Systemic corticosteroids (severe cases)

ADDITIONAL THERAPIES

- If secondarily infected, use topical or oral antibiotics against *Staphylococcus* and *Streptococcus* spp. (i.e., cephalexin, tetracycline, doxycycline, clindamycin, topical mupirocin).
- Epinephrine for anaphylaxis
- Professional extermination may be necessary.
- The CDC recommends a comprehensive integrated pest management program—remove clutter, seal cracks, heat treatment, vacuum, and nonchemical pesticides.
- New approaches (more research necessary) include xenointoxication (oral arthropodicidal agent) toxic to the bed bugs.

COMPLEMENTARY & ALTERNATIVE MEDICINE

- Bed bugs may be eradicated with heat.
- Tropical bed bugs (*C. hemipterus*) require a higher average temperature to eradicate.

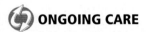 ## ONGOING CARE

FOLLOW-UP RECOMMENDATIONS

- Not necessary as disease is self-limited
- May need specific care in extreme cases or if anaphylactoid reactions
- Consider behavioral health consultation depending on the severity of the patient's emotional reaction to the infestation.

Patient Monitoring

Tips for travel:

- Inspect rooms by checking mattresses and luggage racks (best done with a flashlight).
- Reduce clutter.
- Keep luggage and bags off the bed and bedding.

PATIENT EDUCATION

- Avoid scratching to prevent superinfection.
- Inspect bedding, furniture, and luggage regularly.
- CDC: https://www.cdc.gov/parasites/bedbugs/
- EPA: http://www.epa.gov/bedbugs
- Myth 1: *Bed bugs are invisible*. They are nocturnal and hide during the daytime. Adult bugs are ~1/4-inch long, and eggs are the size of a pin head.
- Myth 2: *Bed bugs reproduce rapidly*. Their life cycle is 4 to 5 weeks, longer than the housefly.
- Myth 3: *Bed bugs can live without feeding*. Bugs can live 3 to 5 months without a blood meal.
- Tips to prevent and control bed bugs
  - Ensure infestation is bed bugs (not fleas, other insects, and/or ticks).
  - Regularly wash and heat dry your clothing and bedding, especially if it touches the floor.
  - EPA tips: https://www.epa.gov/bedbugs/top -ten-tips-prevent-or-control-bed-bugs

COMPLICATIONS

- Bed bug dermatitis, allergic reactions, asthma exacerbations, anaphylaxis
- Significant psychological distress (insomnia, depression, anxiety, delusional parasitosis)
- Secondary bacterial infections
- Transmission of blood-borne diseases (rare)

REFERENCES

1. Leung AKC, Lam JM, Barankin B, et al. Bed bug infestation: an updated review [published online ahead of print April 6, 2023]. *Curr Pediatr Rev*. 2023.
2. Shipman KE, Weaving G, Shipman AR. Bedbugs: how to diagnose and manage cases of infestations. *Clin Exp Dermatol*. 2023;48(5):453–461.

ADDITIONAL READING

National Pesticide Information Center: http://npic.orst.edu/

 ## SEE ALSO

United States Environmental Protection. Do-it-yourself bed bug control. https://www.epa.gov/bedbugs/do-it -yourself-bed-bugf-control. Accessed August 5, 2023.

 ## CODES

ICD10

- S00.96XA Insect bite (nonvenomous) of unspecified part of head, initial encounter
- S10.96XA Insect bite of unspecified part of neck, initial encounter
- S40.269A Insect bite (nonvenomous) of unspecified shoulder, initial encounter

CLINICAL PEARLS

- 90% of infestations occur within 3 feet of bedding.
- Wash bedding/clothing regularly in hot water and vacuum carpet daily or steam clean daily.
- Inspect furniture, bedding, and luggage regularly.
- Bed bugs are largely resistant to over-the-counter (OTC) pesticide products (permethrin, cyfluthrin, bifenthrin, and deltamethrin or fluvalinate and esfenvalerate).

BEHAVIORAL PROBLEMS, PEDIATRIC

Sahil Mullick, MD • Sudeshna Dutta, MD

BASICS

DESCRIPTION
Behavior that disrupts at least one area of psycho-social functioning; commonly reported behavioral problems are as follows:

- Noncompliance: active or passive refusal to do as requested by parent/authority figure
- Temper tantrums: loss of internal control that leads to crying, whining, breath holding, or aggressive behavior
- Sleep problems: difficulty going to sleep or staying asleep, nightmares, night terrors
- Nocturnal enuresis: bed-wetting that occurs in children >5 years of age for ≥3 months with no medical problems
  - Primary: children who have never been dry at night
  - Secondary: children previously dry at night for at least 6 months
  - Monosymptomatic enuresis: only have bed-wetting
  - Nonmonosymptomatic enuresis: bed-wetting in addition to daytime incontinence, urgency, voiding difficulties or voiding <4 or >7 times per day
- Functional encopresis: repeated involuntary fecal soiling that is not caused by organic defect or illness; can be retentive (associated with functional constipation 80%) or nonretentive (20%)
- Problem eating: "picky eating," difficult mealtime behaviors
- Thumb-sucking: can be problematic if persists past eruption of primary teeth (Teeth alignment may be impacted.)

EPIDEMIOLOGY
- Noncompliance issues: manifest as children develop autonomy; slightly more common in males; decreases with age
- Temper tantrums: 5–7% of children 1 to 3 years of age have tantrums lasting at least 15 minutes ≥3 times per week; 20% of 2-year-olds, 18% of 3-year-olds, and 10% of 4-year-olds have at least one tantrum every day (1).
- Sleep problems
  - Night waking in 25–50% of infants 6 to 12 months old
  - Bedtime refusal in 10–30% of toddlers
  - Nightmares in 10–50% of preschoolers; peak age: 6 to 10 years
  - Night terrors in 1–6.5% early childhood; peak age: 4 to 12 years
  - Sleepwalking frequently in 3–5%; peak age: 4 to 8 years (2)
- Nocturnal enuresis: Common, 5–10% of 7-year-olds and 3% of teenagers wet the bed (3).
  - Monosymptomatic nocturnal enuresis is twice as common among boys than girls.
  - Resolves spontaneously at a rate of approximately 15% per year

- Functional encopresis: rare before age 3 years, affects approximately 1–4% of 4-year-olds and 1–2% of children aged ≥7 years; more common in boys (3)
- Problem eating: Prevalence peaks at 50% at 24 months of age; no relation to sex/ethnicity/income (4)
- Thumb-sucking: decreases with age; most children spontaneously stop between 2 and 4 years of age (4).

ETIOLOGY AND PATHOPHYSIOLOGY
Genetics
Nocturnal enuresis: 45% risk if one parent has history and 75% if both parents have history after 5 years of age

COMMONLY ASSOCIATED CONDITIONS
- Noncompliance: If excessive or aggressive, rule out depression, compulsive patterns, adjustment disorder, and inappropriate discipline.
- Temper tantrums: difficult child temperament, stress, normal development
- Sleep problems: inconsistent bedtime routine/sleep schedule, stimulating bedtime environment; can be associated with hyperactive behavior, poor impulse control, and poor attention in young children; acute or chronic anxiety is associated with insomnia. Long-acting stimulant medications may disturb sleep quality.
- Enuresis: associated with constipation, obstructive sleep apnea (OSA), neurodevelopmental conditions such as autism spectrum disorder and ADHD
- Functional encopresis: enuresis, ADHD, emotional stressors

DIAGNOSIS

HISTORY
- Noncompliance: history from caregivers and teachers; direct observation of child or child–caregiver interaction
  - Criteria: problematic for at least some adults, leading to difficult interactions for at least 6 months
  - Reduces child's ability to take part in structured activities
  - Creates stressful relationships with other children
  - Disrupts academic progress; places child at risk for physical injury
- Temper tantrums: may consist of stiffening limbs and arching back, dropping to floor, shouting, screaming, crying, pushing/pulling, stomping, hitting, kicking, throwing, or running away (1)[C]
- Sleep disorders: Ask about sleep and bedtime routine, bedtime problems, excessive daytime sleepiness, awakenings during the night, regularity and duration of sleep, and snoring (BEARS) screen (2)[C].
- Nocturnal enuresis: onset and duration; dry overnight previously; daytime wetting or any associated genitourinary symptoms; fluid intake and voiding patterns, family history of enuresis; medical, developmental, and psychosocial history; constipation; sleep problems; child and caregiver's motivation for treatment; voiding diary (5)[C]

- Encopresis: fecal continence ever attained; triggering event; how often and where the child stools; pain or blood with defecation; how much stool passed accidentally; history of trauma or abuse; rectal prolapse; prior surgery (3)[C]
- Problem eating: review of child's diet, growth curves, nutritional needs, and caregiver's response to behavior (4)

PHYSICAL EXAM
- Nocturnal enuresis: generally normal; inquire about signs of poor growth, tonsillar hypertrophy, constipation, or occult spinal dysraphism (5)[C].
- Functional encopresis: abdominal exam for masses or tenderness; rectal exam for tone, size of rectal vault, fecal impaction, masses, fissures, hemorrhoids; back for dimpling or hair tufts (3)[C]

DIFFERENTIAL DIAGNOSIS
- Temper tantrums: language deficits, autism, or disruptive mood dysregulation disorder (DMDD)—distinguishable because of baseline irritable mood between outbursts and older age (6 to 18 years)
- Nocturnal enuresis: bladder dysfunction, UTI, kidney disease or structural abnormality, OSA, diabetes insipidus, spinal dysraphism
- Functional encopresis: neurologic disorders, ectopic anus, Hirschsprung disease

DIAGNOSTIC TESTS & INTERPRETATION
Initial Tests (lab, imaging)
- Enuresis: urinalysis to rule out UTI, inability to concentrate urine, and glycosuria (5)[C]
- Functional encopresis: TSH; rule out celiac disease if poor growth or family history; urinalysis and culture if enuresis or features of UTI
- Spine imaging if evidence of spinal dysraphism or if both encopresis and daytime enuresis; barium enema if suspect Hirschsprung disease (3)[C]

Follow-Up Tests & Special Considerations
- Sleep disorders: Sleep studies if history of snoring and/or observed apnea to evaluate for OSA; daytime ADHD-type symptoms may be present (2)[C].
- Nocturnal enuresis: urodynamics (bladder dysfunction), renal ultrasound (kidney disease), MRI (spinal dysraphism)

Diagnostic Procedures/Other
- Pediatric Symptom Checklist: https://www.bright futures.org/mentalhealth/pdf/professionals/ped _sympton_chklst.pdf
- National Initiative for Children's Healthcare Quality (NICHQ) Vanderbilt Assessment (ADHD screen): https://www.myadhd.com/vanderbiltparent6175.html
- Child Sexual Behavior Inventory: completed by female caregiver to assist with differentiation of normative versus abnormal behaviors particularly those related to sexual abuse: https://www.nctsn .org/measures/child-sexual-behavior-inventory

TREATMENT

GENERAL MEASURES
- Educate caregiver about specific behavioral problem.
- Parent management training programs and techniques are effective for many child behavior problems.
- Noncompliance: For extreme disobedience, consider parent training programs; may need formal screening for ADHD, obsessive-compulsive disorder (OCD), oppositional defiant disorder (ODD), or conduct disorder (CD)
- Temper tantrums: Remind the caregiver that this is a normal development.
  - The child is experiencing fatigue, anger, or frustration with no other means to cope.
  - Usually occur to get what they want, to avoid or escape doing something they do not want to do, or to seek parental attention
  - Identify triggers such as hunger, overtiredness, or changing activities and try to prevent tantrums.
  - Other methods for dealing with a tantrum include one of the following:
    - Ignore the tantrum; place child in time-out (1 minute for each year of age); hold/restrain child until calm; provide child with clear, firm, and consistent instructions and enough time to obey (1)[C].
- Sleep problems: Educate caregiver at well-child checks about importance of bed routine and consistency and consistency in response to sleep disruptions. Specific recommendations may also include:
  - Graduated extinction: Ignore cries for specified period; check in at increasing intervals.
  - Fading: gradual decrease in direct contact with the child as they fall asleep; the goal is for the child to fall asleep independently.
  - If fearful, special routines or aromatherapy sprays so child feels more secure (2)[C]
- Nocturnal enuresis
  - Ensure that the family and the child know that this is not caused by poor parenting skills or under the child's control.
  - Waking the child to void and limiting fluids are not supported by evidence. Voiding prior to bedtime can be helpful.
  - Nonmonosymptomatic: aggressive treatment of constipation when accompanying enuresis; generally treat daytime symptoms first; may require referral
  - Monosymptomatic: positive reinforcement for dry nights; enuresis alarm used nightly; discontinue after 6 weeks if no progress; if helpful, use until 14 consecutive dry nights is achieved (5)[C].
- Functional encopresis
  - Disimpaction: manually, with enemas or polyethylene glycol solution
  - Maintenance therapy: No quick fix, results take months to achieve, and relapses are common.
    - Medical: polyethylene glycol, increased dietary fiber and fluids, lactulose, sorbitol, magnesium citrate (for retentive type)
    - Behavior modification: toileting after meals for 10 minutes 2 to 3 times a day, star charts, and rewards (3)[C]

- Problem eating
  - Avoid punishment, prodding, or rewards. Offer a variety of healthy foods at every meal; limit milk to 24 oz per day and decrease juice (4)[C].
- Normative sexual behavior: no treatment needed; caregivers should not punish; gently redirect behavior in public setting.
  - Curiosity about sex characteristics is common in children as young as 2 to 5 years old, including interest in looking at others, intruding on physical boundaries, and touching their mother's breasts. Sexual play such as "doctor" is common; 60–80% of children engage in sexual play before age 13 years.
- Thumb-sucking: Praise children when not sucking their thumb, offer alternatives that are soothing (e.g., stuffed toys), and use negative reinforcement such as a bandage around or bitters on the thumb (4).

MEDICATION
Most pediatric behavioral issues respond well to nonpharmacologic therapy:
- Sleep disorders: Cognitive-behavioral therapy and sleep hygiene are first-line treatment; no recommended pharmacotherapy
  - After behavioral methods are exhausted, melatonin 0.5 to 10.0 mg PO can be tried in concert with behavior modification. However, this is not approved by the FDA for children (2)[C].
- Encopresis: laxatives, rectal suppositories, enema for constipation
- Nocturnal enuresis
  - First line: Desmopressin decreases urine production. One-third are dry with med, one-third have no benefit, and one-third have intermediate response; safe for long-term use and few side effects; chronic polydipsia can lead to hyponatremia and is only a contraindication. Give 1- to 2-week trial. Dosing: 0.2 to 0.4 mg 1 hour before bedtime
  - Second line: tricyclic antidepressants (e.g., imipramine) used by specialists (5)[C]
  - Third line: anticholinergics (e.g., oxybutynin) given before bedtime; side effects can be dry mouth, headache, or constipation.

ISSUES FOR REFERRAL
- Tantrums that are severe, occur after the age of 5 years, or those who exhibit self-injurious behaviors, slow recovery time from tantrums, more tantrums in the home than outside the home, or more aggressive behaviors toward others may require referral to a psychologist or psychiatrist (1)[C].
- Children with chronic insomnia or anxiety: Refer to psychologist or psychiatrist (2)[C].
- With enuresis and OSA symptoms, refer for sleep study. Surgical correction of airway obstruction often improves/cures enuresis and daytime wetting (5)[C].
- Must distinguish sexual behavior problems: Developmentally inappropriate behaviors—greater frequency or earlier age than expected—becomes a preoccupation, recurs after adult intervention/corrective efforts. If abuse is not suspected, consider referral to a child psychologist. If abuse is suspected, must report to child protective services.

- If disimpaction by either manual or medical methods is unsuccessful, consult gastroenterology or general surgery. Patients who show no improvement after 6 months of maintenance medical therapy should be referred to gastroenterology (3)[C].
- Thumb-sucking resistant to behavioral intervention and threatening permanent dentition and bite may be evaluated by a pediatric dentist for use of habit-breaking dental appliances (4)[C].

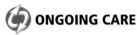

ONGOING CARE

DIET
Nutrition is very important in behavioral issues. Avoiding high-sugar foods and caffeine and providing balanced meals have been shown to decrease aggressive and noncompliant behaviors in children.

PATIENT EDUCATION
- See *Parent Training Programs: Insight for Practitioners* at: https://www.cdc.gov/violence prevention/pdf/Parent_Training_Brief-a.pdf
- Karp H. *The Happiest Baby Guide to Great Sleep: Simple Solutions for Kids from Birth to 5 Years*. New York, NY: HarperCollins Publishers; 2012.

REFERENCES

1. Daniels E, Mandleco B, Luthy KE. Assessment, management, and prevention of childhood temper tantrums. *J Am Acad Nurse Pract*. 2012;24(10):569–573.
2. Bhargava S. Diagnosis and management of common sleep problems in children. *Pediatr Rev*. 2011;32(3):91–99.
3. Har AF, Croffie JM. Encopresis. *Pediatr Rev*. 2010;31(9):368–374.
4. Nasir A, Nasir L. Counseling on early childhood concerns: sleep issues, thumb-sucking, picky eating, school readiness, and oral health. *Am Fam Physician*. 2015;92(4):274–278.
5. Nevéus T, Fonseca E, Franco I, et al. Management and treatment of nocturnal enuresis—an updated standardization document from the International Children's Continence Society. *J Pediatr Urol*. 2020;16(1):10–19.

 CODES

ICD10
- F91.9 Conduct disorder, unspecified
- F91.1 Conduct disorder, childhood-onset type
- F91.2 Conduct disorder, adolescent-onset type

CLINICAL PEARLS

- Well-child visits provide opportunities for screening for these common conditions.
- In extreme disobedience, child may need to be screened for ADHD, OCD, ODD, or CD.
- Parental education, including a review of age-appropriate discipline, is a key component of treatment.
- Temper tantrums in toddlers are common, often occurring at least one per day.

BELL PALSY

Daniel R. Matta, MD • Paul McFarlane, MBBS

BASICS

DESCRIPTION
An acute, usually unilateral, self-limiting peripheral (lower motor neuron) facial nerve (cranial nerve VII) palsy; Bell Palsy is largely idiopathic. It results in the inability to voluntarily move the facial muscles of the affected side. It is associated with edema and compression of CN VII.

EPIDEMIOLOGY
- No race, geographic, or gender predominance
- Affects all ages, with the highest incidence being in patients aged 15 to 45 years
- Occurs with equal frequency on the left and right sides of the face

Incidence
Global studies have demonstrated annual incidence of up to 53 per 100,000.

ETIOLOGY AND PATHOPHYSIOLOGY
- Inflammation of cranial nerve VII causes edema of perineurium and subsequent compression and possibly degeneration of both the nerve and the associated vasa nervorum.
- Activation of latent herpesvirus (herpes simplex virus type 1 and herpes zoster virus) in cranial nerve ganglia thought to account for many cases of Bell palsy.

RISK FACTORS
- Pregnancy, with increased risk seen in patients with chronic hypertension, maternal obesity, and severe preeclampsia
- Immunosuppression
- Diabetes mellitus
- Upper respiratory infection with viruses such as influenza A
- Chronic hypertension
- Obesity
- Extremes of temperature (1)

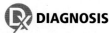

DIAGNOSIS

The diagnosis is based on a thorough history and examination.

HISTORY
- Onset: typically rapid (over 24 to 48 hours)
- Typically unilateral (very rarely bilateral) lower motor neuron-type facial weakness, with no other neurological or systemic signs; a patient may present for medical attention as he or she may complain of inability to close the eyelid or find liquids leaking from the affected side of the mouth.
- Course is progressive, peaking at up to 3 weeks after onset. Symptoms may take up to several months to improve.
- Although strokes may present with facial weakness, it is not usually the presenting symptom. Furthermore, stroke lesions (affecting the ipsilateral facial nerve nucleus or facial nerve tract in the pons) that can mimic Bell palsy is rare.

- Associated symptoms
  - Mastoid or postauricular pain
  - Hyperacusis
  - Dysgeusia: alteration of taste on the ipsilateral anterior 2/3 of the tongue (chorda tympani branch of the facial nerve)
  - Numbness on the ipsilateral side of the face
  - Decreased lacrimation or salivation
- Asking the patient about a travel history (or if the patient lives in a Lyme disease endemic area) or presence of skin rashes may help to elicit a more likely cause for the patient's facial nerve weakness (such as herpes zoster, Lyme disease, or sarcoidosis).

PHYSICAL EXAM
- Neurologic
  - Flaccid paralysis of muscles on the affected side, including the forehead
    - Impaired ability to raise the ipsilateral eyebrow
    - Impaired closure of the ipsilateral eye
    - Impaired ability to smile, grin, or purse the lips
    - Bell phenomenon: upward diversion of the eye with attempted closure of the lid
- Determine if the weakness is caused by either a central (upper motor neuron) or peripheral (lower motor neuron) lesion.
  - In contrast to low motor neuron lesions, the forehead muscles are usually spared in upper motor neuron lesions.
  - Patients may complain of numbness, but no deficit is present on sensory testing.
  - Subtle deficits in other cranial nerves, especially trigeminal, glossopharyngeal, and hypoglossal, may be present, but if these signs are prominent, the diagnosis of Bell palsy is doubtful.
- Head, ears, eyes, nose, and throat
  - Carefully examine to exclude a space-occupying lesion.
- Skin: Examine for erythema migrans (Lyme disease) and vesicular rash (herpes zoster virus).
- House-Brackmann (H-B) Scale used to assess severity of Bell Palsy (2)
  - Grade I: normal function
  - Grade II: slight weakness on close inspection, slight synkinesis, complete eyelid closure with minimal effort
  - Grade III: moderate severity: obvious but not disfiguring facial asymmetry; synkinesis is noticeable but not severe; may have hemifacial spasm or contracture; complete eyelid closure with effort; mouth is slightly weak with maximal effort.
  - Grade IV: moderately severe: disfiguring facial asymmetry or obvious facial weakness; forehead cannot move; incomplete eyelid closure; mouth is asymmetrical with maximal effort.
  - Grave V: total paralysis

DIFFERENTIAL DIAGNOSIS
- Up to 50% of cases of peripheral facial nerve palsy may not be due to Bell palsy.
- Consider other differentials if any of the following "red flags" exist:
  - Gradual onset over weeks to months
  - Concomitant vertigo or hearing loss
  - Constitutional symptoms and/or cervical lymphadenopathy

  - Evidence of Lyme disease
  - Failure of improvement within 3 months or worsening of weakness over several months
- Facial cranial nerve palsy etiologies include:
  - Congenital causes: genetic syndromes, birth-related trauma, developmental hypoplasia of facial muscles
  - Acquired causes: infective (Ramsay Hunt Syndrome, Lyme, TB, HIV), inflammatory (vasculitis, sarcoidosis, autoimmune), neoplastic (benign, malignant), cerebrovascular (stroke, aneurysm), and traumatic
- Clinical approach based on facial palsy pattern:
  - Recurrent, ipsilateral palsy: neoplasm of the nerve (schwannoma) or adjacent structures (parotid, temporal bone, or cerebellopontine angle [CPA])
  - Bilateral palsy: neurologic (Guillain-Barré syndrome, particularly if patient presents with ophthalmoplegia and ataxia) or associated with neoplasm (lymphoma, disseminated carcinomatosis, malignant pachymeningitis); rare: cryptococcal meningitis associated with HIV, autoimmune (MS, myasthenia gravis, Sjögren syndrome), sarcoidosis, granulomatosis with polyangiitis
  - Palsy at birth: segmental developmental palsy (associated with synkinesis, recovers spontaneously)
  - Facial palsy syndromes: Ramsay Hunt (rash in the ear [zoster oticus] and/or mouth caused by VZV); Melkersson-Rosenthal (orofacial edema, recurrent facial palsy, and fissured tongue); Heerfordt-Waldenström (parotid enlargement, anterior uveitis, facial palsy, and fever)

DIAGNOSTIC TESTS & INTERPRETATION
Bell palsy is a clinical diagnosis. Routine lab testing or diagnostic imaging in new-onset Bell palsy is not necessary. However, further testing may be considered in:
- Atypical presentation of facial palsy
- Recurrent facial palsy or symptoms for >2 months; magnetic resonance imaging of the head, orbits, face, or neck, with and without intravenous contrast
- Slowly progressive disease >3 weeks
- Lack of improvement after 4 months

Initial Tests (lab, imaging)
Depending on the clinical scenario, blood testing that may be considered include:
- CBC, CRP/ESR to rule out inflammatory process
- Rapid plasma reagin (RPR), Lyme serology, and/or HIV test if indicated
- Titers for VZV; rubella; cytomegalovirus; hepatitis A, B, and C
- Polymerase chain reaction (PCR) for HSV-1 or herpes zoster virus

Follow-Up Tests & Special Considerations
- Facial radiographs to evaluate for fractures
- Contrast-enhanced CT: to evaluate for stroke or temporal bone fracture
- MRI: to evaluate for brain or parotid neoplasms
- Invasive diagnostic procedures are not indicated because biopsy could further damage the nerve.

Diagnostic Procedures/Other
- Electrodiagnostic studies may be offered to patients with complete paralysis for prognostic purposes, but it does not change the management.
- Parotid gland biopsy: considered if no recovery with negative imaging at 7 months

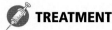 TREATMENT

GENERAL MEASURES
- Artificial tears should be used frequently to lubricate the cornea.
- The ipsilateral eye should be patched or taped shut at night to avoid drying and infection.

MEDICATION
- Recovery from Bell palsy is possible without treatment, particularly in patients who do not have a complete palsy.
- Corticosteroids decrease inflammation and limit nerve damage, thereby increase the number of patients who make full recovery and reduce disabling sequelae (NNT = 10).
- Antiviral alone has no benefit over placebo (3); hence, the use of antivirals as a monotherapy in new-onset Bell palsy is not recommended.
- According to a 2012 Guideline from the American Academy of Neurology (AAN), for patients with new-onset Bell palsy, antivirals (in addition to steroids) might be offered to increase the probability of recovery of facial function (Level C evidence). Patients offered antivirals should be counseled that a benefit from antivirals has not been established, and, if there is a benefit, it is likely to be modest at best (3)[B].
- Corticosteroids
  - Recommended in all cases
  - Should be started within 72 hours of symptoms onset
  - A 10-day course of oral steroids is recommended. This may be either:
    o Prednisolone 50 mg PO daily for 10 days or
    o Prednisone 60 mg daily for 5 days and then tapering dose (by 10 mg/day) the next 5 days
  - Precautions: Use with discretion in patients with peptic ulcer disease and diabetes.
  - Contraindications: documented hypersensitivity, preexisting infections (TB, systemic mycosis)
- If antiviral is being used, consider valacyclovir 1,000 mg PO TID for 7 days or acyclovir 400 mg 5 times per day for 10 days.

Pregnancy Considerations
Steroids should be used cautiously during pregnancy. Acyclovir and valacyclovir are considered category B drugs in pregnancy by the U.S. FDA.

ISSUES FOR REFERRAL
- Refer to ophthalmologist for persistent weakness in eyelid closure.
- Patients with no improvement or progression of symptoms should be referred to ENT and may require neuroimaging to rule out neoplasms.
- If bilateral, recurrent, or prolonged symptoms, refer to neurology.
- In children, refer to neurologist or neurosurgery if condition is associated with trauma, age <2 years, and/or symptoms lasting >4 weeks.

ADDITIONAL THERAPIES
- In patients who make an incomplete recovery following the use of steroids with or without antiviral therapy, consider botulinum toxin to treat facial asymmetry, facial tightness, and synkinesis resulting from Bell palsy.
- Physical therapy should be offered to patients with severe paralysis (H-B grade V or VI) or persistent paralysis (>3 months).

SURGERY/OTHER PROCEDURES
- There is an insufficient evidence to decide whether surgical intervention is beneficial or harmful in the management of Bell palsy.
- Decompression surgery should not be performed >14 days after the onset of paralysis because severe degeneration of the facial nerve is likely irreversible after 2 to 3 weeks.

 ONGOING CARE

FOLLOW-UP RECOMMENDATIONS
Patient Monitoring
- Start steroid treatment immediately.
- Patients who do not recover complete facial nerve function should be referred to ENT and/or ophthalmology for further management.

PATIENT EDUCATION
FamilyDoctor.org from AAFP: https://familydoctor.org/condition/bells-palsy

PROGNOSIS
- Most patients achieve complete spontaneous recovery within 2 weeks. >80% recover within 3 months.
- 85% of untreated patients will experience the first signs of recovery within 3 weeks of onset.
- Up to 30% of patients do not recover facial function completely.
- 7% may have recurrence, which may be on the affected or opposite side.
- 5% experience severe sequelae, and a small number of patients experience permanent facial weakness and dysfunction.
- Poor prognostic factors include the following:
  - Age >60 years
  - History of recurrence
  - Complete facial weakness
  - Diabetes mellitus; hypertension
  - H-B grade >II
- Treatment with corticosteroids and the Sunnybrook score are significant factors for predicting nonrecovery at 1 month.

COMPLICATIONS
- Corneal abrasion or ulceration
- Steroid-induced hyperglycemia, psychological disturbances; avascular necrosis of the hips, knees, and/or shoulders.
- Chronic spasm of facial muscles (synkinesia) or blepharospasm due to aberrant regeneration of facial nerve

REFERENCES
1. Zhang W, Xu L, Luo T, et al. The etiology of Bell's palsy: a review. *J Neurol*. 2020;267(7):1896–1905.
2. Dalrymple SN, Row JH, Gazewood J. Bell palsy: rapid evidence review. *Am Fam Physician*. 2023;107(4):415–420.
3. Gagyor I, Madhok VB, Daly F, et al. Antiviral treatment for Bell's palsy (idiopathic facial paralysis). *Cochrane Database Syst Rev*. 2019;9(9):CD001869.

ADDITIONAL READING
- Baugh RF, Basura GJ, Ishii LE, et al. Clinical practice guideline: Bell's palsy. *Otolaryngol Head Neck Surg*. 2013;149(Suppl 3):S1–S27.
- Madhok VB, Gagyor I, Daly F, et al. Corticosteroids for Bell's palsy (idiopathic facial paralysis). *Cochrane Database Syst Rev*. 2016;7(7):CD001942.
- Peitersen E. The natural history of Bell's palsy. *Am J Otol*. 1982;4(2):107–111.
- Shinn JR, Nwabueze NN, Du L, et al. Treatment patterns and outcomes in botulinum therapy for patients with facial synkinesis. *JAMA Facial Plast Surg*. 2019;21(3):244–251.

 SEE ALSO

Amyloidosis; Diabetes Mellitus, Type 1; Diabetes Mellitus, Type 2; Herpes Simplex; Herpes Zoster (Shingles); Lyme Disease; Sarcoidosis; Sjögren Syndrome

 CODES

ICD10
G51.0 Bell's palsy

CLINICAL PEARLS
- Look closely at the voluntary movement on the upper part of the face on the affected side; in Bell palsy, all of the muscles are involved (weak or paralyzed), whereas in a stroke, the upper muscles (forehead) are spared (because of bilateral innervation).
- No need to obtain routine labs or diagnostic imaging in a typical new-onset Bell palsy.
- Initiate steroids immediately following the onset of symptoms.
- Protect the affected eye with lubrication and taping.
- In areas with endemic Lyme disease, consider Lyme until proven otherwise.

BIPOLAR I DISORDER
Wendy K. Marsh, MD, MSc

BASICS

DESCRIPTION
- An episodic mood disorder of at least one manic or mixed (mania and depression) episode that causes marked impairment, psychosis, and/or hospitalization
- Symptoms are not caused by a substance or general medical condition.

Geriatric Considerations
In new onset in older patients (>50 years of age), a workup for organic or chemically induced pathology is recommended.

Pediatric Considerations
Need for clarity of symptoms is critical to differentiate between attention deficit hyperactivity disorder (ADHD), oppositional defiant disorder (ODD), disruptive mood dysregulation, and other diagnoses with overlapping symptoms that are common in childhood.

Pregnancy Considerations
- Pregnancy does not reduce the risk of mood episodes.
- Need to weigh risk of fetal and maternal exposure to mood episode to that of medication
- Avoid divalproex (Depakote) due to high teratogenicity risk.
- Postpartum carries high risk of severe acute episode with psychosis and/or infanticidal ideation.

EPIDEMIOLOGY
Onset usually between 15 and 30 years of age, average of 25 years

Prevalence
- 1–1.6% lifetime prevalence
- Manic episodes more common in men; depressive episodes more common in women

ETIOLOGY AND PATHOPHYSIOLOGY
- Dysregulation of biogenic amines or neurotransmitters (particularly serotonin, norepinephrine, and dopamine)
- MRI findings suggest abnormalities in prefrontal cortical areas, striatum, and amygdala that predate illness onset (1)[C].

Genetics
- Monozygotic twin concordance 40–70%; dizygotic 5–25%
- 50% have at least one parent with a mood disorder.

GENERAL PREVENTION
Treatment adherence and education help to prevent relapses.

COMMONLY ASSOCIATED CONDITIONS
Substance abuse (60%), ADHD, anxiety disorders (~50%), and eating disorders

DIAGNOSIS

The diagnosis of BP-I requires at least one manic or mixed episode (simultaneous mania and depression). Although a depressive episode is not necessary for the diagnosis, 80–90% of people with BP-I also experience depression. Refer to the *DSM-5* for additional information.

HISTORY
- Collateral information makes diagnostics more complete and is often necessary for a clear history.
- History: safety concerns (e.g., Suicidal/homicidal ideation? Safety plan? Psychosis present?), physical well-being (e.g., Number of hours of sleep? Weight change? Substance abuse?), personal history (e.g., Talkative? Risky driving? Excessive spending? Credit card debt? Promiscuity? Other risk-taking behavior? Legal trouble?), substance use (e.g., Did the mood change precede or occur subsequent to substance use?)

PHYSICAL EXAM
- Mental status exam in acute mania
  - General appearance: disorganized or discombobulated, psychomotor agitation, bright clothing, excessive makeup
  - Speech: pressured, difficult to interrupt
  - Mood/affect: euphoria, irritability, expansive, labile
  - Thought process: flight of ideas (streams of thought occur to patient at rapid rate), easily distracted
  - Thought content: grandiosity, paranoia, hyperreligiosity
  - Perceptual abnormalities: 3/4 of manic patients experience delusions, grandiose, or paranoia.
  - Suicidal/homicidal ideation: aggression toward self or others; suicidal ideation is common with mixed episode.
  - Insight/judgment: poor/impaired
- With mixed episodes, patients may exhibit a combination of manic and depressive mental states.

DIFFERENTIAL DIAGNOSIS
- Other psychiatric considerations: unipolar depression ± psychotic features, schizophrenia, schizoaffective disorder, personality disorders (particularly antisocial, borderline, histrionic, and narcissistic), ADD ± hyperactivity, substance-induced mood disorder
- Medical considerations: epilepsy (e.g., temporal lobe), brain tumor, infection (e.g., AIDS, syphilis), stroke, endocrine (e.g., thyroid) disease, multiple sclerosis
- In children, consider ADHD and ODD.

DIAGNOSTIC TESTS & INTERPRETATION
- The Mood Disorder Questionnaire is a self-assessment screen for history of mood elevation (thus presumed bipolar diagnosis) (sensitivity 73%, specificity 90%).
- Patient Health Questionnaire-9 helps to determine the presence and severity of a depressive episode.

Initial Tests (lab, imaging)
- TSH, CBC, BMP, B12, LFTs, RPR, HIV, ESR
- Drug/alcohol screen with each presentation
- Consider brain imaging (CT, MRI) with initial onset of mania to rule out organic cause (e.g., tumor, infection, or stroke), especially with onset in elderly and if psychosis is present.

Diagnostic Procedures/Other
Consider EEG if presentation suggests temporal lobe epilepsy (hyperreligiosity, hypergraphia).

TREATMENT

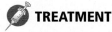

GENERAL MEASURES
- Ensure safety; daily schedule especially sleep, clean from substances, avoid blue light (screens) in evening, exercise, a healthy diet
- Psychotherapy for depression (e.g., cognitive-behavioral therapy, social rhythm, interpersonal) in conjunction with medications

MEDICATION
- Acute mania (2),(3)[B]
  - First line
    - Lithium monotherapy
    - Atypical antipsychotic: quetiapine, risperidone/paliperidone, aripiprazole, asenapine, or cariprazine monotherapy
    - Divalproex
    - Lithium or divalproex plus atypical antipsychotic
  - Second line
    - Olanzapine; carbamazepine; lithium plus divalproex; lithium or divalproex plus olanzapine; ziprasidone; haloperidol; cariprazine
    - Electroconvulsive therapy (ECT)
- Acute bipolar I depression (3)
  - First line
    - Quetiapine
    - Lithium, lamotrigine, lurasidone, cariprazine
  - Second line
    - Divalproex, lumateperone
    - Bupropion adjunctive
    - Olanzapine* + fluoxetine
    - ECT
- *Side effects concerns: Weight gain, metabolic syndrome, and extrapyramidal symptoms (EPS) warrant vigilance and monitoring by the clinician.
- Treatment mood stabilizer(s) or other psychotropic medications; when combining, use different classes (e.g., an atypical antipsychotic and/or an antiseizure medication and/or lithium).
  - Lithium: 600 to 1,200 mg/day divided BID–QID; start 600 to 900 mg/day divided BID–TID; titrate based on blood levels. *Warning*: caution in kidney and heart disease; use can lead to diabetes insipidus or thyroid disease over time. Pregnancy requires close monitoring and risks to fetus (Ebstein anomaly). *Monitor*: Check ECG for those aged >40 years, TSH, BUN, creatinine, electrolytes at baseline and every 6 months; check level 5 to 7 days after initiation or dose change, then every 2 weeks × 3, and then every 3 months (plasma range: 0.8 to 1.2 mmol/L).

- Anticonvulsants
  - Divalproex sodium, valproic acid: Start 250 to 500 mg BID–TID; maximum of 60 mg/kg/day; black box warnings: hepatotoxicity, pancreatitis, thrombocytopenia, pregnancy Category D (high risk for multiple major malformations) Rec. avoiding in reproductive age women. Monitor CBC and LFTs at baseline and every 6 months; check level 5 days after initiation and dose changes (plasma range: 50 to 125 μg/mL).
  - Carbamazepine: 800 to 1,200 mg/day PO divided BID–QID; start 100 to 200 mg PO BID and titrate up to lowest effective dose. *Warning*: Do not use with tricyclic antidepressant (TCA) or within 14 days of an MAOI. Caution in kidney/heart disease; risk of aplastic anemia/agranulocytosis, enzyme inducer; pregnancy Category D; monitor CBC and LFTs at baseline and every 3 to 6 months; check level 4 to 5 days after initiation and dose changes (plasma range: 4 to 12 μg/mL).
  - Lamotrigine: 200 to 400 mg/day; start 25 mg/day for 2 weeks, then 50 mg/day for 2 weeks, then 100 mg/day for 1 week, and then 150 mg/day. *Warning*: Titrate slowly (risk of Stevens-Johnson syndrome); caution with kidney/liver/heart disease; pregnancy relative safety but needs close
  - Oxcarbazepine: 300 mg PO QD; titrate to 1,800 to 2,400/day max.
- Atypical antipsychotics
  - Side effects: orthostatic hypotension, metabolic side effects (glucose and lipid dysregulation, weight gain), tardive dyskinesia, neuroleptic malignant syndrome (NMS), prolactinemia, increased risk of death in elderly with dementia-related psychosis, pregnancy growing data on relative safety, watch for metabolic AE above
  - Monitor LFTs, lipids, glucose at baseline, 3 months and annually; check for EPS with Abnormal Involuntary Movement Scale (AIMS) and assess weight (with abdominal circumference) at baseline; at 4, 8, and 12 weeks; and then every 3 to 6 months; monitor for orthostatic hypotension 3 to 5 days after starting or changing dose.
  - Aripiprazole: 15 to 30 mg/day; IM preparation available; for mania and maintenance
  - Asenapine: 5 to 10 mg sublingual BID
  - Cariprazine: 1.5 to 3 mg/day for depression; 3 to 6 mg/day for mood elevation
  - Lumateperone: 42 mg QD for depression
  - Lurasidone: 20 to 60 mg/day for depression
  - Olanzapine: 5 to 20 mg/day; most likely to cause metabolic side effects (weight gain, diabetes); for mania and maintenance
  - Paliperidone: 6 mg every morning; may cause agranulocytosis, cardiac arrhythmias; IM preparation available
  - Quetiapine: formania, 200 to 400 mg BID; for bipolar depression, 50 to 300 mg QHS; XR dosing 50 to 400 mg QHS for mania, depression, and maintenance
  - Risperidone: 1 to 6 mg/day divided QD–QID; IM preparation available (q2wk) for mania and maintenance
  - Ziprasidone: 40 to 80 mg BID; less likely to cause metabolic side effects for mania and maintenance
- Avoid TCAs and serotonin norepinephrine reuptake inhibitor (SNRI) that increase risk of mood cycling.

ISSUES FOR REFERRAL
Patients benefit from a multidisciplinary team, including a primary care physician, psychiatrist, and therapist.

ADDITIONAL THERAPIES
- Modest evidence supports full spectrum 10,000 lux midmorning light, transcranial magnetic stimulation, ketamine infusion, ar/modafinil, sleep deprivation, and levothyroxine bipolar depression.
- Blue-blocking glasses or dark therapy for mania
- A regular sleep and wake-up schedule is helpful.

ADMISSION, INPATIENT, AND NURSING CONSIDERATIONS
- To admit involuntarily, the patient must have a psychiatric diagnosis (e.g., BP-I) and present a danger to self or others, or the mental disease must be inhibiting the person from obtaining basic needs (e.g., food, clothing, shelter).
- Nursing: Alert staff to potentially dangerous or agitated patients. Acute suicidal threats need continuous observation.

 ## ONGOING CARE

FOLLOW-UP RECOMMENDATIONS
- Regularly scheduled visits support adherence with treatment.
- Frequent communication among primary care doctor, psychiatrist, and therapist

Patient Monitoring
Mood charts are helpful to monitor symptoms.

DIET
Omega three fatty acids and probiotics; data limited

PATIENT EDUCATION
- National Alliance on Mental Illness (NAMI): https://www.nami.org/
- National Institute of Mental Health (NIMH): https://www.nimh.nih.gov/
- International Bipolar Foundation (IBPF): https://ibpf.org/

PROGNOSIS
- Frequency and severity of episodes are related to medication adherence, consistency with therapy, quality of sleep, and support systems.
- 40–50% of patients experience another manic episode within 2 years of first episode.
- 25–50% attempt suicide, and 15% die by suicide.
- Substance abuse, unemployment, psychosis, depression, and male gender are associated with a worse prognosis.

REFERENCES
1. American Psychiatric Association. *Diagnostic and Statistical Manual of Mental Disorders*. 5th ed. Arlington, VA: American Psychiatric Association; 2013.
2. Parikh SV, LeBlanc SR, Ovanessian MM. Advancing bipolar disorder: key lessons from the Systematic Treatment Enhancement Program for Bipolar Disorder (STEP-BD). *Can J Psychiatry*. 2010;55(3):136–143.
3. Yatham LN, Kennedy SH, Parikh SV, et al. Canadian Network for Mood and Anxiety Treatments (CANMAT) and International Society for Bipolar Disorders (ISBD) 2018 guidelines for the management of patients with bipolar disorder. *Bipolar Disord*. 2018;20(2):97–170.

 ## SEE ALSO
Algorithm: Depressive Episode, Major

CODES

ICD10
- F31.9 Bipolar disorder, unspecified
- F31.10 Bipolar disorder, current episode manic without psychotic features, unspecified
- F31.30 Bipolar disord, crnt epsd depress, mild or mod severt, unsp

CLINICAL PEARLS
- BP-I is characterized by at least one manic or mixed episode that causes marked impairment; major depressive episodes usually occur but are not necessary.
- 25–50% of BP-I patients attempt suicide, and 15% die by suicide.
- There is no known way to prevent BP-I, but treatment adherence and education help reduce further episodes.
- The goal of treatment is to decrease the intensity, length, and frequency of episodes as well as greater duration of euthymia (healthy mood) between episodes.

BIPOLAR II DISORDER
Wendy K. Marsh, MD, MSc

BASICS

DESCRIPTION
A mood disorder characterized by at least one episode of major depression (with or without psychosis) and at least one episode of hypomania, a nonsevere mood elevation

Geriatric Considerations
In new onset in older patients (>50 years of age), a workup for organic or chemically induced pathology is strongly recommended.

Pediatric Considerations
Need for clarity of symptoms is critical to differentiate between attention deficit hyperactivity disorder (ADHD), oppositional defiant disorder (ODD), disruptive mood dysregulation, and other diagnoses with overlapping symptoms that are common in childhood.

Pregnancy Considerations
- Pregnancy does not protect against risk of mood episodes.
- Need to weigh risk of exposure to mood episode to that of medication
- Avoid divalproex (Depakote) due to high teratogenicity risk.
- Postpartum caries high risk of severe acute episode with psychosis and/or infanticidal ideation

EPIDEMIOLOGY
Onset usually between 15 and 30 years of age

Prevalence
- 0.5–1% lifetime prevalence
- More common in women

ETIOLOGY AND PATHOPHYSIOLOGY
Dysregulation of biogenic amines or neurotransmitters (particularly serotonin, norepinephrine, and dopamine)

Genetics
Heritability estimate: >77%

RISK FACTORS
Genetics, major life stressors, or substance misuse

GENERAL PREVENTION
Treatment adherence and education can help to prevent further episodes.

COMMONLY ASSOCIATED CONDITIONS
Substance misuse, ADHD, anxiety disorders, and eating disorders

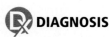
DIAGNOSIS

DSM-5 criteria: one hypomanic episode and at least one major depressive episode; mood elevation symptoms cause unequivocal change in functioning noticed by others but not severe enough to cause marked impairment (1)[C].

- Hypomania is a distinct period of persistently elevated, expansive, or irritable mood, different from usual euthymic mood, including increase in activity or energy lasting at least 4 days:
  - The episode must include at least three of the "DIG FAST" symptoms *plus increased energy* below (four if the mood is only irritable):
    ○ Distractibility
    ○ Insomnia, decreased need for sleep
    ○ Grandiosity or inflated self-esteem
    ○ Flight of ideas or racing thoughts
    ○ Agitation or increase in goal-directed activity (socially, at work or school, or sexually)
    ○ Speech pressured/more talkative than usual
    ○ Taking risks: excessive involvement in pleasurable activities that have high potential for painful consequences (e.g., sexual or financial)
- Major depression: Depressed mood or diminished interest and four or more of the "SIG E CAPS" symptoms are present during the same 2-week period:
  - Sleep disturbance (e.g., trouble falling asleep, early-morning awakening)
  - Interest: loss or anhedonia
  - Guilt (or feelings of worthlessness)
  - Energy, loss of
  - Concentration, loss of
  - Appetite changes, increase or decrease
  - Psychomotor changes (retardation or agitation)
  - Suicidal/homicidal thoughts
  - Rapid cycling is ≥4 mood episodes in 12 months (major depression or hypomania).
  - Mixed specifier: when three or more symptoms of opposite mood pole are present during primary mood episode, for example, hypomania with mixed features (of depression)
- Note: If symptoms have *ever* met the criteria for a full manic episode, for example, hospitalization was necessary secondary to manic/mixed symptoms or psychosis was present, then the diagnosis is BP-I.

HISTORY
- Collateral information makes diagnostics more complete and is often necessary for a clear history.
- History: safety concerns (e.g., Suicidal/homicidal ideation? Safety plan? Psychosis present?), physical well-being (e.g., Number of hours of sleep? Substance abuse?), personal history (e.g., Risky driving? Excessive spending? Credit card debt? Promiscuity? Other risk-taking behavior? Legal trouble?), substance use (e.g., Did the mood change precede or occur subsequent to substance use?)

PHYSICAL EXAM
- Mental status exam in hypomania
  - General appearance: usually appropriately dressed; may be bright colors or eye-catching style, often with psychomotor agitation
  - Speech: may be pressured, talkative, difficult to interrupt
  - Mood/affect: euphoria, irritability, congruent, or expansive
  - Thought process: may be easily distracted; difficulty concentrating on one task
  - Thought content: usually positive, with "big" plans
  - Perceptual abnormalities: none
  - Suicidal/homicidal ideation: low incidence of homicidal or suicidal ideation
  - Insight/judgment: usually stable/may be impaired by distractibility or grandiosity

- Mental status exam in depression
  - General appearance: unkempt, psychomotor retardation, poor eye contact
  - Speech: low, soft, monotone
  - Mood/affect: sad, depressed/congruent, flat
  - Thought process: ruminating thoughts, generalized slowing
  - Thought content: preoccupied with negative or nihilistic ideas
  - Perceptual abnormalities: 15% of depressed patients experience hallucinations or delusions.
  - Suicidal/homicidal ideation: Suicidal ideation is very common.
  - Insight/judgment: often impaired

DIFFERENTIAL DIAGNOSIS
- Other psychiatric considerations: BP-I disorder, unipolar depression, personality disorders (particularly borderline, antisocial, and narcissistic), ADHD, substance-induced mood disorder
- Medical considerations: epilepsy (e.g., temporal lobe), brain tumor, infection (e.g., AIDS, syphilis), stroke, endocrine (e.g., thyroid disease), multiple sclerosis, autoimmune

DIAGNOSTIC TESTS & INTERPRETATION
- Mood Disorder Questionnaire, self-assessment screen for history of mood elevation (thus presumed bipolar diagnosis)
- Hypomania Checklist-32 distinguishes between BP-II and unipolar depression (sensitivity 80%, specificity 51%) (2)[B].
- Patient Health Questionnaire-9 helps to determine the presence and severity of depression.

Initial Tests (lab, imaging)
- Rule out organic causes of mood disorder during initial episode.
- Drug/alcohol screen is prudent with each presentation.
- With initial presentation: Consider CBC, chem 7, TSH, LFTs, ANA, B_{12}, RPR, HIV, and ESR.
- Consider brain imaging (CT, MRI) with initial onset of hypomania to rule out organic cause, especially with onset in the elderly.

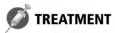
TREATMENT

GENERAL MEASURES
- Ensure safety.
- Psychotherapy for depression, stress reduction (e.g., CBT, social rhythm, interpersonal, family focused) in conjunction with medications
- Regular circadian rhythm/daily sleep and activity schedule, exercise, a healthy diet
- Sobriety, substance free

MEDICATION
- Acute mood elevation (3),(4)[C]
  - First line
    ○ Quetiapine; lithium
    ○ Atypical, other: cariprazine, risperidone, aripiprazole, ziprasidone, asenapine
    ○ Divalproex (avoid in reproductive age women)
  - Second line
    ○ Haloperidol; paliperidone, olanzapine, cariprazine
    ○ Lithium plus divalproex
    ○ Lithium or divalproex plus atypical

- Acute bipolar II depression (4)
  - First line
    - Quetiapine, lumateperone
  - Second line
    - Lithium; lamotrigine; lurasidone; cariprazine
    - Bupropion adjunct
    - ECT
- When combining, use different classes (e.g., an atypical antipsychotic and/or an antiseizure medication and/or lithium) (2)[A].
  - Lithium: 600 to 1,200 mg/day divided BID–QID; start 600 to 900 mg/day divided BID–TID and titrate based on blood levels. *Warning*: caution in kidney and heart disease; use can lead to diabetes insipidus or thyroid disease. Pregnancy requires close monitoring. *Monitor*: Check ECG for ages >40 years, TSH, BUN, creatine, and electrolytes at baseline every 6 months. Check the level 5 to 7 days after initiation or dose change, then every 2 weeks × 3, and then every 3 months (goal: 0.6 to 1.2 mmol/L).
  - Anticonvulsants
    - Divalproex sodium, valproic acid: Start 250 to 500 mg BID–TID; maximum of 60 mg/kg/day; black box warnings: hepatotoxicity, pancreatitis, thrombocytopenia, pregnancy Category D; monitor CBC and LFTs at baseline and every 6 months; check level 5 days after initiation and dose changes (goal: 50 to 125 μg/mL).
    - Lamotrigine: 200 to 400 mg/day; start 25 mg/day for 2 weeks, then 50 mg/day for 2 weeks, then 100 mg/day for 1 week, and then 150 mg/day. (Note: Use half dosing if adjunct to valproate.) *Warning*: Titrate slowly (risk of Stevens-Johnson syndrome); caution with kidney/liver/heart disease; depression prevention indication does not treat mood elevation.
  - Atypical antipsychotics
    - Side effects: orthostatic hypotension, metabolic side effects (glucose and lipid dysregulation, weight gain), tardive dyskinesia, neuroleptic malignant syndrome (NMS), akathisia, prolactinemia (except aripiprazole), sedation, increased risk of death in elderly with dementia-related psychosis
    - Monitor LFTs, lipids, glucose at baseline, 3 months and annually; check for EPS with Abnormal Involuntary Movement Scale (AIMS), and assess weight (with abdominal circumference) at baseline; at 4, 8, and 12 weeks; and then every 3 to 6 months; monitor for orthostatic hypotension 3 to 5 days after starting or changing dose.
    - Aripiprazole: 10 to 30 mg/day; less likely to cause metabolic side effects, IM dosing once a month to once every 6 months for hyptompania and maintentance
    - Asenapine: 5 to 10 mg sublingual BID
    - Lumateperone: 42 mg QD for depression, less likely to cause metabolic side effects
    - Cariprazine: 1.5 mg to 3.0 mg for depression, up to 6 mg for mood elevation
    - Lurasidone: 20 to 60 mg/day for depression
    - Paliperidone: 6 mg every morning; may cause agranulocytosis and cardiac arrhythmias; for hypomania and maintenance

- Quetiapine: 200 to 400 mg BID for hypomania; 50 to 600 mg for bipolar depression QHS; XR dosing 50 to 400 mg QHS, high sedation and metabolic profile
- Risperidone: 1 to 6 mg/day divided QD–QID; IM preparation available (q2wk); watch for hyperprolactinemia and abnormal involuntary muscle movements; for hypomania and maintenance
- Ziprasidone: 40 to 80 mg BID; less likely to cause metabolic side effects; for hypomania and maintenance
- Unipolar antidepressants
  - Bupropion (Wellbutrin): dosing: 150 to 300 mg PO QD; not FDA-approved; use only with antimanic agent.
  - Avoid TCAs and SNRIs—increases mood cycling risk

ISSUES FOR REFERRAL
Patients benefit from a multidisciplinary team, including a primary care physician, psychiatrist, and therapist.

ADDITIONAL THERAPIES
- Modest evidence supports full spectrum bright light, transcranial magnetic stimulation, vagus nerve stimulation, ketamine infusion, sleep deprivation, and hormone therapy (e.g., thyroid) in bipolar depression.
- Blue-blocking glasses or dark therapy for mood elevation, regular sleep–wake cycle, awakening the same time every morning

ADMISSION, INPATIENT, AND NURSING CONSIDERATIONS
- To admit involuntarily, the patient must have a psychiatric diagnosis (e.g., BP-I) and present a danger to self or others, or the mental disease must be inhibiting the person from obtaining basic needs (e.g., food, clothing).
- Nursing: Alert staff to potentially dangerous or agitated patients. Acute suicidal threats need continuous observation.

ONGOING CARE

FOLLOW-UP RECOMMENDATIONS
Regular scheduled visits support adherence with treatment.

Patient Monitoring
Mood charts are helpful to monitor symptoms.

DIET
May benefit from omega 3 fatty acids and probiotics; data limited

PATIENT EDUCATION
- National Alliance on Mental Illness (NAMI): https://www.nami.org/
- National Institute of Mental Health (NIMH): https://www.nimh.nih.gov/index.shtml
- International Bipolar Foundation (IBPF): https://ibpf.org/

PROGNOSIS
- Frequency and severity of episodes are related to medication adherence, consistency with therapy, quality of sleep, and support systems.
- 25–50% attempt suicide, and 15% die by suicide.
- Substance abuse, unemployment, psychosis, depression, and male gender are associated with a worse prognosis.

REFERENCES
1. American Psychiatric Association. *Diagnostic and Statistical Manual of Mental Disorders*. 5th ed. Arlington, VA: American Psychiatric Association; 2013.
2. Ostacher MJ, Tandon R, Suppes T. Florida best practice psychotherapeutic medication guidelines for adults with bipolar disorder: a novel, practical, patient-centered guide for clinicians. *J Clin Psychiatry*. 2016;77(7):920–926.
3. Parikh SV, LeBlanc SR, Ovanessian MM. Advancing bipolar disorder: key lessons from the Systematic Treatment Enhancement Program for Bipolar Disorder (STEP-BD). *Can J Psychiatry*. 2010;55(3):136–143.
4. Yatham LN, Kennedy SH, Parikh SV, et al. Canadian Network for Mood and Anxiety Treatments (CANMAT) and International Society for Bipolar Disorders (ISBD) 2018 guidelines for the management of patients with bipolar disorder. *Bipolar Disord*. 2018;20(2):97–170.

 SEE ALSO

Algorithm: Bipolar Disorder I

CODES

ICD10
F31.81 Bipolar II disorder

CLINICAL PEARLS
- BP-II is characterized by at least one episode of major depression and one episode of hypomania.
- Patients may not recognize symptoms and/or decline treatment during a hypomanic episode; they may enjoy the elevated mood and productivity.
- Patients with BP-II are at great risk of both attempting and completing suicide.

BITES, ANIMAL AND HUMAN

Kellie Wang, PharmD • Brian J. Kimbrell, MD, FACS

BASICS

DESCRIPTION
Animal bite rates vary by species: dogs (60–90%), cats (5–20%), rodents (2–3%), humans (2–3%), and (rarely) other animals, including snakes.

EPIDEMIOLOGY
All ages, but children > adults

Incidence
- 3 to 6 million animal bites per year in the United States; account for 1% of all injury-related ED visits
- 1–2% will require hospital admission, and 20 to 35 victims die from dog bite complications, annually.

ETIOLOGY AND PATHOPHYSIOLOGY
- Dog bites are more common than cat bites; most dog bites are from a known domestic pet; ~90% of cat bites are provoked.
- Human bite wounds are typically incurred by striking another in the mouth with a clenched fist; human bites also occur incidentally (e.g., paronychia, thumb-sucking, or bites to the face, breasts, or genital areas).
- Animal bites can cause tears, punctures, scratches, avulsions, or crush injuries.
- Contamination by oral flora leads to infection.

RISK FACTORS
- Clenched-fist human bites are frequently associated with the use of alcohol or drugs.
- Patients presenting >8 hours following the bite are at greater risk for infection.

GENERAL PREVENTION
- Instruct about animal hazards.
- Educate pet owners.

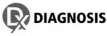

DIAGNOSIS

HISTORY
- Detailed history of the incident (provoked or unprovoked), type of animal, site of the bite, animal's vaccine status, whereabouts of animal, and geographic setting
- Underlying patient medical history—particularly comorbid diseases and immunosuppression
- Ascertain patient immunization history (tetanus and rabies, in particular).

PHYSICAL EXAM
- Dog bites
  - Hands and face are the most common sites of injury in adults and children, respectively; more likely to have associated crush injury
- Cat bites
  - Predominantly involve the hands, followed by lower extremities, face, and trunk; more often puncture-type wound
- Human bites
  - Intentional bite: semicircular or oval area of erythema and bruising, with/without break in skin
  - Clenched-fist injury: wounds over the metacarpophalangeal joints from striking the fist against another's teeth

- Signs of wound infection include fever, erythema, swelling, tenderness, purulent drainage, and lymphangitis.
- Signs of tenosynovitis (hand/finger bites): finger held in flexion, fusiform swelling, pain along tendon sheath, pain with active/passive extension of the affected digit
- Document neurovascular status.

Pediatric Considerations
Human bite marks on a child with an intercanine distance >3 cm are likely from an adult and should raise concerns about child abuse.

DIFFERENTIAL DIAGNOSIS
Evaluate for other possible causes of trauma.

DIAGNOSTIC TESTS & INTERPRETATION
Initial Tests (lab, imaging)
- Gram stain and culture wound drainage; 85% of bite wounds will yield a positive culture; most are polymicrobial.
- Obtain aerobic and anaerobic blood cultures before starting antibiotics if bacteremia is suspected.
- Plain radiograph or CT scan for suspected foreign body or bone or joint injury (Baseline imaging is also helpful for later comparison if osteomyelitis is suspected, especially in clenched-fist injuries.)

> **ALERT**
> Cat bites are twice as likely to become infected as dog bites and have higher risks of osteomyelitis, tenosynovitis, and septic arthritis.

Follow-Up Tests & Special Considerations
- Plain radiograph and/or MRI for suspected osteomyelitis
- CT scan for severe skull bites
- Ultrasound can detect abscess formation.
- If wound fails to heal, culture for atypical pathogens (e.g., fungi, *Nocardia*, and mycobacteria); keep bacterial cultures for 7 to 10 days (some pathogens are slow-growing).

Diagnostic Procedures/Other
Surgical exploration may be needed to determine the extent of injuries or to drain deep infections (e.g., tendon sheath), especially in severe hand wounds.

Test Interpretation
Most common microorganisms include the following:
- Dog bites (1)
  - *Pasteurella* spp. present in 50% of bites
  - Streptococci spp., *Staphylococcus aureus*, *Staphylococcus intermedius*, *Neisseria* spp. *Capnocytophaga canimorsus*, *Bacteroides* spp., *Fusobacterium* sp.
- Cat bites
  - *Pasteurella* spp. in 75% of bites
  - *Streptococcus* spp. (including *Streptococcus pyogenes*), *Staphylococcus* spp. (including methicillin-resistant *S. aureus* [MRSA]), *Neisseria* spp., *Moraxella* spp., *Porphyromonas* spp., *Fusobacterium* spp., *Bacteroides* spp.

- Human bites
  - *Eikenella corrodens* (15–29%), *Streptococcus* spp., *S. aureus* (including MRSA), and various anaerobic bacteria (e.g., *Fusobacterium*, *Peptostreptococcus*, *Prevotella*, and *Porphyromonas* spp.)
  - Although rare, case reports suggest transmission of viruses (hepatitis B/C, HIV, and herpes simplex).
- Aquatic bites
  - *S. aureus*, *Streptococcus* spp., *Vibrio* spp. (saltwater, brackish water), *Aeromonas* spp. (freshwater), *Mycobacterium* spp., *Pseudomonas* spp.
- Reptile bites
  - *Pseudomonas aeruginosa*, *Proteus* spp., *Salmonella*, *Bacteroides fragilis*, and *Clostridium* spp.
- Rodent bites
  - *Streptobacillus moniliformis* or *Spirillum minus*, which causes rat-bite fever
- Ungulate (hooved animal) bites
  - Pigs are the most likely to bite; commonly polymicrobial infections (*Staphylococcus* and *Streptococcus* spp, *Haemophilus influenzae*, *Pasteurella*, *Actinobacillus*, and *Flavobacterium* spp.)

> **ALERT**
> Asplenic patients and those with underlying hepatic disease are at risk for bacteremia and fatal sepsis after dog bites infected with *C. canimorsus*.

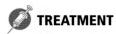

TREATMENT

GENERAL MEASURES
- Elevate the injured extremity to prevent swelling.
- Copious irrigation of the wound with normal saline via a catheter tip to reduce risk of infection
- Complete and submit bite report per local policy.
- Contact local health department to determine rabies prevalence in biting species: https://www.cdc.gov/rabies/resources/contacts.html

MEDICATION
- Prophylactic antibiotics are recommended only for human bites and high-risk wounds (deep puncture, crush injury, venous or lymphatic compromise, hands or near joint, face or genital area, immunocompromised hosts, requiring surgical repair, asplenic, advanced liver, edema).
- Duration of antibiotic therapy: preemptive, 3 to 5 days; treatment of cellulitis/skin abscess, 5 to 10 days
- Refer to the most common microbial organisms to determine appropriate antibiotic coverage for unusual animals.
- Determine the need for antirabies therapy: rabies immunoglobulin and rabies vaccine for those bitten by wild animals (primary vector in the United States is bat or raccoon), rabid pets, unvaccinated pets depending on detail of the incident, or in situations where the animal cannot be quarantined for 10 days.
- Consider tetanus toxoid (Td) for previously immunized with >10 years since their last dose (2)[C]; tetanus, diphtheria, and pertussis (Tdap) formulation is generally preferred to Td (2)[C].

> **ALERT**
> - Anti-HBs negative patients bitten by HBsAg-positive individuals should receive both hepatitis B immunoglobulin (HBIG) and hepatitis B vaccine.

- HIV postexposure prophylaxis is generally not recommended for human bites unless there is significant blood exposure to broken skin
- Snake bite: If venomous, transport for appropriate evaluation and antivenom; be sure the patient is stable for transport.
- Monkey bite: All monkey bites can transmit rabies; bites of macaque monkeys may transmit herpes B virus, which is potentially fatal. Contact CDC and consider an antiviral, such as valacyclovir, that is active against herpes B virus.

First Line
- For prophylactic and empiric antibiotic treatment, amoxicillin clavulanate is first-line antibiotic (2)[B].
  - Adults: amoxicillin and clavulanate 875/125 mg PO BID
  - Children: amoxicillin and clavulanate (dose is based on amoxicillin component) 45 mg/kg/day divided q12h; maximum of 875 mg per dose
- Patients with deep or severe wound infections, systemic infections requiring IV therapy, and the immunocompromised:
  - Adults: ampicillin and sulbactam 3 g IV q6h *or* piperacillin and tazobactam 3.375 g IV q6h (2)
  - Children: ampicillin and sulbactam (dose on ampicillin component) 200 mg/kg/day IV divided q6h; maximum of 3 g per dose

Second Line
- Alternative oral regimens
  - Adults: clindamycin (300 mg PO TID) plus either trimethoprim-sulfamethoxazole (TMP-SMX; 1 DS tablet PO BID) or ciprofloxacin (500 to 750 mg PO BID)
  - Children: clindamycin (25 to 30 mg/kg/day PO in 3 divided doses; maximum of 400 mg per dose) plus TMP-SMX (8 to 10 mg/kg/day of TMP PO in 2 divided doses; maximum of 160 mg TMP per dose)
- Alternative IV regimens
  - Adults: ciprofloxacin 400 mg IV q12h or levofloxacin 750 mg IV QD with metronidazole 500 mg IV q8h

ALERT
- Consider community-acquired MRSA as a possible pathogen (from human skin or colonized pet); if high suspicion, doxycycline or TMP-SMX provide good coverage.
- Avoid 1st-generation cephalosporins (e.g., cephalexin), penicillinase-resistant penicillins (e.g., dicloxacillin), and clindamycin (when not administered with another agent) because they lack activity against *Pasteurella multocida* (dog/cat bites) and *E. corrodens* (human bites).

Pregnancy Considerations
Pregnant women who cannot take penicillins or cephalosporins due to severe allergy: Consider azithromycin and observe closely due to increased risk of treatment failure.

ISSUES FOR REFERRAL
- Consider surgical consultation for deep, severe, or complex bite wounds.
- Deep wounds to the hand and face should be referred to a hand surgeon or plastic surgeon.
- Bites from primates or unusual species of animals should be referred to infectious disease specialist.

SURGERY/OTHER PROCEDURES
- Débride devitalized tissue; débridement of puncture wounds is not advised.
- Consider primary closure if the irrigated wound is clean, the bite is <12 hours old, and in bites to the face (cosmesis).
- Infected wounds and those at high risk for infection (cat bites, human bites, bites to the hand, crush injuries, presentation >12 hours from injury) should be left open.
- Delayed primary closure in 3 to 5 days is an option for infected wounds; large, gaping wounds should be reapproximated with widely spaced sutures or adhesive strips.

ADMISSION, INPATIENT, AND NURSING CONSIDERATIONS
Patients with deep or severe wound infections, systemic infections requiring IV therapy, and immunosuppression generally require inpatient admission.

 ## ONGOING CARE

FOLLOW-UP RECOMMENDATIONS
Patient Monitoring
- Recheck for infection in 24 to 48 hours.
- Base revisions of antibiotic therapy on culture results and clinical response.

PATIENT EDUCATION
Educate patients about how to be safe around animals and avoid animal bites.

PROGNOSIS
Wounds should improve and close over 7 to 10 days.

COMPLICATIONS
- Death (rare)
- Endocarditis
- Extensive soft tissue injuries with scarring, gas gangrene
- Hemorrhage
- Meningitis, osteomyelitis
- Posttraumatic stress disorder
- Sepsis, septic arthritis

REFERENCES

1. Baxter M, Denny KJ, Keijzers G. Antibiotic prescribing in patients who presented to the emergency department with dog bites: a descriptive review of current practice. *Emerg Med Australas.* 2020;32(4):578–585.
2. Stevens DL, Bisno AL, Chambers HF, et al. Practice guidelines for the diagnosis and management of skin and soft tissue infections: 2014 update by the Infectious Disease Society of America. *Clin Infect Dis*. 2014;59(2):e10–e52.

ADDITIONAL READING

Elcock KL, Reid J, Moncayo-Nieto OL, et al. Biting the hand that feeds you: management of human and animal bites. *Injury*. 2022;53(2):227–236.

 ## SEE ALSO

Bartonella Infections; Cellulitis; Rabies

CODES

ICD10
- S61.459A Open bite of unspecified hand, initial encounter
- S01.85XA Open bite of other part of head, initial encounter
- S20.97XA Other superficial bite of unspecified parts of thorax, initial encounter

CLINICAL PEARLS
- Cleanse, débride, and culture animal and human bites.
- Antibiotic prophylaxis is recommended for human bites and high-risk wounds.
- Consider rabies and tetanus vaccination.
- Animal and human bites require close follow-up to assess for signs of infection or other complications.

BLADDER CANCER

Jon S. Parham, DO, MPH, FAAFP • Sandra N. New, DNP

BASICS

A primary cancer tumor originating in cells lining the urinary bladder lumen

DESCRIPTION
- Bladder cancer (BC) cell types: urothelial carcinoma (formerly named transitional cell) and others (squamous cell and adenocarcinoma)
  - Urothelial carcinoma comprises >90% of all cases in the USA and Europe.
- The spectrum BC relates to tumor penetration into muscularis propria layer or not:
  - Nonmuscle invasion (NMIBC)
  - Muscle invasion (MIBC)
  - Metastatic disease (MIBC plus spread beyond the bladder)
- Very rarely, uroepithelial carcinoma or rhabdomyosarcoma of the bladder in children

EPIDEMIOLOGY
Primarily white men aged >55 years who smoke tobacco

Incidence
- Estimated 4.2% of all new cancer cases in 2023
- Increases with age (median age at diagnosis is 73 years)
- Two times more common in Whites than in other races
  - Incidence rate in Asia is predicted to rise 74% from 2020 to 2024, compared to 52% in North America.
- Male > female (3 to 4:1); but in smokers, risk is 1:1.
  - Fourth most common cancer in men and the eighth most common cause of cancer death in United States
  - Lifetime risk: 1 in 28 for men, 1 in 91 for women
  - Women are diagnosed in more advanced stages than men (hematuria mimicking gynecologic illnesses).
- Decreased incidence rate primarily in men in 2004–2020
- 15.8/100,000 new cases age-adjusted rate for all in 2020, the United States

Prevalence
- Lifetime risk is 2.3% overall based on 2017–2020 data in United States.
- In 2020, 725,549 cases in the United States, far exceeding the population of Wyoming or Vermont.

ETIOLOGY AND PATHOPHYSIOLOGY
Unknown, other than related to risk factors
- 70% is nonmuscle invasive, longer survival.
- 30% of tumors are muscle invasive at presentation, prognosis worse.

Genetics
- Same-sex, monozygotic twins have 10% increase risk.
- Patient with Lynch syndrome has up to 20% lifetime risk due to altered DNA mismatch repair genes.

RISK FACTORS
- Male sex
- Advanced age, greatest single risk factor, due to prolonged exposure time to risky substances
- Tobacco smoking is the single greatest modifiable risk factor.

- 50% cases attributed to personal smoking.
- Secondhand tobacco smoke exposure or e-cigarettes contain carcinogenic compounds.
- Other risk factors:
  - Occupational exposures to benzidine; magenta, auramine dyes; aluminum and rubber production; certain paints, plastics, carbon black dust (printing ink), petroleum, and diesel exhaust; and soot from chimneys
  - Arsenic exposure in drinking water
  - History of bladder radiation, pelvic irradiation, or certain chemotherapy drugs like cyclophosphamide or ifosfamide
  - Chronic lower UTI or chronic indwelling urinary catheter
  - Pioglitazone (diabetes), aristolochic acid (herbal supplement), cyclophosphamide, and chlornaphazine

ALERT
Microscopic (≥3 RBC/hpf) or gross hematuria found in a smoker needs cystoscopy and axial upper tract imaging, regardless of anticoagulation or antiplatelet status, unless there is a documented UTI with urgency and frequency that responds to UTI treatment or if related to a gynecologic or other non-malignant genitourinary cause.

GENERAL PREVENTION
- Avoid tobacco smoke exposure.
- https://www.cdc.gov/tobacco/quit_smoking/index.htm or 800-QUIT NOW (800-784-7669)
- Counseling of avoidance in individuals with risky occupational exposure
- Prompt follow-up for individuals with hematuria, regardless of anticoagulation or antiplatelet status

DIAGNOSIS

HISTORY
- Painless hematuria: most common symptom of BC
  - 4% BC risk with microhematuria; 16.5% BC risk with gross hematuria (1)[C]
- Urinary symptoms persisting (frequency, urgency, dysuria, decreased urine flow)
- Occupational exposures or pelvic radiation
- Chemotherapy with cyclophosphamide or ifosfamide
- Abdominal or pelvic pain in advanced disease
- Prolonged indwelling urinary catheter

PHYSICAL EXAM
Normal in early cases; pelvic or abdominal mass in advanced disease; wasting in systemic disease

DIFFERENTIAL DIAGNOSIS
- UTI; nephrolithiasis
- Noninfectious hemorrhagic cystitis
- Urinary tract trauma; renal cell carcinoma
- Interstitial cystitis/nephritis
- Papillary urothelial hyperplasia
- Other urinary tract neoplasms

DIAGNOSTIC TESTS & INTERPRETATION
Core testing: Urinalysis/microscopy, cystoscopy, upper tract imaging

Initial Tests (lab, imaging)
- Urinalysis with microscopy in patients with gross or microscopic hematuria or irritating urinary symptoms
- Cystoscopy and axial upper tract imaging in all with hematuria, except in the presence of a benign cause or low risk, asymptomatic, microhematuria patients with shared decision-making to repeat urinalysis with microscopy in 6 months
- Endoscopic transurethral resection of bladder tumor (TURBT) is diagnostic for histologic grade, tumor depth, and possibly therapeutic. Repeat TURBT needed in 4 to 6 weeks in certain stages or if detrusor muscle is not sampled.
- Renal ultrasound may be used with low- and intermediate-risk microscopic hematuria patients
- Urogram (CT or MRI) if gross hematuria or high-risk microhematuria, or renal ultrasound or retrograde pyelogram (1)[C]
- Because tumor invasion of detrusor muscle is poorly seen in regular CT urography, dual energy CT recommended then
- T2-weighted and functional sequenced MRI views are most revealing if obtained before TURBT or at least 2 weeks after TURBT.
- MRI without contrast can be used in special situations:
  - Severe renal dysfunction or severe contrast allergy
  - Detrusor muscle invasion seen poorly on CT, or if need to avoid radiation (2)[C]
- Urine cytology for gross hematuria or posttreatment follow-up is low in sensitivity (37%) but high in specificity (95%).
- Urine tumor markers are NOT accurate enough to replace cystoscopy.
- Enhanced cystoscopy, narrowband or blue light types improved sensitivity and specificity in diagnosis and resection (1)[B]

Follow-Up Tests & Special Considerations
Vesicle imaging-reporting and data system (VI-RADS) reports a schemata for multiparametric MRI.
- Sensitivity: 83–90%, specificity: 90–97% with level 3 as threshold
- Estimating likelihood of tumor invasion of muscle wall
- Diffusion-weighted and dynamic-contrast enhanced MRI and dual-energy spectral CT scan are options for use in diagnosis and staging of bladder tumors (2)[C].
- For invasive disease, metastatic workup should include chest x-ray and PET scan.
- For metastatic disease suspicion:
  - Liver function tests and alkaline phosphatase (AP) blood testing
  - Nuclear medicine bone scan if the patient has bone pain or if AP is elevated.

Test Interpretation
- TURBT: characterized as superficial (NMIBC) or invasive (MIBC)
- Superficial cancer (70%)
  - Ta: noninvasive papillary carcinoma, low grade, tend to recur
  - Tis: CIS; flat lesion, high grade
  - T1: extends into submucosa, lamina propria; usually high grade

- Invasive cancer (30%)
  - T2: invasion into: muscle, superficial (pT2a); deep (pT2b)
  - T3: invasion into: perivesical fat, microscopic (pT3a); macroscopic (pT3b)
  - T4: invasion into adjacent organs
    - T4a: invades prostate, uterus, vagina, or bowel
    - T4b: invades abdominal wall, pelvic wall, or other organs
- N1–N3: invades lymph nodes
- M: metastasis to bone or soft tissue (1)[C]

 ## TREATMENT

- NMIBC, risk group:
  - Low:
    - Solitary Ta ≤3 cm diameter
      - Primary: TURBT: enhanced cystoscopy, in <24 hr single-dose chemotherapy (1)[B], reject adjuvant intravesical therapy, may fulgurate small lesions (1)[C]
  - Intermediate:
    - Recurrence <1 year, low-grade Ta, or solitary low-grade Ta >3 cm diameter, or multifocal low-grade Ta, or high-grade Ta ≤3 cm diameter, or low-grade T1
    - Primary: TURBT: enhanced cystoscopy, in T1 restage TURBT at 4 to 6 weeks, <24 hours single-dose chemotherapy, or consider induction intravesical therapy (chemotherapy or bacille Calmette-Guérin [BCG]) (1)[B], or do maintenance chemotherapy or BCG for 1 year in responders (1)[C]
    - Alternatives: if persistent or recurrent disease/cytology after intravesical therapy, do prostatic urethra and upper tract evaluation; or offer repeat induction course of BCG; or pembrolizumab in BCG-failure patients or offer clinical trial (1)[C]
  - High:
    - T1 high-grade; or any high-grade recurrent Ta; or Ta >3 cm high-grade or multifocal; or any carcinoma in situ (CIS); or any high-grade disease, BCG failure; or any variant histology; or any lymphovascular invasion (LVI); or any prostatic urethral involvement that is high-grade
    - Primary: TURBT: enhanced cystoscopy (1)[B]; in high-grade Ta restage TURBT at 4 to 6 weeks (1)[C], or in T1 restage TURBT at 4 to 6 weeks, or induction BCG, or in responders, maintenance BCG for 3 years (1)[B]
    - Alternatives: Consider radical cystectomy in high-grade T1 persistently or T1 with variant histology, LVI, or CIS; or recurrent or persistent disease after intravesical therapy do prostatic urethra evaluation; offer second BCG induction course; or if failed BCG, use pembrolizumab; or offer clinical trial (1)[C].
- MIBC, nonmetastatic: primary and alternative treatment
  - Cisplatin ineligible: initial radical cystectomy
  - Cisplatin eligible: neoadjuvant cisplatin-based chemotherapy (i.e., dose-dense methotrexate), vinblastine, doxorubicin, and cisplatin (ddMVAC) or gemcitabine plus cisplatin followed by radical cystectomy or chemoradiation and concurrent maximal TURBT
  - If patient declines primary, alternative is partial cystectomy or in ideal patients, maximal TURBT.

- MIBC, metastatic: primary and alternative treatment:
  - Cisplatin ineligible: If tumor expresses PD-L1 or patient is ineligible for any platin-based therapy, try atezolizumab/pembrolizumab; or if negative PD-L1, try combination carboplatin-based chemotherapy; or gemcitabine with or without paclitaxel; or ifosfamide, gemcitabine, doxorubicin.
  - Cisplatin eligible: chemotherapy (gemcitabine + cisplatin vs. ddMVAC)
  - Alternative treatment:
    - Postplatinum failure: pembrolizumab (preferred); or atezolizumab versus nivolumab versus durvalumab versus avelumab; or erdafitinib
    - Postplatinum and checkpoint inhibitor immunotherapy failure: enfortumab vedotin (1)[C]

MEDICATION
See above listed treatment, by category

ISSUES FOR REFERRAL
Microscopic hematuria, delayed referral to urologist

ADDITIONAL THERAPIES
Radiosensitization in BCG-unresponsive NMIBC may have a role to preserve bladder (2)[C].

SURGERY/OTHER PROCEDURES
Surgery is definitive therapy:

- Superficial cancer: TURBT
- Invasive cancer: radical cystectomy, full pelvic lymphadenectomy and exenteration, plus urine diversion
- Meticulous lymph node dissection is prognostic, therapeutic, and essential in curative treatment (1)[B].

 ## ONGOING CARE

FOLLOW-UP RECOMMENDATIONS
- NMIBC
  - Urine cytology alone has NOT been shown to be sufficient for follow-up.
  - Low risk: cystoscopy at 3 to 4 months, 6 to 9 months, then annually for 5 years; no upper tract imaging, no urinary biomarkers if normal cystoscopy
  - Intermediate/high risk: cystoscopy with cytology at 3 to 4 months, then each 3 to 6 or 4 months for 2 years, then each year/6 months ongoing; upper tract imaging each 1 to 2 years; urinary biomarker may indicate response to BCG or to resolve equivocal cytology
- Follow-up for invasive cancers depends on the metastasis and approach to treatment but involves cystoscopy (if no cystectomy), urine cytology, advanced imaging urography or renal ultrasound in years 5 to 10, chest imaging (x-ray or CT), FDG-PET/CT (if no metastasis), serum laboratory tests (1)[C].

Patient Monitoring
BCG patients require lifelong follow-up.

DIET
Continue adequate fluid intake.

PATIENT EDUCATION
- Smoking cessation, occupational exposures
- Cancer.NET: https://www.cancer.net/cancer-types/bladder-cancer

PROGNOSIS
- Death rates, 2016–2020, men 7.1, women 2 per 100,000 age-adjusted to 2000 U.S. standard population
- NMIBC
  - 5-year relapse-free survival at risk level: low, 43%; intermediate, 33%; high, 23%
  - 5-year progression-free survival at risk level: low, 93%; intermediate, 74%; high, 54%
  - BCG treatment decreases risk of recurrence and progression in high-risk superficial lesions (1)[B].
- MIBC and advanced BC
  - Nonmetastatic: 36–48% overall survival rate at 5 years
  - Metastatic disease: regional, 36%; distant, 5% relative survival rate at 5 years (1)[C]

COMPLICATIONS
Neobladder patients at risk for azotemia (absorption of ammonium chloride) and metabolic acidosis (bicarb loss) (1)[C]

REFERENCES
1. Lenis AT, Lec PM, Chamie K, et al. Bladder cancer: a review. *JAMA*. 2020;324(19):1980–1991.
2. Compérat E, Amin MB, Cathomas R, et al. Current best practice for bladder cancer: a narrative review of diagnostics and treatments. *Lancet*. 2022;400(10364):1712–1721.

ADDITIONAL READING
Jubber I, Ong S, Bukavina L, et al. Epidemiology of bladder cancer in 2023: a systematic review of risk factors. *Eur Urol*. 2023;84(2):176–190.

 ## SEE ALSO

- Hematuria
- Algorithm: Hematuria

 ## CODES

ICD10
- C67.8 Malignant neoplasm of overlapping sites of bladder
- C67 Malignant neoplasm of bladder
- C67.6 Malignant neoplasm of ureteric orifice

CLINICAL PEARLS
- Painless hematuria should be evaluated with cystoscopy when there is no benign explanation, especially in non–low-risk, patient, regardless of anticoagulation or antiplatelet use.
- The U.S. Preventive Services Task Force does NOT recommend routine screening for BC.

BORDERLINE PERSONALITY DISORDER

Daniel John Majarwitz, MD • Parvathi Perumareddi, DO

 BASICS

DESCRIPTION

Borderline personality disorder (BPD) is a psychiatric disorder characterized by a consistent and pervasive pattern of emotional dysregulation including: distorted sense of self, rapidly labile mood, unstable sense of self, impulsivity, and volatile or chaotic interpersonal relationships. It is often manifested during adolescence but is typically diagnosed in early adulthood (1).

- Diagnostic criteria must include at least five of the following (1),(2):
  - Significant discordant sense of identity and values
  - Unstable interpersonal relationships including "splitting," alternating between idealizing and devaluing
  - Impulsive behavior including excessive spending, substance abuse, unsafe sex, binge-eating, precipitous driving, or other reckless behaviors (need at least two domains, does not include self-mutilation as separate category below)
  - Recurrent suicidal actions or threats, including self-harm
  - Chronic feelings of emptiness
  - Extreme, out of proportion anger, or difficulty managing anger
  - Rapid and intense emotional shifts (usually hours)
  - Dissociative symptoms or paranoia, often transient and associated with stress
  - Frantic efforts to avoid perceived abandonment
- Patients may overuse of emergency department services due to nature of symptoms.
  - Overuse of emergency department services

EPIDEMIOLOGY

Onset during adolescence or early adulthood; however, may go undiagnosed for years

Prevalence

- 1.6% of general population (1),(2)
- 6% of primary care population
- 10% of outpatient psychiatric visits
- 20% of inpatient psychiatric milieu

ETIOLOGY AND PATHOPHYSIOLOGY

Undetermined but generally accepted that BPD is multifactorial in etiology including (1),(2),(3):

- Genetic transmission
- Environmental factors (i.e., history of childhood sexual and/or physical abuse, history of childhood neglect, ongoing conflict in home, maladaptive parenting styles)
- Neuroimaging studies have shown hyperactivity of the amygdala, decreased prefrontal cortex activation, and decreased brain volumes/white matter connectivity in frontal and limbic structures.
- Dysregulation of various neurotransmitter systems, including serotonin, oxytocin, and endogenous opiates, may also play a role.

Genetics

First-degree relatives are at greater risk for this disorder (1).

RISK FACTORS

- Childhood trauma, that is, sexual and/or physical abuse and neglect
- Lack of secure parental attachment beginning in early childhood
- External social stressors may exacerbate BPD.

GENERAL PREVENTION

Children, caregivers, and significant others should have some time and activities away from the borderline individual and set strict boundaries, which may protect their well-being.

COMMONLY ASSOCIATED CONDITIONS

High rate of associated comorbid psychiatric disorders such as depression, anxiety, panic disorder, and substance abuse (1),(2)

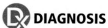 **DIAGNOSIS**

- A starting screening test may include McLean Screening instrument for BPD (2)
- The comprehensive evaluation should identify:
  - Comorbid conditions
  - Functional impairments
  - Adaptive/maladaptive coping styles

- Psychosocial stressors
- Patient strengths
- Patient needs/goals

HISTORY

- Obtain collateral information (i.e., from family, partner) about patient behaviors.
- History of interpersonal difficulties, affective instability, and impulsivity
- History of self-injurious behavior, possibly with suicidal threats or attempts

PHYSICAL EXAM

- Perform a physical exam and consider laboratory workup as indicated.
- Rule out personality changes due a physiologic etiology from a medical condition.
- Physical exam may show signs of self-mutilation such as cutting or burning.

DIFFERENTIAL DIAGNOSIS

- Mood disorders:
  - Screen for or differentiate between generalized anxiety disorder, depression, PTSD, and/or substance abuse.
- Psychotic disorder
  - Though auditory and visual hallucinations may be present (1), they typically are in the context of situational crises and are not accompanied by disordered thoughts, bizarre delusions, flat affect, or other negative symptoms.
- Attention deficit hyperactivity disorder (ADHD)
- BPD has more severe emotional dysregulation with rapid mood cycling.
- General medical conditions (GMCs)
- Substance use disorder (SUD)

DIAGNOSTIC TESTS & INTERPRETATION

- Consider age of onset—to meet criteria for BPD, borderline pattern of behaviors will be present from adolescence or early adulthood.
- Formal psychological testing
- Rule out personality change due to a medical condition (1)[C].

Initial Tests (lab, imaging)

Can consider obtaining labs such as Thyroid-stimulating hormone (TSH) and urine drug screen to rule out GMC and SUD

Diagnostic Procedures/Other

According to *Diagnostic and Statistical Manual of Mental Disorders, 5th edition, Text Revision* (*DSM-5-TR*) criteria, patients must meet at least five of the nine criteria, present in various situations, and with symptoms starting in early adulthood. The criteria are listed in the "Description" section earlier (1)[C].

 ## TREATMENT

- Dialectical behavioral therapy (DBT) psychotherapy for BPD appears to be the most established treatment, although other psychotherapy modalities have shown some benefit (3)[C]:
  - DBT combines cognitive behavioral techniques for emotional regulation and processes including distress tolerance, acceptance, and self-awareness.
- Other empirically supported treatments to consider include transference-focused (psychodynamic) psychotherapy, cognitive behavioral therapy (CBT), mentalization, schema-focused therapy, and mindfulness-based therapies.
- It is important to note that BPD is not curable and often requires longitudinal therapy.

GENERAL MEASURES

Focus on patient management rather than on "fixing" behaviors:

- Schedule consistent appointment follow-ups to alleviate patient anxiety.
- Use team-based communication to avoid splitting of team by patient and to be aware of the potential for splitting.
- Set appropriate boundaries for communication and expectations between the provider and patient.
- Treatment is usually most effective when consistent psychotherapy is used.
- Medications may aid in symptom management if comorbid conditions are present.

MEDICATION

- Although no specific medications are approved by the FDA to treat BPD, pharmacotherapy can be used for symptom management and to help with comorbid psychiatric disorders (3)[A].
  - Antidepressants appear to have the least benefit on BPD symptoms compared to antipsychotics and mood stabilizers.

- There is some evidence for the use of second-generation antipsychotics (SGAs), including aripiprazole and olanzapine, to target specific BPD symptoms, including mood dysregulation, psychotic-like symptoms, and anger. However, effects such as cardiometabolic changes may limit use.
- There is some evidence for the use of mood stabilizers, including valproic acid, lamotrigine, and topiramate, for managing specific symptom domains of BPD; however, a larger systematic review stated insufficient evidence.
- There is some evidence for the use of omega-3 fatty acids, especially on depressive symptoms.
- The overall evidence in support of use of psychopharmacologic interventions is minimal, with no evidence showing overall improvement of BPD severity. Future studies are needed to continue to assess the efficacy of such medications.
- Consider risk of self-harm and suicidal behavior when prescribing.

ADMISSION, INPATIENT, AND NURSING CONSIDERATIONS

- Hospitalizations should be limited and of short duration to adjust medications, implement psychotherapy for crisis intervention, and stabilize patients from psychosocial stressors.
- Extended inpatient hospitalization should be considered for the following reasons:
  - Persistent/severe suicidal ideation or risk of harm to others
  - Comorbid substance use and/or nonadherence to outpatient or partial hospitalization treatments
  - Severe comorbid disorders (i.e., eating disorders, mood disorders)

 ## ONGOING CARE

FOLLOW-UP RECOMMENDATIONS

- Schedule visits that are short, more frequent, and focused to relieve patients' anxiety about relationships with their physician/provider and to help reduce risk of provider burnout.
- Emphasize importance of healthy lifestyle modifications (i.e., exercise, rest, sleep, nutrition, stress management).

Patient Monitoring

Monitor for suicidal ideation/behaviors or other self-harm behaviors.

PATIENT EDUCATION

Include patients in the treatment plan so that they are aware of their behavior and its impact.

PROGNOSIS

Borderline behaviors may decrease with age.

REFERENCES

1. American Psychiatric Association. *Diagnostic and Statistical Manual of Mental Disorders*. 5th ed., text rev. Arlington, VA: American Psychiatric Association; 2022.
2. Mendez-Miller M, Naccarato J, Radico JA. Borderline personality disorder. *Am Fam Physician*. 2022;105(2):156–161.
3. Nathan PE, Gorman JM. *A Guide to Treatments That Work*. Oxford University Press: 2015.

CODES

ICD10

F60.3 Borderline personality disorder

CLINICAL PEARLS

- BPD is a chronic condition with one of the characteristic features being mood dysregulation in which individuals react out of proportion to stressors, often stemming from a lack of self-identity and a feeling of emptiness.
- Clear boundaries should be established with the treatment team.
- Pharmacology is not the mainstay of treatment, whereas frequent psychotherapy (such as DBT) sessions can be useful.

BRAIN INJURY, TRAUMATIC

Corey J. Costanzo, DO, MPH, MS

BASICS

DESCRIPTION
- Traumatic brain injury (TBI) is defined as an alteration in brain function caused by an external force.
- System(s) affected: neurologic; psychiatric; cardiovascular; endocrine/metabolic; gastrointestinal; pulmonary
- Synonym(s): head injury, concussion

EPIDEMIOLOGY
Incidence
- 801,700 ED visits and 326,600 hospitalizations per year in the United States
- 61,000 deaths per year; ~30% of all injury-related deaths

ETIOLOGY AND PATHOPHYSIOLOGY
- Centers for Disease Control and Prevention (CDC) TBI data in 2017, mechanism of injury of hospitalized patients (male vs. female percentage)
  - Unintentional falls (35.6 vs. 23.9)
  - Motor vehicle crashes (22.5 vs. 10.8)
  - Unintentionally being struck by or against an object (2.3 vs. 0.9)
  - Intentional self-harm (0.8 vs. 0.3)
  - Assault (7.5 vs. 1.7)
  - Children aged 0 to 17 years
    - Falls (7.7)
    - Motor vehicle crashes (6.8)
- Contact sports account for 45% of TBI emergency room visits for children related to sports and recreation.
- Mechanical damage with actuation of complex cellular and molecular cascades that promote cerebral edema, ischemia, and apoptotic cell death

RISK FACTORS
Alcohol and drug use, prior/recurrent head injury, contact sports, seizure disorder, ADHD, male sex

Geriatric Considerations
Subdural hematomas (SDH) are common after a fall or blow in elderly; symptoms may be subtle and not present until days after trauma.

GENERAL PREVENTION
- Safety education and fall prevention
- Seat belts; bicycle and motorcycle helmets
- Protective headgear for contact sports

Pediatric Considerations
Child abuse: Consider if dropped or fell <4 feet (e.g., off bed, couch), suspicious history, significant injury present, or any retinal hemorrhages.

DIAGNOSIS

HISTORY
- Loss of consciousness (LOC), headache, vomiting, amnesia, confusion, dizziness, sensitivity to light
- Epidural hemorrhage from blunt trauma: 30% with a "lucid interval" (initial LOC followed by recovery of consciousness and then LOC recurs and persists)

PHYSICAL EXAM
- Neurologic and cognitive testing is important.
- Repeat neurologic exams every 30 minutes until 2 hours after Glasgow Coma Scale (GCS) reaches 15, then hourly for 4 hours, and then every 2 hours.
- Evidence of increased intracranial pressure (ICP) (elevated BP, decreased pulse rate, or slow/irregular breathing [Cushing triad]—only 30% have all three)
- Signs of basilar skull fracture: raccoon eyes, Battle sign, hemotympanum, CSF rhinorrhea or otorrhea

DIFFERENTIAL DIAGNOSIS
Other causes of altered mental status (e.g., toxicologic, infectious, metabolic, vascular)

DIAGNOSTIC TESTS & INTERPRETATION
Initial Tests (lab, imaging)
- Mild TBI and concussions cognitive screening tests
- Evaluate for coagulopathy.
- Perform drug and alcohol screening.
- Noncontrasted head CT is the study of choice to review bone windows, tissue windows, and subdural space.

Pediatric Considerations
Skull radiographs are not indicated unless abuse is suspected, in which case they can detect fractures not seen under CT; no return to activity until they are asymptomatic and return to school should precede return to sport/physical activity

TREATMENT

GENERAL MEASURES
Acute management depends on injury severity. Most patients need no interventions.

- Immediate goal: Determine who needs further therapy, imaging studies (CT), and hospitalization to prevent further injury.
- For the mildly injured patient
  - Early education is beneficial for recovery.
  - Graduated return to cognitive and physical activity when there are no evident signs or symptoms (physical, cognitive, emotional, or behavioral) on neuropsychological and clinical evaluation

- For the moderate to severely injured patient
  - Avoid hypotension or hypoxia. Head injury causes increased ICP secondary to edema, and cerebral perfusion pressure (CPP) should be maintained between 60 and 70 mm Hg (1)[A].
  - 30-degree head elevation decreases ICP and improves CPP.
  - Hyperventilation (hypocapnia) for patients with impending herniation while preparing for definitive treatment or intraoperatively
  - Mild systematic hypothermia lowers ICP but leads to increased rates of pneumonia.
  - 3% hypertonic saline and mannitol effectively reduce ICP.
- Seizure prophylaxis with phenytoin or levetiracetam for 1 week postinjury or longer for patients with early seizures, dural-penetrating injuries, multiple contusions, and/or SDHs requiring evacuation

MEDICATION
First Line
- Individuals with severe brain injuries who can't communicate may benefit from using the Nociception Coma Scale (NCS) to assess pain.
- Increased ICP
  - Hypertonic saline: 2 mL/kg IV decreases ICP without adverse hemodynamic status; preferred agent
  - Mannitol: 0.25 to 2.0 g/kg (0.25 to 1.0 g/kg in children) given over 30 to 60 minutes in patients with adequate renal function. Prophylactic use is associated with worse outcomes.
- Sedation
  - Propofol: preferred due to short duration of action; avoid high doses to prevent propofol infusion syndrome. When combined with morphine, it can also effectively decrease ICP and decrease use of other medications.
  - Midazolam: similar sedating effect to propofol but may cause hypotension
- Seizures
  - Phenytoin (Dilantin): 15 mg/kg IV (1 mg/kg/min IV, not to exceed 50 mg/min); stop infusion if QT interval increases by >50%.

ALERT
Avoid corticosteroid use because it increases mortality rates and risk of developing late seizures.

ISSUES FOR REFERRAL
Consult neurosurgery for penetrating head trauma, abnormal head CT that meet BIG-3 criteria as discussed in "Admission, Inpatient, and Nursing Considerations" section.

SURGERY/OTHER PROCEDURES

- Early evacuation of trauma-related intracranial hematoma decreases mortality especially with GCS <6 and CT evidence of hematoma, cerebral swelling, or herniation.
- CSF drainage reduces ICP but has not been demonstrated to have a long-term benefit.
- CSF leakage often resolves in 24 hours with bed rest, but if not, it may require surgical repair.

COMPLEMENTARY & ALTERNATIVE MEDICINE

Music therapy in conjunction with multimodal stimulation improves awareness in comatose TBI patients.

ADMISSION, INPATIENT, AND NURSING CONSIDERATIONS

TBI severity can be defined by the Brain Injury Guidelines as BIG-1, BIG-2, or BIG-3. Criteria and therapeutic plan listed below (2):

- BIG-1:
  - Normal neurologic exam
  - Not intoxicated
  - Any of the following non-contrast CT head findings: SDH <4 mm, epidural hematoma (EDH) <4 mm, intraparenchymal hemorrhage (IPH) <4 mm in one location, traced subarachnoid hematoma (SAH), no intraventricular hemorrhage (IVH)
  - No skull fracture
  - Negative history of anticoagulation or antiplatelet use
  - Repeat neurologic physical exam check every 2 to 4 hours.
  - Observation for 6 hours, only repeat head noncontrast CT for neurologic changes; otherwise, no need for repeat head CT.
  - Can be discharged if neurologic exam at baseline after 6-hour observation
  - Neurosurgical consultation is not required.
- BIG-2:
  - Normal neurologic exam
  - Any of the following noncontrast CT head findings: SDH 5 to 7 mm, EDH 5 to 7 mm, IPH 3 to 7 mm in two locations, localized SAH, no IVH
  - Nondisplaced skull fracture
  - Negative history of anticoagulation or antiplatelet use
  - Repeat neurologic exam every 2 hours.
  - Inpatient admission is required.
  - Only repeat head noncontrast CT for neurologic changes; otherwise, no need for repeat head CT.
  - Neurosurgical consultation is not required.

- BIG-3:
  - Abnormal neurologic exam
  - Any of the following noncontrast CT head findings: SDH >8 mm, EDH >8 mm, IPH >8 mm in multiple locations, scattered SAH, presence of IVH
  - Displaced skull fracture
  - Positive history of anticoagulation or antiplatelet use
  - Repeat neurologic exam hourly.
  - Inpatient admission is required; consider ICU admission.
  - Neurosurgery consult required
- C-spine immobilization should be considered in all head trauma.
- Use normal saline for resuscitation fluid.

 ONGOING CARE

FOLLOW-UP RECOMMENDATIONS

- Schedule regular follow-up within a week to determine return to activities.
- Rehabilitation indicated following a significant acute injury; set realistic goals.
- For patients on anticoagulants, net benefit to restarting therapy after discharge despite increased bleeding risk
- Screen for depression and PTSD after TBI as the prevalence of these conditions are higher in those with history of TBI (3).

PATIENT EDUCATION

Patient should be discharged to the care of a competent adult with clear instructions on signs and symptoms that warrant immediate evaluation (e.g., changing mental status, worsening headache, focal findings, or any signs of distress). Patients should be monitored but not awakened from sleep.

PROGNOSIS

- Gradual improvement may continue for years.
- Mortality rate for TBI is 30 per 100,000 annually in the United States.
- Poor prognostic factors: low GCS on admission, nonreactive pupils, old age, comorbidity, midline shift, nonambulatory
- 50% of patients with mild TBI will return to work by 1 month after injury and >80% by 6 months.

COMPLICATIONS

- Chronic SDH, which may follow even "mild" head injury, especially in the elderly; often presents with headache and decreased mentation
- Seizures: incidence of late seizures after TBI, >30 years is 2% for mild injuries, 4% for moderate injuries, and >15% for severe injuries

REFERENCES

1. Tsang KK, Whitfield PC. Traumatic brain injury: review of current management strategies. *Br J Oral Maxillofac Surg*. 2012;50(4):298–308.
2. Joseph B, Obaid O, Dultz L, et al; for AAST BIG Multi-institutional Study Group. Validating the brain injury guidelines: results of an American Association for the Surgery of Trauma prospective multi-institutional trial. *J Trauma Acute Care Surg*. 2022;93(2):157–165.
3. McCrory P, Meeuwisse W, Dvořák J, et al. Consensus statement on concussion in sport—the 5th international conference on concussion in sport held in Berlin, October 2016. *Br J Sports Med*. 2017;51(11):838–847.

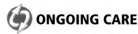 CODES

ICD10

- S06.9X0A Unsp intracranial injury w/o loss of consciousness, init
- S06.5X0A Traum subdr hem w/o loss of consciousness, init
- S06.6X0A Traum subrac hem w/o loss of consciousness, init

CLINICAL PEARLS

- TBI involves two distinct phases: the primary mechanical insult and secondary dysregulation of the cerebrovascular system with cerebral edema, ischemia, and cell-mediated death.
- Indications for imaging include evidence of skull fracture, altered consciousness, neurologic deficit, persistent vomiting, scalp hematoma, abnormal behavior, coagulopathy, and age >65 years.

BREAST ABSCESS

Kelley V. Lawrence, MD, IBCLC • Emily Valentin-Mendez, MD • Lauren A. Griffin, DO

 BASICS

DESCRIPTION
- Breast abscess: localized accumulation of infected fluid within the breast parenchyma
- Mastitis: breast inflammation with or without infection; this can be associated with lactation (puerperal) or nonlactational.
- Associated with lactation or fistulous tracts secondary to squamous epithelial neoplasm or duct occlusion
- System(s) affected: skin/exocrine, immune
- Synonym(s): mammary abscess; peripheral breast abscess; subareolar abscess; puerperal abscess

Pregnancy Considerations
Most commonly associated with postpartum lactation

EPIDEMIOLOGY
- Most common benign breast problem during pregnancy and puerperal period (1)
- Predominantly reproductive age and perimenopausal (between ages 18 and 50 years)
  - Puerperal abscess: lactational
  - Subareolar abscess: reproductive age through postmenopause (2)
    - 90% of nonlactational breast abscesses are subareolar (1).
- Predominant sex: female
- Higher incidence in African American, diabetic, tobacco use, or obese women

Incidence
Ranges between 3% and 11% of women with mastitis (1),(3)

Prevalence
Transient condition usually as a complication of mastitis; mastitis prevalence ranges between 1% and 10% (1).

ETIOLOGY AND PATHOPHYSIOLOGY
- Puerperal abscesses:
  - Associated with hyperlactation and dysbiosis (disrupted milk microbiome); these can lead to ductal narrowing and inflammation and subsequently to reduced milk flow, obstruction, plugged lactiferous duct causing stasis, microbial growth, and infection (3).
  - Mammary dysbiosis is a consequence of multiple factors including genetic, breastfeeding-related, medical, and microbial (3).
  - Likely that bacteria (often from infants oral flora) gain entry through cracks/fissures in the nipple (1)
  - Insufficient treatment of mastitis
  - Unattended postpartum engorgement and other situations leading to breast milk stasis (3)
- Subareolar abscess:
  - Associated with squamous metaplasia of the lactiferous duct epithelium, keratin plugs, ductal ectasia, and fistula formation (2)

- Microbiology
  - *Staphylococcus aureus* is the most common cause of lactational abscesses (1),(2).
  - Methicillin-resistant *S. aureus* (MRSA) is a significant cause (1).
  - Other common causes include coagulase-negative staphylococci and *Streptococcus* spp. (2),(3).
  - Less common causes (1):
    - *Escherichia coli*, *Enterobacteriaceae*, *Corynebacterium*, and *Pseudomonas*
    - Anaerobes
    - May be polymicrobial

Genetics
Maternal genetics may play a role as protective and predisposing factors for mammary dysbiosis, which is associated with the pathophysiology (3).

RISK FACTORS
- Smoking, maternal age >30 years
- Primiparous, pregnancy ≥41 weeks' gestation
- Diabetes and obesity
- African American
- Nipple piercing
- Milk stasis:
  - Infrequent or missed feeds
  - Poor latch, weak or uncoordinated suckling
  - Damage or irritation of the nipple, nipple inversion or retraction
  - Inefficient removal of milk (by baby or pump), oversupply of milk
  - Illness in mother or baby, rapid weaning, plugged duct
  - Pressure on the breast (i.e., tight bra, car seatbelt)
  - Maternal stress and fatigue
- Medically related risk factors
  - Steroids
  - Breast implants
  - Lumpectomy with radiation
  - Inadequate antibiotics to treat mastitis
  - Topical antifungal medication used for mastitis

GENERAL PREVENTION
- Frequent breast emptying with on-demand feeding and/or pumping to prevent mastitis
- Early treatment of mastitis with milk expression, antibiotics, and compresses
- Smoking cessation to minimize occurrence/recurrence

COMMONLY ASSOCIATED CONDITIONS
Lactation, mastitis, weaning

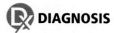 **DIAGNOSIS**

HISTORY
- Tender breast lump, usually unilateral
- Breastfeeding, weaning, or returning to work
- Decreased breast milk supply on affected breast
- Perimenopausal/postmenopausal
- Systemic malaise (usually less than with mastitis)
- Localized erythema, warmth, edema, pain
- Fever, nausea, vomiting
- Spontaneous nipple drainage
- Prior breast infection
- Diabetes
- Smoking
- Recent or recurrent mastitis

PHYSICAL EXAM
- Fever, tachycardia (not always present)
- Erythema of overlying skin
- Palpable mass, sometimes fluctuant
- Tenderness on palpation
- Induration
- Local edema
- Draining pus or skin ulceration
- Nipple and/or skin retraction
- Regional lymphadenopathy
- Puerperal abscesses are generally peripheral; nonlactational abscesses are more commonly found in periareolar/subareolar region.

DIFFERENTIAL DIAGNOSIS
- Engorgement, plugged milk duct, mastitis
- Galactocele (sometimes referred to as a milk lake)
- Fibrocystic breasts
- Fat necrosis
- Tuberculosis (may be associated with HIV infection), sarcoid; granulomatous mastitis
- Syphilis
- Foreign body reactions (e.g., to silicone and paraffin)
- Mammary duct ectasia
- Carcinoma (inflammatory or primary squamous cell)

DIAGNOSTIC TESTS & INTERPRETATION
Initial Tests (lab, imaging)
- Ultrasound helps identify fluid collection (1),(3).
- Elevated WBC, elevated ESR
- Culture of expressed breast milk or aspirate to identify pathogen
  - The presence of pathogenic bacteria or high bacteria count (e.g., > 10^3/mL) indicates mastitis; low predictive value; clinical context is needed (1)[C],(3).

Follow-Up Tests & Special Considerations
Mammogram to rule out malignancy (generally not done during acute phase)

Diagnostic Procedures/Other
- Aspiration (+/− ultrasound guided) for culture
  - Can be diagnostic and therapeutic
  - Does not exclude malignancy
  - Cytology (particularly in nonlactating patient)
- Mammography has limited value in the acute assessment of breast abscesses or mastitis (1)[C].

Test Interpretation
- Abscesses on ultrasound can be hypoechoic, well-circumscribed, and/or macrolobulated (1)
  - If ultrasound is negative for pocket of fluid, consider alternative diagnoses.
  - If multiloculated on imaging, refer to breast surgical/interventional specialist.
- Use culture sensitivities to guide antibiotic therapy when possible.

 TREATMENT

GENERAL MEASURES
- Cold and/or warm compresses for pain control (3)[C]
- Continue to breastfeed or express milk to drain the affected breast (3)[A].
- Drainage of abscess with antibiotics; without drainage, antibiotics are ineffective (2),(3)[A].
  - Acceptable to start antibiotics while working to get patient to drainage/aspiration

MEDICATION
First Line
- Drainage for source control and culture; adjust antibiotics if indicated based on culture and sensitivities (2)[C].
- First line for nonsevere and no MRSA risk factors (3)[C]:
  - Dicloxacillin or flucloxacillin 500 mg QID for 10 to 14 days
  - Cephalexin 500 mg QID for 10 to 14 days
- If risk factors for MRSA, including past MRSA infection, recent hospitalization in the last 12 months, antibiotic use in the last 6 months, or severe β-lactam hypersensitivity (3)[C]:
  - Clindamycin 300 to 450 mg PO TID for 10 to 14 days
  - Trimethoprim-sulfamethoxazole (TMP-SMZ) 1 to 2 tabs PO BID for 10 to 14 days
- Mothers should continue breastfeeding (3)[A].

Second Line
- Clindamycin 300 mg QID for 10 to 14 days (3)[C]
- TMP-SMZ DS BID for 10 to 14 days (3)[C]
  - Not recommended for mothers of children with G6PD deficiency; use with caution in mothers with premature infants or infants with hyperbilirubinemia, especially <30 days old.
- Consult infectious disease specialist if inadequate response to antibiotic treatment plus drainage.

ISSUES FOR REFERRAL
If showing signs of hemodynamic instability, patient should be referred for inpatient stabilization and care (rare).

ADDITIONAL THERAPIES
- NSAIDs for analgesia, anti-inflammatory effect, and/or antipyresis (3)[B]
- Rest, adequate fluid intake, good nutrition (3)[B]
- Application of heat to the breast just prior to feeding/milk expression may help with adequate milk flow (3)[C].
- Cold packs applied after a feeding/milk expression can reduce pain and edema (3)[C].

SURGERY/OTHER PROCEDURES
- Current best practice recommendation suggests:
  - Aspiration (using 18- to 21-gauge needle) with or without ultrasound guidance for abscesses <3 cm (1),(2)[B] (Serial aspirations may be necessary.)
    - Ultrasound-guided aspiration of breast abscess is preferred to incision and drainage (I&D) in most cases due to better cosmesis and faster recovery.
  - Consider ultrasound-guided percutaneous catheter placement if abscess >3 cm (2)[B].
  - Consider I&D using a no. 15 blade scalpel if abscess is >5 cm, recurrent, or chronic (2)[B].
- Biopsy nonpuerperal abscesses to rule out malignancy; remove all fistulous tracts in nonlactating patients as well (2)[C].

COMPLEMENTARY & ALTERNATIVE MEDICINE
- Lecithin supplementation
- Probiotics
- Acupuncture may help with breast engorgement and prevention of breast abscess.
- Breast lymphatic massage may ease engorgement.
- Judicious use of cabbage leaves applied over affected area (to decrease inflammation and milk production)

ADMISSION, INPATIENT, AND NURSING CONSIDERATIONS
- Outpatient, unless systemically immunocompromised, septic, or requiring inpatient antibiotic treatment
- Hospital-grade breast pump should be made available to patient from time of admission.

 ONGOING CARE
- If lactating, continue effective milk removal to prevent recurrence.
- If planning to wean from breastfeeding, avoid abrupt discontinuation of feeding.
- Consider smoking cessation to decrease risk of nonlactational abscess recurrence.

FOLLOW-UP RECOMMENDATIONS
Patient Monitoring
- Ensure complete resolution to exclude malignancy.
- Close outpatient follow-up until resolution as abscesses may require serial aspirations or drainage

DIET
No dietary patterns have been associated with breast abscess formation; however, these can affect the microbiome (3).

PATIENT EDUCATION
- Wound care, rest, breast milk emptying
- Continue with breastfeeding or pumping (if breastfeeding is not possible due to location of abscess; infant mouth not to come in contact with affected tissue) to prevent engorgement.

PROGNOSIS
- Drained abscess heals from inside out (in 8 to 10 days).
- Subareolar abscesses frequently recur, even after I&D and antibiotics; may require surgical removal of ducts

COMPLICATIONS
- Fistula: mammary duct or milk fistula
- Poor cosmetic outcome
- Early cessation of breastfeeding

REFERENCES
1. Boakes E, Woods A, Johnson N, et al. Breast infection: a review of diagnosis and management practices. *Eur J Breast Health*. 2018;14(3):136–143.
2. Lam E, Chan T, Wiseman SM. Breast abscess: evidence based management recommendations. *Expert Rev Anti Infect Ther*. 2014;12(7):753–762.
3. Mitchell KB, Johnson HM, Rodríguez JM, et al; for the Academy of Breastfeeding Medicine. Academy of Breastfeeding Medicine Clinical Protocol #36: the mastitis spectrum, revised 2022. *Breastfeed Med*. 2022;17(5):360–376.

CODES

ICD10
- N61 Inflammatory disorders of breast
- O91.13 Abscess of breast associated with lactation
- O91.12 Abscess of breast associated with the puerperium

CLINICAL PEARLS
- Up to 11% of cases of puerperal mastitis progress to abscess formation (most often due to inadequate therapy).
- Risk factors for mastitis and breast abscess include a combination of genetic, microbial, breastfeeding, and medical factors.
- Treat abscesses not associated with lactation with antibiotics that cover anaerobic bacteria and work up for malignancy.
- The treatment of choice for most breast abscesses is the combination of antibiotics plus aspiration.
- Ultrasound-guided aspiration of breast abscess is preferred to I&D in most cases due to better cosmesis and faster recovery.
- If abscess is <5 cm, surgical I&D is recommended.
- If lactating, continue to empty the breast (feeding, pumping, or expression of breast milk).

BREAST CANCER

Anne Campbell Larkin, MD

BASICS

Most commonly diagnosed cancer (CA) in women and the second most common cause of CA death for U.S. women; females have a ~2.5% or 1 in 39 chance of dying from breast cancer (BC) in the United States.

DESCRIPTION
- Malignant neoplasm of cells native to the breast—epithelial, glandular, or stroma
- Types: ductal carcinoma in situ (DCIS), infiltrating ductal carcinoma, infiltrating lobular carcinoma, Paget disease, phyllodes tumor, inflammatory BC, angiosarcoma
- Molecular subtypes: luminal A (ER+/PR+/HER2−), triple negative (ER−/PR−/HER2−), luminal B (ER+/HER−), luminal B-like (ER+/HER2+), HER2-enriched (ER−/PR−/HER2+)

EPIDEMIOLOGY
Incidence
Estimated in 2023: ~297,790 new cases of invasive BC, ~55,720 DCIS; ~43,700 deaths from BC in U.S women; increased by ~0.5% per year since mid-2000s

Prevalence
>3.8 million BC survivors in the United States (1)

ETIOLOGY AND PATHOPHYSIOLOGY
- Genes such as *BRCA1* and *BRCA2* function as tumor suppressor genes, and mutation leads to cell cycle progression and limitations in DNA repair.
- Mutations in estrogen/progesterone induce cyclin D1 and *c-Myc* expression, leading to cell cycle progression.
- Additional tumors (33%) may cross talk with estrogen receptors and epidermal growth factor receptors (EGFRs), leading to similar abnormal cellular replication.

Genetics
- Criteria for additional risk evaluation/gene testing in affected BC individual
  - BC at age ≤50 years
  - BC at any age and
    - ≥1 family member with BC (≤50 years of age or in men) or ovarian/fallopian tube/primary peritoneal CA at any age
    - ≥2 family members with BC or pancreatic CA any age
    - Population at increased risk (e.g., Ashkenazi Jewish descent)
  - Triple-negative BC (ER−, PR−, HER2−)
  - Second primary BC (not recurrence of first), ovarian/fallopian tube/primary peritoneal CA
  - ≥1 family member with BC and CA of thyroid, adrenal cortex, endometrium, pancreas, central nervous system (CNS), diffuse gastric, aggressive prostate (Gleason score of >7), leukemia, lymphoma, sarcoma, dermatologic manifestations, and/or macrocephaly, gastrointestinal (GI) hamartomas
  - Male BC
- Criteria for additional risk evaluation/gene testing in unaffected BC individual
  - First- or second- relative with BC ≤45 years of age
  - ≥2 breast primaries in one individual
  - ≥1 ovarian/fallopian tube/primary peritoneal CA from same side of family
  - ≥2 with breast primaries on same side of family
  - ≥1 family member with BC and CA of thyroid, adrenal cortex, endometrium, pancreas, CNS, diffuse gastric, aggressive prostate, leukemia, lymphoma, sarcoma, dermatologic manifestations, and/or macrocephaly, GI hamartomas

- Ashkenazi Jewish descent with BC/ovarian CA at any age
  - Male BC
- 5–10% of BCs are associated with genetic mutations and are thus hereditary.
  - *BRCA1* and *BRCA2* are inherited in an autosomal fashion and account for
  - Syndromes associated with BC: Cowden syndrome (PTEN), Li-Fraumeni syndrome (TP53), ataxia-telangiectasia (ATM), and Peutz-Jeghers (STK11), hereditary diffuse gastric CA (CDH1); other BC genes include PALB2 and CHEK2.

RISK FACTORS
- National Cancer Institute Breast Cancer Risk Assessment Tool. https://bcrisktool.cancer.gov
- Female sex; increased age
- Hormone replacement therapy (combination estrogen-progesterone and estrogen only agents [but not vaginal estrogen]) during perimenopause increases BC risk for 10 years after medication is discontinued.
- Age >65 years, biopsy confirmed atypical hyperplasia, DCIS, lobular carcinoma in situ (LCIS)
- *BRCA* mutation, Ashkenazi Jewish descent
- Personal or family history of BC at a younger age
- Postmenopausal
- History of radiation or diethylstilbestrol (DES) exposure (especially at a young age)
- Increased alcohol use
- Proliferative breast disease without atypia (fibroadenoma or ductal hyperplasia)
- Dense breasts (>50%)
- Reproductive factors
  - Nulliparous, no history of full-term pregnancy or breastfeeding
  - Early menarche (<12 years old), late menopause (>55 years old), first pregnancy at >35 years old
- Obesity
- Tall stature
- History of endometrial or ovarian CA

GENERAL PREVENTION
- Maintain healthy weight/body mass index (BMI)—obesity increases BC risk.
- Limit alcohol use—≤1 serving of alcohol per day is recommended.
- High serum 25-OH vitamin D levels correlate with lower BC risk; consider vitamin D supplementation.
- Medication: U.S. Preventive Services Task Force (USPSTF) recommends that clinicians offer to prescribe risk-reducing medications, such as tamoxifen, raloxifene, or aromatase inhibitors (AIs), to women who have a >3% risk for BC and low risk for adverse medication effects (B grade recommendation).
- Breast self-exams (BSEs): no longer recommended
- Clinical breast exam (CBE): USPSTF: insufficient evidence to assess clinical benefits and harms; American Cancer Society (ACS): no clear benefit
- Mammography (MMG):
  - USPSTF: Women should undergo biennial mammogram starting at age 40 years until age 74 years (B grade recommendation).
  - ACS: Women annual mammograms starting at age 45 to 54 years and then women >55 years old biennial mammograms or yearly screening if desired (1); age 40 to 44 years, optional mammograms yearly

COMMONLY ASSOCIATED CONDITIONS
- Li-Fraumeni and Cowden disease
- History of atypical ductal hyperplasia (ADH), atypical lobular hyperplasia (ALH), and LCIS
- Obesity

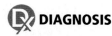

DIAGNOSIS

HISTORY
- Painless lump in breast or axilla; swelling, thickening, redness, or dimpling of the skin
- Nipple discharge (serous, serosanguineous, or bloody), erosion, or retraction

PHYSICAL EXAM
- Visualize breasts with patient sitting and supine looking for skin dimpling, peau d'orange, and asymmetry.
- Palpation of all four breast quadrants and regional lymph node exam: cervical, supraclavicular, infraclavicular, axillary

DIFFERENTIAL DIAGNOSIS
- Benign breast disease:
  - Fibrocystic disease, fibroadenoma
  - Intraductal papilloma (bloody nipple discharge), duct ectasia
  - Simple cyst, galactocele
  - Sclerosing adenosis, fat necrosis (history of serial/parallel breast trauma)
- Infection: abscess, cellulitis, mastitis

DIAGNOSTIC TESTS & INTERPRETATION
Initial Tests (lab, imaging)
- MMG Breast Imaging–Reporting and Data System (BI-RADS): BI-RADS is a quality assurance (QA) method published by the American College of Radiology.
  - BI-RADS has been extended to breast US and MRI interpretation as well.
  - Components of BI-RADS report:
    - Overall breast composition, including breast density
      - A—breasts are almost entirely fatty tissue; B—scattered areas of fibroglandular density; C—heterogenously dense; D—extremely dense
  - Final BI-RADS assessment category:
    - BI-RADS 0: incomplete; additional imaging evaluation needed and/or prior imaging for comparison
      - Commonly occurs on screening studies
    - BI-RADS 1: negative; continue with current screening guidelines.
    - BI-RADS 2: benign; no further action needed
    - BI-RADS 3: probably benign, possibility of malignancy is ≤2%
      - Follow-up imaging in 6 months for 1 year; consider imaging every 6 to 12 months for 2 to 3 years.
      - Can consider biopsy if patients is anxious or follow-up is uncertain
    - BI-RADS 4: suspicious—Patient and clinician should discuss possible management plans and likely a biopsy.
    - BI-RADS 5: highly suggestive of malignancy, possibility of malignancy ≥95%—diagnostic imaging needed with follow-up and biopsy
    - BI-RADS 6: known biopsy—proven malignancy; includes patients with biopsy-proven CAs that have yet to be surgically removed

- Calcifications on screening MMG requires diagnostic mammogram (Dx MMG) and stereotactic-guided biopsy.
- Palpable masses on exam should be evaluated with Dx MMG and US ± biopsy.
  - Palpable mass ≥30 years: Obtain Dx MMG and US to determine cystic versus solid.
    ○ If BI-RADS 1 to 3, then get US ± biopsy. If BI-RADS 4 to 6, then get core needle biopsy ± surgical excision.
- Palpable mass <30 years: Obtain US ± Dx MMG ± biopsy; if low clinical suspicion, observe for 1 to 2 menstrual cycles for resolution.
- Spontaneous, reproducible nipple discharge: Obtain Dx MMG ± US; if negative, then consider ductogram or MRI ± surgical excision.
- Asymmetric thickening/nodularity <30 years: Obtain US ± Dx MMG ± biopsy.
- Asymmetric thickening/nodularity ≥30 years: Obtain Dx MMG + US ± biopsy.
- Skin changes, peau d'orange: Obtain Dx MMG ± US ± biopsy for underlying mass; if no mass, then perform punch biopsy of skin change.
- Palpable lymph nodes: Obtain CT scan of chest, abdomen/pelvis, and bone scan.
- All newly diagnosed BC should be offered multidisciplinary care including genetic and fertility counseling.

Follow-Up Tests & Special Considerations
- Advanced disease (stage IIIA or higher): chest CT, abdominal ± pelvis CT, FDG positron emission tomography (PET)/CT scan, bone scan or sodium fluoride PET/CT if FDG-PET/CT indeterminate
- Breast MRI if: indeterminant BC (particularly in dense breasts), invasive BC not captured on mammographic projections
- Most common metastasis: lungs, liver, bone, brain
- Bone scan if localized bone pain or elevated alkaline phosphate
- Abdominal ± pelvis CT if abdominal symptoms, elevated alkaline phosphate, abnormal LFTs
- Chest CT if pulmonary symptoms present
- Brain/spine MRI if CNS/spinal cord symptoms

Diagnostic Procedures/Other
- Primary tumor: fine-needle aspiration (FNA), US-guided core needle biopsy, stereotactic-guided core-needle biopsy, MRI-guided biopsies for abnormalities only visualized on breast MRI
- US of axillary lymph nodes during workup and core-needle biopsy or FNA if suspicious nodes are identified

Test Interpretation
Surgical pathology results should note ductal/lobular/other, tumor size, inflammatory component, invasive/noninvasive, margins, nodal involvement, and tumor receptor status: ER, PR, HER2 assay.

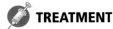 TREATMENT

MEDICATION
- Neoadjuvant chemotherapy: locally advanced (large tumor and/or positive lymph nodes), early operable BC to facilitate breast conservation surgery, triple negative BC and tumor size >0.5 cm, HER2 (+) tumors ≥2 cm with positive lymph nodes
- Consider 21-gene PT-PCR assay in ER/PR(+) tumors with (−) nodes to potentially assess risk of recurrence; not validated to predict chemotherapy response; can determine if chemotherapy indicated in the adjuvant setting

- Cytotoxic therapy: anthracyclines, taxanes, alkylating agents, antimetabolites: higher risk patients with nonmetastatic operable tumors, patients with high risk of recurrence after local treatment (status post surgery ± radiation)
- Dose-dense chemotherapy demonstrates overall survival advantage in early BC: doxorubicin/cyclophosphamide (AC) weekly or every 2 weeks paclitaxel for HER2 negative BC.
- Anti-HER2/neu antibody (e.g., trastuzumab with or without pertuzumab) in HER2/neu-positive patients; given with other chemotherapy agents in the neoadjuvant or adjuvant setting

ISSUES FOR REFERRAL
Cardiology for trastuzumab-induced cardiomyopathy

ADDITIONAL THERAPIES
- Radiation therapy (RT)
  - Upon completion of surgery ± chemotherapy, whole breast radiation should be offered for patients undergoing breast conservation therapy (BCT) prior to starting endocrine therapy.
  - Postmastectomy RT is offered if tumor >5 cm, ≥1 lymph nodes are involved, chest wall/skin involvement, unable to obtain clear margins.
- ASA once per week
- General prevention for high-risk lesions (LCIS, ALH, ADH); tamoxifen 20 mg QD for 5 years
- Hormone therapy for ER+ tumors
  - DCIS:
    ○ Tamoxifen 200 mg QD for 5 years
    ○ Age <60 years and postmenopausal: may consider use of AIs
    ○ Age >60 years: selective estrogen receptor modulator (SERM) or AI equally effective
  - Invasive CA:
    ○ SERM (tamoxifen 20 mg QD): premenopausal at diagnosis: 5-year treatment and consider for additional 5 years; avoid during lactation, pregnancy, or with history of deep venous thrombosis/pulmonary embolism.
    ○ AIs (anastrozole 1 mg QD, letrozole 2.5 mg QD, and exemestane 25 mg QD): postmenopausal women, 5-year treatment following endocrine therapy for 4.5 to 6 years, or endocrine therapy for up to 10 years
    ○ Ovarian ablation or suppression with luteinizing hormone–releasing hormone agonists: premenopausal women
- Neoadjuvant endocrine therapy should be continued following surgery as adjuvant endocrine therapy.
- Advanced disease: hormone and cytotoxic therapy, bisphosphonates, anti-vascular endothelial growth factor (anti-VEGF) antibody, anti-HER2/neu antibody in select HER2/neu-positive patients
- Incomplete response to neoadjuvant therapy: Administer adjuvant capecitabine or ado-trastuzumab emtansine if pembrolizumab was used in the neoadjuvant setting

Pregnancy Considerations
- Mastectomy or breast conservation: BCT can be offered at any point in pregnancy but may require delay in adjuvant RT with sentinel lymph node biopsy (SLNB)
- Lymphoscintigraphy is safe in pregnancy with radioactive colloid alone.
- Chemotherapy: appropriate in 2nd and 3rd trimesters; trastuzumab contraindicated; RT: avoid until after delivery

SURGERY/OTHER PROCEDURES
- Breast-conserving therapy (lumpectomy) offered if negative margins and the patient will also receive adjuvant RT.
- Mastectomy indicated for multicentric disease, large tumor to breast size ratio, inflammatory BC, T4 disease, contraindication to RT, and/or patient preference
- Axillary nodes: preoperative US and biopsy for all patients with axillary nodes; if biopsy is positive, axillary node dissection

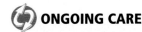 ONGOING CARE

FOLLOW-UP RECOMMENDATIONS
- Every 4 to 6 months for 5 years and then annually
- No evidence for routine complete blood count, LFTs, "tumor markers," bone scan, chest x-ray, liver US, CT scans, MRI, PET
- Mammogram 6 to 12 months postsurgery or postradiation then annually
- Annual pelvic exam on endocrine therapy; bone mineral density at baseline and follow-up when on AIs or with ovarian failure secondary to treatment

PROGNOSIS
5-year relative survival (SEER 18, all races, females): localized 99%, regional 86%, distant 30%, all stages 91%

COMPLICATIONS
- Surgery: lymphedema, wound infections, seroma, hematoma, chronic pain, limited range of motion, poor cosmesis
- Chemotherapy: immunosuppression, neuropathy, cardiotoxicity
- Radiation: skin breakdown, fibrosis, chronic pain, long-term increased risk of malignancy
- Endocrine therapy: osteoporosis, endometrial CA, and deep venous thrombosis

REFERENCE
1. American Cancer Society. About breast cancer. https://www.cancer.org/cancer/breast-cancer/about.html. Accessed January 26, 2023.

 CODES

ICD10
- C50.52 Malignant neoplasm of lower-outer quadrant of breast, male
- C50.929 Malignant neoplasm of unspecified site of unspecified male breast
- C50.812 Malignant neoplasm of overlapping sites of left female breast

CLINICAL PEARLS
- U.S. women; 1 in 8 develop BC in within their lifetime, of those 1 in 3 become metastatic
- Alcohol consumption, high BMI after menopause, and physical inactivity are modifiable risk factors of BC.
- Normal MMG does not exclude the possibility of CA with a palpable mass.

BREASTFEEDING

Angelia Leipelt, BA, IBCLC, ICCE, CLE • Ronald G. Chambers Jr., MD, FAAFP

BASICS

- Breastfeeding/chestfeeding is the natural process of feeding human milk directly from the breast.
- Breast milk is the preferred nutritional source and the normal and physiologic way to feed all newborns and infants.
- Breast milk contains over 200 active components which provide nutrition, fight pathogens, promote healthy gut microbiome, and aid in maturity of immune system.
- The American Academy of Pediatrics (AAP), the American Academy of Family Physicians (AAFP), and the American Congress of Obstetricians and Gynecologists (ACOG) recommend exclusive breastfeeding for 6 months, with continuation of breastfeeding for ≥2 year as desired by birth parent and infant (1).

DESCRIPTION

- Maternal benefits (as compared with those who do not breastfeed/chestfeed) include the following:
  - Rapid involution/decreased postpartum bleeding
  - Decreased risk of postpartum depression and increased bonding
  - Postpartum weight loss
  - Decreased risk of breast cancer and association of decreased risk of pre- and postmenopausal ovarian cancer (2), decreased risk of type 2 diabetes, hypertension, hyperlipidemia, rheumatoid arthritis, and cardiovascular disease
  - Decreased risk of prematurity
  - Increased bone density
- Infant benefits include the following:
  - Ideal food: easily digestible, nutrients well absorbed, less constipation
  - Lower rates of virtually all infections via maternal antibody protection
    ○ Fewer respiratory and GI infections
    ○ Decreased risk of ear infections, bacterial meningitis, pneumonia, and sepsis
    ○ Decreased incidence of otitis media and necrotizing enterocolitis
  - Decreased incidence of obesity and type 1 and 2 diabetes
  - Decreased incidence of allergies, clinical asthma, and atopic dermatitis in childhood
  - Decreased risk of developing celiac disease and inflammatory bowel disease
  - Decreased risk of childhood leukemia
  - Decreased risk of sudden infant death syndrome (SIDS)
  - Enhanced neurodevelopmental performance including intelligence (3)
  - Increased attachment between birth parent and baby

EPIDEMIOLOGY

Incidence

- According to CDC's Breastfeeding Scorecard, U.S. breastfeeding rates are on the rise in 2019: any breastfeeding: 83.2% (however, differs among different sociodemographic and culture)
- Breastfeeding at 6 months: 55.8%
- Breastfeeding at 12 months: 35.9%
- Exclusive breastfeeding at 3 months: 45.3%
- Exclusive breastfeeding at 6 months: 24.9%

ETIOLOGY AND PATHOPHYSIOLOGY

- The mechanism of milk production is based on several hormones: Prolactin triggers milk production and oxytocin releases milk based on supply and demand. Endocrine control system triggers making of colostrum at 5 months' gestation.
- Alveoli make milk in response to hormone prolactin. Sucking stimulates secretion of prolactin, which triggers milk production.
- Stimulation of areola causes secretion of oxytocin. Oxytocin is responsible for let-down reflex when myoepithelial cells contract and milk is ejected into milk ducts.
- Endocrine/metabolic: Cystic fibrosis, diabetes, galactosemia, phenylketonuria, and thyroid dysfunction may cause delayed lactation or decreased milk.

GENERAL PREVENTION

Most vaccinations can be given to breastfeeding mothers, including COVID-19 immunization. The CDC recommends that the diphtheria-tetanus-acellular pertussis, hepatitis B, inactivated influenza virus (as opposed to live attenuated), measles-mumps-rubella (MMR), and inactivated polio and varicella vaccines can be given. The CDC recommends avoiding the yellow fever or smallpox vaccine in breastfeeding mothers.

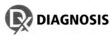 DIAGNOSIS

PHYSICAL EXAM

Breast/chest examination during pregnancy; assess for scars, lumps, or flat/inverted nipples. Confirm history of infertility, endocrine disorders, breast and hormonal pathology, overall health and psychosocial concerns, perinatal complications, and previous breastfeeding problems.

ALERT

A breast lump should be followed to complete resolution or worked up if present and not just attributed to changes from lactation.

 TREATMENT

GENERAL MEASURES

Breast/chest feeding initiation

- Initiate breast/chest feeding immediately after birth, ideally placing the infant naked on birth parent's chest uninterrupted skin-to-skin *in first hour.*
- As baby opens wide, bring baby close, tucking baby in "belly to belly." Line baby's nose to nipple, baby tilts its head back with wide-open mouth, bring baby close as baby latches to ensure baby's gum takes in more of the areola.
- Baby's lips are flanged, rounded cheeks, no clicking or popping sounds, and absence of nipple pain when latched.
- Feed baby 2 to 8 times for the first 24 hours and 8 or more times per 24 hours, feeding 10 or more minutes.
- Observation of a nursing session by an International Board Certified Lactation Consultant (IBCLC), nurse, or experienced physician

- Avoid supplementation with infant formula or water and/or artificial nipples unless medically indicated.
- Contraindications to breastfeeding are few (WHO).
  - Maternal HIV (in industrialized world) or human T-cell leukemia virus (HTLV) infection
  - Active untreated tuberculosis
  - Active herpes simplex virus (HSV) lesions on the breast
  - Substances of abuse without evaluation and discontinuation of use
  - Review medications that will pass into human milk.
  - Infants with galactosemia or maple syrup urine disease should not be fed with breast milk. Infants with phenylketonuria may be fed breast milk under close observation.
  - Mothers who develop varicella 5 days before through 2 days after delivery
  - Suspected or confirmed Ebola virus disease
  - Maternal hepatitis is *not* a contraindication.

ISSUES FOR REFERRAL

- Refer to IBCLC, experienced nurse, or physician for inpatient and/or outpatient teaching.
- Frequent follow-up if having problems with latching, nipple/breast pain, breast infection, overactive let down, oversupply or inadequate milk production

COMPLEMENTARY & ALTERNATIVE MEDICINE

Galactagogues

- Metoclopramide, domperidone, fenugreek, goat's rue, and milk thistle have mixed results in improving milk production, but efficacy and safety data are lacking in literature.

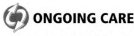 ONGOING CARE

FOLLOW-UP RECOMMENDATIONS

See mother and baby within 3 to 5 days of hospital discharge, especially if first time breastfeeding.

- Risk factors for suboptimal initiation
  - Breast surgery or reduction surgery prior to pregnancy may disrupt breast milk production.
  - Severe postpartum hemorrhage may lead to Sheehan syndrome associated with difficulty breastfeeding due to poor milk production.
  - Other factors: delivery mode, duration of labor, gestational age, maternal infection, parity, culture, birth parent–baby separation, maternal anxiety, use of artificial nipple or use of non–breast milk fluids

Patient Monitoring

- Monitor maternal breast milk supply concerns.
- Monitor infant's weight, behavior, and output closely.
- Supplementation with pumped milk and/or infant formula if infant has lost ≥10% of birth weight.
- Supplementation without persistent breast stimulation with frequent feedings or breast pump use will decrease milk production and decrease breastfeeding success.

DIET

- For chestfeeding/breastfeeding parent:
  - Healthy choices from protein-rich foods, vegetables, fruits, and whole grains; drink plenty of fluids to satisfy thirst and optimal hydration.
  - Breastfeeding/chestfeeding parent may require ~500 more calories per day.
  - Limit caffeine to <300 mg/day.
  - Alcohol should be avoided. Possible long-term effects of alcohol in maternal milk remain unknown.
- For infants:
  - In 2008, the AAP increased its recommended daily intake of vitamin D for infants from 200 to 400 IU. For exclusively breastfed babies, this will require taking a vitamin supplement, such as Poly-Vi-Sol or Vi-Daylin vitamin drops, 0.5 mL/day, beginning in the first few days of life.
  - In 2010, the AAP recommended adding supplementation for breastfed infants with oral iron of 1 mg/kg/day, beginning at age 4 months.
    - Preterm infants fed by human milk should receive an iron supplement of 2 mg/kg/day by 1 month of age, and this should be continued until the infant is weaned to iron-fortified formula or begins eating complementary foods that supply the 2 mg/kg of iron.

PATIENT EDUCATION

- Support measures to normalize breastfeeding have been shown to be successful with respect to infant/child and maternal health outcomes.
  - Emphasize the importance of exclusive breastfeeding for the first 6 weeks of life to allow adequate buildup of sufficient milk supply.
  - Regular promotion of the advantages of breastfeeding/risks of not breastfeeding
- Milk usually transitions to mature milk about 3–5 days postpartum.
- Signs of adequate nursing
  - Baby feeding on demand (8 to 12 feedings per 24 hours by day 2)
  - Baby should have 6 to 8 wet diapers per day and 3 to 4 bowel movements per day by day 6 to 8.
  - Proper latching and positioning
  - Baby satisfied; appropriate weight gain (average of 1 oz/day in first few months)
- Weaning
  - Solid food may be introduced at 4 months with continuation of breastfeeding.
  - Breast/chest-feeding parent returning to work/school should begin alternative feeding methods 1 to 2 weeks prior. Initiate breast pumping plan.
- Family planning
  - Options include lactational amenorrhea method (LAM), barrier methods, implants, medroxyprogesterone (Depo-Provera), oral contraception, and intrauterine devices (IUDs). ACOG recommends that progesterone-only pills be used 2 to 3 weeks postpartum and that medroxyprogesterone (Depo-Provera), IUDs, combined OCPs, and etonogestrel implant (Implanon) can be used 6 weeks, postpartum.
  - Monitor for changes in milk supply after starting a contraceptive.

COMPLICATIONS

- Breast milk jaundice should be considered if jaundice persists for >1 week in an otherwise healthy, well-hydrated newborn. It peaks at 10 to 14 days.
- Plugged duct
  - Mother is well except for sore lump in one or both breasts and is without fever. Use moist, hot packs on lump prior to, and during, nursing; more frequent nursing on affected side
- Mastitis (see "Mastitis")
  - Sore lump in one or both breasts plus maternal fever and/or redness on skin overlying lump
  - Use warm or cool compress on lump prior to nursing to reduce pain and inflammation.
  - Antibiotics covering for *Staphylococcus aureus* (most common organism)
  - Other possible sources of fever should be ruled out, that is, endometritis and pyelonephritis.
  - Mother should get increased rest; use acetaminophen (Tylenol) PRN.
  - Fever should resolve within 48 hours or consider changing antibiotics. Lump should resolve. If it continues, an abscess may be present, requiring surgical drainage.
- Milk supply inadequate
  - Review health concerns; breast changes; infant weight loss; signs of adequate supply; technique, frequency, and duration of nursing; or use of non-breast milk fluids.
- Sore nipples
  - Check technique and improve latch-on.
  - Baby should be taken off the breast by breaking the suction with a finger in the mouth.
  - Check for signs of thrush in baby and on mother's nipple. If affected, treat both.
  - Check for evidence of ankyloglossia (tongue-tie) in the infant. Correction of ankyloglossia may lead to decreased nipple soreness and improved breastfeeding.
  - Nipple bleb (a blister on the nipple that can be filled with serous fluid or another fluid) due to improper positioning; moist heat and improve latching techniques.
- Flat or inverted nipples
  - When stimulated, inverted nipples will retract inward; flat nipples remain flat; check for this on initial prenatal physical. Assess latch if using nipple shield to aid in latching and review rationale for use with breastfeeding.
- Engorgement
  - Develops after milk transitions by day 3 or 4, resolves within a day or 2
  - Signs are warm, hard, sore breasts.
    - Frequent nursing; breastfeed long enough to empty breasts.
    - Pump to relieve discomfort.
    - Explore reasons for ongoing problems.

REFERENCES

1. Johnston M, Landers S, Noble L, et al. Breastfeeding and the use of human milk. *Pediatrics*. 2012;129(3):e827–e841.
2. Westerfield KL, Koenig K, Oh R. Breastfeeding: common questions and answers. *Am Fam Physician*. 2018;98(6):368–373.
3. Horta BL, Loret de Mola C, Victora CG. Breastfeeding and intelligence: a systematic review and meta-analysis. *Acta Paediatr*. 2015;104(467):14–19.

ADDITIONAL READING

- American Academy of Pediatrics, American College of Obstetricians and Gynecologists. *Breastfeeding Handbook for Physicians*. 3rd ed. Elk Grove Village, IL: American Academy of Pediatrics; 2023.
- Mitchell KB, Johnson HM, Rodríguez JM, et al. Academy of Breastfeeding Medicine clinical protocol #36: the mastitis spectrum, revised 2022. *Breastfeed Med*. 2022;17(5):360–376.
- National Library of Medicine. *Drugs and lactation database: COVID-19 vaccines*. Bethesda, MD: National Library of Medicine; 2006. https://www.ncbi.nlm.nih.gov/books/NBK565969/. Updated August 15, 2023. Accessed September 16, 2023.

 ## CODES

ICD10

Z39.1 Encounter for care and examination of lactating mother

CLINICAL PEARLS

- Support systems improve duration of breastfeeding.
- Almost all can breastfeed with accurate information, support from family, health care system, and society at large.
- Breast milk is the optimal food for infants, with myriad health benefits for the chestfeeder/breastfeeder and for the child being fed.

BRONCHIECTASIS

Evan R. Locke, MD • Michael J. Kim, MD, FAAFP

 BASICS

DESCRIPTION

Bronchiectasis is an irreversible syndrome with symptoms of chronic productive cough and recurrent exacerbations and with characteristic findings on cross-sectional imaging of bronchial wall dilation and thickening.

EPIDEMIOLOGY

Prevalence

- Overall estimated prevalence of bronchiectasis in the United States is 701 per 100,000 (1).
- Prevalence is higher among women than men and increases with age.

ETIOLOGY AND PATHOPHYSIOLOGY

- Bronchiectasis often arises as a complication of inherited or acquired disease states but may arise as an isolated diagnosis.
- Vicious cycle hypothesis (1):
  - An initial pulmonary insult causes airway inflammation, dysfunction, and structural disease.
  - Dysfunctional airways are further impaired in their ability to clear infections.
  - A pattern of lung damage/inflammation and progressive airway dysfunction is established, leading to clinical decline.
- Neutrophil extracellular traps (NETs) levels and neutrophil elastase activity correlate with disease activity and may serve as potential therapeutic targets (1).

GENERAL PREVENTION

- Routine immunization against respiratory infections (pertussis, measles, *Haemophilus influenzae* type B [HIB], influenza, and *Streptococcus* pneumonia).
- Early recognition and treatment of respiratory disease, inflammatory disease, and other predisposing conditions
- Genetic counseling for patients with inheritable conditions which predispose to bronchiectasis who wish to conceive
- Encourage and support smoking cessation in all patients who smoke

COMMONLY ASSOCIATED CONDITIONS

- Many cases are idiopathic, and bronchiectasis may be an isolated pulmonary diagnosis.
- Acquired conditions associated with bronchiectasis:
  - Pneumonia
  - GERD
  - Asthma/chronic obstructive pulmonary disease (COPD)
  - Rheumatologic conditions (rheumatoid arthritis, IBD)
  - Tuberculosis (TB)
  - Allergic bronchopulmonary aspergillosis (ABPA)
  - Chronic rhinosinusitis
  - Focal airway obstruction
- Inherited conditions associated with bronchiectasis:
  - Cystic fibrosis
  - Primary ciliary dyskinesia
  - Congenital abnormalities of the airways (e.g., tracheobronchomalacia, Mounier-Kuhn syndrome)
  - α1-Antitrypsin deficiency

 DIAGNOSIS

HISTORY

- Symptoms are commonly present for many years and include the following:
  - Cough
  - Sputum production most days of the week
  - Dyspnea
  - Fatigue
  - Rhinosinusitis
- Patients often report a history of recurrent exacerbations of symptoms, defined as a deterioration in ≥3 of the following symptoms for at least 48 hours *and* if a clinician determines that a change in treatment is needed (2):
  - Cough
  - Sputum volume/consistency
  - Sputum purulence
  - Breathlessness or exercise intolerance
  - Fatigue or malaise for at least 48 hours
  - Hemoptysis

PHYSICAL EXAM

- Basal, coarse rales, and wheezing may be present.
- Assess for physical exam features, which might suggest an alternative diagnosis.

DIFFERENTIAL DIAGNOSIS

Differential diagnosis primarily consists of other causes of chronic cough (e.g., COPD, asthma, chronic rhinosinusitis, lung cancer, GERD).

DIAGNOSTIC TESTS & INTERPRETATION

Initial Tests (lab, imaging)

For patients in which bronchiectasis is expected, consider ordering the following studies (2):

- Pulmonary function testing to detect chronic obstructive or restrictive lung disease
  - Normal or obstructive pattern on spirometry is most commonly seen in bronchiectasis.
- Chest x-ray is used primarily to evaluate for alternative or comorbid diagnoses.
  - In moderate to severe disease, chest radiographs may show atelectasis, dilated airways, and/or peripheral opacifications.
- Computed tomography (CT) with slice thickness ≤1 mm is the test of choice to diagnosis bronchiectasis.

Follow-Up Tests & Special Considerations

- Current guidelines suggest that the following tests should be considered in all patients with confirmed bronchiectasis (2):
  - CBC with differential
  - Quantitative serum immunoglobulins
  - ABPA testing (skin prick testing, Aspergillus-specific IgE antibodies)
- Recommended testing in children with suspected bronchiectasis includes the following (3):
  - High-resolution MDCT chest for diagnostic confirmation
  - Sweat chloride testing
  - Pulmonary function tests (if old enough to perform spirometry)

- CBC with differential
- Quantitative serum immunoglobulins and specific antibodies to vaccine antigens
- Sputum smear and cultures for bacteria, mycobacteria, and fungi
- Consider testing for TB, HIV, primary ciliary dyskinesia, GERD, airway aspiration, and immunodeficiencies.

Test Interpretation

- CT chest findings suggesting bronchial dilation are required to diagnose bronchiectasis (one or more of the following) (1):
  - Broncoarterial ratio >1 (inner or outer airway diameter to adjacent pulmonary artery)
  - Lack of tapering of the airways
  - Radiographically visible airways in the perimeter within 1 cm of costal pleural surface or touching mediastinal pleura
- Other CT chest findings commonly associated with bronchiectasis may include mucus plugging, bronchial wall thickening, "tree in bud" nodularity, and mosaic perfusion.
- Location of disease may suggest but not prove etiology (1).
  - Predominantly upper lobe disease is seen in CF-associated bronchiectasis.
  - Centrally located disease is common in ABPA.
  - Right middle lobe disease is associated with nontuberculous mycobacterial (NTM) infection.

TREATMENT

- In adults, existing guidelines recommend stepwise treatment based on severity (2):
  - Step 1 (initial treatment):
    - Treat the underlying cause.
    - Educate on airway clearance techniques and consider referral for pulmonary rehabilitation.
    - Recommend pneumococcal polysaccharide vaccine and annual influenza vaccination.
    - Create a self-management plan with patients.
  - Step 2 (if ≥3 exacerbations/year despite adherence to step 1):
    - Evaluate adequacy of physiotherapy.
    - Consider trial of mucolytics in appropriate patients (notable difficulties with sputum expectoration).
    - Ensure patient is referred to a specialist team if not already followed.
  - Step 3 (if ≥3 exacerbations/year despite adherence to step 2)
    - Initiate long-term antibiotics based on review of sputum cultures.
  - Step 4 (if ≥3 exacerbations/year despite adherence to step 3)
    - Long-term macrolide and long-term inhaled antibiotics are recommended.
  - Step 5 (if ≥3 exacerbations/year despite adherence to step 4)
    - IV antibiotics every 2 to 3 months should be considered.

- At all stages, obtain sputum cultures and treat exacerbations with prompt administration of empiric antibiotics.
  – Recommended duration of antibiotics is 14 days (2).
- Different guidelines exist for treatment of bronchiectasis in children/adolescents (3).
  – All patients should be seen by a pediatric chest physiotherapist for education on airway clearance techniques.
  – Exacerbations of bronchiectasis should be treated with a 14-day course of appropriate antibiotics.
  – Eradication therapy should be considered for children/adolescents with a new detection of *Pseudomonas aeruginosa*.
  – Children/adolescents with ≥3 exacerbations per year should receive long-term macrolides.

MEDICATION

First Line

- First-line antibiotics are selected based on sputum microbiology (2).
  – Amoxicillin 500 mg TID (*S. pneumoniae*, *H. influenzae* β-lactamase negative)
  – Amoxicillin with clavulanic acid 625 mg TID (*H. influenzae* β-lactamase positive, *Moraxella catarrhalis*)
  – Flucloxacillin 500 mg QID (*Staphylococcus aureus*)
  – Ciprofloxacin 500 to 750 mg BID (*P. aeruginosa*)
- Duration of antibiotics for treatment of exacerbations is 14 days (2).
- Eradication therapy should be considered for patients with new sputum isolation of *P. aeruginosa* (2).
  – Eradication: oral fluoroquinolone for 2 weeks followed by inhaled antibiotics for a total duration of 3 months

Second Line

Second-line antibiotics (2)
- Doxycycline 100 mg BID (*Streptococcus pneumoniae*, *H. influenzae* β-lactamase negative/positive)
- Clarithromycin 500 mg BID (*M. catarrhalis*, *S. aureus*)

ISSUES FOR REFERRAL

Indications for specialty referral include the following (2):
- ≥3 exacerbations per year
- Positive sputum cultures for *P. aeruginosa*, MRSA, or NTM; or diagnosis or ABPA
- Patients on long-term antibiotics (≥3 months)
- Rapidly deteriorating condition (or other indication for lung transplantation)

ADDITIONAL THERAPIES

- Mucoactive medications can be considered in patients who have difficulty with sputum expectoration despite airway clearance techniques (2).
  – Dry powder mannitol 320 to 400 mg BID
  – Nebulized hypertonic saline
- Long-acting bronchodilators may benefit some patients with significant breathlessness.
- Pulmonary rehabilitation should be considered for patients with symptomatic breathlessness.
- Support/encourage optimization of nutrition, exercise, and psychological support.

SURGERY/OTHER PROCEDURES

- Patients with localized bronchiectasis and frequent exacerbations despite adequate treatment may need surgery.
- Lung transplantation may be indicated in patients experiencing rapidly progressive deterioration.
- Patients with refractory issues with sputum expectoration may benefit from bronchial aspiration or bronchial wash.

ADMISSION, INPATIENT, AND NURSING CONSIDERATIONS

Factors which may prompt inpatient admission for treatment of bronchiectasis may include need for supplemental oxygen or other vital sign instability, need for IV medications, or outpatient treatment failure.

ONGOING CARE

FOLLOW-UP RECOMMENDATIONS

Children and adults with CF and non–CF-related bronchiectasis should be treated by comprehensive interdisciplinary chronic disease management programs.

Patient Monitoring

See patients in clinic at least every 3 to 6 months for the following:
- Assess adherence to respiratory physiotherapy/pulmonary rehabilitation regimen, and consider rereferral if additional education is required.
- Routine monitoring of sputum cultures every 6 to 12 months
- Consideration of repeat testing (i.e., pulmonary function testing, CT imaging) based on individual clinical factors
- Consideration of adjunctive therapies (i.e., mucolytics, bronchodilators)

PATIENT EDUCATION

Bronchiectasis, American Lung Association: https://www.lung.org/lung-health-diseases/lung-disease-lookup/bronchiectasis

PROGNOSIS

- Validated symptoms severity scores can be used to aid in determination of short- and long-term prognosis.
  – Bronchiectasis Severity Index: https://bronchiectasis.com.au/assessment/medical/bronchiectasis-severity-index
  – FACED Score: https://bronchiectasis.com.au/assessment/medical/faced-score
- *Pseudomonas* infection, low body mass index, and advanced age are associated with poorer prognosis.

COMPLICATIONS

Hemoptysis, pneumothorax, sepsis, lung abscesses, pulmonary hypertension, cor pulmonale

REFERENCES

1. O'Donnell AE. Bronchiectasis—a clinical review. *N Engl J Med*. 2022;387(6):533–545.
2. Polverino E, Goeminne PC, McDonnell MJ, et al. European Respiratory Society guidelines for the management of adult bronchiectasis. *Eur Respir J*. 2017;50(3):1700629.
3. Chang AB, Fortescue R, Grimwood K, et al. European Respiratory Society guideline for the management of children and adolescents with bronchiectasis. *Eur Respir J*. 2021;58(2):2002990.

 CODES

ICD10
- Q33.4 Congenital bronchiectasis
- A15.0 Tuberculosis of lung
- J47.0 Bronchiectasis with acute lower respiratory infection

CLINICAL PEARLS

- Symptoms of bronchiectasis include chronic productive cough, wheezing, and dyspnea often accompanied by repeated respiratory infections.
- A chest x-ray has poor sensitivity and specificity for the diagnosis; a noncontrast multidetector chest CT is the most important diagnostic tool.
- Current practice guidelines recommend treating acute exacerbations with a 14-day course of antibiotics. Frequent exacerbations may be treated with prolonged and aerosolized antibiotics.

BRONCHIOLITIS
Dennis E. Hughes, DO, FACEP

 BASICS

DESCRIPTION
- Inflammation and obstruction of small airways and reactive airways generally affecting infants and young children; manifests as an upper respiratory infection (URI) prodrome followed by increased respiratory effort, crackles, and wheezing
- Usual course: insidious, acute, progressive with a variable duration; some experience persistent symptoms (primarily cough) for 14 to 21 days.
- Leading cause of hospitalizations in infants and children in most Western countries; it is the most common cause of lower respiratory tract infections (LRTI) in children <24 months of age.
- Predominant age: newborn to 2 years (peak age <6 months); neonates are not protected despite transfer of maternal antibody.
- Predominant sex: male > female

EPIDEMIOLOGY
Incidence
- Accounts for ~$1.7 billion in health care costs in the United States; incidence is estimated at 3.2/1,000. Almost 100% of children experience RSV infection by two seasons.
- Usually seasonal (October to May in the Northern Hemisphere) and often occurs in epidemics—in subtropical regions; RSV is endemic year-round.
- Responsible for 18.8% (90,000 annually) of all pediatric hospitalizations (excluding live births) in children aged <2 years
- Incidence is increasing since 1980 (with concomitant increase in relative rate of hospitalization from 2002 to 2007); of those <12 months of age with condition, the hospitalization rate is ~2–3%.

Prevalence
There is a 21–25% prevalence of bronchiolitis in children <12 months of age, decreasing to 13% from 12 to 24 months of age in the United States.

ETIOLOGY AND PATHOPHYSIOLOGY
RSV accounts for 70–85% of all cases (children <12 months of age), but rhinovirus, parainfluenza virus, metapneumovirus, adenovirus, influenza virus, *Mycoplasma pneumoniae*, and *Chlamydophila pneumoniae* have all been implicated (1):
- Infection results in necrosis and lysis of epithelial cells and subsequent release of inflammatory mediators.
- Edema and mucus secretion, which combined with accumulating necrotic debris and loss of cilia clearance, result in airflow obstruction.
- Ventilation/perfusion mismatching, which may result in hypoxia
- Air trapping is caused by dynamic airways narrowing during expiration, which increases work of breathing.
- Bronchospasm appears to play little or no role.

RISK FACTORS
- Secondhand cigarette smoke
- Low birth weight, premature birth (especially those infants born <35 weeks' gestation)
- Immunodeficiency—both congenital and acquired
- Formula-fed infants
- Contact with infected person (primary mode of spread)
- Children in daycare environment
- Congenital cardiopulmonary disease
- Comorbid neurologic disorder
- <12 weeks of age

GENERAL PREVENTION
- Hand washing or use of alcohol-based hand rubs (preferred)—this simple exercise has been estimated to have the largest impact on prevention of transmission.
- Contact isolation of infected babies
- Persons with colds should keep contact with infants to a minimum.
- Breastfeeding of infants for at least 6 months has been associated with reduced morbidity of disease.
- Palivizumab (Synagis), a monoclonal product, administered monthly, October to May, 15 mg/kg IM; used for RSV prevention only in high-risk patients (see American Academy of Pediatrics [AAP] recommendations) (2)

Pediatric Considerations
Prior infection does not seem to confer subsequent immunity.

COMMONLY ASSOCIATED CONDITIONS
- Upper respiratory congestion
- Conjunctivitis
- Pharyngitis
- Otitis media
- Diarrhea

 DIAGNOSIS

History and physical examination should be the basis for the diagnosis of bronchiolitis; ancillary testing is only indicated if clinical picture is unclear (no single group of tests is confirmatory for bronchiolitis).

HISTORY
- Irritability
- Anorexia
- Fever
- Noisy breathing (due to rhinorrhea)
- Cough
- Grunting
- Cyanosis
- Apnea
- Vomiting

PHYSICAL EXAM
- Tachypnea
- Retractions (increased work of breathing)
- Rhinorrhea
- Wheezing
- Upper respiratory findings: pharyngitis, conjunctivitis, otitis

DIFFERENTIAL DIAGNOSIS
- Other pulmonary infections such as pertussis, croup, or bacterial pneumonia
- Aspiration
- Vascular ring
- Foreign body
- Asthma
- Heart failure
- Gastroesophageal reflux
- Cystic fibrosis

DIAGNOSTIC TESTS & INTERPRETATION
Laboratory and other ancillary testing (including chest x-ray) are not required if clinical diagnosis is bronchiolitis. Recent meta-analysis found no single history or physical factor that predicted air-space disease on chest radiograph.

Initial Tests (lab, imaging)
- Arterial oxygen saturation by pulse oximetry; results are need to be interpreted in clinical context. Transient hypoxemia is a common phenomenon in healthy infants (2); capnography not found to aid in prediction of disease severity or need for hospitalization; AAP guidelines (2014/2019), 2013 Choosing Wisely Campaign, and 2020 BEEP suggest intermittent verses continuous pulse oximetry be considered.
- Rapid respiratory viral antigen testing is not necessary during RSV season because the disease is managed symptomatically but may be useful for epidemiologic, hospital cohorting, or in the very young to reduce unnecessary other workup; also indicated in infants admitted while receiving palivizumab prophylaxis (If positive, prophylaxis may be discontinued as recent data suggests there is no benefit in using palivizumab prophylaxis during active disease.)
- The AAP does not recommend routine RSV testing in infants and children with bronchiolitis.
- Chest x-ray findings are variable and may include atelectasis, peribronchial cuffing, hyperinflation, and perihilar infiltrates (AAP and others do not recommend routine chest radiographs in clinical picture of acute bronchiolitis) (2).

Diagnostic Procedures/Other
Point-of-care ultrasound (POCUS) is being used to assist with diagnosis of pneumonia in bronchiolitis with accuracy comparable to radiographs. Also, use of a POCUS-derived scoring system may prognosticate patients who need escalation of therapy.

TREATMENT

- The cornerstone of therapy is supportive to include upper airway suctioning, prevention of significant and prolonged hypoxia, and dehydration.
- Positive-pressure ventilation (PPV) in the form of continuous positive airway pressure (CPAP) can be used in cases of respiratory failure. There is limited clinical evidence other than observational studies.
- Recent clinical practice guidelines do not support the routine use of corticosteroids, bronchodilators, or epinephrine. Despite these recommendations against such treatments, some estimated 50% of patients receive some combination of medication or other treatments during their course. Many experienced clinicians feel that trials of therapy (other than supportive care) are warranted based on clinical appearance (i.e., bronchodilators in wheezing patients).
- Parental education and support is vital (2)[A].

GENERAL MEASURES

To prevent the transmission of RSV (most common infectious etiology of bronchiolitis), it is recommended that caregivers disinfect their hands with alcohol-based skin cleaners both before and after contact with patients. Family should also be instructed on similar measures to reduce transmission.

MEDICATION

First Line

- Humidified oxygen for hypoxia of <90% (many feel that transient pulse oximetry in 85–90% range during sleeping in clinically well-appearing infant may be observed) (2)[C]
- Nebulized hypertonic saline (3%) can be effective in reducing LOS in hospitalized patients but not recommended for use in the ED (more recent literature review shows some signal of benefit) (2).
- Antibiotics only if secondary bacterial infection present (rare); not indicated for routine use (2)[B]
- High-flow nasal cannula oxygen is widely used in various settings to improve oxygen saturation with resultant reduction in end-tidal CO_2 ($ETCO_2$) and respiratory rate, but overall effectiveness remains unproven to date. Recent RCT indicates that high-flow oxygen therapy is effective in treating those potentially needing escalated therapy.

Second Line

Consider NG or IV fluids in those infants or children unable to maintain intake and adequate hydration due to work of breathing.

ADDITIONAL THERAPIES

- Ribavirin and palivizumab for patients at high risk (for prophylaxis per CDC/AAP guidelines)
- Heliox therapy (70% helium and 30% oxygen) may be of benefit early in moderate to severe bronchiolitis to reduce degree of respiratory distress due to air flow restriction, but Cochrane Review found little evidence of sustained benefit at 24 hours.
- Although not routinely recommended, inhaled β-agonists (albuterol) can be effective in selected cases (particularly in patients with a history of bronchospasm). Many clinicians will attempt an empiric trial of bronchodilators in a primary presentation to judge the clinical response (some argue that this condition maybe asthma equivalent).

ADMISSION, INPATIENT, AND NURSING CONSIDERATIONS

- Bronchiolitis can be associated with apnea in children <6 weeks of age.
- Respiratory rate >45 breaths/min with respiratory distress or apnea
- Hypoxia is common, so clinical criteria are more helpful (sustained pulse oximetry <94% used by many as cutoff).
- Ill or toxic appearance
- Underlying heart condition, respiratory condition, or immune suppression
- High risk for apnea (aged <30 days, preterm birth [<37 weeks])
- Dehydrated or unable to feed (<50% of normal intake suggested as threshold for hospitalization consideration)
- Uncertain home care
- Use of respiratory distress assessment instrument may aid in determining admission. The five best predictors of admission, age, respiratory rate, heart rate, oxygen saturation, and duration of symptoms, were recently incorporated into a scoring instrument.
- Supplemental oxygen for pulse oximetry <94% on room air if clinically indicated (i.e., retractions, increased WOB, etc.); AAP recommends O_2 saturation >90% if infant is otherwise well.
- IV fluids indicated only if tachypnea precludes oral feeding; weight-based maintenance rate plus insensible losses
- Discharge criteria
  - Normal respiratory rate and no oxygen requirement: Recent small studies suggest that after a period of observation, children can be safely discharged on home oxygen with home health follow-up. Despite reassuring appearance, the clinical course is unpredictable, so follow-up and parental education is important.

ONGOING CARE

FOLLOW-UP RECOMMENDATIONS

Patient Monitoring

- Hospitalization is usually required only if oxygen is a requirement or unable to feed/drink.
- For a hospitalized patient, monitor as needed depending on the severity of the infection.
- If the patient is receiving home care, follow daily by telephone call for 2 to 4 days; the patient may need frequent office visits.

PATIENT EDUCATION

- American Academy of Pediatrics: http://www.aap.org
- American Academy of Family Physicians: http://www.familydoctor.org

PROGNOSIS

- Recovery time is variable. 40% can have symptoms at 14 days and 10% at 4 weeks.
- Mortality statistics differ but probably <1%.
- High-risk infants (bronchopulmonary dysplasia, congenital heart disease) may have a prolonged course.

COMPLICATIONS

- Bacterial superinfection
- Bronchiolitis obliterans
- Apnea
- Respiratory failure
- Death
- Increased incidence of development of reactive airway disease (asthma)

REFERENCES

1. Manti S, Staiano A, Orfeo L, et al. UPDATE—2022 Italian guidelines on the management of bronchiolitis in infants. *Ital J Pediatr.* 2023;49(1):19.
2. Ralston SL, Lieberthal AS, Meissner HC, et al. Ralston SL, Lieberthal AS, Meissner HC, et al. Clinical practice guideline: the diagnosis, management, and prevention of bronchiolitis. *Pediatrics.* 2014;134(5):e1474–e1502. *Pediatrics.* 2015;136(4):782.

ADDITIONAL READING

Joseph MM, Edwards A. Acute bronchiolitis: assessment and management in the emergency department. *Pediatr Emerg Med Pract.* 2019;16(10):1–24.

CODES

ICD10

- J21.9 Acute bronchiolitis, unspecified
- J21.0 Acute bronchiolitis due to respiratory syncytial virus
- J21.8 Acute bronchiolitis due to other specified organisms

CLINICAL PEARLS

- Bronchiolitis is the leading cause of hospitalizations in infants and children—especially <3 months of age.
- Diagnosis is a clinical one of children in the first 2 years of life, associated with rhinorrhea, cough, labored breathing, and irritability.
- RSV causes the majority of bronchiolitis. CXR is not indicated.
- Parental education and support is essential.
- Treatment: nasal and upper airway suctioning mainstay of treatment

BRONCHITIS, ACUTE
Ghazaleh Bigdeli, MD, FCCP

BASICS

- Acute bronchitis is a common clinical condition characterized by an acute onset but persistent cough, with or without sputum production. It is typically self-limited, resolving within 1 to 3 weeks. Symptoms result from inflammation of the lower respiratory tract and are most frequently due to viral infection.
- Treatment is focused on patient education and supportive care. Antibiotics are not needed for the great majority of patients with acute bronchitis but are greatly overused for this condition. Reducing antibiotic use for acute bronchitis is a national and international health care priority.

DESCRIPTION

- Acute bronchitis is a lower respiratory tract infection that causes reversible bronchial inflammation, involving the large airways, without evidence of pneumonia, that occurs in the absence of chronic obstructive lung disease.
- Cough, the predominant symptom, may last as long as 3 weeks (1).
- Generally self-limited, with complete healing and full return of function (1)
- Most infections are viral if no underlying cardiopulmonary disease is present (1).
- Synonym(s): tracheobronchitis

Geriatric Considerations
Can be serious, particularly if part of influenza, with underlying COPD or CHF

Pediatric Considerations
- Usually occurs in association with other conditions of upper and lower respiratory tract (Trachea is usually involved.)
- If repeated attacks occur, child should be evaluated for anomalies of the respiratory tract, immune deficiencies, or for asthma.
- Acute bronchitis caused by RSV may be fatal.
- Antitussive medication is not indicated in patients aged <6 years (1).

EPIDEMIOLOGY

- Predominant age: all ages
- Predominant gender: male = female

Incidence
It accounts for approximately 10% of ambulatory care visits in the United States or 100 million visits per year. The incidence of acute bronchitis is highest in late fall and winter when transmission of respiratory viruses peaks (1),(2).

ETIOLOGY AND PATHOPHYSIOLOGY

- Viruses are the most commonly identified pathogens in patients with acute bronchitis (about 60%). The most common viral causes of acute bronchitis include the following (1):
  - Influenza A and B
  - Parainfluenza
  - Coronavirus types 1 to 3
  - Rhinoviruses
  - Respiratory syncytial virus
  - Human metapneumovirus
- Bacteria account for 6% of cases.
- The bacteria most commonly associated with acute bronchitis include *Mycoplasma pneumoniae*, *Chlamydophila pneumoniae*, and *Bordetella pertussis*.

- Approximately 10% of patients presenting with a cough lasting at least 2 weeks have evidence of *B. pertussis* infection.
- Possible fungal infections
- Chemical irritants
- Acute bronchitis causes an injury to the epithelial surfaces, resulting in an increase in mucus production and thickening of the bronchiole wall.

Genetics
No known genetic pattern

RISK FACTORS

- Infants
- Elderly
- Air pollutants
- Smoking
- Secondhand smoke
- Environmental changes
- Chronic bronchopulmonary diseases
- Chronic sinusitis
- Tracheostomy or endobronchial intubation
- Bronchopulmonary allergy
- Hypertrophied tonsils and adenoids in children
- Immunosuppression
  - Immunoglobulin deficiency
  - HIV infection
  - Alcoholism
- Gastroesophageal reflux disease (GERD)

GENERAL PREVENTION

- Avoid smoking and secondhand smoke.
- Control underlying risk factors (i.e., asthma, sinusitis, and reflux).
- Avoid exposure, especially daycare.
- Pneumovax, influenza immunization

COMMONLY ASSOCIATED CONDITIONS

- Allergic rhinitis
- Sinusitis
- Pharyngitis
- Epiglottitis (rare but can be rapidly fatal)
- Coryza
- Croup
- Influenza
- Pneumonia
- Asthma
- COPD/emphysema
- GERD

DIAGNOSIS

- Acute bronchitis should be suspected in patients with an acute onset but persistent cough (often lasting 1 to 3 weeks) who do not have clinical findings suggestive of pneumonia (e.g., fever, tachypnea, rales, signs of parenchymal consolidation) and do not have COPD.
- In most cases, the diagnosis can be made based on the history and physical examination.
- Testing is generally reserved for cases in which pneumonia is suspected, clinical diagnosis is uncertain, or when results would change management.

HISTORY

- Cough for >5 days and no evidence of pneumonia, asthma, exacerbation of COPD
- Cough is initially dry and nonproductive, then productive; later, mucopurulent sputum, which may indicate secondary infection

- Cough lasts >5 days.
- Dyspnea, wheeze, and fatigue may occur.
- Possible contact with others who have respiratory infections
- Fever may suggest pneumonia or influenza infection.

PHYSICAL EXAM

- Fever
- Tachypnea
- Pharynx injected
- Rhonchi, wheezing
- No evidence of pulmonary consolidation, rales, etc.

DIFFERENTIAL DIAGNOSIS

- Pneumonia
- COVID-19
- Postnasal drip syndrome
- Common cold
- Acute sinusitis
- Bronchopneumonia
- Influenza
- Bacterial tracheitis
- Bronchiectasis
- Asthma
- Reactive airway dysfunction syndrome (RADS)
- Allergy
- Eosinophilic pneumonitis
- Aspiration
- Retained foreign body
- Inhalation injury
- Cystic fibrosis
- Bronchogenic carcinoma
- Heart failure
- GERD
- Chronic cough
- ACE inhibitor use

DIAGNOSTIC TESTS & INTERPRETATION

Initial Tests (lab, imaging)

- None normally needed; diagnosis is based on history and physical exam showing no postnasal drip or rales.
- For a complicated picture, consider the following:
  - CBC with differential
  - Influenza titers (if appropriate for time of year)
  - Viral panel/testing for SARS-CoV-2 (COVID-19) is recommended for all patients during the COVID-19 pandemic.
- No testing needed unless concerned about pneumonia
- Pulse oximetry if underlying pulmonary disease is present
- CXR are only indicated if:
  - Dyspnea, bloody sputum, or rusty sputum color
  - Pulse >100 beats/min
  - Respiratory rate >24 breaths/min
  - Oral body temperature >100°F (37.8°C)
  - Focal consolidation, egophony, or fremitus on chest examination

Follow-Up Tests and Special Considerations

- Arterial blood gases: hypoxemia (rarely)
- Pulmonary function tests (seldom needed during acute stages): increased residual volume, decreased maximal expiratory rate (1)
- Sputum culture in those patients intubated or with tracheostomy
- Procalcitonin

B

TREATMENT

GENERAL MEASURES
- Outpatient treatment unless elderly or complicated by severe underlying disease
- Rest
- Stop smoking and avoid secondhand smoke.
- Steam inhalations
- Vaporizers
- Adequate hydration
- Antitussives (1 tbsp of honey every 2 to 3 hours PRN)
- Antibiotics are not recommended (2)[A].
- Treat associated illnesses (e.g., GERD).

MEDICATION

ALERT
Antibiotics are not recommended unless a treatable pathogen has been identified or significant comorbidities are present. This should be explained to patients who likely expect an antibiotic to be prescribed.

First Line
- Supportive; increased fluids (Cough results in increased fluid loss.)
- Antipyretic analgesic such as aspirin, acetaminophen, or ibuprofen
- Decongestants if accompanied by sinus symptoms or postnasal drip
- Cough suppressant for troublesome cough (not with COPD); nonpharmacologic therapy: honey (1 tbsp every 2 to 4 hours PRN), throat lozenges, hot tea; smoking cessation and avoidance of secondhand smoke is a reasonable first step.
- Pharmacologic therapy: benzonatate (Tessalon), guaifenesin with dextromethorphan; not indicated in children aged <6 years (1)[C]
- Mucolytic agents are not recommended.
- Inhaled β-agonist (e.g., albuterol) or in combination with high-dose inhaled corticosteroids for cough with bronchospasm in those with known airflow obstruction (1),(3)[B]
- If influenza is highly suspected and symptom onset is <48 hours: oseltamivir (Tamiflu), zanamivir (Relenza) (1)[B], IV peramivir (Rapivab) or baloxavir marboxil (Xofluza)
- In case of positive COVID-19 infection, patients can be treated with antiviral medications or monoclonal antibodies based on the National Institute of Health (NIH) COVID-19 treatments. Nirmatrelvir with ritonavir (Paxlovid) is the first-choice treatment for mild-to-moderate COVID-19 in patients with a higher risk of severe illness.
- Antibiotics ONLY if a treatable cause (i.e., pertussis) is identified (1)[A].
  - Doxycycline: 100 mg/day × 10 days if *Moraxella, Chlamydia,* or *Mycoplasma* is suspected
  - Quinolone for more serious infections or other antibiotic failure or in elderly or patients with multiple comorbidities
  - Clarithromycin (Biaxin): 500 mg q12h or azithromycin (Zithromax [Z-Pak]) for atypical or pertussis infection
- Contraindication(s): Doxycycline and quinolones should not be used during pregnancy or in children.

- Precautions:
  - Multiple antibiotics have the potential to interfere with the effectiveness of oral contraceptives.
  - Antibiotic use can be associated with *Clostridium difficile* infections.
  - Cough and cold preparations should not be used in children aged <6 years (1)[B].

ISSUES FOR REFERRAL
- Complications such as pneumonia or respiratory failure
- Comorbidities such as COPD
- Cough lasting >3 months

ADDITIONAL THERAPIES
- Antipyretic for fever (e.g., acetaminophen or ibuprofen)
- Inhaled β-agonist (e.g., albuterol) or in combination with high-dose inhaled corticosteroids for cough with bronchospasm (1)[B]
- Oral corticosteroids probably not indicated with exception in COVID-19 infection (1)

ADMISSION, INPATIENT, AND NURSING CONSIDERATIONS
- Hypoxia—may require supplemental oxygen
- Respiratory failure that may require CPAP/bilevel ventilation
- Severe bronchospasm
- Exacerbation of underlying disease
- Bronchodilators if patient is bronchospastic
- IV fluids may be helpful if patient is dehydrated.
- Ensure patient comfort and monitor for signs of deterioration, especially if underlying lung disease exists.
- May need to follow oxygen saturation in patients with underlying lung disease
- Discharge criteria: improvement in symptoms and comorbidities

ONGOING CARE

FOLLOW-UP RECOMMENDATIONS
- Usually a self-limited disease not requiring follow-up
- Cough may linger for several weeks.
- In children, if recurrent, need to consider other diagnoses, such as asthma (2)

Patient Monitoring
- Oximetry until no longer hypoxemic
- Recheck for chronicity.

DIET
Increased fluids (3 to 4 L/day) while febrile

PATIENT EDUCATION
- For patient education materials favorably reviewed on this topic, contact the American Lung Association: https://www.lung.org
- American Academy of Family Physicians: https://www.familydoctor.org
- The NIH provides COVID-19 treatment guidelines.

PROGNOSIS
- Usual: complete resolution
- Can be serious in the elderly or debilitated
- Cough may persist for several weeks after an initial improvement.
- Postbronchitic reactive airways disease (rare)
- Bronchiolitis obliterans and organizing pneumonia (rare)

COMPLICATIONS
- Superinfection such as bronchopneumonia
- Bronchiectasis
- Hemoptysis
- Acute respiratory failure
- Chronic cough

REFERENCES

1. Albert RH. Diagnosis and treatment of acute bronchitis. *Am Fam Physician*. 2010;82(11):1345–1350.
2. Gonzales R, Anderer T, McCulloch CE, et al. A cluster randomized trial of decision support strategies for reducing antibiotic use in acute bronchitis. *JAMA Intern Med*. 2013;173(4):267–273.
3. Becker LA, Hom J, Villasis-Keever M, et al. Beta2-agonists for acute cough or a clinical diagnosis of acute bronchitis. *Cochrane Database Syst Rev*. 2015;(9):CD001726.

SEE ALSO

- Asthma; Chronic Obstructive Pulmonary Disease and Emphysema
- Algorithm: Cough, Chronic

CODES

ICD10
- J20.9 Acute bronchitis, unspecified
- J68.0 Bronchitis and pneumonitis due to chemicals, gases, fumes and vapors
- B97.0 Adenovirus as the cause of diseases classified elsewhere

CLINICAL PEARLS
- Acute bronchitis is a common and generally self-limited disease.
- Treat cough with honey (1 tbsp every 2 to 4 hours as needed), benzonatate (Tessalon), guaifenesin with dextromethorphan
- It does not require treatment with antibiotics. This needs to be explained to patients who expect antibiotics to be prescribed.
- Cough may linger for several weeks after the resolution of other symptoms.
- Recurrent or seasonal episodes may suggest another disease process, such as asthma.
- Fever is uncommon and should prompt investigation for pneumonia or influenza.

BULIMIA NERVOSA
Matthew J. Kor, MD

BASICS

DESCRIPTION
An eating disorder which includes binge eating and inappropriate compensatory behaviors; symptoms include the following:

- Episodes of binge eating (approximately 2,000 kcal), lack of self-control for eating at least once a week for 3 months
- Inappropriate compensations
  - For example, caloric restriction (most common), excessive exercise, self-induced vomiting, inappropriate laxative or diuretics use
- Alternating binge eating and compensations for prolonged time not during anorexia nervosa
- Distorted self body image
- *DSM-5* classifies severity based on inappropriate compensatory behaviors per week:
  - Mild (1 to 3), moderate (4 to 7), severe (8 to 13), extreme (≥14)
- System(s) affected: oropharyngeal, endocrine/metabolic, gastrointestinal, dermatologic, cardiovascular, pulmonary, psychiatric

EPIDEMIOLOGY
- Mean age of onset: 18 to 21 years
- Predominant sex: female > male (13:1)

Prevalence
Approximately 0.5% of females and 0.08% males in their lifetime in the United States

ETIOLOGY AND PATHOPHYSIOLOGY
Combination of biologic, psychological, environmental, and social factors

Genetics
Heritability estimated to be up to 41%

RISK FACTORS
- Female gender
- History of obesity and dieting
- Body dissatisfaction; critical comments about weight, body shape, or eating; low self-esteem
- Depression, social anxiety, severe life stressor
- Poor impulse control, substance abuse
- Family history of substance abuse, affective disorders, eating disorder, or obesity
- Diabetes
- Childhood trauma (sexual or physical abuse, neglect)

GENERAL PREVENTION
- Realistic and healthy weight management strategies and attitudes
- Decrease body dissatisfaction and promote self-esteem.
- Reduce focus on thin as ideal.

COMMONLY ASSOCIATED CONDITIONS
- Major depression, dysthymia, anxiety, obsessive-compulsive and bipolar disorders
- Substance use disorder
- Personality disorders: borderline, schizotypal, antisocial (1)
- Nonsuicidal self injury (33%) and suicidal attempts (21%) (2),(3)

DIAGNOSIS

HISTORY
- Patients are unlikely to self-identify binge eating or purging behaviors; corroborate with parent/relative.
- Unhappiness and/or preoccupation with weight and diet attempts
- Pattern of binge eating and compensatory behaviors
  - Binging
  - Vomiting (often with little effort)
  - Vigorous aerobic exercise
  - Distress/shame related to loss of control
  - Use of diuretics, laxatives without medical indication
- Depressed mood and self-depreciation following the binges
- Other possible signs and symptoms
  - Requesting weight loss help and mildly underweight to overweight
  - Diet pill, diuretic, laxative, ipecac, and thyroid medication use/abuse, frequent fluctuations in weight
  - Menstrual disturbances or amenorrhea
  - Fatigue and lethargy
  - Abdominal pain, bloating, constipation, diarrhea, rectal prolapse
  - Sore throat and thermal tooth sensitivity
  - Omission/underdosing insulin in diabetes patients

PHYSICAL EXAM
- Often with normal/fluctuating weight or overweight range
- Tachycardia
- Erosion of dental enamel (8.33%)
- Perimylolysis, cheilosis, gingivitis
- Sialadenosis (parotid gland swelling and/or asymptomatic, noninflammatory parotid gland enlargement)
- Epigastric tenderness to palpation
- Russell sign: scars, calluses, abrasions, bruising on hand, thumb
- Peripheral edema

DIFFERENTIAL DIAGNOSIS
- Anorexia, binge eating/purging type; distinguished by body mass index (BMI) <18.5 kg/m²
- Major depressive disorder/borderline personality disorder
- Other metabolic disorders: Addison disease, celiac disease, diabetes mellitus, hyperthyroidism, hypothyroidism, hyperpituitarism
- Genetic syndromes: Kleine-Levin syndrome, Prader-Willi syndrome
- Pregnancy

DIAGNOSTIC TESTS & INTERPRETATION
- All lab results may be within normal limits and are unnecessary for diagnosis.
- Psychological self-report screening tests may be helpful but tend to increase false positives.
- SCOFF Questionnaire is recommended by United States Preventative Task Force (sensitivity of 0.86 and specificity of 0.83) (4).
- Eating disorder screen for primary care
- Primary Care Evaluation of Mental Disorders Patient Health Questionnaire

Initial Tests (lab, imaging)
- Complete blood count, comprehensive metabolic panel, and liver function tests
  - Hypokalemia, hyponatremia, hypochloremia, hypocalcemia, hypomagnesemia, hypophosphatemia, hypoproteinemia, hypoglycemia
  - Serum amylase levels and pH derangements
  - Elevated blood urea nitrogen
- Urinalysis: increased urine specific gravity

Diagnostic Procedures/Other
- Pregnancy test
- Electrocardiogram: bradycardia or arrhythmias, conduction defects, depressed ST segment due to hypokalemia

TREATMENT

Cognitive-behavioral therapy (CBT) and nutritional rehabilitation should be considered as first-line treatment (5),(6). Combination treatment with CBT and medications are more effective than psychotherapy alone, and psychotherapy alone is more effective than medication alone.

GENERAL MEASURES
- Multidisciplinary team (primary care clinician, behavioral health provider, nutritionist)
- CBT for bulimia nervosa (6)
- Family therapy for adolescents
- Nutritional education, relaxation techniques

MEDICATION

First Line

- Selective serotonin reuptake inhibitors (SSRIs) (7)[A], particularly fluoxetine (Prozac) titrated by 20 mg/day every week to 60 mg/day, are effective in reducing symptoms. Higher doses than standard doses for depression are often needed.
  - Maintain full therapeutic dose for at least 6 to 12 months after remission (8).
- If there is no adequate response to treatment, evaluate for medical nonadherence or adjust the treatment every 4 to 8 weeks.

Second Line

- Select different SSRIs (sertraline, escitalopram, and fluvoxamine). Paroxetine is not often used for increased risk of weight gain.
- Third-line therapies include TCAs, MAOIs, and trazodone.
- The anticonvulsant topiramate may help to diminish binge-purge episodes.
- Ondansetron (Zofran) 4 to 8 mg TID between meals may decrease nausea and vomiting.
- Bupropion is contraindicated due to association with seizures with electrolyte abnormalities.

ISSUES FOR REFERRAL

A multidisciplinary approach should be used, which include a primary care physician, behavioral health provider, and nutritionist.

COMPLEMENTARY & ALTERNATIVE MEDICINE

Bright light therapy is potentially effective at improving disordered eating and mood (9).

ADMISSION, INPATIENT, AND NURSING CONSIDERATIONS

- Admission to a specialized eating disorders unit for one or more of the following:
  - ≤75% ideal BMI for age and sex
  - Dehydration; electrolyte disturbance (hypokalemia, hyponatremia, hypophosphatemia)
  - EKG abnormalities (e.g., prolonged QTc or severe bradycardia)
  - Severe bradycardia (<50 beats/min during daytime; <45 beats/min at night)
  - Hypotension (systolic <90 mm Hg)
  - Hypothermia (body temperature <96.0°F [35.6°C])
  - Orthostasis
  - Acute food refusal, uncontrollable bingeing and purging
  - Acute medical complications of malnutrition (e.g., syncope, seizures, cardiac failure, pancreatitis)
  - Comorbid psychiatric or medical condition that prohibits or limits appropriate outpatient treatment (e.g., severe depression, suicidal ideation, obsessive-compulsive disorder, type 1 diabetes mellitus) (10)
- During admission:
  - Supervised meals and bathroom privileges
  - Gradually shift control to patients as they demonstrate improvement.

 ONGOING CARE

FOLLOW-UP RECOMMENDATIONS

Patient Monitoring

- Binge-purge activity, including antecedents and consequences, level of exercise activity
- Self-esteem, comfort with body and self, rumination and depressive symptoms
- Repeat any abnormal lab values weekly until stable.

DIET

- Balanced diet, normal eating pattern
- Nutritional rehabilitation aims to restore a structured and consistent meal pattern: three meals and two snacks per day

PATIENT EDUCATION

National Alliance on Mental Illness: https://www.nami.org/Learn-More/Mental-Health-Conditions/Eating-Disorders/Overview

PROGNOSIS

- An estimated 45–70% will have a full recovery or improvement of symptoms, and 20–30% may experience relapse (11).
- Positive prognostic factors: younger age at presentation, shorter duration of illness, less frequent symptoms, absence of laxative use, close social relationships, and a good therapeutic response within the first month of treatment
- Negative prognostic factors: overemphasis on body shape and weight, history of physical abuse, disturbed family relationships, poor motivation, self-injurious behaviors, and presence of a personality disorder (11)

COMPLICATIONS

- Substance use disorder
- Osteopenia/osteoporosis/stress fracture
- Gastric dilatation/Boerhaave syndrome/Mallory-Weiss tears
- Spontaneous pneumomediastinum
- Potassium depletion, cardiac arrhythmia, cardiac arrest
- Suicide
- Pharmacotherapy and psychotherapy, alone, can relieve depressive symptoms, however, combination therapy has high rates of improvement

REFERENCES

1. Udo T, Grilo CM. Psychiatric and medical correlates of DSM-5 eating disorders in a nationally representative sample of adults in the United States. *Int J Eat Disord*. 2019;52(1):42–50.
2. Cucchi A, Ryan D, Konstantakopoulos G, et al. Lifetime prevalence of non-suicidal self-injury in patients with eating disorders: a systematic review and meta-analysis. *Psychol Med*. 2016;46(7):1345–1358.
3. Mandelli L, Arminio A, Atti AR, et al. Suicide attempts in eating disorder subtypes: a meta-analysis of the literature employing DSM-IV, DSM-5, or ICD-10 diagnostic criteria. *Psychol Med*. 2019;49(8):1237–1249.
4. Kutz AM, Marsh AG, Gunderson CG, et al. Eating disorder screening: a systematic review and meta-analysis of diagnostic test characteristics of the SCOFF. *J Gen Intern Med*. 2020;35(3):885–893.
5. Linardon J, Wade TD, de la Piedad Garcia X, et al. The efficacy of cognitive-behavioral therapy for eating disorders: a systematic review and meta-analysis. *J Consult Clin Psychol*. 2017;85(11):1080–1094.
6. Hay PP, Bacaltchuk J, Stefano S, et al. Psychological treatments for bulimia nervosa and binging. *Cochrane Database Syst Rev*. 2009;(4):CD000562.
7. Bacaltchuk J, Hay P, Trefiglio R. Antidepressants versus psychological treatments and their combination for bulimia nervosa. *Cochrane Database Syst Rev*. 2001;(4):CD003385.
8. Yager J, Devlin MJ, Halmi KA, et al. Guideline watch (August 2012): practice guideline for the treatment of patients with eating disorders, 3rd edition. *FOCUS*. 2014;12(4):416–431.
9. Beauchamp MT, Lundgren JD. A systematic review of bright light therapy for eating disorders. *Prim Care Companion CNS Disord*. 2016;18(5).
10. Golden NH, Katzman DK, Sawyer SM, et al; for Society for Adolescent Health and Medicine. Position Paper of the Society for Adolescent Health and Medicine: medical management of restrictive eating disorders in adolescents and young adults. *J Adolesc Health*. 2015;56(1):121–125.
11. Castillo M, Weiselberg E. Bulimia nervosa/purging disorder. *Curr Probl Pediatr Adolesc Health Care*. 2017;47(4):85–94.

 CODES

ICD10
F50.2 Bulimia nervosa

CLINICAL PEARLS

- Asking "Are you satisfied with your eating patterns?" and/or "Do you worry that you have lost control over how much you eat?" may help to screen for an eating problem.
- Screening with SCOFF is recommended for eating disorders.
- Utilize a multidisciplinary team approach when resources are available.
- SSRIs, particularly fluoxetine (60 mg/day), is a useful first line medication and/or s adjunctive treatment with CBT.
- Pharmacotherapy alone is reasonable if specialized nutritional rehabilitation and psychotherapy are not available.

BUNION (HALLUX VALGUS)

Jennifer G. Chang, MD

 BASICS

DESCRIPTION

- Lateral deviation of the great toe ("Hallux abducto valgus" derives from the Latin for "big toe askew.")
- Associated medial deviation of the 1st metatarsal, leading to a medial prominence of the 1st metatarsophalangeal (MTP) joint (also known as "bunion")
- Progressive subluxation of the 1st MTP joint in later stages
- System(s) affected: musculoskeletal/skin

EPIDEMIOLOGY

- Predominant age: more common in adults
- Gender difference: Female > male by ~2:1
- More common in shoe-wearing populations
- Commonly bilateral

Incidence

Unknown and difficult to assess

Prevalence

- Prevalence increases with age, particularly in females.
- Adults (aged 18 to 65 years): estimated prevalence of 23%
- Elderly (>65 years) adults: estimated prevalence of 36%
- Juvenile hallux valgus: more common in girls (>80% of cases)

ETIOLOGY AND PATHOPHYSIOLOGY

Multifactorial and controversial. Contributing factors may include underlying anatomy and repetitive external forces:

- Absence of muscles that directly stabilize the 1st MTP allows relatively unopposed forces to influence lateral deviation of the proximal phalanx and medial deviation of the 1st metatarsal head.
- Medial MTP joint capsule and medial collateral ligament are chronically stretched and may eventually rupture, decreasing stability and causing progressive subluxation of the 1st MTP joint.
- Lateral joint capsule and collateral ligaments also contract
- Lateral and plantar migration of abductor hallucis muscle moves the great toe into plantar flexion and lateral pronation.

Genetics

- Cohort and twin studies suggest heritability.
- Genome-wide association studies suggest sex-specific differences in genetic mechanisms.

RISK FACTORS

- Genetic predisposition
- Abnormal biomechanics (i.e., flexible flat feet)
- Foot deformities: joint laxity, hindfoot pronation, Achilles tendon tightness, pes planus (fallen arches), metatarsus primus varus
- Amputation of 2nd toe
- Inflammatory joint disease
- Neuromuscular disorders (cerebral palsy, stroke)
- Improper footwear (high heels; narrow toe box)

GENERAL PREVENTION

Proper footwear may decrease the progression of the disease.

COMMONLY ASSOCIATED CONDITIONS

- Medial bursitis of the 1st MTP joint (most common)
- Hammertoe deformity of the 2nd phalanx
- Plantar callus
- Metatarsalgia
- Degeneration of cartilage covering the 1st metatarsal head and sesamoids
- Pronated feet; ankle equinus
- Onychocryptosis (ingrown toenail)
- Entrapment of the medial dorsal cutaneous nerve
- Synovitis of the MTP joint

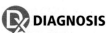 DIAGNOSIS

- Based on clinical exam
- Radiographs are used for staging.

HISTORY

- Painful MTP joint (most common symptom in adults)
- Abnormal position of great toe
- Enlargement of the MTP joint medially (patients complain of a "bump")
- Shoes do not fit properly.
- Pain with ambulation
- Skin irritation, blister, or callus at the 1st MTP

PHYSICAL EXAM

- Observe gait; may be antalgic due to pain
- Medial prominence at the MTP joint
- Skin changes: erythema, blistering, callus, or ulceration at the MTP joint
- Great toe over- or underriding the 2nd toe
- Examine the entire 1st metatarsal and toe for:
  - 1st MTP range of motion
  - 1st tarsometatarsal (TMT) mobility
  - Neurovascular integrity
  - Degenerative osteoarthritis

DIFFERENTIAL DIAGNOSIS

- Trauma: turf toe; sesamoiditis; stress fracture
- Infection: osteomyelitis; septic arthritis
- Joint disorder: osteoarthritis; rheumatoid arthritis; pseudogout; gout
- Tendon disorder: tendinosis; tenosynovitis; tendon rupture
- Other: bursitis; ganglion cyst; foreign body granuloma

DIAGNOSTIC TESTS & INTERPRETATION

Initial Tests (lab, imaging)

- Weight-bearing AP and lateral radiographs (sesamoid view optional) to assess:
  - Joint congruency and degenerative changes
  - Lateral sesamoid bone displacement
  - Rounded 1st metatarsal head
  - Longer 1st metatarsal
- Radiographic parameters include but are not limited to:
  - Hallux valgus angle (HVA): Long axis of the 1st MT and proximal phalanx is normally <15 degrees.
  - Intermetatarsal angle (IMA): Between long axis of 1st and 2nd metatarsal is normally <9 degrees.
  - Distal metatarsal articular angle (DMAA): Between 1st metatarsal long axis and line through base of distal articular cap is normally <8 degrees.
  - Hallux valgus interphalangeal angle (IPA): Between long axis of distal phalanx and proximal phalanx is normally <10 degrees.

 TREATMENT

- Primary indication for treatment is pain.
- There are conservative (nonoperative) and surgical approaches.
- Only surgical approaches can correct the hallux valgus deformity.
- Surgical treatment is generally more effective in improving pain but has attendant risks.

GENERAL MEASURES

Nonoperative treatment options may improve pain and delay the progression of hallux valgus deformity, although high-quality evidence is limited (1)[B]:

- Proper fitting footwear: low-heeled, wide-toe shoes to decrease stress on MTP joint
- Orthotics: correct foot alignment (pes planus and overpronation). Improving gait may prevent bunion formation and reduce pressure on the MTP.

- Splinting: in theory, stabilizes and balances soft tissue structures around the MTP. Limited evidence shows improvement in degree of angulation in mild hallux valgus. Dynamic splint use may reduce pain.
- Foot mobilization and exercise, combined with a toe separator, may improve pain scores, strength, and range of motion in moderate hallux valgus (2)[B].
- Pads/spacers: Pads decrease friction on the MTP joint. A toe spacer in the 1st interdigital space may reduce pain.

MEDICATION

- Topical (NSAIDs) and oral medications (NSAIDs, acetaminophen) can be used to relieve pain. Other topical options include capsaicin cream.
- Corticosteroid injections may improve pain (rarely used outside of postoperative setting).

ISSUES FOR REFERRAL

Surgery is indicated for patients with severe pain, dysfunction, or persistent symptoms that do not abate with conservative therapy.

SURGERY/OTHER PROCEDURES

- >150 different surgical techniques exist to treat hallux valgus.
- No single technique is proven superior; no universally accepted standard exists for procedure selection.
- Minimally invasive techniques continue to evolve and may achieve better outcomes than open techniques (3)[B].
- Choice of technique depends on disease severity, radiographic findings, and patient/surgeon-specific factors:
  - Arthrodesis: fusion of the 1st MTP joint; used for severe and/or recurrent hallux valgus; fusion of the 1st TMT joint (modified Lapidus) is considered for TMT joint hypermobility.
  - Arthroplasty: removing the joint or replacing it with a prosthesis; high revision rates
  - Exostectomy/bunionectomy: removing the medial bony prominence of the MTP joint (less common now)
  - Soft tissue realignment: alters the function of surrounding ligaments and tendons; used for minor deformities or as an adjunct to bony correction techniques

  - Osteotomy and realignment: common and includes wide variety of techniques:
    - Distal: used for mild to moderate deformity (e.g., distal chevron osteotomy)
    - Proximal: used more often to correct severe deformity
  - Mini TightRope procedure: use of a FiberWire to correct misalignment
- Some patients may have little to no improvement in symptoms despite interventions. Providers should establish realistic expectations prior to surgery.
- In pediatric patients, surgery should generally be delayed until skeletal maturity.

COMPLEMENTARY & ALTERNATIVE MEDICINE

Marigold ointment may reduce pain and soft tissue swelling related to bunion.

 ONGOING CARE

FOLLOW-UP RECOMMENDATIONS

- Postoperative treatment includes physical therapy, physiotherapy, supportive footwear, continuous passive motion, or manual manipulation.
- Time until full weight-bearing depends on the surgical procedure.

PROGNOSIS

Patient outcome varies depending on biomechanical factors, severity of the deformity, and treatment modality used. Recurrence after surgery is common (25%) and increases with degree of preoperative HVA and IMA and postoperative HVA and sesamoid position.

COMPLICATIONS

- Risks associated with surgery include infection, persistent pain, and poor cosmetic result.
- Additional risks vary with the surgical procedure.
- Other complications may include:
  - Early swelling
  - Hallux varus
  - Recurrence of bunion
  - Metatarsal fracture
  - Decreased sensation over the 1st metatarsal or phalanx

REFERENCES

1. Hurn SE, Matthews BG, Munteanu SE, et al. Effectiveness of nonsurgical interventions for hallux valgus: a systematic review and meta-analysis. *Arthritis Care Res (Hoboken)*. 2022;74(10):1676–1688.
2. Abdalbary SA. Foot mobilization and exercise program combined with toe separator improves outcomes in women with moderate hallux valgus at 1-year follow-up: a randomized clinical trial. *J Am Podiatr Med Assoc*. 2018;108(6):478–486.
3. Ji L, Wang K, Ding S, et al. Minimally invasive vs. open surgery for hallux valgus: a meta-analysis. *Front Surg*. 2022;9:843410.

ADDITIONAL READING

- Arbeeva L, Yau M, Mitchell BD, et al. Genome-wide meta-analysis identified novel variant associated with hallux valgus in Caucasians. *J Foot Ankle Res*. 2020;13(1):11.
- Barnish MS, Barnish J. High-heeled shoes and musculoskeletal injuries: a narrative systematic review. *BMJ Open*. 2016;6(1):e010053.
- Kwan MY, Yick KL, Yip J, et al. Hallux valgus orthosis characteristics and effectiveness: a systematic review with meta-analysis. *BMJ Open*. 2021;11(8):e047273.

CODES

ICD10
- M20.10 Hallux valgus (acquired), unspecified foot
- M20.11 Hallux valgus (acquired), right foot
- M20.12 Hallux valgus (acquired), left foot

CLINICAL PEARLS

- Avoid footwear with high heels, pointed toe boxes, or inadequate toe space to reduce development or progression of bunions.
- Surgery generally results in superior outcomes for pain relief in appropriately selected patients.
- No single surgical method has shown to be superior for long-term pain relief.
- Establish realistic expectations prior to surgery to improve patient satisfaction with surgical outcomes.

BURNS

Grant Wei, MD, FACEP • Chirag N. Shah, MD • Chelsea Leigh Bunce, DO

 BASICS

DESCRIPTION
- Tissue injuries caused by application of heat, chemicals, electricity, or irradiation
- Extent of injury (depth of burn) is a result of intensity and duration of exposure.
  - Superficial burn (formerly 1st degree) involves superficial layers of epidermis.
  - Partial-thickness burn (formerly 2nd degree) involves varying amounts of epidermis (with blister formation) and part of the dermis.
  - Full-thickness burn (formerly 3rd degree) involves destruction of all skin elements (full thickness) with coagulation of subdermal plexus.
- System(s) affected: endocrine/metabolic, pulmonary, skin/exocrine

Geriatric Considerations
- Prognosis is worse for severe burns.
- Patients >60 years of age account for 11% of all burns.

Pediatric Considerations
Consider child abuse or neglect when dealing with hot water burns in children; abuse accounts for 15% of pediatric burns. Special concerns are sharply demarcated wounds, immersion injuries, and suspect stories. Involve child welfare services early.

EPIDEMIOLOGY
- Fourth most common trauma worldwide
- Predominant age: 20 to 30 years; 13% are infants; 11% are >60 years of age.
- Predominant gender: Males account for 70%.

Incidence
Per year in the United States
- 1.2 to 2.0 million burns; 700,000 emergency room visits; 45,000 to 50,000 hospitalizations; 3,900 deaths from burn-related complications
- In children: 250,000 burns, 15,000 hospitalizations, 1,100 deaths
- Estimated total cost of $2 billion annually for burn care
- House fires cause 75% of deaths.
- Burn deaths are decreasing nationally due to improved prevention and treatment.
- Increase in burns from the illegal production of methamphetamines. Patients can present with a combination of chemical burn, thermal burn, and explosion injury.

ETIOLOGY AND PATHOPHYSIOLOGY
- Open flame and hot liquid are the most common causes of burns (heat usually ≥45°C): flame burns are more common in adults; scald burns are more common in children.
- Caustic chemicals or acids (may show little signs or symptoms for the first few days)
- Electricity (may have significant injury with very little damage to overlying skin)
- Excess sun exposure

RISK FACTORS
- Water heaters set too high
- Workplace exposure to chemicals, electricity, or irradiation
- Young children and older adults with thin skin are more susceptible to injury.

- Carelessness with burning cigarettes: related to 18% of fatal fires in 2006
- Inadequate or faulty electrical wiring
- Lack of smoke detectors: Lacking or nonfunctioning smoke alarms are implicated in 63% of residential fires.
- Arson: cause of 12.4% of fires that resulted in fatalities in 2012
- Low socioeconomic status has been associated with an increased risk of unintentional injury and mortality.

GENERAL PREVENTION
Home safety education should be a key mechanism for injury prevention.
- Families educated on home safety were more likely to have safe hot water temperatures.
- Safety education results in more families having functioning smoke alarms and increased use of fireguards.

COMMONLY ASSOCIATED CONDITIONS
Smoke inhalation syndrome
- May involve thermal burn to respiratory mucosa (e.g., trachea, bronchi) as well as carbon monoxide inhalation
- Occurs within 72 hours of burn
- Should be suspected in all burns occurring in an enclosed space or exposure to explosions

 DIAGNOSIS

HISTORY
History of source of burn. In children or elderly: Check for consistency between the history and the burn's physical characteristics.

PHYSICAL EXAM
- Superficial: erythema of involved tissue, skin blanches with pressure; skin may be tender.
- Partial thickness: Skin is red and blistered; skin is very tender.
- Full thickness: Burned skin is tough and leathery; skin is nontender.
- Rule of 9s
  - Each upper extremity: adult and child 9%
  - Each lower extremity: adult 18%; child 14%
  - Anterior trunk: adult and child 18%
  - Posterior trunk: adult and child 18%
  - Head and neck: adult 10%; child 18%
- Quick estimate: The surface area of the patient's hand (palmar surface plus fingers) is 1% of the body surface area (BSA).
- Careful documentation of the extent of burn and the estimated depth of burn
- Check for any signs suggestive of potential airway involvement: singed nasal hair, facial burns, carbonaceous sputum, progressive hoarseness, inflamed oropharynx, circumferential burns around the neck, tachypnea.

DIAGNOSTIC TESTS & INTERPRETATION
- Children: glucose (hypoglycemia may occur in children because of limited glycogen storage) (1)[B]
- Smoke inhalation: arterial blood gas, carboxyhemoglobin
- Electrical burns: ECG, urine myoglobin, creatine kinase isoenzymes
- Electrolyte abnormalities may occur which can cause seizures or arrhythmias (1)[B].

Initial Tests (lab, imaging)
- Labs: hematocrit; type and crossmatching; electrolytes, including BUN and creatinine; urinalysis
- Imaging: chest radiograph; xenon scan is useful in suspected smoke inhalation.

Diagnostic Procedures/Other
Bronchoscopy may be necessary for smoke inhalation to evaluate lower respiratory tract.

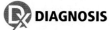 **TREATMENT**

- Prehospital care (1)[B]
  - Remove the patient from the source of the burn and extinguish and remove all burning clothing.
  - Room-temperature water may be poured onto the burn but only in the first 15 minutes following burn exposure.
  - Wrap the patient to prevent hypothermia.
  - All patients to receive 100% oxygen via face mask
- Hospitalization for all serious burns (2)[B]
  - Partial-thickness burns >10% of BSA
  - Any full-thickness burn
  - Burns of hands, feet, face, or perineum
  - Electrical or lightning burns
  - Inhalation injury
  - Chemical burns
  - Circumferential burn
- Transfer to burn center for (2)[B]
  - Partial- and full-thickness burns >10% of BSA in patients aged <10 years and >50 years of age
  - Partial-thickness burns >20% of BSA and full-thickness burns >5% of BSA in any age range
  - Full-thickness burns in any age group
  - Burns of hands, feet, face, or perineum
  - Electrical or lightning burns
  - Inhalation injury
  - Chemical burns
  - Circumferential burn
  - Burns in patients with additional trauma (fractures, etc.) in which the burn is the more severe injury; otherwise, send to trauma center for stabilization.
  - Burn injuries in patients with medical comorbidities that could affect management, mortality, or recovery (3)[A]

GENERAL MEASURES
- Based on depth of burns and accurate estimate of total BSA involved (rule of 9s) (4)[C]
- Tetanus prophylaxis (if not current)
- Remove all rings, watches, and other items from injured extremities to avoid tourniquet effect.
- Remove clothing and cover all burned areas with dry sheets.
- Flush area of chemical burn (for ~2 hours).
- For all major burns, use 100% oxygen administration; consider early intubation.
- Do not apply ice to burn site.
- Nasogastric tube (high risk of paralytic ileus)
- Foley catheter
- Analgesia
- ECG monitoring in first 24 hours following electrical burn
- Daily or BID cleansing with dressing changes

- Burn fluid resuscitation (4)[C]
  - Calculate fluid resuscitation from the time of burn, not from the time treatment begins.
  - 2 to 4 mL of Ringer lactate × body weight (kg) × % total BSA burn (50% fluid given in first 8 hours, remaining 50% in the next 16 hours); in children, this is given in addition to maintenance fluids and is adjusted according to urine output and vital signs. Protocol-based resuscitation leads to superior outcomes.
  - Colloid solutions are not recommended during the first 12 to 24 hours of resuscitation.
  - Other: Use of biologic membranes or skin substitutes may be indicated for burn coverage.
- Inhalation injury
  - Intubation, ventilation with positive end-expiratory pressure assistance. Employ lung protective ventilation strategies.
  - Hyperbaric oxygen treatment may be useful in patients with carbon monoxide levels >25%; patients with coma, focal neurologic deficit, ischemic ECG changes; and pregnant patients.
  - Prophylactic antibiotics and steroids are not indicated.

MEDICATION

First Line

- IV morphine or hydromorphone (Dilaudid) for severe pain (2)[C]
- Oral analgesics, such as acetaminophen (Tylenol) with codeine, acetaminophen with oxycodone (Percocet), or acetaminophen with hydrocodone (Lortab) for moderate pain (2)[C]
- Neosporin or bacitracin ointment
- Use of silver sulfadiazine dressing has been shown to have poorer healing outcomes than alternative dressings (5)[A].
- Mupirocin: has potent inhibitory activity against methicillin-resistant *Staphylococcus aureus* (MRSA) (5)[A]
- Acticoat A.B. (a dressing consisting of two sheets of high-density polyethylene mesh coated with nanocrystalline silver) has a more controlled, prolonged release of silver, allowing less frequent dressing changes.
- Electrical burn with myoglobinuria will require alkalinization of urine and mannitol.
- Consider H_2 blockers (e.g., famotidine) or proton pump inhibitors (e.g., lansoprazole, pantoprazole) for stress ulcer prophylaxis in severely burned patients.
- Tetanus toxoid/tetanus immunoglobulin
- There is no clear indication for prophylactic systemic antibiotics.
- Use of negative pressure wound therapy may result in a low-protease environment with higher levels of angiogenic factor (vascular endothelial growth factor [VEGF]) during wound healing, leading to a more chaotic, hyperkeratinized, thickened epidermis when compared with a standard hydrocolloid dressing (1)[B].

Second Line

- Mafenide (Sulfamylon) for full-thickness burn, best against *Pseudomonas* (*caution*: metabolic acidosis, painful)
- Silver nitrate 0.5% (messy, leeches electrolytes from the burn, causes water toxicity)

- Povidone-iodine (Betadine) may result in iodine absorption from burn and "tan eschar," making débridement more difficult (5)[A].
- Travase (enzymatic débridement)

SURGERY/OTHER PROCEDURES

- Escharotomy may be necessary for constricting circumferential burns of extremities or chest due to compartment syndrome (3)[A].
- Tangential excision with split-thickness skin grafts: Early excision of burns results in a significant reduction in mortality (excluding patients with inhalational injury) and a significant decrease in hospital length of stay (3)[A].
- Various dressings (e.g., biosynthetic, biologic) are available to help reduce the number of dressing changes and promote healing (5)[A].

🔋 ONGOING CARE

FOLLOW-UP RECOMMENDATIONS

Early mobilization is the goal.

DIET

- High-protein, high-calorie diet when bowel function resumes
- Nasogastric tube feedings may be required in early postburn period.
- Total parenteral nutrition if NPO is expected for >5 days
- Early initiation of enteral nutrition in the first 24 hours of admission results in shorter intensive care unit (ICU) stay and lower wound infection rates.

PATIENT EDUCATION

- Use of sunscreen: Skin grafts or newly epithelialized skin is highly sensitive to sun exposure and thermal extremes.
- Isolate household chemicals.
- Use low-temperature setting for water heater (<54°C).
- Household smoke detectors with special emphasis on maintenance
- Family/household evacuation plan
- Proper storage and use of flammable substances
- Burn management: http://www.aafp.org/afp/2000/1101/p2029.html
- Burn prevention: http://www.aafp.org/afp/2000/1101/p2032.html

PROGNOSIS

- Superficial burn: complete resolution
- Partial-thickness burn: epithelialization in 10 to 14 days (deep partial-thickness burns probably will require skin graft)
- Full-thickness burn: no potential for reepithelialization; skin graft is required.
- Baux score (sum of age and total BSA burned) and Denver 2 score (pulmonary score ranging 0 to 3, using PaO_2/FiO_2 cutoffs of 100, 175, and 250), renal score (0 to 3, using creatinine cutoffs of 1.8, 2.5, and 5 mg/dL), hepatic score (0 to 3, using bilirubin cutoffs of 2, 4, and 8 mg/dL), and cardiac score (0 to 3, based on number and dosage of inotropes) can be used to estimate mortality.

- Length of hospital stay and need for ICU care depend on extent of burn, smoke inhalation, comorbidities, and age.
- Burn size is correlated to complications; >60% total BSA burned in children and >40% in adults are at increased risk for mortality and morbidity.
- A 50% survival rate can be expected with a 62% burn in patients aged 0 to 14 years, 63% burn in patients aged 15 to 40 years, 38% burn in patients aged 40 to 65 years, and 25% burn in patients >65 years of age.
- 90% of survivors can be expected to return to an occupation comparable to their preburn employment.

COMPLICATIONS

- Gastroduodenal ulceration (Curling ulcer)
- Marjolin ulcer: malignant squamous cell carcinoma developing in old burn site
- Infection (discoloration, green fat, edema, eschar separation). Biopsy is the best to diagnose wound infection.
- Burn wound sepsis: most commonly *S. aureus* (including MRSA), vancomycin-resistant enterococci, and gram-negative organisms.
- Decreased mobility with possibility of future flexion contractures. Hypertrophic scarring common with burns.

REFERENCES

1. Roshangar L, Rad JS, Kheirjou R, et al. Skin burns: review of molecular mechanisms and therapeutic approaches. *Wounds*. 2019;31(12):308–315.
2. Jeschke MG, van Baar ME, Choudhry MA, et al. Burn injury. *Nat Rev Dis Primers*. 2020;6(1):11.
3. Miroshnychenko A, Kim K, Rochwerg B, et al. Comparison of early surgical intervention to delayed surgical intervention for treatment of thermal burns in adults: a systematic review and meta-analysis. *Burns Open*. 2021;5(2):67–77.
4. Regan A, Hotwagner D. *Burn Fluid Management*. Treasure Island (FL): StatPearls Publishing; 2022. https://www.ncbi.nlm.nih.gov/books/NBK534227. Updated June 23, 2022. Accessed December 10, 2022.
5. Jiang Q, Chen ZH, Wang SB, et al. Comparative effectiveness of different wound dressings for patients with partial-thickness burns: study protocol of a systematic review and a Bayesian framework network meta-analysis. *BMJ Open*. 2017;7(3):e013289.

CODES

ICD10

- T23.029A Burn of unspecified degree of unspecified single finger (nail) except thumb, initial encounter
- T23.039A Burn of unspecified degree of unspecified multiple fingers (nail), not including thumb, initial encounter
- T23.079A Burn of unspecified degree of unspecified wrist, initial encounter

BURSITIS, PES ANSERINE (PES ANSERINE SYNDROME)
Jennifer Schwartz, MD

 BASICS

DESCRIPTION
- The pes anserinus is the combined insertion of the sartorius, gracilis, and semitendinosus tendons on the anteromedial tibia (approximately 5 cm distal to the medial joint line).
  - The sartorius, gracilis, and semitendinosus muscles help flex the knee and also protect the knee against valgus and rotational stresses.
- The pes anserine bursa lies deep to the pes anserinus and the medial collateral ligament (MCL).
- *Pes anserine tendino-bursitis (PATB)* is due to irritation of the bursa and/or tendons in this area. Clinically, it is difficult to distinguish pes anserine tendonitis from pes anserine bursitis due to proximity of the structures.

ETIOLOGY AND PATHOPHYSIOLOGY
PATB is thought to occur due to the following:
- Excessive valgus and rotational stresses on the knee (due to overuse or underlying biomechanical factors)
- Degenerative changes
- Direct trauma

RISK FACTORS
- More common in middle age, overweight females
- Other risk factors include the following:
  - Pes planus; genu valgum
  - Long distance/hill running, cycling, swimming ("breaststroker's knee")
  - Sports with side-to-side/cutting activity (soccer, basketball, racquet sports)

GENERAL PREVENTION
- Avoid repetitive valgus/rotational stresses to the knee and treat underlying biomechanical risk factors
- Control weight
- Adequate hamstring stretching

COMMONLY ASSOCIATED CONDITIONS
- Osteoarthritis (OA)
  - Increased incidence of PATB in patients with symptomatic OA; PATB commonly contributes to knee pain in patients with OA.
  - Higher grades of OA are associated with a thicker pes anserine bursa and a larger area of bursitis.
- Medial meniscal tear
- Type 2 diabetes, rheumatoid arthritis, gout (chronic PATB)

 DIAGNOSIS

Largely a clinical diagnosis (although sensitivity and specificity of clinical findings may be low and PATB can be confused with other medial sided knee pathologies) (1)[C]

HISTORY
- Medial knee pain at the pes anserine insertion
  - Pain is located 4 to 6 cm below the medial joint line on the anteromedial aspect of the tibia.
- Pain is exacerbated by knee flexion:
  - Going up or down stairs
  - Getting up out of a chair or from a sitting position
  - Sitting cross-legged

PHYSICAL EXAM
- Tenderness to palpation or localized swelling at the pes anserine insertion
  - Caution: Many patients without PATB will have tenderness to deep palpation in this area. Be sure to examine both sides and correlate physical exam with history before making a diagnosis.
- Pain worsens with flexion of the knee against resistance.
- Findings that suggest an alternative diagnosis: joint effusion, tenderness directly over the joint line, locking of the knee, systemic signs such as fever

DIFFERENTIAL DIAGNOSIS
- Medial compartment OA
- MCL injury
- Medial meniscal injury
- Medial plica syndrome
- Tibial stress fracture
- Septic arthritis

DIAGNOSTIC TESTS & INTERPRETATION
Initial Tests (lab, imaging)
- Primarily a clinical diagnosis
- Lab work not indicated; imaging is not routinely indicated unless there is a concern for underlying bony injury/fracture, ligamentous injury, or meniscal tear.

Follow-Up Tests & Special Considerations
- X-ray
  - Can demonstrate underlying OA.
- Ultrasound (US)
  - Can demonstrate focal edema within the pes anserine bursa but this may not correlate with clinical findings
  - Many patients with a clinical diagnosis of PATB have no morphologic changes of the pes anserine complex on US.
- MRI: T2-weighted axial images are preferred.
  - May see fluid in the pes bursa on MRI in a subset of asymptomatic patients
  - No large studies have evaluated the correlation between a clinical diagnosis of PATB and radiographic evidence of pes anserine pathology on MRI.

TREATMENT
- Pes anserine bursitis is often self-limited, but it can recur.
- Conservative therapy is preferred:
  - Relative rest and activity modification to avoid offending movements (especially knee flexion)
  - Ice to the affected area
  - NSAIDs for pain control
  - Physical therapy (PT) for knee strengthening and treatment of other underlying pathology
  - Kinesio taping
    - One study found kinesio taping to be more effective than PT + naproxen (Naprosyn) to decrease pain from PATB (2)[C].
  - Corticosteroid injection
    - Steroid injections and PT found to be equally effective for acute pain in PATB. Steroid injections may be preferred in some cases due to immediate results or risk of low PT compliance. However, symptom improvement from steroid injection alone may be less sustained than those from PT.
    - When considering intra-articular steroid injection for symptomatic OA, also consider steroid injection at the pes anserine bursa. PATB also contributes to pain in patients with OA and intra-articular injection alone may not be sufficient.

– Extracorporeal shock wave therapy (ECSWT)
  ○ ECSWT is also a safe and effective treatment for PATB. ECSWT may have a longer lasting effect and lead to more consistent symptom improvement (vs. steroid injection) (3)[C].
– Weight loss to improve biomechanical forces at the knee

MEDICATION

First Line

- NSAIDs: that is, ibuprofen (800 mg PO TID) or naproxen (500 mg PO BID)
- Corticosteroid injection combined with local anesthetic:
  – Inject at the point of maximal tenderness using standard aseptic technique.
  – ~2 mL of anesthetic (i.e., 1% lidocaine) and 1 mL of steroid (i.e., 40 mg of methylprednisolone) are injected into the bursa using a small (e.g., 25-gauge, 1-inch) needle.
  – Insert needle perpendicular to the skin until bone is felt and then withdraw slightly before injecting.
  – Avoid injecting directly into the tendon.
- US-guided injection superior to blind injection

Second Line

Platelet-rich plasma injections can also provide pain relief.

ADDITIONAL THERAPIES

- Hamstring and Achilles stretching
- Quadriceps and adductor strengthening

SURGERY/OTHER PROCEDURES

- No role for surgery in routine isolated cases
- Drainage or removal of bursa may be used in severe/refractory cases.

 ONGOING CARE

Physical therapy with home exercise program focusing on flexibility and strengthening

DIET

Consider dietary changes as part of a comprehensive weight-loss program if obesity is a contributing factor.

PROGNOSIS

Most cases of pes anserine syndrome respond to conservative therapy. Recurrence is common, and multiple treatments may be required.

REFERENCES

1. Atici A, Ulger FEB, Akpinar P, et al. Poor accuracy of clinical diagnosis in pes anserine tendinitis bursitis syndrome. *Indian J Orthop*. 2021;56(1):116–124.
2. Homayouni K, Foruzi S, Kalhori F. Effects of kinesiotaping versus non-steroidal anti-inflammatory drugs and physical therapy for treatment of pes anserinus tendino-bursitis: a randomized comparative clinical trial. *Phys Sportsmed*. 2016;44(3):252–256.
3. Majidi L, Saeb F, Alaei B, et al. Comparison of the effectiveness of local corticosteroid injection and extracorporeal shockwave therapy in patients with pes anserine bursitis: an open-label randomized clinical trial. *Med J Islam Repub Iran*. 2023;37:10.

ADDITIONAL READING

- Alvarez-Nemegyei J. Risk factors for pes anserinus tendinitis/bursitis syndrome: a case control study. *J Clin Rheumatol*. 2007;13(2): 63–65.
- Khosrawi S, Taheri P, Ketabi M. Investigating the effect of extracorporeal shock wave therapy on reducing chronic pain in patients with pes anserine bursitis: a randomized, clinical-controlled trial. *Adv Biomed Res*. 2017;6:70.
- Sarifakioglu B, Afsar SI, Yalbuzdag SA, et al. Comparison of the efficacy of physical therapy and corticosteroid injection in the treatment of pes anserine tendino-bursitis. *J Phys Ther Sci*. 2016;28(7):1993–1997.

 CODES

ICD10

M70.50 Other bursitis of knee, unspecified knee

CLINICAL PEARLS

- Consider pes anserine syndrome in patients presenting with medial knee pain, especially those with persistent symptoms associated with medial sided OA.
- Tenderness over the insertion of the pes anserine tendon on the medial aspect of the tibia 4 to 6 cm distal to the joint line is common in asymptomatic patients as well—correlation of the entire clinical picture is necessary for accurate diagnosis.
- Treatment is typically conservative and PT or kinesio taping can be helpful. A local steroid/anesthetic injection may provide pain relief and enhance rehabilitation and is a more temporary option. Also, consider ECSWT.

CANDIDIASIS, MUCOCUTANEOUS

Karlynn Sievers, MD • Tonya M. Cook, PharmD

 BASICS

DESCRIPTION
- Heterogeneous group of mucocutaneous infections with commensal *Candida* species
- Characterized by superficial infection of the skin, mucous membranes, and nails
- >20 *Candida* species cause infection in humans. *Candida albicans* is responsible for 70% of fungal infections worldwide.
  - *Candida auris* is an emerging global pathogen with a high propensity to develop drug resistance (1).
- Candidiasis affects:
  - Aerodigestive system
    ○ Oropharyngeal candidiasis (thrush): mouth, pharynx
    ○ Angular cheilitis: corner of the mouth
    ○ Esophageal candidiasis
    ○ Gastritis and/or ulcers, associated with thrush; alimental or perianal
  - Other systems
    ○ Candida vulvovaginitis: vaginal mucosa and/or vulvar skin
    ○ Candidal balanitis: glans of the penis
    ○ Candidal paronychia: nail bed or nail folds
    ○ Interdigital candidiasis: webs of the digits
    ○ Candidal diaper dermatitis and intertrigo (within skin folds)
- *Synonym(s): monilia; thrush; yeast; intertrigo*

ALERT
Vaginal antifungal creams and suppositories can weaken condoms and diaphragms.

Pregnancy Considerations
- Vaginal candidiasis is common during pregnancy—extend treatment (typically a full 7-day course).
- Vaginal yeast infection at birth increases the risk of newborn thrush but is of no overall harm to baby.

EPIDEMIOLOGY
- Common in the United States; particularly with immunodeficiency and/or uncontrolled diabetes
- Age considerations
  - Infants and seniors: thrush and cutaneous infections (infant diaper rash)
  - Women (prepubertal through postmenopausal): yeast vaginitis

Incidence
Unknown—mucocutaneous candidiasis is common in immunocompetent patients. Complication rates are low.

Prevalence
Candida species are normal flora of oral cavity, GI tract that are present in >70% of the U.S. population.

ETIOLOGY AND PATHOPHYSIOLOGY
C. albicans (responsible for 80–92% vulvovaginal and >80% of oral isolates); altered cell–mediated immunity against *Candida* species (either transient or chronic) increases susceptibility to infection.

Genetics
Chronic mucocutaneous candidiasis is a heterogeneous, genetic syndrome that typically presents in infancy.

RISK FACTORS
- Immune suppression (antineoplastic treatments, transplant patients, cellular immune defects, HIV/AIDS)
- Malignant diseases
- Corticosteroid use
- Smoking and alcoholism
- Hyposalivation (Sjögren disease, drug-induced xerostomia, radiotherapy)
- Broad-spectrum antibiotic therapy
- Douches, chemical irritants, birth control pills, intrauterine devices, and concurrent vaginitides
- Denture wear, poor oral hygiene
- Endocrine alterations (diabetes mellitus, pregnancy, renal failure, hypothyroidism)
- Uncircumcised men at higher risk for balanitis

GENERAL PREVENTION
- Use antibiotics and steroids judiciously; rinse mouth after using inhaled steroids.
- Minimize perineal moisture (wear cotton underwear; frequent diaper changes; avoid douching).
- Clean dentures often; use well-fitting dentures and remove them during sleep.
- Optimize glycemic control in diabetics.
- Preventive regimens during cancer treatments, especially in patients with hematologic malignancies
- Treat with HAART in HIV-infected patients; antifungal prophylaxis is not recommended unless HIV-infected adults have frequent or severe recurrences.

COMMONLY ASSOCIATED CONDITIONS
HIV, diabetes mellitus, cancer, and other immunosuppressive conditions

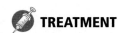 **DIAGNOSIS**

HISTORY
- Infants/children
  - Oral: adherent white patches on oral mucosae or on the tongue that do not wipe away easily
  - Perineal: erythematous rash with characteristic satellite lesions; painful if skin layer eroded
  - Angular cheilitis: painful fissures at mouth corners
- Adults
  - Vulvovaginal lesions; whitish "curd-like" discharge; pruritus; burning
  - Balanitis: erythema, erosions, scaling; dysuria
- Immunocompromised hosts
  - Oral: white, raised, painless, distinct patches; red, slightly raised patches/petechiae
  - Esophagitis: dysphagia, odynophagia, retrosternal pain; usually concomitant thrush
  - GI symptoms: abdominal pain
  - Folliculitis: follicular pustules

PHYSICAL EXAM
- Infants/children
  - Oral: white, raised, distinct patches within the mouth; when wiped off, reveals red base
  - Perineal: erythematous maculopapular rash with satellite pustules or papules
  - Angular cheilitis: tender fissures in mouth corners, often cracked and bleeding
- Adults
  - Vulvovaginal: thick, whitish, cottage cheese–like discharge; vagina or perineum erythema
  - Balanitis: erythema, linear erosions, scaling
  - Interdigital: redness, excoriation at base and web spaces of fingers and/or toes, possible maceration
- Immunocompromised hosts
  - Oral: white, raised, nontender, distinct patches; red, slightly raised patches; thick, dark-brownish coating; deep fissures
  - Esophagitis: Often, oral thrush is visible.
  - Folliculitis: follicular pustules

DIFFERENTIAL DIAGNOSIS
- For oral candidiasis, consider leukoplakia; lichen planus; geographic tongue; herpes simplex; erythema multiforme; pemphigus, burning mouth syndrome
- Baby formula or breast milk can mimic thrush—easier to remove than thrush.
- Hairy leukoplakia: does not rub off; dorsum and lateral margins of tongue
- Angular cheilitis from vitamin B or iron deficiency, staphylococcal infection, or edentulous overclosure
- Bacterial vaginosis and *Trichomonas vaginalis* tend to have more odor, itch, and a different discharge.

DIAGNOSTIC TESTS & INTERPRETATION
Initial Tests (lab, imaging)
- 10% KOH slide preparation: mycelia (hyphae) or pseudomycelia (pseudohyphae) yeast forms
- Associated with normal vaginal pH (<4.5)

Diagnostic Procedures/Other
- If first-line treatment fails, obtain samples for culture.
- Esophagitis or hyperplastic candidiasis may require endoscopy with biopsy (if suspicious for cancer).

Test Interpretation
Biopsy: epithelial parakeratosis with polymorphonuclear leukocytes in superficial layers; periodic acid–Schiff staining reveals candidal hyphae.

TREATMENT

GENERAL MEASURES
Screen for immunodeficiency (diabetes, HIV, autoimmune disease).

MEDICATION

First Line
- Vaginal (choose 1)
  - Miconazole (Monistat) 2% cream: one applicator or 200 mg (one suppository), intravaginally QHS for 7 days
  - Clotrimazole (Gyne-Lotrimin, Mycelex): intravaginal suppository (100 mg QHS for 7 days; 200 mg QHS for 3 days; 500 mg daily for 1 day) or 2% cream (one applicator QHS for 3 days)
  - Fluconazole: 150 mg PO single dose
- Oropharyngeal
  - Mild disease
    ○ Clotrimazole (Mycelex): oral 10-mg troche; 20 minutes 5 times daily for 7 to 14 days
    ○ Nystatin suspension: 100,000 U/mL swish and swallow 400,000 to 600,000 U QID
    ○ Nystatin pastilles: 200,000 U each, QID for 7 to 14 days (2)
    ○ Denture wearers
      ■ Nystatin ointment: 100,000 U/g under denture and corners of mouth for 3 weeks
  - Moderate to severe disease
    ○ Fluconazole: 200 mg load and then 100 to 200 mg (>14 days of age: 6 mg/kg × 1 dose and then 3 mg/kg q24h × 7 to 14 days [max of 100 mg/day])
- Esophagitis
  - Fluconazole: PO 400 mg load and then 200 to 400 mg/day for 14 to 21 days or IV 400 mg (6 mg/kg) daily
  - Alternative options are available if fluconazole is not tolerated; systemic antifungal therapy is always required (3).

Pregnancy Considerations
2% miconazole cream, intravaginally, for 7 days in uncomplicated candidiasis; systemic amphotericin B for invasive candidiasis

Second Line
- Vaginal
  - Topical antifungals, with no one preferred agent recommended (3)
  - Alternatively, fluconazole 150 mg in a single dose (3)
  - For recurrent cases (≥4 symptomatic episodes in 1 year): induction therapy with 10 to 14 days of topical or oral azole and then fluconazole 150 mg once per week for 6 months
    ○ In HIV patients: Concerns with this regimen include emergence of drug resistance.
- Oropharyngeal
  - Miconazole oral gel (20 mg/mL): QID, swish and swallow.
  - Itraconazole (Sporanox) suspension: 200 mg (20 mL) daily; swish and swallow for 7 to 14 days.
  - Posaconazole (Noxafil) oral suspension: 400 mg BID for 3 days and then 400 mg daily for up to 28 days
  - Amphotericin B (Fungizone) oral suspension (100 mg/mL): 1 mL QID daily, swish and swallow; use between meals.

- Esophagitis
  - Amphotericin B (variable dosing) IV dose of 0.3 to 0.7 mg/kg daily or an echinocandin should be used for patients who cannot tolerate oral therapy.
  - For refractory disease:
    ○ Could consider amphotericin B, itraconazole, posaconazole, voriconazole, isavuconazole (2)
  - Echinocandins (may be first choice in severe disease in patients with immunodeficiency) (2)
  - Several new agents are under investigation (2).
- Continue treatments for 2 days after infection is gone:
  - Contraindications
    ○ Ketoconazole, itraconazole, or nystatin (if swallowed): severe hepatotoxicity
    ○ Amphotericin B: can cause nephrotoxicity
- Precautions
  - Miconazole: can potentiate the effect of warfarin but drug of choice in pregnancy
  - Fluconazole: renal excretion; rare, hepatotoxicity; resistance frequent
  - Posaconazole: can cause GI discomfort or QT prolongation (2)
  - Voriconazole: transient visual disturbances; clinical hepatitis, cholestasis, and fulminant liver failure (rare) (2)
- Possible interactions (rarely seen with topical treatment)
  - Fluconazole
    ○ Rifampin and tolbutamide: decreased fluconazole concentrations
    ○ Warfarin, phenytoin, cyclosporine: altered metabolism; check levels.
  - Itraconazole: potent CYP3A4 inhibitor. Carefully assess all coadministered medications.

ISSUES FOR REFERRAL
- Evaluate patients with recurrent superficial candidal infections for immunodeficiency.
- GI candidiasis

ADDITIONAL THERAPIES
- For infants with thrush: Boil pacifiers and bottle nipples; assess mother's breasts/nipples for *Candida* infection.
- For denture-related candidiasis: Remove dentures at night. Disinfect dentures (using soak solution of white vinegar, 2% chlorhexidine gluconate solution, or 0.1% hypochlorite solution) and treat orally.

COMPLEMENTARY & ALTERNATIVE MEDICINE
Probiotics: *Lactobacillus* and *Bifidobacterium* may inhibit *Candida* spp.

ADMISSION, INPATIENT, AND NURSING CONSIDERATIONS
Proper oral hygiene; protocols for brushing, denture care, and oral cavity moistening reduce oral candidiasis.

 ## ONGOING CARE

FOLLOW-UP RECOMMENDATIONS
Patient Monitoring
Immunocompromised persons benefit from regular evaluation and screening.

DIET
Active culture yogurt or other live lactobacillus may decrease colonization; indeterminate evidence

PATIENT EDUCATION
- Advise patients at risk for recurrence about potential for overgrowth with antibacterial therapy.
- Oral "azole" medications should be avoided in the 1st trimester. Thereafter, only give orally when benefits outweigh risks.

PROGNOSIS
Benign prognosis in immunocompetent patients; may have significant morbidity in immunosuppressed persons

COMPLICATIONS
In HIV patients, moderate immunosuppression (e.g., CD4 200 to 500 cells/mm^3) may be associated with chronic candidiasis. With more severe immunosuppression (e.g., CD4 <100 cells/mm^3), esophagitis or systemic fungal infections are possible.

REFERENCES
1. Hendrickson JA, Hu C, Aitken SL, et al. Antifungal resistance: a concerning trend for the present and future. *Curr Infect Dis Rep.* 2019;21(12):47.
2. Quindós G, Gil-Alonso S, Marcos-Arias C, et al. Therapeutic tools for oral candidiasis: current and new antifungal drugs. *Med Oral Patol Oral Cir Bucal.* 2019;24(2):e172–e180.
3. Denison HJ, Worswick J, Bond CM, et al. Oral versus intra-vaginal imidazole and triazole antifungal treatment of uncomplicated vulvovaginal candidiasis (thrush). *Cochrane Database Syst Rev.* 2020;8(8):CD002845.

ADDITIONAL READING
Nambiar M, Varma SR, Jaber M, et al. Mycotic infections—mucormycosis and oral candidiasis associated with Covid-19: a significant and challenging association. *J Oral Microbiol.* 2021;13(1):1967699.

 ## SEE ALSO

Candidiasis, Invasive; HIV/AIDS

CODES

ICD10
- B37.9 Candidiasis, unspecified
- B37.2 Candidiasis of skin and nail
- B37.89 Other sites of candidiasis

CLINICAL PEARLS
- Candidiasis is typically a clinical diagnosis. KOH preparations are a simple confirmatory office test. Culture and biopsy are rarely needed.
- Person-to-person transmission is rare.
- Obtain a biopsy if there is a concern for oral cancer.
- Oral antifungal medications are hepatically metabolized and may have serious side effects.

CAPACITY (COMPETENCE) DETERMINATION AND INFORMED CONSENT

Sandra N. New, DNP

BASICS

- Personal autonomy in decision-making is a fundamental personal freedom.
- Capacity determination is an inherent element of the informed consent process.
- It is universally presumed that patients aged ≥18 years (or an emancipated minor under individual state laws) have legal and clinical capacity to give informed consent for health care testing, interventions, and treatment or to refuse same no matter the harm or benefit until proven otherwise.

DESCRIPTION

- Capacity:
  – Involves a clinical evaluation by a credentialed health care provider
  – Focuses on perceived ability of patient to participate and understand the process of informed consent
- Competence:
  – A legal determination of abilities, performed by a court judge
  – Involves medical information but does not need to be limited to only medical issues
- Capacity is the currently preferred term to competence: legal capacity and medical capacity.
- A capacity determination is needed when arriving at a health care decision for testing, treatment, or an intervention involving risk of harm or no improvement.
  – Any treating health care provider can evaluate capacity, including the provider also obtaining informed consent (although a psychiatrist or neuropsychiatric consultant is often asked to weigh in, other health care providers can determine capacity).
- Medical capacity is determined by:
  – Clinical observation and response to questions
  – Capacity assessment tool(s)
  – Cognitive assessment tool(s)
  – Interviews with a guardian or designated health care power of attorney (if indicated)

- The four "C"s of capacity are:
  – Context: comprehension of their health status
  – Choices: able to describe options
  – Consequences: able to explain possible outcomes
  – Consistency: continuity of choice selection
- Adequate cognition is a fundamental component but not the sole determinant of capacity (1).

EPIDEMIOLOGY

Most adults in the United States do not have an advanced directive—population studies show approximately 1/3 have completed an advanced directive (2).

Incidence

Need for capacity determination has been increased due to:

- Increasingly older population
- Prolonged chronic disease states
- Better patient rehabilitation opportunities
- Safer anesthetics and advanced postsurgery care

Prevalence

Prevalence varies based on the patient risk factors (pretest probability) and physician experience:

- ~3% of healthy outpatient seniors lack capacity.
- Highest rate of incapacity (68%) is in learning disabled patients.

ETIOLOGY AND PATHOPHYSIOLOGY

- Dementia is the most common reason individuals are found incapable of making health care decisions in the outpatient setting.
- Capacity is a dynamic state; reassessment is necessary with each significant health care decision and informed consent.

RISK FACTORS

- For incapacity:
  – Longevity, multiple comorbidities, hospitalized for medical reasons
  – Never married, never worked outside home

- Insufficient informed consent:
  – Patient factors:
    ○ Health illiteracy
    ○ Excessive information
  – Provider factors:
    ○ Inexperience with process (house staff for example)
    ○ Insufficient discussion time

GENERAL PREVENTION

Early assessment and periodic reassessment of capacity in:

- Dynamic patient conditions, like electrolyte imbalance, closed head injuries, delirium states
- After procedures with anesthesia or analgesics
- Enhancement and dissipation of mind-altering substances

COMMONLY ASSOCIATED CONDITIONS

- Dementia/Alzheimer disease, Parkinson disease, and traumatic brain injury
- Schizophrenia, depression, and substance abuse
- Acute illness, metabolic derangement

DIAGNOSIS

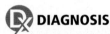

In patients without capacity, physicians are unable or unwilling to recognize the incapacity 42% of the cases (1)[C].

HISTORY

Family or frequent observers are resources regarding behavior patterns and reasoning displayed by patients.

- Engage in a deliberate approach, initially assessing for:
  – Communication barriers: physical impairments, lack of language fluency, medical jargon
  – Reversible causes of incapacity: metabolic derangements, medication side effects, serious illness, delirium
  – Health belief system; cultural differences; religious, political viewpoints, or adverse historical events

PHYSICAL EXAM
Verbal patient responses, facial expression, and body language often confirm capacity or suggest "warning signs" to obtain more formal evaluation.

DIAGNOSTIC TESTS & INTERPRETATION
Initial Tests (lab, imaging)
Screening for capacity occurs with:
- Informal patient conversations
- Discussions inherent to medical history taking
- Informed consent discussions

Follow-Up Tests & Special Considerations
- Four common tools for the formal evaluation of capacity
  - MacArthur Competence Assessment Tool for Treatment (MacCAT-T)—gold standard
    - Assesses understanding, reasoning, appreciation, and expression of choice
    - Semistructured interview; 20 minutes
  - Aid to Capacity Evaluation (ACE)
    - Semistructured interview; seven questions
    - Found predictive for medical and psychiatric patients, except for schizophrenic patients (3)[A]
  - Assessment of Capacity for Everyday Decision-Making (ACED)
    - Semistructured interview
    - Used with cognitively impaired seniors to measure capacity to perform independent activities of daily living
  - Capacity Assessment Tool (CAT)
    - Structured interview
    - Assesses capacity to discern between two intervention choices
- Special situation/considerations for assessment of capacity for informed consent
  - Communication impairments
    - Translators of all languages, including for deaf/mute and blind combined with deafness
    - Health literacy level accommodation
  - Patient participation in research or experimental intervention protocols
  - Patient refusal to participate in informed consent
  - Child or adolescent as patient

Diagnostic Procedures/Other
Cognitive screening (e.g., Mini-Mental State Examination) can contribute to (but not substitute for) capacity determination.

Test Interpretation
Capacity definition is state specific. Capacity determination in the informed consent process is determined by the treating provider (1)[C].

 ## TREATMENT

GENERAL MEASURES
Steps to take if a patient fails to have capacity or fails to display ability to participate in informed consent:
- Determine the acuity of the need for decision-making: (e.g., decisions regarding emergency care—"loss of life or limb"—are made by the treating provider).
- Correct any reversible causes of impaired capacity (e.g., electrolyte rebalance or language translation).
- Reframe questions that help determine capacity or simplify the explanation in informed consent.
- Seek out next of kin to become a proxy decision maker with understanding of patient's values.
- Court appointed guardian process is lengthy and usually is not necessary.

ISSUES FOR REFERRAL
Specialist consultation is not usually necessary to determine capacity for medical decision-making. As indicated, consider consulting with the following expert services:
- Psychiatry; neuropsychiatry; medical ethics; health care attorney

 ## ONGOING CARE

The following, in rank order, have responsibility for medical decision-making/informed consent if patient lacks capacity:
- Spouse (unless legally separated)
- Adult child
- A parent
- An adult sibling
- An adult who has provided unique care and has a special knowledge of the patient's values and is accessible (4)[C].

FOLLOW-UP RECOMMENDATIONS
Reassessment of patients is a provider responsibility:
- At each significant medical decision point
- If the patient shows signs of change in capacity

REFERENCES
1. Barstow C, Shahan B, Roberts M. Evaluating medical decision-making capacity in practice. *Am Fam Physician*. 2018;98(1):40–46.
2. Yadav KN, Gabler NB, Cooney E, et al. Approximately one in three US adults completes any type of advanced directives for end-of-life care. *Health Aff (Millwood)*. 2017;36(7):1244–1251.
3. Downey LVA, Zun L. Who has the ability to consent? *Prim Care Companion CNS Disord*. 2020;22(4):20m02619.
4. Weiss BD, Berman EA, Howe CL, et al. Medical decision-making for older adults without family. *J Am Geriatr Soc*. 2012;60(11):2144–2150.

CLINICAL PEARLS
- Use a structured approach in assessing decision-making capacity, including an assessment of language barriers, identification and remediation of reversible causes of incapacity, and a comprehensive interview to assess the ability to consent. Include appropriate formal assessment tools.
- Capacity is dynamic. Reassess at new (or changing) significant health care decision/informed consent points.
- The order of succession for decision-making is spouse, adult child, parent, adult sibling, and adult with close relationship.
- Integrate formal assessment with individual patient context to determine capacity.

C

CARBON MONOXIDE POISONING

Michael Gray, MD

 BASICS

DESCRIPTION

Carbon monoxide (CO) is an odorless, tasteless, colorless gas produced during the incomplete combustion of carbon-based compounds. If inhaled, CO may cause nonspecific symptoms and is potentially fatal (1).

- CO inhalation leads to displacement of oxygen (O_2) from binding sites on hemoglobin to form carboxyhemoglobin (COHb). The formation of COHb leads to tissue hypoxia from decreased O_2 carrying capacity and a left shift of the oxyhemoglobin dissociation curve (resulting in less O_2 delivery to a tissue at a given arterial O_2 pressure). CO binds to mitochondrial cytochrome oxidase, impairing adenosine triphosphate (ATP) production. It also binds to myoglobin, resulting in decreased contractility and vascular smooth muscle relaxation.

Pregnancy Considerations
Tissue hypoxia, due to CO poisoning, may cause significant fetal abnormalities because CO has a stronger affinity and a longer half-life when bound to fetal hemoglobin. The fetus is, therefore, susceptible to adverse outcomes even if the mother is unaffected.

EPIDEMIOLOGY

Incidence
- CO poisoning is the third leading cause of poisoning death in the United States. There were 481 deaths in 2020, a decrease of 8% from 2019.
- Accounts for 50,000 ER visits annually (16 cases per 100,000 population); 1–3% are fatal.
- Approximately 15,000 intentional poisoning occur per year, accounting for 2/3 reported deaths (10-fold higher than unintentional poisonings); results in approximately 1,200 to 1,600 deaths a year in the United States due to fire and non–fire-related poisoning.
- Vague symptoms may cause patients to not seek care, leading to underdiagnosis.
- May have concurrent co-exposures such as cyanide poisoning or intoxicants.

Prevalence
- More prevalent during the winter months in areas with colder climate.
- Occupational exposure to methylene chloride, found in industrial solvents such as paint remover, is metabolized to CO in the liver and can result in exposure and toxicity.

ETIOLOGY AND PATHOPHYSIOLOGY

- CO is rapidly absorbed through the lungs, binding hemoglobin with 210 to 240 times the affinity of O_2. This stabilizes hemoglobin in the relaxed high affinity state (R state), reducing O_2-carrying capacity and delivery, leading to left shift of the oxyhemoglobin dissociation curve. CO inactivates cytochrome oxidase. This leads to decreased ATP production, especially in tissues with high metabolic demands (brain, heart). The electron transport chain continues, generating superoxide radicals, leading to further damage.
- CO displaces nitric oxide (NO) from platelets, leading to platelet activation and aggregation. Oxidative stress, lipid peroxidation, and apoptosis are additional effects. NO also causes vasodilation and profound hypotension.

- Mitochondrial dysfunction and hypoxia leads to myocardial stunning and injury. Proteases released from neutrophil degranulation interact with xanthine hydrogenase forming xanthine oxidase. This inhibits endogenous defense against oxidative stress.
- CO also initiates an inflammatory cascade that can lead to oxidative degradation of nervous system lipids and delayed neurologic damage.

RISK FACTORS
- Alcohol and tobacco use
- Patients with severe COPD regardless of current tobacco smoke exposure; closed or improperly ventilated spaces
- Fires and fire-related injuries; high-risk vocations: coal miners, auto mechanics, paint stripping, work in the solvent industry; exposure to exhaust from motor vehicles, faulty furnaces, stoves, generator use (power outages and storms), and other fuel burning devices

GENERAL PREVENTION
- Appropriate ventilation around fuel-burning devices; installation of in-home CO monitors or alarms
- Postexposure determination of CO source to limit future exposures, eliminate source, and initiate treatment
- Public policy to ensure building code safety; limiting occupational exposures for those who work with automobiles, paint, solvents, or mines

COMMONLY ASSOCIATED CONDITIONS
- CO and cyanide poisoning often occur simultaneously after smoke inhalation and have synergistic effects.
- Intentional poisoning often occurs in the context of coingestion of other substances (~40%).
- Up to 50–75% of fire-related injuries have a component of CO poisoning.

 DIAGNOSIS

- Clinical triad of (i) relevant symptoms, (ii) history of CO exposure, (iii) and elevated COHb levels (2)
- An elevated COHb level of >5% in a nonsmoker and >10% in smokers; people living in high pollution areas and heavy tobacco users may have higher levels at baseline (1).
- The COHb level does not correlate with the severity of the illness or long-term prognosis but is necessary for the diagnosis (2),(3). Older pulse oximeters do not differentiate COHb from oxyhemoglobin, with normal oximeter readings in a hypoxic patient.

HISTORY
- The diagnosis of CO poisoning is dependent on duration and mechanism of exposure. No single symptom is sensitive or specific. A high index of suspicion is necessary.
- Common symptoms include:
  - Headache (91% of patients), dizziness (77%) and weakness (53%) are the most common symptoms; confusions/impaired judgment (1)
  - Nausea/vomiting, fatigue, chest pain, and shortness of breath
- Patients may also present with visual disturbances, seizures, syncope, arrhythmias, rhabdomyolysis, and loss of consciousness.

- Some patients may present with cardiopulmonary symptoms such as chest pain, palpitations, or shortness of breath.
- Long-term (subacute) exposure is defined as >24 hours and occurs with repeated exposure to low concentrations of CO. Symptoms include chronic fatigue, emotional distress, memory deficits, difficulty working, sleep disturbances, vertigo, neuropathy, recurrent infections, polycythemia, paresthesia, abdominal pain, and diarrhea.
- Delayed neurologic symptoms can appear 2 to 40 days later and is a poorly defined syndrome with incidence of 1–47% after CO exposure and can be manifested with a wide variety of neurologic complications (4).
- Exclude pregnancy in all female patients.

PHYSICAL EXAM
- Pulse oximetry does not distinguish between oxygenated hemoglobin, deoxygenated hemoglobin, COHb and methemoglobin. Therefore, patients exposed to CO must have COHb levels measured with a co-oximeter or blood gas analysis; respiratory depression or tachypnea, and cyanosis; tachycardia, hypotension, cardiac dysrhythmias (2)
- Findings vary. Patients often report confusion or have altered mental status.
- Classically described "cherry red" skin coloring of lips and skin is rare (<1% of cases).
- Examine for signs of burns of the skin and oropharynx (enclosed space fires) or other secondary injuries
- Full neurologic and mental status examinations; confusion/CNS depression, ataxia, visual field defects, papilledema, and nystagmus
- Respiratory depression or tachypnea, and cyanosis; tachycardia, hypotension, cardiac dysrhythmias

DIFFERENTIAL DIAGNOSIS
- Cyanide toxicity (also co-existent); methylene chloride (dichloromethane) inhalation or ingestion
- Viral syndromes
- Behavioral and mental health disorders (major depressive disorder)
- Infections (meningitis or encephalitis); metabolic causes (hypoglycemia, electrolyte impairment)
- Alcohol intoxication, opiates, acetylsalicylic acid (ASA) overdose; trauma; CNS lesions; coingestion of other substance

DIAGNOSTIC TESTS & INTERPRETATION

Initial Tests (lab, imaging)
- Diagnosis requires a recent history of CO exposure, consistent symptoms, and demonstration of an elevated COHb level.
- Chronic CO intoxication is more difficult to diagnose due to a lack of a clear eliciting event.
- Noninvasive COHb measurement should not be used to diagnose CO poisoning (3)[A].
- Arterial or venous blood gas:
  - COHb levels of >5% in nonsmokers, >10% in smokers. COHb may be low despite significant poisoning (e.g., treatment with O_2 or significant time elapses before the level is drawn).
  - Significant metabolic acidosis; anion gap >16; elevated lactate confers worse prognosis and should prompt consideration of cyanide toxicity PaO_2 tends to be normal because O_2 dissolved in blood is not affected by CO.

- Serum chemistries, CBC, troponin, lactic acid, chest x-ray
- ECG in all patients: cardiac enzymes in patients with moderate or severe poisoning; if elevated, there is an increased risk of mortality in all patients (~24%) and is even higher in patients aged >65 years and those with cardiac disease (3)[B]
- Pregnancy test in all women of childbearing age
- Toxicology screen (particularly important in intentional poisoning); CK to evaluate for rhabdomyolysis
- Head CT/MRI scan can help to rule out other neurologic causes; may also show infarction due to hypoxia/ischemia: The most common CT finding is bilateral globus pallidus lesions and diffuse white matter changes; however, the presence of bilateral globus pallidus changes is not pathognomonic for CO poisoning and can be seen with other intoxications as well (4).

Follow-Up Tests & Special Considerations
- Consider CO poisoning in younger patients with chest pain or symptoms suggestive of ischemia.
- Consider the diagnosis in afebrile patients with vague or "flulike" symptoms. CO poisoning and the flu are both common during the winter time. Patients may present as a group (coworkers, family members, school children) with similar symptoms. Patients with intentional poisoning should undergo behavioral evaluation when stable.
- Implement suicide precautions if appropriate.

 TREATMENT

GENERAL MEASURES
- Prompt removal from the CO source and initiation of O_2 therapy to displace CO.
- Supportive care as necessary; intubation and mechanical ventilation may be necessary for severe intoxication, particularly if the patient is unable to protect their airway or if there are signs of respiratory failure.
- Poison Control: 1-800-222-1222 (United States)

MEDICATION
First Line
100% O_2 via nonrebreathing reservoir facemask until COHb is normal (<3%) and patient is asymptomatic, regardless of O_2 saturation or PO_2.
- CO has a half-life of 250 to 320 minutes in room air and this half-life is reduced to 90 minutes with O_2 therapy via a nonrebreather mask.
- Consider high-flow nasal cannula, especially in patients unable to tolerate nonrebreather facemask.
- Concurrent treatment of associated disorders such as cyanide poisoning, intentional overdose, etc.

Second Line
Hyperbaric oxygen (HBO_2) therapy (not always readily available)

ADDITIONAL THERAPIES
- HBO_2 is associated with lower long- and short-term mortality rates and long-term neuropsychiatric symptoms, although criteria for starting therapy remains unclear (5).
- NBO_2 and HBO_2 reduce the elimination half-life of COHb to ~85 minutes and 20 minutes, respectively (2).
- If HBO_2 is unavailable, administer NBO_2 until CO has normalized and symptoms have resolved (3).

- HBO_2 therapy may reduce permanent neurologic deficit by reversing inflammatory response and mitochondrial dysfunction (2)[C].
- Optimal HBO_2 protocols are unclear (time to initiate HBO_2, depth, length of time, frequency) (1).
- HBO_2 currently recommended for exposure >24 hours; CO levels >25% (>20% if pregnant); altered mental status; cardiovascular ischemia; severe acidosis; HBO_2 not as likely to be helpful if >24 hours since exposure; greatest benefit occurs if initiated as early as possible, goal is within 6 hours of exposure; however, American College of Medical Toxicology and American Academy of Clinical Toxicology have not published guidelines (1).
- Empirically treat patients for cyanide poisoning who present with CO poisoning from a house fire, if the pH is <7.2 or plasma lactate is >10 mmol/L (2).
- Expert consensus favors HBO_2 therapy for pregnant women.
- Locating a HBO_2 chamber in the United States through the Undersea and Hyperbaric Medical Society Web site (https://www.uhms.org/) or via the Divers Alert Network Emergency Hotline (+1-919-684-9111) but are not always available 24/7.
- Estimated only 75 chambers available for high acuity emergency basis within the United States (4)

ADMISSION, INPATIENT, AND NURSING CONSIDERATIONS
- Patients whose symptoms do not improve after 4 to 5 hours of 100% O_2 should be transported to the nearest HBO_2 facility. Hospitalize patients with severe poisoning, ECG or laboratory evidence of end-organ damage, and those with concerning medical or social factors. Admit unconscious patients with CO poisoning to ICU following intubation.
- Patients with accidental poisoning and mild symptoms that resolve in the ED can be safely discharged.

 ONGOING CARE

FOLLOW-UP RECOMMENDATIONS
- All patients treated for acute CO poisoning should follow up in 1 to 2 months after discharge (2).
- If there are behavioral or cognitive concerns, pursue neuropsychological evaluation, particularly following intentional CO poisoning. Long-term cognitive, psychiatric, speech, occupational, and physical rehab may be necessary.

Patient Monitoring
Repeat measurement of COHb levels with arterial blood gases.

PATIENT EDUCATION
- Professional installation and maintenance of combustion devices
- CO detector in bedrooms and by potential CO sources; avoid use of combustion engines indoors; periodic furnace inspection
- Centers for Disease Control and Prevention: https://www.cdc.gov/

PROGNOSIS
Although most patients completely recover, chronic neuropsychiatric impairment is described in 12–68% of patients.

COMPLICATIONS
- High-activity metabolic tissues are at higher risk.
- Cardiac: myocardial ischemia/infarction; left ventricular dysfunction; dysrhythmia (prolonged QT)
- Pulmonary: inhalation injury; pulmonary edema; pneumonia; acute respiratory failure
- Neurologic: encephalopathy; vestibulomotor defects; hippocampal atrophy; cognitive dysfunction; parkinsonism
- Behavioral: depression, anxiety, irritability, moodiness, violent behavior

Geriatric Considerations
Increased number of comorbid leading to possibility of complications and worse outcomes

REFERENCES
1. Chenoweth JA, Albertson TE, Greer MR. Carbon monoxide poisoning. *Crit Care Clin.* 2021;37(3):657–672.
2. Rose JJ, Wang L, Xu Q, et al. Carbon monoxide poisoning: pathogenesis, management, and future directions of therapy. *Am J Respir Crit Care Med.* 2017;195(5):596–606.
3. Wolf SJ, Maloney GE, Shih RD, et al; for American College of Emergency Physicians Clinical Policies Subcommittee (Writing Committee) on Carbon Monoxide Poisoning. Clinical policy: critical issues in the evaluation and management of adult patients presenting to the emergency department with acute carbon monoxide poisoning. *Ann Emerg Med.* 2017;69(1):98–107.e6.
4. Nañagas KA, Penfound SJ, Kao LW. Carbon monoxide toxicity. *Emerg Med Clin North Am.* 2022;40(2):283–312.
5. Huang CC, Ho CH, Chen YC, et al. Hyperbaric oxygen therapy is associated with lower short- and long-term mortality in patients with carbon monoxide poisoning. *Chest.* 2017;152(5):943–953.

 CODES

ICD10
- T58.0 Toxic effect of carbon monoxide from motor vehicle exhaust
- T58.2 Toxic effect of carbon monoxide from incomplete combustion of other domestic fuels
- T58.9 Toxic effect of carbon monoxide from unspecified source

CLINICAL PEARLS
- CO poisoning warrants a high index of suspicion. Consider in patients exposed to fire; during the winter months, in young patients with chest pain; and when patients present as a group.
- Noninvasive pulse oximeters are not reliable for the diagnosis of CO poisoning.
- If CO poisoning is suspected, remove individuals from the source and immediately administer 100% O_2.
- Although not required in all cases, consider HBO_2 for the treatment of CO poisoning if it is available.

CARDIOMYOPATHY

Pawan Daga, MD

 BASICS

DESCRIPTION
- Cardiomyopathies are myocardial diseases which result in structural and functional heart abnormalities in the absence of coronary artery disease, congenital heart disease, valvular disease, or hypertension which could sufficiently explain the clinical myocardial dysfunction.
- Results in 5–10% of cases of heart failure
- Classification of cardiomyopathies
  – Primary (mainly involves the heart)
    ○ Genetic
      ▪ Hypertrophic cardiomyopathy (HCM)
      ▪ Arrhythmogenic right ventricular cardiomyopathy/dysplasia (ARVC/D)
      ▪ Left ventricular (LV) noncompaction (LVNC)
      ▪ Glycogen storage (Danon type, PRKAG2)
      ▪ Conduction defects
      ▪ Mitochondrial myopathies
      ▪ Ion channel disorders: long QT syndrome (LQTS), Brugada syndrome, short QT syndrome, and catecholaminergic polymorphic ventricular tachycardia (CPVT)
    ○ Mixed (genetic and nongenetic)
      ▪ Dilated cardiomyopathy (DCM)
      ▪ Restrictive (nonhypertrophied and nondilated)
    ○ Acquired
      ▪ Myocarditis, stress cardiomyopathy, peripartum, tachycardia induced, infants of type 1 diabetic mothers
  – Secondary (multiorgan involvement; see list)
    ○ Specific: ischemic, valvular, hypertensive, and congenital heart disease

EPIDEMIOLOGY
Incidence
DCM: 5 to 8 new cases per 100,000 population annually

Prevalence
- DCM: roughly 1:2,500; most common reason for heart transplantation
- HCM: 1:500 of the adult population; 50% sporadic and rest are familial

ETIOLOGY AND PATHOPHYSIOLOGY
- HCM: hypertrophied (>15 mm), nondilated left and/or right ventricle which is disproportionate to hemodynamic stress on the heart
- ARVC/D: involves the right ventricle with progressive loss of myocytes and fatty/fibrofatty tissue replacement; can be associated with myocarditis (adenovirus or enterovirus)
- LVNC: congenital cardiomyopathies with "spongy" appearance of the LV myocardium
- LQTS: most common ion channelopathy with prolonged ventricular repolarization and QTc
- DCM: Ventricular chamber enlargement and systolic dysfunction with normal LV wall thickness result in progressive heart failure and further complications; strong genetic component with infectious and toxic etiologies
- RCM: normal/decreased ventricular volume with restrictive physiology, biatrial enlargement, and impaired ventricular filling
- Myocarditis: acute or chronic inflammation of the myocardium produced by toxins, drugs, or infectious causes
- Peripartum cardiomyopathy (PPCM): a form of DCM with LV systolic dysfunction and heart failure of unknown etiology
- Stress cardiomyopathies: triggered by profound psychological stress resulting in acute but rapidly reversible LV systolic dysfunction
- Endocrine: diabetes mellitus, hyperthyroidism, hypothyroidism, hyperparathyroidism, pheochromocytoma, acromegaly
- Nutritional deficiencies: beriberi, pellagra, scurvy, selenium, carnitine, kwashiorkor
- Autoimmune/collagen: systemic lupus erythematosus, dermatomyositis, rheumatoid arthritis, scleroderma, polyarteritis nodosa
- Infectious causes
  – Viral (e.g., HIV, coxsackievirus, adenovirus)
  – Bacterial and mycobacterial (e.g., diphtheria, rheumatic fever)
  – Parasitic (e.g., toxoplasmosis, *Trypanosoma cruzi*)

- Infiltrative (1): amyloidosis, Gaucher disease, Hurler disease, Hunter disease, Fabry disease
- Storage: hemochromatosis, glycogen storage disease (type II, Pompe), Niemann-Pick disease
- Neuromuscular/neurologic: Duchenne and Emery-Dreifuss muscular dystrophies, Friedreich ataxia, myotonic dystrophy, neurofibromatosis, tuberous sclerosis
- Toxic: alcohol, drugs and chemotherapy (anthracyclines, cyclophosphamide, trastuzumab [Herceptin]), radiation, heavy metal, chemical agents
- Inflammatory (granulomatous): sarcoidosis
- Idiopathic
- Endomyocardial: endomyocardial fibrosis, hypereosinophilic syndrome (Loeffler endocarditis)

Genetics
- Genetic causes well recognized in HCM; less common in DCM
- Most familial cardiomyopathies are inherited in autosomal dominant pattern.
- Involves mutations in sarcomere contractile proteins.

RISK FACTORS
Same as etiology

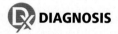 **DIAGNOSIS**

HISTORY
- Dyspnea at rest or with exertion, paroxysmal nocturnal dyspnea, orthopnea
- Right upper quadrant pain or bloating, edema
- Chest pain

PHYSICAL EXAM
- Tachypnea
- Cheyne-Stokes breathing
- Low pulse pressure
- Cool extremities
- Jugular venous distention
- Bibasilar rales
- Tachycardia

- Displaced point of maximal impulse (PMI)
- S_3 gallop
- Blowing systolic murmur
- Hepatosplenomegaly
- Ascites
- Edema

DIFFERENTIAL DIAGNOSIS
- Severe pulmonary disease
- Primary pulmonary hypertension
- Recurrent pulmonary embolism
- Constrictive pericarditis
- Some advanced forms of malignancy
- Anemia

DIAGNOSTIC TESTS & INTERPRETATION
Initial Tests (lab, imaging)
- ECG: LV hypertrophy, interventricular conduction delay, atrial fibrillation (Afib), evidence of prior Q-wave infarction
- Chest radiograph: cardiomegaly, increased vascular markings to the upper lobes, pleural effusions
- Echocardiography
  - In DCM: four-chamber enlargement and global hypokinesis; mural thrombi may be seen.
  - In HCM: Severe LV hypertrophy is present; systolic anterior motion of mitral valve, MR, dynamic flow obstruction (2)
  - In RCM: low voltage, pseudoinfarction pattern
- Cardiac MRI (3)
  - Useful to characterize certain nonischemic cardiomyopathies like myocarditis or infiltrative disease
  - In HCM: hypertrophy + patchy delayed enhancement
- Stress myocardial perfusion imaging (MPI): useful to rule out ischemia

Follow-Up Tests & Special Considerations
Genetic tests, genetic counselling

Diagnostic Procedures/Other
Cardiac catheterization: to rule out ischemia

 ## TREATMENT

MEDICATION
First Line
- Treat associated heart failure (2). See "Heart Failure, Chronic."
- If nonobstructive physiology: transplant evaluation
- If refractory: Options include surgical myectomy and alcohol septal ablation.
- Caution with use of diuretics (decrease in preload can worsen output) and digoxin (increased contractility can worsen obstruction)
- Negative ionotropes/chronotropes: β-blockers, CCB
- Implantable cardioverter-defibrillator (ICD): if VT/VF/SCD prevention; consider if family history of SCD
- Counsel to prevent dehydration and extreme exertion.
- If associated Afib: anticoagulation, rate control with β-blocker
- Immunosuppression: in cases of DCM associated with myocarditis, collagen vascular disease
- Tafamidis (TTR binder): for restrictive cardiomyopathy associated with TTR amyloid

ISSUES FOR REFERRAL
- Management by a heart failure team improves outcomes and facilitates early transplant referral.
- Refer for transplant evaluation if refractory to medical management.

 ## ONGOING CARE

DIET
Low fat, low salt, fluid restriction

PROGNOSIS
~20–40% of patients in NYHA FC IV die within 1 year. With a transplant, 1-year survival is as high as 94%.

COMPLICATIONS
Worsening congestive heart failure syncope, renal failure, arrhythmias, or sudden death

REFERENCES
1. Seward JB, Casaclang-Verzosa G. Infiltrative cardiovascular diseases: cardiomyopathies that look alike. *J Am Coll Cardiol.* 2010;55(17):1769–1779.
2. Elliott PM, Anastasakis A, Borger MA, et al; for Authors/Task Force members. 2014 ESC guidelines on diagnosis and management of hypertrophic cardiomyopathy: the Task Force for the Diagnosis and Management of Hypertrophic Cardiomyopathy of the European Society of Cardiology (ESC). *Euro Heart J.* 2014;35(39):2733–2779.
3. Japp AG, Gulati A, Cook SA, et al. The diagnosis and evaluation of dilated cardiomyopathy. *J Am Coll Cardiol.* 2016;67(25):2996–3010.

 ## SEE ALSO

- Alcohol Use Disorder (AUD); Alcohol Withdrawal; Amyloidosis; Diabetes Mellitus, Type 1; Diabetes Mellitus, Type 2; Hypertension, Essential; Hypertrophic Cardiomyopathy; Hypothyroidism, Adult; Protein–Energy Malnutrition; Rheumatic Fever; Sarcoidosis
- Algorithm: Congestive Heart Failure: Differential Diagnosis

 ## CODES

ICD10
- I42.9 Cardiomyopathy, unspecified
- I42.0 Dilated cardiomyopathy
- I42.5 Other restrictive cardiomyopathy

CLINICAL PEARLS
- Cardiomyopathy represents the end-stage of a large number of disease processes involving the heart muscle.
- Ischemic, hypertensive, postviral, familial, alcoholic, and incessant tachycardia-induced are the most common cardiomyopathy varieties seen in the United States.
- Core therapy for heart failure applies salt restriction, diuretics, ACE inhibitors, β-blockers, digoxin, and electrical treatments, such as cardiac resynchronization and implantable defibrillators, as appropriate.

CAROTID SINUS HYPERSENSITIVITY

Afsha Rais Kaisani, MD • Tasaduq Hussain Mir, MD, FAAFP • Niyomi De Silva, MD

 BASICS

Carotid sinus hypersensitivity (CSH) is an exaggerated response to stimulation or pressure applied to the carotid sinuses that results clinically as syncope or presyncope.

DESCRIPTION

- The carotid sinuses play a central role in maintaining blood pressure (BP) homeostasis.
- The carotid sinuses are located near the bifurcation of the internal and external carotid arteries and contain baroreceptors that are responsive to changes in arterial pressure.
- An endogenous increase in BP or external pressure applied to a carotid sinus can cause an increase in the baroreceptor firing rate and activate vagal efferents and/or inhibit the sympathetic discharge to the heart and blood vessels which results in a slowing of the heart rate and drop in BP.
- In CSH, stimulation of one or both carotid sinuses, (such as mechanical forces with turning the neck) causes an exaggerated baroreceptor response that can result in dizziness or syncope.
- There are three definitions for CSH (1):
  – Standard criteria: a pause in heart rate of ≥3 s in response to carotid sinus massage (CSM) and/or ≥50 mm Hg drop in systolic BP or both of the above
  – Krediet criteria: a pause in heart rate of ≥6 s in response to CSM and/or a fall in MAP to a value <60 mmHg for ≥6 s
  – Kerr criteria: a pause in heart rate in response to CSM >95th percentile of the population response (7.3 s asystole), and/or vasodepression in response to CSM >95th percentile of the population response (>77 mmHg fall in systolic BP), or both
- CSH is generally divided into three subtypes, based on response to CSM:
  – Cardioinhibitory (70–75%): asystole for at least 3 seconds
  – Vasodepressive (5–10%): fall in systolic BP of at least 50 mm Hg
  – Mixed (20–25%): combination of the first 2 subtypes
- Carotid sinus syndrome (CSS) typically (but not consistently) refers to CSH *with syncope and may be classified as*:
  – Spontaneous CSS: syncope after accidental mechanical manipulation (trigger) of the carotid sinuses (e.g., shaving, tight collars, or tumors)
  – Induced CSS: syncope diagnosed by CSM although no mechanical trigger is found

EPIDEMIOLOGY

- Disease of elderly; most often occurs in male patients >65 years.
- Associated with a history of coronary artery disease (CAD) and hypertension (HTN), with right CSH > left CSH

Prevalence

- In 2006, CSH was found in 39% of unselected adults >65 years of age using standard diagnostic criteria and found to be comparable with 2019 review of prevalence data (2).
- CSH may be a cause of the symptoms in 30% of elderly patients with unexplained syncope.

ETIOLOGY AND PATHOPHYSIOLOGY

- The exact site that causes the hypersensitivity response remains unknown. Changes in any part of the reflex arc or the target organs may give rise to this condition. It may be a part of a generalized autonomic disorder associated with autonomic dysregulation.
- Associated with resting sympathetic overactivity and increased baroreflex sensitivity
- Bradycardia and asystole seen in cardioinhibitory and mixed CSH subtypes appear to be mediated by vagal efferents, whereas vasodilatation and arterial hypotension in the vasodepressor and mixed subtypes are attributed to decrease sympathetic tone.
- Symptomatic CSH has been shown to be associated with impaired cerebral autoregulation and found to be normal in asymptomatic CSH.
- Atherosclerosis may diminish carotid sinus compliance, resulting in a reduction in afferent impulse traffic in the baroreflex pathway.
- CSH is often idiopathic but can be caused by:
  – Carotid body tumors
  – Inflammatory and malignant lymph nodes in the neck
  – Extensive scarring from prior neck surgery in the area of the carotid sinus
  – Metastatic cancer

RISK FACTORS

- Advanced age, male gender
- CAD
- HTN
- DM

COMMONLY ASSOCIATED CONDITIONS

- Carotid sinus syncope, Sick sinus syndrome
- Atrioventricular block
- CAD
- HTN
- Orthostatic hypotension
- Vasovagal syncope
- Alzheimer disease
- Parkinson disease

DIAGNOSIS

HISTORY

- Recurrent syncope: usually sudden, unexplained, of short duration, seemingly spontaneous, and with complete recovery, although fractures and other injuries may occur
- Unexplained falls: Evidence of a causal relationship is suggested between falls and the cardioinhibitory subgroup.

- Dizziness: manifests as transient light-headedness or presyncope but not usually as true vertigo; associated more with vasodepressor and mixed subtypes
- Syncope may be associated with prodrome or retrograde amnesia.
- Causative or exacerbating factors
  – Any CSM-like maneuver such as shaving, wearing tight collars, or turning one's head sharply
  – Neck tumors, extensive neck scarring secondary to radical dissection or radiation fibrosis, and neck trauma
  – Certain medications can potentiate symptoms associated with CSH:
    ○ Digoxin or β-blockers (especially with cardioinhibitory subtype)
    ○ Physostigmine, morphine, methacholine increase vagal sensitivity and may predispose to cardioinhibitory subtype of CSH

PHYSICAL EXAM

Normal unless carotid baroreceptor is stimulated, then

- Bradycardia
- Hypotension
- Pallor
- Diaphoresis

DIFFERENTIAL DIAGNOSIS

- Neurocardiogenic syncope
- Postural hypotension
- Situational syncope
- Postural tachycardia syndrome (POTS)
- Primary autonomic insufficiency
- Hypovolemia
- Dysrhythmias
- Sick sinus syndrome
- Cerebrovascular insufficiency
- Other causes of syncope (e.g., metabolic, psychogenic)
- ECG may demonstrate sinus pause(s) or atrial-ventricular block.
- Carotid duplex scan to rule out carotid stenosis in presence of a bruit (see the following section)

DIAGNOSTIC TESTS & INTERPRETATION

Diagnostic Procedures/Other

- CSM is indicated in patients >40 years of age with syncope of unknown etiology after a negative initial evaluation.
- Commonly accepted technique for accurate diagnosis involves the following steps:
  – Patient in supine position for 5 minutes with continuous BP monitoring and ECG (on footplate-type tilt table for increased diagnostic accuracy); baseline BP and ECG are recorded.
  – For 5 to 10 seconds, apply firm longitudinal massage over the right carotid sinus (between the superior border of the thyroid and the angle of the mandible) at the site of maximal pulsation:
    ○ Note that light pressure over the carotid sinus will not reliably produce a hypersensitivity response.
    ○ Record symptoms and BP and note ECG changes.
    ○ Discontinue if asystole ≥3 seconds.
  – If initial test nondiagnostic, apply pressure to the left carotid sinus while the patient remains supine; if still nondiagnostic, repeat in 70-degree head-up tilt (first on the right then, if necessary, the left), allowing time for hemodynamic adjustment to the head-up position.

- Evidence behind the testing strategy
  - Right side first: Up to 66% with CSH have positive response on the right; if a positive right response, no need to repeat test on the left side.
  - 30% of CSM exams are found to be nondiagnostic in the supine position; positive predictive value increases from 77% to 96% with a specificity of 93% by performing CSM in the 70-degree position.
- Absolute contraindications for CSM testing
  - Carotid bruit present: must examine via carotid ultrasound with Doppler first:
    ○ No testing if >70% stenosis
    ○ Supine only testing if 50–70% stenosis
  - Myocardial infarction, transient ischemic attack, or stroke within the past 3 months
- Relative contraindications to CSM testing
  - History of ventricular tachycardia or ventricular fibrillation
  - False-positive results with CSM are relatively common in the elderly. Care should be taken to exclude other causes of syncope.
  - Neurologic and cardiovascular complications have been reported during CSM. Cardiovascular complications (primarily arrhythmia) are extremely rare. Transient neurologic symptoms and signs occur in up to 0.9% of patients. Persistent neurologic deficits are extremely rare following CSM. Correctly performed CSM should be considered a safe, low-risk procedure.

Test Interpretation

Standard positive response criteria (asystole ≥3 seconds and/or drop in systolic BP ≥50 mm Hg) is based on historical observations, although expert review of more recent data suggest these criteria may be too sensitive (3)[C].

- Specificity of the CSM technique increases if reproduction of a patient's syncope is demonstrated during a test (3)[B].

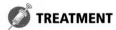

TREATMENT

GENERAL MEASURES

- No treatment is required for isolated CSH in asymptomatic individuals. Educate patients about CSH and monitoring and avoidance of triggers.
- High-dietary salt intake and increased fluid intake may be helpful to maintain intravascular volume in patients with vasodepressor subtype and absence of other cardiovascular disease.
- Evaluation for driving restrictions.

MEDICATION

First Line

No single agent has demonstrated long-term effectiveness for treatment of recurrent and symptomatic CSH.

Second Line

- Fludrocortisone or midodrine may be used to improve orthostatic symptoms in patients with vasodepressor subtype (not approved by FDA for this indication). However, fludrocortisone causes sodium and water retention and should be used with caution in elderly patients with heart disease. An adverse effect with midodrine is that it increases mean ambulatory BP.
- Atropine may be used in the acute setting in patients with cardioinhibitory subtype with bradycardia.
- Some evidence of benefit from sertraline and fluoxetine in patients unresponsive to pacemakers

SURGERY/OTHER PROCEDURES

- 2017 ACC/AHA/HRS Guideline for the Evaluation and Management of Patients With Syncope notes that evidence is very limited and thus recommendation strength not high. Available evidence does not support the use of pacing for reflex-mediated syncope beyond patients with recurrent vasovagal syncope and asystole documented by implantable loop recorder.
- Permanent pacing may reduce the frequency of symptoms but may not completely eliminate them.
- Surgery for patients with CSH secondary to mass effect from tumor burden
- Carotid sinus denervation by surgery or radiation therapy is no longer recommended because of the high rate of complications.

 ONGOING CARE

PATIENT EDUCATION

- Avoid precipitating maneuvers (as described above) that place pressure on the neck, such as tight collars and neckties.
- With syncope, restrict driving or other potentially hazardous activities until the patient is cleared by the physician
- Avoid precipitating medications like vasodilators and those temporally related to symptoms.
- Teach patient to assume supine position if prodromal symptoms or presyncope occurs.
- Explain diagnosis, provide reassurance, and explain risk of recurrence.

PROGNOSIS

- The presence of CSH has not been demonstrated to confer an independent mortality risk.
- Untreated CSS patients have a syncope recurrence rate as high as 62% within 4 years.
- Patients with cardioinhibitory CSH who received a pacemaker had a significant reduction in their mean number of falls, from 9.3 to 4.1 falls in a 1-year follow-up period.

COMPLICATIONS

CSH, according to Kerr criteria, is associated with increased mortality. Further evaluation is needed to predict future falls, syncope, and ability of criteria to identify patients who would benefit from pacing (1)[B].

REFERENCES

1. McDonald C, Pearce MS, Newton JL, et al. Modified criteria for carotid sinus hypersensitivity are associated with increased mortality in a population-based study. *Europace*. 2016;18(7):1101–1107.
2. Kadermuneer P, Sandeep R, Haridasan V, et al. Prevalence and one-year outcome of carotid sinus hypersensitivity in unexplained syncope: a prospective cohort study from South India. *Indian Heart J*. 2019;71(1):1–6.
3. Runser LA, Gauer RL, Houser A. Syncope: evaluation and differential diagnosis. *Am Fam Physician*. 2017;95(5):303–312.

ADDITIONAL READING

- Amin V, Pavri BB. Carotid sinus syndrome. *Cardiol Rev*. 2015;23(3):130–134.
- Kapoor JR. Carotid sinus hypersensitivity: a diagnostic pearl. *J Am Coll Cardiol*. 2009;54(17):1633.
- Varosy PD, Chen LY, Miller AL, et al. Pacing as a treatment for reflex-mediated (vasovagal, situational, or carotid sinus hypersensitivity) syncope: a systematic review for the 2017 ACC/AHA/HRS guideline for the evaluation and management of patients with syncope: a report of the American College of Cardiology/American Heart Association Task Force on Clinical Practice Guidelines and the Heart Rhythm Society. *Circulation*. 2017;136(5):e123–e135.

 SEE ALSO

Syncope

 CODES

ICD10

G90.01 Carotid sinus syncope

CLINICAL PEARLS

- Consider CSH as a potential cause for syncope, dizziness, or unexplained falls, especially in the elderly.
- Diagnose CSH via CSM (using firm pressure for 5 to 10 seconds), producing asystole of at least 3 seconds and/or a drop in systolic BP of at least 50 mm Hg.
- Remember to auscultate for carotid artery bruit prior to considering CSM.
- Consider dual-chamber pacemaker in patients with recurrent syncope and cardioinhibitory or mixed CSH subtypes.
- The finding of CSH does not exclude other causes of syncope.

CAROTID STENOSIS
Rade N. Pejic, MD

BASICS

Carotid stenosis may be caused by atherosclerosis, intimal fibroplasia, vasculitis, adventitial cysts, or vascular tumors. However, atherosclerosis is the most common etiology.

DESCRIPTION
- Narrowing of the carotid artery lumen is typically due to atherosclerotic changes in the vessel wall. Atherosclerotic plaques are responsible for 90% of extracranial carotid lesions and up to 30% of all ischemic strokes.
- A "hemodynamically significant" carotid stenosis produces an internal carotid artery peak systolic velocity (PSV) >125 cm/s on carotid duplex imaging.
- Carotid lesions are classified by the following:
  - Symptom status
    ○ Asymptomatic: homogenous and stable
    ○ Symptomatic: heterogeneous and unstable; present with stroke or transient cerebral ischemic attack
  - Degree of stenosis
    ○ Total occlusion: No detectable patent lumen
    ○ Near occlusion: Markedly narrow lumen on color Doppler ultrasound (US)
    ○ High grade: PSV >230 cm/s; 70–99% stenosis
    ○ Moderate grade: PSV 125 to 230 cm/s; 50–69% stenosis
    ○ Low grade: PSV <125 cm/s with visible plaque or intimal thickening; <50% stenosis
    ○ Normal: PSV <125 cm/s and no visible plaque or intimal thickening

EPIDEMIOLOGY
More common in men and with increasing age (see "Risk Factors")

Incidence
Unclear (Asymptomatic patients often go undiagnosed.)

Prevalence
- Moderate stenosis
  - Age <50 years: men 0.2%, women 0%
  - Age >80 years: men 7.5%, women 5%
- Severe stenosis
  - Age <50 years: men 0.1%, women 0%
  - Age >80 years: men 3.1%, women 0.9%

ETIOLOGY AND PATHOPHYSIOLOGY
- Atherosclerosis at the carotid bifurcation begins during adolescence. The carotid bulb has unique blood flow dynamics. Hemodynamic disturbances cause endothelial injury and dysfunction. Plaque formation in vessel wall results and stenosis then ensues.
- Initial cause is not well understood, but certain risk factors are frequently present (see "Risk Factors"). Tensile stress on the vessel wall, turbulence, and arterial wall shear stress seem to be involved.

Genetics
- Increased incidence among family members
- Genetically linked factors
  - Diabetes mellitus (DM), race, hypertension (HTN), family history, obesity, hyperlipidemia
  - In a recent single nucleotide polymorphism study, the following genes were strongly associated with worse carotid plaque: *TNFSF4*, *PPARA*, *TLR4*, *ITGA2*, and *HABP2*.

RISK FACTORS
- Nonmodifiable factors: advanced age (>65 years old), male sex, family history, coronary artery disease (CAD), peripheral artery disease, aortic aneurysmal disease, congenital arteriopathies
- Modifiable factors: smoking, diet, dyslipidemia, physical inactivity, obesity, HTN, DM
- Possible factors: *Chlamydia pneumoniae* and *Cytomegalovirus*

GENERAL PREVENTION
- Antihypertensive treatment to maintain BP <140/90 mm Hg; see "Hypertension, Essential."
- Smoking cessation to reduce the risk of atherosclerosis progression and stroke
- Lipid control: plaque stabilization and regression of carotid atherosclerotic lesions seen with statin therapy

COMMONLY ASSOCIATED CONDITIONS
- Transient ischemic attack (TIA)/stroke
- CAD/myocardial infarction (MI)
- Peripheral vascular disease (PVD)

DIAGNOSIS

Screening for carotid stenosis is not recommended for asymptomatic low-risk patients (1). However, screening should be considered for asymptomatic high-risk patients and in the setting of symptoms suggestive of stroke or TIA.

HISTORY
- Identification of modifiable and nonmodifiable comorbidities (See "Risk Factors.")
- History of cerebral ischemic event
- Stroke, TIA, amaurosis fugax (monocular blindness), aphasia
- CAD/MI
- Peripheral arterial disease
- Review of systems, with focus on risk factors for
  - Cardiovascular disease
  - Stroke (HTN and arrhythmias)

PHYSICAL EXAM
- Lateralizing neurologic deficits: contralateral motor and/or sensory deficit
- Amaurosis fugax: ipsilateral transient visual obscuration from retinal ischemia
- Visual field defect
- Dysarthria, aphasia (in the case of dominant hemisphere involvement, usually left)
- Carotid bruit (low sensitivity and specificity)

DIFFERENTIAL DIAGNOSIS
- Aortic valve stenosis
- Aortic arch atherosclerosis
- Arrhythmia with cardiogenic embolization
- Migraine
- Brain tumor
- Metabolic disturbances
- Functional/psychological deficit
- Seizure

DIAGNOSTIC TESTS & INTERPRETATION
Initial Tests (lab, imaging)
Workup for suspected TIA/stroke may include the following:
- CBC with differential
- Basic metabolic panel
- ESR (if temporal arteritis is a consideration)
- Glucose/hemoglobin A1c
- Fasting lipid profile
- Duplex ultrasonography is the recommended initial diagnostic test in patients with known or suspected carotid stenosis. Duplex US identifies ≥50% stenosis, with 98% sensitivity and 88% specificity.

Follow-Up Tests & Special Considerations
Other noninvasive imaging techniques can add detail to duplex results:
- CT angiography
  - 88% sensitivity and 100% specificity
  - Requires IV contrast with risk for subsequent renal morbidity
- MR angiography
  - 95% sensitivity and 90% specificity but tends to overestimate the degree of stenosis
  - Evaluates cerebral circulation (extracranial and intracranial) as well as aortic arch and common carotid artery
  - The presence of unstable plaque can be determined.

Diagnostic Procedures/Other
Cerebral digital subtraction angiography is the gold standard for diagnosis:
- Delineates the anatomy pertaining to aortic arch and proximal vessels
- The procedure is invasive and has multiple risks:
  - Contrast-induced renal dysfunction (1–5% complication rate)
  - Thromboembolic-related complications (1–2.6% complication rate) and neurologic complications
  - Should be used only when other tests are not conclusive

Test Interpretation
- Stenosis consistently occurs at the carotid bifurcation with plaque formation most often at the level of the proximal internal carotid artery:
  - Plaque is thickest at the carotid bifurcation.
  - Plaque occupies the intima and inner media and avoids outer media and adventitia.
- Plaque histology
  - Homogenous (stable) plaques seldom hemorrhage or ulcerate:
    ○ Fatty streak and fibrous tissue deposition
    ○ Diffuse intimal thickening
  - Heterogenous (unstable) plaques may hemorrhage or ulcerate:
    ○ Presence of lipid-laden macrophages, necrotic debris, cholesterol crystals
    ○ Ulcerated plaques
  - Soft and gelatinous clots with platelets, fibrin, and red and white blood cells

TREATMENT

Therapeutic lifestyle modifications, smoking cessation, blood pressure (BP) control, glycemic control, statins, and antiplatelet medications are the primary treatments for both asymptomatic and symptomatic carotid stenosis.

GENERAL MEASURES
- Therapeutic lifestyle modifications: heart-healthy diet, weight loss, and exercise of 30 min/day at least 5 days/week
- Patients should be advised to quit smoking and offered smoking cessation intervention.

MEDICATION
- Control of HTN with antihypertensive agents to maintain BP <140/90 mm Hg; in carefully selected individuals, tighter BP control might reduce cerebrovascular events but this remains uncertain.
- Antihypertensive treatment with an ACE-I or ARB reduces the stroke risk in individuals with diabetes.
- Glycemic control in diabetic patients using lifestyle modifications, metformin, SGLT-2 inhibitors, and GLP-1 agonists
- Statin therapy using the maximally tolerated statin dosage
- Aspirin: 75 to 325 mg/day
- If the patient has sustained a TIA or ischemic stroke, antiplatelet therapy with
  - Aspirin alone (75 to 325 mg/day) *or*
  - Clopidogrel alone (75 mg/day), *or*
  - Aspirin plus extended-release dipyridamole (25 and 200 mg BID, respectively)
  - A combination of clopidogrel plus aspirin is NOT recommended within 3 months post-TIA or CVA.

ISSUES FOR REFERRAL
- For acute symptomatic stroke, order imaging and consult neurology.
- For known carotid stenosis, some suggest duplex imaging every 6 months if stenosis is >50% and the patient is a surgical candidate.

SURGERY/OTHER PROCEDURES
- Symptomatic carotid stenosis (history of ischemia ipsilateral to stenosis)
  - Carotid endarterectomy (CEA) is of some benefit in 50–69% symptomatic stenosis, highly beneficial for those with 70–99% stenosis without near occlusion, and has no benefit in people with carotid near-occlusion or total occlusion (2).
  - CEA is recommended for patients with a life expectancy of at least 5 years. The anticipated rate of perioperative stroke or mortality must be <6%.
  - Treatment with aspirin (81 to 325 mg/day) is recommended for all patients who are having CEA. Aspirin should be started prior to surgery and continued for at least 3 months postsurgery but may be continued indefinitely.
  - Carotid artery stenting (CAS) provides similar long-term outcomes as CEA.
    - CAS has an increased risk of adverse cerebrovascular events in the elderly compared to the young but has a similar mortality risk.
    - CAS is suggested in selected patients with neck anatomy unfavorable for arterial surgery and those with comorbid conditions that greatly increase the risk of anesthesia and surgery.
    - Dual antiplatelet therapy with aspirin (81 to 325 mg/day) plus clopidogrel (75 mg/day) is recommended for 30 days post-CAS.
  - Transcarotid artery revascularization (TCAR) appears to avoid the pitfalls of CAS with similar outcomes to CEA (3).
- Asymptomatic patients: As compared with CAS, CEA is the preferred option for the management of asymptomatic carotid stenosis if a surgical option is chosen although TCAR is now an alternative in select patients. CAS has the potential for increased risks of periprocedural stroke and periprocedural death (4)[A].

ADMISSION, INPATIENT, AND NURSING CONSIDERATIONS
- Any patient with a presentation of acute symptomatic carotid stenosis should be hospitalized for further diagnostic workup and appropriate therapy.
- Rapid evaluation for symptoms compatible with TIA should be obtained in the emergency department (ED) or inpatient setting.
- Discharge criteria: 24 to 48 hours post-CEA, if ambulating, taking adequate PO intake, and neurologically intact

 ONGOING CARE

FOLLOW-UP RECOMMENDATIONS
Patient Monitoring
- Duplex at 2 to 6 weeks postoperatively
- Duplex every 6 to 12 months
- Reoperative CEA or CAS is reasonable, if there is rapidly progressive restenosis.
- Patients with any of the following: renal failure, heart failure, diabetes, and age >80 years have a high readmission rate following CEA; thus, intensive medical therapy and rigorous follow-up is recommended.

DIET
Heart-healthy diet low in saturated fat and no trans fat

PATIENT EDUCATION
For patient education materials on this topic, consult the following: https://medlineplus.gov/carotidarterydisease.html

COMPLICATIONS
- Untreated: TIA/stroke (risk of ipsilateral stroke approximately 1.68% per year)
- Postoperative (status post-CEA)
  - Perioperative (within 30 days)
    - Stroke/death, cranial nerve injury, hemorrhage, hemodynamic instability, MI
  - Late (>30 days postoperatively)
    - Recurrent stenosis, false aneurysm at the surgical site

REFERENCES
1. Krist AH, Davidson KW, Mangione CM, et al; for US Preventive Services Task Force. Screening for asymptomatic carotid artery stenosis: US Preventive Services Task Force recommendation statement. *JAMA*. 2021;325(5):476–481.
2. AbuRahma AF, Avgerinos ED, Chang RW, et al. Society for vascular surgery clinical practice guidelines for management of extracranial cerebrovascular disease. *J Vasc Surg*. 2022;75(1S):4S–22S.
3. Columbo JA, Martinez-Camblor P, Stone DH, et al. Procedural safety comparison between transcarotid artery revascularization, carotid endarterectomy, and carotid stenting: perioperative and 1-year rates of stroke or death. *J Am Heart Assoc*. 2022;11(19):e024964.
4. Moresoli P, Habib B, Reynier P, et al. Carotid stenting versus endarterectomy for asymptomatic carotid artery stenosis: a systematic review and meta-analysis. *Stroke*. 2017;48(8):2150–2157.

 SEE ALSO

Algorithms: Stroke; Transient Ischemic Attack and Transient Neurologic Defects

 CODES

ICD10
- I65.29 Occlusion and stenosis of unspecified carotid artery
- I65.21 Occlusion and stenosis of right carotid artery
- I65.22 Occlusion and stenosis of left carotid artery

CLINICAL PEARLS
- Atherosclerosis is responsible for 90% of all cases of carotid artery stenosis.
- Duplex US is the best initial imaging modality.
- Antiplatelet therapy and aggressive treatment of vascular risk factors are the mainstays of medical therapy.
- Compared with CEA, CAS increases the risk of any stroke but decreases the risk of MI. For every 1,000 patients opting for stenting rather than endarterectomy, 19 more patients would have strokes and 10 fewer would have MIs.
- TCAR appears to avoid the pitfalls of CAS with similar outcomes to CEA.

CARPAL TUNNEL SYNDROME

Rahul Kapur, MD • Kelly S. Thao, MD

 BASICS

DESCRIPTION
- Symptomatic compression neuropathy of the median nerve
- Increased pressure within the carpal tunnel leads to compression of the median nerve and characteristic motor-sensory findings.
- The dorsal aspect of the carpal tunnel is composed of the carpal bones. The transverse carpal ligament defines the palmar boundary.
  - The carpal tunnel contains nine flexor tendons and the median nerve.
- Symptoms most commonly affect the dominant hand; >50% of patients will experience bilateral symptoms.
- Most expensive upper extremity musculoskeletal disorder; >$2 billion per year
- Carpal tunnel release (CTR) is one of the most frequently performed hand/wrist procedures, with approximately 600,000 CTR procedures per year.
- Median time lost by U.S. workers with carpal tunnel syndrome (CTS) = 28 days
- System(s) affected: musculoskeletal, nervous

ALERT
Increased incidence during pregnancy (up to 20–45%) and chronic hemodialysis (2–31%)

EPIDEMIOLOGY
Predominant age: 40 to 60 years; predominant sex: female > male (3:1 to 10:1)

Incidence
- Two peaks: late 50s (women), late 70s (both genders)
- Incidence up to 276/100,000 has been reported.
- Incidence increases with age.

Prevalence
- About 3% of the population (4% in women and 2% in men); 50 cases per 1,000 individuals per year in the United States
- 14% in diabetics without neuropathy and 30% in patients with diabetic neuropathy

ETIOLOGY AND PATHOPHYSIOLOGY
- Combination of mechanical trauma, inflammation, increased pressure, and ischemic injury to the median nerve within the carpal tunnel
- Acute CTS caused by rapid and sustained pressure in carpal tunnel, usually secondary to trauma, may require urgent surgical decompression.
- Distal radius fractures and volar lunate dislocations increase risk.
- Chronic CTS divided into four categories:
  - Idiopathic: combination of edema and fibrous hypertrophy without inflammation
  - Anatomic: persistent median artery, ganglion cyst, infection, space-occupying lesion in carpal tunnel
  - Systemic: associated with conditions such as obesity, diabetes, hypothyroidism, rheumatoid arthritis, amyloidosis, scleroderma, renal failure, and drug toxicity
  - Exertional: repetitive use of hands and wrists, repeated palmar impact, use of vibratory tools

Genetics
- Unknown; however, a familial type has been reported.
- More likely to experience CTS if there is a first-degree relative with CTS

RISK FACTORS
- Prolonged postures in extremes of wrist flexion and extension including activities such as gardening, cycling, or tennis; repetitive exposure to vibration (motorcycle riding)
  - There is an insufficient evidence to implicate computer use in the development of CTS.
  - Jobs most at risk for CTS: use of vibratory tools, food processing and packing, dairy and poultry workers, and assembly workers
- Alterations of fluid balance: pregnancy, rheumatoid arthritis, obesity, renal failure, hypothyroidism, congestive heart failure, hemodialysis
  - CTS is the most common neuropathy in patients with rheumatoid arthritis.
- Neuropathic factors: diabetes, alcoholism, vitamin deficiency, or exposure to toxins
- More common in patients with concomitant migraine headaches

GENERAL PREVENTION
There is no known prevention for CTS. It is recommended to take occasional (e.g., hourly) breaks when doing repetitive work involving hands or if prolonged occupational exposure to vibratory tools.

COMMONLY ASSOCIATED CONDITIONS
- Diabetes, obesity; pregnancy; hypothyroidism
- Osteoarthritis of small joints of hand and wrist
- Hyperparathyroidism, hypocalcemia
- Hemodialysis

DIAGNOSIS

HISTORY
- Nocturnal pain, numbness, and tingling of the thumb, index, long, and radial portion of the ring fingers. Symptoms characteristically are relieved by shaking or rubbing the hands known as a positive Flick sign. This has a sensitivity of 93% and specificity of 96%.
- Hand weakness during tasks such as opening jars is often noted early in the disorder.
- Atypical presentation involves paresthesias in radial digits, with pain radiating proximally along median nerve to elbow and sometimes the shoulder.
- During waking hours, symptoms occur when driving, talking on the phone, and occasionally when using the hands for repetitive maneuvers.

PHYSICAL EXAM
- Durkan compression test: Direct compression of median nerve at carpal tunnel for 30 seconds elicits symptoms (87% sensitivity, 90% specificity).
- Positive Phalen sign: Holding the wrist in fully flexed position for 60 seconds precipitates paresthesias, numbness, or pain (68% sensitivity, 73% specificity).

- Positive Tinel sign: Tapping over the palmar surface of the wrist proximal to the carpal tunnel may produce an electric sensation along the distribution of the median nerve (50% sensitivity, 77% specificity).
- Square-sign test: positive if measurement of wrist width/height ≥0.7 (53% sensitivity, 80% specificity)
- Hand elevation test: hands held above head for 1 to 2 minutes; positive if symptoms are reproduced (85% sensitivity, 95% specificity)
- Loss of two-point discrimination
- Decreased sensation to pain
- Wasting of thenar musculature is a late sign and should not be used to rule out CTS (16% sensitivity, 94% specificity).

DIFFERENTIAL DIAGNOSIS
- Cervical spondylosis (carpal tunnel may also occur with cervical spine disease; "double crush")
- Generalized peripheral neuropathy
- Brachial plexopathy, in particular upper trunk
- CNS disorders (multiple sclerosis, cerebral infarction)
- Thoracic outlet syndrome
- Pronator syndrome (median nerve compression at the elbow)
- Anterior interosseous syndrome
- Ulnar nerve compression
- Musculoskeletal disorders of the wrist:
  - Trauma or distal radius fracture
  - Degenerative joint disease
  - Rheumatoid arthritis
  - Ganglion cyst
  - de Quervain tenosynovitis
  - CMC arthritis
- Scleroderma
- Raynaud syndrome

DIAGNOSTIC TESTS & INTERPRETATION
- The most accurate screening forms are the CTS-6, Kamath and Stothard questionnaire, and Katz and Stirrat hand symptom diagram.
- No laboratory test is diagnostic.
  - TSH, HbA1c, ESR, and serum chemistries help exclude secondary conditions associated with CTS.
- The most sensitive indicator is median sensory distal latency, which is prolonged in CTS.

Initial Tests (lab, imaging)
- X-rays of the wrist to evaluate for degenerative joint disease but are not necessary to diagnose CTS; magnetic resonance imaging is of limited benefit.
- Ultrasound—rapid, noninvasive, painless modality; sensitivity 87%; specificity 91%; hypoechoic median nerve cross-sectional area ≥11.5 mm

Diagnostic Procedures/Other
Electrodiagnostic studies
- Sensitivity 85%; specificity 95%
- Most useful with low pretest probability and suspicion of alternate peripheral neuropathy, radiculopathy, or "double-crush" phenomenon with compression at multiple locations
- Nerve conduction studies compare latency and amplitude of median nerve signals across the carpal tunnel.

TREATMENT

GENERAL MEASURES

- Strong evidence supports immobilization (brace/splint/orthosis) and the use of local steroid (methylprednisolone) injection in improving patient-reported outcomes.
- Strong evidence indicates that surgical treatment of CTS results in better functional improvements at 1 year compared with nonoperative treatment.
- A trial of nonoperative management is generally recommended for patients with mild to moderate CTS symptoms.

MEDICATION

First Line

Mainstay treatments for mild to moderate CTS include night splinting (12 weeks) and local corticosteroid injection or oral nonsteroidal anti-inflammatory agents.

- Local corticosteroid injection is effective for treatment of mild and moderate CTS with benefits lasting up to 6 months and a reduced need for surgery up to 12 months (1).
- Recent research has shown significantly improved outcomes in pain, function, and remission of nocturnal paresthesia with a single local corticosteroid injection compared with night splints at 1-, 3-, and 6-month follow-up.
- NSAIDs have demonstrated conflicting evidence of long-term benefit.
- Splinting remains as a first line due to its simplicity, affordability, and tolerability.
- It's unclear if a splint optimally worn full time or only at night time, or long-term use is better than short-term use, but low certainty evidence suggests that benefits manifest in the long term.
- No evidence supports multiple trials of injection; thus, surgery should be considered for those with refractory or recurrent symptoms.
- Those with moderate to severe disease benefit from early surgery.

Second Line

- Oral corticosteroids are less effective than local corticosteroid injection but more effective than placebo in the short term; long-term benefits of oral corticosteroid use have not been shown.
  - The long-term risks of even a short course of steroids should be balanced with the limited potential benefit of symptom improvement.
- Gabapentin is shown to be effective in managing CTS symptoms.
  - 300 mg daily has been shown to be more effective than 100 mg daily while maintaining minimal to no side effects.
- Hand therapy has been shown to improve patient function (2)[B].

ISSUES FOR REFERRAL

Preoperative electrodiagnostic studies are generally obtained prior to any surgical intervention.

SURGERY/OTHER PROCEDURES

- Completely dividing the transverse carpal ligament provides symptom relief in >95% of patients.
- Surgical decompression is an outpatient procedure performed under local or regional anesthesia.
- Incisional healing generally takes 2 weeks; an additional 2 weeks may be required before using the affected hand for tasks requiring strength.
- Complete resolution of numbness in 93.8% of patients with severe CTS by EMG at follow-up of 9.3 years
- The approach should be based on surgeon and patient preference.
  - Endoscopic surgery results in higher patient satisfaction rates, greater key pinch strength, earlier return to work times, and lower incidence of scar-related complications.
  - Patients undergoing endoscopic release are at greater risk of transient nerve injury, but this effect is not permanent.

COMPLEMENTARY & ALTERNATIVE MEDICINE

- No evidence to support the use of vitamin B_6 in the prevention or treatment of CTS
- Acupuncture shown to be as effective as short-term oral prednisolone therapy and may be used as an alternative therapy or as an adjuvant
- No data to support chiropractic therapy as a treatment for CTS

ADMISSION, INPATIENT, AND NURSING CONSIDERATIONS

Outpatient

ONGOING CARE

FOLLOW-UP RECOMMENDATIONS

Patient Monitoring

- Patients treated nonoperatively (splinting, injections) require follow-up over 4 to 12 weeks to ensure adequate progress.
- There is only limited, low-quality evidence to suggest that rehabilitation exercises such as wrist immobilization, ice therapy, and multimodal hand rehabilitation are beneficial.
- 7–20% of patients treated surgically may experience recurrence.

PROGNOSIS

- Approximately 85% of patients that initially respond to conservative therapy will experience reemergence of symptoms within 4 years.
- A positive Phalen test and thenar wasting are factors that have been associated with poorer outcomes with conservative management.
- Patients with severe CTS may not recover completely after surgical release. Paresthesias and weakness may persist, but nighttime symptoms generally resolve.
- If untreated, more severe cases of CTS can lead to numbness and weakness in the hand, atrophy of the thenar muscles, and permanent loss of median nerve function.

COMPLICATIONS

- Injury to the median nerve or its recurrent (motor) branch
- Pillar pain (tenderness adjacent to the actual ligament release sites of the trapezial ridge and hook of hamate) in the months following CTR (prevalence of 6–36%)

REFERENCES

1. Ashworth NL, Bland JDP, Chapman KM, et al. Local corticosteroid injection versus placebo for carpal tunnel syndrome. *Cochrane Database Syst Rev*. 2023;2(2):CD015148.
2. Ostergaard PJ, Meyer MA, Earp BE. Non-operative treatment of carpal tunnel syndrome. *Curr Rev Musculoskelet Med*. 2020;13(2):141–147.

ADDITIONAL READING

Dabbagh A, MacDermid JC, Yong J, et al. Diagnosing carpal tunnel syndrome: diagnostic test accuracy of scales, questionnaires, and hand symptom diagrams—a systematic review. *J Orthop Sports Phys Ther*. 2020;50(11):622–631.

SEE ALSO

- Arthritis, Rheumatoid (RA); Hypoparathyroidism; Lupus Erythematosus, Systemic (SLE); Scleroderma
- Algorithms: Carpal Tunnel Syndrome; Pain in Upper Extremity

CODES

ICD10

- G56.0 Carpal tunnel syndrome
- G56.01 Carpal tunnel syndrome, right upper limb
- G56.02 Carpal tunnel syndrome, left upper limb

CLINICAL PEARLS

- Paresthesias associated with CTS are confined to the thumb, index, long, and radial 1/2 of the ring fingers of the affected hand.
- Thenar atrophy is a late finding, indicating nerve damage, and is associated with a higher likelihood of failure with conservative management.
- The Durkan (carpal compression) test is superior to Tinel sign (tapping on median nerve over carpal tunnel) and Phalen maneuver (holding wrists in flexion) for the clinical diagnosis of CTS. The Flick sign has the highest sensitivity and specificity.
- Steroid injection and night splinting are mainstays of treatment for mild to moderate CTS.
- Surgical release of the carpal tunnel is >90% effective long-term.

CATARACT

Yasir Ahmed, MD • Ingrid U. Scott, MD, MPH

BASICS

DESCRIPTION
- A cataract is any opacity or discoloration of the lens, localized or generalized; the term is usually reserved for changes that affect visual acuity (1).
- Etymology: from Latin *cataracta*, for "waterfall"; named after foamy appearance of opacity
- Leading cause of blindness worldwide, estimated 20 million people (1)
- Types include the following:
  - Age related: approximately 90% of cases
  - Metabolic (diabetes via accelerated sorbitol pathway, hypocalcemia, Wilson disease)
  - Congenital (1/250 newborns; 10–38% of childhood blindness)
  - Systemic disease associated (myotonic dystrophy, atopic dermatitis [AD])
  - Secondary to associated eye disease, so-called complicated (e.g., uveitis associated with juvenile rheumatoid arthritis or sarcoid, tumor such as melanoma or retinoblastoma)
  - Traumatic (e.g., heat, electric shock, radiation, concussion, perforating eye injuries, intraocular foreign body)
  - Toxic/nutritional (e.g., corticosteroids)
- Morphologic classification:
  - Nuclear: exaggeration of normal aging changes of *central* lens nucleus, often associated with myopia due to increased refractive index of lens (Some elderly patients consequently may be able to read again *without spectacles*, so-called "second sight.")
  - Cortical: outer portion of lens; may involve anterior, posterior, or equatorial cortex; radial, spoke-like opacities
  - Subcapsular: Posterior subcapsular cataract has more profound effect on vision than nuclear or cortical cataract; patients particularly troubled under conditions of miosis; near vision frequently impaired more than distance vision
- System(s) affected: nervous

Geriatric Considerations
Some degree of cataract formation is expected in all people >70 years of age.

Pediatric Considerations
See congenital cataract discussion on "Surgery/Other Procedures" section; may present as leukocoria

Pregnancy Considerations
See congenital cataract discussion on "Surgery/Other Procedures" section (i.e., medications, metabolic dysfunction, intrauterine infection, and malnutrition)

EPIDEMIOLOGY
Incidence
- ~48% of the 37 million cases of blindness worldwide result from cataracts (1).
- Leading cause of treatable blindness and vision loss in developing countries (1)

Prevalence
An estimated 50% of people 65 to 74 years of age and 70% of people >75 years of age have age-related cataract.

ETIOLOGY AND PATHOPHYSIOLOGY
- Age-related cataract:
  - Continual addition of layers of lens fibers throughout life creates hard, dehydrated lens nucleus that impairs vision (nuclear cataract).
  - Aging alters biochemical and osmotic balance required for lens clarity; outer lens layers hydrate and become opaque, adversely affecting vision.
- Congenital:
  - Usually unknown etiology
  - Drugs (corticosteroids in 1st trimester, sulfonamides)
  - Metabolic (diabetes in mother, galactosemia in fetus)
  - Intrauterine infection during 1st trimester (e.g., rubella, herpes, mumps)
  - Maternal malnutrition
- Other cataract types:
  - Common feature is a biochemical/osmotic imbalance that disrupts lens clarity.
  - Local changes in lens protein distribution lead to light scattering (lens opacity).

Genetics
Congenital (e.g., chromosomal disorders [Down syndrome])

RISK FACTORS
- Aging
- Cigarette smoking
- Ultraviolet (UV) sunlight exposure
- Diabetes
- Prolonged high-dose steroids
- Positive family history
- Alcohol

GENERAL PREVENTION
- Use of UV protective glasses
- Avoidance of tobacco products
- Effective control of diabetes
- Care with high-dose, long-term steroid use (systemic therapy > inhaled treatment)
- Protective methods using pharmaceutical intervention (e.g., antioxidants, acetylsalicylic acid [ASA], hormone replacement therapy [HRT]) show no proven benefit to date.

COMMONLY ASSOCIATED CONDITIONS
- Diabetes (especially with poor glucose control)
- Myotonic dystrophy (90% of patients develop a visually innocuous change in 3rd decade; becomes disabling in 5th decade)
- AD (10% of patients with severe AD develop cataracts in 2nd to 4th decades; often bilateral)
- Neurofibromatosis type 2

- Associated ocular disease or "secondary cataract" (e.g., chronic anterior uveitis, acute [or repetitive] angle-closure glaucoma or high myopia)
- Drug induced (e.g., steroids, chlorpromazine)
- Trauma

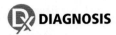

DIAGNOSIS

HISTORY
- Age-related cataract:
  - Decreased visual acuity, blurred vision, distortion, or "ghosting" of images (1)
  - Problems with visual acuity in any lighting condition
  - Falls or accidents; injuries (e.g., hip fracture)
- Congenital: often asymptomatic; leukocoria; parents notice child's visual inattention or strabismus.
- Other types of cataract:
  - May also present with decreased visual acuity
  - Appropriate clinical history or signs to help with diagnosis

PHYSICAL EXAM
- Visual acuity assessment for all cataracts
  - Glare testing allows further assessment of visual dysfunction.
- Age-related cataract: lens opacity on eye examination
- Congenital:
  - Lens opacity present at birth or within 3 months of birth
  - Leukocoria (white pupil), strabismus, nystagmus, signs of an associated syndrome (as with Down or rubella syndrome)
  - *Note*: must always rule out ocular tumor; early diagnosis and treatment of retinoblastoma may be lifesaving.
- Other types of cataract: may present with decreased visual acuity associated with characteristic physical findings (e.g., metabolic, trauma)

DIFFERENTIAL DIAGNOSIS
- An opaque-appearing eye may be due to opacities of the cornea (e.g., scarring, edema, calcification), lens opacities, tumor, or retinal detachment. Biomicroscopic examination (slit lamp) or careful ophthalmoscopic exam should provide a diagnosis.
- In the elderly, visual impairment is often due to multiple factors such as cataract and macular degeneration, both contributing to visual loss.
- Age-related cataract is significant if symptoms and ophthalmic exam support cataract as a major cause of vision impairment.
- Congenital lens opacity in the absence of other ocular pathology may cause severe amblyopia.
- *Note*: Cataract *does not* produce a relative afferent pupillary reaction defect. Abnormal pupillary reactions mandate further evaluation for other pathology.

DIAGNOSTIC TESTS & INTERPRETATION
- Visual quality assessment: Glare testing, contrast sensitivity is sometimes indicated.
- Retinal/macular function assessment: potential acuity meter testing
- Workup of the underlying process

Diagnostic Procedures/Other
- Optical biometry to measure the eye's axial length and corneal keratometry for placement of intraocular lens
- Corneal topography to measure corneal curvature and power

 TREATMENT

- Outpatient (usually)
- ~1.64 million cataract extractions in the United States yearly (2)

GENERAL MEASURES
Eye protection from UV light

MEDICATION
There are currently no medications to prevent or slow the progression of cataracts.

ISSUES FOR REFERRAL
If the patient has cataracts and symptoms do not seem to support recommendation for surgery, a second opinion by another ophthalmologist may be indicated.

SURGERY/OTHER PROCEDURES
- Age-related cataract:
  - Surgical removal is indicated if visual impairment producing symptoms are distressing to the patient, interfering with lifestyle or occupation, or posing a risk for fall or injury (2)[A].
  - Because significant cataracts may develop gradually, the patient may not be aware of how it has changed their lifestyle. The physician may note a significant cataract, and the patient reports "no problems." Thus, evaluation requires an effective physician–patient relationship.
  - Preoperative evaluation: by the primary care physician:
    ○ Patients on anticoagulants may need to be temporarily discontinued 1 to 2 weeks before surgery if possible (but usually not necessary, thus need to discuss with ophthalmologist).
    ○ Patients who have ever taken an α-blocker such as tamsulosin (Flomax) should alert their ophthalmologist due to increased risk of intraoperative floppy iris syndrome [IFIS] even in patients who no longer use these drugs.
  - Anesthesia: usually topical with sedation and monitoring of vital signs, sometimes local injection as well

- Surgical technique: cataract extraction via phacoemulsification through small incisions created by blade or laser, followed by implantation of a prosthetic intraocular lens; lenses have power calculated based on the size of the eye and curvature of the cornea usually to correct for distance vision; surgery performed on one (usually worse) eye, with contralateral surgery after recovery and if deemed necessary
  ○ Laser-assisted cataract surgery: Laser allows automated completion of certain steps of cataract surgery such as incisions, opening the lens capsule, and breaking up the cataract before surgical removal with phacoemulsification (3).
- Postoperative care: usually protective eye shield as directed, topical antibiotic, NSAIDs, and steroid ophthalmic medications; avoid lifting or bending for at least a week; keeping eye protected in general
- Congenital cataract:
  - Treatment is surgical removal of cataract. Newborns may require surgery within days to reduce the risk of severe amblyopia. The use of lens implants is controversial because the eyes are growing.
  - Postoperative care: long-term patching program for the good eye to combat amblyopia; refractive correction of operative eye, with multiple repeat examinations; challenging for physician and parents

 ONGOING CARE

FOLLOW-UP RECOMMENDATIONS
Patient Monitoring
- As the cataract progresses, the glasses or contact lens prescription may change to maintain vision. When this is no longer successful and interferes with patient's activities of daily living, surgery is indicated.
- Following surgery, spectacle correction may still be required to maximize near and/or far visual acuity. Refraction is usually prescribed several weeks after surgery.

PATIENT EDUCATION
MedlinePlus on cataracts at: https://medlineplus.gov/cataract.html

PROGNOSIS
- Ocular prognosis is good after cataract removal if no prior or coexisting ocular disease: 94.3% of otherwise healthy eyes achieve best-corrected visual acuity of 20/40 or better. Success rates are lower with comorbidities such as diabetes and glaucoma (4).
- Posterior capsular opacification can occur after cataract surgery and can cause a decrease in vision (14.7–42.7% of eyes, usually treated with Nd:YAG laser capsulotomy in the office with a rate of 4–25.3%).
- In congenital cataracts, prognosis is often poorer because of the high risk of amblyopia.

COMPLICATIONS
- Vary widely from delay in visual recovery or protracted visual discomfort to blindness and loss of the eye
- Complications are uncommon in general (<2% of eyes). Among the complications, a posterior capsular rupture is significant as it may require additional steps during surgery (5)[B].
- Poor preoperative visual acuity is related to surgical complications.

REFERENCES
1. Asbell PA, Dualan I, Mindel J, et al. Age-related cataract. Lancet. 2005;365(9459):599–609.
2. Riaz Y, Mehta JS, Wormald R, et al. Surgical interventions for age-related cataract. Cochrane Database Syst Rev. 2006;2006(4):CD001323.
3. Kolb CM, Shajari M, Mathys L, et al. Comparison of femtosecond laser-assisted cataract surgery and conventional cataract surgery: a meta-analysis and systematic review. J Cataract Refract Surg. 2020;46(8):1075–1085.
4. Biber JM, Sandoval HP, Trivedi RH, et al. Comparison of the incidence and visual significance of posterior capsule opacification between multifocal spherical, monofocal spherical, and monofocal aspheric intraocular lenses. J Cataract Refract Surg. 2009;35(7):1234–1238.
5. Lundström M, Barry P, Henry Y, et al. Visual outcome of cataract surgery; study from the European Registry of Quality Outcomes for Cataract and Refractive Surgery. J Cataract Refract Surg. 2013;39(5):673–679.

 SEE ALSO

- Floppy Iris Syndrome
- Algorithm: Cataracts

 CODES

ICD10
- H26.049 Anterior subcapsular polar infantile and juvenile cataract, unspecified eye
- H26.069 Combined forms of infantile and juvenile cataract, unspecified eye
- H26.231 Glaucomatous flecks (subcapsular), right eye

CLINICAL PEARLS
- Cataracts are the leading cause of blindness worldwide; most cataracts are age-related.
- The primary indication for cataract surgery is visual impairment leading to significant lifestyle changes for the patient.
- For congenital cataracts, always consider ocular tumor because early diagnosis and treatment of retinoblastoma may be lifesaving.

CELIAC DISEASE

Michelle E. Duffelmeyer, MD • Chelsea E. Robitaille, MS, PA-C

 BASICS

DESCRIPTION

- A non–IgE-mediated immune reaction to gliadin, a protein component of dietary gluten (found in wheat, barley, rye, and other grains) primarily affecting the small intestine in genetically predisposed individuals
- Presentations
  - Typical
    - Diarrheal illness characterized by villous atrophy with symptoms of malabsorption (steatorrhea, weight loss, vitamin deficiencies, anemia); resolves with a gluten-free diet (GFD)
    - <50% of adults present with gastrointestinal (GI) symptoms.
  - Atypical
    - Minor GI symptoms, with a myriad of extraintestinal manifestations (e.g., anemia, elevated LFTs, dental enamel defects, neurologic symptoms, infertility)
  - Asymptomatic (silent) disease
    - Found when screening first-degree relatives
    - Positive laboratory tests and genetics, without signs/symptoms; normal histology on biopsy
- System(s) affected: GI
- Synonym(s): celiac sprue; gluten-sensitive enteropathy; nontropical sprue

EPIDEMIOLOGY

Incidence
- 1 to 13/100,000 worldwide (1)
- 6.5/100,000 in the United States (2)
- Primarily affects those of Northern European ancestry
- Predominant sex: female > male (3:2)

Prevalence
- 0.7% in the United States; an estimated 3 million Americans have celiac disease.
- 1% worldwide (1)

ETIOLOGY AND PATHOPHYSIOLOGY

Sensitivity to gluten, specifically gliadin protein fraction; tissue transglutaminase (tTG) modification of the gliadin protein leads to immunologic cross-reactivity, inflammation, and tissue damage (villous atrophy) with subsequent GI symptoms and malabsorption.

Genetics
Homogenicity for *HLA-DQ2/DQ8* increases risk of celiac disease and enteropathy-associated T-cell lymphoma.

RISK FACTORS
- First-degree relatives: 5–20% incidence (1)
- Second-degree relatives

Pediatric Considerations
No other risk factors (e.g., grain processing, genetically modified organisms, hygiene and illness during childhood, breastfeeding, time of introduction of solid foods, pollution, tobacco use, and medication) definitively explain why some susceptible individuals develop celiac disease, whereas others do not.

COMMONLY ASSOCIATED CONDITIONS
- *Dermatitis herpetiformis* (*DH*): 85% of patients with DH have celiac disease. All patients with DH should follow a GFD (1).
- Secondary lactase deficiency
- Osteopenia and osteoporosis
- Thyroid disease: Hashimoto thyroiditis
- Type 1 diabetes: 3–10% of patients with type 1 diabetes also have celiac disease (1).
- Symptomatic iron deficiency: 10–15% have celiac disease.
- Elevated AST and ALT (with no direct cause)
- Hyposplenism
- Oral aphthous ulcers
- Irritable bowel syndrome (IBS)
- Restless leg syndrome
- Celiac disease is associated with an increased risk for adenocarcinoma and lymphoma of the small bowel.
  - The risk of lymphoproliferative malignancies depends on small intestinal histopathology.
  - Little to no increased risk in latent celiac disease (seropositive but normal biopsy)
- Associated autoimmune conditions (type 1 diabetes, autoimmune thyroiditis, primary biliary cirrhosis, autoimmune hepatitis, psoriasis, Sjögren disease)
- Associated genetic conditions (Down syndrome, IgA deficiency, Turner syndrome, Williams syndrome)

Pregnancy Considerations
- Prevalence of celiac disease: 2.5 to 3.5 times higher in women with unexplained infertility
- Up to 19% of men with celiac disease have androgen resistance. Semen quality and likelihood of pregnancy increase with GFD.
- Higher rates of low birth weight, prematurity, spontaneous abortions, intrauterine growth restriction, and stillbirths

Pediatric Considerations
Children with type 1 diabetes, Down syndrome, Turner syndrome, Williams syndrome, IgA deficiency, and autoimmune thyroid disease are at risk for celiac disease (3)[C].

DIAGNOSIS

HISTORY
- Diarrhea and cramping are the most common GI symptoms.
- Other symptoms: steatorrhea (fatty stools); abdominal pain or distension; nausea, vomiting, flatulence; weight loss, weakness, fatigue; muscle cramps; bone and joint pain; paresthesias in hands and feet; constipation
- Clinical signs: delayed puberty; iron deficiency anemia; recurrent aphthous stomatitis; dental enamel hyperplasia; anxiety, depression; migraines; anorexia; encopresis
- In children, malabsorption may manifest as failure to thrive, short stature, or chronic fatigue (3).

PHYSICAL EXAM
Physical examination is often normal. Findings can include:
- Cardiovascular: orthostatic hypotension, peripheral edema
- Oropharynx: aphthous stomatitis, glossitis, angular cheilitis
- Skin: dermatitis herpetiformis (symmetric erythematous papules and blisters on elbows, knees, buttocks, and back), pallor
- Abdomen: distention

DIFFERENTIAL DIAGNOSIS
- Gluten allergy–type II allergic reaction with signs of anaphylaxis
- Nonceliac gluten sensitivity—GI symptoms and/or systemic symptoms improved by GFD but without biomarkers characteristic of celiac disease
- Short bowel syndrome; small intestinal bacterial overgrowth
- Lactose intolerance; gastroesophageal reflux disease (GERD)
- Pancreatic exocrine insufficiency; Crohn disease; Whipple disease
- Tropical sprue; intestinal lymphoma
- Microscopic colitis; autoimmune enteropathy
- HIV enteropathy
- Acute enteritis; radiation enteritis; eosinophilic gastroenteritis
- Giardiasis
- IBS; dyspepsia

DIAGNOSTIC TESTS & INTERPRETATION
Tissue biopsy is the gold standard for diagnosis.

Initial Tests (lab, imaging)
- Biopsy and histologic examination of duodenal bulb during routine upper endoscopy increase the diagnostic yield of celiac disease. A sampling of the duodenal bulb and the distal duodenum is recommended to improve histologic confirmation of celiac disease. Do not base diagnosis solely on serology in adults. Patients with symptoms highly suggestive of celiac disease or those with positive serologies should undergo endoscopy for small bowel biopsy while on a gluten-containing diet.
- IgA anti-tTG is the preferred serologic test in patients aged >2 years (1).
- Total serum IgA to screen for IgA deficiency

ALERT
Positive IgA tTG has high sensitivity and specificity (sensitivity, 95–98%; specificity, 95%) if on a normal (non–gluten-free) diet for at least 4 weeks.

- IgA-deficient patients have false-negative IgA anti-tTG antibodies.
- IgA deficiency is 10 to 15 times more prevalent in patients with celiac disease.
- The tTG antibody test is the preferred test (over the deamidated gliadin peptide [DGP] antibody).

Follow-Up Tests & Special Considerations

- If the patient is IgA deficient *or* if IgA anti-tTG is negative, follow up with anti-DGP IgA and IgG.
  - Sensitivity, 94%; specificity, 99% (~anti-tTG)
- Do not use HLA DQ serotyping for initial diagnosis. Consider if discrepant serology–histology results in patients unable to test on GFD and children with Down syndrome (1).
- Consider bone mineral density testing at the time of diagnosis and after 1 year (if osteopenia/osteoporosis on initial testing) or 2 years (if normal initially and patient still symptomatic or nonadherent to diet).
- Younger age on diagnosis, less severe initial histologic damage, and male gender increase the likelihood of achieving mucosal recovery.
- Members of a family who have more than one individual with CD are at higher risk. Screen family members, including second-degree relatives (1).

Pediatric Considerations

- Test symptomatic pediatric patients with IgA and IgA anti-tTG antibodies.
- Periodic monitoring with IgA anti-tTG Ab can assess dietary adherence.
- Negative serology cannot rule out CD.
- Consider HLA for high-risk children with negative serology.
- Limit IgA anti-endomysial antibodies to patients with illnesses that increase false-positive tTG Ab, such as type I diabetes or autoimmune liver disease.

Diagnostic Procedures/Other

- Endoscopy with a minimum of four biopsies of distal duodenum and two of duodenal bulb at the time of initial evaluation correctly diagnose 95% of children (1).
- Video capsule endoscopy is a promising alternative with a sensitivity and specificity of 80% and 95%; particularly helpful if antibody screening and clinical picture are consistent with celiac disease despite nondiagnostic duodenal biopsies

Test Interpretation

Small-bowel biopsy

- Villous atrophy, hyperplasia and lengthening of crypts, infiltration of plasma cells, and intraepithelial lymphocytosis in lamina propria
- Villous atrophy is also caused by Crohn disease, radiation enteritis, Giardia, and other food intolerances.

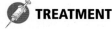 ## TREATMENT

GENERAL MEASURES

- GFD—avoid wheat, barley, rye, and other grains that contain gluten.
  - Rice, corn, and nut flour are safe and palatable substitutes (1).
  - Grains: uncontaminated oats, rice, corn, tapioca, quinoa, amaranth, sorghum
- Levels of IgA antigliadin normalize with gluten abstinence.
- *Lifelong* abstinence is required; immune response to gluten will recur with the resumption of gluten intake.

MEDICATION

First Line

Usually, no medications; GFD is the primary treatment.

Second Line

- In refractory disease, consult with GI to consider the choice, dosing, and duration of second-line treatment with steroids or immunomodulators.
- Depending on disease severity, patients may develop nutritional deficiencies that require appropriate supplementation.

ISSUES FOR REFERRAL

- Additional nutritional support with a qualified dietitian
- Refractory celiac disease
- Child with positive celiac serology

COMPLEMENTARY & ALTERNATIVE MEDICINE

- Many alternative therapies are under development. Future treatment may include predigestion of gluten with peptidase, tight junction blockade, transglutaminase 2 or HLA-DQ2/DQ8 blockers, and induction of immune tolerance.
- Patients with celiac disease are at increased risk for pneumococcal infection. Pneumococcal vaccination should be considered, especially for those between the ages of 15 and 64 years who may not have received vaccination.

 ## ONGOING CARE

FOLLOW-UP RECOMMENDATIONS

- Consultation with a registered dietitian
- Screen for osteoporosis and treat accordingly.
- Follow-up with GI at 3 to 6 months for serology and 12 months for repeat biopsy, if indicated

Patient Monitoring

- Repeat EGD if no clinical response to GFD or relapse in symptoms (1).
- Follow anti-tTG IgA or deaminated antigliadin antibodies to measure response/compliance with diet (vs. antigliadin IgA or IgG).

DIET

- Remove gluten: wheat, rye, barley, and products with gluten additives (processed food/meat, medications, hygiene products).
- Dietary change is challenging (especially identifying sources of "hidden" gluten) and should be coordinated with a skilled registered dietitian.

PATIENT EDUCATION

- Discuss how to recognize gluten in various products; highlight potential complications and outcomes of failing to follow a GFD; support groups and self-education
- Celiac Disease Foundation: https://www.celiac.org/; Quick Start: Gluten-Free Diet Guide for Celiac Disease & Non-Celiac Gluten Sensitivity. https://celiac.org/wp-content/uploads/2013/12/quick-start-guide.pdf
- National Celiac Association: https://nationalceliac.org/; Beyond Celiac: https://www.beyondceliac.org/

PROGNOSIS

- Good prognosis if adherent to GFD
- Patients should see improvement within 7 days of dietary modification.
- Symptoms usually resolve in 4 to 6 weeks.

COMPLICATIONS

- Malignancy: Untreated and refractory patients have increased cancer risk, but successful treatment decreases risk to population baseline (1).
- Refractory disease (rare ~1–2% of all patients)
  - May respond to prednisone
  - May need total parenteral nutrition
- Osteoporosis, dehydration, electrolyte depletion, vitamin deficiencies

REFERENCES

1. Husby S, Murray JA, Katzka DA. AGA clinical practice update on diagnosis and monitoring of celiac disease—changing utility of serology and histologic measures: expert review. *Gastroenterology.* 2019;156(4):885–889.
2. McDermid JM, Almond MA, Roberts KM, et al. Celiac disease: an Academy of Nutrition and Dietetics evidence-based nutrition practice guideline. *J Acad Nutr Diet.* 2023;123(12): 1793–1807.e4.
3. Bingham SM, Bates MD. Pediatric celiac disease: a review for non-gastroenterologists. *Curr Probl Pediatr Adolesc Health Care.* 2020;50(5):100786.

 ## SEE ALSO

Algorithms: Diarrhea, Chronic; Malabsorption Syndrome

 ## CODES

ICD10

K90.0 Celiac disease

CLINICAL PEARLS

- Screen for celiac disease in patients with nonspecific GI symptoms, presumed IBS, dermatitis herpetiformis, unexplained transaminitis, or unexplained iron deficiency anemia.
- Test total IgA levels along with IgA anti-tTG antibodies in patients >2 years of age (1). Positive serology is not definitive.
- Complete diagnostic testing while on a gluten-containing diet.
- Endoscopic biopsy with histologic examination of the intestinal mucosa is the gold standard for diagnosis.
- Standard of treatment is a GFD. Patient symptoms should improve in 7 days if fully compliant.

CELLULITIS

Karl T. Clebak, MD, MHA, FAAFP • Huong N. Nguyen, DO, MS • Jarrett Keller Sell, MD, FAAFP, AAHIVS

 BASICS

Skin and soft tissue infections (SSTIs) are a common health burden with approximately a quarter of infected patients requiring hospital treatment leading to >650,000 admissions per year in the United States.

DESCRIPTION
- An acute bacterial infection of the dermis and subcutaneous tissue
- Types and locations:
  - Periorbital cellulitis: bacterial infection of the eyelid and surrounding tissues
  - Orbital cellulitis: infection of the eye posterior to the septum; sinusitis is the most common risk factor.
  - Facial cellulitis: preceded by upper respiratory infection or otitis media
  - Buccal cellulitis: infection of cheek in children associated with bacteremia (common before *Haemophilus influenzae* type B vaccine)
  - Peritonsillar cellulitis: common in children; associated with fever, sore throat, and "hot potato" speech
  - Perianal cellulitis: sharply demarcated, bright, perianal erythema
  - Necrotizing cellulitis: gas-producing bacteria in the lower extremities; more common in diabetics

EPIDEMIOLOGY
- Predominant sex: male = female
- Seasonality increased hospitalizations for cellulitis in the summer with fewer in the winter months

Incidence
1.5 to 24.6 per 1,000 person years with recurrent cellulitis with an incidence rate ranging from 16% to 53% within 3 years.

Prevalence
Visits to U.S. ambulatory practices for purulent SSTI range from 5.4 to 11.3 million visits annually.

ETIOLOGY AND PATHOPHYSIOLOGY
Cellulitis is caused by bacterial penetration through a compromise in the epidermis, the protective barrier of the skin into the deep dermis and subcutaneous tissues.
- Microbiology
  - β-Hemolytic streptococci (groups A, B, C, G, and F), staphylococci (*Staphylococcus aureus*, including MRSA), and gram-negative aerobic bacilli are most common.
  - *S. aureus* seen in periorbital and orbital cellulitis and people who inject IV drugs
  - *Pseudomonas aeruginosa* seen in diabetics and other immunocompromised patients
  - *H. influenzae* causes buccal cellulitis.
  - Clostridia and non–spore-forming anaerobes: necrotizing cellulitis (crepitant/gangrenous)
  - *Streptococcus agalactiae*: cellulitis following lymph node dissection
  - *Pasteurella multocida* and *Capnocytophaga canimorsus*: cellulitis preceded by bites
  - *Streptococcus iniae*: immunocompromised hosts
  - Rare causes: *Mycobacterium*, fungal (mucormycosis, aspergillosis)

Genetics
No genetic pattern

RISK FACTORS
- Disruption of skin barrier from trauma, infection, insect bites, injection drug use, body piercing, maceration, ulcerations, chronic wounds, fissured toe webs
- Inflammation from excoriating skin disorders or radiation therapy
- Edema due to venous insufficiency; lymphatic obstruction due to surgery or congestive heart failure
- Advanced age, male gender, diabetes, hypertension, cancer, obesity
- Dermatomycosis, tinea pedis, onychomycosis, presence of *S. aureus* and/or streptococci in the toe webs
- Previous episode of cellulitis
- Recurrent cellulitis:
  - Cellulitis recurrence score (predicts recurrence of lower extremity cellulitis based on presence of lymphedema, chronic venous insufficiency, peripheral vascular disease, and deep venous thrombosis)
  - Recurrent cellulitis is seen in immunocompromised patients (HIV/AIDS), steroids and TNF-α inhibitor therapy, diabetes, hypertension, cancer, peripheral arterial or venous diseases, chronic kidney disease, dialysis, IV or SC drug use.

GENERAL PREVENTION
- Good skin hygiene keeping skin well hydrated to avoid dryness and cracking
- Management of edema including elevation, compression stockings, pneumatic pressure pumps
- Maintain glycemic control and proper foot care in diabetic patients.

COMMONLY ASSOCIATED CONDITIONS
Abscess, lymphedema, venous insufficiency, stasis dermatitis, obesity

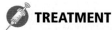 **DIAGNOSIS**

Clinical diagnosis presenting as an area of local inflammation consisting of pain, swelling, and/or erythema which may be associated with a systemic inflammatory response.

HISTORY
- Disruptions of the skin barrier such as previous trauma, surgery/vein stripping, animal/human/insect bites, dermatitis, IVDU, and fungal infection are portals of entry.
- Pain, itching, and/or burning
- Fever, chills, and malaise

PHYSICAL EXAM
- Assess vital signs for hemodynamic stability.
- Localized pain and tenderness with erythema (often poorly demarcated), induration, swelling, and warmth. May include signs of lymphangitis (streaking)
- Regional lymphadenopathy
- Purulent drainage
- Orbital cellulitis: proptosis, globe displacement, limitation of ocular movements, vision loss, diplopia
- Facial cellulitis: malaise, anorexia, vomiting, pruritus, burning, anterior neck swelling

DIFFERENTIAL DIAGNOSIS
Toxic shock syndrome, venous stasis dermatitis, deep vein thrombosis, thrombophlebitis, bursitis, dermatitis, herpes zoster, osteomyelitis, malignancy, drug reaction, sunburn, insect bites, erythema nodosum

DIAGNOSTIC TESTS & INTERPRETATION
Initial Tests (lab, imaging)
- If there are signs of systemic disease (fever, heart rate >100 beats/min, or systolic blood pressure <90 mm Hg): CBC, blood cultures, CPK, CRP, ESR. Consider serum lactate levels.
- Swab breaks in skin, ulcerations, blister fluid for culture. Microbiologic diagnosis is generally not needed.
- Plain radiographs, CT, and MRI are useful if osteomyelitis, fracture, necrotizing fasciitis, retained foreign body.
- MRI and ultrasound are most useful for evaluation of potential underlying abscesses.
- Gallium-67 scintigraphy helps detect cellulitis superimposed on chronic limb lymphedema.
- Procalcitonin is not useful in diagnosing early cellulitis.

Diagnostic Procedures/Other
Consider lumbar puncture in children with *H. influenzae* type B or if meningeal signs and facial cellulitis.

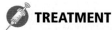 **TREATMENT**

GENERAL MEASURES
- Immobilize/elevate involved limb to reduce swelling.
- Sterile saline dressings or cool aluminum acetate compresses for pain relief
- Edema: compression stockings, pneumatic pumps; diuretic therapy for CHF patients
- Mark the borders of erythema to monitor progression and response to therapy.
- Tetanus immunization if needed

MEDICATION
First Line
- Target treatment if known pathogen and/or with certain exposures (animal bites)
- Empiric antibiotic selection:
  - Nonpurulent cellulitis
    - With nonpurulent drainage, target treatment toward β-hemolytic streptococci and MSSA.
    - Outpatient: treatment duration of 5 to 10 days (1)[C]; shorter courses of 5 days have been shown to be as effective as longer courses, although duration may be extended if there is no or slow clinical improvement.
      - Oral: for mild cellulitis
        - Cephalexin 500 mg PO q6h; children: 25 to 50 mg/kg/day in 3 to 4 doses (max 4,000 mg/day)
        - Dicloxacillin 500 mg PO q6h; children: 25 to 50 mg/kg/day in 4 doses
        - Clindamycin 300 to 450 mg PO q6–8h; children: 20 to 30 mg/kg/day in 4 doses (max 1.8 g/day)

- IV: for rapidly progressing cellulitis
  - Cefazolin 1 to 2 g IV q8h; children: 100 mg/kg/day IV in 2 to 4 divided doses (max 6 g/day)
  - Oxacillin 2 g IV q4h; children: 150 to 200 mg/kg/day IV in 4 to 6 doses (max 12 g/day)
  - Nafcillin 2 g IV q4h; children: 150 to 200 mg/kg/day IV in 4 to 6 doses (max 12 g/day)
  - Clindamycin 600 to 900 mg IV q8h; children: 25 to 40 mg/kg/day IV in 3 to 4 doses (max 4.8 g/day)
- Purulent cellulitis (probable CA-MRSA)
  - Culture purulent wounds and follow-up in 48 hours
  - Start trimethoprim-sulfamethoxazole (TMP-SMX), clindamycin, doxycycline, minocycline, 3rd- or 4th-generation fluoroquinolone for patients with cellulitis likely caused by CA-MRSA (2)[A].
  - Incise and drain abscesses and start empiric antibiotic therapy. Modify based on culture results; tailor duration based on clinical response (3)[C]:
    - Oral
      - Clindamycin 300 to 450 mg PO; children: 40 mg/kg/day in 3 to 4 doses, max 1.8 g/day
      - TMP-SMX 1 DS tab PO BID; children: dose based on TMP at 8 to 12 mg/kg/day divided in 2 doses
      - Doxycycline 100 mg PO BID; children >8 years of age: ≤45 kg: 4 mg/kg/day divided in 2 doses; >45 kg: 100 mg PO BID
      - Minocycline 200 mg PO once and then 100 mg PO BID; children >8 years old: 4 mg/kg PO once and then 4 mg/kg PO BID, max 400 mg/day
      - Linezolid 600 mg PO BID; children aged <12 years: 10 mg/kg/dose (max 600 mg/dose) PO TID; ≥12 years: 600 mg PO BID, limit tyramine food content <100 mg/meal
      - Tedizolid 200 mg PO once daily; children aged >12 years: 200 mg PO daily. Dosing is not established.
    - IV
      - Vancomycin 20 to 35 mg/kg one time loading dose then 15 to 20 mg/kg/dose IV every 8 to 12 hours, adjusted based on blood levels
      - Daptomycin 4 mg/kg/dose IV once daily for moderate infection; if bacteremia is present or suspected: 8 to 10 mg/kg IV once daily
      - Linezolid 600 mg IV q12h
      - Tedizolid 200 mg IV q daily
      - Ceftaroline 600 mg IV q12h
      - Tigecycline 100 mg IV once, thereafter 50 mg IV q12h
- Necrotizing cellulitis: requires broad-spectrum coverage to cover aerobic and anaerobic species including MRSA: ampicillin-sulbactam 1.5 to 3.0 g q6–8h IV or piperacillin-tazobactam 3.37 g q6–8h IV plus ciprofloxacin 400 mg q12h IV plus clindamycin 600 to 900 mg q8h IV; consider intensive care and emergent surgical consultation.

- Freshwater exposure: penicillinase-resistant: penicillin plus gentamicin or fluoroquinolone; salt water exposure: doxycycline 200 mg IV in 2 divided doses
- Bites: The combination of amoxicillin and clavulanic acid is recommended for human and dog bites. Ticarcillin and clavulanic acid or the combination of a 3rd-generation cephalosporin (i.e., ceftriaxone) plus metronidazole provides adequate parenteral therapy for animal or human bites. If allergic to penicillin, use fluoroquinolone plus metronidazole.
- Facial cellulitis in adults: ceftriaxone IV
- Diabetic foot infection:
  - Mild/moderate: cephalexin or cephalexin plus doxycycline or TMP-SMX plus amoxicillin clavulanate
  - Severe: ampicillin-sulbactam or imipenem-cilastatin or meropenem; alternative: combinations of targeting anaerobes as well as gram-positive and gram-negative aerobes
- If severe infection, toxicity, immunocompromised patients, or worsening infection despite empirical therapy, admit for empiric antibiotic therapy covering MRSA.
- Recurrent streptococcal cellulitis: penicillin 250 mg BID, or if penicillin-allergic, use erythromycin 250 mg BID
- Dalbavancin, a 2nd-generation lipoglycopeptide antibiotic with MRSA coverage, can be used to treat cellulitis and be administered rarely as once a week (3)[C].

Pediatric Considerations
- Avoid doxycycline in children ≤8 years old and during pregnancy.
- The Melbourne ASSET tool is helpful in determining the need for IV antibiotics in pediatric populations (sensitivity 60%, specificity 93%).

SURGERY/OTHER PROCEDURES
- Débridement for gas and purulent matter
- Intubation or tracheotomy may be needed for cellulitis of the head or neck.

ADMISSION, INPATIENT, AND NURSING CONSIDERATIONS
- Severe infection, suspicion of deeper or rapidly spreading infection, tissue necrosis, or severe pain
- Marked systemic toxicity or worsening symptoms that do not resolve after 24 to 48 hours of therapy
- Patients with underlying risk factors or severe comorbidities

 ONGOING CARE

FOLLOW-UP RECOMMENDATIONS
Patient Monitoring
- Repeat relevant labs if patient is toxic or not improving.
- Symptomatic improvement usually occurs in 24 to 48 hours, but visible improvement may take 72 hours.

DIET
Glucose control in diabetics

PATIENT EDUCATION
Good skin hygiene including moisturizing to prevent skin barrier breakdown

PROGNOSIS
Older age, higher BMI, and diabetes mellitus have been shown to lower early response to antibiotics.

COMPLICATIONS
- Local abscess
- Bacteremia, sepsis
- Superinfection with gram-negative organisms
- Lymphangitis
- Thrombophlebitis or venous thrombosis
- Bacterial meningitis
- Gangrene

REFERENCES
1. Stevens DL, Bisno AL, Chambers HF, et al. Practice guidelines for the diagnosis and management of skin and soft tissue infections: 2014 update by the Infectious Diseases Society of America. *Clin Infect Dis*. 2014;59(2):147–159.
2. Clebak KT, Reedy-Cooper A, Partin MT, et al. A guide to the Tx of cellulitis and other soft-tissue infections. *J Fam Pract*. 2021;70(5):214–219.
3. Bender S, Oakden K. New developments and treatment options of cellulitis in the hospital. In: Conrad K, ed. *Clinical Approaches to Hospital Medicine: Advances, Updates and Controversies*. Cham, Switzerland: Springer; 2018:77–87.

ADDITIONAL READING
- Ibrahim LF, Hopper SM, Donath S, et al. Development and validation of a cellulitis risk score: the Melbourne ASSET Score. *Pediatrics*. 2019;143(2):e20181420.
- Kaye KS, Petty LA, Shorr AF, et al. Current epidemiology, etiology, and burden of acute skin infections in the United States. *Clin Infect Dis*. 2019;68(Suppl 3):S193–S199.
- Webb E, Neeman T, Bowden FJ, et al. Compression therapy to prevent recurrent cellulitis of the leg. *N Engl J Med*. 2020;383(7):630–639.

CODES

ICD10
- L03.032 Cellulitis of left toe
- L03.312 Cellulitis of back [any part except buttock]
- L03.211 Cellulitis of face

CLINICAL PEARLS
- *S. aureus* and group A *Streptococcus* are the most common organisms causing cellulitis.
- Consider MRSA if cellulitis does not respond to antibiotics within 48 hours or if purulence present.
- Rapid expansion of infected area with discoloration and severe pain may suggest necrotizing fasciitis, requiring urgent surgical evaluation.
- Venous stasis dermatitis often mimics cellulitis leading to improper use of antibiotics.

CELLULITIS, ORBITAL

Frances J. Boly, DO • Hillary Kieran Deveaux, MBBS

 BASICS

DESCRIPTION
- Acute, severe, vision-threatening infection of orbital contents posterior to the orbital septum; preseptal (previously referred to as periorbital) cellulitis is anterior to the septum. Location determines the appropriate workup and treatment.
- Synonym(s): postseptal cellulitis

EPIDEMIOLOGY
- No difference in frequency between genders in adults. Higher incidence in boys in childhood; more common in children
- Orbital cellulitis is much less common than preseptal cellulitis (1).

Incidence
The incidence of orbital cellulitis has declined since introduction of routine *Haemophilus influenzae* type b (Hib) vaccination.

ETIOLOGY AND PATHOPHYSIOLOGY
- Sinusitis is classically associated with orbital cellulitis. Local skin conditions surrounding the eyelids and lashes are typically associated with preseptal cellulitis. The ethmoid sinus is separated from the orbit by the lamina papyracea ("layer of paper"), a thin bony separation, and is often the source of contiguous spread of infection to the orbit. The ethmoid sinus is present at birth. The orbital septum is a connective tissue barrier that extends from the skull into the lid and separates the preseptal from the orbital space.
- Cellulitis in the closed bony orbit causes proptosis, globe displacement, orbital apex syndrome (mass effect on the cranial nerves), optic nerve compression, and vision loss.
- Cultures of surgical specimens in adults often grow multiple organisms. In over 1/3 of cases, no pathogen is recovered. Blood cultures typically do not grow an organism.
- Most common organisms: *Staphylococcus aureus*, *Streptococcus pneumoniae*, *Streptococcus anginosus*
- *Haemophilus* is no longer the leading cause of orbital cellulitis. MRSA is increasingly a consideration.

Genetics
No known genetic predisposition

RISK FACTORS
- Sinusitis (present in 80–100% of cases); pansinusitis is often observed in adults (1).
- Orbital trauma, retained orbital foreign body (FB), ophthalmic surgery, and/or history of sinus surgery (1)
- Dental, periorbital, skin, or intracranial infection; acute dacryocystitis (inflammation of the lacrimal sac) and acute dacryoadenitis (inflammation of the lacrimal gland)
- Immunosuppressed patients are at increased risk of adverse outcomes.

GENERAL PREVENTION
Routine Hib vaccination; appropriate treatment of bacterial sinusitis; proper wound care and perioperative monitoring of orbital surgery and trauma; avoid trauma to the sinus and orbital regions

COMMONLY ASSOCIATED CONDITIONS
- Sinusitis, especially pansinusitis in adults; trauma and intraorbital FB; preseptal cellulitis
- Adverse outcomes include neutropic keratitis, secondary glaucoma, septic uveitis or retinitis, exudative retinal detachment, meningitis, cranial nerve palsies, panophthalmitis, inflammatory or infectious neuritis, retinal vein occlusion, central retinal artery occlusion, orbital abscess, subperiosteal abscess, orbital apex syndrome, subdural or brain abscess, and death.

DIAGNOSIS

HISTORY
- Complaints of acute onset red, swollen, tender eye or eyelid, and pain with eye movements
- History of surgery, trauma, sinus or upper respiratory infection, dental infection
- Malaise, fever, stiff neck, mental status changes
- Specific signs of orbital cellulitis include the following:
  - Proptosis, double vision, ophthalmoplegia, vision loss (or decreased field of vision), pain with eye movement, decreased color vision (differentiating green and red)

ALERT
- Differentiating orbital from preseptal cellulitis is the critical diagnostic step. Preseptal cellulitis can be identified by exam or following CT scan.
- Both preseptal and orbital cellulitis present with a red, swollen painful eye or eyelid.
- Diplopia, ophthalmoplegia, painful extraocular movements, proptosis, vision loss, and fever suggest orbital involvement.
- Contrast CT is the imaging method of choice and must be done for suspicion of orbital cellulitis (2).
- Treat with immediate IV antibiotics, hospital admission, and ophthalmology referral.
- Monitor frequently for vision loss, cavernous sinus thrombosis, abscess, and meningitis.

PHYSICAL EXAM
Vital signs
- Assess visual acuity (with glasses if required).
- Lid exam and palpation of the orbit; pupillary reflex for afferent pupillary defect
- Extraocular movements; assess for pain with eye movement—if present, then concerning for orbital cellulitis.
- Red desaturation: Patient views red object with one eye and compares to the other; reduced red color may indicate optic nerve involvement.
- Proptosis; pain with palpation; confrontation visual field testing

DIFFERENTIAL DIAGNOSIS
- Preseptal cellulitis
  - Eyelid erythema with or without conjunctival erythema, afebrile, no pain on eye movement, no diplopia, normal eye exam, vision intact
- Metastatic tumors and autoimmune inflammation may masquerade as orbital cellulitis in rare cases; usually present with painless slow onset of symptoms
- Idiopathic orbital inflammatory disease (orbital pseudotumor); orbital FB
- Arteriovenous fistula (carotid-cavernous fistula)
- Cavernous sinus thrombosis; acute thyroid orbitopathy; orbital tumor; trauma, insect bite, ruptured dermoid cyst
- Clinical signs help distinguish preseptal from orbital cellulitis. Preseptal infection causes erythema, induration, and tenderness of the eyelid and/or periorbital tissues, and patients rarely show signs of systemic illness. Local skin trauma, lacerations, or bug bites can be seen. Extraocular movements and visual acuity are intact.
- Orbital cellulitis also presents with red, swollen, painful eye or eyelid. More specific symptoms include proptosis, conjunctival edema, ophthalmoplegia, painful eye movements, and decreased visual acuity.

DIAGNOSTIC TESTS & INTERPRETATION
- CBC with differential, C-reactive protein, ESR; inflammatory markers can be higher with orbital cellulitis versus preseptal. An elevated neutrophil-to-lymphocyte ratio (NLR) suggests infection.
- Swab cultures of eye secretions or nasopharyngeal aspirates are often contaminated by normal flora but may identify causative organism(s).
- Blood cultures (usually negative) should be obtained prior to initiation of antibiotic therapy in ill-appearing or febrile patients.

Initial Tests (lab, imaging)
- CT scan of orbits and sinuses with axial and coronal views, with and without contrast, is imaging modality of choice. US and MRI are alternatives.
  - Thin section (2 mm) CT, coronal and axial views with bone windows to differentiate preseptal from orbital cellulitis, confirm extension into orbit, detect coexisting sinus disease, and identify orbital or subperiosteal abscesses that may require surgery; deviation of medial rectus indicates intraorbital involvement.
- MRI offers superior soft tissue resolution for identification of cavernous sinus thrombosis but is less effective for bone imaging.
- US is used to rule out orbital myositis; locate FBs or abscesses, and follow progression of drained abscess.

Follow-Up Tests & Special Considerations
- Frequent eye exam and vital signs (q4h)
- Identify associated conditions, such as meningitis or orbital abscess.

Diagnostic Procedures/Other
Consult ophthalmology for slit lamp and dilated funduscopic exam to evaluate proptosis, color vision, automated visual field and the need for surgery.

TREATMENT
Admit patients with orbital cellulitis for monitoring and treatment with broad-spectrum IV antibiotics.

MEDICATION
- Empiric antibiotic therapy to cover pathogens associated with acute sinusitis (*S. pneumoniae*, *H. influenzae*, *Moraxella catarrhalis*, *Streptococcus pyogenes*), as well as for *S. aureus*, *S. anginosus*, and anaerobes
- Modify IV antibiotic treatment when culture and sensitivity results are available. Duration of IV therapy is usually a week. Additional PO therapy depends on response.
- PO antibiotic therapy for 2 to 3 weeks or longer (3 to 6 weeks) is recommended for patients with severe sinusitis and bony destruction.

First Line
Intravenous (IV) therapy (preferred initially)
- Vancomycin
  - For MRSA coverage
    - Children: 40 to 60 mg/kg per day IV divided into 3 or 4 doses; maximum daily dose of 4 g
    - Adults: 15 to 20 mg/kg per day IV q8–12h; maximum of 2 g for each dose
  - Plus one of the following:
    - Ceftriaxone
      - Children: 50 mg/kg per dose IV QD or BID; maximum daily dose of 4 g/day
      - Adults: 2 g IV per day
    - Cefotaxime
      - Children: 150 to 200 mg/kg per day in 3 doses; maximum daily dose of 12 g
      - Adults: 2 g IV q4h
    - Ampicillin-sulbactam
      - Children: 300 mg/kg per day in 4 divided doses; maximum daily dose of 8 g of ampicillin
      - Adults: 3 g IV q6h
    - Piperacillin-tazobactam
      - Children: 240 mg/kg per day in 3 divided doses; maximum daily dose of 16 g of piperacillin
      - Adults: 4.5 g IV q6h
    - Metronidazole
      - For anaerobic
        - Adults: 500 mg IV or 500 mg PO q8h daily
  - If allergic to penicillin, treat with a combination of vancomycin plus:
    - Ciprofloxacin
      - Adults: 400 mg IV BID or 500 to 750 mg PO BID
      - Children: 20 to 30 mg/kg per day divided q12h; maximum dose of 1.5 g PO daily or 800 mg IV daily
    - Levofloxacin
      - Adults: 500 to 750 mg IV or PO QD
      - Children aged ≥5 years: 10 mg/kg per dose q24h; maximum of 500 mg/day
      - Children aged ≥5 years: 10 mg/kg per dose q12h

- Oral therapy (if good response)
- Clindamycin (alone)
  - Adults: 300 mg q8h
  - Children: 30 to 40 mg/kg per day in 3 to 4 divided doses; maximum of 1.8 g per day
- Clindamycin or trimethoprim-sulfamethoxazol
  - Adults: 1 to 2 DS tablets q12h
  - Children: 10 to 12 mg/kg per day of trimethoprim divided q12h
- Plus one of the following:
  - Amoxicillin
    - Adults: 875 mg PO q12h
    - Children: 45 mg/kg per day in divided doses q12h or 80 to 100 mg/kg per day in divided doses q8h; maximum dose of 500 mg per dose
  - Amoxicillin-clavulanic
    - Adults: 875 mg q12h
    - Children: 40 to 45 mg/kg per day in divided doses q8–12h or 90 mg/kg per day divided q12h (600 mg/5 mL suspension)
  - Cefpodoxime
    - Adults: 400 mg q12h
    - Children: 10 mg/kg per day divided q12h, not to exceed 200 mg per dose
  - Cefdinir
    - Adults: 300 mg BID
    - Children: 7 mg/kg BID, not to exceed 600 mg/day

ALERT
In severe orbital cellulitis, in suspected or proven MRSA infection, vancomycin remains the parenteral drug of choice. Use in conjunction with agents to cover gram-negative bacteria.

- Vancomycin: 1 g IV q12h for adults; 40 mg/kg/day IV divided q8–12h; maximum daily dose of 2 g for children

Second Line
Any number of antibiotic regimens have been reported as successful. There is no definitive consensus for best choice (1).

ISSUES FOR REFERRAL
Always admit to the hospital and consult with ophthalmology. Consider consultation with ID and ENT for orbital cellulitis; neurology/neurosurgery if intracranial spread is suspected

ADDITIONAL THERAPIES
- Steroid use is controversial. PO steroids as an adjunct to IV antibiotics for orbital cellulitis may speed resolution of inflammation.
- Nasal decongestants are often recommended.
- Topical erythromycin or nonmedicated ophthalmic ointment protects the cornea from exposure in cases with severe proptosis.
- Children may be treated with amoxicillin/clavulanate 20 to 40 mg/kg/day divided TID or in adults 250 to 500 mg TID.

SURGERY/OTHER PROCEDURES
- IV antibiotic therapy is the initial therapy. 80–90% of cases respond to medical therapy without surgery.
- Surgical intervention warranted for visual loss, complete ophthalmoplegia, well-defined large abscess (>10 mm) on presentation or no clinical improvement after 24 to 48 hours of antibiotic therapy

ADMISSION, INPATIENT, AND NURSING CONSIDERATIONS
Patients with orbital cellulitis should be admitted for IV antibiotics and serial eye exams to evaluate progression of infection or involvement of optic nerve.

ONGOING CARE

FOLLOW-UP RECOMMENDATIONS
Patient Monitoring
Serial visual acuity testing and slit lamp exams

ALERT
Bedside exam q4h is indicated, as complications can develop rapidly.

PATIENT EDUCATION
Maintain proper hand washing and good skin hygiene. Avoid skin or lid trauma.

PROGNOSIS
Historically, blindness occurred in 20% and death in 17% of cases before antibiotics. Vision loss occurs in 3–11% of cases (1).

COMPLICATIONS
- Vision loss, CNS involvement, and death
- Permanent vision loss
- CNS complications: intracranial abscess, meningitis, cavernous sinus thrombosis

REFERENCES
1. El Mograbi A, Ritter A, Najjar E, et al. Orbital complications of rhinosinusitis in the adult population: analysis of cases presenting to a tertiary medical center over a 13-year period. *Ann Otol Rhinol Laryngol.* 2019;128(6):563–568.
2. Khan SA, Hussain A, Phelps PO. Current clinical diagnosis and management of orbital cellulitis. *Expert Review of Ophthalmology.* 2021;16(5): 387–399.

 CODES

ICD10
- H05.019 Cellulitis of unspecified orbit
- H05.011 Cellulitis of right orbit
- H05.012 Cellulitis of left orbit

CLINICAL PEARLS
- Most cases of orbital cellulitis arise from sinusitis.
- CT of orbits and sinuses with axial and coronal views with and without contrast is diagnostic modality of choice.
- Patients with orbital cellulitis must be admitted for visual monitoring and IV antibiotic therapy.
- Older age (>10 years) and diplopia predict the need for surgical intervention in children.
- Ophthalmoplegia, mental status changes, contralateral cranial nerve palsy, or bilateral orbital cellulitis raise suspicion for intracranial involvement.

C

CELLULITIS, PERIORBITAL

Mark B. Stephens, MD, MS, FAAFP • Fozia Akhtar Ali, MD, FAAFP • Khorshid Amirkhosravi, MD

BASICS

DESCRIPTION
- An acute bacterial infection of the skin and subcutaneous tissue anterior to the orbital septum; does not involve the orbital structures (globe, fat, and ocular muscles)
- Synonym(s): preseptal cellulitis

ALERT
It is essential to distinguish periorbital cellulitis from orbital cellulitis. Orbital cellulitis is a potentially life-threatening condition. *Orbital cellulitis is posterior to the orbital septum; symptoms include restricted eye movement, pain with eye movement, proptosis, and vision changes.*

EPIDEMIOLOGY
- Occurs more commonly in children; mean age 21 months
- 3 times more common than orbital cellulitis

Incidence
Increased incidence in the winter months (due to increased cases of sinusitis)

ETIOLOGY AND PATHOPHYSIOLOGY
- The anatomy of the eyelid distinguishes periorbital (preseptal) from orbital cellulitis:
  - A connective tissue sheet (orbital septum) extends from the orbital bones to the margins of the upper and lower eyelids; it acts as a barrier to infection of deeper orbital structures.
  - Infection of tissues anterior to the orbital septum is periorbital (preseptal) cellulitis.
  - Infection deep to the orbital septum is orbital (postseptal) cellulitis.
- Periorbital cellulitis typically arises from a contiguous infection of soft tissues of the face.
  - Sinusitis (via lamina papyracea) extension
  - Local trauma; insect or animal bites
  - Foreign bodies
  - Dental abscess extension
  - Hematogenous seeding
- Common organisms
  - *Staphylococcus aureus*, typically MSSA (MRSA is increasing.)
  - *Staphylococcus epidermidis*
  - *Streptococcus pyogenes*
- Atypical organisms
  - *Acinetobacter* spp.; *Nocardia brasiliensis*
  - *Bacillus anthracis*; *Pseudomonas aeruginosa*
  - *Neisseria gonorrhoeae*; *Proteus* spp.
  - *Pasteurella multocida*; *Mycobacterium tuberculosis*; *Trichophyton* sp. (ringworm)
- Since vaccine introduction, the incidence of *Haemophilus influenzae* disease has decreased (should still be suspected in unimmunized or partially immunized patients).

Genetics
No known genetic predisposition

RISK FACTORS
- Contiguous spread from upper respiratory infection
- Acute sinusitis
- Conjunctivitis
- Blepharitis
- Dental infection
- Local skin trauma/puncture wound
- Insect bite
- Bacteremia

GENERAL PREVENTION
- Avoid trauma around the eyes.
- Avoid swimming in fresh or salt water with facial skin abrasions.
- Routine vaccination: particularly *H. influenzae* type B and *Streptococcus pneumoniae*

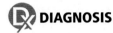

DIAGNOSIS

HISTORY
- Induration, erythema, warmth, and/or tenderness of periorbital soft tissue, usually with normal vision and normal eye movements
- Chemosis (conjunctival swelling), proptosis; pain with extraocular eye movements can occur in severe cases of periorbital cellulitis and are concerning for orbital cellulitis.
- Fever (not always present)

ALERT
Pain with eye movement, fever, and conjunctival swelling raise the suspicion for orbital cellulitis.

PHYSICAL EXAM
- Vital signs and general appearance (Patients with orbital cellulitis often appear systemically ill.)
- Inspect eyes and surrounding structures—eyelids, lashes, conjunctiva, and skin.
- Erythema, swelling, and tenderness of eyelids without orbital congestion
  - Violaceous discoloration of eyelid is more commonly associated with *H. influenzae*.
- Evaluate for skin breakdown.
- Look for vesicles to rule out herpetic infection.
- Inspect nasal vaults and palpate sinuses for signs of acute sinusitis.
- Examine oral cavity for dental abscesses.
- Test ocular motility and visual acuity.

DIFFERENTIAL DIAGNOSIS
- Orbital cellulitis
  - Orbital cellulitis may have the same signs and symptoms as periorbital cellulitis, with fever, proptosis, chemosis, ophthalmoplegia, decreased visual acuity.
- Abscess
- Dacryocystitis
- Hordeolum (stye)
- Allergic inflammation
- Orbital or periorbital trauma
- Idiopathic inflammation from orbital pseudotumor
- Orbital myositis
- Rapidly progressive tumors
  - Rhabdomyosarcoma
  - Retinoblastoma
  - Lymphoma
- Leukemia

DIAGNOSTIC TESTS & INTERPRETATION
Initial Tests (lab, imaging)
- CBC with differential diagnosis
- Blood cultures (low yield) (1)[C]
- Wound culture of purulent drainage (if present)
- Imaging is indicated if there is suspicion for orbital cellulitis (marked eyelid swelling, fever, and leukocytosis or failure to improve on appropriate antibiotics within 24 to 48 hours).
- CT to evaluate the extent of infection and detect orbital inflammation or abscess:
  - CT with contrast, thin sections (2 mm); coronal and axial views with bone windows
  - The classic sign of orbital cellulitis on CT scan is bulging of the medial rectus.

Follow-Up Tests & Special Considerations
- Children with periorbital or orbital cellulitis often have underlying sinusitis.
- If a child is febrile, <15 months old, and appears toxic, admit for blood cultures, antibiotic therapy, and consider lumbar puncture.

TREATMENT

MEDICATION

- Treat periorbital cellulitis with oral antibiotics and ensure close follow-up.
- Empiric antibiotic treatment should cover the most likely organisms (*Staphylococcus* and *Streptococcus*).
- Observe local prevalence of MRSA to determine need for coverage.
- No evidence that IV antibiotics are more effective than PO in reducing recovery time or preventing secondary complications in simple periorbital cellulitis
- No evidence for benefit of steroid use

First Line

- Uncomplicated posttraumatic periorbital cellulitis
  - Usually due to skin flora, including *Staphylococcus* and *Streptococcus*
  - Cephalexin 500 mg PO q6h or dicloxacillin 500 mg PO q6h
  - Clindamycin 300 mg PO TID, doxycycline 100 mg PO BID, or trimethoprim-sulfamethoxazole (TMP-SMX) 1 to 2 DS tablets PO q12h if MRSA is suspected
- Extension from sinusitis
  - Amoxicillin-clavulanate 875 mg/125 mg PO BID
  - 3rd-generation cephalosporin (e.g., cefdinir 300 mg PO BID)
- Dental abscess
  - Amoxicillin-clavulanate 875 mg/125 mg PO BID or clindamycin 300 mg PO TID
- Bacteremic cellulitis
  - May be associated with meningitis
  - Ceftriaxone 1 g IV q24h plus vancomycin 15 mg/kg/dose IV q8–12h or clindamycin 600 to 900 mg IV q8h to cover MRSA
  - Duration of therapy: A 10- to 14-day course is usually sufficient. Follow patients treated with oral antibiotics for presumed periorbital cellulitis closely (daily follow-up until improvement occurs), for response to antibiotics, and possible progression to orbital cellulitis. If symptoms do not improve within 24 hours, reevaluate for IV antibiotic therapy.

ISSUES FOR REFERRAL

Consult ENT and ophthalmology if there is concern for orbital cellulitis or if patients do not respond quickly to first-line treatment.

SURGERY/OTHER PROCEDURES

- Usually not indicated in uncomplicated cases
- If there is an abscess or potential compromise of critical structures, orbital surgery is indicated.
- Diplopia is the strongest clinical predictor for surgery.

ADMISSION, INPATIENT, AND NURSING CONSIDERATIONS

- If the patient is stable and there are no systemic signs of toxicity, mild cases in adults and children >1 year of age can be safely managed on an outpatient basis.
- Consider hospitalization and IV antibiotics:
  - If patient appears systemically ill
  - Children <1 year of age (2)[C]
  - Patients not immunized against *S. pneumoniae* or *H. influenzae*
  - If patients do not improve or deteriorate within 24 hours of oral antibiotics
  - High suspicion for orbital cellulitis (eyelid swelling with reduced vision, diplopia, abnormal light reflexes, or proptosis)
- No strict guidelines indicate when to switch from parenteral to PO therapy. In general, a switch from IV to oral antibiotics is reasonable once eyelid edema and erythema have significantly improved.
- A 10- to 14-day course of antibiotics is indicated.

 ONGOING CARE

FOLLOW-UP RECOMMENDATIONS

Patient Monitoring

Follow for signs of orbital involvement, including decreased visual acuity or painful/limited ocular motility.

PATIENT EDUCATION

- Maintain good skin hygiene.
- Avoid skin trauma.
- Report early skin changes (swelling, redness, and pain) if recurrent after a course of therapy.

PROGNOSIS

- With timely treatment, patients do well.
- Recurrent periorbital cellulitis occurs with ≥3 periorbital infections in 1 year with at least 1 month of in between episodes; must be differentiated from treatment failure due to antibiotic resistance

COMPLICATIONS

- Orbital cellulitis; orbital abscess formation
- Scarring
- Vision loss
- Cavernous sinus thrombosis
- Osteomyelitis

REFERENCES

1. Baring DEC, Hilmi OJ. An evidence based review of periorbital cellulitis. *Clin Otolaryngol*. 2011;36(1):57–64.
2. Williams KJ, Allen RC. Paediatric orbital and periorbital infections. *Curr Opin Ophthalmol*. 2019;30(5):349–355.

ADDITIONAL READING

Ekhlassi T, Becker N. Preseptal and orbital cellulitis. *Dis Mon*. 2017;63(2):30–32.

CODES

ICD10
L03.211 Cellulitis of face

CLINICAL PEARLS

- Periorbital (preseptal) and orbital (postseptal) cellulitis occur most commonly in children.
- CT scan of sinuses and orbits can differentiate periorbital cellulitis from orbital cellulitis.
- Orbital cellulitis typically has fever, pain with eye movement, diplopia, and/or proptosis.
- Prompt imaging and consultation is necessary if there is a concern for orbital cellulitis.

CEREBRAL PALSY
Tony Cha Her, MD

BASICS

DESCRIPTION
Cerebral palsy (CP) is a group of clinical syndromes characterized by motor and postural dysfunction due to permanent and nonprogressive disruptions in the developing brain. Motor impairment resulting in activity limitation is necessary for this diagnosis. CP is classified by the nature of the movement disorder and its functional severity.

EPIDEMIOLOGY
Incidence
- Overall, 1.5 to 3.0/1,000 live births
- Incidence increases as gestational age (GA) at birth decreases:
  – 146/1,000 for GA of 22 to 27 weeks
  – 62/1,000 for GA of 28 to 31 weeks
  – 7/1,000 for GA of 32 to 36 weeks
  – 1/1,000 for GA of ≥37 weeks
- Incidence increases as birth weight decreases (1).

ETIOLOGY AND PATHOPHYSIOLOGY
- Multifactorial; CP results from static injury or lesions in the developing brain, occurring prenatally, perinatally, or postnatally.
- Cytokines, free radicals, and inflammatory response are likely contributing factors.
- Spastic CP is most common, usually related to premature birth, with either periventricular leukomalacia or germinal matrix hemorrhage.

Genetics
There are reports of associations between CP and polymorphisms of certain genes: thrombophilic, cytokines, and apolipoprotein E.

RISK FACTORS
- Prenatal: congenital anomalies, multiple gestation, in utero stroke, intrauterine infection (cytomegalovirus [CMV], varicella), intrauterine growth retardation (IUGR), clinical and histologic chorioamnionitis, antepartum bleeding, maternal factors (cognitive impairment, seizure disorders, hyperthyroidism), abnormal fetal position (e.g., breech)
- Perinatal: preterm birth, low birth weight, periventricular leukomalacia, perinatal hypoxia/asphyxia, intracranial hemorrhage/intraventricular hemorrhage, neonatal seizure or stroke, hyperbilirubinemia
- Postnatal: traumatic brain injury or stroke, sepsis, meningitis, encephalitis, asphyxia, and progressive hydrocephalus

GENERAL PREVENTION
- Effective prevention strategies include antenatal corticosteroids, magnesium sulfate, and neonatal hypothermia (2).
- Treating mothers with magnesium sulfate during preterm delivery is neuroprotective for fetus and may reduce the risk of CP. Effect on term fetus is unknown (3)[B].
- Term-born infants who experience intrapartum hypoxia have benefit from therapeutic hypothermia (4).

COMMONLY ASSOCIATED CONDITIONS
- Seizure disorder
- Intellectual and speech and language impairments
- Behavioral problems
- Hearing and visual impairments
- Feeding impairment, swallowing dysfunction, and aspiration: when severe, may require gastrostomy feedings
- Poor dentition, excessive drooling
- GI conditions: constipation (59%), vomiting (22%), gastroesophageal reflux
- Decreased linear growth and weight abnormalities (underweight and overweight)
- Osteopenia
- Bowel and bladder incontinence
- Orthopedic: contractures, hip subluxation/dislocation, scoliosis (60%)

DIAGNOSIS

- Guidelines for early and accurate diagnosis (5):
  – International guidelines for early diagnosis of CP before 12 months of age: The tools for detection include neuroimaging and Prechtl General Movements Assessment (GMA) (6) before 5 months and the use of the Hammersmith Infant Neurologic Examination (HINE) (7) in a longitudinal fashion between 3 and 12 months.
- A clinical diagnosis including
  – Delayed motor milestones
  – Abnormal tone
  – Abnormal neurologic exam suggesting a cerebral etiology for motor dysfunction
  – Absence of regression (not losing function)
  – Absence of underlying syndromes or alternative explanation for etiology
- Although the pathologic lesion is static, clinical presentation may change as the infant grows and develops.

HISTORY
Ask about prenatal, perinatal, and postnatal risk factors.
- Neurobehavioral signs (poor feeding/frequent vomiting/irritability)
- Timing of motor milestones
- Abnormal spontaneous general movements
- Asymmetry of movements such as early hand preference
- Regression of motor skills does not occur with CP.

PHYSICAL EXAM
- Spasticity: increased tone/reflexes/clonus
- Dyskinesia: abnormal movements
- Hypotonia: decreased tone
- Ataxia: abnormal balance/coordination
- Tone: may be increased or decreased
- Trunk and head control: often poor but may be advanced due to high tone
- Reduced strength and motor control
- Persistence of primitive reflexes

- Asymmetry of movement or reflexes
- Decreased joint range of motion and contractures
- Brisk deep tendon reflexes, clonus
- Delayed motor milestones: serial exams most effective
- Gait abnormalities: scissoring, toe-walking
- CP is classified by the following:
  – Spasticity
    ○ Unilateral: hemiplegic
    ○ Bilateral: diplegic (lower extremity [LE] > upper extremity [UE] involvement) or quadriplegic (UE ≥ LE involvement)
  – Dystonia: hypertonia and reduced movement
  – Choreoathetosis: irregular spasmodic involuntary movements of the limbs or facial muscles
  – Ataxia: loss of orderly muscular coordination
  – The Manual Ability Classification System (MACS) can be used to assess UE and fine motor function.

DIFFERENTIAL DIAGNOSIS
Benign congenital hypotonia, brachial plexus injury, familial spastic paraplegia, dopa-responsive dystonia, transient toe-walking, muscular dystrophy, metabolic disorders (e.g., glutaric aciduria type 1), mitochondrial disorders, genetic disorders (e.g., Rett syndrome)

DIAGNOSTIC TESTS & INTERPRETATION
Laboratory testing is not needed to make diagnosis, but it can help to exclude other etiologies.
- Testing for metabolic and genetic syndromes (8)[C]
  – Considered if no specific etiology is identified by neuroimaging or if there are atypical features in clinical presentation
  – Detection of certain brain malformations may warrant genetic or metabolic testing to identify syndromes.
- Diagnostic testing for coagulopathies should be considered in children with hemiplegic CP with cerebral infarction identified on neuroimaging (8)[C].

Initial Tests (lab, imaging)
- Neuroimaging is not essential, but it is recommended in children with CP for whom the etiology has not been established (8)[C].
- MRI is preferred to CT (8)[C].
- Abnormalities found in 80–90% of patients: brain malformation, cerebral infarction, intraventricular or other intracranial hemorrhage, periventricular leukomalacia, ventricular enlargement, or other CSF space abnormalities

Diagnostic Procedures/Other
- Screening for comorbid conditions: developmental delay/intellectual impairment, vision/hearing impairments, speech and language disorders, feeding/swallowing dysfunction, or seizures
- Electroencephalograms (EEGs) should only be obtained if there is a history of suspected seizures.

TREATMENT

Focuses on control of symptoms; treatments reduce spasticity to prevent painful contractures, manage comorbid conditions, and optimize functionality and quality of life.

GENERAL MEASURES
- Early intervention for children aged 0 to 3 years (6)[A]
- Various therapies enhance function:
  – Physical therapy to improve posture stability and gait, motor strength and control, and prevent contractures
  – Occupational therapy to increase functional activities of daily living
  – Speech therapy for verbal and nonverbal speech and to aid in feeding
- Equipment optimizes participation in activities:
  – Orthotic splinting (ankle–foot orthosis)
  – Spinal bracing (body jacket) may slow down scoliosis.
  – Augmentative communication with pictures, switches, or computer systems for nonverbal individuals
  – Crutches, walkers, gait trainers, and wheelchairs for mobility and standers for weight bearing

MEDICATION
First Line
- Diazepam (7)[A]
  – A γ-aminobutyric acid-A (GABA$_A$) agonist that facilitates CNS inhibition at spinal and supraspinal levels to reduce spasticity
  – Used for short-term treatment for generalized spasticity; insufficient evidence on motor function
  – Adverse effects: ataxia and drowsiness
  – Adult dose: 2 to 12 mg/dose PO q6–12h
  – Pediatric dose (<12 years and <15 kg): <8.5 kg: 0.5 to 1.0 mg HS; 8.5 to 15.0 kg: 1 to 2 mg HS; children 5 to 16 years of age and ≥15 kg: 1.25 mg TID
- Botulinum toxin type A (7)[A]
  – Acts at neuromuscular junction to inhibit the release of acetylcholine to reduce tone
  – Injected directly into muscles of interest for localized spasticity; insufficient evidence on motor function
  – Higher functional benefit when combined with occupational therapy
  – Lasts for 12 to 16 weeks following injection

Second Line
- Baclofen (7)[A]
  – A GABA$_B$ agonist, facilitates presynaptic inhibition of monosynaptic and polysynaptic reflexes
  – Adverse effects: drowsiness and sedation
  – Abrupt withdrawal symptoms: spasticity, hallucinations, seizures, confusion, hyperthermia

  – Adults: Initial dose is 5 mg TID; increase dosage every 3 days to an average maintenance dose of 20 mg TID, 80 mg/day maximum.
  – Pediatric dose (>2 years): initially, 10 to 15 mg/day; titrate to effective dose (maximum of 40 mg/day); <8 years old: 60 mg/day maximum; >8 years old: 60 mg/day maximum
- Intrathecal baclofen (baclofen pump) (9)[A]
  – Continuous intrathecal route allows greater maximal response with smaller dosage to reduce spasticity.
  – May help ambulatory individuals with gait but no improvement seen in nonambulatory patients
  – Adverse effects: infection, catheter malfunction, CSF leakage

ADDITIONAL THERAPIES
Multidisciplinary care including ophthalmology; neurology; orthopedics; physiatry along with physical, occupational, and speech therapists

SURGERY/OTHER PROCEDURES
- Dorsal root rhizotomy selectively cuts dorsal rootlets from L1–S2; decreases spasticity in lower limbs when done in conjunction with physiotherapy but associated with adverse effects; evidence is lacking as to long-term outcomes.
- Surgical treatment of joint dislocations/subluxation, scoliosis management, tendon lengthening, gastrostomy

COMPLEMENTARY & ALTERNATIVE MEDICINE
- Therapeutic horse riding or hippotherapy improves postural control and balance.
- Aquatherapy improves gross motor function in patients with various motor severities.

 ONGOING CARE

PROGNOSIS
Reduced lifespan strongly associated with level of functional impairment and intellectual disability

REFERENCES
1. Sadowska M, Sarecka-Hujar B, Kopyta I. Cerebral palsy: current opinions on definition, epidemiology, risk factors, classification and treatment options. *Neuropsychiatr Dis Treat*. 2020;16:1505–1518.
2. Novak I, Morgan C, Fahey M, et al. State of the evidence traffic lights 2019: systematic review of interventions for preventing and treating children with cerebral palsy. *Curr Neurol Neurosci Rep*. 2020;20(2):3.
3. Nguyen TMN, Crowther CA, Wilkinson D, et al. Magnesium sulphate for women at term for neuroprotection of the fetus. *Cochrane Database Syst Rev*. 2013;(2):CD009395.
4. Badawi N, Mcintyre S, Hunt RW. Perinatal care with a view to preventing cerebral palsy. *Dev Med Child Neurol*. 2021;63(2):156–161.
5. Maitre NL, Burton VJ, Duncan AF, et al. Network implementation of guideline for early detection decreases age at cerebral palsy diagnosis. *Pediatrics*. 2020;145(5):e20192126.
6. Spittle A, Orton J, Anderson P, et al. Early developmental intervention programmes post-hospital discharge to prevent motor and cognitive impairments in preterm infants. *Cochrane Database Syst Rev*. 2012;(12):CD005495.
7. Delgado MR, Hirtz D, Aisen M, et al; for the Quality Standards Subcommittee of the American Academy of Neurology, Practice Committee of the Child Neurology Society. Practice parameter: pharmacologic treatment of spasticity in children and adolescents with cerebral palsy (an evidence-based review): report of the Quality Standards Subcommittee of the American Academy of Neurology and the Practice Committee of the Child Neurology Society. *Neurology*. 2010;74(4): 336–343.
8. Ashwal S, Russman BS, Blasco PA, et al; for the Quality Standards Subcommittee of the American Academy of Neurology, Practice Committee of the Child Neurology Society. Practice parameter: diagnostic assessment of the child with cerebral palsy: report of the Quality Standards Subcommittee of the American Academy of Neurology and the Practice Committee of the Child Neurology Society. *Neurology*. 2004;62(6):851–863.
9. Pin TW, McCartney L, Lewis J, et al. Use of intrathecal baclofen therapy in ambulant children and adolescents with spasticity and dystonia of cerebral origin: a systematic review. *Dev Med Child Neurol*. 2011;53(10):885–895.

 CODES

ICD10
- G80.9 Cerebral palsy, unspecified
- G80.1 Spastic diplegic cerebral palsy
- G80.2 Spastic hemiplegic cerebral palsy

CLINICAL PEARLS
- Management should focus on maximizing functioning and quality of life using multidisciplinary team approach.
- Regression of motor skills does not occur with CP.

CERVICAL HYPEREXTENSION INJURIES

Daniel R. Matta, MD • Elias Moreno, DO

BASICS

DESCRIPTION

- Class of neck injuries typically seen in rapid, forceful extension of the cervical spine
- Flexion–extension injuries ("whiplash") are usually from motor vehicle accidents (MVAs), typically side-impact or rear-end collisions.
- Other causes include falls, violence, or sports-related injuries (1).
- May involve:
  - Injury to vertebral and paravertebral structures: fractures, dislocations, ligamentous tears, and disc disruption/subluxation
  - Spinal cord injury (SCI): traumatic central cord syndrome (CCS) secondary to cord compression or vascular insult, SCI without radiologic abnormality (SCIWORA)
  - Blunt cerebrovascular injury (BCVI): vertebral artery or carotid artery dissection
  - Soft tissue injury: cervical strain/sprain (i.e., whiplash), cervical stingers (See "Brachial Plexopathy.")

EPIDEMIOLOGY

- Predominant age: SCI average age of injury is 43 years; CCS average age is 53 years.
- High-energy trauma (e.g., road accidents) and sports injuries are more common in young adults (average age is 29 years), whereas low-energy trauma (e.g., falls) are usually implicated in the >65 years age group
- Most (~80%) new SCI cases are male (1).

Incidence

In the United States

- Cervical fractures: 2 to 5/100 blunt trauma patients
- CCS: 4/100,000 people/year
- BCVI: estimated 1/1,000 of hospitalized trauma patients; incidence increased with cervical spine or thoracic injury
- Cervical strain: 3 to 4/1,000 people/year
- Whiplash is the most common injury in MVAs and accounts for 28% of all ED visits for MVAs.
- Incidence of whiplash is 70 to 328/100,000 with rates highest in 20- to 24-year-old females.
- 2–6% of patients with blunt trauma have SCI. 80% are below the C2 level (2).
- The incidence of traumatic SCI is approximately 54 cases per million population per year (1).

ETIOLOGY AND PATHOPHYSIOLOGY

Blunt trauma due to MVAs, falls, sports injuries, and violence (primarily gunshot wounds)

RISK FACTORS

- Whiplash: initial injury, no seat belt use, low neck rest, female gender (thinner necks)
- Chronic pain and/or disability: litigation, previous neck pain or injury, female gender, report of headache/low back pain at onset, low education level (3)[C]
- Fractures: osteoporosis, conditions predisposing to spinal rigidity, such as ankylosing spondylitis or other spondyloarthropathies
- CCS: preexisting spinal stenosis present in >50%
  - Acquired: prior trauma, spondylosis
  - Congenital: Klippel-Feil syndrome (congenital fusion of any two cervical vertebrae)

GENERAL PREVENTION

Seat belts, rule changes, proper technique, and proper use of protective equipment for sports activities can prevent or minimize injury.

COMMONLY ASSOCIATED CONDITIONS

Closed head injuries, whiplash-associated disorders (WADs), SCI, soft tissue trauma

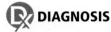

DIAGNOSIS

HISTORY

Usually acute presentation with mechanism of cervical hyperextension and complaints of neck pain, stiffness, or headaches ± neurologic symptoms

PHYSICAL EXAM

- External signs of trauma on the head and neck such as abrasions, lacerations, or contusions provide clues to mechanism and associated injuries.
- Presence, severity, and location of neck tenderness help localize involved structure(s):
  - Posterior, midline bony tenderness raises concern for underlying fracture.
  - Paraspinal or lateral soft tissue tenderness suggests muscular/ligamentous injury.
  - Anterior tenderness concerning for vascular injury
- Carotid bruit raises concern for carotid dissection.
- Trauma patients presenting with Glasgow Coma Scale (GCS) <15 warrant close attention and reassessment.
- Neurologic exam: paresthesias; weakness suggests SCI or stroke secondary to BCVI:
  - CCS often presents as
    - Distal > proximal symptom distribution, upper extremity > lower extremity
    - Extremity weakness/paralysis predominates
    - Variable sensory changes below level of lesion (including paresthesias and dysesthesia)
    - Bladder/bowel incontinence may occur.

DIFFERENTIAL DIAGNOSIS

- Acute or chronic disc pathology (herniation or internal disruption)
- Osteoarthritis
- Cervical radiculopathy
- For CCS
  - Bell cruciate palsy
  - Bilateral brachial plexus injuries
  - Carotid or vertebral artery dissection

DIAGNOSTIC TESTS & INTERPRETATION

Initial Tests (lab, imaging)

- Low-risk patients can be cleared clinically (without imaging) using either the Canadian C-Spine Rule (CCR) or the National Emergency X-Ray Utilization Study (NEXUS) criteria:
  - CCR: stable and alert (GCS>15) trauma patient with no history of cervical spine disease/surgery can be cleared if all the following conditions are met:
    - Able to actively rotate neck 45° left and right
    - No dangerous mechanism or extremity paresthesias

- Age <65 years
- At least one "low-risk factor" (i.e., simple rear-end MVA, ambulatory at any time, no midline cervical tenderness, delayed onset of neck pain, or sitting position in the ED)
  - NEXUS C-Spine Rule: clinically cleared if all the following conditions are met:
    - No midline tenderness
    - No evidence of intoxication
    - Normal level of alertness
    - No focal neurologic deficit
    - No distracting injury
  - Reported sensitivity/specificity: CCR (99.4%/45.1%), NEXUS (90.7%/36.8%)
- In patients with high-risk mechanism or concerning historical/physical exam, recommend imaging based on the suspected injury and level of clinical suspicion:
  - Plain radiographs: in some patients who cannot be cleared clinically but are still in low-suspicion category: sensitivity for C-spine injury 31.6%:
    - Dynamic: flexion–extension injuries; only if asymptomatic and no neurologic deficits or mental impairment, poor identification of ligamentous injury, limited diagnostic value
  - Axial CT scan from occiput to T1 with coronal and sagittal reconstructions has replaced plain radiography as the test of choice for cases with moderate to high clinical suspicion of C-spine injury, given high sensitivity (90–100%).
  - MRI: test of choice in CCS with direct visualization of traumatic cord lesions (edema or hematomyelia), soft tissue compressing cord, and/or stenosis of canal; detects ligamentous injury and abnormalities of intervertebral discs and soft tissues; MRI is less helpful for fractures.
  - CT angiography: visualization of cervical and cerebral vascular structures to detect BCVI, sensitivity approaches 100% when a ≥16-slice CT scanner is used. MR angiography is an alternative, although sensitivity of 47–50% limits utility.

Test Interpretation

- CCS: thought to be due to white matter axonal disruption of the lateral column, particularly the corticospinal tracts
- BCVI: intimal disruption, leading to thrombosis and embolization
- Acute cervical strain/sprain: Models suggest myofascial tearing, edema, and inflammation.

Geriatric Considerations

- Degenerative changes of the C-spine may be confused with acute traumatic change; osteopenia may limit fracture visualization on x-ray—CT is more accurate.
- Degenerative disease and osteopenia increase risk of upper cervical spine injuries (even with low-velocity trauma).

Pediatric Considerations

SCIWORA: high incidence at age <9 years accounting for up to 50% of pediatric cervical spine injuries; MRI helps detect injury

TREATMENT

GENERAL MEASURES
- Whiplash/WAD
  - Limited or no benefit to cervical collar; if provided, use for <72 hours.
  - No advantage to engaging early multiprofessional intervention (e.g., pain management and psychology)
  - No outcome differences with physical therapy (PT) versus passive (immobilization, rest) treatment; advance activity levels as tolerated
  - No preferred approach to treatment in absence of fracture
- Fractures
  - Stability determined by imaging
  - Decompression and stabilization are indicated for:
    - Incomplete SCIs with spinal canal compromise
    - Clinical deterioration or failure to improve despite conservative management
  - Hangman fracture: traumatic spondylolisthesis of C2 with bilateral fractures through C2 pedicles, often with anterior subluxation of C2 over C3; can be unstable:
    - Managed with halo vest immobilization for 12 weeks until flexion–extension films normal
  - Odontoid fractures: treat according to type:
    - I: through apex; usually stable; external immobilization with a cervical collar (less often halo vest) for up to 12 weeks
    - II: most common, at base of dens, usually unstable; nonunion rates of up to 67% with halo immobilization alone, especially with dens displacement >6 mm or age >50 years
    - III: through C2 body, usually stable; immobilization in halo or cervical collar for 12 to 20 weeks
  - Hyperextension teardrop fractures
    - If stable, rigid collar or cervicothoracic brace for 8 to 14 weeks
    - If unstable, halo brace for up to 3 months
- CCS: neck immobilization with cervical collar, PT/occupational therapy (OT)
- Cervical strain: no difference in outcomes with active (PT) versus passive (immobilization, rest) treatment; may use soft cervical collar for 10 days for symptomatic relief and then mobilize and increase activity as tolerated; no clear EBM guidelines

MEDICATION
- Fractures: pain control with analgesics
- CCS: Within 8 hours of injury, consider methylprednisolone 30 mg/kg IV over 15 minutes and then continuous infusion 5.4 mg/kg/hr IV for 23 hours. Further improvement in motor function recovery may be seen if infusion is continued for 48 hours, especially if initial bolus administration is delayed after injury.
- BCVI: anticoagulation with IV heparin, followed by warfarin therapy for 3 to 6 months and then long-term antiplatelet therapy; antiplatelet agent as sole initial therapy in patients with contraindications to anticoagulation
- Cervical strain: NSAIDs or acetaminophen; there is a little benefit to adding cyclobenzaprine for acute cervical strain.

ISSUES FOR REFERRAL
- If cervical spine injury is suspected, immobilize patient and send to ED for evaluation and clearance.
- Emergent consultation from a spine surgeon for any concern for unstable fracture or SCI

SURGERY/OTHER PROCEDURES
- Fractures
  - Hangman fracture: surgical fixation for excessive angulation or subluxation, disruption of intervertebral disc space, or failure to obtain alignment with external orthosis
  - Odontoid fractures
    - Type II: Early surgical stabilization is recommended in setting of age >50 years, dens displacement >5 mm, and specific fracture patterns.
    - Type III: Surgical intervention is often reserved for cases of nonunion/malunion after trial of external immobilization.
- CCS: Surgical decompression/fixation is indicated in setting of unstable injury, herniated disc, or when neurologic function deteriorates.
- BCVI: Surgical and/or angiographic intervention may be required if there is an evidence of pseudoaneurysm, total occlusion, or transection of the vessel.

ADMISSION, INPATIENT, AND NURSING CONSIDERATIONS
- Varies by injury; clinical judgment, imaging findings, concomitant injuries, and need for operative intervention
- Advanced trauma life support protocol with backboard and collar

ONGOING CARE

FOLLOW-UP RECOMMENDATIONS
Patient Monitoring
Follow patients with known injuries using serial imaging under the care of a specialist.

PATIENT EDUCATION
ThinkFirst National Injury Prevention Foundation: https://www.thinkfirst.org

PROGNOSIS
- Presenting neurologic status is the most important factor in determining prognosis.
- Fractures
  - Hangman fracture: Healing rates with conservative treatment decrease sequentially from type I to type III fractures (100% to approximately 40%)
  - Odontoid fracture, fusion rate by type: type I, ~100% with external immobilization alone; type II, nonunion rates of up to 67% with halo immobilization alone, especially with dens displacement >6 mm or age >50 years; type III, 85% with external immobilization, 100% with surgical fixation
- BCVI
  - Patients have fewer neurologic sequelae with early diagnosis and antithrombotic therapy. There is unequal efficacy of anticoagulation and antiplatelet agents in preventing stroke.

- CCS
  - Spontaneous recovery of motor function in >50% over several weeks; younger patients are more likely to regain function.
  - Leg, bowel, and bladder functions return first, followed by upper extremities.
- WAD: Prognostic factors for development of late whiplash syndrome (>6 months of symptoms affecting normal activity) include increased initial pain intensity, pain-related disability, and cold hyperalgesia.

COMPLICATIONS
- Fractures: instability or malunion/nonunion necessitating second operation, reactions, and infection related to orthosis
- BCVI: embolic ischemic events and pseudoaneurysm formation

REFERENCES
1. Jara-Almonte G, Pawar C. Emergency department management of cervical spine injuries. *Emerg Med Pract*. 2021;23(10):1–28.
2. Masson de Almeida Prado R, Masson de Almeida Prado JL, Ueta RHS, et al. Subaxial spine trauma: radiological approach and practical implications. *Clin Radiol*. 2021;76(12):941.e1–941.e10.
3. Godek P. Whiplash injuries. Current state of knowledge. *Ortop Traumatol Rehabil*. 2020;22(5):293–302.

ADDITIONAL READING
- Astrup J, Gyntelberg F. The whiplash disease reconsidered. *Front Neurol*. 2022;13:821097.
- Usman S. Management of head and neck injuries by the sideline physician. *Am Fam Physician*. 2022;106(5):543–548.

CODES

ICD10
- S13.4XXA Sprain of ligaments of cervical spine, initial encounter
- S13.101A Dislocation of unspecified cervical vertebrae, init encntr
- S14.109A Unsp injury at unsp level of cervical spinal cord, init

CLINICAL PEARLS
- Use NEXUS or CCR to determine the need for imaging in every patient with a potential neck injury.
- Always perform imaging if clinical judgment suggests the need to do so.
- Inquire about preexisting cervical spine conditions, especially in the elderly, because this may increase risk of injury or change radiographic interpretation.
- Suspect SCI until fully cleared through exam and imaging.
- Consider BCVI when neurologic deficits are inconsistent with level of known injury or in the setting of a significant mechanism of injury.

CERVICAL MALIGNANCY

Hansaa Gopalakrishnan, MD • Jeremy Golding, MD, FAAFP

BASICS

DESCRIPTION
Cervical cancer is a malignant neoplasm arising from the cells of the uterine cervix. Most cervical cancers, almost 90%, are squamous cell carcinomas and begin in the squamocolumnar junction where the exocervix and endocervix meet, also known as the transformation zone. A small percentage of cervical cancers are adenocarcinomas and begin in the glandular cells of the endocervix.

EPIDEMIOLOGY
Incidence
- According to the American Cancer Society (ACS), the annual incidence of cervical cancer in the United States between 2015 and 2019 was 7.7 cases per 100,000 person-years.
- According to the World Health Organization (WHO), cervical cancer is the fourth most common cancer in women worldwide, with 604,000 new cases and 342,000 deaths in 2020, 90% of which were in low and middle income countries.
- In the United States, cervical cancer is most frequently diagnosed in the 35 to 44 years age group, with average age at diagnosis being 50 years. Women >20 years of age rarely get cervical cancer. However, >20% of cervical cancer cases are in women >65 years of age.

Prevalence
In 2023, the ACS estimates 13,960 new cases of invasive cervical cancer and 4,310 deaths due to cervical cancer in the United States.

ETIOLOGY AND PATHOPHYSIOLOGY
- Human papillomavirus (HPV) infection with high-risk (HR) serotypes, especially HPV 16 and HPV 18, is the most important etiologic factor.
- HPV infection has high prevalence with most sexually active adults having it at one point in their lives.
- HR HPV accounts for 99% of all cervical cancer.

Genetics
There is a broad separation of HPV types, and the HR types that can be tested include HPV 16, 18, 31, 33, 35, 39, 45, 51, 52, 56, 58, 59, 66, and 68.

RISK FACTORS
- Persistent HPV infection is the primary risk factor for developing cervical cancer.
- Other risk factors include lack of or decreased access to health care and ability to obtain regular Pap tests, early coitarche especially before the age of 18 years, multiple sexual partners, unprotected sex, a history of sexually transmitted infections (STIs), low socioeconomic status, first birth prior to age of 20 years, high parity (≥3 full-term deliveries), cigarette smoking (doubles the risk), immunosuppression (HIV/AIDS, chemotherapy), diethylstilbestrol (DES) exposure in utero, oral contraceptive use of ≥5 years (risk back to baseline after ≥10 years of nonuse), family history of cervical cancer

GENERAL PREVENTION
- The cornerstone of prevention includes not only routine screening with a Pap test (or HPV test) but also vaccination against HR-HPV.
- The three FDA-approved vaccines are four-serotype Gardasil 4, nine-serotype Gardasil 9, and two-serotype (HPV 16 and 18) Cervarix, but only Gardasil 9 is currently distributed.
- Vaccination is recommended for:
  - Everyone through the age of 26 years
  - Girls and boys ages 11 or 12 years in 2 doses, 6 to 12 months apart. It can also be given as early as 9 years of age.
  - Children aged ≥15 years should receive 3 doses over the course of 6 months.
  - Immunocompromised patients ages 9 to 26 years, men who have sex with men, and the LGBTQ community
- Current guidelines from the US Preventive Services Task Force (USPSTF) recommend screening as follows:
  - Women aged 21 to 29 years: cytology alone every 3 years
  - Women aged 30 to 65 years: cytology alone every 3 years, HR-HPV testing (using an assay specifically approved by the FDA for HPV-screening-only testing) alone every 5 years, or cytology plus HR-HPV cotesting every 5 years
- An alternative screening algorithm using a risk-based strategy and specific FDA-approved high-risk HPV tests followed by cytology for positive screens is a recommended alternative.

COMMONLY ASSOCIATED CONDITIONS
Condyloma acuminata, preinvasive/invasive lesions of the vulva, vagina, oral, anal, and oropharyngeal cancers

DIAGNOSIS

HISTORY
- Patients with HPV infection may be asymptomatic. Early stages can be discovered incidentally as a result of cervical cancer screening.
- The most common symptoms of cervical cancer are irregular or heavy bleeding, postcoital vaginal bleeding, unusual discharge, pain with sex, and pelvic pain.

PHYSICAL EXAM
- A thorough pelvic exam is essential. Many patients have a normal exam, especially with microinvasive disease. Lesions may be exophytic, endophytic, polypoid, papillary, ulcerative, or necrotic.
- In women with symptoms of cervical cancer, bimanual and rectovaginal examination should be performed to evaluate uterine size, vaginal wall, rectovaginal septum, and parametrial, uterosacral, and pelvic sidewall involvement.
- Enlarged supraclavicular or inguinal lymphadenopathy, lower extremity edema, ascites, or decreased breath sounds with lung auscultation may indicate metastases or advanced stage disease.

DIFFERENTIAL DIAGNOSIS
- Cervical condyloma, leiomyoma, or polyp
- Metastasis from endometrial carcinoma or gestational trophoblastic neoplasia

DIAGNOSTIC TESTS & INTERPRETATION
Initial Tests (lab, imaging)
- Pap test
- Colposcopy with directed biopsies and/or biopsy of gross lesions are the definitive means of diagnosis.
- In advanced disease, may need to check CBC, UA, BUN, creatinine, and liver function tests (LFTs)
- Computed tomography (CT) scan of the chest, abdomen, and pelvis and/or a positron emission tomography (PET) scan for metastatic workup
- 2018 FIGO staging recommendations emphasize MRI of the pelvis to image extent of tumor and nodal involvement in patients who are surgical candidates or for planning radiation therapy.

Follow-Up Tests & Special Considerations
- Exam under anesthesia may be helpful in determining clinical stage, disease extent, and suitability for surgery.
- Endocervical curettage and cervical conization as indicated to determine depth of invasion and presence of lymphovascular involvement
- Cystoscopy to evaluate bladder invasion, proctoscopy for invasion into rectum

TREATMENT

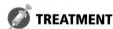

GENERAL MEASURES
Improve nutritional state, correct anemia (Hb <12 g/dL), and treat pelvic infections. Lymph node evaluation is key to staging and treatment. Correction of urinary tract obstruction is important prior to beginning chemoradiation. Pretreatment evaluation should be done prior to chemotherapy for lymph nodes involvement using PET/CT scan.

MEDICATION
- Chemoradiation with a cisplatin-containing regimen is the preferred treatment for certain stages of cervical cancer.
- Neoadjuvant chemotherapy may improve survival for early and locally advanced tumors. Adjuvant chemotherapy after chemoradiation may improve progression-free survival in patients who receive primary chemoradiation for stages IIB to IVA tumors.
- The addition of the antiangiogenesis drug bevacizumab to standard combination chemotherapy (cisplatin/topotecan or cisplatin/paclitaxel) for recurrent, persistent, or metastatic disease has been shown to improve overall survival.

First Line

- Chemoradiation is the primary treatment of choice for stages IB3 to IVA. The preferred regimen is weekly cisplatin or cisplatin with 5-fluorouracil along with radiation. If cisplatin is not a good option, then carboplatin can be used.
- The preferred first-line treatment for recurrent or metastatic disease is a combination of cisplatin/carboplatin/paclitaxel/bevacizumab/topotecan.

Second Line

Other alternative medications include docetaxel (Taxotere), ifosfamide (Ifex), 5-fluorouracil (5-FU), irinotecan (Camptosar), gemcitabine (Gemzar), and mitomycin. Bevacizumab (Avastin) can also be added to chemo regimen.

ISSUES FOR REFERRAL

Multidisciplinary management of patients as needed and in a timely fashion

ADDITIONAL THERAPIES

- Chemoradiation (without surgery) is the first-line therapy for tumors stage IB3 and higher. Combination of external-beam pelvic radiation and brachytherapy is usually employed.
- If para-aortic lymph node metastases are suspected, extended-field radiation or lymph node dissection prior to radiation therapy may be performed.

SURGERY/OTHER PROCEDURES

- Removal of precursor lesions (cervical intraepithelial neoplasia [CIN]) by loop electrosurgical excision procedure (LEEP), cold knife conization, laser ablation, or cryotherapy
- Open hysterectomy is superior to laparoscopic hysterectomy for cervical cancer treatment for patients with stages IA1 and IB1.
- Stage IA2 (lesions with >3-mm but ≤5-mm depth): option of radical hysterectomy with lymph node dissection or radiation depending on clinical setting; robotic radical hysterectomy (RRH) has demonstrated to be superior to laparoscopic radical hysterectomy and open radical hysterectomy in intraoperative blood loss, length of hospital stay, and intraoperative and postoperative complications; RRH can be regarded as a safe and effective therapeutic procedure for the management of cervical cancer.
- Stages IA2 to IB1: Fertility-sparing radical trachelectomy may be considered in selected patients.
- Stages IB1 to IIA (gross lesions without obvious parametrial involvement): option of radical hysterectomy with lymph node sampling or primary chemoradiation with brachytherapy and teletherapy, depending on clinical setting (1); in stage IB, when comparing adjuvant radiotherapy with no adjuvant radiotherapy, there is no significant difference in survival at 5 years between women who received radiation and those who received no further treatment (risk ratio [RR] = 0.8, 95% confidence interval [CI] 0.3–2.4). However, women who received radiation had a significantly lower risk of disease progression at 5 years (RR 0.6, 95% CI 0.4–0.9).
- Stage IVA (lesions limited to central metastasis to the bladder and/or rectum): Primary pelvic exenteration may be feasible.
- Stage IVB (lesions spread to distant organs): Treatment goal is palliation; therefore, early referral to palliative care should be made.

Pregnancy Considerations

- Management is guided by consideration of stage of lesion, gestational age, and maternal assessment of risks and benefits from treatment. Abnormal cytology is best followed up by colposcopy with directed biopsies.
- In pregnant women with early stages (IA1, IA2, IB) diagnosed before 3 months' gestation, treatment may be delayed to allow for fetal maturity.
- In pregnant women diagnosed with stage 1 cervical cancer in 2nd or 3rd trimester, a cold knife conization or radical trachelectomy may be suggested with plan for early C-section delivery.
- In pregnant women with advanced disease (stage 2 or higher) diagnosed in 2nd or 3rd trimester, chemotherapy may be recommended. Cisplatin, carboplatin, and paclitaxel usually do not harm the fetus if given in the 2nd or 3rd trimester but could possibly cause early labor or low-birth weight.

ADMISSION, INPATIENT, AND NURSING CONSIDERATIONS

- Admission may be needed for active bleeding, dehydration, treatment complications, and ureteral blockage (with hydronephrosis or urosepsis).
- Active vaginal bleeding can be controlled with timely vaginal packing and radiation therapy.

 ONGOING CARE

FOLLOW-UP RECOMMENDATIONS

Patient Monitoring

- With completion of definitive therapy and based on individual risk factors, patients are evaluated with physical/pelvic examinations: every 3 to 6 months for 2 years, every 6 to 12 months until the 5th year, and yearly thereafter.
- Pap smears may be performed yearly but have a low sensitivity for detecting recurrence.
- CT and PET scan are useful in locating metastases when recurrence is suspected; preferably 3 to 4 months posttreatment
- Signs of recurrence include vaginal bleeding, unexplained weight loss, leg edema, and pelvic or thigh pain.

PATIENT EDUCATION

The Society of Gynecologic Oncology: https://www.sgo.org/; the Foundation for Women's Cancer: https://www.foundationforwomenscancer.org

PROGNOSIS

- If detected early, invasive cervical cancer can be treated successfully. Survival rates were calculated based on women diagnosed with cervical cancer between the years of 2012 and 2018. Rates were calculated for each Surveillance, Epidemiology, and End Results (SEER) stage.
  - The 5-year survival rate for localized disease is estimated at 92%.
  - The 5-year survival rate for regional disease is estimated at 59%.
  - The 5-year survival rate for distant disease is estimated at 17%.
  - The 5-year survival rate for all SEER stages combined is estimated at 67%.

- An elevated squamous cell carcinoma antigen (SCC-Ag) serum levels estimated by ELISA technique can be used to predict the clinical response to neoadjuvant chemotherapy and residual disease. Persistently elevated SCC-Ag level at 2 to 3 months after RT had a significantly higher incidence of treatment failure. Serum SCC-Ag levels are also useful for monitoring treatment efficacy, disease progression, recurrence, and poor prognosis in SCCs. The combination of clinical pelvic examination and SCC-Ag levels provides useful information for the further need of treatment.

COMPLICATIONS

- Loss of ovarian function from radiotherapy or indication for bilateral oophorectomy
- Hemorrhage, pelvic infection, genitourinary fistula, bladder dysfunction, sexual dysfunction
- Ureteral obstruction with renal failure, bowel obstruction, pulmonary embolism, lower extremity lymphedema

REFERENCE

1. World Health Organization. Cervical cancer. https://www.who.int/news-room/fact-sheets/detail/cervical-cancer. Accessed October 23, 2023.

ADDITIONAL READING

- American Cancer Society. Information and resources about for cancer: breast, colon, lung, prostate, skin. https://www.cancer.org/. Accessed October 23, 2023.
- Tewari KS, Monk BJ. Evidence-based treatment paradigms for management of invasive cervical carcinoma. *J Clin Oncol.* 2019;37(27):2472–2489.

 SEE ALSO

Abnormal Pap and Cervical Dysplasia

CODES

ICD10

- C53.9 Malignant neoplasm of cervix uteri, unspecified
- C53.0 Malignant neoplasm of endocervix
- C53.1 Malignant neoplasm of exocervix

CLINICAL PEARLS

Cervical cancer is the second most common malignancy in women worldwide. Improving access to screening is likely to have the greatest impact in the reduction of the burden of disease. With HPV immunization and screening, the disease should be almost completely preventable.

CHILD ABUSE

Sasha Svendsen, MD

BASICS

DESCRIPTION
- Types of abuse: neglect (most common and highest mortality), physical abuse, emotional/psychological abuse, sexual abuse, and sexual exploitation
- Neglect includes physical (e.g., failure to provide necessary food or shelter or lack of appropriate supervision), medical (e.g., failure to provide necessary medical or mental health treatment), educational (e.g., failure to educate a child or attend to special education needs), and emotional (e.g., inattention to a child's emotional needs, failure to provide psychological care, or permitting the child to use alcohol or other drugs).
- System(s) affected: gastrointestinal (GI), endocrine/metabolic, musculoskeletal, nervous, renal, reproductive, skin/exocrine, pulmonary, cardiac, immune, and psychiatric
- Synonym(s): nonaccidental trauma; child maltreatment; inflicted injury

EPIDEMIOLOGY
Prevalence
Children's Bureau report for federal fiscal year (FFY) 2021 (1):
- Child Protective Services agencies received an estimated 3.9 million referrals alleging maltreatment, with a national screened-in referral rate of 27.6 referrals per 1,000 children.
- Approximately 3 million children received either an investigation or alternative response. Of those investigated, 588,229 children (8.1 per 1,000) were found to be victims of abuse or neglect.
- Neglect is the most common type of reported maltreatment at 76%, followed by physical abuse at 16% and sexual abuse at 10.1%.
- The overall rate of child fatalities was 2.46 deaths per 100,000 children in the national population. The rate of child fatalities is slightly higher in boys compared to girls.
- The majority of perpetrators are the parents of their victims (76.8%).

RISK FACTORS
- American Indian or Alaska Native children had the highest rates of victimization.
- Children from birth to 1 year of age had the highest rate of victimization with 25.3 per 1,000 infants and had the highest rate of mortality.
- Females have a slightly higher rate of victimization versus males.
- Military families are at risk, especially with deployment.
- Child risk factors: chronic illness, physical/congenital disability, developmental delay, preterm, unintended pregnancy
- Caregiver risk factors: poverty, substance misuse, lower educational status, parental history of abuse, parental mental health issues, young and/or unmarried mother, poor support network, and domestic violence

GENERAL PREVENTION
- Screen for risk factors at prenatal, postnatal, and pediatric visits.
- Physicians can educate parents on a range of normal behaviors to expect in infants and children: for example, anticipatory guidance on ways to handle crying infants; methods of discipline for toddlers

COMMONLY ASSOCIATED CONDITIONS
Failure to thrive, prematurity, developmental delays, poor school performance, poor social skills, low self-esteem, anxiety or depression

DIAGNOSIS

- Relatively minor skin injuries, frenulum tears, or bruising in precruising infants may be the first indications of child physical abuse; these relatively minor, unexplained injuries have been termed "sentinel injuries."
- 27.5% had a sentinel injury (80% had a bruise), 41.9% of those cases, HCW was aware of the injury.
- Infants with injuries caused by child abuse often present with vague complaints.
- Documentation
  - Critical elements include the following:
    - Brief statement of child's disclosure or caregiver's explanation, including any alternate explanations offered (Use direct quotations when possible.)
    - Time the incident occurred and date/time of disclosure
    - Whether witnesses were present
    - Developmental abilities of child
    - Objective medical findings
    - Other at-risk children in the household (siblings)
- DO NOT use terms such as "rule out," "R/O," and "alleged." Clearly state objective findings and medical provider's opinion.
- Obtain history from caregiver separately from child.
- Any description of abuse given by the child should be documented word for word using quotation marks in the child's own language and attributed to the child whenever possible.
- The child should not be rewarded after a disclosure (e.g., "Tell me what happened, and you can go back to your mom. . .").
- Documentation should include disposition of patient and record any report made to child welfare.

HISTORY
- Use nonjudgmental, open-ended questions (ask: who, what, when, and where; NEVER why).
- Document past medical history, developmental history, child's temperament, and thorough social history including objective documentation of family interactions.
- History of a sentinel injury should prompt consideration of abuse.

- The following historical elements may suggest abusive injury:
  - History that is inconsistent with the injury or with the child's developmental level
  - No explanation offered for the injury or the injury is blamed on sibling or another child.
  - Important detail of explanation changes dramatically.
  - Different witnesses provide different history.
  - There is a delay in seeking treatment.
  - Denial of trauma in a child with injury
- Nonspecific symptoms of abuse:
  - Behavior changes; self-destructive behavior; anxiety and/or depression
  - Sleep disturbances, night terrors; school problems

PHYSICAL EXAM
- Examine the child in a comfortable setting:
  - Explain what the exam will involve and why procedures are needed.
  - Allow the child to choose who will be in the room.
  - Completely undress the child and have them wear a gown to perform a complete physical examination, including thorough skin exam.
- Complete a general assessment for signs of physical abuse, neglect, and self-injurious behaviors:
  - Measurements, photographs, and careful objective descriptions are critical for accurate diagnosis.
- A thorough physical exam may include:
  - Skin (completely undress, including diaper to visualize buttocks)
  - Head (including fontanels), eyes, ears, nose, and mouth (including frenulum)
  - Chest/abdomen
  - Anogenital area (visualization of external genital structures with labial separation and traction—no speculum)
  - Extremities
  - Review growth charts
- Physical abuse findings
  - Skin markings (e.g., lacerations, burns, bruises, patterned injuries, bites)
  - Immersion injuries with clearly demarcated borders
  - Oral trauma (e.g., torn frenulum, loose teeth)
  - Ear bruising
  - Eye trauma (e.g., hyphema, subconjunctival hemorrhage)
  - Head/abdominal blunt trauma
  - Fractures
  - Patterns suggestive of abuse:
    - Bruises seen away from bony prominences (e.g., face, back, abdomen, arms, buttocks, ears, hands)
    - Multiple bruises in clusters or uniform shape
    - Patterned injuries (such as bite marks or the imprint of an object like a hand, belt, or cord) should be considered highly concerning for inflicted injury.
    - TEN-4-FACESp method to identify bruises suggestive of child abuse:
      - T: torso; E: ear; N: neck
      - 4: any bruise, anywhere on a child aged ≤4 months
      - F: frenulum; A: angle of jaw; C: cheeks; E: eyelids; S: subconjunctivae; p: patterned bruising

- Sexual abuse findings
  - Unexplained penile, vaginal, hymenal, perianal, or anal injuries/bleeding/discharge
  - Pregnancy or sexually transmitted infections (STIs)
- Neglect findings
  - Low-growth parameter trends, unclean, unkempt, rashes
  - Fearful or overly trusting
  - Abnormal development or growth parameters

DIFFERENTIAL DIAGNOSIS
- Physical trauma mimics
  - Accidental injury; toxic ingestion
  - Bleeding disorders (e.g., von Willebrand disease, hemophilia)
  - Metabolic or congenital conditions
  - Conditions with skin manifestations (e.g., congenital dermal melanocytosis, Henoch-Schönlein purpura, meningococcemia, erythema multiforme, hypersensitivity, staphylococcal scalded skin syndrome, varicella, impetigo)
  - Cultural practices (e.g., cupping, coining)
- Neglect mimics
  - Endocrinopathies (e.g., diabetes mellitus), constitutional growth delay
  - GI (clefts, malabsorption, irritable bowel), seizure disorder
- Skeletal trauma mimics
  - Obstetrical trauma, nutritional (scurvy, rickets)
  - Infection (congenital syphilis, osteomyelitis)
  - Osteogenesis imperfecta

DIAGNOSTIC TESTS & INTERPRETATION
Initial Tests (lab, imaging)
- Directed by history and physical exam findings:
  - Urinalysis (abdominal/flank/back/genital trauma)
  - Complete blood count, coagulation studies
  - Electrolytes, creatinine, blood urea nitrogen, glucose
  - Liver and pancreatic function tests (abdominal trauma)
  - Guaiac stool (abdominal trauma)
- In cases of suspected neglect:
  - Stool exam, calorie count, purified protein derivative and anergy panel, sweat test, lead and zinc levels
- In cases of suspected sexual abuse:
  - STI testing:
    - Urine NAAT: gonorrhea, chlamydia, *Trichomonas*
    - Serum: HIV, hepatitis B and C serologies, syphilis
  - Urine/serum pregnancy test
- In cases of suspected physical abuse:
  - Skeletal survey: 22 radiographs surveying each bone of the body, examining for evidence of acute or healing fractures
    - Recommended for:
      - Infants aged <6 months with bruising, regardless of pattern
      - Children aged <2 years with bruising concerning for abuse or domestic violence (See TEN-4-FACESp in Physical Exam section.)
      - All children aged <2 years with fractures and poorly explained injuries
      - All children aged <2 years who live with an abused child should be evaluated.
      - May also consider for any age child in which the patient has impaired mobility or communication skills

- Noncontrast head CT:
  - Consider brain magnetic resonance imaging (MRI) of head/neck/spine for further evaluation of more subtle findings, brain parenchyma, intracerebral edema, or hemorrhage.
  - All abused children with skull fracture found on skeletal survey
  - All infants aged <6 months (perhaps aged <1 year) when any physical abuse is suspected
  - All infants in whom nonaccidental head injury is suspected.
- CT scan of abdomen with IV contrast:
  - Children with clinical concern for abdominal injury (abdominal bruising, peritonitis, or a positive abdominal ultrasound) or history of blunt abdominal trauma and abdominal tenderness
- Dilated fundoscopic exam: Presence of retinal hemorrhages is highly concerning for abusive head trauma.
  - For any child with intracranial hemorrhage; within 24 to 72 hours of initial presentation
- High risk imaging findings:
  - Fractures in nonambulatory patients (Children who are not walking or cruising rarely have bruising or fractures from "short falls.")
  - Corner or bucket-handle fractures
  - Posterior rib fractures in infants
  - Injury to liver/spleen/pancreas in blunt abdominal trauma

Follow-Up Tests & Special Considerations
In cases of sexual abuse where there is a concern for exposure to body fluids, forensic evidence kit collection may be indicated up to 120 hours postassault.

 TREATMENT

MEDICATION
First Line
- Consider antibiotics postexposure prophylaxis in postpubertal children as indicated for STIs. Of note, do not prophylactically treat prepubertal children with antibiotics for STIs.
- If exposure to body fluids is of concern, consider HIV postexposure prophylaxis.

ALERT
Emergency contraception reduces rate of pregnancy after sexual assault:

- Levonorgestrel (Plan B): single dose of 1.5 mg or two 0.75-mg doses taken together or 12 hours apart; effective up to 72 hours OR
- Ulipristal (Ella): 30-mg single dose as soon as possible; effective up to 120 hours

ISSUES FOR REFERRAL
When responding to possible abuse, consider:
- The child's safety
  - Is the child at imminent risk for additional harm if sent back to the environment where the possible perpetrator has access to the child?
  - Are there other children in the home/environment who may also be at risk?

- Work with child welfare to ensure the family is complying with a plan of safe care that may include the following:
  - Mental health referrals for the victim and other family members, including siblings
  - Any follow-up with medical subspecialties, as needed
  - Continue to support the caregivers through the process when possible

ADMISSION, INPATIENT, AND NURSING CONSIDERATIONS
Admission if moderate/severe injuries, psychological trauma, inability to coordinate safe discharge plan

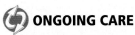 ONGOING CARE

PATIENT EDUCATION
- National Child Abuse Hotline: 1.800.4.A.CHILD
- National Toll-Free Crisis Hotline Numbers: www.childwelfare.gov/pubs/reslist/tollfree/
- Trauma resources: National Child Traumatic Stress Network (NCTSN): https://www.nctsn.org/

PROGNOSIS
Without intervention, child abuse is often a chronic and escalating phenomenon.

COMPLICATIONS
Sexual, physical, and emotional abuse in childhood are risk factors for poorer adult mental and physical health. This includes maltreatment, depression, substance misuse, suicide attempts, and risky sexual behaviors.

REFERENCE
1. U.S. Department of Health & Human Services, Administration for Children and Families, Administration on Children, Youth and Families, Children's Bureau. Child maltreatment 2021. https://www.acf.hhs.gov/cb/report/child-maltreatment-2021. Accessed September 17, 2023.

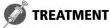 CODES

ICD10
- T74.12XA Child physical abuse, confirmed, initial encounter
- T74.32XA Child psychological abuse, confirmed, initial encounter
- T74.22XA Child sexual abuse, confirmed, initial encounter

CLINICAL PEARLS
- Mandated reporting is required for suspected child abuse and neglect; the medical provider does not have to prove abuse before reporting.
- When a bruise is present, it should be considered as a potential sentinel injury for physical abuse if no plausible explanation is given.
- Vague complaints and repeated visits to the office and/or ED should prompt further consideration.
- Neglect is the most common and lethal form of abuse.

CHLAMYDIA INFECTION (SEXUALLY TRANSMITTED)

Casandra Cashman, MD, FAAFP

BASICS

DESCRIPTION
- *Chlamydia trachomatis* is an intracellular membrane-bound prokaryotic organism. Chlamydia derives from the Greek word for "cloak."
- Chlamydia is the most common bacterial sexually transmitted infection (STI) in the United States.
- Transmitted through vaginal, anal, or oral sex; transmitted vertically during vaginal delivery
- Most cases are asymptomatic, especially in people with female anatomy. Untreated disease can lead to pelvic inflammatory disease (PID), ectopic pregnancy, and infertility.
- System(s) affected: reproductive

Pregnancy Considerations
Perinatal acquisition may result in neonatal pneumonia and/or conjunctivitis.

EPIDEMIOLOGY
Incidence
- Mandatory reporting started in 1985; there has generally been a steady increase in incidence since then.
- 1.64 million cases reported in 2020; ~1.8 million *reported* cases in 2019; incidence had been steadily increasing until 2020; lower reported numbers likely reflect reduced screening during COVID-19 pandemic rather than true decrease in actual infections.
- Swedish new variant of *C. trachomatis* (nvCT) first reported in 2006; often produces false-negative tests; largely confined to Nordic countries

Prevalence
- 495/100,000 people in the United States
- Young females, ethnic minorities most affected
- Highest prevalence in ages 20 to 24 years, followed by ages 15 to 19 years
- Predominant sex: females > males; females have twice the reported incidence and prevalence than males, likely reflecting increased testing in females. The use of highly sensitive nucleic acid amplification test (NAAT) urine screening may increase identification in males.
- Estimated ~2% of young sexually active individuals in the United States are affected.

ETIOLOGY AND PATHOPHYSIOLOGY
C. trachomatis serotypes D to K associated with genital tract infections. Chlamydia is an obligate intracellular organism. Chlamydia has biphasic life cycle. Extracellular elementary body (EB) is metabolically inactive and infectious. Once taken up by host cell (columnar epithelium of the genital tract), the EB prevents lysosomal phagocytosis and transforms to reticulate body (RB) which uses energy from host cell to synthesize RNA, DNA, and proteins. EBs are released and infect neighboring cells or spread through sexual contact.

RISK FACTORS
Risk correlates with:
- Number of lifetime sexual partners and number of concurrent sexual partners
- No use of barrier contraception during intercourse
- Black/Hispanic/Native American and Alaskan Native ethnicity
- Men who have sex with men (MSM) may be at higher risk for rectal and pharyngeal chlamydia than other groups; consider testing with NAAT when appropriate (1).

GENERAL PREVENTION
- Screening is recommended if new or >1 sex partner in the past 6 months; attending an adolescent clinic, family planning clinic, STD or abortion clinic, or attending a jail or other detention center clinic; screen if rectal pain, discharge or tenesmus, testicular pain occurs; test all individuals with urethral or cervical discharge.
- All sexually active women ≤25 years of age should be screened at least yearly. Repeat testing in ~3 months is recommended for those who screen positive because reinfection rate is high regardless of whether the sexual partner is treated (2)[A].
- Consider screening sexually active men ≤25 years of age particularly in high-risk populations.
- Screen high-risk MSM annually with genital and extragenital screening (3)[A].
- NAAT is the preferred screening test in all circumstances except child sexual abuse involving boys or rectal/oropharyngeal testing in prepubescent girls. For these situations, culture and susceptibility testing is preferred (3)[A].
- Acceptable to screen women for chlamydia on same day as intrauterine device (IUD) insertion—treat if positive (no need to remove IUD in this circumstance)
- Doxycycline postexposure prophylaxis (Doxy-PEP) is an emerging prevention strategy for prevention of chlamydia, syphilis, and possibly gonorrhea; currently best studied in MSM and transgender women with a history of bacterial STI within the past year

COMMONLY ASSOCIATED CONDITIONS
- Individuals with female anatomy
  - PID: ~10% develop PID within 12 months if untreated.
  - Infertility, ectopic pregnancy
  - Chronic pelvic pain
  - Urethral syndrome (dysuria, frequency, and pyuria in the absence of infection)
  - Arthritis (less common)
  - Spontaneous abortion
- Individuals with male anatomy
  - Epididymitis and nongonococcal urethritis
  - Reiter syndrome (HLA-B27)
  - Proctitis
- Neonates
  - Inclusion conjunctivitis (occurs in ~40% of exposed neonates)
  - Otitis media
  - Pneumonia
  - Pharyngitis
- Diseases caused by other chlamydial species
  - Lymphogranuloma venereum (LGV): *C. trachomatis* serotypes L1 to L3
  - Trachoma: *C. trachomatis* serotypes A to C

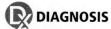

DIAGNOSIS
Many patients are asymptomatic.

Pregnancy Considerations
- Test all patients at first prenatal visit.
- Obtain repeat testing 3 to 4 weeks after treatment for all pregnant patients with confirmed chlamydial infection. Test again after 3 months.
- Repeat screening in 3rd trimester in high-risk patients (2)[A].

HISTORY
- Thorough sexual history, including number of sex partners (lifetime and past year), prior history of STIs, use of barrier protection, commercial sex work, oral or anal receptive intercourse, and partner fidelity
- In females, the most common symptoms are:
  - Mucopurulent vaginal discharge, dysuria (urethral syndrome), bartholinitis, abdominopelvic pain (endometritis, salpingitis/PID), right upper quadrant pain (Fitz-Hugh–Curtis syndrome)
- In males, the most common symptoms are:
  - Dysuria, urethral discharge (urethritis), scrotal pain (epididymitis), rectal pain or discharge (proctitis), acute arthritis (Reiter syndrome)

PHYSICAL EXAM
- All patients: external genitalia (rash, lesions), urethral discharge, inguinal lymphadenopathy, pharyngeal exudate, and perianal lesions
- People with female anatomy: cervix (discharge, motion tenderness), bimanual examination for cervical motion tenderness, uterine, ovarian/adnexal tenderness or mass
- LGV (*C. trachomatis* serovars L1, L2, or L3): Primary lesion is a small papule that may ulcerate at the site of transmission after an incubation period of 3 to 30 days; unilateral tender lymphadenopathy; with rectal transmission, LGV causes an invasive proctocolitis.

DIFFERENTIAL DIAGNOSIS
- *Neisseria gonorrhoeae*: urethritis, proctitis, epididymitis, cervicitis, PID, Bartholin abscess
- *Mycoplasma* or *Ureaplasma urealyticum*: urethritis, epididymitis, Reiter disease, PID
- *C. trachomatis* (serotypes L1 to L3): LGV, proctitis
- Trichomoniasis

DIAGNOSTIC TESTS & INTERPRETATION
Initial Tests (lab, imaging)
- NAAT: sensitivity >95%; specificity >99%
- Urine test is similarly sensitive to cervical swabs but preferably is collected on first catch urine. Self-collected vaginal swabs are most sensitive (3)[A].
- Lab result may remain positive for 3 weeks after successful treatment.
- Test for concurrent STIs, including gonorrhea, HIV, and syphilis; perform cervical cancer (Pap smear) screening according to recommended guidelines.

Follow-Up Tests & Special Considerations
See "Patient Monitoring."

TREATMENT

GENERAL MEASURES
- Offer patients concurrent testing for gonorrhea, HIV (after counseling and consent), and possibly syphilis. Ensure women are up-to-date with recommended cervical cancer screening.
- Consider treating gonorrhea empirically.
- Test and treat all partners (most recent partner and all partners within the past 60 days).

MEDICATION
First Line
- https://www.cdc.gov/std/treatment-guidelines/chlamydia.htm
- Treatment of chlamydial urethritis, cervicitis, proctitis, and pharyngitis
- Doxycycline 100 mg PO BID for 7 days (preferred)
  - Alternative regimens: azithromycin 1 g PO × 1 *or* levofloxacin 500 mg PO daily for 7 days
- First-line PID treatment (outpatient)
  - Ceftriaxone 250 mg IM × 1 *plus* doxycycline 100 mg PO for 14 days with or without metronidazole 500 mg PO BID for 14 days *or (Please note updated uncomplicated gonorrhea treatment guidelines published December 2020, which recommend 500 mg of ceftriaxone IM for patients <150 kg, and 1 g for patients >150 kg.)*
  - Cefoxitin 2 g IM × 1 with probenecid 1 g PO × 1 *plus* doxycycline 100 mg PO for 14 days with or without metronidazole 500 mg PO BID for 14 days
- Azithromycin and ceftriaxone may be given simultaneously in the office to treat both chlamydia and gonorrhea. This reduces nonadherence.
- Doxy-PEP after condomless sex for MSM and transgender women; 200 mg as soon as possible after sex (and within 3 days)

ALERT
Use azithromycin with caution in patients with known QT prolongation, hypokalemia, hypomagnesemia, bradycardia, or who are currently treated with antiarrhythmics.

Pregnancy Considerations
- Tetracyclines (doxycycline) and quinolones (levofloxacin) are contraindicated in pregnant people.
- Consider the following:
  - Azithromycin 1 g PO *or*
  - Amoxicillin 500 mg PO TID for 7 days *or*
  - Erythromycin base 500 mg PO QID for 7 days

ALERT
Tetracyclines and quinolones are contraindicated in young children:

- <45 kg: erythromycin base or ethinyl succinate 500 mg/kg/day PO QID for 14 days
- >45 kg but <8 years: azithromycin 1 g PO once
- >8 years: adult regimen
- Investigate possible sexual abuse in children with chlamydial infections.

Second Line
For chlamydial urethritis/cervicitis
- Erythromycin base 500 mg PO QID for 7 days *or* erythromycin ethylsuccinate 800 mg PO QID for 7 days
- Levofloxacin 500 mg PO daily for 7 days *or* ofloxacin 300 mg PO BID for 7 days

ADDITIONAL THERAPIES
Patient-delivered partner therapy (PDPT) or expedited partner therapy (EPT): Provide medications or prescriptions to take to sexual partners of persons infected with STIs without clinical assessment.
- EPT reduces recurrence more effectively than traditional partner referral.
- http://www.cdc.gov/std/ept/legal/

ADMISSION, INPATIENT, AND NURSING CONSIDERATIONS
- Inpatient treatment of PID: pregnancy, lack of response or intolerance to oral medicines, suspicion of poor compliance, severe clinical illness, pelvic abscess, and possible need for surgical intervention
- Otherwise, treat PID as outpatient unless moderately or severely ill.

ONGOING CARE

FOLLOW-UP RECOMMENDATIONS
Abstain from sexual contact for at least 7 days after treatment (single-dose treatment such as azithromycin) or until completion of the full course of other antibiotics (doxycycline, levofloxacin).

Patient Monitoring
- Test of cure is not routinely recommended except in pregnancy. Do not repeat NAAT <3 weeks after testing; may be falsely positive due to nonviable organisms
- Test of cure in 3 to 4 weeks in pregnancy as well as test for reinfection in 3 months
- Consider rescreening higher risk pregnant people in 3rd trimester even if initial screening is negative.
- Test for reinfection (not cure) 3 months after treatment or, if not possible, then at next presentation to medical care if within 12 months.
- Sexual partners should be treated. Some states allow for EPT.

PATIENT EDUCATION
- Counsel regarding safe sexual practices, barrier protection, and abstinence.
- Complete antibiotic course (patient and partners).

PROGNOSIS
Prognosis is good following therapy.

COMPLICATIONS
- Both sexes: Chlamydial infection enhances transmission of and susceptibility to HIV.
- People with female anatomy: tubal infertility (most common cause of acquired infertility), tubal (ectopic) pregnancy, chronic pelvic pain
  - Annual screening of sexually active women would prevent 61% of chlamydia-related PID.
- People with male anatomy: transient oligospermia and postepididymitis urethral stricture (rare)

REFERENCES

1. Centers for Disease Control and Prevention. Sexually transmitted disease surveillance 2021: Chlamydia. https://www.cdc.gov/std/statistics/2021/overview.htm#Chlamydia. Accessed May 10, 2023.
2. Centers for Disease Control and Prevention. Sexually transmitted infections treatment guidelines, 2021. https://www.cdc.gov/std/treatment-guidelines/chlamydia.htm. Accessed May 10, 2023.
3. Luetkemeyer AF, Donnell D, Dombrowski JC, et al; for the DoxyPEP Study Team. Postexposure doxycycline to prevent bacterial sexually transmitted infections. *N Engl J Med*. 2023;388(14):1296–1306.

ADDITIONAL READING
He W, Jin Y, Zhu H, et al. Effect of *Chlamydia trachomatis* on adverse pregnancy outcomes: a meta-analysis. *Arch Gynecol Obstet*. 2020;302(3):553–567.

SEE ALSO

Cervicitis, Ectropion, and True Erosion; Epididymitis; Gonococcal Infections; HIV/AIDS; Pelvic Inflammatory Disease; Syphilis; Urethritis

CODES

ICD10
- A56.8 Sexually transmitted chlamydial infection of other sites
- A56.01 Chlamydial cystitis and urethritis
- A56.02 Chlamydial vulvovaginitis

CLINICAL PEARLS
- *C. trachomatis* is common in young sexually active individuals. Annual screening is recommended in sexually active women ≤25 years of age and in other individuals with known risk factors.
- To prevent recurrence, treat patients and their partners concurrently.
- Doxycycline is the most effective treatment for rectal chlamydia.
- Test of cure is only recommended for pregnant patients 3 to 4 weeks after treatment for an identified chlamydia infection. Test for reinfection 3 months afterward. Repeat screens in 3rd trimester for high-risk patients regardless of initial test results.
- Postexposure prophylaxis with 200 mg of doxycycline (Doxy-PEP) in MSM has been shown to significantly reduce the incidence of gonorrhea, chlamydia, and syphilis.

C

CHOLELITHIASIS
Hongyi Cui, MD, PhD

BASICS

DESCRIPTION
- The presence of cholesterol, pigment, or mixed stones (calculi) within the gallbladder
- Synonym(s): gallstones

Pediatric Considerations
Uncommon in children aged <10 years. Most gallstones in children are pigment stones associated with blood dyscrasias.

EPIDEMIOLOGY
Incidence
Increases with age ~1–3% per year; peaks at 7th decade of life; 2% of the U.S. population develops gallstones annually.

Prevalence
- 8–10% of the U.S. population with gallstones; 20% >65 years of age
- Female > male (2 to 3:1)

ETIOLOGY AND PATHOPHYSIOLOGY
- Gallstone formation is a complex process mediated by genetic, metabolic, immune, and environmental factors. Gallbladder sludge (a mixture of cholesterol crystals, calcium bilirubinate granules, and mucin gel matrix) serves as the nidus for gallstone formation. Bile supersaturated with cholesterol (cholesterol stones) precipitates as microcrystals that aggregate and expand. Stone formation is enhanced by biliary stasis or impaired gallbladder motility.
- Decrease in bile phospholipid (lecithin) or decreased bile salt secretion
- Excess unconjugated bilirubin in patients with hemolytic diseases; passage of excess bile salt into the colon with subsequent absorption of excess unconjugated bilirubin in patients with inflammatory bowel disease (IBD) or after distal ileal resection (black or pigment stones)
- Hydrolysis of conjugated bilirubin or phospholipid by bacteria in patients with biliary tract infection or stricture (brown stones or primary bile duct stones; rare in the Western world and common in Asia)

RISK FACTORS
- Age peaks in patients 60 to 80 years of age; female gender, pregnancy, multiparity, obesity, and metabolic syndrome
- Caucasian, Hispanic, or Native American descent
- High-fat diet rich in cholesterol
- Cholestasis or impaired gallbladder motility in association with prolonged fasting, long-term total parenteral nutrition (TPN), following vagotomy, long-term somatostatin therapy, and rapid weight loss
- Hereditary (p.D19H variant for the hepatic canalicular cholesterol transporter ABCG5/ABG8); short gut syndrome, terminal ileal resection, IBD; hemolytic disorders (hereditary spherocytosis, sickle cell anemia, etc.), cirrhosis (black/pigment stones)
- Medications (birth control pills, estrogen at high doses, long-term corticosteroids)
- Viral hepatitis, biliary tract infection, and stricture (promotes intraductal formation of pigment stones)

GENERAL PREVENTION
- Regular exercise and dietary modification may reduce the incidence of gallstone formation.
- Lipid-lowering drugs (statins) may prevent cholesterol stone formation by reducing bile cholesterol saturation.
- Ursodiol (Actigall) taken during rapid weight loss helps prevent gallstone formation.

COMMONLY ASSOCIATED CONDITIONS
90% of people with gallbladder carcinoma have gallstones and chronic cholecystitis.

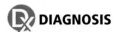**DIAGNOSIS**

HISTORY
- Most patients are asymptomatic (80%): 2% become symptomatic each year. Over their lifetime, <50% of patients with gallstones develop symptoms.
- Episodic right upper quadrant or epigastric pain lasting >15 minutes and sometimes radiating to the back (biliary colic—due to transient cystic duct obstruction); pain is usually postprandial, particularly following a fatty meal but sometimes awakens patients from sleep; most patients develop recurrent symptoms after a first episode of biliary colic.
- Other symptoms include nausea, vomiting, indigestion or bloating sensation, and fatty food intolerance.
- Gallstone-related complications (such as gallstone pancreatitis [GP]) may be the first manifestation of gallstone disease.

PHYSICAL EXAM
- Physical exam is *usually normal* in patients with cholelithiasis in the absence of an acute attack.
- Epigastric and/or right upper quadrant tenderness (Murphy sign) is a traditional physical finding associated with acute cholecystitis. Murphy sign has limited sensitivity and specificity.
- Charcot triad: fever, jaundice, right upper quadrant pain historically associated with cholangitis
- Reynolds pentad: fever, jaundice, right upper quadrant pain, hemodynamic instability, mental status changes; also classically associated with ascending cholangitis
- Flank and periumbilical ecchymoses (Cullen sign and Grey Turner sign) in patients with acute hemorrhagic pancreatitis
- Courvoisier sign: palpable mass in the right upper quadrant in patient with obstructive jaundice most commonly due to malignant tumors within the biliary tree or pancreas

DIFFERENTIAL DIAGNOSIS
- Peptic ulcer diseases and gastritis; hepatitis
- Pancreatitis; cholangitis; gallbladder cancer; gallbladder polyps
- Acalculous cholecystitis; biliary dyskinesia; choledocholithiasis

DIAGNOSTIC TESTS & INTERPRETATION
Ultrasound (US) is the preferred diagnostic modality for cholelithiasis (high sensitivity and specificity).

Initial Tests (lab, imaging)
- Leukocytosis and elevated C-reactive protein level are common in acute calculus cholecystitis.
- US is the preferred imaging modality. US detects gallstones in 97–98% of patients.
- Thickening of the gallbladder wall (≥5 mm), pericholecystic fluid, and direct tenderness when the probe is pushed against the gallbladder (sonographic Murphy sign) are associated with acute cholecystitis.
- CT scan has no advantage over US except for detecting distal common bile duct (CBD) stones.
- MR cholangiopancreatography (MRCP) is reserved for cases of suspected CBD stones. However, MRCP has no therapeutic value, and preoperative MRCP is not more cost-effective than initial cholecystectomy with cholangiography in the diagnosis of patients with suspected CBD stones and patients with mild to moderate GP.
- Endoscopic US is as sensitive as endoscopic retrograde cholangiopancreatography (ERCP) for detection of CBD stones in patients with GP.
- Hepatobiliary iminodiacetic acid (HIDA) scan is useful in diagnosing acute cholecystitis secondary to cystic duct obstruction. It is also useful in differentiating acalculous cholecystitis from other causes of abdominal pain. False-positive tests can result from a fasting state, insufficient resistance of the sphincter of Oddi, and gallbladder agenesis.
- Cholecystokinin (CCK)-HIDA is specifically used to diagnose gallbladder dysmotility (biliary dyskinesia).
- 10–30% of gallstones are radiopaque calcium or pigment-containing gallstones (visible on plain x-ray). A "porcelain gallbladder" is a calcified gallbladder (also visible by x-ray) associated with chronic cholecystitis and gallbladder cancer.

Test Interpretation
Pure cholesterol stones are white or slightly yellow. Pigment stones may be black or brown. Black stones contain polymerized calcium bilirubinate, most often secondary to cirrhosis or hemolysis; these almost always form within the gallbladder. Brown stones are associated with biliary tract infection, caused by bile stasis, and as such primarily form in the bile ducts.

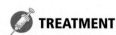**TREATMENT**

GENERAL MEASURES
- Treat symptomatic cholelithiasis.
- Conservative therapy is preferred during pregnancy; surgery in the 2nd trimester if necessary
- Prophylactic cholecystectomy for patients with calcified (porcelain) gallbladder (risk for gallbladder cancer), patients with large stones (≥3 cm), patients with sickle cell disease, children with gallstones, patients planning an organ transplant, and patients with recurrent pancreatitis due to microlithiasis

- In morbidly obese patients, cholecystectomy may be performed in combination with bariatric procedures to reduce subsequent stone-related comorbidities.
- Consider prophylactic cholecystectomy for gallstones discovered incidentally during open abdominal surgery.

Geriatric Considerations
Gallstones are more common in the elderly. Age alone should not alter the therapeutic plan.

MEDICATION
First Line
- Analgesics for pain relief
  - NSAIDs are the first-choice treatment for pain control which is equivalent to opioid therapy.
  - Opioids are an option for patients who cannot tolerate or fail to respond to NSAIDs.
- Antibiotics for patients with acute cholecystitis
- Prophylactic antibiotics in low-risk patients do not prevent infections during laparoscopic cholecystectomy (LC).

ISSUES FOR REFERRAL
Patients with retained or recurrent bile duct stones following cholecystectomy should be referred for ERCP.

SURGERY/OTHER PROCEDURES
- Surgery should be considered for patients who have symptomatic cholelithiasis or gallstone-related complications (e.g., cholecystitis) or in asymptomatic patients with immune suppression, calcified gallbladder, giant gallstones (≥3 cm), or family history of gallbladder cancer.
- Open and LC have similar mortality and complication rates. LC is the current gold standard.
- In well-selected patients, robotic cholecystectomy (RC) is an alternative to LC. RC is associated with higher cost and has not been shown to be superior to LC in terms of pain and risk of complication.
  - Conversion to open procedure is based on clinical judgment.
  - In 10–15% of patients with symptomatic cholelithiasis, CBD stones are detected by intraoperative cholangiogram (IOC). CBD stone(s) can be removed by laparoscopic CBD exploration or postoperative ERCP.
  - IOC helps delineate bile duct anatomy when dissection is difficult. Routine use of IOC is controversial and may be associated with decreased incidence and severity of bile duct injury.
- Early LC (<24 hours after diagnosis of biliary colic) decreases hospital stay and operating time. For patients with acute cholecystitis, early LC (<7 days of clinical presentation) is safe and may shorten the total hospital stay versus delayed LC (>6 weeks after index admission with acute cholecystitis) (1)[A].
- Percutaneous cholecystostomy (PC) is used for high-risk patients with cholecystitis or gallbladder empyema. Interval cholecystectomy is recommended.

- Symptomatic patients who are not candidates for surgery or those who have small gallstones (5 mm or smaller) in a functioning gallbladder with a patent cystic duct are candidates for oral dissolution therapy (ursodiol [Actigall]). The recurrence rate is >50% once medication is discontinued.
- Cystic duct stenting via ERCP is a viable option for managing severe acute cholecystitis, gallbladder hydrops, or empyema in patients unfit for surgery. It can be used as a bridge to LC.
- Extracorporeal shock wave lithotripsy is a non-invasive therapeutic alternative for symptomatic patients who are not candidates for surgery. It helps break down large bile duct stones before ERCP. Complications include biliary pancreatitis, hepatic hematoma, incomplete ductal stone clearance, and recurrence.

ADMISSION, INPATIENT, AND NURSING CONSIDERATIONS
For patients with symptomatic cholelithiasis, LC is typically an outpatient procedure. For patients with complications (i.e., cholecystitis, cholangitis, pancreatitis), inpatient care is necessary; acute phase: NPO, IV fluids, and antibiotics; adequate pain control with narcotics and/or NSAIDs

 ## ONGOING CARE

FOLLOW-UP RECOMMENDATIONS
Patient Monitoring
- Follow for signs of symptomatic cholelithiasis.
- Follow patients on oral dissolution agents with serial liver enzymes, serum cholesterol, and imaging.

DIET
A low-fat diet may help.

PATIENT EDUCATION
- Change in lifestyle (e.g., regular exercise) and dietary modification (low-fat diet and reduction of total caloric intake) may reduce gallstone-related hospitalizations.
- Patients with asymptomatic gallstones should be educated about the typical symptoms of biliary colic and gallstone-related complications.

PROGNOSIS
- <50% of patients with gallstones become symptomatic.
- Cholecystectomy-related mortality is <0.5% in elective cases and 3–5% in emergency cases; morbidity is <10% in elective cases and 30–40% in emergency cases. ~10–15% of patients have associated choledocholithiasis. After cholecystectomy, stones may recur within the biliary tree in patients with associated risk factors.

COMPLICATIONS
- Acute cholecystitis (90–95% secondary to gallstones)
- GP; ERCP ± sphincterotomy offers no clear benefit in patients with mild GP but reduces complications in those with severe GP (2)[A].
- CBD stones with obstructive jaundice and acute cholangitis. In patients undergoing ERCP for CBD stones, early LC reduces the risk of recurrent biliary events (2)[B]; biliary-enteric fistula and gallstone ileus
- Gallbladder cancer; Mirizzi syndrome (extrinsic bile duct obstruction caused by gallstones lodged in gallbladder or cystic duct)

REFERENCES
1. Chung AYA, Duke MC. Acute biliary disease. *Surg Clin North Am.* 2018;98(5):877–894.
2. Garcia-Pagan JC, Francoz C, Montagnese S, et al. Management of the major complications of cirrhosis: beyond guidelines. *J Hepatol.* 2021;75(Suppl 1):S135–S146.

 ## SEE ALSO

Cholangitis, Acute; Choledocholithiasis

 ## CODES

ICD10
- K80.20 Calculus of gallbladder w/o cholecystitis w/o obstruction
- K80.21 Calculus of gallbladder w/o cholecystitis with obstruction
- K80.01 Calculus of gallbladder w acute cholecystitis w obstruction

CLINICAL PEARLS
- Most gallstones are asymptomatic.
- Transabdominal US is the imaging modality of choice for cholelithiasis (sensitivity, 97%; specificity, 95%).
- LC is the preferred surgical procedure for symptomatic cholelithiasis and gallstone-related complications.
- Acute acalculous cholecystitis is associated with bile stasis and gallbladder ischemia.
- Prophylactic cholecystectomy is not routinely indicated in patients with asymptomatic gallstones.

CHRONIC COUGH

Liz Buck, MD

BASICS

DESCRIPTION

- Chronic cough is defined as a cough that persists for >8 weeks in adults.
- In children, chronic cough is often defined as a cough of >4 weeks in duration.
- Subacute cough describes a cough lasting 3 to 8 weeks.
- Patients present because of fear of the causative illness (e.g., cancer), annoyance, self-consciousness, and hoarseness.
- System(s) affected: gastrointestinal (GI), pulmonary

EPIDEMIOLOGY

- Predominant age: all age groups
- Predominant sex: male = female, with females more likely to seek out medical attention

Incidence

Persistent unexplained cough occurs in up to 10% of patients presenting with chronic cough and up to 46% referred to specialty cough clinics.

Prevalence

Chronic cough is one of the most common reasons for primary care visits.

ETIOLOGY AND PATHOPHYSIOLOGY

Varies with findings and disorders implicated

- Often multiple etiologies, but most are related to bronchial irritation. Frequent etiologies (account for >90% of cases) in nonsmokers include the following:
  - Upper airway cough syndrome (UACS) and other upper airway abnormalities, including allergic and vasomotor rhinitis syndromes
  - Chronic rhinitis with postnasal drip (allergic, nonallergic, chronic sinusitis, etc.)
  - Postviral cough
  - Asthma
  - Gastroesophageal reflux disease (GERD)
- Other causes:
  - ACE inhibitors
  - Chronic smoking or exposure to smoke or pollutants
  - Aspiration
  - Bronchiectasis
  - Infections (e.g., pertussis, tuberculosis)
  - Nonasthmatic eosinophilic bronchitis (NAEB)
  - Cystic fibrosis
  - Sleep apnea
  - Restrictive lung diseases
  - Neoplasms: bronchogenic or laryngeal
  - Psychogenic (habit cough)
- Cough hypersensitivity syndrome defines a syndrome of cough with characteristic trigger symptoms not adequately explained by other medical conditions.

- Etiologies of chronic cough in young children differ from those in older children and adults with asthma, protracted bacterial bronchitis, and UACS as most common causes (1),(2).

RISK FACTORS

Although various conditions may contribute to chronic cough, the main causes include smoking and pulmonary diseases.

COMMONLY ASSOCIATED CONDITIONS

Patients with UACS, asthma, and GERD may present with chronic cough as the only symptom and not the usual symptoms associated with the diagnoses.

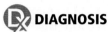**DIAGNOSIS**

HISTORY

- Patient's age, associated signs/symptoms, medical history, medication history (i.e., ACE inhibitors), environmental and occupational exposures, potential for aspiration, and smoking history may make some causes more likely.
- The character of cough or description of sputum quality is rarely helpful in predicting the underlying cause.
- Cough diaries have not correlated well with objective measures.
- Hemoptysis or signs of systemic illness preclude empiric therapy.

PHYSICAL EXAM

- Signs and symptoms are variable and related to the underlying cause; usually, a nonproductive cough with no other signs or symptoms
- Possible signs and symptoms of UACS, sinusitis, GERD, congestive heart failure, chronic stressors
- Absence of additional signs/symptoms of a particular condition not necessarily helpful
  - For example, 5% of patients with GERD have no other signs or symptoms and sometimes have poor response to empiric proton pump inhibitor (PPI) trials.

DIAGNOSTIC TESTS & INTERPRETATION

- Evaluation often starts with empiric therapy directed at likely underlying etiology and/or simple testing such as a chest x-ray (CXR).
- Extensive testing only if indicated by the history and physical

Pediatric Considerations

Children with chronic cough not responsive to an inhaled β-agonist and without overt stressors should undergo spirometry (if age-appropriate) and foreign body evaluation (CXR).

Initial Tests (lab, imaging)

- Evaluation will be dictated by findings in the comprehensive history and physical.
- Evaluation of peak flow may be indicated.
- If considering neoplasm, heart failure, or infectious etiologies, CXR or B-type natriuretic peptide (BNP) may be indicated.
- In cases of failure to respond to initial trial of empiric therapy, CXR may also be beneficial.

Follow-Up Tests & Special Considerations

- Examples:
  - If considering chronic obstructive pulmonary disease (COPD), asthma, or restrictive lung disease: spirometry
  - If suspicious of cystic fibrosis: sweat chloride testing
  - If suspicious of hypereosinophilic syndrome, tuberculosis, or malignancy: sputum for eosinophils and cytology
- If abnormal CXR, suspected neoplasm, or underlying pulmonary disorder, consider a chest CT.
- Consider pulmonary consultation.
- Consider specialist cough clinic.
- Refer to gastroenterologist for endoscopy.

Diagnostic Procedures/Other

If diagnosis suggested and inadequate response to initial measures, other procedures can be considered:

- Pulmonary function testing
- Purified protein derivative (PPD) skin testing
- Allergen testing
- 24-hour esophageal pH monitor
- Bronchoscopy, if history of hemoptysis or smoking with normal CXR
- Endoscopic or video fluoroscopic swallow evaluation or barium esophagram
- Sinus CT
- Ambulatory cough monitoring and cough challenge with citric acid, capsaicin, or other bronchodilator (at specialized cough clinic)
- Echocardiogram

Test Interpretation

Specific to underlying cause

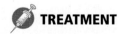**TREATMENT**

GENERAL MEASURES

- With chronic cough, empiric treatment should be directed at the most common causes as clinically indicated (UACS, asthma, GERD) (2)[C].
- Empiric trial of nasal steroids and/or antihistamines should be considered if allergic symptoms or postnasal drip is present.

- With concomitant complaints of heartburn and regurgitation, GERD should be considered as a potential etiology (2)[C].
- In patients with cough associated with the common cold, nonsedating antihistamines were not found to be effective in reducing cough (2)[C].
- Many patients will have resolution of cough after smoking cessation.
- When indicated, ACE inhibitor therapy should be switched in patients in whom intolerable cough occurs. It may take several days or weeks for cough to resolve after stopping ACE inhibitor therapy.
- Empirically treat postnasal drip and GERD.
- Empiric PPI are not recommended in children or adults in the absence of a GERD diagnosis (2)[C].
- Multimodality speech pathology therapy had a positive benefit on cough severity in some adults.
- Attempt maximal therapy for single most likely cause for several weeks and then search for coexistent etiologies.

MEDICATION
- Treatments (nasal steroids, classic antihistamines, antacids, bronchodilators, inhaled corticosteroids, PPIs, antibiotics) should be directed at the specific cause of cough.
- If history and physical exam suggest GERD, may want to trial empiric PPI therapy prior to further diagnostic testing
- The FDA issued a public health advisory stating that OTC cough and cold medicines, including antitussives, expectorants, nasal decongestants, antihistamines, or combinations, should not be given to children aged <2 years. Subsequently, manufacturers have changed labeling to state "do not use" in children aged <4 years. In 2017, the FDA issued a contraindication to codeine for cough treatment in children aged <12 years.
- Routine empiric treatment of children with chronic cough with leukotriene receptor antagonists lacks evidence and cannot be recommended.

First Line
In adults:
- Nasal steroids: fluticasone, budesonide, others, 1 spray BID for those with allergic rhinitis symptoms or postnasal drip or an empiric trial of PPI (omeprazole, others) once a day

Second Line
- A peripherally acting antitussive agent has been used:
  – In patients aged >10 years, benzonatate (Tessalon Perles) 100 to 200 mg PO TID as needed (maximum of 600 mg/day)
- Gabapentin was evaluated in a randomized, double-blind, placebo-controlled trial of patients with refractory chronic cough. Gabapentin demonstrated improved cough-specific quality of life compared to placebo. Nausea and fatigue occurred in 31%. A therapeutic trial with a risk-benefit assessment at 6 months is suggested.

- A comparative effectiveness review of 49 studies with common opioid and nonanesthetic antitussives stated that there is some efficiency for treating cough in adults, but evidence is limited (3)[C].
- Studies evaluating inhaled corticosteroid use in chronic cough for patients without additional indication such as asthma did not show consistent benefits.

ISSUES FOR REFERRAL
Patients with chronic cough may benefit from evaluation by pulmonary, gastroenterology, ear/nose/throat (ENT), and/or allergy specialists. Consider specialist cough clinic.

SURGERY/OTHER PROCEDURES
Fundoplication may be effective for cough secondary to refractory GERD.

 ONGOING CARE

FOLLOW-UP RECOMMENDATIONS
Consider stepwise withdrawal of medications after resolution of cough.

Patient Monitoring
Frequent follow-up is necessary to assess the effectiveness of treatment.

DIET
Dietary modification: Patients with GERD may benefit by avoiding ethanol, caffeine, nicotine, citrus, tomatoes, chocolate, and fatty foods.

PATIENT EDUCATION
- Reassure patient that most cases of chronic cough are not life-threatening and that the condition can usually be managed effectively.
- Counsel that several weeks to a month may be needed for significant reduction or elimination of cough.
- Prepare the patient for the possibility of multiple diagnostic tests and therapeutic regimens because the treatment is very often empiric.

PROGNOSIS
- >80% of patients can be effectively diagnosed and treated using a systematic approach.
- Cough from any cause may take weeks to months until resolution, and resolution depends greatly on efficacy of treatment directed at underlying etiology.

COMPLICATIONS
- Cardiovascular: arrhythmias, syncope
- Stress urinary incontinence
- Abdominal and intercostal muscle strain
- GI: emesis, hemorrhage, herniation

- Neurologic: dizziness, headache, seizures
- Respiratory: pneumothorax, laryngeal, or tracheo-bronchial trauma
- Skin: petechiae, purpura, disruption of surgical wounds
- Medication side effects
- Other: negative impact on quality of life

REFERENCES
1. Chang AB, Oppenheimer JJ, Weinberger M, et al; and CHEST Expert Cough Panel. Etiologies of chronic cough in pediatric cohorts: CHEST guideline and expert panel report. *Chest*. 2017;152(3):607–617.
2. Michaudet C, Malaty J. Chronic cough: evaluation and management. *Am Fam Physician*. 2017;96(9):575–580.
3. Yancy WS Jr, McCrory DC, Coeytaux RR, et al. Efficacy and tolerability of treatments for chronic cough: a systematic review and meta-analysis. *Chest*. 2013;144(6):1827–1838.

 SEE ALSO

- Asthma; Bronchiectasis; Eosinophilic Pneumonias; Gastroesophageal Reflux Disease; Laryngeal Cancer; Lung, Primary Malignancies; Pertussis; Pulmonary Edema; Rhinitis, Allergic; Sinusitis; Tuberculosis
- Algorithm: Cough, Chronic

 CODES

ICD10
- R05 Cough
- J44.9 Chronic obstructive pulmonary disease, unspecified
- J41.0 Simple chronic bronchitis

CLINICAL PEARLS
- Chronic cough is defined as a cough that persists for >8 weeks in adults.
- In patients with chronic cough, most frequent etiologies include a history of smoking, asthma, UACS, and GERD.
- The FDA issued a public health advisory stating that OTC cough and cold medicines should not be given to children aged <2 years. OTC cough expectorant and suppressant product labels state "do not use" in children aged <4 years. Codeine is contraindicated for cough treatment in children aged <12 years.

CHRONIC KIDNEY DISEASE

Ramanpreet Grewal, MD

BASICS

Chronic kidney disease (CKD) is defined as structural or functional abnormalities of the kidney, as determined by either pathologic abnormalities or markers of damage (abnormalities in blood or urine tests, histology, imaging studies) or a glomerular filtration rate (GFR) <60 mL/min/1.73 m². Findings present for ≥3 months. CKD is classified based on the cause, GFR category (G1 to G5), and albuminuria category (A1 to A3).

DESCRIPTION
- Kidney Disease: Improving Global Outcomes (KDIGO) categories by GFR estimation (in mL/min/1.73 m²): G1: kidney damage with normal or increased GFR ≥90; G2: mild ↓ GFR 60 to 89; G3a: mild to moderate ↓ GFR 45 to 59; G3b: moderate to severe ↓ GFR 30 to 44; G4: severe ↓ GFR 15 to 29; G5: kidney failure: GFR <15 or dialysis
- CKD per albumin-to-creatinine ratio (ACR) category: A1: normal to mildly increased: <30 mg/g or <3 mg/mmol; A2: moderately increased: 30 to 300 mg/g or 3 to 30 mg/mmol; A3: severely increased: >300 mg/g or >30 mg/mmol

EPIDEMIOLOGY
- African Americans are 3.6 times more likely to develop CKD than Caucasians.
- Similar in both sexes; however, rate of end-stage renal disease (ESRD) is 1.6 times higher in males than females.

Incidence
Estimated annual incidence of 1,700/1 million population

Prevalence
Overall prevalence of CKD (stages 1 to 5) is 14.8%. Unadjusted prevalence/incidence rates of ESRD (stage 5) are 1,752 and 362/1 million, respectively. Numbers do not reflect the burden of earlier stages of CKD (stages 1 to 4), which are estimated to affect 13.1% of the population in the United States. Prevalence increases with age and peaks after 70 years.

ETIOLOGY AND PATHOPHYSIOLOGY
Progressive destruction of kidney nephrons; GFR will drop gradually, and plasma creatinine (Cr) values will approximately double, with 50% reduction in GFR and 75% loss of functioning nephrons mass. Hyperkalemia usually develops when GFR falls to <20 to 25 mL/min/1.73 m². Anemia develops from decreased renal synthesis of erythropoietin.

- Renal parenchymal/glomerular
  - Nephritic: hematuria, red blood cell (RBC) casts, hypertension (HTN), variable proteinuria
    - Focal proliferative: IgA nephropathy, systemic lupus erythematosus (SLE), Henoch-Schönlein purpura, Alport syndrome, proliferative glomerulonephritis, crescentic glomerulonephritis
    - Diffuse proliferative: membranoproliferative glomerulonephritis, SLE, cryoglobulinemia, rapidly progressive glomerulonephritis (RPGN), Goodpasture syndrome
  - Nephrotic: proteinuria (>3.5 g/day), hypoalbuminemia, hyperlipidemia, and edema
    - Minimal change disease, membranous nephropathy, focal segmental glomerulosclerosis
    - Amyloidosis, diabetic nephropathy

- Vascular: HTN, thrombotic microangiopathies, vasculitis (granulomatosis with polyangiitis), scleroderma, crush injury
- Interstitial tubular: infections, obstruction, toxins, allergic interstitial nephritis, multiple myeloma, connective tissue disease, cystic disease, nephrolithiasis
- Postrenal: obstruction (benign prostatic hyperplasia [BPH]), neoplasm, neurogenic bladder

Genetics
- Alport syndrome, Fabry disease, sickle cell anemia, SLE/autoimmune disease, and autosomal dominant polycystic kidney disease can lead to CKD.
- Polymorphisms in gene that encodes for podocyte nonmuscle myosin IIA are more common in African Americans than Caucasians and appear to increase risk for nondiabetic ESRD.

RISK FACTORS
Type 1 or 2 diabetes mellitus (DM) (most common), age >60 years, low socioeconomic status, obesity, smoking, drug use, chronic infection (hepatitis B and C, HIV), cardiovascular disease (CVD) (HTN, renal artery stenosis, atherosclerosis), prior kidney transplant, BPH, autoimmune disease, vasculitis, connective tissue disease, nephrotoxic drugs (nonsteroidal anti-inflammatory drugs [NSAIDs], lithium, sulfonamide, aminoglycosides, vancomycin, PPIs, allopurinol, loop diuretics, chemotherapeutic agents), congenital anomalies, obstructive uropathy, renal aplasia/hypoplasia/dysplasia/reflux nephropathy)

GENERAL PREVENTION
The U.S. Preventive Services Task Force has concluded that the evidence is insufficient to recommend screening asymptomatic adults for CKD (1)[C].

DIAGNOSIS

HISTORY
Patients with CKD stages 1 to 3 are usually asymptomatic; can present with oliguria, nocturia, polyuria, change in urinary frequency, bone disease, edema, HTN, dyspnea, fatigue, depression, weakness, pruritus, ecchymosis, anorexia, nausea, vomiting, hyperlipidemia, claudication, erectile dysfunction, decreased libido, amenorrhea

PHYSICAL EXAM
Check for volume status (pallor, BP/orthostatic; edema; jugular venous distention; weight), skin for sallow complexion or uremic frost, ammonia-like odor, murmurs, bruits, pericarditis, pleural effusions, enlarged prostate, CNS changes such as asterixis, confusion, seizures, coma, and peripheral neuropathy.

DIAGNOSTIC TESTS & INTERPRETATION
Initial Tests (lab, imaging)
GFR can be estimated using the Modification of Diet in Renal Disease (MDRD) and Chronic Kidney Disease-Epidemiology Collaboration (CKD-EPI) equations, Cr clearance using the Cockcroft-Gault formula to determine medication dosage, UA to assess for evidence of damage (WBC casts in pyelonephritis, RBC casts in glomerulonephritis/vasculitis, Na, Cr, urea, albuminuria), US (initial imaging test of choice to assess for cysts, masses, hydronephrosis, kidney size)

Follow-Up Tests & Special Considerations
- Hematology: normochromic, normocytic anemia; increased bleeding time
- Chemistry: elevated BUN, Cr, hyperkalemia, metabolic acidosis, increased parathyroid hormone (PTH), hyperlipidemia, hyperphosphatemia, decreased 25-(OH) vitamin D, hypocalcemia, decreased albumin
- Serology: antinuclear antibody (ANA); double-stranded DNA, antineutrophil cytoplasmic antibody; complements (C3, C4, CH50); antiglomerular basement membrane (anti-GBM) antibodies; hepatitis B and C; and HIV screening
- Serum and urine immunoelectrophoresis

ALERT
Drugs that may alter lab result:
- Cimetidine: inhibits Cr tubular secretion
- Trimethoprim: inhibits Cr and K^+ secretion and may cause/worsen hyperkalemia
- Cefoxitin and flucytosine: increases serum Cr
- Diltiazem and verapamil (like angiotensin-converting-enzyme inhibitors [ACE-Is]/angiotensin receptor blockers [ARBs]) have significant antiproteinuric effects in patients with CKD.

Diagnostic Procedures/Other
- Biopsy: hematuria, proteinuria, acute/progressive renal failure, nephritic or nephrotic syndrome
- In patients with an estimated GFR <60 mL/min/1.73 m², there is some evidence for a one-time cystatin-C GFR estimation.
- ECG: assess for abnormal heart rhythms due to electrolyte imbalances

TREATMENT

MEDICATION
- HTN: Adults with elevated blood pressure and CKD G1 to G3 should be treated to a target systolic blood pressure of 120 mm Hg using standardized office measurements. Renal transplant patients should have a target blood pressure of <130/80 mm Hg (2)[C].
  - ACE-I or ARB recommended for diabetic and nondiabetic adults with albumin excretion >30 mg/24 hr based on evidence of benefits.
    - An ACE-I or ARB can still be considered in patients with no albuminuria. Those patients, however, are at less risk of CKD progression.
    - Avoid combining ACE-I, ARB, and DRI therapy in diabetic and nondiabetic patients with CKD.
    - Advise contraception in women who are receiving ACE-I or ARB therapy and discontinue in women who are considering pregnancy or have become pregnant (3)[C].
  - CCB or ARB is first line in adult kidney transplant patients for prevention of allograft failure and minimization of possible drug-induced side effects.
  - In children with CKD, 24-hour mean arterial pressure by ABPM should be lowered to <50th percentile for age, sex, and height. In this population, an ACE-I or ARB is first line.
  - A combination between a low-sodium diet plus the use of an ACE-I or ARB leads to a significant reduction in proteinuria (4)[C].

- Secondary hyperparathyroidism
- For GFR <45 mL/min/1.73 m^2, monitor for hyperphosphatemia, hypocalcemia, and vitamin D deficiency if intact PTH is elevated.
- Calcimimetic agents (oral cinacalcet or IV etelcalcetide) are not FDA approved for use in patients with CKD not on dialysis. These should be reserved for ESRD patients (4)[C].
- Hyperphosphatemia: Maintain normal serum phosphate levels using the following:
  – Stages 3 to 5 CKD (not on dialysis): Restrict dietary phosphate to 800 to 1,000 mg/day.
  – Noncalcium phosphate binders (with meals): sevelamer, lanthanum
  – Calcium binders have not been associated with improvement in mortality or cardiovascular outcomes (4)[C].
  – Vitamin D: inactive vitamin D$_2$ (ergocalciferol) or vitamin D$_3$ (cholecalciferol), calcitriol (active vitamin D 1,25 [OH]): Vitamin D may increase absorption of phosphate by intestines and should not be started until serum phosphate concentration is controlled.
- Anemia: Treat with iron replacement therapy with or without erythropoietin-stimulating agents (ESAs). Consider ESA if Hb >9 g/dL and <10 g/dL. ESA initiation not recommended for Hb >10 g/dL. If using ESA, goal Hb range 10 to 11 g/dL, not to exceed 11.5 g/dL.
- Hyperlipidemia: statins with low-density lipoprotein (LDL) goal <70 mg/dL
- Glycemic control: Goal HbA1c range 6.5–8.0%. HbA1c may be falsely low in patients with decreased RBC; glucose logs may be more accurate reflection of glycemic control. Metformin use should be reviewed for GFR between 30 and 44 mL/min/1.73 m^2 and discontinued if GFR <30 mL/min/1.73 m^2. Use SGLT2 inhibitors along with metformin in patients with type II DM and GFR >30 mL/min/1.73 m^2 (3)[C]. SGLT2 inhibitors can be used for patients with and without DM to control disease progression.
- Metabolic acidosis: Start treatment with sodium bicarb when bicarbonate <22 mEq/L with goal to maintain in normal range.

ISSUES FOR REFERRAL

- Nephrology consult:
  – GFR <15 mL/min/1.73 m^2: immediate, GFR 15 to 29 mL/min/1.73 m^2: urgent, GFR 30 to 59 mL/min/1.73 m^2: nonurgent referral, GFR 60 to 89 mL/min/1.73 m^2: not required unless with comorbidities
  – Rapid decline of eGFR (>5 mL/min/1.73 m^2 per year), nondiabetics with heavy proteinuria (24-hour urine protein >500 mg, urine PCR >0.5, urine ACR >300, diabetics with >3 g proteinuria or hematuria, management of complications (metabolic management, electrolyte abnormalities, acidosis, etc.)
- Urology consult for hematuria, renal masses, complex renal cysts, symptomatic nephrolithiasis, hydronephrosis
- Registered Dietitian/psychology/social work/physical therapy/occupational therapy consultation to assist with dietary options, behavioral modification, access to food resources, and mobility
- Renal replacement: Prepare for dialysis or transplant when GFR <30 mL/min/1.73 m^2.

ADDITIONAL THERAPIES

- Aspirin for secondary prevention for patients with established CVD
- For mild pain associated with CKD, acetaminophen is considered first-line therapy. Oral, parental, and even topical NSAIDs are generally not recommended.
- For moderate to severe pain, opioids may be indicated, but the risk of overdose or toxicity is increased because many are renally excreted. Oxycodone, fentanyl, and methadone are preferred, but dose adjustment is still recommended. Meperidine is contraindicated in CKD. Codeine and morphine should be used with caution.
- Chronic pain syndromes may be treated with anticonvulsants and gabapentinoids, which should be renally dosed.

COMPLEMENTARY & ALTERNATIVE MEDICINE

Caution with herbal supplements as these are generally not regulated and may contain excessive amounts of potassium and phosphorus. They may also interact with metabolism of prescription drugs. Ginseng, turmeric, feverfew, alfalfa, garlic leaf, Japanese honeysuckle, lemongrass, papaya, milk thistle, flaxseed, coriander leaf, sunflower seeds, evening primrose, yohimbe, goldenrod, licorice root, and creatine should all be avoided.

ADMISSION, INPATIENT, AND NURSING CONSIDERATIONS

- For use of contrast in imaging, patients should have eGFR > 30 mL/min/1.73 m^2. Volume expansion with IV isotonic saline prior to and following iodinated contrast is recommended.
- Metformin should be held prior to iodinated contrast imaging and resumed after 48 hours.

ONGOING CARE

FOLLOW-UP RECOMMENDATIONS
Patient Monitoring

- Monitor for changes in blood pressure, serum Cr, and serum potassium within 2 to 4 weeks of initiation of ACE-I or ARB. If >30% increase in Cr, correct AKI, reassess medications, and reduce/stop the current ACE-I or ARB dose. Discontinue therapy in the setting of symptomatic hypotension or uncontrolled hyperkalemia.
- For patients taking metformin, monitor eGFR annually and vitamin B$_{12}$ levels after taking metformin >4 years.
- Monitor Cr levels in pregnant patients with CKD closely.
- Monitor Hgb annually for GFR 30 to 59 mL/min/1.73 m^2 and biannually for GFR <30 mL/min/1.73 m^2, calcidiol levels, HbA1c 2 to 4 times a year, volume status, electrolytes, kidney function (urine albumin, GFR, serum Cr).
- Calcium, phosphate, PTH, alkaline phosphatase beginning at CKD stage G3

DIET
<2 g Na per day; limit processed foods, refined carbohydrates, and sweetened beverages. Restrict potassium and phosphorus if indicated. In CKD stages 3 to 5, restrict protein to 0.6g/kg/day if non-diabetic and 0.8g/kg/day if diabetic. Mediterranean diet is generally recommended. Restrict fluids depending on volume status; can consider iron and vitamin D supplementation (5)[C]

PROGNOSIS
Progression is defined as 25% decrease in GFR from baseline. Rapid progression is decrease in GFR by >5 mL/min/1.73 m^2/year. Patients with CKD gradually progress to ESRD.

COMPLICATIONS
HTN, anemia, secondary hyperparathyroidism, renal osteodystrophy, sleep disturbances, infections, malnutrition, electrolyte imbalances, platelet dysfunction/bleeding, pseudogout, gout, metabolic calcification, sexual dysfunction

REFERENCES

1. Moyer VA; for U.S. Preventive Services Task Force. Screening for chronic kidney disease: U.S. Preventive Services Task Force recommendation statement. *Ann Intern Med*. 2012;157(8):567–570.
2. Kidney Disease: Improving Global Outcomes (KDIGO) Blood Pressure Work Group. KDIGO 2021 clinical practice guideline for the management of blood pressure in chronic kidney disease. *Kidney Int*. 2021;99(3S):S1–S87.
3. Kidney Disease: Improving Global Outcomes (KDIGO) Diabetes Work Group. KDIGO 2020 clinical practice guideline for diabetes management in chronic kidney disease. *Kidney Int*. 2020;98(4S):S1–S115.
4. U.S. Department of Veterans Affairs. VA/DoD clinical practice guideline: management of chronic kidney disease. https://www.healthquality.va.gov/guidelines/CD/ckd/VADoDCKDCPGFinal5082142020.pdf. Accessed November 3, 2023.
5. Ikizler TA, Burrowes JD, Byham-Gray LD, et al. KDOQI clinical practice guideline for nutrition in CKD: 2020 update. *Am J Kidney Dis*. 2020; 76(3 Suppl 1):S1–S107.

CODES

ICD10
- N18.9 Chronic kidney disease, unspecified
- Q63.9 Congenital malformation of kidney, unspecified
- N18.3 Chronic kidney disease, stage 3 (moderate)

CLINICAL PEARLS

- ACE-I and ARB are first line for HTN treatment in CKD with albuminuria.
- Consider nonurgent nephrologist referral for GFR ≤59 mL/min/1.73 m^2 and urgent nephrologist referral for GFR ≤29 mL/min/1.73 m^2.
- Restrict sodium in diet (<2 g/day) and potassium, phosphorus if indicated; in CKD stages 3 to 5, restrict protein to 0.6 g/kg/day if nondiabetic and 0.8 g/kg/day if diabetic.
- CKD progression should be monitored closely and managed by a multidisciplinary team to ensure proper nutrition, pain control, mobility, and access to care.

CHRONIC OBSTRUCTIVE PULMONARY DISEASE AND EMPHYSEMA

Jasmine S. Beria, DO, MPH

 BASICS

DESCRIPTION
- The 2023 Global Initiative for Chronic Obstructive Lung Disease (GOLD) defines COPD as follows:
  - COPD is a heterogenous lung condition characterized by chronic respiratory symptoms (dyspnea, cough, sputum production and/or exacerbations) due to abnormalities of the airways (bronchitis, bronchiolitis) and/or alveoli (emphysema) that cause persistent, often progressive, airflow obstruction (1).
- COPD is ranked among the top causes of death in the United States, it was the third leading cause of death worldwide prior to the COVID-19 pandemic. Given its prevalence and chronicity, it causes a high resource utilization with multiple hospitalizations due to acute exacerbations, frequent office visits, and the need for chronic therapy. Globally, there are around 3,000,000 deaths annually due to COPD.

EPIDEMIOLOGY
Incidence
The incidence of COPD is 8.9/1,000 person-years.

Prevalence
Global prevalence of COPD based on the Burden of Obstructive Lung Diseases (BOLD) program is 10.3%

ETIOLOGY AND PATHOPHYSIOLOGY
Exposure to noxious gasses or particles leading to pathologic processes in the lung:
- Impaired gas (carbon dioxide [CO_2] and oxygen) exchange, persistent airway obstruction, destruction of lung parenchyma

Genetics
α_1-Antitrypsin deficiency is a rare, inherited disorder due to two autosomal codominant alleles.

RISK FACTORS
- Smoking tobacco or marijuana: including passive smoking and water pipe
- History of severe childhood respiratory infections
- Aging—including healthy aging as well as the cumulative summation of lung exposure over time
- Lower level of education and lower socioeconomic status
- Asthma and airway hyperreactivity
- Indoor air pollution (especially indoor biomass cooking worldwide)
- Occupational organic or inorganic dusts, chemical agents and fumes (i.e., high doses of pesticides)

GENERAL PREVENTION
Smoking cessation and general avoidance of noxious material are the most important preventative measures.

COMMONLY ASSOCIATED CONDITIONS
- Pulmonary: lung cancer, chronic respiratory failure, acute bronchitis, sleep apnea, pulmonary hypertension (HTN), asthma
- Cardiac: coronary artery disease, arrhythmia
- Ear/nose/throat (ENT): chronic sinusitis, laryngeal carcinoma

DIAGNOSIS

The diagnosis of COPD requires 3 features:
- A post-bronchodilator forced expiratory volume in 1 second (FEV_1)/forced vital capacity (FVC) ratio of <0.7, which confirms the presence of persistent airflow limitation.
- Appropriate symptoms including dyspnea, chronic cough, sputum production, and/or wheezing
- Significant exposure to noxious stimuli, such as history of smoking cigarettes or environmental exposures

HISTORY
- Discuss patient's use of tobacco and/or cannabis.
- Consider environmental history of indoor pollution and occupational exposures.
- Review possible causes of exacerbation (e.g., cold weather, recent upper respiratory infection, pneumonia, sick contacts, noncompliance with medications).
- Exacerbation: A new definition of COPD exacerbation is included in the 2023 GOLD guidelines; it focuses on dyspnea or cough and sputum that worsen during ≤14 days, with associated inflammation due to airway infections, pollution, or other insult to the airways.

PHYSICAL EXAM
- Prolonged expiration, wheezing
- Barrel chest, diminished breath sounds, distant heart sounds
- Accessory muscle use, pursed lip breathing, cyanosis, exertional dyspnea
- Clubbing not typical for COPD, however, may indicate another process (e.g., lung cancer, bronchiectasis, or interstitial lung disease)

DIFFERENTIAL DIAGNOSIS
- Asthma (including occupational), reactive airways dysfunction syndrome (RADS)
- Respiratory infection (tuberculosis)
- Interstitial lung disease, bronchiectasis, primary alveolar hypoventilation, bronchiolitis obliterans
- Lung cancer
- Chronic pulmonary embolism
- Sleep apnea, congestive heart failure (CHF), gastroesophageal reflux disease
- Cystic fibrosis
- Vasculitis (i.e., granulomatosis with polyangiitis)

DIAGNOSTIC TESTS & INTERPRETATION
Initial Tests (lab, imaging)
- Spirometry
- Arterial blood gases (ABGs) may show hypercapnia and hypoxia.
- CBC to evaluate eosinophilia; may reveal polycythemia, reflecting chronic hypoxia
- BMP may reveal elevated CO_2, indicative of chronic CO_2 retention.
- Imaging (CXR, CT chest) to rule out other conditions; CXR—hyperinflation, flat diaphragms, and possibly bullous changes

Follow-Up Tests & Special Considerations
- Pulse oximetry to assess need for oxygen, both at rest and with exertion
- α_1-Antitrypsin screening for those with COPD aged <45 years, have a blood relative with this disease, or spirometry out of proportion to tobacco use
- Chest CT may show parenchymal destruction and bullae.

Diagnostic Procedures/Other
Pulmonary function testing without/with bronchodilator
- Decreased postbronchodilator FEV_1/FVC ratio <0.7; this is the diagnostic criteria for airway obstruction; repeat spirometry recommended if between 0.6 and 0.8
- Reduced FEV_1
- Normal or increased FVC
- Normal or increased total lung capacity
- Increased residual volume and functional residual capacity
- Diffusing capacity is normal or reduced.
- Typically not bronchodilator responsive (change in FEV_1 or FVC of ≥12% and change in volume of ≥200 mL)

Test Interpretation
- Staging: GOLD criteria staging in the presence of FEV_1/FVC <0.7 (1)
  - Grade 1: FEV_1 ≥80% predicted
  - Grade 2: FEV_1 50–80% predicted
  - Grade 3: FEV_1 30–50% predicted
  - Grade 4: FEV_1 <30% predicted
- Symptom severity assessments:
  - COPD Assessment Test (CAT), which is an 8-item questionnaire worth 5 points each (overall score ranges from 0 to 40) that determine disease-specific, health-related quality of life
  - Modified Medical Research Council (mMRC) questionnaire, which evaluates breathlessness based on scale of 0 (breathless with strenuous exercise) to 4 (too breathless to leave the house or breathless when dressing or undressing)
  - GOLD severity assessment based on symptom burden and risk of exacerbation
- The ABE assessment tool incorporates severity of patient's symptoms and exacerbation history.
  - Group A: low risk, less symptoms: 0 to 1 exacerbation per year and no prior hospitalization for exacerbation; and CAT score <10 or mMRC grade 0 to 1
  - Group B: low risk, more symptoms: 0 to 1 exacerbation per year and no prior hospitalization for exacerbation; and CAT score ≥10 or mMRC grade ≥2
  - Group E: high risk, more or less symptoms: ≥2 exacerbations per year or ≥1 hospitalization for exacerbation; and CAT score <10 or ≥10 or mMRC grade 0 to grade ≥2

TREATMENT

GENERAL MEASURES
- GOLD severity assessment based on symptom burden and risk of exacerbation in conjunction with:
  - COPD Assessment Test (CAT Score: https://www.researchgate.net/figure/Evaluative-questions-from-the-COPD-Assessment-Test-CAT-COPD-Assessment-Test-and-the_fig1_244482870)
  - Modified Medical Research Council Dyspnea Scale (mMRCD): https://www.ncbi.nlm.nih.gov/books/NBK559281/figure/article-26083.image.f5/
- Treatment is based on GOLD Severity Assessment (see "First Line").
- Smoking cessation: This is the most important intervention to decrease risk of disease progression.
- Home oxygen: in patients with severe resting chronic hypoxemia (PaO$_2$ ≤55 mm Hg or <60 mm Hg if there is cor pulmonale or secondary polycythemia), long-term oxygen therapy improves survival.
- All patients should receive COVID-19, pneumococcal, influenza, and pertussis vaccines, and those aged >50 years should also receive the varicella zoster vaccine.
- Inhaler techniques need to be assessed regularly.
- Pulmonary rehabilitation
- Noninvasive positive-pressure ventilation (NPPV) may decrease mortality and prevent rehospitalization.

MEDICATION
First Line
- GOLD group A: one or no moderate exacerbations requiring systemic steroids and/or antibiotics with no hospitalizations or ED visits for COPD exacerbations *and* dyspnea with exercise or walking uphill (CAT score <10 or mMRC grade 0 to 1): short- or long-acting bronchodilator
  - Short-acting β-agonists: albuterol, levalbuterol
- GOLD group B: one or no moderate exacerbations requiring systemic steroids and/or antibiotics with no hospitalizations or ED visits for COPD exacerbations *and* dyspnea with simple walking, needing stop to catch breath (CAT score ≥10 or mMRC grade ≥2)
  - Combined long-acting β-agonists (LABAs)–long-acting muscarinic antagonists (LAMAs) rather than steroids
    ○ LABA: formoterol, arformoterol, salmeterol
    ○ LAMA: tiotropium, aclidinium, umeclidinium, glycopyrrolate
- GOLD group E: two or more moderate exacerbations requiring systemic steroids and/or antibiotics, or a hospitalization or ED visit for a COPD exacerbation (former groups C and D are now merged into Group E)
  - Combined long-acting β-agonists (LABA)–long-acting muscarinic antagonists (LAMA) rather than steroids.
    ○ LABA: formoterol, arformoterol, salmeterol
    ○ LAMA: tiotropium, aclidinium, umeclidinium, glycopyrrolate
    ○ Add to LABA/LAMA an inhaled corticosteroid (ICS) if blood eosinophil count is ≥100 cells/μL
  - For those on a LABA/LAMA and ICS who continue to have exacerbations, consider adding a macrolide (azithromycin) or roflumilast.

- Acute COPD exacerbations: mild to moderate exacerbations can be treated with short-acting bronchodilators and possibly short courses of steroids and/or antibiotics (5 to 7 days). Severe exacerbations require inpatient admission (see below).

Second Line

 ALERT
Precautions:
- β-Agonists: sinus tachycardia, arrhythmias in susceptible patients; can consider levalbuterol
- Anticholinergics: minimal systemic absorption in inhaled form; urinary retention possible
- ICS: increased risk of pneumonia; oral candidiasis
- Corticosteroids: weight gain, diabetes, adrenal suppression, osteoporosis, infection (pneumonia)
- Macrolides: Long-term use can possibly lead to bacterial resistance and hearing impairment (monitor QTC interval).

ISSUES FOR REFERRAL
Severe exacerbation, frequent hospitalizations, rapid progression, weight loss, or surgical evaluation

ADDITIONAL THERAPIES
Pulmonary rehabilitation program for patients with high symptom burden

SURGERY/OTHER PROCEDURES
Lung reduction surgery, bronchoscopic lung reduction, surgical bullectomy, lung transplantation

ADMISSION, INPATIENT, AND NURSING CONSIDERATIONS
- Severe acute exacerbation: Maintain oxygenation, short-acting inhaled β-agonists/inhaled anticholinergic agents, and oral or IV corticosteroids prednisone (up to 1 mg/kg/day commonly 40 mg/day for 5 days); antibiotics for moderate/severe exacerbations with increased sputum volume or sputum purulence; optimal antibiotic therapy has not been determined; NPPV if necessary
- May lead to acute or acute on chronic respiratory failure requiring ICU admission and intubation
- Prior to discharge: Assess proper inhaler use, prescribe proper maintenance inhalers, and ensure understanding; assess the need for home oxygen; schedule pulmonary follow-up close after discharge.

ALERT
If not already in place, have patient delineate an advance directive.

 ONGOING CARE

FOLLOW-UP RECOMMENDATIONS
- May taper or stop oral steroids as outpatient
- Pulmonary rehabilitation program for patients with high symptom burden and risk of exacerbations

Patient Monitoring
Initially within 4-week period and at 12 weeks after an exacerbation; review symptoms, medication compliance, and the need for oxygen. Consider spirometry at 12 weeks.

PATIENT EDUCATION
American Lung Association: https://www.lung.org/lung-health-diseases

PROGNOSIS
- Supplemental oxygen, when indicated, is shown to increase survival (may only require at night).
- Smoking cessation improves prognosis.
- For severe upper lobe disease and poor control or poor post-rehabilitation exercise capacity, lung volume reduction surgery may be considered.
- For very severe disease unresponsive to all interventions, patient may be a candidate for lung transplant.
- 4-year mortality estimates range from 28% for mild-to-moderate COPD to 62% for moderate-to-severe COPD.

COMPLICATIONS
- Malnutrition, poor sleep quality, infections, secondary polycythemia
- Acute or chronic respiratory failure, bullous lung disease, pneumothorax
- Arrhythmias, cor pulmonale, pulmonary HTN

REFERENCE
1. Global Initiative for Chronic Obstructive Lung Disease. Global strategy for the diagnosis, management, and prevention of chronic obstructive pulmonary disease: 2023 report. https://goldcopd.org/2023-gold-report-2/. Accessed November 4, 2023.

SEE ALSO

Bronchitis, Acute

CODES

ICD10
- J44.9 Chronic obstructive pulmonary disease, unspecified
- J43.9 Emphysema, unspecified
- J42 Unspecified chronic bronchitis

CLINICAL PEARLS
- Smoking cessation remains the most important intervention to prevent disease or delay disease progression.
- Consider screening PFTs on any high-risk patient.
- Home oxygen evaluation is important because supplemental oxygen improves mortality.
- Regularly reevaluate disease burden to titrate short- and long-acting medication regimen.
- Influenza/pneumococcal vaccines should be current.
- Discuss advance directives before the patient becomes seriously ill.

C

CHRONIC PAIN MANAGEMENT: AN EVIDENCE-BASED APPROACH

Carolyn Murphy, MD

 BASICS

- Chronic pain persists beyond the time anticipated for normal tissue healing (usually >3 months).
- Over time, neuroplastic changes in the CNS transform pain into a chronic experience with emotional, psychological, and cognitive dimensions.
- An epidemic of undertreated pain coexists with an epidemic of prescription drug abuse in the United States.
- People of color, especially African Americans, are often undertreated.
- Opioid medications should be prescribed using an evidence/systems-based approach and used only when indicated for chronic, nonmalignant pain.

EPIDEMIOLOGY

Incidence
- Chronic pain has been reported by as many as 20–40% of patients in primary care.
- The annual economic cost of chronic pain in the United States is estimated at $560 to $635 billion.

Prevalence
In the United States, an estimated 20% (50 million) of adults report some level of chronic pain on cross-sectional household surveys. The prevalence is higher among women and those with lower socioeconomic status (https://www.cdc.gov/mmwr/volumes/67/wr/mm6736a2.htm).

ETIOLOGY AND PATHOPHYSIOLOGY
- With intense, repeated, or prolonged stimulation of damaged or inflamed tissues, the threshold for activating primary afferent pain fibers is lowered, the frequency of firing is higher, and there is an increased response to noxious and/or normal stimuli (peripheral and central sensitization). The amygdala, prefrontal cortex, and cortex relay emotions related to the pain experience, and these areas undergo structural and functional changes over time.
- Patients often have an identifiable etiology, but pain levels can be worse than observable tissue injury. Many patients have no obvious source of chronic pain.

Genetics
A genetic polymorphism in opioid receptors may affect patient's response to individual opioids.

RISK FACTORS
- Traumatic: motor vehicle accidents, repetitive motion injuries, falls
- Postsurgical: back surgeries, amputations, thoracotomies
- Psychiatric comorbidities: substance abuse, depression, posttraumatic stress disorder (PTSD)

GENERAL PREVENTION
- Prevent work-related injuries through ergonomic workplace design.
- Varicella vaccine and rapid treatment of shingles to lower risk of postherpetic neuralgia
- Tight glycemic control for diabetic patients, prevention of alcohol abuse, smoking cessation

COMMONLY ASSOCIATED CONDITIONS
Any chronic disease and/or its treatment can cause chronic pain.

 DIAGNOSIS

Two general categories of pain:
- Nociceptive pain (response to tissue damage):
  – *Somatic*: skin, bone, soft tissue disease; described as well localized, sharp, stabbing, aching
  – *Visceral*: visceral inflammation/injury; described as poorly localized, dull, aching; may refer to sites remote from lesion; can wax and wane
- Neuropathic pain: damaged peripheral or central nerves; described as burning, tingling, and/or numbness
  – Sympathetically mediated pain: Peripheral nerve injury can cause severe burning pain, swelling of the affected limb, and focal changes in sweat production and skin appearance (e.g., complex regional pain syndrome).

HISTORY
- Pain history: location, onset, intensity, duration, quality, temporal pattern, exacerbating agents, alleviators, prior treatments
- Assess and document how pain affects patient's functioning and quality of life. Screen for personal or family history of substance abuse (including tobacco addiction), mental health conditions, and/or sexual abuse.
- Standardized tools: pain severity—Brief Pain Inventory (short form); mood—Patient Health Questionnaire-9 (PHQ-9; https://www.apa.org/depression-guideline/patient-health-questionnaire.pdf); substance abuse—Screener and Opioid Assessment for Patients with Pain (SOAPP; https://www.mcstap.com/docs/SOAPP-5.pdf)
- Stratify patients according to risk of chronic opioid therapy and need for increased monitoring; a positive screen does not automatically exclude patients from opioid therapy.

PHYSICAL EXAM
Exam is guided by history and includes functional and behavioral assessments.

DIFFERENTIAL DIAGNOSIS
Aberrant drug-taking behaviors could be related to:
- Inadequate analgesia ("pseudoaddiction"), disease progression, opioid-resistant pain, opioid-induced hyperalgesia, opioid tolerance, substance use disorder, self-medication of nonpain symptoms, criminal intent (diversion), and poor health literacy

DIAGNOSTIC TESTS & INTERPRETATION
Base testing on history, exam, and differential diagnosis.

Initial Tests (lab, imaging)
- Urine drug screen: qualitative analysis for drugs of abuse and quantitative analysis for individual drugs
- Most tests are immunoassays, which detect morphine and heroin but often not other opioids.

Follow-Up Tests & Special Considerations
For chronic opioid therapy, consider random urine drug screens.

Diagnostic Procedures/Other
Consider interventional pain clinic for complex injections and nerve blocks.

Test Interpretation
There is a possibility of false-positive urine drug screen due to commonly prescribed medications. Laboratory-based chromatography/spectrometry can identify specific drugs.

 TREATMENT

- The goals of treatment are to restore function and decrease pain.
- Treatment should always include exercise, cognitive-behavioral therapy (CBT), patient and family education, yoga, massage, relaxation techniques, support groups, mindfulness, meditation, and acupuncture.
- For complex regional pain syndrome, sympathetic block may decrease risk of chronic pain.
- Evidence on use of cannabis for chronic pain is low quality and controversial (1)[A].

GENERAL MEASURES
- Keep a pain and function diary; record medication use.
- CDC: Summary of the 2022 Clinical Practice Guideline for Prescribing Opioids for Pain | Opioids | CDC: https://www.cdc.gov/opioids/patients/guideline.html
- AAPM: https://academic.oup.com/painmedicine/article/21/7/1331/5817092
- VA: https://www.healthquality.va.gov/guidelines/Pain/cot/

MEDICATION

- Management varies depending on type of pain (neuropathic vs. nociceptive).
- Use sequential time-limited trials of medications; start at low doses, and gradually increase until effect or dose-limiting side effects are reached.
- Combination of acetaminophen/NSAID products with opioids can lead to serious acetaminophen/NSAID toxicities if patients exceed recommended doses.
- Note: Be aware of implicit bias. Minority patients (particularly people of color) are at greatest risk for undertreatment regardless of pain type (traumatic or not) or type of analgesia (opioids or not).
- For mild to moderate chronic noncancer pain
  - Acetaminophen: daily dose not to exceed a total of 4 g in healthy adults and 2 g in elderly patients with hepatic disease or current/past alcohol use.
  - NSAIDs: Use COX-2 selective inhibitors with caution because of cardiac risks (may have less gastric risk). If high cardiac risk, consider nonselective COX inhibitor (naproxen) with or without gastric prophylaxis.
  - Topical agents: NSAIDs (diclofenac gel 1–3% BID), lidocaine (4% gel OTC is less effective but more affordable than 5% patch), ketamine 0.5–10% BID–QID, capsaicin 0.035–0.1% QD–QID
  - Tramadol: An opioid analgesic with weak serotonin-norepinephrine reuptake inhibitor (SNRI) may be helpful in neuropathic pain but has ceiling dose, risk of seizures, and requires dose adjustment for renal and hepatic failure (initial dose of 50 mg q6h PRN, ceiling dose of 400 mg/day or 300 mg/day for older adults).
- For neuropathic pain
  - Classes of medications include (i) tricyclic antidepressants (desipramine [25 to 100 mg QD but start with 10 mg QD in frail elderly] and nortriptyline [25 to 100 mg QD but start with 10 mg QD in frail elderly]); (ii) SNRI antidepressants (duloxetine 30 to 60 mg BID); (iii) anticonvulsants (α2-δ ligands, gabapentin [initial dose of 300 mg/day and titrate to max of 3,600 mg/day in 3 divided doses], and pregabalin [100 to 300 mg/day in 2 to 3 divided doses]); and (iv) last line is opioids, including tramadol.
- For moderate to severe chronic pain
  - Morphine, oxycodone, hydromorphone, oxymorphone, fentanyl; check institutional opioid equianalgesic table.
    - Avoid morphine in patients with renal insufficiency.
    - Methadone should only be prescribed by experienced providers due to many drug interactions and risk of potentially fatal cardiac arrhythmias.
  - No evidence supports any of these opioids as superior to other or having improved side effect profile.
  - Buprenorphine has been found to reduce pain intensity for patients with chronic pain and can be more effective in patients without a history of opioid use disorder.

- Once stable dose of opioids is established, change to sustained-release formulations if pain is constant or frequent; short-acting formulations for breakthrough/episodic pain only
- Common side effects: constipation: senna should be coprescribed with opioids; also nausea, sedation, mental status changes, and pruritus
- Coprescribe nasal naloxone for patients on chronic opioids (see "Ongoing Care").

ALERT
Patients on chronic opioid therapy must agree to monitoring. Use universal precautions (see "Ongoing Care").

SURGERY/OTHER PROCEDURES
Consider interventional procedures, including joint injections, nerve blocks, spinal cord stimulation, and intrathecal medication among others, as needed.

COMPLEMENTARY & ALTERNATIVE MEDICINE
- For adults with chronic low back pain, consider mindfulness-based stress reduction (MBSR) or CBT.
- Yoga is as effective as standard physical therapy for moderate to severe chronic low back pain (2)[A].

 ## ONGOING CARE

FOLLOW-UP RECOMMENDATIONS
Patient Monitoring
- Maintain a nonjudgmental approach.
- Assess and document benefits, risks, pain levels, functioning, and quality of life.
- *Universal precautions*:
  - Informed consent for opioid therapy; written agreement between patient and clinician
  - One prescriber and one pharmacy; no after-hours prescriptions or early refills
  - Mandatory police reporting for medication thefts; random urine drug tests, pill/patch counts
  - Continue with physical therapy, counseling, and psychiatric medications.
  - Participate in state's prescription drug monitoring program: https://www.cdc.gov/drugoverdose/pdmp/index.html.
  - Taper and discontinue medications if patient does not benefit, if side effects outweigh benefits. If medications are abused or diverted, more rapid taper is appropriate. If addiction is suspected, always offer treatment for substance abuse.
  - Tapering opioids should involve shared decision-making between patient and clinician with an individualized taper plan to each patient based on risks and benefits (3)[C].
  - Patients on long-term opioid therapy may see improvement in pain, function, and quality of life with voluntary dose reductions.
- Nasal naloxone
  - Naloxone kit: two 1 mg/mL prefilled syringes with intranasal mucosal atomization device; takes effect in 2 to 5 minutes, lasts 30 to 90 minutes

PATIENT EDUCATION
American Chronic Pain Association: https://theacpa.org

COMPLICATIONS
- Rate of addiction in chronic pain patients is ~3–19%; aberrant medication-taking behaviors is ~5%–24%.
- Definitions
  - Addiction: chronic biopsychological disease characterized by impaired control over drug use, compulsive use, and continued use despite harm
  - Physical dependence: withdrawal syndrome produced by abrupt cessation or rapid dose reduction
  - Tolerance: state of adaptation when a drug induces changes that diminish its effects over time
  - Diversion: selling drugs or giving them to persons other than for whom they are prescribed

REFERENCES
1. Fisher E, Moore RA, Fogarty AE, et al. Cannabinoids, cannabis, and cannabis-based medicine for pain management: a systematic review of randomised controlled trials. *Pain*. 2021;162(Suppl 1):S45–S66.
2. Saper RB, Lemaster C, Delitto A, et al. Yoga, physical therapy, or education for chronic low back pain: a randomized noninferiority trial. *Ann Intern Med*. 2017;167(2):85–94.
3. Dowell D, Ragan KR, Jones CM, et al. CDC clinical practice guideline for prescribing opioids for pain—United States, 2022. *MMWR Recomm Rep*. 2022;71(3):1–95.

ADDITIONAL READING
Nicola M, Correia H, Ditchburn G, et al. Defining pain-validation: the importance of validation in reducing the stresses of chronic pain. *Front Pain Res (Lausanne)*. 2022;3:884335.

CODES

ICD10
- G89.29 Other chronic pain
- G89.21 Chronic pain due to trauma
- G89.28 Other chronic postprocedural pain

CLINICAL PEARLS
- Start with the foundational belief that a patient's pain is *real*.
- Emphasize that a pain-free life may not be possible—better function and quality of life are shared goals.
- Use a multidisciplinary approach with nonpharmacologic therapies and thoughtful medication use with clear goals, expectations, and documentation of care plan.
- Universal precautions are a systems-based approach for opioid prescription in cases of chronic pain.

CIRRHOSIS OF THE LIVER

Liam P. Burke, MD

BASICS

DESCRIPTION
A chronic inflammatory disease with hepatocellular dysfunction, fibrosis, necrosis, and vascular remodeling possibly leading to liver failure and/or cancer

EPIDEMIOLOGY
- Diagnosis: typically at 40 to 60 years old; male > female
- Liver disease and cirrhosis are the 12th leading cause of death in the United States.
- Nonalcoholic steatohepatitis (NASH) is an increasingly common cause of cirrhosis.

Incidence
~≥30,000 new cases of cirrhosis per year

Prevalence
- 0.3% of Americans are diagnosed with cirrhosis (~630,000) and 2% with chronic liver disease (CLD).
- Highest in non-Hispanic blacks, Mexican Americans, and those living below the poverty level

ETIOLOGY AND PATHOPHYSIOLOGY
- Chronic hepatitis C virus (HCV) (26%); alcohol abuse (21%); NASH (~10%) and increasing; hepatitis B virus (HBV) plus hepatitis D infection (15%); other (~25%): hemochromatosis, autoimmune hepatitis, primary biliary cirrhosis (PBC), secondary biliary cirrhosis, biliary atresia, idiopathic biliary fibrosis, primary sclerosing cholangitis, Wilson disease, α_1-antitrypsin deficiency, granulomatous disease (e.g., sarcoidosis); drug-induced liver disease (e.g., methotrexate, α-methyldopa, amiodarone); venous outflow obstruction (e.g., Budd-Chiari syndrome, veno-occlusive disease)
- Hepatocellular injury results in cellular hyperplasia (regenerating nodules), fibrous changes, and angiogenesis. Distortions in blood flow result in portal hypertension.

Genetics
Hereditary hemochromatosis, Wilson disease, and α_1-antitrypsin deficiency in adults are associated with cirrhosis.

RISK FACTORS
Alcohol abuse, intravenous drug abuse, obesity

GENERAL PREVENTION
- Mitigate risk factors (e.g., screen for and address hepatitis C and alcohol overuse); >80% of CLD is preventable.
- Advise weight loss in overweight or obese patients.

COMMONLY ASSOCIATED CONDITIONS
HCV, alcohol and drug abuse, diabetes, depression, obesity

DIAGNOSIS

HISTORY
- Review risk factors (alcohol use, viral hepatitis, and family history of primary liver cancer, liver disease, or autoimmune disease).
- Symptoms
  - Fatigue, malaise, weakness, anorexia, weight loss (weight gain if ascites/edema)
  - Right upper abdominal pain; tea-colored urine, clay-colored stools
  - Edema, abdominal swelling/bloating, pruritus; bruising, bleeding, hematemesis, hematochezia, melena
  - Absent/irregular menses, chronic anovulation; diminished libido, erectile dysfunction

PHYSICAL EXAM
Physical exam may be normal until end-stage disease—many relate to manifestations of portal hypertension and/or hyperestrinism.
- Skin changes: spider angiomas, palmar erythema, jaundice, scleral icterus, ecchymoses, caput medusa, hyperpigmentation, decreased body hair, facial telangiectasias
- Hepatomegaly, splenomegaly, abdominal fluid wave, shifting dullness
- Gynecomastia, Dupuytren contractures
- Pretibial/presacral pitting edema, and clubbing (mostly in hepatopulmonary syndrome [HPS])
- Asterixis, altered mental status (AMS)(hepatic encephalopathy [HE]), muscle wasting, fetor hepaticus

DIFFERENTIAL DIAGNOSIS
Steatohepatitis, other causes of portal hypertension (e.g., portal vein thrombosis, lymphoma); metastatic or multifocal cancer in the liver; vascular congestion (e.g., cardiac cirrhosis); acute alcoholic hepatitis

DIAGNOSTIC TESTS & INTERPRETATION
Fibrosis-4 (FIB-4) index: age; aspartate aminotransferase (AST); alanine aminotransferase (ALT); platelet count (1)

Initial Tests (lab, imaging)
- AST/ALT is often mildly elevated, typically AST > ALT; enzymes may normalize as cirrhosis progresses; elevated alkaline phosphatase (ALP), γ-glutamyl transpeptidase (GGT), and total/direct bilirubin; anemia from hemolysis, folate deficiency, or splenomegaly
- Thrombocytopenia (<110; 95% specific for cirrhosis); FIB-4 <1.45 or AST to platelet ratio index <0.7 is unlikely cirrhotic; FIB-4 >3.25 likely indicates cirrhosis.
- Impaired synthetic liver function: hypoalbuminemia, low cholesterol, prolonged prothrombin time (PT) and partial thromboplastin time (PTT), elevated international normalized ratio (INR)
- Hyperammonemia, elevated BUN, hyperkalemia, and hyponatremia indicate progression.
- Hepatorenal syndrome (HRS): creatinine clearance <40 mL/min (or serum creatinine >1.5) with urine volume <500 mL/day and urine sodium <10 mEq/L
- Abdominal ultrasound to screen for hepatocellular carcinoma (HCC) and to assess parenchyma and hepatic and portal veins; elastography evaluates parenchymal scarring/fibrosis.

Follow-Up Tests & Special Considerations
Consider:
- Hepatitis serologies; ethanol and GGT if alcohol abuse is suspected; antimitochondrial antibody to screen for primary biliary cirrhosis; anti-smooth muscle and antinuclear antibodies to screen for autoimmune hepatitis
- Transferrin saturation (>50%) and ferritin (markedly increased) to screen for hemochromatosis; if abnormal, check hemochromatosis (HFE) genetics/mutation analysis; α_1-antitrypsin phenotype screen; ceruloplasmin to screen for Wilson disease; if low, check copper excretion (serum copper plus 24-hour urine copper); α-fetoprotein level to screen for HCC

Diagnostic Procedures/Other
- Liver biopsy: recommended if noninvasive markers incongruent with imaging; percutaneous if INR <1.5 and no ascites
- Endoscopy (EGD) if esophageal varices/portal hypertensive gastropathy
- Known liver nodularity or splenomegaly on MRI or CT indicates cirrhosis.
- Magnetic resonance elastography: in obese or nonalcoholic fatty liver disease (NAFLD)

Test Interpretation
Fibrous bands and regenerative nodules are classic biopsy features of cirrhosis.

TREATMENT

Outpatient care for all acute and chronic HCV patients, except during major GI bleeding, altered mental status, sepsis/infection, rapid hepatic decompensation, or renal failure

GENERAL MEASURES
- Abstain from alcohol, drugs, hepatotoxic medicines, and herbs; pneumococcal-20, hepatitis A/B, and influenza vaccinations; weight loss, exercise, and control of lipids/glucose
- Determine if uncompensated disease: ascites; spontaneous bacterial peritonitis (SBP); HE, coagulopathy, variceal hemorrhage

MEDICATION
First Line
Treat the underlying cause first (note prescribing precautions in decompensated cirrhosis) to delay progression of disease.
- HCV: treatment with direct acting antivirals (DAAs) to eradicate viral RNA are recommended if without cirrhosis (e.g., FIB-4 <3.25, FibroScan <12.5 kPa, normal biopsy, or platelet count >150,000) with glecaprevir-pibrentasvir for 8 weeks in genotypes 1 to 6, or sofosbuvir-velpatasvir for 12 weeks in genotypes 1, 2, 4, 5, and 6; if cirrhosis, past treatment failure, eGFR <30 mL/min/m², pregnancy, hepatitis B, HIV, suspected HCC, then specialty referral; monitor INR for those taking warfarin and for hypoglycemia diabetes.
- HBV: When no cirrhosis with PCR DNA >20,000 and ALT >2 × ULN, the goal of treatment is to reduce HCC and decompensation risk. First line is entecavir 0.5 to 1 mg PO daily and then tenofovir 300 mg PO or telbivudine 600 mg PO daily; often prescribed indefinitely without return to HBeAg-negative status; alternatively, PEG-IFN α-2a 180 μg weekly injection used for 48 weeks can be used in absence of cirrhosis.

- NAFLD: Weight loss of 3–5% of body weight reduces steatosis, and >10% loss with improved fitness up to >150 min/week of physical activity reduces NASH and fibrosis. Minimize saturated fats, carbohydrate-laden beverages, and refined carbohydrates. Consider glucagon-like peptide-1 receptor antagonists, SGLT-2 inhibitors, or pioglitazone in diabetes mellitus +/− NASH.
- Alcoholic hepatitis: treat alcohol withdrawal; Maddrey Discriminant Function score >32 indicates poor prognosis; patients may benefit from prednisolone of 40 mg/day for 28 days with 2 to 4 weeks; taper to reduce short-term mortality; pentoxifylline for patients who cannot tolerate steroids
- Hereditary hemochromatosis: phlebotomy every 1 to 2 weeks until serum ferritin is 50 to 100 μg/L and then 2 to 6 times per year as needed; deferoxamine 40 mg/kg/day over 8 to 12 hours for 5 to 7 days in dyserythropoietic syndrome and chronic hemolytic anemia to reduce iron overload quickly
- Primary biliary cirrhosis: ursodeoxycholic acid (ursodiol) 13 to 15 mg/kg PO divided BID with food; for pruritus, if ursodiol is ineffective, then cholestyramine 4 to 8 g PO BID is the next therapy, followed by antihistamines, rifampin 150 to 300 mg PO BID or naltrexone 50 mg/day; evaluate for fat-soluble vitamin deficiencies, metabolic bone disease, hypercholesterolemia, hypothyroidism, and anemia.
- Wilson disease: initial treatment with penicillamine 1,000 to 1,500 mg/day PO BID–QID or trientine 750 to 1,500 mg/day PO BID–TID on an empty stomach; trientine 750 to 1,500 mg/day PO BID–TID is better tolerated; after 1 year, zinc acetate 150 mg/day PO BID–TID for maintenance; zinc for presymptomatic, pregnant, and pediatric populations
- Autoimmune hepatitis: Treat if AST or ALT >10 times ULN, or if either >5 times ULN and γ globulins >2 times ULN with prednisone 30 mg/day for 1 week, then 20 mg/day for 1 week, then 10 mg/day for 2 weeks with maintenance of 5 mg/day; at outset test for TPMT activity, and if not low or negative, add azathioprine (AZA) 50 to 100 mg/day throughout; treat to normal transaminases. At 24 months of remission trial, withdrawal of steroids with AZA maintenance × 3 months then trial AZA taper by 50 mg q3mo.
- Esophageal varices: variceal bleed prophylaxis with propranolol >40 mg, carvedilol 6.25 mg, or nadolol 40 mg PO daily, to lower heart rate to 55 to 60 beats/min; PPI indicated when varices require banding and for portal hypertensive gastropathy
- Ascites/edema: low-sodium (<2 g/day) diet and spironolactone 100 to 400 mg/day with or without furosemide 40 to 160 mg/day PO; torsemide as substitute for furosemide. If serum sodium <120 mmol/L, then 1.0 to 1.5 L/day water restriction; if new onset, rule out SBP. If prior SBP, consider SBP prophylaxis with TMP-SMX DS or norfloxacin 400 mg PO daily.
- HE: lactulose 15 to 45 mL BID; titrate to induce 2 to 3 loose bowel movements daily to resolve AMS. Add rifaximin 550 mg PO BID if needed.
- Renal insufficiency: Stop NSAIDs, diuretics, and nephrotoxic drugs; normalize electrolytes; and hospitalize for plasma expansion or dialysis.
- Prophylactic antibiotics for invasive procedures, GI bleeding, or history of SBP

Second Line
HBV: adefovir 10 mg PO daily second line; lamivudine is not recommended as first-line agent due to resistance.

ISSUES FOR REFERRAL
Evaluate for liver transplant at onset of ascites, variceal bleeding, HE, jaundice, liver lesion suggestive of HCC, or when evidence of hepatic dysfunction develops (Child-Turcotte-Pugh [CTP] >7 and Model for End-Stage Liver Disease [MELD] >10).

SURGERY/OTHER PROCEDURES
Varices: endoscopic ligation, 4 to 6 treatments (if acute bleed, use pre-esophagogastroduodenoscopy [EGD] octreotide as vasoconstrictor); transjugular intrahepatic portosystemic shunt (TIPS) second-line or salvage therapy for acute bleed; ascites: if tense, therapeutic paracentesis every 2 weeks PRN; caution if pedal edema is absent; fulminant hepatic failure: liver transplantation; HCC: curable if small with radiofrequency ablation or resection and transplant

COMPLEMENTARY & ALTERNATIVE MEDICINE
- Zinc sulfate 220 mg BID for dysgeusia and appetite; adjunct for HE
- Milk thistle may lower transaminases and improve symptoms.
- Vitamin E 800 IU daily in NASH with caution and monitoring for vitamin K dependent antagonism diathesis

ADMISSION, INPATIENT, AND NURSING CONSIDERATIONS
Major GI bleeding, AMS, sepsis/infection, rapidly progressing hepatic decompensation, renal failure

 ## ONGOING CARE
- Monitor liver enzymes, sodium, creatinine, platelets, and PT q6–12mo; calculate MELD score.
- Serial α-fetoprotein and liver ultrasound screening q6–12mo in patients with cirrhosis. Patients aged >55 years with chronic HBV or HCV, elevated INR, or low platelets are at highest risk for HCC. MRI with contrast is the best follow-up test for HCC if α-fetoprotein is elevated and/or liver mass is found on ultrasound. EGD at cirrhosis diagnosis and every 3 years (compensated) and every 1 year (decompensated) to screen for varices

FOLLOW-UP RECOMMENDATIONS
Regular physical conditioning may help with fatigue.

Patient Monitoring
- Monitor for fatigue, weakness, reduced appetite, and/or itchy skin at each visit.
- AMS, jaundice, or abdominal pain are major concerns.

DIET
Protein (1.2 to 1.5 g/kg body weight daily), high fiber, multivitamin (without iron), sodium restriction (<2 g/day), combined with fluid restriction, essential if ascites/edema

PATIENT EDUCATION
- Educate about when to seek emergency care (e.g., hematemesis, AMS).
- Drug, alcohol, and smoking cessation (no cannabis)
- Update required immunizations; HCV transmission precautions

PROGNOSIS
- 5 to 20 years of asymptomatic disease from time of initial diagnosis.
- After onset of complications, death is typically within 5 years without transplant.
- 5% per year develop HCC. 50% develop ascites over 10 years; 50% 5-year survival after ascites develop. Acute variceal bleeding is the most common fatal complication; 30% mortality; median survival after complications (ascites, variceal bleeding, HE) is 1.5 years. With transplant, 85% survive 1 year; after transplant, ~5% annual mortality; <25% of eligible patients receive a transplant due to organ shortage.

COMPLICATIONS
Ascites, edema, infections, HE, GI bleeding, esophageal varices, gastropathy, colopathy, HRS, HPS, HCC, hepatic failure

REFERENCE
1. Ginès P, Krag A, Abraldes JG, et al. Liver cirrhosis. *Lancet.* 2021;398(10308):1359–1376.

ADDITIONAL READING
- Sharma R, Zhao W, Zafar Y, et al. Serum hepcidin levels in chronic liver disease: a systematic review and meta-analysis [published online ahead of print August 7, 2023]. *Clin Chem Lab Med.* 2023.
- Volk ML, Clarke C, Asrani SK, et al. Cirrhosis Quality Collaborative. *Clin Gastroenterol Hepatol.* 2022;20(5):970–972.

 ## SEE ALSO

Algorithm: Cirrhosis

CODES

ICD10
- K74.60 Unspecified cirrhosis of liver
- K70.30 Alcoholic cirrhosis of liver without ascites
- K74.69 Other cirrhosis of liver

CLINICAL PEARLS
- 80% of CLD is preventable (primarily alcohol abuse, hepatitides).
- After diagnosis of cirrhosis, abdominal ultrasound every 6–12 months for early detection of HCC.
- Update necessary immunizations and treat underlying cause (e.g., HCV, alcohol, etc.).
- Always rule out SBP in patients presenting with initial episode of ascites.

CLOSTRIDIUM DIFFICILE INFECTION

Eileen Ly, MD

 BASICS

DESCRIPTION
- A gram-positive, spore-forming, anaerobic bacillus that releases toxins to produce clinical disease
- Associated with antibiotic use, recent hospitalization, residence at long-term care facilities, weakened immune system, and age >65 years
- Severity of infection ranges from asymptomatic carrier to diarrhea, colitis, sepsis, perforation, and death.
- Typically person-to-person transmission of spores via the fecal-oral route but may also occur through exposure to contaminated surfaces or equipment
- System(s) affected: gastrointestinal
- Synonym(s): *Clostridioides difficile* infection, *C. difficile*–associated disease or diarrhea (CDAD); *C. difficile* infection; *C. difficile* colitis; *C. diff*

EPIDEMIOLOGY
Incidence
- Colonization with *C. difficile* found in:
  - 2–10% of community, 3–18% of inpatients, 4–20% of long-term residents (1)
- Global estimated incidence of *C. difficile* infection 50/100,000/year; hospitalization rates are increasing (2).
- National incidence of health care–associated *C. difficile* infection 73/100,000 persons
- National incidence of community acquired *C. difficile* infection 52/100,000 persons

Prevalence
- *C. difficile* accounted for 12% of health care–associated infections in 2010
- >2 million cases of CDAD in U.S. hospitals from 1993 to 2005

ETIOLOGY AND PATHOPHYSIOLOGY
- Is an anaerobic toxin-producing, gram-positive bacillus bacteria existing in vegetative and spore forms
- Has a 1-week incubation period with spores that can survive for 5 months in harsh conditions and outside the body
- Spread by fecal-oral contact; acid-resistant spores pass through stomach to reside mostly in the colon.
- Colonic colonization causes disruptions in barrier functions of the normal microbiome.
- *C. difficile* is noninvasive. Toxins mediate disease: Toxins A (enterotoxin) and B (cytotoxin) attract neutrophils and monocytes, degrading colonic epithelial cells and causing clinical disease.
- The hypervirulent strain BI/NAP1/027 of *C. difficile* is associated with higher rates of colectomy and death.

Genetics
No known genetic factors

RISK FACTORS
- Host risk factors
  - Age >65 years; hospitalization or long-term health care facility
  - Comorbidities, including inflammatory bowel disease, immunosuppression, chronic liver disease, and end-stage renal disease
  - Enteral feeding; previous *C. difficile* infection

- Factors that disrupt normal colonic microbiota:
  - Exposure to antibiotics (including perioperative prophylaxis)
  - Commonly implicated antibiotics: ampicillin, amoxicillin, clindamycin (most common), cephalosporins, and fluoroquinolones
  - Chronic acid suppression
- Recurrence from prior infection: Recurrence rates are ~25%; recurrence more likely with each additional episode
- Community-acquired *C. difficile* infections (no overnight admission in >12 weeks) are more frequent in patients without other risk factors (younger, no recent antibiotic exposure).
- Risk increases with length of hospital stay, duration of antibiotics exposure, and number of antibiotics used (3).

Geriatric Considerations
C. difficile is the most common cause of acute diarrheal illness in long-term care facilities.

Pediatric Considerations
- Neonates have a higher rate of *C. difficile* colonization (25–80%) but are generally less symptomatic than adults.
- Frequently serve as carrier for infection in adults

GENERAL PREVENTION
- Antibiotic stewardship programs decrease the incidence of *C. difficile* infection.
- Society for Healthcare Epidemiology of America (SHEA)/Infectious Diseases Society of America (IDSA) guidelines for prevention:
  - For health care workers, patients, and visitors
    - Contact precautions, including gloves and gowns, on entry to room; alcohol-based hand sanitizers are not effective. Hand washing with soap and water before and after patient interaction is recommended.
    - Accommodate patients with *C. difficile* infection in private rooms if possible.
  - Environmental cleaning and disinfection
    - Disinfect with hypochlorite or other spore-killing solution.
    - Identify and reduce environmental sources of *C. difficile*.
  - Antimicrobial restrictions: Minimize the frequency and duration of antibiotic therapy.

COMMONLY ASSOCIATED CONDITIONS
Pseudomembranous colitis, toxic megacolon, sepsis, colonic perforation

DIAGNOSIS

HISTORY
- Common presenting symptoms include diarrhea and abdominal cramping or pain.
- Age and underlying comorbidities
- Recent antibiotic (risk of *C. difficile* infection may persist for 3 months after antibiotic is discontinued); proton pump inhibitor or H_2-receptor blocker use
- Diarrhea (defined as >3 stools in 24 hours) that is watery, foul-smelling, and sometimes bloody (1)

- Fever (<10%), anorexia, nausea
- Recent hospitalization or stay at nursing facility

PHYSICAL EXAM
- Abdominal exam: look for tenderness, increasing distension, diminished bowel sounds, peritoneal signs
- Initial presentation can be fulminant and rapidly fatal; assessment of severity is key to management.
- Look for signs of systemic illness including fever, tachycardia, hypotension, and dehydration.

DIFFERENTIAL DIAGNOSIS
- Infectious causes: *Salmonella*; *Shigella*; *Campylobacter*; Shiga toxin–producing *Escherichia coli* infection
- Noninfectious causes
  - Intestinal obstruction; ischemic bowel disease; inflammatory bowel disease: ulcerative colitis, Crohn disease
  - Gastrointestinal cancer; drug-associated diarrhea; foodborne illness
  - Other antibiotic-associated diarrhea (75% of antibiotic diarrhea not associated with *C. difficile*)

DIAGNOSTIC TESTS & INTERPRETATION
Initial Tests (lab, imaging)
- CBC, BMP, lactate to evaluate leukocytosis and serum creatinine, aids in assessment of severity of disease
- Several stool tests are available for diagnosis
  - Glutamate dehydrogenase (GDH) assay (sensitivity, 85–95%; specificity, 89–99%)
  - Enzyme immunoassays which detect toxin A or toxin B, (sensitivity, 63–94%)
  - Nucleic acid amplification tests (NAATs)
  - Cell culture cytotoxicity assays (gold standard)
- Stepwise approach to testing often used may vary by facility; for example, GED plus toxin assay with NAAT testing for discrepant results
- Repeat testing during the same episode of diarrhea is not recommended. Stool carriage persists for 3 to 6 weeks after successful treatment and can remain positive in 60% of patients.
- Routine radiologic examination is not recommended in the absence of signs of systemic disease or clinical suspicion for complicated/severe disease.
  - Plain films may show thumbprinting and colonic distension.
  - CT may show mucosal thickening, colonic wall thickening, pericolonic inflammation, or signs of complicated infection in severe cases (i.e., extraluminal air).

Diagnostic Procedures/Other
Endoscopy can evaluate for presence of pseudomembranes and exclude other conditions.
- Although not all patients with *C. difficile* infection have pseudomembranes, their presence is pathognomonic.
- Flexible sigmoidoscopy may miss 15–20% of pseudomembranes (from the proximal colon).

Test Interpretation
SHEA/IDSA guidelines
- Mild or moderate disease: leukocytosis with white blood cell (WBC) count <15,000 cells/μL and a serum creatinine level <1.5 times the premorbid level
- Severe, uncomplicated disease: leukocytosis with WBC count >15,000 cells/μL or a serum creatinine level >1.5 times the premorbid level
- Severe, complicated disease: hypotension, sepsis, markedly elevated WBC count, lactic acidosis, hypoalbuminemia, and imaging findings of complicated disease

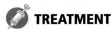 TREATMENT

GENERAL MEASURES
- Antimotility agents are contraindicated.
- Avoid indiscriminate use of antibiotics.
- Proton pump inhibitors are associated with recurrent infection but have not been shown to be causal.
- Discontinue offending antibiotic, whenever possible.

MEDICATION
First Line
- Initial episode (nonsevere or severe disease):
  - First line: fidaxomicin PO 200 mg BID × 10 days; vancomycin PO 125 mg QID × 10 days
  - Second line: metronidazole PO 500 mg TID × 10 days
  - If patient is unable to take oral medications, then intravenous (IV) metronidazole or intraluminal (PO) vancomycin can be used.
- First recurrence
  - Fidaxomicin: 200 mg PO BID × 10 days *or* 200 mg PO BID × 5 days, followed by once every other day × 20 days
  - Alternative vancomycin: 125 mg PO TID × 10 to 14 days, then 125 mg PO BID × 7 days, then 125 mg PO once daily × 7 days, and then 125 mg PO q2–3d for 2 to 8 weeks *or* 125 mg PO TID × 10 days
- Second recurrence
  - Fidaxomicin: 200 mg PO BID × 10 days *or* 200 mg PO BID × 5 days, followed by once every other day × 20 days
  - Alternative vancomycin: 125 mg PO QID × 10 to 14 days, then 125 mg PO BID × 7 days, then 125 mg PO once daily × 7 days, and then 125 mg PO q2–3d × 2 to 8 weeks *or* 125 mg PO QID × 10 days, then rifaximin PO 400 mg TID × 20 days
- Fulminant infection (hypotension, shock, ileus, megacolon): Consider surgical and critical care consultation.
  - Vancomycin 500 mg PO QID or by nasogastric tube; if ileus or PO is not an option, consider vancomycin 500 mg rectally *and* intravenously administered metronidazole (500 mg q8h).

ALERT
- When using vancomycin to treat *C. difficile* infection, use oral or rectal formulations. IV formulations (not excreted into the colonic lumen) are ineffective.
- Monitor creatinine levels very closely.

Second Line
- Oral metronidazole
- 500 mg PO TID for 10 to 14 days
- Vancomycin: for patients who cannot tolerate or have failed metronidazole therapy and for pregnancy
- Fecal transplant: stool from healthy, screened donor; either rectal or oral; effective for recurrent infections (80–90% cure rate) after offending antibiotic stopped; recipient gut flora transformed in as few as 3 days

SURGERY/OTHER PROCEDURES
- Severe abdominal pain or signs of hemodynamic instability should prompt consultation.
- Perforation of the colon (4)

ALERT
BI/NAP1/027 strain is associated with fulminant colitis.

COMPLEMENTARY & ALTERNATIVE MEDICINE
- Adjunctive IV immunoglobulin (IVIG) has shown promise; more data needed before routine use
- Probiotics *Lactobacillus acidophilus* and *Saccharomyces boulardii* have inhibitory effects on *C. difficile* and can help prevent *C. difficile* infection and should be prescribed when started on antibiotics.
- Other investigational treatments:
  - Newer antibiotics (rifalazil, tolevamer, and ramoplanin); monoclonal antibodies to modulate toxin effects
  - Vaccine form of *C. difficile* antitoxin antibody

ADMISSION, INPATIENT, AND NURSING CONSIDERATIONS
- Admission criteria/initial stabilization: hypovolemia; inability to keep up with enteric losses; hematochezia; electrolyte disturbances
- IV fluids to maintain volume status
- Discharge criteria: decreased diarrhea severity and frequency; tolerating oral diet and medications

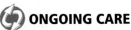 ONGOING CARE

FOLLOW-UP RECOMMENDATIONS
Do not repeat testing for toxins because patients may shed for weeks following an acute infection.

Patient Monitoring
- Relapses of colitis occur in 15–30%.
- Relapses typically occur 2 to 10 days after discontinuing antibiotics.

DIET
- Regular diet
- NPO if severe colitis and surgical evaluation pending

PATIENT EDUCATION
Educate patients about *C. difficile* transmission, the importance of hand washing with soap and water and not relying on alcohol-based sanitizers, and avoidance of unnecessary use of antibiotics.

PROGNOSIS
- Most patients improve with conservative management and oral antibiotics.
- 1–3% of patients develop severe/fulminant colitis requiring emergency colectomy.

REFERENCES
1. Guh AY, Kutty PK. *Clostridioides difficile* infection. *Ann Intern Med*. 2018;169(7):ITC49–ITC64.
2. Balsells E, Shi T, Leese C, et al. Global burden of *Clostridium difficile* infections: a systematic review and meta-analysis. *J Glob Health*. 2019;9(1):010407.
3. McDonald LC, Gerding DN, Johnson S, et al. Clinical practice guidelines for *Clostridium difficile* infection in adults and children: 2017 update by the Infectious Diseases Society of America (IDSA) and Society for Healthcare Epidemiology of America (SHEA). *Clin Infect Dis*. 2018;66(7):e1–e48.
4. Giles J, Roberts A. *Clostridioides difficile*: current overview and future perspectives. *Adv Protein Chem Struct Biol*. 2022;129:215–245.

 CODES

ICD10
- A04.7 Enterocolitis due to Clostridium difficile
- A04.71 Enterocolitis due to Clostridium difficile, recurrent
- A04.72 Enterocolitis due to Clostridium difficile, not specified as recurrent

CLINICAL PEARLS
- *C. difficile* is spread by fecal-oral contact
- Alcohol-based hand sanitizers are ineffective against *C. difficile*. Wash hands thoroughly with soap and water
- Testing and treatment of asymptomatic patients is not recommended
- *C. difficile* and organismal by-products (e.g., toxin) are identifiable from stool samples
- Patients may shed organism or toxin for weeks after treatment. Repeat toxin assays following treatment are not helpful
- Vancomycin and fidaxomicin are first-line treatments Consider metronidazole if neither of these are viable options.
- Consider probiotic use when prescribing antibiotics to potentially decrease risk of development of *C. difficile* infection

COLIC, INFANTILE

Daniel T. Lee, MD, MA • Phillip Charles Brown, MD • Orly Bell, MD, MPH

 BASICS

DESCRIPTION

- Colic is defined as excessive crying in an otherwise healthy infant.
- A commonly used criteria is the Wessel criteria or the Rule of Three, when crying lasts for:
  - >3 hr/day
  - >3 days/week
  - Persists >3 weeks
- Many clinicians do not strictly adhere to the criterion of persistence for >3 weeks because few parents or clinicians will wait that long before evaluation or intervention.
- The Rome IV criteria refined the criteria for clinical purposes and for research purposes.
- For Rome IV clinical diagnostic criteria, must include all the following:
  - An infant who is <5 months when symptoms start and stop
  - Recurrent and prolonged periods of crying, fussing, or irritability without obvious cause and unable to console
  - No evidence of failure to thrive, fever, or illness
- Additional Rome IV criteria for clinical research purposes:
  - Caregiver reports crying/fussing for ≥3 hr/day during ≥3 days within a week.
  - Total daily crying is ≥3 hours when measured by at least one prospectively kept 24-hour diary.
- Colic usually peaks at 6 weeks of life.
- Some clinicians consider that colic represents the extreme end of the spectrum of normal crying, whereas most consider colic a distinct clinical entity.

EPIDEMIOLOGY

Incidence
- Predominant age group is between 2 weeks and 4 months of age.
- Equal predominance among males and females, breast-fed versus formula fed, full term versus preterm, and first-born versus subsequent-born.
- Possibly more common in industrialized countries and in white infants

Prevalence
- Wide range from 8% to 40% of infants; however, more likely affects 10–25% of infants
- Causes 10–20% of pediatric visits during the early weeks of an infant's life

Pediatric Considerations
This is a problem during infancy.

ETIOLOGY AND PATHOPHYSIOLOGY
The cause is unknown. Factors that may play a role include the following:
- Infant gastroesophageal reflux disease
- Intolerance to cow's milk, soy milk, or breast milk protein
- Intolerance to lactose and functional lactose overload (i.e., breast milk with lower lipid content can have faster transit time in the intestine, leading to more lactose fermentation in the gut and hence gas and distension)

- Intestinal immaturity leading to incomplete absorption of carbohydrates in the small intestine, which result in excessive gas when the unabsorbed carbohydrate is fermented by colonic bacteria
- Alterations in intestinal or fecal microflora
- Swallowing air during the process of crying, feeding, or sucking
- Overfeeding or feeding too quickly; underfeeding has also been proposed.
- Inadequate burping after feeding
- Family tension and/or stress
- Parental anxiety, depression, and/or fatigue
- Parent–infant interaction mismatch
- Infant's inability to console himself or herself when dealing with stimuli
- Hypersensitivity after exposure to prolonged environmental stimuli
- Fruit juice intolerance
- Increases in the gut hormone motilin, causing hyperperistalsis
- Tobacco smoke and nicotine exposure
- Immature motor regulation
- Increased serotonin concentration
- Possible early manifestation of childhood migraine

RISK FACTORS
- Physiologic predispositions in an infant may play a role, but no definitive risk factors have been established.
- Maternal smoking or exposure to nicotine replacement therapy during pregnancy is associated with higher incidence of infantile colic.
- Infants with a maternal history of migraine headaches are twice as likely to have colic.

GENERAL PREVENTION
Colic is generally not preventable.

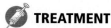 **DIAGNOSIS**

HISTORY
- Evaluation for Wessel criteria or Rome IV criteria
- Thorough history to rule out organic causes
- Episodes usually have a clear beginning and end and generally occur more often in the afternoon and evening.
- The crying is generally spontaneous, without preceding events triggering the episodes.
- The crying is typically different from normal crying. Colicky crying may be louder, more turbulent, variable in pitch, and appears more like screaming.
- Episodes of colic may be associated with hypertonia, which may include facial flushing, circumoral pallor, tense abdomen, arching of the back, tightening of the arms, clenching of the fingers, or drawing up of the legs.
- The infant may be difficult to soothe or console despite all the parents' efforts.
- The infant acts normally when not colicky.
- Assess the support system of caregivers and families, including coping skills.

PHYSICAL EXAM
- A comprehensive physical exam is normal.
- Because excessive crying may be a risk factor for abuse, be sure to examine the child carefully for signs of shaken baby syndrome or other types of child abuse.

DIFFERENTIAL DIAGNOSIS
Organic causes account for <5% of cases of inconsolable crying in infants. These may include:
- Infectious causes such as meningitis, sepsis, otitis media, diaper rash, thrush, or UTI
- Inadequate feeding or difficulty feeding due to causes such as tongue-tie
- Gastrointestinal causes such as gastroesophageal reflux disease, intussusception, lactose intolerance, constipation, anal fissure, or strangulated hernia
- Trauma, which includes foreign body, corneal abrasion, occult fracture, digit or penile hair tourniquet, or child abuse

DIAGNOSTIC TESTS & INTERPRETATION
Initial Tests (lab, imaging)
Infantile colic is a clinical diagnosis. No lab or imaging testing is typically performed unless clinical symptoms imply other causes (UTI, weight loss or poor weight gain, abnormal physical exam, etc.).

Diagnostic Procedures/Other
A thorough history and physical exam should be performed to rule out other causes. Otherwise, no diagnostic procedures are indicated.

TREATMENT

GENERAL MEASURES
- Soothe by holding and rocking the baby (1)[B].
- Use a pacifier (1)[B].
- Use gentle rhythmic motions (e.g., strollers, infant swings, car rides) (1)[B].
- Use white noise (e.g., vacuum cleaner, clothes dryer, white noise machine) (1)[B].
- Crib vibrators or car ride simulators have not proven to be helpful.
- Provide a warm bath (1)[B].
- Increased carrying or use of infant carriers has not been shown to improve colic (1)[B].
- Frequent burping does not significantly lower colic events (and may increase rate of regurgitation).
- Rubbing the infant's abdomen
- Employ the 5 S's (need to be done concurrently):
  - Swaddling: tight wrapping with blanket (with arms snug and straight and hips loose); may be especially beneficial in infants <8 weeks old
  - Side/stomach: holding baby on side or stomach
  - Shushing: loud white noise
  - Swinging: rhythmic, jiggle motion while supporting baby's head and neck
  - Sucking: on a nipple, finger, or pacifier
  - "Stay calm." The baby may not understand what is being said but rather how it is said (e.g., "Everything will be fine; I am here now.").

MEDICATION

- No medication has been found to be universally beneficial in treating infantile colic.
- Probiotics are safe, and some studies have suggested their efficacy. Their use is discussed in the "Complementary & Alternative Medicine" section.
- Dicyclomine (Bentyl) may have some benefit, but potential serious adverse effects, such as apnea, seizures, and syncope, have precluded its use. Furthermore, the manufacturer has made the medication contraindicated for infants <6 months (2)[B].
- Simethicone has not been shown to be beneficial (2)[B].
- Proton pump inhibitors and H_2 receptor antagonists have not been shown to be beneficial.

ISSUES FOR REFERRAL

Excessive vomiting, poor weight gain, recurrent respiratory diseases, or bloody stools should prompt referral to a specialist.

COMPLEMENTARY & ALTERNATIVE MEDICINE

- There is no clear evidence that probiotics are effective at preventing infantile colic.
- Limited studies on *Lactobacillus reuteri* DSM 17938 and *Bifidobacterium* strains (in particular *Bifidobacterium breve* and *Bifidobacterium animalis* subsp. *lactis* BB-12) as probiotics suggest they may decrease daily crying times in breastfed infants (more studies need to be conducted in formula-fed infants) (3).
- There is anecdotal evidence that car rides, both real and simulated, can be effective. You can find a 10-hour recording of a simulated car ride at the following link: https://www.youtube.com/watch?v=8KAXmle-T_4.
- Providing "white noise," such as running a vacuum cleaner, clothes dryer, white noise generator, or infant sound machine may also help. Avoid excessively loud and/or prolonged noise to minimize potential adverse effects on hearing or auditory development.
- Herbal teas and supplements may help but are not recommended because of limited, inconclusive evidence.
  - Herbal teas containing mixtures of chamomile, vervain, licorice, and balm-mint used up to TID may be beneficial. However, the study used high dosages, raising clinical concerns that this therapy may impair needed milk consumption in infants and be impractical to administer. In addition, preparations used in the study may not be commercially available in the United States.
  - There is an evidence supporting the effectiveness of different preparations of fennel, such as oils, teas, and herbal compounds, in treating infantile colic.
  - Medications described as "soothing" that include activated charcoal are growing in popularity but are not recommended at this time and also have their own risks.
- A home-based intervention focusing on reducing infant stimulation and synchronizing infant sleep-wake cycles with the environment, as well as on parental support, has been shown to be effective.

- Use of music may help.
- Chiropractic treatment, craniosacral therapy, and acupuncture have not been shown to be effective.
- Infant massage has not been shown to be helpful.

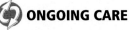 ## ONGOING CARE

FOLLOW-UP RECOMMENDATIONS

Frequent outpatient visits as needed for parental reassurance, education, monitoring, and to ensure the health of the infant and parents.

Patient Monitoring

Follow for proper feeding, growth, and development.

DIET

- If breastfeeding:
  - Continue breastfeeding; switching to formula unlikely to help
  - Low likelihood of therapeutic benefit from eliminating milk products, eggs, wheat, nuts, soy, and/or fish from the diet of breastfeeding mothers, but this may be beneficial if the mother is atopic or if the infant has symptoms of cow's milk allergy (1)[B].
- If formula feeding:
  - Feeding the infant in a vertical position using a curved bottle or bottle with a collapsible bag may help to reduce air swallowing.
  - If no intervention or dietary change has been effective, consider a 1-week trial of hypoallergenic formulas such as whey hydrolysate (e.g., Good Start) or casein hydrolysate (e.g., Alimentum, Nutramigen, Pregestimil) (1)[B],(2)[C].
  - Adding fiber to formula also has not been shown to be helpful (1)[B].
- Supplementing with sucrose solution may be helpful, but the effect may be short-lived (<1 hour) (1),(2)[B].
- Switching to soy protein formula is unlikely to be helpful.
- Despite the proposed mechanism of functional lactose overload, use of lactase enzymes in formula or breast milk or given directly to the infant has no therapeutic benefit (1)[B].

PATIENT EDUCATION

- Caregiver support, in the form of reassurance and education, is critical.
- Reassure parents that colic is not the result of something they are doing or not doing.
- Reassure parents that colic is normal and that the infant is not sick.
- Advise parents about having proper rest breaks, adequate sleep, help in caring for the infant, and even a rescue plan in case parents become overwhelmed.
- Parents need to develop their own personal coping strategies to deal with colic episodes to avoid risk of harm to infant.
- Explain the spectrum of crying behavior.
- Avoid overfeeding or underfeeding.

- Instruct parents regarding beneficial feeding techniques such as improved bottles (low air, curved) and sufficient burping after feeding.
- Information for parents of colicky infants can be found at the following link from the American Academy of Family Physician: https://www.aafp.org/afp/2004/0815/p741.html.

PROGNOSIS

- Colic usually subsides by 3 to 5 months of age.
- Despite apparent abdominal pain, colicky infants eat well and gain weight normally.
- A few studies in toddlers up to 4 years old indicate temper tantrums may be more common among formerly colicky infants.
- Colic has no bearing on the baby's intelligence or future development.

COMPLICATIONS

- Colic is self-limiting, and there are no proven lasting effects to the infant.
- There may be associations with increased risk/incidence of postpartum depression among either or both parents, child abuse, caregiver burnout, and early cessation of breastfeeding.

REFERENCES

1. Johnson JD, Cocker K, Chang E. Infantile colic: recognition and treatment. *Am Fam Physician*. 2015;92(7):577–582.
2. Wade S, Kilgour T. Extracts from "clinical evidence": infantile colic. *BMJ*. 2001;323(7310):437–440.
3. Pereira AR, Rodrigues J, Albergaria M. Effectiveness of probiotics for the treatment of infantile colic. *Aust J Gen Pract*. 2022;51(8):573–576.

ADDITIONAL READING

- Anheyer D, Frawley J, Koch AK, et al. Herbal medicines for gastrointestinal disorders in children and adolescents: a systematic review. *Pediatrics*. 2017;139(6):e20170062.
- Gelfand AA, Thomas KC, Goadsby PJ. Before the headache: infant colic as an early life expression of migraine. *Neurology*. 2012;79(13):1392–1396.

 ## CODES

ICD10

R10.83 Colic

CLINICAL PEARLS

- Colic is defined as excessive crying in an otherwise healthy infant (>3 hr/day, >3 days/week, persists >3 weeks).
- Colic usually subsides spontaneously by 3 to 5 months of age.
- Provide advice, support, and reassurance to parents.
- Prevent caregiver burnout by advising parents to get proper rest breaks, sleep, and help in caring for the infant.

COLITIS, ISCHEMIC

Marie L. Borum, MD, EdD, MPH • *Samuel A. Schueler, MD* • *Luke Thomas Chmielecki, MD*

 BASICS

Ischemic colitis (IC) results from decreased blood flow to the colon with resultant inflammation and tissue damage.

DESCRIPTION
- More common in the elderly; can affect patients of all ages
- IC is self-limited and reversible in 80% of patients:
  – 20% of patients progress to full-thickness necrosis requiring surgical intervention.
- Most commonly, ischemia is related to a nonocclusive reduction in blood flow.
- Presentation varies, but patients with acute IC typically present with localized abdominal pain and tenderness. Frequent loose, bloody stools may be seen within 12 to 24 hours of onset.
- Laboratory and radiographic findings are nonspecific and must be correlated with clinical presentation.
- Colonoscopy is the gold standard for diagnosis of IC.
- Most patients recover with supportive care (IV fluids, bowel rest, and clinical monitoring).

EPIDEMIOLOGY
- More common in women (57–76%—particularly after age 69 years) (1)
- Evidence of IC is seen in 1 of every 100 endoscopies.

Geriatric Considerations
Rare in patients <60 years old; average age at diagnosis is 70 years.

Incidence
Approximately 23 cases per 100,000 person-years (ranges from 4.5 to 44) in the general population (may be underestimated due to nonspecific clinical manifestations)

Prevalence
19 cases per 100,000 in the general population

ETIOLOGY AND PATHOPHYSIOLOGY
- Local colonic hypoperfusion compromises the ability to meet metabolic demands. Reperfusion injury may also play a role.
- The colon is perfused by both the superior and inferior mesenteric arteries (SMAs and IMAs) and branches of the internal iliac arteries. Occlusion of larger branches of the SMA or IMA rarely leads to ischemic consequences due to extensive collateral circulation.
- Watershed areas of the colon (splenic flexure and rectosigmoid junction) are supplied by narrow terminal branches of the SMA and IMA, respectively, and are most susceptible to ischemic damage.
- The left colon is more commonly affected than the right; isolated right-sided disease has the worst prognosis.
- The rectum is often spared because of additional blood supply from the internal iliac arteries.
- Type I: unidentified etiology
  – Likely small vessel disease; treat supportively.

- Type II: etiology identified
  – Treat the underlying cause (1).
    ○ Hypoperfusion from shock, trauma
    ○ Embolic occlusion of mesenteric vessels
    ○ Hypercoagulable states, vasculitis; sickle cell disease
    ○ Arterial thrombosis; venous thrombosis
    ○ Mechanical obstruction of the colon (e.g., tumor, adhesions, hernia, volvulus, prolapse, diverticulitis)
    ○ Surgical complications
    ○ Medications (intestinally active vasoconstrictive substances, medications that induce hypotension and thus, hypoperfusion); cocaine abuse
    ○ Aortic dissection
    ○ Strenuous physical activity (e.g., long-distance running)
- Repeated episodes of ischemia and inflammation may result in chronic colonic ischemia, possible stricture formation, recurrent bacteremia, and sepsis. These patients may have unresolving areas of colitis and require segmental colonic resection.

Genetics
- Various coagulopathies have been related to IC including deficiencies of protein C, protein S, antithrombin III, and factor V Leiden mutation.
- Routine coagulation testing is not justified except in younger patients and patients with recurrent IC (1).

RISK FACTORS
- Age >60 years (90% of patients)
- Smoking (most common cause of recurrent IC) (1)
- Hypertension, diabetes mellitus (1)
- Rheumatologic disorders/vasculitis
- Cerebrovascular disease, ischemic heart disease (1)
- Atherosclerotic disease
- Recent abdominal surgery (i.e., ileostomy)
- Constipation, constipation-inducing medications (1)
- History of vascular surgery (1)
- Chronic obstructive pulmonary disease
- Hypoalbuminemia; hemodialysis
- Hypercoagulability, oral contraceptive (1)
- NSAID use
- Immunomodulators (1)
- IBS (1)

GENERAL PREVENTION
Standard practices, counseling and treatment of risk factors as indicated.

℞ DIAGNOSIS
- Diagnosis is based on history, risk factors, and physical examination (1)[A].
- Laboratory values and radiographic findings are usually nonspecific but may help predict severity (1)[A].
- Colonoscopy is diagnostic (1)[A].

HISTORY
- Abdominal pain is the most common symptom (2). Pain may be out of proportion to physical examination findings.
- Sudden-onset, mild to moderate abdominal pain with tenderness over the affected segment of bowel (3)
- Sudden urge to defecate followed by passage of either bright red or maroon stool typically within 12 to 24 hours of abdominal pain onset (3)
- Lower GI bleeding is rarely heavy.

PHYSICAL EXAM
- Individual signs and symptoms are poorly predictive of IC (4)[C].
- Vital signs: hypotension; tachycardia
- Tenderness over the involved segment of bowel (3)
- Abdominal distention with vomiting (due to possible associated ileus)
- In the uncommon setting of transmural ischemia, patients may develop peritoneal signs (1)[A].

DIFFERENTIAL DIAGNOSIS
- Infectious colitis (1)[A]
- Inflammatory bowel disease (ulcerative colitis, Crohn disease) (1)[A]
- Colon cancer, diverticulitis (1)[A]
- Pseudomembranous colitis (4)[A]

DIAGNOSTIC TESTS & INTERPRETATION
- Depends on clinical presentation, extent of colonic involvement, transmural involvement, acuity
- CT scan is the initial diagnostic test for patients with nonspecific abdominal pain (4)[A].
- Colonoscopy for definitive diagnosis (1)[A]
- Radiographic tests and laboratory values are otherwise nonspecific (4)[A].

Initial Tests (lab, imaging)
- The following lab markers of ischemia are not specific to IC but can help determine disease severity (4)[A]:
  – CBC (leukocytosis) (4)[A]
  – BMP, ABG (signs of metabolic acidosis) (4)[A]
  – Lactate, LDH, CPK, amylase (4)[A]
  – Alkaline phosphatase (4)[A]
  – Albumin (3)
- Abdominal plain film:
  – Rarely may see thumbprinting and mural thickening; may predict more severe disease (1)[A]
- Abdominal CT scan with contrast (1)[A]:
  – Thickening of the colonic wall and pericolonic fat stranding (3)
  – Other findings include hyperdense mucosa, submucosal edema, and mesenteric inflammation.
  – Pneumatosis, pneumoperitoneum, and free peritoneal fluid suggest advanced ischemia.
  – Double halo sign is highly suggestive of IC but is rarely present (1)[A].
- Multiphasic CTA should be performed for suspected right-sided IC or if acute mesenteric ischemia cannot be excluded (3)[B].

Follow-Up Tests & Special Considerations

- Stool cultures, fecal leukocytes, stool ova, and parasites to rule out infection (4)[A]
- Patients undergoing aortic surgery may benefit from postoperative colonoscopy within 2 to 3 days to look for signs of IC (3).
- If indicated, cardiac workup including electrocardiogram, Holter monitoring, or transthoracic echocardiogram to exclude cardiogenic embolism (4)[A]
- Drug and toxicology screening (3)
- If colon cancer screening is indicated, perform several weeks following recovery from the ischemic insult (1).

Diagnostic Procedures/Other

- Colonoscopy is gold standard; sigmoidoscopy is used to evaluate postoperative left-sided ischemia.
- Cyanotic hemorrhagic tissue and edematous mucosa suggest ischemia (3).
  - Segmental distribution (watershed), hemorrhagic nodules, and rectal sparing (3)
  - "Colon single-stripe sign" is a single line of erythema, with a 75% histopathologic yield (3).
  - Routine biopsy no longer advised, as results are typically nonspecific
- In cases of isolated right IC, noninvasive vascular imaging studies are recommended to evaluate acute SMA occlusion (3).

Test Interpretation

Biopsied specimens reveal mucosal infarction and ghost cells, which show normal cellular outlines but lack intracellular contents.

TREATMENT

- Treatment depends on disease severity.
- In the absence of colonic necrosis or perforation, most patients respond to supportive care (1)[A]:
  - Bowel rest (3)
  - IV fluids to maintain hemodynamic stability (3)
  - Avoid intestinally active vasoconstrictive medications (3)[A].
  - Avoid systemic corticosteroids—may worsen ischemia and increase risk of perforation.
- If ileus is present, place nasogastric tube.
- If radiographic abnormalities are present, serial abdominal x-rays help follow improvement (3)[A].
- If signs of clinical deterioration are present despite supportive care (increased abdominal pain, peritoneal signs, persistent diarrhea, bleeding, or sepsis), consider surgery.

MEDICATION

Specific medications have been associated with IC, including (1)[B]:

- Constipation-inducing medications (i.e., opioids)
- Immunomodulators (anti-TNFα inhibitors, type 1 interferon-α/β)
- Illicit drugs (cocaine, amphetamines)

First Line

Consider broad-spectrum antibiotics covering aerobic and anaerobic bacteria to avoid bacterial translocation secondary to colonic mucosal damage (3).

- Ciprofloxacin 400 mg IV BID or 500 mg PO BID
- Metronidazole 500 mg PO/IV TID

Second Line

A third-generation cephalosporin may be used instead of a fluoroquinolone.

ISSUES FOR REFERRAL

- If cardiac workup reveals CHF or cardiac arrhythmias, initiate appropriate treatment (3).
- If signs of clinical deterioration are present despite supportive care (increased abdominal pain, peritoneal signs, persistent diarrhea, bleeding, or sepsis), consider surgery.

SURGERY/OTHER PROCEDURES

- 20% of patients require surgical intervention (2).
- Surgery may be indicated for:
  - Peritoneal signs, increased abdominal tenderness, new-onset shock, lactic acidosis, or acute renal failure
  - Pneumatosis intestinalis, portal vein air, or free peritoneal air
  - Diarrhea, lower GI bleeding, or exudative colitis persisting past 14 days
- Most common surgical intervention is colectomy with end ileostomy (4)[A].
  - Cholecystectomy may prevent resuscitation-related acute acalculous cholecystitis.

COMPLEMENTARY & ALTERNATIVE MEDICINE

- *Ginkgo biloba* extract has been studied as an adjunct to general treatment.
- Weight loss supplements/herbal supplements (ephedra, ma huang, bitter orange, white willow bark) have been implicated in cases of IC.

ADMISSION, INPATIENT, AND NURSING CONSIDERATIONS

- ICU patients represent a difficult population to diagnose IC given the concurrent comorbidities and clinical care (sedation/ventilation) that can mask the characteristic signs and symptoms.
- Consider bedside colonoscopy in critically ill patients.

ONGOING CARE

FOLLOW-UP RECOMMENDATIONS

Patient Monitoring

- Vital sign monitoring depending on initial presentation
- Observation for further episodes of bloody stool or melena
- Consideration of serial CBCs
- Serial abdominal exams

DIET

- Bowel rest until symptoms resolve
- Parenteral nutrition for patients needing prolonged bowel rest who have contraindications to surgery

PATIENT EDUCATION

Risks of IC with the use of weight loss medications/herbal supplements

PROGNOSIS

- In most patients, IC symptoms resolve in 24 to 48 hours.
- Radiographic or endoscopic resolution within 2 weeks
- Right-sided IC is the most significant predictor of outcome. Right-sided IC has a 2-fold increase in mortality and a 4-fold increase in morbidity (3).
- Secondary cardiovascular prevention minimizes recurrence.
- Male gender, low hemoglobin, low serum albumin, high BUN, and presence of metabolic acidosis are poor prognostic factors (1).
- Chronic kidney disease, chronic obstructive pulmonary disease, and long-term care facilities increase mortality in IC (1).

COMPLICATIONS

20–30% of patients develop chronic IC with persistent diarrhea or stricture formation requiring surgery.

REFERENCES

1. Brandt LJ, Feuerstadt P, Longstreth GF, et al. ACG clinical guideline: epidemiology, risk factors, patterns of presentation, diagnosis, and management of colon ischemia (CI). *Am J Gastroenterol*. 2015;110(1):18–45.
2. Huber TS, Björck M, Chandra A, et al. Chronic mesenteric ischemia: clinical practice guidelines from the Society for Vascular Surgery. *J Vasc Surg*. 2021;73(1S):87S–115S.
3. Maimone A, De Ceglie A, Siersema PD, et al. Colon ischemia: a comprehensive review. *Clin Res Hepatol Gastroenterol*. 2021;45(6):101592.
4. Ahmed M. Ischemic bowel disease in 2021. *World J Gastroenterol*. 2021;27(29):4746–4762.

CODES

ICD10

- K55.9 Vascular disorder of intestine, unspecified
- K55.0 Acute vascular disorders of intestine
- K55.1 Chronic vascular disorders of intestine

CLINICAL PEARLS

- Suspect IC in patients with multiple risk factors who present with abdominal pain and loose bloody stools.
- Risk factors include advanced age, smoking, hypertension, diabetes mellitus, cardiovascular or rheumatologic disease, recent abdominal surgery, medications (such as constipation-inducing, NSAIDs, and immunomodulators), IBS, hemodialysis, and chronic obstructive pulmonary disease.
- Colonoscopy is the diagnostic gold standard.
- Most often, IC is self-limited and responds well to conservative management with IV fluids, bowel rest, and empiric broad-spectrum antibiotics.
- Peritoneal signs or lack of clinical improvement suggests more extensive ischemia and the need for surgical intervention.

COLON CANCER

Kento Sonoda, MD • Mako Wakabayashi, MD

BASICS

DESCRIPTION

- Colon and rectal cancers (CRCs) are often grouped together but are two distinct clinical entities that differ in their prognosis, presentation, staging, and management.
- CRC is the third leading cause of cancer-related deaths in men and women in the United States.

EPIDEMIOLOGY

Incidence

- Estimated that in 2023 in the United States, there are 106,970 new cases of colon cancer and 46,050 new cases of rectal cancer per the American Cancer Society (ACS).
- The annual incidence of colorectal cancer was 33% higher in men than women from 2015 to 2019.
- Colorectal cancer is expected to cause about 52,550 deaths during 2022.
- Internationally, CRC is the third most common cancer and the second leading cause of cancer death.

Prevalence

The lifetime risk of developing colorectal cancer in the United States is about 1 in 23 (4.3%) for men and 1 in 26 (3.9%) for women.

ETIOLOGY AND PATHOPHYSIOLOGY

- Progression from the first abnormal cells to colon cancer occurs over 10 to 15 years.
- High-risk polyps: multiple polyps, villous or dysplastic polyps, and larger polyps; hyperplastic polyps are less likely to evolve into CRC.
- Both genetic and environmental factors are linked to CRC.

Genetics

- <10% of CRC cases are linked to an inherited gene. Patients with early-onset CRC have a higher percentage of genetic causes, suggesting family members to have an early screening.
  - Many of these are inherited in an autosomal dominant fashion:
    - *APC*, a tumor-suppressor gene, is altered in familial adenomatous polyposis (FAP).
    - Genes encoding DNA mismatch repair (MMR) enzymes are implicated in hereditary nonpolyposis colon cancer (HNPCC), formerly known as Lynch syndrome, including *hMLH1, hMSH2, hMSH6, hPMS2, EPCAM,* and others.
    - *STK11*, a tumor-suppressor gene, is altered in Peutz-Jeghers syndrome.
  - A smaller portion of patients with familial CRC may have a recessive gene.
    - MUTYH defects lead to issues with the base excision repair gene. This MUTYH-associated polyposis (MAP) may present as a variant form of FAP.
- Sporadic cases of CRC have been linked to oncogenes: *KRAS, PIK3CA, APC, TP53, BRCA1, BRCA2, BRAF*.

RISK FACTORS

- Age
  - The incidence of colon cancer starts to increase significantly between the age of 40 and 50 years old. ~87% of those with new CRC diagnosis will be ≥50 years old.

- Younger patients are more likely to have advanced disease at the time of diagnosis.
- Personal history of colorectal polyps
  - The risk increases with multiple polyps, villous polyps, larger polyps (>1 cm), and presence of dysplasia.
- Personal history of cancer
  - 30% increase in risk of developing metachronous (new primary tumors unrelated to the patients' previous cancers) colon cancer
  - 2–4% incidence of local recurrence with colon cancer, 3–5% incidence of synchronous colon cancer
  - History of radiation therapy to the abdomen/pelvis
- Personal history of inflammatory bowel disease (IBD)
  - The risk of CRC begins approximately 8 years after the onset. Prevalence of CRC in ulcerative colitis and Crohn disease is ~3%, with a cumulative risk of CRC of 2% at 10 years, 8% at 20 years, and 18% at 30 years.
  - Ulcerative colitis with pancolitis up to 10-fold risk of CRC, 8 to 10 years after initial diagnosis.
- Family history of CRC
  - Having a single first-degree relative with a history of CRC increases risk by ~1.7-fold.
  - The risk is more than double for those who have a history of CRC or polyps in:
    - Any first-degree relative <50 years of age
    - ≥2 first-degree relatives, regardless of age
    - One first-degree relative and one second-degree relative
- Inherited syndromes
  - HNPCC
    - Often develops at young age (The average age of diagnosis of CRC is 48 years.)
    - Often presents with right-sided lesions and cancer often recurs
    - Lifetime risk of CRC is 52–69%; also associated with endometrial and other cancers
    - Accounts for ~3% of all CRCs
  - FAP
    - Affected individuals develop hundreds to thousands of polyps in colon and rectum, typically presenting during childhood.
    - CRC usually present by age 40 years in untreated patients; however, most have prophylactic colectomies.
    - Accounts for <1% of CRCs
    - Variants include Gardner and Turcot syndromes as well as attenuated FAP (AFAP).
  - Peutz-Jeghers syndrome
    - Individuals may have hyperpigmented mucocutaneous lesions (mouth, hands, feet) and large polyps in GI tract discovered as an adolescent.
    - 81–93% risk for cancers including CRC, cancers of pancreas, breast, cervix, testes, and lung
  - BRCA1 and BRCA2 syndromes
    - Some data suggest that carriers of *BRCA1* may have increased risk for early CRC; however, more evidence is needed to recommend early screening.
- Race and ethnicity
  - African Americans have the highest CRC incidence and mortality rates in the United States; likely due to social determinants of health
- Lifestyle factors
  - Smoking, obesity, sedentary activity, insulin resistance, high-fat and low-fiber diet, red and processed meat, excessive alcohol consumption, and potentially microbiota

GENERAL PREVENTION

- Lifestyle factors and medications that may reduce the risk:
  - Regular physical activity, diet high in fiber, and fruits/vegetables
  - There is conflicting evidence on folic acid, calcium, vitamin D, magnesium, NSAIDs, fish oil, and statins.

ALERT

The U.S. Preventive Services Task Force (USPSTF) states that all adults aged ≥45 year should be offered with screening regardless of the presence of the risk factors (the recommendation for 45 to 49 years old is Grade B and Grade A for 50 to 75 years old). ACS and American College of Gastroenterology (ACG) also recommend initiating screening at the age of 45 years in average-risk individuals (1). For persons ages 76 to 85 years old, screening should be based on overall health status and life expectancy and should involve shared decision-making between the patients and health professionals.

- Screening methods:
  - Visualization-based tests:
    - Flexible sigmoidoscopy every 10 years with a high-sensitivity fecal immunochemical test (FIT) yearly
    - Flexible sigmoidoscopy every 5 years
    - Colonoscopy every 10 years
  - Stool-based tests:
    - FIT annually
    - High-sensitivity guaiac-based fecal occult blood test (gFOBT) annually
    - Stool DNA-FIT every 1 to 3 years (e.g., Cologuard)
  - Imaging-based tests:
    - CT colonography every 5 years
  - For patients who have a positive FIT, gFOBT, or stool DNA-FIT test, a colonoscopy is recommended.
- ACG guideline recommends a colonoscopy or a FIT as a primary CRC screening method, and other methods are reserved for those unwilling or unable to undergo a colonoscopy or a FIT (1).
- Colonoscopy:
  - People with a history of polyps need frequent colonoscopy screening, with the interval depending on polyp number, size, and histology.
  - People who have a first-degree relative or two second-degree relatives with CRC or advanced polyps before age 60 years should begin colonoscopy at the age of 40 years or 10 years younger than the youngest age of the affected relative at cancer diagnosis, whichever is earlier.
  - Patients with IBD should start surveillance colonoscopies every 1 to 2 years 8 to 10 years after diagnosis.
  - Genetic testing may be appropriate for individuals with a strong family history of CRC or polyps:
    - Family members of a person with HNPCC should start colonoscopy at the age of 20 to 25 years or 2 to 5 years prior to the youngest age of the affected relative at the time of cancer diagnosis, whichever occurs first. This screening should be repeated every 1 to 2 years.
    - Individuals with suspected FAP should have colonoscopy every 1 to 3 years, beginning at the age of 10 to 14 years.

- Frequency of follow-up of polyps:
  - <1 year:
    - Following piecemeal (unable to remove with single loop) removal of a large polyp ≥20 mm
  - 1 year:
    - Known FAP or at risk based on family history
    - >10 adenomatous polyps
  - 1 to 2 years:
    - IBD (Crohn disease or ulcerative colitis)
  - 3 years:
    - 5 to 10 tubular adenomas <10 mm
    - 5 to 10 sessile serrated polyps
    - Tubular adenoma ≥10 mm
    - Sessile serrated polyp ≥10 mm
    - Adenoma with villous or tubulovillous histology and/or high-grade dysplasia
    - Sessile serrated polyp with dysplasia
    - Traditional serrated adenoma
  - 3 to 5 years:
    - 3 to 4 sessile serrated polyp <10 mm without dysplasia
    - 3 to 4 adenomas <10 mm
    - Hyperplastic polyps ≥10 mm
    - History of colon cancer s/p surgery if initial 1 year follow-up is normal
  - 5 to 10 years:
    - 1 to 2 sessile serrated polyp <10 mm without dysplasia
  - 7 to 10 years:
    - 1 to 2 adenomas <10 mm
  - 10 years:
    - Normal screening colonoscopy with no polyps
    - ≤20 Hyperplastic polyps in rectum or sigmoid colon, <10 mm
    - ≤20 Hyperplastic polyps proximal to sigmoid colon, <10 mm

COMMONLY ASSOCIATED CONDITIONS
- HNPCC, Gardner, Crail (Turcot), FAP, Peutz-Jeghers, and juvenile polyposis syndromes
- IBDs including Crohn disease and particularly ulcerative colitis with pancolitis

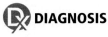 # DIAGNOSIS

HISTORY
- Microcytic, iron-deficiency anemia (IDA) in men of any age, and postmenopausal women should prompt a diagnostic colonoscopy.
- Symptoms may indicate an advanced disease.
  - Abdominal pain or cramping
  - Change in bowel habits or in the caliber of stool (tenesmus, constipation, diarrhea)
  - Rectal bleeding, dark stools, or blood in stool
  - Weakness or fatigue
  - Unintentional weight loss

PHYSICAL EXAM
- Signs of anemia (pallor, systolic flow murmurs, etc.)
- Weight loss
- Palpable abdominal mass (late presentation)
- Hepatomegaly, ascites, and lymphadenopathy can be present in metastatic cases.

DIFFERENTIAL DIAGNOSIS
>95% of colon cancers are adenocarcinomas. Others include carcinoid tumors, lymphomas, gastrointestinal stromal tumors (GIST), and Kaposi sarcoma in HIV.

DIAGNOSTIC TESTS & INTERPRETATION
Initial Tests (lab, imaging)
- If you suspect CRC, colonoscopy should be performed because it can be both diagnostic and therapeutic.
- Although CRC is commonly associated with IDA, the absence of IDA doesn't exclude CRC.
- Tumor marker CEA has a low value for diagnosis of cancer due to its low sensitivity and specificity. However, CEA levels can be useful in predicting prognosis and monitoring patients with a confirmed diagnosis of CRC.

Follow-Up Tests & Special Considerations
- Contrasted CT of chest, abdomen, and pelvis to evaluate for metastatic disease
- Intraoperative ultrasound may be used to evaluate solid organs (e.g., the liver) after tumor resection.
- Positron emission tomography (PET) may be used to detect metastatic disease.
- Staging of colon cancer
  - The SEER staging
    - Localized: no signs with spread outside the colon or rectum
    - Regional: signs with spread outside the colon or rectum but only to nearby structures
    - Distant: signs with spread to distant sites of the body (i.e., the liver, lungs, or distant lymph nodes)

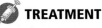 # TREATMENT

ADDITIONAL THERAPIES
Adjuvant chemotherapy is most clearly beneficial for stage III (node-positive) disease, in which improvements of 30% can be achieved in both disease recurrence and overall survival, compared with untreated controls. Chemotherapeutic regimens for metastatic disease may extend overall survival from 6 months to 2 years. Often used therapies are FOLFOX (folinic acid, 5-fluorouracil, oxaliplatin), FOLFIRI (folinic acid, leucovorin, 5-fluorouracil, irinotecan) or CAPEOX (capecitabine, oxaliplatin). Neoadjuvant chemotherapy, immuno therapy, and targeted therapy (bevacizumab, ramucirumab, ziv-aflibercept, pembrolizumab, panitumumab, cetuximab, nivolumab, regorafenib, encorafenib) can also be used.

SURGERY/OTHER PROCEDURES
- Localized cancer
  - Surgery is the primary treatment with regional lymph node dissection.
  - Primary anastomosis can be possible for local cancers;
    - Obstructing lesions tend to require resections with diversion followed by colectomy with regional lymphadenectomy.

- Locally advanced cancers: multivisceral resection
- Metastatic cancer: it can be reasonable to aggressively resect metastatic lesions isolated to the liver/lungs in addition to the primary tumors.

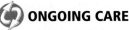 # ONGOING CARE

FOLLOW-UP RECOMMENDATIONS
Patient Monitoring
- Stage T1/T2 with no distant spread: colonoscopy in a year; if normal, repeat in 3 years and then every 5 years.
- Stage T3/T4 or lesser stage with positive lymph nodes: CEA and H&P every 3 to 6 months for 2 years, then every 6 months for a total of 5 years; chest, abdominal, and pelvic CT every year for 5 years; colonoscopy in a year; if normal, repeat in 3 years and then every 5 years.

PATIENT EDUCATION
Centers for Disease Control and Prevention: https://www.cdc.gov/cancer/colorectal/basic_info/screening/tests.htm

PROGNOSIS
- Overall 5-year relative survival rate: 65%
- 5-year relative survival rate: (localized) 90.9%, (regional) 73.4%, (distant) 15.6%

COMPLICATIONS
- Chemotherapy: hair loss, nausea, vomiting, diarrhea, easy bruising, fatigue, skin change, and increased risk for infections
- Radiation therapy: skin irritation, nausea, rectal pain, incontinence, bladder irritation, fatigue, sexual problems, scarring, fibrosis, and adhesion

REFERENCE
1. Shaukat A, Kahi CJ, Burke CA, et al. ACG clinical guidelines: colorectal cancer screening 2021. *Am J Gastroenterol.* 2021;116(3):458–479.

 # CODES

ICD10
- C18.9 Malignant neoplasm of colon, unspecified
- C18.2 Malignant neoplasm of ascending colon
- C18.8 Malignant neoplasm of overlapping sites of colon

CLINICAL PEARLS
Microcytic, iron deficiency anemia in men and postmenopausal women is CRC until proven otherwise, and colonoscopy should be performed.

COLONIC POLYPS

Maximos Attia, MD, FAAFP • Marcelle Meseeha, MD

 BASICS

DESCRIPTION
- Intraluminal colonic tissue growth; most commonly sporadic or part of polyposis syndromes
- Generally slow growing with low malignant potential; due to high prevalence in population; however, resection is generally recommended to eliminate risk.
- Size classification:
  – Diminutive: ≤5 mm; small: 6 to 9 mm; large: ≥10 mm
- Morphologic classification:
  – Depressed, flat, sessile, or pedunculated
- Clinical significance:
  – >95% of colonic adenocarcinomas arise from polyps.

EPIDEMIOLOGY
Colorectal polyps are more common in non-Caucasian men in Western countries.

Incidence
Incidence increases with age.

Prevalence
- 15–20% of all adults
- 30% of U.S. population aged >50 years
- 6% of children
- 12% of children with lower GI bleed

ETIOLOGY AND PATHOPHYSIOLOGY
- Mucosal
  – Neoplastic
    ○ Adenomatous polyps (tubular >80%, villous 5–15%, tubulovillous 5–15%)
    ○ Serrated polyps
    ○ Sessile serrated polyps (SSPs) are common, more in proximal colon, with low malignant potential if no dysplasia and significant malignant potential if dysplastic.
    ○ Traditional serrated adenoma is uncommon, more often noted in distal colon, with significant malignant potential.
  – Nonneoplastic polyps (hyperplastic, juvenile polyps, hamartomas, inflammatory pseudopolyps)
    ○ Hyperplastic polyps are very common, more in distal colon, with very low malignant potential.
    ○ Juvenile polyps are common in childhood, benign hamartomas, more in rectosigmoid, and not premalignant.
- Submucosal (lipomas, lymphoid aggregates, carcinoids)

Genetics
- Inactivation of tumor suppressor genes as adenomatous polyposis coli (APC) or mismatch repair genes (*MLH1*) causes polyps to grow into cancer.
- Familial adenomatous polyposis (FAP) is autosomal dominant. By age 40 years, almost all patients develop colorectal cancer (CRC).

- MUTYH-associated polyposis (MAP) is autosomal recessive caused by biallelic mutations in MUTYH gene.
- Juvenile polyposis syndrome (JPS) is autosomal dominant. 50–60% of patients have a mutation in the SMAD4 or BMPR1A gene. By age 35 years, 20% of patients develop CRC.

RISK FACTORS
- Family history of intestinal polyposis, polyps, or CRC
- Advancing age; male
- High-fat, low-fiber diet; tobacco use
- Excessive alcohol intake: more than eight drinks a week
- Inflammatory bowel disease is associated with a decreased prevalence of colon polyps (but with higher risk of colon cancer).

GENERAL PREVENTION
- Low-fat, high-fiber diet
- Avoid smoking.
- Decrease alcohol intake.
- Use of NSAIDs and calcium is associated with decreased incidence and recurrence of polyps.
- No lower rates of CRC with azathioprine, 6-mercaptopurine, folate, calcium, multivitamins, or statins

COMMONLY ASSOCIATED CONDITIONS
Hereditary polyposis syndromes:
- Adenomatous
  – FAP
    ○ Classic (CFAP), attenuated (AFAP)
  – MAP
  – FAP variants:
    ○ Gardner syndrome, Turcot syndrome
- Hamartomatous
  – Peutz-Jeghers syndrome (PJS), JPS, Cowden syndrome

ALERT
JPS imposes a higher risk of CRC, although juvenile polyps are not premalignant.

 DIAGNOSIS

HISTORY
- Generally asymptomatic
- Painless rectal bleeding, bright or dark red, mixed with stools, dripping, or on wiping
- Diarrhea or mucous stool
- Abdominal pain
- Constipation
- Chronic bleeding, resulting in iron-deficiency anemia
- McKittrick–Wheelock syndrome; large hypersecretory rectosigmoid villous adenoma, resulting in persistent severe diarrhea, electrolyte disorder, dehydration, and prerenal acute renal failure
- Social and family history

PHYSICAL EXAM
- Usually normal
- Rectal polyps noted as prolapsed or palpated on digital rectal examination (DRE)
- Fecal occult blood test (FOBT) by DRE is less effective than FOBT by stool passed spontaneously.

DIAGNOSTIC TESTS & INTERPRETATION
Initial Tests (lab, imaging)
- CBC; anemia with chronic bleeding
- Basic metabolic panel; electrolyte disorder with hypersecretory adenomas
- FOBT, insensitive screening test, because small polyps don't usually bleed:
  – Guaiac (gFOBT)—uses a chemical indicator with color change in presence of blood
  – Immunochemical (iFOBT) or fecal immunochemical test (FIT)—uses antibodies against human hemoglobin
- Stool DNA test is more sensitive and less specific than FIT.

Diagnostic Procedures/Other
- Colonoscopy is the gold-standard test for detection of polyps and allows for concurrent polypectomy; not a perfect screening test, with increased miss rate with right-sided colon polyps, smaller polyp size, low quality of colon prep, less endoscopist experience
- Computed tomographic colonography (CTC) is less sensitive with flat polyps and requires excellent bowel preparation.
- Double-contrast barium enema
- Colon capsule endoscopy
- Enhanced optical technologies can potentially differentiate between neoplastic and nonneoplastic colonic lesions (1)[A].
- Enhanced optical technologies include the following:
  – Narrowed spectrum endoscopy (narrow-band imaging [NBI])
  – Image-enhanced endoscopy (i-scan)
  – Fujinon intelligent chromoendoscopy (FICE)
  – Confocal laser endomicroscopy (CLE)
- Patients with >10 colorectal adenomas should undergo genetic testing for APC and MUTYH.

Test Interpretation
- Tubular adenoma
  – Gross: tends to be polypoid
  – Micro: dysplastic epithelium, tubular architecture
- Villous adenoma:
  – Gross: tends to be sessile
  – Micro: dysplastic epithelium, fingerlike projections
- Tubulovillous adenomas have a combination of tubular and villous architecture.
- Hyperplastic polyps are composed of hyperplastic colonic mucosa.
- Hamartomatous polyps include muscularis mucosa.
- Juvenile polyp
  – Gross: pedunculated, smooth red mass, 1 to 3 cm

TREATMENT

SURGERY/OTHER PROCEDURES
- Colonic polypectomy; diagnostic, therapeutic:
  - Snare polypectomy with electrocautery for pedunculated polyps
  - Endoscopic mucosal resection for sessile polyps
  - Endoscopic submucosal dissection
- Colorectal surgery; prophylactic in FAP and MAP and when there are numerous polyps or persistent bleeding:
  - Total colectomy ileorectal anastomosis
  - Proctocolectomy ileal pouch anal anastomosis
- Chemoprevention: NSAIDs and calcium may reduce incidence and recurrence of polyps in patients with FAP and MAP (2).

ONGOING CARE

FOLLOW-UP RECOMMENDATIONS
Follow-up colonoscopy in: (3)
- 10 years if no polyps or distal small hyperplastic polyps (<10 mm) (3)[B]
- 3 to 5 years in hyperplastic polyps ≥10 mm (3)[C]
- 7 to 10 years if 1 to 2 small tubular adenomas (<10 mm) (3)[B]
- 3 to 5 years if 3 to 4 small tubular adenomas (<10 mm) (3)[C]
- 3 years if 5 to 10 small tubular adenomas (<10 mm) (3)[B]
- 1 year if >10 adenomas (3)[C]
- 3 years if one or more adenomas ≥10 mm (3)[A]
- 3 years if one or more adenomas with tubulovillous or villous features of any size or with HGD (3)[B]
- 6 months if adenoma ≥20 mm or SSP ≥20 mm, with piecemeal resection (3)[B]
- 5 to 10 years if 1 to 2 small SSPs (<10 mm) (3)[C]
- 3 to 5 years if 3 to 4 small SSPs (<10 mm) (3)[C]
- 3 years if 5 to 10 small SSPs (<10 mm) (3)[C]
- 3 years if SSP ≥10 mm or with dysplasia or traditional serrated adenoma (3)[C]
- Different consideration is given for polyps that meet the criteria for serrated polyposis syndrome (3)[B]

Patient Monitoring
- Colonoscopy for CRC screening starts at age 45 years (earlier for at-risk patients). The U.S. Preventive Services Task Force, American College of Gastroenterology (ACG), and the American Cancer Society (ACS) recommend that people at average risk of CRC start screening at age 45 years through age of 75 years, may extend to 85 years, based on life expectancy and overall health.
- Stop screening if life expectancy is <10 years.
- In CFAP and AFAP, screen for extracolonic manifestations: thyroid cancer, desmoid tumors, and gastroduodenal polyposis (every 6 months to 5 years).

- In families, lifetime screening for mutation carriers:
  - In CFAP: with sigmoidoscopy or colonoscopy, every 1 to 2 years starting at age of 10 to 11 years
  - In AFAP and MAP: with colonoscopy, every 1 to 2 years starting at age of 18 to 20 years
- After colorectal surgery, surveillance of the rectum (every 6 to 12 months) or pouch (every 6 months to 5 years) is indicated.
- First-degree relatives of patients with JPS require screening by colonoscopy and upper endoscopy after age 12 years.
- Genetic evaluation is recommended for any patient with >10 adenomas cumulatively over lifespan (3).

DIET
Low-fat, high-fiber diet (insufficient evidence)

PATIENT EDUCATION
Importance of colonoscopy as a screening tool

PROGNOSIS
- Regression or no change in size, more with small hyperplastic polyps and with patients on NSAIDs
- Recurrence: Juvenile polyps recur in 45% of children with multiple polyps and 17% with solitary polyps.
- Risk factors for colon cancer:
  - Polyp pathology
    - Adenomàtous
    - Serrated
    - With HGD
    - With >25% villous histology
    - Polyp size >1 cm in diameter
    - Polyps located in proximal colon
    - More than three polyps
- Recurrence rates <10% postpolypectomy
- Ineffective endoscopic resection of precancerous lesions results in lingering cancer.

COMPLICATIONS
- Polyps: progression to cancer
- Polypectomy: bleeding 2–11%, perforation 0–1%, higher with endoscopic submucosal dissection
- Colonoscopy: complications related to anesthesia and procedure itself

REFERENCES

1. Shaukat A, Kahi CJ, Burke CA, et al. ACG clinical guidelines: colorectal cancer screening 2021. *Am J Gastroenterol*. 2021;116(3):458–479.
2. Ichkhanian Y, Zuchelli T, Watson A, et al. Evolving management of colorectal polyps. *Ther Adv Gastrointest Endosc*. 2021;14:26317745211047010.
3. Gupta S, Lieberman D, Anderson JC, et al. Recommendations for follow-up after colonoscopy and polypectomy: a consensus update by the US Multi-Society Task Force on Colorectal Cancer. *Gastrointest Endosc*. 2020;91(3):463.e5–485.e5.

ADDITIONAL READING

- Kaltenbach T, Anderson JC, Burke CA, et al. Endoscopic removal of colorectal lesions: recommendations by the US Multi-Society Task Force on Colorectal Cancer. *Gastrointest Endosc*. 2020;91(3):486–519.
- Rex DK, Boland CR, Dominitz JA, et al. Colorectal cancer screening: recommendations for physicians and patients from the U.S. Multi-Society Task Force on Colorectal Cancer. *Gastroenterology*. 2017;153(1):307–323.
- Wolf AMD, Fontham ETH, Church TR, et al. Colorectal cancer screening for average-risk adults: 2018 guideline update from the American Cancer Society. *CA Cancer J Clin*. 2018;68(4):250–281.

SEE ALSO

Colon Cancer; Rectal Cancer

CODES

ICD10
- K63.5 Polyp of colon
- D12.6 Benign neoplasm of colon, unspecified
- K51.40 Inflammatory polyps of colon without complications

CLINICAL PEARLS
- Colonoscopy is the gold standard for diagnosing polyps.
- Biopsy small hyperplastic polyps to differentiate adenomatous and serrated polyps.
- The use of NSAIDs and calcium is associated with decreased incidence and recurrence of polyps.
- The progression from normal mucosa through polyp to carcinoma takes years to develop.

COMMUNITY ACQUIRED METHICILLIN-RESISTANT *STAPHYLOCOCCUS AUREUS* (CA-MRSA) SKIN INFECTIONS

Stephen A. Martin, MD, EdM • Paul P. Belliveau, PharmD

 BASICS

DESCRIPTION

- Community-acquired methicillin-resistant *Staphylococcus aureus* (CA-MRSA) has unique properties that allow the organism to cause skin and soft tissue infections (SSTIs) in healthy hosts:
  - CA-MRSA has a different virulence and disease pattern than hospital-acquired MRSA (HA-MRSA).
- CA-MRSA infections generally impact patients who have not been recently (<1 year) hospitalized or had a medical procedure (e.g., dialysis, surgery, catheters).
- Incidence of CA-MRSA increased in the United States from 2000 until 2010 to 2013 when it plateaued for adults and decreased for children.
- CA-MRSA typically causes mild to moderate SSTIs (abscesses, furuncles, and carbuncles).
- Severe or invasive CA-MRSA disease is less frequent but can include:
  - Osteomyelitis
  - Sepsis
  - Septic thrombophlebitis
  - Necrotizing fasciitis
  - Necrotizing pneumonia with abscesses
- Although less frequent, HA-MRSA can still cause SSTIs in the community.
- System(s) affected: skin, soft tissue

EPIDEMIOLOGY

- Predominant age: all ages, generally younger
- Predominant sex: female > male

Incidence

- SSTI incidence for adult ambulatory care peaked in 2010 at 35 per 1,000 population and has since plateaued.
- SSTI incidence for pediatric ambulatory care visits peaked in 2011 at 26 per 1,000 population, decreasing to 13 per 1,000 in 2015.
- The incidence of MRSA-related hospitalizations decreased from 2010 to 2014.
- Among people who inject drugs, the incidence of MRSA-related skin abscesses is increasing. Patients should receive substance misuse disorder care and be linked with syringe exchange programs.

Prevalence

- Local epidemiology patterns vary.
- 25–30% of U.S. population colonized with *S. aureus*; up to 7% are colonized with MRSA.
- CA-MRSA isolated in ~60% of SSTIs presenting to emergency departments (range 15–74%)
- CA-MRSA accounts for up to 75% of all community staphylococcal infections in children.

ETIOLOGY AND PATHOPHYSIOLOGY

- First noted in 1980; current epidemic began in 1999. The USA300 clone is predominant.
- CA-MRSA is distinguished from HA-MRSA by:
  - Lack of a multidrug-resistant phenotype
  - Presence of exotoxin virulence factors
  - Type IV staphylococcal cassette cartridge (contains the methicillin-resistant gene *mecA*)

RISK FACTORS

~50% of patients have no obvious risk factor. Recognized risk factors include:

- Antibiotic use in the past month, particularly cephalosporins and fluoroquinolones
- Abscess; reported "spider bite"
- Intravenous (IV) or intradermal drug use, HIV infection
- Hemodialysis catheter presence, history of MRSA infection
- Close contact with a similar infection; children, particularly in daycare centers
- Resident in long-term care facility, competitive athletes, incarceration

GENERAL PREVENTION

- Colonization (particularly of the anterior nares) is a risk factor for subsequent *S. aureus* infection. It is unclear whether this is similar for CA-MRSA. Oropharyngeal and inguinal colonization are equally prevalent.
- CA-MRSA is transmitted easily through environmental and household contact.
- CDC guidance for prevention of MRSA in athletes: http://www.cdc.gov/mrsa/community /team-hc-providers/advice-for-athletes.html

COMMONLY ASSOCIATED CONDITIONS

Many patients are otherwise healthy.

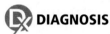 DIAGNOSIS

HISTORY

- Review risk factors.
- "Spider bite" is commonly confused with MRSA—patients often report a history of spider bite.
- Prior CA-MRSA skin infection
- Risk factors alone cannot rule in or rule out a CA-MRSA infection.

PHYSICAL EXAM

- Abscess, sometimes with surrounding cellulitis; nonsuppurative cellulitis is a much less common presentation of CA-MRSA.
- Erythema, warmth, tenderness, swelling; fluctuance; folliculitis, pustular lesions; tissue necrosis

DIFFERENTIAL DIAGNOSIS

SSTIs due to other organisms

DIAGNOSTIC TESTS & INTERPRETATION

Initial Tests (lab, imaging)

- Wound cultures establish definitive diagnosis. Culture a purulent lesion if there are systemic signs of illness or if the patient is immunocompromised (1)[B].
- Susceptibility testing; many labs use oxacillin instead of methicillin.
- "D-zone disk-diffusion test" evaluates for inducible clindamycin resistance if CA-MRSA is resistant to erythromycin.

- Ultrasound may help identify abscesses versus a non-drainable phlegmon; evidence suggests abscesses shallower than 0.4 cm may not need incision and drainage (I&D) (2).
- Look for fascial plane edema on CT or MRI if necrotizing fasciitis is suspected. DO NOT DELAY surgical intervention to obtain imaging in such cases.

Diagnostic Procedures/Other

I&D for purulent lesions; needle aspiration is not recommended (1). An effective alternative to I&D is the loop drainage technique.

 TREATMENT

- For purulent infections, surgical drainage for abscesses, wound culture, and narrow-spectrum antimicrobials
- See "Alert" section regarding the use of antibiotics in uncomplicated cases.
- Use antibiotics active against HA-MRSA for patients with abscesses if no response to initial antibiotic treatment, impaired host defenses, or systemic inflammatory response syndrome (SIRS) and hypotension (1).
- Packing may not improve outcomes. Moist heat may work for small abscesses.
- Extended antibiotic coverage for CA-MRSA is not warranted for nonsuppurative cellulitis.
- Routine elimination of MRSA colonization is not recommended in patients with active infection or for their close contacts.
- Most CA-MRSA infections are localized SSTIs and do not require hospitalization or vancomycin.
- Base initial antibiotic coverage on local CA-MRSA prevalence and individual risk factors.
- CDC guidance: https://www.cdc.gov/mrsa/pdf /Flowchart_pstr.pdf

GENERAL MEASURES

- Modify therapy based on culture and susceptibility.
- Treat underlying conditions that may predispose susceptibility to bacterial infection (e.g., tinea pedis).
- Restrict contact (e.g., sports competition) if wound cannot be covered.
- Elevate affected area.

MEDICATION

ALERT

Studies have shown a role for narrow-spectrum antibiotics in addition to surgical drainage. Clindamycin or trimethoprim/sulfamethoxazole (TMP/SMX) for abscesses <5 cm results in improved cure rates at 7 to 14 days (number needed to treat is 7 to 14).

First Line

Antibiotics for CA-MRSA SSTIs: 7- to 14-day course (depends on severity and clinical response):

- TMP/SMX: DS (160 mg TMP and 800 mg of SMX) 1 to 2 tablet(s) PO q12h; children, 8 to 12 mg/kg/day PO of trimethoprim component in 2 divided doses

- Doxycycline or minocycline: 100 mg PO q12h; children, >8 years and <45 kg, 2 to 5 mg/kg/day PO in 1 to 2 divided doses, not to exceed 200 mg/day; >8 years and >45 kg, use adult dosing; taken with a full glass of water
- Clindamycin: 300 to 450 mg PO q6h; children, 30 to 40 mg/kg/day PO in 3 divided doses; taken with full glass of water; check D-zone test in erythromycin-resistant, clindamycin-susceptible *S. aureus* isolates (a positive test indicates induced resistance—choose a different antibiotic).
- CA-MRSA is resistant to β-lactams (including oral cephalosporins and antistaphylococcal penicillins) and often macrolides, azalides, and quinolones.
- Although most CA-MRSA isolates are susceptible to rifampin, this drug should *never* be used as a single agent because of concerns regarding resistance. The role of combination therapy with rifampin in CA-MRSA SSTIs is not clearly defined.
- There has been increasing resistance to clindamycin, both initial (~33%) and induced.
- Although CA-MRSA isolates are susceptible to vancomycin, oral vancomycin cannot be used for CA-MRSA SSTIs due to limited absorption.

Second Line
Treat severe CA-MRSA SSTIs requiring hospitalization and HA-MRSA SSTIs using:

- Vancomycin: generally, 1 g IV q12h (30 mg/kg/day IV in 2 divided doses); children: 40 mg/kg/day IV in 4 divided doses; vancomycin-like antibiotics that require only 1 or 2 doses are also available.
- Linezolid: 600 mg IV/PO q12h; children, uncomplicated: <5 years of age, 30 mg/kg/day IV/PO in 3 divided doses; 5 to 11 years of age, 20 mg/kg/day IV/PO in 2 divided doses; >11 years, use adult dosing; children, complicated: birth to 11 years, 30 mg/kg/day IV/PO in 3 divided doses; for older children, use adult dosing.
  – Linezolid seems to be more effective than vancomycin for treating people with SSTIs, but current studies have high risk of bias.
- Clindamycin: 600 mg IV q8h; children, 10 to 13 mg/kg/dose IV q6–8h up to 40 mg/kg/day
- Daptomycin: 4 mg/kg/day IV; children, 1 to <2 years, 10 mg/kg IV once daily; 2 to 6 years, 9 mg/kg IV once daily; 7 to 11 years, 7 mg/kg IV once daily; 12 to 17 years, 5 mg/kg IV once daily; ≥18 years, adult dosing
  – Do not use if pulmonary involvement.
- Ceftaroline: 600 mg IV q12h; children, 0* to <2 months, 6 mg/kg IV q8h; 2 months to <2 years, 8 mg/kg IV q8h; ≥2 years to <18 years and ≤33 kg, 12 mg/kg IV q8h; ≥2 years to <18 years and >33 kg, 400 mg IV q8h OR 600 mg IV q12h; ≥18 years, adult dosing.
  – *Gestational age ≥34 weeks and postnatal age ≥12 days

Pediatric Considerations
- Tetracyclines are not recommended for patients aged <8 years for CA-MRSA (in contrast with their position as treatment of choice in tickborne rickettsial diseases).
- TMP/SMX is not recommended for patients aged <2 months.

- Daptomycin is not recommended in pediatric patients <1 year of age (risk of potential muscular, neuromuscular, and/or nervous system side effects).
- Daptomycin dosage adjustment for pediatric patients with renal impairment has not been established.
- Ceftaroline dosage adjustment for pediatric patients with CrCl ≤50 mL/min/1.73 m² has not been established.

Pregnancy Considerations
- Tetracyclines are contraindicated.
- TMP/SMX not recommended in 1st or 3rd trimester

Geriatric Considerations
A recent review notes no prospective trials in this age group and recommends the use of general adult guidelines.

ISSUES FOR REFERRAL
Consider consultation with infectious disease specialist if:
- Refractory CA-MRSA infection; plan to attempt decolonization.

SURGERY/OTHER PROCEDURES
Concern for serious SSTIs (including necrotizing fasciitis) mandates prompt surgical evaluation.

ADMISSION, INPATIENT, AND NURSING CONSIDERATIONS
- Consider admission if:
  – Systemically ill; extensive soft tissue involvement; comorbidities that may delay or complicate resolution of SSTI; immunocompromised status; failure to improve despite appropriate oral antibiotic therapy
  – Presence of SSTI complications (sepsis, necrotizing fasciitis) and comorbidities
- Alternatives to inpatient admission include observation units and outpatient parenteral antimicrobial therapy (OPAT) in carefully selected cases.
- Nursing: contact precautions
- If admitted for IV therapy, assess the following before discharge:
  – Afebrile for 24 hours; clinically improved; able to take oral medication
  – Has adequate social support and is available for outpatient follow-up

 ONGOING CARE

Patients who present with IV drug use should be effectively connected to ongoing substance use disorder care.

FOLLOW-UP RECOMMENDATIONS
Patient Monitoring
For outpatients: Promptly return for care with systemic symptoms, worsening local symptoms, or failure to improve within 48 hours. Consider a follow-up within 48 hours of initial visit to assess response and review culture.

PATIENT EDUCATION
- Cover draining wounds with clean, dry bandages.
- Clean hands regularly with soap and water or alcohol-based gel; hot soapy shower daily
- Do not share items that may be contaminated (including razors or towels). Clean clothes, towels, and bed linens.
- CDC MRSA education: https://www.cdc.gov/mrsa/
- A mixture of 1/4 cup household bleach diluted in 1 gallon of water cleans potentially contaminated surfaces.

PROGNOSIS
In outpatients, improvement should occur within 48 hours.

COMPLICATIONS
- Necrotizing pneumonia or empyema (after an influenza-like illness); necrotizing fasciitis
- Sepsis syndrome; pyomyositis and osteomyelitis
- Purpura fulminans
- Disseminated septic emboli; endocarditis

REFERENCES
1. Stevens DL, Bisno AL, Chambers HF, et al; for Infectious Diseases Society of America. Practice guidelines for the diagnosis and management of skin and soft tissue infections: 2014 update by the Infectious Diseases Society of America. *Clin Infect Dis*. 2014;59(2):e10–e52.
2. Howarth K, Thoppil J, Salazar GA. Emergency department management of cellulitis and other skin and soft-tissue infections. *Emerg Med Pract*. 2022;24(5):1–24.

ADDITIONAL READING
Yueh CM, Chi H, Chiu NC, et al. Etiology, clinical features, management, and outcomes of skin and soft tissue infections in hospitalized children: a 10-year review. *J Microbiol Immunol Infect*. 2022;55(4):728–739.

CODES

ICD10
- A49.02 Methicillin resis staph infection, unsp site
- A41.02 Sepsis due to Methicillin resistant Staphylococcus aureus
- J15.212 Pneumonia due to Methicillin resistant Staphylococcus aureus

CLINICAL PEARLS
- Incise and drain abscesses and send purulent material for culture and sensitivity.
- Local susceptibility patterns of CA-MRSA should guide empiric antibiotic treatment.
- Expect clinical improvement within 48 hours.
- TMP/SMZ; doxycycline and clindamycin are first line oral agents for uncomplicated CA-MRSA infections

COMPLEMENTARY AND ALTERNATIVE MEDICINE

Kelley V. Lawrence, MD, IBCLC • Mollie R. Lerner, DO, MS • Lauren A. Griffin, DO

BASICS

DESCRIPTION

Complementary and alternative medicine (CAM) are systems, practices, and products that are used in conjunction with or in place of conventional medicine.

- Integrative medicine is the coordinated combination of complementary medicine with conventional medicine.
- Examples:
  - Meditation, mindfulness, relaxation
  - Yoga
  - Specialized diets
  - Herbal supplements
  - Massage
  - Osteopathic manipulative therapy
  - Chiropractic therapy
  - Ayurveda
  - Qigong
  - Tai chi
- Common reasons patients choose CAM
  - Additive therapy to address issues not covered by conventional medical treatment
  - Conventional medicine has been unsuccessful in fully addressing the ailment.
  - Preventative health care and/or a desire for a more holistic/natural/noninvasive approach to well-being
  - Concern about medication side effects
  - Cultural or familial belief systems

EPIDEMIOLOGY

- The most common use is among 30- to 69-year-old females (1).
- CAM is most frequently used to treat musculoskeletal issues; 59–90% of patients claim that the use of alternative therapy helped their chronic pain (1).

Prevalence

Estimated 70% of North Americans have tried at least one form of CAM.

COMMONLY ASSOCIATED CONDITIONS

Acute/chronic pain, osteoarthritis, fibromyalgia, insomnia, fatigue, cancer-related symptoms and treatment side effects, headaches, irritable bowel syndrome (IBS), depression/anxiety, low libido, weight loss, asthma, eczema, tinnitus, autoimmune disease

DIAGNOSIS

HISTORY

- Impact of medical condition on patient's life
- Patient's beliefs and goals
- Patient's attitudes and experiences with conventional and alternative medical treatments
- All drugs being taken, including prescription drugs, vitamins, herbals, supplements, and over-the-counter medications
- Nutritional habits, exercise regimen, sleep hygiene
- Social interactions, support system, mood, spirituality

PHYSICAL EXAM

- Focused physical exam based on patient presentation
- If indicated, osteopathic structural exam: Observe gait and posture; screen for somatic dysfunctions, focusing on tissue texture changes, asymmetry, motion restriction, and tenderness.

DIAGNOSTIC TESTS & INTERPRETATION

Consider PHQ-9 and GAD-7 for behavioral health evaluation.

TREATMENT

Variable evidence supports the safety and efficacy of:

- Back pain: chiropractic therapy (2), OMT, massage therapy
- Nausea, including that associated with chemotherapy: ginger (2)
- Migraine prophylaxis: petasites (butterbur extract), riboflavin, CoQ10, magnesium (2)
- Anxiety, depression, and stress: music therapy, meditation, mindfulness-based stress reduction, yoga, massage therapy, relaxation techniques, acupuncture, exercise, light therapy (2),(3)
- Fatigue: qigong, acupuncture, ginseng (2),(3)

ISSUES FOR REFERRAL

- Patient preception of medical professional stigma toward CAM
- Minimal provider education and training in CAM
- Confirm certification and training of CAM providers when referring a patient.

ADDITIONAL THERAPIES

Herbal supplements may help with anxiety, depression, migraines, and cognitive impairment in patients with dementia.

- Anxiety:
  - Kava kava 50 to 70 mg PO up to 3 times daily
  - Ashwagandha 300 mg PO BID
- Depression:
  - St. John's wort 300 mg PO up to 3 times daily
  - 5-HTP 150 to 300 mg PO daily
  - SAMe 200 mg PO BID
  - Omega-3 1 g PO daily
- Migraines:
  - Magnesium 500 to 1,000 mg QHS
  - Riboflavin 200 mg PO BID with meals
  - CoQ10 150 to 300 mg daily
- Cognitive impairment in patients with dementia:
  - Ginkgo 240 mg PO daily
- Yoga, exercise, and light therapy help with depression.
  - Light therapy: 10,000 lux for 30 minutes in the early morning
  - Exercise: 30-minute moderate intensity 3 times per week
  - Yoga: 2 to 4 sessions weekly

ONGOING CARE

FOLLOW-UP RECOMMENDATIONS
Maintain contact and share records between primary care provider and CAM providers.

Patient Monitoring
When discussing current medication regimen, ask specifically for over-the-counter and herbal supplements.

PATIENT EDUCATION
- The National Center for Complementary and Integrative Health: https://nccih.nih.gov/
- Cleveland Clinic: Complementary medicine: what is it, types & health benefits: https://my.clevelandclinic.org/health/articles/16883-complementary-therapy

COMPLICATIONS

ALERT
- Patients may delay seeking medical care or consider replacement of curative conventional treatment.
- Ginkgo, goldenseal, and St. John's wort account for most reported herb–drug interactions.
- Herbs with possible adverse effects (3)
  – Black cohosh (*Actaea racemosa*) reduces the effectiveness of statins.
  – Ginkgo (*Ginkgo biloba*): increased bleeding time
  – Goldenseal (*Hydrastis canadensis*) interferes with many prescription medications.
  – Licorice (*Glycyrrhiza* spp.): Long-term use depletes serum potassium.
  – Senna (*Cassia angustifolia*): depletes serum potassium
  – St. John's wort (*Hypericum perforatum*): numerous drug interactions; induces CYP3A4 pathway, increasing metabolism: cyclosporine, tacrolimus, warfarin, protease inhibitors, theophylline, venlafaxine, digoxin, oral contraceptives
  – Wormwood (*Artemisia absinthium*): elevates serotonin level; may raise blood pressure
  – Yohimbe (*Pausinystalia yohimbe*): elevates blood pressure

Geriatric Considerations
- *Ginkgo biloba* can help improve cognition in patients with dementia; notably, ginkgo commonly interacts with warfarin.
- Incorporating integrative medicine into palliative care may be beneficial.
- Tai chi and yoga may reduce the risk/fear of falls and improve mobility in the elderly. Gentle chair yoga, as well as massage, acupuncture, and reiki, may be beneficial for fatigue in elderly cancer patients.

Pediatric Considerations
- Carob bean juice and preparations including *Matricaria chamomilla* and apple pectin were shown to significantly reduce the duration of diarrhea.
- Peppermint oil can decrease the duration, frequency, and severity of pain in children suffering from undifferentiated functional abdominal pain.
- Different fennel preparations were found to be useful in treating infantile colic.
- Iron is a leading cause of accidental poisoning in children <6 years of age.
- Vitamin A is the most common cause of hypervitaminosis.

REFERENCES

1. Urits I, Schwartz RH, Orhurhu V, et al. A comprehensive review of alternative therapies for the management of chronic pain patients: acupuncture, tai chi, osteopathic manipulative medicine, and chiropractic care. *Adv Ther*. 2021;38(1):76–89.
2. Ng JY, Liang L, Gagliardi AR. The quantity and quality of complementary and alternative medicine clinical practice guidelines on herbal medicines, acupuncture and spinal manipulation: systematic review and assessment using AGREE II. *BMC Complement Altern Med*. 2016;16(1):425.
3. Berman S, Mischoulon D, Naidoo U. Complementary medicine and natural medications in psychiatry: a guide for the consultation-liaison psychiatrist. *Psychosomatics*. 2020;61(5):508–517.

ADDITIONAL READING

- American Osteopathic Association. Tenets of osteopathic medicine. https://osteopathic.org/about/leadership/aoa-governance-documents/tenets-of-osteopathic-medicine. Accessed November 25, 2023.
- Rakel D. *Integrative Medicine*. 4th ed. Philadelphia, PA: Elsevier; 2017.

 CODES

ICD10
Z76.89 Persons encountering health services in other specified circumstances

CLINICAL PEARLS
- CAM allows clinicians to take a holistic approach to health, by focusing on treating the patient and not just the disease.
- Outcomes of CAM are best measured in terms of the patient's symptom relief, satisfaction, and functional status.
- OMT, chiropractic therapy, massage, tai chi, and acupuncture may help with chronic pain.
- Yoga, light therapy, and exercise are helpful for depression.
- Peppermint oil can help with abdominal pain associated with IBS.
- Ginkgo, goldenseal, and St. John's wort account for most herb–drug interactions.
- Tai chi can help with balance and reduce the risk of falls in the elderly. Tai chi is also an effective adjuvant therapy for fibromyalgia.

C

COMPLEX REGIONAL PAIN SYNDROME

Dennis E. Hughes, DO, FACEP

 BASICS

DESCRIPTION

- Complex regional pain syndrome (CRPS) is a pain syndrome that can be chronic and debilitating. It is divided into two subtypes and can result in significant physical and psychosocial short- and long-term disability. Most cases are a result of a physical insult to an extremity such as trauma or surgery. The lack of a dermatomal distribution (i.e., the pain is regional) distinguishes CPRS from other pain syndromes.
  - Type I: no nerve injury (reflex sympathetic dystrophy [RSD])
  - Type II: associated with a demonstrable nerve injury (causalgia)
- Synonym(s): traumatic erythromelalgia; Weir Mitchell causalgia; causalgia; RSD; posttraumatic neuralgia; sympathetically maintained pain

EPIDEMIOLOGY

- Peak age: 50 to 70 years
- Predominant gender: female > male (3:1, 60–81%), with postmenopausal women affected disproportionally.
- Rarely seen in pediatrics—cases in this age group predominantly involve lower extremities in females.
- Recent studies found 3.8% occurrence after wrist fracture and 7% occurrence after intra-articular ankle fracture—both independent strong risk for CRPS. Fractures and sprains are associated in ~60% of cases, the remaining 40% have less precise or no recognized inciting event. Upper extremities are more commonly involved.
- CPRS is more prevalent in patients who report higher than commonly expected pain in early phases of trauma. Latency depends on normal injury recovery time—prolonged pain (>2 months) after injury hints at diagnosis.

Incidence

Incidence of 5.46 to 26.2/100,000 for type I and 0.82/100,000 for type II in the United States

ETIOLOGY AND PATHOPHYSIOLOGY

- Poorly understood activation of abnormal sympathetic reflex that lowers pain threshold. The process is multifactorial and involves both central and peripheral nervous systems.
  - Increased excitability of nociceptive neurons in the spinal cord; "central sensitization"
  - Exaggerated responses to normally nonpainful stimuli (hyperalgesia, allodynia)
  - The exaggerated inflammatory response results in afferent neurons releasing increased amounts of neuropeptides (1).
- Type II is associated with physical injury to nerve. This represents a minority of cases.
- Emerging information reveals CNS changes (functional, anatomic, biochemical) in addition to spinal level changes. Increased levels of immunomodulators suggest autoimmune component. The lack of a definitive pathophysiologic mechanism has led to suggest that CRPS is a "functional neurologic syndrome."

Genetics

No known genetic pattern

RISK FACTORS

- Minor or severe trauma (upper extremity fracture—particularly distal radius noted in a significant number of those with CRPS)
- Surgery (particularly carpal tunnel release)
- Lacerations, burns, frostbite
- Casting/immobilization after extremity injury
- Penetrating injury (case reports of CRPS developing after snakebites)
- Polymyalgia rheumatica
- Myocardial infarction, cerebral vascular accident
- Reports of CRPS development after "innocuous" events such as IV catheters and IM injections

GENERAL PREVENTION

- Early mobilization and avoiding prolonged immobilization has proven to benefit in reducing incidence of CRPS.
- One study of wrist fractures found that addition of 500 mg/day of vitamin C lowered the rates of CRPS.
- There is evidence that limiting use of tourniquets, liberal regional anesthetic use, and ensuring adequate perioperative analgesia can reduce the incidence of CRPS-I.

COMMONLY ASSOCIATED CONDITIONS

- Serious injury to bone and soft tissue
- Herpes zoster postherpetic neuralgia results from partial or complete damage to afferent nerve pathways that occurs in a dermatomal distribution.
- Signal exists for patients having comorbid painful conditions or psychiatric diagnosis at increased risk of developing CRPS.

DIAGNOSIS

Unprovoked pain is the hallmark of the condition, and the diagnosis of CRPS is excluded by the existence of conditions that would otherwise account for the degree of symptoms. Budapest clinical diagnostic criteria can aid in establishing diagnosis:

- Continuing pain which is disproportionate to any inciting event
- At least one symptom in three of the four following categories:
  - Sensory: hyperalgesia and/or allodynia
  - Vasomotor: skin, temperature, color asymmetry
  - Sudomotor/edema: edema, sweating changes, or sweating asymmetry
  - Motor/trophic: decreased range of motion or motor dysfunction and/or trophic changes (hair, nail, skin)
- Must display one sign at the time of the evaluation in two or more of the following:
  - Sensory: hyperalgesia (to pinprick) or allodynia (to light touch, pressure, or joint movement)
  - Vasomotor: evidence of temperature, skin, color asymmetry

  - Sudomotor/edema: evidence of edema or sweating changes or asymmetry
  - Motor/trophic: decreased range of motion; motor dysfunction; or trophic changes in hair, nails, skin
- There is no other diagnosis that explains the signs and symptoms.

HISTORY

The patient commonly complains of persistent burning pain, swelling, and poor function after extremity injury. The severity of the preceding injury may vary from fracture to relatively minor trauma.

PHYSICAL EXAM

- The affected extremity appears swollen with erythematous, shiny skin with brittle nails, and reduced hair.
- The patient usually exhibits limited range of motion—both active and passive in the affected extremity.

DIFFERENTIAL DIAGNOSIS

- Infection
- Hypertrophic scar
- Neuroma
- CNS tumor or syrinx
- Deep vein thrombosis or thrombophlebitis
- Thoracic outlet syndrome
- Connective tissue disorder
- Factitious

DIAGNOSTIC TESTS & INTERPRETATION

The diagnosis of CRPS does not require any specific testing—it is a clinical diagnosis. It is a symptom-based diagnosis of exclusion. Testing is performed to rule out other potential etiologies of clinical symptoms (2).

Initial Tests (lab, imaging)

- CBC, erythrocyte sedimentation rate (ESR)
- Plain radiographs may show patchy demineralization within 3 to 6 weeks of onset of CRPS that are more pronounced than would be seen from disuse alone.
- Three-phase bone scanning has varying sensitivity but is most accurate for support of the diagnosis when there is diffuse activity (especially on phase 3).
- Bone density

Diagnostic Procedures/Other

- Electromyography (EMG) shows nerve injury with type II CRPS.
- Sudomotor function testing (resting sweat testing, resting skin temperature, quantitative sudomotor axon reflex testing; all related to increased autonomic activity of the affected limb)

Test Interpretation

- Partial or complete damage to afferent nerve pathways and probably reorganized central pain pathways
- Nerves most commonly involved are median and sciatic.
- Atrophy in affected muscles
- Incomplete nerve plexus lesion

TREATMENT

GENERAL MEASURES

Discourage maladaptive behaviors (pain medication seeking, secondary gain). Principal of functional restoration is a stepwise and multidisciplinary approach. Early and aggressive mobilization seems to lessen the duration. Avoidance of opiates cannot be overemphasized.

MEDICATION

First Line

- NSAIDs are recommended early in course but have mixed support in literature. The following have literature support of a suggestive benefit in treatment of CRPS-I:
  – Corticosteroids (prednisone 30 mg/day × 2 to 12 weeks with taper) are the only class of drugs that have direct clinical trial support early in the course. A recent retrospective case review found that patients showed significant improvement with various measurable physical parameters after treatment with prednisolone (30 mg starting dose tapering by 5 mg every 3 days for a total of 3 weeks treatment).
  – Gabapentin 600 to 1,800 mg/day for 8 weeks following diagnosis
  – DMSO 50% cream applied to affected extremity up to 5 times daily
  – N-Acetylcysteine 600 mg TID
  – Bisphosphonates (alendronate) at 40 mg/day (however, optimal dose uncertain)
  – Nifedipine 20 mg/day showed benefit early in the course of the condition.
- Although many have advocated the use of tricyclic antidepressants in the treatment of CRPS, there is no credible evidence of improvement of pain. They may be helpful in controlling depressive symptoms that develop with disease progression.

ISSUES FOR REFERRAL

- After 2 months of the illness, psychological evaluation generally is indicated to identify and treat any comorbid conditions. Depressive symptoms frequently develop.
- Physical therapy and occupational therapy early for guided motor and mirror therapy

ADDITIONAL THERAPIES

Type I
- Physical and occupational therapy (beneficial to the overall prognosis for recovery) and should be initiated early in the course of treatment
  – "Mirror therapy" has shown good results.
  – Case reports of patients responding favorably to passive ROM treatment under sedation followed by multiple physical therapy sessions
- Transcutaneous nerve stimulation

- Psychotherapy
- Use of subdissociative (0.2 to 0.5 mg/kg) infusions of ketamine has shown some promise, but effects seem to be time limited; systemic literature review failed to find a high-quality support for ketamine treatment.

SURGERY/OTHER PROCEDURES

- Type II responds more favorably to nerve-directed treatment.
  – Sympathetic blocks
  – Cervicothoracic or lumbar sympathectomies have little data to support their use and should be used judiciously and after all other therapies have failed.
- Anesthetic blockade (chemical or surgical) of sympathetic nerve function
  – Transient relief suggests that chemical or surgical sympathectomy will be helpful.
  – Little in the way of quality clinical trials exist to support local sympathetic blockage as the gold standard of therapy.
- IV regional sympathetic block with guanethidine or reserpine by pain specialist or anesthetist
- Transcutaneous electric nerve stimulation (controversial)
- Inject myofascial painful trigger points.
- Dorsal root ganglion (DRG) stimulation higher rate of success than spinal cord stimulation in recent comparative study; more specific target as DRG home of soma of sensory neurons
- Intrathecal analgesia
- Amputation as a last resort in severe cases, with patients reporting improved quality of life
- Single case study of topical 5% lidocaine revealed significant pain reduction and improved range of motion and function.
- Osteopathic manipulation (case report literature)

COMPLEMENTARY & ALTERNATIVE MEDICINE

- Vitamin C (500 mg/day) may help to prevent CRPS in those with wrist fracture.
- Cognitive behavioral therapy
- Acupuncture
- Hypnosis and guided imagery have been successful in improving pain scores.
- Relaxation training (alternate muscle relaxing and contracting)
- Biofeedback
- Whirlpool baths

ADMISSION, INPATIENT, AND NURSING CONSIDERATIONS

Only for proposed surgical therapy

 ONGOING CARE

FOLLOW-UP RECOMMENDATIONS

Weekly, to monitor progress and initiate additional modalities as needed

PATIENT EDUCATION

- Counsel to remain active physically.
- Reflex Sympathetic Dystrophy Syndrome Association: http://rsds.org/; 203-877-3790

PROGNOSIS

Most improve with early treatment, but symptoms may be lifelong if there is limited response to initial treatments.

COMPLICATIONS

- Depression
- Disability
- Opioid dependence

REFERENCES

1. Prasad A, Chakravarthy K. Review of complex regional pain syndrome and the role of the neuroimmune axis. *Mol Pain*. 2021;17:17448069211006617.
2. Mesaroli G, Hundert A, Birnie KA, et al. Screening and diagnostic tools for complex regional pain syndrome: a systematic review. *Pain*. 2021;162(5):1295–1304.

ADDITIONAL READING

Eldufani J, Elahmer N, Blaise G. A medical mystery of complex regional pain syndrome. *Heliyon*. 2020;6(2):e03329.

 CODES

ICD10

- G90.52 Complex regional pain syndrome I of lower limb
- G90.523 Complex regional pain syndrome I of lower limb, bilateral
- G56.4 Causalgia of upper limb

CLINICAL PEARLS

- A pain syndrome disproportioned to injury
- Pain control and early mobility are the key to recovery.
- Avoid use of opiate analgesics.
- Use a multidisciplinary approach.

CONDYLOMATA ACUMINATA

Megan Ann Christopher, MD, MPH • Victoria Shepard, MD

BASICS

DESCRIPTION

- Condylomata acuminata are soft, skin-colored, fleshy lesions (commonly called genital warts) that are caused by human papillomavirus (HPV). Warts appear singly or in groups (a single wart is a "condyloma"; multiple warts are "condylomas" or "condylomata"); small or large; typically appear on the anogenital skin (penis, scrotum, introitus, vulva, perianal area); and may occur in the anogenital tract (vagina, cervix, rectum, urethra, anus); also conjunctival, nasal, oral, and laryngeal warts
- System(s) affected: skin/exocrine, reproductive, occasionally respiratory

Pediatric Considerations
- Consider sexual abuse if seen in children, although children can be infected by other means (e.g., transfer from wart on another child's hand or prolonged latency period) (1).
- American Academy of Pediatrics recommends all school-aged children who present with lesions be evaluated for abuse and screened for other STDs (1).

Pregnancy Considerations
- Warts often grow larger, increase in number, and become more friable in pregnancy (2). They can regress spontaneously after delivery.
- Neonatal infection is thought to occur through vertical transmission. Incidence remains controversial.
- Few documented cases of laryngeal papillomas due to HPV transmission at the time of delivery. Although rare, the condition is life-threatening. Cesarean section solely to prevent transmission of HPV to the newborn is not indicated (2).
- Cervical infection has been found to be a risk factor for preterm birth.
- HPV vaccination is contraindicated in pregnancy.
- Treatment during pregnancy is somewhat controversial because it can be incomplete, but accepted treatments are trichloroacetic acid (TCA), cryotherapy, electrocautery, or surgical excision.
- The safety of sinecatechins, podophyllin, and podofilox in pregnant women has not been established, and these agents are not recommended for use during pregnancy (2).There is an emerging data that shows imiquimod is low risk in pregnancy.

EPIDEMIOLOGY
- HPV types 6 and 11 are associated with 90% of condylomata acuminata. Types 16, 18, 31, 33, and 35 may be found in warts and may be associated with high-grade intraepithelial dysplasia in immuno-compromised states such as HIV.
- Highly contagious; incubation period may be from 1 to 8 months. Initial infections may very well go unrecognized, so a "new" outbreak may be a relapse of an infection acquired years prior.
- Predominant age: 15 to 30 years
- Predominant sex: 1:1 male to female
- Most infections are transient and clear spontaneously within 2 years.

Incidence
One study population demonstrated that from 2007 to 2010, with the introduction of HPV vaccines, the incidence of genital warts decreased 35% (from 0.94% per year to 0.61% per year) in females aged <21 years and decreased 19% in males aged <21 years.

Prevalence
- Most common viral sexually transmitted infection (STI) in the United States; most sexually active men and women will have acquired a genital HPV infection, usually asymptomatic, at some time.
- Estimated 6.2 million Americans become infected with genital HPV each year.
- Peak prevalence in ages 17 to 33 years
- 10–20% of sexually active women may be actively infected with HPV. Studies in men suggest a similar prevalence.
- Pregnancy and immunosuppression favor recurrence and increased growth of lesions.

ETIOLOGY AND PATHOPHYSIOLOGY
HPV is a circular, double-stranded DNA molecule. There are >120 HPV subtypes. HPV types that cause genital warts do not cause anogenital cancers.

RISK FACTORS
- Usually acquired by unprotected sexual activity
  - Young adults and adolescents
  - Multiple sexual partners; short interval between meeting new sex partner and first intercourse
  - Not using protective barriers
  - Young age of commencing sexual activity
  - History of other STI
- Immunosuppression (particularly HIV)
- Cigarette smoking
- Use of oral contraceptives
- Radiation therapy

GENERAL PREVENTION
- Sexual abstinence or monogamy
- HPV vaccination is for prevention of HPV infections and HPV-associated cancers. This vaccine is targeted to adolescents before the period of their greatest risk for exposure to HPV. The vaccine does not treat previous infections:
  - The Advisory Committee on Immunization Practices (ACIP) recommends routine vaccination at age 11 or 12 years for females (since 2006) and males. Vaccination can start at as early as 9 years old.
  - A 2-dose schedule (0, 6 to 12 months) will have efficacy equivalent to a 3-dose schedule (0, 1 to 2, 6 months) if the HPV vaccination series is initiated before the 15th birthday.
  - For any immunocompromised patient regardless of age, a 3-dose schedule (0, 1 to 2, and 6 months) is recommended (2).
  - The 9-valent HPV (9vHPV; Gardasil 9) vaccine protects against the two most common HPV serotypes (types 6 and 11, which cause most anogenital warts) and the two most cancer-promoting types (16 and 18) as well as 31, 33, 45, 52, and 58.
  - Bivalent HPV, quadrivalent HPV (4vHPV), and 9vHPV vaccines (Gardasil and Gardasil 9) are licensed for use in females and males aged 9 through 45 years, but as of late 2016, only the 9vHPV vaccines are distributed in the United States.
- Use of condoms is partially effective, although warts may be easily spread by lesions not covered by a condom (e.g., 40% of infected men have scrotal warts).
- After treatment, encourage abstinence until treatment is completed.

COMMONLY ASSOCIATED CONDITIONS
- >90% of cervical cancer associated with HPV types 16, 18, 31, 33, and 35
- 60% of oropharyngeal and anogenital squamous cell carcinomas are associated with HPV.
- STIs (e.g., gonorrhea, syphilis, chlamydia), AIDS

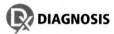

DIAGNOSIS

HISTORY
- Explore sexual history, contraception use, and other lifestyle topics.
- Most warts are asymptomatic, but symptoms include pruritus, burning, redness, pain, bleeding, and vaginal discharge, and large warts may cause obstructive symptoms in the anus (with defecation) or vaginal canal (with intercourse or childbirth).

PHYSICAL EXAM
- Lesions often have a typical rough, warty appearance with multiple fingerlike projections but may be soft, sessile, and smooth.
- Large lesions are cauliflower-like and may grow to >10 cm.
- Most common sites: penis, vaginal introitus, and perianal region
- May be seen anywhere on the anogenital epithelium or in the anogenital tract
- Warts often occur in clusters.
- Bleeding or irritation of the lesions may be noted.

DIFFERENTIAL DIAGNOSIS
- Condylomata lata (flat warts of syphilis), lichen planus
- Normal sebaceous glands, seborrheic keratosis
- Molluscum contagiosum, keratomas, micropapillomatosis
- Scabies, skin tags, melanocytic nevi
- Vulvar intraepithelial neoplasia, squamous cell carcinoma

DIAGNOSTIC TESTS & INTERPRETATION
- Diagnosis is usually clinical, made by unaided visual examination of the lesions; biopsy if needed
- Acetowhitening test: Subclinical lesions can be visualized by applying moistened gauze soaked with 5% acetic acid (vinegar) to the affected area for 5 minutes. Using a 10× hand lens or colposcope, warts appear as tiny white papules. A shiny white appearance of the skin represents foci of epithelial hyperplasia (subclinical infection), but because of low specificity, the CDC recommends against routine use of this test to screen for HPV mucosal infection.

Initial Tests (lab, imaging)
- Usually not required for diagnosis; serologic tests for syphilis may be helpful to rule out condylomata lata.
- Other testing for STIs; Pap smear may be indicated.

Follow-Up Tests & Special Considerations
Because squamous cell carcinoma may resemble or coexist with condylomata, biopsy may be considered for lesions refractory to therapy.

Diagnostic Procedures/Other
- Biopsy with highly specialized identification techniques, such as HPV DNA detected through polymerase chain reaction, is rarely useful.
- Colposcopy, antroscopy, anoscopy, and urethroscopy may be required to detect anogenital tract lesions.
- Screening men who have sex with men (MSM) with anal Pap smears is controversial.

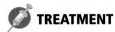 TREATMENT

GENERAL MEASURES
- Approximately, 30% resolve spontaneously in 4 months.
- Change therapy if no improvement after three treatments, clearance not complete after six treatments, or therapy's duration or dosage exceeds manufacturer's recommendations.
- Appropriate screening/counseling of partners
- HIV considerations: Treatment of external genital warts should not be different for HIV-infected persons.
  - Lesions may be larger or more numerous.
  - May not respond as well to therapy as immunocompetent persons

MEDICATION
First Line
- No single therapy for genital warts is ideal for all patients or clearly superior to other therapies.
- Recommendations for external genital warts, patient applied:
  - Podofilox (Condylox) (2)[A]: may be the most effective topical (3)[A]; antimitotic action; apply 0.5% solution or gel to warts twice daily (allowing to dry) for 3 consecutive days at home followed by 4 days of no therapy; may repeat up to 4 total cycles; maximum of 0.5 mL/day or area <10 cm².
  - Imiquimod (Aldara) (2)[A]: immune enhancer; self-treatment with a 5% cream applied once daily at bedtime 3 times weekly until warts resolve for up to 16 weeks. Wash off with soap and water 6 to 10 hours after application. Imiquimod has been noted to weaken condoms and diaphragms; therefore, patients should refrain from sexual contact while the cream is on the skin.
  - Sinecatechins (Veregen) (2): immune enhancer and antioxidant, extract from green tea; apply a 0.5-cm strand of ointment 3 times daily for up to 16 weeks. Do not wash off after.

- Recommendations for external genital warts, provider applied:
  - Cryotherapy: liquid nitrogen applied to warts for two bursts of approximately 10 seconds (or whatever time is needed to freeze the wart without extension significantly deep or lateral to the wart) with thawing in between; usually requires 2 to 3 weekly sessions (2)[A]
  - Podophyllin 10–25% in tincture of benzoin; apply directly to warts and air-dry in office before coming into contact with clothes. Wash off in 1 to 4 hours. Repeat every 7 days in office until gone (2)[A].
  - TCA: 80% solution; apply only to warts; powder/talc to remove unreacted acid; repeat in office at weekly intervals; ideal for isolated lesions in pregnancy (2)[A]
- Recommendations for cervical warts: cryotherapy, surgical removal, TCA or bichloroacetic acid (BCA); for exophytic cervical warts: biopsy to exclude high-grade squamous intraepithelial lesion (HSIL) prior to starting treatment (2)[A]
- Recommendations for vaginal warts: cryotherapy, surgical removal, TCA or BCA 80–90% (2)[A]
- Recommendations for urethral meatus warts: cryotherapy or surgical removal (2)[A]
- Recommendations for anal warts: cryotherapy, TCA or BCA 80–90%, or surgery; specialty consultation for intra-anal warts (2)[A]

Pregnancy Considerations
Cryotherapy, surgery, or TCA; medications contraindicated in pregnancy: podophyllin, podophyllotoxin, sinecatechins, interferon, and imiquimod (2)[C]

Second Line
Podophyllin resin, intralesional interferon, photodynamic therapy, topical cidofovir (2)[A]

SURGERY/OTHER PROCEDURES
- Larger warts may require surgical excision, laser treatment, or electrocoagulation (including infrared therapy). Precaution: Laser treatment may create smoke plumes that contain HPV. CDC recommendation is for the use of a smoke evacuator no >2 inches from the surgical site. Masks are recommended; N95 is the most efficacious.
- Intraurethral, external (penile and perianal), anal, and oral lesions can be treated with fulgurating CO_2 laser. Oral or external penile/perianal lesions can also be treated with electrocautery or surgery.

 ONGOING CARE

FOLLOW-UP RECOMMENDATIONS
No restrictions, except for sexual contact

Patient Monitoring
- Patients should be seen every 1 to 2 weeks until lesions resolve.
- Patients should follow up 3 months after completion of treatment.
- Persistent warts require biopsy.
- Sexual partners require monitoring.

PATIENT EDUCATION
- Provide information on HPV, STI prevention, and condom use.
- Explain to patients that it is difficult to know how or when a person acquired an HPV infection; a diagnosis in one partner does not prove sexual infidelity in the other partner.
- Emphasize the need for women to follow recommendations for regular Pap smears.

PROGNOSIS
- Asymptomatic infection persists indefinitely.
- Treatment has not clearly been shown to decrease transmissible infectivity.
- Warts may clear with treatment or resolve spontaneously. However, recurrences are frequent, particularly in the first 3 months, and may necessitate repeated treatments.

COMPLICATIONS
- Cervical dysplasia (probably does not occur with type 6 or 11, which cause most warts)
- Malignant change: Progression of condylomata to cancer rarely, if ever, occurs, although squamous cell carcinoma may coexist in larger warts.
- Urethral, vaginal, or anal obstruction from treatment
- The prevalence of high-grade dysplasia and cancer in anal canal is higher in HIV-positive than in HIV-negative patients, probably because of increased HPV activity.

REFERENCES
1. Unger ER, Fajman NN, Maloney EM, et al. Anogenital human papillomavirus in sexually abused and nonabused children: a multicenter study. *Pediatrics*. 2011;128(3):e658–e665.
2. Workowski KA, Bachmann LH, Chan PA, et al. Sexually transmitted infections treatment guidelines, 2021. *MMWR Recomm Rep*. 2021;70(4):1–187.
3. Barton S, Wakefield V, O'Mahony C, et al. Effectiveness of topical and ablative therapies in treatment of anogenital warts: a systematic review and network meta-analysis. *BMJ Open*. 2019;9(10):e027765.

CODES

ICD10
A63.0 Anogenital (venereal) warts

CLINICAL PEARLS
- The majority of sexually active men and women will have acquired a genital HPV infection, usually asymptomatic, at some time.
- No single therapy for genital warts is ideal for all patients or clearly superior to other therapies.
- 9vHPV vaccine is effective in preventing HPV infection, particularly if administered prior to the onset of engaging in sexual activity. Gardasil is approved and recommended for use in males and females aged 9 to 45 years.

CONJUNCTIVITIS, ACUTE

Frances Yung-tao Wu, MD

BASICS

DESCRIPTION
Inflammation of the bulbar and/or palpebral conjunctiva of <4 weeks' duration

Geriatric Considerations
- Suspect bacterial, autoimmune, or irritative process.
- If purulent, risk of bacterial cause increases with age and long-term care facility residence, with age >65 years and bilateral lid adherence. Risk for bacterial infection is >70%.

Pediatric Considerations
Neonatal conjunctivitis may be gonococcal, chlamydial, irritative, or related to dacryocystitis. Children <5 years of age are more likely to have bacterial involvement than adults, but most self-resolve in 2 to 5 days. Despite lack of evidence, some daycare regulations may require a child with presumed conjunctivitis to be treated with a topical antibiotic before returning.

EPIDEMIOLOGY
- Predominant age
  - Pediatric: viral, bacterial, irritant; adult: bacterial, viral, allergic, irritant
- Predominant sex: male = female

Incidence
1–2% of ambulatory office visits, up to 3% of ER visits

ETIOLOGY AND PATHOPHYSIOLOGY
- Viral
  - Adenovirus (common cold), coxsackievirus; enterovirus (acute hemorrhagic conjunctivitis); herpes simplex; herpes zoster or varicella; measles, mumps, or influenza; SARS-CoV-2
- Bacterial
  - *Staphylococcus aureus*, MRSA or *Staphylococcus epidermidis*; *Streptococcus pneumoniae*; *Haemophilus influenzae* (children)
  - *Pseudomonas* spp. or anaerobes (contact lenses users); *Acanthamoeba*-contaminated contact lenses solution (rare; ~30 cases/year in the United States); *Neisseria gonorrhoeae*; *Chlamydia trachomatis*: gradual onset 1 to 4 weeks
- Allergic
  - Hay fever, seasonal allergies, atopy
- Nonspecific
  - Irritative: topical medications, wind, dry eye, UV light exposure, smoke, chlorine
  - Autoimmune: Sjögren syndrome, pemphigoid, Wegener granulomatosis, Reiter syndrome, sarcoid

RISK FACTORS
- History of contact with infected persons; sexually transmitted disease (STD) contact: gonococcal, chlamydial, syphilis, or herpes; contact lenses: pseudomonal or acanthamoeba keratitis
- Epidemic bacterial (streptococcal) conjunctivitis reported in school settings, epidemic adenoviral transmission in crowded settings, MRSA in long-term care facilities

GENERAL PREVENTION
- Wash hands frequently.
- Eyedropper technique: while eye is closed and head back, several drops over nasal canthus and then open the eyes to allow liquid to enter; never touch the tip of the dropper to skin or eye.

COMMONLY ASSOCIATED CONDITIONS
Viral infection (e.g., common cold); possible sexually transmitted infection

DIAGNOSIS

HISTORY

ALERT
Red flag: Any decrease in visual acuity is not consistent with conjunctivitis alone; must document normal vision for diagnosis of true isolated conjunctivitis

- Viral: contact or travel; may start with one eye and then both; if herpetic, recurrences or vesicles on skin
- Bacterial: difficult to distinguish from viral; assume bacterial in contact lenses wearer, unless cultures are negative. If recent STD, suspect chlamydia/gonococcus. Nursing home residents may have MRSA conjunctivitis—obtain culture.
- Allergic: itching, atopy, seasonal, dander
- Irritative: feels dry, exposure to wind, tear-film deficit may persist 30 days after acute conjunctivitis, chlorine from pools. Medications: atropine, aminoglycosides, iodide, phenylephrine, antivirals, bisphosphonates, retinoids, topiramate, chamomile, COX-2 inhibitors, immune modulators
- Foreign body: Redness may persist 24 hours after removal.

PHYSICAL EXAM
- Must document normal visual acuity
- General: common to all types of conjunctivitis
  - Red eye, conjunctival injection; foreign-body sensation
  - Eyelid sticking or crusting, discharge; normal visual acuity and pupillary reactivity
- Viral
  - Pharyngitis, preauricular lymphadenopathy, and/or recent infectious contact makes viral diagnosis much more likely.
  - Hemorrhagic coxsackievirus, adenoviral epidemics seen in health care facilities and community
  - Severe viral: herpes simplex or zoster: burning sensation, rarely itching; unilateral, dermatomal distribution herpetic skin vesicles in zoster; palpable preauricular node
- Bacterial (non-STD): may be epidemic
  - Mucopurulent discharge or concomitant otitis media make bacterial diagnosis twice as likely (1)[A].
  - Conjunctival chemosis/edema
  - If contact lenses user, must rule out pseudomonal (or other bacterial) keratitis. If long-term care resident, culture to rule out MRSA.
- Bacterial: gonococcal (or meningococcal) hyperacute infection
  - Rapid onset 12 to 24 hours; severe purulent discharge; chemosis/conjunctival/eyelid edema
  - Rapid growth of superior corneal ulceration; preauricular adenopathy; signs of STDs (chlamydia, GC, HIV, etc.)
- Allergic
  - Itching predominant, chemosis, edema; seasonal or animal dander allergies
- Nonspecific irritative
  - Dry eyes, intermittent redness, chemical/drug exposure
  - Foreign body: may have redness and discharge 24 hours after removal
- Cornea should be clear and without fluorescein uptake. Cloudy or ulcerated cornea signifies keratitis; consult ophthalmologist. Fluorescein stain exam is recommended. Evert lid to inspect for foreign bodies.

- Skin: Look for herpetic vesicles, nits on lashes (lice), scaliness (seborrhea), lid inflammation (blepharitis, rosacea, or styes).
- Limbal flush at corneal margin if uveitis. If pupil is irregular (i.e., penetrating foreign body), emergent referral is warranted.
- Discharge on lid margin but no conjunctival injection: blepharitis

DIFFERENTIAL DIAGNOSIS
- Punctate keratitis due to prolonged contact lenses wear; uveitis (iritis, iridocyclitis, choroiditis): limbal flush, hazy anterior chamber, and decreased visual acuity
- Acute glaucoma (emergency): headache, corneal clouding, poor visual acuity; corneal ulcer, keratitis, or foreign body: lesions or tear-film deficits on fluorescein exam; dacryocystitis: tenderness and swelling over tear sac (below medial canthus); scleritis and episcleritis: red injected vessels radially oriented; pingueculitis: inflammation of a yellow nodular or wedge-like area of chronic conjunctival degeneration (pinguecula)
- Ophthalmia neonatorum: neonates in the first 2 days of life (gonococcal; 5 to 12 days of life): chlamydial, herpes simplex virus (HSV); blepharitis: Lid margins are inflamed producing itching, scale, or discharge but no conjunctival injection.
- Giant fornix syndrome: an elderly patient with recurrent or chronic conjunctivitis due to accumulation of infected material in enlarged fornices (2)

DIAGNOSTIC TESTS & INTERPRETATION
Usually not needed initially for most common causes, if COVID-19 epidemic related, consider viral PCR or antigen. Culture swab if STD suspected severe symptoms, contact lenses user, or failed prior treatment.

Diagnostic Procedures/Other
Fluorescein exam to rule out corneal ulcer, herpes zoster or abrasion. Remove small, superficial foreign bodies with irrigation or moistened swab. Refer cases of prolonged symptoms (>7 days).

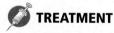

TREATMENT

GENERAL MEASURES
Viral conjunctivitis does not require antibiotics, most resolve spontaneously. Clean external eyelid with wet cloth up to 4 times per day. Stop use of contact lenses as long as eye is red. Eye patching is not beneficial.

MEDICATION
First Line
- Viral (nonherpetic)
  - Artificial tears for symptomatic relief; vasoconstrictor/antihistamine (e.g., naphazoline/pheniramine) QID for severe itch; may consider topical antibiotic (see bacterial below) if return to daycare requires treatment
  - Adenoviral conjunctivitis course may be shortened by one dose of 5% povidone-iodine (3)[B].
  - If very severe or prolonged, refer to ophthalmologist for possible steroid
- Viral (herpetic) (with ophthalmology consultation)
  - Ganciclovir gel: 0.15%, 5 times per day for 7 days
  - Acyclovir: PO 400 mg 5 times per day for HSV; 800 mg for zoster for 7 days

- Bacterial (nonsexually transmitted): 3 days of cool compresses to allow for self-resolution before starting antibiotic reduces unnecessary antibiotic use.
  – If preferred, may use topical antibiotics (NNT 7 by day 6) (immediate topical antibiotics may allow for earlier return to school for some children)
  – Bacitracin ophthalmic ointment (over the counter [OTC]): Apply 3 to 4 times per day for 5 to 7 days.
  – Povidone-iodine 1.25% ophthalmic solution (antimicrobial lubricant OTC) 1 gtt 4 times per day for 5 to 7 days (1)[A]
  – Polymyxin B-trimethoprim solution 1 gtt 6 times per day for 5 to 7 days; erythromycin ophthalmic ointment: 1/2 inch 2 to 4 times per day for 5 days; sodium sulfacetamide (Bleph-10) (10% solution): 2 drops q4h (while awake) for 5 days; tobramycin or gentamicin: 0.3% ophthalmic drops/ointment q4h (drops) to q8h (ointment) for 7 days
- Bacterial (gonococcal)
  – Neonates: Hospitalize for IV ceftriaxone or cefotaxime.
  – Adults: ceftriaxone: 1 g IM as single dose and topical bacitracin ophthalmic ointment 1/2 inch QID; neonates: 25 to 50 mg/kg IV or IM, not to exceed 125 mg, as a single dose. Chlamydia in neonates requires oral erythromycin: 50 mg/kg/day divided q6h PO for 14 days, max of 3 g/day.
- Allergic and atopic: OTC medications are efficacious, no definitive evidence favoring one over another, cost varies widely.
  – Ketotifen (Zaditor, Alaway, and other generics OTC): 0.25% 1 drop 2 times per day; ketorolac (Acular): 0.1% 1 drop 4 times per day; lodoxamide (Alomide) 0.1% 1 drop 4 times a day; cetirizine (Zerviate): 0.24% 1 drop 2 times per day; olopatadine (Pataday, Patanol): 0.1% 1 drop 2 times per day or 0.2% 1 drop daily; cromolyn (Opticrom): 4% 1 drop 4 times per day; naphazoline (Vasocon-A, Naphcon-A, Opcon-A, Visine-A: OTC) 1 drop 4 times a day; azelastine (Astelin): 0.05% 1 drop 2 times per day; nedocromil (Alocril): 2% 1 drop 2 times per day
  – Alcaftadine (OTC): 0.25% 1 drop daily; epinastine 0.05% 1 drop 2 times per day; bepotastine (Bepreve) 1.5% 1 drop 2 times per day (3)
  – Oral nonsedating antihistamines (cetirizine [Zyrtec] 10 mg/day, fexofenadine [Allegra] 60 mg BID, etc.) may treat nasal symptoms but cause ocular drying; oral antihistamine (e.g., diphenhydramine 25 mg TID) in severe itching
- Contraindications: steroids *not* beneficial in treatment of bacterial keratitis; any topical steroid requires baseline and periodic specialist's exam; topical immune modulators (tacrolimus, cyclosporine) for specialist use only
- Precautions
  – Do not allow dropper to touch the eye; case reports of eye irritation from gentamicin in infants, moxifloxacin in adults, sulfacetamide in allergic individuals; vasoconstrictor/antihistamine: rebound vasodilation after prolonged use

Second Line

- Viral and allergic: numerous OTC products, oral montelukast 10 mg daily
- Bacterial: second line (quinolones used as postoperative or for known resistant organisms)
  – Ofloxacin: 0.3% 1 gtt QID for 7 days; Ciprofloxacin: 0.3% 1 gtt QID for 7 days
  – Levofloxacin: 0.3% 1 gtt QID for 7 days; Azithromycin: 1.5% BID for 3 days

ISSUES FOR REFERRAL

Refer to ophthalmology for decreased visual acuity, suspected herpetic keratitis/contact lenses–related conjunctivitis, or immunocompromised (HIV). Refer for prolonged symptoms or worsening >7 days (concern for severe adenoviral keratitis).

COMPLEMENTARY & ALTERNATIVE MEDICINE

Usually benign and self-limited; saline flushes, cool compresses, and similar treatments help.

ADMISSION, INPATIENT, AND NURSING CONSIDERATIONS

Acute gonococcal conjunctivitis (or very rare case of meningococcal conjunctivitis) requires inpatient treatment with ceftriaxone 50 mg/kg IV every day (pediatric), 1 g IM for one (adult) along with ophthalmologic consultation.

 ## ONGOING CARE

FOLLOW-UP RECOMMENDATIONS

- If not resolved within 5 to 7 days, reconsider diagnosis or consult specialist.
- Children may be excluded from school until the eye is no longer red, depending on school policy. Allergic conjunctivitis (noncontagious) should return to school with doctor's note.

Patient Monitoring

Patient should follow up in 1 day if any worsening.

PATIENT EDUCATION

- No contact lenses until eyes are fully healed (~1 week). Discard current contact lenses.
- Adenovirus may persist on surfaces up to 28 days; practice soap hand-washing and hypochlorite surface wipe use.
- Discard old eye makeup, especially mascara. Cool, moist compresses can ease irritation and itch.

PROGNOSIS

- Viral: 5 to 10 days of symptoms for pharyngitis with conjunctivitis, 2 weeks with adenovirus
- Herpes simplex: 2 to 3 weeks of symptoms
- Most common bacterial—*H. influenzae*, *Staphylococcus*, *Streptococcus*: self-limited; 74–80% resolution within 7 days, whether treated or not

COMPLICATIONS

- Corneal scars with herpes simplex; lid scars, conjunctival scars, symblepharon or entropion may occur with varicella zoster and chlamydia or any severe inflammation; corneal ulcers or perforation; hypopyon: pus in anterior chamber
- Chlamydial neonatal (ophthalmic): could have concomitant pneumonia; otitis media may follow *H. influenzae* conjunctivitis. Very rarely *N. meningitidis* conjunctivitis may be followed by meningitis.

REFERENCES

1. Johnson D, Liu D, Simel D. Does this patient with acute infectious conjunctivitis have a bacterial infection?: The rational clinical examination systematic review. *JAMA*. 2022;327(22):2231–2237.
2. Commiskey P, Bowers E, Dmitriev A, et al. Bilateral, chronic, bacterial conjunctivitis in giant fornix syndrome. *BMJ Case Rep*. 2022;15(1):e245460.
3. Labib BA, Chigbu DI. Therapeutic targets in allergic conjunctivitis. *Pharmaceuticals (Basel)*. 2022;15(5):547.

 ### SEE ALSO

- Rhinitis, Allergic
- Algorithm: Eye Pain

CODES

ICD10

- H10.30 Unspecified acute conjunctivitis, unspecified eye
- H10.33 Unspecified acute conjunctivitis, bilateral
- H10.32 Unspecified acute conjunctivitis, left eye

CLINICAL PEARLS

- Conjunctivitis does *not* cause decreased acuity or photophobia. If visual acuity is decreased or if there is pain with ocular movements, consider more serious ophthalmic disorders.
- Culture discharge in all *contact lenses wearers and nursing home residents*. Consider referral, discard current lenses, and use spectacles for visual correction until eyes are fully healed.
- Antibiotics are of no value in viral conjunctivitis (most cases of infectious conjunctivitis).
- Cool compresses for 3 days before using any antibiotic is appropriate for treating conjunctivitis in healthy adults and children >1 month of age.

CONSTIPATION

Daniel R. Matta, MD • Jeremy Maxwell, MBBS

BASICS

- Unsatisfactory defecation characterized by infrequent stools, difficult stool passage, or both
- Characteristics include <3 bowel movements a week, hard stools, excessive straining, prolonged time spent in the restroom, a sense of incomplete evacuation, and abdominal discomfort/bloating.

DESCRIPTION

Geriatric Considerations
Consider new-onset constipation after age 50 years a "red flag" for colorectal neoplasms. Use warm water enemas (instead of sodium phosphate enemas) for impaction in geriatric patients. Sodium phosphate enemas in older adults have been associated with hypotension, volume depletion, EKG changes (prolonged QT interval), and severe electrolyte disturbances.

Pediatric Considerations
Consider Hirschsprung disease in cases of pediatric constipation. This accounts for 25% of all newborn intestinal obstructions and can present as milder cases diagnosed in older children with chronic constipation, abdominal distension, and decreased growth. Hirschsprung has a 5:1 male-to-female ratio and is associated with inherited conditions (e.g., Down syndrome).

Pregnancy Considerations
Constipation is common in pregnancy due to progesterone slowing GI motility, gravid pressure of uterus on colon, iron supplementation, and decreased physical activity.

EPIDEMIOLOGY
- More pronounced in children and elderly
- Predominant sex: female > male (2:1)
- Nonwhites > whites

Incidence
- 5 million office visits annually
- 100,000 hospitalizations

Prevalence
- 16% of adults >18 years of age, rising to 33% of adults >60 years of age
- 3% of pediatric visits relate to constipation.

ETIOLOGY AND PATHOPHYSIOLOGY
Defecation reflex is a reflex that can be inhibited by voluntarily contracting the external sphincter or facilitated by straining to contract the abdominal muscles while voluntarily relaxing the anal sphincter. Rectal distention initiates the defecation reflex. The urge to defecate occurs with an increase in rectal pressure. Distention of the stomach also initiates rectal contractions and a desire to defecate (gastrocolic reflex).

RISK FACTORS
- Extremes of age
- Female sex
- Polypharmacy
- Sedentary lifestyle or condition
- Low-fiber diet and inadequate fluid intake
- Increased stress or history of abuse

GENERAL PREVENTION
High-fiber diet, adequate fluids, exercise, and training to "obey the urge" to defecate

COMMONLY ASSOCIATED CONDITIONS
- General debilitation (disease or aging)
- Dehydration
- Hypothyroidism
- Electrolyte abnormalities: hypokalemia, hypercalcemia

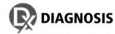

DIAGNOSIS

ALERT
Red flags:
- New onset after age of 50 years
- Fever
- Nausea/vomiting
- Hematochezia/melena
- Unintentional weight loss >10 lb (>4.5 kg)
- Change in bowel habits/narrowing of the stool
- Family history of colon cancer or inflammatory bowel disease
- Abdominal pain
- Fatigue
- Iron deficiency anemia
- Neurologic deficits

HISTORY
- Assess onset of symptoms, number of bowel movements per week, straining, completeness of evacuation, and the use of manual manipulation.
- Identify red flags; evaluate diet, lifestyle, prescription and OTC medication use; identify reversible causes; ask about history of sexual abuse, opioid use; identify any systemic or neurologic disorders that affect colonic motility.
- Bristol Stool Form Scale—seven categories of consistency (1)
- A diary of dietary intake and bowel patterns may help to identify causative agents, to quantify the severity of the constipation, and to measure treatment response.
- Rome IV criteria (1):
  - At least two of the following for 12 weeks in the previous 6 months:
    ○ <3 stools per week
    ○ Straining at least 1/4 of the time
    ○ Hard stools (Bristol Stool Form Scale 1 to 2) at least 1/4 of time
    ○ Need for manual assist at least 1/4 of time
    ○ Sense of incomplete evacuation at least 1/4 of time
    ○ Sense of anorectal blockage at least 1/4 of time
  - Loose stools rarely seen without use of laxatives
  - Does not meet irritable bowel syndrome (IBS) criteria
  - Although there can be overlap, the history of primary constipation differs from constipation-predominant IBS.
    ○ In primary constipation, pain and bloating are relieved by adequate defecation. In IBS, pain and bloating predominate and are not readily relieved by defecation.
- Bowel Function Index—for opioid-induced constipation (OIC)
- Assessment tools such as the Constipation Assessment Scale, Constipation Scoring System, and Patient Assessment of Constipation-Symptoms questionnaire could be used to assess severity.

PHYSICAL EXAM
- Vital signs
- Abdominal exam, previous surgical scars, distention, hypoactive bowel sounds, tenderness, and masses
- Gynecologic exam: Evaluate for masses and rectocele.
- External anorectal examination: excoriations, scars, fistulas, fissures, hemorrhoids, rectal prolapse, and anal wink
- Digital rectal exam: Evaluate for structural lesions: masses, stool, fissures, and hemorrhoids; assess for pelvic floor dyssynergia and sphincter tone, strictures as noted by inability to insert, or difficulty inserting finger into anal canal.
- Neurologic exam

DIFFERENTIAL DIAGNOSIS
- Primary constipation (primary problem is within the GI tract) has four subtypes (2).
  - Normal colonic transit time most common subtype; can be difficult to differentiate from constipation-predominant IBS (IBS-C)
  - Slow colonic transit time
  - Pelvic floor/anal sphincter dysfunction (defecatory disorders)
  - Combination pelvic floor/anal sphincter dysfunction and slow transit
- Secondary constipation (outside the GI tract)
  - Endocrine dysfunction
    ○ Diabetes mellitus, hypothyroidism, hyperparathyroidism
  - Metabolic disorders
    ○ Chronic kidney disease and electrolyte abnormalities (hypercalcemia, hypokalemia, hypomagnesemia)
  - Mechanical
    ○ Colonic stricture or obstruction: inflammation, ischemia, postradiation
  - Neurologic disorders
    ○ Central: multiple sclerosis, spinal cord injuries, Parkinson disease, dementia, traumatic brain injury
    ○ Peripheral: diabetes, Hirschsprung disease, Chagas disease
  - Myopathy
  - Pregnancy
  - Psychiatric/psychosocial
    ○ Abuse, anorexia nervosa, depression
  - Congenital
    ○ Hirschsprung disease/syndrome; hypoganglionosis; congenital dilation of the colon; small left colon syndrome
  - Medication effect
    ○ Opioids/NSAIDs; tricyclic antidepressants; antipsychotics; antacids (calcium, aluminum)
    ○ Calcium channel blockers: nifedipine and verapamil
    ○ Iron and multivitamins with iron; diuretics
    ○ Overuse of antidiarrheal medications
    ○ 5-HT3 antagonists: ondansetron
    ○ Antihistamines
    ○ Chemotherapy agents: cyclophosphamide and vincristine

DIAGNOSTIC TESTS & INTERPRETATION
Identify red flags, secondary causes, and reversible conditions. If none present, go to first-line treatment. Routine use of lab studies or imaging, including colonoscopy, is not recommended in the absence of red flags.

Initial Tests (lab, imaging)
- CBC to screen for iron deficiency anemia
- Consider toxicology screen if illicit opioid use is suspected.
- Electrolytes, calcium, creatinine, glucose, and thyroid function testing (TSH) based on history and exam
- If red flags are present and due for colorectal cancer screening, should be referred for a colonoscopy

Diagnostic Procedures/Other
- Anorectal manometry (ARM)
- Balloon expulsion testing (BET)
- Surface electromyelography
- Barium or magnetic resonance defecography
- Radio-opaque markers and scintigraphy

Test Interpretation
- ARM and BET are recommended for all refractory cases; if negative, barium or magnetic resonance defecography to evaluate transit time
- Consider biofeedback with pelvic floor therapy.

 TREATMENT

GENERAL MEASURES
In patients with no known secondary causes, conservative nonpharmacologic treatment is recommended.
- Eliminate medications that cause constipation.
- Increase fluid intake.
- Increase soluble fiber (25 to 30 g/day) in diet.
- Encourage regular defecation attempts after eating.
- Regular exercise

MEDICATION
First Line
Bulking agents (accompanied by adequate fluids) (2)
- Osmotic laxatives
  – Polyethylene glycol (PEG) (MiraLAX) 17 g/day PO dissolved in 4 to 8 oz of beverage (current evidence shows PEG to be superior to lactulose)
  – Lactulose (Chronulac, Enulose) 15 to 60 mL PO QHS (flatulence, bloating, cramping)
  – Sorbitol: 15 to 60 mL PO QHS (as effective as lactulose)
  – Magnesium salts (milk of magnesia): 15 to 30 mL PO once daily; avoid in renal insufficiency.
- Hydrophilic colloids (bulk-forming agents)
  – Psyllium (Konsyl, Metamucil, Perdiem Fiber): 1 tbsp (approximately 3.5 grams fiber) in 8-oz liquid PO daily up to TID
  – Methylcellulose (Citrucel): 1 tbsp (approximately 2 grams fiber) in 8-oz liquid PO daily up to TID
  – Polycarbophil (Mitrolan, FiberCon): 2 caplets (500 mg fiber per tab) with 8-oz liquid PO up to QID
  – Wheat dextrin (Benefiber): 2 tsp (1.5 gram fiber per tsp) up to TID

Second Line
- Stimulants (irritate bowel, causing muscle contraction; usually combined with a softener; work in 8 to 12 hours)
  – Senna/docusate (Senokot-S, Ex-lax, Peri-Colace): 1 to 2 tablets or 15 to 30 mL PO at bedtime
  – Bisacodyl (Dulcolax, Correctol): 1 to 3 tablets PO daily

- Suppositories
  – Osmotic: sodium phosphate
  – Lubricant: glycerin
  – Stimulatory: bisacodyl
  – Enemas: saline (Fleet enema)
- Long-term prescription agents
  – Lubiprostone (Amitiza)
  – Prucalopride (Motegrity); increased incidence of suicidal ideation reported in clinical trials
- Guanylate cyclase-C agonists (adult use only)
  – Plecanatide (Trulance): dose: 3 mg PO once daily
  – Linaclotide (Linzess): dose: 145 μg PO once daily; can use lower dose 72 μg once daily
- OIC (1)
- Trial of laxatives first followed by peripherally acting μ-opioid receptor antagonists
  – Methylnaltrexone (Relistor): dose: 38 to <62 kg: 8 mg; 62 to 114 kg: 12 mg SC every other day PRN
  – Naloxegol (Movantik): dose: 12.5 to 25.0 mg PO daily; discontinue other laxatives for 3 days when initiating naloxegol; avoid in patients on strong CYP3A4 inhibitors due to increased naloxegol levels and risk of opioid withdrawal
  – Naldemedine (Symproic): dose: 0.2 mg PO daily; monitor for opioid withdrawal in patients on strong CYP3A4 inhibitors or P-gp inhibitors.
- Linaclotide (Linzess): dose 145 μg PO once daily; can use lower dose 72 μg once daily
- Prokinetic agents (partial 5-HT4 agonists): cisapride (Propulsid) has been withdrawn due to cardiac side effects; only available via IND protocols; tegaserod (Zelnorm) available for IBS-C; side effects include cardiac events, ischemic colitis, and suicidal ideation.

ADDITIONAL THERAPIES
- Biofeedback
- Behavior therapy
- Acupuncture: initial randomized trial effective at 20 weeks; longer term trials needed

SURGERY/OTHER PROCEDURES
Surgery rarely indicated; sometimes required for anatomic findings (rectocele or enterocoele) and in whom nonsurgical management has been ineffective.
- Abdominal colectomy and ileorectal anastomosis

ADMISSION, INPATIENT, AND NURSING CONSIDERATIONS
- Toxic megacolon
- Manual disimpaction occasionally required in chronic refractory cases

 ONGOING CARE

DIET
Increase soluble fiber (bloating and gas can be problematic with insoluble fiber):
- Gradually increase intake to 25 g/day over a 6-week period.
- Oat bran, peas, onions, lentils, beans, seeds, nuts, and fruits- including bananas, apples, and strawberries
- Encourage liberal intake of fluids.

PATIENT EDUCATION
- Occasional mild constipation is normal.
- Bowel training: the best time to move bowels is in the morning, after eating breakfast, when the normal bowel transit and defecation reflexes are functioning.

PROGNOSIS
- Occasional constipation responds well to simple measures.
- Habitual constipation can be a lifelong nuisance.
- Patients with neurologic compromise can suffer from obstipation, impaction, and toxic megacolon.
- No evidence for laxative dependence or harm from stimulant use; melanosis coli may develop but is a benign condition.

COMPLICATIONS
- Volvulus; toxic megacolon
- Acquired megacolon in severe, long-standing cases
- Fluid and electrolyte depletion: laxative abuse
- Rectal ulceration (stercoral ulcer) related to recurrent fecal impaction; anal fissures; rectal prolapse; hemorrhoids

REFERENCES
1. Sadler K, Arnold F, Dean S. Chronic constipation in adults. *Am Fam Physician*. 2022;106(3):299–306.
2. Bharucha AE, Lacy BE. Mechanisms, evaluation, and management of chronic constipation. *Gastroenterology*. 2020;158(5):1232–1249.e3.

 CODES

ICD10
- K59.00 Constipation, unspecified
- K59.01 Slow transit constipation
- K59.09 Other constipation

CLINICAL PEARLS
- Consider new-onset constipation after age 50 years a "red flag" for colorectal neoplasms
- Consider Hirschsprung disease in cases of newborn/infant constipation
- In patients with no known secondary causes, conservative nonpharmacologic treatment is recommended.
- Bulking agents and adequate hydration are important first-line steps in management

CONTRACEPTION
Jeremy Golding, MD, FAAFP • Katharine L. Neff, DO

BASICS

DESCRIPTION
- Medications or procedures that control timing of pregnancies and prevent unintended pregnancies
- Options are divided into two major categories: hormonal and nonhormonal.

EPIDEMIOLOGY
Incidence
45% of pregnancies in the United States are unintended. Unintended pregnancies are associated with increased risk of adverse maternal and infant outcomes.

RISK FACTORS
Unintended pregnancy: higher rates among women ages 18 to 24 years and >40, unmarried women, women with less than a college education, and minority women

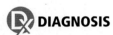**DIAGNOSIS**

HISTORY
- Review past medical, family, social, obstetric, and gynecologic histories including menstrual history, prior contraceptive use, and prior sexually transmitted infections (STIs).
- Screen for hypertension.
- In family history of thrombophilia, consider testing before initiation of estrogen-containing contraception.
- Contraindications: See CDC medical eligibility criteria (MEC) (1) and chart (2) or app (3).
  - Estrogen-progestin contraceptives
    - Common absolute: age ≥35 years and smoking ≥15 cigarettes per day, <21 days postpartum, SBP ≥160 mm Hg or DBP ≥100 mm Hg, current/prior venous thromboembolism (VTE), thrombophilia, long-standing/complicated diabetes, ischemic heart disease, systemic lupus erythematosus, migraine with aura, breast cancer
    - Common relative: age ≥35 years and smoking <15 cigarettes per day, breastfeeding <42 days postpartum, SBP 140 to 159 mm Hg or DBP 90 to 99 mm Hg (or well-controlled on medications), bariatric surgery, migraines without aura but ≥35 years, breast cancer history
  - Progestin-only (pill/Depo-Provera/implant)
    - Absolute: current breast cancer
    - Common relative: bariatric surgery, heart disease, stroke, lupus, migraine with aura
  - Levonorgestrel—intrauterine device (IUD)
    - Common absolute: postseptic abortion, postpartum sepsis, current breast cancer, distorted uterine cavity
    - Absolute contraindications for initiation but do not require discontinuation: cervical/endometrial cancer, PID, known untreated chlamydia or gonorrhea infection
    - Common relative: heart disease, lupus
  - Copper IUD (ParaGard)
    - Absolute: same as levonorgestrel IUD, ok to use in breast cancer
    - Absolute contraindications for initiation but not continuation: same as levonorgestrel IUD
    - Relative: thrombocytopenia, solid organ transplant

DIAGNOSTIC TESTS & INTERPRETATION
Initial Tests (lab, imaging)
- Consider pregnancy test. Consider testing for gonorrhea and chlamydia prior to IUD insertion.
- Pap smear if indicated; contraception should not be withheld pending a Pap smear.

TREATMENT

GENERAL MEASURES
Method(s) should be selected based on patient preference, effectiveness, need for STI prevention, side effects, and contraindications.

MEDICATION
- Estrogen-progestin contraceptives
  - Mechanism of action: suppression of ovulation, thickening of cervical mucus, and endometrial changes
  - Efficacy: failure rate of 9% (~8 pregnancies per 100 women per year) with typical use and 0.3% with perfect use at 1 year
  - Side effects: irregular bleeding, nausea, headaches, mastalgia, depression; all estrogen-containing methods increase risk of venous thrombosis from approximately 2 per 10,000 users per year to 7 to 10 per 10,000 users per year (4).
  - Combined oral contraceptives (COCs)
    - COCs mostly contain ethinyl estradiol (EE) but differ in the amount (10 to 50 μg) and type of progestin.
    - Dosing
      - Most have 21 active days and 7 placebo days.
      - Alternatively, active pills can be taken continuously with scheduled withdrawal bleeds.
    - Initiation
      - Recommended: "quick start" (Begin pill on the day medication is obtained.)
      - Alternative: Begin the pill on the 1st day of menses or first Sunday. Note: If not starting pill within 5 days of start of menses, back-up contraception is recommended for 7 days.
    - Nextstellis (estetrol 14.2 mg, drospirenone 3 mg): new plant-derived estrogen with mixed agonist/antagonist properties; similar efficacy to other COC; expensive (brand-only); monitor potassium.
- Weekly hormonal patch
  - Applied transdermally and changed weekly for 3 weeks; no patch worn during week 4 for withdrawal bleeding, unless user prefers fewer yearly periods (continuous cycling)
  - Ortho Evra, Xulane:
    - 20 μg/day EE and 150 μg/day norelgestromin
    - Produces higher serum estrogen levels than oral 20-μg pill (slightly increased risk of VTE)
    - Application site irritation; reduced efficacy in women >90 kg
  - Twirla:
    - 30 μg/day of EE and 120 μg/day of levonorgestrel
    - Common adverse reactions: application site disorders, nausea, headache, weight gain
    - Contraindicated in women with a BMI ≥30 kg/m²; reduced effectiveness in women with a BMI ≥25 to <30 kg/m²

- Vaginal contraceptive ring
  - Ring is inserted in the vagina and remains in place; adverse reactions: headaches, nausea and vomiting, vulvovaginal mycotic infection, vaginal discharge, UTI
  - NuvaRing: in vagina for 3 weeks followed by 1 week of ring-free interval; may also use continuous cycling for 4 weeks and then immediately replaced with a new ring (off-label)
    - 15 μg/day of EE and 120 μg/day of etonogestrel absorbed via vaginal wall
    - Although systemic exposure to estrogen is about 50% of exposure with COCs, the risk of VTE is similar.
  - Annovera: Single ring is cleaned and used for up to 1 year; not adequately evaluated in females with a BMI >29 kg/m²
- Progestin-only birth control
  - Mechanism of action: Primary mechanism is ovulation inhibition with possible secondary benefit from thickening of cervical mucus and thinning of endometrial lining.
  - Progestin-only pills (POPs)
    - Norethindrone 0.35 mg (Micronor, etc.); efficacy: failure rate of about 0.3% with perfect use, 9% with typical use at 1 year
      - Can be used in some women with contraindications to estrogen, including (for example) breastfeeding women
      - Dosing: 1 pill at the same time daily, no placebo days; side effects: irregular/unscheduled bleeding (common)
    - Drospirenone 4 mg (Slynd); efficacy similar to COC; expensive (brand-only)
      - Progestin with antiandrogen and antimineralocorticoid effect; may be particularly useful for PCOS and other high-androgen conditions; potassium levels may need to be monitored periodically.
      - 24 active pills, 4 placebo per pack; less menstrual irregularity than norethindrone
    - Norgestrel (Opill): first OTC contraceptive pill approved by FDA (2023), available in 2024
      - Dosing: 1 pill at the same time daily, no placebo days; side effects: irregular/unscheduled bleeding (common)
      - Pregnancy rate is 2% in trials, likely >7 per 100 women-years in real-world use.
- Injectable contraceptive (medroxyprogesterone acetate, DMPA) (Depo-Provera)
  - Efficacy: failure rate of 0.2% with perfect use, 6% with typical use at 1 year
  - Dosing: one injection every 3 months; contraceptive levels of hormone persist for up to 4 months.
  - Side effects: irregular bleeding, weight gain (average of 5 lb/year of use), amenorrhea, depression
- LARCs: IUDs and implantable devices
  - Mirena, Liletta, generic (52-mg levonorgestrel-releasing IUD):
    - Primary mechanism of action: produces sterile inflammatory reaction due to foreign body that is toxic to sperm and ova, thickens cervical mucus
    - Efficacy: failure rate of 0.2% with both perfect and typical use at 1 year (1 pregnancy per 400 to 500 users per year)

○ Release: 20 μg/day initially; reduces to 10 μg/day (FDA approved for 8 years)
○ Safe and recommended in nulliparous women/teenagers
○ Can be inserted immediately postpartum or immediately following D&C for miscarriage or abortion, although with higher rates of expulsion compared to delayed placement (6 to 10 weeks); may be used as postcoital contraception up to 5 days after intercourse (limited data)
○ Side effects: irregular bleeding for first 3 to 6 months that usually resolves; may see amenorrhea after 1 year
○ Side effect management: Consider NSAIDs, COCs, or POPs for spotting and cramps.
– Kyleena (19.5-mg levonorgestrel-releasing IUD): releases 17.5 μg/day initially; reduced to 7.5 μg/day (approved for 5 years)
– Skyla (13.5-mg levonorgestrel-releasing IUD): smaller insertion tube; more bleeding days than Mirena; release: 14 μg/day initially; reduces to 5 μg/day (approved for 3 years)
– Copper IUD (ParaGard): approved for 10 years, effective for longer (especially in women aged >30 years)
○ Primary mechanism of action: produces sterile inflammatory reaction
○ Efficacy: failure rate of 0.6% with perfect use, 0.8% with typical use at 1 year
○ May be used as postcoital contraceptive within 5 to 7 days of intercourse (solid data)
○ Side effects: increased menstrual bleeding and cramping (common)
– Nexplanon (etonogestrel implant):
○ Mechanism of action: inhibits ovulation
○ Efficacy: failure rate of 0.05% with perfect use, 0.3% with typical use at 1 year (1 pregnancy per 400 to 500 users/year)
○ Dosing: semirigid plastic rod containing 68 mg of etonogestrel; initially 60 to 70 μg/day; subsequently 25 to 30 μg/day
○ FDA approved for 3 years, evidence-based efficacy to 4 to 5 years
○ Inserted only by certified providers but technique is simple to learn
○ Side effects: menstrual irregularities (very common for 6 to 12 months, may persist for 3 years)
• Emergency contraception: initiated as soon as possible after unprotected intercourse; copper IUD and levonorgestrel-releasing IUD are the most effective, followed by ulipristal, levonorgestrel, and Yuzpe method.
– Copper and 42-mg levonorgestrel-releasing IUD (Mirena, Liletta) (IUD): up to 5 days after intercourse; 0.04–0.19% failure rate
– Ulipristal acetate (Ella): 30 mg once; selective progesterone modulator, up to 5 days after intercourse 2% failure rate
– Levonorgestrel: 1.5 mg taken as two 0.75-mg tablets (Plan B) or one 1.5-mg tablet (Plan B One-Step); most effective within 72 hours; 1.1–2.4% failure rate; less nausea than "Yuzpe regimen"; available over the counter; likely ineffective for women with BMI >30 kg/m²
– "Yuzpe regimen" 50 μg/0.25 mg, 2 tablets q12h (4 tablets total); any OCP may be used as long as the dose of estrogen component ≥100 μg/dose; 3.2% failure rate. *Note:* Antiemetic should be given 1 to 2 hours.

ADDITIONAL THERAPIES

• Male condoms: failure rate of 2% with perfect use, 18% with typical use at 1 year
• Spermicides: All contain nonoxynol-9; may alter vaginal flora and mucosal barrier; failure rate: 28% with typical use at 1 year
• Sponge (Today Sponge): Soft foam disk contains nonoxynol-9. Moisten with water before use; effective for 24 hours; must leave in for 6 hours after use; failure rate: 12–24% with typical use
• Diaphragm: latex or silicone dome-shaped device with flexible spring-activated rim, prevents sperm from entering cervix; used with spermicides; failure rate: 12% with typical use, 6% with perfect use at 1 year
• Phexxi: nonhormonal spermicidal prescription contraceptive; combination of lactic and citric acids and potassium bitartrate indicated as an on demand method of contraception. Administer single-dose applicator vaginally immediately before or up to 1 hour prior to each episode of intercourse. May be used with other methods except vaginal ring. Avoid use in women with a history of recurrent UTIs or urinary tract abnormalities. Common side effects: discomfort, mycotic infection, UTI, and bacterial vaginosis; failure rate: 13.7%

SURGERY/OTHER PROCEDURES

Permanent sterilization

• Female: tubal ligation; failure rate: 0.5% at 1 year
• Male: vasectomy; failure rate: 0.15% at 1 year

COMPLEMENTARY & ALTERNATIVE MEDICINE

• Fertility awareness methods; failure rate: 24% at 1 year typical use (~20 pregnancies per 100 women per year)
• Withdrawal method: Failure rate: 22% at 1 year
• Lactational amenorrhea method: effective only if the infant is <6 months old and exclusively breastfeeding and the mother has not resumed regular menses; failure rate: 7% at 1 year typical use

Pediatric Considerations

AAP and ACOG recommend LARCs as first-line agents.

 ONGOING CARE

FOLLOW-UP RECOMMENDATIONS

Patient Monitoring

• 1 to 3 months postinitiation to assess tolerance
• Consider IUD string-check 1 month after insertion; spontaneous expulsion rate highest in the 1st month
• BP check within 3 months of initiating on estrogen-containing methods

DIET

St. John's wort may alter estrogen levels.

PATIENT EDUCATION

• Diaphragm: Insert before intercourse using spermicide per manufacturer's recommendations.
• Male condom: Describe proper use.
• IUD: Patient may wish to check strings monthly.

• STI prevention
• Useful patient education materials: https://www.reproductiveaccess.org/contraception/ and https://www.cdc.gov/reproductivehealth/contraception/

COMPLICATIONS

• Estrogen-progestin contraceptives: serious (requires discontinuation): stroke, thromboembolism, hypertension, myocardial infarction, and cholestatic jaundice
• Injectable DMPA: decreased bone mineral density (BMD) if used for ≥2 years; mostly recovers after discontinuation; consider calcium/vitamin D supplementation if prolonged use.
• Nexplanon: insertion site reaction including pain, bleeding, paresthesias, and infection
• IUDs: uterine perforation (4); absolute risk of ectopic pregnancy is reduced with IUD, but if pregnancy does occur, there is a higher risk that it will be ectopic.
• Sponge and diaphragm: toxic shock syndrome

REFERENCES

1. Centers for Disease Control and Prevention. U.S. Medical Eligibility Criteria (US MEC) for Contraceptive Use. https://www.cdc.gov/reproductivehealth/contraception/mmwr/mec/summary.html. Accessed November 6, 2023.
2. Centers for Disease Control and Prevention. Summary Chart of U.S. Medical Eligibility Criteria for Contraceptive Use. https://www.cdc.gov/reproductivehealth/contraception/pdf/summary-chart-us-medical-eligibility-criteria_508tagged.pdf. Accessed November 6, 2023.
3. Centers for Disease Control and Prevention. Reproductive Health. Contraception app. https://www.cdc.gov/reproductivehealth/contraception/contraception-app.html. Accessed November 6, 2023.
4. Teal S, Edelman A. Contraception selection, effectiveness, and adverse effects: a review. *JAMA.* 2021;326(24):2507–2518.

CODES

ICD10
• Z30.9 Encounter for contraceptive management, unspecified
• Z30.41 Encounter for surveillance of contraceptive pills
• Z30.431 Encounter for routine checking of intrauterine contracep dev

CLINICAL PEARLS

LARC methods provide very high efficacy and convenience for patients.

CORNEAL ABRASION AND ULCERATION

Jon S. Parham, DO, MPH, FAAFP • Luke T. Hentrich, PharmD

BASICS

As the most anterior eye structure, a cornea is unique: mechanical and immunologic eye protector, light refractor/transmitter, and conduit for nutrients and oxygen via tears to the eye.

DESCRIPTION

- Corneal injuries via: a foreign body (most commonly abrasion), ultraviolet (UV) burns, or chemical contact burns.
  - Corneal abrasions: result from any single or repetitive violation by cutting or scratching the thin, protective, clear coat of the exposed corneal epithelium.
  - Corneal stromal ulceration: any violation of the epithelial layer of the cornea leading to direct exposure of the underlying corneal stromal layer, may result (especially with delay in diagnosis/ treatment) in infectious keratitis which may lead to an infected corneal ulcer.
  - Superficial ulcers, limited to loss of the corneal epithelium, are the most common form of ulceration.
  - Peripheral ulcerative keratitis (PUK) is noninfectious, complicating many autoimmune diseases with corneal ulceration.
- UV burns of the cornea (photokeratitis) occur when exposed to intense sunlight, tanning booth light, halogen lamp, welding torch, or close lightening flash with unprotected or inadequate UV eye protection.
  - Strictly involve a 6- to 12-hour latency of acute, intense pain in a photophobic red eye
- Chemicals directly on the cornea may cause serious, extensive damage to the epithelial or deeper layers.
- Corneal abrasion and keratitis/ulceration can each cause scarring which may lead to impaired vision or permanent vision loss.

EPIDEMIOLOGY

All unprotected eyes are vulnerable to corneal injuries.

Incidence

- Corneal abrasions:
  - Eight percent of total ER visits are eye trauma-related; 64% of these eye complaints are abrasions via direct minor trauma.
  - Twelve percent of corneal abrasions relate to contact lenses, particularly in young people.
  - Only conjunctivitis and subconjunctival hemorrhage surpass corneal abrasion as a cause of red eye complaints.
- Worldwide, infectious keratitis and ulceration is 5th leading cause of blindness.
- Chemical ocular injuries: 67% occur in men at work, aged 20 to 30 years old; 33% occur by assault incidents in United Kingdom.
- In United States, 1 million ER and clinic visits per year result in a keratitis diagnosis.

ETIOLOGY AND PATHOPHYSIOLOGY

- Corneal abrasions: usually caused by mechanical scratching, from various foreign bodies or chemical and flash (UV) burns
- Recurring: Acute corneal injuries or spontaneous defects can cause corneal scarring and permanent vision loss.

- Corneal ulcers: The injury precedes keratitis and infectious corneal ulceration.
  - Contact lenses use, impaired immunity (HIV), corneal trauma or abrasion, and ocular surface disease can promote keratitis or cause corneal ulceration. Ischemia of the cornea induces edema which plays a significant role in epithelial dysfunction. Trauma, ischemia, and increased intraocular pressure can result from edema which then itself can promote further edema.
- Pathogens causing ulcerations include the following:
  - Gram-positive bacteria ~20–69%; *Staphylococcus aureus* and coagulase-negative *Streptococcus* are common.
  - Gram-negative bacteria ~21–35%; *Pseudomonas* sp. most common, especially contact lenses users
  - Herpes simplex (most common viral cause) with or without bacterial superinfection; herpes zoster
  - Fungal: Fusarium, Aspergillus, Curvularia, and Candida; rank order varies geographically.
  - Parasites: Acanthamoeba is very, very rare in United States, but 85% are in contact lenses users
- Autoimmune disorders: Sjögren, PUK, rheumatoid arthritis, inflammatory bowel disease
- Corneal ulceration is more common in immunocompromised: cancer, HIV, and diabetes mellitus (DM).
- Ocular surface diseases: Chronic blepharitis, entropion, Graves eye disease, and dry eyes/corneal dystrophy/bullous keratopathy/mucous membrane pemphigoid promote ulceration.

RISK FACTORS

- Acute eye trauma: direct contact trauma, chemical burn, UV overexposure
- Contact lenses use:
  - The most common contributing factor for bacterial keratitis in United States
  - Risky handling of contact lenses (poor hand and lenses hygiene)
  - Extended wear lenses, excessive wear times
- Perioperative time: sedation and general anesthesia
- Lack of proper eye protection
- Males, age 20 to 34 years old
- Manufacturing, construction, agricultural work (equatorial especially)

GENERAL PREVENTION

- Strong, face/periorbital, skin contact-fitting eyewear during:
  - Work (auto mechanics, metalworkers, miners, etc.) or anywhere hammering, grinding, sawing
  - Contact sports
- Occupational Safety and Health Administration mandates safety standards for at risk employees; see https://www.osha.gov/laws-regs/regulations /standardnumber/1926/1926.102.

COMMONLY ASSOCIATED CONDITIONS

- Xerophthalmia (common) or exophthalmos (occasional); allergic eye disease (common)
- Severe vitamin A deficiency (associated with corneal keratitis—rare)
- Neuropathy of cranial nerve V1, the ophthalmic branch (rare)

- DM (occasional), immunocompromise (e.g., HIV), connective tissue disease: bacterial (occasional) or fungal (rare) ulcers
- Critically ill or patients under anesthesia with impaired blink reflex or lagophthalmos and those on intermittent positive pressure ventilation (occasional)

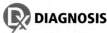

DIAGNOSIS

Key historical questions and a systematic eye examination keenly focus the diagnosis.

HISTORY

- Ask about recent significant ocular trauma, and if so, consider penetrating injury.
- Acute corneal foreign bodies: minor abrasions: abrupt foreign body sensation, severe photophobia/ pain; but abrasions *without* foreign body sensation suggests acute keratitis or current erosion syndrome.
- Excessive UV or welding exposure: 6- to 12-hour *delay* in usually severe, *bilateral* symptoms: significant pain, scleral injection, photophobia, facial erythema (UV)
- Contact lenses misuse: pain and photophobia on awakening or interrupted sleep by searing eye pain: "classic" for recurrent erosion syndrome
- Other symptoms include red eye, pain with extraocular muscle movement, eye twitching, excessive tearing, blurred or decreased vision, nausea, and headache.
- Past medical/surgical history: diabetes, immunosuppression, contact lenses use/misuse, or refractive surgery, last tetanus shot date

PHYSICAL EXAM

- First, 1 drop of ophthalmic topical ocular anesthetic (TOA) facilitates best exam.
- Survey: orbit (palpation), eyelids, globe surface, pupils, and extraocular muscles
- Document far or near visual acuity by Snellen chart, wall or hand held: A two-line decrease is significant; if only hand motion or light seen in a usually normal eye, then same day call to ophthalmologist.
- Slit lamp is ideal or otoscope or ophthalmoscope or even penlight exam of cornea/associated structures.
- Evert the upper lid and then retract lower lid to inspect for foreign body.
- Fluorescein stain exam with Wood's light for corneal surface defects: retention of yellow/green color at abrasion or full cornea in UV keratitis

DIFFERENTIAL DIAGNOSIS

- Corneal abrasion: acute angle-closure glaucoma, acute conjunctivitis, adult blepharitis, corneal ulcer, infective keratitis, uveitis, iritis, entropion, epidemic keratoconjunctivitis
- Corneal ulceration: contact lenses mechanical trauma; keratoconjunctivitis: atopic or sicca; keratitis: interstitial or infectious or neurotrophic or PUK; band keratopathy; and HLA-B27 syndromes

DIAGNOSTIC TESTS & INTERPRETATION
An "eye tray": instruments and meds; lights

Initial Tests (lab, imaging)
- Corneal ulcer: uncommon to culture (corneal scrape) but need same day discussion with ophthalmologist
- Usually avoid prereferral definitive treatment with topical antibiotics; may obscure true culture findings
- If suspicious for high-impact foreign body or direct injury: fluorescein (generous amount) stain exam with Wood's lamp or slit lamp for ocular surface exam—if blue/green color flows from surface, it indicates corneal or scleral penetration (positive Siedel test)
- If penetrating injury suspicious for retained foreign body: ocular CT if metallic or MRI if nonmetallic (1)[C]

Diagnostic Procedures/Other
- 1–2 drops 0.5% proparacaine or tetracaine ophthalmic solution topical anesthetic for pain control
- Tonometry for intraocular pressure testing (8 to 21 = normal) if need to rule out acute open-angle glaucoma
- Evert the upper lid and retract the lower lid to inspect and sweep (with sterile, wet, cotton swab) for foreign body removal
- Slit or Wood's lamp exam, after fluorescein strip saturated with sterile: saline, water, or TOA, to stain cornea and identify abrasions, ulcerations, keratitis/infiltrates
- Corneal trauma/foreign body/infection effects have planar geographic shape or more linear stains; contact lenses cause several punctate or curvilinear shape stains, and herpetic dendrites with terminal bulb pattern (atypical herpetic lesion may appear as >4 mm abrasion) (2)[C].

Test Interpretation
Scraping culture: fungal, bacterial identifies bacteria, yeast to help identify specific infection

 ## TREATMENT

Goals: Control pain, prevent infection, and teach patient daily self-monitoring (vision degradation, excess pain).

GENERAL MEASURES
- Normal saline irrigation of ocular surface and both fornices may flush away foreign body.
- If patient is cooperative, adherent epithelial foreign body without stain may be removed with sterile moist cotton swab or 25-gauge needle by experienced operator.
- Give tetanus booster as indicated for eye abrasions/punctures (1)[C].
- Patching is *not* recommended (fails to reduce pain, delays healing, more risk of infection) (2)[C].

MEDICATION
- *Oral* analgesic: narcotics, acetaminophen, or NSAIDs
- Topical anesthetics include proparacaine hydrochloride 0.5%, tetracaine hydrochloride 0.5%.
  – Tetracaine does not require refrigeration; proparacaine does.
  – Patients should *not* use TOAs as overuse can cause superimposed infections or scaring, nor topical steroids.

- If photophobia and pain, meiosis and limbal flush: topical cycloplegic agents like 1% cyclopentolate 1 drop every 8 hours for 1–2 days.
- Ophthalmic NSAIDs: Diclofenac 0.1% 1 drop QID reduces moderate pain; limit to 1- to 2-day use as it may impair healing or rarely damage cornea (3)[C].
- Caution: Frequent use of artificial tears may dilute other medications.

First Line
- Topical ophthalmic antibiotics to prevent corneal infection, especially in contact lenses users, fingernail or plant matter involvement
- Some ophthalmic antibiotics include polymyxin B/trimethoprim 1 drop q3h for 7 days for lower risk abrasions or erythromycin 0.5% ointment 1 ribbon q3h for 7 days.
  – Broad spectrum: polymyxin B/trimethoprim 1 drop q3h for 7 days or erythromycin ointment for lower risk abrasions
  – Higher risk abrasions (involving: contact lenses user, fingernail or plant matter) gram-negative coverage/antipseudomonals: ofloxacin 0.3% solution 1–2 drop q2–3h for 2 days, then same QID for 3 days or ciprofloxacin 0.3% solution, same dose/duration.
- Fungal keratitis: if suspected, <24 hours, referral to ophthalmologist for antifungal—topical antifungal agents
- Herpetic keratitis: <24 hours, referral to ophthalmologist for confirmation or may start (after phone consult ophthalmologist): trifluridine 1% solution 1 drop q2h while awake (2)[C]

ISSUES FOR REFERRAL
- Lack of improvement by 24 hours or worsening symptoms
- Any chemical burn
- Any corneal ulcer or infiltrate
- Any symptoms or incomplete healing by 3 to 4 days
- Retained foreign body or any stain/ring
- Any penetrating globe injury
- Any hyphema (blood) or hypopyon (pus)
- Anytime a vision loss of more than two lines on Snellen chart or abrupt decline to hand or light recognition only (2)[C]

ADDITIONAL THERAPIES
Novel approaches: amniotic membrane/fluid, autologous blood tears; proposed: topical insulin and substance P (3)[C]

 ## ONGOING CARE

FOLLOW-UP RECOMMENDATIONS
Patient Monitoring
It is best to follow up *all* corneal abrasions in 24 hours; especially lesions ≥4 mm, or decreased vision, or abrasions due to contact lenses, strict follow-up within 24 hours.

PATIENT EDUCATION
Corneal Abrasion and Erosion (English and Spanish versions by American Academy Ophthalmology [AAO]) (https://www.aao.org/eye-health/diseases/what-is-corneal-abrasion). See if you qualify for a no-cost eye exam from AAO's EyeCare America program.

PROGNOSIS
- Minor corneal abrasions <4 mm heal within 24 to 72 hours; larger ones, maximum of 5 days.
- Among extended wear contact lenses users, risk of microbial keratitis is 15 times nonusers.
- Daily wear contact users occasionally wearing through the night have 9 times risk for nonusers for microbial keratitis (2)[C].

COMPLICATIONS
- Recurrence of abrasion or ulcer by reinjury or spontaneously
- Conversion of abrasion to keratitis/ulcer
- Scarring of the cornea may produce vision loss.
- Exogenous endophthalmitis, risk loss of vision or eye

REFERENCES
1. Ambikkumar A, Arthurs B, El-Hadad C. Corneal foreign bodies. *CMAJ*. 2022;194(11):E419.
2. Amed F, House RJ, Feldman BH. Corneal abrasions and corneal foreign bodies. *Prim Care*. 2015;42(3):363–375.
3. Dang DH, Riaz KM, Karamichos D. Treatment of non-infectious corneal injury: review of diagnostic agents, therapeutic medications and future targets. *Drugs*. 2022;82(2):145–167.

ADDITIONAL READING
Arbabi EM, Kelly RJ, Carrim ZI. Corneal ulcers in general practice. *Br J Gen Pract*. 2018;68(666):49–50.

 ## CODES

ICD10
- S05.00XA Inj conjunctiva and corneal abrasion w/o fb, unsp eye, init
- H16.009 Unspecified corneal ulcer, unspecified eye
- H16.049 Marginal corneal ulcer, unspecified eye

CLINICAL PEARLS
- Visual acuity testing is *the* vital sign at the beginning of every eye visit.
- When corneal abrasion is healed and asymptomatic, contact lenses use may restart.
- Eye patching is *not* recommended for corneal ulcerations or abrasions.
- Consider topical NSAIDs and/or oral analgesics a maximum of 3 days for symptom control.
- Treatment usually involves frequent topical antimicrobial application.
- Prompt referral to an ophthalmologist should be made with suspicion of any ulcer (same-day phone), recurrence of abrasion, retained foreign body (same-day consult), hyphema or hypopyon (same day), viral keratitis (<24 hours), significant visual decrease (same-day phone), or lack of prompt improvement despite therapy (next day).

CORNS AND CALLUSES

Sandra N. New, DNP • Jon S. Parham, DO, MPH, FAAFP

BASICS

DESCRIPTION

- Corns and calluses are pressure-generated hyperkeratotic skin conditions of the feet or hands.
- A callus (tyloma [Greek]) is a diffuse area of hyperkeratosis, usually without a distinct border. Typically, callus is the result of exposure to repetitive forces, including friction and mechanical pressure. They tend to occur on the palms of hands and soles of feet.
- A corn (heloma [Greek]) is a circumscribed hyperkeratotic lesion with a central conical core of keratin that causes pain and inflammation. The conical core in a corn is a thickening of the stratum corneum. Corns typically occur at pressure points or result from poor-fitting shoes or an underlying bone lesion/spur.
- Hard corn or heloma durum (more common): often on toe surfaces, especially on the 5th toe (proximal interphalangeal [PIP] joint)
- Soft corn or heloma molle: commonly in the interdigital space
- Digital corns are also known as clavi or heloma durum.
- Intractable plantar keratosis is usually located under a metatarsal head (1st and 5th are the most common), is typically more difficult to resolve, and often is resistant to usual conservative treatments.

EPIDEMIOLOGY

Corns and calluses are the most prevalent of all foot disorders.

Incidence

- Incidence of corns and calluses are more common in elderly.
- Less common in pediatric patients
- Women are affected slightly more often than men, possibly due to ill-fitting fashionable shoes.
- Blacks report corns and calluses 30% more often than whites.

Prevalence

- Corns and calluses represent 46% of foot disorders presenting to podiatric clinics and affect about 9.2 million Americans.
- About 38 per 1,000 people are affected.

ETIOLOGY AND PATHOPHYSIOLOGY

Corns and calluses are symptoms, not a disease entity themselves. Repetitive, accumulated, or excessive friction and mechanical trauma on external skin produces a natural, protective dermal response of hyperkeratosis on hands and feet, particularly over bony prominences.

- Calluses typically form diffusely over bony prominences or deformities where there are repetitive forces and/or frequent weight-bearing forces. Examples include metatarsal head deformities or from ill-fitting shoes on normal bony anatomy. Corns rarely form on the hands. Although calluses may frequently form on palmar surfaces, symptoms are rare because these surfaces are nonweight bearing.
- Hard corns are an extreme form of callus with a keratin-based core. Often found on the digital surfaces and commonly linked to bony protrusions, causing skin to rub against shoe surfaces.
- Soft corns arise from increased moisture from perspiration leading to skin maceration, along with mechanical irritation, especially between toes.

Genetics

No genetic basis

RISK FACTORS

- Extrinsic factors producing pressure, friction, and local stress
  - Poorly fitting shoes with narrow toe box or with abrasive surfaces
  - Absence of socks or gloves for protection
  - Repetitive activities: sports, guitar playing, labor
  - Walking barefoot or wearing thin-soled shoes offering no support
- Intrinsic factors
  - Bony malformations such as hammertoes, bunions
  - Neuropathy such as frequently seen in diabetic patients
  - Gait disturbances

GENERAL PREVENTION

Reduce mechanical pressure or friction by wearing protective shoes, socks, or gloves.

Geriatric Considerations

Regular foot exams, more frequently for diabetic and/or peripheral vascular disease patients, to assess for skin integrity, neuropathy, and pressure points are paramount.

COMMONLY ASSOCIATED CONDITIONS

- Foot ulcers in vascularly compromised individuals due to history of smoking and poor circulation or secondary to diabetes with microangiopathy and neuropathy
- Infection, local or regional symptoms/signs:
  - Pain, increasing size, redness, or swelling
  - Purulent discharge
  - Fever
  - Color changes: pale, red, black
  - Excessive heat or coolness of skin to touch

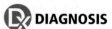

DIAGNOSIS

- Visual examination of entire foot and focal lesion(s)
- History of activities that incite focal pain
- Examination of footwear typically worn for excessive wear areas

HISTORY

- Engage patient in identification of friction sites corresponding with pain.
- Inquire if patient has vascular or neurologic health issues such as smoking history or diabetes.
- Ask what has been done thus far to treat the hyperkeratotic lesions.

PHYSICAL EXAM

- Calluses
  - Assess skin area of complaint for plantar hyperkeratosis and areas of pain.
  - Inspect feet and hands for areas of friction; palpate for focal, excessive hyperkeratosis and tenderness.
  - Identify skin color changes.
  - Assess sensory response in area of complaint.
- Corns
  - Hard corns
    - Assess the dorsum of feet and toes for hard corns and note distinct, circumscribed borders.
    - Identify central core mass and focal, marked tenderness to perpendicular pressure on direct palpation.
  - Soft corns
    - Inspect between toes for maceration and discoloration of hyperkeratotic lesion, commonly at the 4th to 5th intertriginous space.
    - Evaluate the painfulness of corn—usually severely painful.

DIFFERENTIAL DIAGNOSIS
- Plantar warts—viral origin with blood capillary dots visible (often after débridement) and pain with bilateral compression to lesion
- Porokeratosis (small nodule[s] from occluded sweat gland)
- Skin pressure (dark-colored) eschar overlying a pathologic wound, commonly affecting feet in diabetics and elderly

DIAGNOSTIC TESTS & INTERPRETATION
Rarely indicated

Initial Tests (lab, imaging)
- Radiographs are warranted if no external cause is found. Look for abnormalities in foot structure and bone spurs.
- Use of metallic radiographic marker (BB taped over skin lesion) and weight-bearing films often highlight the relationship between the callus and bony prominence.

Follow-Up Tests & Special Considerations
Evaluate chronic conditions such as diabetes, arterial insufficiency, and recurrent infections (tinea pedis) that could worsen symptoms.

Diagnostic Procedures/Other
Biopsy with microscopic evaluation only in atypical appearing cases

Test Interpretation
Abnormal accumulation of keratin in epidermis, stratum corneum (1)[C]

TREATMENT
Local débridement of hyperkeratosis and focal pressure/friction alleviation are the key steps.

GENERAL MEASURES
- Management can be done in home:
  - Soak affected skin areas in warm water.
  - Use pumice stones or coarse sandpaper to reduce the thickened skin.
- In office: Tangential-skin shaving to reduce the stratum corneum thickness using a size 15 (or 10 for larger areas) blade is usually very helpful.
- Adding foam padding or silicon sleeve can reduce the friction area over bony prominences.
- Wear socks or gloves (for hands) regularly.
- Cutouts of padding corresponding to pressure points may off-load bony prominences.
- Choose low-heeled shoes with soft upper and deep, wide toe boxes (1)[C].
- Shoe repair shops can stretch shoes made of certain materials to prevent friction point(s) (2)[C].

- Avoidance of chronic, friction-generating activities
- The use of prefabricated or custom orthotics may be helpful in some cases.
- Silicone sleeves for toes, foam toe spacers, and small pieces of lamb's wool or adhesive felt strategically placed can significantly reduce "shoe to skin" friction areas, example, dorsum and/or tip of hammer toes (1)[C]

MEDICATION
Keratolytic agents may be used in certain cases but usually avoided in elderly (1)[C].

Geriatric Considerations
- The use of salicylic acid corn plasters can cause skin breakdown and ulceration in patients with thin, atrophic skin (diabetics and those with vascular compromise).
- Aggressive use of pumice stones can also lead to excessive skin breakdown, especially surrounding the callus (1)[C].

ISSUES FOR REFERRAL
- If initial changes/treatments are not effective, a podiatrist referral is indicated.
- Bony foot abnormalities—may require referral to a podiatrist or orthopedic surgeon for bony prominence débridement

SURGERY/OTHER PROCEDURES
- Surgical treatment of hammer toe, claw toe, or mallet toe to reduce bony abnormalities may correct stress friction points if reasonable conservative measures have failed.
- Orthotic footwear may off-load pressure and reduce reformation of calluses or corns.
- Shaving a callus using a scalpel is usually indicated. An 11 type scalpel is used to "core" out corn's keratin core in the office (1)[C].

COMPLEMENTARY & ALTERNATIVE MEDICINE
- May benefit from urea-based lotions, creams, or ointments
- Warm water/Epsom salt soaks prior to pumice stone débridement (2)[C]

ADMISSION, INPATIENT, AND NURSING CONSIDERATIONS
- Admission very rarely indicated-unless progression to ulcerated lesion with signs of severe infection, gangrene, or sepsis
- Chronic venous-related edema or arterial insufficiency of feet requires a vascular surgery referral
- Nursing
  - Wound care, dressing changes for infected lesions, teaching signs and symptoms to report such as fever, increased pain, redness, swelling
  - Shoe choice teaching: wide toe box, low-heel shoes with support, and wearing of diabetic socks by all at-risk persons

ONGOING CARE
Periodic assessment of feet for signs of corns or calluses, hyperkeratosis, and general skin/nail health by patient or professional

FOLLOW-UP RECOMMENDATIONS
Daily foot skin care with over the counter skin emollients can prevent dry skin, which is more sensitive to pressure points.

PATIENT EDUCATION
- General information: http://www.mayoclinic.org/diseases-conditions/corns-and-calluses/symptoms-causes/syc-20355946
- American Academy of Dermatology Association: https://www.aad.org/public/everyday-care/injured-skin/burns/treat-corns-calluses
- American Podiatric Medical Association: http://www.apma.org

PROGNOSIS
Complete cure is possible if all factors causing pressure or injury are eliminated.

COMPLICATIONS
Ulceration; infection if simple calluses and corns are not properly addressed and sources of friction eliminated

REFERENCES
1. Freeman DB. Corns and calluses resulting from mechanical hyperkeratosis. *Am Fam Physician*. 2002;65(11):2277–2280.
2. Bailey J. Nail and foot procedures. *Prim Care*. 2022;49(1):63–83.

ADDITIONAL READING
- American College of Foot and Ankle Surgeons: http://www.acfas.org
- Theodosat A. Skin diseases of the lower extremities in the elderly. *Dermatol Clin*. 2004;22(1):13–21.

CODES

ICD10
L84 Corns and callosities

CLINICAL PEARLS
- Most therapy for corns and calluses can be done as self-care at home using débridement, then padding over the affected area, and friction/pressure source correction of the shoe.
- Cryotherapy may worsen discomfort and is not advised for treatment.

CORONARY ARTERY DISEASE AND STABLE ANGINA

Jeremy Golding, MD, FAAFP

 BASICS

DESCRIPTION

- Coronary artery disease (CAD) refers to the atherosclerotic narrowing of the epicardial coronary arteries. It may manifest insidiously as angina pectoris or as an acute coronary syndrome (ACS).
- Stable angina is a chest discomfort due to myocardial ischemia that is predictably reproducible at a certain level of exertion or emotional stress.
- The spectrum of ACS includes unstable angina (UA), non–ST elevation myocardial infarction (NSTEMI), and ST elevation myocardial infarction (STEMI). See "Acute Coronary Syndromes: NSTE-ACS (Unstable Angina and NSTEMI)."
- Definitions
  - Typical angina: exhibits three classical characteristics: (i) substernal chest pressure, pressure or heaviness that may radiate to the jaw, back, or arms and generally lasts from 2 to 15 minutes; (ii) occurs at a certain level of myocardial oxygen demand from exertion, emotional stress, or increased sympathetic tone; and (iii) relieved with rest or sublingual nitroglycerin
  - Atypical angina: exhibits two of the above typical characteristics
  - Noncardiac chest pain: exhibits ≤1 of the above typical characteristics
  - Anginal equivalent: Patients may present without chest discomfort but with nonspecific symptoms such as dyspnea, diaphoresis, fatigue, belching, nausea, light-headedness, or indigestion that occur with exertion or stress.
  - UA: anginal symptoms that are new or more frequent, more severe, or occurring with lessening degrees of myocardial demand; considered ACS but do not present with cardiac biomarker elevation.
  - NSTEMI: elevation of cardiac biomarker (troponin I or T) with either anginal symptoms, ischemic ECG changes other than ST elevation, or both.
  - STEMI: presents with typical symptoms as mentioned above with ST elevations noted on ECG; generally caused by acute plaque rupture and complete obstruction of culprit vessel and may present prior to laboratory detection of troponin.

Geriatric Considerations
The elderly may present with atypical symptoms. Physical limitations may delay recognition of angina until it occurs with minimal exertion or at rest. Maintain a high degree of suspicion during evaluation of dyspnea and other nonspecific complaints.

EPIDEMIOLOGY

- CAD is the leading cause of death for adults both in the United States and worldwide, causing about 1 in 5 deaths in the United States. The cost of CAD in the United States is estimated at between $240 billion (Centers for Disease Control and Prevention) and $378 billion (American Heart Association [AHA]) annually for 2017 to 2019.
- ~80% of CAD is preventable with a healthy lifestyle.

Incidence
In the United States, the lifetime risk of a 40-year-old developing CAD is 49% for men and 32% for women.

Prevalence
In the United States, about 5% of adults have CAD.

ETIOLOGY AND PATHOPHYSIOLOGY
Anginal symptoms occur during times of myocardial ischemia caused by a mismatch between coronary perfusion and myocardial oxygen demand. Atherosclerotic narrowing of the coronary arteries is the most common etiology of angina, but it may also occur in those with significant aortic stenosis, pulmonary hypertension, hypertrophic cardiomyopathy, coronary spasm, or volume overload.

RISK FACTORS

- Traditional risk factors: hypertension, ↑ LDL cholesterol, smoking, diabetes, premature CAD in first-degree relatives (men <55 years old; women <65 years old), age (>45 years for men; >55 years for women), ↓ HDL
- Nontraditional risk factors: obesity, sedentary lifestyle, chronic inflammation, abnormal ankle-brachial indices, renal disease

GENERAL PREVENTION

- Smoking cessation
- Regular aerobic exercise program and weight loss for obese patients (goal body mass index [BMI] <25 kg/m^2); a plant-based or a Mediterranean-like diet is recommended.
- Blood pressure (BP) control (goal <140/90 mm Hg; consider <130/80 mm Hg for those with 10-year ASCVD risk ≥10%.)
- Type 2 diabetes management: Consider more aggressive hemoglobin A1c (HbA1c) goal of 6.5–7% in younger, recently diagnosed individuals.
- At least moderate-intensity statin therapy for those with diabetes aged 40 to 75 years and those with 10-year ASCVD risk ≥7.5–20% (Recommendations of advisory organizations vary. Caution: American College of Cardiology [ACC]/AHA risk calculator overestimates risk in many by as much as 50–100%.)
- Low-dose aspirin should not be recommended for routine primary prevention of myocardial infarction (MI) without objective evidence of CAD. It may be used for those with high clinical suspicion in the interim prior to stress testing/catheterization.

COMMONLY ASSOCIATED CONDITIONS
Hyperlipidemia, peripheral vascular disease, cerebrovascular disease, hypertension, obesity, diabetes

DIAGNOSIS

HISTORY

- Pain may be described with a clenched fist over the center of the chest (Levine sign). Episodes of angina are generally of the same character and in the same location as previous episodes. Dyspnea on exertion may present as the only symptom.
- May present with symptoms similar to gastric reflux or GI upset (indigestion, nausea, diaphoresis). Atypical symptoms are more likely in women, elderly, and diabetic patients.

PHYSICAL EXAM

- Normal cardiac exam does not exclude the diagnosis of angina or CAD.
- Cardiac exam may reveal dysrhythmias, heart murmurs indicative of valvular disease, gallops, or signs of congestive heart failure.

DIFFERENTIAL DIAGNOSIS

- Vascular: aortic dissection, pericarditis, myocarditis, MI, vasospasm
- Pulmonary: pleuritis, pulmonary embolism, pneumothorax
- Gastroesophageal: gastric reflux, esophageal spasm, peptic ulcer
- Musculoskeletal: costochondritis, arthritis, muscle strain, rib fracture
- Other: anxiety, psychosomatic, cocaine abuse

DIAGNOSTIC TESTS & INTERPRETATION

Initial Tests (lab, imaging)

- Serial cardiac troponins for those presenting acutely with symptoms
- Complete blood count, lipid profile, and HbA1c for risk stratification, basic metabolic panel
- ECG—should be obtained unless there is a clearly noncardiac cause of the chest pain; may be normal or may show signs of ischemia; left bundle branch block or ventricular pacing makes interpretation for ischemia difficult.
- Chest x-ray may identify other causes of pain.

Follow-Up Tests & Special Considerations

- The goal is to detect high-risk coronary lesions where intervention would improve long-term mortality or alleviate anginal symptoms. Various algorithms exist depending on pretest risk and test results.
- Stress testing is most helpful for patients at intermediate risk of CAD; exercise testing for those who can physically exercise (≥5 metabolic equivalents [METs]): standard exercise ECG for those with normal baseline ECG (i.e., without left bundle branch block or ventricular pacing); exercise stress testing with echo or perfusion imaging for those with abnormal baseline ECG and for those with intermediate-high pretest probability; for those who cannot tolerate exercise, consider pharmacologic stress testing. Stress testing may also be useful to evaluate effectiveness of the PT's therapeutic regimen.
- CT coronary angiography or cardiac MRI can be considered as a supplement/alternative to stress testing in patients with continued symptoms despite negative stress testing, inconclusive stress testing, or if there is a need for better anatomic definition of disease.

Diagnostic Procedures/Other

- Cardiac catheterization with coronary angiography is the gold standard for confirmation and delineation of coronary disease and direction of interventional therapy or surgery. It is indicated if noninvasive testing suggests a high-risk lesion or if patient fails to respond to appropriate medical management.
- Significant CAD is defined as ≥50% stenosis of the left main coronary artery or ≥70% stenosis of other major coronary arteries by angiography.

TREATMENT

GENERAL MEASURES
- AHA/ACC-recommended BP control goal for most patients with significant CAD: <130/80 mm Hg
- Smoking cessation goal: complete cessation, no exposure to secondhand smoke or e-cigarettes
- Physical activity goal: 30 to 60 minutes of moderate aerobic activity, at least 5 (preferably 7) days/week

MEDICATION

First Line
- β-Blockers: decrease myocardial oxygen demand by lowering heart rate (HR), BP, and contractility and can improve angina; they also decrease mortality in patients with MI or heart failure and should be used as initial therapy. Metoprolol (25 to 400 mg/day [succinate] or divided BID [tartrate]) or carvedilol (3.125 to 25 mg BID) is preferred. Adjust doses according to clinical response. Maintain resting HR 50 to 60 beats/min.
- Calcium channel blockers (CCBs): cause arterial vasodilation, decreased myocardial oxygen demand, and improved coronary blood flow; similar effectiveness to β-blockers; may be used instead of or in addition to β-blockers; only long-acting CCBs should be used:
  - Dihydropyridine CCBs: Nifedipine (30 to 90 mg/day), amlodipine (5 to 10 mg/day), or felodipine (2.5 to 10 mg/day) works predominantly on arterial vasodilation and can improve coronary blood flow.
  - Nondihydropyridine CCBs: Diltiazem (120 to 480 mg/day) or verapamil (120 to 480 mg/day) also has negative inotropic effects and should not be used in those with ejection fracture <40% because they may precipitate heart failure.
- Nitrates: dilate systemic veins and arteries (including coronary vessels) and cause decreased preload; at higher doses, they decrease BP. Side effects include headache and hypotension but tend to improve with continued usage.
  - Sublingual nitroglycerin (0.4 mg every 5 minutes for up to 3 doses) used for acute anginal episodes
  - Long-acting nitrates such as isosorbide mononitrate (30 to 240 mg/day [extended release]) can be used for angina prophylaxis.
- Lipid-lowering agents:
  - High-intensity statin therapy is indicated for all patients with CAD regardless of lipid levels.
  - Atorvastatin (40 to 80 mg/day) and rosuvastatin (20 to 40 mg/day) are high-intensity statins.
  - Statins reduce risk of MI and revascularization need. Side effects include myalgias, transaminitis, rhabdomyolysis (rare), and impaired glucose tolerance. Evidence for benefit in primary prevention after age 75 years is sparse.

- Ezetimibe may be added to statin therapy if LDL is not at goal after maximally tolerated dose of statin, especially in secondary prevention.
- Proprotein convertase subtilisin/kexin type 9 inhibitors further reduce LDL levels when used in combination with statins for high-risk patients and reduce cardiovascular events in highly selected patients but are expensive.
- Antiplatelets: decrease risk of thrombosis
  - Aspirin (75 to 162 mg/day) decreases risk of first MI and reduces adverse cardiovascular events in those with stable angina.
  - Clopidogrel (75 mg/day) may be used in patients with contraindications to aspirin.
  - Dual antiplatelet therapy with aspirin + clopidogrel, prasugrel, or ticagrelor is indicated after MI or percutaneous coronary intervention (PCI) (use prasugrel only after PCI. Do not use in patient with CVA history) for a period of time determined by the particular circumstances (1)[C].
- Angiotensin-converting enzyme inhibitors (ACEIs): act on the renin-angiotensin-aldosterone system to reduce BP and afterload. They also have effects on cardiac remodeling after MI.
  - ACEIs such as lisinopril (5 to 40 mg/day) and enalapril (2.5 to 20.0 mg BID) have been shown to reduce both cardiovascular death and MI in patients with CAD and left ventricular systolic dysfunction.
  - Angiotensin receptor blockers such as candesartan (4 to 32 mg/day) may be used in patients intolerant to ACEIs.
  - Side effects include cough (ACEIs predominantly), hyperkalemia, and angioedema.

Second Line
- Ranolazine (500 to 1,000 mg BID) decreases calcium overload in myocytes, acting as an antianginal/antiischemic agent. It does not affect HR or BP and may be used as an adjunctive therapy when symptoms persist despite optimal dose of other antianginals.
- Low dose colchicine (0.5 to 0.6 mg/day) improves outcomes in those with established CAD.

SURGERY/OTHER PROCEDURES
- Revascularization should be considered if optimal medical therapy is inadequate to control symptoms. Coronary artery bypass graft (CABG) is preferred over PCI for those with severe left main coronary stenosis, significant lesions in ≥3 major coronary arteries, and for lesions not amenable to PCI.
- PCI with balloon angioplasty and/or stent placement is performed for significant lesions, especially for those whose angina is not adequately controlled by optimal medical therapy. Additional techniques include laser therapy and atherectomy. PCI does not appear to decrease mortality or risk of MI versus aggressive medical management in those with stable angina (2)[A].

ONGOING CARE

FOLLOW-UP RECOMMENDATIONS
Lifestyle modifications should be aggressively stressed at every visit.

DIET
Plant-based or Mediterranean-like diet is recommended and shown to lower all-cause mortality compared to standard diet. Eating fatty fish like salmon is recommended (but not omega-3 supplements).

PROGNOSIS
Variable; depends on severity of symptoms, extent of CAD, and left ventricular function

COMPLICATIONS
ACS, arrhythmia, cardiac arrest, heart failure

REFERENCES
1. Lawton JS, Tamis-Holland JE, Bangalore S, et al. 2021 ACC/AHA/SCAI guideline for coronary artery revascularization: a report of the American College of Cardiology/American Heart Association Joint Committee on Clinical Practice Guidelines. *Circulation*. 2022;145(3):e18–e114.
2. Maron DJ, Hochman JS, Reynolds HR, et al; for ISCHEMIA Research Group. Initial invasive or conservative strategy for stable coronary disease. *N Engl J Med*. 2020;382(15):1395–1407.

SEE ALSO

Algorithm: Chest Pain/Acute Coronary Syndrome

CODES

ICD10
- I25.119 Athscl heart disease of native cor art w unsp ang pctrs
- I25.118 Athscl heart disease of native cor art w oth ang pctrs
- I20.9 Angina pectoris, unspecified

CLINICAL PEARLS
- Maximize antianginal therapy combining β-blockers, CCBs, and nitrates as tolerated, along with high-intensity statin therapy and anti-platelet therapy.
- PCI may be considered for those with stable ischemic heart disease who continue to have angina on maximally tolerated medical therapy. PCI is first-line treatment for those with UA/NSTEMI/STEMI.

COSTOCHONDRITIS

Smriti Ohri, MD

BASICS

DESCRIPTION
- Anterior chest wall pain and tenderness of the costochondral and costosternal regions, most often affecting the 2nd to the 5th costal cartilages
- System(s) affected: musculoskeletal
- Synonym(s): costosternal syndrome; parasternal chondrodynia; anterior chest wall syndrome

EPIDEMIOLOGY
- Predominant age: 40 to 50 years
- Predominant gender: female

Incidence
- 30% emergency room visits for chest pain
- 13% primary care visits for chest pain

ETIOLOGY AND PATHOPHYSIOLOGY
Although not fully understood, inflammation can be caused by pulling from adjoining muscles at costochondral or costosternal regions.

RISK FACTORS
- Unusual physical activity or upper extremity overuse
- Recent trauma (including motor vehicle accident, domestic violence) or new-onset physical activity
- Recent upper respiratory infection (URI) with coughing

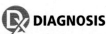DIAGNOSIS

- Pain is usually sharp, achy, or pressure-like, involving multiple (and mostly unilateral 2nd to 5th) costal cartilages.
- Exacerbated by upper body movements and exertional activities
- Reproduced by palpation of the affected cartilage segments
- Chest tightness is often associated with the pain.

HISTORY
- A complete and thorough history (including a cardiac risk stratification with validated clinical prediction rules) is mandatory for an accurate diagnosis (1).
- Social history: careful screening and evaluation for domestic violence and substance abuse

PHYSICAL EXAM
- A thorough cardiopulmonary exam to exclude other conditions presenting with chest pain
  - Cardiac rhythm, murmurs, gallops, rubs
  - Adventitious lung sounds—rales, rhonchi, wheezes, rubs
- Tenderness over the costochondral junctions is necessary to establish the diagnosis but does not completely exclude other causes of chest pain.
- If swelling or redness of costal cartilage is present, the presentation is often termed Tietze syndrome (also an inflammatory condition generally involving single costal cartilage of ribs 2 or 3, typically unilateral presentation).
- Movement of upper extremity of the same side may reproduce the pain.

Pediatric Considerations
- Consider psychogenic chest pain in children who perceive family discord.
- Consider slipping rib syndrome in children with chronic chest and abdominal pain (2).

Geriatric Considerations
Consider herpes zoster in elderly patients.

DIFFERENTIAL DIAGNOSIS
- Consider alternate diagnosis if presence of other signs and symptoms, like shortness of breath, dyspnea on exertion, cough, fever, tachycardia, and hypotension
- Cardiac
  - Coronary artery disease (CAD); acute coronary syndrome (ACS)
  - Cardiac contusion from trauma
  - Aortic aneurysm
  - Pericarditis
  - Myocarditis
- Gastrointestinal
  - Gastroesophageal reflux
  - Peptic esophagitis
  - Esophageal spasm
  - Cholecystitis
- Musculoskeletal (2)
  - Fibromyalgia
  - Slipping rib syndrome
  - Costovertebral arthritis
  - Painful xiphoid syndrome
  - Rib trauma
- Psychogenic
  - Panic attacks
- Respiratory
  - Pulmonary embolism
  - Pneumonia
  - Chronic cough
  - Pneumothorax
- Other
  - Domestic violence and abuse
  - Herpes zoster
  - Spinal tumor
  - Metastatic cancer
  - Substance abuse (cocaine)

DIAGNOSTIC TESTS & INTERPRETATION
- Primarily a clinical diagnosis
- Laboratory exams and imaging to rule out other diagnoses

Initial Tests (lab, imaging)
Imaging is not indicated for the diagnosis of costochondritis.

Diagnostic Procedures/Other
None indicated for the diagnosis of costochondritis. Diagnostic tests should be directed toward ruling out other etiologies based on history and exam. For example:
- Consider ECG in patients aged >35 years and for patients with history of or at risk for CAD (3)[C].
- Consider chest x-ray in patients with appropriate cardiopulmonary symptoms (3)[C].
- Consider CT imaging if high suspicion of aortic dissection, infectious or neoplastic process (3)[C].
- Consider spiral CT for pulmonary embolism and D-dimer if history or risk factors are present.

TREATMENT

Reassurance of benign nature of condition and potential for long, slow recovery from pain

GENERAL MEASURES
- Rest, local application of heat (or ice), massage
- Stretching exercises
- Minimize symptom-provoking activities (e.g., reduce frequency or intensity of exercise/work activity).

MEDICATION
- Pain relief with NSAIDs (oral or topical), acetaminophen, lidocaine patches, capsaicin cream
- The use of skeletal muscle relaxants may be beneficial if associated with muscle spasm.
- Refractory cases can be treated with local injections of combined lidocaine/corticosteroid into costochondral areas; rarely necessary (2)[C]

ISSUES FOR REFERRAL
- Consider referral to physical therapy for pain reduction and improvement in function in patients with prolonged symptoms (4)[B].
- Consider referral to gastroenterology or cardiology if an alternate diagnosis meriting special input is suspected.

COMPLEMENTARY & ALTERNATIVE MEDICINE
Limited data but may be safely tried if patient is interested
- Chiropractic manipulation; exercise prescription
- Dry needling by properly trained providers (5)[C]
- Acupuncture (6)[C]
- Massage

ADMISSION, INPATIENT, AND NURSING CONSIDERATIONS
Only if cardiac or other serious etiology of chest pain is being considered

 ONGOING CARE

FOLLOW-UP RECOMMENDATIONS
Follow-up within 1 week if diagnosis is unclear or symptoms do not abate with conservative treatment

PATIENT EDUCATION
- Educate regarding the self-limited (although potentially recurrent) nature of the illness.
- Instruct patient on proper physical activity regimens to avoid overuse syndromes.
- Avoid sudden, significant changes in activity.

PROGNOSIS
- Self-limited illness lasts for weeks to months and usually abates by 1 year.
- Often recurs

COMPLICATIONS
May be refractory or recurrent

REFERENCES

1. Mott T, Jones G, Roman K. Costochondritis: rapid evidence review. *Am Fam Physician*. 2021;104(1):73–78.
2. Ayloo A, Cvengros T, Marella S. Evaluation and treatment of musculoskeletal chest pain. *Prim Care*. 2013;40(4):863–887, viii.
3. Proulx AM, Zryd TW. Costochondritis: diagnosis and treatment. *Am Fam Physician*. 2009;80(6): 617–620.
4. Zaruba RA, Wilson E. Impairment based examination and treatment of costochondritis: a case series. *Int J Sports Phys Ther*. 2017;12(3):458–467.
5. Westrick RB, Zylstra E, Issa T, et al. Evaluation and treatment of musculoskeletal chest wall pain in a military athlete. *Int J Sports Phys Ther*. 2012;7(3):323–332.
6. Lin K, Tung C. Integrating acupuncture for the management of costochondritis in adolescents. *Med Acupunct*. 2017;29(5):327–330.

ADDITIONAL READING

Collins RA, Ray N, Ratheal K, et al. Severe post-COVID-19 costochondritis in children. *Proc (Bayl Univ Med Cent)*. 2021;35(1):56–57.

 CODES

ICD10
M94.0 Chondrocostal junction syndrome [Tietze]

CLINICAL PEARLS
- A common disorder, accounting for up to 30% of all cases of chest pain
- Diagnosis is primarily clinical. Obtain lab and other testing to exclude other conditions based on patient risk.
- Self-limited (potentially recurrent) condition; activity modification helps prevent recurrence.

COUNSELING TYPES

Akanksha Samal, DO

BASICS

DESCRIPTION

- Psychotherapeutic and counseling interventions play an important role in the management of chronic and acute-onset diseases and disorders. They are typically the primary initial mode of evaluation and/or treatment for most mild to moderate psychiatric disorders that reach criteria using the *DSM-5* (1) or *ICD-11* diagnostic classification systems.
- Treatment and successful control of either medical or psychological conditions typically benefit from some form of professional counseling. Best outcomes occur when they are employed by a skilled practitioner. However, psychotherapy differs from generic counseling, which can take many forms and is delivered commonly in nonmedical settings. In recent years, attempts to integrate counseling and psychotherapy within primary care practices have increased.
- Counseling approaches are usually tailored to the specific presenting problem or issue and serve educational and emotional support functions. Typically, counseling in medical settings will be time-limited and problem-focused and often not intended to lead to major medical symptom relief or major behavioral changes but to improve patient coping.
- The goals of psychotherapy range from increasing individual psychological insight and motivation for change to reduction of interpersonal conflict in the marriage or family, reduction of chronic or acute emotional suffering, or reversal of dysfunctional or habitual behaviors. There are several general classes of psychotherapy, starting with individual, marital, or family approaches. In addition, a number of psychological theories guide various methods and treatment philosophies. The following is a brief overview of commonly used psychotherapeutic and counseling methods.
- Psychodynamic therapy: Unconscious conflict manifests as patient's symptoms/problem behaviors:
  - Short term (4 to 6 months) and long term (≥1 year)
  - The focus is on increasing insight of underlying conflict or processes to initiate symptomatic change.
  - Therapist actively helps patient identify patterns of behavior stemming from existence of an unconscious conflict or beliefs and motivations that may not be accurately perceived by the individual.
- Cognitive-behavioral therapy (CBT): Patterns of thoughts and behaviors can lead to development and/or maintenance of symptoms. Thought patterns may not accurately reflect reality and may lead to psychological distress:
  - CBT aims at modifying thought patterns by increasing cognitive flexibility and changing dysfunctional behavioral patterns.
  - CBT encourages patient self-monitoring of symptoms and the precursors or results of maladaptive behavior.
  - Uses therapist-assisted challenges to patient's basic beliefs/assumptions
  - May use *exposure*, a procedure derived from basic learning theories, which encourages gradual steps toward change, at a speed that is tolerated by the patient

- CBT can be offered in group or individual formats, for adults or children.
  - A CBT practitioner attempts to combine practical interventions with emotional supports.
- Dialectical behavior therapy (DBT): Techniques such as social skills training, mindfulness, and problem solving are used to modulate impulse control and affect management:
  - DBT is a therapy approach that derives from CBT but emphasizes emotional control in relationships.
  - Originally used in treatment of patients with self-destructive behaviors (e.g., cutting, suicide attempts)
  - Seeks to change rigid patterns of cognitions and behaviors that have been maladaptive
  - Uses both individual and group treatment modalities
  - The DBT therapist takes an active role in interpretation and support.
- Interpersonal psychotherapy: Interpersonal relationships in a patient's life are linked to symptoms. Therapy seeks to alleviate symptoms and improve social adjustment through exploration of patient's relationships and experiences. The focus is on one of four potential problem areas:
  - Grief or loss
  - Interpersonal role disputes
  - Role transitions
  - Interpersonal deficits: Therapist works with the patient in resolving the problematic interpersonal issues to facilitate change in symptoms.
- Family therapy: focuses on the family as a unit of intervention
  - Uses psychoeducation to increase patient's and family's insight
  - Teaches communication and problem-solving skills
- Motivational interviewing (MI): focuses on motivation as a key to successful change process
  - Short-term and problem-focused; many therapists use MI prior to initiating other therapies.
  - Focuses on identifying discrepancies between goals and behavior, and the patient's desire to change
  - "5 A's" model is a brief counseling framework developed specifically for physicians to effect behavioral change in patients:
    - ○ Assess for a problem.
    - ○ Advise making a change.
    - ○ Agree on action to be taken.
    - ○ Assist with self-care support to make the change.
    - ○ Arrange follow-up to support the change.
- Supportive and informational counseling (heterogeneous treatment)
  - Often focuses on situational factors maintaining symptoms
  - Often encourages the use of community resources
- Behavioral therapy: relatively nontheoretical approach to behavioral change or symptom reduction/eradication through application of principles of stimulus and response; MI is often performed at the onset of behavioral and parenting counseling or therapy.

Pediatric Considerations

- Important distinctions are made between psychotherapy and counseling for children/teens compared to adults/couples.
- The focus of evaluation must include attention to parent and family processes and factors. Interventions typically include interactions and sessions with parents as well as collateral work with teachers and other school personnel.
- Younger children will often be evaluated and diagnosed through behavioral descriptions provided by parents and other adults who know them well as well as through direct observation and/or play techniques. Children of all ages should be screened using behavioral checklists that are standardized and norm-referenced for age and gender.
- Any child or teenager who requests counseling should be interviewed initially by the primary care provider and referred appropriately. Most referrals will be in response to parental request, however.
- Psychotherapeutic interventions with the strongest empirical basis with children include behavior therapy/modification, CBT, and family/parenting therapy. Play therapy has the least empirical support but has been found to be useful for developing rapport and for treating trauma in younger children. Insight-oriented therapies appear to be more effective with older children (age ≥10 years).
- There is a controversy regarding the efficacy of psychopharmacologic treatment in preadolescents, although clear benefits have been demonstrated in some studies as well as clinical practice. Treatment guidelines for mild to moderate depressed mood and/or anxiety disorders typically recommend pediatric CBT initially, and studies have typically supported this approach in preteen and milder cases. Medications should be considered in more severe presentations.

EPIDEMIOLOGY

- 19 million adults suffer from clinical depression, and >20 million adults have a diagnosable anxiety disorder in the United States.
- One in four Americans report seeking some form of mental health treatment in their adult life. This includes generic counseling in nonmedical settings such as work, clergy, or school settings and also includes visits to primary care providers. It is estimated that between 3.5% and 5% of adults in the United States participate in formal mental health psychotherapy annually. Recent estimates emerging from the COVID-19 pandemic suggest these rates have increased since spring 2020.
- Public health experts report that the majority of those adults with diagnosable psychiatric disorders do not receive professional mental health services. This is due to multiple factors, including failure to identify, noncompliance with psychiatric referral, regional shortages of providers, economic or insurance barriers, and excessive time duration from referral to an available service.

RISK FACTORS

The need for psychotherapy or counseling services is associated with a host of socioeconomic and biogenetic factors, including the general effects of poverty, family or marital dysfunction, life stressors, medical diseases or conditions, and individual biologic predisposition to mental health disorders.

GENERAL PREVENTION

It is generally assumed that early identification and intervention of child and adolescent psychopathology increases the likelihood of reducing the risk for adult psychopathology, but this has not been sufficiently validated in all categories of psychological disorders. Data support such claims in disorders such as childhood ADHD, anxiety disorders, and habit disorders of childhood, however. A range of evidence-based therapies now exist that are designed for children and adults.

 TREATMENT

GENERAL MEASURES

There is an evidence of a "dose effect" in psychotherapy outcomes research, with some investigators suggesting that 6 to 8 sessions are necessary to yield positive initial effects in adults, and upward of 15 to 20 sessions for longer term, sustainable therapeutic effects. This dose effect may not be applicable to counseling services with primarily informational or emotional/supportive functions. Also, long-term therapy should be evaluated at 3- to 6-month intervals to determine efficacy.

MEDICATION

- Psychotherapy is most likely to be accompanied by use of pharmaceutical adjuncts in moderate to severe cases of psychological dysfunction that do not respond to other therapies or in cases of extremely poor quality of life or high risk. The most common examples are in cases of clinical depression or anxiety that clearly incapacitates the patient or significantly reduces his or her quality of life. Patients at risk for suicide or who represent a danger to others are also candidates for acute psychopharmacotherapy. Studies suggest that verbal and behaviorally oriented therapies can add efficacy to medication treatment in both depression and anxiety and reduce the risk of relapse.
- There is a controversy in the research field regarding the efficacy of medication alone versus psychotherapy alone versus combined treatments. The most recent consensus has been that combined treatments in moderate to severe psychological dysfunction are most likely to render positive short-term results and increase the likelihood that such effects can be sustained over time. Many patients in mental health settings do not require psychotropic medications.

ADDITIONAL THERAPIES

- Anxiety disorders
  - Panic disorder with and without agoraphobia: CBT, psychodynamic therapy
  - Generalized anxiety disorder: CBT

  - Obsessive-compulsive disorder: CBT
  - Posttraumatic stress disorder: CBT, play therapy with children
  - Specific phobia: CBT
  - Social phobia: CBT
- Mood disorders
  - Unipolar depression: CBT, interpersonal therapy, psychodynamic therapy
  - Bipolar disorder: family therapy, interpersonal therapy, CBT/DBT
  - Schizophrenia: psychodynamic therapy, family therapy, CBT/DBT
- Eating disorders
  - Binge eating disorder: CBT/DBT, interpersonal therapy, behavior modification
  - Bulimia nervosa: CBT/DBT, interpersonal therapy, behavior modification
- Personality disorders
  - Borderline: DBT, CBT
- Substance use disorders
  - Alcohol: counseling, CBT, MI
  - Cocaine, heroin, opioids, cannabis: CBT, counseling
  - Smoking: MI, behavioral modification with evidence-based medications

COMPLEMENTARY & ALTERNATIVE MEDICINE

A host of nonempirically based psychological and nutritional therapies can be found outside of mainstream medicine and psychological science. Very little or no evidence exists to support many experimental therapies, but all have the considerable power of the placebo effect fueling their anecdotal supports or claims. Placebo effects are also thought to be powerfully enhanced by the use of ingested or applied substances that create real physiologic, although not therapeutic, changes in the patient. If it makes them feel different, they are more likely to believe it helps. Placebo alone accounts for moderate amounts of perceived symptom improvement in a range of psychiatric medications, as well as nonregulated supplements.

 ONGOING CARE

FOLLOW-UP RECOMMENDATIONS

Patient Monitoring

There is an evidence of a "dose effect" in psychotherapy outcomes research, with investigators suggesting upward of 20 sessions for sustainable therapeutic effects. This dose effect may not be applicable to counseling services with primarily informational or emotional/supportive functions. Because many patients cease attendance to psychotherapy sessions after one or a few sessions, most interventions of this type cannot be accurately evaluated by the referring provider. Long-term therapy should also be evaluated for effectiveness at regular periods. Patients at suicidal risk need to be monitored more often and in-person.

REFERENCE

1. American Psychiatric Association. *Diagnostic and Statistical Manual of Mental Disorders.* 5th ed. Arlington, VA: American Psychiatric Association; 2013.

ADDITIONAL READING

- Bortolotti B, Menchetti M, Bellini F, et al. Psychological interventions for major depression in primary care: a meta-analytic review of randomized controlled trials. *Gen Hosp Psychiatry*. 2008;30(4):293–302.
- Eddy KT, Dutra L, Bradley R, et al. A multidimensional meta-analysis of psychotherapy and pharmacotherapy for obsessive-compulsive disorder. *Clin Psychol Rev*. 2004;24(8):1011–1030.
- Furukawa TA, Watanabe N, Churchill R. Combined psychotherapy plus antidepressants for panic disorder with or without agoraphobia. *Cochrane Database Syst Rev*. 2007;2007(1):CD004364.
- Hunot V, Churchill R, Silva de Lima M, et al. Psychological therapies for generalised anxiety disorder. *Cochrane Database Syst Rev*. 2007;2007(1):CD001848.

CODES

ICD10

- Z71.9 Counseling, unspecified
- Z71.89 Other specified counseling
- Z63.9 Problem related to primary support group, unspecified

CLINICAL PEARLS

- Combined medication and psychotherapeutic treatments in moderate to severe psychological dysfunction are most likely to render positive short-term results and increase the likelihood that such effects can be sustained over time.
- Relapse is common over time and/or as treatments are discontinued or not reevaluated.
- Children aged <10 years may benefit significantly from counseling or behavior therapy alone for symptom relief.
- Older children and those with more severe symptoms typically require psychopharmacologic options in concert with counseling and/or CBT approaches.

C

CROHN DISEASE

Samir A. Shah, MD, FACG, FASGE, AGAF • Eric J. Mao, MD

BASICS

DESCRIPTION
- A chronic, progressive inflammatory GI tract disorder, most commonly involving the terminal ileum (80%)
- Hallmark features of Crohn disease (CD)
  - Transmural inflammation that can result in fibrotic strictures, fistulas, fissures, or abscesses; noncaseating granulomas (30%); skip lesions: diseased mucosa interspersed with normal mucosa; can be continuous, mimicking ulcerative colitis (UC); rectal sparing; diverse presentations: ileitis (1/3), ileocolitis (1/3); isolated colitis (1/3)

EPIDEMIOLOGY
Incidence
3 to 20 cases per 100,000 person-years in North America; incidence is rising globally. Bimodal age distribution: Predominant age is 15 to 30 years, with a second smaller peak at 50 to 80 years. Women are slightly more affected than men; increased incidence in northern climates

Prevalence
247 cases per 100,000 persons

ETIOLOGY AND PATHOPHYSIOLOGY
- General: Clinical manifestations result from activation of inflammatory cells and subsequent tissue injury.
- Multifactorial: Genetics, environmental triggers, commensal microbial antigens, and immunologic abnormalities result in inflammation and tissue injury.

Genetics
- 15% of CD patients have a first-degree relative with inflammatory bowel disease (IBD); first-degree relative of an IBD patient has 3- to 30-fold increased risk of developing IBD by the age of 28 years.
- Associated genetic syndromes: Turner and Hermansky-Pudlak syndromes, glycogen storage disease type 1b

RISK FACTORS
Environmental factors:
- Cigarette smoking doubles the risk of CD; tobacco cessation reduces flares and relapses.
- Dietary factors: higher incidence if diet is high in refined sugars, animal fat or protein, processed or ultraprocessed foods

COMMONLY ASSOCIATED CONDITIONS
- Extraintestinal manifestations
  - Arthritis (20%): seronegative, small and large joints (ankylosing spondylitis [AS] or sacroiliitis [SI], associated with HLA-B27); skin disorders (10%): erythema nodosum, pyoderma gangrenosum, psoriasis; ocular disease (5%): uveitis (associated with HLA-B27), iritis, episcleritis
  - Kidney stones: calcium oxalate stones (from steatorrhea and diarrhea) or uric acid stones (from dehydration and metabolic acidosis); osteopenia and osteoporosis; hypocalcemia; hypercoagulability: venous thromboembolism prophylaxis essential in hospitalized patients; gallstones: cholesterol stones resulting from impaired bile acid reabsorption; primary sclerosing cholangitis (PSC) (5%)

- Conditions associated with increased disease activity
  - Peripheral arthropathy (not SI and AS); episcleritis (not uveitis); oral aphthous ulcers and erythema nodosum
- Complications: GI bleed, toxic megacolon, bowel obstruction, bowel perforation, peritonitis, malignancy, intra-abdominal fistula, perianal disease

DIAGNOSIS

HISTORY
Hallmarks: crampy abdominal pain (+/− bleeding), prolonged diarrhea, fatigue, weight loss, fever, perianal disease; children may present with failure to thrive.
- Factors exacerbating CD: concurrent infection, smoking, NSAIDs, antibiotics, stress

PHYSICAL EXAM
Presentation varies with location of disease and severity
- General: signs of sepsis/disease activity (fever, tachycardia, hypotension) or wasting/malnutrition
- Abdominal: focal or diffuse tenderness, distension, rebound/guarding, rectal bleeding, palpable mass
- Perianal: fistula, fissures, abscess
- Skin: erythema nodosum, pyoderma gangrenosum; psoriasis

DIFFERENTIAL DIAGNOSIS
- Acute, severe abdominal pain: perforated viscus, pancreatitis, appendicitis, diverticulitis, bowel obstruction, kidney stones, ovarian torsion
- Chronic diarrhea with crampy pain (colitis-like): UC, radiation colitis, infection, drugs, ischemia, microscopic colitis, celiac disease, malignancy (lymphoma, carcinoma), carcinoid, segmental colitis associated with diverticulosis
- Wasting illness: malabsorption, malignancy

DIAGNOSTIC TESTS & INTERPRETATION
Initial Tests (lab, imaging)
- CBC, serum chemistries, LFTs, erythrocyte sedimentation rate (ESR), C-reactive protein (CRP), serum iron, vitamin B$_{12}$, vitamin D-25 OH, stool calprotectin
- If diarrhea, stool specimen for routine culture, *Clostridium difficile*, and ova and parasites in at risk populations
- With severe flares, KUB to rule out toxic megacolon
- Ileocolonoscopy provides the greatest diagnostic sensitivity and specificity; biopsy normal and abnormal mucosa (1)[C]
- Upper endoscopy for patients with upper GI signs or symptoms (1)[C]
  - Endoscopic signs of upper GI CD: antral narrowing, segmental stricturing, inflammatory mucosa
- Small bowel: sensitivity of CT or magnetic resonance enterography (MRE) better than small bowel follow through; MRE has no radiation exposure (important in younger patients). Capsule endoscopy allows small bowel visualization only.
  - Signs of small bowel disease: narrowed lumen with nodularity (string sign); bowel loop separation (transmural inflammation); increased bowel wall enhancement or thickening suggests inflammation.

- Perianal disease: endoscopic ultrasound (EUS) or MRI pelvis, exam under anesthesia
- Contraindications to endoscopy: perforated viscus, recent myocardial infarction, severe diverticulitis, toxic megacolon
- In some cases, unprepared limited sigmoidoscopy allows adequate visualization to assess severity, extent, aspirate stool for *C. difficile*, obtain biopsies to assess histologic severity, and exclude other disorders (e.g., cytomegalovirus) in distal colonic CD.

Follow-Up Tests & Special Considerations
- Evidence of complications
  - Stricture: obstructive signs—nausea, vomiting, abdominal pain, weight loss, diarrhea, or inability to pass gas/feces
  - Abscess/inflammatory mass: localized abdominal peritonitis with fever and abdominal pain; diffuse peritonitis suggests perforation or abscess rupture (may be masked by steroids, opiates).
  - Fistula: enteroenteric: asymptomatic or a palpable, commonly indolent, abdominal mass; enterovesicular: pneumaturia, recurrent UTI; retroperitoneal: psoas abscess, ureteral obstruction; enterovaginal: vaginal passage of gas or feces; clear, nonfeculent drainage from ileal fistula (may be misdiagnosed as primary vaginal infection)
- Treatment goals
  - Steroid-free clinical remission; biochemical (CRP and ESR) and biologic (calprotectin) remission
  - Radiologic response by cross-sectional or ultrasound imaging; endoscopic response and remission (2)
  - Symptoms may not correlate with disease activity, so objective testing (biomarkers, imaging, endoscopy) is crucial.

Diagnostic Procedures/Other
How to distinguish CD from UC:
- CD: small bowel or colonic disease, rectal sparing; skip lesions; granulomas, perianal fistula or abscess; RLQ pain; rectal bleeding is uncommon.
- UC: continuous colonic involvement including the rectum; LLQ pain; rectal bleeding is common.

ALERT
CD can mimic UC with continuous bowel involvement; 10–15% of cases are difficult to differentiate.

TREATMENT

- Disease activity: Harvey Bradshaw Index or Crohn Disease Activity Index (CDAI)
- Disease severity: risk stratification for rapidly progressive disease
  - Risk factors for high-risk disease: age at diagnosis <30 years, extensive anatomic involvement, perianal or severe rectal disease, deep ulcers/ severe endoscopic disease, prior surgical resection, stricturing/penetrating behavior, extraintestinal manifestation
- Disease severity considers longitudinal factors and prognosis, whereas disease activity is a one-time assessment of symptoms; disease severity/risk assessment should drive therapy decisions.

- Low-risk disease: budesonide or prednisone taper with or without immunomodulator
- Moderate-/high-risk disease: biologic monotherapy or biologic combination therapy with immunomodulator

MEDICATION
- Mild to Moderate CD
  - Asymptomatic with mild endoscopic disease: observation alone; no role for mesalamine in CD (1)[A]
  - Antibiotics are not recommended (1)[C].
  - Induction: controlled ileal release budesonide (9 mg/day for 8 weeks and then discontinued over 2-week taper) for distal ileum and/or right colon involvement or prednisone taper
  - Maintenance: Stop therapy and observe or consider immunomodulator/biologic therapy.
- Moderate to severe CD
  - Induction: biologic as initial induction agent to avoid corticosteroids; may need budesonide 6 to 9 mg or prednisone 40 to 60 mg/day for short term to alleviate symptoms (1)[C]
  - Maintenance: no role for mesalamine; if steroids are required for induction, consider biologic and/or immunomodulator.
- Immunomodulators:
  - Thiopurines: azathioprine or 6-mercaptopurine (6MP) for maintenance but not induction (1)[C]
  - Methotrexate (SC or IM): effective for induction and maintenance of steroid-dependent CD (1)[C]; take with folic acid 1 mg/day.
- Anti-tumor necrosis factor (anti-TNF): infliximab, adalimumab, certolizumab pegol for induction and maintenance (1)[A],(3)[A]
  - Test for TB and HBV infection prior to anti-TNF initiation.
- Combination therapy: anti-TNF and immunomodulator
  - Combination therapy with standard dose immunomodulator is more effective than either alone. Combining anti-TNF with low-dose immunomodulator reduces immunogenicity against anti-TNF.
- Antileukocyte trafficking: vedolizumab for induction and maintenance (1)[A],(3)[B]
  - Gut-selective; no risk of progressive multifocal leukoencephalopathy (PML)
- Anti–IL-12/IL-23: ustekinumab for induction and maintenance (1)[A],(3)[B]
- Anti-IL-23: risankizumab for induction and maintenance
- Janus kinase (JAK) inhibitor: upadacitinib 45 mg once a day for 12 weeks followed by maintenance at dose of 30 mg or 15 mg per day; must have failed an anti-TNF before using a JAK inhibitor per FDA label; shingles vaccine is paramount as JAK inhibition carries increased risk of shingles.

First Line
For moderate to severe CD patients naive to biologic drugs:
- Infliximab, adalimumab, or ustekinumab recommended over certolizumab to induce remission (3)[A]
- Vedolizumab recommended over certolizumab to induce remission (3)[C]

Second Line
- For moderate to severe CD patients who never responded to anti-TNFα (primary nonresponse):
  - Ustekinumab is recommended to induce remission (3)[A].
  - Vedolizumab is recommended over no therapy to induce remission (3)[C].
  - Upadacitinib is recommended over no therapy to induce remission.
- For moderate to severe CD patients who previously responded to anti-TNFα (secondary nonresponse):
  - Adalimumab or ustekinumab is recommended to induce remission (3)[A].
  - Vedolizumab is recommended over no therapy to induce remission (3)[C].
  - Upadacitinib is recommended over no therapy to induce remission.

ADDITIONAL THERAPIES
- Oral lesions: triamcinolone acetonide in benzocaine and carboxymethyl cellulose or topical sucralfate for aphthous ulcers, cheilitis
- Gastroduodenal CD: Case reports show success of anti-TNF therapy; symptomatic relief possible from proton pump inhibitors, H_2 receptor blockers, and/or sucralfate

SURGERY/OTHER PROCEDURES
Multidisciplinary care with colorectal surgery, gastroenterology, nutrition, radiology, pathology, etc. helps optimize outcomes.

ADMISSION, INPATIENT, AND NURSING CONSIDERATIONS
DVT prophylaxis on admission

 ONGOING CARE

FOLLOW-UP RECOMMENDATIONS
- Monitor CBC, BMP, and LFTs every 3 to 4 months.
- Actively monitor disease with CRP and/or calprotectin every 6 months.
- With azathioprine or 6MP therapy, check TPMT/NUDT15 genotype/activity prior to initiation and thiopurine metabolites 1 month afterwards
- With infliximab or biosimilars of infliximab, consider proactive therapeutic drug monitoring.

Patient Monitoring
- Vaccinations
  - Check titers; avoid live vaccines (MMR, varicella zoster vaccine) in patients on immunosuppressive therapy.
  - Regardless of immunosuppression: HPV, influenza, pneumococcal, meningococcal, hepatitis A and B, Tdap, and varicella zoster for those aged ≥18 years
  - COVID-19 vaccine is recommended for all IBD patients.
  - Zoster vaccine (Shingrix) is recommended for immunosuppressed patients aged >18 years.
- Cancer prevention
  - Colonoscopy with targeted biopsies every 1 to 5 years after 8 to 10 years of CD with colonic involvement; consider chromoendoscopy; in PSC patients, annual screening colonoscopy is recommended.

- Annual Pap smears if immunocompromised
- Annual skin exam
- Bone health
  - Calcium and vitamin D supplementation with each course of corticosteroids or if vitamin D deficient
  - Bone density assessment if previous steroid use, maternal history of osteoporosis, malnourished, amenorrheic, postmenopausal

DIET
Mediterranean diet

PATIENT EDUCATION
- CrohnsandColitisFoundation.org
- IBDandMe.org

REFERENCES
1. Lichtenstein GR, Loftus EV, Isaacs KL, et al. ACG clinical guideline: management of Crohn's disease in adults. Am J Gastroenterol. 2018;113(4): 481–517.
2. Colombel JF, D'haens G, Lee WJ, et al. Outcomes and strategies to support a treat-to-target approach in inflammatory bowel disease: a systematic review. J Crohns Colitis. 2020;14(2):254–266.
3. Feuerstein JD, Ho EY, Shmidt E, et al; for American Gastroenterological Association Institute Clinical Guidelines Committee. AGA clinical practice guidelines on the medical management of moderate to severe luminal and perianal fistulizing Crohn's disease. Gastroenterology. 2021;160(7):2496–2508.

ADDITIONAL READING
Miglioretto C, Beck E, Lambert K. A scoping review of the dietary information needs of people with inflammatory bowel disease [published online ahead of print October 8, 2023]. Nutr Diet. doi:10.1111/1747-0080.12843.

CODES

ICD10
- K50.0 Crohn's disease of small intestine
- K50.113 Crohn's disease of large intestine with fistula
- K50.011 Crohn's disease of small intestine with rectal bleeding

CLINICAL PEARLS
- Cigarette smoking doubles the risk of CD; tobacco cessation reduces flares and need for surgery.
- MRE allows assessment of luminal and extraluminal CD without radiation exposure.
- Assess for TB and HBV infection prior to initiating biologic therapy.
- Test for C. difficile infection when evaluating diarrhea in all CD patients.
- Hospitalized CD patients require deep vein thrombosis prophylaxis.
- Anti-TNF therapy is effective in delaying or preventing postoperative recurrence in CD.
- Disease severity rather than disease activity should drive therapy decisions.

CROUP (LARYNGOTRACHEOBRONCHITIS)

Afsha Rais Kaisani, MD • Tasaduq Hussain Mir, MD, FAAFP • Amulya Sajja, MD

BASICS

Croup is a self-limited upper respiratory tract infection causing inflammation and edema, leading to obstruction of the larynx and subglottic airway. It presents with barking cough and inspiratory stridor. Although usually mild, croup can cause significant respiratory distress and even death.

DESCRIPTION
- The spectrum of croup includes laryngotracheitis (LT), laryngotracheobronchitis (LTB), and laryngo-tracheobronchopneumonitis. It is often a result of a viral infection and most common cause of airway obstruction in young children.
- May occur in absence of viral prodrome, known as spasmodic croup, occurring in older children; rapid onset and resolution and often has a recurrent course

EPIDEMIOLOGY
- Most commonly affects children aged 6 months to 3 years of age, peaks at 18 months; although rare, croup can affect children as young as 3 months and as old as 6 to 7 years.
- Predominant sex: male > female
- Most often occurs in the fall and early winter but may present year-round

Incidence
- Accounts for 1.3% of emergency department cases
- The vast majority are considered mild cases, but 3–7% of cases require hospitalization.
- <3% require laryngoscopic or airway procedures.
- 4.4% of children returned to the emergency department within 48 hours (1).

Prevalence
60% of barking cough are resolved within 48 hours, and only 2% have symptoms persisting for >5 nights (1).

ETIOLOGY AND PATHOPHYSIOLOGY
- Infection of the larynx, trachea, and bronchi, causing narrowing of the airway secondary to inflammation and edema
- Children have narrow airway, and negative-pressure inspiration pulls airway walls closer together, creating inspiratory stridor.
- Typically, caused by viruses that infect oropharyngeal mucosa and migrates inferiorly; most common pathogen is parainfluenza virus, responsible for >80% of cases
  - Types 1 and 2 are the most common.
  - Type 3 is affiliated with bronchiolitis and pneumonia in young infants and children.
  - Type 4 (subtypes 4A and 4B) are associated with milder illness.
- Other viruses: RSV, paramyxovirus, influenza virus type A or B, adenovirus, rhinovirus, enteroviruses (coxsackie and echo), reovirus, measles virus where vaccination is not common, and metapneumovirus
- *Mycoplasma pneumoniae* and *Corynebacterium diphtheriae* have been reported but are rare.

- Bacterial croup is commonly caused by *Staphylococcus aureus*, *Streptococcus pneumoniae*, *Haemophilus influenzae*, and *Moraxella catarrhalis*.
- Spasmodic croup cause is unclear, possibly allergy, airway hyperactivity, and gastroesophageal reflux.

Genetics
Congenital subglottic stenosis, which is a narrowing of the lumen of the cricoid region, can present as recurrent croup.

RISK FACTORS
Prior intubations, structural airway abnormality, prematurity, and age <3 years increase the risks for recurrent croup (more than two episodes per year) (2).

GENERAL PREVENTION
Croup spreads through droplets. Children should be considered contagious up to 3 days after the start of illness and/or until afebrile. There is no specific vaccine for croup, but seasonal influenza vaccine may contribute to decreased risk.

COMMONLY ASSOCIATED CONDITIONS
- Some evidence suggests croup hospitalization may be associated with future development of asthma.
- If recurrent (more than two episodes in a year) or during the first 90 days of life, consider host factors or allergic factors.
- Underlying anatomic abnormality (e.g., subglottic stenosis, paradoxical vocal cord dysfunction)
- Consider gastroesophageal reflux disease diagnostic consideration for patients with recurrent croup symptoms.
- COVID-19—a potential viral agent in patients with croup

DIAGNOSIS

- Croup is a clinical diagnosis; most children present with acute onset of classic "seal-like" barking cough, inspiratory stridor, hoarseness, and chest wall indrawing.
- Low-to-moderate grade fever but absence of fever should not reduce suspicion for croup.
- Severity is determined by clinical inspection for signs of respiratory distress: nasal flaring, retractions, tripoding, sniffing position, abdominal breathing, and tachypnea. Although uncommon, hypoxia, cyanosis, and fatigue are late signs of severity.
- For cases presenting with more severe symptoms or not improving as rapidly as expected, SARS-CoV-2 testing should be considered (3).
- Westley Croup Severity Score is the commonly used scoring system. It looks at five clinical features, and the scores are as follows: ≤2 mild; 3 to 7 moderate; 8 to 11 severe; ≥12 impending respiratory failure.
  - Level of consciousness: normal, including sleep = 0; disoriented = 5
  - Cyanosis: none = 0; with agitation = 4; at rest = 5
  - Stridor: none = 0; with agitation = 1; at rest = 2
  - Air entry: normal = 0; decreased = 1; markedly decreased = 2
  - Retractions: none = 0; mild = 1; moderate = 2; severe = 3

HISTORY
Croup is primarily a clinical diagnosis characterized by abrupt onset of barking cough, inspiratory stridor, and hoarseness (2).

PHYSICAL EXAM
- Vital signs can demonstrate tachypnea and tachycardia.
- Pulse oximetry often is normal as there is no disturbance of alveolar gas exchange; however, oxygen saturation might be decreased in severe cases.
- Visual inspection: Nasal flaring, retraction, and/or cyanosis indicate high suspicion for croup.
- Breathing sounds and voice are important for diagnosis; typically, the patient will present with hoarseness, stridor, and/or inspiratory wheezing to auscultation.
  - Stridor can be present at rest and aggravated by agitation.
  - Substantial wheezing, rhonchi, and rales should prompt alternative diagnosis.
- Decreased breath sounds and respiratory effort may indicate the child is progressing into respiratory failure and less able to mount an effort to move air (2).

DIFFERENTIAL DIAGNOSIS
- Foreign body aspiration
- Bacterial tracheitis: high fever, barking cough, respiratory distress, and rapid deterioration
- Retropharyngeal or peritonsillar abscess: similar septic appearance with dysphonia
- Allergic reaction (acute angioneurotic edema) includes spasmodic croup with classic nocturnal exacerbations.
- Epiglottitis: rapid onset, high fever, dysphonia, drooling, and prototypical posture of extended chin and leaning forward; the incidence of epiglottitis has significantly decreased with widespread vaccination against *H. influenzae* being replaced by strep and staph organisms.
- Others: subglottic stenosis, thermal injury/smoke inhalation, hemangioma, airway anomalies (e.g., tracheo-/laryngomalacia), neoplasm, other anatomic obstructions (2)
- SARS-CoV-2 presents with more severe symptoms, and response to treatment is not as rapid as expected (3).

DIAGNOSTIC TESTS & INTERPRETATION
- Croup is a clinical diagnosis and does not require confirmatory testing.
- Blood work is not required; if done, WBC counts may be mildly elevated with a predominance of lymphocytes.
  - An elevated WBC shift to the left (bandemia) would suggest bacterial etiology (epiglottitis, bacterial tracheitis, peritonsillar, and/or retropharyngeal abscess).
- Rapid antigen or viral culture tests should be reserved for patients in whom initial treatment is ineffective.

- If imaging were to be done, posteroanterior and lateral neck films will show funnel-shaped subglottic region with normal epiglottis: "steeple" or "pencil point" sign (present in 40–60% of children with croup).
  - A steeple sign can be seen in patients without croup warranting other considerations.
  - Monitor all patients during imaging as airway obstruction may occur rapidly.
- When suspecting an alternative diagnosis, the following findings can be appreciated:
  - Retropharyngeal abscess: bulging of posterior pharyngeal wall
  - Epiglottitis: thumb sign, which is a thickened epiglottis
- Polymerase chain reaction testing from nasopharyngeal mucosa is used when SARS-CoV-2 is suspected as the cause of croup (3).

Initial Tests (lab, imaging)
Radiographic imaging is not routinely indicated. CT of the neck can be considered for patients with suspected abscess, tumor, or foreign body aspiration (2).

Follow-Up Tests & Special Considerations
Recurrent croup needs evaluation to check for other underlying predisposing conditions (e.g., asthma, gastroesophageal reflux, anatomical airway abnormalities).

Diagnostic Procedures/Other
Laryngoscopy should be reserved for atypical presentations or when alternate diagnosis is suspected (2). Specifically, those that are hospitalized but not intubated or those with a history of intubation and <36 months of age.

TREATMENT
- Treatment is supportive; severity of illness may dictate additional measurements.
- Outpatient patients with severe croup or impending respiratory failure should be transported via ambulance to the nearest hospital for management.
- The limited experience with COVID-19 croup suggests cases can present with severe pathology and may not improve as rapidly as with typical croup.

GENERAL MEASURES
- Symptomatic treatment
- Minimize lab tests, imaging, and procedures that upset the child; agitation worsens tachypnea and can be detrimental.
- Pulse oximetry and oxygen should be administered for hypoxemia or respiratory distress.
- Frequent clinical checks may be more sensitive in identifying worsening disease.
- Heliox is a helium and oxygen mixture used for respiratory conditions, and it improves airflow resistance by decreasing gas density; data are limited on its benefits for croup (2)[B].

MEDICATION
Treatment is based on Wesley Croup Severity Score: mild (0 to 2): give 1 dose of dexamethasone; moderate to severe (≥3): give nebulized epinephrine in addition to dexamethasone.

First Line
- Corticosteroids: Oral corticosteroids should be used in patients with any severity. They provide faster resolution and decrease hospital admission by decreasing laryngeal mucosa edema.
  - Dexamethasone is the preferred corticosteroid due to its easy single dosing and ability to give orally, intramuscularly, and intravenously. It is also the least expensive steroids. Optimal dosage is unclear, but 0.6 mg/kg is the most commonly used range—maximum of 16 mg.
  - Other steroids (betamethasone, budesonide, prednisolone) are beneficial. In randomized trials comparing prednisolone to dexamethasone, the latter is more commonly used in the emergency department, but they have no difference in efficacy in the community.
- Nebulized epinephrine; racemic or L-epinephrine (equal efficacy and side effect profiles); reserved for moderate-to-severe cases with stridor at rest
  - Racemic epinephrine is dosed at 0.05 mL/kg of 2.25% (max of 0.5 mL) solution nebulized in normal saline to total volume of 3 mL.
  - L-epinephrine is dosed at 0.5 mL/kg (max of 5 mL) of a 1:1,000 via nebulizer. Onset of action is within 1 to 5 minutes, and duration is of approximately 2 hours. Repeat as necessary as long as side effects are tolerated. Observe the child for 2 hours to ensure no recurrence after epinephrine wears off.
- Antitussives and decongestants are not recommended.
- Antibiotics when suspecting a primary or secondary bacterial infection
- Oxygen as needed
- Humidified air without clinical benefit in croup (2)

SURGERY/OTHER PROCEDURES
- Intubation is rarely required; tube 0.5 to 1.0 mm smaller than normal
- Intubation may be required for fatigue due to work of breathing or obstruction.

ADMISSION, INPATIENT, AND NURSING CONSIDERATIONS
- Outpatient care for mild cases
- In most cases, observation in the emergency room after medical management is sufficient.
- Admission criteria: poor response to therapy or recurrent stridor at rest after epinephrine wears off, increased oxygen requirement, pneumonia, or other serious conditions
- Discharge criteria
  - At least 2 hours since last epinephrine
  - Received dose of steroids
  - No stridor at rest, no difficulty breathing
  - Able to tolerate oral fluids
  - Normal air entry, color, and consciousness
  - Has home management and outpatient follow up established

ONGOING CARE

DIET
- Cool, liquid diet is better tolerated.
- Frequent small feedings

PATIENT EDUCATION
- Croup is usually a self-limited and mild disease, but some will need hospital care.
- Avoid agitation, which may worsen symptoms; use antipyretics as needed. Keep hydrated with liquids, ice pops, etc.

- Emergency ambulance for cyanosis, lethargy, struggling to breathe, drooling and unable to swallow
- It is contagious in the first few days; good hand hygiene is very important.
- The cough may linger for a few weeks.
- Parents of patients with COVID-19–related croup should be counseled on quarantine guidelines.

PROGNOSIS
- Prognosis is usually good. The few cases that are severe respond to intensive respiratory management.
- Recurrence is rare in viral-mediated disease. If croup recurs, consider an anatomic, allergic, or obstructive etiology.

COMPLICATIONS
- Subglottic stenosis in intubated patients
- Bacterial tracheitis
- Cardiopulmonary arrest
- Pneumonia (2)

REFERENCES
1. Hanna J, Brauer PR, Morse E, et al. Epidemiological analysis of croup in the emergency department using two national datasets. *Int J Pediatr Otorhinolaryngol*. 2019;126:109641.
2. Smith DK, McDermott AJ, Sullivan JF. Croup: diagnosis and management. *Am Fam Physician*. 2018;97(9):575–580.
3. Venn AMR, Schmidt JM, Mullan PC. Pediatric croup with COVID-19. *Am J Emerg Med*. 2021;43:287.e1–287.e3.

ADDITIONAL READING
Quraishi H, Lee DJ. Recurrent croup. *Pediatr Clin North Am*. 2022;69(2):319–328.

CODES

ICD10
- J05.0 Acute obstructive laryngitis [croup]
- J20.9 Acute bronchitis, unspecified
- J38.5 Laryngeal spasm

CLINICAL PEARLS
- Croup outbreaks are most common in fall and winter seasons in ages 6 months to 3 years.
- Inspiratory stridor is the clinically evident and should raise suspicion of croup.
- Symptoms often occur at night.
- Clinical diagnosis, medical management, and stabilization of the patient take priority over lab testing or radiographic images.
- Recurrence requires further evaluation.
- Consider other diagnoses in acute presentations with a toxic appearance: epiglottitis, abscess, and bacterial tracheitis.
- Be aware of severity if the child becomes less noisy; less air movement can be sign of respiratory failure.
- Foundation of treatment is corticosteroid; supplemental oxygen as needed and epinephrine for moderate-to-severe cases

CRYPTORCHIDISM
Pamela Ellsworth, MD

BASICS

DESCRIPTION
- Incomplete or improper descent of one or both testicles; also called *undescended testes* (UDT) (1)
- Normally descent is in month 7 to 8 of gestation. The cryptorchid testis may be palpable or nonpalpable.
- Can be congenital or acquired
- Types of cryptorchidism
  - Prescrotal: at or above scrotal inlet
  - Abdominal: testis located inside the internal inguinal ring
  - Canalicular: testis located between the internal and external inguinal rings
  - Ectopic: located outside the normal path of testicular descent; may be ectopic to perineum, femoral canal, superficial inguinal pouch (most common), suprapubic area, or opposite hemiscrotum
  - Retractile: fully descended testis that moves freely between the scrotum and the groin
  - Iatrogenic: Previously descended testis becomes undescended due to scar tissue after inguinal surgery.
  - Also may be referred to as palpable versus nonpalpable (1)
- System(s) affected: reproductive
- Synonym(s): UDT

EPIDEMIOLOGY
Incidence
Predominant age: newborn, more common in premature newborns

Prevalence
- In the United States, cryptorchidism occurs in 1–3% of full-term and 15–30% of premature newborn males (2).
- Spontaneous testicular descent occurs by age 1 to 3 months in 50–70% of full-term males.
- Descent at 6 to 9 months of age is rare (1).

ETIOLOGY AND PATHOPHYSIOLOGY
- Not fully understood, may involve alterations in
  - Mechanical factors (gubernaculum, length of vas deferens and testicular vessels, groin anatomy, epididymis, cremasteric muscles, and abdominal pressure), hormonal factors (gonadotropin, testosterone, dihydrotestosterone, and müllerian-inhibiting substance), and neural factors (ilioinguinal nerve and genitofemoral nerve)
  - Insulin-like growth factor 3 (IGF-3) or androgen receptor gene (1)
  - Environmental factors acting as endocrine disruptors
- Major regulators of testicular descent are the Leydig cell–derived hormones, testosterone, and IGF-3.
- Risk of ascent as high as 32% in retractile testis

Genetics
Increased risk of UDT in first-degree relatives suggests a genetic etiology.

RISK FACTORS
- Family history: highest risk if brother had UDT, followed by uncle and then father
- Low birth weight, prematurity, and small for gestational age (1)
- Retractile testes are at increased risk for ascent.
- Maternal smoking and diabetes during gestation

COMMONLY ASSOCIATED CONDITIONS
- Anatomic anomalies: inguinal hernia/hydrocele, abnormalities of vas deferens and epididymis, hypospadias, meningomyelocele
- Endocrine disorders: intersex abnormalities, hypogonadotropic hypogonadism, germinal cell aplasia
- Genetic disorders: Prune-belly syndrome, Prader-Willi syndrome, Kallmann syndrome, cystic fibrosis
- Wilms tumor

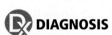DIAGNOSIS

HISTORY
≥1 testicles in a site other than the scrotum

PHYSICAL EXAM
- Performed with warm hands, with child in sitting, standing, and squatting position
- A Valsalva maneuver and applied pressure to lower abdomen may help to identify the testes, especially a gliding testis.

- Failure to palpate a testis after repeated exams suggests an intra-abdominal or atrophic testis.
- An enlarged contralateral testis in the presence of a nonpalpable testis suggests testicular atrophy/absence.
- Testes should be palpated for quality and position at each recommended well-child visit (1)[B].

DIFFERENTIAL DIAGNOSIS
- Retractile testis (hypermobile testis): a normally descended testis that ascends into the inguinal canal because of an active cremasteric reflex (more common in males 4 to 6 years of age)
- Atrophic testis: may occur as a result of neonatal torsion
- Vanished testis may be the result of a lack of development or in utero torsion.

DIAGNOSTIC TESTS & INTERPRETATION
Initial Tests (lab, imaging)
- If only single testis not palpable in an otherwise normal male, no need for lab tests or imaging
- In phenotypic male newborn with bilateral, nonpalpable UDTs, hormone levels help determine whether the testes are ectopic or absent (1)[A].
  - Luteinizing hormone (LH), follicle-stimulating hormone (FSH), MIS, testosterone, serum electrolytes, karyotype
- If bilateral nonpalpable testes presents at >3 months of age, evaluate for disorders of sexual development (3) and evaluate for congenital adrenal hyperplasia.
- Ultrasound or other imaging should not delay referral to a specialist, as they are rarely needed in decision-making (1)[B].

Follow-Up Tests & Special Considerations
In infants <6 months of age, periodic examination to determine if testis becomes palpable prior to further intervention (1)

Pediatric Considerations
Without spontaneous testicular descent by 6 months (gestational age adjusted), infant should be referred to urology, and surgery should be performed within 1 year (1)[B].
- In children with retractile testes, yearly examinations to rule out subsequent ascent (1)[B]

Diagnostic Procedures/Other
Laparoscopy can confirm presence or absence of testis when nonpalpable and determine the feasibility of performing a standard orchidopexy.

Test Interpretation

Higher incidence of carcinoma in UDT and alterations in spermatogenesis; histologic changes occur by 1.5 years of age (4).

 TREATMENT

GENERAL MEASURES

- Rule out retractile testis.
- American Urological Association (AUA) guidelines on cryptorchidism do not recommend use of hormonal therapy to induce testicular descent due to low response rate and lack of evidence for long-term efficacy (1).

MEDICATION

Medical therapy is not indicated in the United States per the AUA guidelines on cryptorchidism in 2014 (1).

ISSUES FOR REFERRAL

- ≥1 testes not descended by 6 months age (1)[B]
- Bilateral nonpalpable UDTs (1)
- Newly diagnosed cryptorchidism after 6 months of age (1)[B]

SURGERY/OTHER PROCEDURES

- Benefits: avoids torsion, averts trauma, decreases but does not eliminate risk of malignancy, and prevents further alterations in spermatogenesis
- If no spontaneous testicular descent by 6 months of age (gestational age adjusted), surgery should be performed within 1 year (1)[B].
- Prepubertal orchidopexy decreases risk of testicular cancer (1).
- Laparoscopy/abdominal exploration is performed first if testis is nonpalpable.
- If palpable, an inguinal approach is usually performed. If low-lying, a single-incision scrotal approach can also be considered but may increase the risk of hernia.

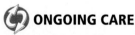 **ONGOING CARE**

FOLLOW-UP RECOMMENDATIONS

- Initial follow-up within 1 month of surgery and periodically thereafter to assess testicular size/growth
- Patients with retractile testes should be examined at least annually to monitor for secondary ascent until testis is no longer retractile (1)[B].

Patient Monitoring

- Patients should be followed after surgery to evaluate testicular growth.
- Testicular tumors occur mainly during or after puberty; thus, these children should be taught self-examination.

DIET

No restrictions

PATIENT EDUCATION

Discuss with parents about causes, treatments, patient's reproductive potential, and increased risk for testicular cancer.

PROGNOSIS

- Disorder is usually corrected with surgical therapy; however, there are possible lifelong consequences.
- If testicle is absent or orchiectomy is required, may consider placement of testicular prosthesis.
- Early orchidopexy may decrease risk of testicular damage and risk of malignancy.

COMPLICATIONS

- Paternity rates are similar to the general population for men with a unilateral UDT; however, lower (33–65%) for men with bilateral UDT
- Abnormalities also have been identified in the contralateral descended testis, suggesting that unilateral cryptorchidism is a bilateral disease.

REFERENCES

1. Kolon TF, Herndon CDA, Baker LA, et al; for American Urological Association. Evaluation and treatment of cryptorchidism: AUA guideline. *J Urol*. 2014;192(2):337–345.
2. Sijstermans K, Hack WWM, Meijer RW, et al. The frequency of undescended testis from birth to adulthood: a review. *Int J Androl*. 2008;31(1):1–11.
3. Docimo SG, Silver RI, Cromie W. The undescended testicle: diagnosis and management. *Am Fam Physician*. 2000;62(9):2037–2044, 2047–2048.
4. Park KH, Lee JH, Han JJ, et al. Histological evidences suggest recommending orchiopexy within the first year of life for children with unilateral inguinal cryptorchid testis. *Int J Urol*. 2007;14(7):616–621.

ADDITIONAL READING

- Braga LH, Lorenzo AJ. Cryptorchidism: a practical review for all community healthcare providers. *Can Urol Assoc J*. 2017;11(1–2 Suppl 1):S26–S32.
- Fantasia J, Aidlen J, Lathrop W, et al. Undescended testes: a clinical and surgical review. *Urol Nurs*. 2015;35(3):117–126.

 CODES

ICD10

- Q53.9 Undescended testicle, unspecified
- Q53.20 Undescended testicle, unspecified, bilateral
- Q53.10 Unspecified undescended testicle, unilateral

CLINICAL PEARLS

- If testicular descent does not occur by 6 months of age, it is unlikely to occur. Refer to urologist at 6 months.
- Children with bilateral, nonpalpable UDTs require laboratory evaluation to determine if viable testicular tissue is present and to rule out disorder of sexual differentiation.
- Radiologic imaging has no role in the initial evaluation of cryptorchidism.
- The risk of infertility is increased with bilateral UDTs.

CUSHING DISEASE AND CUSHING SYNDROME

Dana M. Vlachos, DO • Adora Ilochonwu, MD

 BASICS

DESCRIPTION
- Cushing syndrome is defined as excessive gluco-corticoid exposure from exogenous sources (such as steroids) or less commonly from endogenous sources (pituitary, adrenal, pulmonary, etc.).
- The most common cause of endogenous Cushing syndrome is Cushing disease, which is characterized by excessive adrenocorticotropic hormone (ACTH) secretion from a benign pituitary adenoma.
  - Cushing syndrome from excess endogenous sources may also be caused by a benign or malignant nonpituitary corticotropin secreting tumor (known as ectopic Cushing Syndrome).
- System(s) affected: endocrine/metabolic, musculoskeletal, skin/exocrine, cardiovascular and neuropsychiatric

Pediatric Considerations
- Rare in infancy and childhood
- The most common presenting symptom is lack of growth and weight gain.

Pregnancy Considerations
Pregnancy may exacerbate the disease.

EPIDEMIOLOGY
Incidence
The estimated incidence of Cushing syndrome attributable to endogenous production of cortisol ranges from about 2 to 3 per million people annually to 8 per million people annually.

Prevalence
- An estimated 10 to 15 cases per million people are affected yearly.
- Cushing disease most commonly affects adults 20 to 50 years old and is more prevalent in females.
- 2–5% prevalence reported in difficult-to-control diabetics with obesity and hypertension (HTN)

ETIOLOGY AND PATHOPHYSIOLOGY
- Cortisol is a steroid hormone produced by the zona fasciculata of the adrenal cortex. It is classically a catabolic hormone released during periods of stress. Excess levels of cortisol causes increased free glucose, insulin resistance, immunosuppression, neurocognitive changes, bone disorders such as osteoporosis, and mood disorders such as depression and protein catabolism.
- Prolonged glucocorticoid use such as in asthma and COPD is the most common exogenous source.
- Endogenous cause is either ACTH-dependent or ACTH-independent.
  - ACTH is typically secreted by the anterior pituitary gland and stimulates the adrenal glands to release cortisol. As such, release of ACTH from any source will result in increased cortisol levels.

Genetics
- Multiple endocrine neoplasia (MEN) syndrome
- McCune-Albright syndrome (mutation of *GNAS1* gene)

RISK FACTORS
Prolonged use of corticosteroids

GENERAL PREVENTION
Avoid corticosteroid exposure.

COMMONLY ASSOCIATED CONDITIONS
Psychiatric disorders, diabetes, HTN, hypokalemia, infections, dyslipidemia, osteoporosis, and poor physical fitness

DIAGNOSIS
- The most common age at diagnosis ranges from ages 30 to 49 years, but Cushing Syndrome can be diagnosed from the ages of 5 to 75 years.
- Symptoms may include facial plethora, round face, dorsocervical fat pads, easy bruising, purple striae, thin skin, fragility fractures, and muscle weakness.

HISTORY
- Weight gain: 95%
- Decreased libido: 90%
- Menstrual irregularity: 80%
- Depression/emotional lability: 50–80%
- Easy bruising: 95%
- Diabetes or glucose intolerance: 90%

PHYSICAL EXAM
- Obesity (usually central): 95%
- Facial plethora: 90%
- Moon face (facial adiposity): 90%
- Thin skin: 85%
- HTN: 75%
- Hirsutism: 75%
- Proximal muscle weakness: 90%
- Purple striae on the skin
- Increased adipose tissue in neck and trunk, supraclavicular fat pads, buffalo hump
- Acne
- Skeletal growth retardation in children (epiphyseal plates remain open): 70–80%

DIFFERENTIAL DIAGNOSIS
- Obesity; type 2 diabetes mellitus (T2DM); HTN
- Polycystic ovarian disease
- Pseudo-Cushing syndrome (e.g., alcoholism, physical stress, severe major depression)

DIAGNOSTIC TESTS & INTERPRETATION
Initial testing includes midnight salivary cortisol measurement, 1 mg overnight dexamethasone suppression test, and 24-hour urinary free cortisol (UFC).

Initial Tests (lab, imaging)
- Endocrine Society guidelines (1)[C] recommend testing for Cushing syndrome with the following:
  - Adrenal incidentaloma
  - Unusual features for age such as early osteoporosis and HTN
  - Abnormal growth and increased weight in children
  - Screening tests
  - Documenting loss of diurnal variation: late-night salivary cortisol with at least two measurements
    - Cortisol secretion is highest in the morning and lowest between 11 PM and midnight.

- The nadir of serum cortisol is maintained in pseudo-Cushing syndrome but not in Cushing syndrome. Sensitivity and specificity are >90–95%.
- Cortisol levels may vary day-to-day, and a single UFC or late-night salivary cortisol may not reflect the extent of cortisol exposure.
- Endocrine Society guidelines recommend biochemical diagnosis based on three different approaches:
  - Assessing daily cortisol excretion: measuring 24-hour UFC level:
    - Measure concomitant 24-hour urinary creatinine excretion to verify adequacy of collection as results may be falsely low if renal impairment (GFR <60 mL/min).
    - Overall sensitivity and specificity: 90–97% and 85–99%, respectively
    - Avoid drinking excessive amounts of water due to the risk of false-positive values.
    - Most widely used tests are the late-night salivary cortisol, 24-hour UFC, or low-dose dexamethasone suppression testing.
- It is important to differentiate Cushing from pseudo-Cushing syndrome (e.g., obesity, alcoholism, depression) by documenting loss of feedback inhibition of cortisol on hypothalamic-pituitary-adrenal (HPA) axis: low-dose dexamethasone suppression testing:
  - Dexamethasone 1 mg given between 11 PM and midnight, and fasting plasma cortisol is measured between 8 and 9 AM the following morning.
  - A serum cortisol level <1.8 μg/dL excludes Cushing syndrome, but specificity is limited.
  - Test of choice in subclinical Cushing syndrome (those with subtle increase in cortisol without signs of overt hormonal excess; follow such patients for possible progression)
  - The presence of pseudo-Cushing syndrome states (depression, obesity, etc.), hepatic or renal disease, or any drug that induces cytochrome P450 enzymes may cause a false result. Measuring a concomitant dexamethasone level may be helpful.
  - Localization tests: once the diagnosis of Cushing syndrome is confirmed:
    - Morning ACTH levels:
      - <10 pg/mL: ACTH-independent Cushing
      - >20 pg/mL: ACTH-dependent Cushing
      - 10 to 20 pg/mL: Corticotropin-releasing hormone (CRH) stimulation test is recommended to differentiate between the two forms.
  - High-dose suppression test: 8 mg of oral dexamethasone is given at 11 PM, with measurement of an 8-AM cortisol level the next day.
    - A baseline 8-AM cortisol measurement is also obtained the morning prior to ingesting dexamethasone. Suppression of serum cortisol level to <50% of baseline is suggestive of a pituitary source of ACTH rather than ectopic ACTH or primary adrenal disease. Sensitivity and specificity are 95% and 100%, respectively.
    - Another approach is to measure 8-AM cortisol level after 8-mg dexamethasone given the night before: Cushing disease: cortisol suppressed to <5 μg/dL.

- Imaging:
  - Confirm Cushing diagnosis before imaging studies due to the possibility of both pituitary and adrenal incidentalomas.
    - Dotatate PET/CT, a high-resolution diagnostic tool, is quite useful in identifying tumors missed by other forms of imaging, with a sensitivity of around 90–91%.
    - Up to 19% of ectopic ACTH-secreting tumors can remain occult despite conventional body imaging and modalities of nuclear imaging such as scintigraphy/SPECT.
    - Octreotide scintigraphy to look for occult ACTH-secreting tumor
    - Chest CT scan if ectopic ACTH secretion is suspected
    - Abdominal CT scan if adrenal disease is suspected
    - Pituitary MRI scan if pituitary tumor is suspected (all patients with ACTH-dependent hypercortisolism)

ALERT
- Antiepileptic drugs, progesterone, oral contraceptives, rifampin, and spironolactone may cause a false-positive dexamethasone suppression test.
- Pregnancy: UFC is recommended instead of dexamethasone in the initial evaluation of pregnant women (or on birth control pills). Only UFC in the 2nd or 3rd trimester >3 times the upper limit of normal is suggestive of Cushing syndrome.

Diagnostic Procedures/Other
Testing for associated findings can be useful, including:
- Thyroid function, T2DM, osteoporosis
- Polycystic ovarian syndrome/hyperandrogenism
- Oligomenorrhea/hypogonadism
- Hypercoagulable state/venous thromboembolism
- Metastases from malignant tumors
- Atrial fibrillation
- Hypokalemia
- Growth hormone reduction

TREATMENT
- For patients with endogenous Cushing Syndrome, the primary aim of therapy is complete resection of the underlying tumor.
- For patients with Cushing Disease, the primary therapy is transsphenoidal pituitary surgery with selective adenomectomy.

MEDICATION
- Medical therapy is usually ineffective for long-term treatment and is typically used in preparation for surgery or as adjunctive therapy after surgery or pituitary radiotherapy.
- Metyrapone, ketoconazole, and mitotane lower cortisol levels by directly inhibiting synthesis and secretion in the adrenal gland. Replacement glucocorticoid therapy is often required (2).

- Metyrapone is notable for rapid onset of action as the nadir of cortisol levels after a single dose is 2 hours. Mitotane inhibits steroidogenic enzymes in the adrenal gland, inducing a chemical adrenalectomy. It has a long half-life due to accumulation in adipose tissue. Ketoconazole inhibits enzymes in the adrenal gland, leading to a nadir of cortisol in 2 to 3 days of treatment.
- Etomidate (IV) inhibits adrenal corticosteroid synthesis and is effective in rapidly lowering cortisol levels in severe Cushing syndrome.
- Mifepristone is a potent glucocorticoid receptor antagonist. It is FDA approved to control hyperglycemia in adults with endogenous Cushing syndrome who have T2DM or glucose intolerance secondary to hypercortisolism that has not responded to (or who are not candidates for) surgery.
- Pasireotide is a somatostatin receptor ligand that is approved for the treatment of Cushing disease when surgery is not successful or cannot be performed (3). Hyperglycemia is a common and significant adverse side effect.
- Osilodrostat (a CYP11B1 and CYP11B2 inhibitor) inhibits steroidogenesis. Comparable to Metyrapone, and superior to Ketoconazole, in inhibition of cortisol production (4)[B].
- Also, pituitary tumor–directed agents such as retinoic acid, silibinin (inhibitor of heat shock protein overexpressed in Cushing disease tumors), and roscovitine (cyclin-dependent kinase inhibitor) may be effective in managing Cushing disease.

ONGOING CARE

FOLLOW-UP RECOMMENDATIONS
Patient Monitoring
- Once treated, the physical signs/symptoms of Cushing disease/syndrome gradually disappear over a period of 2 to 12 months. Obesity, HTN, glucose intolerance, and osteoporosis may remain even after treatment. Treatment of these secondary signs/symptoms is recommended until complete resolution.
- In children, bone density and growth rate increase after treatment although likely not to normal rates.

PATIENT EDUCATION
Education about diet and monitoring daily weight, early treatment of infections and emotional lability

PROGNOSIS
- Generally chronic course with cyclic exacerbations and rare remissions
- Recurrence rate is 20% for adrenal tumors.
- Poor with small-cell carcinoma of the lung producing ectopic hormone
- After surgery, a drop in cortisol level is a predictor.
- Some patients may need supraphysiologic steroid replacement postsurgery, tapered over months.

COMPLICATIONS
Untreated Cushing syndrome is often fatal secondary to cardiovascular, thromboembolic, and infectious causes.

REFERENCES
1. Nieman LK, Biller BMK, Findling JW, et al; for Endocrine Society. Treatment of Cushing's syndrome: an Endocrine Society clinical practice guideline. *J Clin Endocrinol Metab*. 2015;100(8):2807–2831.
2. Nieman LK, Ilias I. Evaluation and treatment of Cushing's syndrome. *Am J Med*. 2005;118(12):1340–1346.
3. Ferriere A, Tabarin A. Cushing's syndrome: treatment and new therapeutic approaches. *Best Pract Res Clin Endocrinol Metab*. 2020;34(2):101381.
4. Creemers SG, Feelders RA, de Jong FH, et al. Osilodrostat is a potential novel steroidogenesis inhibitor for the treatment of Cushing syndrome: an in vitro study. *J Clin Endocrinol Metab*. 2019;104(8):3437–3449.

 SEE ALSO

Algorithm: Cushing Syndrome

 CODES

ICD10
- E24.9 Cushing's syndrome, unspecified
- E24.0 Pituitary-dependent Cushing's disease
- E24.2 Drug-induced Cushing's syndrome

CLINICAL PEARLS
- Cushing disease is due to excessive ACTH secretion from a pituitary tumor.
- Cushing syndrome is due to excessive corticosteroid exposure from exogenous sources (medications) or endogenous sources (pituitary, adrenal, pulmonary, etc.) or tumor.
- Depression, alcoholism, medications, eating disorders, and other conditions can cause mild clinical and laboratory findings similar to those in Cushing syndrome (pseudo-Cushing syndrome).
- Symptoms may include facial plethora, round face, dorsocervical fat pads, easy bruising, purple striae, thin skin, fragility fractures, and muscle weakness.

CUTANEOUS DRUG REACTIONS

Mark A. Gardon, DO, MS • Kasey M. Scott, MD

 BASICS

DESCRIPTION
- An adverse cutaneous reaction in response to administration of a drug. Rashes are the most common form of adverse drug reaction (ADR).
- Severity can range from mild eruptions that resolve within 24 hours after the removal of the inciting agent, to severe skin damage with multiorgan involvement.
- Morbilliform and urticarial eruptions are the most common, accounting for approximately 94% of cutaneous drug reactions.
- Approximately 2% are severe and life-threatening.

EPIDEMIOLOGY
- All ages affected; immunosuppressed individuals at increased risk
- Increased likelihood of severe cutaneous and systemic reactions in geriatric population; unclear if due to polypharmacy or change in drug metabolism
- Difficult to distinguish from viral exanthems in pediatric patients

Incidence
In the United States, incidence of 1–3% in hospitalized patients; estimated 1/1,000 hospitalized patients has had a severe cutaneous reaction.

ETIOLOGY AND PATHOPHYSIOLOGY
Two classifications of ADR:
- Predictable (type A): dose dependent, known pharmacologic effect of drug, and drug–drug interaction
- Unpredictable (type B): drug intolerance, drug idiosyncrasy secondary to abnormality in metabolism, drug allergy, and drug pseudoallergy
- Immunologically mediated reaction: immunoglobulin (Ig) E–mediated reaction (type I hypersensitivity), cytotoxic/IgG/IgM induced (type II), immune complex reactions (type III), and delayed-type hypersensitivity (type IV) with T cells, eosinophils, neutrophils, and monocytes
- The most common medications causing adverse cutaneous reactions are carbamazepine and phenytoin.
- >700 drugs are known to cause cutaneous drug reactions.

Genetics
Genetics may play a role because certain HLA antigens have been associated with increased predisposition to specific drug eruptions:
- *HLA-B*5801*, *HLA-B*5701*, and *HLA-B*1502* have been linked to allopurinol-induced and carbamazepine-induced SJS/TEN, respectively; CYP2C9*3 variants linked to phenytoin-induced SJS/TEN
- HLA-DQB1*0301 allele found in 66% of patients of erythema multiforme compared with 31% of control subjects

GENERAL PREVENTION
Always ask the patients about prior adverse drug events. Be aware of medications with higher incidence of reactions as well as drug–drug reaction.

DIAGNOSIS

HISTORY
Develop a timeline documenting the onset and duration of all drugs, dosages, and onset of cutaneous eruption.

PHYSICAL EXAM
May present as a number of different eruption types, including, but not limited to the following:
- Morbilliform eruptions (exanthems)
  - Most frequent cutaneous reaction (75–95%); difficult to distinguish from viral exanthem; often secondary to an antibiotic
  - Starts on trunk as pruritic red macules and papules, then extends symmetrically to extremities in confluent fashion, sparing face, palms, soles, and mucous membranes
- Urticaria
  - Pruritic erythematous wheals distributed anywhere on the body, including mucous membranes
  - Lesions can vary in size and shape (e.g., round oval, rhomboid) and may change over time.
  - Angioedema, a related manifestation, may appear as asymmetric soft tissue swelling which can compromise airway and be life-threatening.
  - Individual lesions usually fade within 24 hours, but new lesions may develop.
- Acneiform eruptions
  - Folliculocentric, monomorphous pustules typically involving the face, trunk, and proximal extremities can also present in areas atypical of acne vulgaris such as forearms and legs.
  - Distinguished from acne vulgaris by absence of comedones
- Fixed drug eruptions
  - Solitary/few, sharply demarcated, round and/or oval erythematous plaques with dusky center that may leave postinflammatory hyperpigmentation; occur on skin or on mucous membrane
  - Onset usually 30 minutes to 8 hours after administration of drug
- Acute generalized exanthematous pustulosis (AGEP)
  - Rapidly appearing multiple nonfollicular sterile pustules on erythematous background typically involving intertriginous areas
  - Usually resolves within 1 to 3 days after removal of offending drug leaving a desquamation pattern
  - AGEP often causes fever and marked leukocytosis with neutrophilia and/or eosinophilia.
- Drug rash with eosinophilia and systemic symptoms (DRESS) syndrome
  - Drug-induced, multiorgan inflammatory response which may be life-threatening
  - Presentation can involve cutaneous eruptions (typically pruritic erythematous papules and patchy erythematous macules), fever, eosinophilia, hepatic dysfunction, renal dysfunction, and lymphadenopathy.
  - Onset usually 2 to 8 weeks after drug exposure
  - Symptoms and organ involvement may worsen after discontinuation of offending agent and persist for months.
  - Mucosal involvement rare

- Erythema multiforme
  - Acute, immune-mediated, mucocutaneous condition
  - Most commonly associated with herpes simplex virus (HSV) and other viral/bacterial etiologies (i.e., *Mycoplasma*); less likely secondary to drug exposure (<10% of cases)
  - Palpable classic target lesions and/or two-zone atypical target lesions with localized erythema
  - Most commonly distributed symmetrically on extensor surfaces of acral extremities; may involve mucus membrane (25–60%)
- SJS/TEN
  - Classification and distinction between SJS and TEN determined by affected body surface area (BSA); SJS: <10% BSA; SJS–TEN overlap: 10–30% BSA; TEN: >30% BSA
  - TEN strongly associated with drug intake (>95%); SJS less strongly associated (~50%)
  - Onset is usually 4 to 28 days but as delayed as 8 weeks after starting offending drug: flat atypical two-zone target lesions and erythematous macules that are truncal and generalized with mucosal involvement
  - May develop confluent areas of bullae, erosions, and necrosis; significant risk for infection and sepsis
  - SJS: 1–5% mortality; TEN: 25–35% mortality
- Lichenoid eruptions
  - Eruption of violaceous, pruritic polygonal papules symmetrically distributed favoring extensor surfaces/sun-exposed areas
  - Chronic lesions persist for weeks/months after the drug discontinued.
- Photosensitivity reaction
  - Phototoxic reactions: usually occur within minutes to hours after sunlight exposure with exaggerated sunburn reaction
  - Photoallergic reactions: more pruritic than painful; photodistributed sparing scalp, submental, and periorbital areas
- Hypersensitivity vasculitis
  - Nonblanching petechiae/palpable purpura which commonly present on lower extremities
  - Onset usually 7 to 21 days after drug exposure
  - Biopsy shows inflammation and necrosis of vessel walls.
- Sweet syndrome
  - Fever; neutrophilia; tender, edematous violaceous papules, plaques, or nodules, with or without pustules/vesicles that spontaneously resolve
  - Classically seen in young women after a mild respiratory illness or GI infection
- Exfoliative dermatitis/erythroderma
  - Severe end-stage dermatosis that develops from other drug reactions; commonly associated with systemic manifestations such as fever and chills
  - Generalized erythema with exfoliation and/or fine desquamation of large confluent areas
  - Increased risk of secondary infection and insensible fluid and temperature loss with hemodynamic instability

DIFFERENTIAL DIAGNOSIS
- Viral exanthem: Presence of fever, lymphocytosis, and other systemic findings may help in narrowing differential.
- Primary dermatosis (e.g., pustular psoriasis): Correlation of drug withdrawal to rash resolution may clarify diagnosis; skin biopsy is helpful.
- Bacterial infection: Cultures of pustules may distinguish primary infection from AGEP and acneiform eruptions.

DIAGNOSTIC TESTS & INTERPRETATION
Initial Tests (lab, imaging)
Selection of initial tests should be guided by clinical history and physical exam findings. CBC with differential; significant eosinophilia may be seen in DRESS and other drug-induced allergic reactions. LFT, urinalysis, and serum creatinine to assess for internal organ involvement; chest x-ray if suspected vasculitis

Diagnostic Procedures/Other
Special tests depend on suspected mechanism:
- Type I: skin/intradermal testing, radioallergosorbent test (RAST)
- Type II: direct/indirect Coombs test
- Type III: ESR, C-reactive protein, ANA, complement components, cryoglobulin assays
- Type IV: patch testing, lymphocyte proliferation assay (investigational)
- Anaphylaxis/nonimmunologic mast and basophil cell reaction: plasma histamine, serum tryptase levels, 24-hour urine N-methylhistamine

Test Interpretation
SJS/TEN: partial or full-thickness necrosis of the epidermis necrotic keratinocytes, vacuolization leading to subepidermal blister at basal membrane zone

 TREATMENT

GENERAL MEASURES
Do not rechallenge with drugs causing urticaria, bullae, angioedema, DRESS, anaphylaxis, or erythema multiforme.

MEDICATION
- Immediate withdrawal of offending drug; depending on the type of eruption, symptomatic treatment may be useful, but most require no additional therapy except cessation of the offending agent.
- Anaphylaxis or widespread urticaria: epinephrine 0.1 to 0.5 mg (1:1,000 [1 mg/mL] solution) IM in the mid-outer thigh every 5 to 15 min; prednisone PO 1 mg/kg in tapering doses may be given for severe refractory cases.
- Acute urticaria (<6 weeks) and chronic urticaria (>6 weeks): 2nd-generation antihistamines (preferred, less sedating): cetirizine 10 to 20 mg daily, loratadine 10 to 20 mg daily, fexofenadine 180 mg daily; H₂ antagonists: ranitidine 150 mg BID

- Erythema multiforme: Treatment is generally supportive with management of suspected underlying infection. Recurrent, HSV associated: prophylaxis with acyclovir 400 mg BID, valacyclovir 500 mg BID, or famciclovir 250 mg BID; "magic mouthwash" and oral antiseptic are helpful for mucosal erosions; consider ophthalmology consult for severe ocular involvement.
- SJS/TEN: Treatment is supportive. Consult with a dermatologist, ophthalmologist, and gynecologist as applicable. Systemic corticosteroid use remains controversial. Consider IVIG 2 to 3 g/kg for severe disease, although limited studies have not shown survival benefits in adults. In pediatric SJS/TEN patients, IVIG and systemic glucocorticoids appear to improve outcome; varied success rates reported with use of antitumor necrosis factor-α agents, cyclosporine, cyclophosphamide, and plasmapheresis. Avoid debridement and consider using detached epidermis as natural biologic dressing to minimize risk for hypertrophic scars.
- DRESS syndrome: systemic corticosteroid therapy recommended in early stages of DRESS diagnosis with prednisolone 1 mg/kg/day. Abrupt discontinuation commonly induces relapse; therefore, tapering oral prednisolone should be done gradually for 6 to 8 weeks to 3 months. Topical corticosteroids, systemic antihistamines, and emollients for rashes reduce relapse and hospitalization in mild cases.
- AGEP: Topical corticosteroid use has been correlated with a decreased median duration of hospitalization; systemic steroid use is generally not recommended, given the benign course.

ADMISSION, INPATIENT, AND NURSING CONSIDERATIONS
Hospitalization is indicated with certain signs of severity present:
- Cutaneous: skin surface >60%, erythema confluence, facial edema, skin pain, palpable purpura, skin necrosis, bullae or epidermal detachment, positive Nikolsky sign, mucosal erosions, urticaria, and/or tongue edema
- General: high fever, lymphadenopathy, arthralgia or arthritis, expiratory dyspnea, hypotension
- Biologic: eosinophilia >1,000/mm³, lymphocytosis with atypical lymphocytes, liver function abnormalities

 ONGOING CARE

FOLLOW-UP RECOMMENDATIONS
Patient Monitoring
- Patients with anaphylaxis/angioedema should be given EpiPens to be kept at home, work, and in the car for secondary prevention and a Med-Alert bracelet; label the patient's medical record with the agent and reaction.
- If the patient needs to take the inciting drug (e.g., antibiotic) in the future, induction of drug tolerance or graded challenge procedures may be necessary.

PROGNOSIS
- Majority of cases are self-limiting on removal of offending drug.
- Anaphylaxis, angioedema, DRESS, SJS/TEN, and bullous reactions are potentially fatal.
- Severity-of-illness score for toxic epidermal necrolysis (SCORTEN), a prognostic scoring system, can be used to guide management of hospitalized patients of SJS/TEN; also, may be helpful when discussing prognosis

ADDITIONAL READING
- Ahmed AM, Pritchard S, Reichenberg J. A review of cutaneous drug eruptions. *Clin Geriatr Med.* 2013;29(2):527–545.
- Dodiuk-Gad RP, Chung WH, Valeyrie-Allanore L, et al. Stevens-Johnson syndrome and toxic epidermal necrolysis: an update. *Am J Clin Dermatol.* 2015;16(6):475–493.

CODES

ICD10
- L27.1 Loc skin eruption due to drugs and meds taken internally
- L50.0 Allergic urticaria
- R21 Rash and other nonspecific skin eruption

CLINICAL PEARLS
- Virtually, any drug can cause a rash; antibiotics, anticonvulsants, and anti-inflammatory medications are the most common culprits that cause cutaneous drug reactions.
- Usually self-limited after withdrawal of offending agent
- Symptoms such as tongue swelling/angioedema, skin necrosis, blisters, high fever, dyspnea, and mucous membrane erosions signify more severe drug reactions.
- Useful resources: Drug Eruption Reference Manual by Jerome Litt; http://www.drugeruptiondata.com

CYSTIC FIBROSIS

Ryan D. Lurtsema, MD • Nica E. Lurtsema, MD, MPH

 BASICS

DESCRIPTION

- Cystic fibrosis (CF) is an autosomal recessive mutation that primarily affects the pulmonary and pancreatic systems but may involve any organ system (1).
- Due to improvements in medical care leading to a dramatic increase in survival, adults living with CF now outnumber children.

EPIDEMIOLOGY

Although CF is the most common lethal inherited disease in Caucasians, it is found in every racial group.

Incidence

- 1 in 3,200 Caucasians
- 1 in 10,000 Latin Americans
- 1 in 10,500 Native Americans
- 1 in 15,000 African Americans
- 1 in 30,000 Asian Americans

Prevalence

There are >30,000 patients with CF living in the United States and 70,000 worldwide, with a median predicted survival in the United States of 46.2 years (95% CI 45.2–47.6) (1)

ETIOLOGY AND PATHOPHYSIOLOGY

- Abnormal function of an epithelial chloride channel protein encoded by CF transmembrane conductance regulator (*CFTR*) gene on chromosome 7q31.2 affects the activity of chloride and sodium channels on the cell surface, leading to abnormally viscous secretions that alter organ function.
- Obstruction, infection, and inflammation negatively affect lung growth, structure, and function, leading to decreased mucociliary clearance, intense neutrophilic response with infection, and eventual degradation of supporting tissues, leading to bronchiectasis and eventual failure.

Genetics

- CF is an autosomal recessive, single-gene disorder. There exists >1,500 mutations in the CFTR gene that can cause varying severity of phenotypic CF. Most common is the deltaF508 mutation, which accounts for 85.3% of cases in the United States, followed by the G542X (4.5%) and G551D (4.3%) mutations.
- The severity of disease can also be affected by modifier genes (CFTM1 for meconium ileus), GERD, severe respiratory infection, or environmental factors such as smoke exposure.

GENERAL PREVENTION

Preconception counseling

- American College of Obstetricians and Gynecologists recommends preconception or 1st/2nd trimester genetic analysis for all North American couples.
- Newborn screening has been integral in early diagnosis, with 62.4% of new CF cases in 2019 identified by this method.
- Diagnosis prior to onset of symptoms leads to better lung function and nutritional outcomes.

COMMONLY ASSOCIATED CONDITIONS

- CF-related diabetes (CFRD)
  - May present as steady decline in weight, lung function, or increased frequency of exacerbation
  - Leading comorbid complication (20.7%)
  - Result of progressive insulin deficiency
  - Early screening and treatment may improve survival.
- Upper respiratory
  - Rhinosinusitis is seen in up to 100% of patients with CF.
  - Nasal polyps are seen in up to 86% of patients.
- The GI tract
  - Pancreatic exocrine insufficiency (85–90%)
  - Malabsorption of fat, protein, and fat-soluble vitamins (A, D, E, and K)
  - Hepatobiliary disease (12.6%) including focal biliary cirrhosis and cholelithiasis
  - Meconium ileus at birth (10–15%)
  - Distal intestinal obstruction syndrome (DIOS): (5.3%)
  - GERD (32.7%)
- Endocrine
  - Bone mineral disease (16.6%)
  - Joint disease (3%)
  - Hypogonadism
  - Frequent low testosterone levels in men
  - Menstrual irregularities
- Reproductive organs—congenital bilateral absence of the vas deferens with obstructive azoospermia in 98% of males
- Depression (12.8%)

Pregnancy Considerations

- Pulmonary disease may worsen during pregnancy.
- CF may cause increased incidence of preterm delivery, IUGR, and cesarean section.
- Advances in fertility treatments now allow men with CF to father children.

DIAGNOSIS

Criteria for diagnosis of CF

- At least one of the following:
  - One or more typical phenotypic features of CF:
    ○ Chronic pulmonary disease
    ○ Chronic sinusitis
    ○ Characteristic GI and nutritional abnormalities
    ○ Salt loss syndromes
    ○ Obstructive azoospermia
  - History of CF in a sibling
  - Positive newborn screening test
- *Plus* at least one of the following:
  - Elevated sweat chloride concentration on two or more occasions
  - Two mutations known to cause CF on separate alleles
  - Abnormalities in nasal potential difference (NPD) testing that are typical of CF

HISTORY

- History during prenatal period:
  - Routine prenatal ultrasonography indicates hyperechogenic bowel.
    ○ The risk is highest if there is an evidence of meconium peritonitis, bowel dilatation, or absent gallbladder. Parents should be offered CF carrier screening if these findings are present.
- History during neonatal period:
  - Meconium ileus (20%) (generally considered pathognomonic for CF)
  - Prolonged jaundice
- History during infancy:
  - Failure to thrive
  - Chronic diarrhea
  - Anasarca/hypoproteinemia
  - Pseudotumor cerebri (vitamin A deficiency)
  - Hemolytic anemia (vitamin E deficiency)
- History during childhood:
  - Recurrent endobronchial infection
  - Bronchiectasis
  - Chronic pansinusitis
  - Steatorrhea
  - Poor growth
  - Distal intestinal obstruction syndrome (DIOS)
  - Allergic bronchopulmonary aspergillosis (ABPA)
- History during adolescence and adulthood (7% diagnosed >18 years old):
  - Recurrent endobronchial infection
  - Bronchiectasis
  - ABPA
  - Chronic sinusitis
  - Hemoptysis
  - Pancreatitis
  - Portal hypertension
  - Azoospermia
  - Delayed puberty
- Suspect with failure to thrive, steatorrhea, and recurrent respiratory problems
  - Chronic/recurrent respiratory symptoms, including airway obstruction and infections
  - Persistent infiltrates on chest x-rays (CXRs)
  - Hypochloremic metabolic acidosis

PHYSICAL EXAM

- Respiratory: rhonchi or crackles, hyperresonance on percussion, and nasal polyps
- GI: hepatosplenomegaly if cirrhotic
- Other: digital clubbing, growth retardation, and pubertal delay

DIFFERENTIAL DIAGNOSIS

- Immunologic
  - Severe combined immunodeficiency
- Pulmonary
  - Difficult-to-manage asthma
  - Chronic obstructive pulmonary disease
  - Recurrent pneumonia
  - Chronic/recurrent sinusitis
  - Primary ciliary dyskinesia
- GI
  - Celiac disease
  - Protein-losing enteropathy
  - Pancreatitis of unknown etiology
  - Shwachman-Diamond syndrome

DIAGNOSTIC TESTS & INTERPRETATION

Initial Tests (lab, imaging)
- Newborn screening tests blood levels of immunoreactive trypsin (IRT).
- Sweat test (gold standard)
  - Sweat chloride (<40 mmol/L is normal.): >60 mmol/L on two occasions is positive for CF.
- CFTR mutation analysis
  - Allele-specific PCR identifies >90% of mutations; finite chance of false-negative
  - Full-sequence testing is more costly and time consuming.
- NPD (when sweat test and DNA testing inconclusive)
- CXR

Follow-Up Tests & Special Considerations
To further investigate the presence of CF-related complications, these tests are generally ordered:
- Sputum culture (common CF organisms)
- Pulmonary function tests (PFTs)
- 72-hour fecal fat, stool elastase
- Oral glucose tolerance test annually after the age of 10 years
- Head CT: Abnormal sinus CT findings are nearly universal in CF.
- Chest CT: after abnormal CXR
- Referral to CF facility within the first 24 to 72 hours of diagnosis is recommended.

Diagnostic Procedures/Other
Flexible bronchoscopy with bronchoalveolar lavage

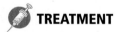 **TREATMENT**

GENERAL MEASURES
- Cystic Fibrosis Foundation guidelines call for:
  - Four office visits, four respiratory cultures, PFTs q6mo, and at least one evaluation by a multidisciplinary team, including dietitian, GI, and social worker per year
  - PFT goals: >75% predicted for adults, >100% predicted for children <18 years old
  - Annual screening for ABPA for patients aged >6 years with total serum IgE concentration
  - Annual influenza vaccination for all CF patients aged >6 months
  - Screen all adults and children aged >8 years with risk factors for osteoporosis with a DEXA scan.
  - Annual measurement of fat-soluble vitamins to rule out vitamin deficiencies
  - Annual LFTs
  - Decrease exposure to tobacco smoke.
  - COVID-19 vaccination for all eligible age groups
  - Telehealth with home-based spirometry is a viable option for disease monitoring.
- All patients should be followed in a CF center (accredited sites listed at https://www.cff.org/).
- Infant care:
  - Monthly visits for the first 6 months of life and then every 2 months until 1 year of life
  - Fecal elastase testing and salt supplementation
  - Consider palivizumab for RSV prophylaxis in infants with CF aged <2 years.

MEDICATION
- Pathogens for pulmonary infections: MRSA and MSSA, *Stenotrophomonas maltophilia*, *Pseudomonas aeruginosa*, *Burkholderia cepacia*, nontuberculous mycobacteria
  - Antibiotics should be targeted to most likely pathogen with most courses lasting 2 weeks.
  - Significant antibiotic resistance in *Staphylococcus aureus* has been observed, particularly with clindamycin and erythromycin.
- Pulmonary infections:
  - Antibiotics, oral
    - *S. aureus*: Bactrim (MRSA), doxycycline (MRSA), or cephalexin
    - *P. aeruginosa*: fluoroquinolones
  - Antibiotics, inhaled
    - Tobi (tobramycin): For *P. aeruginosa*, nebulize twice daily for 28 days; stop for 28 days and then resume use.
    - Cayston (aerosolized aztreonam)
  - Antibiotics, IV
    - *S. aureus*: cefazolin or nafcillin
    - MRSA: vancomycin or linezolid
    - *P. aeruginosa*: piperacillin and tazobactam (Zosyn) or ceftazidime plus aminoglycoside (tobramycin)
- Medications recommended for chronic use in pulmonary disease:
  - Recombinant human DNase (dornase alfa)
  - Hypertonic saline (7%)
  - High-dose ibuprofen in patients 6 to 17 years old with $FEV_1 \geq 60$ PPV
- Up to four CF modulator drugs now exist, including Orkambi, which can be used between ages 1 and 2 years, and Trikafta for those aged ≥6 years; which may improve lung function, respiratory symptoms, BMI, and prevent irreversible progression of disease (2).
  - Trikafta decreases systemic and airway inflammation, improves glycemic control in those with CFRD, and improves sleep
- Inhaled steroids are not recommended for chronic use in the absence of asthma or ABPA.
- Insufficient evidence for chronic use of inhaled β-agonist, inhaled anticholinergics, leukotriene modifiers, inhaled colistin
- Pancreatic enzymes, often combined with H_2 blockers or PPI to increase effectiveness
- Fat-soluble vitamin supplementation (A, D, E, and K)
- Ursodeoxycholic acid has not been proven effective for cholestasis.

ADDITIONAL THERAPIES
- High-frequency chest wall oscillation vest is the most widely used airway clearance technique, with aerobic exercise being a useful adjunct.
- CF-related bone disease: Consider bisphosphonate therapy.

SURGERY/OTHER PROCEDURES
- Timing for lung transplantation (bilateral) is polyfactorial. Key indications for referral are:
  - FEV_1 <50% predicted for those with a rapidly declining FEV_1 (>20% relative decline within 12 months)
  - FEV_1 <40% predicted with additional markers of shortened survival
  - FEV_1 <30% predicted for all others
- 5-year posttransplant survival is up to 62%.
  - Concerns for drug–drug interaction between Trikafta and tacrolimus, so dose adjustments may be necessary

- Liver transplantation is reserved for progressive liver failure ± portal hypertension with GI bleeding.
- Nasal polypectomy in 4.5% of CF patients

ADMISSION, INPATIENT, AND NURSING CONSIDERATIONS
- Pulmonary exacerbation (most common reason for admission)
- Bowel obstruction
- Pancreatitis in pancreatic-sufficient patients
- Always admit on contact precautions and to private rooms.
- Increased salt loss increases risk of hyponatremic hypochloremic dehydration.
- Cautious use of IV fluids with worsening lung disease

 ONGOING CARE

FOLLOW-UP RECOMMENDATIONS
- On discharge for a pulmonary exacerbation, follow-up with CF specialist within 2 to 4 weeks.
- Routine clinic visits every 3 months with airway cultures and PFTs as indicated
- Annual comprehensive nutritional evaluation

DIET
High-calorie, high-fat diet titrated to specific BMI goals established by the Cystic Fibrosis Foundation. If not meeting nutritional goals, consider referral to dietitian, pancreatic enzymes, or supplemental tube feeds

PATIENT EDUCATION
Cystic Fibrosis Foundation: https://www.cff.org

PROGNOSIS
- Median survival is 48.4 years.
- Progression of lung disease usually determines length of survival.

REFERENCES
1. Dickinson KM, Collaco JM. Cystic fibrosis. *Pediatr Rev*. 2021;42(2):55–67.
2. Nichols DP, Paynter AC, Heltshe SL, et al; PROMISE Study group. Clinical effectiveness of elexacaftor/tezacaftor/ivacaftor in people with cystic fibrosis: a clinical trial. *Am J Respir Crit Care Med*. 2022;205(5):529–539.

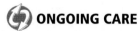 **CODES**

ICD10
- E84.9 Cystic fibrosis, unspecified
- E84.11 Meconium ileus in cystic fibrosis
- E84.0 Cystic fibrosis with pulmonary manifestations

CLINICAL PEARLS
- Meconium ileus is pathognomonic for CF
- When sweat test is equivocal, CFTR genetic testing is diagnostic
- Consider CF in any child with chronic diarrhea, especially with poor growth or failure to thrive
- All children with nasal polyps, digital clubbing, or bronchiectasis should be evaluated
- A rapid decline in pulmonary function suggests resistant organisms (e.g., *B. cepacia*), CFRD, ABPA, or GERD

C

DE QUERVAIN TENOSYNOVITIS

Lee A. Mancini, MD, CSCS*D, CSN • Nicholas R. Martin, MD • Michael J. Maddaleni, MD

 BASICS

DESCRIPTION
- First identified in 1895 by Fritz De Quervain, de Quervain tenosynovitis is a painful condition due to stenosis of the tendon sheath in the 1st dorsal compartment of the radial aspect of the wrist.
- Caused by repetitive motion of the extensor pollicis brevis (EPB) and abductor pollicis longus (APL) over the radial styloid with resultant metaplastic changes of the surrounding tendon sheath

EPIDEMIOLOGY
- The predominant age range is 30 to 50 years.
- Women are affected more commonly than men (1).
- With new occupational and professional demands, the prevalence of this condition is increasing gradually.

Incidence
- The overall incidence of de Quervain tenosynovitis is 0.9/1,000 person-years.
- For patients aged >40 years, the incidence is 1.4/1,000 person-years compared with 0.6/1,000 person-years for those aged <20 years.
- Women have an incidence rate ratio of 2.8/1,000 person-years compared with 0.6/1,000 person-years in men.
- The incidence ratio rate of de Quervain tenosynovitis is 1.3/1,000 person-years in black people and 0.8/1,000 person-years in white people (1).

Prevalence
Currently, estimated at 1.3% in females and 0.5% in males

ETIOLOGY AND PATHOPHYSIOLOGY
- Repetitive motions of the wrist and/or thumb result in microtrauma, metaplastic thickening of the tendons (EPB, APL), and narrowing of the surrounding tendon sheath.
- EPB and APL movement is resisted as they glide over the radial styloid, causing pain with movements of the thumb and wrist.
- Among individual undergoing release of the 1st dorsal compartment, histopathology of the tendon sheaths was characterized by myxoid degeneration with dense fibrous tissue and mucopolysaccharide accumulation.
- Cadaveric analyses have identified an additional septum within the 1st dorsal compartment in 34–44% of individuals and subcompartmentalization has been reported in 86–94% of patients with de Quervain tenosynovitis (2).

RISK FACTORS
- Women aged 30 to 50 years
- Pregnancy (primarily 3rd trimester and postpartum)
- Black race
- Systemic diseases (e.g., rheumatoid arthritis)
- Participation in activities that include repetitive motion or forceful grasping with thumb and wrist deviation such as golf, fly-fishing, racquet sports, rowing, or bicycling, video gaming, and more recently text messaging

- Repetitive movements with the hand/thumb requiring forceful grasping with wrist involving ulnar/radial deviation; dental hygienists, musicians, carpenters, assembly workers, and machine operators
- Recent analyses suggest anatomic variability including tendon insertion variation and subcompartmentalization of the 1st dorsal compartment may be the greatest risk factors.

GENERAL PREVENTION
Avoid overuse or repetitive movements of the wrist and/or thumb associated with forceful grasping and ulnar/radial deviation.

 DIAGNOSIS

HISTORY
- Repetitive motion activity; overuse of wrist or thumb
- Gradually worsening pain along the radial aspect of the thumb and wrist with certain movements, particularly ulnar deviation of the wrist
- Pregnancy
- Sports, leisure, and occupational history
- Trauma (rare)

PHYSICAL EXAM
- Pain over the radial styloid exacerbated when patients move the thumb or make a fist
- Crepitus with movement of the thumb
- Swelling over the radial styloid and base of the thumb
- Decreased range of motion of the thumb
- Pain over the 1st dorsal compartment on resisted thumb abduction or extension
- Tenderness may extend proximally or distally along the tendons with palpation or stress.
- Finkelstein test: Ask the patient to actively ulnar deviate off the edge of a table and the examiner grasps the affected thumb and passively continues to deviate the hand in the ulnar direction. A positive test occurs when there is a pain along the distal radius.
- Eichhoff test: Patient grasps a flexed thumb, and the examiner deviates the wrist in an ulnar direction.
- Finkelstein test is more sensitive for determining tenosynovitis of the APL and EPB tendons (3)[A].

DIFFERENTIAL DIAGNOSIS
- Scaphoid fracture
- Scapholunate ligament tear
- Dorsal wrist ganglion
- Osteoarthritis of the 1st carpometacarpal (CMC) joint
- Flexor carpi radialis tendonitis
- Infectious tenosynovitis
- Tendonitis of the wrist extensors
- Intersection syndrome
- Trigger thumb

DIAGNOSTIC TESTS & INTERPRETATION
Initial Tests (lab, imaging)
- Primarily a clinical diagnosis
- Radiographs of the wrist to rule out other pathology, such as CMC arthritis, if the diagnosis is in question
- MRI is the imaging test of choice to rule out coexisting soft tissue injury or wrist joint pathology.

Follow-Up Tests & Special Considerations
- Ultrasound can help to detect anatomic variations in the 1st dorsal extensor compartment of the wrist and target corticosteroid injections (4),(5).
- Ultrasound imaging has been reported as 100% sensitive for detection of pathology (2).

Test Interpretation
Inflamed and thickened retinacular sheath of the tendon

 TREATMENT

- Most cases of de Quervain tenosynovitis are self-limited.
- Rest and NSAIDs (3)[A]
- Ice (15 to 20 minutes 5 to 6 times a day)
- Immobilization with a thumb spica splint (3)[A]
- Occupational therapy
- Acupuncture
- Corticosteroid injection (preferably ultrasound guided)
- Consider surgery if conservative measures fail >6 months.

GENERAL MEASURES
- If full relief is not achieved, a corticosteroid injection of the tendon sheath can improve symptoms.
- Anatomic variation, including subcompartmentalization of the 1st dorsal compartment or the EPB tendon traveling in a separate compartment, may complicate treatment. Ultrasound can distinguish these variants and improve anatomic accuracy of injections (4).
- Surgical release may be indicated after 3 to 6 months of conservative treatment if symptoms persist. Surgery is highly effective and has a relatively low rate of complications.

MEDICATION
First Line
Splinting, rest, and NSAIDs

Second Line
- Corticosteroid injection of the tendon sheath has shown significant cure rates. Additional injections are sometimes required.
- Corticosteroid injection plus immobilization is more effective than immobilization alone (6)[B].
- Ultrasound-guided percutaneous tenotomy, retinaculum release, and/or injection of platelet-rich plasma are newer techniques that show promise for treatment of de Quervain tenosynovitis.

ISSUES FOR REFERRAL

Referral to a hand surgeon is indicated if there is no improvement with conservative therapy.

ADDITIONAL THERAPIES

- Hand therapy, along with iontophoresis/phonophoresis, may help improve outcomes in persistent cases.
- Patients may use thumb-stretching exercises as part of their rehabilitation.

SURGERY/OTHER PROCEDURES

- Indicated for patients who have failed conservative treatment
- Endoscopic release may provide earlier relief, fewer superficial radial nerve complications, and greater patient satisfaction with resultant scar compared to open release (6)[B].

ADMISSION, INPATIENT, AND NURSING CONSIDERATIONS

Hospitalization for care associated with surgical treatment

 ONGOING CARE

FOLLOW-UP RECOMMENDATIONS

- Additional corticosteroid injection may be performed at 4 to 6 weeks if symptoms persist. Caution with repeat steroid injections.
- Avoid repetitive motions and activities that cause pain.

DIET

As tolerated

PATIENT EDUCATION

Activity modification: Avoid repetitive movement of the wrist/thumb and forceful grasping.

PROGNOSIS

- Extremely good with conservative treatment
- Complete resolution can take up to 1 year.
- 95% success rates have been shown with conservative therapy >1 year.
- Up to 1/3 of patients will have persistent symptoms.

COMPLICATIONS

- Most complications are secondary to treatment. These include GI, renal, and hepatic injury secondary to NSAID use.
- Nerve damage may occur during surgery.
- Hypopigmentation, fat atrophy, bleeding, infection, and tendon rupture have been reported as potential adverse events from corticosteroid injection. Ultrasound guidance reduces the rate of complications.
- If not appropriately treated, thumb flexibility may be lost due to fibrosis.

REFERENCES

1. Wolf JM, Sturdivant RX, Owens BD. Incidence of de Quervain's tenosynovitis in a young, active population. *J Hand Surg Am*. 2009;34(1):112–115.
2. Dunn JC, Polmear MM, Nesti LJ. Dispelling the myth of work-related de Quervain's tenosynovitis. *J Wrist Surg*. 2019;8(2):90–92.
3. Huisstede BMA, Coert JH, Fridén J, et al; for European HANDGUIDE Group. Consensus on a multidisciplinary treatment guideline for de Quervain disease: results from the European HANDGUIDE study. *Phys Ther*. 2014;94(8):1095–1110.
4. Lee KH, Kang CN, Lee BG, et al. Ultrasonographic evaluation of the first extensor compartment of the wrist in de Quervain's disease. *J Orthop Sci*. 2014;19(1):49–54.
5. Di Sante L, Martino M, Manganiello I, et al. Ultrasound-guided corticosteroid injection for the treatment of de Quervain's tenosynovitis. *Am J Phys Med Rehabil*. 2013;92(7):637–638.
6. Kang HJ, Koh IH, Jang JW, et al. Endoscopic versus open release in patients with de Quervain's tenosynovitis: a randomised trial. *Bone Joint J*. 2013;95-B(7):947–951.

ADDITIONAL READING

- Ali M, Asim M, Danish SH, et al. Frequency of de Quervain's tenosynovitis and its association with SMS texting. *Muscles Ligaments Tendons J*. 2014;4(1):74–78.
- Ashraf MO, Devadoss VG. Systematic review and meta-analysis on steroid injection therapy for de Quervain's tenosynovitis in adults. *Eur J Orthop Surg Traumatol*. 2014;24(2):149–157.
- Cavaleri R, Schabrun SM, Te M, et al. Hand therapy versus corticosteroid injections in the treatment of de Quervain's disease: a systematic review and meta-analysis. *J Hand Ther*. 2016;29(1):3–11.
- Goel R, Abzug JM. de Quervain's tenosynovitis: a review of the rehabilitative options. *Hand (N Y)*. 2015;10(1):1–5.
- Kume K, Amano K, Yamada S, et al. In de Quervain's with a separate EPB compartment, ultrasound-guided steroid injection is more effective than a clinical injection technique: a prospective open-label study. *J Hand Surg Eur Vol*. 2012;37(6):523–527.
- Kwon BC, Choi SJ, Koh SH, et al. Sonographic identification of the intracompartmental septum in de Quervain's disease. *Clin Orthop Relat Res*. 2010;468(8):2129–2134.
- Orlandi D, Corazza A, Fabbro E, et al. Ultrasound-guided percutaneous injection to treat de Quervain's disease using three different techniques: a randomized controlled trial. *Eur Radiol*. 2015;25(5):1512–1519.

- Pagonis T, Ditsios K, Toli P, et al. Improved corticosteroid treatment of recalcitrant de Quervain tenosynovitis with a novel 4-point injection technique. *Am J Sports Med*. 2011;39(2):398–403.
- Peters-Veluthamaningal C, van der Windt DAWM, Winters JC, et al. Corticosteroid injection for de Quervain's tenosynovitis. *Cochrane Database Syst Rev*. 2009;(3):CD005616.
- Rousset P, Vuillemin-Bodaghi V, Laredo JD, et al. Anatomic variations in the first extensor compartment of the wrist: accuracy of US. *Radiology*. 2010;257(2):427–433.
- Scheller A, Schuh R, Hönle W, et al. Long-term results of surgical release of de Quervain's stenosing tenosynovitis. *Int Orthop*. 2009;33(5):1301–1303.
- Walker-Bone K, Palmer KT, Reading I, et al. Prevalence and impact of musculoskeletal disorders of the upper limb in the general population. *Arthritis Rheum*. 2004;51(4):642–651.

 SEE ALSO

Algorithm: Pain in Upper Extremity

 CODES

ICD10

M65.4 Radial styloid tenosynovitis [de Quervain]

CLINICAL PEARLS

- Repetitive movements of the wrist and thumb, and activities that require forceful grasping, are the most common causes of de Quervain tenosynovitis.
- Anatomic variations of the 1st dorsal compartment and metaplastic changes are identified in a majority of cases.
- Initial treatment is typically conservative.
- Corticosteroid injections are helpful and have lower complication rates if done under ultrasound guidance.
- Combined orthosis/corticosteroid injection approaches are more effective than either intervention alone.
- Ultrasound-guided percutaneous retinacular release and endoscopic surgery are helpful for recalcitrant cases.

DEEP VEIN THROMBOPHLEBITIS

Naureen Bashir Rafiq, MD, FAAFP

BASICS

DESCRIPTION

- Development of blood clot within the deep veins of the body, usually as a result of surgery or trauma to blood vessels, accompanied by inflammation of the vessel wall
- Major clinical consequences are embolization (usually to the lung), recurrent thrombosis, and postphlebitic syndrome.

EPIDEMIOLOGY

- Age- and gender-adjusted incidence of venous thromboembolism (VTE) is 100 times higher in the hospital than in the community. Almost half of all VTEs occur either during or soon after discharge from a hospital stay or surgery.
- 10–30% of patients diagnosed with deep venous thrombosis (DVT) and/or pulmonary embolism (PE) will die within 1 month of diagnosis.
- 1/3 (about 33%) of people with DVT/PE will have a recurrence within 10 years.
- Of patients with VTE, 20% are complicated with PE. The 28-day DVT fatality rate is 5.4%; at 1 year, 20%; at 3 years, 29%.

Incidence
- In the United States, VTE incidence is 50.4/100,000 person per year.
- Increased incidence in Caucasian and African American populations and with aging
- Most common site: lower extremity DVT
- Incidence in pregnancy: ~0.5 to 3/1,000
- 1–5% of central venous catheters are complicated by thrombosis.

Prevalence
- Variable; depends on medical condition or procedure
- At the time of DVT diagnosis, as many as 40% of patients also have asymptomatic PE; conversely, 30% of patients diagnosed with PE do not have a demonstrable source.
- Present in 11% of patients with acquired brain injury entering neurorehabilitation

ETIOLOGY AND PATHOPHYSIOLOGY
Factors involved may include venous stasis, endothelial injury, and hypercoagulability (Virchow triad).

Genetics
- Factor V Leiden, the most common thrombophilia, is found in 5% of the population and in 10–65% of all VTE events and increases VTE risk 3- to 6-fold.
- Prothrombin G20210A is found in 3% of Caucasians; increases the risk of thrombosis ~3-fold

RISK FACTORS
- Acquired: COVID-19 infection (up to 3 months after acute infection), previous DVT, cancer, immobilization, trauma, traumatic brain injury, recent major surgery, medications (oral/transdermal contraceptives, estrogens, tamoxifen, glucocorticoids), obesity, smoking, antiphospholipid syndrome, acute infectious process, thrombocytosis, pregnancy/puerperium, central venous catheters, inflammatory bowel disease
- Hereditary: deficiencies of protein C, protein S, or antithrombin III; factor V Leiden R506Q, prothrombin G20210A mutation, dysfibrinogenemia, elevated factor VIII activity, hyperhomocysteinemia

GENERAL PREVENTION
- Mechanical thromboprophylaxis for patients with high bleeding risk
- For acutely ill and for critically ill hospitalized patients at increased risk of thrombosis, low-molecular-weight heparin (LMWH), low-dose unfractionated heparin, or fondaparinux is recommended.

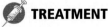**DIAGNOSIS**

HISTORY
- Higher clinical suspicion in patient with risk factors (See "Risk Factors" section.)
- DVT is classified as provoked or idiopathic based on underlying risk factors.
- Clinical assessment of bleeding risk (bleeding with the previous history of anticoagulation, history of liver disease, recent surgeries, history of GI bleed) is important prior to initiating treatment.
- Modified Wells criteria, a validated clinical prediction rule, is useful to determine the pretest probability of having a DVT.
  - Active cancer (treatment ongoing or within last 6 months) (+1 point)
  - Calf swelling >3 cm when compared to the asymptomatic leg (+1 point)
  - Collateral superficial veins (nonvaricose) (+1 point)
  - Pitting edema in the symptomatic leg (+1 point)
  - Previous documented DVT (+1 point)
  - Swelling of the entire leg (+1 point)
  - Localized tenderness along deep venous system (+1 point)
  - Paralysis, paresis, or recent cast immobilization of lower extremities (+1 point)
  - Recently bedridden >3 days or major surgery in past 4 weeks (+1 point)
  - Alternative diagnosis at least as likely (−2 points)
- Interpretation: score of 0, DVT unlikely; score of 1 to 2, moderate risk; score of ≥3, DVT likely; D-dimer testing and/or ultrasound should follow based on Wells criteria score.

PHYSICAL EXAM
- Symptoms may present as pain, swelling, tenderness, or discoloration but may be nonspecific or absent.
- Edema, due to swelling of collateral veins, is the most specific symptom.
- Resistance to dorsiflexion of the foot (Homan sign) is unreliable and nonspecific.

DIFFERENTIAL DIAGNOSIS
Cellulitis, fracture, ruptured synovial cyst (Baker cyst), lymphedema, calf muscle strain/tear/hematoma, Achilles tendon tear, extrinsic compression of vein (e.g., by tumor/enlarged lymph nodes), compartment syndrome, and localized allergic reaction

DIAGNOSTIC TESTS & INTERPRETATION
Initial Tests (lab, imaging)
- Routine laboratory testing (CBC, metabolic panel, coagulation studies) is not useful for diagnosis.
- D-dimer (sensitive but not specific; has high negative predictive value [NPV]), indicated in patients with a low and moderate pretest probability of DVT or PE but not indicated in high pretest probability patients; false positives in liver disease, inflammation, malignancy, trauma, pregnancy, and recent surgery; D-dimer should be adjusted for patients aged >50 years, and cut-off value is calculated by multiplying the patient's age by 10.

- Patients with a prior DVT and those with malignancy have higher rates of VTE, which decreases the NPV of Wells criteria.
- Compression ultrasound (CUS): first-line imaging for DVT due to its noninvasive nature and ease of use
- In patients with suspected DVT, the diagnosis process should be guided by the assessment of the pretest probability.
  - Low pretest probability: high-sensitivity D-dimer assay sufficient to exclude DVT if negative; if positive, follow with CUS.
  - Moderate pretest probability: high-sensitivity D-dimer assay preferred as an initial test; if positive, follow with CUS.
  - High pretest probability: CUS initial test; if positive CUS, then treat DVT. If negative, no further testing is necessary; if continued concern, may repeat CUS in 24 hours
- Other imaging modalities, such as CT venography and magnetic resonance venography, are rarely used but maybe better than CUS for demonstrating new from old thrombosis.
- Contrast venography and impedance plethysmography are now rarely used.

Follow-Up Tests & Special Considerations
- In young patients and/or those of concern or with idiopathic/recurrent VTE, consider thrombophilia testing (factor V Leiden mutation, prothrombin G20210A genetic assay, ATIII functional assay, protein C functional assay, protein S antigen, and functional assay and free S, phospholipid-dependent tests and anticardiolipin antibodies, lupus anticoagulant [drawn before initiation of heparin]).
- The risk of an underlying malignancy is more likely if recurrent VTE, risk 3.2 (95% CI 2.0–4.8). Unprovoked VTE, 4.6 times higher (vs. secondary); upper extremity DVT, not catheter-associated; odds ratio (OR) 1.8, abdominal DVT; OR 2.2 (1), bilateral lower extremity DVT, OR 2.1 (1)

TREATMENT

MEDICATION
Consider starting therapy before diagnosis confirmation in patients with high pretest probability and acceptable risk of bleeding.

- Anticoagulation is the mainstay of therapy. For patients with PE or proximal DVT, long-term therapy (at least 3 months) is recommended. Duration of therapy after 3 months is case-by-case basis.
- Indefinite anticoagulation is considered if there is a low risk of bleeding if index event is unprovoked PE and/or if D-dimer is positive 1 month after stopping anticoagulation.
- Direct oral anticoagulants (dabigatran, rivaroxaban, apixaban, or edoxaban) are recommended instead of vitamin K antagonists for the first 3 months of treatment in patients with lower extremity DVT or PE and no cancer (1)[B]
- The use and choice of anticoagulation should be considered based on the patient's history, bleeding risk, cost, and ease of compliance.

First Line
- Unfractionated heparin
  - IV drip: initial dose of 80 U/kg followed by continuous infusion of 18 U/kg/hr; target aPTT ratio >1.5 times control. Monitor aPTT every 6 hours and adjust infusion rate accordingly until two successive values are within the therapeutic range.
- LMWH
  - Enoxaparin (Lovenox): 1 mg/kg/dose SC q12h or 1.5 mg/kg daily
  - Dalteparin (Fragmin): 200 U/kg SC q24h or 100 U/kg SC q12h
- Direct and indirect factor Xa inhibitors
  - Fondaparinux (Arixtra): 5 mg (body weight <50 kg), 7.5 mg (body weight = 50 to 100 kg), or 10 mg (body weight >100 kg) SC once daily
  - Rivaroxaban (Xarelto): 15 mg PO twice daily with food for the first 3 weeks and then 20 mg PO every day with food
  - Apixaban (Eliquis): 10 mg PO twice daily for 1 week followed by 2.5 to 5.0 mg PO twice daily
  - Edoxaban (Savaysa): Initially give parenteral anticoagulants for 5 to 10 days and then transition to 60 mg PO daily (>60 kg) or 30 mg PO daily (≤60 kg).
- Thrombin inhibitors
  - Dabigatran (Pradaxa): Initially give parenteral anticoagulants for 5 to 10 days and then transition to 150 mg PO twice daily for creatinine clearance >30 mL/min.
- Vitamin K antagonists
  - Warfarin (Coumadin): Start with 2 to 5 mg/day. Adjust to a target INR of 2 to 3; overlap with a parenteral anticoagulant for a minimum of 5 days until therapeutic INR is sustained ≥24 hours.
- Adverse effects
  - All anticoagulants increase the risk of bleeding.
  - Heparin and LMWH can also cause heparin-induced thrombocytopenia (HIT) (LMWH has a lower risk) and injection site irritation.
  - Warfarin is teratogenic.
  - Dosage adjustments may be required for patients with decreased creatinine clearance.

Second Line
Heparin can be given by intermittent SC self-injection.

Pregnancy Considerations
- Warfarin (Coumadin) is a teratogen. It is contraindicated in pregnancy but is safe during breastfeeding.
- LMWH is recommended over unfractionated heparin for treatment of acute DVT and PE in pregnancy.
- Enoxaparin, dalteparin, fondaparinux, and apixaban are pregnancy Category B.
- Dabigatran, rivaroxaban, edoxaban are pregnancy Category C.

SURGERY/OTHER PROCEDURES
- In selected patients with proximal DVT (acute iliofemoral DVT <14 days, good functional status, >1 year of life expectancy), may consider catheter-directed thrombolysis/open thrombectomy
- Thrombolysis (systemic or catheter-directed) reduces the incidence of a postthrombotic syndrome (PTS) after a proximal (iliofemoral or femoral) DVT by 1/3.

- Thrombectomy is recommended in patients with limb-threatening ischemia due to iliofemoral venous outflow obstruction.
- IVC filter
  - Not routinely inserted in patients with acute DVT, except with DVT or PE with absolute contraindication to anticoagulation or recurrent embolism despite adequate anticoagulation
  - Special considerations can be given to patients who are chronically immobile, such as spinal cord injury patients.

ADMISSION, INPATIENT, AND NURSING CONSIDERATIONS
- In patients with acute PE, if the following criteria are met, then hospital admission is not necessary. Patients who meet these criteria but are admitted may be discharged early (<5 days of inpatient treatment) (1):
  - The patient is clinically stable with good cardiopulmonary reserve.
  - No recent bleeding, severe renal or liver disease, or severe thrombocytopenia <70,000
  - Expected to be compliant
  - The patient feels well enough to be treated at home.
- Admission for respiratory distress, elevated cardiac biomarkers, right ventricular dysfunction, candidate for thrombolysis, active bleeding, renal failure, phlegmasia alba dolens, phlegmasia cerulea dolens, history of HIT
- In medically stable and properly anticoagulated patients, an overlap of anticoagulation and warfarin monitoring may be done as an outpatient.
- Limb elevation and graduated compression stockings for symptomatic relief

 ONGOING CARE

FOLLOW-UP RECOMMENDATIONS
- Resumption of normal activity with avoidance of prolonged immobility
- Compression stockings are not routinely recommended for the prevention of PTS after acute DVT (1)[B] but can be used for patients who already present with symptoms of PTS.

Patient Monitoring
- Monitor platelet counts while on heparin, LMWH, and fondaparinux for HIT.
- An anti-Xa activity level may help guide LMWH titration of therapy.
- Investigate significant bleeding (e.g., hematuria or GI hemorrhage) because anticoagulant therapy may unmask a preexisting lesion (e.g., cancer, peptic ulcer disease, or arteriovenous [AV] malformation).

PATIENT EDUCATION
Dietary habits should be discussed when warfarin is initiated to ensure that intake of vitamin K–rich foods are monitored.

PROGNOSIS
- 20% of untreated proximal (iliofemoral, femoral, or popliteal) lower extremity DVTs progress to PE, and 10–20% of those are fatal. However, with anticoagulant therapy, mortality is decreased 5- to 10-fold.
- DVT confined to the infrapopliteal veins has a small risk of embolization but can propagate proximally.
- Up to 75% of patients with symptomatic DVT present with PTS after 5 to 10 years.

COMPLICATIONS
PE (fatal in 10–20%), arterial embolism (paradoxical embolization) with AV shunting, chronic venous insufficiency, PTS, treatment-induced hemorrhage, soft tissue ischemia associated with massive clot and high venous pressures; phlegmasia cerulea dolens (rare but a surgical emergency)

REFERENCE
1. Kearon C, Akl EA, Ornelas J, et al. Antithrombotic therapy for VTE disease: CHEST guideline and expert panel report. *Chest*. 2016;149(2):315–352.

 SEE ALSO

Antithrombin Deficiency; Factor V Leiden; Protein C Deficiency; Protein S Deficiency; Prothrombin 20210 (Mutation); Pulmonary Embolism

CODES

ICD10
- I80.209 Phlbts and thombophlb of unsp deep vessels of unsp low extrm
- I80.299 Phlebitis and thombophlb of deep vessels of unsp low extrm
- I80.10 Phlebitis and thrombophlebitis of unspecified femoral vein

CLINICAL PEARLS
- Many cases of VTE are asymptomatic.
- At the time of DVT diagnosis, as many as 40% of patients also have asymptomatic PE.
- Wells criteria are useful to determine the pretest probability of a DVT, but follow-up testing and/or imaging should be done if moderate to high probability.
- Choice of anticoagulant therapy should be individualized based on patient's history and compliance.

D

DEHYDRATION

Stephen W. Line, DO, CAQ-SM • Calli M. Fry, DO • Greg Bowlin, MD

 BASICS

DESCRIPTION
- Dehydration is a deficiency in total body water (1).
- The two types of dehydration:
  - Water loss
  - Salt and water loss (combination of dehydration and hypovolemia)

EPIDEMIOLOGY
Dehydration is associated with increased mortality and morbidity and is prevalent in the health-care setting and in the community (1); responsible for 10% of all pediatric hospitalizations United States (2)

Incidence
In the United States, admission rate for dehydration and related diagnosis has remained stable at approximately 130 per 100,000 for the general population. Two observational studies in Europe have shown that 37–46% of patients aged >65 years presented to major hospitals with dehydration (1).

Prevalence
Several retrospective studies have sought to evaluate the prevalence of dehydration occurring after hospital admission, with current estimates of 2–3.5% of patients meeting dehydration criteria (1).

ETIOLOGY AND PATHOPHYSIOLOGY
- Body water can be lost through the skin, lungs, kidneys, and gastrointestinal tract.
- Negative fluid balance occurs when ongoing fluid losses exceed fluid intake.
- Fluid losses can be insensible (sweat, respiration), obligate (urine, stool), or abdominal (diarrhea, vomiting, osmotic diuresis in diabetic ketoacidosis).
- Negative fluid balance can lead to hypovolemia (severe intravascular volume depletion) and end-organ damage from inadequate perfusion.
- "Third spacing" of fluids can occur in patients with effusions, ascites, capillary leaks (e.g., burns), or sepsis.

Geriatric Considerations
The elderly are at increased risk as kidney function, urine concentration, thirst sensation, aldosterone secretion, release of vasopressin, and renin activity all significantly decline with age.

Genetics
Some cases of dehydration have a genetic component (diabetes), whereas others do not (gastroenteritis).

RISK FACTORS
- Children <5 years of age at highest risk (2)
- Elderly
- Acute or chronic illness
- Decreased cognition or mental status
- Lack of access to water
- Increased exertion in high temperature
- Taking certain medications (e.g., diuretics)

GENERAL PREVENTION
- Patient and/or parent education on early signs of dehydration
- Provide preferred beverages (especially in illness).
- Universal precautions (including hand hygiene)

Clinical Finding	Mild	Moderate	Severe
Dehydration: children	5–10%	10–15%	>15%
Dehydration: adults	3–5%	5–10%	>10%
General condition: infants	Thirsty, alert, restless	Lethargic/drowsy	Limp, cold, cyanotic extremities, may be comatose
General condition: older children	Thirsty, alert, restless	Alert, postural dizziness	Apprehensive, cold, cyanotic extremities, muscle cramps
Quality of radial pulse	Normal	Thready/weak	Feeble or impalpable
Quality of respiration	Normal	Deep	Deep and rapid/tachypnea
BP	Normal	Normal to low	Low (shock)
Skin turgor	Normal skin turgor	Reduced skin turgor, cool skin	Skin tenting, cool, mottled, acrocyanotic skin
Eyes	Normal	Sunken	Very sunken
Tears	Present	Absent	Absent
Mucous membranes	Moist	Dry	Very dry
Urine output	Normal	Reduced	None passed in many hours
Anterior fontanelle	Normal	Sunken	Markedly sunken

COMMONLY ASSOCIATED CONDITIONS
- Hyponatremia
- Hypernatremia
- Hypokalemia
- Hyperglycemia
- Hypovolemic shock
- Renal failure
- Rhabdomyolysis
- Heat illness

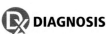 **DIAGNOSIS**

- Assessment of a patient's hydration status is complex and accounts for the patient's history, clinical assessment, and laboratory values.
- Several clinical variables are used to measure dehydration (see table).
- Calculate percent dehydration = (preillness weight − illness weight)/preillness weight × 100.

HISTORY
- Fever
- Intake (including description and amount)
- Diarrhea (including duration, frequency, consistency, ± mucus/blood)
- Vomiting (including duration, frequency, consistency, ± bilious/nonbilious)
- Urination pattern
- Sick contacts or recent illness
- Medication history (e.g., diuretics, laxatives, steroids)
- Heat exposure

PHYSICAL EXAM
- Vitals: pulse, BP, temperature
- Orthostatic vital signs
- Weight loss: <5%, 10%, or >15%
- Mental status (Assess for lethargy.)
- Evaluate the eyes for sunken appearance and tear production.
- Mucous membranes appear tacky, dry, or parched.
- Capillary refill may be prolonged (i.e., >3 seconds).
- Urine output: normal, reduced, or none passed in many hours

Pediatric Considerations
In children, prolonged capillary refill time, abnormal skin turgor, and abnormal respiratory pattern are red flags for dehydration. In infants, a sunken anterior fontanelle is an additional sign of poor volume status. Pay special attention to the number and weight of wet/soiled diapers produced as this can provide valuable objective evidence (2).

DIFFERENTIAL DIAGNOSIS
- Decreased intake: ineffective breastfeeding, inadequate thirst response, anorexia, malabsorption, metabolic disorder, obtunded state
- Excessive losses: gastroenteritis, diarrhea, febrile illness, diabetic ketoacidosis, hyperglycemia, hyperosmolar hyperglycemic state, diabetes insipidus, intestinal obstruction, sepsis

DIAGNOSTIC TESTS & INTERPRETATION

Initial Tests (lab, imaging)
- For mild dehydration, serum or urine studies are generally not necessary.
- For moderate to severe dehydration:
  - Plasma osmolality (gold standard for determining dehydration) (1)
  - Urinalysis (specific gravity, hematuria, glucosuria) and urine osmolality
  - Serum creatinine, BUN, and BUN/creatinine
- Imaging is typically not needed to diagnose or manage dehydration, but some adult patient populations may benefit from assessment of inferior vena cava collapsibility using bedside ultrasound evaluation.

Follow-Up Tests & Special Considerations
Infants and the elderly may not concentrate urine maximally, making urinalysis and urine specific gravity less helpful.

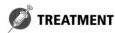 **TREATMENT**

GENERAL MEASURES
Oral rehydration therapy (ORT) is the first-line treatment in dehydrated adults and children. Intravenous, nasogastric, and intraosseous (IO) rehydration may be considered in moderate to severe dehydration cases.

MEDICATION

First Line

- ORT
  - Preferred first-line treatment for mild to moderately dehydrated patients
  - Oral rehydration solution should be given as soon as possible to patients who are able to drink and sit upright. The goal should be to take small, frequent sips at a rate of 100 mL every 5 minutes until symptoms stabilize.
  - When oral rehydration solution is not available, then water or broth should be consumed. Sports drinks are also an option but may worsen volume loss in some patients with infectious volume losses with diarrhea.
- Intravenous, nasogastric, and/or IO rehydration therapy
  - Second-line treatment for mild dehydration but often needed in cases of moderate to severe dehydration or when patients are unable to drink adequately.
  - For moderate to severe hypovolemia in adults:
    - Step I: IV crystalloid fluid bolus for volume resuscitation
      - Give 20 mL/kg/hr until vital signs normalize.
    - Step II: Replace fluid deficit; start maintenance fluids; account for losses.
      - Fluid deficit (mL) = [preillness weight (kg) − illness weight (kg)] × 1,000
      - 4-2-1 formula:
        - 0 to 10 kg: + 4 mL/kg/hr
        - 10 to 20 kg: + 2 mL/kg/hr
        - >20 kg: + 1 mL/kg/hr
        - Example: maintenance fluids for a 50-kg patient
          - 10 kg(4 mL/kg/hr) + 10 kg(2 mL/kg/hr) + 30 kg(1 mL/kg/hr) = 90 mL/hr
  - For moderate to severe dehydration in children:
    - Step I: ORT with NG tube or begin IV fluids
      - IV crystalloid fluid bolus for volume resuscitation: give 10 to 20 mL/kg; may repeat up to 60 mL/kg
    - Step II: Replace fluid deficit; start maintenance fluids; account for losses.
      - Typically, deficit is replaced over 24 to 48 hours.
- IV Fluid Considerations
  - The choice of crystalloid fluid should be customized to the patient.
    - Most common crystalloid fluids are:
      - Isotonic saline (0.9% NaCl; NS)
      - Lactated Ringer (LR) solution
      - D5 1/2 NS + 20 mEq KCl/L
  - In patients with dehydration and severe hyponatremia, there is a risk of rapid rise in sodium with too quick of volume administration which can lead to central pontine myelinolysis.
  - Caution should be exercised in patients with increased age, heart failure, and advanced kidney disease. These patients require smaller volume boluses and frequent reassessments.
  - Consider nasogastric administration of fluids in young children as an alternative to IV fluids (3).

Second Line

- If the patient is experiencing excessive vomiting, consider using an antiemetic.
  - Ondansetron (PO, SL, IV): 4 to 8 mg every 4 to 8 hours as needed
    - May be effective in decreasing the rate of emesis and can improve success rate of oral hydration (3)
    - Risk of QT prolongation, constipation, and headaches
  - Promethazine (PO, PR, IM, IV): 12.5 to 25.0 mg every 4 to 6 hours as needed (max of 50 mg/day)
    - Contraindicated in children <2 years old due to risk of fatal respiratory depression
    - Caution with IM/IV administration due to elevated risk of severe tissue injury
  - Other antiemetics are also available
- Loperamide may reduce the duration of diarrhea compared with placebo in children with mild to moderate dehydration.

Pediatric Considerations

Given a higher risk for serious adverse events, loperamide is not indicated for children <3 years of age with acute diarrhea.

ISSUES FOR REFERRAL

- For severe dehydration, critical care referral and ICU-level care may be warranted.
- Surgical consultation for acute abdominal issues if needed

SURGERY/OTHER PROCEDURES

For specific underlying causes of dehydration, such as intestinal obstruction or appendicitis

ADMISSION, INPATIENT, AND NURSING CONSIDERATIONS

- Admission criteria:
  - Intractable vomiting/diarrhea
  - Electrolyte abnormalities
  - Hemodynamic instability
  - Inability to tolerate ORT
- Inpatient management considerations:
  - Stabilize airway, breathing, and circulation.
  - Mild dehydration:
    - Begin ORT. If unsuccessful, then initiate IV/IO/NG fluids.
    - The Holliday-Segar method can be used to determine maintenance ORT in children.
  - Moderate to severe dehydration or hemodynamic instability:
    - Obtain IV access and begin IV fluid resuscitation immediately.
  - Strict inputs and outputs should be monitored while assessing fluid volume status.
    - Input: all oral intake and parenteral medications and fluids
    - Output: all urine and stool excretion; any procedural fluid loss or body fluid drainage.
- Discharge criteria
  - Recovery of volume status to euvolemia and tolerating an oral diet/fluids
  - Underlying etiology is treated and improving.

ONGOING CARE

DIET

- Bland food bananas, rice, applesauce, toast (BRAT) diet.
- Small frequent sips of room temperature liquids.
- Oral rehydration solutions are available commercially.

Pediatric Considerations

Continue breastfeeding ad lib. If diarrhea is present, lactose-free feeds may reduce the duration of diarrhea in children with mild to severe dehydration.

PATIENT EDUCATION

- Patients should seek medical care if they (or their child) feel faint or dizzy when rising from a sitting or lying position, become lethargic and/or confused, or complain of a rapid HR.
- Patients should call their physician if they are unable to keep down any fluids, vomiting has been going on >24 hours in an adult or >12 hours in a child, diarrhea has lasted >2 days in an adult/child, or an infant/child is much less active than usual or is very irritable.

PROGNOSIS

Self-limited if treated early; potentially fatal if untreated and persistent

COMPLICATIONS

Seizures, renal failure, cardiovascular arrest

REFERENCES

1. Lacey J, Corbett J, Forni L, et al. A multidisciplinary consensus on dehydration: definitions, diagnostic methods and clinical implications. *Ann Med.* 2019; 51(3–4):232–251.
2. Santillanes G, Rose E. Evaluation and management of dehydration in children. *Emerg Med Clin North Am.* 2018;36(2):259–273.
3. Colletti JE, Brown KM, Sharieff GQ, et al; for ACEP Pediatric Emergency Medicine Committee. The management of children with gastroenteritis and dehydration in the emergency department. *J Emerg Med.* 2010;38(5):686–698.

ADDITIONAL READING

https://5minuteconsult.com/collectioncontent/3-195944/patient-handouts/dehydration

SEE ALSO

Oral Rehydration

CODES

ICD10

- E86.0 Dehydration
- E87.1 Hypo-osmolality and hyponatremia
- E86.1 Hypovolemia

CLINICAL PEARLS

- Dehydration is the result of a deficiency in total body water leading to a negative fluid balance.
- Dehydration and its sequelae are the common causes of hospitalization in adults, children, and elderly.
- Begin by assessing the level of dehydration, determining the underlying cause, and calculating necessary replacement needs.
- Treatment is directed at treating the underlying cause while restoring fluid balance via oral rehydration (preferred) or IV/IO/NG fluids (if necessary).

DELIRIUM

Dongsheng Jiang, MD, MSc • Joseph P. Wiedemer, MD, FAAFP • Juan Qiu, MD, PhD

BASICS

DESCRIPTION
- A temporary neurocognitive complication of illness and/or medication(s) manifested by new confusion and impaired attention
- Requires evaluation to decrease morbidity and mortality

EPIDEMIOLOGY
- Predominant age: older persons
- Predominant sex: male = female

Incidence
- >50% in older ICU patients
- 11–51% in postoperative patients
- 19% after intracranial surgery and 42% after neurovascular surgery
- 10–40% in hospitalized older patients
- 20–22 % in nursing home/post–acute care patients

Prevalence
- 1–2% in outpatients
- 8–17% in older ED patients

ETIOLOGY AND PATHOPHYSIOLOGY
- Multifactorial: believed to result from a decline in physiologic reserves with aging, resulting in a vulnerability to new stressors
- Often interaction between predisposing and precipitating risk factors

RISK FACTORS
- Predisposing risk factors
  - Advanced age, >70 years
  - Preexisting cognitive impairment
  - Functional impairment
  - Dehydration
  - History of alcohol abuse
  - Malnutrition
  - Hearing or vision impairment
  - Multiple comorbidities
- Precipitating risk factors
  - Severe illness in any organ system
  - Medical devices (urinary catheter, restraints)
  - Polypharmacy (≥5 medications)
  - Specific medications, especially benzodiazepines, opioids, anticholinergics diphenhydramine, high-dose neuroleptics
  - Pain
  - Any iatrogenic event
  - Surgery
  - Sleep deprivation

COMMONLY ASSOCIATED CONDITIONS
Multiple but most common are the following:
- Medication changes
- Infections (especially lung, urine, and bloodstream, but consider meningitis as well)
- Toxic metabolic (especially low sodium, elevated calcium, renal failure, and hepatic failure)
- Heart attack or stroke
- Alcohol or drug withdrawal
- Preexisting cognitive impairment increases risk.

DIAGNOSIS

- Delirium is a diagnosis of exclusion made using a careful history, behavioral observation, and cognitive assessment.
- *Diagnostic and Statistical Manual of Mental Disorders*, 5th edition diagnostic criteria include:
  - Disturbance in attention and awareness
  - Change in cognition not due to dementia or coma
  - Presence of an additional disturbance in cognition (e.g., memory deficit, language, visuospatial ability, disorientation, or perception)
  - Onset over short period (hours to days) and fluctuates during course of day
  - Evidence from history, exam, or lab that disturbance is caused by physiologic consequence of medical condition, intoxicating substance, medication use, or more than one cause
- The Confusion Assessment Method (CAM) is the most well-validated and tested clinical tool (sensitivity of 94–100% and specificity of 90–95%) and has been adapted for ICU setting in adults (CAM-ICU) and children (pediatric CAM-ICU [pCAM-ICU]).

ALERT
- Four key diagnostic features of the CAM:
  - Acute change in mental status
  - Fluctuating course
  - Inattention
  - Disorganized thinking or altered level of consciousness
- Several nondiagnostic symptoms may be present:
  - Short- and long-term memory problems
  - Sleep–wake cycle disturbances
  - Hallucinations and/or delusions
  - Emotional lability
  - Tremors and asterixis
- Subtypes based on level of consciousness
  - Hyperactive delirium (15%): Patients are loud, agitated, restless, and disruptive.
  - Hypoactive delirium (20%): quietly confused; sleepy; may sit and not eat, drink, or move
  - Mixed delirium (50%): features of both hyperactive and hypoactive delirium
  - Normal consciousness delirium (15%): still displays disorganized thinking, along with acute onset, inattention, and fluctuating mental status
  - Subsyndromal delirium (23%): some delirium symptoms but does not progress to full delirium

HISTORY
- Time course of mental status changes
- Recent medication changes
- Symptoms of infection
- New neurologic signs
- Abrupt change in functional ability

PHYSICAL EXAM
- Comprehensive cardiorespiratory exam is essential.
- Focal neurologic signs are usually absent.
- Mini-Mental State Examination (MMSE) is the most well-known and studied cognitive screen, but it may not be the most appropriate in an acute care setting; shorter cognitive screens have been studied in delirious patients (i.e., Short Blessed Test [SBT], Brief Alzheimer Screen [BAS], and Ottawa 3DY) and may be helpful if performed serially over time.
- Gastrointestinal/genitourinary exam for constipation/urinary retention

DIFFERENTIAL DIAGNOSIS
- Depression (disturbance of mood, normal level of consciousness, fluctuates weeks to months)
- Acute stress disorder (disturbance of mood, normal level of consciousness, precipitated by traumatic event)
- Bipolar disorder, manic episode (pressured speech, impulsivity, fluctuates weeks to months, rarely sudden onset in older adults)
- Dementia (insidious onset, memory problems, normal level of consciousness, fluctuates days to weeks)
- Psychosis (rarely sudden onset in older adults)
- Seizure disorders (i.e., nonconvulsive status epilepticus)

DIAGNOSTIC TESTS & INTERPRETATION

Initial Tests (lab, imaging)
- Labs: guided by history and physical exam
  - Complete blood count (CBC), comprehensive metabolic panel (CMP), urinalysis (UA), urine culture, blood culture
  - Medication levels (digoxin, theophylline, antiepileptics) where applicable
- Chest radiograph
- Electrocardiogram as necessary

Follow-Up Tests & Special Considerations
- If preliminary lab tests do not indicate a precipitator of delirium, consider:
  - Venous blood gases
  - Troponin
  - Toxicology screen
  - Thyroid-stimulating hormone (TSH)
  - Thiamine, B12
- Noncontrast-enhanced head CT scan if
  - Recent fall
  - Receiving anticoagulants
  - New focal neurologic signs
  - Ruling out mass before lumbar puncture

Diagnostic Procedures/Other
- Lumbar puncture (rarely necessary)
- Electroencephalogram (rarely necessary)

TREATMENT

- Establish a comprehensive and well-coordinated multidisciplinary team to include physicians, nurses, pharmacists, psychologists, speech therapists, dieticians, physical/occupational therapists, spiritual/religious specialists, and social workers and to design and fine-tune treatment strategy according to each patient's unique situation (1).
- There is a strong evidence for multicomponent nonpharmacologic interventions.
- A2F bundle strategy (2):
  - A—Assess, prevent, and manage pain.
  - B—Both spontaneous awakening and spontaneous breathing trials
  - C—Choice of analgesic and sedation
  - D—Delirium: assess, prevent, and manage
  - E—Early mobility and exercise
  - F—Family engagement

- The Hospital Elder Life Program (HELP) is a widely used approach (3):
  - Address acute medical issues (e.g., treat underlying disorder, stabilize vitals, maintain hydration).
  - Reorientation strategies:
    ○ Use orientation boards, clocks, and calendars.
    ○ Provide eyeglasses, hearing aids, interpreters; encourage family involvement.
  - Optimize hydration and nutrition.
  - Early mobilization
  - Avoid restraints.
  - Encourage self-care.
  - Normalize sleep–wake cycle (discourage napping, open curtains during day, prioritize uninterrupted sleep).
  - Pain control with nonopioids
  - Drug adjustments (Avoid or reduce psychoactive drugs and anticholinergic medications; prioritize nonpharmacologic approaches.)
- Pharmacologic management of symptoms (reserve for severe circumstances)
- Addressing six risk factors (i.e., cognitive impairment, sleep deprivation, dehydration, immobility, vision impairment, and hearing impairment) in at-risk hospitalized patients can reduce the incidence of delirium by 33%.

GENERAL MEASURES
- De-escalation skill training for care staff
- Look for underlying causes: hypotension, hypoxia, hypoglycemia, drug overdose or withdrawal, and others.
- Remove unnecessary tubes/catheters.
- Actively involve family members in care.
- Postoperative patients should be monitored for
  - Myocardial infarction/ischemia
  - Infection (i.e., pneumonia, urinary tract infection)
  - Pulmonary embolism
  - Urinary or stool retention (attempt catheter removal by postoperative day 2)
  - Anemia/bleeding
- Anesthesia route (general vs. epidural) may affect the risk of delirium. Depth of anesthesia likely affects risk of delirium.
- ICU sedation and avoidance of benzodiazepines may reduce risk.
- Multifactorial treatment: identify contributing factors and provide preemptive care to avoid iatrogenic problems, with special attention to
  - CNS oxygen delivery (attempt to attain):
    ○ $SaO_2 > 90\%$ with a goal of $SaO_2 > 95\%$
    ○ Systolic BP <2/3 of baseline or >90 mm Hg
    ○ Hematocrit >30%
  - Fluid/electrolyte balance
    ○ Sodium, potassium, and glucose normal (glucose <300 mg/dL in diabetics)
    ○ Treat fluid overload or dehydration.
  - Treat pain
    ○ Scheduled acetaminophen with PRN morphine for breakthrough pain for example

ALERT
Any change with patient's medication can lead to delirium.

- Eliminate unnecessary medications.
  - Investigate new symptoms as potential medication side effects (i.e., Beers medications).
- Constipation and urinary retention can cause delirium, so monitor and regulate bowel/bladder function.
  - Bowel movement for at least every 48 hours
  - Screen for urinary retention.
- Prevent major hospital-acquired problems.
  - Use a pressure-reducing mattress.
  - Avoid urinary catheters.
  - Encourage incentive spirometry.
  - Venous thromboembolism (VTE) prophylaxis if bedbound
  - Early mobilization
  - Environmental stimulation
    ○ Glasses and hearing aids
    ○ Clock and calendar
    ○ Soft lighting with curtains open during the day
    ○ Music and television, if desired
  - Sleep
    ○ Quiet and dark environment
    ○ Soft music
    ○ Therapeutic massage
- Restraints increase risk of delirium and falls/injury.
  - Use as a last resort for patients at risk for self-injury or risk for injuring caregivers. Remove as soon as possible.

MEDICATION
- Nonpharmacologic approaches are preferred for initial treatment, but medication may be needed for severe agitation and injurious behaviors, especially in the ICU setting.
- No FDA-approved medication for delirium treatment
- No medication can prevent delirium.

First Line
- For symptomatic management of intolerable agitation, delusion, or hallucinations:
  - Antipsychotics (in alphabetical order)
    ○ Aripiprazole (Abilify) 2 to 5 mg PO daily to BID
    ○ Haloperidol (Haldol): initially, 0.25 to 0.50 mg PO/IM; reevaluate and potentially redose hourly until symptoms are controlled and then use effective dose up to QID PRN. Critical care guidelines do not support use of antipsychotics for prevention of ICU delirium.
    ○ Olanzapine (Zyprexa) 2.5 to 5.0 mg PO daily to BID
    ○ Quetiapine (Seroquel) 12.5 to 25.0 mg PO BID–TID
    ○ Risperidone (Risperdal) 0.25 to 0.50 mg PO daily
- Precautions: Antipsychotics may cause extrapyramidal effects and increase fall risk; avoid in patients with parkinsonism.
- Antipsychotics may prolong the QT interval. Aripiprazole (Abilify) has minimal or no QT prolonging effect.

- For management of sedation in ICU patients
  - Alpha 2-agonist dexmedetomidine is preferred for sedation in ICU patients and is the only medication that has been found to possibly shorten delirium duration. The primary adverse effects of this medication include hypotension and bradycardia. Some studies have also found the use of clonidine as an oral bridge off of dexmedetomidine.
- Melatonin and melatonin agonists are gaining interest as sleep aids in ICU patients.

Second Line
- Benzodiazepines should generally be avoided except in alcohol withdrawal, or if patient takes regularly at baseline, or when antipsychotic is contraindicated. Benzodiazepines can cause delirium; lorazepam (Ativan): initially, 0.25 to 0.50 mg PO/IM/IV TID–QID PRN; may need to adjust to effect
- Cholinesterase inhibitors should be avoided.

REFERENCES
1. Kotfis K, van Diem-Zaal I, Roberson SW, et al. The future of intensive care: delirium should no longer be an issue. *Crit Care*. 2022;26(1):200.
2. Stollings JL, Kotfis K, Chanques G, et al. Delirium in critical illness: clinical manifestations, outcomes, and management. *Intensive Care Med*. 2021;47(10):1089–1103.
3. Bellelli G, Brathwaite JS, Mazzola P. Delirium: a marker of vulnerability in older people. *Front Aging Neurosci*. 2021;13:626127.

 SEE ALSO

- Dementia; Depression; Substance Use Disorders
- Algorithm: Delirium

 CODES

ICD10
- R41.0 Disorientation, unspecified
- F19.931 Oth psychoactive substance use, unsp w withdrawal delirium
- F10.231 Alcohol dependence with withdrawal delirium

CLINICAL PEARLS
- The criteria for delirium include an acute onset of fluctuating mental status, inattention, and either disorganized thinking or altered level of consciousness.
- Primary treatment for delirium is to identify and treat the underlying causes.
- Nonpharmacologic measures are preferable.
- Delirium may not resolve as soon as the treatable contributors resolve; may take weeks or months
- Team building and teamwork is critical in delirium prevention, early diagnosis, and treatment.

DEMENTIA

Hammad Mohsin, MD

BASICS

DESCRIPTION

Dementia refers to cognitive decline from previous level of performance in various cognitive domains (attention, executive function perceptual-motor, social cognition, language, and memory) interfere significantly with ADLs in the absence of delirium or any other mental disorder.

- *DSM-5* classifies dementias under neurocognitive disorders (major and mild) and specifies the cause of neurocognitive decline secondary to the following:
  – Alzheimer dementia (AD)
  – Vascular dementia (VaD)
  – Lewy body dementia
  – Parkinson disease dementia
  – Frontotemporal dementia
  – Creutzfeldt-Jakob disease (CJD)
  – HIV dementia
  – Substance-/medication-induced neurocognitive disorder

EPIDEMIOLOGY

Incidence

- In 2011, average annual incidence for AD was 0.4% in ages 65 to 74 years, 3.2% in ages 75 to 84 years, and 7.6% in ages ≥85 years.
- Annual incidence of Alzheimer and other dementias expected to double by 2050

Prevalence

- In patients aged ≥65 years
  – AD: 11.3% (5.3% in ages 65 to 74 years, 13.8% in ages 75 to 84 years, 34.6% in ages ≥85 years)
  – VaD: 1.6%
  – Other: 13%
- Estimated 5 to 6 million Americans living with dementia
- Expected to increase to 14 million by 2050

ETIOLOGY AND PATHOPHYSIOLOGY

- AD: involves β-amyloid protein accumulation and/or neurofibrillary tangles (NFTs), synaptic dysfunction, neurodegeneration, and eventual neuronal loss
- Age, genetics, systemic disease, smoking, and other host factors may influence the β-amyloid accumulation and/or the pace of progression toward the clinical manifestations of AD.
- VaD: cerebral atherosclerosis/emboli with clinical/subclinical infarcts

Genetics

- AD: positive family history in 50%, but 90% of AD is sporadic: *APOE4* increases risk but full role unclear.
- Familial/autosomal dominant AD accounts for <5% of AD: amyloid precursor protein (APP), presenilin-1 (PSEN-1), and presenilin-2 (PSEN-2).

RISK FACTORS

- Age is the strongest factor.
- Sex: female > male
- Genetic predisposition
- Hypertension: AD, VaD
- Hypercholesterolemia: AD, VaD
- Diabetes: VaD
- Obesity: VaD
- Cigarette smoking: VaD
- Endocrine/metabolic abnormalities:
  – Hypothyroidism, Cushing syndrome; thiamine and vitamin B_{12} deficiency
- Chronic alcoholism, other drugs

- Lower educational status
- Head injury early in life
- Sedentary lifestyle

GENERAL PREVENTION

- Treat reversible causes of dementia, such as drug-induced, alcohol-induced, and vitamin deficiencies.
- Treat hypertension, hypercholesterolemia, and diabetes.
- No evidence for statins (or any other specific medication) to prevent onset of dementia (1)[A]
- BP control and low-dose aspirin may prevent or lessen cognitive decline in VaD.
- Maintain or increase physical activity and exercise.
- Continue cognitively stimulating activities and social interactions.

COMMONLY ASSOCIATED CONDITIONS

- Anxiety and major depression
- Psychosis (delusions; delusions of persecution are common)
- Delirium
- Behavioral disturbances (agitation, aggression)
- Sleep disturbances

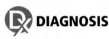

DIAGNOSIS

Clinical diagnosis

HISTORY

Requires a family member or someone who knows the patient well to describe changes in the patient's cognition and behavior

- Probable diagnosis in AD (2):
  – Age between 40 and 90 years (usually >65 years)
  – Progressive cognitive decline of insidious onset
  – No disturbances of consciousness
  – Deficits in areas of cognition
  – No other explainable cause of symptoms
  – Specifically rule out thyroid disease, vitamin deficiency (B_{12}), grief reaction, and depression.
  – Supportive factors: family history of dementia

PHYSICAL EXAM

Clinical assessment

- Physical exam to assess for neurologic deficits, motor and gait abnormalities, tremors, etc.
- No disturbances of consciousness
- Can start with brief initial screening tests for cognitive impairment
  – Mini-Cog test
  – General Practitioner Assessment of Cognition
  – Ascertain Dementia Eight-item Informant Questionnaire
- If screening is positive, should be screened for depression (such as with PHQ-2 and PHQ-9, and geriatric depression scale) and can be assessed by other cognitive assessment tools
- Cognitive decline demonstrated by standardized instruments, including the following:
  – Mini-Mental State Examination (MMSE)
  – Montreal Cognitive Assessment (MoCA) test
  – ADAS-Cog
  – Use caution in relying solely on cognition scores, especially in those with learning difficulty, language barriers, or similar limitations.
- Neuropsychological testing extensively evaluates multiple cognitive domains and can help discriminate between normal aging and dementia. This may be useful in difficult situations when history and mental status examination do not agree and most useful when repeated over time.

DIFFERENTIAL DIAGNOSIS

- Major depression
- Medication side effect
- Chronic alcohol use
- Delirium
- Subdural hematoma
- Normal pressure hydrocephalus
- Brain tumor
- Thyroid disease
- Parkinson disease
- Vitamin B_{12} deficiency
- Toxins
  – Aromatic hydrocarbons, solvents, heavy metals, marijuana, opiates, sedative-hypnotics

DIAGNOSTIC TESTS & INTERPRETATION

Initial Tests (lab, imaging)

- Used to rule out causes
  – CBC, CMP
  – Thyroid-stimulating hormone
  – Vitamin B_{12} level
- Select patients based on clinical suspicion
  – HIV, rapid plasma reagin (RPR)
  – Erythrocyte sedimentation rate (ESR)
  – Folate
  – Heavy metal and toxicology screen
- Research studies with cerebrospinal fluid (CSF) biomarkers in patient with confirmed AD have shown decreased β-amyloid (1 to 42) and increased τ and p-τ levels, which are specific features of AD, and CSF τ proteins are increased in CJD (3)[A].
- Neuroimaging (CT/MRI of brain):
  – Routine neuroimaging generally recommended to evaluate for dementia and can help to distinguish specific types of dementia with structural imaging finding
  – Early age of onset (<65 years), rapid progression, focal neurologic deficits, cerebrovascular disease risk, or atypical symptoms: neuroimaging (CT/MRI) to rule out other causes
- Important findings
  – AD: Diffuse cerebral atrophy starting in association areas, hippocampus (hippocampal atrophy may be the earliest sign), and amygdala.
  – VaD: old infarcts, including lacunar

Follow-Up Tests & Special Considerations

- Genetic testing for dementia is not recommended, such as testing for *APOE4* for Alzheimer, unless there are multiple family members diagnosed with AD at a young age.
- LP and CSF analysis can be considered in atypical presentations to identify infectious, inflammatory, or neoplastic etiologies.

Diagnostic Procedures/Other

PET scan not routinely recommended; has been approved to differentiate between AD and frontotemporal dementia

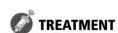

TREATMENT

GENERAL MEASURES

- Daily schedules and written directions
- Emphasis on nutrition, personal hygiene, accident-proofing the home, safety issues, sleep hygiene, and supervision
- Socialization (adult daycare)
- Sensory stimulation (display of clocks and calendars) in the early to middle stages
- Occupational training and structured physical exercise program

- Discussion with the family concerning support and advance directives

MEDICATION
- Cognitive dysfunction
- Medications for AD (4)[A] show a small improvement in some cognitive measures, but it remains unclear if the improvement is clinically significant and associated with side effects.
- Cognitive dysfunction, mild
  – Cholinesterase inhibitors: donepezil (Aricept), 5 to 10 mg/day; rivastigmine (Exelon), 1.5 to 6.0 mg BID, transdermal system 4.6 mg/24 hr and 9.5 mg/24 hr; galantamine (Razadyne), 4 to 12 mg BID, extended release 8 to 24 mg/day
    ○ Adverse events: nausea, vomiting, diarrhea, anorexia, nightmares, bradycardia/syncope
    ○ Galantamine warning: associated with mortality in patients with mild cognitive impairment in clinical trial
    ○ It is suggested to consider cholinesterase inhibitor for patients with mild to moderate dementia (MMSE 10 to 26). Responses may be quite variable.
    ○ Start drug with lowest acquisition cost; also consider adverse event profile, adherence, medical comorbidity, drug interactions, and dosing profiles.
- Cognitive dysfunction, moderate to severe
  – Cholinesterase inhibitors
  – Memantine (Namenda), NMDA receptor antagonist, 5 to 20 mg/day
    ○ Adverse events: dizziness, confusion, headache, constipation
    ○ Generally well tolerated with fewer side effects compared to cholinesterase inhibitors
    ○ Not shown to be beneficial in milder forms of AD
  – Combination cholinesterase inhibitor and memantine
    ○ In patients with moderate to advanced dementia (MMSE <17), recommendations are to add memantine (10 mg BID) to a cholinesterase inhibitor or to use memantine alone in patients who do not tolerate or benefit from a cholinesterase inhibitor.
    ○ In patients with severe dementia (MMSE <10), it is suggested to continue memantine. However, in advanced dementia, medications can be discontinued to maximize quality of life and patient comfort.
  – Monoclonal antibodies, anti–β-amyloid
    ○ Aducanumab (Aduhelm)—FDA granted accelerated approval for Alzheimer Disease for patients with mild cognitive impairment or mild dementia stage disease
    ○ Lecanemab-irmb (Leqembi)—indicated for Alzheimer Disease with mild cognitive impairment or mild dementia stage disease.
- Commonly associated conditions
  – Psychosis and agitation/aggressive behavior:
    ○ Look for precipitating factors (infection, pain, depression, medications).
    ○ Nonpharmacologic therapies (behavioral interventions, music therapy, etc.) are preferred as first-line treatment.
    ○ Mood stabilizers (valproic acid, carbamazepine) have been used, although evidence is lacking.
    ○ For moderate/severe symptoms; antipsychotics: Initiate low doses, risperidone 0.25 to 1 mg/day; olanzapine 1.25 to 5 mg/day; quetiapine 12.5 to 50 mg/day; aripiprazole 5 mg/day; ziprasidone 20 mg/day
    ○ Atypical antipsychotic, quetiapine, is often first line due to decreased extrapyramidal side effect.
    ○ Novel antipsychotic, pimavanserin (selective 5-HT2A receptor inverse agonist), has shown to effectively treat Parkinson disease psychosis with minimal risk of worsening motor function associated with other treatment (5)[B].

ALERT
Black box warning on antipsychotics due to increased mortality in elderly with dementia

Geriatric Considerations
- Initiate pharmacotherapy at low doses and titrate slowly up if necessary.
- Benzodiazepines are potentially inappropriate for older adults, yet their use persists.

ALERT
Benzodiazepine use is associated with increased fall risk (6)[A].

- Watch decreased renal function and hepatic metabolism.

First Line
Nonpharmacologic management: environmental modifications, caregiver training, music therapy, exercise, pet therapy

Second Line
- Cholinesterase inhibitors, memantine, atypical antipsychotics, antidepressants, mood stabilizers, methylphenidate, benzodiazepines, melatonin
- Antidepressants not clearly superior to placebo in treating depression (HTA-SADD)

ISSUES FOR REFERRAL
Neuropsychiatric evaluation helpful in early stages or mild cognitive impairment

ADDITIONAL THERAPIES
Behavioral modification
- Socialization, such as adult daycare, to prevent isolation and depression
- Sleep hygiene program as alternative to pharmaceuticals for sleep disturbance
- Scheduled toileting to prevent incontinence

ADMISSION, INPATIENT, AND NURSING CONSIDERATIONS
Psychiatry admission may be required because of safety concerns (self-harm/harm to others), self-neglect, aggressive behaviors, or other behavioral issues.

ONGOING CARE

FOLLOW-UP RECOMMENDATIONS
Patient Monitoring
- Progression of cognitive impairment by use of standardized tool (e.g., MMSE, ADAS-Cog)
- Development of behavioral problems
  – Sleep, depression, psychosis, aggression
- Adverse events of pharmacotherapy
- Nutritional status
- Caregiver evaluation of stress

PATIENT EDUCATION
- Advance care planning
  – Discuss safety, management of finances, medical decision-making, and possible skilled facility placement; legal guardianship, if necessary
- Advance directives and health care proxy should be established early on if possible.
- National Institute on Aging: https://www.nia.nih.gov/health/topics/dementia

PROGNOSIS
- AD: usually steady progression leading to profound cognitive impairment; average survival about 10 years
- VaD: incrementally worsening dementia, but cognitive improvement is unlikely

- Secondary dementias: Treatment of the underlying condition may lead to improvement; commonly seen with normal pressure hydrocephalus, hypothyroidism, and brain tumors
- Late-stage dementia: Palliative and hospice care can be beneficial.

COMPLICATIONS
- Wandering
- Sundowner syndrome is common in older people (who are sedated) and also in people who have dementia (can have adverse reaction to even small dose of psychoactive substances).
- Falls with injury
- Neglect and abuse
- Caregiver burnout

REFERENCES
1. McGuinness B, Craig D, Bullock R, et al. Statins for the prevention of dementia. *Cochrane Database Syst Rev.* 2009;(2):CD003160.
2. Blass DM, Rabins PV. In the clinic. Dementia. *Ann Intern Med.* 2008;148(7):ITC4-1–ITC4-16.
3. van Harten AC, Kester MI, Visser PJ, et al. Tau and p-tau as CSF biomarkers in dementia: a meta-analysis. *Clin Chem Lab Med.* 2011;49(3):353–366.
4. Birks J. Cholinesterase inhibitors for Alzheimer's disease. *Cochrane Database Syst Rev.* 2006;2006(1):CD005593.
5. Cummings J, Isaacson S, Mills R, et al. Pimavanserin for patients with Parkinson's disease psychosis: a randomised, placebo-controlled phase 3 trial. *Lancet.* 2014;383(9916):533–540.
6. Seppala LJ, Wermelink AMAT, de Vries M, et al; for EUGMS Task and Finish Group on Fall-Risk-Increasing Drugs. Fall-risk-increasing drugs: a systematic review and meta-analysis: II. Psychotropics. *J Am Med Dir Assoc.* 2018;19(4):371.e11–371.e17.

ADDITIONAL READING
Lyketsos CG, Colenda CC, Beck C, et al; for Task Force of American Association for Geriatric Psychiatry. Position statement of the American Association for Geriatric Psychiatry regarding principles of care for patients with dementia resulting from Alzheimer disease. *Am J Geriatr Psychiatry.* 2006;14(7):561–572.

SEE ALSO
Algorithm: Dementia

CODES
ICD10
- F03 Unspecified dementia
- G30.9 Alzheimer's disease, unspecified
- F01.50 Vascular dementia without behavioral disturbance

CLINICAL PEARLS
- Medications for AD show a small, statistically significant improvement in some cognitive measures, but it remains unclear if the improvement is clinically significant.
- Do not forget the role of adult protective services in case of elderly abuse—Elder Abuse Hotline: 800-922-2275.
- A particular concern in nursing homes relates to finding alternatives to the use of physical restraints and antipsychotic medications.

DEMENTIA, VASCULAR

Birju B. Patel, MD, FACP

 BASICS

Vascular dementia is a heterogeneous disorder caused by the sequelae of cerebrovascular disease that manifests in cognitive impairment affecting memory, thinking, learning, language, behavior, judgment, and executive dysfunction.

DESCRIPTION
- Vascular dementia (previously known as multi-infarct dementia) was first mentioned by Thomas Willis in 1672. Later, it was further described in the late 19th century by Binswanger and Alzheimer as a separate entity from dementia paralytica caused by neurosyphilis. This concept has evolved tremendously since the advent of neuroimaging modalities.
- Synonym(s): vascular cognitive impairment (VCI); vascular cognitive disorder (VCD); Binswanger disease; *Diagnostic and Statistical Manual of Mental Disorders*, 5th edition (*DSM-5*) categorizes vascular dementia as mild or major VCD.

EPIDEMIOLOGY
Common cause of dementia in the elderly, and it frequently overlaps with Alzheimer dementia

Incidence
About 6 to 12 cases per 1,000/person aged >70 years

Prevalence
- ~1.2–4.2% in those aged >65 years
- 14–32% prevalence of dementia after a stroke

ETIOLOGY AND PATHOPHYSIOLOGY
No set pathologic criteria exist for the diagnosis of vascular dementia such as those that exist for Alzheimer dementia. Pathology includes the following:
- Large vessel disease: cognitive impairment that follows a stroke
- Small vessel disease (subcortical) includes white matter changes, subcortical infarcts, and incomplete infarction. This is usually the most common cause of multi-infarct dementia. Lacunar infarcts and deep white matter changes are typically included in this category.
- Transient ischemic attack (TIA)/stroke
- Vascular, demographic, genetic factors
  – Vascular disease (i.e., hypertension [HTN], peripheral vascular disease [PVD], atrial fibrillation, hyperlipidemia, diabetes) (1)[B],(2)[C]

Genetics
- Cerebral autosomal dominant arteriopathy with subcortical infarcts and leukoencephalopathy (CADASIL) is caused by a mutation in the *NOTCH3* gene on chromosome 19 that results in leukoencephalopathy and subcortical infarcts. This is clinically manifested in recurrent strokes, migraine with aura, and vascular dementia.
- *Apolipoprotein E* (*ApoE*) gene type: Those with ApoE4 subtypes are at higher risk of developing both vascular and Alzheimer dementia.
- Amyloid precursor protein (APP) gene: leads to a form of vascular dementia called heritable cerebral hemorrhage with amyloidosis

RISK FACTORS
- Age (risk doubles every 5 years)
- Previous stroke
- Tobacco use
- Diabetes (especially with frequent hypoglycemia)
- Atherosclerotic heart disease; HTN; atrial fibrillation; PVD
- Hyperlipidemia
- Metabolic syndrome
- Low socioeconomic status (3)[C]

GENERAL PREVENTION
- Optimization and aggressive treatment of vascular risk factors, such as HTN, diabetes, and hyperlipidemia
- HTN is the single most modifiable risk factor, and the treatment for it must be optimized.
- Smoking is associated with white matter changes on imaging, which may be associated with small vessel disease and vascular dementia progression.
- Lifestyle modification: weight loss, physical activity, smoking cessation
- Hearing loss should be corrected.
- Depression and social isolation should be evaluated.
- Cognitively stimulating activity can be beneficial.
- Medication management for vascular risk reduction: aspirin usage, statin therapy for hyperlipidemia, antihypertensive therapy (4)[B]

COMMONLY ASSOCIATED CONDITIONS
- CADASIL
- Cerebral amyloid angiopathy (CAA) causes ischemic white matter damage due to amyloid deposition in penetrating cortical vessels.

 DIAGNOSIS

Differentiation between Alzheimer dementia and vascular dementia can be difficult, and significant overlap is seen in the clinical presentation of these two dementias. The diagnosis of vascular dementia is a clinical diagnosis. Memory impairment is less prominent in vascular dementia versus Alzheimer dementia. The neuropsychological pattern observed in vascular dementia is impaired recall, relatively intact recognition, less severe forgetfulness with greater benefit from cues and more executive dysfunction.

HISTORY
- Gradual, stepwise progression is typical with multi-infarct dementia.
- Ask about onset and progression of cognitive impairment and the specific cognitive domains involved.
- Ask about vascular risk factors and previous attempts to control these risk factors.
- Ask about medication compliance.
- Ask about urinary incontinence and gait disturbances. Abnormal gait and falls are strong predictors of development of vascular dementia, particularly unsteady, frontal, and hemiparetic types of gait.

- Look for early symptoms, including difficulty performing cognitive tasks, memory, mood, and assessment of instrumental activities of daily living (IADLs).
- History may include TIAs, cerebrovascular accidents (CVAs), coronary atherosclerotic heart disease, atrial fibrillation, hyperlipidemia, and/or PVD. Small vessel disease usually presents with executive dysfunction. Large vessel disease usually presents with gait, visuospatial, and language dysfunction.

PHYSICAL EXAM
- Screen for HTN. Average daily home blood pressure is associated with progression of cerebrovascular disease and cognitive decline in the elderly.
- Focal neurologic deficits may be present.
- Gait assessment is important, especially looking at gait initiation, gait speed, and balance (5).
- Check for carotid bruits as well as abdominal bruits and assess for presence of PVD.
- Do a thorough cardiac evaluation that includes looking for arrhythmias (i.e., atrial fibrillation).

DIFFERENTIAL DIAGNOSIS
- Alzheimer dementia
- Depression
- Delirium
- CNS tumors
- Hypothyroidism/hyperthyroidism
- Vitamin B$_{12}$ deficiency

DIAGNOSTIC TESTS & INTERPRETATION
- Cognitive testing, such as Saint Louis University Mental Status (SLUMS) exam and Montreal Cognitive Assessment (MoCA), provides more definitive information in terms of cognitive deficits, especially executive function, which may be lost earlier in vascular dementia.
- Neuropsychological testing may also be beneficial, especially in evaluating multiple cognitive domains and their specific involvements and deficits.

Initial Tests (lab, imaging)
As appropriate, consider complete blood count, comprehensive metabolic profile, lipid panel, thyroid function, hemoglobin A1C, and vitamin B$_{12}$.
- Cognitive deficits observed clinically do not always have to correlate with findings found on neuroimaging studies.
- MRI is the gold standard of imaging (6).
- White matter changes and specific location of these changes can be associated with executive dysfunction and episodic memory impairment.

Follow-Up Tests & Special Considerations
Consider referral to a cognitive specialist for complex cases.

 TREATMENT

Prevention is the real key to treatment:
- Control of risk factors, including HTN, hyperlipidemia, and diabetes
- Avoidance of tobacco and smoking cessation
- Healthy, low-cholesterol diet

MEDICATION

- Clinical evidence for use of acetylcholinesterase inhibitors and memantine reveals limited benefit in vascular dementia but may slow cognitive decline in patients with mixed Alzheimer and vascular dementia.
- Controlling BP with any antihypertensive medications, treatment of dyslipidemia (e.g., statins), and treatment of diabetes are very important.
- Selective serotonin reuptake inhibitors (SSRIs) may be of benefit for agitation and psychosis in vascular dementia.

ADDITIONAL THERAPIES

- Limit alcohol drink intake to ≤1/day in women and 2/day in men.
- Preventing new CVAs is the key in managing vascular dementia; aspirin and other antiplatelet agents may be useful if no contraindications.

SURGERY/OTHER PROCEDURES

Patients with symptomatic carotid artery stenosis should be referred to a vascular surgeon to be evaluated for carotid endarterectomy. Carotid endarterectomy is recommended over carotid artery stenting in patients >70 years of age if perioperative morbidity/mortality is <6%.

COMPLEMENTARY & ALTERNATIVE MEDICINE

Ginkgo biloba should be avoided due to increased risk of bleeding, especially in CAA.

ADMISSION, INPATIENT, AND NURSING CONSIDERATIONS

- Remain sensitive to functional assessment and avoidance of pressure ulcers after CVAs.
- Avoid Foley catheter usage unless necessary due to increased risk of infection.
- Nonpharmacologic approaches to behavior management should be attempted prior to medication usage.
- Providing optimal sensory input to patients with cognitive impairment is important during hospitalizations to avoid delirium and confusion. Patients should be given frequent cues to keep them oriented to place and time. They should be informed of any changes in the daily schedule of activities and evaluations. Family and caregivers should be encouraged to be with patients with dementia as much as possible to further help them from becoming confused during hospitalization. Recreational, physical, occupational, and music therapy can be beneficial during hospitalization in avoiding delirium and preventing functional decline.
- Depression can present as "pseudodementia" with worsening confusion during hospitalization and is a treatable condition.

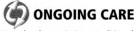 ONGOING CARE

Vascular dementia is a condition that should be followed with multiple visits in the office setting with goals of optimizing cardiovascular risk profiles for patients. Future planning and advanced directives should be addressed early. Family and caregiver evaluation and burden should also be evaluated.

FOLLOW-UP RECOMMENDATIONS

Perform regular follow-up with a primary care provider or geriatrician for risk factor modification and education on importance of regular physical and mental exercises as tolerated.

Patient Monitoring

Appropriate evaluation and diagnosis of this condition, need for future planning, optimizing vascular risk factors, lifestyle modification counseling, therapeutic interventions

DIET

- The American Heart Association diet and Dietary Approaches to Stop Hypertension (DASH) diet is recommended for optimal BP and cardiovascular risk factor control.
- Low-fat, decreased concentrated sweets and carbohydrates, especially in those with metabolic syndrome

PATIENT EDUCATION

- Lifestyle modification is important in vascular risk reduction (smoking cessation, exercise counseling, dietary counseling, weight-loss counseling).
- Optimizing vascular risk factors via medications (i.e., HTN, diabetes, atrial fibrillation, PVD, heart disease)
- Avoiding smoking, including secondhand smoke
- Home BP monitoring and glucometer testing of blood sugars if HTN, impaired glucose tolerance, and/or diabetes is present

PROGNOSIS

- Vascular dementia results in shortened life expectancy and those with previous CVA have a worse prognosis.
- Lost cognitive abilities that persist after initial recovery of deficits from stroke do not usually return. Some individuals can have intermittent periods of self-reported improvement in cognitive function.
- Risk factors for progression of cognitive and functional impairment poststroke include age, prestroke cognitive abilities, depression, polypharmacy, and decreased cerebral perfusion during acute stroke.
- Unsteady or frontal gait can be a predictor for risk of development of vascular dementia.

COMPLICATIONS

- Behavioral abnormalities (delusions, hallucinations, etc.)
- Depression
- Falls
- Frequent hospitalizations
- Aspiration pneumonia
- Physical disability from stroke
- Severe cognitive impairment
- Caregiver stress and burnout

REFERENCES

1. Kalaria RN. The pathology and pathophysiology of vascular dementia. *Neuropharmacology*. 2018;134(Pt B):226–239.
2. Dichgans M, Leys D. Vascular cognitive impairment. *Circ Res*. 2017;120(3):573–591.
3. Sundbøll J, Horváth-Puhó E, Adelborg K, et al. Higher risk of vascular dementia in myocardial infarction survivors. *Circulation*. 2018;137(6):567–577.
4. White WB, Wolfson L, Wakefield DB, et al. Average daily blood pressure, not office blood pressure, is associated with progression of cerebrovascular disease and cognitive decline in older people. *Circulation*. 2011;124(21):2312–2319.
5. Montero-Odasso M, Verghese J, Beauchet O, et al. Gait and cognition: a complementary approach to understanding brain function and the risk of falling. *J Am Geriatr Soc*. 2012;60(11):2127–2136.
6. Iadecola C, Duering M, Hachinski V, et al. Vascular cognitive impairment and dementia: JACC Scientific Expert Panel. *J Am Coll Cardiol*. 2019;73(25):3326–3344.

 SEE ALSO

Alzheimer Disease; Depression; Mild Cognitive Impairment

 CODES

ICD10

- F01.50 Vascular dementia without behavioral disturbance
- F01.51 Vascular dementia with behavioral disturbance

CLINICAL PEARLS

- Executive dysfunction and gait abnormalities are often seen early and are more pronounced in vascular dementia as opposed to Alzheimer dementia.
- Memory is relatively preserved in vascular dementia when compared with Alzheimer dementia in the early stages of this disease.
- Stepwise progression, as opposed to progressive decline in Alzheimer dementia, is typical. History from a caregiver or family member is important in assessing this decline.
- Considerable overlap exists between vascular dementia and Alzheimer dementia in clinical practice, and classification into one of these categories is often difficult. Patients can have mixed etiologies as well.

DENTAL INFECTION

Alicia Leandra Olowu, DO • Meenu Prasad, DO

 BASICS

DESCRIPTION

- Pain ± swelling in the head and neck region with odontogenic (teeth and supporting structures) origin of infection; if left untreated, it can lead to serious and potentially life-threatening illnesses.
- Assume any head and neck infection or swelling to be odontogenic in origin until proven otherwise.
- Antibiotics should be prescribed as an adjunct to proper dental intervention. Antibiotics should be prescribed for acute infections for 3 to 7 days.
- Gingivitis and periodontal disease may be treated with oral antibiotics. Soft tissue infections may require IV antibiotic treatment.

EPIDEMIOLOGY

~20% of Americans have untreated dental caries. 75% have had at least one dental restoration. 35% of Americans between the ages of 30 to 90 years have periodontal disease. 1 in 2,600 hospital admissions are related to dental infection. The presence of odontogenic disease is closely linked to socioeconomic status as fewer Americans have dental insurance than health insurance.

Incidence

- Overall incidence of dental caries in children is ~47%.
- Rates of untreated dental caries are highest in Latino and non-Latino black individuals below the poverty line (up to 58%).

Prevalence

- Dental caries are the most common chronic disease worldwide.
- 90% of adults aged 20 to 64 years have had dental caries in their permanent teeth.

ETIOLOGY AND PATHOPHYSIOLOGY

- >90% of all head and neck infections have an odontogenic origin.
- Caries or trauma can lead to death of the tooth pulp, which can lead to infection and/or abscess of adjacent tissues via direct or hematogenous bacterial colonization.
- Caries (tooth decay; "cavity") represent a contagious bacterial infection causing demineralization and destruction of the tooth tissue (enamel, dentin, and cementum).
- *Streptococcus mutans* is easily transmitted to newly dentate infants by caregivers.
- Acidic secretions from *S. mutans* are implicated in early caries.
- Typical oral microbiome includes numerous anaerobic bacteria. The most common pathologic aerobic bacteria is *Streptococcus* spp.
- Anaerobic bacteria are more common with infections near the tooth base (1).

RISK FACTORS

- Low socioeconomic status
- Smoking
- Parent and/or sibling with history of caries or existing untreated dental caries (especially in past 12 months)
- Previous dental caries
- Poor access to dental/health care; lack of dental insurance; fear of dentist
- Poor oral hygiene; poor nutrition, including diet containing high level of sugary foods and drinks
- Trauma to the teeth or jaw
- Inadequate access to and use of fluoride
- Gingival recession (increased risk of root caries)
- Physical and mental disabilities
- Poorly controlled systemic diseases (e.g., diabetes)
- Decreased salivary flow (e.g., use of anticholinergic medications, immunologic diseases, radiation therapy to head and neck)

GENERAL PREVENTION

- Most dental problems can be avoided through flossing/use of interdental brushes; brushing with fluoride toothpaste, systemic fluoride (fluoridated bottled water; fluoride supplements for high-risk patients and in non-fluoridated areas); fluoride varnish for all children aged <6 years and moderate- to high-risk patients; regular dental cleanings (2),(1)[B]
- Prevent transmission of *S. mutans* from mother/caregiver to infant by improving maternal dentition, chlorhexidine gluconate rinses, and the use of xylitol products for mother especially during the first 2 years of a child's life. Avoid smoking, which is linked to severe periodontal disease.
- Good control of systemic diseases (e.g., diabetes) and changes in lifestyle (e.g., smoking cessation)
- Fluoride varnish provided by dental or medical primary care providers twice per year

COMMONLY ASSOCIATED CONDITIONS

- Extensive caries, crowding, multiple missing teeth
- Periapical and periodontal abscess
- Soft tissue cellulitis
- Periodontitis (deep inflammation ± infection of gingiva, alveolar bone support, and ligaments)

DIAGNOSIS

HISTORY

- Pain of involved tooth; can be referred to ears, jaw, cheek, neck, or sinuses; unexplained headaches
- Hot/cold sensitivity
- Pain can be unprovoked, intermittent, and/or constant.
- Pain with biting or chewing

- Trismus (inability to open the mouth)
- Bleeding or purulent drainage from gingival tissues
- When severe infection (systemic)
  - Fever
  - Difficulty breathing or swallowing
  - Raspy voice
  - Mental status changes
- Evaluate children aged <4 years with stiff neck, sore throat, and dysphagia for retropharyngeal abscess.

PHYSICAL EXAM

- Gingival edema and erythema
- Cheek (extraoral) or vestibular (intraoral) swelling
- Fluctuant mass at involved site
- Suppuration of gingival margin
- Submandibular or cervical lymphadenopathy
- Severe (systemic) infection may present with dysphagia, fever, and signs of airway compromise.

DIFFERENTIAL DIAGNOSIS

- Bacterial or viral pharyngitis
- Pericoronitis (inflammation ± infection of gum flap over mandibular last molar, typically 3rd molars)
- Otitis media or externa; sinusitis
- Headache/migraine
- Viral (HSV1, herpangina, hand-foot-mouth disease) or aphthous stomatitis
- Temporomandibular joint (TMJ) dysfunction (myofascial pain, ± internal derangement of TMJ)
- Parotitis
- Jaw pain can be anginal equivalent, especially in women and especially in lower left side of the jaw.

DIAGNOSTIC TESTS & INTERPRETATION

Initial Tests (lab, imaging)

- No initial labs needed, unless patient looks acutely ill
- If acutely ill
  - Consider CBC with differential.
  - If abscess present, drain/aspirate pus and culture for aerobes and anaerobes.
  - Typically polymicrobial infections with anaerobic gram-negative rods and anaerobic gram-positive cocci
- Individual films of suspected teeth, including root apices; test with palpation, percussion, and cold sensitivity.
- Panoramic film or CT scan of the teeth and jaw to evaluate the extent of infection

Follow-Up Tests & Special Considerations

- Panoramic radiograph, particularly if trismus is present
- CT/MRI scan can be helpful if facial swelling extends below inferior border of mandible or into infraorbital space. This helps to locate for potential incision and drainage by oral and maxillofacial surgeon or ENT.

TREATMENT

- Early disease (gingivitis, periodontitis) does not typically warrant antibiotic use.
- Antibiotics should be prescribed for acute infections with local/systemic spread or when drainage/débridement is not possible.
- All antibiotics should be prescribed for the shortest duration possible, which is typically 3 to 7 days.
- Consider IV antibiotics only in the case of severe disease such as local infiltration or systemic infection.
- Appropriate pain control: anti-inflammatory agents are first line; short-course opioids in some cases
- Refer to oral health provider for definitive treatment: root canal, extraction, gum therapy.
- If infection is severe (soft tissue infiltration, systemic symptoms), consider hospitalization with IV antibiotics until stable; will likely require intraoral or extraoral incision and drainage; definitive treatment (extraction or root canal therapy) necessary to prevent progression or recurrence

GENERAL MEASURES
- Ibuprofen 600 to 800 mg (pediatrics: 10 mg/kg) q6h or acetaminophen 650 to 1,000 mg (pediatrics: 10 to 15 mg/kg) q4–6h PRN for pain
- For more severe pain, consider acetaminophen with ibuprofen (synergistic effect) + short course of opioids.
- Local nerve block with long-acting anesthetic (bupivacaine); avoid penetrating infection to avoid tracking infection.

MEDICATION
First Line
- Amoxicillin: 500 mg PO TID, 1,000 mg IV BID; in children, 40 to 60 mg/kg/day divided TID
- Penicillin: 250 to 500 mg PO QID, 1.2 to 2.4 million units IM/IV daily
- Amoxicillin/clavulanic acid: 500/125 mg PO TID or 875/125 mg PO BID, 1,000 to 2,000 mg IV TID
- Clindamycin: 300 mg PO TID, 600 mg IV TID (1),(3)

Second Line
If no response to first-line treatment or inability to tolerate above medications
- Ciprofloxacin: 500 mg PO BID
- Azithromycin: 500 mg PO daily for at least 3 consecutive days
- Gentamycin: 3 to 5 mg/kg/day IM/IV daily
- Metronidazole: 500 to 750 mg PO TID; prescribe with antibiotic such as amoxicillin or clindamycin for aerobic coverage

ISSUES FOR REFERRAL
Referral to oral health provider should almost always be done in order to determine the degree of infection and to treat local niduses of infection.

SURGERY/OTHER PROCEDURES
- Incise and drain large, fluctuant abscesses.
- Root canal or extraction is definitive treatment.

ADMISSION, INPATIENT, AND NURSING CONSIDERATIONS
Criteria for hospital admission: swelling involving deep spaces of the neck, floor of the mouth, or infraorbital region; deviation of the airway; unstable vital signs; fever (>101°F); chills; raspy voice; confusion or delirium; or evidence of invasive infection or cellulitis
- Ensure secure airway.
- IV fluid resuscitation if necessary
- Initiate antibiotics as recommended above.
- Ensure good oral hygiene.
- Rinse or swab the mouth with chlorhexidine gluconate BID.
- Use warm saltwater rinses several times per day, especially after incision and drainage; ice packs to decrease swelling and encourage drainage
- Discharge patient when
  – Airway not compromised
  – Abscess and sepsis eliminated
  – Able to take PO intake and ambulate

 ONGOING CARE

Educate regarding proper oral hygiene, need for follow-up dental care, and potential medical complications that arise due to lack of dental care.

FOLLOW-UP RECOMMENDATIONS
- Follow up with oral health provider within 24 hours.
- Ensure adequate PO intake, including protein.

DIET
- Maintain a healthy diet; bacteria thrive on refined sugar and starch.
- Avoid sugary foods that stick between the teeth.
- Avoid the use of sugary/carbonated drinks throughout day; water as beverage of choice between meals

Pediatric Considerations
In children, limit the frequency of sugary drinks and advise against sleeping with a bottle; fluoride varnish twice a year (more for higher risk children) for children aged <6 years

PATIENT EDUCATION
- Control caries and periodontal disease.
- Brush at a minimum of twice daily and use floss/interdental brush daily; brushing/flossing after every meal may further improve oral health.
- Fluoride supplementation is critical if primary water source is fluoride-deficient.
- Biannual dental visits at a minimum for oral care and fluoride varnish, beginning when first primary tooth comes in (3)
  – Limit the frequency of sugar/carbonated drinks and sugary or sticky foods.

- In young children, avoid sleeping with a bottle to decrease the chance of dental caries.
- Avoid milk, formula, or juice in bottles in children whose teeth have started to erupt.

PROGNOSIS
Prognosis is excellent with proper treatment.

COMPLICATIONS
- Ludwig angina
- Retropharyngeal and mediastinal infection
- Osteomyelitis
- Endocarditis/cardiac tamponade
- Submental infection
- Submandibular infection
- Can cause unstable diabetes in diabetics/worsen preexisting heart disease
- Brain abscess/death

REFERENCES
1. Oberoi SS, Dhingra C, Sharma G, et al. Antibiotics in dental practice: how justified are we. *Int Dent J.* 2015;65(1):4–10.
2. Fleming E, Afful J. *Prevalence of Total and Untreated Dental Caries Among Youth: United States, 2015–2016. NCHS Data Brief, No. 307.* Hyattsville, MD: National Center for Health Statistics; 2018.
3. Stephens MB, Wiedemer JP, Kushner GM. Dental problems in primary care. *Am Fam Physician.* 2018;98(11):654–660.

ADDITIONAL READING
Clark MB, Douglass AB, Maier R, et al. *Smiles for Life: A National Oral Health Curriculum.* 3rd ed. Leawood, KS: Society of Teachers of Family Medicine; 2010. https://www.smilesforlifeoralhealth.com/buildcontent.aspx?tut=555&pagekey=62948&cbreceipt=0. Accessed October 16, 2023.

 CODES

ICD10
- K02.9 Dental caries, unspecified
- K04.7 Periapical abscess without sinus
- K12.2 Cellulitis and abscess of mouth

CLINICAL PEARLS
- Do not ignore tooth pain.
- Treat patients with local signs of soft tissue infection aggressively because infections can spread quickly, leading to significant morbidity or even death.
- Prevention (oral hygiene, fluoride, dental visits) is the key to avoid odontogenic infections.
- When indicated, amoxicillin and clindamycin are generally the antibiotics of choice for odontogenic infections.

DEPRESSION

Afsha Rais Kaisani, MD • Tasaduq Hussain Mir, MD, FAAFP • Michael A. Armstrong, MD

 BASICS

DESCRIPTION
Primary mood disorder characterized by a sustained feeling of sadness and/or decreased interest in all or most activities once enjoyed, which represents a change from previous state

EPIDEMIOLOGY
Prevalence
- Lifetime prevalence of major depressive disorder (MDD) is 20.6% (1).
- Low risk before early teens; highest prevalence in teens and young adults; average age of onset is 30 years.

ETIOLOGY AND PATHOPHYSIOLOGY
Pathophysiology is poorly understood.

Genetics
Twin studies suggest 37% concordance.

RISK FACTORS
- Female > male (2:1)
- Adverse life events (2)
- First-degree relative or spouse with depression, bipolar, suicide, substance abuse
- Presence of comorbid medical conditions including neurodegenerative diseases

GENERAL PREVENTION
Physical activity lowers the risk of depression (3).

COMMONLY ASSOCIATED CONDITIONS
Bipolar disorder, cyclothymic disorder, grief reaction, anxiety disorders, somatoform disorders, schizophrenia/schizoaffective disorders, conduct disorder, substance abuse

 DIAGNOSIS

DSM-5 requires the following criteria for MDD:
- Criterion A: ≥5 of the following symptoms present nearly every day during the same 2-week period, with at least 1 being either depressed mood or loss of interest or pleasure:
  – Dysphoria: subjective or observation by others of depressive mood most of the day
  – Anhedonia: decreased interest or pleasure in previously enjoyable activities most of the day either by subjective report or observation from other people
  – Notable change in appetite or unintentional significant weight loss
  – Insomnia or hypersomnia
  – Fatigue or energy loss
  – Agitation, restlessness, or slowed speech or body movements observable by others
  – Diminished thinking/concentration, poor memory
  – Worthlessness, inappropriate guilty feelings
  – Recurrent thoughts of death/harm, suicidal ideations, or suicide attempt or a devised plan for suicide
- Criterion B: Symptoms cause social, occupational, or functional distress.
- Criterion C: symptoms not attributable to substance effects or other medical conditions.
- Minor depression: 2 to 4 of the following symptoms of Criteria A plus B and C as above and:
  – Persistent depressive disorder (dysthymia) and cyclothymic disorder not present
  – The mood disturbance does not occur exclusively during a psychotic disorder.

HISTORY
- The presence of four "SIGECAPS" symptoms plus depressed mood suggests depression.
  – Sleep: changes in sleep habits from baseline; excessive sleep, early waking, or inability to fall asleep
  – Interest: loss of interest in previously enjoyable activities
  – Guilt: excessive or inappropriate guilt that may or may not be related to a specific problem or circumstance
  – Energy: perceived lack of energy
  – Concentration: inability to concentrate on specific tasks
  – Appetite: an increase or decrease in appetite
  – Psychomotor: restlessness and agitation or the perception that everyday activities are too strenuous to manage
  – Suicidality: the desire to end one's life or hurt oneself, harmful thoughts directed internally, or recurrent thoughts of death or homicide
- Depression may present differently between men and women. Women may report physical ailments: headache, myalgias, and/or GI distress; men may report aggression, substance use, and/or risky behavior (2).

Pediatric Considerations
May present with somatic symptoms (headaches, GI upset), irritability, difficulty with concentration, frequent absences from school, or sudden change in grades

Geriatric Considerations
Difficult to diagnose due to medical comorbidities; may present as memory difficulties; geriatric Depression Scale (GDS 15) improves the rate of diagnosis.

PHYSICAL EXAM
Comprehensive physical and mental status examination
- Level of consciousness and orientation
- Appearance: hygiene, posture, clothing
- Attitude: hostility, apathy
- Behavior: eye contact, psychomotor agitation
- Mood: depressed, anxious, angry, tearful, etc.
- Affect: mood-congruent, flat, labile, manic
- Memory: immediate, recent, and remote
- Speech: fluency, repetition, comprehension
- Thought process: delusions, hallucinations, suicidal/homicidal thoughts, flight of ideas, grandiosity, obsessions/compulsions
- Insight: understanding of own illness
- Judgment: ability to make rational decisions

DIFFERENTIAL DIAGNOSIS
- Depressed phase of bipolar disorder
- Adjustment disorder with depressed mood
- Medical comorbidity: adrenal disease, hypothyroidism, diabetes, liver or renal failure, malignancy, sleep disorders, chronic fatigue syndrome, fibromyalgia, vitamin deficiencies

DIAGNOSTIC TESTS & INTERPRETATION
- The Patient Health Questionnaire-9 (PHQ-9) if PHQ-2 is positive; other tools: Beck Depression Inventory, Zung Self-Rating Depression Scale, or GDS 15
- Screen postpartum women using Edinburgh Postnatal Depression Scale (EPDS).
- Assess for suicidal/homicidal ideation.

Initial Tests (lab, imaging)
Laboratory test to exclude other conditions: compete blood count, electrolytes, kidney and liver function, thyroid-stimulating hormone, rapid plasma reagin test, HIV test, toxicology screen, vitamin levels (D, B_{12}, folate); consider pregnancy test in all reproductive-aged women.

Diagnostic Procedures/Other
CT/MRI of brain should be considered for organic brain syndrome or hypopituitarism.

 TREATMENT

American Psychiatric Association (APA) treatment guidelines recommend the following:
- Acute phase (first 3 months of treatment)
  – Full evaluation, including risk to self and others, with selection of appropriate treatment setting; the goal should be symptom remission and recovery of function.
  – Offer either psychotherapy or second-generation antidepressant (selective serotonin reuptake inhibitors [SSRIs] or serotonin-norepinephrine reuptake inhibitors [SNRIs]) or combined therapy in severe cases (3).
  – Follow up 2 to 4 weeks of starting medication, q2wk until improvement, and then monthly.
  – Continue to increase dosage q3–4wk until remission; the full effect is achieved in 4 to 6 weeks. May need second medication.
  – ≥6 visits are recommended for monitoring (younger patients, those at high suicide risk, see within 1st week, and follow frequently).
- Continuation phase (4 to 9 months of treatment)/maintenance phase (>9 months of treatment)
  – Monitor for relapse; q3–6mo if stable
  – Use depression rating scales and patient reports to monitor response.
  – Add psychotherapy for patients without response to medication alone.
  – Continue the dosage for at least 6 to 9 months to reduce relapse once the remission is achieved. Cognitive-behavioral therapy (CBT) is effective in reducing relapse (visits are typically q2wk).
  – Taper medication gradually (weeks to months) to allow the detection of recurring symptoms and minimize discontinuation syndrome. Taper dose by 25% q4wk (3).

GENERAL MEASURES
Pharmacotherapy and psychotherapy, alone, can relieve depressive symptoms. Combination therapy has high rates of improvement, increased quality of life, and better treatment compliance. Psychotherapy methods include the following:
- CBT: combines cognitive psychotherapy with behavioral therapy; proven effective
- Interpersonal psychotherapy (IPT): identifies a trigger of the depressive episode, facilitates mourning, promotes recognition of affects, resolves role disputes and role transitions, and builds social skills
- Psychodynamic psychotherapy: helps identify unconscious thoughts leading to behavior
- Family and marital therapy: addresses family or relationship-oriented problems
- Problem-solving therapy: combines elements of CBT and IPT into a brief treatment lasting 6 to 12 sessions; may have a role in those with mild symptoms of depression

- Supportive psychotherapy: improves self-esteem, psychological functioning, and adaptive skills by focusing on current, problematic relationships or maladaptive patterns of behavior and/or emotional responses.
- APA recommends CBT or IPT with second-generation antidepressants if combination therapy is offered (3).

MEDICATION

Start at the lowest available dose and maintain the highest effectively tolerated FDA-approved dose for at least 4 to 6 weeks before deeming ineffective. Effectiveness is comparable between and within drug classes. Selection should be based on provider familiarity and patient characteristics/preferences.

First Line
- SSRIs
  - Citalopram (Celexa): 20 mg/day; 20 to 40 mg/day; escitalopram (Lexapro): 10 mg/day; 10 to 20 mg/day (both with risk of QTc prolongation)
  - Fluoxetine (Prozac): 20 mg/day; 20 to 40 mg/day (FDA approved for teens); paroxetine (Paxil): 20–40 mg/day or paroxetine (Parxil-CR) 50–62.5 mg/day; avoid use of both in elderly.
  - Sertraline (Zoloft): 50 mg/day; 50 to 200 mg/day (associated with higher rates of diarrhea)
  - Adverse effects: sexual dysfunction, GI upset, dizziness, insomnia, headache, weight gain; typically resolve within the 1st week
  - Abrupt discontinuation may cause withdrawal symptoms (i.e., dizziness, nausea, headache, paresthesia).
- SNRIs
  - Desvenlafaxine (Pristiq): 25 to 50 mg/day; duloxetine (Cymbalta): 30 to 60 mg/day; venlafaxine XR (Effexor XR): 37.5 to 225 mg/day (higher rate of sexual dysfunction and drowsiness)
- Serotonin modulators (starting dose): trazodone (Desyrel): 100 mg/day; vilazodone (Viibryd): 10 mg qHS titrated to 20 mg qHS in week 2 (take with food); vortioxetine (Trintellix): 5 to 10 mg/day; common adverse effects: somnolence, dizziness, constipation/diarrhea, sexual dysfunction
- Pregnancy: Most medication are Category C.
  - Fluoxetine and sertraline are often used but there is an increased risk of pulmonary HTN, mild transient neonatal syndrome of CNS, motor, respiratory, and GI signs if used after 20 weeks' of gestation.
  - Paroxetine (Category D): risk of congenital cardiac defects and other anomalies in 1st trimester

Second Line
- Tricyclic antidepressants (TCAs)
  - Amitriptyline* (Elavil): 25 to 50 mg every bedtime (qHS); imipramine* (Tofranil): 25 mg qHS or 150 mg/day (serotonin > norepinephrine reuptake inhibitor)
  - Desipramine* (Norpramin): 25 mg/day; doxepin* (Sinequan): 25 mg qHS up to 150 mg/day
  - Nortriptyline (Pamelor): 25 mg qHS; (norepinephrine > serotonin reuptake inhibitor) *Drugs that are highly sedating and associated with weight gain

- Relative contraindications: arrhythmias, significant cardiac disease, seizures, osteoporosis, glaucoma
- Common adverse effects: orthostatic hypotension, dry mouth, blurred vision, constipation, urinary retention, tachycardia, confusion/delirium
- Atypical antidepressants
  - Bupropion (Wellbutrin): 100 mg BID (dose varies for SR and XL; lower rates of sexual dysfunction)
  - Mirtazapine (Remeron): 15 mg/day, 45 mg/day (max dose; associated with weight gain, used off-label for appetite stimulation)
- Monoamine oxidase inhibitors (MAOIs)
  - Phenelzine (Nardil): 15 mg/day titrated to 15 mg TID over 2 to 3 days; Selegiline transdermal (Eldepryl): 6 mg patch/24 hr
  - Allow 14-day period off of all antidepressants before starting MAOIs; common adverse effects: hypotension, sexual dysfunction, sleep disturbance

ALERT
- Black box warning: increased risk of suicidality in children, adolescents, and young adults who are treated with antidepressants
- Serotonin syndrome: rare but potentially lethal complication from rapid increase in dose or addition of new medication with serotonergic effects
- Antidepressants can precipitate manic episodes in those with bipolar disorder.
- Antidepressant discontinuation syndrome: symptoms (FINISH mnemonic): flu-like symptoms, insomnia, nausea, imbalance, sensory disturbances, and hyperarousal; up to 50% of patients (3)

ISSUES FOR REFERRAL
Depression complicated by psychosis or treatment resistant depression

ADDITIONAL THERAPIES
Electroconvulsive therapy for severe refractory depression; novel therapies are being developed for major depression and treatment of resistant depression: repetitive transcranial magnetic and deep brain stimulation, ketamine, anti-inflammatory agents, and psilocybin (4).

COMPLEMENTARY & ALTERNATIVE MEDICINE
- Conditional recommendation for use: exercise monotherapy and St. John's wort; if neither acceptable nor available, consider bright-light therapy, yoga, and adding acupuncture to antidepressant medication.
- Insufficient evidence for monotherapy recommendation: tai chi, acupuncture, omega-3-fatty acids monotherapy, S-adenosyl methionine

ADMISSION, INPATIENT, AND NURSING CONSIDERATIONS
Admit if there is a risk of harm to self or others.

 ## ONGOING CARE

PATIENT EDUCATION
- Medications may take 2 to 4 weeks before beneficial effect is noted. Recommend exercise, good sleep hygiene, nutrition, and avoid tobacco and alcohol use.
- The National Suicide Prevention Lifeline: 800-273-TALK (8255)

PROGNOSIS
Complete remission is not common; partial remission can be achieved. Relapse is common.

REFERENCES
1. Hasin DS, Sarvet AL, Meyers JL, et al. Epidemiology of adult DSM-5 major depressive disorder and its specifiers in the United States. *JAMA Psychiatry*. 2018;75(4):336–346.
2. Maurer DM, Raymond TJ, Davis BN. Depression: screening and diagnosis. *Am Fam Physician*. 2018;98(8):508–515.
3. Kovich H, Kim W, Quaste AM. Pharmacologic treatment of depression. *Am Fam Physician*. 2023;107(2):173–181.
4. Marwaha S, Palmer E, Suppes T, et al. Novel and emerging treatments for major depression. *Lancet*. 2023;401(10371):141–153.

 ## SEE ALSO

Depression, Geriatric; Depression, Pediatric; Depression, Postpartum; Depression, Treatment Resistant; Suicide; Suicide, Pediatric

 ## CODES

ICD10
- F32.9 Major depressive disorder, single episode, unspecified
- F33.9 Major depressive disorder, recurrent, unspecified
- F34.1 Dysthymic disorder

CLINICAL PEARLS
- Pharmacotherapy and psychotherapy, alone, can relieve depressive symptoms; however, combination therapy has high rates of improvement.
- Provide close follow-up and education for monitoring of depression.

D

DEPRESSION, ADOLESCENT

Lovella Kanu, MD, FAAFP, Dipl. ABOM • Emily N. Hernandez, DO

 BASICS

DESCRIPTION
- Major depressive disorder (MDD) is a primary mood disorder characterized by sadness and/or irritable mood with impairment of functioning; abnormal psychological development; and a loss of self-worth, energy, and interest in typically pleasurable activities.
- Adolescents with depression are likely to suffer broad functional impairment across social, academic, family, and occupational domains, along with a high incidence of relapse and a high risk for substance abuse and other psychiatric comorbidity.

EPIDEMIOLOGY
Incidence
- 6–12% of adolescents; it is twice as common in females as males (1).
- During adolescence, the cumulative probability of depression ranges from 5% to 20%.

ETIOLOGY AND PATHOPHYSIOLOGY
- Neurobiologic changes can contribute (HPA axis overactivity, serotonergic modulation of emotional processing pathways, decreased dopaminergic reward processing).
- External factors may contribute such as substance use, adverse childhood events, or inadequate social network.

Genetics
- Offspring of parents with depression have 3 to 4 times increased rates of depression.
- Family studies indicate that anxiety in childhood tends to precede adolescent depression.

RISK FACTORS
- Prior depressive episodes
- History of insomnia, anxiety disorders, attention deficit hyperactivity disorder (ADHD), body dysmorphic disorder, chronic childhood illness, and/or learning disabilities
- Increased screen time (2)
- Female gender
- General stressors: adverse life events, difficulties with peers, loss of a loved one, academic difficulties, abuse, chronic illness, tobacco abuse, and low socioeconomic status
- LGBTQ identified

GENERAL PREVENTION
- Child and adolescent mental health may be improved by successfully treating maternal depression.
- The United States Preventive Services Task Force (USPSTF) recommends the screening of adolescents (12 to 18 years of age) for MDD with systems in place to ensure accurate diagnosis, appropriate treatment, and follow-up. Current evidence is insufficient to assess benefits and harms for screening children aged ≤11 years.

COMMONLY ASSOCIATED CONDITIONS
Generalized anxiety disorder, behavioral disorders, substance abuse, and eating disorders

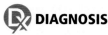 DIAGNOSIS

HISTORY
- Adolescents may present with medically unexplained somatic complaints (fatigue, irritability, headache).
- The below symptoms have to be present for at least 2 weeks and there has to be change from previous functioning.
  - At least 5 symptoms have to be present with one being either a depressed mood or loss of pleasure or interest. These symptoms have to occur nearly every day during the same 2-week period.
    - Feeling sad or depressed mood
    - Loss of interest or pleasure in all activities
    - Presence of unintentional weight loss of >5% in 1 month
    - Inability to sleep (insomnia) or excessive sleepiness (hypersomnia)
    - Psychomotor retardation or agitation observed by others
    - Loss of energy or fatigue
    - Feelings of rejection or being unloved (worthlessness) or inappropriate or excessive feeling of guilt
    - Decreased ability to concentrate, think, and make choices
    - Recurrent thoughts of death and suicidal ideation or plan
  - Above symptoms usually cause significant impairment in social, occupational, or other areas of functioning. Substance effects and other medical conditions need to be ruled out.
  - Symptoms when present should not be attributable to schizophreniform, schizoaffective, or delusional disorders and no history of manic or hypomanic episodes.
- Family history may be notable for mood disorders.

PHYSICAL EXAM
- Concentration, speech, affect, psychomotor activity, and other nonverbal cues may be assessed in clinical interview.
- Assess for signs of self-injury (such as wrist lacerations) or abuse.

DIFFERENTIAL DIAGNOSIS
- Normal bereavement
- Substance-induced mood disorder
- Bipolar disorder
- Adjustment disorder with depressed mood
- Mood disorder secondary to a medical condition (thyroid, anemia, vitamin deficiency, diabetes)
- Infectious mononucleosis or other viral diseases
- ADHD, posttraumatic stress disorder (PTSD), eating disorders, and anxiety disorders
- Sleep disorder

DIAGNOSTIC TESTS & INTERPRETATION
Initial Tests (lab, imaging)
May be used to rule out reversible or other underlying biologic diagnoses (i.e., CBC, TSH, glucose, vitamin B_{12}, folate, mono spot, and urine drug testing)

Diagnostic Procedures/Other
- Depression is primarily diagnosed after a formal interview, with supporting information from caregivers and teachers.
- Standardized tests are useful as screening tools and to monitor response to treatment but should not be used as the sole basis for diagnosis:
  - Beck Depression Inventory II (BDI-II): ages 13 to 18 years
  - Child Depression Inventory 2 (CDI2): ages 7 to 17 years
  - Center for Epidemiologic Studies Depression Scale for Children (CES-DC): ages 6 to 17 years
  - Patient Health Questionnaire-9 (PHQ-9): ages 11 to 17 years
- The evaluation of adolescents who screen positive for depression should include assessment of potential for harm to self and others using structured screening and interview tools (3).

 TREATMENT

GENERAL MEASURES
- Initial management should include education regarding the presentation, prognosis, and interpersonal impact of depression.
- Psychotherapy and/or pharmacotherapy should be considered based on the severity, duration, comorbidities, and biopsychosocial context of the depression.
- Social domains (family/school environments) can impact treatment efficacy and should therefore be incorporated into the patient's management plan (i.e., learning plans/accommodations, interpersonal family counseling).
- Patient's safety should also be addressed if there is concern for self-harm or suicidality. Assess home safety and access to weapons. In outpatient settings, consider making a safety plan with the patient and family.
- A Cochrane review showed that there was no significant difference between remission rates for adolescents treated with cognitive-behavioral therapy (CBT) versus medication or combination therapy immediately postintervention (4)[A].
- A multitreatment meta-analysis showed that combined fluoxetine/CBT had higher efficacy than monotherapies, but other selective serotonin reuptake inhibitors (SSRIs), such as sertraline and escitalopram, were better tolerated (5)[A].

MEDICATION

First Line

- Fluoxetine: for depression in age >8 years; starting dose of 10 mg/day; effective dose of 10 to 60 mg/day; the most studied SSRI and with the most favorable effectiveness and safety data has the longest half-life of the SSRIs and is not generally associated with withdrawal symptoms between doses or on discontinuation (4)[A].
- Escitalopram: for depression in age >12 years; starting dose of 5 mg/day; effective dose of 10 to 20 mg/day (4)[A].
- Citalopram: for depression in age >12 years; starting dose of 10 mg/day; effective dose of 10 to 40 mg/day (4)[A].
- Sertraline: for depression in age >12 years; starting dose of 25 mg/day; effective dose of 50 to 200 mg/day (4)[A]
- Can titrate dose every 1 to 2 weeks if no significant adverse effects emerge (headaches, GI upset, insomnia, agitation, behavior activation, suicidal thoughts) (4)[A]

ALERT
SSRI black box warning to monitor for worsening condition, behavior changes, and suicidal thoughts (4)[A]

- Closely monitor for suicidality and other adverse effects after initiating pharmacotherapy. Follow-up in 2 weeks is recommended.
- Given their rates of increased drug metabolism, adolescents may be at higher risk for withdrawal symptoms from SSRIs than adults; if these are present, twice-daily dosing may be considered (5)[A].
- All other SSRIs except fluoxetine should be slowly tapered when discontinued (4)[A].

Pediatric Considerations
- Tricyclic antidepressants (TCAs) have not been proven to be effective in adolescents and should not be used (4)[A].
- Paroxetine (SSRI): avoid use due to short half-life, associated withdrawal symptoms, and higher association with suicidal ideation

ISSUES FOR REFERRAL
Collaborative care interventions between mental health and primary care have a greater improvement in depressive symptoms after 12 months (4)[B].

SURGERY/OTHER PROCEDURES
Electroconvulsive therapy has been shown to be effective in treating persistent adolescent MDD (6)[A].

COMPLEMENTARY & ALTERNATIVE MEDICINE
- Physical exercise and light therapy may have a mild to moderate effect (7)[B].
- St. John's wort, acupuncture, S-adenosylmethionine, and 5-hydroxytryptophan have not been shown to have an effect or have inadequate studies to support use in adolescent depression.

ADMISSION, INPATIENT, AND NURSING CONSIDERATIONS
If severely depressed, psychotic, suicidal, or homicidal, inpatient management is indicated.

 ## ONGOING CARE

- Antidepressant treatment should be continued for 6 to 12 months at full therapeutic dose after the resolution of symptoms at the same dosage.
- After resolution of symptoms, monitor monthly for 6 months and then regularly for the next 18 months (4).

FOLLOW-UP RECOMMENDATIONS

Patient Monitoring
- SSRI medications include black box warning to monitor for worsening condition, behavior changes, and suicidal thoughts (4)[A].
- Systematic and regular tracking of goals and outcomes from treatment should be performed, including assessment of depressive symptoms and functioning in home, school, and peer settings (4)[A].
- Diagnosis and initial treatment should be reassessed if no improvement is noted after 6 to 8 weeks of treatment (4)[A].
- The goals of treatment should be sustained symptom remission and restoration of full function.

PROGNOSIS
- 60–90% of episodes remit within 1 year.
- Depression in adolescence predicts mental health disorders in adult life, psychosocial difficulties, and ill health (1)[A].

COMPLICATIONS
- Treatment-induced mania, aggression, or lack of improvement in symptoms
- School failure/refusal
- 1/3 of adolescents with suicidal ideation go on to make an attempt (5).

REFERENCES

1. American Psychiatric Association. *Diagnostic and Statistical Manual of Mental Disorders*. 5th ed. Arlington, VA: American Psychiatric Association; 2013.
2. Liu M, Wu L, Yao S. Dose-response association of screen time-based sedentary behaviour in children and adolescents and depression: a meta-analysis of observational studies. *Br J Sports Med*. 2016;50(20):1252–1258.
3. Lewandowski RE, Acri MC, Hoagwood KE, et al. Evidence for the management of adolescent depression. *Pediatrics*. 2013;132(4):e996–e1009.
4. Cheung AH, Zuckerbrot RA, Jensen PS, et al; for GLAD-PC STEERING GROUP. Guidelines for adolescent depression in primary care (GLAD-PC): part II. Treatment and ongoing management. *Pediatrics*. 2018;141(3):e20174082.
5. Nock MK, Green JG, Hwang I, et al. Prevalence, correlates, and treatment of lifetime suicidal behavior among adolescents: results from the National Comorbidity Survey Replication Adolescent Supplement. *JAMA Psychiatry*. 2013;70(3): 300–310.
6. Lima NN, Nascimento VB, Peixoto JA, et al. Electroconvulsive therapy use in adolescents: a systematic review. *Ann Gen Psychiatry*. 2013;12(1):17.
7. Larun L, Nordheim LV, Ekeland E, et al. Exercise in prevention and treatment of anxiety and depression among children and young people. *Cochrane Database Syst Rev*. 2006;(3):CD004691.

 ## CODES

ICD10
- F32.9 Major depressive disorder, single episode, unspecified
- F33.9 Major depressive disorder, recurrent, unspecified
- F32.8 Other recurrent depressive disorders

CLINICAL PEARLS

- Adolescent depression is underdiagnosed and often presents with irritability and anhedonia.
- Fluoxetine is the most studied FDA-approved for treatment of adolescent depression.
- Escitalopram, citalopram, and sertraline are also FDA-approved antidepressants.
- CBT combined with fluoxetine is efficacious for adolescents with major depression.
- Paroxetine and TCAs should not be used to treat adolescent depression.
- Referral to a child psychiatrist is appropriate for complex cases or treatment-resistant depression.
- Monitor all adolescents with depression for suicidality, especially during the 1st month of treatment with an antidepressant.

DEPRESSION, GERIATRIC
Benjamin Cottrell, DO • Rose Katherine Appel, DO

BASICS

DESCRIPTION
A primary mood disorder characterized by a depressed mood and/or a markedly decreased interest or pleasure in normally enjoyable activities most of the day, almost every day for at least 2 weeks, and causing significant distress or impairment in daily functioning; the geriatric population can have variable presentations and comorbid conditions that present different challenges than treating depression in the younger population.

EPIDEMIOLOGY
Incidence
- 2–10% of community-dwelling elderly
- 5–10% seen in primary care clinics
- 10–37% of hospitalized elderly patients
- 12–27% of nursing home residents

Prevalence
- The Global Burden of Disease Study (2015) estimated the prevalence of depressive disorders among older adults (>60 years old) of 4–6% among males and 5–8% among females.
- Suicide is the 11th leading cause of death in the United States for all ages. The elderly account for 24% of all completed suicides with the highest rates for males aged >85 years.

ETIOLOGY AND PATHOPHYSIOLOGY
- A complex interaction between heritable, biologic, psychological, and environmental factors
- Abnormalities in neurotrophins, neurogenesis, neuroimmune systems, and neuroendocrine systems

Genetics
Possible mechanisms, including genetic influences on monoamine transmission and associated transcriptional and translational activity and dysregulation in biological processes and proteostasis involving C-peptide, FABP-liver, and ApoA-IV proteins

RISK FACTORS
- Female sex
- Lower socioeconomic status
- Widowed, divorced, or separated marital status
- Chronic physical health conditions
- History of mental health conditions
- Chronic or uncontrolled pain
- Family history of depression
- Death of a loved one
- Being a caregiver
- Functional/cognitive impairment
- Lack/loss of social support/social isolation
- Significant loss of independence
- Insomnia/sleep disturbance

GENERAL PREVENTION
Limited but growing body of evidence suggest these interventions to prevent depression in the elderly:
- Following traditional dietary patterns (e.g., Mediterranean, Japanese, or Norwegian)
- Increasing the consumption of foods rich in omega-3 polyunsaturated fatty acids (e.g., salmon, tuna, sardine, mackerel)
- Engaging in regular physical activity and exercise
- Provision/participation in social or group activities, including those focused on elderly populations

COMMONLY ASSOCIATED CONDITIONS
Chronic disease (e.g., coronary artery diseases [CADs], cerebrovascular diseases [CVDs], cancer, Parkinson disease)

DIAGNOSIS
Refer to *Diagnostic and Statistical Manual of Mental Disorders*, 5th Edition (DSM-5) criteria.

HISTORY
- Depressed mood most of the day, nearly every day, and/or loss of interest/pleasure in life for at least 2 weeks
- Other common symptoms include the following:
  – Feeling hopeless, helpless, or worthless
  – Insomnia and loss of appetite/weight (alternatively, hypersomnia with increased appetite/weight in atypical depression)
  – Fatigue and loss of energy
  – Somatic symptoms (headaches, chronic pain)
  – Neglect of personal responsibility or care
  – Psychomotor retardation or agitation
  – Diminished concentration, indecisiveness
  – Thoughts of death or suicide
- Screening with "SIGECAPS"
  – **S**leep: changes in sleep habits from baseline, including excessive sleep, early waking, or inability to fall asleep
  – **I**nterest: loss of interest in previously enjoyable activities (anhedonia)
  – **G**uilt: excessive or inappropriate guilt that may or may not focus on a specific problem or circumstance
  – **E**nergy: perceived lack of energy
  – **C**oncentration: inability to concentrate on specific tasks
  – **A**ppetite: increase/decrease in appetite
  – **P**sychomotor: restlessness and agitation or the perception that everyday activities are too strenuous to manage
  – **S**uicidality: desire to end one's life or hurt oneself, harmful thoughts directed internally, recurrent thoughts of death or thoughts of homicidality

PHYSICAL EXAM
Mental status examination, focused neurologic and physical examination to rule out other underlying conditions

DIFFERENTIAL DIAGNOSIS
Concurrent medical conditions, cognitive disorders, and medications may cause symptoms that mimic depression:
- Medical conditions: hypothyroidism, vitamin B_{12} or folate deficiency, liver or renal failure, cancers, stroke, sleep disorders, electrolyte imbalances, Cushing disease, chronic fatigue syndrome
- Cognitive disorders: delirium, dementia, and other neurodegenerative disorders

- Medications: interferon-α, β_2-blockers, isotretinoin, benzodiazepines, glucocorticoids, GnRH agonists, levodopa, clonidine, H_2 blockers, baclofen, phenobarbital, topiramate, triptans, varenicline, metoclopramide, reserpine
- Other psychiatric disorders

DIAGNOSTIC TESTS & INTERPRETATION
Initial Tests (lab, imaging)
Initial laboratory evaluation to rule out potential medical factors that could be causing symptoms
- Thyroid-stimulating hormone (hypothyroidism)
- CBC with differential (anemia, infection)
- Vitamin B_{12}, folic acid (deficiencies)
- Urinalysis (urinary tract infection, glucosuria)
- Comprehensive metabolic panel
- Urine toxicology screen
- 24-hour urine free cortisol (Cushing disease)

Follow-Up Tests & Special Considerations
Additional testing for possible confounding medical disorders, as warranted (e.g., sleep study)

Diagnostic Procedures/Other
Validated screening tools and rating scales (1)[A]:
- Geriatric Depression Scale (GDS): 15- or 30-point scales
- Patient Health Questionnaire (PHQ-2 and PHQ-9)
- Hamilton Depression Rating Scale (HDRS): 17- or 21-item, clinician-administered scale
- Beck Depression Inventory (BDI): 21- or 13-item, self-report rating
- Cornell Scale for Depression in Dementia

Test Interpretation
Refer to appropriate scoring and interpretation instructions.

TREATMENT
Although 50% reduction in symptoms alone is considered clinically meaningful, the goal is to treat the patient to the point of remission (i.e., essentially the absence of depressive symptoms).

GENERAL MEASURES
- Lifestyle modifications:
  – Improve nutrition.
  – Encourage social interactions/activities.
  – Exercise and physical activity
- Psychotherapy:
  – Cognitive-behavioral therapy (CBT)
  – Psychodynamic psychotherapy

MEDICATION
Conservative initial dosing of antidepressants in the elderly, starting with 1/2 of the usual initiation dose and titrating dose every 2 to 4 weeks, as tolerated, to reach an adequate treatment dose

First Line
- Selective serotonin reuptake inhibitors (SSRIs) have been found to be effective in treating depression in the elderly and are considered first line for pharmacotherapy.
- No single SSRI clearly outperforms others in the class; choice of medication often reflects side effect profile or practitioner familiarity (2)[A]:
  - Citalopram: Start at 10 mg/day; treatment ranges from 10 to 20 mg/day.
  - Sertraline: Start at 25 mg/day; treatment ranges from 50 to 200 mg/day.
  - Escitalopram: Start at 5 to 10 mg/day; treatment ranges from 10 to 20 mg/day.
  - Fluoxetine: Start at 10 mg/day; treatment ranges from 20 to 60 mg/day.
  - Paroxetine: Start at 10 mg/day; treatment ranges from 20 to 40 mg/day.
- SSRIs should not be used concomitantly with monoamine oxidase inhibitors (MAOIs).
- Common side effects: increased risk of falls, nausea, diarrhea, sexual dysfunction

Second Line
Atypical antidepressants: more effective than placebo in the treatment of depression in the elderly, although additional studies are needed to better delineate patient factors that determine response:

- Bupropion: Start at 150 mg/day. Increase dose in 3 to 4 days. Treatment ranges from 300 to 450 mg/day. Avoid in patients with elevated seizure risk, tremors, or anxiety (3)[A].
- Venlafaxine: Start at 37.5 mg/day extended-release and titrate weekly. Treatment ranges from 150 to 225 mg/day; monitor BP at higher doses (3)[C].
- Duloxetine: Start at 20 to 30 mg/day. Treatment ranges from 60 to 120 mg/day; may also be associated with elevated BP (3)[A]
- Mirtazapine: Start at 7.5 to 15.0 mg nightly. Treatment ranges from 30 to 45 mg/day; may be associated with dry mouth, weight gain, sedation, and cognitive dysfunction (3)[A]
- Desvenlafaxine: 50 mg/day in the morning; higher doses do not confer additional benefit; 50 mg every other day if CrCl <30 mL/min (3)[A]

ISSUES FOR REFERRAL
Depression with suicidal ideation, psychotic depression, bipolar disorder, comorbid substance abuse issues, polypharmacy, severe or refractory illness

ADDITIONAL THERAPIES
For patients who have not responded to initial SSRI trial:

- Try a different SSRI medication, switch to an atypical antidepressant, or augment initial antidepressant with bupropion.
- 2nd-generation antipsychotic agents (3)[C]:
  - Aripiprazole: 2 to 5 mg/day. Treatment ranges from 5 to 15 mg/day; can produce sedation, weight gain
  - Used for augmentation in conjunction with other antidepressant medications

- Tricyclic antidepressants (TCAs):
  - Nortriptyline: 25 to 50 mg nightly. Treatment ranges from 75 to 150 mg nightly; anticholinergic effects, weight gain, increase risk of falls (3)[C]
  - TCAs have been shown to be effective in treating depression; however, difficult for elderly patients to tolerate due to side effect profile and are potentially lethal in overdose, limiting their use as initial agents (1)[A]
- MAOIs are effective in the treatment of depression in the elderly. They are not used frequently in clinical practice due to potential side effects and necessary dietary restrictions (1)[A].
- Although not FDA-approved, buspirone, lithium, or triiodothyronine is used off-label to augment a primary antidepressant.
- Evidence for benefit of antidepressants in the treatment of depression in patients with dementia is equivocal. Consideration should be made for a limited trial with close monitoring for symptom improvement or side effects and is used only in patients with severe symptoms.
- Electroconvulsive therapy (ECT) has been shown to produce remission of depressive symptoms in the elderly. However, due to lack of consistent evidence, it should only be considered as an option for patients with severe or psychotic depression.

COMPLEMENTARY & ALTERNATIVE MEDICINE
- St. John's wort may have minimal benefit but has many drug interactions to consider.
- Tryptophan and 5-hydroxytryptophan: 150 to 300 mg/day; possible efficacy

ADMISSION, INPATIENT, AND NURSING CONSIDERATIONS
Inpatient care is indicated if imminent safety risk is present (e.g., acutely suicidal) or if unable to adequately care for themselves due to depression.

ONGOING CARE

FOLLOW-UP RECOMMENDATIONS
Due to the delay of benefit following the initiation of antidepressant therapy, it is necessary to ensure open communication with the patient to prevent premature discontinuation of therapy. An adequate explanation of potential side effects with instructions to call the office before discontinuing therapy is imperative.

Patient Monitoring
- A patient with severe depression who exhibits suicidality will require admission.
- Monitor for worsening anxiety symptoms or increase in suicidality especially in the week following initiation or switching of antidepressants.

DIET
Patients taking MAOIs need to avoid foods high in tyramine (i.e., certain cheeses and wines).

PATIENT EDUCATION
- Depression is a treatable illness.
- Medications need to be taken for 2 to 4 weeks before any beneficial effect is noted, and it may take 6 to 8 weeks to reach maximum efficacy.
- Depression is often a recurring illness.
- National Suicide Prevention Lifeline at 1-800-273-TALK (8255) is a free, 24-hour hotline available.

PROGNOSIS
Estimates vary for initial clinical response and remission (between 30% and 70%).

COMPLICATIONS
- Impairment in social, occupational, or interpersonal functioning
- Difficulty performing activities of daily living and self-care
- Increase in medical services utilization and increased costs of care
- Increased risk of suicide

REFERENCES
1. Taylor WD. Clinical practice. Depression in the elderly. *N Engl J Med*. 2014;371(13):1228–1236.
2. Ruhé HG, Huyser J, Swinkels JA, et al. Switching antidepressants after a first selective serotonin reuptake inhibitor in major depressive disorder: a systematic review. *J Clin Psychiatry*. 2006;67(12):1836–1855.
3. Nelson JC, Delucchi K, Schneider LS. Efficacy of second generation antidepressants in late-life depression: a meta-analysis of the evidence. *Am J Geriatr Psychiatry*. 2008;16(7):558–567.

 SEE ALSO

Algorithms: Depressed Mood Associated with Medical Illness; Depressive Episode, Major

CODES

ICD10
- F32.9 Major depressive disorder, single episode, unspecified
- F03 Unspecified dementia
- F43.21 Adjustment disorder with depressed mood

CLINICAL PEARLS
- Late-life depression (LLD) is not a normal part of aging.
- Depression in the elderly may be difficult to diagnose due to medical and cognitive comorbidities.
- Depression may present primarily with cognitive dysfunction, and this may improve with treatment of the depression.
- SSRIs are considered as first-line therapy. A full remission may take upward of 12 weeks of treatment.
- A multidisciplinary approach to the treatment of depression is often the most efficacious.

DEPRESSION, POSTPARTUM
Jennifer E. Cavin, MD

 BASICS

DESCRIPTION
- Major depressive disorder (MDD) that recurs or has its onset in the postpartum period
- Postpartum depression (PPD) is similar to non-pregnancy depression (sleep disorders, anhedonia, psychomotor changes, etc.); it most often has its onset within the first 12 weeks postpartum; yet, it can occur in the antepartum period or within 1 year after delivery.
- Different from postpartum "blues" (sadness and emotional lability), which is experienced by 30–70% of women and has an onset and resolution within first 10 days postpartum

EPIDEMIOLOGY
Incidence
9–14% of women experience depression during the postpartum period (1).

Prevalence
>50% of women with PPD enter pregnancy depressed or have an onset during pregnancy (2).

ETIOLOGY AND PATHOPHYSIOLOGY
- May be related to sensitivity in hormonal fluctuations, including estrogen; progesterone; and other gonadal hormones as well as neuroactive steroids; cytokines; hypothalamic–pituitary–adrenal (HPA) axis hormones; altered fatty acid, oxytocin, and arginine vasopressin levels; and genetic and epigenetic factors
- Multifactorial including biologic–genetic predisposition in terms of neurobiologic deficit, destabilizing effects of hormone withdrawal at birth, inflammation, and psychosocial stressors

RISK FACTORS
- Previous episodes of PPD, history of MDD, or anxiety and depression during pregnancy
- History of premenstrual dysphoria, family history of depression
- Poor pregnancy outcomes (preterm birth, stillbirth, neonatal death, major malformations)
- Substance use, unwanted or unplanned pregnancy, multiple psychosocial stressors, lack of social support, intimate partner violence
- Young maternal age, multiple births; African Americans and Hispanics may have higher rates of PPD.
- Postpartum pain, sleep disturbance, and fatigue
- Recent immigrant status, history of adverse childhood experiences
- Decision to decrease antidepressants during pregnancy

GENERAL PREVENTION
- Universal screening, using validated rating scales, during pregnancy and postpartum year for better detection; evidence suggests that screening pregnant and postpartum women for depression reduces depressive symptoms in women with depression and reduces the prevalence of depression in a given population. Evidence for pregnant women was less robust but is also consistent with the evidence for postpartum women regarding the benefits of screening, the benefits of treatment, and screening instrument accuracy (3)[A].
- Psychotherapy/counseling, particularly using cognitive behavioral therapy (CBT) and interpersonal therapy (IPT) based interventions, has been shown to be effective in small randomized trials in the prevention of PPD in at-risk individuals, but the USPSTF concludes that further research is needed (4)[A].
- The use of SSRIs, specifically sertraline, may be effective in preventing PPD in women at high risk for PPD (4)[A].

COMMONLY ASSOCIATED CONDITIONS
- Bipolar mood disorder, depressive disorder not otherwise specified, dysthymic disorder, cyclothymic disorder, MDD
- Postpartum blues

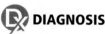 **DIAGNOSIS**

HISTORY
- Decreased interest in formerly compelling or pleasurable activities, depressed/low mood, guilt, low self-esteem
- Increased/decreased sleep, decreased energy, decreased concentration, increased/decreased appetite
- Psychomotor agitation or retardation, suicidal ideation

DIFFERENTIAL DIAGNOSIS
- Baby blues: not a psychiatric disorder; mood lability resolves within days.
- Postpartum psychosis: a psychiatric emergency
- Postpartum anxiety/panic disorder
- Postpartum obsessive-compulsive disorder
- Hypothyroidism
- Postpartum thyroiditis: can occur in up to 5.7% of patients in the United States and can present as depression
- Bipolar disorder, depressive episode

DIAGNOSTIC TESTS & INTERPRETATION
Initial Tests (lab, imaging)
No blood testing is necessary, but selective tests based on history and symptoms might include complete blood count (CBC), thyroid-stimulating hormone (TSH), vitamin B_{12} level

Follow-Up Tests & Special Considerations
Urine analysis, urine drug screen

Diagnostic Procedures/Other
- Edinburgh Postnatal Depression Scale is a validated screening tool. A score of >11 indicates likely PPD.
- The Patient Health Questionnaire-9 (PHQ-9) is a validated commonly used screening tool.
- Edinburgh Postnatal Depression Scale (partner version): to be completed by mother's partner to obtain his/her view of mother's depression

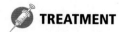 **TREATMENT**

GENERAL MEASURES
- Assess for the presence of suicidal ideation.
- Assess for the presence of homicidal ideation and thoughts of harming the baby (infanticide).
- Assess for symptoms of psychosis including delusions and hallucinations.
- Suicidal ideation, homicidal ideation, or infanticide ideation may require immediate hospitalization.
- Psychotherapy is considered first-line treatment for mild depressive episodes.
- Strongly consider pharmacotherapy when symptoms of depression are moderate to severe.
- Outpatient individual psychotherapy in combination with pharmacotherapy may be beneficial.

MEDICATION
First Line
- For nonbreastfeeding women, selection of antidepressants is similar to nonpostpartum patients.
- Selective serotonin reuptake inhibitors (SSRIs) are generally effective and safe. Paroxetine has been associated with fetal cardiac defects when used during pregnancy:
  – Sertraline (Zoloft): 50 to 200 mg/day PO; fluoxetine (Prozac): 20 to 60 mg/day PO
  – Paroxetine (Paxil): 20 to 50 mg/day PO given at bedtime (associated with very small increase in risk of cardiovascular defects with 1st trimester use); citalopram (Celexa): 20 to 40 mg/day PO; escitalopram (Lexapro): 10 to 20 mg/day PO
- Serotonin-norepinephrine reuptake inhibitors (SNRIs):
  – Venlafaxine (Effexor XR): 75 to 225 mg/day PO; desvenlafaxine (Pristiq): 50 to 100 mg/day PO
  – Duloxetine (Cymbalta): 60 to 120 mg/day PO
- Atypical antidepressants:
  – Bupropion (Wellbutrin): 150 to 450 mg/day PO (no sexual dysfunction, activating)
  – Mirtazapine (Remeron): 15 to 45 mg/day PO at bedtime (increases appetite and is sedating at lower doses, no sexual dysfunction)
- Tricyclic antidepressants (TCAs), particularly nortriptyline, have been shown to be as effective as SSRIs; yet, they are more lethal in overdose and have increased rates of unfavorable side effects; nortriptyline: 75 to 150 mg/day PO given at bedtime

- Bipolar disorder requires treatment with mood stabilizer.
- Among breastfeeding mothers: Breastfeeding should generally not preclude treatment with antidepressants.
  – SSRIs and some other antidepressants are considered reasonable options during breastfeeding.
  – All antidepressants are excreted in breast milk but are generally compatible with lactation.
  – Sertraline and paroxetine have the lowest translactal passage and are considered most compatible with breastfeeding.
  – Avoid fluoxetine, citalopram (5)[B], and venlafaxine due to increased translactal passage.
  – Start with low doses and increase slowly. Minimize polypharmacy. Attempt to maximize use of only one psychotropic medication at a time. Monitor the infant for adverse side effects.
  – Continuing an efficacious medication is preferred over switching antidepressants to avoid exposing the mother and infant to the risks of untreated PPD (5)[B].
  – Consider negative effects of untreated PPD on infant and child development.
  – Discuss the treatment options with the patient and her partner when possible. Take into account the patient's personal psychiatric history and previous response to treatment, the risks of no treatment or undertreatment, available data about the safety of medications during breastfeeding, and her individual expectations and treatment preferences.
  – For further information: https://www.ncbi.nlm .nih.gov/books/NBK501922/?report=classic

Second Line
Consider switching to a different antidepressant if patient has a lack of response. Augmentation may be necessary in the setting of treatment-resistant PPD. Electroconvulsive therapy (ECT) is an option for depressed postpartum women who do not respond to antidepressant medications, have severe or psychotic symptoms, cannot tolerate antidepressant medications, are actively engaged in suicidal self-destructive behaviors, or have a previous history of response to ECT.

ISSUES FOR REFERRAL
- Obtain psychiatric consultation for patients with psychotic symptoms.
- Strongly consider immediate hospitalization if delusions or hallucinations are present.
- Hospitalization is indicated if mother's ability to care for self and/or infant is significantly compromised.

ADDITIONAL THERAPIES
- CBT and IPT are evidence-based treatments shown to effectively treat PPD.
- Psychoeducation, listening visits (nondirective counseling), and psychodynamic psychotherapy may also improve symptoms of PPD.

SURGERY/OTHER PROCEDURES
Brexanolone was approved by the FDA in March 2019 for PPD. It is a rapidly acting steroid related to progesterone, with antidepressant effects. It is administered as a continuous IV infusion over a period of 60 hours. There is a restricted access to this medication. It is only administered at sites enrolled in the Risk

Evaluation and Mitigation Strategy Program, and it is very expensive (>$35,000 for a course of treatment). Consider in women with severe PPD who refuse or do not respond to ECT (6).
- Requires constant monitoring with pulse oximetry
- FDA recommends that providers monitor patient at least every 2 hours for excessive sedation and loss of consciousness.
- Side effects include dry mouth, hot flashes/flushing, diarrhea, dyspepsia, excessive sedation, loss of consciousness, and dizziness.

COMPLEMENTARY & ALTERNATIVE MEDICINE
- Breastfeeding has been associated with reduced stress and improved maternal mood.
- Infant massage, infant sleep intervention, exercise, and bright light therapy may be beneficial.

ADMISSION, INPATIENT, AND NURSING CONSIDERATIONS

ALERT
Obtain psychiatric consultation for patients with refractory depression or psychotic symptoms. If delusions or hallucinations are present, strongly consider immediate hospitalization. The psychotic mother should *not* be left alone with the baby.

- Admission criteria/initial stabilization: presence of suicidal or homicidal ideation and/or psychotic symptoms and/or thoughts of harming the baby and/or inability to care for self or infant; severe weight loss
- Discharge criteria: Absence of suicidal or homicidal ideation and/or psychotic symptoms and/or thoughts of harming the baby; the mother must be able to care for self and infant.

 ONGOING CARE

FOLLOW-UP RECOMMENDATIONS
Patient Monitoring
- Collaborative care approach, including primary care visits and case manager follow-ups
- Consultation with the infant's doctor, particularly if the mother is breastfeeding while taking psychotropic medications

DIET
- Good nutrition and hydration, especially when breastfeeding
- Mixed evidence to support the addition of multivitamin with minerals and omega-3 fatty acids

PATIENT EDUCATION
- *This Isn't What I Expected: Overcoming Postpartum Depression* by Karen R. Kleiman and Valerie Davis Raskin
- Web resources:
  – Postpartum Support International: https://www .postpartum.net/
  – La Leche League: https://www.llli.org/
  – Center for Women's Mental Health: https://www .womensmentalhealth.org/

PROGNOSIS
- Treatment of maternal depression to remission has been shown to have a positive impact on children's mental health.
- Some patients, particularly those with undertreated or undiagnosed depression, may develop chronic depression requiring long-term treatment.
- Untreated maternal depression is linked to impaired mother–infant bonding and cognitive and language development delay in infants and children.
- Postpartum psychosis is associated with tragic outcomes such as maternal suicide and infanticide.

COMPLICATIONS
- Suicide, self-injurious behavior, psychosis
- Neglect of baby, harm to the baby
- Preterm and low-birth-weight baby

REFERENCES
1. Liu X, Wang S, Wang G. Prevalence and risk factors of postpartum depression in women: a systematic review and meta-analysis. *J Clin Nurs*. 2022;31(19–20):2665–2677.
2. Wisner KL, Sit DKY, McShea MC, et al. Onset timing, thoughts of self-harm, and diagnoses in postpartum women with screen-positive depression findings. *JAMA Psychiatry*. 2013;70(5):490–498.
3. O'Connor E, Rossom RC, Henninger M, et al. Primary care screening for and treatment of depression in pregnant and postpartum women: evidence report and systematic review for the US Preventive Services Task Force. *JAMA*. 2016;315(4):388–406.
4. O'Connor E, Senger CA, Henninger ML, et al. Interventions to prevent perinatal depression: evidence report and systematic review for the US Preventive Services Task Force. *JAMA*. 2019;321(6):588–601.
5. Gavin NI, Gaynes BN, Lohr KN, et al. Perinatal depression: a systematic review of prevalence and incidence. *Obstet Gynecol*. 2005;106(5 Pt 1):1071–1083.
6. Leader LD, O'Connell M, VandenBerg A. Brexanolone for postpartum depression: clinical evidence and practical considerations. *Pharmacotherapy*. 2019;39(11):1105–1112.

CODES

ICD10
- F53 Puerperal psychosis
- O90.6 Postpartum mood disturbance

CLINICAL PEARLS
- Universal screening for depression is recommended during the 1st and 3rd trimesters and at regular intervals during the postpartum period.
- Early diagnosis and treatment are vital, as untreated PPD can lead to developmental difficulties for the infant and prolonged disability and suffering for the mother.
- Psychotherapy may be an effective monotherapy for mild to moderate depressive systems. In severe PPD, the use of medications is strongly urged.
- Antidepressant treatment is safe during pregnancy and breastfeeding, and the treatment should be individualized for each mom (5)[B].

DEPRESSION, TREATMENT RESISTANT
Bliss Puthenpurayil, MD • Nida Zahra, MD, FAAFP

BASICS

DESCRIPTION
- Major depressive disorder (MDD) that has failed to respond to ≥2 adequate trials of antidepressant therapy in ≥2 different classes is considered to be "treatment resistant."
- Individual antidepressants must be given for 6 weeks at standard doses before being considered a failure.

EPIDEMIOLOGY
- Depression affects >16 million people in the United States and >350 million people worldwide.
- The average adult has a 16% lifetime risk of MDD, with majority experiencing onset before the age of 30 years.
- Approximately 1/3 of patients with MDD will develop treatment-resistant depression.

Incidence
Among patients with unipolar major depression who receive initial treatment, the estimated incidence for treatment resistance ranges from 45% to 46%.

ETIOLOGY AND PATHOPHYSIOLOGY
- Unclear. Low levels of neurotransmitters (serotonin, norepinephrine, dopamine, and γ-aminobutyric acid [GABA]) have been indicated.
- Serotonin has been linked to irritability, hostility, and suicidal ideation.
- Norepinephrine has been linked to low energy.
- Dopamine may play a role in low motivation and depression with psychotic features.
- GABA can help with feelings of anxiety, stress, and fear.
- Environmental stressors such as abuse and neglect may affect both the function and levels of neurotransmitters.
- Inflammation and oxidative stress in the brain can contribute to treatment-resistant depression.

Genetics
A genetic abnormality in the serotonin transporter gene (5-HTTLPR) may increase risk for treatment-resistant depression.

RISK FACTORS
- Suicidal thoughts and behavior, severity of disease
- Early age of onset of major depression
- Recurrent depressive episodes
- Mislabeling bipolar patients as depressed
- Comorbid medical disease (including chronic pain)
- Comorbid personality disorder
- Comorbid anxiety disorder
- Comorbid substance use disorder
- Genetic familial predisposition to poor response to antidepressants
- Loss of employment and low socioeconomic status

GENERAL PREVENTION
- Medication adherence in combination with psychotherapy
- Maintenance electroconvulsive therapy (ECT) may prevent relapse.

COMMONLY ASSOCIATED CONDITIONS
- Suicide
- Bipolar disorder
- Substance use disorders
- Anxiety disorders
- Dysthymia
- Eating disorders
- Somatic symptom disorders

DIAGNOSIS

HISTORY
- Symptoms are the same as in MDD. However, patients do not respond to standard form of treatment.
- Important to screen for suicidality in treatment-resistant depression
- Screening with SIGECAPS
  - Sleep: too much or too little
  - Interest: inability to enjoy activities
  - Guilt: excessive and uncontrollable
  - Energy: poor
  - Concentration: inability to focus on tasks
  - Appetite: too much or too little
  - Psychomotor changes: restlessness/agitation or slowing/lethargy noted by others
  - Suicidality: desire to end life or feeling hopeless

PHYSICAL EXAM
Mental status exam may reveal poor hygiene, limited eye contact, poor relatedness, restricted affect, tearfulness, weight loss or gain, psychomotor retardation or agitation, and suicidal thoughts.

DIFFERENTIAL DIAGNOSIS
- Bipolar disorder
- Persistent depressive disorder
- Posttraumatic stress disorder
- Dementia
- Early-stage Parkinson disease
- Personality disorder
- Medical illness such as malignancy, thyroid disease, HIV, anemia
- Substance use disorders

DIAGNOSTIC TESTS & INTERPRETATION
Initial Tests (lab, imaging)
Used to rule out medical factors that could be causing/contributing to treatment resistance
- CBC, complete metabolic profile
- Urine drug screen
- Thyroid-stimulating hormone (TSH)
- 25-OH vitamin D, vitamin B_{12}, folate
- Urinalysis
- FSH, LH if applicable
- HCG, if applicable
- Testosterone, if applicable
- CT or MRI of the brain if neurologic disease, tumor, or dementia is suspected

Follow-Up Tests & Special Considerations
Delirium and dementia often look like depression.

Diagnostic Procedures/Other
Depression is a clinical diagnosis, and other diagnosis such as bipolar depression and dysthymic disorder should be ruled out. Use validated depression rating scales to assist:
- Beck Depression Inventory
- Hamilton Depression Rating Scale
- Patient Health Questionnaire 9 (PHQ-9)
- Edinburgh Postnatal Depression Scale if pregnant or postpartum

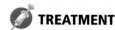

TREATMENT

MEDICATION
First Line
Please see "Depression" topic. When those fail, augmentation and combination strategies are as follows:
- Antidepressants in combination
  - Citalopram (start 20 mg/day; max dose 40 mg/day) + bupropion (start 100 mg BID; max dose 450 mg total) (1),(2)[B]
  - Tricyclic antidepressants (TCAs) and selective serotonin reuptake inhibitors (SSRIs) may be used in combination. Proceed with caution due to risk of serotonin syndrome; citalopram (start 20 mg/day; max dose 40 mg/day) + nortriptyline (start 25 mg at bedtime; max dose 150 mg at bedtime)
  - Serotonin-norepinephrine reuptake inhibitors (SNRI) and noradrenergic and specific serotonergic antidepressant (NaSSA) may also be used in combination such as venlafaxine extended release (start 75 mg/day; max dose 225 mg/day) and mirtazapine (start 15 mg/day; max dose 45 mg/day)
- Antidepressants + antipsychotics
  - Citalopram (start 20 mg/day; max dose 40 mg/day) + aripiprazole (start 2 mg/day; up to 20 mg/day, different mechanism of action at higher doses) *or* + risperidone (start 0.5 to 1.0 mg at bedtime; max dose 6 mg/day) *or* + quetiapine (start 50 mg at bedtime; titrate to 100 to 300 mg at bedtime; max dose 600 mg/day) (1)[A],(2)
  - Olanzapine/fluoxetine combination (start 3 mg/25 mg to 12 mg/50 mg at bedtime) (1)[A],(2)
- Antidepressant + lithium
  - TCA: nortriptyline (start 25 mg at bedtime; max dose 150 mg at bedtime) + lithium (start 300 mg at bedtime; max dose 900 mg BID)
  - SSRI: citalopram (start 20 mg/day; max dose 40 mg QD) + lithium (start 300 mg at bedtime; max dose 900 mg BID) (1)[A],(2)
- In all combinations, citalopram (Celexa) can be replaced with other SSRIs such as fluoxetine (Prozac) 20 to 80 mg/day, sertraline (Zoloft) 50 to 200 mg/day, and escitalopram (Lexapro) 10 to 20 mg/day, vortioxetine (Trintellix) 5 to 20 mg/day or with SNRIs duloxetine (Cymbalta) 30 to 120 mg/day, venlafaxine XR (Effexor XR) 75 to 225 mg/day, or desvenlafaxine (Pristiq) 50 to 100 mg/day, or with a NaSSA mirtazapine (Remeron) 15 to 45 mg at bedtime.
- Maximum doses for medication in treatment-resistant cases may be higher than in treatment-responsive cases.

Second Line

- Citalopram (start 20 mg/day; max dose 40 mg/day) + triiodothyronine (T3; 12.5 to 50.0 μg/day) (1),(2)[B]
- Citalopram (start 20 mg/day; max dose of 40 mg/day) + buspirone (start 7.5 mg BID; max dose of 30 mg BID) (1),(2)[B]
- Citalopram (start 20 mg/day; max dose 40 mg/day) + lisdexamfetamine (Vyvanse) (20 to 50 mg every morning) (1)[B],(2)
- Antidepressant in combination with therapy, particularly, cognitive-behavioral therapy (CBT) (3)[A]
- Monoamine oxidase inhibitor (MAOI)
  - Tranylcypromine (Parnate): Start 10 mg BID and increase 10 mg/day every 1 to 3 weeks; max dose 60 mg/day
  - Selegiline transdermal (Emsam patch): Apply 6-mg patch daily and increase 3 mg/day; max dose 12 mg/day
  - Side-effect profile (e.g., hypertensive crisis), drug–drug interactions, and dietary restrictions make MAOIs less appealing. Patch version does not require dietary restrictions at lower doses.
  - High risk of serotonin syndrome if combined with another antidepressant. 2-week washout period is advised.

ISSUES FOR REFERRAL

Treatment-resistant depression should be managed in consultation with a psychiatrist.

ADDITIONAL THERAPIES

- First line
  - ECT: brief administration of electrical stimulation to the brain via superficial electrode placement
    - Safe and cost-effective option for treatment-resistant and life-threatening depression, with a 66.6% response rate (4)[A]
    - Known to rapidly relieve suicidality, psychotic depression, and catatonia
    - Cognitive side effects during treatment can occur but are more likely with bilateral lead placement
- Second line
  - Deep brain stimulation (DBS): surgical implantation of intracranial electrodes, connected to an impulse generator implanted in the chest wall:
    - Reserved for those who have failed medications, psychotherapy, and ECT
    - Preliminary data are promising, showing 40–70% response rate and 35% remission rate. Further trials are being done.
  - Transcranial magnetic stimulation (TMS): noninvasive brain stimulation technique that is generally safe
    - Currently, only FDA-approved for less severe forms of the illness
  - Vagus nerve stimulation (VNS): surgical implantation of electrodes onto left vagus nerve
    - Use has become limited in recent years.

- Ketamine (0.5 mg/kg single-dose infusion over 40 minutes): Studies show evidence of rapid improvement in mood and suicidal thinking; currently used off-label for treatment-resistant depression (2)[B],(4); esketamine, an intranasal spray, in conjunction with an oral antidepressant, has been FDA-approved for treatment-resistant depression. Dosing is 28 mg, 56 mg, or 84 mg twice a week for 1 to 4 weeks, followed by taper and/or maintenance treatment.
  - The effects of ketamine and esketamine appear temporary, usually lasting days to weeks (5). Continued studies are focusing on dosing and frequency of administration to maintain longer lasting response and remission.
- Stanford neuromodulation therapy (SNT) (under investigation):
  - SNT: new TMS technique in which patients get 10 sessions daily of high-dose TMS for 5 consecutive days
  - 79% remission rate with SNT (n = 14) versus 13% remission rate with sham (n = 15)
- Psilocybin (under investigation):
  - Psilocybin: psychedelic compound isolated from species of Psilocybe mushrooms
  - 32.9% response rate and 26.6% remission rate at week 12 after a single dose of 25 mg psilocybin (n = 79)
  - 58% response rate up to 3 months after 2 doses, an initial low dose and a subsequent high dose of 25 mg psilocybin (n = 12).

ADMISSION, INPATIENT, AND NURSING CONSIDERATIONS

- Inpatient care is indicated for severely depressed, psychotic, catatonic, or suicidal patients.
- Discharge criteria: symptoms improving, no longer suicidal, psychosocial stressors addressed

ONGOING CARE

FOLLOW-UP RECOMMENDATIONS

- Frequent visits (i.e., every month)
- During follow-up, evaluate side effects, dosage, and effectiveness of medication as well as the need for referral for ECT or ketamine/esketamine treatment.
- Patients who have responded to ECT or ketamine/esketamine treatment may need maintenance treatments (q2–12 wk) to prevent relapse.
- Combination of lithium/nortriptyline after ECT appears to be as effective as maintenance ECT in reducing relapse.

DIET

Patients on MAOIs need a dietary restriction on foods that are rich in tyramine.

PATIENT EDUCATION

- Educate patients that depression is a medical illness, not a character defect.
- Review signs and symptoms of worsening depression and when patient needs to come in for further evaluation.
- Discuss safety plan to address suicidal thoughts.

PROGNOSIS

With medication adherence, close follow-up, improved social support, and psychotherapy, prognosis improves.

COMPLICATIONS

- Suicide
- Disability
- Poor quality of life

REFERENCES

1. McIntyre RS, Filteau MJ, Martin L, et al. Treatment-resistant depression: definitions, review of the evidence, and algorithmic approach. *J Affect Disord*. 2014;156:1–7.
2. Taylor RW, Marwood L, Oprea E, et al. Pharmacological augmentation in unipolar depression: a guide to the guidelines. *Int J Neuropsychopharmacol*. 2020;23(9):587–625.
3. Wiles NJ, Thomas L, Turner N, et al. Long-term effectiveness and cost-effectiveness of cognitive behavioural therapy as an adjunct to pharmacotherapy for treatment-resistant depression in primary care: follow-up of the CoBalT randomised controlled trial. *Lancet Psychiatry*. 2016;3(2):137–144.
4. Ross EL, Zivin K, Maixner DF. Cost-effectiveness of electroconvulsive therapy vs pharmacotherapy/psychotherapy for treatment-resistant depression in the United States. *JAMA Psychiatry*. 2018;75(7):713–722.
5. Sanacora G, Frye MA, McDonald W, et al; for American Psychiatric Association (APA) Council of Research Task Force on Novel Biomarkers and Treatments. A consensus statement on the use of ketamine in the treatment of mood disorders. *JAMA Psychiatry*. 2017;74(4):399–405.

CODES

ICD10

- F32.9 Major depressive disorder, single episode, unspecified
- F33.9 Major depressive disorder, recurrent, unspecified

CLINICAL PEARLS

- Treatment-resistant depression is common, affecting 1/3 of patients with MDD.
- Combination and augmentation strategies with antidepressants, antipsychotics, therapy, and mood stabilizers can be helpful.
- ECT and ketamine/esketamine treatment should be considered in severe and life-threatening cases. DBS, TNS, and psilocybin are still experimental but they are showing excellent promise.

DERMATITIS HERPETIFORMIS

Faraz Yousefian, DO • Sujitha Yadlapati, MD

BASICS

DESCRIPTION
- Dermatitis herpetiformis (DH) is an autoimmune disease that presents as a chronic, relapsing, polymorphous, intensely pruritic, erythematous papulovesicular eruption with symmetrical distribution primarily involving extensor skin surfaces of the elbows, knees, buttocks, back, and scalp.
- DH is associated with autoimmune diseases, especially celiac disease, in addition to gluten sensitivity with genetic, environmental, and immunologic influences.
- DH is distinguished from other bullous diseases by characteristic histologic and immunologic findings as well as associated gluten-sensitive enteropathy (GSE).
- System(s) affected: skin
- Synonym(s): Duhring disease, Duhring-Brocq disease

EPIDEMIOLOGY
- Occurs most frequently in those of Northern European origin
- Rare in persons of Asian or African American origin
- Predominant age: most common in the 4th decade of life but may present at any age
- Equal male-to-female incidence, in comparison to celiac disease which is female dominant.
- >90% have evidence of GSE, whereas only 20% are symptomatic of celiac disease.

Incidence
As high as 2.6/100,000 people per year (1)

Prevalence
As high as 39.2/100,000 people (1)

ETIOLOGY AND PATHOPHYSIOLOGY
- Evidence suggests that epidermal transglutaminase (eTG) 3, is the autoantigen in DH. eTG is highly homologous with tissue transglutaminase (tTG), which is the antigenic target in celiac disease and GSE.
- The initiating event for DH is presumed to be the interaction of wheat peptides with tTGs, which results in the formation of an autoantigen with high affinity for particular class II major histocompatibility complex (MHC) molecules. Presentation of the autoantigen leads to activation of T cells and the humoral immune system.
- IgA antibodies against tTG cross-react with eTG and result in IgA-eTG immune complexes that are deposited in the papillary dermis. Subsequent activation of complement and recruitment of neutrophils to the area result in inflammation and microabscesses. Skin eruption may be delayed up to 5 to 6 weeks after exposure to gluten.
- Gluten applied directly to the skin does not result in eruption, whereas gluten taken by mouth or rectum does. This implies necessary processing by the GI system; thought to be immune complex-mediated disease

Genetics
- High association with human leukocyte antigen (HLA)-DQ2 (95%), with remaining patients being positive for DQ8, DR4, or DR3 (1)
- Strong association with a combination of alleles DQA1*0501 and DQB1*0201/0202, DRB1*03 and DRB1*05/07, or DQA1*0301 and DQB1*0302 (2)

RISK FACTORS
- GSE: >90% of those with DH will have GSE, which may be asymptomatic (1),(3).
- Family history of DH or celiac disease

GENERAL PREVENTION
A gluten-free diet (GFD) results in the improvement of DH and reduces dependence on medical therapy. GFD also may reduce the risk of lymphomas associated with DH.

COMMONLY ASSOCIATED CONDITIONS
- Hypothyroidism, hyperthyroidism, thyroid nodules, thyroid cancer
- Celiac disease, GSE, gluten ataxia
- Gastric atrophy, hypochlorhydria, pernicious anemia
- GI lymphoma, non-Hodgkin lymphoma
- IgA nephropathy
- Autoimmune disorders, including systemic lupus erythematosus, dermatomyositis, Sjögren syndrome, rheumatoid arthritis, sarcoidosis, Raynaud phenomenon, insulin-dependent diabetes mellitus, myasthenia gravis, Addison disease, vitiligo, alopecia areata, primary biliary cirrhosis, and psoriasis

DIAGNOSIS

Diagnosis of DH involves a clinicopathologic correlation between clinical presentation, histologic and direct immunofluorescence (DIF) evaluation, serology, and response to therapy or dietary restriction (2),(3).

HISTORY
Waxing and waning, intensely pruritic eruption with papules and tiny vesicles; eruption may worsen with gluten intake. GI symptoms may be absent or may not be reported until prompted.

PHYSICAL EXAM
- The classic lesions of DH are described as symmetric, grouped, erythematous papules, and vesicles. Isolated vesicles are rarely seen due to intense itching.
- More commonly presents with erosions, excoriations, lichenification, hypopigmentation, and/or hyperpigmentation secondary to scratching and healing of old lesions
- Areas involved include extensor surfaces of elbows (90%), knees (30%), shoulders, buttocks, and sacrum. The scalp is also frequently affected. Oral lesions are rare.
- In children, purpura may be visible on digits and palmoplantar surfaces.
- Adults with associated enteropathy are most often asymptomatic, with about 20% experiencing steatorrhea and <10% with findings of bloating, diarrhea, or malabsorption. Children with associated enteropathy may present with abdominal pain, diarrhea, iron deficiency, and reduced growth rate.

DIFFERENTIAL DIAGNOSIS
- In adults
  - Bullous pemphigoid: linear deposition of C3 and IgG at the basement membrane zone
  - Linear IgA disease: homogeneous and linear deposition of IgA at the basement membrane zone, absence of GSE
  - Prurigo nodularis
  - Urticaria: wheals, angioedema, dermal edema
  - Erythema multiforme

- In children
  - Atopic dermatitis: face and flexural areas
  - Scabies: interdigital areas, axillae, genital region
  - Papular urticaria: dermal edema
  - Impetigo

DIAGNOSTIC TESTS & INTERPRETATION

Initial Tests (lab, imaging)
- Serum IgA tTG antibodies: Detection of tTG antibodies was noted to be up to 95% sensitive and >90% specific for DH in patients on unrestricted diets (2),(3).
- Serum IgA eTG antibodies: Antibodies to eTG, the primary autoantigen in DH, were shown to be more sensitive than antibodies to tTG in the diagnosis of patients with DH on unrestricted diets (95% vs. 79%) but are not widely available in all labs (2),(3).
- Serum IgA endomysial antibodies (EMA): Antibodies to EMA have a sensitivity between 50% and 100% and a specificity close to 100% in patients on unrestricted diets but are more expensive, time-consuming, and operator-dependent than tTG (2),(3).

Follow-Up Tests & Special Considerations
- Serologic assessment of anti-tTG and anti-eTG correlate with intestinal involvement of disease and in conjunction with anti-EMA may be useful in monitoring major deviations from GFD.
- Genetic testing for haplotypes HLA-DQ2 and HLA-DQ8 can also be offered to patients to determine genetic susceptibility, to screen patients with a high risk of CD, or if the diagnosis is not clear (2),(3).

Diagnostic Procedures/Other
- The gold standard test to establish a diagnosis of DH is DIF of the perilesional skin that demonstrate characteristic granular IgA deposits in dermal papillae and/or basement membrane. It is this key diagnostic feature that differentiates this blistering skin condition from all other dermatologic diseases (2),(3).
- DIF has a sensitivity and specificity of close to 100%. In patients with high suspicion for DH with a negative DIF, another perilesional skin biopsy should be obtained from a different site. Histopathology of these lesions with routine staining reveals neutrophilic microabscesses in the tips of the dermal papillae and may show subepidermal blistering.

TREATMENT

GENERAL MEASURES
GFD is the mainstay of treatment in DH and can lead to the complete resolution of symptoms (2),(3). Typically, it requires 18 to 24 months of strict adherence to GFD prior to the resolution of skin lesions without any additional treatment. Lesions can recur within 12 weeks of reintroduction of gluten. Once prolonged remission has been obtained, some gluten may be tolerated in a subset of patients to build tolerance with immunologic response modification.

MEDICATION

Dapsone, sulfapyridine, and topical steroids are useful for immediate symptom management but should only be used as an adjunct to dietary modification.

First Line

- Dapsone is a widely used FDA-approved medication (2).
- Initial dosing of 25 to 50 mg/day on a strict GFD typically results in improvement of symptoms within 24 to 72 hours.
- It is recommended to use a minimum effective dose with slow titration based on the patient's response and tolerability. The average maintenance dose is 1 mg/kg/day (50 to 150 mg/day) and can be increased up to 300 mg to obtain better symptom control (2).
- Minor outbreaks on the face and scalp are common even with treatment; not ideal for long-term use in DH
- Dapsone works by inhibiting neutrophil recruitment and IL-8 release, inhibiting the respiratory burst of neutrophils, and protecting cells from neutrophil-mediated injury, thereby suppressing the skin reaction. It has no role in preventing IgA deposition or mitigating the immune reaction in the gut (2).
- Precautions: See product labeling.
  - Common side effects include nausea, vomiting, headache, dizziness, weakness, and hemolysis.
  - A drop in hemoglobin of 1 to 2 g is characteristic with dapsone 100 mg/day.

ALERT

- Monitor for potentially fatal dapsone-induced sulfone syndrome: fever, jaundice and hepatic necrosis, exfoliative dermatitis, lymphadenopathy, methemoglobinemia, and hemolytic anemia.
- Can occur 48 hours or 6 months after treatment, most often 5 weeks after initiation

Pediatric Considerations

- <2 years: Dosing is not established.
- >2 years: 0.5 to 1.0 mg/kg/day

Pregnancy Considerations

- Category C: Safety during pregnancy is not established.
- Secreted in breast milk and will produce hemolytic anemia in infants
- Adherence to a strict GFD 6 to 12 months before conception should be considered with the hope of eliminating the need for dapsone during pregnancy due to its side effects profile (2).

Second Line

- High-potency topical steroids can be used acutely to control symptoms until dapsone becomes effective (2).
- Sulfapyridine (1 to 2 g/day) is FDA-approved for use in DH and is thought to be the active metabolite in sulfasalazine (2 to 4 g/day). Common side effects include nausea, vomiting, and anorexia. The enteric-coated form may reduce side effects. Other side effects include agranulocytosis, hypersensitivity reactions, hemolytic anemia, proteinuria, and crystalluria (2).

- Topical steroids and 3rd-generation antihistamines can be used to provide relief from symptoms of pruritus and itching.
- Recently, JAK inhibitors such as tofacitinib have shown improvement in DH (4).

ISSUES FOR REFERRAL

Over time, the management of DH warrants an interdisciplinary treatment that includes providing a referral to a dermatologist, gastroenterologist, and registered dietitian.

ONGOING CARE

FOLLOW-UP RECOMMENDATIONS

Patient Monitoring

- Every 6 to 12 months by a physician and a dietitian to evaluate GFD adherence and recurrence of symptoms.
- Adherence to GFD can be monitored with serologic levels of anti-tTG, anti-eTG, and EMA levels.
- Patients on dapsone require lab monitoring weekly for the 1st month, biweekly for 2 months, and then every 3 months for the duration of medication use (2).

DIET

- Grains that should be avoided: wheat (including spelt, Kamut, semolina, and triticale), rye, and barley (including malt)
- Safe grains (gluten-free): rice, amaranth, buckwheat, corn, millet, quinoa, sorghum, teff (an Ethiopian cereal grain), and oats
- Care should be taken to avoid gluten-free grains that are contaminated with sources of gluten during processing such as oats.
- Sources of gluten-free starches that can be used as flour alternatives
  - Cereal grains: amaranth, buckwheat, corn, millet, quinoa, sorghum, teff, rice (white, brown, wild, basmati, jasmine), and Montina
  - Tubers: arrowroot, jicama, taro, potato, and tapioca
  - Legumes: chickpeas, lentils, kidney beans, navy beans, pea beans, peanuts, and soybeans
  - Nuts: almonds, walnuts, pistachios, chestnuts, hazelnuts, and cashews
  - Seeds: sunflower, flax, and pumpkin

PATIENT EDUCATION

- Patients started on dapsone should be made aware of potential hemolytic anemia and the signs associated with methemoglobinemia (2).
- American Academy of Dermatology, 930 N. Meacham Road, P.O. Box 4014, Schaumberg, IL 60168-4014; (708) 330-0230
- The University of Chicago Celiac Disease Center, 5841 S. Maryland Ave., Mail Code 4069, Chicago, IL 60637; (773) 702-7593; http://www.celiacdisease.net/ or https://www.cureceliacdisease.org/
- Gluten Intolerance Group of North America, 31214-124 Ave. SE, Auburn, WA 98092; (206) 246-6652; fax (206) 246-6531; https://gluten.org/
- Commercial source for gluten-free products https://glutenfreemall.com

PROGNOSIS

- DH is a chronic disease with an excellent prognosis, provided strict adherence to a GFD which is the only sustainable method of eliminating cutaneous and GI disease.
- 10- to 15-year survival rates do not seem to differ from general population.
- Remission in 10–15%
- Skin disease responds readily to dapsone. Occasional new lesions (2 to 3 per week) are to be expected and are not an indication for altering the daily dosage (2).
- The risk of lymphoma may be decreased in those who maintain a GFD.

COMPLICATIONS

- The majority of complications are associated with GSE.
- Malnutrition, weight loss, anemia (folate, vitamin B_{12}, iron nutritional deficiencies)
- Abdominal pain, dyspepsia
- Osteoporosis, dental abnormalities
- Autoimmune diseases (especially hypothyroidism)
- Increased risk of enteropathy-associated T-cell lymphoma

REFERENCES

1. Bolotin D, Petronic-Rosic V. Dermatitis herpetiformis. Part I. Epidemiology, pathogenesis, and clinical presentation. *J Am Acad Dermatol.* 2011;64(6):1017–1026.
2. Bolotin D, Petronic-Rosic V. Dermatitis herpetiformis. Part II. Diagnosis, management, and prognosis. *J Am Acad Dermatol.* 2011;64(6):1027–1034.
3. Reunala T, Salmi TT, Hervonen K. Dermatitis herpetiformis: pathognomonic transglutaminase IgA deposits in the skin and excellent prognosis on a gluten-free diet. *Acta Derm Venereol.* 2015;95(8):917–922.
4. Kahn JS, Moody K, Rosmarin D. Significant improvement of dermatitis herpetiformis with tofacitinib. *Dermatol Online J.* 2021;27(7).

 SEE ALSO

- Celiac Disease
- Algorithm: Rash

CODES

ICD10

L13.0 Dermatitis herpetiformis

CLINICAL PEARLS

DH is a chronic, relapsing, intensely pruritic rash that has a strong association with GSE.

DERMATITIS, ATOPIC
Dennis E. Hughes, DO, FACEP

BASICS

DESCRIPTION
- A chronic, relapsing, inflammatory, intensely pruritic skin disease
- Early-onset cases have coexisting allergen sensitization more often than late-onset cases.
- Clinical phenotypical presentation is highly variable, suggesting multifactorial pathophysiology.
- May have significant effect on quality of life for patient and family—recurrent symptoms affect lifestyle and mental health

EPIDEMIOLOGY
- 45% of all cases begin in the first 6 months of life with 80–95% onset prior to age of 5 years.
- 50–66% of affected children will have a spontaneous remission before adolescence.
- Also, may have late-onset dermatitis in adults or relapse of childhood condition—primarily hand eczema
- Darker pigmented individuals are affected more often than whites.
- 60% incidence if one parent is previously affected and rises to 80% if both parents are previously affected. Monozygotic twins have 80% concordance for the disorder.

Incidence
Varies worldwide, but all countries' populations are affected. The only consistent signal favored lower incidence in rural versus urban locations (exceptions are Canada and Mexico).

Prevalence
Approaching 20% prevalence in children and 10% in young adults; still present in later adulthood 2%

ETIOLOGY AND PATHOPHYSIOLOGY
- Current understanding is atopic dermatitis (AD) is a systemic T-helper cell driven disorder.
- Alteration in stratum corneum results in transepidermal water loss and defect in barrier function.
- Epidermal adhesion is reduced either as a result of (i) genetic mutation resulting in altered epidermal proteins or (ii) defect in immune regulation causing an altered inflammatory response.
- Interleukin-31 (IL-31) upregulation is thought to be a major factor in pruritus mediated by cytokines and neuropeptides rather than histamine excess.

Genetics
- Recent discovery of association between AD and mutation in the filaggrin gene (*FLG*), which codes for a skin barrier protein
- Both epidermal and immune coding are likely involved.

RISK FACTORS
- "Itch–scratch cycle" (stimulates histamine release)
- Skin infections
- Emotional stress
- Irritating clothes and chemicals
- Excessively hot or cold climate

- Food allergies may be seen in association with AD, but there is no conclusive common origin. Studies of breastfeeding conveying decreased risk versus increased risk are mixed in conclusion.
- Exposure to tobacco smoke
- Some evidence suggests that repeated exposure to water high in mineral content may exacerbate the condition.
- Family history of atopy
  - Asthma
  - Allergic rhinitis

COMMONLY ASSOCIATED CONDITIONS
- Food sensitivity/allergy in many cases. Strong association with asthma and allergic rhinitis; atopic march—clinical succession of AD with subsequent development of allergic rhinitis followed by asthma (1)
- Association with both cutaneous and extra-cutaneous infections: URI, OM, UTI, cellulitis, erysipelas, zoster, endocarditis, both methicillin-resistant and susceptible stains of *Staphylococcus aureus*, pharyngitis, and rarely sepsis
- Hyper-IgE syndrome (Job syndrome)
  - AD
  - Elevated IgE
  - Recurrent pyodermas
  - Decreased chemotaxis of mononuclear cells

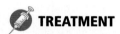

DIAGNOSIS

Clinical diagnosis

HISTORY
- Presence of major symptoms including relapsing of condition, family history, typical distribution, and morphology necessary to make diagnosis of AD
- Most prevalent symptoms: itch (54%), dryness and scaling (19.6%), inflamed skin (7.2%), skin pain (8.2%), sleep disturbance (11.4%)

PHYSICAL EXAM
Primarily skin manifestations
- Distribution of lesions
  - Infants: trunk, face, and extensor surfaces; diaper-sparing
  - Children: antecubital and popliteal fossae, wrists and ankle locations
  - Adults: hands, feet, face, neck, upper chest, and genital areas as well as flexor surfaces
- Morphology of lesions
  - Infants: erythema and papules; may develop oozing, crusting vesicles
  - Children and adults: Lichenification and scaling are typical with chronic eczema as a result of persistent scratching and rubbing (lichenification is rare in infants).
- Associated signs
  - Facial erythema, mild to moderate
  - Perioral pallor
  - Infraorbital fold (Dennie–Morgan fold)—atopic pleat

- Dry skin progressing to ichthyosis
- Increased palmar linear markings
- Pityriasis alba (hypopigmented asymptomatic areas on face and shoulders)
- Keratosis pilaris

DIFFERENTIAL DIAGNOSIS
- Photosensitivity rashes
- Contact dermatitis (especially if only the face is involved)
- Scabies
- Seborrheic dermatitis (especially in infants)
- Psoriasis or lichen simplex chronicus if only localized disease is present in adults
- Rare conditions of infancy
  - Histiocytosis X
  - Wiskott-Aldrich syndrome
  - Ataxia-telangiectasia syndrome
- Ichthyosis vulgaris

DIAGNOSTIC TESTS & INTERPRETATION
Initial Tests (lab, imaging)
- No test is diagnostic.
- Serum IgE levels are elevated in as many as 80% of affected individuals, but test is not routinely ordered or indicated.
- Eosinophilia tends to correlate with disease severity.
- Scoring AD (SCORAD) is a scoring system for AD, comprising scores for area, intensity, and subjective symptoms.

TREATMENT

GENERAL MEASURES
- Minimize flare-ups and control the duration and intensity of flare-up.
- Avoid agents that may cause irritation (e.g., wool, perfumes).
- Minimize sweating.
- Lukewarm (not hot) bathing. No evidence significantly guides frequency of bathing, but a minimum of twice weekly and when hygiene dictates for with postbath skin emollients.
- Avoid alkaline soaps. Use hypoallergenic cleansers with a slightly acidic (pH 5 to 6) with gentle mechanical removal of crusts, scale, and bacterial skin contaminants.
- Sun exposure may be helpful.
- Humidify the house.
- Avoid excessive contact with water.
- Avoid lotions that contain alcohol.
- If very resistant to treatment, search for a coexisting contact dermatitis.

Pediatric Considerations
Chronic potent fluorinated corticosteroid use may cause striae, hypopigmentation, or atrophy, especially in children.

MEDICATION

First Line

- Frequent systemic lubrication with thick emollient creams (e.g., Eucerin, Vaseline) over moist skin is the mainstay of treatment before any other intervention is considered. The "soak and seal" method is recommended.
- Infants and children: short-course and moderate-potency steroids such as hydrocortisone valerate 0.2% for flares followed by 0.5–1% topical hydrocortisone creams or ointments (Use the "fingertip unit [FTU]" dosing.)
- Adults: higher potency topical corticosteroids in areas other than face and skin folds
- Short-course, higher potency corticosteroids for flares; then, return to the lowest potency that will control dermatitis.
- Topical immunomodulators (tacrolimus or pimecrolimus) may be considered as first-line therapy for AD in children aged >2 years. They may be used in combination with topical corticosteroids (2).
- Antihistamines for pruritus (e.g., hydroxyzine 10 to 25 mg at bedtime and as needed); limited benefit as sole treatment

Second Line

- Crisaborole, a PDE-4 inhibitor, decreases itching, inflammation, excoriation, and lichenification. It is FDA-approved for moderate-to-severe AD in patients ≥3 months. It is a 2% topical ointment applied twice daily. It is expensive.
- Plastic occlusion in combination with topical medication to promote absorption (not to be used on face)
- Topical tricyclic doxepin, as a 5% cream, may decrease pruritus.
- Modified Goeckerman regimen (tar and ultraviolet light)
- Topical antibiotics promptly at the first sign of secondary skin infection
- Dupilumab, a biologic that targets mediators of inflammation (IL-22, IL-17, IFN-γ), is FDA-approved for moderate-severe AD in patients ≥6 months of age. It is injected weekly and is the only biologic agent approved for the treatment of AD. It is extremely expensive.
- American Academy of Dermatology's "choosing wisely" campaign recommends against routine antibiotic use unless there is clear evidence of secondary bacterial infection; use of oral/injectable corticosteroids; skin prick testing or radioallergosorbent blood testing (1)

ISSUES FOR REFERRAL

- Ophthalmology evaluation for persistent vernal conjunctivitis
- If using topical steroids around the eyes for extended periods, ophthalmology follow-up for cataract evaluation
- For consideration of systemic immunotherapy (cyclosporine, azathioprine, methotrexate) in the most severe cases and when associated mental health affects quality of life

ADDITIONAL THERAPIES

- Methods to reduce house-mite allergens (micropore filters on heating, ventilation, and air-conditioning systems; impermeable mattress covers)
- Behavioral relaxation therapy to reduce scratching
- Bleach baths may reduce staph colonization, but the definitive evidence for benefit in the condition is lacking. Recommend 1/2 cup of standard 6% household bleach for a full tub of water and soak for 5 to 10 minutes, blotting the skin dry upon leaving the bath.

COMPLEMENTARY & ALTERNATIVE MEDICINE

- Evening primrose oil (includes high content of fatty acids)
  - May decrease prostaglandin synthesis
  - May promote conversion of linoleic acid to ω-6 fatty acid
- Probiotics may reduce the severity of the condition, thus reducing the medication use.

 ONGOING CARE

FOLLOW-UP RECOMMENDATIONS

Patient Monitoring

Evaluate to ensure that secondary bacterial or fungal infection does not develop as a result of disruption of the skin barrier. Most patients with AD are colonized by *S. aureus*. There is a little evidence for the routine use of antimicrobial interventions to reduce skin bacteria, but the treatment of clinical infection with coverage for *S. aureus* is recommended.

DIET

- Trials of elimination may find certain "triggers" in some patients.
- Breastfeeding in conjunction with maternal hypoallergenic diets may decrease the severity in some infants (varying opinions).

PATIENT EDUCATION

- American Academy of Dermatology Association: http://www.aad.org/skin-conditions/dermatology -a-to-z/atopic-dermatitis
- National Eczema Association: www.nationaleczema.org

PROGNOSIS

- Chronic disease
- Declines with increasing age
- 90% of pediatric patients have spontaneous resolution by puberty.
- Localized eczema (e.g., chronic hand or foot dermatitis, eyelid dermatitis, or lichen simplex chronicus) may continue in some adults.

COMPLICATIONS

- Cataracts are more common in patients with AD.
- Skin infections (usually *S. aureus*); sometimes subclinical
- Eczema herpeticum
  - Generalized vesiculopustular eruption caused by infection with herpes simplex or vaccinia virus
  - Causes acute illness requiring hospitalization
- Atrophy and/or striae if fluorinated corticosteroids are used on face or skin folds
- Systemic absorption may occur if large areas of skin are treated, particularly if high-potency medications and occlusion are combined.

REFERENCES

1. Frazier W, Bhardwaj N. Atopic dermatitis: diagnosis and treatment. *Am Fam Physician*. 2020;101(10):590–598.
2. Berkey F, Wiedemer J. Atopic dermatitis: more than just a rash. *J Fam Pract*. 2021;70(1):13–19.

 SEE ALSO

Algorithm: Rash

 CODES

ICD10

- L20.9 Atopic dermatitis, unspecified
- L20.89 Other atopic dermatitis
- L20.83 Infantile (acute) (chronic) eczema

CLINICAL PEARLS

- Institute early and proactive treatment to reduce inflammation. Use the lowest potency topical steroid that controls symptoms.
- Monitor for secondary bacterial infection.
- Frequent systemic lubrication with thick emollient creams (e.g., Eucerin, Vaseline) over moist skin is the mainstay of treatment before any other intervention is considered.

DERMATITIS, CONTACT

Konstantinos E. Deligiannidis, MD, MPH, FAAFP

BASICS

DESCRIPTION
- A cutaneous reaction to an external substance
- Each type has a different mechanism, whereas the clinical presentation is the same (1).
- Primary irritant dermatitis (ID) is a result of direct damage to the stratum corneum by chemicals or physical agents that occurs faster than the skin is able to repair itself, which results in an inflammatory nonimmunologic cutaneous reaction. Prior sensitization is not required (2). ID occurs immediately or within 48 hours of exposure.
- Allergic contact dermatitis (ACD) affects only individuals previously sensitized to a substance. It represents a delayed hypersensitivity reaction, requiring several hours or days for the cascade of cellular immunity to manifest itself (2).
- System(s) affected: skin/exocrine
- Synonym(s): dermatitis venenata

EPIDEMIOLOGY
Common

Incidence
Occupational contact dermatitis accounts for up to 70% of occupational skin disease occurrences and affects 20.5/100,000 workers per year in one Australian study.

Prevalence
- Florists, hairdressers, cooks, beauticians, health care workers, and metal-working machine operators have the highest incidence.
- Predominant sex: male = female
  - Variations due to differences in exposure to offending agents as well as normal cutaneous variations between males and females (eccrine and sebaceous gland function and hair distribution)

Geriatric Considerations
Increased incidence of ID secondary to skin dryness

Pediatric Considerations
Increased incidence of positive patch testing due to better delayed hypersensitivity reactions (3)

ETIOLOGY AND PATHOPHYSIOLOGY
Hypersensitivity reaction to a substance generating cellular immunity response
- Plants
  - Urushiol (allergen): poison ivy, poison oak, poison sumac
  - Primary contact: plant (roots/stems/leaves)
  - Secondary contact: clothes/fingernails (not blister fluid—the established eruption is not itself contagious or transmissible)

- Chemicals
  - Nickel: jewelry, zippers, hooks, and watches (4)
  - Potassium dichromate: tanning agent in leather
  - Paraphenylenediamine: hair dyes, fur dyes, and industrial chemicals
  - Turpentine: cleaning agents, polishes, and waxes
  - Soaps and detergents
- Topical medicines
  - Neomycin: topical antibiotics
  - Thimerosal (Merthiolate): preservative in topical medications
  - Anesthetics: benzocaine
  - Parabens: preservative in topical medications
  - Formalin: cosmetics, shampoos, and nail enamel

Genetics
Increased frequency of ACD in families with allergies

RISK FACTORS
- Occupation
- Hobbies
- Travel
- Cosmetics
- Jewelry

GENERAL PREVENTION
- Avoid causative agents.
- Use of protective gloves (with cotton lining) may be helpful.

DIAGNOSIS

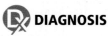

HISTORY
- Itchy rash
- Assess for prior exposure to irritating substance.

PHYSICAL EXAM
- Acute
  - Papules, vesicles, bullae with surrounding erythema
  - Crusting and oozing
  - Pruritus
- Chronic
  - Erythematous base
  - Thickening with lichenification
  - Scaling
  - Fissuring
- Distribution
  - Where epidermis is thinner (eyelids, genitalia)
  - Areas of contact with offending agent (e.g., nail polish)
  - Palms and soles relatively more resistant, although hand dermatitis is common
  - Deeper skin folds spared

- Linear arrays of lesions
- Lesions with sharp borders and sharp angles are pathognomonic.
- Well-demarcated area with a papulovesicular rash

DIFFERENTIAL DIAGNOSIS
- Based on clinical impression
  - Appearance, periodicity, and localization
- Groups of vesicles
  - Herpes simplex
- Diffuse bullous or vesicular lesions
  - Bullous pemphigoid
- Photodistribution
  - Phototoxic/allergic reaction to systemic allergen
- Eyelids
  - Seborrheic dermatitis
- Scaly eczematous lesions
  - Atopic dermatitis
  - Nummular eczema
  - Lichen simplex chronicus
  - Stasis dermatitis
  - Xerosis
- ID reaction (see chapter "ID Reaction")

DIAGNOSTIC TESTS & INTERPRETATION
Diagnostic Procedures/Other
Consider patch tests for suspected allergic trigger (systemic corticosteroids or recent, aggressive use of topical steroids may alter results).

Test Interpretation
- Intercellular edema
- Bullae

TREATMENT

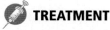

GENERAL MEASURES
- Identify and remove offending agent (5)[C]:
  - Avoidance
  - Work modification
  - Protective clothing
  - Barrier creams, especially high-lipid content moisturizing creams (e.g., Keri lotion, petrolatum, coconut oil)
- Topical soaks with cool tap water, Burow solution (1:40 dilution), saline (1 tsp/pt water), or silver nitrate solution
- Lukewarm water baths
- Aveeno oatmeal baths
- Emollients (white petrolatum, Eucerin)

MEDICATION

First Line

- Topical medications (4)[C]
  - Lotion of zinc oxide, talc, menthol 0.15% (Gold Bond), phenol 0.5%
  - Corticosteroids for ACD as well as ID
    - High-potency steroids: fluocinonide (Lidex) 0.05% gel, cream, or ointment TID–QID
    - Use high-potency steroids only for a short time and then switch to low- or medium-potency steroid cream or ointment. Avoid long-term daily use (6)[C].
    - Caution regarding face/skin folds: Use lower potency steroids (4)[C] and avoid prolonged usage. Switch to lower potency topical steroid once the acute phase is resolved.
- Calamine lotion for symptomatic relief
- Topical antibiotics for secondary infection (bacitracin, erythromycin)
- Systemic
  - Antihistamine
    - Hydroxyzine: 25 to 50 mg PO QID, especially useful for itching
    - Diphenhydramine: 25 to 50 mg PO QID
    - Cetirizine: 10 mg PO BID–TID
- Corticosteroids
  - Prednisone: Taper starting at 60 to 80 mg/day PO, over 10 to 14 days, occasionally 21 days.
  - Used for moderate to severe cases, particularly involving face or genitals
  - Little published evidence to compare appropriate length of treatment, but clinical experience suggests that short courses of therapy (i.e., 5 to 7 days) are not adequate to prevent rebound dermatitis.
  - Treatment for up to 21 days for severe/extensive rash resulting from exposure to potent allergens like urushiol (e.g., poison ivy) is commonly recommended to prevent reemergence of dermatitis on taper (rebound), although 14 days is usually adequate.
  - May use burst dose of steroids for up to 5 days for less persistent immunogens or less severe dermatitis
- Antibiotics for secondary skin infections
  - Dicloxacillin: 250 to 500 mg PO QID for 7 to 10 days
  - Amoxicillin-clavulanate: 500 mg PO BID for 7 to 10 days
  - Cephalexin: 500 mg PO QID for 7 to 10 days
  - Trimethoprim-sulfamethoxazole (Bactrim DS): 160 mg/800 mg (1 tablet) PO BID for 7 to 10 days (suspected resistant *Staphylococcus aureus*)
- Precautions
  - Antihistamines may cause drowsiness.
  - Prolonged use of potent topical steroids may cause local skin effects (atrophy, stria, telangiectasia).
  - Use tapering dose of oral steroids if using >5 days.

Second Line

Other topical or systemic antibiotics, depending on organisms and sensitivity

Pregnancy Considerations

Usual caution with medications

ISSUES FOR REFERRAL

May need referral to a dermatologist or allergist if refractory to conventional treatment

COMPLEMENTARY & ALTERNATIVE MEDICINE

The use of complementary and alternative treatment is a supplement and not an alternative to conventional treatment.

ADMISSION, INPATIENT, AND NURSING CONSIDERATIONS

Rarely needs hospital admission

 ONGOING CARE

FOLLOW-UP RECOMMENDATIONS

Stay active, but avoid overheating.

Patient Monitoring

- As necessary for recurrence
- Patch testing for etiology after resolved

DIET

No special diet

PATIENT EDUCATION

- Avoidance of irritating substance
- Cleaning of secondary sources (nails, clothes)
- Fallacy of blister fluid spreading disease

PROGNOSIS

- Self-limited
- Benign
- 55% of patients still had contact dermatitis at 2 years after diagnosis.
- Improvement in rash less likely for those who remain in the same or similar profession
- Increased length of exposure and atopy are poor prognostic indicators.

COMPLICATIONS

- Generalized eruption secondary to autosensitization
- Secondary bacterial infection

REFERENCES

1. Al-Otaibi ST, Alqahtani HAM. Management of contact dermatitis. *J Dermatol Dermatol Surg*. 2015;19(2):86–91.
2. Tan CH, Rasool S, Johnston GA. Contact dermatitis: allergic and irritant. *Clin Dermatol*. 2014;32(1):116–124.
3. Admani S, Jacob SE. Allergic contact dermatitis in children: review of the past decade. *Curr Allergy Asthma Rep*. 2014;14(4):421.

4. Usatine RP, Riojas M. Diagnosis and management of contact dermatitis. *Am Fam Physician*. 2010;82(3):249–255.
5. Fonacier L, Bernstein DI, Pacheco K, et al; for American Academy of Allergy, Asthma & Immunology; American College of Allergy, Asthma & Immunology; and Joint Council of Allergy, Asthma & Immunology. Contact dermatitis: a practice parameter-update 2015. *J Allergy Clin Immunol Pract*. 2015;3(3 Suppl):S1–S39.
6. Nassau S, Fonacier L. Allergic contact dermatitis. *Med Clin North Am*. 2020;104(1):61–76.

ADDITIONAL READING

- Pelletier JL, Perez C, Jacob SE. Contact dermatitis in pediatrics. *Pediatr Ann*. 2016;45(8):e287–e292.
- Rashid RS, Shim TN. Contact dermatitis. *BMJ*. 2016;353:i3299.

 SEE ALSO

Algorithm: Rash

 CODES

ICD10

- L25.9 Unspecified contact dermatitis, unspecified cause
- L23.9 Allergic contact dermatitis, unspecified cause
- L25.5 Unspecified contact dermatitis due to plants, except food

CLINICAL PEARLS

- Commonly occurs on hands and face
- Anyone exposed to irritants or allergic substances is predisposed to contact dermatitis, especially in occupations that have high exposure to chemicals.
- The most common allergens causing contact dermatitis are plants of the *Toxicodendron* genus (poison ivy, poison oak, poison sumac).
- Poison-ivy dermatitis typically requires 10 to 14 days (occasionally more) of topical or oral steroid therapy to prevent recurrent eruption.
- Worldwide, nickel is the number one patch-tested allergen causing ACD.
- The usual treatment for contact dermatitis is avoidance of the allergen or irritating substance and temporary use of topical steroids.
- A contact dermatitis eruption presents in a nondermatomal geographic fashion due to the skin being in contact with an external source.

DERMATITIS, DIAPER
Dennis E. Hughes, DO, FACEP

 BASICS

DESCRIPTION
- Diaper dermatitis is a rash occurring under the covered area of a diaper (named for typical location, not etiology). It is usually initially a contact irritant dermatitis but can be caused by or contributed by systemic conditions.
- Rarely, a serious condition, but patient discomfort and caregiver anxiety are considerations.
- System(s) affected: skin/exocrine
- Synonym(s): diaper rash; nappy rash; napkin dermatitis

Geriatric Considerations
Incontinence is a significant cofactor in the elderly population.

EPIDEMIOLOGY
Incidence
- The most common dermatitis is found in infancy.
- Peak incidence: 7 to 12 months of age and then decreases
- Lower incidence is reported in breastfed babies due to lower pH, urease, protease, and lipase activity.

Prevalence
Prevalence has been variably reported from 4–35% in the first 2 years of life. Upward of 75% of infants will have episodes of varying duration and severity in United States. Severity varies: 58% slight symptoms; 34% moderate; 8% severe. Underreporting contributes to difficulty in determining impact of condition.

ETIOLOGY AND PATHOPHYSIOLOGY
- Immature infant skin with histologic, biochemical, functional differences compared to mature skin
- Wet skin is central in the development of diaper dermatitis, as prolonged contact with urine or feces results in susceptibility to chemical, enzymatic, and physical injury; wet skin is also penetrated more easily.
- Fecal proteases and lipases are irritants.
- Superhydrase urease enzyme found in the stratum corneum liberates ammonia from cutaneous bacteria.
- Fecal lipase and protease activity are increased by acceleration of GI transit; thus, a higher incidence of irritant diaper dermatitis is observed in babies who have had diarrhea in the previous 48 hours.

- Once the skin is compromised, secondary infection by *Candida albicans* is common. 40–75% of diaper rashes that last >3 days are colonized with *C. albicans*.
- Bacteria may play a role in diaper dermatitis through reduction of fecal pH and resulting activation of enzymes.
- Allergy is exceedingly rare as a cause in infants.

RISK FACTORS
- Infrequent diaper changes
- Improper laundering (cloth diapers)
- Family history of dermatitis
- Hot, humid weather
- Recent treatment with oral antibiotics
- Diarrhea (>3 stools per day increases the risk.)
- Dye allergy
- Eczema may increase the risk.

GENERAL PREVENTION
Most effectively managed by prevention including rigorous attention to hygiene

COMMONLY ASSOCIATED CONDITIONS
- Contact (allergic or irritant) dermatitis
- Seborrheic dermatitis
- Psoriasis
- Candidiasis
- Atopic dermatitis

 DIAGNOSIS

Correct diagnosis is key. The initial presentation of diseases other than contact irritant dermatitis may be in the diaper area. Avoid assuming that all diaper-area dermatitis is simple contact/irritant dermatitis by performing an appropriate general skin examination.

HISTORY
- Onset, duration, and change in the nature of the rash
- Presence of rashes outside the diaper area
- Associated scratching or crying
- Contact with infants with a similar rash
- Recent illness, diarrhea, or antibiotic use
- Fever
- Pustular drainage
- Lymphangitis

PHYSICAL EXAM
- Mild forms consist of shiny erythema ± scale.
- Margins are not always evident.
- Moderate cases have areas of papules, vesicles, and small superficial erosions.
- It can progress to well-demarcated ulcerated nodules that measure ≥1 cm in diameter.
- It is found on the prominent parts of the buttocks, medial thighs, mons pubis, and scrotum.
- Skin folds are spared or involved last (skin fold involvement suggests secondary infection with candida sp or *Staphylococcus aureus*).
- *Tidemark dermatitis* refers to the bandlike form of erythema of irritated diaper margins.
- Diaper dermatitis can cause an id reaction (autoeczematous) outside the diaper area.

DIFFERENTIAL DIAGNOSIS
- Contact dermatitis
- Seborrheic dermatitis
- Candidiasis
- Atopic dermatitis
- Scabies
- Acrodermatitis enteropathica (deficiency in zinc)
- Letterer-Siwe disease
- Congenital syphilis
- Child abuse
- Streptococcal/staphylococcal infection
- Kawasaki disease
- Biotin deficiency
- Psoriasis
- HIV infection

DIAGNOSTIC TESTS & INTERPRETATION
Initial Tests (lab, imaging)
Rarely needed

Follow-Up Tests & Special Considerations
- Consider a culture of lesions or a potassium hydroxide (KOH) preparation.
- The finding of anemia in association with hepatosplenomegaly and the appropriate rash may suggest a diagnosis of Langerhans cell histiocytosis or congenital syphilis.
- Finding mites, ova, or feces on a mineral oil preparation of a burrow scraping can confirm the diagnosis of scabies.

Test Interpretation
- The need for biopsy is rare.
- Histology may reveal acute, subacute, or chronic spongiotic dermatitis.

 TREATMENT

Prevention is the key to treatment of this condition.

GENERAL MEASURES
- Expose the buttocks to air as much as possible.
- Use mild, slightly acidic or neutral pH cleanser with water; no rubbing and pat dry.
- Avoid impermeable waterproof pants during treatment (day or night); they keep the skin wet and subject to rash or infection.
- Change diapers frequently, even at night, if the rash is extensive.
- Superabsorbent diapers are beneficial (1), as they wick urine away from skin and still allow air to permeate. Manufacturer-associated data indicate diapers with a mesh-like top sheet construction may be superior in allowing stool to separate from skin.
- Discontinue using baby lotion, powder, ointment, or baby oil (except zinc oxide).
- The use of appropriately formulated baby wipes (alcohol and fragrance-free) is safe and as effective as water. Those baby wipes are commercially marketed as safe for sensitive skin appear to be generally equally effective.
- Apply zinc oxide ointment (1) or other barrier cream to the rash at the earliest sign and BID or TID (e.g., Desitin or Balmex). Thereafter, apply to clean, thoroughly dried skin.
- Cornstarch can reduce friction. Avoid talcum-containing products.

MEDICATION
First Line
- For a pure contact dermatitis, a low-potency topical steroid (hydrocortisone 0.5–1% TID for 3 to 5 days) and removal of the offending agent (urine, feces) should suffice.
- If candidiasis is suspected or diaper rash persists, use an antifungal such as miconazole nitrate 2% cream, miconazole powder, econazole (Spectazole), clotrimazole (Lotrimin), or ketoconazole (Nizoral) cream at each diaper change. Candida superinfection is common in persistent dermatitis in the moist diaper area.

- If inflammation is prominent, consider a very low-potency steroid cream such as hydrocortisone 0.5–1% TID along with an antifungal cream ± a combination product such as clioquinol–hydrocortisone (Vioform–Hydrocortisone) cream.
- If a secondary bacterial infection is suspected, use an antistaphylococcal oral antibiotic or mupirocin (Bactroban) ointment topically.
- Precautions: Avoid high- or moderate-potency steroids often found in combination of steroid antifungal mixtures—these should never be used in the diaper area.

Second Line
- Sucralfate paste for resistant cases
- Recent study suggests that the use of hydrocolloid dressings can speed the healing of rash.
- Case reports support the use of immune modulators such as topical tacrolimus (0.03%) in refractory cases; however, it is not approved for children <2 year of age. Recent literature review by American Academy of Allergy and American College of Allergy found no findings to suggest harm.

ISSUES FOR REFERRAL
Consider if a systemic disease such as Langerhans cell histiocytosis, acrodermatitis enteropathica, or HIV infection is suspected.

ADMISSION, INPATIENT, AND NURSING CONSIDERATIONS
- Admission criteria/initial stabilization
  - Febrile neonates
  - Recalcitrant rash suggestive of immunodeficiency
  - Toxic-appearing infants
- Assist first-time parents with hygiene education.

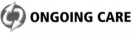 **ONGOING CARE**

FOLLOW-UP RECOMMENDATIONS
Patient Monitoring
Recheck weekly until clear and then at times of recurrence.

PATIENT EDUCATION
Patient education is vital to the treatment and prevention of recurrent cases.

PROGNOSIS
- Quick, complete clearing with appropriate treatment
- Secondary candidal infections may last a few weeks after treatment has begun.

COMPLICATIONS
- Secondary bacterial infection (Consider community-acquired methicillin-resistant *S. aureus* [MRSA] in pustular dermatitis that does not respond to normal therapy.)
- Rare complication is inoculation with group A β-hemolytic *Streptococcus* resulting in necrotizing fasciitis.
- Secondary yeast infection

REFERENCE
1. Burdall O, Willgress L, Goad N. Neonatal skin care: developments in care to maintain neonatal barrier function and prevention of diaper dermatitis. *Pediatr Dermatol*. 2019;36(1):31–35.

ADDITIONAL READING
Chadha A, Jahnke M. Common neonatal rashes. *Pediatr Ann*. 2019;48(1):e16–e22.

 SEE ALSO

Algorithm: Rash

 CODES

ICD10
- L22 Diaper dermatitis
- B37.2 Candidiasis of skin and nail

CLINICAL PEARLS
- Hygiene is the main preventative measure.
- Look for secondary infection in persistent cases (especially candida and Staph sp).

D

DERMATITIS, SEBORRHEIC
Shane L. Larson, MD • Briana Lindberg, MD, CAQSM

 BASICS

DESCRIPTION
Chronic, superficial, recurrent inflammatory skin disorder affecting sebum-rich, hairy regions of the body, especially the scalp, eyebrows, and face and to lesser extent, chest, and back

EPIDEMIOLOGY
Incidence
- Predominant age: adolescence, followed by infancy and adulthood (1)
- Predominant sex: male > female

Prevalence
- Affects 2–5% of the global population; up to 83% in immunosuppressed, HIV-positive individuals (2)
- Infantile seborrheic dermatitis (SD) is common in the first 3 months of life, affecting all ethnicities in all climates.

ETIOLOGY AND PATHOPHYSIOLOGY
- Skin surface yeast such as *Malassezia* may be a contributing factor.
- Genetic and environmental factors: Flares are common with stress/illness.
- Parallels increased sebaceous gland activity in infancy and adolescence or as a result of some acnegenic drugs.
- SD is more common in immunosuppressed patients, suggesting that immune mechanisms are implicated in the pathogenesis of the disease, although the mechanisms are not well-defined.

Genetics
Positive family history; no genetic markers have been identified to date.

RISK FACTORS
- Immunosuppressed conditions such as HIV/AIDS (2)
- Parkinson disease, neurologic disorders, facial paralysis (1)
- Emotional stress (2)
- Obesity (2)
- Oily skin (2)
- Acne (2)
- Down syndrome (1)
- Medications may cause flares/induce SD: buspirone, chlorpromazine, cimetidine, ethionamide, griseofulvin, haloperidol, interferon-α, methyldopa, psoralen, and IL-2 (2).

GENERAL PREVENTION
Seborrheic skin should be washed more often than usual to soften the affected areas.

COMMONLY ASSOCIATED CONDITIONS
- Parkinson disease
- HIV/AIDS
- Facial paralysis
- Down syndrome

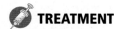 **DIAGNOSIS**

Diagnosis of SD is usually made by history and physical exam. If unclear, a punch biopsy of the skin will confirm the diagnosis.

HISTORY
- Intermittent active phases manifest with burning, scaling, and itching, alternating with inactive periods; activity is increased in winter and early spring, with remissions commonly occurring in summer.
- Infants
  - Cradle cap: greasy scaling of the scalp with occasional erythema
  - Diaper and/or axillary rash
  - Age of onset: ~1 month
  - Usually self-resolves by 8 to 12 months
- Adults
  - Red, greasy, scaling rash consisting of macules and plaques with indistinct margins
  - Red, smooth, glazed appearance in skin folds
  - Hypopigmented, scaling macules on skin of color
  - Minimal pruritus
  - Chronic waxing and waning course
  - Bilateral and symmetric
  - Most commonly located in hairy skin areas: scalp and scalp margins, eyebrows and eyelid margins, nasolabial folds, ears and retroauricular folds, presternal area, middle to upper back, buttock crease, inguinal area, genitals, and armpits

PHYSICAL EXAM
- Scalp appearance varies from mild, patchy scaling to widespread, thick, adherent crusts. Plaques are rare.
- SD can spread onto the forehead, the posterior part of the neck, and the postauricular skin, as in psoriasis.
- Skin lesions manifest as brawny or yellow greasy scaling over red, inflamed skin.
- Hypopigmentation can be seen in skin tones of color.
- Infectious eczematoid dermatitis, with oozing and crusting, suggests secondary infection.
- Seborrheic blepharitis may occur independently.

DIFFERENTIAL DIAGNOSIS
- Atopic dermatitis: Distinction may be difficult in infants.
- Psoriasis
  - More common on the extensor surfaces of the knees and elbows, and the nail beds are usually involved.
  - Scalp psoriasis will be more sharply demarcated than SD with crusted, infiltrated plaques rather than mild scaling and erythema.
- *Candida*
- Tinea cruris/capitis: Suspect these when usual medications fail or hair loss occurs.
- Eczema of auricle/otitis externa
- Rosacea
- Discoid lupus erythematosus: Skin biopsy will be beneficial.
- Histiocytosis X: may appear as seborrheic-like eruption
- Dandruff: scalp only, noninflammatory
- Drug eruption

DIAGNOSTIC TESTS & INTERPRETATION
Diagnostic Procedures/Other
- Consider biopsy if:
  - Usual therapies fail.
  - Petechiae are noted.
  - Histiocytosis X is suspected.
- Consider fungal cultures if:
  - Refractory to treatment
  - Pustules and alopecia are present.

Test Interpretation
Nonspecific changes
- Hyperkeratosis, acanthosis, accentuated rete ridges, focal spongiosis, and parakeratosis are characteristic.
- Parakeratotic scale around hair follicles and mild superficial inflammatory lymphocytic infiltrate

TREATMENT

GENERAL MEASURES
- Increase frequency of shampooing.
- Sunlight in moderate doses may be helpful.
- Infants (cradle cap)
  - As above, increasing frequency of shampooing with a mild, nonmedicated shampoo may help.
  - Remove thick scale by applying warm mineral oil and then wash off 1 hour later with a mild soap and a soft-bristle toothbrush or terrycloth washcloth.
- Adults
  - Wash all affected areas with antiseborrheic shampoos. Start with over-the-counter products (i.e., selenium sulfide), allowing shampoo/lotion to remain on the skin for several minutes before washing off, and increase to more potent preparations (those containing coal tar, sulfur, or salicylic acid) if no improvement is noted.
  - For dense scalp scaling, 10% liquor carbonic detergents in Nivea oil may be used at bedtime, covering the head with a shower cap. This should be done nightly for 1 to 3 weeks.

MEDICATION
First Line
- Cradle cap: Use a coal tar shampoo or ketoconazole shampoo if the nonmedicated shampoo is ineffective. Massage in and keep on for several minutes before removing.
- Adults
  - Topical antifungal agents
    - Ketoconazole 2% or miconazole 2% shampoo twice a week (allow to remain on scalp for several minutes before washing off) for clearance and then once a week or every other week for maintenance (2)[A]
    - Ketoconazole 2% or sertaconazole 2% cream may be used to clear scales in other areas (2)[A].
    - Ciclopirox 1% shampoo twice weekly (2)[A]
    - Facial hair can also be treated with ketoconazole 2% shampoo.

– Topical corticosteroids
  - Begin with 1% hydrocortisone and advance to more potent (fluorinated) steroid preparations daily for 2 to 4 weeks (1)[C].
    - Avoid continuous use of potent steroids to reduce the risk of skin atrophy, hypopigmentation, and/or systemic absorption (especially in infants, children, and elderly).
    - Precautions: Fluorinated corticosteroids and higher concentrations of hydrocortisone (e.g., 2.5%) may cause atrophy or striae if used on the face or on skin folds.
– Other topical agents
  - Coal tar 1% shampoo twice a week
  - Selenium sulfide 2.5% shampoo twice a week
  - Zinc pyrithione 1% shampoo twice a week
  - Lithium gluconate/succinate 8% ointment/gel twice a week (1)
- Once controlled, washing with zinc soaps or using selenium sulfide lotion with periodic use of steroid cream may help to maintain remission.

Second Line
- Calcineurin inhibitors (3)[C] (not linked to skin atrophy and hypopigmentation; just as effective as topical steroids; potentially more side effects)
  – Pimecrolimus 1% cream BID
  – Tacrolimus 0.1% ointment
- Systemic antifungal therapy
  – For severe or recalcitrant SD (1)
    - Terbinafine: 250 mg/day × 4 to 6 weeks or pulse therapy 250 mg/day × 12 days per month for 3 months (1)[C]
    - Itraconazole: 200 mg/day, effective with good safety profile (1)[C]
      - Daily regimen for 1 week followed by 2 days per month for the following 2 months *or*
      - 150 to 200 mg/day once a week for a period of 2 to 3 months
    - Monitor potential hepatotoxic effects.
- Low-molecular-weight hyaluronic acid (1)
  – Hyaluronic acid sodium salt gel 0.2% BID

ISSUES FOR REFERRAL
- No response to first-line therapy and concerns regarding systemic illness (e.g., HIV)
- Resistant SD in adults should prompt testing for HIV.

COMPLEMENTARY & ALTERNATIVE MEDICINE
- Honey, antifungal, antioxidant and antibacterial: effective in remission and prevention of relapses of SD (3)
- Aloe vera, anti-inflammatory and antifungal: reduction in pruritus and scaling associated with SD (3)

- Borage oil containing essential amino acid γ-lineolic acid (GLA): may be effective in infantile SD (3)
- Tea-tree essential oil, antifungal, anti-inflammatory and antioxidant: effective in mild to moderate cases (3)
- Quassia amara extract, anti-inflammatory and antifungal, especially against *Malassezia* yeast: outperformed topical 2% ketoconazole and 1% ciclopiroxolamine (3)

ONGOING CARE

Individuals with coiled hair or hair that is heated and/or chemically treated will need less drying agents to prevent hair breakage compared to those with straighter hair who may prefer drying agents. Applying shampoos and other topical treatments directly to scalp instead of hair shaft can decrease the risk of hair damage.

FOLLOW-UP RECOMMENDATIONS
Patient Monitoring
Every 2 to 12 weeks depending on the disease severity and the patient's response to therapy

PATIENT EDUCATION
Seborrheic dermatitis: http://familydoctor.org/familydoctor/en/diseases-conditions/seborrheic-dermatitis.html

PROGNOSIS
- In infants, SD usually remits after 6 to 8 months.
- In adults, SD is usually chronic and relapsing, with exacerbations and remissions. The disease is usually controlled with shampoos and topical steroids.
- Erythema or hypopigmentation typically resolves with treatment (1).

COMPLICATIONS
- Skin atrophy/striae are possible from fluorinated corticosteroids, especially if used on the face.
- Glaucoma and/or cataracts can result from use of fluorinated steroids around the eyes.
- Photosensitivity is caused occasionally by tar-containing products.
- Herpes keratitis is a rare complication of herpes simplex: Instruct the patient to stop eyelid steroids if herpes simplex develops.

REFERENCES

1. Dall'Oglio F, Nasca MR, Gerbino C, et al. An overview of the diagnosis and management of seborrheic dermatitis. *Clin Cosmet Investig Dermatol*. 2022;15:1537–1548.
2. Okokon EO, Verbeek JH, Ruotsalainen JH, et al. Topical antifungals for seborrhoeic dermatitis. *Cochrane Database Syst Rev*. 2015;(5):CD008138.
3. Borda LJ, Perper M, Keri JE. Treatment of seborrheic dermatitis: a comprehensive review. *J Dermatolog Treat*. 2019;30(2):158–169.

ADDITIONAL READING

- Victoire A, Magin P, Coughlan J, et al. Interventions for infantile seborrhoeic dermatitis (including cradle cap). *Cochrane Database Syst Rev*. 2019;3(3):CD011380.
- Kastarinen H, Oksanen T, Okokon EO, et al. Topical anti-inflammatory agents for seborrhoeic dermatitis of the face or scalp. *Cochrane Database Syst Rev*. 2014;(5):CD009446.

SEE ALSO

Algorithm: Rash

CODES

ICD10
- L21.9 Seborrheic dermatitis, unspecified
- L21.1 Seborrheic infantile dermatitis
- L21.0 Seborrhea capitis

CLINICAL PEARLS
- Search for an underlying systemic disease in a patient who is unresponsive to usual therapy.
- In infants, SD is usually self-limited.
- In adults, SD is usually chronic, with exacerbations and remissions. Disease is usually easily controlled with shampoos and topical steroids.

DERMATITIS, STASIS
Pooja Mira Jayaprakash, MD

BASICS

DESCRIPTION
- Chronic, eczematous, scaling, erythematous plaques, and patches to the lower extremities accompanied by cycle of scratching, excoriations, weeping, crusting, and inflammation in patients with chronic venous insufficiency (CVI) and edema; clinical skin manifestation of CVI usually appears late in the disease; may present as a solitary lesion most often starting on medial ankle; can be associated with venous leg ulcers on bony prominences
- System(s) affected: skin/exocrine
- Synonym(s): gravitational eczema; varicose eczema; venous dermatitis

EPIDEMIOLOGY
Incidence
In the United States: common in patients aged >50 years (6–7%); predominant age: adult, geriatric; predominant sex: female > male

Geriatric Considerations
Common in this age group: estimated to affect 15 to 20 million patients aged >50 years in the United States

ETIOLOGY AND PATHOPHYSIOLOGY
- Due to venous hypertension from venous incompetence (valve dysfunction and reflux) or obstruction (thrombosis or stenosis) of superficial, perforating, or deep veins
- Inflammatory changes include microvascular abnormalities (leaking capillaries with fibrin cuffs, thickened venules, microthrombosis) and increased leukocytes (macrophages, T lymphocytes, mast cells).
- Usually with chronic dependent edema; inflamed, edematous skin may be more susceptible to trauma.
- Itch may be caused by inflammatory mediators (from mast cells, monocytes, macrophages, or neutrophils) liberated in the microcirculation and endothelium. Abnormal leukocyte–endothelium interaction is proposed to be a major factor. A cascade of biochemical events leads to ulceration.

Genetics
Familial link probable

RISK FACTORS
- Atopy, chronic edema, superimposition of itch–scratch cycle
- Old age, obesity
- Cigarette use
- Previous DVT, previous pregnancy, hx vein stripping, vein harvesting for coronary artery bypass graft surgery
- Prolonged standing
- Trauma
- Low-protein diet
- High-estrogen states
- Genetic propensity (familial history of congenital disease)

GENERAL PREVENTION
- Treat lower extremity edema with compression stockings, exercise, and leg elevation. This will mobilize the interstitial lymphatic fluid from the region of stasis dermatitis and also following DVT.

- Consider early treatment of venous insufficiency with specialist care and interventional procedures as indicated.
- Use topical emollients twice a day to prevent fissuring and itching.

COMMONLY ASSOCIATED CONDITIONS
Varicose veins, venous insufficiency, other eczematous disease, hyperhomocysteinemia, venous HTN

DIAGNOSIS

HISTORY
- Skin itching, pain, and burning may precede visible skin changes.
- Lower extremity edema (often initially around ankles) preceding skin eruption, insidious onset, usually bilateral
- Description may include aching/heavy legs.
- Erythema and scaling of lower extremities with later development of hyperpigmentation
- Symptoms may worsen in the evening with dependent edema

PHYSICAL EXAM
- Evaluation of the lower extremities characteristically reveals:
  - Bilateral scaly, eczematous patches, papules, and/or plaques
  - Violaceous (sometimes brown), erythematous lesions due to deoxygenation of venous blood (postinflammatory hyperpigmentation and hemosiderin deposition within the cutaneous tissue)
- Distribution: medial aspect of ankle, with frequent extension onto the foot and lower leg, occasionally lateral side of ankle
- Early signs include prominent superficial veins and pitting ankle edema.
- Brawny induration, swelling, and warmth
- Venous ulcers (frequently accompany stasis dermatitis) often over bony prominences secondary to minor trauma; varicosities are often associated with ulcers.
- In later stages excoriations, weeping, and crusting
- Skin changes are more common in the lower 1/3 of the extremity and medially.
- May present as a solitary lesion mimicking a neoplasm
- Can present with comorbid atrophie blanche (hypopigmented patches with punctate red from microthrombosis) and/or lipodermatosclerosis (fibrosing panniculitis which can bind skin to subcutaneous tissues)
- May also develop contact sensitization to topical agents locally and/or autosensitization dermatitis (similar skin changes at a remote cutaneous site)

DIFFERENTIAL DIAGNOSIS
- Other eczematous diseases: atopic dermatitis, uremic dermatitis, contact dermatitis (due to topical agents used to self-treat), neurodermatitis, arterial insufficiency, sickle cell disease causing skin ulceration, cellulitis, erysipelas
- Tinea dermatophyte infection
- Pretibial myxedema
- Nummular eczema

- Lichen simplex chronicus
- Xerosis
- Asteatotic eczema
- Amyopathic dermatomyositis
- Psoriasis
- Actinic keratoses
- Skin cancer (squamous or basal cell carcinoma, rarely can mimic Kaposi sarcoma)

DIAGNOSTIC TESTS & INTERPRETATION
Initial Tests (lab, imaging)
Duplex ultrasound (US) imaging helps establish diagnosis and location(s) of venous insufficiency.

Follow-Up Tests & Special Considerations
- Can consider cross-sectional (CT or MR) venography if equivocal US results; be aware that these are performed with contrast.
- Special consideration: Skin biopsy may help confirm stasis dermatitis in unclear cases; however, perform with extreme caution due to possibility of co-existing arterial insufficiency, which could result in nonhealing wound at biopsy site.

Diagnostic Procedures/Other
- Rule out arterial insufficiency. Check peripheral pulses; ankle brachial pressure index (ABPI or ABI)
- Screen for diabetes.
- Interventionalist may perform catheter-based venography to verify venous outflow obstruction prior to procedural management.

Test Interpretation
- Duplex US retrograde/reversed flow >0.5 second is diagnostic of reflux in superficial/perforating veins.
- Duplex US retrograde/reversed flow >1 second is diagnostic of reflux in deep veins.
- ABPI <0.8 is suggestive of arterial insufficiency.
- ABPI can be elevated, >1.2 in diabetic patients and others with distal small vessel calcifications.
- Arterial duplex US and angiography are the gold standards for arterial insufficiency diagnosis.

TREATMENT

GENERAL MEASURES
Primary role of treatment is to reverse effects of venous HTN. Appropriate care:
- Outpatient:
  - Reduce edema:
    - Leg elevation: legs above the level of heart for 30 minutes, 3 to 4 times daily; avoid prolonged dependent position.
    - Compression therapy: This is the mainstay of treatment of venous stasis ± ulcers. Compression bandages can be safely applied in patients with ABI of 0.8 to 1.2.
    - Elastic bandage wraps: Ace bandages or Unna paste boot (zinc gelatin) or compression stockings
    - Graduated elastic compression of 30 to 40 mm Hg at the ankle improves ulcer healing rate and may prevent ulcer recurrence (1)[A].

○ Compression bandages containing both elastic and inelastic components (mixed component systems) are as effective as four-layer bandages, are easier to apply, and have less slippage and associated with favorable quality of life outcomes.

○ High compression is contraindicated in arterial insufficiency.

○ Pneumatic compression devices are beneficial, especially in nonambulatory patients and those with a component of arterial insufficiency (2)[B].

- Improvement of lipodermatosclerosis:
  – Activity:
    ○ Avoid standing still for prolonged periods.
    ○ Stay active and exercise regularly.
    ○ Elevate foot of bed unless contraindicated.
- Inpatient, for endovascular radiofrequency ablation, vein stripping, sclerotherapy, or skin grafts:
  – Venous ulcer treatment: Treat infection: Débride the ulcer base of necrotic tissue (surgical necrotomy if possible, or enzymatic débridement with collagenase).

  ○ Autolytic: Modern wound dressings (hydrogel, hydrocolloids, alginate, foam bandages, plain nonadherent dressing) are better than traditional wet to dry dressing because they maintain moist wound environment, with less tissue damage on removal, and less frequent changing requirement (2)[A]. However, there is no difference in healing rate of venous stasis ulcers by use of hydrocolloid dressing versus simple nonadherent dressing when used beneath compression.

  ○ Biologic: Topical application of granulocyte-macrophage colony-stimulating factor promotes healing of ulcers (insufficient evidence).

  ○ Mechanical: wet to dry dressings, hydrotherapy, and irrigation

  ○ Surgical: modifying cause of venous HTN (by venous ligation, valvuloplasty, and endoscopic perforator vein surgery); treat ulcer by graft.

MEDICATION

First Line
- Pentoxifylline 400 mg TID is effective in treating venous leg ulcer.
- The use of low-dose aspirin because the adjuvant treatment for venous leg ulcers is not supported.
- In light of increasing bacterial resistance to antibiotics, current guidelines recommend the use of antibacterial preparations only for clinical infection (cellulitis, increased pain, warmth, malodorous exudate), not for bacterial colonization (3)[A].
- If secondary infection, treat with PO antibiotics for *Staphylococcus* or *Streptococcus* organisms (e.g., dicloxacillin 250 mg QID, cephalexin 500 mg BID, or levofloxacin 500 mg daily).
- If MRSA suspected, clindamycin 300 mg QID, doxycycline 100 mg BID, TMP/SMX or IV vancomycin
- There is no reliable evidence in the effectiveness of topical antiseptics such as povidone-iodine, peroxide-based preparations, mupirocin, chlorhexidine (3)[A].

- Uncomplicated stasis dermatitis can be treated with short courses (about 2 weeks) of topical steroids (2)[B] (topical triamcinolone 0.1% cream/ointment BID).
- Topical antipruritic: pramoxine, camphor, menthol, and doxepin
- Topical anesthetic (lidocaine/prilocaine) may reduce pain during débridement.
- Silver sulfadiazine (SSD) has a positive effect in wound healing (2)[A].
- Currently, there is insufficient evidence to recommend routine use of other phlebotonic medications to treat venous insufficiency.

Second Line
- Consider antibiotics on basis of culture results of exudate from infected ulcer craters.
- Lubricants when dermatitis is quiescent
- Chronic stasis dermatitis can be treated with topical emollients (e.g., white petroleum).
- Antipruritic medications (e.g., diphenhydramine, cetirizine hydrochloride)
- Hydrocolloid or a foam dressing may reduce ulcer pain; no evidence that ibuprofen dressings offer pain relief

ISSUES FOR REFERRAL
Consider referral for nonhealing ulcer, arterial insufficiency, uncertain diagnosis, patch testing to evaluate for contact dermatitis, associated venous insufficiency disease (e.g., symptomatic varicose veins)

ADDITIONAL THERAPIES
Consider discontinuation of medications causing iatrogenic edema (such as amlodipine, gabapentin, etc.) as appropriate.

SURGERY/OTHER PROCEDURES
Sclerotherapy, ablation, vein stripping, and skin grafting may be required for associated disease.

 ## ONGOING CARE

FOLLOW-UP RECOMMENDATIONS
Patient Monitoring
- If Unna boot compression is used: Cut off and reapply boot once a week. Unna boots reduce edema by compression and prevent scratching.
- Regular use of high-compression stockings reduces chance of recurrent venous ulcer (4)[A].

DIET
Lose weight, if overweight.

PATIENT EDUCATION
- Encourage staying active to keep circulation and leg muscles in good condition. Walking is ideal. Keep legs elevated while sitting or lying.
- Do not wear girdles, garters, or pantyhose with tight elastic tops. Do not scratch.
- Elevate foot of bed with 2- to 4-inch blocks. Apply compression stockings prior to getting out of bed when less edema is present. Regular use of high-compression stockings may prevent recurrence of venous ulcers.

PROGNOSIS
- Chronic course with intermittent exacerbations and remissions
- The healing process for ulceration is often prolonged and may take months.

COMPLICATIONS
- Sensations of itching, pain, and burning have negative impact on the quality of life.
- Secondary bacterial infection
- Contact sensitization to topical agents and superimposed contact dermatitis; auto sensitization rash in remote areas
- Bleeding at dermatitis sites
- Squamous cell carcinoma in edges of long-standing stasis ulcers
- Scarring, which in turn leads to further compromise to blood flow and increased likelihood of minor trauma

REFERENCES
1. O'Meara S, Cullum N, Nelson EA, et al. Compression for venous leg ulcers. *Cochrane Database Syst Rev*. 2012;11(11):CD000265.
2. Evidence-based (S3) guidelines for diagnostics and treatment of venous leg ulcers. *J Eur Acad Dermatol Venereol*. 2016;30(11):1843–1875.
3. O'Meara S, Al-Kurdi D, Ologun Y, et al. Antibiotics and antiseptics for venous leg ulcers. *Cochrane Database Syst Rev*. 2014;(1):CD003557.
4. Nelson EA, Bell-Syer SEM. Compression for preventing recurrence of venous ulcers. *Cochrane Database Syst Rev*. 2012;(8):CD002303.

 ## SEE ALSO
- Varicose Veins
- Algorithm: Rash

CODES

ICD10
- I83.10 Varicose veins of unsp lower extremity with inflammation
- I83.11 Varicose veins of right lower extremity with inflammation
- I83.12 Varicose veins of left lower extremity with inflammation

CLINICAL PEARLS
- Treatment of edema associated with stasis dermatitis via elevation, exercise, and/or mechanical compression (stockings, bandages, or pneumatic devices) is essential for optimal results.
- No difference in healing rate of venous stasis ulcers by use of hydrocolloid dressing versus simple nonadherent dressing when used beneath compression. Decision about the dressing should be based on local cost and patient or physician's preferences.

DIABETES MELLITUS, TYPE 1
Vicente T. San Martin, MD • David T. Broome, MD

 BASICS

DESCRIPTION
- Type 1 diabetes mellitus (T1DM) is a chronic disease caused by insulin deficiency following β-cell destruction.
- Results in hyperglycemia and potential end-organ complications
- Features include:
  - Usually rapid onset
  - Absolute insulin dependence
  - Polyphagia, polydipsia, polyuria, and nocturia
  - Ketosis or diabetic ketoacidosis (DKA)
  - Body habitus: usually normal or thin physique at diagnosis
- System(s) affected: endocrine, metabolic, cardiovascular, neurologic, renal, ocular

Pregnancy Considerations
- T1DM confers maternal and fetal risk (spontaneous abortion, fetal anomalies, preeclampsia, fetal demise, macrosomia, neonatal hypoglycemia, and neonatal hyperbilirubinemia).
- Preconception counseling should address the importance of glycemic control as close to normal as safely possible to reduce congenital anomalies.
- Glycemic targets during pregnancy: fasting <95 mg/dL, and 1-hour postprandial <140 mg/dL, or 2-hour postprandial <120 mg/dL
- Glycated hemoglobin (HbA1c) is slightly lower during pregnancy due to increased RBC turnover. The HbA1c target should ideally be <6% if achieved without hypoglycemia but can be relaxed to <7% if necessary to prevent hypoglycemia (1)[B].
- Dilated eye examinations should occur before pregnancy or in the 1st trimester and monitored every trimester and 1-year postpartum (1)[B].
- Women with T1DM should be prescribed with low-dose aspirin 60 to 150 mg/day (usual dose 81 mg/day) by the end of the 1st trimester in order to lower the risk of preeclampsia (if no contraindication) (1)[C].

EPIDEMIOLOGY
Age of presentation is bimodal: at 4 to 6 years of age and at 10 to 14 years of age (early puberty) (2).

Incidence
- In the United States, incidence is 23.6/100,000 in non-Hispanic white children and adolescents.
- Lower rates in other racial and ethnic groups

Pediatric Considerations
In infants and toddlers, symptoms of T1DM may be subtle or masquerade as an intercurrent illness.

ETIOLOGY AND PATHOPHYSIOLOGY
There are two main categories of T1DM: immune-mediated and idiopathic diabetes (1):
- Immune-mediated diabetes: cellular-mediated autoimmune destruction of β-cells of the pancreas (markers: autoantibodies to insulin, GAD65, tyrosine phosphatases IA-2 and IA-2β, including zinc transporter 8 autoantibody [ZnT8A]); obtain three antibody tests (GAD65, IA-2A, ZnT8) to rule out MODY-monogenic diabetes.
- Idiopathic diabetes: no known etiology for permanent insulinopenia; prone to ketoacidosis but have no evidence of autoimmunity
- At least one autoantibody is present in 85–90% of individuals (1).

Genetics
- HLA associations, with linkage to the DQA and DQB genes, and it is influenced by the DRB genes (HLA-DQA1, HLA-DQB1, and DLA-DRB1). These antibodies can be predisposing or protective (1).
- The major susceptibility locus maps to the HLA class II genes at 6p21 (accounting for 30–50% of genetic T1DM), but there are >40 loci (3).

RISK FACTORS
- Risk factors: viral infections, vitamin D deficiency, perinatal factors (maternal age, history of preeclampsia, neonatal jaundice), high birth weight for gestational age, and lower gestational age at birth
- Increased susceptibility to T1DM is inheritable:
  - T1DM in monozygous twins with long-term follow-up is >50%.
  - Among first-degree relatives, siblings are at a higher risk (5–10% risk by age 20 years) than offspring.
  - Offspring of fathers with diabetes are at a higher risk (~12%) than offspring of mothers with diabetes (~6%) (3).

GENERAL PREVENTION
Although there is currently a lack of accepted screening programs, providers should consider referring relatives of those with T1DM for risk assessment in a clinical research study (https://www.trialnet.org/) (1).

COMMONLY ASSOCIATED CONDITIONS
Autoimmune diseases, such as primary adrenal insufficiency (Addison disease), celiac disease, autoimmune hepatitis, pernicious anemia, myasthenia gravis, vitiligo, Graves disease, and Hashimoto hypothyroidism

 DIAGNOSIS

HISTORY
New-onset polyuria and polydipsia
- Polyuria may present as nocturia, bed-wetting, or incontinence in a previously continent child.
- Polyuria may be difficult to appreciate in diaper-clad children.
- Polyuria occurs when serum glucose concentration rises >180 mg/dL (10 mmol/L).

PHYSICAL EXAM
- Weight loss, increased fatigue, lethargy, muscle cramps
- Ketosis/DKA leads to abdominal discomfort and nausea.
- Vision changes, such as blurriness (3)

DIFFERENTIAL DIAGNOSIS
- Type 2 diabetes
- Monogenic diabetes considered when (1):
  - Diabetes diagnosed before 6 months of age should have immediate genetic testing.
  - Strong family history of diabetes without classic features of type 2 diabetes
  - Nonobese diabetic child with negative autoantibodies

- Secondary diabetes
  - Pancreatic disease (chronic pancreatitis, cystic fibrosis, hereditary hemochromatosis)
  - Endocrine-associated diabetes: acromegaly, Cushing syndrome, pheochromocytoma, glucagonoma, neuroendocrine tumors
  - Drug- or chemical-induced diabetes: glucocorticosteroids, HIV protease inhibitors, atypical antipsychotics, tacrolimus, cyclosporine, immune checkpoint inhibitors
- Acute poisonings (Salicylate poisoning can mimic DKA.)

DIAGNOSTIC TESTS & INTERPRETATION
Initial Tests (lab, imaging)
- Criteria for the diagnosis of diabetes:
  - Fasting (>8 hours) glucose ≥126 mg/dL (7 mmol/L) on more than one occasion
  - Random glucose of ≥200 mg/dL (11.1 mmol/L) in a patient with classic symptoms of hyperglycemia
  - Oral glucose tolerance test (OGTT): plasma glucose ≥200 mg/dL 2 hours after a glucose load of 1.75 g/kg (max dose of 75 g)
  - HbA1c level ≥6.5%
- Other tests to consider:
  - Urinalysis for glucose, ketones, and albuminuria (urine albumin:creatinine ratio)
  - Pancreatic autoantibodies: islet cell, IAA, GAD, IA2A, and ZnT8A
  - Serum β-hydroxybutyrate (BHB) and urine ketones
  - Fructosamine
  - Continuous glucose monitoring (CGM)
- C-peptide level if needed to differentiate from type 2 diabetes because low or no C-peptide indicates insulinopenia

Follow-Up Tests & Special Considerations
Screen for thyroid disease on diagnosis and periodically thereafter (1)[C].

Test Interpretation
In the absence of unequivocal hyperglycemia, results should be confirmed by repeat testing.

 TREATMENT

GENERAL MEASURES
Insulin is the mainstay of therapy with education regarding matching of mealtime insulin dose to carbohydrate intake, premeal blood glucose level, and anticipated activity.
- Premeal blood glucose goal: 90 to 130 mg/dL (5 to 7.2 mmol/L)
- Bedtime/overnight blood glucose levels goal: 90 to 150 mg/dL (5.0 to 8.3 mmol/L)
- Pediatric A1c goal: <7.5% (A1c <7% is reasonable if achieved without excessive hypoglycemia.)
- Adult A1c goal: <7% (A1c <6.5% is reasonable in select individuals); less stringent A1c goals (such as <8%) may be appropriate for elderly patients and other special populations.
- If using a CGM, most individuals should aim for a time in range (70 to 180 mg/dL) of at least 70% of readings; for those with frailty or at high risk of hypoglycemia, a target of >50% time in range with <1% time below range is recommended.

MEDICATION

- Most treated with multiple daily injections (MDI) of prandial insulin and basal insulin, or continuous subcutaneous insulin infusion (CSII)
- Use rapid-acting insulin analogs to reduce hypoglycemia risk.
- Types of injectable insulin:
  – Long-acting insulin analogs: insulin glargine/glargine-yfgn/glargine-aglr, insulin detemir, and insulin degludec; these should not be mixed with other insulins in the same syringe.
  – Intermediate-acting insulin (e.g., NPH) can be mixed with other insulins.
  – Short-acting (regular) insulin
  – Rapid-acting insulin analogs: insulin lispro, insulin aspart, and insulin glulisine

First Line

- Flexible intensive insulin therapy is the gold standard.
- Total initial dose is 0.2 to 0.4 units/kg/day for insulin-naive patients (up to 1.0 unit/kg/day in puberty).
- ~50% of total dose given as basal insulin, with the rest as bolus insulin.
- MDI regimen (1):
  – Basal, long-acting insulin once or twice a day
  – Prandial, short-acting insulin based on number of carbohydrate portions (e.g., 1:10, meaning 1 U of insulin for every 10 g of carbohydrates)
  – Correctional short-acting mealtime insulin based on premeal blood glucose level and sensitivity factor (e.g., 1 U for every 50 mg/dL over 150 mg/dL, where 50 mg/dL is the sensitivity factor)
- CSII regimen:
  – CSII and CGM should be encouraged when there is active patient/family participation (1).

Second Line

- Twice-daily injections with NPH along with regular or rapid-acting insulin (not physiologic, but lower cost and fewer injections)
- Pramlintide: delays gastric emptying, blunts pancreatic secretion of glucagon, and enhances satiety

ISSUES FOR REFERRAL

New and established diagnoses of T1DM would benefit from endocrinology referral.

ADDITIONAL THERAPIES

- Inhaled rapid acting insulin may be used for mealtime coverage.
- Pancreatic and islet transplantation have been shown to normalize glucose levels but require lifelong immunosuppression; reserved for simultaneous renal transplantation, recurrent DKA, or severe hyperglycemia
- Donislecel: allogeneic pancreatic islet cellular therapy; approved for the treatment of adults with T1DM who are unable to approach target HbA1c because of current repeated episodes of severe hypoglycemia despite intensive management

- Bionic pancreas: bihormonal (insulin and glucagon), fully automated delivery system
- Investigational therapies (not yet FDA-approved for T1DM): insulin icodec (ultra-long-acting insulin), metformin, GLP-1 receptor agonists, DPP-4 inhibitors, SGLT-1/SGLT-2 inhibitors, do-it-yourself automated insulin delivery systems (DIY AID) (1)[C]

SURGERY/OTHER PROCEDURES

- All patients with T1DM should always have basal insulin continued if not eating prior to a procedure.
- If patients are not eating on the morning prior to a procedure/surgery, prandial insulin should be held.

ADMISSION, INPATIENT, AND NURSING CONSIDERATIONS

Newly diagnosed patients with T1DM may require hospitalization during initiation of insulin therapy.

 ONGOING CARE

FOLLOW-UP RECOMMENDATIONS

Regular aerobic exercise with care to avoid hypoglycemia by lowering basal requirements (temporary basal rate if using an insulin pump) or be advised to eat/drink 15 to 30 g of carbohydrates prior to vigorous exercise

Patient Monitoring

- Blood pressure (BP) checks at every routine visit with a goal BP of <130/80 mm Hg
- Home blood glucose monitoring with home blood glucose meter or CGM: Glucose checks should be done at least 4 to 6 times/day.
- Comprehensive foot exam at least annually
- Quarterly measurement of HbA1c
- For patients of all ages with diabetes and atherosclerotic cardiovascular disease (ASCVD), high-intensity statin therapy should be added to lifestyle therapy.
- For patients with diabetes aged 40 to 75 years and aged >75 years without ASCVD, use moderate-intensity statin in addition to lifestyle therapy.
- Annual screenings:
  – Albuminuria for earliest signs of possible nephropathy (urine albumin:creatinine ratio)
  – Initial dilated comprehensive eye exam within 5 years of diagnosis and then every 1 to 2 years
  – Monofilament testing with pinprick, temperature, and vibration sensation for screening of peripheral neuropathy 5 years after diagnosis and then annually
- Vaccines: annual influenza, pneumococcal pneumonia, hepatitis B, COVID-19 vaccination

DIET

- American Diabetes Association diet: https://diabetes.org/food-nutrition
- Carbohydrate counting using insulin-to-carbohydrate ratio with all meals and snacks allows patient flexibility in eating.

PATIENT EDUCATION

Patient education of their diagnosis, carbohydrate counting, nutritional recommendations is important.

PROGNOSIS

- Initial remission or 3 to 6 month "honeymoon phase" with decreased insulin needs and easier control
- Prognosis improves with careful blood glucose monitoring, improvement in insulin delivery regimens, and appropriate glycemic control.

COMPLICATIONS

- Microvascular disease (retinopathy, nephropathy, neuropathy)
- Macrovascular disease (coronary and cerebral artery disease)
- Chronic foot ulcers/amputations
- Hypoglycemia (recommend checking glucose before driving)
- DKA
- Excessive weight gain
- Increased risk of serious infection
- Increased risk of preeclampsia and preterm delivery

REFERENCES

1. ElSayed NA, Aleppo G, Aroda VR, et al; for American Diabetes Association. Introduction and methodology: standards of care in diabetes—2023. *Diabetes Care*. 2023;46(Suppl 1):S1–S4.
2. Felner EI, Klitz W, Ham M, et al. Genetic interaction among three genomic regions creates distinct contributions to early- and late-onset type 1 diabetes mellitus. *Pediatr Diabetes*. 2005;6(4):213–220.
3. Steck AK, Rewers MJ. Genetics of type 1 diabetes. *Clin Chem*. 2011;57(2):176–185.

CODES

ICD10

- E10.319 Type 1 diabetes mellitus with unspecified diabetic retinopathy without macular edema
- E10.321 Type 1 diabetes mellitus with mild nonproliferative diabetic retinopathy with macular edema
- E10.351 Type 1 diabetes mellitus with proliferative diabetic retinopathy with macular edema

CLINICAL PEARLS

- The age of presentation of T1DM is bimodal: one peak at 4 to 6 years of age and a second peak at 10 to 14 years of age.
- Therapy with MDI or CSII and the use of a multidisciplinary team care approach are associated with improved glycemic control, resulting in better long-term outcomes.
- Adult A1c goal is <7.0%; less stringent A1c goals may be appropriate for elderly patients and other special populations.

D

DIABETES MELLITUS, TYPE 2

Samir Malkani, MD, MRCP–UK • Sanaa Ayyoub, MD

BASICS

DESCRIPTION
Diabetes mellitus (DM) type 2 is due to a progressive insulin secretory defect in the setting of insulin resistance.

Geriatric Considerations
Monitor for hypoglycemia; adjust doses for renal/hepatic dysfunction and cognitive function; less aggressive glucose targets than younger patients

Pediatric Considerations
Incidence is increasing and parallels obesity epidemic.

Pregnancy Considerations
- Diet, metformin, glyburide, and insulin are all options for treatment of gestational diabetes.
- In gestational diabetes, screen for diabetes/prediabetes with oral glucose tolerance test (OGTT) 6 to 12 weeks postpartum and every 3 years.

EPIDEMIOLOGY
Prevalence
Estimated 37.3 million Americans (11.3% of the population); 90–95% are likely type 2.

ETIOLOGY AND PATHOPHYSIOLOGY
- Peripheral insulin resistance and defective insulin secretion with increased hepatic gluconeogenesis
- Obesity and visceral adiposity
- Associated with dyslipidemia, hypertension, and gut microbiome changes
- Drug or chemical induced (e.g., glucocorticoids, antiretroviral therapy, atypical antipsychotics, organ transplant immunosuppressants)

Genetics
- Family history is strongly predictive of risk.
- Polygenic; rarely monogenic (e.g., peroxisome proliferator–activated receptor [PPAR] γ and insulin gene mutations)

RISK FACTORS
- Parental history of type 2 diabetes
- Gestational diabetes or history of baby with birth weight ≥4 kg (≥9 lb)
- Polycystic ovarian syndrome (PCOS)
- Hypertriglyceridemia or low high-density lipoprotein (HDL)
- Ethnicity: African American, Latino, Native American, Asian, and Pacific Islander
- Sedentary lifestyle, visceral obesity

GENERAL PREVENTION
- Maintenance of normal weight, or weight loss of 7% body weight, decrease intake of carbohydrates and overall calories; moderate-intensity exercise (150 min/week)
- Metformin, α-glucosidase inhibitors, thiazolidinediones (TZDs), and glucagon-like peptide-1 receptor agonist (GLP-1 RA) in prediabetes

COMMONLY ASSOCIATED CONDITIONS
Hypertension, dyslipidemia, metabolic syndrome, fatty liver disease, PCOS, acanthosis nigricans, hemochromatosis

DIAGNOSIS

HISTORY
Polyuria, polydipsia, polyphagia, weight loss, fatigue, blurry vision, neuropathy, and frequent infections; many individuals are asymptomatic.

PHYSICAL EXAM
BMI, waist circumference, funduscopic exam, oral exam, cardiopulmonary exam, abdominal exam for hepatomegaly, focused neurologic exam, and diabetic foot exam

DIFFERENTIAL DIAGNOSIS
- Type 1 DM—low or absent insulin, C-peptide, positive β-cell autoantibodies, ketosis
- DM is one of the features of Cushing syndrome, acromegaly, and glucagonoma.

DIAGNOSTIC TESTS & INTERPRETATION
Initial Tests (lab, imaging)
Criteria for diagnosis
- HbA1c ≥6.5% *or*
- Hyperglycemic symptoms and random plasma glucose ≥200 mg/dL (11.1 mmol/L) *or*
- Fasting plasma glucose (FPG) ≥126 mg/dL (7 mmol/L) *or*
- 2-hour plasma glucose ≥200 mg/dL (11.1 mmol/L) during OGTT with 75-g glucose load
- If equivocal, perform different test on the same sample or repeat the test.

TREATMENT

Tight glucose control prevents long-term microvascular complications, but the benefits on macrovascular outcomes are less apparent. Individuals likely to benefit from a more aggressive target are those without preexisting DM complications, with recent diagnoses of DM, and with long life expectancy.
- Use patient-centered approach.
- Dietary modification, regular exercise, control of cardiovascular risk factors (blood pressure [BP] and lipids)
- HbA1c targets—ADA recommendations (1) and ACP targets differ (2).
  – HbA1c <7.0: long life expectancy, no cardiovascular disease (CVD), short duration of DM, no history of hypoglycemia
  – HbA1c <8.0%: limited life expectancy, advanced micro- or macrovascular complications, extensive comorbidities, history of severe hypoglycemia or long-standing DM where lower goal is difficult to attain.
  – The ACP recommends an HbA1c between 7% and 8% in most patients (2).
  – ADA recommends preprandial glucose 80 to 130 mg/dL; postprandial glucose <180 mg/dL

- For cardiorenal risk reduction in high-risk patients, initiate therapy with GLP-1 RA or SGLT2 inhibitor with proven CVD benefit. SGLT2 inhibitors have proven benefit in patients with heart failure and CKD with GFR <60 or albuminuria with albumin-to-creatinine ratio >30 mg/g. Metformin to be used in combination to maintain HbA1c goal (1).
- Always consider side effect profile, CV benefit, renal benefit, and cost.

GENERAL MEASURES
- Regular foot exam
- Nephropathy: annual urine microalbumin-to-creatinine ratio and plasma creatinine (eGFR)
- Retinopathy: annual diabetic eye exam
- If 40 to 75 years old, prescribe moderate-to-high intensity statin.
- Hypertension: goal BP <140/80 mm Hg

MEDICATION
First Line
Metformin—500 to 2,000 mg in divided doses BID or extended release QD
- Reduces hepatic gluconeogenesis and multiple other mechanisms of action
- Preferred due to high efficacy in lowering glucose, good safety profile, low hypoglycemia risk, low cost; weight neutral
- Avoid in severe acute illnesses (e.g., liver disease, cardiogenic shock, pancreatitis, hypoxia) due to risk of lactic acidosis.
- Caution with acute heart failure, alcohol abuse, elderly; associated with vitamin B_{12} deficiency
- Severe diarrhea in 10% of patients, requiring switch to another agent
- In CKD for eGFR 30 to 45, reduce dose to ≤1,000 mg; stop if eGFR <30.

Second and Third Line
- General principles
  – If patient has CAD, heart failure, or CKD, consider drugs that improve outcomes with these conditions as first-line agents.
  – Consider drug-specific side effects such as weight gain or hypoglycemia.
  – Cost of drug is an important consideration.
- GLP-1 RA (incretins)
  – Exenatide (Byetta): 5 to 10 μg SC BID or exenatide ER (Bydureon) 2 mg/week
  – Liraglutide (Victoza): 0.6 to 1.8 mg/day; improved CV outcomes (3)
  – Dulaglutide (Trulicity): 0.75 to 4.50 mg weekly; improved CV outcomes (3)
  – Lixisenatide (Adlyxin): up to 20 μg SC QD
  – Semaglutide injection (Ozempic): 0.25 to 2.00 mg weekly; improved CV outcomes (3); oral (Rybelsus) 3 to 14 mg/day neutral CV risk (4)
  – Reduced risk of atherosclerotic CVD events
  – Low hypoglycemia risk, promotes weight loss
  – Small risk of acute pancreatitis; use cautiously in CKD ≥ stage 4; may exacerbate gastroparesis
  – Contraindicated in personal/family history of medullary thyroid cancer or multiple endocrine neoplasia (MEN) type 2

- GLP-1/GIP RA—tirzepatide (Mounjaro): 2.5 to 15 mg weekly injection
  - Trials showed doses of 5 mg, 10 mg, and 15 mg had clinically meaningful HbA1c reduction compared to placebo (5) and superior HbA1c/weight reductions when compared to semaglutide (6) and titrated insulin degludec.
  - Similar side effect profile as GLP-1 RAs
- SGLT2 inhibitors
  - Canagliflozin (Invokana): 100 to 300 mg/day
  - Dapagliflozin (Farxiga): 5 to 10 mg/day
  - Empagliflozin (Jardiance): 10 to 25 mg/day
  - Ertugliflozin (Steglatro): 5 to 15 mg/day
  - Inhibit renal glucose reabsorption, cause weight loss, no hypoglycemia risk
  - Canagliflozin, dapagliflozin, and empagliflozin reduce CV mortality; slow progression of renal disease (3)
  - Risk of genital mycotic infections and UTI; higher risk of euglycemic diabetic ketoacidosis (DKA); higher fracture risk; relatively expensive
    - Can be used in patients with GFR >20 mL/min up until dialysis or renal transplant
  - Dipeptidyl peptidase-4 (DPP-4) inhibitors
    - Alogliptin 25 mg/day
    - Saxagliptin 5 mg/day
    - Linagliptin 5 mg/day
    - Sitagliptin 100 mg/day
    - Inhibit DPP-4 enzyme, which deactivates endogenous GLP-1 and GIP
    - Low risk for hypoglycemia; reduce dose in renal impairment except linagliptin.
    - Weight neutral
    - No evidence for CV risk reduction
  - Sulfonylureas
    - Glipizide (Glucotrol): 2.5 to 40.0 mg/day
    - Glipizide extended-release: 5 to 20 mg/day
    - Glyburide (DiaBeta, Micronase): 1.25 to 20.0 mg/day, Glynase: 0.75 to 12.00 mg/day
    - Glimepiride (Amaryl): 1 to 8 mg/day
    - Stimulate β-cell production of insulin
    - Caution with renal or liver disease, sulfa allergy, creatinine clearance <50 mL/min
    - Potentiate weight gain, high hypoglycemia risk
    - Inexpensive
  - TZD—pioglitazone (Actos): 15 to 45 mg/day; rosiglitazone (Avandia): 4 to 8 mg/day
    - Increases insulin sensitivity; activates PPARs
    - Pioglitazone reduces triglycerides; low cost
    - Can worsen heart failure symptoms
    - Increased risk of fractures/low bone mass
  - Insulin
    - Increases glucose disposal, inhibits hepatic glucose production
    - Consider as initial therapy if HbA1c >10%, catabolic symptoms, ketosis.
    - Use as additional therapy after dual/triple therapy has been tried.
    - Weight gain and hypoglycemia risk
    - Analogs have lower hypoglycemia risk than NPH and regular insulin but more expensive.

- Basal insulin: Start with 0.1 to 0.3 U/kg/day. Titrate up for desired result. Add mealtime (rapid/short-acting) insulin if postmeal glucose is high. Mealtime starting dose can be 4 U or 10% of basal dose.
  - Rapid-acting analogs—lispro (Humalog), aspart (Novolog), glulisine (Apidra): duration of action 3 to 5 hours; ultrarapid (Fiasp and lispro-aabc) quicker onset
  - Inhaled insulin (Afrezza): rapid onset of action; duration of action 4.5 hours
  - Short-acting insulin—human regular (Humulin R/Novolin R/ReliOn R): duration of action 6 to 8 hours
  - Intermediate-acting insulin—human NPH (Humulin N/Novolin N/ReliOn N): duration of 13 to 20 hours; human regular U-500 (Humulin R U-500): duration of 6 to 10 hours
  - Basal insulin analogs—glargine U-100 (Lantus, Basaglar): duration of 22 to 24 hours; glargine U-300 (Toujeo): duration of 36 hours; detemir (Levemir): duration of 21.5 hours; degludec U-100, U-200 (Tresiba): duration of 42 hours
  - Premixed insulin products—NPH/regular 70/30 (Novolin 70/30, Humulin 70/30), 70/30 and 50/50 aspart mix (Novolog mix), 75/25 and 50/50 lispro mix (Humalog mix)
- Amylinomimetic—pramlintide (Symlin): 60 to 120 μg SC premeal
  - Delays gastric emptying, blunts glucagon, enhances satiety and weight loss
- α-Glucosidase inhibitors—acarbose (Precose): 25 to 100 mg TID; miglitol (Glyset): 25 to 100 mg TID
  - Slows intestinal carbohydrate digestion, reduced postmeal hyperglycemia
  - Avoid in renal insufficiency and bowel diseases.
- Meglitinides—repaglinide (Prandin): 0.5 to 4.0 mg TID; nateglinide (Starlix): 60 to 120 mg TID
  - Take at beginning of meals.
  - Mechanism similar to SU but much shorter duration of action
- Combination therapy with drugs from different classes with complementary mechanisms of actions can be helpful.

SURGERY/OTHER PROCEDURES
Consider bariatric surgery if BMI >35 kg/m².

 ## ONGOING CARE

PATIENT EDUCATION
Diabetes self-management

PROGNOSIS
Normal lifespan with good management

COMPLICATIONS
- ASCVD, peripheral vascular disease, stroke, foot ulcers, Charcot joints
- Microvascular: neuropathy, retinopathy, diabetic CKD
- GI: fatty liver disease, gastroparesis

REFERENCES

1. ElSayed NA, Aleppo G, Aroda VR, et al; for American Diabetes Association. 17. Diabetes advocacy: standards of care in diabetes—2023. *Diabetes Care*. 2023;46(Suppl 1):S279–S280.
2. Qaseem A, Wilt TJ, Kansagara D, et al; for Clinical Guidelines Committee of the American College of Physicians. Hemoglobin A1c targets for glycemic control with pharmacologic therapy for nonpregnant adults with type 2 diabetes mellitus: a guidance statement update from the American College of Physicians. *Ann Intern Med*. 2018;168(8):569–576.
3. Sim R, Chong CW, Loganadan NK, et al. Comparative effectiveness of cardiovascular, renal and safety outcomes of second-line antidiabetic drugs use in people with type 2 diabetes: a systematic review and network meta-analysis of randomised controlled trials. *Diabet Med*. 2022;39(3):e14780.
4. Husain M, Birkenfeld AL, Donsmark M, et al. Oral semaglutide and cardiovascular outcomes in patients with type 2 diabetes. *N Engl J Med*. 2019;381(9):841–851.
5. Min T, Bain SC. The role of tirzepatide, dual GIP and GLP-1 receptor agonist, in the management of type 2 diabetes: the SURPASS clinical trials. *Diabetes Ther*. 2021;12(1):143–157.
6. Frías JP, Davies MJ, Rosenstock J, et al; for SURPASS-2 Investigators. Tirzepatide versus semaglutide once weekly in patients with type 2 diabetes. *N Engl J Med*. 2021;385(6):503–515.

 ## SEE ALSO

- Diabetes Mellitus, Type 1; Diabetic Ketoacidosis; Hypertension, Essential
- Algorithms: Type 2 Diabetes, Treatment; Weight Loss, Treatment

CODES

ICD10
- E11.329 Type 2 diabetes mellitus with mild nonproliferative diabetic retinopathy without macular edema
- E11.331 Type 2 diabetes mellitus with moderate nonproliferative diabetic retinopathy with macular edema
- E11.359 Type 2 diabetes mellitus with proliferative diabetic retinopathy without macular edema

CLINICAL PEARLS

- Individualize HbA1c targets based on life expectancy and comorbidities.
- Hypoglycemia poses more short-term danger than hyperglycemia.

DIABETIC KETOACIDOSIS
Daniel R. Matta, MD • Amanda Kimberley Davis, MD, MBBS

 BASICS

DESCRIPTION
- A life-threatening medical emergency which most commonly occurs in patients with type 1 diabetes
- Characterized by a biochemical triad of hyperglycemia, ketosis, and high anion gap metabolic acidosis
- Rarely, it can occur in the absence of hyperglycemia (i.e., euglycemic diabetic ketoacidosis [DKA]) during pregnancy and in individuals taking sodium-glucose cotransporter-2 (SGLT2) inhibitors (1).
- System(s) affected: endocrine/metabolic, neurologic

EPIDEMIOLOGY
Incidence
Incidence by age group: 1 to 17 years (10.1%), 18 to 44 years (53.3%), 45 to 64 years (27.1%), 65 to 84 years (8.7%), and ≥85 years (0.8%)

ETIOLOGY AND PATHOPHYSIOLOGY
- Impaired glucose utilization secondary to insulin deficiency, leading to the activation of counter regulatory mechanisms (gluconeogenesis, glycogenolysis, proteolysis) which further increase blood glucose level and trigger ketone bodies production; resulting ketonemia and hyperglycemia lead to osmotic diuresis, dehydration, electrolytes disturbances and acidosis.
- Leading causes include medication noncompliance and infection. Other precipitating factors are:
  - First presentation of DM
  - Myocardial infarction (MI); cerebrovascular accident (CVA)
  - Medications (corticosteroids, sympathomimetics [e.g., dobutamine, terbutaline], atypical antipsychotics, SGLT2 inhibitors)
  - Alcohol and illicit drugs (cocaine)
  - Trauma; surgery
  - Emotional stress and psychiatric comorbidities
  - Pregnancy

RISK FACTORS
- Type 1 DM
- Ketosis-prone type 2 DM (Hispanic and African American ethnicity, G6PD deficiency)
- Euglycemic ketoacidosis specially with SGLT2 inhibitor drug use
- COVID-19 infection

GENERAL PREVENTION
- Close monitoring of glucose during periods of stress, illness, and trauma with "sick day" management instructions
- Careful insulin control and regular monitoring of blood glucose levels along with education on symptom recognition

COMMONLY ASSOCIATED CONDITIONS
>30% of patients have features of both DKA and hyperosmolar hyperglycemic syndrome (HHS).

 DIAGNOSIS

- Diagnostic criteria (1)[C]
  - Hyperglycemia (usually 250 to 800 mg/dL) as rapidly assessed on fingerstick glucose testing and confirmed on serum chemistry
  - Low bicarbonate (HCO_3) (usually ≤18 mEq/L)
  - Metabolic acidosis on arterial blood gases (ABGs) (pH <7.3)
  - Anion gap = serum sodium − (serum chloride + HCO_3); >10 mmol
  - Positive β-hydroxybutyrate (B-OHB) in serum is highly sensitive and specific.
- Diagnosis can be stratified into three levels of severity depending on laboratory findings and physical exam, most importantly the mental status.
  - Mild: pH 7.25 to 7.30; bicarbonate 10 to 18 mEq/L; alert moderate: pH 7.10 to 7.24; bicarbonate 5 to 9 mEq/L; alert or drowsy
  - Severe: pH <7.1; bicarbonate <5 mEq/L; stupor
- Individualization of treatment based on clinical and laboratory assessment is needed (1).

HISTORY
- Recent illness, injury, or surgery
- Changes in diet or medications; missed insulin doses/noncompliance, insulin pump failure
- Polyuria, polydipsia, polyphagia, weight loss
- Generalized weakness, malaise, fatigue, lethargy, nausea, vomiting, abdominal pain
- Anorexia or increased appetite

PHYSICAL EXAM
- Vital signs: hypotension, tachycardia, fever or hypothermia
- Tachypnea, hyperpnea, Kussmaul respirations
- Fruity odor of ketotic breath (acetone smell)
- Abdominal tenderness, decreased bowel sounds
- Dry mucous membranes, poor skin turgor, dehydration
- Decreased reflexes
- Altered mental status, coma

DIFFERENTIAL DIAGNOSIS
- HHS
- Alcoholic ketoacidosis, starvation ketosis, lactic acidosis
- Metabolic encephalopathy
- Toxic ingestions (e.g., salicylates, methanol, ethylene glycol)
- Uremia/chronic renal failure
- Sepsis
- Acute pancreatitis

DIAGNOSTIC TESTS & INTERPRETATION
Initial Tests (lab, imaging)

ALERT
- Important labs:
  - β-OHB is the predominant ketone produced and is preferred over serum ketones. β-OHB >3 mg/dL is abnormal and should be decreased to <1.5 mg/dL within 12 to 24 hours.
  - ABG or venous blood gases (VBG) for pH assessment: VBG pH correlates with 0.03 lower than ABG pH.
  - Urinalysis: ketonuria, glycosuria
  - Creatinine and BUN: Markedly increased serum ketones may cross-react and cause a falsely high serum creatinine.
  - Electrolytes derangements: hypomagnesemia, hypophosphatemia, base deficit with high anion gap
  - Decreased total body K^+: Severe acidosis causes an artificially elevated K^+ level.
  - Pseudohyponatremia secondary to hyperglycemia or hypertriglyceridemia: It is now accepted to correct Na+ concentration by adding 2.4 mmol/L to measured Na+ for every 100 mg/dL increase in serum glucose >100 mg/dL.
  - Calculate serum osmolality: if calculated osmolality <320 mOsm/kg, consider etiologies other than DKA especially in patients with altered mentation.
  - Glycosylated hemoglobin (HbA1c) helps assess long-term history of diabetic control.
  - CBC: Consider DKA-related leukocytosis versus infection.
- Other tests
  - Blood and urine culture, chest x-ray, and lumbar puncture based on clinical suspicion for infection
  - ECG: frequently shows nonspecific sinus tachycardia, changes consistent with electrolyte abnormalities, and/or ischemic changes with MI as a precipitation factor
  - Troponin
  - Head CT scan if CVA or cerebral edema suspected

Follow-Up Tests & Special Considerations
Elevated lipase and amylase might not be reliable for diagnosis of pancreatitis in DKA.

TREATMENT

- Restore circulatory volume and tissue perfusion
- Gradual reduction of glucose level and osmolality
- Resolution of anion gap acidosis and ketosis
- Correction of electrolytes imbalance
- Identify and treat precipitating cause(s)

GENERAL MEASURES
- Severe DKA requires an ICU setting.
- Fluid resuscitation: Start isotonic crystalloid solution (e.g., 0.9% saline, or lactated Ringer bolus).
- Check serum glucose every hour along with serum electrolytes, BUN, creatinine, venous pH, and glucose every 2 to 4 hours until stable.

MEDICATION
First Line
- Intravenous fluid (IVF) is a priority (1)[C]
  - Start fluid of choice at 15 to 20 mL/kg of body weight or 1,000 mL to 1,500 mL in the first hour of treatment.
  - After the first hour, IVF infusion rate should be adjusted based on hemodynamics and electrolytes (usually 250 to 500 mL/hour in patients without cardiac, renal, or hepatic compromise).
  - Consider use of 0.45% NaCl in patients with normal to high corrected Na+ concentration after initial fluid resuscitation. Although continuous 0.9% NaCl is not contraindicated, risk of hyperchloremic metabolic acidosis should also be considered.
  - When glucose is 200 mg/dL, change to 5% dextrose with 0.45% NaCl at same rate to prevent hypoglycemia.
    - The "two bag method" is a feasible management alternative with two bags of 0.45% NaCl, one with and another without dextrose 10% being infused simultaneously. Infusion rates are adjusted based on hourly glucose level to maintain a total infusion rate of 250 mL/hr. This method has been associated with earlier correction of acidosis compared to conventional fluid replacement (1).
- Insulin: Start IV infusion after initial IVF resuscitation and correction of hypokalemia (<3.3 mg/dL) (1)[C].
  - Optional initial bolus 0.1 U/kg IV and then continuous infusion at 0.1 U/kg/hr (Do not use initial insulin bolus in children.)
  - If bolus not given, 0.14 U/kg/hr continuous infusion is recommended (1).
  - Aim for rate of serum glucose reduction of 50 to 75 mg/dL/hr in the first hour; adjust infusion rate hourly until steady decline is achieved.
  - ADA recommends reducing infusion rate to 0.02 to 0.05 U/kg/hr IV to maintain serum glucose between 150 to 200 mg/dL until correction of acidosis.
  - Use of subcutaneous (SC) basal insulin (glargine 0.25U/kg SC) within 12 hours of starting treatment may result in reduction of time to gap closure, shorter hospital stay, and less rebound hyperglycemia (1).
  - Overlap and continue IV insulin infusion for 2 to 4 hours after SC insulin is initiated to prevent recurrence of ketoacidosis and rebound hyperglycemia (2).
  - No significance difference has been found in outcomes for mild to moderate DKA treated with SC insulin combined with aggressive fluid management compared to continuous IV insulin infusion (2).
- Potassium: Start replacement with 20 to 30 mEq/L of K+ in 1 L IV fluids when serum K+ ≤5.2 mg/dL and if urine output is adequate.
  - Hold insulin if K+ ≤3.3 mg/dL; give IV potassium 20 to 30 mEq/hr with fluids until >3.3 mg/dL to prevent cardiac arrhythmia. For each 0.1 unit of pH, serum K+ will change by ~0.6 mEq in opposite direction.

- Phosphorus: Routine replacement is not recommended because it may lead to hypocalcemia; if very low (<1.0 mg/dL), give 20 to 30 mEq/L of K-Phos in fluids.
- Sodium bicarbonate (NaCHO$_3$): Available evidence does not support its use in patients with pH 6.9 or higher (1). Patients with pH <6.9 or life-threatening hyperkalemia are at increased risk of poor outcome; therefore, slow administration of 100 mEq NaCHO$_3$ over 2 hours can be considered in such cases. NaCHO$_3$ use may increase risk of cerebral edema, especially in children.
- Magnesium (Mg): If Mg ≤1.2 mg/dL or ≤1.8 and patient is symptomatic, Mg treatment should be considered.
- Precautions
  - If glucose does not fall by 10% in first hour, give regular insulin 0.14 U/kg IV bolus and then continuous infusion at previous rate.
  - If using bicarbonate NaCHO$_3$, add 100 mmol or 2 ampules of sodium bicarbonate to 400 mL isotonic solution with 20 mEq KCL >200 mL/hr for 2 hours until venous pH is >7.0 and then stop infusion.

Second Line
- Rapid acting subcutaneous insulin can be considered for patients who are alert, tolerating oral intake, serum bicarbonate > 10 mEq/L, and pH >7.0.
- Load with 0.3 U/kg SC, followed by 0.1 to 0.2 U/kg q1–2h. Once glucose <200 mg/dL, reduce dosing to 0.05 to 0.10 U/kg q1–2h till resolution of ketoacidosis.

Pediatric Considerations
- Initial insulin infusion rates of 0.05 to 0.1 U/kg/hr are recommended (3)[C].
- Cerebral edema is a rare complication (~1%) but has a mortality of 20–50%. Treatment should be started as soon as suspected clinically and not delayed for neuroimaging.

Pregnancy Considerations
- DKA per se is not an indication for emergency delivery; imperative to stabilize mother first.
- Euglycemic DKA

ADMISSION, INPATIENT, AND NURSING CONSIDERATIONS
- Admission criteria: blood glucose >250 mg/dL; pH <7.3; HCO$_3$ ≤15 mEq/L; ketones in urine; ICU setting for severe DKA
- Discharge when DKA has resolved anion gap <12, glucose <200 mg/dL; pH >7.3; bicarbonate >18 mEq/L. Patient must be tolerating PO intake and able to resume home medication regimen.

 ONGOING CARE

FOLLOW-UP RECOMMENDATIONS
Follow up within 1 to 2 weeks

DIET
- NPO initially, advance diet when nausea and vomiting are controlled
- Avoid foods with high glycemic index (e.g., soft drinks, fruit juice, white bread, added sugar).

PATIENT EDUCATION
- Self-monitoring of glucose, glucose, goals, and when to call PCP
- Recognition and prevention of hypoglycemia
- Healthy nutritional choices
- Sick day management
- Proper use of insulin syringes/needles

PROGNOSIS
- Worse in the extremes of age and in the setting of coma and hypotension
- Overall DKA mortality of 0.5–2%

COMPLICATIONS
- Cerebral edema (most common cause of death in children with DKA)
- Pulmonary edema, respiratory distress, MI
- Vascular thrombosis
- Hypokalemia, hyperkalemia, hypophosphatemia
- Cardiac dysrhythmia (secondary to hypokalemia or acidosis)
- Acute renal failure
- Late hypoglycemia (secondary to treatment)
- Infection

REFERENCES
1. Karslioglu French E, Donihi AC, Korytkowski MT. Diabetic ketoacidosis and hyperosmolar hyperglycemic syndrome: review of acute decompensated diabetes in adult patients. *BMJ.* 2019;365:I1114.
2. ElSayed NA, Aleppo G, Aroda VR, et al; for American Diabetes Association. 16. Diabetes care in the hospital: standards of care in diabetes—2023. *Diabetes Care.* 2023;46(Suppl 1):S267–S278.
3. Cashen K, Peterson T. Diabetic ketoacidosis. *Pediatric Rev.* 2019;40(8):412–420.

CODES

ICD10
- E10.11 Type 1 diabetes mellitus with ketoacidosis with coma
- E10.10 Type 1 diabetes mellitus with ketoacidosis without coma
- E13.11 Other specified diabetes mellitus with ketoacidosis with coma

CLINICAL PEARLS
- DKA is defined by a classic clinical triad of hyperglycemia, ketosis, and high anion gap metabolic acidosis.
- Admit if blood glucose >250 mg/dL, pH <7.3, HCO$_3$ ≤15 mEq/L, and ketones in urine.
- Potassium is falsely elevated due to acidosis; start replacement when K+ ≤5.2 mg/dL and urine output is adequate.

DIABETIC POLYNEUROPATHY

Samir Malkani, MD, MRCP–UK

BASICS

DESCRIPTION
Peripheral nerve dysfunction seen in diabetes; several patterns described:
- Symmetric polyneuropathy
  - Distal sensory or sensorimotor
- Mononeuropathy, radiculopathy, and polyradiculopathy
  - Cranial neuropathy
  - Focal limb or truncal neuropathy
  - Radiculoplexus neuropathy (diabetic amyotrophy)
- Acute painful small fiber neuropathy
- Autonomic neuropathies
- Chronic inflammatory demyelinating polyneuropathy (CIDP)

EPIDEMIOLOGY
Prevalence
- Generalized polyneuropathy
  - 10–30% at diabetes diagnosis
  - In diabetes, 50% at 10 years
  - Prevalence is higher in type 2 diabetes than type 1 diabetes.
- Autonomic neuropathy: 16.7% in a United Kingdom study

ETIOLOGY AND PATHOPHYSIOLOGY
- Metabolic derangement due to hyperglycemia and dyslipidemia
  - Aldose reductase converts excess glucose to sorbitol, which causes nerve damage.
  - Nonenzymatic glycation of neural proteins and lipids forms damaging advanced glycosylation end products.
  - Protein kinase C activation causes vascular endothelial changes.
  - Oxidative stress from excessive production of reactive oxygen species
  - Mitochondrial dysfunction and impaired mitochondrial trafficking within the neurons
- Vasculopathy causing nerve ischemia: predominant factor in mononeuropathies

RISK FACTORS
- Poor glycemic control
- Duration of diabetes
- Hypertension
- Dyslipidemia
- Obesity
- Tobacco and alcohol consumption

GENERAL PREVENTION
- Maintenance of normal blood sugar
- Exercise and appropriate diet

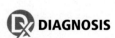

DIAGNOSIS

HISTORY
- Most common form (typical): symmetric distal sensory or sensorimotor polyneuropathy
  - Distressing numbness, tingling, pain of legs/feet, usually worse at night; allodynia; hyperalgesia
  - Often silent sensory loss; the patient is unaware.
- Ataxia and falls due to proprioceptive loss
  - Neuropathic foot ulcers due to analgesia and repetitive injury
  - Neuropathic degeneration of foot joints
  - Hands involved late
  - Distal muscle involvement, usually mild
- Symmetric proximal polyneuropathy
  - Proximal leg weakness and wasting
  - Muscles of shoulder girdle are rarely involved.
  - Pain and sensory changes are less prominent.
- Focal cranial or limb mononeuropathy
  - May involve 3rd, 4th, 6th, or 7th cranial nerve
  - Femoral, sciatic, or peroneal neuropathy: weakness or pain in nerve distribution
  - Any major peripheral nerve can be involved.
- Truncal neuropathies: painful radiculopathy over dermatomes
- Lumbar radiculoplexus neuropathy (diabetic amyotrophy)
  - Unilateral hip and thigh pain
  - Pelvic girdle and thigh weakness with atrophy
  - Recovery over months
- Diabetic autonomic neuropathy
  - GI: nocturnal diarrhea, sometimes alternating with constipation; gastroparesis with postprandial fullness; nausea and vomiting
  - Cardiovascular: postural dizziness, exercise intolerance
  - Urogenital: urinary hesitancy, overflow incontinence, erectile dysfunction, vaginal dryness, sexual dysfunction
  - Sudomotor: anhidrosis or hyperhidrosis; gustatory sweating of head and upper body
- CIDP: progressive, severe motor loss
- Diabetic cachexia: painful small fiber neuropathy with prominent weight loss and depression

PHYSICAL EXAM
- Symmetric distal polyneuropathy
  - "Stocking-and-glove" distal sensory loss
  - Large-fiber neuropathy: loss of perception of vibration and light touch (10-g monofilament)
  - Small fiber involvement: loss of temperature and pinprick
  - Absent ankle reflexes
  - Wasting, weakness of small muscles in foot; changes in arch of foot or clawing of toes
  - With small fiber involvement, there may be lack of objective sensory deficit despite pain.
- Symmetric proximal polyneuropathy
  - Proximal leg, arm wasting, and weakness
  - Loss of patellar reflexes
- Focal cranial or limb mononeuropathy
  - 3rd cranial nerve palsy: painful ophthalmoplegia and ptosis; preserved pupillary reflexes (in contrast to compressive palsies)
  - 6th cranial nerve: lateral gaze palsy
  - Femoral neuropathy: weakness of lower leg extension, hip flexion, quadriceps wasting, absent patellar reflex, sensory loss in anterior thigh
  - Sciatic neuropathy: pain or sensory loss in back of thigh and leg; weakness of hamstrings and lower leg muscles
  - Peroneal neuropathy: foot drop

- Truncal neuropathies: sensory loss along dermatome
- Lumbar radiculoplexus neuropathy (diabetic amyotrophy)
  - Weakness and wasting pelvic girdle and thigh
  - Sensory loss in L2–L3
  - Absent patellar reflex
- Autonomic neuropathy
  - Cardiovascular: resting tachycardia; orthostatic hypotension
  - Gastroparesis: postprandial distension; gastric splash
- CIDP: motor weakness

DIFFERENTIAL DIAGNOSIS
- Metabolic
  - Uremia, hypothyroidism
- Drug-induced
  - Antineoplastic drugs: cisplatin, vincristine
  - Isoniazid
  - Amiodarone
  - Alcohol
- Toxic
  - Chronic arsenic poisoning
  - n-Hexane, methyl-n-butyl ketone
- Nutritional deficiency
  - Vitamin B_{12}, pyridoxine, thiamine
- Paraneoplastic polyneuropathy

DIAGNOSTIC TESTS & INTERPRETATION
Initial Tests (lab, imaging)
- Fasting plasma glucose, 2-hour glucose tolerance test or hemoglobin A1c for diagnosis and to assess glycemic control; may occur in "prediabetes"
- Serum vitamin B_{12}
- Thyroid function
- Creatinine and BUN
- Syphilis and HIV testing
- Serum protein electrophoresis
- In mononeuropathy/mononeuritis multiplex, test for vasculitis, paraproteinemia, Lyme disease, and sarcoidosis.
- In radiculopathy or mononeuropathy, imaging studies to exclude compressive lesions

Diagnostic Procedures/Other
- Bedside testing of vibration perception with 128-Hz tuning fork, monofilament perception of 10-g filament, pinprick, and temperature testing
- Quantitative sensory testing for vibratory and thermal thresholds
  - Standardized measures for assessing severity and risk of foot ulceration
- Electromyogram nerve conduction velocity
  - Useful to confirm mononeuropathy and entrapment syndromes
  - Sensitive but nonspecific index of presence and severity of diabetic polyneuropathy
  - In small unmyelinated fiber painful neuropathy, test may be normal.
- Lumbar puncture
  - In CIDP, elevation of spinal fluid protein
- Skin biopsy with epidermal nerve fiber density
  - Enables direct study of small nerve fibers that are difficult to assess electrophysiologically
- Corneal confocal microscopy
  - Noninvasive approach; loss of corneal innervation correlates with neuropathy

Test Interpretation

- In nerve biopsy of peripheral nerve, Wallerian degeneration, focal axonal swellings containing neurofilaments, axonal atrophy, and demyelination are seen.
- Thick neural capillary basement membrane and endothelial proliferation
- Obliterative microvascular lesions and perivascular inflammation

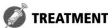

TREATMENT

GENERAL MEASURES

- Maintain blood glucose control.
- Provide appropriate footwear to prevent pressure damage to insensate feet.

MEDICATION

Specific treatment to reverse nerve damage, other than improved glucose control, is not available. Current therapies target pain relief. Combination of agents from different classes may be more effective when a single medication is ineffective.

First Line

Management of pain and sensory neuropathy

- Calcium channel modulators: pregabalin (1),(2),(3)
  - Binds same calcium channel as gabapentin
  - Linear pharmacokinetics and quicker onset of action compared to gabapentin
  - Usual dose: 150 to 600 mg/day; NNT ~4 to 10
  - Adverse effects are drowsiness, dizziness, and edema.
- Duloxetine (1),(2),(4)
  - Selective serotonin-norepinephrine reuptake inhibitor
  - Usual dose is 30 to 60 mg/day; NNT ~4 to 9
  - Adverse effects are nausea and dizziness.
- Management of autonomic neuropathy
  - Orthostatic hypotension
    - Fludrocortisone (off-label)
    - Midodrine (off-label)
  - Gastroparesis
    - Metoclopramide or domperidone
    - Erythromycin (off-label)
  - Diabetic diarrhea
    - Loperamide
    - Clonidine (off-label)
    - Octreotide (off-label)
    - Antibiotics for bacterial overgrowth
  - Hyperhidrosis
    - Propantheline (off-label)
    - Topical glycopyrrolate

Geriatric Considerations

Anticholinergic effects of TCAs may cause urinary retention and cardiac arrhythmias.

Second Line

- Calcium channel modulators: gabapentin (1),(2),(3) (off-label)
  - Binds Ca^{2+} channel–associated protein α_2-δ; inhibits neurotransmitter release
  - Dose range of 300 to 1,200 mg TID; NNT ~4 to 8
  - Reduce dose in renal insufficiency.
  - Adverse effects: dizziness, fatigue, edema

- TCAs (1),(2),(4) (off-label)
  - Analgesia may be related to effects on sodium channels; NNT ~2 to 5, NNH ~3 to 16
  - Amitriptyline 25 to 150 mg at bedtime
  - Nortriptyline (25 to 150 mg); desipramine (25 to 200 mg) is less sedating than amitriptyline but limited trial data
  - Anticholinergic effects and cardiac arrhythmias may occur; use with caution in patients with ischemic heart disease.
- Venlafaxine (2),(4) (off-label)
  - 75 to 225 mg daily; NNT ~2 to 5
  - Serotonin-norepinephrine reuptake inhibitor
- Topical therapies
  - Capsaicin (1),(2),(4),(5) 0.075% cream applied TID, 8% long-acting patch applied by health care professional in office
    - Depletes C fibers in skin of substance P
    - Limited data on efficacy
  - Lidocaine (2),(4),(5) 5% (700 mg) patches applied daily to feet (off-label):
    - Causes sodium channel blockade
- Opiate analgesia
  - Tramadol (1),(2),(4) (off-label): 100 to 400 mg/day; NNT ~3 to 9
    - Binds opiate receptors; also inhibits reuptake of norepinephrine and serotonin; fewer opiate side effects
  - Tapentadol (1),(2),(4)
    - Binds to μ-opiate receptor and inhibits norepinephrine uptake

ISSUES FOR REFERRAL

If CIDP is suspected, refer to neurologist for investigation and treatment.

ADDITIONAL THERAPIES

- Transcutaneous electrical nerve stimulation
- Percutaneous nerve stimulation
- Electrical spinal cord stimulation
- Actovegin, dextromethorphan with quinidine

SURGERY/OTHER PROCEDURES

Electrical spinal cord stimulation 10 kHz (1)

COMPLEMENTARY & ALTERNATIVE MEDICINE

Acupuncture, Reiki, electromagnetic field treatment: no convincing trial data

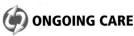

ONGOING CARE

PROGNOSIS

- Generalized symmetric polyneuropathies
  - Usually slow, chronic progression
  - Insensitive but painless foot as pain lessens
- Focal neuropathies
  - Recovery over months to years

COMPLICATIONS

- Claw foot deformity
- Neurotropic ulceration
  - Painless ulcers on weight-bearing area
  - Callus formation is a precursor to ulceration.
- Neuropathic arthropathy
  - Results in complete disorganization of joint structure in foot, Charcot joint

REFERENCES

1. Pop-Busui R, Ang L, Boulton AJM, et al. *Diagnosis and Treatment of Painful Diabetic Peripheral Neuropathy.* Arlington, VA: American Diabetes Association; 2022.
2. Gandhi M, Fargo E, Prasad-Reddy L, et al. Diabetes: how to manage diabetic peripheral neuropathy. *Drugs Context.* 2022;11:2021-10-2.
3. Derry S, Bell RF, Straube S, et al. Pregabalin for neuropathic pain in adults. *Cochrane Database Syst Rev.* 2019;1(1):CD007076.
4. Alam U, Sloan G, Tesfaye S. Treating pain in diabetic neuropathy: current and developmental drugs. *Drugs.* 2020;80(4):363–384.
5. Azmi S, Alam U, Burgess J, et al. State-of-the-art pharmacotherapy for diabetic neuropathy. *Expert Opi Pharmacothe.* 2021;22(1):55–68.

ADDITIONAL READING

- Elafros MA, Andersen H, Bennett DL, et al. Towards prevention of diabetic peripheral neuropathy: clinical presentation, pathogenesis and new treatments. *Lancet Neuro.* 2022;21(10):922–936.
- Patel K, Horak H, Tiryaki E. Diabetic neuropathies. *Muscle Nerve.* 2021;63(1):22–30.
- Vinik AI. Clinical practice. Diabetic sensory and motor neuropathy. *N Engl J Med.* 2016;374(15):1455–1464.

 SEE ALSO

Diabetes Mellitus, Type 1; Diabetes Mellitus, Type 2

 CODES

ICD10

- E10.42 Type 1 diabetes mellitus with diabetic polyneuropathy
- E11.42 Type 2 diabetes mellitus with diabetic polyneuropathy
- E13.42 Oth diabetes mellitus with diabetic polyneuropathy

CLINICAL PEARLS

- Occasionally, when glycemic control improves dramatically, as can occur when treatment for diabetes is initiated, there may be a worsening of neuropathic symptoms (described as treatment-induced neuropathy). Symptoms usually stabilize and gradually improve as glycemic control is maintained.
- It is common to combine agents with different mechanisms of action in the management of neuropathic pain. Topical therapies can be combined with systemic therapies. There is limited evidence-based data to support combination oral therapy.

DIARRHEA, ACUTE

Marie L. Borum, MD, EdD, MPH • Ankit Patel, MD • Ivan Berezowski, MD

BASICS

DESCRIPTION
- An abnormal increase in stool water content, volume, or frequency (≥3 stools above baseline in 24 hours) for <14 days duration
- Most commonly secondary to infectious etiology; often self-limited
- Acute viral diarrhea (50–70%)
  - Most common cause of infectious diarrhea; noninflammatory (watery)
  - Frequently presents with associated nausea and/or vomiting
  - Symptoms usually develop after an incubation period of ~1 day and last for 1 to 3 days; typically self-limited
- Bacterial diarrhea (15–20%)
  - Most common infectious cause of inflammatory (bloody) diarrhea
  - Incubation period variable; diarrhea is caused by preformed enterotoxin presents within 1 to 6 hours of contaminated food ingestion, whereas bacterial infection typically presents within 1 to 3 days.
  - Symptoms usually resolve in 1 to 7 days; antibiotic use attenuates length and/or severity of disease.
  - Suspect when concurrent illness in others who have shared potentially contaminated food.
- Protozoal infections (10–15%)
  - Typically cause noninflammatory (watery) diarrhea
  - Long incubation period and prolonged disease course; symptoms develop approximately 7 days after exposure and commonly last >7 days.
  - Suspect when outbreaks of watery diarrhea in areas with contaminated water or food supply
- Traveler's diarrhea (TD) typically begins 3 to 7 days after arrival in foreign location and resolves within 5 days; rapid onset, generally self-limited

EPIDEMIOLOGY
- In resource-limited countries, acute diarrhea is more common in children; no age predilection in resource-rich countries
- Acute diarrhea accounts for >128,000 U.S. hospital admissions and ~2.5 million annual deaths worldwide (1).
- The WHO categorizes acute diarrhea (symptoms <14 days) into watery and bloody (dysentery) subtypes.

Prevalence
- Fourth leading cause of death in children aged <5 years and eighth leading cause of death among all ages worldwide
- Affects 11% of the general population
- In resource-rich countries, acute diarrhea is largely due to contaminated food and water.

ETIOLOGY AND PATHOPHYSIOLOGY
- Bacterial
  - *Escherichia coli, Salmonella, Shigella, Campylobacter jejuni*
  - *Vibrio parahaemolyticus, Vibrio cholerae, Yersinia enterocolitica*
  - *Clostridium difficile, Staphylococcus aureus*
  - *Bacillus cereus, Clostridium perfringens*
  - *Listeria monocytogenes*
  - *Mycobacterium avium complex* (in immuno-compromised), *Mycobacterium tuberculosis* (in immunocompromised)

- Viral
  - *Rotavirus* and *Norovirus* (most common)
  - Adenovirus
  - Astrovirus
  - *Cytomegalovirus* (CMV) (in immunocompromised)
- Protozoal
  - *Giardia lamblia, Entamoeba histolytica*
  - *Cryptosporidium* (in immunocompromised)
  - *Cystoisospora belli*
  - *Cyclospora, Microspora* (in immunocompromised)
- Pathophysiology (1)
  - Noninflammatory: most commonly viral; increased intestinal secretions without disruption of intestinal mucosa; watery character
  - Inflammatory: generally invasive or toxin-producing bacteria; disrupts mucosal integrity with subsequent tissue invasion/damage; bloody character
- Viral diarrhea: changes in small intestine cell morphology, including villous shortening, increased number of crypt cells, and increased cellularity of the lamina propria
- Bacterial diarrhea: Bacterial invasion of colonic wall leads to mucosal hyperemia, edema, and leukocytic infiltration.

RISK FACTORS
- Travel to resource-limited countries
- Failure to observe food/water precautions
- Immunocompromised host (HIV, malignancy, chemotherapy)
- Recent hospitalization
- Antibiotic use
- Proton pump inhibitor (PPI) use
- Daycare exposure
- Fecal-oral sexual contact
- Nursing home residence
- Pregnancy (12-fold increase for listeriosis) (1)

GENERAL PREVENTION
- Frequent hand washing reduces incidence of diarrhea by approximately 30%.
- Proper food and water precautions, particularly during foreign travel—"boil it, peel it, cook it, or forget it"
- Avoid undercooked meat, raw fish, and unpasteurized milk.
- Rotavirus vaccine (for infants)
- Typhoid fever and cholera vaccine (for travel to endemic areas)
- TD prevention:
  - Pretravel counseling on high-risk food/beverage
  - Consider daily prophylaxis with bismuth subsalicylate (BSS) in all travelers (can reduce the risk of TD by up to 60%); usual dosing of 2 tablets (262 mg each) or 2 oz (60 mL) liquid formulation 4 times daily
  - Do not use routine antibiotic prophylaxis.
  - When indicated (immunocompromised), the Infectious Disease Society of America recommends chemoprophylaxis with fluoroquinolones: norfloxacin 400 mg/day or ciprofloxacin 500 mg orally once or twice daily; otherwise, avoid given increasing global resistance to fluoroquinolones
  - Probiotics, prebiotics, and synbiotics have unclear benefit as prophylaxis.

COMMONLY ASSOCIATED CONDITIONS
- Inflammatory bowel disease (IBD)
- Immunocompromised (HIV, malignancy, chemotherapy)

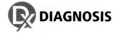

DIAGNOSIS

HISTORY
- Duration of symptoms <14 days
- Historical clues for dehydration: orthostatic hypotension, dizziness, increased thirst, decreased urine output, or altered mental status
- Description of stool—characteristics and output
  - Frequency; quantity; consistency; character: presence of mucus, blood, or fat; floating
  - *Giardia* associated with pale, greasy stools
- Weight loss
- Associated symptoms: change in appetite, abdominal pain or bloating, nausea/vomiting, or fever
- Risk factors of acute diarrhea (See "Risk Factors.")
- Cirrhosis (associated with *Vibrio*)
- Hemochromatosis (associated with *Yersinia*)

PHYSICAL EXAM
- Assess degree of dehydration (1); ill-appearing, dry mucous membranes, tachycardia, orthostatic hypotension, decreased skin turgor, delayed capillary refill, altered mental status; can be absent in early dehydration
- Fever is more suggestive of inflammatory diarrhea.
- Thyroid: Assess for enlargement or nodules.
- Abdomen: Assess for distention, rigidity, and rebound tenderness.
- Rectum: blood, tenderness, stool consistency

Geriatric Considerations
Fecal impaction or obstructing neoplasm can cause overflow diarrhea with chronic constipation.

DIFFERENTIAL DIAGNOSIS
- IBD; malabsorption
- Medications (cholinergic agents, magnesium-containing antacids, chemotherapy, antibiotics)
- Diverticulitis, ischemic colitis; spastic (irritable) colon
- Fecal impaction
- Endocrinopathies: thyroid disease
- Neoplasia

DIAGNOSTIC TESTS & INTERPRETATION
Initial Tests (lab, imaging)
- Reserve laboratory testing for patients with persistent fever, moderate-severe disease characterized by passage of ≥6 stools per day, duration of >72 hours, dysentery, profuse watery diarrhea, immunosuppression, or if suspected outbreak (2).
- Complete blood count (CBC)
  - Leukocytosis, anemia (blood loss), eosinophilia (parasite infection), thrombocytopenia (hemolytic-uremic syndrome [HUS])
- Basic metabolic panel (BMP)
  - Serum electrolytes, BUN and creatinine (may elevate with volume depletion), nonanion gap metabolic acidosis

- Stool sample
  - Occult blood (IBD, bowel ischemia, and certain bacterial infections)
  - Fecal leukocytes: useful to distinguish inflammatory diarrhea from noninflammatory but should not be used to determine the infectious cause of diarrhea
  - Stool ova and parasites
  - Stool culture
  - Multiplex stool testing (PCR testing for bacterial, viral, and parasitic causes of diarrhea) if dysentery, moderate to severe disease, and symptoms lasting >7 days
  - *C. difficile* toxin (especially IBD, recently hospitalized or recent antibiotic use) (3)[C]
  - *G. lamblia* antigen ELISA kit >90% sensitive in at-risk population
- Abdominal radiographs (flat plate and upright) if severe abdominal pain or concern for obstruction
- Abdominal CT scan is preferred to evaluate intra-abdominal disease.

Diagnostic Procedures/Other
- Consider sigmoidoscopy or colonoscopy in patients with persistent diarrhea, when there is no clear diagnosis after routine blood and stool tests, and if empiric or supportive therapy is ineffective.
- Consider colonoscopy in immunocompromised patients to evaluate for CMV colitis.

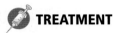

TREATMENT

GENERAL MEASURES
- Oral rehydration and electrolyte management are key to successful treatment.
  - Oral intake, as tolerated—"if the gut works, use it"
  - IV fluids if patient cannot tolerate oral rehydration or presents with severe dehydration
- Balanced electrolyte rehydration solutions recommended in elderly and profuse, watery TD (2)

MEDICATION

First Line
- Consider empiric antibiotics (fluoroquinolones or macrolides) in patients with signs and symptoms of systemic infection, severe disease, or clear cases of TD (2).
  - Fever; bloody diarrhea; fecal leukocytes
  - Immunocompromised host
  - Signs of severe volume depletion
- Tailor antibiotics to stool culture results.
  - *Giardia*: metronidazole 250 mg PO TID for 5 to 7 days, tinidazole 2 g PO once
  - *E. histolytica*: metronidazole 500 to 750 mg PO TID for 7 to 10 days, tinidazole 2 g PO daily for 3 to 5 days
  - *Shigella*: ciprofloxacin 500 mg PO BID for 3 to 5 days or ceftriaxone 1 to 2 g IM/IV daily for 5 days
  - *Campylobacter*: azithromycin 500 mg PO daily for 3 to 5 days or erythromycin 500 mg PO QID for 5 days
  - *C. difficile*: The Infectious Disease Society of America now recommends fidaxomicin 200 mg PO BID for 10 days as first-line therapy. Vancomycin 125 to 500 mg PO QID for 10 to 14 days can be used as alternative; consider fecal microbiota transplant in recurrent mild to moderate *C. difficile* infections.

- TD: ciprofloxacin 500 mg PO BID for 1 to 3 days, azithromycin (if suspicion of quinolone resistant pathogens) 500 mg PO daily or 1 g PO daily for 1 to 3 days, rifamycin SV 388 mg PO BID for 3 days or rifaximin 200 mg PO TID for 3 days (noninvasive strains of E.coli); can combine with loperamide; loperamide or BSS may be used alone in cases of mild TD.
- General considerations
  - Antibiotics are not recommended in *Salmonella* infections unless caused by *Salmonella typhosa* or if the patient is febrile or immunocompromised.
  - Avoid antibiotics in patients with *E. coli* O157:H7 due to risk for HUS.
  - Antibiotics are not indicated for foodborne toxigenic diarrhea.
  - Avoid antimotility agents (e.g., loperamide) in patients with febrile or bloody diarrhea or antibiotic-associated colitis due to risk of toxic megacolon.
  - Antimotility agents used with antibiotics may speed recovery from TD.
  - Antibiotics are not recommended for the treatment of mild TD.

COMPLEMENTARY & ALTERNATIVE MEDICINE
- BSS may help control rate of diarrhea stools (2).
- Probiotics are recommended for prevention of antibiotic-associated diarrhea and *C. difficile* infection recurrence and for treatment of acute infectious diarrhea in setting of symptomatic irritable bowel syndrome (IBS).
- Probiotic use >10^{10}/g may help in patients with antibiotic-associated diarrhea.
- Avoid probiotics in immunocompromised patients.

ADMISSION, INPATIENT, AND NURSING CONSIDERATIONS
Outpatient management, except for patients who are severely ill with signs of volume depletion

ONGOING CARE

DIET
- Early oral refeeding is encouraged. Regular diets are as effective as restricted diets.
- The traditional bananas, rice, applesauce, toast (BRAT) diet has little evidence-based support (despite heavy clinical use) and may result in suboptimal nutrition.
- During periods of active diarrhea, coffee, alcohol, dairy products, fruits, vegetables, red meats, and heavily seasoned foods may exacerbate symptoms.

PATIENT EDUCATION
See "General Prevention."

PROGNOSIS
Acute diarrhea is rarely life-threatening if adequate hydration is maintained.

COMPLICATIONS
- Volume depletion, shock, sepsis
- HUS with *E. coli* O157:H7
- Guillain-Barré syndrome with *C. jejuni*
- Reactive arthritis with *Salmonella*, *Shigella*, and *Yersinia*
- Functional bowel disorders (e.g., postinfectious IBS [PI-IBS])

REFERENCES

1. Hamilton KW, Cifu AS. Diagnosis and management of infectious diarrhea. *JAMA*. 2019;321(9): 891–892.
2. Ferris A, Gaisinskaya P, Nandi N. Approach to diarrhea. *Prim Care*. 2023;50(3):447–459.
3. Khanna S, Shin A, Kelly CP. Management of *Clostridium difficile* infection in inflammatory bowel disease: expert review from the Clinical Practice Updates Committee of the AGA Institute. *Clin Gastroenterol Hepatol*. 2017;15(2):166–174.

ADDITIONAL READING
- da Cruz Gouveia MA, Lins MTC, da Silva GAP. Acute diarrhea with blood: diagnosis and drug treatment. *J Pediatr (Rio J)*. 2020;96(Suppl 1):20–28.
- Florez ID, Niño-Serna LF, Beltrán-Arroyave CP. Acute infectious diarrhea and gastroenteritis in children. *Curr Infect Dis Rep*. 2020;22(2):4.

 SEE ALSO

Botulism; Cholera; Food Poisoning, Bacterial

 CODES

ICD10
- R19.7 Diarrhea, unspecified
- A09 Infectious gastroenteritis and colitis, unspecified
- A08.4 Viral intestinal infection, unspecified

CLINICAL PEARLS
- Viruses are the most common causes of acute diarrheal illness in the United States.
- Consider broad infectious etiologies if patients are immunocompromised (CMV, *Cryptosporidium*, *Cyclospora*, *Microspora*, *M. avium complex*, and *M. tuberculosis*).
- Oral rehydration is the most important and effective treatment for acute diarrhea.
- Avoid antimotility agents (e.g., loperamide) in febrile patients, bloody diarrhea, and antibiotic-associated colitis.
- Routine stool culture is not recommended, unless patients present with bloody diarrhea, fever, severe dehydration, signs of inflammatory disease, persistent symptoms >7 days, or have a history of immunosuppression.
- Start empiric antibiotics in patients who are severely ill or immunocompromised.

DIARRHEA, CHRONIC

Marie L. Borum, MD, EdD, MPH • Reid Evan Schalet, DO, BA

BASICS

DESCRIPTION
- Chronic diarrhea refers to a sustained change in stool consistency, characterized by loose stools (consistency between types 5 and 7 on the Bristol stool chart), and an increase in frequency of defecation (typically >3 loose stools per day) for >4 weeks (1),(2).
- Etiologies include osmotic, secretory, malabsorptive, inflammatory, infectious, and hypermotility (2).

EPIDEMIOLOGY
Incidence
Difficult to estimate as definitions vary

Prevalence
Varies by etiology; worldwide prevalence is ~3–20% (2). U.S. prevalence is ~6.6%.

ETIOLOGY AND PATHOPHYSIOLOGY
Disturbances in luminal water and electrolytes cause increased water volume in the stool.
- Osmotic (fecal osmotic gap >100 mOsm/kg) (3); resolves with fasting (2); less voluminous than secretory diarrhea
  - Carbohydrate malabsorption: disaccharides (e.g., lactose), monosaccharides (e.g., fructose), and polyols (sugar substitutes); Mg, citrates, phosphate, and sulfate ingestion
- Secretory (fecal osmotic gap <50 mOsm/kg) (1),(4); does not resolve with fasting (2); characterized by watery stools that persist at night and during fasting
  - Alcoholism, stimulant laxative ingestion; bacterial enterotoxins (i.e., cholera); postcholecystectomy/ ileal resection <100 cm: Excessive intestinal bile salts cause choleretic diarrhea.
  - Disordered motility: postvagotomy, autonomic neuropathy, hyperthyroidism
  - Neuroendocrine tumors: VIPoma; carcinoid syndrome, gastrinoma, somatostatinoma
  - Metastatic medullary thyroid cancer; adrenal insufficiency
  - Noninvasive infection: giardiasis, cryptosporidiosis
  - Microscopic colitis; protein-losing enteropathy
- Fatty diarrhea: characterized by bulky, foul-smelling stools
  - Hepatobiliary disorders, cystic fibrosis (CF), chronic pancreatitis, diabetes mellitus
- Malabsorptive (1),(4): characterized by higher than average stool volumes
  - Celiac disease, Whipple disease; tropical sprue, giardiasis, amyloidosis
  - Chronic mesenteric ischemia, lymphatic obstruction (e.g., heart failure, lymphoma)
  - Short bowel syndrome: Ileal resection of >100 cm leads to insufficient bile salts.
  - Small intestinal bacterial overgrowth (SIBO); pancreatic exocrine insufficiency
- Inflammatory (1),(4): characterized by loose liquid stool with occasional blood
  - Inflammatory bowel disease (IBD)—ulcerative colitis; Crohn disease
  - Microscopic colitis; diverticulitis; vasculitis; radiation enterocolitis
  - Infections: *Clostridium difficile*, *Entamoeba histolytica*, cytomegalovirus, tuberculosis, salmonella
  - Neoplasms: colon cancer, lymphoma
- Hypermotility (normal fecal osmotic gap; 50 to 100 mOsm/kg) (1)
  - Irritable bowel syndrome (IBS); functional diarrhea (Pain differentiates IBS from functional diarrhea.) (2),(3)
- Drugs (1),(4): confirmed by resolution of symptoms following withdrawal of medication
  - NSAIDs, PPIs, colchicine, metformin, digoxin, ACE inhibitors, β-blockers, gliptins, theophyllines, antibiotics, SSRIs, antineoplastic agents, excessive laxative use (factitious diarrhea)
  - Herbal products: St. John's wort, echinacea, garlic, saw palmetto, ginseng, etc.
- Infectious (1)
  - Bacterial: *C. difficile*, *M. avium intracellulare*; viral: cytomegalovirus; parasitic: *Giardia lamblia*, *Cryptosporidium*, *Isospora*, *E. histolytica*, *Strongyloides*
- Food allergies (1)

Genetics
- Celiac disease is associated with HLA-DQ2 and HLA-DQ8 haplotypes (3).
- IBD is polygenic. First-degree relative of IBD patients have 10-fold increased risk (3).
- CF transmembrane conductance regulator (CFTR) mutation contributes in CF.

RISK FACTORS
- Osmotic
  - Excess ingestion of nonabsorbable carbohydrates (i.e., artificial sweeteners); magnesium-containing antacids (3)
  - Excess ingestion poorly absorbed ions (phosphate, sulfate, magnesium) (1)
  - Lactose intolerance, celiac disease
  - Medications (i.e., citrates, phosphates, sulfates, magnesium-containing laxatives, sugar alcohols)
- Secretory (1)
  - Postsurgical: small bowel resection/ileal surgery, vagotomy, bile acid malabsorption; history of neuroendocrine disease or stimulant laxative abuse; dysmotility syndromes
  - Medications (i.e., NSAIDs, caffeine, metformin, colchicine, carbamazepine, antibiotics, calcitonin) (3)
- Malabsorptive
  - CF; chronic alcohol abuse, celiac disease
  - Chronic pancreatitis/pancreatic insufficiency (fat malabsorption); medications (e.g., orlistat, acarbose, aminoglycosides, thyroid supplements)
- Inflammatory
  - IBD, NSAID use, antibiotics, radiation; HIV/AIDS, colorectal cancer, invasive infection (tuberculosis, *Yersinia*)
  - Pseudomembranous colitis (*C. difficile*)
  - Antineoplastic drugs (i.e., 5-fluorouracil, methotrexate, irinotecan), radiation
  - Immunosuppressant therapy
- Hypermotility
  - Psychosocial stress, preceding infection
  - Stimulant medications (i.e., macrolides, metoclopramide, senna, bisacodyl [Dulcolax]) (3)
- Genetic predisposition

ALERT
Diabetes mellitus and cholecystectomy can cause secretory and osmotic diarrhea.

GENERAL PREVENTION
Varies by etiology; treat the underlying cause.

COMMONLY ASSOCIATED CONDITIONS
- Extraintestinal manifestations of IBD include arthralgias, aphthous stomatitis, uveitis/episcleritis, erythema nodosum, pyoderma gangrenosum, perianal fistulas, rectal fissures, ankylosing spondylitis, and PSC.
- Celiac disease is associated with dermatitis herpetiformis, T1DM, and IgA deficiency.
- Latex-food allergy syndrome: allergies to latex, banana, avocado, kiwi, and walnut (1)

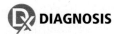

DIAGNOSIS

HISTORY
- Detailed history: stooling onset, pattern, frequency, characteristics (greasy, floating, watery), volume, travel, diet, medications, family history, urgency, fecal incontinence
- Alarm features: rectal bleeding, weight loss, fever, nocturnal symptoms, onset after the age of 50 years
- Skin changes (rashes), arthritis, ocular problems, heat intolerance, polyuria/polydipsia, fever, flushing, alcohol use
- Food allergies (1)
- Flatus and bloating are predominant features of carbohydrate malabsorption (1).
- Risk factors: history of STIs, prior gastrointestinal surgeries, diabetes, radiation, family history of colorectal cancer (2),(4)
- IBS or functional diarrhea by Rome IV criteria (2),(3),(4):
  - IBS: recurrent abdominal pain at least 1 day/week in the preceding 3 months (symptoms >6 months) associated with ≥2 of the following criteria: related to defecation, change in frequency of stool, change in form of stool
  - Functional diarrhea: ≥25% loose or watery stools without abdominal pain or bloating for >3 months (symptoms >6 months); normal abdominal, oral, and skin examinations; lack of alarm features

PHYSICAL EXAM
- General: volume depletion, nutritional status, recent weight loss, anasarca (1),(2)
- Skin: flushing (carcinoid), erythema nodosum (IBD), pyoderma gangrenosum (IBD), ecchymoses (vitamin K deficiency), dermatitis herpetiformis (celiac disease), hyperpigmentation (Addison disease) (1),(2)
- HEENT: iritis/uveitis/episcleritis (IBD), lid lag (hyperthyroid); exophthalmos (hyperthyroid); neck: goiter (hyperthyroid), lymphadenopathy (Whipple disease), oral ulcerations (IBD), aphthous stomatitis (IBD)
- Cardiovascular: tachycardia (hyperthyroid), heart murmur (carcinoid syndrome) (2),(4)
- Pulmonary: wheezing (carcinoid)
- Abdomen: hyperactive bowel sounds (IBD), distension, and/or diffuse tenderness (IBD/IBS), anorectal fistulas or anal fissures (IBD), fecal impaction (overflow incontinence)
- Extremities: arthritis (IBD); neurologic: tremor (hyperthyroid), spondylitis (IBD)

DIFFERENTIAL DIAGNOSIS
See "Etiology and Pathophysiology," "Commonly Associated Conditions," and "Risk Factors."

DIAGNOSTIC TESTS & INTERPRETATION
Initial Tests (lab, imaging)
Test patients with alarm symptoms or persistent symptoms and no identifiable cause.

- Blood: CBC, electrolytes (Mg, P, Ca), total protein, albumin, thyroid-stimulating hormone, free T_4, erythrocyte sedimentation rate, C-reactive protein (CRP), iron studies (1),(4)
  - Normal CRP (<10mg/L) or fecal calprotectin (<50 μg/g) level effectively rules out IBD for patients who meet Rome IV diagnostic criteria for IBS without alarm features (3)[A].
- Stool: fecal WBC, lactoferrin/calprotectin (preferred), culture, ova and parasite, *Giardia* antigen, *C. difficile* toxin, electrolytes, occult blood, osmolality, qualitative fecal fat (Sudan stain) (1)
  - Fecal osmotic gap = 290 mOsm/kg—2(Na[feces] + K[feces])
  - *C. difficile* testing only in diarrheal stools (3)[C]
- CT or MRI to evaluate the GI tract structure (i.e., IBD, malignancy, chronic pancreatitis) (1)

Follow-Up Tests & Special Considerations
- Celiac disease: antiendomysial antibody IgA, anti-TTG IgA (sensitivity and specificity >90%) in patients without IgA deficiency, serum IgA level (10% of celiac patients have IgA deficiency—may cause false-negative results.)
  - IgA TTG positive result should be confirmed by duodenal biopsy (2).
- Pancreatic insufficiency: fecal elastase, fecal chymotrypsin, serum trypsinogen (1)[C]
- Protein-losing enteropathy: fecal α_1-antitrypsin (1)[C]
- Microscopic colitis: colonic biopsy from normal-appearing mucosa (3)[C],(4)[C]
- Carbohydrate malabsorption: fecal pH (<7.0) and hydrogen breath test
- SIBO: hydrogen breath test and proximal jejunal aspirate with >10^5 CFU/mL coliform bacteria (3)
- Recent hospitalization or antibiotics: *C. difficile* toxin
- HIV ELISA, *Isospora/Cryptosporidium* stains (1)[C]
- Consider testing for protozoa, atypical infections, *Strongyloides*, *E. histolytica*, *Giardia*, *Cyclospora*, *Microsporidium* and tropical sprue if indicated (1)[C].
- Allergy testing (1)[C]
- Laxative abuse: stool osmotic gap (4)[C]
- Neuroendocrine tumor: chromogranin A, somatostatin, VIP, gastrin, calcitonin; urine: 5-HIAA, histamine; CT or MRI abdomen (3)

Diagnostic Procedures/Other
- Ileocolonoscopy with biopsies: IBD, microscopic or CMV colitis, and colorectal cancer
- Flexible sigmoidoscopy: if pregnant, with comorbidities, or if left-sided symptoms predominate (tenesmus and urgency)
- Esophagogastroduodenoscopy (EGD) with biopsies if malabsorption or small bowel enteropathy is suspected
- MRCP if chronic pancreatitis is suspected
- CT or magnetic resonance enterography (1)

Test Interpretation
- Celiac disease: intraepithelial lymphocytosis, crypt hyperplasia, villous atrophy
- Crohn disease: cobblestoning, creeping fat, strictures, linear ulcerations, skip lesions, noncaseating granulomas, lymphoid aggregates

- Ulcerative colitis: crypt abscesses, continuous rectal lesion, loss of haustra ("lead pipe" sign)
- Lactose Intolerance: normal-appearing villi, lactase deficiency
- Lymphocytic colitis: high intraepithelial lymphocytes, inflammatory cells in the lamina propria, normal mucosa
- Melanosis coli suggests laxative abuse (1).

 TREATMENT

GENERAL MEASURES
Volume resuscitation, electrolyte repletion; if stable, outpatient treatment (1)[C]

MEDICATION
First Line
- Lactose intolerance: lactose-free diet; postcholecystectomy, abdominal radiation therapy or ileal resection: cholestyramine or colestipol 2 to 16 g/day PO split BID; diabetes: glucose control; hyperthyroidism: methimazole 5 to 20 mg/day PO, propylthiouracil (PTU) 100 to 150 mg/day PO divided; thyroid ablation; *C. difficile*: 10 days of vancomycin 125 mg PO q6h or metronidazole (Flagyl) 500 mg PO q8h or fidaxomicin 200 mg PO BID; *G. lamblia*: metronidazole 250 mg PO q8h × 5 to 7 days, nitazoxanide 500 mg PO q12h × 3 days (1)[A]
- Whipple disease: ceftriaxone 2 g IV for 14 days or penicillin 2 MU IV every 4 hours for 2 weeks and then trimethoprim and sulfamethoxazole (Bactrim DS) 160/800 mg PO BID for 1 to 2 years
- SIBO: rifaximin 550 mg PO BID, fluoroquinolones 250 to 750 mg PO BID, metronidazole 500 mg PO q6–8h
- Pancreatic insufficiency: pancrelipase; HIV/AIDS: antiretroviral therapy (HAART)
- Microscopic colitis: budesonide 9 mg/day PO, mesalamine 800 mg PO TID, bismuth subsalicylate (Pepto-Bismol) 786 mg PO TID; IBD: 5-ASA, short courses of corticosteroids and/or antibiotics, immunomodulators, anti-TNF therapy, cholestyramine; neuroendocrine tumor: octreotide 100 to 600 g/day SC (1)[C]
- Celiac disease: gluten-free diet; IBS diarrhea predominant: rifaximin 550 mg PO TID × 14 days, alosetron 0.5 to 1.0 mg PO BID, peppermint oil, eluxadoline 100 mg PO BID; TCAs may also be considered (1)[C].
- Symptom relief: loperamide 4 to 8 mg/day (if infection ruled out), diphenoxylate-atropine 1 to 2 tabs BID–QID, activated charcoal, fiber supplementation, bismuth subsalicylate 525 to 1,050 mg every 0.5 to 1 hour (1)[C]

ISSUES FOR REFERRAL
Gastroenterology referral for suspected inflammatory diarrhea or endoscopy/biopsy

SURGERY/OTHER PROCEDURES
- Resection of neuroendocrine tumors; intestinal resection for refractory IBD
- Fecal transplant for recurrent *C. difficile*

ADMISSION, INPATIENT, AND NURSING CONSIDERATIONS
Consider hospitalization if hemodynamically unstable, severe electrolyte abnormalities, dehydration, malnutrition, AKI, or unable to tolerate oral intake.

 ONGOING CARE

DIET
Elimination diet: Avoid gluten-containing foods, nonabsorbable carbohydrates, lactose-containing products, and food allergens. Low FODMAP diet helps symptoms in up to 75% of IBS patients (1),(2).

PATIENT EDUCATION
- Chronic diarrhea is generally defined as three or more loose bowel movements per day for over 4 weeks.
- Wide variation in "normal" bowel habits; restrict colon stimulants.

PROGNOSIS
Varies according to etiology

COMPLICATIONS
- Fluid and electrolyte imbalances, AKI; malnutrition, anemia, weight loss
- Malignancy (colon cancer [IBD], lymphoma [IBD therapies], small bowel cancer [celiac disease, Crohn disease]); infection with immunosuppressive therapies for IBD

REFERENCES
1. Schiller LR, Pardi DS, Sellin JH. Chronic diarrhea: diagnosis and management. *Clin Gastroenterol Hepatol*. 2017;15(2):182–193.e3.
2. Chu C, Rotondo-Trivette S, Michail S. Chronic diarrhea. *Curr Probl Pediatr Adolesc Health Care*. 2020;50(8):100841.
3. Burgers K, Lindberg B, Bevis ZJ. Chronic diarrhea in adults: evaluation and differential diagnosis. *Am Fam Physician*. 2020;101(8):472–480.
4. Schiller LR. Evaluation of chronic diarrhea and irritable bowel syndrome with diarrhea in adults in the era of precision medicine. *Am J Gastroenterol*. 2018;113(5):660–669.

ADDITIONAL READING
Tripathi PR, Srivastava A. Approach to a child with chronic diarrhea [published online ahead of print June 27, 2023]. *Indian J Pediatr*. doi: 10.1007/s12098-023-04587-9.

 SEE ALSO

Algorithm: Diarrhea, Chronic

 CODES

ICD10
K52.9 Noninfective gastroenteritis and colitis, unspecified

CLINICAL PEARLS
- A comprehensive medical history guides the appropriate workup and avoids unnecessary testing.
- Consider IBS, IBD, malabsorption syndromes, celiac disease, prescribed or OTC medication use, herbal product use, and chronic infections (immunocompromised) in the differential diagnosis.
- Treatment is based on the underlying cause.

DIVERTICULAR DISEASE

Brianna Stadsvold, MD • Davis M. O'Brien, MD • Adel M. Abuzeid, MBBS

BASICS

DESCRIPTION
Diverticulum (single) or diverticula (multiple) are outpouchings of the colonic wall. Diverticular disease is a spectrum of diseases impacting the entire GI tract (except the rectum):
- Asymptomatic diverticulosis: common incidental finding on routine colonoscopy or imaging
- Symptomatic diverticulosis: also known as symptomatic uncomplicated diverticular disease (SUDD); recurrent abdominal pain attributed to diverticulosis without colitis or diverticulitis (1)
- Acute diverticulitis: diverticular disease with associated inflammation and/or infection
  - Uncomplicated diverticulitis: abdominal pain and leukocytosis without peritoneal signs or systemic toxicity
  - Complicated diverticulitis: secondary abscess formation, bowel obstruction, perforation, peritonitis, fistula, or stricture in the setting of diverticular inflammation
- Diverticular bleeding
  - Accounts for >40% of lower GI bleeds; often presents as painless hematochezia unless associated with active diverticulitis; bleeding is more common with right-sided diverticula.

EPIDEMIOLOGY
Incidence
- Diverticular disease accounts for ~300,000 hospitalizations per year in the United States.
- Diverticulitis occurs in 1–2% of the general population and in 4% of patients with diverticulosis (1). Diverticular bleeding occurs in 3–5% of patients with diverticulosis.

Prevalence
- Prevalence of diverticulosis and the number of diverticula increase with age.
  - Diverticulosis occurs in 20% of those aged 40 years, 60% of those aged 60 years, and 70% by the age of 80 years.
  - Incidence of diverticulitis increased from 62 to 75/100,000 people from 1998 to 2005; largest increase in patients <45 years of age—mostly due to changes in diet
- Male = female overall; more common in men <65 years of age and more common in women aged >65 years

ETIOLOGY AND PATHOPHYSIOLOGY
Diverticula form at points of weakness along the intestinal wall where small blood vessels (vasa recta) penetrate through the muscular layer of the colon.
- Age-related degeneration of the mucosal wall; increased intraluminal pressure from dense, fiber-depleted stools; and abnormal colonic motility contribute to diverticulosis.
- Most right-sided diverticula are true diverticula (involves all layers of the colonic wall).
- Most left-sided diverticula are pseudodiverticula (outpouchings of the mucosa and submucosa only).
- Diverticulitis occurs when local inflammation and infection contribute to tissue necrosis with risk for mucosal micro- or macroperforation.
- Alterations in intestinal microbiota contribute to chronic inflammation (1).
- Thinning of the vasa recta over the neck of the diverticula increases susceptibility to bleeding.
- Diverticular disease and irritable bowel syndrome (IBS) may represent the same disease continuum.

Genetics
- Although genetics may play a role, there is no known genetic pattern.
- Asian and African populations have lower overall prevalence but develop diverticular disease with adoption of a Western lifestyle.

RISK FACTORS
- Age >40 years; low-fiber diet
- Sedentary lifestyle, obesity; previous diverticulitis; risk rises with the number of diverticula.
- Smoking increases the risk of perforation (1).
- Risk of diverticular bleeding increases with NSAIDs, steroids, and opiate analgesics. Calcium channel blockers and statins protect against diverticular bleeding.

GENERAL PREVENTION
- High-fiber diet or nonabsorbable fiber (psyllium)
- Regular physical activity

COMMONLY ASSOCIATED CONDITIONS
Colon cancer, connective tissue diseases, obesity, IBS, and inflammatory bowel disease

DIAGNOSIS

HISTORY
- Diverticulosis
  - 80–85% of patients are asymptomatic. Of the 15–20% with symptoms, 1–2% will require hospitalization, and 0.5% undergo surgery.
  - The most common symptom is dull, colicky abdominal pain, typically in the LLQ. Pain can be exacerbated by eating and by passing bowel movement or flatus. Diarrhea or constipation is common.
- Acute diverticulitis: uncomplicated (85%) and complicated (15%)
  - Abdominal pain: acute onset, typically in LLQ; fever and/or chills
  - Anorexia, nausea (20–62%), or vomiting; constipation (50%) or diarrhea (25–35%)
  - Dysuria and urinary frequency suggest bladder or ureteral irritation.
  - Pneumaturia and fecaluria if associated with a colovesical fistula
- Diverticular bleeding
  - Melena, hematochezia (0.5/1,000 person-years); painless rectal bleeding
- Immunocompromised patients may not present with fever or leukocytosis and are at higher risk for perforation and abscess formation.

PHYSICAL EXAM
- Diverticulosis
  - Exam is usually normal.
  - May have intermittent distension or tympany
  - May have heme + stools
- Acute diverticulitis
  - Bowel sounds hypoactive (high-pitched/intermittent with obstruction); abdominal tenderness (usually LLQ); abdominal distension and tympany
  - Rebound tenderness, involuntary guarding, or rigidity suggests perforation and/or peritonitis; palpable mass in LLQ (20%)
  - Rectal exam may reveal tenderness or a mass.
  - Colovaginal, colovesical, and perirectal fistulae are rarely the initial presentation.

DIFFERENTIAL DIAGNOSIS
Urinary tract infection, nephrolithiasis, IBS, lactose intolerance, carcinoma, inflammatory bowel disease, fecal impaction, bowel obstruction, angiodysplasia, ischemic colitis, acute appendicitis, ectopic pregnancy

DIAGNOSTIC TESTS & INTERPRETATION
Initial Tests (lab, imaging)
- Diverticulosis: no labs or imaging needed
- Acute diverticulitis
  - WBC count is normal in up to 45% of cases. As diverticulitis worsens, WBC count becomes elevated with left shift.
  - Hemoglobin normal (unless bleeding); ESR elevated
  - Urinalysis may show microscopic pyuria or hematuria; urine culture: usually normal; persistent infection is suspicious for colovesical fistula.
  - Blood cultures positive in systemic cases
  - Plain films of the abdomen (acute abdominal series—supine and upright) to assess for free air under the diaphragm (bowel perforation) and signs of bowel obstruction (dilated loops of bowel)
  - CT scan with IV, oral, and/or rectal contrast (sensitivity: 98%, specificity: 99%) to stage disease and determine treatment plan (2)[A]
  - Ultrasound and MRI (sensitivity: 94%, specificity: 92%) are useful alternatives.
  - Barium enema is not recommended due to risk of peritoneal extravasation.
- Diverticular bleeding
  - Anemia with bleeding; obtain coagulation panel.

Diagnostic Procedures/Other
Diverticular bleeding
- Endoscopy to evaluate GI bleeding; NG lavage to exclude upper GI bleeding
- Angiography if bleeding obscures endoscopy or when endoscopy cannot visualize a source; 99mTcpertechnetate–labeled RBC scan (more sensitive) with follow-up angiography to localize bleeding

TREATMENT

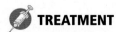

GENERAL MEASURES
- Diverticulosis: outpatient therapy with fiber supplementation and/or bulking agents (psyllium) (>30 g/day) (2)[A]
- Uncomplicated diverticulitis: outpatient therapy (see exceptions below) with or without oral antibiotics; 1–2% of subjects require hospitalization for toxicity, septicemia, peritonitis, or failure of symptoms to resolve. Up to 30% of patients may require surgery at first episode of diverticulitis.

- Complicated diverticulitis: hospitalization, bowel rest, and IV antibiotics; Hinchey classification (severity):
  - Stage I: diverticulitis + confined paracolic abscess; stage II: diverticulitis + distant abscess; stage III: diverticulitis + purulent peritonitis; stage IV: diverticulitis + fecal peritonitis
- Symptomatic improvement is expected within 2 to 3 days. Antibiotics should be continued for 7 to 10 days.
- Diverticular bleeding: 80% of cases resolve spontaneously.

MEDICATION

First Line

- Symptomatic diverticulosis: cyclical rifaximin 400 mg PO BID for 7 days every month or continuous mesalamine 800 mg PO BID (2)[C]
- Acute diverticulitis
  - The routine use of antibiotics in uncomplicated diverticulitis is controversial (2),(3)[C].
  - Outpatient oral antibiotics: Cover for anaerobes and gram-negative bacteria with:
    - A fluoroquinolone (ciprofloxacin 750 mg BID or levofloxacin 750 mg QD) *plus* metronidazole 500 mg TID (may use clindamycin if metronidazole intolerant) or
    - Trimethoprim/sulfamethoxazole DS BID *plus* metronidazole 500 mg TID
    - Treat for 7 to 10 days.
  - Inpatient: Use IV antibiotics.
    - Monotherapy with a β-lactam/β-lactamase inhibitor: piperacillin/tazobactam (3,375 g IV QID) or ampicillin/sulbactam 3 g IV q6h or ertapenem (1 g IV QD)
    - Penicillin-allergic patient: quinolone (levofloxacin 750 mg IV QD *plus* metronidazole 500 mg IV TID)
    - Unresponsive or severe disease: imipenem or meropenem
  - Recurrences of acute diverticulitis may be decreased by using mesalamine ± rifaximin or probiotics.
- Diverticular bleeding
  - Consider vasopressin 0.2 to 0.3 U/min through selective intra-arterial catheter.
- Precautions
  - Avoid morphine and other opiates that may increase intraluminal pressure or promote ileus.
  - Increased fiber intake is not recommended in the acute management of diverticulitis.

Second Line

- Outpatient: amoxicillin/clavulanate monotherapy (875/125 mg BID) (contraindicated in patients with clearance <30 mL/min) or moxifloxacin (400 mg PO QD) *plus* metronidazole (500 mg PO TID)
- Severely ill inpatients: ampicillin (500 mg IV q6h) + metronidazole (500 mg IV TID) + a quinolone *or* ampicillin + metronidazole + an aminoglycoside

ISSUES FOR REFERRAL

- Acute diverticulitis patients should follow up with a gastroenterologist or surgeon after resolution of diverticulitis (6 to 8 weeks) for colonoscopy to exclude malignancy, fistula, strictures, or inflammatory bowel disease (2).
- Acute complicated diverticulitis should have appropriate surgical and critical care/infectious disease consultations.

SURGERY/OTHER PROCEDURES

- Acute diverticulitis
  - Indications for emergent surgery: peritonitis, uncontrolled sepsis, perforation, obstruction
  - Hinchey I and II: consultation to interventional radiology to drain large abscesses (>4 cm)
  - Hinchey III or IV: frequently requires surgery during the same hospital admission
  - Elective colon resection in recurrent diverticulitis is a case-by-case decision and is typically performed during the quiescent phase following appropriate nonoperative treatment (2).
  - Immunocompromised patients are more likely to present with acute complicated diverticulitis, fail medical management, and have complications from elective surgery.
- Diverticular bleeding
  - Endoscopy and hemostasis via epinephrine injection, electrocautery, or clipping
  - Angiography is preferred over endoscopy in unstable patients to identify/embolize the bleeding source.
  - Massive or recurrent bleeding requires surgery to control hemorrhage.

COMPLEMENTARY & ALTERNATIVE MEDICINE

Probiotics have been used to prevent recurrence with mixed success.

ADMISSION, INPATIENT, AND NURSING CONSIDERATIONS

- Admit for systematic toxicity, sepsis, and/or peritonitis (complicated diverticulitis).
- Consider admitting patients with uncomplicated diverticulitis and the following: elderly, immunocompromised, evidence of microperforation, marked leukocytosis, temperature >39°C, intolerance of PO intake, severe abdominal pain, or unreliable follow up.

 ONGOING CARE

FOLLOW-UP RECOMMENDATIONS

Patient Monitoring

- Follow-up outpatients 2 to 3 days after initiating antibiotic therapy and then weekly thereafter until symptom resolution.
  - Repeat imaging and/or inpatient therapy may be required if there is a disease progression at follow-up.
- Colonoscopy should be performed in 6 to 8 weeks (unless done within the past year).

DIET

- Bowel rest with NPO during acute diverticulitis; advance diet as tolerated as bowel function returns
- Patients with known diverticulosis or a history of diverticulitis should consume a high-fiber diet to prevent recurrence (3).
- Avoiding nuts and popcorn is not necessary (3).

PROGNOSIS

- Good with early detection and prompt treatment
- After first episode of diverticulitis, there is a 33% chance of recurrence. After a second episode, there is a 66% chance of further recurrence. Rebleeding occurs in up to 6%.
- Most complications occur during first bout of diverticulitis. Younger patients are more likely to have recurrence.

COMPLICATIONS

Hemorrhage, perforation, peritonitis, obstruction, abscess, or colovesicular/colovaginal fistula

REFERENCES

1. Tursi A, Scarpignato C, Strate LL, et al. Colonic diverticular disease. *Nat Rev Dis Primers*. 2020;6(1):20.
2. Eckmann JD, Shaukat A. Updates in the understanding and management of diverticular disease. *Curr Opin Gastroenterol*. 2022;38(1):48–54.
3. Peery AF, Shaukat A, Strate LL. AGA clinical practice update on medical management of colonic diverticulitis: expert review. *Gastroenterology*. 2021;160(3):906–911.e1.

CODES

ICD10

- K57.92 Diverticulitis of intestine, part unspecified, without perforation or abscess without bleeding
- K57.13 Diverticulitis of small intestine without perforation or abscess with bleeding
- K57.21 Diverticulitis of large intestine with perforation and abscess with bleeding

CLINICAL PEARLS

- Diverticulosis is common in elderly patients with a sedentary lifestyle who consume a Western diet.
- Patients with diverticulosis benefit from a high-fiber diet.
- Antibiotics may not be necessary for low-risk patients with acute uncomplicated diverticulitis.
- Not all patients with recurrent diverticulitis require surgical intervention (colectomy).
- Dietary restrictions do not prevent recurrent diverticulitis.
- After an episode of diverticulitis, patients should undergo colonoscopy to rule out malignancy.
- Diverticular disease is a common cause of GI bleeding.

DOWN SYNDROME

Brian G. Skotko, MD, MPP • Michele Roberts, MD, PhD

BASICS

DESCRIPTION
- Down syndrome (DS) is a congenital condition associated with intellectual disability and an increased chance of multisystem medical problems.
- Synonym: trisomy 21

Pediatric Considerations
A multidisciplinary evaluation is warranted (1).

Geriatric Considerations
Life expectancy has increased to ~60 years.

Pregnancy Considerations
The American College of Obstetricians and Gynecologists (ACOG) and the Society for Maternal-Fetal Medicine (SMFM) acknowledge that any women may choose noninvasive prenatal screening (NIPS). American College of Medical Genetics and Genomics (ACMG) recommends all women be offered with NIPS (2),(3).

EPIDEMIOLOGY
Incidence
In the United States, 1/772 live births, ~5,100 births per year

Prevalence
~217,000 persons in the United States

ETIOLOGY AND PATHOPHYSIOLOGY
- Etiology: presence of all or part of an extra chromosome 21
- Trisomy 21: 95% of DS, an extra chromosome 21 is found in all cells due to nondisjunction, usually in maternal meiosis.
- Translocation DS: 3–4% of DS, extra chromosome 21q material is translocated to another chromosome (usually 13, 14, or 21); ~25% have parental origin.
- Mosaic trisomy 21: 1–2% of DS, manifestations may be milder.

Genetics
- Online Mendelian Inheritance in Man (OMIM) 190685
- Inheritance: most commonly sporadic nondisjunction resulting in trisomy 21
- Chance of having another child with DS is
  - 1% (or age risk, whichever is greater) after conceiving a pregnancy with nondisjunction trisomy 21
  - 10–15% for mothers/sisters and 3–5% for fathers/brothers who carry balanced translocation with chromosome 21
  - 100% if the parental balanced translocation is 21;21 (45,t[21;21])
  - Unclear after child with mosaic DS but ~1%

RISK FACTORS
- DS is believed to occur in all races and ethnicities with equal frequency, although live birth prevalence may differ based on different elective termination rates.
- Chance of having an infant with DS increases with mother's age

GENERAL PREVENTION
Preimplantation diagnosis with in vitro fertilization (IVF), prenatal diagnosis followed by elective termination, and adoption are current options for expectant parents who do not wish to raise a child with DS.

COMMONLY ASSOCIATED CONDITIONS
- Cardiac
  - Congenital heart defects (40–50%)
- GI/growth
  - Feeding problems are common in infancy.
  - Structural defects (~12%)
  - Gastroesophageal reflux
  - Constipation
  - Celiac disease (~5%)
- Pulmonary
  - Tracheal stenosis/tracheoesophageal fistula
  - Pulmonary hypertension
  - Obstructive sleep apnea (50–75%)
- Genitourinary
  - Cryptorchidism, hypospadias
- Hematologic/neoplastic
  - Transient myeloproliferative disorder (~10%): generally resolves spontaneously; can be preleukemic (acute megakaryoblastic leukemia [AMKL]) in 20–30%
  - Leukemia (AMKL or acute lymphoblastic leukemia [ALL]) in 0.5–1%
  - Decreased risk of most solid tumors; increased risk of germ cell tumors/testicular cancer
- Endocrine
  - Hypothyroidism: congenital or acquired (13–63%)
  - Diabetes
- Skeletal
  - Atlantoaxial instability (15%): ~2% symptomatic
  - Short stature is common.
  - Scoliosis (Some cases have adult onset.)
  - Hip problems (1–4%)
- Immune/rheumatologic
  - Abnormal immune function with increased rate of respiratory infections
  - Increased risk of autoimmune disorders, including Hashimoto thyroiditis, celiac disease, and alopecia
- Neurologic
  - Intellectual ability ranging from mild to severe disability; average is moderate intellectual disability.
  - Autism spectrum disorder (<18%)
  - Hypotonia
  - Seizures (8%): typically occurring <1 year of age (infantile spasms) or >30 years of age
  - Alzheimer disease: At least 40% at age 40 years develop signs of dementia; percentage increases with age.
- Psychiatric
  - Attention deficit hyperactivity disorder (ADHD), obsessive-compulsive disorder (OCD), and autism spectrum disorder increased frequency in children.
  - Generalized depression and anxiety with increased frequency in young adults/adults
  - Down syndrome regression disorder is a very rare clinical regression syndrome that can occur in adolescents or young adults.
- Sensory
  - Hearing loss (75%): mostly conductive due to high frequency of asymptomatic middle ear effusion; otitis media (50–70%)
  - Visual impairment (60%): strabismus (refractive errors, 15%), myopia, hyperopia, nystagmus, cataracts (15%)
- Dermatologic
  - Xerosis, eczema, palmoplantar hyperkeratosis, atopic or seborrheic dermatitis, onychomycosis, syringomas, furunculosis/folliculitis, hidradenitis suppurativa

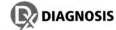

DIAGNOSIS

HISTORY
~85% of mothers of infants with DS learn about the diagnosis postnatally, although this is changing with the availability of prenatal screening such as NIPS.

PHYSICAL EXAM
- In November 2015, DS-specific growth charts were released. These charts do not represent "optimal" growth of children with DS; 50% BMI on the DS-specific growth curves corresponds to the 85% (overweight) on the standard NCHS growth curves (4).
- Infants and children
  - Brachycephaly (100%)
  - Hypotonia (80%)
  - Small ears, often low set and simplified
  - Upslanting palpebral fissure (90%)
  - Epicanthic folds (90%)
  - Brushfield spots
  - Depressed nasal bridge
  - Short neck, often with increased nuchal folds
  - Single palmar crease, single flexion crease on 5th finger
  - Increased space between toes 1 and 2, 5th finger clinodactyly, brachydactyly

DIAGNOSTIC TESTS & INTERPRETATION
Initial Tests (lab, imaging)
- Maternal prenatal screening includes the following:
  - 1st trimester: combined screen (maternal age, β-human chorionic gonadotropin [β-hCG], pregnancy-associated plasma protein A [PAPP-A], and nuchal translucency)
  - 2nd trimester: quad screen (α-fetoprotein, β-hCG, estriol, inhibin A)
  - Sequential screen (combined screen in 1st trimester, if abnormal, obtain amniocentesis or await 2nd trimester quad screening)
  - Integrated screen (combined screening in 1st trimester plus quad screen in 2nd trimester)
  - NIPS with cell-free DNA (beginning ~10 weeks' gestation) (2),(3)
- Prenatal diagnosis includes the following:
  - Chorionic villus sampling: 1st trimester, ~99% accurate, ~1% miscarriage
  - Amniocentesis: 2nd trimester, ~99% accurate, ~0.25% miscarriage rate

- Postnatal diagnosis
  - Fluorescence in situ hybridization (FISH) can be performed at time of clinical suspicion, but karyotype should always be done to differentiate genetic type of DS.
  - Parental (and adult-aged sibling) karyotype is indicated only if translocation DS is found in child.
- Workup for newborns (1)
  - Echo, with or without murmur
  - CBC with differential (to look for transient myelo-proliferative disorder)
  - Thyroid-stimulating hormone (TSH) test
  - Audiogram
  - Ophthalmologic exam to assess for cataracts (Look for red reflex.)
  - Swallowing study for those with feeding difficulties
  - Car-seat test

Follow-Up Tests & Special Considerations
- After delivering a prenatal diagnosis, the clinician should offer "Understanding a Down Syndrome Diagnosis" (https://understandingdownsyndrome.org).
- If the diagnosis is postnatal, the new parent and partner, if present, should be informed of the diagnosis promptly by a physician (preferably the obstetrician and pediatrician or family physician) on the basis of clinical observations and before the karyotype is available but with consideration of extenuating circumstances (e.g., birth parent's medical condition). The spouse/partner and infant should be present unless this would cause an undue delay. The meeting should be private. Refer to the baby by name.
- In the postnatal setting, the clinician should be knowledgeable on the subject of DS and should conduct a discussion with content that is current, respectful, balanced, informative, and realistic but not overly pessimistic, concentrating on what is relevant to the 1st year of life.
- Cardiac follow-up, as indicated

TREATMENT

ISSUES FOR REFERRAL
- Lactation consultant
- Physical/occupational/speech therapy (early intervention)
- Pediatric cardiologist, if indicated

SURGERY/OTHER PROCEDURES
Repair of congenital anomalies as needed.

COMPLEMENTARY & ALTERNATIVE MEDICINE
- There is no evidence to support the use of supplements in children with DS.
- Craniosacral manipulation is dangerous due to potential atlantoaxial instability.

ADMISSION, INPATIENT, AND NURSING CONSIDERATIONS
If the social situation indicates adoption, consider the National Down Syndrome Adoption Network (NDSAN) (http://www.ndsan.org/)—a national registry for families seeking to adopt a child with DS.

ONGOING CARE

FOLLOW-UP RECOMMENDATIONS
Patient Monitoring
- Children with DS: the American Academy of Pediatrics recommends ongoing assessment and review, at least annually, with the following surveillance (1):
  - Vision: Assess for strabismus, cataracts, and nystagmus by ophthalmologist by 6 months, annually between ages 1 and 5 years, every 2 years between ages 5 and 13 years, and every 3 years between ages 13 and 21 years.
  - Hearing: neonatal screen with auditory brainstem response (ABR) or otoacoustic emissions (OAE), then audiogram every 6 months until age 3 years, and then annually
  - Thyroid: initial newborn screen. Repeat TSH test at 6 months, 12 months, and then annually (4)[C].
  - Screening for celiac disease (total IgA and tissue transglutaminase [tTG]-IgA) annually, if symptomatic
  - Three-view cervical spine films if patient is symptomatic, beginning at 3 to 5 years of age
  - Hemoglobin test annually to screen for iron-deficiency anemia
  - Repeat echocardiogram in teens if with murmur or fatigue
  - Sleep: Obtain a sleep study for everyone with DS between 3 and 5 years of age, given the high prevalence of obstructive sleep apnea.
- Adults with DS: A comprehensive approach to medical care is also necessary (5).

DIET
- No special diet, but caloric needs are lower in adolescents/adults with DS than their peers.
- Obesity is prevalent at all ages.

PATIENT EDUCATION
- Down Syndrome Clinic to You (DSC2U), an online health and wellness portal for patients with DS and their caregivers and primary care providers; https://www.dsc2u.org
- National Down Syndrome Congress: 800-232-NDSC; https://www.ndsccenter.org/
- National Down Syndrome Society: 800-221-4602; https://www.ndss.org/
- The LuMind IDSC Down Syndrome Foundation provides information on the latest research for people with DS: https://www.lumindidsc.org.
- Lettercase provides peer-reviewed booklet for parents who have received a prenatal diagnosis of DS and have not yet made a decision about their pregnancy: https://www.lettercase.org/.

- Down Syndrome Pregnancy provides free downloadable books and articles for expectant mothers who have decided to continue their pregnancies after a prenatal diagnosis of DS: http://downsyndromepregnancy.org/.
- Understanding a Down Syndrome Diagnosis provides an overview of DS and select resources: http://understandingdownsyndrome.org/.

PROGNOSIS
- 99% of young adults/adults with DS report being happy with their lives.
- Life expectancy is ~60 years.

REFERENCES
1. Bull MJ, Trotter T, Santoro SL, et al; for Council on Genetics. Health supervision for children and adolescents with Down syndrome. *Pediatrics.* 2022;149(5):e2022057010.
2. Rose NC, Kaimal AJ, Dugoff L, et al. Screening for fetal chromosomal abnormalities: ACOG Practice Bulletin, Number 226. *Obstet Gynecol.* 2020;136(4):e48–e69.
3. Dungan JS, Klugman S, Darilek S, et al. Noninvasive prenatal screening (NIPS) for fetal chromosome abnormalities in a general-risk population: an evidence-based clinical guideline of the American College of Medical Genetics and Genomics (ACMG). *Genet Med.* 2023;25(2):100336.
4. Zemel BS, Pipan M, Stallings VA, et al. Growth charts for children with Down syndrome in the United States. *Pediatrics.* 2015;136(5):e1204–e1211.
5. Tsou AY, Bulova P, Capone G, et al. Medical care of adults with Down syndrome: a clinical guideline. *JAMA.* 2020;324(15):1543–1556.

ADDITIONAL READING
- Antonarakis SE, Skotko BG, Rafii MS, et al. Down syndrome. *Nat Rev Dis Primers.* 2020;6(1):9.
- Bull MJ. Down syndrome. *N Engl J Med.* 2020;382(24):2344–2352.

SEE ALSO

Algorithm: Intellectual Disability

CODES

ICD10
- Q90.0 Trisomy 21, nonmosaicism (meiotic nondisjunction)
- Q90 Down syndrome
- Q90.1 Trisomy 21, mosaicism (mitotic nondisjunction)

CLINICAL PEARLS
- 99% of young adults/adults with DS report being happy with their lives.
- DS specialty clinics, including virtual ones like DSC2U, may improve medical outcomes.

DRUG ABUSE, PRESCRIPTION

Moez K. Sumar, MD, BSc • Ned Francis Nasr, MD, FASA • Rishi Gaiha, MD

BASICS

Controlled substances are prone to misuse and diversion. Cautious prescribing should be considered in all cases and monitoring all patients prescribed controlled substances to identify substance use disorder (SUD) is the key. Patients with SUD should be offered treatment (and/or referred as needed).

DESCRIPTION
- Prescription drug abuse behaviors exist on a continuum and can include:
  - Use of medication for medical reasons other than what the prescriber intended
  - Use of medication for nonmedical reasons such as to get high (dissociative effects) or to enhance performance
  - Use of medication for any reason by someone other than the person it was intended for
- Commonly abused prescription medications include opioid analgesics, stimulants, central nervous system depressants, and barbiturates.
- *Diversion* is a term used to describe the rerouting of medications from prescriptions or other legitimate supplies for recreational use or criminal activity, such as selling prescription medication for personal profit.

EPIDEMIOLOGY
- From 2013 to 2018, substance use–related emergency department (ED) visits increased from 2.926 million to 4.132 million.
- The number of drug overdose deaths quadrupled from 1999 to 2019 and >932,000 deaths have been attributed to drug overdose.
- In 2020, >91,000 drug overdose deaths occurred in the United States in which opioids were responsible for 78.4% of those deaths.

Incidence
- Predominant sex: males > females
- 1 in 4 patients on long-term opioid therapy in primary care settings struggles with opioid addiction.
- Predominant age: highest among adults aged 18 to 25 years (mean 22 years), then adolescents and teens aged 12 to 17 years, followed by adults aged ≥26 years

Prevalence
In 2017, 191 million opioid prescriptions were issued, and 11.5 million Americans were reported misusing opioid medications.

ETIOLOGY AND PATHOPHYSIOLOGY
Opioids, benzodiazepines, stimulants, and barbiturates produce euphoria, tolerance, and dependence, leading to misuse and addiction.

Genetics
Variant alleles affect the expression and function of opioid, dopamine, acetylcholine, serotonin, and γ-aminobutyric acid, helping to explain susceptibility to different forms.

RISK FACTORS
- Sociodemographic, psychiatric, pain, drug-related factors, genetics, sex, environment, and family history
- Ongoing opioid prescription (≥3 months) greatly increases risk of opioid-related overdose at 1 year (4-fold) and 5 years (30-fold).

GENERAL PREVENTION
- Try all available nonopioid treatments for pain before prescribing opioids for chronic pain.
- Limit/avoid prescribing controlled medications on the first visit and limit quantity of opioid pain medication prescribed to a few days (1)[A].
- Screen by asking questions about unhealthy drug use (including prescription drugs, USPSTF-B recommendation).
- Conduct thorough history, review records (prescription monitoring programs [PMPs]), and perform urine drug screens (UDSs) before deciding if a controlled substance is indicated.
- Avoid prescribing benzodiazepines in the treatment of anxiety. Try cognitive-behavioral therapy, mindfulness, selective serotonin reuptake inhibitors, PRN antihistamines (anti-H1), or buspirone.
- Support the use of CDC guidelines for prescribing controlled substances for chronic pain while integrating quality improvement measures, making these standard practice.
- Wean/stop prescription of analgesics for chronic pain if ineffective for improving pain and function, if aberrant behaviors suggesting opioid use are present, or if patient overdoses.
- Dose reduction of chronic opioids can decrease risk while improving pain, function, and quality of life.
- Prescribe intranasal naloxone to all patients prescribed chronic opioids, provide education to patient and family members on proper use in case of overdose, and increase access to SUD services.
- Identify and treat underlying SUD.

COMMONLY ASSOCIATED CONDITIONS
- Opioids: tolerance, opioid-induced hyperalgesia, dependence, addiction (which can lead to loss of savings, job, close relationships and incarceration, hepatitis C virus or HIV infection, etc.), overdose/death, depression, constipation, low testosterone, and sexual dysfunction
- Benzodiazepines and barbiturates: dependence (withdrawal can cause seizures, delirium tremens, death), psychosis, anxiety, sleep driving, blackout states, cognitive impairment, impaired driving; increased fall risk and mortality in elderly patients
- Stimulants: dependence, hypertension, tachyarrhythmias, myocardial ischemia, seizures, hypothermia, psychosis, hallucinations, paranoia, anxiety

DIAGNOSIS
- Initial screening: "How many times in the past year have you used an illegal drug or used a prescription medication for nonmedical reasons?"; primary care setting sensitivity of 100% and specificity of ~75%
- Other screening tools: Drug Abuse Screening Test (DAST) helps determine involvement with drugs over the past year. Assess alcohol use with CAGE or Alcohol Use Disorders Identification Test (AUDIT); SUD diagnostic criteria as per *DSM-5*

HISTORY
Patients may show hostile/threatening, impulsive, or flattering behavior. Patients may ask for dose/quantity increase, fabricate false stories, ask for early refills, ask for specific drugs by name, make appointments near the end of the day, and also try to establish care after clinic hours.

PHYSICAL EXAM
- Monitor patients for signs of sedation, confusion, or intoxication (can include slurred speech and unsteady gait in case of benzodiazepines). Patient may have unkept or disheveled appearance.
- Physical exam findings of opioid withdrawal including dilated pupils, frequent yawning, tachycardia, elevated blood pressure, and piloerection. In benzodiazepine withdrawal, symptoms include tachycardia, elevated blood pressure, and tremors.
- There are often no physical exam findings when a patient is misusing a prescription medication; other objective findings such as urine drug testing should be used in monitoring.

DIFFERENTIAL DIAGNOSIS
Depression, anxiety, mania, psychosis

DIAGNOSTIC TESTS & INTERPRETATION
UDSs are recommended to ensure safe use of medication and to prevent diversions (2)[C]. Assessing baseline CBC, electrolytes, renal function, liver function, thyroid function, fasting plasma glucose, and lipid panel along with testing for communicable diseases (HIV, hepatitis, and syphilis) may help rule out other pathologic states.

Initial Tests (lab, imaging)
- UDSs: Ensure the panel includes semisynthetics (hydrocodone, hydromorphone, oxycodone) and synthetics (methadone, fentanyl, propoxyphene, meperidine) along with tramadol and buprenorphine. Test for other drugs of abuse such as benzodiazepines (clonazepam, alprazolam, and lorazepam are ordered individually), cocaine, amphetamine, alcohol metabolites, marijuana, and consider other drugs that may be highly prevalent in your area (such as gabapentin, PCP, and barbiturates).
- Codeine will be positive for codeine plus morphine.
- Morphine will be positive for morphine.
- Oxycodone (OxyContin) will be positive for oxycodone and oxymorphone.
- Hydrocodone will be positive for hydrocodone and hydromorphone.
- Buprenorphine will be positive for buprenorphine and norbuprenorphine.
- Diazepam will be positive for nordiazepam, oxazepam, and temazepam.
- Chlordiazepoxide will be positive for nordiazepam and oxazepam.
- Alprazolam will be positive for α-hydroxyalprazolam.
- Clonazepam will be positive for 7-aminoclonazepam.
- Lorazepam will be positive for lorazepam glucuronide.

Follow-Up Tests & Special Considerations
Random pill counts are useful for identifying patients who are taking more controlled substance than prescribed. Random urine drug testing can also be concurrently collected. Ancillary services such as rehab may help improve outcomes.

Test Interpretation

- Screening drug tests (by enzyme-linked immuno-sorbent assay method) may result in false positives from interactions with other commonly prescribed medications or substances people are frequently exposed to (e.g., poppy seeds [opioid], hemp food products [marijuana], diet pills, and energy drinks [amphetamines]); treatment decisions should be based on highly specific confirmation testing (such as by gas chromatography/mass spectrometry).
- Results are positive if drugs (or metabolites of drugs) that are not prescribed are present; positive in presence of illicit drugs (e.g., cocaine)
- Suspect diversion when negative for prescribed drug at a time when the patient reported taking it.

 TREATMENT

The general approach to treatment includes inpatient, residential, or outpatient detoxification as required; counseling and intensive counseling as needed; and ongoing medication-assisted treatment (MAT) with buprenorphine or injectable naltrexone.

- Buprenorphine/naloxone: Begin taper to initiate discontinuation whenever there is an evidence of prescription opioid abuse (2)[C]. Some situations indicate immediate discontinuation rather than taper (e.g., diversion or plan to switch to buprenorphine/naloxone treatment).
- Opioid discontinuation through interdisciplinary pain care programs, buprenorphine-assisted or methadone programs, and detoxification programs have achieved opioid discontinuation rates >85%.
- Benzodiazepines cannot be stopped abruptly for risk of seizures and death; therefore, discontinue via slow taper.
- Amphetamines can be stopped abruptly without risk of severe withdrawal or death.

GENERAL MEASURES

Multiple treatments are available including inpatient programs (detoxification and induction into MAT), outpatient programs (MAT and behavioral health), and peer-led support services.

MEDICATION

Short-term opioid detoxification programs use clonidine, buprenorphine, or methadone under the direction of an addiction specialist. Long-term MAT with buprenorphine/naloxone, methadone, or naltrexone is more effective than short-term detoxification.

- Buprenorphine and naloxone MAT
  - Any provider (MD, DO, NP, or PA) may prescribe buprenorphine/naloxone after completing training. For details, see Substance Abuse and Mental Health Services Administration: https://www.samhsa.gov/medication-assisted-treatment/become-buprenorphine-waivered-practitioner.
  - Buprenorphine/naloxone titrated to the maximum of 24 mg/day for patients who continue to use opioids
  - Naloxone-based formulations discourage misuse (such as by sniffing or IV) because naloxone displaces buprenorphine binding to opioid receptors when taken parenterally.

- Buprenorphine available as a monthly long-acting injectable administered by a nurse at clinic, eliminating the need for daily dosing and diversion-related issues while creating an opportunity to offer support
- Naltrexone is (oral or long-acting injectable) an opioid antagonist that reduces cravings for opioids and opioid-euphoria when ingested; started after a person has been off opioids for 7 days to avoid acute, severe withdrawal
- Buprenorphine/naloxone and methadone are similarly effective when used in long-term opioid maintenance therapy.
- Methadone
  - Dispensed by addiction specialists for treatment of opioid use disorder at a certified opioid treatment program

First Line

Multiple modalities including MAT, support groups, etc., tailored to specific patient needs

ISSUES FOR REFERRAL

Enlist the help of chemical dependency groups/addiction specialists/pain management and psychiatry/psychology when polysubstance abuse suspected and to treat underlying psychiatric disorders.

ADDITIONAL THERAPIES

- Behavioral health support or Smart Recovery and 12-step programs such as AA and NA
- Residential treatment programs (short-term vs. long-term rehabilitation, transitional support programs, crisis stabilization units)
- Al-Anon/Alateen and Learn to Cope provide helpful free support groups for family members.

COMPLEMENTARY & ALTERNATIVE MEDICINE

Mindfulness and meditation, acupuncture, or yoga may help with stress reduction.

ADMISSION, INPATIENT, AND NURSING CONSIDERATIONS

Consider additional support if continued use of opioids despite outpatient treatment, concomitant alcohol and benzodiazepine dependence (increased risk of seizures), mental confusion/delirium, history of seizures, psychosis, suicidal ideation, serious, or absence of social support.

 ONGOING CARE

Treatment with MAT should continue for as long as the patient benefits from it.

FOLLOW-UP RECOMMENDATIONS

Expert opinion suggests high-frequency visits (such as weekly) when a patient begins MAT.

Patient Monitoring

Monitor patients with in-person check-ins, drug testing, and review of the PMP.

DIET

If concern for opioid-induced constipation, tapering dose to complete cessation with increase in high-fiber diet, stool softeners, stimulant laxative, and increased hydration

PATIENT EDUCATION

- Controlled medication should be inaccessible to others (ideally in locked box/bag). Diverting medication may result in legal charges.
- Address "red flags"; dose escalation when necessary; provide support and strategies for managing stress, cravings, preoccupation about the next dose, and abuse identification

PROGNOSIS

The majority of patients with SUD are able to achieve remission.

COMPLICATIONS

Misuse of opioids and benzodiazepines may lead to overdose and death. Misuse of stimulants may lead to psychosis and cardiac conditions such as myocardial infarction and arrhythmias.

REFERENCES

1. Onwuchekwa Uba R, Ankoma-Darko K, Park SK. International comparison of mitigation strategies for addressing opioid misuse: a systematic review. *J Am Pharm Assoc (2003)*. 2020;60(1):195–204.
2. Manchikanti L, Abdi S, Atluri S, et al; for American Society of Interventional Pain Physicians. American Society of Interventional Pain Physicians (ASIPP) guidelines for responsible opioid prescribing in chronic non-cancer pain: part I—evidence assessment. *Pain Physician*. 2012;15(Suppl 3):S1–S65.

 SEE ALSO

- https://www.cdc.gov/drugoverdose/pdf/pdo_checklist-a.pdf
- https://www.cdc.gov/drugoverdose/strategies/index.html

CODES

ICD10

- F19.10 Other psychoactive substance abuse, uncomplicated
- F11.10 Opioid abuse, uncomplicated
- F15.10 Other stimulant abuse, uncomplicated

CLINICAL PEARLS

- Addiction is a treatable chronic disease. Most licensed physicians and nurse practitioners may now provide MAT with buprenorphine without the requirement of special certification.
- Discontinue the prescription of opioid analgesics if pain or functionality does not improve or if there is evidence of abuse or diversion (e.g., positive UDSs, driving while intoxicated [DWI], overdose, early refills).
- PMPs reduce doctor shopping but not ED visits for overdose and prescription drug abuse—related deaths.

D

DUCTAL CARCINOMA IN SITU

Anne Campbell Larkin, MD

 BASICS

DESCRIPTION

- Ductal carcinoma in situ (DCIS) is a heterogeneous group of premalignant lesions that have the presence of neoplastic, clonal proliferation of *noninvasive* epithelial cells confined to ducts and lobules.
- Comprises 1 in 4 cases of all newly diagnosed breast cancers
- Mortality from DCIS with subsequent progression to invasive breast carcinoma (IBC) is low (<1%), regardless of histologic type or treatment.

EPIDEMIOLOGY

Incidence

- Average annual percentage increase of ~1%
- Estimated 55,720 new diagnoses of DCIS for U.S women in 2023 (1)
- Estimated 51,400 new diagnoses of DCIS for U.S women in 2022
- DCIS accounts for ~80–85% of in situ breast carcinomas (lobular carcinoma in situ [LCIS] accounts for approximately 15–20%) and ~26% of all new breast cancers.
- Increase in incidence with increase in age; rate of DCIS doubles from age range of 40 to 49 years to 70 to 84 years

ETIOLOGY AND PATHOPHYSIOLOGY

Genetics

- Low-grade DCIS typically expresses estrogen receptor (ER) and progesterone receptor (PR), without HER2 protein overexpression or amplification.
- High-grade DCIS not consistently ER+ or PR+
- *BRCA1* and *BRCA2* associations observed

RISK FACTORS

- Female sex, nulliparity, late age at first birth or menopause, first-degree relative with breast cancer, long-term use of postmenopausal combined estrogen and progestin therapy, history of atypical ductal hyperplasia (ADH), dense breast tissue
- Associations with age, BMI, age at menarche, lactation history, oral contraceptive use, and modifiable lifestyle factors (alcohol and smoking) remain unclear.

GENERAL PREVENTION

- Screening may result in overdiagnosis with little or no reduction in the incidence of advanced cancers.
- General screening guidelines—U.S. Preventive Services Task Force (USPSTF):
  - Biennial mammography (MMG) for women aged 40 to 74 years (B recommendation)
  - Screening MMG in women aged <40 years should be based on risk factors.
  - Insufficient evidence regarding benefits and harms of screening MMG if ≥75 years old

- Insufficient evidence to assess the benefits and harms of digital breast tomosynthesis (DBT) as a primary screening method (I statement)
- Insufficient evidence to assess the balance of benefits and harms of adjunctive screening using breast ultrasonography, magnetic resonance imaging (MRI), DBT, or other methods in women identified to have dense breasts on an otherwise negative screening mammogram (I statement)
- Clinical breast exam (CBE):
  - USPSTF evidence is insufficient to assess benefits and harms when added to MMG screening for women aged ≥40 years.
  - WHO states CBE may be beneficial in settings with weak health settings (MMG not accessible) for women 50 to 69 years old.
- Risk reduction:
  - Limit alcohol intake to <1 drink per day, exercise, maintain a healthy diet, and weight control.
  - Calcium (1,000 mg) plus vitamin D (1,000 IU) may lower risk of DCIS.
  - Hormonal risk reduction agents recommended in certain high-risk women ≥35 years old; tamoxifen for premenopausal women and raloxifene for postmenopausal women
  - Anastrozole (an aromatase inhibitor) may significantly decrease incidence of DCIS in postmenopausal women.

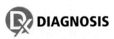 **DIAGNOSIS**

PHYSICAL EXAM

- CBE with patient in upright and supine position; evaluating for asymmetry, spontaneous discharge, skin changes (peau d'orange, erythema, scaling); nipple retraction/excoriation (Paget disease)
- Palpation of all breast quadrants, including lymph nodes (axillary, supraclavicular and cervical)
- Positive clinical findings: Refer for diagnostic imaging and/or surgical evaluation unless <30 years old with a low clinical suspicion (observe 1 to 2 menstrual cycles; refer if clinical findings persist).

DIFFERENTIAL DIAGNOSIS

Usual ductal hyperplasia, columnar cell changes, flat epithelial atypia, ADH, LCIS, microinvasive carcinoma, intraductal papilloma, mucinous breast lesions

DIAGNOSTIC TESTS & INTERPRETATION

Initial Tests (lab, imaging)

- MMG Breast Imaging–Reporting and Data System (BI-RADS): BI-RADS is a quality assurance (QA) method published by the American College of Radiology.
  - BI-RADS has been extended to breast US and MRI interpretation as well.

- Components of BI-RADS report:
  - Indication for study and type of examination
  - Overall breast composition, including breast density
    - A—Breasts are almost entirely fatty tissue.
    - B—scattered areas of fibroglandular density
    - C—heterogenously dense
    - D—extremely dense
  - Description of abnormalities and important findings
    - Uses standard BI-RADS descriptors
  - Comparison to prior images and summary report, including final BI-RADS assessment category
- Final BI-RADS assessment category and screening recommendations:
  - BI-RADS 0: incomplete; additional imaging evaluation needed
    - Commonly occurs on screening studies, consider diagnostic workup
  - BI-RADS 1: negative
    - Continue with current screening guidelines.
  - BI-RADS 2: benign
    - No further action needed; continue current screening guidelines.
  - BI-RADS 3: probably benign; possibility of malignancy is <2%.
    - Follow-up imaging should occur in 6 months for 1 year; consider imaging every 6 to 12 months for 2 to 3 years.
    - Can consider biopsy if patients is anxious or follow-up is uncertain
  - BI-RADS 4: suspicious
    - Patient and clinician should discuss possible management plans and likely a biopsy.
  - BI-RADS 5: highly suggestive of malignancy
    - Diagnostic imaging needed with follow-up and biopsy
  - BI-RADS 6: known biopsy—proven malignancy
    - Includes patients with biopsy-proven cancers that have yet to be surgically removed
- DCIS most often seen as clustered microcalcifications

Follow-Up Tests & Special Considerations

- Sensitivity of breast MRI screening > MMG; with decreased specificity resulting in increased number of false positives
- Screening MRI only recommended in certain women:
  - *BRCA* mutation—*commence at age 25 to 29 years*
  - First-degree relative of *BRCA* carrier—*commence at age 25 to 29 years*
  - ≥20% lifetime risk of breast cancer defined by models that are largely based on family history—*annual breast MRI to begin 10 years prior to the youngest family member but not prior to age 25 years*

– Thoracic radiation between the ages of 10 and 30 years—*annual breast MRI to begin 10 years after radiation therapy but not prior to age 25 years*
– Presence of Li-Fraumeni, *PTEN*, or Bannayan-Riley-Ruvalcaba syndrome in patient or first-degree relative
– ≥20% risk of breast cancer based on gene and/or risk level: ATM, CDH1, CHEK2, PALB2, PTEN, STK11, TP53
• Pathology
– Tissue is necessary for diagnosis: typically core-needle (CN) or vacuum-assisted (VA) biopsy (mammographic/stereotactic, US, or MRI guided).
– Fine-needle aspiration (FNA) is not adequate for specific diagnosis of DCIS; however, it can suggest the presence of neoplastic cells.
– Histologic classification
  ○ Classification is subjective; however, traditionally classified as either low, intermediate, or high grade based on architectural patterns (comedo, solid, cribriform, clinging, papillary, and micro-papillary), nuclear grade (I, II, or III), and the absence or presence of necrosis
  ○ Ductal intraepithelial neoplasia (DIN) is an alternative histologic classification incorporating size as a discriminating factor.
  ○ Grade is more important for prognosis, risk for progression, and local recurrence.
  ○ Comedo-type necrosis (necrosis filling central portion of involved duct) is typically seen in high-grade DCIS, with varying degrees of necrosis in other types of DCIS.
– Determination of ER and PR status

 TREATMENT

MEDICATION
Secondary chemoprevention following breast-conserving surgery for ER+ DCIS:
• Tamoxifen for premenopausal patients or tamoxifen or an aromatase inhibitor for postmenopausal patients for 5 years
• There may be some advantage for aromatase inhibitor therapy in patients <60 years old or patients with concerns for thromboembolism.
• Considered in lumpectomy patients with or without whole breast radiation
• Adjuvant chemotherapy is not indicated.

SURGERY/OTHER PROCEDURES
• Surgery is the primary treatment option.
– Options for surgery are based on risk of recurrence, anatomic location, extent of disease, and the ability to achieve "negative" margins.
• Surgical options include the following:
– Breast conservation (lumpectomy) without lymph node procedure, with or without breast radiation therapy
– A sentinel lymph node biopsy may be considered if the lumpectomy is in an anatomic location compromising the performance of a future sentinel lymph node procedure.

– Patients not amenable to margin-free lumpectomy should have total mastectomy.
– Mastectomy with or without sentinel node biopsy plus optional breast reconstruction
– A complete axillary lymph node dissection should not be performed in the absence of evidence of invasive cancer and proven axillary metastatic disease.
– Long-term cause-specific survival seems to be equivalent to lumpectomy with whole breast radiation.
• Radiation considerations:
– Radiation decreases recurrence rates by about 50% but with no overall survival benefit.
– Side effects include burden of daily treatments, slight increase in secondary cancers, inability to receive radiation therapy again in ipsilateral breast.
• DCIS recurrence considerations:
– Recurrence generally requires mastectomy; rates of recurrence for DCIS and IBC are similar:
  ○ ~50% of recurrences are pure DCIS; ~50% are IBC.
• Secondary chemoprevention following breast-conserving surgery for ER+ DCIS:
– Tamoxifen for premenopausal patients or tamoxifen or an aromatase inhibitor for postmenopausal patients for 5 years
– There may be some advantage for aromatase inhibitor therapy in patients <60 years old or patients with concerns for thromboembolism.

 ONGOING CARE

FOLLOW-UP RECOMMENDATIONS
• History and physical exam should occur every 6 to 12 months for the first 5 years and then annually after that.
• MMG every 12 months (first mammogram 6 to 12 months after breast conservation therapy)
• If treated with tamoxifen or an aromatase inhibitor, monitor per consensus guidelines for breast cancer risk reduction.

PROGNOSIS
• 10-year breast cancer–specific survival rates of >95%; mortality of treated DCIS >98%
• Risk of local recurrence after mastectomy 1–2%
• Higher risk of local recurrences after breast-conserving therapy occurs in:
– Age <40 years, larger tumor size, high nuclear grade, comedo-type necrosis, close/positive margin status (related to DCIS volume)
• ER+ tumors are associated with lower risk for recurrence.
• There is interest in identifying subsets of patients who have low rates of ipsilateral breast tumor recurrence such that they might safely forgo radiation.
– The Oncotype DX DCIS test may help clinicians in selecting which patients with DCIS might safely forgo radiation therapy after breast-conserving surgery.

  ○ The test results in an Oncotype DX DCIS score, with the following risk categories:
    ▪ *DCIS score <39*—low risk of recurrence
      □ Radiation therapy benefits are likely to be small and will not outweigh the risks of side effects.
    ▪ *DCIS score 39 to 54*—intermediate risk of recurrence
      □ Radiation therapy benefits are unclear relative to the risks of side effects.
    ▪ *DCIS score 55 to 100*—high risk of recurrence
      □ Radiation therapy benefits are likely to be greater than the risks of side effects.

REFERENCE
1. American Cancer Society. Cancer Statistics Center. https://cancerstatisticscenter.cancer.org. Accessed May 14, 2023.

 SEE ALSO

Breast Cancer

 CODES

ICD10
• D05.10 Intraductal carcinoma in situ of unspecified breast
• D05.11 Intraductal carcinoma in situ of right breast
• D05.12 Intraductal carcinoma in situ of left breast

CLINICAL PEARLS
• DCIS is a heterogeneous group of *noninvasive* neoplastic breast ductal epithelial cell lesions.
• The incidence of DCIS has continued to increase in women with increase in age; more stable incidence in women >50 years of age
• Increased incidence, including for women <50 years of age, attributable to advancements in screening MMG
• The primary goal of DCIS treatment is to prevent recurrence and progression to IBC.
• The Oncotype DX DCIS score may help clinicians in selecting which patients with DCIS who may safely forgo radiation therapy after breast-conserving surgery.
• Current standard of care is local treatment with breast-conserving therapy or mastectomy, with consideration for postoperative whole breast radiation therapy and/or postsurgical tamoxifen or aromatase inhibitor therapy, unless otherwise contraindicated.
• With appropriate therapy, the overall prognosis of pure DCIS is excellent.

DUPUYTREN CONTRACTURE

Karl T. Clebak, MD, MHA, FAAFP • Morgan Lee Chambers, MD, MEd • Shawn Phillips, MD

 BASICS

DESCRIPTION
- Palmar fibromatosis; caused by progressive fibrous proliferation and tightening of the fascia of the palms, resulting in flexion deformities and loss of function
- Not the same as "trigger finger," which is caused by thickening of the distal flexor tendon
- Similar change rarely occurs in plantar fascia, usually appearing simultaneously.
- System(s) affected: musculoskeletal
- Dupuytren diathesis is an aggressive heritable form associated with age of onset <40 years; bilateral presentation to include radial digits, plantar fibromatosis (Ledderhose disease), and penile fibromatosis (Peyronie disease) (1).
- Synonyms: morbus Dupuytren; Dupuytren disease; "Celtic hand;" Viking disease; palmar fascial fibromatosis, contracture of palmar fascia

EPIDEMIOLOGY
Prevalence
- Increases with age; mean prevalence in Western countries: 12%, 21%, and 29% at ages 55, 65, and 75 years, respectively; Norway: 30% of males aged >60 years; Spain: 19% of males aged >60 years
- More common in Caucasian men of Scandinavian or Northern European ancestry
- Mean age of onset is 60 years with typical age-range of onset between 40 and 80 years.

ETIOLOGY AND PATHOPHYSIOLOGY
- Definitive etiology unknown; possibly oxidative stress, altered wound repair, and/or abnormal immune response
- Occurs in three stages (Luck classification) (1):
  - Proliferative phase: proliferation of myofibroblasts with nodule development on palmar surface
  - Involutional stage: Myofibroblasts spread along palmar fascia to fingers with cord development via production of more type 3 collagen.
  - Residual phase: Fibroblasts are predominant with dense collagen leading to cord tightening and contracture formation

Genetics
- Autosomal dominant with incomplete penetrance:
  - Siblings with 3-fold risk
- 68% of male relatives of affected patients develop disease at some time.
- Possible association with HLA alleles

RISK FACTORS
- Smoking (mean 16 pack-years, odds ratio: 2.8)
- Increasing age
- Male/Caucasian; male > female (range 3.5:1 to 9:1)
- Vibration exposure and manual work—risk doubles if regular (weekly) exposure
- Diabetes mellitus (DM) (Increases with duration of DM, usually mild; middle and ring finger are involved.)
- Excessive alcohol consumption
- Northern European ethnicity
- Family history
- Hand trauma
- Low body weight and BMI

COMMONLY ASSOCIATED CONDITIONS
- Alcoholism
- Epilepsy (inconstant data)
- DM
- Chronic lung disease
- Occupational hand trauma (vibration)
- Hypercholesterolemia
- Carpal tunnel syndrome
- Peyronie disease
- HIV
- Cancer
- Adhesive capsulitis of shoulder

 DIAGNOSIS

Diagnosis is largely clinical, based on history and physical exam.

HISTORY
- Caucasian male aged 40 to 80 years
- Family history and additional risk factors as listed above.
- Commonly report loss of ability to complete iADLs (1)
- Gradual onset of initially painless nodule of the palm
- Progression to include:
  - Pain of palpable nodule
  - Loss of function of affected finger
- Ring finger or middle finger is the most common, but any digit can be involved (1).
- Metacarpophalangeal (MCP) joint is most commonly affected; proximal and distal interphalangeal joints are rarely affected (1).

PHYSICAL EXAM
- Visual inspection and palpation of the affected region of the palm to assess for nodule or cordlike band
- Earliest sign is triangular "puckering" over the flexor tendon proximal to flexor crease
- Assess for contracture of the affected finger.
  - More common in ulnar digits
  - Hueston table top test—ask patient to lay hands flat on table, positive if patient is unable to lie fingers flat
  - Garrod nodes—callous over knuckles, associated with severe disease progression
- Tubiana's Staging (2)
  - 0: no extension deficit, no disease
  - N: no extension deficit, nodule present on exam
  - I: 1 to 45 degrees of extension deficit (surgical referral warranted)
  - II: 46 to 90 degrees of extension deficit
  - III: 91 to 135 degrees of extension deficit
  - IV: >135 degrees of extension deficit

DIFFERENTIAL DIAGNOSIS
- Camptodactyly: early teens; tight fascial bands on ulnar side of small finger
- Diabetic cheiroarthropathy: all four fingers
- Volkmann ischemic contracture
- Trigger finger (thickening of the distal flexor tendon)
- Ganglion cyst

DIAGNOSTIC TESTS & INTERPRETATION
Initial Tests (lab, imaging)
Diagnosis is based on history and physical; testing is not routinely indicated. MRI can assess cellularity of lesions that correlate with recurrence after surgery.

 TREATMENT

No definitive cure exists, and all treatments are palliative. Patients must be educated that risk for recurrence exists with all treatment, surgical and nonsurgical (3).

GENERAL MEASURES
- Observation for mild disease is reasonable.
- Extension splinting
- Physical therapy for range of motion
- See indications for surgical referral below.

MEDICATION

First Line

- Clostridial collagenase injections (FDA-approved 2010):
  - Degrades collagen to allow manual rupture of diseased cord
  - Best for isolated cord of MCP joint
  - 5-year recurrence rate of 47%; comparable with surgical recurrence rates
  - More rapid recovery of hand function compared to limited fasciectomy with fewer serious adverse events
  - Complications: injection site reaction, skin tear
  - Can do two cords concurrently
  - Can be effective for postsurgical recurrence
- Steroid injection:
  - Can treat acute nodules or painful knuckle pads
  - Serial triamcinolone injections improved long-term outcomes when combined with needle aponeurotomy.
  - Steroid alone is associated with 50% recurrence in 1 to 3 years.

Second Line

Extracorporeal shockwave treatment

ISSUES FOR REFERRAL

Indications for orthopedic surgery referral:

- Any involvement of PIP joints
- MCP joints contracted >30 degrees
- Impaired function
- Disabling deformity

ADDITIONAL THERAPIES

Percutaneous and needle fasciotomy:

- Best for MCP joint; improvement of 93% for MCP joint versus improvement of 57% for PIP joint
- Recurrence common; 50%
- Shown to be effective for recurrent disease
- Better for MCP joints in patients with comorbid conditions; lower complication rate but higher recurrence
- At 3 months and 1 year, outcomes of needle fasciotomy and collagenase injections are the same.

SURGERY/OTHER PROCEDURES

- Dermofasciectomy/limited fasciectomy/segmental aponeurectomy:
  - Greater initial correction over nonincisional treatment; higher complication rates; superior long-term advantages over collagenase injections and needle fasciotomy
  - Percutaneous aponeurotomy and lipofilling (PALF) is a new, minimally invasive procedure that appears to have shorter convalescence, less long-term complications, similar operative contraction correction, and no significant difference at 1 year in results versus limited fasciectomy.

- Indications:
  - Any involvement of the PIP joints
  - MCP joints contracted at least 30 degrees
  - Positive Hueston table top test (Patient is unable to lay palm flat on a table.)
- May require skin grafts for wound closure with severe cutaneous shrinkage
- 80% have full range of movement with early surgery.
- Amputation of 5th digit if severe and deforming
- MCP joints respond better to surgery than PIP joints, especially if contracted >45 degrees.

 ## ONGOING CARE

FOLLOW-UP RECOMMENDATIONS

Patient Monitoring

Regular follow-up every 6 months to 1 year

PATIENT EDUCATION

- Avoid risk factors (alcohol, vibratory exposure, etc.), especially if there is a strong family history.
- Mild disease: Passively stretch the digits twice a day and avoid recurrent gripping of tools.

PROGNOSIS

- Unpredictable but usually slowly progressive; without any treatment, progression is observed in about 50% over 6 years.
- 10% may regress spontaneously.
- Dupuytren diathesis predicts aggressive course. Features include ethnicity (Nordic), family history, bilateral lesions outside of palm, age <50 years—all factors with 71% risk of recurrence compared to baseline 23% without any risk factors.
- Prognosis is better in MCP joint versus PIP joint after surgery and collagenase injection.

COMPLICATIONS

- Complex regional pain syndrome
- Operative nerve injury
- Postoperative recurrence in 46–80%
- Postoperative hand edema and skin necrosis
- Digital infarction
- Limited hand function

REFERENCES

1. Dutta A, Jayasinghe G, Deore S, et al. Dupuytren's contracture—current concepts. *J Clin Orthop Trauma*. 2020;11(4):590–596.
2. Mella JR, Guo L, Hung V. Dupuytren's contracture: an evidence based review. *Ann Plast Surg*. 2018;81(6S Suppl 1):S97–S101.
3. Wong CR, Huynh MNQ, Fageeh R, et al. Outcomes of management of recurrent Dupuytren contracture: a systematic review and meta-analysis. *Hand (N Y)*. 2022;17(6):1104–1113.

ADDITIONAL READING

- Eaton C. Evidence-based medicine: Dupuytren contracture. *Plast Reconstr Surg*. 2014;133(5):1241–1251.
- Lanting R, Broekstra DC, Werker PMN, et al. A systematic review and meta-analysis on the prevalence of Dupuytren disease in the general population of Western countries. *Plast Reconstr Surg*. 2014;133(3):593–603.
- Obed D, Salim M, Scholottmann F, et al. Short-term efficacy and adverse effects of collagenase clostridium histolyticum injections, percutaneous needle fasciotomy and limited fasciectomy in the treatment of Dupuytren's contracture: a network meta-analysis of randomized controlled trials. *BMC Musculoskele Disord*. 2022;23(1):939.

CODES

ICD10

M72.0 Palmar fascial fibromatosis [Dupuytren]

CLINICAL PEARLS

- Dupuytren contracture is a fixed flexion deformity of (most commonly) the 4th and 5th digits due to palmar fibrosis. 90% of cases are progressive. It is not the same as "trigger finger," which is due to thickening of the distal flexor tendon
- Refer patients with involvement of the PIP joints or MCP joints involvement with contractures of >30 degrees.
- Both surgical and enzymatic fasciotomy have high rate of recurrence.

D

DYSHIDROSIS
Robyn Lee Reese, DO • LaRae L. Seemann, MD

BASICS

DESCRIPTION
- Common, chronic dermatitis involving the palms and soles. The precise definition is frequently debated, with many terms used interchangeably. Efforts are being made to define "dyshidrosis" more specifically, and literature supports the presence of several classes within the family "dyshidrosis."
- Dyshidrotic eczema
  - Common, chronic, or recurrent; nonerythematous; symmetric, fluid filled, vesicular eruption primarily of the palms, soles, and interdigital areas
  - Associated with burning, itching, and pain
- Pompholyx (from Greek "bubble")
  - Rare condition characterized by abrupt onset of large bullae
  - Often used interchangeably with dyshidrotic eczema (small vesicles); however, may be a distinct entity
- Lamellar dyshidrosis
  - Fine, spreading, exfoliation of the superficial epidermis in the same distribution as described above
- System(s) affected: dermatologic, exocrine, immunologic
- Synonym(s): cheiropompholyx, keratolysis exfoliativa, vesicular palmoplantar eczema, desquamation of interdigital spaces pompholyx, acute and recurrent vesicular hand dermatitis, recurrent vesicular palmoplantar dermatitis

EPIDEMIOLOGY
Incidence
- Mean age of onset is ≤40 years.
- Male = female
- Comprises 5–20% of hand eczema cases

Prevalence
20 cases/100,000 people

ETIOLOGY AND PATHOPHYSIOLOGY
- Exact mechanism is unknown; thought to be multifactorial (allergies, genetics, and dermatophyte infection implicated)
- Dermatopathology: intraepidermal spongiosis without effect on eccrine sweat glands
- Vesicles remain intact due to thickness of stratum corneum of palmar/plantar skin (1).
- Immunologic reaction: theorized that rapid rise in immunoglobulin levels may precipitate vesicle formation
- Aggravating factors (debated)
  - Hyperhidrosis (in 40% of patients with the condition)
  - Detergents/solvents
  - Increased water exposure (e.g., florists, hair stylists, health care workers)
  - Climate: hot/cold weather; humidity
  - Contact sensitivity (in 30–67% of patients with the condition) (2)
  - Metals: nickel, cobalt, and chromate sensitivity (may include implanted orthopedic or orthodontic metals) (1)
  - Stress
  - Dermatophyte infection (present in 10% of patients with the condition) (2)
  - Prolonged wear of occlusive gloves
  - Cement workers

- IV immunoglobulin therapy
- Smoking
- Sunlight/UVA radiation

Genetics
- Atopy: 50% of patients with dyshidrotic eczema have atopic dermatitis (1).
- Rare autosomal dominant form of pompholyx found in Chinese population maps to chromosome 18q22.1–18q22.3 (2)

RISK FACTORS
- Many risk factors are disputed in the literature, with none being consistently associated.
- Atopy
- Other dermatologic conditions
  - Atopic dermatitis (early in life)
  - Contact dermatitis (later in life)
  - Dermatophytosis
- Sensitivity to
  - Foods
  - Drugs: neomycin, quinolones, acetaminophen, and oral contraceptives
  - Contact and dietary: nickel (more common in young women), chromate (more common in men), and cobalt (1)
  - Smoking

GENERAL PREVENTION
- Control emotional stress.
- Avoid excessive sweating.
- Avoid exposure to irritants.
- Avoid diet high in metal salts (chromium, cobalt, nickel).
- Avoid smoking.

COMMONLY ASSOCIATED CONDITIONS
- Atopic dermatitis
- Allergic contact dermatitis
- Parkinson disease
- HIV (2)

DIAGNOSIS

HISTORY
- Episodes of pruritic rash
- Recent emotional stress
- Familial or personal history of atopy
- Exposure to allergens or irritants
  - Occupational, dietary, or household
  - Cosmetic and personal hygiene products
  - Vesicular eruption typically occurs 24 hours after allergen challenge (1).
- Costume jewelry use
- IV immunoglobulin therapy
- HIV
- Smoking

PHYSICAL EXAM
- Transient, often recurrent, symmetrical vesicular eruptions located on volar and plantar surfaces and lateral fingers; lesions may not heal completely between flares (1).
- Prodrome: Intense pruritus may occur prior to vesicular eruption.
- Early findings
  - 1 to 2 mm, clear, nonerythematous, deep-seated vesicles (lasting 2 to 3 weeks)
  - Has a "tapioca pudding" appearance

- Late findings
  - Unroofed vesicles with inflamed bases
  - Desquamation (terminal phase)
  - Peeling, rings of scale, or lichenification is common.

DIFFERENTIAL DIAGNOSIS
- Vesicular tinea pedis/manuum
- Vesicular id reaction
- Contact dermatitis (allergic or irritant)
- Scabies
- Chronic vesicular hand dermatitis
- Drug reaction
- Dermatophytid
- Bullous disorders: dyshidrosiform bullous pemphigoid, pemphigus, bullous impetigo, epidermolysis bullosa
- Pustular psoriasis
- Acrodermatitis continua
- Erythema multiforme
- Herpes simplex infection
- Pityriasis rubra pilaris
- Vesicular mycosis fungoides
- Palmoplantar pustulosis (PPP)

DIAGNOSTIC TESTS & INTERPRETATION
Follow-Up Tests & Special Considerations
- Skin culture in suspected secondary infection (most commonly, *Staphylococcus aureus*) (3)
- Consider antibiotics based on culture results and severity of symptoms.

Diagnostic Procedures/Other
- Diagnosis is based on clinical exam.
- Potassium hydroxide (KOH) wet mount (if concerned about dermatophyte infection)
- Patch test (if suspecting allergic cause) (3)

Test Interpretation
- Fine, 1- to 2-mm spongiotic, intraepidermal vesicles with little to no inflammatory change
- No eccrine glandular involvement
- Thickened stratum corneum
- Pompholyx may be confused with PPP but will contain the following distinguishing histopathologic features that PPP will not: vesicles with spongiosis and neutrophils only on the top, without microabscesses on the edges of vesicles.

TREATMENT

GENERAL MEASURES
- Avoid possible inciting factors: stress, direct skin contact with irritants, nickel, occlusive gloves, household cleaning products, smoking, sweating.
- Use moisturizers/emollients for symptomatic relief and to maintain effective skin barrier (3).
- Skin care
  - Avoid shoes with known irritants (e.g., leather, rubber soles).
  - Wear socks and gloves made of cotton and change frequently.
  - Wash infrequently in lukewarm water, carefully dry, and then apply emollient.
  - Avoid direct contact with fresh fruit.

MEDICATION

First Line

- Mild cases: topical steroids (high potency) (2)[C]
  - Considered cornerstone of therapy but limited published evidence
  - Steroid use limited to 2 weeks each episode due to risk of infection (3)[C]
- Moderate to severe cases
  - Ultra high-potency topical steroids with occlusion over treated area (3)[C]
  - Prednisone 40 to 100 mg/day tapered after blister formation ceases (2)[C]
    ○ Limited use due to significant side effects (3)[B]
  - Psoralens plus ultraviolet (UV)-A (PUVA) therapy, either systemic/topical or immersion in psoralens (2)[C]
- Recurrent cases (3)[C]
  - Systemic steroids at onset of itching prodrome
  - Prednisone 60 mg PO for 3 to 4 days

Second Line

- Topical calcineurin inhibitors (Mitigate the long-term risks of topical steroid use.)
  - Topical tacrolimus
  - Topical pimecrolimus
  - May not be as effective on plantar surface
- Other therapies (typically with dermatology consultation)
  - Oral cyclosporine (3)[C]; monitor for hypertension and renal injury.
  - Injections of botulinum toxin type A (BTXA)
    ○ Newer topical forms of BTXA currently being developed show promise.
    ○ Painful, requires nerve block
  - Systemic alitretinoin (teratogenic)
  - Topical bexarotene (a teratogenic retinoid X receptor agonist approved for use in cutaneous T-cell lymphoma)
  - Methotrexate (significant side effects including GI intolerance and hepatotoxicity) (3)[C]
  - Azathioprine (1)[C] (6- to 8-week onset of action; must monitor for GI side effects, liver toxicity, blood dyscrasia)
  - Disulfiram or sodium cromoglycate in nickel-allergic patients (1)[C]
  - Mycophenolate mofetil (2)[C] (GI side effects; benefit: no hepatotoxicity with long-term use) (3)[B]
  - Tap water iontophoresis (2)[C]

ISSUES FOR REFERRAL

- Allergist (if allergen testing required)
- Psychologist (if stress modification needed)

ADDITIONAL THERAPIES

- Other oral agents
  - Thalidomide (do not use in pregnancy/no available studies on efficacy)
  - Dapsone 100 to 150 mg daily (also limited literature on efficacy; may be used in combination with steroids) both significant side effects; very limited use (3)[C]
- High-dose UVA1 radiation therapy (1)[C]
- UV-free phototherapy
- Treat underlying dermatophytosis (1).
- BTXA in those in which excessive sweating is an exacerbating factor (3)[C]

COMPLEMENTARY & ALTERNATIVE MEDICINE

- Conservative management:
  - Antihistamines: hydroxyzine, cetirizine, loratadine
  - Soaks/cold compresses of weak solutions of potassium permanganate, Burow solution (aluminum acetate), or vinegar 15 minutes, 4 times daily (3)[C]
- Exposure to sunlight as maintenance therapy, 12 minutes every other day, 10 to 15 exposures
- Dandelion juice (not for atopic patients)
- Cognitive relaxation techniques (3)[C]

 ## ONGOING CARE

FOLLOW-UP RECOMMENDATIONS

Patient Monitoring

- Dyshidrotic Eczema Area and Severity Index (DASI); useful in assessing severity and effect of therapy, but not studied in large cohorts (1)
- Parameters used in the DASI score
  - Number of vesicles per square centimeter
  - Erythema
  - Desquamation
  - Severity of itching
  - Surface area affected
- Grading: mild (0 to 15), moderate (16 to 30), severe (31 to 60)
- Monitor BP and glucose in patients receiving systemic corticosteroids.
- Monitor for adverse effects of medications.

DIET

- Consider diet low in metal salts if history of nickel sensitivity (3)[B].
- Updated recommendations for low-cobalt diet are available (1).

PATIENT EDUCATION

- Instructions on self-care, complications, and avoidance of triggers/aggravating factors
- American Academy of Dermatology: dyshidrotic eczema at https://www.aad.org/public/diseases/eczema/types/dyshidrotic-eczema

PROGNOSIS

- Condition is benign.
- Usually heals without scarring
- Lesions may spontaneously resolve.
- Recurrence is common.

COMPLICATIONS

- Quality of life impact: skin tightening, pain, and decreased dexterity
- Secondary bacterial infections with or without steroid use (*S. aureus* most common)
- Dystrophic nail changes
- Fissures and ulcerations
- Psychological distress
- Lymphedema

REFERENCES

1. Veien NK. Acute and recurrent vesicular hand dermatitis. *Dermatol Clin*. 2009;27(3):337–353.
2. Wollina U. Pompholyx: a review of clinical features, differential diagnosis, and management. *Am J Clin Dermatol*. 2010;11(5):305–314.
3. Lofgren SM, Warshaw EM. Dyshidrosis: epidemiology, clinical characteristics, and therapy. *Dermatitis*. 2006;17(4):165–181.

ADDITIONAL READING

- Agner T, Aalto-Korte K, Andersen KE, et al; for European Environmental and Contact Dermatitis Research Group. Classification of hand eczema. *J Eur Acad Dermatol Venereol*. 2015;29(12):2417–2422.
- Calle Sarmiento PM, Chango Azanza JJC. Dyshidrotic eczema: a common cause of palmar dermatitis. *Cureus*. 2020;12(10):e10839.
- Molin S, Diepgen TL, Ruzicka T, et al. Diagnosing chronic hand eczema by an algorithm: a tool for classification in clinical practice. *Clin Exp Dermatol*. 2011;36(6):595–601.

 ## SEE ALSO

Algorithm: Rash

 ## CODES

ICD10

L30.1 Dyshidrosis [pompholyx]

CLINICAL PEARLS

- Dyshidrosis is a transient, recurrent, vesicular eruption, most commonly of the palms, soles, and interdigital areas.
- Etiology and pathophysiology are unknown but are most likely related to a combination of genetic and environmental factors.
- Best prevention is effective skin care and limiting exposure to irritating agents.
- Treatment is based on disease severity; preferred treatments include topical steroids, oral steroids, and calcineurin inhibitors.
- Although benign and self-healing, this condition can be chronic and debilitating with major concern for superimposed bacterial infection that may be avoided by preventive measures, early treatment, and recognition.

D

DYSMENORRHEA
Maggie C. Wertz, MD

BASICS

DESCRIPTION
- Pelvic pain occurring at/around time of menses; a leading cause of absenteeism for women <30 years old
- Primary dysmenorrhea: pelvic pain without pathologic physical findings; diagnosis of exclusion
- Secondary dysmenorrhea: often more severe, results from specific pelvic pathology; often resistant to typical treatments for dysmenorrhea; severity based on activity impairment
- Mild: painful, rarely limits daily function, rarely requires analgesics
- Moderate: daily activity affected, rare absenteeism, requires analgesics
- Severe: daily activity affected, likelihood of absenteeism increased, limited benefit from analgesics
- System affected: reproductive
- Synonym(s): menstrual cramps

EPIDEMIOLOGY
- Predominant age
  - Primary: onset 6 to 12 months after the start of menarche, teens to early 20s
  - Secondary: 20s to 30s
- Predominant sex: women only

Prevalence
- Up to 90% of menstruating females have experienced primary dysmenorrhea (1).
- Up to 42% lose days of school/work monthly due to dysmenorrhea
- Up to 20% reported impairment in daily activities and/or sleep

ETIOLOGY AND PATHOPHYSIOLOGY
- Primary: Elevated prostaglandin (PGF2α) production through indirect hormonal control (decrease in progesterone at start of menses leads to increase in prostaglandins) causes nonrhythmic hypercontractility and increased uterine muscle tone with vasoconstriction and resultant uterine ischemia. Ischemia results in hypersensitization of type C pain nerve fibers; intensity of cramps is directly proportional to amount of PGF2α released (1).
- Secondary: endometriosis (most common cause); adenomyosis; congenital abnormalities of uterine/vaginal anatomy; cervical stenosis; pelvic inflammatory disease; ovarian cysts; pelvic tumors, especially leiomyomata (fibroids) and uterine polyps

Genetics
Not well studied

RISK FACTORS
- Primary (1),(2)
  - Cigarette smoking
  - Alcohol use
  - Early menarche (age <12 years)
  - Age <30 years
  - Family history of dysmenorrhea
  - Irregular/heavy menstrual flow
  - Nonuse of oral contraceptives
  - Sexual abuse/history of sexual assault
  - Psychological symptoms (depression, anxiety, increased stress, etc.)
  - Nulliparity

- Secondary
  - Pelvic infection
  - Use of intrauterine device (IUD) in the few months following insertion
  - Structural pelvic malformations
  - Family history of endometriosis in first-degree relative

GENERAL PREVENTION
- Primary: regular exercise; early childbirth and higher parity; use of hormonal contraceptives
- Secondary: Reduce risk of sexually transmitted infections (STIs)

Pediatric Considerations
Onset with first menses raises probability of genital tract anatomic abnormality (i.e., transverse vaginal septum, imperforate or minimally perforated hymen, uterine anomalies).

COMMONLY ASSOCIATED CONDITIONS
- Irregular/heavy menstrual periods
- Longer menstrual cycle length/duration of bleeding
- Anxiety/depression
- Decreased quality of life

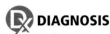

DIAGNOSIS

Typically, a clinical diagnosis is based on characteristic symptom history of suprapubic/low back cramping/pain occurring at or near menstrual flow onset lasting for 8 to 72 hours (2).

HISTORY
- Primary: onset once ovulatory cycles are established in adolescents; 6 to 12 months after menarche on average
- Patients may have associated nausea, vomiting, diarrhea, headache, fatigue, insomnia, pain radiating into the low back or inner thighs, and rarely syncope and fever. These are all considered to be secondary to prostaglandin release.
- Recurrence at or just before the onset of the menstrual flow
  - Pelvic pain occurring between menstrual periods is not likely to be dysmenorrhea.
  - Present with most menstrual periods (cyclic)
- Acute relief associated with the following:
  - Use of analgesics, especially NSAIDs
  - Local topical heat application
  - Orgasm
- Response to NSAIDs helps confirm diagnosis.
- Impact of symptoms on daily activities can help determine severity.
- Secondary: can be associated with chronic pelvic pain, midcycle pain, dyspareunia, abnormal uterine bleeding, typical onset after age 25 years, nonmidline pain, progression of severity, lack of response to NSAIDs/hormonal treatment and infertility.

PHYSICAL EXAM
- Primary: Physical exam is typically normal. Examine to rule out secondary dysmenorrhea only if the history is inconsistent with primary dysmenorrhea. Pelvic exam is recommended if patient is sexually active to rule out infection.
- Secondary: Evaluate for cervical discharge, uterine enlargement, tenderness, irregularity, or fixation.

DIFFERENTIAL DIAGNOSIS
- Primary: History is characteristic.
- Secondary: Endometriosis (most common), pelvic/genital infection; complication of pregnancy; missed/incomplete abortion; ectopic pregnancy; uterine/ovarian neoplasm; UTI; complication with IUD use; congenital uterine or cervical anomaly; adenomyosis; leiomyomata (fibroids); pelvic adhesions; inflammatory bowel disease; irritable bowel syndrome; chronic pelvic pain (idiopathic)

DIAGNOSTIC TESTS & INTERPRETATION
Initial Tests (lab, imaging)
All tests should only be performed if indicated based on history or if patient has symptoms refractory to first-line therapies; most cases of primary dysmenorrhea can be diagnosed on history alone.
- Pregnancy test
- Urine testing for infection
- Gonorrhea/chlamydia cervical testing, especially in women aged <25 years and in high-prevalence areas
- Primary: Consider pelvic ultrasound to rule out secondary abnormalities.
- Secondary: ultrasound and/or laparoscopy to define anatomy for severe/refractory cases. MRI may be useful as second-line noninvasive imaging if ultrasound is nondiagnostic and fibroids, ovarian torsion, deep endometriosis, or adenomyosis is suspected.

Follow-Up Tests & Special Considerations
Counsel regarding appropriate preventive measures for STI and pregnancy.

Diagnostic Procedures/Other
Laparoscopy is rarely needed and is usually only considered in cases of suspected endometriosis or pelvic adhesions not definitively identified on transvaginal ultrasound.

Test Interpretation
- Primary: none
- Secondary: Specific anatomic abnormalities may be noted (see "Differential Diagnosis").

Pregnancy Considerations
Consider ectopic pregnancy when pelvic pain occurs with vaginal bleeding in a patient with a positive pregnancy test.

TREATMENT

- Reassure the patient that treatment success is very likely with adherence to recommendations.
- Relief may require the use of several treatment modalities at the same time.

GENERAL MEASURES
- Regular exercise (1),(3)[A] and topical local heat (1)[C] are noninvasive general measures to relieve pain. Local heat in conjunction with the use of an NSAID is superior to an NSAID alone (1)[C].
- High-frequency transcutaneous electrical nerve stimulation (TENS) has been found to be beneficial (1),(4). Low-frequency TENS is not recommended because it is not superior to placebo.
- Secondary dysmenorrhea: treatment of suspected/confirmed underlying cause of pain

MEDICATION

First Line

- NSAIDs: inhibit the peripheral production of prostaglandins. No NSAID has been found to be superior to others. Medication should be taken on scheduled dosing starting 1 to 2 days prior to onset of menses and continued for 2 to 3 days (1),(2). If one NSAID preparation does not work, another NSAID preparation should be tried. Each preparation should be taken as prescribed for at least 3 menstrual cycles prior to determining effectiveness.
  - Ibuprofen 400 mg PO q8h
  - Naproxen sodium 500 mg PO q12h
  - Celecoxib 400 mg PO × 1 and then 200 mg PO q12h
  - Mefenamic acid 500 mg PO × 1 and then 250 mg PO q6h (not to exceed 3 days)
- Hormonal contraceptives: recommended for primary dysmenorrhea in women desiring contraception (2)[C]. Directly suppresses ovulation and limits endometrial growth resulting in reduced prostaglandin production, intrauterine pressure, and uterine contractions. Continuous rather than cyclic dosing has been found to be superior for pain control (4). Amenorrhea by any means can improve symptoms of dysmenorrhea. Estrogen-containing contraceptives are recommended first-line medications for secondary dysmenorrhea due to endometriosis, although progestin-only methods have been shown to be just as or even more effective (5).
  - Low- and high-dose combined oral contraceptives (COCs) along with transdermal and intravaginal combined contraceptives have all been found to be superior to placebo (1)[C].
  - Levonorgestrel IUDs are just as effective as COCs (4)[C].
  - Progestin-only contraceptives including subcutaneous and subdermal preparations appear to decrease primary dysmenorrhea but to a lesser extent than combined options and IUDs (1),(2)[B].
- Potential contraindications to NSAIDs and COCs
  - Platelet disorders
  - Gastric ulceration or gastritis
  - Personal and family history of thromboembolic disorders
  - Vascular disease
  - Migraines with aura
  - Active smoking
- Precautions for first-line options
  - GI irritation
  - Lactation
  - Coagulation disorders
  - Impaired renal function
  - Heart failure
  - Liver dysfunction
  - Pregnancy
  - Hypertension
- Significant possible interactions
  - Coumadin-type anticoagulants
  - Aspirin with other NSAIDs

Second Line

- Acetaminophen and acetaminophen with caffeine are superior to placebo and have less potential side effects than NSAIDs (1)[B].
- Behavioral interventions, such as relaxation exercises including yoga, may help alleviate pain in primary dysmenorrhea (5).
- Nifedipine may be effective in some women and may be used in women trying to conceive (pregnancy Category C).

SURGERY/OTHER PROCEDURES

Laparoscopic uterosacral nerve ablation and presacral neurectomy have been shown to relieve pain at 6 and 12 months, respectively, but are still reserved for patients with pain resistant to all other first- and second-line treatments (1),(4)[B]. Hysterectomy is effective for dysmenorrhea but should only be considered in very rare occasions and when all desired childbearing is complete (1).

COMPLEMENTARY & ALTERNATIVE MEDICINE

- Chinese herbal medicine shows promising evidence of decreasing pain, but more evidence is needed.
- Acupuncture treatments have been shown to decrease pain in dysmenorrhea, but further randomized, well-designed studies are needed. Additionally, these treatments must be frequent and timely for effectiveness.
- Acupoint stimulation, particularly noninvasive stimulation (acupressure), has been found to reduce pain scores but is inferior to NSAIDs (5).
- Aromatherapy abdominal massage performed daily for 10 minutes, 7 days prior to onset of menses can decrease primary dysmenorrhea.
- Further research needed to determine benefit and safety for regular use of oral fennel, oral ginger, oral fenugreek, oral valerian, extracorporeal magnetic innervation, vitamin K_1 injection into the spleen-6 acupuncture point, use of high-frequency vibratory stimulation tampon, transdermal nitroglycerin, and vaginal sildenafil.

ADMISSION, INPATIENT, AND NURSING CONSIDERATIONS

Both primary and secondary dysmenorrhea are usually managed in the outpatient setting.

- Primary: outpatient care
- Secondary: usually outpatient care

ONGOING CARE

FOLLOW-UP RECOMMENDATIONS

Normal

DIET

Insufficient evidence for any specific dietary changes

PATIENT EDUCATION

Reassure the patient that primary dysmenorrhea is treatable with the use of NSAIDs, COCs, IUDs, exercises, or local heat and that it will usually abate with age and parity.

PROGNOSIS

- Primary: reduced with age and parity
- Secondary: likely to require therapy based on underlying cause

COMPLICATIONS

- Primary: anxiety and/or depression
- Secondary: infertility from underlying pathology

REFERENCES

1. Burnett M, Lemyre M. No. 345—primary dysmenorrhea consensus guideline. *J Obstet Gynaecol Can.* 2017;39(7):585–595.
2. Osayande AS, Mehulic S. Diagnosis and initial management of dysmenorrhea. *Am Fam Physician.* 2014;89(5):341–346.
3. Brown J, Brown S. Exercise for dysmenorrhoea. *Cochrane Database Syst Rev.* 2010;(2):CD004142.
4. Oladosu FA, Tu FF, Hellman KM. Nonsteroidal antiinflammatory drug resistance in dysmenorrhea: epidemiology, causes, and treatment. *Am J Obstet Gynecol.* 2018;218(4):390–400.
5. McKenna KA, Fogleman CD. Dysmenorrhea. *Am Fam Physician.* 2021;104(2):164–170.

ADDITIONAL READING

- Ryan SA. The treatment of dysmenorrhea. *Pediatr Clin North Am.* 2017;64(2):331–342.
- Woo HL, Ji HR, Pak YK, et al. The efficacy and safety of acupuncture in women with primary dysmenorrhea: a systematic review and meta-analysis. *Medicine (Baltimore).* 2018;97(23):e11007.

 SEE ALSO

- Dyspareunia; Endometriosis; Menorrhagia (Heavy Menstrual Bleeding); Premenstrual Syndrome (PMS) and Premenstrual Dysphoric Disorder (PMDD)
- Algorithm: Pelvic Pain

CODES

ICD10

- N94.6 Dysmenorrhea, unspecified
- N94.4 Primary dysmenorrhea
- N94.5 Secondary dysmenorrhea

CLINICAL PEARLS

- Dysmenorrhea is a leading cause of absenteeism for women aged <30 years.
- In women who desire contraception, hormonal contraceptives are the preferred treatment.
- All NSAIDs studied have been found to be equally effective in the relief of dysmenorrhea and should be initiated 1 to 2 days prior to onset of menses with scheduled dosing for at least 2 to 3 days with each menstrual cycle.

D

DYSPAREUNIA

Bindusri Paruchuri, MD • Whitney Green, MD

 BASICS

The information presented in this chapter pertains to female dyspareunia.

DESCRIPTION

- Recurrent and persistent genital or pelvic pain associated with sexual activity, which is not exclusively due to intensity of intercourse, lack of lubrication or vaginismus, or an involuntary contraction of vaginal muscles
  - May be superficial, causing pain with attempted vaginal insertion, or deep
  - Complex, multifactorial disorder involving psychosocial and physical conditions (1)
- Dyspareunia and vaginismus were previously viewed as separate conditions but are now combined into genito-pelvic pain and penetration disorder as described by the *DSM-5* (1).
- Individuals whose sexual activity do not involve penetration can still have this disorder if they have pain interfering with sexual function.

EPIDEMIOLOGY

- Predominant age: all ages
- Predominant sex: female > male

Incidence

>50% of all sexually active women will report dyspareunia at some time.

Geriatric Considerations

Up to 50% of menopausal women are affected by symptoms associated with genitourinary syndrome of menopause which includes a constellation of genital, sexual, and urinary symptoms associated with decreased estrogen levels.

Prevalence

10–20% of U.S. women are affected, varying by age and population (2).

ETIOLOGY AND PATHOPHYSIOLOGY

Female

- Vulva and vagina
  - Dermatologic diseases: lichen sclerosus, lichen planus, contact dermatitis
  - Inadequate lubrication: premature ovarian failure, bilateral oophorectomy, menopause, pituitary tumors, postpartum status, diabetes mellitus, chemotherapy/radiation therapy, and medications (listed below)
  - Pelvic floor dysfunction
  - Vaginal atrophy
  - Vaginismus
  - Vaginitis
  - Vulvodynia
- Bladder
  - Interstitial cystitis
- Uterus and adnexa
  - Ovarian masses
  - Uterine retroversion
- Pelvis
  - Adhesions or chronic pelvic inflammatory disease
  - Endometriosis

- Iatrogenic
  - Hysterectomy
  - Dilation and curettage
- Postpartum
  - Obstetric trauma: perineal tears, episiotomy, instrumented delivery, cesarean delivery
  - Breastfeeding
- Genitourinary syndrome of menopause
- Medications such as gonadotropin-releasing hormone agonists, selective estrogen receptor modulators, tamoxifen, aromatase inhibitors, progestogens, and danazol
- Female genital mutilation
- Trauma
- Psychological disorders
  - Anxiety
  - Depression
  - PTSD
  - History of sexual abuse

RISK FACTORS

- Demographic risk factors: younger age, white race, lower socioeconomic status, and being in postpartum, perimenopausal, or postmenopausal period.
- Psychosocial risk factors: depression, anxiety, low sexual satisfaction, and history of sexual abuse
- Other etiologies: irritable bowel syndrome, musculoskeletal disorders, and fibromyalgia

Pregnancy Considerations

- Pregnancy has a potent influence on sexuality; dyspareunia is common in late pregnancy and postpartum.
  - Breastfeeding, perineal pain, fatigue, and stress can be risk factors in postpartum period.
- Vacuum-assisted or forceps vaginal delivery or have had pelvic floor surgery is at increased risk.
- Episiotomies do not have a protective effect. Women who experience delivery interventions including episiotomy are at greater risk than women who deliver over an intact perineum or who have an unrepaired laceration.

COMMONLY ASSOCIATED CONDITIONS

- Vaginismus: involuntary contraction of pelvic floor muscles with attempted vaginal penetration
- Vulvodynia: chronic genital pain of at least 3 months duration with no known etiology

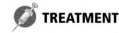 **DIAGNOSIS**

- For women, the diagnosis of dyspareunia is made with the persistent or recurrent presence of one or more of the following symptoms per the *DSM-5*:
  - Difficulty having intercourse
  - Marked vulvovaginal or pelvic pain during intercourse or penetration attempts
  - Marked fear or anxiety about vulvovaginal or pelvic pain anticipating, during, or resulting from vaginal penetration
  - Marked tensing or tightening of the pelvic floor muscles during attempted vaginal penetration

- Symptoms have persisted for a minimum of 6 months and cause clinically significant distress in the individual not better explained by nonsexual mental health disorder, intimate partner violence, or substance/medications (3).

HISTORY

Obtain a detailed sexual history including, but not limited to, number of partners and their gender, temporality of symptoms and their evolution with time, presence and degree of personal distress, alleviating factors, personal health problems, medication use, substance use, past or current abuse or violence experienced, number of pregnancies, menstrual status, physical activity, and injuries related to genito-pelvic area.

PHYSICAL EXAM

- A complete exam, including a focused pelvic exam, to identify pathology
  - Exam must include inspection and palpation of urethra, vulva, and vaginal areas; palpation of the uterine, bladder, and adnexal structures; rectovaginal exam; penis, scrotum, pelvic floor muscles, and digital rectal exam.
  - Assess for atrophy, discoloration, lesions, or trauma
  - Sensory mapping with a cotton-tipped applicator to localize sensitive and painful areas; document location with reference to the "clock face" by starting on vestibule.
  - It may be beneficial for patients to contribute to the exam with the use of a mirror (2).
  - Musculoskeletal evaluation will help rule out associated etiologies such as pelvic muscle overactivity or myofascial disorders (3). Palpation of pelvic floor muscles: levator ani, obturator internus, and piriformis can help localize.
    - Tenderness of vaginal muscles during single-digit exam can indicate pelvic floor dysfunction (2).
- Because examination often reproduces the pain, examiner should be cautious and sensitive to patient's anxiety.

DIFFERENTIAL DIAGNOSIS

- Refer to section on etiology.
- Many conditions can cause dyspareunia, and individuals can experience more than one type of sexual dysfunction.

DIAGNOSTIC TESTS & INTERPRETATION

- Typically, none necessary for diagnosis unless an undiagnosed, underlying medical condition is suspected
- Cultures, biopsy, or microscopy can be considered as indicated based on history and exam findings to rule out organic causes of pain.

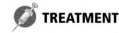 **TREATMENT**

GENERAL MEASURES

- Initiate specific treatment when initial evaluation identifies an organic cause (2).
- Once organic causes are ruled out, treatment is a multidimensional and multidisciplinary approach.

- Nonpharmacologic measures
  - Psychologic interventions
    - Sexual skills training
    - Cognitive-behavioral therapy
    - Mindfulness
    - Couples therapy
  - Pelvic floor physical therapy
  - Self-dilation enabled by prescription and OTC-based products can alleviate vaginismus and pelvic floor trigger points (1).
  - Education on genital hygiene, avoidance of harsh detergents or perfumed products (2)
- Lubrication-associated etiology: use of vaginal moisturizers several times per week with lubricants during intercourse
- Genitourinary syndrome of menopause: Vaginal estrogen is most effective if symptomatic.

MEDICATION

First Line
Depends on the etiology (2)

- Antibiotics, antifungals, or antivirals, as indicated, for infection
- Water- and silicone-based vaginal lubricants or moisturizers containing hyaluronic acid and polycarbophil products can be used several times per week for vaginal dryness.
- Low-dose vaginal estrogen as cream, rings, and tablets is preferred for genitourinary syndrome of menopause; they have been shown to provide faster relief than systemic estrogen.
- Nonestrogen intravaginal treatments like ospemifene or prasterone can be recommended as an alternative for women with history of breast cancer (2).
- SSRIs to treat underlying depression
- Analgesics like NSAIDs and topical anesthetics for pain
- Neuropathic pain associated with vulvar vestibulitis/vulvodynia may respond to tricyclic antidepressants (amitriptyline or nortriptyline) or gabapentin.
- Trigger point injections with local anesthetics or botox.
- In observational studies, pain with ejaculation improved or resolved completely with tamsulosin (1).

ISSUES FOR REFERRAL
Referral for long-term therapy with consultants with expertise in treating sexual dysfunction should be considered such as pelvic floor physical therapy.

SURGERY/OTHER PROCEDURES
- Consideration of surgical interventions for dyspareunia due to altered anatomy, uterine position, fibroids, or prior pelvic surgery
  - Laparoscopic excision of endometriotic lesions or pelvic adhesions
  - Surgical vestibulectomy can be considered if medical measures fail with vulvar vestibulitis.
  - Fractional CO_2 laser treatments demonstrate improvement in symptoms of vulvovaginal atrophy (although this should only be used in a research setting).
- FDA warns against the use of medical devices for unapproved uses including "vaginal rejuvenation" procedures.

COMPLEMENTARY & ALTERNATIVE MEDICINE
- Sitz baths may relieve painful inflammation.
- Perineal massage
- Antioxidants may improve symptoms associated with endometriosis.

 ONGOING CARE

FOLLOW-UP RECOMMENDATIONS
Patient Monitoring
- Outpatient follow-up depends on therapy.
- Every 6 to 12 months once resolved

DIET
A high-fiber diet may help if constipation is a contributing cause.

PATIENT EDUCATION
- Norsigian J; for Boston Women's Health Book Collective. *Our Bodies, Ourselves*. New York, NY: Touchstone; 2011.
- Kegel exercise information
- Provide couples with information about sexual arousal techniques.

PROGNOSIS
Depends on underlying cause but most patients will respond to treatment

REFERENCES

1. American College of Obstetricians and Gynecologists' Committee on Practice Bulletins—Gynecology. Female sexual dysfunction: ACOG practice bulletin clinical management guidelines for obstetrician–gynecologists, number 213. *Obstet Gynecol*. 2019;134(1):e1–e18.
2. Hill DA, Taylor CA. Dyspareunia in women. *Am Fam Physician*. 2021;103(10):597–604.
3. American College of Obstetricians and Gynecologists' Committee on Gynecologic Practice and American Society for Colposcopy and Cervical Pathology. Committee Opinion No. 673: persistent vulvar pain. *Obstet Gynecol*. 2016;128(3):e78–e84.

ADDITIONAL READING
Sorensen J, Bautista KE, Lamvu G, et al. Evaluation and treatment of female sexual pain: a clinical review. *Cureus*. 2018;10(3):e2379.

 SEE ALSO

- Endometriosis; Genito-Pelvic Pain/Penetration Disorder (Vaginismus); Pelvic Inflammatory Disease; Sexual Dysfunction in Women; Vulvovaginitis, Estrogen Deficient; Vulvovaginitis, Prepubescent
- Algorithms: Dyspareunia; Vaginal Discharge

CODES

ICD10
- N94.1 Dyspareunia
- F52.6 Dyspareunia not due to a substance or known physiol cond

CLINICAL PEARLS
- Thorough history to determine if patient feels pain before, during, or after intercourse will help identify the cause.
- Genito-pelvic pain and penetration disorder includes one or more of the following symptoms: tightening of the vaginal muscle with decreased ability or inability to accommodate penetration; tension, pain, or burning felt when penetration is attempted; a decrease in or no desire to have intercourse; avoidance of sexual activity; intense phobia or fear of pain (2).
- A complete history and pelvic exam is needed for appropriate diagnosis.
- Low-dose vaginal estrogen is the preferred hormonal treatment for female sexual dysfunction (1).
- Psychologic interventions are recommended as part of treatment (1).
- Pelvic floor physical therapy is recommended to restore muscle function (1).
- Episiotomy does not offer any benefit in the prevention of dyspareunia; an episiotomy in fact may cause more future discomfort.

D

DYSPEPSIA, FUNCTIONAL

Tya-Mae Y. Julien, MD

BASICS

DESCRIPTION
- The presence of bothersome postprandial fullness, early satiety, or epigastric pain/burning in the absence of causative structural disease (to include normal upper endoscopy) for at least 1 to 3 days per week for the preceding 3 months, with initial symptom onset at least 6 months prior to diagnosis (Rome IV criteria)
- Rome IV criteria divide patients into two subtypes:
  – Postprandial distress syndrome (PDS)
  – Epigastric pain syndrome (EPS)
- System(s) affected: GI
- Synonym(s): idiopathic dyspepsia; nonulcer dyspepsia; nonorganic dyspepsia; PDS; and EPS

EPIDEMIOLOGY
Incidence
Unknown; accounts for 70% of patients with dyspepsia and ~5% of primary care visits

Prevalence
- 10–20% prevalence worldwide (varies based on criteria)
- Overall more common in Western cultures
- PDS subtype may be more common in Eastern cultures.
- Predominant age: adults (can be seen in children)
- Predominant gender: female > male

ETIOLOGY AND PATHOPHYSIOLOGY
Unknown but proposed mechanisms or associations include gastric motility disorders, visceral pain hypersensitivity, *Helicobacter pylori* infection, alteration in upper GI microbiome, postinfectious complications, immune activation, inflammation, and gut-brain axis disorders

Genetics
Possible link to G-protein β_3 subunit 825 CC genotype, serotonin transport genes, and/or cholecystokinin-A-receptor gene polymorphisms

Geriatric Considerations
Patients aged >60 years with new-onset dyspepsia should undergo endoscopy.

Pediatric Considerations
Be alert for family system dysfunction.

Pregnancy Considerations
Pregnancy may exacerbate symptoms.

RISK FACTORS
- Other functional disorders: fibromyalgia, temporo-mandibular joint pain, chronic fatigue syndrome
- Anxiety/depression, psychosocial stressors (e.g., divorce; unemployment; history of physical, sexual, or emotional trauma/abuse)
- Smoking
- Female gender
- NSAID use

GENERAL PREVENTION
Avoid modifiable risk factors.

COMMONLY ASSOCIATED CONDITIONS
Other functional bowel disorders

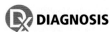DIAGNOSIS

HISTORY
- Postprandial fullness
- Early satiety
- Epigastric pain
- Epigastric burning
- Symptoms for 3 months
- Alarm features include (1),(2):
  – Unintended weight loss
  – Progressive dysphagia
  – Odynophagia
  – Persistent vomiting
  – GI bleeding
  – Family history of upper GI cancer
  – Age ≥60 years

PHYSICAL EXAM
- Document weight status and vital signs.
- Examine for signs of systemic illness.
  – Murphy sign for cholecystitis
  – Rebound and guarding for ulcer perforation
  – Palpate during muscle contraction to assess for abdominal wall pain (Carnett sign).
  – Jaundice
  – Thyromegaly

DIFFERENTIAL DIAGNOSIS
- Peptic ulcer disease; gastroesophageal reflux disease
- Cholecystitis; choledocholithiasis
- Gastric or esophageal cancer; esophageal spasm
- Malabsorption syndromes; celiac disease
- Pancreatic cancer; pancreatitis
- Inflammatory bowel disease; carbohydrate malabsorption; gastroparesis
- Ischemic bowel disease
- Intestinal parasites
- Irritable bowel syndrome
- Ischemic heart disease
- Diabetes mellitus; thyroid disease; connective tissue disorders
- Medication effects

DIAGNOSTIC TESTS & INTERPRETATION
Initial Tests (lab, imaging)
- Functional dyspepsia is a diagnosis of exclusion. Order labs based on clinical suspicion.
- Test for *H. pylori* (stool antigen or urea breath test) in areas of high *H. pylori* prevalence (2)[A].
- CBC (if anemia or infection are suspected)
- Liver-associated enzymes/right upper quadrant ultrasound (if hepatobiliary disease is suspected)
- Pancreatic enzymes (if pancreatic disease is suspected)
- Upper endoscopy for patients aged >60 years or with alarm symptoms to rule out malignancy (2)[C]
- Upper endoscopy is unlikely to change outcomes or management (3).
- Self-report questionnaires can track symptoms (1).

Diagnostic Procedures/Other
- Esophageal manometry or gastric accommodation studies are infrequently needed (1)[C].
- Motility studies are unnecessary, unless gastroparesis is strongly suspected (2)[C].

Test Interpretation
None (By definition, this is a functional disorder.)

TREATMENT

GENERAL MEASURES
- Reassurance/physician support is helpful (1)[C].
- Treatment is based on presumed etiologies.
- Discontinue offending medications (1)[C].
- Routine endoscopy not recommended in dyspeptic patients aged <60 years without alarm features (2)[B]

MEDICATION

First Line
- Treat *H. pylori* if confirmed on testing (1),(2)[A].
- Trial of once daily proton pump inhibitor (PPI) medication (e.g., omeprazole 20 mg PO QD) or H_2 receptor antagonist for up to 8 weeks in patients without alarm symptoms—most effective for patients with EPS (1),(2),(3)
- Prokinetics have been proposed as first-line agents in PDS, although efficacy data for metoclopramide 5 to 10 mg PO TID 30 minutes before meals (only agent approved in the United States) are limited. Prokinetics should be prescribed at the lowest effective dose to avoid potential side effects (2)[C]. Use with caution due to side effects of tardive dyskinesia, parkinsonian symptoms, and QT prolongation.

Second Line
- Trial of tricyclic antidepressant (TCA) medication is more helpful for EPS than PDS (e.g., amitriptyline 25 mg PO QD, can up titrate to 50 mg PO QD), with an NNT of 6 (2)[A]. Caution in elderly. There is insufficient data to support the use of SSRIs/SNRIs.
- Trazodone 25 mg at bedtime is an alternative (3). Consider buspirone or mirtazapine if no response or if contraindications to TCA.
- Gabapentin 300 mg twice daily can be a useful adjunct, particularly for treatment of gastrointestinal pain symptoms.

ADDITIONAL THERAPIES
- Stress reduction (3)
- Psychotherapy and/or cognitive behavioral therapy effective in some patients (1),(2)[B]
- Patients should be given a positive diagnosis and reassured of benign prognosis.

COMPLEMENTARY & ALTERNATIVE MEDICINE
Alternative medicine approaches show promise but need further study and are not currently recommended (2)[C].

- STW 5 (Iberogast) shown to be helpful in some studies
- Probiotics have theoretical benefit but lack consistent trial data to support routine use.
- Hypnotherapy may help.
- Transcutaneous electroacupuncture may help (1)[B].

 ONGOING CARE

FOLLOW-UP RECOMMENDATIONS

Patient Monitoring
- Provide ongoing support and reassurance.
- Consider upper endoscopy if persistent symptoms.
- Change medications if no difference in symptoms after 4 weeks (1)[C].
- Discontinue medications once symptoms resolve (1)[C].

DIET
- Limited data to support dietary modification, including restricting high fermentable oligosaccharides, disaccharides, monosaccharides, and polyols (FODMAP) foods
- Consider limiting fatty foods (3).
- Avoid foods that exacerbate symptoms: wheat and cow milk proteins, peppers or spices, coffee, tea, and alcohol (3).

PATIENT EDUCATION
Reassurance and stress reduction techniques

PROGNOSIS
Long-term/chronic symptoms with symptom-free periods

COMPLICATIONS
Iatrogenic, from evaluation to rule out serious pathology

REFERENCES
1. Lacy BE, Cangemi DJ. Updates in functional dyspepsia and bloating. *Curr Opin Gastroenterol*. 2022;38(6):613–619.
2. Moayyedi PM, Lacy BE, Andrews CN, et al. ACG and CAG clinical guideline: management of dyspepsia. *Am J Gastroenterol*. 2017;112(7):988–1013.
3. Gwee KA, Lee YY, Suzuki H, et al. Asia-Pacific guidelines for managing functional dyspepsia overlapping with other gastrointestinal symptoms. *J Gastroenterol Hepatol*. 2023;38(2):197–209.

ADDITIONAL READING
- Jamshidfar N, Hamdieh M, Eslami P, et al. Comparison of the potency of nortriptyline and mirtazapine on gastrointestinal symptoms, the level of anxiety and depression in patients with functional dyspepsia. *Gastroenterol Hepatol Bed Bench*. 2023;16(1):468–477.
- Jones MP, Guthrie-Lyons L, Sato YA, et al. Factors associated with placebo treatment response in functional dyspepsia clinical trials. *Am J Gastroenterol*. 2023;118(4):685–691.
- Marasco G, Maida M, Cremon C, et al. Meta-analysis: Post-COVID-19 functional dyspepsia and irritable bowel syndrome. *Aliment Pharmacol Ther*. 2023;58(1):6–15.

 SEE ALSO

- Irritable Bowel Syndrome
- Algorithm: Dyspepsia

CODES

ICD10
K30 Functional dyspepsia

CLINICAL PEARLS
- Dyspepsia without underlying organic disease is classified as functional or idiopathic.
- Consider empiric acid suppression therapy as first line for functional dyspepsia.
- Extensive diagnostic testing is not recommended, unless alarm symptoms are present.

DYSPHAGIA

Felix B. Chang, MD, DABMA, ABIHM, ABIM

BASICS

Subjective sensation of difficulty or abnormality of swallowing

DESCRIPTION
- Oropharyngeal: difficulty transferring food bolus from oropharynx to proximal esophagus
- Esophageal: difficulty moving food bolus through the body of the esophagus to the pylorus

EPIDEMIOLOGY
5–8% of the general population >50 years of age

Incidence
- Esophageal food impaction 25 per 100,000 persons per year
- Males to female (1.5:1)

Prevalence
- 14–33% among community-dwelling individuals ≥65 years old
- Up to 40% in hospital settings
- 29–32% of patients in nursing homes
- 44% in patients in geriatrics acute care
- 60% in older patients that are institutionalized

ETIOLOGY AND PATHOPHYSIOLOGY
- Oropharyngeal (transfer dysphagia):
  - Functional motor disorder in the oropharynx
  - Mechanical: pharyngeal and laryngeal cancer, acute epiglottitis, carotid body tumor, pharyngitis, tonsillitis, strep throat, lymphoid hyperplasia of lingual tonsil, lateral pharyngeal pouch, hypopharyngeal diverticulum
  - Neuromyogenic: stroke, head trauma, Parkinson disease, amyotrophic lateral sclerosis (ALS), myasthenia, polymyositis, dermatomyositis, muscular dystrophies, thyrotoxicosis, hypothyroidism, amyloidosis, Cushing syndrome
  - Esophageal:
    - Mechanical: carcinomas, diverticula, webs, Schatzki ring, structures (peptic, chemical, trauma, radiation), foreign body; eosinophilic esophagitis
    - Extrinsic mechanical: peritonsillar abscess, thyroid disorders, tumors, vascular compression (enlarged left atrium, aberrant subclavius, aortic aneurysm), adenopathy, duplication cyst
- Neuromuscular: achalasia, spasm, hypertonic sphincter, scleroderma, CVA, Alzheimer disease, Huntington chorea, Parkinson disease, multiple sclerosis, polymyositis, dermatomyositis, neuromuscular junction disease (myasthenia gravis, Lambert-Eaton syndrome, botulism), hyperthyroidism and hypothyroidism, Guillain-Barré syndrome, SLE, ALL, amyloidosis, diabetic neuropathy, brainstem tumors, Chagas disease
  - Infections: diphtheria, meningitis, tertiary syphilis, Lyme disease, rabies, poliomyelitis, CMV, esophagitis (*Candida*, herpetic)

RISK FACTORS
- Children: hereditary and/or congenital malformations
- Adults: age >50 years; elderly: GERD, stroke, COPD, chronic pain
- Medications: quinine, potassium chloride, vitamin C, tetracycline, trimethoprim (Bactrim), clindamycin, NSAIDs, procainamide, anticholinergics, bisphosphates, seizure meds: phenobarbital, carbamazepine, and phenytoin; antihistaminics, TCA's: amitriptyline, imipramine, anti-psychotics: haloperidol, phenothiazine, butyrophenone, thioxanthene; oxybutynin; opiates; rizatriptan; ACE, ARB, calcium channel blockers, β-blockers, α_2-agonist; HCTZ and chlorothiazide; cytotoxic, (antineoplastics; interferon-α, ribavirin); sibutramine; β_2-agonist bronchodilators, muscle relaxants
  - Xerostomia: ACE inhibitors, antiarrhythmics, antiemetics, diuretics, SSRI, sunitinib everolimus
  - Neurologic: CVA, myasthenia gravis, multiple sclerosis, Parkinson disease, ALS, Huntington chorea, dementia; HIV patients with CD4 cell count <100 cells/mm³
- Trauma or irradiation of head, neck, and chest; mechanical lesions; extrinsic mechanical lesions: lung, thyroid tumors, lymphoma, metastasis; iron deficiency
- Smoking, excess alcohol intake, obesity

GENERAL PREVENTION
Liquid and soft food diet as appropriate

COMMONLY ASSOCIATED CONDITIONS
Peptic structure, esophageal webs and rings, carcinoma, history of stroke, dementia, pneumonia

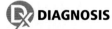

DIAGNOSIS

HISTORY
- Oropharyngeal dysphagia presents as difficulty initiating the swallowing process. Dysphagia for solids that progresses to involve liquids more likely reflects mechanical obstruction.
- Progressive dysphagia is usually caused by cancer or a peptic stricture. Intermittent dysphagia is most often related to a lower esophageal ring.
- Inquire about heartburn, weight loss, hematemesis, coffee ground emesis, anemia, regurgitation of undigested food particles, and respiratory symptoms.
- Inquire about regurgitation, aspiration, or drooling immediately after swallowing as this may represent oropharyngeal dysphagia, smoking, alcohol abuse.

- Does the food bolus feel stuck?
  - Upper sternum or back of throat may represent oropharyngeal dysphagia, whereas sensation over the lower sternum is typical of esophageal dysphagia.
- Is odynophagia (pain) present?
  - Inflammation, achalasia, diffuse esophageal spasm, esophagitis, pharyngitis, pill-induced esophagitis, cancer
  - Globus sensation ("lump in the throat")?
    - Cricopharyngeal or laryngeal disorders
  - History of sour taste in the back of the throat or chronic heartburn suggests GERD.
- Symptoms: Weight loss or chest pain? Double aortic arch, right aortic arch with retroesophageal left subclavian artery, and left ligamentum arteriosum
- Halitosis: Rule out diverticulum and tissue disorder.
- Changes in speech, hoarseness, weak cough, dysphonia? Rule out neuromuscular dysfunction.

PHYSICAL EXAM
- Skin: telangiectasia, sclerodactyly, calcinosis (rule out autoimmune disease); Raynaud phenomenon, sclerodactyly may be found in CREST syndrome or systemic scleroderma; stigmata of alcohol abuse (palmar erythema; telangiectasia)
- Head, eye, ear, nose, throat (HEENT):
  - Oropharyngeal: pharyngeal erythema/edema, tonsillitis, pharyngeal ulcers or thrush, odynophagia (bacterial, viral, fungal infections); tongue fasciculations (ALS)
  - Neck: masses, lymphadenopathy, neck tenderness (thyroiditis), goiter
- Neurologic:
  - Cranial nerve exam: sensory: cranial nerves V, IX, and X; motor: cranial nerves V, VII, X, XI, and XII
  - CNS, mental status exam, strength testing, Horner syndrome, ataxia, cogwheel rigidity

DIFFERENTIAL DIAGNOSIS
The first step is to distinguish between oropharyngeal and esophageal pathology.

DIAGNOSTIC TESTS & INTERPRETATION

There is a low threshold of referral for patients with oropharyngeal symptoms for EGD to rule out esophageal pathology (1)[C].

- EGD is recommended for the initial assessment of patient with esophageal dysphagia; barium esophagography is recommended as an adjunct if EGD findings are negative (1)[C].
- For accurate diagnosis of eosinophilic esophagitis, biopsies from normal-appearing mucosa in the midthoracic and distal esophagus should be requested for all patients with unexplained solid food dysphagia (1)[B].
- Older patients with chronic illness or recent pneumonia should be screened for dysphagia; if it is present, the physician and patient should discuss goals of care (1)[C]. The diagnosis of eosinophilic esophagitis is established by upper endoscopy and esophageal biopsy, with an increase of eosinophils >15 per high-power field. Biopsies from normal-appearing mucosa in the midthoracic and distal esophagus should be requested (1),(2)[A].

Initial Tests (lab, imaging)
- CBC (infection and inflammation).
- Antiacetylcholine antibodies (myasthenia)
- TSH, free T_4 cobalamin levels, LFT

Diagnostic Procedures/Other
- Video fluoroscopic swallowing as initial assessment for detection of aspiration (1)[A]
- Patients with persistent oropharyngeal symptoms and a negative initial workup should be referred for EGD to rule out esophageal pathology.

 TREATMENT

GENERAL MEASURES
- Exclude cardiac disease.
- Ensure airway patency and adequate pulmonary function.
- Assess nutritional status; speech therapy

MEDICATION
Modify medications taken by patient according to patient functional swallowing ability.

First Line
Patients with GERD symptoms, esophagitis, or peptic stricture should undergo acid suppression therapy with standard doses of proton pump inhibitors for 8 to 12 weeks (1)[A].

- Older patients with chronic illness or recent pneumonia should be screened for dysphagia; if it is present, the physician and patient should discuss goals of care (1)[C].

ISSUES FOR REFERRAL
Swallow and speech, nutritional evaluation

ADDITIONAL THERAPIES
Self-expanded metal stent is safe, effective, and quicker in palliation.

SURGERY/OTHER PROCEDURES
- Esophageal dilatation (pneumatic or bougie) for achalasia; esophageal stent; laser for cancer palliation
- Need for enteral feeding; hospitalization with total or near-total obstruction of esophageal lumen

 ONGOING CARE

Swallow therapy may reduce the incidence of chest infections or pneumonia after stroke.

FOLLOW-UP RECOMMENDATIONS
In patients with progressive conditions, the goal is to maintain current state.

Patient Monitoring
Medications should be reviewed.

DIET
See "General Prevention."

PATIENT EDUCATION
- Drink using small sips of liquids, without any gulping.
- Sit upright at 90 degrees and avoid drinking or eating when lying down or slouched.
- Eat slowly, small bites of food, chew food completely before swallowing

PROGNOSIS
- 45% reported mortality within 12 months in nursing home residents with oropharyngeal dysphagia and aspiration.
- Swallowing treatment reduced the incidence of pneumonia, no difference in swallow quality of life scores

COMPLICATIONS
Oropharyngeal: pneumonia, lung abscess, aspiration pneumonia, airway obstruction; malnutrition and dehydration

REFERENCES

1. Wilkinson JM, Codipilly DC, Wilfahrt R. Dysphagia: evaluation and collaborative management. *Am Fam Physician*. 2021;103(2):97–106.
2. Malagelada JR, Bazzoli F, Boeckxstaens G, et al. World gastroenterology organisation global guidelines: dysphagia—global guidelines and cascades update September 2014. *J Clin Gastroenterol*. 2015;49(5):370–378.

ADDITIONAL READING

Choosing Wisely Campaign: https://www.choosingwisely.org

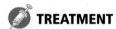 CODES

ICD10
- R13.10 Dysphagia, unspecified
- R13.12 Dysphagia, oropharyngeal phase
- R13.14 Dysphagia, pharyngoesophageal phase

CLINICAL PEARLS

Dysphagia warrants prompt evaluation to define the cause and appropriate treatment.

ECTOPIC PREGNANCY

Kristina Gracey, MD, MPH • Nicole D. Somes, MD • Jeremy Golding, MD, FAAFP

BASICS

DESCRIPTION
Ectopic: pregnancy implanted outside the uterine cavity; subtypes include:
- Tubal—pregnancy implanted in the fallopian tube
- Abdominal—pregnancy implanted intra-abdominally, usually after tubal abortion or rupture of tubal ectopic pregnancy
- Heterotopic pregnancy—implanted intrauterine pregnancy (IUP) AND a separate pregnancy implanted outside the uterine cavity
- Ovarian—implantation of pregnancy in ovarian tissue
- Cervical—implantation of pregnancy in cervix
- Intraligamentary—implantation of pregnancy within the broad ligament

EPIDEMIOLOGY
Incidence
- Incidence is around 2 per 100 pregnancies in the United States (1). About 1 in 10 first-trimester pregnancies presenting to the emergency department with pain and/or bleeding are due to ectopic pregnancy. In the United States, ectopic pregnancy is the leading cause of first-trimester maternal deaths.
- Heterotopic pregnancy, although rare (1:30,000), occurs with greater frequency (1/1,000) in women undergoing in vitro fertilization (IVF); increasing incidence of nontubal, and particularly cesarean scar ectopic pregnancies, due in part to more cesarean sections and more IVF
- ~33% recurrence rate if prior ectopic pregnancy

ETIOLOGY AND PATHOPHYSIOLOGY
95–97% of ectopic pregnancies occur in the fallopian tube: 55–80% in the ampulla, 12–25% in the isthmus, and 5–17% in the fimbria. One cause of tubal pregnancy is impaired movement of the fertilized ovum to the uterine cavity due to dysfunction of the tubal cilia, scarring, or narrowing of the tubal lumen.

RISK FACTORS
- History of pelvic inflammatory disease (PID), endometritis, or current gonorrhea/chlamydia infection, pelvic adhesive disease (infection or prior surgery)
- Previous ectopic pregnancy, history of tubal surgery (~33% of pregnancies after tubal ligation are ectopic.)
- Use of an intrauterine device (IUD): IUD reduces absolute risk (and therefore number) of ectopic pregnancies, but in a patient with an IUD in place presenting with a pregnancy, there is an increased likelihood that the pregnancy is ectopic, compared with a patient without an IUD.
- Use of assisted reproductive technologies
- Tobacco use; patients with disorders that affect ciliary motility may be at increased risk (e.g., endometriosis, Kartagener syndrome).

GENERAL PREVENTION
Reliable contraception (especially long-acting reversible contraception [LARC] methods)

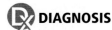**DIAGNOSIS**

HISTORY
In >50% of presenting cases, patients have sudden-onset abdominal pain coupled with cessation of/or irregular menses and acute vaginal bleeding (the classic triad). Other common symptoms include nausea and/or vomiting, vaginal bleeding, and pain referred to the shoulder (from hemoperitoneum).

PHYSICAL EXAM
- Abdominal tenderness ± rebound tenderness associated with vaginal bleeding
- Palpable mass on pelvic exam (adnexal or cul-de-sac fullness), cervical motion tenderness
- In cases of rupture and significant intraperitoneal bleeding, signs of shock such as pallor, tachycardia, and hypotension may be present.

DIFFERENTIAL DIAGNOSIS
Missed, threatened, inevitable, or completed abortion (miscarriage), gestational trophoblastic neoplasia ("molar pregnancy"); appendicitis; salpingitis; PID; ruptured corpus luteum or hemorrhagic cyst; ovarian tumor, benign or malignant; ovarian torsion; cervical polyp; cancer; trauma; or cervicitis

DIAGNOSTIC TESTS & INTERPRETATION
Initial Tests (lab, imaging)
- CBC and ABO type and antibody screen
- Transvaginal US (TVUS) is the gold standard for diagnosis:
  – Failure to visualize a normal intrauterine gestational sac when serum human chorionic gonadotropin (hCG) is above the discriminatory level (>1,500 to 2,000 IU/L) suggests (but is not definitively diagnostic of) an abnormal pregnancy. TVUS is often inconclusive, and the pregnancy is then called "pregnancy of unknown location" (PUL).
  – An hCG level of 3,500 IU/L is associated with a 99% probability of detecting a normal intrauterine gestational sac in clinical practice.
  – These values are not validated for multiple gestations.
- If TVUS unavailable or inconclusive for IUP, check hCG (1)[C]: Serial quantitative serum levels normally increase by 35–53% every 48 hours. Higher initial HCG levels increase less than lower initial levels (1). Abnormal rise (<35%) should prompt workup for gestational abnormalities. Clinical impression of acute abdomen/intraperitoneal bleeding concurrent with a positive hCG level is indicative of ectopic pregnancy until proven otherwise.
- MRI may also be useful but costly and rarely used if TVUS is available; benefits particularly for abdominal or cesarean scar pregnancy

Follow-Up Tests & Special Considerations
Serum progesterone level: >20 mg/mL associated with lower risk of ectopic pregnancy, but levels are generally not helpful (1).

Diagnostic Procedures/Other
In the setting of an undesired pregnancy, uterine aspiration or D&C can identify the presence/absence of intrauterine chorionic villi. When an IUP has been evacuated, hCG levels should drop by 50% within 48 hours. Historically, culdocentesis was performed to confirm suspected hemoperitoneum prior to surgical management. Currently, TVUS quantification of pelvic fluid is sufficient.

Test Interpretation
Products of conception (POC; especially chorionic villi) outside the uterine cavity

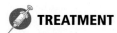**TREATMENT**

MEDICATION
- Methotrexate (MTX): treatment for unruptured tubal pregnancy or for remaining POCs after laparoscopic salpingostomy; methotrexate inhibits DNA synthesis via folic acid antagonism by inactivating dihydrofolate reductase. If TVUS is suggestive but not diagnostic, in the hemodynamically stable, patient who qualifies for medical management, confirm suspected US findings with 2 hCG levels drawn 48 hours apart. Rise <35% is consistent with non-viable pregnancy. MTX is most effective when pregnancy is <3 cm diameter, hCG <5,000 mIU/mL, and no fetal heart activity is seen. Success rate is 88% if hCG <1,000 mIU/mL, 71% if hCG 1,000 to 2,000 mIU/mL, 38% if 2,000 to 5,000 mIU/mL. All regimens require following quant HCG to 0.
  – Three main dosage regimens exist (1) and require a reliable, hemodynamically stable patient. The single-dose regimen is preferred for simplicity, safety, and comparable effectiveness to multidose regimens (2)[A]:
    ○ Single: IM methotrexate 50 mg/m² of body surface area (BSA); may repeat once if <15% decline in hCG between days 4 and 7; follow hCG weekly.
    ○ Two dose: methotrexate 50 mg/m² of BSA once and then repeated on day 4; if <15% decline in hCG between days 4 and 7, may repeat third dose on day 7. Repeat hCG as needed on days 11 and 14 until decreases >15% in the interval and then weekly. If not dropping by day 14, refer for surgical management; may be somewhat more effective for higher initial HCG levels than in the single dose regimen
    ○ Multidose: methotrexate 1 mg/kg IM/IV every other day, with leucovorin 0.1 mg/kg IM rescue in between; maximum of 4 doses until hCG drop below 15%; course may be repeated 7 days after last dose if necessary
  – Contraindications: hemodynamic instability or any evidence of rupture, moderate to severe anemia, severe hepatic or renal dysfunction, immunodeficiency
  – Relative contraindications: fetal heart activity seen, large gestational sac (>3 to 4 cm, less effective), noncompliance or limited access to hospital or transportation, hCG >5,000 mIU/mL

- Precautions: immunologic, hematologic, renal, GI, hepatic, and pulmonary disease, or interacting medications
- Pretreatment testing: serum hCG, CBC, liver and renal function tests, blood type and screen
- Patient counseling: During therapy, refrain from use of alcohol, aspirin, NSAIDs, and folate supplements (decreases efficacy of methotrexate); avoid excessive sun exposure due to risk of sensitivity. Adherence to scheduled follow-up appointments is critical. Increased abdominal pain may occur during treatment; however, severe pain, nausea, vomiting, bleeding, dizziness, or light-headedness may indicate treatment failure and require urgent evaluation.
- Rupture of ectopic pregnancy during methotrexate treatment ranges from 7% to 14%.
- Side effects include stomatitis; conjunctivitis; abdominal cramping; and rarely neutropenia, pneumonitis, or alopecia (2).
- Systemic methotrexate may be offered in some kinds of nontubal ectopic pregnancies, but data is limited.

ISSUES FOR REFERRAL
Consider gynecologic consultation if not experienced in medical management, and for surgical care.

ADDITIONAL THERAPIES
- Physician or patient may elect for surgical treatment as primary method and then postop hCG should guide need for supplemental methotrexate.
- After evidence of medical failure or tubal rupture, surgery is necessary.
- Treatment of cervical, ovarian, abdominal, or other ectopic pregnancy is complicated and requires immediate specialist referral.
- Offer anti-D Rh prophylaxis at a dose of 50 μg to all Rh-negative women who have a surgical procedure to manage an ectopic pregnancy or if there has been significant bleeding or abdominal pain.
- Expectant management of ectopic (confirmed on TVUS) may be offered to women who are clinically stable and have low and decreasing hCG level initially <1,500 mIU/mL (3)[B].
- Expectant management to allow for spontaneous resolution of PUL is acceptable in asymptomatic patients with no evidence of rupture or hemodynamic instability coupled with an appropriately low hCG and no extrauterine mass suggestive of ectopic. Ruptured tubal pregnancies may occur even with extremely low hCG levels (<100 mIU/mL).
- With expectant management of PUL, repeat TVUS weekly (or when hCG above discriminatory zone) until location is confirmed or clinical picture is unstable.

SURGERY/OTHER PROCEDURES
- Indications include ruptured ectopic pregnancy, inability to comply with medical follow-up, previous tubal ligation, known tubal disease, current heterotopic pregnancy, and desire for permanent sterilization at time of diagnosis.
- Laparoscopy is the first-line surgical management (3)[C].

- Salpingectomy (tubal removal) is preferred and is indicated for uncontrolled bleeding, recurrent ectopic pregnancy, severely damaged tube, large gestational sac, or patient's desire for sterilization (3)[C]. Salpingostomy (preservation of tube) is considered in patients who wish to maintain fertility particularly if contralateral tube is damaged/absent (3)[C]. No difference in recurrence rate compared to salpingectomy. Persistent trophoblastic tissue with salpingostomy remains in the fallopian tube in 4–15% of cases; will need to follow weekly hCG
- Surgical treatment is first line for cesarean and cornual pregnancies.

ADMISSION, INPATIENT, AND NURSING CONSIDERATIONS
- Fails criteria for methotrexate management, suspicion of rupture, orthostatic, shock, and severe abdominal pain requiring IV narcotics
- Inpatient observation in the setting of an uncertain diagnosis, particularly with an unreliable patient, may be appropriate.
- Surgical emergency: Two large-bore IV access lines should be placed immediately if suspicion of rupture; aggressive resuscitation as needed; blood product transfusion if necessary en route to OR; in cases of shock, pressors and cardiac support may be necessary.
- IV fluids are unnecessary for a stable ectopic pregnancy being medically treated but are critical for a surgical patient who is bleeding.
- Strict input/output, hourly vitals, orthostatics if mobile, frequent abdominal exams, serial hematocrit, pad counts if heavy vaginal bleeding
- Discharge criteria: afebrile, abdominal pain resolving or resolved, diagnosis established, surgical treatment, and recovery is complete

ONGOING CARE

FOLLOW-UP RECOMMENDATIONS
Patient Monitoring
- Serial serum quantitative hCG until level drops to zero: After methotrexate administration, a strict monitoring protocol should be followed. Following salpingostomy, weekly levels are appropriate. Following salpingectomy, further follow-up may be unnecessary.
- Pelvic US for persistent or recurrent masses
- Pain control: brief course of narcotics usually necessary with medical or surgical management
- Liver and renal function tests weekly following methotrexate administration if repeat dosing is required
- Delay of subsequent pregnancy for at least 3 months after treatment with methotrexate due to teratogenicity (3)[C]

DIET
During treatment, avoid alcohol and foods and vitamins high in folate (leafy greens, liver, edamame) due to interaction with methotrexate efficacy.

PATIENT EDUCATION
- Signs and symptoms of ectopic pregnancy should be reviewed.
- Patients should be encouraged to plan subsequent pregnancies and seek early medical care on discovery of future pregnancies.

PROGNOSIS
- Chronic ectopic pregnancies are rare and treated with surgical removal of the fallopian tube.
- Future fertility depends on fertility prior to ectopic pregnancy and degree of tubal compromise. In women with normal fertility, treatment options make no differences in future fertility rates. In women with subfertility, expectant or medical treatments confer better future fertility (3)[C].
- ~66% of women with a history of ectopic pregnancy will have a future IUP if they are able to conceive.
- If infertility persists >12, the fallopian tubes should be evaluated.

COMPLICATIONS
Hemorrhage and hypovolemic shock, persistent trophoblastic tissue after medical or surgical management, infection, infertility, blood transfusions with associated infections/transfusion reaction, disseminated intravascular coagulation in the setting of massive hemorrhage

REFERENCES
1. Tonick S, Conageski C. Ectopic pregnancy. *Obstet Gynecol Clin North Am*. 2022;49(3):537–549.
2. Yuk JS, Lee JH, Park WI, et al. Systematic review and meta-analysis of single-dose and non-single-dose methotrexate protocols in the treatment of ectopic pregnancy. *Int J Gynaecol Obstet*. 2018;141(3):295–303.
3. Diagnosis and management of ectopic pregnancy: Green-top Guideline No. 21. *BJOG*. 2016;123(13):e15–e55.

ADDITIONAL READING
Hajenius PJ, Mol F, Mol BWJ, et al. Interventions for tubal ectopic pregnancy. *Cochrane Database Syst Rev*. 2007;2007(1):CD000324.

CODES

ICD10
- O00.9 Ectopic pregnancy, unspecified
- O00.1 Tubal pregnancy
- O00.0 Abdominal pregnancy

CLINICAL PEARLS
- 97% of ectopic pregnancies occur in the fallopian tube.
- Diagnosis requires high clinical suspicion in the setting of abdominal pain and a positive pregnancy test until IUP is confirmed.

EJACULATORY DISORDERS

Payam Sazegar, MD

BASICS

DESCRIPTION

- Group of dysfunctions involving altered time and control (premature ejaculation [PE], delayed ejaculation [DE]), presence (anejaculation [AE]), direction (retrograde ejaculation [RE]), volume (perceived ejaculate volume reduction [PEVR]), or force (decreased force of ejaculation [DFE]) of ejaculation
- PE is defined as a persistent/recurrent pattern of ejaculation occurring during partnered sexual activity within 1 minute following vaginal penetration and before the individual wishes it + present for 6 months + causing significant distress for individual.
  - Natural biologic response is to ejaculate within 2 to 5 minutes after vaginal penetration.
  - Ejaculatory control is an acquired behavior that increases with experience.
  - Comorbidities common (diabetes, hypertension, sexual desire disorder, erectile dysfunction [ED])
- DE: prolonged time to ejaculate (>30 minutes) despite desire, stimulation, and erection
- Aspermia (lack of sperm in the ejaculate):
  - AE: lack of emission or contractions of bulbospongiosus muscle
  - RE: partial or complete ejaculation of semen into the bladder
  - Obstruction: ejaculatory duct obstruction or urethral obstruction
- Also:
  - Painful ejaculation: genital or perineal pain during or after ejaculation
  - Ejaculatory anhedonia: normal ejaculation lacking orgasm or pleasure
  - Hematospermia: presence of blood in the ejaculate (often not a serious condition)

EPIDEMIOLOGY

Prevalence

- PE is common; reported prevalence in U.S. males is 5 to 20%.
- DE is reported in 5–8% of men aged 18 to 59 years, but <3% have the problem for >6 months.
- Predominant age: all sexually mature age groups

ETIOLOGY AND PATHOPHYSIOLOGY

Male sexual response:

- Erection mediated by parasympathetic nervous system
- Normal ejaculation consists of three phases:
  - Emission phase: Semen is deposited into urethra by contraction of prostate, seminal vesicles, vas deferens; under autonomic sympathetic control
  - Ejaculation phase: semen forcibly propelled out of urethra by rhythmic contractions of the bulbospongiosus and ischiocavernosus muscles. This is mediated by the somatic nervous system on the motor branches of the pudendal nerve. Bladder neck contracture by α-adrenergic receptors ensures anterograde ejaculation.
  - Orgasm: the pleasurable sensation associated with ejaculation (cerebral cortex); smooth muscle contraction of accessory sexual organs; release of pressure in posterior urethra

- PE:
  - Hypersensitivity/hyperexcitability of glans penis
  - 5-hydroxytryptamine (5-HT) receptor sensitivity
  - Psychogenic (inexperience, anxiety/guilt, low frequency of sex, relationship problems)
  - Urologic (ED, prostatitis, urethritis)
  - Endocrine (hyperthyroid, obesity, diabetes)
  - Lack of physical or sexual activity
  - Withdrawal or detox from prescription or illicit drugs (e.g., opioids)
- DE:
  - Rarely due to underlying painful disorder (e.g., prostatitis, seminal vesiculitis)
  - Often has a psychogenic component
  - Sometimes associated with low testosterone levels
  - Sexual performance anxiety and other psychosocial factors
  - Drugs or medications may impair ejaculation (e.g., MAOIs, SSRIs, α- and β-blockers, thiazides, antipsychotics, tricyclic antidepressants, NSAIDs, opiates, alcohol, cannabis).
- AE:
  - Never has ejaculate: congenital structural disorder (müllerian duct cyst, Wolffian abnormality)
  - Acquired causes: surgery (radical prostatectomy, retroperitoneal lymph node [LN] dissection), spinal cord injury or other sympathetic nerve injury (especially T10–T12 level), diabetes mellitus with neuropathy, and medications (α- and β-blockers, benzodiazepines, SSRIs, MAOIs, TCAs, antipsychotics, aminocaproic acid)
- RE:
  - Transurethral resection of the prostate (25%) or other prostate resection procedures
  - Surgery on the neck of the bladder
  - Extensive pelvic surgery
  - Retroperitoneal LN dissection for testicular cancer (also may produce failure of emission)
  - Neurologic disorders (multiple sclerosis [MS], DM)
  - Medications (tamsulosin, other α-blockers, SSRIs, antipsychotics)
  - Urethral stricture (may be posttraumatic)
- Painful ejaculation:
  - Infection or inflammation (orchitis, epididymitis, prostatitis, urethritis)
  - Ejaculatory duct obstruction
  - Seminal vesicle calculi
  - Obstruction of the vas deferens
  - Psychological/functional
- Hematospermia (often unable to find cause):
  - Usually not a serious condition
  - Inflammation/infection
  - Calculi: bladder, seminal vesicle, prostate, urethra
  - Trauma to genital area (cycling, constipation, masturbation)
  - Obstruction
  - Cyst
  - Tumor (1–3% prostate cancers present with hematospermia)
  - Arteriovenous malformations
  - Iatrogenic
  - Hypertension

RISK FACTORS

ED: pudendal neuralgia; substance use; psychological distress or relationship issue.

GENERAL PREVENTION

Screen for sexual transmitted infections (STIs).

COMMONLY ASSOCIATED CONDITIONS

- Neurologic disorders (e.g., MS)
- Diabetes
- Prostatitis
- Ejaculatory duct obstruction
- Urethral stricture
- Psychological disorders
- Endocrinopathies
- Relationship/interpersonal difficulties

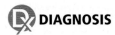

DIAGNOSIS

HISTORY

Detailed sexual history, including:

- Time frame of the problem
- Quality of patient's sexual response
- Sense of ejaculatory control and sexual distress
- Overall assessment of the relationship
- Detailed history of recent and current medications
- History of past trauma or recent infections
- Past surgical history with particular attention to genitourinary (GU) surgeries
- Supplements and alternative therapies tried
- Many men do not distinguish initially between problems related to erection and ejaculation.
- Include the sexual partner in the interview, especially if the patient expresses a belief that he is not meeting his partner's needs.
- In review of systems, elicit any evidence of testosterone deficiency or prolactin excess, especially if anhedonia present.

PHYSICAL EXAM

- Check vitals. Look for focal neurologic signs (MS, spinal cord injury) and psychiatric disorders.
- Thorough GU exam, including:
  - Size and texture of testes and epididymis
  - Verification of the presence of the vas deferens
  - Location and patency of urethral meatus
  - Digital rectal examination to evaluate prostate consistency, size, and possible midline lesions

DIAGNOSTIC TESTS & INTERPRETATION

- Fasting glucose or HbA1c to rule out diabetes
- Postorgasmic urinalysis will confirm RE. Semen fructose level, sperm count, and viscosity can be measured.
- AE will have fructose negative, sperm negative, and nonviscous postorgasmic urinalysis.
- In painful ejaculation, urinalysis and urine culture needed to rule out infection
- If prostate cancer is considered, check prostate-specific antigen (PSA).
- In anhedonia, consider checking testosterone, prolactin, glucose, TSH.
- In hematospermia, painful ejaculation, or if ejaculatory duct obstruction is considered, transrectal ultrasound (TRUS)
- TRUS-guided seminal vesicle aspiration if ejaculatory duct obstruction is present
- If suspicious of anatomic abnormality, can get scrotal US and/or MRI

Initial Tests (lab, imaging)

Consider CBC, HbA1c, PSA, TSH, testosterone, urine studies. Often, no workup is needed for PE. For hematospermia, check CBC, coagulation tests, urine culture, chem panel, STI screening, semen analysis, STI screening, condom test.

Follow-Up Tests & Special Considerations

Scrotal US or MRI or TRUS. Most patients do not require these tests.

 TREATMENT

GENERAL MEASURES

- Identifying any medical cause (even if not reversible) helps patient accept condition.
- Improve partner communication.
- Psychological counseling for patient and partner
- Reduce performance pressure through reassurance.
- PE:
  - Use sensate focus therapy (gradual progression of nonsexual contact to sexual contact).
  - Quiet vagina: Female partner stops moving just prior to ejaculation.
  - Techniques to learn ejaculatory control (e.g., coronal squeeze technique [squeezing the glans penis until ejaculatory urge ceases] or start-and-stop technique [cessation of penile stimulation when ejaculation approaches and resumption of stimulation when ejaculatory feeling ends])
- DE:
  - Change to antidepressant less likely to cause DE (citalopram, fluvoxamine, nefazodone) (1)[C]
- AE/RE:
  - Discontinue offending medications.
  - Improve diabetic control.
  - If urethral obstruction present, refer to urology.
  - RE may be helped if intercourse occurs when bladder is full.
  - Consider penile vibratory stimulation (effective in spinal cord injuries >T10) or electroejaculation (place on monitor if lesions above T6 because autonomic dysreflexia may result) to collect sperm in AE cases.
- Painful ejaculation:
  - Rule out infection. Counseling may be beneficial.
  - If seminal vesicle stones are possible, refer to urology.
- Hematospermia:
  - Often benign and resolves spontaneously, without known cause. Reassure initially.
  - May try empiric antibiotic, but little evidence to support
  - If persistent or high degree of suspicion for abnormality, refer to urologist.

MEDICATION

- PE:
  - Treat underlying ED (a common comorbidity) with PDE5 inhibitors
  - First line:
    - Antidepressants "on demand": clomipramine 20 to 50 mg 4 to 24 hours before intercourse, sertraline 50 mg 4 to 8 hours before intercourse, and paroxetine 20 mg 3 to 4 hours before intercourse (1)[A].
    - Daily dosing of clomipramine 20 to 50 mg, sertraline 25 to 200 mg, fluoxetine 5 to 20 mg, or paroxetine 10 to 40 mg can delay ejaculation within 1 to 3 weeks of starting (1)[A].
    - PDE5 inhibitor with or without SSRI.
  - Second Line:
    - Topical anesthetic gel (e.g., 2.5% prilocaine ± 2.5% lidocaine [EMLA]) 2.5 g applied under a condom for 30 minutes prior to intercourse (2)[B]
    - Tramadol 5 to 50 mg used "on demand" 2 hours before sex; also available in spray form (2)[B]
    - Modafinil, behavioral/sex therapy, pelvic floor muscle therapy (1),(3)[B]
- DE:
  - No FDA-approved pharmacotherapy
  - Patients who must continue SSRIs may respond to bupropion and buspirone (2)[C].
  - Sex therapy, self-stimulation therapies (2)[C]
  - Consider oxytocin, pseudoephedrine, and midodrine (1),(2)[C].
- AE and RE:
  - First line: sympathomimetics (pseudoephedrine 60 mg PO daily to QID) or anticholinergics (imipramine 25 to 75 mg PO BID) that enhance bladder outlet resistance (2)[B].
  - Second line: for RE, can try postejaculation bladder harvest of sperm (if fertility desired); for AE, can try midodrine, penile vibratory stimulation, or electroejaculation
  - α-Agonists and antihistamines can be helpful but are not approved by the FDA.
- Painful ejaculation:
  - Treat underlying infection/inflammatory process.
  - No specific pharmacotherapy (2)[C]

ISSUES FOR REFERRAL

Refer to a urologist:

- Ejaculatory duct obstruction
- Seminal vesicle or prostatic stones
- Urethral obstruction
- Vas deferens obstruction
- Calculi
- Persistent or severe hematospermia

SURGERY/OTHER PROCEDURES

Transurethral resection of the ejaculatory ducts (if duct obstruction present)

COMPLEMENTARY & ALTERNATIVE MEDICINE

Daily caffeine consumption and folic acid supplementation may be beneficial.

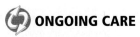 **ONGOING CARE**

PATIENT EDUCATION

See "General Measures."

PROGNOSIS

PE often improves with therapy and counseling.

COMPLICATIONS

Psychological impact on some males: signs of severe inadequacy, self-doubt, additional anxiety, and guilt

REFERENCES

1. Shindel AW, Althof SE, Carrier S, et al. Disorders of ejaculation: an AUA/SMSNA guideline. *J Urol*. 2022;207(3):504–512.
2. Chen T, Mulloy EA, Eisenberg ML. Medical treatment of disorders of ejaculation. *Urol Clin North Am*. 2022;49(2):219–230.
3. Haghighi M, Jahangard L, Meybodi AM, et al. Influence of modafinil on early ejaculation—Results from a double-blind randomized clinical trial. *J Psychiatr Res*. 2022;146:264–271.

 SEE ALSO

Erectile Dysfunction

 CODES

ICD10

- F52.4 Premature ejaculation
- N53.11 Retarded ejaculation
- N53.14 Retrograde ejaculation

CLINICAL PEARLS

- If ED is contributing to ejaculatory difficulty, management of ED should precede attempted management of ejaculatory disorders.
- Medications should always be thoroughly reviewed because they may be the primary cause of ejaculatory disorders.
- PE and DE generally have both psychogenic and physical causes, whereas AE and RE are due to organic neurogenic/autonomic dysfunction.
- A multidisciplinary approach, including the primary care physician, urologists, psychologists, and other appropriate health care professionals, is essential to the proper treatment of ejaculatory disorders.

E

ELDER ABUSE

Thomas Triantafillou, MD • Vivian Nnenna Chukwuma, MD

BASICS

DESCRIPTION
Elder abuse (EA) is a public health concern (autonomy, wellbeing). Defined as: (i) intentional actions that cause harm or create a serious risk of harm to a vulnerable elder (financial, physical, emotional, impaired capacity for self-care or self-protection risk) by a caregiver or other person who stands in a trust relationship, or (ii) failure by a caregiver to satisfy the elder's basic needs or to protect the elder from harm (National Academy of Sciences, 2003). In 2009, the estimated cost was approximately $2.9 billion, a 12% increase from the preceding year (National Committee for the Prevention of Elder Abuse).

EPIDEMIOLOGY
Incidence
The global incidence of EA is around 16% (World Health Organization [WHO]). In the United States, it is estimated that 10% of the population are victims of EA and as many as 5 million elders are affected each year.

Prevalence
EA in both the community and in institutions has increased during the COVID-19 pandemic (WHO). The estimated annual prevalence per 1,000 people of key forms of violence is: 22 for physical and sexual abuse, 17 for intimate partner violence, fatal suicide 0.17, nonfatal self-harm 0.27, and 9.7 to 32.6 for violence by older adults with dementia against others (1).

ETIOLOGY AND PATHOPHYSIOLOGY
The etiology of EA involves biopsychosocial factors in combination with increased dependence on the care-giver by the victim in a suboptimal environment with poor behavioral coping methods, further compounded by increased stress.

RISK FACTORS
The victim: advanced age; female gender; low socio-economic status; exploitable resources; social isolation; lack of purpose; PTSD in veterans; poor self-perceived health; loss of sense of control; health care insecurity; prior history of abuse in life; functional dependence; cognitive impairment; mental illness or substance use; polyvictimization (victim's perception of EA, protecting the offender, perpetrator influence on the victim). The abuser: early child abuse; history of violence; mental illness or substance use; high stress or poor coping; poor physical or cognitive health; inadequate training or supervision; poor prior relationship between the care-giver and the victim; financial dependency on the victim.

GENERAL PREVENTION
Complete annual wellness visits to discuss advanced care plan, power of attorney for health or finances, goals of care (GOC), degree of self-sufficiency, the role of the caregiver, the risk of caregiver burnout. Assess caregiver stress and burden (meet without patient). Screen for risk or presence of mood disorders (depression: PHQ-2 or PHQ-9; anxiety: General Anxiety Disorder-7 (GAD-7); loneliness: 3-item UCLA) or cognitive impairment (Folstein Mini-Mental State Examination [MMSE], Montreal Cognitive Assessment [MoCA], Saint Louis University Mental Status [SLUMS]). Encourage socialization. Refer to community programs: Department of Aging, Adult Protective Services (APS), Alzheimer's Association.

COMMONLY ASSOCIATED CONDITIONS
Conditions commonly associated with EA can be risk factors. They include social isolation, increased dependence for activities of daily living/instrumental activities of daily living (ADLs/IADLs), depression, cognitive impairment, and aggressive behavior.

DIAGNOSIS
There is no golden standard for EA screen. The U.S. Preventive Services Task Force has not recommended screening for EA. However, when there is a high clinical suspicion, EA should be considered. Types of EA: physical or sexual, violation of personal rights, material exploitation, neglect (includes abandonment), financial, and psychological. The context can vary from self-neglect, institutional (nursing home, assisted living), or domestic (home). Most commonly, the abuser in a domestic environment is a family member. Screening tools (2),(3): (i) hospital: Elderly Indicators of Abuse (E-IOA); (ii) emergency department: Elder Abuse Instrument (EAI), ED Senior Abuse Identification (AID); (iii) nursing home: Elder Psychological Abuse Scale (EPAS); and (iv) general: Elder Abuse Suspicion Index (EASI); Hwalek-Sengstock Elder Abuse Screening Test (H-S/EAST); Vulnerability Abuse Screening Scale (VASS); Lichtenberg Financial Decision Screening Scale (LFDSS)

HISTORY
Use a culture-sensitive history with a focus on prior or current advance care plan. Do a review of living arrangements, degree of physical or cognitive function, who the caregivers are, and if there is evidence of caregiver burnout.

PHYSICAL EXAM
- It is important to document positive and negative findings in your physical exam and to be detailed because they can be admissible in court. Assess for unexplained fractures.
- General overall appearance: cachexia; hygiene and clothing; if bedbound, record integrity of mattress and sheets; evidence of falls, including broken eyeglasses
- Oral exam: dentition, oral ulcers
- Skin exam: large bruises (>5 cm) located at the face, lateral arm, back, or inner thighs
  - Patterned injury suggesting inappropriate restraint such as bite marks, ligature marks around wrists, ankles, or neck
  - Burn marks in patterns inconsistent with unin-tentional injury e.g., stocking and glove pattern suggesting forced immersion
  - Open wounds, cuts, punctures, untreated injuries in various stages of healing, traumatic alopecia, or scalp swelling
  - Check for pressure ulcers on the bony promi-nences of the patient.

DIFFERENTIAL DIAGNOSIS
- Dementia (FAST 6 or 7), or dementia in a withdrawn or malnourished patient
- Elderly with Alzheimer, mixed, or lewy body demen-tia (LBD) can present with delusions.

- Psychosis
- Substance use disorders
- Parkinson disease resulting in fractures or bruises
- Coagulopathy with advanced malignancy or other conditions
- Antiplatelet therapy associated with bruising
- Wasting from malignancy, infections, or chronic disease
- Delirium due to electrolyte, trauma, infection, heart disease, urine retention, constipation, end-of-life
- Thyroid disorder associated with altered mental status, delirium, depression, frailty, or anxiety
- Fixed drug reaction, fragile photo-aged skin, steroid purpura, allergic reaction
- Fracture from osteoporosis

DIAGNOSTIC TESTS & INTERPRETATION
Initial Tests (lab, imaging)
CBC, CMP, UA, vitamin B_{12}, folic acid, RPR, TSH, PT/INR (if bruising)

Follow-Up Tests & Special Considerations
- Anemia: iron, TIBC, ferritin
- Change in mental status: vitamin B_1, vitamin B_6; con-sider toxicology; consider encephalopathy panel.
- Trauma: image to assess for new or old fractures. Consider CT head imaging to look for hemorrhage (e.g., subdural).

Diagnostic Procedures/Other
- Use tools to assess for cognitive impairment such as MMSE (proprietary), MoCA (forgetfulness, MCI), SLUMS
- Depression screening tools such as the Geriatric Depression Scale, PHQ2 or PHQ9, and GAD-7
- Documentation
  - Can document "suspected mistreatment" but avoid making definitive diagnosis of EA (or dementia) in your initial assessment, unless it is obvious. Document the abuser's name, relation-ship, and contact information.
  - Pictures need to include the patient's name, medi-cal number, date and time taken, a ruler (used for measurement), name of witnesses that took image. Take pictures of torn clothes.
- Include anatomical diagrams.
- In some states, reporting is only mandated when the patient cannot (i.e., for cognitive or physical reasons) do so. The law protects those who report in "good faith." The identity of the reporter shall not be disclosed except with the written permission of the reporter or by order of a court.

TREATMENT
- Most states require all health care providers to report suspected EA to a local agency such as the APS (https://www.preventfamilyviolence.org/adult-protective-services-numbers) with limited evi-dence on effectiveness of other interventions (4).
- The treatment plan should be centered around action items related but not limited to: the vulner-able older adult, trusted other, or context (Abuse Intervention Model: domain I/II/III) (5).

- Domain I—vulnerable older adult (victim): Consider virtual education interventions (Elder Abuse Training Institute Island; Ejaz et al). Consider a Family-Based Cognitive Behavioral Social Work (FBCBSW) approach to reduce emotional and financial neglect.
  - Impaired physical function: Assess need for assist devices or physical therapy.
  - Impaired cognition: Make recommendations for a healthy diet, activity, and sleep habits customized to the patient's capabilities.
  - Emotional distress or mental illness: Assess presence of depression (PHQ-2 or PHQ-9), anxiety (GAD-7). When appropriate, use medications for mood or mental illness.
- Domain II—trusted others (perpetrator)
  - Dependence on the vulnerable elder: Share with the perpetrator resources to support financial planning to allow mitigation of dependence on the victim.
  - Mood or substance use or pathologic personality traits: Ask the perpetrator to follow with their clinical provider. Report to law enforcement entities if the patient's life is threatened.
- Domain III—context of abuse (circumstances)
  - Social isolation: Provide resources to expand a patient's social network. Can consider a trial of care at assisted living or a nursing home. Work closely with social work (clinic; home health).
  - Low-quality relationship between victim-perpetrator: Seek help from social work or psychologist.
  - Cultural norms: Address taboos related to diagnosis such as dementia in a culture-sensitive manner and customize the plan of care to the patient.

MEDICATION
None

ISSUES FOR REFERRAL
Mood or behavior concern: behavioral health services; cognitive assessment: neurocognitive specialist

ADDITIONAL THERAPIES
Physical and occupational therapy for ambulation, safety assessment, cognition assessment

COMPLEMENTARY & ALTERNATIVE MEDICINE
Relaxation or well-being techniques

ADMISSION, INPATIENT, AND NURSING CONSIDERATIONS
- Victims of abuse should not be transferred or discharged without reliable follow-up, including:
  - A home visit either by PCP or by APN, combined with home health services
  - Report to the state's APS or a designated alternative (e.g., if patient resides in nursing home, then report to that state's regulatory entity, public health department, and Ombudsman). With physical harm, report to local law enforcement.
  - Follow-up with appropriate mental health care
- Manage uncontrolled chronic conditions due to neglect (i.e., wound care from ulcers or infections).
- Hospital security may need to be notified if restricted visitor access to a patient is required.
- Locations for disposition: friend or family member, nursing home, assisted living facility

 ONGOING CARE

FOLLOW-UP RECOMMENDATIONS
- Although evidence is unclear on a change in outcomes from any education intervention, information about responsibilities should be shared with the person responsible for the patient.
- Educate caregivers on signs and effects of caregiver burnout matched with resources for home aid services.
- Review your state requirements on reporting: http://www.napsa-now.org/wp-content/uploads/2014/11/Mandatory-Reporting-Chart-Updated-FINAL.pdf.
- Contact the APS. A helpful resource is http://www.napsa-now.org/get-help/help-in-your-area/.
- Contact the Department of Aging to request an assessment at home including a review of services that can support the patient to be independent in the community.
- ED providers should report to the Long-Term Care Ombudsman.

Patient Monitoring
The patient should have frequent home or clinic visits.

DIET
Mediterranean, or MIND diet

PATIENT EDUCATION
- For EA resources in your state, https://ncea.acl.gov, or call 800-677-1166
- Other useful resources for families
  - Eldercare locator, 800-677-1116, https://eldercare.acl.gov/Public/Index.aspx
  - Alzheimer's Association, 800-272-3900
  - National Organization for Victim Assistance, https://www.trynova.org/

PROGNOSIS
EA and self-neglect are associated with an overall increased risk in mortality.

COMPLICATIONS
Associated outcomes: mortality; hospitalizations; functional health decline; loneliness; depression

REFERENCES
1. Rosen T, Makaroun LK, Conwell Y, et al. Violence in older adults: scope, impact, challenges, and strategies for prevention. *Health Aff (Millwood)*. 2019;38(10):1630–1637.
2. Van Royen K, Van Royen P, De Donder L, et al. Elder abuse assessment tools and interventions for use in the home environment: a scoping review. *Clin Interv Aging*. 2020;15:1793–1807.
3. Ries NM, Mansfield E. Elder abuse: the role of general practitioners in community-based screening and multidisciplinary action. *Aust J Gen Pract*. 2018;47(4):235–238.
4. Baker PRA, Francis DP, Hairi NN, et al. Interventions for preventing abuse in the elderly. *Cochrane Database Syst Rev*. 2016;2016(8):CD010321.
5. Mosqueda L, Burnight K, Gironda MW, et al. The Abuse Intervention Model: a pragmatic approach to intervention for elder mistreatment. *J Am Geriatr Soc*. 2016;64(9):1879–1883.

ADDITIONAL READING
- American Bar Association Commission on Law and Aging. Adult protective services reporting chart (laws current as of December 2019). https://www.americanbar.org/content/dam/aba/administrative/law_aging/2020-elderabuse-reporting-chart.pdf. Published December 2019. Accessed January 3, 2022.
- Cooper C, Katona C, Finne-Soveri H, et al. Indicators of elder abuse: a crossnational comparison of psychiatric morbidity and other determinants in the Ad-HOC study. *Am J Geriatr Psychiatry*. 2006;14(6):489–497.
- Hoover RM, Polson M. Detecting elder abuse and neglect: assessment and intervention. *Am Fam Physician*. 2014;89(6):453–460.

 SEE ALSO

- Tools on EA for clinicians from Weill Cornell Medicine: https://elderabuseemergency.org/ElderWP/
- National Council on Aging: https://www.ncoa.org

 CODES

ICD10
- T74.11XA Adult physical abuse, confirmed, initial encounter
- T74.21XA Adult sexual abuse, confirmed, initial encounter
- T74.01XA Adult neglect or abandonment, confirmed, initial encounter

CLINICAL PEARLS
- To reduce the risk of EA, strengthen the patients' social support, address depression, provide the patient with assistive devices, screen for cognitive impairment with a trial of medication if possible, and identify caregiver burnout.
- Refer to the Department of Aging for services such as home aid when ADLs or IADLs are impaired.
- Patient with capacity: The APS cannot act if a patient has the capacity to make decisions and elects not to report the abuse. Patient with impaired capacity: A medicolegal process along with guidance from the APS can lead to guardianship.

ENCOPRESIS
Parul Chaudhri, DO

BASICS

DESCRIPTION
- Defined by *DSM-5* and Rome IV diagnostic criteria as repetitive and inappropriate passage of feces
- Diagnostic criteria: chronological and developmental age of at least 4 years; repeated passage of stool in inappropriate places—floors, clothes; symptoms mostly involuntary but may be intentional; at least one event per month for 3 months; behavior can't be explained by other medical conditions or use of substances (e.g., laxatives); excludes mechanisms involving constipation
- Categories:
  - With constipation and overflow incontinence (functional constipation or retentive encopresis)—more common
  - Without constipation (nonretentive fecal soiling or nonretentive fecal incontinence)
- Constipation is passing delayed or infrequent hard stools with pain and straining.

EPIDEMIOLOGY
Incidence
There is no clear difference in the incidence of functional constipation between women and men. Constipation in children accounts for 3% of primary care visits and 25% referrals to pediatric gastroenterology. Functional constipation is the cause of 95% of all constipation in children and adolescents with median age of onset ~2.3 years of age and often coinciding with transition to solid foods, toilet training, or start of school.

Prevalence
Occurs in 1–3% of children 4 years of age and 25% of children with functional constipation go on to have adult GI issues.

ETIOLOGY AND PATHOPHYSIOLOGY
- In 90% of cases, encopresis develops as a consequence of chronic constipation, with resulting overflow incontinence (retentive encopresis). The other 10% are caused by specific organic etiologies.
- Constipation causes pain with defecation which causes further stool withholding. Stool withholding increases colonic water absorption, making stools harder and more difficult to pass.
- Withholding behaviors such as hiding, rocking back and forth, or fidgeting when feeling the urge to defecate can be confused with signs of straining to defecate. Many children voluntarily withhold stool for fear of pain or a preoccupation with not interrupting social activities.
- Chronic constipation with irregular and incomplete evacuation results in progressive rectal distension and stretching of the internal/external anal sphincters.
- Chronic rectal distension causes habituation, leading to the loss of sensing the normal urge to defecate causing abdominal pain, nausea, and bloating. Eventually, soft or liquid stool leaks around the retained fecal mass.
- Psychological: stool withholding, fear, anxiety; difficulty with toilet training, including unusual anxiety or conflict with parent; resistance to using public toilet facilities, such as school bathrooms or outdoor toilets; associated with abuse; developmental delay

- Anatomic: rectal distension and desensitization, anal fissure or painful defecation; muscle hypotonia, slow intestinal motility; Hirschsprung disease, cystic fibrosis; spinal cord defects (e.g., spina bifida), congenital anorectal malformations; anal stenosis, anterior displacement of the anus, postoperative stricture of anus or rectum; pelvic mass, neurofibromatosis
- Dietary or metabolic: inadequate dietary fiber; excessive protein or milk intake; inadequate water intake; hypothyroidism; hypercalcemia; hypokalemia; diabetes insipidus; diabetes mellitus; Food allergy; gluten enteropathy
- Medication side effects

Genetics
None known; although incidence may be higher in children with family history of constipation

RISK FACTORS
Transition of foods: breast milk to formula or cow's milk or start of solid foods; parental conflicts or divorce; new sibling; history of constipation; painful defecation; difficulty with bowel training, including social pressure related to early daycare placement; organic/anatomic causes; anxiety and depression; insufficient fluid or fiber intake; fear of using bathrooms/public restrooms; attention deficit; history of abuse; medications (particularly opiates, ADD/ADHD medications, antidepressants)

GENERAL PREVENTION
Family education: toilet training when ready; optimize fluid and fiber intake.

COMMONLY ASSOCIATED CONDITIONS
Constipation, developmental and behavioral diagnoses, urinary incontinence, cow's milk protein allergy, autism and ADHD, psychosocial or neurological conditions—especially nonretentive fecal incontinence, UTI

DIAGNOSIS

Functional constipation is a clinical diagnosis above (see "Basics") no additional testing or labs in children with no red flag symptoms

HISTORY
- Stool pattern, consistency, and interval; abdominal pain that improves with stool passage; hiding while defecating before child is toilet-trained; avoiding use of the toilet
- Signs/symptoms of constipation: hard, large caliber stools, <3 defecations per week, pain or discomfort with stool passage, withholding stool, blood on stool or in diaper/toilet bowl
- Diet low in fiber or fluids, high in dairy products
- No stool passage in the first 48 hours of life
- Urinary symptoms: recurrent UTIs or enuresis
- General symptoms: decreased appetite fevers/chills
- Stressors, family, social and family history of constipation or medication use: opiates or antidepressants
- Abrupt onset after age 5 years is more likely to be associated with psychological trauma.

PHYSICAL EXAM
- Neurologic exam of lower extremities and perineal area, with attention to S1–S4 distribution, perineal sensation, cremasteric reflex, anal sphincter tone, and evidence of neural tube defects
- Genital examination and digital rectal exam: Assess for anal fissures, sphincter tone, rectal distension/impaction, and occult or visible blood.
- Abdominal exam: bowel sounds, percussion note (tympany), abdominal distension; palpate for stool (most common in left lower quadrant); strength/laxity of abdominal musculature
- Growth parameters: height, weight, head circumference
- Insufficient evidence of doing digital rectal exam in the absence of specific clinical indications

DIFFERENTIAL DIAGNOSIS
Irritable bowel syndrome, celiac disease, hypothyroidism, Down syndrome, anal fissures, trauma, Hirschsprung disease, cerebral palsy, hypercalcemia, neuromuscular disease

DIAGNOSTIC TESTS & INTERPRETATION
Most cases diagnosed by history and physical

Initial Tests (lab, imaging)
Used only to rule out organic causes: UA/urine culture: UTI/glucosuria; thyroid function tests: hypothyroidism; electrolyte panel, including calcium: hypokalemia, hypercalcemia, or hyperglycemia; abdominal plain films if impaction is suspected and otherwise not confirmed by physical exam

Follow-Up Tests & Special Considerations
Failure to pass meconium within 48 hours of birth, failure to thrive, bloody diarrhea, or bilious vomiting in a neonate should be promptly evaluated to exclude aganglionic megacolon; constipation and diarrhea, rash, failure to thrive, or recurrent pneumonia—consider cystic fibrosis; patients with abdominal distension or ileus should be evaluated for possible obstruction.

TREATMENT

GENERAL MEASURES
- Four key elements: dietary modification, behavior modification, medications, disimpaction (if needed)
- Anticipatory toilet training advice about when children should reduce reliance on diapers or use pull-ups during the daytime hours (average age for toilet training in girls is 29 months; 31 months for boys)
- Eliminate impaction prior to initiating any maintenance therapy.
- Once stools are regular in frequency, child should sit on toilet BID at the same time each day for 10 to 15 minutes and for 10 to 15 minutes after meals. Incorporate positive reinforcement for successful bowel movements.
- Juices containing sorbitol (e.g., apple, pear, prune) increase water content and promote stool softness.
- Recommended daily fluid intake: ages 1 to 3 years: 4 cups; ages 4 to 8 years: 5 cups; age >8 years: 7 to 8 cups

- Recommended fiber intake: A rough guide in children is to add 5 g to child's age in years.
- Children may experience shame, bullying, and rejection. Adolescents may have depression, anxiety, and social problems. Parents of children with these issues may need extra education. They may also feel shame, blame, and/or dismissal.
- 50%–60% recovery rate after 1 year of intensive treatment

MEDICATION
- Remove impaction and start maintenance treatment.
- No RCTs have compared methods of disimpaction: can use oral agents, enemas, and rectal suppositories; oral agents are least traumatic. Glycerin suppositories are best option for infants.

First Line
- Disimpaction with polyethylene glycol (PEG): Give 17 g (240 mL) water or juice: 1.0 to 1.5 g/kg/day for 3 days for disimpaction (may occasionally need higher doses via NG in hospital setting if at home treatment fails). Use 0.4 to 0.8 g/kg/day for maintenance.
- Disimpaction with mineral oil for child aged >1 year; give 15 to 30 mL/year of age to a maximum of 240 mL; for maintenance: 1 to 3 mL/kg/day or divided BID; may mix with orange juice to make palatable; avoid in infants to avoid aspiration pneumonia.
- Disimpaction with saline enema: 5 to 10 mL/kg once/day for 3 to 6 days up to 5 yo
- Other maintenance regimens include the following: Milk of Magnesia (MOM) 400 mg (5 mL): 1 to 2 mL/kg/day BID; magnesium citrate: 4 mL/kg/day; lactulose 10 g (15 mL): 1 to 3 mL/kg/day divided BID; Senna syrup 8.8 g sennoside (5 mL): ages 2 to 6 years: 2.5 to 7.5 mL/day divided BID; ages 6 to 12 years: 5 to 15 mL/day divided BID; bisacodyl suppository 10 mg: 0.5 to 1.0 suppository once or twice per day—children >2 years old; sorbitol containing juices: 1 to 3 mL/kg BID in infants
- Continue maintenance medications for 1 to 2 months after symptom resolution or until after toilet training is achieved.

ISSUES FOR REFERRAL
- No improvement after 6 months of treatment; refer to pediatric gastroenterology.
- Refer to psychologist or use combination of medical and behavior therapy if no improvement in 3 months.

ADDITIONAL THERAPIES
Behavioral treatment and counseling; caregiver education

SURGERY/OTHER PROCEDURES
If refractory symptoms, consider anorectal manometry to evaluate for internal anal sphincter achalasia (or ultrashort-segment Hirschsprung disease). If present, this condition can be treated successfully in most patients with an internal sphincter myectomy.

COMPLEMENTARY & ALTERNATIVE MEDICINE
- Children who receive combination of behavioral and medication treatment are more likely to have resolution of encopresis at 3 and 6 months than with medication alone.
- No evidence that biofeedback training adds benefit to conventional treatment
- Behavioral interventions combined with laxative therapy (rather than laxative therapy alone) improve continence in children with functional fecal incontinence associated with constipation.
- No evidence for effectiveness of either probiotics or increased physical activity

ADMISSION, INPATIENT, AND NURSING CONSIDERATIONS
- Admission criteria/initial stabilization: continued soiling and recurrent impaction on outpatient medical therapy; decreased intake leading to malnutrition or dehydration, recalcitrant vomiting or concern for obstruction; involve appropriate agencies if concern for abuse; hospital admission and abdominal films may be necessary to ensure complete removal of impaction; this may include direct gastric administration of balanced electrolyte–PEG solutions if the patient cannot tolerate by mouth. Serial abdominal films and observation of rectal effluent can help determine treatment adequacy.
- IV fluids if the patient is dehydrated and has difficulty tolerating oral intake
- Nursing to document stool output and character
- Discharge criteria: Stools that are looser in consistency and clearer in appearance are a successful inpatient end point; abdominal radiograph showing less fecal loading (compared with a pretreatment x-ray) with improving serial abdominal exams

ONGOING CARE

Record bowel movements successfully passed as well as soiling episodes as well as incorporating a reward system to promote continued efforts at sitting on the toilet regularly. Open communication and close follow-up are essential in the long run.

FOLLOW-UP RECOMMENDATIONS
Follow-up monthly at first with clinician to review the patient's stooling regimen, conduct a physical exam and readjust the home regimen as needed to ensure continued progress and remission of symptoms.

Patient Monitoring
- Continue maintenance treatment for 6 months to 2 years with visits every 4 to 10 weeks for support and to ensure compliance; more frequent visits with oppositional or anxious children
- Treat recurrences of impaction promptly and emphasize compliance with medication and regular bathroom visits.
- Refer children for mental health evaluation and counseling if no progress with comprehensive behavior plan.

DIET
Adequate fluid and fiber intake; reduce cow's milk products. Avoid excessive consumption of bananas, rice, apples, and gelatin.

PATIENT EDUCATION
- Demystify defecation.
- Carefully explain the treatment plan including medications and dietary changes.
- Avoid punishment for inadvertent soiling.
- In children >4 years of age, explain to parents how overreliance on diapers and pull-ups (although convenient) can prolong the problem.
- Always attempt to use positive reinforcement for successful toilet sits and medication compliance.
- If positive approach is unsuccessful, consider removing desired privileges (e.g., TV, video games) for noncompliance with behavioral plan. Some children respond well to a token economy (earned privileges) to promote desired behavior.
- Encourage regular physical activity.

PROGNOSIS
- Many children exhibit a good response and relapse due to parental noncompliance.
- From 30% to 50% of children may still have encopresis after 5 years of treatment.
- Children with psychosocial or emotional problems preceding the encopresis are more recalcitrant to treatment.

COMPLICATIONS
- Colitis due to excessive enema/suppository
- Perianal dermatitis
- Anal fissure

ADDITIONAL READING
- Baird DC, Bybel M, Kowalski AW. Toilet training: common questions and answers. *Am Fam Physician.* 2019;100(8):468–474.
- Constipation Guideline Committee of the North American Society for Pediatric Gastroenterology, Hepatology and Nutrition. Evaluation and treatment of constipation in infants and children: recommendations of the North American Society for Pediatric Gastroenterology, Hepatology and Nutrition. *J Pediatr Gastroenterol Nutr.* 2006;43(3):e1–e13.
- LeLeiko NS, Mayer-Brown S, Cerezo C, et al. Constipation. *Pediatr Rev.* 2020;41(8):379–392.
- Lu PL, Mousa HM. Constipation: beyond the old paradigms. *Gastroenterol Clin North Am.* 2018;47(4):845–862.

CODES

ICD10
- R15.9 Full incontinence of feces
- R15.1 Fecal smearing
- F98.1 Encopresis not due to a substance or known physiol condition

CLINICAL PEARLS
- 90% of encopresis results from chronic constipation.
- Address toddler constipation early by decreasing excessive milk intake, increasing fruits/vegetables intake, and ensuring adequate fluid and fiber intake.
- Eliminate fecal impaction before initiating maintenance therapy.

ENDOCARDITIS, INFECTIVE
Theodore B. Flaum, DO • Kaitlin Unser, DO

 BASICS

Infective endocarditis (IE) is an infection of the inner layer of the heart including the valves (native/prosthetic), interventricular septum, intracardiac devices, chordae tendineae, and mural endocardium. IE occurs worldwide and is generally fatal if left untreated.

DESCRIPTION
- An infection of the valvular (primarily) and/or mural (rarely) endocardium
- System(s) affected: cardiovascular, endocrine/metabolic, hematologic/lymphatic, immunologic, pulmonary, renal/urologic, skin/exocrine, neurologic
- Synonym(s): bacterial endocarditis; subacute bacterial endocarditis (SBE); acute bacterial endocarditis (ABE)

EPIDEMIOLOGY
More common in males (range is 3:2 to 9:1); >50% of cases in the United States occur in individuals >60 years of age.

Incidence
- Incidence at ~15 in 100,000, increasing from previous years
- The predominant form of IE is community associated. Up to one-third of cases are health care-acquired in resource-rich countries.
- Increasing incidence of cardiovascular device-related infections due to a higher frequency of implantable devices
- Can be community- or hospital-acquired
- Most commonly affects the mitral valve and aortic valve (increased left-sided pressures and turbulent flow).

ETIOLOGY AND PATHOPHYSIOLOGY
IE is most commonly caused by a nonbacterial thrombus that adheres to an endocardial surface, coupled with a bacterial source sufficient to seed the thrombus. This can occur from direct bacterial invasion or valvular trauma:
- Native valve endocarditis
  - Acute: *Staphylococcus aureus*; *Streptococcus* groups A, B, C, G; *Streptococcus pneumoniae*; *Staphylococcus lugdunensis*; *Enterococcus* spp.; *Haemophilus influenzae* or *parainfluenzae*; *Neisseria gonorrhoeae*
  - Subacute: α-hemolytic streptococci, *Streptococcus bovis*, *Enterococcus* spp., *S. aureus*, *Staphylococcus epidermidis*; HACEK organisms
- Intravenous drug abuse endocarditis (IVDA) (most commonly tricuspid valve): *S. aureus*, *Enterococcus* spp.; *Pseudomonas aeruginosa*, *Burkholderia cepacia*, other bacilli (gram-negative); *Candida* spp.
- Prosthetic valve endocarditis
  - Early (≤12 months after valve implantation): *S. aureus*, *S. epidermidis*; gram-negative bacilli; *Candida* spp., *Aspergillus* spp.
  - Late (>12 months after valve implantation): α-hemolytic streptococci, *S. aureus*, *Enterococcus* spp., *S. epidermidis*, *Candida* spp., *Aspergillus* spp.
- Culture-negative endocarditis: 10% of cases; *Bartonella quintana* (homeless); *Brucella* spp., fungi, *Coxiella burnetii* (Q fever), *Chlamydia trachomatis*, *Chlamydophila psittaci*, HACEK organisms
- Device-related endocarditis: coagulase-negative staphylococci or *S. aureus*

RISK FACTORS
- Injection drug use, IV catheterization, certain malignancies (colon cancer), poor dentition/infection, chronic hemodialysis, age >60 years, male sex, implantable devices
- Highest risk with (1):
  - Previous IE
  - Prosthetic cardiac valves (including transcatheter-implanted prostheses and homografts)
  - Cardiac transplant with valvular regurgitation
  - Prosthetic material used for cardiac valve repair (such as annuloplasty rings or chords)
  - Congenital heart disease (CHD): unrepaired cyanotic CHD or repaired CHD residual shunts of valvular regurgitation at the site of or adjacent to the site of a prosthetic patch or prosthetic device

GENERAL PREVENTION
- Good oral hygiene
- Antibiotic prophylaxis is only recommended in patients with a high risk of adverse outcomes if IE were to occur—(see "Risk Factors"). Administer 30 to 60 minutes prior to the procedure (exception vancomycin which should be administered 120 minutes prior to the procedure).
- In high-risk patients, consider antibiotic prophylaxis for dental procedures involve manipulation of gingival tissue, manipulation of the periapical region of teeth, or perforation of the oral mucosa.
- *Procedures requiring prophylaxis*
  - Oral/upper respiratory tract procedures/biopsies: Amoxicillin 2 g PO 30 to 60 minutes before procedure or ampicillin 2 g IV/IM are the first-line prophylactic choices. Clindamycin is no longer recommended for dental prophylaxis because it is associated with more frequent and severe adverse effects (i.e., *Clostridium difficile* infection).
  - GI/GU: Only consider coverage for *Enterococcus* (with penicillin, ampicillin, piperacillin, or vancomycin) for patients with an established infection undergoing procedures.
  - Cardiac valvular surgery or placement of prosthetic intracardiac/intravascular materials: perioperative cefazolin 1 to 2 g IV 30 minutes preoperative or vancomycin 15 mg/kg (max of 1 g) (penicillin-allergic patients) 60 minutes preoperative
  - Skin/soft tissue: incision and drainage of infected tissue; use agents active against skin pathogens (e.g., cefazolin 1 to 2 g IV q8h or vancomycin 15 mg/kg q12h; max of 1 g) if penicillin-allergic or if methicillin-resistant *S. aureus* (MRSA) is suspected.

COMMONLY ASSOCIATED CONDITIONS
Most patients with IE have preexisting conditions (see "Risk Factors").

DIAGNOSIS
- Modified Duke Criteria (clinical criteria for IE (1): 2 major criteria, or 1 major and 3 minor criteria, or 5 minor criteria; possible IE: 1 major and 1 minor or 3 minor criteria; rejected diagnosis: firm alternative diagnosis explaining evidence of IE, or resolution of IE after ≤4 days with antibiotic therapy, or does not meet criteria for possible IE as seen above)

- Major clinical criteria
  - Positive blood culture: isolation of typical microorganism for IE from two separate blood cultures or persistently positive blood culture
  - Single positive blood culture for *C. burnetii* or anti–phase-1 IgG antibody titer >1:800
  - Positive echocardiogram: presence of vegetation, abscess, or new partial dehiscence of prosthetic valve
  - New valvular regurgitation (change in preexisting murmur not sufficient)
- Minor criteria
  - Predisposing heart condition or IV drug use
  - Fever ≥38°C (100.4°F)
  - Vascular phenomena: arterial emboli, septic pulmonary infarcts, mycotic aneurysm, intracranial hemorrhage, conjunctival hemorrhage, Janeway lesions
  - Immunologic phenomena: glomerulonephritis, Osler nodes, Roth spots, rheumatoid factor (RF)
  - Microbiologic evidence

HISTORY
- Fever (>38°C), chills, cough, dyspnea, orthopnea; especially in subacute endocarditis: night sweats, weight loss, fatigue
- Review risk factors.
- Symptoms of transient ischemic attack, cerebrovascular accident (CVA), or myocardial infarction (MI) on presentation

PHYSICAL EXAM
- Most patients with IE have new murmur/change to an existing murmur. Signs of heart failure are common if valve function is compromised.
- Peripheral stigmata of IE: splinter hemorrhages in fingernail beds, Osler nodes, Roth spots, Janeway lesions, palatal/conjunctival petechiae, splenomegaly, hematuria
- Neurologic findings consistent with CVA

DIFFERENTIAL DIAGNOSIS
Vasculitis, temporal arteritis, fever of unknown origin, infected central venous catheter, marantic endocarditis, connective tissue diseases, rheumatic fever, salmonellosis, brucellosis, Lyme disease, malignancy, tuberculosis, atrial myxoma, septic thrombophlebitis

DIAGNOSTIC TESTS & INTERPRETATION
- If not critically ill; three sets of blood cultures drawn >2 hours apart from different sites *before administration* of *antibiotics* with repeat cultures in 48 to 72 hours until bacterial clearance
- If acutely ill, draw three sets of blood cultures over 1 hour *prior to empiric therapy*.
- Leukocytosis; anemia; decreased C3, C4, CH50; and +RF in subacute endocarditis
- ESR, C-reactive protein (CRP)
- Hematuria
- Consider serologies for *Chlamydia*, Q fever, *Legionella*, and *Bartonella* in "culture-negative" endocarditis.
- Transthoracic (TTE) or transesophageal echocardiogram (TEE [preferred])
- CT scan

Initial Tests (lab, imaging)

Routine laboratory findings are often nonspecific and often are a manifestation of secondary sequelae of IE.

- Laboratory findings:
  - Nonspecific
    - Elevated inflammatory markers; leukocytosis, +RF; normochromic normocytic anemia
  - Findings related to secondary system involvement
    - RBC casts; microscopic hematuria, proteinuria, pyuria
- Imaging
  - ECG: New/evolving signs of conduction disease (atrioventricular blocks and/or bundle branch blocks) are often a sign of paravalvular and/or myocardial involvement.
  - TTE/TEE: new or worsening valvular regurgitation, new partial dehiscence of prosthetic valve, new intracardiac shunting, presence of vegetations

Follow-Up Tests & Special Considerations

If indicated, follow-up imaging to evaluate for secondary system involvement or to rule out other causes:

- Chest x-ray: may reveal evidence of septic pulmonary emboli or signs of congestive heart failure
- CT chest/abdomen/pelvis: Evaluate distal sites of infections and/or infarction.

TREATMENT

GENERAL MEASURES

In general, antibiotic therapy for IE should be targeted to the organism isolated from blood cultures. The duration of therapy should be calculated from the first day of the negative blood cultures.

MEDICATION

First Line

- Start empiric treatment after three sets of blood cultures have been drawn. Results guide treatment.
  - Native valves: ampicillin-sulbactam IV with gentamicin IV/IM; if penicillin-allergic, use vancomycin IV with gentamicin IV/IM and with ciprofloxacin PO/IV.
  - Prosthetic valves: vancomycin IV with gentamicin IV/IM and rifampin PO, if <12 months postsurgery; if >12 months, use native valve regimen.
- Penicillin-susceptible viridans streptococci or *S. bovis*
  - Native valve: penicillin G IV continuously or ceftriaxone IV/IM for 4 weeks
  - Prosthetic valve: penicillin G IV for 6 weeks or ceftriaxone IV/IM ± gentamicin IV/IM for 2 weeks
- Penicillin-resistant viridans streptococci or *S. bovis*
  - Native valve: penicillin G IV + gentamicin IV/IM
  - Prosthetic valve: penicillin G IV or ceftriaxone IV/IM for 6 weeks + gentamicin IV/IM for 2 weeks

- Penicillin-susceptible *Staphylococcus*
  - Native valve: oxacillin or nafcillin IV for 6 weeks; for the oxacillin-resistant strains, use vancomycin IV for 6 weeks.
  - Prosthetic valve: oxacillin or nafcillin IV + rifampin IV/PO for 6 weeks, + gentamicin IV for the first 2 weeks; for oxacillin-resistant strains, use vancomycin IV, + rifampin IV/PO, both for 6 weeks, + gentamicin IV/IM for the first 2 weeks.
- Penicillin-resistant *Staphylococcus*
  - Native valve: vancomycin for 6 weeks or daptomycin IV for 6 weeks
  - Prosthetic valve: vancomycin + rifampin IV/PO + gentamicin IV/IM for 2 weeks
- Penicillin-sensitive *Enterococcus*
  - Native or prosthetic valve: ampicillin IV or penicillin G IV + gentamicin IV for 4 to 6 weeks
- *HACEK* organisms: ceftriaxone IM or IV for 4 weeks *or* ampicillin-sulbactam IV for 4 weeks *or* ciprofloxacin PO or IV for 4 weeks

SURGERY/OTHER PROCEDURES

Surgery is required in 50% of IE cases. Indications:

- Heart failure due to aortic or mitral valve disease
  - Prevention of embolism: aortic or mitral valve vegetations >10 mm with prior embolic episodes; isolated very large vegetation >15 mm; in patients with major ischemic stroke, surgery is delayed for at least 4 weeks, if possible.
- Uncontrolled infection: persistent fever and positive cultures >7 to 10 days; infection caused by fungi or resistant organism; presence of abscess, fistula, false aneurysm, or enlarging vegetations
- Early prosthetic valve IE

ONGOING CARE

FOLLOW-UP RECOMMENDATIONS

Patient Monitoring

- Baseline ECG; monitor ECG for conduction disturbances/MI in initial weeks of therapy.
- TTE at the conclusion of therapy
- Blood cultures q48h until negative

PROGNOSIS

The 1-year mortality of IE is 30%. Late complications contribute to poor prognosis. These include heart failure, reinfection, and cerebral emboli. The 10-year survival is 60–90%.

COMPLICATIONS

- Cerebral complications are the most frequent and severe, occurring in 15–20% of patients. Neurologic events are the most frequent complications in patients with IE requiring ICU admission. Ischemic stroke is the presenting symptom of IE in 20% of cases.

- Emboli: arterial, infectious (e.g., abscesses of heart, lung, brain, meninges, bone, pericardium)
- Inflammatory/immune disorders (e.g., arthritis, myositis, glomerulonephritis)
- Other complications: congestive heart failure, ruptured valve cusp, sinus of Valsalva aneurysm, arrhythmia, and mycotic aneurysms

REFERENCE

1. McDonald EG, Aggrey G, Aslan AT, et al. Guidelines for diagnosis and management of infective endocarditis in adults: a WikiGuidelines Group consensus statement. *JAMA Netw Open*. 2023;6(7):e2326366.

ADDITIONAL READING

- Cimmino G, Bottino R, Formisano T, et al. Current views on infective endocarditis: changing epidemiology, improving diagnostic tools and centering the patient for up-to-date management. *Life (Basel)*. 2023;13(2):377.
- Hussein H, Montesinos-Guevara C, Abouelkheir M, et al. Quality appraisal of antibiotic prophylaxis guidelines to prevent infective endocarditis following dental procedures: a systematic review. *Oral Surg Oral Med Oral Pathol Oral Radiol*. 2022;134(5):562–572.

CODES

ICD10

- I33.0 Acute and subacute infective endocarditis
- I39 Endocarditis and heart valve disord in dis classd elswhr
- A54.83 Gonococcal heart infection

CLINICAL PEARLS

- Preprocedural antibiotic prophylaxis is recommended for patients with artificial heart valves, a previous history of IE, CHD, and cardiac transplants with valvulopathy.
- TEE/TTE and blood cultures are the mainstays for diagnosing IE.
- The most commonly identified organisms are viridans *Streptococcus* spp. and *Staphylococcus*.
- Valves most commonly involved: (i) mitral valve, (ii) aortic valve, (iii) combination of aortic and mitral valves, (iv) tricuspid valve, (v) pulmonic valve

ENDOMETRIOSIS
Kenneth A. Ballou, MD

 BASICS

DESCRIPTION
- Endometriosis is a common and potentially painful, debilitating estrogen-dependent gynecologic condition predominately affecting women of reproductive age.
- Symptoms and signs generally consist of pelvic and/or abdominal pain, pelvic mass, and/or decreased fertility.
- Due to estrogen-dependent implants of endometrial tissue found outside the uterus; although endometriomas have been recorded in liver, bowel, umbilicus, lung, and other tissue, the most common pathologic sites are:
  - Peritoneum (bladder, cul-de-sac, pelvic walls, ligaments, and fallopian tubes)
  - Ovaries
  - Rectovaginal septum
- Ectopic endometrial implants proliferate and slough with the menstrual cycle.
- Stage I (minimal) to IV (severe). Staging is useful in therapeutic planning but does not correlate with pain severity.

EPIDEMIOLOGY
Prevalence
- Biologic females only
- Affects 6–10% of fertile women
- Found in 21–40% of infertile women
- Found in 70–90% of women with chronic pelvic pain

Pediatric Considerations
Endometriosis may begin with puberty, as endometrial implants are dependent on ovarian hormones. This can lead to debilitating pelvic pain and severe dysmenorrhea associated with missed school and family/social activities.

Pregnancy Considerations
The presence of endometriosis decreases fecundability from 15–20% per month to 2–10% per month. 21–40% of infertile women have endometriosis. However, pelvic endometriosis generally improves during pregnancy.

Geriatric Considerations
Although menopause often results in a resolution of symptoms, pelvic endometriosis may extend into menopause and may be exacerbated by hormone replacement therapy (HRT).

ETIOLOGY AND PATHOPHYSIOLOGY
- Not fully understood; several factors are believed to play a role, including immunologic changes and genetic predisposition in the presence of abnormal proliferating endometrial tissue implants causing chronic peritoneal inflammation.
- Theories include:
  - Sampson theory: Retrograde menstruation results in peritoneal implantation and disease.
  - Halban theory: Distant disease is probably caused by hematogenous/lymphatic dissemination or metaplastic transformation.
  - Coelomic metaplasia: Coelomic epithelium remains undifferentiated in the peritoneal cavity and differentiates to form functioning endometrium.

- Endometrial-associated infertility is multifactorial:
  - Pelvic inflammation
  - Anatomic disruption of pelvic structures (Involvement of the fallopian tube may cause isthmic tubal obstruction.)
  - Proliferation and activation of peritoneal macrophages (may predispose to gamete phagocytosis)
  - Alteration in eutopic endometrium

Genetics
Odds ratio of symptomatic endometriosis with a first-degree affected relative is 7.2. Those with affected first-degree relatives have a 26% chance of severe manifestations versus 12% if no first-degree affected relatives.

RISK FACTORS
- Family history
- Prolonged lifetime exposure to menstruation and ovulation (early menarche, late menopause)
- Delayed childbirth/nulliparity
- Low body mass index
- Prolonged menstruation (>5 days)/shorter menstrual cycles (<28 days)

GENERAL PREVENTION
- Suppression of heavy menstruation and ovulation with oral contraceptives during adolescence may delay sequelae.
- Some factors are considered protective:
  - Fruits, green vegetables, n-3 long-chain fatty acids
  - Regular aerobic exercise (>4 hours per week)
- Early diagnosis and treatment might help prevent sequelae.

COMMONLY ASSOCIATED CONDITIONS
Infertility, dysmenorrhea, ovarian cysts, dyspareunia, chronic abdominal/pelvic pain syndrome, pelvic inflammatory disease, and irritable bowel disease

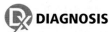 **DIAGNOSIS**

HISTORY
- Dysmenorrhea (50–90% of cases) due to deep infiltrating endometrial implants
- Dyspareunia with or without postcoital bleeding due to lesions of the cul-de-sac, uterosacral ligaments, and posterior vaginal fornix
- Dyschezia due to involvement of the rectosigmoid colon and rectovaginal regions
- Chronic pelvic pain (≥6 months) that worsens with time and begins 1 to 2 days prior to menstrual cycles
- Hematochezia
- Cyclic nausea, abdominal distention
- Infertility (late finding)
- History of pelvic pain, infertility, and hysterectomy in first- or second-degree relative

PHYSICAL EXAM
- Focal pain/tenderness on pelvic exam is associated with endometriosis in 66% of patients.
- Pelvic mass may be present.
- Immobile pelvic organs (frozen pelvis)
- Rectovaginal exam revealing uterosacral nodules, beading, or tenderness
- Exquisite tenderness in the region of the uterosacral ligament is found in severe cases.

DIFFERENTIAL DIAGNOSIS
Differential diagnosis of pelvic pain includes all causes of acute abdomen and
- Pelvic adhesions
- Nonspecific dysmenorrhea
- Acute salpingitis/pelvic inflammatory disease
- Ovarian cyst/hydrosalpinges
- Uterine leiomyomas
- Adenomyosis
- Irritable bowel syndrome
- Inflammatory bowel disease
- Intraabdominal adhesions
- Pelvic malignancy
- Complications of intrauterine/ectopic pregnancy
- Urinary tract infection/interstitial cystitis
- Anal fissures
- Psychosexual pain syndrome, vaginal atrophy, vulvodynia, infectious vaginitis or cervicitis
- Chronic pain syndrome

DIAGNOSTIC TESTS & INTERPRETATION
Initial Tests (lab, imaging)
- Initial diagnosis is primarily clinical.
- Labs are only useful to rule out other diagnoses; there are no reliable labs to rule in endometriosis.
- CA-125 levels are not recommended due to low sensitivity.
- If history and physical exam reveal adnexal pain or tenderness with/without fullness on pelvic exam
  - Transvaginal ultrasound (US) is the modality of choice; MRI may be useful for evaluating deeper retrosigmoid and ureteral infiltrating lesions but generally has lower sensitivity (1).
  - Both modalities are poor in detecting peritoneal implants and adhesions.

Diagnostic Procedures/Other
Definitive diagnosis is made only by microscopic characteristics of tissue biopsied during laparoscopy or laparotomy.

Test Interpretation
- Laparoscopically visualized red and blue-black lesions described as "powder-burns," adhesions, and "chocolate cysts" on the ovarian and peritoneal surfaces
- Histologically described endometrial glands and stroma on analysis of biopsied lesions

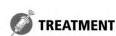 **TREATMENT**

GENERAL MEASURES
Management is dependent on multiple factors:
- Age and reproductive desires of the patient
- The certainty of the diagnosis
- The degree of degradation on quality of life due to pain and infertility
- The threat to other organ systems: GI tract, bladder

MEDICATION
Medications are used to improve the patient's quality of life through symptom relief and to prevent progression of the disease and its potential to cause organ dysfunction. Unfortunately, few studies of medical therapy report patient-relevant outcomes. Many patients gain only limited or intermittent benefit from medical therapies.

First Line

Patients found to have endometriomas during incidental surgery or studies may not need any treatment. Others with minimal symptoms may find sufficient relief with NSAID medications. Increased exercise, especially aerobic, may help others.

- Cyclic combined oral contraceptive pills (OCPs) suppress ovulation (2).
- NSAIDs initiated at the beginning or just before menses. Evidence is inconclusive on effectiveness.

Second Line

- Combination of OCPs or low-dose progestin-only medications with recommendations to switch from cyclic to continuous combined contraception for 3 to 6 months if symptoms persist or if there is chronic, noncyclic pelvic pain
- Levonorgestrel intrauterine device (IUD) (Mirena) found to decrease recurrence of painful menstruation
- Medroxyprogesterone acetate 150 mg IM every 3 months; prolonged use may lead to loss of bone mineral density of uncertain clinical significance.
- Gonadotropin-releasing hormone (GnRH) agonists: inhibit pituitary gonadotropin synthesis and induce a hypoestrogenic state
- Norethindrone acetate 5 mg PO once daily plus conjugated equine estrogen 0.625 mg PO once daily

Third Line

If symptoms and signs continue, physicians should be experienced in the use and side effects of GnRH analogues prior to their use (symptoms return in as many as 70% of treated patients):

- Leuprolide acetate (Lupron Depot) 3.75 mg IM each month or 11.25 mg IM every 3 months (gluteal)
- Nafarelin (Synarel) intranasal one spray (200 μg) in one nostril each morning and the other nostril each evening (start between days 2 and 4 of menstrual cycle)
- Goserelin (Zoladex) implant 3.6 mg SC in upper abdominal wall every 28 days
- Danazol: also effective, with side effects similar to GnRH analogs
- Aromatase inhibitors (anastrozole and letrozole) prolong the remission induced by GnRH medications.

ALERT

Calcium (1,000 to 1,500 mg/day) with vitamin D 1,000 to 2,000 IU daily or low-dose estrogen with progestogen is recommended when using GnRH agonists to prevent calcium loss.

ISSUES FOR REFERRAL

- Refer early to a gynecologist with expertise in medical and surgical treatment of endometriosis, especially if the patient desires to conceive in the future.
- Indications for referral to include the following:
  - Need for definitive diagnosis
  - Failure to respond to a conservative or first-line therapy
  - Chronic pelvic pain
  - Delayed fertility

ADDITIONAL THERAPIES

Regular exercise and counseling for pain-management strategies; narcotics are contraindicated for chronic pain.

SURGERY/OTHER PROCEDURES

Surgery (laparoscopy or laparotomy) is both diagnostic and therapeutic (first line or when conservative measures fail):

- Peritoneal endometriosis: laser ablation/excision/fulguration
- Ovarian endometriosis (endometriomas) >3 to 4 cm: ablation, excision, drainage
- Lysis of adhesions (LOA)
- Hysterectomy with bilateral salpingo-oophorectomy may be considered for debilitating symptoms refractory to other medical or surgical treatments in patients who do not desire pregnancy:
  - Relieves pain in 80–90%, but pain recurs in 10% within 1 to 2 years after surgery
  - Postoperative HRT should include estrogen and progestogen or progesterone.
- Interruption of nerve pathways: Laparoscopic ablations and presacral neurectomy improve dysmenorrhea.
- Fertility procedures: Ablation or excision of lesions with LOA is recommended to treat infertility in stages I and II disease:
  - Spontaneous conception should be attempted for 1 year prior to assisted reproduction techniques.
  - Disease does not endanger in vitro fertilization (IVF) pregnancies.

ALERT

Surgery for endometriomas may decrease ovarian reserve in advanced disease.

COMPLEMENTARY & ALTERNATIVE MEDICINE

- Osteopathic manipulative therapy found to improve quality of life
- Postsurgical use of Chinese herbal medicine has been found to be effective.
- Acupuncture may be effective in relieving pain (3)
- Botulinum toxin injections have been used to control pain.

 ONGOING CARE

FOLLOW-UP RECOMMENDATIONS

Routine gynecologic care

Patient Monitoring

Symptomatic and asymptomatic pelvic masses (http://www.acog.org/)

PROGNOSIS

- Excellent, especially if diagnosis and treatment plans are initiated early in disease course
- Poor for recovery of fertility if the disease has progressed to stage III/IV
- Symptoms and signs improve after bilateral oophorectomy.

COMPLICATIONS

Sequelae include chronic pelvic pain, reduced quality of life, repetitive surgical intervention, depression, medication side effects and costs, and infertility.

REFERENCES

1. Kiesel L, Sourouni M. Diagnosis of endometriosis in the 21st century. *Climacteric*. 2019;22(3):296–302.
2. Chauhan S, More A, Chauhan V, et al. Endometriosis: a review of clinical diagnosis, treatment, and pathogenesis. *Cureus*. 2022;14(9):e28864.
3. Mira TAA, Buen MM, Borges MG, et al. Systemic review and meta-analysis of complementary treatments for women with symptomatic endometriosis. *Int J Gynaecol Obstet*. 2018;143(1):2–9.

ADDITIONAL READING

- Mistry M, Simpson P, Morris E, et al. Cannabidiol for the management of endometriosis and chronic pelvic pain. *J Minim Invasive Gynecol*. 2022;29(2):169–176.
- Rossi V, Tripodi F, Simonelli C, et al. Endometriosis-associated pain: a review of quality of life, sexual health and couple relationship. *Minerva Ostet Gynecol*. 2021;73(5):536–552.
- Zondervan KT, Becker CM, Missmer SA. Endometriosis. *N Engl J Med*. 2020;382(13):1244–1256.

CODES

ICD10

- N80.2 Endometriosis of fallopian tube
- N80.5 Endometriosis of intestine
- N80.0 Endometriosis of uterus

CLINICAL PEARLS

- Endometriosis should be considered in patients of reproductive age with chronic pelvic/abdominal pain, dysmenorrhea, and/or delayed fertility.
- Initial diagnosis is clinical; no reliable diagnostic lab tests are available, although transvaginal US may be helpful.
- First-line treatments include NSAIDs and oral birth control medications.
- Refer to Gynecology if fertility is desired or if symptoms are refractory to first-line treatments (see above).

ENDOMETRITIS AND OTHER POSTPARTUM INFECTIONS

Justin P. Lavin Jr., MD, FACOG • Annemarie Newark, MD

 BASICS

DESCRIPTION
- Endometritis (infection of the endometrium) is the most common postpartum infection.
- Bacterial infection of genital tract, manifesting after delivery with a peak incidence at postpartum day 7. It can occur as late as 6 weeks postpartum.
- Postpartum infections of the myometrium and parametrial tissues are less common. Vaginal and cervical cellulitis, perianal cellulitis, pelvic cellulitis, pelvic abscess, septic pelvic vein thrombophlebitis, and parametrial phlegmon are other (generally rare) postpartum infections of the pelvic region.
- System(s) affected: reproductive
- Synonym(s): postpartum infection; endometritis; endoparametritis; endomyometritis; myometritis; endomyoparametritis; metritis; metritis with pelvic cellulitis

EPIDEMIOLOGY
Prevalence
- Occurs after 1–3% of all births
- 10 times more likely after cesarean section
  - 2–15% of infections begin prior to labor.
  - 30–35% occur after labor in absence of appropriate antibiotic prophylaxis; 2–15% occur after labor with appropriate prophylaxis.
  - Fifth leading cause of maternal mortality, accounting for 11% of maternal deaths

ETIOLOGY AND PATHOPHYSIOLOGY
- Endometritis is more common in labors complicated by chorioamnionitis.
- Other infections follow trauma to the perineum, vagina, cervix, and uterus.
- Postpartum infections are typically polymicrobial, involving organisms ascending from the lower genital tract:
  - Aerobic isolates (70%): *Streptococcus faecalis, Streptococcus agalactiae, Streptococcus viridans, Staphylococcus aureus, Escherichia coli*
  - Anaerobic isolates (80%): *Peptococcus* sp., *Peptostreptococcus* sp., *Clostridium* sp., *Bacteroides bivius, Bacteroides fragilis, Fusobacterium* sp.
- Other genital *Mycoplasma*
- Consider herpes simplex virus and cytomegalovirus, particularly in immunocompromised patients failing to improve on appropriate antibiotics.
- Thrombosis of any pelvic vein, including vena cava
- Phlegmon on leaves of the broad ligament

RISK FACTORS
- Cesarean delivery is the primary risk factor.
- Chorioamnionitis
- Bacterial vaginosis, group B streptococcal colonization of genital tract
- HIV infection
- Prolonged labor, prolonged rupture of membranes; heavily meconium-stained amniotic fluid
- Multiple vaginal examinations, internal fetal monitoring during labor
- Episiotomy, 3rd or 4th degree perineal laceration, or other perineal trauma
- Operative vaginal delivery; manual extraction of the placenta; intrauterine balloon tamponade, care in a teaching hospital
- Inappropriately timed or delayed prophylactic antibiotics
- Low socioeconomic status, obesity, anemia

GENERAL PREVENTION
- Intrapartum prophylaxis for group B colonization of genital tract
- Vaginal delivery
  - Avoid unnecessary vaginal examinations.
  - Treat chorioamnionitis during labor.
  - Avoid manual placental extraction and retained placental products.
  - Aseptic technique for operative vaginal delivery
  - Consider prophylaxis with amoxicillin and clavulanic acid for operative vaginal delivery (1)[B].
  - Antibiotic prophylaxis for manual removal of the placenta has not been demonstrated to be effective.
- Cesarean delivery
  - Preoperative paint and scrub with 10% povidone-iodine or an alcohol-based solution decreases puerperal infection by up to 38%.
  - Prophylactic antibiotics before both emergency and scheduled cesarean deliveries prior to skin incision reduce postpartum infection (2)[A].
    ○ Administer antibiotics within 1 hour of the start of surgery (3). Repeat for lengthy procedures or excessive blood loss (3). Appropriate administration of antibiotics results in a 40% reduction in postpartum maternal infections without any increase in neonatal infections (2)[A],(3).
  - Extended coverage with cephalosporin and azithromycin further decreases infection risk and is cost-effective (3)[A].
  - Vaginal preparation with povidone-iodine solution or chlorhexidine-alcohol solutions immediately before cesarean delivery reduces the risk of postoperative endometritis.
  - Weight-based antibiotic dosage helps ensure appropriate tissue concentrations prior to skin incision.

COMMONLY ASSOCIATED CONDITIONS
- Chorioamnionitis
- Wound infection

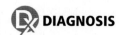 **DIAGNOSIS**

HISTORY
- History of cesarean delivery or chorioamnionitis
- Fever and chills
- Malaise
- Headache
- Anorexia
- Abdominal pain
- Heavy vaginal bleeding or foul smelling lochia

PHYSICAL EXAM
- Oral temperature >38°C (100.4°F)
- Tachycardia
- Uterine tenderness on exam (key finding)
- Other localized abdominopelvic tenderness on exam
- Purulent or malodorous lochia
- Heavy vaginal bleeding
- Ileus

DIFFERENTIAL DIAGNOSIS
- "5 Ws": Wind (pneumonia); Water (UTI); Wound infection; Wow (mastitis); Wonder drug (medication-related fever)
- Viral syndrome; dehydration
- Pelvic abscess, thrombophlebitis
- Thyroid storm
- Appendicitis

DIAGNOSTIC TESTS & INTERPRETATION
Initial Tests (lab, imaging)
- CBC: Interpret with care. (Physiologic leukocytosis may be as high as 20,000 WBCs.)
- CMP
- Diagnosis often made on clinical grounds. Potential testing includes the following:
  - Genital tract cultures and rapid test for group B streptococci (may be done during labor)
  - Amniotic fluid Gram stain: usually polymicrobial
  - Uterine tissue cultures: Prep the cervix with disinfectant and use a shielded specimen collector as samples are very difficult to obtain without contamination.
- If the patient meets criteria for SIRS and/or suspected sepsis, follow institution guidelines (i.e., serum lactate, fluid resuscitation, two sets of blood cultures, and timely administration of broad spectrum antibiotics).

- If patient not responding to antibiotics in 24 to 48 hours:
  - Ultrasound for retained products of conception, pelvic abscess, or mass
  - CT or MRI looking for pelvic vein thrombophlebitis, abscess, or deep-seated wound infection

Diagnostic Procedures/Other
Paracentesis/culdocentesis with culture rarely necessary

Test Interpretation
- Superficial layer of infected necrotic tissue in microscopic sections of uterine lining
- >5 neutrophils per high-power field in superficial endometrium; ≥1 plasma cell in endometrial stroma

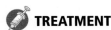

TREATMENT

MEDICATION
First Line
- Clindamycin 900 mg IV q8h + gentamicin 5 mg/kg IV q24h
  - Potential side effects include nephrotoxicity, ototoxicity, pseudomembranous colitis, or diarrhea (in up to 6%).

Second Line
- Ampicillin/sulbactam 3 g IV q6h
- Metronidazole 500 mg IV or PO q8–12h + penicillin 5,000,000 U IV q6h, or
- Ampicillin 2 g IV q6h + gentamicin 5 mg/kg IV q24h
- Cefoxitin 2 g IV q6h. Add ampicillin 2 g IV q6h, if clinical failure after 48 hours.
- Cefotetan 2 g IV q12h. Add ampicillin 2 g IV q6h, if clinical failure after 48 hours.
- Note: Base therapy on cultures, sensitivities, and clinical response.
- Contraindications
  - Drug allergy, renal failure (aminoglycosides)
  - Avoid sulfa, tetracyclines, and fluoroquinolones before delivery and if breastfeeding. Metronidazole is relatively contraindicated if breastfeeding.
- Precautions:
  - Clindamycin and other antibiotics occasionally cause pseudomembranous colitis.
  - Antibiotic-associated diarrhea (Clostridium difficile)
  - Gentamicin can cause renal injury.
- Note: Consider adding a macrolide antibiotic (for chlamydia coverage) and/or ampicillin (for coverage of enterococci) for infections persisting after 48 hours.
- Note: In regions with high levels of group B streptococcal resistance to clindamycin consider adding ampicillin.
- Note: Heparin typically indicated for septic pelvic vein thrombophlebitis; requires 10 days of full anticoagulation

SURGERY/OTHER PROCEDURES
- Ultrasound to look for retained products of conception if not responsive to initial therapy
- Curettage for retained products of conception
- Surgery or image-guided drainage to drain abscess

ADMISSION, INPATIENT, AND NURSING CONSIDERATIONS
- Inpatient care is recommended for postpartum infections.
- Many infections occur after hospital discharge. Therefore, education regarding the importance of fever, pain, heavy vaginal bleeding, foul-smelling lochia, or other signs of infection should occur prior to discharge (1).
- IV antibiotics and close observation for severe infections
- Open and drain infected wounds.
- Optimize fluid status.

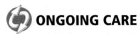

ONGOING CARE

FOLLOW-UP RECOMMENDATIONS
Patient Monitoring
- Individualize according to severity.
- IV antibiotics can be stopped when the patient is afebrile for 24 to 48 hours.
- Oral antibiotics on discharge are not necessary, unless patient was bacteremic; then continue oral antibiotics to complete a 7-day course.

DIET
As tolerated, although may be limited by ileus

PATIENT EDUCATION
- Advise patient to contact physician with fever >38°C (100.4°F) postpartum, heavy vaginal bleeding, foul-smelling lochia, or other symptoms of infection.
- Information available at http://www.healthline.com/health/pregnancy/complications-postpartum-endometritis

PROGNOSIS
With supportive therapy and appropriate antibiotics, most patients improve quickly and recover without complication.

COMPLICATIONS
- Resistant organisms, peritonitis, pelvic abscess
- Septic pelvic thrombophlebitis, ovarian vein thrombosis
- Sepsis, death

REFERENCES

1. Knight M, Chiocchia V, Partlett C, et al. Prophylactic antibiotics in the prevention of infection after operative vaginal delivery (ANODE): a multicentre randomised controlled trial. Lancet. 2019;393(10189):2395–2403.
2. Bollig C, Nothacker M, Lehane C, et al. Prophylactic antibiotics before cord clamping in cesarean delivery: a systematic review. Acta Obstet Gynecol Scand. 2018;97(5):521–535.
3. Committee on Practice Bulletins-Obstetrics. ACOG Practice Bulletin No. 199: use of prophylactic antibiotics in labor and delivery. Obstet Gynecol. 2018;132(3):e103–e119.

ADDITIONAL READING
Carter EB, Temming LA, Fowler S, et al. Evidence-based bundles and cesarean delivery surgical site infections: a systematic review and meta-analysis. Obstet Gynecol. 2017;130(4):735–746.

 SEE ALSO

Algorithm: Pelvic Pain

 CODES

ICD10
- O86.12 Endometritis following delivery
- O86.4 Pyrexia of unknown origin following delivery
- O86.13 Vaginitis following delivery

CLINICAL PEARLS
- Postpartum endometritis follows 1–3% of all births.
- Infections are typically polymicrobial and involve organisms ascending from the lower genital tract.
- Evidence supports antibiotic prophylaxis prior to skin incision for all cesarean deliveries but not for operative vaginal deliveries.
- Clindamycin 900 mg IV q8h and gentamicin 5 mg/kg q24h are recommended as first-line therapy for endometritis. Treat until the patient is afebrile for 24 to 48 hours and stop antibiotics completely (unless there is documented bacteremia, which requires a 7-day course of therapy).
- If no improvement occurs on antibiotics, consider retained placental products, abscess, wound infection, hematoma, cellulitis, phlegmon, or septic pelvic vein thrombosis.

E

ENURESIS

Hermione Gaw, MD • Nancy V. Nguyen, DO

BASICS

DESCRIPTION
- Classification
  - Primary nocturnal enuresis (NE): 80% of all cases; person who has never established urinary continence on consecutive nights for a period of ≥6 months
  - Secondary NE: 20% of cases; resumption of enuresis after at least 6 months of urinary continence
- NE: intermittent nocturnal incontinence after the anticipated age of bladder control (age 5 years)
  - Primary monosymptomatic NE (PMNE): bedwetting with no history of bladder dysfunction or other lower urinary tract (LUT) symptoms
  - Nonmonosymptomatic NE (NMNE): bed-wetting with LUT symptoms such as frequency, urgency, daytime wetting, hesitancy, straining, weak or intermittent stream, post-urination dribbling, lower abdominal or genital discomfort, or sensation of incomplete emptying

ALERT
Adult-onset NE with absent daytime incontinence is a serious symptom; complete urologic evaluation and therapy are warranted.

- System(s) affected: nervous, renal/urologic
- Synonym(s): bed-wetting; sleep enuresis; nocturnal incontinence; primary NE

EPIDEMIOLOGY
Incidence
- Depends on family history
- Spontaneous resolution: 15% per year

Prevalence
- Very common; 5 to 7 million children in the United States
- 10% of 7-year-olds; 3% of 11- to 12-year-olds; 0.5–1.7% at 16 to 17 years old (1)
- 2 to 3 times more common in males than females
- Nocturnal > daytime (3:1)

Geriatric Considerations
Infrequent; often associated with daytime incontinence (formerly referred to as diurnal enuresis)

ETIOLOGY AND PATHOPHYSIOLOGY
- A disorder of sleep arousal, a low nocturnal bladder capacity, and nocturnal polyuria are the three factors that interrelate to cause NE.
- Both functional and organic causes (below); many theories, none absolutely confirmed
- Detrusor instability
- Deficiency of arginine vasopressin (AVP); decreased nocturnal AVP or decreased AVP stimulation secondary to an empty bladder (Bladder distension stimulates AVP.)
- Maturational delay of CNS
- Severe NE with some evidence of interaction between bladder overactivity and brain arousability: association with children with severe NE and frequent cortical arousals in sleep
- Organic urologic causes in 1–4% of enuresis in children: urinary tract infection (UTI), occult spina bifida, ectopic ureter, lazy bladder syndrome, irritable bladder with wide bladder neck, posterior urethral valves, neurologic bladder dysfunction

- Organic nonurologic causes: epilepsy, diabetes mellitus, food allergies, obstructive sleep apnea, chronic renal failure, hyperthyroidism, pinworm infection, sickle cell disease
- NE occurs in all stages of sleep.

Genetics
Most commonly, NE is an autosomal-dominant inheritance pattern with high penetrance (90%).
- 1/3 of all cases are sporadic.
- 75% of children with enuresis have a first-degree relative with the condition.
- Higher rates in monozygotic versus dizygotic twins (68% vs. 36%)
- If both parents had NE, risk in child is 77%; 44% if one parent is affected. Parental age of resolution often predicts when child's enuresis should resolve.

RISK FACTORS
- Family history
- Stressors (emotional, environmental) common in secondary enuresis (e.g., divorce, death)
- Constipation and/or encopresis
- Organic disease: 1% of monosymptomatic NE (e.g., urologic and nonurologic causes)
- Psychological disorders
  - Comorbid disorders are highest with secondary NE: depression, anxiety, social phobias, conduct disorder, hyperkinetic syndrome, internalizing disorders.
  - Association with ADHD; more pronounced in ages 9 to 12 years
- Altered mental status or impaired mobility

COMMONLY ASSOCIATED CONDITIONS
- Obstructive sleep apnea syndrome (10–54%) (2): Atrial natriuretic factor inhibits renin-angiotensin-aldosterone pathway leading to diuresis.
- Constipation (33–75%) (2)
- Behavioral problems (specifically ADHD in 12–17%) (2)
- Overactive bladder or dysfunctional voiding (up to 41%) (2)
- UTI (18–60%) (2)

DIAGNOSIS

HISTORY
- LUT symptoms
- Daily intake patterns; voiding and stooling patterns (voiding diary); constipation issues
- Psychosocial history (patient, parental, school/bullying, etc.)
- Family history of enuresis

PHYSICAL EXAM
- ENT: evaluation for adenotonsillar hypertrophy (associated with sleep apnea)
- Abdomen: enlarged bladder, kidneys, fecal masses
- Back: dimpling, tufts of hair on sacrum
- Genitourinary exam
  - Males: meatal stenosis, hypospadias, epispadias, phimosis
  - Females: vulvitis, vaginitis, labial adhesions, ureterocele at introitus; evidence of abuse
- Rectal exam: tone, fecal soiling, fecal impaction. In adult males, DRE for prostate enlargement.
- Neurologic exam, especially lower extremities

DIFFERENTIAL DIAGNOSIS
- Primary NE
  - Delayed physiologic urinary control
  - UTI (both primary and secondary)
  - Spina bifida occulta
  - Obstructive sleep apnea (both primary and secondary)
  - Idiopathic detrusor instability
  - Previously unrecognized myelopathy or neuropathy (e.g., multiple sclerosis, tethered cord, epilepsy)
  - Anatomic urinary tract abnormality (e.g., ectopic ureter)
- Secondary NE
  - Acute situational stress (most common cause)
  - Bladder outlet obstruction
  - Neurologic disease, neurogenic bladder (e.g., spinal cord injury)

DIAGNOSTIC TESTS & INTERPRETATION
Initial Tests (lab, imaging)
- Only obligatory test in children is urinalysis.
- Urinalysis and urine culture: UTI, pyuria, hematuria, proteinuria, glycosuria, and poor concentrating ability (low specific gravity) may suggest organic etiology, especially in adults.
- Urinary tract imaging is usually not necessary.
- If abnormal clinical findings: renal and bladder ultrasound.
- IV pyelogram, voiding cystourethrogram (VCUG), or retrograde pyelogram is rarely indicated.
- MRI if spinal dysraphism is suspected

Follow-Up Tests & Special Considerations
- Secondary enuresis: (if no psychosocial factors identified) serum glucose, BUN, creatinine, thyroid-stimulating hormone (TSH), urine culture
- In children, imaging and urodynamic studies are helpful for significant daytime symptoms, history of UTIs, suspected structural abnormalities, and in refractory cases.

Diagnostic Procedures/Other
Urodynamic studies may be beneficial.

TREATMENT

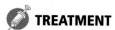

GENERAL MEASURES
- Use nonpharmacologic approaches as first line before prescribing medications (2)[A].
- Simple behavioral interventions (e.g., scheduled wakening, positive reinforcement, bladder training, diet changes) are effective, although less so than alarms or medications (2)[B]; found to achieve dryness in 15–20% of cases (1)
  - Patient education (fragmented sleep, low nocturnal bladder capacity, and increased nocturnal urine production)
  - Encourage normal daytime drinking and reduction of intake 2 hours prior to sleep.
  - Voiding before bed and scheduled waking for nighttime voiding
  - Nightlights to light the way to the bathroom
  - Reward system for dry nights

- Use pull up over regular underwear or cloth underwear with built in waterproof barrier.
- "Cleanliness training": child helps with changing wet bedding
- Do not shame or punish bed-wetting; have child participate in removing/laundering soiled bedding.
- Treat underlying constipation.
- Secondary enuresis:
  - Referral for behavioral counseling if suspicion
  - Stool softeners and cathartics if constipation present
- If behavioral interventions alone have no success, combined therapy (e.g., enuresis alarm, bladder training, motivational therapy, and pelvic floor muscle training) is more effective than each component alone or than pharmacotherapy (2)[A].
- Enuresis alarms (bells or buzzers)
  - 66–70% success rate; must be used nightly for 2 to 4 months; offers cure; significant parental involvement
  - If successful, it should be used until 14 consecutive dry nights are achieved.

MEDICATION

First Line

Desmopressin (DDAVP): synthetic analogue of vasopressin that decreases nocturnal urine output (1)[A]

- Intranasal DDAVP: adults only, 20 mg (2 sprays) intranasally at bedtime
  - FDA recommends against use in children due to reports of severe hyponatremia resulting in seizures and deaths in children using intranasal formulations of desmopressin.
- Oral DDAVP: safe in children; available in tablet or fast-melting oral lyophilisate form (not available in the United States). Begin with 0.2-mg tablet taken at bedtime on empty stomach; after 14 days of inefficient treatment, can titrate up to 0.4 mg (1).
  - Maximally effective in 1 hour; effect lasts from 8 to 10 hours.
  - If treatment is successful, can be continued for 3 months, then stop for 2 weeks for test of dryness
  - High relapse rate after discontinuation without a structured withdrawal program. If relapse occurs, oral desmopressin can continue to be prescribed in 3-month blocks.
  - Important side effects: water intoxication and hyponatremia, presenting as headache, nausea, vomiting, and convulsions. Fluid intake in the evening can be restricted to 200–250 mL and no drinks during the night to avoid excessive fluid intake. Suspend the dose in children who display symptoms.
  - 60–70% success; 30% of children have full response and 40% have partial response.
  - Long-lasting curative effect is low.

Pediatric Considerations

FDA recommends against using intranasal formulations of desmopressin in children due to reports of severe hyponatremia resulting in seizures and deaths (2)[A].

Second Line

- Anticholinergics: Monotherapy is not recommended in children. Before considering, screen for constipation and residual urine.
  - Oxybutynin (Ditropan, Ditropan XL, Oxytrol patch): anticholinergic; smooth muscle relaxant, antispasmodic; may increase functional bladder capacity and aids in timed voiding
    - 30–50% success; 50% relapse after stopped
    - Ditropan: adults: 5 mg PO TID–QID; children >5 years old with overactive bladder who have failed alarm therapy and desmopressin can try 5 mg at bedtime
    - Ditropan XL: adults: 5 mg/day PO; increase to 30 mg/day PO (5- to 10-mg tablet).
    - Oxytrol patch: one patch every 3 to 4 days (3.9 mg/patch) (Periodic trials of the medication, i.e., weekends or weeks at a time, will help determine efficacy and resolution of primary disturbance.)
  - Other anticholinergics (may be used in adults; not yet approved for label use in children): tolterodine 2 to 4 mg/day, fesoterodine 4 to 8 mg/day, solifenacin 5 to 10 mg/day.
- Imipramine (Tofranil): tricyclic antidepressant, anticholinergic effects; increases bladder capacity, antispasmodic properties
  - Dose: adults, 25 to 75 mg and children aged >6 years, 10 to 25 mg PO given 1 hour before bedtime; increase by 10 to 25 mg at 1- to 2-week intervals; treat for 2 to 3 months and consider drug holiday for 2 weeks before restarting. When discontinuing, taper by halving dosage every 1 to 2 weeks.
  - Desmopressin may be added if the effect is incomplete.
  - 40% success rate but relapses after discontinuation are high (1)
  - Pretreatment ECG recommended identifying underlying rhythm disorders such as long QT syndrome.
- Precautions
  - Oxybutynin: glaucoma, myasthenia gravis, GI or genitourinary obstruction, ulcerative colitis, constipation, megacolon; use a decreased dose in the elderly.
  - Tolterodine: urinary retention, gastric retention, constipation, uncontrolled narrow-angle glaucoma; significant drug interactions with CYP2D6, CYP3A3/4 substrates
  - Desmopressin: Avoid in patients at risk for electrolyte changes or fluid retention (congestive heart failure [CHF], renal insufficiency). Stop during gastroenteritis or other acute illness with risk of dehydration.
  - Imipramine: Do not use with monoamine oxidase inhibitors (MAOIs), hypotension, and arrhythmias; low-toxic therapeutic ratio.
- Combination therapy with DDAVP and oxybutynin has better results than individual use.

ISSUES FOR REFERRAL

- Primary NE: persistent enuresis despite nonpharmacologic and pharmacologic therapies
- Diurnal incontinence or nonmonosymptomatic enuresis with voiding dysfunction or underlying medical condition

COMPLEMENTARY & ALTERNATIVE MEDICINE

Acupuncture has small amounts of supportive data.

 ## ONGOING CARE

FOLLOW-UP RECOMMENDATIONS

Patient Monitoring

- With nonpharmacologic treatment, reassess every 1 to 3 months.
- With enuresis alarm, reassess in 1 to 3 weeks.
- With DDAVP, reassess in 1 to 2 weeks, then every 3 months.
- With imipramine, reassess in 1 month (monitor for UTI or constipation).

DIET

Limit fluid and caffeine intake 1 to 2 hours before sleep.

PATIENT EDUCATION

- http://www.hypnoticworld.com/hypnosis-scripts/habits-disorders/enuresis; http://wetstop.com; www.dri-sleeper.com; www.nitetrain-r.com; https://bedwettingstore.com
- App Store for free bed-wetting diary apps (e.g., My Dryness Tracker, Bedwetting Tracker, HapPee Time)

PROGNOSIS

In children, NE is usually self-limiting; 1% will persist as adult; evaluate for organic causes.

COMPLICATIONS

UTI, perineal excoriation, psychological disturbance (especially in children)

REFERENCES

1. Kuwertz-Bröking E, von Gontard A. Clinical management of nocturnal enuresis. *Pediatr Nephrol*. 2018;33(7):1145–1154.
2. Baird DC, Seehusen DA, Bode DV. Enuresis in children: a case based approach. *Am Fam Physician*. 2014;90(8):560–568.

 ## SEE ALSO

- Incontinence, Urinary Adult Female; Incontinence, Urinary Adult Male
- Algorithm: Enuresis, Secondary

 ## CODES

ICD10

- N39.44 Nocturnal enuresis
- R32 Unspecified urinary incontinence
- F98.0 Enuresis not due to a substance or known physiol condition

CLINICAL PEARLS

- Behavioral and lifestyle interventions are the first-line treatment for PMNE; alarms and desmopressin are the most effective treatments.
- Secondary enuresis: most often due to psychosocial factors

EPICONDYLITIS

Julie A. Creech, DO • Caleb Weiss Kiesow, MD, BS

BASICS

DESCRIPTION
- Tendinopathy of the elbow characterized by pain and tenderness at the myotendinous junctions or tendinous insertions of the wrist flexors/extensors at the humeral epicondyles
- Although commonly known as medial and lateral epicondylitis, without microscopic histologic examination, the more appropriate term is medial epicondyle tendinopathy (MET) and lateral epicondyle tendinopathy (LET).
- Most commonly secondary to chronic (overuse) pathology, although acute (traumatic) etiology can occur
- Two types
  - MET/common flexor tendinopathy (CFT) ("golfer's elbow")
    ○ Involves the wrist flexors and pronators, which have proximal attachment at the medial epicondyle
  - LET/common extensor tendinopathy (CET) ("tennis elbow")
    ○ Involves the wrist extensors and supinators, which have proximal attachment at the lateral epicondyle
    ○ Most commonly involves the extensor carpi radialis brevis (ERCB) tendon
- May be caused by various different athletic or occupational activities
- Common in carpenters, plumbers, gardeners, and overhead athletes
- 75% of cases involve the dominant arm.

EPIDEMIOLOGY
- Predominant age: >40 years
- Predominant sex: male = female

Incidence
- Common overuse injury
- Lateral > medial
- Estimated between 1% and 3%

Prevalence
- MET: 0.4%
- LET: 1.3%

ETIOLOGY AND PATHOPHYSIOLOGY
- Acute (tendonitis)
  - Rare, uncommon pathology
  - Inflammatory response to injury or sudden, violent contraction
- Chronic (tendinosis or tendinopathy)
  - Overuse injury
  - Repetitive wrist flexion (MET) or extension (LET) places strain across enthesis of flexor or extensor group, respectively.
  - Degeneration, calcium deposition, fibroblast proliferation, microvascular proliferation, hyaline cartilage destruction, diminished restorative inflammatory response
- Aggravating activities
  - Tool/racquet griping
  - Shaking hands
  - Occupational (painters, mechanics, cooks)
  - Sports (golf, tennis, archery, pitchers)

RISK FACTORS
- Repetitive wrist motions
  - Flexion/pronation: medial epicondyle tendinopathy
  - Extension/supination: lateral epicondyle tendinopathy
- Smoking
- Obesity
- Forceful activities of the upper extremity

GENERAL PREVENTION
- Limit overuse of the wrist flexors, extensors, pronators, and supinators.
- Use proper technique when working with hand tools or playing racquet sports.
- Use lighter tools and smaller grips.

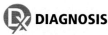**DIAGNOSIS**

HISTORY
- Insidious onset
- Pain localized to lateral or medial elbow, at or just distal to bony epicondyle
- Aching pain, often radiates from epicondyle to forearm or wrist
- Pain with gripping
- Sensation of mild forearm weakness

PHYSICAL EXAM
- Localized pain at or just distal to the affected epicondyle
- MET
  - Tenderness at origin of wrist flexor tendons
  - Increased pain with resisted wrist flexion and pronation
  - Normal elbow range of motion
  - Increased pain with gripping
- LET
  - Tenderness at origin of wrist extensors
  - Increased pain with resisted wrist extension and supination
  - Normal elbow range of motion
  - Increased pain with gripping

DIFFERENTIAL DIAGNOSIS
- Arthritis, such as posterior osteophytes
- Epicondylar fractures
- Posterior interosseous nerve entrapment (lateral elbow pain)
- Radial tunnel syndrome (lateral elbow pain)
- Ulnar neuropathy (medial elbow pain)
- Pronator syndrome (anteromedial elbow pain)
- Synovitis
- Thoracic outlet syndrome
- Medial collateral ligament injury
- Referred pain from shoulder or neck

DIAGNOSTIC TESTS & INTERPRETATION
Initial Tests (lab, imaging)
No imaging is required for initial evaluation and treatment of a classic overuse injury.

Follow-Up Tests & Special Considerations
- Anterior-posterior (A-P)/lateral radiographs if decreased range of motion, trauma, or no improvement with initial conservative therapy; assess for fractures or signs of arthritis.
- For recalcitrant cases
  - Musculoskeletal ultrasound (US) reveals abnormal tendon appearance (e.g., hypoechoic, tendon thickening, partial tear at tendon origin, calcifications, hyperemia). US can also guide injections of prolotherapy, platelet-rich plasma (PRP), steroid and/or anesthetic.
  - MRI can show intermediate or high T2 signal intensity within the common flexor or extensor tendon or the presence of peritendinous soft tissue edema.

Diagnostic Procedures/Other
Infiltration of local anesthetic with subsequent resolution of symptoms supports the diagnosis if clinically in doubt.

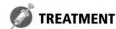**TREATMENT**

GENERAL MEASURES
Initial treatment consists of activity modification, counterforce bracing, oral or topical NSAIDs, ice, and physical therapy.

- If left untreated, symptoms typically last between 6 months and 2 years. For patients with good function and minimal pain, consider conservative management using a "wait and see" approach based on patient's preference.
- Modify activity, encourage relative rest, and correct faulty biomechanics.
- Bracing
  - Splinting is not recommended except for severe cases, as it is associated with higher rates of limited duty, more medical visits, higher charges, and longer duration of treatment than those managed without splints.
  - Counterforce bracing with a forearm strap is easy and inexpensive. Systematic reviews are inconclusive about overall efficacy, but initial bracing may improve the ability to perform daily activities in the first 6 weeks.
- Ice frequently after activities
- Physical therapy
  - Infiltration of local anesthetic can reduce pain and may permit better participation in physical therapy.
  - Eccentric strength training and stretching program
  - Therapeutic US
  - Corticosteroid iontophoresis
  - Dry needling

MEDICATION

First Line

- Topical NSAIDs: Low-quality evidence suggests topical NSAIDS are significantly more effective than placebo with respect to pain and number needed to treat to benefit (NNT = 7) in the short term (up to 4 weeks) with minimal adverse effects (1)[A].
- Oral NSAIDs: unclear efficacy with respect to pain and function, but may offer short-term pain relief; associated with adverse GI effects (1)[A]

Second Line

Corticosteroid injections: short-term (≤8 weeks) reduction in pain; no benefits found for intermediate or long-term outcomes (2)[A]. Corticosteroid injections demonstrated favorable outcomes compared with local PRP treatments for lateral elbow epicondylitis during the short-term follow-up period (4 weeks and 8 weeks posttreatment). Otherwise, at the long-term follow-up (24 weeks posttreatment), PRP injections had improved pain and function more effectively than corticosteroid injections (3)[A].

ISSUES FOR REFERRAL

Failure of conservative therapy

ADDITIONAL THERAPIES

Given the mechanism of injury, many new treatments are targeted at strengthening the underlying tendon rather than strict palliation of pain. High-quality evidence is limited for many of these interventions.

- Glyceryl trinitrate (GTN) transdermal patch
  - Nitric oxide (NO) is a small free radical generated by NO synthesis. NO is expressed by fibroblasts and is postulated to aid in collagen synthesis. Topical application of GTN theoretically improves healing by this mechanism. One-fourth of a 5-mg/24-hr GTN transdermal patch is applied once daily for up to 24 weeks.
  - Significant decreases in pain are seen at 3 weeks and 6 months compared to placebo patch.
- Extracorporeal shock wave therapy (ESWT) is a noninvasive, nonelectrical therapy found to be 89% effective in treating LET in some studies and is noted to be as effective as WES (4)[B].
- Prolotherapy
  - Injection of a dextrose solution into and around the tendon attachment stimulates a localized inflammatory response, leading to increased blood flow to stimulate healing.
- PRP injections
  - Injection of supraphysiologic autologous PRP leads to a local inflammatory response. Platelets degranulate, release growth factors, and stimulate the physiologic healing cascade.
  - PRP treatment of chronic LET significantly reduces pain and increases function. The benefit exceeds that of corticosteroid injection even after a follow-up of 1 year.
- US-guided percutaneous needle tenotomy
  - Injection of a local anesthetic followed by US-guided tendon fenestration, aspiration, and abrasion of the underlying bone; thought to break apart scar tissue and stimulate inflammation and healing
  - Usually requires referral to sports medicine or orthopedic physician with specific equipment and training

- Autologous tenocyte injection (ATI)
  - Two-step process
  - Small number of tenocytes are harvested, often from patellar tendon, and cultured.
  - Cultured tenocytes are then injected into tendon to help stimulate regeneration.
- Botulinum toxin A for chronic LET
  - Injections into the forearm extensor muscles (60 U) can be performed in the outpatient setting.

SURGERY/OTHER PROCEDURES

- Surgical intervention required in only 2.8% of patients
- Elbow surgery may be indicated in refractory cases:
  - Involves débridement and tendon release
  - Can be performed open or arthroscopically
  - Improvements in VAS, DASH scores, and grip strength seen in 5-year study (5)[B]
- Denervation of the lateral humeral epicondyle
  - Transection of the posterior cutaneous nerve of the forearm with implantation into the triceps may help with chronic symptoms and pain.

COMPLEMENTARY & ALTERNATIVE MEDICINE

Acupuncture: effective for short-term pain relief for lateral epicondyle pain

 ONGOING CARE

PROGNOSIS

Good: Majority resolve with conservative care.

REFERENCES

1. Pattanittum P, Turner T, Green S, et al. Non-steroidal anti-inflammatory drugs (NSAIDs) for treating lateral elbow pain in adults. *Cochrane Database Syst Rev*. 2013;2013(5):CD003686.
2. Krogh TP, Bartels EM, Ellingsen T, et al. Comparative effectiveness of injection therapies in lateral epicondylitis: a systematic review and network meta-analysis of randomized controlled trials. *Am J Sports Med*. 2013;41(6):1435–1446.
3. Li A, Wang H, Yu Z, et al. Platelet-rich plasma vs corticosteroids for elbow epicondylitis: a systematic review and meta-analysis. *Medicine (Baltimore)*. 2019;98(51):e18358.
4. Aydın A, Atiç R. Comparison of extracorporeal shock-wave therapy and wrist-extensor splint application in the treatment of lateral epicondylitis: a prospective randomized controlled study. *J Pain Res*. 2018;11:1459–1467.
5. Han SH, Lee JK, Kim HJ, et al. The result of surgical treatment of medial epicondylitis: analysis with more than a 5-year follow-up. *J Shoulder Elbow Surg*. 2016;25(10):1704–1709.

ADDITIONAL READING

- Cullinane FL, Boocock MG, Trevelyan FC. Is eccentric exercise an effective treatment for lateral epicondylitis? A systematic review. *Clin Rehabil*. 2014;28(1):3–19.
- Dingemanse R, Randsdorp M, Koes BW, et al. Evidence for the effectiveness of electrophysical modalities for treatment of medial and lateral epicondylitis: a systematic review. *Br J Sports Med*. 2014;48(12):957–965.
- Green S, Buchbinder R, Barnsley L, et al. Acupuncture for lateral elbow pain. *Cochrane Database Syst Rev*. 2002;(1):CD003527.
- Lin YC, Wu WT, Hsu YC, et al. Comparative effectiveness of botulinum toxin versus non-surgical treatments for treating lateral epicondylitis: a systematic review and meta-analysis. *Clin Rehabil*. 2018;32(2):131–145.
- Mattie R, Wong J, McCormick Z, et al. Percutaneous needle tenotomy for the treatment of lateral epicondylitis: a systematic review of the literature. *PM R*. 2017;9(6):603–611.
- Ozden R, Uruç V, Doğramaci Y, et al. Management of tennis elbow with topical glyceryl trinitrate. *Acta Orthop Traumatol Turc*. 2014;48(2):175–180.

 SEE ALSO

Algorithm: Pain in Upper Extremity

 CODES

ICD10

- M77.00 Medial epicondylitis, unspecified elbow
- M77.10 Lateral epicondylitis, unspecified elbow
- M77.01 Medial epicondylitis, right elbow

CLINICAL PEARLS

- MET (golfer's elbow) is characterized by pain and tenderness at the tendinous origins of the wrist flexors on the medial epicondyle.
- LET (tennis elbow) is characterized by pain and tenderness at the tendinous origins of the wrist extensors on the lateral epicondyle.
- Left untreated, symptoms typically last between 6 months and 2 years.
- Most patients improve using conservative treatment with oral NSAIDs, activity modification, and physical therapy.
- Newer therapies such as ATI, PRP, prolotherapy, and tenotomy are directed toward tendon regeneration.

E

EPIDIDYMITIS
Jarrett Keller Sell, MD, FAAFP, AAHIVS • Michael T. Partin, MD

BASICS

DESCRIPTION
- Inflammation (infectious or noninfectious) of the epididymis resulting in scrotal pain and swelling, induration of the posterior epididymis, involvement of the adjacent testicle, and possible hydrocele formation
- Acute epididymitis: scrotal pain for <6 weeks
- Chronic epididymitis: scrotal pain for ≥6 weeks
- Epididymitis with involvement of the testis is named epididymo-orchitis
- Classification: infectious (bacterial, viral, fungal, parasitic) versus noninfectious (chemical, traumatic, autoimmune, idiopathic, industrial, vaso-epididymal reflux syndrome)
- System(s) affected: reproductive

EPIDEMIOLOGY
- Predominant age: generally younger, sexually active men or older men with UTIs and bladder outlet obstruction (e.g., benign prostatic hyperplasia [BPH])
- Predominant sex: male only

Pediatric Considerations
Epididymitis is found to be the most common cause of acute scrotal pain in prepubertal boys—more common than testicular torsion.

Incidence
- Common (600,000 cases annually in the United States) (1)
- 1 in 1,000 adult males per year
- 1.2 in 1,000 boys aged 2 to 13 years per year (2),(3)

Prevalence
Common

ETIOLOGY AND PATHOPHYSIOLOGY
- Infectious epididymitis
  - Retrograde passage of urinary bacteria from the prostate or urethra to the epididymis via the ejaculatory ducts and the vas deferens; rarely, hematogenous spread
  - Causative organism is identified in 80% of patients and varies according to patient age.
- Noninfectious epididymitis
  - Often, no etiology is found; however, can be instigated by trauma, autoimmune disease, or vasculitis
  - Likely secondary to reflux of sterile urine causing a chemical inflammation
  - Can develop as sequelae of strenuous exercise with a full bladder when urine is pushed through internal urethral sphincter (located at proximal end of prostatic urethra) or prolonged periods of sitting
  - Reflux of urine through orifice of ejaculatory ducts at verumontanum may occur with history of urethritis/prostatitis because inflammation may produce rigidity in musculature surrounding orifice to ejaculatory ducts, holding them open.
  - Exposure of epididymis to foreign fluid may produce inflammatory reaction within 24 hours.
- <14 years of age
  - Cause largely unknown, although likely from anatomic abnormalities resulting in urine reflux such as vesicoureteral reflux, ectopic ureter, or anorectal malformation (rectourethral fistula)
  - May also result from postinfectious syndrome from *Mycoplasma pneumoniae*, enterovirus, or adenovirus
  - Henoch-Schönlein purpura may present as acute scrotal pain.

- 14 to 35 years of age
  - Usually *Chlamydia trachomatis*, *Neisseria gonorrhoeae*, or *Mycoplasma genitalium* in sexually active males
  - With anal intercourse, likely enteric pathogens (e.g., *Escherichia coli*)
- >35 years
  - Commonly enteric bacteria but occasionally *Staphylococcus aureus* or *Staphylococcus epidermidis*
  - In elderly men, often with distal urinary tract obstruction, BPH, UTI, or catheterization
  - Tuberculosis (TB), if sterile pyuria, nodularity of vas deferens (hematogenous spread), and recent infection. TB is the most common granulomatous disease affecting the epididymis.
  - Sterile urine reflux after transurethral prostatectomy
  - Granulomatous reaction following BCG intravesical therapy for bladder cancer
- Amiodarone may cause a dose-dependent noninfectious epididymitis; usually resolves with decreasing drug dosage (<200 mg/day)
- Syphilis, blastomycosis, coccidioidomycosis, and cryptococcosis are rare causes, but brucellosis can be a common cause in endemic areas.

RISK FACTORS
- UTI
- Prostatitis
- Indwelling urethral catheter
- Urethral instrumentation or transurethral surgery
- Urethral or meatal stricture
- Transrectal prostate biopsy
- Prostate brachytherapy (seeds) for prostate cancer
- Anal intercourse
- High-risk sexual activity
- Strenuous physical activity
- Prolonged sedentary periods
- Bladder obstruction (BPH, prostate cancer)
- HIV-immunosuppressed patient
- Severe Behçet disease
- Presence of foreskin
- Constipation
- Increased intra-abdominal pressure (due to frequent physical strain)
  - Military recruits, especially who begin physically unprepared
  - Laborers; restaurant kitchen workers
  - Full bladder during intense physical exertion

GENERAL PREVENTION
- Safer sexual practices
- Mumps vaccination
- Antibiotic prophylaxis for urethral manipulation
- Early treatment of prostatitis/BPH
- Vasectomy or vasoligation during transurethral surgery
- Avoid vigorous rectal exam with acute prostatitis.
- Emptying the bladder prior to physical exertion
- Physically conditioning the body prior to engaging in regular intense physical exertion
- Treat constipation.

COMMONLY ASSOCIATED CONDITIONS
- Prostatitis/urethritis/orchitis
- Hematospermia
- Constipation
- UTI

DIAGNOSIS

HISTORY
- Gradual onset of scrotal pain, sometimes radiating to the groin region over 1 to 2 days
- Urethral discharge or symptoms of UTI, such as urinary frequency, dysuria, cloudy urine, or hematuria
- Detailed sexual history, especially new exposures
- Fever only in 11–19% (3)
- Progresses from the posterior-lying epididymis to the body/head of epididymis
- Entire hemiscrotum may become swollen and red; the testis becomes indistinguishable from the epididymis; the scrotal wall becomes thick and indurated, and reactive hydrocele may occur.
- Noninfectious epididymitis
  - Unilateral scrotal pain/swelling preceded by prolonged intense physical exertion with full bladder
  - No symptoms of infection

Pediatric Considerations
- Bacteremia from *Haemophilus influenzae* infection may produce acute epididymitis.
- Must rule out testicular torsion (with scrotal ultrasound [US]) in adolescent males particularly aged >13 years.
- History not helpful in distinguishing epididymitis from testicular torsion

Geriatric Considerations
Patients with diabetic neuropathy may have no pain despite severe infection/abscess.

PHYSICAL EXAM
- Epididymis is markedly tender to palpation.
- The tail of the epididymis is larger in comparison with the contralateral side.
- Elevation of the testis in epididymis reduces the discomfort (Prehn sign).
- Absence of a cremasteric reflex should raise suspicion for testicular torsion.

DIFFERENTIAL DIAGNOSIS
- Testicular/testicular appendage torsion
- Urethritis/orchitis
- Testicular trauma
- Epididymal congestion following vasectomy
- Testicular malignancy
- Epididymal cyst
- Inguinal hernia
- Spermatocele
- Hydrocele
- Hematocele
- Varicocele
- Epididymal adenomatoid tumor
- Epididymal rhabdomyosarcoma
- Vasculitis (Henoch-Schönlein purpura)

DIAGNOSTIC TESTS & INTERPRETATION
Initial Tests (lab, imaging)
- All suspected cases should be evaluated for objective evidence of inflammation by one of the following:
  - Urinalysis/urine culture preferably on first-void urine to evaluate for positive leukocyte esterase and bacteriuria
  - Urine culture/Gram stain urethral discharge; ≥2 WBC per oil immersion field; evaluate for gonococcal infection.
  - Microscopic examination of sediment from a spun first-void urine with ≥10 WBC per high-power field
- Urine gonorrhea and chlamydia testing for all suspected cases

- Elevated CRP level can help distinguish epididymitis from testicular torsion (2).
- A clear urinalysis and negative culture suggest noninfectious epididymitis.
- If testicular torsion/mass cannot be excluded (especially in children), Doppler US is test of choice (2),(3).

Pediatric Considerations
Further radiographic imaging in children should be done to rule out anatomic abnormalities.

Diagnostic Procedures/Other
This is a clinical diagnosis.

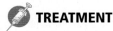 ## TREATMENT

GENERAL MEASURES
- Bed rest or restriction of activity
- Scrotal elevation, athletic scrotal supporter
- Ice pack wrapped in towel
- Avoid constipation
- Spermatic cord block with local anesthesia in severe cases
- If noninfectious epididymitis:
  – No strenuous physical activity and avoidance of any Valsalva maneuvers for several weeks
  – Empty bladder prior to strenuous exercises.

MEDICATION
First Line
- Sexually active adults aged <35 years: doxycycline 100 mg PO BID for 10 days (C. trachomatis coverage) plus ceftriaxone 500 mg IM × 1 or 1 g IM if weigh >150 kg (N. gonorrhoeae coverage). Treat all sexual partners within last 60 days (2)[C],(4)
- Aged ≥35 years, not suspecting STD with enteric etiology (i.e., bacteriuria due to bladder outlet obstruction, prostate biopsy, urinary instrumentation, systemic disease, and/or immunosuppression)
  – Levofloxacin 500 mg/day PO for 10 days (4)
  – Note: 2016 FDA black box warning on fluoroquinolones due to disabling and potentially permanent side effects. Consider trimethoprim-sulfamethoxazole for milder infections.
- Men who practice insertive anal intercourse: ceftriaxone 500 mg IM × 1 plus fluoroquinolone as above. If HIV positive, usually no difference in treatment (2)[C].
- Analgesia:
  – NSAIDs (e.g., naproxen or ibuprofen) for mild to moderate pain
  – Consider steroid if patient cannot tolerate NSAID.
  – Acetaminophen with codeine or oxycodone for moderate to severe pain
- Septic or toxic patient
  – 3rd-generation cephalosporin or aminoglycoside
- For Behçet, sarcoid, Henoch-Schönlein purpura
  – Steroids, such as methylprednisolone, 40 mg/day recommended
- Chronic epididymitis: 2-week course of NSAIDs, scrotal icing/elevation; if no improvement, may add TCA or neuroleptic (2)

Second Line
- Trimethoprim-sulfamethoxazole (Bactrim, Septra) double strength PO BID for 10 to 14 days; increasing bacterial resistance may limit effectiveness.
- Add rifampin (rifampicin) or vancomycin, as required.

Pediatric Considerations
- May be postinfectious inflammatory condition; treat with anti-inflammatories and analgesics.
- Antibiotic therapy can be reserved for young infants until positive urine cultures (2).

ISSUES FOR REFERRAL
- If suspicion is high for testicular torsion, then urgent US or referral to emergency department for possible surgery (1)[C]
- Epididymitis in ages <14 years requires a urology referral due to high incidence of associated urogenital abnormalities.
- If medical management fails, should be referred to urologist to rule out anatomic abnormality or chemical epididymitis
- If HIV positive, CMV, salmonella, toxoplasmosis, Ureaplasma urealyticum, Corynebacterium sp., Mycoplasma sp., and Mima polymorpha must also be considered.

SURGERY/OTHER PROCEDURES
- Vasostomy to drain infected material if severe or refractory case
- Scrotal exploration if unable clinically to distinguish between epididymitis and testicular torsion
- Drainage of abscesses, epididymectomy (acute suppurative), or epididymo-orchidectomy in severe cases refractory to antibiotics
- Surgery to correct underlying anatomic abnormality or obstruction

ADMISSION, INPATIENT, AND NURSING CONSIDERATIONS
- Intractable pain
- Sepsis
- Abscess
- Persistent vomiting
- Scheduled surgery
- Purulent drainage
- Most cases can be managed with outpatient care.

 ## ONGOING CARE

FOLLOW-UP RECOMMENDATIONS
Patient Monitoring
- Routine follow-up in 1 week. Follow up within 72 hours if symptoms fail to improve with treatment for reevaluation of diagnosis and therapy.
- Swelling and tenderness after antibiotic course should be evaluated for abscess, tumor, infarction, cancer, TB, and fungal epididymitis.
- In noninfectious epididymitis, follow up in 4 weeks to assess efficacy of NSAIDs and lifestyle changes.

DIET
If constipation is contributing to pain or chemical epididymitis, then consider constipation prevention (high-fiber diet) and/or treatment.

PATIENT EDUCATION
- Stress completing course of antibiotics, even when asymptomatic.
- Early recognition and treatment of UTI or prostatitis
- Safer sexual practices. Avoid sex until antibiotic course completed and partner treated if likely STI.
- Repeat STI testing in 3 months to evaluate for reinfection if STI identified.

- If treated for STI, refer sexual partners for evaluation of N. gonorrhoeae or C. trachomatis and empirically treat sexual contacts within 60 days preceding onset of symptoms.
- If noninfectious epididymitis, then educate on noninfectious etiology and proper lifestyle changes.

PROGNOSIS
- Pain improves within 1 to 3 days, but induration may take several weeks/months to completely resolve.
- If bilateral involvement, sterility may result.
- In noninfectious epididymitis, symptoms usually resolve in <1 week.

COMPLICATIONS
- Recurrent epididymitis
- Infertility
- Oligospermia
- Testicular necrosis or atrophy
- Secondary abscess formation
- Fournier gangrene (necrotizing synergistic infection)

REFERENCES
1. Trojian TH, Lishnak TS, Heiman D. Epididymitis and orchitis: an overview. Am Fam Physician. 2009;79(7):583–587.
2. McConaghy JR, Panchal B. Epididymitis: an overview. Am Fam Physician. 2016;94(9):723–726.
3. Tekgül S, Dogan HS, Kocvara R, et al; for European Society for Paediatric Urology and European Association of Urology. EAU Guidelines on Paediatric Urology. Arnhem, The Netherlands: European Association of Urology; 2016.
4. Workowski KA, Bachmann LH, Chan PA, et al. Sexually transmitted infections treatment guidelines, 2021. MMWR Recomm Rep. 2021;70(4):1–187.

ADDITIONAL READING
Somekh E, Gorenstein A, Serour F. Acute epididymitis in boys: evidence of a post-infectious etiology. J Urol. 2004;171(1):391–394.

CODES

ICD10
- N45.1 Epididymitis
- N45.2 Orchitis
- N45.3 Epididymo-orchitis

CLINICAL PEARLS
- With epididymitis, pain is gradual in onset, and the tenderness is mostly posterior to the testis. With testicular torsion, the symptoms are quite rapid in onset, the testis will be higher in the scrotum and may have a transverse lie, and the cremasteric reflex will be absent. The absence of leukocytes on urine analysis and decreased blood flow on scrotal US with Doppler will suggest torsion.
- Prostatic massage is contraindicated in epididymitis because of the risk for worsening local infection. The potential for sepsis is increased with acute prostatitis.
- Noninfectious epididymitis is a clinical diagnosis of exclusion, and infectious causes are much more common but must be considered in certain occupations, such as soldiers and laborers.

EPISCLERITIS

Dongsheng Jiang, MD, MSc • Juan Qiu, MD, PhD

BASICS

- Episcleritis is irritation and inflammation of the episclera, a thin layer of vascular connective tissue between the conjunctiva and sclera.
- Usually a benign self-limited condition, typically resolving without treatment within 3 weeks
- Topical lubricants and/or topical corticosteroid treatment may relieve symptoms while awaiting for spontaneous resolution.

DESCRIPTION
- Edema and injection confined to the episcleral tissue
- Two types
  - Simple episcleritis: diffuse scleral involvement—more common
  - Nodular episcleritis: focal area(s) of involvement—less common

EPIDEMIOLOGY
Slight female predominance (~60–65%)

Incidence
- May occur at any age
- Peak incidence in 40s to 50s
- Community incidence is not well known (~20 to 50 cases per 100,000 person-years).

Prevalence
Not historically well-known; a recent community study found a prevalence of 53 cases per 100,000 person-years.

ETIOLOGY AND PATHOPHYSIOLOGY
- Etiology: It is usually idiopathic, but up to one-third of the patients can have systemic autoimmune conditions (1).
- Pathophysiology:
  - Nonimmune (e.g., dry eye syndrome, with histology showing widespread vasodilation, edema, lymphocytic infiltration)
  - Immune (systemic vasculitis or rheumatologic disease)

COMMONLY ASSOCIATED CONDITIONS
- Usually not associated with another condition
- Less commonly associated conditions include the following: In rare cases, episcleritis can be the initial symptom of a systemic condition.
  - Rheumatoid arthritis
  - Vasculitis
  - Inflammatory bowel disease
  - Ankylosing spondylitis
  - Psoriatic arthritis
  - Systemic lupus erythematosus
  - Gout
  - Herpes zoster
  - Hypersensitivity disorders
    - Rosacea
    - Contact dermatitis
    - Penicillin sensitivity
    - Erythema multiforme
- It can be an uncommon manifestation of other ocular infectious conditions

DIAGNOSIS

- Episcleritis is a clinical diagnosis.
- Phenylephrine test (2):
  - It is used to differentiate episcleritis from scleritis.
  - Apply 10% phenylephrine drops.
    - Blanching = episcleritis (superficial blood vessels)
    - Nonblanching = scleritis (deeper vessels)

HISTORY
- History should elicit potential causative factors, recurrence, or associated systemic disease.
- A detailed reviewed of systems should be performed on all patients on the first visit.
- Pain: absent or mild and localized to the eye
- Mild tearing may be present.

PHYSICAL EXAM
- Check visual acuity; decreased vision is very unusual with episcleritis, and its presence should raise suspicion for another condition such as scleritis.
- The white sclera will have a pink or purplish hue.
- Focal hyperemia
- Pupils are equal and reactive.
- Superficial episcleral vascular dilation
- Episcleral edema
  - Diffuse in simple episcleritis
  - Focal in nodular episcleritis
- Tenderness over involved area may be present, but it is usually absent.
- Superficial episcleral vascular hyperemia blanches with topical phenylephrine.

ALERT
Recurrent episodes, difficulty confirming the diagnosis, or worsening symptoms should prompt an ophthalmology referral.

DIFFERENTIAL DIAGNOSIS
- Scleritis
- Bacterial or viral conjunctivitis
- Uveitis
- Herpes (ulcerative) keratitis
- Superficial keratitis
- Increased intraocular pressure (ocular hypertension)

DIAGNOSTIC TESTS & INTERPRETATION
Most patients do not require extensive lab work or diagnostic studies unless episcleritis progresses to scleritis or is refractory to treatment (1). May consider:
- Labs: CBC, CMP, ESR, CRP, RF, ANA, ANCA test, complements 3 and 4, RPR, HLA B27, ACE, UA
- TB screening: PPD or T-SPOT.TB test
- Imaging: CXR, chest CT

TREATMENT

- Simple episcleritis is usually self-limited (up to 21 days), but it can recur.
- Nodular type can be prolonged and painful.

MEDICATION

Treatment for episcleritis typically consists of symptomatic relief. The goal is to suppress the inflammation, which will, in turn, relieve the discomfort or pain (1).

First Line

Topical lubricants such as artificial tears are typically used for initial management of symptomatic episcleritis.

Second Line

- Topical NSAIDs such as Diclofenac 0.1% and Ketorolac 0.5%
- Topical corticosteroids are useful when discomfort is not sufficiently controlled by conservative measures (1).
  - Fluorometholone drops 4 times daily; if not effective, may increase frequency
  - Prednisolone 0.5–1% eye drops
- Refractory episcleritis may be treated with oral NSAIDs or COX inhibitors such as indomethacin or ketorolac (1).

ISSUES FOR REFERRAL

Ophthalmology referral is advised:

- If prescribing corticosteroid eye drops
- Recurrent episodes, uncertain diagnosis, and/or worsening symptoms
- If concern for progression to scleritis

ADDITIONAL THERAPIES

- Topical NSAIDs have not been shown to have a significant benefit over artificial tears.
- When episcleritis results from viral infection, appropriate antiviral therapy is indicated.

 # ONGOING CARE

FOLLOW-UP RECOMMENDATIONS

Episcleritis is usually self-limited (up to 21 days) and does not typically require follow-up.

PROGNOSIS

Most patients have no ocular complications and make a full recovery.

COMPLICATIONS

Associated complications are rare.

- Anterior uveitis may occur in 4–16% of cases.
- Decreased vision may occur in 0–4% of cases.
- Ocular hypertension has been reported in 0–3.5% of cases.

REFERENCES

1. Diaz JD, Sobol EK, Gritz DC. Treatment and management of scleral disorders. *Surv Ophthalmol*. 2016;61(6):702–717.
2. Miller JR, Hanumunthadu D. Inflammatory eye disease: an overview of clinical presentation and management. *Clin Med (Lond)*. 2022;22(2):100–103.

 # CODES

ICD10

- H15.109 Unspecified episcleritis, unspecified eye
- H15.129 Nodular episcleritis, unspecified eye
- H15.102 Unspecified episcleritis, left eye

CLINICAL PEARLS

- Episcleritis is the irritation and inflammation of the episclera, a thin layer of vascular connective tissue between the conjunctiva and sclera.
- A benign, self-limited disorder, usually resolving within 3 weeks of symptom onset
- Often not painful and presents without decrease in visual acuity
- Although treatment is often not needed, when employed, the goal is symptomatic relief while awaiting for spontaneous resolution.
- Topical lubricants and/or topical corticosteroid treatment may relieve symptoms.
- Associated complications are uncommon and not severe but may include anterior uveitis, decreased vision, and ocular hypertension.
- Episcleritis can be an early presentation of scleritis, which is more severe. Accurate diagnosis of episcleritis is important.

E

EPISTAXIS
Christopher R. Heron, MD, BS • Lawrence Go, MD

BASICS

DESCRIPTION
- Hemorrhage from the nares, nasal cavity, or nasopharynx involving either the anterior or posterior mucosal surfaces
- Intractable or refractory epistaxis: recurrent or persistent despite appropriate packing or multiple episodes during a short period, each requiring medical attention
- Synonym(s): nosebleed

EPIDEMIOLOGY
Incidence
- Bimodal, with peaks in children up to 15 years old and in adults aged >50 years, particularly ages 70 to 79 years
- Most common in males aged <49 years
- Rare in children aged <2 years
- ~6% of patients require medical or surgical intervention; accounts for ~1 in 200 ER visits

Prevalence
Estimated lifetime prevalence: ~60%

ETIOLOGY AND PATHOPHYSIOLOGY
- Most nosebleeds are due to local causes as opposed to systemic disease.
- Anterior: 90–95% of all cases (Kiesselbach plexus)
- Posterior: 5–10% of cases (Woodruff plexus); usually branches of sphenopalatine arteries: may be asymptomatic or may present with other symptoms (hematemesis, hemoptysis)
- Trauma
  - Epistaxis digitorum (nose picking)
  - Foreign bodies
  - Septal perforation
  - Nasal fracture
  - Nasal surgery
  - Barotrauma
- Local inflammation, irritation, and insult
  - Infection (viral URI, sinusitis, TB, syphilis)
  - Irritant inhalation (smoking, rhinitis, current or past cocaine use)
  - Topical steroid or antihistamine use
  - Chronic and excessive use of nasal vasoconstrictors
  - Septal deviation (disproportionate, unilateral air movement)
  - Low humidity, nasal oxygen use, CPAP
  - Tumors: benign, malignant
  - Vascular malformations, especially in context of prior trauma (e.g., carotid artery aneurysm)
- Systemic
  - Thrombocytopenia
  - Congenital or acquired coagulopathies
  - Liver or renal disease
  - Chronic alcohol abuse
  - Leukemia
  - Anticoagulant drug use
  - CHF
  - Hereditary hemorrhagic telangiectasia (HHT)

- Collagen abnormalities
- Mitral valve stenosis
- Multiple myeloma
- Polycythemia vera
- HIV

RISK FACTORS
- Local irritation from multiple causes
- Medications/supplements including aspirin, clopidogrel, ginseng, garlic, ginkgo biloba, sildenafil, warfarin, and other anticoagulants
- Prior septoplasty/turbinate procedures, anemia, and thrombocytopenia are risk factors for recurrent epistaxis

GENERAL PREVENTION
- Humidification at night
- Cut fingernails and minimize picking
- For topical-nasal medication users, direct spray laterally away from septum. Use opposite hand to spray (i.e., right hand to spray in left nostril).
- Petroleum jelly to prevent anterior mucosal drying

COMMONLY ASSOCIATED CONDITIONS
- Vascular malformation/telangiectasia (HHT)
- Neoplasm (rare; consider if persistent and unilateral)
- Systemic conditions:
  - Coagulopathy: primary or iatrogenic; thrombocytopenia
  - Cirrhosis; renal failure; alcohol misuse
- No proven association with hypertension but may make control of bleeding more difficult

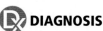

DIAGNOSIS

HISTORY
- Assess for symptoms of anemia and cardiovascular compromise.
- Determine the side on which bleeding began as well as its severity and duration.
- Identify and define trauma (including nose picking) and other possible precipitants (e.g., cocaine use).
- Ask about previous episodes of epistaxis and their frequency (if applicable).
- Identify comorbid conditions (e.g., cardiovascular compromise symptoms, cirrhosis, primary coagulopathies).
- Review current medications, including nasal sprays, anticoagulants, antiplatelets, and attempted treatments.
- Assess for nausea, hematemesis, and hemoptysis, which may indicate a posterior and more severe bleed.

PHYSICAL EXAM
- Assess for airway patency and cardiovascular stability.
- Focus on localizing site of bleeding to anterior versus posterior nasal cavity. Most cases are due to anterior nasal septal bleeding.

- When formally examining the nasal cavity, have patient seated in an upright or semi-upright position.
- Utilize a nasal speculum, if available, with a reliable light source to increase visualization of the nasal cavities.
- Between exams, have the patient lean forward and pinch their nose (or use nasal clips) to avoid blood from draining into the posterior pharynx.

DIFFERENTIAL DIAGNOSIS
- Diagnosis usually apparent; the differential for the etiology is key.
- Posterior bleeding must be included in the differential for any chronic blood loss.

DIAGNOSTIC TESTS & INTERPRETATION
Lab testing and imaging are not indicated in most uncomplicated cases in which bleeding is easily controlled.

Initial Tests (lab, imaging)
- Mild cases, responsive to pressure: no labs
- For recurrent or intractable cases
  - CBC, PT/PTT, BMP
  - PT/PTT if on warfarin or other medications affecting coagulation
  - Cross-match when appropriate.
- Toxicology screen when nasal use of illicit drugs is suspected
- For most cases, imaging is not indicated.

Follow-Up Tests & Special Considerations
Consider evaluation for neoplasia if recurrent unilateral epistaxis, especially if not responding to treatment.

Diagnostic Procedures/Other
Nasal endoscopy (1)

Pediatric Considerations
More likely anterior, idiopathic, and recurrent

Geriatric Considerations
More likely to be posterior bleed

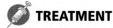

TREATMENT

- Most cases are managed as outpatient (1)[B].
- Home use—Nosebleed QR: a nonprescription powder of hydrophilic polymer with potassium salt; induces scab formation
- Patient applies direct pressure by pinching the lower part of the nose (nasal ala) for 5 to 20 minutes without a break. This stops bleeding in most patients.
- Cleanse nasal cavity of blood clots by blowing nose.
- An ice pack placed over the dorsum of the nose may help with hemostasis.
- Inspect the nasal septum for the bleeding site.

GENERAL MEASURES

Resuscitation, as indicated. Use universal "airway/breathing/circulation (ABC)" approach.

MEDICATION

First Line

If general measures fail, affected naris may be sprayed with topical vasoconstrictor, such as (2):

- Oxymetazoline: 0.05%
- Phenylephrine: 0.5–1%
- Epinephrine: 1:1,000
- Cocaine: 4%

Second Line

- Chemical (silver nitrate) or electrical cautery
- Nasal packing: ribbon gauze, nasal tampons, nasal balloon catheter
- For intractable/refractory: Consider surgical ligation, endoscopic ligation/cautery, endovascular embolization.

ISSUES FOR REFERRAL

- Posterior bleeding frequently requires an otolaryngology (ENT) consultation.
- Anterior bleeding that fails conservative measures, packing, and cauterization
- Recurrent episodes
- HHT patients should establish care with ENT.
- Concurrent anticoagulation
  - If bleeding stops with packing and INR is therapeutic, may continue same dose of warfarin. If INR supratherapeutic, manage appropriately.
  - If bleeding persists despite packing, stop anticoagulation and administer vitamin K (10 mg IV × 1), recheck INR in 30 minutes. If still >1.5, give prothrombin complex concentrate (PCC).
  - Novel anticoagulation agents may be associated with lower rates of epistaxis than warfarin. When epistaxis occurs, it may be harder to control.

ADDITIONAL THERAPIES

- Nasal packing: either with ribbon gauze or preformed nasal tampons. Systemic prophylactic antibiotics are unnecessary in the majority of patients with nasal packs; topical antibiotics may be as effective and cheaper (3)[B].
- Floseal: A biodegradable hemostatic sealant (a thrombin-type gel) in one study is more effective and better tolerated than packing (2)[C].
- Local application of tranexamic acid may reduce bleeding time as compared to anterior packing.
- If an actively bleeding anterior septal site is visualized, this may be treated with gentle silver nitrate cautery for ~10 seconds for definitive treatment; 75% silver nitrate is preferred. Apply in a spiral fashion, starting around the bleeding vessel, moving inward.
- Limit cautery (silver nitrate) to one side of septum, or wait 4 to 6 weeks in between treatments to reduce risk of perforation.
- Posterior: Posterior packing or tamponade with balloon devices (Foley catheters have been used). Inpatient monitoring is generally required in these cases.

- Recurrent epistaxis: Cochrane review in children shows no difference in effectiveness between antiseptic nasal cream, petroleum jelly, silver nitrate cautery, or no treatment.

SURGERY/OTHER PROCEDURES

- Packing, anterior bleed
  - Layering of Vaseline ribbon gauze (1/2 inch)
    ○ For gauze packing, be certain that both ends of the ribbon gauze protrude from the nostril.
    ○ Packing is layered from the floor upward.
    ○ Secure packing with gauze across the outside of the nostril.
  - Nasal tampon may be used after lubricating the tip with KY Jelly or antibiotic cream or ointment.
  - Additional saline may be needed to expand the tampon if the bleeding has slowed.
  - Merocel and Rapid Rhino packs are easier to use than gauze packing and are usually well tolerated.
- Packing, posterior bleed
  - In the emergent setting, this may be attempted utilizing a Foley catheter or a specific posterior packing balloon.
  - With both methods, the tubing is introduced through the nose similar to the passage of a nasogastric tube. Once it reaches the posterior oral pharynx, the balloon is inflated and the tubing is pulled back outward to tamponade the posterior bleeding source.
    ○ If using a Foley catheter (10 to 14F catheter), the balloon can be inflated with 10 mL of saline.
    ○ Traction is maintained with an umbilical cord clamp with adequate padding between the clip and the nose to avoid injury.

ADMISSION, INPATIENT, AND NURSING CONSIDERATIONS

- Consider hospitalization for elderly or for patients with posterior bleeding or coagulopathy; may also consider if significant comorbidities
- Admission criteria/initial stabilization
  - Posterior bleed
  - Intractable vomiting
  - Hemodynamic changes
  - Clotting dysfunction
  - Universal ABC approach. Stop blood loss.

 ONGOING CARE

FOLLOW-UP RECOMMENDATIONS

Patient Monitoring

- Hemodynamic monitoring if severe blood loss
- 24-hour minimum for leaving packing in place; some recommend 3 to 5 days. Rebleed usually occurs between 24 and 48 hours. Longer durations of packing have increased risk of mucosal injury and toxic shock syndrome.

PATIENT EDUCATION

- Demonstrate proper pinching pressure techniques.
- Avoidance of trauma or irritants is key.
- Management of systemic illness and proper use of medication

PROGNOSIS

- Most are self-limited.
- Good results with proper treatment.

COMPLICATIONS

- Septal perforation
- Pressure-induced tissue necrosis of the nasal mucosa
- Toxic shock syndrome with packing
- Arrhythmias triggered by packing (particularly posterior)

REFERENCES

1. Tunkel DE, Anne S, Payne SC, et al. Clinical practice guideline: nosebleed (epistaxis) executive summary. Otolaryngol Head Neck Surg. 2020;162(1):8–25.
2. Gottlieb M, Long B. Managing Epistaxis. Ann Emerg Med. 2023;81(2):234–240.
3. Biggs TC, Nightingale K, Patel NN, et al. Should prophylactic antibiotics be used routinely in epistaxis patients with nasal packs? Ann R Coll Surg Engl. 2013;95(1):40–42.

CODES

ICD10

R04.0 Epistaxis

CLINICAL PEARLS

- Most epistaxis is anterior and responds well to timed pressure over the anterior nares for 5 to 20 minutes.
- Most nosebleeds are idiopathic or as a result of digital trauma (nose picking).
- Posterior nosebleeds can be asymptomatic or present with nausea, hematemesis, or heme-positive stool.
- Consider evaluation for neoplasm in cases of recurrent unilateral epistaxis.

ERECTILE DYSFUNCTION

Christine M. Van Horn, MD, MS • Jennifer Fantasia, MD

 BASICS

DESCRIPTION

- Erectile dysfunction (ED): the consistent or recurrent inability to acquire and/or sustain an erection of sufficient rigidity and duration for sexual intercourse
- In the past, ED was assumed to be a symptom of the aging process in men. It is more often the result of concurrent medical conditions of the patient or from medications that patients may be taking to treat those conditions.
- Sexual problems are frequent among older men and have a detrimental effect on their quality of life but are infrequently discussed with their physicians.
- Synonym(s): impotence

EPIDEMIOLOGY

Incidence
>600,000 new cases of ED diagnosed annually in the United States; ED is vastly underreported.

Prevalence
Overall prevalence for some degree of ED:
- 52% in men aged 40 to 70 years
- Age-related increase ranging from 12.4% in men aged 40 to 49 years up to 46.6% in men aged 50 to 69 years

ETIOLOGY AND PATHOPHYSIOLOGY
- Erections are neurovascular events.
  - With stimulation, there is a release of nitrous oxide, which increases production of cyclic guanosine 3',5'-monophosphate (cGMP).
  - This leads to relaxation of cavernous smooth muscle, leading to increased blood flow to penis.
  - As cavernosal sinusoids distend with blood, there is passive compression of subtunical veins, which decreases venous outflow, and this leads to an erection.
- Alterations in any of these events lead to ED.
- ED may result from problems with systems required for normal penile erection.
- Vascular: diseases that compromise blood flow (peripheral vascular disease, diabetes, arteriosclerosis, essential hypertension, and some medications that treat hypertension)
- Neurologic: diseases that impair nerve conduction to brain or penile vasculature (spinal cord injury, stroke, diabetes)
- Endocrine: diseases associated with changes in testosterone, luteinizing hormone, prolactin levels
- Structural: phimosis, lichen sclerosis, congenital curvature
- Psychological: patients suffering from depression, performance anxiety, premature ejaculation
- Smoking or excessive alcohol intake
- Medications
- Prostate cancer treatment
- Structural injury or trauma (bicycling accident)

RISK FACTORS
- Advancing age
- Cardiovascular disease (CVD)
- Diabetes mellitus
- Metabolic syndrome
- Sedentary lifestyle
- Cigarette smoking
- Pelvic surgery, radiation, trauma/injury to pelvic area or spinal cord
- Medications that induce ED: SSRIs, β-blockers, clonidine, digoxin, spironolactone, antiandrogens, corticosteroids, H_2 blockers, anticonvulsants
- Central neurologic and endocrinologic conditions
- Substance abuse (alcohol, cocaine, opioids, marijuana)
- Psychological conditions: stress, anxiety or depression, sexual abuse, relationship problems

GENERAL PREVENTION
- Healthy lifestyle: exercise, limiting alcohol, not smoking
- Treating existing health problems: diabetes, heart disease, etc.

ALERT
Aging alone is not a cause.

COMMONLY ASSOCIATED CONDITIONS
- CVD:
  - There is a documented two-way relationship between ED and CVD, and ED has been identified as an independent risk marker for CVD with ED found to confer a 25% increased 10-year risk of CVD in the QRISK model (1). Men with ED have a greater likelihood of having angina, myocardial infarction, stroke, transient ischemic attack, congestive heart failure, or cardiac arrhythmia compared to men without ED.
- Diabetes
- Neurologic and psychiatric conditions
- Metabolic syndrome

 DIAGNOSIS

HISTORY
- Identify concurrent medical illnesses or surgical procedures, history of trauma, and a list of current medications (e.g., antihypertensive meds).
- Psychosocial history: smoking, alcohol intake, recreational drug use, anxiety and depression, satisfaction with current relationship
- Presence or absence of morning erections
- Speed of onset and duration of symptoms
- Relationship of symptoms to libido
- Detailed sexual history is important to rule out premature ejaculation, as this is frequently confused with ED.
- International Index of Erectile Function (IIEF) patient questionnaire is a useful tool in the clinical assessment and measurement of effectiveness of ED treatments.

PHYSICAL EXAM
- Signs and symptoms of hypogonadism: gynecomastia, small testicles, decreased body hair
- Penile plaques (Peyronie disease)
- Detailed examination of the cardiovascular, neurologic, and genitourinary systems
  - Blood pressure, waist circumference, body mass index (BMI)
  - Check femoral and lower extremity pulses to assess vascular supply to genitals.
  - Check anal sphincter tone and genital reflexes, including cremasterics and bulbocavernosus. (Note: Absence of the bulbocavernosus reflex can be present in up to 30% of normal patients.)
  - DRE is not required but should be considered as BPH/LUTS can be comorbid with ED and considered before testosterone supplementation (1).

DIFFERENTIAL DIAGNOSIS
- Premature ejaculation
- Decreased libido
- Anorgasmia
- Acute versus chronic ED

DIAGNOSTIC TESTS & INTERPRETATION
Vascular and/or neurologic assessment and monitoring of nocturnal erections may be indicated in selected patients but not for routine workup.

Initial Tests (lab, imaging)
- HbA1c, lipid panel, CBC, BMP, TSH
- Morning total and free testosterone level (1)[C]
- Specialized testing may be indicated in men with ED who have a more complex history (young, lifelong dysfunction, prior pelvic trauma, etc.). Doppler ultrasound, angiogram, and cavernosogram are available radiologic modalities but not recommended in routine practice for the diagnosis of ED.

Diagnostic Procedures/Other
Questionnaires to assess the severity of ED, including the IIEF and the Sexual Health Inventory for Men (SHIM)

TREATMENT
- Lifestyle modifications and managing medications contributing to ED is first-line therapy for ED.
- Cardiovascular risk stratification and risk-factor management is recommended in all men with vasculogenic ED (1).
- Current smoking is significantly associated with ED, and smoking cessation has a beneficial effect on the restoration of erectile function (2)[A].
- Men should be counseled on all options for management of ED, including phosphodiesterase type 5 (PDE-5) inhibitors, vacuum erection devices (VEDs), intraurethral alprostadil, intracavernosal injections, and penile prosthesis implantation (1).

GENERAL MEASURES
- Psychosexual therapy alone or in combination with psychoactive drugs may be helpful in men whose ED is related to depression or anxiety.
- Weight loss and increased physical activity for obese men with ED; men with metabolic syndrome should be counseled to make lifestyle modifications to reduce the risk of cardiovascular events and ED (2)[B].

MEDICATION

First Line

PDE-5 inhibitors are effective in the treatment of ED in many men, including those with diabetes mellitus and spinal cord injury and sexual dysfunction associated with antidepressants. Choice should be based on patient's preference (cost, ease of use, and adverse effects). There is insufficient evidence to support the superiority of one agent over the others:

- Sildenafil (Viagra): usual daily on-demand dose: 50 to 100 mg at least 1 hour and up to 4 hours prior to sexual intercourse
- Vardenafil (Levitra): usual daily on-demand dose: 10 mg within at least 1 hour prior to sexual intercourse
- Vardenafil (Staxyn): (oral-dissolving tablet) usual daily on-demand dose: 10 mg within at least 1 hour prior to sexual intercourse
- Tadalafil (Cialis): usual daily dose of 2.5 to 5.0 mg/day regardless of activity or on-demand dosing of 5 to 20 mg at least 30 minutes and up to 36 hours prior to sexual intercourse
- Avanafil (Stendra): usual daily on-demand dose: 50 to 200 mg at least 15 to 30 minutes prior to sexual intercourse, no more than once daily
- Adverse effects of PDE-5 inhibitors: headache, facial flushing, dyspepsia, nasal congestion, dizziness, hypotension, increased sensitivity to light (sildenafil), vision changes, lower back pain (tadalafil), and priapism
- Sildenafil and vardenafil should be taken on an empty stomach for maximum effectiveness. Tadalafil can be taken with or without food.

Geriatric Considerations

Use doses at the lower end of the dosing range for elderly patients and evaluate exercise tolerance before prescribing.

- Sildenafil 25 mg/day
- Vardenafil 5 mg/day

Second Line

Intraurethral and intracavernosal injectables are shown to be effective and should be administered based on patient's preference (1),(2)[B]. Intraurethral suppositories are a less invasive treatment option than intracavernosal injections; however, they are not as effective. Alprostadil, also known as prostaglandin E1, causes smooth muscle relaxation of the arterial blood vessels and sinusoidal tissues in the corpora:

- Intraurethral alprostadil (Muse): Intraurethral suppository: 125- and 250-μg pellets; administer 5 to 50 minutes before intercourse. No >2 doses in 24 hours are recommended.
- Intracavernosal alprostadil (available in 2 formulations):
  - Alprostadil (Caverject): usual dose: 10 to 20 μg, with max dose of 60 μg; injection should be made at right angles into one of the lateral surfaces of the proximal 3rd of the penis using a 0.5-inch, 27- or 30-gauge needle. Do not use >3 times a week or more than once in 24 hours.
  - Alprostadil may also be combined with papaverine (Bimix) plus phentolamine (Trimix), plus atropine (Quadmix).

- VED: noninvasive option, available over the counter
- Penile prosthesis

ALERT

- Initial trial dose of intracavernosal therapies should be administered under supervision of a specialist or primary care physician with expertise in these therapies.
- Patient should notify physician if erection lasts >4 hours for immediate attention.
- Do not use vacuum devices in men with sickle cell anemia or blood dyscrasias.
- Testosterone supplementation in men with hypogonadism improves ED and libido.
- Do not prescribe testosterone to men with ED who have normal testosterone levels (2).
- Contraindications: nitroglycerin (or other nitrates) and phosphodiesterase inhibitors: theoretical potential for severe hypotension
- Precautions/side effects:
  - Testosterone: *precautions*: Exogenous testosterone reduces sperm count and thus do not use in patients wishing to keep fertility; *side effects*: acne, sodium retention
  - Intraurethral suppository: local penile pain, urethral bleeding, dizziness, and dysuria
  - Intracavernosal injection: penile pain, edema and hematoma, palpable nodules or plaques, and priapism
  - PDE-5 inhibitors: Use caution with congenital prolonged QT syndrome, class Ia or II antiarrhythmics, nitroglycerin, α-blockers (e.g., terazosin, tamsulosin), retinal disease, unstable cardiac disease, liver and renal failure
- Significant possible interactions
  - PDE-5 inhibitor concentration is affected by CYP3A4 inhibitors (e.g., erythromycin, indinavir, ketoconazole, ritonavir, amiodarone, cimetidine, clarithromycin, delavirdine, diltiazem, fluoxetine, fluvoxamine, grapefruit juice, itraconazole, nefazodone, nevirapine, saquinavir, and verapamil). Serum concentrations and/or toxicity may be increased. Lower starting doses should be used in these patients.
  - PDE-5 inhibitor concentration may be reduced by rifampin and phenytoin.

ADDITIONAL THERAPIES

- Men with relationship difficulties who received therapy plus sildenafil had more successful intercourse than those who received only sildenafil (3)[A].
- A topical over-the-counter therapy, composed of a hydroalcoholic gel (MED3000) was recently FDA approved for treatment of ED. It is already available in the United Kingdom over-the-counter.

SURGERY/OTHER PROCEDURES

Penile prosthesis (inflatable and malleable/semirigid options)

COMPLEMENTARY & ALTERNATIVE MEDICINE

Trazodone, yohimbine, and herbal therapies are not recommended for the treatment of ED; not proven to be efficacious; low-intensity shock wave treatment is not FDA approved but may be effective.

ONGOING CARE

FOLLOW-UP RECOMMENDATIONS

Patient Monitoring

Treatment should be assessed at baseline and after the patient has completed at least 1 to 3 weeks of a specific treatment: Monitor the quality and quantity of penile erections and monitor the level of satisfaction patient achieves.

DIET

Diet and exercise to achieve a normal BMI; limit alcohol.

PROGNOSIS

- All commercially available PDE-5 inhibitors are equally effective. In the presence of sexual stimulation, they are 55–80% effective.
  - Lower success rates with diabetes mellitus and radical prostatectomy patients who suffer from ED
- Overall effectiveness is 70–90% for intracavernosal alprostadil and 43–60% for intraurethral alprostadil.
- Penile prostheses are associated with an 85–90% patient satisfaction rate.

REFERENCES

1. Burnett AL, Nehra A, Breau RH, et al. Erectile dysfunction: AUA guideline. *J Urol*. 2018;200(3): 633–641.
2. Rew KT, Heidelbaugh JJ. Erectile dysfunction. *Am Fam Physician*. 2016;94(10):820–827.
3. Melnik T, Soares BGO, Nasselo AG. Psychosocial interventions for erectile dysfunction. *Cochrane Database Syst Rev*. 2007;2007(3):CD004825.

CODES

ICD10

- N52.03 Combined arterial insufficiency and corporo-venous occlusive erectile dysfunction
- N52.2 Drug-induced erectile dysfunction
- F52.21 Male erectile disorder

CLINICAL PEARLS

- Nitrates should be withheld for 24 hours after sildenafil or vardenafil administration and for 48 hours after use of tadalafil. PDE-5 inhibitors are contraindicated in patients taking concurrent nitrates of any form (regular or intermittent nitrate therapy), as it can lead to severe hypotension and syncope.
- Reserve surgical treatment for patients who do not respond to drug treatment.
- The use of PDE-5 inhibitors with α-adrenergic antagonists may increase the risk of hypotension. Tamsulosin is the least likely to cause orthostatic hypotension.
- ED may be a marker for subclinical CVD. Thoroughly assess patients with nonpsychogenic ED for cardiovascular risks.

ERYSIPELAS
Barbara M. Kiersz Mueller, DO

BASICS

DESCRIPTION
- Distinct form of cellulitis: an acute, well-demarcated, superficial bacterial skin infection (most commonly on face or leg) with lymphatic involvement almost always caused by *Streptococcus pyogenes*
- Usually acute, but a chronic recurrent form can also exist
- Nonpurulent
- System(s) affected: skin, exocrine

EPIDEMIOLOGY
- Predominant age: infants, children, and adults aged >45 years
- Greatest in elderly (aged >75 years)
- No gender/racial predilection

Incidence
- Erysipelas occurs in ~24/1,000 persons/year (1).
- Incidence on the rise since the 1980s

Prevalence
Unknown

ETIOLOGY AND PATHOPHYSIOLOGY
- Group A streptococci induce inflammation and activation of the contact system, a proinflammatory pathway with antithrombotic activity, releasing proteinases and proinflammatory cytokines.
- The generation of antibacterial peptides and the release of bradykinin, a proinflammatory peptide, increase vascular permeability and induce fever and pain.
- The M proteins from the group A streptococcal cell wall interact with neutrophils, leading to the secretion of heparin-binding protein, an inflammatory mediator that also induces vascular leakage.
- This cascade of reactions leads to the symptoms seen in erysipelas: fever, pain, erythema, and edema.
- Group A β-hemolytic streptococci primarily; commonly *Streptococcus pyogenes*, occasionally, other *Streptococcus* groups C/G
- Rarely, group B streptococci/*Staphylococcus aureus* may be involved.

RISK FACTORS
- Disruption in the skin barrier (surgical incisions, insect bites, eczematous lesions, local trauma, abrasions, dermatophytic infections, intravenous drug user [IVDU])
- Chronic diseases (diabetes, malnutrition, nephrotic syndrome, heart failure)
- Immunocompromised (HIV)/debilitated
- Fissured skin (especially at the nose and ears)
- Toe-web intertrigo and lymphedema
- Leg ulcers/stasis dermatitis
- Venous/lymphatic insufficiency (saphenectomy, varicose veins of leg, phlebitis, radiotherapy, mastectomy, lymphadenectomy)
- Alcohol abuse
- Morbid obesity
- Recent streptococcal pharyngitis
- Varicella

GENERAL PREVENTION
- Good skin hygiene
- It is recommended that predisposing medical conditions, such as tinea pedis and stasis dermatitis, be appropriately managed first.
- Men who shave within 5 days of facial erysipelas are more likely to have a recurrence.
- With recurrences, search for other possible sources of streptococcal infection (e.g., tonsils, sinuses).
- Compression stockings should be encouraged for patients with lower extremity edema.
- Consider suppressive prophylactic antibiotic therapy, such as penicillin, in patients with >2 episodes in a 12-month period.

Pediatric Considerations
Group B *Streptococcus* may be a cause of erysipelas in neonates/infants.

DIAGNOSIS

Prodromal symptoms before the skin eruption of erysipelas may include:
- Moderate- to high-grade fever
- Chills
- Headache
- Malaise
- Anorexia, usually in the first 48 hours
- Vomiting
- Arthralgias

ALERT
It is important to differentiate erysipelas from a methicillin-resistant *S. aureus* (MRSA) infection, which usually presents with an indurated center, significant pain, and later evidence of abscess formation.

PHYSICAL EXAM
- Vital signs: moderate- to high-grade fever with resultant tachycardia. Hypotension may occur.
- The presence of a fever in erysipelas can be considered a differentiating factor from other skin infections.
- Headache and vomiting may be prominent.
- Acute onset of intense erythema; well-demarcated painful plaque (2)
- Peau d'orange appearance
- Milian ear sign (Erythema involves skin of ear as well as face implies erysipelas.)
- Vesicles and bullae may form but are not uniformly present.
- Desquamation may occur later.
- Lymphangitis
- Location (most commonly unilateral; bilateral presentation should prompt consideration of alternative diagnosis)
  - Lower extremity 70–80% of cases
  - Face involvement is less common (5–20%), especially nose and ears.
  - Chronic form usually recurs at site of the previous infection and may recur years after initial episode.

- Patients on systemic steroids may be more difficult to diagnose because signs and symptoms of the infection may be masked by anti-inflammatory action of the steroids.
- Systemic toxicity resolves rapidly with treatment; skin lesions desquamate on days 5 to 10 but usually heal without scarring.
- In geriatric patients, facial involvement presents in a butterfly pattern. Pustules are characteristically absent, and regional lymphadenopathy with lymphangitic streaking is seen.

Pediatric Considerations
- Abdominal involvement is more common in infants, especially around umbilical stump.
- Face, scalp, and leg involvement are common in older children due to the excoriations when scratching in atopic dermatitis, allowing an easy port of entry.

Geriatric Considerations
- Fever may not be as prominent.
- 80% of cases affect the lower extremities. The rest is usually on the face.
- High-output cardiac failure may occur in debilitated patients with underlying cardiac disease.
- More susceptible to complications

DIFFERENTIAL DIAGNOSIS
- Cellulitis (Margins are less clear and do not involve ear.)
- Necrotizing fasciitis (systemic illness and more pain)
- Skin abscess (feel for area of fluctuance)
- DVT (needs to rule out if clinically suspected)
- Acute gout (Check patient history.)
- Insect bite (Check patient history.)
- Dermatophytes
- Impetigo (blistered/crusted appearance; superficial)
- Ecthyma (ulcerative impetigo)
- Herpes zoster (dermatomal distribution)
- Erythema annulare centrifugum (raised pink-red ring/bull's-eye marks)
- Contact dermatitis (no fever, pruritic, not painful)
- Giant cell urticaria (transient, wheal appearance, severe itching)
- Angioneurotic edema (no fever)
- Scarlet fever (widespread rash with indistinct borders and without edema; rash is most common early in skin folds; develops generalized "sandpaper" feeling as it progresses)
- Toxic shock syndrome (diffuse erythema with evidence of multiorgan involvement)
- Lupus (of the face; less fever, positive antinuclear antibodies)
- Polychondritis (Common site is the ear.)
- Other bacterial infections to consider:
  - Meat, shellfish, fish, and poultry workers: *Erysipelothrix rhusiopathiae* (known as erysipeloid)
  - Human bite: *Eikenella corrodens*
  - Cat/dog bite: *Pasteurella multocida/Capnocytophaga canimorsus*
  - Salt water exposure: *Vibrio vulnificus*
  - Fresh/brackish water exposure: *Aeromonas hydrophila*

DIAGNOSTIC TESTS & INTERPRETATION
Reserve diagnostic tests for severely ill, toxic patients, patients who failed initial antibiotic therapy, or those who are immunosuppressed.

Initial Tests (lab, imaging)
- Leukocytosis
- Blood culture (<5% positive)
- Elevated erythrocyte sedimentation rate (ESR) and C-reactive protein (CRP)
- Streptococci may be cultured from exudate/noninvolved sites.

Test Interpretation
Biopsy is not needed; however, skin findings would show
- Dermal and epidermal edema, extending into the subcutaneous tissues
- Peau d'orange appearance caused by edema in the superficial tissue surrounding the hair follicles
- Vasodilation and enlarged lymphatics
- Mixed interstitial infiltrate mainly consisting of neutrophils and mononuclear cells
- Endothelial cell swelling
- Gram-positive cocci in lymphatics and tissue with rare invasion of local blood vessels
- Fibrotic thickening of lymphatic vessel walls with possible luminal occlusion may be seen in recurrent erysipelas.

 ## TREATMENT

GENERAL MEASURES
- Symptomatic treatment of myalgias and fever
- Adequate fluid intake
- Local treatment with cold compresses
- Elevation of affected extremity
- Appropriate therapy for any underlying predisposing condition

MEDICATION
- Antibiotics cure 50–100% of infections, but which regimen is most successful is unclear.
- Antibiotics may be as effective when given orally versus intravenously unless systemic symptoms are present (fever, chills).
- A 5-day course of antibiotics may be as effective as a 10-day course at curing.

First Line
- Adults
  - Extremities, nondiabetic
    - Primary
      - Penicillin G: 1 to 2 million U IV q6h *or* cefazolin 1 g IV q8h
    - Alternative (if penicillin allergic)
      - Vancomycin 15 mg/kg IV q12h
      - When afebrile, change to oral regimen of trimethoprim-sulfamethoxazole (TMP-SMX) or clindamycin

  - Total 10 days, diabetics
    - Early mild:
      - TMP-SMX DS: 1 to 2 tabs PO BID and penicillin VK 500 mg PO QID *or* cephalexin 500 mg PO QID
    - Severe disease
      - MP or MER or ERTA IV and linezolid 600 mg IV/PO BID *or* vancomycin IV or daptomycin 4 mg/kg IV q24h
  - Facial
    - Primary
      - Vancomycin: 15 mg/kg (actual weight) IV q8–12h with target trough 15 to 20
    - Alternative
      - Daptomycin 4 mg/kg IV q24h or linezolid 600 mg IV q12h
- Children
  - Penicillin G
    - 0 to 7 days, <2,000 g = 50,000 U/kg q12h
    - 8 to 28 days, <2,000 g = 75,000 U/kg q8h
    - 0 to 7 days, >2,000 g = 50,000 U/kg q8h
    - 8 to 28 days, >2,000 g = 50,000 U/kg q6h
    - >28 days = 50,000 U/kg/day
  - Cefazolin
    - 0 to 7 days, <2,000 g = 25 mg/kg q12h
    - 8 to 28 days, <2,000 g = 25 mg/kg q12h
    - 0 to 7 days, >2,000 g = 25 mg/kg q12h
    - 8 to 28 days, >2,000 g = 25 mg/kg q8h
    - >28 days = 25 mg/kg q8h
- No reported group A streptococci resistance to β-lactam antibiotics
- In chronic recurrent infections, prophylactic treatment after the acute infection resolves:
  - Penicillin G benzathine: 1.2 million U IM q4wk *or* penicillin VK 500 mg PO BID or azithromycin 250 mg PO QD
- If staphylococcal infection is suspected or if patient is acutely ill, consider a β-lactamase-stable antibiotic.
- Consider community-acquired MRSA, and depending on regional sensitivity, may treat MRSA with TMP-SMX DS 1 tab PO BID *or* vancomycin 1 g IV q12h *or* doxycycline 100 mg PO BID.

ISSUES FOR REFERRAL
Recurrent infection, treatment failure

ADDITIONAL THERAPIES
For patients with worsening skin symptoms after initiation of antibiotics, a trial of topical 1% hydrocortisone may be considered.

ADMISSION, INPATIENT, AND NURSING CONSIDERATIONS
- Admission criteria/initial stabilization
  - Patient with systemic toxicity
  - Patient with high-risk factors (e.g., elderly, lymphedema, postsplenectomy, diabetes)
  - Failed outpatient care
- IV therapy if systemic toxicity/unable to tolerate PO
- Discharge criteria: no evidence of systemic toxicity with resolution of erythema and swelling

 ## ONGOING CARE

FOLLOW-UP RECOMMENDATIONS
Bed rest with elevation of extremity during acute infection and then activity as tolerated

PROGNOSIS
- Patients should recover fully if adequately treated.
- May experience deepening of erythema after initiation of antibiotics
- Most respond to therapy after 24 to 48 hours.
- Mortality is <1% in patients receiving appropriate treatment.
- Bullae formation suggests longer disease course and often indicates a concomitant *S. aureus* infection that may require antibiotic coverage for MRSA.
- Chronic edema/scarring may result from chronic recurrent cases.
- Rarely, obstructive lymphadenitis may result from chronic recurrent cases.

COMPLICATIONS
- Recurrent infection
- Abscess (suggests staphylococcal infection)
- Necrotizing fasciitis
- Lymphedema (most prominent risk factor for recurrence) (3)
- Bacteremia, which may lead to sepsis
- Pneumonia (due to sepsis/toxin-producing organism)
- Meningitis (due to sepsis/toxin-producing organism)
- Embolism
- Gangrene
- Bursitis, septic arthritis, tendinitis, or osteitis

REFERENCES
1. Jendoubi F, Rohde M, Prinz JC. Intracellular streptococcal uptake and persistence: a potential cause of erysipelas recurrence. *Front Med*. 2019;6:6.
2. Breen JO. Skin and soft tissue infections in immunocompetent patients. *Am Fam Physician*. 2010;81(7):893–899.
3. Inghammar M, Rasmussen M, Linder A. Recurrent erysipelas—risk factors and clinical presentation. *BMC Infect Dis*. 2014;14:270.

 ## CODES

ICD10
A46 Erysipelas

CLINICAL PEARLS
- Athlete's foot is the most common portal of entry.
- Erysipelas is distinguished from cellulitis by its sharp, shiny, fiery-red, raised border.
- In recurrent cases, search for other possible source of streptococcal infection (e.g., tonsils, sinuses, intertrigo).
- Most erysipelas infections now occur on the legs, rather than the face.

ERYTHEMA MULTIFORME

James R. Yon, MD • Justin D. Leavitt, MD

BASICS

- Erythema multiforme (EM) is an uncommon, self-limiting, immune-mediated, mucocutaneous disease.
  - Approximately 90% of cases are triggered by infectious agents (herpes simplex virus [HSV] is most common, up to 50%), or less commonly, by drugs and vaccinations (1).
  - Characteristic skin lesions are acrally distributed, distinct, targetoid papules with concentric color variation (3 zones), occasionally accompanied by oral, genital, or ocular mucosal involvement.
  - EM needs to be differentiated from Steven-Johnson syndrome (SJS) and toxic epidermal necrolysis (TEN), which are characterized by truncal, flat lesions with or without blisters which can result in significant mortality (1).
- There are no universal diagnostic criteria, but clinical history, clinical examination, skin biopsy, laboratory studies, and special consideration of persistent EM are all helpful in making a diagnosis.
- Treatment focuses on supportive care in addition to treating the underlying etiology and discontinuing causative agents (1).

DESCRIPTION

- There are two subtypes of EM: erythema multiforme minor (EMm) which involves ≤1 mucosal site and erythema multiforme major (EMM), which involves ≥2 mucosal sites. EMM is now separate from SJS and TEN. Skin lesions that are predominantly truncal, flat (macular, nonpalpable), and atypical (less sharply demarcated with only two concentric zones) with or without blisters are more suggestive of SJS or TEN (1).
- Recurrent EM is defined as ≥3 episodes but has a mean number of 6 episodes per year and a mean duration of 6 to 10 years.

EPIDEMIOLOGY

Incidence
Annual U.S. incidence is estimated at <1% (1).

Prevalence
Predominant in young adults from age 20 to 40 years; rare in <3 years and >50 years of age (1). Slight female predominance is observed. There is no apparent race predilection (1).

ETIOLOGY AND PATHOPHYSIOLOGY

- Etiology (1)
  - Viral infections: HSV-1 (most common etiology) and HSV-2, Epstein-Barr, hepatitis C, coxsackievirus, echovirus, varicella, mumps, poliovirus, cytomegalovirus, HIV, molluscum contagiosum, COVID-19
  - Bacterial infections: *Mycoplasma pneumoniae* (2nd most common etiology), *Treponema pallidum*, *Mycobacterium tuberculosis*, and *Gardnerella vaginalis*
  - Drugs: NSAIDs, anti-epileptics, antibiotics (penicillin, sulfonamides, erythromycin, nitrofurantoin, tetracyclines), statin, tumor necrosis factor (TNF)-α inhibitors, and barbiturates

- Vaccines: stronger association with HPV, MMR, and small pox vaccines, but also associated with hepatitis B, meningococcal, pneumococcal, varicella, influenza, diphtheria-pertussis-tetanus, *Haemophilus influenzae*, and COVID-19
  - Other causes: occupational exposures: herbicides (alachlor and butachlor), iodoacetonitrile, heavy metals; radiation therapy; premenstrual hormone changes; malignancy (e.g., lymphoma); inflammatory bowel disease
- Pathogenesis of EM
  - In HSV-associated EM, peripheral mononuclear cells that phagocytose the virus transport fragmented HSV DNA to keratinocytes. Within the keratinocytes, the HSV DNA polymerase gene (pol) leads to a TH-1 mediated immune response. Activation of the HSV-specific CD4+ TH-1 cells then produces cytokines such as interferon (IFN)-γ and triggers an inflammatory cascade which leads to the mucocutaneous findings.
  - Development of EM from other inciting factors such as drugs and vaccinations is not completely understood, but it appears that the pathway involves TNF-α, perforin, and granzyme B rather than IFN-γ.

Genetics
Genetic susceptibility may play a role in some patients with EM. There is a strong association with the HLA-DQB1*0301 allele found among patients with herpes-associated EM. In recurrent EM, there is an association with HLA-B35, -B62, and -DR53 alleles.

RISK FACTORS
Previous history of EM, age 20 to 40 years, use of causative agents or infection with causative pathogens

GENERAL PREVENTION
- Known etiologic agents or those with potential for cross-reactivity should be avoided.
- Oral acyclovir or valacyclovir may help prevent herpes-related recurrent EM (2).

COMMONLY ASSOCIATED CONDITIONS
See "Etiology and Pathophysiology."

DIAGNOSIS

- Diagnosis is based on history and clinical findings, and most cases do not require further work-up.
- In unclear cases, histopathologic analysis including immunofluorescence microscopy and other laboratory studies can help in making a diagnosis (1).

HISTORY
- Acute, self-limiting episodic course.
- Prodromal symptoms are usually absent, but common in cases with mucosal involvement
- Signs and symptoms of infections associated with EM such as an HSV eruption (10 to 15 days prior to onset of EM lesions) or respiratory symptoms suggestive of *M. pneumoniae*
- History of new medication use or vaccination
- Exposure to other causative agents like radiation, herbicides, heavy metals, etc.

PHYSICAL EXAM
- Thorough skin exam should be completed, including of mucous membranes.
  - Typical cutaneous lesions with erythematous, papular, and targetoid appearance that has three concentric zones of varied color: central portion of epidermal necrosis (dusky or blistered) surrounded by a dark red inflammatory zone followed by an outer lighter edematous ring
  - Acral lesions with symmetric distribution and predilection for extensor surfaces
- Mucosal involvement
  - Oral involvement manifests as erythema, erosions, bullae, and ulcerations on both nonkeratinized and keratinized mucosal surfaces and on the vermilion of the lips
  - Minimal involvement in EMm, but if present, most commonly involves the mouth
  - At least two mucosal sites involved in EMM, including eyes (conjunctivitis, keratitis); mouth (stomatitis, cheilitis, characteristic blood-stained crusted erosions on lips); and probable trachea, bronchi, GI tract, or genital tract (balanitis and vulvitis)

DIFFERENTIAL DIAGNOSIS
- SJS
  - Medications are the most frequent cause.
  - Generalized distribution of lesions; concentrated on the trunk
  - Targetoid lesions are less sharply demarcated and atypical. Atypical signifies macular (flat and nonpalpable) with only two concentric zones
  - Blisters and skin detachment <10% of the total body surface area
  - Nikolsky sign may be positive—applying gentle pressure to what appears to be intact skin will extend sloughing of epidermis.
  - 90% of patients have mucosal involvement, commonly at ≥2 sites.
  - Presence of constitutional symptoms with presence of high fever (>38.5°C)
  - Can be associated with anemia, lymphadenopathy, high C-reactive protein levels (>10 mg/dL), and hepatic dysfunction
  - ~10% mortality
- TEN: similar to SJS but has full-thickness skin necrosis and skin detachment >30% of the total body surface area; up to 50% mortality rate
- Urticaria: pruritic wheal-and-flare skin lesion; each lesion is transient, lasting <24 hours, unlike in EM
- Fixed drug eruption
- Broad additional ddx: Bullous pemphigoid, paraneoplastic pemphigoid, Sweet syndrome, Rowell syndrome, polymorphous light eruption, cutaneous small-vessel vasculitis, mucocutaneous lymph node syndrome, erythema annulare centrifugum, acute hemorrhagic edema of infancy, subacute cutaneous lupus erythematosus, contact dermatitis, pityriasis rosea, tinea corporis, secondary syphilis, dermatitis herpetiformis, herpes gestationis, septicemia, serum sickness, Rocky Mountain spotted fever, viral exanthem, meningococcemia, lichen planus, Behçet syndrome, recurrent aphthous ulcers, herpetic gingivostomatitis

DIAGNOSTIC TESTS & INTERPRETATION

Laboratory studies and skin biopsies are not required for diagnosis. However, they can be useful in determining inciting factors, ruling out other conditions, and confirming a diagnosis of EM (1).

Initial Tests (lab, imaging)

- Because HSV is the most common cause of EM, every patient should be evaluated for an underlying infection. Evaluation can include serologic tests or checking skin biopsy samples for HSV infection by direct immunofluorescence (DIF), direct fluorescent antibody (DFA), polymerase chain reaction (PCR), viral culture, or Tzanck smear (1).
- No imaging studies are indicated unless there is suspicion for *M. pnuemoniae* in which case work-up should include CXR, PCR testing of throat swab, and serologic tests.

Follow-Up Tests & Special Considerations

- Antinuclear antibodies, rheumatoid factor, and anti-Ro and anti-La antibodies can be ordered if suspicious for Rowell syndrome. Presence of IgM antibodies or greater than 2-fold increase in IgG antibodies can confirm the diagnosis.
- Antibody staining to IFN-γ and TNF-α to differentiate HSV from drug-associated EM
- Serum complement levels should be checked in cases of persistent EM as they are likely to be low.
- Erythrocyte sedimentation rate, white blood cell count, and liver function enzymes should be checked in severe cases with mucosal involvement as they are likely to be elevated.

Diagnostic Procedures/Other

- Skin biopsy: Histopathologic analysis of lesional and perilesional tissue can help with diagnosis in equivocal conditions.
- DIF and indirect immunofluorescence (IIF) can be used to differentiate EM from other vesiculobullous diseases. DIF is performed on a biopsy of perilesional tissue, and IIF is performed on a blood sample.

Test Interpretation

- Histopathology of EM lesions may demonstrate the following:
  - Spongiosis (intercellular edema)
  - Necrotic keratinocytes resulting in dermal interface bullae formation
  - Inflammatory infiltrate including lymphocytes in the dermal-epidermal junction with perivascular accentuation
- DIF and IIF findings are usually either negative or nonspecific in EM. It may show lichenoid inflammatory infiltrate and epidermal necrosis including circulating immune complexes, deposition of C3, IgM, and fibrin around the dermal blood vessels.

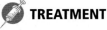 ## TREATMENT

GENERAL MEASURES

- Treatment will depend on disease severity, underlying cause, and course of the disease.
- Determine the level of care: outpatient versus inpatient

- Determine the cause of EM
  - Drug-induced EM: Discontinue the inciting factor and avoid reexposure to the same drug or exposure to other drugs with potential for cross-reactivity.
  - Infectious: Treat the underlying condition as indicated.
- Some cases may require close follow-up.

MEDICATION

- Acute EM
  - Discontinue inciting factors and treat the underlying disease
    - *M. pneumoniae*–associated EM: may require antibiotics
    - HSV-induced EM: Most recent sources report no proven effect on the course of EM using antivirals with acute mild EM.
  - Mild cutaneous involvement
    - Medium potency topical steroids for lesions on trunk and extremities (1)[C]
    - Low potency topical steroids for lesions on the face and intertriginous skin (1)[C]
    - Oral antihistamines for pruritic lesions (1)[C]
- Mucous membrane EM
  - Ocular involvement—Urgent ophthalmology consultation (1)[C]. Ophthalmic preparations such as nonpreserved dexamethasone 0.1% and lubricants such as nonpreserved hyaluronate should be used under the guidance of ophthalmologists.
  - Oral involvement
    - Nondisabling
      - High-potency topical corticosteroid gel (e.g., fluocinonide 0.05% gel applied 2 to 3 times per day) (1)[C]
      - Mouthwashes that contain a combination of lidocaine 2%, antacids, and diphenhydramine 12.5 mg/5 mL (e.g., Maalox, swish and spit as needed up to 4 times per day) (1)[C]
    - Disabling
      - Hospitalization may be required for pain control and to ensure adequate hydration and nutrition if insufficient oral intake.
      - Systemic corticosteroids may be used for severe symptoms, but controlled studies have not been performed to validate efficacy of this approach (e.g., prednisone 40 to 60 mg per day, tapered over 2 to 4 weeks).
- Recurrent EM
  - First-line treatment with HSV-associated and idiopathic recurrent EM is antiviral prophylaxis for at least 6 months. Options include: acyclovir 400 mg BID, valacyclovir 500 mg BID, famciclovir 250 mg BID. If the patient is unresponsive to one antiviral, can double the dose or switch to a different antiviral regimen.
  - Second-line therapy includes: dapsone (100 to 150 mg/day), azathioprine (100 to 150 mg/day), mycophenolate mofetil (1,000 to 1,500 mg BID), thalidomide (100 to 200 mg/day), tacrolimus (0.1% ointment daily), hydroxychloroquine (400 mg/day), levamisole (75 to 200 mg/week)

ALERT

Levamisole can cause agranulocytosis, although the incidence is low (1–2%). The agranulocytosis is dose-dependent, hence, initiation of treatment with a lower dose and regular monitoring during treatment is recommended. Once in remission, therapy should be continued for 6 to 12 months followed by a taper over 2 to 4 months to the lowest effective dose or cessation.

ISSUES FOR REFERRAL

Consider appropriate referrals when concerned about etiologies such as autoimmune disorders, recurrent HSV infections, or possible malignancy.

ADMISSION, INPATIENT, AND NURSING CONSIDERATIONS

Determining the level of care:

- Most cases can be managed outpatient.
- However, if lesions involve the oral mucosa thereby preventing sufficient oral intake, patients need to be hospitalized for IV hydration, electrolyte repletion, nutrition, and pain control. Wound care may also be indicated for cases with epidermal detachment.

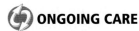 ## ONGOING CARE

FOLLOW-UP RECOMMENDATIONS

Patient Monitoring

The disease is self-limiting. Complications are rare, with no mortality.

PATIENT EDUCATION

Avoid any identified etiologic agents.

PROGNOSIS

Rash evolves over 1 to 2 weeks and subsequently resolves within 2 to 6 weeks, generally without scarring or sequelae, although there may be postinflammatory hyper- or hypopigmentation.

COMPLICATIONS

Secondary infection, scarring, eye damage

REFERENCES

1. Trayes KP, Love G, Studdiford JS. Erythema multiforme: recognition and management. *Am Fam Physician.* 2019;100(2):82–88.
2. de Risi-Pugliese T, Sbidian E, Ingen-Housz-Oro S, et al. Interventions for erythema multiforme: a systematic review. *J Eur Acad Dermatol Venereol.* 2019;33(5):842–849.

 ## SEE ALSO

Cutaneous Drug Reactions; Dermatitis Herpetiformis; Pemphigoid Gestationis; Stevens-Johnson Syndrome; Toxic Epidermal Necrolysis; Urticaria

 ## CODES

ICD10

- L51.0 Nonbullous erythema multiforme
- L51.1 Stevens-Johnson syndrome
- L51.3 Stevens-Johnson syndrome-toxic epidermal necrolysis overlap syndrome

CLINICAL PEARLS

EM is diagnosed clinically. No lab tests are required for the diagnosis. Typical lesions are targetoid or "iris." Lesions are symmetrical. Recurrent cases often due to HSV, and antiviral therapy may benefit.

E

ERYTHEMA NODOSUM

Faraz Yousefian, DO • Sujitha Yadlapati, MD

 BASICS

DESCRIPTION
- A delayed-type IV hypersensitivity reaction to various antigens, or an autoimmune reaction presenting as a panniculitis (1) that affects subcutaneous fat
- The clinical pattern of multiple, bilateral, erythematous, tender nodules in a typically anterior pretibial distribution that undergo a characteristic pattern of color changes, similar to that seen in bruises. Unlike erythema induratum, the lesions of erythema nodosum (EN) do not typically ulcerate.
- Occurs most commonly on the shins; less commonly on the thighs, forearms, trunk, head, or neck
- Often associated with nonspecific prodrome including fever, weight loss, and arthralgia
- Often idiopathic but may be associated with a number of clinical entities
- Usually remits spontaneously in weeks to months without scarring, atrophy, or ulceration
- Uncommon to have recurrences after the initial presentation
- Divided into acute (more common) and chronic (rare)

Pregnancy Considerations
May have repeat outbreaks during pregnancy

Pediatric Considerations
A rare pediatric variant has lesions only on palms or soles, often unilateral; typically has a shorter duration in children than in adults

EPIDEMIOLOGY
Frequently observed in women aged 18 to 34 years (2)

Incidence
- 1 to 5/100,000/year
- Predominant age: 20 to 30 years
- Predominant sex: female > male (6:1) in adults

Prevalence
- Varies geographically depending on the prevalence of disorders associated with EN
- Reported 1 to 5/100,000

ETIOLOGY AND PATHOPHYSIOLOGY
- Idiopathic: up to 55%
- Infectious: 44%; streptococcal pharyngitis (most common), mycobacteria, mycoplasma, chlamydia, mycoplasma, coccidioidomycosis, rarely can be caused by *Campylobacter* spp., rickettsiae, *Salmonella* spp., psittacosis, syphilis
- Sarcoidosis: 11–25%
- Drugs: 3–10%; sulfonamides amoxicillin, oral contraceptives, bromides, azathioprine, vemurafenib

- Pregnancy: 2–5%
- Enteropathies: 1–4%; ulcerative colitis, Crohn disease, Behçet disease, celiac disease, diverticulitis
- Rare causes: <1% (3)
  - Fungal: dermatophytes, coccidioidomycosis, histoplasmosis, blastomycosis, Kerion of Celso
  - Viral/chlamydial: infectious mononucleosis; lymphogranuloma venereum; paravaccinia; HIV; hepatitis B, C
  - Malignancies: lymphoma/leukemia, sarcoma, myelodysplastic syndrome
  - Sweet syndrome
  - Sorafenib, pembrolizumab, dupilumab
  - COVID-19 virus, SARS-CoV-2 vaccine (4)

RISK FACTORS
See "Etiology and Pathophysiology."

COMMONLY ASSOCIATED CONDITIONS
See "Etiology and Pathophysiology."

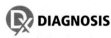 **DIAGNOSIS**

HISTORY
- Often a prodrome 1 to 3 weeks prior to the onset of lesions; can consist of malaise, fever, weight loss, cough, and arthralgia
- Increasingly tender nodules on the legs, usually over the shins
- Fever, malaise, chills, fatigue
- Headache
- Can precede systemic process by weeks

PHYSICAL EXAM
- Lesions initially present as warm, tender, erythematous firm nodules and plaques and become fluctuant, gradually fading to resemble a bruise >1 to 2 months (erythema contusiformis).
- Classically on anterior pretibial, although can extend proximally to involve thighs or trunk (atypically can involve extensor surface of forearms), rarely on the face
- Diameter varies from 1 to 10 cm with poor demarcation.

DIFFERENTIAL DIAGNOSIS
- Nodular vasculitis or erythema induratum (warm ulcerating calf nodules)
- Superficial thrombophlebitis
- Cellulitis
- Weber-Christian disease (violaceous, scarring nodules)
- Lupus panniculitis
- Cutaneous polyarteritis nodosa

- Sarcoidal granulomas
- Cutaneous T-cell lymphoma
- EN leprosum (clinically similar to EN but shows vasculitis on histopathology)
- Subcutaneous infection (including *Staphylococcus*, *Sporothrix schenckii*, *Nocardia brasiliensis*, *Mycobacterium marinum*, *Leishmania braziliensis*)

DIAGNOSTIC TESTS & INTERPRETATION
Diagnosis is made clinically, with support of testing.
- ESR or C-reactive protein (CRP): often elevated but can be normal in up to 40% (5)[C]
- CBC: mild leukocytosis (5)
- Urine pregnancy test (5)
- Throat culture, antistreptolysin O titer (5)
- Blood and/or stool culture, stool ova and parasites (O&P)
- Tuberculin skin testing (5)
- Seronegative rheumatoid factor

Initial Tests (lab, imaging)
CXR for hilar adenopathy or infiltrates related to sarcoidosis or tuberculosis (5)[C]

Diagnostic Procedures/Other
- Deep-incisional or excisional skin biopsy including subcutaneous tissue; rarely necessary except in atypical cases with ulceration, duration >12 weeks, or absence of nodules overlying lower limbs (6)
- Histology commonly reveals acute inflammation of the dermo-hypodermic junction and interlobular septa of the subcutaneous fat, developing without signs of necrosis or sequelae. Tissue culture should be considered in biopsy cases.
- Recently, cutaneous ultrasound can also be used to detect mixed lobular/septal panniculitis (7).

Test Interpretation
- Septal panniculitis without vasculitis
- Neutrophilic infiltrate in septa of fat tissue early in course
- Actinic radial (Miescher) granulomas, consisting of collections of histiocytes around a central stellate cleft, may be seen.
- Fibrosis, paraseptal granulation tissue, lymphocytes, and multinucleated giant cells predominate late in course (8).

 TREATMENT

- Condition usually self-limited within 1 to 2 months
- All medications listed as treatment for EN are off-label uses of the medications. There are no specific FDA-approved medications.

GENERAL MEASURES

- Mild compression bandages and leg elevation may reduce pain (wet dressings, hot soaks, and topical medications are not useful).
- Discontinue potentially causative drugs.
- If specific cause is identified, treatment of the condition typically leads to resolution of EN.
- Indication for treatment is poorly defined in literature; hence, therapy specifically for EN is directed toward symptom management.

MEDICATION

First Line

- NSAIDs:
  - Ibuprofen 400 mg PO q4–6h (not to exceed 3,200 mg/day)
  - Indomethacin 25 to 50 mg PO TID
  - Naproxen 250 to 500 mg PO BID
- Precautions
  - GI upset/bleeding (avoid in Crohn or ulcerative colitis)
  - Fluid retention
  - Renal insufficiency
  - Dose reduction in elderly, especially those with renal disease, diabetes, or heart failure
  - May mask fever
  - NSAIDs can increase cardiovascular (CV) risk.
- Significant possible interactions
  - May blunt antihypertensive effects of diuretics and β-blockers
  - NSAIDs can elevate plasma lithium levels.
  - NSAIDs can cause significant elevation and prolongation of methotrexate levels.

Second Line

- Potassium iodide 400 to 900 mg/day divided BID or TID for 3 to 4 weeks (for persistent lesions); need to monitor for hyperthyroidism with prolonged use; pregnancy class D (9)[B]
- Corticosteroids for severe, refractory, or recurrent cases in which an infectious workup is negative. Prednisone 1 mg/kg/day for 1 to 2 weeks is the recommended dose/duration. Potential side effects include hyperglycemia, hypertension, weight gain, worsening gastroesophageal reflux disease, mood changes, bone loss, osteonecrosis, and proximal myopathy (3).
- For EN related to Behçet disease, one can also consider colchicine 0.6 to 1.2 mg BID. Potential side effects include GI upset and diarrhea (10)[B].

ADMISSION, INPATIENT, AND NURSING CONSIDERATIONS

Occasionally, admission may be needed for the antecedent illness (e.g., tuberculosis).

 ONGOING CARE

FOLLOW-UP RECOMMENDATIONS

- Keep legs elevated.
- Elastic wraps or support stockings may be helpful when patients are ambulating.

Patient Monitoring

Monthly follow-up or as dictated by underlying disorder

DIET

No restrictions

PATIENT EDUCATION

- Lesions will resolve over a few weeks to months.
- Scarring is unlikely.
- Joint aches and pains may persist.
- <20% recur.

PROGNOSIS

- Individual lesions resolve generally within 2 weeks.
- Total time course of 6 to 12 weeks but may vary with underlying disease
- Joint aches and pains may persist for years.
- Lesions do not scar.
- Recurrences: occurs over variable periods, averaging several years; seen most often in sarcoid, streptococcal infection, pregnancy, and oral contraceptive use. If medication induced, avoid recurrent exposure.

COMPLICATIONS

- Vary according to underlying disease
- None expected from lesions of EN

REFERENCES

1. Chowaniec M, Starba A, Wiland P. Erythema nodosum—review of the literature. *Reumatologia*. 2016;54(2):79–82.
2. Laborada J, Cohen PR. Tuberculosis-associated erythema nodosum. *Cureus*. 2021;13(12):e20184.
3. Schwartz RA, Nervi SJ. Erythema nodosum: a sign of systemic disease. *Am Fam Physician*. 2007;75(5):695–700.
4. Xie Y, Yin B, Shi X. Erythema nodosum following SARS-CoV-2 vaccine. *J Eur Acad Dermatol Venereol*. 2022;36(10):e752–e753.
5. Cribier B, Caille A, Heid E, et al. Erythema nodosum and associated diseases. A study of 129 cases. *Int J Dermatol*. 1998;37(9):667–672.
6. Requena L, Yus ES. Erythema nodosum. *Dermatol Clin*. 2008;26(4):425–438.
7. Nazzaro G, Maronese CA, Passoni E. Ultrasonographic diagnosis of erythema nodosum. *Skin Res Technol*. 2022;28(2):361–364.
8. Yus ES, Sanz Vico MD, de Diego V. Miescher's radial granuloma. A characteristic marker of erythema nodosum. *Am J Dermatopathol*. 1989;11(5):434–442.
9. Horio T, Imamura S, Danno K, et al. Potassium iodide in the treatment of erythema nodosum and nodular vasculitis. *Arch Dermatol*. 1981;117(1):29–31.
10. Yurdakul S, Mat C, Tüzün Y, et al. A double-blind trial of colchicine in Behçet's syndrome. *Arthritis Rheum*. 2001;44(11):2686–2692.

ADDITIONAL READING

Mustin DE, Cole EF, Blalock TW, et al. Dupilumab-induced erythema nodosum. *JAAD Case Rep*. 2021;19:41–43.

 CODES

ICD10

- L52 Erythema nodosum
- A18.4 Tuberculosis of skin and subcutaneous tissue

CLINICAL PEARLS

- Lesions of EN appear to be erythematous patches, but when palpated, their underlying nodularity is appreciated.
- Evaluation for a concerning underlying etiology is necessary in EN, but most cases are idiopathic.
- EN in the setting of hilar adenopathy may be seen with multiple etiologies and does not exclusively indicate sarcoidosis.
- In patients with a history of Hodgkin lymphoma, EN may be an early sign of recurrence.

E

ESOPHAGEAL VARICES

Maximos Attia, MD, FAAFP • Marcelle Meseeha, MD

BASICS

DESCRIPTION
- Dilated submucosal esophageal veins connecting the portal and systemic circulations
- Most commonly results from portal hypertension (usually a result of cirrhosis)
- Variceal rupture: most common fatal complication of cirrhosis; severity of liver disease correlates with presence of varices and risk of bleeding.

EPIDEMIOLOGY
Incidence
- 30% of cirrhotic patients have varices at the time of diagnosis; 90% of cirrhotic patients will have varices at 10 years.
- 1-year rate of first variceal bleeding is 5% for small varices and 15% for large varices.

Prevalence
- 50% of patients with esophageal varices experience bleeding at some point.
- Variceal bleeding: 10–20% mortality in the 6 weeks following the episode
- Gender: male > female

ETIOLOGY AND PATHOPHYSIOLOGY
- Portal hypertension causes the formation of portacaval anastomoses to decompress the portal circulation. This leads to a congested submucosal venous plexus with tortuous dilated veins, particularly in the distal esophagus. Variceal rupture results in hemorrhage.
- Pathophysiology of portal hypertension:
  – Increased resistance to portal flow at the level of hepatic sinusoids caused by:
    ○ Intrahepatic vasoconstriction due to decreased nitric oxide production and increased release of endothelin-1 (ET-1), angiotensinogen, and eicosanoids
    ○ Sinusoidal remodeling causes disruption of blood flow.
  – Increased portal flow caused by hyperdynamic circulation due to splanchnic arterial vasodilation through mediators such as nitric oxide, prostacyclin, and TNF
- Causes of portal hypertension:
  – Prehepatic:
    ○ Extrahepatic portal vein obstruction
    ○ Massive splenomegaly with increased splenic vein blood flow
  – Posthepatic:
    ○ Severe right-sided heart failure, constrictive pericarditis, and hepatic vein obstruction (Budd-Chiari syndrome)
  – Intrahepatic:
    ○ Cirrhosis (accounts for most cases of portal hypertension)
  – Less frequent causes are schistosomiasis, massive fatty change, diseases affecting portal microcirculation as nodular regenerative hyperplasia, and diffuse fibrosing granulomatous disease as sarcoidosis.

Genetics
Cirrhosis is rarely hereditary.

RISK FACTORS
- Cirrhosis. In cirrhotic patients, thrombocytopenia and splenomegaly are independent predictors of esophageal varices.
- Noncirrhotic portal hypertension. Increased bleeding risk for known varices is associated with varix size, endoscopic signs (red wale marks, cherry-red spots), vessel wall thickness, and abrupt increase in variceal pressure (i.e., Valsalva maneuver).
- MELD/Child-Pugh score; presence of portal vein thrombosis; high hepatic venous pressure gradient (HVPG)

GENERAL PREVENTION
Prevent underlying causes: Prevent alcohol abuse, administer hepatitis B vaccine, needle hygiene, IV drug use (needle exchange programs reduce risk of hepatitis); specific screening and therapy for hepatitis B and C, hemochromatosis

COMMONLY ASSOCIATED CONDITIONS
- Portal hypertensive gastropathy; varices in stomach, duodenum, colon, rectum (causes massive bleeding, unlike hemorrhoids); rarely at umbilicus (caput medusae) or ostomy sites
- Isolated gastric varices can occur due to splenic vein thrombosis/stenosis from hypercoagulability/contiguous inflammation (most commonly, chronic pancreatitis).
- Other complications of cirrhosis: hepatic encephalopathy, ascites, hepatorenal syndrome, spontaneous bacterial peritonitis, hepatocellular carcinoma

DIAGNOSIS

- First indication of varices is often GI bleeding: hematemesis, hematochezia, and/or melena.
- Occult bleeding (anemia): uncommon

HISTORY
- Underlying history of cirrhosis/liver disease. Variceal bleed can be initial presentation of previously undiagnosed cirrhosis.
- Alcohol abuse, exposure to blood-borne viruses through intravenous drug use or sexual practices
- Hematemesis, melena, or hematochezia
- Rapid upper GI bleed can present as rectal bleeding.

PHYSICAL EXAM
- Assess hemodynamic stability: hypotension, tachycardia (active bleeding).
- Abdominal exam—liver palpation/percussion (often small and firm with cirrhosis)
- Splenomegaly, ascites (shifting dullness; fluid shift; puddle splash—physical maneuvers have limited sensitivity)
- Visible abdominal periumbilical collateral circulation (caput medusae)
- Peripheral stigmata of alcohol abuse: spider angiomata on chest/back, palmar erythema, testicular atrophy, gynecomastia
- Rectal varices
- Hepatic encephalopathy; asterixis
- Blood on rectal exam

DIFFERENTIAL DIAGNOSIS
- Upper GI bleeding: 10–30% are due to varices.
  – In patients with known varices, as many as 50% bleed from nonvariceal sources.
  – Peptic ulcer; gastritis; gastric/esophageal malignancy
  – Congestive gastropathy of portal hypertension; arteriovenous malformation
  – Mallory-Weiss tears; aortoenteric fistula
  – Hemoptysis; nosebleed
- Lower GI bleeding
  – Rectal varices; hemorrhoids
  – Colonic neoplasia
  – Diverticulosis/arteriovenous malformation
  – Rapidly bleeding upper GI site
- Continued/recurrent bleeding risk: actively bleeding/large varix, high Child-Pugh severity score, infection, renal failure

DIAGNOSTIC TESTS & INTERPRETATION
Initial Tests (lab, imaging)
- Anemia: Hemoglobin may be normal in active bleeding; may require 6 to 24 hours to equilibrate; other causes of anemia are common in patients with cirrhosis.
- Thrombocytopenia: most sensitive and specific parameter, correlates with portal hypertension, large esophageal varices
- Abnormal aspartate aminotransferase (AST), alanine aminotransferase (ALT), alkaline phosphatase, bilirubin; prolonged PT; low albumin suggests cirrhosis.
- BUN, creatinine (BUN often elevated in GI bleed)
- Sodium level; may drop in patients treated with terlipressin
- Noninvasive tests are preferred to rule out high-risk varices (HRVs) in patients with compensated cirrhosis (1)[B].
- Esophagogastroduodenoscopy
  – Can identify actively bleeding varices as well as large varices and stigmata of recent bleeding
  – Can be used to treat bleeding with esophageal band ligation (preferred to sclerotherapy); prevent rebleeding; detect gastric varices, portal hypertensive gastropathy; diagnose alternative bleeding sites
  – Can identify and treat nonbleeding varices (protruding submucosal veins in the distal third of the esophagus)

Diagnostic Procedures/Other
- Transient elastography (TE) for identifying CLD patients at risk of developing clinically significant portal hypertension (CSPH)
- HVPG >10 mm Hg: gold standard to diagnose CSPH (normal: 1 to 5 mm Hg)
- HVPG response of ≥10% or to ≤12 mm Hg to intravenous propranolol identifies responders to nonselective β-blocker (NSBB) and is linked to a decreased risk of variceal bleeding (2)[A].
- Video capsule endoscopy screening as an alternative to traditional endoscopy
- Doppler sonography (second line): demonstrates patency, diameter, and flow in portal and splenic veins, and collaterals; sensitive for gastric varices; documents patency after ligation or transjugular intrahepatic portosystemic shunt (TIPS)

- CT- or MRI-angiography (second line, not routine): demonstrates large vascular channels in abdomen, mediastinum; demonstrates patency of intrahepatic portal and splenic vein
  - Venous-phase celiac arteriography: demonstrates portal vein and collaterals; hepatic vein occlusion
  - Portal pressure measurement using retrograde catheter in hepatic vein

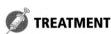 **TREATMENT**

GENERAL MEASURES
- Treat underlying cirrhotic comorbidities.
- Variceal bleeding is often complicated by hepatic encephalopathy and infection.
- Active bleeding (1)
  - IV access, hemodynamic resuscitation
  - Type and crossmatch packed RBCs. Overtransfusion increases portal pressure and increases rebleeding risk.
  - Treat coagulopathy as necessary. Fresh frozen plasma may increase blood volume and increase rebleeding risk.
  - Avoid sedation, monitor mental status, and avoid nephrotoxic drugs and β-blockers acutely.
  - IV octreotide to lower portal venous pressure as adjuvant to endoscopic management; IV bolus of 50 μg followed by drip of 50 μg/hr
  - Terlipressin (alternative): 2 mg q4h IV for 24 to 48 hours and then 1 mg q4h
  - Erythromycin 250 mg IV 30 to 120 minutes before endoscopy
  - Urgent upper GI endoscopy for diagnosis and treatment
    - Variceal band ligation preferred to sclerotherapy for bleeding varices; also for nonbleeding medium-to-large varices to decrease bleeding risk
    - Ligation: lower rates of rebleeding, fewer complications, more rapid cessation of bleeding, higher rate of variceal eradication
- Repeat ligation/sclerosant for rebleeding.
- If endoscopic treatment fails, consider self-expanding esophageal metal stents or per oral placement of Sengstaken-Blakemore–type tube up to 24 hours to stabilize patient for TIPS.
- As many as 2/3 of patients with variceal bleeding develop an infection, most commonly spontaneous bacterial peritonitis, UTI, or pneumonia; antibiotic prophylaxis with oral norfloxacin 400 mg or IV ceftriaxone 1 g q24h for up to a week
- In active bleeding, avoid β-blockers, which decrease BP and blunt the physiologic increase in heart rate during acute hemorrhage.
- Prevent recurrence of acute bleeding.
  - Vasoconstrictors: terlipressin, octreotide (reduce portal pressure)
  - Endoscopic band ligation (EBL): if bleeding recurs/portal pressure measurement shows portal pressure remains >12 mm Hg
  - TIPS: second-line therapy if above methods fail; TIPS decreases portal pressure by creating communication between hepatic vein and an intrahepatic portal vein branch.

MEDICATION
Primary prevention of variceal bleeding
- Endoscopy: assesses variceal size, presence of red wale sign (longitudinal variceal reddish streak that suggests either a recent bleed or a pending bleed) to determine risk stratification.
  - Primary prophylaxis: (i) NSBB, (ii) endoscopic variceal ligation (EVL)
  - Endoscopy every 2 to 3 years if cirrhosis but no varices; every 1 to 2 years if small varices and not receiving β-blockers (2)[A]

First Line
- Not actively bleeding. NSBB reduces portal pressure and decreases risk of first bleed from 25% to 15% when used as primary prophylaxis; beneficial in cirrhosis with small varices and increased hemorrhage risk as well as cirrhosis with medium-to-large varices (2)
- Carvedilol: 6.25 mg daily (2)[A] is more effective than NSBB in dropping HVPG.
  - Propranolol: 20 mg BID increase until heart rate decreased by 25% from baseline
  - Nadolol 80 mg daily; increase as above
  - Contraindications: severe asthma
- Chronic prevention of rebleeding (secondary prevention): NSBBs and EBL reduce rate of rebleeding to a similar extent, but β-blockers reduce mortality, whereas ligation does not.

Second Line
Obliterate varices with esophageal ligation if not tolerant of medication prophylaxis.
- During ligation: proton pump inhibitors, such as lansoprazole 30 mg/day, until varices obliterated
- Management of Budd-Chiari syndrome: anticoagulation, angioplasty/thrombolysis, TIPS, and orthotopic liver transplantation
- Management of EHPVO: anticoagulation; mesenteric-left portal vein bypass (Meso-Rex procedure)

ISSUES FOR REFERRAL
Refer for endoscopy, liver transplant, and interventional radiology for TIPS.

ADDITIONAL THERAPIES
Pneumococcal and hepatitis A/B vaccine (HAV/HBV)

SURGERY/OTHER PROCEDURES
- Esophageal transection: in rare cases of uncontrollable, exsanguinating bleeding
- Liver transplantation

 ONGOING CARE

FOLLOW-UP RECOMMENDATIONS
Patient Monitoring
- EVL, every 1 to 4 weeks, until varices eradicated
- Endoscopic screening in patients with known cirrhosis every 2 to 3 years; yearly in patients with decompensated cirrhosis
- Patients with a liver stiffness <20 kPa and with platelets >150,000 can avoid endoscopic screening and may follow up by annual TE and platelet count.

PATIENT EDUCATION
National Institute of Diabetes and Digestive and Kidney Diseases (https://www.niddk.nih.gov/health-information/) or American Liver Foundation (http://liverfoundation.org/)

PROGNOSIS
- In cirrhosis, 1-year survival is 50% for those who survive at least 2 weeks following a variceal bleed.
- In-hospital mortality remains high and is related to severity of underlying cirrhosis, ranging from 0% in Child-Pugh class A disease to 32% in Child-Pugh class C disease.
- Prognosis in noncirrhotic portal fibrosis is better than for cirrhotic portal fibrosis.

COMPLICATIONS
- Formation of gastric varices after eradication of esophageal varices
- Esophageal varices can recur.
- Hepatic encephalopathy, renal dysfunction, hepatorenal syndrome
- Infections after banding/ligation of varices

REFERENCES
1. Jakab SS, Garcia-Tsao G. Evaluation and management of esophageal and gastric varices in patients with cirrhosis. *Clin Liver Dis.* 2020;24(3):335–350.
2. Simonetto DA, Liu M, Kamath PS. Portal hypertension and related complications: diagnosis and management. *Mayo Clin Proc.* 2019;94(4):714–726.

ADDITIONAL READING
Mauro E, Gadano A. What's new in portal hypertension? *Liver Int.* 2020;40(Suppl 1):122–127.

 CODES

ICD10
- I85.0 Esophageal varices
- I85 Esophageal varices
- I85.1 Secondary esophageal varices

CLINICAL PEARLS
- Thrombocytopenia is the most sensitive marker of increased portal pressure and large esophageal varices.
- Roughly half of all patients with cirrhosis will have esophageal varices. One in three of those patients with varices will experience a variceal bleed. The risk of bleeding relates directly to the size and appearance of the esophageal varices.
- β-Blockers (nadolol, propranolol, carvedilol) act to reduce pressure in the portal circulation and are the preferred pharmacologic choice for primary prevention of variceal bleeding.
- In acute bleeding, avoid β-blockers, and overtransfusion can elevate portal pressure and increase bleeding risk.

ESSENTIAL TREMOR SYNDROME

Jennifer E. Svarverud, DO

 BASICS

DESCRIPTION

- Essential tremor is a postural (occurring with voluntary maintenance of a position against gravity) or kinetic (occurring during voluntary movement) flexion–extension tremor that is slow and rhythmic and primarily affects the hands, forearms, head, or voice with a frequency of 4 to 12 Hz. Older patients tend to have lower frequency tremors, whereas younger patients exhibit frequencies in the higher range.
- The disease may be familial, sporadic, or associated with other movement disorders. Incidence and prevalence increase with age, but symptom onset can occur at any age. The tremor can be intermittent and exacerbated by emotional or physical stressors, fatigue, and caffeine.
- System(s) affected: neurologic, musculoskeletal, ear/nose/throat (ENT) (voice)

EPIDEMIOLOGY

Essential tremor is the most common pathologic tremor in humans.

Incidence

Can occur at any age, but bimodal peaks exist in the 2nd and 6th decades. Incidence rises significantly after age 49 years.

Prevalence

The overall prevalence for essential tremor has been estimated between 0.4% and 0.9% but is increased in older patients with an estimated prevalence of 4.6% at age 65 years and up to 22% at age 95 years.

ETIOLOGY AND PATHOPHYSIOLOGY

- Suspected to originate from an abnormal oscillation within thalamocortical and cerebello-olivary loops, as lesions in these areas tend to reduce essential tremor
- Essential tremor is not a homogenous disorder. Many patients have other motor manifestations and nonmotor features, including cognitive and psychiatric symptoms.

Genetics

- Positive family history in 50–70% of patients; autosomal dominant inheritance is demonstrated in many families with poor penetrance. Twin studies suggest that environmental factors are also involved.
- A link to genetic loci exists on chromosomes 2p22–2p25, 3q13, and 6p23. In addition, a Ser9Gly variant in the dopamine D_3 receptor gene on 3q13 has been suggested as a risk factor.

COMMONLY ASSOCIATED CONDITIONS

- Can be present in 10% of patients with Parkinson disease (PD); characteristics of PD that distinguish it from essential tremor include 3- to 5-Hz resting tremor; accompanying rigidity, bradykinesia, or postural instability; and no change with alcohol consumption
- Patients with essential tremor have a 4% risk of developing PD.
- Resting tremor, typically of the arm, may be seen in up to 20–30% of patients with essential tremor. Although action tremor is the hallmark feature of essential tremor, it is commonly found in patients with PD as well.

 DIAGNOSIS

HISTORY

- Core criteria for diagnosis
  - Bilateral action or postural or kinetic tremor (occurs with voluntary muscle contraction) of the hands and forearms
  - Absence of other neurologic signs with the exception of cogwheel phenomenon
  - May have tremor in other locations to include head, voice, or lower limbs
  - Symptoms present for at least 3 years' duration
- Secondary criteria include positive family history and beneficial response to alcohol.

PHYSICAL EXAM

- Tremor can affect upper limbs (~95% of patients).
- Less commonly, the tremor affects head (~34%), lower limbs (~30%), voice (~12%), tongue (~7%), face (~5%), and trunk (~5%).

DIFFERENTIAL DIAGNOSIS

- PD
- Enhanced physiologic tremor
- Wilson disease
- Hyperthyroidism
- Multiple sclerosis
- Dystonic tremor
- Cerebellar tremor
- Asterixis
- Psychogenic tremor
- Orthostatic tremor
- Drug-induced or enhanced physiologic tremor (amiodarone, cimetidine, lamotrigine, itraconazole, valproic acid, SSRIs, steroids, lithium, cyclosporine, β-adrenergic agonists, ephedrine, theophylline, tricyclic antidepressants [TCAs], antipsychotics)

DIAGNOSTIC TESTS & INTERPRETATION

Initial Tests (lab, imaging)

- No specific biologic marker or diagnostic test is available.
- Ceruloplasmin and serum copper to rule out Wilson disease
- Thyroid-stimulating hormone to rule out thyroid dysfunction
- Serum electrolytes, BUN, creatinine
- Brain MRI usually is not necessary or indicated unless Wilson disease is found or exam findings imply central lesion.

Diagnostic Procedures/Other

- Accelerometry evaluates tremor frequency and amplitude; >95% of PD cases exhibit frequencies in the 4- to 6-Hz range, and 95% of essential tremor cases exhibit frequencies in the 5- to 8-Hz range.
- Surface electromyography is less helpful in distinguishing essential tremor from PD.

Test Interpretation

Posture-related tremor seen on exam

 TREATMENT

MEDICATION

Pharmacologic treatment should be considered when tremor interferes with activities of daily living (ADLs) or causes psychological distress.

First Line

- Propranolol 60 to 320 mg/day in divided doses or in long-acting formulation reduces limb tremor magnitude by ~50%, and almost 70% of patients experience improvement in clinical rating scales. There is insufficient evidence to recommend propranolol for vocal tremor. Single doses of propranolol, taken before social situations that are likely to exacerbate tremor, are useful for some patients.
- Primidone 25 mg at bedtime, gradually titrated to 150 to 300 mg at bedtime, improves tremor amplitude by 40–50%. Maximum dose is 750 mg/day, with doses >250 mg/day typically divided to BID or TID. Low-dose therapy (<250 mg/day) is just as effective as high-dose (750 mg/day) therapy.
- Propranolol and primidone have similar efficacy when used as initial therapy for limb tremor; both carry a level A recommendation (1)[A].
- 30–50% of patients will not respond to either propranolol or primidone.

Second Line

- Topiramate in doses up to 400 mg/day decreases tremor and is recommended as second line by the American Academy of Neurology (AAN) (1)[B].
- Gabapentin up to 400 mg TID (1)[B]
- Sotalol, nadolol, and atenolol are alternative β-blockers; each has less evidence than propranolol to support use.
- Clonazepam and alprazolam should be used with caution because of potential abuse.
- Clozapine has shown efficacy at doses of 6 to 75 mg/day but is recommended only for refractory cases of limb tremor because of a 1% risk of agranulocytosis. The AAN indicates that insufficient evidence exists to support or refute the efficacy of clozapine for chronic use (1)[A].
- Memantine, in a pilot study using doses up to 40 mg/day, showed significant benefit in a small subset of the study group. Adverse events at this dose included dizziness, somnolence, and poor energy (2)[B].
- Pramipexole, at a dose of 2.1 mg/day, demonstrated moderate efficacy in reducing severity of tremor in a pilot study of 29 patients. Immediate- and extended-release formulations were equally effective (3)[B].
- Levetiracetam and 3,4-diaminopyridine are probably ineffective at reducing limb tremor and should not be considered according to the AAN (1)[A].
- Other medications that have been evaluated for treatment of essential tremor, with limited data to support their use, include acetazolamide, clonidine, flunarizine, methazolamide, nimodipine, olanzapine, phenobarbital, pregabalin, quetiapine, sodium oxybate, and zonisamide (1)[A].
- Alcohol may provide transient improvement in symptoms, but its brief duration of action, subsequent rebound, and associated risk of developing alcohol addiction make it a less attractive option for longer term treatment. Alcohol may be an appropriate option for short-term, situation-specific improvement in symptoms.
- Botulinum toxin A injections should be offered as a treatment option for cervical dystonia (level A recommendation from AAN) and may be offered for blepharospasm, focal upper extremity dystonia, adductor laryngeal dystonia, and upper extremity essential tremor (1)[B].

SURGERY/OTHER PROCEDURES

- Deep brain stimulation provides a magnitude of benefit that is superior to all available medications and may be used to treat medically refractory limb tremor; it has fewer adverse effects than thalamotomy.
- Bilateral thalamic ventral intermediate nucleus stimulation is effective in reducing tremor and functional disability; however, paresthesias and dysarthria are possible complications.
- Unilateral thalamotomy may be used to treat limb tremor that is refractory to medical management.
- Bilateral thalamotomy is not recommended because of adverse side effects.
- There is growing interest in development of external neuromodulator devices for the treatment of essential tremor to include exoskeletons, orthosis, and biomechanical loading. Currently, evidence for these devices is limited and of low quality, and further research is needed.

COMPLEMENTARY & ALTERNATIVE MEDICINE

Physical therapy may be considered for strengthening and training in use of weighted utensils to help offset the tremor. Although strength training has not been shown to have improvement in functional ability, no negative effects have been reported.

ONGOING CARE

DIET
Avoid caffeine.

PATIENT EDUCATION
Although essential tremor can cause significant impairment in daily functioning, it does not decrease life expectancy.

PROGNOSIS
Tremor tends to worsen with age, increasing in amplitude.

REFERENCES

1. Zesiewicz TA, Elble RJ, Louis ED, et al. Evidence-based guideline update: treatment of essential tremor: report of the Quality Standards Subcommittee of the American Academy of Neurology. *Neurology*. 2011;77(19):1752–1755.
2. Handforth A, Bordelon Y, Frucht SJ, et al. A pilot efficacy and tolerability trial of memantine for essential tremor. *Clin Neuropharmacol*. 2010;33(5):223–226.
3. Herceg M, Nagy F, Pál E, et al. Pramipexole may be an effective treatment option in essential tremor. *Clin Neuropharmacol*. 2012;35(2):73–76.

ADDITIONAL READING

- Buijink AWG, Contarino MF, Koelman JHTM, et al. How to tackle tremor—systematic review of the literature and diagnostic work-up. *Front Neurol*. 2012;3:146.
- Deuschl G, Raethjen J, Hellriegel H, et al. Treatment of patients with essential tremor. *Lancet Neurol*. 2011;10(2):148–161.

CODES

ICD10
G25.0 Essential tremor

CLINICAL PEARLS

- Core criteria for diagnosis of essential tremor include bilateral action or postural tremor of the hands, forearm, and/or head without a resting component present for at least 3 years.
- Beneficial response to alcohol and positive family history help to differentiate essential tremor from PD (PD is characterized by tremor at rest, bradykinesia, and rigidity, and it does not improve with alcohol use).
- 10% of patients with PD will have both resting tremors of PD and essential tremor.
- Wilson disease, thyroid disease, and medication effect should be ruled out.
- Brain MRI is usually not necessary or indicated.
- First-line treatments include propranolol and primidone. 30–50% of patients will not benefit from these first-line treatments.

EUSTACHIAN TUBE DYSFUNCTION

Roland W. Newman II, DO

 BASICS

The eustachian tube (ET), also known as the auditory or pharyngotympanic tube, connects the posterior nasopharynx to the middle ear. The proximal two-thirds of the ET is composed of cartilage, whereas the distal third closest to the middle ear is made of bone. Its primary function is to equilibrate pressure within the middle ear to atmospheric pressure. It also ventilates and drains the middle ear space which prevents and clears infection and debris. When the ET malfunctions by either becoming too dilated (patulous dysfunction) or occluded (obstructive dysfunction), it results in ET dysfunction (ETD).

DESCRIPTION

- A spectrum of disorders involving impairment of the functional valve of the ET
- ETD can be classified as *patulous dysfunction*, in which the ET is excessively open, or *dilatory dysfunction*, in which there is failure of the tubes to dilate (i.e., open) appropriately.
- Pathophysiology related to pressure dysregulation, impaired protection secondary to reflux of irritating material into the middle ear, or impaired clearance by the mucociliary system
- May occur in the setting of pressure changes (e.g., scuba diving or air travel) or acute upper airway inflammation (e.g., allergic or infectious rhinosinusitis, acute otitis media [OM])
- Chronic ETD may lead to a retracted tympanic membrane, recurrent serous effusion, recurrent OM, adhesive OM, chronic mastoiditis, or cholesteatoma.
- Synonym(s): auditory tube dysfunction; ET disorder; blocked ET; patulous ET

ALERT
Sudden sensorineural hearing loss (SSNHL) can be misdiagnosed as ETD.
- A simple 512-Hz tuning fork test lateralizes to the opposite ear in SSNHL and to the affected ear in ETD with conductive hearing loss.
- Any SSNHL is a medical emergency and should be referred to an otolaryngologist immediately.

EPIDEMIOLOGY
Adults: >2 million health care visits annually
- Median age: 48
- Females > Males
- Most common comorbidity is acute rhinitis.

Prevalence
Greater in children than in adults (0.77 adult visits to every 1 pediatric visit) (1)

ETIOLOGY AND PATHOPHYSIOLOGY
- Under normal circumstances, the ET is closed, opening to release a small amount of air to equilibrate middle ear pressure with surrounding atmospheric pressure.
- ETD is failure of the ET, palate, nasal cavities, and nasopharynx to regulate middle ear and mastoid pressure.

- ET functions:
  - Ventilation/regulation of middle ear pressure
  - Protection from nasopharyngeal secretions
  - Drainage of middle ear fluid
  - ET is closed at rest and opens with yawning, swallowing, and chewing.
- Cycle of dysfunction: structural or functional obstruction of the ET:
  - Negative pressure develops in middle ear.
  - Serous exudate is drawn to the middle ear by negative pressure or refluxed into the middle ear if the ET opens momentarily.
  - Infection of static fluid causes edema and release of inflammatory mediators, exacerbating the cycle of inflammation and obstruction.
- In children, a horizontal and shorter ET predisposes to difficulties with ventilation and drainage.
- Adenoid hypertrophy can block the torus tubarius (proximal opening of the ET).
- In adults, paradoxical closing of the ET with swallowing occurs in a majority of affected patients.
- Tumors that impair/occlude the ET or that invade the tensor veli palatini to impair normal swallow regulation, can also lead to dysfunction.

Genetics
Twin studies show a genetic component. Specific genetic cause is undefined.

RISK FACTORS
Adult and pediatric:
- Allergic rhinitis, tobacco exposure, GERD, chronic sinusitis, adenoid hypertrophy or nasopharyngeal mass, neuromuscular disease, altered immunity
- Prematurity and low birth weight, young age, daycare, crowded living conditions, low socioeconomic status, prone sleeping position, prolonged bottle use, craniofacial abnormalities (e.g., cleft palate, Down syndrome)

Pregnancy Considerations
ETD may be exacerbated by rhinitis of pregnancy; symptoms resolve postpartum.

GENERAL PREVENTION
- Control of upper airway inflammation: allergies, infectious rhinosinusitis, GERD
- Autoinsufflation of middle ear (i.e., blow gently against pinched nostril and closed mouth)
- Avoid atmospheric pressure changes (e.g., plane flight, scuba diving) in the setting of acute allergy exacerbation or URI.
- Avoid exposure to environmental irritants: tobacco smoke and pollutants.

COMMONLY ASSOCIATED CONDITIONS
- Hearing loss
- OM: acute, chronic, and serous; chronic mastoiditis; cholesteatoma
- Allergic rhinitis, chronic sinusitis/URI, adenoid hypertrophy
- GERD
- Cleft palate, Down syndrome
- Obesity
- Nasopharyngeal carcinoma or other tumor

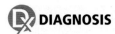 **DIAGNOSIS**

HISTORY
- Symptoms of ear pain, fullness, "plugging," hearing loss, tinnitus, popping or snapping noises, and vertigo
  - Unilateral or bilateral. Evaluate adults with persistent unilateral symptoms for nasopharyngeal tumor.
  - History of previous ear infections, surgeries, head trauma, recent flying or diving
  - Voice change (hypo- or hypernasal voice, consider NP mass or palatal dysfunction)
  - Differentiate patulous dysfunction, in which patient's own voice and breath sounds are amplified (autophony), from dilatory dysfunction, in which patient complains more of ear pain, "plugged" ear, hearing loss, and tinnitus.
- ETDQ-7 is a questionnaire that attempts to quantify ETD in adult patients. Based on presence and intensity of symptoms in past 1 month, severity is rated on 1 to 7 scale. A total score >14.5 categorizes patient as having ETD (2)[B].
  - Pressure in ears in past 1 month?
  - Pain in ears in past 1 month?
  - A feeling that ears are clogged or "under water"?
  - Ear symptoms when you have cold or sinusitis?
  - Crackling or popping sounds in the ears?
  - Ringing in ears?
  - A feeling that your hearing is muffled?

PHYSICAL EXAM
- Pneumatic otoscopy: retracted tympanic membrane, effusion, decreased drum movement
- Toynbee maneuver: View changes of the drum while patient autoinsufflates against closed lips and pinched nostrils; may show various degrees of retraction
  - Entire drum may be retracted and "lateralize" with insufflation.
  - Posterosuperior quadrant (pars flaccida) may form a retraction pocket.
- Tuning fork tests: 512-Hz fork placed on the forehead lateralizes to affected ear (Weber test); the fork will be louder behind the ear on the mastoid than in front of the ear (bone conduction > air conduction, Rinne test) in conductive hearing loss.
- Nasopharyngoscopy: adenoid hypertrophy or nasopharyngeal mass
- Anterior rhinoscopy: deviated nasal septum, polyps, mucosal hypertrophy, turbinate hypertrophy

DIFFERENTIAL DIAGNOSIS
- SSNHL (a medical emergency)
- Tympanic membrane perforation
- Barotrauma
- Temporomandibular joint disorder
- Ménière disease
- Superior semicircular canal dehiscence

DIAGNOSTIC TESTS & INTERPRETATION
Initial Tests (lab, imaging)
- No routine radiologic studies needed if clinical signs/symptoms suggest ETD
- CT scan (not necessary) may show changes related to OM or middle ear/mastoid opacification.
- Functional MRI might determine cause of ETD (in recalcitrant cases), as the ET opening can be visualized during Valsalva.

Diagnostic Procedures/Other
- Audiogram may show conductive hearing loss.
- Tympanometry: Type B or C tympanograms indicate fluid or retraction, respectively; negative middle ear peak pressures seen even with normal (type A) tympanograms

 ## TREATMENT
- Due to limited high-quality evidence, it is difficult to recommend any one treatment option/intervention as superior.
- Use of a "nasal balloon" shown effective for clearing OM with effusion; unclear of benefit for ETD
- General principle is to remove or fix the underlying cause (e.g., infection, tumor, perforation of tympanic membrane, restore tensor palatini muscle) and reduce or eliminate the cycle of infection/inflammation
- Although no evidence exists, some consider antibiotics for acute OM; decongestants, nasal steroids, antihistamines (if allergic rhinitis is present), and surgery/procedures for recalcitrant cases
- Tympanostomy tubes ± adenoidectomy when indicated for recurrent ear infections or severe progressive retractions

MEDICATION
- Antibiotics only if infection is suspected as cause of ETD
- Few data support pharmacologic treatments such as decongestants, nasal steroids, or antihistamines for ETD.
- Medications treat comorbid conditions.
- Decongestants, topical, oral
  – Avoid prolonged use (>3 days); can cause rhinitis medicamentosa
  – Decongestants are most useful for acute ETD related to a resolving URI.
  – Decongestants are not typically used for relief of chronic ETD in children.
    ○ Phenylephrine
    ○ Pseudoephedrine
    ○ Oxymetazoline
- Nasal steroids (may be beneficial for those with allergic rhinitis)
  – Beclomethasone (Beconase, Vancenase)
  – Budesonide (Rhinocort)
  – Fluticasone propionate (Flonase)
  – Mometasone (Nasonex)
  – Triamcinolone (Nasacort)
- 2nd-generation H1 antihistamines (may be beneficial for those with ETD and chronic rhinitis)
  – Cetirizine (Zyrtec) (tablets, chewable tablets, liquid)
  – Desloratadine (Clarinex) (tablets, RediTabs, liquid)
  – Fexofenadine (Allegra) (tablets, RediTabs, liquid)
  – Levocetirizine (Xyzal) (tablets, liquid)
- Antihistamine nasal sprays (may be beneficial for those with ETD and chronic rhinitis)
  – Azelastine (Astepro or Astelin)
  – Olopatadine (Patanase)

ADDITIONAL THERAPIES
- Any activity that promotes swallowing, such as chewing gum, eating or drinking, can open the ET and promote relief of symptoms.
- Patients with ETD should refrain from flying during times of nasal congestion or ear infection. If the patient must fly, advise them to take oral and intranasal decongestants an hour prior to take off.
- Patients should refrain from scuba diving.

SURGERY/OTHER PROCEDURES
- Myringotomy and pressure equalization tube placement to ventilate middle ear, relieve pressure, and prevent sequelae of chronically retracted drum
- Patients with ETD during pressure changes may benefit from minimally invasive laser eustachian tuboplasty.
- Balloon tuboplasty (limited data in terms of efficacy, safety, and long-term outcomes)
- Microwave ablation (MWA) targeting hypertrophic tissue at the orifice of the ET (3)
- Adenoidectomy if hypertrophied tissue is present
  – In children, first set of tubes are typically placed alone. Adenoidectomy is performed with second set of tubes if problems recur.
  – Some advocate adenoidectomy even in absence of excess tissue; reduces frequency and number of subsequent tubes

COMPLEMENTARY & ALTERNATIVE MEDICINE
Osteopathic manipulative treatment (OMT) can be utilized in the treatment of ETD.
- Galbreath technique
- Modified Muncie technique

 ## ONGOING CARE

FOLLOW-UP RECOMMENDATIONS
- Monitor pressure equalization tubes every 6 to 8 months in children and every 6 to 12 months in adults.
- Monitor tympanic membrane retraction pocket for progression every 6 to 12 months to allow for early intervention for progression in hearing loss, obvious ossicular erosion, or cholesteatoma.

DIET
Breastfeeding is associated with lower incidence of ETD and OM.

PROGNOSIS
If symptoms of ETD persist beyond age 7 years, patient is more likely to have long-term problems and require regular monitoring.

COMPLICATIONS
Morbidity related to hearing compromise or associated sequela of chronic ear infections

REFERENCES
1. Hamrang-Yousefi S, Ng J, Andaloro C. *Eustachian Tube Dysfunction*. In: StatPearls [Internet]. Treasure Island, FL: StatPearls Publishing; 2023. https://www.ncbi.nlm.nih.gov/books/NBK555908/. Updated February 13, 2023. Accessed September 21, 2023.
2. Van Roeyen S, Van de Heyning P, Van Rompaey V. Value and discriminative power of the seven-item Eustachian Tube Dysfunction Questionnaire. *Laryngoscope*. 2015;125(11):2553–2556.
3. Bal R, Deshmukh P. Management of eustachian tube dysfunction: a review. *Cureus*. 2022;14(11):e31432.

 ## SEE ALSO

Algorithm: Ear Pain/Otalgia

 ## CODES

ICD10
- H69.90 Unspecified Eustachian tube disorder, unspecified ear
- H69.00 Patulous Eustachian tube, unspecified ear
- H68.109 Unspecified obstruction of Eustachian tube, unspecified ear

CLINICAL PEARLS
- ETD can be acute or chronic. Treatment is based on the underlying etiology.
- Rule out SSNHL (medical emergency), which can be misdiagnosed as ETD, especially in patients with unilateral symptoms.

FACTOR V LEIDEN

Frank J. Domino, MD • Elyas Parsa, DO

BASICS

DESCRIPTION

- Factor V Leiden (FVL) is a genetic point mutation in the F5 gene at the activated protein C (APC) cleavage site on the factor V and Va molecule leading to increase in thrombin and as a result leads to clot formation. This is the most common form of inherited thrombophilia.
- System(s) affected: cardiovascular, gastrointestinal, hemo/lymphatic/immunologic, nervous, pulmonary, reproductive
- Synonym(s): FVL thrombophilia; FVL mutation, hereditary APC resistance

Pediatric Considerations
- The incidence of venous thrombosis in healthy children is extremely low (0.07/100,000 per year).
- There is a weak, however significant, association between procoagulant states (including FVL) and coronary events in younger patients.

Pregnancy Considerations
- Recurrent pregnancy loss is a possible complication.
- Increased thrombotic risk in pregnancy and postpartum (additive) especially in homozygous state
- Possible increased risk of IUGR, preeclampsia, placental abruption: evidence mixed
- Women with a history of adverse pregnancy outcomes should be tested for thrombophilia if they are planning a future pregnancy (1).

EPIDEMIOLOGY
Prevalence
- ~5–8% occurrence of heterozygosity in Caucasians, Hispanic Americans ~2%, African Americans ~1%, and Asian Americans ~0.45% of those heterozygous for FVL small percentage of individuals develop VTE, estimated 5–10%
- General population 4–5% without history of venous thromboembolism (VTE); 12–14% reported in parts of Greece, Sweden, and Lebanon. No reports seen in Chinese or Japanese

ETIOLOGY AND PATHOPHYSIOLOGY
- Factor V is a protein that is part of the clotting cascade that circulates in the plasma. When exposed to tissue factor, factor V amplifies the production of thrombin, which further promotes clotting by activating factor V into procoagulant factor Va.
- For balance, thrombin also promotes APC production, which will cleave and inactivate factors V, Va, and VIII, thereby keeping the clotting cascade in check (negative feedback loop).
- In FVL, a point mutation at the binding site of APC (Arg506Glu) renders it less able to cleave factor V or Va. This reduces the anticoagulant role of factor V as a cofactor to APC and increases the *procoagulant* role of activated factor V because there is now 20-fold slower degradation of factor Va.

RISK FACTORS
- Risk for VTE is ~7-fold in heterozygous and ~80-fold in homozygous factor V Leiden individuals, compared with individuals without the mutation. This risk is compounded/increased by the presence of the following:
  - Having non-O blood type (A, B, or AB): 2- to 4-fold
  - Oral contraceptives: homozygotes up to 100-fold; heterozygotes, 35-fold. The increased risk is halved when the patient uses desogestrel-containing oral contraceptives.

  - Hormone replacement therapy (HRT) and selective estrogen receptor modulators (SERMs) both increase the risk of thrombosis; in patients with FVL, that risk is compounded.
  - In men with an underlying thrombophilia, testosterone therapy can promote VTE.
  - Pregnancy and *homozygous* FVL increase the risk of thrombosis 7- to 16-fold during pregnancy and the puerperium.
  - Those with combined thrombophilias and end-stage renal disease are at risk for developing calciphylaxis.
  - 30% of patients with VTE is attributed to FVL and prothrombin mutation G20210A; however, the risk is weaker compared to antithrombin III, protein C and protein S deficiency, which is around 1% in the general population.
- FVL versus general population, a modest increase in the recurrence risk of VTE is seen.

GENERAL PREVENTION

> **ALERT**
> Patients with FVL without thrombosis do not require prophylactic anticoagulation.

COMMONLY ASSOCIATED CONDITIONS
Venous thrombosis

DIAGNOSIS

HISTORY
- It is critical to differentiate between provoked and unprovoked VTE and determine family history, risk factors, detailed symptoms.
- In up to 70% of patients suffering from VTE, a provoking factor is present.
- Isolated PE without evidence of DVT, however, is less common than general population; this phenomenon is known as "FVL paradox."
- There is no clinical feature specific for FVL. Most patient are asymptomatic until they develop thrombosis.
- Recurrent pregnancy loss
- Family history of thrombosis
- Family history of FVL mutation

PHYSICAL EXAM
- Findings suggestive of VTE in any form (DVT, PE, cerebral thrombosis): 10–26% of patients with VTE are carriers of the FVL mutation.
- Test individuals who develop VTE in unusual location (e.g., portal vein, cerebral vein, or recurrent VTE) especially <50 years old.

DIFFERENTIAL DIAGNOSIS
- Protein C deficiency
- Protein S deficiency
- Antithrombin deficiency
- Other causes of APC resistance (e.g., antiphospholipid antibodies)
- Dysfibrinogenemia
- Dysplasminogenemia
- Homocystinemia
- Prothrombin mutation G20210A
- Elevated factor VIII levels

DIAGNOSTIC TESTS & INTERPRETATION
Initial Tests (lab, imaging)
- For VTE diagnosis, tests, and imaging, refer to DVT/PE chapters.
- NICE guidelines specifies the only clear indication for thrombophilia testing including FVL is when the consideration is being given to discontinuing anticoagulation therapy after an unprovoked VTE event.
- FVL thrombophilia should be suspected in individuals with the following:
  - A history of first and recurrent VTE manifest as deep vein thrombosis (DVT) or pulmonary embolism (PE), especially in women with a history of VTE during pregnancy or in association with use of estrogen-containing contraceptives
  - A family history of recurrent thrombosis
- FVL molecular genetic test: DNA-based for factor V mutation, will be unaffected by anticoagulation and other drugs; recommended in individuals on direct thrombin inhibitors or direct factor Xa inhibitors, those with strong lupus inhibitors, and significantly prolonged baseline aPTT
- Functional assay for APC resistance: plasma-based coagulation assay using factor V–deficient plasma to which patient plasma is added along with purified APC. The relative prolongation of the aPTT is used to assay for the defect. Heparin, direct thrombin inhibitors, and factor Xa inhibitor may cause false-negative results. In the absence of exposure to anticoagulants, functional testing is preferred to genetic testing due to cost and time to diagnosis.

Follow-Up Tests & Special Considerations
- For individuals with family history of FVL, genetic testing is preferred, especially if they have concomitant antiphospholipid syndrome or who are receiving anticoagulant—this will elucidate potential source of test interference for direct thrombin inhibitor or direct factor Xa inhibitor.
- Inherited genetic factors such as FVL, prothrombin mutation G20210A, antithrombin, protein C or protein S deficiencies, non-O blood group, as well as CYP2C9*2 and the rs4379368 mutations, have been shown to be genetic predictive risk factors for VTE in women. Therefore, consider testing for mutations prior implementing combined oral contraception and monitor for potential thrombogenicity induced by COC therapy.

Diagnostic Procedures/Other
- Thrombophilia testing in pediatric patients with recurrent central venous catheter (CVC)-related VTE.
- If thrombophilia is suspected in children with VTE, include testing: FVL mutation, prothrombin mutation G20210A, antithrombin deficiency, protein C deficiency, protein S deficiency, and antiphospholipid
- The thrombophilia screen consists of antithrombin III, protein C and S deficiency, PCR for FVL mutation and prothrombin mutation G20210A, testing for antiphospholipid antibodies and homocysteine level.

TREATMENT

Only indicated if with thrombotic event. For asymptomatic patients (no thrombotic event), prophylaxis is not recommended.

GENERAL MEASURES
- Initiation of anticoagulation therapy for acute venous thrombosis should be the same in patients with and without FVL or other inherited thrombophilia.
- The treatment for first VTE in patients with FVL or any other thrombophilias does not differ from those without it.
- VTE treatment should be a minimum of 3 months for the first episode.
- For those patients with recurrence, the risks and benefits of indefinite anticoagulation need to be assessed and considered.

MEDICATION
First Line
- First-line treatment for first VTE is the same for a patient with and a patient without FVL.
- In patients with proximal DVT or PE, anticoagulation therapy is recommended over no therapy (Grade 1B).
- In patients with DVT or PE and no cancer, anticoagulation suggested are dabigatran, rivaroxaban, apixaban, or edoxaban over vitamin K antagonist (all Grade 2B).
- In patients with cancer-associated thrombosis, low molecular weight heparin (LMWH) is recommended.
- LMWH:
  - Enoxaparin (Lovenox): SubQ: 1 mg/kg every 12 hours (preferred) or 1.5 mg/kg once every 24 hours; Note: In select low-risk patients, may consider outpatient treatment using 1 mg/kg every 12 hours for the remainder of the course after first dose administered in hospital or urgent care center
  - Fondaparinux (Arixtra): 5 mg (body weight <50 kg), 7.5 mg (body weight 50 to 100 kg), or 10 mg (body weight >100 kg) SC daily
  - Tinzaparin (Innohep): 175 anti-Xa IU/kg SC daily for minimum of 5 days and patient is adequately anticoagulated with warfarin (INR of at least 2.0 for 2 consecutive days)
  - Dalteparin (Fragmin): 200 IU/kg SC daily
- Oral anticoagulant
  - Apixaban (Eliquis): treatment dose: 10 mg BID × 7 days and then 5 mg BID × 3 to 6 months
  - Rivaroxaban (Xarelto): treatment dose: 15 mg BID × 7 days and then 20 mg daily × 3 to 6 months
  - Dabigatran (Pradaxa): After at least 5 days of initial therapy with a parenteral anticoagulant, transition to dabigatran in hemodynamically stable patients: 150 mg BID
- Contraindications
  - Active bleeding precludes anticoagulation.
  - Risk of bleeding is a relative contraindication to long-term anticoagulation.

- Precautions
  - Observe patient for signs of embolization, further thrombosis, or bleeding.
  - Avoid IM injections. Periodically check stool and urine for occult blood; monitor CBCs, including platelets.
  - LMWH: Adjust dosage in renal insufficiency; may also need dose adjustment in pregnancy
- Significant possible interactions
  - Agents that intensify the response to oral anticoagulants: alcohol, allopurinol, amiodarone, anabolic steroids, androgens, many antimicrobials, cimetidine, chloral hydrate, disulfiram, all NSAIDs, sulfinpyrazone, tamoxifen, thyroid hormone, vitamin E, ranitidine, salicylates, acetaminophen
  - Agents that diminish the response to anticoagulants: aminoglutethimide, antacids, barbiturates, carbamazepine, cholestyramine, diuretics, griseofulvin, rifampin, oral contraceptives

Second Line
- Heparin 80 mg/kg IV bolus followed by 18 g/kg/hr continuous infusion
- Oral anticoagulant
  - Warfarin (Coumadin) PO with dose adjusted to an INR of 2.0 to 3.0
  - Contraindications
    ○ Active bleeding precludes anticoagulation.
    ○ Risk of bleeding is a relative contraindication to long-term anticoagulation.
    ○ Warfarin is contraindicated in patients with history of warfarin skin necrosis.
    ○ Warfarin is contraindicated in pregnancy.
  - Precautions
    ○ Heparin: thrombocytopenia and/or paradoxical thrombosis with thrombocytopenia
    ○ Warfarin: necrotic skin lesions (typically breasts, thighs, or buttocks)

ISSUES FOR REFERRAL
- Recurrent thrombosis on anticoagulation
- Difficulty anticoagulating
- Genetic counseling
- Homozygous state in pregnancy

SURGERY/OTHER PROCEDURES
Recommendations are against routine use of inferior vena cava filter in addition to anticoagulation, except when there is contraindication for anticoagulation.

ONGOING CARE

FOLLOW-UP RECOMMENDATIONS
Patient Monitoring
Warfarin use requires periodic (~monthly after initial stabilization) INR measurements, with a goal of 2.0 to 3.0.

DIET
Large amounts of foods rich in vitamin K may interfere with anticoagulation with warfarin.

PATIENT EDUCATION
- Patients should be educated about the following:
  - Use of oral anticoagulant therapy
  - Avoidance of NSAIDs while on anticoagulation
- The role of family screening is unclear because most patients with this mutation do not have thrombosis. In a patient with a family history of FVL, consider screening during pregnancy or if considering oral contraceptive use.

PROGNOSIS
- Most patients heterozygous for FVL do not have thrombosis.
- Homozygotes have about a 50% lifetime incidence of thrombosis.
- Recurrence rates after a first thrombosis are not clear; some estimate as high as 5%.
- FVL does not increase overall mortality.

COMPLICATIONS
- Recurrent thrombosis
- Bleeding on anticoagulation

REFERENCE
1. Dłuski D, Mierzyński R, Poniedziałek-Czajkowska E, et al. Adverse pregnancy outcomes and inherited thrombophilia. *J Perinat Med*. 2018;46(4):411–417.

SEE ALSO

Deep Vein Thrombophlebitis

CODES

ICD10
D68.51 Activated protein C resistance

CLINICAL PEARLS
- Extremely rare in Asian and African populations
- Asymptomatic patients with FVL do not need anticoagulation.
- For pregnant women homozygous for FVL but no prior history of VTE, postpartum prophylaxis with prophylactic or intermediate-dose LMWH or vitamin K antagonists with target INR 2.0 to 3.0 for 6 weeks is recommended. Antepartum prophylaxis is added if there is positive family history of VTE.

FAILURE TO THRIVE
Durr-e-Shahwaar Sayed, DO

 BASICS

DESCRIPTION
- Failure to thrive (FTT) is not a diagnosis but a sign of inadequate nutrition in young children manifested by a failure of physical growth, usually affecting weight. In severe cases, decreased length and/or head circumference may develop.
- It is commonly defined as either weight or BMI for age below the 5th percentile on more than one occasion or weight that drops two or more major percentile lines on standard growth charts *or* weight-for-length that falls below the 5th percentile.
- A combination of anthropometric criteria rather than one criterion should be used to identify children at risk of FTT.

Pediatric Considerations
- Children with genetic syndromes, intrauterine growth restriction (IUGR), or prematurity follow different growth curves.
- 25% of children will decrease their weight or height crossing ≥2 major percentile lines in the first 2 years of life. These children are failing to reach their genetic potential or demonstrating a constitutional growth delay (slow growth with a bone age < chronologic age). After shifting down, these infants grow at a normal rate along their new percentile and do not have FTT.

EPIDEMIOLOGY
Incidence
- Predominant age: 6 to 12 months; 80% <18 months
- Predominant sex: male = female

Prevalence
- As many as 10% of children seen in primary care have signs of growth failure.
- 1–5% of pediatric inpatient admissions are for FTT.
- Occurs more frequently in children living in poverty

ETIOLOGY AND PATHOPHYSIOLOGY
- Often grouped into four major categories:
  - Inadequate caloric intake (most frequent)
  - Inadequate caloric absorption
  - Excessive caloric expenditure
  - Defective utilization
- Causes of FTT can be grouped by pathophysiology (including examples):
  - Inadequate caloric intake: breastfeeding difficulty, incorrect formula preparation, poor transition to food (6 to 12 months), poor feeding habits (e.g., excessive juice, restrictive diets), mechanical problems (e.g., oromotor dysfunction, congenital anomalies, GERD, CNS, or PNS anomalies), oral aversion, poverty, neglect/abuse, poor parent–child interaction, caregiver feeding style
  - Inadequate caloric absorption: necrotizing enterocolitis, short bowel syndrome, biliary atresia, liver disease, cystic fibrosis, celiac disease, milk protein allergy, vitamin/mineral deficiency, environmental enteric dysfunction

- Increased expenditure: hyperthyroidism, congenital/chronic cardiopulmonary disease, HIV, immunodeficiencies, malignancy, renal disease, obstructive sleep apnea
- Defective utilization: metabolic disorders, congenital infections (TORCH: toxoplasmosis, other agents, rubella, cytomegalovirus, herpes simplex)

RISK FACTORS
- Psychosocial risks (1)
  - Poverty, parent(s) with mental health disorder or cognitive impairment, ineffective parenting skills or hypervigilant parents, families with unique health/nutritional beliefs, physical or emotional abuse, substance abuse, and social isolation
- Medical risks (1)
  - Intrauterine exposures, history of IUGR (symmetric or asymmetric), congenital abnormalities, oromotor dysfunction, premature or sick newborn, infant with physical deformity, acute or chronic medical conditions, developmental delay, lead poisoning, anemia

GENERAL PREVENTION
- Educate the parents on normal feeding and parenting skills.
- Access to supplemental feeding programs (Women, Infants, and Children [WIC])

DIAGNOSIS

HISTORY
- Successful treatment of FTT is almost always accomplished by a careful and detailed history because most cases are due to underfeeding or inappropriate feeding.
- Prenatal and developmental history/prenatal exposures
- Past medical history: acute/chronic disease affecting caloric intake, digestion, absorption, or causing increased energy need or defective utilization
- Medication history, including complementary and alternative medications
- Family history: stature of parents and growth trajectories of siblings, chronic diseases, genetic disorders, developmental delay, consanguinity
- Diet history from birth: breastfeeding or formula feeding; timing and introduction of solids; who feeds the child, when, and how often; placement of child during feeds; amounts consumed/caloric intake; beverages consumed; snacking; vomiting or stooling associated with feeds; oral aversions or unusual behaviors during feeding
- Social history: family composition, socioeconomic status, hygiene practices, child-rearing beliefs, stressors, parental depression, parental substance abuse, caretaker's personal history of abuse/neglect
- Review of systems: anorexia, activity level, mental status, fevers, dysphagia, vomiting, gastroesophageal reflux, stooling pattern/consistency, dysuria, urinary frequency

PHYSICAL EXAM
- A combination of anthropometric criteria, rather than one criterion, should be used, and measurements over time are required for diagnosis.
- Accurate measurement of height, weight, and head circumference from the National Center for Health Statistics (NCHS) (https://www.cdc.gov/growthcharts/)
- The World Health Organization (WHO) growth charts may be more appropriate for breastfed infants (https://www.who.int/childgrowth/standards/en/).
- Exam should assess for the following:
  - Signs of dehydration or severe malnutrition
    - Severity of malnutrition estimated via Gomez classification: Compare current weight for age with expected weight for age (50th percentile): severe, <60% of expected; moderate, 61–75%; mild, 76–90%.
  - Dysmorphic features
  - Mental status (alert, responsive to stimuli)
  - Any signs of physical abuse and/or neglect
- Observe the interaction with caregivers and feeding techniques, specifically the bonding and social/psychological cues.

DIFFERENTIAL DIAGNOSIS
Differentiate based on growth patterns.
- FTT classically presents as low weight for age, with normal linear growth and head circumference *or* low weight for age, followed by decreased linear growth *or* low weight for age, leading to decreased linear growth and decreased head circumference (without neurologic signs).
- If low linear growth with normal weight for length *or* low linear growth and proportionately low weight and decreased head circumference:
  - Consider genetic potential (constitutional short stature or growth delay), genetic syndromes, teratogens, and endocrine disorders.
- If microcephaly with prominent neurologic signs, with poor growth secondary to presumed neurologic disorder:
  - Consider TORCH infections, genetic syndromes, teratogens, and brain injury (i.e., hypoxic/ischemic).

DIAGNOSTIC TESTS & INTERPRETATION
- Labs are useful only in ~1% of cases and are generally not recommended.
- A period of addressing nutritional causes is preferable prior to extensive labs and other workup.

Initial Tests (lab, imaging)
- Tests are often considered in initial evaluation:
  - CBC with differential, ESR, lead level
  - Electrolytes, BUN/creatinine, liver function tests, TSH, free T4
  - Urinalysis and urine culture
- Other tests as dictated by the history and exam:
  - Amylase/lipase, serum zinc level, iron studies, IGF-1, karyotype, genetic testing, sweat chloride test, stool for ova and parasite or fat/reducing substances, guaiac, α_1-antitrypsin and elastase, radioallergosorbent test for IgE food allergies, tissue transglutaminase and total IgA (celiac sprue), p-ANCA and fecal calprotectin (for inflammatory bowel disease [IBD]), TB test, HIV, hepatitis A and B, other infections
  - X-ray of hand/wrist to assess bone age and for skeletal dysplasia

Follow-Up Tests & Special Considerations

- Prospective 3-day food diary for accurate record of caloric intake should be obtained.
- Home visit by a clinician/visiting nurse to observe infant feeding, interaction of caretakers, and home environment
- Observe breastfeeding and/or formula preparation to ensure adequacy and offer instruction.

Diagnostic Procedures/Other

Can consider
- Skeletal survey if suspicion of physical abuse
- Bone age if possible endocrine disorder
- Swallowing studies, small bowel follow-through if possible oromotor dysfunction, GERD, structural abnormalities
- Brain imaging if microcephalic and/or neurologic findings on examination
- Echocardiogram if murmur is auscultated

 TREATMENT

GENERAL MEASURES

- Caregiver and infant interaction should be evaluated in infants and children with FTT.
- Age-appropriate nutritional counseling should be provided.
  - The goal is to improve nutrition to allow catch-up growth (weight gain 2 to 3 times > average for age).
- Calculate energy needs based on recommended energy intake for age and then increase by 50%.
- Alternatively, may calculate caloric requirements for infants to achieve catch-up growth
  - kcal/kg/day required = RDA for age (kcal/kg) × ideal weight for height/actual weight, where ideal weight for height is the median weight for the patient's height
- Try various strategies to increase caloric intake, such as the following:
  - Optimize breastfeeding support; consider supplementation.
  - Higher calorie formulas
  - Addition of rice cereal or fats to current foods
  - Limit intake of milk to 24 to 32 oz/day.
  - Avoid juice and soda.
  - Vitamin and/or nutritional supplements
  - Take into account cultural differences in food preparation
  - Assist with social determinants of health and offer referrals to address poverty and food insecurity (WIC, food stamps, and other transitional assistance).
- Rapid high-calorie intake can cause diarrhea, malabsorption, hypokalemia, and hypophosphatemia. Therefore, increasing formulas >24 kcal/oz is not recommended.
- The target energy intake should be slowly increased to goal over 5 to 7 days.
- Catch-up growth should be seen in 2 to 7 days.
- Accelerated growth should be continued for 4 to 9 months to restore weight and height.
- Consider visiting nurse referral, early childhood intervention referral, and social services evaluation to determine services that the family may qualify for.

MEDICATION

No specific medication is recommended.

ISSUES FOR REFERRAL

Multidisciplinary clinics may be of benefit for children with complicated situations, failure to respond to initial treatment, or when the PCP does not have access to specialized services such as nutrition, psychology, PT/OT, and speech therapy.

SURGERY/OTHER PROCEDURES

In severe cases, nasogastric tube feedings or gastrostomy may be considered.

ADMISSION, INPATIENT, AND NURSING CONSIDERATIONS

- Hospitalization should be considered if:
  - Outpatient management fails.
  - There is evidence of severe dehydration or malnutrition.
  - There are signs of abuse or neglect.
  - There are concerns that the psychosocial situation presents harm to child.
  - During catch-up growth, some children will develop nutritional recovery syndrome:
    ○ Symptoms include sweating, increased body temperature, hepatomegaly (increased glycogen deposits), widening of cranial sutures (brain growth > bone growth), increased periods of sleep, fidgetiness, and mild hyperactivity.
  - There may also be an initial period of malabsorption with resultant diarrhea.
- Catch-up growth should be seen in 2 to 7 days. If this is not seen, reevaluation of causes is needed.

 ONGOING CARE

FOLLOW-UP RECOMMENDATIONS

- Close (every 2 to 4 weeks at first and then 1 to 2 months if there is a good progress), long-term follow-up with frequent visits
- Children with history of FTT are at increased risk of recurrent FTT.
- If the family fails to comply, child protection authorities must be notified.

DIET

Nutritional requirements for a "normal" child:
- Infant
  - 120 kcal/kg/day, decreased to 95 kcal/kg/day at 6 months; if breastfed, ensure appropriate frequency and duration of feeding.
  - Between 6 and 12 months, continue the same amount of breast milk and/or formula with puréed foods consumed several times a day.
- Toddler
  - Three meals plus two nutritional snacks, 16 to 32 oz of whole milk per day; stop all juice and soda; feed in a social environment.
  - Rate of weight gain expected for age:
  - 0 to 3 months: 26 to 31 g/day
  - 3 to 6 months: 17 to 18 g/day
  - 6 to 9 months: 12 to 13 g/day
  - 9 to 12 months: 9 g/day
  - 1 to 3 years: 7 to 9 g/day

PATIENT EDUCATION

- Counsel the parents regarding the need to avoid "food battles," which can worsen the problem.
- Educate the parents regarding the infant's social and physiologic cues, formula/food preparation, proper feeding techniques, and importance of relaxed and social mealtimes.
- "Failure to Thrive: What This Means for Your Child" available from AAFP at: https://www.aafp.org/pubs/afp/issues/2011/0401/p837.html
- WIC provides grants to states for supplemental foods, health care referrals, and nutrition education for low-income pregnant, breastfeeding, and nonbreastfeeding postpartum women and to infants and children up to age 5 years at nutritional risk: https://www.fns.usda.gov/wic/women-infants-and-children-wic.

PROGNOSIS

- Many children with FTT show adequate improvement in dietary intake with intervention (1)[B].
- Children with FTT are at increased risk for future undernutrition, overnutrition, and eating disorders.

COMPLICATIONS

- Complications can be related to the underlying cause, thus identifying and treating growth failure early on is important.
- Developmental delays, behavioral problems, problems in school and shorter stature later in life are all potential complications.

REFERENCE

1. Black MM, Tilton N, Bento S, et al. Recovery in young children with weight faltering: child and household risk factors. *J Pediatr.* 2016;170:301–306.

ADDITIONAL READING

- Homan GJ. Failure to thrive: a practical guide. *Am Fam Physician.* 2016;94(4):295–299.
- Tang MN, Adolphe S, Rogers SR, et al. Failure to thrive or growth faltering: medical, developmental/behavioral, nutritional and social dimensions. *Pediatr Rev.* 2021;42(11):590–603.

CODES

ICD10
- R62.7 Adult failure to thrive
- R62.51 Failure to thrive (child)
- P92.6 Failure to thrive in newborn

CLINICAL PEARLS

- FTT is a sign of inadequate nutrition. It is rarely due to a medical condition.
- Underlying medical and/or social issues are generally suggested by history and physical exam, and extensive laboratory or imaging tests are rarely needed.
- A multidisciplinary team approach to diagnosis and treatment is critical to help children with FTT and their families.

F

FEMALE ATHLETE TRIAD

Rahul Kapur, MD • Alex T. Fredrickson, MD

 BASICS

Syndrome of three interrelated clinical entities: low energy availability (LEA) (with or without disordered eating [DE]), menstrual dysfunction (MD), and low bone mineral density (LBMD)

DESCRIPTION
- Female athlete triad first described in 1992 to include DE, amenorrhea, osteoporosis
- In 2007, the American College of Sports Medicine (ACSM) updated the definition to: components including LEA (with or without DE), MD, and LBMD with each component representing an inter-related spectrum ranging from health to dysfunction.
- LEA is fundamental to the triad, and full recovery is not possible without correction of it.
- 2014 Female Athlete Triad Coalition (TC) Consensus Statement largely agreed with the ACSM's update and included many recommendations (as later briefly outlined in this review).
- 2014 International Olympic Committee's position statement from 2014 deviated to consider "Relative Energy Deficiency in Sport" (RED-S) (1).
  - Focus on energy deficiency and its broader physiologic effects beyond bone and menstrual health, ranging from growth to cardiovascular.
  - Emphasized similar syndrome in males
- Since then, debate has ensued between the classic TC model and RED-S. TC authors assert that RED-S movement is simply "rebranding" >30 years worth of triad research.
- TC authors have since released papers introducing the concept of the Male Athlete Triad; consisting of LEA, functional hypothalamic hypogonadism, and LBMD.
- Concept of energy deficiency in men involving reproductive and bone abnormalities
  - Men seem to be more resilient to the effects of LEA compared to women, requiring more severe energetic perturbations before alterations are observed. Recovery of the hypothalamic pituitary gonadal axis can be observed more quickly in men than in women.
  - Male triad needs to be further evaluated.

EPIDEMIOLOGY
Prevalence
- Overall prevalence: 3/3 criteria (LEA, MD, LBMD): 0–16%; 2/3 criteria: 3–27%; 1/3 criteria: 16–60%.
- DE higher than general population
- MD: Prevalence of secondary amenorrhea is as high as 60% in female athletes compared to 2–5% in the general population.
- LBMD: Using the WHO criteria for LBMD, prevalence of osteopenia (T-score between −1 and −2) ranges from 0% to 40% in female athletes, as compared to ~12% in the general population.
- Full triad is more prevalent in lean sports (1.5–6.7%), including swimming and cross country, versus non-lean sports (0–2%), including volleyball and softball.
- Increasing recognition that LEA prevalence is very difficult to measure accurately due to variability in methods used for measurement.

ETIOLOGY AND PATHOPHYSIOLOGY
- Energy availability is defined by energy intake minus exercise energy expenditure.
  - LEA can occur either intentionally or inadvertently. Examples include increasing training or DE (1).
- When there is an LEA, energy is shunted from reproduction to more critical functions, such as thermoregulation cellular maintenance.
- Specifically, LEA leads to suppression of luteinizing hormone (LH) pulse frequency and thus MD.
  - This process suppresses ovulation and estrogen concentrations, which can lead to decreased bone formation and increased bone resorption, ultimately leading to LBMD.
- Triad elements exist along a bidirectional continuum of severity, ranging from "healthy" to "unhealthy." Importantly, elements exist as a triad, although there is unidirectionally implication from one to another.
  - LEA (with or without an eating disorder) can lead to both MD and LBMD.
- MD (via hypoestrogenemia) can lead to LBMD.
- Other effects of LEA seem to include endothelial dysfunction and altered lipid profiles.
- RED-S considers LEA to lead to broader physiologic effects including metabolic rate, growth and development, immunity, protein synthesis, hematologic, gastrointestinal, cardiovascular, and psychological.
- TC authors hold that there may be a basis for RED-S, but it is insufficiently supported by evidence at the present time.

RISK FACTORS
- History of menstrual irregularities and amenorrhea; history of stress fractures and recurrent or nonhealing injuries; history of critical comments about eating or weight from parent or coach; history of depression; history of dieting; personality factors including perfectionism and/or obsessiveness, overtraining, and inappropriate coaching behaviors
- Lean physique sports with an aesthetic component (ballet, figure skating, gymnastics, distance running, diving, and swimming) or sports with weight classifications (martial arts and wrestling); frequent weigh-ins, consequences for weight gain, and win-at-all-cost attitude all increase risk.
- A lack of family or social support; intense training hours; social isolation or entering a new environment (boarding school or college); an athlete with comorbid psychological conditions (anxiety, depression, and/or obsessive-compulsive disorder)
- Age: A Japanese study found stress fracture in teenagers with the Triad but no stress fractures in athletes in their 20s.

GENERAL PREVENTION
- Education of athletes (middle school through college), coaches, trainers, parents, and physicians. Young athletes are extremely impressionable and may turn negative comments and unhealthy advice into maladaptive eating and exercising habits.
- General screening during preparticipation exam (PPE) and annual physicals are endorsed by AAP, AAFP, ACSM, AOSSM, and AMSSM.
- TC has 11-question screening to use during PPE.

- Screen athletes presenting with "red flag" conditions such as fractures, weight changes, fatigue, amenorrhea, bradycardia, orthostatic hypotension, syncope, arrhythmias, electrolyte abnormalities, or depression.
- Screen for other conditions that may accelerate bone loss, including steroid use, tobacco use, alcohol use, and hyperthyroidism.

COMMONLY ASSOCIATED CONDITIONS
- Anorexia nervosa, bulimia nervosa, avoidant or restrictive food intake disorder, and other psychological disorders, including low self-esteem, depression, and anxiety
- LBMD predisposes athletes to stress fractures and may not be fully reversible. This may lead to a higher rate of fractures after menopause.

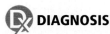 **DIAGNOSIS**

The female athlete triad is a clinical diagnosis based primarily on patient's history; screening for the female athlete triad at annual sports physicals or during routine exams and acute visits if there are concerns

HISTORY
- Assess menstrual history (including hormonal contraceptive use), fracture history, and symptoms of depression. Assess dietary practices, eating behaviors, and history of weight changes.
- Dietary intake logs and a nutritional assessment by a sports dietitian can help. Assess body image, fear of weight gain, fluctuations in weight, history of DE, and use of laxatives, diet pills, or enemas.

PHYSICAL EXAM
- Height, weight, body mass index (BMI) $<17.5 \text{ kg/m}^2$, <85% of expected body weight in adolescents, or ≥10% weight loss in 1 month
- Common findings include bradycardia, orthostatic hypotension, hypothermia, cold or cyanotic extremities, lanugo, parotid gland enlargement or tenderness, epigastric tenderness, eroded tooth enamel, and knuckle or hand calluses (Russell sign).
- Patients with amenorrhea should undergo a pelvic exam to verify the presence of a uterus and evaluate for outflow tract abnormalities. Vaginal atrophy may be present if the patient is in a low estrogen state.

DIFFERENTIAL DIAGNOSIS
Screen for anorexia nervosa, bulimia nervosa, avoidant/restrictive food intake disorder, and rumination disorder using the *DSM-5* criteria. Rule out the following in amenorrheic patients:
- Pregnancy
- Endocrine abnormalities: thyroid dysfunction, Cushing syndrome
- Hypothalamic dysfunction: psychological stress-induced amenorrhea, medication-induced amenorrhea, Kallmann syndrome
- Pituitary dysfunction: prolactinoma, Sheehan syndrome, sarcoidosis, empty sella syndrome
- Ovarian dysfunction: polycystic ovarian syndrome, premature ovarian failure, menopause, gonadal dysgenesis, Turner syndrome, ovarian neoplasm, autoimmune disease
- Uterine dysfunction: Asherman syndrome, absence of uterus

DIAGNOSTIC TESTS & INTERPRETATION
Initial Tests (lab, imaging)
- Basic metabolic panel, magnesium, phosphorus, albumin, CBC with differential, ESR, thyroid-stimulating hormone (TSH), calcium, 25-OH vitamin D, and urinalysis
- Evaluation for secondary amenorrhea includes urine hCG and serum FSH, LH, prolactin, and TSH.
- Consider adding an alkaline phosphatase in patients with multiple metatarsal fractures to evaluate for possible underlying hypophosphatasia.
- Pelvic ultrasound in patients with hyperandrogenism to exclude polycystic ovaries or virilizing ovarian tumors
- ECG to rule out prolonged QT interval

Follow-Up Tests & Special Considerations
- BMD testing by DEXA is based on a risk stratification model. Risk factors include DE, eating disorders >6 months, hypoestrogenism, amenorrhea, oligomenorrhea, and/or in patients with a history of stress fractures or fractures from minimal impact.
- If components of the triad persist, ISCD 2013 guidelines suggest reevaluation by the same DEXA machine every 1 to 2 years.

 TREATMENT

- A multidisciplinary team including a physician, registered dietitian, and behavioral health provider. Build open lines of communication with coaches, trainers, and family.
- Cognitive behavioral therapy (CBT) may have a role in treating LEA itself.
- Physically active females should strive for an EA of >45 kcal/kg of fat-free muscle mass per day.
- Nonpharmacologic measures should be taken first and followed for at least 1 year.
- First step is optimizing nutritional status to increase energy intake, which often encourages weight gain and increased BMI.
- Goal is body weight associated with normal menses (proving return of acceptable estrogen levels). This often correlates with BMI >18.5 kg/m² or >90% predicted weight.
- Encourage real food with proper balance of macronutrients/micronutrients over supplements if possible.
- Calcium intake with a goal of 1,000 to 1,300 mg/day. Encourage calcium-rich foods; supplementation to reach goal if dietary intake is insufficient
- A minimum of 600 IU of vitamin D should be consumed/supplemented; may require 1,500 to 2,000 IU to keep serum levels between 32 and 50 ng/ml.

- There may be a role for iron, at least in athletes with iron-deficiency anemia if not others.
- Treat maladaptive behavioral disorders.

MEDICATION
First Line
First-line medication for failed nutrition intervention and/or worsening symptoms (particularly fractures): nonoral estrogen, specifically transdermal estrogen with oral cyclic progestin.

Second Line
- Other postmenopausal medications, including bisphosphonates and denosumab, should not be recommended in reproductive-aged women due to potential teratogenic effect.
- Experimental medications: recombinant insulin-like growth factor (rhIGF-1) and metreleptin (synthetic leptin analogue).

ADMISSION, INPATIENT, AND NURSING CONSIDERATIONS
Evaluate patients with eating disorders for potentially life-threatening conditions requiring hospital admission, including bradycardia, severe orthostatic hypotension, significant electrolyte imbalances, hypothermia, arrhythmias, or prolonged QT interval.

 ONGOING CARE

- Patients should have regular follow-up with a multidisciplinary treatment team.
- Intermittent training: (2 weeks on, 2 weeks off) training may be a safe, enjoyable way to build strength without exacerbating features of the Triad.
- The Female Athlete TC consensus statement provided the first evidence-based clearance and return to play guidance, which considers the following factors: LEA (with emphasis on DE), BMI, delayed menarche, oligo/amenorrhea, LBMD, stress fracture.
- RED-S released a clinical assessment tool (CAT) in 2014 (updated in 2015), which considers similar criteria as compared to the TC clearance guide, although classifies them into "green, yellow, red" categories.
- Both groups continue to debate the validity of the other group's CAT.

PATIENT EDUCATION
All young female patients should be counseled on the importance of proper nutrition, calcium and vitamin D intake, and the benefits of regular weight-bearing exercise. Patients presenting with ≥1 components of the triad should be educated about the short- and long-term effects of LBMD.

PROGNOSIS
- The short- and long-term prognosis for patients with female athlete triad depends on time of diagnosis and response to treatment.
- It is estimated that amenorrheic women will lose 2–3% of bone mass per year without intervention.
- With early diagnosis and treatment using a multidisciplinary team, the prognosis for patients with the female athlete triad is good. Patients regain normal menstrual cycling and increase BMD.
- Because the triad often occurs within the age window of optimal bone strengthening, patients with a prolonged disease course may suffer from complications of decreased BMD throughout their adolescent and adult life.
- Patients with DE behaviors often require long-term therapy to manage their disease.

REFERENCE
1. Mountjoy M, Sundgot-Borgen J, Burke L, et al. The IOC consensus statement: beyond the Female Athlete Triad—Relative Energy Deficiency in Sport (RED-S). *Br J Sports Med*. 2014;48(7):491–497.

ADDITIONAL READING
Williams NI, Koltun KJ, Strock NCA, et al. Female athlete triad and relative energy deficiency in sport: a focus on scientific rigor. *Exerc Sport Sci Rev*. 2019;47(4):197–205.

 SEE ALSO

Algorithms: Amenorrhea, Primary (Absence of Menarche by Age 16 Years); Amenorrhea, Secondary; Weight Loss, Unintentional

 CODES

ICD10
- F50.9 Eating disorder, unspecified
- N91.2 Amenorrhea, unspecified
- R53.83 Other fatigue

CLINICAL PEARLS
- The female athlete triad consists of LEA (with or without DE), MD, and LBMD.
- Early intervention by a multidisciplinary team, including physicians, registered dietitians, mental health professionals, coaches, trainers, and parents, is the most successful strategy to minimize further bone loss, recover BMD, and regain normal menstrual function.

F

FEVER OF UNKNOWN ORIGIN (FUO)

Daniel R. Matta, MD • Nicholas Smith, MD

 BASICS

DESCRIPTION
- Classic definition
  - Repeated fever >38.3°C
  - Fever duration at least 3 weeks
  - Diagnosis remains uncertain (1) after 1 week of study in the hospital.
- Categories of fever of unknown origin (FUO): infection, neoplasia, inflammatory (rheumatologic or connective tissue disease), miscellaneous disease, and undiagnosed illness
- Often an atypical presentation of a common disease versus a rare disease; 75% of cases resolve without reaching a definitive diagnosis.

EPIDEMIOLOGY
Incidence
The exact incidence is not known.

Prevalence
The definition of fever with unresolved cause (true FUO) is difficult, as it is a moving target, given the constant advancement of imaging and biomarker analysis. Therefore, the prevalence of FUO is unknown.

ETIOLOGY AND PATHOPHYSIOLOGY
- True FUO are uncommon; most frequently, FUO is an atypical presentation of a common condition.
- Spectrum of causes varies widely.
  - Higher percentage of infectious causes in developing countries compared to developed countries
  - Although infection is the most common cause of FUO in developed countries, there is a higher incidence of noninfectious inflammatory disease when compared to developing countries.
- Infection
  - Abdominal or pelvic abscesses; amebic hepatitis
  - Catheter infections
  - Cytomegalovirus
  - Dental abscesses
  - Endocarditis/pericarditis
  - HIV (advanced stage)
  - Mycobacterial infection (often with advanced HIV)
  - Osteomyelitis
  - Pyelonephritis or renal abscess
  - Sinusitis
  - Wound infections
  - Other miscellaneous infections
- Neoplasms
  - Atrial myxoma
  - Colorectal cancer and other GI malignancies
  - Hepatoma
  - Lymphoma; leukemia
  - Solid tumors (renal cell carcinoma)
- Noninfectious inflammatory disease
  - Connective tissue diseases
    ○ Adult Still disease
    ○ Rheumatoid arthritis
    ○ Systemic lupus erythematosus
  - Granulomatous disease
    ○ Crohn disease
    ○ Sarcoidosis
  - Vasculitis syndromes
    ○ Giant cell arteritis
    ○ Polymyalgia rheumatica

- Other causes
  - Alcoholic hepatitis
  - Cerebrovascular accident
  - Cirrhosis
  - Medications
    ○ Allopurinol, captopril, carbamazepine, cephalosporins, cimetidine, clofibrate, erythromycin, heparin, hydralazine, hydrochlorothiazide, isoniazid, meperidine, methyldopa, nifedipine, nitrofurantoin, penicillin, phenytoin, procainamide, quinidine, sulfonamides
    ○ Medication reactions include hypersensitivity, serotonin syndrome, adrenergic fever, neuroleptic malignant syndrome, malignant hyperthermia, anticholinergic fever, DRESS syndrome, chemotherapy/infusion-related reaction, and mitochondrial uncoupling (pesticides/toxins) (1).
  - Endocrine disease
  - Factitious/fraudulent fever
  - Occupational causes
  - Periodic fever
  - Pulmonary emboli/deep vein thrombosis
  - Thermoregulatory disorders
- In up to 20–30% of cases, the cause of the fever is never identified despite a thorough workup.

RISK FACTORS
- Recent travel (malaria, enteric fevers, tick-borne illness)
- Exposure to biologic or chemical agents
- HIV infection (particularly in acute infection and advanced stages)
- Elderly, drug abuse, immigrants
- Young, (typically) female health care workers (factitious fever)

Geriatric Considerations
In geriatric populations aged >65 years, noninfectious multisystem diseases, such as polymyalgia rheumatica, giant cell arteritis, and other vasculitides have a higher incidence than infection. Common infectious causes in the elderly are intra-abdominal abscess, urinary tract infections, tuberculosis (TB), and endocarditis. Other common causes of FUO in patients aged >65 years include malignancies (particularly hematologic cancers) and drug-induced fever.

Pediatric Considerations
- 1/3 are self-limited undefined viral syndromes. ~50% of FUO in pediatric cases are infectious. Collagen vascular disease and malignancy are the next most common.
- Inflammatory bowel disease is a common cause of FUO in older children and adolescents.

DIAGNOSIS

The initial approach should include a comprehensive history and physical examination, as well as laboratory testing. The decision of what further testing should be gathered should be guided by the resulting information (2).

HISTORY
- Onset and pattern of fever
- Constitutional symptoms:
  - Chills, night sweats, myalgias, weight loss with an intact appetite (infectious etiology)
  - Arthralgias, myalgias, fatigue (inflammatory etiology)
  - Fatigue, night sweats, weight loss with loss of appetite (neoplastic etiology)

- Past medical history: chronic infections, abdominal diseases, transfusion history, malignancy, psychiatric illness, and recent hospitalization
- Past surgical history: type of surgery performed, postoperative complications, and any indwelling foreign material
- Comprehensive medication history, including over-the-counter and herbal products
- Family history, such as hereditary causes, periodic fever syndromes, and recent febrile illnesses in close contacts
- Social history: travel, animal exposure (e.g., pets, occupational, farms), living environment, sexual activity, recreational drug use

ALERT
Obtain a thorough travel, psychosocial, occupational, sexual, medication, and recreational drug use history.

PHYSICAL EXAM
Physical findings with high diagnostic yield generally involve skin, eyes, lymph nodes, liver, and spleen. Helpful clues can be found with:
- Funduscopic exam for choroid tubercles or Roth spots
- Temporal artery tenderness
- Oral-mucosal lesions
- Cardiac auscultation for bruits and murmurs
- Pulmonary exam: consolidation or effusion
- Abdominal palpation for masses or organomegaly and tenderness or peritoneal signs
- Rectal examination for blood, fluctuance, and/or tenderness
- Testicular examination
- Lymph node examination
- Skin and nail bed exam for clubbing, nodules, lesions, and erosions
- Focal neurologic signs
- Musculoskeletal exam for tenderness or effusion
- Serial exams help identify evolving physical signs (e.g., findings associated with endocarditis).

DIAGNOSTIC TESTS & INTERPRETATION
Initial Tests (lab, imaging)
- CBC, C-reactive protein, ESR, ANA, peripheral blood smear
- Electrolytes, BUN, and creatinine; LFT; calcium; lactate dehydrogenase; creatine phosphokinase
- Heterophile antibody testing
- Hepatitis, RPR, and HIV testing
- Three blood cultures drawn from different sites, within hours, without administering antibiotics
- Urinalysis and urine culture
- Chest x-ray, CT, or MRI of abdomen and pelvis (with directed biopsy, if indicated)

Follow-Up Tests & Special Considerations
- Rheumatoid factor and antinuclear antibody test
- Serologies: Epstein-Barr, Lyme disease, Q fever, cytomegalovirus, brucellosis, amebiasis, coccidioidomycosis, histoplasmosis
- Serum ferritin; serum protein electrophoresis
- AFB smear; sputum and urine cultures for TB

- TB testing
  - Tuberculin skin test
    - May not be helpful if anergic or acute infection
    - If test negative, repeat in 2 weeks.
  - Interferon-γ release assay (IGRA)
    - Preferred in those likely to be infected with TB and/or who are BCG-vaccinated
- Thyroid function tests
- Technetium-based scan (infection tumor)
- FDG-PET/CT scan if infectious process, inflammatory process, or tumor suspected; PET scans have a high negative predictive value and good sensitivity (but may have false positives).
- Ultrasound of abdomen and pelvis (with directed biopsy, if indicated) if renal obstruction or biliary pathology suspected
- Echocardiogram if endocarditis, atrial myxomas, or pericardial effusion is suspected
- Lower extremity Doppler ultrasound if deep vein thrombosis/pulmonary embolism suspected
- CT scan of chest if pulmonary embolism suspected
- Indium-labeled leukocyte scanning if inflammatory process or occult abscess suspected
- Bone scan if osteomyelitis or metastatic disease suspected

Diagnostic Procedures/Other
- Liver biopsy if granulomatous disease suspected
- Temporal artery biopsy, particularly in the elderly
- Lymph node, muscle, or skin biopsy, if clinically indicated
- Bone marrow aspiration biopsy with smear, culture, histologic examination, and flow cytometry
- Lumbar puncture, if clinically indicated
- Endoscopy procedures can be helpful for IBD or sarcoidosis

 ## TREATMENT

GENERAL MEASURES
- Treatment depends on the specific etiology.
- Consider discontinuation of recently started or potentially offending medications.
- Empiric therapy is not recommended in patients with prolonged fever because it may camouflage and therefore delay diagnosis and subsequently also hamper correct treatment decisions.
- Therapeutic trials are a last resort and should be as specific as possible based on available clinical evidence. Avoid "shotgun" approaches because they obscure the clinical picture, have untoward effects, and do not provide a diagnostic solution.
- Empiric therapy is prudent in a few difficult-to-diagnose life-threatening cases, for example, CNS or miliary TB, or giant cell arteritis/temporal arteritis.

MEDICATION
First Line
- Antipyretic therapy as a symptomatic approach is a special form of empiric therapy, as it does not necessarily require understanding the cause of fever.
- First-line drugs depend on the diagnosis.
- Evidence does not support isolated treatment of fever.

Second Line
Consider a therapeutic trial only if the patient has localizing symptoms associated with the fever or continues to decline. Consultation with appropriate specialists (infectious disease, rheumatology) is recommended in this case (3).
- Antibiotic trial based on patient's history and suspected culture negative endocarditis
- Antituberculous therapy if there is a high risk for TB pending definitive culture results
- Corticosteroid trial based on patient's history (once occult malignancy is ruled out) if temporal arteritis is suspected

ALERT
- Empiric antibiotic therapy has not been shown to be effective unless the patient is neutropenic, immunocompromised, or critically ill (2).
- If a steroid trial is initiated, patient may have a relapse after treatment or if certain conditions (e.g., TB) have been undiagnosed.

ADDITIONAL THERAPIES
Febrile patients have increased caloric and fluid demands.

SURGERY/OTHER PROCEDURES
The need for exploratory laparotomy has been largely eliminated with the advent of more sophisticated tests and imaging modalities.

ADMISSION, INPATIENT, AND NURSING CONSIDERATIONS
- Reserved for the ill and debilitated
- Consider if factitious fever has been ruled out or an invasive procedure is indicated.

 ## ONGOING CARE

FOLLOW-UP RECOMMENDATIONS
Patient Monitoring
If the etiology of the fever remains unknown, repeat the history, physical exam, and screening lab studies.

DIET
No specific dietary recommendations have been shown to ameliorate undiagnosed fever.

PATIENT EDUCATION
Maintain an open line of communication between physician and patient/family as the workup progresses:
- The extended time required in establishing a diagnosis can be frustrating.

PROGNOSIS
- Depends on etiology, age, and time to diagnosis
  - Patients with HIV have the highest mortality.
- Spontaneous remission is not uncommon in patients with unknown cause of FUO after a thorough workup including a negative FDG-PET/CT scan.
- 1-year survival rates (reflecting deaths due to all causes)
  - <35 years of age is 91%, 35 to 64 years of age is 82%, >64 years of age is 67%

COMPLICATIONS
Depends on etiology

Pregnancy Considerations
Fever increases the risk of neural tube defects in pregnancy and can also trigger preterm labor.

REFERENCES
1. Haidar G, Singh N. Fever of unknown origin. *N Engl J Med*. 2022;386(5):463–477.
2. David A, Quinlan JD. Fever of unknown origin in adults. *Am Fam Physician*. 2022;105(2):137–143.
3. Cunha BA, Lortholary O, Cunha CB. Fever of unknown origin: a clinical approach. *Am J Med*. 2015;128(10):1138.e1–1138.e15.

ADDITIONAL READING
van Rijswijk ND, IJpma FFA, Wouthuyzen-Bakker M, et al. Molecular imaging of fever of unknown origin: an update. *Semin Nucl Med*. 2023;53(1):4–17.

 ## SEE ALSO

Algorithms: Fever in First 60 Days of Life; Fever of Unknown Origin

 ## CODES

ICD10
R50.9 Fever, unspecified

CLINICAL PEARLS
- A sequential approach to FUO based on a careful history, physical examination, with targeted testing and imaging typically yields an appropriate diagnosis and avoids excessive nontargeted testing.
- Empiric therapy is indicated only for carefully defined circumstances.
- FUO cases that defy precise diagnosis after intensive investigation and prolonged observation generally have a favorable prognosis.
- FUO in older persons often presents as an atypical presentation of a common disease.
- The most common causes of FUO in high-income countries are noninfectious inflammatory diseases and idiopathic causes.

FIBROCYSTIC CHANGES OF THE BREAST

Sharon L. Koehler, DO, FACS

BASICS

DESCRIPTION

- Benign epithelial lesions are common findings in women and can be divided into nonproliferative and proliferative and with and without atypia.
- Fibrocystic changes (FCC) are not a disease but refers to a group of benign, nonproliferative histologic findings. It is the most frequent female benign epithelial lesion.
- FCC are seen clinically in up to 50% and histologically in up to 90% of women.
- FCC may also be described as aberrations of normal development and evolution.
- The most common symptoms are cyclic pain, tenderness, swelling, and fullness.
- The breast tissue may feel dense with areas of thicker tissue having an irregular, nodular, or ridge-like surface.
- Women may experience sensitivity to touch with a burning sensation. For some, the pain is so severe that it limits exercise or the ability to lie prone; usually affects both breasts, most often in the upper outer quadrant where most of the milk-producing glands are located
- The sensitivity may be associated with monthly hormonal fluctuations.
- Histologically, in addition to macrocysts and microcysts, FCC may contain solid elements including adenosis, sclerosis, apocrine metaplasia, stromal fibrosis, and epithelial metaplasia and hyperplasia.
  - Depending on the presence of epithelial hyperplasia, FCC are classified as nonproliferative, proliferative without atypia, or proliferative with atypia (1).
  - Nonproliferative lesions are generally not associated with an increased risk of breast cancer.
- System(s) affected: endocrine/metabolic, reproductive
- Synonym(s): diffuse cystic mastopathy; fibrocystic disease; chronic cystic mastitis; or mammary dysplasia

EPIDEMIOLOGY

FCC occur with great frequency in the general population. It affects women between the ages of 25 and 50 years, and it is rare below the age of 20 years.

Incidence

Unknown but very frequent

Prevalence

Up to 1/3 of women aged 30 to 50 years have cysts in their breasts (1). It most commonly presents in the 3rd decade, peaks in the 4th decade when hormonal function is at its peak, and sharply diminishes after menopause. With hormone replacement therapy, FCC may extend into menopause.

ETIOLOGY AND PATHOPHYSIOLOGY

- FCC originate from an exaggerated response of breast stroma and epithelium to a variety of circulating and locally produced hormones (mainly estrogen and progesterone) and growth factors.
- Cysts may form due to dilatation of the lobular acini possibly due to imbalance of fluid secretion and resorption or due to obstruction of the duct leading to the lobule.

RISK FACTORS

- In many women, methylxanthine-containing substances (e.g., coffee, tea, cola, and chocolate) can potentiate symptoms of FCC, although a direct causality has not been established.
- Diet high in saturated fats may increase risk of FCC.

COMMONLY ASSOCIATED CONDITIONS

FCC categorized as proliferative with atypia confers a higher risk of breast cancer.

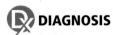

DIAGNOSIS

HISTORY

- Obtain personal history of breast biopsy and family history of breast disease (benign or malignant). It is important to ascertain if the patient has a known family history of *breast, ovarian, and other cancers*.
- Determine (if known) if there is a family history of deleterious mutations: *BRCA1, BRCA2, PALB2, CHEK2, CDH1, PTEN, STK11, PT53,ATM, BARD1, BRIP1, CASP8, CTLA4, CYP19A1, FGFR2, H19, LSP1, MAP3K1, MRE11A, NBN, RAD51,* and *TERT*.
- Inquire regarding pertinent signs/symptoms, such as breast pain, swelling, nipple discharge, palpable lumps, retractions, skin changes, and tenderness. Symptomatically, the condition is manifested as premenstrual cyclic mastalgia, with pain and tenderness to touch.

PHYSICAL EXAM

- The patient should be examined in the following positions while disrobed down to the waist:
  - With the patient standing with arms at sides, observe for elevation of the level of a nipple, dimpling, bulging, and peau d'orange.
  - With the patient's arms raised above her head, observe for dimpling and elevation/retraction of the nipple (may accentuate a mass fixed to the pectoral fascia). If so, have the patient push her hands down against her hips to flex and tense the pectoralis major muscles; move the mass to determine fixation to the underlying fascia.
  - If the patient has large and pendulous breasts, ask her to lean forward, so that her breasts hang free from the chest wall (retraction and masses may become more evident).
  - Axillary lymph nodes are evaluated with the patient sitting up, the arm is supported by the examiner's arm while finger pads gently palpate the axilla from the posterior axillary line to the pectoralis.
  - With the patient laying supine, palpate with the pads of the three middle fingers (with varying pressures from light, to medium, to deep), rotating the fingers in small circular motions and moving in vertical overlapping passes from rostral to caudal and then back caudal to rostral in the next pass. The lateral half of the breast is best palpated with the patient rolled onto the contralateral hip and the medial half with the patient laying supine, both with the ipsilateral hand behind the head. The entire breast from the 2nd to 6th rib and from the left sternal border to the midaxillary line must be palpated against the chest wall.

- Be certain to examine the creases under and between the breasts. If the patient has noted a lump, ask her to point it out; always palpate the opposite breast first.
- Patients with FCC have clinical breast findings that range from mild alterations in texture to dense, firm breast tissue with palpable masses.

DIFFERENTIAL DIAGNOSIS

- Pain
  - Mastitis
  - Costochondritis
  - Pectoralis muscle strain
  - Neuralgia
  - Breast cancer
  - Angina pectoris
  - Gastroesophageal reflux (GERD)
  - Superficial phlebitis of the thoracoepigastric vein (Mondor disease)
- Masses
  - Breast cancer
  - Sebaceous cyst
  - Fibroadenoma
  - Lipoma
  - Fat necrosis
  - Phyllodes tumor
  - Granuloma
- Skin changes
  - Breast cancer (peau d'orange: thickened skin similar to peel of an orange)
  - Eczema
  - Infection
  - Fungus
  - Paget disease

DIAGNOSTIC TESTS & INTERPRETATION

- Evaluation should focus on excluding breast cancer.
- Testing may be conducted based on a level of clinical suspicion.
- FCC can be evaluated with mammogram, although dense breast tissue may appear normal in women <35 years of age.
- Ultrasound (US) is the most useful method for assessing a cyst.

Initial Tests (lab, imaging)

- On mammogram, FCC appear as nodular densities of breast tissue; solitary cysts can appear as round or ovoid or well-circumscribed masses, usually with low to intermediate density. FCC may also contain calcifications.
- On US, if a simple cyst is demonstrated as an anechoic structure with imperceptible wall and posterior acoustic enhancement, benign diagnosis is confirmed and no further imaging or intervention is indicated. However, if the cyst appears to be thick-walled and/or contains internal echoes, differential diagnosis should include a complicated cyst, an abscess, a galactocele, or a focal duct ectasia in the appropriate clinical contexts.
- MRI is indicated in patients with *BRCA1, BRCA2,* or other related deleterious mutation, or in any woman with ≥25% lifetime risk for breast cancer. Additionally, MRI may be indicated for extremely dense breasts as well as inconclusive findings on other breast imaging.
- On MRI, cystic changes are well-circumscribed lesions of high-signal intensity on T2-weighted sequences and of low-signal intensity on T1-weighted images (1).

Diagnostic Procedures/Other

- Fine-needle aspiration (FNA) biopsy:
  - Allows differentiation of cystic and solid lesions
  - Aspirate may be straw-colored, dark brown, or green.
  - Cells sent for cytology can reveal cancer with high accuracy.
  - Low morbidity
- If the lesion disappears, no further evaluation is necessary (including cytologic evaluation of aspirated fluid).
- On the basis of the presence and degree of epithelial hyperplasia, FCC are comprised of nonproliferative (approximately 65% of the total), proliferative without atypia (approximately 30% of the total), and proliferative with atypia (approximately 5–8% of the total) (2).

Test Interpretation

Certain histologic changes in the setting of FCC confer an increased risk for breast cancer:

- Nonproliferative changes: relative risk of 1.2 to 1.4
- Proliferative disease (PD) without atypia: relative risk of 1.7 to 2.1
- PD with atypia: relative risk ≥4

 TREATMENT

- After ruling out malignancy by means of examination and/or imaging and diagnostic procedures, FCC may not require treatment and often resolves with time.
- Cool compresses, avoiding trauma, and around-the-clock wearing of a well-fitting, supportive brassiere may be useful for symptom relief.
- Reduction in caffeine, additional supplementation with vitamin E, and/or evening primrose oil have been advocated. Trials have not proven the benefit (1).

MEDICATION

First Line

Analgesics and anti-inflammatory drugs are used to reduce cyclic breast pain and swelling. This includes oral and topical NSAIDs or acetaminophen.

- Acetaminophen: 1,000 mg every 6 to 8 hours; maximum daily dose of 3,000 mg unless directed by health care provider
- Ibuprofen: 400 mg every 4 to 6 hours as needed
- Naproxen: 500 mg every 12 hours as needed

Second Line

- Oral contraceptives (OCPs) may be useful in modulating symptoms or in preventing the development of new changes in females with cyclic symptoms.
- For severe pain, consider the following (3)[A]:
  - Danazol is effective for reducing breast pain and tenderness but has androgenic effects and is associated with hepatotoxicity and teratogenicity, which limits its use. This drug is administered orally at a dosage of 100 to 400 mg/day in 2 divided doses.

- Tamoxifen 10 mg/day for 3 to 6 months; along with teratogenicity, this selective estrogen receptor modulator (SERM) can increase the risk of thromboembolism and endometrial carcinoma in treated females.
- Several other medications, such as bromocriptine and GnRH agonists have been studied but are associated with toxicities.

ISSUES FOR REFERRAL

- If discrete palpable lesion in a woman aged <30 years: US, then consider referral to a surgeon, especially if not a simple cyst/lesion resolving at follow-up in a different phase of menstrual cycle
- If discrete palpable lesion in a woman aged >30 years: diagnostic mammography ± US, then refer to surgeon

SURGERY/OTHER PROCEDURES

- Breast cyst aspiration can be both diagnostic and therapeutic.
- Core-needle biopsies performed under stereotactic guidance with vacuum assistance has similar accuracy in distinguishing between malignant and benign lesions compared to open surgical biopsy (4)[A].
- Biopsy results must be assessed for concordance.

COMPLEMENTARY & ALTERNATIVE MEDICINE

- The use of vitamin E has shown effectiveness in treating breast pain due to FCC.
- Anecdotal evidence supports the use of evening primrose oil for FCC.

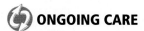 ONGOING CARE

FOLLOW-UP RECOMMENDATIONS

Condition is benign, chronic, and recurrent.

Patient Monitoring

- Follow-up times are variable, depending on the clinical situation and pertinent family history.
- US is useful to differentiate cysts from solid lesions and in evaluating women <35 years of age for FCC but is not useful for screening.
- Screening mammograms: Refer to the USPSTF, ACOG, or ACS recommendations for screening schedules.

DIET

The role of caffeine consumption in the development and treatment of FCC has never been proven; however, some patients report relief of symptoms after abstinence from coffee, tea, and chocolate.

PATIENT EDUCATION

- Patient information on fibrocystic breasts from the Mayo Foundation for Medical Education and Research: https://www.mayoclinic.com/health/fibrocystic-breasts/DS01070

- Information on breast cancer prevention from the National Cancer Institute: https://www.cancer.gov
- Information on fibrocystic breasts from the American Cancer Society: https://www.cancer.org/cancer/types/breast-cancer/non-cancerous-breast-conditions/fibrosis-and-simple-cysts-in-the-breast.html

REFERENCES

1. Pearlman M, Griffin J, Swain M, et al; for American College of Obstetricians and Gynecologists' Committee on Practice Bulletins—Gynecology. Practice Bulletin No. 164: diagnosis and management of benign breast disorders. *Obstet Gynecol*. 2016;127(6):e141–e156.
2. Hartmann LC, Sellers TA, Frost MH, et al. Benign breast disease and the risk of breast cancer. *N Engl J Med*. 2005;353(3):229–237.
3. Srivastava A, Mansel RE, Arvind N, et al. Evidence-based management of mastalgia: a meta-analysis of randomised trials. *Breast*. 2007;16(5):503–512.
4. Bruening W, Fontanarosa J, Tipton K, et al. Systematic review: comparative effectiveness of core-needle and open surgical biopsy to diagnose breast lesions. *Ann Intern Med*. 2010;152(4):238–246.

ADDITIONAL READING

- Hafiz SP, Barnes NLP, Kirwan CC. Clinical management of idiopathic mastalgia: a systematic review. *J Prim Health Care*. 2018;10(4):312–323.
- Salzman B, Collins E, Hersh L. Common breast problems. *Am Fam Physician*. 2019;99(8):505–514.

 CODES

ICD10

- N60.19 Diffuse cystic mastopathy of unspecified breast
- N60.09 Solitary cyst of unspecified breast
- N60.29 Fibroadenosis of unspecified breast

CLINICAL PEARLS

- FCC of the breast comprise a spectrum of histopathologic changes are a common finding in reproductive-aged women. The former term of fibrocystic disease is a misnomer.
- Atypia, as demonstrated histopathologically, confers an increased cancer risk and may require additional diagnostic workup.
- NSAIDs are the first-line treatment.
- OCPs, danazol, and tamoxifen are second-line treatments, the latter two with considerable adverse effects.
- Consultation with a breast specialist is recommended for symptomatic disease refractory to simple measures or for diagnostic issues.

F

FIBROMYALGIA

F. Stuart Leeds, MD, MS

BASICS

DESCRIPTION
- Chronic, widespread noninflammatory musculoskeletal pain syndrome with multisystem manifestations; although the specific pathophysiology has not been fully elucidated, it is generally thought to be a disorder of altered central pain regulation.
- Synonym(s): FMS; fibrositis, fibromyositis (misnomers)

EPIDEMIOLOGY
Incidence
- Predominant sex: female (70–90%) > male
- Predominant age range: 20 to 65 years
Prevalence
2–5% of adult U.S. population; 8% of primary care patients

ETIOLOGY AND PATHOPHYSIOLOGY
- Current consensus is that fibromyalgia is a primary disorder of central pain processing (central sensitization) with increased sensitivity to multiple classes of painful sensation (nociceptive, nociplastic, and neuropathic)
- Alterations in neuroendocrine, neuromodulation, neurotransmitter, neurotransporter, biochemical, and neuroreceptor function/physiology
- Sleep abnormalities—α-wave intrusion
- Systemic inflammation is not a feature of fibromyalgia, although localized immunologic and inflammatory processes in the CNS may play a role. There may be a distinctive cytokine profile in patients with fibromyalgia.

Genetics
- Genetics
  - High familial aggregation
  - Inheritance is unknown but likely polygenic.
  - Odds ratio may be as high as 8.5 for a first-degree relative of a familial proband.
- Environmental—several triggers have been described:
  - Physical trauma or severe illness
  - Stressors (e.g., work, family, life events, and physical or sexual abuse)
  - Viral and bacterial infections

RISK FACTORS
- Female gender
- Poor functional status
- Negative/stressful life events
- Low socioeconomic status

GENERAL PREVENTION
No known strategies for prevention

COMMONLY ASSOCIATED CONDITIONS
- Often a comorbid condition with other rheumatologic or neurologic disorders
- Psychiatric comorbidities, including depression, anxiety, and posttraumatic stress disorder (PTSD) occur in 2/3 of patients—similar to findings in other chronic pain conditions.
- Obesity is common and associated with increased severity of symptoms.

DIAGNOSIS

- Original 1990 ACR criteria, still widely used: (i) pain in all four quadrants >3 months, (ii) axial (neck/spine) involvement, (iii) tender points (TPs) ≥11
- 2010/2011 ACR criteria, revised in 2016 (1)
  - Based on Widespread Pain Index (WPI) and Symptom Score (SS)
    ○ Generalized pain present in 4/5 body regions
    ○ Must have WPI ≥7 + SS ≥5, or WPI 4 to 6 and SS ≥9
    ○ Symptoms for >3 months
    ○ Fibromyalgia may be diagnosed irrespective of other active disease entities (i.e., it need not be the only explanation for the patient's symptoms).
- WPI/SS patient scoring and diagnosis tool
- The revised Fibromyalgia Impact Questionnaire (FIQr) or the simpler Visual Analogue Scale Fibromyalgia Impact Questionnaire (VASFIQ) should be used for initial and serial assessments of patient's functional status and response to therapy.

HISTORY
- Invariant symptoms include
  - Chronic widespread pain ≥3 months: bilateral limbs and in the axial skeleton
  - Fatigue and sleep disturbances
- Often present:
  - Mood disorders, including depression, anxiety, panic symptoms, and PTSD
  - Cognitive impairment: qualitatively different from that seen in isolated mood disorders ("fibro fog")
  - Headaches: typically tension and migraine types
  - Other regional pain syndromes, such as irritable bowel syndrome, chronic pelvic pain, vulvodynia, and interstitial cystitis
  - Small-fiber neuropathies and "nonanatomic" paresthesias
  - Exercise intolerance, dyspnea, and palpitations
  - Sexual dysfunction
  - Ocular dryness
  - "Multiple chemical sensitivity" and an increased tendency to report drug reactions
  - Impaired social/occupational functioning
  - Symptoms can wax and wane on a day-to-day basis, varying in quality, intensity, and location. Emotional distress can both trigger and aggravate symptoms.

PHYSICAL EXAM
- Classic fibromyalgia TPs: 9 symmetric pairs (5 anterior, 4 posterior)
- The presence of ≥11 TPs carries a sensitivity of 88% and specificity of 81% for the disease.
- TPs in fibromyalgia are distinct from the "trigger points" found in myofascial pain syndromes and are not sites for therapeutic injection.
- Examine joints for swelling, tenderness, erythema, decreased range of motion, crepitus, and cystic or mass lesions. These are typically absent in fibromyalgia.

- Document absence of inflammatory features (e.g., no synovitis, enthesopathy, dermatologic, or ocular findings).
- Neurologic exam: may demonstrate generalized or "nonanatomic" dysesthesia, hyper- or hypesthesia; Focal neurologic findings suggest alternative or additional diagnoses.

DIFFERENTIAL DIAGNOSIS
- RA, SLE, sarcoidosis, and other inflammatory connective tissue disorders
- Diffuse/advanced OA, seronegative spondyloarthropathies (AS, psoriatic arthritis, etc.)
- Polymyalgia rheumatica; drug-induced, endocrine, and inflammatory myopathies
- Post–COVID-19 conditions (PCC; "long COVID"); viral/postviral polyarthralgia syndromes
- Anemia and iron deficiency, sickle-cell disease and variants
- Electrolyte disturbances: Mg, Na, K, Ca; vitamin deficiencies: D, B_{12}, B_6
- Obstructive sleep apnea; restless leg syndrome; joint hypermobility syndromes (Ehlers-Danlos et al.)
- Complex regional pain syndromes (CRPS), opioid-induced hyperalgesia
- Hypothyroidism; hyperparathyroidism
- Lyme disease, hepatitis B and C (chronic)
- Generalized muscular deconditioning, peripheral vascular disease
- Central poststroke pain syndromes
- Multiple sclerosis, spinal cord syndromes, inflammatory polyneuropathies (AIDP, CIDP, etc)
- Malignancies: metastatic and paraneoplastic syndromes
- Somatic symptom disorder and other psychiatric conditions with associated somatization symptoms
- Overlap syndromes
  - Chronic fatigue syndrome/chronic fatigue immune dysfunction syndrome (ME/CFS, CFIDS)
  - Myofascial pain syndrome (more anatomically localized than fibromyalgia but these may co-occur)

DIAGNOSTIC TESTS & INTERPRETATION
Initial Tests (lab, imaging)
- CBC with differential, ESR or CRP, CPK, TSH, comprehensive metabolic profile; consider 25-OH vitamin D, Mg, vitamin B_{12}, folate, and urine drug screen.
- ANA, RF, Lyme titers, and other rheumatologic labs are generally unnecessary, unless there are specific or localizing symptoms suggestive of inflammatory or infectious disease.
- Imaging is not generally indicated, except to exclude other specific diagnoses.

Diagnostic Procedures/Other
- Sleep studies may be indicated to rule out obstructive sleep apnea or narcolepsy.
- Consider psychiatric or neuropsychiatric evaluation for comorbid mood disorders and cognitive disturbances.

TREATMENT

Evidence-based interventions:

- Includes both medication and nonpharmacologic interventions (2); a multimodal approach using safe combinations of mutually reinforcing therapies, both pharmacologic and nonpharmacologic, provides the best results. In general, a partial or complete remission can only be achieved with committed changes in lifestyle, including regular exercise, proper sleep hygiene, and smoking cessation.
- Nonpharmacologic
  - Educate about diagnosis, signs, symptoms, and treatment options: Online resources include:
    ○ https://www.fmaware.org
    ○ https://www.fibromyalgiaforums.org/
    ○ https://www.fibro.org/
  - VASFIQ for initial assessment and interval evaluation during treatment
  - Cognitive-behavioral therapy (CBT) improves mood, energy, pain, and functional status (2)[A].
  - Acceptance and Commitment Therapy (ACT)
  - Aerobic exercise: moderately intense, with gradual titration to minimize symptom exacerbation ("start low and slow") (2)[A]
  - Strength/resistance training—mild to moderate; tai chi—equal or superior to aerobic exercise
  - Aquatic exercise training; mixed exercise training (combined aerobic, resistance, flexibility)
  - Weight loss may augment the benefits of exercise.
  - Sleep hygiene
  - Mitigate/eliminate tobacco, alcohol, and substance use.
- Pharmacologic
  - Three FDA-approved drugs: duloxetine, milnacipran, and pregabalin; others are off-label. Recent studies suggest that these agents, when used as monotherapy, only benefit a minority of responders.
  - **Caution**: Fibromyalgia patients are frequently treated with multidrug regimens; monitor closely for drug interactions, and especially for "stacked" sedative, serotonergic, and anticholinergic effects.

MEDICATION

First Line

- Amitriptyline 10 to 50 mg PO at bedtime to treat pain, fatigue, and sleep disturbances; TCAs that are secondary amines (e.g., desipramine, nortriptyline) may be similarly effective and less sedating.
- Duloxetine initially 30 mg/day for 1 week and then increase to 60 mg/day as tolerated; taper if discontinued (2)[A].
- Milnacipran day 1: 12.5 mg/day; days 2 to 3, begin dividing doses: 12.5 mg BID; days 4 to 7: 25 mg BID; after day 7: 50 mg BID; max dose of 100 to 200 mg BID. Taper if discontinued (2)[A]
- Pregabalin: Start with 75 mg BID, titrate over 1 week to 150 mg BID; max dose of 450 mg/day (some authorities recommend up to 600 mg/day) divided BID–TID (2)[A].
- Cyclobenzaprine 5 mg qHS; titrate to 10 mg BID–TID as tolerated (2)[A].

Second Line

- Gabapentin: Start at 300 mg HS, titrate to 1,200 to 2,400 mg/day divided BID–TID; max dose of 3,600 mg/day
- Venlafaxine XR 37.5 to 225.0 mg; likely to be as effective as other SNRIs (duloxetine, milnacipran)
- Tramadol 50 to 100 mg q6h; likely more effective in combination with acetaminophen (2)[B]
- Quetiapine 25 to 100 mg qHS
- Several agents have shown some promise of benefit, albeit with limited evidence, including pramipexole, memantine, low-dose naltrexone, medical cannabis (especially with higher CBD:THC ratios), and hyperbaric O_2 therapy.
- Cholecalciferol may be beneficial in patients with low 25-OH vitamin D levels.

ISSUES FOR REFERRAL

In cases of unclear diagnosis or poor response to therapy, refer to rheumatology, neurology, and/or pain management.

ADDITIONAL THERAPIES

- Trigger point (not TP) injections for regional myofascial dysfunction may provide relief.
- Multidisciplinary rehab (specialized clinic with physical medicine and therapy, occupational therapy, and integrated pain management)
- Ineffective or dangerous treatment modalities (2)
  - NSAIDs, full-agonist opioids (except in refractory cases), benzodiazepines, SSRIs (although may have efficacy in combination therapy with TCAs or pregabalin), magnesium, guaifenesin, thyroxine, corticosteroids, DHEA, growth hormone, valacyclovir, interferon, calcitonin, nabilone, and antiepileptic agents (other than those listed above)
  - Fibromyalgia often presents concurrently with other pain syndromes that may respond to NSAIDs, corticosteroids, opioids, and other agents.

COMPLEMENTARY & ALTERNATIVE MEDICINE

- The following have evidence-based support for their efficacy and safety:
  - Acupuncture and electroacupuncture, biofeedback, hypnotherapy
  - Balneotherapy (mineral-rich baths)
  - Yoga, tai chi, and qi gong
  - Mindfulness-based meditation
  - Repetitive transcranial magnetic (rTMS) and direct current stimulation (tDCS) therapies
- Low-level laser therapy (LLLT)
- Limited double-blind trials have shown effectiveness of supplementation with S-adenosyl-L-methionine and acetyl-L-carnitine.
- Likely to be ineffective: chiropractic treatment, multivitamin therapy, homeopathy

ONGOING CARE

FOLLOW-UP RECOMMENDATIONS

Patient Monitoring

- For efficacy of initial therapy: at 2- to 4-week intervals, then every 1 to 6 months, tailored to patient's needs
- Advance exercise gradually and as tolerated.

DIET

Patient should make healthy choices and address negative dietary habits. Caloric or carbohydrate restriction may be helpful in obese patients. Reduction in pain has been reported in patients following hypocaloric and vegan diets, as well as diets low in fermentable saccharides and polyols (FODMAPs).

PATIENT EDUCATION

It is important to make a clear diagnosis of fibromyalgia and communicate it to the patient (1).

PROGNOSIS

- A chronic, fluctuating course is characteristic of the disease; 50% with partial remission after 2 to 3 years of therapy; complete remission possible but uncommon
- Poorer outcomes tied to greater duration and severity of symptoms, depression, obesity, insufficient engagement and "ownership" of the treatment plan, advanced age, and lack of social support

REFERENCES

1. Wolfe F, Clauw DJ, Fitzcharles MA, et al. 2016 Revisions to the 2010/2011 fibromyalgia diagnostic criteria. *Semin Arthritis Rheum*. 2016;46(3):319–329.
2. Macfarlane GJ, Kronisch C, Dean LE, et al. EULAR revised recommendations for the management of fibromyalgia. *Ann Rheum Dis*. 2017;76(2): 318–328.

ADDITIONAL READING

- Häuser W, Fitzcharles MA. Facts and myths pertaining to fibromyalgia. *Dialogues Clin Neurosci*. 2018;20(1):53–62.
- Ovrom EA, Mostert KA, Khakhkhar S, et al. A comprehensive review of the genetic and epigenetic contributions to the development of fibromyalgia. *Biomedicines*. 2023;11(4):1119.

 SEE ALSO

Algorithm: Fatigue

CODES

ICD10

M79.7 Fibromyalgia

CLINICAL PEARLS

- Fibromyalgia is a disease of nociplastic pain and central sensitization. It is not a somatoform disorder, and is not merely a manifestation of depression or anxiety. As with all chronic pain syndromes, however, fibromyalgia is frequently associated with comorbid mood and anxiety disorders that must also be assessed and treated.
- Use 1990 or 2010–2016 ACR criteria to formally diagnose fibromyalgia.
- The best clinical outcomes occur in patients who understand their illness and actively participate in a multimodal treatment regimen that includes exercise, sleep hygiene, and lifestyle modifications, along with appropriate combination pharmacotherapy and CBT.

FOLLICULITIS

David C. Cadena Jr., MD • Mayra A. Perez, DO

 BASICS

DESCRIPTION

- Common skin condition involving inflammation of the hair follicle
- Most frequent symptom is pruritus.
- Painless or tender pustules, vesicles, or pink/red papulopustules up to 5 mm in size
- Most commonly infectious in etiology:
  - *Staphylococcus aureus* bacteria
  - *Pseudomonas aeruginosa* infects areas of the body exposed to poorly sanitized hot tubs, pools, or contaminated water.
  - Fungal (dermatophytic, *Pityrosporum*, *Candida*)
  - Viral (VZV, herpes simplex virus [HSV])
  - Parasitic (*Demodex* mites, schistosomes)
- Noninfectious types
  - Acneiform folliculitis
  - Actinic superficial folliculitis
  - Acne vulgaris
  - Keloidal folliculitis
  - Folliculitis decalvans
  - Perioral dermatitis
  - Fox-Fordyce disease
  - Pruritus folliculitis of pregnancy
  - Toxic erythema of the newborn
  - Eosinophilic folliculitis (seen in HIV positive/immunocompromised)
  - Follicular mucinosis
- Skin disorders that may produce a follicular eruption:
  - Pseudofolliculitis barbae: similar in appearance; occurs after shaving; commonly known as razor bumps, occurs more frequently in black men
  - Atopic dermatitis
  - Follicular psoriasis
  - Rosacea

EPIDEMIOLOGY

Affects persons of all ages, gender, and race; those who shave or have chronic conditions such as diabetes or those who are immunocompromised are at increased risk.

Incidence

Superficial folliculitis is most commonly a self-limited condition; therefore, the exact incidence is not known.

Prevalence

Folliculitis is a relatively common skin condition; prevalence rate in the United States is 8 per 1,000.

ETIOLOGY AND PATHOPHYSIOLOGY

Predisposing factors to folliculitis

- Chronic staphylococcal carrier
- Diabetes mellitus
- Malnutrition
- Pruritic skin disease (e.g., scabies, eczema)
- Exposure to poorly chlorinated swimming pools/hot tubs
- Occlusive corticosteroid use (for multiple hours)
- Bacteria
  - Most frequently due to *S. aureus* (increasing number of methicillin-resistant *S. aureus* [MRSA] cases)
  - Also due to *Streptococcus* species, *Pseudomonas* (following exposure to water contaminated with the species), or *Proteus*
  - May progress to furuncle and carbuncle

- Fungal
  - Dermatophytic (tinea capitis, tinea corporis, tinea pedis)
  - *Pityrosporum* (Pityrosporum orbiculare) commonly affecting teenagers and men, predominantly on upper chest and back
- Viral
  - HSV
  - Molluscum contagiosum
- Parasitic
  - *Demodex* mites (commonly *Demodex folliculorum*), common around nasolabial area
  - Schistosomes (swimmer's itch)
- Acneiform type commonly drug induced (systemic and topical corticosteroids, lithium, isoniazid, rifampin), EGFR inhibitors
- Severe vitamin C deficiency
- Actinic superficial type occurs within 24 to 48 hours of exposure to the sun, resulting in multiple follicular pustules on the shoulders, trunk, and arms.
- Acne vulgaris
- Keloidal folliculitis is a chronic condition affecting mostly black patients; involves the neck and occipital scalp, resulting in hypertrophic scars and hair loss; usually consequence of uncontrolled folliculitis barbae
- Folliculitis decalvans is a chronic folliculitis that leads to progressive scarring and alopecia of the scalp.
- Rosacea consists of papules, pustules, and/or telangiectasias of the face; individuals are genetically predisposed; *can be confused with folliculitis*
- Fox-Fordyce disease affects the skin containing apocrine sweat glands (i.e., axillae), resulting in follicular papules.
- Eosinophilic pustular folliculitis has three variants: classic (Ofuji disease), associated with HIV infection, and infantile.
- Toxic erythema of the newborn is a self-limiting pustular eruption usually appearing during the first 3 to 4 days of life and subsequently fading in the following 2 weeks.
- *Malassezia* infections

Genetics

No known genetic predisposition

RISK FACTORS

- Hair removal (shaving, plucking, waxing, epilating agents)
- Other pruritic skin conditions: eczema, scabies
- Occlusive dressing or clothing
- Sweating
- Personal carrier or contact with MRSA-infected persons
- Diabetes mellitus
- Immunosuppression (medications, chemotherapy, HIV)
- Use of hot tubs or saunas
- Use of EGFR inhibitors
- Chronic antibiotic use (gram-negative folliculitis)
- Tattoo recipient

GENERAL PREVENTION

- Good hygiene practices
  - Wash hands frequently with antimicrobial soap.
  - Wash towels, clothes, and linens frequently with hot water to avoid reinfection.
- Good hair removal practices
  - Exfoliate beforehand.
  - Use witch hazel, alcohol, or Tend Skin afterward.
  - Shave in direction of hair growth; use shaving gel and moisturizer.
  - Decrease frequency of shaving.
  - Use clippers primarily or single-blade razors if straight shaving is desired.

COMMONLY ASSOCIATED CONDITIONS

Impetigo, scabies, acne, follicular psoriasis, eczema, xerosis, *Staphylococcus*/MRSA colonization

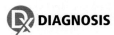 **DIAGNOSIS**

HISTORY

- Recent use of hot tubs, swimming pools, topical corticosteroids, certain hairstyling and shaving practices, antibiotics or systemic steroids
- HIV status
- History of STDs (specifically syphilis)
- MRSA exposures/carrier status
- Home and work environment (risk/exposure potential)
- Pityrosporum folliculitis occurs more often in warm, moist climates.
- Inquire about the timeline in which the lesions have occurred, including previous similar episodes.

PHYSICAL EXAM

- Characteristic lesions are 1- to 5-mm–wide vesicles, pustules, or inflamed papules with surrounding erythema.
- Rash occurs on hair-bearing skin, especially the face (beard), proximal limbs, scalp, and pubis.
- Pseudomonal folliculitis appears as a widespread rash, mainly on the trunk and limbs.
- In pseudofolliculitis barbae, the growing hair curls around and penetrates the skin at shaved areas.

DIFFERENTIAL DIAGNOSIS

- Acne vulgaris/acneiform eruptions
- Arthropod bite
- Contact dermatitis
- Perioral dermatitis
- Cutaneous candidiasis
- Milia
- Atopic dermatitis
- Follicular psoriasis
- Hidradenitis suppurativa

DIAGNOSTIC TESTS & INTERPRETATION

Initial Tests (lab, imaging)

- Diagnosis can be made clinically, taking risk factors, history, and locations of lesions into account.
- Culture and Gram stain may be done for larger lesions lancing or unroofing the pustule.

- KOH preparation as well as Wood lamp fluorescence to identify *Candida* or yeast
- Tzanck smear where suspicion of herpetic simplex viral folliculitis is high
- Ultrasound can be performed for questionably deeper seeding infections.

Follow-Up Tests & Special Considerations
- If risk factors or clinical suspicion exist, consider serologies for HIV or syphilis.
- If recurrent, consider HIV testing and A1C/fasting blood sugar testing to evaluate for diabetes.
- Consider punch biopsy with uncertain diagnosis.
- Treat positive bacterial culture according to sensitivities.
- Positive HIV serology: Follow up with CD4 count and punch biopsy to rule out eosinophilic folliculitis.

TREATMENT

GENERAL MEASURES
- Lesions usually resolve spontaneously.
- Avoid shaving or waxing affected areas (1)[C].
- Warm compresses may be applied TID.
- Systemic antibiotics are typically unnecessary.
- Topical mupirocin may be used in presumed *S. aureus* infection (2).
- Topical antifungals for fungal folliculitis
- Preventive measures:
  - Antibacterial soaps (Dial soap, chlorhexidine, or benzoyl peroxide wash when showering/bathing)
  - Bleach baths (1/2 cup of 6% bleach per standard bathtub and soak for 5 to 15 minutes followed by water, rinse 1 to 2 times a week)
  - Keep skin intact; daily skin care with noncomedogenic moisturizers; avoid scratching.
  - Avoid trauma to skin: Use an electric razor as able.
  - Clean shaving instruments daily or use disposable razor, disposing after one use (1).
  - Change washcloths, towels, and sheets daily.

MEDICATION
Antiseptic and supportive care is usually enough. Systemic antibiotics may be used for severe or persistent infection but have questionable efficacy, and available evidence is of generally low quality (3)[A].

First Line
- Staphylococcal folliculitis
  - Topical mupirocin ointment applied TID for 10 days
  - Cephalosporin (cephalexin): 250 to 500 mg PO QID for 7 to 10 days
  - Dicloxacillin: 250 to 500 mg PO QID for 7 to 10 days
- For MRSA
  - Bactrim DS: 1 to 2 tablets (160 mg/800 mg) BID PO for 5 to 10 days
  - Clindamycin: 300 mg PO TID for 10 to 14 days
  - Minocycline: 200 mg PO initially and then 100 mg BID for 5 to 10 days
  - Doxycycline: 50 to 100 mg PO BID for 5 to 10 days

- *Pseudomonas* folliculitis
  - Topical dilute acetic acid baths
  - Ciprofloxacin: 500 to 750 mg PO BID for 7 to 14 days for severe infections
- Eosinophilic folliculitis/eosinophilic pustular folliculitis
  - HAART treatment for HIV-positive–related causes
  - High-potency topical corticosteroids for inflammation
  - Antihistamines (hydroxyzine, cetirizine) to control itching
  - Can consider: tacrolimus topically BID *or*
  - Isotretinoin 0.5 mg/kg/day PO with caution
  - Itraconazole or metronidazole
- Fungal folliculitis
  - Topical antifungals: ketoconazole 2% cream or shampoo or selenium sulfide shampoo daily *or*
  - Econazole cream applied to affected area BID for 2 to 3 weeks
    - Systemic antifungals for relapses fluconazole (100 to 200 mg/day for 3 weeks) *or* itraconazole (200 mg/day for 1 week) *or* griseofulvin (500 mg/day for 2 to 4 weeks)
    - Do not use oral ketoconazole due to risk of liver failure.
- Parasitic folliculitis
  - 5% permethrin: Apply to affected area, leave on for 8 hours, and wash off.
  - Ivermectin: 200 μg/kg PO and repeat in 1 to 2 weeks if topical application unsuccessful
- Herpetic folliculitis
  - Valacyclovir: 500 mg PO TID for 5 to 10 days or
  - Famciclovir: 500 mg PO TID for 5 to 10 days or
  - Acyclovir: 200 mg PO 5 times daily for 5 to 10 days

ISSUES FOR REFERRAL
Unusual or persistent cases should be biopsied and referred to dermatology.

ADDITIONAL THERAPIES
- Stay informed: Testing strips can be used to test hot tubs and pools. This will help determine proper chlorine levels.
- Both hot tubs and pools should have a pH level of 7.2 to 7.8.

SURGERY/OTHER PROCEDURES
Incision and drainage are unlikely to be necessary and typically not preferred due to potential for scar formation unless secondary abscess has formed. If isolated abscess has developed, it may be treated with incision and drainage alone.

ONGOING CARE

FOLLOW-UP RECOMMENDATIONS
Patient Monitoring
- Resistant cases should be followed every 2 weeks until cleared.
- Consider prompt system therapy for worsening cases.

DIET
Caloric monitoring for obese patients; weight reduction will decrease risk of skin trauma and distension.

PATIENT EDUCATION
- Avoid shaving in involved areas.
- Monitor hot tub and pools.

PROGNOSIS
- Usually resolves with treatment; however, *S. aureus* carriers may experience recurrences.
- Mupirocin nasal treatment for carrier status and for family/household members might be helpful.
- Resistant or severe cases may warrant testing for diabetes mellitus or immunodeficiency (HIV).

COMPLICATIONS
- Primary complication is recurrent folliculitis.
- Extensive scarring with hyperpigmentation
- Progression to furunculosis or abscess

REFERENCES
1. Khanna N, Chandramohan K, Khaitan BK, et al. Post waxing folliculitis: a clinicopathological evaluation. *Int J Dermatol*. 2014;53(7):849–854.
2. Sartelli M, Guirao X, Hardcastle TC, et al. 2018 WSES/SIS-E consensus conference: recommendations for the management of skin and soft-tissue infections. *World J Emerg Surg*. 2018;13:58.
3. Lin HS, Lin PT, Tsai YS, et al. Interventions for bacterial folliculitis and boils (furuncles and carbuncles). *Cochrane Database Syst Rev*. 2021;2(2):CD013099.

 SEE ALSO

Algorithm: Rash

 CODES

ICD10
- L73.9 Follicular disorder, unspecified
- L66.2 Folliculitis decalvans
- L73.8 Other specified follicular disorders

CLINICAL PEARLS
- Folliculitis lesions are typically 1- to 5-mm clusters of pruritic erythematous papules and pustule surrounding hair follicles.
- Most commonly due to *S. aureus*; if community has increased incidence of MRSA, consider anti-MRSA treatment.
  - It is extremely important to educate patients on proper hygiene and skin care techniques to prevent chronic or recurrent cases.
- If not improving after 2 weeks, consider oral antibiotics or biopsy for confirmation.

FOOD ALLERGY
Brian P. Vickery, MD • Idil D. Ezhuthachan, MD, MS • Melinda M. Rathkopf, MD, MBA

 BASICS

Food allergies are adverse health effects arising from a specific immune response that occurs reproducibly on exposure to a given food. Immune responses can be IgE mediated or non-IgE mediated. This review focuses on IgE-mediated food allergy.

DESCRIPTION
- A reproducible hypersensitivity reaction related to certain food exposures mediated by IgE
- System(s) affected: gastrointestinal (GI), hematologic/lymphatic/immunologic, pulmonary, skin, cardiovascular
- Synonym(s): IgE-mediated food reactions, food hypersensitivity, anaphylaxis

EPIDEMIOLOGY
- Predominant age: all ages; traditionally thought to affect infants and young children more commonly; however, recent data show increasing prevalence in adults (1).
- Predominant sex: male > female in children, female > male in adults
- Although it is difficult to discern the exact effects of socioeconomic and racial differences on food allergy prevalence, disproportionate impact on underserved and minority patients have been reported (2),(3).

Incidence
Egg allergy incidence has been reported as 1.23% in infants, whereas this number for cow's milk allergy was 0.54%.

Prevalence
- The prevalence of IgE-mediated food allergy assessed by food challenge, the diagnostic gold-standard, is 3%.
- The self-reported prevalence of food allergy is >10%, with 1 in 10 adults and 1 in 12 children being affected (1).
- In children, the most common food allergies are cow's milk (2%), egg (0.6–0.8%), peanut (1.2–2%), and tree nuts (approximately 1%) (4).
- Adults more commonly have allergies to shellfish (2.9%), milk (1.9%), peanuts (1.8%), tree nuts (1.2%), and fish (0.9%) (3).
- Most will outgrow their milk and egg allergy, but only 20% of children with peanut allergy may outgrow their sensitivity by school age.

ETIOLOGY AND PATHOPHYSIOLOGY
- Food allergic reactions are a result of failure of immunologic tolerance to food proteins and result in immune-mediated responses to specific foods.
- Any ingested substance can cause allergic reactions:
  - 90% of food allergies in the United States involve cow's milk, egg white, wheat, soy, peanut, tree nuts (e.g., walnut, cashew, and pecan), fish, and shellfish. Food dyes and additives are rare causes of allergy.

Genetics
- HLA alleles have been identified as genetic determinants for peanut allergy.
- Food allergy screening is currently not recommended for siblings of food allergy patients.

RISK FACTORS
- Sex (male children, female adults); race/ethnicity (Asian and black children at higher risk)
- Allergic or atopic predisposition (particularly eczema)
- Family history of food hypersensitivity

GENERAL PREVENTION
- High-risk infants who are regularly fed with peanut protein (6 g/week) have an 80% risk reduction in developing peanut allergy by the age of 5 years.
- Current recommendations for food allergy prevention through nutrition include:
  - Introduce peanut and egg to all infants around 6 months of age but not before 4 months.
  - Do not deliberately delay the introduction of other allergenic foods.
- Have epinephrine autoinjectors for patients at risk for anaphylaxis.

COMMONLY ASSOCIATED CONDITIONS
- Food protein-induced enterocolitis syndrome (FPIES); eosinophilic esophagitis
- Atopic dermatitis; asthma; allergic rhinitis

 DIAGNOSIS

HISTORY
- Symptoms after food ingestion/exposure—usually within minutes
- Document a temporal relationship between symptoms and suspected food.
- Differentiate true food allergy/hypersensitivity from food intolerance.
- Inquire about cofactors—exercise, sleep deprivation, NSAID use, alcohol consumption, illness
- IgE-mediated food allergic reactions can present with: GI: nausea, vomiting, diarrhea, abdominal pain; skin: urticaria/angioedema, pallor, flushing, contact rashes; respiratory: allergic rhinitis, asthma, bronchospasm, stridor, cough; other: anaphylaxis, ocular injection

PHYSICAL EXAM
- Vital signs; growth parameters
- Signs of allergic disease—pulmonary, skin exam in particular
- Other exam findings based on clinical presentation

DIFFERENTIAL DIAGNOSIS
- Nonimmune food intolerance such as enzyme deficiencies (e.g., lactose intolerance)
- Toxic food exposures (e.g., scombroid fish, bacterial food poisoning)

- GI: irritable bowel syndrome, celiac disease, dumping syndrome, inflammatory bowel diseases
- Dermatologic: chronic/recurrent urticaria
- Psychiatric: generalized anxiety disorder, psychosomatic manifestations
- Other immune-mediated reactions to food:
  - Oral allergy syndrome
    - Commonly causes oral pruritus and possibly edema; rarely progresses or causes anaphylaxis
  - Galactose-α-1,3-galactose (α-gal)
    - Following a lone star tick bite, susceptible patients may develop an IgE sensitivity to α-gal which manifests as delayed anaphylaxis 3 to 6 hours after ingestion of mammalian meat; confirmed by IgE specific to α-gal
  - Food-dependent exercise-induced anaphylaxis
    - Ingestion of certain foods results in anaphylaxis if followed by exercise; diagnosed through history and food-specific IgE (skin or serum IgE test)
  - Eosinophilic esophagitis
    - Chronic inflammation of the esophagus leading to feeding difficulties, dysphagia, chest pain, food impaction
  - FPIES
    - A GI food hypersensitivity presenting with lethargy, repetitive vomiting, diarrhea; symptoms usually occur within 2 to 4 hours of food ingestion.
  - Food protein-induced allergic proctocolitis
    - Allergic inflammation of the distal colon in infants; presents in the first months of life with rectal bleeding, most commonly associated with cow's milk and soy proteins

DIAGNOSTIC TESTS & INTERPRETATION
Initial Tests (lab, imaging)
- Allergy tests are confirmatory (not diagnostic). Interpretation depends on history of exposure and specific symptoms.
- Epicutaneous (prick or puncture) allergy skin tests document IgE-mediated immunologic hypersensitivity (especially useful in testing for fruits and vegetables).
- Skin testing using the suspect food can be helpful. If negative on skin test, food allergy is unlikely. If positive, an oral challenge may aid in diagnosis.
  - Skin testing has a high sensitivity (low false-negative rate) *but* a low specificity (high false-positive rate).
- Food-specific IgE assays (fluorescent enzyme immunoassay [FEI]) detect specific IgE antibodies to offending foods.
  - Test only for specific IgE to foods based on patient history.
- Periodic monitoring of food-specific IgE levels every 1 to 2 years may be helpful. If the levels are decreasing over time, this may be indicative of remission. A supervised oral challenge can help confirm resolution.

- Component-resolved diagnosis (CRD) measures specific allergenic food proteins to identify specific IgE.
- Widespread allergy skin testing or serum IgE tests are *not* recommended (4).
- Unproven diagnostic procedures that are not recommended include IgG testing, leukocytotoxic assay, provocative neutralization, lymphocyte stimulation, hair analysis, and applied kinesiology (4).

Diagnostic Procedures/Other
Double-blind, placebo-controlled oral food challenges are the research gold standard in food allergy diagnosis.

- Oral challenges should be delayed in patients with history of anaphylaxis until IgE sensitivity declines or disappears.
- Most allergic reactions occur within 30 minutes to 2 hours after challenge.

 TREATMENT

GENERAL MEASURES
- Food avoidance is the mainstay of treatment. Patients with severe food allergy should meticulously avoid their offending foods and carry an epinephrine auto-injector.
- Immunotherapy may be effective for certain food allergies.
- Subcutaneous immunotherapy or hyposensitization (e.g., "allergy shots") with food extracts are not recommended.

MEDICATION
- Patients with significant type 1, IgE-mediated hypersensitivity should have epinephrine available.
- Monitor patients receiving epinephrine for a systemic anaphylactic reaction to a food (~20% may require another dose).
- Symptomatic treatment for milder reactions with nonsedating antihistamines is generally adequate.
- For patients aged 4 to 17 years with allergic sensitivity to peanut protein, oral immunotherapy with peanut (*Arachis hypogaea*) allergen powder (Palforzia) is available to reduce the risk for anaphylaxis after accidental peanut protein exposure.
- Cromolyn is not recommended for use in most patients with food allergy.

COMPLEMENTARY & ALTERNATIVE MEDICINE
Benefits of herbal medicines, probiotics and prebiotics in food allergy are inconclusive.

 ONGOING CARE

FOLLOW-UP RECOMMENDATIONS
Patient Monitoring
Follow-up skin tests and/or serum IgE studies as clinically indicated

DIET
- Strict avoidance of offending food
- Dietary counseling to maintain a nutritionally sound diet while avoiding offending foods

PATIENT EDUCATION
- Food Allergy Research & Education: 800-929-4040; https://www.foodallergy.org
- https://www.allergyasthmanetwork.org, https://college.acaai.org, and https://www.aaaai.org

PROGNOSIS
- Many children will outgrow food hypersensitivity within the 1st or 2nd decade of life:
  - Significant reductions in skin test wheal size and serum specific IgE can indicate the development of tolerance.
  - Food allergy is frequently a transient phenomenon; ≥50% of the children diagnosed with milk, egg, or wheat allergy have resolution of their allergy later on in childhood. 20% of peanut allergies resolve by the age of 5 years.
- Adults with food hypersensitivity (particularly to milk, fish, shellfish, or nuts) tend to maintain their allergy for many years (4).

COMPLICATIONS
- Anaphylaxis; angioedema; asthma; environmental allergies
- Decreased quality of life; anxiety; depression

REFERENCES

1. Warren CM, Jiang J, Gupta RS. Epidemiology and burden of food allergy. *Curr Allergy Asthma Rep*. 2020;20(2):6.
2. Coulson E, Rifas-Shiman SL, Sordillo J, et al. Racial, ethnic, and socioeconomic differences in adolescent food allergy. *J Allergy Clin Immunol Pract*. 2020;8(1):336–338.e3.
3. Gupta RS, Warren CM, Smith BM, et al. Prevalence and severity of food allergies among US adults. *JAMA Netw Open*. 2019;2(1):e185630.
4. Bird JA, ed. *Food Allergy, an Issue of Immunology and Allergy Clinics of North America*. Philadelphia, PA: Elsevier Health Sciences; 2017.

ADDITIONAL READING

Fleischer DM, Chan ES, Venter C, et al. A consensus approach to the primary prevention of food allergy through nutrition: guidance from the American Academy of Allergy, Asthma, and Immunology; American College of Allergy, Asthma, and Immunology; and the Canadian Society for Allergy and Clinical Immunology. *J Allergy Clin Immunol Pract*. 2021;9(1):22–43.e4.

 SEE ALSO

Anaphylaxis; Celiac Disease; Irritable Bowel Syndrome

 CODES

ICD10
- T78.1XXA Oth adverse food reactions, not elsewhere classified, init
- T78.00XA Anaphylactic reaction due to unspecified food, init encntr
- L27.2 Dermatitis due to ingested food

CLINICAL PEARLS

- Up to 20% of children with peanut allergy may outgrow their sensitivity. Most other common childhood food allergies are outgrown by adulthood.
- Oral itching following ingestion of fresh fruit suggests oral allergy syndrome.
- Maternal dietary restrictions during pregnancy and lactation do not prevent atopic disease in infants.
- Breastfeeding is recommended for the first 6 months of life, particularly with a family history of atopy or food allergy.
- Delaying introduction of solid foods beyond 6 months does not prevent development of allergies.
- Introduce peanut and egg around 6 months of age (not before 4 months). Consider skin testing in high-risk infants.

F

FOOD POISONING, BACTERIAL

Irfan H. Siddiqui, MD • Chris Para, MD • Matthew E. Posen, DO

BASICS

DESCRIPTION
- Food poisoning or foodborne illness is caused by the consumption of food or water that is contaminated with bacterial, parasitic, or viral pathogens. Other causes can result from ingestion of molds, toxin, contaminants, and/or allergens.
- Symptoms are most commonly gastrointestinal in nature and are typically self-limited. Some cases can lead to severe dehydration and critical illness.

EPIDEMIOLOGY
- The cause is unclear in up to 80% of cases. Most foodborne illnesses are secondary to viral causes, with *Norovirus* being the most common. Other viral causes include hepatitis A, rotavirus, and adenovirus.
- *Campylobacter* and nontyphoidal *Salmonella* are the most common causes of bacterial foodborne illness in the United States; other less common pathogens include Shiga toxin-producing *Escherichia coli* (STEC), *Shigella*, *Cyclospora*, *Yersinia*, *Listeria*, and *Vibrio*.
- *Salmonella* (nontyphoidal) infections are the most dangerous of the bacterial foodborne illnesses as they are most commonly associated with hospitalizations and deaths (1).

Incidence
Roughly 1 in 6 Americans (56 million) and 1 in 10 (33 million) across the world become ill from foodborne illness each year. Approximately 128,000 hospitalizations and 3,000 deaths occur per year in America (2). Worldwide, diarrhea associated with foodborne illness is estimated to cause 2.2 million deaths every year (1).

Prevalence
Due to the acute nature of food poisoning, the prevalence and incidence are similar as above.

ETIOLOGY AND PATHOPHYSIOLOGY
- *Staphylococcus aureus*: timing: 1 to 6 hours; symptoms: sudden onset of severe nausea and vomiting; abdominal cramps and fever; sources: unrefrigerated or improperly refrigerated meats and potato, mayonnaise and egg salads
- *Bacillus cereus*: timing: symptom onset: 10 to 16 hours; symptoms: sudden onset of severe nausea; vomiting and watery diarrhea, nausea and cramps; sources: soil, improperly cooked rice/fried rice and red meats
- *Clostridium perfringens*: timing: 8 to 16 hours; symptoms: watery diarrhea, nausea, cramps; sources: dry/precooked or undercooked meats, poultry, home-canned goods
- *Clostridium botulinum*: timing: 12 to 72 hours; symptoms: vomiting, diarrhea, slurred speech, diplopia, dysphagia, and descending muscle weakness/flaccid paralysis; source: commercially canned or improperly home-canned foods
- Enterohemorrhagic *E. coli* (e.g., 0157:H7): timing: 1 to 8 days; symptoms: severe diarrhea that often becomes bloody, abdominal pain, vomiting; sources: undercooked ground beef, juice, unpasteurized milk, raw produce, and contaminated water
- Enterotoxigenic *E. coli* ("traveler's diarrhea"): timing: 1 to 3 days; symptoms: watery diarrhea, abdominal cramps, tenesmus, fecal urgency, and vomiting; sources: food or water contaminated by human feces

- *Salmonella*, nontyphoidal: timing: 6 to 48 hours; symptoms: small volume, mucopurulent/bloody diarrhea; fever; cramps; vomiting; food sources: contaminated eggs, poultry; unpasteurized milk or juice, cheese; contaminated raw fruit and vegetables; and contaminated peanut butter
- *Campylobacter jejuni*: timing: 2 to 5 days; symptoms: diarrhea (bloody), cramps, vomiting, fever; food sources: raw and undercooked poultry, unpasteurized milk, and contaminated meats
- *Shigella*: timing: 4 to 7 days; symptoms: abdominal cramps, fever, mucopurulent and bloody diarrhea; food sources: contaminated water, raw produce, uncooked foods, foods handled by infected food workers
- *Vibrio parahaemolyticus*: timing: 4 to 96 hours; symptoms: nausea, vomiting, diarrhea, abdominal pain; food source: undercooked or raw seafood, especially shellfish
- *Vibrio vulnificus*: timing: 1 to 7 days; symptoms: vomiting, diarrhea, abdominal pain, bacteremia, wound infections; can be fatal in patients with liver disease or those who are immunocompromised; food source: undercooked or raw seafood, particularly oysters
- *Yersinia enterocolitica*: timing: 4 to 7 days; symptoms: abdominal pain, fever, diarrhea (possibly bloody), vomiting; food sources: undercooked beef and pork, unpasteurized dairy products, tofu, contaminated water; additionally, can be due to exposure to house pets with diarrhea
- *Listeria monocytogenes*: timing: 4 to 48 hours; symptoms: nausea, vomiting, fever, watery diarrhea; pregnant women may have a flulike illness leading to premature delivery or stillbirth; immunocompromised patients may develop meningitis and bacteremia; food sources: unpasteurized/contaminated milk, soft cheese, and processed deli meats

RISK FACTORS
Recent travel to developing countries; food handlers, daycare attendees, nursing home residents, recently hospitalized patients, or patients recently exposed to antibiotics; altered immunity due to underlying disease or use of certain medications, including antacids, H_2 blockers, and proton pump inhibitors; cross-contamination and subsequent ingestion of improperly prepared and stored foods; pregnancy; children aged <5 years and adults aged >65 years; immunocompromised patients

GENERAL PREVENTION
- When preparing food: Wash hands, cutting boards, and preparation surfaces. Wash fresh produce thoroughly before consuming. Keep raw meat, poultry, fish, and their juices away from other food (e.g., salad). Wear gloves when handling raw meat (3). Thoroughly cook the meat. Refrigerate leftovers within 2 to 3 hours in clean, shallow, covered containers. If the temperature is >90°F, refrigerate within 1 hour.
- When traveling to underdeveloped countries: Eat only freshly prepared food. Avoid beverages and foods prepared with nonpotable water. Bottled, carbonated, and boiled beverages are safe to drink. Chemoprophylaxis for traveler's diarrhea is recommended for high-risk travelers (e.g., immunocompromised).

COMMONLY ASSOCIATED CONDITIONS
- Botulism—symmetric neurologic deficits and changes in mental status due to ingestion of toxin types A, B, and E produced by *C. botulinum*; outbreaks typically involve home-canned foods such as fruits, vegetables, and meats (3).
- Neonatal meningitis—immunocompromised hosts, particularly neonates (<29 days old), can contract meningitis from systemic *L. monocytogenes* infection (3).
- Hemolytic uremic syndrome (HUS)—microangiopathic hemolytic anemia, renal impairment, and thrombocytopenia caused by both *Shigella* and STEC (3)
- Guillain-Barré syndrome—ascending paralysis strongly associated with *C. jejuni* infection (3)
- Reactive arthritis—can occur after severe infections with *Salmonella*, *Shigella*, *Yersinia*, or *Campylobacter* species (3).
- Irritable Bowel Syndrome—can occur after infections with Campylobacter, Salmonella, Shigella, STEC, and Giardia (1).

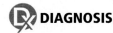

DIAGNOSIS

HISTORY
- Onset, duration, frequency, severity, and character (i.e., watery, bloody, mucus-filled, etc.) of diarrhea
- Diarrhea is >3 or more unformed stools daily or the passage of >250 g of unformed stool per day (1).
- Suspect bacterial food poisoning when multiple persons have rapid onset of symptoms after eating the same meal; high fever, blood, or mucus in stool; severe abdominal pain; signs of dehydration; or recent travel to a foreign country
- Further evaluation and treatment of patients with high fever (≥101.3°F), ≥6 stools per day, blood in the stools, elevated white blood cell count, signs of dehydration, or diarrheal illness that lasts >2 to 3 days

PHYSICAL EXAM
- Key signs of dehydration: delayed capillary refill, decreased skin turgor, dry mucous membranes, and orthostatic hypotension (1).
- Fever may suggest invasive or toxin-producing bacteria
- Abdominal exam: Assess for pain, peritoneal signs, and bowel activity to differentiate from other acute abdominal processes; rectal exam for blood, rectal pain, stool consistency.

DIFFERENTIAL DIAGNOSIS
- Inflammatory/autoimmune
  - Inflammatory bowel disease (Crohn disease, ulcerative colitis, microscopic colitis), celiac disease
- Infectious
  - Cholecystitis, choledocholithiasis, cholangitis, hepatitis, small intestinal bacterial overgrowth, diverticulitis, *Helicobacter pylori*, appendicitis
- Structural
  - Short bowel syndrome, tube feeding
- Other
  - Mesenteric ischemia

DIAGNOSTIC TESTS & INTERPRETATION
Initial Tests (lab, imaging)
- For mild, self-limiting illness, a stool culture is not typically necessary and is unlikely to change management unless there are signs of fever, blood, or severe diarrhea.
- Testing for fecal leukocytes and fecal occult blood is not necessary unless patients have fever or bloody diarrhea (3) and consider ova and parasites if dehydration, history of foreign travel, or symptoms lasting >2 weeks.
- CBC, basic metabolic profile for severe cases with dehydration, inpatient, and nursing home exposure. Abdominal CT may be helpful when intraabdominal pathology is in the differential and the clinical presentation is unclear.

Follow-Up Tests & Special Considerations
Epidemiologic investigation may be warranted. Reporting requirements vary by state and organism.

Diagnostic Procedures/Other
Consider endoscopic evaluation for severe cases. Have a low threshold for endoscopy among patients with AIDS and persistent diarrhea (3).

 TREATMENT

Most cases of food poisoning are self-limited.

MEDICATION
First Line
- Oral rehydration is the first-line therapy (3).
- Empiric antibiotic therapy is not recommended unless traveler's diarrhea is suspected (1).

Second Line
- Consider antibiotics for patients with severe illness requiring hospitalization, patients with fever (>101.3°F) and signs of invasive disease (hematochezia, fecal WBC); if symptoms are severe and last for >1 week or >8 liquid stools a day, stool testing should be completed. Empiric antibiotic choice is a fluoroquinolone in adults or trimethoprim/sulfamethoxazole in children.
- Pathogen-specific therapy:
  - B. cereus: supportive care only
  - C. jejuni: mild: supportive care only; severe: erythromycin 500 mg BID for 5 days or azithromycin 500 mg on day 1, with 250 mg/day for days 2 to 5; fluoroquinolones are no longer recommended.
  - C. botulinum: supportive care only; antitoxin can be helpful early during illness.
  - C. perfringens: supportive care only
  - Enterohemorrhagic E. coli (e.g., 0157:H7): supportive care; closely monitor renal function, hemoglobin, and platelets. Antibiotics may increase risk of HUS.
  - Enterotoxigenic E. coli (common cause of traveler's diarrhea): generally self-limited; antibiotics shorten course of illness (1). Ciprofloxacin 500 mg BID for 3 days; azithromycin 500 mg/day on day 1 with 250 mg/day for days 2 to 5; or trimethoprim-sulfamethoxazole 160/800 mg BID for 3 to 7 days

  - Salmonella (nontyphoidal): no therapy for mild disease; moderate: ciprofloxacin 500 mg BID for 5 to 7 days; or azithromycin 500 mg on day 1 and then 250 mg on days 2 to 5; severe diarrhea, immunocompromised, systemic signs, positive blood cultures: IV ceftriaxone 1 to 2 g/day for 5 to 7 days
  - Shigella: azithromycin (drug of choice secondary to quinolone resistance) 500 mg on day 1 and then 250 mg/day on days 2 to 5 or ciprofloxacin 500 mg BID 3 days
  - S. aureus: supportive care only
  - Noncholera Vibrio: Not indicated in mild, noninvasive, disease. Severe: ceftriaxone and doxycycline.
  - Vibrio cholerae: doxycycline 300 mg 1-time dose in most cases; alternative treatment includes azithromycin 1,000 mg as single dose or 500 mg/day for 3 days, ceftriaxone, or ciprofloxacin.
  - Yersinia: Usually, supportive care only; trimethoprim-sulfamethoxazole 160/800 mg BID for 5 days; or ciprofloxacin 500 mg BID for 7 to 10 days

ADDITIONAL THERAPIES
- For severe nausea and vomiting, promethazine is effective for adults. Ondansetron is effective in children.
- Loperamide 4 mg initially and then 2 mg after each loose stool to a maximum of 8 mg in a 24-hour period may be used unless high fever, bloody diarrhea, and/or severe abdominal pain present (signs of enteroinvasion).
- Bismuth subsalicylate 525 mg QID is moderately effective in traveler's diarrhea.
- Evidence for the effectiveness of probiotics and prebiotics is limited and inconsistent.

ADMISSION, INPATIENT, AND NURSING CONSIDERATIONS
If patient is not able to be orally rehydrated, then admission should be considered for IV fluids.

 ONGOING CARE

FOLLOW-UP RECOMMENDATIONS
Patient Monitoring
Certain states require reporting of specific causes of bacterial foodborne illness to local CDC agencies. These infections include but are not limited to hepatitis A, botulism, Salmonella, Shigella, STEC, Listeria, and Vibrio.

DIET
- Modify food intake when nausea is present or vomiting prevents intake. As nausea subsides, drink adequate fluids; add in bland, low-fat meals; and rest. Avoid alcohol, coffee, nicotine, and spicy foods.
- Breastfeed nursing infants on demand. Infants and older children should be offered the usual food.
- For diarrhea, consider a bland diet. Limiting dairy to 24 hours after the last diarrhea episode may assist in symptom reduction.

PATIENT EDUCATION
When traveling to regions with high incidence of foodborne illness, do not drink local water nor ice that was not purified before drinking. Thoroughly cook food and avoid reheated rice.

PROGNOSIS
Most infections are self-limited. Antibiotics for moderate to severe traveler's diarrhea shorten duration by several days.

REFERENCES
1. Sell J, Dolan B. Common gastrointestinal infections. *Prim Care*. 2018;45(3):519–532.
2. Lee H, Yoon Y. Etiological agents implicated in foodborne illness world wide. *Food Sci Anim Resour*. 2021;41(1):1–7.
3. Wang B, Wang H, Lu X, et al. Recent advances in electrochemical biosensors for the detection of foodborne pathogens: current perspective and challenges. *Foods*. 2023;12(14):2795.

ADDITIONAL READING
Tao D, Hu R, Zhang D, et al. A novel foodborne illness detection and web application tool based on social media. *Foods*. 2023;12(14):2769.

 SEE ALSO

Appendicitis, Acute; Botulism; Brucellosis; Dehydration; Diarrhea, Acute; Guillain-Barré Syndrome; Hypokalemia; Intestinal Parasites; Salmonella Infection; Typhoid Fever

 CODES

ICD10
- A05.9 Bacterial foodborne intoxication, unspecified
- A02.0 Salmonella enteritis
- A04.5 Campylobacter enteritis

CLINICAL PEARLS
- Consider bacterial food poisoning when multiple patients present with fever and blood/mucus in stool after ingesting the same food or having recently returned from a developing nation.
- Consider culture and antibiotics if there is persistent fever with blood/mucus in stool, concern for sepsis, and/or for symptoms lasting >7 days.
- Withhold antispasmodics and antidiarrheal agents if there is a concern for enteroinvasion (high prolonged fever, bloody diarrhea, severe pain, septicemia).
- Consider empiric antibiotic therapy for traveler's diarrhea in cases of moderate to severe disease.

F

FROSTBITE

Sangili Chandran, MD • Teresa M. Chirayil, MD • Rahim Shareef, DO

BASICS

DESCRIPTION
- A severe localized injury due to cold exposure, causing tissue to freeze, resulting in direct cellular injury and progressive dermal ischemia (most commonly of exposed hands, feet, face, and ears)
- Systems affected: integumentary, vascular, muscular, skeletal, nervous
- Synonym: dermatitis congelationis; freezing cold injury (FCI)

EPIDEMIOLOGY
- Predominantly adults but can affect all ages
- Predominant sex: male ≤ female, potentially more common in females due to increased surface area in conjunction with less body mass although exposure rates in males may be higher (1)

ETIOLOGY AND PATHOPHYSIOLOGY
- Prolonged exposure to cold
- Ice crystals form intracellularly and extracellularly. Vasoconstriction reduces blood flow, and microvascular endothelial injury leads to ischemia. Cellular dehydration leads to abnormal electrolyte concentrations and cell death.
- In severe cases, tissue injury extends to muscle and bone leading to necrosis and mummification. Rewarming injured endothelium results in edema and bullae as the ice crystals melt. Inflammatory mediators such as prostaglandins and thromboxane A2 induce vasoconstriction and platelet aggregation, worsening ischemia.
- In severe frostbite, the chronic inflammation can result in an imbalance of proinflammatory and anti-inflammatory macrophages, which can lead to delayed healing (2).
- If refreezing occurs after thawing, cascade of events are more extreme (1).

RISK FACTORS
- Prolonged exposure to below freezing temperatures, especially combined with wind and/or water exposure
- High-altitude activities, such as mountaineering
- Military operations in cold environments
- Constricting or wet clothing with inadequate insulation
- Altered mental status due to alcohol, drugs, or psychiatric illness
- The experience of homelessness
- Previous cold-related injury
- Dehydration and/or malnutrition
- Conditions that interfere with total heat production and/or thermoregulation (i.e., endocrine abnormalities) (1)
- Conditions that promote loss of body heat including chronic skin conditions, hyperhidrosis, burns (including sunburns) (1)
- Hypothermia
- Any condition that results in decreased vasoconstriction and/or vascular pathology as in (1):
  – Smoking; Raynaud phenomenon; peripheral vascular disease; diabetes

GENERAL PREVENTION
- Dress in layers with appropriate cold weather gear and avoid clothing that is too constricting.
- Cover exposed areas and extremities appropriately.
- Stay dry; avoid alcohol and minimize wind exposure.
- Ensure adequate hydration and caloric intake.
- Use supplemental oxygen at very high altitudes (>7,500 meters).
- Exercise can protect against frostbite by increasing core and peripheral temperatures. Note: Caution should be made that the exercise will not lead to exhaustion and inability to seek for shelter/warmth.
- Appropriate use of chemical or electric hand and foot warmers can help maintain peripheral warmth.
- Recognize expected temperatures and take into consideration wind chills prior to exposure and, if possible, avoid exposure.
- Avoid emollients on the skin as they can lead to a false sense of protection (1).
- Avoid alcohol, caffeine, and other medications that can cause vasoconstriction (1).

COMMONLY ASSOCIATED CONDITIONS
- Hypothermia
- Alcohol or drug abuse

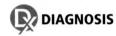

DIAGNOSIS

HISTORY
- Significant cold exposure—determine length and severity.
- Throbbing pain
- Paresthesias
- Numbness
- Loss of coordination and dexterity

PHYSICAL EXAM
- Hands, feet, face, and ears are most commonly affected.
- Before rewarming, skin may be insensate, white or grayish-yellow in color, cyanotic, or hard and waxy to touch.
- After rewarming, immediate physical exam findings can be categorized as:
  – Grade 1: no cyanosis on the extremity
  – Grade 2: cyanosis isolated to the distal phalanx
  – Grade 3: intermediate and proximal phalangeal cyanosis
  – Grade 4: cyanosis over the carpal or tarsal bones
- Frostbite can alternatively be categorized into four degrees (similar to burn injuries):
  – 1st degree: numbness and erythema; a white or yellow, firm, slightly raised plaque develops. No gross tissue infarction occurs; there may be slight epidermal sloughing. Mild edema is common.
  – 2nd degree: superficial skin vesiculation; a clear or milky blisters, surrounded by erythema and edema
  – 3rd degree: deeper hemorrhagic blisters
  – 4th degree: extends through the dermis to involve subcutaneous tissues, with necrosis extending into muscle and bone
  – 1st- and 2nd-degree injuries are superficial.
  – 3rd- and 4th-degree injuries are deep (3)[C].

DIFFERENTIAL DIAGNOSIS
- Frostnip: a superficial cold injury that resolves spontaneously without tissue loss
- Chilblains (pernio): a localized inflammatory reaction to cold and wet exposure without tissue freezing; typically presents as edematous, erythematous to violaceous skin lesions
- Immersion foot (trench foot): inflammatory reaction of the feet to prolonged exposure to cold and moisture
- COVID toes, a SARS-CoV-2 phenomenon related to pernio/chilblains (4)

DIAGNOSTIC TESTS & INTERPRETATION
Initial Tests (lab, imaging)
- Baseline labs: CBC, CMP, UA for myoglobinuria, culture wound if suspected infection
- Radiography can be an initial imaging to identify extent of soft tissue involvement versus bone involvement (2).
- Technetium (Tc)-99m scintigraphy can identify tissue viability at early stage and identify candidates for thrombolytic therapy.
- MRI/MRA, duplex ultrasonography, and standard or digital subtraction angiography are occasionally used.
- Consider serial photographs at time of injury, at 24 hours, and every several days until hospital discharge.
- For severe frostbite especially, angiography and bone scans, as well as MRI/MRA, US, and infrared thermal imaging, are useful to determine need for thrombolysis versus amputation (2).
- Angiography and bone scans can be used to determine effectiveness of thrombolysis if done before and after treatment (2).
- There is some evidence that angiography has been shown to accurately determine the need for amputation, whereas bone scans cannot reveal this information (caution with angiography with renal insufficiency).
- SPECT/CT should be used to reveal clinical prognosis (2).

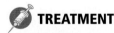

TREATMENT

GENERAL MEASURES
- Correct hypothermia.
- Assess for additional injuries.
- Remove jewelry from affected extremities.
- Initiate rewarming of affected body part only if there is no risk of refreezing. Warm affected parts of body in 37–39°C water for approximately 30 minutes until the involved part takes on a red or purple appearance and becomes pliable to touch. A whirlpool bath can help with rewarming and antiseptic. Avoid using other heat sources, such as a fire or space heater, to rewarm affected parts avoided.
- Apply topical aloe vera gel before dressing.
- Selectively drain clear or cloudy blisters; leave hemorrhagic blisters intact.
- Splint and elevate the affected extremity.

- Tetanus prophylaxis
- Oral hydration if patient is alert and has no GI symptoms; otherwise, IV hydration with warm normal saline in small boluses
- Daily bathing in warm water with active and passive mobilization
- Dry, loose bulky dressings, including in between fingers/toes (3)[C]
- Pain control (1)
- Antibiotics only if infectious complications become apparent (1)

ALERT
- Avoid rubbing the affected area as this can lead to further tissue damage.
- Patients should avoid weight bearing on frostbitten limbs prior to definitive care.

MEDICATION
First Line
- Tissue plasminogen activator (tPA) for deep injury (grades 3 and 4) (5) administered (either IV or intra-arterially) within 24 hours of injury may prevent damage from microvascular thrombosis and may reduce amputation rates; if administered, should be done so immediately after rewarming (5)
- **Precaution**: tPA should not be used with history of recent bleeding, stroke, peptic ulcer, or recent surgery.
- Heparin is recommended as adjunctive therapy in tPA protocols. Heparin is not recommended as monotherapy.
- Consider low-molecular-weight dextran in patients not given other systemic treatments (e.g., tPA) (3)[C].
- Iloprost plus rTPA has little supporting evidence. Buflomedil has been withdrawn from use (5).
- Update tetanus toxoid (3)[C].
- Ibuprofen 400 mg q12h (inhibit prostaglandins) (3)[C]
- NSAIDs for mild to moderate pain; narcotic analgesia for moderate to severe pain
- Use systemic antibiotics for proven infection. Prophylactic antibiotics are not recommended (3)[C].

Second Line
Pentoxifylline 400 mg q8h

ADDITIONAL THERAPIES
- Heated oxygen
- Warm IV fluids
- Botulinum toxin injections to improve sequelae including chronic pain

SURGERY/OTHER PROCEDURES
- Urgent surgery is rarely needed.
- Fasciotomy is indicated if the patient develops elevated compartment pressures (3)[C].
- Surgical débridement, as needed, to remove necrotic tissue
- Amputation only if tissues are necrotic: may take 4 to 12 weeks for the demarcation of tissue necrosis to become definitive
- Consider imaging with 99 mTc bone scan and/or MRA in severe cases to determine extent of injury; assess viability of surrounding tissue and determine need for surgery.

ADMISSION, INPATIENT, AND NURSING CONSIDERATIONS
- Hospitalization is generally recommended unless no blisters are present after rewarming (e.g., grade 1/1st-degree frostbite) (3)[C].
- Patients are typically best cared for in a hospital with experience treating frostbite injuries (trauma center or burn unit).
- Administer tPA in intensive care setting.
- Ensure proper hydration and nutrition.
- Treat pain (often requires narcotic analgesia).
- Wound care—clean dressings and twice daily whirlpool baths
- Apply aloe vera gel every 6 to 8 hours through resolution of blisters.
- Elevate injured extremities above heart level to minimize edema.
- Physical therapy and early mobilization
- If patient cannot tolerate oral fluids or has altered mental status, give warmed normal saline in small boluses (3)[C].

 ONGOING CARE

FOLLOW-UP RECOMMENDATIONS
- Protect injured body parts.
- Continue physical therapy.
- Avoid smoking and alcohol.
- Avoid recurrent cold exposure.
- Ensure properly fitting clothing and footwear.

Patient Monitoring
- Follow up for physical therapy progress, infection, and other complications listed below.
- Monitor growth of affected extremity in pediatric patients.

DIET
- As tolerated
- Warm oral fluids

PATIENT EDUCATION
Provide education on:
- Protection from cold injuries
- Risk factors for frostbite
- Early signs and symptoms of frostbite
- Field treatment of cold injuries
- Wound care grade 1: no amputation and no sequelae

PROGNOSIS
- Grade 2: potential soft tissue amputation and nail sequelae
- Grade 3: potential bone amputation of the digit and functional sequelae
- Grade 4: potential bone amputation of the limb with functional sequelae
- Other factors that attribute to poor prognosis include the following:
  – Severity of injury as seen above
  – Longer duration of exposure
  – Concomitant substance abuse

COMPLICATIONS
- Tissue loss: distal parts of an extremity may undergo spontaneous amputation; tissue necrosis requiring amputation
- Gangrene; hyperhidrosis due to nerve injury; decreased hair and nail growth
- Raynaud phenomenon
- Frostbite arthropathy and osteoarthritis
- Chronic regional pain; neuropathy
- Localized osteoporosis
- Premature closure of epiphyses in pediatric patients

REFERENCES
1. Fudge J. Preventing and managing hypothermia and frostbite injury. *Sports Health*. 2016;8(2): 133–139.
2. Gao Y, Wang F, Zhou W, et al. Research progress in the pathogenic mechanisms and imaging of severe frostbite. *Eur J Radiol*. 2021;137:109605.
3. McIntosh SE, Hamonko M, Freer L, et al; for Wilderness Medical Society. Wilderness Medical Society practice guidelines for the prevention and treatment of frostbite. *Wilderness Environ Med*. 2011;22(2):156–166.
4. Volansky R. Diagnosing "COVID toes" and other challenges in the derm-rheum overlap. https://www.healio.com/news/rheumatology /20210818/diagnosing-covid-toes-and-other -challenges-in-the-dermrheum-overlap. Accessed November 18, 2023.
5. Hickey S, Whitson A, Jones L, et al. Guidelines for thrombolytic therapy for frostbite. *J Burn Care Res*. 2020;41(1):176–183.

 SEE ALSO

- Hypothermia
- Algorithm: Hypothermia

CODES

ICD10
- T33.90XA Superficial frostbite of unspecified sites, init encntr
- T34.90XA Frostbite with tissue necrosis of unsp sites, init encntr
- T33.829A Superficial frostbite of unspecified foot, initial encounter

CLINICAL PEARLS
- Frostbite is a tetanus-prone injury. Provide appropriate tetanus prophylaxis.
- Avoid rewarming en route to the hospital if there is a chance of refreezing; rewarm only with water.
- Assess for additional injuries to areas which may be insensate.
- tPA can reduce amputation rates. Use within 24 hours of injury in appropriate clinical settings.
- Early assessment of the degree of tissue involvement is difficult. Delay surgery until a definite tissue demarcation of necrosis occurs (may take 4 to 12 weeks).

F

FURUNCULOSIS

Zoltan Trizna, MD, PhD

BASICS

DESCRIPTION
- Acute bacterial abscess of a hair follicle (often *Staphylococcus aureus*)
- System(s) affected: skin/exocrine
- Synonym(s): boils

EPIDEMIOLOGY
Incidence
- Predominant age
  - Adolescents and young adults
  - Clusters have been reported in teenagers living in crowded quarters, within families, or in high school athletes.
- Predominant sex: male = female

Prevalence
Exact data are not available.

ETIOLOGY AND PATHOPHYSIOLOGY
- Infection spreads away from hair follicle into surrounding dermis.
- Pathogenic strain of *S. aureus* (usually); most cases in United States are now due to community-acquired methicillin-resistant *S. aureus* (CA-MRSA), whereas methicillin-sensitive *S. aureus* (MSSA) is most common elsewhere (1)[A].

Genetics
Unknown

RISK FACTORS
- Carriage of pathogenic strain of *Staphylococcus* sp. in nares, skin, axilla, and perineum
- Rarely, polymorphonuclear leukocyte defect or hyperimmunoglobulin E–*Staphylococcus* sp. abscess syndrome
- Diabetes mellitus, malnutrition, alcoholism, obesity, atopic dermatitis
- Primary immunodeficiency disease and AIDS (common variable immunodeficiency, chronic granulomatous disease, Chédiak–Higashi syndrome, C3 deficiency, C3 hypercatabolism, transient hypogammaglobulinemia of infancy, immunodeficiency with thymoma, Wiskott-Aldrich syndrome)

- Secondary immunodeficiency (e.g., leukemia, leukopenia, neutropenia, therapeutic immunosuppression)
- Medication impairing neutrophil function (e.g., omeprazole)
- The most important independent predictor of recurrence is a positive family history.

GENERAL PREVENTION
Patient education regarding self-care (see "General Measures"); treatment and prevention are interrelated.

COMMONLY ASSOCIATED CONDITIONS
- Usually normal immune system
- Diabetes mellitus
- Polymorphonuclear leukocyte defect (rare)
- Hyperimmunoglobulin E–*Staphylococcus* sp. abscess syndrome (rare)
- See "Risk Factors."

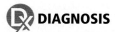
DIAGNOSIS

HISTORY
- Located on hair-bearing sites, especially areas prone to friction or repeated minor traumas (e.g., underneath belt, anterior aspects of thighs, nape, buttocks)
- No initial fever or systemic symptoms
- The folliculocentric nodule may enlarge, become painful, and develop into an abscess (frequently with spontaneous drainage).

PHYSICAL EXAM
- Painful erythematous papules/nodules (1 to 5 cm) with central pustules
- Tender, red, perifollicular swelling, terminating in discharge of pus and necrotic plug
- Lesions may be solitary or clustered.

DIFFERENTIAL DIAGNOSIS
- Folliculitis
- Pseudofolliculitis
- Carbuncles
- Ruptured epidermal cyst
- Myiasis (larva of botfly/tumbu fly)

- Hidradenitis suppurativa
- Atypical bacterial or fungal infections

DIAGNOSTIC TESTS & INTERPRETATION
Initial Tests (lab, imaging)
Obtain culture if with multiple abscesses marked by surrounding inflammation, cellulitis, systemic symptoms such as fever, or if immunocompromised.

Follow-Up Tests & Special Considerations
- Immunoglobulin levels in rare (e.g., recurrent or otherwise inexplicable) cases
- If culture grows gram-negative bacteria or fungus, consider polymorphonuclear neutrophil leukocyte functional defect.

Test Interpretation
Histopathology (although a biopsy is rarely needed)
- Perifollicular necrosis containing fibrinoid material and neutrophils
- At deep end of necrotic plug, in SC tissue, is a large abscess with a Gram stain positive for small collections of *S. aureus.*

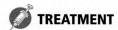
TREATMENT

GENERAL MEASURES
- Moist, warm compresses (provide comfort, encourage localization/pointing/drainage) 30 minutes QID
- If pointing or large, incise and drain: Consider packing if large or incompletely drained.
- Routine culture is not necessary for localized abscess in nondiabetic patients with normal immune system.
- Sanitary practices: Change towels, washcloths, and sheets daily; clean shaving instruments; avoid nose picking; change wound dressings frequently; do not share items of personal hygiene (2)[B].

MEDICATION
First Line
- Systemic antibiotics usually *unnecessary*, unless extensive surrounding cellulitis or fever. Other indications include a single abscess >2 cm, immunocompromise.
- If suspecting MRSA, see "Second Line."

- If multiple abscesses, lesions with marked surrounding inflammation, cellulitis, systemic symptoms such as fever, or if immunocompromised: Place on antibiotic therapy directed at *S. aureus* for 10 to 14 days.
  - Dicloxacillin (Dynapen, Pathocil) 500 mg PO QID *or* cephalexin 500 mg PO QID *or* clindamycin 300 mg TID, if penicillin-allergic

Second Line
- Resistant strains of *S. aureus* (MRSA): clindamycin 300 mg q6h or doxycycline 100 mg q12h or trimethoprim-sulfamethoxazole (TMP-SMX DS) 1 tab q8–12h or minocycline 100 mg q12h
- If known or suspected impaired neutrophil function (e.g., impaired chemotaxis, phagocytosis, superoxide generation), add vitamin C 1,000 mg/day for 4 to 6 weeks (prevents oxidation of neutrophils).
- If antibiotic regimens fail:
  - May try PO pentoxifylline 400 mg TID for 2 to 6 months (inhibits neutrophil activation and adhesion)
  - Contraindications: recent cerebral and/or retinal hemorrhage; intolerance to methylxanthines (e.g., caffeine, theophylline); allergy to the particular drug selected
  - Precautions: prolonged prothrombin time (PT) and/or bleeding; if on warfarin, frequent monitoring of PT

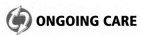 ## ONGOING CARE

FOLLOW-UP RECOMMENDATIONS
Patient Monitoring
Instruct patient to see physician if compresses are unsuccessful.

DIET
Unrestricted

PROGNOSIS
- Self-limited: usually drains pus spontaneously and will heal with or without scarring within several days
- Recurrent/chronic: may last for months or years

- If recurrent, usually related to chronic skin carriage of staphylococci (nares or on skin). Treatment goals are to decrease or eliminate pathogenic strain *or* suppress pathogenic strain.
  - Culture nares, skin, axilla, and perineum (culture nares of family members)
  - Mupirocin 2%: Apply to both nares BID for 5 days each month.
  - Culture anterior nares every 3 months; if failure, retreat with mupirocin or consider clindamycin 150 mg/day for 3 months.
  - Long-term efficacy of strategies to eliminate carrier state (decolonization) remains unclear.
- Especially in recurrent cases, wash entire body and fingernails (with nailbrush) daily for 1 to 3 weeks with povidone-iodine (Betadine), chlorhexidine (Hibiclens), or hexachlorophene (pHisoHex soap), although all can cause dry skin.

COMPLICATIONS
- Scarring
- Bacteremia
- Seeding (e.g., septal/valve defect, arthritic joint)

REFERENCES

1. Lin H-S, Lin P-T, Tsai Y-S, et al. Interventions for bacterial folliculitis and boils (furuncles and carbuncles). *Cochrane Database Syst Rev*. 2021;2(2):CD013099.
2. Fritz SA, Camins BC, Eisenstein KA, et al. Effectiveness of measures to eradicate *Staphylococcus aureus* carriage in patients with community-associated skin and soft-tissue infections: a randomized trial. *Infect Control Hosp Epidemiol*. 2011;32(9):872–880.

ADDITIONAL READING

- Balakirski G, Hischebeth G, Altengarten J, et al. Recurrent mucocutaneous infections caused by PVL-positive *Staphylococcus aureus* strains: a challenge in clinical practice. *J Dtsch Dermatol Ges*. 2020;18(4):315–322.
- Ibler KS, Kromann CB. Recurrent furunculosis— challenges and management: a review. *Clin Cosmet Investig Dermatol*. 2014;7:59–64.

- Nowicka D, Grywalska E. *Staphylococcus aureus* and host immunity in recurrent furunculosis. *Dermatology*. 2019;235(4):295–305.

 ## SEE ALSO

Folliculitis; Hidradenitis Suppurativa

 ## CODES

ICD10
- L02.92 Furuncle, unspecified
- L02.12 Furuncle of neck
- L02.429 Furuncle of limb, unspecified

CLINICAL PEARLS

- Pathogens may be different in different localities. Keep up-to-date with the locality-specific epidemiology.
- If few, furuncles/furunculosis do not need antibiotic treatment. If systemic symptoms (e.g., fever), cellulitis, or multiple lesions occur, oral antibiotic therapy is used.
- Other treatments for MRSA include linezolid PO or IV and IV vancomycin.
- Folliculitis, furunculosis, and carbuncles are parts of a spectrum of pyodermas.
- Other causative organisms include aerobic (e.g., *Escherichia coli, Pseudomonas aeruginosa,* and *Streptococcus faecalis*), anaerobic (e.g., *Bacteroides, Lactobacillus,* and *Peptostreptococcus*), and *Mycobacteria*.
- Decolonization (treatment of the nares with topical antibiotic) is only recommended if the colonization was confirmed by cultures because resistance is common and treatment is of uncertain efficacy.

F

GALACTORRHEA

Kelley V. Lawrence, MD, IBCLC • Madeleine Cutrone, MD • Ryan Accomazzo, MD, MPH

 BASICS

DESCRIPTION
- Milky nipple discharge not associated with lactation, defined as >1 year after pregnancy or cessation of breastfeeding.
- Does not include serous, purulent, or bloody nipple discharge
- System(s) affected: endocrine/metabolic, nervous, reproductive

Pediatric Considerations
Can occur in infants secondary to maternal estrogen exposure

Pregnancy Considerations
Milk production often begins during the second trimester; milk leakage that occurs during pregnancy is not pathophysiologic galactorrhea.

EPIDEMIOLOGY
- Predominant age: 15 to 50 years (reproductive age), most commonly ages 20 to 35 years
- Third most common breast complaint in women

Incidence
Marked variability reported

Prevalence
Approximately 20–25% of women experience galactorrhea in their lifetime.

ETIOLOGY AND PATHOPHYSIOLOGY
- Oxytocin stimulates the anterior pituitary to secrete prolactin, which induces lactation.
- Prolactin secretion is inhibited by dopamine produced in the hypothalamus.
- Galactorrhea results either from prolactin overproduction or loss of inhibitory regulation by dopamine.
- Physiologic galactorrhea can be due to pregnancy, nipple stimulation, nipple piercing, exercise, or sexual activity.
- Hyperprolactinemia can be due to overproduction by malignancy or mass effect, most commonly prolactinoma.
- Hyperprolactinemia secondary to systemic diseases:
  – Hypothyroidism
  – Chronic renal failure (reduced clearance of prolactin leading to elevated serum levels)
  – Cirrhosis
  – Adrenal insufficiency
- Medications/substances:
  – Cardiovascular (α-methyldopa, reserpine, verapamil, spironolactone)
  – GI (domperidone, metoclopramide)
  – Herbal (anise [licorice], barley, blessed thistle, fenugreek seed, fennel, goat's rue)
  – Illicit (cocaine, marijuana)
  – Antimicrobials (isoniazid, protease inhibitors)
  – Opioids
  – Psych/neuro (neuroleptics, antipsychotics, stimulants, SSRIs, tricyclic antidepressants, MAOIs)
  – Reproductive (estrogens, copper IUD)
  – DMARDs (azathioprine)

GENERAL PREVENTION
- Avoid frequent nipple stimulation.
- Avoid medications that can suppress dopamine.

COMMONLY ASSOCIATED CONDITIONS
- Commonly associated with hypothyroidism, chronic kidney disease, hypogonadism, and pituitary adenoma
- Rarely associated with adrenal insufficiency, chest wall conditions/trauma, post-breast reduction surgery, acromegaly

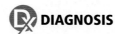 DIAGNOSIS

HISTORY
- Usually bilateral milky nipple discharge that may be spontaneous or induced by stimulation
- Determine possibility of pregnancy or recent discontinuation of lactation.
- Association with initiation of new medication or supplement
- Signs of hypogonadism related to hyperprolactinemia (oligomenorrhea, amenorrhea, anovulation, infertility, decreased libido, erectile dysfunction, hot flashes)
- Mass effects from pituitary enlargement (headache, vision changes)

PHYSICAL EXAM
- Breast examination should be performed with attention to the presence of spontaneous or induced nipple discharge (with gentle hand expression).
- Should observe bilateral, milky white, or brown nipple discharge
- Perform formal visual field testing if pituitary adenoma suspected.

DIFFERENTIAL DIAGNOSIS
- Pregnancy-induced lactation or recent weaning (Average duration of lactation after weaning is 40 days but can be longer in cases of prolonged duration of breastfeeding.)
- Nonmilky (straw colored, gray, yellow, green, brown) nipple discharge: intraductal papilloma, fibrocystic disease
- Purulent breast discharge: typically due to infection; may see breast redness, pain, warmth, and edema. Possible diagnoses include mastitis, breast abscess, impetigo, eczema.
- Bloody breast discharge: If palpable mass, edema, or axillary lymphadenopathy, consider malignancy (Paget disease, breast cancer).

DIAGNOSTIC TESTS & INTERPRETATION
Initial Tests (lab, imaging)
- Start with urine hCG testing to rule out pregnancy and physiologic lactation in premenopausal women.
- If negative hCG, measure prolactin level. Normal prolactin level in nonpregnant women is up to 30 ng/mL, although values may vary with different laboratories. During pregnancy, serum prolactin ranges 200 to 500 ng/mL (1)[C].
- If prolactin is elevated, evaluate thyroid, liver, and renal function (TSH, free T4, hepatic panel, BMP) for possible underlying etiology.
- Prolactin levels fluctuate (highest in early morning) and may be falsely elevated by a recent breast examination, vigorous exercise, or sexual activity. Elevated and borderline levels should be confirmed with repeat level drawn in a fasting, nonexercised state, with no breast stimulation (2)[C].
- If a breast mass is palpated, consider evaluation with mammogram and/or ultrasound.

Follow-Up Tests & Special Considerations
- Follicle-stimulating hormone and luteinizing hormone if amenorrheic
- Growth hormone levels if acromegaly suspected
- Measure adrenal steroids if signs of Cushing disease present.
- Consider formal visual field testing.
- Pituitary MRI with gadolinium if the serum prolactin level is significantly elevated (>200 ng/mL) or if a tumor is otherwise suspected

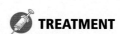 TREATMENT

GENERAL MEASURES
- Identify and treat the underlying cause.
- Idiopathic galactorrhea (normal prolactin levels) does not require treatment (3)[C].
- Avoid excess nipple stimulation.
- Discontinue causative medications, if possible.
- Conservative treatment may also include nursing pads to manage nipple discharge.

MEDICATION

- Dopamine agonists (cabergoline and bromocriptine) are first-line therapy for hyperprolactinemia, whether idiopathic or caused by prolactinoma (3)[C].
  - Dopamine agonists work to reduce prolactin levels and shrink tumor size. Therapy is not curative (3)[C].
- Contraindications are similar for all and include the following:
  - Uncontrolled hypertension
  - Sensitivity to ergot alkaloids
- Precautions
  - Dopamine agonists may cause nausea, vomiting, psychosis, or dyskinesia.
  - Discontinue therapy if a patient becomes pregnant.
- Significant possible drug interactions: serotonergic agents, ergot derivatives, antipsychotic agents
- Therapy should be continued for at least 2 years. If prolactin level has normalized, can consider tapering treatment at that time.

First Line
Cabergoline (Dostinex)
- Start at 0.25 mg PO twice weekly and increase by 0.25 mg monthly until prolactin levels normalize. Usual dose ranges from 0.25 to 3.00 mg PO weekly.
- Equally efficacious and better tolerated than bromocriptine (3)[C]
- Check ESR and serum creatinine at baseline and every 6 to 12 months.
- Monitor prolactin monthly until normalized and then every 3 months during treatment.

Second Line
Bromocriptine
- Start at 1.25 mg QHS PO with food and increase every 3 to 7 days by 2.5 mg/day until therapeutic response achieved (usually 2.5 to 15.0 mg/day).
- Check creatinine, CBC, hepatic panel, HbA1c, at least twice yearly; pregnancy test every 4 weeks during amenorrheic periods.
- Monitor prolactin monthly until normalized and then every 3 months during treatment.

ISSUES FOR REFERRAL
Dependent on underlying pathology; neurology, endocrinology, and breast surgeon as indicated.

SURGERY/OTHER PROCEDURES
For tumors >10 mm, patients may require surgery or radiotherapy.

COMPLEMENTARY & ALTERNATIVE MEDICINE
Alternative modalities used to cease milk production include ingestion of peppermint, parsley, and/or sage on a regular basis and topical application of cabbage leaves over the breast tissue.

 ONGOING CARE

FOLLOW-UP RECOMMENDATIONS
Patient Monitoring
- Check prolactin levels every month until normalized. After levels normalize, check again every 3 months while on dopamine agonist therapy. After discontinuation, prolactin should be checked every 3 months for the first year and then yearly discontinuation of therapy (3)[C].
- Monitor visual fields and/or MRI at least yearly until stable for prolactinoma.

DIET
No restrictions; may include peppermint, parsley, and sage in diet for symptom management

PATIENT EDUCATION
- Caution patient about symptoms of mass enlargement in pituitary (vision changes, headaches).
- Inform patient that offending medications should be discontinued long-term.
- Educate new moms that this condition can be normal in infants due to exposure to maternal hormones.

PROGNOSIS
- Symptoms can recur after discontinuation of a dopamine agonist.
- Surgery can have 50% recurrence.
- Prolactinomas <10 mm can resolve spontaneously.

COMPLICATIONS
- If enlarging pituitary adenoma, risk of permanent visual field loss
- Osteoporosis if amenorrhea persists without estrogen replacement (1)[C]
- Hyperprolactinemia does not increase breast cancer risk.

REFERENCES

1. Majumdar A, Mangal NS. Hyperprolactinemia. *J Hum Reprod Sci*. 2013;6(3):168–175.
2. Huang W, Molitch ME. Evaluation and management of galactorrhea. *Am Fam Physician*. 2012;85(11):1073–1080.
3. Melmed S, Casanueva FF, Hoffman AR, et al. Diagnosis and treatment of hyperprolactinemia: an Endocrine Society Clinical Practice guideline. *J Clin Endocrinol Metab*. 2011;96(2):273–288.

ADDITIONAL READING
- Bruehlman RD, Winters S, McKittrick C. Galactorrhea: rapid evidence review. *Am Fam Physician*. 2022;106(6):695–700.
- DiVasta AD, Weldon CB, Labow BI. The breast: examination and lesions. In: Emans SJ, Laufer MR, DiVasta AD, eds. *Emans, Laufer, Goldstein's Pediatric & Adolescent Gynecology*. 7th ed. Philadelphia, PA: Wolters Kluwer, 2020:781.

 CODES

ICD10
- N64.3 Galactorrhea not associated with childbirth
- N64.52 Nipple discharge

CLINICAL PEARLS
- Galactorrhea is a common disorder, affecting up to 50% of reproductive-aged women.
- Galactorrhea is defined as bilateral milk production, usually milky, but can be varied.
- Common causes include idiopathic, nipple stimulation, dopamine-suppressing medications, systemic disease, or pituitary prolactinoma.
- Evaluate prolactin >200 ng/mL (or signs of suspicion for a pituitary macroadenoma) with a gadolinium-enhanced MRI.
- First-line medication treatment is cabergoline; second-line is bromocriptine.

G

GASTRITIS

Marie L. Borum, MD, EdD, MPH • Nouf O. Turki, MD

 BASICS

DESCRIPTION
- Inflammation of the gastric mucosa
- Classified by duration:
  - Acute: neutrophilic infiltration on histology
  - Chronic: mixture of mononuclear cells, lymphocytes, macrophages on histology
- Subtypes include:
  - Erosive gastritis
    - Mucosal injury by a noxious agent (especially nonsteroidal anti-inflammatory drugs [NSAIDs] or alcohol)
    - Vascular congestion due to portal hypertension (HTN) or gastric antral vascular ectasia (GAVE)
  - Reflux gastritis—a reaction to protracted reflux exposure to biliary and pancreatic fluid
  - Hemorrhagic gastritis (stress ulceration)—a reaction to hemodynamic disorder (e.g., hypovolemia or hypoxia [shock]); common in intensive care unit (ICU) patients, particularly after severe burns and trauma
  - Infectious gastritis
    - Acute and/or chronic: *Helicobacter pylori* infection (most common cause of gastritis). *H. pylori* has been linked with gastric cancer.
    - Viral systemic infection caused by cytomegalovirus (CMV) or Epstein-Barr virus (EBV)
    - Phlegmonous gastritis: rapidly progressive and frequently fatal bacterial infection of the gastric wall
  - Atrophic gastritis
    - Metaplastic atrophic gastritis: autoimmune primary (pernicious) anemia
    - Frequent in elderly and prolonged proton pump inhibitor (PPI) use (long-standing *H. pylori* infections)
    - Major risk factor for gastric cancer
  - Others—granulomatous disease: sarcoidosis or Crohn disease

Geriatric Considerations
Persons aged >60 years often harbor *H. pylori* infection.

Pediatric Considerations
Gastritis rarely occurs in infants or children. Most common etiology for pediatric gastritis is *H. pylori* infection.

EPIDEMIOLOGY
- Predominant age: all adult ages, prevalence increases with age (more common in elderly)
- Predominant sex: male = female; autoimmune gastritis is female > male

Incidence
1.8 to 2.1 million annual visits in the United States

Prevalence
- Roughly 50% of people aged >60 years are infected with *H. pylori* vs. 20% of people aged <40 years.
- In 2018, ~27% of U.S. adults were found to be infected with *H. pylori*.
  - Rates of infection are higher in minority groups, immigrants, and lower socioeconomic status.

ETIOLOGY AND PATHOPHYSIOLOGY
- Noxious agents cause a breakdown in the gastric mucosal barrier, exposing underlying epithelial tissue to injury.
- Infection: *H. pylori* (most common), *Staphylococcus aureus* exotoxins, and viral infections (EBV, CMV)
- Alcohol via cell DNA damage and subsequent pyroptosis
- Aspirin and other NSAIDs through inhibition of protective prostaglandin synthesis
- Bile reflux, pancreatic enzyme reflux
- Portal HTN gastropathy, causing erosion
- Emotional stress due to cortisol production
- Crohn disease–related gastritis; focally enhanced histiocytes, lymphocytes, and granulomatous inflammation
- Hemodynamic instability (hypoxemia)

Genetics
There is difference in opinion regarding genome studies between the association of toll-like receptor 1 (TLR1) causing inflammation in *H. pylori*–infected gastric mucosa. Further research is warranted.

RISK FACTORS
- Age >60 years
- Exposure to potentially noxious drugs or chemicals (e.g., alcohol or NSAIDs, tobacco use)
- Hypovolemia, hypoxia (shock), burns, head injury, complicated postoperative course
- Autoimmune diseases (thyroiditis, type 1 diabetes mellitus, Addison disease, vitiligo, erosive oral lichen planus)
- Family history of *H. pylori* and/or gastric cancer
- Radiation, chemotherapy, pernicious anemia, gastric mucosal atrophy

GENERAL PREVENTION
- Avoid injurious drugs or chemical agents, alcohol, and tobacco.
- Patients with hypovolemia or hypoxia (especially ICU patients) should receive prophylaxis with H_2 antagonists, PPIs, prostaglandins, or sucralfate.
- Consider testing for *H. pylori* in patients on long-term NSAID therapy, diagnosed with idiopathic thrombocytopenic purpura (ITP), or from endemic regions.

COMMONLY ASSOCIATED CONDITIONS
- Gastric or duodenal peptic ulcer
- Primary (pernicious) anemia—atrophic gastritis
- Portal HTN, hepatic failure
- Mucosa-associated lymphoid tissue (MALT) lymphoma

DIAGNOSIS

HISTORY
- Burning epigastric pain or discomfort, often aggravated by eating
- Unintentional weight loss, anorexia
- Nausea, with or without vomiting
- Significant bleeding is unusual except in hemorrhagic gastritis.
- Rectal bleeding/melena
- Hiccups, belching, bloating or fullness
- Neurologic symptoms related to vitamin B_{12} deficiency if atrophic gastritis
- History of smoking, alcohol use, NSAID use, radiotherapy, gallbladder disorders, autoimmune disorders, IBD, vasculitis or eosinophilic disorders
- Can be asymptomatic

PHYSICAL EXAM
- Vital signs to assess hemodynamic stability
- Abdominal exam often normal; mild epigastric tenderness
- May have heme-positive stool
- Stigmata of chronic alcohol abuse
- May have pallor, slowing of capillary refill if anemic

DIFFERENTIAL DIAGNOSIS
- Functional abdominal pain (dyspepsia)
- Peptic ulcer disease, viral gastroenteritis
- Gastric cancer (elderly), cholecystitis
- Pancreatic disease (inflammation vs. tumor)

DIAGNOSTIC TESTS & INTERPRETATION
Initial Tests (lab, imaging)
Usually normal
- Evaluate for iron deficiency anemia.
- Stool analysis for fecal *H. pylori* antigen
  - 95% specificity and sensitivity
  - Can be used for diagnosis and eradication
- ^{13}C-urea breath test for *H. pylori*—95% specificity and sensitivity
- *H. pylori*, serology serum IgG
  - Inexpensive; 85% sensitivity, 79% specificity
  - Positive in history of colonization or prior infections; *cannot be used to assess eradication*
- Gastric acid analysis may be abnormal but is not a reliable indicator of gastritis.
- Patients with autoimmune chronic gastritis may have antibodies to intrinsic factor (IF) or parietal cells (the latter being the most sensitive), elevated serum fasting gastrin, elevated serum pepsinogen 1 (PGI), and elevated PGI to PGII ratio.
- Patients with pernicious anemia may have macrocytic anemia with low serum B_{12} levels and IF autoantibodies.
- Drugs that may alter lab results: Antibiotics, PPIs, and bismuth-containing compounds may affect urea breath test for *H. pylori*.
  - Hold PPIs for 2 weeks, H_2 antagonists for 24 hours, and antibiotics for 4 weeks prior to stool or breath tests (1)[B].

Follow-Up Tests & Special Considerations
Endoscopy for *H. pylori*: Obtain multiple biopsies in body and antrum for culture; polymerase chain reaction (PCR); histology with H&E plus second staining; rapid urease testing

Diagnostic Procedures/Other
- Gastroscopy with biopsy is first line in:
  - Age >50 years with new-onset symptoms
  - Weight loss, persistent vomiting, or GI bleed
- Consider for patients aged <50 years who are *H. pylori*–negative.
- Gastric biopsies recommended if there is a poor response to treatment. *Patients must discontinue PPIs for 2 weeks prior to endoscopy to improve diagnostic accuracy.*

Test Interpretation
Inflammatory infiltrate in gastric mucosa, often with distortion or erosion of adjacent epithelium; presence of *H. pylori* often confirmed on biopsy. Ulcers or bleeding may be present.

 TREATMENT

GENERAL MEASURES
- *H. pylori* treatment is required to relieve symptoms.
- Parenteral fluid and electrolyte supplements if unable to tolerate oral intake
- Discontinue NSAID use; abstinence from alcohol; smoking cessation

MEDICATION
First Line
- Antacids: liquid form, 30 mL 1 hour after meals and at bedtime
- H$_2$ receptor antagonists oral cimetidine (Tagamet) 300 mg q6h or famotidine (Pepcid) 20 mg BID or nizatidine (Axid); 150 mg BID not shown to be clearly superior to antacids
- Sucralfate (Carafate): 1 g q4–6h on an empty stomach; rationale uncertain but empirically helpful
- Prostaglandins (misoprostol [Cytotec]): can help allay gastric mucosal injury; dosage 100 to 200 µg QID
- PPIs if no response to antacids or H$_2$ antagonists (omeprazole or esomeprazole 20 mg daily or BID)
- *H. pylori*: Treatment will depend on penicillin (PCN) allergy, previous macrolide exposure, or clarithromycin resistance of >15%.
  - Clarithromycin triple therapy (CTT)—75–80% eradication
    - Short course (14 days) of amoxicillin 1 g BID, PPI BID (omeprazole 20 mg BID, etc.), and clarithromycin 500 mg BID
    - *If PCN allergic:* Substitute amoxicillin with metronidazole 500 mg TID.
    - Alternative: Prevpac combination pill (lansoprazole, amoxicillin, and clarithromycin)
  - Bismuth quadruple therapy (BQT)—75–90% eradication
    - PPI BID (omeprazole 20 mg), bismuth salicylate (Pepto-BismolT) 30 mL liquid or 2 tablets QID, metronidazole 250 mg QID, tetracycline 500 mg QID for 10 to 14 days (2)[A]
    - Use as initial therapy in areas of high clarithromycin resistance (>15%) or PCN-allergic patients.
    - Alternative: Pylera combination pill (bismuth subcitrate, metronidazole, and tetracycline)
- *H. pylori* treatment failure: Use a different regimen; avoid clarithromycin (unless confirmed susceptibility):
  - BQT for 7 to 14 days (3)[A]
  - Consider levofloxacin 250 mg BID, amoxicillin 1 g BID, and standard-dose PPI BID for 14 days in those who fail twice (2)[A].
  - In PCN-allergic, consider levofloxacin quadruple therapy with levofloxacin 500 mg QD, omeprazole QD 40 mg, nitazoxanide 500 mg BID, and doxycycline 100 mg QD for 7 to 10 days (3)[A].

- Consider probiotics in known symptomatic *H. pylori*; may decrease severity of gastritis, peptic ulcers; and possibly slow progression toward atrophic gastritis and gastric adenocarcinoma (4)[A]
  - Probiotics alone likely do not eradicate *H. pylori*.
  - Possible regimens as used in trials: *Bifidobacterium* spp. BID × 14 days
- Contraindications: hypersensitivity
- Precautions: Bismuth may turn stool black.

Pregnancy Considerations
- Avoid sodium carbonate and magnesium trisilicate containing antacids.
- Women with hyperemesis gravidarum (HG) have a higher prevalence of *H. pylori* infection. Treatment can be deferred until after delivery. Routine testing for *H. pylori* is not recommended in those with HG.

SURGERY/OTHER PROCEDURES
Surgical intervention is not necessary, except in the case of phlegmonous gastritis or gastritis with high-grade dysplasia.

COMPLEMENTARY & ALTERNATIVE MEDICINE
Studies suggest cranberry, garlic, curcumin, ginger, and Pistacia gum may prevent and/or reduce *H. pylori* infection due to potent anti-inflammatory properties.

ADMISSION, INPATIENT, AND NURSING CONSIDERATIONS
Prophylaxis in ICU patients

 ONGOING CARE

FOLLOW-UP RECOMMENDATIONS
Confirm *H. pylori* eradication >4 weeks after treatment.

Patient Monitoring
- Consider repeat endoscopy after 6 weeks if gastritis was severe or if poor treatment response.
- Surveillance endoscopy in patients with mild to moderate atrophic gastritis not currently recommended. Patients with advanced atrophic gastritis should receive endoscopy with biopsy sampling every 3 years.
- 25% of patients with high-grade dysplasia may progress to adenocarcinoma within a year, although this number is strongly influenced by geography, ethnicity, race, and family history—recommend endoscopic resection.
- Surveillance may be suspended when two or more endoscopies are negative for dysplasia.

DIET
Diet restrictions (e.g., bland, light, soft foods) depend on symptom severity. In general, avoid caffeine, spicy foods, alcohol, peppermint, carbonated beverages, and high-fat content food.

PATIENT EDUCATION
- Smoking cessation; limit alcohol, dietary changes
- Relaxation therapy; avoid NSAIDs.

PROGNOSIS
Phlegmonous gastritis has a 40–50% mortality even with treatment.

COMPLICATIONS
- Bleeding from extensive mucosal erosion or ulceration
- Gastric outlet obstruction due to edema
- Gastric intestinal metaplasia, which puts patient at a 10-fold increase of developing gastric cancer.
- Clearing *H. pylori* before the development of chronic gastritis may prevent development of gastric cancer.
- Chronic autoimmune gastritis has increased risk for development of gastric neuroendocrine tumors and adenocarcinoma due to dysplasia.

REFERENCES
1. Yang H, Guan L, Hu B. Detection and treatment of *Helicobacter pylori*: problems and advances. *Gastroenterol Res Pract*. 2022;2022:4710964.
2. Malfertheiner P, Megraud F, O'Morain CA, et al; for the European Helicobacter and Microbiota Study Group and Consensus panel. Management of *Helicobacter pylori* infection—the Maastricht V/Florence consensus report. *Gut*. 2017;66(1):6–30.
3. Chey WD, Leontiadis GI, Howden CW, et al. ACG clinical guideline: treatment of *Helicobacter pylori* infection [published correction in *Am J Gastroenterol*. 2018;113(7):1102]. *Am J Gastroenterol*. 2017;112(2):212–239.
4. Buzás GM, Birinyi P. Newer, older, and alternative agents for the eradication of *Helicobacter pylori* infection: a narrative review. *Antibiotics (Basel)*. 2023;12(6):946.

 CODES

ICD10
- K29.5 Unspecified chronic gastritis
- K29.40 Chronic atrophic gastritis without bleeding
- K29.50 Unspecified chronic gastritis without bleeding

CLINICAL PEARLS
- *H. pylori* is the most common cause of gastritis; >50% of adult patients are colonized with *H. pylori* by age 60 years.
- *H. pylori* antibodies decline in the year after treatment and should not be used to determine eradication.
- *H. pylori* stool antigen tests can be used before and after therapy to assess for eradication and reinfection.
- Several courses of therapy may be necessary to eradicate *H. pylori*.
- In cases of suspected gastritis, discontinue PPI 2 weeks prior to endoscopy to improve diagnostic accuracy.

G

GASTROESOPHAGEAL REFLUX DISEASE

Bliss Puthenpurayil, MD • Amrutha Pavle, MD • Nida Zahra, MD, FAAFP

BASICS

DESCRIPTION
- Changes of the esophageal mucosa resulting from reflux of gastric contents into the esophagus
- Often described as "heartburn," "acid indigestion," and "acid reflux"

EPIDEMIOLOGY
Incidence
Incidence: 5/1,000 person-years
Prevalence
- The prevalence of GERD in North America is ~15% (95% CI, 10.7–20.9%) (1).
- There is no association between sex and symptoms of GERD in North America.
- Advanced age increases your risk of GERD; >50 versus <50 years old, odds ratio (OR) of 1.32 (95% CI, 1.46–2.06) of having GERD (1)
- Pediatric population: Regurgitation occurs in nearly 50% of newborn infants, resolving spontaneously in 90% of children by age 1 year (1).

ETIOLOGY AND PATHOPHYSIOLOGY
- Stomach acid contacts the squamous mucosal lining of the esophagus, which is less acid resistant than gastric columnar mucosa, followed by release of chemokines and cytokines causing symptoms and disease.
- GERD can be the result of one or a combination of the following: lower esophageal sphincter (LES) dysfunction, esophageal hypersensitivity, delayed gastric emptying, and increased gastroesophageal junction distensibility.
- Patients with severe GERD often have evidence of a hiatal hernia which can trap acid, impair acid emptying, reduce LES pressure, and increase retrograde acid flow.

Genetics
Genetic heterogeneity may account for 31–43% of the predisposition to develop GERD (2).

RISK FACTORS
- Obesity; OR of 1.7 (95% CI, 1.4–2.1) (1)
  - Higher prevalence of hiatal hernia; increased intra-abdominal pressure; increased estrogen, bile, and pancreatic enzymes
- Tobacco use; OR of 1.2 (95% CI, 1.04–1.5) (1)
- Hiatal hernia
- Pregnancy
- Diet; alcohol use
- Scleroderma; neuromuscular disorders

GENERAL PREVENTION
- Weight loss (1)[A],(2)[A]
- Tobacco cessation (1)[B]
- Change of diet: Decrease consumption of spicy, acidic and fatty foods, alcoholic and carbonated beverages, chocolate, and caffeine (2)[C].
- Elevate head of bed at night for selected patients (2)[C].
- Avoid meals within 2 to 3 hours of bedtime (2)[C].

- Smaller portions
- Staying upright during and after meals
- Infants: Use car seat for 2 to 3 hours after meals, thickened feedings, burp frequently while feeding

COMMONLY ASSOCIATED CONDITIONS
- Nonerosive and erosive esophagitis, the latter occurs in 18–25% of patients with GERD (1).
- Barrett esophagus: prevalence of 7% (95% CI, 5%–9%) in patients with GERD (1)
- Esophageal adenocarcinoma
- Peptic ulcer disease (PUD)
- Peptic esophageal stricture
- Extraesophageal reflux: asthma, aspiration, chronic cough, laryngitis, vocal cord granuloma, sinusitis, otitis media
- Halitosis

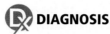DIAGNOSIS

HISTORY
- Typical symptoms: acid regurgitation, heartburn, dysphagia (mostly postprandial)
- Extraesophageal signs and symptoms: chronic cough, bronchospasm, wheezing, hoarseness, sore throat, throat clearing
- Atypical symptoms: epigastric fullness/pressure/pain, dyspepsia, nausea, bloating, belching, chest pain, lump in throat
- Heartburn: retrosternal burning sensation
- Regurgitation; sour or acid taste in mouth
- Symptoms worse with bending or lying down
- Diet, alcohol and tobacco use

PHYSICAL EXAM
Often benign but look for potential
- Epigastric tenderness or palpable epigastric mass
- Dental erosions

DIFFERENTIAL DIAGNOSIS
- Angina/coronary artery disease
- Infectious esophagitis (*Candida*, herpes, HIV, cytomegalovirus)
- Chemical esophagitis; pill-induced esophagitis; eosinophilic esophagitis
- PUD; biliary tract disease
- Achalasia or other upper gastrointestinal motility disorders
- Esophageal stricture or anatomic defect (ring, sling)
- Gastrointestinal malignancy

DIAGNOSTIC TESTS & INTERPRETATION
Previously based on symptoms and history but this has been proven to be erroneous. Society of American Gastrointestinal and Endoscopic Surgeons (SAGES) diagnose GERD with one or greater of the following (1)[A]:
- A mucosal break observed on endoscopy in a patient with typical symptoms
- Barrett esophagus on biopsy
- A peptic stricture in the absence of malignancy
- Positive pH measurement

Initial Tests (lab, imaging)
- Formal diagnosis requires an esophagogastroduodenoscopy (EGD) with biopsy and pH probe. As these are invasive procedures and require expertise, a PPI test can be appropriate (2)[B].
  - PPI is given daily for 8 weeks, and symptoms are monitored. If symptoms completely resolve, most likely diagnosis is GERD with a sensitivity of 78% and specificity of 54% (2).
- No lab studies are needed for initial workup of GERD (1).
- Appropriately evaluate patients who present with symptoms suspicious for cardiac disease.

Follow-Up Tests & Special Considerations
If patient fails the PPI challenge, then an EGD, pH monitoring, and manometry should take place (1).

Diagnostic Procedures/Other
- Upper endoscopy
  - Recommended for those with alarm signs such as dysphagia, bleeding, anemia, weight loss, recurrent vomiting
  - Recommended if uncontrolled persistent symptoms after twice-daily PPI for 4 to 8 weeks
  - Recommended if at risk for Barrett esophagus (or with know history requiring surveillance)
- High resolution manometry (HRM)
  - Helpful in refractory cases, can evaluate peristaltic function, record LES pressure, and diagnose motility disorders
  - HRM helps with placement of pH probes, operative planning for surgical, or endoscopic antireflux procedures.
  - Used for patients unresponsive to PPI with inconclusive pH monitoring
- Ambulatory reflux (pH) monitoring
  - Evaluate excessive acid exposure in those with GERD symptoms, normal endoscopy, and no response to PPI.
  - Used to document frequency of reflux
  - Discontinue PPI for 7 days prior to test.
  - Measured for 24 to 96 hours depending on placement technique
  - Calculate SI or SAP; both are a ratio of event to time to objectify GERD. If SAP >85% or SI >50%, test is positive (2).
- Barium swallow: not used for GERD diagnosis; used to evaluate complaints of dysphagia or to outline anatomic abnormalities (hiatal hernia)

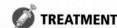TREATMENT

GENERAL MEASURES
Lifestyle changes are first-line intervention, reviewed in the "General Prevention" section.
- Step-wise approach to therapy
  - Phase I: lifestyle and diet modifications, antacids plus H_2 blockers or PPIs
    - PPI > H_2 blockers > Placebo (1)[A]
  - Phase II: If symptoms persist, consider endoscopy.
  - Phase III: If symptoms still persist, consider surgery.
    - Laparoscopic preferred over open fundoplication (1)[A]

MEDICATION

First Line

- H₂ blockers in equipotent oral doses (e.g.,famotidine 20 mg BID, nizatidine 150 mg BID, cimetidine 800 mg BID or 400 mg QID); ranitidine pulled from U.S. market
  - Block histamine receptors in parietal cells of stomach, thereby reducing acid production.
  - Renally excreted and will need dose adjustments
  - Less effective than PPIs (1),(2)
  - Can be used in conjunction to PPI for bedtime relief (2)[C]
- PPIs in equipotent oral doses (e.g., pantoprazole 40 mg/day, dexlansoprazole 30 mg/day)
  - Irreversibly bind proton pump (H⁺/K⁺ ATPase), effective onset within 4 days
  - Complete symptom relief at 4 weeks in 70–80% of patients with EE (2).
  - PPIs are more effective than H₂ blockers and prokinetics for healing erosive and nonerosive esophagitis (2)[A].
  - PPIs increase risk of clostridium difficile infections and have a theoretical risk of hypomagnesemia, bone fracture, vitamin B₁₂ deficiency, and community-acquired pneumonia (2).
  - Dose 30 to 60 minutes before meals except dexlansoprazole (2)
  - GERD relief and healing rates vary minimally among PPIs (2).
- Reevaluate symptoms after 4 to 8 weeks of treatment (1).
- Discontinuation of long-term PPI can cause potential rebound acid hypersecretion due to high levels of gastrin, which can be reduced by tapering PPI dose before stopping (2)[C].
- Blood dyscrasias and anemia may occur with PPIs and H₂ blockers.
- Tachyphylaxis may occur with H₂ blockers.

Pregnancy Considerations

- Trial lifestyle changes first; if that fails, antacids and sucralfate are first-line options (2).
- H₂ blockers (category B) and all PPIs are category B except omeprazole (category C) (2).

Pediatric Considerations

Antacids or liquid H₂ blockers and PPIs are available. Prokinetics have a minimal role due to safety concerns and limited efficacy.

Second Line

- Sucralfate is a mucosal barrier agent.
  - Limited data, could be as efficacious as H₂RA (2)[C]
  - Dose: 1 g PO QID 1 hour before meals and at bedtime for 4 to 8 weeks
- Prokinetics: metoclopramide
  - Increase LES pressure, esophageal peristalsis, and gastric emptying.
  - Can be used as adjunct, limited data (2)[C]
  - Dose: 5 to 10 mg before meals
  - Metoclopramide is a dopamine blocker; risk of dystonia and tardive dyskinesis

ISSUES FOR REFERRAL

Treatment resistant, persistent, severe disease or advanced esophageal disease (e.g., dysplasia, Barrett esophagus) should be referred to a specialist.

SURGERY/OTHER PROCEDURES

- Laparoscopic fundoplication, wrapping gastric fundus around distal esophagus, decreases reflux into esophagus by improving function of GE junction.
  - Partial and total fundoplications have similar outcomes, but partial has less complications (1).
  - GERD remission is similar between PPI and fundoplication (1).
  - Surgery has higher risk of severe adverse events (1).
- Bariatric surgery
  - BMI >35 kg/m², prevalence of GERD increases up to 6-fold (2)
  - Obesity increases risk of complications or failure of fundoplication.
  - Gastric sleeve or Roux-en-Y gastric bypass is beneficial for the obese patient with GERD (1),(2).
  - Manometry to rule out esophageal dysmotility, achalasia, or scleroderma prior to surgery
- Ablative endoscopic techniques, radiofrequency ablation to levels below and above the LES, results in thickening of the sphincter, decreases transient relaxation rate, and reduces esophageal exposure to gastric acid (1).
  - Contradicting results in multiple studies (2)
- Transoral incisionless fundoplication (TIF), endoscopically suturing serosa to serosa creating a valve around esophagogastric junction, reducing acid reflux.
  - Contradicting results in multiple studies (1),(2)

 ## ONGOING CARE

FOLLOW-UP RECOMMENDATIONS

Patient Monitoring

- Monitor symptoms over time. Consider additional workup and/or treatment if symptoms fail to improve after 8 weeks of PPI treatment.
- Repeat endoscopy in 4 to 8 weeks if there is a poor symptomatic response to medical therapy, especially in older patients.
- Monitoring recommendations changes depending on level of disease and dysplasia.

PATIENT EDUCATION

Lifestyle and dietary modifications per "General Prevention" section.

PROGNOSIS

- Two-thirds of patients with nonerosive esophagitis have symptoms relapse when PPI stopped (2).
  - Maintenance PPI should be considered among those with GERD complications as relapse is common.
  - Los Angeles (LA) classification is endoscopic scoring system, and the two categories are mild (grades A and B) and severe (grades C and D). Patients with LA grade C or D EE will need long-term PPI therapy to heal (2)[A].
- Intermittent PPI therapy or as needed can successfully manage noncomplicated GERD (2)[C].
- Medical and surgical therapy are equally effective for symptom reduction (1).
- Laparoscopic fundoplication has a 6.9% reoperation rate within 10 years (1).

COMPLICATIONS

- Peptic stricture: 10–15%
- Risk of Barrett esophagus, progression to adenocarcinoma:
  - Men are at greater risk than women.
  - Annual incidence of adenocarcinoma with Barrett esophagus and low-grade dysplasia is 0.54% (95% CI, 0.32–0.76%) (1).
  - Annual incidence of adenocarcinoma with Barrett esophagus and high-grade dysplasia is 1.73% (95% CI, 0.99–2.47%) (1).
- Bleeding due to mucosal injury

Geriatric Considerations

- Complications from PPI use more likely (e.g., enteric infection), higher risk for side effects from medical management
- Increased risk of adenocarcinoma

REFERENCES

1. Maret-Ouda J, Markar SR, Lagergren J. Gastroesophageal reflux disease: a review. *JAMA*. 2020;324(24):2536–2547.
2. Katz PO, Dunbar KB, Schnoll-Sussman FH, et al. ACG clinical guideline for the diagnosis and management of gastroesophageal reflux disease. *Am J Gastroenterol*. 2022;117(1):27–56.

ADDITIONAL READING

Newberry C, Lynch K. Using diet to treat diseases of esophagus: back to the basics. *Gastroenterol Clin North Am*. 2021;50(4):959–972.

 ## SEE ALSO

Algorithms: Abdominal Pain, Upper; Dyspepsia

 ## CODES

ICD10

- K21.9 Gastro-esophageal reflux disease without esophagitis
- K21.0 Gastro-esophageal reflux disease with esophagitis

CLINICAL PEARLS

- Formal diagnosis can be achieved with a combination of endoscopy, biopsy, and pH monitoring.
- Consider GERD in nonsmokers with a chronic cough (>3 weeks).
- PPIs provide the most rapid symptomatic relief and healing of esophagitis.
- Consider additional workup and/or treatment if symptoms fail to improve after 8 weeks of PPI treatment.
- Endoscopy is recommended for patients with alarm symptoms, has risk factors for Barrett esophagus, or continued symptoms despite adequate PPI trial.

G

GAY HEALTH

Stacy P. Rubin, MD

BASICS

- Men who have sex with men, or MSM, is a clinical term that refers to sexual behavior alone, regardless of sexual orientation, as MSM may include men who identify as gay, bisexual, or heterosexual. Sexual orientation is independent of gender identity.
- MSM are less likely to access health care and are disproportionately impacted by mental health issues, substance use and abuse, and sexually transmitted infections (STI).
- Health disparities exist between patients in the LGBTQ community and those of heterosexual orientation. Sexual minority groups tend to fare worse across all realms.

DESCRIPTION

- Structural barriers of an unwelcoming health care system and minority stress (e.g., fear, stigma, internalized homophobia) experienced by LGBTQ people likely contribute to health disparities.
- LGBTQ individuals may hide their orientation out of fear of stigma and discrimination, so it is important to ask all patients about sexual orientation and behavior in a nonjudgmental environment.
- Although this chapter reviews the important topics that effect this population disproportionately, primary care of MSM foremost is about delivering the same level of care to all patients, regardless of sexual orientation.

GENERAL PREVENTION

- The majority of screening guidelines are the same for MSM as they are for non-MSM age- and sex-matched populations.
- Centers for Disease Control and Prevention (CDC) and the United States Preventative Services Task Force (USPSTF) suggest at least annual screening for HIV, syphilis, gonorrhea, and chlamydia as detailed below, with increased frequency and other screening tests based on the level of risk of the patient's behavioral practices.
- CDC recommends testing for hepatitis B serology at least at the initial visit and vaccination for MSM who are seronegative or for whom vaccination status cannot be ascertained (1)[A]. However, in 2022, the Advisory Committee on Immunization Practices (ACIP) expanded hepatitis B vaccination recommendations to include all adults aged 19 to 59 years.
- Screening for hepatitis C is recommended in all patients between the ages of 18 and 79 years at least once in a lifetime. Annual screening for hepatitis C is only recommended in MSM with HIV.
- Screening for hepatitis A is not recommended. However, hepatitis A vaccination is recommended for MSM.
- Annual digital anorectal examination (DARE) is recommended as a screening for anal cancer, but there is insufficient evidence to recommend obtaining anal cytology in all MSM patients.

- ACIP recommends routine vaccination schedules be followed for MSM patients, including vaccination against (i) hepatitis A and B viruses; (ii) human papillomavirus (HPV) for all patients between 11 and 26 years old with additional consideration for MSM patients outside this age category; (iii) serogroup B meningococcal vaccine (MenB) and quadrivalent meningococcal vaccine against serogroups A, C, W, and Y (MenACWY); and (iv) smallpox monkeypox virus, live nonreplicating, if high prevalence in geographical area.
- Cultivating a nonjudgmental, welcoming environment is the cornerstone of prevention of disease for the LGBTQ community. Consider accessing community or web-based resources to create an LGBTQ safe zone for clinical practice sites.

DIAGNOSIS

- STIs
  - Taking a detailed sexual history is of paramount importance in LGBTQ individuals. The CDC suggest the 5Ps approach (partners, practices, protection from STI, past history of STI, and pain/pleasure) when obtaining a patient's sexual history.
  - Physicians should screen for behaviors placing patients at increased risk of STI such as:
    - Anonymous sexual encounters
    - Multiple active sex partners (or partners with multiple active partners or a history of multiple partners)
    - Inconsistent barrier protection (condom) use
    - Substance use during and around sex, including exchanging sex for drugs or money
    - History of or current STI
    - Receptive and insertive anal intercourse, with receptive having higher risk of STI transmission
  - Screening of all sexually active MSM should include at least annual screening for HIV, syphilis, chlamydia, and gonorrhea at all sites of contact (urethra, rectum, and pharynx). Hepatitis C should be performed at the initial visit and conducted annually in HIV-infected patients. Screening for STI can be performed more frequently (every 3–6 months) based on risk of sexual practices.
  - MSM are at risk of sexual transmission of enteric pathogens such as *Shigella*, *E. coli*, *Campylobacter*, hepatitis A, and parasitic infections such as *Giardia lamblia* and *Entamoeba histolytica* through oral-anal contact or through contact with fecally contaminated fingers or objects.
  - Recently, outbreaks of monkeypox in the United States were almost exclusively identified in the MSM community.
  - Postexposure prophylaxis (PEP) and preexposure prophylaxis (PrEP) regimens for non-HIV STI are on the horizon for chlamydial and gonorrheal infections, but none have been approved by the FDA or recommended in CDC guidelines yet due to limitations in sample size of studies (2)[C].

- HIV
  - 69% of new cases of HIV diagnosed in 2018 were among MSM. These disproportionately affected Black and Latinx MSM, young MSM, and transgender women. Up to 44% of MSM may not know their HIV status (1).
  - When patients are adherent to drug regimens, PrEP has a >90% efficacy in preventing HIV transmission in patients with detectable drug levels.
  - Indications for PrEP:
    - HIV negative (confirm with RNA viral load if exposed within last 4 weeks)
    - Sexually active but not with a monogamous HIV-negative partner
    - Male sex partner within last 6 months
    - And at least one of the following: (i) insertive or receptive anal sex without condoms in the past 6 months, (ii) any STI in the last 6 months, or (iii) in a sexual relationship with an HIV-positive partner
  - Prior to initiating PrEP, clinicians must exclude acute or chronic HIV infection, assess renal function, and screen for hepatitis B and C. Patients should be vaccinated for hepatitis B virus if appropriate.
  - There are three FDA-approved regimens for PrEP in MSM patients, two oral and one injection-based (3)[A]. The oral regimens are daily fixed-dose single-pill combinations and have similar efficacy.
- Combination tenofovir disoproxil fumarate (TDF)/emtricitabine (FTC); should not be used if CrCl <60 mL/min
- Combination tenofovir alafenamide (TAF)/FTC (only FDA-approved for MSM and transgender women). TAF is a version of tenofovir with less impact on bone and renal integrity than TDF; should not be used with CrCl <30 mL/min
- Cabotegravir (CAB) intramuscular injection once every 2 months, with or without oral lead-in therapy, was FDA-approved in late 2021; may be used in renal impairment with CrCl ≥15 mL/min
- Alternative dosing, "on-demand" dosing, or "2-1-1 PrEP" means patients take 2 doses of TDF/FTC within 2 to 24 hours before sex and 1 dose daily for 2 days afterward. Presently, this regimen is not approved by FDA or recommended by CDC. On-demand use of TAF/FTC has not been studied.
- Patients need follow-up while on PrEP to screen for HIV and other STI every 3 months. Creatinine clearance should be monitored every 6 months, and lipids and weight should be reviewed annually (3)[A].
- PEP is indicated after exposure to a known HIV-positive partner ≤72 hours prior through mucous membranes, which includes sexual exposure via oral, anal, and vaginal sex.
- PEP generally involves a 28-day course of highly active antiretroviral therapy (HAART) in a three-drug combination of two nucleoside reverse transcriptase inhibitors (NRTI) and an integrase strand transfer inhibitor (INSTI) or a protease inhibitor (PI).
- Selection of medications is based on side effect profiles, patient adherence, and patient convenience.

- "Preferred" PEP regimens are TDF/FTC OR TDF/lamivudine (3TC) *plus* raltegravir *or* dolutegravir in patients with CrCl ≥60 mL/min. Adjust dose of TDF/FTC or TDF/3TC for patients with CrCl <60 mL/min.
- Alternative PEP regimens include the following:
  – Combination elvitegravir (EBG)/cobicistat (COBI)/FTC/TDF fixed dose; cannot use with CrCl <70 mL/min
  – TDF/FTC *plus* darunavir *and* ritonavir in patients with normal renal function. Provide renally adjusted dose of TDF-containing medication for CrCl <60 mL/min.
- Counsel on safer sex and risk reduction for repeated exposures, including immediate transition to PrEP after completing PEP.
- Hepatitis C
  – MSM have a slightly higher prevalence of hepatitis C infection than the general population. However, MSM who are HIV-positive are at much higher risk of hepatitis C infection compared to both MSM who are HIV-negative and patients who are not MSM.
  – Screening for hepatitis C is recommended in all MSM patients at initial visit and then more frequently based on risk assessments.
  – Annual screening for hepatitis C is recommended in MSM with HIV.
- Anal cancer
  – The annual incidence of anal cancer is 5 times higher in MSM who are HIV-negative than the general population. This risk increases to between 78- and 168-times higher in MSM who are HIV-positive.
  – Anal carcinoma has been linked to certain high-risk subtypes of HPV, specifically types 16 and 18.
  – Screening for anal dysplasia with anal cytology may be considered for at-risk populations, especially HIV-infected MSM, but further research is needed for appropriate screening intervals. Anal cytology only should be performed if there is the potential for referral for high-resolution anoscopy and subsequent treatment, if indicated.
  – HPV vaccine is recommended for all patients aged 11 to 26 years (can start at age 9 years) to reduce the risk of HPV-related anal cancer. Providers can consider giving HPV vaccination above age 26 years given high incidence and prevalence of HPV-related anal cancers in MSM patients.
- Substance use and substance use disorders
  – MSM have significantly higher rates of use of nearly all substances as well as higher rates of substance use disorders than men who do not identify as MSM.
  – "Chem sex" refers to use of drugs in conjunction with sexual intercourse by MSM. Inhaled nitrites ("poppers"), stimulants (methamphetamine and cocaine), GHB, ketamine, and alcohol are often used during or around sexual encounters to increase pleasure and performance.
  – Chem sex may be associated with unprotected intercourse and other high-risk sexual behaviors, which may increase risk of HIV and STI transmission.

– Substance abuse treatment programs implementing cognitive behavioral intervention from a harm reduction perspective are beneficial in reducing stimulant use and sexual risk-taking behavior.
– Most MSM do not report substance use or abuse. It is important to avoid inadvertently introducing or contributing to stigma in the clinical environment by not assuming that all MSM engage in high-risk behaviors.
- Mental health
  – Rates of mental illness or serious mental illness among MSM are 2 to 3 times as high as rates among other men.
  – Risk of deliberate self-harm is also increased especially among MSM youth due to stressors such as having an identity different from family and peers, isolation, bullying, family rejection, and self-nonacceptance.
- Intimate partner violence (IPV) (domestic violence)
  – A recent study reported ~21% of sexual minority men have a history of physical abuse and ~50% have a history of psychological abuse; the highest rates were reported among bisexual men.
  – Providers can stigmatize same-gender IPV as not being serious, especially when wounds may not be overt or physical strength of both partners may be considered equal.
  – Clinicians should screen for IPV with patients alone and respond with compassion and connection to local LGBTQ welcoming resources.

Pediatric Considerations
- Normalizing nonheterosexual identities and behaviors during regular screening of sexual development during adolescent well-visits may reduce stigma and decrease risk for negative mental health outcomes.
- Regular assessments of mental health and suicide risk should include questions about family and peer support, experiences of stigma, connection to an LGBTQ community, and self-acceptance.
- Same-gender parenting
  – There is no causal relationship between parents' sexual orientation and children's emotional, psychosocial, and behavioral development.
  – Pathways to parenting for same-gender couples include adoption, fostering, IVF, and surrogacy.

ONGOING CARE

- Establish with patients that information related to sexual orientation is asked confidentially of all patients to assist in providing them the best care.
- Take an inclusive and complete sexual history and individualize regular discussions about substance abuse, HIV/STI, mental health, and IPV.
- Create a welcoming environment by displaying LGBTQ-friendly symbols and using intake forms, waiting room, and marketing materials inclusive of same-gender couples and sexual identities.
- Avoid labeling patients as gay, lesbian, bisexual, or transgender unless prompted by the patients. Many patients may not choose to label at all.
- Understand the significance of terms used in LGBTQ communities, such as "bottom" partner (receptive sex) and "top" partner (insertive sex) and use that language with patients.

PATIENT EDUCATION
- Educate patients on risk-reduction strategies for safer sex such as condoms, PrEP, and PEP, and avoiding or limiting substance use around sex.
- Educate patients on LGBTQ-specific or welcoming resources in your community for substance use and abuse, IPV, mental health, and suicide prevention.

REFERENCES
1. Workowski KA, Bachmann LH, Chan PA, et al. Sexually transmitted infections treatment guidelines, 2021. *MMWR Recomm Rep*. 2021;70(4):1–187.
2. Centers for Disease Control and Prevention. Men who have sex with men (MSM). https://www.cdc.gov/std/treatment-guidelines/msm.htm. Accessed July 30, 2023.
3. Centers for Disease Control and Prevention. US Public Health Service: Preexposure prophylaxis for the prevention of HIV infection in the United States—2021 Update: a clinical practice guideline. https://www.cdc.gov/hiv/pdf/risk/prep/cdc-hiv-prep-guidelines-2021.pdf. Accessed July 30, 2023.

ADDITIONAL READING
- Compton WM, Jones CM. Substance use among men who have sex with men. *N Engl J Med*. 2021;385(4):352–356.
- PEP to prevent HIV infection. AIDS Institute Clinical Guidelines. https://www.hivguidelines.org/pep-for-hiv-prevention/pep/. Accessed July 30, 2023.

 SEE ALSO

- GLAAD: https://www.glaad.org/
- Safe Zone Project: https://thesafezoneproject.com/

 CODES

ICD10
- Z11.59 Encounter for screening for other viral diseases
- Z11.4 Encounter for screening for human immunodeficiency virus
- Z72.52 High risk homosexual behavior

CLINICAL PEARLS
- Provide MSM patients with the same comprehensive primary care delivered to all patients.
- All sexually active MSM should be offered annual screening for HIV, syphilis, rectal and urethral gonorrhea and chlamydia, and pharyngeal gonorrhea.
- Screen for hepatitis C virus annually in HIV-positive MSM.
- Counsel patients on risk-reduction strategies for safer sex such as condoms, PrEP, a PEP, and avoiding or limiting substance use around sex.

GENITO-PELVIC PAIN/PENETRATION DISORDER (VAGINISMUS)

Jeffrey D. Quinlan, MD, FAAFP

BASICS

Genito-pelvic pain/penetration disorder is the name of the conditions formally known as vaginismus and dyspareunia. Vaginismus results from involuntary contraction of the vaginal musculature. Primary vaginismus occurs in women who have never been able to have penetrative intercourse. Women with secondary vaginismus were previously able to have penetrative intercourse but are no longer able to do so.

DESCRIPTION
- Persistent or recurrent difficulties for 6 months or more with at least one of the following:
  - Inability to have vaginal intercourse/penetration on at least 50% of attempts
  - Marked genito-pelvic pain during at least 50% of vaginal intercourse/penetration attempts
  - Marked fear of vaginal intercourse/penetration or of genito-pelvic pain during intercourse/penetration on at least 50% of vaginal intercourse/penetration attempts
  - Marked tensing or tightening of the pelvic floor muscles during attempted vaginal intercourse/penetration on at least 50% of occasions
- The disturbance causes marked distress or interpersonal difficulty.
- Dysfunction is not as a result of:
  - Nonsexual mental disorder
  - Severe relationship stress
  - Other significant stress
  - Substance or medication effect
- Specify if with a general medical condition (e.g., lichen sclerosus, endometriosis)

Pregnancy Considerations
May first present during evaluation for infertility
- Pregnancy can occur in patients with genito-pelvic pain/penetration disorder when ejaculation occurs on the perineum.
- Vaginismus may be an independent risk factor for cesarean delivery.

EPIDEMIOLOGY
Incidence
The incidence of vaginismus is thought to be about 1–17% per year worldwide. In North America, 12–21% of women have genito-pelvic pain of varying etiologies (1).

Prevalence
- True prevalence is unknown due to limited data/reporting.
- Population-based studies report prevalence rates of 0.5–30%.
- Affects women in all age groups
- Approximately 15% of women in North America report recurrent pain during intercourse.

ETIOLOGY AND PATHOPHYSIOLOGY
Most often multifactorial in both primary and secondary vaginismus
- Primary
  - Psychological and psychosocial issues
    - Negative messages about sex and sexual relations in upbringing may cause phobic reaction.
    - Poor body image and limited understanding of genital area
    - History of sexual trauma
  - Abnormalities of the hymen
  - History of difficult gynecologic examination
- Secondary
  - Often situational
  - Often associated with dyspareunia secondary to:
    - Vaginal infection
    - Inflammatory dermatitis
    - Surgical or postdelivery scarring
    - Endometriosis
    - Inadequate vaginal lubrication
    - Pelvic radiation
    - Estrogen deficiency
  - Conditioned response to pain from physical issues previously listed

RISK FACTORS
- Most often idiopathic
- Although the exact role in the condition is unclear, many women report a history of abuse or sexual trauma.
- Often associated with other sexual dysfunctions

COMMONLY ASSOCIATED CONDITIONS
- Marital stress, family dysfunction
- Anxiety
- Vulvodynia/vestibulodynia

DIAGNOSIS

DSM-5 has combined vaginismus and dyspareunia in a condition called genito-pelvic pain/penetration disorder.

HISTORY
- Complete medical history
- Full psychosocial and sexual history, including the following:
  - Onset of symptoms (primary or secondary)
  - If secondary, precipitating events, if any
  - Relationship difficulty/partner violence
  - Inability to allow vaginal entry for different purposes
    - Sexual (penis, digit, object)
    - Hygiene (tampon use)
    - Health care (pelvic examination)
  - Infertility
  - Traumatic experiences (exam, sexual, etc.)
  - Religious beliefs
  - Views on sexuality

PHYSICAL EXAM
- Pelvic examination is necessary to exclude structural abnormalities or organic pathology.
- Educating the patient about the examination and giving her control over the progression of the examination is essential because genital/pelvic examination may induce varying degrees of anxiety in patients.
- Referral to a gynecologist, family physician, or other provider specializing in the treatment of sexual disorders may be appropriate.
- Contraction of pelvic floor musculature in anticipation of examination may be seen.
- Lamont classification system aids in the assessment of severity:
  - First degree: perineal and levator spasm relieved with reassurance
  - Second degree: perineal spasm maintained throughout the pelvic exam
  - Third degree: levator spasm and elevation of buttocks
  - Fourth degree: levator and perineal spasm and elevation with adduction and retreat

DIFFERENTIAL DIAGNOSIS
- Vaginal infection
- Vulvodynia/vestibulodynia
- Vulvovaginal atrophy
- Urogenital structural abnormalities
- Interstitial cystitis
- Endometriosis

DIAGNOSTIC TESTS & INTERPRETATION
No laboratory tests are indicated unless signs of vaginal infection are noted on examination. When diagnosing of this disorder has been conducted, five factors should be considered.
- Partner factors
- Relationship factors
- Individual vulnerability factors
- Cultural/religious factors
- Medical factors

Test Interpretation
Not available; may be needed to check for secondary causes

TREATMENT
- Genito-pelvic pain/penetration disorder may be successfully treated (1)[B].
- Meta-analysis of RCTs documented a trend toward higher efficacy of active treatment versus controls, whereas the meta-analysis of observational studies indicated that women with vaginismus benefit from a range of treatments in almost 80% of cases (2)[A].

- Another meta-analysis of level 1 evidence found that 2/3 of the treatment effect for female sexual dysfunction is accounted for by placebo (3)[A]. These findings suggest that the current treatments for female sexual dysfunction are, overall, minimally superior to placebo, which emphasizes the ongoing need for more efficacious treatment for female sexual dysfunction.
- Outpatient care is appropriate.
- Treatment of physical conditions, if present, is first line (see "Secondary" under "Etiology and Pathophysiology" section).
- Most begin with pelvic floor physical therapy and myofascial release
- Some evidence suggests that cognitive-behavioral therapy may be effective, including desensitization techniques, such as gradual exposure, aimed at decreasing avoidance behavior and fear of vaginal penetration (4)[A].
- Based on a Cochrane review, a clinically relevant effect of systematic desensitization cannot be ruled out (5)[A].
- Evidence suggests that sex therapy may be effective (5)[B].
  - Involves Kegel exercises to increase control over perineal muscles
  - Stepwise vaginal desensitization exercises
    ○ With vaginal dilators that the patient inserts and controls
    ○ With woman's own finger(s) to promote sexual self-awareness
    ○ Advancement to partner's fingers with patient's control
    ○ Coitus after achieving largest vaginal dilator or three fingers; important to begin with sensate-focused exercises/sensual caressing without necessarily a demand for coitus
    ○ Female superior at first; passive (nonthrusting); female-directed
    ○ Later, thrusting may be allowed.
- Topical anesthetic or anxiolytic with desensitization exercises may be considered.
- Patient education is an essential component of treatment (see "Patient Education" section).

MEDICATION

- Antidepressants and anticonvulsants have been used with limited success. Low-dose tricyclic antidepressant (amitriptyline 10 mg) may be initiated and titrated as tolerated (4)[B].
- Topical anesthetics or anxiolytics may be used in combination with either cognitive-behavioral therapy or desensitization exercises as noted above (5)[B].
- Botulinum neurotoxin type A injections may improve vaginismus in patients who do not respond to standard cognitive behavioral and medical treatment for vaginismus (6)[B].
  - Dosage: 20, 50, and 100 to 400 U of botulinum toxin type A injected in the levator ani muscle have been shown to improve vaginismus (5)[B].
- Intravaginal botulinum neurotoxin type A injection (100 to 150 U) followed by bupivacaine 0.25% with epinephrine 1:400,000 intravaginal injection (20 to 30 mL) while the patient is anesthetized may facilitate progressive placement of dilators and ultimately resolution of symptoms (6)[B].

ISSUES FOR REFERRAL

For diagnosis and treatment recommendations, the following resources may be consulted:

- Obstetrics/gynecology
- Pelvic floor physical therapy
- Psychiatry
- Sex therapy
- Hypnotherapy

SURGERY/OTHER PROCEDURES

Contraindicated

COMPLEMENTARY & ALTERNATIVE MEDICINE

- Biofeedback
- Functional electrical stimulation

 ## ONGOING CARE

FOLLOW-UP RECOMMENDATIONS

Desensitization techniques of gentle, progressive, patient-controlled vaginal dilation

Patient Monitoring

General preventive health care

DIET

No special diet

PATIENT EDUCATION

- Education about pelvic anatomy, nature of vaginal spasms, normal adult sexual function
- Handheld mirror can help the woman to learn visually to tighten and loosen perineal muscles.
- Important to teach the partner that spasms are not under conscious control and are not a reflection on the relationship or a woman's feelings about her partner
- Instruction in techniques for vaginal dilation
- Resources
  - American College of Obstetricians and Gynecologists (ACOG), 409 12th St., SW, Washington, DC 20024-2188; 800-762-ACOG. http://www.acog.org/
  - Valins L. *When a Woman's Body Says No to Sex: Understanding and Overcoming Vaginismus.* New York, NY: Penguin; 1992.

PROGNOSIS

Favorable, with early recognition of the condition and initiation of treatment

REFERENCES

1. Landry T, Bergeron S. How young does vulvovaginal pain begin? Prevalence and characteristics of dyspareunia in adolescents. *J Sex Med.* 2009;6(4):927–935.
2. Maseroli E, Scavello I, Rastrelli G, et al. Outcome of medical and psychosexual interventions for vaginismus: a systematic review and meta-analysis. *J Sex Med.* 2018;15(12):1752–1764.
3. Weinberger JM, Houman J, Caron AT, et al. Female sexual dysfunction and the placebo effect: a meta-analysis. *Obstet Gynecol.* 2018;132(2):453–458.
4. Crowley T, Goldmeier D, Hiller J. Diagnosing and managing vaginismus. *BMJ.* 2009;338:b2284.
5. Melnik T, Hawton K, McGuire H. Interventions for vaginismus. *Cochrane Database Syst Rev.* 2012;12(12):CD001760.
6. Pacik PT. Vaginismus: review of current concepts and treatment using Botox injections, bupivacaine injections, and progressive dilation with the patient under anesthesia. *Aesthetic Plast Surg.* 2011;35(6):1160–1164.

ADDITIONAL READING

- Basson R, Wierman ME, van Lankveld J, et al. Summary of the recommendations on sexual dysfunctions in women. *J Sex Med.* 2010;7(1 Pt 2):314–326.
- Pacik PT. Understanding and treating vaginismus: a multimodal approach. *Int Urogynecol J.* 2014;25(12):1613–1620.
- Simons JS, Carey MP. Prevalence of sexual dysfunctions: results from a decade of research. *Arch Sex Behav.* 2001;30(2):177–219.
- ter Kuile MM, van Lankveld JJDM, de Groot E, et al. Cognitive-behavioral therapy for women with lifelong vaginismus: process and prognostic factors. *Behav Res Ther.* 2007;45(2):359–373.

 ## SEE ALSO

Dyspareunia; Sexual Dysfunction in Women

CODES

ICD10

- N94.2 Vaginismus
- N94.1 Dyspareunia

CLINICAL PEARLS

- In a patient with suspected genito-pelvic pain/penetration disorder, a complete medical history, including a comprehensive psychosocial and sexual history and a patient-centric, patient-controlled educational pelvic exam should be conducted.
- This condition can be treated effectively. Further research into the most effective methods is needed.
- Cognitive-behavioral therapy may be effective for the treatment of this condition.
- Botox injection therapy is in the experimental stages but looks promising for the treatment of vaginismus. Bupivacaine and dilation under general anesthesia has also been tried as a treatment for vaginismus.

G

GERIATRIC CARE: GENERAL PRINCIPLES

Zahra Sardar Sheikh, MD, MPH, CMD

BASICS

DESCRIPTION
"First do no harm"; many well-intended diagnostic and therapeutic interventions (with efficacy established in younger patients) may not benefit the elder. Geriatric care, more than many other medical specialties, focuses on preserving and improving function and comfort, rather than on life extension.

EPIDEMIOLOGY
The percentage of the U.S. population anticipated to be >65 years old by the year 2050 exceeds 20%, and the percentage of those who are >85 years old may reach 24%.

ETIOLOGY AND PATHOPHYSIOLOGY
Physiology of aging
- The aging process is not pathologic but part of the developmental continuum. However, physiologic changes associated with aging tend to diminish the body's compensatory reserve and increase susceptibility to disease.
  - Aging increases body fat and decreases total body water and lean body mass. This results in hydrophilic drugs having a smaller apparent volume of distribution. Lipophilic drugs will have an increased volume of distribution and longer half-life.
  - Aging decreases renal elimination of drugs.
  - Declines in lung capacity, oxygen uptake, cardiac output, muscle mass, glomerular filtration rate as well as blood flow to the brain, liver, and kidneys are associated with aging and must be considered in the diagnosis and treatment of elderly patients.

RISK FACTORS
Access to care
- Despite Medicare, persistent barriers to care include but not limited to lack of provider responsiveness, medical bills, and transportation.
- Barriers tend to be more prevalent in the female population and with increasing age.
- Alternatives to the traditional face-to-face visit have become more possible since the COVID-19 pandemic. These could enhance access to care, and these include:
  - Encrypted email or home telehealth for those who are technologically equipped
  - Phone visits for those with adequate hearing
  - Nurse visits at home to evaluate and plan care by reporting to provider

GENERAL PREVENTION
- Vaccination schedule for seniors: https://www.vaccines.gov/who_and_when/seniors/index.html
- Function is the heart of geriatric care. Assess and promote function at each encounter as changes in functional independence are common. Assess activities of daily living (ADLs) and instrumental ADLs (IADLs) (ability to use equipment such as a phone).
- Hearing assessment via hearing
  - Handicapped inventory
- Depression via:
  - Geriatric Depression Scale: https://consultgeri.org/try-this/general-assessment/issue-4.pdf
- Cognition via Mini Cognitive Assessment Instrument (https://www.alz.org/media/Documents/mini-cog.pdf) and Montreal Cognitive Assessment (https://mocacognition.com/#)

- Falls: Those with two or more falls in the past year, fall with injury requiring medical treatment, or fear of falling due to difficulty with gait or balance require a full fall risk assessment: https://www.cdc.gov/steadi/pdf/STEADI-Algorithm-508.pdf and https://www.cdc.gov/steadi/materials.html.
- Urinary incontinence: Inquire if patient has lost urine >5 times in past year.
- Polypharmacy
  - Use of five or more medications is polypharmacy.
  - Use pill bottles, pharmacy records, and patient and caregiver input to reconcile medication lists.
  - Ask about use of over-the-counter and alternative medications.
  - Reconcile medications at each visit.
  - Make an attempt to simplify medications at each encounter.
  - Engage patients and their caregivers in discussions regarding prescribing cascade and polypharmacy disadvantages.
- Substance use: CAGE criteria: https://www.mdcalc.com/cage-questions-alcohol-use
- Advanced care planning

ALERT
Completion of an advanced directive is critically important.

- Definition: Advanced directives are documents a person completes while still in possession of decisional capacity to ensure their values are reflected when considering how treatment decisions should be made on her or his behalf in the event she or he loses the capacity to make such decisions.
- Instruments:
  - Durable power of attorney: Patient (called the principal) appoints an agent to handle specific health, legal, and financial responsibilities.
  - Health care proxy: a durable power of attorney specifically for health care decisions; their role is to express the patient's wishes and make health care decisions if the patient cannot speak for themselves.
  - Living will: a legal document that allows patients to express their wishes for end-of-life medical care, in case they become unable to communicate their decisions
  - Discussions and completion of orders pertaining to end of life care, referred to as physician order for life-sustaining treatment (POLST) in most states and medical orders for life-sustaining treatment (MOLST) in some northeastern states

DIAGNOSIS

HISTORY
Optimizing communication
- Speak directly to your patient unless directed toward their surrogate.
- Assess and manage emotionally charged interactions. Refrain from taking negative energy personally.
- Assess patient and caregiver health literacy and adjust explanations accordingly.
- Gauge the degree of social and financial support.
- Establish patient's values, preferences, and goals of care.

PHYSICAL EXAM
Geriatric-specific considerations:
- Orthostatic hypotension: contributes to poor energy, diminished functional status, increased risk of falls, and decline in renal function due to ineffective organ perfusion
- Hypothermia/hyperthermia: increased susceptibility in the elderly; less likely to mount a fever in the setting of infection; consider thyroid derangement.
- Weight loss: Assess access to food; may be presenting feature in mood disorder, thyroid derangement, dementia, malignancy
- Hearing: Check for cerumen impaction; perform Whisper Test: https://www.youtube.com/watch?v=PzRzpW6JKzQ
- Gait, balance, and proximal muscle strength: assessed via Timed Get up and Go Test (https://www.cdc.gov/steadi/materials.html), functional reach test, and Tinetti balance assessment tool (https://www.uclahealth.org/sites/default/files/documents/2a/tinetti-gait-and-balance.pdf?f=4b27bebf and other sites)

DIFFERENTIAL DIAGNOSIS
Geriatric-specific presentations:
- Coronary artery disease: Elderly patients with coronary heart disease often present with atypical symptoms, including exertional dyspnea. Silent myocardial ischemia is also common.
- Constipation: In older adults, constipation due to slow transit is very common and may be associated with fecal impaction and overflow fecal incontinence.
- Delirium: Nearly 30% of older patients experience delirium at some time during hospitalization.
- Urinary tract infection (UTI): UTI is the most common infectious illness in adults aged ≥65 years, but diagnosis of UTI is fraught with difficulty because of the high prevalence of asymptomatic bacteriuria and pyuria, neither of which should be treated unless symptomatic. Asymptomatic bacteriuria is a marker for debility, but treatment does not improve outcomes and may cause harm.
- Depression: It is more common in elderly females. If left untreated, is often the precursor of overt dementia.
- Insomnia: Late-life insomnia is often persistent and may prompt self-medication with over-the-counter sleep aids or alcohol.
- Hearing difficulties: Some studies showed increased incidence of dementia in patient with hearing difficulties.
- Visual impairment: Macular degeneration, glaucoma and cataracts are the most commonly encountered causes and a yearly eye exam is important.

DIAGNOSTIC TESTS & INTERPRETATION
Informed decision-making
- Decision-making capacity: Evaluate in four areas: ability to understand information about treatment, ability to appreciate how that information applies to their situation, ability to reason with that information, and ability to make a choice and express it: http://www.aafp.org/afp/2001/0715/p299.html
- Surrogate decision maker
  - Patient-identified agent (durable power of attorney for health care, medical power of attorney, health care agent)
  - Court-appointed surrogate (legal guardian or conservator)

Diagnostic Procedures/Other
- Avoid unnecessary patient/caregiver burden if results will not significantly enhance the plan of care. Consider risks/harms, cost, time, travel, pain/discomfort, anxiety, and recovery time for all testing under consideration.
- Take into consideration renal function for imaging studies involving contrast.
- Many lab results require comparison with age-specific reference values (e.g., thyroid-stimulating hormone, A1c, prostate-specific antigen, D-dimer).

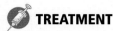 **TREATMENT**

GENERAL MEASURES
- Optimize nonpharmacologic options first.
- Align with patients' goals of care.
- Feasibility for patient and caregivers: Assess cost, availability, travel burden, and adherence.
- Compliance
- Nonpharmacologic (1)
  - Occupational therapy, physical therapy, speech therapy, hearing aids
  - Walking assist devices
  - Nonpharmacologic treatment of depression and insomnia
- Pharmacologic
  - Start low and go slow.
  - Adjust dose for renal and hepatic function, volume of distribution, decreased protein binding (more free/active drug available).
  - Be cognizant of pill burden, drug–drug interactions, and risks of polypharmacy. Anticoagulants and hypoglycemic medication (particularly insulin and sulfonylureas) are high-risk drugs in the elderly.
  - Beers criteria: assists in selecting medications with the best geriatric benefit-to-risk ratio; https://geriatricscareonline.org/ProductAbstract/american-geriatrics-society-updated-beers-criteria-for-potentially-inappropriate-medication-use-in-older-adults/CL001#
- Deprescribing: AGA and Choosing Wisely suggest:
  - Don't recommend percutaneous feeding tubes in patients with dementia; instead, offer oral-assisted feeding. Feeding tubes do not prolong life and may worsen suffering and thirst in this population.
  - Avoid antipsychotics as the first choice to treat behavioral and psychological symptoms of dementia.
  - Nonpharmacologic interventions are more efficacious than pharmacologic interventions for reducing aggression and agitation in adults with dementia. Antipsychotic medications increase risk of death. They may have a role in a carefully considered overall palliative plan that focuses on nonpharmacologic means of soothing agitation. And in individuals who are being cared for at home and lack of antipsychotics may add caregiver burden and hence hasten placement.
  - In diabetes care, meticulously avoid hypoglycemia, which is of far greater potential harm to the patient than is hyperglycemia. Metformin is generally safe. The major goal, especially in care of the older or more debilitated population is maintenance of glucose levels below those that cause symptomatic polyuria and polydipsia. This is not a specific A1c target.
- Don't use benzodiazepines or other sedative hypnotics in older adults for insomnia, agitation, or delirium.
  - Don't use antimicrobials to treat bacteriuria in older adults unless specific urinary tract symptoms are present. Delirium in patients seen in the ED and hospital is not likely caused by bacteriuria or lower UTI but usually by other causes.
  - Don't prescribe cholinesterase inhibitors for dementia without periodic assessment for perceived cognitive benefits and adverse gastrointestinal effects.
  - Don't recommend screening for breast, colorectal, prostate, or lung cancer without considering life expectancy and the risks of testing, overdiagnosis, and overtreatment.
  - Avoid using prescription appetite stimulants or high-calorie supplements for treatment of anorexia or cachexia in older adults; instead, optimize social supports, discontinue medications that may interfere with eating, provide appealing food and feeding assistance, and clarify patient goals and expectations.
  - Don't prescribe any medication without conducting a drug regimen review. Deprescribe when possible.
  - Don't use physical restraints to manage behavioral symptoms of hospitalized older adults with delirium.
- Geriatric pain management:
  - Stepwise care, nonpharmacologic interventions (PT, massage, environmental changes [e.g., music and aromatherapy], followed by cautious use of medication as necessary). NSAIDs involve significant risks in the elderly (renal, GI, cardiovascular). Use low doses of naproxen or ibuprofen preferentially, with GI-protective medication (e.g., omeprazole) if chronic therapy is needed.
  - Pharmacologic: Consider Beers criteria. Many commonly used medications (e.g., gabapentin) offer little benefit and significant potential for harm.
- Assess the home environment: Visiting Nurse Association (VNA) evaluation (social worker, PT/OT). Home visitation, social activity, and group support may be of particular value. Consider adult day program enrollment.

MEDICATION
First Line
Acetaminophen is the safest when used in <3 g dose over 24 hours

Second Line
Use caution with tramadol, narcotics, and NSAIDs.

ADMISSION, INPATIENT, AND NURSING CONSIDERATIONS
Inpatient prevention measures:
- Falls, acute delirium, skin breakdown, pain management, infections

 ONGOING CARE

FOLLOW-UP RECOMMENDATIONS
- Realistic expectations
- Carefully review medications, eliminate hospital-prescribed unnecessary medications.

Patient Monitoring
Use team members optimally: home health/VNA, social services.

DIET
A well-balanced diet should be encouraged and caloric intake should be optimal.

PATIENT EDUCATION
- Resources for caregivers:
  - Support group: Alzheimer's Association 800-272-3900
  - Respite care: It is important for caregivers to seek occasional respite from their responsibilities.
  - Local agency on aging (Councils on Aging)
- Elder mistreatment: Be aware of warning signs such as bruises and lacerations, fractures, malnutrition, and dehydration; can also screen using: Brief Abuse Screen for the Elderly (BASE).
  - Elder Assessment Instrument (EAI): pressure ulcers, signs of sexual abuse, change in the ability to manage and control finances (be alert for signs of financial exploitation).
- Consider referral for palliative care evaluation.
  - A philosophy of care for those with serious illnesses that focuses on symptom, pain, and stress relief with a goal of optimizing functional status and quality of life
- Consider referral for hospice, a model of end-of-life care, that provides physical, emotional, and spiritual support to patients with <6 months life expectancy to maintain optimal quality of life and die with dignity.

REFERENCE
1. Abraha I, Cruz-Jentoft A, Soiza RL, et al. Evidence of and recommendations for non-pharmacological interventions for common geriatric conditions: the SENATOR-ONTOP systematic review protocol. *BMJ Open*. 2015;5(1):e007488.

 CODES

ICD10
Z71.89 Other specified counseling

CLINICAL PEARLS
- Establish patient goals of care and align all clinical decisions within the context of these goals.
- Use an interdisciplinary team approach to optimize holistic care for elders and their caregivers.

G

GIARDIASIS

Marie L. Borum, MD, EdD, MPH • Nouf O. Turki, MD

BASICS

DESCRIPTION
- *Giardia lamblia* (also known as *Giardia duodenalis* or *Giardia intestinalis*) is a protozoan pathogen that leads to intestinal infection and is one of the most common causes of diarrhea worldwide.
- The life cycle consists of cysts and trophozoite stages. Transmission occurs via ingestion of infective cysts, followed by excystation in the duodenum with the release of trophozoites, leading to symptoms.
  - Trophozoites pass to the large intestine, where they revert to the infectious cyst form, which are excreted in the stool back into the environment.
- Most infections result from ingestion of unfiltered surface water (e.g., contaminated swimming areas) or fecal-oral transmission; less commonly acquired through contaminated food

EPIDEMIOLOGY
- Age
  - Most commonly children <5 years old and adults aged 25 to 44 years (1)
- Gender
  - More common in males
- Minimal seasonal variability: slight increase in cases reported in summer and early fall
- The highest risk areas include South and Southeast Asia, North Africa, the Caribbean, and South America (1).

Pediatric Considerations
- Most common in early childhood
- Chronic infection in children can lead to intestinal malabsorption (may also be associated with growth restriction/failure to thrive).

Incidence
- Estimated to cause 280 million diarrheal infections annually (2)
- In 2019, 14,887 cases were reported in the United States (~6 cases per 100,000) (3).
- In the United States, giardiasis affects 1.2 million individuals annually, resulting in 3,584 hospitalizations per year (4).
- The actual rate of giardiasis infection is likely much higher due to underreporting.

Prevalence
Occurs in about 2% of adults and 6–8% of children in developed countries, whereas 33% of people in developing countries have had giardiasis (4)

ETIOLOGY AND PATHOPHYSIOLOGY
Giardia trophozoites colonize the surface of the proximal small intestine.
- Cellular attachment to host enterocytes via the ventral suction disc and the excretion of parasite products results in structural damage compromising intestinal epithelial cells and inhibiting the function of brush border enzymes. This causes electrolyte imbalances and increased intestinal permeability, leading to the production of diarrhea (2).

Genetics
G. lamblia has eight defined genotypes (referred to as assemblages A–H), but only A and B are known to infect humans (2).

RISK FACTORS
- Daycare centers
- Anal intercourse
- Wilderness camping
- Travel to developing countries
- Children adopted from developing countries
- Drinking untreated water from lakes, streams, or wells
- Swimming in contaminated recreational water (pools, lakes, streams, rivers)
- Pets with *Giardia* infection/diarrhea
- Eating raw produce

GENERAL PREVENTION
- Hand hygiene
- Water purification when camping and when traveling to developing countries; boiling is the most effective.
- Properly cook all foods.
- Protect public water supply from fecal contamination.
- Sanitary disposal of feces
- Barrier protection during anal intercourse

COMMONLY ASSOCIATED CONDITIONS
Hypogammaglobulinemia, common variable immunodeficiency, IgA deficiency, and immunosuppression are associated with prolonged course of the disease and treatment failures.

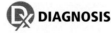

DIAGNOSIS

HISTORY
- Acute giardiasis
  - 50–75% of infected people are asymptomatic (4).
  - Symptomatic infections occur more frequently in children than adults (4).
  - Symptoms usually appear 1 to 2 weeks after exposure and may last 1 to 4 weeks.
  - Diarrhea (90%)
  - Malaise (86%)
  - Foul-smelling and fatty stools (75%)
  - Flatulence (75%)
  - Abdominal cramps and bloating (71%)
  - Nausea (69%)
  - Weight loss (66%)
  - Vomiting (23%)
  - Fever (15%)
  - Constipation (13%)
  - Urticaria (10%)
- Chronic giardiasis
  - Loose stools, steatorrhea
  - Profound weight loss, malabsorption, stunted growth
  - Malaise, fatigue
  - Depression
  - Abdominal cramping, borborygmi, flatulence, burping

PHYSICAL EXAM
- Vital signs are typically normal.
- Nonspecific; abdominal exam; may have bloating, tenderness, or increased bowel sounds
- Assess for weight loss, signs of dehydration, malabsorption, or failure to thrive in children.

DIFFERENTIAL DIAGNOSIS
- Cryptosporidiosis, microsporidiosis, strongyloidiasis, cyclosporiasis, amebiasis, *Dientamoeba fragilis* infection
- Viral gastroenteritis or traveler's diarrhea is caused by a range of pathogens, including *Escherichia coli* and *Campylobacter* spp.
- Other causes of malabsorption include lactose intolerance, celiac sprue, tropical sprue, bacterial overgrowth syndromes, and Crohn disease.
- Irritable bowel syndrome (diarrhea without weight loss)

DIAGNOSTIC TESTS & INTERPRETATION
Initial Tests (lab, imaging)
- Light microscopy of stool for ova and parasites:
  - Three serial stool specimens are collected every 2 to 3 days; single stool specimen examination has 50–70% sensitivity, whereas three serial specimens increase sensitivity to >90% (4).
  - Cysts in fixed or fresh stools, and occasionally trophozoites, are found in fresh diarrhea stools.
  - Test limitations: labor-intensive; experienced operator for interpretation; intermittent shedding means that ova may not be present in the stool sample.
- When available, gold-standard tests for diagnosis are direct fluorescent antibody (DFA) tests, which detect intact organisms with 92–100% sensitivity and 100% specificity, and ELISA, which detects soluble antigens in the stools with sensitivity 85–100% and specificity ≥95% (1). These two methods have increased turnaround time compared to stool microscopy (4)[B].
- PCR assays have replaced routine microscopy in some developed countries, showing sensitivity of 98% and specificity of 100% (4).
- Serologic tests for circulating IgG and IgM antibodies to *Giardia* are not appropriate for clinical diagnosis (1).

Follow-Up Tests & Special Considerations
String test (entero-test):
- A gelatin capsule on a string is swallowed and left in the duodenum for several hours or overnight. The string is removed and evaluated for the presence of trophozoites by microscopy.
- String test is being replaced by sensitive PCR stool assays but may still be useful if antigen assays are not available (1).

Diagnostic Procedures/Other
Esophagogastroduodenoscopy (EGD) with biopsy and a sample of small intestinal fluid

Test Interpretation
Intestinal biopsy shows flattened, mild lymphocytic infiltration and trophozoites on the surface.

TREATMENT

Outpatient for mild cases; inpatient if symptoms are severe enough to cause dehydration warranting parenteral fluid replacement

GENERAL MEASURES
- No treatment is required in asymptomatic patients.
- Prophylactic therapy is indicated for asymptomatic patients in close contact with pregnant or immunocompromised individuals and asymptomatic food handlers.
- Fluid replacement is the first line for dehydration.

MEDICATION
First Line
Drugs of choice
- Tinidazole: 2 g PO single dose (4)[A] and for age ≥3 years: 50 mg/kg PO single dose
- Nitazoxanide: 500 mg PO BID for 3 days (4)[A]

Second Line
Alternative agents
- Metronidazole: 250 mg PO TID for 5 to 7 days or 500 mg PO BID for 5 to 7 days (4)[A]
- Albendazole: 400 mg PO daily for 5 days
- Mebendazole: 200 mg PO TID for 5 days
- Paromomycin: 10 mg/kg PO TID for 5 to 10 days
- Furazolidone: 100 mg PO QID for 7 to 10 days
- Quinacrine: 100 mg PO TID for 5 days

Precautions
- Consumption of alcohol while on treatment with tinidazole or metronidazole has been associated with a disulfiram-like effect (diaphoresis, palpitations, facial flushing, nausea, vertigo, hypotension, and tachycardia) (4).
- Patient with refractory giardiasis who fail monotherapy may warrant combination therapy, high-dose therapy, and/or longer courses of therapy (4).
  - Confirmation of treatment failure is best provided by PCR (1).
  - Treatment failure might be due to host factors or to true drug resistance, which is increasingly common, particularly in travelers returning from South and Southeast Asia (1).

Pregnancy Considerations
- For patients with mild giardiasis, delay of treatment until 2nd trimester may be reasonable to avoid adverse drug effects to the fetus.
- Medications to treat giardiasis are relatively contraindicated during pregnancy.
- Paromomycin is a nonaminoglycoside recommended in pregnancy due to lower risk of teratogenicity because systemic absorption is low; cure rate, however, is about 60%, which is lower than most other agents (4).

Pediatric Considerations
- For children <12 months of age, metronidazole is the drug of choice.
- For children 12 to 36 months of age, nitazoxanide is preferred.
- For children ≥36 months of age, tinidazole is preferred.

ISSUES FOR REFERRAL
Patients with treatment failure should be discussed with or referred to a specialist, who should exclude underlying problems such as celiac disease, inherited disaccharidase deficiency, and immunodeficiency disorders, particularly of total and IgA antibody production (1).

ADDITIONAL THERAPIES
Fluids to prevent dehydration

COMPLEMENTARY & ALTERNATIVE MEDICINE
Zinc and vitamin A have been associated with protective effect against giardiasis among children.

 ONGOING CARE

FOLLOW-UP RECOMMENDATIONS
Patient Monitoring
Monitor symptoms, weight, and stool exams, particularly if patients fail to improve.

DIET
Low-lactose/lactose-free diet for at least 1 month; low-fat diet is generally helpful.

PATIENT EDUCATION
- Hand washing is more important than water purification to prevent transmission in outdoor enthusiasts.
- Lactose intolerance may follow *Giardia* infection and cause persistent diarrhea posttreatment. Recommend patients to adhere to a low-lactose/lactose-free diet to mitigate symptoms.
- CDC facts about *Giardia* and swimming pools: https://www.cdc.gov/healthywater/pdf/swimming/resources/giardia-factsheet.pdf
  - Don't swim if you have diarrhea.
  - Wash hands with soap after changing diapers before returning to the pool.
  - Do not ingest pool, lake, or river water.
  - Use chlorine to kill *Giardia* in water used for recreational activities.

PROGNOSIS
- Generally, prognosis is excellent; most patients are asymptomatic.
- Majority of infections resolve within a few weeks; occasionally may last for months and persist as chronic infections; patients with underlying immunodeficiency may experience more severe and prolonged illness.
- Mortality is rare, except in those cases of extreme dehydration that are untreated or inadequately treated, which occurs mainly in infants or malnourished children (4).

COMPLICATIONS
Malabsorption, impaired growth development, hypersensitivity reactions, weight loss, postinfectious IBS, and lactose intolerance; more rarely cholecystitis, cholangitis, granulomatous hepatitis, impaired exocrine pancreatic function

ALERT
Reportable disease to the CDC

REFERENCES
1. Minetti C, Chalmers RM, Beeching NJ, et al. Giardiasis. *BMJ*. 2016;355:i5369.
2. Adam RD. Giardia duodenalis: biology and pathogenesis. *Clin Microbiol Rev*. 2021;34(4):e0002419.
3. Centers for Disease Control and Prevention. *Giardiasis Summary Report—National Notifiable Disease Surveillance System, United States, 2019*. Atlanta, GA: Centers for Disease Control and Prevention; 2021.
4. Leung AKC, Leung AAM, Wong AHC, et al. Giardiasis: an overview. *Recent Pat Inflamm Allergy Drug Discov*. 2019;13(2):134–143.

ADDITIONAL READING
Fink MY, Singer SM. The intersection of immune responses, microbiota, and pathogenesis in giardiasis. *Trends Parasitol*. 2017;33(11):901–913.

 SEE ALSO

Algorithm: Diarrhea, Chronic

G

 CODES

ICD10
A07.1 Giardiasis [lambliasis]

CLINICAL PEARLS
- Daycare facilities and public swimming pools are common sources of *Giardia* transmission (a history of camping or recent travel is not required for the diagnosis).
- Abdominal bloating and loose, foul-smelling stool are common presenting symptoms.
- First-line treatment is tinidazole and nitazoxanide. Metronidazole is also highly effective (but less well tolerated).
- Most treatment failures may warrant combination therapy, high-dose therapy, and/or longer courses of therapy.
- DFA testing is the gold standard for diagnosis.

GILBERT SYNDROME

Jared Morphew, MD • Astrud S. A. Villareal, MD, FAAFP

 BASICS

Also known as Meulengracht disease

DESCRIPTION
A benign, inherited syndrome in which mild, intermittent unconjugated hyperbilirubinemia occurs in the absence of hemolysis or liver dysfunction

Pediatric Considerations
Rare for the disorder to be diagnosed before puberty

Pregnancy Considerations
The relative fasting that may occur with morning sickness can elevate bilirubin level.

EPIDEMIOLOGY
- Predominant age: present from birth but most often presents in the 2nd or 3rd decade of life
- Predominant sex: male > female (2 to 7:1)

Prevalence
The reported prevalence of Gilbert syndrome (GS) is between 5–10% in different populations, with most presentations during or after adolescence (1).

ETIOLOGY AND PATHOPHYSIOLOGY
Indirect hyperbilirubinemia in GS results from impaired hepatic bilirubin clearance (<30% of normal) due to decreased levels of the enzyme uridine diphospho-glucuronate-glucuronosyltransferase (UDPGT). Hepatic bilirubin conjugation (glucuronidation) is thus reduced, although this may not be the only defect.

Genetics
- Inherited defects within the promoter region of the gene that encodes the enzyme UDPGT yields reduced conjugation of bilirubin with glucuronic acid. In particular, patients with GS have a mutation in the UGT1A1 gene (1).
- Once considered as an autosomal dominant condition, GS is now thought to be inherited in an autosomal recessive manner.

RISK FACTORS
- Male gender
- Family history; particularly first-degree relatives

COMMONLY ASSOCIATED CONDITIONS
GS is part of a spectrum of hereditary disorders that includes types I and II Crigler-Najjar syndrome. However, bilirubin levels in these cases will be >6 mg/dL. There is an associated increased risk of cholelithiasis in certain populations. A neonatal presentation may lead to breast milk jaundice in the 2nd week of life.

DIAGNOSIS

HISTORY
- In patients with GS, a nonpruritic jaundice can occur in the setting of stressors like fasting, dehydration, infection, lack of sleep, physical exertion or overexertion, menstruation, or surgery. Other symptoms that may present during an episode of jaundice, including fatigue, are caused by the triggering factor and are not directly a result of GS.
- Some medications may also trigger episodes of jaundice in patients with GS due to abnormal metabolism. These include drugs that inhibit glucuronyl transferase (i.e., gemfibrozil) as well as selective protease inhibitors (i.e., atazanavir and indinavir). There is some evidence that tocilizumab, a monoclonal antibody used to treat rheumatoid arthritis, and ribavirin, an antiviral for hepatitis C treatment, may also induce jaundice. Note, the aforementioned drugs have not been associated with causing liver toxicity in patients with GS.

PHYSICAL EXAM
The physical exam is usually normal. Occasional mild jaundice precipitated by the aforementioned triggers may be seen. Careful attention should be paid for the stigmata of chronic liver disease, which should be absent.

DIFFERENTIAL DIAGNOSIS
- Hemolysis
- Ineffective erythropoiesis (megaloblastic anemias, certain porphyrias, thalassemia major, sideroblastic anemia, severe lead poisoning, congenital dyserythropoietic anemias)

- Cirrhosis
- Chronic persistent hepatitis
- Pancreatitis
- Biliary tract disease

DIAGNOSTIC TESTS & INTERPRETATION
Initial Tests (lab, imaging)
- Bilirubin: elevated but <6 mg/dL (103 μmol/L) and usually <3 mg/dL (51 μmol/L), virtually all unconjugated (indirect), with conjugated bilirubin within the normal range and/or <20% of the total bilirubin
- CBC with peripheral smear is normal.
- Reticulocyte count, haptoglobin, and lactate dehydrogenase levels are normal.
- Liver function tests (LFTs) (aspartate aminotransferase [AST], alanine transaminase [ALT], alkaline phosphatase, and γ-glutamyl transpeptidase [GGT]) are normal.
- Direct Coombs test is normal.
- Up to 60% of patients with GS have a clinically insignificant mild hemolysis that frequently can only be detected with sophisticated red cell survival studies.
- Drugs that may alter lab results: Bilirubin level may be raised by nicotinic acid and some other medications and lowered by phenobarbital. Administration of corticosteroids can reduce the plasma bilirubin concentrations as steroids increase the hepatic uptake of bilirubin.
- Disorders that may alter lab results: Bilirubin levels increase during fasting and may increase during a febrile illness.

Follow-Up Tests & Special Considerations
GS should be suspected if unconjugated hyperbilirubinemia persists in the absence of hemolysis or other liver dysfunction. A definitive diagnosis may be reported after 3 to 12 months of follow-up if the exam and diagnostic workup is otherwise normal.

Diagnostic Procedures/Other

- A presumptive diagnosis can be made in patients who have:
  - Unconjugated hyperbilirubinemia on repeated testing
  - Normal CBC, blood smear, and reticulocyte count
  - Normal plasma aminotransferases and alkaline phosphatase
- Confirmatory testing is rarely necessary. When patients continue to have normal lab studies apart from the plasma bilirubin elevation in the next 12 to 18 months, GS can be definitively diagnosed. Regarding possible additional testing (2):
  - A 48-hour fast is impractical and nonspecific for GS.
  - Provocation testing with rifampin could be employed if there is significant diagnostic doubt:
    - After 12 hours of fasting, an increase of total bilirubin to >1.9 mg/dL 2 hours after an oral dose of rifampin 900 mg distinguishes patients with GS with a sensitivity of 100% and a specificity of 100%.
  - Genetic testing is available in the form of polymerase chain reaction (PCR) or DNA-fragment sequencing for DNA mutations in the *UGT1A1* gene.

ALERT
A liver biopsy is not usually needed to exclude other diagnoses, unless concomitant liver disease is present.

 TREATMENT

- Outpatient
- Avoid unnecessary testing and procedures.
- Specific treatment is not necessary.
- Discussing mode of inheritance with patients and family members is important to prevent unnecessary testing and worry for family members.

 ONGOING CARE

FOLLOW-UP RECOMMENDATIONS
Patient Monitoring
Once GS has been confidently diagnosed, no further monitoring is required.

PATIENT EDUCATION
- Reassure patients that GS is benign.
- Educate patients on common triggers for jaundice.
- Recommend patients to inform medical providers of their diagnosis.
- Instruct patients to seek medical help if severe or prolonged jaundice occurs because these may be signs of a separate disease process.

PROGNOSIS
- GS is benign with an excellent prognosis.
- Patients with GS are able to serve as donors for right lobe of liver for transplantation.
- Preliminary evidence suggests that patients with GS may have protective properties against cardiovascular disease, type 2 diabetes mellitus, some cancers such as Hodgkin lymphoma, and all-cause mortality.

COMPLICATIONS
There are no known complications from GS.

ALERT
- Caution before using irinotecan in patients with GS. Once metabolized, this colorectal cancer treatment affects the enzyme responsible for GS, significantly increasing risk of toxicity.
- The impact of UGT1A1 mutations on the metabolism of chemotherapy agents should be taken into consideration in patients with known or suspected GS; however, there are no current recommendations on specific dose adjustments to minimize the risk of toxicity.

REFERENCES
1. Wagner KZ, Shiels RG, Lang CA, et al. Diagnostic criteria and contributors to Gilbert's syndrome. *Crit Rev Clin Lab Sci*. 2018;55(2):129–139.
2. Kwo PY, Cohen SM, Lim JK. ACG clinical guideline: evaluation of abnormal liver chemistries. *Am J Gastroenterol*. 2017;112(1):18–35.

 CODES

ICD10
- E80.4 Gilbert syndrome
- E80.6 Other disorders of bilirubin metabolism

CLINICAL PEARLS

- GS is a benign, inherited syndrome, in which mild, intermittent unconjugated hyperbilirubinemia causing jaundice occurs with otherwise normal liver function.
- Reduced hepatic bilirubin conjugation (glucuronidation) occurs due to altered *UDPGT1A1* gene promotion.
- GS is diagnosed when a mild, persistent, or recurrent elevation in unconjugated hyperbilirubinemia persists in the absence of hemolysis or other liver dysfunction.
- Confirmatory tests are not frequently needed, and a liver biopsy is not recommended, unless there is a serious concern for concomitant liver disease.
- Patient education and reassurance is essential, and unnecessary testing and procedures should be avoided.

G

GINGIVITIS

Karlynn Sievers, MD • Stephanie Vaux Voyles, MD

 BASICS

DESCRIPTION
Gingivitis is a reversible form of inflammation of the gingiva. It is a mild form of periodontal disease. Classification includes the following:
- Plaque induced
- Not plaque induced (bacterial, viral, or fungal; e.g., necrotizing ulcerative gingivitis, Vincent disease ["trench mouth"], denture related)
- Modified by systemic factors (e.g., pregnancy, puberty, HIV/AIDS, diabetes, smoking, leukemia)
- Modified by medications (calcium channel blockers, antipsychotics, antiepileptics, antirejection medications, hormones)
- Modified by malnutrition (vitamin deficiencies)
- Acute or chronic
- System(s) affected: gastrointestinal; ears, nose, throat; dental
- Synonym(s): mild periodontal disease; gum disease

Geriatric Considerations
More frequent in this age group

Pediatric Considerations
Cases of plaque-induced gingivitis are common in children (most common form of pediatric periodontal disease) and usually require no specific interventions other than improved oral hygiene.

Pregnancy Considerations
- Very common in pregnant women; hormonal effect
- Self-limited

EPIDEMIOLOGY
- Predominant age: children, teenagers, and young adults
- 42% of adults in the United States have periodontal diseases.

ETIOLOGY AND PATHOPHYSIOLOGY
Inflammation of the marginal gingiva; this can progress to deeper, destructive inflammation; if involving supporting bone, classified as periodontitis, not gingivitis
- Inadequate plaque removal
- Medication induced (e.g., oral contraceptives, antiepileptics)
- Nutritional deficiencies
- Vasoconstriction (nicotine, methamphetamine)
- Endocrine/hormonal variations
  - Pregnancy, menses, menarche
- Chronic debilitating disease
- Vincent disease, necrotizing ulcerative gingivitis
  - Synergistic infection with fusiform bacillus (*Fusobacterium* spp.) and spirochete (*Borrelia vincentii*)
- Pathology
  - Acute or chronic inflammation
  - Hyperemic capillaries
  - Polymorphonuclear infiltration
  - Papillary projections in subepithelial tissue
  - Fibroblasts

Genetics
Possible genetic link (up to 30% of population); rare condition called hereditary gingival fibromatosis, where severe gingival hyperplasia covers teeth, associated with hirsutism

RISK FACTORS
- Poor dental hygiene/plaque formation
- Pregnancy
- Uncontrolled diabetes mellitus
- Malocclusion, dental crowding, faulty dental restorations
- Smoking
- Mouth breathing
- Xerostomia
- HIV-positive; AIDS
- Vitamin C deficiency; coenzyme Q10 deficiency
- Dental appliances (dentures, braces)
- Necrotizing ulcerative gingivitis
  - Stress
  - Lack of sleep
  - Malnutrition
  - Viral illness
  - Typically, teens and young adults
- Bronchial asthma and other respiratory diseases
- Rheumatoid arthritis
- Epilepsy

GENERAL PREVENTION
- Good oral hygiene
  - Adults
    - Regular twice-daily brushing with fluoride toothpaste
    - Powered toothbrushes, especially the oscillating-rotating type, improve gingivitis (1).
    - Daily "high-quality" flossing (studies show that flossing only helps when it is done correctly), water jets, and interdental brushes (1)
    - Chlorhexidine with oral hygiene (2)
      - Use in acute phase.
  - Pediatrics
    - Regular twice-daily brushing with fluoride toothpaste under parental supervision until full manual dexterity (~8 years of age)
    - Regular flossing if no spaces between teeth
- Cleaning by a dentist or hygienist every 6 months or more frequently, as indicated
- Mouth rinse with essential oils (menthol, thymol, eucalyptol; e.g., Listerine) combined with brushing (1),(2)

COMMONLY ASSOCIATED CONDITIONS
- Periodontitis
- Glossitis
- Pedunculated growths (pyogenic granulomata)

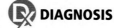 **DIAGNOSIS**

HISTORY
- Gingival erythema, edema, and bleeding
- Gingiva is tender to touch but otherwise painless.

- Bleeding of gingiva when brushing, flossing, or eating
- Inquire about HIV risk, pregnancy, nutritional deficiencies, diabetes, and other risk factors as indicated (see "Risk Factors").
- Smoking history
- Poor oral hygiene, infrequent dental visit history

PHYSICAL EXAM
- Normal gums should appear pink, firm, stippled, and scalloped.
- Gingivitis—marginal gingiva edematous with blunted papilla (usually painless, except to touch)
- Gingiva erythema: bright red or red-purple appearance
- Bleeding with manipulation of gingiva
- Biofilm of plaque (soft) and calculus (calcified, not easily removed)
- Edema of interdental papillae
- HIV gingivitis
  - Also called linear gingival erythema
  - Narrow band of bright red inflamed gum surrounding neck of tooth
  - Painful
  - Bleeds easily
  - Rapid destruction of gingival tissue and can progress to periodontitis with destruction of underlying support tissues (periodontal ligament, supporting alveolar bone)
- Vincent disease/necrotizing ulcerative gingivitis
  - Ulcers
  - Fever
  - Malaise
  - Regional lymphadenopathy
  - Pain
  - Mouth odor

DIFFERENTIAL DIAGNOSIS
- Periodontitis (deeper inflammation, causing destruction to connective tissue, ligaments, and alveolar bone)
- Glossitis
- Desquamative gingivitis (painful, persistent, usually middle-aged women)
- Pericoronitis (gum flap traps food and plaque over partially erupted 3rd molar), common in adolescence
- Gingival ulcers (aphthous, herpetic, malignancy, TB, syphilis)
- Specific forms of gingivitis: See "Description," including acute necrotizing ulcerative gingivitis (Vincent disease) and HIV gingivitis (linear gingival erythema), adrenal crisis, and leukemia.

DIAGNOSTIC TESTS & INTERPRETATION
Initial Tests (lab, imaging)
- No tests usually needed
- Possible smear or culture to identify causative agent (HIV gingivitis includes gram-negative anaerobes, enteric strains, and yeast—*Candida*.)
- Labs for contributing conditions (HIV, pregnancy, diabetes, nutritional deficiencies)
- Increase in C-reactive protein

TREATMENT

GENERAL MEASURES
- Stop any contributing medications.
- Remove irritating factors (plaque, calculus, faulty dental restorations, or partial dentures).
- Good oral hygiene (See "General Prevention.")
- Regular dental checkups (for scaling and polishing if plaque and/or tartar are present)
- Smoking cessation
- Special needs patients: use of tray-applied 10% carbamide peroxide gels

MEDICATION
First Line
- Chlorhexidine rinses or varnishes may be used. (Note: Prolonged use of chlorhexidine can lead to blackening of the tongue and taste alterations/metallic.) (3)
- Essential oil mouthwash (EOMW) may be equally effective to chlorhexidine for reduction of gingival inflammation (1),(2),(3).
- Antibiotics indicated *only* for acute necrotizing ulcerative gingivitis (Vincent disease):
  – Penicillin V: pediatric dose, 25 to 50 mg/kg/day divided q6h; adult dose, 250 to 500 mg q6h *or*
  – Metronidazole: pediatric dose, 30 mg/kg/day PO/IV divided q6h; maximum 4 g/day; adult dose, 500 mg BID or TID for 10 days *or*
  – Amoxicillin-clavulanic acid: pediatric dose, 30 mg/kg/day PO divided q12h; information: use 125 mg/31.25 mg/5 mL suspension; adult dose, 875 mg/125 mg PO BID for 10 days
  – Erythromycin: pediatric dose, 30 to 40 mg/kg/day divided q6h; adult dose, 250 mg q6h
  – Clindamycin: penicillin allergy; pediatric dose, 8 to 20 mg/kg/day in 3 to 4 divided doses as hydrochloride; adults, 300 mg q6h (maximum 1.8 g/day)
  – Doxycycline: adult dose, 100 mg BID on 1st day and then QD for 10 days
- Topical corticosteroids
  – Triamcinolone 0.1% in Orabase (spray or ointment), applied locally TID, QID
- Precautions
  – Erythromycin frequently causes GI issues.

Second Line
- Acetaminophen or ibuprofen for pain
- Other antibiotics or antifungal rinses or systemic according to culture or smear

---

- Decapinol oral rinse (surfactant that acts as a physical barrier, making it harder for bacteria to stick to the polysaccharide pellicle on tooth and mucosal surfaces) to reduce bacteria (not recommended for pregnant women or children aged <12 years); should be used in conjunction with traditional oral hygiene practices when those practices alone are not enough

ISSUES FOR REFERRAL
- Dental referral for acute gingivitis and routine cleanings and further treatment, as needed
- If gingivitis becomes periodontitis, deep root scaling, root planing, and antibiotics may be indicated.

SURGERY/OTHER PROCEDURES
- Débridement for acute necrotizing gingivitis
- Minor surgery may be necessary to correct tissue overgrowth for gingivitis caused by medicines/hereditary gingival fibromatosis.

COMPLEMENTARY & ALTERNATIVE MEDICINE
- Bilberry: potentially helpful in reducing inflammation and stabilizing collagen tissue
- Coenzyme Q10: topically, to restore coenzyme Q10 deficiency
- Replace any nutritional deficiencies (e.g., vitamins A, B$_{12}$, C).

 ONGOING CARE

FOLLOW-UP RECOMMENDATIONS
Patient Monitoring
Until clear; dental follow-up for continued cleanings and secondary prevention

DIET
- Well-balanced diet that includes fruits, vegetables, and vitamin C
- Avoid sugary snacks and drinks, which contribute to plaque formation.
- Soft foods during flare, if significant inflammation/bleeding

PATIENT EDUCATION
- Good oral hygiene, including twice-daily brushing with circular oscillating electric brush, fluoridated toothpaste, and daily flossing; regular dental visits
- Printable and viewable patient information available from the American Dental Association at https://www.mouthhealthy.org/en.org/en/, and the American Academy of Periodontology under "For Patients" at https://www.perio.org/, and National Institute of Dental and Craniofacial Research at https://www.nidcr.nih.gov/oralhealth/Topics/GumDiseases/PeriodontalGumDisease.htm

---

PROGNOSIS
- Usual course: acute, relapsing, intermittent; chronic
- Prognosis: generally favorable, responds well to appropriate treatment
- Left untreated, may progress to periodontitis (controversial), which is a major cause of tooth loss

COMPLICATIONS
Severe periodontal disease (which is associated with supporting bone loss, tooth loss, heart disease, diabetes, dementia, and preterm birth)

REFERENCES
1. Kumar S. Evidence-based update on diagnosis and management of gingivitis and periodontitis. *Dent Clin North Am.* 2019;63(1):69–81.
2. Karamani I, Kalimeri E, Seremidi K, et al. Chlorhexidine mouthwash for gingivitis control in orthodontic patients: a systematic review and meta-analysis. *Oral Health Prev Dent.* 2022;20(1):279–294.
3. Figuero E, Roldán S, Serrano J, et al. Efficacy of adjunctive therapies in patients with gingival inflammation: a systematic review and meta-analysis. *J Clin Periodontol.* 2020;47(Suppl 22):125–143.

 SEE ALSO

- Dental Infection; Glossitis
- Algorithm: Bleeding Gums

G

CODES

ICD10
- K05.10 Chronic gingivitis, plaque induced
- K05.11 Chronic gingivitis, non-plaque induced
- K05.00 Acute gingivitis, plaque induced

CLINICAL PEARLS
- Gingivitis may be prevented and treated with regular dental cleanings, good oral hygiene, and use of certain mouth rinses including chlorhexidine.
- Untreated, gingivitis may progress to periodontitis, a possible contributor to systemic inflammation and its consequences (e.g., coronary artery disease and uncontrolled diabetes).
- New-onset or difficult-to-treat gingivitis, consider differential of etiology: pregnancy, HIV, diabetes, medications, and vitamin deficiencies.

GLAUCOMA, PRIMARY CLOSED-ANGLE

Richard W. Allinson, MD • Hunter Grey, OD

 BASICS

DESCRIPTION
- Glaucoma is a progressive decline in vision from damage to the optic nerve and is usually associated with elevated intraocular pressure (IOP) in the eye. Angle-closure is a mechanical blockage of the trabecular meshwork (TM) by the peripheral iris.
- In primary angle-closure (PAC), there is an anatomic predisposition with no identifiable secondary pathologic condition.
- In secondary angle-closure, there is an identifiable pathologic cause, such as iris neovascularization or an enlarged cataractous lens.
- Angle-closure can be classified as the following:
  - Primary angle-closure suspect (PACS) is >180 degrees of iridotrabecular contact (ITC) but no evidence of TM or optic nerve damage
  - PAC is >180 degrees of ITC with peripheral anterior synechiae (PAS) or elevated IOP but with no optic neuropathy.
  - Primary angle-closure glaucoma (PACG) is PAC with glaucomatous optic neuropathy.
  - Acute primary angle-closure (APAC) or acute angle-closure crisis (AACC) is when the angle is occluded with symptomatic high IOP. It is a medical emergency requiring prompt treatment.
  - Chronic angle-closure (CAC) may develop after APAC in which synechial closure persists. It can also develop when the angle gradually closes and the angle function becomes progressively compromised leading to a slow rise in IOP. Vision loss may be the presenting complaint because of the asymptomatic nature of the condition.

Geriatric Considerations
Increased risk with age and cataracts

Pregnancy Considerations
Majority of IOP-lowering medications are within class C, and the risk of adverse effects to the fetus must be balanced with risk of vision loss in the mother.

EPIDEMIOLOGY
- Female sex. PAC is 2 to 4 times more common in women than in men. Women tend to have smaller anterior segments and shorter axial lengths.
- More likely in those of Inuit and East or South Asian descent

Prevalence
The prevalence of PACG in patients >40 years varies depending on race and ethnicity. The prevalence is 0.1–0.2% in blacks, 0.1–0.6% in whites, 0.3% in the Japanese, 0.4–1.4% in other East Asians, and 2.1–5.0% in the Inuit. The burden of PACG is greater in Asian countries.

ETIOLOGY AND PATHOPHYSIOLOGY
- PAC happens when iris touches the TM in the anterior chamber angle. ITC causes obstruction of aqueous humor outflow through the TM, which causes elevation in IOP. Prolonged ITC can cause scarring, with formation of PAS.

- Most common underlying mechanism of angle-closure is pupillary blockage of the aqueous flow from posterior to anterior chamber. This causes increase in pressure in the posterior chamber as compared to the anterior chamber. The buildup of pressure in the posterior chamber leads to anterior bowing of the iris and closing of the angle.
  - One of the most important factors in closing the angle in an anatomically predisposed eye is dilation of the pupil. Dilation leading to closure of the angle may occur as a result of a variety of causes including darkness, emotion, and medications that can cause the pupil to dilate. Pupillary block is maximal when the pupil is in the mid-dilated position.
- Plateau iris syndrome is an atypical configuration of the anterior chamber angle that can result in acute or chronic PAC. Angle-closure in plateau iris is most often caused by anteriorly positioned ciliary processes that narrow the anterior chamber recess by pushing the peripheral iris forward. A component of pupillary block is often present.

Genetics
First-degree relatives have a 1–12% increased risk in whites; 6 times greater risk in Chinese patients with positive family history

RISK FACTORS
- Age >50 years
- Female gender
- Family history of angle-closure
- Hyperopia
- Anterior positioned lens
- Drugs that can induce angle-closure by dilating the pupil include:
  - Adrenergic agonists (albuterol, phenylephrine), anticholinergics (oxybutynin, atropine), antihistamines, antidepressants including selective serotonin reuptake inhibitors (SSRIs) and tricyclic antidepressants (TCAs), and cocaine
- Drugs that can induce angle-closure by causing a uveal effusion include:
  - Topiramate and other sulfonamides

GENERAL PREVENTION
- Routine eye exam with gonioscopy for high-risk populations
- Prophylactic laser peripheral iridotomy (LPI) may be considered in PACS patients for preventing PACG.
- Argon laser peripheral iridoplasty for plateau iris syndrome

COMMONLY ASSOCIATED CONDITIONS
- Cataract
- Hyperopia

℞ DIAGNOSIS

HISTORY
- Patient may be asymptomatic as in PACS or may have acute symptoms as in APAC.
- Acute symptoms commonly include unilateral:
  - Severe eye pain
  - Blurred vision
  - Eye redness
  - Halos around lights/objects
  - Headache
  - Nausea and vomiting

- Patients with PACG can be asymptomatic, have subacute symptoms (intermittent subacute attacks), or compromised peripheral vision.
- Family history of acute angle-closure glaucoma
- Obtain history of prescription, over-the-counter, and herbal medications.

PHYSICAL EXAM
Includes, but is not limited to, the following in the undilated eye:
- Visual acuity with refractive error (hyperopic eyes especially in older phakic patients)
- Visual field testing
- Pupil size and reactivity (mid-dilated, asymmetric or oval, minimally reactive, and may have relative afferent pupillary defect)
- Slit-lamp examination demonstrates conjunctival hyperemia (in acute cases), central and peripheral anterior chamber shallowing, corneal edema, iris abnormalities (diffuse and focal iris atrophy, posterior synechiae), and lens changes (cataract and glaukomflecken-patchy localized anterior subcapsular lens opacities).
- IOP elevation. During an acute attack, the IOP may be high enough to cause glaucomatous optic nerve damage, ischemic nerve damage, and/or retinal vascular occlusion.
- The Van Herick assessment (VHA) is a noncontact estimate of the angle configuration based on comparison of peripheral anterior chamber depth to peripheral corneal thickness using a thin slit lamp beam of light. Even when performed by experienced ophthalmologists, VHA misses a substantial proportion of angle-closure.
- Gonioscopy allows visualization of anatomy of the angle of both eyes. Look for ITC and PAS.
- Anterior segment imaging with ultrasound (US) biomicroscopy and anterior segment optical coherence tomography (AS-OCT) to understand the angle anatomy

DIFFERENTIAL DIAGNOSIS
- Secondary angle closure due to iris membranes:
  - Neovascularization of the iris
  - Iridocorneal endothelial (ICE) syndrome
- Secondary pupillary block due to the following:
  - Uveitis with secondary posterior synechiae leading to iris bombe
  - Lens-related disorders, such as ectopia lentis or malpositioned intraocular lenses (IOLs)
- Retinal conditions leading to the forward shift of the lens-iris diaphragm (uveal effusion, hemorrhagic choroidal detachment, intraocular tumors
- Topiramate is an oral medication prescribed for the treatment of epilepsy, depression, and headaches. In some patients, this medication may cause a syndrome characterized by acute myopic shift and acute bilateral angle closure. Treatment involves immediate discontinuation of the medication and initiation of medical therapy to lower the IOP. Cycloplegia may deepen the anterior chamber and relieve the attack. Because pupillary block is not an underlying mechanism of this syndrome, an LPI is not indicated.
- Malignant glaucoma (also called aqueous misdirection) is a rare form of glaucoma that usually presents following ocular surgery. Miotics can make malignant glaucoma worse and should not be used; instead, use cycloplegics.

DIAGNOSTIC TESTS & INTERPRETATION
Initial Tests (lab, imaging)
- Gonioscopy
- US biomicroscopy
- AS-OCT

Test Interpretation
Narrow or closed anterior chamber angle

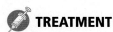 TREATMENT

ALERT
For patients with acute symptoms (severe eye pain, blurred vision, eye redness, halos around lights/objects, headache, nausea and vomiting) and asymmetric pupillary response, obtain immediate consultation with ophthalmology.

GENERAL MEASURES
Goals of treatment are to reverse or prevent angle-closure process, to control IOP, and to prevent damage to the optic nerve.

MEDICATION
- During acute attack, medical therapy lowers IOP to relieve symptoms and clear corneal edema so that LPI can be performed as soon as possible.
- Medical therapy aims at:
  - Reduction of aqueous production:
    - Carbonic anhydrase inhibitors (CAIs): acetazolamide 250 to 500 mg IV or 250 mg tab × 2 PO at once; topical CAI such as dorzolamide 2%; CAIs are contraindicated in sulfa allergy and hepatic insufficiency.
    - Topical β-blockers such as timolol 0.5%; use with caution in patients with lung disease.
    - Topical α_2-agonists such as brimonidine 0.2%
  - Prostaglandin analogues such as latanoprost 0.005% enhance uveoscleral outflow and increase aqueous outflow.
  - Pupillary constriction to open the chamber angle: topical pilocarpine 1% or 2% q15min × 3. Miotic therapy may be ineffective when IOP is markedly elevated due to iris sphincter ischemia.
  - Topical steroid such as prednisolone acetate 1% q15–30min × 4 and then hourly to treat the inflammation
  - Hyperosmotic agents which reduce the vitreous volume, which in turn reduces IOP:
    - Glycerin 50% solution administered orally, dosage is 1 to 1.5 g/kg. Use with caution if patient has nausea or emesis. To improve the taste, the solution may be mixed with a small amount of orange juice and poured over crushed ice.
    - Mannitol 20% solution, administered IV at 1.5 to 2 g/kg of body weight over 30 minutes to 60 minutes
      - Hyperosmotic agent should be used with caution in patients with heart and kidney disease. Glycerin can increase blood sugar level and should not be given to diabetic patients.

- During acute attack, acetazolamide 500 mg IV is given followed by 500 mg PO BID. Topical therapy is initiated with 0.5% timolol maleate and 0.2% brimonidine drops 1 minute apart. Reduction of inflammation is accomplished with frequent topical steroids. In addition, systemic therapy with mannitol 20% 1.5 to 2.0 g/kg infused over 30 to 60 minutes or oral glycerol (Osmoglyn) (50%) 6 oz PO may be needed. Treat pain and nausea with analgesic and antiemetics. Initiate treatment with 3 doses of 1% or 2% pilocarpine drops administered 15 minutes apart to cause miosis in an attempt to open the angle.

SURGERY/OTHER PROCEDURES
- Definitive therapy for PAC, PACG, and AACC is Nd:YAG or argon LPI. LPI can be performed temporally or superiorly. Location of the LPI does not seem to influence the occurrence of new postoperative dysphotopsias.
- Surgical iridectomy may be performed if cornea is cloudy and laser iridotomy cannot be performed.
- Plateau iris syndrome may be initially treated by either LPI or lensectomy if a cataract is present. Eyes with plateau iris syndrome remain predisposed to angle closure despite a patent iridotomy or lensectomy.
  - Argon laser peripheral iridoplasty may be needed to flatten and thin the peripheral iris.
- Growing evidence shows cataract extraction alone can lower IOP and reduce the risk of lens-induced angle closure. This can be considered as a treatment option in appropriate cases. Other procedures to reduce IOP include argon laser peripheral iridoplasty (especially for plateau iris syndrome), anterior chamber paracentesis, goniosynechialysis, and trabeculectomy.
  - APAC patients who underwent phacoemulsification with an IOL had better IOP control, deeper anterior chambers, and required less glaucoma medications than those who underwent LPI alone. Performing phacoemulsification weeks to months after the initial LPI did not appear to adversely affect outcomes compared to early phacoemulsification (1)[B].
  - Clear lens extraction (CLE) can be considered for first-line treatment of eyes with more advanced angle-closure disease, such as APAC eyes with an IOP >30 mmHg (2)[C].

 ONGOING CARE

FOLLOW-UP RECOMMENDATIONS
Patient Monitoring
Half of the other eye of patients with APAC will develop APAC within 5 years. Hence, prophylactic LPI should be performed in the other eye as soon as possible.

PATIENT EDUCATION
- Advise patient to seek emergency attention if experiencing a change in visual acuity, blurred vision, eye pain, or headache.
- PACS patients and no LPI; avoid use of decongestants, motion sickness medications, adrenergic agents, antipsychotics, antidepressants, and anticholinergic agents.

PROGNOSIS
- Prognosis depends on ethnicity, underlying eye disease, and time to treatment.
- After LPI, most PACS subjects can be expected to have no further treatment.
- Many PAC and APAC eyes and most PACG eyes are given additional treatment to control IOP after LPI.

COMPLICATIONS
- Chronic angle closure
- Iris atrophy; cataract; optic atrophy
- Malignant glaucoma
- Central retinal artery/vein occlusion
- Permanent decrease in visual acuity; blindness
- Fellow (contralateral) eye attack

REFERENCES
1. Lin YH, Wu CH, Huang SM, et al. Early versus delayed phacoemulsification and intraocular lens implantation for acute primary angle-closure. *J Ophthalmol*. 2020;2020:8319570.
2. Tanner L, Gazzard G, Nolan WP, et al. Has the EAGLE landed for the use of clear lens extraction in angle-closure glaucoma? And how should primary angle-closure suspects be treated? *Eye (Lond)*. 2020;34(1):40–50.

CODES

ICD10
- H40.20X0 Unsp primary angle-closure glaucoma, stage unspecified
- H40.219 Acute angle-closure glaucoma, unspecified eye
- H40.2290 Chronic angle-closure glaucoma, unsp eye, stage unspecified

CLINICAL PEARLS

For patients with acute symptoms (severe eye pain, blurred vision, eye redness, halos around lights/objects, headache, nausea and vomiting) and asymmetric pupillary response, obtain immediate consultation with ophthalmology.

G

GLAUCOMA, PRIMARY OPEN-ANGLE

Bethany P. Marshall, PharmD • Frederick C. Stone Jr., MD, MPH

 BASICS

DESCRIPTION

Primary open-angle glaucoma (POAG) is a chronic, progressive optic neuropathy which causes loss of the optic nerve rim and retinal nerve fiber layer (RNFL) with associated visual field defects. POAG is associated with increased intraocular pressure (IOP). Normal IOP is 10 to 21 mm Hg. However, early glaucoma can be present even with normal IOP, which can make early detection very difficult.

Pregnancy Considerations
Prostaglandins should be avoided during pregnancy in the treatment of POAG.

EPIDEMIOLOGY
Prevalence
- Prevalence in persons >40 years of age is ~3.5%.
- POAG is the second leading cause of blindness and the leading cause of blindness of people of African descent in the United States.

ETIOLOGY AND PATHOPHYSIOLOGY
- Aqueous humor is produced by the ciliary epithelium of the ciliary body and is secreted into the posterior chamber of the eye. The purpose of aqueous humor is to maintain the shape and function of the eye as well as provide nourishment. Aqueous humor then flows through the pupil and enters the anterior chamber to be drained by the trabecular meshwork (TM) in the iridocorneal angle of the eye. It then drains into the Schlemm canal and passes into the episcleral venous system. 5–10% of the total aqueous humor outflow leaves via the uveoscleral pathway.
- IOP is maintained by a balance of aqueous humor production in the ciliary body and drainage by the TM.
- Impaired aqueous humor outflow through the TM leads to greater resistance in the aqueous humor drainage system and causes an increase in IOP.
- IOP varies with blood pressure and respirations as well as throughout the day with lower IOP observed in the evenings.
- Increase in IOP above normal values over time can damage the optic nerve, eventually leading to vision loss. Typically, peripheral vision is lost before central vision, which allows POAG to go undiagnosed for longer.

Genetics
- TMCO1 genotype has been found to increase the risk of developing glaucoma among non-Hispanic whites.
- The myocilin (MYOC) gene was the first gene associated with POAG.

RISK FACTORS
- Myopia
- Diabetes mellitus, hypothyroidism, hypertension
- African descent
- Positive family history
- Prolonged use of corticosteroids
- Systemic calcium channel blockers
- High coffee consumption

- Prior history of pars plana vitrectomy
- Obstructive sleep apnea

GENERAL PREVENTION
Higher dietary nitrate and green leafy vegetable intake has been associated with a lower POAG risk. Evidence suggests that nitrate, a precursor of nitric oxide, is beneficial for blood circulation.

 DIAGNOSIS

HISTORY
Painless, slowly progressive visual loss; patients are generally unaware of the visual loss until late in the disease. Central visual acuity remains unaffected until late in the disease.

PHYSICAL EXAM
- Visual acuity and visual field assessment
- Ophthalmoscopy to assess optic nerve for glaucomatous damage
- Tonometry to measure IOP; the IOP may be elevated or within the normal range.
- CDR score of >0.5: Normal eyes show a characteristic configuration for disc rim thickness of inferior ≥ superior ≥ nasal ≥ temporal (ISNT rule).
- Earliest visual field defects are paracentral scotomas and peripheral nasal steps.

DIFFERENTIAL DIAGNOSIS
- Normal-tension glaucoma
- Optic nerve pits
- Anterior ischemic optic neuropathy
- Compressive lesions of the optic nerve or chiasm

DIAGNOSTIC TESTS & INTERPRETATION
Initial Tests (lab, imaging)
Optical coherence tomography (OCT) can be useful in the detection of glaucoma.
- The RNFL is thinner in patients with glaucoma.
- OCT angiography (OCTA) demonstrates a decrease in macular vessel density in eyes with POAG. OCTA shows that parapapillary choroidal microvasculature dropout (MvD) is associated with progressive RNFL thinning in POAG. Macular, peripapillary, and choroidal vessel density measurements may complement visual field and structural OCT measurements (1)[A].

Diagnostic Procedures/Other
- Visual field testing: perimetry
- Tonometry to measure IOP: Thicker corneas resist the deformation inherent in most methods of tonometry, which may result in an overestimation of the IOP. Thinner corneas may give an artificially low reading.

Test Interpretation
- Atrophy and cupping of optic nerve
- Macular ganglion cell-inner plexiform layer (mGCIPL) OCT thickness is effective for predicting glaucoma progression regardless of the presence of high myopia (2)[B]. The peripapillary RNFL of highly myopic eyes tends to be thinner than that of normal eyes.

 TREATMENT

GENERAL MEASURES
- Early Manifest Glaucoma Trial compared observation to treatment with betaxolol combined with argon laser trabeculoplasty (ALT) and found that early treatment delays progression, with the magnitude of initial IOP reduction influencing disease progression.
- Ocular Hypertension Treatment Study of patients with increased IOP of 24 to 32 mm Hg were treated with topical ocular hypotensive medication with a ~20% reduction in IOP. At 5 years, treatment reduced the incidence of POAG by >50%: 9.5% in the observation group versus 4.4% in the medication-treated group.
- Advanced Glaucoma Intervention Study randomized patients to laser trabeculoplasty or filtering surgery when medical therapy failed. In follow-up, if IOP was always <18 mm Hg, visual fields tended to stabilize. When IOP was >17 mm Hg, more than half of the time, patients tended to have worsening of visual fields.
- Collaborative Initial Glaucoma Treatment Study demonstrated that both initial medical and surgical (trabeculectomy) treatment achieved significant IOP reduction, and both had little visual field loss over time.
- The selective laser trabeculoplasty (SLT) versus eye drops for first-line treatment of ocular hypertension and glaucoma trial showed a reduction in IOP in SLT compared to medical treatment over a 3-year period.

MEDICATION
More than one medication, with different mechanisms of action, may be needed. Categories include the following:

- Prostaglandin analogues: generally used as first-line treatment; enhance uveoscleral outflow and increase aqueous humor outflow through the TM: latanoprost 0.005% 1 drop at bedtime; travoprost 0.004% 1 drop at bedtime; bimatoprost 0.01% 1 drop at bedtime
  - Latanoprostene bunod, 0.024% solution; this is a combination drug with one of the actions being the release of nitric oxide. Instill 1 drop at bedtime.
  - Contraindications/precautions
    - Prostaglandin analogues may cause increased pigmentation of the iris and periorbital tissue.
    - Increased pigmentation and growth of eyelashes
    - Should be used with caution in active intraocular inflammation (iritis/uveitis)
    - Caution is also advised in eyes with risk factors for herpes simplex, iritis, and cystoid macular edema.
    - Macular edema may be a complication associated with treatment.
    - Avoid during pregnancy.

- β-Adrenergic antagonists (nonselective and selective): decrease aqueous humor formation; best when used as an add-on therapy: timolol 0.25% (initial) to 0.5% 1 drop in affected eye q12h; gel-forming solution (0.25% or 0.5%) 1 drop in affected eye once daily (nonselective); betaxolol 0.5% 1 drop in affected eye BID (selective)
  - Nonselective β-adrenergic antagonists: Avoid in asthma, chronic obstructive pulmonary disease (COPD), 2nd- and 3rd-degree atrioventricular (AV) block, and decompensated heart failure. Betaxolol is a selective β-adrenergic antagonist and is safer in patients with pulmonary disease.
  - β-Adrenergic antagonists: caution in patients taking calcium antagonists because of possible AV conduction disturbances, left ventricular failure, or hypotension
- Adrenergic agonists (selective α_2-adrenergic agonists)
  - Brimonidine tartrate 0.2%: 1 drop TID (α_2-adrenergic agonist) decreases aqueous humor formation and increases uveoscleral outflow.
    - Brimonidine should not be used in infants and young children because of the risk of CNS depression, apnea, bradycardia, and hypotension.
    - Monoamine oxidase inhibitors and tricyclic antidepressants may interfere with the metabolism of brimonidine and result in toxicity.
- Carbonic anhydrase inhibitors (oral, topical) decrease aqueous humor formation.
  - Acetazolamide: 250 mg PO 1 to 4 times per day
  - Dorzolamide 2%: 1 drop TID
  - Brinzolamide 1%: 1 drop TID
  - Carbonic anhydrase inhibitors
    - Do not use with sulfa drug allergies.
    - Do not use if patient has cirrhosis because of the risk of hepatic encephalopathy.
- Rho kinase (ROCK) inhibitors increase aqueous humor outflow through the trabecular outflow pathway by decreasing actomyosin-driven cellular contraction and reducing production of fibrotic extracellular matrix proteins.
  - Netarsudil 0.02%: 1 drop once daily in the evening
  - Corneal verticillata, or whorl keratopathy, can occur with its usage.
- Parasympathomimetics (miotics) including direct-acting cholinergic agonists increase aqueous humor outflow.
  - Pilocarpine 1–4%: 1 drop in affected eye BID–QID (direct-acting cholinergic agonist)
  - Parasympathomimetics (miotics): cause pupillary constriction and may cause decreased vision in patients with a cataract; may cause eye pain or myopia due to increased accommodation; all miotics break down the blood–aqueous humor barrier and may induce chronic iridocyclitis.
- Hyperosmotic agents: increase blood osmolality, drawing water from the vitreous cavity; these can be especially helpful in acute emergencies when awaiting evaluation by specialist or awaiting surgical intervention.
  - Mannitol 20% solution is administered IV at 0.5 to 2 g/kg of body weight over a period of 45 minutes.

- Glycerin 50% solution is administered orally; dosage is 1.0 to 1.5 g/kg, this is usually 4 to 7 oz. To improve the taste, the solution may be mixed with a small amount of orange juice and poured over crushed ice.
- Hyperosmotic agents: caution in diabetics; dehydrated patients; and those with cardiac, renal, and hepatic disease
- Contact lens wearers: Many glaucoma drops contain benzalkonium chloride; remove contact lens prior to administration and wait 15 minutes before reinsertion.

SURGERY/OTHER PROCEDURES
- ALT
  - Improves aqueous humor outflow
- Selective 532-nm Nd:YAG laser trabeculoplasty (SLT)
  - As effective as ALT in lowering IOP
  - May be repeated if necessary
- Trabeculectomy (glaucoma filtering surgery)
  - Usually reserved for patients needing better IOP control after maximal medical therapy and who may have previously undergone an ALT/SLT
- Shunt (tube) surgery (e.g., Molteno, Ahmed devices)
  - Reserved for difficult glaucoma cases in which conventional filtering surgery has failed or is likely to fail
  - Tube Versus Trabeculectomy (TVT) study showed after 5 years of follow-up, both procedures were associated with similar IOP reduction and the number of glaucoma medications needed.
- Ciliary body ablation: indicated to lower IOP in patients with poor visual potential or those who are poor candidates for filtering or shunt procedures
- Minimally invasive glaucoma surgery (MIGS) is frequently combined with cataract surgery; currently targeted at patients with mild to moderate glaucoma
  - Schlemm canal, suprachoroidal, or subconjunctival stents
  - The Kahook Dual Blade performs an excisional goniotomy by removing a strip of TM.
  - Cataract extraction can decrease IOP in patients with ocular hypertension.

ONGOING CARE

FOLLOW-UP RECOMMENDATIONS
Patient Monitoring
- Monitor vision and IOP every 3 to 6 months.
- Optic nerve evaluation every 3 to 18 months, depending on POAG control
- A worsening of the mean deviation by 2 dB on the Humphrey field analyzer and confirmed by a single test after 6 months had a 72% probability of progression.

PATIENT EDUCATION
POAG is a silent robber of vision, and patients may not appreciate the significance of their disease until much of their visual field is lost. Patients should ensure compliance with any prescribed medications if diagnosed with POAG.

PROGNOSIS
- With standard glaucoma therapy, the rate of visual field loss in POAG is slow.
- Patients still may lose vision and develop blindness, even when treated appropriately.
- The structure of the mGCIPL was better preserved in surgically treated eyes than in medically treated eyes, even when the IOPs were similar during follow-up in cases of advanced glaucoma.

COMPLICATIONS
Blindness

REFERENCES
1. WuDunn D, Takusagawa HL, Sit AJ, et al. OCT angiography for the diagnosis of glaucoma: a report by the American Academy of Ophthalmology. *Ophthalmology*. 2021;128(8):1222–1235.
2. Shin JW, Song MK, Sung KR. Longitudinal macular ganglion cell-inner plexiform layer measurements to detect glaucoma progression in high myopia. *Am J Ophthalmol*. 2021;223:9–20.

ADDITIONAL READING
Weinreb RN, Khaw PT. Primary open-angle glaucoma. *Lancet*. 2004;363(9422):1711–1720.

G

CODES

ICD10
H40.1190 Primary open-angle glaucoma, unspecified eye, stage unspecified

CLINICAL PEARLS
- Painless, slowly progressive visual loss; patients generally are unaware of the visual loss until late in the disease. Central visual acuity remains unaffected until late in the disease.
- Patients still may lose vision and develop blindness, even when treated appropriately.
- Topical or system steroids can cause the IOP to increase.

GLOMERULONEPHRITIS, ACUTE

Lewjain Sakr, MD

BASICS

DESCRIPTION
- Acute glomerulonephritis (GN) is an inflammatory or immune-mediated process involving the glomerulus of the kidney, resulting in a clinical syndrome consisting of sudden-onset of hematuria, proteinuria, and renal insufficiency.
- Acute GN may be caused by primary glomerular disease or secondary to systemic disease.
- Clinical severity ranges from self-limited asymptomatic microscopic or gross hematuria to a rapidly progressive loss of kidney function over days to weeks.

ALERT
Urgent investigation and treatment are required to avoid irreversible loss of kidney function and subsequent progression to chronic kidney disease and end-stage renal disease.

EPIDEMIOLOGY
- Infection-related GN
  - Postinfectious GN most commonly manifests children and occurs about 2 weeks after resolution of group A β-hemolytic *Streptococcus* infection.
  - Can also occur as a result of other bacterial infections, such as infective endocarditis, VP shunt nephritis, or less commonly with viral, helminthic, or parasitic infections
- IgA nephropathy
  - Most common primary GN in the world
  - Most common in the 2nd and 3rd decades
  - Incidence differs geographically: Asia > United States
  - HSP, the form with extrarenal manifestations, typically occurs in children <10 years old.
- Anti-GBM disease
  - Goodpasture syndrome: a notable cause of pulmonary–renal syndrome
  - Peak distribution in 3rd and 6th decades
- ANCA-associated GN
  - Often has a relapsing and remitting course
  - Four disease presentations:
    - Granulomatosis with polyangiitis (GPA), formerly Wegener granulomatosis
    - Microscopic polyangiitis (MPA)
    - Isolated pauci-immune GN—when isolated to kidneys
    - Eosinophilic GPA, formerly Churg-Strauss disease—GN relatively common but renal involvement rarely severe
- MPGN
  - May be primary or secondary to systemic diseases
  - Epidemiology varies depending on the mechanism of injury and is more often a subacute or chronic presentation
- Lupus nephritis
  - About 60% of systemic lupus erythematosus patients will have renal involvement.
  - Incidence of lupus nephritis is higher among black and Hispanic populations in comparison to white populations.

- 6 classes
  - Minimal mesangial disease
  - Mesangial proliferation
  - Focal proliferative (active) and/or sclerosing (chronic) disease
  - Diffuse segmental or global proliferative (active) and/or sclerosing (chronic) disease
  - Membranous lupus nephritis
  - Advanced sclerosis lupus nephritis
- Cryoglobulin-associated vasculitis
  - 80% of cases with hepatitis C virus (HCV) infection
  - May also be associated with autoimmune disease or dysproteinemia

Prevalence
- In patients >65 years of age, with an average age of 75 years, about 1.2% of people are affected by either primary or secondary GN.
- In patients between the ages of 37 and 65 years, GN was much less commonly seen, with only about 0.12% of people affected by either primary or secondary GN (1).
- The incidence and prevalence of GN in children is unknown. Acute postinfectious GN is the most common type, but has diminished over the years.

ETIOLOGY AND PATHOPHYSIOLOGY
- Systemic and/or local immune activation causes glomerular injury.
- Immune complex mediated: antigen–antibody formation and deposition in the kidneys; immune complexes are seen on immunofluorescence.
  - Postinfectious GN
  - IgA nephropathy
  - MPGN
    - Cryoglobulin-associated GN
  - Lupus nephritis
- Direct antibody-mediated injury, linear staining on immunofluorescence
  - Anti-GBM disease
- Pauci-immune GN, not seen on immunofluorescence staining
  - ANCA-associated GN
- Alternative complement pathway dysregulation
  - C3 glomerulopathy

RISK FACTORS
- Epidemics of nephritogenic strains of streptococci are triggers for postinfectious GN.
- Anti-GBM disease has been associated with prior pulmonary injury and inhalation exposures, such as hydrocarbon solvents.
- ANCA-associated GN may be drug induced (e.g., hydralazine, levamisole-contaminated cocaine) and is also associated with environmental exposures such as silica.
- Hepatitis B is associated with MPGN. Hepatitis C is associated with both MPGN and cryoglobulinemic GN.

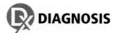**DIAGNOSIS**

HISTORY
- Symptoms: cola- or tea-colored urine, decreased urine volume, blurry vision, dizziness, light-headedness, headache, altered mental status, edema, dyspnea, generalized malaise
- Timing
  - Poststreptococcal GN typically occurs 1 to 3 weeks after pharyngitis or 2 to 6 weeks after skin infection.
  - IgA nephropathy may present within several days after an acute infection.
- Patients may also present with complaints more specific to the associated disease:
  - Lupus nephritis: joint pain or rash
  - Pulmonary–renal syndromes: hemoptysis (see "Physical Exam")
  - ANCA-associated GN: sinusitis, pulmonary infiltrates, arthralgias
  - IgA–HSP: abdominal or joint pain and purpura
  - Cryoglobulinemia-associated GN: purpura and skin vasculitis

PHYSICAL EXAM
- Majority of patients will have normal exam, but can often present with hypertension and signs of fluid overload.
- Sinus disease: ANCA-associated GN/GPA
- Pharyngitis or impetigo: postinfectious GN or IgA nephropathy
- Pulmonary hemorrhage (pulmonary–renal syndrome): anti-GBM disease/Goodpasture syndrome, ANCA-associated GN, or lupus nephritis
- Hepatomegaly or liver tenderness: cryoglobulinemia-associated GN or IgA nephropathy
- Purpura: ANCA-associated GN or HSP/IgA nephropathy

DIFFERENTIAL DIAGNOSIS
Nonglomerular hematuria: trauma, prostate diseases, urologic cancer, cystitis, nephrolithiasis, renal cysts, thrombotic microangiopathy

DIAGNOSTIC TESTS & INTERPRETATION
Initial Tests (lab, imaging)
- Urinalysis
  - Dysmorphic red blood cells (RBCs) or RBC casts on urine microscopy indicate glomerular hematuria and strongly suggest the diagnosis of an acute GN.
  - Pyuria and white blood cell casts may also be present.
- Proteinuria: 24-hour collection or random urine protein-to-creatinine ratio
- Electrolytes, blood urea nitrogen, creatinine, complete blood count
- Serologies may help clarify etiology:
  - Antistreptolysin O titer, streptozyme
  - Complement levels (C3, C4)
  - Antinuclear antibody (ANA) to rule out lupus nephritis
  - ANCA screen: myeloperoxidase and anti-proteinase 3 antibodies

– Anti-GBM antibody
– Hepatitis B surface antigen and antibody
– Hepatitis C antibody
– Cryoglobulins
– Rheumatoid factor
– HIV testing
– Serum free light chain to assess for monoclonal gammopathies

- Renal ultrasound to rule out structural causes of glomerular disease
- Chest x-ray in the setting of hemoptysis or a suspected infiltrate

Diagnostic Procedures/Other
Definitive diagnosis is made via renal biopsy.

Test Interpretation
Renal biopsy

- Light microscopy
  – Diffuse hypercellularity suggests a proliferative disease such as IgA nephropathy, lupus nephritis, or postinfectious GN.
  – Presence of glomerular crescents correlates with RPGN and disease severity.
  – Significant overlap between endothelial, mesangial, and epithelial cell proliferation
- Immunofluorescence
  – Pattern of IgG, IgA, IgM, C3, and C4 staining may aid in characterizing the GN.
  – Lupus nephritis typically positive for all immunoglobulins and complements
  – Isolated mesangial IgA staining is pathognomonic for IgA nephropathy.
  – Crescentic GN in absence of immune complex staining suggests ANCA-associated GN.
  – Crescentic GN with linear staining of IgG is characteristic of anti-GB
- Electron microscopy: The location of immunoglobulin deposits is useful in pointing to a particular diagnosis.

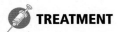

TREATMENT

GENERAL MEASURES
Treat the underlying condition if able.

MEDICATION
First Line
- Diuretics
- Calcium channel blockers
- Avoid ACE inhibitors or ARBs if acute renal dysfunction is present.

Second Line
- Supportive care is typically adequate in postinfectious GN.
- Crescents on renal biopsy may be an indication for steroids in postinfectious GN and, in other cases, are often an indication for additional potent immunosuppressive medications (2)[C].
- Treatment with antiviral therapy for nephritic syndromes that have been shown to be secondary to underlying viral infections such as HCV and hepatitis B virus (HBV).

- Commonly used immunosuppressive medications include:
  – Corticosteroids—may consider initiation in high doses even prior to kidney biopsy (2)[C]
  – Cyclophosphamide
  – Mycophenolate-mofetil (MMF)
  – Calcineurin inhibitors (cyclosporine, tacrolimus)
  – Rituximab
- Choice of immunosuppressive agent depends on patient characteristics and the disease process.
- Plasmapheresis may also be considered in some cases for RPGN or ANCA-associated renal disease with diffuse pulmonary hemorrhage (2)[C],(3),(4)[A].
- Dialysis may be needed for uremia, hyperkalemia refractory to medical management, intractable acidosis, and diuretic-resistant pulmonary edema.

ISSUES FOR REFERRAL
- Consultation with a nephrologist is usually required to assist with renal biopsy to confirm diagnosis and assist with management.
- Consultation with a rheumatologist may also be helpful in cases with systemic manifestations.

ADMISSION, INPATIENT, AND NURSING CONSIDERATIONS
- Consider admission for patients with no urine output, rapidly deteriorating renal function, significant hypertension, and suspicion of pulmonary hemorrhage or fluid overload that is compromising heart or respiratory function.
- Hemodynamically stable patients without complications may be managed as outpatients.

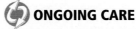 ONGOING CARE

FOLLOW-UP RECOMMENDATIONS
Patient Monitoring
- Regular blood pressure checks and urinalysis to detect recurrence, assessment of renal function to detect acute or follow chronic renal disease as a result of the primary event, and regular clinical assessment to detect suspicious symptoms that may herald a recurrence (i.e., rash, joint complaint, hemoptysis)
- Periodic reassessment of serology tests to follow asymptomatic individuals

DIET
- Salt-restricted diet (<2 g/day) and fluid restriction until edema and hypertension clear
- Avoid foods that are high in potassium and phosphorus if significant renal dysfunction is present.

PATIENT EDUCATION
National Kidney Foundation: https://www.kidney.org/atoz/content/glomerul

PROGNOSIS
- The GN may be self-limited or part of a chronic disease that makes the possibility of recurrence of acute disease likely, with the potential for progressive loss of renal function over time.
- Some forms of acute GN (including ANCA-associated and severe lupus) require long-term immunosuppression to prevent recurrence.

COMPLICATIONS
- Hypertensive retinopathy and encephalopathy
- Microscopic hematuria may persist for years.
- Chronic kidney disease
- Nephrotic syndrome (~10%)

REFERENCES
1. Wetmore JB, Guo H, Liu J, et al. The incidence, prevalence, and outcomes of glomerulonephritis derived from a large retrospective analysis. *Kidney Int*. 2016;90(4):853–860.
2. Beck L, Bomback AS, Choi MJ, et al. KDOQI US commentary on the 2012 KDIGO clinical practice guideline for glomerulonephritis. *Am J Kidney Dis*. 2013;62(3):403–441.
3. Walters G, Willis NS, Craig JC. Interventions for renal vasculitis in adults. *Cochrane Database Syst Rev*. 2008;(3):CD003232.
4. Jayne DRW, Gaskin G, Rasmussen N, et al; for European Vasculitis Study Group. Randomized trial of plasma exchange or high-dosage methyl-prednisolone as adjunctive therapy for severe renal vasculitis. *J Am Soc Nephrol*. 2007;18(7): 2180–2188.

 SEE ALSO

- Glomerulonephritis, Postinfectious; Henoch-Schönlein Purpura; Hyperkalemia; Hypertensive Emergencies; IgA Nephropathy; Lupus Nephritis; Nephrotic Syndrome; Vasculitis
- Algorithm: Acute Kidney Injury (Acute Renal Failure); Hematuria

 CODES

ICD10
- N00.9 Acute nephritic syndrome with unsp morphologic changes
- N00.2 Acute nephritic syndrome w diffuse membranous glomrlneph
- N00.8 Acute nephritic syndrome with other morphologic changes

CLINICAL PEARLS
- Dysmorphic RBCs and RBC casts are key components of the urinalysis in GN.
- Postinfectious GN in children is typically a self-limited disease.
- Searching for other organ involvement is useful in establishing a definitive diagnosis.
- With the discovery of a GN, monitor the initial renal function labs frequently to identify an RPGN.
- Clinical course and treatment strategies depend on the underlying disease process.

G

GLOMERULONEPHRITIS, POSTINFECTIOUS

Theodore B. Flaum, DO • Kaitlin Unser, DO

BASICS

DESCRIPTION
Postinfectious glomerulonephritis (PIGN) is an immune complex disease associated with nonrenal infection by certain strains of bacteria, most commonly *Streptococcus* and *Staphylococcus*. The most common form of PIGN, poststreptococcal glomerulonephritis (PSGN), is preceded by infection with *Streptococcus* spp. and predominantly affects children. The clinical presentation can be asymptomatic or with an acute nephritic syndrome, characterized by gross hematuria, proteinuria, edema, hypertension (HTN), and acute kidney injury.

EPIDEMIOLOGY
PIGN is declining globally, especially in developed countries, in large part due to better hygiene and a decreased incidence of streptococcal skin infections. There are an estimated 470,000 new cases per annum of PSGN worldwide, and it remains the most common cause of acute nephritis in children globally, with 97% of cases occur in developing countries. PSGN is primarily a pediatric disease, but a recent increase in cases has been seen in nonstreptococcal GN in adults.

ETIOLOGY AND PATHOPHYSIOLOGY
- Glomerular immune complex disease induced by specific nephritogenic strains of bacteria:
  - >95% of cases are caused by group A β-hemolytic *Streptococcus* (GAS) (1)
  - *Staphylococcus* (predominantly *Staphylococcus aureus*; more commonly methicillin-resistant *S. aureus* [MRSA], occasionally coagulase-negative *Staphylococcus*)
  - Gram-negative bacteria including *Escherichia coli*, *Yersinia*, *Pseudomonas*, and *Haemophilus* (2)
  - Occasionally viral, fungal, helminthic or protozoal causes
- Proposed mechanisms for the glomerular injury (3) relates to the deposition of circulating immune complexes with streptococcal or staphylococcal antigens—although these complexes can be detected in patients with streptococcal- or staphylococcal-related GN, they do not correlate to disease activity. IgG is the most frequent immunoglobulin in PSGN (2).
- These glomerular immune complexes result in complement activation and inflammation:
  - Nephritis-associated plasmin receptor (NAPlr): activates plasmin; contributes to activation of the alternative complement pathway
  - Streptococcal pyrogenic exotoxin B (SPE B): binds plasmin and acts as a protease; promotes the release of inflammatory mediators
- Activation of the alternative complement pathway causes initial glomerular injury as evidenced by C3 deposition and decreased levels of serum C3. The lectin pathway of complement activation has also been recently implicated in glomerular injury (1).

RISK FACTORS
- Children 5 to 12 years of age
- Older patients (>65 years of age) with immuno-compromising comorbid conditions such as diabetes and alcohol abuse

GENERAL PREVENTION
- Early antibiotic treatment for streptococcal and staphylococcal infections, although efficacy in preventing GN is uncertain
- Improved hand hygiene and respiratory etiquette
- Prophylactic penicillin treatment to be used in closed communities and household contacts of index cases in areas where PIGN is prevalent

COMMONLY ASSOCIATED CONDITIONS
Streptococcal or staphylococcal infection

DIAGNOSIS

HISTORY
- Usually history of antecedent GAS skin/throat infection
- Patients present with acute nephritic syndrome, characterized by sudden onset of hematuria associated with edema and HTN for 1 to 2 weeks after an infection.
- A triad of edema (usually generalized), gross hematuria, and HTN is classic but not always seen.
- Urine described as "tea-colored" or "cola-colored"
  - Gross hematuria: present in 25–60% of patients
  - Microscopic hematuria: subclinical cases of PIGN
  - Oliguria: present in 18–51% of patient
- The latent period between GAS infection and PIGN depends on the site of infection: 1 to 3 weeks following GAS pharyngitis and 3 to 6 weeks following GAS skin infection.
- Adult PIGN most commonly follows staphylococcal infections (3 times more common than streptococcal infections) of the upper respiratory tract, skin, heart, lung, bone, or urinary tract. Studies show 7–16% of cases of adult PIGN have no preceding evidence of infection and, in 24–59%, the offending microorganism cannot be identified.

PHYSICAL EXAM
- Constitutional:
  - Fever: 40–50% of patients
- Cardiovascular:
  - Edema: present in ~2 of 3 adult patients due to sodium and water retention; less common in pediatric patients
  - HTN: present in 80–90% of patients and varies from mild to severe; secondary to fluid retention. Hypertensive encephalopathy is an uncommon but serious complication.
- Pulmonary:
  - Respiratory distress: due to pulmonary edema (rare)
- Neurological:
  - Encephalopathy and seizures are rare.

DIFFERENTIAL DIAGNOSIS
The diagnosis of PIGN is generally accomplished by history once the diagnosis of acute nephritis is made, with documentation of a recent infection and nephritis beginning to resolve 1 to 2 weeks after presentation. However, with progressive disease (>2 weeks, persistent hematuria/HTN >4 to 6 weeks, or no adequate documentation of a GAS or other infection) the differential diagnosis of GN needs to be considered and renal biopsy performed:
- Membranoproliferative glomerulonephritis (MPGN): Patients with MPGN have persistent nephritis and hypocomplementemia beyond 4 to 6 weeks. Patients with PIGN tend to have resolution of their disease and a return to normal C3 and CH50 levels within 2 to 4 weeks.
- Secondary causes of GN: Lupus nephritis and Henoch-Schönlein purpura nephritis have similar features to PIGN. Hypocomplementemia is not characteristic of Henoch-Schönlein purpura, and the hypocomplementemia that occurs in lupus nephritis usually results in reductions in both C3 and C4, whereas C4 levels are normal in PIGN.
- IgA nephropathy often presents after an upper respiratory infection. It can be distinguished from PIGN based on a shorter time frame between the upper respiratory illness and onset of hematuria, as well as history of gross hematuria, as PIGN recurrence is rare. IgA nephropathy is a chronic illness and will recur. Patients with IgA nephropathy have normal C3/C4 levels.
- IgA-dominant acute PIGN: a recently recognized form of PIGN occurring in poststaphylococcal GN. This differs from primary IgA nephropathy in that these patients do not have a history of renal disease (2)[A].
- Pauci-immune crescentic GN: In elderly with severe renal failure and active urine sediment, this is much more common, so antineutrophil cytoplasmic antibody (ANCA) testing should be done (2)[A].

DIAGNOSTIC TESTS & INTERPRETATION
Initial Tests (lab, imaging)
- Urinalysis
  - Hematuria with possible dysmorphic red cells
    - Gross hematuria: present in 25–60% of patients
    - Microscopic hematuria: subclinical cases of PIGN
  - With/without RBC casts and pyuria
  - Proteinuria ~90% of patients (nephrotic range proteinuria is uncommon in children)
- Renal function
  - Decreased GFR with elevated creatinine to the point of renal insufficiency in 25–83% of cases, more commonly in adults (83%)

Follow-Up Tests & Special Considerations

- Culture: PSGN usually presents weeks after a GAS infection; only ~25% of patients will have either a positive throat or skin culture.
- Complement: 90% of pediatric patients (slightly fewer adult patients) will have depressed C3 and CH50 levels in the first 2 weeks of the disease, whereas C2 and C4 levels remain normal. C3 and CH50 levels return to normal within 4 to 8 weeks after presentation.
- Serology: Elevated titers of antibodies support evidence of a recent GAS infection. Streptozyme test measuring antistreptolysin O (ASO), antihyaluronidase (AHase), antistreptokinase (ASKase), anti–nicotinamide-adenine dinucleotidase (anti-NAD), and anti-DNAse B antibodies: positive in >95% of patients with PSGN due to pharyngitis and 80% with skin infections. In pharyngeal infection, ASO, anti-DNAse B, anti-NAD, and AHase titers are elevated. In skin infections, only the anti-DNAse and AHase titers are typically elevated.

Diagnostic Procedures/Other

Renal biopsy is rarely done in children; recommended in most adults to confirm the diagnosis and rule out other glomerulopathies

Test Interpretation

- Light microscopy: diffuse proliferative glomerulonephritis with prominent endocapillary proliferation and numerous neutrophils within the capillary lumen. Deposits may also be found in the mesangium ("starry sky"). Severity of involvement varies and correlates with clinical findings. Crescent formation is uncommon and is associated with a poor prognosis.
- Immunofluorescence microscopy: deposits of C3 and IgG distributed in a diffuse granular pattern
- Electron microscopy: dome-shaped subepithelial electron-dense deposits that are referred to as "humps." These deposits are immune complexes, and they correspond to the deposits of IgG and C3 found on immunofluorescence. Rate of clearance of these deposits affects recovery time.

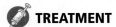

TREATMENT

MEDICATION

- No specific therapy exists for PIGN, and no randomized controlled trials indicate that aggressive immunosuppressive therapy has a beneficial effect in patients with rapidly progressive crescentic disease. Despite this, patients with >30% crescents on renal biopsy are often treated with steroids.
- Older patients often require hospitalization to treat complications of heart failure (HF) from volume overload (2).

- Management is mainly supportive, with focus on treating the clinical manifestations of PIGN (HTN; pulmonary edema):
  - Salt and water restriction and loop diuretics
  - Calcium channel blockers/angiotensin-converting enzyme (ACE) inhibitors may be used in cases of severe HTN.
- Patients with evidence of persistent bacterial infection should be given a course of antibiotic therapy.

SURGERY/OTHER PROCEDURES

Acute dialysis is required in approximately 50% of elderly patients (1),(2).

ADMISSION, INPATIENT, AND NURSING CONSIDERATIONS

Admission may be necessary for elderly at risk for complications such as new onset or exacerbation of preexisting CHF (2).

 ONGOING CARE

FOLLOW-UP RECOMMENDATIONS

Patient Monitoring

- Repeat urinalysis to check for clearance of hematuria and/or proteinuria.
- Consider other diagnosis if no improvement within 2 weeks.

DIET

Renal diet if requiring instances of dialysis

PROGNOSIS

- Most children with PIGN have an excellent outcome, with >90% of cases achieving full recovery of renal function.
- Elderly patients, especially adults, develop HTN, recurrent proteinuria, and renal insufficiency long after the initial illness. Adults with multiple comorbid factors have the worst prognosis and highest incidence of chronic renal injury following PIGN (2).
- Complete remission in adult PIGN is only 26–56%. This has declined since the 1990s, suggesting prognosis is worsening.
- The presence of diabetes, higher creatinine levels, and more severe glomerular disease (e.g., crescents) on biopsy are all risk factors for developing end-stage renal disease (2).

COMPLICATIONS

Complications related to PIGN are primarily due to volume overload. These complications can include HTN and, less commonly, pulmonary edema. Patients may also develop recurrent proteinuria and renal insufficiency; however, this is rare.

REFERENCES

1. Hunt EAK, Somers MJG. Infection-related glomerulonephritis. *Pediatr Clin North Am*. 2019;66(1):59–72.
2. Nasr SH, Radhakrishnan J, D'Agati VD. Bacterial infection-related glomerulonephritis in adults. *Kidney Int*. 2013;83(5):792–803.
3. Nadasdy T, Hebert LA. Infection-related glomerulonephritis: understanding mechanisms. *Semin Nephrol*. 2011;31(4):369–375.

ADDITIONAL READING

- Balasubramanian R, Marks SD. Post-infectious glomerulonephritis. *Paediatr Int Child Health*. 2017;37(4):240–247.
- Ramdani B, Zamd M, Hachim K, et al. Acute postinfectious glomerulonephritis [in French]. *Nephrol Ther*. 2012;8(4):247–258.
- Wen Y-K. Clinicopathological study of infection-associated glomerulonephritis in adults. *Int Urol Nephrol*. 2010;42(2):477–485.

CODES

ICD10

- N05.9 Unsp nephritic syndrome with unspecified morphologic changes
- N00.9 Acute nephritic syndrome with unsp morphologic changes

CLINICAL PEARLS

- PIGN is an immune complex disease occurring after infection with certain strains of bacteria, most commonly group A *Streptococcus pyogenes*.
- The clinical presentation can be asymptomatic or with an acute nephritic syndrome, characterized by gross hematuria, proteinuria, edema, HTN, and acute kidney injury.
- Treatment is primarily supportive and includes treating HTN and edema, along with antibiotics for any ongoing bacterial infection.
- Persistent nephritis and low C3 levels for >2 weeks should prompt evaluation for other causes of GN, such as MPGN or systemic lupus erythematosus nephritis.

G

GLUCOSE INTOLERANCE

Robert A. Baldor, MD, FAAFP

 BASICS

DESCRIPTION
- Glucose intolerance is an intermediate stage between a normal glucose metabolism and diabetes. It occurs due to a gradual decline in β-cell function.
- Individuals with impaired fasting glucose (IFG) and/or impaired glucose intolerance (IGT) have been referred to as having prediabetes:
  - IFG: 100 to 125 mg/dL
  - IGT: 140 to 199 mg/dL 2 hours after ingestion of 75 g oral glucose load
  - Hemoglobin A1c (HbA1c) 5.7–6.4% (1)

EPIDEMIOLOGY
- As of 2010, it is estimated that one of every three U.S. adults ≥20 years of age have prediabetes (2).
- In the United States, an estimated 88 million people aged ≥18 years are living with prediabetes as of 2020, based on The National Diabetes Statistics Report.
- Only 11% of people with prediabetes are aware of their condition (3).
- Prediabetes has a 34.5% prevalence among adults >18 years old and 51% of adults ≥65 years old in the United States (4).

Incidence
- Systematic review indicates a 5-year cumulative incidence of developing diabetes of 9–25% for people with an HbA1c of 5.5–6% and 25–50% for people with an HbA1c of 6–6.5% (1).
- Highest incidence in American Indians/Alaska Natives, non-Hispanic blacks, and Hispanics (2)

Prevalence
As of 2020, prevalence of prediabetes in the United States was 34.5% in adults >20 years old and 51% in adults >65 years old. According to ADA, in 2015, 84.1 million Americans >18 years old had prediabetes. As of 2010, worldwide prevalence was 8%.

ETIOLOGY AND PATHOPHYSIOLOGY
Progressive loss of insulin secretion on the background of insulin resistance (1)

Genetics
- Genetic heterogeneity is established by family, twin, immunologic, and HLA disease association studies.
- Variants in 11 genes have been shown to be significantly associated with future development of type 2 diabetes and IFG. Variants in 8 of these genes have been associated with impaired β-cell function.

RISK FACTORS
- Body mass index (BMI) ≥25: overweight
- History of gestational diabetes mellitus (GDM)
- Sedentary lifestyle
- Medications

GENERAL PREVENTION
- Lifestyle modification with weight reduction and increased physical activity
- A decrease in excess body fat provides the greatest risk reduction.

Pregnancy Considerations
- Screening for diabetes in pregnancy is based on risk factor analysis:
  - High risk: first prenatal visit
  - Average risk: 24 to 28 weeks' gestation
- Women with GDM should be screened for diabetes 6 to 12 weeks' postpartum with 75-g OGTT and then every 1 to 3 years via any method (5).

COMMONLY ASSOCIATED CONDITIONS
- Obesity (abdominal and visceral obesity)
- Dyslipidemia with high triglycerides (TG)
- PCOS
- GDM
- Congenital diseases (Down, Turner, Klinefelter, and Wolfram syndromes)

 DIAGNOSIS

Who to screen
- BMI ≥25 or ≥23 for Asian Americans (1)[B]
- Age ≥45 years (1)[B]
- First-degree relative with diabetes
- High TG >250 mg/dL
- Low HDL <35 mg/dL
- HTN: BP >140/90 mm Hg or on treatment
- History of GDM
- History of cardiovascular disease
- Ethnic group at increased risk (non-Hispanic black, Native American, Hispanics, Asian American, Pacific Islander)
- PCOS
- Conditions associated with insulin resistance such as severe obesity or acanthosis nigricans

HISTORY
- No clear symptoms
- Polyuria
- Polydipsia
- Weight loss
- Blurred vision
- Polyphagia

PHYSICAL EXAM
- General physical exam
- BMI assessment

DIFFERENTIAL DIAGNOSIS
- Type A insulin resistance
- Leprechaunism
- Rabson-Mendenhall syndrome
- Lipoatrophic diabetes
- Pancreatitis
- Cushing syndrome
- Glucagonoma
- Pheochromocytoma
- Hyperthyroidism
- Somatostatinoma
- Aldosteronoma
- Drug-induced hyperglycemia
  - Thiazide diuretics (high doses)
  - β-Blockers
  - Corticosteroids (including inhaled corticosteroids)
  - Thyroid hormone
  - α-Interferon
  - Pentamidine
  - Protease inhibitors
  - Atypical antipsychotics
  - Selective serotonin reuptake inhibitors

DIAGNOSTIC TESTS & INTERPRETATION

Initial Tests (lab, imaging)
- Fasting glucose, 2-hour OGTT, or HbA1c is equally appropriate (1)[B].
- Repeat screen at 3-year intervals with normal results, sooner depending on risk status (1)[C].

Follow-Up Tests & Special Considerations
- Fasting lipid profile
- Creatinine and GFR
- Urinalysis
- Microalbumin-to-creatinine ratio
- Thyroid-stimulating hormone with free T_4
- Periodic measurement of vitamin B_{12} levels for patients on long-term metformin therapy especially those with anemia or peripheral neuropathy

 TREATMENT

- Therapeutic lifestyle modification to include physical activity focused on weight loss and medical nutrition therapy (preferably via a registered dietitian)
- Mediterranean diet and diets high in fiber-rich foods such as vegetables, fruits, whole grains, seeds, and nuts plus white meat sources are protective against type 2 diabetes (6)[B].
- Consider referring patients with prediabetes to an intensive diet and physical activity behavioral counseling program adhering to the tenets of the Diabetes Prevention Program targeting a loss of 7% of body weight and should increase their moderate-intensity physical activity (such as brisk walking to at least 150 min/week) (6)[A].

- Resistance training and endurance exercise both reduce diabetes risk.
- Interrupt prolonged sitting every 30 minutes with short bouts of physical activity (6)[B].
- Diabetes prevention programs are cost-effective and often covered by third-party payers (6)[B].
- Screen and treat modifiable risk factors for cardiovascular disease (6)[B].
- Diabetes self-management education and support systems are appropriate venues for people with prediabetes to receive education and support to develop and maintain behaviors that can prevent or delay the onset of diabetes (6)[B].
- Technology-assisted tools including internet-based social networks, distance learning, DVD-based content, and mobile applications can be useful elements of effective lifestyle modification to prevent diabetes (6)[B].

MEDICATION

Consider metformin therapy for prevention of type 2 diabetes, especially in those with BMI >35, those aged <60 years, and women with prior GDM and/or rising HbA1c despite lifestyle intervention (6)[C].

First Line

Metformin (drug of choice): started at 500 mg BID or 500 mg XR. Observational data suggest that it can be used safely down to GFR of 30 to 45 but may require dose adjustments.

Second Line

- Acarbose: started at 50 mg PO once daily and titrated to 100 mg PO TID; GI upset is common.
- GLP-1 Agonists: Recent clinical trials in primarily obese patients, GLP-1 agonists have shown various benefits including weight loss, improvement in β-cell function, and a return to a normal glycemic state. Overall prediabetes incidence decreased by 84–96%. However, no GLP-1 inhibitors are FDA approved for prediabetes as of 2020 (7)[A].

ISSUES FOR REFERRAL

- Diabetes educator/registered dietitian on diagnosis
- Exercise physiologist
- Lifestyle coaching
- Obesity Specialist

ADDITIONAL THERAPIES

Alternative/botanical therapy:

- Although studies lack large sample size and ideal design, there is some evidence that fenugreek, bitter melon, and cinnamon can reduce hyperglycemia and improve insulin sensitivity (7).

 ONGOING CARE

FOLLOW-UP RECOMMENDATIONS

Patient Monitoring

- At least annual monitoring for development of diabetes with HbA1c, 2-hour OGTT, or fasting glucose
- BP should be routinely measured.
- Annual testing for lipid abnormalities and microalbuminuria (for detection and therapy modification of incipient diabetic nephropathy)
- Monitoring of BMI

DIET

- Mediterranean diet has been shown to be beneficial. One small cohort study showed that the addition of about 10 g of extra virgin olive oil to meals improved the postprandial glucose by reducing DPP4 activity and increasing insulin and GLP-1. It also showed a significant decrease in TG and apolipoprotein B-48.
- Limit high glycemic carbohydrates and sucrose-containing foods.
- Diets high in fiber, vegetables, nuts, seeds, and whole grains
- Intermittent fasting has shown benefit in improving fasting glucose as well as postprandial hyperglycemia (8)[C].

PROGNOSIS

- Individuals with IFG and/or IGT have high risk for the future development of diabetes.
- Prediabetes increases the risk of developing type 2 diabetes, heart disease, and stroke.
- 20–70% of individuals with prediabetes who do not lose weight, change their dietary habits, and/or engage in moderate physical activity will progress to type 2 diabetes within 3 to 6 years.
- Lifestyle intervention reduced 3-year diabetes incidence by 58% compared to 31% with metformin.

COMPLICATIONS

- Cardiovascular and peripheral artery disease
- Stroke: 2 to 4 times higher risk
- Ketoacidosis
- Sexual dysfunction
- Gastroparesis
- Nephropathy and potential for renal failure
- Retinopathy and potential for loss of vision
- Peripheral and autonomic neuropathy

REFERENCES

1. American Diabetes Association. 2. Classification and diagnosis of diabetes. *Diabetes Care*. 2017;40(Suppl 1):S11–S24.
2. Centers for Disease Control and Prevention. *National Diabetes Statistics Report, 2014: Estimates of Diabetes and Its Burden in the United States*. Atlanta, GA: U.S. Department of Health and Human Services; 2014.
3. Centers for Disease Control and Prevention. Awareness of prediabetes—United States, 2005–2010. *MMWR Morb Mortal Wkly Rep*. 2013;62(11):209–212.
4. Centers for Disease Control and Prevention. Prediabetes. https://www.cdc.gov/diabetes/basics/prediabetes.html. Accessed December 27, 2022.
5. American Diabetes Association. 13. Management of diabetes in pregnancy. *Diabetes Care*. 2017;40(Suppl 1):S114–S119.
6. American Diabetes Association. 5. Prevention or delay of type 2 diabetes. *Diabetes Care*. 2017;40(Suppl 1):S44–S47.
7. Deng R. A review of the hypoglycemic effects of five commonly used herbal food supplements. *Recent Pat Food Nutr Agric*. 2012;4(1):50–60.
8. Arnason TG, Bowen MW, Mansell KD. Effects of intermittent fasting on health markers in those with type 2 diabetes: a pilot study. *World J Diabetes*. 2017;8(4):154–164.

ADDITIONAL READING

Papaetis GS. Incretin-based therapies in prediabetes: current evidence and future perspectives. *World J Diabetes*. 2014;5(6):817–834.

 CODES

ICD10

- E74.39 Other disorders of intestinal carbohydrate absorption
- R73.09 Other abnormal glucose
- R73.01 Impaired fasting glucose

CLINICAL PEARLS

- Patient education and lifestyle reinforcement should be emphasized in all clinical encounters as lifestyle optimization is essential for all patients with prediabetes.
- Research shows that you can lower your risk for type 2 diabetes by 58% by losing 7% of your body weight (or 15 lb if you weigh 200 lb).
- Recommend exercising moderately (such as brisk walking) 30 min/day, 5 days a week.
- Consider concurrent cardiovascular risks and further workup as indicated clinically.

G

GONOCOCCAL INFECTIONS

Alicia Leandra Olowu, DO • Nelly Singh, DO • Kliment Todosov, MD

BASICS

DESCRIPTION
A sexually or vertically transmitted bacterial infection caused by *Neisseria gonorrhoeae*:

- *N. gonorrhoeae* is a fastidious gram-negative intracellular diplococcus (1).
- Presents as conjunctival, pharyngeal, urogenital, or anorectal infection; urogenital infections are the most common.
- Hematogenous dissemination leads to fever, cutaneous lesions, arthralgias, purulent or sterile arthritis, tenosynovitis, endocarditis, or (rarely) meningitis (1).
- Asymptomatic carrier states occur in men and women (more often in women) (1).
- In newborns of infected mothers, gonococcal ophthalmia neonatorum, a purulent conjunctivitis, may occur after vaginal delivery; can lead to potential blindness if not treated promptly (1),(2)[A]
- System(s) affected: cardiovascular, musculoskeletal, nervous, reproductive, skin/exocrine
- Synonym(s): gonococcal infection; clap

EPIDEMIOLOGY
- Predominant age: 15- to 44-year-olds account for 92% of cases; highest rate among those aged 20 to 24 years
- Predominant sex: men 213/100,000; women 146/100,000

Incidence
Centers for Disease Control and Prevention (CDC) 2021: 710,151 reported cases

Prevalence
Incidence and prevalence are roughly equal. The true prevalence is higher due to asymptomatic cases (2)[A]:
- Rates peaked in mid-1970s and fell 74% over the next 20 years with national control program. Rates have been slowly increasing since 2012 (2)[A].
- Rates in men now higher than women (2)[A]

ETIOLOGY AND PATHOPHYSIOLOGY
Infection requires four steps: (i) mucosal attachment—bacterial proteins bind to receptors on host cells, (ii) local penetration/invasion, (iii) local proliferation, (iv) inflammatory response or dissemination. *N. gonorrhoeae* spreads most commonly through sexual contact.

Genetics
Deficiency of late components of complement cascade (C7–C9) predisposes to disseminated disease.

RISK FACTORS
- History of previous gonorrhea infection or other STIs
- Age ≤25 years
- Sexual exposure to an infected individual without appropriate use of barrier protection (condom)
- New/multiple sexual partners
- Men who have sex with men (MSM)
- Inconsistent condom use
- Commercial sex work or drug use
- Infants: infected mother
- Children: sexual abuse by infected individual
- Autoinoculation (finger to eye)

GENERAL PREVENTION
- Condoms offer partial protection and must be used appropriately during oral, anal, and vaginal sex.
- Treat sexual contacts; consider expedited partner therapy (EPT) (2)[A].

COMMONLY ASSOCIATED CONDITIONS
Other STIs: *Chlamydia*, syphilis, HIV, hepatitis B, herpes (2)[A]

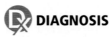

DIAGNOSIS

HISTORY
- Sexual history
  - Number of partners; age of onset of sexual activity; STI history
  - New/recent change in sexual partners
  - Contact with commercial sex workers
  - Condom use
  - Menses and possibility of pregnancy
- 10% of men and 20–40% of women are asymptomatic (2)[A].
- If symptomatic, explore onset, context, duration, timing, severity, and associated symptoms:
  - Symptoms (when present) typically appear within 1 to 14 days after exposure (1).
- Ocular symptoms: discharge, itch, redness (1)
- Pharyngeal symptoms: asymptomatic infection (98%), sore throat (1)
- GI symptoms: acute diarrhea (1)
- Urinary symptoms: frequency, urgency, dysuria (1)
- Urethral symptoms: discharge (1),(2)[A]
  - Males: scant to copious purulent urethral discharge (82%), dysuria (53%), asymptomatic (10%), testicular pain (1%), proctitis
  - Females: endocervical discharge (96%), asymptomatic cervical infection (20%), vaginal discharge, Bartholin gland swelling, dysmenorrhea, menometrorrhagia, abdominal pain/tenderness, dyspareunia, cervical motion tenderness, rebound, infertility, chronic pelvic pain
- Either sex, with receptive anal intercourse: rectal discharge, tenesmus, rectal burning; can also be asymptomatic
- Disseminated syndromes (1),(2)[A]
  - Fever, chills, malaise, skin rash, arthralgia/arthritis
  - Endocarditis: high fevers
  - Meningitis: meningeal signs, headache, skin lesions, fever, altered mental status

PHYSICAL EXAM
- General: fever, chills (1)
- Ocular: purulent discharge, conjunctivitis, chemosis, eyelid edema, corneal ulceration (1)
- Pharynx: exudative pharyngitis (<1%)
- GI: acute diarrhea, hyperactive bowel sounds (1)
- Genitourinary (GU) (1)
  - Males: urethral discharge, testicular tenderness
  - Females: endocervical discharge, Bartholin gland abscess, abdominal pain/tenderness, cervical motion tenderness, rebound tenderness

- Either sex, for receptive anal intercourse: rectal discharge; rectal exam may be normal (1).
- Disseminated syndromes (1):
  - Fever, chills, malaise, tenosynovitis, maculopapular–pustular rash, polyarthralgia—typically large joints (knee, wrist, ankle), purulent arthritis
  - Endocarditis: rapid cardiac valve destruction, heart murmurs, high fevers
  - Meningitis: meningeal signs, headache, skin lesions, fever, altered mental status

DIFFERENTIAL DIAGNOSIS
Chlamydia trachomatis, UTIs, other vaginitis, or urethritis (bacterial, viral, or parasitic)

DIAGNOSTIC TESTS & INTERPRETATION

Initial Tests (lab, imaging)
- The nucleic acid amplification test (NAAT) is the most sensitive and specific test for *N. gonorrhoeae* (2)[A].
- Other options:
  - Genital culture
  - Add pharyngeal culture in adolescents.
  - Gram stain (diagnostic for symptomatic urethritis in men)
  - Urethral smear, sensitivity in symptomatic male: ≥95%; sensitivity of endocervical smear in infected woman: 40–60%; specificity: 100%
- DNA probes and polymerase chain reaction (PCR) sensitivity: 92–99% dependent on population; specificity: >97%; can replace culture
- Blood culture is 50% sensitive in disseminated disease. Joint fluid culture is 50% sensitive in septic arthritis. Screen for additional STIs, especially chlamydia, syphilis, and HIV.
- Imaging is not generally recommended.

Follow-Up Tests & Special Considerations
- Test of cure is unnecessary for persons with uncomplicated urogenital or rectal gonorrhea who are treated with any of the recommended or alternative regimens: Individuals treated for pharyngeal gonorrhea should have test of cure 7 to 14 days after treatment with NAAT or culture (3)[A].
- Reinfection within 12 months occurs in 7–12% of persons treated for gonorrhea. Patients should be retested 3 months after treatment regardless of whether they believe their sex partners were treated. If retesting at 3 months is not possible, clinicians should retest within 12 months after initial treatment (3)[A].

Diagnostic Procedures/Other
Culdocentesis may demonstrate free purulent exudate and provide material for Gram staining and culture. Gram staining material from unroofed skin lesions may show typical organisms. Pelvic ultrasound or CT scan may demonstrate thick, dilated fallopian tubes or abscess formation.

Test Interpretation
- Gram-negative intracellular diplococci
- Nonpathologic gram-negative diplococci may be found in extragenital locations. For this reason, Gram stain of pharyngeal or rectal swabs is not recommended.

TREATMENT

GENERAL MEASURES
- STI counseling and condom use
- In children and adolescents, suspect sexual abuse.

MEDICATION
- Dual therapy is no longer recommended (3)[A].
- Quinolones are not recommended (2),(4)[A].
- *If treatment fails, check culture and sensitivities and report to CDC through local health authorities* (2)[A].
- Treat with regimen that is also effective against uncomplicated genital chlamydial infection if chlamydial infection has not been ruled out (3)[A].

First Line
- Uncomplicated urogenital, anorectal, and pharyngeal gonorrheal infection (3)[A]
  - Ceftriaxone 500 mg IM in a single dose; for persons weighing ≥150 kg (300 lb), use 1 g IM in a single dose.
    - If IM ceftriaxone is not available, cefixime 800 mg PO once is an alternative. Cefixime has limited treatment efficacy for pharyngeal gonorrhea.
  - If chlamydial infection has not been excluded, also give doxycycline 100 mg PO twice a day for 7 days.
  - Alternative: gentamicin 240 mg IM once *plus* azithromycin 2 g PO once
- Conjunctivitis: ceftriaxone, 1 g IM single dose; consider saline solution lavage of infected eye (1),(2)[A].
- Arthritis and arthritis–dermatitis syndrome (1),(2)[A]
  - Ceftriaxone 1 g IM or IV q24h until 24 to 48 hours after improvement begins then switch to PO agent; complete at least 1 week of antibiotic treatment.
  - Alternative regimens:
    - Cefotaxime 1 g IV q8h until 24 to 48 hours after improvement begins and then switch to PO agent. Complete at least 1 week of antibiotic treatment.
    - Ceftizoxime 1 g IV q8h until 24 to 48 hours after improvement begins and then switch to PO agent. Complete at least 1 week of antibiotic treatment
- Meningitis and endocarditis (1),(2)[A]: ceftriaxone 1 to 2 g IV q12–24h 10 to 14 days for meningitis; 4 weeks for endocarditis
- Contraindications: Doxycycline is contraindicated in pregnancy and young children.

Pediatric Considerations
- Children >45 kg: same dosing as adults (1),(2)[A]
  - Bacteremia or arthritis: ceftriaxone 1 g IM or IV in single daily dose every 24 hours for 7 days
- Children <45 kg: uncomplicated urethral, cervical, rectal, or pharyngeal gonococcal infections (1),(2)[A]
  - Ceftriaxone 25 to 50 mg/kg IV or IM in a single dose, not to exceed 125 mg IM
  - Disseminated infections: ceftriaxone 50 mg/kg IV or IM daily (max dose of 1 g) in single dose; bacteremia or arthritis: 7 days; meningitis: 10 to 14 days; endocarditis: 4 weeks
- Ophthalmic neonatorum prophylaxis: single application of erythromycin 0.5% ophthalmic ointment to each eye immediately after delivery (2)[A]

- Neonatal conjunctivitis: ceftriaxone 25 to 50 mg/kg IV or IM in a single dose (not to exceed 125 mg) (1),(2)[A]
- *Conjunctival exudates should be cultured for definitive diagnosis* (1),(2)[A].
- Scalp abscesses (from scalp electrodes) (1),(2)[A]
  - Ceftriaxone 25 to 50 mg/kg/day IV or IM in a single daily dose for 7 days; treat for a duration of 10 to 14 days if meningitis is documented.
  - Alternative: cefotaxime 25 mg/kg IV or IM q12h for 7 days; treat for a duration of 10 to 14 days if meningitis is documented.
- Asymptomatic infants born to mothers with untreated gonorrhea (1),(2)[A]: ceftriaxone 25 to 50 mg/kg IV or IM, not to exceed 125 mg in a single dose

Pregnancy Considerations
- Pregnant women should be treated with the same treatments as listed above (2)[A]. For uncomplicated urogenital, anorectal, and pharyngeal gonorrheal infection, if chlamydial infection has not been excluded, add azithromycin 1 g single dose orally or add alternative of amoxicillin 500 mg orally 3 times daily for 7 days.
- An alternative is treatment with spectinomycin. If spectinomycin or other regimens are not possible, consultation with an infectious disease specialist is recommended (2)[A].

Second Line
- A single 2-g oral dose of azithromycin has been used in the past, although it should be avoided due to the potential to develop macrolide resistance (2)[A].
- For additional treatment options, see CDC STD treatment guidelines: https://www.cdc.gov/std /treatment-guidelines/default.htm

ADMISSION, INPATIENT, AND NURSING CONSIDERATIONS
- Hematogenously disseminated infection
- Pneumonia or eye infection in infants

 ONGOING CARE

FOLLOW-UP RECOMMENDATIONS
Patient Monitoring
- U.S. Preventive Services Task Force (USPSTF) (5)[A]
  - Screen all sexually active women ≤24 years of age and in older women at increased risk for infection for chlamydia and gonorrhea: grade B recommendation.
  - Insufficient evidence to recommend for or against screening for chlamydia and gonorrhea in men: grade I recommendation
  - Report cases of gonorrhea to public health (5)[A].
- CDC: Screen all MSM annually at sites of contact (urethra, rectum, pharynx), regardless of condom use. Increase screening to every 3 to 6 months if at increased risk.

PATIENT EDUCATION
- Counseling concerning risk reduction, condom use, future fertility, and full STI testing
- Encourage patient to notify partners (from past 60 days); consider EPT.
- Encourage patient to abstain from sex until 7 days after patient and all partners have been treated.
- Encourage retesting 3 months after treatment given high prevalence of reinfection (2).

PROGNOSIS
Complete cure with return to normal function with adequate and timely treatment

COMPLICATIONS
Pelvic inflammatory disease, infertility, ectopic pregnancy, urethral stricture, corneal scarring, destruction of joint articular surfaces, cardiac valvular damage

Pediatric Considerations
Vertical transmission is a significant risk among patients with gonococcal infection at the time of delivery (2)[A].

REFERENCES
1. Mahapure K, Singh A. A review of recent advances in our understanding of Neisseria gonorrhoeae. *Cureus.* 2023;15(8):e43464.
2. Centers for Disease Control and Prevention. Sexually transmitted infections treatment guidelines, 2021: gonococcal infections among adolescents and adults. https://www.cdc.gov/std /treatment-guidelines/gonorrhea-adults.htm. October 9, 2023.
3. St. Cyr S, Barbee L, Workowski KA, et al. Update to CDC's treatment guidelines for gonococcal infection, 2020. *MMWR Morb Mortal Wkly Rep.* 2020;69(50):1911–1916.
4. Committee on Gynecologic Practice. ACOG Committee Opinion No. 645: dual therapy for gonococcal infections. *Obstet Gynecol.* 2015;126(5):e95–e99.
5. U.S. Preventive Services Task Force. Final recommendation statement: chlamydia and gonorrhea: screening. http://www.uspreventiveservicestask force.org/Page/Document/UpdateSummaryFinal /chlamydia-and-gonorrhea-screening. Accessed October 9, 2023.

 SEE ALSO

Chlamydia Infection (Sexually Transmitted); HIV/AIDS; Pelvic Inflammatory Disease; Syphilis

CODES

ICD10
- A54.9 Gonococcal infection, unspecified
- A54.03 Gonococcal cervicitis, unspecified
- A54.31 Gonococcal conjunctivitis

CLINICAL PEARLS
- Gonococcal antibiotic resistance is a significant clinical problem.
- Treatment for uncomplicated gonorrhea should include two drugs, one of which is effective against chlamydia.
- Screen patients with gonorrhea for chlamydia, syphilis, HIV, and hepatitis.

G

GOUT

Sangili Chandran, MD • Katherine Metropulos, DO • Alqasem Alsaqri, MD

 BASICS

DESCRIPTION
- An inflammatory arthritis leading to an acutely red, hot, swollen joint, which can progress to a chronic tophaceous joint that is associated with pain, nodule formation, and cutaneous compromise
- Characterized by deposition of monosodium urate (MSU) crystals in joints and soft tissues, resulting in acute and chronic arthritis, soft-tissue masses called tophi, urate nephropathy, and uric acid nephrolithiasis
- The long limb, foot, ankle, and knee are preferentially involved, with the 1st metatarsophalangeal joint (podagra) characteristically affected.
- Flares are usually monoarticular. Polyarticular flares can be associated with pronounced systemic symptoms, including fever, chills, and delirium.
- Gout is related to a hyperuricemia (serum uric acid level >6.8 mg/dL).

EPIDEMIOLOGY
Prevalence
- Ranges between 0.68% and 3.9% in adults
- Gout has a higher incidence in males than females.

ETIOLOGY AND PATHOPHYSIOLOGY
Four pathophysiologic stages:
- Development of hyperuricemia (from uric acid overproduction and/or renal underexcretion)
- Deposition of MSU crystals (Changes in uric acid solubility caused by local temperature decrease, trauma, or acidosis may precipitate out of solution and accumulate as crystals in joints and soft tissues.)
- Clinical presentation of gout flares due to an acute inflammatory response to deposited crystals
- Clinical presentation of advanced disease characterized by tophi and joint damage

Genetics
Consider *HLA-B*5801* mutation genotyping for people in Asian origin.

RISK FACTORS
- Age >40 years
- Excessive purine consumption from diet (alcohol [especially beer], red meat, seafood, sugar-sweetened beverages)
- Diabetes mellitus, metabolic syndrome, obesity
- Congestive heart failure, chronic kidney disease (CKD), dyslipidemia, hypertension
- Smoking
- Urate-elevating medications: thiazide diuretics, loop diuretics (less of a risk vs. thiazides), niacin, aspirin
- Transplant-associated gout can happen in immunosuppressed solid organ transplant recipients on low-dose prednisolone and calcineurin inhibitors (cyclosporine and tacrolimus) as these medications increase uric acid (1).
- Hyperuricemia from rapid cell turnover/tumor lysis syndrome (e.g. hemolysis, chemotherapy)

GENERAL PREVENTION
- Diet modification: Avoid purine-rich foods like red meat and shellfish. Reduce alcohol consumption (beer and liquor).
- Maintain fluid intake and avoid dehydration.

COMMONLY ASSOCIATED CONDITIONS
- Nontraumatic joint disorders
- Renal disease

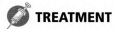 **DIAGNOSIS**

HISTORY
- Typical first presentation of gout (2):
  - Intensely painful acute inflammatory arthritis, usually a gout flare, affecting a lower limb joint, which can be self-limited over a period of 7 to 14 days if goes untreated
  - Lower limb and monoarticular arthritis are common early in course of disease—gout flares can occur in the joints or periarticular tissues (e.g., bursae, tendons, entheses), whereas upper extremity and polyarticular presentations are usually seen in chronic cases.
  - The joint may be swollen, warm, erythematous, and exquisitely tender to touch. The pain can be described as stabbing, gnawing, burning, or throbbing.
  - There is a substantial limitation in using the affected areas such as difficulty walking and fear of even minimal physical contact.
  - Often awakes patients from sleep due to an intolerance to contact with clothing or bedsheets
  - There is a rapid onset of intense pain, often progressing rapidly over 12 to 24 hours.
  - Acute attacks are usually precipitated by infection, injury, dehydration, or excess alcohol or purine intake.
  - Fever can be present.
  - Subcutaneous or intraosseous nodules, referred to as tophi, can be seen after many recurrent attacks.
- Chronic manifestations of gout:
  - Subcutaneous tophi located in joints, ears, olecranon bursae, finger pads, tendon
  - Tophi are firm and hard, vary in size, can become acutely inflamed but are usually not tender.
  - Can ulcerate with thick/white discharge and superimposed infections

PHYSICAL EXAM
- Examine the joint(s) for tenderness, swelling, and range of motion (ROM).
- Tophi can be found in the affected joints, the helix of the ear, over the olecranon process, or on the Achilles tendon.

DIFFERENTIAL DIAGNOSIS
Septic arthritis, calcium pyrophosphate deposition disease (formerly known as "pseudogout"), cellulitis, osteoarthritis, rheumatoid arthritis and bursitis, traumatic arthritis, hemarthrosis

DIAGNOSTIC TESTS & INTERPRETATION
- Diagnostic compound score for patients presenting with monarthritis in primary care settings (<4 of below ruled out gout in 97%) (3):
  - Male sex
  - Previous patient-reported arthritis attack
  - Onset within 1 day
  - Joint redness
  - 1st metatarsophalangeal joint involvement
  - Hypertension or cardiovascular disease
  - High serum urate
- Initial acute gout episode
  - Uric acid (may be normal or low), CBC (WBC maybe elevated), ESR/CRP
  - Synovial fluid analysis: urate crystals (negatively birefringent under polarizing microscopy), cell count (WBC usually 2,000 to 5,000 cells/mm³); gram stain and culture to rule out infection
  - 24-hour urine to screen for uric acid overproduction (>800 mg/24 hours) in those with onset before the age of 25 years or with a history of urolithiasis

Follow-Up Tests & Special Considerations
- Radiographs/plain x-rays are normal early in disease, but they can reveal periarticular erosions with periosteum overgrowth in chronic gout.
- Ultrasonography can show a double contour sign (reflecting MSU crystal deposition on the surface of hyaline articular cartilage), intra-articular or intra-bursal tophi, and a snowstorm appearance.
- Dual energy CT (DECT) imaging can show urate deposition at articular or periarticular sites.

TREATMENT

GENERAL MEASURES
Supportive care—ice packs, rest, mobility assistance, and adequate nutrition and hydration

First Line
- Treatment should be initiated within 12 to 24 hours of acute gout attack and continued for 1 to 2 days after attack has subsided (1).
  - Urate-lowering therapy should not be interrupted during an acute gout attack.
  - Mild/moderate gout severity (≤6 of 10 on Visual Analog Pain Scale, particularly for an attack involving only one or a few small joints or 1 to 2 large joints)
  - NSAIDs:
    ○ Naproxen: 500 mg BID
    ○ Meloxicam: 7.5 to 15 mg/day
    ○ Indomethacin: 50 to 150 mg/day (generally less well tolerated than others)
    ○ Diclofenac: 75 mg BID
    ○ Ibuprofen: 800 mg q8h
  - Oral/intra-articular/intramuscular/intravenous corticosteroids
    ○ Corticosteroids are useful in patients with acute gout flare who cannot tolerate NSAIDs or have contraindications to NSAIDs and colchicine such as CKD.

- When monotherapy is insufficient for acute flares, a combination of NSAIDs with either intra-articular corticosteroid, oral steroid, or colchicine may be used.
  - Oral corticosteroids—medium dose (15 to 20 mg/day) to high dose (30 to 35 mg/day) for 5 days
- Intra-articular/intramuscular/intravenous preparation—triamcinolone acetonide, dexamethasone, methylprednisolone
- Colchicine: used for gout attacks where the onset was <36 hours prior to treatment initiation
  - Begin a loading dose of 1.0 to 1.2 mg followed by 0.5 to 0.6 mg 1 hour later, after 12 hours, resume 0.5 to 0.6 mg q8h with no >6 mg per course, and at least 3 days between courses.
- Severe gout (≥7 of 10 pain scale, involving four or more joints with arthritis involving more than one region or involving three separate large joints)
  - Initial combination therapy is an option, and it includes the use of full doses of the following:
    - Colchicine and NSAIDs
    - PO corticosteroids and colchicine
    - Intra-articular steroids
- Chronic treatment includes using urate-lowering therapies for a serum uric acid <6 mg/dL (may need <5 mg/dL to improve symptoms).
  - Urate-lowering agents can be prescribed during an acute attack provided that effective anti-inflammatory prophylaxis has been initiated first such as the following:
    - Low-dose NSAIDs: naproxen 250 mg PO BID
    - Low-dose colchicine: 0.5 to 0.6 mg once or twice daily
    - If colchicine and NSAIDs are contraindicated or ineffective:
    - Low-dose prednisone at ≤10 mg/day
    - Treatment duration of at least 6 months or 3 months after achieving serum urate target.
  - Urate-lowering agents:
    - Allopurinol: xanthine oxidase inhibitor—does not reduce number of acute attacks
      - Start no higher than 100 mg/day (50 mg/day in stage 4 or 5 CKD).
      - Titrate dose upward q2–5wk to a maximum dose.
      - Monitor serum uric acid level and renal function every 3 months in the 1st year and annually thereafter.
      - Monitor for allopurinol hypersensitivity syndrome (AHS), pruritus, rash, elevated hepatic transaminases, and eosinophilia. HLA-B*5801 allele for AHS should be performed in those of Korean, Chinese, or Thai.
    - Febuxostat: selective xanthine oxidase inhibitor
      - Start 40 mg/day; titrate to 80 mg/day.
    - Probenecid: uricosuric agent
      - Alternative if xanthine oxidase inhibitor is contraindicated.
      - May be used in addition to allopurinol or febuxostat if serum urate target is not achieved
      - Increased risk of urolithiasis with this agent
      - Not recommended if CrCl is <50 or if there is a history of urolithiasis
      - Start 250 mg BID; titrate to 2,000 mg/day.

Second Line
- If not responding to initial pharmacologic monotherapy, add a second agent.
- IL-1 inhibitors: for patients who have intolerable side effects or have contraindications to first-line anti-inflammatory therapy
  - Anakinra 100 mg SQ daily for 5 days
  - Canakinumab 150 mg SQ × 1 dose (Monitor for adverse events, including serious infections.)

ADDITIONAL THERAPIES
- Losartan possesses uricosuric properties; consider for hypertensive patients.
- Fenofibrate also possesses uricosuric properties and may be useful with lipid disorders.

SURGERY/OTHER PROCEDURES
Large tophi that are infected or interfering with joint motion may need to be surgically removed.

COMPLEMENTARY & ALTERNATIVE MEDICINE
Vitamin C (>500 mg QD) has been shown to reduce serum uric acid levels (1)[C].

 ## ONGOING CARE

FOLLOW-UP RECOMMENDATIONS
Patient Monitoring
- Serum uric acid measurements q2–5wk while titrating urate-lowering treatment to goal
- Regularly monitor CBC, renal function, liver function test, and urinalysis.

DIET
- Avoid:
  - Organ meats high in purine content (sweetbreads, liver, kidney)
  - High-fructose corn syrup–sweetened sodas, other beverages, or foods (reducing fructose to <1 g/kg/day)
  - Alcohol overuse (>2 drinks per day for men and >1 drink per day for women)
- Limit:
  - Beef, lamb, pork, and seafood with high purine content such as sardines and shellfish
  - Servings of naturally sweetened fruit juices
  - Sugar, sweetened beverages, and desserts
  - Table salt, including in sauces and gravies
  - Alcohol (particularly beer) in all patients (<1 to 2 drinks per day)
- Encourage:
  - Coffee intake of >4 cups per day reduced the risk of gout by 57%.
  - Foods that are rich in dietary fiber, folate, and vitamin C decreased the incidence of gout.
  - Higher intake of dairy products has been associated with lower serum uric acid levels (4).
  - Cherry consumption may be of benefit in gout prophylaxis (5)[C].
  - Weight loss in overweight patients; increased adiposity and weight gain are risk factors for incident gout (6).

PATIENT EDUCATION
Explain to patients that they may have increased acute flare-ups with the initiation of urate-lowering therapy, presumably due to liberation of crystals from dissolving urate collections.

PROGNOSIS
Usually successfully managed with proper treatment and lifestyle modifications

COMPLICATIONS
- Inflammatory arthritis and joint destruction
- Uric acid nephropathy and renal stones

REFERENCES
1. Abhishek A, Roddy E, Doherty M. Gout—a guide for the general and acute physicians. *Clin Med (Lond)*. 2017;17(1):54–59.
2. Rogenmoser S, Arnold MH. Chronic gout: Barriers to effective management. *Aust J Gen Pract*. 2018;47(6):351–356.
3. Neogi T, Jansen TLTA, Dalbeth N, et al. 2015 Gout classification criteria: an American College of Rheumatology/European League Against Rheumatism collaborative initiative. *Arthritis Rheumatol*. 2015;67(10):2557–2568.
4. daSilva MT, de Fátima Haueisen Sander Diniz M, Coelho CG, et al. Intake of selected foods and beverages and serum uric acid levels in adults: ELSA-Brasil (2008–2010). *Public Health Nutr*. 2020;23(3):506–514.
5. Lamb KL, Lynn A, Russell J, et al. Effect of tart cherry juice on risk of gout attacks: protocol for a randomised controlled trial. *BMJ Open*. 2020;10(3):e035108.
6. Choi HK, Atkinson K, Karlson EW, et al. Obesity, weight change, hypertension, diuretic use, and risk of gout in men: the health professionals follow-up study. *Arch Intern Med*. 2005;165(7):742–748.

 ## CODES

ICD10
- M10.269 Drug-induced gout, unspecified knee
- M10.161 Lead-induced gout, right knee
- M10.221 Drug-induced gout, right elbow

CLINICAL PEARLS
- Acute gouty arthritis can affect more than one joint; the 1st metatarsophalangeal joint is most commonly involved at presentation (podagra).
- MSU crystals found in synovial fluid aspirate are pathognomonic for gout.
- Pharmacologic treatment should begin within 24 hours of acute gout flare. NSAIDs and/or corticosteroids are effective for mild/moderate attacks.
- Asymptomatic hyperuricemia does not require treatment.

GRANULOMA, PYOGENIC

Michelle Moran McDonough, MD • Keith L. Stelter, MD

 BASICS

DESCRIPTION
- Pyogenic granulomas (PG) are benign vascular pro-liferations that appear most commonly on the skin and mucus membranes. Most common sites are the head and neck, the lips and oral cavity, the trunk, and the extremities (1),(2).
- Described as rapidly growing erythematous to viola-ceous nodules that develop into pedunculated masses with erosive surface that are friable and tend to bleed profusely due to the vascular nature of the lesion
- Less commonly presents as a sessile lesion
- Rarely regress completely without intervention (2)
- Synonym(s): lobular capillary hemangioma, granu-loma telangiectaticum, granuloma gravidarum

EPIDEMIOLOGY
- The peak incidence of PG occurs in children and young adults (2).
- Commonly seen in early pregnancy
- Conflicting evidence from prior studies regarding male or female predominance; overall, seems to have a male predominance in childhood through adolescence and female predominance during reproductive years before the age of 40 years

Prevalence
- Up to 1 in 25,000 adults are diagnosed with an intraoral PG in their lifetime (2).
- Cutaneous pyogenic granulomas account for 0.5% of childhood skin nodules (2).

ETIOLOGY AND PATHOPHYSIOLOGY
- Definitive cause unknown
- Thought to be associated with capillary proliferation resulting from aberrant healing response to minor trauma
- Associated with peripheral nerve injury, inflamma-tory systemic diseases, and drugs (retinoids, systemic steroids, protease inhibitors, epidermal growth factor receptor inhibitors)

- May be related to hormonal changes in pregnancy
- Not considered a hemangioma or neoplasm; no true granulomatous histology present

RISK FACTORS
- Pregnancy
- Trauma
- Intraoral trauma or surgery
- Inflammatory systemic diseases
- Medications such as retinoids, systemic steroids, protease inhibitors, epidermal growth factor receptor inhibitors

GENERAL PREVENTION
Good oral hygiene may be helpful.

COMMONLY ASSOCIATED CONDITIONS
Inflammatory systemic diseases

DIAGNOSIS

HISTORY
- Solitary lesion that develops rapidly from days to weeks after minor trauma
- Tends to bleed easily
- Grows early in pregnancy and partially regresses postpartum

PHYSICAL EXAM
- Most commonly located at the head, neck, and upper extremities, especially in children
- Among oral lesions, gingiva is the most common location.
- Usually a bright red, friable papule; can also be purple, yellow, or brown
- Moist and sometimes scaly-appearing surface with serosanguineous crusting and sharp demarcation
- Usually <1 cm but ranges from a few millimeters to 2 to 3 cm in diameter
- Giant lesions may occur on areas such as the foot (rare).

- Soft; pedunculated or sessile
- Solitary red papule, grows rapidly, forming a stalk, may bleed, and ulcerate
- Dermoscopy exam: red structureless, homogenous area surrounded by a white collarette intersected by white lines

DIFFERENTIAL DIAGNOSIS
- Benign lesions
  - Cherry/infantile hemangioma (3)
  - Fibrous papule (1),(3)
  - Bacillary angiomatosis, from *Bartonella* spp. (1)
  - Carbuncle or furuncle
- Malignant lesions
  - Basal cell carcinoma (1)
  - Squamous cell carcinoma (1)
  - Amelanotic melanoma (1)
  - Kaposi sarcoma (1)
  - Cutaneous metastases (1)

DIAGNOSTIC TESTS & INTERPRETATION
Initial Tests (lab, imaging)
No labs are necessary for the diagnosis.

Diagnostic Procedures/Other
- Excisional/shave biopsy
- Send for pathology

Test Interpretation
Microscopic examination reveals the following:
- Small, endothelial-lined vascular spaces
- Loose/dense connective tissue stroma
- Acute and chronic inflammatory cells
- No true granuloma formation
- Abundant mitotic activity
- Resembles granulation tissue in an edematous matrix, showing immature capillaries with interspersed tissue

TREATMENT

Full thickness surgical excision is best to yield material for histopathologic analysis and avoid recurrence (4)[C]. Excision must be adequate to avoid recurrence. Even a small fragment of tissue left behind may lead to recurrence.

MEDICATION
First Line
- Topical imiquimod (4)[C]
- Silver nitrate (5)[A]
- Topical timolol or propranolol (4)[C]
- Topical 1.5% phenol solution may be used for periungual lesion (5)[C].

SURGERY/OTHER PROCEDURES
- Shave biopsy can be used for pedunculated lesions; can combine with cautery (5)[C]
- Punch biopsy acceptable for small lesions
- Electrosurgery: electrodesiccation and curettage (5)[B]
- CO_2 laser ablation results in less pain and allows for superficial dermal ablation (4)[C].
- Cryotherapy with liquid nitrogen (recur 2%) (5)[C]
- Pulsed dye laser or CO_2 laser (5)[C]

 ONGOING CARE

PATIENT EDUCATION
Patient should avoid trauma to area following excision.

PROGNOSIS
- Some lesions spontaneously resolve on their own (usually within 6 months).
- With treatment, recurrence rates are between 4% and 5% (2).

COMPLICATIONS
Recurrence: After removal or destruction of solitary lesion, multiple satellite lesions can form around original treatment site.

REFERENCES
1. Lin RL, Janniger CK. Pyogenic granuloma. *Cutis.* 2004;74(4):229–233.
2. Borden A, Harrington JW. Pyogenic granuloma: an overview of pathogenesis, diagnosis, and management. *Consultant.* 2018;58(6):e181.
3. Pagliai KA, Cohen BA. Pyogenic granuloma in children. *Pediatr Dermatol.* 2004;21(1):10–13.
4. Plachouri KM, Georgiou S. Therapeutic approaches to pyogenic granuloma: an updated review. *Int J Dermatol.* 2019;58(6):642–648.
5. Lee J, Sinno H, Tahiri Y, et al. Treatment options for cutaneous pyogenic granulomas: a review. *J Plast Reconstr Aesthet Surg.* 2011;64(9):1216–1220.

ADDITIONAL READING
- Gilmore A, Kelsberg G, Safranek S. Clinical inquiries. What's the best treatment for pyogenic granuloma? *J Fam Pract.* 2010;59(1):40–42.
- Greene AK. Management of hemangiomas and other vascular tumors. *Clin Plast Surg.* 2011;38(1):45–63.
- Hinen HB, Trenor CC III, Wine Lee L. Childhood vascular tumors. *Front Pediatr.* 2020;8:573023.
- Koo MG, Lee SH, Han SE. Pyogenic granuloma: a retrospective analysis of cases treated over a 10-year. *Arch Craniofac Surg.* 2017;18(1):16–20.

- Losa Iglesias ME, Becerro de Bengoa Vallejo R. Topical phenol as a conservative treatment for periungual pyogenic granuloma. *Dermatol Surg.* 2010;36(5):675–678.
- Zaballos P, Llambrich A, Cuéllar F, et al. Dermoscopic findings in pyogenic granuloma. *Br J Dermatol.* 2006;154(6):1108–1111.
- Zalaudek I, Kreusch J, Giacomel J, et al. How to diagnose nonpigmented skin tumors: a review of vascular structures seen with dermoscopy: part II. Nonmelanocytic skin tumors. *J Am Acad Dermatol.* 2010;63(3):377–386.

 CODES

ICD10
- L98.0 Pyogenic granuloma
- K06.8 Oth disrd of gingiva and edentulous alveolar ridge
- K13.4 Granuloma and granuloma-like lesions of oral mucosa

CLINICAL PEARLS
- Benign, vascular tumor, usually rapidly growing, that involves exposed areas, such as distal extremities and face, as well as in the oral cavity
- Excision must be adequate to avoid recurrence.
- Excisional biopsy recommended to ensure proper diagnosis and rule out malignancy
- Excision with primary closure is superior to shave excision with cautery in terms of recurrence risk, but both are effective.

G

GRANULOMA ANNULARE

Sarah E. Nickolich, MD • Kyle Burke, DO

 BASICS

DESCRIPTION
Granuloma annulare (GA) is a benign skin condition characterized by groups of skin-colored to erythematous papules that are usually in an annular (ring-like) pattern and typically located on the dorsal aspects of the hands and feet. There are five types of GA: localized, generalized, subcutaneous, patch, and perforating.

EPIDEMIOLOGY
Incidence
- GA is a relatively common, noninfectious granulomatous disease. Incidence is reported to be 0.04% per year within the United States (1).
- Although most lesions resolve spontaneously within 2 years, some persist for ≥10 years.
- Predominant sex: female > male (3:1) (1)
- Onset of symptoms occurs at <30 years old in 2/3 of all patients. Typical ages for onset of each subtype are as follows:
  – Localized: <30 years old
  – Generalized: bimodal: <10 years old, 30 to 60 years old
  – Subcutaneous: 2 to 14 years old
  – Patch: >30 years old
  – Perforating: children and young adults
- Distribution of subtypes:
  – Localized: 75%
  – Generalized: 10–15%
  – Subcutaneous: <5%
  – Patch type: <5%
  – Perforating: <5%

Prevalence
Prevalence is reported to be highest in the 5th decade of life (1).

ETIOLOGY AND PATHOPHYSIOLOGY
The etiology of GA remains unknown; however, recent studies have helped to further elucidate its underlying cause. It is hypothesized to be related to upregulation of T-helper (Th) 1 and Th2 pathways in GA lesions. Increased cytokine expression was subsequently noted to include tumor necrosis factor alpha (TNF-α), interleukin (IL)-1β, IL-4, interferon (IFN)-γ, IL-12/IL-23p40, and IL-31. Janus kinase/signal transducer and activator of transcription (JAK/STAT) pathways were also found to be activated in GA. Response by "M1" and "M2" macrophages was described, which can be related to histopathologic findings of collagen degradation followed by tissue remodeling and mucin deposition, respectively.

Genetics
There is some evidence for a genetic predisposition. Two studies reported an increased frequency of HLA-Bw35 in patients with generalized GA. Of note, HLA-Bw35 has also been associated with thyroid disease.

RISK FACTORS
No definite risk factors have been identified. There are reported associations between GA and diabetes mellitus (DM), autoimmune thyroid disease, dyslipidemia, HIV, Epstein-Barr virus, herpes simplex virus, systemic lupus erythematosus, tuberculosis, and hepatitis B and C, among others. There have also been associations with interferon-α therapy, trauma, sun exposure, insect bites, borreliosis, and malignancies (most commonly lymphoma).

GENERAL PREVENTION
There are no known preventive measures for GA.

COMMONLY ASSOCIATED CONDITIONS
- DM: The association between GA and DM remains controversial, but there is increasing evidence of an association. Early studies from the 1980s showed a possible link, and a recent large, retrospective cohort study (51,169 patients with GA) showed that 21% of patients had both GA and DM, whereas 13.3% of matched controls had DM (1).
- Autoimmune thyroid disease: Multiple case reports have linked thyroid disease with both generalized and localized GA. In one case-control study, 24 women with localized GA were compared to 100 age-matched women with non-GA dermatologic disease. A statistically significant increase in the incidence of autoimmune thyroid disease among those with localized GA as compared with those with other non-GA cutaneous disease was identified (12% vs. 1%, $p = .022$) (2),(3).
- Malignancy: There is no definitive relationship between GA and malignancy. A review of the literature found in 14 case reports and two correlation studies in which patients who had one or more malignancies also had GA. In a majority of these cases, the malignancies were hematologic, primarily lymphoma (2),(3).
- Dyslipidemia: Dyslipidemia may be associated with GA. A single case-control study ($n = 140$) demonstrated a statistically significant increase in hyperlipidemia among patients with GA compared to controls (79.3% vs. 51.9%, $p < .001$). Further studies, including the large, retrospective cohort study noted above, have demonstrated significant associations with GA and hyperlipidemia.
- Infectious: Among patients with GA, those who also have HIV appear more likely to have the generalized subtype. In one study of 34 patients with GA and HIV, 20 (59%) had generalized GA (2). Additional viral triggers have been suggested to include SARS-CoV-2, Epstein-Barr virus, and varicella zoster virus. There has been recent data showing evidence of potential bacterial triggers, including *Chlamydiales* spp. and *Borrelia* spp. (1).
- Iatrogenically-induced: Several drugs have been implicated in triggering GA: acetazolamide, anti-TNFα agents, amlodipine, allopurinol, botulinum toxin, desensitization injections, immune checkpoint inhibitors, immunizations, levetiracetam, paroxetine, topiramate, and phototherapy (1).

- Note: Conclusions regarding associations between GA and various diseases, including those mentioned earlier, are limited by both design and power. Consequently, in the absence of new research, definitive associations between GA and other diseases cannot be made.

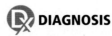 DIAGNOSIS

HISTORY
Cutaneous lesions of GA are generally asymptomatic. Lesions often persist for months or years, especially in patients who have generalized GA. In most cases, regardless of subtype, GA resolves spontaneously but may thereafter recur without obvious trigger.

PHYSICAL EXAM
- Localized: asymptomatic, flesh-colored or erythematous annular, or arciform plaque with a moderately firm, rope-like border and central clearing, ranging from 5 mm to 5 cm in diameter. Small 1- to 2-mm papules may be noted peripheral to the primary lesion. The most common locations are the dorsal aspects of the distal upper and lower extremities; involvement of palms is rare. It is common to have multiple lesions at the time of presentation.
- Generalized: Lesions have the same morphology as localized GA lesions but tend to be larger, greater in number (usually >10), persist for a longer period of time, and are more widespread.
- Subcutaneous: firm, nontender nodules that tend to grow rapidly; usually solitary but may occur in groups; the most common location is scalp and/or anterior aspect of the lower extremities, followed by upper extremities and buttocks.
- Patch: Erythematous macules and patches are distributed symmetrically on the extremities and trunk. The typical annular configuration may or may not be present; often involves proximal extremities
- Perforating: Damaged collagen from dermis is extruded onto skin surface. Papules may be up to 4 mm in diameter and display yellowish umbilication, crusting, or scale. Lesions are often widely distributed on the body and cause scaring.

DIFFERENTIAL DIAGNOSIS
- Localized: tinea corporis, annular lichen planus, necrobiosis lipoidica, pityriasis rosea, erythema migrans, leprosy
- Generalized: sarcoidosis, lichen planus, cutaneous metastases, mycosis fungoides (cutaneous T-cell lymphoma)
- Patch type: erythema migrans
- Subcutaneous: rheumatoid nodules
- Perforating: molluscum contagiosum, sarcoidosis, insect bites

DIAGNOSTIC TESTS & INTERPRETATION

Initial Tests (lab, imaging)

- Diagnosis is typically established by history and physical examination; laboratory investigations are rarely needed. Microscopic evaluation of skin cells using potassium hydroxide (KOH) preparation may be useful to exclude a fungal process.
- Consider laboratory testing to evaluate comorbid dyslipidemia, DM, thyroid disease, HIV, hepatitis B/C, and malignancy as clinically indicated.

Diagnostic Procedures/Other

Punch biopsy and histologic evaluation may aid in confirming the diagnosis and identifying the subtype. Immunohistochemical streptavidin-biotin–horseradish peroxidase (HRP) analysis for CD68/KP-1 (a marker for histiocytic differentiation) may also aid in the diagnosis. Ultrasound evaluation has been shown to assist in diagnosis of subcutaneous GA, which may be beneficial in the pediatric population (1).

Test Interpretation

Dermal infiltrate demonstrating foci of degenerative collagen associated with palisading granulomas around an anuclear dermis with mucin deposition. Mucin deposition is a strong indicator of a GA diagnosis. Histologic variants include interstitial (histiocytic infiltrate between collagen fibers), classic (palisading dermal granulomas), and epithelioid (tuberculoid and sarcoidal granulomas).

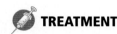 TREATMENT

GENERAL MEASURES

GA is a self-limited condition that is likely to regress spontaneously. The clinician's primary role after making the diagnosis is to educate the patient about the natural history of GA and to consider screening for conditions that may be associated with this disease. No specific treatment has been satisfactorily studied in reliable randomized controlled trials with most recommendations based on case reports, case series, and retrospective reviews.

MEDICATION

- The trauma induced by biopsy alone can cause involution of lesions through an unknown mechanism.
- Given the self-limited nature of the disease, it is incumbent on providers to assess the risk/benefit ratio of treatment. Reassurance is often all that is required for localized, asymptomatic disease.
- The following therapies have been tried with variable success. Duration of therapy is often undefined and is based on clinical response.

First Line

Topical and intralesional corticosteroids

- High-potency topical (class I or II), with or without occlusion (1)[C],(3)[C]
- Intralesional triamcinolone: concentration of 2.5 to 5 mg/mL (3)[C]; technique: Insert the needle into the dermis at the elevated border and slowly inject while withdrawing the needle, with enough volume to cause the lesion to begin to blanch. Take care to avoid allowing the tip of the needle to push through to inserting the needle through the lesion.

Second Line

- Doxycycline: 100 mg/day for 8 to 10 weeks (1)[C], (3)[C]
- Pimecrolimus cream: 1% BID (3)[C]
- Tacrolimus ointment: 0.1% BID (3)[C]
- Chloroquine: 250 mg/day (1)[C],(3)[C]
- Hydroxychloroquine: 9 mg/kg/day for 2 months, 6 mg/kg/day for month 3, 2 mg/kg/day for month 4 (3)[C]
- Isotretinoin: 0.5 to 0.75 mg/kg/day (3)[C]
- Rifampin 600 mg, ofloxacin 400 mg, with minocycline 100 mg once daily (1)[C],(3)[C]
- Dapsone: 100 mg/day for mean duration of 9.8 months (1)[C],(3)[C]
- Cyclosporine: 3 to 4 mg/kg/day (3)[C]
- Methotrexate: 10 mg IM weekly for 11 months (1)[C]
- Niacinamide: 500 mg TID (3)[C]
- Fumaric acid esters: variable dosing schemes (3)[C]
- Interferon gamma 1b: intralesional injection, 2.5 × 10^5 IU per lesion for 7 consecutive days followed by 3 times per week for 2 weeks (3)[C]
- TNF-α inhibitors, such as infliximab 5 mg/kg IV at weeks 0, 2, and 6, then variable or adalimumab 80 mg SC at week 0 and then 40 SC at week 1 and every other week or etanercept 50 mg twice weekly (3)[C]
- Photodynamic therapy (1)[C]
- Pentoxifylline 400 mg TID (1)[C]

ADDITIONAL THERAPIES

- Cryotherapy (one 10- to 60-second freeze thaw cycle) (3)[C]
- Fractional thermolysis (e.g., YAG fractionated laser) (3)[C]
- 585- to 595-nm pulsed dye laser (3)[C]
- Narrowband ultraviolet B (NBUVB)
- Psoralen ultraviolet A (PUVA)
- Surgical excision (for subcutaneous GA) (2)[C]
- Apremilast: phosphodiesterase-4 inhibitor (1)[C]
- Tofacitinib: JAK inhibitor (1)[C]
- Control of comorbidities such as DM and hyperlipidemia (1)[C]

 ONGOING CARE

FOLLOW-UP RECOMMENDATIONS

Routine follow-up is not required unless treatment is initiated. In such situations, follow-up is recommended to monitor for possible adverse effects of treatment. Referral to a dermatologist is prudent for patients who have generalized GA, cosmetic concerns, and for patients whose lesions persist despite conservative therapy.

PATIENT EDUCATION

Patients should be educated that GA is a benign, self-limited condition that may persist for months to years, spontaneously resolve, and spontaneously recur. Additionally, patients may benefit from knowing that GA is not thought to be of an infectious etiology and is not transmissible to others.

PROGNOSIS

>50% of cases resolve spontaneously within 2 months to 2 years after onset, although recurrence, typically at the original site, is common (>40%). Patients aged <39 years tend to have a shorter duration of illness.

COMPLICATIONS

Complications of treatment are much more likely than complications from GA.

REFERENCES

1. Joshi TP, Duvic M. Granuloma annulare: an updated review of epidemiology, pathogenesis, and treatment options. *Am J Clin Dermatol*. 2022;23(1):37–50.
2. Piette EW, Rosenbach M. Granuloma annulare: pathogenesis, disease associations and triggers, and therapeutic options. *J Am Acad Dermatol*. 2016;75(3):467–479.
3. Keimig EL. Granuloma annulare. *Dermatol Clin*. 2015;33(3):315–329.

 CODES

ICD10
L92.0 Granuloma annulare

CLINICAL PEARLS

- GA is a benign, self-limited condition. Consider risk-to-benefit ratio when partnering with patients to determine treatment.
- When initiating therapy for localized GA, start with high-dose topical corticosteroids or intralesional corticosteroids followed by cryotherapy or other listed topical therapies. For widespread disease, consider initiating treatment with antimalarials or phototherapy.
- Consider GA in the differential diagnosis of lesions that appear to be tinea, especially when these lesions lack scale and are KOH-negative.
- Consider fasting lipid panel, fasting blood glucose or HbA1C, TSH, free T4, thyroid antibodies, hepatitis B and C panel, HIV screening test, and age-appropriate cancer screening, especially in those with generalized or atypical presentations of GA.

G

GRAVES DISEASE

Juan Perez, DO

BASICS

DESCRIPTION
Autoimmune disease in which thyroid-stimulating hormone (TSH) receptor activation by thyrotropin receptor antibodies (TRAb) cause increased thyroid hormone secretion; most common cause of hyperthyroidism; classic findings are thyrotoxicosis, diffuse goiter, ophthalmopathy (orbitopathy), and occasionally localized dermopathy (pretibial myxedema).

EPIDEMIOLOGY
Incidence
- Annual incidence of 20 to 50 cases per 100,000 persons
- Peaks between 30 and 50 years of age
- Occurs in 0.2% of pregnancies, of which 95% is due to Graves disease
- Graves disease accounts for 60–80% of all cases of hyperthyroidism.

Prevalence
Has been reported to affect 1–1.5% of the world population

ETIOLOGY AND PATHOPHYSIOLOGY
- Excessive production of TSH receptor antibodies from B cells primarily within the thyroid, likely due to genetic clonal lack of suppressor T cells
- Binding of these antibodies to TSH receptors in the thyroid activates the receptor, stimulating thyroid hormone synthesis and secretion as well as thyroid growth (leading to goiter)
- Binding to similar antigen in retro-orbital connective tissue causes ocular symptoms.

Genetics
- Higher risk with personal or family history of any autoimmune disease, especially Hashimoto thyroiditis
- Twin studies show concordance rate as high as 20%.

RISK FACTORS
- Female gender (5 to 10 times more than men)
- Postpartum period
- Family history (15% of patients with Graves disease have an affected relative.)
- Medications: iodine, selenium, amiodarone, lithium, highly active antiretroviral therapy (HAART); rarely, immune-modulating medications (e.g., interferon therapy)
- Smoking (higher risk of developing ophthalmopathy)
- Low vitamin D levels
- Bacterial/viral infections

GENERAL PREVENTION
Screening TSH in asymptomatic patients is not recommended.

COMMONLY ASSOCIATED CONDITIONS
- Mitral valve prolapse
- Type 1 diabetes mellitus
- Addison disease, hypokalemic periodic paralysis
- Vitiligo, alopecia areata
- Other autoimmune disorders

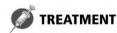 DIAGNOSIS

HISTORY
- Tachycardia, palpitations
- Tremor, restlessness
- Hyperactivity, anxiety, emotional lability, insomnia, poor concentration
- Sweating, heat intolerance
- Pruritus, skin changes
- Weight loss with increased appetite
- Fatigue, dyspnea (due to muscle weakness)
- Oligo-/amenorrhea (women), loss of libido, erectile dysfunction (men), gynecomastia
- Loose, frequent stools
- Blurred vision or diplopia, lacrimation, photophobia, gritty sensation in eyes (ocular dryness), retro-orbital discomfort, painful eye movement, loss of color vision or visual acuity
- Worsening of chronic medical conditions (anxiety, bipolar disorder, glucose intolerance, heart failure, or angina)

Geriatric Considerations
Elderly patients may present with atrial fibrillation, weight loss, or shortness of breath

PHYSICAL EXAM
- Ophthalmologic (present in 50% of cases): Grittiness/discomfort in the eyes, retrobulbar pressure/pain, lid lag/retraction, proptosis, ophthalmoplegia, papilledema, and loss of color vision may signify optic neuropathy.
- Thyroid: enlarged (goiter), nontender, and without nodules; possible bruit (increased blood flow)
- Integumentary: fine hair, warm skin, onycholysis, palmar erythema, brittle nails, clubbing of the fingers, possible pretibial myxedema (orange peel appearance), possible hyperpigmented plaques (dermopathy)
- Cardiac: resting tachycardia, hyperdynamic circulation, possible atrial fibrillation
- Extremities: fine tremor, hyperreflexia, proximal myopathy; rarely, soft tissue edema of extremities and clubbing of digits (acropachy)

DIFFERENTIAL DIAGNOSIS
- Toxic multinodular goiter and toxic adenoma
- Hashimoto thyroiditis
- Iatrogenic: Iodine, medications (amiodarone) induced or thyroid hormone overreplacement
- Tumors: adenoma, human chorionic gonadotropin (hCG)-producing tumors, struma ovarii, or metastatic thyroid cancer

DIAGNOSTIC TESTS & INTERPRETATION
Initial Tests (lab, imaging)
- TSH is initial test: suppressed (low or undetectable)
- TSH <0.1 mIU/L has >98% sensitivity and >92% specificity in confirming suspected thyroid disease. Elevated free T_4 with low TSH confirms hyperthyroidism.
- T_3 maybe elevated as well in conjunction with free T_4 or isolated elevation, known as T_3 toxicosis.

Follow-Up Tests & Special Considerations
Thyroid peroxidase (TPO) antibodies (present in 70–80% of patients with Graves disease) and TSH receptor antibodies (thyroid binding inhibitory immunoglobulin) may be useful in differentiating between Graves disease and toxic multinodular goiter. If both TRAb and TPO antibodies are absent, then nonautoimmune causes are likely.

Pregnancy Considerations
Increase in serum T_4-binding globulin concentration and initial stimulation of TSH by hCG results in a total T_4 and T_3 rise during first half of pregnancy. The TSH level is decreased throughout pregnancy and should be compared to the trimester-specific ranges for pregnancy. Measurement of TRAb is positive in 95% of patients with Graves disease and should be used if diagnosis is unclear in pregnancy (1)[A].

Diagnostic Procedures/Other
- Biochemical, immunologic, and clinical findings are usually sufficient to diagnose Graves disease. In cases where thyroid antibodies are negative or where there is nodularity of the thyroid gland to palpation, imaging should be pursued.
- After confirming suppressed TSH and high T_4, perform radioactive iodine uptake (RAIU) and scan. Patients with Graves disease will have diffuse, elevated RAIU (vs. localized/nodular elevated uptake in adenoma and multinodular goiter and decreased uptake in thyroiditis or exogenous thyroid hormone).
- Thyroid ultrasound may be used to distinguish nodular forms of Graves disease from nodular nonautoimmune causes of hyperthyroidism.

TREATMENT

GENERAL MEASURES
The goal is to correct the hypermetabolic state with the fewest side effects and lowest incidence of post-treatment hypothyroidism.

MEDICATION
First Line
- Antithyroid drugs: methimazole (MMI) and propylthiouracil (PTU)
  - Compete with the thyroid for iodine, thereby decreasing the synthesis of thyroid hormone; PTU blocks peripheral conversion of T_4 to T_3.
  - Treatment of choice for children and for adults who refuse RAI
  - May use as pretreatment for older or cardiac patients before RAI or surgery
  - Methimazole is now almost exclusively used except during the 1st trimester of pregnancy. It has longer duration of action, allowing for once daily dosing, more rapid efficacy, and lower incidence of side effects (2)[A].
  - Lowest effective dose of methimazole should be used (1)[B].

– Minor side effects (<5% incidence): controlled by switching from one agent to another: skin rash (3–5%), fever, arthralgias, GI side effects

– Major side effects necessitating change in treatment: polyarthritis (1–2%), idiopathic granulocytopenia (0.5%), and cholestasis/jaundice (rare)

– Optimal duration of antithyroid drugs is 12 to 18 months; no increased benefit to treatment >18 months

– Relapse rates up to 50% in patients who respond initially; higher rates if smoker, large goiter, or positive thyroid-stimulating antibodies at end of treatment

• Radioactive iodine (RAI)

– Concentrates in the thyroid gland and destroys thyroid tissue

– Treatment of choice for definitive therapy of hyperthyroidism, in the absence of moderate or severe orbitopathy (1)[A]

– Risks: side effects (neck soreness, flushing, decreased taste); worsening ophthalmopathy (15% incidence, higher in smokers); posttreatment hypothyroidism (80% incidence, not dosage dependent); radiation thyroiditis (1% incidence); need to adhere to safety precautions until radiation is eliminated from the body

– Pretreatment with antithyroid medication should be considered in patients with severe disease and the elderly, to reduce risk of posttreatment transient hyperthyroidism and posttreatment radiation thyroiditis

– May be repeated in as soon as 3 months if minimal response or after 6 months if not euthyroid (2)[A]

Second Line

Thyroidectomy is indicated with relapsed thyrotoxicosis, in the presence of goiter, when orbitopathy is present, when thyroid cancer is suspected, or in pregnant women in the 2nd trimester of pregnancy.

ISSUES FOR REFERRAL

• Endocrinologist for RAI therapy; if patient is pregnant or breastfeeding
• Ophthalmologist for Graves ophthalmopathy
• Surgeon if failed drug therapy or refusing RAI; obstruction or cosmesis

ADDITIONAL THERAPIES

• Graves hyperthyroidism

– β-Blockers provide prompt control of adrenergic symptoms; start while workup is in progress (2)[A]. Long-acting propranolol is used most commonly and titrated to symptom control (40 to 160 mg/day).

– Symptom control may be achieved with iodides, which block the conversion of T_4 to T_3 and inhibit TSH release. Use for pregnant patients who do not tolerate antithyroid medication or in conjunction with antithyroid medications; should not be used long term (may cause a paradoxical increase in TSH release) or in combination with RAI

– IV corticosteroids are used when rapid control of thyrotoxicosis is needed; they inhibit deiodinase type 2, thereby inhibiting conversion of T_4 to T_3 (3).

– Bile acid sequestrants are used as adjuncts with antithyroid drugs; their mechanism is binding of thyroid hormones in the enterohepatic circulation (3).

• Graves ophthalmopathy

– For corneal protection: tinted glasses when outdoors, artificial tears, patching/taping the lids at night

– For orbitopathy: Mild cases can be treated with lubricants, nocturnal ointments, botulinum toxin injection for upper lid retraction, and smoking cessation. Moderate to severe cases should be treated with pulse-dose IV glucocorticoid if no contraindications. Alternative is PO steroid (prednisone 60 to 80 mg/day for 2 to 4 weeks and then taper off).

– Newly approved by the FDA is the use of teprotumumab, which is a fully humanized monoclonal antibody inhibitor of insulin-like growth factor 1 receptor in patients with moderate to severe ophthalmopathy (3),(4).

– Compressive optic neuropathy is a medical emergency managed with a combination of IV glucocorticoid, orbital irradiation, and surgical decompression (3),(4).

• Graves dermopathy

– For dermopathy, use medium- to high-potency topical corticosteroids with occlusive dressing.

SURGERY/OTHER PROCEDURES

Indications for thyroidectomy include persistent or recurrent thyrotoxicosis, diffusely enlarged thyroid with compressive symptoms, concurrent hyperparathyroidism or thyroid cancer, nodular thyroid, active Graves ophthalmopathy, and 2nd-trimester pregnancy (3),(4).

ADMISSION, INPATIENT, AND NURSING CONSIDERATIONS

ICU for severe thyrotoxicosis with hemodynamic compromise (thyroid storm)

 ONGOING CARE

FOLLOW-UP RECOMMENDATIONS

Patient Monitoring

Check TSH and T_4 levels every 1 to 2 months for the first 6 months after treatment, then every 3 months for a year, and then every 6 to 12 months thereafter. For patients on treatment with PTU and methimazole, check CBC and liver function yearly. Also, check anti-TSH receptor antibodies at 12 months of treatment to determine possibility of discontinuing medication. Remission is much more likely in the context of a normal value for anti-TSH receptor antibodies.

Pregnancy Considerations

• RAI is contraindicated in pregnancy and during breastfeeding
• PTU is preferred in 1st trimester of pregnancy due to teratogenic effects of methimazole. Switch to methimazole in 2nd and 3rd trimesters due to risk of PTU-induced hepatotoxicity.
• Postpartum exacerbation of hyperthyroidism is common for women not currently under treatment, so TSH and symptoms should be monitored.

PROGNOSIS

• Generally good with treatment, although may have irreversible ocular, cardiac, and psychiatric consequences
• Increased morbidity and mortality due to osteoporosis, atherosclerotic disease, insulin resistance and obesity, and endothelial cell dysfunction (thromboembolic risk)

COMPLICATIONS

The percentage of patients with Graves disease who become hypothyroid within the 1st year after treatment varies with treatment modality.

REFERENCES

1. Ren Z, Qin L, Wang JQ, et al. Comparative efficacy of four treatments in patients with Graves' disease: a network meta-analysis. *Exp Clin Endocrinol Diabetes*. 2015;123(5):317–322.
2. Bahn Chair RS, Burch HB, Cooper DS, et al; for American Thyroid Association, American Association of Clinical Endocrinologists. Hyperthyroidism and other causes of thyrotoxicosis: management guidelines of the American Thyroid Association and American Association of Clinical Endocrinologists. *Thyroid*. 2011;21(6):593–646.
3. Kotwal A, Stan M. Current and future treatments for Graves' disease and Graves' ophthalmopathy. *Horm Metab Res*. 2018;50(12):871–886.
4. Dosiou C, Kossler AL. Thyroid eye disease: navigating the new treatment landscape. *J Endocr Soc*. 2021;5(5):bvab034.

ADDITIONAL READING

Lane LC, Wood CL, Cheetham T. Graves' disease: moving forwards. *Arch Dis Child*. 2023;108(4):276–281.

 SEE ALSO

Algorithms: Anxiety; Cardiac Arrhythmias; Weight Loss, Unintentional

 CODES

ICD10

• E05.00 Thyrotoxicosis w diffuse goiter w/o thyrotoxic crisis
• E05.01 Thyrotoxicosis w diffuse goiter w thyrotoxic crisis or storm
• E05.20 Thyrotoxicosis w toxic multinod goiter w/o thyrotoxic crisis

CLINICAL PEARLS

• Graves disease accounts for 60–80% of all cases of hyperthyroidism.
• Potential morbidities of hyperthyroidism include ophthalmopathy, atrial fibrillation, congestive heart failure (CHF), stroke, seizure, and osteopenia/osteoporosis.

G

GYNECOMASTIA

Franklyn C. Babb, MD, FAAFP

 BASICS

DESCRIPTION

- Benign glandular proliferation of male breast tissue
- Increase in estrogen activity relative to androgen leads to the development of gynecomastia.
- Gynecomastia can be transient and may represent the normal physiologic changes that occur in utero or in adolescence. However, gynecomastia presenting or persisting in adulthood is typically pathologic in nature.
- Pseudogynecomastia which is lipomastia (subareolar fat)

EPIDEMIOLOGY

- 60–90% of infants and 50–60% of pubertal males have transient gynecomastia.
- Up to 70% of men between 50 and 69 years of age report gynecomastia.

Incidence

A study out of Bulgaria in 2007 put the incidence of pubertal gynecomastia at 3.9% in Caucasian boys aged 10 to 19 years.

Prevalence

Prevalence in adolescents varies from 22% to 69% and in adult males ranges from 36% to 57% (1).

ETIOLOGY AND PATHOPHYSIOLOGY

Multiple factors can alter the estrogen to androgen ratio and precipitate gynecomastia:

- Decrease in androgen production
- Increase in estrogen production
- Increase in peripheral conversion to estrogen
- Inhibition of the androgen receptor
- Increase in the level of sex hormone–binding globulin (SHBG) or the affinity of androgens to SHBG (decreases free or bioavailable testosterone)
- Displacement of estrogen relative to testosterone from SHBG due to medications

RISK FACTORS

Gynecomastia can be physiologic or pathologic in nature.

- Physiologic gynecomastia presents in infants and adolescent boys and resolves spontaneously.
  - Neonatal gynecomastia: The placenta converts dehydroepiandrosterone (DHEA) and dehydroepiandrosterone sulfate (DHEA-S) to estrone and estradiol, resulting in transient gynecomastia.
  - Adolescent gynecomastia: Transient increases in estradiol levels at the onset of puberty lead to gynecomastia.
- Pathologic gynecomastia: persistent or adult-onset gynecomastia. 25% of cases are idiopathic, most secondary to age-associated decline in free testosterone and adipose tissue–mediated aromatase activity.

ALERT

- Illicit drugs: marijuana, heroin, methadone, alcohol, amphetamines, and over-the-counter bodybuilding supplements
- Hormones: androgens, anabolic steroids, estrogens, estrogen agonist, and human chorionic gonadotropin (hCG)
- Antiandrogens or inhibitors of androgen synthesis: bicalutamide, flutamide, nilutamide, cyproterone, and GnRH agonists (leuprolide and goserelin)
- Anti-infectives: metronidazole, ketoconazole, minocycline, isoniazid
- Antiulcer medications: cimetidine, ranitidine, metoclopramide, and proton pump inhibitors
- Cytotoxic agents: methotrexate, alkylating agents, and vinca alkaloids
- Cardiovascular drugs: Digoxin, spironolactone, calcium channel blockers, ACE inhibitors, amiodarone, methyldopa, reserpine, minoxidil, and recently statins can be added to this list.
- Psychoactive drugs: antidepressants, benzodiazepines, phenothiazines, antipsychotics (typical and atypical) (i.e., haloperidol and risperidone)
- Medications: HIV medications like efavirenz, phenytoin, penicillamine, sulindac, or theophylline
- Causes to rule out:
  - Primary hypogonadism: androgen insensitivity syndromes (defect in the androgen receptor), Klinefelter syndrome
  - Testicular tumor: germ cell (secretes hCG), Leydig cell (secretes estrogen), Sertoli cell (excessive aromatization to estrogens)
  - Adrenal tumors (secrete DHEA-S and estrogens)
  - Ectopic hCG tumors (hepatoblastoma, gastric tumors, renal cell carcinomas)
  - Cirrhosis
  - Secondary hypogonadism: Kallmann syndrome or prolactinemia, which can also stimulate milk production in breast tissue
  - Hyperthyroidism
  - Renal disease or dialysis
  - Malnutrition/starvation
  - Rare (true hermaphroditism [both testicular and ovarian tissue present])

Pediatric Considerations

Transient gynecomastia is seen in neonates or pubertal boys; typically resolves within 6 to 24 months

Geriatric Considerations

Medications and age-associated decline in testosterone production and increase in SHBG production leads to low free testosterone levels. The increased ratio of fat mass to lean mass leads to adipose tissue–mediated peripheral conversion of androgens to estrogen.

COMMONLY ASSOCIATED CONDITIONS

- Prostate carcinoma—treatment estrogen and antiandrogen leads to gynecomastia in 50–75% of patients.
- Cirrhosis
- Primary hypogonadism; especially Klinefelter syndrome—primary hypogonadism; at risk for breast cancer
- Testicular tumors; Leydig or Sertoli cell tumors especially when associated with Peutz-Jeghers syndrome or Carney complex

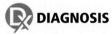 **DIAGNOSIS**

HISTORY

- If suspicious of hypogonadism, ask about erectile dysfunction, muscle mass, and decreased shaving frequency and libido.
- Obtain a family history including Carney complex and Peutz-Jeghers syndrome.
- Review medication list extensively and inquire about the use of illicit substances.
- Herbal supplements, marijuana use, and over-the-counter cimetidine or other H_2 antagonist use

PHYSICAL EXAM

- Careful breast exam to evaluate characteristics:
  - Firm, concentric glandular tissue beneath the nipple and areola palpable by pinching the thumb and forefinger together from either side of the breast toward the nipple; diameter of this tissue for diagnostic purposes ranges from >0.5 to >2 cm, but the most recent large study recommended 1 cm as the diagnostic criteria. Patients are most often classified using Simon's or similar criteria.
  - Grade I: small; visible breast enlargement, no skin redundancy
  - Grade IIa: moderate; breast enlargement without any skin redundancy
  - Grade IIb: moderate; breast enlargement with skin redundancy
  - Grade III: marked; breast enlargement with marked skin redundancy (i.e., pendulous female breasts) (2)
  - May involve one or both breasts
  - Usually asymptomatic but may be painful or tender if it is of recent onset
  - Off center, hard, fixed mass is concerning for malignancy, although palpation of subareolar fat is more consistent with pseudogynecomastia.
  - Breast discharge should raise concern for malignancy or prolactinemia. In the latter, the discharge is typically clear or milky.
- Thyroid exam
- Abdominal exam (Evaluate for masses and liver size.)
- Genitourinary exam (Evaluate for testicular size, hair pattern, and presence of ovary or uterus.)
- Visual field exam (Evaluate for peripheral field defect.)

DIFFERENTIAL DIAGNOSIS

- Pseudogynecomastia—fat deposition without glandular proliferation often seen in obesity
- Breast cancer—typically unilateral; firm; eccentric to the nipple; skin dimpling, nipple retraction/discharge, and lymphadenopathy
- Lipomas, sebaceous cyst, dermoid cyst, mastitis, hematoma, hamartoma

DIAGNOSTIC TESTS & INTERPRETATION

Laboratory and radiologic investigations should be tailored to fit history and physical exam findings.

Initial Tests (lab, imaging)

- Luteinizing hormone (LH)—elevated in primary hypogonadism and decreased in secondary hypogonadism
- Morning total and free testosterone—decreased testosterone level in hypogonadism
- hCG—elevated in germ cell tumors and ectopic hCG tumors
- Estradiol—elevated in Leydig cell tumors, Sertoli cell tumors, adrenal tumors, and with increased aromatase activity
- DHEA-S levels, which can be increased in adrenal tumors
- Urine for drugs of abuse (UDA)
- Other tests to consider include creatinine, liver function test, thyroid function tests, and prolactin.

Diagnostic Procedures/Other

Consider biopsy to rule out malignancy (i.e., off center, hard, fixed, discharge).

Test Interpretation

- Elevated hCG: Check testicular ultrasound. If positive for a mass, likely a testicular germ cell tumor; if the ultrasound is negative, consider extragonadal germ cell tumor or hCG-secreting neoplasm and order a CXR and CT abdomen.
- Elevated LH: if in relation to low testosterone, likely primary hypogonadism; if elevated in relation to high testosterone, check thyroid-stimulating hormone (TSH) and free thyroxine (FT_4); if FT_4 is elevated and TSH is suppressed, likely hyperthyroidism; if TSH and FT_4 are normal, likely androgen resistance
- Normal or decreased LH in relation to low testosterone: Check prolactin level; if prolactin is elevated, likely due to a prolactin-secreting pituitary tumor (need MRI); if normal, likely due to secondary hypogonadism
- Normal or decreased LH in relation to increased estradiol: Check testicular ultrasound; if positive for a mass, likely Leydig or Sertoli cell tumor; if negative for mass, check CT abdomen to evaluate the adrenals; if mass is present, possible adrenal neoplasm versus adenoma; if no mass is detected, then likely due to increased aromatase activity in extraglandular tissue

 TREATMENT

GENERAL MEASURES

- Gynecomastia usually regresses spontaneously within 6 months of onset. Monitor for the first 6 months.
- Neonatal and pubertal gynecomastia spontaneously resolves within 6 to 24 months. Persistent pubertal gynecomastia (>24 months) occurs in 8% of pubertal boys. In adult males, 75% of gynecomastia is secondary to persistent pubertal gynecomastia, medications, and idiopathic conditions. Only 25% is related to an underlying medical condition.
- All illicit drug use and offending medications should be stopped if appropriate.
- Treat underlying medical conditions (i.e., testosterone replacement for hypogonadal men, dopamine agonist for prolactinoma, appropriate treatment for thyrotoxicosis, and tumor resection).

MEDICATION

There are no U.S. Food and Drug Administration–approved medications for the treatment of gynecomastia.

- SERMs: Clinical trials of both tamoxifen (10 to 20 mg/day) and raloxifene (60 mg/day) showed partial reduction in pubertal gynecomastia and successful resolution of idiopathic gynecomastia in 90% of study participants after 3 to 9 months.
- Aromatase inhibitors block peripheral conversion of androgens to estrogens. In prostate cancer patients, anastrozole prevented the development of gynecomastia in patients undergoing androgen deprivation therapy.

ADDITIONAL THERAPIES

In clinical trials, prophylactic radiotherapy prevented the development of gynecomastia in prostate cancer patients on androgen deprivation therapy.

SURGERY/OTHER PROCEDURES

Surgery can be recommended if gynecomastia does not regress within 12 months either spontaneously or after medical therapy, significant discomfort (i.e., pain, tenderness), it causes embarrassment or anxiety, or if biopsy is suspicious for malignancy. Multiple surgical techniques are available, and studies indicate good patient satisfaction overall (2).

 ONGOING CARE

FOLLOW-UP RECOMMENDATIONS

Patient Monitoring

Every 3 to 6 months for 24 months; consider medical therapy (i.e., tamoxifen) if severe, painful symptoms persist after 6 to 12 months and surgery if symptoms persist after 12 to 24 months. In individuals with asymptomatic or mild disease, routine yearly breast and physical exam is recommended.

PATIENT EDUCATION

Patients should be reassured of the benign nature of gynecomastia in almost all cases.

PROGNOSIS

- Good in physiologic cases because they often regress spontaneously within 3 to 6 months
- Majority of patients experience regression once underlying disorder is treated or offending agents are eliminated.
- The majority of patients, who undergo surgery, are satisfied with the postoperative cosmetic appearance.

REFERENCES

1. Kanakis GA, Nordkap L, Bang AK, et al. EAA clinical practice guidelines-gynecomastia evaluation and management. *Andrology*. 2019;7(6):778–793.
2. Burger A, Sattler A, Grünherz L, et al. Scar versus shape: patient-reported outcome after different surgical approaches to gynecomastia measured by modified BREAST Q®. *J Plast Surg Hand Surg*. 2023;57(1–6):1–6.

 SEE ALSO

Algorithm: Gynecomastia

 CODES

ICD10

N62 Hypertrophy of breast

CLINICAL PEARLS

- Gynecomastia can be transient and may represent normal physiologic changes in neonates or adolescents. Gynecomastia presenting or persisting in adulthood is pathologic.
- Lab and radiologic studies associated with gynecomastia including thyrotoxicosis, prolactinemia, hypogonadism, testicular tumors, adrenal tumors, and ectopic hCG tumors.
- ~25% of gynecomastia is idiopathic in nature, and treatment should focus on symptom control.
- Clinical trials of SERMs, aromatase inhibitors, and radiation therapy seem promising. Surgery is the treatment of choice for refractory gynecomastia.

G

HAMMER TOES
Neil Feldman, DPM

BASICS

Contraction deformities of the toes

DESCRIPTION

- Hammer toes include three distinct types of deformity.
  - Hammer toe (as defined) involves a plantar flexion deformity of the proximal interphalangeal (PIP) joint with varying degrees of hyperextension of the metatarsophalangeal (MTP) and distal interphalangeal (DIP) joint, primarily in sagittal plane (1).
  - Claw toe involves a plantar flexion deformity of the PIP and DIP joint with varying degrees of hyperextension of the MTP.
  - Mallet toe involves a plantar flexion deformity of the DIP joint only.
- Each can be flexible, semirigid, or fixed.
  - Flexible: passively correctable to neutral position
  - Semirigid: partially correctable to neutral position
  - Fixed: not correctable to neutral position without intervention

EPIDEMIOLOGY

Most common deformity of lesser digits, typically affecting only one or two toes:

- Second toe is the most commonly involved.
- *Hallux malleus* is term used when the great toe (hallux) is involved.

Incidence

- Undefined
- Increases with age, duration of deformity (from flexible to rigid)

Prevalence

- Predominant sex: female > male (2)
  - Female predominance from 2.5:1 to 9:1, depending on age group
- Can range from 1% to 20% of population studied
- Blacks are more often affected than whites (2).

ETIOLOGY AND PATHOPHYSIOLOGY

- Can be congenital or acquired
- Three categories of acquired hammer toes:
  - Flexor stabilization (most common cause and occurs in pronated foot/foot with pes planus). The flexor digitorum longus (FDL) muscle remains overactive, overusing the toes to assist in relative foot instability.
  - Extensor substitution (most common with pes cavus)—occurs during the swing phase of gait. The extensor digitorum longus (EDL) muscle remains overactive, substituting for dysfunctional hip and ankle extensors.
  - Flexor substitution—the least common cause and seen commonly with pes cavus. The FDL muscle remains overactive with relative weakness/dysfunction to the Achilles and flexor hallucis longus (FHL), which are the main plantar flexors of the foot.
- Biomechanical dysfunction results in muscle/tendon imbalance between the EDL tendon at the PIP joint and the FDL tendon at the MTP joint; the imbalance at the MTP joint level leads to the altering of the stabilizing force of the intrinsic muscles inserting into the extensor sling and wing apparatus of the MTP joint. In the case of classic hammer toes, the toe(s) sublux dorsally as the MTP hyperextends. This results in plantar flexion of the PIP joint and hyperextension of the MTP joint (2).

- Specific pathomechanics vary by etiology:
  - Toe length discrepancy or narrow footwear toe box induces PIP joint flexion by forcing digit to accommodate shoe.
    - May also lead to MTP joint synovitis secondary to overuse, with elongation of plantar plate and MTP joint hyperextension
    - 4th and 5th toes commonly assume an adductovarus attitude, which can make the toes appear to sit on their side and in advanced cases can cause one toe to sit directly under another toe.
  - Rheumatoid arthritis (RA) causes MTP joint destruction and resultant subluxation.
  - Any condition that compromises intra-articular and periarticular tissues, first ray instability with or without a bunion deformity, an anatomically long 2nd metatarsal, inflammatory joint disease, neuromuscular conditions, improper-fitting shoes, and trauma
  - Damage to joint capsule, collateral ligaments, or synovia leads to unstable PIP joint or MTP joint.

Genetics

- Significant heritability rates of 49–90%
- Specific genetic markers are not identified.

RISK FACTORS

- Pes cavus, pes planus
- Hallux valgus
- Metatarsus adductus
- Ankle equinus
- Neuromuscular disease (rare)
- Trauma; improperly fitted shoes (narrow toe box) and/or tight hosiery
- Abnormal metatarsal and/or digit length
- Inflammatory joint disease (e.g., RA)
- Connective tissue disease
- Diabetes mellitus

GENERAL PREVENTION

- Proper fitting of shoes. Use of pressure-dispersive footwear, shoes with soft uppers, and extra-depth toe boxes can help reduce pain and irritation from rubbing.
- Foot orthoses modulate biomechanical dysfunction and muscular imbalance, preventing progression (2).
- Limiting use of shoes in the growing foot. Use of zero drop shoes when necessary. Traditional shoes have an elevated heel relative to the ball of the foot (MTP joints). Therefore, at rest, the toes are positioned in dorsal subluxation at the MTP joints and forced to be contracted (termed toe spring).
- Perform toe strengthening exercises, which will help with prevention of imbalance between the extrinsic muscles of the calf and the intrinsic muscles of the foot.
- Control of predisposing factors (e.g., inflammatory joint disease) may also slow progression.

COMMONLY ASSOCIATED CONDITIONS

- Hallux valgus
- Cavus foot (pes cavus)
- Flat foot (pes planus)
- Metatarsus adductus
- Dorsal callus

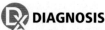

DIAGNOSIS

History and physical exam are typically sufficient for diagnosis of hammer toes. Additional tests are available to exclude other conditions.

HISTORY

- Location, duration, severity, and rate of progression of foot deformity
- Type, location, duration of pain
  - Patients often relate sensation of lump on plantar aspect of MTP joint.
- Degree of functional impairment
- Improving/exacerbating factors
- Type of footwear and hosiery worn
- Peripheral neurologic symptoms
- Any prior treatment rendered

PHYSICAL EXAM

- Note MTP joint hyperextension, PIP joint flexion, and DIP joint extension or flexion.
- Observe any adjacent toe deformities (e.g., hallux valgus, flexion contractures).
- Assess degree of flexibility and reducibility of deformity in both weight-bearing and non–weight-bearing positions (2).
- Note any hyperkeratosis over the joint, ulcers, clavi (dorsal PIP joint, metatarsal head), adventitious bursa, erythema, or skin breakdown or ulceration (2).
- Palpate for pain over dorsal aspect of PIP joint or MTP joint.
- Drawer test of MTP joint
- Palpate web spaces to exclude interdigital neuroma.
- Neurovascular evaluation (e.g., pulses, sensation, muscle bulk)

DIFFERENTIAL DIAGNOSIS

- Hammer toe: hyperextension of the MTP and DIP joints and plantar flexion of the PIP joint
- Claw toe: dorsiflexion of MTP joint and plantar flexion of the DIP joint
- Mallet toe: fixed or flexible deformity of the DIP joint of the toe
- Overlapping 5th toe
- Interdigital neuroma
- Plantar plate rupture
- Nonspecific synovitis of MTP joint
- Fracture; exostosis
- Arthritis (e.g., rheumatoid, psoriatic)

DIAGNOSTIC TESTS & INTERPRETATION

Initial Tests (lab, imaging)

- Not required unless clinically indicated to rule out suspected metabolic or inflammatory arthropathies (2)[C]: rheumatoid factor, antinuclear antibodies (ANA), HLA-B27 serologies for inflammatory disease
- Weight-bearing x-rays of affected foot in anteroposterior (AP), lateral, and oblique views (2)[C]:
  - AP view superior for assessing transverse plane MTP subluxation or dislocation
  - Lateral view is best for the evaluation of hammer toe.

Follow-Up Tests & Special Considerations

MRI or bone scan if osteomyelitis is suspected

Diagnostic Procedures/Other

- Nerve conduction studies or EMG if neurologic disorder is suspected
- Doppler or plethysmography if impaired circulation and surgery is considered
- Computerized weight-bearing pressure testing is indicated only in setting of neuromuscular deficiencies.

Test Interpretation

Histologic evaluation is not necessary before treatment.

TREATMENT

- Goal of treatment is to relieve symptoms and help patients return to their normal activity level.
- Surgical and nonsurgical interventions are available.
- Mild and asymptomatic cases may not require treatment.

GENERAL MEASURES

Nonsurgical (conservative) treatments include

- Shoe modifications (wider and/or deeper toe box) to accommodate the deformity and decrease the pressure over osseous prominences. Avoid high-heeled shoes (2)[C].
- Toe sleeve or orthodigital padding of the hammer toe prominence
- Metatarsal pads in reducible deformities and crest pads in nonreducible deformities
- Dynamic toe splints for MTP joint subluxations or dislocations with (semi)reducible deformity
- Hammer toe–straightening orthotics or taping to reduce flexible deformities
- Débridement of hyperkeratotic lesions can reduce symptoms. Topical keratolytics may be helpful (2)[C].
- In-shoe foot orthotics can mitigate abnormal biomechanics.
- Physical therapy for stretching and strengthening of the toes helps preserve flexibility, which include intrinsic muscle strengthening (short foot exercises).

MEDICATION

First Line

NSAIDs may be helpful in managing symptoms of pain and joint inflammation.

ISSUES FOR REFERRAL

If nonsurgical (conservative) treatment is unsuccessful and/or impractical or patient has combined deformity of MTP joint, PIP joint, and/or DIP joint, refer to podiatric physician/surgeon or orthopedic surgeon.

SURGERY/OTHER PROCEDURES

- Surgical procedures for the correction of hammer toes depend on the degree and flexibility of the contracture(s) and related abnormalities.
- Surgical interventions for *flexible* hammer toes include (1)
  - PIP joint arthroplasty or arthrodesis (most common)
  - Flexor tenotomy for reducible or mallet toe deformities with distal ulceration

- Extensor tendon lengthening/tenotomy/MTP joint capsulotomy
- Flexor tendon transfer with digital arthrodesis
- Exostosectomy
- Implant arthroplasty
- Surgical interventions for semirigid/rigid hammer toes include (1)
  - PIP joint resection arthroplasty or arthrodesis
  - Girdlestone-Taylor flexor-to-extensor transfer
  - Metatarsal shortening (Weil osteotomy)
  - Exostosectomy
  - Middle phalangectomy (more common in 5th toe)
  - Soft tissue releases/lengthening
  - Diaphysectomy of the proximal phalanx (less common)
  - Phalangeal base resection as part of Hoffman-Clayton procedure for RA mutilans

ONGOING CARE

FOLLOW-UP RECOMMENDATIONS

- Obtain radiographs immediately following surgery or at the first postoperative visit; subsequent x-rays as needed
- Full weight-bearing in a postoperative (surgical) shoe or other device based on the procedure(s) performed and the individual patient
- Pinning often used across the MTP joint, which often requires patient to be non–weight-bearing to the forefoot for 3 to 5 weeks
- Elevate the foot to minimize swelling.
- Return to regular shoe wear after pain is controlled, swelling has subsided, and wounds have healed.
- Role and efficacy of postoperative physical therapy unclear

PATIENT EDUCATION

- Patients should be aware of mild to moderate swelling and plantar foot discomfort that may persist for many (1 to 6) months after surgery and may limit footwear options until resolved.
- MTP joint and PIP joint may remain stiff for extended periods of time.
- "Molding" of the operative toe (assuming the contours of adjacent toes) is common.
- Encourage patients to wear shoes of adequate size with "roomy" (rounded or squared) toe box.

PROGNOSIS

- Nonoperative (conservative) treatment in mild deformities usually alleviates pain; however, the deformity may progress.
- Surgical treatment of flexible hammer toe deformity reliably corrects the deformity and alleviates pain. Recurrence and progression are common, especially if the patient continues to wear ill-fitting shoes.
- Surgical treatment of fixed hammer toe deformity provides reliable deformity correction and pain relief. Recurrence is less common; however, adjacent toes can subsequently develop deformities.

COMPLICATIONS

- Common complications specific to digital surgery include but are not limited to
  - Persistent edema
  - Recurrence of deformity
  - Residual pain
  - Excessive stiffness
  - Metatarsalgia
- Less common complications include
  - Numbness (e.g., digital nerve palsy)
  - Flail toe
  - Symptomatic osseous regrowth
  - Malposition of toe
  - Malunion/nonunion
  - Infection
  - Sausage toe
  - Vascular impairment (e.g., toe ischemia, gangrene)

REFERENCES

1. Shirzad K, Kiesau CD, DeOrio JK, et al. Lesser toe deformities. *J Am Acad Orthop Surg*. 2011;19(8):505–514.
2. Thomas JL, Blitch EL IV, Chaney DM, et al; for Clinical Practice Guideline Forefoot Disorders Panel. Diagnosis and treatment of forefoot disorders. Section 1: digital deformities. *J Foot Ankle Surg*. 2009;48(3):418.e1–418.e9.

ADDITIONAL READING

Richie D. Exposing the myths about metatarsalgia. *Podiatry Manage*. September 2022:57–63.

SEE ALSO

Algorithm: Foot Pain

CODES

ICD10

- M20.40 Other hammer toe(s) (acquired), unspecified foot
- M20.41 Other hammer toe(s) (acquired), right foot
- M20.42 Other hammer toe(s) (acquired), left foot

CLINICAL PEARLS

- Hammer toe is a plantar flexion deformity of the PIP joint. Claw and mallet toes are additional types of hammer toes.
- Initial management of hammer toe deformity is conservative. Consider surgery if pain persists or the deformity worsens.
- Properly fitting footwear helps minimize recurrence. Patients should be aware of mild to moderate swelling and plantar foot discomfort that may persist for months after surgery and may limit footwear options until resolved.

H

HAND-FOOT-AND-MOUTH DISEASE

Sahil Mullick, MD • Farzad Effan, MBBS

BASICS

DESCRIPTION
- Common clinical syndrome caused by several enterovirus serotypes
- Classic appearance of oral enanthem along with exanthem of hands and feet (classically) and potentially located elsewhere
- Exanthem (rash) may be macular, maculopapular, and/or vesicular.
- Synonym(s): herpangina (when affecting oral mucosa and posterior pharynx)

EPIDEMIOLOGY
- Self-limiting illness resolves in 7 to 10 days.
- Moderately contagious
- Infection is spread by direct contact with nasal secretions, saliva, blister fluid, or stool.
- Infected individuals are most contagious during the 1st week of the illness but may continue to spread illness for days to weeks after. Some exposed individuals (especially adults) may be asymptomatic but still contagious.
- The viruses that cause hand-foot-and-mouth disease (HFMD) can persist for weeks after symptoms have resolved, most commonly in stool, allowing transmission following resolution of symptoms.
- The incubation period is 3 to 7 days.

Incidence
- Children <5 years of age are most commonly affected, especially in daycare facilities.
- Can occur as isolated cases, outbreaks, or epidemics
- Occurs worldwide
- Vertical transmission is possible.
- Most large outbreaks occur in Southeast Asia.

ETIOLOGY AND PATHOPHYSIOLOGY
- HFMD is not the same as foot (hoof) and mouth disease found in cattle, and there is no cross species infectious concern.

- Transmission by the fecal–oral route or contact with skin lesions or oral secretions; caused by viruses that belong to the Enterovirus genus and replicated in the GI tract, most commonly coxsackievirus A16 and enterovirus 71 (previously caused outbreaks)
- Also coxsackie viruses A5, A7, A9, A10, B2, B5
- More severe cases are associated with enterovirus 71 (1).

GENERAL PREVENTION
- Handwashing, especially around food handling or diaper changes
- Exclusion of children from group settings during the first few days of the illness in the presence of open lesions in the mouth or on the skin may reduce the spread of infection.
- Hand hygiene measures are effective in reducing transmission.
- Pregnant woman should avoid contact with infected individuals.
- Clinical trials with monovalent and polyvalent vaccines have shown promise in decreasing incidence and prevalence (2).

DIAGNOSIS

HISTORY
- 1- to 2-day prodrome of fever, anorexia, malaise, abdominal pain, upper respiratory symptoms
- Progression of disease divided into 5 stages: rash, neurological dysfunction, early cardiopulmonary failure, cardiopulmonary failure, recovery; most patients only develop rash (2)[C]
- Maculopapular rash on hands, feet, and mouth. Oral lesions may precede skin.
- Fever may last 3 to 4 days. Sore throat follows fever.
- Often history of sick contacts

PHYSICAL EXAM
- Oral enanthem along with tender vesicles becoming ulcers on buccal mucosa, sides of tongue, and palate
- May persist for up to 1 week
- Cutaneous vesicles 3 to 5 mm in diameter start as painful maculopapular eruptions, occur typically on dorsal aspect of fingers and toes.
- May also occur on the palms, soles, buttocks, and groin
- Adults are less likely to have cutaneous findings.
- Nail dystrophies are not uncommon and may persist for weeks following the acute infection.
- Be mindful of central nervous system (CNS) symptoms. Although rare, CNS involvement is possible.

DIFFERENTIAL DIAGNOSIS
- Herpetic gingivostomatitis
- Aphthous stomatitis
- Scabies
- Chickenpox
- Measles
- Rubella
- Scarlet fever
- Roseola infantum
- Fifth disease
- Other enteroviral infections
- Kawasaki disease
- Viral pharyngitis
- Varicella
- Rickettsial infection (RFSF)
- Behcet syndrome
- Pemphigus vulgaris
- Stevens-Johnson syndrome

DIAGNOSTIC TESTS & INTERPRETATION
Clinical diagnosis is typically adequate.

Initial Tests (lab, imaging)

Although not typically performed, culture for responsible virus (virus isolation) can be obtained from oral lesions, cutaneous vesicles, nasopharyngeal swabs, stool, and CSF. Polymerase chain reaction (PCR) of throat swabs and vesicle fluid is the most efficient test if enterovirus 71 is suspected.

TREATMENT

- Symptomatic
- No current specific antiviral treatments
- Avoid spicy or acidic foods to limit oral pain.
- IV fluids may be required in more severe cases of dehydration.

GENERAL MEASURES

Isolation of patients to avoid cross-infection

MEDICATION

- Symptomatic care using ibuprofen or acetaminophen for pain from oral ulcers or fever
- Soothing mouthwashes ("magic mouthwash") containing lidocaine are not recommended as they do not appear to be superior to placebo and have risk of side effects when absorbed systemically (3)[B].
- Antiviral treatments are not available.

Pediatric Considerations

Avoid aspirin use in treating febrile illness in children due to concern of Reye syndrome—an encephalopathy associated with aspirin use in viral illness in children.

ADMISSION, INPATIENT, AND NURSING CONSIDERATIONS

- Patients with CNS manifestations or autonomic dysregulation should require hospitalization.
- Admit those with dehydration unable to maintain adequate oral hydration.
- Intravenous immunoglobulin is not recommended.

ONGOING CARE

DIET

- Encourage cold liquids (e.g., ice cream, popsicles) to prevent dehydration.
- Avoid acidic, salty, and spicy foods, as they will increase pain.

COMPLICATIONS

- Dehydration most common due to painful oral ulcerations
- CNS involvement (i.e., aseptic meningitis) is a rare complication, although it is on the rise globally, particularly in severe cases.
- Fever >3 days and lethargy are associated with CSF pleocytosis.
- Enterovirus 71 has caused outbreaks and has been implicated in more severe disease associated with CNS infection.
- Cardiopulmonary complications include myocarditis, pneumonitis, and pulmonary edema.
- Nail dystrophies and desquamation (loss of nails, Beau lines) are common.

REFERENCES

1. Saguil A, Kane SF, Lauters R, et al. Hand-foot-and-mouth disease: rapid evidence review. *Am Fam Physician*. 2019;100(7):408–414.
2. Zhu P, Ji W, Li D, et al. Current status of hand-foot-and-mouth disease. *J Biomed Sci*. 2023;30(1):15.
3. Hopper SM, McCarthy M, Tancharoen C, et al. Topical lidocaine to improve oral intake in children with painful infectious mouth ulcers: a blinded, randomized, placebo-controlled trial. *Ann Emerg Med*. 2014;63(3):292–299.

ADDITIONAL READING

Jones E, Pillay TD, Liu F, et al. Outcomes following severe hand foot and mouth disease: a systematic review and meta-analysis. *Eur J Paediatr Neurol*. 2018;22(5):763–773.

CODES

ICD10

- B08.4 Enteroviral vesicular stomatitis with exanthem
- B34.1 Enterovirus infection, unspecified
- B08.5 Enteroviral vesicular pharyngitis

CLINICAL PEARLS

- Most common: May to October
- Children <5 years of age tend to have worse symptoms than older children.
- HFMD is the most common cause of mouth sores in pediatric patients.
- Dehydration is a common problem secondary to swallowing aversions.
- Usually self-limiting, resolving in 7 to 10 days
- Careful handwashing to limit dissemination
- Counsel parents that nail desquamation may occur in the weeks following the infection.

H

HEADACHE, CLUSTER

Samuel C. Wang, MD • Anna Sophia Fields, MD

 BASICS

DESCRIPTION

- A primary headache disorder characterized by circadian and circannual episodes consisting of multiple attacks of severe, unilateral, sharp, searing, or piercing pain typically localized to the periorbital and/or temporal areas
- It is the most common headache among trigeminal autonomic cephalgias (TACs).
- Accompanied by signs of ipsilateral parasympathetic autonomic activation as well as restlessness or agitation
- Autonomic symptoms: signs of parasympathetic hyperactivity (ipsilateral lacrimation, eye redness, nasal congestion) and sympathetic hypoactivity (ipsilateral ptosis and miosis)
- Individual attacks occur from once every other day up to 8 times per day and can last 15 to 180 minutes per day if untreated.
- Attacks usually occur in series (cluster periods) that are often seasonal, lasting for weeks or months, and are separated by remission periods usually lasting months to years.
- About 10–15% of patients have chronic symptoms without remissions (i.e., chronic cluster headache [cCH]).

EPIDEMIOLOGY

Prevalence

1 year prevalence: 53/100,000

- Gender: male > female; 4.3:1 overall
- Mean age of onset: 30 years; women often develop CH earlier in life (20s).
- Episodic/chronic ratio: 6:1

ETIOLOGY AND PATHOPHYSIOLOGY

Complex and incompletely understood, possible mechanisms include the following:

- Activation of the trigeminovascular system, which leads to the release of vasodilatory peptides including substance P, neurokinin, and calcitonin gene-related peptide (CGRP)
- Posterior hypothalamus activation and the hypothalamic-brainstem-cerebellar interconnections may trigger an attack by activating trigeminal nociceptive pathways through increased parasympathetic outflow.
- Alterations in the descending pain modulation network and disordered pain modulation during cluster periods

Genetics

- Autosomal dominant in 5% of cases; otherwise, recessive or multifactorial
- First-degree relatives are 18 times more likely, and second-degree relatives are 1 to 3 times more likely to be affected by cluster headaches.
- >50% with migraine and 18% with CH in family history

RISK FACTORS

- Age: 70% onset before age 30 years
- Cigarette smoking or childhood exposure to cigarette smoke
- History of head trauma

COMMONLY ASSOCIATED CONDITIONS

- Depression (24%) with increased risk of suicide
- History of migraine, frequently in female patients; medication-overuse headache
- Asthma (9%)
- Sleep apnea (30–80%)

 DIAGNOSIS

International Classification of Headache Disorders (3rd edition, 2018) criteria

- At least five attacks of severe or very severe unilateral orbital, supraorbital, and/or temporal pain lasting from 15 to 180 minutes if untreated
- Either one or both of the following:
  – At least one of the following symptoms ipsilateral to the headache:
    ○ Conjunctival injection and/or lacrimation
    ○ Nasal congestion and/or rhinorrhea
    ○ Eyelid edema
    ○ Forehead and facial sweating/flushing
    ○ Miosis and/or ptosis
  – Restlessness or agitation during acute attack
- Attack frequency: one every other day to eight per day for more than half of the time during cluster periods
- Episodic CH (eCH): at least two cluster periods lasting 7 days to 1 year, separated by a pain-free interval of ≥3 months (80–90% of cases)
- cCH: occurring for ≥1 year without remission period, or remission period lasting <3 months, for at least 1 year

HISTORY

- Episodic periods of recurring headaches, described as excruciating, unilateral, sharp, searing, or piercing pain typically localized to the periorbital and/or temporal area
- Conjunctival injection, tearing, nasal congestion, rhinorrhea, sweating
- Timing of headaches is often circadian in nature, often occurring at the same time each day (usually at night).
- Patients often pace the floor during an acute attack because lying down seems to exacerbate the pain.
- Presence of triggers such as vasodilators (e.g., alcohol, nitroglycerin, sildenafil), histamine, or strong odors
- Seasonal pattern of cluster periods, often recurring around the same time of the year

PHYSICAL EXAM

Exam is often unremarkable, unless having an acute attack:

- Distress, crying spells, restlessness, and/or agitation
- Ipsilateral lacrimation, conjunctival injection, eyelid edema, ptosis, and miosis
- Edematous nasal mucosa or rhinorrhea

DIFFERENTIAL DIAGNOSIS

- Other TACs (e.g., paroxysmal hemicrania; short-lasting, unilateral, neuralgiform headache attacks with conjunctival injection and tearing [SUNCT]; hemicrania continua), hypnic headaches, trigeminal and other facial neuralgias, migraine, temporal arteritis, herpes zoster, acute angle closure glaucoma
- Secondary CH:
  – Vascular causes: vertebral or carotid artery dissection, brain arteriovenous malformations, intracranial artery aneurysms
  – Tumors: pituitary tumors/meningiomas/carcinomas, cavernous hemangioma
  – Infections/inflammation: sinusitis, herpes zoster ophthalmicus, inflammation of the cavernous sinus (i.e., Tolosa-Hunt syndrome)
  – Ophthalmic causes: glaucoma, orbital pseudotumor

DIAGNOSTIC TESTS & INTERPRETATION

Diagnosis is primarily clinical and often delayed (>40% report 5-year delay in diagnosis).

Initial Tests (lab, imaging)

Neuroimaging (head MRI/CT with detailed study of pituitary and cavernous sinus) is recommended for all TACs in order to exclude other intracranial conditions that may mimic TACs.

 TREATMENT

Many of the medications discussed are used off-label in the treatment of CH (1).

GENERAL MEASURES

- Avoid major changes in sleep habits.
- Stop smoking.
- Avoid use of alcohol during cluster period.
- Avoid exposure to chemical agents or other known triggers.

MEDICATION

- Avoid narcotic analgesics, for acute attacks.
- The goal is abortion of acute attack and transitional prophylaxis for expected duration of the cluster period.
- Long-term prophylaxis should be used for cCH.
- Assess cardiovascular risk before instituting vasoactive drugs, such as triptans or ergot derivatives.

First Line

Abortive therapy:

- Oxygen: 100% at 12 to 15 L/min via nonrebreather mask or demand valve oxygen mask while sitting or standing provides relief within 15 minutes; high flow used if resistant to lower-flow oxygen; excellent side effect profile (2)[A]
- Sumatriptan
  – SubQ: 6 mg, up to 12 mg/24 hr with at least 1 hour between injections is the most effective medication for acute attacks; NNT = 2.4 and 3.3 for headache relief and pain free in 15 minutes, respectively
  – Intranasal: 20 mg once in single nostril contralateral to the side of the headache; may repeat in 2 hours, max dose of 40 mg/24 hr; NNT = 3.2 for headache relief at 30 minutes (2)[A]

- Zolmitriptan
  - Intranasal: 5- and 10-mg dosage both effective; may repeat in 2 hours, max of 2 times per day; NNT = 12 and 4.9 for headache relief in 15 minutes for 5 and 10 mg, respectively
  - PO: 5- and 10-mg dosage both effective; may repeat in 2 hours, max dose of 10 mg/24 hr; NNT = 6.7 and 4.5 for headache relief in 30 minutes for 5 and 10 mg, respectively (2)[A]
- Noninvasive vagus nerve stimulation (nVNS)
  - FDA approved durable medical device that delivers electrical stimulation positioned on the neck overlying the vagus nerve. Modest efficacy in short-term pain reduction for eCH was demonstrated in two double-blind, sham controlled trials (ACT-1 and ACT-2); NNT = 5 and 3, respectively

ALERT
Adverse effects of triptans: paresthesias, flushing, tingling, chest pain, neck tightness ("triptan sensations"). triptans are contraindicated in ischemic cardiac disease, stroke, uncontrolled hypertension, Prinzmetal angina, basilar migraine, hemiplegic migraine, ischemic bowel disease, and peripheral vascular disease.

Second Line
Abortive treatment:
- Lidocaine: 1 mL of 4–10% lidocaine solution administered intranasally on ipsilateral side of symptoms; no well-controlled randomized controlled trials (RCTs) done
- Octreotide: SubQ 100 μg; can be considered in patients when triptans are contraindicated; main side effect is GI upset.

ISSUES FOR REFERRAL
Consider a neurology or headache center referral for complicated patients.

ADDITIONAL THERAPIES
- Transitional therapy:
  - Used to rapidly reduce attack frequency until the effectiveness of longer term preventive treatment is reached; longer term maintenance agents are started concurrently.
  - Suboccipital nerve or greater occipital nerve steroid injections (preferred option): 3.75 mg of cortivazol injected into the suboccipital area on the ipsilateral side of the headache; single injection or series of three injections, given 48 to 72 hours apart, reduce attack frequency during cluster period when used as add-on therapy to verapamil; NNT = 2.5 (3)[A]
  - Steroids: prednisone 60 to 100 mg daily for 5 days with a taper no longer than 18 days to avoid side effects; several open studies suggested benefit but no rigorous trials to prove efficacy; adverse effects for short-term use: insomnia, psychosis, hyponatremia, edema, hyperglycemia, peptic ulcer

- Prophylactic therapy should be used as soon as possible at the start of a cluster period:
  - First line:
    - Verapamil: Start at 80 mg TID and increase by 80 mg/week to 480 mg and then 80 mg every 2 weeks if needed; short- or long-acting equivalent; most patients respond to daily dose of 200 to 480 mg, but up to 960 mg/day may be needed; NNT = 1.2 (2)[A]
    - Galcanezumab: 300 mg subQ injection every month until cluster period ends; only FDA-approved medication for eCH prophylaxis; most common side effects are nasopharyngitis, hepatic enzyme elevation, and local injection site reaction and pain; NNT = 5.2 (4)[B]
  - Second line:
    - Lithium: Start 300 mg BID; titrate to therapeutic range of 600 to 1,500 mg/day. In a head-to-head trial with verapamil, lithium was shown to be comparable; must monitor drug levels and liver, renal, and thyroid function; caution with nephrotoxic drugs and diuretics; monitor for CNS side effects.
    - Topiramate: 25 to 100 mg BID showed efficacy in several small, open-label trials. Can be used as an add-on therapy with verapamil
    - Gabapentin: For refectory cCH, 1,000 to 1,800 mg showed efficacy in small, open-label observational series.
    - nVNS: FDA approved for preventive treatment of cCH and eCH. One prospective, open-label RCT (PREVA study) showed greater reduction from baseline in number of CH per week in nVNS + standard of care than standard of care alone; NNT = 4

Pregnancy Considerations
- Collaboration between headache specialist, obstetrician, and lactation specialist is recommended (5)[C].
- For acute treatment, oxygen is the most appropriate first-line therapy. Intranasal triptans (pregnancy Category C), intranasal lidocaine (pregnancy Category B), and/or subcutaneous sumatriptan (pregnancy Category C) can be used as second-line therapy.
- For transitional therapy, steroids (pregnancy Category C/D) can be used, but systemic use should be avoided in 1st trimester.
- As prophylactic therapy, verapamil (pregnancy Category C) remains the preferred option. The use of SC or intranasal sumatriptan and zolmitriptan (pregnancy Category C) should be limited as much as possible. Avoid ergotamines (pregnancy Category X).

SURGERY/OTHER PROCEDURES
- No evidence for hyperbaric oxygen treatment or CPAP
- Botox shows conflicting results in two small open-label trials. An RCT is ongoing.
- Surgery or gamma knife radiation may be considered for refractory patients
- Neuromodulation: although a promising area of continuing research is invasive, expensive, and should be considered only for refractory patients

COMPLEMENTARY & ALTERNATIVE MEDICINE
For prophylaxis:
- Melatonin: 10 mg regular-release tablet in late evening has shown reduction in headache frequency versus placebo in small RCT.

ADMISSION, INPATIENT, AND NURSING CONSIDERATIONS
- Intractable, severe pain
- Suicidal ideation

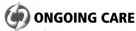 ONGOING CARE

FOLLOW-UP RECOMMENDATIONS
Patient Monitoring
- Anticipate cluster bouts, and initiate prophylaxis early.
- Monitor for depression and suicidal ideation, especially in those with cCH.

DIET
Avoid alcohol consumption.

PROGNOSIS
- Unpredictable but often chronic course
- Attack frequency often decreases with increasing age.
- Possibility of transformation of eCH to cCH

COMPLICATIONS
Depression and suicide

REFERENCES
1. Diener HC, May A. Drug treatment of cluster headache. *Drugs*. 2022;82(1):33–42.
2. Robbins MS, Starling AJ, Pringsheim TM, et al. Treatment of cluster headache: the American Headache Society evidence-based guidelines. *Headache*. 2016;56(7):1093–1106.
3. Gordon A, Roe T, Villar-Martínez MD, et al. Effectiveness and safety profile of greater occipital nerve blockade in cluster headache: a systematic review. *J Neurol Neurosurg Psychiatry*. 2023;jnnp-2023-331066.
4. Yuan H, Spare NM, Silberstein SD. Targeting CGRP for the prevention of migraine and cluster headache: a narrative review. *Headache*. 2019;59(Suppl 2):20–32.
5. Bjørk MH, Kristoffersen ES, Tronvik E, et al. Management of cluster headache and other trigeminal autonomic cephalalgias in pregnancy and breastfeeding. *Eur J Neurol*. 2021;28(7): 2443–2455.

 CODES

ICD10
- G44.009 Cluster headache syndrome, unspecified, not intractable
- G44.019 Episodic cluster headache, not intractable
- G44.029 Chronic cluster headache, not intractable

CLINICAL PEARLS
- Patients are often agitated and restless during acute attacks.
- High-flow oxygen and triptans, not narcotics, are first-line therapy for acute attacks.
- Among triptans, injected forms are more effective than nasal sprays, which are more effective than oral tablets.
- Abortive, transitional, and prophylactic treatment must all be considered.

HEADACHE, MIGRAINE

Karly Pippitt, MD • Seniha Ozudogru, MD

BASICS

DESCRIPTION
Recurrent headache disorder manifesting in attacks lasting 4 to 72 hours; typically: unilateral location, pulsating quality, moderate to severe intensity, and associated nausea and/or photophobia and phonophobia (1)

- Most frequent subtypes of migraine (1):
  - Without aura: defines >80% of migraines, vomiting, photophobia, and/or phonophobia
  - With aura: visual or other (motor, sensory or brainstem symptoms, including previously known as basilar or hemiplegic migraine); fully reversible neurologic phenomenon, develop gradually over 5 minutes and last up to 60 minutes
  - Chronic migraine: >15 migraine days/month, >4 hours/attack, for ≥3 months
  - Menstrual migraine: migraine attacks in a menstruating person, onset of 1 to 2 days prior to menses or up to day 3 of menstruation, occurring in 2 of 3 menstrual cycles and at no other time during cycle
  - Menstrually related migraine: menstrual migraine plus migraine attacks at other times during cycle
- Rare but important subtypes (1):
  - Status migrainosus: debilitating migraine lasting >72 hours
  - Prolonged aura: Aura symptoms of >60 minutes (can last up to 7 days) should prompt consideration of secondary causes.
  - Ocular: repeated attacks of monocular visual disturbance, including scintillations, scotomata, or blindness, with migraine
  - Vertiginous: migraine with vertigo or dizziness
  - Acephalgic migraine (migraine aura without headache): typical aura symptoms not followed by a migraine headache

EPIDEMIOLOGY
- Female > male (3:1)
- Affects >28 million Americans

ETIOLOGY AND PATHOPHYSIOLOGY
- Trigeminovascular hypothesis: Hyperexcitable trigeminal sensory neurons in brainstem are stimulated and release neuropeptides, such as substance P and calcitonin gene-related peptide (CGRP), leading to vasodilation and neurogenic inflammation.
- Cortical spreading depression: mainly accepted hypotheses for migraine with aura; change in electrical activity with reduction of blood flow, leading to aura

Genetics
>80% of patients have a family history.

RISK FACTORS
- Female sex (menstrual cycle)
- Positive family history of migraine
- Triggers:
  - Sleep pattern disruption
  - Diet: skipped meals (48%), alcohol (32%), chocolate (20%), cheese (13%), caffeine overuse (14%), monosodium glutamate (MSG) (12%), and artificial sweeteners
  - Medications: estrogens, vasodilators

GENERAL PREVENTION
- Lifestyle modifications are the cornerstone: sleep hygiene, stress management, healthy diet, adequate hydration, and regular exercise.
- Prophylactic medication for frequent attacks

COMMONLY ASSOCIATED CONDITIONS
- Depression, anxiety, PTSD
- Sleep disturbance (e.g., sleep apnea)
- Cerebral vascular disease
- Seizure disorders
- Irritable bowel syndrome
- Other pain syndromes (cervical spine disease, endometriosis)

DIAGNOSIS

Clinical diagnosis; recommend thorough history and neurologic examination

HISTORY
- Validated migraine screening tool: ID migraine (2)
- In the last 3 months, did you have the following symptoms with your headaches: Nauseated or sick to your stomach? Light bothered you (more than when you didn't have a headache)? Headaches limited your ability to work, study, or do what you needed for a day?
  - Yes to 2 questions: 81% migraine probability; yes to 3 questions increases probability of migraine to 93% (2)
- Headache usually begins with mild pain escalating into unilateral (30–40% bilateral), throbbing (40% nonthrobbing) pain lasting 4 to 72 hours. If side locked headache, never shifts sides, or there are potential secondary causes (e.g., tumor, systemic illnesses); this should prompt evaluation for alternative diagnosis.
- Intensified by movement and associated with nausea, vomiting, diarrhea, photophobia, phonophobia, muscle tenderness, light-headedness, and vertigo
- May be preceded by aura
  - Visual disruptions most common: scotoma, hemianopsia, fortification spectra, geometric visual patterns, and occasionally hallucinations
  - Somatosensory disruption in face or arms
  - Speech difficulties
- Headache diary: episodes per month, HA days per month, frequency, and amount and effect of medications used
- Identify possible triggers (e.g., stress, sleep disturbance, food, caffeine, alcohol).
- Migraine disability assessment (MiDAS) is a useful tool to assess level of disability and correlates well with headache diaries.

PHYSICAL EXAM
Neurologic exam, including funduscopy, to rule out other causes:
- Gait abnormalities, other cerebellar findings
- Loss of gross and/or fine motor function
- Altered mental status
- Short-term memory loss
- Papilledema

DIFFERENTIAL DIAGNOSIS
- Other primary headache syndromes (e.g., idiopathic intracranial hypertension [IIH], trigeminal autonomic cephalgia [TAC])
- Secondary headaches: medication overuse headache (MOH), tumor, infection, inflammation, vascular pathology, drug use

DIAGNOSTIC TESTS & INTERPRETATION
- Neuroimaging is appropriate with suspicious symptomatology and/or abnormal exam (3)[C]. Red flags include the following:
  - New onset after 50 years of age
  - Change in established headache pattern
  - Atypical pattern or unremitting/progressive neurologic symptoms
  - Prolonged or different/change in typical aura
- Appropriate workup includes the following:
  - Head CT for concern of brain bleed; brain MRI more common imaging study
  - EEG is *not* indicated unless evaluating LOC and AMS.
  - Consider systemic disease (i.e., hypothyroidism, SLE, and vitamin deficiencies) in appropriate clinical scenario and evaluate accordingly.

Pediatric Considerations
- NSAIDs and triptans are effective for acute treatment; NSAIDs first line
- Rizatriptan is FDA-approved for children aged >6 years; sumatriptan succinate, almotriptan, and zolmitriptan nasal spray FDA-approved for age >12 years (4)[A]

Pregnancy Considerations
- Frequency may decrease in 2nd and 3rd trimesters.
- For new-onset headaches in pregnancy, consider preeclampsia and venous sinus thrombosis.
- No migraine drug has FDA approval in pregnancy and breastfeeding.
  - Acetaminophen, antiemetics, and short-acting opioids can be considered for acute headaches.
  - Data does not find increased teratogenicity with triptans (most data for sumatriptan). When triptans are compellingly needed, they are acceptable.
  - Ergotamines are contraindicated.
  - Avoid herbal remedies.
  - β-Blockers and calcium channel blockers are effective prophylaxis.
  - Occipital nerve blocks and trigger point injections (lidocaine and bupivacaine) are safe.

TREATMENT

GENERAL MEASURES
- Consistent sleep hours and eating habits
- Cold compresses to area of pain

MEDICATION

- First-line abortive treatments
  - Mild to moderate attacks:
    - Acetaminophen is effective; when combined with metoclopramide has relief rates similar to triptans (5)[A]
    - NSAIDs are effective in up to 60% of cases (5)[B].
    - Aspirin–acetaminophen–caffeine (Excedrin Migraine) (5)[B]
  - Moderate to severe attacks:
    - Triptans when OTC agents fail for mild to moderate attacks *or* first line for moderate to severe attacks (5)[C]
      - Sumatriptan 100 mg PO, can repeat after 2 hours, max of 200 mg/24 hr; sumatriptan 3 or 4 or 6 mg SC, can repeat after 1 hour; max of 12 mg/24 hr; rapid onset, should consider for wake up headache and migraine with severe GI upset; sumatriptan intranasal 20 mg, can repeat after 2 hours, max of 40 mg/24 hr
      - Rizatriptan 10 mg PO (dose is 5 mg if using propranolol for prophylaxis); can repeat after 2 hours; max of 30 mg/24 hr
      - Naratriptan 2.5 mg PO; can repeat after 4 hours; max of 5 mg/24 hr
      - Zolmitriptan 2.5 mg PO; 5 mg intranasal; can repeat after 2 hours; max of 5 mg for oral, 10 mg for nasal spray/24 hr
      - Frovatriptan 2.5 mg PO; can repeat after 4 hours; max of 5 mg/24 hr
      - Eletriptan 40 mg PO; can repeat after 2 hours; max of 80 mg/24 hr
        □ Frovatriptan and naratriptan have slow onset but long half-lives—ideal for long migraine duration and menstrual migraine.
    - Antiemetics: dopamine antagonists add-ons (5)[B]
  - Contraindications: Avoid triptans and ergots in coronary artery or uncontrolled hypertension.
  - Precautions
    - Frequent use of acute-treatment drugs can result in MOH (especially Excedrin, triptans, butalbital).
    - Triptan common adverse reactions: chest pain, flushing, weakness, dizziness, and paresthesias; recommend trying more than one triptan before considered a class failure.
- Second-line abortive treatment
  - Ubrogepant 50 and 100 mg: can repeat after 2 hours; max of 200 mg/24 hr
  - Rimegepant 75 mg ODT: 1 daily PRN dose; max of 75 mg/24 hr
  - Dihydroergotamine: drug of choice in status migrainosus and triptan resistance or failure; ergotamine oral tablets and dihydroergotamine nasal sprays are more convenient and safer than intramuscular injections.
  - Lasmiditan 50 and 100 mg: 5-HT1F receptor agonist; schedule V controlled substancet should not drive following 8 hours; safe with CV risk factors

- First-line preventive treatment (6)[A]: lifestyle modifications, trigger reduction, CBT
  - Consider prophylactic treatment if:
    - Quality of life is severely impaired
    - ≥6 headache days per month, ≥4 headache days per month of moderate severity, or ≥2 headache days per month of severe impairment
    - Migraines not responding to abortives
    - Frequent, long, or uncomfortable auras
- Preventive treatment of *migraine*: divalproex, topiramate, metoprolol, and propranolol to reduce frequency; amitriptyline, venlafaxine, lisinopril, and candesartan are other options (6)[A].
  - NSAIDs can be effective prevention if predictable triggers (menses, etc.)
  - CGRP monoclonal antibodies:
    - Erenumab-aooe 70 and 140 mg, complete CGRP receptor antagonist; 1 SC/month
    - Fremanezumab-vfrm partial CGRP receptor antagonist; 225 mg monthly SC injections or 675 mg quarterly SC injections
    - Galcanezumab-gnlm partial CGRP receptor antagonist; 240 mg loading dose and then 120 mg monthly SC injections
    - Eptinezumab-jjmr 100 mg/mL: Dilute with 0.9% NaCl; infuse over 30 minutes.
  - CGRP small molecule antagonists:
    - Rimegepant 75 mg ODT: 1 tablet every other day
    - Atogepant 10, 30, and 60 mg: 1 tablet daily
  - For *chronic migraine*, onabotulinumtoxinA (Botox) injections every 3 months (6)[A]

ISSUES FOR REFERRAL

Obscure diagnosis, unresponsive to usual treatment, significant comorbid medical diagnoses

COMPLEMENTARY & ALTERNATIVE MEDICINE

- Riboflavin (vitamin B$_2$): 400 mg/day (6)[B]
- Magnesium: 400 mg/day (6)[B]
- MIG-99 (Feverfew): 6.25 mg TID (6)[B]
- Acupuncture maybe effective

 ## ONGOING CARE

FOLLOW-UP RECOMMENDATIONS
Patient Monitoring
- Quarterly or more frequent appointments when headaches not well controlled
- Monitor frequency of attacks and medication usage via headache diary.
- Migraine (especially with aura) is a risk factor for stroke; consider lipid assessment and other risk reduction such as tobacco cessation. Women with migraine with aura should avoid estrogens due to increased risk of stroke (2)[A].

PATIENT EDUCATION
- Trigger identification and modification can significantly improve headache frequency.
- Setting expectations critical, especially with prophylactic medications where success is 50% reduction in severity of headaches or decrease in disability from headaches
- Benefits may be seen from prophylactic medications after many weeks of treatment.

PROGNOSIS
- With increasing age (including menopause), there is a reduction in severity, frequency, and disability.
- Most attacks subside within 72 hours.

COMPLICATIONS
- Status migrainosus (>72 hours)
- MOH: headache ≥10 days per month for >3 months due to regular overuse of a rescue headache medication; likelihood with butalbital > opiates > triptans > NSAIDs
- Cerebral ischemic events (rare)

REFERENCES

1. Headache Classification Committee of the International Headache Society (IHS). The International Classification of Headache Disorders, 3rd edition. *Cephalalgia*. 2018;38(1):1–211.
2. Sacco S, Merki-Feld GS, Ægidius KL, et al; for European Headache Federation, European Society of Contraception and Reproductive Health. Hormonal contraceptives and risk of ischemic stroke in women with migraine: a consensus statement from the European Headache Federation (EHF) and the European Society of Contraception and Reproductive Health (ESC). *J Headache Pain*. 2017;18(1):108.
3. Loder E, Weizenbaum E, Frishberg B, et al; for American Headache Society Choosing Wisely Task Force. Choosing wisely in headache medicine: the American Headache Society's list of five things physicians and patients should question. *Headache*. 2013;53(10):1651–1659.
4. Patterson-Gentile C, Szperka CL. The changing landscape of pediatric migraine therapy: a review. *JAMA Neurol*. 2018;75(7):881–887.
5. Becker WJ. Acute migraine treatment in adults. *Headache*. 2015;55(6):778–793.
6. Loder E, Burch R, Rizzoli P. The 2012 AHS/AAN guidelines for prevention of episodic migraine: a summary and comparison with other recent clinical practice guidelines. *Headache*. 2012; 52(6):930–945.

 SEE ALSO

Algorithm: Headache, Chronic

CODES

ICD10
- G43.909 Migraine, unsp, not intractable, without status migrainosus
- G43.109 Migraine with aura, not intractable, w/o status migrainosus
- G43.409 Hemiplegic migraine, not intractable, w/o status migrainosus

CLINICAL PEARLS

- Migraine is a chronic headache disorder of unclear etiology often characterized by unilateral, throbbing pain that may be associated with additional neurologic symptoms.
- Consider OTC analgesics for mild attacks; migraine-specific treatments for more severe attacks or those not responding to OTC medications
- Avoid opiates and barbiturates or frequent (>8 per month) triptan or NSAID use to avoid MOH.
- Counsel on lifestyle modifications and trigger identification.
- Consider prophylactic treatment if frequent or debilitating migraines.

H

HEADACHE, TENSION

Gregory John Ferenchak, MD • Sophia R. Barber, DO

BASICS

DESCRIPTION
- A bilateral mild to moderate, nonthrobbing head pain or pressure, without other associated symptoms
- Tension-type headache (TTH) replaced the older terms muscle contraction headache; stress, ordinary, or essential headache; idiopathic headache; and psychogenic headache.

EPIDEMIOLOGY
It is the most common type of primary headache and the second-most prevalent disorder in the world.

Prevalence
- Peak age of prevalence in the United States: the 4th decade
- Prevalence of episodic TTH decreases with age, whereas the prevalence of chronic TTH increases with age.

ETIOLOGY AND PATHOPHYSIOLOGY
- Not well understood, multifactorial etiology with both peripheral and central nervous system mechanisms triggering TTH
- Activation of peripheral nociceptors leads to myofascial pain in episodic TTH.
- Prolonged stimulation of nociceptors sensitizes the central pain pathways leading to chronic TTH.
- Nitric oxide may play an important role in TTH.

RISK FACTORS
Associated with triggers/precipitating factors:
- Stress (mental or physical)
- Change in sleep regimen
- Skipping meals, dehydration
- Certain foods (caffeine, alcohol, chocolate)
- Environmental factors (sun glare, odors, smoke, noise, lighting)
- Female hormonal changes
- Medications (e.g., nitrates, SSRIs, antihypertensives)
- Overuse of abortive headache medication

GENERAL PREVENTION
Lifestyle factors to promote headache prevention include avoiding triggers, increasing exercise, regular sleep patterns, decreasing caffeine and alcohol, and staying adequately hydrated.

COMMONLY ASSOCIATED CONDITIONS
- 83% of patients with migraine headaches also suffer from TTHs.
- Possible increased prevalence of comorbid anxiety and depression

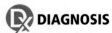 DIAGNOSIS

HISTORY
Obtain a thorough pain history to rule out other headache disorders, including onset, location, radiation, quality of pain, severity, associated symptoms; concurrent medical conditions and medications; and recent trauma or other procedures.
- Diagnosis is based on clinical assessment
- Pain may be described in many ways, such as "dull," "band-like," "pressure."

- Diagnostic criteria by the International Headache Society (ICHD-3) (1):
  – Episodic TTH: ≥10 headache episodes that meet all of the following criteria:
    ○ Headache lasting 30 minutes to 7 days
    ○ At least two of the following:
      ■ Bilateral location
      ■ Pressing/tightening (nonpulsating) quality
      ■ Mild or moderate intensity
      ■ Not aggravated by routine physical activity
    ○ Not associated with:
      ■ Nausea or vomiting
      ■ No more than one of photophobia or phonophobia
    ○ Headache not due to another ICHD-3 diagnosis
  – Chronic TTH: ≥15 days per month (on average) for >3 months that meet all of the following criteria:
    ○ Headache lasting hours to days, or unremitting
    ○ At least two of the following:
      ■ Bilateral location
      ■ Pressing/tightening (nonpulsating) quality
      ■ Mild or moderate intensity
      ■ Not aggravated by routine physical activity
    ○ Both of the following:
      ■ No more than one of photophobia, phonophobia, or mild nausea
      ■ Neither moderate or severe nausea nor vomiting
- Must assess and rule out "red flag" symptoms that suggest secondary headache causes such as:
  – Thunderclap headache, fever, meningismus, focal neurologic deficit, pregnancy, age >50 years, neoplasm history, positional exacerbation of headache, worsened by sneezing/coughing, painful eye and vision changes

PHYSICAL EXAM
- Assess vital signs, looking for elevated blood pressure.
- Usually unremarkable clinical exam
- Head and neck: palpation of myofascial tissues for pericranial muscle tenderness including the cervical paraspinal muscles, trapezius, muscles of mastication, and for pain near the jaw around the temporomandibular joint
- Neurologic exam: mental status, pupillary responses, motor-strength testing, deep tendon reflexes, sensation, cerebellar function, gait testing, signs of meningeal irritation

DIFFERENTIAL DIAGNOSIS
- Migraine or cluster headache
- Ischemic cerebrovascular disease, cerebral venous thrombosis, intracranial hemorrhage
- Temporal arteritis
- Arterial hypertension (HTN), benign intracranial HTN
- Intracranial neoplasm
- Infection such as meningitis, encephalitis, sinusitis, and acute otitis media
- Medication (nonprescription analgesic dependency, nitrates)
- Caffeine dependency
- Metabolic disorders (hypoxia, hypercapnia, hypoglycemia)
- Temporomandibular joint syndrome
- Eyes: glaucoma, refractive errors

- Cervical spondylosis
- Severe anemia or polycythemia
- Paget disease of bone

DIAGNOSTIC TESTS & INTERPRETATION
- Most primary headaches with typical features do not require lab testing or diagnostic imaging, and recommendations regarding TTH and neuroimaging are not well-defined.
- MRI/CT imaging is rarely revealing for chronic or recurrent headaches with normal neurologic findings (see "Additional Reading").

Initial Tests (lab, imaging)
Labs and neuroimaging (CT or MRI) should be considered when a secondary cause is suspected:
- Atypical pattern of headache (does not fit specific category such as migraine, cluster, or tension)
- Rapid increase in frequency
- Unexplained focal neurologic findings
- New onset after age 35 years
- Sudden onset or worsening with exertion

Follow-Up Tests & Special Considerations
Some may find that a headache diary is useful to track symptoms, triggers, and response to treatment.

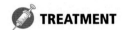 TREATMENT

GENERAL MEASURES
Relief measures include relaxation routines; rest in quiet, dark room; hot bath or shower; massage of back of neck and temples.

MEDICATION
- Nonsteroidal anti-inflammatory drugs (NSAIDs), aspirin or acetaminophen, are effective for short-term relief of episodic TTH (2)[B].
- Amitriptyline should be considered first line for prophylaxis of chronic TTH (2)[B].

First Line
- For acute treatment in episodic TTH:
  – NSAIDs:
    ○ Ibuprofen (Motrin, Advil): 200 to 400 mg; may repeat q8h PRN (max 3.2 g/day)
    ○ Naproxen sodium (Naprosyn): 220 to 550 mg BID PRN (max 1,250 mg base per day)
    ○ Contraindications: aspirin or NSAID allergy or bronchospasm, renal disease, bleeding disorders, increased risk of cardiovascular events (myocardial infarction [MI], stroke, new onset or worsening of HTN)
    ○ Drug interactions: antihypertensives, anticoagulants, antiplatelet drugs, aspirin, lithium, methotrexate
    ○ Adverse effects: epigastric distress, peptic ulcer
  – Aspirin: 650 to 1,000 mg; may repeat q6h PRN (max 4 g/day):
    ○ Contraindication: aspirin or NSAID allergy or bronchospasm, bleeding disorders, peptic ulcer
    ○ Drug interactions: anticoagulants, antiplatelet drugs, ACE inhibitors, β-blockers, corticosteroids, NSAIDs, sulfonylureas
    ○ Adverse effects: GI irritation/bleeding, thrombocytopenia

- Acetaminophen (Tylenol): 1,000 mg; may repeat q6h PRN (max 3 to 4 g/day):
  - Adverse effects (rare): rash, pancytopenia, liver damage
  - Precaution: hepatic impairment, consumption of ≥3 per day alcoholic beverages
- For prophylaxis in frequent episodic and chronic TTH:
  - Tricyclic antidepressants (TCAs): amitriptyline (Elavil): Start at 10 mg, may slowly up-titrate to 100 mg QHS.
    - Not FDA-approved for chronic TTH, but there is high quality evidence that TCAs have moderate benefit and are superior to placebo (3)[A].
    - Consider if patient has depression, anxiety, or insomnia.
    - Contraindications: acute recovery phase (within 30 days) of MI, use of monoamine oxidase inhibitors (MAOIs) within 14 days
    - Drug interactions: clonidine, MAOIs, quinolone antibiotics, SSRIs, sympathomimetics, azole antifungals, valproic acid
    - Adverse effects: weight gain, drowsiness, dry mouth, tachycardia, heart block, blurred vision, urinary retention, seizure

Second Line

- For acute treatment in episodic TTH:
  - Caffeine combinations: 130 mg caffeine with 500 mg acetaminophen and/or 500 mg aspirin q6h PRN (2)[C]
  - Ketorolac: 60 mg IM once, for severe episodes
  - Opioids (e.g., codeine), butalbital, or their combination are not recommended. Consider secondary causes of headache or secondary gain such as drug-seeking behavior for personal use or diversion/sale.
- For prophylaxis in frequent episodic and chronic TTH:
  - Mirtazapine: 15 to 30 mg/day (not FDA-approved for chronic TTH) (2)[B]
  - Venlafaxine 150 mg/day (2)[B]

ALERT

Use of abortive agents >2 days/week may lead to medication-overuse headaches; must withdraw acute treatment to diagnose.

ADDITIONAL THERAPIES

- The combination of stress management therapy and a TCA (amitriptyline) may be most effective for chronic TTH.
- Topiramate: 100 mg/day (limited clinical evidence for prevention of chronic TTH; not FDA-approved for chronic TTH)
- Alternative TCAs with evidence of benefit (3)[B]:
  - Nortriptyline (Pamelor): 25 to 50 mg/day (mild-moderately sedating, causes weight gain)
  - Protriptyline (Vivactil): 25 mg/day (nonsedating, causes weight loss)
- Tizanidine has conflicting clinical evidence for use in chronic TTH and thus should not be considered.

SURGERY/OTHER PROCEDURES

Trigger point lidocaine injections may reduce headache frequency, whereas Botox injections have conflicting evidence to support their use in TTH.

COMPLEMENTARY & ALTERNATIVE MEDICINE

Many complementary and alternative medicine treatment modalities have been investigated with varying degrees of success, though quality evidence remains limited (4). Some modalities include the following:

- Tiger Balm or peppermint oil applied topically to the forehead
- Cognitive-behavioral therapy
- Electromyography (EMG) biofeedback with or without relaxation therapy
- Physical therapy, including positioning, ergonomic instruction, massage, transcutaneous electrical nerve stimulation, and application of heat/cold
- Exercise, primarily upper-limb resistance training (5)
- Chiropractic spinal manipulation has equivocal evidence in the management of episodic and chronic TTH.
- Cervical manual therapy, particularly soft-tissue and trigger-point therapies
- Acupuncture (6)

ONGOING CARE

DIET

- Identify and avoid dietary triggers.
- Regulate meal schedule.

PATIENT EDUCATION

- National Headache Foundation: http://www.headaches.org/resources
- Family Doctor by American Academy of Family: https://familydoctor.org/condition/headaches

PROGNOSIS

Most cases are intermittent and decrease with age.

COMPLICATIONS

- Medication-overuse headache
- GI bleeding from NSAID use
- Dependence/addiction to narcotic analgesics

REFERENCES

1. Headache Classification Committee of the International Headache Society (IHS) The international classification of headache disorders, 3rd edition. *Cephalalgia*. 2018;38(1):1–211.
2. Becker WJ, Findlay T, Moga C, et al. Guideline for primary care management of headache in adults. *Can Fam Physician*. 2015;61(8):670–679.
3. Jackson JL, Mancuso JM, Nickoloff S, et al. Tricyclic and tetracyclic antidepressants for the prevention of frequent episodic or chronic tension-type headaches in adults: a systematic review and meta-analysis. *J Gen Intern Med*. 2017;32(12):1351–1358.
4. Sun-Edelstein C, Mauskop A. Complementary and alternative approaches to the treatment of tension-type headache. *Curr Pain Headache Rep*. 2012;16(6):539–544.
5. Varangot-Reille C, Suso-Martí L, Dubuis V, et al. Exercise and manual therapy for the treatment of primary headache: an umbrella and mapping review. *Phys Ther*. 2022;102(3):pzab308.
6. Linde K, Allais G, Brinkhaus B, et al. Acupuncture for the prevention of tension-type headache. *Cochrane Database Syst Rev*. 2016;4(4):CD007587.

ADDITIONAL READING

Viera AJ, Antono B. Acute headache in adults: a diagnostic approach. *Am Fam Physician*. 2022;106(3):260–268.

 SEE ALSO

Algorithm: Headache, Chronic

CODES

ICD10

- G44.209 Tension-type headache, unspecified, not intractable
- G44.219 Episodic tension-type headache, not intractable
- G44.229 Chronic tension-type headache, not intractable

CLINICAL PEARLS

- Typical characteristics include bilateral mild to moderate, nonthrobbing head pain or pressure, without other associated symptoms.
- First-line therapy for TTH includes NSAIDs. For preventive therapy, TCAs have benefit, but they are not FDA-approved for this indication.
- Consider secondary causes and obtain further testing, such as neuroimaging, if there are unexplained focal neurologic signs, atypical presentation, late onset (>50 years of age), or when usual treatment fails.
- Chronic TTH is difficult to treat, and it can lead to medication-overuse headaches if abortive therapy is used more than 2 days per week.
- Avoid the use of opioids or butalbital-containing medications as first-line treatment for recurrent headaches.

H

HEARING LOSS
Sabina M. Constantine, DO

BASICS

Hearing impairment is one of the most common chronic conditions in older adults affecting at least 29 million Americans. Hearing loss has a prevalence ranging from 20.6% in adults aged 48 to 59 years old to 90% in adults >80 years old. The severity of this condition has been shown to be associated with a poorer quality of life, communication difficulties, impaired activities of daily living, dementia, and cognitive dysfunction.

DESCRIPTION
- Decrease in the ability to perceive and comprehend sound; it can be partial, complete, unilateral, and/or bilateral.
- Typically, defined as a deficit of >25 dB
- Types of hearing loss include conductive hearing loss (CHL or air–bone gap), sensorineural hearing loss (SNHL), or mixed hearing loss.
- System(s) affected: auditory; outer and middle ear (CHL) or inner ear, auditory nerve, and/or brainstem (SNHL)
- Sudden hearing loss is defined as rapid-onset, subjective sensation of hearing impairment in one or both ears (1).

EPIDEMIOLOGY
- All ages affected; common in children (CHL) and elderly (SNHL)
- Usually more severe at an earlier age in men

Incidence
- Increases with age
- Sudden sensorineural hearing loss (SSHL) occurs in 5 to 27 per 100,000 persons per year.

Prevalence
Geriatric Considerations
- 24.7% of 60- to 69-year-olds in the United States have bilateral speech-frequency hearing loss.
- ~80% of people aged >85 years have hearing loss.
- Hearing impairment is an independent and modifiable risk factor for cognitive decline in the elderly and may lead to emotional distress and physical risk secondary to the loss of communication (2).
- Consider auditory rehabilitation (facing people when talking, improving lighting, minimizing background noise).

Pediatric Considerations
- Early diagnosis and treatment improves outcome.
- 60% of childhood hearing loss is secondary to preventable causes.
- Screen newborns with otoacoustic emission (OAE) and auditory brainstem response (ABR) testing.

ETIOLOGY AND PATHOPHYSIOLOGY
- CHL: Hearing loss can result from middle ear effusion or obstruction of the auditory canal (chronic otitis media, eustachian tube dysfunction, cerumen/foreign body, osteomas/exostoses, cholesteatoma, tumor), loss of continuity (ossicular discontinuity), stiffening of the components (myringosclerosis, tympanosclerosis, and otosclerosis), and loss of the pressure differential across the tympanic membrane (TM) (perforation) (3).

- SNHL: acoustic damage from vascular/metabolic insult, mass effect, infection and inflammation, and acoustic trauma
  - Noise-induced hearing loss is caused by acoustic insult that affects outer hair cells in the organ of Corti, causing them to be less stiff. Over time, severe damage occurs with fusion and loss of stereocilia. Eventually, this may progress to inner hair cells and auditory nerve as well.
- Large vestibular aqueduct or superior canal dehiscence: Third mobile window shunts acoustic energy away from cochlea.

Genetics
- Nonsyndromal genetic hearing loss is the most common; connexin 26 (13q11–13q12) (4)
- Otosclerosis: frequently familial
- Congenital syndromes (e.g., Alport syndrome, Stickler syndrome)

RISK FACTORS
- Loud noise/acoustic trauma
- Medications (aminoglycosides, loop diuretics, aspirin, nonsteroidal anti-inflammatory drugs (NSAIDs), quinine, chemotherapeutic agents, especially cisplatin, vancomycin)
- Tobacco, alcohol use
- Vestibular schwannoma/skull base neoplasm
- Previous ear surgery
- Sensorineural, pediatric specific
  - Perinatal asphyxia
  - Congenital infections (toxoplasmosis, other agents, rubella, cytomegalovirus, herpes simplex [TORCH] syndrome)
  - Toxemia of pregnancy; maternal diabetes; Rh incompatibility
  - Prematurity or birth weight <1,500 g
  - Severe hyperbilirubinemia; exchange transfusions
  - Anomalous temporal bone (Mondini dysplasia or large vestibular aqueduct)
  - Infectious diseases (chickenpox, measles, encephalitis, influenza, mumps, Zika virus infection, bacterial meningitis, etc.)

GENERAL PREVENTION
- Limit noise exposure; use hearing protection.
- Avoid or limit ototoxic medications.

COMMONLY ASSOCIATED CONDITIONS
Tinnitus: common for patients to experience both tinnitus and hearing loss

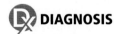

DIAGNOSIS

HISTORY
- Social problems and comments from friends and family are often the first presentation of presbycusis (age-related hearing loss); patients are often not aware of the degree of hearing loss they experience and how it affects their lives; insidious onset and progression
- Difficulty hearing
  - Rapid versus gradual decline: Rapid loss (<3 days) is a medical emergency. Urgent ear/nose/throat referral and steroid therapy are recommended.
  - Difficulty with discrimination of sounds, hearing in crowds, or turning up the volume of television sets

  - Frequently having to ask speakers to repeat
  - Friends/family complain of hearing loss
- Tinnitus, bilateral or unilateral
- Otalgia
- Otorrhea, clear or purulent
- Dizziness or vertigo
- Aural fullness
- Autophony (hearing own voice louder or echoing)
- History of ear infections or ear surgeries
- History of trauma or noise exposure
- Family history of hearing loss
- History of recent viral infection

PHYSICAL EXAM
- Whispered voice test: A whisper heard from ~2 feet away is a good screen for intact hearing. Patients with SNHL have difficulty with this because their hearing loss is usually in the high frequency range.
- A simple 512-Hz tuning fork test lateralizes to the unaffected ear in sudden SNHL (emergency) and lateralizes to the affected ear in CHL (not an emergency).
- 512-Hz tuning fork tests:
  - Sensorineural loss
    - Placed on the forehead: lateralizes to unaffected ear (Weber test)
    - Base of tuning fork placed on the mastoid and then fork end placed next to ear; heard louder next to ear—air conduction > bone conduction (positive Rinne test)
  - Conductive loss
    - Placed on the forehead or teeth lateralizes to affected or symptomatic ear
    - Placed on the mastoid and then next to ear; heard louder behind the ear on the side of conductive deficit bone conduction > air conduction (negative Rinne test)
- Otoscopy: assess for deformity, canal patency, and otorrhea; TM integrity/retraction/mobility with insufflation, canal, or middle ear mass, cerumen impaction
- Facial symmetry
- Cranial nerve exam
- Nasopharyngoscopy: adenoid hypertrophy or nasopharyngeal mass (mandatory in adult patient with new unilateral serous effusion)

DIFFERENTIAL DIAGNOSIS
- Conductive loss secondary to mechanical issues (e.g., cerumen impaction/foreign body, perforation of TM, acoustic neuroma)
- Sensorineural loss:
  - Presbycusis (age-related hearing loss)
  - Noise-induced (recreational, occupational)
  - Ménière disease
  - Ototoxicity (aspirin, NSAIDs, aminoglycosides)
  - Viral labyrinthitis
  - Cerebellopontine angle (CPA) tumor
  - Temporal bone fracture
  - Metabolic (hyperthyroidism/hypothyroidism)
  - Paget disease
  - Perilymphatic (inner ear) fistula
  - Vasculitis (including giant cell arteritis, Takayasu arteritis, polyarteritis nodosa, granulomatosis with polyangiitis, microscopic polyangiitis, eosinophilic granulomatosis with polyangiitis, systemic lupus erythematosus, immune-complex associated vasculitis, and others)

DIAGNOSTIC TESTS & INTERPRETATION

Consider as clinically indicated:

- MRI of the brain and brainstem with gadolinium to evaluate SNHL in congenital, early onset, and asymmetric hearing loss
- Fine-cut CT temporal bones without contrast may help in the evaluation of CHL.
- Newborn screening with OAE and/or ABR
- Consider genetic testing for connexin 26, mitochondrial studies for children with SNHL.
- TORCH screening (congenital infection)
- Rapid plasma reagin (RPR) or venereal disease research laboratory (VDRL) confirmed by fluorescent treponemal antibody absorption (FTA-ABS)
- Lyme titer in endemic areas
- Antinuclear antibodies and sedimentation rate as a screen for autoimmune disease
- Pendred syndrome (goiter, mental retardation + SNHL): perchlorate test, thyroid function tests
- Alport syndrome (nephritis + SNHL): urinalysis, renal function tests
- Jervell and Lange-Nielsen syndrome (syncope, family history of sudden death + profound SNHL): ECG

Diagnostic Procedures/Other

- Audiometry: pure tone (air and bone), speech testing, and impedance (middle ear pressure) testing
- Tympanometry: Type B or C tympanograms indicate fluid or retraction, respectively. Negative middle ear peak pressures were seen even with normal (type A) tympanograms.
- Other tests: ABR, OAEs: "echo" of the cochlea, behavioral audiometry for children 6 months to 5 years old
- Myringotomy and tubes can be considered for persistent fluid with hearing loss

TREATMENT

MEDICATION

- Clinical practical guidelines for sudden hearing loss include the following:
  - Distinguishing SNHL from CHL; testing for bilateral sudden hearing loss in patients with unilateral sudden hearing loss; obtaining an MRI, ABR, or audiometric follow-up to evaluate for retrocochlear pathology; offer intratympanic steroid perfusion for refractory cases after initial management fails to treat idiopathic sudden SNHL (ISSNHL).
  - May offer corticosteroids as initial therapy to patients with ISSNHL and hyperbaric oxygen therapy (HBOT) within 2 weeks of onset; may consider HBOT within 1 month of onset as salvage therapy
  - Recommend against prescribing antivirals, thrombolytics, vasodilators, vasoactive substances, or antioxidants to patients with ISSNHL.
  - Recommend against routine laboratory tests in patients with ISSNHL.

- Treatment should begin ASAP, within 1 to 2 weeks of onset with high-dose oral steroids: 1 mg/kg or 60 to 100 mg/day prednisone or 12 to 16 mg/day dexamethasone for 7 to 14 days, followed by a taper (5).
- Intratympanic steroids show similar efficacy to oral steroids and reduce systemic side effects.
- Some studies suggest benefit of combined oral and intratympanic steroids for first-line treatment of sudden SNHL.

ISSUES FOR REFERRAL

- Failure of newborn screen
- Audiology for suspected hearing loss for formal evaluation
- Speech therapist: if speech delay or speech impediment is present
- Neurology and neurosurgery: CPA lesion, intracranial complication of middle ear disease

ADDITIONAL THERAPIES

- Aural rehabilitation: interdisciplinary approach involving audiologists, speech language pathologists, otologist, family physician, and other members of health care team as needed
- HBOT: Limited data shows improved outcomes in patients with SSHL who do not respond to steroids.

SURGERY/OTHER PROCEDURES

- Surgical options for CHL include tympanostomy and tube placement, tympanoplasty, mastoidectomy, ossicular chain reconstruction, stapedectomy/stapedotomy, and canaloplasty.
- Surgical options for SNHL include cochlear implantation (in those with profound, bilateral hearing loss).

ONGOING CARE

FOLLOW-UP RECOMMENDATIONS

Patient Monitoring

Audiogram and clinical exam are the primary means of monitoring patients.

DIET

- Salt restriction to 2 g/day is helpful for patients with Ménière disease.
- Reduce alcohol consumption.

PATIENT EDUCATION

- Avoid excessive and prolonged noise exposure.
- Use protective devices.
- National Institute on Deafness and Other Communication Disorders (NIDCD): https://www.nidcd.nih.gov/health/hearing/Pages/Default.aspx

PROGNOSIS

- SNHL is usually permanent and may be progressive.
- ISSNHL may recover spontaneously in 32–70% of cases, but urgent referral and treatment is recommended to maximize recovery.

COMPLICATIONS

Acute middle ear problems may become chronic (perforations, cholesteatoma).

REFERENCES

1. Michels TC, Duffy MT, Rogers DJ. Hearing loss in adults: differential diagnosis and treatment. *Am Fam Physician*. 2019;100(2):98–108.
2. Bisogno A, Scarpa A, Di Girolamo S, et al. Hearing loss and cognitive impairment: epidemiology, common pathophysiological findings, and treatment considerations. *Life (Basel)*. 2021;11(10):1102.
3. Shapiro SB, Noij KS, Naples JG, et al. Hearing loss and tinnitus. *Med Clin North Am*. 2021;105(5):799–811.
4. Mitchell CO, Morton CC. Genetics of childhood hearing loss. *Otolaryngol Clin North Am*. 2021;54(6):1081–1092.
5. Rahne T, Plontke S, Keyßer G. Vasculitis and the ear: a literature review. *Curr Opin Rheumatol*. 2020;32(1):47–52.

 CODES

ICD10

- H91.11 Presbycusis, right ear
- H91 Other and unspecified hearing loss
- H91.09 Ototoxic hearing loss, unspecified ear

CLINICAL PEARLS

- In sudden hearing loss, if a 512-Hz tuning fork test (Weber test) lateralizes to the *unaffected ear*, suspect sensorineural causes (emergent evaluation needed), but if it lateralizes to the *affected* ear, the diagnosis is CHL (not an emergency).
- ~80% of people aged >85 years have hearing loss; encourage screening and treatment, especially in patients with early dementia.
- Best way to prevent noise-induced hearing loss is to protect against noise exposure.
- Consider auditory rehabilitation in all patients.

H

HEART FAILURE, ACUTELY DECOMPENSATED

Muhammad I. Durrani, DO, MS • Carla Dugas, DO • Clifford M. Chang, MD

 BASICS

DESCRIPTION

Acute decompensated heart failure (ADHF) is a heterogenous group of syndromes characterized by new onset or recurrence of structural or functional cardiac pump impairment severe enough for patients to seek medical attention. Symptoms of ADHF are most often due to worsening dysfunction of the myocardium or heart valves; however, it can also arise from complications related to the pericardium or endocardium. The pathophysiology is characterized by either impaired ventricular filling or decreased ejection of blood resulting in pulmonary vascular and/or systemic venous congestion. In severe cases, it can cause tissue hypoperfusion and present as cardiogenic shock. ADHF can be a new diagnosis or represent worsening of preexisting heart failure (HF). A number of terms have been used to describe this pathology including acute HF and acute decompensation of chronic HF.

EPIDEMIOLOGY

Incidence

Incidence, prevalence, and costs of HF are discussed in the chapter on "Heart Failure, Chronic." HF is one of the most common causes of admission and readmission in the United States in those >65 years of age, responsible for >1 million annual hospitalizations.

Prevalence

HF is primarily a disease of the elderly. About half of people who have HF die within 5 years of diagnosis, and 90% of patients who have HF die within 10 years. See Heart Failure: Chronic.

ETIOLOGY AND PATHOPHYSIOLOGY

- Two main pathophysiologic conditions lead to the clinical findings of HF, namely, systolic and/or diastolic dysfunction. See "Heart Failure, Chronic." Systolic dysfunction is an *inotropic* abnormality, while diastolic dysfunction is a *compliance* abnormality
  - The terms HF with reduced, midrange (also called mildly reduced), preserved, or improved LVEF (HFrEF, HFmrEF, HFpEF, and HFimpEF, respectively) have been adopted recently.
  - Recent American HF guidelines have also described three clinical profiles of patients with ADHF that take into account the patient's clinical manifestations, hemodynamics, and systemic perfusion:
    - Patients with volume overload: evidenced by pulmonary vascular and/or systemic venous congestion and often triggered by an acute hypertensive crisis
    - Patients with depression of cardiac output: evidenced by hypotension, renal hypoperfusion, and/or shock
    - Patients with signs and symptoms of both volume overload and shock
- ADHF can result from the following conditions:
  - Myocardial disease: Exacerbation of preexisting chronic HF can be triggered by medication noncompliance, diet, or some other acute insult such as coronary artery disease (CAD) and myocardial infarction (MI), immune-mediated and inflammatory damage, infiltrative diseases, metabolic derangements, toxins, and genetic abnormalities.

  - Abnormal ventricular filling: elevated afterload and hypertension (HTN), valvular and myocardial structural defects, pericardial and endomyocardial pathologies, high-output states, volume overload
  - Arrhythmias: atrial fibrillation, tachyarrhythmias, high-grade heart block, bradyarrhythmias

Genetics
See "Heart Failure, Chronic."

RISK FACTORS
See "Heart Failure, Chronic."

GENERAL PREVENTION
See "Heart Failure, Chronic."

COMMONLY ASSOCIATED CONDITIONS
Dysrhythmia followed by pump failure is the leading cause of death in ADHF. Most patients have >5 comorbidities (especially CAD, chronic kidney disease, and diabetes) and take >5 medications.

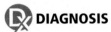 **DIAGNOSIS**

See Heart Failure: Chronic.

HISTORY
Patients typically have a history of HF, MI, uncontrolled HTN, and other risk factors mentioned above. Dyspnea on exertion and orthopnea are the only symptoms with high sensitivity but suffer from low specificity. Other symptoms: See "Heart Failure, Chronic."

PHYSICAL EXAM
- S_3 has the highest likelihood ratio (LR) in respect to PE with positive LR ranging from 1.6 to 13.0. No PE finding has sensitivity >70%.
- Lung exam: rales (crackles) and sometimes wheezing, Cheyne-Stokes respirations

DIFFERENTIAL DIAGNOSIS
Rule out life-threatening diagnoses first: pulmonary embolism, MI, tamponade, pneumothorax, acute respiratory distress syndrome (ARDS), sepsis, chronic obstructive pulmonary disease (COPD), pneumonia, constrictive pericarditis, high-output states (anemia, hyperthyroidism).

DIAGNOSTIC TESTS & INTERPRETATION
Laboratory data are adjunctive and help with prognostication and clinical course.

Initial Tests (lab, imaging)
- See also "Heart Failure, Chronic." Assess blood pressure (BP) and other vital signs to rule out hemodynamic instability and signs of cardiogenic shock.
- ECG and cardiac troponins to evaluate for ACS; note that elevated troponins are detected in the majority of HF patients, often without obvious myocardial ischemia.
- BUN, creatinine, electrolytes, liver function tests, TSH (new onset), UA, iron studies (new onset), glucose, and CBC
- Transthoracic echocardiogram: recommended immediately in hemodynamically unstable ADHF patients and within 48 hours when cardiac structure and function are either not known or may have changed since previous studies

- BNP and/or N-terminal fragment pro-BNP (NT-proBNP): Measurement of BNP or NT-proBNP is recommended in all patients with acute dyspnea and suspected ADHF when the cause of dyspnea is unclear and may be related to ADHF. BNP <100 essentially will rule out HF with negative LR of 0.2 and sensitivity of 93.5%. BNP >500 has a specificity of 89.8%. BNP 100 to 400 is an intermediate range and may indicate HF but also other cardiac, noncardiac (e.g., pulmonary), or multiple conditions.
- NT-proBNP values >450 pg/mL for people aged <50 years, >900 pg/mL for aged 50 to 75 years, and >1,800 pg/mL for aged >75 years are highly suggestive of HF (sensitivity of 90%, specificity of 84%) in the correct clinical setting.
- Chest x-ray: to assess for pulmonary congestion and to detect other cardiac or noncardiac diseases that may cause or contribute to the patient's symptoms
- Lung ultrasound (LUS): emerging as a diagnostic tool for ADHF with a positive LUS defined by the presence of >3 B lines in two bilateral lung zones yielding a specificity of 92.7% and LR of 7.4%

Follow-Up Tests & Special Considerations
Please see "Heart Failure, Chronic."

Diagnostic Procedures/Other
Cardiac catheterization may be considered when CAD is suspected. Pulmonary artery catheterization had previously been performed to guide therapy in severe cases with cardiogenic shock but is falling out of favor.

Test Interpretation
Cardiac pathology depends on the etiology of HF. Please refer to "Heart Failure, Chronic" topic.

 TREATMENT

The initial goals of treatment are to improve hemodynamics and organ perfusion, to alleviate symptoms, to limit cardiac and renal damage, and to restore oxygenation. Once stabilized, the goal is to identify the inciting cause or precipitating factors, to decrease hospital length of stay, and to optimize as well as educate the patient to prevent future exacerbations. Below recommendations are all derived from the 2022 ACC guideline for the management of heart failure (1)[C].

MEDICATION

ALERT
- Although many therapies in the acute phase do not improve long-term mortality, prompt and evidence-based treatment of ADHF can lead to improved patient centered outcomes including avoidance of mechanical ventilation, symptomatic and functional improvement, and decreased length of stay.
- Vital signs and physical exam should guide the initial triage and resuscitation of critically ill patients with suspected ADHF. Critically ill, hypertensive patients (typically systolic blood pressure (SBP) >180 mm Hg) in ADHF may benefit from afterload reduction with vasodilators such as nitrates, whereas those who are hypotensive or demonstrating signs of shock may benefit from the addition of vasopressors and/or ionotropes. In either case, respiratory support with the early use of noninvasive positive pressure ventilation (NIPPV) such as CPAP/bilevel positive airway pressure (BIPAP) has been associated with improved outcomes.

- Once stabilized, diuretics are given for symptom control in parallel to guideline-directed medical therapies (GDMTs) that have been shown to improve long-term survival. As tolerated, a full GDMT regimen includes four components: ACE inhibitors (also, ARBs/ARNIs), β-receptor blockers, mineralcorticoid receptor antagonists (MRA), and sodium-glucose cotransporter 2 inhibitors. ICD placement for select patient populations has also been associated with improved survival. Use of a new agent ivabradine has also been used in select patients but has not been shown to reduce cardiovascular mortality. It should be noted that there are no class IA drug recommendations for ADHF.
- In conjunction with GDMT, risk factor modification with antihypertensives, statins, and glycemic agents should be considered. Education must be provided—see "Heart Failure, Chronic."

First Line
- Vasodilators: Consider in ADHF with SBP >90 mm Hg. Patients with hypertensive ADHF should receive IV vasodilators as initial therapy to improve hemodynamics if no contraindications exist. Vasodilators lower ventricular filling pressure and systemic vascular resistance to indirectly improve cardiac function. Use in chronic HF is not effective.
  - IV nitroglycerin decreases preload and afterload by relaxing the smooth muscle in peripheral venous capacitance and arterial resistance vessels, respectively (IV 10 to 20 μg/min, increase up to 200 μg/min).
  - IV nitroprusside: Administer with caution, start with 0.3 μg/kg/min, and increase up to 5.0 μg/kg/min.
  - IV ACE inhibitors: Evidence is unclear, and recommendations vary. They are thought to work by reducing both preload and afterload.
- IV loop diuretics are recommended for all patients with ADHF and symptoms of fluid overload in hemodynamically stable patients (contraindicated if SBP <90 mm Hg, severe hyponatremia, acidosis); be cautious of electrolyte abnormalities and if kidney disease is present. Diuresis should be instituted early in ADHF, continuous infusion is no better than bolus, and high dose is not significantly better than low dose. Furosemide is the most commonly used diuretic. Torsemide has better pharmacokinetics and pharmacodynamics and should be considered first line.
  - Furosemide (Lasix): New-onset ADHF patients should get boluses of 20 to 40 mg IV. If on furosemide chronically, initial IV dose should be equal or exceed chronic oral daily dose (1.0 to 2.5 times home dose). Monitor for appropriate urine output.
  - Torsemide is more potent and more bioavailable than furosemide; initial doses of 10 to 20 mg IV, doubled every 2 hours if needed; IV bumetanide is an alternative.
  - When congestion fails to improve with initial diuretic therapy, consideration should be given to addition of second type of diuretic orally (metolazone or spironolactone) or intravenously (chlorothiazide).

- Patients with renal insufficiency or renal hypoperfusion may suffer from ineffective dieresis. If diuresis is refractory to single agent loop agents, either a thiazide or MRA can be considered. Common thiazides for this indication include hydrochlorothiazide 25 mg PO or metolazone 2.5 to 20.0 mg/day PO. MRAs include spironolactone or eplerenone (25 to 50 mg PO).
- NPPV with BIPAP or CPAP decreases symptom severity, rate of intubation, and early mortality in ADHF. NPPV improves hemodynamics by increasing intrathoracic pressure which serves in turn to decrease preload and has an indirect ionotropic effect. Cochrane Review shows that one death can be avoided for every 14 ADHF patients treated with NPPV and one death for every 9 ADHF patients treated with CPAP (level A evidence).

Second Line
- Tolvaptan for severe hypervolemic hyponatremia refractory to water restriction and medical therapy is being studied.
- Inotropes: reserved for patients with severe systolic dysfunction occurring most often in hypotensive ADHF.
  - Phosphodiesterase inhibitors (milrinone, enoximone) decrease pulmonary resistance; may be used for patients on β-blockers but may increase medium-term mortality in CAD patients; milrinone specifically produces ionotropic and vasodilatory effects without β-adrenergic stimulation of the heart.
  - Dobutamine infusion 2.5 to 20.0 μg/kg/min requires close BP monitoring; avoid in patients with cardiogenic shock or tachyarrhythmias. Low-dose dopamine infusion may be considered (3 to 5 μg/kg/min).
- Vasopressors: Consider in patients with cardiogenic shock despite treatment with another inotrope.
- Generally not recommended: nesiritide, ultrafiltration renal replacement therapy, levosimendan
- Extracorporeal membrane oxygenation (ECMO): venoarterial ECMO for the sickest cohort of ADHF patients; ECMO has traditionally been viewed as a bridge to transplant; however, there is a sizeable cohort of patients on long-term mechanical support.

ADDITIONAL THERAPIES
- Oxygen: Begin treatment early; ideally titrate to an arterial oxygen saturation >92% (88–92% if COPD). Treat anemia with transfusion: conservative trigger Hgb <8; target Hgb 10.
- See "Heart Failure, Chronic" for maintenance treatments.

SURGERY/OTHER PROCEDURES
Heart valve surgery if valvular disease is responsible, PCI/CABG for patients with CAD/MI if applicable; for more rare diagnosis, consider disease-specific approaches such as pericardiectomy for constrictive pericarditis.

ADMISSION, INPATIENT, AND NURSING CONSIDERATIONS
- Admission criteria considerations:
  - Evidence of severely decompensated HF: hypotension, worsening renal function, altered mental status, dyspnea at rest, concomitant arrhythmia, acute coronary syndrome, decreased functional status
  - Consider observation unit stay for stable patients with preexisting HF and the following: no acute interventions needed for comorbid condition, SBP >120 mm Hg, RR <32 breaths/min, BUN <40 mg/dL, creatinine <3.0 mg/dL, no evidence of ischemia or elevated troponins, and BNP <1,000, N-type pro-BNP <5,000, and the clinical impression that the patient could be discharged in the next 24 hours.
- 1.5 to 2.0 L/day fluid restriction may be useful to reduce congestive symptoms.
- Discharge criteria: improved symptoms, SBP normalized at 100 to 120 mm Hg, good urine output, serum sodium >135 mEq/L, HF outpatient education

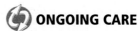 ONGOING CARE

FOLLOW-UP RECOMMENDATIONS
Patient Monitoring
Early follow-up and multidisciplinary care to reduce hospitalization and mortality

DIET
See "Heart Failure, Chronic" (1).

PATIENT EDUCATION
Monitoring and self-care; teach: medication, activity, daily weight (and how to adjust diuretic). See "Heart Failure, Chronic."

PROGNOSIS
See "Heart Failure, Chronic."

COMPLICATIONS
Arrhythmia, pulmonary edema, hyponatremia, death

REFERENCE
1. Heidenreich PA, Bozkurt B, Aguilar D, et al. 2022 AHA/ACC/HFSA guideline for the management of heart failure: a report of the American College of Cardiology/American Heat Association Joint Committee on clinical practice guidelines. *Circulation.* 2022;145(18):e895–e1032.

 CODES

ICD10
- I50.9 Heart failure, unspecified
- I50.21 Acute systolic (congestive) heart failure
- I50.31 Acute diastolic (congestive) heart failure

CLINICAL PEARLS
Look for an underlying cause of each episode of ADHF.

H

HEART FAILURE, CHRONIC

Afsha Rais Kaisani, MD • Tasaduq Hussain Mir, MD, FAAFP • Tamanna Vir, DO

 BASICS

DESCRIPTION

Heart failure (HF) results from inability of the heart to fill and/or pump blood sufficiently to meet tissue metabolic needs. Occurs when adequate cardiac output can be achieved only at the expense of elevated filling pressures. It is the principal complication of heart disease. For acute HF, see "Heart Failure, Acutely Decompensated." HF is the preferred term to congestive HF as patients are not always congested (fluid overloaded).

- Can involve the left heart, the right heart, or be biventricular. It is progressive and manifested by remodeling (altered heart anatomy). The AHA/ACC uses a staging system to delineate the one-way progression of HF: stage A: at risk for HF, no structural disease; stage B: structural disease, no HF symptoms; stage C: structural disease, HF symptoms; stage D: end-stage disease.
- The New York Heart Association (NYHA) classification is a subjective grading scale used for classifying a patient's functional status: NYHA I: asymptomatic; NYHA II: symptomatic with moderate exertion; NYHA III: symptomatic with mild exertion and may limit activities of daily living; NYHA IV: symptomatic at rest.

EPIDEMIOLOGY

HF accounts for close to 1 million hospitalizations a year, with 25% readmission in 30 days.

Incidence

In the United States, 550,000 new cases are diagnosed annually with >250,000 deaths/year. Incidence in the US is stable; however, incidence of HF with preserved ejection fraction (HFpEF) continues to rise accounting for 50% of HF cases (1).

Prevalence

Estimated 23 million individuals have HF worldwide. ~6.5 million people in the United States have HF; <1% in those age <50 years, increasing to 10% of those age >80 years. Primarily a disease of the elderly; 75% of hospital admissions for HF are for persons >65 years of age.

ETIOLOGY AND PATHOPHYSIOLOGY

- Two physiologic components explain the clinical findings of HF and result in four categories:
  - HF with reduced ejection fraction (HFrEF): an *inotropic* abnormality, often from myocardial infarction (MI) or dilated cardiomyopathy (CM), resulting in diminished systolic emptying (EF ≤40%)
  - HF with mildly reduced EF (HFmrEF): mild systolic dysfunction with EF of 41–49%, clinically behaves like HFpEF
  - HF with improved EF (HFimpEF): previously HFrEF, with improvement in systolic function now EF >40%
  - HFpEF: a *compliance* abnormality, often due to hypertensive CM, in which the ventricular relaxation is impaired (EF ≥50%)

- Most common etiologies: coronary artery disease (CAD)/MI and hypertension (HTN). Others include the following:
  - Myocarditis and CM: alcoholic, viral, drugs, muscular dystrophy, infiltrative (e.g., amyloidosis, sarcoidosis), postpartum, infectious (e.g., Chagas disease, HIV), hypertrophic CM (HCM), inherited familial dilated CM
  - Valvular and vascular abnormalities: valvular stenosis or regurgitation, rheumatic heart; renal artery stenosis, usually bilateral, may cause recurrent "flash" pulmonary edema.
  - Chronic lung disease and pulmonary HTN
  - Arrhythmias: atrial fibrillation (AFib), other tachyarrhythmias, high-grade heart block, frequent PVCs
  - Other: high-output states: hyperthyroidism, anemia; cardiac depressants (β-blocker overdose), stress induced; iatrogenic volume overload (extreme overload in patients with normal hearts and kidneys); idiopathic: 20–50% of idiopathic dilated CM are familial.

Genetics

Multiple genetic abnormalities responsible for a variety of phenotypes have been identified. Consider genetic screening for first-degree relatives of HCM and arrhythmogenic RV dysplasia.

RISK FACTORS

CAD/MI, HTN, valvular heart disease, diabetes, cardiotoxic medications, obesity, older age

GENERAL PREVENTION

Control HTN and other risk factors.

 DIAGNOSIS

The Framingham criteria can be used during initial evaluation of suspected HF. Two major criteria or one major and two minor criteria must be met. Major criteria include acute pulmonary edema, cardiomegaly, hepatojugular reflex, neck vein distension, PND/orthopnea, rales, or S3. Minor criteria include ankle edema, DOE, hepatomegaly, nocturnal cough, pleural effusion, or HR >120 beats/min. The H$_2$FPEF score may help determine the likelihood diagnosis of HFpEF (1).

HISTORY

- Dyspnea on exertion: *cardinal sign of left-sided HF*. Deteriorating exercise capacity: easy fatigued, general weakness; nocturnal nonproductive cough, orthopnea, and paroxysmal nocturnal dyspnea; sometimes frothy or pink sputum; wheezing, especially nocturnal, in absence of history of asthma or infection (cardiac asthma); Cheyne-Stokes respirations
- Anorexia and/or fullness or dull pain in right upper quadrant (hepatic congestion); nausea and poor appetite may indicate right-sided HF or advanced HF.

PHYSICAL EXAM

- Increased filling pressures: rales and sometimes wheezing, peripheral edema, S$_3$ gallop, hepatomegaly, jugular venous distention, hepatojugular reflux, ascites
- Remodeling: enlarged or displaced point of maximal impulse
- Poor cardiac output: hypotension, pulsus alternans, tachycardia, narrow pulse pressure, cool extremities, cyanosis

DIFFERENTIAL DIAGNOSIS

Simple dependent edema, pulmonary embolism, exertional asthma, cardiac ischemia, asthma/chronic obstructive pulmonary disorder, constrictive pericarditis, nephrotic syndrome, cirrhosis, venous occlusive disease

DIAGNOSTIC TESTS & INTERPRETATION

Diagnosis should be primarily clinical, with laboratory data and imaging as adjunctive and indicative of complications.

Initial Tests (lab, imaging)

- β-Type natriuretic peptide (BNP) and N-terminal pro-BNP (NT-proBNP): helpful in acute setting to differentiate the cause of dyspnea (<100 pg/mL essentially rules out HF, >800 pg/mL confirms HF). BNP level can help predict development of symptomatic HF in those with risk factors for developing HF or with structural heart disease but asymptomatic; elevated BNP: pulmonary embolism, renal failure, and acute coronary syndromes; sacubitril/valsartan can raise BNP levels, less impact on NT-proBNP levels; obesity may lower BNP levels; BNP-guided therapy in chronic HF is not well established; a predischarge BNP can predict risk of readmission and survival.
- Lab findings: respiratory alkalosis, azotemia, decreased erythrocyte sedimentation rate, proteinuria, elevated creatinine (cardiorenal syndrome), dilutional hyponatremia (poor prognosis), hyperbilirubinemia, electrolyte imbalance, thyroid disorders
- Chest x-ray (changes lag clinical symptoms): increased heart size, vascular redistribution (cephalization) with "butterfly" pattern of pulmonary edema, interstitial and alveolar edema, Kerley B lines, and pleural effusions
- Echocardiogram: evaluates heart function and anatomical abnormalities; critical for proper diagnosis and characterization of HF, RV function, diastolic dysfunction, ventricular size, wall thickness, and valvular abnormalities; repeat if change suspected in underlying cardiac status; usually transthoracic, but transesophageal is possible for evaluation.
- 12-lead ECG: Evaluate for underlying causes and create baseline for prognosis of HF.

Follow-Up Tests & Special Considerations

Monitor and manage comorbidities: HTN, diabetes, CKD, COPD, arrhythmia, asthma, hyperlipidemia, ischemic heart disease. Screen first-degree relatives of patients with genetic CM leading to HF.

Diagnostic Procedures/Other

- Nuclear imaging: estimates ventricular size, assess for ischemia or infarction, amyloidosis, and systolic function
- Cardiac MRI: suspicion of cardiac sarcoidosis, arrhythmogenic RV CM, acute myocarditis, amyloidosis, hemochromatosis
- Cardiac catheterization: important for excluding CAD as etiology considering risk factors
- Endomyocardial biopsy: for special circumstances (e.g., suspected giant cell myocarditis)

Test Interpretation

Echo LVEF: HFrEF <40%; HFmrEF 40–49%; HFpEF >50%

TREATMENT

GENERAL MEASURES
Focus on comorbidities and risk stratification, improving hemodynamics, nonpharmacological management, and blocking neurohormonal response to improve survival and symptoms (1).

MEDICATION
- Diuretics and nitrates are used for acute HF.
- Angiotensin-converting enzyme inhibitors (ACEi) and aldosterone antagonists (especially for HFrEF) can be added at any time.
- Start β-blocker once acute HF resolved.
- Sodium-glucose cotransporter-2 inhibitors (SGLT-2i): recommended for reducing hospitalization and cardiovascular (CV) death across all HF subgroups (2)[A]
- Avoid nonsteroidal anti-inflammatory drugs, which worsens HF; avoid diltiazem and verapamil with systolic dysfunction due to increase mortality and negative inotropic effects.

First Line
First line consist of ACEi/angiotensin receptor blockers (ARB), β-blocker, mineralocorticoid receptor antagonist (MRA), and SGLT-2i (2)[A]. Add diuretics as needed (3)[C].

- ACEi: decrease afterload, increase survival, improve symptoms and exercise capacity in all NYHA classifications; greatest benefit for patients with systolic dysfunction and post-MI. All ACEi are considered equally effective. Initiate at low doses, titrate as tolerated to targeting doses. Starting dose: captopril: 6.25 mg PO TID; enalapril: 2.5 mg PO BID; lisinopril: 2.5–5 mg daily; ramipril: 1.25 mg daily
- ARB: indicated if intolerant to ACEi. Avoid combination of ACEi and ARB. Starting dose: candesartan: 4–8 mg PO daily; losartan: 25–50 mg PO daily; valsartan: 20–40 mg PO BID
- β-Blockers: used in systolic or diastolic HF; initiate in hemodynamically stable/compensated patients at low dose, titrate upward slowly; decrease mortality in systolic HF; evidence for titration to heart rate (HR) rather than specific dose. Starting dose: carvedilol: 3.125 mg PO BID; metoprolol succinate ER: 12.5 mg/day PO; bisoprolol: 1.25 to 10 mg once daily
- Sacubitril/valsartan (Entresto): an angiotensin receptor and neprilysin inhibitor (ARNI) and ARB; reduces the risk of CV death and HF hospitalizations in patients with HFrEF. Recommended dose: 24/26 mg or 49/51 mg PO BID to a target of 97/103 PO BID. In patients with HFrEF and NYHA class II and III who tolerate an ACE-I or ARB with CrCl >30, replacement by an ARNI is recommended to reduce morbidity and mortality (NNT to prevent one CV death over 3.5 years: 31). ACEi should be discontinued at least 36 hours prior to starting ARNIs.
- SGLT-2i (dapagliflozin and empagliflozin): shows improvement in worsening HF or CV death in patients with EF≤40% and NYHA II/IV, irrespective of diabetes. May decrease overall death (NNT 50 to 60/year). Recommended dose: 10 mg PO daily (2)[A].
- Diuretics help manage volume overload/reduce preload.
  - Torsemide (Demadex): 10 to 200 mg/day PO likely more effective than furosemide; furosemide (Lasix): 40 to 120 mg/day PO; bumetanide (Bumex): 0.5 to 10 mg/day IV/PO
  - Metolazone (Zaroxolyn): 2.5 to 20 mg/day PO; hydrochlorothiazide: 12.5 to 100 mg/day PO; chlorothiazide (Diuril): 250 to 2,000 mg/day IV/PO

- MRA, also known as aldosterone antagonist: Spironolactone, eplerenone (improve mortality when added to standard therapy in NYHA class II to IV + EF <35%): spironolactone 12.5–25 mg/day PO; max 50 mg/day PO; eplerenone 25–50 mg/day; caution regarding hyperkalemia and chronic kidney disease (CKD). Eplerenone less likely to cause gynecomastia.
- Combination of isosorbide dinitrate and hydralazine (20 mg/37.5 mg PO TID): effective for improving survival and reducing hospitalizations in African Americans; can be used if the patient is unable to take an ACEi/ARB

Second Line
- Vericiguat, a guanylate cyclase simulator, shown to reduce the risk of death from CV causes or hospitalization for HF. Starting dose: 2.5 mg QD. FDA approved in patients with an EF ≤45%, recent HF hospitalization, or need for IV diuretics
- Ivabradine (Corlanor): considered in NYHA II and III HF, EF ≤35%, on maximally tolerated β-blockers with HR >70 beats/min to reduce hospitalization. Do not give to patients currently in AFib and discontinue if AFib develops.
- Digoxin: reduces symptoms, without positive effect on mortality; considered as an add-on strategy at low doses, in patients with preserved renal function (CrCl >50 mL/min).

ISSUES FOR REFERRAL
Cardiology referral: Patients who remain symptomatic despite maximal standard HF regimen.

ADDITIONAL THERAPIES
Device therapy including implantable cardioverter-defibrillators (ICDs) and cardiac resynchronization therapy (CRT) are shown to improve outcomes.

- CRT recommended: sinus rhythm with a QRS width ≥150 ms due to left bundle-branch block (LBBB), LVEF ≤35%, persistent mild-to-moderate HF despite guideline-directed medical therapy (GDMT), chronic RV pacing or bradyarrhythmias and anticipated need for pacemaker
- Consider CRT: LVEF ≤35%, sinus rhythm, QRS width >150 ms, non-LBBB pattern, NYHA II or ambulatory NYHA IV symptoms, and QRS width >150 ms due to LBBB pattern in ambulatory NYHA class IV patients
- ICD recommended: primary prevention in patients with nonischemic and ischemic CM, at least 40 days post-MI; LVEF ≤35%, NYHA class II or III HF and LVEF ≤30%, on optimal medical therapy and >1 year estimated survival; generally not indicated in end-stage HF

SURGERY/OTHER PROCEDURES
- Heart valve surgery for defective heart valve; mitral valve repair if mitral regurgitation is the primary issue and not functional
- Biventricular pacemaker: EF 35% or less with NYHA class III to IV and QRS >150 ms on ECG
- Cardiac transplantation and LV assist device (LVAD) implantation

ADMISSION, INPATIENT, AND NURSING CONSIDERATIONS
Admission: hemodynamic/respiratory compromise, mental status change, acute renal injury, volume overload, electrolyte abnormalities. Discharge: euvolemia, stable vitals, outpatient education performed.

 ## ONGOING CARE

FOLLOW-UP RECOMMENDATIONS
Close outpatient follow-up after hospitalization to decrease frequency of readmission

Patient Monitoring
Monitor for leg edema and sudden weight changes, which indicates fluid overloaded state.

DIET
Reduce sodium load; fluid restriction: 1,500 to 1,800 mL

PATIENT EDUCATION
Educate patient on management of weight gain or new edema. Recommend daily exercise, assist with smoking cessation.

PROGNOSIS
After diagnosis: 1-year survival ~75%, 5-year survival <50%, and 10-year survival <25%

COMPLICATIONS
Sudden death, progressive pump failure

REFERENCES
1. Kittleson MM, Panjrath GS, Amancherla K, et al. 2023 ACC Expert Consensus Decision Pathway on management of heart failure with preserved ejection fraction: a report of the American College of Cardiology Solution Set Oversight Committee. *J Am Coll Cardiol*. 2023;81(18):1835–1878.
2. Cardoso R, Graffunder FP, Ternes CMP, et al. SGLT2 inhibitors decrease cardiovascular death and heart failure hospitalizations in patients with heart failure: a systematic review and meta-analysis. *EClinicalMedicine*. 2021;36:100933.
3. Heidenreich PA, Bozkurt B, Aguilar D, et al. 2022 AHA/ACC/HFSA guideline for the management of heart failure: a report of the American College of Cardiology/American Heart Association Joint Committee on Clinical Practice Guidelines. *J Am Coll Cardiol*. 2022;79(17):e263–e421.

 ## SEE ALSO
Algorithm: Congestive Heart Failure: Differential Diagnosis

 ## CODES

ICD10
- I50.9 Heart failure, unspecified
- I50.1 Left ventricular failure
- I50.22 Chronic systolic (congestive) heart failure

CLINICAL PEARLS
- Core medications for management: β-blockers, ACEi/ARB, and aldosterone antagonists
- Have patients weigh themselves and report weight gains of >2 lb in a day or 5 lb above dry weight.

H

HEAT ILLNESS: HEAT EXHAUSTION AND HEAT STROKE

Sean C. Robinson, MD, CAQSM • Sherilyn DeStefano, MD

BASICS

DESCRIPTION
- A continuum of increasingly severe illness caused by dehydration, electrolyte losses, and failure of thermoregulatory mechanisms when exposed to elevated environmental temperatures
  - Heat exhaustion is a mild to moderate form of heat illness displaying dehydration-type symptoms with a normal to elevated temperature (1).
  - Heat stroke is characterized by an elevated core temperature >104°F with central nervous system (CNS) abnormalities and is a true medical emergency (1),(2).
- Can be exertional (related to activity) or non-exertional
- System(s) affected: endocrine/metabolic, nervous, hepatic, hematologic
- Synonym(s): heat illness; heat injury; hyperthermia; heat collapse; heat prostration

Geriatric Considerations
Elderly persons are more susceptible.

Pediatric Considerations
Children are more susceptible.

Pregnancy Considerations
Pregnant women may be more susceptible to volume depletion with heat stress.

EPIDEMIOLOGY
- Predominant age: more likely in children or elderly
- Predominant sex: male = female

Incidence
- Depends on intensity of heat; estimate of 20/100,000 persons per season
- Concern for increasing incidence because ambient environmental temperatures continue to rise

Prevalence
- Depends on predisposing conditions in combination with environmental factors
- Roughly 600 deaths per year in the United States

ETIOLOGY AND PATHOPHYSIOLOGY
- Excess heat has direct cellular toxicity. Excess heat also leads to an imbalance between inflammatory and anti-inflammatory cytokines, vascular endothelial damage, and end-organ dysfunction.
- Interplay between failure of heat-dissipating mechanisms, an overwhelming heat stress, and an exaggerated acute-phase inflammatory response

RISK FACTORS
- Poor acclimatization to heat
- Poor physical conditioning
- Salt or water depletion
- Obesity
- Acute febrile or GI illnesses
- Chronic illnesses: uncontrolled diabetes mellitus, hypertension, cardiac disease
- Alcohol and other substance abuse
- High heat and humidity, poor environmental air circulation
- Heavy, restrictive clothing
- Nutritional supplements (e.g., ephedra) (2)
- Medications (α-adrenergics, anticholinergics, antihistamines, antipsychotics, benzodiazepines, β-blockers, calcium channel blockers, clopidogrel, diuretics, laxatives, neuroleptics, phenothiazines, thyroid agonists, tricyclic antidepressants) (1)

GENERAL PREVENTION
- The most important factor in preventing heat illness is prevention. Activity modification and adequate fluid replacement are key preventive measures.
- Allow acclimatization through proper conditioning and activity modification.
- Dress appropriately with loose-fitting, open-weaved, light-colored clothing.
- Consume a proper volume of fluids, particularly during physical activity in hot environments.
- Never leave children (or pets) unattended in cars during hot weather.
- Try to gain access to air-conditioned environments during hot weather.

DIAGNOSIS

- Heat exhaustion: Symptoms are milder than in heat stroke, and there are no CNS derangements:
  - Fatigue, lethargy, weakness, dizziness, nausea, vomiting, myalgias, headache, profuse sweating, tachycardia, hypotension, thirst, hyperventilation
  - Core temperature usually elevated but can be normal; if elevated, <104°F (40°C)
- Heat stroke: marked by mental status changes and elevated core temperature
  - *Classic (nonexertional)*: caused by environmental exposure, primarily in elderly or chronically ill patients, and may develop gradually over days
    - Delirium
    - Confusion
    - Coma
    - Core temperature >104°F (>40°C)
    - Hot, flushed, dry skin

- *Exertional*: typically younger, active patients; rapid onset
  - Exhaustion
  - Confusion, disorientation
  - Delirium
  - Coma
  - Hot, flushed skin, typically with sweating
  - Core temperature >104°F (>40°C) (1),(2)

HISTORY
- Heat cramps: sweating; muscle cramps/spasms
- Heat exhaustion: sweating; fatigue, light-headedness/dizziness; cramping; nausea, vomiting; headache
- Heat stroke: altered mental status

PHYSICAL EXAM
- Rectal temperature (*Don't rely on oral temperature.*)
- Heat exhaustion: tachycardia; cool/clammy skin
- Heat stroke: rectal (core temperature) elevated (>103°F); hot/dry skin (compensatory sweating impaired)

DIFFERENTIAL DIAGNOSIS
- Febrile illnesses, sepsis
- Drug-induced fluid loss
- Cardiac arrhythmia or infarction
- Acute cocaine intoxication
- Neuroleptic malignant syndrome
- Malignant hyperthermia (an autosomally inherited disorder of skeletal and cardiac muscle in which patients have abnormal muscle metabolism on exposure to halothane or skeletal muscle reactants)

DIAGNOSTIC TESTS & INTERPRETATION
Detect end-organ damage.

Initial Tests (lab, imaging)
- Creatinine, BUN, electrolytes (sodium in particular)
- Liver enzymes, muscle enzymes (creatine phosphokinase)
- CBC—hemoconcentration
- Urinalysis: increased urine specific gravity
- Drugs that may alter lab results: diuretics

TREATMENT

GENERAL MEASURES
- For heat stroke: immediate body immersion in ice water to cool core temperature; monitor hemodynamics and airway status (1).
- Careful fluid and electrolyte replacement with normal saline; avoid hypotonic fluids. Follow serum sodium (1),(2)[C].

- Consider CVP monitoring.
- For heat exhaustion, consider:
  - Evaporative cooling: spraying water over the patient and using fans to facilitate evaporative and convective heat loss (1)
  - Immerse hands and forearms in cold water.
  - Ice or cold packs on the neck, groin, and axillae (1),(2)[C]
- No clear superiority of any one method for heat exhaustion (1)

MEDICATION

First Line
- No medications are required in the initial management. Use isotonic saline solution to rehydrate.
- Do not use antipyretics to lower core temperature in heat illness.

Second Line
- For severely ill, consider immunomodulators such as corticosteroids (patients in ICU setting).
- Iced gastric, bladder, or peritoneal lavage
- If disseminated intravascular coagulation (DIC), consider appropriate replacement therapy.

ADMISSION, INPATIENT, AND NURSING CONSIDERATIONS
- *Cool patient immediately* (prior to transport even) if heat stroke is suspected or once diagnosed.
- Rapid cooling: remove clothing, wet patient down, and apply ice packs.
- Emergency treatment; best in a hospital setting

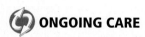 ONGOING CARE

FOLLOW-UP RECOMMENDATIONS
Rest with legs elevated.

Patient Monitoring
- Rectal temperature monitoring: Cooling may be discontinued when the core temperature drops to 102°F (38.9°C) and stabilizes.
- Heat stroke patients may require airway management, hemodynamic monitoring, and careful fluid and electrolyte administration and monitoring.
- Consider CVP monitoring.

DIET
- Cool or cold clear liquids only (noncarbonated)
- Avoid caffeine.
- Unrestricted sodium

PATIENT EDUCATION
- Proper hydration is the key to prevention.
- Proper conditioning and acclimatization
- Recognize signs and symptoms of heat stress—fatigue and headache.
- Skin exposure facilitates heat loss in hot, humid conditions (use proper sun protection).

PROGNOSIS
- If mental function is not altered and serum chemistries are normal, the prognosis is good and recovery within 24 to 48 hours is typical.
- The mortality rate for heat stroke (10–80%) is directly related to the duration and intensity of hyperthermia as well as to the speed and effectiveness of diagnosis and treatment.
- The priority in heat-related illness is early recognition and intervention. The faster the patient is cooled to <40°C, the lower the patient mortality (3).

COMPLICATIONS
- May involve failure of any major organ system
- Cardiac arrhythmias or infarction
- Pulmonary edema, acute respiratory distress syndrome
- Coma, seizures
- Acute renal failure
- Rhabdomyolysis
- DIC
- Hepatocellular necrosis

REFERENCES

1. Roberts WO, Armstrong LE, Sawka MN, et al. ACSM expert consensus statement on exertional heat illness: recognition, management, and return to activity. *Curr Sports Med Rep*. 2021;20(9):470–484.
2. Gauer R, Meyers BK. Heat-related illnesses. *Am Fam Physician*. 2019;99(8):482–489.
3. Bouchama A, Abuyassin B, Lehe C, et al. Classic and exertional heatstroke. *Nat Rev Dis Primers*. 2022;8(1):8.

ADDITIONAL READING

- Armstrong LE, Casa DJ, Millard-Stafford M, et al; for American College of Sports Medicine. American College of Sports Medicine position stand. Exertional heat illness during training and competition. *Med Sci Sports Exerc*. 2007;39(3):556–572.
- Atha WF. Heat-related illness. *Emerg Med Clin North Am*. 2013;31(4):1097–1108.
- O'Connor FG. Sports medicine: exertional heat illness. *FP Essent*. 2019;482:15–19.

 CODES

ICD10
- T67.5XXA Heat exhaustion, unspecified, initial encounter
- T67.0XXA Heatstroke and sunstroke, initial encounter
- T67.3XXA Heat exhaustion, anhydrotic, initial encounter

CLINICAL PEARLS

- Exertional heat stroke is a life-threatening medical emergency that requires immediate whole body cooling (cold/ice water immersion preferred).
- The diagnosis of heat stroke includes an elevated core temperature and signs of CNS dysfunction (e.g., mental status changes, irritability, ataxia, confusion, seizures, coma).
- Start the cooling process immediately when heat exhaustion is recognized, beginning with wetting the skin with a cool mist and giving oral rehydration solutions if the patient is alert and oriented.
- If in the field (e.g., sporting events, wilderness), cooling should begin immediately (prior to transport if possible).
- Do not rely on oral temperature—a rectal temperature is always preferred.

H

HEMATURIA

Sahil Mullick, MD • Sreelakshmi Surendran Pillai, MD

BASICS

DESCRIPTION
Gross (visible) or microscopic (nonvisible) blood in urine, either symptomatic or asymptomatic

EPIDEMIOLOGY
Prevalence
Children: gross: 0.13%; asymptomatic microscopic hematuria (AMH): 0.4–4.1%; adults: AMH: 0.9–17%

ETIOLOGY AND PATHOPHYSIOLOGY
- Trauma
  - Exercise-induced (resolves within 24 hours of ceasing activity)
  - Abdominal trauma or pelvic fracture with renal, bladder, or ureteral injury
  - Iatrogenic from abdominal or pelvic surgery, indwelling catheters, or foreign body
  - Physical/sexual abuse
- Neoplasms
  - Urologic malignancies or benign tumors
  - Endometriosis of the urinary tract (suspect in females with cyclic hematuria)
- Inflammatory/infectious causes
  - UTI: most common cause of hematuria in adults
  - Renal diseases: radiation nephritis and cystitis, acute/chronic tubulointerstitial nephritis (due to drugs, infections, systemic disease)
  - Glomerular disease
    - Goodpasture syndrome (antiglomerular basement membrane disease; autoimmune; associated pulmonary hemorrhage)
    - IgA nephropathy
    - Lupus nephritis
    - Henoch-Schönlein purpura
    - Membranoproliferative, poststreptococcal, or rapidly progressive glomerulonephritis (GN)
    - Wegener granulomatosis
  - Endocarditis/visceral abscesses
  - Infections: schistosomiasis, TB, syphilis
- Metabolic causes
  - Stones (85% have hematuria.)
    - Hypercalciuria: a common cause of gross and microscopic hematuria in children
    - Hyperuricosuria
    - Drugs that cause calculi such as acyclovir
- Congenital/familial causes
  - Cystic disease: polycystic kidney disease, solitary renal cyst
  - Benign familial hematuria or thin basement membrane nephropathy (autosomal dominant)
  - Alport syndrome (X-linked in 80%; hematuria, proteinuria, hearing loss, corneal abnormalities)
  - Fabry disease (X-linked recessive inborn error of metabolism; vascular kidney disease)
  - Nail–patella syndrome (autosomal dominant; nail and patella hypoplasia; hematuria in 33%)
  - Renal tubular acidosis type 1 (autosomal dominant or autoimmune)
- Hematologic causes
  - Bleeding dyscrasias (e.g., hemophilia)
  - Sickle cell anemia/trait (renal papillary necrosis)

- Vascular causes
  - Hemangioma
  - Arteriovenous malformations (rare)
  - Nutcracker syndrome: compression of left renal vein, renal parenchymal congestion
  - Renal artery/vein thrombosis
  - Arterial emboli to kidney
- Chemical causes
  - Aminoglycosides, cyclosporine, analgesics, oral contraceptives, Chinese herbs, cyclophosphamide, anticoagulants warfarin ([Coumadin], apixaban [Eliquis], rivaroxaban [Xarelto]), sulfa drugs, penicillins
- Obstruction
  - Strictures or posterior urethral valves
  - Hydronephrosis from any cause
  - Benign prostatic hyperplasia: Rule out other causes of hematuria.
- Other causes: loin pain hematuria (most often in young women on oral contraceptives)

RISK FACTORS
- Smoking
- Occupational exposures (dyes, rubber, or tire manufacturing, petrochemicals)
- Medications (e.g., cyclophosphamide, pioglitazone therapy >1 year)
- Pelvic radiation
- Chronic infection, especially with calculi
- Recent upper respiratory tract infection
- Positive family history of stones, GN, or cancer
- Chronic indwelling foreign body

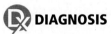

DIAGNOSIS

HISTORY
Considerations
- Burning, urgency, frequency: UTI
- Dark cola-colored urine: glomerular origin
- Clots: extraglomerular bleeding
- Arthritis/arthralgias/rash: lupus, vasculitis, Henoch-Schönlein purpura
- Flank pain: stones, infarction, pyelonephritis
- Recent upper respiratory infection (URI): poststreptococcal GN, membranoproliferative GN
- Concurrent URI: IgA nephropathy
- Excessive vitamin use: stones
- Marathon runner: traumatic, rhabdomyolysis
- Travel: schistosomiasis, TB
- Painless hematuria, weight loss: malignancy
- Family history: Alport disease (hereditary nephritis), sickle cell, polycystic, IgA nephropathy, thin basement membrane disease, von Willebrand disease
- Any episode of visible hematuria (VH) in the urine, even if transient, is associated with an OR of 7.2 for urologic cancers.

PHYSICAL EXAM
Considerations
- Elevated BP, edema, and weight gain: glomerular disease
- Fever: infection
- Palpable kidney: neoplasm, polycystic
- Genitalia: Look for meatal erosion and lesions.

DIFFERENTIAL DIAGNOSIS
Menstrual/vaginal bleeding, rectal bleeding; drugs (rifampin and phenazopyridine) can turn urine into orange or red, mistaking for hematuria.

DIAGNOSTIC TESTS & INTERPRETATION
A hematuria risk index may assist in stratifying patients at risk for urothelial malignancies requiring intensive testing. High-risk indicators are VH, age >50 years, male gender, family history of urologic malignancies, and smoking.

Initial Tests (lab, imaging)
- If acute cystitis/UTI is ruled out, guidelines recommend evaluating AMH with upper urinary tract imaging and cystoscopy; none recommend cytology or urine markers for initial AMH evaluation (1)[C]
- Urine dipstick (sensitivity of 91–100% and specificity of 65–99%)
  - False negatives are rare, but they can be caused by high-dose vitamin C.
  - False positives: oxidizers used to cleanse the perineum, alkaline urine (>9), semen; free hemoglobin (hemolysis) and myoglobin (rhabdomyolysis)
  - Heme-negative red urine: Food dyes, beets, blackberries, rhubarb, porphyria, rifampin, phenytoin, and phenazopyridine may discolor the dipstick, making interpretation difficult.
  - Any proteinuria >2+ raises concern for glomerular disease.
- Microscopic urinalysis should always be done to confirm dipstick findings and to quantify RBCs (1)[C].
  - American Urological Association (AUA) defines clinically significant microscopic hematuria as ≥3 RBCs/HPF on a properly collected urinary specimen when there is not an obvious benign cause (1).
  - Positive dipstick but a negative microscopic exam should be followed by three repeat tests. If anyone is positive, proceed with a workup (1).
  - Exclude factitious or nonurinary causes, such as menstruation, mild trauma, exercise, poor collection technique, or chemical/drug causes, through cessation of activity/cause and a repeat urinalysis (1)[C].
  - RBC casts are pathognomonic for glomerular origin; dysmorphic cells are suggestive.
- Renal function tests (eGFR, BUN, creatinine), albumin, and electrolytes to differentiate intrinsic renal disease and to evaluate for risks for imaging with contrast (1)[C]
  - Indicators of renal disease are significant (>500 mg/day) proteinuria, red cell casts, dysmorphic RBCs, increased creatinine, and albumin:creatinine ratio ≥30 mg/mmol (1).
- Urine culture if suspected infection/pyuria
- Multidetector CT urography (MDCTU); sensitivity of 95% and specificity of 92%
  - The initial imaging of choice in nonpregnant adults without contraindications to contrast or radiation with unexplained hematuria per AUA and the American College of Radiology (ACR) (1)
  - Normal does not obviate the need for cystoscopy, particularly in high-risk patients
  - Presence of calculi on noncontrast does not exclude another diagnosis or need for contrast phase.

- CT
  - Noncontrast CT is the preferred first line in adult patients with acute flank pain suspicious of stones.
  - Use unenhanced helical CT for suspected stone disease in children if US is negative.
  - Perform CT abdomen and pelvis with contrast in children with traumatic hematuria.
- Renal and bladder US (RBUS)
  - Best for differentiating cystic from solid masses
  - Sensitive for hydronephrosis; point of care US may help avoid CT with suspected stones.
  - No radiation or iodinated contrast exposure and cost-efficient
  - US can be used as first line in patients with contraindications to CTU or at low risk of malignancy.
  - Sensitivity and negative predictive value (NPV): for renal cancer = 85.7% and 99.9%, respectively; for upper tract urothelial cancer = 14.3% and 99.7%, respectively
  - Poor sensitivity for renal masses <3 cm
  - The main disadvantage is inability to fully evaluate the urothelium for transitional cell cancer.
- Magnetic resonance urography (MRU)
  - High sensitivity/specificity for renal parenchyma; less useful for collecting system or stones
  - Can be used in patients with contraindications to MDCTU
- MRI
  - Similar to CT in sensitivity for renal masses
  - No radiation exposure, least cost-efficient
  - Limited ability to reliably detect urinary tract calcifications
  - Can be combined with retrograde pyelogram (RPG) for patients who cannot tolerate MDCTU or MRU

Follow-Up Tests & Special Considerations
- Other tests depend on suspected etiology: STD testing, antineutrophil cytoplasmic antibody (ANCA), C3, C4, antistreptolysin O (ASO) titer, hemoglobin electrophoresis, PT/INR for patients on warfarin.
- Consider genetic testing in patients suspected of having familial hematuria.
- Voided urine cytology (sensitivity of 43.5%, specificity of 95.7%, positive predictive value of 47.6%, negative predictive value of 94.9%)
  - Not recommended for routine evaluation of AMH; consider in those with significant risk factors for urinary malignancy (1).
- Insufficient evidence to recommend routine use of urinary tumor markers
- Malignancies are more likely in patients with VH than in patients with nonvisible hematuria (13.8% vs. 3.1%).
- Summary positive predictive value of VH for bladder/renal cancer in age >15 years is 5.1%; risk increases with age and male gender.
- VCUG in children with frequent UTIs

Diagnostic Procedures/Other
- Flexible cystoscopy (sensitivity of 62% and specificity of 43–98%)
  - Best for evaluation of bladder, especially small urothelial lesions; NPV for bladder tumors is 99%.
  - AUA recommends all patients with hematuria who are ≥35 years of age and all patients with risk factors for bladder cancer regardless of age to receive cystoscopy in addition to imaging (1).

- Renal biopsy
  - Not routine but may be necessary to diagnose GN or in the face of increasing renal insufficiency
- RPG
  - Reserved when MDCTU equivocal or in addition to US or noncontrast studies in patients who are contraindicated for contrast or MRI
  - Sensitive for small lesions of supravesicular collecting system
  - Requires cystoscopy
- Ureteroscopy/pyeloscopy
  - For visualization of suspected supravesical collecting system lesions
  - Biopsy, excision, fulguration, or extraction of lesions/stones possible
  - Requires anesthesia and cystoscopy
  - Risk of injury to collecting system

Pregnancy Considerations
US is the initial imaging choice for pregnant patients. MRU or RPG combined with either MRI or US are alternatives.

Pediatric Considerations
- Consider UTI, GN, Wilms tumor, child abuse, hyperuricemia, hypercalciuria, and familial causes.
- The AAP recommends workup for hematuria should not be initiated for hematuria in a pediatric patient before repeating a dipstick urinalysis. In patients with persistent ASM, the most common diagnoses on renal biopsy are hypercalciuria (30–35%), hyperuricemia (5–20%), and glomerulonephritides, such as IgAN and thin basement membrane disease.
- Gross or symptomatic hematuria needs a full workup.
  - If eumorphic RBCs, consider UTI; hypercalciuria; familial causes; or masses, stones, or dx cysts. Obtain a family history, urine culture, US, and urinary Ca:Cr ratio. Urine Ca:Cr ratio >0.2 (mg/mg) is suggestive of hypercalciuria in children >6 years of age.
  - If dysmorphic RBCs, with proteinuria, elevated BP, edema, or a positive family history, consider renal consult.
- Renal US identifies the most congenital and malignant conditions; CT is reserved for cases of suspected trauma (with contrast) or stones (without contrast).

 TREATMENT

MEDICATION
First Line
Treatment of the underlying cause of hematuria; discontinue drugs that cause hematuria.

ISSUES FOR REFERRAL
- Nephrology referral for proteinuria, red cell casts, elevated serum creatinine, and albumin:creatinine ratio ≥30 mg/mmol
- Urology referral for stones, vascular/anatomic anomalies, or nutcracker syndrome

ADDITIONAL THERAPIES
Surgery for removal of endometriosis if causing hematuria with symptoms

 ONGOING CARE

Close follow-up by specialists indicated based on the underlying cause

FOLLOW-UP RECOMMENDATIONS
May repeat urinalysis in 12 months if initial testing is negative (2); if repeat is positive, then may need further evaluation.

Patient Monitoring
Some experts still recommend periodic urinalysis; recent literature suggests that after thorough initial negative investigations (imaging, cystoscopy), no follow-up is indicated for the patient with AMH unless symptoms or frank hematuria develop. AUA recommends annual urinalyses in these patients, until two consecutive tests are negative and the consideration for a repeat workup at 3 to 5 years if hematuria is persistent (1).

DIET
Increased fluids for stones or clots

PROGNOSIS
- Excellent for common causes of hematuria
- Poorer for malignant tumors and certain types of nephritis
- Persistent AMH is associated with an increased risk of end-stage renal disease in patients aged 16 to 25 years.

REFERENCES
1. Linder BJ, Bass EJ, Mostafid H, et al. Guideline of guidelines: asymptomatic microscopic haematuria. *BJU Int*. 2018;121(2):176–183.
2. Barocas DA, Boorjian SA, Alvarez RD, et al. Microhematuria: AUA/SUFU guideline. *J Urol*. 2020;204(4):778–786.

 SEE ALSO

Algorithm: Hematuria

 CODES

ICD10
- R31.9 Hematuria, unspecified
- R31.1 Benign essential microscopic hematuria
- R31.0 Gross hematuria

CLINICAL PEARLS
- Screening asymptomatic patients for microscopic hematuria is an "I" recommendation from the USPSTF.
- AMH and hematuria persisting after treatment of UTIs must be evaluated.
- Patients with bladder cancer can have intermittent microscopic hematuria; a thorough evaluation in high-risk patients is needed after just one episode.
- In patients with AMH, a history of anticoagulant use does not preclude the need for an evaluation, and any new hematuria in patients on anticoagulants requires full evaluation including imaging and cystoscopy (1)[C].
- Signs of underlying renal disease indicate the need for a nephrologic workup, but a urologic evaluation is still needed in the presence of persistent hematuria.

H

HEMOCHROMATOSIS

Alethea Y. Turner, DO, FAAFP • Leslie Shelton, DO

 BASICS

DESCRIPTION

Hereditary hemochromatosis (HH) is a common genetic disease with autosomal recessive inheritance that results in iron overload and subsequent deposition into various tissues.

- HH includes at least four types of iron overload conditions, which involve gene mutations that alter iron metabolism.
- There is no mechanism to excrete excess iron, so the surplus is stored in tissue, including the liver, pancreas, and heart, eventually resulting in severe damage to the affected organ(s).
- Patients are often asymptomatic, but late effects may include diabetes, liver cirrhosis, hypermelanotic pigmentation of the skin, cardiac issues, and other complications.
- Synonym(s): bronze diabetes; Troisier-Hanot-Chauffard syndrome

EPIDEMIOLOGY

Incidence

- Predominant age: Metabolic abnormality is congenital, but symptoms typically present between the 3rd and 5th decades for HH types 1, 3, and 4; type 2 juvenile hemochromatosis typically presents between the 1st and 3rd decades of life, and neonatal presentation is exceedingly rare.
- Predominant sex: Gene frequency is equal between male and female, although clinical signs are more frequent in men.

Prevalence

- Prevalence in the United States for carrying an *HFE* gene mutation (type 1 HH) is 5.4% for the *C282Y* gene and 13.5% for the *H63D* gene; prevalence for homozygosity is 0.3% for *C282Y* and 1.9% for *H63D* (1).
- Type 1 accounts for >90% of HH cases in the United States and primarily occurs in people of northern European descent; ~1 in 200 white adults in the United States are *C282Y* homozygous (1).

Pediatric Considerations

Juvenile (type 2) HHC is rare but can present in young patients (between 1st and 3rd decades of life) with hypogonadism and cardiomyopathy.

ETIOLOGY AND PATHOPHYSIOLOGY

- HH type 1 is caused by mutations in the *HFE* gene (most frequently *C282Y* and/or *H63D*), and it is the most common form of HH overall. Other variations include type 2 which is caused by mutations in either the *HJV* or *HAMP* gene, type 3 by mutations in the *TFR2* gene, and type 4 by mutations in the *SLC11A3* gene.
- Types 1 to 3 involve a deficiency in an iron-regulating hormone named hepcidin, which causes increased intestinal absorption of iron through excessive expression of ferroportin (a transmembrane protein that transports iron out of the cell and into the bloodstream).

- Type 4 is caused by an insensitivity of ferroportin to hepcidin (4a) or an inactivity of ferroportin itself (4b); the latter leads to iron accumulation within mesenchymal tissue.
- Other rare types of HH exist as a result of different gene mutations.
- Increased plasma iron and transferrin saturation (TS) leads to elevated levels of unbound iron, which are then absorbed into various tissue, eventually causing organ dysfunction.

Genetics

- Genetically heterogeneous disorder of iron overload; types 1, 2, and 3 are autosomal recessive; type 4 is autosomal dominant.
- Biochemical penetrance is incomplete and expressivity is variable; in type 1 HH, the penetrance for developing clinically significant iron overload is rare, but approximately 75% of men with type 1 HH and 50% of women will have an increase in TS (with or without elevated serum ferritin [SF]) (2).
- Factors contributing to variable expressivity include different mutations in the same gene, mitigating or exacerbating genes, and environmental factors.

RISK FACTORS

- Family history
- White men between the ages of 30 and 50 years (particularly for HFE-related HH)
- Loss of blood, such as that which occurs during menstruation and pregnancy, delays the onset of symptoms in women
- Alcohol consumption because it increases the absorption of iron and synergistically damages the liver along with the oxidative effects of iron

GENERAL PREVENTION

- First-degree relatives of those with HH should be screened; typically, with fasting TS and ferritin levels.
- Children of a diagnosed parent, HFE testing of the other parent is recommended with no further testing required if the results are normal.

ALERT

Screening of the general population is *not* recommended because only a small subset of patients with HH will develop symptoms or advanced disease (2).

DIAGNOSIS

HISTORY

- Fatigue, weakness
- Arthralgias
- Abdominal pain
- Loss of libido or impotency
- Symptoms of diabetes
- Skin pigmentation or blistering

PHYSICAL EXAM

- Hepatomegaly and/or splenomegaly
- Increased skin pigmentation
- Hepatic tenderness and/or jaundice
- Peripheral edema and/or ascites
- Gynecomastia
- Testicular atrophy

DIFFERENTIAL DIAGNOSIS

- Inflammatory syndromes
- Various causes of hepatitis
- Biliary or alcoholic cirrhosis
- Repeated transfusions
- Sideroblastic anemia
- β-Thalassemia major

DIAGNOSTIC TESTS & INTERPRETATION

Initial Tests (lab, imaging)

There is currently no evidence to support a concrete relationship between symptoms and the degree of iron overload (1).

- SF: ≥300 μg/L for men and postmenopausal women and 200 μg/L for premenopausal women (2); may be elevated for a number of other reasons including but not limited to inflammation (consider checking inflammatory markers); if elevated with suspicion of hemochromatosis, obtain fasting TS.
- Fasting TS (serum iron concentration ÷ total iron-binding capacity × 100) is the earliest biochemical marker to be increased in HH: ≥45% is suspicious for HH but warrants further evaluation because it can be elevated in other disease processes including chronic anemias.
- Confirmatory testing should be done through HFE gene mutation analysis.

Follow-Up Tests & Special Considerations

- After the diagnosis is established, check ALT, AST, hematocrit, and hemoglobin to determine the need for phlebotomy.
- Assess for complications of HH and order appropriate testing when necessary.
- Consider screening for osteoporosis in patients >50 years with additional risk factors (i.e., alcohol or tobacco use).
- Test for other causes of hepatitis if transaminitis exists to rule out concomitant disease.
- Consider monitoring for liver lesions with an abdominal ultrasound if severe liver fibrosis or cirrhosis is present.

Diagnostic Procedures/Other

- Hepatic MRI should be done to measure liver iron content if hepatomegaly is present, SF is >1,000 μg/L, and/or ALT/AST are elevated.
- Consider liver biopsy only if there is a need to determine the degree of liver fibrosis for staging or to confirm the etiology of liver damage (2).

Test Interpretation
- Hepatic MRI without contrast (T2-weighted imaging) can effectively rule out iron overload within the liver (negative predictive value 0.88) and diagnose it as well but with slightly less accuracy (positive predictive value 0.74) (2)[B].
- Liver biopsy will reveal increased hepatic parenchymal iron stores and evidence of any fibrosis or cirrhosis.

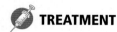 ## TREATMENT

GENERAL MEASURES
Due to a lack of evidence-based data, there is debate regarding when treatment should be initiated (particularly in asymptomatic patients) as well as what the target serum indices and frequency of phlebotomy should be. American and European liver associations recommend initiating treatment when SF is above the normal limit (see "Initial Tests [lab, imaging]"). The American College of Gastroenterology further outlines their recommendations regarding initiation of treatment based on whether the patient is C282Y homozygote or C282Y/H63D heterozygote (2). If HH diagnosis is confirmed, there is no liver involvement, SF remains normal, and the patient is asymptomatic, it is reasonable to monitor SF at least annually.

- Phlebotomy (~500 mL per session) is the mainstay of therapy and is performed once or twice weekly in the initial treatment phase and may take up to 2 to 3 years to deplete iron stores (1),(2).
- When the patient finally becomes iron deficient, a lifelong maintenance program of ~2 to 6 phlebotomies a year is required to keep iron storage normal or below normal (2).
- Erythrocytapheresis (~600 mL per session) is an alternative to phlebotomy and only removes red cells from the blood; it is expensive and not widely available. However, there is limited evidence that erythrocytapheresis in the maintenance phase of treatment can reduce the frequency of treatments (1.9 vs 3.3 treatments annually when compared to phlebotomy) (2)[B].
- Adverse effects of phlebotomy and erythrocytapheresis are mild and are typically secondary to hypovolemia, so prehydration is recommended.

MEDICATION
- If phlebotomy is not feasible or if it is contraindicated (severe anemia or heart failure), a second-tier option is chelation therapy with parenteral deferoxamine (monitor patients for auditory or visual changes), oral deferasirox (contraindicated in renal or hepatic failure, and can increase risk of gastrointestinal hemorrhage in some patients) or oral deferiprone (can cause agranulocytosis and neutropenia); of these options, deferoxamine is preferred in most patients (2)[C].
- Proton pump inhibitor (PPI) use for a minimum of 1 year may reduce the absorption of iron in patients with HH and decrease the overall number of phlebotomies needed. Consider adding a PPI as adjunct therapy to phlebotomy.
- Testosterone replacement in men with HH may improve symptoms of erectile dysfunction and decreased libido, but risks of hepatotoxicity must be considered.

- Hepatitis A and B immunizations should be provided if there is no evidence of previous exposure.
- Pneumococcal vaccination should be given if cirrhosis is present.

ALERT
Caution is advised for prescribing androgens in the setting of hypogonadism secondary to risk of hepatotoxicity.

ISSUES FOR REFERRAL
Refer to a gastroenterologist if liver biopsy is indicated and for the management of concomitant liver disease.

 ## ONGOING CARE

FOLLOW-UP RECOMMENDATIONS
Patient Monitoring
- Measure hemoglobin and hematocrit before each phlebotomy; skip phlebotomy if hemoglobin is <11 g/dL (2).
- During the initiation phase of treatment, check SF every 1 to 3 months (2).
- Once iron stores are depleted, the maintenance phase of treatment should include phlebotomy every 1 to 6 months (adjusted based on patient's need) to maintain SF levels near 50 μg/L (2).
- During maintenance therapy, measure TS and SF yearly.

DIET
- Avoid consumption of iron-fortified foods, oysters, uncooked shellfish, vitamin C supplements, and iron-containing supplements. Natural food sources of vitamin C and iron are considered safe.
- Black tea chelates iron and may be consumed with meals.
- Minimize alcohol use; consumption of >60 g/day (4 U.S. drinks) increases the risk of developing cirrhosis by 9-fold (2).

PATIENT EDUCATION
- Adequate hydration prior to phlebotomy is recommended.
- Blood collected through phlebotomy may be donated.
- http://www.hemochromatosis.org/

PROGNOSIS
- The presence or absence of cirrhosis is a critical factor for prognosis (2).
- Type 2 HH is associated with earlier onset and increased disease severity that type 1 HH (2).
- SF <1,000 μg/L, normal AST, and the absence of hepatomegaly have a negative predictive value of 95% for severe fibrosis or cirrhosis (2).
- Patients diagnosed and treated before the development of cirrhosis or diabetes have a normal life expectancy.
- Cirrhosis is associated with an increased risk of hepatocellular carcinoma (annual incidence of 3–4%) and mortality.
- Cirrhosis is irreversible; diabetes, arthralgias and symptoms of hypogonadism may not improve with phlebotomies, but other complications and symptoms may be averted with successful management (2).

COMPLICATIONS
Complications develop as a result of untreated HH.
- Arthritis and chondrocalcinosis sometimes requiring joint replacement surgery
- Osteoporosis
- Diabetes mellitus
- Hypogonadism
- Arrhythmia
- Congestive heart failure
- Cirrhosis (prevalence of 20–45% in C282Y homozygotes with SF >1,000 μg/L)
- Hepatocellular carcinoma (one study suggests carcinoma risk is higher in men with p.C282y homozygosity).
- Infection from Listeria monocytogenes, Escherichia coli, Yersinia enterocolitica, or Vibrio vulnificus is rare, but those with iron overload are at increased risk (2).

REFERENCES
1. Buzzetti E, Kalafateli M, Thorburn D, et al. Interventions for hereditary haemochromatosis: an attempted network meta-analysis. Cochrane Database Syst Rev. 2017;3(3):CD011647.
2. Kowdley KV, Brown KE, Ahn J, et al. ACG clinical guideline: hereditary hemochromatosis. Am J Gastroenterol. 2019;114(8):1202–1218.

 ## CODES

ICD10
- E83.110 Hereditary hemochromatosis
- E83.118 Other hemochromatosis
- E83.111 Hemochromatosis due to repeated red blood cell transfusions

CLINICAL PEARLS
- Screening of the general population for hemochromatosis is not recommended, but testing is recommended if there is clinical suspicion or family history.
- Many patients with iron overload remain asymptomatic.
- An elevated TS is the earliest abnormality in hemochromatosis. Ferritin is a sensitive measure of iron overload but can be elevated in a variety of infectious and inflammatory conditions without iron overload being present. Genetic testing is recommended to confirm HH.
- Patients with HH who have hepatomegaly, transaminitis, and/or serum transferrin >1,000 μg/L should be evaluated for liver iron content via hepatic MRI or sometimes liver biopsy.
- Initiate once or twice weekly phlebotomy when SF levels are elevated especially when symptoms or clinical findings are present and recommend hydration prior to phlebotomy.
- Goal is to achieve and then maintain SF levels near 50 μg/L without causing anemia below a hemoglobin of 11 g/dL.

H

HEMORRHOIDS
Donna I. Meltzer, MD

BASICS

DESCRIPTION
- Varicosities of the hemorrhoidal venous plexus
- External hemorrhoids
  - Located below (distal to) the dentate line; somatic innervation (painful)
  - Covered by squamous epithelium
- Internal hemorrhoids
  - Located above (proximal to) the dentate line; visceral innervation (painless)
  - Covered by columnar epithelium
  - Classification of internal hemorrhoids:
    - Grade I: Hemorrhoid vessel bulges without prolapse.
    - Grade II: Hemorrhoid prolapses with straining but reduces spontaneously.
    - Grade III: Hemorrhoid prolapses with straining and requires manual reduction.
    - Grade IV: chronically prolapsed—cannot be reduced
- Internal and external hemorrhoids often coexist.
- Although often asymptomatic, hemorrhoids can present with itching, bleeding, soilage, prolapse, or pain.
- Pain and thrombosis are more common with external than internal hemorrhoids.

Geriatric Considerations
Hemorrhoids and rectal prolapse are more common in elderly.

Pediatric Considerations
- Uncommon in infants and children; most common cause is chronic liver failure; other findings (rectal polyps, skin tags, condyloma) often misdiagnosed as hemorrhoids
- In adolescents, chronic constipation and prolonged toilet time can result in hemorrhoids.

Pregnancy Considerations
- Common in pregnancy
- Often resolve after delivery
- No treatment required, unless extremely painful

EPIDEMIOLOGY
- Predominant age: adults; peak from 45 to 65 years old (1)
- Predominant sex: male = female

Incidence
Common; >3.5 million office visits in United States per year are related to hemorrhoidal disease.

Prevalence
- ~4–5% in general population in the United States
- 39% prevalence on routine screening colonoscopy (1)

ETIOLOGY AND PATHOPHYSIOLOGY
- Exact pathophysiology is unknown.
- There are three primary hemorrhoidal cushions—typically located in left lateral, right anterior, and right posterior positions. Hemorrhoidal cushions augment anal closing pressure and protect the anal sphincter during stool passage. During Valsalva, increased intra-abdominal pressure raises pressure within the hemorrhoidal cushions. Mechanisms implicated in symptomatic hemorrhoidal disease include the following:
  - Dilated veins of hemorrhoidal plexus
  - Tight internal anal sphincter
  - Abnormal distention of the arteriovenous anastomosis
  - Prolapse of the cushions and the surrounding connective tissues

Genetics
No known genetic pattern

RISK FACTORS
- Pregnancy
- Pelvic space-occupying lesions
- Liver disease; portal HTN
- Constipation (prolonged straining)
- Occupations that require prolonged sitting
- Loss of perianal muscle tone due to old age, rectal surgery, birth trauma/episiotomy, anal intercourse
- Obesity
- Chronic diarrhea

GENERAL PREVENTION
- Avoid constipation by consuming high-fiber diet (>30 g/day) and ensuring proper hydration.
- Avoid prolonged sitting or straining on the toilet.

COMMONLY ASSOCIATED CONDITIONS
- Liver disease; cirrhosis, ascites
- Pregnancy
- Constipation

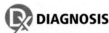

DIAGNOSIS

Diagnosis is typically straightforward through history and inspection of the perineum, rectal exam, and anoscopy.

HISTORY
- Symptoms
  - Bleeding (~60%)
  - Classically, bright red blood per rectum, may range from scant blood on toilet paper to copious blood in the toilet bowl
  - Pruritus (~55%)
  - Perianal discomfort (~20%)
  - Soiling (~10%)
  - Constipation or diarrhea
  - Straining with defecation
- More extensive internal hemorrhoids
  - Feeling of incomplete evacuation
- External hemorrhoids
  - Episodic bleeding on stool or toilet paper, pruritus, and irritation from compromised hygiene and pain
- Thrombosed hemorrhoids present as acute painful mass.
- Ask about diet (fiber, fluid intake), bowel patterns (frequency, consistency, incontinence), bowel habits (prolonged sitting), change in stools, and systemic symptoms (weight loss, pain, fever).
- Ask about past medical history and family history (gastrointestinal disease, colorectal cancer).

PHYSICAL EXAM
- Visual anorectal inspection at rest and with Valsalva maneuver in left lateral or lithotomy or knee-chest position
- Digital rectal exam: Check sphincter tone and tenderness.
- Anoscopy
  - Internal hemorrhoid appears as purple mass on lumen wall.
  - Examine for additional anorectal pathology (skin tags, mass, abscess, fissure, fistula).
- Abdominal exam to exclude mass
- Peripheral stigmata of cirrhosis and portal HTN (caput, telangiectasias, palmar erythema)

DIFFERENTIAL DIAGNOSIS
- Rectal or anal neoplasia
- Condyloma, skin tag
- Inflammatory bowel disease
- Anal fistula, fissure, or abscess
- Rectal polyp, rectal prolapse

DIAGNOSTIC TESTS & INTERPRETATION
Initial Tests (lab, imaging)
Not indicated unless anemia is suspected

Diagnostic Procedures/Other
Sigmoidoscopy or colonoscopy depending on risk factors for malignancy in patients with rectal bleeding

TREATMENT

Prevention
- Fiber supplements and adequate fluid intake
- Stool softeners
- Anal hygiene

GENERAL MEASURES
- Hemorrhoids are a recurrent disease, even after surgical excision. Preventive measures should be continued indefinitely.
- For mild symptoms or prevention
  - Avoid prolonged sitting during bowel movements; effect of squatting is unknown. Avoid straining.
  - Avoid constipation by eating a high-fiber diet or by taking fiber supplements (psyllium husks); if necessary, take regular stool softeners.
  - Regular exercise, weight loss if indicated
- Pruritus or mild discomfort after stooling might respond to topical corticosteroid ointment, anesthetic ointments or sprays, and warm sitz baths.
- Constipation relief, anal hygiene, local ointments, and sitz baths are effective through the stage of easy reduction (grade II). More severe stages often require ligation or surgery.

MEDICATION
First Line
- Dietary modification with adequate fluid (generally ≥2 L water per day) and high fiber (25 to 35 g/day) is first-line, nonoperative therapy for symptomatic hemorrhoids (1).
- Fiber supplementation helps relieve overall symptoms and bleeding (2)[A].
- Stool softener or bulk-forming laxative to soften stool
- Topic anesthetics (benzocaine, lidocaine, pramoxine), steroids, emollients to alleviate symptoms; these over-the-counter (OTC) products have been traditionally used but lack strong evidence for long-term use.
  - Local anesthetics for relief of pain and itch; applied to perianal area (not inserted into rectum)
  - Dibucaine 1% ointment (Nupercainal), lidocaine 5% (Preparation H, Tucks), pramoxine 1% foam, ointment, wipe (Proctofoam); benzocaine 20% spray, ointment
- Anti-inflammatory agents (corticosteroids) to decrease swelling and itch
  - Hydrocortisone ointment, cream (0.25–2.5%) (Anusol HC, Cortifoam); rectal suppositories are for short-term use only.

- Astringents to help cleanse and soothe skin
  - Witch hazel solution, wipes, pads (Preparation H, Tucks) after stooling
- Vasoconstrictors to shrink hemorrhoids and ameliorate bleeding, pain, itch
  - 0.25% phenylephrine ointment, suppository, gel (Preparation H)

Second Line
Treatment for special cases

- Acute thrombosed external hemorrhoids: If present within 72 hours after pain onset, recommend incision and clot evacuation or excision of hemorrhoid complex. Early surgical excision may resolve symptoms faster and lower incidence of recurrence (2)[C].
- Strangulated hemorrhoid: Untreated irreducible hemorrhoid can progress to thrombosis and necrosis. Treatment requires urgent or emergent hemorrhoidectomy.
- Acute hemorrhoidal bleeding associated with portal HTN: Treatment depends on degree of hemorrhoids and amount of bleeding. Differentiate from more serious anorectal varices which require medical management (correct coagulopathy) and surgical interventions (suture ligation and shunts if necessary).

SURGERY/OTHER PROCEDURES
- Indications: failure of medical and nonoperative therapy, symptomatic grade III or IV hemorrhoids in presence of a concomitant anorectal condition requiring surgery, or patient's preference
- Office-based procedures for patients with grade I or II (or III) internal hemorrhoids who have failed conservative management
  - Rubber band ligation (RBL) is the most common and most effective office-based procedure for symptomatic internal (not external) hemorrhoids. Avoid if on anticoagulants (2)[A].
  - Infrared photocoagulation causes necrosis within hemorrhoid; similar or slightly higher recurrence rates compared to RBL; less postoperative pain and fewer complications (1)[A],(2)[B]
  - Sclerotherapy: submucosal injections causing local thrombosis; might be best for patients at increased bleeding risk (anticoagulated, advanced liver disease); care must be taken to inject proper site; not for advanced disease or if evidence of infection, inflammation, or ulceration
  - Cryotherapy is no longer recommended due to high rate of complications.
- Surgery for patients with symptomatic grade III or IV disease or for those who have failed nonoperative treatments (2)[A]
  - Conventional hemorrhoidectomy to treat internal and external hemorrhoidal disease
    - Closed hemorrhoidectomy—closure of mucosal defect, more often used to treat internal hemorrhoids
    - Open hemorrhoidectomy—tissue removed and mucosal defect left open
  - Different technologies are now used to excise hemorrhoidal tissue: diathermy, lasers, ultrasonic dissectors; associated with less pain

- Other techniques reduce surgical time, early postoperative pain, urinary retention, and time to return to normal activity.
  - Doppler guided hemorrhoidal artery ligation (HAL): anoscope or proctoscope with Doppler probe to identify and ligate hemorrhoidal artery; faster return to work than open hemorrhoidectomy (3)[A]
  - Stapled hemorrhoidopexy—for advanced internal hemorrhoidal disease; shorter recovery but more recurrent disease than conventional hemorrhoidectomy (1),(3)[A]
  - LigaSure hemorrhoidectomy: electrosurgical technique to coagulate vessels; reduces operating time, is superior in terms of patient tolerance, and is equal to conventional hemorrhoidectomy in long-term symptom control (1)[A]
  - Laser treatment for grades II and III hemorrhoids has acceptable outcomes with less postoperative pain and bleeding compared to open hemorrhoidectomy (3)[A].
- No gold standard surgical treatment; need to individualize based on symptoms and risks/benefits of each procedure

COMPLEMENTARY & ALTERNATIVE MEDICINE
- Oral bioflavonoids have shown beneficial effect on bleeding, pruritus, and recurrence (2)[A].
- Topical nifedipine (compounded by pharmacist) can relieve pain of thrombosed hemorrhoids.
- Topical nitroglycerin (0.4%) has been used to decrease anal sphincter spasm in thrombosed hemorrhoids; headache is the primary side effect.
- Botulinum toxin injection into anal sphincter to relieve spasm and pain of thrombosed hemorrhoid
- Aloe vera cream on the surgical site after hemorrhoidectomy reduces postoperative pain and decreases healing time and analgesic requirements.

 ## ONGOING CARE

FOLLOW-UP RECOMMENDATIONS
- Encourage physical fitness, weight management, and dietary compliance.
- Avoid prolonged sitting and straining on the toilet.

Patient Monitoring
As needed, depending on treatment

DIET
High fiber with a target of 30 g of insoluble fiber per day through sources such as wheat bran cereals, oatmeal, peanuts, artichokes, beans, corn, peas, spinach, potatoes, apples, apricots, berries, prunes, pears, bananas; adequate fluid; avoid excessive caffeine.

PATIENT EDUCATION
Increasing dietary fiber: https://familydoctor.org/fiber-how-to-increase-the-amount-in-your-diet/

PROGNOSIS
- Spontaneous resolution
- Recurrence

COMPLICATIONS
- Thrombosis
- Ulceration
- Incontinence
- Pelvic sepsis following hemorrhoidectomy

REFERENCES
1. Mott T, Latimer K, Edwards C. Hemorrhoids: diagnosis and treatment options. *Am Fam Physician*. 2018;97(3):172–179.
2. Davis BR, Lee-Kong SA, Migaly J, et al. The American Society of Colon and Rectal Surgeons clinical practice guidelines for the management of hemorrhoids. *Dis Colon Rectum*. 2018;61(3):284–292.
3. Aibuedefe B, Kling SM, Philp MM, et al. An update on surgical treatment of hemorrhoidal disease: a systematic review and meta-analysis. *Int J Colorectal Dis*. 2021;36(9):2041–2049.

ADDITIONAL READING
- Ng KS, Holzgang M, Young C. Still a case of "no pain, no gain"? An updated and critical review of the pathogenesis, diagnosis, and management options for hemorrhoids in 2020. *Ann Coloproctol*. 2020;36(3):133–147.
- Sandler RS, Peery AF. Rethinking what we know about hemorrhoids. *Clin Gastroenterol Hepatol*. 2019;17(1):8–15.

 ## SEE ALSO

Colon Cancer; Portal Hypertension; Rectal Cancer

CODES

ICD10
- K64.9 Unspecified hemorrhoids
- K64.4 Residual hemorrhoidal skin tags
- K64.1 Second degree hemorrhoids

CLINICAL PEARLS
- Hemorrhoids are common. Internal hemorrhoids are typically painless. External hemorrhoids are typically painful.
- Many cases can be managed conservatively.
- All patients should be encouraged to consume 25 to 35 g of fiber per day.
- More advanced hemorrhoidal disease requires intervention with ligation or surgery.

H

HENOCH-SCHÖNLEIN PURPURA

Shani H. Cunningham, DO, MEd, FAAP • Emerald Russell-Nathan, MD

BASICS

Increasingly referred to as immunoglobulin-A vasculitis (IgAV)

DESCRIPTION
- Henoch-Schönlein purpura (HSP) is a nonthrombocytopenic, predominantly IgA-mediated, small vessel vasculitis that affects multiple organ systems and occurs in both children and adults.
- HSP is often self-limited, with the greatest morbidity and mortality attributable to long-term renal damage.
- Characterized by a tetrad of purpuric skin lesions, arthralgia, abdominal pain, and nephropathies

EPIDEMIOLOGY
Incidence
- Annual incidence: estimated 29.9/100,000 children and 0.1 to 1.8/100,000 adults
- Peak incidence: age 4 to 6 years; 90% of patients with HSP are <10 years of age; however, has been reported in patients aged 6 months to 75 years old
- Gender: Male-to-female ratio is between 1.2:1 and 1.8:1.
- Race/ethnicity: most common in Caucasians and Asians; less common among African Americans

Prevalence
Annual prevalence: 10 to 22/100,000 persons; more common in fall and winter

ETIOLOGY AND PATHOPHYSIOLOGY
- Autoimmune disorder in which IgA production is increased in response to trigger(s), IgA1 immune complexes then activate the complement pathway, leading to production of inflammatory cytokines and chemokines.
- IgA-containing immune complex deposition results in small vessel inflammation which leads to fibrosis and necrosis within skin, intestinal mucosa, joints, and kidneys.
- No single etiologic agent has been identified; however, there are some associations (listed below) and a popular theory is one of a multihit model leading to HSP-associated glomerulonephropathy.
  - Infections are suggested by prevalence in the fall/winter and a common upper respiratory infection (URI) prodrome. Associated pathogens include (but are not limited to) group A *Streptococcus* (may be present in up to 30% of HSP-associated nephritis), parvovirus B19, *Bartonella henselae*, *Helicobacter pylori*, *Haemophilus parainfluenzae*, coxsackievirus, adenovirus, hepatitis A and B viruses, Mycoplasma, Epstein-Barr virus, herpes simplex, varicella, *Campylobacter*, and methicillin-resistant *Staphylococcus aureus*.
  - Drugs are most often associated with adults with HSP: acetaminophen, angiotensin-converting enzyme inhibitors (ACEI), angiotensin II receptor antagonists (ARB), some antibiotics including clarithromycin quinolones, etanercept, codeine, nonsteroidal anti-inflammatory drugs.
  - Vaccinations are rarely associated with HSP; MMR, pneumococcal, meningococcal, influenza and hepatitis B

Genetics
Associated with α_1-antitrypsin deficiency, familial Mediterranean fever, HLA-A2, HLA-A11, HLA-B35, HLA-DRB1, renin-angiotensin, and nitric oxide synthetase polymorphisms

COMMONLY ASSOCIATED CONDITIONS
- Rare association is with solid tumors, lymphoma, prostate cancer, non–small cell lung cancer, multiple myeloma.
- Possible relationship with *H. pylori* infection and immune-related disorders (food allergy, drug allergy, inflammatory bowel disease)

DIAGNOSIS

Palpable purpura/petechiae (mandatory criteria)—without thrombocytopenia and *at least one* of the following:
- Diffuse abdominal pain
- Biopsy with predominant IgA deposition
- Arthralgia or arthritis
- Renal involvement (hematuria or proteinuria)
- Direct immunofluorescence showing IgA deposition (negative staining does not exclude IgAV)

HISTORY
- Exposure to possible trigger, including recent infection (particularly URI) or offending drug
- Rash (most common presenting symptom): purpuric, palpable; predominant distribution often symmetric on dependent areas (lower extremities and buttocks); may spread elsewhere, typical duration 3 to 10 days with no definitive temporal association with other symptoms.
- Gastrointestinal (GI) (about 50–75% of cases)
  - Nausea/vomiting
  - Abdominal pain (diffuse, colicky, may be transient or constant)
  - Hematochezia/melena
- Polyarthritis (about 75% of cases)
  - Often symmetric involvement of knees and ankles
- Renal (about 20–55% of cases)
  - Gross hematuria (higher in adults than children)
  - Oliguria or anuria
- Fatigue
- Low-grade fever
- Rare symptoms: periorbital or scrotal swelling, headache, seizures, neuropathy, behavioral changes, hemoptysis

PHYSICAL EXAM
- Rash (96% of cases, 74% primary presenting symptom):
  - May start as urticaria, develops into nonblanching, palpable purpura, with or without petechiae, ecchymoses and bullae
  - Distribution usually symmetric, most commonly involving the lower extremities but may involve the face and trunk
- Abdominal tenderness (66% of cases, 12% primary presenting symptom):
  - Evidence of GI hemorrhage (28% of cases), recommend rectal examination to assess for hematochezia.

- Joint tenderness (64% of cases, 15% primary presenting symptom):
  - Mainly affects knees or ankles; may have associated warmth and limited range of motion, less commonly effusion; erythema is absent; nonmigratory, transient; lower extremity edema
- Orchitis (5%):
  - Presents as scrotal swelling and tenderness, may have associated torsion
- Renal disease (<1% primary presenting symptom):
  - Hypertension may be present.
- Rarely, patients present with central nervous system (CNS) or pulmonary involvement

DIFFERENTIAL DIAGNOSIS
- Infection:
  - Meningococcemia
  - Rocky Mountain spotted fever
  - Bacterial endocarditis
  - Rheumatic fever
  - Epstein-Barr virus
  - Sepsis
- Vasculitides:
  - Polyarteritis nodosa
  - Granulomatosis with polyangiitis
  - Microscopic polyangiitis
  - Systemic lupus erythematosus
  - Kawasaki disease
  - Urticarial vasculitis
  - Cryoglobulinemia-associated vasculitis
- Other:
  - Acute poststreptococcal glomerulonephritis
  - Inflammatory bowel disease
  - Idiopathic thrombocytopenic purpura/thrombotic thrombocytopenic purpura
  - Juvenile idiopathic arthritis/mixed connective tissue disease/juvenile dermatomyositis
  - Leukemia/lymphoma
  - Hereditary hemorrhagic telangiectasia
  - Acute surgical abdomen
  - Child abuse

DIAGNOSTIC TESTS & INTERPRETATION
- Histological analysis of skin/renal biopsies, revealing leukocytoclastic vasculitis of postcapillary venules
- Labs directed toward excluding other illnesses and assessing degree of renal involvement

Initial Tests (lab, imaging)
- Complete blood count:
  - Leukocytosis and thrombocytosis may occur. Eosinophilia is common. Thrombocytopenia indicates an alternative cause of purpura; anemia if GI hemorrhage occurs.
- Blood culture if sepsis is a concern.
- Basic serum chemistry panel: Evaluate renal function.
- Urinalysis/estimated glomerular filtration rate, hematuria
- Prothrombin time/international normalized ratio and partial thromboplastin time:
  - Normal in HSP. Abnormal coagulation studies may indicate an alternative cause of purpura.
- Acute phase reactants (erythrocyte sedimentation rate (ESR)/C-reactive protein)
- IgA level: often elevated, nonspecific, and nonsensitive

- Complement levels: normal; sometimes decreased
- Antistreptolysin-O titer: evaluates for preceding streptococcal infection
- Imaging not routine for HSP but may be performed to rule out alternative etiologies or complications
  - Abdominal radiographs for free air and US intussusception (most serious and common GI manifestation)
  - CT arteriography may be necessary to identify the location of bleeding in patients with GI hemorrhage.

Diagnostic Procedures/Other
- Renal biopsy: Obtain if diagnosis is uncertain or if urinalysis shows nephrotic range proteinuria. Biopsy may show mesangial IgA deposition, mesangial proliferation, or, in severe cases, crescentic glomerulonephritis.
- Skin biopsy of purpura: IgA deposition in the dermis on immunofluorescence
- Endoscopy for hemorrhage as symptomatic overlap of HSP with inflammatory bowel disease
- Barium enema may be therapeutic for intussusception.

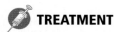 TREATMENT

GENERAL MEASURES
Rest and elevation of affected areas may limit purpura. Hydration and nutrition play a supportive role in treatment.

MEDICATION
- In the absence of renal dysfunction or complication, HSP is usually self-limited and best managed with supportive care as it resolves in 94% of children and 89% of adults.
- NSAIDs effective for symptomatic joint pain. Caution is advised in cases of renal involvement and consider acetaminophen as an alternative.
- Steroids useful early in disease for patients with severe joint and abdominal pain, cerebral vasculitis, pulmonary hemorrhage, orchitis, and in those with glomerulonephritis with severe renal involvement. Oral prednisone (1 to 2 mg/kg/day) or pulsed intravenous methylprednisolone (10 to 30 mg/kg/day) may decrease both duration of abdominal pain and severity of joint pain. This may have benefit in preventing GI bleeding and causes of surgical abdomen, including intussusception, may benefit dermatologic and renal complications.
  - Early steroids have no effect on prevention or development of renal involvement after 1 year.

- Immunosuppressive (cyclosporine [Sandimmune] and mycophenolate [CellCept]) therapy may be beneficial for patients with evidence of severe renal involvement and those with steroid-resistant disease. There have been many small case studies and case reports showing benefit in these patients. High-dose IV pulse steroids, cyclophosphamide, rituximab, mycophenolate, and plasmapheresis have all been described in small studies. Consensus for when to definitively use these agents is still controversial and the subject of further research (1)[B].
- ACEI or ARB may be helpful in patients with HSP and persistent proteinuria.

ISSUES FOR REFERRAL
Nephrology referral for renal biopsy if nephrotic range proteinuria at any time or proteinuria >100 mg/mmol for 3 months after diagnosis

ADMISSION, INPATIENT, AND NURSING CONSIDERATIONS
Admission criteria/initial stabilization
- Insufficient oral intake, renal insufficiency
- Severe abdominal pain, severe GI bleeding
- Altered mental status
- Mobility restriction due to arthritis
- HTN, nephrotic syndrome

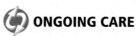 ONGOING CARE

FOLLOW-UP RECOMMENDATIONS
Patient Monitoring
- Seen weekly during the acute illness with history, physical exam (include BP measurement), and urinalysis.
- Because ~100% of patients who develop renal involvement will do so within 6 months of HSP diagnosis, all patients should be followed at least monthly with BP and urinalysis for a duration of at least 6 months.
- Women with a history of HSP should be monitored for proteinuria and HTN during pregnancy.
- Consider workup for occult malignancy in patients with adult-onset HSP.

PATIENT EDUCATION
National Kidney and Urologic Diseases Information Clearinghouse (NKUDIC): IgAV

PROGNOSIS
- Long-term prognosis heavily dependent on presence and severity of nephritis
- HSP is self-limited in 94% of children and 89% of adults.
- Most cases of HSP resolve within 4 weeks of diagnosis. Recurrence rate within 6 months of diagnosis is 33%.

- Factors associated with poorer prognosis include age >8 years, fever at presentation, purpura above the waist, elevated ESR or IgA concentration, low initial proteinuria, and increasing severity of renal histology grade.
- Chronic renal disease occurs in up to 20% of children with nephritic and nephrotic syndrome compared with 50% of adults who had any renal involvement. Risk of long-term renal failure is ≤5%.
- Risk factors that may result in renal failure include old age, HTN, elevated serum creatinine, and nephrotic and mixed nephritic–nephrotic syndrome at the onset of disease.

COMPLICATIONS
- Nephrotic/nephritic syndrome and renal failure, HTN
- Hemorrhagic cystitis, ureteral obstruction
- Intestinal infarction, perforation, obstruction, stricture
- GI hemorrhage, intussusception
- Alveolar hemorrhage
- CNS complications, including cerebral hemorrhage and seizure
- Anterior uveitis
- Myocarditis
- Orchitis, testicular torsion

REFERENCE
1. Pohl M. Henoch-Schönlein purpura nephritis. *Pediatr Nephrol*. 2015;30(2):245–252.

ADDITIONAL READING
Kawasaki Y. The pathogenesis and treatment of pediatric Henoch-Schönlein purpura nephritis. *Clin Exp Nephrol*. 2011;15(5):648–657.

 CODES

ICD10
D69.0 Allergic purpura

CLINICAL PEARLS
- HSP is a systemic small vessel vasculitis characterized by clinical tetrad of palpable purpura, abdominal pain, arthralgia, and renal dysfunction.
- The main form of treatment is supportive care, but oral corticosteroids may be beneficial if there appears to be severe renal involvement.
- In all patients with HSP, regardless of renal involvement at presentation, it is reasonable to check BP and urinalysis at weekly to monthly intervals for at least 6 months after diagnosis to monitor for developing renal dysfunction.

H

HEPATIC ENCEPHALOPATHY

Walter M. Kim, MD, PhD • Sloan F. Miler, MD

 BASICS

DESCRIPTION

- Reversible altered mental and neuromotor functioning in association with acute or chronic liver disease and/or portosystemic shunting
- Wide spectrum of neurologic/psychiatric abnormalities ranging from subclinical alterations to coma: Prominent features are confusion, impaired arousability, and a "flapping tremor" (asterixis).

EPIDEMIOLOGY

Male = female (reflects prevalence of underlying liver disease)

Incidence

- The risk of first episode of overt hepatic encephalopathy (HE) is 5–25% within 5 years of cirrhosis diagnosis.
- Posttransjugular intrahepatic portosystemic shunt (TIPS), median cumulative 1-year incidence of overt HE is 10–50%

Prevalence

- May occur at any age; parallels the age predominance of fulminant liver disease: peaks in the 40s (Cirrhosis peaks in the late 50s.)
- Occurs in all cases of fulminant hepatic failure or acute liver failure (ALF); overt HE occurs in 30–45% of cirrhotic patients; present in ~50% of patients requiring liver transplantation

ETIOLOGY AND PATHOPHYSIOLOGY

- There is no defined pathophysiology for the development of HE. However, elevated serum levels of ammonia (hyperammonemia) correlate with the severity of HE, suggesting a central role of ammonia as a neurotoxin.
- Classifications based on four factors have been proposed:
  - According to the underlying disease:
    - Type A: resulting from ALF; type B: resulting from portosystemic bypass or shunting in absence of inherent liver disease; type C: resulting from cirrhosis
  - According to severity of manifestation:
    - West Haven classification: Convert to grades I to IV (see "Physical Exam" section).
  - According to time course:
    - Episodic HE; recurrent HE = >1 episode occurring within 6 months; persistent HE = persistent behavioral alterations interspersed with relapses of overt HE
  - According to precipitating factors:
    - Nonprecipitated; precipitated
- Several metabolic factors implicated in HE based on the failure of the liver to detoxify noxious CNS agents (e.g., ammonia, mercaptan, octopamine, tyramine, fatty acids, lactate, manganese)
- Increased aromatic and reduced branched chain amino acids in blood may act as false neurotransmitters, possibly interacting with the γ-aminobutyric acid (GABA) receptor to cause clinical symptoms
- HE presents most commonly in patients with long-standing cirrhosis and spontaneous shunting of intestinal blood through collateral vessels or surgical portacaval shunts.

- Asterixis is the inability to maintain a particular posture due to metabolic encephalopathy. Abnormal diencephalic function leads to the characteristic liver flap noted when the arms and wrists are held in extension.

Genetics

- Unknown/unclear
- Conditions that predispose an individual to developing chronic liver disease such as cystic fibrosis, α_1-antitrypsin deficiency, hemochromatosis, and Wilson disease can contribute to the development of HE.
- A glutaminase gene variation that increases enzyme activity may predispose patients to develop HE.

RISK FACTORS

In patients with underlying liver disease, precipitating factors include the following:

- Electrolyte disturbance (Na^+, K^+, Mg^{2+} most common); infection (overt or occult, including spontaneous bacterial peritonitis [SBP]); GI hemorrhage
- Use of sedative (e.g., benzodiazepines) or opiate drugs; fluid abnormalities including from diuretic overuse
- TIPS—a radiologically inserted shunt to lower portal pressure—elderly patients and those with worse liver function are at increased risk of developing HE following TIPS.

GENERAL PREVENTION

- Recognize early signs and seek prompt treatment. Avoid nonessential medications, particularly opiates, benzodiazepines, and sedatives. Consider lactulose therapy as secondary prophylaxis for recurrence of overt HE.
- For patients who have already experienced bouts of overt HE while on lactulose, lactulose + rifaximin is the best-documented agent to maintain remission (1).

COMMONLY ASSOCIATED CONDITIONS

- Cirrhosis; portal hypertension; may occur as a complication of acute fatty liver of pregnancy
- Occurs rarely in patients with a portacaval shunt accompanied by normal liver function

 DIAGNOSIS

HISTORY

Preexisting liver disease; altered mental status, confusion; impaired arousability; constipation

PHYSICAL EXAM

- Age <10 years
  - Signs of underlying liver disease are prominent; fulminant hepatic failure or advanced cirrhosis; progression is very rapid, often over hours. Wilson disease can imitate HE.
- Ages 10 to 60 years
  - Five grades of confusion and degree of obtundation (West Haven criteria):
    - Minimal (Covert): psychometric or neuropsychological alterations without mental status changes
    - Grade I: lack of awareness, anxiety, shortened attention span, impaired arithmetic, altered sleep rhythm

---

  - Grade II (Overt): asterixis, lethargy, disorientation to time, personality change, inappropriate behavior
  - Grade III: somnolence to stupor, confusion, gross disorientation, bizarre behavior
  - Grade IV: coma
  - Prominent signs of underlying liver disease (50%); jaundice is most common; ascites is second most common.
  - GI bleeding with hematemesis or melena (20%)
  - Systemic infection, urinary tract infection, or pulmonary infection (20%)
- Age >60 years
  - Signs of underlying liver disease diminish (25%); confusion is more prominent
  - Precipitating GI hemorrhage or infection is less often identified. Progression is slower.
- Vital signs:
  - Bradycardia; increased blood pressure suggestive of increased intracranial pressure (ICP)
- Jaundice, ascites, other correlates of liver disease (e.g. spider telangiectasias, muscle wasting)
- CNS exam: Assess short-term memory and presence of asterixis ("liver flap"—a flapping of the wrist when arms and wrists are extended). Use Glasgow Coma Scale in patients with grades III to IV West Haven criteria of HE severity (1).
- Pupillary reaction regresses from normal to sluggish and then absent with worsening HE.

DIFFERENTIAL DIAGNOSIS

- Metabolic encephalopathy related to anoxia, hypoglycemia, hypokalemia, hypo- or hypercalcemia, or uremia
- Head trauma, concussion, subdural hematoma; transient ischemic attack (TIA), ischemic stroke
- ICP, intracranial hemorrhage (ICH)
- Alcohol intoxication; alcohol withdrawal syndrome; confusion due to medications or illicit drugs
- Meningitis, encephalitis; Wilson disease without cirrhosis; Reye syndrome; Wernicke-Korsakoff syndrome

DIAGNOSTIC TESTS & INTERPRETATION

- Clinical findings are diagnostic in 80% of cases.
- Response to treatment often confirms the diagnosis.
- EEG (limited utility): symmetric slowing of basic (α) rhythm (also common with other metabolic encephalopathies)
- Number connection test (NCT), line drawing test, critical flicker frequency (CFF) test, digit symbol test (DST), continuous reaction time (CRT) test, inhibitory control test (ICT), repeatable battery for the assessment of neuropsychological status (RBANS), and other psychometric tests may be used to assess minimal HE.
- Use Glasgow Coma Scale in patients with more severe HE (grades III to IV).

Initial Tests (lab, imaging)

- Serum ammonia level is elevated in 90% of patients with HE—it is *not*, however, diagnostic for HE.
- Serum ammonia level on presentation appears to correlate with HE severity (2).

- Liver function tests, including aspartate aminotransferase (AST), alanine aminotransferase (ALT), and serum albumin
- Prothrombin time (PT) and international normalized ratio (INR) often elevated reflecting liver dysfunction
- Complete blood count (CBC): anemia and leukocytosis; complete metabolic profile (CMP) to identify hypokalemia, hyperbilirubinemia, altered calcium concentration, hypomagnesemia, and hypoglycemia; BUN: Creatinine >20 suggests dehydration or GI bleeding.
- Diagnostic paracentesis to rule out SBP in setting of ascites
- Blood, urine, sputum, and ascitic fluid cultures to identify infection, ABG to assess acid-base as clinically indicated
- Toxicology screen; head CT to identify frontal cortical atrophy and/or edema as well as to rule out other causes of altered mental status
- MRI is more sensitive than CT.

Follow-Up Tests & Special Considerations
Clinicians should not rely on serial monitoring of serum ammonia levels when evaluating severity of HE.

Test Interpretation
- Cerebral edema is seen in 100% of fatal cases.
- Glial hypertrophy in chronic encephalopathy

TREATMENT

GENERAL MEASURES
- Identify and treat precipitating causes: electrolyte imbalance, GI bleeding, infection
- Avoid sedatives, benzodiazepines, opiates, diphenoxylate, and atropine.
- Grade I or higher: Ensure adequate fluid and caloric ≥1,000 kcal (4.19 MJ) intake; avoid hypoglycemia.
- Consider lactulose enema for patients without diarrhea.
- If clumsiness and poor judgment are prominent, institute fall precautions.

MEDICATION
First Line
- Lactulose syrup (nonabsorbable disaccharide with laxative action that decreases colonic transit time and bacterial digestion that acidifies the colon to promote conversion of ammonia [NH_3] to ammonium [NH_4^+] which decreases ammonia absorption and reduces serum ammonia levels): 30 to 45 mL PO up to every hour for goal of 3 to 6 bowel movements per day; decrease to 15 to 30 mL BID when ≥3 bowel movements per day are observed.
- Lactulose enema (for patients who cannot tolerate oral lactulose or have suspected ileus): 300 mL lactulose plus 700 mL tap water, retained for 1 hour
- If worsening HE occurs acutely or there is no improvement in 2 days, add rifaximin: 400 mg PO TID or 550 mg PO BID (nonabsorbable antibiotic); highly effective in reversing minimal HE
- Contraindications: total ileus; hypersensitivity reaction; precautions: hypokalemia; other electrolyte imbalance; dehydration and renal failure

Second Line
- Neomycin: 1 to 2 g/day PO divided q6–8h, if renal function is within normal limits
- Polyethylene glycol as an alternative to lactulose
- Metronidazole and vancomycin are alternative antibiotics, although use is limited by adverse side effect profile and risk of antimicrobial resistance.
- Flumazenil may be of benefit in select patients.

ISSUES FOR REFERRAL
Refer early to experienced transplant center, especially if refractory to drug therapies.

ADDITIONAL THERAPIES
Branched-chain amino acids, probiotics, and IV L-ornithine L–aspartate; supporting evidence is controversial.

SURGERY/OTHER PROCEDURES
- Artificial liver perfusion devices are useful in fulminant hepatic failure as a bridge to transplantation.
- Liver failure with recurrent, intractable overt HE is indication for liver transplant.
- Consider liver transplant in patients with grades II to IV HE.

COMPLEMENTARY & ALTERNATIVE MEDICINE
Probiotics and prebiotics have been associated with improvement of HE through modulation of gut flora.

ADMISSION, INPATIENT, AND NURSING CONSIDERATIONS
- Monitor clinical status closely in grades I and II when diagnosis is clear, and watch for progression.
- Evaluate patients with grades II to IV HE in fulminant hepatic failure for liver transplantation.

ONGOING CARE

FOLLOW-UP RECOMMENDATIONS
Activity as tolerated once resolved; after the first HE episode, start secondary prophylaxis with nonabsorbable disaccharides (lactulose or lactitol) at 20 mL of syrup or equivalent in granules twice daily and modulate dose for 2 to 3 soft stools per day. If HE recurs (one or more HE episodes within 6 months), then add rifaximin.

Patient Monitoring
- Asterixis and using the trail-making test (ask patient to connect-the-dots according to numbers) helps monitor HE patients. Periodic evaluation helps determine maintenance treatment and diet. Test daily at first and then at each visit when changes in drugs and diet are made.
- See patients biweekly if there are changes on the trail-making test. Stable patients should be seen monthly.
- NCT or line drawing test at each office visit can also help with patient monitoring.
- In cirrhosis, evaluate for transplantation and periodically monitor Model for End-Stage Liver Disease (MELD) score.
- Uncontrolled diabetes and malnutrition are associated with precipitation of overt HE in cirrhotic patients.

DIET
- Weight loss with sarcopenia may worsen HE.
- Regular protein diet (1.2 to 1.5 g/kg/day); protein-limited diets are avoided as patients are typically malnourished. Vegetable protein diets are better tolerated than animal protein diets in patients with advanced cirrhosis; special IV/enteral formulations with increased branched chain amino acids are available.
- Patients with grades III to IV HE require nutritional support by parenteral nutrition or jejunal feeds.

PATIENT EDUCATION
American Association for the Study of Liver Diseases: https://www.aasld.org/

PROGNOSIS
- With appropriate treatment and monitoring, acute HE often resolves.
- Chronic liver disease
  - HE recurs with variable frequency. With each recurrence, HE is more difficult to treat—the degree of improvement with treatment is reduced, and the mortality rate approaches 80%.

COMPLICATIONS
- Recurrence; with many recurrences, permanent basal ganglion injury (non-Wilsonian hepatolenticular degeneration)
- Hepatorenal syndrome

REFERENCES
1. European Association for the Study of the Liver. EASL clinical practice guidelines on the management of hepatic encephalopathy. *J Hepatol.* 2022;77(3):807–824.
2. Shalimar, Sheikh MF, Mookerjee RP, et al. Prognostic Role of Ammonia in Patients With Cirrhosis. *Hepatology.* 2019;70(3):982–994.

ADDITIONAL READING
Acharya C, Bajaj JS. Current management of hepatic encephalopathy. *Am J Gastroenterol.* 2018;113(11):1600–1612.

 SEE ALSO

Algorithm: Delirium

CODES

ICD10
- K72.91 Hepatic failure, unspecified with coma
- K72.11 Chronic hepatic failure with coma
- K70.40 Alcoholic hepatic failure without coma

CLINICAL PEARLS
- HE includes a spectrum of neuropsychiatric findings that occur in patients with significant alterations in hepatic function.
- Lactulose is the cornerstone of therapy for HE.
- Asterixis ("liver flap") is the classic physical finding associated with HE.
- Serum ammonia level is not diagnostic for HE; however, correlation with severity has been suggested.

H

HEPATITIS A

Marie L. Borum, MD, EdD, MPH • Gabriel J. Diaz, CRNP-BC, MS

 BASICS

DESCRIPTION
Caused by the hepatitis A virus (HAV) and is a small nonenveloped single stranded RNA virus; HAV infections are common worldwide primarily involving the liver.

EPIDEMIOLOGY
Incidence
- 1.5 million cases globally each year; since the release of the HAV vaccine in 1995, the incidence of HAV in the United States has decreased significantly. Regional outbreaks contribute to ongoing disease.
- As many as 1/2 of current HAV infections in the United States are acquired during travel to endemic countries.

Prevalence
- Serologic evidence of prior HAV infection is present in approximately 1/3 of the U.S. population.
- Seroprevalence for HAV has been decreasing in many parts of the world; however, it remains very high in developing countries where HAV tends to occur within the first few years of life.

Pediatric Considerations
Often, milder or asymptomatic in children; severity increases with age. Asymptomatic infections with lack of jaundice development occur in 70% of children aged <6 years.

Pregnancy Considerations
Increased risk of complications; vertical transmission has been reported; fecal-oral transmission during birth is possible. Breastfeeding is not contraindicated.

ETIOLOGY AND PATHOPHYSIOLOGY
- HAV is a single-stranded linear RNA enterovirus of the Picornaviridae family. Infection is limited to hepatocytes and macrophages. HAV is excreted into the bile and then stool, providing major route of spread. Humans are the only known natural reservoir. Transmission is primarily through fecal-oral route; however, HAV is also transmitted through sexual intercourse (particularly anal-oral contact) and intravenous drug use. Incubation is 2 to 6 weeks with a mean of 4 weeks.
- Disease course is divided in two phases: prodromal phase, which is associated with the development of symptoms (fever, malaise, weakness, anorexia, nausea, vomiting), and convalescent period (jaundice develops).
- Greatest infectivity period is 2 weeks before the appearance of jaundice or elevation of liver enzymes coinciding with peak in viral stool concentration.
- Virus is stable in water and on surfaces but is easily killed with high heat or cleaning agents.
- HAV is not a chronic disease.

Genetics
Autoimmune hepatitis is rarely associated with HLA class II DR3 and DR4 after infection with HAV.

RISK FACTORS
- Person-to-person contact:
  - Intimate exposure, particularly anal-oral contact; residential institutional transmission; employment in health care; household exposure; child care centers, schools

- Contaminated food or water contact: Travel to developing countries accounts for >50% of cases in North America and Europe; consumption of raw/undercooked shellfish, vegetables, or other foods; consumption of improperly handled food or contaminated water
- Other modes of transmission: injection of illicit drugs; blood exposure or transfusion (rare); no identifiable risk factor in 50% of cases

GENERAL PREVENTION
- Proper sanitation and personal hygiene (hand washing), especially for food handlers, health care, and daycare workers
- Active immunization HAV vaccines: Havrix and Vaqta or Twinrix—combination HAV and HBV; vaccine provides protection for >20 years (1).
- Vaccine is recommended for:
  - All children aged 12 to 23 months, with catch-up administration until 18 years old; all travelers to countries with high endemic rate of hepatitis A (parts of Africa, Central and South America, and South and Southeast Asia)
  - Men who have sex with men; individuals using (primarily illicit) injection and noninjection drugs; individuals with occupational risks; pregnant women, if risk of infection or severe outcomes is present; all individuals ≥1 year of age with HIV
  - Chronic liver disease (including pre– and post–liver transplant patients); household members and close contacts of children adopted from countries with a high HAV prevalence (prior to arrival); individuals experiencing homelessness or unstable housing; unvaccinated individuals exposed during an outbreak
- Routine vaccination is no longer recommended for those receiving blood products to treat clotting disorders.
- HAV is *not* killed by freezing; HAV is killed by heating surfaces, supplies, or food to >185°F for 60 seconds; direct contact with chlorine is also virucidal.

COMMONLY ASSOCIATED CONDITIONS
HAV can sometimes be associated with rare extrahepatic manifestations.

DIAGNOSIS

- Case definition for acute hepatitis A (1)
- Clinical criteria
  - An acute illness with a discrete onset of any sign or symptom consistent with acute viral hepatitis (e.g., fever, headache, malaise, anorexia, nausea, vomiting, diarrhea, abdominal pain, or dark urine) *and* (i) jaundice or elevated total bilirubin levels ≥3 mg/dL *or* (ii) elevated serum alanine aminotransferase (ALT) levels >200 IU/L *and* (iii) the absence of a more likely diagnosis
- Laboratory criteria for diagnosis confirmatory laboratory evidence:
  - Immunoglobulin M (IgM) antibody to hepatitis A virus (anti-HAV) positive *or* nucleic acid amplification test (NAAT; such as polymerase chain reaction [PCR] or genotyping) for hepatitis A virus RNA positive

- Case classification—meets the clinical criteria and is IgM anti-HAV positive *or* a case that has hepatitis A virus RNA detected by NAAT (such as PCR or genotyping) *or* a case that meets the clinical criteria and occurs in a person who had contact (e.g., household or sexual) with a laboratory-confirmed hepatitis A case 15 to 50 days prior to onset of symptoms

HISTORY
- Onset is often abrupt. Common initial symptoms include nausea, emesis, diarrhea, and headache. Symptom severity increases with age. Pediatric cases (<6 years) are frequently asymptomatic.
- Other presenting historical findings: fever, malaise, fatigue, myalgias, anorexia, joint pain, dark urine (bilirubinuria), right upper abdominal pain, pruritus (can suggest cholestasis)

PHYSICAL EXAM
- Fever (variable); jaundice and icterus present in >70% of adults and older children
- Hepatomegaly and right upper quadrant tenderness are common. Splenomegaly is less common.
- Rare symptoms include lymphadenopathy (especially cervical), arthritis, or rash.
- Asterixis suggests acute hepatic failure.

DIFFERENTIAL DIAGNOSIS
- Hepatitis B, C, D, E; HIV infection, drug-induced hepatitis; toxin-induced hepatitis, alcoholic hepatitis; autoimmune hepatitis; hemochromatosis (adults) or Wilson disease
- Malarial infection; adenovirus infection; Epstein-Barr virus (EBV), cytomegalovirus (CMV), herpes simplex virus, yellow fever; primary or secondary hepatic malignancy; ischemic hepatitis or Budd-Chiari syndrome

DIAGNOSTIC TESTS & INTERPRETATION
Initial Tests (lab, imaging)
- Anti-HAV IgM: positive at time of onset of symptoms sensitivity and specificity >95%; primary test used to diagnose acute infection; anti-HAV IgG: appears soon after IgM and generally persists from years to lifetime
- AST/ALT elevated ~500 to 5,000: ALT usually > AST; alkaline phosphatase: mildly elevated
- Bilirubin: conjugated and unconjugated fractions usually increased; bilirubin rises typically following rise in ALT/AST, consistent with hepatocellular injury pattern.
- Prothrombin time and partial thromboplastin time usually remain normal or near normal. Significant rises should raise concern for acute hepatic failure or coexisting chronic liver disease.
- CBC: mild leukocytosis; aplasia and pancytopenia; thrombocytopenia may predict illness severity.
- Albumin, electrolytes, and glucose to evaluate for hepatic and renal function (rare renal failure)
- Urinalysis (not clinically necessary): bilirubinuria
- Consider ultrasound (US) to rule out biliary obstruction only if lab pattern is cholestatic.

Follow-Up Tests & Special Considerations
Illness usually resolves within 4 weeks of onset. Repeat labs are not indicated unless symptoms persist or new symptoms develop.

Diagnostic Procedures/Other
Abdominal ultrasonography can rule out thrombosis, cirrhosis, and other intra-abdominal pathology.

Test Interpretation
- Positive serum markers in hepatitis A
  - Acute disease: anti-HAV IgM only; recent disease (last 6 months): anti-HAV IgM and IgG positive
  - Previous disease or prior vaccination: anti-HAV IgM negative and IgG positive
- If liver biopsy is obtained, it will show portal inflammation; immunofluorescent stains for HAV antigen positive

 ## TREATMENT

GENERAL MEASURES
- Maintain appropriate nutrition/hydration; avoid alcohol especially during the acute phase.
- Universal precautions to prevent spread (e.g., washing hands, proper handling of food and water)
- Monitor coagulation defects, fluid, electrolytes, acid–base imbalance, hypoglycemia, and renal function; laboratory evaluation including coagulation factors to rule out hepatic failure; refer to liver transplant center for fulminant failure (rare).
- Report cases to public health department.

MEDICATION
- Preexposure vaccination per recommended guidelines; both hepatitis A vaccines in the United States (Havrix, Vaqta) require 2 doses at least 6 months apart (2)[C].
- The ACIP recommends administering the first dose as soon as possible in travelers to endemic areas.
  - For healthy individuals aged 12 months to 40 years, administer a single dose as soon as possible and complete the series within the recommended time frame. In addition, consider concurrent immunoglobulin administration to those aged >40 years, with chronic liver disease, or with immunosuppression if <2 weeks from planned departure. Complete vaccine series within recommended time frame.
  - For patient with contraindications, those refusing vaccination, or those <6 months should receive immunoglobulin therapy (IG).
- Give postexposure prophylaxis to persons who have not previously received HAV vaccine within 2 weeks of exposure to HAV.
  - Administer hepatitis A vaccine series as soon as possible to healthy persons between the ages of 1 and 40 years. Consider IG coadministration for individuals >40 years of age. A second dose of vaccine is not needed if patient has previously received at least 1 dose of vaccine. Administer IG (0.1 mL/kg) to persons <1 year of age.
  - Administer vaccine and IG to individuals with significant comorbidities (immunosuppression, liver disease) not previously vaccinated. A second dose of vaccine is not needed if the patient has previously received at least 1 dose of vaccine.
- Vaccination with same manufacturer is preferred.

- >95% of adults achieve protective antibodies after first vaccine administration and most achieve 100% after receiving their second dose.
- Hepatitis A vaccination is safe during pregnancy.

First Line
No antiviral medications indicated; spontaneous resolution occurs in nearly 99% of patients. Symptom management is recommend. Use caution with acetaminophen; if used, limit to ≤2 g/day. Avoid hepatotoxic agents.

Second Line
- Antiemetics (e.g., ondansetron); IV fluids if patient is presenting with signs of dehydration
- Pruritus: diphenhydramine 50 mg PO IM q6h; consider cholestyramine 4 g BID if cholestasis.

ISSUES FOR REFERRAL
Dictated by severity of illness; hepatic failure, refer to a high-volume liver transplant program

SURGERY/OTHER PROCEDURES
Liver transplant in fulminant hepatic failure—only rare indications

COMPLEMENTARY & ALTERNATIVE MEDICINE
Avoid potentially hepatotoxic botanicals including barberry, comfrey, golden ragwort, groundsel, huang qin, kava kava, pennyroyal, sassafras, senna, valerian, wall germander, and wood sage.

ADMISSION, INPATIENT, AND NURSING CONSIDERATIONS
Treatment is usually outpatient unless signs of liver failure; dictated by severity of illness; treat dehydration and electrolyte imbalances; enteric isolation; private rooms, gowns, and masks are not necessary. 1:100 bleach dilution can be used to clean surfaces; frequent hand washing; use gloves when handling potentially contaminated material.

 ## ONGOING CARE

FOLLOW-UP RECOMMENDATIONS
Return to work/school 10 to 14 days after onset of symptoms. Maintain hygiene as patients remain infectious for up to 4 weeks from symptom onset.

Patient Monitoring
Coagulation defects, fluid and electrolytes, acid–base imbalance, hypoglycemia, renal function

DIET
Adequate balanced nutrition with increased fluid intake; avoid alcohol.

PATIENT EDUCATION
Segregate food handlers with HAV. HAV immunity persists after infection.

PROGNOSIS
- Excellent; case-fatality ratio ranges from 0.1% to 5.4% depending on age and study.
- Risk increased with underlying chronic liver disease and in the elderly (1.8% mortality aged >50 years)

COMPLICATIONS
- Risk of liver failure is higher in patients >50 years of age and those with preexisting liver diseases.
- Relapsing hepatitis—patient can experience symptoms during the 6 months following initial infection. Relapsing phase can last between 3 weeks and 12 months. Present with elevated aminotransferases and persistence of serum anti-HAV IGM antibodies.
- Prolonged cholestasis: characterized by prolonged periods of jaundice, malaise, and pruritus (>3 months); resolves spontaneous
- Autoimmune hepatitis: can be seen after HAV infection; however, responds well to steroids (3)

REFERENCES
1. Centers for Disease Control and Prevention. Hepatitis A questions and answers for health professionals. https://www.cdc.gov/hepatitis/hav/havfaq.htm. Accessed October 30, 2023.
2. Desai AN, Kim AY. Management of hepatitis A in 2020–2021. *JAMA*. 2020;324(4):383–384.
3. Pati I, Cruciani M, Candura F, et al. Hyperimmune globulins for the management of infectious diseases. *Viruses*. 2023;15(7):1543.

ADDITIONAL READING
Yang J, Wang D, Li Y, et al. Metabolomics in viral hepatitis: advances and review. *Front Cell Infect Microbiol*. 2023;13:1189417.

 ## SEE ALSO

- Hepatitis B; Hepatitis C
- Algorithms: Cirrhosis; Hyperbilirubinemia and Jaundice

CODES

ICD10
B15.9 Hepatitis A without hepatic coma

CLINICAL PEARLS
- HAV vaccine is indicated for all children, travelers (particularly to endemic areas), those at elevated risk of disease, and patients with liver impairment.
- Check HAV IgG in all HIV-positive patients; provide HAV vaccine if results are negative.
- HAV disease severity directly correlates with age; children are often asymptomatic.
- Treatment of acute HAV is supportive.
- Eligible patients should receive postexposure prophylaxis within 14 days of exposure.

H

HEPATITIS B

Afsha Rais Kaisani, MD • Tasaduq Hussain Mir, MD, FAAFP • Oregon J. McDiarmid, MD

BASICS

DESCRIPTION
Hepatitis B infection (HBV), caused by a DNA virus, is often transmitted by body fluids (blood, semen, and vaginal secretions). HBV is a serious global health care concern due to the spectrum of liver disease; it can cause ranging from acute hepatitis to cirrhosis and/or hepatocellular carcinoma (HCC).

EPIDEMIOLOGY

Incidence
- Infects patients of all ages; 80% of cases are in persons aged 30 to 59 years (1).
- Predominant sex: fulminant HBV: male > female (2:1)
- Confirmed approximately 3,000 new cases of hepatitis B in United States every year, although it is estimated to be closer to approximately 20,000 new cases that go unconfirmed
- Lower incidence in the United States compared to Asia and Africa due to better access to health care, use of vaccinations, and preventive measure

Prevalence
- During 2020, a total of 11,635 newly identified cases of chronic hepatitis B were reported to CDC, corresponding to a rate of 5 cases per 100,000 people.
- New reported cases of chronic hepatitis B among Asian/Pacific Islander persons (17.6 cases per 100,000 people) were almost 12 times the rate among non-Hispanic white persons (1.5 cases per 100,000 people).
- Chronic HBV worldwide: affects approximately 296 million people, including >6 million children aged <5 years
  - Contributes to an estimated 820,000 deaths every year
  - 25% of chronic hepatitis B infections progress to liver cancer.

ETIOLOGY AND PATHOPHYSIOLOGY
HBV is a DNA virus of the Hepadnaviridae family; two modes of transmission:
- Horizontal: mucosal surface contact with infectious bodily fluids
- Vertical: maternal-to-newborn perinatal

Genetics
Family history of HBV and/or HCC

RISK FACTORS
- The following high-risk groups should be screened for HBV with HBsAg. If HBsAg is positive, test for antibodies to HBsAg (anti-HBs) and hepatitis B core antigen (anti-HBc) to distinguish between infection and immunity. Vaccinate if seronegative (2):
  - Household or sexual contacts with hepatitis B; persons born in regions with increase prevalence (Asia, Africa, Eastern Europe); HIV- and HCV-positive patients
  - Persons born in the United States who were not vaccinated as infants or whose parents are from regions of high prevalence
  - Individuals with chronic liver disease; pregnant women; residents in carceral facilities
- Additional risk factors:
  - Donors and recipients of blood/products; persons on hemodialysis or immunosuppressive therapy; needle stick/occupational exposure; intranasal drug use; body piercing/tattoos; survivors of sexual assault; infants born to mothers positive for hepatitis B surface antigen

Pediatric Considerations
- Shorter acute course; fewer complications
- 90% of vertical/perinatal infections become chronic.

Pregnancy Considerations
- Screen for HBsAg at first prenatal visit (2)[A].
- If HBsAg (+), obtain HBV DNA.
- Consider treating patients with high viral load at 28 weeks or history of previous HBV (+) infant with oral nucleos(t)ide medication beginning at 32 weeks to reduce perinatal transmission. Infants born to HBV-infected mothers require hepatitis B immune globulin (HBIg) and HBV vaccine within 12 hours of birth, completing the vaccine series and serologic testing for infection and immunity by 9 to 12 months.
- Breastfeeding is safe if HBIg and HBV vaccines are administered and the areolar complex is without fissures or open sores. Avoid oral nucleos(t)ide medications during lactation.
- Continue treatment while pregnant to decrease viral load and decrease the chances of vertical transmission.

GENERAL PREVENTION
- Vaccination
  - Three IM injections at 0, 1, and 6 months in infants or healthy adults
  - Indicated for all medically stable infant weighing ≥2,000 g (4 lb, 6 oz) within 24 hours of birth; unvaccinated infants, children, and adults; all at-risk patients; health care and public safety workers; sexual contacts; and household contacts of HBsAg carriers
  - CDC does not recommend administration of >2 complete hepatitis B series except for certain cases related to patients on hemodialysis.
- Other preventive measures
  - Proper hygiene/sanitation by health care workers, IVDUs, and tattoo/piercing artists; barrier precautions, needle disposal, sterilize equipment, cover open cuts; do not share personal items exposed to blood (e.g., nail clipper, razor, toothbrush).
  - Safe sexual practices (condoms)
  - HBsAg carriers cannot donate blood or tissue.
  - Postexposure (e.g., needle stick):
    ○ HBIg 0.06 mL/kg in <24 hours in addition to vaccination (no more than 7 days after exposure)
    ○ Second dose of HBIg should be administered 30 days after exposure.

COMMONLY ASSOCIATED CONDITIONS
- HIV, hepatitis C coinfection
- Extrahepatic manifestations include:
  - Serum sickness-like syndrome (fever, erythematous rash, myalgias, arthralgias, fatigue); glomerulonephritis (membranous or membranoproliferative glomerulonephritis, IgA-mediated nephropathy)
  - Polyarteritis nodosa (primary systemic necrotizing vasculitis, high fever, weakness, malaise, loss of weight and appetite); dermatologic conditions (bullous pemphigoid, lichen planus, Gianotti-Crosti syndrome); cryoglobulinemia (Raynaud phenomenon, arthritis, sicca syndrome)
  - Neurologic/psychological condition (Guillain-Barré syndrome, altered mental status, depression/psychosis)

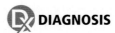

DIAGNOSIS

HISTORY
Exposure: detailed family history, such as HBV infection and liver disease, vaccinations status, and social history including alcohol use, drug use, and sexual history
- Acute HBV
  - Fever, fatigue, arthralgias, myalgias, anorexia, nausea, vomiting, right upper quadrant (RUQ) abdominal pain
  - Jaundice/scleral icterus, dark urine, pale stools
- Chronic HBV: typically asymptomatic

PHYSICAL EXAM
Evaluate for stigmata of chronic liver disease: jaundice/scleral icterus, RUQ tenderness, hepatomegaly, palmar erythema, ascites, spider nevi, hepatic encephalopathy.

DIFFERENTIAL DIAGNOSIS
- Epstein-Barr virus (EBV); cytomegalovirus (CMV); hepatitis A, C, D, or E
- Drug-induced, alcoholic, or autoimmune hepatitis
- Wilson disease; hemochromatosis; HIV

DIAGNOSTIC TESTS & INTERPRETATION

Initial Tests (lab, imaging)
- AST/ALT: markedly elevated in acute HBV, ALT typically higher than AST
  - Transaminases may be normal or mildly elevated in chronic HBV; may increase before bilirubin
- Bilirubin (conjugated/unconjugated): normal to markedly elevated in acute HBV; last test to normalize as acute infection resolves
- Alkaline phosphatase: mild elevation
- HBcAb IgM may be the only early finding ("window period" before HBsAg is positive).
- For acute hepatitis:
  - PT/INR, albumin, electrolytes, glucose, and CBC; if severe acute HBV, check for superinfection with hepatitis D (HDV Ag and HDV Ab); hepatitis B serologic markers
- Hepatitis B e-antigen (HBeAg+) indicates high replication/infectivity; confirmed with high HBV DNA ($\geq 10^5$ copies/mL); benefit from medical therapy
- Screen for HDV, HIV, HCV, and immunity to hepatitis A virus (HAV Ab total/IgG).
  - Acute HBV and HDV coinfection tends to be more severe than acute HBV infection alone.
  - 10% of patients with HIV have coinfection/chronic HBV, making treatment of each more complex.
- Ultrasound to document ascites, organomegaly, signs of portal hypertension, hepatic or portal obstruction, and screen for HCC

Follow-Up Tests & Special Considerations
- Chronic HBV: HBsAg+ persistence >6 months; has five distinct phases based on HBsAg, HBeAg, HBV DNA, ALT, liver inflammation: immune tolerant, immune reactive HBeAg positive, inactive carrier, HBeAg negative, and occult hepatitis B
  - Measure HBV DNA level and ALT q3–6 mo.
  - If aged >40 years and ALT borderline or mildly elevated, consider liver biopsy.
  - Measure baseline AFP.
  - Follow HBeAg for elimination q6–12mo.
- Screening for HCC (2)
  - HCC surveillance recommended for all patients with viral load >100,000 copies/mL
  - Abdominal ultrasound and α-fetoprotein testing every 6 months as screening for HCC; if ultrasound is abnormal, CT or MRI of the liver is recommended.
  - Continue surveillance even after treatment.

Marker	Acute Infection	Chronic Infection	Inactive Carrier	Resolved Infection	Susceptible to Infection	Vaccinated
HBsAg	+	+	+	−	−	−
Anti-HBs	−	−	−	+	−	+
Anti-HBc	+IgM	−IgM; +total/IgG	+	+	−	−
HBeAg	+	±	−	−	−	−
Anti-HBe	−	±	+	±	−	−
HBV DNA	Present	Present	Low negative	−	−	−
ALT	Marked elevation	Normal to mildly elevated	Normal	Normal	Normal	Normal

 TREATMENT

GENERAL MEASURES
- Vaccinate for HBV if seronegative.
- Monitor CBC, coagulation, electrolytes, glucose, and renal function. Monitor ALT and HBV DNA; increased ALT and reduced DNA imply response to therapy. Screen for HCC if HBsAg+.
- High risk for developing HCC with chronic HBV infection—needs routine monitoring

MEDICATION
Goals of therapy: loss of HBsAg with sustained HBV DNA suppression, improvement in patient-oriented outcomes, HBeAg loss/seroconversion, and ALT normalization

First Line
- Acute HBV
  - Supportive care; spontaneously resolves in 95% of immunocompetent adults
  - Antiviral therapy is not indicated except for fulminant liver failure or immunosuppressed.
  - Treat patients with severe or protracted course and those with acute liver failure.
  - Treatment options include monotherapy with tenofovir or entecavir.
- Chronic HBV: treatment per HBeAg status:
  - FDA-approved drugs: lamivudine 100 mg, adefovir 10 mg, entecavir* 0.5 to 1.0 mg, telbivudine 600 mg, or tenofovir alafenamide* 25 mg, all given PO every day (dose based on renal function and age); pegylated interferon (peg-IFN) α2a (Pegasys)*, α2b SC weekly for 48 weeks (2)[A]
  - *Recommended as first-line treatment options for chronic hepatitis B

- Extended oral regimens are indicated (2)[A].
  - If HBeAg+, treat 6 to 12 months post disappearance of antigen and gain of antibody.
  - If HBeAg−, treat indefinitely or until clearance of antigen with antibody development.
- Change/add drug based on resistance; confirm medication adherence prior to assuming drug resistance.
- Precautions:
  - Oral drugs: renal insufficiency
  - Peg-IFN: coagulopathy, myelosuppression, depression/suicidal ideation

ISSUES FOR REFERRAL
Referral to hepatology and transplant for all persistent HBsAg+ patients, fulminant acute hepatitis, end-stage liver disease, or HCC.

SURGERY/OTHER PROCEDURES
Liver transplantation, operative resection, radiofrequency ablation for HCC

 ONGOING CARE

FOLLOW-UP RECOMMENDATIONS
Patient Monitoring
- Serial ALT and HBV DNA: high ALT + low HBV DNA associated with favorable therapy response
- WBC and platelets if on interferon therapy
- Monitor HBV DNA q3–6mo during therapy:
  - Undetectable DNA at week 24 of oral therapy associated with low resistance at year 2
- Monitor for complications (ascites, encephalopathy, variceal bleed) in cirrhosis.
- Vaccination status
- Ultrasound q6–12mo to screen for HCC starting at age 40 years in men and age 50 years in women (2)[B]

DIET
Alcohol increases risk of cirrhosis or HCC.

PATIENT EDUCATION
- Acute HBV: Review transmission precautions.
- Chronic HBV, alcohol and tobacco use accelerate progression. Emphasize medication compliance to prevent flare.
- Counsel chronic HBV carriers regarding risk of transmission to others.
- Immunizations, especially against hepatitis A

PROGNOSIS
Chronic hepatitis B:
- Once HBV is diagnosed, the 5-year cumulative incidence of developing cirrhosis is ~8–20% in those with untreated chronic HBV. Of patients with chronic HBV, 2–5% will progress to HCC with or without presence of cirrhosis.

COMPLICATIONS
- Hepatic necrosis; cirrhosis; hepatic failure; HCC (all chronic HBV are at risk)
- Severe flare of chronic HBV with corticosteroids and other immunosuppressants
- Reactivation of infection if immunosuppressed; premedicate prophylactically if HBsAg+ or if HBcAb+ and receiving systemic chemotherapy.

REFERENCES
1. Schillie S, Vellozzi C, Reingold A, et al. Prevention of hepatitis B virus infection in the United States: recommendations of the Advisory Committee on Immunization Practices. *MMWR Recomm Rep*. 2018;67(1):1–31.
2. Wilkins T, Sams R, Carpenter M. Hepatitis B: screening, prevention, diagnosis, and treatment. *Am Fam Physician*. 2019;99(5):314–323.

ADDITIONAL READING
Centers for Disease Control and Prevention. 2019 Viral hepatitis surveillance report. https://www.cdc.gov/hepatitis/statistics/2019surveillance/index.htm. Accessed November 8, 2023.

 SEE ALSO

Cirrhosis of the Liver; Hepatitis A; Hepatitis C

 CODES

ICD10
- B19.10 Unspecified viral hepatitis B without hepatic coma
- B16.9 Acute hepatitis B w/o delta-agent and without hepatic coma
- B18.1 Chronic viral hepatitis B without delta-agent

CLINICAL PEARLS
- Screen all patients born in countries with endemic disease for HBV infection using HBsAg.
- Chronic HBV is present if HBsAg persists >6 months. Patients with chronic HBV need lifetime monitoring for disease progression and HCC.
- Acute HBV is diagnosed with HBsAg and IgM anti-HBc; treatment is supportive.
- Antiviral therapy is based on the presence or absence of cirrhosis, the ALT level, and HBV DNA levels.

Chronic Hepatitis B Therapy (2)

HBeAg	HBV DNA Viral Load	ALT[a]	Recommend
+	≥20,000 IU/mL	Elevated	Treat with antiviral or interferon.
+	≥20,000 IU/mL	Elevated but <2 × ULN	Monitor every q3–6mo; treat if biopsy shows moderate fibrosis.
+	≥20,000 IU/mL	Normal	Observe q6mo; consider treatment if ALT is elevated. Biopsy if aged >40 years or if ALT is high normal to mild elevation.
−	≥2,000 IU/mL	Elevated	Treatment is indicated.
−	≥2,000 IU/mL	Elevated but <2 × ULN	Consider biopsy or serum fibrosis marker and treatment if findings are concerning.
−	≥2,000 IU/mL	Normal	Monitor q3mo.
−	≤2,000 IU/mL	Normal	Monitor q3–6mo.
Cirrhosis	Any	Any	Treat with mono or combination treatment.
Liver failure	Any	Any	Treat and refer for transplant.

[a]ALT elevated if >2 × ULN; ULN for male = 30 IU/mL and for female = 19 IU/mL

HEPATITIS C

Matthew Nodelman, MD • Morgan Adams Rhodes, PharmD

BASICS

DESCRIPTION
Systemic viral infection involving the liver

EPIDEMIOLOGY
Geriatric Considerations
Patients aged >60 years may be less responsive to therapy, as they are more likely to have advanced fibrosis or cirrhosis at time of diagnosis (1).

Pregnancy Considerations
- Routine prenatal HCV testing
- For HCV-infected mothers, retest HCV RNA postpartum to evaluate for spontaneous clearance.

Pediatric Considerations
- Test children born to HCV-positive mothers (at 18 months of age).
- HCV-positive children have no restrictions for participation in regular childhood activities.
- Treatment starts ≥3 years of age (1),(2)

Incidence
- Incidence of acute hepatitis C has more than doubled since 2013.
- IV drug use accounts for ~60–70% of new cases.

Prevalence
- HCV is the most common cause of chronic liver disease and transplantation in the United States.
- There are eight known genotypes (GT) with 86 subtypes. GT 1 is the predominant form, 75% in the United States and ~46% worldwide. GT predicts response to treatment (1).

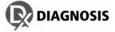 DIAGNOSIS

HISTORY
- Determine exposure risk: detailed social history, including alcohol and IV drug use, psychiatric and medical comorbidities, and coinfections.
- Chronic HCV: Most cases are mildly symptomatic (nonspecific fatigue, depression) or asymptomatic (isolated elevation in ALT, AST).
- Acute HCV: typically asymptomatic, but may result in mild illness
  - Average onset of symptoms (if present) is 2 to 12 weeks postexposure.
  - Fatigue, jaundice, dark urine, steatorrhea, nausea, abdominal pain, low-grade fevers, myalgias, arthralgias (1),(2)

PHYSICAL EXAM
- May have RUQ tenderness/hepatomegaly and/or jaundice
- Signs of advanced fibrosis/cirrhosis: spider angioma, caput medusa, palmar erythema, jaundice, gynecomastia, Terry nails
- HCV-associated conditions with pertinent physical exam findings: arthralgias/myalgias, neuropathy (decreased sensation), sun-exposed skin blisters (PCT), livedo reticularis, lichen planus (palpable purpura), acanthosis nigricans, enlarged lymph node

DIFFERENTIAL DIAGNOSIS
Hepatitis A or B; EBV, CMV; alcoholic hepatitis; non-alcoholic steatohepatitis (NASH); hemochromatosis; Wilson disease, α_1-antitrypsin deficiency; ischemic, drug-induced, or autoimmune hepatitis

DIAGNOSTIC TESTS & INTERPRETATION
Initial Tests (lab, imaging)
Screening
- One-time, routine HCV antibody (Ab) screening for all adults aged 18 to 79 years
- Screen patients <18 years of age or >79 years of age if high risk (see above) or if persistently elevated ALT.

Follow-Up Tests & Special Considerations
- Anti-HCV Ab
  - If nonreactive, no further action unless exposure within the last 6 months (Test with HCV RNA.)
  - If reactive, test for HCV RNA.
    - If not detected, no current HCV infection and no further action required
    - If detected, current HCV infection confirmed
- Anti-HCV Ab detected 4 to 10 weeks after infection
  - ~97% of patients with HCV will develop antibodies by 6 months after exposure.
- HCV RNA detected as early as 1 to 2 weeks after infection

Pretreatment Testing and Assessment
- Recommend CBC, liver function tests, INR, and eGFR within 6 months of starting HCV treatment.
- Screening for HIV coinfection
- Hepatitis B infection or immunity status
  - Hep B surface antigen (+ means coinfection)
  - Hep B core antibody
  - Hep B surface antibody

Diagnostic Procedures/Other
Evaluate for hepatic fibrosis:
- AASLD/IDSA guidelines recommend calculating FIB-4 score prior to initiation of treatment.
- Liver imaging: ultrasound (US), CT scan, MRI, transient US elastography, MR elastography
- Liver biopsy (gold standard)

Test Interpretation
- FIB-4 scoring: https://www.hepatitisc.uw.edu/page/clinical-calculators/fib-4
  - Score >3.25 indicates advanced fibrosis.
- Sustained virologic response (SVR): undetectable HCV RNA after 12 weeks; considered a virologic cure of HCV infection

TREATMENT

GENERAL MEASURES
- Goal is to achieve SVR, reduce adverse events (including progression to cirrhosis and hepatocellular carcinoma) and all-cause mortality.
- Report acute HCV to state health department.
- Treat all patients with virologic evidence of HCV.
- Exceptions: children <3 years of age, pregnancy, short life expectancy

MEDICATION
First Line
- Patients are first divided into those without cirrhosis and those with compensated cirrhosis.
- There are two treatment algorithms for simplified treatment or nonsimplified treatment. Simplified treatment does not require a genotype in most cases to guide treatment.
- Simplified treatment guidelines for patients without cirrhosis (https://www.hcvguidelines.org/treatment-naive/simplified-treatment) and with compensated cirrhosis (https://www.hcvguidelines.org/treatment-naive/simplified-treatment-compensated-cirrhosis)

- For all treatments, review all patient medications (including over-the-counter medications and supplements) for drug interactions with HCV treatment (https://www.hep-druginteractions.org/).
- Screen for hepatitis B infection as all medications for hepatitis C carry a black box warning for hepatitis B reactivation.

Second Line
If a patient fails initial DAA treatment, alternative regimens can be considered for treatment experienced patients, such as:
- Sofosbuvir (400 mg)/velpatasvir (100 mg)/voxilaprevir (100 mg) (SOF/VEL/VOX) +/− weight-based ribavirin
- Glecaprevir (300 mg)/pibrentasvir (120 mg) plus daily sofosbuvir (400 mg) and weight-based ribavirin

ISSUES FOR REFERRAL
- Referral to gastroenterology, hepatology or infectious disease specialists if a patient fails to achieve SVR with initial first-line treatment
- Refer to liver transplant program if fulminant acute hepatitis, complication of end-stage disease, decompensated cirrhosis or HCC.

ADDITIONAL THERAPIES
Chronic HCV treatment with traditional agents, pegylated interferon (PEG-IFN) and ribavirin, is often poorly tolerated and less effective than DAA treatments, which limits consideration as first-line treatment. Patients previously treated with PEG-IFN and ribavirin can be treated with first-line options.

SURGERY/OTHER PROCEDURES
See "Follow-Up Recommendations."

COMPLEMENTARY & ALTERNATIVE MEDICINE
Patients should be counseled to avoid supplements and over-the-counter medications while taking hepatitis C treatments to avoid the potential for drug interactions.

ADMISSION, INPATIENT, AND NURSING CONSIDERATIONS
Standard precautions

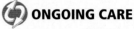 ONGOING CARE

FOLLOW-UP RECOMMENDATIONS
- Serial viral loads are normally not required, unless a patient has inadequate medication adherence, but all patients treated should have a viral load completed 12 weeks after therapy completion.
- AASLD and IDSA recommend an abdominal US every 6 months for patients with cirrhosis, with or without serum α-fetoprotein (AFP) to monitor for HCC.
- If cirrhosis is present, patients need endoscopic screening for varices.
  - Compensated cirrhosis without known varices: endoscopic evaluation every 2 to 3 years
  - Cirrhosis with known varices: endoscopic surveillance every 1 to 2 years (2)

Patient Monitoring
- 8- to 12-week course of therapy
- No routine monitoring while on treatment, except to assess medication adherence
- SVR12: Undetectable HCV RNA 12 weeks after completing therapy generally translates to long-term cure (goal of therapy).
- If no evidence of cirrhosis, once SVR is achieved, there is no recommendation for continued surveillance. The AASLD and IDSA guidelines currently recommend treating the patient as if they have never had HCV.

Medications	Abbreviation	Standard Dose	Common Side Effects (>10%); Contraindications
A: Elbasvir-grazoprevir (Zepatier)	ELB/GZR	50 mg/100 mg daily	Fatigue, headaches; avoid with OATP1B1/3 inhibitors or CYP3A inducers.
B: Glecaprevir-pibrentasvir (Mavyret)	GLEC/PIB	300 mg/120 mg daily	Fatigue, headaches, nausea, diarrhea, pruritus; must take with food; take 3 tablets at the same time each day.
C: Ledipasvir-sofosbuvir (Harvoni)	LED/SOF	90 mg/400 mg daily	Fatigue, headaches, weakness, irritability, insomnia, dizziness, depression, nausea, diarrhea, myalgias, cough
D: Sofosbuvir-velpatasvir (Epclusa)	SOF/VEL	400 mg/100 mg daily	Fatigue, headaches, irritability, insomnia, depression, rash, nausea, weakness

Simplified regimen for noncirrhotic patients:
- **B for 8 weeks OR D for 12 weeks**

Simplified regimen for compensated cirrhotic patients:
- **For GT 1–6: regimen B for 8 weeks**

OR

- **For GT 1, 2, 4, 5, 6: regimen D for 12 weeks**
- **For GT 3—NS5A RAS testing results dictate treatment regimen:**
  - **If NO Y93H: can be treated with regimen D for 12 weeks**

Genotype-Directed Nonsimplified Treatment Regimens for Treatment-Naive Patients (Genotype, Regimen, Duration, Evidence):

Without Cirrhosis

Genotype 1a	Genotype 1b	Genotype 2	Genotype 3	Genotype 4	Genotypes 5 or 6
GLEC/PIB × 8 weeks (1A)	GLEC/PIB × 8 weeks (1A)	GLEC/PIB × 8 weeks (1A)	GLEC/PIB × 8 weeks (1A)	GLEC/PIB × 8 weeks (1A)	GLEC/PIB × 8 weeks (1A)
LED/SOF × 12 weeks (1A)	SOF/VEL × 12 weeks (1A)	SOF/VEL × 12 weeks (1A)	SOF/VEL × 12 weeks (1A)	SOF/VEL × 12 weeks (1A)	SOF/VEL × 12 weeks (1B)
SOF/VEL × 12 weeks (1A)	ELB/GZR × 12 weeks (1A)			ELB/GZR × 12 weeks (1A)	LED/SOF × 12 weeks (IIaB)
LED/SOF × 8 weeks (HIV-uninfected, HCV viral load <6 million IU/mL) (1B)	LED/SOF × 12 weeks (1A)			LED/SOF × 12 weeks (1A)	
	LED/SOF × 8 weeks (HIV-uninfected, HCV viral load <6 million IU/mL) (1B)				

With Compensated Cirrhosis

Genotype 1a	Genotype 1b	Genotype 2	Genotype 3	Genotype 4	Genotype 5 or 6
SOF/VEL × 12 weeks (1A)	SOF/VEL × 12 weeks (1A)	SOF/VEL × 12 weeks (1A)	SOF/VEL × 12 weeks (1A)[†]	SOF/VEL × 12 weeks (1A)	GLEC/PIB × 8 weeks (1A)
LED/SOF × 12 weeks (1A)	ELB/GZR × 12 weeks (1A)	GLEC/PIB × 8 weeks (1B)	GLEC/PIB × 8 weeks (1B)	GLEC/PIB × 8 weeks (1B)	SOF/VEL × 12 weeks (1B)
GLEC/PIB × 8 weeks (1B)	LED/SOF × 12 weeks (1A)			ELB/GZR × 12 weeks (IIa, B)	LED/SOF × 12 weeks (IIa, B)
	GLEC/PIB × 8 weeks (1B)			LED/SOF × 12 weeks (IIa, B)	

[†]Must complete NS5A resistance-associated substitutions (RASs) for Y93H.

- SVR decreases risk of portal hypertension, hepatic decompensation, and HCC. Monitor for decompensation (low albumin, ascites, encephalopathy, GI bleed, etc.).
- Monitor for HBV reactivation while on medication if the patient has history of HBV infection (DAA side effect).

DIET
- Low-fat, high-fiber diet and exercise to treat obesity/fatty liver
- Avoid alcohol.

PATIENT EDUCATION
- Avoid alcohol, tobacco, and illicit drugs (including marijuana); refer to rehabilitation, 12-step or other program, and monitor for relapse as appropriate.
- Education on risk of transmission to sexual partners and with sharing personal hygiene items
- Caution with nutritional supplements and herbal medications (may contain hepatotoxins and/or have drug interactions with HCV medications)

PROGNOSIS
- Only about 50% of patients with chronic HCV are diagnosed and aware of infection and, despite simple and well-tolerated treatments available, many of those diagnosed patients are not linked to care and treatment.
- Modern treatment regimens have SVR of >95% in most circumstances.

- Approximately 5–25% of patients with chronic HCV develop cirrhosis in 10 to 20 years.
- Patients with HCV and cirrhosis have a 1–4% annual risk of HCC and 3–6% annual risk of hepatic decompensation.
- Following successful SVR, there is an approximate 70% reduction in risk of HCC and 90% reduction in risk of liver-related mortality and liver transplantation (1),(2).

COMPLICATIONS
- Fibrosis and cirrhosis typically develop within the first 5 to 10 years of infection if untreated.
- Risk factors for cirrhosis: age, white race, hypertension, alcohol use, anemia; risk for decompensation: diabetes, hypertension, anemia

REFERENCES
1. Schillie S, Wester C, Osborne M, et al. CDC recommendations for hepatitis C screening among adults—United States, 2020. *MMWR Recomm Rep.* 2020;69(2):1–17.
2. Ghany MG, Morgan TR. Hepatitis C guidance 2019 update: American Association for the Study of Liver Diseases–Infectious Diseases Society of America recommendations for testing, managing, and treating hepatitis C virus infection. *Hepatology.* 2020;71(2):686–721.

SEE ALSO

- Cirrhosis of the Liver; Hepatitis A; Hepatitis B; HIV/AIDS
- Algorithm: Hyperbilirubinemia and Jaundice
- www.hcvguidelines.org

CODES

ICD10
- B19.20 Unspecified viral hepatitis C without hepatic coma
- B17.10 Acute hepatitis C without hepatic coma
- B18.2 Chronic viral hepatitis C

CLINICAL PEARLS
- HCV is the most common cause of HCC in the western world. Genotype 1 is the most common GT in the United States.
- 1 of 10 patients with HCV has no identifiable risk factors; 15–25% of HCV-infected persons clear the infection without specific treatment.
- One-time routine HCV screening in all adults aged 18 to 79 years and HCV testing as part of routine prenatal care are recommended. Screen other patients if high risk.
- Half of all patients with acute HCV develop chronic HCV; 25% of those develop cirrhosis within 20 years.

H

HERNIA
Cecile T. Robes, DO

BASICS

DESCRIPTION
Areas of weakness or disruption of the abdominal wall through which structures can pass
- Types
  - Inguinal
    - Direct: acquired; herniation through defect in transversalis fascia of abdominal wall medial to inferior epigastric vessels; increased frequency with age as fascia weakens
    - Indirect: congenital; herniation lateral to the inferior epigastric vessels through internal inguinal ring into inguinal canal; a "complete hernia" descends into the scrotum, and an "incomplete hernia" remains in the inguinal canal.
  - Pantaloon: combination of direct and indirect inguinal hernia with protrusion of abdominal wall on both sides of the epigastric vessels
  - Femoral: herniation descending through the femoral canal deep to the inguinal ligament; has a narrow neck and is especially prone to incarceration and strangulation
  - Incisional or ventral: herniation through a defect in the anterior abdominal wall at the site of a prior surgical incision
  - Congenital: herniation through defect in abdominal wall fascia due to collagen deficiency disease
  - Umbilical: defect at umbilical ring
  - Epigastric: protrusion through the middle line above the level of the umbilicus
  - Spigelian hernia: herniation through Spigelian line (lateral border of the rectus abdominis) for a lateral ventral hernia result
  - Sports hernia (not a true hernia): strain or tear of soft tissue of groin or lower abdomen
  - Others: obturator, sciatic, perineal
- Definitions
  - Reducible: Extruded sac and its contents can be returned to intra-abdominal position spontaneously or with gentle manipulation.
  - Irreducible/incarcerated: Extruded sac and its contents cannot be returned to original intra-abdominal position.
  - Strangulated: Blood supply to hernia sac contents is compromised.
  - Richter: Partial circumference of the bowel is incarcerated or strangulated. Partial wall damage may occur, increasing potential for bowel rupture and peritonitis.
  - Sliding: Wall of a viscus forms part of the wall of the inguinal hernia sac (i.e., right side–cecum, left side–sigmoid colon).

Geriatric Considerations
Abdominal wall hernias increase with advancing age, with significant increase in risk during surgical repair.

Pregnancy Considerations
- Increased intra-abdominal pressure and hormone imbalances with pregnancy may contribute to increased risk of abdominal wall hernias.
- Umbilical hernias are associated with multiple, prolonged deliveries.

EPIDEMIOLOGY
Incidence
- 75–80% groin hernias: inguinal and femoral
- 2–20% incisional/ventral, depends if prior surgery was associated with infection or contamination
- 3–10% umbilical, considered congenital

- Groin
  - 6–27% lifetime risk in adult men
  - Two peaks: Most inguinal hernias present between the ages of 0 to 5 and 75 to 80 years.
  - ~50% of children aged <2 years have a patent processus vaginalis (this decreases to 40% after the age of 2 years). Only between 25% and 50% are clinically significant.
  - Inguinal hernia in <5% of newborns male-to-female ratio 10:1
  - Increased incidence in premature infants
  - Increased incidence in patients with abdominal aortic aneurysms
  - Femoral <10% of all groin hernias, 40% present as a surgical emergency
- Incisional/ventral: ~10–23% of abdominal surgeries complicated by an incisional hernia, most common in upper midline incisions; females have a higher risk of strangulation and incarceration.
- Incidence ratio: male = female
- Umbilical: 10–20% of newborns; most close by age 5 years

Prevalence
- Groin and inguinal hernias are more prevalent in men; femoral and umbilical more prevalent in women
- Most inguinal hernias are indirect in men and women.
- Incisional/ventral hernias (IVH) are more prevalent in smokers and obese individuals.

ETIOLOGY AND PATHOPHYSIOLOGY
Loss of tissue strength and elasticity (especially with aging or congenital defect in abdominal fascia) results in a fascial defect of the abdominal wall. Most pediatric hernias are congenital (e.g., patent processus vaginalis). Most adult hernias are a result of acquired weakness in the tissues of the anterior abdominal wall.

Genetics
No known genetic pattern

RISK FACTORS
- Increased abdominal pressure, coughing, heavy lifting, constipation, pregnancy, ascites, prostatism, open prostatectomy (carries 4 times of risk), obesity, advancing age (loss of tissue turgor), smoking, steroid use, low birth weight, prematurity
- Age: Femoral and scrotal hernias, along with recurrent groin hernias, are associated with increased risk for acute hernia surgery.

COMMONLY ASSOCIATED CONDITIONS
Obesity, chronic obstructive pulmonary disease, multiple abdominal surgeries, pregnancy, advanced age, Ehlers-Danlos syndrome, Marfan syndrome, polycystic kidney disease (PKD), osteogenesis imperfecta, Down syndrome, abdominal aortic aneurysm

DIAGNOSIS

HISTORY
- May observe protrusion through abdominal wall during increased intra-abdominal pressure (Valsalva maneuver or cough)
- Pain, nausea, vomiting, bloating; relieved with reclining; may signal complication (e.g., strangulation)

PHYSICAL EXAM
- Examine initially with patient standing. During palpation, the patient should cough, strain, or perform Valsalva maneuver to determine the extent of intracavitary content movement. Repeat the exam with patient in supine position.
- Inguinal (superior to inguinal ligament)
  - Direct inguinal hernia: Finger in inguinal canal finds defect of the transversalis fascia as a deep (posterior to anterior) bulge palpated with increased intra-abdominal pressure.
  - Indirect inguinal hernia: Finger in inguinal canal finds a persistent process vaginalis as a bulge (lateral to medial) that may extend into scrotum.
- Femoral (inferior to inguinal ligament): bulge in upper middle thigh; neck of the sac protrudes lateral to and below a finger placed on the pubic tubercle.
- Umbilical: palpable protrusion at umbilicus
- Incisional/ventral: palpable protrusion at site of prior abdominal incision or midline superior to the umbilicus
- Epigastric: palpable protrusion off midline above umbilicus

DIFFERENTIAL DIAGNOSIS
Lymphadenopathy, hydrocele, lipoma, varices, cryptorchidism, abscess, tumor, sports hernia (athletic pubalgia), pelvic fractures, adductor tears, omphalomesenteric duct, urachal cyst

DIAGNOSTIC TESTS & INTERPRETATION
Imaging rarely required; reserve for suspected abdominal hernia or unclear diagnosis; plain radiographs to rule out obstruction
- Ultrasound (US) is the best initial imaging modality for identifying occult inguinal hernia.
- CT or tangential radiography for incisional and abdominal wall hernias and postsurgical patients with complaints of abdominal pain
- If there is difficulty with routine imaging, MRI with Valsalva is an option.
- Herniography is no longer recommended.

Follow-Up Tests & Special Considerations
Patients in whom an occult inguinal hernia is suspected should undergo MRI definitive examination (1)[A],(2).

TREATMENT

- Elective
- Three options for elective inguinal hernia repair: open, laparoscopic, and robotic
- Elective surgical repair is associated with significantly lower morbidity and mortality.
- Acute setting
  - Pain management for symptomatic hernias
  - Strangulated hernias should be surgically repaired early to prevent complications such as necrosis and viscus perforation.
  - Manual reduction of incarcerated hernias improves outcomes by allowing for elective repair after swelling and inflammation subside.
  - Complication rate is greater with emergent pediatric inguinal hernia repairs compared to elective procedures.

- Acute hernia repair carries a higher morbidity and lower survival rate.
- Laparoscopic repair of IVH is safe and has fewer complications, shorter hospital stays, and possibly a shorter surgical time. Postoperative pain and recurrence rates are similar to open repair.
- For patients undergoing repair, operative times are shorter for extraperitoneal laparoscopic repair compared to open mesh repair with no difference in complication rates (2)[B].
- Mesh is generally preferred for hernia repairs; there have been numerous FDA product recalls in the past—primarily related to complications of bowel perforation and obstruction (https://www.fda.gov/medicaldevices/productsandmedical procedures/implant).

MEDICATION

- Antibiotics: Prophylaxis does not reduce wound infections after groin hernia repairs.
- Antibiotics are recommended for uncomplicated inguinal or femoral hernia repairs using mesh or if there are other risks for infection (2)[B].
- Pain: Local anesthetic during surgical repair results in significant reduction of postoperative pain. Tension-free procedures (e.g., Lichtenstein) may be performed under local anesthesia.

ISSUES FOR REFERRAL

Warn patients of symptoms or signs of incarceration or strangulation (acute abdominal pain, fever, bloody bowel movements), which mandate immediate evaluation.

ADDITIONAL THERAPIES

Geriatric Considerations

Use of a truss (external supportive device) for direct inguinal hernias is common; this is primarily for pain control.

SURGERY/OTHER PROCEDURES

Inguinal hernias should be surgically repaired. Watchful waiting in asymptomatic patients is safe if the patient has significant comorbidities that may compromise urgent repair.

- Incarceration and strangulation are absolute indications for hernia repair.
- Contraindications: patients who are not surgical candidates based on risk factors
  - Avoid elective repair in pregnant patients or patients with active infections.
- Special considerations
  - Umbilical hernias <0.5 cm can usually be followed clinically.
  - Umbilical hernias in children aged 2 to 4 years typically close spontaneously.
  - Operative times and complication rates are similar when comparing single-incision laparoscopic inguinal hernia repair versus traditional multiport laparoscopic repair (3)[B].
  - "Watchful waiting" is recommended in pregnancy. Elective postpartum repair has similar outcomes and no increased risk of incarceration or strangulation before or during delivery.
  - Women have lower recurrence rates using laparoscopic compared with open method.
  - Ascites is not a strict contraindication for repair.

- Gold standard
  - Inguinal hernia
    - Open: Lichtenstein with mesh (37%): decreased recurrence rates
    - Laparoscopic (14%) with mesh: decreased hospital stay and postoperative pain
      - Requires general anesthesia
      - Transabdominal preperitoneal (TAPP) versus total extraperitoneal (TEP)
      - Robotic repair can be a consideration although the procedure is longer than open or laparoscopic and may have 30-day operative complications of ~5% versus ~1% for other techniques (4)[B].
    - Pediatric: Laparoscopic percutaneous repair is an efficient, safe, and effective alternative to open repair. It is associated with reduced operative times and no increase in complication or recurrence rates. Avoid mesh in pediatric patients (4)[B].
  - Incisional/ventral
    - Laparoscopic repair is effective for most patients with primary or recurrent ventral hernias; there is <10% recurrence rate.
  - Umbilical
    - Pediatric: open excision with suture closure
    - Adult: Open repair with mesh may reduce hernia recurrence.
- Complications
  - Recurrence
  - Seromas
  - Postoperative pain, temporary or chronic: less with laparoscopic versus open technique
  - Wound infection
  - Injury to cord structures in inguinal herniorrhaphy; with nerve injury, most symptoms will resolve.

 ## ONGOING CARE

PATIENT EDUCATION

Cleveland Clinic: https://my.clevelandclinic.org/health/diseases/15757-hernia

PROGNOSIS

- Groin (pediatric): low recurrence rates (<3%) with surgery; may spontaneously resolve in infants
- Groin (adult): ≥1% per year risk of bowel strangulation without surgical treatment; 0–10% postoperative recurrence rates, depending on surgeon experience and procedure type
- Incisional/ventral: 3–5% postoperative occurrence: 2–17% postrepair recurrence, increased to 20–46% in larger hernias
- Umbilical (pediatric)
  - High rate of spontaneous resolution
  - Hernia less likely to close further in older children and in children with larger defects
- Umbilical (adult): up to 11% postoperative recurrence
- Epigastric: most ultimately become incarcerated and/or strangulated without surgical treatment. Recurrence is high due to frequency of missed defects during repair.

REFERENCES

1. Orelio CC, van Hessen C, Sanchez-Manuel FJ, et al. Antibiotic prophylaxis for prevention of postoperative wound infection in adults undergoing open elective inguinal or femoral hernia repair. *Cochrane Database Syst Rev*. 2020;4(4):CD003769.
2. Lockhart K, Dunn D, Teo S, et al. Mesh versus non-mesh for inguinal and femoral hernia repair. *Cochrane Database Syst Rev*. 2018;9(9):CD011517.
3. Buckley FP III, Vassaur H, Monsivais S, et al. Comparison of outcomes for single-incision laparoscopic inguinal herniorrhaphy and traditional three-port laparoscopic herniorrhaphy at a single institution. *Surg Endosc*. 2014;28(1):30–35.
4. Timberlake MD, Sukhu TA, Herbst KW, et al. Laparoscopic percutaneous inguinal hernia repair in children: review of technique and comparison with open surgery. *J Pediatr Urol*. 2015;11(5): 262.e1–262.e6.

ADDITIONAL READING

- Berger D. Evidence-based hernia treatment in adults. *Dtsch Arztebl Int*. 2016;113(9):150–157.
- Pereira JA, López-Cano M, Hernández-Granados P, et al; for Spanish National Registry of Incisional Hernia (EVEREG). Initial results of the National Registry of Incisional Hernia. *Cir Esp*. 2016;94(10):595–602.
- Schmidt L, Öberg S, Andresen K, et al. Recurrence rates after repair of inguinal hernia in women: a systematic review. *JAMA Surg*. 2018;153(12): 1135–1142.

 SEE ALSO

Algorithms: Abdominal Pain, Lower; Intestinal Obstruction; Pelvic Pain

CODES

ICD10

- K46.9 Unspecified abdominal hernia without obstruction or gangrene
- K40.90 Unil inguinal hernia, w/o obst or gangr, not spcf as recur
- K41.90 Unil femoral hernia, w/o obst or gangrene, not spcf as recur

CLINICAL PEARLS

- Inguinal hernias are either direct or indirect:
  - Direct: acquired herniation through defect in transversalis fascia of abdominal wall medial to inferior epigastric vessels
  - Indirect: congenital herniation lateral to the inferior epigastric vessels; a "complete hernia" descends into the scrotum; an "incomplete hernia" remains within the inguinal canal.
- Femoral: descends through the femoral canal deep to the inguinal ligament
- Umbilical: Defect occurs at umbilical ring tissue. Most pediatric umbilical hernias close spontaneously within the first few years of life.
- Incarceration and strangulation are the primary complications associated with hernias.
- For hernias in women and bilateral hernias, a laparoscopic endoscopic procedure is preferable.

H

HERPES EYE INFECTIONS

Stephanie L. Conway-Allen, PharmD, RPh • Kathleen A. Barry, MD

BASICS

DESCRIPTION
- Eye infection (blepharitis, conjunctivitis, keratitis, stromal keratitis, uveitis, retinitis, glaucoma, or optic neuritis) caused by herpes simplex virus (HSV) types 1 or 2 or varicella-zoster virus (VZV, also known as human herpes virus type 3 [HHV3])
  - HSV: most often affects the cornea (herpes keratoconjunctivitis); HSV1 > HSV2; can be further divided into primary and recurrent
  - VZV: When VZV is reactivated and affects the ophthalmic division of the 5th cranial nerve, this is known as herpes zoster ophthalmicus (HZO)—a type of shingles.
- System(s) affected: eye, skin, central nervous system (CNS) (neonatal)

EPIDEMIOLOGY
Predominant age: HSV—mean age of onset 37.4 years but can occur at any age, including primary infection in newborns; VZV—usually advancing age (>50 years)

Incidence
- HSV keratitis: In Europe, North America, and South America, approximated at 12.5 to 31.5 new or recurrent cases per 100,000 person-years (1)
- VZV: 1 million new cases of shingles per year in the United States; 25–40% develop ophthalmic complications. Temporary keratitis is most common.

Prevalence
VZV: Prevalence of herpes zoster infection is 20–30%. Ocular involvement in 50% if not treated with antivirals; overall lifetime prevalence of HZO: 1%

ETIOLOGY AND PATHOPHYSIOLOGY
- HSV and VZV are herpesviridae dsDNA viruses.
- HSV: primary infection from direct contact with infected person via saliva, genital contact, or birth canal exposure (neonates)
  - Primary infection may lead to severe disease in neonates, including eye, skin, CNS, and disseminated disease.
  - Recurrent infection is more common overall cause of herpetic eye infections.
- VZV: Primary infection from direct contact with infected person may cause varicella ("chickenpox") and/or lead to a latent state within trigeminal ganglia.
  - Reactivation of the virus may affect any dermatome (resulting in herpes zoster or "shingles"), including the ophthalmic branch (HZO).

RISK FACTORS
- HSV: personal history of HSV or close contact with HSV-infected person
  - General risk factors for reactivation: stress, trauma, fever, UV light exposure, other viral infections
  - Risk factors for HSV keratitis: UV laser eye treatment, some topical ocular medications such as prostaglandin analogues, and primary/secondary immunosuppression
- HZO
  - History of varicella infection, advancing age (>50 years), sex (female > male), acute/painful prodrome, trauma, stress, immunosuppression (2)

GENERAL PREVENTION
- Contact precautions with active lesions (HSV and VZV)
- VZV can be spread to those who have not had chickenpox, are not immunized, or are not immune.
- Varicella recombinant zoster vaccine (Shingrix) (VZV only): 2 doses 2 to 6 months apart recommended by the CDC for all persons aged ≥50 years
  - Do not give varicella vaccine during an acute infection.
- Acyclovir can be used prophylactically to prevent recurrence of ocular HSV.

Pregnancy Considerations
- Pregnant women without history of chickenpox should avoid contact with persons with active zoster.
- Pregnancy increases risk of recurrence of HSV/VZV.
- Shingrix is contraindicated during pregnancy.

COMMONLY ASSOCIATED CONDITIONS
Primary and secondary immunocompromised states

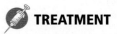DIAGNOSIS

HISTORY
- Varies according to the virus and the ocular structures involved
- History of varicella or herpes simplex infection
- Acute onset, eye pain, headache, photophobia, tearing, ocular redness, decreased or blurry vision (2)
- May present with a prodromal period of fever, malaise, headache, and eye pain before skin eruptions and eye lesions (HZO) (2)

PHYSICAL EXAM
- Varies according to the virus and ocular structures involved
  - HSV most commonly affects the corneal epithelium.
  - VZV most commonly affects corneal stroma and uvea (2).
- Typically unilateral in presentation
  - HZO presents as early as 1 to 2 days after unilateral vesicular eruption in a dermatomal pattern (2).
- Decreased visual acuity
- Conjunctival injection near the limbus
- Decreased corneal sensation
- Dendritic pattern seen with conjunctival florescence staining

DIFFERENTIAL DIAGNOSIS
- Any other cause of red, painful eye
  - Bacterial, fungal, allergic, or other viral conjunctivitis
  - Acute angle-closure glaucoma
- Corneal abrasion, recurrent corneal erosion, toxic conjunctivitis
- Temporal arteritis; trigeminal neuralgia

DIAGNOSTIC TESTS & INTERPRETATION
Initial Tests (lab, imaging)
Typically none needed, as diagnosis is based on history and physical exam (2)[C]
- Corneal swab for HSV DNA by polymerase chain reaction (PCR) (PPV = 96%)
- If vesicle present, can perform a Tzanck smear for VZV or HSV (multinucleated giant cells)
- Antibody titers to assess exposure only; direct fluorescent antibody (DFA); tissue culture

TREATMENT

GENERAL MEASURES
- Avoid contact with nonimmune people.
- No contact lenses should be worn during treatment period.
- Cool compresses, artificial tears, oral pain medications

MEDICATION
First Line
- HSV corneal epithelial disease
  - Trifluridine 1%: Apply 1 drop q2h while awake to a max of 9 drops daily until reepithelialization occurs and then 1 drop q4h for an additional 7 days.
  - Acyclovir: 400 mg PO 5 times per day for 10 days
  - Ganciclovir: 0.15% gel: Apply 1 drop in eye q3h while awake, ~5 times per day, until reepithelialization occurs and then 1 drop q8h for 7 days.
  - Trifluridine and acyclovir cure about 90% of treated eyes within 2 weeks with no significant differences in effectiveness (3)[A].
  - Evidence is conflicting whether ganciclovir is as good as or better than acyclovir (3)[A].
  - Epithelial débridement by an ophthalmologist: may accelerate healing in combination with treatment as above (3)[A]
  - Avoid topical steroids.
- Utility of PO antivirals unclear HSV stromal keratitis or uveitis (without epithelial disease): combination of antiviral and steroid treatment; requires ophthalmology evaluation
  - Prednisolone acetate: 1% drops QID with slow taper (1)[A]
  - Consider systemic steroids in severe uveitis (1)[A].
  - Trifluridine: 1% drops QID for prophylaxis while on topical steroids

- HZO
  - Valacyclovir (Valtrex) 1 g PO TID for 7 to 10 days or famciclovir (Famvir) 500 mg PO TID for 7 to 10 days or acyclovir 800 mg PO 5 times a day for 7 to 10 days
  - Valacyclovir and famciclovir result in significant reduction in PHN compared to acyclovir (number needed to treat [NNT] = 3) with equivalent efficacy (4)[A].
  - Topical antibiotic ophthalmic ointment to protect ocular surfaces (e.g., bacitracin, polymyxin B): 0.5-inch ribbon BID to TID for 7 to 10 days (5)[C]
  - If immunocompromised: acyclovir 10 to 15 mg/kg IV q8h for 10 days
  - Prednisolone acetate: 1% drops QID with slow taper with an ophthalmologist (5)[C]
- Cycloplegic agent if anterior uveitis present; intraocular pressure-lowering agent if necessary

Second Line
- HSV: acyclovir 2 g/day PO in divided doses over 10 days in patients who are intolerant of topical antivirals
- Topical idoxuridine, acyclovir, and brivudine, although approved internationally, are not approved for use in the United States.
- Concomitant treatment with interferon may also improve outcomes, but it is not currently available.

ALERT
HZO: Antiviral therapy is most effective within the first 72 hours of rash onset but should still be initiated >72 hours after onset because of the possible complications of HZO (6)[C].

- Topical antiviral agents
  - Toxic to corneal epithelium, especially after 10 to 14 days of continuous use
- Acyclovir: Reduce dosage in renal insufficiency.
- Topical steroids
  - Prescribe only in consultation with an ophthalmologist.
  - Contraindicated with active corneal epithelial disease, which is best monitored with a slit lamp
  - Can increase intraocular pressure; cause corneal thinning; and, with long-term use, cause cataracts
- Prednisone: caution in immunocompromised patients

ISSUES FOR REFERRAL
Emergent or urgent ophthalmology referral, depending on severity of disease

ADDITIONAL THERAPIES
- Recurrent HSV requires suppressive therapy.
- HZO leading to PHN is common and can be treated with gabapentin or pregabalin, TCAs, opioids, and/or lidocaine gel.

SURGERY/OTHER PROCEDURES
Corneal transplantation for severe scarring or perforation

ADMISSION, INPATIENT, AND NURSING CONSIDERATIONS
- Severe systemic VZV disease
- Systemic HSV in neonates—see "Herpes Simplex Virus, Pediatric."

 ## ONGOING CARE

FOLLOW-UP RECOMMENDATIONS
Patient Monitoring
- Monitor with slit-lamp exam q1–2d until improvement and then q3–4d until epithelial defect resolves.
- Weekly after epithelial disease resolves until off topical antivirals

PATIENT EDUCATION
Educate about the importance of early recognition of recurrent symptoms and need for prompt evaluation and treatment.

PROGNOSIS
- Many cases are self-limited but, depending on the ocular structure involved, can lead to permanent blindness, especially in the setting of recurrent disease.
- Ocular HSV is the number one cause of infectious blindness worldwide.
- Recurrent ocular HSV
  - HSV epithelial disease without treatment
  - Without sequelae, 40% resolve.
  - With treatment, 90–95% resolve without complication.

Pediatric Considerations
- Neonatal primary HSV often disseminated, with high mortality rate; 37% develop vision worse than 20/200.
- Pediatric cases are more likely to be bilateral (26%), recurrent (48% in 15 months old), and may cause amblyopia.

COMPLICATIONS
- Recurrence
- Corneal neovascularization and scarring resulting in poor vision
- Neurotrophic ulcer with perforation
- Secondary bacterial or fungal infection
- Secondary glaucoma in 10%
- PHN in 20–40% with VZV, typically longer lasting in older patients
- Vision loss from optic neuritis or chorioretinitis

REFERENCES

1. Knickelbein JE, Hendricks RL, Charukamnoetkanok P. Management of herpes simplex virus stromal keratitis: an evidence-based review. *Surv Ophthalmol.* 2009;54(2):226–234.
2. Liesegang TJ. Herpes zoster ophthalmicus natural history, risk factors, clinical presentation, and morbidity. *Ophthalmology.* 2008;115(2)(Suppl):S3–S12.
3. Wilhelmus KR. Antiviral treatment and other therapeutic interventions for herpes simplex virus epithelial keratitis. *Cochrane Database Syst Rev.* 2015;1(1):CD002898.
4. McDonald EM, de Kock J, Ram FSF. Antivirals for management of herpes zoster including ophthalmicus: a systematic review of high-quality randomized controlled trials. *Antivir Ther.* 2012;17(2):255–264.
5. Dworkin RH, Johnson RW, Breuer J, et al. Recommendations for the management of herpes zoster. *Clin Infect Dis.* 2007;44(Suppl 1):S1–S26.
6. Carter WP III, Germann CA, Baumann MR. Ophthalmic diagnoses in the ED: herpes zoster ophthalmicus. *Am J Emerg Med.* 2008;26(5):612–617.

 ## SEE ALSO

- Herpes Simplex; Herpes Simplex Virus, Pediatric; Herpes Zoster (Shingles)
- Algorithm: Eye Pain

 ## CODES

ICD10
- B00.50 Herpesviral ocular disease, unspecified
- B02.30 Zoster ocular disease, unspecified
- B00.52 Herpesviral keratitis

CLINICAL PEARLS

- HSV and VZV can lead to a wide array of ocular manifestations, ranging from self-limited disease to potentially vision-threatening disease and complications.
- An exam with fluorescein stain should be performed on all patients with possible HSV keratitis or HZO.
- Topical antiviral treatment is appropriate for HSV, but systemic PO antiviral treatment is necessary for HZO.
- An ophthalmologist should be consulted before prescribing topical steroids. All HZO patients should be referred to an ophthalmologist.
- Hutchinson sign (vesicular lesion on nose from VZV) is a strong indicator of HZO.
- Shingrix is effective at preventing zoster and HZO as well as decreasing the duration of PHN.

HERPES SIMPLEX
Naureen Bashir Rafiq, MD, FAAFP

 BASICS

DESCRIPTION
- Characteristic vesicular rash primarily located in oral and genital regions caused by infection with HSV-1 and HSV-2
- Historically, HSV-1 and HSV-2 caused infection in different areas. HSV-1 in the lips, mouth, face, and eyes and HSV-2 in the genitals. At present, primary genital infection with HSV-1 is as common as with HSV-2.
- Wide range of sequelae, impacted by age and immune status of host, whether the infection is primary or recurrent, and the degree of dissemination
- Viral shedding is typically greatest in the first (primary) infection and lessens with recurrences.

EPIDEMIOLOGY
Affects all ages; most HSV-1 is acquired in childhood, and most HSV-2 is acquired in young–middle adulthood.

Incidence
>1 million new cases of HSV per year

Prevalence
- Widespread; 1–25% of adults may shed HSV-1 or HSV-2. Many are unaware of their infection status.
- HSV-1 about 49% and HSV about 12% (1)
- Prevalence of antibodies to HSV-1 is 90% by adulthood in the general population; 33% of the population infected by age 5 years
- 30% of adults have antibodies to HSV-2.
- According to the WHO, about 417 million people worldwide, ages 15 to 49 years are affected by HSV-1.
- 400 million people have genital herpes caused by HSV-2.
- 1 in 5 pregnant women are seropositive for HSV-2.

ETIOLOGY AND PATHOPHYSIOLOGY
HSV-1 and HSV-2 are double-stranded DNA viruses from the family *Herpesviridae*. HSV-1 and HSV-2 are transmitted by contact with infected skin during periods of viral shedding. Transmission can occur vertically during childbirth.

RISK FACTORS
- Immunocompromised state: advanced age, chemotherapy, malignancy, or chronic diseases such as diabetes or AIDS
- Atopic eczema, especially in children
- Sexual intercourse with infected person (Condoms minimize transmission, but lesions outside condom-protected areas can spread virus.)
- Occupational exposure: dental professionals at higher risk for HSV-1 and resulting herpetic whitlow
- Neonatal herpes simplex: usually via vaginal birth; greatest risk with primary genital herpes infection; incubation is usually from 5 to 7 days (rarely 4 weeks); cutaneous, mucous membrane, or ocular signs seen in only 70%
- Herpes gladiatorum: contact with abrasion sites, often acquired through high-contact sports (such as rugby and wrestling)

GENERAL PREVENTION
- If active lesions are present, avoid direct contact with immunocompromised people, elderly, and newborns.
- Hand hygiene

- Avoid kissing, sharing beverages, sharing utensils, and sharing toothbrushes.
- Genital herpes: Avoid sexual contact if active lesions are present (transmission can occur when disease appears inactive); discuss condom benefits and limits, and encourage safe sex; and consider antiviral therapy to reduce viral shedding.

COMMONLY ASSOCIATED CONDITIONS
- Erythema multiforme: 50% of cases associated with HSV-1 or HSV-2
- Herpetic whitlow, Bell palsy
- Screen all severe, treatment-resistant, or unusual HSV for concurrent HIV infection.

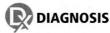 **DIAGNOSIS**

HISTORY
- Many patients are unaware of a known exposure.
- Prodrome of fatigue, low-grade fever, itching, tingling for several days prior to primary outbreak
- Prodrome of pain, burning, tingling, and itching occurs 6 to 48 hours before vesicles in subsequent outbreaks.
- Outbreak precipitated by sunlight, fever, trauma, menses, and stress

PHYSICAL EXAM
- Vesicles are often clustered and become painful ulcerated lesions with erythematous base.
- For more information on genital herpes: See "Herpes, Genital."
- Primary herpetic gingivostomatitis and pharyngitis: early childhood; incubation from 2 to 12 days, followed by fever, sore throat, pharyngeal edema, and erythema
  - Small vesicles on pharynx rapidly ulcerate, and multiply to involve soft palate, buccal mucosa, tongue, floor of mouth, lips, and cheeks; bleeding gums; cervical adenopathy; fever, poor oral intake, and excess salivation; autoinoculation of other sites may occur; resolves in 10 to 14 days
- Primary herpes keratoconjunctivitis: unilateral conjunctivitis with regional adenopathy, blepharitis with vesicles on eyelid; lasts 2 to 3 weeks; systemic involvement prolongs process.
- Eczema herpeticum: painful diffuse pox-like eruption complicating atopic dermatitis; sudden appearance of lesions in typical atopic areas; high fever, localized edema, adenopathy
- Herpetic whitlow: localized painful/itchy infection of a finger, followed by vesicles that may coalesce with swelling and erythema; mimics pyogenic paronychia; neuralgia and axillary adenopathy are possible; heals in 2 to 3 weeks
- Congenital infection (transplacental transmission): jaundice, hepatosplenomegaly, disseminated intravascular coagulation (DIC), encephalitis, seizures, temperature instability, chorioretinitis, and conjunctivitis with/without vesicles
- Recurrent diseases from endogenous reactivation
  - Herpes labialis: recurrent lesions with HSV-1; usually <1 recurrence/6 months, but 5–25% may have >1 attack/month; vesicles vermilion border, ulcerate and crust within 48 hours; heal within 8 to 10 days; may have local adenopathy
  - Ocular herpes: may recur as keratitis, blepharitis, or keratoconjunctivitis; dendritic ulcers, decreased corneal sensation, decreased visual acuity; uveitis may cause permanent visual loss.

DIFFERENTIAL DIAGNOSIS
Impetigo: honey-crusted vesicles; aphthous stomatitis: grayish, shallow erosions with ring of hyperemia of anterior in mouth and lips; herpes zoster: unilateral dermatome distribution; syphilitic chancre: painless genital ulcer; folliculitis: "shave bumps" in genital area; herpangina: vesicles on anterior tonsillar pillars, soft palate, uvula, and oropharynx but not more anteriorly on lips/gums (usually caused by group A coxsackievirus); Stevens-Johnson syndrome: fungal infection; secondary bacterial infection; lymphogranuloma venereum

DIAGNOSTIC TESTS & INTERPRETATION
Initial Tests (lab, imaging)
- Usually a clinical diagnosis; testing should be reserved for atypical presentation and immunocompromised patients.
- Tzanck smear test shows multinucleated giant cells often with eosinophilic intranuclear inclusions (scrape material from lesion to slide, fix with ethanol/methanol, stain with Giemsa or Wright stain)
- HSV culture: gold standard of diagnosis; unroof vesicle, soak swab with fluid, and use swab to scrape the base of the vesicle; must have correct viral swab and media; highest yield if swab collected within 48 hours of outbreak; can take up to 6 days to be positive; highly specific (reliable if positive) but has 20% false-negative rate
- HSV type–specific antibody tests distinguish between HSV-1 and HSV-2
  - 3 weeks after infection, 50% of infected test positive; 70%, 6 weeks after infection; by 16 weeks, nearly all infected test positive
- HSV IgM testing is not clinically useful; can be positive during initial or recurrent infection

Follow-Up Tests & Special Considerations
- No follow up for HSV is needed if adequately treated
- Screen for other sexually transmitted infections (STIs) in patients with primary genital herpes (HIV, gonorrhea, chlamydia, syphilis)

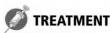 **TREATMENT**

GENERAL MEASURES
- Symptom management while lesions heal
- Cool dressings moistened with aluminum acetate solution
- For genital lesions: Pour a cup of warm water over genitals or sit in a warm bath (sitz bath) while urinating if lesions cause urinary difficulty.
- Children with gingivostomatitis who resist oral intake or have extensive skin disease (eczema herpeticum) may require IV hydration.

MEDICATION
First Line
- Treat promptly, preferably in prodrome
- For episodic treatment of recurrent HSV infection, start treatment within 1 day of symptom onset.
- Offer suppressive therapy to those with severe psychological distress, severe physical pain, or pregnant women after 36 weeks' gestation.
- Topical therapy: penciclovir (Denavir): 1% cream; apply to oral lesions q2h during waking hours for 4 days.

- Acyclovir (generic)
  - Mucocutaneous (or genital) HSV
    - Primary/first infection: 400 mg 5 times per day for 5 days
    - If severe, start with IV q8h dosing for the first few days and then complete 10-day course PO route.
    - Recurrence:
      - 200 mg PO 5 times daily for 5 days
      - 400 mg PO 3 times daily for 5 days
      - 800 mg PO BID for 5 days
      - 800 mg PO 3 times daily for 2 days
    - Suppression: 400 mg BID daily (2)[B]
    - Keratitis HSV: 400 mg PO 5 times per day; topical treatment is preferred as first line.
  - Pediatric dosing: neonatal herpes simplex or encephalitis: 60 mg/kg/day IV divided q8h for 14 to 21 days
    - Older (>3 months of age) immunocompetent is weight-based dosing (40 to 80 mg/kg/day [max of 1,000 mg/day] divided q8h for 5 to 7 days).
  - Safe in pregnancy and lactation—Category B (3),(4)[B]
- Valacyclovir (Valtrex)
  - Herpes labialis: 2,000 mg PO q12h for 1 day
  - Primary genital herpes: 1 g PO BID for 10 days, started within 48 hours of symptoms
  - Recurrent genital herpes: 500 mg PO BID for 3 days, started within 24 hours of symptoms; 500 to 1,000 mg PO daily
  - Suppression: 500 to 1,000 mg/day dose
- Famciclovir (Famvir)
  - Primary genital herpes: 250 mg PO TID for 7 to 10 days
  - Recurrence: 125 mg PO BID for 5 days or 1,000 mg PO BID for 1 day
  - Suppression: 250 mg PO BID
- Precautions
  - Renal dosing for all oral antivirals
  - Significant interactions: Probenecid with IV acyclovir or valacyclovir may reduce renal clearance and elevate antiviral drug levels.

Second Line
- Foscarnet
  - Drug of choice for acyclovir resistance in immunocompromised persons with systemic HSV
  - 40 mg/kg IV q8h (Assume valacyclovir and famciclovir resistance also if acyclovir resistance occurs.)
- Other topicals
  - Ophthalmic preparations: acyclovir, vidarabine (Vira-A), ganciclovir, trifluridine
  - Topical acyclovir and penciclovir improve recurrent herpes labialis healing times by ~10% (3)[B].
  - Topical analgesics: Lidocaine 2% or 5% helps reduce pain associated with vulvar and penile outbreaks.
- Over-the-counter topical antivirals: docosanol

ISSUES FOR REFERRAL
Refer recurrent cases of herpes keratoconjunctivitis to an ophthalmologist.

ADMISSION, INPATIENT, AND NURSING CONSIDERATIONS
Pregnancy Considerations
- Cesarean section and/or acyclovir are indicated if any active genital lesions (or prodrome) present at time of delivery; consider cesarean delivery if primary genital herpes is suspected within previous 4 weeks.
- Daily oral antivirals after 36 weeks of pregnancy with history of genital herpes help to prevent outbreak at the time of delivery.
- Avoid fetal scalp electrodes, forceps, vacuum extractor, and artificial rupture of membranes if mother has history of genital HSV.
- Risk of viral shedding at delivery from asymptomatic recurrent genital HSV is low (~1.6%).
- Primary maternal HSV-1 or HSV-2 infection carries a 60% risk of neonatal infection at time of delivery.

Pediatric Considerations
Neonates with likely exposure at birth or those who exhibit signs of HSV infection should have body fluids cultured and immediately start treatment (IV acyclovir).

 ## ONGOING CARE

FOLLOW-UP RECOMMENDATIONS
- Follow-up not usually necessary; lesions and symptoms resolve within 10 days. Extensive cases should be rechecked in 1 week; monitor for secondary bacterial infections.
- Consider long-term suppression.

DIET
If oral lesions are present, avoid salty, acidic, or sharp foods (e.g., snack chips, orange juice).

PATIENT EDUCATION
- Discuss the natural course of the virus, that timing of exposure is difficult to determine, and that the virus will remain in the body indefinitely. Acknowledging psychological impact helps to reduce stigmatization.
- Emphasize personal hygiene to avoid self-spreading to other body areas or exposing others. Frequent hand washing; avoid scratching; cover active, moist lesions.
- Reinforce safe sexual practices.
- Inform sex partners of infection before starting sexual relationship.

PROGNOSIS
- Usual duration of primary disease is 5 days to 14 days.
- Antiviral treatment shortens duration, reduces complications, and mitigates recurrences (if used for suppression).
- Viral shedding during recurrence is briefer than with primary disease; frequency of recurrence varies depending on individual host factors.

- Newborns/immunocompromised individuals are at highest risk for major morbidity/mortality.
- HSV remains dormant in dorsal root ganglia and can reactivate, causing recurrent symptoms.

COMPLICATIONS
- People with HSV-2 have a higher risk of HIV infection due to open ulcers, facilitating HIV infection during sexual contact.
- Herpes encephalitis; herpes pneumonia, pneumonitis
- Hepatitis; disseminated herpes; acute urinary retention; neonatal infection

REFERENCES
1. McQuillan G, Kruszon-Moran D, Markowitz LE, et al. Prevalence of HPV in adults aged 18–69: United States, 2011–2014. NCHS Data Brief. 2017;(280):1–8.
2. Sauerbrei A. Optimal management of genital herpes: current perspectives. Infect Drug Resist. 2016;9:129–141.
3. Rahimi H, Mara T, Costella J, et al. Effectiveness of antiviral agents for the prevention of recurrent herpes labialis: a systematic review and meta-analysis. Oral Surg Oral Med Oral Pathol Oral Radiol. 2012;113(5):618–627.
4. Sawleshwarkar S, Dwyer DE. Antivirals for herpes simplex viruses. BMJ. 2015;351:h3350.

ADDITIONAL READING
Groves MJ. Genital herpes: a review. Am Fam Physician. 2016;93(11):928–934.

 ## SEE ALSO

- Herpes, Genital
- Algorithm: Genital Ulcers

 ## CODES

ICD10
- B00 Herpesviral [herpes simplex] infections
- B00.0 Eczema herpeticum
- B00.1 Herpesviral vesicular dermatitis

CLINICAL PEARLS
- 25–30% of the U.S. population has serologic evidence of genital herpes (HSV-2), and >80% is seropositive for HSV-1.
- Most individuals are unaware they are infected, allowing for asymptomatic viral transmission.
- Viral suppression for patients with frequent recurrences reduces transmission and decreases outbreak frequency.

H

HERPES ZOSTER (SHINGLES)

Loreal Dolar, DO • Rose Katherine Appel, DO

BASICS

DESCRIPTION
- Results from reactivation of latent varicella-zoster virus (VZV) (human herpesvirus type 3) infection
- Postherpetic neuralgia (PHN) is defined as pain persisting at least 1 month after rash has healed. The term *zoster-associated pain* is more clinically useful.
- Herpes zoster ophthalmicus (HZO) is an important complication involving branch of the trigeminal nerve.
- Zoster usually presents as a painful unilateral vesicular eruption with a dermatomal distribution.
- System(s) affected: nervous; integumentary; exocrine
- Synonym(s): shingles

EPIDEMIOLOGY
Incidence
- Incidence increases with age—2/3 of cases occur in adults aged ≥50 years. Incidence is increasing overall as the U.S. population ages.
- Herpes zoster: 4/1,000 person-years
- PHN: 18% in adult patients with herpes zoster; 33% in patients ≥79 years of age
- Individual lifetime risk of 30% in the United States

Prevalence
~1 million new cases of herpes zoster annually in the United States

Pregnancy Considerations
May occur during pregnancy

Geriatric Considerations
- Increased incidence of zoster outbreaks
- Increased incidence of PHN

Pediatric Considerations
- Occurs less frequently in children
- Has been reported in newborns infected in utero

ETIOLOGY AND PATHOPHYSIOLOGY
Reactivation of VZV from dorsal root/cranial nerve ganglia; on reactivation, the virus replicates within neuronal cell bodies, and virions are carried along axons to dermatomal skin zones, causing local inflammation and vesicle formation.

RISK FACTORS
- Increasing age
- Immunosuppression (malignancy or chemotherapy)
- Physical trauma
- Female

- HIV infection
- Spinal surgery

GENERAL PREVENTION
- Shingrix recombinant herpes zoster vaccination is the preferred vaccine. It is recommended for adults who previously received Zostavax.
- Patients with active zoster may transmit disease-causing varicella virus—typically through direct contact.

COMMONLY ASSOCIATED CONDITIONS
Immunocompromised states, HIV infection, posttransplantation, immunosuppressive drugs, and malignancy

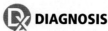

DIAGNOSIS

HISTORY
- Prodromal phase (sensory changes over involved dermatome prior to rash)
  - Tingling, paresthesias
  - Itching
  - Boring "knife-like" pain
  - Allodynia and hyperalgesia
- Acute phase
  - Constitutional symptoms (e.g., fatigue, malaise, headache, low-grade fever) are variable.
  - Dermatomal rash

PHYSICAL EXAM
- Acute phase
  - Rash: initially erythematous and maculopapular; evolves to characteristic grouped vesicles usually in one dermatome but may affect two to three adjacent dermatomes
  - Thoracic and lumbar dermatomes are the most commonly involved sites.
  - Vesicles become pustular and/or hemorrhagic in 3 to 4 days.
  - Weakness in distribution of rash (1%)
  - Rash crusts and resolves by 14 to 21 days.
- Possible sine herpete (zoster without rash) and other chronic disorders associated with VZV without the typical rash
  - HZO; vesicles on tip of the nose (Hutchinson sign) indicate involvement of the external branch of cranial nerve V and are associated with increased incidence of HZO.
- Chronic phase
  - PHN is the most common complication (15% overall; increases with age).

- 1–5% of cases may affect the motor nerves, causing weakness (*zoster motorius*), facial nerve involvement (Ramsay Hunt syndrome), and spinal motor radiculopathies.
- Lesions usually heal 2 to 4 weeks after onset, but scarring and pigmentation changes are common (1).

DIFFERENTIAL DIAGNOSIS
Rash
- Herpes simplex virus
- Coxsackievirus
- Contact dermatitis
- Superficial pyoderma

DIAGNOSTIC TESTS & INTERPRETATION
Initial Tests (lab, imaging)
Rarely necessary; clinical appearance is distinct.

Follow-Up Tests & Special Considerations
- Viral culture
- Tzanck smear (does not distinguish from herpes simplex, and false-negative results occur)
- Polymerase chain reaction
- Immunofluorescent antigen staining
- Varicella-zoster–specific IgM

Test Interpretation
- Multinucleated giant cells with intralesional inclusion
- Lymphatic infiltration of sensory ganglia with focal hemorrhage and nerve cell destruction

TREATMENT

GENERAL MEASURES
- Treat to control symptoms and prevent complications.
- Antiviral therapy decreases viral replication, lessens inflammation and nerve damage, and reduces the severity and duration of long-term pain.
- Prompt analgesia may shorten the duration of zoster-associated pain.
- Calamine and colloidal oatmeal may help reduce itching and burning.

MEDICATION
First Line
- Acute treatment
  - Antiviral agents initiated within 72 hours of skin lesions help relieve symptoms, speed resolution, and prevent or mitigate PHN (2).

- Antivirals do not significantly reduce the incidence of PHN (3).
  - Valacyclovir: 1,000 mg PO TID for 7 days
  - Famciclovir: 500 mg PO TID for 7 days
  - Acyclovir: 800 mg q4h (5 doses daily) for 7 days
  - In children, oral acyclovir is the drug of choice.
- Analgesics (acetaminophen, NSAIDs)
- Corticosteroids do not prevent PHN but may accelerate resolution of acute neuritis.
  - Tricyclic antidepressants (TCAs); amitriptyline 10 to 25 mg at bedtime and other low-dose TCAs relieve pain acutely and may reduce pain duration; dose may be titrated up to 75 to 150 mg/day as tolerated.
  - Lidocaine patch 5% (Lidoderm) applied over painful areas (limit three patches simultaneously or trim a single patch) for up to 12 hours may be effective.
  - Gabapentin: 300 to 600 mg TID for pain; limited by adverse effects
  - Capsaicin cream and other analgesics may be useful adjuncts. Use opioids sparingly.
  - Pregabalin: 150 to 300 mg/day divided BID or TID reduces pain; use is limited by side effects.
- Prevention of PHN and zoster-associated pain: There are no treatments to prevent PHN. Treatment may, however, shorten duration and/or reduce severity of symptoms.
  - Antiviral therapy with valacyclovir, famciclovir, or acyclovir given during acute skin eruption may decrease the duration of pain.
  - Low-dose amitriptyline (25 mg at bedtime) started within 72 hours of rash onset and continued for 90 days may reduce PHN incidence/duration.
  - Paravertebral blockade: Nerve blocks during the acute phase shorten the duration of pain; somatic blocks, paravertebral blocks, and repeated/continuous epidural blocks can be used to prevent PHN (1).
  - Insufficient evidence to suggest that corticosteroids reduce incidence, severity, or duration of PHN
- Precautions
  - Assess renal function prior to using valacyclovir, famciclovir, acyclovir, gabapentin, and pregabalin.
  - Valacyclovir, famciclovir, and acyclovir are pregnancy Category B.

COMPLEMENTARY & ALTERNATIVE MEDICINE
Cupping therapy (traditional Chinese medicine) shows potential benefit. Definitive evidence is lacking.

ADMISSION, INPATIENT, AND NURSING CONSIDERATIONS
- Outpatient treatment, unless disseminated or occurring as complication of serious underlying disease requiring hospitalization
- Consultation with ophthalmology for ophthalmic involvement (VZO)

 ONGOING CARE

FOLLOW-UP RECOMMENDATIONS
Refer to ophthalmology if concern that ophthalmic branch of the trigeminal nerve is involved.

Patient Monitoring
Follow duration of symptoms—particularly PHN. Consider hospitalization if symptoms are severe; patients are immunocompromised; >2 dermatomes are involved; serious bacterial superinfection, disseminated zoster, ophthalmic involvement, or meningoencephalitis develops.

DIET
No special diet

PATIENT EDUCATION
- The rash typically lasts 2 to 3 weeks.
- Encourage good hygiene and proper skin care.
- Warn of potential for dissemination (dissemination must be suspected with constitutional illness signs and/or spreading rash).
- Warn of potential PHN.
- Warn of potential risk of transmitting illness (chickenpox) to susceptible persons.
- Seek medical attention if any eye involvement.

PROGNOSIS
- Immunocompetent individuals should experience spontaneous and complete recovery within a few weeks.
- Acute rash typically resolves within 14 to 21 days.
- PHN may occur in patients despite antiviral treatment.

COMPLICATIONS
- PHN
- HZO: 10–20%
- Superinfection of skin lesions
- Meningoencephalitis
- Disseminated zoster
- Hepatitis; pneumonitis; myelitis
- Cranial and peripheral nerve palsies
- Acute retinal necrosis

REFERENCES
1. Patil A, Goldust M, Wollina U. *Herpes zoster: a review of clinical manifestations and management. Viruses*. 2022;14(2):192.
2. Tsatsos M, Athanasiadis I, Myrou A, et al. Herpes zoster ophthalmicus: a devastating disease coming back with vengeance or finding its nemesis? *J Ophthalmic Vis Res*. 2022;17(1):123–129.
3. Harbecke R, Cohen JI, Oxman MN. Herpes zoster vaccines. *J Infect Dis*. 2021;224(12 Suppl 2):S429–S442.

ADDITIONAL READING
- Forbes HJ, Bhaskaran K, Grint D, et al. Incidence of acute complications of herpes zoster among immunocompetent adults in England: a matched cohort study using routine health data. *Br J Dermatol*. 2021;184(6):1077–1084.
- Tseng HF, Bruxvoort K, Ackerson B, et al. The epidemiology of herpes zoster in immunocompetent, unvaccinated adults ≥50 years old: incidence, complications, hospitalization, mortality, and recurrence. *J Infect Dis*. 2020;222(5):798–806.

 SEE ALSO

- Bell Palsy; Chickenpox (Varicella Zoster); Herpes Eye Infections; Herpes Simplex
- Algorithm: Genital Ulcers

 CODES

ICD10
- B02.9 Zoster without complications
- B02.29 Other postherpetic nervous system involvement

CLINICAL PEARLS
- Initiate antiviral therapy within 72 hours of rash onset for maximal effect.
- Patients with active herpes zoster can transmit clinically active disease (chickenpox) to susceptible individuals.
- Shingrix (recombinant) is the recommended vaccine for healthy adults aged ≥50 years, including those who previously received Zostavax (live attenuated), to prevent shingles and related complications.
- HZO is a potentially debilitating complication.

H

HERPES, GENITAL

Sahil Mullick, MD • Sreelakshmi Surendran Pillai, MD

BASICS

DESCRIPTION
- Chronic, recurrent herpes simplex virus (HSV) type 1 or 2 infection of any area innervated by the sacral ganglia
- HSV-1 causes anogenital and orolabial lesions; HSV-2 causes anogenital lesions.
- Primary episode: occurs in the absence of preexisting antibodies to HSV-1 or HSV-2 (may be asymptomatic)
- First episode, nonprimary: initial genital eruption; preexisting antibodies are present.
- Reactivation: recurrent episodes
- Synonym(s): herpes genitalis

EPIDEMIOLOGY
- Most commonly infected from age 15 to 30 years; prevalence increases with age due to cumulative likelihood of exposure.
- Predominant sex: female > male
- Predominant race: non-Hispanic blacks

Incidence
True incidence is unknown because genital herpes is not reportable. Studies estimate the incidence in the United States to be ~572,000 to 1.6 million new cases per year; highest in 18- to 24-year-olds.

Prevalence
- Overall prevalence of HSV-2 is 10–40% in the general population and up to 60–95% in the HIV-positive population (1).
- Between the ages of 14 and 49 years, the prevalence of HSV-1 in the United States is ~48%, and the prevalence of HSV-2 is ~12%.
- Up to 90% of those who are seropositive lack formal diagnosis.
- Globally, it is estimated that HSV-1 infects 3.7 billion people versus 140 million for HSV-2.

ETIOLOGY AND PATHOPHYSIOLOGY
- HSV is a double-stranded DNA virus of the *Herpetoviridae* family (1).
- Spread via genital-to-genital contact, oral-to-genital contact, and via maternal–fetal transmission (2)
- Incubation is 4 to 7 days after exposure.
- Risk of transmission is highest when lesions are present.
- Viral shedding is possible in the absence of lesions, increasing the risk of transmission (precautions—abstinence, condom use—may not be followed). Viral shedding occurs intermittently, unpredictably, and more commonly with HSV-2.
- HSV infection increases the risk for HIV.

RISK FACTORS
- Risk increases with age, number of lifetime partners, history of sexually transmitted infections (STIs—particularly HIV), sexual encounters before the age of 17 years, and partner with HSV-1 or HSV-2.
- Infection with HSV-1 confers 3-fold risk of infection with HSV-2.
- Immunosuppression, fever, stress, and trauma increase risk of reactivation.

GENERAL PREVENTION
- Use barrier contraception and avoid sexual contact when symptoms/lesions are present.
- Abstinence is the only means of complete protection.

COMMONLY ASSOCIATED CONDITIONS
Syphilis, HIV/AIDS, chlamydia, gonorrhea, other STIs

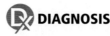

DIAGNOSIS

HISTORY
- Many patients are asymptomatic (74% for HSV-1, 63% for HSV-2) or do not recognize clinical manifestations of infection (2).
- Symptoms that are present during primary episode are often more severe, longer in duration, and associated with constitutional symptoms.
- Common presenting symptoms (primary episode): multiple genital ulcers, dysuria, pruritus, fever, tender inguinal lymphadenopathy, headache, malaise, myalgias, cervicitis/dyspareunia, urethritis (watery discharge)
- Common presenting symptoms for recurrent episodes: prodrome of tingling, burning, or shooting pain (2 to 24 hours before lesion appears); single ulcer; lesion can be atypical in appearance; dysuria; pruritus (lasting 4 to 6 days on average)
- Recurrent episodes are more frequent with HSV-2 than with HSV-1, especially in the 1st year after infection. Recurrences are less frequent over time. An increasing proportion of anogenital herpetic infections have been attributed to HSV-1, which is especially prominent among young women and MSM.
- Less common presentations: constipation (from anal involvement causing tenesmus), proctitis, stomatitis, pharyngitis, sacral paresthesias

PHYSICAL EXAM
- Lesions around groin/perineum and within anus, vagina, and on cervix
- Lesion may appear in various stages as papular, vesicular, pustular, ulcerated, or crusted
- Inguinal lymphadenopathy
- Extragenital manifestations include meningitis, recurrent meningitis (Mollaret syndrome), sacral radiculitis/paresthesias, encephalitis, transverse myelitis, and hepatitis.

Pediatric Considerations
- Neonatal infection occurs in 20 to 50/100,000 live births; 80% of infections result from asymptomatic maternal viral shedding during an undiagnosed primary infection in the 3rd trimester.
- Transmission ranges from 30% to 50% if the primary episode is near the time of delivery. This risk is higher with HSV-1 than with HSV-2. Neonatal disease is associated with high morbidity and mortality.
- Suspect sexual abuse with genital lesions in children.

DIFFERENTIAL DIAGNOSIS
- HIV; syphilis; chancroid; herpes zoster
- Ulcerative balanitis, granuloma inguinale; lymphogranuloma venereum
- Cytomegalovirus, Epstein-Barr virus
- Drug eruption, trauma
- Behçet syndrome
- Ulcus vulvae acutum (Lipschütz ulcer)
- Neoplasia

DIAGNOSTIC TESTS & INTERPRETATION
Initial Tests (lab, imaging)
- Laboratory testing can be used to confirm clinical diagnosis.
- Viral isolation (swab or scraping) for culture or PCR
  - Use Dacron or polyester-tipped swabs with plastic shafts (cotton tips/wood shafts inhibit viral growth and/or replication) (1).
  - Culture by unroofing vesicle to obtain fluid sample; specificity >99%; sensitivity per sample: 52–93% for vesicle, 41–72% for ulcer, and 19–30% for crusted lesion (1)
  - Culture requires timely transport of live virus to the laboratory in appropriate medium at 4°C.
  - PCR has the greatest sensitivity (98%) and specificity (>99%) but is also expensive and not readily available. It can increase detection rates by up to 70%; used primarily for CSF (1)
- Type-specific serologic assays
  - Seroconversion occurs 10 days to 4 months after infection. *Antibody testing is not necessary if a positive culture or PCR has been obtained.*
  - *IgM antibody testing to determine a primary episode (especially during pregnancy) if IgM is positive and IgG is negative.*
  - Western blot (gold standard) and type-specific IgG antibody (glycoprotein G) enzyme-linked immunosorbent assay (ELISA) are used to discriminate between HSV-1 and HSV-2.
  - Western blot is >97–99% sensitive and specific but is labor intensive and not readily available (1).
  - ELISA is 81–100% sensitive; 93–100% specific (1) for HSV-2 but lower for HSV-1 detection; false positives are possible.
  - Screening with type-specific antibody is not generally recommended for:
    ○ Asymptomatic patients with HIV infection
    ○ Discordant couples (one partner with known HSV, the other without)
    ○ Recurrent symptoms but no active lesions

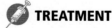

TREATMENT

GENERAL MEASURES
- Ice packs to perineum, sitz baths, topical anesthetics
- Analgesics, NSAIDs

MEDICATION
Start antiviral medications within 72 hours of onset of symptoms (including prodrome). After 3 days, antivirals may help if new lesions form or for significant pain. Persons with HIV will require higher doses for longer duration.

First Line

- Acyclovir: the most studied antiviral in genital herpes; decreases pain, duration of viral shedding, and time to full resolution
  - Primary episode
    - 400 mg PO TID for 7 to 10 days, extend duration if lesion not completely healed at 10 days
  - Episodic therapy
    - 800 mg BID for 5 days
    - 800 mg TID for 2 days
    - For immunocompromised persons and those with HIV, 400 mg TID for 5 to 10 days
  - Daily suppression
    - 400 mg BID
    - For immunocompromised persons and those with HIV, 400 to 800 mg 2 to 3 times per day
  - Severe, complicated infections (IV therapy)
    - 5 to 10 mg/kg/dose q8h until clinical improvement; switch to PO therapy to complete a 10-day course (14 days for CNS involvement).
  - Precautions
    - Modify dose in renal insufficiency.
- Valacyclovir (Valtrex): prodrug of acyclovir, improved bioavailability, less frequent dosing
  - Primary episode
    - 1 g PO BID for 7 to 10 days, extend duration if lesion not completely healed at 10 days
  - Episodic therapy
    - 500 mg PO BID for 3 days
    - 1 g PO daily for 5 days
    - For immunocompromised persons and those with HIV, 1 g PO daily for 5 to 10 days
  - Daily suppression
    - 500 mg PO daily
    - 1 g PO daily
    - For immunocompromised persons and those with HIV, 500 mg PO BID
- Famciclovir (Famvir)
  - Primary episode
    - 250 mg PO TID for 7 to 10 days, extend duration if lesion not completely healed at 10 days
  - Episodic therapy
    - 125 mg PO BID for 5 days
    - 1 g PO BID for 1 day
    - 500 mg PO once, followed by 250 mg PO BID for 2 days
    - For immunocompromised persons and those with HIV, 500 mg PO BID for 5 to 10 days
  - Daily suppression 250 mg PO BID
    - 250 mg PO BID
    - For immunocompromised persons and those with HIV, 500 mg PO BID

ISSUES FOR REFERRAL

For acyclovir-resistant HSV, in consultation with infectious disease specialist:

- Foscarnet: 40 to 80 mg/kg/dose IV q8h until clinical resolution
  - First-line treatment
  - Associated with significant nephrotoxicity
- Cidofovir: 5 mg/kg IV qwk

Pregnancy Considerations

ACOG clinical management guidelines:

- Screening: Pregnant women negative for HSV-1 and HSV-2 antibodies should avoid sexual contact in the 3rd trimester if their partner is antibody-positive.
- Suppressive therapy: Pregnant women with a history of genital herpes should be offered suppression treatment starting at 36 weeks' gestation until delivery to decrease reactivation rate and reduce the risk of neonatal infection:
  - Acyclovir 400 mg PO TID
  - Valacyclovir 500 mg PO BID
- Monitor for outbreaks during pregnancy. C-section is recommended if prodromal symptoms or lesions are present at onset of labor.

Pediatric Considerations

- High-risk infants include those with active symptoms or lesions, those delivered vaginally with maternal lesions present, and those born during a primary maternal episode. Monitor closely and obtain diagnostic laboratory specimens (HSV PCR and ocular, nasal, anal, and oral cultures). If symptomatic, require prolonged treatment:
  - Acyclovir 20 mg/kg IV q8h for 14 days if skin or mucosal lesions, 21 days if disseminated or CNS disease
- Low-risk infants who are asymptomatic can be observed while obtaining serum HSV PCR and ocular, nasal, anal, and oral cultures.
- Infants with possible HSV infection should be isolated from other neonates; maternal separation is not necessary, and breastfeeding is not contraindicated.

 ONGOING CARE

Counsel persons with genital herpes and their sex partners with goal of helping patients cope with the infection and preventing sexual and perinatal transmission.

FOLLOW-UP RECOMMENDATIONS

Patient Monitoring

Test for HIV and other STIs.

PATIENT EDUCATION

- Patient education helps in treatment of subsequent outbreaks and in reducing risk of transmission:
  - Options include daily suppressive therapy and episodic therapy.
  - Alert partners of history prior to sexual activity.
  - Avoid sexual contact when symptoms or lesions are present.
  - Viral shedding and transmission can occur when symptoms/lesions are NOT present.
    - Shedding increased with HSV-2 and HIV.
  - 100% condom use reduces HSV-2 transmission risk by 30%.
  - Sexual activity between concordant couples (i.e., both partners with the same type of herpes [HSV-1 or HSV-2]) does not increase risk of outbreaks.
  - Ensure that maternity care team knows HSV status.
- American Sexual Health Association: https://www.ashasexualhealth.org/stdsstis/herpes/
- Centers for Disease Control and Prevention: https://www.cdc.gov/std/herpes/stdfact-herpes.htm

PROGNOSIS

- Resolution of signs/symptoms: 3 to 21 days
- Average recurrence rate is 1 to 4 episodes per year (2).
- Antivirals can reduce transmission, shedding, and outbreaks.

Pediatric Considerations

Neonatal infection survival rates: localized >95%, CNS 85%, systemic 30%

COMPLICATIONS

- Behavioral issues include lowered self-esteem, guilt, anger, depression, fear of rejection, and fear of transmission to partner.
- The risk of being infected with HIV is 2- to 3-fold with HSV-2.
- Hepatitis with disseminated HSV, especially in pregnancy
- HSV-2 meningitis is a rare complication of HSV-2 genital herpes infection that affects women more than men.

REFERENCES

1. Nath P, Kabir MA, Doust SK, et al. Diagnosis of herpes simplex virus: laboratory and point-of-care techniques. *Infect Dis Rep*. 2021;13(2):518–539.
2. Rogan SC, Beigi RH. Management of viral complications of pregnancy: pharmacotherapy to reduce vertical transmission. *Obstet Gynecol Clin North Am*. 2021;48(1):53–74.

ADDITIONAL READING

- Management of genital herpes in pregnancy: ACOG practice bulletin, number 220. *Obstet Gynecol*. 2020;135(5):e193–e202.
- Spicknall IH, Flagg EW, Torrone EA. Estimates of the prevalence and incidence of genital herpes, United States, 2018. *Sex Transm Dis*. 2021;48(4):260–265.

 SEE ALSO

Algorithm: Genital Ulcers

 CODES

ICD10

- A60 Anogenital herpesviral [herpes simplex] infections
- A60.02 Herpesviral infection of other male genital organs
- A60.0 Herpesviral infection of genitalia and urogenital tract

CLINICAL PEARLS

- HSV-1 and/or HSV-2 cause genital herpes.
- Many seropositive individuals are unaware that they are infected.
- Most primary episodes are asymptomatic.
- Viral shedding occurs in the absence of lesions.
- Meticulous (100%) condom use decreases transmission of HSV.

H

HICCUPS

Tya-Mae Y. Julien, MD

 BASICS

DESCRIPTION

- Hiccups are caused by a repetitive sudden involuntary contraction of the inspiratory muscles (predominantly the diaphragm) with the abrupt closure of the glottis, which stops the inflow of air and produces a characteristic sound.
- Hiccups are classified based on their duration: Hiccup bouts last up to 48 hours; persistent hiccups last >48 hours but <1 month; intractable hiccups last for >1 month.
- System(s) affected: nervous, pulmonary
- Synonym(s): hiccoughs; singultus

Geriatric Considerations
Can be a serious problem, particularly among the elderly

Pregnancy Considerations
- Fetal hiccups are rhythmic fetal movements (confirmed sonographically) that can be confused with contractions.
- Fetal hiccups are a sign of normal neurologic development.

EPIDEMIOLOGY
- Predominant age: all ages (including fetus)
- Predominant sex: male > female (4:1)

Incidence
Overall incidence in the general population is uncertain.

Prevalence
Self-limited hiccups are extremely common, as are intraoperative and postoperative hiccups.

ETIOLOGY AND PATHOPHYSIOLOGY
- Results from stimulation of ≥1 limbs of the hiccup reflux arc (vagus and phrenic nerves) with a "hiccup center" located in the upper spinal cord and brain (1)
- In men, >90% have an organic basis; in women, psychogenic causes are more common.
- Specific underlying causes include the following:
  - CNS disorders: vascular lesions (AV malformation), infectious causes (meningitis, encephalitis), structural lesions (intracranial/brainstem mass lesions, multiple sclerosis, hydrocephalus, syringomyelia), posterior inferior cerebellar artery (PICA) aneurysm; seizure disorder
  - Diaphragmatic irritation (tumors, pericarditis, eventration, splenomegaly, hepatomegaly, peritonitis)
  - Irritation of the tympanic membrane
  - Nerve irritation: pharyngitis, laryngitis, neck tumors
  - Mediastinal and other thoracic lesions (pneumonia, aortic aneurysm, tuberculosis [TB], myocardial infarction [MI], lung cancer, rib exostoses)
  - Esophageal lesions (reflux esophagitis, achalasia, *Candida* esophagitis, carcinoma, obstruction)
  - Gastrointestinal (GI) disorders (gastritis, GERD, PUD, distention, cancer)
  - Hiccups have been reported as an initial presentation of COVID-19.
  - Cardiovascular disorders (MI, pericarditis)
  - Hepatic lesions (hepatitis, hepatoma); pancreatic lesions (pancreatitis, pseudocysts, cancer)
  - Inflammatory bowel disease; cholelithiasis, cholecystitis
  - Prostatic disorders
  - Appendicitis; postoperative, particularly with abdominal procedures
  - Metabolic causes (uremia, hyponatremia, gout, diabetes)
  - Drug-induced (dexamethasone, methylprednisolone, anabolic steroids, benzodiazepines, α-methyldopa, propofol, levofolinate, oxaliplatin, fluorouracil, carboplatin, cisplatin, tramadol)
  - Toxic (alcohol-induced)
  - Psychogenic causes (anorexia, conversion, grief, malingering, schizophrenia, stress)
  - Idiopathic

RISK FACTORS
- Overeating
- Consuming carbonated beverages
- Excessive alcohol consumption
- Excitement or emotional stress
- Changes in ambient or GI temperature

GENERAL PREVENTION
- Identify and correct relevant underlying cause(s).
- Avoid gastric distention.
- Acupuncture shows promise compared to chronic drug therapy for controlling hiccups.

 DIAGNOSIS

- Hiccup attacks usually occur at brief intervals and last seconds or minutes. Persistent bouts lasting >48 hours often imply an underlying physical or metabolic disorder.
- Intractable hiccups may occur continuously for months or years (2).
- Hiccups usually have a frequency of 4 to 60 per minute (2).
- Persistent and intractable hiccups warrant further evaluation.

HISTORY
- Severity and duration of hiccup bouts
- Associated medical conditions that could be causative—GI, cardiac, neurologic, or pulmonary disorders
- Recent surgery (especially genitourinary)
- Behavioral health history
- Review of medications
- Alcohol and illicit drug use

PHYSICAL EXAM
- Correlate exam with potential etiologies (e.g., rales with pneumonia; organomegaly with splenic or hepatic disease).
- Examine the ear canal for foreign bodies.
- Head and neck masses and lymphadenopathy
- Complete neurologic exam

DIFFERENTIAL DIAGNOSIS
Hiccups are rarely confused with burping (eructation).

DIAGNOSTIC TESTS & INTERPRETATION
- When an underlying etiology is suspected, consider condition-specific testing (e.g., CBC, electrolytes, BUN, creatinine, LFTs, amylase/lipase, metabolic panel, chest x-ray) for hiccups lasting longer than 48 hours.
- Fluoroscopy can evaluate hemidiaphragm movement.

Diagnostic Procedures/Other
- Upper endoscopy; CT scan (or other imaging) of brain, thorax, abdomen, and pelvis to look for underlying causes
- Head MRI with contrast, lumbar puncture
- The extent of the workup is often in proportion to the duration and severity of the hiccups (1).

 TREATMENT

- Outpatient (usually)
- Inpatient (if elderly, debilitated, or intractable hiccups)
- Many hiccup treatments are purely anecdotal.

GENERAL MEASURES
- Evaluate frequent bouts or persistent hiccups.
- Treat underlying cause when identified (1),(2)[C].
  - Dilate esophageal stricture or obstruction.
  - Treat ulcers or reflux disease.
  - Remove hair or foreign body from ear canal.
  - Bitters for alcohol-induced hiccups
  - Catheter stimulation of pharynx for operative and postoperative hiccups
  - Antifungal treatment for *Candida* esophagitis
  - Correct electrolyte imbalance.
- Medical measures
  - Relieve gastric distention (gastric lavage, nasogastric aspiration, induced vomiting).
  - Cautious counterirritation of the vagus nerve (supraorbital pressure, carotid sinus massage, digital rectal massage)
  - Respiratory center stimulants (breathing 5% CO_2)
  - Behavioral health modification (hypnosis, meditation, paced respirations)
  - Phrenic nerve block or electrical stimulation (or pacing) of the dominant hemidiaphragm
  - Acupuncture
  - Miscellaneous (cardioversion)

MEDICATION

First Line

- Physical maneuvers: breath holding, Valsalva maneuver, breathing into a bag, fright, ice water gargles
- Others: swallowing granulated sugar, hard bread, or peanut butter; biting on a lemon, pulling knees to chest, or leaning forward to compress chest
- Drug therapy if physical maneuvers have failed or treatment is directed toward a specific cause of hiccups
- Pharmacologic therapy
  - Chlorpromazine (FDA-approved for hiccups): 25 to 50 mg PO/IV TID
  - Metoclopramide: 5 to 10 mg PO QID
  - Baclofen: 5 to 10 mg PO TID (1),(2)[B]
  - Haloperidol: 2 to 5 mg PO/IM followed by 1 to 2 mg PO TID
  - Phenytoin: 200 to 300 mg PO HS
  - Nifedipine: 10 to 20 mg PO daily to TID
  - Amitriptyline: 10 mg PO TID
  - Viscous lidocaine 2%: 5 mL PO daily to TID
  - Gabapentin (Neurontin): 300 mg PO HS; may increase up to 1,800 mg/day PO in divided doses (2)[B]; 1,200 mg/day PO for 3 days and then 400 mg/day PO for 3 days in patients undergoing stroke rehabilitation or in the palliative care setting where chlorpromazine adverse effects are undesirable (2)[B]
  - Combination of lansoprazole 15 mg PO daily, clonazepam 0.5 mg PO BID, and dimenhydrinate 25 mg PO BID
  - Contraindications: Refer to manufacturer's literature.
    - Chlorpromazine is not recommended in elderly patient with dementia.
  - Baclofen is not recommended in patients with stroke or other cerebral lesions or in severe renal impairment. Avoid abrupt withdrawal of baclofen.
- Other possible drug therapies (1)
  - Amantadine, carbidopa and levodopa in Parkinson disease
  - Steroid replacement in Addison disease
  - Antifungal agent in *Candida* esophagitis
  - Ondansetron in carcinomatosis with vomiting
  - Nefopam (a nonopioid analgesic with antishivering properties related to antihistamines and antiparkinsonian drugs) is available outside the United States in both IV and oral formulations.
  - Olanzapine 10 mg QHS or chlorpromazine 25 mg PO TID in combination with olanzapine 5 mg PO daily (3)
  - Pregabalin 375 mg/day

ISSUES FOR REFERRAL

For acupuncture or phrenic nerve crush, block, or electrostimulation; continuous cervical epidural block; cardioversion

SURGERY/OTHER PROCEDURES

- Phrenic nerve crush or transaction or electrostimulation of the dominant diaphragmatic leaflet
- Resection of rib exostoses

COMPLEMENTARY & ALTERNATIVE MEDICINE

- Acupuncture is increasingly used to manage persistent or intractable hiccups, especially in cancer patients (2)[A].
- Home remedies (none of which are universally effective) (1)
  - Swallowing a spoonful of sugar
  - Sucking on hard candy or swallowing peanut butter
  - Holding breath and increasing pressure on diaphragm (Valsalva maneuver)
  - Tongue traction
  - Lifting the uvula with a cold spoon
  - Inducing fright
  - Smelling salts
  - Rebreathing into a paper (not plastic) bag
  - Sipping ice water
  - Rubbing a wet cotton-tipped applicator between hard and soft palate for 1 minute

ADMISSION, INPATIENT, AND NURSING CONSIDERATIONS

Most patients can be managed as outpatients; those with severe intractable hiccups may require rehydration, pain control, IV medications, or surgery.

⚡ ONGOING CARE

FOLLOW-UP RECOMMENDATIONS

Patient Monitoring
Until hiccups cease

DIET
Avoid gastric distension from overeating, carbonated beverages, and aerophagia.

PATIENT EDUCATION
See "General Measures."

PROGNOSIS

- Hiccups often cease during sleep.
- Most acute benign hiccup bouts resolve spontaneously or with home remedies.
- Intractable hiccups may last for years or decades.
- Hiccups have persisted despite bilateral phrenic nerve transection.

COMPLICATIONS

- Inability to eat
- Weight loss
- Exhaustion, debility
- Insomnia
- Cardiac arrhythmias
- Wound dehiscence
- Death (rare)

REFERENCES

1. Leung AKC, Leung AAM, Wong AHC, et al. Hiccups: a non-systematic review. *Curr Pediatr Rev.* 2020;16(4):277–284.
2. Thompson DF, Brooks KG. Gabapentin therapy of hiccups. *Ann Pharmacother.* 2013;47(6):897–903.
3. Srinivasan M, Yadav G, Singh Y, et al. Comparison of efficacy of combination therapy with chlorpromazine and olanzapine with chlorpromazine alone for treatment of hiccups in traumatic brain injury patients—a randomised control trial. *J Clin Diagn Res.* 2022;16(9):28–31.

ADDITIONAL READING

- Hosoya R, Uesawa Y, Ishii-Nozawa R, et al. Analysis of factors associated with hiccups based on the Japanese Adverse Drug Event Report database. *PLoS One.* 2017;12(2):e0172057.
- Moretto EN, Wee B, Wiffen PJ, et al. Interventions for treating persistent and intractable hiccups in adults. *Cochrane Database Syst Rev.* 2013;2013(1):CD008768.
- Steger M, Schneemann M, Fox M. Systemic review: the pathogenesis and pharmacological treatment of hiccups. *Aliment Pharmacol Ther.* 2015;42(9):1037–1050.

CODES

ICD10
- R06.6 Hiccough
- F45.8 Other somatoform disorders

CLINICAL PEARLS

- Most hiccups resolve spontaneously.
- An organic cause is more likely in men and individuals with intractable hiccups.
- Rule out foreign body in the ear canal as a trigger.
- Baclofen and gabapentin are the only pharmacologic agents proven to be clinically effective.
- Acupuncture may be effective for persistent hiccups.

HIDRADENITIS SUPPURATIVA

Kelsey R. Henry, MD • Donna R. Potts, MD

BASICS

DESCRIPTION
- Chronic inflammatory skin disease manifested as recurrent inflammatory nodules, abscesses, sinus tracts, and complex scar formation
- Areas affected are tender, malodorous, often with exudative drainage.
- Has higher risk of concomitant decrease in quality of life secondary to physical, emotional, and psychological stress
- Common in intertriginous skin regions: axillae, groin, perianal, perineal, inframammary skin
- System(s) affected: skin, psychosocial
- Synonym(s): acne inversa; Verneuil disease; apocrinitis; hidradenitis axillaris

EPIDEMIOLOGY
- Predominant sex: female > male (3:1)
- African Americans

Incidence
Peak onset during 2nd and 3rd decades of life but can be found from puberty until age 40 years

Prevalence
1–4% (1)

ETIOLOGY AND PATHOPHYSIOLOGY
- Not fully understood; previously considered a disorder of apocrine glands but more recently thought to be due to a follicular epithelium defect; deregulation of the local immune system may also play a role.
- Hormonally induced ductal keratinocyte proliferation leads to a failure of follicular epithelial shedding, causing follicular occlusion.
- Mechanical stress on skin (intertriginous regions) precipitates follicular rupture and immune response.
- Bacterial involvement is a secondary event.
- Rupture and reepithelialization cause sinus tracts to form.

Genetics
- Familial occurrences suggest single gene transmission (autosomal dominant), but the condition may also be polygenic.
- Estimated 40% of patients have an affected family member.

RISK FACTORS
- Obesity
- Smoking
- Hyperandrogenism
- Lithium may trigger onset of or exacerbate this condition.

GENERAL PREVENTION
- Lose weight if overweight or obese.
- Smoking cessation
- Avoid constrictive clothing/synthetic fabrics, frictional trauma, heat exposure, excessive sweating, shaving, depilation, and deodorants.
- Use of antiseptic soaps

COMMONLY ASSOCIATED CONDITIONS
- Acne vulgaris, acne conglobate
- Perifolliculitis capitis abscedens et suffodiens (dissecting cellulitis of scalp)
- Pilonidal disease
- Metabolic syndrome/obesity
- Polycystic ovary syndrome (PCOS) and androgen dysfunction
- Thyroid disease
- Arthritis and spondyloarthritis (seronegative)
- Inflammatory bowel disease
- Squamous cell carcinoma
- PAPASH syndrome (pyogenic arthritis, pyoderma gangrenosum, acne, and suppurative hydradenitis)
- Type 2 diabetes mellitus

DIAGNOSIS

HISTORY
- Diagnostic criteria adopted by the 2nd International Conference on Hidradenitis Suppurativa, 2009
- All three criteria (morphology, location, progression) must be present for diagnosis:
  - Typical lesions: painful nodules, abscesses, draining sinus, bridged scars, and "tombstone" double-ended pseudocomedones in secondary lesions
  - Typical topography: axillae, groins, perineal and perianal region, buttocks, infra- and intermammary folds
  - Chronicity and recurrences, commonly refractory to initial treatments

PHYSICAL EXAM
- Tender dome-shaped nodules 0.5 to 3.0 cm in size are present.
  - Location corresponds with the distribution of apocrine-related mammary tissue and terminal hair follicles dependent on low androgen concentrations.
  - Sites ordered by frequency of occurrence: axillary, inguinal, perianal and perineal, mammary and inframammary, buttock, pubic region, chest, scalp, retroauricular, eyelid
  - Large lesions are often fluctuant; comedones may be present.
- Possible malodorous discharge
- Hurley clinical staging system
  - **Stage I**: nodule/abscess formation without sinus tracts or scarring
  - **Stage II**: more than one lesion widely spaced with tract and scar formation
  - **Stage III**: diffuse, multiple interconnected tracts and abscesses with scarring
- Sartorius clinical staging system (points attributed)
  - Anatomic region involved
  - Quantity and quality of lesions
  - Distance between lesions
  - Presence or absence of normal skin between lesions
- Other scoring tools include IHS4, HiSCR, and HASI-R which include more information including response to treatment and changes in severity.

DIFFERENTIAL DIAGNOSIS
- Acne vulgaris, conglobate
- Furunculosis/carbuncles
- Infected Bartholin or sebaceous cysts
- Lymphadenopathy/lymphadenitis
- Cutaneous Langerhans cell histiocytosis
- Actinomycosis
- Granuloma inguinale
- Lymphogranuloma venereum
- Apocrine nevus
- Crohn disease with anogenital fistula(s) (may coexist with hidradenitis suppurativa [HS])
- Fox-Fordyce disease

DIAGNOSTIC TESTS & INTERPRETATION
Initial Tests (lab, imaging)
- Cultures of skin or aspirates of boils are most commonly negative. When positive, cultures are often polymicrobial and commonly grow *Staphylococcus aureus* and *Staphylococcus epidermidis*.
- May note increased erythrocyte sedimentation rate (ESR), leukocytosis, decreased serum iron, normocytic anemia, or changes in serum electrophoresis pattern

Follow-Up Tests & Special Considerations
- Consider biopsy of concerning lesions due to increased risk of squamous cell carcinoma.
- If the patient is female, overweight, and/or hirsute, consider evaluating the following: testosterone, dehydroepiandrosterone sulfate, sex hormone–binding globulin, and progesterone
- Incidence is rare after menopause and before puberty (consider premature adrenarche).
- If pregnant, do not use isotretinoin or tetracyclines for teratogenicity.

Diagnostic Procedures/Other
- Incision and drainage, culture and biopsy
- Ultrasound may be useful in planning an excision to identify the full extent of sinus tracts.

Test Interpretation
- Dermis shows granulomatous inflammation and inflammatory cells, giant cells, sinus tracts, subcutaneous abscesses, and extensive fibrosis.
- Hair follicular dilatation and occlusion by keratinized stratified squamous epithelium

TREATMENT

Despite the prevalence of this condition, most trials have been small and underpowered. Evidence is therefore generally of poor quality. Treatment goals: Reduce extent of disease, prevent new lesions, remove chronic disease, and limit scar formation.

- Conservative treatment includes all items under "General Prevention," plus use of warm compresses, sitz baths, topical antiseptics for inflamed lesions, and nonopioid analgesics.
- Weight loss and smoking cessation result in marked improvement (2).
- Corticosteroids, isotretinoin, and zinc gluconate
- For stages I and II, attempt medical treatment.
- Short medical trial may be appropriate in stage III prior to moving on to surgical therapies.
- Only FDA-approved medication for this condition is adalimumab (3). Other biologics may be effective. No medications are curative; relapse is almost inevitable, but the disease may be controlled; usually must fail other treatments before starting biologics; they can be a costly option.

GENERAL MEASURES
- Education and psychosocial support
- Appropriate hygiene including avoidance of shearing stress to skin (light clothing), daily cleansing with antibacterial soap
- Diet: Avoid dairy, high glycemic loads.
- Symptomatic treatment for acute lesions, especially pain control
- Improve environmental factors that cause follicular blockage (see "General Prevention").
- Smoking cessation and weight loss

MEDICATION
First Line
- Stage I disease (mild-to-moderate disease): Consider either systemic or topical antibiotics.
  - Skin cleansers (i.e., chlorhexidine 4% solution) are part of first line; however, no data exists on efficacy for specific agents and have very limited data, mostly expert opinion (4).
  - Keratolytic agents could be considered; however, it can cause irritant dermatitis (4).
  - Topical antibiotics (clindamycin was studied in clinical trials) (2)[B]
    - Clindamycin 0.1% solution BID for 12 weeks with benzoyl peroxide 5–10% solution was shown to reduce the rates of S. aureus resistance (4).
  - Systemic antibiotics
    - For mild-to-moderate HS, tetracycline medications were recommended for a 12-week course for maintenance (i.e., doxycycline 100 mg q12h or clindamycin 300 mg BID) (5)[B].
    - Dapsone 50 to 150 mg daily (recommended for 3-month course, not as effective in Hurley stage III disease)
  - Intralesional corticosteroids: limited evidence; possible reduction in pain, erythema, edema, and lesion size (2) (triamcinolone acetonide 10 mg/mL usually 0.2 to 2.0 mL injection)
- Stages II and III disease
  - Should be treated with first-line interventions to decrease severity; consider immediate referral to dermatology if disease is severe.
  - Biologic medications (i.e., TNF-α inhibitors such as adalimumab 40 mg weekly) can improve disease severity and quality of life in those with moderate-to-severe HS (3).
  - Minor surgical procedures (punch débridement, local unroofing) to treat individual lesions or sinus tracts

Second Line
- Clindamycin and rifampin combination treatment could be effective in mild-to-moderate disease or adjunct in severe disease.
- Hormonal agents have mixed data and efficacy but can be considered in patients with comorbidities.
- Retinoids should be used as a second- or third-line medication due to the limited and mixed result data.
- Limited and weak evidence for immunosuppressants such as methotrexate, azathioprine, colchicine/minocycline, cyclosporine

- Short courses of pulse steroids can be considered for acute flares or long-term (the lowest appropriate dose) corticosteroids for severe HS treatment.
- IV ertapenem 1 g for 6-week course has been shown to be highly effective; however, it should only be used as a bridge to surgery, given concern for antibiotic resistance and cost prohibitive home infusion costs.

ISSUES FOR REFERRAL
- Lack of response to treatment, stages II and III disease, or concern for malignancy
- If significant psychosocial stress exists secondary to disease, refer for stress management or psychiatric evaluation.
- Suspicion of hyperandrogenic states (e.g., PCOS) should prompt investigation or referral.
- Severe perianal/perivulvar disease or otherwise very extensive disease may prompt referral to plastic surgeon or reconstructive urologist.

SURGERY/OTHER PROCEDURES
- Important mode of treatment; necessary if wanting to permanently remove tunnels and scarring
- Could be used in conjunction with antibiotics or if first-line therapy fails
- Various surgical approaches have been used for stages II and III disease.
- Laser therapy for Hurley stages I and II disease (rarely used); no consensus on the benefit
- Cryotherapy and photodynamic therapy have shown variable results; they are not routinely recommended.

 ## ONGOING CARE

FOLLOW-UP RECOMMENDATIONS
Follow-up monthly or sooner to evaluate progress and to assist with symptom management.

DIET
- Avoid dairy and high glycemic loads.
- Healthy diet that promotes weight loss
- May benefit from zinc supplementation

PATIENT EDUCATION
- Severity can range from only two to three papules per year to extensive draining sinus tracts.
- Medications are temporizing measures, rarely curative. Attempts at local surgical "cures" do not affect recurrence at other sites.
- Smoking cessation and weight loss can improve symptoms significantly.
- Hidradenitis Suppurativa Foundation: https://www.hs-foundation.org/

PROGNOSIS
- Individual lesions heal slowly in 10 to 30 days.
- Recurrences may last for several years.
- Relentlessly progressive scarring and sinus tracts are likely with severe disease.
- Radical wide-area excision, with removal of all hair-bearing skin in the affected area, shows the greatest chance for cure.
- Increased all-cause mortality

COMPLICATIONS
- Contracture and stricturing of the skin after extensive abscess rupture, scarring, and healing; or at sites of surgical excisions
- Lymphatic obstruction, lymphedema
- Psychosocial: anxiety, malaise, depression, self-injury
- Anemia, amyloidosis, and hypoproteinemia (due to chronic suppuration)
- Lumbosacral epidural abscess, sacral bacterial osteomyelitis
- Squamous cell carcinoma may develop in indolent sinus tracts.
- Disseminated infection or septicemia (rare)
- Urethral, rectal, or bladder fistula (rare)

REFERENCES
1. Seyed Jafari SM, Hunger RE, Schlapbach C. Hidradenitis suppurativa: current understanding of pathogenic mechanisms and suggestion for treatment algorithm. *Front Med (Lausanne)*. 2020;7:68.
2. Saunte DML, Jemec GBE. Hidradenitis suppurativa: advances in diagnosis and treatment. *JAMA*. 2017;318(20):2019–2032.
3. Lim SYD, Oon HH. Systematic review of immunomodulatory therapies for hidradenitis suppurativa. *Biologics*. 2019;13:53–78.
4. Alikhan A, Lynch PJ, Eisen DB. Hidradenitis suppurativa: a comprehensive review. *J Am Acad Dermatol*. 2009;60(4):539–563.
5. Wang SC, Wang SC, Sibbald RG. Hidradenitis suppurativa: a frequently missed diagnosis, part 1: a review of pathogenesis, associations, and clinical features. *Adv Skin Wound Care*. 2015;28(7):325–334.

ADDITIONAL READING
Jemec GBE. Clinical practice. Hidradenitis suppurativa. *N Engl J Med*. 2012;366(2):158–164.

 ## CODES

ICD10
L73.2 Hidradenitis suppurativa

CLINICAL PEARLS
- Chronic inflammatory disease of the skin, often difficult to control with behavior changes and medication alone
- First-line treatment for mild disease is topical and/or systemic antibiotics.
- For patients with refractory or severe disease, wide local excision provides the only chance at a cure. Success rates depend on the location and extent of excision.
- This is a difficult to treat disease that can greatly affect the patient's quality of life.

H

HIRSUTISM

Jarrett Keller Sell, MD, FAAFP, AAHIVS

 BASICS

DESCRIPTION
- Presence of excessive terminal (coarse, pigmented) hair of body and face, in a male pattern
- May be present as an ethnic characteristic or may develop as a result of androgen excess
- Often seen in polycystic ovary syndrome (PCOS) which is characterized by hirsutism, acne, menstrual irregularities, and obesity
- System(s) affected: dermatologic, endocrine, metabolic, reproductive

EPIDEMIOLOGY
Prevalence
5–10% of reproductive age women

ETIOLOGY AND PATHOPHYSIOLOGY
- Due to increased androgenic hormones, either from increased peripheral binding (idiopathic) or increased production from the ovaries, adrenals, or body fat
- Exogenous medications
- Can be a symptom of multiple etiologies such as clinical evidence of PCOS, androgen secreting tumors, virilizing disorders, or androgenic medication use

Genetics
Multifactorial

RISK FACTORS
- Family history/ethnicity (e.g., Ashkenazi Jews and Mediterranean backgrounds)
- Obesity

GENERAL PREVENTION
Women with late-onset congenital adrenal hyperplasia (CAH) should be counseled that they may be carriers for the severe early-onset childhood disease.

COMMONLY ASSOCIATED CONDITIONS
- PCOS: the most common cause of premenopausal hirsutism
- Prolonged amenorrhea and anovulation, common
- Acne, common
- Central obesity
- Virilization (rapid onset, clitoromegaly, balding, deepening voice) (1)

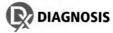 **DIAGNOSIS**

HISTORY
- Severity, time course, and age of onset of hirsutism
- Weight, BMI
- Psychosocial impact on patient
- Menstrual and fertility history, anovulation (defined as ovulatory cycle >35 days)
- Severe acne, especially if treatment resistant
- Presence of virilization
- Medication history: Look for use of valproic acid, testosterone, danazol, glucocorticoids, topical androgen use by partner, and athletic performance drugs.
- The presence of galactorrhea

PHYSICAL EXAM
- Increased hair growth in premenopausal women, particularly over the chin, neck, sideburns, lower back, sternum, areola, abdomen, shoulders, buttocks, perineal area, and inner thighs
- Check the skin for acne, striae, and acanthosis nigricans (velvety black skin in the axillae or neck).
- Virilization: deep voice, male pattern balding, increased muscle mass, and clitoromegaly
- The Ferriman-Gallwey scale (an instrument that rates hair growth in nine areas on a scale of 0 to 4, with >8 being positive) may be used for diagnosis but may underrate patient's perception of hirsutism and can be altered by previous cosmetic treatment. Scores between 8 and 15 are considered to be mild hirsutism, 16 to 25 moderate, and >25 severe (1),(2).

DIFFERENTIAL DIAGNOSIS
- PCOS (72–82%)—irregular menses, elevated androgens, polycystic ovaries on US, infertility, insulin resistance
- Idiopathic hyperandrogenemia (6–15%)—hirsutism with normal ovaries on US, elevated androgen levels, no other explainable cause
- Idiopathic hirsutism (4–7%)—hirsutism with normal menses, androgen levels, and ovaries on ultrasonography, no other explainable cause
- Late-onset or non-classic CAH (2–4%), a genetic enzyme deficiency presents in adolescence with severe hirsutism and irregular menses.
- Androgen-secreting tumor (0.2%)—ovaries (benign or malignant) or adrenals (commonly malignant)
- Thyroid dysfunction, most commonly presents with menstrual irregularity and not common as isolated hirsutism
- Hyperprolactinemia, if accompanied by galactorrhea or amenorrhea
- Rare endocrine disorders—Cushing syndrome, acromegaly
- Medication side effects (e.g., cyclosporine, danazol, glucocorticoids, minoxidil, testosterone)

DIAGNOSTIC TESTS & INTERPRETATION
- Assess androgen levels. Guidelines recommend screening hyperandrogenemic women for non-classical congenital adrenal hyperplasia (NCCAH) due to 21-hydroxylase deficiency by measuring early morning 17-hydroxyprogesterone levels (1).
- PCOS diagnosed with two out of three signs: menstrual dysfunction, clinical or biochemical hyperandrogenemia, polycystic ovaries on US (1)[C]
- Lab testing can be considered to rule out underlying tumor and pituitary diseases (rare) if suggested by history, physical, or initial testing.

Initial Tests (lab, imaging)
- Random total testosterone level is usually sufficient as an initial screen (1)[C].
- Normal upper limit for serum total testosterone in adult women is approximately 40 to 60 ng/dL (1.4 to 2.1 nmol/L). Patients who have clinical features consistent with PCOS but have normal total testosterone should have repeat testing, with an early morning serum free testosterone level calculated from sex hormone–binding globulin (SHBG). A morning free testosterone is 50% more sensitive (3).
- If testosterone is >150 (some use 200) ng/dL, consider US for ovarian tumor and CT scan for adrenal tumor (1).

- The workup for PCOS recommended by the American College of Obstetricians and Gynecologists (ACOG) includes the above tests plus:
  - Screening for metabolic syndrome with a fasting and 2-hour glucose after 75-g glucose load, lipid panel, waist circumference, and blood pressure (4)
- Ovarian US to look for polycystic ovaries
- If the patient is amenorrheic, check prolactin, FSH, LH, TSH, and a pregnancy test (5). An LH/FSH ratio >2 is consistent with PCOS.

Follow-Up Tests & Special Considerations
- 17α-Hydroxyprogesterone (17α-OHP)
  - Best evaluated during the follicular phase or on a random day in women with infrequent menses or amenorrhea
  - Elevations of 17α-OHP (>300) can indicate late-onset CAH.
  - Consider in patients with onset in early adolescence or high-risk group (Ashkenazi Jews) (1)[C].
  - If elevated, order corticotropin stimulation test.
- If prolactin level is high, consider MRI of the pituitary if medication causes not suspected
- If PCOS is diagnosed, ACOG recommends screening for dyslipidemia and DM type 2 (4).
- Suggest against testing for elevated androgen levels in eumenorrheic women with unwanted local hair growth.
- Dehydroepiandrosterone sulfate (DHEA-S) should be checked in virilization (2).
  - Levels >700 may indicate adrenal tumor.

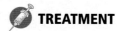 **TREATMENT**

GENERAL MEASURES
- Treatment depends on patient's preference and psychosocial effect.
- The treatment goal is to decrease new hair growth and improve metabolic disorders.
- If patient desires pregnancy, induction of ovulation may be necessary.
- Provide contraception, as needed.
- A calorie-restricted diet is recommended in all overweight patients with PCOS. Weight loss has positive effects on fertility and metabolic profile, and it may improve hirsutism (5).
- Treat accompanying acne.

MEDICATION
First Line
- Direct hair removal or pharmacologic therapy is recommended for mild hirsutism (1)[B].
- Oral contraceptives are first line to manage menstrual abnormalities and hirsutism/acne (2),(3)[A]; they will suppress ovarian androgen production and increase SHBG, improve metabolic syndrome, and slow but not reverse hair growth.
  - Doses of 20 to 35 μg ethinyl estradiol effectively decrease ovarian androgen production. Those containing the progestins, norgestimate, desogestrel, or drospirenone have more androgen-blocking effects, but desogestrel and drospirenone are associated with more DVTs especially in severely obese patients (3).

- They take 6 months to show effect and are continued for years.
  - Oral preparations, compared to vaginal or transdermal, are better at controlling hirsutism and acne; by passing through the liver, they induce SHBG production.
  - For patients with high risk for VTE, it is recommended to use the lowest dose of an ethinyl estradiol–based oral contraceptive and a low-risk, progesterone based-oral contraceptive (1).
- Progesterone (depot or intermittent oral) can be used if estrogens are contraindicated.
- Eflornithine (Vaniqa) HCl cream: Apply BID at least 8 hours apart; reduces facial hair in 40% of women (must be used indefinitely to prevent regrowth); only FDA-approved hirsutism treatment; may be costly and not covered by insurance
- Laser therapy with eflornithine cream shown to have a more rapid response
- Combination of oral contraceptives and antiandrogen is contraindicated first line unless those with severe hirsutism and significant emotional distress or no success with oral contraceptives alone (failure of therapy after 6 months) (1)[B].

Second Line

- Antiandrogenic drugs will further reduce hirsutism to 15–25%. Usually begin 6 months after first-line therapy if results are suboptimal; must be used in combination with oral contraceptives to prevent menorrhagia and potential fetal toxicity; all should be avoided in pregnancy (1).
  - Spironolactone, 50 to 200 mg/day: Onset of action is slow; use with oral contraceptives to prevent menorrhagia. Watch for hyperkalemia, especially with drospirenone-containing OCP (Yasmin); avoid use in pregnancy.
  - Finasteride: 2.5 to 7.5 mg/day decreases androgen binding; not approved by FDA; use with contraception (pregnancy Category X).
  - Cyproterone, not available in the United States: 12.5 to 100.0 mg/day for days 5 to 15 of cycle combined with ethinyl estradiol 20 to 50 μg for days 5 to 25 of cycle
  - Leuprolide, 3.75 mg IM monthly, can cause bone loss, vaginal dryness and hot flashes; avoid use in pregnancy.
  - Flutamide is not recommended due to potential hepatotoxicity (1)[C].
  - Topical antiandrogen therapy is not recommended.
- It is suggested against using insulin-lowering drugs as the sole indication of treating hirsutism (1),(2).
- Steroids: used in late-onset CAH
  - Dexamethasone: 2 mg/day
- Cosmetic treatment: includes many methods of hair removal
  - Temporary: shaving, chemical depilation, plucking, waxing
  - Permanent: Laser epilation and photoepilation are preferred to electrolysis (2).
  - For direct hair removal, electrolysis rather than photoepilation is recommended in women with blonde or white hair (2).
  - Pharmacologic therapy is suggested to minimize regrowth.

Pregnancy Considerations

- May have related infertility
- As hormone balance improves, fertility may increase; provide contraception, as needed.
- Several medications used for treatment are contraindicated in pregnancy.

COMPLEMENTARY & ALTERNATIVE MEDICINE

Glycyrrhiza uralensis (Chinese liquorice) and *Paeonia lactiflora* in combination with *Glycyrrhiza* spp. in single-arm trials have been shown to lower androgen levels in women (6).

 ## ONGOING CARE

FOLLOW-UP RECOMMENDATIONS
Patient Monitoring
Monitor for known side effects of medications.

DIET
Diet consisting of low-calorie, low-glycemic index foods improve fertility and metabolic parameters in patients with PCOS who are overweight (5).

PATIENT EDUCATION
- Hormonal treatment stops further hair growth and will improve but not reverse present hair.
  - Treatment takes 6 months to take effect and may need to be lifelong.
- Cosmetic measures may be needed for the already present hair.

PROGNOSIS
- Good (with long-term therapy) for halting further hair growth
- Moderate to poor for reversing current hair growth

COMPLICATIONS
- If PCOS is present, dysfunctional uterine bleeding may lead to anemia.
- If PCOS is present, anovulation may increase endometrial hyperplasia and uterine cancer risk.
- Androgenic excess may adversely affect lipid status, cardiac risk, and bone density.

REFERENCES

1. Martin KA, Anderson RR, Chang RJ, et al. Evaluation and treatment of hirsutism in premenopausal women: an endocrine society clinical practice guideline. *J Clin Endocrinol Metab*. 2018;103(4):1233–1257.
2. Matheson E, Bain J. Hirsutism in women. *Am Fam Physician*. 2019;100(3):168–175.
3. Goodman NF, Cobin RH, Futterweit W, et al; for American Association of Clinical Endocrinologists, American College of Endocrinology, Androgen Excess and PCOS Society. American Association of Clinical Endocrinologists, American College of Endocrinology, and Androgen Excess and PCOS Society disease state clinical review: guide to the best practices in the evaluation and treatment of polycystic ovary syndrome—part 1. *Endocr Pract*. 2015;21(11):1291–1300.
4. American College of Obstetricians and Gynecologists' Committee on Practice Bulletins—Gynecology. ACOG practice bulletin no. 194: polycystic ovary syndrome. *Obstet Gynecol*. 2018;131(6):e157–e171.
5. Williams T, Moore JB, Regehr J. Polycystic ovary syndrome: common questions and answers. *Am Fam Physician*. 2023;107(3):264–272.
6. Arentz S, Abbott JA, Smith CA, et al. Herbal medicine for the management of polycystic ovary syndrome (PCOS) and associated oligo/amenorrhoea and hyperandrogenism; a review of the laboratory evidence for effects with corroborative clinical findings. *BMC Complement Altern Med*. 2014;14:511.

ADDITIONAL READING

- Teede HJ, Misso ML, Costello MF, et al; International PCOS Network. Recommendations from the international evidence-based guideline for the assessment and management of polycystic ovary syndrome. *Fertil Steril*. 2018;110(3):364–379.
- van Zuuren EJ, Fedorowicz Z, Carter B, et al. Interventions for hirsutism (excluding laser and photoepilation therapy alone). *Cochrane Database Syst Rev*. 2015;2015(4):CD010334.

SEE ALSO

Acne Vulgaris; Infertility; Polycystic Ovarian Syndrome (PCOS)

 ## CODES

ICD10
- L68.0 Hirsutism
- E28.2 Polycystic ovarian syndrome

CLINICAL PEARLS

- PCOS is the most common cause of hirsutism (diagnosed with two out of three: menstrual dysfunction, clinical or biochemical hyperandrogenemia, polycystic ovaries on US).
- Diagnosis is based on androgen level in all women with abnormal hirsutism score; total testosterone and TSH for initial testing
- Virilization (clitoromegaly, balding, deepening voice): Suspect if testosterone >150 ng/dL; look for adrenal and ovarian tumor.
- Lifestyle modification and OCPs are first-line therapy for hirsutism, menstrual irregularities, and acne.

H

HIV/AIDS

Pamela R. Hughes, MD • Gregorio Climaco, MD

 BASICS

DESCRIPTION

- HIV is a retrovirus (subgroup lentivirus) that integrates into CD4 T lymphocytes, altering cell-mediated immunity and causing cell death, severe immunodeficiency, opportunistic infections, and malignancies if not treated.
- The natural history of untreated HIV infection includes viral transmission, acute retroviral syndrome, recovery and seroconversion, asymptomatic chronic HIV infection, and symptomatic HIV infection or AIDS.
- Without treatment, the average patient progresses to AIDS ~10 years after acquiring HIV. Without treatment, people living with full-blown AIDS typically survive about 3 years.

EPIDEMIOLOGY

Incidence

- ~30,500 people aged >13 years were diagnosed with HIV in the United States during 2020. The incidence decreased by 8% from 2016 to 2019.
- There were approximately 1.5 million new cases of HIV worldwide in 2020 (1).

Prevalence

- As of 2019, ~1.2 million persons in the United States have HIV; ~13% are not aware that they are infected (1).
- As of 2020, ~38 million people are living with HIV worldwide. ~45% of new diagnoses are in Eastern and Southern Africa (1).
- In 2020, ~680,000 people died from AIDS-related illnesses (1).

ETIOLOGY AND PATHOPHYSIOLOGY

- HIV primarily infects CD4+ cells. HIV is a single-stranded, positive-sense, enveloped RNA virus. After entering target cells, viral RNA is transcribed to DNA (through reverse transcription), imported to the host cell nucleus, and incorporated into host DNA. The virus can become latent or produce new viral RNA with proteins that are released to infect other CD4+ cells. Host CD8+ cells are activated as part of the seroconversion response.
- There are two types of HIV. HIV-1 causes the majority of HIV infections. HIV-2 is less infectious and seen primarily in West Africa.

RISK FACTORS

- Sexual activity (>90% of transmission): Receptive anal sex is the highest risk. Ulcerative urogenital lesions promote transmission (1).
- Injection drug use
- Children of HIV-infected women: Maternal HIV-1 RNA level predicts transmission.
  - HIV can also be transmitted in breast milk. HIV+ women should not breastfeed, unless there is no alternative. In this case, consider antiretroviral therapy (ART).
- Recipients of blood products prior to 1985
- Occupational exposure (health care workers)

GENERAL PREVENTION

- Primary prevention: behavioral counseling for all sexually active people with high risk of STIs (2)
  - Avoid unprotected, high-risk sex, and injection drug use, especially shared needle
  - Condom use reduces risk of transmission by 77–80%.
- Preexposure prophylaxis (PrEP) is recommended by WHO and USPSTF for persons at high risk of acquiring HIV.
  - General guidelines for PrEP: (i) exclude acute or chronic HIV infection before initiating therapy, (ii) repeat HIV testing every 3 months during therapy, (iii) renal and liver function testing at baseline, 2 to 8 weeks after initiating PrEP, and every 6 months
- Postexposure prophylaxis (PEP) should be started within 72 hours of exposure and continued for 28 days with a three-drug regimen.
- For HIV+ patients using ART, maintaining HIV RNA levels <200 copies/mL prevents risk of transmission to sexual partners (treatment as prevention) (3)[A].
- CDC recommends screening for HIV at least once in patients aged 13 to 64 years.
- Pregnant women should be tested at the initial prenatal visit and again during the 3rd trimester (2).
- At least annual screening is recommended for patients at higher risk (2).

COMMONLY ASSOCIATED CONDITIONS

- Other sexually transmitted infections
- Syphilis, tuberculosis, and hepatitis (B or C) can be more aggressive in HIV-infected persons.
- Increased risk for cervical cancer, lymphoma, and skin malignancies

DIAGNOSIS

- Acute retroviral syndrome: CD4 lymphocyte count declines with increase in viral load 1 to 4 weeks after transmission; confirmed by high-HIV RNA in the absence of HIV antibody
  - Presents as an influenza-like syndrome: fever, lymphadenopathy, pharyngitis, rash, myalgias/arthralgias
- Clinical latency (asymptomatic): variable duration (average is 8 to 10 years) accompanied by a gradual decline in CD4 cell counts and relatively stable HIV RNA levels; patients often develop persistent generalized lymphadenopathy and may develop fever, weight loss, myalgias, and gastrointestinal problems if unrecognized.
- AIDS is defined by a CD4 cell count <200, a CD4 cell percentage of total lymphocytes <14%, or an AIDS-related opportunistic infection: *Pneumocystis jiroveci (carinii)* pneumonia, cryptococcal meningitis, recurrent bacterial pneumonia, *Candida* esophagitis, CNS toxoplasmosis, TB, non-Hodgkin lymphoma (NHL), progressive multifocal encephalopathy, HIV nephropathy, Kaposi sarcoma, Hodgkin lymphoma, and invasive cervical cancer
- Advanced HIV disease: CD4 cell count <50; most AIDS-related deaths occur at this time.

HISTORY

- Complete medical history, including risk exposures; sexual, social, and occupational histories; injection drug use; receipt of blood products (prior to 1985); prior use of PrEP or PEP; and medications
- Comprehensive review of systems
- Review immunizations record.

PHYSICAL EXAM

- No physical examination findings are specific to HIV.
- Focus on weight; skin exam; funduscopic (retinal) exam; oropharynx, lymph nodes, lung, liver, spleen, mental status, neurologic, genital, and rectal examinations.

DIFFERENTIAL DIAGNOSIS

Burkitt lymphoma, candidiasis, CMV, coccidioidomycosis, *Cryptococcus*, EBV, herpes simplex, influenza, lymphoma, mononucleosis, TB, toxoplasmosis

DIAGNOSTIC TESTS & INTERPRETATION

Initial Tests (lab, imaging)

- Rapid HIV testing available (lower negative predictive value)
- HIV testing combines antibody/antigen immunoassay for HIV-1/HIV-2 (3)[A].
  - Can be positive within 2 to 3 weeks of exposure
- Obtain HIV RNA if acute HIV infection is suspected using quantitative PCR; detects infection within 12 days of exposure
- CD4 cell count and percentage (3)[A]
- Plasma HIV RNA viral load (3)[A]
- CBC with differential, lipid levels, fasting blood glucose, creatinine (Cr), blood urea nitrogen (BUN), chemistry, transaminase levels, total bilirubin
- Screen for hepatitis A/B/C, chlamydia, gonorrhea, and syphilis.
- Cervical cytology and HPV testing if aged ≥30 years
- PPD or interferon-γ release assay (IGRA) to screen for latent TB infection; chest x-ray (CXR) if pulmonary symptoms or positive PPD
- HLA-B*5701 testing if abacavir planned for treatment (3)[A]
- Genotypic tests for resistance to antiretrovirals for patients with pretreatment HIV RNA level <1,000 copies/mL; transmitted resistance to at least one drug seen in 6–16% of patients (3)[A]

Follow-Up Tests & Special Considerations
PEP

- Nonoccupational PEP (nPEP) is recommended if care sought within 72 hours of possible exposure and substantial risk of exposure:
  - Source known to be HIV+; exposure to blood, semen, vaginal, or rectal secretions; breast milk
- 28 days of a three-drug regimen should be started if nPEP indicated.
  - Tenofovir disoproxil fumarate 300 mg + emtricitabine 200 mg/day plus:
    ○ Raltegravir 400 mg BID *or* dolutegravir 50 mg/day
- Counsel patients with more than one course of nPEP on prevention and consider PrEP.

- For nPEP: Complete HIV, hepatitis B, and hepatitis C testing at baseline, 4 to 6 weeks, 3 months, and 6 months after exposure.
- For persons exposed via sexual contact: Test for syphilis, gonorrhea, and chlamydia at time of presentation and 4 to 6 weeks after exposure; syphilis serology 6 months postexposure

 ## TREATMENT

- Initiate ART and then select/change regimens based on resistance testing.
- Consider dosing frequency, pill burden, adverse toxic effect profiles, comorbidities, and drug interactions (including OTC supplements).
- Pregnancy, AIDS-defining conditions, acute opportunistic infections, CD4 count <200, HIV-associated nephropathy, acute/early infection, hepatitis B or C coinfection, rapidly declining CD4 counts (>100 cells/mm³ per year), and high viral loads (>100,000 copies/mL) increase urgency for immediate therapy (3)[A].

GENERAL MEASURES
- The goal of ART is to reduce viral load (below limits of detection: HIV RNA <200) and delay immune suppression. Viral load is the most important indicator of response to ART.
- Assess drug resistance and recommend genotypic testing to guide therapy (3).
- Assess substance abuse, economic factors (unstable housing, food insecurity), social support, mental illness, comorbidities, and high-risk behaviors.

MEDICATION
- PrEP:
  - For patients without HIV who may be exposed to HIV
  - HIV-negative individuals whose partner is HIV+ with detectable or unknown viral load
  - IV drug use with shared needles
- Prior to providing PrEP:
  - Ensure that the patient does not have HIV through confirmatory testing.
  - Screen for chlamydia, gonorrhea, syphilis, and HBV.
  - Obtain baseline kidney function (CrCl).
- Medication regimens approved by the FDA:
  - Emtricitabine 200 mg + tenofovir disoproxil fumarate 300 mg PO daily (F/TDF)
  - Emtricitabine 200 mg + tenofovir alafenamide 25 mg PO daily (F/TAF)
  - Cabotegravir 600 mg IM q2mo (preferred in patients with CrCl <30 mL/min)
- PrEP prevention of HIV transmission via sexual route is 99% effective and >74% effective for transmission via IV drug use.

First Line
Recommended regimens for most people with HIV (3)[A]

- Integrase strand transfer inhibitor plus two nucleoside reverse transcriptase inhibitors:
  - Bictegravir/tenofovir alafenamide/emtricitabine (50 mg/25 mg/200 mg PO daily)
  - Dolutegravir/abacavir/lamivudine (50 mg/600 mg/300 mg PO daily)—only for patients who are HLA-B*5701 negative

- Dolutegravir (50 mg PO daily) plus tenofovir disoproxil fumarate (300 mg PO daily) or tenofovir alafenamide (25 mg PO daily) plus emtricitabine (200 mg PO daily) or lamivudine (300 mg PO daily)
- Integrase strand transfer inhibitor plus one nucleoside reverse transcriptase inhibitors
  - Dolutegravir/lamivudine (50 mg/300 mg PO daily) except if HIV RNA >500,000, hepatitis B coinfection or genotypic resistance testing results not available
  - Dolutegravir is the preferred treatment for women who are pregnant or trying to conceive (3)[A].

ADDITIONAL THERAPIES
Prophylactic antimicrobials and vaccines:

- *P. jiroveci* prophylaxis: trimethoprim/sulfamethoxazole (TMP-SMX) if CD4 <200 cells/mm³, prior *P. jiroveci*, thrush, or unexplained fever for >2 weeks
- *Mycobacterium tuberculosis*: Treat for latent TB if positive PPD or positive IGRA if no prior prophylaxis or treatment, negative CXR, no recent TB contact, and no history of inadequately treated TB.
- *Toxoplasma gondii* prophylaxis when CD4 <100 cells/mm³: TMP-SMX 1 DS tab daily
- *Mycobacterium avium* complex prophylaxis when CD4 <50 and no ART; azithromycin 1,200 mg PO weekly
- Influenza vaccine annually (no live vaccine), hepatitis A and B vaccines, human papillomavirus vaccine, *Streptococcus* pneumonia series, and at least three Tdap vaccines in lifetime and Td vaccination every 10 years

 ## ONGOING CARE

FOLLOW-UP RECOMMENDATIONS
Patient Monitoring
- Monitor HIV RNA viral load 2 to 8 weeks after starting therapy; if detectable, repeat testing every 4 to 8 weeks until viral load is suppressed to <200 copies/mL (3).
  - A 3-fold decrease in HIV RNA viral load is considered a significant response.
- Monitor HIV RNA viral load, CD4, and CBC every 3 to 4 months for the first 2 years of ART or if the CD4 count is <300 cells/mm³.
- HIV RNA monitoring can be spaced to every 6 months in patients adherent to ART with consistently suppressed viral load and immunologically stable for >2 years.
- Confirm CD4 count level has increased 50 to 150 cells/mm³ within the 1st year of ART.
- Space CD4 monitoring to 12 months if suppressed viral load and CD4 >300 cells/mm³.
- Once viral load has been suppressed consistently for >2 years and CD4 cell counts are consistently >500/μL, monitoring CD4 cell counts is optional unless virologic failure occurs (or if immunosuppressive treatments or conditions arise).
- Annual fasting lipids and CMP plus urinalysis every 6 months
- Annual cervical cytology (regardless of age) until three negative screens and then every 3 years
- Urinalysis every 6 to 12 months or as indicated

- β-hCG in women of childbearing age at diagnosis and then as clinically indicated
- Test for syphilis, gonorrhea, and chlamydia at initial diagnosis and annually. Women should additionally be tested for trichomonas.

DIET
Encourage good nutrition; avoid raw eggs and unpasteurized dairy products.

PATIENT EDUCATION
Provide nonjudgmental, sex-positive prevention counseling, reviewing high-risk behaviors and viral transmission. Discuss the importance of continual ART and ongoing medical care, even if viral load is undetectable. Discuss importance of communication of HIV status with sexual partners.

PROGNOSIS
- Untreated HIV infection leading to the diagnosis of AIDS has an associated life expectancy of about 3 years. If the patient has an opportunistic infection, the life expectancy is about 1 year.
- AIDS-defining opportunistic infections usually do not develop until CD4 <200.
- Adherence failure is the most common cause of treatment failure.

REFERENCES
1. Centers for Disease Control and Prevention. Statistics overview. https://www.cdc.gov/hiv/statistics/overview/index.html. Accessed May 25, 2023.
2. Centers for Disease Control and Prevention. Sexually transmitted infections treatment guidelines, 2021. https://www.cdc.gov/std/treatment-guidelines/STI-Guidelines-2021.pdf. Accessed May 25, 2023.
3. U.S. Department of Health and Human Services. Guidelines for the use of antiretroviral agents in adults and adolescents living with HIV. https://clinicalinfo.hiv.gov/sites/default/files/guidelines/archive/AdultandAdolescentGL_2021_08_16.pdf. Accessed October 9, 2023.

 ## CODES

ICD10
- Z21 Asymptomatic human immunodeficiency virus infection status
- B20 Human immunodeficiency virus [HIV] disease
- R75 Inconclusive laboratory evidence of human immunodef virus

CLINICAL PEARLS
- Routine screening for HIV should be completed in all adults and adolescents.
- Discuss prevention strategies, including PrEP, with individuals who are at high risk of HIV infection.
- Acute HIV seroconversion illness mimics mononucleosis or influenza and is characterized by fever, sore throat, adenopathy, myalgias, and rash.
- Consider HIV testing in at-risk patients reporting unintended weight loss, fatigue, night sweats, or rash.
- Provide necessary vaccinations and prophylactic antibiotics to HIV+ patients based on clinical history and CD4 count.

H

HODGKIN LYMPHOMA

Prarthna V. Bhardwaj, MBBS • Doyun Park, MD

BASICS

Hodgkin lymphoma (HL) is a neoplasm of the lymphatic system representing one of the common cancers in young adults; characterized by a low number of malignant cells deriving from B lymphocytes and an extensive inflammatory microenvironment

DESCRIPTION
- Historical background:
  - Described first in 1832 by Thomas Hodgkin about a series of six patients with clinical findings different from those with tuberculosis, syphilis, and inflammation
  - German pathologist Carl Sternberg (1898) and American pathologist Dorothy Reed (1902) independently provided accounts of the giant "Reed-Sternberg" (RS) cells—the microscopic hallmarks of Hodgkin disease.
  - Initially treated with herbs, surgery, and arsenic in the 19th century; noted to shrink upon exposure to x-rays in the beginning of the 20th century. Chemotherapy instituted as first-line treatment in the early 1970s.
- Subtypes:
  - Two subtypes:
    ○ Classical HL (cHL)—95% of cases; includes nodular sclerosing, mixed cellularity, lymphocyte rich, and lymphocyte depleted
    ○ Nodular lymphocyte predominant HL (NLPHL)—5% of cases

EPIDEMIOLOGY
- Incidence: 2 to 3 per 100,000 per year
- 11% of all lymphoid malignancies
- Has a bimodal age distribution—between 20 and 40 years and a second peak at around 55 years; typically diagnosed at age 20 to 34 years with median age 39 years at diagnosis given decreasing bimodal age distribution
- 1.3:1 male-to-female ratio

ETIOLOGY AND PATHOPHYSIOLOGY
- cHL is a B-cell lymphoma of germinal center origin that has lost its B-cell phenotype.
- RS cells harbor clonal rearrangements of hypermutated, class-switched immunoglobulin genes resulting in nonfunctional immunoglobulin genes lacking the expression of the cell surface B-cell receptor. In a healthy B cell, this should lead to apoptosis; however, in HL, these cells appear to be "rescued" from apoptosis by additional oncogenic events.
- NLPHL lacks typical RS cells but has lymphocytic and histiocytic cells, characterized by larger cells with folded multilobulated nuclei ("popcorn cells" or LP cells)—show a nucleus with multiple nucleoli that are basophilic and smaller than RS cells.
- Genome-wide association studies identified 19p13.3 at intron 2 of *TCF3*.

Genetics
- First-degree relative: 3 to 9 times risk
- Siblings of younger patients: 7 times risk
- Weak correlation between familial HL and HLA class I regions containing HLA-A1, HLA-B5, HLA-B8, HLA-B18 alleles

RISK FACTORS
- HIV: Increased risk of HL in patients who are HIV positive
- Epstein-Barr virus (EBV): detected in nearly 45% of patients with HL
- Genetic predisposition: significantly increased risk in identical twins indicating role of genetics in HL

GENERAL PREVENTION
Avoid exposure to chemicals such as pesticides, herbicides, and benzene.

COMMONLY ASSOCIATED CONDITIONS
HIV infection

DIAGNOSIS

HISTORY
- Painless lymphadenopathy (cervical/supraclavicular)
- Pel-Ebstein (cyclic) fever—high-grade fever every 7 to 10 days
- Constitutional symptoms or "B symptoms": drenching night sweats, profound weight loss, fatigue, anorexia
- Chronic pruritus may be encountered.
- If mediastinal lymphadenopathy is large, can cause chest pain and shortness of breath
- Can present with a mass on chest radiograph

PHYSICAL EXAM
- Lymphadenopathy 70% (cervical > supraclavicular > axillary)—firm, rubbery, consistency
- Splenomegaly may be present.
- Hepatomegaly may be present.
- Tonsillar enlargement may be present.

DIFFERENTIAL DIAGNOSIS
Non-HL, solid tumor metastases, sarcoidosis, autoimmune disease, drug reaction, and infections like HIV, syphilis, tuberculosis

DIAGNOSTIC TESTS & INTERPRETATION
Initial Tests (lab, imaging)
- CBC with differential—may show eosinophilia, ESR
- Comprehensive metabolic panel, LDH
- HIV, EBV, HCV
- Pregnancy test for women of childbearing age
- Echocardiogram—in anticipation of treatment with anthracycline
- Pulmonary function tests (PFTs)—DLCO measurement in anticipation of treatment with bleomycin
- Chest x-ray
- Computed tomography (CT) with contrast of chest, abdomen, and pelvis
- Positron emission tomography (PET): for initial staging, midtreatment decision making, and end-of-treatment evaluation

Follow-Up Tests & Special Considerations
- Fertility considerations:
  - Semen cryopreservation if chemotherapy or pelvic radiation therapy (RT)
  - In vitro fertilization or ovarian tissue/oocyte cryopreservation

- RT considerations:
  - Splenic RT: pneumococcal, *Haemophilus influenzae*, meningococcal vaccine

Geriatric Considerations
Poorer prognosis if present at age ≥60 years:
- Less likely to tolerate intensive chemotherapy or be included in a trial

Pediatric Considerations
Young females (<30 years of age) treated with thoracic radiation are at high risk for breast cancer, and early breast cancer screening is recommended.

Pregnancy Considerations
Abdominal ultrasonography to detect subdiaphragmatic disease
- Delay until after delivery if asymptomatic and early stage.
- ABVD more likely to cause fetal malformations in 1st trimester; malformation risk is lower when used in 2nd and 3rd trimesters.
- Vinblastine monotherapy to control symptoms

Diagnostic Procedures/Other
- Excisional/incisional lymph node biopsy
- Immunohistochemistry
- Bone marrow biopsy if cytopenia with negative PET
- Lumbar puncture and MRI of the brain if neurologic symptoms

Test Interpretation
- Morphology: RS cells in cHL described as "owl eye" appearance—two nucleoli in two separate nuclear lobes, abundant slightly basophilic cytoplasm; popcorn cells noted in NLPHL
- Immunophenotype: CD15+, CD30+, CD45−, CD3− (T-cell marker), and typically CD20−
- Cytogenetics: no consistent or specific karyotypic findings

TREATMENT

- Ann Arbor staging with Cotswold modification
  - Stage I: single lymph node or of a single extralymphatic organ or site
  - Stage II: ≥2 lymph node regions on the same side of diaphragm alone or with involvement of extralymphatic organ or tissue
  - Stage III: node groups on both sides of the diaphragm
  - Stage IV: dissemination involving extranodal organs (except the spleen, which is considered lymphoid tissue)
  - Subclasses: A = no systemic symptoms; B = systemic symptoms (fever, night sweats, weight loss >10% body weight); X = bulky disease (>1/3 intrathoracic, diameter, or >10-cm nodal mass)
- Intent of treatment: curative
- All subsequent treatment and follow-up care recommendations based on National Comprehensive Cancer Network (NCCN) consensus; please refer to NCCN Practice Guidelines in Oncology for HL.

MEDICATION

First Line

- Early-stage disease: combined modality treatment with chemotherapy/radiotherapy *or* chemotherapy
- Advanced stage disease: chemotherapy
- PET/CT used after cycle 2 (PET-2) to guide either escalation or de-escalation of therapy (1)
- Chemotherapy:
  - ABVD (doxorubicin, bleomycin, vinblastine, dacarbazine):
    - ○ Severe phlebitis—need for central line to administer treatment
    - ○ Highly emetogenic
    - ○ Vinblastine: risk of neuropathy
    - ○ Bleomycin: risk of pulmonary toxicity, death; test dose may be administered prior to first cycle.
    - ○ Doxorubicin: risk of cardiotoxicity; monitor LVEF.
  - AAVD (doxorubicin, brentuximab vedotin [anti-CD30 chimeric antibody conjugated to synthetic antimicrotubule agent monomethyl auristatin E], vinblastine, dacarbazine):
    - ○ Superior to ABVD per ECHELON-1 trial in terms of PFS as well as OS (2)
    - ○ Preferred especially if abnormal PFTs
    - ○ Brentuximab vedotin: peripheral neuropathy, nausea, fatigue, neutropenia, diarrhea
    - ○ AAVD now deemed to be preferred front-line therapy for patients with Stage III or IV HL.

Second Line

- Reserved for patients with relapsed/refractory (R/R) disease
- Therapeutic strategy and sequencing of treatment influenced by: eligibility for ASCT, functional response to salvage chemotherapy, duration of remission, prior therapy and comorbidities.
- Standard: chemotherapy agents not used for initial treatment followed by high-dose therapy with autologous stem cell transplant (HDT/ASCT)
- Pembrolizumab (anti-PD1) FDA approved for patients with R/R cHL who have failed two or more lines of therapy
- Nivolumab (anti-PD1) in a phase 2 study of R/R cHL showed ORR 69% with durable response and favorable safety profile.
- Third-line novel agents undergoing studies: proteosome inhibitors (bortezomib), mammalian target of rapamycin (mTOR) inhibitors (everolimus), immunomodulators (lenalidomide); CART-cell therapy directed to CD30 noted high rates of durable response in heavily pretreated patients.
- Median survival <3 years if failed second-line therapy, including HDT/ASCT
- NLPHL
  - Treated with rituximab + CHOP (CD20 positive)
- Allogeneic stem cell transplant (alloSCT) remains a curative-intent treatment option for patients with R/R cHL, including those who have failed an autologous transplantation.

ADDITIONAL THERAPIES

Radiotherapy used for residual disease after salvage chemotherapy or ASCT for R/R disease

 ONGOING CARE

Patients treated with ABVD become neutropenic. Treatment is continued despite neutropenia with no clear increased risk of infection with or without growth factors.

FOLLOW-UP RECOMMENDATIONS

Patient Monitoring

- During therapy: CBC, nutrition, and hydration
- Restage with PET after 2 cycles of chemotherapy: sensitive prognostic indicator
- Posttreatment surveillance:
  - History and physical: q3–6mo for the first 2 years, then q6–12mo for the next 1 year, and then annually
  - Laboratory studies
    - ○ CBC, platelets, BMP, ESR (if elevated at time of diagnosis), as indicated clinically
    - ○ Thyroid-stimulating hormone (TSH) annually if radiation to neck
  - Imaging:
    - ○ PET-CT to demonstrate negativity within 3 months following completion of treatment to document "Complete Response"; no role for annual surveillance PET
    - ○ CT scans no more often than every 6 months for the first 2 years or as clinically indicated
    - ○ Annual breast mammogram beginning 8 to 10 years after therapy or at the age of 40 years (whichever is first) if chest or axillary irradiation (annual breast MRI as well if initially radiated between ages 10 and 30 years) according to the American Cancer Society
  - Annual influenza vaccine
  - Referral for cancer survivorship with psychosocial support
  - Smoking cessation: Combination of smoking and chest irradiation dramatically increases risk of lung cancer.

PATIENT EDUCATION

- Reproductive impact
- Risks of secondary malignancy

PROGNOSIS

- Cure rate for cHL: 85%
- Relapse or progression of disease rate: 5–20%
- Overall survival rates:
  - 1-year survival: 92%
  - 5-year survival: 87% (93% if localized)
  - 10-year survival: 80%

- International prognostic score for advanced disease:
  - Age >45 years
  - Male gender
  - Albumin <4 g/dL
  - Hemoglobin <10.5 g/dL
  - Lymphocytopenia: <600 lymphocyte cells/dL or lymphocytes <8% of WBC
  - WBC ≥15,000 cells/dL
  - Stage IV disease

COMPLICATIONS

Late complications:

- Peripheral neuropathy after treatment.
- Anthracycline and radiation exposure increase risk of cardiovascular and valvular disease.
- Irreversible pulmonary toxicity due to bleomycin
- Risk of secondary malignancies like myeloid neoplasms (due to alkylating agents) and breast cancer (radiation exposure)

REFERENCES

1. Barrington SF, Kirkwood AA, Franceschetto A, et al. PET-CT for staging and early response: results from the response-adapted therapy in advanced Hodgkin lymphoma study. *Blood.* 2016;127(12):1531–1538.
2. Ansell SM, Radford J, Connors JM, et al. Overall survival with brentuximab vedotin in stage III or IV Hodgkin's lymphoma. *N Engl J Med.* 2022;387(4):310–320.

 CODES

ICD10

- C81.96 Hodgkin lymphoma, unspecified, intrapelvic lymph nodes
- C81.44 Lymphocyte-rich Hodgkin lymphoma, lymph nodes of axilla and upper limb
- C81.75 Other Hodgkin lymphoma, lymph nodes of inguinal region and lower limb

CLINICAL PEARLS

- HL mainly affects young people.
- It is a potentially curable lymphoma. Treatment includes chemotherapy +/− RT.
- If patient develops neutropenia during treatment of HL with ABVD regimen, chemotherapy should be continued provided there is no concern for an infection without delays.
- Long-term effects of chemotherapy should be discussed with patients.
- Close collaboration between oncologist and PCP required for future monitoring

H

HOMELESSNESS

Dana Sprute, MD, MPH, FAAFP • Jenney Vongprathoum, MD

 BASICS

DESCRIPTION
- Lacking a fixed, regular, and adequate nighttime residence
- Chronic homelessness: lacking fixed, regular housing for at least 1 year or at least four episodes of being unhoused in the past 3 years for a combined length of at least 1 year
- People struggling with homelessness often have complex and chronic medical illnesses such as mental illness, substance use disorders, and physical disabilities (1).

EPIDEMIOLOGY
Incidence
- Increasing since 2017 nationwide; 6% overall increase
- The COVID-19 pandemic disrupted accounting of unsheltered people, but conditions during the pandemic may have increased the incidence (1).

Prevalence
In 2022, 0.18% of the U.S. population (approximately 582,462 individuals) experienced homelessness on any given night: 61% in sheltered locations and 39% in unsheltered locations (1).
- 6% are veterans, 28% are families with children, 5% are unaccompanied youth (age <25 years), and 22% are chronically homeless individuals.
- 50% of the homeless population is white.

RISK FACTORS
- Poverty
  - 2023 federal poverty level: $30,000 annual income for four-person household in the lower 48 states and District of Columbia, slightly higher in Alaska and Hawaii (2)
  - In 2021, 11.6% of U.S. population are below federal poverty line.
- Unemployment: U.S. rate of 3.6% in June 2023 (U.S. Bureau of Labor Statistics)
- Lack of affordable health care: In 2022, 8.6% of U.S. population (280 million) were uninsured for the entire calendar year (3).
- Lack of affordable housing: <30% of gross income for housing costs, including utilities; roughly 37.8 million of U.S. households spend >30% on housing costs; 18.2 million households spend ≥50% of income on housing.
- Intimate partner violence (IPV): 12% of overall persons experiencing homelessness and about 20% of families experiencing homelessness report IPV; IPV often involves exertion of psychological and financial control that leaves survivors with poor credit, limited support, and few resources.
- Veterans: decreasing due to policy changes; decreased by 50% over a decade (2010 to 2020) (2)
- Transgender individuals: 0.6% identify as transgender and 0.4% as gender nonconforming (2)
- Addiction disorders: 46% report substance use as a major factor contributing to homelessness (1).
- Psychiatric illness: 25% of adults experiencing homelessness (1)
- Postincarceration: 50,000 people each year enter homeless shelters from jails/prisons (1).

GENERAL PREVENTION
- Policy and funding for community programs to provide emergency/rapid housing, housing stabilization, and case management services; the CARES Act of 2020 and the American Rescue Plan Act of 2021 provide funding for permanent housing. Over the past 5 years, the fastest growing forms of assistance include rapid rehousing and "other permanent housing."
- Increased Medicaid eligibility, expanded home- and community-based services, and case management for people experiencing homelessness
- HUD: increasing permanent supportive housing units; increasing services for veterans, families with children, and those with disabilities
- Social justice policy recommendations: permanent affordable housing; foreclosure and homelessness prevention; increased funds for HUD McKinney-Vento programs (emergency, transitional, and permanent housing) and National Housing Trust Fund, rural homeless assistance, universal health care, universal livable income, employment/workforce services; prevention of hate crimes against the homeless; decriminalization of homelessness

COMMONLY ASSOCIATED CONDITIONS
- Hunger and malnutrition
- Exposure-related conditions (frostbite, heatstroke)
- Substance use disorders and their associated conditions
  - Liver disease (alcohol, hepatitis B and C)
  - Abscesses (IV drug use)
  - Overdose
- Dental problems
- Psychiatric illness
- Trauma (increased risk of assault, victims of hate crime)
- Infectious diseases
  - Skin/nail infection and infestation (lice, bedbugs, and scabies)
  - Tuberculosis, HIV/AIDS, STI
- Worsening of chronic medical conditions; lack of healthy food, places to store medications, or medical equipment; lack of restful sleep; decreased health literacy; limited transportation to appointments

 DIAGNOSIS

HISTORY
- Living conditions: location, access to food, restrooms, place to store medicines, safety
- Prior homelessness: causes and circumstances
- Family members, especially dependent children
- Medications: OTC medication, dietary supplements, medication "borrowed" from others
- Prior providers: oral health, primary and specialty care, current medical home
- Mental health: stress, anxiety, appetite, sleep, concentration, mood, speech, memory, thought process and content, auditory/visual hallucinations, suicidal/homicidal ideation, insight, judgment, impulse control, social interactions; symptoms of brain injury (headaches, seizures, memory loss, irritability, dizziness, insomnia, poor organizational/decision-making skills), trauma history

- Alcohol/nicotine/drug use: amount, frequency, duration
- Gender identity/orientation, behaviors, rape, pregnancies, hepatitis, HIV/AIDS, other STIs
- History of or current abuse: emotional, physical, sexual; patient safety
- Legal problems/violence: history of incarceration
- Activities: routines (treatment feasibility); level of strenuous activity
- Work: previous types of jobs, length held, veteran status, occupational injuries/toxic exposures; vocational skills, interest
- Education: highest level; ever in special education; assess ability to read/language skills/English fluency.
- Nutrition/hydration: diet, food resources, preparation skills, liquid intake
- Cultural heritage/affiliations: family, friends, faith community, other sources of support
- Strengths: coping skills, job skills, resourcefulness, abilities, interests

PHYSICAL EXAM
- Comprehensive exam: height, weight, BMI, especially abdominal, cardiopulmonary, dermatologic, oral, feet, neurologic, mental status
- Focused exams: for patients uncomfortable with full-body, unclothed exam at first visit
- Dental assessment: age-appropriate teeth, obvious caries, dental/referred pain, diabetes, CVD

DIAGNOSTIC TESTS & INTERPRETATION
Initial Tests (lab, imaging)
- Mental health: Patient Health Questionnaire (PHQ-9, PHQ-2), MHS-III, MDQ, GAD-7
- Cognitive assessment: Mini-Mental State Examination (MMSE), Montreal Cognitive Assessment (MOCA), Traumatic Brain Injury Questionnaire (TBIQ), Repeatable Battery for the Assessment of Neuropsychological Status (RBANS)
- Developmental assessment: Ages & Stages Questionnaires, Parents' Evaluation of Developmental Status (PEDS), Denver II, or other screening tool
- Interpersonal violence: IPV, sexual assault, TBI
- Forensic evaluation: if indicated by history
- Baseline labs: as needed to address suspected medical concerns
- TB screening: PPD or T-SPOT.TB test/QuantiFERON-TB Gold if available
- STI screening: HIV/AIDS, chlamydia, gonorrhea, syphilis, hepatitis B, hepatitis C, trichomoniasis
- Substance abuse: Simple Screening Instrument for Alcohol and Other Drugs (SSI-AOD), urine drug screen

Follow-Up Tests & Special Considerations

- Reproductive health care and STIs: Obtain a detailed sexual history (sexual identity, orientation, behaviors/sexual practices, number of partners). Consider patient exploitation, especially if mental illness/developmental disability is suspected. Communicate willingness to initiate contraception on first visit without exam. Genital exam is recommended, but be sensitive to the patient, especially if there is a possible sexual abuse history. If pelvic exam is refused, consider self-collected testing and/or empiric treatment for STI (and possibility of multiple orifice infection). Dispense medications on site; facilitate partner treatment.
- Consider access to facilities, even if residing at a shelter. For example, patient may not have access to restroom for colonoscopy bowel prep.
- Pediatric care: complete exam every visit; use each visit to identify/address problems and provide vaccinations because homeless families may not see a medical provider unless a child is sick. Vision and hearing screening at every visit. Facilitate referrals as able.

 TREATMENT

- Enlist community resources: mental health and substance abuse programs, free clinics, case management
- Health care maintenance: vaccinations (hepatitis A and B, pneumococcal, Tdap, influenza, SARS-CoV-2), cancer and chronic disease screening for adults; Early and Periodic Screening, Diagnosis, and Treatment (EPSDT) program screening and vaccinations for children
- Care plan
  - Basic needs: food, clothing, and housing
  - Patient goals and priorities: immediate/long-term health needs address patient's concerns first.
  - Action plan: simple language, pocket card
  - After hours: extended clinic hours and access
  - Safety plan: violence and abuse; mandatory reporting requirements
  - Emergency plan: location of nearest emergency department (ED), preparation for evacuation
  - Adherence plan: use of interpreter; identification of potential barriers

MEDICATION

- Simple regimen: low pill count, once-daily dosing
- Dispensing: Small amounts on site to promote follow-up, decrease loss/theft/misuse; determine resources for written prescriptions.
- Storage of medications: If no access, avoid medications that are requiring refrigeration.
- Patient assistance: free/low-cost drugs depending on available local options
- Aids to adherence: harm reduction, outreach/case management, directly observed therapy

- Side effects: Primary reason for medication nonadherence are drugs causing diarrhea, polyuria, nausea, and/or disorientation.
- Analgesia/symptomatic treatment: Consider pain contract, single provider for pain medication refills.
- Dietary supplements: multivitamins with minerals, nutritional supplements
- Managed care: generics, if possible; assistance getting prescription filled
- Lab monitoring: Monitor patients on antipsychotic medications for metabolic disorders using available laboratory resources.

ADDITIONAL THERAPIES

- Associated problems/complications
  - Fragmented care: multiple providers; use electronic medical record (EMR) as possible; list prescribed medication on wallet-sized card.
  - Masked symptoms/misdiagnosis: for example, weight loss, dementia, edema, lactic acidosis
  - Focus on immediate concerns, not on possible future consequences.
  - Integrated treatment for concurrent mental illness/substance use disorders
  - Support for parent of child abused by others and for abused parent
  - Large appointment burdens: Specialty care may be difficult to obtain.
- Follow-up
  - Reliable phone/email contact for patient/friend/family/case manager
  - Frequent follow-up, incentives, nonjudgmental care regardless of adherence
  - Anticipate/accommodate unscheduled clinic visits.
  - Provide car fare, tokens, and help with transportation services.
  - Monitor school attendance and address health/developmental problems with family/school.

ADMISSION, INPATIENT, AND NURSING CONSIDERATIONS

- Admission is beneficial if living conditions are not conducive to treatment of medical, psychiatric, and substance use disorders.
- Discharge considerations:
  - Acute or chronic wound care: Bed rest, extended periods of elevation, rest, or icing are not feasible in most instances.
  - Need for durable medical equipment (DME): Portable oxygen tanks and nebulizers may not be covered by the hospital and may be cumbersome to use in absence of stable housing.
  - Medications: It is preferable to fill prescriptions at hospital outpatient pharmacy.
  - Outpatient follow-up: Transportation to appointments should be arranged if possible.

 ONGOING CARE

FOLLOW-UP RECOMMENDATIONS

- Patients with a history of nonadherence need additional support (e.g., case manager, outreach) to succeed in ongoing care after hospital discharge.
- Limited telephone access to schedule appointments; may be unable to receive telephone messages with test results or rescheduled appointment times; some social service agencies will provide phone, mail, email, Internet, and laundry services.
- Arrange appointments prior to discharge.
- Document the best way to contact the individual.
- Work with experienced health care agency designed to address physical/mental health services and substance use treatment.

PATIENT EDUCATION

- National Health Care for the Homeless Council: https://www.nhchc.org/
- National Alliance to End Homelessness: http://www.endhomelessness.org/

PROGNOSIS

Mortality rates are 3 to 4 times higher than general U.S. population.

REFERENCES

1. National Alliance to End Homelessness. State of homelessness: 2023 edition. https://endhomelessness.org/homelessness-in-america/homelessness-statistics/state-of-homelessness/. Accessed July 9, 2023.
2. U.S. Department of Health and Human Services. HHS poverty guidelines for 2023. https://aspe.hhs.gov/topics/poverty-economic-mobility/poverty-guidelines. Accessed July 9, 2023.
3. de Sousa T, Andrichik A, Cuellar M, et al; for Abt Associates. *The 2022 Annual Homeless Assessment Report (AHAR) to Congress. Part 1: Point-in-Time Estimates of Homelessness*: December 2022. Washington, DC: U.S. Department of Housing and Urban Development, Office of Community Planning and Development; 2022.

 CODES

ICD10

- Z59.0 Homelessness
- Z59.1 Inadequate housing
- Z59.8 Other problems related to housing and economic circumstances

CLINICAL PEARLS

- Permanent supportive housing is an important step toward ending homelessness, in accordance with a Housing First approach.
- Assistance in gaining access to benefits or providing help to support basic needs decreases stress, improves therapeutic relationship, and allows individuals to focus on physical and mental health.

H

HORDEOLUM (STYE)

Konstantinos E. Deligiannidis, MD, MPH, FAAFP

BASICS

DESCRIPTION
- An acute inflammation or infection of the eyelid margin involving the sebaceous gland of an eyelash (external hordeolum) or a meibomian gland (internal hordeolum)
- System(s) affected: skin/exocrine
- Synonym(s): internal hordeolum; external hordeolum; zeisian stye; meibomian stye; stye

EPIDEMIOLOGY
- Predominant age: none
- Predominant sex: male = female

Incidence
Unknown: Although external hordeolum is common, internal hordeolum is rare.

ETIOLOGY AND PATHOPHYSIOLOGY
- Bacterial infection of sweat or sebaceous glands, causing an acute inflammatory reaction
- In an internal hordeolum, the meibomian gland may become obstructed, leading to a pustule on the conjunctival surface as opposed to the margin of the eyelid.
- Most commonly caused by *Staphylococcus aureus* (~90–95% of all cases) or by *Staphylococcus epidermidis*
- Seborrhea can predispose to infections of the eyelid.

Genetics
No known genetic pattern

RISK FACTORS
- Poor eyelid hygiene
- Previous hordeolum
- Contact lens wearers
- Application of makeup
- Seborrheic dermatitis
- Predisposing blepharitis (low-grade infections of the eyelid margin)
- Ocular rosacea

GENERAL PREVENTION
Eyelid hygiene

COMMONLY ASSOCIATED CONDITIONS
- Acne
- Seborrhea
- An association may exist between hordeolum during childhood and developing rosacea in adulthood.

DIAGNOSIS

HISTORY
- Localized inflammation (vs. involvement of the entire eyelid or surrounding skin)
- Foreign body sensation in the eye
- Symptoms may start as vague eyelid pain and inflammation and then localize 1 to 2 days later.
- Prior episodes are common.

PHYSICAL EXAM
- Localized inflammation of the eyelashes or a small pustule at the margin of the eyelid
- Localized swelling and tenderness on the internal or external aspect of the eyelid with an opening to either side
- To determine if an internal hordeolum is obstructed, the eyelid should be gently everted to examine for a pustule on the tarsal conjunctiva.
- Itching or scaling of the eyelids; collection of discharge, redness, and irritation leading to localized tenderness and pain
- The size of the swelling usually correlates to the severity of the hordeolum.

DIFFERENTIAL DIAGNOSIS
- Chalazion
- Blepharitis
- Eyelid neoplasms
- Periorbital cellulitis
- Dacryocystitis
- Squamous cell carcinoma

DIAGNOSTIC TESTS & INTERPRETATION
Culture of the eyelid margins usually is not necessary.

Diagnostic Procedures/Other
History and eye exam

Test Interpretation
Bacterial contamination and white cells in eyelid discharge

TREATMENT

GENERAL MEASURES
- The hordeolum should not be expressed.
- Warm compresses to the area of inflammation can help increase blood supply and encourage spontaneous drainage.
- Good personal hygiene with attention to cleansing the eyelids on a daily basis helps to prevent recurrent infections.

MEDICATION

First Line
- A Cochrane review found no evidence for or against nonsurgical treatment of internal hordeolum. External hordeola were not considered (1)[A].
- Usually, a hordeolum spontaneously drains, aided by warm compresses to the area.
- Also, lid scrubs, digital massage, and alternative medicine have been used to reduce healing time and to relieve symptoms.
- Application of an antibiotic ointment (e.g., erythromycin) to the margin of the eyelid after proper cleansing (except in children aged <12 years, in whom there is a risk of blurred vision and amblyopia) helps reduce bacterial proliferation. There is a little evidence that any topical therapy is effective. Erythromycin ophthalmic ointment may be applied up to 6 times per day for 7 to 10 days or an antibiotic ointment containing bacitracin (2),(3)[C],(4)
- Treat underlying dry eye with artificial tears.

Second Line
- Occasionally, the use of an aminoglycoside ophthalmic ointment, such as gentamicin or tobramycin, may be necessary if condition is refractory to simpler treatment (case reports).
- Oral dicloxacillin or cephalexin for 2 weeks if refractory to topical antibiotics

ISSUES FOR REFERRAL
Consider referral if unresponsive to oral antibiotics.

SURGERY/OTHER PROCEDURES
- If the infection becomes localized to a single gland, incision, drainage, or curettage sometimes is necessary. This is an in-office procedure with a local anesthetic: Exercise caution because ocular perforation has been reported with the injection of an anesthetic to an infected lid.
- The use of combined antibiotic ointment (neomycin sulfate, polymyxin B sulfate, and gramicidin) after surgery was not shown to have any statistically significant benefit compared with artificial tears.

COMPLEMENTARY & ALTERNATIVE MEDICINE
- Broncasma Berna is a polyvalent antigen vaccine that may be useful in the treatment of recurrent hordeolum.
- A Cochrane review found low-quality evidence that acupuncture (with or without antibiotics and/or warm compresses) may increase the chance of improvement of hordeolum compared to antibiotics and/or warm compresses (5)[A].

ADMISSION, INPATIENT, AND NURSING CONSIDERATIONS
Outpatient

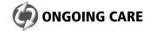 ONGOING CARE

FOLLOW-UP RECOMMENDATIONS
No restrictions

Patient Monitoring
The patient should be seen within several weeks to assess the effectiveness of therapy or should at least call the physician's office with a progress report.

DIET
No special diet

PATIENT EDUCATION
- The patient should be instructed in proper cleansing of the eyelids using a solution of tap water and baby shampoo or a commercially prepared hypoallergenic cleanser.
- The stye should not be squeezed or incised.

PROGNOSIS
- Usually responds well to good hygiene and warm compresses
- Inflammation usually improves within a week.
- Hordeolum tends to recur in some patients, usually due to incomplete elimination of bacteria.

COMPLICATIONS
An internal hordeolum, if untreated, may lead to chalazion, infections of adjacent glands, or generalized cellulitis of the lid.

REFERENCES
1. Lindsley K, Nichols JJ, Dickersin K. Non-surgical interventions for acute internal hordeolum. *Cochrane Database Syst Rev*. 2017;1(1):CD007742.
2. Wald ER. Periorbital and orbital infections. *Pediatr Rev*. 2004;25(9):312–320.
3. Mueller JB, McStay CM. Ocular infection and inflammation. *Emerg Med Clin North Am*. 2008;26(1):57–72, vi.
4. Alsoudi AF, Ton L, Ashraf DC, et al. Efficacy of care and antibiotic use for chalazia and hordeola. *Eye Contact Lens*. 2022;48(4):162–168.
5. Cheng K, Law A, Guo M, et al. Acupuncture for acute hordeolum. *Cochrane Database Syst Rev*. 2017;2(2):CD011075.

ADDITIONAL READING
- Bamford JTM, Gessert CE, Renier CM, et al. Childhood stye and adult rosacea. *J Am Acad Dermatol*. 2006;55(6):951–955.
- Hirunwiwatkul P, Wachirasereechai K. Effectiveness of combined antibiotic ophthalmic solution in the treatment of hordeolum after incision and curettage: a randomized, placebo-controlled trial: a pilot study. *J Med Assoc Thai*. 2005;88(5):647–650.
- Kim JH, Yang SM, Kim HM, et al. Inadvertent ocular perforation during lid anesthesia for hordeolum removal. *Korean J Ophthalmol*. 2006;20(3):199–200.
- Nakatani M. Treatment of recurrent hordeolum with Broncasma Berna. *Eye (Lond)*. 1999;13(Pt 5):692.
- Wald ER. Periorbital and orbital infections. *Infect Dis Clin North Am*. 2007;21(2):393–408, vi.

 CODES

ICD10
- H00.019 Hordeolum externum unspecified eye, unspecified eyelid
- H00.029 Hordeolum internum unspecified eye, unspecified eyelid
- H00.039 Abscess of eyelid unspecified eye, unspecified eyelid

CLINICAL PEARLS
- A hordeolum should not be expressed.
- Warm compresses to the area of inflammation can encourage spontaneous drainage.
- Application of an antibiotic ointment (e.g., erythromycin) to the margin of the eyelid after proper cleansing helps reduce bacterial proliferation but may have no effect on the healing of the stye.
- Good personal hygiene with attention to cleansing the eyelids on a daily basis can prevent recurrent infections.

H

HORNER SYNDROME

Iain W. Decker, DO • Omar B. Saeed, DO, MPH

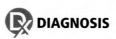 **BASICS**

DESCRIPTION

- A constellation of neurological signs and symptoms manifested as a classic triad of ipsilateral miosis, eyelid ptosis, and anhidrosis of the ipsilateral face and/or neck (with iris heterochromia in children)
- System(s) affected: nervous, skin/exocrine
- Synonym(s): Bernard syndrome

EPIDEMIOLOGY

Incidence

- Estimated incidence of pediatric Horner syndrome is 1.42 per 100,000 in patients <19 years of age with a birth prevalence of 1 in 6,250 for those with congenital onset of Horner syndrome.
- Incidence in adults is not known.

ETIOLOGY AND PATHOPHYSIOLOGY

- A lesion affecting the neurons in the sympathetic chain (first, second, or third order) may produce signs and symptoms of Horner syndrome as a result of a lack of sympathetic input to the orbit.
  - Ptosis: Sympathetic innervation to the Müller muscle in the upper eyelid and the lower eyelid retractors helps to maintain normal eyelid position. When sympathetic innervation to these structures is interrupted, a subtle ptosis of both the upper lid (ptosis) and lower lid (reverse ptosis) may result. This ptosis may be subtle, often ≤2 mm.
  - Meiosis: The radially oriented pupillary dilator muscle produces pupillary dilation in response to stimulation by the sympathetic nervous system. Anisocoria will be more pronounced in dim lighting, reflecting impairment of dilation in the affected eye. The affected eye will constrict normally in response to light but will be slower to dilate than the unaffected pupil.
  - Anhidrosis: When present, anhidrosis may assist in localizing a lesion. Sympathetic fibers innervating sweat glands of the lower face and vasodilatory muscles branch off before the superior cervical sympathetic ganglion and travel along the external carotid artery. Lesions affecting primary and secondary neurons are more likely to produce anhidrosis of both the upper and lower face.
- Etiologies in adults:
  - Arnold-Chiari malformation, basal meningitis (e.g., syphilis), cerebral vascular accident, lateral medullary (Wallenberg) syndrome, cervical cord trauma, cervical spondylosis, demyelinating disease (multiple sclerosis), intrapontine hemorrhage, neck trauma, syringomyelia/syringobulbia, tumor (basal skull, pituitary), unintended subdural placement of lumbar epidural catheter
  - Aneurysm/dissection of aorta, central venous catheterization, chest tubes, 1st rib fracture, lymphadenopathy (Hodgkin lymphoma, leukemia, tuberculosis, sarcoidosis), mandibular tooth abscess, neuroblastoma, Pancoast tumor or infection of the lung apex, proximal common carotid artery dissection, thoracic outlet obstruction (cervical rib, subclavian artery aneurysm), trauma/surgical injury, tumor (thyroid, mediastinum)

- Carotid cavernous fistula or other pathology, carotid endarterectomy or carotid artery stenting, cluster headaches/paroxysmal hemicrania, internal carotid artery dissection, herpes zoster virus infection, lesions of the middle ear (acute otitis media), Lyme disease, tumor (nasopharyngeal, pituitary, paratrigeminal, metastasis, skull base), tonsillectomy, trauma/surgical injury, Raeder paratrigeminal syndrome
- Etiologies in children:
  - Birth trauma/neck trauma (injury to the brachial plexus)—most common; brainstem glioma, neuroblastoma, vascular anomalies, surgical interventions in the neck/chest, idiopathic

Genetics
Rare autosomal dominant inheritance

RISK FACTORS

- Recent trauma to the head/neck/thorax (e.g., motor vehicle accidents)
- Smoking (Pancoast tumor)
- Known aneurysm of the carotid or subclavian arteries
- Known malignancy/tumor/mass
- Previous surgery (neck/thoracic)
- Cluster headache

D̶x̶ DIAGNOSIS

HISTORY

- When did symptoms begin? (acute vs. chronic)
- Any visual symptoms? (blurred vision, field loss, transient visual loss, diplopia)
- Previous ophthalmic history? (eye trauma, surgery, etc.)
- Are symptoms associated with pain? (ipsilateral head/neck/face)
- Recent head/neck trauma?
- Recent surgical procedures?
- Any associated headaches?
- Any other neurologic signs?
- Does the degree of ptosis vary over the course of the day or with fatigue?
- Any sweating abnormalities or flushing on one side of the face?

Pediatric Considerations

- Congenital Horner syndrome will affect the iris color as iris melanocytes require sympathetic innervation to produce melanin; if the innervation is not present at birth, a lighter iris will occur—resulting in heterochromia.
- Loss of facial flushing can be appreciated (Harlequin sign—affected side will appear pale secondary to denervation supersensitivity to circulating adrenaline). This flushing occurs with nursing or crying.

- New onset, nontraumatic Horner syndrome in a child necessitates workup for neuroblastoma.

ALERT
Horner syndrome in the presence of pain merits urgent evaluation.

- Acute-onset, ipsilateral facial or neck pain: Consider carotid artery dissection until proven otherwise, even in the absence of obvious head/neck trauma. Pain from dissection is usually located around the temple and orbit. Patients may also experience amaurosis fugax and dysgeusia. If missed, stroke is a potential complication.
- Axial, shoulder, scapula, arm, or hand pain may be related to Pancoast tumor or cervical cord lesion.
- Paratrigeminal syndromes:
  - Raeder paratrigeminal syndrome type I: orbital pain, miosis, ptosis, with associated ipsilateral lesions of CN III to VI; suspect middle cranial fossa mass or cavernous sinus lesion.
  - Raeder paratrigeminal syndrome type II: episodic retrobulbar or orbital pain, miosis, ptosis with no CN lesions; suspect migraine variant.

PHYSICAL EXAM

- Measure pupillary diameter under both dim and bright lighting to determine the presence of anisocoria. In Horner syndrome, anisocoria will be greater in dim/dark lighting conditions.
- Evaluate pupil reactivity to light and accommodative response.
- A pupillary dilation lag may be present and the affected pupil may gradually dilate 5 to 15 seconds after exposure to light.
- Examine the upper lids for ptosis (often <2 mm).
- A "reverse ptosis" of the lower lid may also be visible in the form of a slight elevation of the lower lid relative to the unaffected eye.
- Additional acute features of sympathetic disruption may include ipsilateral conjunctival injection and nasal congestion.
- Biomicroscopic/slit lamp exam of the eye, including iris structure and color (if available)
- Observe for the presence of nystagmus, facial swelling, lymphadenopathy, or vesicular eruptions.
- A full cranial nerve exam with special attention to extraocular movements.
- Palpation and inspection of the neck for any masses or evidence of trauma
- Neurologic and chest exams for associated physical findings

DIFFERENTIAL DIAGNOSIS

- Physiologic anisocoria (~20% population) varies by <1 mm and may fluctuate throughout the day.
- Neurologic diseases (myasthenia gravis, botulinum toxin)

- Third nerve palsy
- Pharmacologic causes including unilateral use of miotics or mydriatics, acetophenazine, alseroxylon, bupivacaine, butaperazine, carphenazine, chloroprocaine, deserpidine, diacetylmorphine, diethazine, ethopropazine, etidocaine, guanethidine, influenza virus vaccine, levodopa, lidocaine, mepivacaine, mesoridazine, methdilazine, methotrimeprazine, oral contraceptives, perazine, prilocaine, procaine, prochlorperazine, promazine, propoxycaine, reserpine, thioproperazine, thioridazine, trifluoperazine

DIAGNOSTIC TESTS & INTERPRETATION

Initial Tests (lab, imaging)

- Lab: CBC, FTA-ABS, VDRL, purified protein derivative; vanillylmandelic acid (VMA), homovanillic acid (HVA) to rule out neuroblastoma in pediatric patients
- Imaging considerations are unique because of the long pathway traveled by the sympathetic nervous system. A lesion at any point along this pathway, extending from the hypothalamus down to T2, may contribute to the onset of Horner syndrome. Recommended imaging includes the following:
  - In the chronic setting, a neuroimaging study of the oculosympathetic pathway extending from the hypothalamus down to T2 with a contrast-enhanced MRI (MRI of head, neck, and chest) with MRA of the head and neck (chest imaging to evaluate lung apex for Pancoast tumor; MRA to evaluate carotid artery dissection)
  - In the acute setting (or for patients unable to tolerate MRI), an initial CT of the head/neck/chest and CTA of the head/neck followed by HS MRI protocol mentioned in step 3 is recommended if initial CT/CTA are negative. Life-threatening causes of Horner syndrome including carotid artery dissection may be ruled out with this initial CT/CTA to avoid delay in the treatment (1)[B].
  - Consider carotid angiogram if MRA or CTA yield equivocal results.

Pediatric Considerations

In a child of any age without contributory history, MRI of brain, neck, and chest as outlined above is appropriate. Clinicians may consider MRI of abdomen as well if the clinical suspicion of neuroblastoma is high.

Pregnancy Considerations

Most authors believe that pregnant patients may undergo MRI safely, but it should be noted that contrast material (e.g., gadolinium) is FDA category C (1)[B].

Diagnostic Procedures/Other

To diagnose Horner syndrome, a confirmation test is required. The first two of these tests (apraclonidine and cocaine) help to confirm the presence of Horner syndrome, whereas the third (hydroxyamphetamine) attempts to localize the lesion. It is usually not necessary to test with both apraclonidine and cocaine, and most choose apraclonidine due to the challenge associated with obtaining cocaine drops.

- Topical 0.5% apraclonidine drops: (2)[A],(3)[B],(4)[B]
  - Apraclonidine is a strong alpha-2 agonist and weak alpha-1 agonist with little to no effect on the normal pupil. To test for Horner syndrome, 1 drop of apraclonidine is placed in each eye, and the patient is reassessed after 60 minutes. The miotic eye with Horner syndrome should dilate and the anisocoria reverses.

– A positive test result occurs when both pupils become equally sized or if the affected pupil becomes the larger one. NOTE: the apraclonidine test may be negative in cases of acute trauma as there has not been enough time for denervation hypersensitivity to develop (2 to 5 days).

- 4–10% topical cocaine drops:
  - Cocaine blocks reuptake of norepinephrine from the synaptic cleft. To test for Horner syndrome, two drops of 4% or 10% cocaine are instilled in both eyes 5 minutes apart, and after 40 to 60 minutes, the pupils are reevaluated.
  - Cocaine drops will dilate the normal pupil. The miotic pupil in Horner syndrome (regardless of location of lesion) will not dilate or will dilate poorly after 45 minutes because of the absence of norepinephrine at the nerve endings of the third-order neuron (2)[A]. Positive test is anisocoria of ≥1 mm.
- Topical 1% hydroxyamphetamine drops (2)[A]
  - Used to differentiate between preganglionic (first- and second-order neurons) and postganglionic (third-order neuron) Horner syndrome.
  - One hour after the instillation of 1% hydroxyamphetamine drops, the pupils should be evaluated. Dilation of both pupils indicates a lesion of the first- or second-order neurons. Failure of the pupil to dilate, or poor dilation, indicates a third-order neuron lesion (the test is considered positive when anisocoria increases by ≥1 mm).

Pediatric Considerations

Due to transsynaptic degeneration in children, the hydroxyamphetamine test is not reliable.

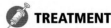

TREATMENT

GENERAL MEASURES

Once life-threatening etiologies have been excluded, cosmesis or functional vision impairment due to ptosis may be addressed if symptoms have persisted for 12 months.

MEDICATION

- Carotid artery dissection: Pharmacologic treatment options include thrombolysis, antithrombotic therapy with anticoagulation, or antiplatelet therapy (5)[C].
- For mild ptosis, oxymetazoline hydrochloride 0.1% can be used. Oxymetazoline is an alpha-adrenergic receptor agonist and selectively activates alpha-adrenergic receptors in the Müller muscle. This can raise the ptotic eyelid by 1 to 1.3 mm (according to two clinical trials). Some patients may get more dramatic effect than others. Oxymetazoline reaches peak effect ~2 hours postinstillation and can last up to 8 hours. In two clinical trials, oxymetazoline significantly improved the superior visual field deficits. Common side effects include instillation site discomfort, headache, and dry eye (6).

ISSUES FOR REFERRAL

Depending on etiology of Horner syndrome, referrals may include neurosurgery, oncology, interventional radiology, pulmonology, neurology/neuro-ophthalmology, and oculoplastic surgery.

SURGERY/OTHER PROCEDURES

- Surgical intervention depending on etiology
- Consider ptosis repair for cosmesis or functional vision impairment secondary to ptosis if symptoms have persisted for 12 months (oculoplastics).

 ONGOING CARE

PROGNOSIS

- Postganglionic: usually benign
- Central and preganglionic: poorer prognosis

COMPLICATIONS

- Chronic pupillary constriction
- Cosmesis

REFERENCES

1. Chen Y, Morgan ML, Palau AEB, et al. Evaluation and neuroimaging of the Horner syndrome. *Can J Ophthalmol.* 2015;50(2):107–111.
2. Antonio-Santos AA, Santo RN, Eggenberger ER. Pharmacological testing of anisocoria. *Expert Opin Pharmacother.* 2005;6(12):2007–2013.
3. Koc F, Kavuncu S, Kansu T, et al. The sensitivity and specificity of 0.5% apraclonidine in the diagnosis of oculosympathetic paresis. *Br J Ophthalmol.* 2005; 89(11):1442–1444.
4. Chen PL, Chen JT, Lu DW, et al. Comparing efficacies of 0.5% apraclonidine with 4% cocaine in the diagnosis of Horner syndrome in pediatric patients. *J Ocul Pharmacol Ther.* 2006;22(3):182–187.
5. Sadaka A, Schockman SL, Golnik KC. Evaluation of Horner syndrome in the MRI era. *J Neuroophthalmol.* 2017;37(3):268–272.
6. Slonim CB, Foster S, Jaros M, et al. "Association of oxymetazoline hydrochloride, 0.1%, solution administration with visual field in acquired ptosis: a pooled analysis of 2 randomized clinical trials." *JAMA Ophthalmol.* 2020;138(11):1168–1175.

 CODES

ICD10

- G90.2 Horner's syndrome
- S14.5XXA Injury of cervical sympathetic nerves, initial encounter

CLINICAL PEARLS

- Horner syndrome triad: ipsilateral miosis, eyelid ptosis, and anhidrosis caused by a lesion of the oculosympathetic pathway
- Red flag: Horner syndrome in the presence of acute-onset, ipsilateral facial or neck pain: Consider carotid artery dissection until proven otherwise.
- Ptosis is mild, usually <2 mm.

H

HYDROCELE

Jared M. Patton, MD, MS

BASICS

DESCRIPTION
A hydrocele is a collection of fluid between the parietal and visceral layers of the tunica vaginalis within the scrotum.

- Communicating hydrocele (patent processus vaginalis)
  – Direct communication between the hydrocele sac and the peritoneal cavity
  – Contains peritoneal fluid
  – Almost always with associated indirect inguinal hernia
  – Decreases in size with recumbent position
- Noncommunicating hydrocele (processus vaginalis is not patent)
  – No direct connection between the hydrocele sac and the peritoneal cavity
  – Fluid contained is from the mesothelial lining.
  – Can be isolated to the cord with the distal and proximal portions of the processus vaginalis closed
- Acute hydrocele: fluid collection resulting from an acute process within the tunica vaginalis, typically involving only the scrotum
- Although this disorder is found nearly exclusively in male patients, there are rare hydroceles into the canal of Nuck in females which result from a fluid collection in an abnormal open pouch of peritoneum extending into the labia majora.
- System(s) affected: urogenital

Pediatric Considerations
Most congenital communicating hydroceles resolve spontaneously by 2 years of age.

EPIDEMIOLOGY
Predominant age: childhood

Incidence
Estimated at 0.7–4.7% of male infants

Prevalence
- 1,000/100,000
- Estimated at 1% of adult men

ETIOLOGY AND PATHOPHYSIOLOGY
- Incomplete closure of the processus vaginalis trapping peritoneal fluid anywhere along the length of the tunica vaginalis
- Failure of closure of the processus vaginalis maintains a communication to the peritoneal cavity.
- Imbalance of the secretion and reabsorption of fluid from the lining of the tunica vaginalis
- Infection
- Tumors
- Trauma
- Ipsilateral renal transplantation (due to disruption of the spermatic cord during the procedure)

RISK FACTORS
- For adult acquired hydroceles:
  – Ventriculoperitoneal shunt
  – Ehlers-Danlos syndrome
  – Peritoneal dialysis
  – History of scrotal surgery (to include varicocelectomy)
- For congenital hydroceles:
  – Exstrophy of the bladder
  – Cloacal exstrophy

GENERAL PREVENTION
None

COMMONLY ASSOCIATED CONDITIONS
For adult acquired hydroceles:
- Testicular tumors
- Scrotal trauma
- Ventriculoperitoneal shunt
- Nephrotic syndrome
- Renal failure with peritoneal dialysis

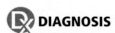

DIAGNOSIS

HISTORY
- Acute, subacute, or chronic swelling of the scrotum or inguinal canal
- Frequent changes in size of the hydrocele with position change or activity (indicative of a communicating hydrocele)

- Usually painless unless acute onset
- Sensation of heaviness or pressure in the scrotum
- Pain radiating to the flank/back

PHYSICAL EXAM
- Swelling in the scrotum or inguinal canal
- Scrotal mass (usually fluctuant)
- Fluctuation in size with change of position (communicating hydrocele)
- Scrotal mass that transilluminates
- A fluctuant mass that is reducible with gentle pressure can identify a communicating hydrocele versus noncommunicating

DIFFERENTIAL DIAGNOSIS
- Indirect inguinal hernia
- Orchitis
- Epididymitis
- Varicocele
- Traumatic testicular injury
- Testicular torsion or torsion of appendix testes
- Testicular neoplasm

DIAGNOSTIC TESTS & INTERPRETATION
Initial Tests (lab, imaging)
- Inguinoscrotal ultrasound (US) can demonstrate the presence of bowel (e.g., distinguish incarcerated hernia from a hydrocele of the cord) as well as the presence of testicular torsion.
- Testicular MRI when US is unable to distinguish etiology
- Doppler US or testicular nuclear scan can identify testicular torsion.

ALERT
Aspiration of a hydrocele for diagnosis is not indicated and may lead to severe complications if herniated bowel is present.

Diagnostic Procedures/Other
Transillumination of the hemiscrotum along with history and exam are usually sufficient in making the diagnosis, but a formal US should be obtained prior to treatment to verify scrotal contents.

TREATMENT

ISSUES FOR REFERRAL
- Urology referral for symptomatic adults or if underlying diagnosis is unclear
- Pediatric urology/surgery referral for children with symptomatic noncommunicating hydrocele
- Pediatric urology/surgery referral if not resolved by 2 years of age

SURGERY/OTHER PROCEDURES
- Children: For congenital hydrocele, surgical treatment is generally deferred until 2 years of age because many hydroceles will spontaneously resolve. Some evidence shows that delaying longer than 2 years may be appropriate and decreases unnecessary surgery (1)[C]. When surgery is indicated, children with communicating hydroceles may undergo either open or laparoscopic approach.
  - Laparoscopic repair offers the benefit of contralateral exploration which may reveal additional defects. It also may have diminished postoperative pain and a lower rate of complications.
  - Open scrotal approach involves ligation and removal of the processus vaginalis. The benefit of this approach is improved cosmesis and decreased operative time (2)[B].
  - Open inguinal approach involves ligation of the processus vaginalis and excision, distal splitting, or drainage of hydrocele sac (in a hydrocele of the cord, the sac can be completely removed).
- Adults: No therapy is needed unless the hydrocele causes discomfort or unless there is a significant underlying cause such as a tumor.
  - Aspiration of the hydrocele with instillation of a sclerosing agent has been successfully used in adults.
  - If resection is indicated, all the open surgical techniques have the same 6% rate of recurrence; however, the overall rate of complications and the rate of postoperative hematoma were lowest with the "Lord's" repair (3)[B].
  - Postoperative complications as well as cost and time to work resumption can be less in treatment by aspiration and sclerotherapy versus resection, but the recurrence rate may be higher.

ADMISSION, INPATIENT, AND NURSING CONSIDERATIONS
- Open inguinal or scrotal approach is typically performed as an outpatient.
- Laparoscopic approach in pediatric patients may require 24-hour admission for postoperative monitoring.
- Sclerotherapy is a same-day office procedure.

 ONGOING CARE

FOLLOW-UP RECOMMENDATIONS
Patient Monitoring
- Depending on method of treatment, initial follow-up is generally in the first 4 to 6 weeks.
- With sclerotherapy, follow-up is for confirmation of resolution or to proceed with retreatment.
- Postoperative follow-up at 2 to 4 weeks and subsequent 2- to 3-month intervals until resolution of any postoperative complications

PROGNOSIS
- Children/infants: As stated above, most congenital hydroceles resolve spontaneously with no intervention by age 2 years. For those who do need treatment, nearly all patients have resolution of symptoms after surgical intervention with very low long-term morbidity.
- Adults: Low risk of long-term morbidity with either treatment method with eventual resolution of symptoms in nearly all cases depending on the underlying etiology (e.g., peritoneal dialysis).

COMPLICATIONS
- Complication rate for a scrotal approach may reach 30%.
- Postoperative traumatic hydrocele is common and usually resolves spontaneously.
- Injury to vas deferens or spermatic vessels
- Suture granuloma
- Hematoma
- Wound infection
- Recurrence

REFERENCES
1. Hall NJ, Ron O, Eaton S, et al. Surgery for hydrocele in children—an avoidable excess? *J Pediatr Surg*. 2011;46(12):2401–2405.
2. Alp BF, Irkilata HC, Kibar Y, et al. Comparison of the inguinal and scrotal approaches for the treatment of communicating hydrocele in children. *Kaohsiung J Med Sci*. 2014;30(4):200–205.
3. Tsai L, Milburn PA, Cecil CL IV, et al. Comparison of recurrence and postoperative complications between 3 different techniques for surgical repair of idiopathic hydrocele. *Urology*. 2019;125:239–242.

 CODES

ICD10
- N43.0 Encysted hydrocele
- N43.3 Hydrocele, unspecified
- N43.2 Other hydrocele

CLINICAL PEARLS
- A hydrocele can usually be diagnosed by physical exam and transillumination. If there is any concern for other underlying process, a formal US is recommended.
- Aspiration alone is not indicated as the primary treatment of a hydrocele due to high recurrence rate.
- Attempted aspiration of an unconfirmed hydrocele could lead to bowel injury in an undiagnosed inguinal hernia and should not be attempted.
- Expectant management of children with hydrocele until >2 years of age is acceptable to allow sufficient time for spontaneous resolution, decreasing the likelihood of an unnecessary procedure.
- In adults, surgical resection costs more and has more complications than aspiration and sclerotherapy, but has a much lower recurrence rate and a much higher patient satisfaction rate.

H

HYDRONEPHROSIS

Pang-Yen Fan, MD • Mwangi Kamau, MD

 BASICS

DESCRIPTION
- Hydronephrosis refers to a structural finding: dilatation of the renal calyces and pelvis.
- Can be accompanied with hydroureter (dilatation of the ureter)
- Hydronephrosis should not be used interchangeably with obstructive uropathy, which refers to the damage to renal parenchyma resulting from urinary tract obstruction (UTO).

EPIDEMIOLOGY
- More common in children than adults due to congenital anomalies.
- Hydronephrosis is more common in women for adults <60 years old and in men for adults >60 years old.

ETIOLOGY AND PATHOPHYSIOLOGY
- Hydronephrosis develops with increased pressure in the urinary collecting system, most commonly from some form of obstruction.
- Nonobstructive hydronephrosis can occur in the setting of very high urinary output such as with diabetes insipidus or as a physiologic change in pregnancy.
- Hydronephrosis may be acute/chronic, partial/complete, and uni-/bilateral.
- Obstruction may occur at an level of the GU system:
  - Kidney: nephrolithiasis, transitional cell carcinoma, sloughed renal papillae, congenital ureteropelvic junction (UPJ) obstruction, blood clot, fungal ball
  - Ureter: nephrolithiasis, transitional cell carcinomas, strictures, sloughed renal papillae, retroperitoneal fibrosis, extrinsic compression
  - Bladder: neurogenic bladder, extrinsic compression, posterior urethral valves
  - Urethra: prostatic hypertrophy or cancer, strictures
- Hydronephrosis in a transplanted kidney is more common than in native kidneys, due to ureteral reflux, strictures, ureteral compression (from peritransplant lymphoceles, hematomas) and bladder dysfunction.

Pediatric Considerations
- Antenatal hydronephrosis is diagnosed in 1–5% of pregnancies, usually by US, as early as the 12th to 14th week of gestation.
- Children with antenatal hydronephrosis are at greater risk of postnatal pathology.
- Postnatal evaluation begins with US exam; further studies, such as voiding cystourethrogram (VCUG), based on the severity of postnatal hydronephrosis
- In neonates, it is the most common cause of abdominal mass.
- Common etiologies in children are VUR, congenital UPJ obstruction, neurogenic bladder, and posterior urethral valves.
- Pediatric diagnostic algorithm differs from adult due to different differential diagnosis necessitating age-appropriate testing.

Pregnancy Considerations
- Physiologic hydronephrosis in pregnancy is more prominent on the right than left and can be seen in up to 80% of pregnant women.
- Dilatation is caused by hormonal effects, external compression from expanding uterus, and intrinsic changes in the ureteral wall.
- Despite high incidence, most cases are asymptomatic.
- If symptomatic and refractory to medical management, ureteric calculus should be considered and urinary infection must be excluded.

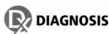 **DIAGNOSIS**

HISTORY
- Symptoms vary according to cause, chronicity, location, and degree of obstruction.
- Although often asymptomatic, hydronephrosis can be associated with pain ranging from vague, intermittent discomfort to severe renal colic.
- Can be associated with hematuria
- Nausea and vomiting may be associated with pain or infection.
- Fever and chills suggest coexisting urinary infection.
- Anuria suggests complete obstruction bilaterally or unilateral obstruction of a solitary kidney.
- Polyuria may occur due to impaired urinary concentration in partial obstruction.
- Symptoms of chronic kidney disease (CKD): anorexia, malaise, weight gain, edema, shortness of breath, mental state changes, tremors from long-standing obstruction
- Symptoms of bladder outlet obstruction: weak urine stream, nocturia, straining to void, overflow incontinence, urgency, and frequency
- General medical and surgical history: malignancy (extrinsic compression), radiotherapy (ureteric stricture/fibrosis), surgery (iatrogenic obstruction), trauma hematoma or fibrosis), gynecologic disease (extrinsic compression from endometriosis, ovarian masses, uterine prolapse), smoking (urothelial cancer), drugs (methysergide-induced retroperitoneal fibrosis)

PHYSICAL EXAM
- General signs
  - Volume overload (edema, rales, hypertension [HTN]) from renal failure
  - Diaphoresis, tachycardia, tachypnea with pain
  - High-grade fever, if infection
- Abdominal exam: CVA tenderness, palpable bladder, rarely palpable abdominal mass (may be visible, particularly in thin children)
- Pelvic exam: pelvic mass, uterine prolapse, palpable enlarged prostate (cancer or benign), urethral meatal stenosis, phimosis

DIAGNOSTIC TESTS & INTERPRETATION
- Urinalysis with microscopy: hematuria, proteinuria, crystalluria, pyuria
- Midstream urine culture and sensitivity: Exclude UTI.
- Basic metabolic panel: Elevated urea and creatinine may indicate obstructive uropathy. Hyperkalemic nonanion gap metabolic acidosis may indicate type 4 distal RTA due to obstruction.
- CBC: anemia of CKD, leukocytosis; if infection, check platelet count prior to considering ureteral instrumentation
- Prostate-specific antigen (PSA): adult males age >50 years or with abnormal digital rectal exam or bladder outlet obstruction signs or symptoms
- Urine cytology: for malignant cells in urothelial malignancies
- US and noncontrast CT scanning are effective in diagnosing presence and cause of obstruction in most cases.
- US: screening test of choice for hydronephrosis
  - Sensitivity 90%, specificity 84.5%. Does not assess function and rarely detects cause and level of obstruction. Degree of hydronephrosis does not correlate with duration or severity of the obstruction.
  - Advantages: detects renal parenchymal disease (decreased renal size, increased cortical echogenicity, cortical thinning, cysts); no exposure to radiation or contrast; safe in pregnancy, contrast allergy, and renal dysfunction
  - False-positive findings 15.5%: normal extrarenal pelvis, parapelvic cysts, VUR, excessive diuresis
  - False-negative findings 10%: dehydration, acute obstruction, calyceal dilatation misinterpreted as renal cortical cysts, and retroperitoneal fibrosis
- Noncontrast helical CT (NHCT): test of choice for suspected nephrolithiasis
  - Reported sensitivity 94–96%, specificity 94–100%. Stone is most commonly found at levels of ureteral luminal narrowing: UPJ, pelvic brim, and the vesicoureteric junction.
  - Typical findings in acute obstruction are hydronephrosis with hydroureter proximal to the level of obstruction, perinephric stranding, and renal swelling. If chronic, renal atrophy may be noted.
  - Advantages: no contrast exposure, time-saving, cost-effective, identifies extraurinary pathology (1)
  - Disadvantages: does not assess function or degree of obstruction; higher radiation exposure, although low radiation dose protocols have shown comparable accuracy
- DTPA or MAG-3 radionuclide renal scan (diuretic renal scintigraphy)
  - Indicated only for evaluation of hydronephrosis without apparent obstruction
  - Determines presence of true obstruction as well as total and split (right vs. left) renal function
  - Furosemide is given 20 minutes after the tracer and the T1/2 for the tracer's washout is measured. T1/2; <10 minutes is unobstructed, >20 minutes

is obstructed, and 10 to 20 minutes is equivocal; some experts consider <15 minutes normal.
– Advantages: no contrast exposure, safe in contrast allergy and renal dysfunction
– False-positive findings: delayed excretion due to renal failure, massive dilatation causing a water-reservoir effect of delayed excretion without obstruction
– False-negative findings: dehydration or inadequate diuretic challenge
• Multiphase contrast-enhanced CT
– Nonenhanced phase detects stones and swelling.
– Parenchymal phase demonstrates decreased enhancement of renal parenchyma with acute obstruction; can identify extraurinary causes of obstruction and determine the relative glomerular filtration rate (GFR) of each kidney with accuracy equal to radionuclide renal scan
– Delayed phase allows visualization of the collecting system and soft tissue filling defects (e.g., urothelial cancer).
• Magnetic resonance urography (MRU): indicated when US and NHCT are nondiagnostic
– Provides anatomic, functional, and prognostic information; sensitivity not superior to US or NHCT for nephrolithiasis (70%) but superior for soft tissue causes including strictures
– Advantages: no radiation exposure, safe in pregnancy
– Disadvantages: more expensive and time-consuming (35 minutes vs. 5 minutes) and less available compared with CT. Gadolinium is contraindicated in renal failure especially when GFR is <30 mL/min due to risk of nephrogenic systemic fibrosis.

Follow-Up Tests & Special Considerations
The presence of fever in the setting of hydronephrosis should be considered a medical emergency due to the risk of bacteremia from urinary infection in an obstructed urinary system.

Diagnostic Procedures/Other
Cystoscopy, retrograde pyelogram ± ureteroscopy, and biopsy are occasionally used to determine the cause of obstruction (e.g., small urothelial cancer missed on imaging) or to confirm a normal distal ureter prior to pyeloplasty. In addition, such procedures are often needed to establish a definitive pathologic diagnosis for mass lesions.

TREATMENT

GENERAL MEASURES
• Medical treatment: correction of fluid and electrolyte abnormalities, pain control, antibiotics as an adjunct to drainage if infection present
• Relief of obstruction: prompt drainage indicated in the presence of UTI, compromised renal function, or uncontrollable/persistent pain
– Bladder outlet obstruction: urethral or suprapubic catheter
– Ureteric obstruction: retrograde (cystoscopic) or antegrade (percutaneous) stenting (2)

• VUR is often managed conservatively with antibiotics; surgical management may be required in severe cases in children or women of childbearing age.
• Medical expulsive therapy (MET) with α-blockers or calcium channel blockers indicated for urethral stones <10 mm in patients with controlled pain, no signs of sepsis, with good renal function (3)[C]

SURGERY/OTHER PROCEDURES
• Hydronephrosis due to obstruction
– Congenital UPJ obstruction: Pyeloplasty (open or laparoscopic) and minimally invasive stricture incision (endopyelotomy) are used with comparable results.
– Nephrolithiasis: Extracorporeal shock wave lithotripsy (ESWL) is the initial treatment of choice for management of impacted upper urethral stones ≤2 cm. Ureteroscopy with or without intracorporeal lithotripsy has lower retreatment but higher complication rates and longer hospital stay; ureteral stenting pre-ESWL or postureteroscopy associated with no additional benefit and more discomfort and morbidity (4)[A],(5)
– Transitional cell cancer: nephroureterectomy
– Idiopathic retroperitoneal fibrosis: ureterolysis (frees ureters from inflammatory mass)
– Prostate disorders: various treatment modalities, including transurethral resection of the prostate (TURP) and radical prostatectomy
• Nonobstructed hydronephrosis
– VUR: ureteric reimplantation, endoscopic subure-thral injection

ADMISSION, INPATIENT, AND NURSING CONSIDERATIONS
Obstruction coexisting with infection (pyonephrosis) is a true urologic emergency requiring urgent drainage. Typically, this requires placement of percutaneous nephrostomy tube(s) because retrograde (cystoscopic) stenting is often difficult, but both are equally effective.

ONGOING CARE

FOLLOW-UP RECOMMENDATIONS
• Serial monitoring of kidney function (electrolytes, BUN, and creatinine) and BP until renal function stabilizes. Frequency of monitoring depends on severity of renal dysfunction.
• Follow-up US after stabilization of renal function to assess for resolution of hydronephrosis. If hydronephrosis persists, consider diuretic radionuclide study to rule out persistent obstruction.

PROGNOSIS
• Recovery of renal function depends on etiology, presence or absence of UTI, and degree and duration of obstruction.
• Significant recovery can occur despite days of complete obstruction, although some irreversible injury may develop within 24 hours. Delays in therapy can lead to irreversible renal damage (6).
• Diagnostic testing is of poor predictive value. Course of incomplete obstruction is highly unpredictable.

COMPLICATIONS
• Urine stasis: increased risk of infection and stones formation
• Obstruction causes progressive atrophy of kidney with irreversible loss of function.
• Spontaneous rupture of a calyx may occur with urine extravasation in the perinephric space.
• Postobstructive diuresis: marked polyuria after relief of obstruction:
– Caused mostly by fluid and solute overload but may be exacerbated by impaired renal tubular concentrating ability. Urine output may be >500 mL/hr.
– Replace urine losses with hypotonic fluid (usually with 0.45% NaCl) and only enough to avoid volume depletion. Replacement of urine output with equal amounts of saline will perpetuate the diuresis.

REFERENCES
1. Worster A, Preyra I, Weaver B, et al. The accuracy of noncontrast helical computed tomography versus intravenous pyelography in the diagnosis of suspected acute urolithiasis: a meta-analysis. *Ann Emerg Med*. 2002;40(3):280–286.
2. Ramsey S, Robertson A, Ablett MJ, et al. Evidence-based drainage of infected hydronephrosis secondary to ureteric calculi. *J Endourol*. 2010;24(2):185–189.
3. Seitz C, Liatsikos E, Porpiglia F, et al. Medical therapy to facilitate the passage of stones: what is the evidence? *Eur Urol*. 2009;56(3):455–471.
4. Aboumarzouk OM, Kata SG, Keeley FX, et al. Extracorporeal shock wave lithotripsy (ESWL) versus ureteroscopic management for ureteric calculi. *Cochrane Database Syst Rev*. 2011;(12):CD006029.
5. Shen P, Jiang M, Yang J, et al. Use of ureteral stent in extracorporeal shock wave lithotripsy for upper urinary calculi: a systematic review and meta-analysis. *J Urol*. 2011;186(4):1328–1335.
6. Cohen EP, Sobrero M, Roxe DM, et al. Reversibility of long-standing urinary tract obstruction requiring long-term dialysis. *Arch Intern Med*. 1992;152(1):177–179.

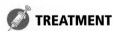 CODES

ICD10
• N13.2 Hydronephrosis with renal and ureteral calculous obstruction
• N13.30 Unspecified hydronephrosis
• Q62.0 Congenital hydronephrosis

CLINICAL PEARLS
• US and noncontrast CT identify most causes of hydronephrosis.
• Relief of obstruction, when present, is the primary treatment.

HYPERCHOLESTEROLEMIA

Michelle Nelson, MD • Egle Klugiene, MD

BASICS

DESCRIPTION
- Elevated cholesterol is a significant risk factor for atherosclerotic cardiovascular disease (ASCVD).
- Lipoprotein subtypes:
  - Low-density lipoproteins (LDL): atherogenic; primary target of therapy
  - High-density lipoproteins (HDL): atheroprotective
  - Triglycerides (TGs)
- System(s) affected: cardiovascular (CV)

EPIDEMIOLOGY
According to the CDC between 2017 and 2020, 10% of U.S. adults aged >20 years old have hypercholesterolemia, and 7% of U.S. children and adolescents between the ages of 6 and 19 years have hypercholesterolemia.

Prevalence
Disease incidence and prevalence increases with age.

ETIOLOGY AND PATHOPHYSIOLOGY
- Pathophysiology
  - Deposition of cholesterol in vascular walls creates fatty streaks that become fibrous plaques.
  - Inflammation causes plaque instability, leading to plaque rupture.
  - Atherosclerosis, inflammation, and vascular reactivity have a multifactorial etiology.
- Etiology of hypercholesterolemia
  - Primary: genetic causes (familial dyslipidemia)
  - Secondary: obesity, diet, excessive alcohol intake, hypothyroidism, diabetes mellitus (DM), inflammatory disease, liver disease, nephrotic syndrome, chronic renal failure, medications (thiazide diuretics, carbamazepine, cyclosporine, progestins, anabolic steroids, corticosteroids, protease inhibitors, antipsychotics, isotretinoin)

Genetics
- Familial hypercholesterolemia (FH)
  - Elevated LDL levels from birth
  - Prevalence is 1:300 worldwide for heterozygous FH.
  - Predisposition to atherosclerotic disease in early adulthood and high coronary heart disease risk at younger ages; individuals with homozygous FH typically die before 20 years old.
  - Early lipid-lowering drug therapy has been shown to reduce ASCVD risk.
- Early lipid screening of first-degree relatives is recommended.

RISK FACTORS
Obesity, physical inactivity, family history, cigarette smoking, excessive alcohol use; the relationship between dietary saturated fat and hypercholesterolemia and coronary artery disease is complex.

GENERAL PREVENTION
Regular physical activity, weight control (see "Ongoing Care"), diet lower in saturated fats (grade 1B)

COMMONLY ASSOCIATED CONDITIONS
Hypertension, DM, obesity

DIAGNOSIS

Screening recommendations:
- U.S. Preventive Services Task Force (USPSTF) (1)[A]: total cholesterol and HDL cholesterol (HDL-C)
  - Men and women aged ≥40 years old
- American Diabetes Association: yearly dyslipidemia screening for patients with DM

Pediatric Considerations
- National Heart, Lung, and Blood Institute: Recommend universal lipid screening on all children between 9 and 11 years old and between 17 and 21 years old. This was endorsed by the American Academy of Pediatrics (2), although pros and cons should be discussed with patients and family as more research is needed on population cost and harms versus benefit of screening.
- Screening is recommended for children with a family history of premature coronary artery disease or familial hypercholesterolemia.

HISTORY
Review possible secondary etiologies and assess other ASCVD risk factors.

PHYSICAL EXAM
Nonspecific findings; may calculate BMI and examine for xanthomas

DIAGNOSTIC TESTS & INTERPRETATION
Initial Tests (lab, imaging)
- Lipid panel (nonfasting preferred); LDL is usually a calculated value and is accurate if TG is <350 mg/dL. Perform fasting labs in hypertriglyceridemia (TG >440 mg/dL) or conditions that can elevated TG such as pancreatitis.
- Consider genetic etiology in very high LDL (>190 mg/dL) or TG (>500 mg/dL).

Follow-Up Tests & Special Considerations
In patients with ASCVD risk factors, the American Heart Association (AHA) recommends glucagon-like peptide-1 receptor agonists (GLP1-RA), regardless if the patient has DM or not.

TREATMENT

ALERT
Multiple guidelines exist. The American College of Cardiology/AHA (ACC/AHA) cholesterol guidelines return to targeting LDL goals. Risk stratifying patients should be reserved for primary prevention as patients with established CV disease should be considered as high-risk (secondary prevention).

- United States: ACC/AHA cholesterol guidelines (3)
  - According to the ACC/AHA, four groups benefit from statin therapy:
    - Primary elevation of LDL-C ≥190 mg/dL: high-intensity statin
    - Patients with DM aged 40 to 75 years with LDL-C ≥70 mg/dL: moderate-intensity statin
    - ASCVD risk based on Pooled Cohort Equations: http://tools.acc.org/ASCVD-Risk-Estimator (see below comment on calculator)
      - 10-year ASCVD risk <5%: lifestyle modifications with Mediterranean diet and exercise
      - 10-year ASCVD risk ≥5–7.5%: moderate-intensity statin; discuss with patient.
      - 10-year ASCVD risk ≥7.5–20%: moderate-intensity statin with a goal to reduce LDL-C by 30–49%
      - 10-year ASCVD risk ≥20%: high-intensity statin with a goal to reduce LDL-C >50%
    - Secondary ASCVD prevention
      - Age ≤75 years: high-intensity statin with a goal to reduce LDL-C ≥50%; add ezetimibe if LDL is ≥70 mg/dL after maximal statin therapy in very high-risk ASCVD patients.*
      - Age >75 years: moderate- or high-intensity statin as tolerated
  - *Definition of very high-risk ASCVD is at least one major ASCVD event and multiple high-risk conditions:
    - Major ASCVD events: acute coronary syndrome or history of myocardial infarction, history of ischemic stroke, symptomatic peripheral arterial disease
    - High-risk conditions: age ≥65 years, heterozygous FH, history of CABG or PCI, DM, HTN, chronic kidney disease, current smoker, history of congestive heart failure, LDL-C >100 mg/dL despite maximum medical therapy
    - Controversy exists regarding the threshold calculated risk with which to treat patients: The Pooled Cohort Equations calculator significantly *overestimates* 10-year ASCVD risk (by ≥50%). Therefore, discuss with patients the benefits and harms of statin therapy—factors in patient longevity.

- United States: USPSTF 2022 statin recommendations (1)[A]
  - Adults aged 40 to 75 years with no history of CVD, one or more CVD risk factors (dyslipidemia, hypertension, DM, or smoking), and a calculated 10-year CVD event risk of ≥10%: low- to moderate-intensity statin (grade B recommendation)
  - Adults aged 40 to 75 years with no history of CVD, one or more CVD risk factors, and a calculated 10-year CVD event risk of 7.5–10%: low- to moderate-dose statin (grade C recommendation)
  - Adults aged ≥76 years with no history of CVD: insufficient evidence to make recommendations

ALERT

In hypertriglyceridemia with TG >500 mg/dL, lowering TG becomes the primary goal until it is <500 mg/dL to prevent acute pancreatitis. Statin therapy is usually recommended as first line unless TGs remain >500. Fibrates may be used cautiously with statins (increased risk of rhabdomyolysis).

MEDICATION

- Therapeutic lifestyle changes are cornerstone therapies to be attempted before drug therapy.
- Available data do not support initiation of statin therapy for primary prevention in most adults aged >75 years (ALLHAT-LLT).
- Check lipid panel 4 to 12 weeks after starting medication to evaluate response and/or adherence. Subsequent monitoring is not generally indicated unless there is a question of patient adherence.

First Line

HMG-CoA reductase inhibitors (statins)

- Categorized based on intensity
  - High intensity (reduces LDL-C by >50%): atorvastatin 40 to 80 mg/day, rosuvastatin 20 to 40 mg/day
  - Moderate intensity (reduces LDL-C by 30–49%): atorvastatin 10 to 20 mg/day, rosuvastatin 5 to 10 mg/day, simvastatin 20 to 40 mg/day, pravastatin 40 to 80 mg/day, lovastatin 40 mg/day, fluvastatin XL 80 mg/day, fluvastatin 40 mg BID, pitavastatin 2 to 4 mg/day
  - Low intensity (reduces LDL-C by <30%): simvastatin 10 mg/day, pravastatin 10 to 20 mg/day, lovastatin 20 mg/day, fluvastatin 20 to 40 mg/day, pitavastatin 1 mg/day
- Effect is greatest in lowering LDL-C; shown to decrease coronary heart disease incidence and all-cause mortality (1)
- Contraindications: pregnancy, lactation, or active liver disease
- Adverse reactions:
  - Mild myalgia is common.
  - Liver transaminase elevations: alanine aminotransferase (ALT) before therapy to establish baseline; if ALT >3 times upper limit of normal, do not start statin; routine monitoring is not recommended.
  - Association with increased cases of DM: 0.1 excess cases of DM per 100 persons on moderate-intensity statin and 0.3 excess cases per 100 persons on high-intensity statin

- Myopathies (considered rare but not well studied):
- Statin intolerance strategies: Consider using a different statin (pravastatin, simvastatin), dose reduction, or alternate day therapy. A majority of patients who had previously discontinued statins due to side effects are able to restart the same or another statin and tolerate them.

ALERT

- U.S. Food and Drug Administration alert: Do not prescribe simvastatin at 80 mg/day due to increased myopathy risk. Patients who have been at this drug dosage for >1 year can continue if no signs of myopathy. Dose restrictions to reduce myopathy risk include the following: Do not exceed simvastatin 10 mg/day with amiodarone, verapamil, and diltiazem. Do not exceed simvastatin 20 mg/day with amlodipine and ranolazine.
- Avoid grapefruit juice with statins as it can increase the risk of statin myopathy.

Pregnancy Considerations

Statins contraindicated during pregnancy, possibly unsafe with lactation

Second Line

- Second-line drugs are now recommended as primary prevention if LDL-C is ≥70 mg/dL on maximal statin therapy.
- Ezetimibe: can be taken by itself or in combination with a statin: monotherapy (10 mg/day) or ezetimibe /simvastatin; effect lowers LDL-C; one randomized controlled trial shows combination therapy with statin has small benefit in reducing CV events and CV-related mortality after acute coronary syndromes.
- Fibrates gemfibrozil, fenofibrate; effect most effective in lowering TG with moderate effect in lowering LDL and raising HDL. More recent studies fail to show mortality benefit in most patients.
- Niacin raises HDL but no evidence for improved outcomes; should not be used routinely
- PCSK9 inhibitors (e.g., alirocumab, evolocumab): monoclonal antibodies; current evidence shows decreased incidence of CVD in secondary prevention without affecting incidence of all-cause mortality; very expensive medications
- Icosapent ethyl, an omega-3 fatty acid as adjunct to statin for hypertriglyceridemia treatment and CV risk reduction
- Bempedoic acid alternative to PCSK9 inhibitors if cost is prohibitive
- Inclisiran for patients who prefer fewer injections
- General strategy: Statin then add ezetimibe if LDL-C is ≥70 mg/dL on maximally tolerated statin therapy; if still not at goal, then add PCSK9 inhibitors.

ADDITIONAL THERAPIES

Antithrombotic therapies for patients with type 2 DM and risk factors for CVD

COMPLEMENTARY & ALTERNATIVE MEDICINE

Omega-3 fatty acids and fish oil intake: sources—fatty fish, plants (flaxseed, canola oil, soybean oil, nuts); they decrease TG and LDL level and increase HDL. Overall CV benefit and mortality reduction is uncertain.

ADMISSION, INPATIENT, AND NURSING CONSIDERATIONS

If lipid panel was checked while inpatient due to myocardial infarction, recommend rechecking a fasting lipid panel in 4 to 12 weeks after discharge as the first lab may not be as accurate.

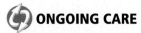 ONGOING CARE

FOLLOW-UP RECOMMENDATIONS

Moderate-intensity exercise for 150 minutes per week: increases HDL, lowers TC, and helps control weight

Patient Monitoring

Routine monitoring of liver function tests is no longer recommended if initial ALT is within normal range.

DIET

Plant-based diets and the Mediterranean diet, which are high in legumes, fruits, vegetables, nuts, fish, and olive oil, reduce the risk of CV disease.

PATIENT EDUCATION

- AHA: https://www.heart.org/en/healthy-living /healthy-eating/eat-smart/nutrition-basics /mediterranean-diet
- American College of Lifestyle Medicine: https://lifestylemedicine.org/project/patient -resources/

COMPLICATIONS

Myocardial infarction, peripheral artery disease, cerebrovascular accident

REFERENCES

1. Mangione CM, Barry MJ, Nickolson WK, et al; for US Preventive Services Task Force. Statin use for the primary prevention of cardiovascular disease in adults: US Preventive Services Task Force recommendation statement. *JAMA.* 2022;328(8):746–753.
2. Berger JH, Chen F, Faerber JA, et al. Adherence with lipid screening guidelines in standard- and high-risk children and adolescents. *Am Heart J.* 2021;232:39–46.
3. Grundy SM, Stone NJ, Bailey AL, et al. 2018 AHA/ ACC/AACVPR/AAPA/ABC/ACPM/ADA/AGS/APhA/ ASPC/NLA/PCNA guideline on the management of blood cholesterol: executive summary: a report of the American College of Cardiology/American Heart Association Task Force on clinical practice guidelines. *J Am Coll Cardiol.* 2019;73(24):3168–3209.

 SEE ALSO

Diabetes Mellitus, Type 2; Hypertension, Essential; Obesity

 CODES

ICD10

E78.0 Pure hypercholesterolemia

CLINICAL PEARLS

- A plant-based diet (Mediterranean diet) and exercise should be tried before pharmaceutical interventions for those with hypercholesterolemia.
- Decision to initiate statins in primary prevention should be based on risk and patient preferences.

HYPEREMESIS GRAVIDARUM

Zachary H. Hicks, DO

BASICS

- Nausea and vomiting in pregnancy is a common condition that affects approximately 70–80% of pregnancies.
- Hyperemesis gravidarum (HG) is a severe form of nausea and vomiting in pregnancy that affects 0.5–2% of pregnancies and can have significant adverse physical and psychological sequela.
- HG is a diagnosis of clinical judgement and is one of the most common indications for hospitalization during pregnancy.
- HG is associated with several adverse fetal outcomes including preterm delivery, low birth weight, small for gestation age, low 5-minute Apgar scores, and neurodevelopmental delay.

DESCRIPTION

- Although morning sickness is common during pregnancy, HG is a rare condition.
- Intractable vomiting in a pregnant woman that interferes with fluid and electrolyte balance as well as nutrition:
  - Usually associated with the first 8 to 20 weeks of pregnancy
  - Associated with high estrogen and human chorionic gonadotropin (hCG) levels
  - Symptoms usually begin ~2 weeks after first missed period, peak around the 12th week, and resolve by the 20th week
- System(s) affected: endocrine/metabolic, gastrointestinal, reproductive

EPIDEMIOLOGY

- Generally affects young women, primiparous, non-smokers, and nonwhite people
- Other risk factors: prior history of hyperemesis, pre-existing diabetes, hyperthyroid disorder, psychiatric illness, asthma, and GI disorders

Incidence
HG occurs in 0.5–2% of pregnancies.

Prevalence
The most common cause of hospitalization in the first half of pregnancy; the second most common cause of hospitalization of all pregnant women

ETIOLOGY AND PATHOPHYSIOLOGY
Etiology is unknown; proposed influences include the following:
- Hyperthyroidism
- Hyperparathyroidism
- Pregnancy hormones
- Liver dysfunction
- Autonomic nervous system dysfunction
- CNS neoplasm
- Addison disease
- Possible psychological factors

Genetics
Increased risk if maternal family history of HG

RISK FACTORS
Nulliparity; multiple gestations; history of migraines; history of motion sickness; black or Asian women; gestational trophoblastic disease; fetus with trisomy 21; female fetus; possible association with *Helicobacter pylori* infection

GENERAL PREVENTION
Guidance regarding dietary habits to avoid dehydration and nutritional depletion
- Small, frequent meals
- Avoid an overly empty or full stomach.
- Avoid greasy, spicy, and fatty foods.
- Eat bland, low-fiber, high-protein snacks.

DIAGNOSIS

Intractable nausea and vomiting in pregnancy leading to dehydration and electrolyte imbalances after the exclusion of other causes of severe nausea and vomiting

HISTORY
- Nausea
- Vomiting with retching >3 times per day
- Decreased urine output
- Fatigue
- Dizziness with standing
- Poor appetite

PHYSICAL EXAM
- >5% weight loss from prepregnancy weight
- Thyroid evaluation
- Signs of dehydration, such as orthostatic hypotension, large ketonuria, high urine specific gravity

DIFFERENTIAL DIAGNOSIS
Other common causes of vomiting must be considered: gastroenteritis, gastritis, reflux esophagitis, peptic ulcer disease, cholelithiasis, cholecystitis, pyelonephritis, appendicitis, pancreatitis, anxiety, hyperparathyroidism, hypercalcemia, thyrotoxicosis, *H. pylori* infection

DIAGNOSTIC TESTS & INTERPRETATION
Initial laboratory studies for HG are used to evaluate maternal clinical status and rule out other possible causes of nausea and vomiting.

Initial Tests (lab, imaging)
- Urinalysis: may see glucosuria, albuminuria, granular casts, and hematuria (rare); ketosis more common
- Thyroid-stimulating hormone (TSH), free T_4
- Electrolytes, BUN, creatinine
- Liver enzymes and bilirubin levels
- Hematocrit
- Hepatitis panel
- Calcium
- Albumin

Diagnostic Procedures/Other
Indicated only if it is necessary to rule out other diagnoses, as listed in the following section:
- Upper abdominal ultrasound if pancreatitis or cholecystitis are suspected
- Abdominal MRI if appendicitis is suspected
- Ultrasound if hydatidiform mole or multiple gestation is suspected

Test Interpretation
- Urinalysis: When positive for ketones and high specific gravity indicate starvation ketosis and volume depletion
- TSH, free T_4: A transient hyperthyroidism (suppressed TSH with normal free T_4) may be present in approximately 50% of HG. If TSH is suppressed with elevated free T_4, further investigation is needed for overt hyperthyroidism.

- Electrolytes, BUN, creatinine: Dehydration can cause low potassium, low sodium, and elevated BUN and creatinine.
- Liver enzymes and bilirubin levels: Mild elevation of AST and ALT occurs in approximately 50% of cases and self-resolves.
- Hematocrit: Dehydration causes increase (volume contraction).
- Hepatitis panel: Hepatitis A, B, and C may present similarly to hyperemesis; consider and rule out.
- Calcium: Hypercalcemia resulting from hyperparathyroidism occurs rarely.
- Albumin: Decreased albumin may indicate malnutrition secondary to nausea and vomiting.

TREATMENT

Pyridoxine and doxylamine (pregnancy Category A) are first-line treatments for HG (1)[C]. This is followed by metoclopramide or ondansetron (pregnancy Category B) and then prochlorperazine (pregnancy Category C), methylprednisolone (pregnancy Category C), or promethazine (pregnancy Category C).

GENERAL MEASURES
- First, treat dehydration and electrolyte imbalances and then treat nausea.
- IV fluids, either normal saline or 5% dextrose normal saline (with consideration for potential thiamine deficiency)
- For severe cases, consider PO thiamine 25 to 50 mg TID or IV 100 mg in 100 mL of normal saline over 30 minutes once weekly and potential parental nutrition if needed.
- Ondansetron carries an FDA warning for QT prolongation. It has unclear risk in the setting of pregnancy. The majority of the current studies shows no increased fetal risk.

MEDICATION
- Pyridoxine (vitamin B_6) 25 mg PO or IV q8h, max dose of 200 mg/day
- Antihistamines (e.g., diphenhydramine [25 to 50 mg q4–6h], doxylamine [12.5 mg PO BID], meclizine [25 mg PO q4–6h], and dimenhydrinate [25 to 50 mg PO q4–6h]) (2)[C]
- Combination product Diclegis (sustained-release pyridoxine 10 mg and doxylamine 10 mg) dosed (start 2 tabs PO QHS; if symptoms persist, increase to 1 tab in AM and 2 QHS; if symptoms still persist, take 1 tab every AM, 1 midday, and 2 QHS; max of 4 tablets/day) or doxylamine 12.5 mg and pyridoxine 25 mg
- Phenothiazines (e.g., promethazine or prochlorperazine): associated with prolonged jaundice, extrapyramidal effects, and hyper- or hyporeflexia in newborns
- Metoclopramide 10 mg PO q6–8h

- Methylprednisolone 16 mg PO/IV q8h for 2 to 3 days and then taper over 2 weeks if initial 3-day treatment is effective; reserved for severe cases with unclear benefit
- Ondansetron 4 to 8 mg PO q8h

First Line
- For women with mild to moderate nausea, pyridoxine (vitamin B$_6$) 10 to 25 mg PO or IV q8h can improve symptoms and has a good safety profile. Maximum dose is 200 mg/day.
- If nausea and vomiting continue, combination doxylamine succinate 12.5 mg and pyridoxine 25 mg PO q8h; this combination is more effective than either drug alone.
- Ginger capsules 350 mg PO TID can be added with refractory vomiting.

Second Line
- Antihistamines such as diphenhydramine, meclizine, and dimenhydrinate; doxylamine-pyridoxine should be discontinued before starting a different antihistamine.
- Metoclopramide 10 mg PO q8h
- Promethazine 12.5 mg PO or rectally q8h
- Ondansetron 4 to 8 mg PO or IV q8h

ISSUES FOR REFERRAL
- Inpatient management required for IV antiemetics and fluids for symptoms refractory to outpatient management
- May also consider psychiatry or psychology referral if psychological assessment is warranted

ADDITIONAL THERAPIES
- Glucocorticoids (methylprednisolone 16 mg IV q8h for 48 to 72 hours) of uncertain benefit but may be considered for severe and refractory cases
- H$_2$ receptor antagonists (cimetidine and ranitidine) as adjunctive therapy to reduce heartburn/acid reflux

SURGERY/OTHER PROCEDURES
Rarely, if all pharmacologic and nonpharmacologic interventions fail and weight loss continues, tube feeding or parenteral nutrition is required. Enteral nutrition, either through a gastric or duodenal route, is preferred to the parenteral route as it may relieve nausea and vomiting.

COMPLEMENTARY & ALTERNATIVE MEDICINE
- Ginger 350 mg PO q6h may help (3)[A].
- Mixed evidence for acupressure and acupuncture; acupressure bands at the Neiguan point are effective adjuvant treatment in severe hyperemesis (4)[A].
- Medical hypnosis may be a helpful adjunct to the typical medical treatment regimen, but further study is needed.

ADMISSION, INPATIENT, AND NURSING CONSIDERATIONS
- In some severe cases, parenteral therapy in the hospital or at home may be required.
- Enteral volume and nutrition repletion may be indicated, but early enteral tube feeding does not improve maternal or perinatal outcomes (5)[A].

ONGOING CARE
Approximately 10% of patients with HG will be affected throughout the pregnancy.

FOLLOW-UP RECOMMENDATIONS
Overall quality of life and future fertility plans can be impacted by severity of nausea and vomiting (6)[B].

Patient Monitoring
- In severe cases, follow-up on a daily basis for weight monitoring
- Special attention should be given to monitor for ketosis, hypokalemia, or acid–base disturbances due to hyperemesis.

DIET
- Bland or liquid diet as tolerated
- For outpatient: a diet rich in carbohydrates and protein, such as fruit, cheese, cottage cheese, eggs, beef, poultry, vegetables, toast, crackers, rice; patients should avoid spicy meals and high-fat foods. Encourage small amounts at a time every 1 to 2 hours.

PATIENT EDUCATION
- Attention should be given to psychosocial issues, such as possible ambivalence about the pregnancy.
- Patients should be instructed to take small amounts of fluid frequently to avoid volume depletion.
- Avoid individual foods known to be irritating to the patient.
- Wet-to-dry nutrients (sherbet, broth, gelatin to dry crackers, toast)

PROGNOSIS
- Self-limited illness with good prognosis if patient's weight is maintained at >95% of prepregnancy weight.
- With complication of hemorrhagic retinitis, mortality rate of pregnant patient is 50%.

COMPLICATIONS
- Maternal complications:
  – Vitamin deficiency, dehydration, and malnutrition
  – In severe cases, Wernicke encephalopathy secondary to thiamine deficiency, coma, and even death
- Fetal complications:
  – Patients with >5% weight loss are associated with intrauterine growth retardation and fetal anomalies.
  – Poor weight gain is associated with slightly increased risk for small for gestational age infant <2,500 g and premature birth <37 weeks (7)[A].
  – Hemorrhagic retinitis
  – Liver damage

REFERENCES

1. Maltepe C, Koren G. The management of nausea and vomiting of pregnancy and hyperemesis gravidarum—a 2013 update. *J Popul Ther Clin Pharmacol*. 2013;20(2):e184–e192.
2. Boelig RC, Barton SJ, Saccone G, et al. Interventions for treating hyperemesis gravidarum. *Cochrane Database Syst Rev*. 2016;2016(5):CD010607.
3. Viljoen E, Visser J, Koen N, et al. A systematic review and meta-analysis of the effect and safety of ginger in the treatment of pregnancy-associated nausea and vomiting. *Nutr J*. 2014;13:20.
4. Adlan AS, Chooi KY, Mat Adenan NA. Acupressure as adjuvant treatment for the inpatient management of nausea and vomiting in early pregnancy: a double-blind randomized controlled trial. *J Obstet Gynaecol Res*. 2017;43(4):662–668.
5. Grooten IJ, Koot MH, van der Post JA, et al. Early enteral tube feeding in optimizing treatment of hyperemesis gravidarum: the Maternal and Offspring outcomes after Treatment of HyperEmesis by Refeeding (MOTHER) randomized controlled trial. *Am J Clin Nutr*. 2017;106(3):812–820.
6. Heitmann K, Nordeng H, Havnen GC, et al. The burden of nausea and vomiting during pregnancy: severe impacts on quality of life, daily life functioning and willingness to become pregnant again—results from a cross-sectional study. *BMC Pregnancy Childbirth*. 2017;17(1):75.
7. Veenendaal MVE, van Abeelen AFM, Painter RC, et al. Consequences of hyperemesis gravidarum for offspring: a systematic review and meta-analysis. *BJOG*. 2011;118(11):1302–1313.

ADDITIONAL READING
- Boelig RC, Barton SJ, Saccone G, et al. Interventions for treating hyperemesis gravidarum: a Cochrane systematic review and meta-analysis. *J Matern Fetal Neonatal Med*. 2018;31(18):2492–2505.
- McParlin C, O'Donnell A, Robson SC, et al. Treatments for hyperemesis gravidarum and nausea and vomiting in pregnancy: a systematic review. *JAMA*. 2016;316(13):1392–1401.

CODES

ICD10
- O21.9 Vomiting of pregnancy, unspecified
- O21.0 Mild hyperemesis gravidarum
- O21.1 Hyperemesis gravidarum with metabolic disturbance

CLINICAL PEARLS
- Do not allow patients to become volume depleted. Once this occurs, it is more difficult to treat.
- Do not be hesitant to use medications for nausea/vomiting, as this may help avoid volume depletion.
- Consider secondary causes of hyperemesis if it develops after 12 weeks of gestation.

H

HYPERKALEMIA
Pooja Gandhi, DO • Tyler D. Sharpe, MD

BASICS

DESCRIPTION
- Hyperkalemia is a common electrolyte disorder defined as a plasma potassium (K) concentration >5.5 mEq/L (>5 mmol/L).
- Hyperkalemia depresses cardiac conduction and can lead to fatal arrhythmias.
- Normal K regulation
  - Ingested K enters portal circulation; pancreas releases insulin in response. Insulin facilitates K entry into cells.
  - K in renal circulation causes renin release from juxtaglomerular cells, leading to activation of angiotensin I, which is converted to angiotensin II in lungs. Angiotensin II acts in adrenal zona glomerulosa to stimulate aldosterone secretion. Aldosterone, at the renal collecting ducts, causes K to be excreted and sodium to be retained.
- Four major causes
  - Increased load: either endogenous from tissue release or exogenous from a high intake, usually in association with decreased excretion or chronic kidney disease (CKD)
  - Decreased excretion: due to decreased glomerular filtration rate (GFR) or impaired aldosterone secretion
  - Cellular redistribution: shifts from intracellular space (majority of K is intracellular) to extracellular space
  - Pseudohyperkalemia: related to red cell lysis during collection or transport of blood sample, thrombocytosis, or leukocytosis

Geriatric Considerations
Increased risk for hyperkalemia because of decreases in renin and aldosterone as well as comorbid conditions

EPIDEMIOLOGY
Incidence
Incidence is higher in patients of older age, male sex, worse kidney function, comorbidities and use of renin angiotensin-aldosterone system inhibitors.

Prevalence
- 1–10% of hospitalized patients
- 2–3% in general population but as high as 50% in patients with CKD

ETIOLOGY AND PATHOPHYSIOLOGY
- Pseudohyperkalemia
  - Hemolysis of red cells in phlebotomy tube (Spurious result is the most common.)
  - Thrombolysis; thrombocytosis
  - Leukocytosis (reverse pseudohyperkalemia)
  - Hereditary spherocytosis
  - Infectious mononucleosis
  - Traumatic venipuncture or fist clenching during phlebotomy (spurious result)
  - Familial pseudohyperkalemia
- Increased K intake (1)
  - Bananas, potatoes, melons, citrus juice, avocados, red meat, nuts, and dried fruits
  - Salt substitutes given to chronic kidney patients
  - Clay ingestion
- Transcellular shift (redistribution)
  - Metabolic acidosis
  - Insulin deficiency
  - Hyperglycemia (diabetic ketoacidosis or hyperosmolar hyperglycemic state)
  - Tissue damage (rhabdomyolysis, tumor lysis syndrome, burns, trauma)
  - Cocaine abuse
  - Exercise with heavy sweating
- Impaired K excretion
  - Renal insufficiency/failure
  - Addison disease
  - Mineralocorticoid deficiency
  - Primary hyporeninemia, primary hypoaldosteronism
  - Type IV renal tubular acidosis (hyporeninemic hypoaldosteronism)
  - Obstructive uropathy
  - Cirrhosis
  - Congestive heart failure (CHF)
  - Sickle cell disease
  - Amyloidosis
  - Gordon syndrome
  - Systemic lupus erythematosus
- Medication-induced (numerous)

Genetics
Associated with some inherited diseases and conditions
- Familial hyperkalemic periodic paralysis
- Congenital adrenal hyperplasia

RISK FACTORS
- Impaired renal excretion of K
- Acidemia
- Massive cell breakdown (rhabdomyolysis, burns, trauma)
- Use of K-sparing diuretics
- Excess K supplementation
- Comorbid conditions: CKD, diabetes, heart failure, liver disease

GENERAL PREVENTION
Low K diet and oral supplement compliance in those at risk

COMMONLY ASSOCIATED CONDITIONS
- Acute kidney injury or CKD, typically with GFR <30 mL/min
- End-stage renal disease (ESRD)
- CHF
- Myocardial infarction (MI)
- Rhabdomyolysis
- Liver disease
- Use of medications such as ACE inhibitors or angiotensin II receptor blockers

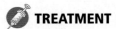 DIAGNOSIS

Serum K level greater than the normal range (3.5 to 5.0 mEq/L); patients may be asymptomatic until >6 mEq/L.

HISTORY
- Neuromuscular cramps, myalgias, muscle weakness or paralysis
- Abdominal pain
- Palpitations
- Numbness
- Arrhythmia or cardiac arrest

PHYSICAL EXAM
- Decreased deep tendon reflexes
- Muscle weakness or flaccid paralysis of extremities

DIAGNOSTIC TESTS & INTERPRETATION
- Serum electrolytes
- Renal function: BUN, creatinine
- Urinalysis: K, creatinine, osmoles (to calculate fractional excretion of K and transtubular K gradient; both assess renal handling of K)
- Disorders that may alter lab results
  - Acidemia: K shifts from the intracellular to extracellular space
  - Insulin deficiency
  - Hemolysis of sample
- Cortisol, aldosterone, and renin levels to check for mineralocorticoid deficiency when other causes are ruled out

Diagnostic Procedures/Other
ECG abnormalities usually occur when K ≥7 mEq/L.
- Peaked T wave with shortened QT interval in precordial leads (most common, usually earliest ECG change; however, neither sensitive nor specific) (2)[C]
- Lengthening of PR interval, loss of P wave, widened QRS
- Sine wave at very high K >8 mEq/L
- Can eventually lead to arrhythmias including bradycardia, ventricular fibrillation, and asystole

TREATMENT

MEDICATION
- Stabilize myocardial membranes; initial treatment with calcium gluconate IV 1,000 mg (10 mL of 10% solution) over 2 to 3 minutes (3)[A]
  - With constant cardiac monitoring
  - Can repeat after 5 minutes if needed
  - Effect begins within minutes, but only lasts 30 to 60 minutes and should be used in conjunction with definitive therapies
  - Can also use calcium chloride (3 times as concentrated; however, central or deep vein administration is necessary to avoid tissue necrosis.)
- If suspected, stop offending agent and address any reversible causes.
- Drive extracellular K into cells.
  - Nebulized albuterol (at 10 to 20 mg/4 mL saline >10 minutes—4 to 8 times bronchodilation dose) and other β-agonists have an additive effect with insulin and glucose (3)[B].
  - Dextrose 50% 1 amp (if plasma glucose <250 mg/dL) and insulin 10 U IV may drive K intracellularly but does not decrease total body K and may result in hypoglycemia (close monitoring advised, especially 1 to 2 hours postinjection) (3)[B].
  - Sodium bicarbonate not routinely recommended but some possible benefits in severe metabolic acidosis (4)[C]

- Remove excess K from body.
  - Cation exchange resins definitive treatment but require several doses and best used with rapidly acting transient therapies above and when dialysis not readily available (5)[A]
  - Gastrointestinal cation exchangers, patiromer calcium (Veltassa), sodium polystyrene sulfonate (Kayexalate) and sodium zirconium cyclosilicate (Lokelma) bind K in the intestinal tract. Patiromer in particular is favored for improved tolerance and decreased side effects in both acute and chronic settings (6)[C]
  - Patiromer calcium (Veltassa): 8.4 g PO daily (dose may vary 4.2 to 16.8 g BID in studies)
    ◦ This requires ~7 to 24 hours to lower K. This may be repeated q12h, if necessary (7)[C].
  - Sodium zirconium cyclosilicate (Lokelma): 10 mg PO TID for up to 48 hours (8)[C].
  - Sodium polystyrene sulfonate (Kayexalate): 15 g PO or 30 g rectally
    ◦ This requires 1 to 4 hours to lower K. This may be repeated q6h, if necessary.
    ◦ Enema has faster effect than PO (3)[C].
  - Loop diuretics (furosemide): 40 mg IV q12h or continuous infusion; may need to give isotonic fluids as well if patient is euvolemic or hypovolemic prior to furosemide (Lasix)
  - Hemodialysis is the definitive therapy when other measures are not effective. This may be required particularly when conditions, such as digitalis toxicity, rhabdomyolysis, ESRD, severe CKD, or acute kidney injury, are present; should watch for postdialysis rebound (3)[A]
  - Little clinical evidence for the use of diuretics (loop and thiazides), however, can consider for control of chronic hyperkalemia (3)[B].
- Chronic hyperkalemia treatment
  - Review medication and discontinue those that can be contributing to hyperkalemia.
  - Dietary counseling of K-rich food
  - Diuretic therapy using thiazide and loop diuretics

ALERT
- Sodium polystyrene sulfonate (Kayexalate) provides a sodium load that may exacerbate fluid overload in patients with cardiac or renal failure.
- Avoid sodium polystyrene sulfonate use in patients who are postoperative or with a bowel obstruction or ileus due to high risk of intestinal necrosis.
- Rapid administration of calcium in patients with suspected digitalis toxicity may result in a fatal dysrhythmia. Calcium should be administered slowly over 20 to 30 minutes in 5% dextrose with extreme caution. Preferred therapy is digoxin-specific antibody fragments.

ADDITIONAL THERAPIES
Mineralocorticoid replacement (9)
- If the patient does not have a contraindication (greater than stage 1 HTN, volume overload, history of heart failure) to mineralocorticoid administration then
  - Consider a trial of fludrocortisone 0.1 mg daily × 3 to 5 days (9) (in patients with moderately advanced CKD, consider maintaining or increasing diuretics in tandem with the assistance of nephrology consulting service).

ADMISSION, INPATIENT, AND NURSING CONSIDERATIONS
- If hyperkalemia is severe, treat first, and then do diagnostic investigations.
- IV calcium to stabilize myocardium (caution in setting of digoxin toxicity/digoxin induced hyperkalemia, as this treatment can induce heart block)
- Insulin (usually 10 U IV, given with 50 mL of 50% glucose [if serum glucose <250 mg/dL] to avoid hypoglycemia); consider repeating if elevation persists.
- Inhaled β_2-agonist (nebulized albuterol)
- Discontinue any medications that may increase K (e.g., K-sparing diuretics, exogenous K).
- Admit for cardiac monitoring if ECG changes are present or if K is >6 mEq/L (6 mmol/L).
- Consider if the patient meets the criteria for emergent hemodialysis.

 ## ONGOING CARE

FOLLOW-UP RECOMMENDATIONS
Patient Monitoring
Serum K levels should be rechecked every 2 to 4 hours until the patient has stabilized, and recurrent hyperkalemia is no longer a threat.

DIET
Dietary K intake is rarely the only culprit, even in CKD. Recommend ≤80 mEq (≤80 mmol) of K per 24 hours if difficult to control hyperkalemia or symptoms while workup ongoing (10). Those that are particularly high in K (>6.4 mEq/serving) include bananas, orange juice, other citrus fruits and their juices, figs, molasses, seaweed, dried fruits, nuts, avocados, lima beans, bran, tomatoes, tomato juice, cantaloupe, honeydew melon, peaches, potatoes, and salt substitutes. Multiple herbal medications can also increase K levels, including alfalfa, dandelion, horsetail nettle, milkweed, hawthorn berries, toad skin, oleander, foxglove, and ginseng.

PATIENT EDUCATION
Consult with a dietitian about a low-K diet.

PROGNOSIS
- Associated with poor prognosis in patients with heart failure and CKD
- Associated with poor prognosis in disaster medicine, with trauma, tissue necrosis, K$^+$ supplementation, metabolic acidosis, if calcium gluconate administered for treatment of hyperkalemia, if AKI, or if prolonged duration of hyperkalemia (4)

COMPLICATIONS
- Life-threatening cardiac arrhythmias
- Potential complications of the use of ion-exchange resins for the treatment of hyperkalemia include volume overload and intestinal necrosis (6)[C].

REFERENCES

1. Palmer BF, Clegg DJ. Diagnosis and treatment of hyperkalemia. *Cleve Clin J Med*. 2017;84(12): 934–942.
2. Wong R, Banker R, Aronowitz P. Electrocardiographic changes of severe hyperkalemia. *J Hosp Med*. 2011;6(4):240.
3. Viera AJ, Wouk N. Potassium disorders: hypokalemia and hyperkalemia. *Am Fam Physician*. 2015;92(6):487–495.
4. Khanagavi J, Gupta T, Aronow WS, et al. Hyperkalemia among hospitalized patients and association between duration of hyperkalemia and outcomes. *Arch Med Sci*. 2014;10(2): 251–257.
5. Sterns RH, Rojas M, Bernstein P, et al. Ion-exchange resins for the treatment of hyperkalemia: are they safe and effective? *J Am Soc Nephrol*. 2010;21(5):733–735.
6. Ingelfinger JR. A new era for the treatment of hyperkalemia? *N Engl J Med*. 2015;372(3): 275–277.
7. Bushinsky DA, Williams GH, Pitt B, et al. Patiromer induces rapid and sustain potassium lowering in patients with chronic kidney disease and hyperkalemia. *Kidney Int*. 2015;88(6):1427–1433.
8. Peacock WF, Rafique Z, Vishnevskiy K, et al. Emergency potassium normalization treatment including sodium zirconium cyclosilicate: a phase II, randomized, double-blind, placebo-controlled study (ENERGIZE). *Acad Emerg Med*. 2020;27(6):475–486.
9. Montford JR, Linas S. How dangerous is hyperkalemia? *J Am Soc Nephrol*. 2017;28(11): 3155–3165.
10. Ramos CI, González-Ortiz A, Espinosa-Cuevas A, et al. Does dietary potassium intake associate with hyperkalemia in patients with chronic kidney disease? *Nephrol Dial Transplant*. 2021;36(11):2049–2057.

 ## SEE ALSO

- Addison Disease; Hypokalemia
- Algorithm: Hyperkalemia

CODES

ICD10
E87.5 Hyperkalemia

CLINICAL PEARLS
- Urgent management of hyperkalemia takes precedence to a thorough diagnostic workup. Urgent treatment includes stabilization of the myocardium with calcium gluconate to protect against arrhythmias and pharmacologic strategies to move K from the extracellular (vascular) space into cells.
- Calcium and dextrose/insulin are only temporizing measures and do not lower total body K levels. Definitive treatment with either dialysis or cation exchange resin (sodium polystyrene sulfonate) is necessary.
- To lower a patient's risk of developing hyperkalemia, recommend a low-K diet, use selective β_1-blockers, such as metoprolol or atenolol, instead of nonselective β-blockers such as carvedilol. Avoid NSAIDs. Concomitant use of kaliuretic loop diuretics may be useful.

HYPERNATREMIA

Pang-Yen Fan, MD • Rajarshi Bhadra, MD

 BASICS

DESCRIPTION
- Defined as serum sodium (Na) concentration >145 mEq/L, which usually represents a state of hypertonicity (1),(2)
- Na concentration reflects balance between total body water (TBW) and total body Na. Hypernatremia occurs from deficit of water relative to Na.
- Dehydration refers to hypernatremia from water loss.
- Hypovolemia refers to concomitant water and salt loss.
- Hypernatremia commonly results from net water loss or, more rarely, from primary Na gain (1).
- Hypernatremia will not develop in patients with intact thirst mechanisms who are able to access water.

EPIDEMIOLOGY
Incidence
- More common in elderly and very young
- Occurs in 1% of hospitalized elderly patients (3)
- Seen in about 9% of ICU patients (3)

ETIOLOGY AND PATHOPHYSIOLOGY
- Due to the powerful effect of the thirst mechanism, hypernatremia typically occurs only in patients who cannot readily access water such as infants, intubated patients, and those with altered mental status or patients with hypodipsia (4).
- Water loss out of proportion to salt loss is the most common cause of hypernatremia. The following conditions lead to excessive water loss:
  - Transdermal loss such as burns or excessive sweating (e.g., fever, infants under radiant heaters, heat exposure, extreme exercise)
  - Urinary loss
    - Nephrogenic diabetes insipidus (DI) (congenital or due to renal dysfunction, hypercalcemia, hypokalemia, medication-related, e.g., lithium)
    - Central DI (due to head trauma, stroke, meningitis) (3)
    - Osmotic diuresis: glucose, urea, and mannitol
    - Post-ATN diuresis
  - Gastrointestinal loss
    - Osmotic diarrhea: lactulose, malabsorption, and some types of infectious diarrhea
    - Enterocutaneous fistula
    - Vomiting, NG suction
- Disorders of the thirst mechanism can result in hypernatremia due to reduced water intake (e.g., intracranial lesions, primary hypodipsia, chronic volume expansion in mineralocorticoid excess).

- Excess Na (increase in total body Na) less commonly leads to hypernatremia. The following condition may result in excessive total body Na:
  - IV infusion of hypertonic NaCl or $NaHCO_3$ during treatment of brain injury, metabolic acidosis, or hyperkalemia (3)
  - Sea water ingestion
  - Excessive use of $NaHCO_3$ antacid
  - Incorrect infant formula preparation, tube feeding
  - Excessive Na in dialysate solutions
- With acute hypernatremia, the rapid decrease in brain volume can cause rupture of the cerebral veins, leading to focal intracerebral and sub-arachnoid hemorrhages and possibly irreversible neurologic damage (2).

Genetics
Some forms of DI may be hereditary.

RISK FACTORS
- Infants/children
- Elderly patients (may also have a diminished thirst response to osmotic stimulation via an unknown mechanism)
- Patients who are intubated/have altered mental status
- Acute gastrointestinal illness
- Poorly controlled diabetes mellitus
- Prior brain injury
- Surgery
- Diuretic therapy, especially loop diuretics
- Lithium treatment

GENERAL PREVENTION
- Treatment/prevention of underlying cause
- Properly prepare infant formula and never add salt to any commercial infant formula.
- Keep patients well hydrated.

COMMONLY ASSOCIATED CONDITIONS
- Gastroenteritis
- Altered mental status
- Burns
- Head injury

DIAGNOSIS

HISTORY
- History of conditions leading to water loss or impaired thirst: nausea, vomiting, diarrhea, polyuria, fever, heat exposure, extreme exercise, brain injury
- Neurologic symptoms are common:
  - Mild: thirst, anorexia
  - Moderate: altered mental status, myalgia, muscle weakness, twitching, lethargy, irritability
  - Severe: seizure (especially if rapid development of hypernatremia), coma

- Severity of symptoms correlate with rapidity of the increase in Na as well as the degree of hypernatremia.
- Severe symptoms are likely to occur with sudden increases in plasma Na levels or at concentrations >160 mEq/L.

PHYSICAL EXAM
- Signs of water or volume loss: tachycardia, hypotension, orthostatic hypotension, dry mucous membranes, poor skin turgor
- Neurologic abnormalities: lethargy, weakness, tremor, focal deficits (in cases of intracerebral bleeding/lesion), confusion, coma, seizures

DIFFERENTIAL DIAGNOSIS
- DI
- Hyperosmotic coma
- Salt ingestion
- Hypertonic dehydration
- Hypothyroidism
- Cushing syndrome

DIAGNOSTIC TESTS & INTERPRETATION
Initial Tests (lab, imaging)
- Serum Na, potassium, BUN, creatinine, glucose, calcium, and osmolality (serum lithium if appropriate)
- Hemoglobin/hematocrit (may be elevated above baseline due to hemoconcentration)
- Urine Na and osmolality
  - Low urine osmolality: urine osmolality (usually <300 mOsm/kg) < serum osmolality suggests DI.
  - Intermediate urine osmolality (300 to 800 mOsm/kg) may be from hypovolemia, osmotic diuresis, partial DI.
  - High urine osmolality (>800 mOsm/kg) suggests extrarenal water loss or, rarely, salt ingestion.
- Urine Na
  - Low urine Na (<10): usually suggests volume depletion, although may also be from dilution in the setting of high urine output with DI
  - Intermediate urine Na may be from osmotic diuresis.
  - High urine Na suggests salt ingestion.

Follow-Up Tests & Special Considerations
- Special tests for DI
  - Antidiuretic hormone (ADH) stimulation: distinguishes central versus nephrogenic DI
    - Urine osmolality does not increase after ADH or desmopressin in nephrogenic DI.
- Head CT/MRI in patients with central DI or hypodipsia to rule out intracranial lesions

TREATMENT

GENERAL MEASURES

- The treatment of hypernatremia involves treating the underlying cause and correcting the water deficit.
- Determine the duration of hypernatremia because speed of correction depends on symptom severity and rate of development of hypernatremia.
- Acute hyponatremia: relatively uncommon, may occur in acute DI, severe hyperglycemia, or salt ingestion
  - D5W infusion at 3 to 6 mL/kg/hr to lower the serum Na by 1 to 2 mEq/L/hr
  - Check serum Na every 1 to 2 hours to confirm correction at desired rate.
  - When serum Na decreases to 145 mEq/L, reduce D5W infusion to 1 mL/kg/hr until serum Na normalizes.
  - Aim to correct hypernatremia in 24 to 48 hours.
- Chronic hypernatremia (>48 hours): Avoid rapid correction to prevent development of cerebral edema.
- D5W infusion at 1.35 mL/kg/hr
- Check serum Na every 4 to 6 hours to determine correction at desired rate.
- Correct at maximum of 0.5 mEq/L/hr or 10 to 12 mEq/L/day.
- Often need to adjust infusion rate to account for ongoing water losses
- Hypernatremia with hyponatremia: Correct severe volume depletion with isotonic IV fluids first and then address hypernatremia:
  - Once hemodynamically stable, can correct hypovolemia and hypernatremia simultaneously with 0.45% saline as every 2 mL of this solution will provide 1 mL of saline and 1 mL of water
- Hypernatremia with hypervolemia: can treat hypervolemia with diuretics while simultaneously correcting hypernatremia
  - Concomitant diuretic treatment will increase urinary water losses and may necessitate increased water repletion.
- Consider oral water repletion for mild hypernatremia.
- High infusion rates of D5W may cause hyperglycemia.
- Hyperglycemia-induced osmotic diuresis will increase urinary water losses and necessitate increased water repletion.
- Dialysis can be considered if acute kidney injury and conventional treatment has failed (5)[B].

MEDICATION

First Line
- See "General Measures" for overall approach because treatment is generally done with water or hypotonic IV fluids rather than medication.
- May use medication in treatment of DI

- Central DI
  - Desmopressin acetate (DDAVP): Use parenteral form for acute symptomatic patients, and use intranasal or oral form for chronic therapy (4).
  - Free water replacement: may use 2.5% dextrose in water if giving large volumes of water in DI to avoid glycosuria
  - May consider sulfonylureas/thiazide diuretics for chronic but not acute treatment
- Nephrogenic DI
  - Treat with diuretics and NSAIDs.
  - Lithium-induced nephrogenic DI: hydrochlorothiazide 25 mg PO BID or indomethacin 50 mg PO TID, or amiloride hydrochloride 5 to 10 mg PO BID

Second Line
- Consider NSAIDs in nephrogenic DI.
- Continuous renal replacement therapy (CRRT): Multiple case reports and case series have shown success and safety in using CRRT to treat hypernatremia in critically ill patients with CHF and severe burns (5).

ISSUES FOR REFERRAL
Underlying renal involvement associated with hypernatremia would benefit from a nephrology referral.

ADMISSION, INPATIENT, AND NURSING CONSIDERATIONS
- Symptomatic patient with serum Na >155 mEq/L requires IV fluid therapy.
- Discharge criteria: stabilization of serum Na level and resolution of symptoms

 ## ONGOING CARE

FOLLOW-UP RECOMMENDATIONS
Patient Monitoring
- Frequent neurologic checks during acute correction
- Daily weight, electrolytes, and blood glucose for a period immediately after correction
- Periodic monitoring of urine osmolality and urine output in DI

DIET
- Ensure proper nutrition during acute phase.
- After resolution of acute phase, may consider Na-restricted diet for patient
- Low-salt, low-protein diet in nephrogenic DI

PATIENT EDUCATION
Patients with nephrogenic DI must avoid salt and drink large amounts of water.

PROGNOSIS
Most recover but neurologic impairment can occur.

COMPLICATIONS
- More common if rapid development of hypernatremia
- CNS thrombosis/hemorrhage
- Seizures
- Chronic hypernatremia: >2 days duration has higher mortality.
- Serum Na >180 mEq/L (>180 mmol/L): often results in residual CNS damage

REFERENCES

1. Adrogué HJ, Madias NE. Hypernatremia. *N Engl J Med*. 2000;342(20):1493–1499.
2. Sterns RH. Disorders of plasma sodium—causes, consequences, and correction. *N Engl J Med*. 2015;372(1):55–65.
3. Bagshaw SM, Townsend DR, McDermid RC. Disorders of sodium and water balance in hospitalized patients. *Can J Anaesth*. 2009;56(2):151–167.
4. Hannon MJ, Finucane FM, Sherlock M, et al. Clinical review: disorders of water homeostasis in neurosurgical patients. *J Clin Endocrinol Metab*. 2012;97(5):1423–1433.
5. Huang C, Zhang P, Du R, et al. Treatment of acute hypernatremia in severely burned patients using continuous veno-venous hemofiltration with gradient sodium replacement fluid: a report of nine cases. *Intensive Care Med*. 2013;39(8):1495–1496.

 ## SEE ALSO

- Diabetes Insipidus
- Algorithm: Hypernatremia

CODES

ICD10
- P74.21 Hypernatremia of newborn
- E87.0 Hyperosmolality and hypernatremia

CLINICAL PEARLS

- Occurs from water deficit in comparison to total body Na stores
- Common causes include dehydration, DI, impaired access to fluids.
- Avoid rapid correction of chronic hypernatremia to prevent development of cerebral edema (goal rate is 10 mEq/L in 24 hours).
- Monitor serum Na and adjust water repletion to achieve desired rate of correction as available formulas for calculating water deficit and estimating ongoing water losses have limited accuracy.

HYPERPARATHYROIDISM

Juan Perez, DO

BASICS

DESCRIPTION
Excess production of parathyroid hormone (PTH)

- Primary hyperparathyroidism (HPT): intrinsic parathyroid gland dysfunction resulting in excessive secretion of PTH with a lack of response to feedback inhibition by elevated calcium
- Secondary HPT: appropriate increased secretion of PTH in response to hypocalcemia and/or hyperphosphatemia; can be caused by vitamin D deficiency, kidney dysfunction, decreased calcium intake or absorption, and/or phosphate loading
- Tertiary HPT: autonomous hyperfunction of the parathyroid gland in the setting of long-standing secondary HPT

EPIDEMIOLOGY
Prevalence
- Primary HPT is 1 in 500 to 1 in 1,000 in the United States.
- Primary HPT is the etiology for 90% of patients with hypercalcemia.
- Predominantly postmenopausal females

ETIOLOGY AND PATHOPHYSIOLOGY
PTH is synthesized by the four parathyroid glands, which are located behind the thyroid gland, and mostly regulated by calcium levels.

- Ectopic (abnormal locations and most common is the thymus) or supernumerary glands (more than four glands)
- PTH releases calcium from bone by osteoclastic stimulation (increasing bone resorption).
- PTH increases reabsorption of calcium in the distal tubules of the kidneys.
- PTH increases phosphorus excretion by decreasing reabsorption in the proximal tubules of the kidneys.
- PTH stimulates conversion of 25-hydroxycholecalciferol (25[OH]D) to 1,25-dihydroxycholecalciferol (1,25[OH]$_2$D or active vitamin D) in the kidneys. 1,25(OH)$_2$D increases calcium and phosphate absorption from the GI tract and kidneys and stimulates osteoclastic activity and bone resorption.
- Primary HPT: unregulated PTH production and release due to the loss of normal feedback control by extracellular calcium, causing increase in serum calcium
  - Solitary adenoma (80–85%)
  - Diffuse parathyroid gland hyperplasia (10–15%), either sporadically or in association with multiple endocrine neoplasia
  - Parathyroid carcinoma (<1%)
- Secondary HPT: adaptive parathyroid gland hyperplasia and hyperfunction from decreased calcium
  - Dietary from vitamin D deficiency causes decreased calcium absorption or calcium deficiency.
  - Chronic renal disease including renal parenchymal loss causing hyperphosphatemia; impaired calcitriol production causing hypocalcemia
- Tertiary HPT: autonomous oversecretion of PTH following prolonged parathyroid stimulation

Genetics
- A genetic basis of primary HPT is identified in about 10% of all cases.
- Patients with multiple gland hyperplasia in the absence of renal disease should be screened for MEN-I gene mutation.

- Neonatal severe primary HPT: infants born without both calcium sensing receptor (CaSR) gene alleles
- HPT—jaw tumor syndrome
- Familial hypocalciuric hypercalcemia (FHH): loss of one CaSR gene allele

RISK FACTORS
Chronic kidney disease, increasing age, poor nutrition, radiation, and/or family history

GENERAL PREVENTION
Adequate intake of calcium and vitamin D may help prevent secondary HPT.

COMMONLY ASSOCIATED CONDITIONS
- Vitamin D deficiency
- Chronic renal failure
- MEN syndromes: MEN type 1 and MEN type 2A

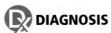

DIAGNOSIS

HISTORY
- History of present illness
  - Almost 80% of patients are asymptomatic.
  - Kidney stones (15–20%)
  - Osteitis fibrosa cystica (<5%) characterized by subperiosteal resorption of phalanges, tapering of distal clavicles, bone cysts, brown tumors of long bones, and "salt and pepper" appearance of the skull
  - Symptoms due to hypercalcemia like mental fogginess, memory impairment, polyuria, polydipsia, constipation, nausea, anorexia, bone pain, decreased concentration, altered mental status, fatigue, and muscle weakness
- Past medical history
  - The following conditions may be associated with HPT:
    o MEN syndrome (MEN type 1 is associated with pituitary adenomas, pancreatic cancers and parathyroid hyperplasia; MEN type 2A is associated with medullary thyroid cancer, pheochromocytoma and parathyroid hyperplasia), nephrolithiasis (in 20–30%), nephrocalcinosis, pancreatitis, gastroduodenal ulcer, hypertension, short QT interval, left ventricular hypertrophy, osteitis fibrosa cystica, cystic bone lesions, spontaneous fracture, vertebral collapse, osteoporosis, gout, pseudogout, anxiety, depression, psychosis, coma, conjunctivitis, band keratopathy, conjunctival calcium deposits
- Medications: hydrochlorothiazide or lithium (decreases parathyroid sensitivity to calcium in small subset of patients)

PHYSICAL EXAM
- Limited usefulness; 70–80% of patients have no obvious symptoms or signs of disease.
- Physical findings related to the underlying cause of HPT may be found.

DIFFERENTIAL DIAGNOSIS
- Increased PTH: Ectopic PTH production is rare. In most of the cases, it establishes the diagnosis of primary HPT, but first rule out:
  - FHH: Rule out FHH with a 24-hour urine calcium: creatinine ratio
  - Drug side effect (thiazide diuretics and lithium)

- Nonparathyroid causes
  - Malignancy: lung (squamous cell) carcinoma, breast carcinoma, multiple myeloma, lymphoma, leukemia, prostate cancer
  - Granulomatous diseases: sarcoidosis, tuberculosis, berylliosis, histoplasmosis, coccidioidomycosis
  - Drugs: vitamin D intoxication, milk-alkali syndrome, thiazide diuretics
  - Endocrine: hyperthyroidism, acute adrenal insufficiency
  - High bone turnover: immobilization, Paget disease

DIAGNOSTIC TESTS & INTERPRETATION
Initial Tests (lab, imaging)
- Often detected by incidental hypercalcemia on routine labs
- Calculate the corrected calcium: [serum calcium in mg/dL + 0.8 × (4 − patient's albumin in g/dL)]. Alternatively, order an ionized calcium level.
- If hypercalcemia is confirmed, follow with intact PTH level (1)[B].
  - PTH-dependent: High or (abnormally) normal PTH suggests primary HPT.
  - PTH-independent: Undetectable or low PTH suggests PTH-independent hypercalcemia.
- Other findings may include low serum phosphate and high 24-hour urine calcium excretion.
- In secondary HPT, an elevated phosphorus suggests chronic renal failure; a low phosphorus suggests another cause, commonly 25(OH)D deficiency. Both are common causes of elevated PTH levels while having normal corrected calcium levels.

Follow-Up Tests & Special Considerations
- A 24-hour urine calcium concentration to creatinine clearance ratio >0.02 suggests primary HPT; a ratio <0.01 may be normal or indicate FHH; an important finding because FHH does not require surgery (1)[C].
- Routine measurement of 25(OH)D levels is recommended in all patients with primary HPT. In case of vitamin D deficiency (<20 ng/mL or <50 nmol/L), defer management decisions until the levels are maintained >20 ng/mL (50 nmol/L) (1)[C].

Diagnostic Procedures/Other
- Imaging is not required for diagnosis. It is required for surgical planning, especially for minimally invasive parathyroidectomy (MIP).
  - Imaging is also indicated to localize hyperplasia or an ectopic parathyroid gland in repeat surgery.
- Imaging options for presurgical localization
  - Technetium-99m sestamibi with or without single-photon emission computed tomography (SPECT): It has the greatest reported success in localizing single parathyroid adenomas but often inaccurate in multigland disease.
  - Neck ultrasound (US): Painless, noninvasive, and does not expose the patient to radiation; however, its accuracy is operator-dependent (2)[C].
  - Four-dimensional CT (4D-CT) may be more effective for primary localization than both US and sestamibi-SPECT (2)[B].
  - Positron emission tomography (PET) using C-methionine (MET-PET) is comparable to US and technetium-99m sestamibi with SPECT in terms of diagnostic use.
  - CT and MRI are mostly used to localize ectopic mediastinal glands.

🩺 TREATMENT

MEDICATION
- Primary HPT: Operative management is curative; indications for surgical intervention are mentioned below. For those awaiting or unable to have surgery:
  - Bisphosphonates (alendronate): reduce bone turnover and help to maintain bone density; avoid in patients with kidney disease (GFR ≤35).
  - Calcimimetics (cinacalcet) (1)[B]: activates CaSR in parathyroid gland thereby inhibiting PTH secretion; FDA-approved for symptomatic patients who are unfit for surgery; no long-term data on its effect on constitutional, neuropsychological symptoms or fractures
  - Selective estrogen receptor modulator therapy (raloxifene): antagonizes PTH-mediated bone resorption
  - Hormone replacement therapy with estrogens is not recommended as first-line treatment; must weigh benefit with risks of known systemic effects
    - Can be used in postmenopausal women who do not undergo or refuse surgery
- Secondary HPT: Treatment is often aimed at underlying etiology:
  - Calcium replacement
  - Vitamin D analogues (paricalcitol and calcitriol)
  - Phosphorus-binding agents (sevelamer)
  - Calcimimetic (cinacalcet)
- Tertiary HPT
  - Medical treatment is not curative and is generally not indicated.

SURGERY/OTHER PROCEDURES
- Operative management is curative for patients with primary HPT in 95–98% of patients. It is the first-line treatment for pediatrics. It is also usually the first-line treatment for young adults up to 50 years of age (3)[C].
- Indications for parathyroidectomy
  - Symptomatic primary HPT
    - Nephrolithiasis
    - Fragility fractures
    - Osteitis fibrosa cystica
  - Asymptomatic primary HPT (1)[C]
    - Serum Ca^+ level >1 mg/dL above normal
    - Age <50 years
    - Creatinine clearance <60 mL/min
    - 24-hour urine for calcium >400 mg/day (>10 mmol/day) and increased stone risk by biochemical stone risk analysis
    - Presence of nephrolithiasis or nephrocalcinosis by x-ray, US, or CT
    - Bone density loss with a T-score <−2.5 at the lumbar spine, femoral neck, total hip, or distal 1/3 radius

- Surgical removal of diseased gland or tissue is the only proven curative therapy for HPT; options include the following:
  - Bilateral open neck exploratory surgery
  - MIP using preoperative sestamibi scan with SPECT/US/4D-CT and intraoperative PTH levels (high sensitivity 79–95% to predict location of single parathyroid adenoma) (4), which result in decreased pain, smaller incisions, improved cosmetic results, lower morbidity, and decreased length of hospital stay when compared with open neck exploratory surgery
- Follow postoperative serum calcium, magnesium, and phosphorus levels; monitor closely for hypocalcemia "hungry bone" syndrome.
- Patients may need IV calcium infusion postoperatively with oral calcitriol and calcium supplementation initially. Hungry pain syndrome can be severe, although less common now.
- Patients are also at risk for bleeding and airway compromise.
- Monitor renal function closely.

ADMISSION, INPATIENT, AND NURSING CONSIDERATIONS
Critical hypercalcemia requires IV fluid rehydration, saline diuresis with IV saline and loop diuretics, IV bisphosphonate therapy, SC calcitonin (4 U/kg q12h), corticosteroids, and hemodialysis (5) for severe symptoms.

⚕️ ONGOING CARE

FOLLOW-UP RECOMMENDATIONS
Asymptomatic patients with primary HPT require serial monitoring of calcium and PTH.

Patient Monitoring
In patients with primary HPT who are asymptomatic, measurement of serum calcium and creatinine annually and bone density scan every 1 to 2 years is sufficient (1)[C].

DIET
- In the presence of hypercalciuria or elevated $1,25(OH)_2D$ levels, dietary calcium restriction is recommended. Otherwise, daily calcium intake should be maintained at up to 1,000 mg.
- Restrict dietary phosphate in secondary HPT.

PATIENT EDUCATION
- Importance of periodic lab testing
- Signs of severe hypercalcemia

PROGNOSIS
Prognosis after surgery is excellent in primary HPT, with resolution of many of the preoperative symptoms.

COMPLICATIONS
Related to high levels of PTH and/or elevated calcium

REFERENCES
1. Bilezikian JP, Brandi ML, Eastell R, et al. Guidelines for the management of asymptomatic primary hyperparathyroidism: summary statement from the Fourth International Workshop. *J Clin Endocrinol Metab*. 2014;99(10):3561–3569.
2. Cheung K, Wang TS, Farrokhyar F, et al. A meta-analysis of preoperative localization techniques for patients with primary hyperparathyroidism. *Ann Surg Oncol*. 2012;19(2):577–583.
3. Markowitz ME, Underland L, Gensure R. Parathyroid disorders. *Pediatr Rev*. 2016;37(12):524–535.
4. Kunstman JW, Kirsch JD, Mahajan A, et al. Clinical review: parathyroid localization and implications for clinical management. *J Clin Endocrinol Metab*. 2013;98(3):902–912.
5. Kulkarni P, Tucker J. Symptomatic versus asymptomatic primary hyperparathyroidism: a systematic review. *J Clin Transl Endocrinol*. 2023;32:100317.

ADDITIONAL READING
- Bilezikian JP. Primary hyperparathyroidism. *J Clin Endocrinol Metab*. 2018;103(11):3993–4004.
- Salvatore M, Arnold A, Belaya Z, et al. Epidemiology, pathophysiology, and genetics of primary hyperparathyroidism. *J Bone Miner Res*. 2022;37(11):2315–2329.

🔢 CODES

ICD10
- E21.3 Hyperparathyroidism, unspecified
- N25.81 Secondary hyperparathyroidism of renal origin
- E21.1 Secondary hyperparathyroidism, not elsewhere classified

CLINICAL PEARLS
- 80% of patients with primary HPT are asymptomatic.
- HPT is often detected by an incidental finding of hypercalcemia on a routine serum chemistry analysis.
- Classic symptoms of HPT include painful bones, renal stones, abdominal pain, and behavioral changes (stones, bones, moans, and groans).
- Repeat calcium (elevated), correct for serum albumin, and obtain intact PTH levels to make an initial diagnosis.
- Secondary HPT is due to excessive secretion of PTH in response to hypocalcemia, which can be caused by vitamin D deficiency or renal failure.
- In patients with primary HPT who are asymptomatic, measurement of serum calcium and creatinine annually and bone density scan every 1 to 2 years is sufficient.

H

HYPERPROLACTINEMIA

William E. Somerall Jr., MD, MAEd • D'Ann Wilson Somerall, FAANP, FNP-BC, DNP, CRNP, MAEd • Robert A. Baldor, MD, FAAFP

 BASICS

DESCRIPTION
Hyperprolactinemia is an abnormal elevation in the serum prolactin (PRL) level from either physiologic or pathologic influences of the lactotroph cells of the pituitary gland.

EPIDEMIOLOGY
Prevalence
- Predominant age: reproductive age
- Predominant sex: female (70%) > male (30%)
- More readily detected in females because a slight elevation in PRL causes changes in menstruation and galactorrhea; men present with headache, visual disturbances, and erectile dysfunction (1)
- Adenomas in men are typically larger because of delayed onset of symptoms (1).

ETIOLOGY AND PATHOPHYSIOLOGY
- PRL, which is produced by lactotrophs in the anterior pituitary, is regulated by:
  - Inhibitory factors, primarily dopamine, are produced in the hypothalamus and delivered via the hypothalamic-pituitary vessels in the pituitary stalk.
  - Stimulatory factors, primarily thyrotropin-releasing hormone (TRH)
- Causes of hyperprolactinemia include the following:
  - Physiologic
    ○ Pregnancy due to increased estrogen
    ○ Breastfeeding or nipple stimulation
    ○ Stress, including postoperative state
    ○ Medications: Concentrations are typically in the 25 to 100 ng/mL range (2)[A].
      ■ Dopamine (D_2) blockers: prochlorperazine, metoclopramide
      ■ Dopamine depleters: α-methyldopa, reserpine
      ■ Antidepressants: tricyclic antidepressants (TCAs); paroxetine (an SSRI) causes transient hyperprolactinemia—usually resolves in 7 to 10 days
      ■ Gastric motility drugs: metoclopramide and domperidone
      ■ Verapamil (but no other calcium channel blockers; thought to decrease the hypothalamic synthesis of dopamine)
      ■ Older antipsychotics (category is the most common cause of medication induced): haloperidol, fluphenazine, risperidone (level of elevation with risperidone greater than with other antipsychotics)
      ■ Newer antipsychotics (asenapine, iloperidone, lurasidone) may cause elevation but less than the older antipsychotics (1).
  - Pathologic
    ○ Hypothyroidism (due to elevated TRH)
    ○ Chest wall conditions such as herpes zoster, trauma, or postthoracotomy

    ○ PRL-secreting adenoma in the anterior pituitary (microadenoma: <1 cm; macroadenoma: >1 cm)
    ○ Pituitary stalk compression/disruption:
      ■ Craniopharyngioma, Rathke cleft cyst
      ■ Meningioma, astrocytoma
      ■ Metastases
      ■ Head trauma
      ■ Infiltrative/inflammatory disorders
    ○ Diminished PRL clearance (chronic renal failure, cirrhosis, cocaine)
  - Idiopathic hyperprolactinemia—a substantial number of cases where the serum levels are between 20 and 100 ng/mL the cause cannot be found (3)[A]

Genetics
Unknown

RISK FACTORS
See causes in "Etiology and Pathophysiology" section.

GENERAL PREVENTION
Avoid offending medications.

COMMONLY ASSOCIATED CONDITIONS
- Infertility
- Osteoporosis
- Amenorrhea
- Gynecomastia

 DIAGNOSIS

Based on clinical history, physical exam, and laboratory findings; symptoms listed below are typically found in premenopausal women. Postmenopausal women are typically diagnosed due to headaches or impaired vision where an incidental finding of a lactotroph adenoma via MRI.

HISTORY
- Galactorrhea
- Amenorrhea or oligomenorrhea
- Infertility
- Osteoporosis/osteopenia
- Decreased libido, impotence
- Weight gain
- Pregnancy
- Chronic kidney disease
- Also, may have signs and symptoms of pituitary enlargement:
  - Headache
  - Visual field impairment (bitemporal hemianopia)
  - Hypopituitarism (secondary to tumor pressure on surrounding structures)
- Also, may have signs and symptoms of associated conditions:
  - Hypothyroidism
  - Cushing disease
  - Acromegaly
  - Multiple endocrine neoplasia (MEN)-1 syndrome

PHYSICAL EXAM
- Visual field testing (bitemporal field loss)
- Cranial nerve exam
- Examination of chest wall for lesions
- Signs of hypothyroidism

DIFFERENTIAL DIAGNOSIS
Macroprolactinemia: Macroprolactin, a polymer of several units of PRL, is detected by immunologically based lab tests but is not biologically active. If the patient is asymptomatic but found to have elevated PRL, consider this diagnosis and notify the lab. No treatment is required.

DIAGNOSTIC TESTS & INTERPRETATION
- Serum PRL (most accurate results if checked fasting, in morning; food only has a small effect on concentrations, thus fasting is not required, but if elevated levels repeat on a fasting specimen) <25 μg/L normal; >25 μg/L abnormal; >30 in postmenopausal women; >250 μg/L often indicates a prolactinoma (4)[A].
- Pregnancy test
- Thyroid-stimulating hormone (TSH)
- Luteinizing hormone (LH)/follicle-stimulating hormone (FSH) if amenorrheic
- Chem panel

Initial Tests (lab, imaging)
A single measurement of serum PRL (levels drawn prior to a breast exam)—a level above the upper limit of normal confirms the diagnosis.
- Pituitary MRI: single-best imaging

Follow-Up Tests & Special Considerations
Formal visual field testing if pituitary adenoma is suspected

Diagnostic Procedures/Other
CT scan if MRI is contraindicated

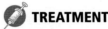 TREATMENT

GENERAL MEASURES
- Discontinue offending medications, if any (4)[A].
- Treat underlying causes (4)[A].
- For asymptomatic patients with mild PRL elevations, observation alone may be considered (4)[A],(5)[A].
- Medications indicated for (4)[A]:
  - Symptoms of hypogonadism, such as decreased libido
  - Galactorrhea (if bothersome to patient)
  - Restoration of fertility
  - Pituitary adenoma
  - Prevention of osteoporosis

MEDICATION

First Line

- Dopamine agonists: decrease serum PRL concentrations and decrease the size of the most lactotroph adenomas
- Cabergoline (Dostinex): This is now the first-line choice due to efficacy and favorable side effect profile (4)[A],(6)[A]: dosed 0.25 mg twice weekly or 0.50 once a week. Although more expensive, cabergoline was more effective than bromocriptine in reducing persistent hyperprolactinemia, galactorrhea, and amenorrhea/oligomenorrhea (5)[A]; has recently been reported to be associated with significant improvements in the body mass index, total HDL and LDL cholesterol levels, and insulin sensitivity (7); decrease in proinflammatory markers; and carotid intima-media thickness, indicated with bromocriptine failure or resistance; has been shown to reduce erectile dysfunction in hyperprolactinemic men (4)[A]
  - Adverse effects (better tolerated if start with low dose, slow titration, given at night with food):
    - Nausea/vomiting
    - Headache, dizziness, fatigue
    - Postural hypotension (5)[A]
  - Contraindications
    - Uncontrolled hypertension
    - Cardiac valvular disorders
    - Pulmonary, pericardial, or retroperitoneal fibrotic disorders
- Bromocriptine (Parlodel): This has the longest clinical history: dosed BID; begin at 1.25 mg once at bedtime or after dinner for 1 week and then increase to BID; preferred by some clinicians when infertility is an indication for treatment (2)[A],(5)[A]
- Both are effective for reducing tumor size and improving symptoms (5)[A].
- SE less with cabergoline than bromocriptine (5)[A]

Second Line

Pergolide (Permax) is no longer used in the United States. If patient is still on this medication, do not withdraw abruptly.

ADDITIONAL THERAPIES

Patients with medically and surgically refractory prolactinomas; radiotherapy produced a reduction in PRL levels in nearly all patients and normalization in over a quarter of patients with low complication rates (5)[A].

SURGERY/OTHER PROCEDURES

- For adenomas, medical treatment will be successful in 80–90% of patients. In some cases, surgery is indicated (4):
  - Intolerance or resistance to medical treatment
  - Headache
  - Visual field loss
  - CSF leak due to tumor apoplexy or shrinkage
  - Cranial nerve deficit
- Risks include a high recurrence rate (up to 40%), CSF leakage, meningitis, pituitary insufficiency, and transient diabetes insipidus (6).

 ONGOING CARE

FOLLOW-UP RECOMMENDATIONS

Reevaluate lab levels after 1 month; if normal, continue the initial dose. If lab levels do not decrease but patient experiences no side effects, increase cabergoline to 1.25 mg 2 to 3 times/week or bromocriptine to 5 mg twice a day.

Patient Monitoring

- After at least 2 years of treatment, no tumor, and PRL levels normal may consider decreasing and stopping medication; must be followed closely, as the tumor may grow back (4)
- Consider:
  - Formal visual field testing yearly (2)[A]
  - Serial MRIs if clinically indicated (2)[A]

Pregnancy Considerations

- If pregnancy is desired in a woman with hyperprolactinemia, dopamine agonists are not approved during pregnancy and should be discontinued once pregnancy is confirmed, but their use is recommended if neurologic findings are present (4)[A].
- With microprolactinoma: Treat with bromocriptine if symptomatic; monthly pregnancy tests; discontinue bromocriptine when pregnancy is confirmed.
- With macroprolactinomas: A definitive, individualized plan is made. Options include discontinuation of bromocriptine at conception and careful monitoring of PRL levels and VS, with or without MRI scan evidence of tumor enlargement; prepregnancy transsphenoidal surgery with debulking of tumor; continuation of bromocriptine throughout gestation, with a risk to the fetus.
- Careful monitoring of visual fields in each trimester; no need to monitor PRL levels, as they are normally high due to pregnancy (4)[A]

PATIENT EDUCATION

Discuss risks of untreated hyperprolactinemia:

- Headache
- Visual field loss
- Decreased bone density
- Infertility

PROGNOSIS

- Following treatment for 1 to 2 years, if PRL levels have remained normal, consider stopping meds.
- 5–10% of macroadenomas may progress to macroadenomas.
- Follow-up imaging not needed unless signs or symptoms of enlarging tumor
- >10 years, 7% chance of progression of prolactin-secreting microadenoma (2)

COMPLICATIONS

- If pituitary adenoma, risk of permanent visual field loss
- For patients with high doses of cabergoline, suggest cardiac US every 2 years.

REFERENCES

1. Somerall WE Jr, Somerall DW. Hyperprolactinemia: the ABCs of diagnosis and management. *Women's Healthcare*. 2020;8(6):6–12.
2. Casanueva FF, Molitch ME, Schlechte JA, et al. Guidelines of the Pituitary Society for the diagnosis and management of prolactinomas. *Clin Endocrinol (Oxf)*. 2006;65(2):265–273.
3. Inder WJ, Castle D. Antipsychotic-induced hyperprolactinaemia. *Aust N Z J Psychiatry*. 2011;45(10):830–837.
4. Hoffman AR, Melmed S, Schlechte J. Patient guide to hyperprolactinaemia diagnosis and treatment. *J Clin Endocrinol Metab*. 2011;96(2):35A–36A.
5. Wang AT, Mullan RJ, Lane MA, et al. Treatment of hyperprolactinemia: a systematic review and meta-analysis. *Syst Rev*. 2012;1:33.
6. Bloomgarden E, Molitch ME. Surgical treatment of prolactinomas: cons. *Endocrine*. 2014;47(3):730–733.
7. Inancli SS, Usluogullari A, Ustu Y, et al. Effect of cabergoline on insulin sensitivity, inflammation, and carotid intima media thickness in patients with prolactinoma. *Endocrine*. 2013;44(1):193–199.

ADDITIONAL READING

Klibanski A. Clinical practice. Prolactinomas. *N Engl J Med*. 2010;362(13):1219–1226.

 CODES

ICD10

E22.1 Hyperprolactinemia

CLINICAL PEARLS

- If a cause for hyperprolactinemia cannot be found by history, examination, and routine laboratory testing (>250 μg/L often indicates a prolactinoma), an intracranial lesion might be the cause and brain MRI with specific pituitary cuts and intravenous contrast media should be performed.
- Treatment of hyperprolactinemia should be targeted at correcting the cause (hypothyroidism, discontinuation of offending medications, etc.).
- There is a difference among antipsychotics in influencing PRL levels. In general, those with the highest potency D_2 antagonism are most likely to elevate PRL levels. Among the newer atypical antipsychotics, risperidone has been identified as more likely to elevate PRL.
- High PRL levels decrease testosterone by inhibiting gonadotropin-releasing hormone (GnRH), LH, and FSH secretion and by decreasing central dopamine activity, both of which are important in mediating sexual arousal.

H

HYPERSENSITIVITY PNEUMONITIS

Han Q. Bui, MD, MPH

 BASICS

DESCRIPTION

- Hypersensitivity pneumonitis (HP) is also called extrinsic allergic alveolitis (EAA).
- HP is a diffuse inflammatory disease of the lung parenchyma caused by an immunologic reaction to aerosolized antigenic particles found in a variety of environments. Classification depends on time frame involved:
  - Acute: fever, chills, diaphoresis, myalgias, nausea; cough and dyspnea common but not necessarily present; occurs 4 to 12 hours after heavy exposure to an inciting agent. Symptoms subside within 12 hours to several days after removal from exposure. Complete resolution occurs within weeks.
  - Subacute: mainly caused by continual low-level antigen exposure, could have a low-grade fever in 1st week; cough, dyspnea, fatigue, anorexia, weight loss—develops over days to weeks
  - Chronic: from recurrent exposure either acute or subacute cases; prolonged and progressive cough, dyspnea, fatigue, weight loss; could lead to fibrosis and respiratory failure
- Farmer's lung is an old term of this disease, a type of HP, particular to the farmer population; causative agent is a bacterium found in moldy hay or straw. Farmer's lung now has new and different etiologies due to modernization of farming practices.

EPIDEMIOLOGY

- Not well defined; tends to occur in adults as a result of occupation-related exposure, but some home environmental exposures are also seen
- HP is increasingly recognized as an important cause of fibrotic interstitial lung disease (1).

Incidence

0.9/100,000

Prevalence

- Farmers: 1–19% exposed farmers
- Bird fanciers: 6–20% exposed individuals
- Others: 1–8% exposed

ETIOLOGY AND PATHOPHYSIOLOGY

- Hypersensitivity reaction involving immune complexes: Inhaled antigens bind to IgG, triggering complement cascade (types III and IV immunologic reactions) (1).
- Cellular-mediated reaction: T cell–mediated immune inflammatory response
- Farming, vegetable, or dairy cattle workers
  - Moldy hay, grain, silage: thermophilic actinomycetes, such as *Faenia rectivirgula*
  - Mold on pressed sugar cane: *Thermoactinomyces sacchari, Thymus vulgaris*
  - Tobacco plants: *Aspergillus* sp., *Scopulariopsis brevicaulis*
  - Mushroom worker's lung: *Saccharopolyspora rectivirgula, T. vulgaris, Aspergillus* spp.
  - Potato riddler's lung: thermophilic actinomycetes, *T. vulgaris, F. rectivirgula, Aspergillus* sp.
  - Wine maker's lung: *Mucor stolonifer*
  - Cheese washer's lung: *Penicillium caseifulvum, Aspergillus clavatus*
  - Coffee worker's lung: coffee bean dust
  - Tea grower's lung: tea plants

- Ventilation and water-related contamination
  - Contaminated humidifiers and air conditioners: amoebae, nematodes, yeasts, bacteria
  - Unventilated shower: *Epicoccum nigrum*
  - Hot-tub lung: *Cladosporium* sp., *Mycobacterium avium complex*
  - Sauna taker's lung: *Aureobasidium* sp.
  - Summer-type pneumonitis: *Trichosporon cutaneum*
  - Swimming pool lifeguard's lung: aerosolized endotoxin and *M. avium complex*
  - Contaminated basement pneumonitis: *Cephalosporium* and *Penicillium* spp.
- Bird and poultry handling
  - Bird fancier's lung: droppings, feathers, serum proteins
  - Poultry worker's lung: serum proteins
  - Turkey-handling disease: serum proteins
  - Canary fancier's lung: serum proteins
  - Duck fever: feathers, serum proteins
- Veterinary work and animal handling
  - Laboratory worker's lung: urine, serum, pelts, proteins
  - Pituitary snuff taker's disease: dried, powdered neurohypophysis
  - Furrier's lung: animal pelts
  - Bat lung: bat serum protein
  - Fish meal worker's lung: fish meal
  - Coptic lung: cloth wrapping of mummies
  - Mollusc shell HP: sea snail shell
  - Pearl oyster shell pneumonitis: oyster shells
- Grain and flour
  - Grain measurer's lung: cereal grain, grain dust
  - Miller's lung: *Sitophilus granarius*
  - Malt worker's disease: *Aspergillus fumigatus, A. clavatus*
- Lumber milling, construction, wood stripping, paper, wallboard manufacture
  - Wood dust pneumonitis: *Alternaria* sp., *Bacillus subtilis*
  - Sequoiosis: *Graphium, Pullularia, Trichoderma* sp., *Aureobasidium pullulans*
  - Maple bark disease: *Cryptostroma corticale*
  - Wood trimmer's disease: *Rhizopus* sp., *Mucor* sp.
  - Wood pulp worker's disease: *Penicillium* sp.
  - Suberosis: *Trogon viridis, Penicillium glabrum*
- Plastic manufacturing, painting, electronics, chemicals
  - Chemical HP: diphenyl diisocyanate, toluene diisocyanate
  - Detergent worker's lung: *B. subtilis* enzymes
  - Pauli reagent alveolitis: sodium diazobenzene sulfate
  - Vineyard sprayer's lung: copper sulfate
  - Pyrethrum pneumonitis: *pyrethroids*
  - Epoxy resin lung: phthalic anhydride
  - Bible printer's lung: moldy typesetting water
  - Machine operator's lung: *Pseudomonas fluorescens*, aerosolized metal working fluid
- Textile workers
  - Byssinosis: cotton mill dust
  - Velvet worker's lung: nylon, tannic acid, potato starch
  - Upholstery fabric: aflatoxin-producing fungus, *Fusarium* sp.
  - Lycoperdonosis: puffball spores

Genetics

No evidence of clear genetic susceptibility; possible genetic predisposition involving tumor necrosis factor alpha (TNF-α) and major histocompatibility complex (MHC) class II genes (1)[B]

RISK FACTORS

- Contact with organic antigens increases risk of developing HP. Viral infection at time of exposure may increase risk.
- Nonsmokers have an increased incidence of HP compared with smokers. The mechanisms that account for the "protective" effect of smoking are poorly understood, but nicotine is thought to inhibit macrophage activation and lymphocyte proliferation and function (1).
  - Smokers have a diminished antibody response to inhaled antigens.
  - However, smokers who develop disease tend to have the chronic form, and mortality is higher.

GENERAL PREVENTION

Avoidance of offending antigen and/or use of protective equipment

COMMONLY ASSOCIATED CONDITIONS

Constrictive bronchiolitis

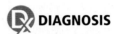 **DIAGNOSIS**

- Diagnosis criteria most widely used but not validated: (i) history and physical and pulmonary function tests (PFTs) indicating restriction or diffusion disease. DL$_{co}$ is the most frequently affected lung parameter but may be normal in up to 22% of patients, (ii) radiologic imaging consent with interstitial lung disease, (iii) exposure to a recognized cause, (iv) proof of sensitization in bronchoalveolar lavage (BAL) fluids (serum precipitins and/or lymphocytosis)
- Six significant predictors: exposure to a known antigen, positive antibodies precipitating, (if identified) recurrent episodes of symptoms, inspiratory crackles, symptoms 4 to 8 hours after exposure, weight loss (1)
- Acute form: develops 4 to 12 hours following exposure. Cough, dyspnea without wheezing, fever, chills, diaphoresis, headache, nausea, malaise, chest tightness. Symptoms last hours to days.
- Sequela (prior subacute, chronic): gradual or progressive productive cough, dyspnea, fatigue, anorexia, weight loss can lead to respiratory failure; develops over days, weeks to months
- Symptomatic improvement when away from work or home

PHYSICAL EXAM

- Acute: fever, tachypnea, diffuse fine rales
- Sequela or chronic: inspiratory crackles, progressive hypoxia, weight loss, diffuse rales, clubbing, rarely wheezing

DIFFERENTIAL DIAGNOSIS

- Acute: acute infectious pneumonia: influenza (or other viral pneumonia), mycoplasma, *Pneumocystis jiroveci* pneumonia, asthma, aspiration
- Chronic: sarcoidosis, chronic bronchitis, chronic obstructive pulmonary disease, tuberculosis, collagen vascular disease, idiopathic pulmonary fibrosis, lymphoma, fungal infections, *P. jiroveci* pneumonia

DIAGNOSTIC TESTS & INTERPRETATION

- Testing for positive precipitating antibodies is NOT diagnostic because up to 40% may have positive antibody without disease; antigens that cover most cases: pigeon and parakeet sera, dove feather, *Aspergillus* sp., *Penicillium*, *S. rectivirgula*, and *Thalassomonas viridans*
- PFTs: Typical profile is a restrictive pattern with low diffusing capacity; could also have an obstructive pattern
- BAL with serum precipitins and lymphocytosis (>50%) and a relative predominance of CD8—low CD4-to-CD8 ratio; findings not unique to HP
- Positive antigen–specific inhalation challenge testing: reexposure to the environment, inhalation challenge to the suspected antigen in a hospital setting, but it lacks standardization (1)
- Chest x-ray (CXR): used to rule out other diseases
  - Acute: ground-glass infiltrates, nodular or striated patchy opacities, interstitial pattern in a variety of distributions in lung field. Up to 20% could be normal.
  - Sequela/chronic: upper lobe fibrosis, nodular or ground-glass opacities, volume loss, emphysematous changes
- CT scan of chest; patterns not specific to HP:
  - Acute: ground-glass opacities, poorly defined centrilobular nodules, and ground-glass opacities and air trapping on expiratory images (1),(2)
  - Chronic: fibrosis, ground-glass attenuation, irregular opacities, bronchiectasis, loss of lung volume, honeycombing, emphysematous changes (1),(2)
- High-resolution CT (HRCT) mid-to-upper zone predominance of centrilobular ground glass or nodular opacities with signs of air trapping (1)
- Usually start with CXR; may progress to HRCT based on findings (1)

Diagnostic Procedures/Other

Lung biopsy:
- Transbronchial: reveals small, poorly formed non-caseating granulomas near respiratory or terminal bronchioles, large foam cells, peribronchial fibrosis
- Open lung biopsy: highest yield in advanced disease; reveals varying patterns of organizing pneumonia, centrilobular and perilobular fibrosis, multinucleated giant cells with clefts

ALERT

HP in farmers must be distinguished from febrile, toxic reactions to inhaled dusts (organic dust toxic syndrome [ODTS]). Nonimmunologic reactions occur 30–50% more commonly than HP in farmers. ODTS is associated with intense exposure occurring on a single day.

 ## TREATMENT

GENERAL MEASURES

- Outpatient, except for acute pneumonitis cases and admission for workup (BAL, lung biopsy)
- Every effort should be made to remove the patient completely from repeated exposure to the causative antigen. This action offers the best outcome of disease.

MEDICATION

First Line

- Avoidance of offending antigen is primary therapy and results in disease regression (1).
- Corticosteroids: help control the symptoms of exacerbations but do not improve long-term outcomes
  - Prednisone: 20 to 50 mg daily (1)
  - For severe symptomatic patients, initial course of 1 to 2 weeks with taper (1)

Second Line

- Bronchodilators and inhaled corticosteroids may symptomatically improve patients with wheeze and chest tightness.
- Oxygen may be needed in advanced cases.
- Lung transplantation may be the last resort in severe cases unresponsive to therapy.

ISSUES FOR REFERRAL

Referral to pulmonologist/immunologist

ADMISSION, INPATIENT, AND NURSING CONSIDERATIONS

Supportive management, as needed, to maintain oxygenation and ventilation:
- Unstable ventilation, oxygen requirement, mental status changes
- Need for invasive evaluation (lung biopsy)

 ## ONGOING CARE

FOLLOW-UP RECOMMENDATIONS

Patient Monitoring

- Initial follow-up should be weekly to monthly, depending on severity and course.
- Follow treatments with serial CXR, PFTs, and circulating antibody levels.

DIET

No dietary restrictions

PATIENT EDUCATION

Note that chronic exposure may lead to a loss of acute symptoms with exposure (i.e., the patient may lose awareness of exposure–symptom relationship).

PROGNOSIS

- Presence of fibrosis is a poor prognosis factor (1).
- Acute: good prognosis with reversal of pathologic findings if elimination of offending antigen early in disease
- Sequela/chronic: Corticosteroids have been found to improve lung function acutely but offer no significant difference in long-term outcome (1)[C].

COMPLICATIONS

- Progressive interstitial fibrosis with eventual respiratory failure
- Cor pulmonale and right-sided heart failure

REFERENCES

1. Spagnolo P, Rossi G, Cavazza A, et al. Hypersensitivity pneumonitis: a comprehensive review. *J Investig Allergol Clin Immunol*. 2015;25(4):237–250.
2. D'souza RS, Donato A. Hypersensitivity pneumonitis: an overlooked cause of cough and dyspnea. *J Community Hosp Intern Med Perspect*. 2017;7(2):95–99.

 ## CODES

ICD10

- J67.9 Hypersensitivity pneumonitis due to unspecified organic dust
- J67.0 Farmer's lung
- J67.2 Bird fancier's lung

CLINICAL PEARLS

- Skin testing is not useful for the diagnosis of HP.
- Diagnosis should be suspected in every patient with unexplained cough and dyspnea on exertion, functional impairment (restriction or diffusion defect), and unclear fever, especially if exposure to potential antigens is known (workplace, domestic bird keeping, moldy walls in the home).
- HP may mimic viral upper respiratory illness or asthma exacerbation. Misdiagnosis has critical therapeutic and prognostic implications because it may delay proper treatment, resulting in significant morbidity, unnecessary hospitalizations, and irreversible fibrosis to the lungs (1).
- Once the disease is established, smoking does not appear to attenuate its severity, and it may predispose to more chronic and severe course.
- Use of protective gear on individual with high-risk exposure occupations can prevent HP.
- Chronic HP is increasingly recognized as an important mimic of other fibrotic lung diseases (1).

H

HYPERTENSION, ESSENTIAL

Ronald N. Adler, MD, FAAFP • Leigh Weatherly, DO • Mukti Kulkarni, MD, MPH

BASICS

DESCRIPTION

- Primary hypertension (HTN) is HTN without an identifiable cause; also known as essential HTN. An importance risk factor for CV disease and other morbidity and mortality, there is persistent controversy regarding recommended thresholds for diagnosis and treatment.
- HTN is defined (Joint National Committee [JNC] 8 and the International Society of Hypertension) as (all pressures in mm Hg) (1):
  - Age <60 years: systolic BP (SBP) ≥140 and/or diastolic BP (DBP) ≥90 at ≥2 visits
  - Age ≥60 years: SBP ≥150 and/or DBP ≥90 at ≥2 visits
  - With diabetes or chronic kidney disease (CKD): SBP ≥140 and/or DBP ≥90
  - The American College of Cardiology (ACC)/American Heart Association (AHA) designates SBP ≥130 and/or DBP ≥80 as "stage 1 hypertension" which should be treated with exercise and lifestyle modification, reserving medication for patients at "higher risk" (defined as age ≥65 years, CKD, diabetes, or known cardiovascular disease [CVD]).

Geriatric Considerations
Isolated systolic HTN is common. Therapy is effective at preventing stroke, CV morbidity and all-cause mortality (2)[A]. Target SBP for seniors is higher than in younger patients (~150 mm Hg systolic), and adverse reactions to medications are more frequent, especially in those who are very old. The benefit of therapy has been conclusively demonstrated in older patients for SBP ≥160. The strongest evidence of benefit has been shown with use of thiazide diuretics.

Pediatric Considerations
Defined as SBP or DBP ≥95th percentile on repeated measurements; measure BP during routine exams beginning at age 3 years; pre-HTN: SBP or DBP between 90th and 95th percentile

Pregnancy Considerations
Elevated BP during pregnancy may represent chronic HTN, pregnancy-induced HTN, or preeclampsia. Preferred agents: labetalol, nifedipine, methyldopa, or hydralazine with angiotensin-converting enzyme inhibitors (ACEI) and angiotensin II receptor blockers (ARBs) being contraindicated. Maternal and fetal mortality are reduced with treatment of severe HTN (see "Preeclampsia and Eclampsia [Toxemia of Pregnancy]").

EPIDEMIOLOGY

Prevalence
32–46% of adults in the United States have HTN; incidence and prevalence higher in men

ETIOLOGY AND PATHOPHYSIOLOGY
>90% of cases of HTN have no identified cause. For differential diagnosis and causes of secondary HTN, see "Hypertension, Secondary and Resistant."

RISK FACTORS
Family history, obesity, alcohol use, excess dietary sodium, stress, physical inactivity, tobacco use, insulin resistance, obstructive sleep apnea (OSA) and other causes of sleep disruption

DIAGNOSIS

- Despite more aggressive guidelines issued by the ACC/AHA in 2017, many experts consider recommendations from JNC 8 (1) to retain primacy.
- Critics of the ACC/AHA guidelines note multiple methodologic concerns. Thresholds of <130/80 (as endorsed by ACC/AHA) compared to JNC 8 would result in the diagnosis of and treatment for HTN of millions more people, with unclear benefits and some inevitable harms.
- This chapter uses JNC 8 as its basis, but recommendations are relevant regardless of the specific guideline being applied. We recommend assessment of overall CV risk and joint decision-making.

HISTORY
HTN is asymptomatic except in extreme cases or after related cardiovascular complications develop. Headache can be seen with higher BP, often present on awakening and occipital in location.

PHYSICAL EXAM
- Weight assessment, waist circumference; measure BP in both arms (correct technique is essential to accurate diagnosis and treatment). Incorrect BP determination is a common cause of overdiagnosis.
- Complete cardiac and peripheral pulse exam: Compare radial and femoral pulse for differences in volume and timing (evaluation for aortic coarctation [especially in young people], subclavian stenosis). Funduscopic exam for arteriolar narrowing, AV compression, hemorrhages, exudates, and papilledema

DIFFERENTIAL DIAGNOSIS
- Secondary HTN: Consider workup only if the history, physical exam, or basic laboratory evaluation suggest a higher likelihood. Also consider for patients who prove nonresponsive to treatment (see "Hypertension, Secondary and Resistant").
- White coat HTN: elevation of BP in office setting and normal BP outside office

DIAGNOSTIC TESTS & INTERPRETATION

ALERT
- Measuring BP: Caffeine, exercise, and smoking should be avoided >30 minutes before measurement. Patient should be seated with back supported quietly for at least 5 minutes with feet on floor and patient's arm supported at heart level. Use correct cuff size. Deflate cuff slowly or use an automated device. Average two or more measurements. May leave patient alone to obtain in-office readings using an automated or patient-activated cuff.
- 2021 United States Preventive Services Taskforce (USPSTF) statement (3)[A]: A diagnosis of HTN should be confirmed with BP measurements outside the clinical setting. Home BP measurements (HBPM) correlate better with CV outcomes than office values and also help to mitigate the errors of clinic measurement. Home BP measurement for diagnosis and for monitoring should be encouraged. For HBPM results, ≥135/85 should be used as a diagnostic threshold, and <135/85 should be the treatment target.
- Ambulatory BP monitoring (ABPM) is the ideal method, but this is not widely available in the United States.

Initial Tests (lab, imaging)
- Hemoglobin or hematocrit or complete blood count; potassium, calcium, creatinine (Cr); urinalysis; lipids; fasting glucose or hemoglobin A1c
- Calculate 10-year ASCVD risk. Consider possibility of sleep apnea particularly in patients with excess weight (2).
- ECG to evaluate possible presence of left ventricular hypertrophy (LVH) or rhythm abnormalities

Follow-Up Tests & Special Considerations
- ABPM or HBPM if "white coat" or masked HTN is suspected, episodic HTN, or autonomic dysfunction; ambulatory measurement may be especially helpful if there is suspected autonomic dysfunction.
- Perform CV risk assessment. The AHA/ACC risk tool overestimates risk (by ≥50%, especially in older patients). A definition of "low risk" excludes patients with a history of CVD, diabetes mellitus, CKD, and familial hypercholesterolemia or familial premature coronary artery disease.

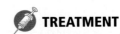

TREATMENT

GENERAL MEASURES
- The treatment discussed follows JNC 8 guidelines. Recent systematic reviews and meta-analyses of randomized trials do not support recommendations for lower-than-standard targets for the average-risk population. Weigh potential harms of therapy against potential benefits, ideally through shared decision-making.
- Treatment goals:
  - Age <60 years: SBP <140 and DBP <90 (for HBPM <135/85)
  - Age ≥60 years: SBP <150 and DBP <90 (for HBPM <140/90)
  - Age ≥60 years with CKD or diabetes: SBP <140 and DBP <90 (for HBPM <135/85)
  - More aggressive treatment may be considered in high-risk patients meeting enrollment criteria for SPRINT because aggressive treatment shows improvement in outcomes, but 61 nondiabetic patients would need to be treated (NNT) for 3 years to a goal SBP of <120 mm Hg to prevent one major cardiovascular outcome, and NNT is 90 over 3 years to prevent one death.
  - Even in secondary prevention, no firm conclusions can yet be drawn regarding the comparative effectiveness of intensive versus standard therapy.
  - Individual treatment goals should be jointly established with patients after discussion of the anticipated potential benefits and harms (shared decision-making) (2).
- Treatment considerations:
  - Review current medications and supplements for potential contributors to HTN.
  - Recommend lifestyle improvements, including diet, exercise, and reducing or eliminating tobacco/alcohol.
  - Benefit of pharmacologic treatment of low-risk patients with class I HTN (140 to 150/90 to 99) remains uncertain, with harms including syncope, kidney injury, and electrolyte abnormalities. Individualize decisions.

– Treating patients with CKD or diabetes to lower-than-standard BP targets, <140/90, does not appear to further reduce mortality or morbidity. Individualize goal for BP based on risk factors and patient preferences.

– The majority of treatment benefit is attained by lowering very high SBP (e.g., from 190 to 150, as compared with the benefit of lowering from 150 to 136). Striving for small additional drops in BP by adding fourth or fifth medications to achieve a "target" is less clinically beneficial and more likely to cause adverse effects. Lower-than-standard JNC-8 DBP targets are not associated with decreased morbidity/mortality.

MEDICATION

- For initial monotherapy, choose from 1 of 4 classes of medications: ACEI, ARBs, dihydropyridine (DHP) calcium channel blockers (CCBs), or thiazide diuretics.
- Sequential monotherapy attempts should be tried with different classes because individual responses vary.
- Many patients will require multiple medications—especially those presenting with BP >20/10 mm Hg above target, for whom it may be appropriate to begin with combination therapy.
- Multiple drugs at submaximal dose may achieve target BP with fewer side effects. However, these benefits must be balanced against adherence challenges associated with increased pill burden and more complicated dosing regimens. Consider combination pills in these scenarios.
- In patients on >1 medication, consider nondiuretic medications at bedtime for better 24-hour antihypertensive effect
- ACEI or ARBs should be used in patients with diabetes, proteinuria, atrial fibrillation, or heart failure with reduced ejection fraction (HFrEF) but *not in pregnancy*.
- α-Adrenergic blockers are not a first choice for monotherapy but are suitable as combination therapy for males with benign prostatic hypertrophy (BPH).
- DHP-CCB could be considered in patients with isolated systolic HTN, atherosclerosis, angina, migraine, or asthma; well-documented to reduce risk of stroke
- β-blockers should be prioritized in patients with ischemic heart disease, atrial fibrillation, CHF, migraine, and patients with history of ST-segment elevation myocardial infarction (STEMI).

First Line

- ACEI: lisinopril: 5 to 40 mg/day; enalapril: 5 to 40 mg/day; ramipril: 2.5 to 20.0 mg/day
- ARBs: losartan: 25 to 100 mg in 1 or 2 doses; has unique but modest uricosuric effect; valsartan: 80 to 320 mg/day; irbesartan: 75 to 300 mg/day; candesartan: 4 to 32 mg/day; renin inhibitor: aliskiren 150 to 300 mg/day
- Thiazide diuretics may not be effective with Cr clearance <30 mL/min.

– Chlorthalidone: 12.5 to 25.0 mg/day (longer half-life and more potent than hydrochlorothiazide but causes more hyponatremia and hypokalemia); strongest evidence base for this medication
– Hydrochlorothiazide: 12.5 to 50.0 mg/day; indapamide: 1.25 to 2.5 mg/day; metolazone: 2.5 to 5.0 mg/day is more effective in patients with impaired renal function than other thiazides, but outcomes studies lacking.

- DHP-CCB: amlodipine: 2.5 to 10 mg/day; nifedipine (sustained release): 30 to 90 mg/day; non-DHP: diltiazem CD: 180 to 360 mg/day; verapamil (sustained release): 120 to 480 mg/day
- Contraindications: Thiazide diuretics may worsen gout. β-Blockers (relative) in asthma, heart block, diabetes, and peripheral vascular disease; likely avoid in patients with metabolic syndrome or insulin-requiring diabetes. Diltiazem or verapamil: Do not use with systolic dysfunction or heart block.

Second Line

- Before escalating therapy, ensure that patient is adherent to prescribed regimen. Choose additional medications with complementary effects (i.e., ACEI/ARBs with diuretic or a vasodilator with a diuretic or β-blocker). Don't combine ACEI and ARB.
- Evidence from the ACCOMPLISH trial suggests that the combination of ACEI/CCB should be prioritized over ACEI/HCTZ to achieve better CV outcomes
- Medication-refractory HTN (see "Hypertension, Secondary and Resistant"): spironolactone 25 to 100 mg/day or eplerenone 50 mg once to twice daily
- β-Blockers may be effective in patients with resting tachycardia. Metoprolol succinate allows for once-daily dosing over a wide dosage range (25 to 400 mg/day). Carvedilol and labetalol combine α- and β-blockade.
- Centrally acting α_2-agonists: clonidine 0.1 to 1.2 mg BID or weekly patch 0.1 to 0.3 mg/day, guanfacine 1 to 3 mg/day, or methyldopa 250 to 2,000 mg BID
- α-Adrenergic antagonists: prazosin 1 to 10 mg BID, terazosin 1 to 20 mg/day, or doxazosin 1 to 16 mg/day
- Vasodilators: hydralazine 10 to 25 mg TID; minoxidil 2.5 mg BID; risk of tachycardia and fluid retention, so generally combined with β-blocker and/or diuretic; minoxidil: rarely used due to adverse effects; may be more effective than other medications in renal failure and refractory HTN
- Metolazone and loop diuretics may be used with more severe renal impairment, but outcomes data are absent; loop diuretics (for volume overload): furosemide 20 to 320 mg/day or torsemide 5 to 100 mg/day
- K^+-sparing diuretics in patients with hypokalemia while taking thiazides: amiloride 5 to 10 mg/day or triamterene 50 to 150 mg/day

COMPLEMENTARY & ALTERNATIVE MEDICINE

Biofeedback and relaxation exercise

 ## ONGOING CARE

FOLLOW-UP RECOMMENDATIONS
Patient Monitoring

ALERT

Repeat electrolytes, BUN/Cr about 3 to 6 weeks after initiating thiazide diuretics, ARB, or ACEI. Reevaluate patients q3–6mo until stable and then q6–12mo. Consider BP self-monitoring; monitor quality-of-life issues including sexual function. Poor medication adherence is a leading cause of apparent medication failure; at least annual Cr and potassium for patients on diuretics, ACEIs, and ARBs

DIET

- ~20% of patients will respond to reduced-salt diet (<6 g NaCl or <2.4 g Na/d). Limit alcohol consumption to <1 oz/day.
- Consider Dietary Approaches to Stop HTN (DASH) diet: https://www.nhlbi.nih.gov/education/dash-eating-plan.

COMPLICATION

Heart and renal failure, LVH, MI, retinal hemorrhage, stroke, dementia or cognitive decline, drug side effects, erectile dysfunction, all-causing mortality

REFERENCES

1. James PA, Oparil S, Carter BL, et al. 2014 Evidence-based guideline for the management of high blood pressure in adults: report from the panel members appointed to the Eighth Joint National Committee (JNC 8). *JAMA*. 2014;311(5):507–520.
2. Qaseem A, Wilt TJ, Rich R, et al. Pharmacologic treatment of hypertension in adults aged 60 years or older to higher versus lower blood pressure targets: a clinical practice guideline from the American College of Physicians and the American Academy of Family Physicians. *Ann Intern Med*. 2017;166(6):430–437.
3. Krist AH, Davidson KW, Mangione CM, et al; for US Preventive Services Task Force. Screening for hypertension in adults: US Preventive Services Task Force reaffirmation recommendation statement. *JAMA*. 2021;325(16):1650–1656.

 ## SEE ALSO

Hypertension, Secondary and Resistant; Hypertensive Emergencies; Polycystic Kidney Disease

 ## CODES

ICD10
I10 Essential (primary) hypertension

CLINICAL PEARLS

- NNT to prevent a major adverse CV events (MACE) ranges from 10 to 50 per year in patients with severe HTN, to 100s or 1000s per year for patients with mild HTN.
- Measure BP outside the office.
- Overly aggressive treatment may cause significant harms, especially in the elderly.
- Many patients are non-responders to specific medication classes; consider sequential monotherapy instead of combination therapy—especially for those within 20/10 mm Hg of target.

H

HYPERTENSION, SECONDARY AND RESISTANT
George Maxted, MD

BASICS

DESCRIPTION
Uncontrolled hypertension (HTN) comprises the following entities (see "Alert" below):

- Resistant HTN: blood pressure (BP) that remains above goal in spite of the concurrent use of three antihypertensive agents of different classes. Ideally, one of the three agents should be a diuretic, and all agents should be prescribed at optimal dose amounts. The diagnosis should not include "white-coat effect" or medication nonadherence, although these are common mimics.
- Secondary HTN: elevated BP that results from an identifiable underlying mechanism
- The 2017 revised ACC/AHA guideline recommends a change in the classification of HTN. For the purposes of this chapter, we are considering stage 2 HTN: systolic blood pressure (SBP) ≥140 mm Hg or diastolic blood pressure (DBP) ≥90 mm Hg. The guideline is quite controversial. See "Hypertension, Essential" topic. Many experts still adhere to the JNC 8 guideline, do not agree with a diagnosis or class of HTN for pressures below 140/90 mm Hg (1)[C].

Geriatric Considerations
- Onset of HTN in adults >60 years of age is a strong indicator of secondary HTN.
- In patients >80 years of age, consider a higher target SBP of ≥150 mm Hg. Be cautious to avoid excessive diastolic lowering. Elderly may be particularly responsive to diuretics and dihydropyridine calcium channel blockers.
- Systolic HTN is particularly problematic in the elderly.
- Secondary causes more common in the elderly include sleep apnea, renal disease, atherosclerotic renal artery stenosis (ARAS), and primary aldosteronism (PA).
- Noncompressible arteries (Osler phenomenon)—mostly in elderly with arteriosclerosis: Brachial and radial artery pulsations are present at high cuff pressures.

ALERT
Pseudoresistance: inaccurate measurement of BP (cuff too small, patient not at rest; sitting quietly for 5 minutes); poor adherence: in primary care settings, this has been estimated to occur in 40–60% of patients with HTN. White coat effect: prevalence 20–40%. Do not make clinical decisions about HTN based solely on measurement in the clinic setting. Home BP monitoring (HBPM), self-monitoring (SBPM), remote monitoring or ambulatory (ABPM) are more reliable.

EPIDEMIOLOGY
- Predominant age: In general, HTN has its onset between ages 30 and 50 years. Patients with resistant HTN are more likely to experience the combined outcomes of death, myocardial infarction, congestive heart failure (CHF), stroke, or chronic kidney disease.
- Depending on etiology, age of onset can vary. Age of onset <20 or >50 years increases likelihood of a secondary cause for HTN.

Prevalence
- Prevalence of resistant HTN is estimated to be 10–15% (2). NHANES: 53% of adults are controlled to a BP of <140/90 mm Hg. The most common cause of apparently resistant HTN is likely medication nonadherence.
- Secondary HTN occurs in about 5–10% of adults with chronic HTN.
- A recent study of secondary HTN among otherwise healthy children with a diagnosis of HTN indicated a prevalence of 3.7%.

ETIOLOGY AND PATHOPHYSIOLOGY
- Obstructive sleep apnea (25–50%)
- Primary hyperaldosteronism (8–20% of resistant HTN cases)
- Chronic renal disease (1–2% of hypertensives)
- Renovascular disease (0.2–0.7%, up to 35% of elderly, 20% of patients undergoing cardiac catheterization)
- Cushing syndrome (<0.1%)
- Pheochromocytoma (0.04–0.1% of hypertensives)
- Other rare causes: hyperthyroidism, hyperparathyroidism, aortic coarctation, intracranial tumor
- Drug-related causes (many)
  - Medications, especially NSAIDs (may also blunt effectiveness of ACE inhibitors), decongestants, stimulants, anorectic agents including herbals (e.g., guarana, ma huang, bitter orange), natural licorice (in some chewing tobacco), glucocorticoids
  - Oral contraceptives (OCP): Cessation of OCP may result in normalization of the BP. Postmenopausal estrogen does not appear to correlate as strongly (2).
  - Cocaine, amphetamines, other illicit drugs; drug and alcohol withdrawal syndromes
- Lifestyle factors: obesity, dietary salt, excessive alcohol, physical inactivity

Genetics
Genetic variants have been detected in patients with resistant HTN but are estimated to account for less than 3% of BP variance (2).

RISK FACTORS
A large cohort study revealed that those with resistant HTN (16.2%) were more likely to be male, Caucasian, older, and diabetic. Factors predictive of resistant or secondary HTN: obesity, diabetes, worsening of control in previously stable hypertensive patient, onset in patients age <20 years or >50 years, lack of family history of HTN, significant target end-organ damage, stage 2 HTN (SBP >160 mm Hg or DBP >100 mm Hg), renal disease, and alcohol or drug use

GENERAL PREVENTION
The prevention of resistant and secondary HTN is thought to be the same as for primary or essential HTN: a Dietary Approaches to Stop Hypertension (DASH) diet, a low-sodium diet, weight loss in obese patients, exercise, limitation of alcohol intake, and smoking cessation. Relaxation techniques may be of help.

COMMONLY ASSOCIATED CONDITIONS
Sleep disorders; obesity

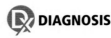

DIAGNOSIS
HTN

HISTORY
- Ask or review at every visit: SANS mnemonic: (i) Salt intake, (ii) Alcohol intake, (iii) NSAID use, (iv) Sleep. These identify the most common causes of poorly controlled HTN.
- Ask about medication adherence. Estimates are that during the 1st year of treatment for HTN, only 20% of patients have sufficiently high adherence to achieve clinical benefit (2).
- Review home BP readings; consider ABMP.
- History varies with etiology of secondary HTN. OSA: loud snoring while asleep, daytime somnolence; pheochromocytoma: episodes of headache, palpitations, sweating; Cushing syndrome: weight gain, fatigue, weakness, easy bruising, amenorrhea; increased intravascular volume: swelling

PHYSICAL EXAM
- Ensure that the BP is measured correctly. The patient should be sitting quietly with back supported for at least 5 minutes before measurement. Proper cuff size: bladder encircling at least 80% of the arm. Support arm at heart level. Minimum of two readings at least 1 minute apart. Check BP in both arms. Also check standing BP for orthostasis.
- The USPSTF recommends "obtaining measurements outside of the clinical setting for diagnostic confirmation." Attention to findings related to possible etiologies: renovascular HTN: systolic/diastolic abdominal bruit; pheochromocytoma: diaphoresis, tachycardia; Cushing syndrome: hirsutism, moon facies, dorsal hump, purple striae, truncal obesity; thyroid disease: enlarged thyroid, tremor, exophthalmos, tachycardia; coarctation of the aorta: upper limb HTN with decreased or delayed femoral pulses.

DIFFERENTIAL DIAGNOSIS
Pseudoresistance

DIAGNOSTIC TESTS & INTERPRETATION
- ECG performed as part of the initial workup; LVH is an important marker of resistant HTN.
- Sleep study if history and physical indicate. The Epworth Sleepiness Scale is recommended.
- Home-based polysomnography has been shown to be accurate in screening for OSA. Overnight oximetry is not helpful.

Initial Tests (lab, imaging)
Initial limited diagnostic testing should include urinalysis, CBC, potassium, sodium, glucose, creatinine, lipids, thyroid-stimulating hormone (TSH), and calcium. 50% of patients with hyperaldosteronism may have normal potassium levels. Urine spot test for microalbuminuria, an important marker of ASCVD risk.

- Imaging tests listed are necessary only if history, physical, or lab data indicate.
- Abdominal US: if renal disease is suspected
- Duplex ultrasonography may be the preferred test for renovascular disease. MR angiography (MRA) of renal vasculature is sensitive but has low specificity and potentially more harmful. Conventional catheter angiography or CT angiography may be required to confirm the diagnosis.

Follow-Up Tests & Special Considerations

Further testing for PA may be considered.

- Empiric treatment with an aldosterone antagonist may be preferable and more clinically relevant: spironolactone or eplerenone. Amiloride may be an option for potassium sparing but has not been shown to affect the aldosterone level.
- Plasma aldosterone-to-renin ratio (ARR) is the preferred lab test, but the test is difficult to perform and interpret properly. Consult your reference lab and interpret results with caution.
  - Further testing (screening) for pheochromocytoma: 30 minutes supine plasma (or 24 hours urinary) metanephrines (consult lab for best local option)
  - Other tests to consider for resistant or secondary HTN: 24-hour urine for free cortisol, calcium, parathyroid hormone (PTH), overnight 1-mg dexamethasone suppression test, urine toxicology screen

Diagnostic Procedures/Other

Consider 24-hour ABPM, especially if white coat effect is suspected. HBPM results predict mortality, stroke, and other target organ damage better than office BP. Optimal protocol involves two paired measurements: morning and evening (four measurements) over 4 to 7 days.

- Oscillometric, electronic, upper arm, fully automatic device with memory: average multiple readings over several days
- Remote BP monitoring devices may be useful in the clinical management of HTN but thus far have not been shown to be more effective than standard monitoring.

 TREATMENT

- Treatment modality depends on etiology of HTN. Please see each etiology listed for information on proper treatment. Empiric trial of aldosterone antagonist is a commonly used initial medication strategy if diagnostic workup does not reveal a specific cause.
- The National Institute for Health Care and Excellence (2) offers a useful management algorithm emphasizing lifestyle modification: diet, less sodium, exercise, alcohol in moderation.
- Emphasize adherence to JNC 8 and/or AHA/ACC guidelines, with emphasis on lifestyle modification (1)[C].
  - Obese patients and elderly may be particularly responsive to diuretics.
  - Tolerance to diuretics may occur: long-term adaptation to thiazides or the "braking effect." Consider increasing the dose of thiazide or adding an aldosterone inhibitor.
- Treatment specific to certain secondary etiologies
  - PA: aldosterone receptor antagonist: spironolactone or eplerenone (latter has less estrogenic effect)
  - Cushing syndrome: aldosterone receptor antagonist

- OSA: continuous positive airway pressure (CPAP) ±; oxygen, surgery, weight loss, upper airway nerve stimulation. A mandibular advancement device (MAD) may be as effective as CPAP for OSA for some.
  - Nocturnal hypoxia: oxygen supplementation
  - Renal sympathetic denervation is controversial as current approaches have largely failed to demonstrate clinical benefit.
- The treatment of ARAS is controversial. Percutaneous stenting may not be effective. ACEi and ARB medications may confer long-term mortality benefit (2)[C].

MEDICATION

- Follow treatment guidelines and algorithms by JNC 8 and AHA/ACC/CDC, understanding the differences between them (1)[C].
- Adding a medication to the regimen may have greater efficacy than increasing the dose of medications.
- Empiric use of aldosterone antagonists is often effective.

ALERT

- Agents specific for treatment of HTN emergencies should be initiated in those situations, in which immediate BP reduction will prevent or limit end-organ damage (see "Hypertensive Emergencies").
- Renovascular HTN: Angioplasty is the treatment of choice for fibromuscular dysplasia of a renal artery.
- CORAL study: In patients with atherosclerotic renovascular disease and HTN, renal artery stenting did not improve outcomes over medical therapy alone.
- Referral to an HTN specialist or clinic: Retrospective studies indicate improved control rates for patients with resistant HTN referred to special HTN clinics.

First Line

- ARB medications may be considered first line for HTN. ACEi and thiazide diuretics may also be considered (3).
- Note: Race-based prescribing has lately been called into question. People of African descent may, however, not respond to ACEi or ARB medications.

Second Line

Combine thiazide diuretic with ACEi, ARB, or CCB or add an aldosterone inhibitor. Beta blockers—especially if compelling indication such as ischemic heart disease or CHF—migraine and tachyarrhythmias may also be indications. Hydralazine and isosorbide mononitrate or dinitrate are options.

Third Line

Add agent not used in second line; if this does not adequately lower BP, initiate workup for secondary causes (chronic NSAID use, alcohol abuse, RAS, etc.).

ISSUES FOR REFERRAL

If control is not successful, consider referral to a HTN center or nephrology.

COMPLEMENTARY & ALTERNATIVE MEDICINE

The University of Wisconsin Integrative Medicine program has an excellent handout and patient information.

ADMISSION, INPATIENT, AND NURSING CONSIDERATIONS

Hypertensive urgency or emergency general measures

 ONGOING CARE

FOLLOW-UP RECOMMENDATIONS

Encourage aerobic activity of 30 min/day, depending on patient's condition.

Patient Monitoring

Remote BP monitoring may be useful in a clinical setting.

DIET

Reduced salt may lower BP in some patients. Recommend the Mediterranean diet or DASH.

PATIENT EDUCATION

HBPM is recommended.

REFERENCES

1. James PA, Oparil S, Carter BL, et al. 2014 Evidence-based guideline for the management of high blood pressure in adults: report from the panel members appointed to the Eighth Joint National Committee (JNC 8). *JAMA.* 2014;311(5):507–520.
2. Carey RM, Calhoun DA, Bakris GL, et al. Resistant hypertension: detection, evaluation, and management: a scientific statement from the American Heart Association. *Hypertension.* 2018;72(5):e53–e90.
3. Chen RJ, Suchard MA, Krumholz HM, et al. Comparative first-line effectiveness and safety of ACE (angiotensin-converting enzyme) inhibitors and angiotensin receptor blockers: a multinational cohort study. *Hypertension.* 2021;78(3):591–603.

 SEE ALSO

Aldosteronism, Primary; Coarctation of the Aorta; Cushing Disease and Cushing Syndrome; Hyperparathyroidism; Hypertension, Essential; Hyperthyroidism; Pheochromocytoma

CODES

ICD10

- I15.9 Secondary hypertension, unspecified
- I15.8 Other secondary hypertension
- I15.0 Renovascular hypertension

CLINICAL PEARLS

- Aldosterone inhibitors should be considered in all cases of resistant HTN.
- HBPM predicts outcomes better than office monitoring of BP.

H

HYPERTHYROIDISM

Anup Sabharwal, MD, MBA, FACE, FASPC, FNLA

BASICS

- Hyperthyroidism or thyrotoxicosis is due to thyroid hormone excess. The former describes excess from the thyroid gland, whereas the latter can also be produced from another source.
- In general, patients with thyrotoxicosis have hyperthyroidism. However, patients could suffer from thyrotoxicosis subacute thyroiditis, exogenous thyrotoxicosis, and radiation-induced thyroiditis.

DESCRIPTION

- Graves disease (GD) is the most common cause with autoantibodies directed at the thyroid-stimulating hormone (TSH) receptors.
- Toxic multinodular goiter (TMNG) is the most common cause of hyperthyroidism in patients >65 years of age; often an insidious onset, frequent in iodine-deficient areas.
- Toxic adenoma (Plummer disease) is seen in younger patients—autonomously functioning nodules.
- TSH-producing adenoma, not to be confused with a resistance to thyroid hormone
- Iodine-induced hyperthyroidism
- Subacute thyroiditis/de Quervain: granulomatous giant cell thyroiditis, benign course; viral infections have been involved.
- Postpartum thyroiditis
- Drug-induced thyroiditis: amiodarone, interferon-α, interleukin-2, lithium
- Subclinical hyperthyroidism: suppressed TSH with normal thyroxine (T_4)
  - Grade 1 reflects a mild suppression of TSH in the range of 0.10 to 0.39 mU/L.
  - Grade 2 reflects a greater suppression with TSH <0.1 mU/L.
- Thyroid storm: fever, tachycardia, gastrointestinal (GI) symptoms, CNS dysfunction (e.g., coma); up to 50% mortality

Geriatric Considerations
- Characteristic symptoms and signs may be absent.
- Atrial fibrillation is common when TSH <0.1 mIU/L (1)[A].

Pediatric Considerations
- Neonates and children are treated with antithyroid medications for 12 to 24 months.
- Radioactive iodine treatment is controversial in children.

Pregnancy Considerations
Propylthiouracil (PTU) is currently the drug of choice during 1st trimester of pregnancy, and methimazole is preferred in the 2nd and 3rd trimesters (2)[A]. Treat with lowest effective dose because PTU can cross the placenta and put the fetus at risk for goiter. Avoid treatment-induced hypothyroidism. Radioiodine therapy is contraindicated.

EPIDEMIOLOGY
- 1.3% of population
- Predominant sex: female > male (7 to 10:1)
- Predominant age: autoimmune thyroid disease (GD) in 2nd and 3rd decades; TMNG is more common in patients aged >40 years.

Prevalence
The prevalence of hyperthyroidism is 1.3% and can increase in older women to 4–5%.

ETIOLOGY AND PATHOPHYSIOLOGY
- GD: autoimmune disease
- TMNG: 60% TSH receptor gene abnormality; 40% unknown
- Toxic adenoma: point mutation in TSH receptor gene with increased hormone production
- Hashitoxicosis: autoimmune destruction of the thyroid; antimicrosomal antibodies present
- Subacute/de Quervain thyroiditis: Granulomatous reaction viruses, such as coxsackievirus, adenovirus, echovirus, and influenza virus, have been implicated.
- Drug-induced thyroiditis: amiodarone, lithium, interferon-α, and interleukin-2
- Postpartum thyroiditis: autoimmune thyroiditis that lasts up to 8 weeks, and in 60% of patients, hypothyroidism manifests in the future.

Genetics
Concordance rate for GD among monozygotic twins is 35%.

RISK FACTORS
- Positive family history, especially in maternal relatives
- Other autoimmune disorders
- Iodide repletion after iodide deprivation, especially in TMNG

COMMONLY ASSOCIATED CONDITIONS
- Autoimmune diseases
- Down syndrome

DIAGNOSIS

HISTORY
- Thyrotoxicosis is a hypermetabolic state in which energy production exceeds needs, causing increased heat production, diaphoresis, and even fever.
- Thyrotoxicosis affects different systems:
  - Constitutional: fatigue, weakness, increased appetite, weight loss
  - Neuropsychiatric: agitation, anxiety, emotional lability, psychosis, coma, and poor concentration and memory
  - GI: increased appetite, hyperdefecation
  - Gynecologic: oligomenorrhea, amenorrhea
  - Cardiovascular: tachycardia (most common) and chest discomfort that mimics angina

Geriatric Considerations
Apathetic hyperthyroidism in the elderly

PHYSICAL EXAM
- Skin: warm, moist, pretibial myxedema (GD only)
- Head, eye, ear, nose, throat (HEENT): exophthalmos, lid lag
- Endocrine: hyperhidrosis, heat intolerance, goiter, gynecomastia, and spider angiomata (males)
- Cardiovascular: tachycardia, atrial fibrillation, cardiomegaly
- Musculoskeletal: fractures
- Neurologic: tremor, proximal muscle weakness, anxiety and lability, brisk deep tendon reflexes
- Rarely: thyroid acropathy (clubbing), localized dermopathy
- Children will have a linear growth acceleration.

DIFFERENTIAL DIAGNOSIS
- Anxiety; depression
- Diabetes mellitus
- Pregnancy; menopause
- Pheochromocytoma; carcinoid syndrome

DIAGNOSTIC TESTS & INTERPRETATION
- 95% have suppressed TSH and elevated free T_4 (3)[A].
- Triiodothyronine (T_3) is elevated in T_3 toxicosis or amiodarone-induced thyrotoxicosis (AIT):
  - TSH, T_4, and T_3 can all be elevated with symptomatology in cases of a TSH-producing pituitary adenoma; however, symptoms may be absent in resistance to thyroid hormone binding.
- Presence of TSH receptor antibody or thyroid-stimulating immunoglobulin is diagnostic of GD.
- Free thyroxine index (FTI): calculated from T_4 and thyroid hormone–binding ratio; corrects for misleading results caused by pregnancy and estrogens
- Inappropriately normal or elevated TSH with high T_4 suspicious for pituitary tumor or thyroid hormone resistance
- Drugs may alter lab results: estrogens, heparin, iodine-containing compounds (including amiodarone and contrast agents), phenytoin, salicylates, and steroids (e.g., androgens, corticosteroids).
- Other findings that can occur: anemia, granulocytosis, lymphocytosis, hypercalcemia, transaminase, and alkaline phosphate elevations

Initial Tests (lab, imaging)
- TSH, free T_4, total T_4, and T_3 will establish the hyperthyroid diagnosis.
- Thyrotropin receptor antibody (TRAb)
- TSH receptor antibodies (TSH-R Abs): The routine assay is the TSH-binding inhibitor immunoglobulin assay (TBII). TSH-R Abs are useful in the prediction of postpartum Graves thyrotoxicosis and neonatal thyrotoxicosis.

- T_4/T_3: The T_4-to-T_3 ratio may be a useful tool when the iodine uptake testing is not available/contra-indicated. ~2% of thyrotoxic patients have "T_3 toxicosis."
- Nuclear medicine uptake and scanning (^{123}I or ^{131}I): The reference-range value for 24-hour radioiodine uptake is between 5% and 25%.
  – Increased thyroid iodine uptake is seen with TMNG, toxic solitary nodule, and GD.
  – GD shows a diffuse uptake and can have a paradoxical finding of high uptake at 4 to 6 hours but normal uptake at 24 hours because of the rapid clearance.
  – TMNG will show a heterogeneous uptake, whereas solitary toxic nodule will show a warm or "hot" nodule.
  – In iodine-deficient areas, an increased uptake is associated with low urine iodine levels.

Diagnostic Procedures/Other
Neck ultrasound will show increased diffuse vascularity in GD.

Test Interpretation
- GD: hyperplasia
- Toxic nodule: nodule formation

TREATMENT

- Observation may be appropriate for patients with mild hyperthyroidism (TSH >0.1 or no symptoms) especially those who are young and with low risk of complications (atrial fibrillation, osteoporosis).
- Treatment for subacute thyroiditis is supportive with NSAIDs and β-blockers. Steroids can be used for 2 to 3 weeks (2).
- GD or TMNG can be managed by either antithyroid medication, radioactive iodine therapy (RAIT), or thyroidectomy.
- Pretreatment with antithyroid drugs is preferred to avoid worsening thyrotoxicosis after RAIT. Methimazole is preferred over PTU as pretreatment because of decreased relapse, but it is held 3 to 5 days before therapy (2)[A].
- Usually, patients become hypothyroid 2 to 3 months after RAIT; therefore, antithyroid medications are continued after ablation.
- Glucocorticoids: reduce the conversion of active T_4 to the more active T_3; in Graves ophthalmopathy, the use of prednisone before and after RAIT prevents worsening ophthalmopathy (2)[B].
- For GD, due to the chance of remission, 12- to 18-month trial of antithyroid medications may be considered prior to offering RAIT.
- For TMNG, the treatment of choice is RAIT. Medical therapy with antithyroid medications has shown a high recurrence rate. Surgery is considered only in special cases (2)[B].
- For AIT type I, the treatment is antithyroid drugs and β-blockers. Thyroidectomy is the last option. AIT type II is self-limited but may use glucocorticoids.
- β-Blockers can aid in mitigating palpitations and reducing heart rate in those with accelerated sinus rhythm.

MEDICATION
First Line
- Antithyroid drugs: Methimazole and PTU are thioamides that inhibit iodine oxidation, organification, and iodotyrosine coupling. PTU can block peripheral conversion of T_4 to active T_3. Both can be used as primary treatment for GD and prior to RAIT or surgery (3)[A].
- Duration of treatment: 12 to 18 months; 50–60% relapse after stopping; treatment beyond 18 months did not show any further benefit on remission rate. The most serious side effects are hepatitis (0.1–0.2%), vasculitis, and agranulocytosis; baseline CBC recommended:
  – Methimazole (preferred): adults: 10 to 15 mg q12–24h; children aged 6 to 10 years: 0.4 mg/kg/day PO once daily
  – PTU: adults (preferred in thyroid storm and 1st trimester of pregnancy): 100 to 150 mg PO q8h, not to exceed 200 mg/day during pregnancy
- β-Adrenergic blocker: Propranolol in high doses (>160 mg/day) inhibits T_3 activation by up to 30%. Atenolol, metoprolol, and nadolol can be used and are also useful in relieving palpitations and in slowing the heart rate in patients with sinus tachycardia.
- Glucocorticoids: reduce the conversion of active T_4 to the more active T_3
- Cholestyramine: anion exchange resin that decreases thyroid hormone reabsorption in the enterohepatic circulation; dose: 4 g QID (3)[B]
- Other agents:
  – Lithium: inhibits thyroid hormone secretion and iodotyrosine coupling; use is limited by toxicity.
  – Lugol solution or saturated solution of potassium iodide (SSKI); blocks the release of hormone from the gland but should be administered at least 1 hour after thioamide was given; otherwise, acts as a substrate for hormone production (Jod-Basedow effect)

ISSUES FOR REFERRAL
Refer patients with Graves ophthalmopathy to an experienced ophthalmologist.

SURGERY/OTHER PROCEDURES
Thyroidectomy for compressive symptoms, masses, and thyroid malignancy may be performed in the 2nd trimester of pregnancy only.

 ONGOING CARE

FOLLOW-UP RECOMMENDATIONS
Smoking cessation in GD patients as this is a risk factor for ophthalmopathy, especially after RAIT

Patient Monitoring
- Repeat thyroid tests q3mo, CBC, and liver function tests (LFTs) on thioamide therapy; continue therapy with thioamides for 12 to 18 months.
- After RAIT, thyroid function tests at 6 weeks, 12 weeks, 6 months, and annually thereafter if euthyroid; TSH may remain undetectable for months even after patient is euthyroid; follow T_3 and T_4.

DIET
Sufficient calories to prevent weight loss

PROGNOSIS
Good with early diagnosis and treatment

COMPLICATIONS
- Surgery: hypoparathyroidism, recurrent laryngeal nerve damage, and hypothyroidism
- RAIT: postablation hypothyroidism
- GD: high relapse rate with antithyroid drug as primary therapy
- Graves ophthalmopathy, worsening heart failure if cardiac condition, atrial fibrillation, muscle wasting, proximal muscle weakness, increased risk of cerebrovascular accident (CVA), and cardiovascular mortality

REFERENCES
1. Cappola AR, Fried LP, Arnold AM, et al. Thyroid status, cardiovascular risk, and mortality in older adults. *JAMA*. 2006;295(9):1033–1041.
2. Bahn RS, Burch HB, Cooper DS, et al. Hyperthyroidism and other causes of thyrotoxicosis: management guidelines of the American Thyroid Association and American Association of Clinical Endocrinologists. *Endocr Pract*. 2011;17(3): 456–520.
3. Bahn Chair RS, Burch HB, Cooper DS, et al. Hyperthyroidism and other causes of thyrotoxicosis: management guidelines of the American Thyroid Association and American Association of Clinical Endocrinologists. *Thyroid*. 2011;21(6):593–646.

CODES

ICD10
- E05.81 Other thyrotoxicosis with thyrotoxic crisis or storm
- E05.80 Other thyrotoxicosis without thyrotoxic crisis or storm
- E05.1 Thyrotoxicosis with toxic single thyroid nodule

CLINICAL PEARLS
- Not all thyrotoxicoses are secondary to hyperthyroidism.
- GD presents with hyperthyroidism, ophthalmopathy, and goiter.
- Thyroid storm is a medical emergency that needs hospitalization and aggressive treatment.
- Serum TSH level may be misleading and remain low in the early period after initiating treatment, even when T_4 and T_3 levels have decreased.

H

HYPERTRIGLYCERIDEMIA

S. Lindsey Clarke, MD, FAAFP • Katherine G. W. Johnson, MD

 BASICS

DESCRIPTION

- Hypertriglyceridemia (HTG) is a common form of dyslipidemia characterized by an excess fasting plasma concentration of triglycerides (TGs).
  - TGs are fatty molecules that occur naturally in vegetable oils and animal fats and are major sources of dietary energy.
  - Absorbed TGs are packaged into very-low-density lipoproteins (VLDL) and chylomicrons.
- HTG is a risk factor for acute pancreatitis at levels ≥500 mg/dL and especially ≥1,000 mg/dL.
  - Risk is 10–20% at these TG levels.
  - Third leading cause of acute pancreatitis
- HTG also is independently associated with cardio-vascular disease (atherosclerotic cardiovascular disease [ASCVD]) at levels ≥175 mg/dL.
  - The American Heart Association (AHA) and the American College of Cardiology (ACC) consider persistent HTG as a risk-enhancing factor.
  - A large Danish population study in 2018 showed that TG ≥264 mg/dL conferred a 10-year risk of major adverse cardiovascular events comparable to that of statin eligible individuals.
  - However, a causal relationship between HTG and ASCVD has not been firmly established.
  - Moreover, lowering TG has not been proven to reduce cardiovascular risk.
- AHA and ACC classify HTG into two categories:
  - Moderate: 175 to 499 mg/dL (2.0 to 5.6 mmol/L), characterized mainly by excess VLDL
  - Severe: ≥500 mg/dL (≥5.6 mmol/L), characterized by excess VLDL and chylomicrons

EPIDEMIOLOGY

- Predominant gender: male > female
- Predominant race: Hispanic, white > black

Prevalence

- 25-33% of U.S. population has TG levels ≥150 mg/dL.
- 1.7% has TG levels ≥500 mg/dL.
- Highest prevalence at age 50 to 70 years
- The most common genetic syndromes with HTG, familial combined hyperlipidemia and familial HTG, each affect ≤1% of general population.

ETIOLOGY AND PATHOPHYSIOLOGY

- Primary
  - Familial
  - Acquired (sporadic)
- Secondary
  - Lifestyle factors
    - Obesity and overweight
    - Physical inactivity
    - Cigarette smoking
    - Excess alcohol intake
    - High-carbohydrate diets (>60% of total caloric intake)
  - Medical conditions
    - Type 2 diabetes mellitus
    - Metabolic syndrome/insulin resistance
    - Hypothyroidism
    - Chronic liver disease
    - Chronic kidney disease, nephrotic syndrome
    - Autoimmune disorders (e.g., systemic lupus erythematosus)
    - Paraproteinemias (e.g., macroglobulinemia, myeloma, lymphoma, lymphocytic leukemia)
    - Pregnancy (usually physiologic and transient)
  - Medications
    - Acitretin
    - β-Blockers
    - Bile acid sequestrants
    - Cyclophosphamide
    - Cyclosporine
    - Glucocorticoids
    - Isotretinoin
    - Oral estrogens
    - Protease inhibitors
    - Second-generation antipsychotics
    - Tamoxifen and raloxifene
    - Thiazides

Genetics

- Familial chylomicronemia (type 1 dyslipidemia): autosomal recessive inheritance of lipoprotein lipase deficiency; 0.0001% population prevalence
- Familial combined hyperlipidemia (type IIb): usually autosomal dominant, caused by overproduction of apolipoprotein (APO) B-100; approximately 1% prevalence
- Familial dysbetalipoproteinemia (type III): usually autosomal recessive, caused by lipoprotein overproduction due to inheritance of two APOE2 variants; 0.01% prevalence
- Familial HTG (type IV): autosomal dominant, caused by an inactivating mutation of the lipoprotein lipase gene; 1% prevalence
- Primary mixed HTG (type V)

RISK FACTORS

- Genetic susceptibility
- Obesity, overweight
- Lack of exercise
- Type 2 diabetes mellitus
- Alcoholism
- Certain medical conditions and drugs (See "Etiology and Pathophysiology.")

GENERAL PREVENTION

- Maintain healthy body weight.
- Moderation of dietary fat and refined carbohydrates
- Regular aerobic exercise
- Avoid excess alcohol.

COMMONLY ASSOCIATED CONDITIONS

- Pancreatitis
- Coronary artery disease
- Type 2 diabetes mellitus and insulin resistance
- Dyslipidemias
- Metabolic syndrome
- Nonalcoholic steatohepatitis (NASH)
- Polycystic ovarian syndrome

DIAGNOSIS

HISTORY

- Usually asymptomatic
- Patients with chylomicronemia syndrome can have memory loss, headache, vertigo, dyspnea, and paresthesias.
- Pancreatitis: epigastric pain, nausea, and vomiting
- Assess for other cardiac risk factors.
- Family history of coronary artery disease

PHYSICAL EXAM

- Obesity, overweight (body mass index ≥25 kg/m^2)
- Eruptive cutaneous, tuberous, and striate palmar xanthomas
- Lipemia retinalis
- Epigastric tenderness in pancreatitis
- Hepatomegaly in NASH and chylomicronemia

DIFFERENTIAL DIAGNOSIS

Primary and secondary HTG

DIAGNOSTIC TESTS & INTERPRETATION

Initial Tests (lab, imaging)

- Serum: turbid with milky supernatant
- Fasting (12 hours) or nonfasting lipid profile
  - USPSTF recommends screening adults aged 40 to 75 years to identify dyslipidemia and to calculate 10-year ASCVD risk; repeat every 5 years.
  - American Academy of Pediatrics recommends screening all children for dyslipidemia at 9 to 11 years and 17 to 21 years of age, but USPSTF found insufficient evidence for screening in children and adolescents.
  - Statin therapy may be indicated for LDL and ASCVD risk reduction in some adults (e.g., clinical ASCVD, diabetes) regardless of lipid levels.
  - Confirm severe HTG with fasting measurement.
- Evaluation for secondary causes
  - Glycosylated hemoglobin A1c (HbA1c), fasting or postprandial glucose for type 2 diabetes mellitus
  - Creatinine, urinary protein measurement for nephrotic syndrome, renal failure
  - Thyroid-stimulating hormone for hypothyroidism
- Pancreatitis: serum lipase; US and/or CT scan of pancreas
- Atherosclerosis: cardiac stress testing, coronary CT angiography, cardiac catheterization, and coronary angiography

Follow-Up Tests & Special Considerations

- Repeat lipid panel after 1 to 3 months of therapy.
- High levels of apolipoprotein B (apoB >130 mg/dL) predict ASCVD in patients whose LDL cannot be calculated due to HTG. But evidence for routine clinical measurement of apoB is lacking.

TREATMENT

GENERAL MEASURES

- Cardiovascular risk reduction through LDL lowering should be prioritized over TG lowering unless patient is at risk for pancreatitis due to severe HTG (TG ≥500 mg/dL) (1)[C].
- Therapeutic lifestyle changes are first-line interventions for all patients and can reduce TG by as much as 50%:
  – Dietary modification (limit carbohydrate intake to 50–60% of calories; restrict sugars and alcohol)
  – Moderate-intensity physical activity can reduce TG by 20–30%.
  – Weight loss of 5–10% can reduce TG by as much as 20%.
  – Persons with severe HTG should abstain from alcohol.
- Search for correctable secondary causes, treat underlying illness, or remove offending drug.
- Improve glycemic control if diabetic.
- Control other cardiac risk factors, such as hypertension, diabetes mellitus, and smoking.
- Primary HTG: Screen other family members.

MEDICATION

First Line

- Statins: preferred for ASCVD risk reduction; primarily affect LDL but also may lower TG 15–30%; USPSTF recommends statins for primary prevention of ASCVD in adults aged 40 to 75 years who have clinical risk factors and 10-year ASCVD risk ≥10%. Dosing depends on intensity of statin desired based on ASCVD risk. See "Coronary Artery Disease and Stable Angina" and "Hypercholesterolemia."
  – Atorvastatin: 10 to 80 mg/day
  – Rosuvastatin: 5 to 40 mg/day
  – Adverse reactions: myalgias, myopathy, rhabdomyolysis (especially if combined with fibrates); contraindicated in pregnancy and lactation
- Fibrates: preferred for reducing risk of pancreatitis in severe HTG; may lower TG up to 50% and may decrease cardiovascular and coronary events but not all-cause mortality (2)[A]:
  – Adverse reactions: GI upset, hepatotoxicity, cholelithiasis, myalgias, rhabdomyolysis (when combined with a statin), gemfibrozil-warfarin interaction (enhanced anticoagulation)
  – Fenofibrate: 30 to 200 mg/day (preferred)
  – Gemfibrozil: 600 mg BID; avoid in combination with statins due to high risk of muscle injury

Second Line

- Icosapent ethyl (Vascepa) 2 g BID: preferred add-on therapy for ASCVD risk reduction in patients with known ASCVD or diabetes mellitus plus additional risk factors and persistent HTG despite statin therapy (3)[C].
  – 2019 REDUCE-IT trial showed 25% reduction in major adverse cardiovascular events in this high-risk population.
  – Adverse reactions: atrial fibrillation/flutter, major bleeding (caution with coagulopathy, anticoagulation or antiplatelet therapy)

- Other marine omega-3 fatty acids
  – Omega-3-acid ethyl esters (Lovaza, other fish oils): 4 g/day or 2 g BID
  – Appropriate for reducing pancreatitis risk but do not improve ASCVD risk
  – May lower TG 30–50%
  – Limited tolerability due to adverse GI effects (diarrhea, nausea, abdominal pain, eructation)

ISSUES FOR REFERRAL

- Severe HTG refractory to treatment
- Familial HTG syndromes

ADMISSION, INPATIENT, AND NURSING CONSIDERATIONS

- Acute pancreatitis
- In acute hypertriglyceridemic pancreatitis with TG >1,000 mg/dL, the following interventions can be used to lower TG rapidly and safely to <500 mg/dL:
  – Apheresis (therapeutic plasma exchange) for 1 to 3 days
  – Insulin infusion
    ∘ Regular insulin 0.1 to 0.3 U/kg/hr IV for 2 to 4 days
    ∘ Administer separate infusion of dextrose 5% if blood glucose is <200 mg/dL.
- Discharge criteria: stabilization of acute complicating illness

 ONGOING CARE

FOLLOW-UP RECOMMENDATIONS

1 to 3 months after initiation or modification of therapy (repeat fasting lipid profile)

Patient Monitoring

- Fasting lipid profile every 6 to 12 months
- Maintain TG <500 to 1,000 mg/dL to reduce risk of acute pancreatitis.
- Hepatic transaminases
- Creatine phosphokinase if patient has myalgias

DIET

- Limit carbohydrates to 50–60% of total caloric intake.
- Increase dietary fiber.
- Avoid sugars and refined carbohydrates.
- Moderate alcohol intake (<1 oz/day) or complete abstinence if TGs are very high.
- Restrict dietary fat to 30% of total caloric intake; restrict further to 15% of caloric intake if TG ≥1,000 mg/dL.
- Increase marine-derived omega-3 polyunsaturated fatty acids. Eat fatty fish such as salmon, mackerel, sardines, and trout.
- Eliminate trans-fatty acids.
- Mediterranean-style diet reduces TG 10–15% more than a low-fat diet.

PATIENT EDUCATION

Smoking cessation for cardiovascular risk reduction

PROGNOSIS

- Good with correction of TG levels
- Patients with primary HTG usually require lifelong treatment.

COMPLICATIONS

- Atherosclerosis
- Chylomicronemia syndrome
- Pancreatitis

REFERENCES

1. Grundy SM, Stone NJ, Bailey AL, et al. 2018 AHA/ACC/AACVPR/AAPA/ABC/ACPM/ADA/AGS/APhA/ASPC/NLA/PCNA guideline on the management of blood cholesterol: a report of the American College of Cardiology/American Heart Association Task Force on clinical practice guidelines. *J Am Coll Cardiol*. 2019;73(24):e285–e350.
2. Jakob T, Nordmann AJ, Schandelmaier S, et al. Fibrates for primary prevention of cardiovascular disease events. *Cochrane Database Syst Rev*. 2016;11(11):CD009753.
3. Orringer CE, Jacobson TA, Maki KC. National Lipid Association scientific statement on the use of icosapent ethyl in statin-treated patients with elevated triglycerides and high or very-high ASCVD risk. *J Clin Lipidol*. 2019;13(6):860–872.

ADDITIONAL READING

- Simha V. Management of hypertriglyceridemia. *BMJ*. 2020;371:m3109.
- Virani SS, Morris PB, Agarwala A, et al. 2021 ACC expert consensus decision pathway on the management of ASCVD risk reduction in patients with persistent hypertriglyceridemia: a report of the American College of Cardiology Solution Set Oversight Committee. *J Am Coll Cardiol*. 2021;78(9):960–993.

 SEE ALSO

- Hypercholesterolemia; Pancreatitis, Acute
- Algorithm: Hypertriglyceridemia

 CODES

ICD10

E78.1 Pure hyperglyceridemia

CLINICAL PEARLS

- HTG is likely a risk factor for atherosclerosis at levels ≥175 mg/dL and for acute pancreatitis at levels ≥500 to 1,000 mg/dL.
- Therapeutic lifestyle interventions (diet and exercise) are recommended for all patients who have HTG and for all patients at risk for ASCVD.
- Address reversible secondary causes of HTG such as uncontrolled diabetes and medications that raise TGs.
- In patients with TG levels <500 mg/dL, the main pharmacologic strategy for cardiovascular risk reduction is statins. Icosapent ethyl can further reduce cardiovascular events in high-risk patients.
- For patients with TG levels ≥500 mg/dL, the greatest amount of TG lowering is achieved with fibrates. But, the magnitude of clinical benefit is uncertain, so statin use is generally recommended first for cardiovascular risk reduction, with cautious addition of fibrates, if needed.

H

HYPOGLYCEMIA, DIABETIC

Afsha Rais Kaisani, MD • Tasaduq Hussain Mir, MD, FAAFP • Christoffer Amdahl, MD

BASICS

According to American Diabetic Association (ADA), hypoglycemia is defined as any blood sugar level <70 mg/dL.

DESCRIPTION
- Abnormally low concentration of glucose in circulating blood of a patient with diabetes mellitus (DM); often referred to as an *insulin reaction*, as classified by the ADA
  - Level 1: hypoglycemia alert value; <70 mg/dL (<3.9 mmol/L) but ≥54 mg/dL (≥3.0 mmol/L): may or may not be accompanied by symptoms; asymptomatic hypoglycemia if symptoms not present
  - Level 2: clinically significant hypoglycemia; <54 mg/dL (<3.0 mmol/L)
  - Level 3: severe hypoglycemia associated with severe cognitive impairment requiring external assistance for recovery
  - Pseudohypoglycemia: typical symptoms but glucose ≥70 mg/dL (≥3.9 mmol/L)
- Hypoglycemia is the leading limiting factor in the glycemic management of type 1 DM (T1DM) and type 2 DM (T2DM). Severe or frequent hypoglycemia requires modification of treatment regimens, including higher treatment goals (1).

EPIDEMIOLOGY
Incidence
- Most commonly found in patients with long-standing T1DM and children aged <7 years
- From the ACCORD study, the annual incidence of hypoglycemia was the following:
  - 3.14% in the intensive treatment group
  - 1.03% in the standard group
  - Increased risk among women, African Americans, those with less than high school education, aged participants, and those who used insulin at trial entry
- RECAP-DM study: Hypoglycemia was reported in 35.8% of patients with T2DM who added a sulfonylurea or thiazolidinedione to metformin therapy during the past year.

ETIOLOGY AND PATHOPHYSIOLOGY
- Loss of hormonal counterregulatory mechanism in glucose metabolism
- Impaired insulin, glucagon, and epinephrine secretion

RISK FACTORS
- Nearly 3/4 of severe hypoglycemic episodes occur during sleep.
- Severe hypoglycemia is associated with comorbid conditions in patients aged ≥65 years.
- Intensive insulin therapy (further lowering HbA1c from 7% to 6%) is associated with higher rate of hypoglycemia.
- Comorbidities: renal/liver disease, congestive heart failure (CHF), hypothyroidism, hypoadrenalism, gastroenteritis, gastroparesis (unpredictable carbohydrate (CHO) delivery), autonomic neuropathy, pregnancy, anxiety, depression, disordered eating behavior, illness/stress, and unplanned life events
- Duration of DM: >5 years
- Young children with T1DM

- Advanced age
- Reduced cognitive function, dementia
- Starvation, prolonged fasting, weight loss, or food insecurity
- Current smokers with T1DM
- Alcohol consumption may increase risk of delayed hypoglycemia, especially if on insulin or insulin secretagogues. Evening consumption of alcohol is associated with an increased risk of nocturnal and fasting hypoglycemia, especially in patients with T1DM.
- Insulin secretagogues: Sulfonylureas (glyburide, glimepiride, glipizide, etc.) and glinide derivatives (repaglinide, nateglinide) stimulate insulin secretion.
- Hypoglycemia is rare in diabetics not treated with insulin or insulin secretagogues.
- Other antidiabetes medications such as dipeptidyl peptidase 4 (DPP-4) inhibitors, glucagon-like peptide-1 (GLP-1) agonists, and sodium-glucose contransporter-2 (SGLT-2) agents carry a lower but present risk of hypoglycemia, which may increase when combining agents from different categories.

Geriatric Considerations
- American Geriatric Society Beers Criteria recommend avoiding glyburide and chlorpropamide due to their prolonged half-life in older adults and risk for prolonged hypoglycemic episodes. Medications should be dosed for age and renal function.
- Individualize pharmacologic therapy in older adults to reduce the risk of hypoglycemia, avoid overtreatment, and simplify complex regimens if possible while maintaining the HbA1c target (1)[A].

Pediatric Considerations
Children may not realize when they have hypoglycemia, needing increased supervision during times of higher activity such as competitive sports. Children may have higher glycemic goals for this reason. Caregivers should be instructed in use of glucagon (2)[A].

Pregnancy Considerations
Hypoglycemia management and avoidance education should be reemphasized and blood glucose monitoring increased due to more stringent glycemic goals and increased risk in early pregnancy (1)[A].

GENERAL PREVENTION
- Maintain routine schedule of diet (consistent CHO intake), medication, and exercise (1)[A].
- Self-monitoring of blood glucose (SMBG) or continuous glucose monitoring (CGM)
  - Particularly helpful for asymptomatic hypoglycemia
  - Use if taking insulin or secretagogue.
  - Use ≥3 times daily testing if multiple injections of insulin, insulin pump therapy, or pregnant diabetic; frequency and timing dictated by needs and treatment goals
- Diabetes treatment and teaching programs (DTTPs) especially for high-risk type 1 patients, which teach flexible insulin therapy to enable dietary freedom
- Hypoglycemia may be decreased with use of insulin analogs, continuous SC insulin infusion (CSII) pumps, and CGM systems (1)[A].

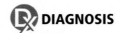

DIAGNOSIS

HISTORY
Discuss timing of episodes, awareness, frequency, and causes (1). Symptoms vary considerably between individuals.
- Adrenergic symptoms: hunger, trembling, pallor, sweating, shaking, pounding heart, anxiety, urinary incontinence
- Neurologic symptoms: dizziness, poor concentration, drowsiness, weakness, confusion, light-headedness, slurred speech, blurred vision, double vision, unsteadiness, poor coordination
  - Hypoglycemia causes a significant deterioration in reading span and subject-verb agreement, demonstrating that language processing is impaired during moderate hypoglycemia.
- Behavioral symptoms: tearfulness, confusion, fatigue, irritability, aggressiveness
- If altered cognition, consider hypoglycemia.
- Surgical history including but not limited to bariatric procedures such as gastric sleeve or Roux-en-Y gastric bypass

PHYSICAL EXAM
- General: confusion, lethargy
- HEENT: diplopia
- Coronary: tachycardia
- Neurologic: tremulousness, weakness, paresthesia, stupor, seizure, or coma
- Mental status: irritability, anxiety, inability to concentrate, or short-term memory loss
- Skin: pale, diaphoresis
- End-organ damage: microvascular, macrovascular, ophthalmologic, neurologic, renal

DIFFERENTIAL DIAGNOSIS
Hypoglycemia not associated with DM may be seen in:
- Chronic alcoholics and binge drinkers
- GI dysfunction causing postprandial hypoglycemia or alimentary reactive hypoglycemia
- Hormonal deficiency states (hormonal reactive hypoglycemia)
- Hypoglycemia of sepsis
- Islet cell tumors
- Factitious hypoglycemia from surreptitious injection of insulin

DIAGNOSTIC TESTS & INTERPRETATION
- Plasma, serum, or whole-blood glucose
- SMBG and CGM are especially useful for asymptomatic hypoglycemia (2)[A].
- Low HbA1c level may be due to chronic hypoglycemia.
- Disorders that may alter lab results: Conditions that affect erythrocyte turnover, such as hemolysis or blood loss, and hemoglobin variants may alter HbA1c (1)[A].

Follow-Up Tests & Special Considerations
A hypoglycemic reading from a CGM sensor should be verified by SMBG fingerstick glucose testing prior to treatment, unless a specific device is approved otherwise.

TREATMENT

Fast-acting CHO at the hypoglycemia alert value of ≤70 mg/dL.

GENERAL MEASURES

- Glucose: pure glucose preferred; any form of CHO that contains glucose should be effective; avoid CHO high in protein for acute treatment or prevention of hypoglycemia (1)[A].
- Glucagon should be prescribed proactively to patients at risk for clinically significant hypoglycemia. People in close contact with these individuals should be instructed in how to use an emergency glucagon kit (1)[A].
- Insulin-treated patients with hypoglycemia unawareness or an episode of clinically significant hypoglycemia should have glycemic targets raised to strictly avoid hypoglycemia (1)[A].
- α-Glucosidase inhibitors (acarbose) prevent digestion of complex CHOs; therefore, hypoglycemia must be treated with monosaccharides, such as glucose tablets.
- Patients with T1DM should use insulin analogs to reduce hypoglycemia risk (1)[A].
- Address medications (i.e., insulin, sulfonylureas, GLP-1 agonists, thiazolidinediones) that may induce hypoglycemia.
- CGM-augmented CSII with automated insulin suspension when blood glucose falls below a threshold value reduces the combined rate of severe and moderate hypoglycemia in T1DM and reduces nocturnal hypoglycemia without increasing HbA1c levels in patients >16 years old (3)[A].

MEDICATION

- Conscious patients (1)[A]
  - Glucose (15 to 20 g) is preferred, although any form of CHO may be used.
    - Any sugar-containing food or beverage that can be rapidly absorbed: juice or nondiet soda (4 to 5 oz), candy (5 to 6 pieces of hard candy), or OTC glucose tablets (4 tablets = 16 g CHO)
    - Takes ~15 minutes for CHOs to be digested and enter bloodstream as glucose
    - "Rule of 15": 15 to 20 g CHO (~60 to 80 calories simple CHO) repeated q15min until blood sugar is ≥70 mg/dL
- Loss of consciousness at home or people unable or unwilling to consume CHO by mouth—administer glucagon (1)[A].
  - IM or SC in the deltoid or anterior thigh; powder that requires reconstitution prior to injection
    - Age <6 years and/or weight <20 to 25 kg: 0.50 mg
    - Age ≥6 years and/or weight >20 to 25 kg: 1 mg
    - May repeat dose in 15 minutes if needed
  - Intranasal glucagon—comes in a ready-to-use fixed-dose autoinjector; does not require active participation from the patient. Place the device in one nostril followed by pressing a plunger (1).
    - Age ≥4 years: 3 mg initial dose; may repeat dose in 15 minutes if needed

- In unconscious, with emergency medical personnel present or patient hospitalized (3)[A]:
  - Give 25 g IV 50% dextrose every 5 to 10 minutes until patient awakens.
  - Then, feed orally and/or administer 5% dextrose IV at level that will maintain blood glucose >100 mg/dL.
  - Patients with hypoglycemia secondary to oral hypoglycemics should be monitored for 24 to 48 hours because hypoglycemia may recur after apparent clinical recovery.

ADMISSION, INPATIENT, AND NURSING CONSIDERATIONS

Admission criteria/initial stabilization

- Any doubt of cause
- Expectation of prolonged hypoglycemia (e.g., caused by sulfonylurea drug)
- Inability to drink/eat
- Treatment has not resulted in prompt sensory recovery.
- Seizures, coma, or altered behavior (e.g., ataxia, disorientation, unstable motor coordination, dysphasia) secondary to documented or suspected hypoglycemia
- Discharge criteria: Normoglycemia and risk of severe hypoglycemia are negligible (1).

ONGOING CARE

FOLLOW-UP RECOMMENDATIONS

Discuss hypoglycemia prevention at all visits.

DIET

- Alcohol consumption may place patients with DM at increased risk for delayed hypoglycemia (1)[A].
- CHO sources high in protein should not be used to treat or prevent hypoglycemia (1)[A].
- Fats may slow absorption of CHOs and may prolong the acute glycemic response (1)[A].
- Food insecurity increases risk of hypoglycemia due to inadequate or erratic CHO consumptions following administration of sulfonylureas or insulin (1)[A].

PATIENT EDUCATION

- Always have access to fast-acting CHO.
- Consider ingestion of added CHO or a reduced insulin dose if preexercise blood sugar is <100 mg/dL.
- Educate patients, their relatives, close friends, teachers, and supervisors of DM diagnosis and signs/symptoms of hypoglycemia and treatment.
- Teach SMBG and self-adjustment for insulin therapy, diet control, and exercise regimen.
- Wear medical alert identification bracelet or necklace.

COMPLICATIONS

- Coma, seizure, myocardial infarction, stroke (especially in elderly)
- Prolonged or severe hypoglycemia may cause permanent neurologic damage and/or cognitive impairment.
- Children with T1DM have a greater vulnerability to neurologic manifestations of hypoglycemia.

REFERENCES

1. ElSayed NA, Aleppo G, Aroda VR, et al; for American Diabetes Association. 6. Glycemic targets: standards of care in diabetes—2023. *Diabetes Care*. 2023;46(Suppl 1):S97–S110.
2. Seaquist ER, Anderson J, Childs B, et al; for American Diabetes Association, Endocrine Society. Hypoglycemia and diabetes: a report of a workgroup of the American Diabetes Association and the Endocrine Society. *J Clin Endocrinol Metab*. 2013;98(5):1845–1859.
3. Cryer PE, Axelrod L, Grossman AB, et al; for Endocrine Society. Evaluation and management of adult hypoglycemic disorders: an Endocrine Society clinical practice guideline. *J Clin Endocrinol Metab*. 2009;94(3):709–728.

ADDITIONAL READING

Allen KV, Pickering MJ, Zammitt NN, et al. Effects of acute hypoglycemia on working memory and language processing in adults with and without type 1 diabetes. *Diabetes Care*. 2015;38(6):1108–1115.

SEE ALSO

- Diabetes Mellitus, Type 1
- Algorithm: Hypoglycemia

CODES

ICD10

- E11.649 Type 2 diabetes mellitus with hypoglycemia without coma
- E10.649 Type 1 diabetes mellitus with hypoglycemia without coma
- E13.649 Oth diabetes mellitus with hypoglycemia without coma

CLINICAL PEARLS

- Abnormally low concentration of glucose in patients with DM; often referred to as an *insulin reaction*
- Treatment includes:
  - Immediate administration of glucose—in form of CHO (oral), IM, IV, or intranasal glucagon
  - Patient education and empowerment—address hypoglycemia in every visit with patients at risk.
  - Frequent SMBG or CGM with flexible insulin (or other drug) regimens
  - Individualized glycemic goals based in part on the risk of hypoglycemia
- Using the "rule of 15" is an easy way to teach patients to manage hypoglycemia at home. "Rule of 15": 15 to 20 g CHO (~60 to 80 calories simple CHO) SMBG and repeated q15min until blood sugar is ≥70 mg/dL

H

HYPOGLYCEMIA, NONDIABETIC

Matthew A. Silva, PharmD, RPh, BCPS • Pablo I. Hernandez Itriago, MD, MHCM, FAAFP

 BASICS

DESCRIPTION

- Hypoglycemia is defined by the Whipple triad as low plasma glucose level (≤60 mg/dL) with hypoglycemic symptoms that are relieved when glucose is corrected.
- Occurs commonly in patients with diabetes receiving insulin secretagogues (sulfonylureas, meglitinides) or insulins; is less common in patients without diabetes
- Hypoglycemia is also seen after GI or bariatric surgery (in association with dumping syndrome).
- Postprandial or reactive hypoglycemia is insulin dependent and occurs in response to a meal, nutrients, drugs, or herbal substances and may occur 2 to 3 hours postprandially or later.
- Spontaneous (fasting) hypoglycemia may be associated with primary conditions including hypopituitarism, Addison disease, myxedema, rare metabolic diseases and inborn errors of metabolism such as glycogen storage disease, critical illness, heart failure, hepatic or renal failure, and sepsis

EPIDEMIOLOGY

Incidence
0.5–8.6% of hospitalized patients aged ≥65 years without diabetes

ETIOLOGY AND PATHOPHYSIOLOGY

- Reactive, postprandial, insulin dependent
  - Alimentary hyperinsulinism
  - Meals including refined or processed carbohydrates, liquid forms of fructose, sucrose, or glucose
  - Certain nutrients, including galactose, leucine
  - Glucose intolerance (prediabetes)
  - GI surgery, especially bariatric surgery (i.e., Roux-en-Y gastric bypass)
- Spontaneous
  - Fasting
  - Restricted food access (i.e., unhoused persons, persons in hospitals, prisons)
  - Alcohol or prescription medication–associated (insulin, sulfonylureas, meglitinides, thiazolidinediones, incretin mimetics, sodium-glucose cotransporter-2 [SGLT 2] inhibitors, DPP-IV inhibitors, angiotensin-converting enzyme-inhibitors, β-blockers, salicylates, quinine, hydroxychloroquine, fluoroquinolones, doxycycline and tetracycline derivatives, linezolid, sertraline, disopyramide, pentamidine, gabapentin, tramadol) (1)
  - Consider medication administration errors as a source of unexplained hypoglycemia in persons without diabetes, especially those with polypharmacy.
  - Poisoning (ethanol, wild-mushroom, β-adrenergic receptor antagonists) and toxidromes (salicylates, NSAIDs, oral hypoglycemics)
  - Nonprescription over-the-counter (OTC) agents, including performance-enhancing agents; adulterated versions of phosphodiesterase inhibitors and performance-enhancing agents are routinely imported and adulterated, containing sulfonylureas and other hypoglycemic agents.

- Natural medicines or herbs (bitter melon, caffeine, cassia cinnamon, chromium, fenugreek, ginseng, guarana, mate, stevia, vanadium)
- Postsurgical (e.g., Roux-en-Y bariatric surgery, gastrectomy) hypoglycemia/dumping syndrome
- Islet cell hyperplasia or tumor (insulinomas), leukemia or other neoplasia-related process (tumor mediated insulin-like growth factor 2 [IGF-2]) and insulin receptor upregulation
- Extrapancreatic insulin-secreting tumors and other large tumors secreting IGF-2
- Autoimmune hypoglycemia (Hirata disease) and insulin receptor mutations
- Heart failure with or without SGLT-2 inhibitors (empagliflozin, dapagliflozin, canagliflozin)
- Hepatic disease or failure; renal disease or failure
- Renal glycosuria
- Glucagon deficiency
- Adrenal insufficiency
- Catecholamine deficiency
- Hypopituitarism
- Hypothyroidism
- Eating disorders
- Exercise or physical activity (i.e., manual labor)
- Pregnancy
- Severe nutrient deficiencies (i.e., selenium)
- Ketotic hypoglycemia of childhood
- Congenital disorders and errors of inborn metabolism, glycogen storage disease
- Sepsis, cachexia, anorexia

Genetics
Monogenic and congenital hyperinsulinism (i.e., channelopathies, enzyme and transport anomalies, transcription factor or enzyme abnormalities) (2)

RISK FACTORS
Prolonged fasting or inability to consume food and nutrition orally, alcohol, medications, pregnancy, critical illness or surgery, endocrine diseases or tumors, excess caffeine, a family history of congenital disorders of inborn metabolism or glycogen storage diseases

GENERAL PREVENTION
- Follow dietary and exercise guidelines.
- Patient recognition of early symptoms and knowledge of corrective action

Pediatric Considerations
- Usually divided into two syndromes:
  - Transient neonatal hypoglycemia
  - Hypoglycemia of infancy and childhood
- Screening infants for hypoglycemia is appropriate when pregnancy was complicated by maternal diabetes.
- Cases of hypoglycemia observed in children taking propranolol for infantile hemangioma
- Associated with indomethacin when treating patent ductus arteriosus
- Consider errors of inborn metabolism, galactosemia, fructose intolerance, and glycogen storage disease in children and young adults.

Geriatric Considerations
- More likely to have underlying disorders or be caused by medications
- Iatrogenic hypoglycemia is common in the hospitalized elderly with renal insufficiency.

COMMONLY ASSOCIATED CONDITIONS
- Heart failure; severe, chronic hepatic and renal disease; alcoholism
- Addison disease; adrenocortical insufficiency
- Myxedema
- Malnutrition (patients with renal failure)
- GI and bariatric surgery
- Panhypopituitarism
- Insulinoma and other neoplastic process

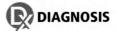 **DIAGNOSIS**

HISTORY
- Adrenergic symptoms are prominent with acute drop in glucose ≤60 mg/dL.
  - Anxiety, tremulousness, dizziness
  - Diaphoresis, flushing
  - Heart palpitations
  - Adrenergic symptoms may be masked by β-receptor antagonists (i.e., metoprolol, propranolol, bisoprolol, carvedilol) or rate-blocking calcium channel antagonists (verapamil, diltiazem)
- CNS (neuroglycopenic) symptoms appear at a serum glucose ≤50 mg/dL.
  - Headache
  - Light-headedness, fatigue, and weakness
  - Visual disturbances
  - Changes in personality, confusion
- GI and cholinergic symptoms
  - Hunger, nausea, belching
  - Diaphoresis, palmar sweating

PHYSICAL EXAM
- CNS (neuroglycopenic) symptoms predominate with gradual glucose reduction:
  - Convulsions, coma
  - Hypotension
- Adrenergic and cholinergic symptoms: more prominent in acute drop in glucose
  - Tremulousness
  - Diaphoresis, flushing
  - Heart palpitations

DIFFERENTIAL DIAGNOSIS
- CNS disorders
- Psychogenic/pseudohypoglycemia: Symptoms of hypoglycemia or self-diagnosis in patients in whom low blood glucose may not be detectable and may be impossible to convince that they do not suffer from hypoglycemia after all tests are found to be normal.

DIAGNOSTIC TESTS & INTERPRETATION

Initial Tests (lab, imaging)
- Blood glucose ≤45 mg/dL (≤2.5 mmol/L) when symptomatic followed by symptom resolution with feeding (3)[C]
- Plasma glucose overnight fasting: ≤60 mg/dL (≤3.33 mmol/L); confirm on two or more occasions (3)[C].
- Plasma glucose 72-hour fasting: ≤45 mg/dL (≤2.5 mmol/L) for females; ≤55 mg/dL (≤3.05 mmol/L) for males; fasting may be ended when Whipple triad is achieved or hypoglycemia is demonstrated (3)[C].
- Imaging (abdominal) using transabdominal ultrasound, CT, MRI, or PET (2)[C]

Follow-Up Tests & Special Considerations
- Misinterpretation of glucose tolerance tests may lead to misdiagnosis of hypoglycemia; ≥1/3 of normal patients have hypoglycemia, with or without symptoms, during the 4-hour glucose tolerance test. These patients may be at future risk for type 2 diabetes.
- If hypoglycemia presents as a primary disorder, consider hyperinsulinism and extrapancreatic tumors.
- C-peptide measurement (3)[C]
- Check liver studies, serum insulin, adrenocorticotropic hormone (ACTH), and cortisol. Serum insulin should be suppressed when glucose is <60 mg/dL (2)[C].
- Serum β-hydroxybutyrate <2.7 mg/dL in the presence of high-serum insulin, C-peptide, and low-serum glucose suggests excessive insulin production (3)[C].
- Insulin radioimmunoassay: Elevated insulin levels suggest islet cell hyperplasia or tumor.
- Drugs that may alter lab results: Many drugs can affect glucose levels. Review drugs individually and refer to drug or laboratory reference.
- Ensure comprehensive medication reconciliation to address medication, supplements, and recreational substances, and consider toxicology workup (i.e., salicylates, NSAIDs, β-receptor antagonists).

Diagnostic Procedures/Other
For definitive diagnosis (2),(3)[C]:
- Document low glucose levels and symptoms with low levels.
- Evidence that symptoms are relieved by ingestion of glucose or food
- Identify the specific type of hypoglycemia (2),(3)[C].

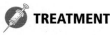

TREATMENT

GENERAL MEASURES
- Oral carbohydrate for alert patient without drug overdose (2 to 3 tbsp of sugar in glass of water or fruit juice, 1 to 2 cups of milk, piece of fruit, or several soda crackers)
- If unable to swallow: Use glucagon IM or SC.

- Discontinue, avoid, or control causative medications/agents.
- Avoid alcohol.
- If triggered by meals: Try high-protein diet with carbohydrate restriction.
- Nonhypoglycemic hypoglycemia or pseudohypoglycemia
- Symptoms may pertain to chronic fatigue and somatic complaints.
- Management difficult; listening is important. Try 120 g carbohydrate diet.
- Counseling may be useful for stress and other problems.

MEDICATION
- Once diagnosis is established, begin therapy that is appropriate for underlying disorder (3)[C].
- If unable to swallow: glucagon 1 mg (1 unit) IV, IM, or SC; if no response, give IV bolus of 25 to 50 g of 50% glucose solution followed by continuous infusion until patient is able to take by mouth; intranasal glucagon is 3 mg (one actuation per device) into a single nostril; may repeat 1 time after 15 minutes if there is no response using a second intranasal device (2)[C]
- Postsurgical gastrectomy patients who are unresponsive to dietary changes may benefit from propantheline, psyllium, fiber, or oat bran to delay gastric emptying.

ISSUES FOR REFERRAL
Refer if suspecting rare inborn errors of metabolism, genetic disorders, fructose intolerance, galactosemia or glycogen storage disease, or refractory to usual treatments

SURGERY/OTHER PROCEDURES
If islet cell tumor (insulinoma) or other insulin-secreting tumor, surgery is treatment of choice; if inoperable, diazoxide may relieve symptoms (2)[C].

ADMISSION, INPATIENT, AND NURSING CONSIDERATIONS
Persistent hypoglycemia unresponsive to oral intake of glucose

 ONGOING CARE

FOLLOW-UP RECOMMENDATIONS
Patient Monitoring
Hypoglycemia from sulfonylureas can last for hours to days depending on half-life and renal function.

DIET
- High protein, high fiber, complex carbohydrates from plant and multigrain sources (whole food) with some fat
- Frequent small feedings (six daily); avoid liquid calories (2)[C].
- Avoid fasting.

PATIENT EDUCATION
- Recognition of early symptoms of hypoglycemia and how to take corrective action
- Exercise routine or daily activity may need to be adjusted.
- Patients with recurrent hypoglycemia should have glucose source at hand for immediate ingestion during symptoms.

PROGNOSIS
Favorable, with appropriate treatment

COMPLICATIONS
- Insulinoma: If tumor is identified and removed, some surgical risk is involved.
- Organic brain syndrome: may occur with extensive, prolonged hypoglycemia

REFERENCES
1. Ben Salem C, Fathallah N, Hmouda H, et al. Drug-induced hypoglycaemia: an update. *Drug Saf*. 2011;34(1):21–45.
2. Kittah NE, Vella A. MANAGEMENT OF ENDOCRINE DISEASE: pathogenesis and management of hypoglycemia. *Euro J Endocrinol*. 2017;177(1):R37–R47.
3. Cryer PE, Axelrod L, Grossman AB, et al. Evaluation and management of adult hypoglycemic disorders: an Endocrine Society clinical practice guideline. *J Clin Endocrinol Metab*. 2009;94(3):709–728.

 SEE ALSO

- Hypoglycemia, Diabetic; Insulinoma
- Algorithm: Hypoglycemia

CODES

ICD10
- E16.2 Hypoglycemia, unspecified
- E16.1 Other hypoglycemia
- P70.4 Other neonatal hypoglycemia

CLINICAL PEARLS
- Symptoms coincide with low blood glucose levels and resolve with PO/IV glucose or glucagon.
- Avoid known agents/nutrients that trigger hypoglycemia.
- Treat the underlying cause.

H

HYPOKALEMIA

Robert A. Baldor, MD, FAAFP • Sibley Strader, MD

BASICS

DESCRIPTION
A serum potassium concentration <3.5 mEq/L (normal range, 3.5 to 5 mEq/L).
- Mild: 3 to 3.5 mEq/L
- Moderate: 2.5 to 3 mEq/L
- Severe: <2.5 mEq/L

EPIDEMIOLOGY
Predominant sex: male = female

Prevalence
- Commonly encountered in clinical practice
- >20% of hospitalized patients (when defined as potassium <3.6 mEq/L)
- >10% of inpatients with alcoholism
- 80% of patients receiving diuretics
- 12–18% of patients with chronic kidney disease
- Higher (5–20%) in individuals with eating disorders
- Higher in patients with AIDS
- Associated risk after bariatric surgery

ETIOLOGY AND PATHOPHYSIOLOGY
Most common causes:
- Decreased intake: deficient diet in alcoholics and elderly; anorexia nervosa
- GI loss: vomiting, diarrhea, nasogastric tubes, laxative abuse, fistulas, colorectal tumor, bowel diversion, ureterosigmoidostomy, malabsorption, chemotherapy, radiation enteropathy, bulimia
- Intracellular shift of potassium: metabolic alkalosis, insulin excess, β-adrenergic catecholamine excess (acute stress, β_2-agonists), hypokalemic periodic paralysis, intoxications (theophylline, caffeine, barium, toluene), refeeding syndrome (1), intensive exercise
- Renal potassium loss
  - Drugs: diuretics especially loop and thiazides, amphotericin B, aminoglycosides, antipseudomonal penicillin (carbenicillin), high-dose penicillin, clay (bentonite)
  - Mineralocorticoid excess: primary hyperaldosteronism (Conn syndrome); secondary hyperaldosteronism (congestive heart failure, cirrhosis, nephrotic syndrome, malignant hypertension, renin-producing tumors); renovascular hypertension
  - Exogenous mineralocorticoids (glycyrrhizic acid in licorice, carbenoxolone, nasal steroids)
  - Osmotic diuresis (e.g., poorly controlled diabetes)
  - Types I and II renal tubular acidosis
- Magnesium depletion
- Glucocorticoid excess: Cushing syndrome, exogenous steroids, ectopic adrenocorticotrophic hormone production, refeeding syndrome
- Diabetic ketoacidosis (DKA) treatment with delayed/inadequate potassium replenishment

Genetics
Some rare, familial disorders that can cause hypokalemia
- 11-β-Hydroxysteroid dehydrogenase deficiency
- Apparent mineralocorticoid excess
- Congenital adrenogenital syndromes
- Familial glucocorticoid resistance
- Familial hypokalemic periodic paralysis
- Familial interstitial nephritis
- Fanconi syndrome
- Geller syndrome
- Sodium channel mutations: Bartter, Gitelman, Liddle syndromes

RISK FACTORS
- Higher systolic BP
- Thiazide/loop diuretic use; ACE
- Low serum cholesterol/low BMI
- Higher albumin-to-creatinine ratio

GENERAL PREVENTION
When initiating a diuretic, monitor potassium level.

COMMONLY ASSOCIATED CONDITIONS
- Acute GI illnesses with severe vomiting or diarrhea
- Increased risk of cardiac arrhythmias
- Predictor of development of severe alcohol withdrawal syndrome

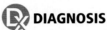

DIAGNOSIS

- Usually asymptomatic until serum potassium is <3.0 mEq/L, unless it falls rapidly or patient has potentiating factor, for example, disposition to arrhythmia
- Signs and symptoms mainly involve neuromuscular, cardiovascular, renal, and endocrine system.

HISTORY
- Diuretic use, malnutrition, vomiting, diarrhea
- Easy fatigability, leg cramps, muscle weakness
- Polyuria, polydipsia, nocturia; hyperglycemia, alkalosis/acidosis
- Heart failure, shortness of breath

PHYSICAL EXAM
- Neuromuscular—skeletal muscle weakness (proximal > distal), ascending paralysis
  - Smooth muscle—GI hypomobility
  - Respiratory muscle—respiratory acidosis, respiratory arrest
- Cardiovascular—hypotension, orthostasis, peripheral edema; auscultate for arrhythmias and rales.
- Renal—metabolic acidosis, rhabdomyolysis, myoglobinuria; chronic kidney disease (tubulointerstitial nephritis, nephrogenic diabetes insipidus, renal cyst)

DIFFERENTIAL DIAGNOSIS
Hypokalemia is a laboratory diagnosis that does not require distinction from other entities once laboratory error has been excluded.

DIAGNOSTIC TESTS & INTERPRETATION
- Serum potassium <3.5 mEq/L (<3.5 mmol/L)
- Disorders that may alter lab results: leukemia and leukocytosis

Initial Tests (lab, imaging)
- ECG
- Start workup if history rules out GI or iatrogenic causes (2).
  - Serum and urinary potassium level to evaluate the severity of hypokalemia
  - Basic metabolic panel (serum sodium, potassium, glucose, chloride, bicarbonate, BUN, creatinine); serum magnesium, calcium, and/or phosphorus to exclude associated electrolyte abnormality especially if alcoholism is suspected.
  - Spot urine electrolytes (potassium and chloride) to differentiate renal versus nonrenal cause.
  - Arterial blood gas to detect metabolic acidosis or alkalosis
  - Urinalysis and urine pH for renal tubular acidosis
  - Serum digoxin level for patient on digitalis
  - Creatine kinase for rhabdomyolysis in severe hypokalemia
  - Clinical suspicion is high: urine/serum drug screen for amphetamines and other sympathomimetic stimulants; TSH in case of tachycardia or suspicion of hypokalemic periodic paralysis

Follow-Up Tests & Special Considerations
- Two major components (2)
  - Urine potassium excretion to distinguish renal loss versus other causes
  - Acid–base status
- 24-hour urinary potassium excretion (best method): >15 mEq/day = inappropriate renal loss; if unavailable:
  - Spot urine potassium-to-creatinine ratio >13 mEq/g (1.5 mEq/mmol) can indicate inappropriate renal loss; or
  - Transtubular potassium gradient (TTKG) >4 can also suggests renal loss
    - TTKG = (urine K^+ / plasma K^+) / (urine Osm/ plasma Osm)
- Metabolic acidosis + low urinary excretion → GI loss
- Metabolic acidosis + urinary potassium wasting → DKA, renal tubular acidosis type 1 or 2
- Metabolic alkalosis + low urinary excretion → vomiting or diuretic use
- Metabolic alkalosis + urine potassium wasting →
  - Normotensive: vomiting (low urine chloride); Gitelman/Bartter syndrome (normal urine chloride), diuretics (Urine chloride varies with types.)
  - Hypertensive: primary aldosteronism, Liddle syndrome, Geller syndrome, glucocorticoid resistance
- If excessive renal potassium loss (>20 mEq/day) and hypertension, obtain plasma renin and aldosterone levels to differentiate adrenal from nonadrenal causes of hyperaldosteronism.

Diagnostic Procedures/Other
Consider imaging in cases with high clinical index of suspicion (2)
- MRI/CT of adrenal gland with suspicion of mineralocorticoid, glucocorticoid, or catecholamine excess
- MRI of pituitary gland to exclude Cushing syndrome
- Abdominal CT for VIPoma

Test Interpretation
ECG
- T-wave flattening, ST-segment changes
- U waves (small, positive deflection after T wave, best seen in V_2 and V_3)
- Arrhythmias include sinus bradycardia, PAC/PVC, paroxysmal atrial or junctional tachycardia, atrioventricular block, ventricular tachycardia or fibrillation.

TREATMENT

- Reduce potassium loss.
- Replenish stored potassium.
- Evaluate potential toxicities.
- Determine cause.

GENERAL MEASURES
Manage underlying disease or eliminate causative factor.

- Discontinue laxative, use potassium-neutral or potassium-sparing diuretics.
- Treat diarrhea and vomiting.
- Use H_2 blockers in patient with nasogastric suction.
- Control hyperglycemia if glucosuria is present.

MEDICATION
- Nonemergent conditions (serum potassium >2.5 mEq/L [>2.5 mmol/L], no cardiac manifestations)
  - Oral therapy preferred: 40 to 120 mEq/day (40 to 120 mmol/day) in divided doses
  - Ensure adequate hydration (100 to 250 mL of water), better if given with or after meal.
  - IV potassium only when oral administration is not feasible (e.g., vomiting, postoperative state)
    - Rate should not exceed 10 mEq/hr, and concentration should not exceed 40 mEq/L to lessen burning and discomfort at IV site and to avoid phlebitis.
    - A central line is recommended for rate >10 mEq/hr; up to 40 mEq in 100 mL can be safely given via central access.
    - Potassium chloride (KCl) is suitable for all forms of hypokalemia.
    - Potassium bicarbonate or precursor (gluconate, acetate, or citrate) in metabolic acidosis
    - Potassium phosphate in phosphate deficiency as in DKA (3)[C]
- Emergent situations (serum potassium <2.5 mEq/L [<2.5 mmol/L], arrhythmias) (2)[A]
  - IV replacement—standard infusion rate: 10 mmol/hr; maximum infusion rate: 20 mmol/hr
  - Central line preferred
- If patient is hypomagnesemic (2)[A]
  - First, give 4 mL MgSO4 50% (8 mmol) in 10 mL of NaCl 0.9% >20 minutes and then start first 40 mmol KCl infusion followed by magnesium replacement.
- Precautions
  - Any form of potassium replacement carries the risk of hyperkalemia.
  - Serum potassium should be checked more frequently in groups at higher risk: the elderly, diabetic patients, and patients with renal insufficiency.
  - Patients receiving insulin for DKA require more timely and aggressive potassium replacement in order to account for the intracellular shift (4)[A].
  - Dietary potassium is almost entire coupled to phosphate, rather than chloride, and does not correct potassium loss from chloride depletion (e.g., diuretics or vomiting).
- Significant possible interactions: Concomitant administration of potassium-sparing diuretics (spironolactone, triamterene, amiloride, ACE inhibitors) magnifies risk of hyperkalemia.

Geriatric Considerations
- Younger patient has a higher prevalence for hypokalemia, but elderly develop hypokalemia more rapidly.
- Low serum potassium can induce limb paralysis, myonecrosis, and increase fall risk.

ISSUES FOR REFERRAL
Patient with unexplained hypokalemia, refractory hyperkalemia, or features suggesting alternative diagnosis (e.g., aldosteronism or hypokalemic periodic paralysis) should be referred to endocrinology or nephrology.

ADMISSION, INPATIENT, AND NURSING CONSIDERATIONS
- Outpatient follow-up is sufficient for asymptomatic patients treated with oral replacement.
- Patients with cardiac manifestations require IV replacement with continuous cardiac monitoring in an inpatient setting.
- Patient with life-threatening complications such as arrhythmias or respiratory failure requires ICU admission.

 ONGOING CARE

FOLLOW-UP RECOMMENDATIONS
Patient Monitoring
- Patients receiving IV therapy should have continuous cardiac monitoring and serum potassium level monitored q4–6h.
- Patients requiring potassium supplements should have serum potassium and magnesium levels repeated at intervals dictated by clinical judgment and patient compliance (5)[C].

DIET
- Ensure adequate intake: potassium-rich food including oranges, bananas, cantaloupes, prunes, raisins, dried beans, dried apricots, and squash
- Reduce sodium intake: High-sodium diet can cause urinary potassium loss.

PATIENT EDUCATION
- Instructions for appropriate diet
- Emphasis the risk of nonadherence to potassium supplement.
- National Institutes of Health, Office of Dietary Supplements "Potassium Fact Sheet for Consumers": https://ods.od.nih.gov/pdf/factsheets/Potassium-Consumer.pdf

PROGNOSIS
- Most hypokalemia will correct with replacement after 24 to 72 hours.
- If primary cause is eliminated, hypokalemia will likely resolve with no further treatment needed.
- Associated with higher morbidity and mortality because of cardiac arrhythmias

COMPLICATIONS
- Hyperkalemia during the course of treatment
- Increased risk of digoxin toxicity
- Increased risk of arrhythmias by increasing myocyte's resting potential and in turn its refractory period

REFERENCES

1. Palmer BF. A physiologic-based approach to the evaluation of a patient with hypokalemia. *Am J Kidney Dis*. 2010;56(6):1184–1190.
2. Kardalas E, Paschou SA, Anagnostis P, et al. Hypokalemia: a clinical update. *Endocr Connect*. 2018;7(4):R135–R146.
3. Asmar A, Mohandas R, Wingo CS. A physiologic-based approach to the treatment of a patient with hypokalemia. *Am J Kidney Dis*. 2012;60(3):492–497.
4. Kovesdy CP, Matsushita K, Sang Y, et al. Serum potassium and adverse outcomes across the range of kidney function: a CKD Prognosis Consortium meta-analysis. *Eur Heart J*. 2018;39(17):1535–1542.
5. Unwin RJ, Luft FC, Shirley DG. Pathophysiology and management of hypokalemia: a clinical perspective. *Nat Rev Nephrol*. 2011;7(2):75–84.

ADDITIONAL READING
- Skogestad J, Aronsen JM. Hypokalemia-induced arrhythmias and heart failure: new insights and implications for therapy. *Front Physiol*. 2018;9:1500.
- Viera AJ, Wouk N. Potassium disorders: hypokalemia and hyperkalemia. *Am Fam Physician*. 2015;92(6):487–495.

 SEE ALSO

- Hyperkalemia
- Algorithm: Hypokalemia

 CODES

ICD10
E87.6 Hypokalemia

CLINICAL PEARLS
- In patients with cardiac ischemia, heart failure, or left ventricular hypertrophy, even mild to moderate hypokalemia can cause arrhythmias. These patients should receive potassium repletion as well as cardiac monitoring.
- Uncorrected hypomagnesemia can hinder the correction of hypokalemia.
- Hypokalemia in an otherwise healthy young woman should prompt evaluation for bulimia nervosa.
- Supplement potassium when prescribing drugs that cause hypokalemia; minimize dosage of non–potassium-sparing diuretics.

H

HYPONATREMIA

Summer Chavez, DO, MPH, MPM

BASICS

DESCRIPTION

- Hyponatremia is a plasma sodium (Na^+) concentration of ≤135 mEq/L.
- Hyponatremia itself does not provide information about the total body water (TBW) state of the patient. Patients with hyponatremia may be hypervolemic, hypovolemic, or euvolemic.
- System(s) affected: endocrine/metabolic, renal, cardiovascular, central nervous system (CNS)

EPIDEMIOLOGY

Prevalence
- Most common electrolyte disorder seen in the general hospital population, affecting 2.5%
- 7.7% outpatients (1)

Geriatric Considerations
Elderly patients have a decreased renal mass placing them at risk for decreased urinary concentration and decreased response to antidiuretic hormone. Presenting symptoms may be frequent falls and gait disturbances. Clinicians should also consider the impact of comorbidities and acute disease.

Pediatric Considerations
Children are at increased risk of brain herniation from cerebral edema.

ETIOLOGY AND PATHOPHYSIOLOGY

- Volume status and serum osmolality must be ascertained to determine etiology in order to direct management (2).
- Normal serum osmolality is 280 to 295 mOsmol/kg.
- Serum osmolality (Osm) (mOsm/kg) = (2 × serum [Na]) + (serum [glucose] / 18) + (blood urea nitrogen [BUN] / 2.8)
- Hypertonic hyponatremia: serum Osm >295 mOsmol/kg
  – Accumulation of solutes that are osmotically active, causing water shifts from intracellular fluid (ICF) to extracellular fluid (ECF), resulting in dilution.
    ○ Unchanged TBW and Na^+
    ○ Causes: hyperglycemia, mannitol, sorbitol, radiologic contrast
- Isotonic hyponatremia ("pseudohyponatremia"): serum Osm 275 to 295 mOsmol/kg
  – Falsely low levels of sodium; actual levels are normal.
  – Osmolality is normal; usually euvolemic
  – Unchanged TBW and Na^+
  – Causes: hyperlipidemia, hyperproteinemia (e.g., multiple myeloma), laboratory artifact, irrigant solutions, hyperglycemia
- Hypotonic hyponatremia: serum Osm <275 mOsmol/kg
  – Subdivided by volume status into hypovolemic, euvolemic, or hypervolemic
  – Hypovolemic hyponatremia: low TBW and low Na^+
- Signs include orthostatic hypotension, decreased skin turgor, dry mucous membranes.
- If urine Na^+ <30 mmol/L, it indicates extrarenal loss such as GI loss (vomiting, diarrhea), third-spacing (pancreatitis, burns), skin loss (burns, cystic fibrosis, sweating), and heat-related illnesses.

- If urine Na^+ >30 mmol/L, it indicates renal loss such as cerebral salt wasting, adrenal insufficiency, diuretics, and osmotic diuresis.
- Euvolemic hyponatremia: mild to moderate increase in TBW, normal Na^+ (most common subtype)
- Signs include a nonedematous state.
- If urine Osm >100 mOsm/kg, causes include syndrome of inappropriate antidiuretic hormone (SIADH), hypothyroidism, adrenal insufficiency, medications (e.g., thiazide diuretics, loop diuretics, carbamazepine, clofibrate, cyclosporine, levetiracetam, oxcarbazepine, SSRIs, TCAs, vincristine, barbiturates, chlorpropamide, opioids).
- If urine Osm <100 mOsm/kg, causes include primary polydipsia, beer potomania, and exercise-induced hyponatremia.
- Hypervolemic hyponatremia: increased TBW and Na^+
- Signs include edematous state.
- Urine Na^+ <30 mmol/L
- Causes include congestive heart failure (CHF), cirrhosis, nephrotic syndrome, hypoalbuminemia, psychogenic polydipsia, and renal failure.

Genetics
Mutations have been associated with nephrogenic syndrome of inappropriate antidiuresis (NSAID; SIADH).

COMMONLY ASSOCIATED CONDITIONS
- Hypothyroidism, hypopituitarism
- Cirrhosis, CHF, nephrotic syndrome
- Adrenocortical hormone deficiency
- SIADH is associated with cancers, pneumonia, tuberculosis, encephalitis, meningitis, head trauma, cerebrovascular accident, and HIV infection.
- Marathon runners in hot environments
- Beer potomania
- Tea-and-toast diet
- Ecstasy use

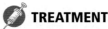**DIAGNOSIS**

- Symptoms are related to the rate of fall in serum Na^+, onset, and degree of hyponatremia (1)[C],(3)[C].
- Acute (≤48 hours): no time for full adaptation, more likely to present with moderate or severe symptoms
- Chronic (>48 hours): develops gradually, organ systems adapt to Na^+ concentration, associated with minimal symptoms
- Mild (serum Na^+ 130 to 135 mEq/L): usually asymptomatic, fatigue, loss of appetite
- Moderate (serum Na^+ 120 to 130 mEq/L): nausea, vomiting, lethargy
- Severe (serum Na^+ 115 to 120 mEq/L): headache, lethargy, restlessness, disorientation
- Severe/rapid decrease in serum Na^+ can cause seizures, coma, brain herniation, respiratory arrest, and may be fatal.
- Other signs and symptoms: headache, dizziness, ataxia, weakness, muscle cramps, anorexia, hiccups, depressed deep tendon reflexes, hypothermia, positive Babinski responses, cranial nerve palsies, orthostatic hypotension

HISTORY
- Symptoms include headache, nausea, vomiting, and muscle cramps.
- Can progress to lethargy or restlessness and disorientation

PHYSICAL EXAM
- Volume status: skin turgor, jugular venous pressure, heart rate, peripheral edema, orthostatic blood pressure measurement
- Evaluate for underlying illness: signs of CHF, cirrhosis, hypothyroidism.
- Decreased reflexes may be seen.
- Evaluate patient's gait for unsteadiness and ataxia. Perform a complete neurologic exam.

DIFFERENTIAL DIAGNOSIS
See "Etiology and Pathophysiology."

DIAGNOSTIC TESTS & INTERPRETATION

Initial Tests (lab, imaging)
- BUN, creatinine, glucose, electrolytes, liver function studies
- Thyroid-stimulating hormone (TSH)
- Lipid panel
- Serum osmolality
- Urine Na^+ and osmolality
- Chest x-ray to rule out pulmonary pathology if SIADH is diagnosed

Follow-Up Tests & Special Considerations
CT scan of head if pituitary problem is suspected or if SIADH from CNS problem is suspected.

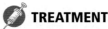**TREATMENT**

GENERAL MEASURES
- Assess all medications that patient is taking.
- Institute seizure precautions.
- Institute fluid restriction for hypervolemic patients.
- Fluid resuscitation in hypovolemic patients. Indications for 3% hypertonic saline versus normal saline solution include: acute hyponatremia, symptomatic hyponatremia, association with intracranial pathology already at risk for cerebral edema (1)[C],(3)[C].

MEDICATION

- Treatment is tailored to etiology, degree of hyponatremia, onset, and symptomatology; some general principles apply:
  - Expected change in serum Na^+ with selected infusate: $\Delta Na = [(\text{infusate } Na^+ + \text{infusate } K^+ - \text{serum } Na^+) / (TBW + 1)]$
  - TBW = a coefficient $\times$ weight (kg) as in the following table:

Total Body Water	
Children and men	$0.6 \times$ weight
Women and elderly men	$0.5 \times$ weight
Elderly women	$0.45 \times$ weight

  - Formula to determine correction available at https://www.mdcalc.com/calc/480/sodium -correction-rate-hyponatremia-hypernatremial
  - Asymptomatic, euvolemic patients can be treated with fluid restriction; etiology must be addressed.
- Severe hyponatremia (<125 mEq/L) 3% hypertonic saline should be given.
  - Done as a 100 to 150 mL bolus, with the goal of increasing the serum Na^+ 2 to 3 mEq/L. The bolus may be given twice if symptoms have not resolved.
  - Done as a continuous infusion of 3% to increase the serum Na^+ 6 to 8 mEq/L, with the goal to not exceed correction of 10 to 12 mEq/L in the first 24 hours.
  - Desmopressin can also be considered, given 1 to 2 μg every 4 to 6 hours.
  - Serum Na^+ should be checked every 2 hours. The infusion rate and fluids should be changed to isotonic saline when appropriate.
  - In patients who do not respond to the aforementioned approach, consider the use of vasopressin V2-receptor antagonists, such as tolvaptan or conivaptan. This class of medications should not be in used in patients with liver disease.
  - For mild to moderate hyponatremia, use isotonic saline solution (0.9%).
  - In patients with severe hyponatremia (euvolemic and hypervolemic state) who do not respond to the aforementioned approach, consider the use of vasopressin V2-receptor antagonists, such as tolvaptan or conivaptan (5)[A]. This class of medications should not be in used in patients with liver disease (2).
  - Patients with hypervolemic hyponatremia caused by cirrhosis, heart failure, or kidney disease benefit from restriction of sodium and fluids, diuretic therapy, and management of the underlying etiology.
  - Treat underlying etiology.
  - Chronic hyponatremia resulting from SIADH (6)[A]: demeclocycline (inhibits ADH action at the collecting duct) if fluid restriction alone is not effective
    - Contraindications: drug allergy, pregnancy, children <8 years old; caution in renal and hepatic disease
    - In doses of 600 to 1,200 mg/day, the drug produces nephrogenic diabetes insipidus.
    - Significant possible interactions: oral anticoagulants, oral contraceptives, penicillin

  - In case of overcorrection, re-lower Na^+ concentration. Begin with infusion of 3 mL/kg of 5% dextrose in water over 1 hour. Repeat Na^+ measurement. Be cautious, dextrose infusion rates >250 to 300 mL/hr can cause significant hyperglycemia in both diabetic and nondiabetic patients and may lead to osmotic diuresis and subsequent free water loss with increased serum Na^+ concentration. Consider 2 to 4 μg IV desmopressin every 8 hours to prevent overcorrection.

ALERT
Caution: If severe, consider hypertonic saline (3% Na^+ chloride) with central line access, exercise extreme caution, and monitor serum Na^+ as frequently as every 1 to 2 hours.

First Line
- Fluid resuscitation (hypovolemia)
- Fluid restriction (euvolemia/hypervolemia)

Second Line
Vasopressin V2-receptor antagonists

ADMISSION, INPATIENT, AND NURSING CONSIDERATIONS
- Admission is mandatory if the patient is symptomatic or has acute hyponatremia (developing over <48 hours), which increases the risk of cerebral edema.
- Admission is advised if patient is asymptomatic and has a serum Na^+ <125 mEq/dL.

 ## ONGOING CARE

DIET
- Euvolemic hyponatremia: Restrict water to 1 to 1.5 L/day.
- Hypervolemic hyponatremia: water and Na^+ restriction

PROGNOSIS
- In hospitalized patients, hyponatremia is associated with an elevated risk of adverse clinical outcomes and higher mortality (1).
- Recently, in community-dwelling, middle-aged, and elderly adults, mild hyponatremia has been shown to be an independent predictor of death.
- Associated with poor prognosis in patients with acute pulmonary embolism
- Associated with poor prognosis in patients with liver cirrhosis and those waiting for liver transplant; it is associated with significant postoperative risk and short-term graft loss.

COMPLICATIONS
- Occult tumor may be present if SIADH is identified.
- Hypervolemia if isotonic saline solution is used
- Osmotic demyelination (central pontine and extrapontine irreversible myelinolysis) if the Na^+ is corrected too quickly (1)
- Hyponatremia is the cause of 30% new-onset seizures in intensive care settings.

- Can cause hyponatremic encephalopathy and brain herniation if severe and untreated, especially in young women and children (3)
- Chronic hyponatremia associated with increased risk of osteoporosis, attention deficit, gait disturbances, falls, and fractures.

REFERENCES
1. Rondon-Berrios H, Agaba EI, Tzamaloukas AH. Hyponatremia: pathophysiology, classification, manifestations and management. *Int Urol Nephrol*. 2014;46(11):2153–2165.
2. Braun MM, Barstow CH, Pyzocha NJ. Diagnosis and management of sodium disorders: hyponatremia and hypernatremia. *Am Fam Physician*. 2015;91(5):299–307.
3. Williams DM, Gallagher M, Handley J, et al. The clinical management of hyponatraemia. *Postgrad Med J*. 2016;92(1089):407–411.
4. Singh TD, Fugate JE, Rabinstein AA. Central pontine and extrapontine myelinolysis: a systematic review. *Eur J Neurol*. 2014;21(12):1443–1450.
5. Rozen-Zvi B, Yahav D, Gheorghiade M, et al. Vasopressin receptor antagonists for the treatment of hyponatremia: systematic review and meta-analysis. *Am J Kidney Dis*. 2010;56(2):325–337.
6. Basu A, Ryder REJ. The syndrome of inappropriate antidiuresis is associated with excess long-term mortality: a retrospective cohort analyses. *J Clin Pathol*. 2014;67(9):802–806.

 SEE ALSO

Algorithm: Hyponatremia

CODES

ICD10
E87.1 Hypo-osmolality and hyponatremia

CLINICAL PEARLS
- Assess all medications that patient is taking because many are associated with hyponatremia.
- Alcohol-dependent individuals with vitamin deficiencies, elderly women taking thiazide diuretics, and people with hypokalemia or burns are at increased risk of central pontine myelinolysis from too rapid correction of hyponatremia. Chronic hyponatremia is also a risk factor.
- Bronchogenic carcinoma and pancreatic, duodenal, and prostate cancer, as well as thymoma, lymphoma, and mesothelioma, are neoplastic diseases associated with SIADH.
- Formulas have been developed (Adrogue and Madias) for safe correction of hyponatremia and are available online (see https://www.mdcalc.com /calc/480/sodium-correction-rate-hyponatremia -hypernatremia).

H

HYPOPARATHYROIDISM

Caroline E. Cox, MD

BASICS

DESCRIPTION
- Deficient or absent secretion of parathyroid hormone (PTH), a major hormone regulator of serum calcium and phosphorus levels in the body (1)
- Acute hypoparathyroidism: tetany that is mild (muscle cramps, perioral numbness, paresthesias of hands and feet) or severe (carpopedal spasm, laryngospasm, heart failure, seizures, stridor)
- Chronic: often asymptomatic; lethargy, anxiety/depression, urolithiasis and renal impairment, dementia, blurry vision from cataracts or keratoconjunctivitis, parkinsonism or other movement disorders, mental retardation, dental abnormalities, and dry, puffy, coarse skin
- System(s) affected: endocrine/metabolic, musculoskeletal, nervous, ophthalmologic, renal

Pediatric Considerations
- May occur in premature infants
- Neonates born to hypercalcemic mothers may experience suppression of developing parathyroid glands.
- Congenital absence of parathyroids
- May appear later in childhood as autoimmune

Geriatric Considerations
Hypocalcemia is fairly common in elderly, however, rarely secondary to hypoparathyroidism.

Pregnancy Considerations
- Use of magnesium as a tocolytic may induce functional hypoparathyroidism.
- For women with hypoparathyroidism, calcitriol requirements decrease during lactation.

EPIDEMIOLOGY
More common in women; affects all ages

Incidence
- Most common after surgical procedure of the anterior neck, particularly when the surgeon performs few anterior neck dissections (<50–100 thyroidectomies/parathyroidectomies per year).
- Transient hyperparathyroidism is common (6.9–46% of thyroidectomies), whereas permanent hypoparathyroidism differs depending on surgeon and facility expertise.

Prevalence
- Affects 24 to 37/100,000 persons per year in the United States (1)
- Genetic disorders account for <10% of all hypoparathyroidism, but represent a large proportion of cases in children.

ETIOLOGY AND PATHOPHYSIOLOGY
- PTH aids in regulating calcium homeostasis:
  - Mobilizes calcium and phosphorus from bone stores
  - Increases calcium absorption from the intestine by stimulating formation of 1,25-dihydroxy vitamin D
  - Stimulates reabsorption of calcium in the distal convoluted tubule and phosphate excretion in proximal tubule
- Reduced or absent PTH action results in hypocalcemia, hyperphosphatemia, and hypercalciuria.

- Acquired hypoparathyroidism
  - Surgical: removal or damage to parathyroid glands or their blood supply/enervation during neck surgery for thyroidectomy/parathyroidectomy, or neck surgery for head and neck cancers (2)
  - Autoimmune: isolated or combined with other endocrine deficiencies in polyglandular autoimmune (PGA) syndrome
  - Deposition of heavy metals in gland: copper (Wilson disease) or iron (hemochromatosis, thalassemias), radiation-induced destruction, and metastatic infiltration
  - Functional hypoparathyroidism: may result from hypomagnesemia or hypermagnesemia because magnesium is crucial for PTH secretion and activation of the PTH receptor
  - Congenital
    - Calcium-sensing receptor (CaSR) abnormalities: hypocalcemia with hypercalciuria
    - HDR or Barakat syndrome: deafness, renal dysplasia
    - Familial: mutations of the *TBCE* gene; abnormal PTH secretions
    - 22q11.2 deletion syndrome
- Autoimmune: genetic gain-of-function mutation in CaSR
- Infiltrative: metastatic carcinoma, hemochromatosis, Wilson disease, granulomas

Genetics
- X-linked or in autosomal recessive mutations in the transcription factor glial cell missing B (GCMB)
- Mutations in transcription factors or regulators of parathyroid gland development
  - Component of a larger genetic syndrome (APS-1 or DiGeorge syndrome) or in isolation (X-linked hypoparathyroidism) (3)
  - May be autosomal dominant (DiGeorge), autosomal recessive (APS-1), or X-linked recessive (X-linked hypoparathyroidism) (3)
  - Congenital syndromes
    - 22q11.2 deletion syndrome, familial hypomagnesemia, hypoparathyroidism with lymphedema (3)
    - Hypoparathyroidism with sensorineural deafness
    - ADHH: mutations gain-of-function of the CaSR gene suppressing the parathyroid gland, without elevation of PTH
  - PGA syndrome type I: mucocutaneous candidiasis, hypoparathyroidism, and Addison disease

RISK FACTORS
Neck surgery and neck trauma, neck malignancies, family history of hypocalcemia, PGA syndrome

GENERAL PREVENTION
Intraoperative identification and preservation of parathyroid tissue

COMMONLY ASSOCIATED CONDITIONS
- DiGeorge syndrome
- Bartter syndrome
- PGA syndrome type I
- Multiple endocrine deficiency autoimmune candidiasis (MEDAC) syndrome
- Juvenile familial endocrinopathy
- Addison disease
- Moniliasis (HAM) syndrome: a polyglandular deficiency syndrome, possibly genetic, characterized by hypoparathyroidism

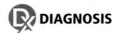

DIAGNOSIS

HISTORY
Often asymptomatic; ask about previous neck trauma or surgery, head or neck irradiation, family history of hypocalcemia, or presence of other autoimmune endocrinopathies.
- Cardinal clinical feature: neuromuscular hyperexcitability
- Also includes: fatigue, circumoral or distal extremity paresthesias, muscle spasm, seizures, neuropsychiatric symptoms

PHYSICAL EXAM
- Surgical scar on neck
- Chvostek sign: ipsilateral twitching of the upper lip on tapping the facial nerve on the cheek. 15% of normocalcemic people have positive sign (1).
- Trousseau sign: painful carpal spasm after 3-minute occlusion of brachial artery with BP cuff. BP cuff inflation to above systolic BP for 3 minutes leads to carpal spasm (flexion of metacarpophalangeal [MCP] joints, extension of interphalangeal [IP] joints, adduction of fingers and thumb).
- Tetany, laryngo- or bronchospasm, cardiac arrhythmias, refractory heart failure, dyspnea, edema
- Dry, coarse, puffy hair; brittle nails
- Loss of deep tendon reflexes
- Dysrhythmias (secondary hypocalcemia)
- Cataracts or ectopic calcifications
- Tooth enamel defects
- Vitiligo

DIFFERENTIAL DIAGNOSIS
- Vitamin D deficiency/resistance
- Pseudohypoparathyroidism, which presents in childhood; kidney and bone unresponsiveness to PTH; characterized by hypocalcemia, hyperphosphatemia, and, in contrast to hypoparathyroidism, elevated rather than reduced PTH concentrations
- Hypoalbuminemia, renal failure, malabsorption, familial hypocalcemia, hypomagnesemia

DIAGNOSTIC TESTS & INTERPRETATION
Initial Tests (lab, imaging)
- Calcium: low ionized and total (Correct serum calcium level for albumin.)
  - Corrected serum calcium = total serum calcium + 0.8 (4 − serum albumin)
- Phosphorus: high
- Intact or "whole" PTH: low; distinguish from pseudohypoparathyroidism or secondary causes
- Magnesium: low or normal
- BUN, creatinine: Monitor renal function, especially in the elderly.
- 25-OH vitamin D level: Vitamin D deficiency can worsen hypoparathyroidism.
- Urinary calcium: normal or high
- Calcium should be monitored after thyroid or parathyroid surgery, including intraoperatively
- Radiographs may show absent tooth roots, calcification of cerebellum, choroid plexus, or cerebral basal ganglia.

Follow-Up Tests & Special Considerations

- ECG: prolongation of ST and QTc intervals, nonspecific repolarization changes, dysrhythmias
- Urine calcium: Creatinine ratio (normal 0.1 to 0.2) may be low before treatment but should be monitored to prevent stones due to hypercalciuria.
- Gene sequencing: Evaluation of other hormone levels may be required to diagnose APS-1.
- Hungry bone syndrome (transient hypoparathyroidism after parathyroid surgery)
  - Hypocalcemia due to hungry bone syndrome may persist despite recovery of PTH secretion from the remaining normal glands. Thus, serum PTH concentrations may be low, normal, or even elevated.
- Osteoblastic metastasis of prostate, breast, or lung cancer; consider appropriate imaging.
- Autoantibodies against NACHT leucine-rich-repeat protein 5 (NALPS) found in 49% of 73 patients with APS-1 and hypoparathyroidisms

 TREATMENT

GENERAL MEASURES

- Monitor ECG during calcium repletion.
- Maintenance therapy: may require lifelong treatment with calcium and calcitriol
  - Maintain serum calcium in low normal range: 8 to 8.5 mg/dL (2.00 to 2.12 mmol/L).
- If hypercalcemia occurs, hold therapy until calcium returns to normal. Treat magnesium deficiency if present.
- Phosphate binders are required if high calcium-phosphate product.
- Thiazide diuretics combined with a low-salt diet may be used to prevent hypercalciuria, nephrocalcinosis, and nephrolithiasis.
- Oral calcium administration and vitamin D supplementation after thyroidectomy may reduce the risk for symptomatic hypocalcemia after surgery.

MEDICATION

- Acute hypoparathyroidism
  - Hypoparathyroid with severe symptoms (tetany, seizures, cardiac failure, laryngospasm, bronchospasm)
    - IV calcium gluconate: 1 or 2 g, each infused over a period of 10 minutes. Central venous catheter is preferred because calcium-containing solutions can irritate surrounding tissues. Follow with infusion of 10 g calcium gluconate in 1 L 5% dextrose water at a rate of 1 to 3 mg calcium gluconate per kg body weight per hour (2)[B].
  - Hypomagnesemia: acutely: 1 to 2 g IV q6h; long-term magnesium oxide tablets (600 mg) once or twice per day
  - Maintenance: See "First Line" treatment for chronic hypoparathyroidism.
- Chronic hypoparathyroidism

First Line

- Adults
  - Oral calcium carbonate: preferred due to high elemental calcium concentration; take with meals and stop PPI for better absorption.
- Oral calcium citrate: preferred for patients on PPI therapy and those with constipation on calcium carbonate
- Starting dose: 1 to 3 g/day of elemental calcium, although doses vary widely; divided doses preferred

- Calcitriol (vitamin D 1, 25-dihydroxycholecalciferol): preferred form of vitamin D replacement; start at 0.25 µg/day; doses 0.5 to 2.0 µg/day are usually required (3)[A].
- For hypercalciuria, consider a thiazide diuretic.
- For phosphate level well above normal (>6.5 mg/dL), use low phosphate diet or phospate binder.
- Children
  - Oral elemental calcium: 25 to 50 mg/kg daily
  - Calcitriol: 0.25 µg daily for age >1 year

ISSUES FOR REFERRAL

- Endocrinologist.
- Refer to nephrologist for renal impairment or recurrent stones; ophthalmologist for eye involvement; geneticist for inherited concerns

ADDITIONAL THERAPIES

PTH peptides 1–34 and 1–84 SC

- rhPTH 1-84—FDA-approved, 50 µg SC daily
- For patients with frequent episodes of hyper- and hypocalcemia, nephrolithiasis, nephrocalcinosis, GFR <60 mL/min, persistently high phosphate (4)[B]
- Treatment goal: Eliminate use of active vitamin D_3, reduce supplemental calcium to 500 mg daily; maintain consistent calcium level in low normal range.
- Improved well-being and increased bone mineral density have been shown for these patients.

SURGERY/OTHER PROCEDURES

Autotransplantation of cryopreserved parathyroid tissue: restores normocalcemia in 23% of cases

ADMISSION, INPATIENT, AND NURSING CONSIDERATIONS

- Admission criteria/initial stabilization: laryngospasm, seizures, tetany, QT prolongation
- Discharge criteria: resolution of hypocalcemic symptoms, patient educated on hypoparathyroidism and treatment

 ONGOING CARE

FOLLOW-UP RECOMMENDATIONS

Patient Monitoring

- Goal is a total corrected serum calcium level in low normal range (8.0 to 8.5 mg/dL or 2.00 to 2.12 mmol/L), 24-hour urine calcium <300 mg, and calcium-phosphate product <55. If calcium <2.0 mmol/L or <8.0 mg/dL, then treat even if asymptomatic (4)[B].
- Outpatient measurement of serum calcium, phosphate, magnesium, and creatinine weekly to monthly during initial management; for changes in medication, check weekly or every other week; when stable, measure every 6 months (4)[B].
- 24-hour urine for calcium and Cr secretion yearly
- If symptoms of renal stone disease or increasing Cr, get renal imaging every 5 years (4)[B].
- Annual slit-lamp and ophthalmologic evaluations are recommended.
- DEXA scan: standard monitoring recommended (4)[B]

DIET

Low-phosphate diet in patients with hyperphosphatemia

PATIENT EDUCATION

https://www.hypopara.org/

PROGNOSIS

Hypoparathyroidism following neck surgery is often transient. Length of required treatment may vary depending on origin.

COMPLICATIONS

- Reversible: due to low calcium levels, most likely to improve with adequate treatment
  - Neuromuscular symptoms: paresthesias (circumoral, fingers, toes), tetany, seizures, parkinsonian symptoms; pseudotumor cerebri has been described.
  - Renal: hypercalciuria, nephrocalcinosis, nephrolithiasis
  - Cardiovascular: heart failure, arrhythmias
- Irreversible: when condition starts early in childhood and will not improve with calcium and vitamin D treatment
  - Stunting of growth
  - Enamel defects and hypoplasia of teeth
  - Atrophy, brittleness, and ridging of nails
  - Cataracts and basal ganglia calcifications

REFERENCES

1. Abate E, Clarke B. Review of hypoparathyroidism. *Front Endocrinol (Lausanne)*. 2017;7:172.
2. Al-Azem H, Khan A. Hypoparathyroidism. *Best Pract Res Clin Endocrinol Metab*. 2012;26(4):517–522.
3. Bilezikian JP, Khan A, Potts JT Jr, et al. Hypoparathyroidism in the adult: epidemiology, diagnosis, pathophysiology, target-organ involvement, treatment, and challenges for future research. *J Bone Miner Res*. 2011;26(10):2317–2337.
4. Brandi M, Bilezikian D, Shoback D, et al. Management of hypoparathyroidism: summary statement and guidelines. *J Clin Endocrinol Metab*. 2016;101(6):2273–2283.

ADDITIONAL READING

- Bollerslev J, Rejnmark L, Marcocci C, et al. European Society of Endocrinology clinical guideline: treatment of chronic hypoparathyroidism in adults. *Eur J Endocrinol*. 2015;173(2):G1–G20.
- Michels TC, Kelly KM. Parathyroid disorders. *Am Fam Physician*. 2013;88(4):249–257.
- Stack BC Jr, Bimston DN, Bodenner DL, et al. American Association of Clinical Endocrinologists and American College of Endocrinology disease state clinical review: postoperative hypoparathyroidism—definitions and management. *Endocr Pract*. 2015;21(6):674–685.

 CODES

ICD10

- E20 Hypoparathyroidism
- E20.8 Other hypoparathyroidism
- E20.0 Idiopathic hypoparathyroidism

CLINICAL PEARLS

Often asymptomatic; consider if hypocalcemic with fatigue and circumoral or distal extremity paresthesias.

- Correct the serum calcium level for albumin level.
- Monitor calcium after thyroid or parathyroid surgery.
- Distinguish hypoparathyroidism from pseudohypoparathyroidism and secondary causes by PTH level.
- Not much clinical difference between 2nd- and 3rd-generation PTH assays
- Serum levels of magnesium and 25-OH should be measured to rule out deficiency that could contribute to reduced serum calcium levels.

H

HYPOTHERMIA
Corey J. Costanzo, DO, MPH, MS

 BASICS

DESCRIPTION
- Accidental hypothermia is the result of an unanticipated environmental exposure to cold temperatures. It is manifested as a core temperature of <35°C (95°F) and it may take hours to days to develop (1).
- Although patients with cold-water immersion may appear dead, they can sometimes be resuscitated; therefore, it is important to evaluate, treat as indicated, rewarm, and reassess (2).
- System(s) affected: all body systems
- Synonym(s): accidental hypothermia

EPIDEMIOLOGY
- Predominant age: young children and elderly
- Predominant sex: male > female

Geriatric Considerations
More common in elderly due to lower metabolic rate, impaired ability to maintain normal body temperature, and impaired ability to detect temperature changes (2)

Incidence
From 1999 to 2011, the CDC reported 16,911 deaths due to hypothermia.

Prevalence
Estimates vary widely; typically a secondary issue

ETIOLOGY AND PATHOPHYSIOLOGY
Core temperature is typically tightly maintained between 36.5 and 37.5°C. Accidental hypothermia is most often the result of overwhelming environmental cold stress. Other contributing factors include the following (1):
- Decreased heat production (e.g., hypopituitarism; hypothyroidism; adrenal insufficiency) (1)
- Increased heat loss (e.g., immersion—this is the most commonly encountered form of hypothermia in emergency situations—or burns) (1)
- Alcohol consumption (contributes in up to 68% of cases) (1)
- Impaired thermoregulation (e.g., stroke, central nervous system [CNS] tumors) (1)

Pediatric Considerations
- Children are at greater risk for hypothermia due to a larger ratio of surface area to body mass (2).
- Young infants cannot increase heat production through shivering and children have limited glycogen stores to maintain heat production.
- Children and infants have a decreased ability to recognize, avoid, or escape hypothermic exposure. Also, the history may not suggest hypothermia. Hypothermia does not require extreme exposure in children. Nonaccidental trauma may contribute.

RISK FACTORS
- Alcohol consumption; drug intoxication
- Bronchopneumonia
- Cardiovascular disease; cardiac arrest
- Cold-water immersion; prolonged environmental exposure
- Dermal dysfunction (burns, erythrodermas)
- Endocrinopathies (myxedema, severe hypoglycemia)
- Excessive fluid loss, malnutrition
- Hepatic failure; renal failure/uremia; sepsis
- Hypothalamic and CNS dysfunction
- Mental illness; Alzheimer disease
- Trauma (especially head) (1),(2)

GENERAL PREVENTION
- Appropriate clothing, with particular attention to head, feet, and hands (1).
- For outdoor activities, carry survival bags with rescue foil blanket and dry clothes for use if stranded or injured.
- Avoid alcohol.
- Remain alert to early symptoms and initiate preventive steps (e.g., drinking warm fluids, getting out of the cold) (1).
- Identify medications that may predispose to hypothermia (e.g., neuroleptics, sedatives, hypnotics, tranquilizers) (1).

COMMONLY ASSOCIATED CONDITIONS
- Addison disease; hypothyroidism; hypopituitarism; diabetes; ketoacidosis (2)
- CNS dysfunction
- Congestive heart failure
- Pulmonary infection; sepsis
- Uremia

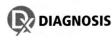 **DIAGNOSIS**

HISTORY
- Presentation varies with temperature of patient.
- The history is often apparent in the setting of outdoor environmental exposures. It may be less clear with cold indoor environments. Patients can present with confusion, dizziness, dyspnea, and altered mental status. Taking a careful history is particularly important in cases of "indoor hypothermia."

ALERT
History of prolonged exposure to cold may make the diagnosis obvious, but hypothermia may be overlooked in other situations, especially in comatose patients. Always obtain a core temperature if hypothermia is suspected.

PHYSICAL EXAM
- Esophageal temperature is most accurate, minimally invasive method of assessing core temperature (1).
  - Must have secure airway
  - Probe inserted into lower 3rd of esophagus
  - Peripheral thermometers are associated with reduced accuracy. The use of rectal thermometors is more accurate.
- Exam findings vary with the temperature of the patient at the time of presentation (2).
  - Mild (32–35°C)
    - Lethargy, shivering, mild confusion
    - Tachypnea, tachycardia, elevated BP
    - Hyperventilation
    - Loss of fine motor coordination
    - Peripheral vasoconstriction
    - Hyperactive reflexes
  - Moderate (28–32°C)
    - Delirium
    - Hypotension, hypoventilation
    - Cyanosis
    - Arrhythmias (bradycardia, prolonged PR interval, AV junctional rhythm, accelerated idioventricular rhythm, prolonged QT interval, altered T waves)
    - CNS depression, slowed reflexes
    - Muscular rigidity
    - Generalized edema

- Severe (<28°C)
  - Very cold skin
  - Rigidity, areflexia, unresponsive
  - Apnea
  - Bradycardia, hypotension
  - No pulse: ventricular fibrillation, asystole
  - Pupils (dilated <27°C; fixed and dilated <27°C)

ALERT
Use specially designed thermometers that can record low temperatures and measure core temperatures.

Pediatric Considerations
- Infants may present with bright red, cold skin, and lethargy.
- A child's body temperature drops faster than an adult does when immersed in cold water.
- Altered mental status is the most important clue to significant hypothermia in children (2).

DIFFERENTIAL DIAGNOSIS
- Cerebrovascular accidents
- Intoxication, drug overdose
- Complications of diabetes, hypothyroidism, hypopituitarism

DIAGNOSTIC TESTS & INTERPRETATION
Initial Tests (lab, imaging)
- Arterial blood gases (correct for temperature)
- CBC with platelet counts
- Serum electrolytes; BUN/creatinine; glucose; calcium; magnesium
- Urinalysis
- Coagulation studies; fibrinogen level
- Blood culture
- Liver function studies; amylase
- Cardiac enzymes
- Alcohol level and toxicology screen
- Cervical spine, chest, and abdomen x-rays, if appropriate
- Bedside ultrasound to assess hemodynamics
- CT of the head for any concern regarding mental status

Follow-Up Tests & Special Considerations
Serum cortisol and TSH if underlying endocrine dysfunction (Hypothalamus stimulates release of hormones in response to hypothermia.)

Diagnostic Procedures/Other
ECG

Test Interpretation
Serum potassium >12 mmol/L in adults is associated with nonsurvival.

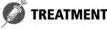 **TREATMENT**

GENERAL MEASURES
- Prehospital (2),(3)
  - Factors to guide treatment (Although helpful, core temperature should not be the sole basis to guide treatment.)
    - Level of consciousness
    - Shivering intensity
    - Cardiovascular stability based on blood pressure and cardiac rhythm

- Treatment (1),(3)
  - Basic life support (1)
  - Remove wet garments; dry the patient (3).
  - Protect against heat loss and wind chill.
  - If mildly hypothermic, with significant endogenous heat production from shivering, will likely be able to rewarm themselves with insulation and a vapor barrier; active rewarming will provide comfort and save energy.
  - For colder, nonshivering patients, add active rewarming—a nonshivering patient will not rewarm spontaneously (1).
    - Warm intravenous fluids before infusion (3).
    - Active rewarming can include warm blankets, heating pads, radiant heat, and forced warm air (3).
    - Give warm, humidified oxygen if available.
    - If far from definitive care, begin active rewarming but do not delay transport.
- See "Admission, Inpatient, and Nursing Considerations."

MEDICATION
- For sepsis or bacterial infections, begin antibiotics.
- For hypoglycemia: D50W at a dose of 1 mg/kg
- Thiamine: 100 mg, if alcoholic or cachectic
- Naloxone: 2 mg if opioid use suspected
- Levothyroxine: 150 to 500 μg for myxedema
- Severe acidosis: Consider sodium bicarbonate.
- Precautions (2)
  - Medications including epinephrine, lidocaine, and procainamide can accumulate to toxic levels if used repeatedly; avoid until core temperature is >30°C:
    - When temperature reaches >30°C, IV medications are indicated. Administer slowly.
  - Consider vasopressors according to standard ACLS algorithm with concurrent rewarming in setting of cardiac arrest.
  - Use all drugs cautiously due to impaired metabolism and renal elimination. Once rewarming has occurred, there is mobilization of depot stores.
  - Routine use of steroids or antibiotics does not increase survival or decrease postresuscitative damage.

ADMISSION, INPATIENT, AND NURSING CONSIDERATIONS
- Rewarming depends on severity of hypothermia and presence of cardiac arrest (1),(2),(3).
  - If no cardiac arrest, consider active external rewarming.
  - If cardiac arrest is present, consider active internal rewarming.
- Warm core first.
  - Don't rewarm frostbitten extremities until core temperature is >34°C (2).
- The rate of rewarming is determined by whether perfusing cardiac output is present.
  - If a perfusing cardiac output is present, 1–2°C/hr is appropriate. If not, use a faster rate of >2°C/hr.
- Monitor core temperature, blood pressure, and cardiac rhythm.
- Correct metabolic acidosis.
- Evaluate for frostbite and other trauma.
- Mild hypothermia
  - Passive rewarming
  - Administration of heated IV solutions
  - Provide warm fluids by mouth if fully alert.

- Moderate hypothermia
  - Active external rewarming
  - Administration of heated IV solutions
- Severe hypothermia (active internal [core] rewarming) (2)
  - Heated IV fluids
  - Heated humidified oxygen
  - Extracorporeal life support (preferred method in cardiac arrest)
    - Cardiopulmonary bypass, extracorporeal membrane oxygenation
  - Body cavity lavage (second options)
    - Thoracic cavity lavage, peritoneal lavage (40–45°C)
    - Continuous arteriovenous rewarming
    - Hemodialysis and hemofiltration
- Cardiac arrhythmias
  - Atrial fibrillation and sinus bradycardia are common—patients usually convert to NSR with rewarming.
  - If ventricular fibrillation is present, treat with one shock. If patient does not respond, consider deferring further attempts until rewarm has occurred.
  - Do not treat transient ventricular arrhythmias.
  - If cardiac pacing required, preferable to use external noninvasive pacemaker
- Admit patients, preferably to the ICU, with underlying disease, physiologic abnormalities, or core temperature <32°C.
- Normal saline is preferred as fluid of choice; IV bolus preferred over infusion when practical
- Heat IVs from 40°C to 42°C if possible—should be no colder than core temperature.

ALERT
- Avoid overheating dextrose solutions; dextrose caramelizes at 60°C (2).
- Avoid fluid overload. Avoid lactated Ringer solution because of decreased lactate metabolism.
- Heart is irritable and susceptible to arrhythmias; take care transporting.
- Electrolytes may fluctuate with rewarming; check electrolytes (particularly potassium) frequently.
- Monitor blood pressure frequently with rewarming as hypotension can develop from severe dehydration and fluid shifts.
- Discharge from emergency department once normothermic, if mild hypothermia and no predisposing conditions or complications and has suitable place to go. All others require admission.

ONGOING CARE

FOLLOW-UP RECOMMENDATIONS
Patient Monitoring
- During acute episode: Monitor cardiac rhythm, urinary output; check electrolytes, blood gases, and glucose frequently.
- Following acute episode: continued therapy for underlying disorder

DIET
Warm fluids only if alert and able to swallow
- Alcohol intake increases risk of becoming hypothermic in cold conditions.
- Refer to social service agency for help with housing, heat, and/or clothing, if appropriate.

PATIENT EDUCATION
Persons with known cardiovascular disease should use caution when exercising outdoors in cold weather.

PROGNOSIS
- Mortality rates are decreasing due to increased recognition and advanced therapy (2).
- Mortality usually depends on age and the severity of underlying cause and comorbidities.
  - Mortality rate in healthy patients is <5%; those with coexisting illness >50%.
  - Mortality rates increase with age. Over half of deaths are seen in patients aged >65 years.

COMPLICATIONS
- Core temperature after drop (2)
- Cardiac arrhythmias
- Hypotension, sepsis
- Hyperkalemia, hypoglycemia, metabolic acidosis
- Rhabdomyolysis
- Pneumonia, pulmonary edema, acute respiratory distress syndrome
- Pancreatitis, peritonitis, GI bleeding, ileus
- Acute tubular necrosis, bladder atony
- Intravascular thromboses/disseminated intravascular coagulation
- Gangrene of extremities
- Compartment syndrome
- Seizures, cerebral ischemia, delirium

REFERENCES
1. Dow J, Giesbrecht GG, Danzl DF, et al. Wilderness Medical Society Clinical Practice Guidelines for the out-of-hospital evaluation and treatment of accidental hypothermia: 2019 update. *Wilderness Environ Med*. 2019;30(4S):S47–S69.
2. Paal P, Gordon L, Strapazzon G, et al. Accidental hypothermia—an update: the content of this review is endorsed by the International Commission for Mountain Emergency Medicine (ICAR MEDCOM). *Scand J Trauma Resusc Emerg Med*. 2016;24(1):111.
3. Haverkamp FJC, Giesbrecht GG, Tan ECTH. The prehospital management of hypothermia—an up-to-date overview. *Injury*. 2018;49(2):149–164.

 CODES

ICD10
- T68.XXXA Hypothermia, initial encounter
- T68.XXXD Hypothermia, subsequent encounter
- T68.XXXS Hypothermia, sequela

CLINICAL PEARLS
- The most common cause of hypothermia in the United States is cold exposure associated with alcohol intoxication.
- With a severely decreased core temperature, begin resuscitation (if possible) unless there are obvious lethal injuries. Continue resuscitation and rewarm to 33–35°C and reassess.
- Hypothermia, coagulopathy, and acidosis are the trauma triad associated with higher rates of death (3).

HYPOTHYROIDISM, ADULT

Faraz Ahmad, MD, MPH • Hiba Ahmad, PharmD, BCOP • Ryan S. Poland, MD

BASICS

DESCRIPTION
- Clinical and metabolic state resulting from decreased levels of free thyroid hormone or from resistance to hormone action
- Classified as primary, central, or peripheral based on pathology in the thyroid, the pituitary or hypothalamus, or peripheral tissue, respectively (1)
- Subclinical: serum TSH above the upper reference limit with a normal free thyroxine (T_4) and normal hypothalamic-pituitary-thyroid axis (2)
- Overt: elevated TSH, typically 4 to 5 mIU/L with a subnormal free T_4

EPIDEMIOLOGY
Incidence
- Women: 3.5/1,000 persons per year
- Men: 0.6/1,000 persons per year

ETIOLOGY AND PATHOPHYSIOLOGY
- Primary: abnormality at the thyroid gland (>95% of cases)
- Most common cause worldwide: environmental iodine deficiency (2)[A]
- Most common cause in the United States: Hashimoto thyroiditis (chronic autoimmune thyroiditis)
  - Hashimoto thyroiditis is characterized by loss of thyroid function secondary to autoimmune-mediated destruction from thyroid antibodies.
  - The typical course of the disease is gradual loss of thyroid function.
- Postablative/posttherapeutic: follows radioactive iodine therapy or total/subtotal thyroidectomy for hyperthyroidism; radiotherapy or surgery for thyroid cancer, benign nodular thyroid disease, or neck malignancies
- Transient hypothyroidism: de Quervain thyroiditis (viral), postpartum, silent thyroiditis (3)
- Drug use: propylthiouracil, methimazole, lithium, amiodarone, antiepileptic drugs, and newer chemotherapeutic agents such as tyrosine kinase inhibitors (sunitinib), interleukin-2, or interferon-α
- Central: hypothyroidism due to insufficient stimulation by TSH of an otherwise normal thyroid gland; can be secondary (level of the pituitary) or tertiary (level of the hypothalamus)
- Consumptive: T_3 and T_4 excessively degraded by ectopically produced type 3 iodothyronine deiodinase (rare)
- Other etiologies include genetic defects, tumors, vascular, empty sella syndrome, inflammatory, infiltrative, iatrogenic, posttrauma, or drug related.

RISK FACTORS
- Personal or family history of autoimmune diseases
- External head or neck irradiation; radioiodine therapy or thyroid surgery
- Abnormal thyroid examination, presence of goiter and/or TPOAb positivity
- Treatment with amiodarone, lithium, interferon-α, sunitinib, or sorafenib
- Down syndrome or Turner syndrome

COMMONLY ASSOCIATED CONDITIONS
- Pernicious anemia
- Celiac disease
- Primary adrenal failure (Addison disease)
- Rheumatoid arthritis, systemic lupus erythematosus
- Depression

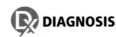
DIAGNOSIS

HISTORY
Symptoms can vary and can be nonspecific.
- Lethargy, fatigue
- Cold intolerance
- Constipation
- Dry skin
- Muscle cramps, arthralgias, paresthesias
- Modest weight gain (4 to 11 lb [1.8 to 5.0 kg])
- Menstrual disturbances, infertility, subfertility
- Depression
- Change in voice (hoarseness)
- Sleep apnea
- Carpal tunnel syndrome

PHYSICAL EXAM
- Dry, thickened skin
- Hair loss/brittle hair
- Periorbital edema
- Nonpitting swelling of hands and feet (myxedema)
- Bradycardia; reduced systolic, increased diastolic BP
- Delayed deep tendon reflex relaxation
- Macroglossia
- Goiter (iodine insufficiency, Hashimoto thyroiditis)

Geriatric Considerations
Frequently nonspecific signs and symptoms

DIFFERENTIAL DIAGNOSIS
- Chronic fatigue syndrome, depression
- Anemia
- Congestive heart failure
- Primary adrenal insufficiency

DIAGNOSTIC TESTS & INTERPRETATION
Initial Tests (lab, imaging)
- Primary hypothyroidism
  - Elevated TSH (>4.5 mIU/L)
  - Decreased serum free T_4 (3)[A]
- Central (secondary or tertiary) hypothyroidism (decreased TSH)
  - Assess free T_4 or free T_4 index (2)[A].
  - Decreased serum free T_4
  - Antithyroid antibodies absent
  - TRH stimulation test, especially if free T_4 and/or TSH is low-normal and patient has hypothalamo-pituitary pathology
  - Imaging of the hypothalamus and pituitary gland
- Subclinical hypothyroidism
  - Elevated serum TSH (>4.5 mIU/L)
  - Normal serum free T_4 (4)[A]
  - Note: Serum free triiodothyronine (T_3) or total T_3 should not be done to diagnose hypothyroidism (2)[A].

Follow-Up Tests & Special Considerations
- Antithyroid antibodies (primarily thyroid peroxidase antibodies and antithyroglobulin antibodies) may define the cause of primary hypothyroidism but are not necessary in all settings.
- Drugs that may alter lab results:
  - Drugs that decrease TSH: thyroid supplement, glucocorticoids, dopamine agonists, octreotide
  - Drugs that increase TSH: phenytoin, amiodarone, dopamine antagonist (metoclopramide/domperidone), oral cholecystographic dyes (sodium ipodate), or estrogen or androgen in excess
  - Drugs that increase free T_4: heparin, high intake of biotin
- Disorders that may alter lab results: any severe illness, pregnancy, chronic protein malnutrition, hepatic failure, or nephrotic syndrome
- TSH has circadian fluctuations, particularly higher levels in the evening.

Test Interpretation
Screening
- Patient with risks factors as described in "Risk Factors" section (2)[A]
- Patient with imaging abnormalities of thyroid or laboratory abnormalities including
  - Substantial hyperlipidemia or change in lipid pattern
  - Hyponatremia, often resulting from inappropriate production of antidiuretic hormone
  - High serum muscle enzyme concentrations
  - Macrocytic anemia
  - Pericardial or pleural effusion
  - Pituitary or hypothalamic disorder
- Pregnant women
  - Personal or family history of thyroid disease
  - Type 1 diabetes mellitus
  - History of recurrent miscarriage, morbid obesity, or infertility; TPO Ab should be considered (2)[A].
  - Universal screening not recommended for pregnant patients or planning pregnancy
- U.S. Preventive Services Task Force found insufficient evidence for or against screening nonpregnant, asymptomatic children or adults (3)[A].
  - ACOG recommends women with history of autoimmune disease or strong family history of thyroid disease should be screened at age 19 years.

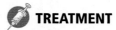
TREATMENT

MEDICATION
First Line
- Levothyroxine (Synthroid, Levothroid)
  - 1.5 to 1.8 μg/kg/day (use ideal body weight) (3)[A]; titrate by 12.5 to 25.0 μg/day q4–8wk until TSH is in normal range.
  - For patients with CAD, multiple comorbidities, or elderly, 12.5 to 25.0 μg is the recommended starting dose despite ideal body weight, titrating as above.
  - Elderly patients may require 2/3 of dose used in young adults because clearance is decreased.

– Dosage requirements may vary with age, gender, residual secretory capacity of thyroid gland, other drugs being taken by patient, and intestinal function (2)[A].

– Use caution when changing between capsule, tablet, and liquid because formulations may be absorbed differently.

– Levothyroxine should be taken on an empty stomach, ideally an hour before breakfast. Administering at bedtime may result in higher levels of T_4 than administering in the morning if taken at least 2 hours after last meal (5)[A].

– Medications that interfere with its absorption should be taken 4 hours after the T_4 dose; these include ferrous sulfate, proton pump inhibitors, calcium carbonate, and bile acid resins.

• Contraindications
  – Overt thyrotoxicosis
  – Uncorrected adrenocorticoid insufficiency
  – MI, acute
  – TSH suppression, preexisting

• Precautions
  – Diabetic patients may need readjustment of hypoglycemic agents with institution of T_4.
  – Dosage of vitamin K antagonists may need adjustment; monitor prothrombin time while initiating treatment.
  – Patients on digoxin may need close monitoring.
  – Elderly patients more susceptible to AFib and osteoporotic fracture with thyroid hormone excess
  – Patients requiring doses that are higher than expected should be evaluated for GI disorders that may lead to decrease thyroid hormone absorption (*Helicobacter pylori*, celiac disease).

• Controversy exists whether subclinical hypothyroidism should be treated. Cochrane Review found no improvement in survival, cardiovascular morbidity, or health-related quality of life. Subclinical hypothyroidism should be treated in patients with iron deficiency anemia and in patients with TSH >10 mIU/L (4),(6)[B],(7).

• If elective surgery: Achieve euthyroid state prior to procedure.

• If urgent surgery: proceed with individualized replacement therapy preoperatively and postoperatively.

• Brand and generic T_4 formulations available; likely equivalent efficacy of preparation when switching between manufactures; can measure serum TSH 6 weeks after changing manufactures if concerns

Pregnancy Considerations

• Replacement therapy may need adjustment; average dose increases from 25% to 50% (7)[A].

• TSH levels should be monitored monthly during first half of pregnancy and at least once in second half; goal TSH of 2.0 to 2.5 mIU/L for 1st trimester and <3 mIU/L for 2nd and 3rd trimesters (7)[A]

• Postpartum: Check TSH levels at 6 weeks (7)[A].

• Painless subacute thyroiditis may occur in postpartum period, leading to transient hypothyroidism lasting 2 weeks to 24 weeks. Treatment with replacement therapy may be warranted. Up to 30% of these individuals develop permanent hypothyroidism.

Second Line

Liothyronine (T_3) or desiccated thyroid hormone (T_3 and T_4) may be an alternative for patients who do not tolerate T_4 alone.

ISSUES FOR REFERRAL

• Children, infants, pregnancy or women planning conception
• Presence of goiter, nodule, or other structural changes in the thyroid gland
• Presence of adrenal or pituitary disorders (2)[C]

ADDITIONAL THERAPIES

There is little evidence for alternative therapies for hypothyroidism

ADMISSION, INPATIENT, AND NURSING CONSIDERATIONS

• Myxedema coma (decompensated severe untreated hypothyroidism)
• Hypotension or potentially fatal arrhythmias
• Pericardial or pleural effusion

 ## ONGOING CARE

FOLLOW-UP RECOMMENDATIONS
Patient Monitoring

• Monitor TSH and free T_4 every 4 to 8 weeks after initiating treatment or after change in dose. Once stabilized, periodic TSH level should be done after 6 months and then at 12-month intervals or more frequently if clinically indicated (2)[B].
• Monitor cardiac function in older patients.
• Check TSH more frequently during pregnancy, initiation of estrogen supplementation, or after large changes in body weight.
• In central hypothyroidism, TSH is unreliable; must monitor free T_4
• Thyroid hormones should not be used to treat obesity in euthyroid patients (2)[A].

PATIENT EDUCATION

• Describe signs of thyrotoxicity.
• Counsel patient on taking medications on empty stomach

PROGNOSIS

• Return to normal state is the rule.
• Relapses will occur if treatment is interrupted.
• If untreated, severe cases may progress to myxedema coma.

COMPLICATIONS

• Mortality and complication rates from surgery are similar between euthyroid patients and patients with mild to moderate hypothyroidism.
• Myxedema coma: mortality of 30–60%
• Increased susceptibility to infection
• Megacolon
• Sexual dysfunction, infertility
• Organic psychosis, depressed mood, apathy
• Hypersensitivity to opiates
• Treatment over long periods can lead to decreased bone mineral density.

• Iatrogenic thyrotoxicosis can lead to AFib and osteoporosis.
• Can precipitate adrenal crisis if levothyroxine initiated prior to steroids in patients with untreated adrenal insufficiency
• Treatment-induced congestive heart failure in people with coronary artery disease (small risk)

REFERENCES

1. Chaker L, Razvi S, Bensenor IM, et al. Hypothyroidism. *Nat Rev Dis Primers*. 2022;8(1):30.
2. Garber JR, Cobin RH, Gharib H, et al; for American Association of Clinical Endocrinologists, American Thyroid Association Taskforce on Hypothyroidism in Adults. Clinical practice guidelines for hypothyroidism in adults: cosponsored by the American Association of Clinical Endocrinologists and the American Thyroid Association. *Endocr Pract*. 2012;18(6):988–1028.
3. Chaker L, Bianco AC, Jonklaas J, et al. Hypothyroidism. *Lancet*. 2017;390(10101): 1550–1562.
4. Cooper DS, Biondi B. Subclinical thyroid disease. *Lancet*. 2012;379(9821):1142–1154.
5. Khandelwal D, Tandon N. Overt and subclinical hypothyroidism: who to treat and how. *Drugs*. 2012;72(1):17–33.
6. Jonklaas J, Bianco AC, Bauer AJ, et al; for American Thyroid Association Task Force on Thyroid Hormone Replacement. Guidelines for the treatment of hypothyroidism: prepared by the American Thyroid Association Task Force on Thyroid Hormone Replacement. *Thyroid*. 2014;24(12):1670–1751.
7. Alexander EK, Marqusee E, Lawrence J, et al. Timing and magnitude of increases in levothyroxine requirements during pregnancy in women with hypothyroidism. *N Engl J Med*. 2004;351(3): 241–249.

H

 ## CODES

ICD10
• E03.9 Hypothyroidism, unspecified
• E06.3 Autoimmune thyroiditis
• E89.0 Postprocedural hypothyroidism

CLINICAL PEARLS

• Screening test: Order TSH levels; serum free T_4 should be obtained only if TSH is abnormal and not as part of initial screening test (2)[A].
• Monitor TSH and free T_4 every 4 to 8 weeks after initiating treatment or after change in dose. Once stabilized, periodic TSH level should be done after 6 months and then at 12-month intervals or more frequently if clinically indicated.

ID REACTION

Sahil Mullick, MD • Diana V. Steau, MD

BASICS

DESCRIPTION
A generalized skin reaction associated with various infectious (fungal, bacterial, viral, or parasitic) or inflammatory cutaneous conditions distant from the primary disease site (1)
- "Id" is often combined with a root to reflect the causative factor (i.e., bacterid, syphilid, and tuberculid). Dermatophytid is the most frequently referenced id reaction. A dermatophytid is an autosensitization reaction in which a secondary cutaneous reaction occurs at a site distant to a primary fungal infection. The eruption typically begins within 1 to 2 weeks of the onset of the main lesion or following exacerbation of the main lesion.
- Most commonly localized vesicular lesions, erythema nodosum, and erythema multiforme; more uncommonly, can cause presence of vesicles and pustules
- System(s) affected: skin/exocrine
- Synonym(s): dermatophytid, trichophytid, autoeczematization

EPIDEMIOLOGY
- Predominant age: all ages
- Predominant sex: male = female
- Predominant race: all races

Incidence
Unknown

Prevalence
Common

ETIOLOGY AND PATHOPHYSIOLOGY
Precise pathophysiology is uncertain. Circulating antigens may react with antibodies at sensitized areas of the skin. An abnormal immune recognition of autologous skin antigens may also occur. Inflammation may lower the irritation threshold of the skin, and hematogenous spread of cytokines from the primary site of inflammation may also play a role (1).
- Etiology
  - Infectious
    - Fungal infections: *Trichophyton mentagrophytes*, *Trichophyton rubrum*, *Epidermophyton floccosum*, and *Candida* spp.
    - Bacterial infections: *Streptococcus pyogenes*, *Staphylococcus aureus*, and *Mycobacterium tuberculosis*
    - Viral infections: HSV, *Molluscum contagiosum*, orf, and milker's nodules
    - Parasitic infections: *Sarcoptes scabiei*, *Leishmania* spp., and *Pediculus humanus capitis*
  - Allergic
    - Id reactions occur in patients with nickel and aluminum allergy or, less commonly, second to concurrent treatment with antibacterial agent and terbinafine.
  - Miscellaneous
    - Id reaction rarely develops due to retained postoperative sutures, cyanoacrylate application, ionizing radiation, blunt trauma, red tattoo ink, postpicosecond laser tattoo removal.
    - Rarely, id reaction has been documented in patients receiving intravesical BCG live therapy for transitional cell carcinoma.

RISK FACTORS
- Fungal infection of the skin, especially tinea pedis
- Stasis dermatitis

GENERAL PREVENTION
- Good skin hygiene (particularly in intertriginous areas) to minimize risk of developing fungal infections
- Promptly treat any developing fungal infection.

COMMONLY ASSOCIATED CONDITIONS
- Primary fungal infection
- Stasis dermatitis

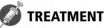

DIAGNOSIS

HISTORY
Itchy rash: Inquire about presence of lesions (typically fungal or bacterial) that could have incited the id reaction in the preceding days to weeks.

PHYSICAL EXAM
- Common
  - Symmetric, pruritic vesicles on the palms and, most commonly, on lateral aspects of fingers
  - Tinea infection on the feet; contact or other eczematous dermatitis; bacterial, fungal, or viral infection of the skin
- Less common
  - Papules
  - Lichenoid eruption
  - Erythema nodosum
- Eczematoid eruption

DIFFERENTIAL DIAGNOSIS
- Pompholyx (dyshidrotic eczema)
- Contact dermatitis
- Drug eruptions
- Pustular psoriasis
- Folliculitis
- Scabies

DIAGNOSTIC TESTS & INTERPRETATION
- Potassium hydroxide (KOH) or fungal culture of primary lesion
- No fungal elements are present at the site of the id reaction.
- Special tests: Skin shows a positive trichophyton reaction. A wheal >10 mm at 20 minutes and induration of >5 mm at 72 hours is a positive response.

Follow-Up Tests & Special Considerations
- The id reaction resolves with successful eradication of the primary skin condition.
- It is important to distinguish dermatophytids from drug-induced allergic reactions because continued treatment is essential to clear the underlying infection.

Test Interpretation
Histology
- Vesicles in the upper dermis
- Superficial perivascular lymphohistiocytic infiltrate with small numbers of eosinophils and increased granular cell layer
- No infectious agents present in biopsy specimen.

TREATMENT

GENERAL MEASURES
- Outpatient treatment of the underlying infection or eczematous dermatitis
- Symptomatic treatment of pruritus with antihistamines and/or topical steroids if needed (may require class 1 or 2 steroid)
- Treatment for secondary bacterial infection
- Stopping causative agent

MEDICATION
First Line
- PO antihistamines for pruritus (2)
  - Chlorpheniramine: 4 mg PO q4–6h PRN; max 24 mg/24 hr (pediatric: 6 to 11 years 2 mg PO q4–6h PRN; max 12 mg/24 hr; ≥12 years, refer to adult dosing)
  - Diphenhydramine: 25 to 50 mg PO q4–6h PRN; max 400 mg/24 hr (pediatric: 5 mg/kg/24 hr divided q6h PRN; 2 to 5 years max 37.5 mg/24 hr; 6 to 11 years max 150 mg/24 hr; ≥12 years, refer to adult dosing)
  - Hydroxyzine: 25 to 100 mg PO q6–8h PRN; max 600 mg/24 hr (pediatric: 2 mg/kg/24 hr divided q6h PRN)

- Topical treatments for pruritus
  - Triamcinolone 0.1% ointment TID
  - Hydrocortisone 0.5%, 1%, 2.5%: up to QID
  - Capsaicin 0.025%, 0.075% cream: Apply TID–QID; EMLA (2.5% lidocaine + 2.5% prilocaine) applied 30 to 60 minutes prior to capsaicin may minimize burning.
  - Doxepin 5% cream: Apply QID for up to 8 days (to max of 10% of the body).
  - Permethrin 5% cream (for scabies)
    - Apply from neck down after bath.
    - Wash off thoroughly with water in 8 to 12 hours.
    - May repeat in 7 days
  - Permethrin 1% cream rinse (for lice)
    - Shampoo, rinse, towel dry, saturate hair and scalp (or other affected area), leave on 10 minutes and then rinse.
    - May repeat in 7 days
  - White petroleum emollients: Apply after short bath/shower in warm (not hot) water.
- Systemic steroids only if reaction is severe or generalized (e.g., prednisone 20 mg)

Second Line
- Topical and/or systemic antifungals for identified associated fungal infection (common)
  - Tinea cruris/corporis
    - Topical azole antifungal compounds econazole (Spectazole) and ketoconazole (Nizoral): usually applied BID for 2 to 4 weeks
    - Terbinafine (Lamisil): over-the-counter (OTC) compound; can be applied daily or BID for 1 to 2 weeks
    - Butenafine (Mentax): applied once daily for 2 weeks; also very effective
  - Tinea capitis
    - PO griseofulvin for *Trichophyton* and *Microsporum* spp.; microsized preparation available; dosage 20 to 25 mg/kg/day divided BID or as a single dose daily for 6 to 12 weeks
    - PO terbinafine can be used for *Trichophyton* spp. at 62.5 mg/day in patients weighing 10 to 20 kg, 125 mg/day if weighing 20 to 40 kg, 250 mg/day if weighing >40 kg, and use for 4 to 6 weeks.

- Topical or systemic antibiotics for any secondary bacterial infection
- Treatment with antiviral agents for erythema multiforme associated with HSV is required.

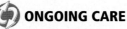 **ONGOING CARE**

PATIENT EDUCATION
Avoid hot, humid conditions that promote fungal growth. Aerate susceptible body areas (e.g., wear sandals or open footwear). If possible, wear loose-fitting clothing and undergarments, dry wet skin after bathing, and use powders and antiperspirants to discourage fungal growth. Treat primary dermatitis promptly.

PROGNOSIS
After appropriate treatment, complete resolution in days to weeks

COMPLICATIONS
- Secondary bacterial infection (cellulitis)
- After resolution of dermatophytid, postinflammatory hyperpigmentation is common and disappears without treatment in 1 month.

REFERENCES
1. Ilkit M, Durdu M, Karakaş M. Cutaneous id reactions: a comprehensive review of clinical manifestations, epidemiology, etiology, and management. *Crit Rev Microbiol*. 2012;38(3):191–202.
2. Cotes MES, Swerlick RA. Practical guidelines for the use of steroid-sparing agents in the treatment of chronic pruritus. *Dermatol Ther*. 2013;26(2):120–134.

ADDITIONAL READING
- Antibacterials/terbinafine: Id reaction in the form of erythema nodosum, tarsal arthritis and abdominal pain: Case report. *Reactions Weekly*. 2020;1785(1):49.
- Elmariah SB, Lerner EA. Topical therapies for pruritus. *Semin Cutan Med Surg*. 2011;30(2):118–126.

- Huerth KA, Glick PL, Glick ZR. Cutaneous id reaction after using cyanoacrylate for wound closure. *Cutis*. 2020;105(3):E11–E13.
- Jordan L, Jackson NA, Carter-Snell B, et al. Pustular tinea id reaction. *Cutis*. 2019;103(6):E3–E4.
- Paulsen LL, Geller DD, Guggenbiller M. Symmetrical vesicular eruption on the palms. *Am Fam Physician*. 2012;85(8):811–812.
- Price A, Tavazoie M, Meehan SA, et al. Id reaction associated with red tattoo ink. *Cutis*. 2018;102(5):E32–E34.
- Sadhasivamohan A, Karthikeyan K, Palaniappan V. Pediculosis capitis with id reaction and plica polonica. *Am J Trop Med Hyg*. 2021;105(4):862–863.
- Stachler RJ, Al-khudari S. Differential diagnosis in allergy. *Otolaryngol Clin North Am*. 2011;44(3): 561–590, vii–viii.
- Veien NK. Acute and recurrent vesicular hand dermatitis. *Dermatol Clin*. 2009;27(3):337–353, vii.
- Wong IT, Cheung LW. Id reaction and allergic contact dermatitis post-picosecond laser tattoo removal: a case report. *SAGE Open Med Case Rep*. 2021;9:2050313X211057934.
- Yosipovitch G, Bernhard JD. Clinical practice. Chronic pruritus. *N Engl J Med*. 2013;368(17):1625–1634.

 CODES

ICD10
- L30.2 Cutaneous autosensitization
- B35.9 Dermatophytosis, unspecified

CLINICAL PEARLS
- When one skin eruption follows another closely in time, consider an id reaction.
- When assessing an itchy rash, inquire about potential fungal or bacterial lesions in the preceding days to weeks as a potential prelude to the id reaction.

IMMUNE THROMBOCYTOPENIA (ITP)

Tara Baney, MS, CRNP

 BASICS

DESCRIPTION
- Immune thrombocytopenia (ITP) is a condition characterized by the immunologic destruction of normal platelets and/or impaired thrombopoiesis in response to an unknown stimulus.
- ITP is defined as a platelet count $<100 \times 10^9$/L, once other causes of thrombocytopenia have been ruled out (1).
- ITP nomenclature:
  - Newly diagnosed (<3 months), persistent (3 to 12 months), and chronic (>12 months)
  - Primary when it presents in isolation; secondary when associated with other disorders
- ITP is a relatively common disease of childhood that typically follows a viral infection. Onset is within 1 week, and spontaneous resolution occurs within 2 months in $>80\%$ of patients.
- In adults, ITP is usually a chronic disease and spontaneous remission is rare.
- Synonym(s): idiopathic thrombocytopenic purpura; immune thrombocytopenic purpura; and Werlhof disease

EPIDEMIOLOGY
- Peak age: pediatric ITP: 2 to 4 years; chronic ITP: >50 years with incidence 2 times higher in persons aged 60 years than those <60 years of age
- Predominant gender: pediatric ITP: male = female; chronic ITP: female > male (1.2 to 1.7:1)

Incidence
- Pediatric acute ITP: 1.9 to 6.4/100,000 children per year; adult ITP: 1.6/100,000 per year (1)
- Peak incidence of ITP in the spring and early summer in temperate climates. This observation supports the notion that viral triggers are an important cause of ITP.

Prevalence
Limited data; in one population (in Oklahoma): Overall prevalence of 11.2/100,000 persons

ETIOLOGY AND PATHOPHYSIOLOGY
- Accelerated platelet uptake and destruction by reticuloendothelial phagocytes results from action of IgG autoantibodies against platelet membrane glycoproteins IIb/IIIa, GP Ib/IX, GP Ia/IIa, and GP VI. There is also cell-mediated platelet destruction by CD8+ T cells.
- Autoantibodies interfere with megakaryocyte maturation, resulting in decreased production.
- Fc-independent desialylated platelet clearance has been proposed as the mechanism of refractoriness to therapies that target the classic Fc-dependent pathway.
- Association in patients receiving immune checkpoint inhibitor therapy

RISK FACTORS
- Autoimmune thrombocytopenia (e.g., Evans syndrome)
- Common variable immunodeficiency (CVID)
- Drug side effect (e.g., quinidine, vancomycin, penicillin, sulfonamides)
- Infections: *Helicobacter pylori*, hepatitis C, HIV, CMV, varicella zoster, measles, rubella, influenza, EBV, Whipple disease

- Vaccination side effect. Live virus vaccinations carry a lower risk than natural viral infection: 2.6/100,000 cases MMR vaccine doses versus 6 to 1,200/100,000 cases of natural rubella or measles infections.
- Bone marrow transplantation side effect
- Connective tissue disease, such as: systemic lupus erythematosus, antiphospholipid antibody syndrome
- Lymphoproliferative disorders

 DIAGNOSIS

A careful history, physical exam, and review of CBC and peripheral blood smear remain the key components of the diagnosis of ITP.

HISTORY
- Often asymptomatic; found incidentally on routine CBC
- Posttraumatic bleeding occurs at counts of 40 to 60×10^9/L.
- With counts $<30 \times 10^9$/L, bruising tendency, epistaxis, menorrhagia, and gingival bleeding are common.
- Spontaneous bleeding may occur with platelet count $<20 \times 10^9$/L.
- Intracerebral bleeding is rare and may occur with counts $<20 \times 10^9$/L and associated trauma or vascular lesions, resulting in neurologic symptoms.
- Female gender and exposure to NSAIDs have been associated with bleeding.

PHYSICAL EXAM
- Ecchymoses, petechiae, epistaxis, and gingivorrhagia are common.
- Abnormal uterine bleeding may be present.
- Hemorrhagic bullae on buccal mucosa reflect acute, severe thrombocytopenia.
- Absence of splenomegaly, hepatomegaly, lymphadenopathy, stigmata of congenital disease

DIFFERENTIAL DIAGNOSIS
- Acute leukemia
- Thrombotic thrombocytopenic purpura, hemolytic uremic syndrome, disseminated intravascular coagulopathy (ITP)
- Factitious: platelet clumping on peripheral smear
- Thrombocytopenia secondary to sepsis
- Myelodysplastic syndrome, particularly in older patients
- Decreased marrow production: malignancy, drugs, viruses, megaloblastic anemia
- Posttransfusion
- Gestational thrombocytopenia
- Isoimmune neonatal purpura
- Congenital thrombocytopenias
- Alcohol-induced thrombocytopenic purpura

DIAGNOSTIC TESTS & INTERPRETATION
Diagnosis of ITP is often a diagnosis of exclusion. Other more worrisome or pathologic causes of thrombocytopenia need to be ruled out.

Initial Tests (lab, imaging)
- CBC with differential and peripheral smear:
  - Isolated decreased platelet count $<100 \times 10^9$/L
  - Giant platelets are usually present.
  - Normal red and white blood cell morphology

- For patients with history, exam, CBC, and peripheral smear typical of ITP, consider the following:
  - PT/PTT is normal.
  - In adults, serologies for hepatitis B and C, and HIV infections are recommended (1)[C].
  - In pediatric ITP, immunoglobulin levels to exclude CVID are commonly obtained (1)[C].
  - Other tests are not necessary for patients with typical ITP presentation: antiplatelet, antinuclear, antiphospholipid antibodies; *H. pylori* testing; thrombopoietin; platelet parameters; direct anti-globulin test; reticulocyte count; urinalysis; and thyroid function tests (1)[C].
- Further studies should be considered if the patient with thrombocytopenia also presents with: fever, arthralgia, lymphadenopathy, family history of bleeding disorder, risk factors for HIV, or abnormalities in other cell lines
- Other tests not currently recommended in the guidelines:
  - Analyzing reticulated platelets or immature platelet function (RP/IPF) to make a differential diagnosis in cases of ITP yields a sensitivity and specificity of 83% and 75%, respectively.
  - In equivocal cases, testing for platelet antibodies such as GPIIb/IIIa and GPIb/IX yield sensitivity and specificity of 90% and 78%, respectively.

Diagnostic Procedures/Other
Imaging is not necessary. Bone marrow aspiration/biopsy: not necessary for diagnosis in children (1)[C] and adults; can be considered for a patient with atypical symptoms, such as fever and weight loss and multiple abnormalities in blood count (1)

Test Interpretation
- Peripheral smear: normal red and white cells with large or giant platelets but diminished in number
- Marrow reveals normal to abundant megakaryocytes with normal erythroid and myeloid precursors.

TREATMENT

GENERAL MEASURES
- Management is based on both platelet count and hemorrhagic manifestations.
- Current evidence-based guidelines recommend treatment should be administered for newly diagnosed patients with a platelet count $<30 \times 10^9$/L (1).
- The main goal is to achieve a platelet count associated with adequate hemostasis, rather than a normal count (1).
- Outpatient management unless patient has platelet count $<20 \times 10^9$/L and is at risk for bleeding
- Admit patients with active bleeding.

MEDICATION
First Line
- Pediatric
  - First-line treatment:
    - For children with no or mild bleeding (bruising and petechiae only with no mucosal bleeding), observation alone regardless of platelet count (1)[C]
    - For children with significant bleeding
      - Single-dose IV immunoglobulin (IVIG) 0.8 to 1.0 g/kg, especially when a more rapid increase in platelet count is desired (1)[C]. Do not administer in patients with IgA deficiencies because of anaphylaxis risk.

- A short course of corticosteroids (e.g., PO prednisone 2 mg/kg/day for 2 weeks with 3 weeks taper) (1)[C]
- Single dose of anti-Rho(D) immunoglobulin (anti-D), 50 to 75 g/kg for non-splenectomized children who are Rh-positive, with negative direct antiglobulin test (1). Do not use in children with low hemoglobin or evidence of hemolysis (1)[C].
  - Second and other treatments for pediatric and adolescent with ITP
    - Splenectomy for chronic or persistent ITP. This is often only completed if all other therapies have failed (1)[C].
    - Rituximab (Rituxan) 375 mg/m^2 weekly for 4 weeks (1)
    - High-dose dexamethasone 0.6 mg/kg/day for 4 days every 4 weeks (1)
    - Others without adequate data: azathioprine, cyclosporin A, danazol, mycophenolate mofetil, anti-CD52 monoclonal antibody, and interferon
    - Phase 3 clinical trials have shown that thrombopoietin receptor agonists induce good response in children with chronic ITP.
- Adult
  - First line, adult ITP
    - Treatment is recommended for newly diagnosed patients with platelet count <30 × 10^9/L (1).
    - 4 days of dexamethasone 40 mg/day for 4 consecutive days is preferred over longer courses of steroids or IVIG, as shorter course of corticosteroids has equivalent efficacy without as many adverse effects.
    - If corticosteroids are contraindicated:
      - IVIG: 1 to 2 g/kg once, repeating as necessary (1), OR
      - Anti-D: 50 to 75 μg/kg once, repeating as necessary for Rh$^+$, nonsplenectomized patients. Risk of severe hemolytic transfusion reactions are possible. Do not use anti-D in patients with low hemoglobin or evidence of hemolysis (1).
  - Second line, adult ITP
    - Splenectomy for patients who failed corticosteroid therapy (1)[C]
    - For patients for whom splenectomy is contraindicated and have risk of bleeding, thrombopoietin receptor agonists: eltrombopag (Promacta), 50 mg/day PO OR romiplostim (Nplate), 1 μg/kg SC weekly
    - Rituximab, 375 mg/m^2 IV weekly for 4 weeks, for patients at high risk of bleeding who have failed one line of therapy or postsplenectomy (1)
    - Others to consider: azathioprine, cyclosporine A, cyclophosphamide, danazol, dapsone, mycophenolate mofetil, and vincristine
    - Asymptomatic patients after splenectomy, with platelet counts >30 × 10^9/L, do not require treatment (1)[C].
    - FDA-approved: avatrombopag (Doptelet), 5 daily doses (60 mg if baseline platelet count below 40 × 10^9/L or 40 mg if 40 to below 50 × 10^9/L) and fostamatinib (Tavalisse), 100 mg twice daily

- ITP in pregnancy
  - Preeclampsia or gestational thrombocytopenia may cause thrombocytopenia unrelated to ITP.
  - Corticosteroids or IVIG are considered safe and are considered first line (1)[C].
  - ITP management at time of delivery is based on maternal bleeding risks, and mode of delivery should be based on obstetric indications. Platelet autoantibodies can cross the placenta and cause neonatal thrombocytopenia.
  - Cesarean section can be considered if platelet count >50 × 10^9/L.
  - Prednisone and/or IVIG may be considered 2 to 3 weeks prior to delivery.
- ITP secondary to HIV: Antivirals should be considered before other treatment (1)[C]. If treatment is required, corticosteroids, IVIG, or anti-D are first-line options, and splenectomy is a second-line option (1).
- ITP secondary to HCV: Antivirals should be considered before other treatment (1). If treatment required, IVIG is initial treatment (1). Based on recent studies, TPO mimetics are approved for HCV-related ITP because they increase platelets to a level required to initiate antiviral therapy.
- ITP and *H. pylori*: Screen for *H. pylori* in patients in whom eradication therapy would be considered if result is positive (1).
- ITP secondary to immune checkpoint inhibitor therapy: When suspected, first, stop the offending agent and treat with first-line therapy for ITP in adults as outlined above.
- Emergency treatment
  - Patients with intracranial or GI bleeding, massive hematuria, internal hematoma, or who need emergent surgery
  - IV corticosteroids (e.g., IV methylprednisolone, 1 g/day for 3 doses) with caution in patients with GI bleeding and/or IVIG 1 g/kg; repeat the following day for count <50 × 10^9/L (1)[C].
  - Platelet transfusions with IVIG may also be considered for significant bleeding (1)[C].
  - Other agents that may be considered: Recombinant factor VIIa not only promotes hemostasis but also increases risk of thrombosis. Efficacy of antifibrinolytic agents, aminocaproic acid and tranexamic acid, is unproved in randomized trials; they may be used as adjunctive treatments only. Emergent splenectomy has been reported.

ISSUES FOR REFERRAL

Hematology consultation is recommended for acute bleeding or for those who fail to respond to first-line therapies.

SURGERY/OTHER PROCEDURES

Splenectomy

- Mortality rate is very low (<1%) even in patients with severe thrombocytopenia. Laparoscopic splenectomy has similar long-term outcomes compared to open splenectomy and has better short-term outcomes in medically suitable patients (1)[C]. Reported 5- to 10-year efficacy is ~65% for all patients.

- Necessary vaccinations prior to splenectomy: polyvalent pneumococcal vaccine and quadrivalent meningococcal vaccine every 3 to 5 years and one-time *Haemophilus influenzae type b* (Hib) vaccine
- Consider lifelong prophylactic antibiotics with penicillin or erythromycin.
- Raise the platelet count to at least 20 × 10^9/L prior to surgery

 ## ONGOING CARE

FOLLOW-UP RECOMMENDATIONS
Patient Monitoring
Platelet counts weekly for patients on steroids and monthly for stable patients are reasonable. If short-course of dexamethasone is selected, platelet counts are recommended after 10 days of initiation of therapy. A second course of short course is recommended if platelet count increment is below target goal.

PATIENT EDUCATION
Modify activity to prevent injury or bruising; avoid contact sports. Avoid anticoagulants, aspirin and other platelet-inhibiting drugs, and NSAIDs.

PROGNOSIS
- Acute ITP: ~80–85% of patients completely recover within 2 months. 15% proceed to chronic ITP.
- Chronic ITP: ~10–20% of the patients recover spontaneously; remainder with diminished platelets for months to years. May see spontaneous remissions (5%) and relapses
- ~10% are refractory (fail medical therapy and splenectomy).

COMPLICATIONS
- Related to thrombocytopenia: 1% mortality due to intracranial hemorrhage and severe blood loss
- Related to treatment: for example, adverse effects from medications

REFERENCE

1. Neunert C, Terrell DR, Arnold DM, et al. American Society of Hematology 2019 guidelines for immune thrombocytopenia. *Blood Adv*. 2019;3(23): 3829–3866.

 ## CODES

ICD10
D69.3 Immune thrombocytopenic purpura

CLINICAL PEARLS

ITP is defined as a platelet count <100 × 10^9/L, once other causes of thrombocytopenia have been ruled out

IMPETIGO
Rade N. Pejic, MD

BASICS

DESCRIPTION
- A contagious, superficial, intraepidermal infection occurring prominently on exposed areas of the face and extremities, most often seen in children
- Primary impetigo (pyoderma): invasion of previously normal skin
- Secondary impetigo (impetiginization): invasion at sites of minor trauma (abrasions, insect bites, underlying eczema)
- Infected patients usually have multiple lesions.
- Cultures are positive in >80% cases for *Staphylococcus aureus* either alone or combined with group A β-hemolytic streptococci; *S. aureus* is the more common pathogen since the 1990s.
- Nonbullous impetigo: most common form of impetigo; formation of vesiculopustules that rupture, leading to crusting with a characteristic of golden appearance; local lymphadenopathy may occur.
- Bullous impetigo: staphylococcal impetigo that progresses from small to large flaccid bullae (newborns/young children) caused by epidermolytic toxin release; ruptured bullae leaving brown crust; less lymphadenopathy; trunk more often affected; <30% of patients
- Folliculitis: considered by some to be *S. aureus* impetigo of hair follicles
- Ecthyma: a deeper, ulcerated impetigo infection often with lymphadenitis
- System(s) affected: skin/exocrine
- Synonym(s): pyoderma; impetigo contagiosa; impetigo vulgaris

EPIDEMIOLOGY
Incidence
- Predominant sex: male = female
- Predominant age: children aged 2 to 5 years

Prevalence
In the United States: not reported but common

Pediatric Considerations
- Poststreptococcal glomerulonephritis may follow impetigo (in young children).
- Impetigo neonatorum may occur due to nursery contamination.

ETIOLOGY AND PATHOPHYSIOLOGY
- Coagulase-positive staphylococci: pure culture ~50–90%; more contagious via contact
- β-Hemolytic streptococci: pure culture only ~10% of the time (primarily group A)
- Mixed infections of streptococci and staphylococci are common; data suggest increasing importance of staphylococci over the past decades.
- Methicillin-resistant *S. aureus* (MRSA) detected in some cases

- Direct contact or insect vector
- Can result from contamination at trauma site
- Regional lymphadenopathy

RISK FACTORS
- Warm, humid environment
- Tropical or subtropical climate
- Summer or fall season
- Minor trauma, insect bites, breaches in skin
- Poor hygiene, poverty, crowding, epidemics, wartime
- Familial spread
- Poor health with anemia and malnutrition
- Complication of pediculosis, scabies, chickenpox, eczema/atopic dermatitis
- Contact dermatitis (*Rhus* spp.)
- Burns
- Contact sports
- Children in daycare
- Carriage of group A *Streptococcus* and *S. aureus*

GENERAL PREVENTION
- Close attention to family hygiene, particularly hand washing among children
- Covering of wounds
- Avoidance of crowding and sharing of personal items
- Treatment of atopic dermatitis

COMMONLY ASSOCIATED CONDITIONS
- Malnutrition and anemia
- Crowded living conditions
- Poor hygiene
- Neglected minor trauma
- Any chronic/underlying dermatitis
- Can occur as coinfection with scabies

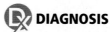 DIAGNOSIS

HISTORY
- Lesions are often described as painful.
- May be slow and indolent or rapidly spreading
- Most frequent on face around mouth and nose or at site of trauma

PHYSICAL EXAM
- Tender red macules or papules as early lesions (contact dermatitis presents with pruritic lesions)
- Thin-roofed vesicles to bullae: usually nontender
- Pustules
- Weeping, shallow, red ulcers
- Honey-colored crusts
- Satellite lesions
- Often multiple sites
- Bullae on buttocks, trunk, face

DIFFERENTIAL DIAGNOSIS
- Nonbullous
  - Contact dermatitis
  - Chickenpox
  - Herpes
  - Folliculitis
  - Erysipelas
  - Insect bites
  - Severe eczematous dermatitis
  - Scabies
  - Tinea corporis
- Bullous
  - Burns
  - Pemphigus vulgaris
  - Bullous pemphigoid
- Stevens-Johnson syndrome

DIAGNOSTIC TESTS & INTERPRETATION
Initial Tests (lab, imaging)
- None usually necessary in typical presentations; cultures of pus/bullae fluid may be helpful if no response to empiric therapy.
  - Culture: taken from the base of lesion after removal of crust; will grow both staphylococci and group A streptococci
  - Antistreptolysin-O (ASO) titer: can be weak positive for streptococci but overall not useful
  - Antideoxyribonuclease B (anti-DNase B) and antihyaluronidase (AHT) response are more reliable than ASO response.
  - Streptozyme: positive for streptococci
- Disorders that may alter lab results: Streptococcal pharyngitis will alter streptococcal enzyme tests.

Follow-Up Tests & Special Considerations
- Monitor for spread of disease and systemic manifestations.
- Serologic testing is helpful in context of impetigo with subsequent poststreptococcal glomerulonephritis.

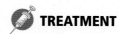 TREATMENT

GENERAL MEASURES
- Treatment speeds healing, improves cosmetic appearance, and avoids spread of disease.
- Prevent with mupirocin ointment TID to sites of minor skin trauma.
- Remove crusts; clean with gentle washing 2 to 3 times daily; and clean with antibacterial soap, chlorhexidine, or Betadine (povidone iodine).
- Washing of entire body may prevent recurrence at distant sites.

MEDICATION

- In 2014, the Infectious Diseases Society of America (IDSA) recommended topical treatment for limited lesions and oral medication when the disease is more severe/extensive (1)[C]. A 2017 Canadian systematic review found that topical mupirocin is equally or more effective than oral treatments for nonextensive impetigo (2)[A]. Penicillin and macrolide therapy is no longer recommended. Fluoroquinolones are not indicated due to resistance patterns and risk of serious adverse events.
- Consult the local hospital or health department for microbial resistance information.
- Nonbullous (minor spread, treat 7 days; widespread, treat 10 days); bullous (treat 10 days)
  - Mupirocin (Bactroban) 2% topical ointment applied TID for 5 to 7 days (nonbullous only); not as effective on scalp as around mouth
  - Retapamulin 1% ointment to be applied BID for 5 days (very expensive) (3)[A]
  - Ozenoxacin 1% cream applied BID for 5 days (very expensive) (3)[A]
  - Dicloxacillin: adult 250 mg PO QID; pediatric <40 kg: 12 to 25 mg/kg/day divided q6h; >40 kg: 125 to 250 mg/kg/day divided q6h
- Dicloxacillin, cephalexin, topical mupirocin, and fusidic acid are effective, unless local staphylococcal strains are resistant. For MRSA infections, treatment options include clindamycin, tetracyclines, or trimethoprim-sulfamethoxazole. Oral doses given for 7 days are usually sufficient (4)[C].
- 1st-generation cephalosporins
  - Children
    - Cephalexin 25 to 50 mg/kg/day divided, q6–12h
    - Cefaclor 20 to 40 mg/kg/day divided q8h
    - Cephradine 25 to 50 mg/kg/day divided q6–12h
    - Cefadroxil 30 mg/kg/day divided BID
  - Adults
    - Cephalexin 250 mg up to QID
    - Cefaclor 250 mg TID
    - Cephradine 500 mg BID
    - Cefadroxil 1 g/day in divided doses
- Clindamycin 300 mg q6–8h
- Severe bullous disease may require IV therapy such as nafcillin or cefazolin.

ISSUES FOR REFERRAL

If resistant or extensive infections occur, especially in immunocompromised patients

ADDITIONAL THERAPIES

Monitor for microbial resistance patterns.

ONGOING CARE

FOLLOW-UP RECOMMENDATIONS

- Athletes are restricted from contact sports.
- School and daycare contagious restrictions
- Children can return to school 24 hours after initiation of antimicrobial treatment.

Patient Monitoring

If not clear within 7 to 10 days, culture the lesions.

PATIENT EDUCATION

Avoidance of infection spread is the key; hand washing is vital, especially for reducing spread in children.

PROGNOSIS

- Complete resolution in 7 to 10 days with treatment
- Antibiotic treatment will not prevent or halt glomerulonephritis, as it will in rheumatic fever.
- If not clear within 7 to 10 days, culture is necessary to find resistant organism.
- Recurrent impetigo: Evaluate for carriage of *S. aureus* in nares (also perineum, axillae, toe web). Apply mupirocin ointment to nares BID for 5 days for decolonization.

COMPLICATIONS

- Ecthyma
- Erysipelas
- Poststreptococcal acute glomerulonephritis
- Cellulitis
- Bacteremia
- Osteomyelitis
- Septic arthritis
- Pneumonia
- Lymphadenitis

REFERENCES

1. Stevens DL, Bisno AL, Chambers HF, et al; for Infectious Diseases Society of America. Practice guidelines for the diagnosis and management of skin and soft tissue infections: 2014 update by the Infectious Diseases Society of America. *Clin Infect Dis*. 2014;59(2):147–159.
2. Edge R, Argáez C. *Topical Antibiotics for Impetigo: A Review of the Clinical Effectiveness and Guidelines*. Ontario, Canada: Canadian Agency for Drugs and Technologies in Health; 2017.
3. Gahlawat G, Tesfaye W, Bushell M, et al. Emerging treatment strategies for impetigo in endemic and nonendemic settings: a systematic review. *Clin Ther*. 2021;43(6):986–1006.
4. Del Giudice P, Hubiche P. Community-associated methicillin-resistant *Staphylococcus aureus* and impetigo. *Br J Dermatol*. 2010;162(4):905–906.

ADDITIONAL READING

- Bowen AC, Mahé A, Hay RJ, et al. The global epidemiology of impetigo: a systematic review of the population prevalence of impetigo and pyoderma. *PLoS One*. 2015;10(8):e0136789.
- Clebak KT, Malone MA. Skin infections. *Prim Care*. 2018;45(3):433–454.
- Koning S, van der Sande R, Verhagen AP, et al. Interventions for impetigo. *Cochrane Database Syst Rev*. 2012;1(1):CD003261.
- Stanley JR, Amagai M. Pemphigus, bullous impetigo, and the staphylococcal scalded-skin syndrome. *N Engl J Med*. 2006;355(17):1800–1810.

SEE ALSO

Algorithm: Rash

CODES

ICD10

- L01.01 Non-bullous impetigo
- L01.03 Bullous impetigo
- L01.00 Impetigo, unspecified

CLINICAL PEARLS

- Superficial, intraepidermal infection
- Predominantly staphylococcal in origin
- Microbial resistance patterns need to be monitored.
- Topical treatment is recommended for limited lesions and oral medication only when the disease is more severe/extensive.

INCONTINENCE, FECAL

Kalyanakrishnan Ramakrishnan, MD

 BASICS

Continuous or recurrent involuntary passage of feces through the anal canal for >1 month in an individual who has previously achieved continence.

- Recurrent, involuntary loss of stool
- Assess rectal tone, voluntary squeeze, and differentiate overflow incontinence from fecal impaction
- Endorectal ultrasound (EUS) is the simplest, most reliable, and least invasive method to detect anal sphincter defects.
- The goal of treatment is to restore continence and/or improve quality of life.

DESCRIPTION
Major incontinence is the involuntary evacuation of feces. Minor incontinence includes passage of flatus and/or occasional seepage of liquid stool. Categories include urge and passive incontinence.

Geriatric Considerations
- Fecal incontinence increases with age and is an important cause for nursing home placement among the elderly.
- Idiopathic fecal incontinence is more common in older women.

EPIDEMIOLOGY
Incidence
Patients are often embarrassed and do not report fecal incontinence unless specifically queried ("silent affliction").

Prevalence
- 7% of adults; 15% of adults aged >90 years; women > men
- 56–66% of hospitalized older patients and >50% of nursing home residents
- 50–70% of patients who have urinary incontinence also suffer from fecal incontinence.

Pregnancy Considerations
Obstetric injury to the pelvic floor may result in either temporary or persistent fecal incontinence.

Geriatric Considerations
Fecal impaction with overflow diarrhea is common in older patients.

ETIOLOGY AND PATHOPHYSIOLOGY
- Continence requires the complex orchestration of pelvic musculature, nerves, and reflex arcs.
- Stool volume/consistency, colon transit time, anorectal sensation, rectal compliance, anorectal reflexes, external/internal sphincter muscle tone, puborectalis muscle function, and mental capacity all play a role in maintaining continence.
- Congenital: spina bifida and myelomeningocele with spinal cord damage
- Trauma: anal sphincter damage from vaginal delivery or surgical procedures
- Medical: diabetes mellitus (most common metabolic disorder causing incontinence through pudendal nerve neuropathy), stroke, spinal cord trauma, neurodegenerative disorders, inflammatory bowel disease (IBD), rectal neoplasia

Genetics
No clear genetic association detected in the genome-wide association study.

RISK FACTORS
- Poor functional status—older age, female sex, obesity, limited physical activity
- Potential association with child abuse and adult sexual abuse
- Neurologic/neuropsychiatric conditions—multiple sclerosis, spinal cord injury, stroke, diabetic neuropathy (dementia, depression)
- Trauma: pelvic surgery, vaginal delivery, radiation. Risk factors during vaginal delivery include occipitoposterior presentation, prolonged second stage of labor, assisted vaginal delivery (forceps or vacuum-assist), and episiotomy.
- Diarrhea, IBD, irritable bowel syndrome (IBS), menopause, smoking, constipation, fecal impaction
- Congenital abnormalities, such as imperforate anus/rectal prolapse

GENERAL PREVENTION
- Behavioral/lifestyle changes: Obesity, limited physical activity/exercise, poor diet, and smoking are modifiable risk factors.
- Post meal bowel regimen—defecate regularly after meals to maximize positive impact of gastrocolic reflex.
- Pelvic floor muscle training during and after pregnancy and pelvic surgery, increase fiber intake (>30 g/day)

COMMONLY ASSOCIATED CONDITIONS
- Increasing age (>65 years)
- Chronic medical conditions—diabetes mellitus, dementia, stroke, spinal cord compression, depression, immobility, chronic obstructive pulmonary disease, IBS, and IBD
- Perineal trauma (obstetric); anorectal surgery; history of pelvic/rectal irradiation; urinary incontinence/pelvic organ prolapse

DIAGNOSIS

Diagnosis is based on history and physical findings.

HISTORY
- Patients seldom volunteer information about fecal incontinence. Direct questioning is important.
- Problem-specific history includes (1)[C]
  - Severity of soiling by liquid stool or gross incontinence of solid stool
  - Onset and duration (recent onset vs. chronic); frequency, presence of constipation/diarrhea
- Review diet; medical, surgical, and obstetric history; lifestyle; and mobility; thorough medication review
- Evaluate for social withdrawal and depression.

PHYSICAL EXAM
- Inspect perineum for dermatitis, hemorrhoids, fistula, surgical scars, skin tags, rectal prolapse, soiling, and ballooning of the perineum (sarcopenia of pelvic musculature). A patulous anal orifice may indicate myopathy or a neurologic disorder.
- Evaluate the external sphincter response to perineal skin stimulation (anal wink). Absence suggests neuropathy.
- Ask the patient to bear down, preferably in standing position, to assess for rectal prolapse.
- Digital rectal exam to assess anal canal pressure sphincter tone, rectal bleeding, hemorrhoids, neoplasm, fecal consistency, and diarrhea/distal fecal impaction
- General neurologic examination, including perianal sensation and mental status evaluation (1)[C]

DIFFERENTIAL DIAGNOSIS
- Anorectal disorders
  - Prolapsed internal hemorrhoids; rectal prolapse
  - Trauma: obstetric, surgical, accidental, sexual
  - Inflammatory/infectious gastrointestinal disorders, ischemic colitis, fistulas, bowel neoplasms, radiation proctitis
- Neurologic disorders
  - Stroke, dementia, neoplasms, spinal cord injury, and/or diseases causing altered level of consciousness
  - Pudendal neuropathy, neurosyphilis, multiple sclerosis, diabetes mellitus
- Miscellaneous causes
  - Infectious diarrhea, fecal impaction and overflow, IBS, laxative abuse, IBD, short bowel syndrome, myopathies, senescence and frailty, collagen vascular disease, psychological and behavioral problems

DIAGNOSTIC TESTS & INTERPRETATION
Diagnostic approach should be individualized, minimally invasive, practical, and feasible. History and physical examination are generally sufficient for diagnosis. If uncertainty remains, consider:
- Plain abdominal x-ray (fecal impaction, constipation)
- Sigmoidoscopy/anoscopy/colonoscopy (hemorrhoids, colitis, neoplasm)

Initial Tests (lab, imaging)
- Stool studies (culture, ova and parasites, *Clostridium difficile* toxin assay)—if travel, antibiotic use, tube feedings, or sepsis
- Thyroid-stimulating hormone (TSH), electrolytes, and BUN in elderly patients
- EUS—most reliable and least invasive test for defining anatomic defects in the external and internal anal sphincters, rectal wall, and the puborectalis muscle (1)[B]. EUS can reliably predict therapeutic response to sphincteroplasty.

Follow-Up Tests & Special Considerations

- Defecography measures anorectal angle, evaluates pelvic descent, and detects occult/overt rectal prolapse. MRI defecography (dynamic MRI) further defines pelvic floor anatomy.
- Anorectal manometry measures maximal resting anal pressure, amplitude/duration of squeeze, rectoanal inhibitory reflex, threshold of conscious rectal sensation, rectal compliance, and anorectal pressures during straining.
- Pudendal nerve terminal motor latency (PNTML) measures neuromuscular integrity between the pudendal nerve and the anal sphincter; is operator-dependent and has poor correlation with clinical and histologic findings
- Electromyography can assess neurogenic/myopathic damage.

 TREATMENT

GENERAL MEASURES

- In ambulatory patients, scheduled (or prompted) defecation is effective, particularly in those with overflow incontinence.
- Kegel exercises to strengthen pelvic floor
- If bed-bound, scheduled osmotic or stimulant laxatives and suppositories promote evacuation and minimize fecal leakage.
- Use of stool deodorants (Peri-Wash, Derifil, Devrom), barrier creams to prevent/treat associated dermatitis

MEDICATION

Limited evidence that antidiarrheals (loperamide, codeine) and drugs enhancing sphincter tone (phenylephrine gel, sodium valproate) are of benefit (2)[B]; cholestyramine, colestipol useful in diarrhea following malabsorption or cholecystectomy; alosetron in diarrhea associated with IBS; amitriptyline in idiopathic fecal incontinence

First Line

Specific treatment of underlying disorder (e.g., infectious diarrhea/IBD) may improve fecal continence.

Second Line

- Stool-bulking agents—high-fiber diet, psyllium products, methylcellulose useful in milder forms of incontinence (1),(3)[B]
- Antidiarrheal agents, such as adsorbents or opium derivatives, may reduce diarrhea-associated incontinence (1),(3)[C].
- Disimpacting patients with fecal impaction/overflow incontinence and using bowel regimens prevent recurrence.

ADDITIONAL THERAPIES

- Biofeedback: initial treatment modality in motivated patients with some voluntary sphincter control (1)[C]; teaches patients to recognize rectal distension and contract the external anal sphincter, keeping intra-abdominal pressure low
- Biofeedback plus electrical stimulation of the anal sphincters is more effective than either measure. Patients with systemic neurologic disorders, anal deformities, or frequent episodes of incontinence respond poorly.

SURGERY/OTHER PROCEDURES

- Surgery should be considered only when nonsurgical approaches have failed. Sphincter repair offered in highly symptomatic patients with a well-defined defect of external anal sphincter (1),(3)[A].
- Tissue-bulking agent such as silicone elastomer or polysaccharide gel injected into the anorectal mucosa or the intersphincteric space is appropriate for patients with internal anal sphincter dysfunction (3),(4)[A].
- Artificial anal sphincter implantation/dynamic graciloplasty (gracilis muscle transposed into anus as modified sphincter) considered in patients with severe fecal incontinence and irreparable sphincter damage (1)[B]
- Colostomy/ileostomy appropriate in patients with disabling fecal incontinence and failed multiple therapeutic options (1)[B]; continent stomas created using the appendix/cecum as entry points enables flushing the colon in these patients
- Anal plugs minimize fecal leakage in patients who do not benefit from other treatment modalities, especially immobilized, institutionalized, or neurologically disabled patients; plugs are often poorly tolerated (1),(3)[B].
- Sacral nerve stimulation (neuromodulation) via implantation of electrodes delivering low-amplitude electrical stimulation to sphincter muscles improves rectal tone, especially in those with a coexistent sphincter defect (3)[B].
- SECCA procedure—temperature-controlled radio-frequency energy delivered to the anorectal junction distal to the dentate line causes scarring and anal canal narrowing; minimally invasive, useful in mild/moderate incontinence (1)[C]
- Magnetic anal sphincter (MAS) devices—series of 14 to 20 interlinked titanium beads with magnetic cores forming a flexible ring encircling the external anal sphincter 3 to 5 cm from the anal verge. During defecation, the beads separate, allowing evacuation after which the beads approximate closing the canal (4)[C], useful in moderate/severe incontinence.
- A vaginally placed bowel control device that the patient inflates to control leakage and deflates to defecate (Eclipse system) is well tolerated and effective (4)[B].
- Percutaneous posterior tibial nerve stimulation at the ankle for 30 minutes weekly for 12 weeks (50% efficacy) and the TOPAS pelvic floor repair system (polypropylene mesh placed behind the anorectum to support the puborectalis) (55% efficacy) are other recent advances in controlling fecal incontinence (4)[B].

COMPLEMENTARY & ALTERNATIVE MEDICINE

Ten weekly acupuncture sessions did improve quality of life, but this modality has not been studied in detail (3)[C].

ADMISSION, INPATIENT, AND NURSING CONSIDERATIONS

- If secondary to fecal impaction, manual evacuation of fecal mass (after lubrication with lidocaine jelly)
- Avoid hot water, soap, or hydrogen peroxide enemas

 ONGOING CARE

FOLLOW-UP RECOMMENDATIONS

Periodic rectal exam

Patient Monitoring

Consider impaction if there is <1 bowel movement every other day in patients with fecal incontinence.

DIET

High fiber (20 to 30 g/day) and at least 1.5 L fluid daily; avoid precipitants (caffeine).

PATIENT EDUCATION

Kegel/sphincter training exercises are helpful but not sufficient for treating fecal incontinence.

PROGNOSIS

- Reimpaction likely if bowel regimen discontinued
- 50% failure rate over 5 years following overlapping sphincteroplasty

COMPLICATIONS

- Depression and social isolation, skin ulcerations
- Artificial bowel sphincter: infection, erosion, mechanical failure

REFERENCES

1. Tjandra JJ, Dykes SL, Kumar RR, et al. Practice parameters for the treatment of fecal incontinence. *Dis Colon Rectum.* 2007;50(10):1497–1507.
2. Omar MI, Alexander CE. Drug treatment for faecal incontinence in adults. *Cochrane Database Syst Rev.* 2013;(6):CD002116.
3. Assmann SL, Keszthey D, Kleijnen J, et al. Guideline for the diagnosis and treatment of faecal incontinence—a URG/ESCP/ESNM/ESPCC collaboration. *United European Gastroenterol J.* 2022;10(3):251–286.
4. Rosenblatt P. New developments in therapies for fecal incontinence. *Curr Opin Obstet Gynecol.* 2015;27(5):353–358.

ADDITIONAL READING

Da Silva G, Sirany A. Recent advances in managing fecal incontinence. *F1000Res.* 2019;8:F1000 Faculty Rev-1291.

 CODES

ICD10

- R15.9 Full incontinence of feces
- R15.2 Fecal urgency
- R15.0 Incomplete defecation

CLINICAL PEARLS

- Scheduled defecation after meals, bulking agents, and scheduled enemas minimize impaction and are helpful in managing mild/moderate fecal incontinence.
- Differentiate true incontinence from pseudoincontinence (overflow or functional incontinence).
- New-onset fecal incontinence may indicate spinal cord compression.

INCONTINENCE, URINARY ADULT FEMALE

Vanessa Joyce M. Evardone, MD, BSMT • Alexander Sasha Rackman, MD

BASICS

- Urinary incontinence (UI): involuntary urine (ur) loss; common in women; few seek care despite effective options; may affect quality of life (QoL)
- UI: transient (acute, <6 months, and reversible if cause addressed) or chronic (have subtypes)

DESCRIPTION

- Stress UI: increased intra-abdominal pressure (coughing, exertion); most common in younger women
- Urge UI: sudden uncontrollable ur loss, preceded or accompanied by urgency; from overactive bladder (OAB) or detrusor overactivity (DO); most common in older adults
- Mixed UI: >1 type of UI, often a combo (stress and urge UIs); overall most common type
- Overflow UI: high-residual volume from inadequate bladder emptying (chronic ur retention), causing frequent dribbling; predisposes to recurrent infections, vesicoureteral reflux, autonomic dysreflexia
- Functional UI: ur loss due to deficits in cognition or mobility with normal ur system function
- Continuous UI: sustained slow leakage in between regular voiding; may have no awareness nor bladder fullness

EPIDEMIOLOGY

Prevalence

- Overall prevalence in women: 10–20% (up to 77% in nursing homes)
- In women, stress UI decreases with age, whereas urge UI increases.

ETIOLOGY AND PATHOPHYSIOLOGY

- Stress UI: 2 types—anatomic (urethral hypermobility from lack of pelvic support) and intrinsic sphincter deficiency (impaired urethral closure); stress UI is secondary to surgical scarring, radiation, hormonal, or age-related changes.
- Urge UI: DO (usual cause) or OAB from neuro causes (SCI), abd trauma, infection, Rx, certain fluids, or idiopathic; DO could be idiopathic or neurogenic (MS).
- Overflow UI: detrusor underactivity ("neurogenic bladder"), increased bladder ur volume (DM or Rx), or bladder outlet obstruction (fibroids, pelvic organ prolapse [POP], masses)
- Mixed UI: aggregate of etiologies from each type of UI present
- Functional UI: cognitive impairment (dementia, delirium, intellectual disabilities); unable to recognize need for toilet; psychological issues and mental illness (decreased awareness); medical conditions (arthritis) and physical disability impairing mobility; poor vision; and environmental barriers
- Continuous UI: constant involuntary ur loss; ectopic ureters in females usually open in urethra distal to sphincter or in the vagina, causing sustained leakage through the urethra or extra-urethral (urogenital fistulas: vesicovaginal [most common], ureterovaginal, and urethrovaginal).

RISK FACTORS

Advanced age, vaginal atrophy (menopause), impaired cognition-function, obesity (BMI >30), medical conditions (DM, chronic obstructive pulmonary disease [COPD]), multiparity, pelvic floor dysfunction (vaginal birth, pelvic surgery or radiation), urethral diverticula, POP, neuro diseases (stroke, MS, Parkinson disease), smoking, constipation, caffeine, and high-impact exercises

DIAGNOSIS

HISTORY

- Age: Onset in childhood indicates congenital cause (ectopic ureter). Stress UI is common in women 19 to 64 years old; mixed UI is common in women >65 years old.
- Nature-duration: Stress UI presents with small spurts of ur loss, typically dry at night in bed, and may have pelvic floor Sx (bulging, dyspareunia, pressure). Urge UI have sudden urge followed by large amounts of ur leakage (use pads), frequency, nocturia, and maybe triggered by sensory stimuli (cold).
- Suprapubic pain with dysuria: infection, interstitial cystitis
- Surgical Hx: Pelvic surgery (gynecologic or bowel) can injure the pelvic floor and affect neuro function.
- Comorbidities: constipation, DM, CHF, COPD, sleep apnea, neuro dysfunction (cognition), depression
- Medication that decreases bladder contractility ⇒ ur retention and overflow (antidepressants, antihistamines, antimuscarinics, anti-Parkinson's, antipsychotics, β-adrenergic agonists, CCBs, opioids, sedative-hypnotics, skeletal muscle relaxants); detrusor irritability or increased Cr clearance (EtOH, caffeine, diuretics); increased urethral sphincter tone ⇒ ur retention and overflow (α-adrenergic agonists, TCAs, amphetamines); and decreased urethral sphincter tone ⇒ stress UI (α-adrenergic antagonists); ACEi ⇒ chronic dry cough (stress UI)
- Tobacco smoking
- 3-day voiding diary (fluid-caffeine intake, ur Sx, situations and timing of UI, patient habits)
- The International Consultation on Incontinence Questionnaire (ICIQ)

PHYSICAL EXAM

- Neuro exam (sensation deficit in perineal–sacral area) and cognitive and functional evaluation.
- Pelvic exam: perineum and external (vaginal atrophy), half speculum vaginal exam (POP), bimanual pelvic exam (masses-cystocele, pelvic floor resting tone-function based on ability to isolate and contract pelvic floor using Oxford Scale), and anorectal exam (fecal impaction, rectocele or posterior vaginal wall prolapse).
- CST: immediate ur leakage on coughing and Valsalva with comfortably full bladder; excellent reliability, sensitivity, and specificity for stress UI versus urodynamics (UDS); increased sensitivity performed in standing position but can be done in supine lithotomy position; PPV: 78–97%

- Cotton swab test (urethral hypermobility): Little diagnostic utility to UDS; may predict response to midurethral sling (MUS) surgery.
- UDS testing: unnecessary in uncomplicated UI; postvoid residual (PVR) if patient reports incomplete voiding, POP past introitus, or for stress UI surgery; PVR (catheterization or sonography) within 10 minutes postmeasured void (normal: <100 mL for adults and <150 mL for older adults for voided volume >200 mL, or 1/3 of total voided volume)

DIFFERENTIAL DIAGNOSIS

- Nocturnal enuresis: idiopathic, DO, neurogenic, cardiogenic, sleep apnea
- Continuous leakage: ectopic ureter, fistulas
- Postvoid dribbling: urethral diverticulum, idiopathic, iatrogenic, surgical
- Pain (dyspareunia): interstitial cystitis, STI
- POP
- Hematuria, recurrent UTIs, or pelvic mass: malignancy
- Functional UI: neurologic, cognitive, psychological, physical impairment
- Mnemonic for causes of UI: TOILETED (DIAPPERS): Thin dry vaginal-urethral epithelium (atrophic urethritis, vaginitis), Obstruction (stool impaction/constipation), Infection, Limited (restricted) mobility, Emotional (psychological, depression), Therapeutic medications (pharmacologic), Endocrine disorders (excessive ur), Delirium

DIAGNOSTIC TESTS & INTERPRETATION

Initial Tests (lab, imaging)

- UA: in all patients (infection, hematuria, proteinuria, glycosuria)
- Ur Cx: if suspicious for infection (Tx of asymptomatic bacteriuria will not improve UI in elderly.)
- Renal function: if concern for renal impairment or obstruction
- TSH: if with constipation
- Imaging is unnecessary in uncomplicated UI; renal US for hydronephrosis if suspicious for obstruction (microhematuria)
- Urodynamic testing: for complicated UI or if surgery is considered.
- Bladder scan if overflow UI is suspected (PVR >200 mL)

Diagnostic Procedures/Other

UDS and cystoscopy: after failing conservative Tx; include cystometric study of detrusor function, pressure flow studies (bladder emptying), and cystoscopy (women with microhematuria or recurrent UTIs).

TREATMENT

GENERAL MEASURES

- Stepwise approach: conservative (first line), Rx-mechanical devices (second line), invasive interventions (third line)
- Tx correctable causes (infection, constipation).

- Stress UI: 6- to 8-week trial of behavioral modification and pelvic floor training; if no improvement, refer to urology.
- Urge UI: behavior modification, pelvic floor muscle training (PFMT), and medication; behavior modification plus medication: > effective versus medication alone
- Mixed UI: directed at predominant Sx (stress or urge UI)

MEDICATION

First Line

Conservative management
- I. Behavioral techniques: (i) bladder training (resist and expanding intervals between voiding); more benefit if supervised by health care provider; (ii) double voiding (voiding then waiting a few minutes trying again to empty bladder completely); (iii) toileting assistance (scheduled q2–4h); (iv) fluid-diet management: less EtOH, caffeine (<1 cup a day), or acidic food; less fluid intake before sleep and <2L/day; diet changes; and wt loss (moderate weight loss improves UI in BMI ≥30 kg/m²); (v) lifestyle changes (more active, stop smoking)
- II. PFMT (Kegel): effective for stress UI (may help urge UI); ± bladder training, manual feedback (palpating pelvic muscle during exercise), biofeedback (vaginal-anal device for visual-audio feedback on pelvic muscle contraction), or electrical stimulation. Pelvic floor therapists improve technique or use of weighted intravaginal cones. Home electrode stimulation Tx (vagina, anus) is a Medicare-covered option (if unable to voluntarily contract pelvic muscle).

Second Line

- I. Medications
  - Stress UI: no FDA-approved Rx
  - Topical estrogen may be beneficial for urgency and frequency Sx in postmenopausal women with vaginal atrophy (transdermal or oral may worsen UI).
  - Urge UI: If behavior Tx is unsuccessful, antimuscarinic agents (selective: darifenacin, solifenacin; nonselective: oxybutynin, tolterodine, trospium) and β3-AR agonists (mirabegron, vibegron) are FDA-approved. Dual Tx (mirabegron and low-dose anticholinergic agents) can be considered.
  - Anticholinergic agents inhibit involuntary detrusor contractions; effective for urge UI and OAB (significant improvement and modest >QoL)
  - No single anticholinergic agents is shown to be overall superior (higher doses: more effective but more side effects); extended release and transdermal prep have fewer side effects (dry mouth and eyes, constipation, impaired cognition). Avoid in narrow-angle glaucoma, ur retention, impaired gastric emptying, long QT (worsening of arrhythmias), and frailty.

- β3-AR agonists: no associated significant cognitive decline; avoided in ESRD, ESLD and uncontrolled HTN (BP check weeks postinitiation)
  - Rx: can be used for both urge and mixed UIs; combo Tx (Rx-behavior) is more effective than either modality alone.
  - OnabotulinumtoxinA for urge UI: similar Sx reduction as antimuscarinic (anticholinergic agents) options, with more Sx resolution; risk of ur retention, incomplete bladder emptying, and UTI
- II. Mechanical devices
  - Vaginal inserts (pessaries, tampons): option for stress UI in pregnancy, in nonsurgical candidates, and in those unresponsive to prior surgeries; compress bladder neck and/or urethra leading to decreased ur loss; pessaries: low cost, low risk, quick results
  - Urethral plugs: prevent UI during activities (running); limited evidence; associated with ADRs (UTI, hematuria, device migration into bladder)

Third Line

Individualized: based on Sx, goals, and expectations. Surgery may be used as first line for moderate to severe stress UI.
- Stress UI
  - Sling procedures: Mesh is the most common and studied for stress UI; better outcomes at 1 year than PFMT. Other options: autologous fascia pubovaginal sling (PVS), Burch colposuspension; POP may unmask UI in 40% of women (repair both during same surgery).
  - Intravesical balloons: more effective than sham Tx; more effective than behavior Tx with neuromodulation
- Periurethral injections (bulking agents: silicone polymers, collagen) leads to increased periurethral resistance (recurrent UI postsurgery or cannot tolerate surgery but often require injections); low-quality evidence: improved outcomes versus no Tx
- Urge UI
  - Neuromodulation (sacral nerve stimulation): invasive (surgically implanted), expensive, frequent complications, and inferior to onabotulinumtoxinA and posterior tibial nerve stimulation (PTNS)
  - OnabotulinumtoxinA (intravesical injection to detrusor via cystoscopy): FDA-approved, well tolerated, and significant improvement in overall OAB and QoL (prior inadequately treated with anticholinergic agents)
  - Bladder augmentation: complex reconstructive surgical procedure leads to increased bladder size and elasticity; after failing all other Tx

Geriatric Considerations

- UI: not a normal part of aging
- Anticholinergic agents used with caution; can worsen cognition and delirium (cumulative effects with use)
- Urethral sling
- Medication list review
- β3-AR agonists increase BP; not used in ESRD or ESLD

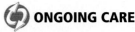 ONGOING CARE

COMPLICATIONS

Skin maceration (nursing home admissions), social isolation and depression, fear of leakage, impaired sexual function/QoL, risk of falls and fractures.

ADDITIONAL READING

Riemsma R, Hagen S, Kirschner-Hermanns R, et al. Can incontinence be cured? A systematic review of cure rates. *BMC Med.* 2017;15(1):63.

CODES

ICD10

- R32 Unspecified urinary incontinence
- N39.3 Stress incontinence (female) (male)
- N39.41 Urge incontinence

CLINICAL PEARLS

- Most UI: diagnosed with Hx and PE in conjunction with CST, PVR, and UA; UDS does not add value in uncomplicated UI.
- Rule out: infection (UTI, STI), hematuria.
- Try lifestyle changes first for all types of UI.
- Pelvic floor training: safe effective first-line Tx for stress and urge UI; can improve QoL; if no improvement in stress UI: mesh sling has high success rates. If no improvement in urge UI, anticholinergic agents (antimuscarinics) and β3-ARs could be used.

I

INCONTINENCE, URINARY ADULT MALE

Jason R. Ramos, MD, FAAFP

 BASICS

DESCRIPTION
- Urinary incontinence (UI) is a pathologic condition of an acute or chronic nature that refers to the involuntary loss of urine leading to medical, financial, social, or hygienic problems. Five main types of UI have been described: stress, urge, mixed, overflow (urinary retention), and functional UI (1).
- Stress incontinence: involuntary urine leaks secondary to increased intra-abdominal pressure being greater than the sphincter can control; may be precipitated by sneezing, laughing, coughing, exertion
- Urge incontinence: Involuntary leakage of urine associated with urgency is believed to be secondary to uncontrolled contraction of the urinary bladder. It is also called detrusor overactivity.
- Mixed incontinence: involuntary leakage of urine with urgency and with stress, such as sneezing, laughing, coughing, exertion
- Overflow incontinence: also known as urinary retention; this occurs with bladder overdistention due to impaired detrusor contraction or bladder outlet obstruction (due to benign prostatic hyperplasia [BPH], bladder stones, bladder tumors, pelvic tumors, urethral strictures, or spasms).
- Functional UI: urine leakage variable, often due to environmental or physical barriers to toileting (i.e., reduced mobility)
- Polyuria is defined by excessive amounts of urine (≥2.5 to 3 L) >24 hours.
- Nocturnal polyuria is where >33% of total daily urine output occurs during sleeping hours.

EPIDEMIOLOGY
- Stress incontinence in men is rare and is often attributable to prostate surgery, neurologic disease, or trauma.
- Reported rates of incontinence range from 1% after transurethral resection to 2–66% after radical prostatectomy and 1–15% following transvesical prostatectomy, although rates decline with time (1).

Prevalence
- 12.4% prevalence of UI in community-dwelling adult men in the United States
- 4.5% reported moderate to severe UI, of which 48.6% experienced urge, 23.5% experienced other UI, 15.4% experienced mixed, and 12.5% experienced stress incontinence as per the NHANES report in 2010 (1).

ETIOLOGY AND PATHOPHYSIOLOGY
- Incontinence secondary to bladder abnormalities
  - Detrusor overactivity results in urge incontinence.
  - Detrusor overactivity commonly is associated with bladder outlet obstruction from BPH.
  - Medications that increase bladder contractility or exacerbate obstructive effects
- Incontinence secondary to outlet abnormalities
  - Sphincteric damage secondary to pelvic surgery or radiation
  - Sphincteric dysfunction secondary to neurologic disease
  - Commonly associated with BPH due to compression of the urethra, affecting urinary flow

- Mixed incontinence is caused by abnormalities of both the bladder and the outlet overflow or by enlarged prostate/bladder neck contracture from prostate surgery.
- Stress incontinence is caused by weakened urethral sphincter and/or pelvic floor weakness.

RISK FACTORS
- Age
- Diseases: diabetes, BPH, hypertension (HTN), major depression, neurologic disease
- History of urinary tract infections (UTIs)
- Pelvic trauma, including prostate surgery
- Polypharmacy

GENERAL PREVENTION
Proper management of conditions, such as symptomatic bladder outlet obstruction caused by BPH early in the course, may prevent continence problems later in life.

COMMONLY ASSOCIATED CONDITIONS
Male UI often has a negative impact in both mental and physical aspects of quality of life. It is an independent risk factor for depression and anxiety, and it may significantly reduce work productivity.

 DIAGNOSIS

HISTORY
- 3 Incontinence Questions tool questionnaire:
  - During the last 3 months, have you leaked urine (even a small amount)? If no, end quiz.
  - During the last 3 months, did you leak urine (check all that apply):
    ○ When you were performing some physical activity, such as coughing, sneezing, lifting, or exercise?
    ○ When you had the urge or the feeling that you needed to empty your bladder, but you could not get to the toilet fast enough?
    ○ Without physical activity and without a sense of urgency?
  - During the last 3 months, did you leak urine most often (check only one):
    ○ When you were performing some physical activity, such as coughing sneezing, lifting, or exercise?
    ○ When you had the urge or the feeling that you needed to empty your bladder, but you could not get to the toilet fast enough?
    ○ Without physical activity and without a sense of urgency?
    ○ About equally as often with physical activity as with a sense of urgency?
- Voiding symptoms
  - Duration and characteristics of incontinence
  - Precipitants, severity, timing, and associated symptoms (BPH, fluid intake, etc.)
  - Use of pads, briefs, diapers
  - Alteration in bowel habits
  - Previous treatments and effect on incontinence
- Transient causes: UTI, delirium, medications, constipation, immobility
- Geriatric patients: Assess cognitive levels (dementia/delirium), psychological disorders, mobility problems.

- Medication use: diuretics, drugs for BPH, opioids, muscle relaxants, anticholinergics, antidepressants
- Alcohol and drug use, including caffeine
- Surgery: pelvic surgery or radiation, bowel, back, genitourinary procedures, abdominoperineal resection, prostatectomy: radical for cancer, open/transurethral for benign disease
- Red flag symptoms requiring rapid referral to specialist management
  - Pain, hematuria, recurrent UTI, history of prostate irradiation, history of radical pelvic surgery (i.e., prostate surgery), constant leakage suggesting fistula, voiding difficulty, suspected neurologic disease

PHYSICAL EXAM
- Abdominal examination
  - Suprapubic tenderness suggests UTI.
  - Surgical scars suggesting prior pelvic surgery
  - Suprapubic mass may be a palpable bladder and suggest retention.
  - Suprapubic mass may also be an abdominal mass applying pressure on a normal bladder.
  - Increased abdominal girth
- Genitourinary examination: external genitalia, DRE (prostate)
- Musculoskeletal (look for neurogenic or functional causes.)
  - Extremities, spine, skeletal deformities, scars from previous spinal surgery
  - Sacral abnormalities may be associated with neurogenic bladder dysfunction.
- Neurologic
  - Motor, sensory, reflexes

DIFFERENTIAL DIAGNOSIS
- Transient (infections, meds, constipation, etc.)
- Chronic
  - Urge incontinence
  - Stress incontinence
  - Mixed incontinence
  - Overflow incontinence
  - Functional UI

DIAGNOSTIC TESTS & INTERPRETATION
Initial Tests (lab, imaging)
- Urinalysis and urine culture to check for glucosuria, pyuria, proteinuria, and/or blood
  - If UTI is present, treat and then reassess need for further workup because this frequently causes UI.
- Voiding diary, the 3 Incontinence Questions (1)[C]
- Pad test if quantity of leakage or objective outcome measure is desired (low sensitivity)
- Postvoid residual (PVR) volume if difficulty voiding or other lower urinary tract symptoms using ultrasound (US) to measure PVR: PVR persistently ≥100 mL indicates voiding dysfunction (1)[C].
- PVR >200 mL suggests overflow incontinence. A patient whose PVR is <200 mL does not have overflow incontinence.
- Uroflowmetry
- PSA only if diagnosis of prostate cancer will influence treatment or if levels can help decision-making for patients at risk for BPH
- Renal function
- Voiding cystogram in select cases

Diagnostic Procedures/Other
- Prostate US and biopsy if indicated by physical exam or PSA level
- Urethrocystoscopy to exclude suspected bladder or urethral pathology or before invasive therapies
- Imaging of upper and lower urinary tract is not routinely indicated as part of UI assessment.

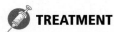

TREATMENT

Conservative, nonmedication interventions, such as behavioral modification, timed voiding, bladder training, and pelvic floor muscle training, should be considered *first-line therapies*, prior to initiating any pharmacologic therapy.

GENERAL MEASURES
- Bladder diaries
- Bladder training and timed voiding are effective.
- Pelvic floor muscle training speeds recovery of continence following radical prostatectomy
- Weight loss may improve UI symptoms.
- Constipation is associated with UI, but treatment may not improve UI.
- Reduction in caffeine intake does not improve UI but may improve urgency and frequency.
- Pads may be used for urine containment in UI as well as external sheaths (1)[B]—external sheaths may have similar rates of UTIs with indwelling catheters but result in better QoL (1)[B].
  - Men with UI should be counseled that leakage is not a normal part of aging and that goals of treatment include elimination of the need for these.

MEDICATION
First Line
- Urge incontinence: There is no consistent evidence that drug therapy is better than behavioral therapy in urge incontinence (1)[B], and behavioral therapy results in higher patient satisfaction (1)[B].
- Antimuscarinic agents are first-line drug therapy in urge incontinence (1)[B], and there is no evidence that any one agent is superior for urge incontinence (1)[A].
- Oxybutynin (Ditropan XL) 5 to 15 mg PO every day
- Tolterodine (Detrol LA) 2 to 4 mg PO every day
- Darifenacin (Enablex) 7.5 to 15 mg PO every day
- Solifenacin (VESIcare) 5 to 10 mg PO every day
- Trospium chloride (Sanctura XR) 60 mg PO every day
- Transdermal oxybutynin (Gelnique) 10% apply daily (EAU Grade B)—no dry mouth
- Fesoterodine (Toviaz) 4 to 8 mg PO every day
- Mirabegron, a β_3-agonist, has been shown in some trials and systematic reviews to be as efficacious as antimuscarinics.
- Mirabegron (Myrbetriq): 25 to 50 mg PO daily; *caution*: HTN
- Review efficacy and side effects 4 to 6 weeks after treatment initiation.
- Most patients will stop antimuscarinic therapy within 3 months due to adverse effects, nonefficacy, or cost.

- Caution in those with bladder outlet obstruction and PVR >250 to 300 mL: In men with urgency associated with BPH, consider α-blockers (i.e., tamsulosin, alfuzosin, silodosin) as monotherapy or in combination with antimuscarinic for residual overactive bladder.
- Stress incontinence
  - No generally accepted drug therapy
  - Mixed stress and urge incontinence; ER formulations are preferred due to reduced side effects.

Second Line
- Urge incontinence
- Tricyclic antidepressants
  - Imipramine 10 to 25 mg PO BID/TID
- Desmopressin (DDAVP) for occasional short-term relief of UI
  - 25 to 50 μg PO or intranasal at bedtime
- Intradetrusor botulinum toxin injections 100 U intravesical injections (not FDA-approved)
- Duloxetine for temporary improvements of incontinence with dose titration (mixed stress/urge)

Geriatric Considerations
Anticholinergics and tricyclics may result in significant cognitive impairment in elderly patients.

ISSUES FOR REFERRAL
- Prior pelvic surgery/invasive procedure or radiation of the prostate or urethra
- PVR >300 mL
- Neurologic disease
- Recurrent bladder or prostate infections
- Pelvic pain
- Severe incontinence requiring multiple heavy pads or diapers each day

ADDITIONAL THERAPIES
- Pelvic floor rehabilitation (Kegel exercises) may significantly reduce both stress and urge incontinence in male patients and should be considered a part of initial management for stress UI.
- Overflow incontinence is usually caused by poor bladder contractility with urinary retention.
  - Indwelling or intermittent catheterization, evaluate for outlet obstruction.

SURGERY/OTHER PROCEDURES
- Urge incontinence
  - Sacral nerve stimulation with behavioral therapy
  - Augmentation cystoplasty and urinary diversion
  - Botulinum toxin injection via cystoscopy
- Stress incontinence
  - Urethral bulking agents: modest success rates with low cure rates
  - Male sling procedures: promising short-term and intermediate results but no long-term studies
  - Artificial urinary sphincter implant has excellent long-term continence rates and is considered gold standard.
    - Success rates have been defined as use of ≤1 pad/day and have ranged from 59% to 90% at follow-up intervals from 1 to 8 years. Surgical intervention has very high patient satisfaction rate, but revision is often required due to urethral erosion, infection, or atrophy. Foley catheter trauma is a common cause of late urethral erosion.

ONGOING CARE

FOLLOW-UP RECOMMENDATIONS
- To assess associated symptoms, severity, and hassles of incontinence, there are:
  - Michigan Incontinence Symptom Index (M-ISI)
- International Consultation on Incontinence Questionnaire–Urinary Incontinence Short Form
- To assess severity of UI, there are:
  - Sadvik questionnaire—used to assess frequency and amount of leakage
  - 24-hour pad weight
  - Bladder diary

COMPLICATIONS
- Dermatitis, candidiasis, skin breakdown
- Social isolation
- Avoidance of sex
- Weight gain

REFERENCE
1. Khandelwal C, Kistler C. Diagnosis of urinary incontinence. *Am Fam Physician*. 2013;87(8): 543–550.

CODES

ICD10
- R32 Unspecified urinary incontinence
- N39.3 Stress incontinence (female) (male)
- N39.41 Urge incontinence

CLINICAL PEARLS
- Think "outside" the lower urinary tract: Comorbid medical illness and impairments are independently associated with UI; treat contributing comorbidities and rule out secondary causes.
- Always check PVR: PVR ≥100 mL indicates voiding dysfunction; ≥200 mL suggests overflow incontinence.

I

INFECTIOUS MONONUCLEOSIS, EPSTEIN-BARR VIRUS INFECTIONS

Dennis E. Hughes, DO, FACEP

 BASICS

DESCRIPTION
- Epstein-Barr virus (EBV) is a member of the gamma herpes virus family; human herpes virus 4.
  - Two subtypes: ST1 predominates in Western Hemisphere, Southeast Asia; ST1 and ST2 equally prevalent in Africa
- Primary infection typically occurs in childhood. The majority of individuals seroconvert by 2 years of age with little clinical manifestation of illness. A second peak occurs in adolescence and young adulthood—this group commonly manifests infection as infectious mononucleosis (IM) (1).
- WHO classified EBV as "tumor virus" (group I carcinogen) due to cancer association.

EPIDEMIOLOGY
Incidence
- Military recruits, college students, and others living in cloistered and crowded populations have highest symptomatic infection rate. Overall rate in the United States is 500/100,000.
- Predominant age of symptomatic primary infection is 15 to 24 years; 200 to 800/100,000 affected
- Incidence increases during the summer months.

Prevalence
- Worldwide, 95% of population has been infected by adulthood. By age 5, 50% of children have been infected; the vast majority of those without manifesting symptoms.
- Seroconversion occurs later in childhood in developed countries; there is suggestion of race/ethnicity disparity in the United States with higher seroprevalence in non-Hispanic black, Asian, and Hispanic populations; also, higher prevalence in larger households and lower levels of parental education (2)

ETIOLOGY AND PATHOPHYSIOLOGY
- After inoculation, the virus replicates in the nasopharyngeal epithelium with resulting cell lysis, virion spread, and viremia. EBV exhibits dual tropism for B-cells and epithelial cells. The reticuloendothelial system is affected, resulting in a host response and the appearance of atypical lymphocytes in the peripheral blood. Viral genome can be detected in the oral cavity 1 week prior to symptoms.
- A polyclonal B-cell proliferative response follows. Relatively few (<0.1%) of circulating lymphocytes are infected by EBV in the acute illness.
- A persistent (asymptomatic) state ensues with the EBV genome invisible to the immune system. The maintenance of the invisible state (to host immunity) is thought to be due to EBV particles, wrapping themselves in host cell-derived membranes and a low rate of viral reproduction (1).
- Either through B-cell stimulation or diminished EBV-specific immune modulation, the previously latent EBV-infected B cells replicate and enter a "lytic" phase, allowing clinical expression of the EBV genome. Risk of this occurrence may be linked to host genetic factors, smoking, increased BMI, and low vitamin D/sunlight exposure. The proteins produced may either modify host response or contribute directly to malignancy (2).
- Immunosuppression (organ transplant/acquired immune deficiency) can result in transformation and lymphoproliferative disorders.

RISK FACTORS
- Age (highest incidence of symptomatic infection in adolescents and young adults)
- Sociohygienic level "crowded conditions"
- Geographic location
- Close, intimate contact; especially "deep kissing" in adolescents and young adults
- Immunosuppression
- Possibly some risk of transmission by fomites (e.g., shared toys)

GENERAL PREVENTION
- Avoid close physical contact with symptomatic EBV/IM patients.
- Meticulous hand washing and hygiene
- General precautions with potential blood exposure (EBV can be transmitted via blood contamination as well as hematopoietic cell and solid organ transplant.)
- EBV vaccines under investigation (Lack of intimate knowledge of mechanism of immune response has impaired the ability to develop an effective vaccine)

COMMONLY ASSOCIATED CONDITIONS
- IM: Symptomatic primary EBV infection is common in otherwise healthy adolescents and young adults.
  - Clinical features vary in severity and duration: In children age <10 years, generally mild; in adolescents and adults, symptoms can be more severe and protracted (are dependent on intensity of T-cell response).
  - Incubation period is 30 to 50 days (extremely long for a viral infection).
- X-linked lymphoproliferative syndrome (XLP—rare, inherited extreme vulnerability to EBV infection)
- Lymphoproliferative syndromes due to EBV infections in transplant recipients
- Lymphomas (B-cell lymphoblastic, T cell)
- Lymphocytic interstitial pneumonitis
- Hairy leukoplakia of the tongue, leiomyosarcoma, and CNS lymphomas in patients with AIDS
- Burkitt lymphoma (most common childhood tumor in Africa and Papua New Guinea where malaria is also endemic and may be a cofactor); much higher prevalence than other areas of the world
- Nasopharyngeal carcinoma (seen worldwide but highest prevalence in Africa and Asia)
- Parotid carcinoma
- Hodgkin lymphoma (most common EBV-associated malignancy in the United States, European Union)
- Postulated to be associated with multiple sclerosis (2 to 3 times incidence in EBV-positive individuals)
- Chronic active EBV (CAEBV) due to loss of host control of viral replication

DIAGNOSIS
Diagnostic accuracy of clinical signs and symptoms varies.

HISTORY
- May be either abrupt or insidious in onset
- Syndrome of fatigue, malaise, and sore throat
- In adults, temperature may rise to 103°F (39.4°C) and gradually fall over a variable period of 7 to 10 days; in severe cases, temperature elevations of 104°F to 105°F (40°C to 40.6°C) may persist for 2 weeks.

- Children typically have low-grade fever or are afebrile.
- Rash, conjunctivitis (3)
- Chest pain (myocarditis and pericarditis)

PHYSICAL EXAM
- Fever, lymphadenopathy, pharyngitis in >50%, with palatal petechiae and hepatosplenomegaly in ~10%
- Diffuse hyperemia and hyperplasia of oropharyngeal lymphoid tissue
- Gelatinous, grayish-white exudative tonsillitis persists for 7 to 10 days in 50%.
- Petechiae at border of hard and soft palates in 60% (LR+1.32–11.4)
- Bilateral upper eyelid edema (Hoagland sign)
- Axillary, epitrochlear, popliteal, inguinal, mediastinal, and mesenteric lymphadenopathy (95% of patients; LR+1.85–4.7)
- Lymph node enlargement subsides over days/weeks.
- Tender lymphadenopathy (cervical nodes are most commonly enlarged); absence of any lymphadenopathy LR-0.37
- Splenomegaly in 50% (LR+1.9–6.6)
- Skin manifestations in 3–16%
  - Erythematous macular/maculopapular rash
  - Petechial and purpuric exanthems reported
  - Rash typically on trunk and upper arms; occasionally, the face and forearms are involved.

DIFFERENTIAL DIAGNOSIS
- Streptococcal pharyngitis and tonsillitis
- Diphtheria
- Blood dyscrasias
- Rubella, measles, viral hepatitis, cytomegalovirus
- Toxoplasmosis
- Acute HIV infection

DIAGNOSTIC TESTS & INTERPRETATION
Initial Tests (lab, imaging)
- CBC with differential
- Lymphocytes and atypical lymphocytes
  - Increased numbers of lymphocytes (especially atypical lymphocytes; may be up to 70% of leukocytes) in peripheral blood
  - In 1st week after onset, WBC count is normal/moderately decreased. Due to EB-related neutrophil fragility, automated processing can result in pseudoneutropenia.
    ○ By week 2, atypical lymphocytosis develops.
  - During early illness, atypical lymphocytes are B cells transformed by the EBV; later, atypical cells are activated CD8 T lymphocytes.
- Antibodies
  - Heterophile antibodies in 80–90% of adults; monospot (latex agglutination) test is highly specific, but its sensitivity varies from 70–90%.
  - Heterophile antibody is an IgM response, which appears during the first 2 weeks of illness; it disappears in 4 to 6 weeks (higher false negative rate in children <4 years of age).
  - In general, agglutinin titer is higher in IM than other disorders; an unabsorbed heterophile titer >1:128 and ≥1:40 is significant.

- Specific antibodies to EBV-associated antigens
  - Develop regularly in IM
  - Viral capsid-specific IgM and IgG are present early in illness.
  - Viral capsid IgM disappears after several weeks; viral capsid IgG persists for life.
- Liver tests: Transaminitis and hyperbilirubinemia are common; jaundice is rare.
- Atypical lymphocytes are not specific for EBV infections and may be present in other clinical conditions, including rubella, infectious hepatitis, allergic rhinitis, asthma, and atypical pneumonia.
- Routine abdominal ultrasound to monitor for splenic enlargement is not necessary.
- Consider ultrasound for those wishing to return to strenuous activity/contact sports at day 21 of illness to exclude splenomegaly.

Follow-Up Tests & Special Considerations
- Abnormal hepatic enzymes persist in 80% of patients for several weeks; hepatomegaly in 15–20%
- In transplant recipients, quantitative polymerase chain reaction (PCR) is used to monitor EBV loads

Diagnostic Procedures/Other
Chest x-ray
- Hilar adenopathy may be observed in IM with extensive lymphoid hyperplasia.

Test Interpretation
- Mononuclear infiltrations of lymph nodes, tonsils, spleen, lungs, liver, heart, kidneys, adrenal glands, skin, and CNS
- Bone marrow hyperplasia with small granuloma formation may be present; these findings are nonspecific and have no prognostic significance.

 TREATMENT
- Treatment is primarily supportive.
- NSAIDs or acetaminophen
- During acute stage, limit activity for 4 weeks to reduce potential complications (e.g., splenic rupture).
- Transplant recipients who develop EBV infection may require alteration of immunosuppressive therapy and administration of monoclonal anti-CD20 (rituximab).

MEDICATION
- In primary infections:
  - Antimicrobial agents (usually penicillin) only if throat culture is positive for group A β-hemolytic streptococci; incidence of rash following β-lactam antibiotic therapy previously is much lower than historically thought.
  - Warm saline gargles for oropharyngeal pain
  - Corticosteroids
    ○ May provide some symptomatic relief but no improvement in resolution of illness; a recent Cochrane review of seven studies provided no support for routine use (4).

○ Consider in severe pharyngotonsillitis with oropharyngeal edema and airway encroachment. Dexamethasone 0.3 mg/kg/day may be used for 1 to 3 days.
○ There is no available evidence to support use in major complications (e.g., hemolytic anemia, thrombocytopenic purpura, neurologic sequelae, myocarditis, pericarditis).
- Antiviral medications (acyclovir) have been found to shorten recovery time and improve subjective symptoms in acute EBV infection in small studies.

ISSUES FOR REFERRAL
Most cases can be managed as an outpatient without the need for specialty referral. Consider referral for complications such as oropharyngeal edema with airway compromise.

SURGERY/OTHER PROCEDURES
- Splenectomy may be necessary with profound thrombocytopenia that is refractory to corticosteroids.
- Only current effective treatment for XLP is hematopoietic stem cell transplantation. There is some use of monoclonal antibody to delay progression pre-HST or treat relapse posttransplant.
- Splenic rupture

 ONGOING CARE

FOLLOW-UP RECOMMENDATIONS

ALERT
Rupture of the spleen may be fatal if not recognized; it requires blood transfusions, treatment for shock, and splenectomy. Occurrence is estimated at 0.1%.

Patient Monitoring
- Avoid contact sports, heavy lifting, and excess exertion until spleen and liver have returned to normal size (ultrasound can verify). Current consensus is that if after 3 weeks and normal exam, no fever, and no constitutional symptoms, patients may return to contact sport activities.
- Eliminate alcohol/exposure to other hepatotoxic drugs until LFTs return to normal.
- Rates of complications are highest during the first 3 weeks of illness.
- Symptoms (malaise, fatigue, intermittent sore throat, lymphadenopathy) may persist for months.

DIET
No restrictions; hydration is important.

PROGNOSIS
- Most recover in ~4 weeks.
- Fatigue may persist for months.

COMPLICATIONS
- Neurologic (rare)
  - Aseptic meningitis, meningoencephalitis
  - Bell palsy, Guillain-Barré syndrome
  - Transverse myelitis, cerebellar ataxia, acute psychosis

- Hematologic (rare)
  - Thrombocytopenia, early in illness
  - Hemolytic anemia with neutropenia (early), hemophagocytic syndrome (splenomegaly, fever, cytopenia)
  - Agammaglobulinemia
- Pneumonitis
- Airway obstruction
- Splenic rupture
  - Rare, but most often occurs in first 21 days of illness

REFERENCES
1. Yu H, Robertson ES. Epstein-Barr virus history and pathogenesis. *Viruses*. 2023;15(3):714.
2. Houen G, Trier NH. Epstein-Barr virus and systemic autoimmune diseases. *Front Immunol*. 2021;11:587380.
3. Cai X, Ebell MH, Haines L. Accuracy of signs, symptoms, and hematologic parameters for the diagnosis of infectious mononucleosis: a systematic review and meta-analysis. *J Am Board Fam Med*. 2021;34(6):1141–1156.
4. Gomes K, Goldman RD. Corticosteroids for infectious mononucleosis. *Can Fam Physician*. 2023;69(2):101–102.

CODES

ICD10
- B27.00 Gammaherpesviral mononucleosis without complication
- B27.09 Gammaherpesviral mononucleosis with other complications
- B27.01 Gammaherpesviral mononucleosis with polyneuropathy

CLINICAL PEARLS
- 98% of patients with acute IM present with some combination of fever, sore throat, cervical node enlargement, and tonsillar hypertrophy.
- False-negative monospot (heterophile antibody) is common in the first 10 to 14 days of illness. 90% will have heterophile antibodies by week 3 of illness.
- Lymphocytosis (not monocytosis) is common in IM.
- Treatment of IM is primarily supportive.

I

INFERTILITY
Sahil Mullick, MD • Sudeshna Dutta, MD

BASICS

DESCRIPTION
Definition: failure to conceive after 12 months of regular sexual intercourse without contraception; evaluation for infertility should begin for failure to conceive after 6 months of regular intercourse without contraception in women >35 years of age. More immediate evaluation is recommended in women >40 years of age. Primary infertility: Couple has never been pregnant. Secondary infertility: Couple has been pregnant.

EPIDEMIOLOGY
Incidence
The incidence of infertility increases with age, with a decline in fertility in the early 30s, accelerating in the late 30s. ~85% of couples will conceive within 12 months of unprotected intercourse. ~95% of couples will conceive within 24 months of unprotected intercourse. In the United States, ~12.7% of women of reproductive age seek infertility treatment each year (1).

Prevalence
- Infertility affects 8.8% of U.S. women between the ages of 15 and 49 (1).
- ~9% of couples between the ages of 15 and 34 years, 25% of couples between the ages of 35 and 39 years, and ~30% of couples between the ages of 40 and 44 years meet the criteria for being infertile, according to the National Survey of Family Growth.
- This may increase as more women delay childbearing.

ETIOLOGY AND PATHOPHYSIOLOGY
- Most cases are multifactorial: Approximately 85% are due to identifiable causes such as tubal disease, ovulatory dysfunction, and male factor infertility (due to abnormal sperm production or delivery). The other 15% have unexplained causes of infertility.
- Acquired: The most common cause of infertility in the United States is pelvic inflammatory disease (PID) secondary to sexually transmitted infections (STIs), followed by endometriosis, polycystic ovary syndrome (PCOS), premature ovarian failure, and increased maternal age. ~25% of infertility diagnoses are due to ovulatory disorders (such as PCOS, hyperprolactinemia, hypothyroidism or hyperthyroidism, primary ovarian insufficiency, ovarian dysgenesis/agenesis, exposure to chemo or radiotherapy, eating disorder, tumors, prior surgery). 70% of women with anovulation have PCOS.
- Diminished ovarian reserve (DOR): low fertility due to insufficient quantity or functional quality of oocytes
- Congenital abnormalities: anatomic (such as undescended testicles, bicornuate uterus, etc.) and genetic

Genetics
There is a higher incidence of genetic abnormalities among the infertile population, including Klinefelter syndrome (47, XXY), Turner syndrome (45X or mosaic), and fragile X syndrome. Y chromosomal microdeletions are associated with isolated defects of spermatogenesis → found in 16% of men with azoospermia/severe oligospermia; cystic fibrosis transmembrane conductance regulator (CFTR) gene mutation causing congenital bilateral absence of vas deferens (CBAVD)

RISK FACTORS
- Female
  - Gynecologic history: irregular/abnormal menses, STIs, dysmenorrhea, fibroids
  - Medical history: advanced age, endocrinopathy, autoimmune disease, undiagnosed celiac disease, collagen vascular diseases, thrombophilia, obesity, and cancer
  - Surgical history: appendicitis, pelvic surgery, intrauterine surgery, tubal ligation
  - Social history: smoking, alcohol/substance abuse, eating disorders, exercise, advanced maternal age
- Male
  - Medical history: STIs, prostatitis, medication use (i.e., β-blockers, calcium channel blockers, antiulcer medication), endocrinopathy, cancer
  - Surgical history: orchiopexy, hernia repair, vasectomy with/without reversal
  - Social history: smoking, alcohol/substance abuse, anabolic steroids, environmental exposures, occupations leading to increased scrotal temperature (frequent use of saunas, hot tubs, or tight underwear), prescription drugs that impair male potency

COMMONLY ASSOCIATED CONDITIONS
Pelvic pathology, endocrine dysfunction, and anovulation (hyperandrogenism, PCOS)

DIAGNOSIS

HISTORY
Complete reproductive history including the age of partners; history of abortion, dilation and curettage, bilateral tubal ligation, vasectomy, or other pelvic/abdominal surgery; age at menarche, regularity of menstrual cycle (i.e., every 21 to 35 days), physical development (Tanner stages), previous methods of contraception, history of abnormal Pap smears and treatment; coital frequency and timing; history of sexual dysfunction; history of STI, endocrine abnormalities, malignancy or chronic illness; family history of reproductive issues; medications: drug abuse, allergies, and exposure to environmental hazards

PHYSICAL EXAM
- Body mass index (BMI), distribution of body fat, and waist circumference
- Female
  - Pubertal development with Tanner staging
  - Signs of PCOS: androgen excess, obesity, signs of insulin resistance like acanthosis nigricans
  - Vaginal exam: Describe rugation, discharge, and anatomic variation.
  - Uterine size/shape, mobility, tenderness
- Male: abnormalities of the penis or urethral meatus; testes: volume, symmetry, masses (varicocele, hydrocele), presence/absence of vas deferens

DIFFERENTIAL DIAGNOSIS
Kallmann syndrome, idiopathic hypogonadotropic hypogonadism, luteinizing hormone (LH) deficiency, follicle-stimulating hormone (FSH) deficiency, growth hormone deficiency, hemochromatosis, endometriosis, thyroid disease, prolactinoma, obesity, PCOS

DIAGNOSTIC TESTS & INTERPRETATION
Initial Tests (lab, imaging)
Evaluation is directed by history:
- Assessment of ovulation
  - Irregular or infrequent menses
  - High LH to FSH ratio suggests PCOS.
  - Basal body temperature (BBT) charting to confirm ovulation is low-cost and may be helpful for some couples to guide the timing of intercourse.
  - LH surge happens 12 to 36 hours before ovulation. Testing usually starts 2 days before the expected ovulation.
  - Follicle size can guide timing of artificial insemination and intercourse.
  - Elevated progesterone level in the blood retrospectively indicates ovulation.
  - Cervical mucosal change (thin mucosa in the proliferative phase versus clear, slippery and stretchy mucosa during ovulation versus thick mucosa in the luteal phase)
  - Endometrial biopsy (invasive procedure) is occasionally used to determine ovulation.
- Assessment of ovarian reserve
  - Women >35 years old need to have ovarian reserve assessed. On day 3 of menses, an FSH >15 to 20 IU/L and estradiol >60 to 80 pg/mL (1) is suggestive of the impaired reserve.
  - Elevated FSH and LH and low estradiol indicate ovarian insufficiency.
  - Anti-müllerian hormone (AMH) and antral follicle counts (AFCs): The number of antral follicles measured by transvaginal ultrasound (US) is termed the "antral follicle count," and a low count is defined as <4 follicles that are between 2 to 10 mm in both ovaries. AMH decreases as a woman approaches menopause. AMH can be measured at any time during the cycle and is not affected by hormones.
  - Clomiphene challenge test: After administration of clomiphene from day 5 to 9, measure FSH of ≥10 mIU/mL on day 10 to help confirm the diagnosis of DOR.
- Semen analysis
  - Warranted in all infertile couples; semen analysis alone is not used to predict male fertility potential.
  - Semen collection: collected after 2 to 7 days of abstinence; repeat the test 2 to 3 times due to inherent variability within the same individual. A repeat analysis with at least a 1-month interval is required to diagnose "abnormal" semen analysis (1).
  - Parameters for normal male values: semen volume ≥1.5 mL, pH 7.2 to 7.8, sperm concentration of ≥15 million spermatozoa per mL, total sperm number of ≥39 million spermatozoa per ejaculate, motility 40% or more forward progressions, sperm morphology (percentage of normal forms) ≥4%, white blood cell count <1 million/microliter
  - Additional labs
    ○ Prolactin, thyroid-stimulating hormone, 17-hydroxyprogesterone, androgen levels
    ○ HIV, herpes simplex virus 1 and 2, chlamydia, gonorrhea, rapid plasma reagin, hepatitis B, and CMV
    ○ Genetic testing based on family history

- Transvaginal US for anatomic abnormality
- Hysterosalpingogram (HSG) to evaluate patency of tubes and contour of the cavity; may be both diagnostic and therapeutic

Follow-Up Tests & Special Considerations
Abnormal imaging may need surgical evaluation.

Diagnostic Procedures/Other
Hysteroscopy is the gold standard used to visualize the endometrial cavity directly; may be indicated to evaluate filling defects on HSG or SHG; laparoscopy is used to directly visualize the peritoneal cavity and may be done to evaluate abnormal findings on HSG such as suspected adhesions causing fallopian tube abnormality. Laparoscopy is the only way to diagnose endometriosis definitively.

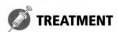 TREATMENT

GENERAL MEASURES
- Lifestyle changes that may improve fertility: achieving an ideal BMI, cessation of smoking, limiting exposure to caffeine and alcohol, coital frequency, and timing (every 1 to 2 days around the expected ovulation period).
- BBT tracking and detection of LH surge may be helpful for some couples. BBT is not as reliable as other methods for ovulation prediction.
- Be mindful of the couple's emotional state: depression, anger, anxiety, and marital discord are common.
- All female fertility patients should be given folate supplementation of 0.4 to 0.8 mg/day by mouth. Dietary carotenoids in males may improve sperm quality.
- In vitro fertilization (IVF) is the most effective infertility treatment available for women with unexplained infertility who have not conceived after 2 years of regular unprotected sexual intercourse:
  - Eggs are removed from the female and fertilized outside the body. The embryo is monitored for 3 to 5 days and then implanted into the uterus on day 3 or 5.
  - Anatomic causes should be referred for IVF. A surgical consult may be required.
  - Fewer complications have been reported for individuals undergoing IVF for anatomic causes rather than ovulatory dysfunction (low APGAR scores, diabetes mellitus).
  - Compared to the general population, an increased risk of preterm birth and low birth weight has also been seen among subfertile women who conceived naturally without IVF.
  - Donor eggs may be obtained.
  - Women <40 years of age or those who have not conceived after 2 years of unprotected intercourse or 12 cycles of artificial insemination should be offered three complete cycles of IVF.
  - Women aged 40 to 42 years with no evidence of previous IVF or low ovarian reserve should be offered one complete cycle of IVF.

- Intrauterine insemination (IUI) without ovarian stimulation can be considered in special circumstances: physical disabilities limiting vaginal intercourse or psychosexual issues, people in same-sex relationships, and so on.
- Male factors
  - IUI: Sperm is placed via a catheter directly in the uterus. IUI effectively increases sperm count to have successful fertilization, but IUI success rate is only 7 to 10% in each cycle.
  - Intracytoplasmic sperm injection (ICSI) is performed in conjunction with IVF for males with severe abnormalities (i.e., <5 million sperm) or those who have failed to conceive with IUI. A single sperm is injected directly into the cytoplasm of the egg. Fertilization occurs ~70% of the time.
  - Donor sperm may be obtained.

MEDICATION
First Line
- Treatment of infertility depends on etiology.
- Women:
  - Anovulation: must determine if HYPOgonadotropic or NORMOgonadotropic
    o Hypogonadotropic patients: Standard treatment to induce ovulation consists of daily injections of both FSH and LH, which need to be carefully monitored to avoid ovarian hyperstimulation syndrome (OHSS).
    o Normogonadotropic patients: most commonly due to PCOS; ovulation induction with letrozole (aromatase inhibitor) is first-line therapy and is found to be superior to clomiphene for patients with PCOS (1).
    o Unexplained infertility: controlled ovarian hyperstimulation, as with clomiphene citrate and IUI; IVF may be recommended as the second line.
  - Coital or cervical problems: IUI
  - Endometriosis: either IVF or surgery
- Male:
  - Lifestyle changes: increasing frequency and timing of intercourse
  - Medication changes to improve sperm count, testicular function, sperm production, and quality by discontinuing or changing certain selective serotonin reuptake inhibitors, calcium channel blockers, and highly active antiretroviral therapy medications
  - Various studies have shown the effectiveness of clomiphene citrate in improving the sperm count.
  - Surgery: reversal of sperm blockage (e.g., vasectomy, varicocele)
  - Sperm retrieval if ejaculation is problematic

Second Line
If clomiphene and letrozole fail to induce ovulation:
- Metformin is beneficial in anovulatory women with PCOS and glucose intolerance; start with 500 mg daily and increase to ~1,500 mg/day; monitor renal function; may take up to 3 months to be effective
- Consider oral contraceptive pills (OCPs) for ≥2 cycles and then retry clomiphene immediately after stopping OCPs.
- Cabergoline or bromocriptine is used if prolactin is elevated or if there is no withdrawal bleeding after progesterone administration. Once pregnancy has occurred, the medication can be stopped.
- Human menopausal gonadotropins (HMGs) or recombinant FSH is indicated if there is a resistance to clomiphene or hypogonadotropic.

ISSUES FOR REFERRAL
Reproductive endocrinology and urology; consider using surrogate pregnancy if the female cannot conceive.

SURGERY/OTHER PROCEDURES
Reproductive surgery may be necessary for those with anatomic causes of infertility; polypectomy, myomectomy, and salpingectomy for hydrosalpinx; consider treatment of varicocele and aspiration of sperm; ovarian drilling/wedge resection in patients with PCOS for reducing ovarian androgen production

 ONGOING CARE

FOLLOW-UP RECOMMENDATIONS
Specialist if not successful after 3 to 6 cycles of oral ovulation induction

DIET
Limit caffeine and alcohol intake.

PATIENT EDUCATION
- American Society for Reproductive Medicine (https://www.asrm.org)
- Resolve: The National Infertility Association (https://www.resolve.org)

PROGNOSIS
Most couples (80–90%) will achieve a pregnancy within 12 months of attempting pregnancy with regular unprotected sexual intercourse. Fecundability progressively decreases over time.

COMPLICATIONS
Anxiety, multiple pregnancies, OHSS, and a slightly increased risk of congenital abnormalities; women diagnosed with infertility and women receiving fertility treatment are at a higher risk of maternal morbidity than are fertile women.

REFERENCE
1. Carson SA, Kallen AN. Diagnosis and management of infertility: a review. *JAMA*. 2021;326(1):65–76.

 SEE ALSO

- Amenorrhea; Endometriosis; Metabolic Syndrome; Pelvic Inflammatory Disease; Polycystic Ovarian Syndrome (PCOS)
- Algorithm: Infertility

 CODES

ICD10
- N97.9 Female infertility, unspecified
- N46.9 Male infertility, unspecified
- N97.1 Female infertility of tubal origin

CLINICAL PEARLS
Infertility is often multifactorial.

INFLUENZA

Susan McDiarmid, EdD, MS, PA-C • Michelle E. Duffelmeyer, MD

 BASICS

DESCRIPTION
Acute, typically self-limited, febrile infection caused by orthomyxovirus influenza types A and B marked by inflammation of nasal mucosa, pharynx, conjunctiva, and respiratory tract

EPIDEMIOLOGY
- Outbreaks of influenza occur annually during the fall–winter months in the Northern and Southern Hemispheres.
- Influenza virus can undergo antigenic shift (abrupt change) leading to viral strains with little immunologic resistance in a population, resulting in pandemic outbreaks. Minor seasonal variations are called *antigenic drift*.
- Persons of all ages are susceptible to infection. Notable demographics at risk for complications and hospitalization include:
  - Those between <2 and >65 years old; immunocompromised states, including pregnancy up to 2 weeks postpartum
  - Individuals with cardiovascular or pulmonary disease, Addison disease, or diabetes; residents of nursing homes or other long-term care facilities

Incidence
Incidence is difficult to ascertain as most individuals do not seek medical care and are therefore not diagnosed.

Prevalence
In the United States, on the 2022–2023 season, the preliminary data reveals an estimated 27 to 54 million confirmed positive cases with 12 to 26 million related medical visits, 300,000 to 650,000 hospitalizations and between 19,000 and 58,000 deaths. Since the introduction of SARS-CoV-2 into the community, influenza rates have decreased as compared to prepandemic. The 2021–2022 season remained historically low with the CDC reporting 9 million flu illnesses, 4 million flu-related medical visits, 100,000 flu-related hospitalizations, and 5,000 flu deaths. Influenza A (H3N2) was the most dominant strain of the season. The number of cases of influenza-associated illness, hospitalizations, and deaths were the lowest since the 2011–2012 season. Rates increased in 2022, likely due in part to changing isolation guidelines (i.e., increased interpersonal contact) in the context of the COVID pandemic.

ETIOLOGY AND PATHOPHYSIOLOGY
Orthomyxovirus (influenza types A [majority] and B); influenza A virus subtypes HxNx based on hemagglutinin and neuraminidase
- Incubation is 1 to 4 days; infected persons are most contagious during peak symptoms. Spread by aerosolized droplets or contact with respiratory secretions, hemagglutinin binds to columnar respiratory epithelium where replication occurs, and neuraminidase protein facilitates spread along respiratory epithelium (1).

RISK FACTORS
- For contracting disease:
  - Crowded environments such as nursing homes, barracks, schools, and correctional facilities
- For complications:
  - Neonates, infants, elderly; pregnancy (including 2 weeks postpartum) especially in 3rd trimester
  - Chronic pulmonary diseases; cardiovascular diseases, including valvular pathology and congestive heart failure
  - Metabolic disease, morbid obesity; hemoglobinopathies; malignancy
  - Immunosuppression; neuromuscular diseases that limit respiratory function and ability to handle secretions

GENERAL PREVENTION
- All persons aged ≥6 months should be vaccinated annually unless contraindication is present.
- Live attenuated influenza vaccine (LAIV) is a quadrivalent intranasal vaccine approved for healthy, nonpregnant individuals between 2 and 49 years of age.
- Inactivated influenza vaccine (IIV) is available either as trivalent (IIV3) or quadrivalent (IIV4) with either three or four strains of influenza. IIV also is available as high-dose, intradermal, cell culture–based (ccIIV3), MF59-adjuvanted (aIIV3), and recombinant hemagglutinin vaccine (RIV3).
- IIV is recommended annually for all persons aged ≥6 months. Vaccine should be administered annually as soon as the vaccine is available. Protection occurs 1 to 2 weeks after immunization. Typically, mild side effects include low-grade fever and local reaction at the vaccination site. Inactivated IM dose: ≥3 years of age: 0.5 mL; children 6 to 35 months of age: 0.25 mL. Intradermal formulation for 18- to 64-year-olds uses a short 30-gauge needle in a single-use prefilled syringe with 0.1 mL vaccine; somewhat higher local reactions when given intradermal; single annual dose except for children <9 years of age, who should receive two doses (4 weeks apart) the 1st year they receive influenza vaccine
- Vaccine contraindication: Severe allergy such as anaphylaxis to IIV components, allergies from eggs are not considered a contraindication; observe all patients for 15 minutes after vaccination; no skin testing with influenza vaccine is needed in egg-allergic patients. RIV is safe in patients with an egg allergy.
- IIV-HD: high-dose quadrivalent IIV contains 4 times the antigen concentration of IIV; licensed for persons ≥65 years of age; results in higher antibody levels but somewhat higher rates of local reactions; Advisory Committee on Immunization Practices does not express a preference for/against IIV-HD.
- Antiviral prophylaxis depends on current resistance patterns each year; see https://www.cdc.gov/flu/ for patterns or check with local health department. In high-risk groups that have not been vaccinated or need additional control measures during epidemics; *not* a substitute for vaccination unless vaccine is contraindicated
  - During influenza season, for those with contraindications to vaccine who have been exposed to the virus
  - For staff and residents in nursing home outbreaks; for immune-deficient persons who are expected not to respond to vaccination after viral exposure

Pediatric Considerations
Vaccinate children 6 months and older annually. Recommend all household members with children aged <6 months be vaccinated. For children who need 2 doses, administer first dose as soon as available for second dose to be given before the end of October. For prophylaxis, oseltamivir dosage varies by weight and is recommended by the CDC for prophylaxis for children aged ≥3 months; zanamivir is approved for prophylaxis for children ≥5 years of age at a dosage of 2 inhalations per day. Prophylaxis treatment duration is 7 days. Currently, amantadine and rimantadine are not recommended due to resistance.

Pregnancy Considerations
- The CDC recommends vaccinating all women who will be pregnant during influenza season. If unvaccinated at the time of flu season, pregnant women should receive IIV or RIV.
- Oseltamivir, zanamivir, peramivir, rimantadine, and amantadine are pregnancy Category C medications.

COMMONLY ASSOCIATED CONDITIONS
Pneumonia, cardiac complications, central nervous system involvement, myositis, rhabdomyolysis, multisystem organ failure

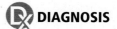 **DIAGNOSIS**

HISTORY
Sudden onset of:
- Fever (37.7–40°C), especially within 3 days of illness onset
- Anorexia; chills, sweats, malaise, myalgia, arthralgia
- Headache; sore throat/pharyngitis
- Nonproductive cough; rhinorrhea, nasal congestion
- Gastrointestinal symptoms of nausea, vomiting, and diarrhea (occur in up to 20% of children)
- Altered mental status (especially in the elderly or immunosuppressed)

PHYSICAL EXAM
- Physical exam is not specific for influenza.
- Physical examination should exclude complications such as otitis media, pneumonia, pharyngitis, sinusitis, and tracheobronchitis.

DIFFERENTIAL DIAGNOSIS
- Respiratory viral infections including, SARS-CoV-2, respiratory syncytial virus, parainfluenza, adenovirus, enterovirus ("influenza-like illness")
- Infectious mononucleosis; coxsackievirus infections; viral or streptococcal tonsillitis
- Atypical mycoplasmal pneumonia; *Chlamydia pneumoniae*; Q fever
- Less likely possibilities include severe acute respiratory syndrome, primary HIV infection, acute myeloid leukemia, tuberculosis, anthrax, and malaria.

DIAGNOSTIC TESTS & INTERPRETATION
Initial Tests (lab, imaging)
During influenza season, decision to pursue diagnostic testing is based on clinical findings. Various testing modalities are discussed below:

- Antigen detection; rapid influenza diagnostic tests (RIDTs); outpatient office based testing detects viral antigens within 10 to 15 minutes; moderate sensitivity (80%), high specificity
- Molecular assay
  - Reverse transcription polymerase chain reaction (RT-PCR); high sensitivity (90–95%) and specificity
- Immunofluorescence
  - Commercial rapid enzyme-linked immunosorbent assay antigen tests are available. Some rapid tests diagnose influenza A, whereas others diagnose A and B. Sensitivity and specificity vary by manufacturer, strain of influenza, and age of patient. False-negative results are common, particularly during peak influenza activity.

Follow-Up Tests & Special Considerations
- In patient with severe symptoms at presentation, consider the additional tests:
  - Complete blood count: typically shows normal WBC count or mild leukopenia. Leukocytosis may indicate bacterial complication. Comprehensive metabolic panel: elevations of liver enzymes or creatinine may indicate severe disease; chest x-ray if pneumonia is suspected
- The concurrent SARS-CoV-2 pandemic poses a diagnostic challenge during the 2022–2023 influenza season given the wide overlap of symptoms. The FDA has granted Emergency Use Authorization for developing commercially available combination tests for both SARS-CoV-2 and influenza A and RSV.

Test Interpretation
Positive and negative predictive values depend on community prevalence. As influenza peaks, a positive test is more likely to reflect true infection, whereas a negative test is more likely to be false.

 TREATMENT

- Symptomatic treatment (saline nasal spray, analgesic gargle, antipyretics, analgesics, expectorants, suppressants)
- Cool-mist or ultrasonic humidifier to increase moisture of inspired air
- Counsel on droplet precautions: wearing a disposable surgical mask around others. Five days is the average period of viral shedding in immunocompetent hosts. Hospitalized patients may require oxygen or ventilatory support.
- Tobacco cessation

MEDICATION
- Antiviral treatment depends on yearly resistance patterns; check https://www.cdc.gov/flu/ or with local health department. Antivirals are most effective if administered within first 48 hours. Antivirals within 48 hours of symptom onset are recommended for patients at risk of complications (i.e., diabetes, CHD, COPD, asthma, etc.). Antivirals are recommended if hospitalized.

- Antivirals include baloxavir, oseltamivir, zanamivir, and peramivir. Amantadine *and* rimantadine *currently are not recommended due to resistance*.
- Consider antivirals for patients whose onset of symptoms is within the past 48 hours and who wish to shorten the duration of illness and further reduce their relatively low risk of complications.
- Symptomatic treatment is preferred for those patients *without risk factors* and *without* signs of lower respiratory tract infection.
- Antiviral effect is 24-hour reduction of symptoms and a reduction in complication rates.
  - Baloxavir dose: oral, 1-time dose
    - 40 to <80 kg, 40 mg; >80 kg, 80 mg; For children >12 years, use adult dosing.
    - Children ≥5 and adolescence <20 kg: Oral suspension: Oral: 2 mg/kg once as a single dose
  - Zanamivir dose: 2 inhalations BID for 5 days (age ≥7 years)
  - Oseltamivir dose: 75 mg PO BID for 5 days (age ≥13 years)
  - Oseltamivir for children ≥1 year of age
    - <15 kg, 30 mg BID; >15 to 23 kg, 45 mg BID; >23 to 40 kg, 60 mg BID; >40 kg, 75 mg BID
  - Oseltamivir for children <1 year of age: 3 mg/kg/dose BID
  - Peramivir dose: 600 mg IV infusion over 15 to 30 minutes for adults ≥18 years of age
- Antipyretics
  - Acetaminophen: in children
- Precautions
  - Zanamivir bronchospasm if the patient has COPD or asthma; have a bronchodilator available
  - Amantadine has anticholinergic properties.
  - Rimantadine may increase the risk of seizures in those with an underlying seizure disorder.
  - Oseltamivir may cause nausea and vomiting; may be less severe if taken with food
  - Peramivir may cause serious skin reactions.
  - Baloxavir may cause diarrhea and hypersensitivity reactions.
- Adjust dose of antivirals if creatinine clearance <60 mL/min.
- Ibuprofen or other NSAIDs for symptomatic relief. Aspirin: should not be used in children aged <16 years due to risk of Reye syndrome; outpatient treatment except for cases with severe complications or in high-risk groups (2).

ADMISSION, INPATIENT, AND NURSING CONSIDERATIONS
Initiate droplet precautions for both confirmed or suspected influenza. Initiate prompt antiviral therapy for patients hospitalized with influenza-related illness, regardless of prior duration of symptoms.

 ONGOING CARE

FOLLOW-UP RECOMMENDATIONS
Mild cases: follow-up typically not required. Moderate/severe: follow up until symptoms and secondary sequelae resolve.

PROGNOSIS
Good

COMPLICATIONS
- Sepsis; pneumonia (primary viral or secondary bacterial)
- Myocarditis; encephalitis; myositis, rhabdomyolysis
- Otitis media; acute sinusitis; croup; bronchitis
- Apnea in neonates Reye syndrome
- Encephalopathy, death

Geriatric Considerations
Complications requiring hospitalization are more likely in elderly patients.

REFERENCES
1. Centers for Disease Control and Prevention. 2022-2023 U.S. flu season: preliminary in-season burden estimates. https://www.cdc.gov/flu/about/burden/preliminary-in-season-estimates.htm. Accessed October 19, 2023.
2. Gaitonde DY, Moore FC, Morgan MK. Influenza: diagnosis and treatment. *Am Fam Physician*. 2019;100(12):751–758.

ADDITIONAL READING
- Committee on Infectious Diseases. Recommendations for Prevention and Control of Influenza in Children, 2022–2023. *Pediatrics*. 2022;150(4)e2022059275.
- Sriwilaijaroen N, Vavricka CJ, Kiyota H, et al. Influenza A virus neuraminidase inhibitors. *Methods in Mol Biol*. 2022;2556:321–353.

 CODES

ICD10
- J10.08 Influenza due to other identified influenza virus with other specified pneumonia
- J11.89 Influenza due to unidentified influenza virus with other manifestations
- J10.81 Influenza due to other identified influenza virus with encephalopathy

CLINICAL PEARLS
- Influenza is an acute, (typically) self-limited, febrile infection caused by influenza virus types A and B.
- All persons aged >6 months should be vaccinated against influenza on an annual basis (there are rare exceptions).
- Recommend concurrent administration of pneumonia vaccine if indicated per CDC guidelines.
- Complications from influenza are most common in the very young, very old, and individuals with comorbid disease.
- Hand hygiene either with soap and water (slightly superior) or with alcohol-based hand rubs and covering coughs are simple ways to reduce the spread of influenza.

INGROWN TOENAIL

William Andrew Pleasant, MD • Daniel Scott Morrison, MD • Chirag N. Shah, MD

 BASICS

DESCRIPTION
- In an ingrown toenail, the distal margin of the nail plate grows into the lateral nail fold, causing irritation, inflammation, and sometimes bacterial or fungal infection:
  - Stage 1 (inflammation): erythema, edema, tenderness to palpation of lateral nail fold
  - Stage 2 (abscess): increased pain, erythema, and edema as well as drainage (purulent or serous)
  - Stage 3 (granulation): Chronic inflammation leads to further erythema, edema, and pain, often with granulation tissue growing over the nail plate and significant nail fold hypertrophy.
- Can reoccur
- Synonym(s): onychocryptosis, unguis incarnatus

EPIDEMIOLOGY
- Great toenail is most often affected.
- Lateral edge of nail is more commonly affected than the medial edge.
- Most common in males aged 14 to 25 years
- Infrequent, but more often in elderly females than in elderly males
- More common in those with lower incomes

Prevalence
- 2.5% of total population
- 5% of population aged > 65 years
- 2:1 male to female ratio

ETIOLOGY AND PATHOPHYSIOLOGY
- Nail plate penetrates the nail fold, causing a foreign body reaction (inflammation).
- Bacteria or fungi may enter through the opening in the nail fold, causing infection and abscess formation.
- The inflamed and infected area leads to granulation tissue and hypertrophy of the nail fold.

RISK FACTORS
- Genetic factors
  - Increased nail fold width
  - Decreased nail thickness
  - Medial rotation of the toe
- Many others proposed; none proven, including the following:
  - Distorted, thickened nail (onychogryphosis)
  - Fungal infection (onychomycosis)
  - Hyperhidrosis
  - Improper trimming of the lateral nail plate
  - Poorly fitting shoes
  - Trauma to nail or nail fold
  - Conditions that predispose to pedal edema (i.e., thyroid dysfunction, diabetes, obesity, heart failure, renal disease)

GENERAL PREVENTION
- Properly fitting shoes
- Proper nail trimming (see "Patient Education")

 DIAGNOSIS

HISTORY
- Patients most often present with pain, redness, and swelling in the toe along one or both sides of the nail.
- Drainage can occur as inflammation and/or infection develop.

PHYSICAL EXAM
- Nail fold tenderness
- Erythema and edema
- Drainage (serous or purulent)
- Granulation tissue
- Lateral nail fold hypertrophy

DIFFERENTIAL DIAGNOSIS
- Cellulitis
- Felon (pulp abscess on plantar aspect of toe)
- Onychogryphosis (gross thickening and hardening of the nail)
- Onycholysis (separation of nail from nail bed)
- Onychomycosis (fungal infection of the nail)
- Osteomyelitis
- Paronychia (infection or inflammation around the nail fold)
- Subungual exostosis (bony projection from distal phalanx)
- Subungual osteochondroma (benign bone tumor)

DIAGNOSTIC TESTS & INTERPRETATION
Initial Tests (lab, imaging)
None usually needed
- Consider x-ray, MRI, or bone scan if osteomyelitis is suspected.
- Consider x-ray if subungual exostosis or osteochondroma is suspected.

TREATMENT

GENERAL MEASURES
- Majority of mild cases (stage 1) respond well to conservative therapy.
- Warm, soapy water or Epsom salt soaks for 10 to 20 minutes 3 times per day until symptoms resolve (1)[C]
- Bluntly insert a cotton wisp or dental floss underneath the ingrown portion of the nail. The patient can continue to replace the insert until the nail grows beyond the fold (2)[C].
- Use tape to pull the lateral nail fold away from the nail plate until the nail grows beyond the fold.
- Stage 2 ingrown nails without significant pain or erythema often respond to conservative treatment, as above, especially cotton wool, or a trial of cryotherapy.

MEDICATION
- NSAIDs are usually adequate for analgesia.
- Topical antibiotic can be applied after soaking.
- Neither oral nor topical antibiotics are useful as an adjunct to surgical treatment (3)[A].

SURGERY/OTHER PROCEDURES
- Surgical interventions are more effective than nonsurgical interventions in preventing recurrence (1)[C],(3)[C].
- Nail avulsion techniques are more effective than nail fold debulking techniques (not described in this topic) (4)[A].
  - Partial avulsion of the nail with phenol nail matrix ablation
    - Obtain surgical consent after explaining the risks, benefits, and alternatives.
    - Achieve local anesthesia with a digital wing or ring block.
    - May consider placing a tourniquet around the base of the toe to assist with hemostasis (caution in patients with diabetes or peripheral vascular disease)
    - Elevate the ingrown part of the nail from the nail bed with a periosteal (Freer) elevator or hemostat.
    - Incise the nail longitudinally with scissors or a nail splitter a few millimeters from the ingrown border, starting at the distal edge and proceeding to the matrix.
    - Grasp, down to the cuticle, the avulsed fragment with a hemostat, and pull this portion gently out with a hemostat, using longitudinal traction, as well as rotation to the lateral nail fold if needed.
    - Remove the tourniquet once hemostasis is attained.
    - Dip a urethral swab in 80–88% phenol solution (phenol use is contraindicated in pregnancy).
    - Apply the phenol 3 times for 30 seconds to the nail matrix under the proximal nail fold. Wash the area with 70% isopropyl (rubbing) alcohol to neutralize phenol.
- Nonsurgical interventions, such as a flexible gutter splint, are another option for treatment of stage 2 or 3 ingrown nails (5)[C].
  - J Flexible gutter splint
    - Cut a 1- to 2-cm long piece of sterilized plastic tube, such as IV tubing, 2 to 3 mm in diameter (alternatively, you may use a cap from a 29-gauge needle).
    - Make a slit in the tubing lengthwise, and cut the end off at an angle.
    - Apply local anesthesia with a digital wing or ring block.
    - Release the ingrown edge of the nail from the nail fold with a hemostat.

- Slide the tube, angled end first, along the ingrown edge of the nail.
- Consider fixing the tube in place with self-curing formable acrylic resin (used for dentures and sculptured nails), tape, or a single suture through the nail plate.
- Leave the tube in place until the nail has grown beyond the nail fold.
- Bilateral partial matricectomy should be considered in patients with severe ingrown toenail or recurrence.
- Permanent destruction of the germinal matrix can be used to prevent recurrence. The use of phenol for nail bed ablation is probably more effective than nail avulsion alone in preventing recurrence (3)[A],(4)[A].
  - Other options for nail bed ablation:
    - Sodium hydroxide (NaOH)
    - Cryotherapy
    - Electrocautery with a special flattened tip coated with Teflon on one side to protect the proximal nail fold
    - Carbon dioxide laser
    - Surgical excision of the nail matrix

 ## ONGOING CARE

FOLLOW-UP RECOMMENDATIONS
- Dress with antibiotic ointment or sterile petroleum jelly; cover with sterile gauze and tube gauze.
- Postop instructions should include the following:
  - Rest and elevate the foot for 12 to 24 hours.
  - Take NSAIDs for discomfort.
  - Change dressing and wash with soap and water at least daily for 1 to 2 weeks following the procedure.
  - Expect a sterile exudate for 2 to 6 weeks.
  - Avulsed nails may take 6 to 12 months to grow completely out (if no matrix ablation).
  - Call for increasing pain, redness, or swelling.
  - Average time to return to normal activities is 2 weeks.
- Patients treated conservatively should be followed up in the office every 7 to 10 days until marked improvement is noted.

PATIENT EDUCATION
- Trim nails straight across perpendicular to long axis of the nail (do not round corners) and not too short.
- Wear properly fitting, comfortable shoes.

COMPLICATIONS
- Cellulitis after surgical procedure (uncommon)
- Damage to fascia or periosteum from overly aggressive matrix ablation
- Damage to nail bed
- Distal toe ischemia due to prolonged use of a tourniquet during surgery (rare)
- Nail plate deformity (due to nail matrix damage)
- Osteomyelitis (rare)
- Permanent narrowing of nail (if partial matrix ablation is performed)
- Persistent postoperative wound drainage particularly with excessive phenolization of adjacent tissues
- Recurrence (40–80% with avulsion alone, 0.6–14% with matrix ablation, 6–13% with gutter splint)

REFERENCES

1. Mayeaux EJ Jr, Carter C, Murphy TE. Ingrown toenail management. *Am Fam Physician*. 2019;100(3):158–164.
2. Thakur V, Vinay K, Haneke E. Onychocryptosis—decrypting the controversies. *Int J Dermatol*. 2020;59(6):656–669.
3. Eekhof JAH, Van Wijk B, Knuistingh Neven A, et al. Interventions for ingrowing toenails. *Cochrane Database Syst Rev*. 2012;(4):CD001541.
4. Park DH, Singh D. The management of ingrowing toenails. *BMJ*. 2012;344:e2089.
5. Nazari S. A simple and practical method in treatment of ingrown nails: splinting by flexible tube. *J Eur Acad Dermatol Venereol*. 2006;20(10):1302–1306.

ADDITIONAL READING

- Bos AMC, van Tilburg MWA, van Sorge AA, et al. Randomized clinical trial of surgical technique and local antibiotics for ingrowing toenail. *Br J Surg*. 2007;94(3):292–296.
- Bryant A, Knox A. Ingrown toenails: the role of the GP. *Aust Fam Physician*. 2015;44(3):102–105.

- Chapeskie H. Ingrown toenail or overgrown toe skin? Alternative treatment for onychocryptosis. *Can Fam Physician*. 2008;54(11):1561–1562.
- Reyzelman AM, Trombello KA, Vayser DJ, et al. Are antibiotics necessary in the treatment of locally infected ingrown toenails? *Arch Fam Med*. 2000;9(9):930–932.
- Richert B. Basic nail surgery. *Dermatol Clin*. 2006;24(3):313–322.
- Woo SH, Kim IH. Surgical pearl: nail edge separation with dental floss for ingrown toenails. *J Am Acad Dermatol*. 2004;50(6):939–940.

 ## SEE ALSO

For a video of this Nail Avulsion and Matrixectomy procedure, go to http://5minuteconsult.com/procedure/1508006.

 ## CODES

ICD10
L60.0 Ingrowing nail

CLINICAL PEARLS
- Nonsurgical interventions are appropriate for patients with stage 1 and mild stage 2 ingrown toenails.
- The most common surgical intervention for treatment of an ingrown toenail is partial nail avulsion with phenol matrix ablation.
- Patients can prevent ingrown toenails by trimming nails properly and wearing properly fitting shoes.
- Oral and topical antibiotics are not useful in the treatment of ingrown nails in conjunction with surgical treatment.

INJURY AND VIOLENCE

Jameson Reich, DO • Breanna Gawrys, DO

 BASICS

DESCRIPTION

- Injury, intentional or not, is often predictable and preventable. Unintentional injuries are no longer considered "accidents" given that most injuries are preventable.
- As of 2020, unintentional injury is the 4th leading cause of death in the United States. Injury is the leading cause of death for people aged 1 to 44 years, accounting for some 80,000 deaths in 2020. It is also a leading cause of disability for people of all ages, regardless of sex, race/ethnicity, or socioeconomic status. Violence-related deaths accounted for >58,000 deaths in the United States in 2020 (>36,000 suicides and >21,000 homicides).

EPIDEMIOLOGY

Incidence

- Children mostly die of unintentional injuries: motor vehicle traffic (MVT), drowning, poisoning, and suffocation.
- MVT is the most common type of unintentional injury deaths in adolescents.

ALERT

Poisoning, which includes drug overdose, has been the leading cause of injury deaths in the United States overall since 2011 and is particularly deadly for persons ages 15 to 64 years, as the leading cause of injury deaths among 25 to 64 years and the second leading cause of unintentional injury deaths for 15 to 24 years.

- Approximately 4.4 million people worldwide die yearly from injuries, of which all forms of violence combine to cause nearly 1/3 of these deaths (World Health Organization [WHO]).
- Unintentional MVT deaths rank third in the United States for overall injury deaths, first in those aged 5 to 24 years and third in those aged 1 to 4 years and 25 to >65 years.
- Among leading causes of injury deaths in the United States, unintentional falls rank third overall. Firearms are related to the fourth and fifth leading causes of injury deaths in the United States, suicide and homicide, respectively.
- Homicide is the second leading cause of death in 2020 for persons aged 15 to 24 years in the United States.

ALERT

Consider homicide as cause of unexplained death in young children.

ETIOLOGY AND PATHOPHYSIOLOGY

Multifactorial

RISK FACTORS

- Motor vehicle accident (MVA):
  - MVT deaths accounted for 40,698 deaths in 2020 with an age-adjusted rate of 11.9 deaths per 100,000 persons (CDC). Each year, approximately 3 million people are nonfatally injured in the United States from motor vehicle crashes (CDC). The leading cause of death for U.S. teens is MVAs (CDC). In the United States, 1 in 3 deaths involved drunk driving and almost 1 in 3 deaths implicated speeding (CDC).
  - Motorcyclists are more likely to die in a motor vehicle crash than car occupants. The risk of death is reduced by 37% with helmets (CDC).
  - Risk factors for involvement in an MVA include high speed, teenage drivers, consumption of alcohol or drugs affecting the central nervous system, fatigue, and distracted driving (handheld mobile phones and inadequate visibility).
  - Increased risk of death by MVA in the United States: not using seat belts, car seats, and booster seats; drunk driving; speeding (CDC)
- Pedestrians:
  - >7,000 pedestrians were killed by motor vehicles and an estimated 104,000 were treated in EDs for nonfatal injuries in the United States (2020; CDC, National Center for Injury Prevention and Control [NCIPC]).
- Bicycles:
  - In the United States, >800 bicyclists died and nearly 357,000 bicycle-related injuries occurred in 2020 (CDC, NCIPC).
  - Risk factors for cyclist injury include age (5 to 19 years for nonfatal injury, 50 to 59 years highest bicycle death rates), male sex, urban area at nonintersection location, and alcohol involvement.
- Sports- and recreation-related injury (CDC):
  - >2.6 million children (0 to 19 years old) are treated in EDs each year.
  - Prevention tips include the following: Use protective gear that is in good condition, fits properly, and worn correctly; sports program and/or school has instituted action plan to teach athletes ways to lower risk of getting a concussion and other injuries; monitor temperature to prevent heat-related injuries; and serve as a role model of safe behavior.
- Drowning: a leading cause of unintentional injury death among all children, particularly those 1 to 4 years of age
  - Children at increased risk include African Americans and those unattended in bathtubs, swimming pools, and recreational water activities (CDC, NCIPC).
- Suffocation: increased risk for children aged <1 year, unsafe sleeping environments (CDC)
- Falls (CDC, NCIPC):
  - The leading cause of nonfatal injuries accounting for >6.5 million nonfatal injuries in the United States in 2020
  - Most common cause of traumatic brain injuries (TBIs)
  - Risk factors for falls include lower body weakness, vitamin D deficiency, difficulties with walking and balance, use of medications (tranquilizers, sedatives, antidepressants, some over-the-counter medicines), vision problems, foot pain or poor footwear, and home hazards (broken/uneven steps, throw rugs, clutter).
- **Violence**: Risk factors include adverse childhood exposures (ACEs); lack of access to social, capital, community organization, and economic resources; familial instability; community and family violence; access to firearms; mental health; personal or household member alcohol and drug use; exposure to suicidal behavior; history of aggressive behavior; cognitive deficits; poor supervision; poor peer-to-peer interaction; academic failure; poverty; and lower socioeconomic class (CDC).

- Homicide and gun violence: Homicide is the second leading cause of death for persons aged 15 to 34 years in the United States (CDC). Most common victims are young males. Firearms are used in more than half of U.S. homicides.
- Suicide: Females are more likely to have suicidal thoughts, but males are 4 times more likely to complete suicide. Most common methods are firearms for males and poisoning for females (CDC, NCIPC).
- Adolescent violence (CDC):
  - In 2019, nearly 8% of students participated in a physical fight at school in the last year.
  - >9% of high schoolers reported not going to school on ≥1 day(s) in the last 30 days because they felt unsafe at school or on their way to or from school.
  - 4% of students have carried a weapon to school; >7% of students have been threatened or injured by a weapon at school.
- Bullying (CDC):
  - In 2020, 20% of students report being bullied on school property in the last year.
  - >15% of students report cyberbullying.
  - Bullying is associated with social, emotional, and academic difficulties.
- Interpersonal and intimate partner violence (IPV):
  - WHO reports about 38% of female homicides globally were killed by male partners, similar to CDC reports of nearly half of female homicide victims in the United States are killed by a current or former male intimate partner.
  - Approximately 1 in 4 women and almost 1 in 10 men have experienced sexual violence, physical violence, and/or stalking in their lifetime from an intimate partner (CDC).
  - Dating violence among teens:
    ○ Almost 1 in 11 female and approximately 1 in 15 male high school students report physical dating violence in the last year (CDC).
    ○ Approximately 1 in 9 female and 1 in 36 male high school students report sexual dating violence in the last year (CDC).
  - Risk factors include individual risk factors (such as low income, young age, heavy alcohol and drug use, depression and suicide attempts, unemployment, being a victim of physical or psychological abuse, witnessing IPV between parents as child, unplanned pregnancy), relationship factors (such as marital conflict, economic stress, association with antisocial and aggressive peers), community factors (such as poverty, low social capital), and societal factors (such as traditional gender norms or gender inequality, societal income inequality).
  - Protective factors include high friendship quality, social support, neighborhood collective efficacy (community cohesiveness, mutual trust, willingness to intervene for the common good), coordination of resources, and services among community agencies.

ALERT

Poisonings (CDC):

- The U.S. epidemic of drug overdoses (poisonings) includes >898,000 deaths from 2001 to 2020 from an overdose involving any opioid (prescription and illicit).
- In 2021, >107,500 drug overdose deaths occurred in the United States.

- Opioids, primarily synthetic fentanyl and fentanyl derivatives, are the main cause of drug overdose deaths. In 2021, opioids were involved in 75% of all drug overdose deaths; two out of three opioid-involved overdose deaths involved synthetic opioids.
- Preventive measures of opioid deaths include improve opioid prescribing, reduce exposure to opioids, prevent misuse, and access to naloxone and treat opioid use disorder.

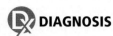

DIAGNOSIS

HISTORY

- Mechanism, timing, and location of injury:
  - Blunt versus penetrating; intentional versus unintentional; others injured versus isolated injury; circumstances (weather, substance use, restrained vs. unrestrained)
  - Does history correlate with level of injury (i.e., level of suspicion for abuse [elderly, child, or partner])?
  - Is further evaluation required (blood and/or urine testing, response to opioid receptor antagonists, imaging)?
- IPV: neurologic deficits, seizures, chronic pain, GI, STI, pregnancy, psychiatric presentations
  - Screen women of childbearing age for IPV and intervene if screening results are positive.

TREATMENT

- Prevention: The primary focus for reducing injury and violence is individually tailored prevention based on risk factors combined with population-level prevention (1).
- Primary (i.e., prevent crash), secondary (i.e., prevent injury from crash), and tertiary (i.e., prevent poor outcomes from injury) prevention (1)[C]
- Motor vehicle injuries (CDC) (2):
  - Infants, toddlers, and children: age-appropriate child safety seats and passenger restraints with distribution programs, education programs for parents and caregivers, safety seat checkpoints, penalties for drivers transporting children under the influence of drugs and/or alcohol, legislation regarding restraint of motor vehicle occupants
  - Adolescents and adults: seat belts, airbags, graduated driver licensing programs, blood alcohol concentration laws, minimum drinking age laws, sobriety checkpoints, ignition interlocks, programs for alcohol servers, zero-alcohol tolerance laws for young drivers, school-based education programs on drinking and driving. Emergency medical services (EMS) response times, engineering cars for rapid extraction, organized trauma systems; collapsible automobile steering columns have been shown to decrease injury mortality and morbidity; texting while driving penalties
  - Older adults: alternative transportation programs, screening for high-risk drivers, gradual curtailment of driving privileges, more frequent license renewal process

- Bicycle helmets can reduce risk of head injury by 63–88%. Canadian helmet legislation decreased mortality by 52%.
  - Pedestrian injury: pedestrian safety education, reflective clothing, use of crosswalks, limit mobile phone use while crossing roads, street lighting for pedestrians, fluorescent clothing for pedestrians and cyclists
  - Cyclists injury: flashing lights and reflectors at night (1)[B], helmet use and laws, cyclists separation for motor vehicles
- Sports-related injuries: proper equipment: Helmets can prevent bicyclist head injuries and mortality; plan of action for dealing with concussion and head injury in young athletes, with guidelines regarding if or when it is safe to return to play (CDC)
- Drowning: improved supervision of young children, especially for those with epilepsy; swimming lessons; trained lifeguard supervision; fencing; locked gates and pool alarms; no use of alcohol in recreation aquatic activities; personal flotation devices and boating safety awareness; parental and caregiver certification in CPR
- Falls:
  - Home safety assessments, installation of handrails and grab bars, removal of tripping hazards, nonslip mats, exercise programs such as tai chi to improve strength and balance, night lights, cataract surgery, gradual withdrawal of psychotropic medication
  - In 2018, United States Preventive Services Task Force (USPSTF) recommends exercise interventions to prevent falls in community-dwelling adults aged ≥65 years who are at increased risk for falls.
- Violence (homicide, suicide, assaults) (CDC):
  - Primary prevention: Most effective strategies focus on younger age groups to change individual attitudes and behaviors.
  - Secondary prevention: Detect and identify violence in early stages. The USPSTF recommends that clinicians should screen women of childbearing age for IPV, such as domestic violence, and provide or refer women who screen positive to intervention services.
  - Gun and school violence prevention among youth: social and emotional learning via CDC Whole School, Whole Community, Whole Child Model (CDC)
  - Tertiary prevention: IPV reduced by alcoholism treatment for partner; intense advocacy interventions of >12 hours
  - Suicide: access to mental health services, improved family and community support, development of healthy coping and problem-solving skills, reduced access to lethal means (CDC)
  - USPSTF recommends screening adults for depression when depression care supports are in place to assure accurate diagnosis, effective treatment, and follow-up.

- Prevent and treat opioid abuse: prescribing practice quality improvement programs; substance abuse counseling and medication for the treatment of opioid use disorders (MOUD) such as buprenorphine and methadone.
- In April 2018, the U.S. Surgeon General issued an advisory emphasizing the importance of the overdose-reversing drug naloxone. *Consider use of naloxone to counter the effects of opioid overdose. Multiple doses of naloxone may be required because the duration of many opioids is greater than that of naloxone.*
- Follow acute care guidelines and call 911; may contact Poison Control Center hotline after discovered ingestion of toxin for recommendations (3)

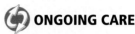

ONGOING CARE

COMPLICATIONS

Social burden of injury: loss of productivity, emotional loss, nonmedical expenditures, reduced quality of life, litigation, rehabilitation, mental health costs, altered family and peer relationships, chronic pain, substance use and abuse, changes in lifestyle (CDC)

REFERENCES

1. Sleet DA, Dahlberg LL, Basavaraju SV, et al; for Centers for Disease Control and Prevention. Injury prevention, violence prevention, and trauma care: building the scientific base. *MMWR Suppl*. 2011;60(4):78–85.
2. Centers for Disease Control and Prevention, National Center for Injury Prevention and Control. Injury prevention and control. https://www.cdc.gov/injury. Accessed January 12, 2023.
3. Mowry JB, Spyker DA, Brooks DE, et al. 2015 Annual report of the American Association of Poison Control Centers' National Poison Data System (NPDS): 33rd annual report. *Clin Toxicol (Phila)*. 2016;54(10):924–1109.

CODES

ICD10

- T14.90 Injury, unspecified
- T14.8 Other injury of unspecified body region
- R29.6 Repeated falls

CLINICAL PEARLS

- Injury and violence are predictable and preventable.
- Unintentional injury is the leading cause of death in the United States.

I

INSOMNIA
Susanne Wild, MD

BASICS

DESCRIPTION
Difficulty initiating or maintaining sleep or non-restorative sleep despite adequate opportunity and circumstances for sleep, resulting in at least one of the following forms of daytime impairment:
- Fatigue or malaise
- Attention, concentration, or memory impairment
- Social or vocational dysfunction or poor school performance
- Mood disturbance or irritability
- Daytime sleepiness
- Motivation, energy, or initiative reduction
- Proneness for errors or accidents at work or while driving
- Tension, headaches, or GI symptoms in response to sleep loss
- Concerns or worries about sleep

EPIDEMIOLOGY
- Predominant age: increases with age
- Predominant sex: female > male (5:1)

Prevalence
- Insomnia (transient and chronic): 5–35% of the population; 10–15% associated with daytime impairment
- Chronic insomnia: 10% middle-aged adults; 1/3 of people aged >65 years

ETIOLOGY AND PATHOPHYSIOLOGY
- Transient/intermittent (<30 days) and short-term (<3 months)
  - Usually caused by an identifiable stressor
  - Stressor can be:
    ○ Physical (e.g., medical illness, high altitude)
    ○ Psychological (e.g., stress, excitement, bereavement)
    ○ Psychosocial (e.g., work deadlines, housing insecurity)
    ○ Interpersonal (e.g., arguments)
- Usually resolves when stressor is removed
- Chronic (>3 months)
  - Usually not due to one single cause
  - Possible contributing factors:
    ○ Medical (e.g., gastroesophageal reflux disease, sleep apnea, chronic pain)
    ○ Psychiatric (e.g., mood, anxiety, psychotic disorders)
    ○ Primary sleep disorder (e.g., idiopathic, psychophysiologic [heightened arousal and learned sleep-preventing associations], paradoxical [sleep state misperception])
    ○ Circadian rhythm disorder (e.g., irregular pattern, jet lag, delayed/advanced sleep phase, shift work)
    ○ Environmental (e.g., lights, noises, movements [partner/young children/pets])
    ○ Behavioral (e.g., poor sleep hygiene, adjustment sleep disorder)
    ○ Substance induced
    ○ Medications (e.g., antihypertensives, antidepressants, corticosteroids, levodopa-carbidopa, phenytoin, quinidine, theophylline, thyroid hormones)

Genetics
No known factors

RISK FACTORS
- Age
- Female gender
- Medical comorbidities
- Unemployment
- Psychiatric illness
- Impaired social relationships
- Shift work
- Separation from spouse or partner
- Drug and substance abuse
- Family or personal history of insomnia

GENERAL PREVENTION
- Practice consistent sleep hygiene:
  - Fixed wake-up times and bedtimes regardless of amount of sleep obtained (weekdays and weekends)
  - Avoid naps. Go to bed only when sleepy.
  - Sleep in a cool, dark, quiet environment.
  - No activities in bedroom associated with anything but sleep or sex
  - 30-minute wind-down time before sleep
  - If unable to sleep within 20 minutes, move to another environment and engage in quiet activity until sleepy.
- Limit caffeine intake to mornings.
- No alcohol after 4 PM
- Fixed eating times
- Avoid medications that interfere with sleep.
- Regular moderate exercise

COMMONLY ASSOCIATED CONDITIONS
- Psychiatric disorders
- Painful musculoskeletal conditions
- Obstructive sleep apnea
- Restless leg syndrome
- Drug or alcohol addiction/dependence

DIAGNOSIS

HISTORY
- Daytime sleepiness and napping
- Unintended sleep episodes (e.g., dozing at a stoplight while driving)
- Insomnia history
  - Duration, time of problem
  - Sleep latency, difficulty in maintaining sleep (repeated awakening), early morning awakening, nonrestorative sleep, or patterns (weekday vs. weekend, with or without bed partner, home vs. away)
- Sleep hygiene
  - Bedtime/wakening time
  - Physical environment of sleep area: LED clocks, TV, room lighting, ambient noise
  - Activity: nighttime eating, exercise, sexual activity
  - Intake: caffeine, alcohol, herbal supplements, diet pills, illicit drugs, prescriptions, over-the-counter (OTC) sleep aids

- Symptoms or history of depression, anxiety, obsessive-compulsive disorder, or other major psychological symptomatology
- Symptoms of restless leg syndrome and periodic limb movement disorder
- Snoring and other symptoms of sleep apnea
- Symptoms of drug or alcohol abuse
- Current medication use
- Chronic medical conditions
- Acute change or stressors such as travel or shift work
- Sleep diary: sleep log for 7 consecutive days

PHYSICAL EXAM
No association with specific findings on physical examination

DIFFERENTIAL DIAGNOSIS
- Obstructive sleep apnea
- CNS hypersomnias (e.g., narcolepsy)
- Circadian rhythm sleep disturbances
- Sleep-related movement disorders (e.g., restless leg syndrome)
- Insomnia due to medical or neurologic disorder
- Mood and anxiety disorders such as depression or anxiety

DIAGNOSTIC TESTS & INTERPRETATION
Diagnostic testing usually not required; consider polysomnography if sleep apnea or periodic limb movement disorder is suspected by history (1)[C].

Initial Tests (lab, imaging)
Testing based on history and exam to evaluate for comorbid conditions

Diagnostic Procedures/Other
Polysomnography or multiple sleep latency test not routinely indicated but may be considered if initial diagnosis is uncertain and interventions have proven unsuccessful.

TREATMENT

- Transient and short-term insomnia
  - May use medications for short-term use only; hypnotic sedatives favored
  - Self-medicating with alcohol can increase awakenings and sleep-stage changes.
- Chronic insomnia
  - Treatment of underlying condition (major depressive disorder, generalized anxiety disorder, medications, pain, substance abuse)
  - Advise good sleep hygiene.
  - Cognitive-behavioral therapy is first-line treatment for chronic insomnia (2).
  - Behavioral therapy is an effective treatment for insomnia and a potentially more effective long-term treatment than pharmacotherapy (3)[B].
  - Ramelteon and doxepin are the only agents without known abuse potential.

MEDICATION

- Reserved for transient and short-term insomnia such as with jet lag, stress reactions, transient medical condition
- Nonbenzodiazepine hypnotics
  - Act on benzodiazepine receptor, so have abuse potential
    - Zaleplon (Sonata) 5 to 20 mg; half-life 1 hour
    - Zolpidem (Ambien) 5 to 10 mg (males); 5 mg (females); half-life 2.5 to 3.0 hours
    - Zolpidem (Ambien CR) 6.25 to 12.50 mg (males); 6.25 mg (females); half-life 2.5 to 3.0 hours
    - Eszopiclone (Lunesta) 1 to 3 mg; half-life 6 hours
- Benzodiazepine hypnotics
  - Short-acting
    - Triazolam (Halcion) 0.25 mg; half-life 1.5 to 5.5 hours
  - Intermediate acting
    - Temazepam (Restoril) 7.50 to 30.0 mg; half-life 8.8 hours
    - Estazolam (Prosom) 1 to 2 mg; half-life 10 to 24 hours
  - Long acting
    - Flurazepam (Dalmane) 15 to 30 mg; half-life 40 to 100 hours
    - Quazepam (Doral) 7.5 to 15.0 mg; half-life 39 hours (parent drug), 73 hours (active metabolite)
- Contraindications/precautions are as follows:
  - Not indicated for long-term treatment due to risks of tolerance, dependency, daytime attention and concentration compromise, incoordination, rebound insomnia
  - Long-acting benzodiazepines associated with higher incidence of daytime sedation and motor impairment
  - Avoid in elderly, pregnant, breastfeeding, substance abusers, and patients with suicidal or parasuicidal behaviors.
  - Avoid in patients with untreated obstructive apnea and chronic pulmonary disease.
- Nonbenzodiazepine receptor agonists may occasionally induce parasomnias (sleepwalking, sleep eating, sleep driving).
- Melatonin receptor agonist
  - Ramelteon (Rozerem) 8 mg; half-life 1.0 to 2.6 hours
    - Effective to reduce sleep time onset for short- and long-term use in adults, without abuse potential; onset may take up to 3 weeks.
- Sedating antidepressants
  - Doxepin (Silenor) 3 to 6 mg; half-life 15 hours (the only antidepressant with FDA approval for insomnia)
  - Trazodone (Oleptro) 25 to 200 mg; half-life 3 to 9 hours
  - Mirtazapine (Remeron) 7.5 to 15.0 mg; half-life 20 to 40 hours
  - Amitriptyline (Elavil) 25 to 100 mg; half-life 10 to 26 hours

- Orexin receptor agonists
  - Suvorexant (Belsomra) 10 to 20 mg; half-life 12 hours
  - Lemborexant (Dayvigo) 5 to 10 mg; half-life 17 to 19 hours
  - Daridorexant (Quviviq) 25 to 50 mg; half-life 8 hours
- Sedating antihistamines are not recommended.
- Antipsychotics should only be prescribed if the patient has a concurrent psychiatric diagnosis warranting their use.

Geriatric Considerations

Caution (risk of falls and confusion) when prescribing benzodiazepines or other sedative hypnotics; if absolutely necessary, use short-acting nonbenzodiazepine agonists at half the dosage or melatonin agonists for short-term treatment.

COMPLEMENTARY & ALTERNATIVE MEDICINE

- Melatonin: particularly effective in patients with delayed sleep phase disorder (e.g., due to jet lag of shift work); decreases sleep latency when taken 30 to 120 minutes prior to bedtime, but there is no good evidence for efficacy in insomnia, and long-term effects are unknown (4)[B]
- Valerian (*Valeriana officinalis*): Inconsistent evidence supporting efficacy and its slow onset of action (2 to 3 weeks) makes it unsuitable for the acute treatment of insomnia.
- Cognitive-behavioral therapy (including relaxation therapy): effective and considered more useful than medications; recommended initial treatment for patients with chronic insomnia; no improvement of efficacy when combined with medication
- Mindfulness awareness practices: improved sleep quality and sleep-related daytime impairment for older adults per small randomized trial
- Behavioral interventions such as stimulus control therapy, sleep restriction, and relaxation training may all be effective.

 ONGOING CARE

FOLLOW-UP RECOMMENDATIONS

- Daily exercise improves quality of sleep and may be more effective than medication.
- Avoid exercise within 4 hours of bedtime.

Patient Monitoring

- Reassess need for medications periodically; avoid standing prescriptions. Treatment response should be measured by using patient self-report (eg: sleep diary); wearable sleep monitors are often inaccurate.
- Caution patients that nonbenzodiazepine agonists (zolpidem, zaleplon, eszopiclone), as well as benzodiazepines, can be habit-forming.

DIET

- Avoid caffeine or reserve for morning only.
- Avoid heavy late-night snacks (light snack at bedtime may help).
- Avoid alcohol within 6 hours of bedtime.

PROGNOSIS

Situational insomnia should resolve with time.

COMPLICATIONS

- Daytime sleepiness, cognitive dysfunction
- Pulmonary hypertension if chronic sleep apnea is left untreated
- Sleep apnea may lead to hypertension, stroke, or cardiac ischemia.

REFERENCES

1. Kushida CA, Littner MR, Morgenthaler T, et al. Practice parameters for the indications for polysomnography and related procedures: an update for 2005. *Sleep*. 2005;28(4):499–521.
2. Qaseem A, Kansagara D, Forciea MA, et al; for Clinical Guidelines Committee of the American College of Physicians. Management of chronic insomnia disorder in adults: a clinical practice guideline from the American College of Physicians. *Ann Intern Med*. 2016;165(2):125–133.
3. Ebben MR, Spielman AJ. Non-pharmacological treatments for insomnia. *J Behav Med*. 2009;32(3):244–254.
4. Verster GC. Melatonin and its agonists, circadian rhythms and psychiatry. *Afr J Psychiatry (Johannesbg)*. 2009;12(1):42–46.

 SEE ALSO

- Anxiety (Generalized Anxiety Disorder); Depression; Fibromyalgia; Sleep Apnea, Obstructive
- Algorithms: Anxiety; Insomnia, Chronic; Restless Legs Syndrome

CODES

ICD10

- G47.00 Insomnia, unspecified
- F51.02 Adjustment insomnia
- F51.01 Primary insomnia

CLINICAL PEARLS

- Treatment of underlying etiology of the insomnia and consistent sleep hygiene are key.
- Most medications are indicated for short-term use only.
- Sedative hypnotics are not recommended in the elderly because risks may outweigh benefits.
- Patients with chronic insomnia benefit from sleep hygiene education and cognitive-behavioral therapy.

INTERSTITIAL CYSTITIS/PAINFUL BLADDER SYNDROME

Dmitry Bisk, MD

BASICS

DESCRIPTION
- A condition characterized by pain, pressure, or discomfort of the bladder or pelvic region associated with one or more of the following urinary symptoms: increased frequency, urgency, or nocturia
- A chronic inflammatory disease of unknown etiology, with associated urinary symptoms for >6 weeks without other identifiable causes such as infection or other pathology
- The symptoms in many patients are insidious, and the disease progresses for years with relapsing and remitting symptoms often before diagnosis is established.
- System(s) affected: renal/urologic
- Synonym(s): urgency frequency syndrome; IC/bladder pain syndrome; chronic cystitis; Hunner ulcer

EPIDEMIOLOGY
- Occurs predominantly among white patients
- Predominant sex: female > male (5:1) in patients 25 to 80 years of age

Incidence
1-year incidence has been reported as
- 21 per 100,000 female patients and 4 per 100,000 male patients

Prevalence
In the United States:
- Prevalence is variable.
- Up to 1.2 million female and 82,000 male patients are affected, but many cases likely are undiagnosed.

ETIOLOGY AND PATHOPHYSIOLOGY
Etiology is unclear, and pathophysiology is likely multifactorial.

RISK FACTORS
Unclear but some reported risks include the following:
- Recent urinary tract infection (UTI)
- Irritable bowel syndrome (IBS)
- Allergies
- History of sexual abuse

COMMONLY ASSOCIATED CONDITIONS
- Fibromyalgia/Chronic fatigue syndrome
- Depression and panic disorder
- Vulvodynia
- Sexual dysfunction
- Sleep disturbance
- Chronic prostatitis
- Chronic pelvic pain and pelvic floor dysfunction
- IBS
- Anal/rectal disease
- Chronic scrotal pain

DIAGNOSIS

- Many diagnostic criteria exist that are dependent on patient's symptoms and the exclusion of other pathology.
- A clinical diagnosis in uncomplicated cases can be characterized by symptoms that have been present for >6 weeks without other causes such as infection or other disorders.
  - Pain, pressure, or discomfort of the bladder or pelvic area and at least one of the following urinary symptoms:
    - Increased daytime frequency, urgency, or nocturia
- Cystoscopy with hydrodistension or urodynamic studies should not be used to establish a diagnosis in uncomplicated presentations, but it can be considered if diagnosis is unclear or if the presentation is complex. Cystoscopy can help identify Hunner lesions, which could change management options (1).

HISTORY
- Thorough history detailing baseline bladder/pelvic pain and urinary symptoms including voiding patterns and alleviating factors
- Common urinary symptoms at presentation are urgency and frequency with small void volumes.
- Symptoms can be variable with flares and remission.
- Episodes may be related to menses, stress, sexual activity, IBS, endometriosis, vulvodynia, fibromyalgia, chronic fatigue syndrome, and autoimmune conditions.
- Medical history of prior pelvic trauma or pelvic surgery
- Use of validated questionnaires:
  - O'Leary/Sant: Voiding and Pain Indices (https://painful-bladder.org/pdf/O'Leary_Sant.pdf)

PHYSICAL EXAM
- Exams findings can be nonspecific; most common: dysphoric mood, bladder neck tenderness, suprapubic tenderness, and levator ani tenderness
- Abdominal exam: Evaluate for masses, hernias, suprapubic tenderness, and costovertebral tenderness.
- Female pelvic exam
  - Findings suggesting interstitial cystitis can include pelvic floor spasms, suprapubic tenderness, rectal spasms, urethral tenderness, and bladder base tenderness when examining the anterior vaginal wall.
- Male digital rectal exam
  - Tenderness of the prostate can occur, but it may lead to a false diagnosis of chronic prostatitis.

DIFFERENTIAL DIAGNOSIS
- UTI
- Acute and chronic prostatitis
- Overactive bladder
- Urge incontinence
- Bladder neoplasm
- Bladder or ureteral stone

- Chronic pelvic pain
- Urogenital prolapse
- Urethral diverticulum
- Neurologic bladder disease
- Nonurinary pelvic disease (STIs, endometriosis, pelvic relaxation, pudendal neuralgia)

DIAGNOSTIC TESTS & INTERPRETATION
Initial Tests (lab, imaging)
- Urinalysis and urine culture to rule out infection
- Gonorrhea and chlamydia testing in patients with pyuria or high risk of STI
- Urine biomarkers and cytology are not recommended unless at increased risk.

Diagnostic Procedures/Other
- Cystoscopy with hydrodistension can be used to help differentiate other pathology but should not be used to establish the diagnosis (1).
- Urodynamic studies are not recommended for routine evaluation but can be used to differentiate other coexisting disorders (overactive bladder, stress urinary incontinence, or voiding dysfunction) (1).
- Intravesical lidocaine (anesthetic bladder challenge) can help to pinpoint the bladder as the source of pain in patients with pelvic pain.
- Potassium sensitivity test is not recommended for clinical use as it is nonspecific, painful, and does not change the treatment approach.
- Bladder biopsy is not recommended for the diagnosis but is performed if there is suspicion for malignancy.

TREATMENT

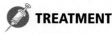

GENERAL MEASURES
- The goal of treatment should be to control symptoms and to increase patient's quality of life.
- There is no universally effective treatment plan. There is also no strong evidence that any treatment method is effective, and more large trials are needed. However, conservative general measures for all patients include the following (1)[C]:
  - Patient education on normal bladder function, disease course, lack of cure, expectant management
  - Diet changes
    - Food and fluid elimination diets with specific focus on common triggers such as caffeine, alcohol, carbonated beverages, high citrus foods, tomatoes, and bananas
  - Meditation, counseling, and stress management
  - Regular exercise
  - Manual physical therapy maneuvers by a trained clinician that improve pelvic, abdominal, and/or hip muscular trigger points; lengthen muscle contractures; and release painful scars should be offered to patients with pelvic floor tenderness. Kegel exercises should be avoided.
  - Avoidance of activity that exacerbates the pain
  - Efficacy of treatment should be periodically reassessed, and infective treatments should be stopped

MEDICATION

- Randomized controlled trials of most medications for interstitial cystitis demonstrate limited benefit over placebo; there are no clear predictors of what will benefit an individual. Prepare the patient that treatment may involve trial and error.
- A systemic review of treatment options including antidepressants, pentosan polysulfate sodium, and neuromuscular blockade did not demonstrate conclusive evidence that they are effective for the treatment of symptoms (2)[A].
- Conservative therapies should be trialed first, and more aggressive therapies can be started based on patient's symptoms and quality of life (1)[C].
- Treatments should be based on symptoms, symptom severity, and patient preferences (1)[C].
- Multiple simultaneous treatments may be considered if it is in the patient's best interest, and patient's symptoms are followed and assessed carefully (1)[C].

First Line

Note: AUA consensus states that patient education, pain management, general relaxation, stress reduction, behavior modification, and self-care are first-line therapy (1)[C].

Second Line

- Patients can be prescribed with analgesic medications (e.g., acetaminophen, NSAIDs) with proper indications and discussion of risks and benefits (1).
- There is no consensus on which medications should be started first. Medication choice should be based on patient's symptoms and preferences. The following treatment methods are considered by the AUA (1)[C].
  - Amitriptyline: 25 to 100 mg/day, most effective at ≥50 mg/day; initiate with lower dose and titrate (1)[C].
  - Cimetidine 400 mg BID; side effects are rare (1)[C].
  - Hydroxyzine 25 to 75 mg QHS; common side effects include drowsiness and xerostomia (1)[C].
  - Pentosan polysulfate 100 mg TID on empty stomach; may take several months (3 to 6) to become effective; (only FDA-approved treatment for interstitial cystitis); side effects can include headache, nausea, diarrhea, dizziness, rash, edema, and hair loss. Patients may need to be counseled on routine eye exams and increased rare atypical maculopathy risk (1)[C].
- Treatment of Hunner lesions if found with laser, electrocautery, and/or injection of triamcinolone (1)[C]

Third Line

- Intravesical treatment (1)[C]
  - Dimethyl sulfoxide (DMSO) q2wk for 6 weeks and then PRN (only FDA-approved intravesical treatment); side effects include pain with instillation, unpleasant odor, and exacerbation of long-term pain.
  - Heparin 10 to 20,000 units in 2 to 5 mL of solution, 3 times a week
  - 1% lidocaine 20 to 30 mL is considered a short-term treatment option.
- Cystoscopy under anesthesia with low-pressure hydrodistention (1)

Fourth Line

Neurostimulation: A permanent neurostimulation device can be placed if other treatments have not been effective in providing the patient with improvement of symptoms or quality of life (1)[C].

ADDITIONAL THERAPIES

- Manual physical therapy (targeted pelvic, hip girdle, abdominal trigger point massage) is considered a second-line therapy by the AUA (1)[C].
- Oral cyclosporine A for Hunner lesions refractory to triamcinolone injection, intravesical hyaluronic acid, and/or intravesical chondroitin sulfate may be offered as a treatment option if other therapies mentioned earlier have not been effective in improving symptoms and quality of life (1)[C].
- Intradetrusor onabotulinumtoxinA may be administered if other treatments have not provided improvement of quality of life. Patients may need to be counseled on the possibility of intermittent self-catheterization risk (1).
- Sildenafil 25 mg; small randomized trial demonstrated urinary symptom improvement after 3 to 6 months.
- Long-term antibiotics and/or long-term systemic oral glucocorticoid should not be used (1).

SURGERY/OTHER PROCEDURES

- Hydraulic distention of bladder under anesthesia: symptomatic but transient relief
- Sacral neuromodulation
- Transurethral electro- or laser fulguration (effective for Hunner lesions); pain relief may persist from several months to years.
- Augmentation cystoplasty to increase bladder capacity and to decrease pressure with or without partial cystectomy can be considered in severe cases that are refractory to other treatments; expected results in severe cases: much improved, 75%; with residual discomfort, 20%; unchanged, 5%
- Urinary diversion with total cystectomy only if disease is completely refractory to medical therapy

COMPLEMENTARY & ALTERNATIVE MEDICINE

- One small trial of 21 patients undergoing hyperbaric oxygen therapy showed a 28% decrease in pain after 3 months.
- There has been a suggested therapy of glycerophosphate and acupuncture, but no clinical trials completed to demonstrate efficacy.

 ## ONGOING CARE

FOLLOW-UP RECOMMENDATIONS

Patient Monitoring

Tailored to severity, duration, and response to intervention

DIET

Dietary modification, elimination diet (caffeine, chocolate, citrus, tomatoes, carbonated beverages, potassium-rich foods, soybean, spicy foods, acidic foods, and alcohol)

PATIENT EDUCATION

- Interstitial Cystitis Association: http://www.ichelp.org/
- Given overlap with chronic pelvic pain syndrome, patients may benefit from home exercises—examples: https://youtu.be/NnqAkM9r2a8 or https://youtu.be/R3Rydb1nZU4

PROGNOSIS

- Patients often report decreased quality of life.
- Potential symptom plateau after approximately 5 years of symptoms
- In mild cases: exacerbations and remissions of symptoms; may not be progressive; does not predispose to other diseases
- In severe cases: progressive problems, often require surgery to control symptoms

REFERENCES

1. Clemens JQ, Erickson DR, Varela NP, et al. Diagnosis and treatment of interstitial cystitis/bladder pain syndrome. *J Urol*. 2022;208(1):34–42.
2. Imamura M, Scott NW, Wallace SA, et al. Interventions for treating people with symptoms of bladder pain syndrome: a network meta-analysis. *Cochrane Database Syst Rev*. 2020;7(7):CD013325.

 ## SEE ALSO

- Urinary Tract Infection (UTI) in Females
- Algorithm: Pelvic Girdle Pain (Pregnancy or Postpartum Pelvic Pain)

CODES

ICD10

- N30.10 Interstitial cystitis (chronic) without hematuria
- N30.11 Interstitial cystitis (chronic) with hematuria

CLINICAL PEARLS

- In most cases, this is a clinical diagnosis that is characterized by symptoms that have been present for >6 weeks without other underlying causes. Symptoms include pain, pressure, or discomfort of the bladder or pelvic area and at least one of the following urinary symptoms: increased daytime frequency, urgency, or nocturia.
- At present, there is no definitive treatment for interstitial cystitis.
- Most patients with severe disease receive multiple treatment approaches. Regular multidisciplinary follow-up, pharmacologic therapy, avoidance of symptom triggers, and psychological and supportive therapy are all important because this disease tends to wax and wane. Monitor patients for comorbid depression.
- Empower the patients to manage their symptoms, to communicate regularly with their physicians, and to learn as much as they can about this disease, which may help them to optimize their outcome.

INTERSTITIAL NEPHRITIS

Touqir Zahra, MD, FACP • Raksha Sharma, MD

BASICS

DESCRIPTION
- Acute and chronic tubulointerstitial diseases result from the interplay of renal cells and inflammatory cells. Injury to renal cells leads to new local antigen expression, inflammatory cell infiltration, and proinflammatory activation. The outcome is acute interstitial nephritis (AIN) or chronic interstitial nephritis (CIN).
- Central component in AIN is altered tubular function, which precedes decrements in filtration rate.
- AIN presents as acute kidney injury (AKI) after the use of offending drugs or agents (OFA) and is associated with proteinuria, hematuria, and white cell casts.

EPIDEMIOLOGY
Incidence
- Accounts for 15–20% of AKI
- Peak incidence in women 60 to 70 years of age

Pediatric Considerations
- Children with history of lead poisoning are more likely to develop CIN as young adults.
- Tubulointerstitial nephritis with uveitis (TINU) presents in adolescent females.

Geriatric Considerations
Compared to younger counterparts, elderly patients (age ≥65 years) tend to develop more severe disease with increased risk of permanent damage, specifically drug-induced AIN (87% vs. 64%), proton pump inhibitor–induced AIN (18% vs. 6%), but less AIN from autoimmune or systemic causes (7% vs. 27%) (1)[B].

ETIOLOGY AND PATHOPHYSIOLOGY
- AIN
  - T cell activation by an antigen leads to delayed drug hypersensitivity reactions, which leads to interstitial inflammatory infiltrates that damage tubules.
  - Renal dysfunction generally is partially or completely reversible.
  - Hypersensitivity to drugs (75%): not dose dependent; the top three were omeprazole (12%), amoxicillin (8%), and ciprofloxacin (8%) (2)[C]; many implicated; NSAIDs, antibiotics, proton pump inhibitors, diuretics, AEDs, antivirals, anticancer drugs, allopurinol, H_2 blockers, diphenylhydantoin, sulfasalazine, and mesalamine
  - Infections (10–15%): streptococci, *Legionella*, *Leptospira*, *Leishmania*, *Escherichia coli*, *Campylobacter*, *Salmonella*, *Treponema pallidum*, *Mycobacterium tuberculosis*, *Histoplasma*, *Coccidioides*, *Toxoplasma*, CMV, EBV, HSV, HIV, and perhaps the SARS-CoV-2 (COVID-19) virus (3)
  - Autoimmune (10–15%): sarcoidosis, SLE, Sjögren syndrome, granulomatosis with polyangiitis, cryoglobulinemia
  - Toxins (e.g., snake bite venom)
  - Idiopathic (5–10%): TINU syndrome and anti–tubular basement membrane (anti-TBM) disease

- CIN
  - Characterized by interstitial scarring, fibrosis, and tubular atrophy, resulting in progressive CKD
  - Follows long-term exposure to OFA (e.g., heavy metals, especially lead)
  - Often found on routine labs
  - Characterized by interstitial scarring, fibrosis, and tubular atrophy, resulting in progressive CKD

GENERAL PREVENTION
- Early recognition and prompt discontinuation of OFA
- Avoid nephrotoxic substances.

COMMONLY ASSOCIATED CONDITIONS
- Chronic pyelonephritis
- Abuse of analgesics
- Lithium use
- Gout and gout therapy
- Immune disorders
- Malignancy (lymphoma, multiple myeloma)
- Amyloidosis
- Exposure to heavy metals (e.g., lead, cadmium)
- Renal papillary necrosis
- Uveitis

DIAGNOSIS

- AIN: suspected in a patient with nonspecific signs and vague systemic symptoms (e.g., malaise/fatigue, fever, nausea, vomiting, rash) with AKI and an abnormal UA
  - AKI: elevated creatinine, BUN, and electrolyte abnormalities; decreased urine output (oliguria in 51%) with signs of fluid overload or depletion
  - Signs of systemic allergy (e.g., fever [27%], maculopapular rash [15%], peripheral eosinophilia [23%], arthralgias [45%], but less commonly found when NSAIDs are the OFA)
  - Urine studies—WBC, RBC, and white cell casts (sterile pyuria, <1 g proteinuria per day except if caused by NSAIDs)
- CIN
  - Hypertension (HTN)
  - Oliguria or polyuria
  - Inability to concentrate urine
  - Polydipsia
  - Hyperkalemia and hyponatremia
  - Proteinuria (<1 g/day), not just albumin but also low molecular proteins like immunoglobulins and microglobulins
  - Non-anion gap metabolic acidosis
  - Anemia
  - Fanconi syndrome

HISTORY
- Medications: Development of AIN following drug exposure ranges from 3 to 5 days to as long as several weeks to many months or even years (the latter more with NSAIDs) (2).
- Infection

- TINU patients present with interstitial nephritis and uveitis.
- Exposure to heavy metals
- Postorgan transplant

PHYSICAL EXAM
- Increased BP
- Fluid retention/extremity swelling/weight gain
- Rash accompanying renal findings in acute AIN
- Lung crackles/rales
- Pericardial rub in uremic pericarditis

DIFFERENTIAL DIAGNOSIS
- AKI secondary to other causes:
  - Prerenal, intrarenal, postrenal
  - Aminoglycosides can cause acute tubular necrosis.
  - NSAIDs can exacerbate prerenal disease.
- CKD secondary to long-standing hypertension, diabetes, and chronic pyelonephritis

DIAGNOSTIC TESTS & INTERPRETATION
Initial Tests (lab, imaging)
- Blood chemistries
  - Elevated creatinine, with 40% requiring dialysis
  - Hyperkalemia and acidosis
- CBC
  - Eosinophilia (80%) but NSAID-induced AIN is associated with eosinophilia in ~15%.
  - Anemia
- Urinalysis with urine electrolytes
  - Hematuria (95%)
  - Mild and variable proteinuria: usually <1 g/24 hr, except AIN associated with NSAIDs where it is higher
  - Urine microscopy: WBC, RBC, white cell casts
  - Eosinophiluria determination can be used but with questionable reliability for diagnosis of AIN due to low specificity (4).
  - Urinary α_1- and β_2-microglobulin, immunoglobulins, TNF-α, and IL-9 may help in the diagnosis and monitoring of tubulointerstitial nephritis.
  - Normal urinalysis does not rule out AIN.
- CXR to evaluate for pulmonary tuberculosis, sarcoidosis, and infections
- Serologies for immunologic disease (e.g., sarcoidosis, Sjögren syndrome, granulomatosis with polyangiitis, Behçet syndrome) or infectious causes
  - Serum levels of ACE and Ca^+ to evaluate for sarcoidosis
  - ANA, anti-dsDNA, and anti-Smith antibodies evaluate for SLE.
  - ANCA to evaluate for granulomatosis with polyangiitis
  - Urinary *Legionella* antigen
  - C3 and C4 to evaluate for SLE and IgG4-related disease
  - Serum protein electrophoresis
  - Anti-Ro/SSA, anti-La/SSB antibodies, CRP, and RF to evaluate for Sjögren syndrome

- Liver function tests elevated in patients with associated drug-induced liver injury
- Renal ultrasound may demonstrate renal architecture and size but no reliable confirmatory ultrasound findings for AIN.
- Studies using IV contrast like IV pyelography and CT are relatively contraindicated given nephrotoxicity and limited diagnostic yield. Gallium-67 imaging has limited sensitivity and specificity for AIN.

Diagnostic Procedures/Other
Renal biopsy is the definitive method of establishing a diagnosis of AIN (contraindicated in bleeding diathesis, solitary kidney, ESRD, uncontrolled hypertension, sepsis, or renal parenchymal infection).

- Patients on an OFA known to cause AIN but have normal UA
- Patients considered for steroid therapy
- Patients not on glucocorticoid therapy and no recovery following cessation of the OFA
- Patients with advanced renal failure with onset <3 months
- Patients with any features (e.g., high-grade proteinuria) that makes AIN diagnosis uncertain

Test Interpretation
- AIN: Biopsy shows marked interstitial infiltrate consisting of T lymphocytes and monocytes. However, eosinophils, plasma cells, and neutrophils may also be found.
- CIN: characterized by tubular atrophy, fibrosis, and cellular infiltration with mononuclear cells

TREATMENT

GENERAL MEASURES
- Discontinue OFA, including topical NSAIDs.
- Reduce exposure to nephrotoxic agents.
- Supportive measures:
  – Maintain adequate hydration.
  – Symptomatic relief for fever and rash
  – Control of BP and correct anemia
  – Correct acidosis and electrolyte imbalances.
  – Short-term dialysis until renal recovery
  – Renally dose meds
- Renal biopsy at 4 to 7 days
- Consider steroid if no improvement within 7 days of removing OFA. For AIN, data on corticosteroids' efficacy have been limited (4), but steroids are commonly used with positive results.

MEDICATION
- First line is supportive therapy.
- If AKI persists after removing OFA, may attempt medication therapy

First Line
- There are no evidence-based guidelines about management of patients with AIN.
- Withdrawal of OFA is the best first step.
- Immunosuppression if no improvement within 3 to 7 days after OFA discontinuation
- Need renal biopsy to confirm AIN and to exclude other etiologies including CIN before starting immunosuppressive therapy or when diagnosis is not clear

- IV pulses of methylprednisolone 125 to 250 mg/day for 3 days followed by oral prednisone 0.5 to 1.0 mg/kg/day PO or equivalent IV (max of 40 to 60 mg/day) starting at day 4, up to 1 to 2 weeks, then gradual taper over 4 to 6 weeks (4). Complete recovery is noted in 49% and partial in 39% (1)[C].
  – Steroids started within 7 days of withdrawal of OFA more likely to recover than those who started later
  – Note: NSAID-induced AIN does not generally respond to steroid therapy.

Second Line
- Limited evidence with treating AIN in patients who are steroid-dependent
- Mycophenolate mofetil may be considered in biopsy-proven AIN patients. Prescription may need to be continued for 1 to 3 years (5)[C].
- Lead toxicity: Chelation may improve function.
  – Succimer 10 mg/kg (max of 500 mg) PO q8h for 5 days, then q12h for 14 days, or
  – EDTA 2 g IV/IM; if IM, use with 2% lidocaine
- SLE nephritis: steroids + cyclophosphamide or azathioprine
- Urate nephropathy: urate-lowering agents
  – Allopurinol starting at 100 mg/day, increasing to 300 mg/day to achieve serum urate level <6 mg/dL
  – Dose need to be adjusted depending on level of renal impairment
  – Note: Allopurinol itself can be a cause of AIN.
  – Discontinue thiazide.
- Lithium-induced nephritis: Use amiloride as adjunct.
- Indinavir-induced nephritis: Use probenecid as adjunct.

ISSUES FOR REFERRAL
Patients presenting with AKI, proteinuria, and acid-base and/or electrolyte disorders require consultation with a nephrologist.

ADMISSION, INPATIENT, AND NURSING CONSIDERATIONS
Patients with AKI and/or with serious electrolyte or acid–base disorders require hospitalization.

ONGOING CARE

FOLLOW-UP RECOMMENDATIONS
Patient Monitoring
If patients must remain on nephrotoxic agents, assess renal function, electrolytes, and phosphorus frequently.

DIET
- Low potassium (<2 g/day), sodium, and protein
- High fiber and DASH diet

PATIENT EDUCATION
National Kidney Disease Education Program, (866) 4-KIDNEY, http://www.niddk.nih.gov/health-information/health-communication-programs/nkdep/Pages/default.aspx

PROGNOSIS
- If AIN is detected early (within 1 week of rise in serum creatinine) and the OFA is discontinued promptly, the long-term outcome is favorable; however, recovery is often incomplete with persistent serum creatinine noted in up to 40% of patients, especially in NSAID-induced AIN.
- Renal biopsy reveals extent of damage.
- For AIN, recovery within weeks to months; 65% recover, whereas 23% remain with long-term impairments.
- Acute dialysis is needed for 1/3 of patients before resolution.
- Progresses to ESRD in 12% of patients
- CIN: can progress to ESRD
- Untreated severe AKI has 45–70% mortality.

COMPLICATIONS
- Chronic tubulointerstitial disease may progress to ESRD, requiring dialysis or transplantation.
- Analgesics increase the risk of transitional cell cancers of the uroepithelium.

REFERENCES
1. Muriithi AK, Leung N, Valeri AM, et al. Clinical characteristics, causes and outcomes of acute interstitial nephritis in the elderly. Kidney Int. 2015;87(2):458–464.
2. Muriithi AK, Leung N, Valeri AM, et al. Biopsy-proven acute interstitial nephritis, 1993–2011: a case series. Am J Kidney Dis. 2014;64(4):558–566.
3. Ng JH, Zaidan M, Jhaveri KD, et al. Acute tubulointerstitial nephritis and COVID-19. Clin Kidney J. 2021;14(10):2151–2157.
4. Caravaca-Fontán F, Fernández-Juárez G, Praga M. Acute kidney injury in interstitial nephritis. Curr Opin Crit Care. 2019;25(6):558–564.
5. Preddie DC, Markowitz GS, Radhakrishnan J, et al. Mycophenolate mofetil for the treatment of interstitial nephritis. Clin J Am Soc Nephrol. 2006;1(4):718–722.

CODES

ICD10
- N12 Tubulo-interstitial nephritis, not spcf as acute or chronic
- N10 Acute tubulo-interstitial nephritis
- N11.9 Chronic tubulo-interstitial nephritis, unspecified

CLINICAL PEARLS
- First step in treatment is to remove OFA. Most common in elderly are NSAIDs, proton pump inhibitors, and antibiotics.
- A renal biopsy is preferred and is the gold standard to confirm AIN.
- Immunosuppressive therapy is initiated if no subsequent improvement within 3 to 7 days after discontinuation of OFA.

INTIMATE PARTNER VIOLENCE

Rhonda A. Faulkner, PhD • Alyssa Jeanne Vest Hart, DO, FAAFP • Melissa Boucher, DO, MPH

BASICS

DESCRIPTION
- Intimate partner violence (IPV) is abuse or aggression that occurs in a romantic relationship between a former or current partner.
- May include physical, sexual, and/or emotional abuse; economic or psychological actions; stalking; or threats of actions that influence another person
- Although women are at greater risk of experiencing IPV, it occurs among patients of any race, age, sexual orientation, religion, gender, and socioeconomic background.
- Synonym(s): domestic violence (DV); spousal abuse; partner abuse; family violence

EPIDEMIOLOGY
Incidence
- In the United States, women experience 4.8 million incidents of physical or sexual assault annually.
- It is estimated that the COVID-19 pandemic has increased the incidence of IPV due to exacerbations of the risk factors that influence perpetrators of IPV.

Prevalence
- About 1 in 4 women and nearly 1 in 10 men experience a form of IPV in their lifetime.
- Over 43 million women and 38 million men have experienced a form of IPV in their lifetime.
- IPV is estimated to cost the U.S. economy >$10.4 billion annually (1).

Geriatric Considerations
About 1 to 2 million U.S. citizens aged >65 years have been injured, exploited, or mistreated by someone caring for them.

Pediatric Considerations
- IPV can occur in adolescence, known as teen dating violence (TDV). TDV affects millions of U.S. teens each year.
- Approximately 1 in 5 female high school students report being physically and/or sexually abused by a dating partner; females between 16 and 24 years of age are more vulnerable to IPV than any other age group.
- About 11 million women and 5 million men reported experiencing IPV before the age of 18 years.
- Children living in violent homes are at increased risk of physical, sexual, and/or emotional abuse; anxiety and depression; decreased self-esteem; emotional, behavioral, social, and/or physical disturbances; and lifelong poor health.

Pregnancy Considerations
- IPV leads to unintended pregnancies, induced abortions, and sexually transmitted infections (STIs). Pregnant women who experience IPV are twice as likely to have an abortion.
- IPV in pregnancy also increases the likelihood of miscarriage, stillbirth, preterm delivery, and low-birth-weight babies.

RISK FACTORS
- Patient/victim risk factors
  - Substance abuse (drug or alcohol), high-risk sexual behavior
  - Poverty/financial stressors/unemployment/less education
  - Recent loss of social support, family disruption and life cycle changes, social isolation
  - Prior history of abusive relationships or experiencing abuse as child
  - Mental or physical disability in family
  - Pregnancy
  - Transgender-identifying women
  - Attempting to leave the relationship
- Perpetrator risk factors
  - Substance abuse, depression, personality disorders
  - Young age
  - Unemployment, recent job loss or instability, low academic achievement
  - Witnessing/experiencing violence as child
  - Threatening to self or others, violence to children or outside the home
  - Owns weapons
- Relational risk factors
  - Marital conflict or instability, economic stress, traditional gender role norms, poor family functioning, obsessive/controlling relationship

Geriatric Considerations
Factors associated with IPV in geriatric populations: female gender, immigration stress, fear, social isolation, low income, poor physical health, low cognitive functioning, absence of social support, depressive symptoms, neglect, caregiver stress, and burden

Pediatric Considerations
Factors associated with IPV in pediatric populations: transgender, adverse childhood experiences, trauma symptoms, depression, gender attitudes, and economic hardship (1)

DIAGNOSIS

- The U.S. Preventive Services Task Force (USPSTF) in 2013 issued guidelines recommending that clinicians screen all women of reproductive age for IPV and provide or refer women to ongoing support services when appropriate (2)[A].
- The U.S. Department of Health and Human Services has recommended that IPV screening and counseling be a core part of women's preventive health visits.

Pregnancy Considerations
The American College of Obstetrics and Gynecologists (ACOG) recommends that physicians screen all women for IPV at periodic intervals, including during obstetric care (at the first prenatal visit, at least once per trimester, at the postpartum checkup), offer ongoing support, and review prevention and referral options.

HISTORY
- Physicians should introduce the subject of IPV in a general way (i.e., "I routinely ask all patients about IPV. Have you ever been in a relationship where you were afraid?").
- Address patient confidentiality prior to screening (i.e., "I want you to know everything you say here is confidential, meaning that I will not talk to anyone else about what is said unless you tell me [insert laws in your state about what is necessary to disclose].").
- Screen patient alone, without partner, parent, or others present.
- Ask screening questions in patient's primary language; do not use children or other family members as interpreters.
- HITS questions: Each HITS question is scored on a 5-point scale (never, rarely, sometimes, fairly often and frequently, with a score of >10 indicating likely victimization; sensitivity 30–100% and specificity 86–99%). "How often does your partner:
  - **H**urt you physically?; **I**nsult or talk down to you?; **T**hreaten you with harm?; **S**cream or curse at you?" (3)
- Partner Violence Scale (sensitivity 35–71%; specificity 80–94%)
  - "Have you ever been hit, kicked, punched, or otherwise, hurt by someone within the past year? If so, by whom?"
  - "Do you feel safe in your current relationship?"
  - "Is there a partner from a previous relationship who is making you feel unsafe now?"
- SAFE questions
  - **S**tress/safety: "Do you feel safe in your relationship?"
  - **A**fraid/abused: "Have you ever been in a relationship where you were threatened, hurt, or afraid?"
  - **F**riends/family: "Are your friends or family aware that you have been hurt? Could you tell them, and would they be able to give you support?"
  - **E**mergency plan: "Do you have a safe place to go and the resources you need in an emergency?"
- Assess pregnancy difficulties such as poor/late prenatal care, low-birth-weight babies, and perinatal deaths as well as repeat abortions (unplanned pregnancy may be a result of sexual assault or reproductive coercion).
- Pelvic and abdominal pain, chronic without demonstrable pathology, gynecologic disorders
- Headaches, back pain
- STIs
- Depression, suicidal ideation, anxiety, fatigue, eating disorders, substance abuse
- Overuse of health services/frequent emergency room visits
- Nonadherence with medication/treatment plan and/or missed appointments

PHYSICAL EXAM
- Clinical presentation/psychological signs and symptoms
  - Delay in seeking treatment, inconsistent explanation of injuries, reluctance to undress
  - Signs of battered woman syndrome and/or posttraumatic stress disorder (PTSD) (flat affect/avoidance of eye contact, evasiveness, heightened startle response, sleep disturbance, traumatic flashbacks)
  - Suspicious partner accompaniment at appointment; overly solicitous partner and/or refusal to leave exam room
- Physical signs and symptoms
  - Tympanic membrane rupture
  - Rectal or genital injury (centrally located injuries with bathing-suit pattern of distribution—concealable by clothing)

- Head and neck injuries (site of 50% of abusive injuries)
- Scrapes, loose or broken tooth, bruises, cuts, or fractures to face or body
- Knife wounds, cigarette burns, bite marks, welts with outline of weapon (such as belt buckle)
- Defensive posture injuries
- Injuries inconsistent with explanation or in various stages of healing
- Malnutrition or pressure ulcers in the elderly

DIAGNOSTIC TESTS & INTERPRETATION
Initial Tests (lab, imaging)
Liver function tests (LFTs), amylase, lipase if abdominal trauma is suspected, BUN and creatinine if malnutrition/dehydration is suspected, pregnancy test and STI testing (HIV Ab/Ag, syphilis screen, gonorrhea and chlamydia NAAT, trichomonas) in cases of sexual abuse, X-ray if suspected fracture, radiographic skeletal survey for children <2 years old if physical abuse is suspected

 # TREATMENT

- Treatment includes initial diagnosis; ongoing medical care; emotional support, counseling, and patient education regarding the DV cycle; referrals to community and supportive services as needed.
- On diagnosis, use the SOS-DoC intervention:
  - **S**: Offer *Support* and assess *Safety*:
    - Support: "You are not to blame. I am sorry this is happening to you. There is no excuse for you to be treated this way."
    - Remind the patient of your commitment to confidential communication.
    - Safety: Listen and respond to safety issues for the patient: "Do you feel safe going home?"; "Are your children safe?"
  - **O**: Discuss *Options*, including safety planning and follow-up:
    - Provide information about IPV and help when needed. Make referrals to local resources.
    - "Do you need or want to access a safety shelter or IPV service agency?"
    - "Do you want police intervention and if so, would you like me to call the police, so they can make a report with you?"
    - Offer numbers to local resources and National IPV Hotline: 1-800-799-SAFE (open 24/7; can provide physicians in every state with information on local resources)
  - **S**: Validate patient's *Strengths*:
    - "It took courage for you to talk with me today. You have shown great strength in very difficult circumstances."
  - **Do**: *Document* observations, assessment, and plans:
    - Use patient's own words regarding injury and abuse. Language should be chosen carefully; "patient reports" as opposed to "patient denies/claims," which may suggest the clinician does not believe the patient
    - Legibly document injuries: Use a body map.
    - If possible, photograph patient's injuries if given consent. Photographs must include the patient's face or identifying features with the injury in order to be useful as legal evidence.
    - Make patient safety plan. Prepare the patient to get away in an emergency:
    - Encourage patient to prepare an emergency kit to keep in a safe place: keys (house and car); important papers (Social Security card, birth certificates, photo ID/driver's license, passport, green card); cash, food stamps, credit cards; medication for self and children; children's immunization records; important phone numbers/addresses (friends, family, local shelters); personal care items (e.g., extra glasses)
    - Encourage patient to arrange a signal with someone to let that person know when she or he needs help.
  - **C**: Offer *Continuity*:
    - Offer a follow-up appointment and assess barriers to access.

GENERAL MEASURES
- Reporting child and elder abuse to protective services is mandatory in most states. Several states have laws requiring mandatory reporting of IPV.
- Contact the local IPV program to gain information out about laws and community resources before they are needed.
- Display resource materials (National Domestic Violence Hotline: 1-800-799-SAFE) in the office, all exam rooms, and restrooms.

ADDITIONAL THERAPIES
- National Domestic Violence Hotline: 1-800-799-SAFE (7233)
- Rape Abuse & Incest National Network (RAINN) Hotline: 1-800-656-HOPE (4673)
- Post resources and posters in both English and Spanish in exam rooms, bathrooms, waiting rooms; available at https://www.thehotline.org/stakeholders/download-and-request-materials/

 # ONGOING CARE

FOLLOW-UP RECOMMENDATIONS
- Schedule prompt follow-up appointment. Inquire about what occurred since last visit. Offer ongoing support and resources.
- IPV often requires multiple interventions over time before it is resolved.

PATIENT EDUCATION
- Counsel patients about nonviolent ways to resolve conflict and about the cycle of violence.
- CDC: https://www.cdc.gov/violenceprevention/intimatepartnerviolence/prevention
- National Domestic Violence Hotline: https://www.thehotline.org/
- National Coalition Against Domestic Violence: https://ncadv.org/
- National Resource Center on Domestic Violence: https://nrcdv.org/

PROGNOSIS
Victims of IPV can suffer from PTSD, anxiety, and depression. Counseling, support, and resources can improve their prognosis.

REFERENCES
1. Kyle J. Intimate partner violence. *Med Clin North Am*. 2023;107(2):385–395.
2. Moyer VA. Screening for intimate partner violence and abuse of elderly and vulnerable adults: U.S. Preventive Services Task Force recommendation statement. *Ann Intern Med*. 2013;158(6):478–486.
3. Dicola D, Spaar E. Intimate partner violence. *Am Fam Physician*. 2016;94(8):646–651.

ADDITIONAL READING
- Perone HR, Dietz NA, Belkowitz J, et al; for Committee on Child Abuse and Neglect and Committee on Injury, Violence, and Poison Prevention. Intimate partner violence: analysis of current screening practices in primary care setting. *Fam Pract*. 2022;39(1):6–11.
- Thackeray JD, Hibbard R, Dowd MD. Intimate partner violence: the role of the pediatrician. *Pediatrics*. 2010;125(5):1094–1100.

CODES

ICD10
- T74.91XA Unspecified adult maltreatment, confirmed, initial encounter
- T74.11XA Adult physical abuse, confirmed, initial encounter
- T74.31XA Adult psychological abuse, confirmed, initial encounter

CLINICAL PEARLS
- Display resource materials in the office (e.g., posting abuse awareness posters/National Domestic Violence Hotline, 1-800-799-SAFE, in both English and Spanish, in all exam rooms and restrooms).
- Given the high prevalence of IPV and the lack of harm and potential benefits of screening, routine screening is recommended.
- For those who screened positive, offer resources, reassure confidentiality, and provide close follow-up.

IRRITABLE BOWEL SYNDROME

Marie L. Borum, MD, EdD, MPH • Joan Elizabeth Smith, DNP • Zeina M. Bani Hani, MBBS

 BASICS

DESCRIPTION
- A gastrointestinal (GI) disorder characterized by chronic and recurrent abdominal pain and altered bowel habits in the absence of an organic cause
- May be characterized as diarrhea-predominant (IBS-D), constipation-predominant (IBS-C), mixed (IBS-M), or unknown (IBS-U); may alternate between symptoms

EPIDEMIOLOGY
Irritable bowel syndrome (IBS) accounts for 25–50% of visits to gastroenterologists and ~2 million primary care visits annually in United States with estimated cost of $1.5 to 10 billion dollars a year.

Incidence
1–2% per year

Prevalence
- Pooled estimate of ~4% globally using Rome IV criteria or 10% globally using Rome III criteria
- Predominant age: 20 to 39 years; if age >50 years, consider other diagnoses. In the United States, it affects 10–15% of the population; in the United States, female > male (3:1); females are more likely to have IBS-C as compared to males.
- More common in low socioeconomic communities

ETIOLOGY AND PATHOPHYSIOLOGY
- The pathophysiology of IBS is unknown; it is associated with abnormalities of intestinal motility, intestinal inflammation, and enhanced sensitivity to visceral stimuli. The trigger may be luminal contractions, prolonged transit time, or environmental.
- PI-IBS (post-infectious) develops in roughly 10% with infectious enteritis. The odds of developing PI-IBS after acute GI infection is increased 6-fold. The cause of bowel symptoms following acute infection is uncertain, but several theories have been suggested such as malabsorption, increase in enteroendocrine cells/lymphocytes, and antibiotic use.
- Food sensitivity, microbiome dysbiosis, genetic, and psychosocial causes including early childhood stress are under investigation. Increase in mast cell and lymphocytic density and activity has been demonstrated on biopsy from terminal ileum, jejunum, colon in patients with IBS and may correlate with visceral hypersensitivity (1).
- Increase in proinflammatory cytokines have been observed and may correlate with intestinal inflammation.
- Current investigation is ongoing regarding low-grade mucosal and neuroinflammation and the contribution of this inflammation in the dysregulation of the "brain-gut" axis (1).
- There is an ongoing investigation of the role of colonic and small intestinal motility.

Genetics
Unknown; IBS tracks in some families; relatives of someone with IBS are 2 to 3 times more likely to have IBS.

RISK FACTORS
Female sex (odds ratio 1.67); other family members with similar GI disorder; psychological factors: stress, abuse history, anxiety, depression, or somatization; somatic factors: GI infection, pain syndromes, obesity, antibiotic use, and abdominal surgery; social factors: socioeconomic status in childhood

Pediatric Considerations
No risk to mother or fetus

GENERAL PREVENTION
See "Diet."

COMMONLY ASSOCIATED CONDITIONS
- Other functional GI disorders (heartburn, dyspepsia, gastroesophageal reflux disease, nausea, diarrhea, incontinence, pelvic floor dyssynergia, and constipation)
- Chronic conditions including migraines, fibromyalgia, chronic pelvic pain, temporomandibular joint dysfunction, chronic fatigue syndrome, sleep disorders, noncardiac chest pain, and overactive bladder
- Psychiatric disorders: major depression, anxiety, somatoform disorders, and posttraumatic stress

 DIAGNOSIS

HISTORY
- Rome IV criteria: recurrent abdominal pain >1 day/week, on average, in the previous 3 months with an onset >6 months before diagnosis associated with at least two of the following:
  - Related to defecation
  - Change in frequency of stools
  - Change in form (appearance) of stools
- Four bowel patterns in the Rome IV classification:
  - IBS-D: diarrhea predominant: >25% diarrhea with Bristol stool types 6 or 7 and <25% constipation
  - IBS-C: constipation predominant: >25% constipation with Bristol stool types 1 or 2 and <25% diarrhea
  - IBS-M: mixed bowel habits: >25% constipation and >25% diarrhea
  - IBS-U: unclassified-symptoms: meets Rome IV criteria but not subtypes
- Patient has no warning signs (red flags):
  - Age >50 years, no previous colon cancer screening and presence of symptoms; recent change in bowel habit; evidence of overt GI bleeding (melena or hematochezia); nocturnal pain or passage of stools; unintentional weight loss (>10% in 3 months); family history of colorectal cancer, inflammatory bowel disease, or celiac disease; palpable abdominal mass or lymphadenopathy; evidence of iron deficiency anemia on blood testing; positive fecal occult blood; fever in association with the bowel symptoms

PHYSICAL EXAM
- Complete exam to exclude other causes including digital rectal exam; vital signs and physical exam typically unremarkable, but patients may have mild abdominal tenderness.
- There is an absence of peritoneal signs, ascites, lymph node enlargement, jaundice, and organomegaly.

DIFFERENTIAL DIAGNOSIS
Inflammatory bowel disease (Crohn and ulcerative colitis); endocrine disorders (hyper/hypothyroidism, Addison disease, diabetes mellitus); lactose intolerance; fructose malabsorption; infections (Giardia lamblia, Entamoeba histolytica, Salmonella, Campylobacter, Yersinia, Clostridium difficile); celiac sprue; microscopic colitis; medication induced: opioid constipation, laxative abuse; magnesium antacids; pancreatic insufficiency; small bowel bacterial overgrowth; somatization; depression; villous adenoma, endocrine tumors (gastrinoma or carcinoid); radiation damage to colon or small bowel

DIAGNOSTIC TESTS & INTERPRETATION
- No definitive diagnostic laboratory test for IBS; use a positive diagnostic strategy, rather than making a diagnosis of exclusion. With a typical history and no warning signs (e.g., anemia, weight loss), obtain CBC and age-appropriate colorectal cancer screening.
- In patients with diarrhea, obtain baseline labs (fecal calprotectin or lactoferrin, basic metabolic profile, stool O&P, fecal leukocytes, Giardia antigen, Clostridium difficile toxin) and begin treatment.
- Plasma anti-cytolethal distending toxin B (anti-CdtB) and anti-vinculin antibodies have been shown to be elevated in IBS-D and IBS-M but not in IBS-C. The diagnostic role of both antibodies is yet to be confirmed.

Initial Tests (lab, imaging)
Rule out pathology specific to the patient's symptoms:
- Diarrhea-predominant: CRP, IgA tissue transglutaminase (rule out celiac disease) with IgA level, fecal calprotectin or fecal lactoferrin, thyroid-stimulating hormone (TSH), and stool for ova and parasites
- Constipation-predominant: TSH, electrolytes, calcium (hyperparathyroidism); abdominal pain: LFTs, lipase or amylase
- In the absence of alarm symptoms, labs such a fecal calprotectin (<40 μg/g) are considered sufficient to effectively rule out inflammatory bowel disease. CRP (<0.5 mg/dL) and fecal lactoferrin (<7 μg/g) can be used as an alternative (2).
- Consider hydrogen breath testing to exclude bacterial overgrowth; in patients who do not respond to treatment, consider further evaluation with imaging (ultrasound or CT), endoscopy, video capsule endoscopy, or sitz marker study. These will generally be unremarkable in IBS.

Follow-Up Tests & Special Considerations
- Consider lactulose breath test to assess for small intestinal bacterial overgrowth associated with IBS.
- Consider colonoscopy in patients at high risk for microscopic colitis (female gender, >60 years old, and more intense diarrhea).

Diagnostic Procedures/Other

- Sigmoidoscopy/colonoscopy with biopsies may be used to rule out inflammatory bowel disease or microscopic colitis, particularly in patients with diarrhea.
- Abdominal radiograph can be considered to assess for severity of stool burden in IBS-C or if concern for a structure lesion. Additional imaging may be considered including pelvic imaging and/or abdominal CT scan.
- Physiologic testing (anorectal manometry and balloon expulsion) can be done to rule out dyssynergic defecation in patients with severe constipation refractory to dietary change and osmotic laxative therapy.

ALERT
Screen all persons >45 years of age (or those with warning signs/red flags) for colorectal cancer.

 TREATMENT

- The main goals of management are to relieve symptoms and improve the quality of life (3). Therapy should be aimed at specific subtype of IBS.
- Psychosocial therapy: goal should be to decrease stress and anxiety; can be achieved through formal counseling, antidepressant or antianxiety medications, support groups
- Lifestyle modification
  - Exercise 3 to 5 times per week decreases severity (3).
  - Food diary to determine triggers (3)

MEDICATION
- Soluble fiber supplementation (psyllium) increases stool bulk; does not typically relieve abdominal pain; may be used for all types (2)[B]; has been shown to improve both constipation and diarrhea in patients with all types of IBS the recommendation is to start with approximately 3 to 4 g of soluble fiber per day.
- For all types of IBS:
  - Antispasmodics such as hyoscyamine 0.125 to 0.250 mg PO/SL q4h PRN and dicyclomine 20 to 40 mg PO BID; adverse effects include dry mouth, dizziness, and blurred vision; used on an as-needed basis
  - TCAs starting at the lowest dose; typically, reserved for patients with IBS-D due to ability to slow intestinal transit time; multimodal mechanism of action in IBS; common adverse effects include dry mouth, insomnia, flushing, and palpitations. Numbers needed to treat (NNT) is 4.5. Numbers need to harm (NNH) ranges from 9 to 18.
  - Probiotics such as *Lactobacillus, Bifidobacterium,* and *Streptococcus* (not routinely recommended)
- IBS-D
  - Loperamide 4 to 8 mg/day divided 1 to 3 times per day as needed to decrease stool frequency and increase stool consistency (use in limited doses and on an as-needed basis for patients with IBS-M); may also use diphenoxylate and atropine
  - Bile acid sequestrants in patients with suspicion of bile acid malabsorption; these include cholestyramine, colestipol, and colesevelam. Common adverse effects include bloating, flatulence, abdominal discomfort, and constipation.

- Rifaximin (2-week course) has been shown to improve bloating, pain, and stool consistency. Favorable safety profile with a NNH of 8,971; reserved for patients who have failed to respond to other therapies
  - Alosetron (Lotronex; 0.5 to 1.0 mg PO BID) is a 5-HT$_3$ antagonist, slows intestinal transit; indicated for women with severe symptoms that have lasted for 6 months and failed therapy with conventional treatment
  - Ondansetron was found to reduce symptoms severity including stool consistency, frequency, and urgency but with no significant improvement in pain.
  - Eluxadoline (75 to 100 mg BID) is a mixed opioid receptor agonist and antagonist; used in patients with severe IBS-D refractory to all other agents
- IBS-C
  - Laxatives such as polyethylene glycol (17 g of powder dissolved in 8 oz of water, QD) may improve stool frequency and constipation but not pain.
  - Antibiotics such as neomycin
  - Lubiprostone (8 μg BID with meals) is a prostaglandin E1 analog with high affinity for type 2 chloride channels, which increases intestinal secretion and peristalsis. NNT of 12.5, adverse effects include nausea and diarrhea.
  - Linaclotide (290 μg QD) is a guanylate cyclase 2C agonist that has been shown to improve bowel function and reduces abdominal pain and overall severity in adults only; NNT of 6
  - Plecanatide (3 mg QD) is approved for patients with IBS-C; acts by increasing intestinal transit and fluid content and is comparable to linaclotide; NNT of 9
  - Tenapanor (50 mg BID) is a NHE3 inhibitor that reduces absorption of sodium and phosphate and increases intestinal fluid volume and transit.
  - Tegaserod is an FDA-approved serotonin 5-HT$_4$ receptor agonist that increases colonic motility and reduces abdominal pain; only approved for women aged <65 years for emergency treatment
- Mixed: Use medications to match symptoms.

ISSUES FOR REFERRAL
- Behavioral health referral may help with management of affective or personality disorders.
- Gastroenterology referral for difficult to control cases

ADDITIONAL THERAPIES
- Probiotics use may result in reducing IBS symptoms and decreasing pain and flatulence. Multistrain probiotics tend to be more effective in symptom improvement than monostrain (4).
- Peppermint oil is used as a first-line therapy for IBS-D in Europe.

COMPLEMENTARY & ALTERNATIVE MEDICINE
A variety of herbal and natural remedies have been advertised for treatment. No evidence clearly supports benefit.

 ONGOING CARE

FOLLOW-UP RECOMMENDATIONS
Patient Monitoring
The IBS Severity Scoring System is validated measure to assess severity response to treatment.

DIET
- A low FODMAP diet: fermentable oligosaccharides, disaccharides, monosaccharides and polyols; avoid large meals, fatty foods, and caffeine, which can exacerbate symptoms.
- Avoid gas-producing foods. Increase fiber slowly to avoid excess intestinal gas production.
- Initially, consider 2 weeks of lactose-free diet to rule out lactose intolerance.
- A gluten-free diet can resolve symptoms for some patients despite negative testing for celiac disease.

PATIENT EDUCATION
IBS is not a psychiatric illness but is a chronic condition with no increased risk of malignancy.

PROGNOSIS
- IBS is a chronic relapsing disorder that reduces quality of life but does not increase mortality.
- Evidence suggests that "symptom shifting" occurs in some patients, whereby resolution of functional bowel symptoms is followed by the development of functional symptoms in another system.

REFERENCES
1. Lacy BE, Pimentel M, Brenner DM, et al. ACG clinical guideline: management of irritable bowel syndrome. *Am J Gastroenterol.* 2021;116(1):17–44.
2. Kurin M, Cooper G. Irritable bowel syndrome with diarrhea: treatment is a work in progress. *Cleve Clin J Med.* 2020;87(8):501–511.
3. Jayasinghe M, Damianos JA, Prathiraja O, et al. Irritable bowel syndrome: treating the gut and brain/mind at the same time. *Cureus.* 2023;15(8):e43404.
4. Dale HF, Rasmussen SH, Asiller ÖÖ, et al. Probiotics in irritable bowel syndrome: an up-to-date systematic review. *Nutrients.* 2019;11(9):2048.

 SEE ALSO

Algorithm: Diarrhea, Chronic

CODES
ICD10
- K58.9 Irritable bowel syndrome without diarrhea
- K58.0 Irritable bowel syndrome with diarrhea
- K58 Irritable bowel syndrome

CLINICAL PEARLS
- Use Rome IV criteria to establish the diagnosis of IBS.
- The goals of treatment are to relieve symptoms and improve the quality of life.
- Many patients can successfully manage their symptoms with attention to their dietary triggers.
- If patients do not respond to initial treatment, consider further evaluation (including imaging and/or referral for endoscopy) to exclude organic pathology.

I

KAWASAKI SYNDROME

Khadija Kabani, DO, FAAFP • Chelsea M. Shine, DO

 BASICS

DESCRIPTION

- Kawasaki syndrome (KS) is a self-limited acute, febrile, systemic vasculitis of small- and medium-sized arteries that predominantly affects patients aged 6 months to 5 years.
- The most prominent cause of acquired coronary artery disease in children in developed countries (1)
- Vasculitis of coronary arteries results in aneurysms/ectasia, myocardial infarction (MI)/ischemia, or sudden death.
- System(s) affected: cardiovascular, gastrointestinal, hematologic/lymphatic/immunologic, musculoskeletal, nervous, pulmonary, renal/urologic, skin/exocrine
- Synonym(s): mucocutaneous lymph node syndrome (MCLS), infantile polyarteritis, Kawasaki disease

ALERT
Consider in any child with extended high fever unresponsive to antibiotics or antipyretics, rash, and nonexudative conjunctivitis.

EPIDEMIOLOGY

Incidence
- Worldwide: affects all races but most prevalent in Asia; Japan annual incidence rate of 265/100,000 in children <5 years old
- In the United States, annual incidence in children aged <5 years is 20/100,000. Compared to white people, African Americans have 1.5 times risk, and Asian Americans have 2.5 times risk. The highest state incidence is in Hawaii.
- Leading cause of acquired heart disease in children in developed countries
  - Predominant age: 1 to 5 years; median age of diagnosis is 1.5 years of age.
  - 85% of cases are children <5 years of age and 50% <2 years of age.
  - Male-to-female ratio = 1.5:1

Prevalence
- Highest to lowest prevalence: Asian > African American > Hispanic > white
- Seasonal variation: peaks in winter and early spring (January to March) in temperate places; peaks in summer in Asia
- Outbreaks at 2- to 3-year intervals

ETIOLOGY AND PATHOPHYSIOLOGY
- Infectious agent triggers abnormal inflammatory reaction in children with genetic predisposition.
- Acute KS causes a necrotizing arteritis in the smooth muscle layer of medium extraparenchymal arteries, destroying arterial walls into the adventitia, especially in coronary arteries.
- Inflammatory cells secrete cytokines (TNF-α), interleukins 1 and 6, and matrix metalloproteases that cause fragmentation of the internal elastic lamina
- As the acute process resolves, active neutrophilic inflammatory cells are succeeded by a subacute/chronic, lymphocytic vasculitis; fibroblasts and monocytes cause tissue repair/remodeling that may cause vascular fibrosis and stenosis.

Genetics
- Populations at higher risk and family link suggest a genetic predisposition.
- Siblings of patients in Japan have a 10- to 30-fold increased risk, and >50% develop KS within 10 days of first case; increased occurrence of KS in children whose parents also had illness in childhood

- Single-nucleotide polymorphisms in six different genes have been implicated in KS (Fcγ receptor 2A, CASP3, HLA class II, B-cell lymphoid kinase, IPTKC, CD40).
- Coronary aneurisms are associated with variants in TGF-β signaling pathways.

RISK FACTORS
- Male to female prevalence 1.5:1 in the United States
- African Americans at 1.5 times risk; Asian Americans at 2.5 times risk
- Sibling with Kawasaki

GENERAL PREVENTION
None

 DIAGNOSIS

- ≥5 days of fever and ≥4 of the following five principal clinical features (1); OR <4 features and presence of coronary artery disease on 2D echocardiography:
  - Bilateral, nonpurulent conjunctival injection with limbic sparing
  - Erythematous changes to mouth, pharynx, tongue, and lips
  - A polymorphous, generalized, erythematous rash
  - Changes in the skin of the peripheral extremities (edema of hands/feet; erythema of palms/soles; desquamation of fingers/toes)
  - Cervical lymphadenopathy (>1 node >1.5 cm in diameter)
- Note: Diagnosis can be made at day 4 of fever in a patient with >4 principal clinical features, especially if redness/swelling of hands/feet is present.

Pediatric Considerations
- Prolonged fever without rash that is treated with antibiotics and followed by a rash may appear to be a drug reaction.
- Incomplete KS (atypical KS)
  - ≥5 days of fever, 2 to 3 principal clinical features, labs indicating systemic inflammation, and exclusion of other diseases
  - Incomplete cases with <4 clinical criteria often occur in infants ≤6 months of age or older children/adolescents. The frequency of coronary artery aneurysms (CAAs) is higher in patients with missed diagnosis/delayed treatment. Therefore, in infants with prolonged fever and few clinical features, consider echocardiography and inflammatory labs.

HISTORY
- Fever is the first sign during the acute phase.
- Symptoms may not occur all at once but usually occur in close proximity.

PHYSICAL EXAM
- High-spiking and remittent fever for ≥5 days
  - Fever is high (102–105°F [39.4–40.5°C]) and unresponsive to antibiotics/antipyretics.
  - May be prolonged up to 10 to 12 days with more rare cases lasting 3 to 4 weeks (1)
- Bilateral, painless, nonpurulent, conjunctival injection without corneal ulceration or edema; limbic sparing
- Changes in lips and oral cavity: redness and swelling of lips in the acute stage; cracking, fissuring, bleeding in subacute phase; strawberry/erythematous tongue

- Extensive erythematous polymorphous rash: within 5 days of fever
  - Morbilliform is most common; may be maculo-papular, scarlatiniform; can resemble erythema multiforme, erythroderma, urticarial exanthem; rarely micropustular
  - Perineal desquamation, especially in skin folds
- Extremity changes: reddened palms and soles on days 3 to 5; edema of hands and feet on days 4 to 7; painful induration; desquamation of fingers and toes that begins in periungual area at 2 to 3 weeks
- Acute, unilateral cervical lymphadenopathy (least common symptom): ≥1 lymph nodes >1.5 cm, firm, nonfluctuant, and slight tenderness
- Cardiac exam: tachycardia, gallop rhythms, hyperdynamic precordium, innocent flow murmurs, depressed contractility
- Other organ system involvement
  - Cardiovascular: myocarditis; pericarditis (often subclinical), CAAs, and other medium-sized arterial aneurysms
  - Gastrointestinal: anorexia, abdominal pain, vomiting/diarrhea, acute gallbladder hydrops, hepatic enlargement, jaundice
  - Renal: proteinuria, sterile pyuria
  - Joints: polyarthritis of small joints in acute phase; weight-bearing joints affected after 10th day from onset of fever
  - Neurologic: aseptic meningitis, peripheral neuropathy (unilateral facial palsy), transient high-frequency hearing loss

DIFFERENTIAL DIAGNOSIS
- Bacterial: scarlet fever, bacterial cervical lymphadenitis, *Mycoplasma* infection, leptospirosis, Lyme disease, Rocky Mountain spotted fever
- Toxin mediated: staphylococcal scalded-skin syndrome, streptococcal scarlet fever, toxic shock syndrome (1)
- Viral: measles, adenovirus, Epstein-Barr virus, SARS-CoV-2; multisystem inflammatory syndrome in children (MIS-C) is an important consideration given similar presentation
- Toxoplasmosis
- Reiter syndrome
- Hypersensitivity drug reactions (erythema multiforme minor, Stevens-Johnson syndrome)
- Juvenile rheumatoid arthritis
- Acrodynia (mercury poisoning)

DIAGNOSTIC TESTS & INTERPRETATION
- Initial workup: CBC with differential, urinalysis (UA)/culture, liver function tests including AST, ALT, and albumin, blood culture; lumbar puncture if signs of meningitis or if <90 days old
  - Leukocytosis (12,000 to 40,000 cells/mm³) with immature and mature granulocytes
  - Anemia: normochromic, normocytic
  - Thrombocytosis (500,000 to >1,000,000/mm³) in 2nd and 3rd week; thrombocytopenia during acute phase is associated with CAA and MI.
- Elevated C-reactive protein (CRP) (>35 mg/L in 80% cases), erythrocyte sedimentation rate (ESR) (>60 mm/hr in 60% cases), and α_1-antitrypsin
- Normal ESR, CRP, and PLTs after day 7 suggest diagnosis other than KS.
- ESR can be artificially high after intravenous immunoglobulin (IVIG) therapy.
- Hyponatremia
- Moderately elevated AST, ALT, GGT, and bilirubin
- Decreased albumin and protein

- CSF pleocytosis may be seen (lymphocytic with normal protein and glucose).
- Nasal swab to rule out adenovirus, coronavirus (SARS-CoV-2)

Initial Tests (lab, imaging)
- If KS is suspected, obtain ECG and echocardiogram.
  - ECG may show arrhythmias, prolonged PR interval, and ST/T wave changes.
  - Echocardiography has a high sensitivity and specificity for detection of abnormalities of proximal left main coronary artery, and right coronary artery may show perivascular brightening, ectasia, decreased left ventricular contractility, pericardial effusion, or aneurysms.
  - Repeat echocardiography frequency determined by degree of abnormal more significant findings should be followed twice weekly until aneurysmal progression halts.
  - Cardiac stress test if CAA seen on echocardiogram
- Baseline chest x-ray may show pleural effusion, atelectasis, and congestive heart failure.

Diagnostic Procedures/Other
- No laboratory study is diagnostic; diagnosis rests on constellation of clinical features and exclusion of other illnesses.
- Magnetic resonance coronary angiography is non-invasive modality to visualize coronary arteries for stenosis, thrombi, and intimal thickening.
- Patients with complex coronary artery lesions (CALs) may benefit from coronary angiography after the acute inflammatory process has resolved; generally recommended in 6 to 12 months

💉 TREATMENT

GENERAL MEASURES
Use antibiotics until bacterial etiologies are excluded (e.g., sepsis or meningitis).

MEDICATION
- Optimal therapy is IVIG 2 g/kg IV over 10 to 12 hours with high-dose aspirin preferably within 7 to 10 days of fever, followed by low-dose aspirin until follow-up echocardiograms indicate a lack of coronary abnormalities.
  - IVIG lowers the risk of CAA and may shorten fever duration.
  - The extreme irritability often resolves very quickly after IVIG is given.
  - CALs develop in 3–5% of children treated with IVIG. CALs develop in up to 25% of untreated children (1).
- Retreatment with IVIG if clinical response is incomplete or fever persists/returns >36 hours after start of IVIG treatment
  - ≥10% of patients do not respond to initial IVIG treatment. 2/3 of nonresponders respond to the second dose of IVIG.
  - Nonresponders tend to have ↑ bands, ↓ albumin, and an abnormal echo.
- Aspirin 80 to 100 mg/kg/day in 4 doses beginning with IVIG administration. Switch to low-dose aspirin (3 to 5 mg/kg/day) when afebrile for 48 to 72 hours, or continue until day 14 of illness. Maintain low dose for 6 to 8 weeks until follow-up echocardiogram is normal and CRP and/or ESR are normal. Continue salicylate regimen in children with coronary abnormalities, long term or until documented regression of aneurysm.
- Aspirin does not appear to reduce CAA.

- Corticosteroids have conflicting evidence for use and:
  - Should not be used as first-line agent in all KS patients; reserve for IVIG resistant cases.
  - Should be used in conjunction with IVIG and aspirin as initial treatment to decrease risk of CAAs in those at highest risk of IVIG failure
- Contraindications
  - IVIG: documented hypersensitivity, IgA deficiency, anti-IgE/IgG antibodies, severe thrombocytopenia, coagulation disorders
  - Aspirin: vitamin K deficiency, bleeding disorders, liver damage, documented hypersensitivity, hypoprothrombinemia
- Precautions
  - High-dose aspirin therapy can result in tinnitus, decreased of renal function, and increased transaminases.
  - Do not use ibuprofen in children with CAAs who are taking aspirin for antiplatelet effects.
  - Aspirin therapy has been associated with Reye syndrome in children who develop viral infections, especially influenza B and varicella. Yearly influenza vaccination is recommended for children requiring long-term treatment with aspirin. Delay any live vaccines for 11 months after IVIG treatment.

First Line
High dose IVIG and aspirin should be instituted promptly on confirmed diagnosis (1).

Second Line
- In patients refractory to IVIG and steroids, consider infliximab or cyclosporine.
- Plasma exchange may decrease likelihood of CAA in IVIG nonresponders.

ISSUES FOR REFERRAL
Pediatric cardiologist if abnormalities on echo or if extensive stenosis

ADDITIONAL THERAPIES
- Treatment and prevention of thrombosis are crucial.
- Antiplatelet agents (clopidogrel, dipyridamole), heparin, low-molecular-weight heparin, or warfarin are sometimes added to the low-dose aspirin regimen, depending on severity of CAAs.
- Clarithromycin given with IVIG may reduce relapse rates and length of hospital stay; does not reduce duration of fever or improve cardiac outcomes

SURGERY/OTHER PROCEDURES
- Rarely needed; coronary artery bypass grafting for severe obstruction/recurrent MI
- Coronary revascularization via percutaneous coronary intervention for patients with evidence of ischemia on stress testing

ADMISSION, INPATIENT, AND NURSING CONSIDERATIONS
- Normal saline (NS) for rehydration and 1/2 NS for maintenance
- Consider discharge if afebrile after IVIG treatment for 24 hours.

⚡ ONGOING CARE

FOLLOW-UP RECOMMENDATIONS
With aneurysms, contact and high-risk sports should be avoided.

Patient Monitoring
- Repeat ECG and echocardiogram at 6 to 8 weeks. If abnormal, repeat at 6 to 12 months.
- Patients with complex CALs may require a combination of β-blockers to decrease oxidative stress and antithrombotic therapy (1). These patients may benefit from coronary angiography at 6 to 12 months and will require close follow-up.
- Patients receiving long-term ASA should be fully immunized. Measles and varicella-containing immunizations are contraindicated for 11 months after IVIG for Kawasaki disease (1).

PROGNOSIS
- Usually self-limited
- Relates entirely to the extent and severity of cardiac disease (1)
- Moderate-sized aneurysms usually regress in 1 to 2 years, resolving in 50–66% of cases.
- Recurrence (3% in Japan, <1% in the United States)
- Sudden death in early adulthood (rare)

COMPLICATIONS
- 15–25% of untreated patients develop CAAs in convalescent phase.
- 2–7% of treated patients develop aneurysms. 1% develop giant aneurysms.
- Risk factors for aneurysm: male, <1 year of age, ↑ ESR >4 weeks, fever >2 weeks, fever >48 hours after IVIG treatment
- Mortality of 0.08–0.17% is due to cardiac disease.

REFERENCE
1. Son MBF, Newburger JW. Kawasaki disease. *Pediatr Rev*. 2018;39(2):78–90.

ADDITIONAL READING
- Most ZM, Hendren N, Drazner MH, et al. Striking similarities of multisystem inflammatory syndrome in children and a myocarditis-like syndrome in adults: overlapping manifestations of COVID-19. *Circulation*. 2021;143(1):4–6.
- Oates-Whitehead RM, Baumer JH, Haines L, et al. Intravenous immunoglobulin for the treatment of Kawasaki disease in children. *Cochrane Database Syst Rev*. 2003;2003(4):CD004000.
- Rife E, Abraham G. Kawasaki disease: an update. *Curr Rheumatol Rep*. 2020;22(10):75.
- Saguil A, Fargo M, Grogan S. Diagnosis and management of Kawasaki disease. *Am Fam Physician*. 2015;91(6):365–371.

CODES

ICD10
M30.3 Mucocutaneous lymph node syndrome [Kawasaki]

CLINICAL PEARLS
- The diagnosis of KS rests on a constellation of clinical features.
- Once KS is suspected, all patients need an inpatient cardiac evaluation, including ECG and echocardiogram.
- Optimal therapy is IVIG 2 g/kg IV over 10 hours, with high-dose aspirin 80 to 100 mg/kg/day in 4 doses.

KERATOACANTHOMA

Andrew J. Richardson, MD

 BASICS

DESCRIPTION

- Most commonly presents as a solitary, rapidly proliferating, dome-shaped, erythematous or flesh-colored papule or nodule with a central keratinous plug, typically reaching 1 to 2 cm in diameter
- Clinically and microscopically resembles squamous cell carcinoma (SCC)
- Other presentations include grouped, multiple, keratoacanthoma (KA) centrifugum marginatum, intraoral, subungual, regressing, nonregressing, and generally eruptive (1).
- Majority are benign and resolve spontaneously, but lesions do have the potential for invasion and metastasis; therefore, treatment is required.
- Three clinical stages of KAs (1):
  - Proliferative: rapid growth of the lesion over weeks to several months
  - Maturation/stabilization: Lesion stabilizes and growth subsides.
  - Involution: spontaneous resolution of the lesion, leaving a hypopigmented, depressed scar; most but not all lesions will enter this stage.
- System(s) affected: integumentary

EPIDEMIOLOGY

- Greatest incidence age >50 years but may occur at any age
- Presentation increases during summer and early fall seasons.
- Most frequently on sun-exposed and hair-bearing skin but may occur anywhere
- Predominant sex: male > female (2:1)
- Most commonly in fair-skinned individuals; highest rates in Fitzpatrick skin type I to III
- 104 cases per 100,000 individuals

ETIOLOGY AND PATHOPHYSIOLOGY

- Derived from an abnormality causing hyperkeratosis within the follicular infundibulum
- Squamous epithelial cells proliferate to extend upward around the keratin plug and proceed downward into the dermis. This process is followed by invasion of elastic and collagen fibers.
- Cellular mechanism responsible for the hyperkeratosis is currently unknown. The role of human papillomavirus (HPV) has been discussed but has no established causality (2).
- Regression may be due to immune cytotoxicity or terminal differentiation of keratinocytes.
- Multiple etiologies have been suggested:
  - UV radiation
  - May be provoked by surgery, cryotherapy, chemical peels, or laser therapy

- Viral infections: HPV or Merkel cell polyomavirus
- Genetic predisposition: Muir-Torre syndrome, xeroderma pigmentosum, Ferguson-Smith syndrome
- Immunosuppression
- BRAF inhibitors (1)
- Chemical carcinogen exposure

Genetics

- Mutation of *p53* or *H-ras*
- Ferguson-Smith syndrome (AD)
- Witten-Zak (AD)
- Muir-Torre syndrome (AD)
- Xeroderma pigmentosum (AR)
- Grzybowski (sporadic)
- Incontinentia pigmenti (XLD)

RISK FACTORS

- UV exposure/damage: outdoor and/or indoor tanning
- Fitzpatrick skin type I to III
- Trauma (typically appears within 1 month of injury): laser resurfacing, surgery, cryotherapy, tattoos
- Chemical carcinogens: tar, pitch, and smoking
- Immunocompromised state
- Discoid lupus erythematosus
- HPV infection

GENERAL PREVENTION

Sun protection measures

COMMONLY ASSOCIATED CONDITIONS

- Frequently, the patient has concurrent sun-damaged skin: solar elastosis, solar lentigines, actinic keratosis, nonmelanoma skin cancers (basal cell carcinoma and SCC).
- In Muir-Torre syndrome, KAs are found with coexisting sebaceous neoplasms and malignancy of the GI and GU tracts; may have sebaceous differentiation known as a seboacanthoma

 DIAGNOSIS

HISTORY

- Lesion typically begins as a small, solitary, pink macule that undergoes a rapid growth phase; classically reaching a diameter of 1 to 2 cm, although size may vary
- Once the proliferative stage has subsided, the lesion size generally remains stable.
- May decrease in size, indicating regression
- Usually asymptomatic, although occasionally tender
- If multiple lesions are present, it is important to elicit a family history and recent therapies or treatments.
- If sebaceous neoplasms are present, must review history for signs/symptoms of GI or GU malignancies

PHYSICAL EXAM

- Firm, solitary, erythematous or flesh-colored, dome-shaped papule or nodule with a central keratin plug, giving a crateriform appearance
- Surrounding skin and borders of lesion may show telangiectasia, atrophy, or dyspigmentation.
- Usually solitary; multiple lesions can occur.
- Most commonly seen on sun-exposed areas: face, neck, scalp, dorsum of upper extremities, and posterior legs
- May also be seen on areas without sun exposure: buttocks, anus, subungual, mucosal surfaces
- Subungual KAs are very painful and are seen on the first 3 digits of the hands.
- Examine for regional lymphadenopathy due to chance of lesion invasion and metastasis.
- Dermoscopy (3)
  - Central keratin highest sensitivity to distinguish from SCC (4)
  - White circles, blood spots; white circles highest specificity (4)
  - Cannot reliably distinguish between KA and SCC

DIFFERENTIAL DIAGNOSIS

- SCC
- Nodular or ulcerative basal cell carcinoma
- Cutaneous horn
- Hypertrophic actinic keratosis
- Amelanotic melanoma
- Merkel cell carcinoma
- Metastasis to the skin
- Molluscum contagiosum
- Prurigo nodularis
- Verruca vulgaris
- Verrucous carcinoma
- Sebaceous adenoma
- Hypertrophic lichen planus
- Hypertrophic lupus erythematosus
- Deep fungal infection
- Atypical mycobacterial infection
- Nodular Kaposi sarcoma

DIAGNOSTIC TESTS & INTERPRETATION

- Excisional biopsy, including the center of the lesion as well as the margin, is the best diagnostic test (2)[C].
- A shave biopsy may be insufficiently deep to distinguish a KA from an SCC.
- If unable to perform an excisional biopsy, a deep shave (saucerization) of the entire lesion, extending into the subcutaneous fat, can be performed.
- Punch biopsies should be avoided because they give an insufficient amount of tissue to represent the entire lesion.

Initial Tests (lab, imaging)
- Subungual KA: radiograph of the digit to monitor for osteolysis (cup-shaped radiolucent defect)
- Aggressive tumors may need CT with contrast for evaluation of lymph nodes and MRI if there is a concern of perineural invasion.
- Most lesions do not require imaging.

Test Interpretation
- Pathology of biopsy: well-demarcated central core of keratin surrounded by well-differentiated, mildly pleomorphic, atypical squamous epithelial cells with a characteristic of glassy eosinophilic cytoplasm
- Histopathology: keratin-filled crater encompassed with epithelial lips
- May see elastic and collagen fibers invading into the squamous epithelium
- Histologic differentiation of a KA from an SCC may be difficult and unreliable, although immunochemical staining for cellular protein Ki-67 may help to do this (4).
- KAs have a greater tendency than SCCs to display fibrosis and intraepidermal abscesses of neutrophils and eosinophils.
- Regressing KA shows flattening and fibrosis at base of lesion.

TREATMENT
- Treatment of choice is an excisional procedure plus electrodesiccation and curettage (ED&C); however, there are several treatment options available (2)[C].
- For aggressive tumors (>2 cm) or lesions in cosmetically sensitive areas (face, digits, genitalia) that require tissue sparing, consider Mohs micrographic surgery.
  - Mohs micrographic surgery is the treatment of choice in cases with perineural or perivascular invasion.
- Small lesions (<2 cm) of the extremities may undergo ED&C.
- Immunocompromised patients should receive immediate surgical treatment.

MEDICATION
- Nonsurgical management is a viable and relatively cost-effective option in select cases not amenable to surgery due to lesion number, size, or location; may also consider for patients with multiple comorbidities who are unwilling or unable to undergo surgery
- Evidence for the following treatments is based on case reports and retrospective reviews:
  - Intralesional methotrexate 12.5 to 25.0 mg in 0.5 mL normal saline q2–3wk for 1 to 4 treatment sessions (5)[B]
    - Monitor for pancytopenia with complete blood count (5)[C].
  - 5% imiquimod cream 3 times per week for 11 to 13 weeks (5)[B]
  - Topical 5% 5-fluorouracil cream daily, 61–92% cure rate (5)[B]
  - Intralesional 5-fluorouracil of 50 mg/mL on a weekly basis for 3 to 8 treatment sessions—98% cure rate (5)[B]
  - Intralesional IFN α-2a or β-2b (83%, 100% cure rate, respectively) (5)[B]
  - Intralesional bleomycin—100% cure rate (5)[B]
  - Isotretinoin oral 0.5 to 1 mg/kg/day

ISSUES FOR REFERRAL
Dermatology referral if lesions are >2 cm, numerous, mucosal, or subungual

ADDITIONAL THERAPIES
- Photodynamic therapy with methyl aminolevulinic acid and red light; successful case reports (1)[B] but also reported aggravation following treatment
- Cryotherapy (1)
- Argon or YAG lasers
- Radiotherapy, primary or adjuvant: KAs may regress with low doses of radiation but may require doses up to 25 to 50 Gy in low-dose (5 to 10 Gy) fractions for possible SCC (1)[B].
- Erlotinib (EGFR inhibitor) 150 mg/day for 21 days, single case report (1)[B]

SURGERY/OTHER PROCEDURES
Excisional and office-based procedures as mentioned earlier

ONGOING CARE

FOLLOW-UP RECOMMENDATIONS
After the surgical site has healed or if the lesion has resolved, patient should be seen every 6 months due to increased risk of developing new lesions or skin cancers; monitor annually at minimum going forward (3)[C].

Patient Monitoring
- Skin self-exams should be routinely performed with detailed instructions (see "Additional Reading").
- If multiple KAs are present in patient or family members, evaluate for Muir-Torre syndrome and obtain a colonoscopy beginning at aged 25 years, as well as testing for genitourinary cancer (3)[C].

PATIENT EDUCATION
- Sun protection measures: sun block with SPF >30, wide-brimmed hats, long sleeves, dark clothing, avoiding indoor tanning
- Arc welding may produce harmful UV radiation, and skin should not be exposed.
- Tar, pitch, and smoking should be avoided.

PROGNOSIS
- Atrophic scarring and hypopigmentation can occur with self-resolution but may be significantly reduced by intervention.
- 52 of 445 cases (12%) spontaneously regressed without treatment and none of these recurred (2).
- 393 (88%) regressed following medical or excisional treatment (2).
- 445 cases are reported with no metastases or deaths attributable to the KA (2).
- 4–8% recurrence
- Mucosal and subungual lesions do not regress; must undergo treatment

REFERENCES
1. Kwiek B, Schwartz RA. Keratoacanthoma (KA): an update and review. *J Am Acad Dermatol.* 2016;74(6):1220–1233.
2. Savage JA, Maize JC Sr. Keratoacanthoma clinical behavior: a systematic review. *Am J Dermatopathol.* 2014;36(5):422–429.
3. Cavicchini S, Tourlaki A, Lunardon L, et al. Amelanotic melanoma mimicking keratoacanthoma: the diagnostic role of dermoscopy. *Int J Dermatol.* 2013;52(8):1023–1024.
4. Scola N, Segert HM, Stücker M, et al. Ki-67 may be useful in differentiating between keratoacanthoma and cutaneous squamous cell carcinoma. *Clin Exp Dermatol.* 2014;39(2):216–218.
5. Chitwood K, Etzkorn J, Cohen G. Topical and intralesional treatment of nonmelanoma skin cancer: efficacy and cost comparisons. *Dermatol Surg.* 2013;39(9):1306–1316.

ADDITIONAL READING
- The American Academy of Dermatology: https://www.aad.org/public/diseases/skin-cancer/types/common
- The Skin Cancer Foundation: http://www.skincancer.org/

SEE ALSO

Squamous Cell Carcinoma, Cutaneous

CODES

ICD10
- D23.9 Other benign neoplasm of skin, unspecified
- D48.5 Neoplasm of uncertain behavior of skin
- L85.8 Other specified epidermal thickening

CLINICAL PEARLS
- Suspect KA with a solitary, dome-shaped, erythematous or flesh-colored papule or nodule with a central keratinous plug.
- If KA is in the differential diagnosis, elicit time frame of onset during patient encounter; rapid onset supports diagnosis.
- Due to the broad differential diagnosis of a suspected KA and unreliable clinical differentiation between these, strongly consider surgical excision as first-line diagnostic test and therapy.
- Medical and radiation therapies are reasonable and effective options available for patients who are not surgical candidates or for lesions that are not amenable for surgery.

K

KERATOSIS, ACTINIC

Zoltan Trizna, MD, PhD

 BASICS

DESCRIPTION

- Common, usually multiple, premalignant lesions of sun-exposed areas of the skin. Many resolve spontaneously, and a small proportion progresses to squamous cell carcinoma (SCC).
- Common consequence of excessive cumulative ultraviolet (UV) light exposure
- Synonym(s): solar keratosis

Geriatric Considerations
Frequent problem

Pediatric Considerations
Rare (if child, look for freckling and other stigmata of xeroderma pigmentosum)

EPIDEMIOLOGY

Incidence
- Rates vary with age group and exposure to sun.
- Predominant age: ≥40 years; progressively increases with age
- Predominant sex: male > female
- Common in those with blonde and red hair; rare in darker skin types

Prevalence
- Age-adjusted prevalence rate for actinic keratoses (AKs) in U.S. Caucasians is 6.5%.
- For 65- to 74-year-old males with high sun exposure: ~55%; low sun exposure: ~18%

ETIOLOGY AND PATHOPHYSIOLOGY
- The epidermal lesions are characterized by atypical keratinocytes at the basal layer with occasional extension upward. Mitoses are present. The histo-pathologic features resemble those of SCC in situ or SCC, and the distinction depends on the extent of epidermal involvement.
- Cumulative UV exposure

Genetics
The p53 chromosomal mutation has been shown consistently in both AKs and SCCs. Many new genes have been shown recently to have similar expression profiles in AKs and SCCs.

RISK FACTORS
- Exposure to UV light (especially long-term and/or repeated exposure due to outdoor occupation or recreational activities, indoor or outdoor tanning)
- Skin type: burns easily, does not tan
- Immunosuppression, especially organ transplantation

GENERAL PREVENTION
Sun avoidance and protective techniques are helpful.

COMMONLY ASSOCIATED CONDITIONS
- SCC
- Other features of chronic solar damage: lentigines, elastosis, and telangiectasias

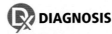 **DIAGNOSIS**

HISTORY
- The lesions are frequently asymptomatic; symptoms may include pruritus, burning, and mild hyperesthesia.
- Lesions may enlarge, thicken, or become more scaly. They also may regress or remain unchanged.
- Most lesions occur on the sun-exposed areas (head and neck, hands, forearms).

PHYSICAL EXAM
- Usually small (<1 cm), often multiple red, pink, or brown macules, papules, or plaques that are rough to palpation, sometimes more easily felt than seen.
- Yellow or brown adherent scale is often present on top of the lesion.
- Several clinical variants exist.
  - Atrophic: dry, scaly macules with indistinct borders and an erythematous base
  - Hypertrophic: Overlying hyperkeratosis (in an extreme form, cutaneous horn) may be impossible to differentiate from SCC clinically.
  - Pigmented: smooth tan/brown plaque, spreading centrifugally
  - Bowenoid: red scaly plaques with distinct borders
  - Actinic cheilitis: inflammatory lesion involving usually the lower lip

DIFFERENTIAL DIAGNOSIS
- SCC (hypertrophic type)
- Keratoacanthoma
- Bowen disease
- Basal cell carcinoma
- Verruca vulgaris
- Less likely: verrucous nevi, warty dyskeratoma, lichenoid keratoses, seborrheic keratoses, poro-keratoses, seborrheic dermatitis or psoriasis (near hairline), lentigo maligna, solar lentigo, discoid lupus erythematosus

DIAGNOSTIC TESTS & INTERPRETATION

Diagnostic Procedures/Other
- The diagnosis is usually made clinically, except where there is a suspicion of carcinoma.
- Skin biopsy is especially recommended if large, ulcerated, indurated, or bleeding, or if the lesions are nonresponsive to treatment.

Test Interpretation
- Dysplastic keratinocytes in lower levels of epidermis with a dermal lymphocytic infiltrate
- Neoplastic cells, mostly found in the lower epidermal layers, are cytologically identical to those of SCCs.
- If neoplastic cells extend throughout entire epider-mis or into the dermis, the lesions will qualify as an SCC in situ or invasive SCC, respectively.
- Malignant cells are sparse except for the bowenoid variety.
- Hypertrophic, atrophic, bowenoid, acantholytic, and pigmented varieties show the corresponding epidermal findings.

 TREATMENT

- First-line treatment is cryotherapy (technically, this is considered surgery, especially by insurance companies) (1). Medical therapy is usually reserved for multiple or extensive AKs ("field therapy").
- Cryotherapy combined with a topical approach resulted in significantly higher complete clearance rates than monotherapy (2)[A].
- A variety of topical therapies and cryosurgery are associated with long-term cure (3)[A].

GENERAL MEASURES
- Sun-protective techniques
- Sunscreens and physical sun protection recommended

MEDICATION

First Line
- Topical treatments target both visible and subclinical lesions.
- With the exception of generic 5-fluorouracil, medica-tion cost is high ($600 to $1,200 per course).

- Topical fluorouracil (Efudex, Carac, Fluoroplex cream, Fluoroplex solution)
  - Every day—BID for 3 to 6 weeks, depending on the brand, concentration, and formulation
  - Can be very irritating
  - Likely the most effective of the topical treatments listed in this section (2)[A],(4)[A]
- Topical imiquimod (Aldara) 5% cream
  - Apply 2 days per week at HS for up to 16 weeks to an area not larger than the forehead or one cheek.
  - Can be irritating
- Topical imiquimod (Zyclara) 3.75% cream
  - Apply once a day for 2 weeks, followed by no treatment for the next 2 weeks, and then apply once a day for another 2 weeks
  - Can be irritating
- Diclofenac (Solaraze) 3% gel
  - Apply BID for 60 to 90 days
  - The least irritating of the topical AK treatments therefore patients tend to be more compliant with it

Second Line
- Topical tretinoin (Retin-A) or tazarotene (Tazorac): may be used to enhance the efficacy of topical fluorouracil
- Systemic retinoids: used infrequently
- Delta aminolevulinate and methyl aminolevulinate combined with laser (photodynamic therapy) (see below)

ADDITIONAL THERAPIES
Close monitoring with no treatment is an appropriate option for mild lesions.

SURGERY/OTHER PROCEDURES
- Cryosurgery ("freezing," liquid nitrogen)
  - Most common method for treating AK
  - Cure rate: 75–98.8%
  - May cause atrophy and hypopigmentation
  - May be superior to photodynamic therapy for thicker lesions
- Photodynamic therapy with a photosensitizer (e.g., aminolevulinic acid) and "blue light"
  - May clear >90% of AKs
  - Less scarring than cryotherapy
  - May be superior to cryotherapy, especially in the case of more extensive skin involvement

- Curettage and electrocautery (electrodesiccation and curettage [ED&C]; "scraping and burning")
- Medium-depth peels, especially for the treatment of extensive areas
- CO_2 laser therapy
- Dermabrasion
- Surgical excision (excisional biopsy)

 ONGOING CARE

FOLLOW-UP RECOMMENDATIONS
Patient Monitoring
Depends on associated malignancy and frequency with which new AKs appear

PATIENT EDUCATION
- Teach sun-protective techniques.
  - Limit outdoor activities between 10 AM and 4 PM.
  - Wear protective clothing and wide-brimmed hat.
  - Proper use (including reapplication) of sunscreens with SPF >30, preferably a preparation with broad-spectrum (UV-A and UV-B) protection
- Teach self-examination of skin (melanoma, squamous cell, basal cell).
- Patient education materials
  - http://dermnetnz.org/lesions/solar-keratoses.html

PROGNOSIS
Very good; a significant proportion of the lesions may resolve spontaneously (5), with regression rates of 20–30% per lesion per year.

COMPLICATIONS
- AKs are premalignant lesions that may progress to SCCs. The rate of malignant transformation is unclear; the reported percentages vary but range from 0.1% to a few percent per year per lesion.
- Patients with AKs are at increased risk for other cutaneous malignancies.
- Approximately 60% of SCCs arise from an AK precursor.

REFERENCES
1. Helfand M, Gorman AK, Mahon S, et al. *Actinic Keratoses: Final Report*. Portland, OR: Oregon Health & Science University; 2001.
2. Heppt MV, Steeb T, Ruzicka T, et al. Cryosurgery combined with topical interventions for actinic keratosis: a systematic review and meta-analysis. *Br J Dermatol*. 2019;180(4):740–748.
3. Steeb T, Wessely A, Petzold A, et al. Evaluation of long-term clearance rates of interventions for actinic keratosis: a systematic review and network meta-analysis. *JAMA Dermatol*. 2021;157(9):1066–1077.
4. Jansen MHE, Kessels JPHM, Nelemans PJ, et al. Randomized trial of four treatment approaches for actinic keratosis. *N Engl J Med*. 2019;380(10):935–946.
5. Criscione VD, Weinstock MA, Naylor MF, et al; for Department of Veterans Affairs Topical Tretinoin Chemoprevention Trial Group. Actinic keratoses: natural history and risk of malignant transformation in the Veterans Affairs Topical Tretinoin Chemoprevention Trial. *Cancer*. 2009;115(11):2523–2530.

 CODES

ICD10
L57.0 Actinic keratosis

CLINICAL PEARLS
- AKs are premalignant lesions, although most will not progress to SCC and many will regress with time.
- Often more easily felt than seen
- Therapy-resistant lesions should be biopsied, especially on the face.

KERATOSIS, SEBORRHEIC
Michael T. Partin, MD • Karl T. Clebak, MD, MHA, FAAFP

BASICS

DESCRIPTION
- Common benign tumor of the epidermis formed from proliferation of keratinocytes
- Frequently appears in multiples on the head, neck, and trunk (sparing the palms and soles) of older individuals but may occur on any hair-bearing area of the body
- Typically presents as multiple, well-circumscribed, yellow to brown raised lesions that feel greasy, velvety, or warty; usually described as having a "stuck-on" appearance
- Clinical variants include the following:
  – Common seborrheic keratosis
  – Dermatosis papulosa nigra
  – Stucco keratosis
  – Flat seborrheic keratosis
  – Pedunculated seborrheic keratosis
- Synonym(s): SK, verruca seborrhoica; seborrheic wart; senile wart; basal cell papilloma; verruca senilis; benign acanthokeratoma; barnacles of aging

EPIDEMIOLOGY
Incidence
- Predominant age: appear most commonly in those aged 31 to 50 years, and incidence increases with age, peaking at age 60 years
- Predominant sex: slightly more common and more extensive involvement in males
- Most common among Caucasians, except for the dermatosis papulosa nigra variant, which usually presents in darker skinned individuals

Prevalence
- 69–100% in patients >50 years of age
- The prevalence rate increases with advancing age.

ETIOLOGY AND PATHOPHYSIOLOGY
- Etiology remains largely unclear with ultraviolet (UV) light and genetics thought to be involved.
- The role of human papillomavirus is uncertain.

Genetics
An autosomal dominant inheritance pattern is suggested.

RISK FACTORS
- Advanced age
- Exposure to UV light and genetic predisposition are the possible factors.

GENERAL PREVENTION
Sun protection methods may help prevent seborrheic keratoses from developing.

COMMONLY ASSOCIATED CONDITIONS
- Sign of Leser-Trélat: a paraneoplastic syndrome characterized by a rapid outbreak of multiple seborrheic keratoses often associated with an internal malignancy, most commonly adenocarcinoma; seborrheic keratosis may resolve with treatment of the malignancy and reappear with neoplasm recurrence.
- Documentation of other cutaneous lesions, such as basal cell carcinoma, malignant melanoma, or squamous cell carcinoma, growing adjacent to or within a seborrheic keratosis, has been reported. The exact relationship between lesions is unclear.

DIAGNOSIS

HISTORY
Generally asymptomatic, but trauma or irritation of the lesion may result in pruritus, erythema, bleeding, pain, and/or crusting.

PHYSICAL EXAM
- Typically begin as oval- or round-shaped, flat, dull, sharply demarcated patches
- As they mature, may develop into thicker, elevated, uneven, verrucous-like papules, plaques, or peduncles with a waxy or velvety surface and appear "stuck on" to the skin
- Commonly appear on sun-exposed areas of the body, predominately the head, neck, or trunk but may appear on any hair-bearing skin
- Surface tends to crumble when scratched
- Vary in color (black, brown, tan, gray to white, or skin-colored) as well as size, ranging from several millimeters to several centimeters, but the average diameter is 0.5 to 1.0 cm
- Usually occur as multiples; patients having >100 is not uncommon.
- If irritated, may be bleeding, inflamed, painful, pruritic, or crusted
- Common clinical variants include:
  – Common seborrheic keratoses: on hair-bearing skin, usually on the face, neck, and trunk; verrucous-like, waxy, or velvety lesions that appear "stuck on" to the skin
  – Dermatosis papulosa nigra: small black papules that usually appear on the face, neck, chest, and upper back; symmetric distribution most common in darker skinned individuals, more common in females; most have a positive family history
  – Stucco keratoses: small gray-white, rough, verrucous papules; usually occur in large numbers on the lower extremities or forearms; more common in men
  – Flat seborrheic keratoses: oval-shaped, tan to brown patches or macules on face, chest, and upper extremities; increases with age
  – Pedunculated seborrheic keratoses: Hyperpigmented peduncles appear on areas of friction (neck, axilla).

DIFFERENTIAL DIAGNOSIS
Consider the following diagnoses if the seborrheic keratosis is:
- Pigmented
  – Malignant melanoma
  – Melanocytic nevus
  – Angiokeratoma
  – Pigmented basal cell carcinoma
- Lightly pigmented
  – Basal cell carcinoma
  – Bowen disease
  – Condyloma acuminatum
  – Fibroma
  – Verruca vulgaris
  – Eccrine poroma
  – Invasive squamous cell carcinoma
  – Acrochordon (skin tag)
  – Acrokeratosis verruciformis of Hopf
  – Follicular infundibulum tumor
- Flat
  – Solar lentigo
  – Verrucae planae juveniles
- Hyperkeratotic
  – Actinic keratosis

DIAGNOSTIC TESTS & INTERPRETATION
Initial Tests (lab, imaging)
Testing is generally not indicated unless diagnosis is unclear or malignancy is suspected.

Diagnostic Procedures/Other
- Diagnosis is generally made clinically.
- Biopsy and histologic exam should be performed if the seborrheic keratosis is atypical or has recently been inflamed or changed in appearance.
- Dermoscopy
  – Can assist in confirmation if diagnosis is uncertain
    ○ Common findings are pigment networks, pigmented globules, streaks, homogenous blue patterns, milia-like cysts, blotches, blue-whitish veils, and hairpin vessels (1).

Test Interpretation
Several histologic variants exist and can include the following:
- Acanthosis and papillomatosis due to basaloid cell proliferation
- "Squamous eddies" or squamous epithelial cell clusters
- Hyperpigmentation
- Hyperkeratosis
- Horn cysts
- Pseudocysts

TREATMENT

- Treatment is typically performed for cosmetic concerns but is usually not required.
- Removal of seborrheic keratoses may be indicated if:
  - They are aesthetically displeasing or undesirable (common patient concern, although removal for this reason is not always covered by insurance).
  - They are symptomatic (e.g., easily irritated, gets caught on clothing or jewelry).
  - There is a concern for their association with malignancy.

MEDICATION
- Generally, medical therapies are not considered first line, with surgical approaches being favored.
- The FDA recently approved HP40 (Eskata) as the first topical treatment for raised seborrheic keratosis, consisting of a 40% hydrogen peroxide solution. The treatment may require two office visits for application, may be less effective than other treatment methods, and has not shown better cosmetic results than other treatments.
- Some reports exist regarding successful treatment of seborrheic keratoses using tazarotene, diclofenac gel, imiquimod, calcitriol, and dobesilate.
- Topical vitamin D analogs do not seem to be effective.

ISSUES FOR REFERRAL
- New seborrheic keratoses that appear abruptly, particularly if many occur within a short time frame concerning for Leser-Trélat sign
- A seborrheic keratosis becomes inflamed or changes in appearance.

SURGERY/OTHER PROCEDURES
- A surgical approach to treatment is generally preferred with the selected therapy depending on physician's preference and availability of the treatment.
- The following procedures can be used in practice:
  - Cryotherapy (liquid nitrogen)
    - Spray flat lesions for 5 to 10 seconds; may require more time or additional treatments if the seborrheic keratosis is thicker
    - Possible complications include scarring, hypopigmentation, and recurrence.
  - Curettage
    - Curette (metal hand tool with small scoop at the tip) is used to scrape off the lesion.
    - Requires local anesthesia

- Electrodessication
  - Tool with needle-like metal tip that uses electric current to destroy affected tissue
  - Requires local anesthesia
- Shave excision
  - Scalpel or flexible razor blade is used to remove lesion.
  - Requires local anesthesia
- Laser
  - Intense beams of light are used to burn and vaporize the lesion.
  - Requires local anesthesia
- Chemical peel
  - An application of chemical solution (e.g., Trichloroacetic acid) is used to remove the top layer of skin.
- In a small study ($n = 25$), a majority of patients preferred cryotherapy over curettage due to decreased wound care after the procedure with no statistically significant differences in patient's ratings of cosmetic appearance between curettage and cryotherapy (2)[B].

 ONGOING CARE

FOLLOW-UP RECOMMENDATIONS
Patient Monitoring
After initial diagnosis, follow-up is not usually required unless
- Inflammation or irritation develops.
- There is a change in appearance.
- New seborrheic keratoses suddenly appear.

PATIENT EDUCATION
- Sun-protective methods may help reduce seborrheic keratosis development.
- Patient education materials
  - https://www.aad.org/public/diseases/bumps-and-growths/seborrheic-keratoses
  - https://www.cdc.gov/cancer/skin/basic_info/prevention.htm

PROGNOSIS
- Seborrheic keratoses generally do not become malignant.
- Sign of Leser-Trélat usually represents a poor prognosis.

COMPLICATIONS
- Irritation and inflammation due to mechanical irritation (e.g., from clothing, jewelry)
- Possible complications of surgical treatment include hypopigmentation, hyperpigmentation, scarring, incomplete removal, and recurrence.
- Misdiagnosis (rare)

REFERENCES
1. Marghoob AA, Usatine RP, Jaimes N. Dermoscopy for the family physician. *Am Fam Physician*. 2013;88(7):441–450.
2. Wood LD, Stucki JK, Hollenbeak CS, et al. Effectiveness of cryosurgery vs curettage in the treatment of seborrheic keratoses. *JAMA Dermatol*. 2013;149(1):108–109.

ADDITIONAL READING
- Higgins JC, Maher MH, Douglas MS. Diagnosing common benign skin tumors. *Am Fam Physician*. 2015;92(7):601–607.
- Krupashankar DS; for IADVL Dermatosurgery Task Force. Standard guidelines of care: CO_2 laser for removal of benign skin lesions and resurfacing. *Indian J Dermatol Venereol Leprol*. 2008; 74(Suppl):S61–S67.

CODES

ICD10
- L82.1 Other seborrheic keratosis
- L82.0 Inflamed seborrheic keratosis

CLINICAL PEARLS
- Seborrheic keratoses are one of the most common benign tumors of the epidermis, and frequency increases with age.
- Although seborrheic keratoses do not need to be removed, there are many options for doing so if patients request this (with surgical methods generally being preferred).
- Underlying internal malignancy should be considered if large numbers of seborrheic keratoses appear suddenly.

K

KNEE PAIN

Lee A. Mancini, MD, CSCS*D, CSN • Emily J. Eshleman, DO, MS • Michael J. Maddaleni, MD

BASICS

DESCRIPTION
A common outpatient complaint with a broad differential
- Knee pain may be acute, chronic, or an acute exacerbation of a chronic condition.
- Trauma, overuse, and degenerative change are the frequent causes.
- A detailed history, including patient's age, pain onset and location, mechanism of injury, and associated symptoms, can help narrow the differential diagnosis.
- A thorough and focused examination of the knee (as well as the back, hips, and ankles) helps to establish the correct diagnosis and appropriate treatment.

EPIDEMIOLOGY
Incidence
- Knee complaints account for 12.5 million primary care visits annually.
- The incidence of knee osteoarthritis (OA) is 240 cases per 100,000 person-years.

Prevalence
- The knee is a common site of lower extremity injury.
  - Patellar tendinopathy and patellofemoral syndrome are the most common causes of knee pain in runners.
- OA of the hip/knee is the 11th cause of global disability and the 38th most common cause of disability-adjusted life years (DALYs).

ETIOLOGY AND PATHOPHYSIOLOGY
- Trauma (ligament or meniscal injury, fracture, dislocation)
- Overuse (tendinopathy, patellofemoral syndrome, bursitis, apophysitis)
- Age (arthritis, degenerative conditions in older patients; apophysitis in younger patients)
- Rheumatologic (rheumatoid arthritis [RA], systemic lupus erythematosus [SLE])
- Crystal arthropathies (gout, pseudogout)
- Infectious (bacterial, postviral, Lyme disease)
- Referred pain (hip, back)
- Vascular (popliteal artery aneurysm, deep vein thrombosis)
- Others (tumor, cyst, plica)

RISK FACTORS
- Obesity
- Malalignment
- Poor flexibility, muscle imbalance, or weakness
- Rapid increases in training frequency and intensity
- Improper footwear, training surfaces, technique
- Activities that involve cutting, jumping, pivoting, deceleration, kneeling
- Previous injuries

GENERAL PREVENTION
- Maintain body mass index <25 kg/m^2.
- Proper exercise technique, volume, and equipment; avoid overtraining.
- Correct postural strength and flexibility imbalances.

COMMONLY ASSOCIATED CONDITIONS
- Fracture, contusion
- Effusion, hemarthrosis
- Patellar dislocation/subluxation
- Meniscal or ligamentous injury
- Tendinopathy, bursitis
- Osteochondral injury
- OA, septic arthritis
- Muscle strain

DIAGNOSIS

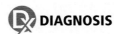

HISTORY
- Pain location, quality, and mechanism of injury guide diagnostic reasoning (also see "Differential Diagnosis"):
  - Diffuse pain: OA, patellofemoral pain syndrome, chondromalacia
  - Pain ascending/descending stairs: meniscal injury, patellofemoral pain syndrome
  - Pain with prolonged sitting, standing from sitting: patellofemoral pain syndrome
  - Mechanical symptoms (locking): meniscal injury
- Mechanism of injury:
  - Hyperextension, deceleration, cutting: anterior cruciate ligament (ACL) injury
  - Hyperflexion, fall on flexed knee, "dashboard injury": posterior cruciate ligament (PCL) injury
  - Lateral force (valgus load): medial collateral injury
  - Twisting on planted foot: meniscal injury
- Effusion:
  - Rapid onset (2 hours): ACL tear, patellar sub-luxation/dislocation, large meniscal tear, tibial plateau fracture; hemarthrosis is common.
  - Slower onset (24 to 36 hours), smaller: meniscal injury, ligament sprain, arthritis
  - Swelling behind the knee: popliteal (Baker) cyst

PHYSICAL EXAM
- Observe gait (antalgia); patellar tracking
- Inspect for malalignment, atrophy, swelling, ecchymosis, or erythema.
- Palpate for effusion, warmth, and tenderness.
- Evaluate active and passive range of motion (ROM) and flexibility of quadriceps and hamstrings.
- Evaluate strength and muscle tone.
- Note joint instability, locking, and catching.
- Evaluate hip ROM, strength, and stability.
- Special tests:
  - Patellar apprehension test: patellar instability; patellar grind test: patellofemoral pain or OA (1)
  - Lachman test (more sensitive and specific), pivot shift, anterior drawer, lever sign: ACL integrity

- Posterior drawer, posterior sag sign: PCL integrity
- Valgus/varus stress test: medial/lateral collateral ligament (MCL/LCL) integrity
- McMurray test, Apley grind test, Thessaly test: meniscal injury
- Ober test: iliotibial band (ITB) tightness
- Dial test: positive with posterolateral corner laxity
- Patellar tilt test and squatting may help suggest patellofemoral pain syndrome.
- Patella facet tenderness suggests OA or patellofemoral pain syndrome (1).

DIFFERENTIAL DIAGNOSIS
- Acute onset: fracture, contusion, cruciate or collateral ligament tear, meniscal tear, patellar dislocation/subluxation; if systemic symptoms: septic arthritis, gout, pseudogout, Lyme disease, osteomyelitis
- Insidious onset: patellofemoral pain syndrome/chondromalacia, ITB syndrome, OA, RA, bursitis, tumor, tendinopathy, loose body, bipartite patella, degenerative meniscal tear
- Anterior pain: patellofemoral pain syndrome, patellar injury, patellar tendinopathy, pre- or suprapatellar bursitis, tibial apophysitis, fat pad impingement, quadriceps tendinopathy, OA (1)
- Posterior pain: PCL injury, posterior horn meniscal injury, popliteal cyst or aneurysm, hamstring or gastrocnemius injury, deep venous thrombosis (DVT)
- Medial pain: MCL injury, medial meniscal injury, pes anserine bursitis, medial plica syndrome, OA
- Lateral pain: LCL injury, lateral meniscal injury, ITB syndrome, OA

DIAGNOSTIC TESTS & INTERPRETATION
Initial Tests (lab, imaging)
- Suspected septic joint, gout, pseudogout:
  - Arthrocentesis with cell count, Gram stain, culture, synovial fluid analysis, erythrocyte sedimentation rate (ESR), CRP
- Suspected RA:
  - CBC, ESR, rheumatoid factor
- Consider Lyme titer.
- Radiographs to rule out fracture in patients with acute knee trauma (Ottawa Rules):
  - Age >55 years *or*
  - Tenderness at the patella or fibular head *or*
  - Inability to bear weight four steps *or*
  - Inability to flex knee to 90 degrees
- Radiographs help diagnose OA, osteochondral lesions, patellofemoral pain syndrome:
  - Weight-bearing, upright anteroposterior, lateral, merchant/sunrise, notch/tunnel views

Follow-Up Tests & Special Considerations
- MRI is "gold standard" for soft tissue imaging.
- Ultrasound may help diagnose tendinopathy, effusions, ligamentous tears, amongst other diagnostic findings.
- CT can further elucidate fracture.

Diagnostic Procedures/Other
Arthroscopy may be beneficial in the diagnosis of certain conditions, including meniscus and ligament injuries.

Geriatric Considerations
OA, degenerative meniscal tears, and gout are more common in middle-aged and elderly populations.

Pediatric Considerations
- 3 million pediatric sports injuries occur annually.
- Look for physeal/apophyseal and joint surface injuries in skeletally immature:
  – Acute: patellar subluxation, avulsion fractures, ACL tear
  – Overuse: patellofemoral pain syndrome, apophysitis, osteochondritis dissecans, patellar tendonitis, stress fracture
  – Others: neoplasm, juvenile RA, infection, referred pain from slipped capital femoral epiphysis

 TREATMENT

GENERAL MEASURES
Acute injury: PRICEMM therapy (**p**rotection, **r**elative rest, **i**ce, **c**ompression, **e**levation, **m**edications, **m**odalities)

MEDICATION
First Line
- Oral medications:
  – Acetaminophen: up to 3 g/day; safe and effective in OA
  – Nonsteroidal anti-inflammatory drugs (NSAIDs):
    ○ Ibuprofen: 200 to 800 mg TID
    ○ Naproxen: 250 to 500 mg BID
      ▪ Useful for acute sprains, strains
      ▪ Useful for short-term pain reduction in OA. Long-term use is not recommended due to side effects.
      ▪ Not recommended for fracture, stress fracture, chronic muscle injury; may be associated with delayed healing; low dose and brief course only if necessary
  – Celecoxib: 200 mg QD may be effective in OA with less GI side effects than NSAIDs (2)[A].
- Topical medications:
  – Topical NSAIDs provide pain relief in OA and may be more tolerable than oral medications (3)[A].
  – Topical capsaicin may be an adjuvant for pain management in OA.
- Injections:
  – Intra-articular corticosteroid injection will likely provide short-term benefit in knee OA stage 2 or 3.
  – Viscosupplementation may reduce pain and improve function in patients with OA. Peak effectiveness is 4 to 6 weeks from 3rd injection.
  – Platelet-rich plasma (PRP) and prolotherapy injections can provide long-term relief.
  – Stem cell therapy with insufficient data

Second Line
Tramadol/opioids: not recommended; can be used with acute injuries for severe pain

ISSUES FOR REFERRAL
- Acute trauma, young athletic patient
- Joint instability
- Lack of improvement with conservative measures
- Salter-Harris physeal fractures (pediatrics)

ADDITIONAL THERAPIES
- Physical therapy is recommended as initial treatment for patellofemoral pain and tendinopathies.
- Muscle strengthening improves outcome in OA.
- Foot orthoses, taping, acupuncture
- May need bracing for stability

SURGERY/OTHER PROCEDURES
- Surgery may be indicated for certain injuries (e.g., ACL tear in competitive athletes or grade IV OA).
- Chronic conditions refractory to conservative therapy may require surgical intervention.

COMPLEMENTARY & ALTERNATIVE MEDICINE
May reduce pain and improve function in early OA:
- Glucosamine sulfate (500 mg TID)
- Chondroitin (400 mg TID)
- Turmeric or curcumin 1,000 mg/day
- Collagen hydrolysates 10 g daily
- S-adenosyl-l-methionine (SAMe), ginger extract, methylsulfonylmethane: less reliable improvement with inconsistent supporting evidence
- Acupuncture: need to do 4 weeks or 10 sessions

 ONGOING CARE

FOLLOW-UP RECOMMENDATIONS
- Activity modification in overuse conditions
- Rehabilitative exercise in OA:
  – Low-impact exercise: walking, swimming, cycling
  – Strength, ROM, and proprioception training

Patient Monitoring
- Rehabilitation after initial treatment of acute injury
- In chronic and overuse conditions, assess functional status, rehabilitation adherence, and pain control at follow-up visit.

DIET
Weight reduction by 10% improved function by 28%.

PATIENT EDUCATION
- Review activity modifications.
- Encourage active role in the rehabilitation process.
- Review medication risks and benefits.

PROGNOSIS
Varies with diagnosis, injury severity, chronicity of condition, patient motivation to participate in rehabilitation, and whether surgery is required

COMPLICATIONS
- Disability
- Arthritis
- Chronic joint instability
- Deconditioning

REFERENCES
1. Hong E, Kraft MC. Evaluating anterior knee pain. *Med Clin North Am*. 2014;98(4):697–717.
2. Bijlsma JWJ, Berenbaum F, Lafeber FPJG. Osteoarthritis: an update with relevance for clinical practice. *Lancet*. 2011;377(9783):2115–2126.
3. Zeng C, Wei J, Persson MSM, et al. Relative efficacy and safety of topical non-steroidal anti-inflammatory drugs for osteoarthritis: a systematic review and network meta-analysis of randomised controlled trials and observational studies. *Br J Sports Med*. 2018;52(10):642–650.

ADDITIONAL READING
Collins NJ, Bisset LM, Crossley KM, et al. Efficacy of nonsurgical interventions for anterior knee pain: systematic review and meta-analysis of randomized trials. *Sports Med*. 2012;42(1):31–49.

 SEE ALSO

Algorithms: Knee Pain; Popliteal Mass

 CODES

ICD10
- M25.569 Pain in unspecified knee
- M17.9 Osteoarthritis of knee, unspecified
- M76.50 Patellar tendinitis, unspecified knee

CLINICAL PEARLS
- A careful history (location/quality of pain and mechanism of injury) targets diagnosis for most causes of knee pain.
- Consider ligamentous injury, meniscal tear, and fracture for patients presenting with acute knee pain.
- Consider OA, patellofemoral pain syndrome, tendinopathy, bursitis, and stress fracture in patients presenting with more chronic symptoms.
- Consider physeal, apophyseal, or articular cartilage injury in young patients presenting with knee pain.
- The presence of an effusion in a patient <30 years of age indicates a significant injury, infection, or inflammatory diagnosis.
- Referred pain from the hip (slipped capital femoral epiphysis, Legg-Calvé-Perthes disease) can present as knee pain.

K

LABYRINTHITIS

Joseph Daniel Hogue, MD, MBA • Nabeel Ali, MD • Scott Rosen, MD

BASICS

DESCRIPTION
- The sudden onset of vertigo, accompanied by sensorineural hearing loss and tinnitus, lasting hours to days, and caused by acute inflammation or infection of the labyrinth of the inner ear
- Can be categorized as suppurative or serous/toxic labyrinthitis (1)
- Labyrinthitis is a clinical diagnosis in absence of neurologic deficits.
- Typically presents with a subjective sense of motion or room-spinning vertigo lasting for hours or days and often sudden unilateral sensorineural hearing loss
- Often associated with vestibular hypofunction of the involved ear; peripheral vertigo improves over time with central compensation. Hearing loss generally improves in the case of serous labyrinthitis but is permanent in the case of suppurative labyrinthitis.
- System(s) affected: nervous, special sensory (auditory and vestibular)

ALERT
- "Vertigo" and "dizziness" are commonly used terms. Clarify the symptoms by giving options of alternative descriptions such as light-headedness, disequilibrium, room-spinning vertigo, or imbalance.
- Hearing loss and duration of symptoms can help narrow the differential diagnosis in patients with vertigo.
- Vestibular neuritis/neuronitis occurs due to inflammation of the vestibular nerve causing vertigo lasting from hours to days without the auditory symptoms of labyrinthitis (2).

EPIDEMIOLOGY
- Most common in 30 to 50 years of age (3)
- 10% of all patients seen for dizziness, if vestibular neuritis is included (4)

Incidence
Estimated incidence of 3.5 per 100,000 if including vestibular neuritis (3)

ETIOLOGY AND PATHOPHYSIOLOGY
- Viral labyrinthitis is the most common etiology with acute inflammation and damage to the labyrinth, involving both the vestibular apparatus and cochlea.
- Common viral: *cytomegalovirus*, mumps, varicella zoster, rubeola, influenza, parainfluenza, herpes simplex, adenovirus, *coxsackievirus*, respiratory syncytial virus, HIV
- Bacterial invasion of the inner ear, either from a middle ear infection or meningitis, occurs in suppurative labyrinthitis (1).
- Common bacterial: *Streptococcus pneumoniae, Haemophilus influenzae, Moraxella catarrhalis, Neisseria meningitidis, Streptococcus* spp., *Staphylococcus* spp., *Borrelia burgdorferi*

RISK FACTORS
- Viral upper respiratory infection
- Otitis media
- Cholesteatoma
- Head trauma
- Meningitis

GENERAL PREVENTION
- Early treatment of acute otitis media to prevent complications
- Scheduled immunizations (to prevent common viral pathogens)
- Prevent maternal transmission of pathogens, including syphilis and HIV.

COMMONLY ASSOCIATED CONDITIONS
- Viral upper respiratory infection
- Otitis media, cholesteatoma
- Head injury

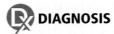

DIAGNOSIS

HISTORY
- Vertigo *AND* sensorineural hearing loss in one ear
- Vertigo is acute in onset and lasts hours to days.
- Nausea and vomiting are common.
- Fullness of affected ear
- Tinnitus of affected ear (roaring, ringing)
- Upper respiratory tract infection symptoms
- Otorrhea or otalgia (not common with viral causes)
- Severe headache, fever, and nuchal rigidity in the setting of meningitis

PHYSICAL EXAM
- Fast-beating nystagmus toward the affected ear during the acute phase and away from the affected ear during the convalescent phase, 48 to 72 hours later
- Symptoms abate with eyes open and visual fixation.
- Otologic exam may be unremarkable in the setting of viral labyrinthitis.
- Serous/purulent effusion may be present in the middle ear.
- Retraction of the tympanic membrane and keratinaceous debris may be present with cholesteatoma.

DIFFERENTIAL DIAGNOSIS
- Benign paroxysmal positional vertigo (BPPV) is the most common cause of vertigo. Unlike labyrinthitis, BPPV is episodic, with severe symptoms lasting <1 minute. BPPV is diagnosed using the Dix-Hallpike maneuver. Unlike labyrinthitis, it is not associated with hearing loss.
- Ménière disease is more episodic than labyrinthitis; it comes and goes, rather than remaining continuous, and is associated with the triad of episodic vertigo, tinnitus, and hearing loss.

- Vestibular migraine is the second most common cause of recurrent vertigo, lasting hours and usually with a history of migraine. Up to 10% of cases can occur without headaches.
- Autoimmune inner ear disease
- Cardiovascular accident (CVA)/brainstem infarct
- Cerebellopontine-angle tumors (e.g., vestibular schwannoma, acoustic neuroma)
- Temporal bone fracture
- Less common etiologies: parainfectious encephalomyelitis or cranial polyneuritis, Ramsay Hunt syndrome, HIV infection, syphilis, temporal lobe epilepsy, perilymphatic fistula, superior canal dehiscence, idiopathic sudden single-sided deafness, multiple sclerosis, vasculitis (cerebral or systemic)

DIAGNOSTIC TESTS & INTERPRETATION
- Routine lab studies are not helpful unless an autoimmune cause is suspected.
- CT of the temporal bone may be indicated in the setting of complicated otitis media or cholesteatoma.
- Consider lumbar puncture only if meningitis is suspected.
- Consider screening for syphilis or HIV when clinically indicated by risk factors or clinical history.
- Imaging is not required for the diagnosis of acute labyrinthitis.
- With acute sensorineural hearing loss or other associated neurologic symptoms, an MRI of the internal auditory canals and/or MRA of the brain and brainstem are recommended.

Initial Tests (lab, imaging)
- Labs and/or imaging is not recommended.
- Profound imbalance or associated focal neurologic signs are not typical and should prompt imaging.

Follow-Up Tests & Special Considerations
Labyrinthitis ossificans is fibrosis of the internal auditory canal following bacterial meningitis and is thought to occur due to a suppurative labyrinthitis. This can occur rapidly, especially after *S. pneumoniae* meningitis.

Diagnostic Procedures/Other
- Audiogram may show varying degrees of both sensorineural hearing loss and discrimination loss.
- Vestibular tests are not typically indicated in the acute setting. If vertigo and dizziness persist after expected resolution of symptoms, videonystagmography should be used.

Test Interpretation
Caloric testing may show relative weakness of the horizontal semicircular canal of the affected side. Sensitivity and specificity of this test are variable within literature.

TREATMENT

- Symptom management and reassurance in the acute phase
- Vestibular suppressants as needed (see "Medication") for severe acute attacks of vertigo only; patients should be advised *NOT* to use these medications as scheduled medications or for prophylaxis without symptoms because this can delay central compensation (2)[B].
- Sudden single-sided sensorineural hearing loss should be managed with high-dose steroids as soon as possible, ideally within 2 weeks. Steroids have not been found to definitively improve vestibular symptoms (5)[B].
- Vestibular rehabilitation is the mainstay of treatment for persistent vertigo and dizziness and has been shown to be safe and effective management for unilateral peripheral vestibular dysfunction (6)[A].
- Patients should begin exercises as soon as the acute phase resolves and movement is tolerable, generally within 2 to 3 days of onset (4).
- For suppurative labyrinthitis, appropriate antibiotics to eradicate infection. Surgical intervention may also be required with tympanostomy tubes or mastoidectomy, depending on the extent of middle ear involvement.

GENERAL MEASURES
Vestibular exercises for prolonged symptoms and unilateral vestibular loss have been shown to alleviate postural control.

MEDICATION
The use of the following drugs should be on a PRN basis. Benzodiazepines can also assist with the anxiety associated with vertigo. No patient should take vestibular suppressants as a chronic medication, because they can block central compensation.

- Vestibular suppressants
  - Lorazepam (Ativan): 0.5 to 2.0 mg SL/PO BID PRN or diazepam (Valium) 2 to 5 mg QID PO PRN
  - Meclizine (Antivert, Bonine, Zentrip [dissolvable]) 12.5 to 25.0 mg PO BID–TID PRN
  - Dimenhydrinate (Dramamine) 25 to 50 mg PO q4–6h PRN
- Antiemetics
  - Ondansetron (Zofran) 4 to 8 mg PO TID PRN or granisetron (Kytril) 1 mg PO TID PRN
  - Meclizine (Antivert, Bonine) 12.5 to 25.0 mg PO q4h PRN
  - Promethazine (Phenergan) 12.5 to 25.0 mg PO/PR QID PRN or prochlorperazine (Compazine) 25 mg PR BID PRN
  - Metoclopramide (Reglan) 10 mg PO TID PRN
- Antivirals
  - Acyclovir 800 mg PO 5 times per day for 7 days can be used in cases associated with herpes.
- Steroids
  - Prednisone 1 mg/kg/day up to a maximum of 60 mg/day for 1 week, followed by 1 week taper
  - Methylprednisolone initially 100 mg PO daily and then tapered to 10 mg PO daily over 3 weeks

- Dexamethasone 0.4 to 0.8 mL of 24 mg/mL strength given via transtympanic injection for three to four sessions; can be used for salvage therapy
- Given early in the setting of bacterial meningitis; may decrease the otologic sequelae, specifically labyrinthitis ossificans
- Used in treatment of labyrinthitis for associated sudden sensorineural hearing loss, ideally within the first 2 weeks

Geriatric Considerations
- Avoid excessive use of scopolamine, meclizine, and other vestibular suppressants following the initial event because this will delay central compensation.
- Benzodiazepines are the preferred vestibular suppressant treatment but do increase the risk of falls in older persons.

Pregnancy Considerations
Dimenhydrinate, diphenhydramine, ondansetron, granisetron, and metoclopramide are pregnancy Category B.

First Line
- Benzodiazepines, which are better vestibular suppressants, are preferred over antihistamine/anticholinergics such as meclizine. Sublingual benzodiazepines are very effective for vertigo and should be considered as first-line therapy.
- Urgent steroid treatment in acute setting

ISSUES FOR REFERRAL
- Consider neurology referral for suspected central causes.
- Consider otolaryngology/neurotology referral for progressive hearing loss and vertigo or in cases of suppurative labyrinthitis requiring surgical intervention.

ADMISSION, INPATIENT, AND NURSING CONSIDERATIONS
Patients with systemic infection or intractable nausea and vomiting may need to be hospitalized.

 ONGOING CARE

FOLLOW-UP RECOMMENDATIONS
Patient Monitoring
Follow hearing loss weekly with audiograms until hearing stabilizes. Acute vertiginous symptoms may last up to 6 weeks. Residual symptoms have been documented to last years.

DIET
Alcohol may exacerbate symptoms.

PATIENT EDUCATION
Opening the eyes with visual fixation should improve symptoms, whereas closing the eyes may make symptoms worse. Minimize rapid head movement until symptoms resolve. Avoid vestibular suppressants for long term because this can inhibit central compensation.

COMPLICATIONS
- Permanent hearing loss, more common with bacterial causes, and chronic impairment of balance
- If bacterial labyrinthitis is not treated sufficiently, there is a risk of developing into mastoiditis.

REFERENCES
1. Kaya S, Schachern PA, Tsuprun V, et al. Deterioration of vestibular cells in labyrinthitis. *Ann Otol Rhinol Laryngol*. 2017;126(2):89–95.
2. Sandhu JS, Rea PA. Clinical examination and management of the dizzy patient. *Br J Hosp Med (Lond)*. 2016;77(12):692–698.
3. Neuhauser HK, Lempert T. Vertigo: epidemiologic aspects. *Semin Neurol*. 2009;29(5):473–481.
4. Wipperman J. Dizziness and vertigo. *Prim Care*. 2014;41(1):115–131.
5. Yoo MH, Yang CJ, Kim SA, et al. Efficacy of steroid therapy based on symptomatic and functional improvement in patients with vestibular neuritis: a prospective randomized controlled trial. *Eur Arch Otorhinolaryngol*. 2017;274(6):2443–2451.
6. McDonnell MN, Hillier SL. Vestibular rehabilitation for unilateral peripheral vestibular dysfunction. *Cochrane Database Syst Rev*. 2015;(1):CD005397.

 SEE ALSO

Ménière Disease; Postconcussion Syndrome (Mild Traumatic Brain Injury); Tinnitus

 CODES

ICD10
- H83.02 Labyrinthitis, left ear
- H83.01 Labyrinthitis, right ear
- H83.09 Labyrinthitis, unspecified ear

CLINICAL PEARLS
- Episodic vertigo tends to be caused by BPPV or Ménière disease, whereas persistent vertigo with sensorineural hearing loss and tinnitus is more consistent with labyrinthitis.
- Ask patients to describe symptoms in their own words; alternative symptoms include light-headedness, vertigo, disequilibrium, or imbalance.
- Benzodiazepines are better vestibular suppressants and are preferred over antihistamine/anticholinergics such as meclizine. Vestibular suppressants should be used for short duration only because these will delay central compensation.
- Vestibular neuritis would be considered if there was no hearing involvement.

L

LACTOSE INTOLERANCE

Nihal K. Patel, MD

 BASICS

DESCRIPTION
- Lactose intolerance is a syndrome of abdominal pain, bloating, and flatulence after the ingestion of lactose.
- Lactose malabsorption results from a reduction in lactase activity in the brush border of the small intestinal mucosa.
- Lactase activity peaks at birth then decreases after the first few months of life, declining continuously throughout life. 75% of adults worldwide exhibit a decline in lactase activity after birth. *Only 50% of lactase activity is needed to digest lactose without causing symptoms of lactose intolerance.*
  – Congenital lactose intolerance: very rare
  – Primary lactose intolerance: common in adults who develop low lactase levels after childhood
  – Secondary lactose intolerance: inability to digest lactose caused by any condition injuring the intestinal mucosa (e.g., infectious enteritis, celiac disease, eosinophilic gastroenteritis, or inflammatory bowel disease) or a reduction of available mucosal surface (e.g., resection)
- Lactose malabsorption may be asymptomatic and is equally common in healthy patients and in those with functional bowel disorders.
- System(s) affected: endocrine/metabolic, gastrointestinal

Pediatric Considerations
- Primary lactose intolerance begins in late childhood.
- No consensus on whether young children (<5 years of age) should avoid lactose following diarrheal illness
- Lactose-free formulas are available.
- Exclude milk protein allergy.

EPIDEMIOLOGY
Incidence
- ≥50% of infants with acute or chronic diarrheal disease have lactose intolerance; particularly common with rotavirus infection
- Lactose intolerance is also common with giardiasis, ascariasis, irritable bowel syndrome (IBS), tropical and nontropical sprue, and AIDS malabsorption syndrome.

Prevalence
- In South America, Africa, and Asia, rates of lactose intolerance are >50%.
- In the United States, the prevalence is 15% among whites, 53% among Hispanics, and 80% among African Americans.
- In Europe, lactose intolerance varies from 15% in Scandinavian countries to 70% in Italy.
- Predominant age:
  – Primary: teenage and adult
  – Secondary: depends on underlying condition
- Predominant sex: male = female

ETIOLOGY AND PATHOPHYSIOLOGY
- Primary lactose intolerance: The normal decline in lactase activity in the intestinal mucosa is genetically determined and permanent after weaning from breast milk.
- Secondary lactose intolerance: associated with gastroenteritis in children; also associated with any gastrointestinal infection or inflammation of the small intestine with resultant lactose malabsorption in both adults and children

Genetics
- In whites, lactase deficiency is associated with a single nucleotide polymorphism (SNP) consisting of a nucleotide switch of T for C 13910 bp on chromosome 2. This results in variants of CC-13910 (lactase nonpersistence) *OR* CT-13910/TT-13910 (lactase persistence) (1). SNP (C/T-13910) is associated with lactase persistence in northern Europeans.
- Other SNPs (G/C-14010, T/G-13915, and C/G-13907) linked to lactase persistence in some of African descent.

RISK FACTORS
- Adult-onset lactase deficiency has wide geographic variation.
- Age:
  – Signs and symptoms usually do not become apparent until after age 6 to 7 years.
  – Symptoms may not be apparent until adulthood, depending on dietary lactose intake and rate of decline of intestinal lactase activity.
  – Lactase activity correlates with age, regardless of symptoms.

GENERAL PREVENTION
Lactose avoidance relieves symptoms. Patients can learn what level of lactose is tolerable in their diet.

COMMONLY ASSOCIATED CONDITIONS
- Tropical or nontropical sprue
- Giardiasis
- IBS or other functional bowel disorders
- Small intestinal bacterial overgrowth (SIBO)
- Celiac disease

🅡 DIAGNOSIS
- Lactose intolerance can be presumed in patients manifesting mild symptoms after ingestion of significant amounts of lactose (such as >2 servings of dairy per day), with resolution of symptoms after avoidance of lactose-containing foods for 1 week.
- A positive lactose hydrogen breath test is confirmatory.
- Lactose intolerance can mimic symptoms of functional gastrointestinal disorders. Lactose intolerance can also be a coexisting condition.

HISTORY
- Assess daily lactose consumption.
- A single dose of lactose (12 g, equivalent to 1 cup of milk) consumed alone produces no or minor symptoms in persons with lactose intolerance.
- Lactose doses of 15 to 18 g are well tolerated with other nutrients. Doses >18 g cause progressively more symptoms, and quantities >50 g elicit symptoms in most individuals.
- Symptoms arise 30 minutes to 2 hours after consumption of lactose-containing products.
- Symptoms include bloating, flatulence, cramping abdominal discomfort, and diarrhea or loose stools. Vomiting may be noted in adolescents.
- Abdominal pain may be crampy in nature and often is localized to the periumbilical area or lower quadrant.
- Stools usually are bulky, frothy, and watery, although diarrhea may be rare in adults.
- Only 20–30% of individuals with lactose malabsorption develop symptoms.

PHYSICAL EXAM
- Vital signs and general appearance are typically normal.
- Audible bowel sounds (borborygmi) on physical examination (may be particularly bothersome to the patient). The exam is otherwise typically normal or nonspecific.

DIFFERENTIAL DIAGNOSIS
- Functional GI disorder (e.g., IBS)
- SIBO
- Celiac disease
- Inflammatory bowel disease
- Infectious enteritis (e.g., giardiasis)
- Drug or radiation induced enteritis
- Sucrase deficiency
- Cow's milk protein allergy

DIAGNOSTIC TESTS & INTERPRETATION
Initial Tests (lab, imaging)
- The lactose breath test (LBT) is a confirmatory for lactose intolerance. It is noninvasive, easy to perform (sensitivity 78%; specificity 98%) (2).
- Intestinal bacteria digest carbohydrates and produce measurable hydrogen and methane in expired breath:
  – Administer lactose when fasting (2 g/kg; max dose 25 g in children; 50 g in adults). Note any symptoms; sample breath hydrogen at baseline and at 30-minute intervals for 3 hours. Compare postlactose and baseline values. A rise in hydrogen concentration value of 20 ppm over baseline is diagnostic for lactose malabsorption. An early peak (15 to 30 minutes) suggests SIBO.
- Small bowel biopsy for histology and direct measurement of lactase activity (rarely needed).
- A positive LBT confirms lactose malabsorption but does not determine etiology.

Diagnostic Procedures/Other

- Lactose tolerance test is an alternative to LBT in adults and measures lactose absorption through serum glucose measurements. Following oral administration of a 50-g test dose in adults (2 g/kg in children), blood glucose levels are monitored at 0, 60, and 120 minutes. An increase in blood glucose of <20 mg/dL (1.1 mmol/L) with the concurrent development of symptoms is diagnostic. False-negative results may occur in patients with diabetes or bacterial overgrowth.
- Stool electrolyte testing, if done, may indicate a stool osmotic gap >125 mOsm/kg, (not specific for lactose intolerance).

Test Interpretation

Low lactase enzyme activity in intestinal mucosa, tested by small bowel biopsy, may be patchy or focal.

 ## TREATMENT

There is insufficient evidence to recommend any particular treatment (including probiotics, colonic adaptation, and other supplements) as definitive first line.

- In the absence of a correctable underlying disease, there are four general treatment principles (3)[B].
  - Avoid milk/dairy products to improve symptoms.
  - Up to 12 to 15 g of lactose can be tolerated in without significant symptoms (1 cup of milk).
  - Gradually reintroduce lactose as symptoms allow. Spreading lactose servings throughout the day improves tolerance.
  - If symptoms persist, substitute fermented and matured milk products for lactose.
- Certain strains, concentrations, and preparations of probiotics may alleviate symptoms.
- Incrementally increasing doses of lactose to induce adaptation have limited success.
- Insufficient evidence to routinely recommend lactose-reduced or hydrolyzed milk, lactase supplements consumed with milk or probiotics
- Maintain calcium and vitamin D intake.

MEDICATION

First Line

Lactase (Lactaid, Lactrase): Effectiveness varies.

- Commercially available "lactase" preparations are bacterial or yeast β-galactosidases.
- Take 1 to 2 capsules or tablets prior to ingesting dairy products.
- Can add tablets or contents of capsules to milk (1 to 2 caps/tabs per quart of milk) before drinking; also commercially available in milk in some areas
- Not effective for all people with lactose intolerance

COMPLEMENTARY & ALTERNATIVE MEDICINE

Certain probiotic formulations taken with meals may alleviate some symptoms of lactose intolerance (4)[B].

 ## ONGOING CARE

DIET

- Reduce or restrict dietary lactose to control symptoms—patient-specific "trial and error."
- Yogurt and fermented products such as hard cheese are often better tolerated than milk.
- Supplement calcium (e.g., calcium carbonate)
- Prehydrolyzed milk (Lactaid) is available.

PATIENT EDUCATION

- Read labels on commercial products—milk sugar is used in many products and may cause symptoms.
- Patients may tolerate whole milk or chocolate milk better than skim milk (slower rate of gastric emptying).
- Lactose consumed with other food products is better tolerated than when consumed with milk alone.
- Primary lactase deficiency is permanent; secondary lactose intolerance usually is temporary, although it may persist for months after the inciting event.
- 20% of prescription drugs and 6% of over-the-counter (OTC) medicines may contain lactose as a base.
- Most patients with lactose intolerance or malabsorption can tolerate 12 to 15 g of lactose per day.

PROGNOSIS

- Normal life expectancy
- Symptoms can be controlled through diet alone if lactase tablets are ineffective.

COMPLICATIONS

Calcium deficiency: Avoidance of milk and other dairy products can lead to reduced calcium intake, which may increase the risk for osteoporosis and fracture.

REFERENCES

1. Jansson-Knodell CL, Krajicek EJ, Savaiano DA, et al. Lactose intolerance: a concise review to skim the surface. *Mayo Clin Proc*. 2020;95(7):1499–1505.
2. Gasbarrini A, Corazza GR, Gasbarrini G, et al; for 1st Rome H2-Breath Testing Consensus Conference Working Group. Methodology and indications of H2-breath testing in gastrointestinal diseases: the Rome Consensus Conference. *Aliment Pharmacol Ther*. 2009;29(Suppl 1):1–49.

3. Shaukat A, Levitt MD, Taylor BC, et al. Systematic review: effective management strategies for lactose intolerance. *Ann Intern Med*. 2010;152(12):797–803.
4. Deng Y, Misselwitz B, Dai N, et al. Lactose intolerance in adults: biological mechanism and dietary management. *Nutrients*. 2015;7(9):8020–8035.

ADDITIONAL READING

- Almeida CC, Lorena SLS, Pavan CR, et al. Beneficial effects of long-term consumption of a probiotic combination of *Lactobacillus casei* Shirota and *Bifidobacterium breve* Yakult may persist after suspension of therapy in lactose-intolerant patients. *Nutr Clin Pract*. 2012;27(2):247–251.
- Facioni MS, Raspini B, Pivari F, et al. Nutritional management of lactose intolerance: the importance of diet and food labeling. *J Transl Med*. 2020;18(1):260.
- Tan-Dy CRY, Ohlsson A. Lactase treated feeds to promote growth and feeding tolerance in preterm infants. *Cochrane Database Syst Rev*. 2013;2013(3):CD004591.

 ## CODES

ICD10

- E73.9 Lactose intolerance, unspecified
- E73.1 Secondary lactase deficiency
- E73.8 Other lactose intolerance

CLINICAL PEARLS

- The diagnosis of lactose intolerance is based on clinical history and confirmed by hydrogen breath testing.
- Most lactose-intolerant patients can tolerate up to 12 to 15 g of lactose per day (equivalent to 1 cup of milk).
- Lactose-intolerant patients may tolerate yogurt and fermented products better than milk and cheese.
- A diary helps identify problematic foods. Patients should read ingredient labels to look for milk, lactose, whey, and curd.
- Lactose-intolerant patients may tolerate whole milk or chocolate milk better than skim milk due to slower gastric emptying.
- Many patients with lactose intolerance unnecessarily avoid all dairy products, potentially causing inadequate intake of calcium and vitamin D.

L

LARYNGITIS

Karlynn Sievers, MD • Bethany Price, DO

BASICS

DESCRIPTION
- Laryngitis is inflammation, erythema, and edema of the mucosa of the larynx and/or vocal cords characterized by hoarseness, loss of voice, throat pain, coughing, and often a negative impact on a person's quality of life and daily activities.
- There is a range of severity, but most cases are acute and are associated with viral upper respiratory infection, irritation, or acute vocal strain.
- System(s) affected: pulmonary; ears, nose, throat (ENT)
- Synonym(s): acute laryngitis; chronic laryngitis; croup or laryngotracheitis (in children)

EPIDEMIOLOGY
Children are more susceptible than adults due to increased risk of symptomatic inflammation from smaller airway.

Prevalence
Common; approximately 1.7% of population have dysphonia with 50% of this being caused by acute laryngitis. Prevalence rates are increasing but difficult to calculate because many patients do not seek medical attention.

ETIOLOGY AND PATHOPHYSIOLOGY
- Misuse or abuse of voice
- Infectious
  - Viral: influenza A, B; parainfluenza; adenovirus; coronavirus; rhinovirus; human papillomavirus; cytomegalovirus; varicella-zoster virus; herpes simplex virus; respiratory syncytial virus; coxsackievirus, COVID-19 (SARS-CoV-2)
  - Fungal: uncommon but thought to be underdiagnosed, potentially accounting for up to 10% of presentations in both immunocompromised and immunocompetent patients; risk factors include recent antibiotic or inhaled corticosteroid use (1): histoplasmosis, blastomycosis, *Coccidioides*, *Cryptococcus*, and *Candida*.
  - Bacterial (uncommon): β-hemolytic streptococcus, *Streptococcus pneumoniae*, *Haemophilus influenzae*, tuberculosis (TB), leprosy, *Moraxella catarrhalis*, *Mycoplasma pneumoniae*, *Chlamydophila pneumoniae*; in patients with chronic laryngitis, methicillin-resistant *Staphylococcus aureus* (MRSA) should be considered as a potential cause.
  - Secondary syphilis if left untreated
  - Leprosy (in 30–55% of those with leprosy, larynx is affected; in tropical and warm countries)
- Irritants
  - Inhalation of irritating substances (e.g., air pollution, cigarette smoke)
  - Aspiration of caustic chemicals
  - Gastroesophageal reflux disease (GERD)/laryngopharyngeal reflux disease (LPRD)
  - Excessively dry environment
  - Allergy exposures (including pollens)
- Anatomic
  - Aging changes: muscle atrophy, loss of moisture in larynx, and bowing of vocal cords
  - Vocal cord nodules/polyps ("singer's nodes")
  - Local cancer

- Iatrogenic: inhaled steroids such as those used to treat asthma, surgical injury, endotracheal intubation injury
- Neuromuscular disorder (e.g., myasthenia gravis); stroke
- Rheumatoid arthritis
- Trauma (e.g., blunt or penetrating trauma to neck)

RISK FACTORS
- Acute:
  - Infection or trauma
  - Upper respiratory tract viral infection (e.g., influenza, rhinovirus, adenovirus, parainfluenza)
  - Voice overuse—excessive talking, singing, or shouting
  - Pneumonia—viral or bacterial
  - Coughing
  - Lack of immunization against pertussis or diphtheria
  - Immunocompromised
  - Recent endotracheal intubation or local surgery
- Chronic (persists beyond 3 weeks):
  - Allergic laryngitis
  - Chronic rhinitis/sinusitis with postnasal drip (PND)
  - Voice abuse
  - GERD/LPRD (1)
  - Smoking: primary or secondhand
  - Excessive alcohol use
  - Autoimmune disorders (e.g., rheumatoid arthritis)
  - Granulomatous diseases (e.g., sarcoidosis)
  - Stroke
  - Environmental pollution; constant exposure to dust or other irritants such as chemicals at workplace
  - Medications: inhaled steroids, anticholinergics, antihistamines, anabolic steroids

Geriatric Considerations
May be more ill, slower to heal; need to consider neoplasm

Pediatric Considerations
- Common
- Consider congenital/anatomic causes.

GENERAL PREVENTION
- Avoid overuse of voice (speech therapy/voice training is helpful for vocal musicians/public speakers).
- Influenza virus vaccine is recommended, as well as other routine vaccines.
- Quit smoking and avoid secondhand smoke.
- Limit or avoid alcohol/caffeine/acidic foods.
- Control GERD/LPRD.
- Maintain proper hydration status.
- Avoid allergens.
- Wear mask around chemical/environmental irritants.
- Good hand washing (infection prevention)

COMMONLY ASSOCIATED CONDITIONS
- Viral pharyngitis
- Diphtheria (rare): Membrane can descend into the larynx.
- Pertussis: larynx involved as part of the respiratory system
- Bronchitis; pneumonitis
- Croup, epiglottitis, in children

DIAGNOSIS

HISTORY
- Hoarseness, throat "tickle," dry cough, and rawness
- Dysphonia (abnormal-sounding voice)
- Constant urge to clear the throat
- Possible fever
- Malaise
- Dysphagia/odynophagia
- Regional cervical lymphadenopathy
- Stridor or possible airway obstruction in children
- Cough may be worse at night in children.
- Hemoptysis
- Laryngospasm or sense of choking
- Allergic rhinitis/rhinorrhea/PND
- Occupation or other reasons for voice overuse
- Smoking history
- Blunt or penetrating trauma to neck
- GERD/LPRD

PHYSICAL EXAM
- Head and neck exam, including airway patency, cervical nodes; cranial nerve exam
- Visualization of the larynx: preferably with a flexible or rigid endoscope or with an indirect mirror examination as a screening technique to dictate further appropriate testing
- Note quality of voice (i.e., hoarse, breathy, wet, "hot potato like," asthenic [weak], strained).

DIFFERENTIAL DIAGNOSIS
- Diphtheria
- Vocal nodules or polyps
- Laryngeal malignancy
- Thyroid malignancy
- Upper airway malignancy
- Epiglottitis
- Pertussis
- Laryngeal nerve trauma/injury
- Foreign body (in children)
- Autoimmune (rheumatoid arthritis)

DIAGNOSTIC TESTS & INTERPRETATION
- Rarely needed
- WBCs elevated in bacterial laryngitis
- Viral culture (seldom necessary)

Follow-Up Tests & Special Considerations
- Barium swallow, only if needed for differential diagnosis
- CT scan if foreign body is suspected
- Do not offer CT imaging before visualization of the larynx with laryngoscopy (2).

Diagnostic Procedures/Other
- Fiber-optic or indirect laryngoscopy: look for red, inflamed, and occasionally hemorrhagic vocal cords; rounded edges and exudate (Reinke edema)
- Consider otolaryngologic evaluation and biopsy: laryngitis lasting >2 weeks in adults with history of smoking or alcohol abuse, to rule out malignancy
- pH probe (24-hour): no difference in incidence of pharyngeal reflux as measured by pH probe between patients with chronic reflux laryngitis and healthy adults
- Fiberoptic laryngoscopy for diagnosis of subtle lesions (e.g., vocal cord nodules or polyps) (1)

TREATMENT

- Limited but good evidence that treatment beyond supportive care is ineffective (1)
- Supportive care consists of hydration, voice rest, humidification, and limitation of caffeine (1).
- Antibiotics appear to have no benefit in acute laryngitis because etiologies are predominantly viral (1). In chronic laryngitis, consider bacterial sources such as MRSA (2).
- Corticosteroids in severe cases of laryngitis to reduce inflammation such as croup
- May need voice training, if voice was overused (2)
- Nebulized epinephrine reduces croup symptoms 30 minutes posttreatment; evidence does not favor racemic epinephrine or L-epinephrine or IPPB over simple nebulization. Racemic epinephrine reduces croup symptoms at 30 minutes, but effect lasts for only 2 hours.
- Botulinum toxin injections for spasmodic dysphonia (2)

GENERAL MEASURES

- Acute:
  - Usually a self-limited illness lasting <3 weeks and not severe
  - Antibiotics of no value
  - Avoid excessive voice use, including whispering.
  - Steam inhalations or cool-mist humidifier
  - Increase fluid intake, especially in cases associated with excessive dryness.
  - Avoid smoking (or secondhand exposure).
  - Warm saltwater gargles
- Chronic:
  - Symptomatic treatment as mentioned earlier
  - Voice therapy (for patients with intermittent dysphagia and vocal abuse)
  - Smoking cessation
  - Reduction or cessation of alcohol intake
  - Occupational change or modification, if exposure driven
  - Allergen avoidance
  - Consider discontinuing offending medication (e.g., inhaled steroids).
- Reflux laryngitis:
  - Elevate head of bed.
  - Diet changes
  - Other antireflux lifestyle change management
  - H_2 blockers or proton pump inhibitors (3)

MEDICATION

Usually none

First Line

- Analgesics
- Antipyretics (rare)
- Cough suppressants
- Throat lozenges
- Plenty of fluids

Second Line

- Inhaled corticosteroids (consider only if allergy induced)
- Oral corticosteroids: only if urgent need in adults (presenter, singer, actor)
- Oral corticosteroids: Evidence of benefit has been studied with single-dose dexamethasone in children ages 6 months to 5 years for moderate-severity croup; reduces symptoms within 6 hours; reduces hospitalizations, hospital length of stay, and revisits to office
- Standard of care is to prescribe proton pump inhibitors for chronic laryngitis if GERD or LPRD is suspected; however, evidence suggests only a modest benefit, if any (3).
- Treat nonviral infectious underlying causes.
- Candidal laryngitis:
  - Mild cases: oral antifungal (fluconazole)
  - Amphotericin B or echinocandin can be given in life-threatening cases.

ISSUES FOR REFERRAL

- Immediate emergency ENT referral for patients with stridor or respiratory distress
- The novel SARS-CoV-2 (COVID-19 pandemic) has become a significant cause of acute viral laryngitis. Case reports have shown higher rates of severe laryngitis with the newer Omicron variant, including reports of fatal upper airway stenosis.
- ENT referral for persistent symptoms (>2 to 3 weeks), especially in those with history of smoking or alcohol abuse to rule out malignancy, or concern for foreign body
- Consider GI consult to rule out GERD/LPRD.

SURGERY/OTHER PROCEDURES

- Vocal cord biopsy of hyperplastic mucosa and areas of leukoplakia if cancer or TB is suspected
- Removal of nodules or polyps if voice therapy fails

COMPLEMENTARY & ALTERNATIVE MEDICINE

Some experts, although not well studied, have recommended barberry, black currant, *Echinacea*, *Eucalyptus*, German chamomile, goldenrod, goldenseal, warmed lemon and honey, licorice, marshmallow, peppermint, saw palmetto, slippery elm, vitamin C, and zinc.

 ONGOING CARE

PATIENT EDUCATION

- Educate on the importance of voice rest, including whispering.
- Provide assistance with smoking cessation.
- Help the patient with modification of other predisposing habits or occupational hazards.

PROGNOSIS

Complete clearing of the inflammation without sequelae

COMPLICATIONS

Chronic hoarseness

REFERENCES

1. Gupta G, Mahajan K. *Acute Laryngitis*. In: StatPearls [Internet]. Treasure Island, FL: StatPearls Publishing; 2022. https://pubmed.ncbi.nlm.nih.gov/30521292/. Accessed September 23, 2023.
2. Francis DO, Smith LJ. Hoarseness guidelines redux: toward improved treatment of patients with dysphonia. *Otolaryngol Clin North Am*. 2019;52(4):597–605.
3. Durazzo M, Lupi G, Cicerchia F, et al. Extra-esophageal presentation of gastroesophageal reflux disease: 2020 update. *J Clin Med*. 2020;9(8):2559.

ADDITIONAL READING

- Carpenter PS, Kendall KA. MRSA chronic bacterial laryngitis: a growing problem. *Laryngoscope*. 2018;128(4):921–925.
- Kimura Y, Hirabayashi E, Yano M, et al. COVID-19 Omicron variant-induced laryngitis. *Auris Nasus Larynx*. 2023;50(4):637–640.
- Reveiz L, Cardona AF. Antibiotics for acute laryngitis in adults. *Cochrane Database Syst Rev*. 2015;2015(5):CD004783.

CODES

ICD10

- J37.0 Chronic laryngitis
- J04.0 Acute laryngitis
- J05.0 Acute obstructive laryngitis [croup]

CLINICAL PEARLS

- Laryngitis is usually self-limited and needs only comfort care. Standard treatment is voice rest, hydration, humidification, and limited caffeine intake.
- Refer to ENT for direct visualization of vocal cords for prolonged laryngitis.
- Corticosteroids have some benefits for children with moderately severe croup.
- Voice training is useful for chronic laryngitis.

L

LEAD POISONING

Jason Chao, MD, MS

 BASICS

DESCRIPTION
- Results from a high body burden of lead (Pb)—an element with no known physiologic purpose
- Synonym(s): Pb poisoning, inorganic

EPIDEMIOLOGY
- Predominant age: 1 to 5 years, adult workers
- Predominant sex: male > female (1:1 in childhood)

Prevalence
- Half of U.S. children have detectable blood Pb levels, and 1.9% have blood Pb levels >5 μg/dL.
- Centers for Disease Control and Prevention (CDC) estimates 2.5% of U.S. children aged 1 to 5 years have blood Pb levels ≥3.5 μg/dL (new blood Pb reference level). Lead levels are highest in children with public health insurance, residing in pre-1950s housing, or poverty.

ETIOLOGY AND PATHOPHYSIOLOGY
- Inhalation of Pb dust or fumes or ingestion of Pb
- Pb replaces calcium in bones. Pb interferes with heme synthesis, causes interstitial nephritis, and interferes with neurotransmitters, especially glutamine. High Pb levels can lead to encephalopathy, seizures, and coma.
- Pb crosses blood–brain barrier by displacing calcium ions. Pb exposure early in life causes methylation changes leading to epigenetic alterations that may predispose to brain dysfunction.

RISK FACTORS
- Children with pica or with iron-deficiency anemia
- Residence in or frequent visitation to deteriorating pre-1978 housing with Pb-painted surfaces or recent renovation
- Soil/dust exposure near older homes, Pb industries, or urban roads
- Sibling or playmate with current or past Pb poisoning
- Dust from clothing of Pb worker or hobbyist
- Pb dissolved in water from Pb or Pb-soldered plumbing (e.g., Flint, Michigan 2014 to 2015)
- Pb-glazed ceramics leachate (especially with acidic food or drink)
- Folk remedies, spices, and cosmetics
  - Latin America: azarcon, greta, litargirio (a topical agent)
  - Asia and Middle East: chuifong tokuwan, payloo-ah, ghasard, bali goli, kandu, ayurvedic herbal medicine from South Asia, kohl (alkohl, ceruse), surma, saoott, cebagin
- Hobbies: target shooting, glazed pottery making, Pb soldering, preparing Pb shot or fishing sinkers, stained-glass making, car/boat repair, home remodeling
- Occupational exposure: plumbers, pipe fitters, Pb miners, auto repairers, glass manufacturers, ship builders, printer operators, plastic manufacturers, Pb smelters and refiners, steel welders or cutters, construction workers, rubber product manufacturers, battery manufacturers, bridge reconstruction workers, firing range workers, military and law enforcement
- Dietary: zinc or calcium deficiency
- Imported toys or jewelry with Pb
- Retained bullet fragments, especially if multiple fragments, associated with fracture, or in joints

Pediatric Considerations
- Children are at increased risk because of incomplete development of the blood–brain barrier prior to 3 years of age (allowing more Pb into the CNS).
- Ingested Pb 40% bioavailable in children (10% in adults)
- Common childhood behaviors such as frequent hand-to-mouth activity and pica (repeated ingestion of nonfood products) increase the risk of Pb ingestion.

Pregnancy Considerations
Cross-sectional studies suggest an association between elevated blood Pb and preeclampsia.

GENERAL PREVENTION
- Counsel families on sources of Pb and how to decrease exposure.
- Screen high-risk children.
- Warn parents about unsafe home renovations.
- Wet mopping and dusting with a high-phosphate solution (e.g., powdered automatic dishwasher detergent with 1/4 cup per gallon of water) helps control Pb-bearing dust. High-phosphate detergent is no longer available in some states.
- If tap water is potentially Pb contaminated, use cold water instead of hot water and run for 30 to 60 seconds to flush pipes. Use Pb-free water source if possible (bottled or distilled water).

COMMONLY ASSOCIATED CONDITIONS
Iron-deficiency anemia

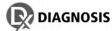 **DIAGNOSIS**

HISTORY
- Often asymptomatic
- Mild-to-moderate toxicity
  - Myalgias, paresthesias, fatigue, irritability, lethargy
  - Abdominal discomfort, arthralgia, difficulty concentrating, headache, tremor, vomiting, weight loss, muscular exhaustibility
- Severe toxicity: three major clinical syndromes:
  - Alimentary type: anorexia, metallic taste, constipation, severe abdominal cramps due to intestinal spasm and sometimes associated with abdominal wall rigidity
  - Neuromuscular type (characteristic of adult plumbism): peripheral neuritis, usually painless and limited to extensor muscles
  - Cerebral type or Pb encephalopathy (more common in children): seizure, coma, and long-term sequelae, including neurologic defects, delayed mental development, and chronic hyperactivity (or other behavioral changes)
- Chronic exposure may cause renal failure.

PHYSICAL EXAM
Often normal but abdominal tenderness may be severe; neurologic exam may reveal neuropathy or encephalopathy.

DIFFERENTIAL DIAGNOSIS
- Alimentary type may present as acute abdomen.
- Neuromuscular type presents similar to other polyneuropathies.
- May be confused with ADD, intellectual disability, autism, dementia, and other causes of seizures

- Elevated erythrocyte protoporphyrin may be caused by iron-deficiency anemia or (less commonly) hemolytic anemia.
- Erythropoietic protoporphyria produces a very high erythrocyte protoporphyrin level.

DIAGNOSTIC TESTS & INTERPRETATION
- Venous blood Pb reference value >3.5 μg/dL (0.17 μmol/L); CDC lowered the reference value from >5 μg/dL (0.24 μmol/L) in 2021 (1)[C]. Confirm screening capillary Pb levels >3.5 μg/dL (0.17 μmol/L) with a venous sample.
- Hemoglobin and hematocrit slightly low; eosinophilia; basophilic stippling on peripheral smear (not diagnostic)
- Renal function is decreased in late stages.
- Abdominal radiograph for Pb particles in gut if recent ingestion is suspected
- Radiograph of long bones may show metaphyseal changes (resulting from growth arrest). Films are not routinely recommended.

Initial Tests (lab, imaging)
Screening questionnaires are only 60% sensitive to identify children with elevated blood levels.

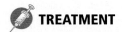 **TREATMENT**

Blood Level (μg/dL)	Time to Confirmation Testing
≥ref value–9	1–3 mo
10–44	1 wk–1 mo
45–59	48 hr
60–69	24 hr
≥70	Urgently as emergency test

ALERT
- For Pb levels >3.5 μg/dL, confirm with repeat testing according to the table.
- For blood Pb levels persistently >15 μg/dL, contact local public health department for home inspection.
- For any elevated level, educate on sources of Pb exposure.
- Pb level 5 to 45 μg/dL: complete history and physical exam, follow-up Pb monitoring; complete inspection of home or workplace to determine source of Pb and Pb-hazard reduction; neurodevelopmental monitoring: iron status, hemoglobin, or hematocrit (2)[C]
- Pb level 45 to 69 μg/dL: treatment to lower level plus free erythrocyte protoporphyrin, oral chelation therapy, or hospitalization if Pb-safe environment cannot be ensured (2)[C]
- Pb >70 μg/dL: Hospitalize for chelation therapy (3)[C].

GENERAL MEASURES
Remove child from source of exposure.

MEDICATION
- Consider oral chelation for asymptomatic and Pb >45 and <70; chelation (preferably parenteral) for Pb >70 or symptomatic Pb <70 (3)[C]
- If evidence of Pb in GI tract, withhold chelation until bowel is decontaminated, because all chelating agents increase absorption of Pb by the gut (2)[C].

First Line

- Oral chelation: succimer (Chemet), dimercaptosuccinic acid (DMSA) 350 mg/m^2 or 10 mg/kg q8h for 5 days and then q12h for 2 weeks; this may be repeated after 2 weeks off if Pb levels are not stabilized at <15 μg/dL (<0.72 μmol/L) (3).
- Parenteral chelation (begin after establishment of adequate urine output):
  - Dimercaprol (British anti-Lewisite [BAL]) 75 mg/m^2 given deep IM and then BAL 450 mg/m^2/day divided q4h for 5 days plus Ca edetate calcium disodium (EDTA) 1,500 mg/m^2/day continuous IV infusion for 5 days; if rebound Pb level ≥45 μg/dL (≥2.17 μmol/L), chelation may be repeated after 2-day interval if symptomatic or after 5-day interval if asymptomatic.
  - Ca EDTA 1,000 mg/m^2/day for 5 days; may be repeated after 5 to 7 days
  - In adults, dimercaprol had greater impact on reducing Pb levels than Ca EDTA.
  - Contraindications: Do not give BAL to patients with a peanut allergy (the drug solution contains peanut oil).
- Diazepam for initial control of seizures; further control maintained with paraldehyde
- Precautions
  - Succimer: GI upset, rash, nasal congestion, muscle pains, elevated liver function tests
  - BAL: nausea, vomiting, fever, headache, transient hypertension, hepatocellular damage
  - Ca EDTA: renal failure; increased excretion of zinc, copper, and iron
- Significant possible interactions
  - Do not give vitamins with minerals while giving chelation.
  - BAL may precipitate hemolytic crisis in a patient with glucose-6-phosphate dehydrogenase deficiency.

Second Line

Oral chelation with penicillamine (D-penicillamine, Depen, Cuprimine) (3)

- Penicillin-allergic patient should not receive penicillamine (cross-sensitivity is common).
- 10 to 15 mg/kg/day given BID mixed in apple juice/sauce on empty stomach (*not* FDA-approved)
- Penicillamine may cause GI upset, renal failure, granulocytopenia, liver dysfunction, iron deficiency, and drug-induced lupus-like syndrome.

ISSUES FOR REFERRAL

Consider consultation if parenteral chelation is required.

ADDITIONAL THERAPIES

- Remove patient from potential source of Pb if Pb level >45 μg/dL until complete home inspection is performed.
- If desired medication is not available due to drug shortage or cost, alternatives include compounded drugs and consulting a poison center or medical toxicologist.

COMPLEMENTARY & ALTERNATIVE MEDICINE

Garlic has been used to treat mild to moderate Pb poisoning in adults.

ADMISSION, INPATIENT, AND NURSING CONSIDERATIONS

- Blood Pb level >70 μg/dL
- If symptomatic, blood Pb level >35 μg/dL
- Outpatient care unless parenteral chelation or immediate removal from contaminated environment is required
- If Pb source is in the home, the patient must reside elsewhere until the abatement process is completed.
- Avoid visit to any site of potential contamination.

 ## ONGOING CARE

Early intervention (before age 3) programs for elevated lead levels improve standardized test performance in elementary school

FOLLOW-UP RECOMMENDATIONS

Patient Monitoring

- Expect rebound after chelation due to release of Pb from bone stores.
- Check for rebound Pb level 7 to 10 days after chelation therapy. Monitor biweekly or monthly thereafter.
- Correct iron or other detected nutritional deficiencies.
- Once Pb <35 μg/dL, repeat testing every 1 to 3 months until level <25 μg/dL is achieved. Then, monitor every 3 to 6 months until level <10 μg/dL. Once <9 μg/dL, test every 6 to 9 months (2)[C].

DIET

- Avoid pica.
- Adequate calcium, iron, zinc, magnesium, and vitamins C and D to reduce absorption of Pb

PATIENT EDUCATION

- United States Environmental Protection Agency: https://www.epa.gov/lead
- National Safety Council: https://www.nsc.org/community-safety/safety-topics/other-poisons/lead-poisoning-prevention?
- CDC, Childhood Lead Poisoning Prevention Program: https://www.cdc.gov/nceh/lead/default.htm

PROGNOSIS

- Symptomatic Pb poisoning without encephalopathy generally improves with chelation, but subtle CNS toxicity may be long lasting or permanent.
- Preschool children with higher Pb levels have lower reading and math scores in elementary school.
- Early childhood high body lead burden is correlated with higher risk of juvenile delinquency and arrest as an adult
- Children with high Pb levels at age 11 years have lower IQ score and socioeconomic status in adulthood.
- With Pb encephalopathy, permanent sequelae (e.g., mental retardation, seizure disorder, blindness, and hemiparesis) occurs in 25–50%.

COMPLICATIONS

- CNS toxicity may be long lasting or permanent.
- Long-term Pb exposure may cause chronic renal failure (Fanconi-like syndrome), gout, or Pb line (blue–black) on gingival tissue.
- Pb exposure in pregnancy is associated with reduced birth weight and premature birth.

REFERENCES

1. Ruckart PZ, Jones RL, Countney JG, et al. Update of the blood lead reference value—United States, 2021. *MMWR Morb Mortal Wkly Rep*. 2021;70(43):1509–1512.
2. Centers for Disease Control and Prevention. Recommended actions based on blood lead levels. https://www.cdc.gov/nceh/lead/advisory/acclpp/actions-blls.htm. Accessed August 5, 2023.
3. Cantor AG, Hendrickson R, Blazina I, et al. Screening for elevated blood lead levels in childhood and pregnancy: updated evidence report and systematic review for the US Preventive Services Task Force. *JAMA*. 2019;321(15):1510–1526.

ADDITIONAL READING

Stingone JA, Sedlar S, Lim S, et al. Receipt of early intervention services before age 3 years and performance on third-grade standardized tests among children exposed to lead. *JAMA Pediatr*. 2022;176(5):478–485.

 ## SEE ALSO

Anemia, Iron Deficiency

CODES

ICD10

- T56.0X4A Toxic effect of lead and its compounds, undetermined, init
- T56.0X1A Toxic effect of lead and its compounds, accidental, init

CLINICAL PEARLS

- Screen children 6 to 11 months of age with ≥1 risk factors
- Children living in high-risk communities (>12% elevated Pb) should be tested annually from 1 to 5 years of age
- CDC updated its blood Pb reference value (BLRV) from 5 μg/dL to 3.5 μg/dL in 2021.
- There is no safe Pb level.
- There are no studies that show benefit of chelation for asymptomatic children with Pb <45. Environmental removal of Pb sources is critical.

L

LEGIONNAIRES' DISEASE

Kenneth A. Ballou, MD

BASICS

DESCRIPTION

- *Legionnaires' disease* was named for an epidemic of lower respiratory tract disease at the 1976 American Legion convention in Philadelphia. The previously unrecognized causative bacterium was isolated, identified, and named *Legionella pneumophila*. The organism primarily causes pneumonia and flulike illness. *Legionella* preferentially colonizes commercial water systems (e.g., hotels, hospitals, apartment buildings, air conditioning cooling towers).
  – It is one of the three most common causes of pneumonias and the most common atypical pneumonia.
- System(s) affected: pulmonary, gastrointestinal (GI)
- Synonym(s): *Legionella* pneumonia; Legionellosis; Pontiac Fever (self-limited flulike illness without pneumonia caused by *Legionella* spp.)

EPIDEMIOLOGY

- Predominant age: 15 months to 84 years; 74–91% of patients are >50 years old.
- Predominant gender: male > female

Incidence

- Cases of Legionnaires' disease have increased 4-fold in the United States since 2000; almost 10,000 cases are reported in 2018.
- Outbreaks are most common in late summer/early fall (1).
- ~2–9% of all cases of pneumonia in the United States; Legionnaires' disease is fatal in 1 of every 10 cases.

ETIOLOGY AND PATHOPHYSIOLOGY

- *L. pneumophila* is a weak gram-negative aerobic saprophytic freshwater bacterium. It is widely distributed in soil and water. Bipolar flagella provide motility; grow optimally at 40–45°C (2)
- Exists in nature as a protozoan parasite, often within fresh water biofilms
- Serogroups 1 to 6 account for clinical disease.
- Serogroup 1 represents 70–92% of all clinical cases of *Legionella* infections in the United States.
- In the lung, *Legionella* infects alveolar macrophages.
- The organism is transmitted by breathing in contaminated water droplets or by aspiration of contaminated water (e.g., contaminated shower water was responsible for the inaugural Philadelphia outbreak).
- Community outbreaks have been associated with whirlpools, spas, fountains, and aboard cruise ships.

RISK FACTORS

- Impaired cellular immunity (*Legionellae* are intracellular pathogens.)
- Male gender
- Smoking; alcohol abuse
- Immunosuppression; HIV; diabetes; organ transplant recipients; chronic or high-dose corticosteroid use
- Chronic cardiopulmonary disease
- Advanced age
- Use of antimicrobials within the past 3 months

GENERAL PREVENTION

- *Not transmitted person to person* (Respiratory isolation is unnecessary.)
- Superheat and flush water systems: Heat water to at least 158°F and flush for 30 minutes.
- Ultraviolet light and copper–silver ionization are bactericidal.
- Monochloramine disinfection of municipal water supplies decreases risk for *Legionella* infection.
- 0.2 micron water filters—must change regularly
- Keep water heaters >140°F; cold water <68°F

DIAGNOSIS

- Illness ranges from asymptomatic seroconversion and mild febrile illness to severe pneumonia.
- Wound infections with *Legionella* are also reported.
- Incubation period is 2 to 14 days.

HISTORY

- Signs and symptoms (with associated percentage):
  – Cough: 92% (typically dry; rarely productive)
  – Fever/chills: 90%
  – Dyspnea: 62%
  – Pleuritic chest pain: 35%
  – Headache: 48%
  – Myalgia/arthralgia: 40%
  – Watery diarrhea: 50%
  – Nausea and vomiting: 49%
  – Neuropsychiatric symptoms include encephalopathy, confusion, disorientation, obtundation, depression, hallucinations, insomnia, and seizure: 53%.
- History of immunosuppression increases risk.

PHYSICAL EXAM

- Fever
- Relative bradycardia (key sign)
  – Temperature ≥102°F with an inappropriately low pulse rate of <100 beats/min (Normal compensatory reaction to fever is >110 beats/min.)
- Rales and signs of consolidation (e.g., pectoriloquy, egophony, tactile fremitus)

DIFFERENTIAL DIAGNOSIS

- Other bacterial pneumonias, especially atypical pneumonias: *Mycoplasma pneumoniae*, Q fever (*Coxiella burnetii*), *Chlamydophila pneumoniae*, *Chlamydophila psittaci*, *Francisella tularensis*
- Viral pneumonias, such as adenovirus, influenza (human, avian, swine), cytomegalovirus (CMV)
- Must be differentiated from COVID-19 pulmonary disease; COVID-19 testing is recommended.

DIAGNOSTIC TESTS & INTERPRETATION

Indications for *Legionella* testing:

- Failed outpatient antibiotic treatment for community-acquired pneumonia (CAP)
- Severe pneumonia, particularly those requiring intensive care; immunocompromised patients with pneumonia

- Patients with a history of traveling away from their home within 10 days of illness onset, especially with a history of commercial lodging such as hotel or cruise-ship stay within the last 2 weeks
- Pneumonia in the setting of a known Legionnaires' disease outbreak; pneumonia beginning ≥48 hours after hospital admission

Initial Tests (lab, imaging)

Diagnosis:

- *Legionella* PCR detects ~100% of all *Legionella* spp from lower respiratory secretions.
- Urinary antigen test (UAT) detects serogroup 1 (which causes 80% of disease). UATs are highly specific (95–100%) but of variable sensitivity.
- *Legionella* culture (gold standard) requires an adequate sputum sample and special media (buffered charcoal yeast extract [BCYE] agar). Culture has variable sensitivity (10–80%) and time delays of up to 7 days for results.
- Other lab abnormalities:
  – Hyponatremia; hypophosphatemia (transient); lymphopenia
  – Mildly elevated serum transaminases; elevated LDH; elevated creatine kinase
  – Microscopic hematuria; highly elevated C-reactive protein (CRP) (>30)
  – Highly elevated ferritin (≥2 times normal)
- Chest radiograph
  – Not specific for *Legionella*
  – Commonly shows unilateral lower lobe patchy alveolar infiltrate with consolidation
  – Cavitation and abscess formation are more common in immunocompromised patients.
  – Pleural effusion occurs in up to 50%. May take 1 to 4 months for radiographic findings to resolve. Progression of infiltrate on x-ray can be seen despite antibiotic therapy.

Diagnostic Procedures/Other

Transtracheal aspiration/bronchoscopy occasionally necessary to obtain sputum/lung samples

Test Interpretation

- Multifocal pneumonia with alveolitis and bronchiolitis and fibrinous pleuritis; may have serous or serosanguineous pleural effusion
- Abscess formation occurs in up to 20% of patients.
- Progression of infiltrates on x-ray (despite appropriate therapy) suggests Legionnaires' disease. Radiographic improvement may not correlate with clinical findings (longer lag times).
- Use of procalcitonin levels of limited value as it is not as sensitive in atypical pathogens such as *Legionella*

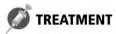

TREATMENT

GENERAL MEASURES

- Supportive care:
  – Oxygenation, hydration, and electrolyte balance with antibiotic therapy

- Extrapulmonary complications and higher mortality may be seen in patients with AIDS and other immunosuppressive conditions.
- In severe pneumonia, start empiric antibiotics to include coverage for *Legionella*.

MEDICATION
First Line
- Antibiotics that achieve high intracellular concentrations (e.g., macrolides, tetracyclines, fluoroquinolones) are most effective; first-line treatment is levofloxacin; no prospective randomized controlled trials have compared fluoroquinolones to macrolides for the treatment of *Legionella*; levofloxacin associated with more rapid defervescence, fewer complications, decreased hospital stay by 3 days, and decreased mortality (4% vs. 10.9%) compared with macrolide antibiotics
- Start antibiotics parenterally if sufficiently ill due to the GI symptoms associated with *Legionella*:
  - Levofloxacin is the preferred agent (3):
    - Levofloxacin 750 mg/day IV daily (switch to PO when patient is afebrile and tolerating PO meds) for 7 to 14 days
  - Azithromycin may also be used first line. It requires a shorter duration of treatment than levofloxacin due to a longer half-life:
    - Azithromycin 500 mg/day IV daily (switch to PO when afebrile/tolerating PO meds) for 7 to 10 days
    - Clarithromycin 500 mg PO BID for 14 to 21 days
- Contraindications: hypersensitivity reactions
- Precautions: liver disease
- Significant drug interactions:
  - Can increase theophylline, carbamazepine, and digoxin levels; can increase activity of oral anticoagulants
  - May decrease the effectiveness of digoxin, quinidine, oral contraceptives, and hypoglycemic agents
- Longer courses of treatment (up to 21 days) may be needed in immunocompromised patients or valvular heart disease.

Second Line
- Doxycycline 200 mg IV/PO as a loading dose and then 100 mg q12h for 14 to 21 days
- Doxycycline should not be used in pregnant patients and is not approved for children aged <8 years.
- Tetracycline 500 mg PO q6h for 14 to 21 days
- Minocycline 100 mg PO q12h for 14 to 21 days
- Caution when using tetracyclines as there are increased rates of resistance in some species of *Legionella* organisms

ADMISSION, INPATIENT, AND NURSING CONSIDERATIONS
- Inability to tolerate oral antibiotics
- Hypoxemia

- Criteria for direct admission to the ICU:
  - Any major criteria for severe CAP:
    - Septic shock requiring vasopressor support
    - Acute respiratory failure requiring intubation and/or mechanical ventilation
  - Three or more minor criteria for severe CAP:
    - RR ≥30 breaths/min, PaO$_2$:FiO$_2$ ratio ≤250, multilobular infiltrates, confusion/disorientation, uremia (BUN ≥20 mg/dL), leukopenia (WBC <4,000 cells/mm^3), thrombocytopenia (PLT <100,000 cells/mm^3), hypothermia (temperature <36°C), hypotension requiring aggressive fluid resuscitation
- Discharge criteria
  - Afebrile; able to tolerate oral antibiotics; return to normal/baseline room-air oxygen saturation

 ONGOING CARE

FOLLOW-UP RECOMMENDATIONS
Patient Monitoring
- Monitor respiratory status, hydration, and electrolyte status closely.
- Chest radiography lags behind the clinical status and may not help with monitoring clinical response.

PATIENT EDUCATION
- Disease prevention: eliminate pathogens from water supplies; low-emission cleaning of cooling towers with control measurements of water and air samples
- *Legionella* is not spread from person to person.

PROGNOSIS
- Improved prognosis when appropriate antibiotics are started early in the disease course
- Recovery is variable:
  - Patients may clinically worsen despite appropriate initial treatment (first 1 to 2 days of therapy).
  - Improvement with defervescence in 3 to 5 days and complete recovery in 6 to 10 days is typical. Some have a more protracted course.
- Mortality in nosocomial infections as high as 15–34%

COMPLICATIONS
- Dehydration; hyponatremia
- Respiratory insufficiency requiring ventilator support
- Bacteremia/lung abscess formation in up to 20%
- Extrapulmonary diseases:
  - Endocarditis (most common extrapulmonary site); cellulitis; sinusitis; pancreatitis; pyelonephritis; encephalitis; pericarditis; perirectal abscess
  - Renal failure; disseminated intravascular coagulation; multiple organ dysfunction syndrome (MODS)
- Death occurs in 8–12% of treated immunocompetent patients and in up to 80% of untreated immunocompromised patients.

REFERENCES
1. Graham FF, Finn N, White P, et al. Global perspective of *Legionella* infection in community-acquired pneumonia: a systematic review and meta-analysis of observational studies. *Int J Environ Res Public Health*. 2022;19(3):1907.
2. Mondino S, Schmidt S, Rolando M, et al. Legionnaires' disease: state of the art knowledge of pathogenesis mechanisms of *Legionella*. *Annu Rev Pathol*. 2020;15:439–466.
3. Viasus D, Gaia V, Manzur-Barbur C, et al. Legionnaires' disease: update on diagnosis and treatment. *Infect Dis Ther*. 2022;11(3):973–986.

ADDITIONAL READING

Metlay JP, Waterer GW, Long AC, et al. Diagnosis and treatment of adults with community-acquired pneumonia: an official clinical practice guideline of the American Thoracic Society and Infectious Diseases Society of America. *Am J Respir Crit Care Med*. 2019;200(7):e45–e67.

 SEE ALSO

Pneumonia, Bacterial

 CODES

ICD10
- A48.2 Nonpneumonic Legionnaires' disease [Pontiac fever]
- A48.1 Legionnaires' disease

CLINICAL PEARLS

- Consider Legionnaires' disease in patients with pneumonia who have GI and other extrapulmonary findings (atypical CAP) and a relative bradycardia. Relative lymphopenia, mildly elevated serum transaminases (aspartate aminotransferase/alanine aminotransferase), highly increased ferritin levels, and hypophosphatemia are other laboratory clues to *Legionella* infection.
- Serology is not useful in early stages of the disease (an increase in *Legionella* antibody titers cannot be detected until 3 to 4 weeks after symptom onset).
- Urine antigen testing and *Legionella* sputum PCR are the most sensitive and practical initial tests. Sputum culture is definitive but can take up to 7 days.
- Consider Legionnaires' disease in cases of nosocomial pneumonia and in any CAP requiring inpatient treatment.
- Levofloxacin and azithromycin are first-line agents.

L

LESBIAN HEALTH

Tina D'Amato, DO

BASICS

DESCRIPTION
- A lesbian is a woman who has her primary emotional and sexual relationships with women.
- Sexual behaviors
  - May be celibate, sexually active only with women or with men, women and/or nonbinary partners
  - ~75% of self-reported lesbians have reported prior or ongoing sexual contact with men.
- Sexual orientation and gender are complex concepts and defining them can be challenging.

EPIDEMIOLOGY
Prevalence
- Estimated to be between 1% and 5%
- Approximately 1.4 million women living in the United States identify as lesbians; another 2.6 million women identify as bisexual
- 2022 Gallup Poll results had 1% of women identifying as lesbian.
- 2022 Gallup Poll shows 2.2% of generation Z and 1.5% of millennials identify as lesbian compared to 0.5% of generation X, 0.7% of boomers, and 0.2% of silent generation.
- 2021 American Community Survey from United States Census Bureau estimates 631,900 households are headed by female same-sex couples.

RISK FACTORS
Higher incidence for the following risk factors compared to heterosexual women:
- Elevated BMI
  - Lesbian women have a higher prevalence of overweight/obesity than all other female sexual orientation groups.
  - Higher prevalence rates of obesity have been found among lesbians who are African American, who live in urban or rural areas, who have lower levels of education, or who have lower socioeconomic status.
- Alcohol use
  - More common use than reported in heterosexual women
  - Age 20 to 34 years is at highest risk for daily use and heavy use of alcohol. Those numbers decline in older age groups, but even one drink per day can increase risks for cancer, hepatic, and heart disease.
- Tobacco use
  - 1.5 to 2 times more likely to smoke than heterosexual women
  - Aggressive marketing by tobacco industry to LGBT individuals
- Sexual minority stress (1)
  - Increased risk for health issues secondary to greater exposure to social stresses related to prejudice and stigma
  - Many of the increased health risks in lesbians can be attributed to behaviors that are the result of dealing with the stress and stigma of homophobia and discrimination.
- The above factors can increase risks for cardiovascular disease (CVD), type 2 diabetes, hepatic disease, and cancers.

GENERAL PREVENTION
Health Access and Outcomes
- Between 2013 and 2018, heterosexual women had significant reductions in delayed/absent medical care due to costs that was not seen in their lesbian peers.
- During 2016 and 2018, lesbian and bisexual women had significantly higher odds of undesirable health outcomes and access to health care compared to their heterosexual peers.

COMMONLY ASSOCIATED CONDITIONS
- Cervical cancer
  - Lesbians are equally at risk for developing cervical cancer compared to heterosexual women.
  - HPV can be transmitted genitally skin to skin, oral to genitals, and digital to genitals.
  - The risk of cervical cancer is highest in lesbians:
    - With prior HPV infection/abnormal Pap smear
    - Who have had a history of heterosexual intercourse
  - Lesbian and bisexual women are 10 times less likely to have had adequate cervical cancer screening compared to heterosexual women.
  - Tobacco use influences cervical cell atypia.
- Breast cancer
  - Risk factors same as heterosexual women
    - Moderate or heavy alcohol consumption
    - Obesity
    - Nulliparity or first child born after age 30 years
  - Mammogram screening rates lower among lesbians
  - Data suggest lesbians have increased mortality rate compared to heterosexual women.
- Ovarian cancer
  - Elevated BMI and tobacco use increase risks.
  - Lesbians less likely to have been on hormonal contraception for ≥5 years
  - Lesbians less likely to have been pregnant or breastfed an infant before age 30 years
  - Lesbians at increased risk for ovarian cancer may want to explore potential benefits of long-term progestin-containing contraception to reduce risk.
- Endometrial cancer
  - Elevated BMI and tobacco use increases risks.
  - Lesbians less likely to have been pregnant
  - Lesbians with polycystic ovarian syndrome should be asked about sustained amenorrhea and consider use of progestin-containing contraception or regular schedule of induced "withdrawal bleeds" to reduce risks.
- CVD
  - Lesbians have higher rates of obesity, alcohol use, smoking, and stress, which increase risks for CVD.
  - A study of French population published in the May 17, 2023 Journal of The American Heart Association identified lesbian and bisexual women as having lower cardiovascular health scores compared to their heterosexual peers

- Mental health diagnoses
  - 2 times more likely to see general physician for mental/emotional complaint compared to heterosexual women
  - More likely to seek care if physician is aware of their sexual orientation
    - Depression
      - Discrimination stress proposed factor
      - Double the rate compared to heterosexual women
    - Suicide
      - "Out" lesbian women are 2 to 2.5 times more likely to have had suicidal ideation in the last 12 months compared to heterosexual women.
      - Lesbian women who were not "out" were more likely to have attempted suicide compared to heterosexual women.
    - Anxiety disorders
      - 3 times risk, multiple diagnoses
      - Higher rates of PTSD, panic, phobia, and 2- to 4-fold higher rate of generalized anxiety disorder
    - Alcohol abuse
      - Greatest in lesbians ages 20 to 34 years
      - Bar culture
      - May not feel comfortable in traditional Alcoholics Anonymous environment
      - Sexual minority females are more likely than heterosexual counterparts to be current alcohol users, binge drinkers, and heavy drinkers.
    - Substance abuse
      - Sexual minority women are at higher rates of all substance abuse compared to heterosexual counterparts.
        □ Bisexual women have highest rates of substance abuse compared to lesbian and heterosexual women.
      - Higher levels of socioeconomic instability were associated with increased odds for substance abuse.
        □ Household Pulse Survey from United States Census Bureau showed how COVID-19 pandemic impacted the LGBTQ population significantly greater than heterosexual counterparts.
- Sexually transmitted infections (STIs)
  - Many lesbians underestimate their STI risks.
  - Difficult to ascertain accurate statistics because of lack of research and the confounding factors of relying on identifiers of sexual orientation versus sexual behaviors
  - Increased risk during menstruation and activities causing friction
  - Lesbian sexual practices include the following:
    - High risk: oral–vaginal contact, genital–genital contact, oral–anal contact, digital stimulation/penetration, and sharing of sex toys
    - Lower risk: kissing, rubbing genitals against partner's body/clothing
- Bacterial vaginosis
  - Higher rate than heterosexual women; estimated 25–52% prevalence
  - Increased incidence with smoking, receptive oral sex, symptomatic partner, and new partner
  - Often found in monogamous lesbian couples suggesting it can be sexually transmitted; consider treating asymptomatic partner especially in recurrent cases.

- Chlamydia, gonorrhea, hepatitis B, syphilis, trichomonas, and herpes can all be transmitted woman to woman (WTW).
- HPV
  - Can be transmitted WTW
  - Up to 30% of women who have sex with women (WSW) have genital HPV.
  - 12% of WSW report genital warts.
  - 25% of WSW report cervical abnormalities.
  - Vaccine rates in WSW have improved significantly but still well below the 80% goal of Healthy People 2020 target. WSW may not get vaccine due to perceived decreased risks.
- HIV—transmission between women is rare but possible. WSW are more likely to have sexual contact with men having sex with men (MSM) than heterosexual women.
- STI screening and prevention
  - Screen based on woman's history.
  - Encourage safer sex practices:
    - Avoid menstrual blood/open sores.
    - Dental dams for oral sex, condoms on sex toys, and cleaning immediately after use
    - Vinyl/latex gloves for manual sex, limit friction with lubricants
- Psychosocial considerations
  - Sexual abuse
    - 3 times more likely than heterosexual women to report having been sexually assaulted
    - 43% of lesbians reported at least one sexual assault in their lifetime.
    - History of childhood sexual abuse can be associated with more complicated and difficult "coming out."
  - Intimate partner violence: National Coalition Against Domestic Violence reports 43.8% of lesbians have experienced rape, physical violence, and/or stalking by an intimate partner.
  - Parenthood: A reported 41% of lesbians desire to have a child. Perinatal depression is common and may be more common than in heterosexual women.
    - >30% have biologic children.
      - Often from previous heterosexual relationship
      - Adoption
      - Assisted reproductive technology/donor insemination
      - Some will engage in high-risk sexual behaviors (MSM, "one-night stand") in an attempt to get pregnant.
      - Providers should discuss parenting with their lesbian patients.
      - Encourage both partners or nonbiologic parent to adopt child to ensure permanent legal relationship to child.
      - Discuss durable power of attorney for health care and finances in the event of death or separation.
      - Adolescents who have been reared in lesbian mother families since birth demonstrate healthy psychological adjustment.
      - Children raised by same-sex parents have similar academic performance levels as their peers raised by different-sex parents.

- Adolescent lesbians
  - Increased risk for eating disorders
  - Higher rates of substance use particularly polysubstance abuse
  - If also having sexual contact with males, higher rates of pregnancy compared to heterosexual counterparts due to (2)
    - High rates of early sexual initiation
    - Greater number of partners
    - Less contraceptive use
  - Higher rates of physical and/or sexual abuse—childhood sexual abuse does not cause children to become LGBTQ.
- Aging lesbians
  - Elders aging "back into the closet"
    - Discrimination by religious and other groups that own nursing homes
    - Fear of discrimination by caregivers/health care workers
    - Few elder care programs specifically directed at LGBT persons

 TREATMENT

GENERAL MEASURES

- Create a safe practice environment for lesbian patients.
  - Have nondiscrimination policy posted where it is visible to patients.
  - Educate staff to be comfortable dealing with the needs of lesbian patients and their families.
  - Brochures/photos should feature both same-sex and heterosexual couples.
  - Intake forms should include options for patient to indicate sexual preference and include options for partnered status.
  - Use "gender-neutral" language. For example, "Do you have a significant other?"
  - Avoid heterosexist assumptions ("What do you use for birth control?" asking instead "Do you plan to become pregnant or have a child? Do you need birth control?").
- Ask about sexual orientation.
  - Many physicians do not ask.
  - Intake/annual physical forms should include questions about orientation/activity.
  - Twice as likely to identify as a sexual minority if questions asked in an indirect way
- Take a detailed sexual history.
  - Sexual identity and sexual behaviors are not always strongly correlated.
  - Ask about behaviors ("Do you have sex with women, men, or both?"); do not just assume current/past sexual activity with women.
  - STI screening based on reported history/activity
  - Address contraception when appropriate.
  - Some physicians may create barriers by believing a patient's sexual self-identity and behaviors are not pertinent to competent care (3).
- Respect the partners.
  - Treat them as you would to any other spouse/partner.
  - Assure access if partner is hospitalized.
  - Recommend durable power of attorney if couple is not legally married.

- Follow same preventive screening guidelines and lifestyle recommendations as for heterosexual women (Pap smear, mammography, colonoscopy screening, safer sex, exercise, diet, alcohol moderation, and tobacco avoidance).
- Legal/U.S. government
  - Healthy People 2010 identified lesbian/gay Americans as 1 of 6 population groups affected by health care disparities.
  - Healthy People 2020 goals are to increase routine data collection efforts on LGBT populations via health care surveys
    - Questions about sexual orientation and gender identity were added to many population surveys.
  - Healthy People 2030 focus is on collecting data on specific health needs of LGBT population and improving health in LGBT adolescents.
    - The goal is to add questions about gender and sexual identity on more state and national surveys.
- Access to health insurance was increased with supreme court decisions on *United States v. Windsor* in 2013 and *Obergefell v. Hodges* in 2015. Some states still recognize same-sex civil union, but access to health insurance varies by state.
- Affordable Care Act (ACA): prohibits discrimination based on sexual orientation in any program receiving federal funds (Medicare/Medicaid); increased emphasis on research and data collections in LGBT population; National Health Interview Survey (NHIS); In 2013, the survey added a question about sexual orientation.

REFERENCES

1. Frost DM, Lehavot K, Meyer IH. Minority stress and physical health among sexual minority individuals. *J Behav Med*. 2015;38(1):1–8.
2. Committee on Adolescence. Office-based care for lesbian, gay, bisexual, transgender, and questioning youth. *Pediatrics*. 2013;132(1):198–203.
3. Knight DA, Jarrett D. Preventive health care for women who have sex with women. *Am Fam Physician*. 2017;95(5):314–321.

 CODES

ICD10
- E66.3 Overweight
- Z72.0 Tobacco use
- F10.10 Alcohol abuse, uncomplicated

CLINICAL PEARLS

Create a safe health care environment for all patients. Use gender-neutral language. Do not assume heterosexuality or sexual practices.

L

LEUKEMIA, ACUTE LYMPHOBLASTIC (ALL) IN ADULTS

Afsha Rais Kaisani, MD • Tasaduq Hussain Mir, MD, FAAFP

 BASICS

Acute lymphoblastic leukemia (ALL) results from abnormal proliferation of hematopoietic stem cells in the bone marrow (1).

DESCRIPTION

ALL in adults is the result of a clonal proliferation, survival, and impaired differentiation of immature lymphocytes. These early lymphoid cells take the place of normal hematopoietic cells in the bone marrow, affecting any organ.

- The World Health Organization (WHO) defines ALL as the presence of ≥25% lymphoblasts in the bone marrow; the US uses ≥20% as the cutoff.
- ALL and lymphoblastic lymphoma (LBL) can arise from the same precursor cell lineage and be considered diseases along the same spectrum:
  - LBL presents as a mass, possibly, but not limited to, the mediastinum, with <25% blasts in the bone marrow.
  - ALL may present with a mass lesion but contains ≥25% bone marrow involvement.

Pregnancy Considerations
Many chemotherapy (CTX) drugs are teratogenic.

Pediatric Considerations
ALL is the most common malignancy in children: accounts for 30% of all pediatric malignancies and 80% of pediatric leukemias (see "Acute Lymphoblastic Leukemia, Pediatric") (1).

Geriatric Considerations
Patients aged >60 years with ALL have a 42% mortality during induction CTX. The cause of death is usually CTX-related complications or relapse. Survival is often reduced due to poor tolerance of CTX; thus, leading to dose reductions and ineffective medication delivery.

EPIDEMIOLOGY
Bimodal distribution: early peak around age of 5 years, second peak at around age of 50 years (2); 80% of cases occur in children, 20% in adults.

Incidence
- Incidence of ALL is 1.7/100,000 per year (2).
- In 2021, 5,690 new cases of ALL in the United States
- Higher incidence in older age, males, whites, those with history of radiation, CTX, or certain genetic disorders

Prevalence
Prevalence of ALL can range from 15% to 50% and increases with age.

ETIOLOGY AND PATHOPHYSIOLOGY
The pathophysiology of ALL involves the abnormal proliferation and differentiation of clonal lymphoid cells. These malignant cells proliferate and replace the bone marrow cells that would normally create red blood cells, neutrophils, and platelets; therefore, resulting in anemia, neutropenia, and thrombocytopenia.

Genetics
- Higher rates in monozygotic and dizygotic twins
- Increased risk of ALL with diseases related to chromosomal instability and inherited chromosomal abnormalities (2).

RISK FACTORS
- Age >70 years, radiation and CTX exposure, and infection with HIV (2).
- Human T-cell lymphotropic virus type 1 is associated with adult T-cell ALL.
- Epstein-Barr virus is associated with mature B-cell ALL.

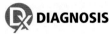 **DIAGNOSIS**

HISTORY
- Symptoms arise from sequelae of bone marrow suppression and/or from leukemic cell organ infiltration.
- B symptoms: fever, weight loss, night sweats
- Anemia: fatigue, shortness of breath, light-headedness, angina, headache, palpitations
- Thrombocytopenia: easy bruising or bleeding
- Neutropenia: fever, infection
- Lymphocytosis: joint pain
- CNS: confusion; meningeal infiltration and cranial nerve involvement occurs in 5%–8% of adults (1).

PHYSICAL EXAM
- Thrombocytopenia: petechiae, ecchymoses, epistaxis, retinal hemorrhages
- Anemia: pallor, flow murmur
- Neutropenia: fever, infections
- Lymphocytosis: lymphadenopathy; hepatosplenomegaly occurs in approximately 20% of adults (1).
- CNS: cranial nerve palsies, meningeal signs
- Extramedullary presentations in testis, skin or mediastinum.

DIFFERENTIAL DIAGNOSIS
- Malignant disorders: other leukemias, AML, chronic myeloid leukemia in lymphoid blast phase, prolymphocytic leukemia, malignant lymphomas; multiple myeloma, bone marrow metastases from solid tumors (breast, prostate, lung, renal), and myelodysplastic syndromes
- Nonmalignant disorders: aplastic anemia, myelofibrosis, autoimmune diseases (Felty syndrome, lupus), infectious mononucleosis, pertussis, autoimmune thrombocytopenic purpura, leukemoid reaction to infection

DIAGNOSTIC TESTS & INTERPRETATION
Initial Tests (lab, imaging)
- CBC with platelets and differential: evidence of leukocytosis, may also present with anemia and thrombocytopenia
- Coagulation studies (PT, PTT, fibrinogen)
- Peripheral blood smear: lymphoblasts (B cell or T cell) that vary in size
- Hepatitis B/C, HIV, CMV, HSV testing
- Pregnancy test in female patients; testicular examination and scrotal US if indicated in male patients
- HLA typing if post-treatment hematopoietic stem cell transplant might be indicated
- CT scan of the neck, chest, abdomen, and pelvis with IV contrast and PET/CT if suspicion of lymphomatous involvement

- CT/MRI of head with contrast if neurologic symptoms are present
- Evaluate patients for opportunistic infections.
- Blood cultures in patients with fever or suspected infection

Follow-Up Tests & Special Considerations
- Immunophenotyping of marrow/blood lymphoblasts: B lineage (CD19, CD20, CD22, CD24), T lineage (CD2, CD3, CD5, CD7), common ALL antigen (CD10); human leukocyte antigen (HLA)-DR, terminal deoxynucleotidyl transferase (TdT), aberrant myeloid antigens (CD13, CD33), and stem cell antigen (CD34).
- Cytochemical stains: myeloperoxidase negative; Sudan black B usually negative; TdT positive; periodic acid–Schiff ± is variable, depending on subtype
- Cytogenetics: Specific chromosomal abnormalities have independent diagnostic and prognostic significance.
- Reverse transcription polymerase chain reaction for rapid diagnosis of BCR/ABL1+ ALL
- Genomic analysis by next-generation sequencing: detection of mutations associated with Ph-like ALL
- HLA typing of patient and siblings for hematopoietic stem cell transplantation

Diagnostic Procedures/Other
- Bone marrow aspiration/biopsy with immunohistochemistry, immunophenotyping, cytogenetics, and molecular diagnostics
- Lymph node biopsy if available
- Lumbar puncture (LP) for CNS involvement and for intrathecal (IT) CTX. First LP should be performed at time of IT CTX unless symptomatic earlier. Repeat LP after bone marrow remission is achieved to evaluate occult CNS involvement.

Test Interpretation
Diagnosis is based on the presence of lymphoblasts (>20%) in the bone marrow. In some cases, the diagnosis can be made based on the presence of certain mutations, even if the percentage of blasts is lower. Bone marrow biopsy typically shows diffuse replacement of marrow and lymph node architecture by sheets of malignant lymphoblasts, T-cell or B-cell lineage determined by CD expression.

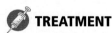 **TREATMENT**

GENERAL MEASURES
- Treatment of ALL determined by patient's age and presence of Philadelphia chromosome
- Three phases to CTX, given with CNS prophylaxis: induction, consolidation, prolonged maintenance

MEDICATION
- Induction; goal: Achieve complete remission and restore normal hematopoiesis.
  - Mainstay of treatment is a regimen called hyper-CVAD (HCVAD) (2)[A]. Hyperfractionated cyclophosphamide, vincristine, anthracycline, and dexamethasone, and is the most widely used regimen.

– HCVAD consists of eight alternating treatment cycles of parts A and B:
  - ○ Part A: HCVAD
  - ○ Part B: high-dose methotrexate and cytarabine
  - ○ Granulocyte colony-stimulating factors given after each cycle to prevent delay in treatment and hasten bone marrow recovery (2)[A].
  - ○ CNS prophylaxis: IT CTX consistent— methotrexate or cytarabine or 6-mercaptopurine (6-MP) (2)[A]
  - ○ CNS leukemia at diagnosis needs twice a week IT therapy until CSF is cleared on three subsequent LPs (2)[A].
- <40 years of age with complete remission after the first induction; the next step is either consolidation CTX or allogeneic stem cell transplant based on risk donor availability.
- Minimal residual disease (MRD), measured by flow cytometry in the US, signifies CTX refractory disease, usually in 8 months from start of treatment with continued CTX. These patients should be evaluated for an allogeneic bone marrow transplant (2)[A].

- Consolidation; goal: Eliminate residual leukemic cells after induction therapy.
  - Induction phase drugs are used; may vary according to treatment regimen selected and patient age
- Maintenance; goal: Prevent relapse and prolong remission.
  - Consist of POMP: daily 6-MP, weekly methotrexate, monthly vincristine, with pulses of prednisone for 2 to 3 years; little benefit has been shown for >3 years of prolonged maintenance (3)[A].
  - Dexamethasone can be substituted for prednisone, also known as DOMP.
- Special considerations
  - Besides HCVAD, some pediatric ALL regimens have shown superior remission outcomes for adults from aged 15 to 39 years. These usually contain vincristine and PEG-asparaginase, nonmyelosuppressive agents.
  - Allogeneic stem cell transplantation is recommended with relapsed ALL during the first remission or for high-risk genetic features.
  - Burkitt leukemia requires 18 weeks of treatment, has better outcomes with methotrexate.
  - Rituximab improves outcomes if CD20 expression is >20% of blast cells in ALL.
  - Immunotherapy: Bispecific anti-CD19/anti-CD3 antibody blinatumomab is approved for relapse/refractory ALL.
  - Ofatumumab: second-generation anti-CD20 monoclonal antibody, is an alternative frontline therapy for CD20+ pre-B-ALL and option for patients who failed a rituximab-based regimen.
  - Ph-positive ALL have improved prognosis with tyrosine kinase inhibitors (TKIs) targeting BCR-ABL1 translocation. Consolidation/maintenance with a TKI may be used instead of allogeneic stem cell transplant.

– Adult T-cell ALL is less common than B-cell ALL and has a relapse rate up to 50% with traditional HCVAD. Nelarabine, a T cell–specific purine nucleoside, is approved for relapsed T-cell ALL, with additional clinical trials studying a combination of HCVAD and nelarabine as part of induction therapy.
– Inotuzumab-ozogamicin (InO) combination: higher rates of complete remission and longer progression free and overall survival in patients with relapsed or refractory ALL compared to standard therapy

ISSUES FOR REFERRAL
Refer to hematologist oncologist for diagnosis confirmation and management (1).

SURGERY/OTHER PROCEDURES
In some centers, patients may undergo surgical placement of a port for CTX. PICC lines are preferred due to easy removal after treatment to decrease the risk of infections, which is important as patients can get neutropenic.

COMPLEMENTARY & ALTERNATIVE MEDICINE
Unproven

ADMISSION, INPATIENT, AND NURSING CONSIDERATIONS
Consider hospital admission in patients with febrile neutropenia.

 ONGOING CARE

Patients on CTX and radiation: annual physical, eye and dental exam; CXR, pulmonary function test, and audiometry as needed; baseline ECG every 2 to 5 years based on CTX used

FOLLOW-UP RECOMMENDATIONS
Age-appropriate vaccinations (avoid live vaccine during CTX); age and sex appropriate cancer screening

Patient Monitoring
- Inpatient admission during induction CTX for continuous infusion and monitoring of complications
- Weekly clinic visits with remission consolidation CTX
- Monthly clinic visits during maintenance therapy; every 3 months thereafter

DIET
Nutritional support; avoid alcohol; calcium/vitamin D for steroid-induced osteoporosis

PATIENT EDUCATION
Neutropenic precautions; physical rehabilitation for deconditioning; smoking cessation

PROGNOSIS
Prognosis is based on age, comorbidities, clinical presentation at time of diagnosis, and cytogenetic findings. Presence of MRD after induction is an independent marker of poor prognosis (2). About 80–90% of adults aged <60 years will achieve a complete remission; however, only 40–50% will remain cured due to relapses. Only 30–40% of adults have a 5-year overall survival as opposed to in children.

COMPLICATIONS
- Hyperleukocytosis: WBC >50,000 to 100,000 can lead to leukostasis, a medical emergency with microvascular white cell plugs; presents with neurologic deficits or respiratory distress, treated with fluids, and cytoreductive therapy
- Tumor lysis syndrome (high uric acid, potassium, and phosphate and low calcium, leading to renal failure and cardiac arrhythmias) may be prevented by administering allopurinol prior to CTX. Doses should be reduced if used with mercaptopurine or azathioprine. Increase fluids; IV urate oxidase (rasburicase) can be used to treat hyperuricemia rapidly (if not G6PD deficient).
- Neutropenia from myelosuppression
- High-dose cyclophosphamide: severe nausea and vomiting; use appropriate antiemetic regimen.
- Vincristine can cause neurotoxicity and ileus.
- Alkylating agents and corticosteroids can cause AVN or osteonecrosis.
- Steroid-induced hyperglycemia
- Anthracyclines causes cardiotoxicity; obtain transthoracic echocardiography before HCVAD initiation and monitor left ventricular ejection fraction during the course of treatment.
- Asparaginase therapy increases risks for deep vein thromboses and veno-occlusive disease.
- Infections (pneumocystis pneumonia, bacterial and fungal pneumonia or sepsis)
- CTX can cause sterility, pancreatitis and liver dysfunction, arachnoiditis and CNS effects.
- Relapse of ALL in marrow or extramedullary sites (CNS, testis)

REFERENCES
1. Gbenjo JTC, McCrary GLM, Wilson SE. Leukemia: what primary care physicians need to know. *Am Fam Physician*. 2023;107(4):397–405.
2. Paul S, Kantarjian H, Jabbour EJ. Adult acute lymphoblastic leukemia. *Mayo Clin Proc*. 2016;91(11):1645–1666.
3. Jabbour E, O'Brien S, Konopleva M, et al. New insights into the pathophysiology and therapy of adult acute lymphoblastic leukemia. *Cancer*. 2015;121(15):2517–2528.

 CODES

ICD10
- C91.00 Acute lymphoblastic leukemia not having achieved remission
- C91.01 Acute lymphoblastic leukemia, in remission
- C91.02 Acute lymphoblastic leukemia, in relapse

CLINICAL PEARLS
- ALL diagnosis is based on the presence of lymphoblasts or characteristic mutations in the bone marrow.
- HCVAD is the main therapy.
- Treatment at an appropriate cancer center for tailored therapy based on mutations in ALL cells.
- Patients need to be monitored closely for CTX toxicities and progression of disease.

L

LEUKEMIA, ACUTE MYELOID

Jan Cerny, MD, PhD

 BASICS

DESCRIPTION

- Acute myeloid leukemia (AML) is characterized by proliferation of abnormal immature myeloid progenitors (blasts) with reduced capacity to differentiate leading to bone marrow failure and a variety of systemic symptoms.
- Historically, the French–American–British (FAB) classification system divided AML based on the cell morphology with the addition of cytogenetics (subtypes M0 to M7).
- The World Health Organization (WHO) classifications attempt to provide more meaningful prognostic information.
  - AML with defining genetic abnormalities:
    - Translocation in t(8;21) RUNX1-RUNX1T1 fusion, t(9;11) KMT2A, t(6;9) DEK-NUP214, t(1;22) RBM15-MRTFA, t(15;17) APL with PML-RARA fusion
    - Inversion in chromosome 16 inv(16) CBFB-MYH11, Inv(3) MECOM
    - Other defined genetic alterations
  - AML, myelodysplasia related: presence of a prior myelodysplastic syndrome (MDS) or myeloproliferative neoplasm (MPN) that transformed into AML
  - Myeloid neoplasms post cytotoxic therapy: AML, MDS, and MDS/MPN exposed to cytotoxic therapy
  - Myeloid neoplasms associated with germline predisposition: Down syndrome, Fanconi anemia, RASopathies
  - Acute leukemias of mixed or ambiguous lineage (*biphenotypic acute leukemia*)
  - Myeloid sarcoma

EPIDEMIOLOGY

- New cases in men and women is 4.1 per 100,000 per year.
- Male ≥ female

Incidence

The incidence of AML increases with age, and median age is 67 years.

Prevalence

~20,050 cases estimated in 2022, making it the most common type of leukemia in adults

ETIOLOGY AND PATHOPHYSIOLOGY

Genetics

- Three risk groups
  - Good risk: inv(16), t(8;21), t(15;17)
  - Standard risk: normal karyotype
  - Poor risk: monosomy 5 and 7 (typically secondary AML), deletion 5q, abnormalities of 11q23 or complex karyotype
- *FLT3* gene mutations, especially internal tandem duplications (FLT3-ITD), have been associated with poor survival in AML. These and growing list of (onco)gene (e.g., *NPM1*, *IDH1/2*, *DNMT3A*, and *P53*) mutations have been studied to further risk-stratify patients (1).

RISK FACTORS

- Genetic predisposition (e.g., Down syndrome); Bloom syndrome (~25% develop AML), Fanconi anemia (52%), neurofibromatosis, Li-Fraumeni syndrome, Wiskott-Aldrich syndrome, Kostmann syndrome, and Diamond-Blackfan anemia
- Radiation exposure

- Immunodeficiency states
- Chemical and drug exposure (nitrogen mustard and alkylating agents; benzene)
- MDS
- Cigarette smoking

GENERAL PREVENTION

Treatment of high-risk MDS with hypomethylating agents (5-azacitidine [Vidaza]) may prolong time to transformation from MDS into AML

COMMONLY ASSOCIATED CONDITIONS

- Disseminated intravascular coagulopathy (DIC) especially in acute promyelocytic leukemia (APL) but may be seen in any AML
- Leukostasis (high blast number and increased adhesive ability of blasts)
- Tumor lysis syndrome (TLS): spontaneous or in response to chemotherapy

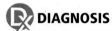 **DIAGNOSIS**

HISTORY

Fatigue (anemia or tumor burden); bleeding (low platelets or DIC); difficulty clearing infections (neutropenia or immune dysregulation)

PHYSICAL EXAM

- Mostly nonspecific and related to marrow or tissue infiltration
  - Fever, bleeding, pallor, splenomegaly, hepatosplenomegaly
  - Lymphadenopathy (usually reactive)
- If CNS is involved, symptoms of increased intracranial pressure can be present.
- Occasionally, patients will present with prominent extramedullary sites of leukemia (e.g., skin infiltration or ultimately as a myeloid sarcoma).

DIFFERENTIAL DIAGNOSIS

- Virus-induced cytopenia, lymphadenopathy, and organomegaly
- Immune cytopenias (including systemic lupus erythematosus [SLE])
- Drug-induced cytopenias
- Other marrow failure and infiltrative diseases (e.g., aplastic anemia, paroxysmal nocturnal hemoglobinuria, MDS, Gaucher disease)

DIAGNOSTIC TESTS & INTERPRETATION

- CBC shows subnormal RBCs, neutrophils, and platelets.
- Bone marrow for histology, flow cytometry, and cytogenetics to establish diagnosis and prognosis
- ESR
- Lactate dehydrogenase (LDH) and uric acid can be elevated (e.g., TLS).
- Coagulation profile can be normal or prolonged (e.g., DIC).
- Lumbar puncture for leukemic cells
- Ultrasonography or CT scan of the abdomen may discover organomegaly.

Diagnostic Procedures/Other

Bone marrow studies are usually necessary to make the diagnosis.

- Aspirates: for cell morphology, cytochemistries, immunophenotyping (can confirm differentiation stage of AML); cytogenetics: chromosomal aberration (prognostic value; see "Genetics")

Test Interpretation

- Marrow is usually hypercellular and the normal architecture effaced; leukemic blast count is ≥20%. Newer updates no longer require >20% blast count for AML type with defining genetic abnormalities.
- Liver and spleen may be infiltrated with leukemic cells.

 TREATMENT

- Classical (cytotoxic) chemotherapy has been the backbone of AML therapy; it consists of induction and consolidation phase ± maintenance (APL), but more recently, other transplant-ineligible AML patients can be treated with hypomethylating agent (oral) azacytidine.
- Bone marrow transplantation (BMT) for high-risk AML
- Relatively modest improvements have been made in AML induction chemotherapy. Supportive care had improved significantly.

GENERAL MEASURES

- Close monitoring of bone marrow, liver, heart, renal function, and coagulation parameters (risk for DIC)
- Supportive therapy with
  - Good hydration
  - Transfusions of packed RBCs and platelets based on patient's needs (threshold as for platelets as low as 5,000); use leukoreduced, irradiated blood products because all patients can be considered for BMT.
  - Avoid antiplatelet agents (e.g., aspirin products).
  - Follow febrile neutropenic guidelines in neutropenic patient who becomes febrile (even low-grade fever).

Geriatric Considerations

- Older patients (>60 to 65 years of age) remain a therapeutic challenge. These patients are offered so-called reduced-intensity or nonmyeloablative BMT.
- Adding growth factors (granulocyte colony-stimulating factor [G-CSF]) may reduce toxicity in older patients (but is not broadly accepted).
- Hypomethylating agent, such as 5-azacitidine or decitabine, with or without venetoclax have been broadly adopted and prolong survival in older adults ineligible for classical chemotherapy.

Pregnancy Considerations

Chemotherapy is a viable option in the 2nd and 3rd trimesters.

MEDICATION

First Line

- APL (APL, AML with t[15;17])
  - All-trans retinoic acid (ATRA) and arsenic trioxide both promote maturation to granulocytes. Their combination can be used in low and intermediate risk APL for (chemotherapy) free treatment.
  - Idarubicin is often added to induction therapy in high-risk group.
  - Monoclonal anti-CD33 (Myelotarg) is being added as well in order to minimize chemotherapy use in this curable leukemia.

- Treatment of AML in younger adults: AML (other than APL)
  - Induction (daunorubicin or idarubicin [anthracycline and cytarabine]): The generally accepted combination is 3 + 7 (anthracycline is given for 3 days and cytarabine for 7 days) or more intensive regimens with high-dose cytarabine (HiDAC) or high dose of anthracycline.
  - Liposomal preparation of daunorubicin and cytarabine (Vyxeos) is now available for AML with MDS changes or therapy-related AML.
- Remission is typically consolidated in younger patients by the following:
  - In good-risk AML, 3 to 4 cycles of HiDAC and BMT are reserved for time of recurrence.
  - In poor-risk patients, 1 to 2 cycles of HiDAC (until donor is identified) are followed by allogeneic BMT.
  - Intermediate-risk AML should be treated based on individual patient's features, donor availability, and access to clinical trials. A meta-analysis showed that even intermediate-risk patients benefit from allogeneic BMT.
- Treatment of AML in older adults (>65 years of age) remains a challenge. These patients have poor performance status, more likely secondary AML, higher incidence of unfavorable cytogenetics, comorbidities, shorter remissions, and shorter overall survival. Liposomal daunorubicin and cytarabine is an agent approved for secondary and therapy-related AML.
  - Intensive chemotherapy may be feasible for patients with good performance status; alternative regimens with mitoxantrone, fludarabine, and clofarabine
  - Newly diagnosed patients who are ≥75 years old or who have conditions that preclude them from receiving intense induction therapy have the following options of novel (targeted) agents:
    - Low-dose cytarabine with glasdegib (DAURISMO, Pfizer Labs)
    - Hypomethylating agents (azacytidine [Vidaza], decitabine [Dacogen]) with ivosideni b (Tibsovo; IDH1 inhibitor)
    - Hypomethylating agents (azacytidine [Vidaza], decitabine [Dacogen]) with venetoclax (Venclexta; BCL-2 inhibitor)
- FLT-3 inhibitors such as midostaurin (Rydapt) are approved as addition to induction and consolidation chemotherapy, and gilteritinib (Xospata) is approved for relapsed/refractory AML.
- Ivosidenib (Tibsovo; IDH1 inhibitor) and enasidenib (Idhifa; IDH2 inhibitor) are approved for relapsed/refractory AML. Both of these agents can cause differentiation syndrome similar to the one seen in ATRA or arsenic-treated APL patients.
- Precautions
  - If organ failure, some drugs may be avoided or dose reduced (e.g., no anthracyclines in patients with preexisting cardiac problems).
  - Patients will be immunosuppressed during treatment. Avoid live vaccines. Administer varicella-zoster or measles immunoglobulin as soon as exposure of patient occurs.

- Significant possible interactions: Allopurinol accentuates the toxicity of 6-mercaptopurine.
- Targeted therapies: midostaurin for AML with FLT3 mutations (both ITD and TKD); ivosidenib (IDH1 inhibitor) and enasidenib (IDH2 inhibitor) for relapsed/refractory AML with respective IDH mutations; gemtuzumab ozogamicin (anti-CD33 monoclonal antibody) for relapsed/refractory AML with CD33 expression

Second Line
- Healthy, younger patients are usually offered reinduction chemotherapy and allogeneic BMT.
- Older patients would receive hypomethylating agent with or without venetoclax or targeted agent (FLT3 or IDH 1/2 inhibitor).

SURGERY/OTHER PROCEDURES
- BMT: Decision between myeloablative and nonmyeloablative approach should be based on patient's performance status, comorbidities, and AML risk factors.
  - Allogeneic BMT is usually indicated in first remission in intermediate- or high-risk AML or in second remission in all other AML patients; matched related donor used to be preferred over matched unrelated donor (lower risk of graft vs. host disease); recent data suggest equal outcomes because allogeneic transplant regimens and post-transplant care have improved significantly.
- Haploidentical transplants and cord blood have emerged as alternative sources of hematopoietic stem cells for adults that show comparable outcomes as well.
- Autologous BMT may be acceptable in specific situations (e.g., no donor is available).

ADMISSION, INPATIENT, AND NURSING CONSIDERATIONS
- Induction treatment for AML requires inpatient care, usually on a specialized ward. Episodes of febrile neutropenia typically require admission and IV antibiotics.
- Appropriate hydration to prevent TLS
- IV may lead to chemical burns in the event of extravasation.

 ## ONGOING CARE

FOLLOW-UP RECOMMENDATIONS
Patient Monitoring
- Repeat bone marrow studies to document remission and also if a relapse is suspected.
- Follow CBC with differential, coagulation studies, uric acid level, and other chemistries related to TLS (creatinine, potassium, phosphate, calcium); monitor urinary function at least daily during induction phase and less frequently later.
- Physical evaluation, including weight and BP, should be done frequently during treatment.

DIET
Total parenteral nutrition (TPN) in case of severe mucositis

PATIENT EDUCATION
Leukemia & Lymphoma Society: https://www.lls.org/leukemia

PROGNOSIS
AML remission rate is 60–80%, with only 20–40% long-term survival. The wide variable prognosis is due to prognostic group (age, cytogenetics, and genetics).

COMPLICATIONS
- Acute side effects of chemotherapy, including febrile neutropenia
- TLS
- DIC
- Late-onset cardiomyopathy in patients treated with anthracyclines
- Chronic side effects of chemotherapy (secondary malignancies)
- Graft versus host disease in patients who have received allogeneic BMT

REFERENCE
1. Döhner H, Wei AH, Appelbaum FR, et al. Diagnosis and management of AML in adults: 2022 recommendations from an international expert panel on behalf of the ELN. *Blood*. 2022;140(12): 1345–1377.

 ### SEE ALSO

Disseminated Intravascular Coagulation; Leukemia, Acute Lymphoblastic (ALL) in Adults; Leukemia, Chronic Myelogenous; Myelodysplastic Syndromes (MDS); Myeloproliferative Neoplasms

CODES

ICD10
- C92.00 Acute myeloblastic leukemia, not having achieved remission
- C92.01 Acute myeloblastic leukemia, in remission
- C92.02 Acute myeloblastic leukemia, in relapse

CLINICAL PEARLS
- AML is a proliferation and accumulation of abnormal immature myeloid progenitors (blasts) with reduced capacity to differentiate into more mature cellular elements. This leads to bone marrow failure and results in a variety of systemic symptoms.
- AML is the most common leukemia in adults.
- Prognosis of leukemia depends on the cytogenetic and molecular profile of the disease.
- Allogeneic transplant remains the only therapy with curative potential for patients with intermediate- and high-risk AML.

L

LEUKEMIA, CHRONIC LYMPHOCYTIC

Jan Cerny, MD, PhD • Michael Haddadin, MD

BASICS

DESCRIPTION
- Chronic lymphocytic leukemia (CLL) is a monoclonal disorder characterized by a progressive accumulation of mature but functionally incompetent lymphocytes.
- Based on percentage of prolymphocytes, the disease may be regarded as CLL (<10% prolymphocytes), prolymphocytic leukemia (PLL; >55%), or CLL/PLL (>10% and <55%).
- Small lymphocytic lymphoma is a lymphoma variant of CLL.
- System(s) affected: hematologic, lymphatic, immunologic

EPIDEMIOLOGY
Incidence
- CLL represents the most common form of leukemia in adults in the United States (2021 incidence of 21,050).
- Second leading cause of death among adults with leukemia in the United States after acute myeloid leukemia
- CLL primarily affects elderly individuals, with median age of diagnosis being 70 years.
- Predominant sex: male > female (1.6:1); higher among Caucasians

ETIOLOGY AND PATHOPHYSIOLOGY
- The cell of origin in CLL is a clonal B cell arrested in the B-cell differentiation pathway, intermediate between pre–B cells and mature B cells. In the peripheral blood, these cells resemble mature lymphocytes.
- Genetic mutations leading to disrupted function and prolonged survival of affected lymphocytes are suspected but are not well known. The BCL2 proto-oncogene (suppressor of apoptosis or programmed cell death) is overexpressed in CLL.

Genetics
Familial cases are rare. CLL does occur at higher frequency among first-degree relatives of patients with the disease, and several somatic gene mutations have been identified at significantly higher rates among CLL patients (1).

RISK FACTORS
Uncertain; possible chronic immune stimulation is suspected; monoclonal B-cell lymphocytosis: 1% risk progression to CLL

COMMONLY ASSOCIATED CONDITIONS
- Immune system dysregulation is common.
- Autoimmune hemolytic anemia (AIHA)
- Immune thrombocytopenia purpura (ITP)
- Pure red cell aplasia (PRCA)

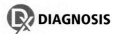**DIAGNOSIS**

HISTORY
- CLL is often discovered incidentally (up to 40% of patients are asymptomatic at the time of diagnosis).
- Others may have the following symptoms:
  - B symptoms: fevers, night sweats, >10% weight loss
  - Fatigue and/or other symptoms of anemia

- Enlarged lymph nodes (lymphadenopathy = LAD)
- Mucocutaneous bleeding and/or petechiae
- Early satiety and/or abdominal discomfort related to an enlarged spleen, rarely enlarged liver
- Recurrent infection(s)

PHYSICAL EXAM
- Lymphadenopathy (localized or generalized)
- Organomegaly (splenomegaly, hepatomegaly)
- Mucocutaneous bleeding (thrombocytopenia)
- Skin: petechiae (thrombocytopenia), pallor (anemia), rash (leukemia cutis)

DIFFERENTIAL DIAGNOSIS
- Infectious:
  - Bacterial (tuberculosis, pertussis)
  - Viral (mononucleosis)
- Neoplastic:
  - Leukemic phase of non-Hodgkin lymphomas
  - Hairy cell leukemia
  - PLL
  - Large granular lymphocytic leukemia
  - Waldenstrom macroglobulinemia

DIAGNOSTIC TESTS & INTERPRETATION
Initial Tests (lab, imaging)
- CBC with differential: B cell absolute lymphocytosis with >5,000 B lymphocytes/μL; often also shows anemia and/or thrombocytopenia in advanced stage
- Blood smear: ruptured lymphocytes ("smudge" cells) and morphologically small mature-appearing lymphocytes
- Confirm with immunophenotyping on peripheral blood via flow cytometry or lymph node biopsy: CLL cells are positive for CD19, CD20 (dim), CD23, and CD5; low levels of surface membrane immunoglobulin (Ig)—either IgM or IgM&D; only a single Ig light chain is expressed (κ or λ) confirming monoclonality. CLL cells are also negative for Cyclin-D1.
- Additional labs:
  - Hemolysis labs (in cases associated with high disease activity or AIHA): high LDH and indirect bilirubin, low haptoglobin, +/− elevated reticulocyte count (bone marrow infiltration)
  - High plasma β_2-microglobulin (poor prognosis)
  - Hypogammaglobulinemia, low IgG level
- Liver/spleen ultrasound: not required for initial workup
- CT scan of chest/abdomen/pelvis: not necessary for staging but may identify compression of organs or internal structures from enlarged lymph nodes
- Positron emission tomography (PET) scan: not recommended unless Richter transformation (RT) is suspected

Diagnostic Procedures/Other
- Bone marrow biopsy: not performed routinely but may be helpful to assess etiology of cytopenia found in conjunction with CLL diagnosis
- Lymph node biopsy: Consider if lymph node(s) begins to rapidly enlarge in a patient with known CLL to assess for transformation to a high-grade lymphoma (RT), especially with fever, weight loss, and painful lymphadenopathy.

Test Interpretation
- Bone marrow biopsy aspirate usually shows >30% lymphocytes.
- Cytogenetics (fluorescence in situ hybridization) may show chromosomal changes, which are prognostic:
  - Unfavorable: del(17p) or TP53 mutation, del(11q), unmutated immunoglobulin heavy-chain variable (IGHV)
  - Neutral: normal, trisomy 12
  - Favorable: del(13q), mutated IGHV

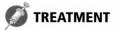**TREATMENT**

GENERAL MEASURES
- Patients with frequent infections due to hypogammaglobulinemia likely to benefit from infusions of intravenous immunoglobulin (IVIG).
- Genetic risk stratification in therapy selection for advanced or symptomatic CLL
  - Very high–risk disease: del(17p) and/or TP53 mutations
  - High-risk disease: IGHV unmutated (without 17p del or TP53 mutation)
  - Standard risk disease: IGHV mutated (without 17p del or TP53 mutation)
- Indications for treatment include constitutional (B) symptoms, cytopenias (thrombocytopenia, or anemia), or AIHA and/or thrombocytopenia poorly responsive to corticosteroids, progressive symptomatic organomegaly (splenomegaly, or lymphadenopathy), absolute lymphocyte doubling time (<6 months), or rarely extranodal involvement.

MEDICATION
First Line
- Standard of care for new diagnosis with no symptoms or early-stage disease: observation
- Low-risk disease, Rai stage 0: observation with periodic follow-up
- Intermediate-risk group, Rai stages I and II: Observe until evidence of disease progression or development of symptoms.
- High-risk patients, Rai stages III and IV: Initiate treatment. Selection of first-line therapy depends on patients' functional status (age, performance status, and medical comorbidities) as well as genetic risk stratification of their CLL (above).
- Main groups of therapeutic agents:
  - Targeted therapies: preferred especially for very high–risk and high-risk patients
    - Bruton tyrosine kinase (BTK) inhibitor: ibrutinib, acalabrutinib, and zanubrutinib
    - BCL2 inhibitor venetoclax
  - Immunotherapy:
    - Monoclonal anti-CD20 antibodies (immunotherapy): rituximab (R), obinutuzumab, ofatumumab
  - Chemotherapy:
    - Alkylators: cyclophosphamide (C), chlorambucil, and bendamustine (B)
    - Purine analogs: fludarabine (F), cladribine, and pentostatin (P)
- Ibrutinib or acalabrutinib (Newer agents have fewer side effects.) (2)

- 1st generation BTK inhibitor (Ibrutinib) is known for a wide variety of cardiac and pulmonary complications and increased risk of bleeding.
- Venetoclax in combination with obinutuzumab offers very effective regimens; fixed duration
- Combinations of BTK inhibitor and venetoclax are being evaluated for the possibility of time-limited treatment for CLL patients that achieved complete response at the molecular level.
- Combination regimens: FC, FR (lower toxicity), BR, PCR, and FCR are used less often, but FCR can offer time-limited and highly effective therapy in IGHV-mutated CLL; such chemotherapy agents increase the risk of myeloid malignancies in the long term.
- Steroids, high dose: useful in autoimmune manifestations of CLL (AIHA, ITP)

Second Line
- Second-line therapy depends on time to progression and previous therapy.
- Early relapse (within 1 year after chemoimmunotherapy, 2 to 3 years after FCR), treatment with targeted therapy is favored.
  – Alternative BTK inhibitor
  – Venetoclax: as monotherapy and with rituximab in relapsed/refractory CLL and in patients with 17p del (2)
  – PI3K kinase inhibitors: idelalisib (PI3Kδ) with rituximab in patients with comorbidities; duvelisib (PI3Kδ and PI3Kγ): approved as single agent for patients (PJP prophylaxis is recommended.) (2)
    ○ PI3K inhibitors are known for many adverse events and are rarely used; hyperglycemia, hepatotoxicity, pneumonitis, and diarrhea; these agents received initially an accelerated approval, and they are currently intensively scrutinized for their safety and long-term outcome.
  – Obinutuzumab alone or with chlorambucil in patients with comorbidities and previously untreated CLL, ofatumumab
- Other options:
  – Lenalidomide, a thalidomide derivative, can be useful in some situations.
- Allogenic (nonmyeloablative conditioning) stem cell transplant (hSCT) may be considered in high-risk and younger patients, particularly those with refractory or RT.
- On the contrary to other non-Hodgkin lymphoma, chimeric antigen receptor T (CAR-T) cells are still in investigational phase as therapies for CLL.

ISSUES FOR REFERRAL
- Surgical consultation for splenectomy in patients with progressive splenomegaly +/− refractory cytopenias
- Radiation oncology consultation for large or bulky lymphadenopathy, particularly those causing compressive symptoms

ADDITIONAL THERAPIES
- Patients at high risk for tumor lysis syndrome (TLS) should be given allopurinol to prevent uric acid nephropathy.
- Patients would require prophylactic antibiotics when they start treatment; PJP and HSV prophylaxis

- Rapid reduction in white blood cell count is sometimes warranted in cases of leukostasis (WBC $>400 \times 10^9$/L).
- Vaccinations (avoid live vaccines):
  – Annual influenza vaccine
  – Pneumococcal vaccine every 5 years
  – Zoster vaccine recombinant, adjuvanted for treatment-naïve patients, or those treated with BTK inhibitor
  – COVID-19 vaccination

ADMISSION, INPATIENT, AND NURSING CONSIDERATIONS
Complications of disease (AIHA) or of therapy (febrile neutropenia, TLS); venetoclax can be associated with TLS and monitoring inpatient may be needed.

ONGOING CARE

FOLLOW-UP RECOMMENDATIONS
Patient Monitoring
Patients with low-risk CLL and/or patients in remission:
- CBC with differential (lymphocytosis), LDH, and β_2-microglobulin every 3 to 6 months
- Physical exam (lymphadenopathy, organomegaly)

PATIENT EDUCATION
Leukemia and Lymphoma Society has educational pamphlets: https://www.lls.org/resource-center/download-or-order-free-publications?language=English&category=Leukemia&sortby=alpha

PROGNOSIS
- Rai system used in the Unites States and Binet system in Europe; International Prognostic Score for Early-Stage CLL (IPS-E) for predicting time to first treatment
- Rai staging system:
  – Stage 0: lymphocytosis only; low-risk status
  – Stage I: lymphocytosis and adenopathy; intermediate-risk status
  – Stage II: lymphocytosis +/− adenopathy and splenomegaly and/or hepatomegaly; intermediate-risk status
  – Stage III: lymphocytosis and anemia (hemoglobin <11 g/dL); high-risk status
  – Stage IV: lymphocytosis and thrombocytopenia (platelets $<100 \times 10^9$/L); high-risk status
- IPS-E is helpful to identify patients who are at risk of needed therapy sooner.
  – The IPS-E score is calculated by giving 1 point for each of the following:
    ○ Unmutated IGHV
    ○ Lymphocytes $>15 \times 10^9$/L
    ○ Palpable lymph nodes
    ○ A score of 0 indicated low risk, 1 intermediate risk, and 2 to 3 high risk of progressing to symptomatic disease requiring treatment. More than half of the high-risk group would require treatment within 5 years of their diagnosis.

- Adverse risk factors:
  – Advanced stage, peripheral lymphocyte doubling time <12 months, diffuse marrow infiltration, increased number of prolymphocytes or cleaved cells, poor response to chemotherapy, high β_2-microglobulin and thymidine kinase levels and low micro RNAs (miRNAs), abnormal karyotyping: del(17p) and del(11q), mutated IGHV genes (expression of ZAP-70 $>20\%$ or CD38 $>30\%$ evaluated by immunophenotyping are surrogate markers.), NOTCH1 mutation (associated with unmutated IGHV), increased Cumulative Illness Rating Scale (CIRS)

COMPLICATIONS
Acute or long-term effects of chemotherapy and targeted therapy, RT, AIHA (fludarabine) slightly increased risk of solid tumors (Kaposi sarcoma, malignant melanoma, laryngeal, lung and colon cancer), increased risk of infections, impaired immune system, membranoproliferative glomerulonephritis (MPGN), leukostasis, and TLS.

REFERENCES
1. Yan H, Tian S, Kleinstern G, et al. Chronic lymphocytic leukemia (CLL) risk is mediated by multiple enhancer variants within CLL risk loci. *Hum Mol Genet*. 2020;29(16):2761–2774.
2. Burger JA. Treatment of chronic lymphocytic leukemia. *N Engl J Med*. 2020;383(5):460–473.

CODES

ICD10
- C91.12 Chronic lymphocytic leukemia of B-cell type in relapse
- C91.11 Chronic lymphocytic leukemia of B-cell type in remission
- C91.10 Chronic lymphocytic leukemia of B-cell type not having achieved remission

CLINICAL PEARLS
- CLL is the most common form of leukemia in adults in the United States.
- CLL primarily affects elderly individuals, median age of diagnosis being 70 years. Incidence continues to rise in those aged >55 years.
- Clinical monitoring of asymptomatic and low-risk patients is a reasonable approach ("watch and wait").
- CLL patients needs to be up-to-date with vaccines for immunocompromised patients and need annual skin surveillance.
- High-risk patients, patients with bulky disease, and patients who fail their first line of treatment typically have a poorer prognoses and may require intensive therapies, including allogeneic hematopoietic stem cell transplantation.
- Several novel agents are being developed to improve therapeutic approaches to CLL.

L

LEUKEMIA, CHRONIC MYELOGENOUS

Jan Cerny, MD, PhD • Erin Thomas, MD, BS

BASICS

DESCRIPTION
- Chronic myelogenous leukemia (CML) is a myeloproliferative neoplasm characterized by clonal proliferation of myeloid precursors in the bone marrow with continuing differentiation into mature granulocytes.
- The hallmark of CML is the Philadelphia chromosome (translocation t[9;22]).
- Natural history of the disease evolves in three clinical phases: a chronic phase, an accelerated phase, and a blast phase or crisis (can transform to acute myeloid leukemia [80%] or acute lymphoblastic leukemia [20%]).

EPIDEMIOLOGY
Incidence
- Per year, 1.9 cases/100,000 persons
- Median age at Diagnosis: 65
- Predominant sex: male > female (1.7:1)

Prevalence
Accounts for 15–20% of adult leukemias

ETIOLOGY AND PATHOPHYSIOLOGY
Philadelphia chromosome is a balanced translocation between *BCR* (on chromosome 22) and *ABL* (on chromosome 9) genes t(9;22)(q34;q11). This fusion gene, *BCR-ABL*, codes for an abnormal, constitutively active tyrosine kinase that affects numerous signal transduction pathways, resulting in uncontrolled cell proliferation and reduced apoptosis.

Genetics
Acquired genomic changes

RISK FACTORS
Ionizing radiation exposure (uncommon)

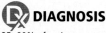

DIAGNOSIS

85–90% of patients present in the chronic phase, and the disease can be found incidentally during routine screening (up to 50%).

HISTORY
- Chronic phase: fatigue, weight loss, night sweats, abdominal fullness owing to enlarged spleen, early satiety, dyspnea, and bleeding; rare: bruising, left upper quadrant abdominal pain, sternal pain (owing to expanding bone marrow), and gouty arthritis; up to 30% of patients are asymptomatic.
- Accelerated phase: progressive splenomegaly and left upper quadrant abdominal pain occasionally referred to the left shoulder (owing to splenic infarction or rupture), progressive weight loss and sweats, unexplained fever or bone pain, chloromas (extramedullary tumors)
- Blast phase: bleeding, bruising, infections, lymphadenopathy, prominent constitutional symptoms

PHYSICAL EXAM
- Splenomegaly (50–90%), hepatomegaly (<10%)
- Less common: splenic friction rub, lymphadenopathy, lower sternal tenderness

DIFFERENTIAL DIAGNOSIS
- Chronic myelomonocytic leukemia, chronic neutrophilic leukemia, chronic eosinophilic leukemia, juvenile myelomonocytic leukemia, infectious mononucleosis, leukemoid reaction, polycythemia vera, and treatment with granulocyte-stimulating factors
- Acute myelogenous leukemia resembles blast crisis with myeloid blasts, and acute lymphoblastic leukemia resembles blast crisis with lymphoid blasts.
- Atypical CML is a chronic myeloproliferative disorder with a clinical hematologic picture similar to CML, but it lacks the Philadelphia chromosome and *BCR-ABL* rearrangement. A hallmark feature is dysplastic granulopoiesis.

DIAGNOSTIC TESTS & INTERPRETATION
- CBC
  - WBC count: markedly increased (50,000 to 100,000/μL), with granulocytes in all stages of maturation, including occasional (<10%) blasts in chronic phase, basophilia, eosinophilia
  - Hematocrit: may be normal, slightly increased, or decreased
  - Platelets: may be normal, elevated, or occasionally low
  - In accelerated phase: anemia, >20% basophils, thrombocytopenia
- Bone marrow biopsy: hypercellular marrow, myeloid hyperplasia; in accelerated phase: 10–19% blasts, ≥20% blasts in blood or marrow indicates blast phase
- Genetics
  - Demonstration of the Philadelphia chromosome, t(9;22), by cytogenetic techniques, fluorescence in situ hybridization (FISH), or reverse transcription-polymerase chain reaction (RT-PCR)
  - Additional cytogenetic abnormalities occur in the accelerated and blast phases (monosomy 7; t[3,21]; trisomies 8 and 19; Philadelphia chromosome duplication; abnormalities of chromosome 17 such as monosomy, trisomy, and isochromosome mutations). These may contribute to resistance to tyrosine kinase inhibitors (TKIs; e.g., imatinib). Further molecular testing (mutations within *BCR-ABL*) is suggested in case of loss of response to therapy.
- Others:
  - Low or absent leukocyte alkaline phosphatase in neutrophils
  - High lactate dehydrogenase (LDH)
  - Elevated uric acid

Initial Tests (lab, imaging)
- CBC, LDH, uric acid, LFTs, bone marrow biopsy and aspiration, cytogenetics on bone marrow, FISH for *BCR-ABL*, and baseline RT-PCR (quantitative as well as qualitative analysis to identify BCR-ABL transcript type)
- Abdominal ultrasound or CT scan shows splenomegaly; not mandatory

Follow-Up Tests & Special Considerations
- Routine CBC with differential until complete hematologic response (CHR)
- Serial monitoring of BCR-ABL by RT-PCR every 3 months to evaluate response to treatment
- Mutation analysis of tyrosine kinase domain of *ABL* kinase can predict resistance to therapy with TKIs.
- HLA-A*02 positive is associated with CML, and a protective effect is seen with the HLA-B*35 allele (pooled odds ratio 0.64, 95% CI 0.48–0.86).

Diagnostic Procedures/Other
Bone marrow aspiration and biopsy

Test Interpretation
Myeloid hyperplasia with elevated myeloid: erythroid ratio, normal maturation, marrow basophilia, and increased reticulin fibrosis

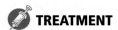

TREATMENT

MEDICATION
- TKIs (e.g., imatinib) provide durable, long-term control of disease.
- The response to TKIs is assessed at specific time points from the beginning of treatment and is categorized as follows:
  - CHR: normalization of peripheral counts, no disease symptoms, no immature cells
  - Complete cytogenetic response (CCR): no Philadelphia-positive metaphases on chromosome analysis
  - Major molecular response (MMR): decreased level of *BCR-ABL* transcript by PCR 3-log
  - Complete molecular response (CMR): *BCR-ABL* transcript is undetectable by PCR.
  - Failure to achieve CHR in 3 months is an indication to change therapy.
  - Hematologic, cytogenetic, and molecular response to TKIs are the most important prognostic indicators or predictors of outcome.

First Line
- Imatinib mesylate (Gleevec), an oral TKI, 400 mg/day
- Side effects: thrombocytopenia, anemia, elevated liver enzymes, edema, GI disturbances, rash
- International Randomized Study of Interferon versus STI571 (IRIS) established imatinib as first-line therapy, and it has shown long-term efficacy after 10-year follow-up (1)[A].
- Imatinib dose can be increased to 600 and 800 mg/day if only suboptimal response is achieved with standard dose.
- 2nd-generation TKIs have shown higher efficacy and fewer side effects and are approved for first-line therapy of chronic phase CML: nilotinib (Tasigna), dasatinib (Sprycel), and bosutinib (Bosulif).

Second Line

- 2nd-generation TKIs; active against most of *BCR-ABL* mutants; not active in *T315I* mutation
  - Dasatinib
    - 100 mg/day in patients resistant or intolerant to imatinib and 70 mg BID or 140 mg/day for patients in accelerated or blastic phase
    - Side effects: pleural effusions, QTc prolongation, cytopenias, pulmonary arterial hypertension
  - Nilotinib
    - 400 mg PO BID in patients resistant or intolerant to imatinib in chronic or accelerated phase
    - Side effects: cytopenias, QTc prolongation, pancreatitis, hyperglycemia, risk of thrombotic events
  - Bosutinib
    - 400 mg PO daily, 500 mg in patients resistant or intolerant to prior therapy in chronic or accelerated phase
    - Side effects: GI toxicity, myelosuppression, hepatotoxicity, fluid retention, pancreatitis
- 3rd-generation TKI
  - Ponatinib has restricted approval due to the risk of thrombotic events, but in addition to omacetaxine (below), they are the only effective agents in patients with *T315I* mutation approved by the FDA.
  - Olverembatinib is showing promise in TKI-resistant chronic phase and accelerated phase patients with *T315I* mutation.
  - Vodobatinib is part of an ongoing phase 2 study for patients refractory to ≥3 TKI including ponatinib.
- Other approved agents or in development:
  - Omacetaxine (protein synthesis inhibitor) is approved for patient with resistance or intolerance to two or more TKIs.
  - Asciminib (a STAMP inhibitor, specifically targeting the ABL myristoyl pocket) is approved for patients with chronic phase CML who have been treated previously with two or more TKIs or who have the *T315I* mutation.
  - If active treatment is required during pregnancy, interferon-α can be used in any trimester without significant risk to the fetus.

ISSUES FOR REFERRAL

All patients with CML should be referred to a hematologist. Patients with inadequate response to TKIs or with *T315I* mutation should consult with a bone marrow transplant (BMT) physician.

ADDITIONAL THERAPIES

Agents targeting leukemic stem cells are being developed for clinical use; emerging agents being studied: PF-114 (4th-generation oral TKI), HQP1351 (3rd-generation oral TKI)

SURGERY/OTHER PROCEDURES

Allogeneic BMT

- It is the only known cure; however, 71% of patients who achieve CCR with imatinib maintain that response beyond 7 years, and no patient progressed on the trial between years 5 and 6 of treatment.
- Most effective in patients <50 years of age who are in the chronic phase

- Initial mortality is higher (related to the use of myeloablative regimens) than medical management but provided higher rates of survival in pre-TKI era.
- Significant improvement in transplant techniques leading to better outcomes, such as alternative sources of stem cells; nonmyeloablative regimens have shown improvements in transplant-related mortality.
- Transplant option should be thoroughly discussed with young patients in chronic phase and considered an alternative to TKIs, especially if the patient does not tolerate TKIs or disease is not responding.
- Can be considered in blast phase CML patients in remission, accelerated phase CML with suboptimal or resistant response to TKIs, and chronic phase patients who fail to achieve CHR by 3 months, have no cytogenetic response or cytogenetic relapse, have *T315I* mutation, or have extramedullary disease with chronic phase CML cells

ADMISSION, INPATIENT, AND NURSING CONSIDERATIONS

- Acute abdominal symptoms (infarcted or ruptured spleen); tumor lysis syndrome owing to initial therapy; complications of BMT
  - Hydroxyurea might be given, with the goal of reduction of the WBC count, but it has minimal impact on patient's response to TKIs.
  - Induction chemotherapy (for acute leukemia) in setting of blastic phase
  - Allopurinol to prevent tumor lysis syndrome in patients with very high counts; however, probably not necessary when TKIs are used
- Discharge criteria: abatement of acute symptoms

 ## ONGOING CARE

FOLLOW-UP RECOMMENDATIONS

- Frequency depends on disease risk at presentation and response to first-line therapy.
- Although splenomegaly persists, avoid contact sports or trauma to abdomen.

Patient Monitoring

- CBC with differential: weekly until blood counts are stable and then every 2 to 4 weeks during CHR; once in CCR and stable, patient can be followed less frequently (3-month intervals).
- Bone marrow cytogenetics (evaluation for clonal evolution) every 6 months while in CHR; every 12 to 18 months while in CCR, MMR, or CMR
- Quantitative RT-PCR every 3 months (peripheral blood)
- ECGs (concern for QT prolongation), LFTs while on TKIs; nilotinib, bosutinib, and ponatinib can cause pancreatitis.
- Blood pressure monitoring because several TKIs have been associated with elevated blood pressure and related cardiovascular complications

PROGNOSIS

- With treatment and good response, the survival is similar to the normal population.
- Without treatment: CML invariably will progress to accelerated phase within 2 to 5 years and blast phase within several months of the accelerated phase.
- Poor prognosis: patients presenting in accelerated or blastic phase or presenting with very large spleen size, platelets >700,000/μL, and patients resistant to TKIs (*T315I* mutation)

COMPLICATIONS

- Splenic infarct or rupture
- Progression to accelerated or blastic phase
- Thrombotic events owing to elevated platelets
- Bleeding owing to low or dysfunctional platelets
- Sequelae of anemia

REFERENCE

1. Hochhaus A, Larson RA, Guilhot F, et al; for IRIS Investigators. Long-term outcomes of imatinib treatment for chronic myeloid leukemia. *N Engl J Med*. 2017;376(10):917–927.

ADDITIONAL READING

- Jabbour E, Kantarjian H. Chronic myeloid leukemia: 2022 update on diagnosis, therapy, and monitoring. *Am J Hematol*. 2022;97(9):1236–1256.
- Senapati J, Sasaki K, Issa GC, et al. Management of chronic myeloid leukemia in 2023—common ground and common sense. *Blood Cancer J*. 2023;13(1):58.

CODES

ICD10
- C92.2 Atypical chronic myeloid leukemia, BCR/ABL-negative
- C92.12 Chronic myeloid leukemia, BCR/ABL-positive, in relapse
- C92.22 Atypical chronic myeloid leukemia, BCR/ABL-negative, in relapse

CLINICAL PEARLS

- CML belongs to the myeloproliferative disorders group.
- The gold standard for diagnosis of CML is the detection of the Philadelphia chromosome or its products, *BCR-ABL* mRNA, and fusion protein.
- TKIs provide durable, long-term control of the disease and have dramatically altered treatment.
- Atypical CML is a form of clinically typical CML but without the presence of the typical *BCR-ABL* translocation.
- Blastic phase (a.k.a. blast crisis) is a form of acute leukemia that is a possible complication of CML.

L

LEUKOPLAKIA, ORAL
Kathya M. Chartre, MD • Christopher Medrano, MD • Justin Ryan Andrada, DO

 BASICS

DESCRIPTION
- Leukoplakia is defined by the World Health Organization (WHO) as "a white plaque of questionable risk having excluded (other) known diseases or disorders that carry no increased risk for cancer."
- System(s) affected: gastrointestinal (GI)
- Hyperplasia of squamous epithelium

EPIDEMIOLOGY
Most common in individuals who use tobacco (smoking and smokeless), heavy alcohol use, and areca nuts (Asian populations).

Incidence
250,000 annual cases worldwide

Prevalence
- Age of onset is >40 years old with peak in the 60s.
- Males are 3 times more likely to be affected than females.
- Smokers are 6 times more likely to be affected than nonsmokers.

Geriatric Considerations
Malignant transformation to carcinoma is more common in older patients.

ETIOLOGY AND PATHOPHYSIOLOGY
Hyperkeratosis or dyskeratosis of the oral squamous epithelium; tissue cell exposure to carcinogens spurs adaptive changes including hyperplasia. Continued irritant exposure can lead to cellular degeneration of the epithelium and eventually apoptosis or malignant transformation.
- Tobacco use in any form
- Alcohol consumption
- Dental restorations/prosthetic appliances/periodontitis
- *Candida albicans* infection
- Human papillomavirus (HPV), types 16 and 18
- Vitamin and combined micronutrient deficiencies
- Syphilis
- Chronic trauma or irritation
- Epstein-Barr virus (EBV) (oral hairy leukoplakia)
- Areca/betel nut (Asian populations)
- Mouthwash/toothpaste containing the herbal root extract sanguinaria
- Hormonal disturbances/estrogen therapy
- Ultraviolet exposure (1)[C]

Genetics
- Dyskeratosis congenital and epidermolysis bullosa increase the likelihood of oral malignancy.
- p53 overexpression; PTEN allelic loss correlates with leukoplakia and particularly squamous cell carcinoma.
- Changes in expression of p53, FGFR1, p16INK4a and 3p, 9p, and 17 (especially TP53) gene mutations can have greater cancer risk (1)[C]. Decreased expression of E-cadherin, hMLH1, and CD1a.
- Biomarkers: IL-6, IL-8, and TNF-α have been detected in leukoplakia, and there is new research showing possible use of Hsp27 and PTHRP/PTHLH as biomarkers (1)[C].

RISK FACTORS
- 70–90% of oral leukoplakia is related to tobacco, particularly smokeless tobacco or areca/betel nut use.
- Alcohol increases risk by 1.5-fold.
- Repeated or chronic mechanical trauma from dental appliances or cheek biting
- Chemical irritation to oral regions
- Diabetes
- Risk factors for malignant transformation of leukoplakia
  - Female
  - Long duration of leukoplakia
  - Nonsmoker (idiopathic leukoplakia)
  - Located on tongue or floor of mouth
  - Size >200 mm^2
  - Nonhomogeneous type
  - Presence of epithelial dysplasia
  - Presence of *C. albicans*
  - Possible shift of oral microbiome in those with malignant transformation

GENERAL PREVENTION
- Avoid tobacco of any kind, alcohol, habitual cheek biting, tongue chewing, and betel nut ingestion.
- Use well-fitting dental equipment.
- Regular dental check-ups to avoid bad restorations
- Diet rich in fresh fruits and vegetables may help to prevent cancer.
- HPV vaccination may be preventive.

COMMONLY ASSOCIATED CONDITIONS
- HIV infection is closely associated with hairy leukoplakia.
- Erythroplakia in association with leukoplakia, "speckled leukoplakia," or erythroleukoplakia is a marker for underlying dysplasia.

 DIAGNOSIS

Leukoplakia is an asymptomatic white patch on the oral mucosa.

HISTORY
- History of tobacco or alcohol use or oral exposure to irritants
- Elicit timing of onset, progression, and presence of pain or sensitivity.
- Identify sources of friction or chronic irritation.

PHYSICAL EXAM
- Location
  - Can develop on any oral mucosal surface
  - Floor of mouth, ventrolateral tongue, and soft palate complex are more likely to have dysplastic lesions.
- Appearance
  - Varies from homogeneous, nonpalpable, faintly translucent white areas to thick, fissured, papillomatous, indurated plaques
  - May feel rough or leathery
  - Lesions can become exophytic or verruciform.
  - Color may be white, gray, yellowish white, or brownish gray.
  - Cannot be wiped or scraped off

- WHO classification
  - Homogeneous refers to color.
    ○ Flat, corrugated, wrinkled, or pumice
  - Nonhomogeneous refers to color and texture (more likely to be dysplastic or malignant).
    ○ Erythroleukoplakia (mixture of red and white)
    ○ Proliferative verrucous leukoplakia (PVL) (multifocal, mostly women)

DIFFERENTIAL DIAGNOSIS
- Geographic tongue
- Developmental/genetic (rare):
  - Cannon white sponge nevus (diffuse bilateral white plaques of buccal mucosa, tongue)
  - Hereditary benign intraepithelial dyskeratosis
  - Pachyonychia congenita; genodermatoses; Darier-White disease
- Reactive/frictional:
  - Leukoedema (delicate gray-white lines, disappear with stretching)
  - Contact desquamation
  - Morsicatio mucosae oris (cheek/gum biting)
  - Benign alveolar ridge keratosis (ill-fitting dentures)
  - Hairy tongue (elongated filiform papillae, may become pigmented from food/bacteria)
  - Nicotinic stomatitis and smokeless tobacco keratosis (South Asian "paan" or "gutka"; American/Swedish snuff; Ethiopian "toombak")
  - Glassblower's white patch
  - Actinic cheilitis
  - Aspirin burn
  - Cinnamon-induced contact stomatitis
  - Epithelial peeling
  - Keratotic lesions
  - Linea alba
- Infectious:
  - Candidiasis
  - Hairy leukoplakia (associated with EBV and HIV-infected individuals)
  - Syphilis
- Immune-mediated:
  - Lichen planus (typically symmetric, bilateral, reticular white lesions)
  - Lichenoid lesions
  - Benign migratory glossitis
- Autoimmune:
  - SLE
  - Chronic graft versus host disease

DIAGNOSTIC TESTS & INTERPRETATION
Biopsy with histopathologic examination to assess presence and grade of dysplasia is the gold standard.

Initial Tests (lab, imaging)
Consider saliva culture if *C. albicans* infection is suspected.

Follow-Up Tests & Special Considerations
- Biopsy is necessary to rule out carcinoma if lesion is persistent, changing, or unexplained.
- Consider CBC and rapid plasma reagin (RPR).

Diagnostic Procedures/Other
- Oral cytology is superior to conventional oral examination.
- Noninvasive brush biopsy and analysis of cells with DNA–image cytometry constitute a sensitive and specific screening method.

- Patients with dysplastic or malignant cells on brush biopsy should undergo more formal excisional biopsy.
- Excisional biopsy is a definitive procedure.

Test Interpretation
- Biopsy specimens range from hyperkeratosis to keratosis of unknown significance (KUS) to dysplasia to invasive carcinoma.
- At initial biopsy, 6% are invasive carcinoma.
- 0.13–6% subsequently undergo malignant transformation.
- Location is important: 60% on floor of mouth or lateral border of tongue are cancerous; buccal mucosal lesions are generally not malignant but require biopsy if not resolving.

 TREATMENT

- All oral leukoplakias should be treated because they are potentially malignant.
- Treatment may include the following:
  - Some small lesions may respond to cryosurgery.
  - For 2 to 3 circumscribed lesions, surgical excision is treatment of choice (2)[C].
  - For multiple or large lesions where surgery would cause unacceptable deformity, consider cryosurgery or laser surgery (2)[C].
- Complete excision is standard treatment for dysplasia or malignancy.
- After treatment, up to 30% of leukoplakia recurs, and some leukoplakia still transforms to squamous cell carcinoma (2)[C].
- Oral hairy leukoplakia may be treated with podophyllin with acyclovir cream.

GENERAL MEASURES
- Abstinence from predisposing habits (alcohol and tobacco)
- Eliminate habitual lip biting.
- Correct ill-fitting dental appliances, bad restorations, or sharp teeth.
- β-Carotene, lycopene, retinoids, and cyclooxygenase-2 (COX-2) inhibitors may cause partial regression.
- For hairy tongue: tongue brushing

MEDICATION
Carotenoids; vitamins A, C, and K; bleomycin; NSAIDs; and photodynamic therapy are ineffective to prevent malignant transformation and recurrence. No generally approved standard systemic pharmacotherapy regimen at this time, but there is a new research being done on chemoprevention.

ISSUES FOR REFERRAL
Consider otolaryngologist or oral surgery referral for extensive disease.

ADDITIONAL THERAPIES
Systemic therapies that may reduce progression include retinoids, COX-2 inhibitors, epidermal growth factor inhibitors, and peroxisome proliferator-activated receptor-γ agonists.

SURGERY/OTHER PROCEDURES
- Scalpel excision, laser ablation, electrocautery, or cryoablation
- Cryotherapy slightly is less effective than photodynamic therapy response and recurrence.
- Biopsy/excision algorithm (1)[C]:
  - KUS that is poorly demarcated and likely frictional: Rebiopsy and follow up.
  - KUS that is well demarcated and >3 cm: Follow up every 3 months; rebiopsy every 12 months.
  - KUS that is <3 cm: Excise/ablate with narrow margins; follow up every 3 months; if recurs, excise with wider margins.
  - PVL: Follow up every 3 months; excise verrucous or nodular areas.
  - Dysplastic/SCC: Excise.

COMPLEMENTARY & ALTERNATIVE MEDICINE
Low or very low evidence for systemic β-carotene, herbal extracts, freeze-dried black raspberry gel, and Bowman-Birk inhibitor

 ONGOING CARE

FOLLOW-UP RECOMMENDATIONS
Patient Monitoring
- Follow-up appointments every 3 to 6 months during the 1st year following surgical removal and then annually thereafter based on anticipated risk and patient's preference
- Biopsy as needed

DIET
Regular

PATIENT EDUCATION
- If biopsy is negative, stress the importance of periodic and careful follow-up.
- Initiate a dental referral to eliminate dental factors.
- Stress the importance of stopping tobacco and alcohol use.
- Encourage participation in smoking cessation program.

PROGNOSIS
- Most leukoplakia is benign.
- Leukoplakia may regress, remain stable, or progress.

- 0.13–6% of initially benign lesions subsequently develop into cancer. Most important predictor of transformation into squamous cell carcinoma is degree of epithelial dysplasia.
- Lack of treatment generally results in malignant development at an annual rate of 2–4%.
- 5-year survival rate of oral cancer is 50%.

COMPLICATIONS
- New lesions may develop after treatment.
- Larger lesions and nonhomogeneous leukoplakia are associated with higher rates of malignant transformation.

REFERENCES
1. Villa A, Woo SB. Leukoplakia—a diagnostic and management algorithm. *J Oral Maxillofac Surg.* 2017;75(4):723–734.
2. Feller L, Lemmer J. Oral leukoplakia as it relates to HPV infection: a review. *Int J Dent.* 2012;2012:540561.

ADDITIONAL READING
Reamy BV, Derby R, Bunt CW. Common tongue conditions in primary care. *Am Fam Physician.* 2010;81(5):627–634.

 SEE ALSO

HIV/AIDS; Infectious Mononucleosis, Epstein-Barr Virus Infections

 CODES

ICD10
- K13.21 Leukoplakia of oral mucosa, including tongue
- K13.3 Hairy leukoplakia

CLINICAL PEARLS
- White plaque or patches on the oral mucosa that cannot be rubbed or easily scrapped off
- Excisional biopsy is indicated for any undiagnosed leukoplakia.
- After treatment, up to 30% of leukoplakia recurs, and some leukoplakia still transforms to squamous cell carcinoma; thus, long-term surveillance is essential.
- To lessen risk of malignant transformation, encourage tobacco and alcohol cessation, HPV vaccination, and consider *C. albicans* eradication.

L

LICHEN PLANUS

Dongsheng Jiang, MD, MSc • Juan Qiu, MD, PhD

BASICS

Lichen planus (LP) is an idiopathic eruption with characteristic shiny, flat-topped (Latin: *planus*, "flat") purple (violaceous) papules and plaques on the skin, often accompanied by characteristic mucous membrane lesions. Itching may be severe.

DESCRIPTION

- Classic (typical) LP is a relatively uncommon inflammatory disorder of the skin and mucous membranes; hair and nails may also be affected.
  - Skin lesions are small, flat, angular, red-to-violaceous, shiny, pruritic papules and/or plaques with overlying fine, white lines (called Wickham striae), or gray-white puncta; most commonly seen on the flexor surfaces of the upper extremities, extensor surfaces of the lower extremities, the genitalia, and on the mucous membranes
  - On the oral mucosa, lesions typically appear as raised white lines in a lacelike pattern seen most often on the buccal mucosa.
  - Onset is abrupt or gradual. Course is unpredictable; may resolve spontaneously, recur intermittently, or persist for many years
- Drug-induced LP
  - Clinical and histopathologic findings may mimic those of classic LP. Lesions usually lack Wickham striae (see in the following text), and oral involvement is rare.
  - There is generally a latent period of months from drug introduction until lesions appear.
  - Lesions resolve when the inciting agent is discontinued, often after a prolonged period.
- LP variants
  - Follicular: also called lichen planopilaris; typically seen on the scalp, can lead to scarring alopecia
  - Annular: papules spread centrifugally as central area resolves; occur on glans penis, axillae, and oral mucosa
  - Linear: may be an isolated finding
  - Hypertrophic: itchy, hyperkeratotic, thick plaques on dorsal legs and feet
  - Atrophic: rare, most often the result of resolved lesions
  - Bullous LP: Intense inflammation in the dermis leads to blistering of epidermis.
  - LP pemphigoides: a combination of LP and bullous pemphigoid (IgG autoantibodies to collagen 17)
  - Nail LP: affects the nail matrix, lateral thinning, longitudinal ridging, and fissuring
- System(s) affected: skin/exocrine
- Synonym(s): lichenoid eruptions

EPIDEMIOLOGY

- Predominant age: 30 to 60 years old; rare in children and the geriatric population
- Predominant sex: female > male

Prevalence

In the United States, 450/100,000

ETIOLOGY AND PATHOPHYSIOLOGY

LP is considered to be a T cell–mediated autoimmune response to self-antigens on damaged keratinocytes.

RISK FACTORS

Exposure to certain drugs or chemicals

- Thiazides, furosemide, β-blockers, sulfonylureas, antimalarials, penicillamine, gold salts, angiotensin-converting enzyme inhibitors, NSAIDs, isoniazid, tetracyclines, and allopurinol

COMMONLY ASSOCIATED CONDITIONS

- Hepatitis C virus infection, particularly in certain geographic regions (Asia, South America, the Middle East, Europe). Hepatitis should be considered in patients with widespread presentations of LP and those with primarily oral disease.
- Chronic active hepatitis, lichen nitidus, and primary biliary cirrhosis
- Dyslipidemia
- Others:
  - Bullous pemphigoid
  - Alopecia areata
  - Myasthenia gravis
  - Vitiligo
  - Ulcerative colitis
  - Graft-versus-host reaction
  - Lupus erythematosus (lupus erythematosus–LP overlap syndrome)
  - Morphea and lichen sclerosus et atrophicus

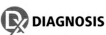DIAGNOSIS

- LP is most commonly diagnosed by its appearance despite its range of clinical presentations.
- Dermoscopy: Most common findings are polymorphic pearly white structures, radial capillaries, and blue-gray granules.
- A skin/mucosal biopsy is recommended.

HISTORY

A minority of patients have a family history of LP. Affected families have an increased frequency of human leukocyte antigen B7 (HLA-B7). A thorough drug history should be performed.

PHYSICAL EXAM

- Skin (often severe pruritus)
  - Papules: 1 to 10 mm, shiny, flat-topped (planar) lesions that occur in crops; lesions may have a fine scale.
  - Evidence of scratching (i.e., crusts and excoriations) is usually absent.
  - Color: violaceous, with white lacelike pattern (Wickham striae) on surface of papules. Wickham striae are best seen after topical application of mineral oil and, if present, are virtually pathognomonic for LP.
  - Shape: polygonal or oval; annular lesions may appear on trunk and mucous membranes. Various shapes and sizes may be noted (polymorphic).
  - Arrangement: may be grouped, linear, or scattered individual lesions
  - Koebner phenomenon (isomorphic response): New lesions may be noted at sites of minor injuries, such as scratches or burns.

- Distribution: ventral surface of wrists and forearms, dorsa hands, glans penis, dorsa feet, groin, sacrum, shins, and scalp; hypertrophic (verrucous) lesions may occur on lower legs and may be generalized.
  - Postinflammatory hyperpigmentation: Lesions typically heal, leaving darkly pigmented macules in their wake.
- Mucous membranes (40–60% of patients with skin lesions; 20% have mucous membrane lesions without skin involvement.)
  - Most commonly asymptomatic, nonerosive, milky-white lines with an elegant, lacy, netlike streaked pattern
  - Usually seen on buccal mucosa but may appear on tongue, gingiva, palate, or lips
  - Less commonly, LP may be erosive; rarely bullous
  - Painful, especially if ulcers present
  - Lesions may develop into squamous cell carcinoma (1–3%).
  - Glans penis, labia minora, vaginal vault, and perianal areas may be involved.
- Hair/scalp
  - LP of the hair follicle (lichen planopilaris) presents with keratotic plugs at the follicle orifice with a violaceous rim; may result in atrophy and permanent destruction of hair follicles (scarring alopecia)
- Nails (10%)
  - Involvement of nail matrix may cause proximal-to-distal linear grooves and partial or complete destruction of nail bed with pterygium formation.

DIFFERENTIAL DIAGNOSIS

- Skin
  - Lichen simplex chronicus
  - Eczematous dermatitis
  - Psoriasis
  - Discoid lupus erythematosus
  - Other lichenoid eruptions (those that resemble LP)
  - Pityriasis rosea
  - Lichen nitidus
  - Self-induced dermatoses
- Oral mucous membranes
  - Leukoplakia
  - Oral hairy leukoplakia
  - Candidiasis
  - Squamous cell carcinoma (particularly in ulcerative lesions)
  - Aphthous ulcers
  - Herpetic stomatitis
  - Secondary syphilis
- Genital mucous membranes
  - Psoriasis (penis and labia)
  - Nonspecific balanitis, Zoon balanitis
  - Fixed drug eruption (penis)
  - Candidiasis (penis and labia)
  - Pemphigus vulgaris, bullous pemphigoid, and Behçet disease (all rare)
- Hair and scalp
  - Scarring alopecia (central centrifugal cicatricial alopecia)

DIAGNOSTIC TESTS & INTERPRETATION
If suggested by history
- Serology for hepatitis
- Liver function tests

Diagnostic Procedures/Other
- Skin biopsy
- Direct immunofluorescence helps to distinguish LP from discoid lupus erythematosus.

Test Interpretation
- Dense, bandlike (lichenoid) lymphocytic infiltrate of the upper dermis
- Vacuolar degeneration of the basal layer
- Hyperkeratosis and irregular acanthosis, increased granular layer
- Basement membrane thinning with "saw-toothing"
- Degenerative keratinocytes, known as colloid or Civatte bodies, are found in the lower epidermis
- Melanin pigment in macrophages

 TREATMENT

Although LP can resolve spontaneously, treatment is usually requested by patients who may be severely symptomatic or troubled by its cosmetic appearance.

GENERAL MEASURES
- The goal is to relieve itching and resolve lesions.
- Discontinue potentially causative medications.
- Asymptomatic oral lesions require no treatment.
- For oral LP (1):
  - No treatment is curative.
  - The goal of treatment is to resolve pain, heal ulcerative lesions, and decrease the risk for oral cancer.

MEDICATION
First Line
- Skin (2),(3)
  - Ultrahigh-potency and high-potency topical steroids: 0.05% clobetasol propionate or 0.1% betamethasone valerate BID for 2 to 4 weeks
  - Triamcinolone acetonide 0.1% or fluocinonide 0.05% under occlusion
  - Intralesional corticosteroids (e.g., triamcinolone [Kenalog] 5 to 10 mg/mL) for recalcitrant and hypertrophic lesions
  - "Soak and smear" technique: can lead to a rapid improvement of symptoms in even 1 to 2 days and may obviate the need for systemic steroids; soaking allows water to hydrate the stratum corneum and allows the anti-inflammatory steroid in the ointment to penetrate more deeply into the skin. Smearing of the ointment traps the water in the skin because water cannot move out through greasy materials.
    - Soaking is done in a bathtub using lukewarm plain water for 20 minutes and then, without drying the skin, the affected area is immediately smeared with a thin film of the steroid ointment containing clobetasol or another superpotent topical steroid.

- Soak and smear may be done for 4 to 5 days or longer, if necessary. The treatments are best done at night because the greasy ointment applied to the skin gets on pajamas (instead of on daytime clothes), and the ointment is on the skin during sleep. A topical steroid cream is applied thereafter during the daytime hours, if necessary.
- Mucous membranes
  - For oral, erosive, painful LP
    - Topical corticosteroids (0.1% triamcinolone [Kenalog] in Orabase) or 0.05% clobetasol propionate ointment BID
    - Intralesional corticosteroids BID

Pediatric Considerations
Children may absorb a proportionally larger amount of topical steroid because of larger skin surface-to-weight ratio.

Second Line
Skin and mucous membranes
- Oral steroids: reserved for acute exacerbation, severe or widespread, or unresponsive to topical steroids; prednisone at 0.5 to 1.0 mg/kg body weight/day (30 to 60 mg/day) for 3 to 6 weeks, taper over 4 to 6 weeks
- Isotretinoin 10 mg, or acitretin 30 mg, or alitretinoin 30 mg PO daily in some refractory cases; observe carefully for resultant dyslipidemia.
- Topical calcineurin inhibitors: 0.1% tacrolimus (Protopic ointment) BID or 1% pimecrolimus (Elidel) cream BID
- Topical retinoids: tretinoin 0.05% BID; isotretinoin 0.1% BID
- Topical calcipotriol
- Other medications used occasionally: metronidazole, sulfasalazine, methotrexate, cyclosporine, hydroxychloroquine, dapsone, thalidomide, griseofulvin, azathioprine, mycophenolate mofetil
- Narrow-band UVB (NBUVB) and broad-band UVB (BBUVB): especially when systemic steroids and immunosuppressive drugs are contraindicated
- Psoralen plus ultraviolet A (PUVA) therapy
- Low-level laser therapy and photodynamic therapy

ALERT
Avoid oral and topical retinoids during pregnancy.

ADDITIONAL THERAPIES
Antihistamines (e.g., hydroxyzine 25 mg PO q6h) have limited benefit for itching but may be helpful for sedation at bedtime.

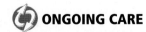 ONGOING CARE

FOLLOW-UP RECOMMENDATIONS
Patient Monitoring
Serial oral examinations for erosive/ulcerative lesions

PATIENT EDUCATION
- Oral, erosive, or ulcerative LP: annual follow-up to screen for malignancy
- Maintain good oral hygiene and dental status.
- Avoid hot, salty, acidic, or spicy foods; alcohol; smoking; and use of tobacco products, especially in patients with atrophic and erosive lesions.
- Avoid mucosal trauma: Avoid dry, crispy foods such as corn chips, pretzels, and toast.

PROGNOSIS
- Spontaneous resolution in weeks is possible, but disease may persist for years, especially oral lesions and hypertrophic lesions on the shins.
- There is a tendency toward relapse.
- Recurrence in 12–20%, especially in those with generalized involvement

COMPLICATIONS
- Alopecia
- Nail destruction
- Squamous cell carcinoma of the mouth or genitals

REFERENCES
1. Rotaru D, Chisnoiu R, Picos AM, et al. Treatment trends in oral lichen planus and oral lichenoid lesions (review). *Exp Ther Med.* 2020;20(6):198.
2. Thandar Y, Maharajh R, Haffejee F, et al. Treatment of cutaneous lichen planus (Part 1): a review of topical therapies and phototherapy. *Cogent Med.* 2019;6(1):1–21.
3. Thandar Y, Maharajh R, Haffejee F, et al. Treatment of cutaneous lichen planus (part 2): a review of systemic therapies. *J Dermatolog Treat.* 2019;30(7):633–647.

 CODES

ICD10
- L43.9 Lichen planus, unspecified
- L43.0 Hypertrophic lichen planus
- L43.1 Bullous lichen planus

CLINICAL PEARLS
- 7 P's of LP: **p**urple, **p**lanar, **p**olygonal, **p**olymorphic, **p**ruritic (not always), **p**apules that heal with **p**ostinflammatory hyperpigmentation
- Serial oral or genital exams are indicated for erosive/ulcerative LP lesions to monitor for the development of squamous cell carcinoma.
- The "soak and smear" technique can lead to a rapid improvement of symptoms in 1 to 2 days and may obviate the need for systemic steroids.

L

LICHEN SIMPLEX CHRONICUS

Dongsheng Jiang, MD, MSc • Joseph P. Wiedemer, MD, FAAFP

 BASICS

DESCRIPTION
- Lichen simplex chronicus (LSC) is a chronic dermatitis resulting from chronic, repeated rubbing or scratching of the skin. Skin becomes thickened with accentuated lines ("lichenification").
- Definition/terminology (1):
  - LSC: localized lichenified plaques often with excoriations
  - Prurigo nodularis (PN): a chronic pruritic condition which is frequently more broadly distributed across multiple regions as nodules
  - Neurodermatitis: include other chronic itchy conditions, such as PN and atopic dermatitis

EPIDEMIOLOGY
Geriatric Considerations
Most common in middle-aged and elderly

Pediatric Considerations
Rare in preadolescents

Incidence
- Peak incidence: ages 35 to 50 years
- Predominant sex: females > males (2:1)

Prevalence
Common—affects 12% of the population

ETIOLOGY AND PATHOPHYSIOLOGY
- Itch–scratch cycle leads to a chronic dermatosis. Repeated scratching or rubbing causes inflammation and pruritus, which leads to continued scratching.
- Primary LSC: scratching secondary to nonorganic pruritus, habit or a conditioned response to stress/anxiety
- Common triggers are excess dryness of skin, heat, sweat, and psychological stress.
- Secondary LSC: begins as a pruritic skin disease that evolves into neurodermatitis, which persists after resolution of the primary condition. Precursor dermatoses include atopic dermatitis, contact dermatitis, lichen planus, stasis dermatitis, psoriasis, tinea, and insect bites.
- There is a possible relation between disease development and underlying neuropathy, particularly radiculopathy or nerve root compression.
- Pruritus-specific C neurons are temperature sensitive, which may explain itching that occurs in warm environments.

RISK FACTORS
- Anxiety disorders
- Dry skin
- Insect bites
- Pruritic dermatosis

GENERAL PREVENTION
Avoid common triggers such as psychological distress, environmental factors such as heat and excessive dryness, skin irritation, and the development of pruritic dermatoses.

COMMONLY ASSOCIATED CONDITIONS
- PN is a nodular variety of the same disease process.
- Atopic dermatitis
- Anxiety, depression, and obsessive-compulsive disorders

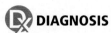 **DIAGNOSIS**

HISTORY
- Gradual onset
- Begins as a localized area of pruritus
- Most patients acknowledge that they respond with vigorous rubbing, itching, or scratching, which brings temporary satisfaction.
- Pruritus is typically paroxysmal, worse at night, and may lead to scratching during sleep.
- Can be asymptomatic with patient scratching at night while asleep

PHYSICAL EXAM
- Well-circumscribed lichenified plaques with varying amounts of overlying excoriation or scaling
- Lichenification: accentuation of normal skin lines
- Hyperpigmentation or hypopigmentation can be seen.
- Scarring is uncommon with typical LSC; can be seen following ulcer formation or secondary infection
- Most commonly involves easily accessible areas
  - Lateral portions of lower legs/ankles
  - Nape of neck (lichen simplex nuchae)
  - Vulva/scrotum/anus
  - Extensor surfaces of forearms
  - Palmar wrist
  - Scalp

- Dermoscopic criteria: (in genital disease) (2)
  - Rich vascularization, linear, serpentine, and dotted in shape
  - Diffuse arrangement
  - White-grayish background

DIFFERENTIAL DIAGNOSIS
- Lichen sclerosis
- Psoriasis
- Atopic dermatitis
- Contact, irritant, or stasis dermatitis
- Extramammary Paget disease
- Lichen planus
- Lichen amyloidosis
- Tinea
- Nummular eczema
- Other systemic disease:
  - T-cell lymphoma
  - Lymphoma
  - Multiple myeloma
  - Lung cancer
  - Leukemia
  - GI tract cancer

DIAGNOSTIC TESTS & INTERPRETATION
Initial Tests (lab, imaging)
- No specific diagnostic test
- Microscopy (i.e., KOH prep) and culture preparation may be helpful in identifying possible bacterial or fungal infection.

Diagnostic Procedures/Other
- Skin biopsy if diagnosis is in question.
- Patch testing may be used to rule out a contact dermatitis.

Test Interpretation
- Hyperkeratosis
- Acanthosis
- Lengthening of rete ridges
- Hyperplasia of all components of epidermis
- Mild to moderate lymphohistiocytic inflammatory infiltrate with prominent lichenification

TREATMENT

GENERAL MEASURES
- Treat underlying causes.
- Patient education is critical.
- Low likelihood of resolution if patient unable to avoid scratching/rubbing. SSRIs may be effective in controlling compulsive scratching resulting from a psychiatric diagnosis such as anxiety disorder or obsessive-compulsive disorder.
- Treatment aimed at reducing inflammation and pruritus

MEDICATION
Treatment is based on disease severity (1):
- Mild disease—options include the following:
  - Emollients
  - High-potency topical steroids
  - Topical calcineurin inhibitors
  - Combination of topical steroids and salicylates
  - Menthol
  - Pramoxine
  - Topical doxepin
  - Topical aspirin with dichloromethane
  - Topical ketamine/amitriptyline/lidocaine
- Moderate disease—below usually combined with a first-line treatment
  - Antidepressants (SSRI, tricyclic antidepressants, i.e., imipramine)
  - Gabapentin
  - For nighttime itch: mirtazapine, sedating antihistamines
  - Topical acetaminophen
  - Cyclosporine
  - Methotrexate
  - Narrowband ultraviolet B
- Severe disease
  - Nemolizumab
  - Dupilumab
  - Janus kinase inhibitors (i.e., tofacitinib)
  - Transcutaneous electrical nerve stimulation
  - Focused ultrasound (in vulvar areas)

First Line

ALERT
High-dose and prolonged treatment with topical steroids can cause dermal/epidermal atrophy as well as pigmentary changes and should not be used on the face, intertriginous areas, or anogenital region. Duration of treatment on other parts of the body should not exceed 3 weeks without close physician supervision.

ISSUES FOR REFERRAL
- No response to treatment
- Presence of signs and symptoms suggestive of a systemic cause of pruritus
- Consultation with a psychiatrist for patients with severe stress, anxiety, or compulsive scratching
- Consultation with an allergist for patients with multisystem atopic symptoms

ADDITIONAL THERAPIES
- Psychotherapy
- Cooling of the skin with ice or cold compresses
- Soaks and lubricants to improve barrier layer function
- Occlusion of lesion with bandages or Unna boots
- Nail trimming
- Silk underwear to decrease friction in genital LSC

COMPLEMENTARY & ALTERNATIVE MEDICINE
- Acupuncture is effective.
- Cognitive-behavioral therapy may improve awareness and help to identify coping strategies.
- Hypnosis may be beneficial in decreasing pruritus and preventing scratching.
- Homeopathic remedies (i.e., thuja and graphite) have been used.

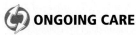 **ONGOING CARE**

FOLLOW-UP RECOMMENDATIONS
Patient Monitoring
Patients should be followed for response to therapy, complications from therapy (especially topical steroids), and secondary infections.

DIET
Regular balanced diet

PATIENT EDUCATION
- Patients should understand the cause of this disease and the critical role they play in its resolution. Emphasize that scratching and rubbing must stop for lesions to heal; medications ineffective if scratching continues.
- Stress reduction techniques can be useful for patients for whom stress plays a role.
- Avoid exposure to known triggers.

PROGNOSIS
- Often chronic and recurrent, can be persistent on genitals
- Good prognosis if the itch–scratch cycle can be broken
- After healing, the skin should return to normal appearance but may also retain accentuated skin markings or post inflammatory pigmentary changes that may be slow to resolve.

COMPLICATIONS
- Secondary infection
- Scarring is rare without ulceration or secondary infection.
- Complications related to therapy, as mentioned in medication precautions
- Squamous cell carcinoma within affected regions is rare.

REFERENCES
1. Ju T, Vander Does A, Mohsin N, et al. Lichen simplex chronicus itch: an update. *Acta Derm Venereol*. 2022;102:adv00796.
2. Borghi A, Virgili A, Corazza M. Dermoscopy of inflammatory genital diseases: practical insights. *Dermatol Clin*. 2018;36(4):451–461.

 CODES

ICD10
L28.0 Lichen simplex chronicus

CLINICAL PEARLS
- LSC is a chronic inflammatory condition that results from repeated scratching and rubbing.
- Primary LSC originates de novo, whereas secondary LSC occurs in the setting of a preexisting pruritic dermatologic condition.
- LSC is a clinical diagnosis based on history and skin examination with biopsy only indicated in difficult or unclear cases.
- Stopping the itch–scratch cycle through patient education, skin lubrication, and topical medications is key.
- Treatment is based on disease severity.

LONG QT INTERVAL

Alec M. Wilhelmi, MD • Leigh A. Romero, MD, CAQSM

BASICS

DESCRIPTION

- QT interval: the interval from the beginning of the QRS complex to the end of the T wave on the surface electrocardiogram (ECG). This represents the period from the onset of ventricular depolarization to completion of repolarization of the ventricular myocardium, or ventricular systole. The QT interval is normal if it is <50% of the RR interval.
- Corrected QT interval (QTc): The QT interval has an inverse relationship with heart rate. The QTc is the QT interval corrected for heart rate, and it estimates the QT interval at a heart rate of 60 beats/min. See formulas.
- Prolonged QTc is generally defined as >450 ms for adult males and >470 ms for adult females:
  – 430 to 450 ms considered borderline in men
  – 450 to 470 ms considered borderline in women (1)
  – 440 to 460 ms considered borderline in children aged 1 to 15 years
- Most cases of prolonged QT are acquired, but several genetic mutations cause inherited long QT syndrome (LQTS) (1).
- Prolonged QTc from any cause can precipitate polymorphic ventricular tachycardia (VT) called torsade de pointes (TdP), leading to dizziness, syncope, and sudden cardiac death from ventricular fibrillation (VF).

EPIDEMIOLOGY

Often presents in childhood, but may present as early as newborn period or go undiagnosed until middle age. The mean onset age is 14 years.

Incidence

Incidence of medication-induced QTc prolongation and TdP varies with medication and a host of other factors. Exact incidences are difficult to estimate but may be 1/2,000 to 1/2,500.

Prevalence

Congenital LQTS is estimated to occur in 1/2,500 to 1/7,000 births. The true incidence of mutations in the population is likely much higher.

ETIOLOGY AND PATHOPHYSIOLOGY

- Acquired
  – Demographics: increasing age, female sex
  – Electrolyte abnormalities: hypokalemia, hypocalcemia, and hypomagnesemia
  – Noncardiac disease: hypothyroidism, renal impairment, and hepatic impairment
  – Cardiac disease: heart failure, LVH, and myocardial ischemia
  – Scenarios: rapid increase in the QT interval >60 ms, conversion from atrial fibrillation/bradycardia
  – Medications (*denotes "high-risk" medication for TdP 25.) (1)
    ○ Antiarrhythmic medications (quinidine, procainamide, dronedarone, dofetilide, sotalol, disopyramide, and amiodarone)
    ○ Antipsychotic medications: especially if given IV (haloperidol*, chlorpromazine*, thioridazine*, pimozide*)
    ○ Antidepressants: most commonly used drugs responsible (SSRIs, SNRIs, trazodone, TCAs)

○ Antibiotics/antivirals/antifungals/antiprotozoals/antimalarials: macrolides (clarithromycin*, erythromycin* also CYP3A4 inhibitors), fluoroquinolones, quinine, and chloroquine
○ Antiemetics: metoclopramide, ondansetron, promethazine
○ Opioids: methadone*, buprenorphine
○ Antihistamines: cetirizine, hydroxyzine, diphenhydramine
○ Decongestants: pseudoephedrine, phenylephrine
○ Stimulants: albuterol, phentermine
○ Misc: chloroquine*, pentamidine*, various antimuscarinics, and anticonvulsants

- Congenital
  – >13 genes have been identified that encode for subunits of various ion membrane channels
  – Mutations of KCNQ1 (LQTS1), KCNH2 (LQTS2), and SCN5A (LQTS3) genes account for >90% of cases.
  – Loss of function mutations in several potassium ion membrane channels or gain of function mutations in the sodium or calcium ion membrane channels in cardiac myocytes
- Pathophysiology
  – Depolarization (phase 0) of the myocardium results from the rapid influx of sodium through sodium channels (I_{Na}) causing myocyte contraction during systole; seen on ECG as the QRS complex
  – Repolarization occurs through the efflux of potassium from the cell (phases 2 and 3) by rapid (I_{Kr}) and slow (I_{Ks}) components of the delayed rectifier; represented by the T wave on an ECG
  – Drug-induced QT prolongation most often due to blockade of the I_{Kr} channel leading to delay in phase 3 rapid repolarization.
  – In both cases, deviation from normal ion channel function leads to transmural dispersion of repolarization currents across the myocardium, triggering early after depolarizations which may devolve into TdP (1).
  – Prolonged QT interval alone does not denote imminent risk for TdP; TdP is often self-limited, but TdP can cause syncope or degrade to VF.

Genetics

- >13 distinct genotypes are linked to LQTS. LQT1 is most common cause of congenital LQTS.
- Penetrance is highly variable making both diagnosis and management challenging (1).

RISK FACTORS

For the feared complication, TdP, risk factors include the following:
- Female (~2 times increased risk), QTc >500 ms (2 to 3 times increased risk), QTc >60 ms over previous baseline (for every 10 ms increase in the QTc, there is a 5–7% increased risk for developing TdP), history of syncope or presyncope, history of TdP, bradycardia, liver or kidney disease (by increasing blood levels of QT-prolonging medications), medications that cause QTc prolongation (high doses, fast infusions, combination of medications), medications that inhibit CYP3A4, electrolyte abnormalities (hypokalemia, hypomagnesemia, hypocalcemia)
- For congenital LQTS
  – Catecholamine surges from exercise, emotional stress, loud noises, postpartum depression.

GENERAL PREVENTION

- Avoid (or use with caution) causative medications, including combinations with potentially additive effects.
- Replete electrolytes (goal: Mg >2 mg/dL, K = 4.5 to 5.0 mEq/L).
- Treat underlying diseases.
- Avoid strenuous sports and other stimulating activities, like amusement park rides or jumping into cold water, in LQTS.
- Avoid sudden loud noises in LQTS (alarm clocks, doorbells, telephones).

COMMONLY ASSOCIATED CONDITIONS

- Illnesses with associated severe vomiting and/or diarrhea leading to electrolyte disturbances
- Eating disorders—anorexia nervosa, bulimia
- Romano-Ward syndrome
- Andersen-Tawil syndrome (LQTS type 7)—prolonged QT interval, muscle weakness, facial dysmorphism
- Timothy syndrome (LQTS type 8)—prolonged QT interval, hand/foot, facial, and neurodevelopment features
- Jervell and Lange-Nielsen syndrome—associated with profound sensorineural hearing loss

DIAGNOSIS

HISTORY

- Incidental finding on ECG in asymptomatic patients
- Evaluate for syncope, presyncopal episodes, palpitations, and associated precipitating events (emotional triggers, swimming, diving).
- Key family history items that increase the likelihood of congenital LQTS include:
  – History of syncope, sudden cardiac death, or other arrhythmic disorders
  – Premature sudden deaths (<40 years of age and autopsy negative)
  – Unexplained motor vehicle accidents
  – Unexplained drownings
  – Generalized seizures (frequently, patients with LQTS have been misdiagnosed with and treated for epilepsy)
- History of seizures in patient or family members (tonic–clonic movement may be due to cerebral hypoperfusion during episodes of ventricular arrhythmia or syncope)
- Detailed medication history
- Congenital deafness

PHYSICAL EXAM

- The physical exam is typically unremarkable because patients with QT syndrome typically have structurally normal hearts.
- May include signs of underlying cardiac disease, hypothyroidism, liver or renal impairment
- Congenital deafness present in many forms of congenital LQTS

DIFFERENTIAL DIAGNOSIS

When evaluating long QT interval, differential should also include: QT-prolonging drugs, hypokalemia, hypomagnesemia, hypocalcemia, neurologic conditions leading to subarachnoid bleed, structural heart disease.

DIAGNOSTIC TESTS & INTERPRETATION
Initial Tests (lab, imaging)
- ECG
- Metabolic panel: especially calcium, magnesium, and potassium; TSH

Follow-Up Tests & Special Considerations
- Echocardiogram to evaluate for cardiomyopathy
- Outpatient cardiac rhythm monitoring (Holter, event loop monitoring, or implantable loop recorder)
- Genetic testing for LQTS mutations is available. Indications to pursue testing include family history of early, unexplained cardiac death, family history of LQTS, or clinical suspicion based on patient's history or examination.

Test Interpretation
- The QT interval is best measured from the onset of the QRS to the completion of the T wave; most commonly measured in lead II or V_2
- QTc calculation can be performed in several ways using RR interval immediately preceding the QT interval for calculation. The Bazett formula is most commonly used method.

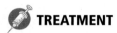 **TREATMENT**

GENERAL MEASURES
- Treat VT, TdP, and VF emergently per ACLS guidelines.
- Withdraw offending agents and correct electrolytes.
- Treat underlying disorder in the setting of gastrointestinal illness, eating disorder, or neurologic conditions involving subarachnoid bleed.
- Avoid triggers, if known.

MEDICATION
First Line
- For TdP: magnesium sulfate 2 g infused over 2 to 5 minutes, followed by continuous infusion of 2 to 4 mg/min if needed. Flushing is a normal side effect of bolus injections. Monitor for magnesium toxicity in those with renal insufficiency.
- For congenital LQTS, to prevent life-threatening arrhythmias: propranolol or nadolol generally regarded as the best β-blockers for management of LQTS, although rigorous studies are lacking.
- β-Blockers are effective in decreasing, but not eliminating the risk of fatal arrhythmias. Patients receiving metoprolol had significantly more breakthrough clinical events (e.g., syncope, aborted cardiac arrest, implantable cardiac defibrillator (ICD) shock, or sudden cardiac death) compared with those receiving propranolol or nadolol (2)[A].

Second Line
- For high-risk patients who remain symptomatic on a β-blocker, ICDs with or without pacemaker may be indicated.
- If no medications are available, an automated external defibrillator is the most useful treatment for any patient with LQTS who converts into a life-threatening arrhythmia.

ISSUES FOR REFERRAL
Refer to cardiologist or electrophysiologist to establish diagnosis, especially for congenital LQTS.

ADDITIONAL THERAPIES
Trials are currently being conducted on medicines that block cardiac sodium channels for LQTS type 3.

SURGERY/OTHER PROCEDURES
- ICD for those with a history of major cardiac events (whether treated with appropriate medical therapy or not).
  - ICDs do not prevent TdP, so patients should continue optimal medical therapy in conjunction to ICD.
- Left cervical—thoracic sympathetic denervation was used for symptomatic LQTS prior to the advent of β-blockers. It is still an option for those patients with LQTS who are refractory to β-blocker therapy (1)[B].

ADMISSION, INPATIENT, AND NURSING CONSIDERATIONS
- Treat TdP, VT, and VF promptly as per ACLS guidelines. Correct electrolytes on an emergent basis. Evaluate for acquired QT prolongation. If no cause is found, consider congenital LQTS.
- Patients with prolonged QTc and syncope/near syncope should be monitored on telemetry.
- Obtain a baseline ECG if initiating or combining medications with QT-prolonging medications, then when the drug reaches steady state, at 30 days, and annually thereafter.
- Avoid QT-prolonging medications in patients with congenital LQTS.
- Monitor electrolytes, urgently treat hypomagnesemia and hypokalemia, and discontinue/change offending medications.

 ONGOING CARE

FOLLOW-UP RECOMMENDATIONS
All patients with LQTS should follow regularly with a cardiologist or electrophysiologist. Classically, patients were limited to low static and low dynamic stresses in the activities they participated in. In 2015, the AHA and ACC released new participation guidelines that allow participation in competitive sports if they meet certain criteria.

Patient Monitoring
- On routine visits, ask about syncope, presyncope, and palpitations in those who have QTc prolongation.
- For pre-participation examinations, ask all participants about these similar symptoms and family history. In individuals responding yes to these questions, have a low threshold to evaluate their QTc with ECG.
- Consider ECG and/or outpatient cardiac rhythm monitoring with medication additions or dosage changes.
- Prompt evaluation is warranted for symptomatic QTc prolongation of any cause.
- Check and correct for electrolyte imbalances.

DIET
- Those with known LQTS often benefit from additional potassium in their diet, whether through diet or supplementation.

- Avoiding caffeinated products, supplements with stimulant properties (such as ginseng), alcohol, and illicit/recreational drugs is also recommended as these can all increase the risk of life-threatening arrhythmias.
- QT prolongation noted in the setting of ketogenic diet and diabetic ketoacidosis irrespective of electrolyte disturbances.

PATIENT EDUCATION
- Educate patients with QTc prolongation about medications side effects and medication interactions.
- Patients with congenital forms of LQTS should be aware of and avoid triggers (depending on their specific gene mutation).
- Consider the emotional and psychological impacts.

PROGNOSIS
Acquired LQTS will resolve after withdrawal of offending agents and normalization of metabolic abnormalities. Patients with underlying cardiovascular disease may be at increased risk of mortality and require further intervention. Prognosis for congenital LQTS if untreated is quite poor.

COMPLICATIONS
TdP resulting in ventricular fibrillation, sudden cardiac death, seizures, loss of consciousness, drowning, and other accidents

REFERENCES
1. Abrams DJ, Macrae CA. Long QT syndrome. *Circulation*. 2014;129(14):1524–1529.
2. Went TR, Sultan W, Sapkota A, et al. A systematic review on the role of beta-blockers in reducing cardiac arrhythmias in long QT syndrome subtypes 1–3. *Cureus*. 2021;13(9):e17632.

 SEE ALSO

Algorithms: Cardiac Arrhythmias; Torsade de Pointes (TdP): Variant Form of Polymorphic Ventricular Tachycardia (VT)

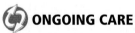 **CODES**

ICD10
I45.81 Long QT syndrome

CLINICAL PEARLS
- Evaluate for acquired causes before making a diagnosis of congenital LQTS.
- Any patient with symptoms of palpitations, syncope, presyncope, any collapse, or with family history of sudden cardiac death should be evaluated with appropriate initial work up, including ECG with QTc evaluation.
- For accurate diagnosis, calculate QTc manually.
- Magnesium sulfate is the treatment of choice during ACLS for TdP.

L

LUNG, PRIMARY MALIGNANCIES

Anila Khaliq, MD • Casey Petronella, DO • Alexandria Quinere, DO, MBS

BASICS

DESCRIPTION

- Primary lung cancers are the leading cause of cancer-related deaths in the United States (estimated 130,180 deaths in 2021 which accounts for 25% of all cancer-related deaths). Lung cancer is mainly diagnosed in older people at average age of diagnosis at 70 years. Lung cancer has the lowest 5-year survival rate at only 18% compared to breast cancer at 90%, prostate cancer at 99%, and colorectal cancer at 65%. Vast majority (85%) of lung cancer is due to smoking, whereas the other 15% is caused by genetics, second hand smoking, asbestos, radon, and other air pollution.
- Divided into two broad categories
  - Non–small cell lung cancer (NSCLC) (85% of all lung cancers)
    ○ Adenocarcinoma (~40% of NSCLC): most common type in the United States and occurs in both smokers and nonsmokers; metastasizes earlier than squamous cell; usually starts from peripheral lung tissue
    ○ Squamous cell carcinoma (SCC) (30% of NSCLC) usually occurs close to large airways.
    ○ Large cell (~10% of NSCLC): named because of the cells' large nuclei
  - Small cell lung cancer (SCLC) (15% of all lung cancers): centrally located, aggressive, and metastasizes very easily through the blood seeding lymph nodes, bones, brain, adrenals, and liver
- Others: mesothelioma and carcinoid tumor
- Staging
  - Both NSCLC and SCLC: staged from I to IV based on primary tumor (T), lymph node status (N), and presence of metastasis (M)
  - SCLC further staged by:
    ○ Limited disease: confined to ipsilateral hemithorax
    ○ Extensive disease: beyond ipsilateral hemithorax (stages IIIB and IV), which may include malignant pleural or pericardial effusion or hematogenous metastases (stage IV)
    ○ Most commonly metastasize to lymph nodes (pulmonary, mediastinal) and then liver, adrenal glands, bones, brain

EPIDEMIOLOGY

Incidence

- There are 236,000 new cases of lung cancer and 130,000 deaths annually in the United States in 2021.
- Overall, lung cancer causes more deaths than breast, prostate, colorectal, and brain cancers combined.
- Average age of diagnosis: 70 years old
- Due to decreases in smoking, lung cancer deaths are declining in the United States.

ETIOLOGY AND PATHOPHYSIOLOGY

Genetics

NSCLC

- Oncogenes: Ras family (H-ras, K-ras, N-ras), EGFR, NTRK, ALK, etc.
- Tumor suppressor genes: retinoblastoma, *p53*
- *Genetics accounts for 8% of lung cancers.*

RISK FACTORS

- Smoking
- Secondhand smoke exposure
- Radon
- Environmental and occupational exposures
  - Air pollution
  - Asbestos exposure (synergistic increase in risk for smokers)
  - Ionizing radiation
  - Mutagenic gases (halogen ethers, mustard gas, aromatic hydrocarbons)
  - Metals (inorganic arsenic, chromium, nickel)
- Lung scarring from tuberculosis
- Radiation therapy to the breast or chest

GENERAL PREVENTION

- Smoking cessation and prevention programs
- As of March 9, 2021, the USPSTF recommends annual screening for lung cancer with low-dose computed tomography (LDCT) in adults aged 50 to 80 years who have a 20 pack-year smoking history and currently smoke or have quit within the past 15 years (1).
- Screening should be discontinued once a person has not smoked for 15 years or develops a health problem that substantially limits life expectancy or the ability or willingness to have curative lung surgery.

COMMONLY ASSOCIATED CONDITIONS

- Paraneoplastic syndromes: hypertrophic pulmonary osteoarthropathy, Lambert-Eaton syndrome (LES), Cushing syndrome, hypercalcemia from ectopic parathyroid hormone–related protein (PTHrP), syndrome of inappropriate antidiuretic hormone (SIADH)
- Hypercoagulable state
- Pancoast syndrome
- Superior vena cava (SVC) syndrome
- Pleural effusion
- Chronic obstructive pulmonary disease (COPD), other sequelae of cigarette smoking

DIAGNOSIS

HISTORY

- May be asymptomatic for most of course
- Respiratory
  - Cough (new or change in chronic cough)
  - Wheezing and stridor
  - Dyspnea
  - Hemoptysis
  - Pneumonitis (fever and productive cough)
- Constitutional
  - Malaise
  - Bone pain (metastatic disease)
  - Fatigue
  - Weight loss, anorexia
  - Fever
  - Anemia
- Other presentations
  - Chest pain (dull, pleuritic), shoulder/arm pain (Pancoast tumors), dysphagia
  - Plethora (redness of face or neck), hoarseness (involvement of recurrent laryngeal nerve)

- Horner syndrome, neurologic abnormalities (e.g., headaches, syncope, weakness, cognitive impairment)
- Pericardial tamponade (pericardial invasion)

PHYSICAL EXAM

- General: fever, chills, night sweats, weight loss
- Head, eye, ear, nose, throat (HEENT): Horner syndrome, dysphonia, stridor, scleral icterus, dysphagia
- Neck: supraclavicular/cervical lymph nodes, mass
- Lungs: effusion, wheezing, airway obstruction, dyspnea
- Abdomen/groin: hepatomegaly or lymphadenopathy
- Extremities: signs of hypertrophic pulmonary osteoarthropathy, deep venous thrombosis (DVT), fingernail clubbing
- Neurologic: headache, syncope, weakness, cognitive impairment

DIFFERENTIAL DIAGNOSIS

COPD (may coexist), asthma, granulomatous (tuberculosis, sarcoidosis), cardiomyopathy/congestive heart failure (CHF)

DIAGNOSTIC TESTS & INTERPRETATION

Initial Tests (lab, imaging)

- Serum
  - Complete blood count (CBC), comprehensive metabolic panel (CMP: Check for hyponatremia (SIADH).
  - Serum calcium: Check for hypercalcemia (paraneoplastic syndrome) and lactate dehydrogenase (LDH).
- Sputum cytology
- Chest x-ray (CXR): nodule or mass, especially if calcified, persistent infiltrate, atelectasis, mediastinal widening, hilar enlargement, pleural effusion
- CT scan of chest (with IV contrast): nodule or mass (central or peripheral), lymphadenopathy
- Biopsy and cytology are definitive diagnosis.
- Evaluation for metastatic disease
  - Positron emission tomography (PET) scan to evaluate metastasis mediastinal lymphadenopathy
  - MRI and CT can also be used to detect mets.

Diagnostic Procedures/Other

- Biopsy with pathology review using
  - Bronchoscopy with transbronchial biopsy (WANG needle); usually for centrally located tumors
  - CT-guided biopsy of lung mass or metastatic site; usually for peripherally located tumors
  - Endobronchial ultrasound (EBUS)-guided fine-needle aspiration
  - Enlarged mediastinal lymph nodes necessitate staging by mediastinoscopy, video-assisted thoracoscopy, and EBUS-guided fine-needle aspiration.
- Video-assisted thoracoscopy (associated pleural disease and suspected mediastinal nodal spread)
- In patients with advanced NSCLC, screening for mutations in EGFR, BRAF, *KRAS G12C*, NTRK, ALK, *ROS1, MET exon 14, and RET* non-SCC (NSCC) or mixed squamous histology
- PD-L1 testing
- Bone marrow aspirate (small cell)

TREATMENT

GENERAL MEASURES
- NSCLC
  - Stage I, stage II, and selected stage III tumors are surgically resectable. Neoadjuvant or adjuvant therapy is recommended for select patients with high-risk IB, II, and IIIA NSCLC. Patients with resectable disease but who are not surgical candidates may receive radiation therapy.
  - Patients with unresectable or N2, N3 disease are treated with concurrent chemoradiation followed by maintenance immunotherapy. Select patients with T3 or N2 disease can be treated effectively with surgical resection and either pre- or postoperative chemotherapy or chemoradiation therapy.
  - Patients with distant metastases (M1B) can be treated with chemotherapy, targeted therapy, immunotherapy, or radiation therapy for palliation or best supportive care alone.
- SCLC
  - Limited stage: concurrent chemoradiation
  - Extensive stage: combination of chemotherapy and immunotherapy
  - Consider prophylactic cranial irradiation (PCI) in patients achieving a complete or partial response.
- Quality-of-life assessments: Karnofsky Performance Status (KPS) scale; Eastern Cooperative Oncology Group (ECOG)
- Discussions with patient and family about end-of-life care

MEDICATION
- Adjuvant chemotherapy following surgery improves survival in patients with fully resected stages II and III NSCLC.
- Comfort measures: oxygen and morphine for shortness or breath, antibiotics for lung infections, diuretics for pulmonary edema, benzodiazepines for anxiety, and corticosteroids for lung obstruction

First Line
- NSCLC
  - Stages II and III: neoadjuvant or adjuvant chemotherapy
    - Cisplatin-based doublets (combination with paclitaxel, etoposide, vinorelbine, docetaxel, gemcitabine)
    - Carboplatin alternative for patients unlikely to tolerate cisplatin
    - Cisplatin plus pemetrexed (NSCC)
  - Unresectable stages IIA and IIIB
    - Concurrent chemoradiation
      - Cisplatin plus etoposide, vinblastine, or pemetrexed (NSCC) plus concurrent radiation
      - Carboplatin plus paclitaxel plus concurrent radiation
      - Carboplatin plus pemetrexed (NSCC) plus concurrent radiation
    - Durvalumab consolidation postchemoradiation for stage III

- Stage IV
  - No chemotherapy regimen can be recommended for routine use.
  - Cisplatin- or carboplatin-based doublets are standard of care in the absence of targetable mutations.
  - Pembrolizumab with pemetrexed and carboplatin for adenocarcinoma without EGFR, ROS, or ALK mutations regardless of PD-L1 expression
  - Pembrolizumab, atezolizumab, or cemiplimab monotherapy for NSCLC with PD-L1 expression ≥50% of tumor cells
  - Osimertinib first line for most patients with EGFR mutations
  - Dabrafenib with trametinib for untreated patients with BRAF V600E mutations
  - Alectinib, lorlatinib, crizotinib, brigatinib, ceritinib, or crizotinib for untreated ALK-positive NSCLC
  - Crizotinib, ceritinib, or entrectinib for patients with ROS1-positive NSCLC
  - Sotorasib for KRAS G12C mutated tumors
  - Larotrectinib or entrectinib for NTRK fusion positive tumors
  - Capmatinib, crizotinib, or tepotinib for tumors with MET exon 14 skipping mutations
  - Selpercatinib, pralsetinib, cabozantinib, or vandetanib for tumors with RET rearrangements
- SCLC
  - Cisplatin or carboplatin plus etoposide with addition of atezolizumab in extensive stage disease

Second Line
- NSCLC
  - Cisplatin-based doublets +/− bevacizumab (NSCC) if not previously used
  - Docetaxel +/− ramucirumab, pemetrexed if not previously used (NSCC), gemcitabine, or nivolumab (squamous cell)
  - Immunotherapy may be considered if progressed during or after first-line platinum-based drug.
- SCLC
  - Lurbinectedin, topotecan, or clinical trial; alternatives include CAV (cyclophosphamide, doxorubicin, vincristine), gemcitabine, docetaxel, paclitaxel, nivolumab, and temozolomide.

ADDITIONAL THERAPIES
- Smoking cessation counseling
- Consider IV bisphosphonates or denosumab in patients with bone metastases to reduce skeletal-related events.

SURGERY/OTHER PROCEDURES
Resection for NSCLC, for stages I, II, and IIIA, if medically fit to undergo surgery

COMPLEMENTARY & ALTERNATIVE MEDICINE
Mind–body therapies
- Creative outlets (e.g., music, art, dance), tai chi, meditation, biofeedback, hypnosis, yoga

 ONGOING CARE

FOLLOW-UP RECOMMENDATIONS
Patient Monitoring
Visits every 3 to 6 months in the first 2 years after surgery with physical exam and CT scan

PATIENT EDUCATION
- National Cancer Institute: https://www.cancer.gov/
- Smokefree.gov: https://smokefree.gov/

PROGNOSIS
- For combined therapy, all types and stages, 5-year survival rate is 18.6%.
- NSCLC 5-year survival
  - Localized disease: for stages IA1, IA2, and IA3 is 92%, 83%, and 77%, respectively; stages IB and IIA is 68% and 60%, respectively
  - Regional disease: for stages IIIA, IIIB, and IIIC is 36%, 26%, and 13%, respectively
  - Distant metastatic disease: for stages IVA and IVB is 10% and <1%, respectively
- SCLC
  - Without treatment: median survival from diagnosis of only 2 to 4 months
  - 5-year survival rate: ranges from 2% (stage IV) to 31% (stage I)
  - Extensive-stage disease: median survival of 6 to 12 months; long-term disease-free survival is rare.

COMPLICATIONS
- Thrombosis
- Paraneoplastic syndromes
- Fatigue, anorexia, weight loss
- Chemotherapy-induced nausea and vomiting
- Neutropenia, anemia
- Neurotoxicities, nephrotoxicities

REFERENCE
1. Krist AH, Davidson KW, Mangione CM, et al; for US Preventive Services Task Force. Screening for lung cancer: US Preventive Services Task Force recommendation statement. *JAMA*. 2021;325(10):962–970.

CODES

ICD10
- C34.90 Malignant neoplasm of unsp part of unsp bronchus or lung
- C34.10 Malignant neoplasm of upper lobe, unsp bronchus or lung
- C34.30 Malignant neoplasm of lower lobe, unsp bronchus or lung

CLINICAL PEARLS
- NSCLC (>85% of all lung cancers); normally originate in periphery
  - Adenocarcinoma (~40% of NSCLC); SCC (~25% of NSCLC); large cell (~10% of NSCLC)
- SCLC centrally located, early metastases, aggressive

L

LUPUS ERYTHEMATOSUS, SYSTEMIC (SLE)

Sahil Mullick, MD • Farzad Effan, MBBS

 BASICS

DESCRIPTION
- Multisystem autoimmune inflammatory disorder with variable presentation, disease course, and prognosis
- Can manifest in any organ system, especially dermatologic, renal, hematologic, musculoskeletal, and cardiovascular
- Synonyms: lupus, systemic lupus erythematosus (SLE)

EPIDEMIOLOGY
Incidence
- 5 to 7 per 100,000 person-years in United States
- Significant variation based on ethnicity: black, 16.0; American Indian/Alaska Native, 7.4; Hispanic, 5.6; Asian/Pacific Islander, 4.6; and white, 3.3 per 100,000 person-years
- Strong female predominance compared to male: 9.8 versus 0.8 per 100,000 person-years (~12-fold higher)
- Peak incidence: 3rd to 7th decades of life for females and 5th to 7th decades of life for males

Prevalence
- Ranges from 70 to 100 cases per 100,000 people in United States.
- Strong female predominance compared to male: 179 versus 21 cases per 100,000 people (~9-fold higher) with highest prevalence in black women: 498 cases per 100,000 people

ETIOLOGY AND PATHOPHYSIOLOGY
Genetic, environmental, immunoregulatory, hormonal, and epigenetic factors all play a role.

Genetics
>90 susceptibility loci for SLE in genome-wide association studies (1)[C]

RISK FACTORS
- Ethnicity: highest risk in black populations; intermediate risk in Asian, Hispanic, and American Indian/Alaska Native populations
- Hormonal: female sex, early menarche/menopause, endometriosis, surgical menopause
- Family history of SLE or autoimmune disease
- Environmental: cigarette smoking, crystalline silica exposure, exogenous female hormones, certain medications (drug-induced lupus)

COMMONLY ASSOCIATED CONDITIONS
Antiphospholipid syndrome, depression, fibromyalgia, thyroid disease, connective tissue disease syndromes (such as rheumatoid arthritis, Sjögren syndrome, systemic sclerosis)

 DIAGNOSIS

- Suspect in multisystem disease including fever, fatigue, and signs of inflammation
- Classification criteria from European League Against Rheumatism/American College of Rheumatology (EULAR/ACR) in 2019: sensitivity 96%, specificity 93% (2)[C]
- Note: Do not exclude clinically appropriate patients from treatment solely based on classification criteria (2)[C].
- Previous criteria from ACR and Systemic Lupus International Collaborating Clinics (SLICC) still used widely in clinical practice

HISTORY
- Common symptoms: fatigue, arthralgia, fever, oral ulcers, hair loss, rash, photosensitivity
- Presentations that may raise suspicion: unprovoked venous thromboembolism (VTE), cerebrovascular accident at young age, acute pericarditis, recurrent pregnancy loss, new-onset seizure or psychosis, unexplained cytopenias, or renal failure

PHYSICAL EXAM
- Constitutional (common): weight loss, fever, lymphadenopathy
- Skin (common)
  - Nonspecific: nonscarring alopecia, painless oral or nasal ulcers, photosensitivity, vasculitis, Raynaud phenomenon
  - Acute cutaneous lupus erythematosus (ACLE)
    ○ Includes classic malar or "butterfly" rash that spares nasolabial folds and generalized maculopapular form that is photodistributed
  - Subacute cutaneous lupus erythematosus (SCLE)
    ○ Annular or papulosquamous eruptions, photo-distributed, frequently found on shoulders, neck, forearms, torso
  - Chronic cutaneous lupus erythematosus (CCLE)
    ○ Includes discoid lupus and erythematous lesions with secondary changes of atrophic scarring and dyspigmentation
  - On scalp, causes follicular hyperkeratosis and plugging and scarring alopecia
  - All have characteristic changes on biopsy
- Musculoskeletal (common):
  - Synovitis, especially symmetric polyarthritis, periarticular involvement (tendons, joint capsule), leading to nonerosive joint deformities (Jaccoud arthropathy)
- Pericarditis/pneumonitis, pleural effusion, VTE
- Edema or anasarca in advanced renal disease; pallor, jaundice, splenomegaly in hematologic disease; seizures, psychosis, delirium, mononeuritis multiplex, peripheral or cranial neuropathies, and cognitive impairment in CNS disease

DIFFERENTIAL DIAGNOSIS
- Extremely broad due to variable presentation and widespread disease manifestations
- Consider other rheumatologic conditions, thyroid disease, fibromyalgia, or organ-specific diagnoses based on presentation
- Consider drug-induced lupus (hydralazine, procainamide, isoniazid, methyldopa, quinidine, chlorpromazine).

DIAGNOSTIC TESTS & INTERPRETATION
Initial Tests (lab, imaging)
- Based on presentation and level of suspicion
- Low suspicion: Limited initial laboratory evaluation may include complete blood count (CBC), complete metabolic panel (CMP), thyroid-stimulating hormone (TSH), and urinalysis; imaging based on signs/symptoms
- Higher suspicion: immunologic testing
  - Lupus-specific
    ○ ANA (titer ≥1:80 by immunofluorescence); sensitivity 97.8%, specificity 74.7%
    ○ Anti-dsDNA (sensitivity 70%, specificity 96%)
    ○ Anti-Smith (sensitivity 39.7%, specificity 98.6%)

- Supporting:
  ○ Complement levels (low C3 and/or C4)
  ○ Anticardiolipin, anti-β2GP1, lupus anticoagulant

Follow-Up Tests & Special Considerations
- 24-hour urine collection or spot protein/creatinine ratio to quantify proteinuria (2)[C]
- Anemia: reticulocyte count, indirect bilirubin, haptoglobin, direct Coombs test to evaluate for hemolysis (2)[C]
- Screen for antiphospholipid syndrome at diagnosis if not already done (3)[C].
- Baseline metabolic labs: lipid panel, fasting glucose or HbA1c, vitamin D level, TSH

Diagnostic Procedures/Other
- Renal biopsy: urine protein >500 mg/day (2)[C]
- Skin biopsy if necessary to confirm clinical findings of cutaneous lupus (2)[C]

Test Interpretation
- Skin biopsy: Interface vacuolar dermatitis consisting of perivascular lymphohistiocytic infiltrate with dermal mucin; may have immune-complex deposition at dermoepidermal junction
- Renal biopsy: per International Society of Nephrology/Renal Pathology Society classification

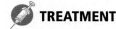 TREATMENT

GENERAL MEASURES
- Requires a multidisciplinary, individualized approach to treatment
- General treatment goals: achieving remission or low disease activity, preventing flares and end-organ damage, increasing survival, improving quality of life (3)[C]
- Supportive measures include sun protection, smoking cessation, adequate exercise, managing cardiovascular risk factors (lipids, glucose, blood pressure, weight)
- Preconception counseling, family planning
- Immunizations: 2019 EULAR guidelines for vaccination

MEDICATION
First Line
- Hydroxychloroquine
  - Recommended for all patients with SLE unless contraindicated (4)[C]
  - Reduces flares, improves skin/musculoskeletal manifestations, reduces thrombosis and bone mass loss, prevents organ damage, increases survival; safe in pregnancy (4)[A]
  - Dosing: 200 to 400 mg/day as single daily dose or 2 divided doses; limit to 5 mg/kg/day (actual body weight) (3)[C]
  - Most common adverse reactions are gastrointestinal (nausea, vomiting, diarrhea, abdominal pain) and cutaneous (rash), and they are usually mild (4)[C].
  - Retinal damage:
    ○ Less common at doses <5 mg/kg/day
    ○ Risk factors: high doses, renal insufficiency, macular disease, tamoxifen use
    ○ Ophthalmologic screening at baseline (3)[C]
    ○ Yearly screening after 5 years in absence of other risk factors (3)[C]

– Cardiomyopathy: conduction abnormalities including prolonged QT interval
– Other adverse reactions include proximal myopathy and neuropathy, neuropsychiatric changes, and hypoglycemia.
– Caution in hepatic and/or renal disease, with insulin and antidiabetic medications, and medication that affects cardiac conduction, especially QT prolonging agents

- Glucocorticoids
  – Dose and route of administration depend on organ involvement and severity.
    ○ Topical steroids are used in cutaneous disease.
    ○ Oral steroids are used for initial management, flares, and/or maintenance therapy.
    ○ Life/organ-threatening flares frequently require pulsed IV methylprednisolone (250 to 1,000 mg/day for 1 to 3 days) (3)[C]
  – Dose of chronic maintenance therapy should be minimized to < 7.5 mg/day and discontinued if possible (3)[C].
  – Early immunomodulatory therapy may help minimize glucocorticoid needs (3)[C].

Second Line
- Choice of agent depends on disease manifestations, patient's characteristics (such as age and childbearing potential), safety, and cost.
- Consider methotrexate, azathioprine, or mycophenolate for patients not controlled on hydroxychloroquine, unable to adequately taper glucocorticoids, or for initial treatment in more severe disease. Consider belimumab add-on for high residual disease activity or frequent flares despite standard treatments. Consider cyclophosphamide or rituximab for severe life-organ-threatening or refractory disease (3)[C].

ISSUES FOR REFERRAL
Mild disease without significant end-organ involvement may be appropriate for treatment in primary care; generally requires multidisciplinary team in coordination with rheumatology; severe disease is best managed in dedicated lupus center.

ADDITIONAL THERAPIES
IVIG has shown to successfully treat cutaneous and neuropsychiatric symptoms of SLE, with reduction in disease activity and daily steroid requirement (5)[A].

SURGERY/OTHER PROCEDURES
Renal transplant for end-stage renal disease

COMPLEMENTARY & ALTERNATIVE MEDICINE
Supplements with some evidence of benefit: vitamin D, omega-3 fatty acids, N-acetylcysteine, and turmeric (6)[C]

ADMISSION, INPATIENT, AND NURSING CONSIDERATIONS
Difficult to differentiate SLE flare from infection; may need to treat both pending full evaluation; IV pulse methylprednisolone (250 to 1,000 mg/day for 1 to 3 days) for organ-threatening flares

ONGOING CARE

FOLLOW-UP RECOMMENDATIONS
Patient Monitoring
- Intensity of monitoring depends on manifestations, severity, medication regimen, and comorbidities.
- Stable, inactive disease without significant organ involvement or comorbidities may be monitored every 6 to 12 months.
- Evaluation should include at least one validated measure of disease activity (i.e., Systemic Lupus Erythematosus Disease Activity Index).
- Vigilant monitoring of kidney function (i.e., every 3 months) in high-risk ethnicity, male sex, juvenile-onset, high serologic activity, positive anti-C1q antibodies (3)[C]
- Atherosclerotic cardiovascular disease (ASCVD)
  – Manage as per established guidelines.
  – Standard ASCVD risk calculators may underestimate risk in SLE—take into account SLE-specific factors (i.e., high disease activity, high doses of glucocorticoids, lupus nephritis, antiphospholipid antibodies).
- Osteoporosis
  – Adequate calcium/vitamin D intake, smoking cessation, weight-bearing exercise, limited alcohol intake
  – Long-term glucocorticoid use: clinical fracture risk assessment +/− bone mineral density measurement
  – 2017 ACR guideline for prevention and treatment
- Ophthalmologic evaluation with hydroxychloroquine (retinal damage) and/or glucocorticoids (cataracts, glaucoma)
- Malignancy: Follow routine cancer-screening guidelines for general population.
- Neuropsychiatric: Consider screening for mood disorders and cognitive impairment.

DIET
Currently, evidence is insufficient to recommend specific dietary pattern for patients with SLE.

PATIENT EDUCATION
- Centers for Disease Control and Prevention: https://www.cdc.gov/lupus/index.htm
- Lupus Foundation of America: https://www.lupus.org/

PROGNOSIS
Permanent, treatment-free remission is rare; 10-year survival ~90%; increased all-cause mortality in SLE compared to general population with standardized mortality ratio (SMR) of 2.6

COMPLICATIONS
Medication toxicity (including osteoporosis and osteonecrosis), obstetric complications, malignancy (especially hematologic, cervical, breast, lung), renal failure, cardiovascular and thromboembolic events, infections, and death

REFERENCES
1. Ameer MA, Chaudhry H, Mushtaq J, et al. An overview of systemic lupus erythematosus (SLE) pathogenesis, classification, and management. *Cureus.* 2022;14(10):e30330.
2. Aringer M, Costenbader K, Daikh D, et al. 2019 European League Against Rheumatism/American College of Rheumatology classification criteria for systemic lupus erythematosus. *Arthritis Rheumatol.* 2019;71(9):1400–1412.
3. Fanouriakis A, Kostopoulou M, Alunno A, et al. 2019 update of the EULAR recommendations for the management of systemic lupus erythematosus. *Ann Rheum Dis.* 2019;78(6):736–745.
4. Ruiz-Irastorza G, Ramos-Casals M, Brito-Zeron P, et al. Clinical efficacy and side effects of antimalarials in systemic lupus erythematosus: a systematic review. *Ann Rheum Dis.* 2010;69(1):20–28.
5. Sakthiswary R, D'Cruz D. Intravenous immunoglobulin in the therapeutic armamentarium of systemic lupus erythematosus: a systematic review and meta-analysis. *Medicine (Baltimore).* 2014;93(16):e86.
6. Furer V, Rondaan C, Heijstek MW, et al. 2019 update of EULAR recommendations for vaccination in adult patients with autoimmune inflammatory rheumatic diseases. *Ann Rheum Dis.* 2020;79(1):39–52.

SEE ALSO
Antiphospholipid Antibody Syndrome

CODES

ICD10
- M32.0 Drug-induced systemic lupus erythematosus
- M32.14 Glomerular disease in systemic lupus erythematosus
- M32.19 Other organ or system involvement in systemic lupus erythematosus

CLINICAL PEARLS
- Multisystem disease, variable presentation—maintain high index of suspicion for diagnosis
- Increased all-cause mortality, particularly with renal disease, infections, cardiovascular disease
- Low threshold for renal biopsy—lupus nephritis is a major risk factor for poor outcomes
- Aggressiveness of therapy should reflect intensity of disease.

LUPUS NEPHRITIS

Neena R. Gupta, MD

BASICS

DESCRIPTION
- Renal disease associated with systemic lupus erythematosus (SLE)
- A kidney biopsy is necessary to confirm the diagnosis (1).
- Clinical manifestations primarily due to immune complex–mediated glomerular disease; tubulointerstitial and vascular involvement often coexist. Diagnosis is based on clinical findings, urine abnormalities, autoantibodies, and renal biopsy.
- Treatment and prognosis depend on severity of disease.
- Early diagnosis improves renal outcomes.

EPIDEMIOLOGY
- Peak incidence of SLE is 15 to 45 years of age. Mean age of diagnosis is between 25 and 30 years of age.
- The lifetime incidence of lupus nephritis (LN) in patients with SLE is 20–60%.
- Predominant sex: female > male (10:1)
- Once SLE develops, LN affects both genders equally; it is more severe in children and men and less severe in older adults.
- More common in African American and Asian populations

Incidence
- SLE: 1 to 22/100,000 people
- Up to 60% of SLE patients develop LN over time; 25–50% of SLE patients have nephritis as the initial presentation.

Pediatric Considerations
LN is more common and more severe in children: 60–80% of children have LN at or soon after SLE onset.

Prevalence
SLE: 7 to 159/100,000 people

ETIOLOGY AND PATHOPHYSIOLOGY
- Immune complex–mediated inflammation injures glomeruli, tubules, interstitium, and vasculature.
- Glomeruli: Varying degrees of mesangial proliferation, crescent formation, and fibrinoid necrosis cause reduced glomerular filtration rate (GFR).
- Persistent inflammation (chronicity) leads to sclerosis and glomerular loss.
- Tubulointerstitial injury (edema, inflammatory cell infiltrate acutely; tubular atrophy in chronic phase) with or without tubular basement membrane immune complex deposition leads to reduced renal function.
- Vascular lesions: immune complex deposition and noninflammatory necrosis in arterioles
- SLE is a multifactorial disease, with multigenic inheritance; exact etiology remains unclear.
- Defective T-cell autoregulation and polyclonal B-cell hyperactivity contribute to dysregulated apoptosis. Impaired clearance of apoptotic cells inhibits self-tolerance to nuclear antigen.
- Anti-DNA, anti-C1q, anti-α-actin, and other nuclear component autoantibodies develop.

- Deposition of circulating immune complexes or autoantibodies attaching to local nuclear antigens leads to complement activation, inflammation, and tissue injury.
- Interaction of genetic, hormonal, and environmental factors leads to great variability in LN severity.

Genetics
- Polygenic inheritance; clustering in families, ~25% concordance in identical twins
- Interaction of general SLE susceptibility genes with more renal-specific genes and epigenetic changes

RISK FACTORS
Younger age, African American or Hispanic race, more ACR criteria for SLE, longer disease duration, hypertension, lower socioeconomic status, family history of SLE, anti-dsDNA antibodies, low albumin to globulin ratio

COMMONLY ASSOCIATED CONDITIONS
Other organ systems often involved in SLE.

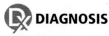

DIAGNOSIS

HISTORY
- Assess for signs/symptoms of SLE.
- Active nephritis is often accompanied by fever, peripheral edema, nausea, vomiting, headache and dizziness.

PHYSICAL EXAM
- Hypertension, fever
- Pleural/pericardial rub (serositis)
- Skin rash
- Edema
- Arthritis
- Alopecia
- Oral ulcers
- Signs of synovitis

DIFFERENTIAL DIAGNOSIS
- Primary glomerular disease
- Secondary renal involvement in other systemic disorders such as antineutrophil cytoplasmic antibody (ANCA)-associated vasculitis, Henoch-Schönlein purpura (HSP), antiglomerular basement membrane disease, polyarteritis nodosa, and viral infections

DIAGNOSTIC TESTS & INTERPRETATION
- Renal biopsy is the gold standard for diagnosing and classifying LN.
- Active urine sediment suggests nephritis.
- Autoantibodies, low C3, C4, and CH50 complement levels support LN.

Initial Tests (lab, imaging)
- Urinalysis, serum electrolytes, BUN, creatinine, albumin, routine serologic markers of SLE such as antinuclear antibody (ANA), anti-dsDNA, anti-Ro, anti-La, anti-RNP, anti-Sm, antiphospholipid (aPL) antibody, C3, C4, CH50, CBC with differential, and C-reactive protein (CRP) (1)[C]
- Renal ultrasound

Follow-Up Tests & Special Considerations
- Monitor disease activity every 3 months (1)[C]: urinalysis for hematuria and proteinuria; blood for C3, C4, anti-dsDNA, serum albumin, and creatinine.
- Manage patients with estimated GFR (eGFR) of <60 mL as per National Kidney Foundation guidelines for chronic kidney disease (CKD): https://kdigo.org/guidelines/ckd-evaluation-and-management/.
- Biomarker panel: α_1-acid glycoprotein (AGP); ceruloplasmin; lipocalin-like prostaglandin synthase (LPGDS); transferring correlates with disease activity in children.

Pregnancy Considerations
- Pregnancy leads to worsening of renal function. Risk factors include renal impairment at baseline, active disease, hypertension, and proteinuria.
- Risk factors for fetal loss include elevated serum creatinine, heavy proteinuria, hypertension, and anticardiolipin antibodies.
- Renin-angiotensin system blockade and mycophenolate mofetil (MMF) are contraindicated in pregnancy; azathioprine can be used, U.S. FDA pregnancy Category D.

Test Interpretation
- On renal biopsy immunofluorescence microscopy: Immune complex deposits consisting of IgG, IgA, IgM, C1q, and C3 ("full house") are highly suggestive of LN.
- Revised ISN/RPS 2003 histologic classification guides therapeutic decisions: https://jasn.asnjournals.org/content/jnephrol/15/2/241.full.pdf?with-ds=yes. Revised 2008 classification awaits endorsement.
- LN is classified as purely mesangial (class I-minimal mesangial LN and II-mesangial proliferative LN), focal proliferative LN: <50% glomeruli (class III), diffuse proliferative LN: ≥50% (class IV), membranous LN (class V), and advanced sclerosis LN (class VI); subdivisions for activity (A) and chronicity (C) in class III/IV and for segmental (S) or global (G) glomerular involvement in class IV (class III A, C, A/C and class IV S[A], G[A], S[A/C], S[C], G[C]); LN class may change with or without therapy.
- Focal and diffuse proliferative LN (classes III and IV) are common and most likely to progress to ESRD.

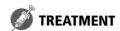

TREATMENT

GENERAL MEASURES
- Monitor bone density; optimize vitamin D and calcium intake, BMI, and regular exercise.
- Low-salt diet
- Avoid sun or ultraviolet light exposure.

MEDICATION
Note: Other than methylprednisolone, prednisone, and belimumab, no other medications listed next are FDA-approved for LN.

First Line
- Class I + II LN: no specific therapy; monitor urine protein-to-creatinine ratio (UPCR); renin-angiotensin system blockade (ACEI or ARB) to manage BP and proteinuria (e.g., lisinopril 5 to 40 mg/day PO, losartan 25 to 100 mg/day PO)
- Proliferative LN (class III or IV [±V]) (1),(2)
- Principles of treatment:
  - Avoid delay; proteinuria reduction of at least 25% by 3 months, 50% by 6 months, and UPCR target below 0.5 to 0.7 by 12 months (2)
  - Patients with baseline nephrotic range proteinuria may need an additional 6 to 12 months.
- INDUCTION: steroids + immunosuppressive agent (for mild class III, high-dose steroids may be sufficient):
  - Glucocorticoids: methylprednisolone pulses, (total dose of 500 to 2,500 mg) followed by oral prednisone (0.3 to 0.5 mg/kg/day) for up to 4 weeks, tapered to ≤7.5 mg/day by 3 to 6 months (2)[A] and
  - Cyclophosphamide: IV cyclophosphamide (low dose = 0.5 g every 2 weeks for a total of 6 doses) or
  - MMF: Target dose of 2 to 3 g/day for 6 months; MMF is as effective as cyclophosphamide in achieving remission with fewer side effects (2)[A].
  - MMF (target dose of 1 to 2 g/day) with calcineurin inhibitor (CNI) is an alternative to patients with nephrotic range proteinuria.
  - High dose IV cyclophosphamide (0.50 to 0.75 g/m²) monthly for 6 doses is an option for patients at high risk for kidney failure.
  - In Asian population, combination of tacrolimus, MMF, and glucocorticoids is found to be superior to cyclophosphamide and glucocorticoids.
- MAINTENANCE:
  - Glucocorticoids: low dose oral prednisone (2.5 to 5.0 mg/day) and
  - MMF 1 to 2 g/day especially if used as initial agent or azathioprine: 2 mg/kg/day PO (2)[A]
  - Optimum duration is unclear but gradual withdrawal (glucocorticoids first) after at least 3 to 5 years therapy in complete clinical response
- Pure class V LN: good prognosis, no standardized treatment
  - MMF (2 to 3 g/day) with IV methylprednisolone pulse (500 to 2,500 mg) followed by oral prednisone (20 mg/day tapered to ≤5 mg/day by 3 months) (2)
  - Options for nephrotic range proteinuria patients include CNI (especially tacrolimus) or IV cyclophosphamide, either as monotherapy or in combination with MMF (2).
- Belimumab in combination with standard initial and subsequent therapy as 10 mg/kg IV every 2 weeks for 3 doses followed by maintenance dosing every 4 weeks for a total of 100 weeks has been shown to improve outcome.
- Hydroxychloroquine: all LN of any class unless contraindicated; maximum daily dose not to exceed 5 mg/kg/day and adjust for GFR with regular ophthalmologic follow-up

Second Line
Refractory LN: no response to initial treatment within 3 to 4 months; multitarget therapy recommended; change either cyclophosphamide to MMF or vice versa, rituximab, obinutuzumab CNI (tacrolimus, voclosporin), belimumab, stem cell transplantation, IVIG, or plasma exchange (3)[C].

ISSUES FOR REFERRAL
Nephrology consults for initial management and relapses.

ADDITIONAL THERAPIES
- RAS blockade is beneficial because of antiproteinuric and antihypertensive effects.
- Vaccination review
- Treat hypertension, dyslipidemia and other modifiable cardiovascular risk factors.
- Low-dose aspirin for high-risk aPL profile

SURGERY/OTHER PROCEDURES
- Renal transplant for ESRD when indicated
- Patient and graft survival rates similar to non-SLE patients
- Recurrent LN ranges between 0% and 30%; graft loss due to recurrence is rare.

ADMISSION, INPATIENT, AND NURSING CONSIDERATIONS
Admission criteria/initial stabilization
- Uncontrolled hypertension, acute kidney injury
- Severe extrarenal manifestation
- Nephrology input for management and renal biopsy

ONGOING CARE

FOLLOW-UP RECOMMENDATIONS
Patient Monitoring
- UPCR, urine microscopy, serum albumin, creatinine, antibody titers (especially anti-dsDNA), C3, C4, BP at least every 3 months for first 2 to 3 years followed by 6 to 12 months if no active disease (1)[C]
- CBC, LFT, and hydration per immunosuppressive regimen

DIET
Low-salt diet; for eGFR <60 mL: Follow National Kidney Foundation guidelines for CKD.

PATIENT EDUCATION
- Medication adherence and self-monitoring for relapse
- Preconception counseling
- Smoking cessation

PROGNOSIS
- 10-year survival of 88% and 94% in SLE patients with and without renal involvement, respectively
- Relapse rate is ~35%; 10–20% of patients progress to ESRD within 10 years.
- 5-year renal survival of class IV LN <30% before 1970 has improved to >80% in the last 2 decades.

- Remission of proteinuria is the best prognostic factor. Others include low baseline proteinuria, normal creatinine, white race, and treatment initiated within 3 months of diagnosis.
- Poor prognosis: crescentic diffuse proliferative LN, higher activity/chronicity index, APOL 1 risk alleles, African American race, lower socioeconomic status, poor response to treatment, high creatinine at baseline, uncontrolled hypertension, and relapse

COMPLICATIONS
- Risks of immunosuppressive therapy: infections, malignancy, GI upset, primary amenorrhea with cyclophosphamide, teratogenic effect of MMF
- Vascular thromboses with aPL antibodies
- About 10–20% of patients develop ESRD requiring dialysis/kidney transplantation.

REFERENCES
1. Kidney Disease: Improving Global Outcomes. KDIGO 2021 clinical practice guideline for the management of glomerular diseases. https://kdigo.org/guidelines/gd/. Accessed September 21, 2023.
2. Fanouriakis A, Kostopoulou M, Cheema K, et al. 2019 Update of the Joint European League Against Rheumatism and European Renal Association—European Dialysis and Transplant Association (EULAR/ERA-EDTA) recommendations for the management of lupus nephritis. *Ann Rheum Dis*. 2020;79(6):713–723.
3. Gasparotto M, Gatto M, Binda V, et al. Lupus nephritis: clinical presentations and outcomes in the 21st century. *Rheumatology (Oxford)*. 2020;59(Suppl 5):v39–v51.

ADDITIONAL READING
- Alforaih N, Whittall-Garcia L, Touma Z. A Review of Lupus Nephritis. *J Appl Lab Med*. 2022;7(6):1450–1467.
- Kidney Disease: Improving Global Outcomes. KDIGO clinical practice guideline for glomerulonephritis. *Kidney Int Suppl*. 2012;2(2):139–274.

CODES

ICD10
M32.14 Glomerular disease in systemic lupus erythematosus

CLINICAL PEARLS
- Early diagnosis, correct classification (based on renal biopsy), and rapid treatment improve renal survival.
- Treat proliferative/progressive LN with a short induction course followed by maintenance therapy using glucocorticoids and immunosuppressants.
- Due to advances in diagnosis and treatment, survival rates for patients have improved dramatically over the past several decades.

L

LYME DISEASE

Brett Lehner, MD

BASICS

Lyme disease is caused by the bacterium *Borrelia burgdorferi*.

DESCRIPTION
- An infection caused by *Borrelia* spirochetes, transmitted primarily by ixodid ticks
- *Ixodes scapularis* (deer ticks) in the Northeast and Great Lakes areas
- *Ixodes pacificus* in the West (black-legged ticks and Western black-legged ticks)

EPIDEMIOLOGY
In 2021, a total of 24,611 confirmed and probable cases of Lyme disease were reported to CDC. Approximately 476,000 people may get Lyme disease each year in the United States.

Incidence
High incidence U.S. states: Connecticut, Delaware, Maine, Maryland, Massachusetts, Minnesota, New Hampshire, New Jersey, New York, Pennsylvania, Rhode Island, Vermont, Virginia, and Wisconsin

Prevalence
Predominant age: most common in children ages 5 to 14 years and in adults aged 55 to 70 years of age

ETIOLOGY AND PATHOPHYSIOLOGY
- Average incubation period of 7 to 10 days after tick bite
- The 1st week of July is the peak week of onset for confirmed and probable cases.
- If a tick is infected, the chance of transmission increases with time attached: 0% at 24 hours, 12% at 48 hours, 79% at 72 hours, and 94% at 96 hours of attachment
- The primary animal reservoir is the white-footed mouse.
- Spirochetes multiply and spread within dermis, resulting in characteristic (erythema multiforme [EM]) rash. Hematogenous dissemination results in involvement of central nervous system (CNS), cardiovascular, or other organ stems.

Genetics
Human leukocyte antigen haplotype DR4 or DR2 increases susceptibility to prolonged arthritis.

RISK FACTORS
Lyme endemic area; ixodid ticks are common on deer; hunters at increased risk

GENERAL PREVENTION
- Wear appropriate clothing when outdoors in endemic areas during times of high tick activity. Clothing should cover the ankles and pretreat clothes, shoes, and tents with 0.5% permethrin.
- "Tick checks": Examine the skin after outdoor activities.
- Remove ticks as soon as possible to limit transmission.
- To prevent of tick bites: N,N-diethyl-meta-toluamide (DEET), picaridin ethyl-3-(N-n-butyl-N-acetyl) aminopropionate (IR3535), oil of eucalyptus (OLE), p-menthane-3,8-diol (PMD), 2-undecanone
- Prophylactic treatment with 1 dose of 200 mg of doxycycline within 72 hours of a tick that has been attached for at least 36 hours is indicated in endemic areas; number needed to treat = 50

COMMONLY ASSOCIATED CONDITIONS
- Coinfection with other tick borne illness (e.g., babesiosis, ehrlichiosis, anaplasmosis)
- Comorbid human granulocytic anaplasmosis and/or babesiosis in patients living in endemic regions

DIAGNOSIS

- Test with a sensitive enzyme immunoassay (EIA) or immunofluorescence assay, which quantifies antibodies against *B. burgdorferi*, and then follow this test with a western immunoblot assay for specimens yielding either a positive or equivocal results in the EIA.
- Both the EIA and Western blot are needed to confirm diagnosis. If the EIA is equivocal the western blot needs to be positive for the diagnosis of Lyme Disease.
- Of note, antibodies can take from 2 to 6 weeks to develop, so if there is a high suspicion for Lyme disease, serum testing can be repeated several weeks following initial presentation.

HISTORY
- History of a tick bite followed by EM and/or illness (fever, fatigue, headache, myalgias)
- EM = round, flat or raised, erythematous bull's-eye lesion that expands in diameter over days to weeks that has an area of central clearing
  - Common sites: axilla, back, abdomen, groin, or popliteal fossa
  - 75–80% presenting with EM having a single lesion
- Early Lyme disease: incubation period of 3 to 30 days; patients may be asymptomatic; fever; headache; myalgias; arthralgias, regional lymphadenopathy
- Early disseminated Lyme disease:
  - Carditis: pleuritic chest pain, palpitations, light headaches, fainting, shortness of breath
  - Facial palsies or other cranial neuropathies
  - Joint pain (polyarthritis/polyarthralgia)
  - Late disease: monoarthritis, iritis, conjunctivitis, migratory musculoskeletal pain
- Late Lyme disease arises months after exposure.
  - Recurrent synovitis; recurrent tendonitis and bursitis
  - Encephalopathic symptoms: severe headaches and neck stiffness; confusion; facial palsy on one or both sides of the face
  - Peripheral nerve involvement: radiculoneuropathy, numbness, tingling, shooting pain, or weakness in the arms or legs
  - Symptoms mimicking other CNS diseases: multiple sclerosis–like symptoms; stroke–like symptoms; transverse myelitis

PHYSICAL EXAM
- Early Lyme disease:
  - EM in 70–80% of patients; expanding erythema arises 3 to 30 days, and the average is about 7 days, after tick detaches. Lesions are often >5 cm, flat or raised, may be homogeneous or have an area of central clearing (classic target session).
- Disseminated Lyme disease:
  - Skin: multiple EM lesions
  - Neurology: facial palsies (uni- or bilateral) or other cranial neuropathies
  - Cardiovascular: irregular pulse, bradycardia (heart block); friction rub (pericarditis)

DIFFERENTIAL DIAGNOSIS
- Other tick-borne illnesses: Rocky Mountain spotted fever (RMSF), ehrlichiosis, babesiosis, anaplasma
- Autoimmune process: juvenile rheumatoid arthritis (RA); systemic lupus erythematosus (SLE); RA
- Viral syndromes
- Contact dermatitis, cellulitis
- Granuloma annulare (mimic EM)
- Syphilis

DIAGNOSTIC TESTS & INTERPRETATION
- A tick bite is considered to be high risk only if the tick bite was from an identified *Ixodes* spp. vector species, it occurs in a highly endemic area, and the tick was attached for ≥36 hours (1)[A].
- Patients who have a typical EM lesion and who live in or have traveled to a Lyme-endemic area can be diagnosed with acute Lyme disease without laboratory testing.
- Serologic testing of patients presenting with EM lesions is not recommended due to insensitivity of serologic assays during the acute stage of infection.
- Health care providers should order Lyme testing only when there is existing clinical and epidemiologic support for diagnosis.

Initial Tests (lab, imaging)
- Potential tick exposure in a Lyme disease endemic area who have one or more skin lesions compatible with EM, recommended clinical diagnosis rather than laboratory testing
- Testing for IgM or IgG-class antibodies to *B. burgdorferi* solely by immunoblot, without a prior positive or equivocal first-tier immunoassay, is strongly discouraged due to an increase frequency of false-positive result.
- CDC recommends two-tier testing.
  - Tier 1 is an antibody screening assay.
  - Tier 2 is an immunoblot.
    - If the immunoassay(s) are negative, no further test is necessary.
    - If the immunoassays are positive or equivocal, reflex testing by immunoblot is required.
    - For patients with symptoms lasting 30 days or less, both IgM and IgG specific anti-B. burgdorferi immunoblots should be performed.
    - For patients with symptoms >30 days, only anti-*B. burgdorferi* Ig immunoblot should be performed.
- Modified two-tiered Lyme disease serologic testing
  - Both tiers are immunoassays, done concurrently or sequentially.
  - Results are faster and simpler to interpret.

Follow-Up Tests & Special Considerations
- Arthritis: Serology + PCR of synovial fluid is both sensitive and specific.
- Neuroborreliosis: serology + CSF pleocytosis (PCR of CSF has a very low sensitivity.)

Diagnostic Procedures/Other
Lumbar puncture when neurologic findings are present

TREATMENT

Prophylactic antibiotic therapy should be given only to adults and children within 72 hours of removal of an identified high-risk tick bite—not for bites that are equivocal risk or low risk (1)[A]; doxycycline 200 mg PO for adults and 4.4 mg/kg up to 200 mg for children (1)[A]

MEDICATION
For people intolerant of amoxicillin, doxycycline, and cefuroxime, macrolides (azithromycin, clarithromycin, or erythromycin) may be used. Macrolides have lower efficacy, so patients treated with them should be monitored to ensure that symptoms resolve.

First Line
- Early Lyme disease (1)[A]: doxycycline 100 mg PO BID for 10 to 14 days (do not use in children <8 years old or in pregnant women); *or* amoxicillin 500 mg PO TID for 14 days (pediatric dose of 50 mg/kg/day); *or* cefuroxime axetil 500 mg PO BID for 14 days; alternative: azithromycin 500 mg QD for 7 to 10 days or clarithromycin 500 mg BID for 14 to 21 days
- Early disseminated Lyme
  - Neurologic disease:
    - In patients aged ≥16 years with acute facial nerve palsy but without other evidence of Lyme disease, corticosteroid treatment should be administered within 72 hours. Treat with appropriate Lyme therapy.
    - Adults: doxycycline 100 mg PO for 14 to 21 days
    - Children: doxycycline 4.4 mg/kg per day divided into 2 doses; 14 to 21 days
    - Lyme meningitis or radiculoneuritis: adults doxycycline 200 mg PO divided into 1 or 2 doses for 14 to 21 days or ceftriaxone 2 g IV once a day for 14 to 21 days or cefotaxime 2 g IV every 8 hours for 14 to 21 days
  - Cardiac disease:
    - Mild (1st-degree AV block, PR <300 ms): adults doxycycline 100 mg PO BID or amoxicillin 500 mg PO TID for 14 to 21 days; children: doxycycline 4.4 mg/kg/day PO, divided BID for 14 to 21 days or amoxicillin 50 mg/kg/day PO, divided TID for 14 to 21 days or cefuroxime 30 mg/kg/day PO, divided BID for 14 to 21 days
    - Severe (symptomatic, 1st-degree AV block with PR interval ≥300 ms, 2nd- or 3rd-degree AV block): adults: ceftriaxone 2 g IV QD for 14 to 21 days; children: ceftriaxone 50 to 75 mg/kg IV QD for 14 to 21 days
  - Arthritis:
    - Adults: doxycycline 100 mg BID PO for 28 days or amoxicillin 500 mg TID PO for 28 days or cefuroxime 500 mg BID PO for 28 days

    - Children ≥8 years old: doxycycline 4.4 mg/kg/day PO, divided BID for 28 days, or amoxicillin 50 mg/kg PO daily divided TID for 28 days or cefuroxime 30 mg/kg/day PO, divided BID for 28 days
    - Children <8 years old: amoxicillin 50 mg/kg/day PO for 28 days or cefuroxime 30 mg/kg/day PO, divided into 2 doses for 28 days
    - Parenteral treatment: adults: ceftriaxone 2 g IV QD for 14 to 28 days; children: ceftriaxone 50 to 75 mg/kg IV QD for 14 to 28 days
- Contraindications:
  - Allergies to specific medications
  - Doxycycline is contraindicated in children and in women who are pregnant or breastfeeding
- Precautions:
  - In ~15% of patients treated with IV therapy, a Jarisch-Herxheimer–type reaction develops within 24 hours.
  - Significant interactions: oral anticoagulants and oral contraceptives

Pregnancy Considerations
Because *B. burgdorferi* can cross the placenta, pregnant patients with active disease should be treated with parenteral antibiotics.

SURGERY/OTHER PROCEDURES
Temporary pacemaker with carditis and high-grade heart block

ADMISSION, INPATIENT, AND NURSING CONSIDERATIONS
Admit patients with Lyme carditis and symptoms of chest pain, syncope, or dyspnea and those with 2nd- or 3rd-degree heart block or 1st-degree heart block of ≥300 ms or symptoms of meningitis.

 ## ONGOING CARE

FOLLOW-UP RECOMMENDATIONS
Do not retest patient to determine whether antibody titers have declined after treatment because seroreactivity often persists for months after treatment of early infection and years after treatment of late infection.

PATIENT EDUCATION
- In endemic areas, protect against tick exposure. Avoid "painting" the tick with nail polish or petroleum jelly, or using heat, detach the ticks from skin.
- Prevention: Use repellents that contain 20–30% DEET. Bathe as soon as possible after coming indoors (within 2 hours) and perform regular tick checks.

PROGNOSIS
Early treatment with antibiotics can shorten the duration of symptoms and prevent later disease. Late-stage disease response to treatment is variable. Symptoms may take weeks to resolve. Untreated rash usually resolves in 3 to 4 weeks; excellent long-term prognosis with early antibiotics; neurologic symptoms arise in about 15% of untreated Lyme disease patients.

COMPLICATIONS
- Posttreatment Lyme disease syndrome (PTLDS): pain, fatigue, or difficulty thinking that last for >6 months after they finish treatment; no proven treatment for PTLDS
- PTLDS: 10–20% lingering symptoms of fatigue, pain, or joint and muscle aches; can last for 6 months
- Lyme carditis >40% syncopal presentation

REFERENCE
1. Lantos PM, Rumbaugh J, Bockenstedt LK, et al. Clinical practice guidelines by the Infectious Diseases Society of America (IDSA), American Academy of Neurology (AAN), and American College of Rheumatology (ACR): 2020 guideline for the prevention, diagnosis and treatment of Lyme disease. *Arthritis Care Res (Hoboken)*. 2021;73(1):1–9.

ADDITIONAL READING
- Association of Public Health Laboratories. Suggested reporting language, interpretation and guidance regarding Lyme disease serologic test results. https://www.aphl.org/aboutAPHL /publications/Documents/ID-2021-Lyme-Disease -Serologic-Testing-Reporting.pdf. Accessed December 1, 2023.
- Branda JA, Steere AC. Laboratory diagnosis of Lyme borreliosis. *Clin Microbiol Rev*. 2021;34(2):e00018–19.

 ## SEE ALSO

https://www.cdc.gov/lyme/index.html

 ## CODES

ICD10
- A69.20 Lyme disease, unspecified
- A69.2 Lyme disease

CLINICAL PEARLS
Steps to prevent Lyme disease include using insect repellent, removing ticks promptly, applying pesticides, and reducing tick habitat. There is no test that can "prove cure." Antibodies can persist long after the infection is gone.

L

LYMPHANGITIS

Sarah Wiggill, MD

BASICS

DESCRIPTION

- Acute or chronic inflammation of lymphatic vessels that typically presents as red, tender streaks rapidly extending proximally to regional lymph nodes
- May be infectious or noninfectious; commonly occurs on an extremity due to skin infection
- Lymphatic filariasis (elephantiasis) most common cause worldwide; bacterial infection most common cause in North America

EPIDEMIOLOGY

Prevalence

Estimated 51 million cases of lymphatic filariasis as of 2018; down from 120 million in 1997

ETIOLOGY AND PATHOPHYSIOLOGY

- Acute infectious lymphangitis
  - Most commonly caused by skin breakdown with secondary infection, typically bacterial
  - *Streptococcus* pyogenes (group A β-hemolytic *Streptococcus*) most common cause in immunocompetent
  - Consider gram-negative bacteria or fungi in immunocompromised patients
  - Less commonly caused by: *Staphylococcus aureus*, *Pasteurella multocida* (cat, dog, or other animal bite), *Bartonella henselae* (cat bite, cat scratch disease), *Erysipelothrix* (fish exposure), *Spirillum minus* (rat bite disease), *Pseudomonas* sp., other *Streptococcus* sp., *Aeromonas hydrophila* (fresh water exposures), *Bacillus anthracis* (cutaneous anthrax), Parapoxvirus (occupational milker's nodule), herpes simplex virus (herpetic whitlow), *Chlamydia trachomatis* (lymphogranuloma venereum)
- Chronic lymphangitis
  - Filarial lymphangitis-typically affects extremities but can result in genital lymphatic involvement
    - Lymphatic filariasis (elephantiasis) most common cause of lymphangitis worldwide
    - Inflammation of lymph vessels due to presence and death of parasite transmitted via mosquito bite
    - Usually caused by nematodes (helminth) *Wuchereria bancrofti*; less commonly, *Brugia malayi* and *Brugia timori*
    - Endemic areas: Asia, Africa, the Western Pacific, the Caribbean, and South America
  - Nodular lymphangitis
    - Also known as sporotrichoid lymphangitis or lymphocutaneous syndrome
    - Painful or painless nodular subcutaneous swellings along lymphatic vessels
    - Lesions may ulcerate with accompanying regional lymphadenopathy

- Usually does not develop as rapidly as acute lymphangitis and may not present with systemic symptoms
- Typical of infections from: *Sporothrix schenckii*, *Nocardia brasiliensis*, *Mycobacterium marinum*, *Leishmania* sp., *Francisella tularensis*, and systemic mycoses (coccidioidomycosis, blastomycosis, histoplasmosis)
- Pathology may show granulomas.
  - Granulomatous intestinal lymphangitis: rare; associated with Crohn disease
  - Lymphangitis secondary to compromised lymphatic drainage
    - Following surgical procedures, trauma, malignancy, or radiation
    - Congenital or acquired anatomic abnormalities-elephantiasis nostras verrucosa (in setting of congestive heart failure and obesity)
  - Cutaneous lymphangitis carcinomatosa or neoplastic lymphangitis: rare presentation of skin metastasis—~5% of all skin metastases; caused by neoplastic occlusion of dermal lymphatic vessels
    - Associated cancers include breast (most common), lung, stomach, pancreas, and rectal.
- Acute noninfectious lymphangitis
  - Sclerosing lymphangitis of the penis: swelling around coronal sulcus of penis as a result of vigorous sexual activity or masturbation
  - Insect or spider bite

RISK FACTORS

- Skin infection—bacterial, viral, fungal
- Impaired lymphatic drainage
- Peripheral venous catheter; IV drug abuse
- Skin trauma including human, animal, insect, or spider bites
- Diabetes mellitus
- Immunocompromising condition
- Residence in filariasis endemic areas

GENERAL PREVENTION

- Proper wound and skin care
- Reduce chronic lymphedema with compression devices or by treating underlying processes.
- Insect repellent; arthropod bite precautions
- Chemoprevention (albendazole, ivermectin, diethyl-carbamazine citrate) in endemic areas for lymphatic filariasis

COMMONLY ASSOCIATED CONDITIONS

- Cellulitis, erysipelas
- Lymphedema
- Filarial infection (*W. bancrofti*)
- Prior lymph node dissection
- Tinea pedis (athlete's foot)
- Sporotrichosis

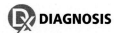 DIAGNOSIS

HISTORY

- Skin breakdown or trauma
- Erythematous streaks that can spread within a few hours
- Systemic symptoms: fever, chills, malaise, loss of appetite, headache, muscle aches
- Travel to filariasis endemic areas

PHYSICAL EXAM

- Erythematous, linear streaks from site of infection proximally toward regional lymph nodes
- Tenderness and warmth over affected skin and/or lymph nodes (lymphadenitis)
- Blistering of affected skin
- Fluctuance, swelling, or purulent drainage
- Nodular lymphangitis can present with subcutaneous swellings along the lymphatic channels
- Sporotrichosis may present with papulonodular lesions that may ulcerate
- Sites may be painless

DIFFERENTIAL DIAGNOSIS

- Superficial thrombophlebitis: thrombus or infection within the thrombosis (septic thrombophlebitis) (1)[C]
- Contact dermatitis
- Cellulitis
- Erysipelas
- Allergic reaction: less likely to be allergic if >24 hours after exposure (e.g., insect bite)

DIAGNOSTIC TESTS & INTERPRETATION

Initial Tests (lab, imaging)

- CBC may show leukocytosis
- Microbiologic investigations—identify potential underlying infectious agent to guide treatment
  - Swab, aspirate, and/or biopsy of primary site, nodule, or distal ulcer for histology and culture
  - Blood cultures if systemic symptoms present
  - Serology (*F. tularensis*, histoplasma)
  - Blood smear (filaria)
  - FNAC for filariasis of testiculoscrotal swelling but not for other superficial locations

Follow-Up Tests & Special Considerations

Imaging: rarely used but can help in identifying anatomic abnormalities in lymphatic vessels—lymphangiography and lymphoscintigraphy

Diagnostic Procedures/Other

Surgical débridement if complicated by necrotizing fasciitis (1)[C]

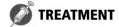 **TREATMENT**

GENERAL MEASURES
- Hot, moist compresses to affected area
- Elevate affected extremity
- Compression devices and weight loss may help lymphedema.
- Abstinence from sexual activity for sclerosing lymphangitis

MEDICATION
- Treat common organisms empirically. Use culture and susceptibility to guide antibiotic treatment (1)[C].
- If mild disease, outpatient oral antibiotics
- If no improvement after 48 hours of oral antibiotics, reassess and consider IV antibiotics and/or hospitalization.
- IV antibiotics if systemically ill
- If necrotizing fasciitis is suspected, treat aggressively with IV antibiotics and surgical intervention.

First Line
- *Streptococcus* pyogenes (group A strep)
  - Amoxicillin—oral antibiotic therapy
    ○ Adults and children ≥40 kg: mild to moderate: 500 mg PO q12h; severe: 875 mg PO q12h or 500 mg PO q8h
    ○ Children <3 months: 30 mg/kg/day PO divided q12h
    ○ Children ≥3 months, ≤40 kg: mild to moderate: 25 mg/kg/day PO divided q12h or 20 mg/kg/day divided q8h; severe: 45 mg/kg/day PO divided q12h or 40 mg/kg/day divided q8h
    ○ Adverse effects:
      ■ Common: nausea, vomiting, diarrhea
      ■ Serious: anaphylaxis, Stevens-Johnson syndrome (SJS), toxic epidermal necrolysis (TEN)
    ○ Drug interactions: methotrexate, venlafaxine, warfarin, hormonal contraceptives
    ○ Contraindications: hypersensitivity to penicillin
  - Ampicillin/sulbactam-IV antibiotic therapy
    ○ Adults and children ≥40 kg: 1.5 to 3.0 g IV/IM q6h
    ○ Children <40 kg: 200 mg/kg/day IV infusion, in divided doses q6h; maximum 8 g ampicillin per day
    ○ Adverse effects:
      ■ Common: diarrhea, injection site pain and reactions
      ■ Serious: anaphylaxis, Stevens-Johnson syndrome (SJS), toxic epidermal necrolysis (TEN), *Clostridium difficile* diarrhea, pseudomembranous enterocolitis

    ○ Drug interactions: hormonal contraceptives
    ○ Contraindications: hypersensitivity to penicillin
- Lymphatic filariasis: diethylcarbamazine, ivermectin, albendazole, and doxycycline
- Acetaminophen or ibuprofen (NSAIDs) for pain and fever

Second Line
- *Streptococcus* pyogenes (group A strep)
  - Oral therapy: cephalexin, macrolides for penicillin and cephalosporin allergic (azithromycin, clarithromycin, erythromycin), clindamycin (for penicillin allergic patients)
  - IV therapy: ceftriaxone, clindamycin (for penicillin allergic patients)
- *S. aureus*—consider risk for methicillin-resistant *S. aureus* (MRSA)
  - Oral therapy: amoxicillin, cephalexin, sulfamethoxazole-trimethoprim, doxycycline, clindamycin, linezolid
  - IV therapy: nafcillin, oxacillin, cefazolin, vancomycin, daptomycin, linezolid

SURGERY/OTHER PROCEDURES
- Incision and drainage (I&D) of abscess if present
- Necrotizing fasciitis requires surgical evaluation and likely débridement
- Nodular lymphangitis may benefit from I&D

ADMISSION, INPATIENT, AND NURSING CONSIDERATIONS
- Admit for signs of serious systemic illness (i.e., sepsis): fluids if in hypotensive shock
- IV antibiotics, ICU, or surgery as indicated
- Discharge on oral antibiotics after systemic symptoms resolve. Home IV antibiotics are an option depending on clinical setting.

 ONGOING CARE

- Routine use of compression devices to reduce lymphedema
- Lymphedema physical therapy

FOLLOW-UP RECOMMENDATIONS
- Elevate affected area
- 48-hour follow-up to ensure improvement
- Work up recurrent lymphangitis to ascertain underlying cause (other infectious organism, anatomic abnormality, etc.)

Patient Monitoring
Close follow-up to ensure response to treatment and decreasing inflammation

PATIENT EDUCATION
- Instruct patients on proper wound and skin care
- Elevate affected extremity
- Use compression devices as recommended

PROGNOSIS
- Good prognosis for uncomplicated cases
- Antimicrobial therapy is effective in 90% of patients
- Untreated, can spread rapidly, especially group A *Streptococcus*

COMPLICATIONS
Sepsis, cellulitis, necrotizing fasciitis, myositis, lymphedema

REFERENCE
1. Kano Y, Momose T. Acute lymphangitis. *Cleve Clin J Med*. 2020;87(3):129–130.

ADDITIONAL READING
Tirado-Sánchez A, Bonifaz A. Nodular lymphangitis (sporotrichoid lymphocutaneous infections). Clues to differential diagnosis. *J Fungi (Basel)*. 2018;4(2):56.

 CODES

ICD10
- I89.1 Lymphangitis
- L03.91 Acute lymphangitis, unspecified
- N48.29 Other inflammatory disorders of penis

CLINICAL PEARLS
- Lymphangitis classically presents with erythematous linear streaks of the skin from site of entry (e.g., bite, cut, abrasion) proximally to regional lymph nodes.
- Patients with prior surgical lymph node dissection are predisposed to lymphangitis.
- Patients with severe systemic symptoms should be admitted for treatment with IV antibiotics.
- Parasitic or fungal infections can cause acute or chronic lymphangitis.
- Treatment of underlying skin infection (such as tinea pedis) may prevent recurrence.

LYMPHEDEMA

Dana M. Vlachos, DO • Rahim Shareef, DO • Natasha E. Scaria, MD

BASICS

DESCRIPTION
- Accumulation of lymphatic fluid in the interstitial tissue causing swelling
- Lymphedema can develop when lymphatic vessels are missing or impaired (primary) or when lymph vessels are damaged or lymph nodes are removed (secondary).
- Most commonly occurs in the lower limb(s) (80% of cases) but also can occur in the arm(s), face, trunk, and external genitalia

EPIDEMIOLOGY
Incidence
- More common in females than in males
- Occurs in 13% of patients with breast cancer treated with surgery and 42% of those treated with surgery and radiation therapy
- Occurs in 25% of patients after gynecologic cancer surgery

Prevalence
- 120 million people worldwide are affected with primary lymphatic filariasis.
- 10 million people are affected by nonfilarial secondary lymphedema in the United States.

ETIOLOGY AND PATHOPHYSIOLOGY
- Primary lymphedema results from inherited conditions affecting the lymph nodes or lymphatic vessels.
- Secondary lymphedema:
  - Postoperative: gradual failure of distal lymphatics, which have to "pump" lymph at a greater pressure through damaged proximal ducts; the risk is higher with postoperative radiation because radiation reduces regrowth of ducts due to fibrous scarring.
  - Other causes include trauma, recurrent infection, malignancy (including metastatic disease), and marked obesity.
  - Most common cause in developing countries is filariasis (*Wuchereria bancrofti*).

Genetics
- Milroy disease is autosomal dominant and is diagnosed either at birth or within the 1st year of life.
- Lymphedema praecox has onset between the ages of 1 and 35 years.
- Lymphedema tarda occurs in those >35 years of age.
- Genetics referral is indicated with primary lymphedema and lymphedema tarda.

RISK FACTORS
- Filariasis: most common cause worldwide
- Lymphadenectomy or radiation therapy of lymph nodes, especially nodes of the underarm, groin, pelvis, and neck regions in cancer treatment (mastectomy, melanoma)
- Prior trauma, serious burns, infection of affected limb
- Obesity (body mass index: >50 kg/m²)
- Inflammatory disorders: arthritis, sarcoidosis, dermatitis

GENERAL PREVENTION
Maintenance of healthy body weight, treatment of congestive heart failure, and early recognition of infection, cancer, and venous insufficiency

COMMONLY ASSOCIATED CONDITIONS
Venous disease, morbid obesity, regional cancer, filarial disease (Africa and Asia)

DIAGNOSIS

HISTORY
- First symptom is often painless swelling.
- Feeling of heaviness in the limb, especially at the end of the day and in hot weather

PHYSICAL EXAM
- Initial: pitting edema, can spread proximally or distally
- Later: nonpitting; after 1st year, does not spread proximally/distally, but spreads radially
- Hyperkeratosis (thicker skin)
- Papillomatosis (rough skin)
- Increase in skin turgor
- Positive Stemmer sign (inability to pinch the skin of the dorsum of the second toe between the thumb and forefinger); false positives are rare.

DIFFERENTIAL DIAGNOSIS
- CHF, renal failure, lipedema
- Hypoalbuminemia, protein-losing nephropathy
- DVT, chronic venous disease
- Postoperative complications following ipsilateral surgery
- Cellulitis, Baker cyst, idiopathic edema

DIAGNOSTIC TESTS & INTERPRETATION
- Lack of response to elevation or diuretic therapy may indicate a lymphatic insufficiency.
- Diuretics increase excretion of salt and water, thereby decreasing plasma volume, venous capillary pressure, and filtration. Diuretics improve filtration edema but do not improve lymph drainage over the long term.
- Some relevant protein biomarkers for lymphedema have been identified and show promise for early- and latent-stage diagnosis.

Initial Tests (lab, imaging)
- Comprehensive chemistry panel to evaluate for hepatic or renal impairment
- TSH to evaluate for hypothyroidism
- Urinalysis to evaluate for protein-losing nephropathy
- Ultrasound evaluates for acute/chronic DVT; also gives information about soft tissue changes but does not inform about truncal anatomy of the lymphatics

Follow-Up Tests & Special Considerations
- Lymphangiogram: direct cannulation of lymphatics through the skin; rarely used and has risk for infection and local inflammation
- Fluorescence microlymphography may be highly sensitive (91.4%) and specific (85.7%), atraumatic, and is without radiation.

- Lymphoscintigraphy: radiolabeled protein technetium-99m–labeled colloid
  - Measures lymphatic function, lymph movement, lymph drainage, and response to treatment
  - Sensitivity, 73–97%; specificity, 100%
  - Best to use 1 hour and delayed images together
- Indocyanine green lymphography: reported
  - Superior to lymphoscintigraphy in early diagnosis of lymphedema of the arm
  - Accurately screens postsurgically for subclinical lymphedema (1)[B]
- CT scan: calf skin thickening, thickening of the SC compartment, increased fat density, thickened perimuscular aponeurosis; typical honeycomb appearance
- MRI: circumferential edema, increased volume of SC tissue, honeycomb pattern above the fascia between the muscle and subcutis; cannot differentiate primary from secondary lymphedema

Test Interpretation
Lymphedema stages:
- Stage 0: no swelling, but can feel that the affected area is heavy or full, or skin is tight
- Stage 1: has swelling of the affected area; will notice increase in size or stiffness of affected area; will notice swelling improves when affected area is raised
- Stage 2: more swelling than stage 1, which does NOT improve when affected area is elevated; will notice that affected area is hard and larger in size than stage 1
- Stage 3: increased swelling compared with stage 2; maybe be to the point that you cannot lift or move the arm or leg on your own; affected can become dry and thick. Fluid can leak from the skin, or blisters can form.

TREATMENT

GENERAL MEASURES
- Seek optimal weight; early treatment of cellulitis; avoid trauma to the affected area (direct injury, venipunctures, inept nail care, extreme heat/cold).
- Achieve mechanical reduction and maintenance of limb size: compression garments or compression pumps.
- Elevate the affected limb/area, but avoid stasis.
- Avoid BP cuffs and other focal constriction in affected limbs.
- Prevent skin infection with daily cleansing, inspection, and skin care (with emollients).
- Nonsurgical treatment of varicose veins in some
- Doubtful that air travel is associated with increased limb volumes

MEDICATION
ALERT
No medications, including diuretics, have been shown to be effective to treat lymphedema.

ISSUES FOR REFERRAL

- Refer to physical therapist with lymphedema training for manual decongestive therapy.
  - In patients with recurrent or metastatic disease, discuss with oncologist prior to initiation of complete decongestive therapy in order not to promote the spread of cancer.
- Provide education for patient/family for self-administration of therapy.
- Education for family about bandaging
- Fitting for compression garments (2)[A]

ADDITIONAL THERAPIES

- Exercise: Lymph flow occurs as a result of inspiratory reduction in the intrathoracic pressure associated with inspiration. The best results are achieved with combination of flexibility, strength, and aerobic training.
- Compression with custom-made elastic stocking (Minimum pressure is 40 mm Hg.)
  - Protection against external incidental trauma
  - Decreases the intrinsic trauma on the skin due to chronically increased interstitial pressures, which cause stretch of the skin and SC tissues
  - No data on preference of custom-made versus prefabricated
  - Replace every 3 to 6 months or when starting to lose elasticity.
- Multilayer bandaging: inner layer of tubular stockinette followed by foam and padding to protect the joint flexures and to even out the contours of the limb so that pressure is distributed evenly; outer layer of at least two short-stretch extensible bandages; more effective than hosiery alone
- Pneumatic pumps develop high pressures like systolic BP and can reduce limb girth significantly; wear a compression sock afterward (2)[A].
- Advanced pneumatic compression devices (APCDs) are programmable, offer a more individualized fit, reduced rates of cellulitis by at least 75%, and reduce early treatment costs by 37–54% depending on health care setting (3)[B].

SURGERY/OTHER PROCEDURES

- Bypass procedures: Creation of lymphatic–venous anastomosis or lymph node transplantation (most effective) via microsurgery showed a reduction in use of conservative compression therapy (4)[C]; reserved for refractory cases only
- Low-level laser therapy in smaller studies was shown to be noninferior to manual lymphatic drainage or in combination in arm volume reduction among breast cancer patients in half the treatment time (4)[C]. This treatment uses lasers to stimulate lymphatic vessel growth, improve lymph fluid flow, and repair skin damage.
- Axillary reverse mapping during axillary node dissection in selected preclinical breast cancer can significantly reduce lymphedema incidence (5)[A].
- Thoracic sympathetic ganglion block for breast cancer–related lymphedema showed better life quality and arm size reduction of >50%, especially in patients with high-grade lymphedema.

- Debulking procedures (Charles procedure): radical excision of SC tissue with primary or staged skin grafting
  - Men had less improvement than women.
  - The main risk is infection and necrosis of the skin graft.
  - Liposuction is cosmetically preferred than debulking (4)[C].

COMPLEMENTARY & ALTERNATIVE MEDICINE

Osteopathic manipulative treatment can be helpful in treatment of lymphedema by removing myofascial and skeletal restrictions to lymphatic flow and also by providing direct encouragement of lymphatic drainage.

ADMISSION, INPATIENT, AND NURSING CONSIDERATIONS

- Systemic signs of infection
  - May admit to specialized rehabilitation unit for combination treatment in patients with heart failure or severe pulmonary disease
  - IV antibiotics for infection; cellulitis is most common.
- Affected extremity positioning with some distal elevation
- Encourage patient mobilization/exercise.
- Patient education for bandaging/wound care
- Discharge criteria
  - Improved signs/symptoms of infection (e.g., elevated WBC count, fever, abnormal vital signs)
  - Clinical improvement in wound appearance

 ONGOING CARE

FOLLOW-UP RECOMMENDATIONS

Lymphedema will return in several days if patient stops wearing compression garments during the day and bandaging at night.

Patient Monitoring

- Daily visit to therapist for acute treatment
- Monthly visits for maintenance care

DIET

Lower sodium, healthy protein, and weight loss-oriented (if needed)

PATIENT EDUCATION

- Use compression garments, especially when exercising.
- Avoid affected limb(s) being dependent for long period of time: Patient should perform daily skin examination.
- National Library of Medicine: http://www.nlm.nih.gov/medlineplus/lymphedema.html

PROGNOSIS

No cure but treatment can produce good results with daily care

COMPLICATIONS

- Infection (local vs. systemic): common
- Risk of wound formation (punctures/abrasions) that are difficult to heal: common
- Lymphangiosarcoma: found in lymphedematous arms of patients following radical mastectomy, also in patients with Milroy disease; treatment is radiotherapy with surgery; reserved for patients with discrete nonmetastatic disease

REFERENCES

1. Keo HH, Husmann M, Groechenig E, et al. Diagnostic accuracy of fluorescence microlymphography for detecting limb lymphedema. *Eur J Vasc Endovasc Surg*. 2015;49(4):474–479.
2. Rogan S, Taeymans J, Luginbuehl H, et al. Therapy modalities to reduce lymphoedema in female breast cancer patients: a systematic review and meta-analysis. *Breast Cancer Res Treat*. 2016;159(1):1–14.
3. Karaca-Mandic P, Hirsch AT, Rockson SG, et al. The cutaneous, net clinical, and health economic benefits of advanced pneumatic compression devices in patients with lymphedema. *JAMA Dermatol*. 2015;151(11):1187–1193.
4. Merchant SJ, Chen SL. Prevention and management of lymphedema after breast cancer treatment. *Breast J*. 2015;21(3):276–284.
5. Han C, Yang B, Zuo WS, et al. The feasibility and oncological safety of axillary reverse mapping in patients with breast cancer: a systematic review and meta-analysis of prospective studies. *PLoS One*. 2016;11(2):e0150285.

ADDITIONAL READING

Choi E, Nahm FS, Lee PB. Sympathetic block as a new treatment for lymphedema. *Pain Physician*. 2015;18(4):365–372.

CODES

ICD10

- I89.0 Lymphedema, not elsewhere classified
- I97.2 Postmastectomy lymphedema syndrome
- Q82.0 Hereditary lymphedema

CLINICAL PEARLS

- Affected skin has a heavy feeling, with painless swelling initially, later nonpitting swelling.
- No medications, including diuretics, are useful.
- Rule out DVT if unilateral limb affected or CHF if bilateral.
- Early referral to lymphedema therapist for manual therapy and placement of compression devices/wrappings
- Aggressive weight loss and health promotion as needed
- High risk for cutaneous-sourced infections, so promote therapeutic skin care
- Lymphoscintigraphy is the standard diagnostic measure if clinical diagnosis is uncertain.
- Refer primary lymphedema and lymphedema tarda to genetics.

L

MACULAR DEGENERATION, AGE-RELATED

Richard W. Allinson, MD • Hunter Grey, OD

BASICS

DESCRIPTION
- Age-related macular degeneration (AMD) is the leading cause of visual loss in older persons.
- Classified as:
  - Atrophic/nonexudative, such as drusen or macular pigmentary changes
  - Neovascular/exudative or neovascular age-related macular degeneration (nAMD)

EPIDEMIOLOGY
- nAMD form is rare in blacks and more common in whites.
- Predominant sex: female

Prevalence
- People 65 to 74 years old: 11%
- People ≥75 years old: 27.9%

ETIOLOGY AND PATHOPHYSIOLOGY
- Atrophic/nonexudative
  - Drusen and/or pigmentary changes in the macula. Drusen are deposits of hyaline material between the RPE and Bruch's membrane (the limiting membrane between the RPE and the choroid).
  - Visible light can result in the formation and accumulation of metabolic by-products in the retinal pigment epithelium (RPE), a pigment layer underneath the retina that normally helps remove metabolic by-products from the retina. Excess accumulation of these metabolic by-products interferes with the normal metabolic activity of the RPE and can lead to the formation of drusen.
- nAMD
  - nAMD stage generally arises from the atrophic stage.
    - In type 1 neovascularization, breaks in Bruch's membrane allow choroidal neovascular membranes (CNVMs) to grow into the sub-RPE space. This corresponds to occult CNVMs. Fluid leakage and bleeding can produce a vascularized serous or fibrovascular RPE detachment.
    - In type 2 neovascularization, the CNVM passes through the RPE and is located in the subretinal space; typically appears as a lacy or gray-green lesion. This corresponds to classic CNVM.
    - Type 3 neovascularization, also known as retinal angiomatous proliferations (RAPS), the neovascularization develops from the deep capillary plexus of the retina and grows downward toward the RPE.
    - Polypoidal choroidal vasculopathy (PCV) is a subtype of nAMD and often presents with multiple, recurrent serosanguineous RPE detachments. An RPE detachment is also known as a pigment epithelial detachment (PED). Optical coherence tomography (OCT) features of PCV include multiple PEDs, sharply peaked PED, notched or multilobulated PED, and a hyperreflective ring surrounding an internal hyporeflective lumen beneath a PED.

Genetics
Complement factor H Y402H genotype is an important susceptibility gene for AMD.

RISK FACTORS
- Obesity
- Cigarette smoking
- *Chlamydia pneumoniae* infection
- Family history
- Excess sunlight exposure
- Blue or light iris color
- Hyperopia
- Short stature

GENERAL PREVENTION
- Ultraviolet (UV) protection for eyes
- Routine ophthalmologic visits

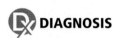

DIAGNOSIS

HISTORY
Patients frequently notice distortion of central vision.

PHYSICAL EXAM
- On Amsler grid testing, the horizontal or vertical lines may become broken, distorted, or missing.
- Atrophic/nonexudative stage: Drusen (small yellowish white lesions)
- nAMD
  - Blood vessels growing underneath the retina from the choroid are called CNVMs or subretinal neovascularization (SRN). The choroid is the vascular layer underneath the RPE.
  - Subretinal fluid or hemorrhage; exudates
- Disciform scar: an advanced stage resulting in a fibrovascular scar

DIFFERENTIAL DIAGNOSIS
- Diabetic or hypertensive retinopathy
- Central serous chorioretinopathy
- Topiramate can cause a macular neurosensory retinal detachment.
- Pentosan polysulfate sodium, which is FDA approved for the treatment of interstitial cystitis, may be associated with the development of a pigmentary maculopathy.

DIAGNOSTIC TESTS & INTERPRETATION
Diagnostic Procedures/Other
- Fluorescein angiography (FA): differentiates between atrophic and nARMD
- Indocyanine green video angiography: may identify occult or hidden CNVMs
- OCT: useful in determining the presence of subretinal fluid, the degree of retinal thickening, and the presence of a PED. Newer generation OCT modalities, including spectral-domain OCT (SD-OCT), swept-source OCT (SS-OCT), and OCT angiography (OCTA), are preferred for evaluating ARMD.

TREATMENT

GENERAL MEASURES
Low-vision aids may be helpful.

MEDICATION
First Line
- Ranibizumab (Lucentis)
  - Antibody fragment that inhibits all active forms of VEGF
  - Injected intravitreally, at a dose of 0.5 mg, every 4 weeks
  - 1 year after treatment, up to 40% of patients treated with ranibizumab gained at least three lines of vision, and ~95% maintained vision.
  - The PrONTO study demonstrated OCT-guided, variable-dosing regimen with ranibizumab resulted in similar results to the MARINA (minimally classic/occult CNVM trial) and ANCHOR (predominantly classic CNVM trial) studies with monthly injections of ranibizumab.
  - When comparing ranibizumab and bevacizumab in a multicenter study, both treatments were effective in stabilizing visual loss, and no difference was found in the visual outcome between the two treatment groups.
    - Visual gains during the first 2 years were not maintained at 5 years. At the 5-year visit, 50% of eyes had vision of 20/40 or better and 20% had vision of 20/200 or worse.
  - Eyes with ≥50% of the lesion composed of blood had a similar visual prognosis compared to other treated eyes in the Comparison of Age-related Macular Degeneration Treatments Trials (CATT). nAMD lesions composed of >50% blood can be managed similarly to those with less or no blood.
  - The treat and extend regimen (TER) is commonly used to decrease the treatment burden. Once no signs of CNVM activity are detected, patient follow-ups and treatments are then extended by intervals of 2 weeks as long as no signs of CNVM activity are present, up to a maximum interval of 12 weeks. If examination shows any sign of recurrence, the interval is shortened by 2 weeks at a time, until the disease is considered to be inactive. Interval extension is then restarted, with the maximum final interval being 2 weeks less than the period when the previous recurrence was observed.
- Aflibercept (Eylea)
  - A VEGF receptor decoy that binds both VEGF and placental-like growth factor
  - Injected intravitreally, at a dose of 2 mg, every 4 weeks for 12 weeks and then every 8 weeks
  - Dosed as needed after the 12-week fixed dosing schedule resulted in a 5.3-letter gain in best corrected visual acuity at 52 weeks.
  - May be beneficial in patients who are not responding to ranibizumab or bevacizumab.

– Anti-VEGF treatment with either ranibizumab or aflibercept has limited efficacy for the complete resolution of PEDs.
  ○ Patients with a PED tend to have worse outcomes when switched from a fixed regimen to a PRN strategy.
• Brolucizumab (Beovu)
  – It is a humanized single-chain antibody fragment that inhibits all isoforms of VEGF-A. It is the smallest of the anti-VEGF antibodies.
  – Injected intravitreally, at a dose of 6 mg monthly for the first 3 doses, followed by one dose every 8 to 12 weeks.
  – A 12-week treatment cycle may be a viable option, which would help reduce the frequency of IVIs. Greater than 50% of brolucizumab treated eyes were maintained on q12wk dosing.
  – There have been some reports of retinal vasculitis and/or retinal vascular occlusion after Beovu was approved by the FDA. There have been cases reported with severe visual loss with brolucizumab treatment.
• Faricimab (Vabysmo) neutralizes angiopoietin-2 and vascular endothelial growth factor A. It has the potential advantage of being administered every 16 weeks. It has recently been approved by the FDA for the treatment of nAMD.
  – 6 mg injected intravitreally, every 4 weeks for the first 4 doses. Then based on clinical outcomes, patients may receive subsequent treatments every 2, 3, or 4 months. Faricimab was noninferior to aflibercept (1)[A].

Second Line
• Bevacizumab (Avastin) is a full-length antibody to VEGF, administered intravitreally at a dose of 1.25 mg; widely used off-label because of its lower cost
• Avacincaptad pegol is an inhibitor of complement C5. Complement is believed to play an important role in retinal degeneration secondary to AMD. Avacincaptad pegol is being investigated for the treatment of GA.

SURGERY/OTHER PROCEDURES
• Laser treatment for CNVMs located ≥200 microns from the center of the macula has been evaluated in the Macular Photocoagulation Study (MPS). Anti-VEGF treatment is first-line therapy for subfoveal CNVMs.
• Vitrectomy has been used to remove CNVMs, but this is generally not recommended.
• CNVMs can bleed spontaneously, leaving blood underneath the retina. Vitrectomy to remove subretinal blood may be of benefit and should be performed within 7 days of the bleed. Tissue plasminogen activator (tPA) instilled into the eye may help remove a subretinal hemorrhage. In some cases, intravitreal gas with or without tPA may displace submacular blood.
  – Intravitreal anti-VEGF monotherapy may be helpful in the treatment of nAMD associated with a submacular hemorrhage.

• Photodynamic therapy (PDT) with verteporfin is not frequently used anymore.
  – Patients should be informed of a <4% risk of acute, severe vision loss after PDT.
  – Ranibizumab has a greater clinical efficacy than PDT.
  – Combination treatment with intravitreal ranibizumab and PDT appears to offer similar gain in visual acuity when compared with ranibizumab monotherapy.

COMPLEMENTARY & ALTERNATIVE MEDICINE
The Age-Related Eye Disease Study (AREDS) found that a high-dose regimen of antioxidant vitamins and mineral supplements reduced progression of AMD in some cases.
• Recommended daily doses: vitamin C 500 mg, vitamin E 400 IU, β-carotene 15 mg, zinc oxide 80 mg, and cupric oxide 2 mg. Exercise caution with β-carotene use in smokers due to potential link to lung cancer.
• The AREDS2 found the addition of lutein with zeaxanthin alone or in combination with omega-3 fatty acids had no overall effect in further reducing the risk of progression to advanced AMD. The recommended daily doses: vitamin C 500 mg, vitamin E 400 IU, lutein 10 mg, zeaxanthin 2 mg, zinc 80 mg. β-carotene was removed from the AREDS2.

 ONGOING CARE

FOLLOW-UP RECOMMENDATIONS
Patient Monitoring
Patients with soft drusen or pigmentary changes in the macula should monitor their vision, by doing daily Amsler grid testing and by following subjective measures of visual acuity, such as reading ability; if no new symptoms, follow-up examination in 6 to 12 months

DIET
• Eating dark green, leafy vegetables (spinach/collard greens), which are rich in carotenoids, may decrease the risk of developing the nAMD.
• Fish consumption with omega-3 fatty acid intake may reduce the risk of AMD.
• A Mediterranean-type diet may reduce the risk of developing AMD (2)[A].

PROGNOSIS
• Patients with bilateral soft drusen and pigmentary changes in the macula, but no evidence of exudation, have an increased likelihood of developing nAMD and subsequent visual loss.
• Patients with bilateral drusen carry a cumulative risk of 14.7% over 5 years of suffering significant visual loss in one eye from nAMD.
• Patients with nAMD in one eye and drusen in the opposite eye are at an annual risk of 5–14% of developing nAMD in the opposite eye with drusen.

• Patients with nAMD with stable preoperative fluid on OCT generally do not have worsening of their nAMD after cataract surgery.
• Aspirin use is not significantly associated with progression to late AMD. When aspirin is medically indicated, patients with ARMD do not need to avoid taking it.
• Anti-VEGF treatment for nAMD was associated with preserved useful vision in almost 20% of patients over their average remaining lifetime (3)[B].

COMPLICATIONS
• Blindness
• The intraocular pressure should be monitored in eyes receiving intravitreal anti-VEGF injections.

REFERENCES

1. Heier JS, Khanani AM, Quezada Ruiz C, et al. Efficacy, durability, and safety of intravitreal faricimab up to every 16 weeks for neovascular age-related macular degeneration (TENAYA and LUCERNE): two randomised, double-masked, phase 3, non-inferiority trials. *Lancet*. 2022;399(10326):729–740.
2. Keenan TD, Agrón E, Mares J, et al. Adherence to the Mediterranean diet and progression to late age-related macular degeneration in the Age-Related Eye Disease Studies 1 and 2. *Ophthalmology*. 2020;127(11):1515–1528.
3. Finger RP, Puth MT, Schmid M, et al. Lifetime outcomes of anti-vascular endothelial growth factor treatment for neovascular age-related macular degeneration. *JAMA Ophthalmol*. 2020;138(12):1234–1240.

ADDITIONAL READING
Keenan TD, Wiley HE, Agrón E, et al. The association of aspirin use with age-related macular degeneration progression in the Age-Related Eye Disease Studies: Age-Related Eye Disease Study 2 Report No. 20. *Ophthalmology*. 2019;126(12):1647–1656.

CODES

ICD10
• H35.32 Exudative age-related macular degeneration
• H35.31 Nonexudative age-related macular degeneration
• H35.3290 Exudative age-related macular degeneration, unspecified eye, stage unspecified

CLINICAL PEARLS
• Patients may notice straight lines appear crooked (e.g., telephone poles).
• The AREDS found that a high-dose regimen of antioxidant vitamins and mineral supplements reduces progression of AMD in some cases.

M

MARFAN SYNDROME

Jana Wei Qiao, MD • Karl T. Clebak, MD, MHA, FAAFP

 BASICS

DESCRIPTION

- Marfan syndrome (MFS) is an inherited disorder of connective tissue.
- Because many features of MFS appear in the general population, diagnostic criteria (Ghent nosology) are useful for diagnosis including features with major and minor criteria (1).
- System(s) affected: musculoskeletal, cardiovascular, ocular, pulmonary, skin/integument, connective tissue (dura)

Pediatric Considerations
Early surgical intervention may reduce the degree of scoliosis. Pectus excavatum deformities can worsen during adolescent growth and may require surgical evaluation for symptomatic or cosmetic concerns.

Pregnancy Considerations
- Consider pregnancy in MFS high risk and consult with a cardiologist; screening transthoracic echocardiogram with serial monitoring
- Consider β-blockers in all pregnancies to minimize risk of aortic dilation.
- Consider elective surgery before pregnancy if aortic root diameter is >47 mm.
  - Type A aortic dissection may require urgent surgical repair; Type B aortic dissection may require medical management over surgical intervention, but treatment should be individualized.
  - Prepartum aortic root diameter 40 to 45 mm may remain stable during pregnancy (2).
- Avoid spinal anesthesia due to risk of dural ectasia.

EPIDEMIOLOGY
- Congenital; although clinical manifestations may be apparent in infancy, affected individuals may not present until adolescence or young adulthood.
- No gender, ethnic, or racial predilection; with advanced paternal age, a slightly increased risk of de novo mutation resulting in MFS in offspring

Incidence
1/5,000 to 1/10,000 live births

ETIOLOGY AND PATHOPHYSIOLOGY
Genetic abnormality; mutations of the fibrillin-1 (*FBN1*) gene.

Genetics
- MFS is an autosomal dominant condition with complete penetrance and variable expressivity.
- *FBN1* mutations have been identified in 92% of patients with MFS.
- Each child of an affected parent has a 50% chance of inheriting MFS and may be more or less severely affected. 25% of cases result from de novo mutation, most of which result from de novo *FBN1* mutation.

RISK FACTORS
Hypertension and increased BMI may increase risk of acute aortic dissection.

GENERAL PREVENTION
Prenatal diagnosis in families with a known mutation

COMMONLY ASSOCIATED CONDITIONS
- Ligamentous laxity, crowded teeth, cataracts, glaucoma, mitral valve prolapse (MVP), aortic regurgitation, and palpitations
- High prevalence of migraines, obstructive sleep apnea in MFS; may be a risk factor for aortic root dilatation

 DIAGNOSIS

- In the revised Ghent (Ghent II) nosology: Diagnosis is made in a person without a known family history of MFS, who has at least one of the following sets of features:
  - An *FBN1* pathogenic variant known to be associated with MFS and aortic root enlargement (Ao) (Z-score ≥2) or ectopia lentis (EL) Z-score calculator for aortic root enlargement: https://www.marfan.org/
  - Demonstration of Ao (Z-score ≥2) and EL or a defined combination of features yielding a systemic score ≥7
- Systemic features, scoring system (see "Physical Exam"):
  - Wrist *and* thumb sign +3; wrist *or* thumb sign +1
  - Pectus carinatum deformity +2; pectus excavatum or chest asymmetry +1
  - Hindfoot deformity +2; pes planus +1
  - Pneumothorax +2; dural ectasia +2
  - Protrusio acetabuli +2 by x-ray, CT, or MRI; reduced elbow extension +1
  - Reduced upper-to-lower segment (US/LS) ratio *and* increased arm/height *and* no severe scoliosis +1
  - Scoliosis or thoracolumbar kyphosis +1
  - Facial features (3/5) +1; myopia >3 diopters +1
  - Skin striae +1
  - MVP (all types) +1
- Maximum: 20 points; score ≥7 indicates systemic involvement. In adults with suggestive findings but who do not meet Ghent criteria, consider alternative diagnoses: EL syndrome, MVP syndrome, MASS (**M**VP, **A**ortic root dilatation, **S**kin, and **S**keletal) phenotype, nonspecific connective tissue disorder. In potential MFS diagnoses, close follow-up is recommended.

PHYSICAL EXAM
- Facial features: dolichocephaly (head length longer than expected compared with width), enophthalmos, down-slanting palpebral fissures, malar hypoplasia, micrognathia; high-arched, narrow palate
- Thumb sign: Distal phalanx of thumb protrudes from clenched fist. Wrist sign: Thumb and 5th digit overlap when circling wrist.
- Pectus carinatum deformity: pectus excavatum or chest asymmetry beyond normal variation
- Hindfoot valgus with forefoot abduction and lowering of the midfoot

- Height may be normal or may be ≥3.3 SD > mean. Increase arm span to height ratio >1.05.
- Reduced US/LS ratio: US is measured from the top of the head to the top of the midpubic bone; LS is measured from the top of the pubic bone to the sole of the foot.
- Scoliosis or thoracolumbar kyphosis is diagnosed if, on bending forward, there is a vertical difference ≥1.5 cm between the ribs of the left and right hemithorax.
- Reduced elbow extension if angle between upper and lower arm measures ≤170 degrees on full extension
- Skin: Striae atrophicae are significant if not associated with significant weight changes (or pregnancy) and if located on mid-back, lumbar region, upper arm, axilla, or thigh.
- Joint hypermobility, high-arched palate, and recurrent or incisional hernias were removed from diagnostic criteria (1).

DIFFERENTIAL DIAGNOSIS
Clinical manifestations overlapping with MFS in cardiovascular, ocular, and skeletal systems:

- EL syndrome: no aortic root dilatation
- MVP syndrome: Limited systemic features may include pectus excavatum, scoliosis, mild arachnodactyly; aortic enlargement and EL preclude this diagnosis.
- MASS phenotype (also *FBN1* mutation): MVP; myopia; borderline, nonprogressive aortic enlargement, nonspecific skeletal and skin involvement. Aortic involvement is usually nonprogressive; some risk for more severe vascular involvement; may be impossible to differentiate from MFS before age 20 years
- Shprintzen-Goldberg, Loeys-Dietz, Ehlers-Danlos, and Stickler syndromes; congenital contractural arachnodactyly; Weill-Marchesani syndrome, multiple endocrine neoplasia syndrome type 2B, fragile X syndrome
- Homocystinuria: marfanoid habitus, thrombosis, mental retardation; urine amino acid analysis is diagnostic; lens dislocates downward.
- Familial thoracic aortic aneurysm
- Aortopathy next generation sequencing (NGS) panel likely to play a more prominent role, especially as variant of unknown significance (VUS) are classified

DIAGNOSTIC TESTS & INTERPRETATION
- Sequencing of *FBN1* is the preferred method for molecular diagnosis. Mutations are found in 95% of patients meeting diagnostic criteria for MFS (1).
- Echocardiography: Measure aortic root at the level of sinuses of Valsalva; check for MVP. Consider CT or MRI to confirm accuracy of echocardiogram.
- Urinary homocysteine to rule out homocystinuria
- Anteroposterior (AP) radiograph: protrusio acetabuli
- Scoliosis: Cobb angle ≥20 degrees on radiographs
- Hindfoot valgus with forefoot abduction and lowering of the midfoot: anterior and posterior views
- MRI or CT to evaluate for dural ectasia if symptomatic (symptoms highly variable, nonspecific, and include lower back pain)

Diagnostic Procedures/Other

- EL is diagnosed on slit-lamp examination after maximal dilatation of the pupil (60%); lens dislocation is most often upward and temporal.
- Myopia: >3 diopters contribute to MFS systemic score.
- Elongated globe, keratoconus, increased risk of vitreous or retinal detachment, glaucoma, and early cataract formation

Test Interpretation

- Cystic medial necrosis of the aorta: descriptive, not pathognomonic
- Myxomatous degeneration of cardiac valves

 ## TREATMENT

Multidisciplinary management: clinical geneticist, cardiologist, ophthalmologist, orthopedist, and cardiothoracic surgeon

MEDICATION

- Prevention of aortic complications: β-blockers; dosage is adjusted to target heart rate (resting heart rate is 60 beats/min, <100 beats/min after submaximal exercise) (1)[C].
- The evidence for β-blocker therapy to reduce morbidity and mortality in MFS is limited to a single small, prospective randomized and nonblinded clinical trial.
- If β-blockers contraindicated: ARBs may slow aortic dilation in children and adolescents.
- Losartan plus β-blockers has been suggested to prevent progressive aortic root dilatation, but clinical trials needed to assess improved outcomes with medication.
- Preliminary evidence suggests calcium channel blockers may increase risk of aortic complications.
- Genetic and molecular factors are likely to influence drug effects but remain unknown. Medical treatment should be individualized, with careful monitoring.

ISSUES FOR REFERRAL

Genetics, cardiology, orthopedics, ophthalmology, pediatric surgery (pectus carinatum deformities)

SURGERY/OTHER PROCEDURES

- When cardiac symptoms develop or aortic root diameter is ≥5 cm, consider surgical intervention. Many patients will ultimately require cardiovascular surgery:
  - Dissection of ascending aorta (type A) is a surgical emergency. Consider prophylactic surgery when diameter of sinus of Valsalva approaches 5 cm, rate of change approaches 1 cm/year, and with progressive aortic regurgitation. Other risk factors: family history, other cardiac pathology, pregnancy
  - Dissection of descending thoracic aorta (type B): Surgical indications include intractable pain, limb or organ ischemia, and aortic diameter >5.5 cm (or rapidly increasing) (1).

- Mitral valve repair: for severe mitral valve regurgitation or progressive LV dilatation or dysfunction or in patients undergoing valve-sparing root replacement (1)
- Lens subluxation: Incidence of glaucoma is high; surgery is performed only if untreatable with corrective lenses; surgical removal of lens for opacity, impending complete luxation, lens-induced glaucoma or uveitis, or anisometropia or refractive error is not amenable to optical correction (1).
- Severe pectus excavatum may interfere with pulmonary or cardiac function. Refer for surgery prior to end of adolescent age.
- Scoliosis: bracing for curves 20 to 40 degrees until growth complete or surgery if >40 degrees
- Surgery for only most severe cases of dural ectasia
- Hip replacement in middle age or later if protrusio acetabuli has led to severe arthritic change.

 ## ONGOING CARE

FOLLOW-UP RECOMMENDATIONS

Exercise restrictions: Avoid sports that can increase aortic root enlargement or pneumothorax. Follow recommendation from the National Marfan Foundation and guidelines from the American Heart Association/American College of Cardiology Task Force.

Patient Monitoring

Exams at least twice per year while patient is growing, with attention to the cardiovascular system and to scoliosis

- Cognitive ability is usually normal, but visual and medical difficulties may interfere with learning (3)[C].
- Cardiac
  - Aortic root dilatation usually progressive; age <20 years, echocardiogram yearly; adults with repeatedly normal aortic root measurements, echocardiogram every 2 to 3 years (1)[C]
  - Consider 6-month repeat imaging following initial surveillance to assess rate of dilatation, more frequent if aortic diameter is increasing rapidly (≥5 cm/year) or approaching surgical threshold (≥4.5 cm in adults)
  - Regular imaging after surgical repair of aorta
- Musculoskeletal
  - Excessive linear growth of long bones, extremities disproportionately long, paucity of muscle mass, peak growth velocity 2 years early. Growth curves for MFS are available (3)[C].
  - Evaluate for scoliosis, joint laxity, and pectus deformity every visit to age 1 year, annually for ages 1 to 5 years, semiannually for ages 6 to 18 years, and yearly thereafter.
  - Bone age in preadolescence: Consider hormonal therapy for large discrepancy (3)[C].
  - Scoliosis or pectus deformity may progress more rapidly than in those without MFS.
  - Excellent prognosis for scoliosis curves <30 degrees; bracing may be effective for curves <35 degrees; rapid progression is likely if curve is >50 degrees (3)[C].

- Annual ophthalmologic evaluation: EL, myopia, cataract, glaucoma, and retinal detachment; myopia is very common with early onset, rapid progression, and high degree of severity; early monitoring and aggressive refraction to prevent amblyopia (1)[C]
- Respiratory: pulmonary function tests (PFTs) with symptoms
- Provide genetic counseling at diagnosis, discuss pregnancy risks in adolescence, and discuss activity restrictions starting age 6 years. Review symptoms of potential catastrophic events: aortic dissection, vision changes, and pneumothorax starting age 6 years.

DIET

Early diagnosis of homocystinuria is important because clinical complications can be minimized with appropriate diet and medication.

PROGNOSIS

Life-threatening complications involve cardiovascular dysfunction. With appropriate diagnosis, treatment, and monitoring, lifespan is nearly normal.

COMPLICATIONS

Bacterial endocarditis, aortic dissection, aortic or mitral valve insufficiency, dilated cardiomyopathy, retinal detachment, glaucoma, pneumothorax

REFERENCES

1. Loeys BL, Dietz HC, Braverman AC, et al. The revised Ghent nosology for the Marfan syndrome. *J Med Genet*. 2010;47(7):476–485.
2. Narula N, Devereux RB, Malonga GP, et al. Pregnancy-related aortic complications in women with Marfan syndrome. *J Am Coll Cardiol*. 2021;78(9):870–879.
3. Tinkle BT, Saal HM; for Committee on Genetics. Health supervision for children with Marfan syndrome. *Pediatrics*. 2013;132(4):e1059–e1072.

 ## CODES

ICD10

- Q87.40 Marfan's syndrome, unspecified
- Q87.43 Marfan's syndrome with skeletal manifestation
- Q87.418 Marfan's syndrome with other cardiovascular manifestations

CLINICAL PEARLS

- Because many features of MFS appear in the general population, diagnostic criteria have been established. Molecular diagnostic testing for *FBN1* mutations will play an increasing role.
- Screen very tall athletes for aortic root dilatation.
- EL and aortic root dilatation are the best discrimination features, but height ≥3.3 *SD* above the mean is a simple discriminant in primary care.

M

MARIJUANA (CANNABIS) USE DISORDER

Jason Edward Lambrecht, MD, FHM, FACP, PharmD • Paul G. Millner, MD • Bradley Devrieze, MD

BASICS

DESCRIPTION

- Marijuana use leading to clinically significant impairment or distress, manifested by two or more of the following symptoms within a 12-month period:
  - Consumption of larger amounts over a longer period of time than intended
  - Persistent desire or inability to cut down or control amount used
  - Inordinate amount of time spent in activities is necessary to obtain, use, or recover from use.
  - Presence of craving for cannabis
  - Recurrent use resulting in failure to fulfill major role obligations at work, school, or home
  - Continued use despite having persistent or recurrent social or interpersonal problems due to cannabis use
  - Important social, occupational, or recreational activities are given up or reduced.
  - Recurrent use in physically hazardous situations
  - Continued use despite knowledge of a persistent physical or psychological problem caused or exacerbated by cannabis
  - Tolerance defined by using increased amounts of cannabis to achieve the desired effect or intoxication or diminished effect with continued use of the same amount
  - Withdrawal occurs following cessation of prolonged use and has at least three behavioral symptoms such as anxiety, restlessness, depression, irritability, insomnia, odd dreams, or physical symptoms such as tremors and/or decreased appetite
- According to *DSM-5*, marijuana or cannabis use disorder (CUD) is defined as being mild, moderate, or severe depending on how many symptoms are present; mild: 2 to 3; moderate: 4 to 5; severe: ≥6

EPIDEMIOLOGY

- The WHO ranks the United States as first among 17 European and North American countries for the prevalence of marijuana use.
- From 2016 to 2020, there was a 4.5 times increase in licensure for medical cannabis with >2.9 million licensures granted in 2020 (1). It is estimated that 4.5 to 7 million persons in the United States met the criteria for CUD annually. There has been an increase from 15% to 32% of cannabis use for symptoms/conditions without a strong evidence base for use (1). Chronic pain remains the most common reason for medical cannabis licensure. 10–30% of lifetime marijuana users met the criteria for CUD; 23% of these individuals met the criteria for severe use.

- Risk of CUD is highest amongst those who start using marijuana before the age of 18 years.
- Cannabinoids have potential for harm especially in vulnerable populations such as adolescents and those with psychiatric disorders. Current evidence is insufficient to support routine prescription of cannabinoids for the treatment of psychiatric disorders. There is also a concern regarding long-term effects on cognitive dysfunction and risk for stroke.
- Approximately 30% of students have used marijuana by the time of college entry. Individuals who use high-potency cannabis are more likely to use cannabis regularly, have cannabis-related problems, use other illicit drugs, and have general anxiety disorder.
- Many states have legalized marijuana in some form. In 1969, only 12% of people approved of legalizing/decriminalizing marijuana; by 2021, >90% of Americans approved of cannabis for medical use.

ETIOLOGY AND PATHOPHYSIOLOGY

- The two most known therapeutically active cannabinoids in marijuana are δ9-tetrahydrocannabinol (THC) and cannabidiol (CBD).
- THC is the psychoactive component responsible for marijuana's analgesic, antiemetic, and intoxicating properties. THC concentrations in marijuana have risen over the past 20 years from 4% to 12–20%.
- CBD is the nonpsychoactive component responsible for marijuana's antianxiety, antidepressant, antipsychotic, antispastic, anticonvulsant, and antineoplastic properties.
- Strains of cannabis vary, with some being THC rich, some CBD rich, and some THC/CBD balanced.
- Smoking marijuana results in 25–50% absorption of THC, which rapidly passes into the circulation. The oral bioavailability of THC is much less (3–10%). Effects of smoked marijuana occur within minutes and last several hours; effects from marijuana consumed in foods or beverages appear more slowly, taking 30 minutes to 2 hours to have an effect.
- Frequent users are likely to experience withdrawal.
- The role of cannabis for treating chronic pain continues to evolve.
- Only 5% of those with CUD seek treatment from a health care provider.

RISK FACTORS

- Young individuals, especially 18- to 29-year-olds, are at more risk for severe CUD.
- Cigarette smokers are at higher risk for CUD compared to nonsmokers.
- Higher potency marijuana use increases risk of CUD and increases severity of symptoms.

- Frequency of use affects the risk of CUD. Monthly users are at 4-fold increased risk, weekly users are at 8-fold increased risk, and daily users are at 17-fold increased risk for developing CUD.
- Family history of chemical dependence
- Comorbid psychiatric disorders (i.e., antisocial personality disorder)
- Other substance use (i.e., alcohol, tobacco)
- Lower educational achievement (rates of dependence are lowest among college graduates); low socioeconomic status
- Ease of acquisition of marijuana
- Among youths with mood disorders, CUD is a risk marker for nonfatal self harm, all-cause mortality, and death by unintentional overdose and homicide.

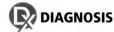 DIAGNOSIS

- USPSTF guidelines encourage screening adults for drug use.
- Ask for frequency and amount used (e.g., "How often do you use marijuana? Daily? Weekly?"; "How long does a typical 'eighth' [1/8 oz] last?").
- Usage is quantified as occasional = 1/8 oz/week, moderate = 1/4 oz/week, and heavy = 1/2 oz/week (1 oz = 28.5 gm which is equivalent to about 50 to 60 cigarettes).
- Unexplained deterioration in school or work performance is a red flag for abuse.
- Problems with, or changes in, social relationships (e.g., spending more time alone or with persons suspected of using drugs) and recreational activities (e.g., giving up activities that were once pleasurable) may also indicate abuse.
- If possible, obtain information from concerned parents or significant others.

HISTORY

- Clinical presentation of acute intoxication:
  - Euphoria, elation, laughter, heightened sensory perception, altered perception of time, increased appetite
  - Poor short-term memory, concentration
  - Fatigue, depression
  - Occasionally, distrust, fear, anxiety, panic
  - With large doses, acute psychosis: delusions, hallucinations, loss of sense of identity
- Withdrawal symptoms include:
  - Irritability; anxiety, restlessness, nausea; weight loss; decreased appetite
  - Insomnia; depressed mood; tremors

PHYSICAL EXAM

- Evaluate for:
  - Conjunctival injection; xerostomia; nystagmus; increased heart rate
  - Decreased coordination; altered mental status
- Withdrawal findings (nonspecific-similar to other drugs of abuse) include:
  - Restlessness/agitation; irritability; tremor; diaphoresis
  - Increased body temperature

DIAGNOSTIC TESTS & INTERPRETATION

Urine drug screen is the preferred sample for screening. Cannabinoids can be detected in urine weeks to months after marijuana use. Blood testing is preferred for interpreting acute effects and levels. In the United States, there is no consensus for acceptable legal limits for marijuana levels while driving. Hair testing can be unreliable and may reflect second-hand exposure. In general, testing identifies cannabis use (not necessarily CUD).

 TREATMENT

- There are no FDA-approved medications for the treatment of CUD. There is an insufficient evidence to recommend for or against pharmacotherapy for CUD (2).
- No specific treatment guidelines for CUD are currently available. No intervention has proved consistently effective for marijuana abuse. Users often have a hard time quitting.
- Behavioral interventions are viable options for initial treatment (2), including:
  - Cognitive-behavioral therapy; motivational interviewing; contingency management
  - Social network behavior therapy; 12-step approach; family-oriented therapy
  - Brief intervention; relapse prevention; community reinforcement approach
- The addition of a comprehensive parenting training curriculum does not enhance efficacy.
- Treating comorbid behavioral health disorders may help reduce use, particularly among heavy users.
- To help manage withdrawal:
  - Reduce amount used before quitting entirely. Delay first use of marijuana until later in the day.
  - Consider nicotine replacement therapy if concomitant tobacco use is present. Avoid cues and triggers associated with use.
- With marked irritability and restlessness, consider very low-dose diazepam for 3 to 4 days.
- Provide the user and family members with information regarding abuse and withdrawal.
- Withdrawal symptoms peak on day 2 or 3 and generally subside by day 7. Vivid dreams can continue for 2 to 3 weeks.

MEDICATION

- No effective medication currently exists to treat marijuana abuse.
- A recent review of medication options for treatment of CUD concluded:
  - SSRI (low strength evidence—did not reduce cannabis use or assist with cravings); antipsychotics (insufficient evidence for benefit); anxiolytics (low strength evidence that buspirone has no benefit over placebo); mood stabilizers (insufficient evidence for any benefit)
  - Gabapentin (insufficient evidence) was not helpful in management.
- Oral FDA-approved cannabinoids such as dronabinol or nabiximols may help abate marijuana withdrawal symptoms in individuals who are trying to quit.
- Options to assist with cravings include naltrexone 50 mg PO daily or N-Acetylcysteine 1,200 mg PO TID.
- Treatment of withdrawal is targeted toward symptom management such as anxiety, insomnia and nausea.

 ONGOING CARE

FOLLOW-UP RECOMMENDATIONS

- Monitor cessation by testing urine over several weeks for the inactive cannabis metabolites (carboxy-THC).
- Drug screening of heavy smokers may remain positive for marijuana up to 6 weeks after last use.

PATIENT EDUCATION

National Institute on Drug Abuse (NIDA): http://www.drugabuse.gov

COMPLICATIONS

- Acute adverse effects:
  - Acute panic or paranoid reactions can occur, especially in drug-naive individuals or those with a history of psychosis or other behavioral health conditions.
  - Marijuana use is an independent risk factor for heart failure.
  - In states where cannabis has been legalized, there has been an increase in ED visits for acute myocardial infarction.
  - Psychotic symptoms with high doses
  - Driving under the influence of marijuana increases the risk for motor vehicle accidents.
  - Adverse long-term effects on cognitive dysfunction and increased risk of stroke
- Chronic adverse effects:
  - Abnormal brain development; diminished lifetime achievement
  - Chronic bronchitis and impaired respiratory function in regular smokers
  - Smoking marijuana is harmful in transplant patients and other immunosuppressed individuals.

- Marijuana use is associated with an increased risk of fibrosis in hepatitis C patients.
- Marijuana may contribute to or result in pancreatitis.
- Psychotic symptoms in heavy users, especially those with a personal or family history of schizophrenia
- Marijuana use increases the risk for addiction to other substances.
- An increased risk of heart failure, hypertension, ischemic stroke, and overall mortality in heavy cannabis users
- Cannabinoid hyperemesis syndrome is characterized by episodes of cyclic nausea and vomiting in association with chronic cannabis use.

REFERENCES

1. Boehnke KF, Dean O, Haffajee RL, et al. U.S. trends in registration for medical cannabis and reasons for use from 2016 to 2020: an observational study. *Ann Intern Med.* 2022;175(7):945–951.
2. Perry C, Liberto J, Milliken C, et al; for VA/DoD Guideline Development Group. The management of substance use disorders: synopsis of the 2021 U.S. Department of Veteran Affairs and U.S. Department of Defense clinical practice guideline. *Ann Intern Med.* 2022;175(5):720–731.

 CODES

ICD10

- F12.10 Cannabis abuse, uncomplicated
- F12.20 Cannabis dependence, uncomplicated
- F12.288 Cannabis dependence with other cannabis-induced disorder

CLINICAL PEARLS

- It is estimated that 4.5 to 7 million persons in the U.S. meet criteria for CUD
- Acute marijuana intoxication is manifested by conjunctival injection, increased heart rate, euphoria, heightened sensory perception, altered perception of time, increased appetite, poor short-term memory and concentration, and fatigue. Large doses may result in acute psychosis, panic or paranoid reactions, delusions, or hallucinations.
- Withdrawal symptoms include weight loss, decreased appetite, insomnia, and depressed mood. These symptoms peak on day 2 or 3 and resolve by day 7.
- Treatment of withdrawal is targeted towards symptom management such as anxiety, insomnia, and nausea.
- Cognitive-behavioral therapy, motivational interviewing, motivational enhancement therapy, and contingency management are four behavioral interventions used to treat marijuana use disorder.

M

MASTITIS

Amena Payami, DO

 BASICS

DESCRIPTION
- Mastitis is an inflammation of the breast parenchyma and possibly associated tissues (areola, nipple, subcutaneous [SC] fat).
- Usually associated with bacterial infection (and milk stasis in the postpartum mother)
- Can be lactational or nonlactational
- Usually an acute condition but can become chronic cystic mastitis

EPIDEMIOLOGY
- Predominantly affects females
- Mostly in the puerperium; epidemic form rare in the age of reduced hospital stays for mothers and newborns
- Neonatal form
- Posttraumatic: ornamental nipple piercing increases risk of transmission of bacteria to deeper breast structures; *Staphylococcus aureus* is the predominant organism.

Incidence
- 3–20% of breastfeeding mothers develop non-epidemic mastitis, with greatest incidence among breastfeeding mothers 2 to 6 weeks postpartum.
- Neonatal form occurs at 1 to 5 weeks of age, with equal gender risk and unilateral presentation.
- Pediatric form occurs at or around or after puberty, with 82% of cases in girls.

ETIOLOGY AND PATHOPHYSIOLOGY
- Microabscesses along milk ducts and surrounding tissues
- Inflammatory cell infiltration of breast parenchyma and surrounding tissues
- Nonpuerperal (infectious) *S. aureus* (including methicillin-resistant *S. aureus* [MRSA]), *Bacteroides* spp., *Peptostreptococcus*, *Staphylococcus* (coagulase negative), *Enterococcus faecalis*, *Histoplasma capsulatum*, *Salmonella enterica*, rare case of *Actinomyces europaeus*
- Puerperal (infectious) *S. aureus* (including MRSA), *Streptococcus pyogenes* (group A or B), *Enterobacteriaceae*, *Corynebacterium* spp., *Bacteroides* spp., *Staphylococcus* (coagulase negative), *Escherichia coli*, *Salmonella* spp. (1)
- Rare secondary site for tuberculosis in endemic areas (1% of mastitis cases in these areas): single breast nodule with mastalgia
- Tuberculosis mastitis in nonendemic areas has also been reported in patients with exposure to TNF-α inhibitors and other immunomodulating compounds.
- *Corynebacterium* sp. associated with greater risk for development of chronic cystic mastitis
- Granulomatous mastitis
  - Idiopathic: predilection for Asian and Hispanic women
    - Association with α_1-antitrypsin deficiency, hyperprolactinemia with galactorrhea, oral contraceptive use, *Corynebacterium* spp. infection, and breast trauma
    - Most women have a history of lactation in the previous 5 years.
    - New cases have been reported in male-to-female transgender patients in setting of exogenous progesterone and estrogen treatment.
  - Lupus; autoimmune

- Puerperal: Retrograde migration of surface bacteria up milk ducts, bacterial trapping behind plugged milk in the ductal outflow tracts. Bacterial migration from nipple fissures to breast lymphatics. Occasionally, secondary monilial infection in the face of recurrent mastitis or diabetes. Seeding from mother to neonate in cyclical fashion may occur.
- Nonpuerperal: a variety of causes including ductal ectasia, breast carcinoma, inflammatory cysts, chronic recurring SC or subareolar infections, parasitic infections (*Echinococcus*, filariasis, guinea worm in endemic areas), herpes simplex, cat-scratch disease, and, in older patients, smoking. Lupus is a rare cause.

RISK FACTORS
- Milk stasis: inadequate emptying of breast (scarring due to previous breast surgery [breast reduction, biopsy, or partial mastectomy], scarring of breast due to prior mastitis), breast engorgement: interruption of breastfeeding, milk oversupply, plugged ducts
- Nipple trauma increases risk of transmission of bacteria to deeper breast structures: *S. aureus* predominant organism.
- Neonatal colonization with epidemic *Staphylococcus*
- Neonatal—occurs more commonly in bottle-fed babies
- Maternal diabetes
- Maternal HIV
- Smoking

GENERAL PREVENTION
Regular emptying of both breasts and nipple care to prevent fissures when breastfeeding; also good hygiene including hand washing and washing breast pumps after each use

COMMONLY ASSOCIATED CONDITIONS
Breast abscess

 DIAGNOSIS

- Fever >38.5°C, malaise, and myalgia
- Nausea ± vomiting
- Localized breast tenderness, firmness, heat, swelling, and redness
- Possible breast mass

HISTORY
Breast pain, "hot cords burning in chest wall"

PHYSICAL EXAM
- Breast tenderness
- Localized breast induration, redness, and warmth
- Peau d'orange appearance to overlying skin

DIFFERENTIAL DIAGNOSIS
- Abscess (bacterial, idiopathic granulomatous mastitis, fungal, tuberculosis)
- Tumor, including inflammatory breast cancer
- Idiopathic granulomatous mastitis
- Wegener granulomatosis
- Sarcoidosis
- Foreign-body granuloma
- Vasospasm (may be presentation for Raynaud): Consider yeast infection if nipple pain and burning and/or infant with thrush.
- Ductal cyst (ductal ectasia)
- Consider monilial infection in lactating mother, especially if mastitis is recurrent.
- Mondor disease—thrombophlebitis of the superficial veins of the breast and anterior chest wall

DIAGNOSTIC TESTS & INTERPRETATION

Initial Tests (lab, imaging)
Mastitis is typically a clinical diagnosis; labs rarely needed; in those ill enough to need hospitalization, consider the following:
- CBC, blood culture
- In epidemic puerperal mastitis: milk leukocyte count, milk culture (or if recurrent outpatient mastitis), neonatal nasal culture
- No imaging required for postpartum mastitis in a breastfeeding mother that responds to antibiotic therapy
- Mammography for women with nonpuerperal mastitis
- Breast ultrasound (US) to rule out abscess formation in women with a mass or fluctuance on palpation; special consideration for this in women with breast implants who have mastitis

Follow-Up Tests & Special Considerations
Lactating mothers produce salty milk from affected side (higher Na and Cl concentrations) as compared with unaffected side. Consider breast milk culture if suspect MRSA. Also consider testing for tuberculosis as may be initial presentation.

Diagnostic Procedures/Other
Options if further progression to abscess formation: needle aspiration, incision and drainage, excisional biopsy, US-guided core needle biopsy is diagnostic method of choice for idiopathic granulomatous mastitis

 TREATMENT

- A Cochrane review found that insufficient evidence exists to confirm or refute the effectiveness of antibiotic therapy for the treatment of lactational mastitis (2)[A]. If present <24 hours and symptoms are mild, conservative management with milk removal and supportive measures is recommended.
- For patients with early idiopathic granulomatous mastitis and mild symptoms or those concerned for surgical scarring, close surveillance or observation alone is acceptable nonsurgical management.

GENERAL MEASURES
- Supportive care including analgesia, warm compress and effective, frequent milk removal from the affected breast via breastfeeding, pumping, or hand expression
- Smoking cessation for patients with periductal mastitis

MEDICATION
- Prioritized on the basis of likelihood of MRSA as etiologic factor and clinical severity of condition; treat for 10 to 14 days.
- For idiopathic granulomatous mastitis and localized infection, usually resolves with antibiotics and drainage

First Line
- Outpatient
  - Effective milk removal is the most important management step.
  - Dicloxacillin 500 mg QID *or* cephalexin 500 mg QID
  - Trimethoprim/sulfamethoxazole (TMP/SMX); DS BID (If mastitis is not improving within 48 hours after starting first-line treatment, consider MRSA.)
  - Doxycycline 100 mg BID; consider MRSA (if clinical course <3 weeks).
  - *Lactobacillus fermentum* or *Lactobacillus salivarius* 9 log 10 CFU/day
- Inpatient
  - Nafcillin 2 g q4h *or* oxacillin 2 g q4h *or* vancomycin 1 g q12h (MRSA possible)
  - Daptomycin 1 g q24h
- If idiopathic granulomatous mastitis, consider corticosteroids ± methotrexate; may consider mycophenolate mofitel in patient refractory to treatment with antibiotics, steroids, and methotrexate

Pediatric Considerations
- TMP/SMX given to breastfeeding mothers with mastitis can potentiate jaundice for neonates.
- Treatment with doxycycline is limited to <3 weeks; long-term therapy (over 3 to 4 weeks) is not recommended because it may cause damage of infant's growth cartilage, teeth discoloration, and imbalance of intestinal flora.

Second Line
- If mastitis is odoriferous and localized under areola, add metronidazole 500 mg TID IV or PO.
- If yeast is suspected in recurrent mastitis, add topical and oral nystatin. Consider testing nipple tissue and milk for presence of yeast. Oral treatment can be considered for mother as well.

ISSUES FOR REFERRAL
- Abscess formation
- Need for breast biopsy (suspected abscess or IGM)

ADDITIONAL THERAPIES
- Warm packs to improve blood flow and milk letdown and/or ice packs to reduce inflammation to affected breast for comfort
- The use of a breast pump may aid in breast emptying, especially if the infant is unable to assist in doing this.
- Wear supporting bra that is not too tight.

SURGERY/OTHER PROCEDURES
In cases of biopsy-proven idiopathic granulomatous mastitis, the most effective and fastest way for complete eradication is surgical removal. The addition of steroids increases the rate of complete remission and decreases remission rate compared to surgery alone; NNT 3.84

COMPLEMENTARY & ALTERNATIVE MEDICINE
- Breast lift technique for lymphatic breast drainage (can reduce engorgement and relieve plugging)
- Cold cabbage leaf compress to be applied up to 15 minutes twice per day (Avoid long or frequent application of cabbage leaves as milk production can be diminished with this.)
- To prevent recurring plugs and mastitis, can use sunflower lecithin 1,200 mg 3 to 4 times per day

ADMISSION, INPATIENT, AND NURSING CONSIDERATIONS
- If a new mother is admitted to the hospital for treatment of her mastitis, rooming-in of the infant with the mother is highly recommended so that breastfeeding can continue. In some hospitals, rooming-in may require hospital admission of the infant.
- Admission criteria/initial stabilization: Failure or outpatient/oral therapy (patient unable to tolerate oral therapy, non-adherent to oral therapy, or severe illness without adequate supportive care at home); neonatal mastitis also requires admission.
  - Administer antibiotics.
  - Empty breasts frequently, if breastfeeding.
  - Give analgesics for pain: ibuprofen or acetaminophen.
  - Breastfeeding/pumping of breasts encouraged; baby and/or breast pump to bedside
- Start infant with feedings on affected side.
- Abscess drainage is not a contraindication for breastfeeding.
- Massage in direction from blocked area toward nipple.
- Positioning the infant at breast with chin or nose pointing to blockage might help drain the affected area.
- Discharge criteria: Patients should be afebrile and tolerating oral antibiotics well.

 ## ONGOING CARE

FOLLOW-UP RECOMMENDATIONS
Patient Monitoring
- Rest for lactating mothers, up to bathroom. Admit to medical floor. If concern for sepsis or hemodynamic instability, admit to intermediate level of care or ICU.
- Follow up with breast imaging such as mammography or US in women >40 years of age after resolution of acute pathology to exclude underlying breast cancer.

DIET
- Encourage oral fluids.
- Multivitamin, including vitamin A

PATIENT EDUCATION
- Encourage oral fluids. Rest is essential.
- Regular emptying/draining of both breasts with breastfeeding
- Nipple care (simply with breast milk or with hypoallergenic nipple balm) to prevent fissures
- Best nipple/areola health comes with optimized latch—seek help with latch if needed from a lactation professional.

PROGNOSIS
- Puerperal
  - Good with prompt (within 24 hours of symptom onset) antibiotic treatment and breast emptying; 96% success rate
  - 11% risk of abscess if left untreated with antibiotics
  - Antibodies develop in breast glands within the first few days of infection, which may provide protection against infection or reinfection.
- Rare risk of abscess formation beyond 6 weeks postpartum if no recurrent mastitis
- Idiopathic granulomatous mastitis recurrence rates high, encourage close follow-up

COMPLICATIONS
Breast abscess 3% of women with puerperal mastitis, recurrent mastitis with resumption of breastfeeding or with breastfeeding after next pregnancy, cessation of breastfeeding, bacteremia, sepsis

REFERENCES
1. Wilson E, Woodd SL, Benova L. Incidence of and risk factors for lactational mastitis: a systematic review. *J Hum Lact*. 2020;36(4):673–686.
2. Jahanfar S, Ng CJ, Teng CL. Antibiotics for mastitis in breastfeeding women. *Cochrane Database Syst Rev*. 2013(2):CD005458.

ADDITIONAL READING

Spencer JP. Management of mastitis in breastfeeding women. *Am Fam Physician*. 2008;78(6):727–731.

 ## SEE ALSO

Algorithms: Breast Discharge; Breast Pain

 ## CODES

ICD10
- O91.11 Abscess of breast associated with pregnancy
- O91.211 Nonpurulent mastitis associated with pregnancy, first trimester
- O91.113 Abscess of breast associated with pregnancy, third trimester

CLINICAL PEARLS
- Emptying/draining of the breasts on a regular schedule (recommend following baby's cues, but going no more than 3 to 4 hours between feeds), avoiding constrictive clothing or bras that might obstruct breast ducts, attention to good latch technique for mom and baby, "adequate rest," and a liberal intake of oral fluids for the mother can all reduce the risk of a breastfeeding mother's developing mastitis.
- Reassure mothers that it is safe (and imperative for healing) to feed baby and/or pump the affected breast.
- Among breastfeeding mothers, if the symptoms of mastitis fail to resolve within several days of appropriate management, including antibiotics, NSAID, and breast emptying, further investigations may be required to confirm resistant bacteria, abscess formation, an underlying mass, or inflammatory or ductal carcinoma.
- More than two recurrences of mastitis in the same location or with associated axillary lymphadenopathy warrant evaluation with US and/or mammography to rule out an underlying mass.

M

MASTOIDITIS
Samantha Carroll, MD • Chantal Soobhanath, MD

 BASICS

Mastoiditis is an inflammatory process of the mastoid bone. It is most commonly seen as a complication of acute otitis media (AOM).

DESCRIPTION
- Clinical manifestations of mastoiditis typically appear days to weeks after the first middle ear symptoms.
- Subdivided according to pathologic stage:
  - Acute mastoiditis with periostitis (incipient mastoiditis): purulent material in the mastoid cavities; symptom duration typically ≤1 month
  - Coalescent mastoiditis (acute mastoid osteitis): destruction of the thin bony septae between air cells; followed by the formation of abscess cavities with pus dissecting into adjacent areas
- Masked mastoiditis (subacute mastoiditis): low grade, persistent infection with destruction of the bony septae between air cells; occurs in patients with persistent middle ear effusion or recurrent episodes of inadequately treated AOM
- Chronic mastoiditis: associated with failed treatment of chronic otitis media; often associated with cholesteatoma; symptoms last for months to years.

EPIDEMIOLOGY
Highest incidence in children aged <2 years
- Similar to population susceptible to AOM (male, daycare attendance)
- Less common if immunizations up-to-date and antibiotics used to treat suppurative AOM

Incidence
1.2 to 3.8 cases per 100,000 children per year in the United States (1)

ETIOLOGY AND PATHOPHYSIOLOGY
- Subclinical stage begins with AOM and inflammation of mastoid air cells.
- Mastoid is part of petrous temporal bone composed of air-filled cells.
- Mastoid aditus and antrum form a narrow connection between middle ear and mastoid air cells.
  - Fluid in the middle ear can cause obstruction at aditus or antrum, blocking outflow tract of mastoid air cells.
  - Edema and accumulation of purulent material most commonly spreads from mastoid air cells to periosteum via mastoid emissary veins with penetration of periosteum (acute mastoiditis with periostitis).
- Increased pressure from fluid within the air cells leads to destruction of bony septae (acute mastoid osteitis/acute coalescent mastoiditis).
- Acute mastoid osteitis can spread to adjacent areas in head and neck with abscess formation.
  - Subperiosteal abscess (most common complication), Bezold abscess, suppurative labyrinthitis, suppurative CNS complications (2)
- AOM: *Streptococcus pneumoniae*, nontypeable *Haemophilus influenzae*
- Acute mastoiditis: *S. pneumoniae* (most common), group A streptococci—*Streptococcus pyogenes*, *Staphylococcus aureus* (including methicillin-resistant *S. aureus* [MRSA]), *H. influenzae*, *Fusobacterium necrophorum*
- Chronic mastoiditis: *Pseudomonas aeruginosa*, *S. aureus*, anaerobic bacteria, polymicrobials (organisms present in external ear canal), rarely *Mycobacterium tuberculosis*

- Abscess: *S. aureus*, mycobacteria, *Aspergillus*
- Increased incidence of penicillin-resistant *S. pneumoniae* infections has gradually lead to higher incidence of mastoiditis as complication of AOM.

Genetics
No known genetic pattern

RISK FACTORS
- Cholesteatoma appears as squamous pearl in antero-superior area of middle ear near tympanic membrane.
- Recurrent AOM or chronic suppurative otitis media
- Immunocompromised state

GENERAL PREVENTION
- Ensure immunizations (particularly pneumococcal vaccine) are up-to-date.
- Referral to ENT for chronic otitis media
- Appropriate diagnosis and treatment of AOM; prevent recurrent AOM.
  - Chemoprophylaxis for AOM is controversial. Historically, consider in children with two episodes of AOM in first 6 months of life or in older children, three episodes in 6 months, or four episodes in 1 year. Chemoprophylaxis is not currently recommended by American Academy of Pediatrics due to concern for multidrug resistance.
- Wear ear plugs when swimming or showering to keep water out of the ears with AOM.
- Treat chronic eustachian tube dysfunction (pressure equalization tubes).
- Early diagnosis of cholesteatoma

COMMONLY ASSOCIATED CONDITIONS
AOM

 DIAGNOSIS

Clinical exam or from CT scan; clinical findings including redness of the mastoid area, with anterior protrusion of the affected ear, ear drainage

HISTORY
- Most common symptoms in infancy
  - Lethargy/malaise/irritability
  - Fever
  - Poor feeding/decreased appetite
- Recent ear infection
- Otorrhea (drainage from an ear infection)
- Otalgia and/or pain on mastoid bone behind the ear
- Swelling or redness over mastoid
- Swelling of the ear lobe
- Headache
- Hearing loss
- Chronic: persistent ear drainage, persistent ear pain
- Chronic: AOM nonresponsive to antibiotic
- Suspicion for mastoiditis increases when symptoms of AOM persist >2 weeks.

PHYSICAL EXAM
- Acute:
  - Fever
  - Erythema, tenderness, and/or edema overlying mastoid (postauricular)
  - Palpable postauricular fluctuance (later finding): most commonly postauricular in children aged >1 year and above ear in children aged <1 year
  - Displaced pinna up and outward in children aged >1 year or down and outward in children aged <1 year
  - Otoscopic exam: AOM present, may have perforation of TM with or without purulent discharge

- Chronic mastoiditis:
  - Persistent or intermittent mucopurulent drainage
  - Decreased hearing
  - May be painless from chronic process
  - Otoscopic exam: may have mucopurulent discharge, perforation of TM

DIFFERENTIAL DIAGNOSIS
- Scalp infection
- Mumps, parotitis
- Severe otitis externa
- Periauricular cellulitis
- Benign neoplasm: aneurysmal bone cyst, fibrous dysplasia
- Malignant neoplasm: acute lymphocytic leukemia, acute myelogenous leukemia, Burkitt lymphoma, non-Hodgkin lymphoma, rhabdomyosarcoma, neuroblastoma
- Deep neck space infections

DIAGNOSTIC TESTS & INTERPRETATION
Initial Tests (lab, imaging)
- CBC with differential: elevated WBC count
- Elevated erythrocyte sedimentation rate (ESR) and C-reactive protein (CRP) in acute but may be normal in chronic
- Blood cultures
- Myringotomy/tympanocentesis: send for cultures, Gram stain, acid-fast stain
- Aspiration if postauricular fluctuance is present: Send for cultures.
- Plain films of mastoid has low diagnostic yield but may show loss of sharpness of mastoid outline, clouding of mastoid air cells, or demineralization of bony septa (3). These changes are not diagnostic and can also be seen in AOM.
- Preferred: CT of the temporal bone (97% sensitivity; 94% positive predictive value for identifying intracranial complications)
  - Clouding/opacification of air cells (also in AOM)
  - Mastoid air cell coalescence
  - Cortical bone erosion
  - Rim-enhancing fluid collections
  - Absence of mastoid opacification excludes the diagnosis.
- Use CT with contrast if complications are suspected (suppurative extension).
- Due to radiation, CT in children should be performed when clinically appropriate. Indications include the following:
  - Neurologic signs
  - Vomiting/lethargy
  - Suspected cholesteatoma
  - Fever after 48 to 72 hours of therapy
- Technetium-99m bone scan is more sensitive to osteolytic changes than CT.
- MRI: partial-to-complete opacification of the mastoid air cells ± middle ear cleft
  - Needed to evaluate for intracranial complications if clinical or radiographic suspicion
- Consider MRA if venous sinus thrombosis is suspected.

Follow-Up Tests & Special Considerations
- Send all cultures for aerobic and anaerobic growth.
- Interpret normal WBC with caution in symptomatic, immunocompromised patients.
- Lumbar puncture if meningitis suspected
- Consider immunologic evaluations in children with recurrent episodes of OM leading to mastoiditis.

Diagnostic Procedures/Other
- Tympanocentesis to obtain middle ear fluid for culture and sensitivity
- Myringotomy with culture (also therapeutic)
- Audiography if hearing loss suspected
- Obtain CSF if intracranial extension is suspected.
- Biopsy tissue protruding through TM or tympanostomy tube

TREATMENT

- IV antibiotics and myringotomy (± tympanostomy tubes) are the preferred treatments for uncomplicated acute mastoiditis (reflecting a shift away from more invasive surgical treatment).
- To avoid intracranial complications, simple mastoidectomy is recommended if patients do not respond to treatment after 3 to 5 days.
- Myringotomy or incision and drainage may be necessary if an abscess is present in mastoid air cells.

GENERAL MEASURES
Inpatient care during acute phase for IV antibiotics

MEDICATION
First Line
- Empiric antibiotics against most common organisms: *S. pneumoniae* (including multiple resistant strains), *S. pyogenes*, *S. aureus* (including MRSA), *P. aeruginosa*
- Use combination therapy with 3rd-generation cephalosporin (ceftriaxone or cefotaxime) plus clindamycin with coverage for resistant strains.
- Ceftriaxone 2 g IV q24h
  – Pediatric dosing: 50 to 75 mg/kg/day IV divided q12–24h
  – Precaution: Adjust dose with renal impairment.
  – Consider levofloxacin 750 mg IV q24h if severe β-lactam allergy.
- Clindamycin for coverage of ceftriaxone-resistant *S. pneumoniae* in pediatric patients:
  – Clindamycin pediatric dosing: 20 to 40 mg/kg/day IV divided q6–8h
- Cefotaxime 1 to 2 g IV q4–8h, depending on severity
  – Pediatric dosing: 100 to 200 mg/kg/day q6–8h
- Add vancomycin 30 to 60 mg/kg/day divided q8–12h if concerned for MRSA or acute on chronic exacerbation:
  – Pediatric dosing: 15 mg/kg/dose q6–8h
  – Precaution: Adjust dose with renal impairment.
- For patients with a history of recurrent AOM or recent antibiotic administration, treat with piperacillin and tazobactam 3.375 g IV q6h:
  – Pediatric dosing: 300 mg/kg/day based on piperacillin component divided q6–8h
- Once culture results are available, target treatment based on antibiotic sensitivities.

Second Line
- Oral antibiotics after 7 to 10 days of IV antibiotics and once myringotomy/blood cultures identify pathogen and sensitivities. Common oral antibiotics:
  – Amoxicillin-clavulanate (Augmentin) or clindamycin + 3rd-generation cephalosporin for 3 weeks or total treatment duration of ≥4 weeks for intracranial complications (4)
- For chronic mastoiditis: Use topical drops, ofloxacin otic solution (0.3%) or neomycin, polymyxin B, hydrocortisone 3 drops, 3 to 4 times per day.

ISSUES FOR REFERRAL
- Consult ENT for mastoiditis in adults and children.
- Consult neurosurgery for intracranial complications.
- Consider infectious disease consult for assistance with antibiotic management.

SURGERY/OTHER PROCEDURES
- Perform tympanocentesis to obtain cultures and guide antibiotic choice.
- Myringotomy and tympanostomy tubes allow for middle ear drainage.
- Clean ear canal under microscopic guidance to ensure pressure-equalization tube patency and adequate drainage of middle ear.
- Simple mastoidectomy is most effective for management of subperiosteal abscesses if trial of conservative therapy (drainage, myringotomy, and IV antibiotics) fails.

COMPLEMENTARY & ALTERNATIVE MEDICINE
No known home remedies

ADMISSION, INPATIENT, AND NURSING CONSIDERATIONS
- Admission criteria/initial stabilization
  – Clinical or imaging evidence of acute mastoiditis
  – Hospitalize patients with acute mastoiditis and start IV antibiotics immediately.
- Avoid getting the affected ear wet.
- Discharge criteria
  – Afebrile for 48 hours before IV antibiotics are discontinued
  – Clinical improvement
  – Able to tolerate oral antibiotics

ONGOING CARE

FOLLOW-UP RECOMMENDATIONS
- Oral antibiotics for 3 weeks following course of IV antibiotics (The total duration of antibiotics is 4 weeks or longer for intracranial complications.)
- For chronic mastoiditis, consider several months of antimicrobial prophylaxis with amoxicillin.

Patient Monitoring
- Assess for hearing loss postoperatively (audiogram) after acute condition has subsided.
- Follow-up with ENT and/or neurosurgery, particularly patients with hearing loss and/or intracranial complications

DIET
No recommended diet modifications necessary for treatment

PATIENT EDUCATION
- Avoid getting the affected ear wet.
- Complete full course of antibiotics.

PROGNOSIS
- Depends on severity and stage of disease
- Most cases of mastoiditis recover fully if diagnosis is made early and treated appropriately.
- Conductive hearing loss may require reconstructive surgery; hearing loss may be permanent.

COMPLICATIONS
Complication rate 5–29% (4)
- Extracranial
  – Subperiosteal abscess (most common); Bezold abscess (abscess of sternocleidomastoid muscle, insidious, risk of mediastinitis); Citelli abscess (osteomyelitis of the calvaria)
  – Osteomyelitis of the temporal bone; suppurative labyrinthitis
  – Permanent hearing loss
  – Facial nerve paralysis
- Intracranial
  – Intracranial abscess: epidural/subdural/cerebral
  – Meningitis/cerebritis/periosteitis
  – Hearing loss
  – Otitis hydrocephalus: decreased venous drainage causes benign intracranial hypertension, manifesting as increased intracranial pressure, headache, papilledema, and sixth nerve palsy
  – Encephalitis; brain abscess
  – Gradenigo syndrome (sixth nerve palsy, severe pain in distribution of fifth nerve, and suppurative OM)
  – Sigmoid sinus thrombophlebitis or thrombosis
  – Lateral sinus thrombosis; central venous sinus thrombosis (3)

REFERENCES
1. Favre N, Patel VA, Carr MM. Complications in pediatric acute mastoiditis: HCUP KID analysis. *Otolaryngol Head Neck Surg*. 2021;165(5): 722–730.
2. Kaufmann MR, Shetty K, Camilon PR, et al. Management of acute complicated mastoiditis: a systematic review and meta-analysis. *Pediatr Infect Dis J*. 2022;41(4):297–301.
3. Loh R, Phua M, Shaw CL. Management of paediatric acute mastoiditis: systematic review. *J Laryngol Otol*. 2018;132(2):96–104.
4. Mansour T, Yehudai N, Tobia A, et al. Acute mastoiditis: 20 years of experience with a uniform management protocol. *Int J Pediatr Otorhinolaryngol*. 2019;125:187–191.

CODES

ICD10
- H70.90 Unspecified mastoiditis, unspecified ear
- H70.009 Acute mastoiditis without complications, unspecified ear
- H70.099 Acute mastoiditis with other complications, unspecified ear

CLINICAL PEARLS
- Suspect mastoiditis if symptoms of AOM persist >2 weeks despite a normal-appearing TM.
- Temporal bone CT is the best diagnostic tool; use only when mastoiditis is suspected to limit radiation exposure in children.
- Hospitalize patients with acute mastoiditis for IV antibiotics. Consult ENT for drainage procedure.
- Treat with broad-spectrum IV antibiotics; collect middle ear fluid cultures to guide-specific therapy. The total duration of antibiotics is ≥4 weeks for intracranial complications.
- If conservative treatment fails after 3 to 5 days, perform mastoidectomy to avoid intracranial complications.

M

MEDIAL TIBIAL STRESS SYNDROME (MTSS)/SHIN SPLINTS

Shane L. Larson, MD • Briana Lindberg, MD, CAQSM

 BASICS

DESCRIPTION
The term medial tibial stress syndrome (MTSS) is pre-ferred to "shin splints." MTSS is an aching pain along the inner edge of the tibial shaft that develops when the musculature and/or periosteum in the (lower) leg become irritated by repetitive activity. The condition is part of a continuum of stress-related injuries to the lower leg and is not related to pain from ischemia (compartment syndrome) or stress fractures.
- Related pathology: tendonitis/periostitis of the medial soleus muscles, anterior tibialis, and posterior tibialis muscles
- Synonyms: tibial stress reaction, anterior muscle syndrome, tibial periostitis, perimyositis, soleus syndrome, shin splints

EPIDEMIOLOGY
Incidence
Common, can account for 4–35% of reported running injuries; frequently occurs bilaterally (1)

Pediatric Considerations
MTSS may account for up to 31% of all overuse injuries in high school athletes.

ETIOLOGY AND PATHOPHYSIOLOGY
- Multifactorial anatomic and biomechanical factors
  - Overuse injuries caused or limited by
    ○ Microtrauma from repetitive motion leading to periosteal inflammation
    ○ Overpronation of the subtalar joint and tight gastrocnemius/soleus complex with increased eccentric loading of musculature inserting along the medial shin
    ○ Interosseous membrane pain
    ○ Periostitis
    ○ Tears of collagen fibers
    ○ Enthesopathy
  - Anatomic structures affected include the following:
    ○ Flexor hallucis longus
    ○ Tibialis anterior
    ○ Tibialis posterior
    ○ Soleus
    ○ Crural fascia
- Pathogenesis is theorized to be due to the following:
  - Calf muscle traction on periosteum
  - Persistent repetitive loading on tibia, which leads to inadequate bone remodeling with subsequent tibial cortex changes
  - Possible microfissures causing pain without evidence of fracture or ischemia

RISK FACTORS
- Intrinsic (personal) risk factors (1):
  - Greater ranges of internal and external (>65 degrees) hip rotation
  - Significant overpronation at the ankle
  - Imbalance of musculature of the ankle and foot (inversion/eversion misbalance)
  - Female gender
  - Lean calf girth
  - Femoral neck anteversion
  - Navicular drop
  - Genu varum
  - History of previous MTSS
- External (environmental) risk factors (1):
  - Lack of physical fitness
  - Inexperienced runners—particularly those with rapid increases in mileage and inadequate prior conditioning
  - Excessive overuse or distance running, particularly on hard or inclined (crowned) surfaces
  - Prior injury
  - Equipment (shoe) failure
- Other risk factors:
  - Elevated BMI
  - Lower bone mineral density
  - Tobacco use
- Those typically affected by MTSS include the following:
  - Runners
  - Military personnel—common in recruit/boot camp
  - Gymnasts, soccer, and basketball players
  - Ballet dancers

GENERAL PREVENTION
- Proper technique for guided calf stretching and lower extremity strength training, although supple-mentary gastrocnemius and soleus stretching has no statistical significance in reducing risk of shin splints
- Rehabilitate prior injuries adequately.
- Other recommendations
  - Gait analysis and retraining, particularly for overpronation
  - Orthotic footwear inserts were found to be preventative in naval recruits.

COMMONLY ASSOCIATED CONDITIONS
Pes planus (flat feet)

> **ALERT**
> Rule out stress fracture and compartment syndrome where pain often persists at rest.

℞ DIAGNOSIS

HISTORY
- Patients typically describe dull, sharp, or deep pain along the lower leg that is resolved with rest.
- Patients are often able to run through the pain in early stages.
- Pain is commonly associated with exercise (also true with compartment syndrome), but in severe cases, pain may persist with rest.

PHYSICAL EXAM
- Tenderness to palpation is typically elicited along the posteromedial border of the middle-to-distal 3rd of the tibia.
- Pain with plantar flexion
- Preservation of neurovascular integrity via palpable distal pulses, intact sensation, reflexes, and muscular strength

DIFFERENTIAL DIAGNOSIS
- Bone
  - Tibial stress fractures
    ○ Typically, pain persists at rest or with weight-bearing activities.
    ○ Focal tenderness over the anterior tibia
    ○ Hopping on involved leg will reproduce pain (less likely with MTSS).
- Muscle/soft tissue injury
  - Strain, tear, tendinopathy
  - Muscle hernia
- Fascial
  - Chronic exertional compartment syndrome (1)
    ○ Pain without direct tenderness on exam
    ○ Pain increases with exertion and resolves at rest.
    ○ Pain is described as cramping or squeezing.
    ○ Pain with possible weakness or paresthesias on exam
  - Interosseous membrane tear
- Nerve
  - Spinal stenosis
  - Lumbar radiculopathy
  - Common peroneal nerve entrapment
- Vascular
  - DVT
  - Popliteal arterial entrapment
    ○ Rare but limb-threatening disease
    ○ History of intermittent unilateral claudication
    ○ MRI reveals compression of the artery by the medial head of the gastrocnemius muscle.
- Infection
  - Osteomyelitis
- Malignancy
  - Bone tumors

DIAGNOSTIC TESTS & INTERPRETATION
Clinical history and exam are considered gold stan-dard in diagnosing MTSS (1).

Initial Tests (lab, imaging)
- Plain radiographs help rule out stress fractures if >2 weeks of symptoms.
- Bone scintigraphy
  - Diffuse linear vertical uptake in the posterior tibial cortex on the lateral view
  - Stress fractures demonstrate a focal ovoid uptake.
- High-resolution MRI reveals abnormal periosteal and bone marrow signals, which are useful for early discrimination of tibial stress fractures.

Follow-Up Tests & Special Considerations

Increased pain and localized tenderness warrant further imaging with MRI due to concern for tibial stress fracture (1).

Diagnostic Procedures/Other

Exclude compartment syndrome using intracompartmental pressure testing.

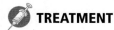 **TREATMENT**

GENERAL MEASURES

- Activity modification with a gradual return to training based on improvement of symptoms
- Running on flat and firm surfaces can help minimize pain.
- Patients should maintain fitness with low-impact activities such as swimming and cycling.
- Continue activity modification until pain free on ambulation.

MEDICATION

- Analgesia with acetaminophen or oral nonsteroidal anti-inflammatory agent
- Cryotherapy (ice massage) is also advised to relieve acute-phase symptoms (1)[C].

ADDITIONAL THERAPIES

- Orthotics may be beneficial.
- Calf stretch, peroneal stretch, TheraBand exercises, and eccentric calf raises may improve endurance and strength (2)[A].
- Compression stockings have been used to treat MTSS with mixed results.
- Structured running programs with warm-up exercises have not been demonstrated to reduce pain in young athletes (3)[B].
- CAM boot for people with significant pain with weight-bearing

SURGERY/OTHER PROCEDURES

- Surgical intervention includes a posterior medial fascial release in individuals with both
  - Severe limitation of physical activity and
  - Failure of 6 months of conservative treatment
    - Counsel patients that complete return of activity to sport may not be always achieved postoperatively. Surgical risks include infection and hematoma formation.
- Extracorporeal shock wave therapy (ESWT) may decrease recovery time when added to a running program (2)[A].

COMPLEMENTARY & ALTERNATIVE MEDICINE

- Individualized polyurethane orthoses may help chronic running injuries.
- Special insoles, low-energy laser treatment, pulsed electromagnetic field, and knee braces have not been shown to improve outcomes (2)[A].
- Ultrasound, acupuncture, aquatic therapy, electrical stimulation, whirlpool baths, cast immobilization, taping, and steroid injection may help improve pain.
- Physical therapy approaches including Kinesio tape and fascial distortion massage may yield quicker return to activity.
- Osteopathic manipulative treatment may yield quicker return to athletic/activity as well.

 ONGOING CARE

FOLLOW-UP RECOMMENDATIONS
Patient Monitoring

- Once well, recommend gradual return to preinjury running pace.
- Maintain stretching and strengthening exercises.
- Identify and correct preinjury training errors.
- Good supportive footwear is recommended as is replacing running shoes every 350 to 450 miles.
- Allow a gradual return to activity dictated by symptoms (pain).

PROGNOSIS

The condition is usually self-limiting, and most patients respond well with rest and nonsurgical intervention.

COMPLICATIONS

- Stress fractures and compartment syndrome
- Undiagnosed MTSS or chronic exertional compartment syndrome can lead to a complete fracture or tissue necrosis, respectively.

REFERENCES

1. Moen MH, Tol JL, Weir A, et al. Medial tibial stress syndrome: a critical review. *Sports Med.* 2009;39(7):523–546.
2. Winters M, Eskes M, Weir A, et al. Treatment of medial tibial stress syndrome: a systematic review. *Sports Med.* 2013;43(12):1315–1333.
3. Moen MH, Holtslag L, Bakker E, et al. The treatment of medial tibial stress syndrome in athletes; a randomized clinical trial. *Sports Med Arthrosc Rehabil Ther Technol.* 2012;4:12.

ADDITIONAL READING

- Abelson B. Tibialis anterior–effective stretching technique. https://www.youtube.com/watch?v=6Z6XM63x2TM. Accessed August 23, 2023.
- Fields KB, Sykes JC, Walker KM, et al. Prevention of running injuries. *Curr Sports Med Rep.* 2010;9(3):176–182.
- Hamstra-Wright KL, Bliven KCH, Bay C. Risk factors for medial tibial stress syndrome in physically active individuals such as runners and military personnel: a systematic review and meta-analysis. *Br J Sports Med.* 2015;49(6):362–369.
- Reinking MF, Austin TM, Richter RR, et al. Medial tibial stress syndrome in active individuals: a systematic review and meta-analysis of risk factors. *Sports Health.* 2017;9(3):252–261.
- Reshef N, Guelich DR. Medial tibial stress syndrome. *Clin Sports Med.* 2012;31(2):273–290.
- Yeung SS, Yeung EW, Gillespie LD. Interventions for preventing lower limb soft-tissue running injuries. *Cochrane Database Syst Rev.* 2011;(7):CD001256.

CODES

ICD10

- S86.899A Other injury of other muscle(s) and tendon(s) at lower leg level, unspecified leg, initial encounter
- S86.891A Other injury of other muscle(s) and tendon(s) at lower leg level, right leg, initial encounter
- S86.892A Other injury of other muscle(s) and tendon(s) at lower leg level, left leg, initial encounter

CLINICAL PEARLS

- MTSS is the preferred term for "shin splints."
- Diagnosis is based on a reliable history of repetitive overuse accompanied by characteristic shin pain; imaging only if strong suspicion for stress fracture
- MTSS pain is typically along the middle and distal 3rd of the posteromedial tibial surface, worsened with activity, and relieved with rest (vs. compartment syndrome or stress fracture, where pain persists with rest).
- Treatment includes ice, activity modification, analgesics, eccentric stretching, gait retraining, and a gradual return to activity.
- Symptoms recur if return to activity is "too much too fast."

M

MEDICAL MARIJUANA
Robert A. Baldor, MD, FAAFP

 BASICS

Medical marijuana or medical cannabis refers to the use of pharmacologic agents derived from the flowering plant genus *Cannabis* to treat disease or alleviate symptoms.

DESCRIPTION
- Marijuana plants contain >100 phytocannabinoids.
- Phytocannabinoids are naturally occurring molecules with an affinity for the mammalian cannabinoid receptors.
- The main cannabinoids that are used for medical marijuana are delta-9-tetrahydrocannabinol (THC) and cannabidiol (CBD). Most of the psychoactive properties come from THC.
- Cannabis interacts with the endocannabinoid system (ECS) in our bodies. The ECS plays critical roles in body homeostasis.
- The ECS has two main receptors:
  - CB1—highly expressed in the central nervous system
  - CB 2—expressed in the periphery including the immune system
- Routes of external cannabinoid administration include inhalation (smoking and vaporized), oral ingestion of edible products, and topical (oral mucosa or skin).

EPIDEMIOLOGY
- In the United States, 36 states and 4 territories allow for the medical use of cannabis products, although it remains illegal under federal law.
- 49 countries worldwide have legalized the medical use of cannabis.

Prevalence
Prevalence of medical cannabis in the U.S. primary care population is estimated at 2% and growing, with 15% of the U.S. population reporting regular use of recreational marijuana.

 TREATMENT

- Conditions that are qualified for medical cannabis vary by state, but most common conditions approved by states include chronic pain, cancer-related weight loss, cancer related nausea and vomiting, and epilepsy.
- Recent reviews of the literature reveal conclusive or substantial evidence that cannabis or cannabinoids are effective for symptom control in (1)[A]:
  - Chronic pain in adults
  - As antiemetics in chemotherapy-induced nausea and vomiting
  - Improving muscle spasticity syndromes in multiple sclerosis (MS)

- Chronic pain (1)[A]
  - Most common condition cited by patients for medical use of cannabis
  - May benefit in refractory pain, neuropathic pain, and pain associated with cancer; in a recent meta-analysis of 27 randomized trials, there is a low-strength evidence that cannabis alleviates neuropathic pain but insufficient evidence in treating other types of pain.
  - Meta-analysis suggests 40% greater improvement in pain with plant derived cannabinoids compared to placebo.
- Chemotherapy-induced nausea and vomiting
  - Conclusive evidence suggests that oral THC preparations are associated with improvements in nausea and vomiting due to chemotherapy (dronabinol and nabiximols) (2)[A].
  - Despite abundant anecdotal evidence of the benefits of plant-based and inhaled preparations for nausea and vomiting, there are no high-quality randomized trials examining this option.
- MS muscle spasticity
  - Substantial evidence that oral cannabinoids are an effective treatment of patient-reported spasticity symptoms but not clinician-measured spasticity (1)[A].
- Anorexia or cachexia due to HIV/AIDS or cancer
  - Low-quality evidence showed some weight gain on dronabinol, although the effect was similar to megestrol (2)[A].
  - Studies done in the 1980s that showed that inhaled cannabis increased caloric intake by 40% have not been replicated due to the difficulties in investigating the cannabis plant (3)[A].
- Posttraumatic stress disorder (PTSD)
  - Single small crossover trial suggests potential benefit from oral cannabinoid, nabilone. This contrasts with nonrandomized trials that showed worsened symptoms of PTSD on plant-based medical cannabis (3)[A].
- Seizures (3)[B]
  - Insufficient evidence to support or refute cannabis as an effective treatment of epilepsy
  - In 2018, FDA-approved cannabidiol oral solution (Epidiolex) for treatment of seizures related to two rare conditions: Lennox-Gastaut syndrome and Dravet syndrome
- Others
  - Limited evidence for cannabis use in acute pain, glaucoma, other neurologic conditions: tremor, Tourette syndrome, Huntington disease, and inflammation

GENERAL MEASURES
- States with medical cannabis laws (4):
  - May require a registry of patients
  - May require patients to carry an ID card
  - May require provider education on the risks and benefits of medical cannabis
- For non–FDA-approved medical cannabis: Certifying providers do not prescribe medical cannabis but only certify the qualifying condition according to state laws.

MEDICATION
FDA-approved medical cannabis products (5):
- THC: dronabinol (Marinol): 2.5 mg BID, max of 20 mg/day
- THC: analog—nabilone (Cesamet): 1 mg BID, max of 6 mg/day
- FDA indications include the following:
  - Refractory chemotherapy-induced nausea and vomiting
  - Anorexia in patients with AIDS
- CBD: cannabidiol (Epidiolex): 2.5 mg/kg BID, max of 20 mg/kg daily
  - FDA indication for Lennox-Gastaut syndrome and Dravet syndrome–associated seizures
- THC/CBD (1:1 ratio): nabiximols (Sativex)—buccal spray: 1 to 14 sprays/day for treating spasticity in MS, cancer-related pain, and neuropathic pain

 ONGOING CARE

FOLLOW-UP RECOMMENDATIONS
Pediatric Considerations
- Between 2000 and 2013, annual rate of poison center calls related to cannabis exposures among children <6 years was 2.82 times higher in states that had legalized medical cannabis compared to those that had not legalized medical cannabis.
- Pediatric cannabis exposure is associated with potentially serious symptoms:
  - Respiratory depression or failure
  - Tachycardia
  - Temporary coma
- Adolescents have increased vulnerability to adverse long-term outcomes (6)[C].
- Brain ECS actively develops during adolescence.
- Initial use during adolescence is associated with long-term brain changes:
  - Increased school dropout
  - Lower IQ
  - Diminished life satisfaction

Pregnancy and Lactation Considerations

- The data on marijuana use during pregnancy is heavily confounded by tobacco use and socio-economic factors but concern for impaired fetal neurodevelopment should be as high as for tobacco use or alcohol use during pregnancy.
- There are no pregnancy indications for medical cannabis.
- Pregnant women should be discouraged from using medical cannabis in any form, around conception, during pregnancy, and throughout breastfeeding.
- There are insufficient data to evaluate the effects of marijuana use (nonmedical or medical) on infants during lactation and breastfeeding. American College of Obstetrics and Gynecology (ACOG) has recommended that marijuana use should be discouraged for breastfeeding mothers (7).

COMPLICATIONS

- Any data on complications of marijuana use is in reference to nonmedical use. There is no data on complications of medical cannabis use. If the route of medical cannabis dosing is inhalation, some inferences could be made because most studies are done in populations of nonmedical cannabis smokers.
- Short-term complications
  - Intoxication and withdrawal
    - Intoxication may cause:
      - Acute physiologic effects including conjunctival injection, orthostatic hypotension, tachycardia, dry mouth, and poor motor coordination
      - Acute psychologic effects relaxation, euphoria, altered sensory perception
    - Withdrawal may cause (mainly psychological symptoms) irritability, depression, restlessness, insomnia, and less likely physiologic symptoms of GI distress, hypertension, chills, and diaphoresis.
  - Increased motor vehicle accidents, relative risk (RR) = 2, compared to RR = 5 for blood alcohol level >0.08
  - Driving under the influence of cannabis as confirmed by presence of THC metabolite was associated with a 20–30% higher odds of having a motor vehicle accident.
- Long-term complications
  - Respiratory (6)[C]:
    - Substantial evidence of worsened respiratory symptoms and more frequent bronchitis in regular cannabis smokers
    - Overall acute cannabis smoking is associated with bronchodilation but any benefit is offset by chronic use.
    - Several studies noted increased FVC in regular cannabis smokers, which is of unclear significance.

- With limited data, it is unclear if there is an association between regular cannabis use and increased risk of developing COPD. Certainly regular cannabis smoking is less significant than regular tobacco smoking in development of COPD.
  - Cardiovascular risk:
    - Limited data to support increased risk of cannabis triggering an acute MI with case study of 9 patients with RR of 3.2
    - A retrospective cohort study showed an RR of acute MI in current users of marijuana was 1.1.
    - Limited quality data that shows small insignificant increase risk of stroke with current use of cannabis
  - Cancer risk
    - Limited quality evidence that shows no statistical evidence of association between cannabis smoking and incidence of lung cancer
    - Recent cohort studies did not find any association between cannabis use and head and neck cancers.
    - Limited quality evidence that shows possible association between chronic cannabis smoking and nonseminoma-type testicular germ cell tumors
    - Insufficient evidence to support or refute an association between cannabis smoking and esophageal cancer
    - Insufficient evidence to support or refute association between cannabis smoking and prostate cancer, cervical cancer, malignant gliomas, non-Hodgkin lymphoma, penile cancer, anal cancer, Kaposi sarcoma, or bladder cancer
  - Psychological (6)[C]:
    - Increased anxiety, psychosis, and depression (noncausal association)
    - Increased risk of schizophrenia in early chronic users
    - Based on data for nonmedical users of cannabis, addiction occurs in 9% of all users, with higher rates among adolescents (17%) and daily users (20–25%). There are no studies that examine the risk of addiction with medical cannabis.
    - Interference with cognitive function and short-term memory results in difficulty learning.
    - "Gateway drug" phenomenon persists even in states where marijuana use is legal.
      - Concurrent use primes brain for enhanced response to other drug
    - Marijuana reduces dopamine activity in reward centers, increasing susceptibility to drug abuse.
  - Gastrointestinal
    - Cannabis-induced hyperemesis syndrome
    - Cannabis use has been associated with hepatotoxicity.

REFERENCES

1. Ebbert JO, Scharf EL, Hurt RT. Medical cannabis. *Mayo Clin Proc*. 2018;93(12):1842–1847.
2. Whiting PF, Wolff RF, Deshpande S, et al. Cannabinoids for medical use: a systematic review and meta-analysis. *JAMA*. 2015;313(24):2456–2473.
3. National Academies of Sciences, Engineering, and Medicine. *The Health Effects of Cannabis and Cannabinoids: The Current State of Evidence and Recommendations for Research*. Washington, DC: The National Academies Press; 2017.
4. National Conference of State Legislatures. State medical marijuana laws. https://www.ncsl.org/health/state-medical-cannabis-laws. Accessed December 2, 2023.
5. Sazeger P. Cannabis essentials: tools for clinical practice. *Am Fam Physician*. 2021;104(6):598–608.
6. Gloss D, Vickrey B. Cannabinoids for epilepsy. *Cochrane Database Syst Rev*. 2014;2014(3):CD009270.
7. American College of Obstetricians and Gynecologists Committee on Obstetric Practice. Committee Opinion No. 637: marijuana use during pregnancy and lactation. *Obstet Gynecol*. 2015;126(1):234–238.

ADDITIONAL READING

- Khalsa JH, Bunt GC, Galanter M, et al. Medicinal uses of cannabis and cannabinoids. In: Miller SC, ed. *The ASAM Principles of Addiction Medicine*. 6th ed. Philadelphia, PA: Wolters Kluwer; 2019:1742–1750.
- Matson TE, Carrell DS, Bobb JF, et al. Prevalence of medical cannabis use and associated health conditions documented in electronic health records among primary care patients in Washington State. *JAMA Netw Open*. 2021;4(5):e219375.

 ## CODES

ICD10

F12.90 Cannabis use, unspecified, uncomplicated

CLINICAL PEARLS

- The clinical evidence supporting benefits of medical cannabis are lacking. Current evidence shows modest benefit in a limited number of conditions.
- In adults with chemotherapy-induced nausea and vomiting, oral cannabinoids are effective antiemetics.
- Medical cannabis may be a useful adjunctive chronic pain medication in selected patients.
- Counseling of medical cannabis users will need to include advice to safeguard against accidental pediatric ingestion.

M

MELANOMA
Anila Khaliq, MD • Nelly Singh, DO

BASICS

DESCRIPTION
- Melanoma is a tumor arising from malignant transformation of pigment-containing cells called melanocytes, which are found in the stratum basale of the epidermis.
  - Most arise in the skin but may also present as a primary lesion in any tissue: ocular (uvea), GI, GU, lymph node, paranasal sinuses, nasal cavity, anorectal mucosa, and leptomeninges.
  - Extracutaneous sites have an adverse prognosis.
  - Metastatic spread to any site in the body
- Types of invasive cutaneous melanomas include the following:
  - Superficial-spreading melanoma: approximately 70% of cases; occurs in sun-exposed areas (trunk, back, and extremities); most <1 mm thick at diagnosis; when seen in younger patients, presents as a flat, slow growing, irregularly bordered lesion
  - Nodular: 15–30% of cases; present in older patients; tendency to ulcerate and hemorrhage; most commonly thick and pigmented; most common melanoma >2 mm
  - Lentigo maligna (subtype of melanoma in situ): slowest growing; older population; occurs in sun-exposed areas (head, neck, forearms); lentigo maligna melanoma (LMM) is its invasive counterpart seen in 10–15% of cases; it is most commonly seen in elderly patients most often in the head and neck regions.
  - Acral lentiginous: <5% of all melanomas; however, most common melanoma in black or Asian patients; found in palmar, plantar, and subungual areas; can mimic other skin abnormalities, including warts, calluses, tinea pedis, or ingrown toenails
    - An important subtype of acral lentiginous melanoma is subungual melanoma. From the nail matrix, presents as dark stripe under the nail plate; Hutchinson nail sign when brown or black pigment extends from the nail to the cuticle and proximal or lateral nail folds
  - Amelanotic melanoma: <5% of cases; can be missed and diagnosed at a later stage because it can mimic benign skin conditions and thus is referred to as a "great pretender"
  - Desmoplastic melanoma: ~1% of cases; "neurotropic melanoma" or "spindled melanoma" with an abundance of fibrous tissue; demonstrates sarcoma-like tendencies with increased hematogenous spread; presents as a slow-growing lesion that is scar-like (no history of injury at the site is noted); often seen in the head and neck
- System(s) affected: skin/exocrine

Geriatric Considerations
Lentigo maligna is most common in elderly patients. This type is usually found on the face, beginning as a circumscribed macular patch of mottled pigmentation showing shades of dark brown, tan, or black.

Pediatric Considerations
Large congenital nevi (>5 cm) are risk factors and have a >2% lifetime risk of malignant conversion. Blistering sunburns in childhood significantly increase risk.

Pregnancy Considerations
No increased risk of melanoma in pregnancy; wait 1 to 2 years after treatment for pregnancy as melanoma can spread to the placenta.

EPIDEMIOLOGY
Incidence
- In 2023, the estimated number of newly diagnosed melanoma cases in Americans are 97,610, with an estimate of 7,990 deaths.
- Predominant age: Median age at diagnosis is 66 years.
- Predominant sex: male > female (1.5 times)
- Melanoma is >20 times more common in whites than in African Americans.
- Minority groups demonstrate increased rates of metastasis, advanced stages at diagnosis, thicker initial lesions, earlier age at diagnosis, and overall poorer outcomes.

Prevalence
- Melanoma is the fifth most common type of cancer in the United States.
- Lifetime risk: men: 1/28; female: 1/4
- 1.2% of all cancer deaths

ETIOLOGY AND PATHOPHYSIOLOGY
- DNA damage by UVA/UVB exposure
- Tumor progression: initially confined to epidermis with lateral growth, vertical growth

Genetics
- Dysplastic nevus syndrome is a risk factor for development of melanoma. Close surveillance is warranted.
- 8–12% of patients with melanoma have a family history of disease.
- Mutations in *BRAF (V600E)* implicated in 50–60% of cutaneous melanomas
- Familial atypical mole malignant melanoma (FAMMM) syndrome characterized by >50 atypical moles, +FH of melanoma (1)

RISK FACTORS
- Genetic predisposition, personal/family history of melanoma
- UVA and UVB exposure
- History of >5 sunburns during lifetime, blistering sunburns in childhood
- Previous pigmented lesions (especially dysplastic melanocytic nevi)
- Fair complexion, freckling, blue eyes, blond/red hair
- Highest predictor of risk is increased number of nevi (>50).
- Tanning bed use: 75% increased risk if first exposure before age 35 years
- Changing nevus (see "ABCDE" criteria)
- Large (>5 cm) congenital nevi
- Chronic immunosuppression (chronic lymphocytic leukemia, non-Hodgkin lymphoma, AIDS, or posttransplant)
- Living at high altitude (>700 meters or 2,300 feet above sea level)
- Occupational exposure to ionizing radiation

GENERAL PREVENTION
- Avoidance of sunburns, especially in childhood
- Use of sunscreen with at least SPF 30 to all exposed skin; reapply regularly and after swimming.
- Avoid tanning beds; class 1 carcinogen by World Health Organization (WHO)
- Any suspicious lesions should be biopsied with a narrow excision with 1- to 3-mm margins that encompass the entire breadth plus sufficient depth of the lesion. Options include elliptical excisions, punch, or deep shave biopsies.

COMMONLY ASSOCIATED CONDITIONS
- Dysplastic nevus syndrome
- >50 nevi; these individuals have higher lifetime risk of melanoma than the general population because 30% of all melanoma arise in preexisting nevi.
- Giant congenital nevus: 6% lifetime incidence of melanoma
- Psoriasis after psoralen-UV-A (PUVA) therapy

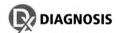DIAGNOSIS

HISTORY
- Change in a pigmented lesion: either hypo- or hyperpigmentation, bleeding, scaling, ulceration, or changes in size or texture
- Family history of skin cancer, occupation, sunbathing, tanning, and other sun exposure

PHYSICAL EXAM
- ABCDE: Asymmetry, Border irregularity, Color variegation (especially red, white, black, blue), Diameter >6 mm, Evolution over time
- Any new and/or changing nevus, bleeding/ulcerated
- Location on Caucasians is primarily back and lower leg; on African Americans, it is the hands, feet, and nails.
- May include mucosal surfaces (nasopharynx, conjunctiva)
- Individuals at high risk for melanoma should have careful ocular exam to assess for presence of melanoma in the iris and retina.

DIFFERENTIAL DIAGNOSIS
- Cutaneous squamous cell carcinoma
- Basal cell carcinoma
- Dysplastic and blue nevi
- Vascular skin tumor
- Pigmented actinic keratosis
- Traumatic hematoma
- Pigmented basal cell carcinomas, seborrheic keratoses, other changing nevi
- Common or atypical melanocytic nevi
- Lentigo
- Pyogenic granuloma

DIAGNOSTIC TESTS & INTERPRETATION
Lactate dehydrogenase (LDH), chest/abdomen/pelvic CT with or without PET/CT at baseline and in monitoring progression in metastatic disease (stage IV); brain MRI if any CNS symptoms or physical findings

Diagnostic Procedures/Other

- Dermoscopy allows for magnification of lesions; evidence limited on utility (1)[C]
- Full-thickness excisional biopsy remains the gold standard for diagnosis. Any suspicious nevus should be excised, either by elliptical excision, punch biopsy, or a scoop shave (saucerization) biopsy.
- Avoid superficial shave of suspicious lesion. Goal for full-thickness excision with 1- to 3-mm margins. Orient excisional biopsy to optimize future treatment.
- Sentinel lymph node biopsy, a staging procedure, remains an important factor for prognosis.

Test Interpretation

- Nodular melanoma is primarily vertical growth, whereas the other three types are horizontal.
- Estimated that 1/10,000 dysplastic nevi become melanoma annually.
- Staging is based on the tumor-node-metastasis (TNM) criteria by current American Joint Committee on Cancer (AJCC) criteria, including:
  - Thickness (mm) and ulceration
  - Number of regional lymph nodes involved
  - Distant metastases and serum LDH

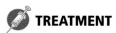

TREATMENT

GENERAL MEASURES

Full surgical excision of melanoma is the standard of care and primary treatment recommended for resectable/nonmetastatic melanomas.

- For stages I to II, surgical excision is curative in most cases.

MEDICATION

- Treatment within the context of a clinical trial always recommended
- FDA-approved first-line medication for unresectable or metastatic melanoma include the following:
  - Anti–PD-1 monotherapy
    - Pembrolizumab (Keytruda)
    - Nivolumab (Opdivo)
  - Anti–PD-1/anti–CTLA-4 therapy
    - Nivolumab with ipilimumab
      - Combo therapy demonstrated 61% response versus ipilimumab alone.
  - If BRAF V600–activating mutation is present, can opt for target therapy with BRAF/MEK inhibitors:
    - Dabrafenib/trametinib
    - Vemurafenib/cobimetinib + atezolizumab (new FDA-approved medications)
    - Encorafenib/binimetinib
- Adjuvant medical therapy for certain high-risk patients after undergoing complete surgical excision with lymph node involvement or metastasis
  - Stage IIIA with sentinel lymph node metastases
    - Pembrolizumab (Keytruda)
    - Dabrafenib/trametinib for BRAF V600–activating mutation
  - Stage IIB/C and IV with nodal recurrence
    - Pembrolizumab (Keytruda)
    - Nivolumab (Opdivo)
    - Dabrafenib/trametinib for BRAF V600–activating mutation

  - Stage IV completely resected
    - Nivolumab (Opdivo)
  - Stage IV with nodal recurrence
    - Ipilimumab recommended only if prior exposure to anti–PD-1 therapy
- Additional active regimens (e.g., dacarbazine [DTIC], temozolomide, paclitaxel, carmustine [BCNU], cisplatin, carboplatin, vinblastine) often limited to those who are not candidates to preferred regimens
- Imatinib (Gleevec) in tumors with c-KIT mutation
- Interferon-α as adjuvant therapy received FDA approval in 1995 (high dose) and 2011 (pegylated) to treat stage IIB to III melanoma; shown to improve 4-year relapse rate but no overall effect on survival; 1/3 of patients will discontinue due to toxicity (granulocytopenia, hepatotoxicity).

First Line

Anti–PD-1 monotherapy, combination anti–PD-1/anti–CTLA-4 therapy, and BRAF/MEK inhibitors

ISSUES FOR REFERRAL

Oncology and surgical specialties may be required based on the extent of nodal and/or metastatic disease, if present.

ADDITIONAL THERAPIES

Local therapy for stage III in-transit disease when resection not possible, prior resection unsuccessful, or refusal of surgery, and seek conservative management including intralesional injections, topical imiquimod, laser ablation, and radiation therapy

- Talimogene laherparepvec (T-VEC) intralesional injections is the recommended option for intralesional injection.
- Other injections include IL-2, BCG, or IFN.

SURGERY/OTHER PROCEDURES

- Standard of care for melanoma includes early surgical excision with the following recommended margins:
  - In situ tumors: 0.5- to 1.0-cm margin
  - Thickness of ≤1 mm (T1): 1-cm margin
  - Thickness of 1.01 to 2.00 mm (T2): 1- to 2-cm margins
  - Thickness of 2.01 to 4.00 mm (T3): 2-cm margins
  - Thickness of ≥4 mm (T4): 2-cm margins
- Sentinel lymph node biopsy is indicated in patients with T1b-, T2-, T3-, and T4-staged melanomas.
  - Not recommended in melanoma in situ or T1a
- Mohs micrographic surgery is being increasingly used for melanoma in situ, but in general, it is not considered a treatment modality for melanoma because it relies on frozen section technique.
- Radiotherapy can be used to treat lentigo maligna in addition to certain head and neck lesions.
- Palliative radiation therapy can be used with metastatic melanoma.
- Stage IIIB/C—intralesional injections in certain cases if limited number of in-transit metastasis or not amenable to complete surgical excision

ONGOING CARE

FOLLOW-UP RECOMMENDATIONS

Patient Monitoring

- Total body photography and dermoscopy should be used for surveillance of skin lesions, most commonly used for patients with >5 atypical nevi.
- For patients with a history of cutaneous melanoma, NCCN guidelines recommend screening every 3 to 12 months depending on recurrence risk, with annual examinations if there is no disease progression for 5 years.
- Surveillance chest x-ray, CT, brain MRI, and/or PET/CT scan every 3 to 12 months for 3 to 5 years at discretion of physician
- Lab and imaging tests after diagnosis and treatment of stages I to II melanoma are low yield, have high false-positive rates, and are not recommended.

PATIENT EDUCATION

Teach all patients to perform regular full-body skin examinations looking for ABCDE criteria, especially those who are at high risk or who have had melanoma.

PROGNOSIS

- Breslow depth (thickness) in millimeters remains among strongest predictors of prognosis.
- Median age at death is 70 years.
- Highest survival seen in women <45 years of age at diagnosis
- Metastatic melanoma has an average survival of 6 to 9 months; 15–20% 5-year survival with current treatment
- Stages I and II, appropriately treated, have 20-year survival rates of 90% and 80%, respectively.

REFERENCE

1. Swetter SM, Tsao H, Bichakjian CK, et al. Guidelines of care for the management of primary cutaneous melanoma. *J Am Acad Dermatol*. 2019;80(1):208–250.

CODES

ICD10

- C43.9 Malignant melanoma of skin, unspecified
- C43.30 Malignant melanoma of unspecified part of face
- C43.4 Malignant melanoma of scalp and neck

CLINICAL PEARLS

- Teach all patients to perform regular full-body skin examinations looking for ABCDE criteria.
- Location on white people is primarily back and lower leg; on black people, it is the hands, feet, and nails.

M

MÉNIÈRE DISEASE

Sangili Chandran, MD • Damini Patel, DO • Shalini Kumar, MD

 BASICS

- An inner ear (labyrinthine) disorder characterized by recurrent attacks of hearing loss, tinnitus, vertigo, and sensations of aural fullness
- Ménière disease is a condition with at least two spontaneous episodes of vertigo lasting >20 minutes but less than 12 hours, an audiogram showing evidence of low to medium frequency sensorineural hearing loss in one ear at any point in time, and fluctuating aural symptoms such as hearing loss, tinnitus, or aural fullness (1).
- Clinically, it involves the triad of:
  – Vertigo lasting 20 minutes to 12 hours
  – Audiometrically documented sensorineural hearing loss (predominantly low frequency)
  – Fluctuating aural symptoms (tinnitus or aural fullness)

DESCRIPTION
- Often unilateral initially; nearly half become bilateral over time.
- Severity and frequency of vertigo may diminish with time, but hearing loss is often progressive and/or fluctuating.
- Usually idiopathic (Ménière disease) but may be secondary to another condition causing endolymphatic hydrops (Ménière syndrome)
- There are five clinical subtypes of both unilateral and bilateral disease (1).
  – Type 1: refers to classic unilateral MD and metachronic bilateral MD (symptom onset in one ear followed by the other)
  – Type 2: refers to delayed unilateral MD (hearing loss onset preceding vertigo onset by months or years) or synchronic bilateral MD (simultaneous symptom onset in both ears)
  – Type 3: familial MD (Most families have bilateral hearing loss, but unilateral patient may coexist in the same family.)
  – Type 4: sporadic MD with migraine
  – Type 5: sporadic MD with an autoimmune disease
- System(s) affected: nervous
- Synonym(s): Ménière syndrome; endolymphatic hydrops

EPIDEMIOLOGY
- Predominant age of onset: 40 to 60 years
- Predominant gender: female > male, but overall fairly equal
- Race/ethnicity: white, Northern European > blacks
- Incidence up to 150/100,000 person-years

ETIOLOGY AND PATHOPHYSIOLOGY
- May be secondary to injury or other disorders (e.g., reduced middle ear pressure, allergy, endocrine disease, lipid disorders, vascular, viral, syphilis, autoimmune)
- Theories include increased pressure of the endolymph fluid due to increased fluid production or decreased resorption. This may be caused by endolymphatic sac pathology, abnormal development of the vestibular aqueduct, or inflammation caused by circulating immune complexes. Increased endolymph pressure may cause rupture of membranes and changes in endolymphatic ionic gradient.
- Others include vascular compromise, cochlear trauma, and viral infection or reactivation

Genetics
Family history in 10% of cases with an autosomal dominant inheritance pattern (2).

RISK FACTORS
May include
- Stress
- Allergy
- Increased intake of salt, caffeine, alcohol, or nicotine
- Chronic exposure to loud noise
- Vascular abnormalities (including migraines)
- Viral exposures (herpes simplex virus)

GENERAL PREVENTION
Reduce known risk factors.

COMMONLY ASSOCIATED CONDITIONS
- Anxiety (secondary to the disabling symptoms)
- Migraines
- Hyperprolactinemia
- Hypothyroidism

 DIAGNOSIS

HISTORY
- Symptomatic episodes are typically spontaneous but may be preceded by an aura of increasing fullness in the ear and tinnitus. These may occur in clusters, with long periods of symptom-free remissions.
- Formal criteria for diagnosis from American Academy of Otolaryngology-Head and Neck Surgery:
  – At least two episodes of vertigo >20 minutes to 12 hours in duration (usually described as rotatory spinning or rocking sensations)
  – Tinnitus or aural fullness; symptoms can fluctuate.
  – Hearing loss: Audiometric testing shows low- to mid-frequency (sensorineural) hearing loss in affected ear on at least one occasion in correlation with an episode of vertigo (3).
  – During severe attacks, pallor, sweating, nausea, vomiting, falling, and prostration may occur (3).

PHYSICAL EXAM
- Physical exam rules out other conditions; no finding is unique to Ménière disease.
- Horizontal nystagmus may be seen during attacks.

- Otoscopy is typically normal.
- Triggering of attacks in the office with Dix-Hallpike maneuver suggests diagnosis of benign paroxysmal positional vertigo (BPPV), not Ménière disease as vertigo is typically of shorter duration and triggered by head movements in BPPV.

DIFFERENTIAL DIAGNOSIS
- Acoustic neuroma or other CNS tumor
- Multiple Sclerosis
- Autoimmune inner ear disease
- Temporal bone fractures
- Syphilis
- Viral labyrinthitis
- Transient ischemic attack (TIA), migraine
- Diabetes or thyroid dysfunction
- Medication side effects

DIAGNOSTIC TESTS & INTERPRETATION
Testing to rule out other conditions

Initial Tests (lab, imaging)
- Consider serologic tests specific for *Treponema pallidum* in at-risk populations.
- Thyroid, fasting blood sugar, and lipid studies
- Consider MRI to rule out acoustic neuroma or other CNS pathology, including tumor, aneurysm, and multiple sclerosis.

Diagnostic Procedures/Other
- Audiometry using pure tone and speech to show low-frequency sensorineural (nerve) loss and impaired speech discrimination; usually shows low-frequency sensorineural hearing loss
- Tuning fork tests (i.e., Weber and Rinne test), ABR, or MRI to rule out acoustic neuroma
- Electrocochleography may be useful to confirm etiology.
- Caloric testing: Reduced activity on either side is consistent with Ménière diagnosis but is not itself diagnostic.
- Head-impulse testing (4)[C]

Test Interpretation
- Cytochemical analysis can reveal altered AQP4 and AQP6 expression in the supporting cell, altered cochlin, and mitochondrial protein expression (5)[B].
- Familial Ménière disease has been associated with DTNA and FAM136A genes (6)[B].

💉 **TREATMENT**

- Medications are primarily for symptomatic relief of vertigo and nausea.
- During attacks, bed rest with eyes closed prevents falls. Attacks rarely last >4 hours.

GENERAL MEASURES
Salt restriction diet has remained the primary first-line treatment, although evidence of its validity remains inconclusive (7).

MEDICATION

First Line

- Acute attack: Initial goal is stabilization and symptom relief; for severe episodes
  - Benzodiazepines (such as diazepam): decrease vertigo and anxiety
  - Antihistamines (meclizine/dimenhydrinate): decrease vertigo and nausea
  - Anticholinergics (transdermal scopolamine): reduce nausea and emesis associated with motion sickness
  - Antidopaminergic agents (metoclopramide, promethazine): decrease nausea, anxiety
  - Rehydration and electrolyte replacement therapies
  - Steroid taper for acute hearing loss
- Maintenance (The goal is to prevent/reduce attacks.)
  - Lifestyle changes (e.g., low-salt diet) are needed.
  - Diuretics may help reduce attacks by decreasing endolymphatic pressure and volume; there is insufficient evidence to recommend routine use:
    - Hydrochlorothiazide; hydrochlorothiazide/triamterene (Dyazide, Maxzide)
    - Acetazolamide (Diamox)
  - Contraindications/warnings:
    - Atropine: cardiac disease, especially supraventricular tachycardia and other arrhythmias; prostatic enlargement
    - Scopolamine: children and elderly, prostatic enlargement
    - Diuretics: electrolyte abnormalities, renal disease
  - Precautions:
    - Sedating drugs should be used with caution, particularly in the elderly. Patients are cautioned not to operate motor vehicles or machinery. Atropine and scopolamine should be used with particular caution.
    - Diuretics: Monitor electrolytes.

Second Line

- Steroids, both intratympanic and systemic (PO or IV), have been used for longer treatment of hearing loss:
  - Addition of prednisone 30 mg/day to diuretic treatment reduced severity and frequency of tinnitus and vertigo in one pilot study.
  - Dexamethasone is practical to use due to better tolerance by patients, as methylprednisolone creates burning sensation in the middle ear mucosa.
- Evidence is lacking for routine use of Famvir (famciclovir); may improve hearing more than balance.

ISSUES FOR REFERRAL

- Consider ear, nose, throat/neurology referral.
- Patients should have formal audiometry to confirm hearing loss.

ADDITIONAL THERAPIES

- Application of intermittent pressures via a myringotomy using a Meniett device has been shown to relieve vertigo (8)[B]:
  - Safe; requires a long-term tympanostomy tube
- Vestibular rehabilitation may be beneficial for patients with persistent vestibular symptoms
  - Safe and effective for unilateral vestibular dysfunction
- International consensus on treatment of MD suggests that vestibular rehabilitation should be offered as treatment option for patients between vertigo crises (9).

SURGERY/OTHER PROCEDURES

- Interventions that preserve hearing:
  - Endolymphatic sac surgery is shown to be effective in controlling vertigo in 75% of patients with Ménière disease who failed medical therapy.
  - Vestibular nerve section (intracranial procedure)
    - More invasive
    - Decreases vertigo and preserves hearing
    - Tympanostomy tube: may decrease symptoms by decreasing the middle ear pressure
- Interventions for patients with no serviceable hearing:
  - Labyrinthectomy: very effective at controlling vertigo but causes deafness
  - Vestibular neurectomy
  - Endoscopic vestibular nerve section
  - Cochlear implantation

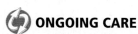 ONGOING CARE

FOLLOW-UP RECOMMENDATIONS

Patient Monitoring

Due to the possibility of progressive hearing loss despite decrease in vertiginous attacks, it is important to monitor changes in hearing and to monitor for more serious underlying causes (e.g., acoustic neuroma).

DIET

Diet is usually not a factor, unless attacks are brought on by certain foods. Consider salt restriction.

PROGNOSIS

- Alert the patients about the nature of alternating attacks and remission.
- Between attacks, patient may be fully active but is often limited due to fear or lingering symptoms. This can be severely disabling.
- 50% resolve spontaneously within 2 to 3 years.
- Some cases last >20 years.
- Severity and frequency of attacks diminish, but hearing loss is often progressive.
- 90% can be treated successfully with medication; 5–10% of patients require surgery for incapacitating vertigo.

COMPLICATIONS

Loss of hearing; injury during attack; inability to work

REFERENCES

1. Borowiec E, Crossley J, Hoa M. Understanding fluctuating hearing loss. *Hear J.* 2020;73(6):12–13.
2. Perez-Carpena P, Lopez-Escamez JA. Current understanding and clinical management of Meniere's disease: a systematic review. *Semin Neurol.* 2020;40(1):138–150.
3. Basura GJ, Adams ME, Monfared A, et al. Clinical practice guideline: Ménière's disease executive summary. *Otolaryngol Head Neck Surg.* 2020;162(4):415–434.
4. Lee SU, Kim HJ, Koo JW, et al. Comparison of caloric and head-impulse tests during the attacks of Meniere's disease. *Laryngoscope.* 2017;127(3):702–708.
5. Ishiyama G, Lopez IA, Sepahdari AR, et al. Meniere's disease: histopathology, cytochemistry, and imaging. *Ann N Y Acad Sci.* 2015;1343:49–57.
6. Frejo L, Giegling I, Teggi R, et al. Genetics of vestibular disorders: pathophysiological insights. *J Neurol.* 2016;263(Suppl 1):S45–S53.
7. Shim T, Strum DP, Mudry A, et al. Hold the salt: history of salt restriction as a first-line therapy for Ménière's disease. *Otol Neurotol.* 2020;41(6):855–859.
8. Ahsan SF, Standring R, Wang Y. Systematic review and meta-analysis of Meniett therapy for Meniere's disease. *Laryngoscope.* 2015;125(1):203–208.
9. Dunlap PM, Holmberg JM, Whitney SL. Vestibular rehabilitation: advances in peripheral and central vestibular disorders. *Curr Opin Neurol.* 2019;32(1):137–144.

 SEE ALSO

- Hearing Loss; Labyrinthitis; Tinnitus
- Algorithm: Dizziness

 CODES

ICD10

- H81.03 Ménière's disease, bilateral
- H81.09 Ménière's disease, unspecified ear
- H81.0 Ménière's disease

CLINICAL PEARLS

- Ménière disease is characterized by vertigo (lasting 20 minutes to 12 hours), with associated hearing loss, tinnitus +/− aural fullness.
- There is a wide differential diagnosis for Ménière disease; therefore, one must fully investigate symptoms.
- Multiple medical, surgical, and rehabilitative treatments are available to decrease the severity and frequency of attacks.

M

MENINGITIS, BACTERIAL
Corey J. Costanzo, DO, MPH, MS

BASICS

DESCRIPTION
Bacterial infection of the meninges resulting in inflammation, pain, and systemic illness

EPIDEMIOLOGY
Predominant age: neonates, infants, and elderly; predominant sex: male = female

Incidence
Varies by age and pathogen
- 18 to 34 years: 0.66/100,000
- 35 to 49 years: 0.95/100,000
- 50 to 64 years: 1.73/100,000
- ≥65 years: 1.92/100,000
- Group B *Streptococcus*: 0.25/100,000; *Neisseria meningitidis*: 0.19/100,00
- *Haemophilus influenzae* type B: 0.08/100,000; *Listeria monocytogenes*: 0.05/100,000

Prevalence
15,000 to 25,000 cases occur annually in the United States.

ETIOLOGY AND PATHOPHYSIOLOGY
Community-acquired bacterial meningitis is most commonly due to *Streptococcus pneumoniae* (50%) and *N. meningitidis* (30%). Nosocomial or postsurgical meningitis occurs after manipulation of the central nervous system (CNS); newborns (<2 months): group B *Streptococcus*, *Escherichia coli*, *L. monocytogenes*; infants and children: *S. pneumoniae*, *N. meningitidis*, *H. influenzae*; adolescents and young adults: *N. meningitidis*, *S. pneumoniae*; immunocompromised adults: *S. pneumoniae*, *L. monocytogenes*, gram-negative bacilli such as *Pseudomonas aeruginosa*; mixed bacterial infection in <1% of cases; older adults: *S. pneumoniae* 50%, *N. meningitidis* 30%, *L. monocytogenes* 5%; 10% gram-negative bacilli: *E. coli*, *Klebsiella*, *Enterobacter*, *P. aeruginosa*

Genetics
Some Native American populations appear to have genetic susceptibility to invasive disease.

RISK FACTORS
Those who are at risk include household or close contacts of case patients; immunocompromised (including HIV, asplenia, or patients taking eculizumab, ravulizumab), alcohol use disorder, diabetes, or chronic disease; neurosurgical procedure/head injury, close living quarters (dormitories or military barracks), and work exposures; neonates: prematurity, low birth weight, premature rupture of membranes, maternal peripartum infection, and urinary tract abnormalities; anatomical abnormality of nasopharynx and subarachnoid space (congenital, trauma), dural fistula; parameningeal source: otitis, sinusitis, mastoiditis, skull fracture; elderly, immunocompromised, and pregnant patients are at risk for listeriosis; complement deficiencies, properdin, factor H, and factor D

GENERAL PREVENTION
- Consider CSF fistula in cases of recurrent meningitis; aseptic techniques for head wounds or skull fractures
- Meningitis caused by *H. influenzae* type B has decreased 55% with routine vaccination. Conjugate vaccines against *S. pneumoniae* may reduce the burden of disease in childhood; chemoprophylaxis for close contacts of meningococcal meningitis patients.

COMMONLY ASSOCIATED CONDITIONS
Factors associated with a worse prognosis: alcohol use disorder, elderly, infancy, diabetes mellitus, multiple myeloma, head trauma, seizures, immunocompromised, coma, sepsis, sinusitis

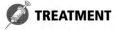
DIAGNOSIS

HISTORY
- Antecedent upper respiratory infection; fever, headache, vomiting, photophobia, seizures, confusion
- Nausea, rigors, sweats, weakness; elderly: subtle findings including confusion
- Infants: irritability, lethargy, poor feeding; altered mental status; food exposures (e.g., *L. monocytogenes*)

PHYSICAL EXAM
95% of patients present with at least two of the following: headache, fever, neck stiffness, and altered mental status.
- Meningismus; focal neurologic deficits
- Meningococcal rash: macular and erythematous at first and then petechial or purpuric; purpura fulminans (Suspect meningococcus.)
- Papilledema
- Brudzinski sign: Passive flexion of neck elicits involuntary flexing of knees in supine position.
- Kernig sign: resistance or pain with passive knee extension following 90-degree hip flexion in supine position
- Late signs and symptoms: hemiparesis, stroke, cognitive impairment, coma, epilepsy, hearing loss, and permanent visual impairment

DIFFERENTIAL DIAGNOSIS
- Bacteremia, sepsis, brain abscess, seizure, other nonbacterial meningitides; aseptic meningitis
- Inflammatory noninfectious: Behçet disease, systemic lupus erythematosus (SLE), sarcoidosis, migraine
- Stroke; viral meningitis, Lyme disease, leptospirosis; subarachnoid hemorrhage; central nervous vasculitides

DIAGNOSTIC TESTS & INTERPRETATION
Initial Tests (lab, imaging)
- Prompt lumbar puncture (1)
  - Head CT first if focal neurologic findings, papilledema, or altered mentation
  - CSF appearance: turbid; CSF Gram stain and cultures
  - Adults: >500 cells/mL WBCs, glucose <40 mg/dL, <2/3 blood-to-glucose ratio, CSF protein >200 mg/dL
    - CSF opening pressure >30 cm; suspect ruptured brain abscess when WBC count is unusually high (>100,000); polymerase chain reaction (PCR) of CSF (particularly in suspected viral meningitis)
- Reserve bacterial antigen tests for cases where initial CSF Gram stain is negative and CSF culture is negative at 48 hours.
- CBC, blood cultures, serum electrolytes, coagulation studies; chest radiograph may reveal pneumonitis or abscess; C-reactive protein (CRP): Normal CRP has high negative predictive value.

- Later in course, head CT if hydrocephalus, brain abscess, subdural effusions, subdural empyema are suspected or if no clinical response after 48 hours of appropriate antibiotics. Elevated CSF protein concentration plus hypoglycorrhachia suggest ventriculitis or meningitis.

Follow-Up Tests & Special Considerations
Consider initiation of empiric antibiotics once the blood cultures are drawn if lumbar puncture is delayed.

Diagnostic Procedures/Other
Lumbar puncture
- Noncontrast head CT is recommended prior to lumbar puncture to assess the risk of herniation if the patient is immunocompromised, has papilledema, a history of CNS disease, focal neurologic deficit on exam, visual field cut, new-onset seizure ≤1 week prior to presentation, or an abnormal level of consciousness.
- Lumbar puncture contraindications: signs of increased intracranial pressure (decerebrate posturing, papilledema), skin infection at site of lumbar puncture, CT or MRI evidence of obstructive hydrocephalus, cerebral edema, herniation
- Symptoms of infection plus positive CSF culture and CSF pleocytosis indicate ventriculitis or meningitis.

Test Interpretation
Bacterial meningitis: opening pressure >180 mm H_2O; CSF protein, usually high; CSF glucose, usually low; cell counts >1 × 10^9/L

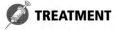
TREATMENT

GENERAL MEASURES
Initiate empiric antibiotic therapy immediately after lumbar puncture. If head CT scan is needed, initiate antibiotic therapy immediately after blood cultures (Abx > CT > lumbar puncture) (1). Watch for seizures and aspiration precautions.

MEDICATION
Empiric antibiotic IV therapy with dexamethasone for known or suspected *S. pneumoniae* meningitis until culture results are available

First Line
- Neonates: ampicillin: 150 mg/kg/day divided q8h and cefotaxime: 150 mg/kg/day divided q8h
- Infants >4 weeks of age: ceftriaxone: 100 mg/kg/day divided q12–24h or cefotaxime 225 to 300 mg/kg/day divided q6–8h and vancomycin: 60 mg/kg/day divided q6h
- Adults (1)
  - Immunocompetent: cefotaxime: 2 g IV q4–6h or ceftriaxone: 2 g IV q12h.
    - In countries with ceftriaxone resistance rates >1%, vancomycin 15 to 20 mg/kg IV q8–12h (target level 15 to 20 μg/mL), plus in adults >50 years of age, ampicillin 2 g IV q4h
  - Immunocompromised: vancomycin 15 to 20 mg/kg IV q8–12h, plus ampicillin 2 g IV q4h, plus either cefepime 2 g IV q8h or meropenem 2 g IV q8h (If meropenem is used, ampicillin is not required.)

- >50 years, add ampicillin: 2 g IV q4h for *Listeria* plus either cefotaxime: 2 g IV q4–6h or ceftriaxone: 2 g IV q12h or meropenem: 2 g IV q8h (ampicillin not needed); if *Listeria* is identified as the causative agent, the regimen should be modified to include ampicillin or penicillin in combination with gentamicin.
  - Penicillin-allergic patients:
    - Without severe β-lactam allergy: Use meropenem instead of ceftriaxone in patients with mild hives to a cephalosporin without other signs of anaphylaxis.
    - Severe allergy: vancomycin: loading dose of 25 to 30 mg/kg IV and then 15 to 20 mg/kg q8–12h (goal trough of 15 to 20) plus moxifloxacin 400 mg IV once daily
- Treatment duration: *S. pneumoniae*: 10 to 14 days (2)[A]
  - *N. meningitidis*, *H. influenzae*: 7 to 10 days; group B *Streptococcus* organisms, *E. coli*, *L. monocytogenes*: 14 to 21 days; neonates: 12 to 21 days or at least 14 days after a repeated culture is sterile
  - No reliable evidence to support using preadmission antibiotics for nonsevere meningococcal disease
- Corticosteroids pediatrics: Corticosteroids are associated with lower rates of hearing loss and neurologic sequelae.
  - Early treatment with dexamethasone (0.15 mg/kg IV q6h for 2 to 4 days) decreases mortality and morbidity for patients >1 month of age with acute bacterial meningitis with no increased risk of GI bleeding.
  - Adults: Initiate in adults and continue only if CSF Gram stain shows gram-positive diplococcus or if blood or CSF positive for *S. pneumoniae*.
    - Associated with increased recurrence of fever (RR 1.27, 95% CI 1.09–1.47); decreased mortality in *S. pneumoniae* (RR 0.8, 95% CI 0.20–0.59) but not in *H. influenzae* or *N. meningitidis* (2)[A]
    - Lower rates of severe hearing loss (RR 0.67, 95% CI 0.51–0.88), any hearing loss (RR 0.74, 95% CI 0.63–0.87), and neurologic sequelae (RR 0.83, 95% CI 0.69–1.00); nonsignificant reduction in mortality (RR 0.90, 95% CI 0.53–1.05); *p* value = .009
  - Dexamethasone: 0.15 mg/kg IV q6h (start 15 to 20 minutes before or with antibiotic) for 2 to 4 days; dexamethasone should only be continued if the CSF Gram stain and/or CSF or blood culture reveal *S. pneumoniae*.

Second Line

Antipseudomonal penicillins should be given in combination with other appropriate agents.

- Aztreonam 2 g IV q6–8h; fluoroquinolones (e.g., ciprofloxacin) IV 400 mg q8–12h; meropenem IV 2 g q8h

ISSUES FOR REFERRAL

Consultation from infectious disease and/or critical care specialist

ADDITIONAL THERAPIES

Chemoprophylaxis in close contacts include household members, roommates/dormitory mates, intimate contacts, contacts at a childcare center, exposed military recruits; travelers who had direct contact with respiratory or oral secretions from an index patient

SURGERY/OTHER PROCEDURES

Postsurgical bacterial meningitis or associated with head trauma or shunt: empiric cover for MRSA and aerobic gram-negative organisms, such as *Pseudomonas* spp., and Enterobacteriaceae (3)[A]

ADMISSION, INPATIENT, AND NURSING CONSIDERATIONS

- Bacterial meningitis requires hospitalization. ICU monitoring may be needed. Patients with suspected meningococcal infection require respiratory isolation for 24 hours.
- Droplet precautions of hospitalized patients as soon as diagnosis is suspected through the first 24 hours of antimicrobial therapy.

ONGOING CARE

FOLLOW-UP RECOMMENDATIONS

Patient Monitoring

- Brainstem auditory—evoked response hearing test for infants before hospital discharge
- Vaccinations
  - **Meningococcal vaccination:**
    - All 11 to 12 years old should get a MenACWY vaccine, with a booster dose at 16 years old. Teens and young adults (16 through 23 years old) may get a MenB Vaccine. CDC recommends meningococcal vaccination for other children and adults who are at increased risk.
    - Routine MenB vaccination for people aged ≥10 years at increased risk for meningococcal disease
  - Pneumococcal vaccination:
    - PCV13: Infants and young children usually need 4 doses of pneumococcal conjugate vaccine, at 2, 4, 6, and 12 to 15 months of age. A dose of PCV13 is recommended for anyone ≥2 years of age with certain medical conditions if they did not already receive PCV13. This vaccine may be given to adults aged ≥65 years based on discussions between the patient and health care provider.
    - Per CDC, PPSV23 for all adults aged ≥65 years; people 2 through 64 years old with certain medical conditions; adults 19 through 64 years old who smoke cigarettes
- Prophylaxis: During 2019 to 2020, 11 meningococcal isolates from U.S. patients had mutations conferring penicillin or ciprofloxacin resistance.
  - Most isolates in the United States are susceptible to recommended antibiotics.
  - Rifampin: 600 mg PO BID for 2 days; ciprofloxacin: 500 mg PO for 1 dose; ceftriaxone: 250 mg IM for 1 dose; azithromycin 500 mg PO single dose for ciprofloxacin-resistance *N. meningitidis* exposure (not first agent); chemoprophylaxis for close contacts of patients with confirmed meningococcal meningitis

DIET

Regular, as tolerated, except with syndrome of inappropriate secretion of antidiuretic hormone (SIADH)

PROGNOSIS

- Mortality: *S. pneumoniae* meningitis 19–37%; meningococcal meningitis: 5%
- Deaths associated with *N. meningitidis* usually occur within 12 to 24 hours of the first symptoms. Mortality rate of untreated disease approaches 100%.

COMPLICATIONS

- Up to 50% develop long-term neurologic complications (cognitive impairment) after pneumococcal meningitis
- Seizures: 20–30% focal neurologic deficit; 15–20% cerebrovascular complications: subdural effusion or empyema, septic sinus thrombosis, intracranial hypertension, cerebral edema, temporal lobe or cerebellar herniation, hydrocephalus
- Cranial nerve palsies (III, VI, VII, VIII) in 10–20% of cases; usually transient; sensorineural hearing loss: 10% in children; permanent visual impairment; neurodevelopmental sequelae: 30% with subtle learning deficits
- Obstructive hydrocephalus, subdural effusion; SIADH; elevated intracranial pressure: herniation, brain swelling
- Purpura fulminans, septic shock
- Meningococcal-induced microvascular thrombosis and DIC; depression, subarachnoid bleed, stroke

REFERENCES

1. Pajor MJ, Long B, Koyfman A, et al. High risk and low prevalence diseases: adult bacterial meningitis. *Am J Emerg Med*. 2023;65:76–83.
2. Tunkel AR, Hartman BJ, Kaplan SL, et al. Practice guidelines for the management of bacterial meningitis. *Clin Infect Dis*. 2004;39(9):1267–1284.
3. Tunkel AR, Hasbun R, Bhimraj A, et al. 2017 Infectious Diseases Society of America's clinical practice guidelines for healthcare-associated ventriculitis and meningitis. *Clin Infect Dis*. 2017;64(6):e34–e65.

CODES

ICD10

- G00.9 Bacterial meningitis, unspecified
- G00.2 Streptococcal meningitis
- G00.8 Other bacterial meningitis

CLINICAL PEARLS

- Monitor prophylaxis failures and antimicrobial resistance among meningococcal isolates to inform prophylaxis recommendations.
- Empiric therapy for suspected meningococcal disease should include an extended-spectrum cephalosporin, such as cefotaxime or ceftriaxone. Once microbiologic diagnosis is established, definitive treatment with penicillin G, ampicillin, or an extended-spectrum cephalosporin is recommended.

M

MENINGITIS, VIRAL
Zoe Foster, MD, FAAFP • Jeffrey Wisinski, DO

BASICS

DESCRIPTION
- A clinical syndrome characterized by fever with signs/symptoms of acute meningeal inflammation (including but not limited to headache, photophobia, neck stiffness, and/or nausea/vomiting)
- Viral meningitis (VM) is the most common cause of aseptic (nonbacterial) meningitis.

EPIDEMIOLOGY
Incidence
- Most common form of meningitis
- Peaks summer to fall in temperate climates (but is year round in subtropical or tropical climates)
  - Nonpolio enteroviruses are the most common cause of viral meningitis; estimated 75,000 VM cases caused by enterovirus annually in the United States

Prevalence
Varies by geographical location and causative pathogen

ETIOLOGY AND PATHOPHYSIOLOGY
- In immunocompetent hosts, VM is a rare complication of an acute viral infection like gastroenteritis, mumps, herpes simplex virus (HSV), varicella-zoster virus (VZV), and arthropod-borne viruses.
  - Case reports in the literature indicate that SARS-CoV-2, rotavirus A, and hepatitis E can cause VM.
  - In immunocompromised hosts, viral pathogens may include cytomegalovirus (CMV) and Epstein-Barr virus (EBV).
- 23–61% of VM cases are caused by nonpolio human enteroviruses, typically transmitted via the fecal-oral route.
- Mosquito-borne viruses include West Nile, Zika, chikungunya, dengue, St. Louis encephalitis, and Eastern equine encephalitis viruses. Tick-borne viruses include Powassan, Colorado tick fever, and tick-borne encephalitis viruses.
- Recurrent benign lymphocytic (Mollaret) meningitis is generally associated with HSV-2 (80% of cases).

Genetics
None identified

RISK FACTORS
- Age (most common in children aged <5 years)
  - Babies <1 month of age are more likely to have severe disease.
- Immunocompromised host (patients more susceptible to CMV, HSV, and EBV)
- Diabetes, chronic renal failure (patients more susceptible to VZV)
- Close contacts of people with VM are unlikely to get VM but may get the primary viral syndrome.

Geriatric Considerations
Cases of VM in the elderly are rare (most common cause is VZV, HSV); consider alternative diagnoses (e.g., cancer, medication-induced aseptic meningitis) (1).

GENERAL PREVENTION
- Hand washing and general hygiene procedures
- Avoid sharing drinks/cups and silverware with others, especially those who are ill.
- Avoid exposure to mosquitos and ticks; if outdoors, recommend use of appropriate clothing, DEET, and mosquito nets.
- Ensure immunizations are up to date.

COMMONLY ASSOCIATED CONDITIONS
Encephalitis; myopericarditis; neonatal enteroviral sepsis; meningoencephalitis; flaccid paralysis

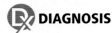

DIAGNOSIS

HISTORY
- Predominant adult symptoms include acute onset (hours to days) of:
  - Fever (incidence varies by virus; 65–83% in enterovirus, 54–98% in mumps, 6–52% in HSV)
  - Headache (prominent early symptom); photophobia (mainly with enterovirus, 79–85% of cases; 33–64% in HSV; 7% in mumps)
  - Myalgias/arthralgias (88% in enterovirus; 50% in HSV; 14–21% in mumps)
  - Nausea/vomiting, malaise
  - Nuchal rigidity (55–69% in enterovirus; 22–71% in HSV; 8–85% in mumps)
    - Altered mental status, seizure, or focal neurologic deficits should prompt consideration of alternative diagnoses.
- In infants, nonspecific symptoms are more common, including poor feeding, vomiting, lethargy, fever (most common), and irritability (most common).
- Additional historical elements:
  - Travel history and outdoor activities; sexual history (e.g., HSV, HIV); immunocompromised host, including solid-organ transplant and HIV (CMV, HSV, adenovirus, West Nile virus); history of VZV infection; immunization status (mumps, influenza, VZV)

PHYSICAL EXAM
- Vital signs: fever, tachycardia, tachypnea, hypotension
- Neurologic:
  - Lack of mental status changes (If present, consider alternative diagnoses.)
  - Photophobia
  - Meningeal signs
    - Nuchal rigidity; Brudzinski sign (neck flexion elicits involuntary hip and knee flexion in supine patient) and Kernig sign (resistance to knee extension following flexion of hips to 90 degrees) are poorly sensitive (~5%) in patients with meningitis
    - Jolt accentuation test: rapid horizontal rotation of the head accentuates headache (of questionable utility in diagnosis of meningitis given low sensitivity and specificity) (2)[C].
  - Asymmetric flaccid paralysis is seen in West Nile virus infection (1)[C].
- HEENT:
  - Parotitis (in mumps infection); herpangina (coxsackievirus A); bulging fontanelle (in infants); generalized lymphadenopathy (EBV, HIV)
- Dermatology:
  - Vesicular rash of hand, foot, and mouth disease (coxsackievirus)
  - Generalized maculopapular rash
    - Presence of a palpable petechial/purpuric rash should prompt consideration of bacterial meningitis (BM).
- Abdomen:
  - Splenomegaly (in EBV); abdominal pain

DIFFERENTIAL DIAGNOSIS
- BM; fungal meningitis (consider if immunocompromised; agents include *Coccidioides* and *Cryptococcus neoformans*) (3)[C]
- Other infectious agents (tuberculosis, syphilis, leptospirosis, Lyme disease, ehrlichiosis, amebiasis) (3)[C]
- Parameningeal infections (e.g., subdural empyema); encephalitis; postinfectious encephalomyelitis; viral syndrome (e.g., influenza)
- Leukemia, lymphoma, or other neoplastic disease (including metastasis)
- Migraine/tension headache; acute metabolic encephalopathy; postoperative aseptic meningitis
- Drug-induced (chemical) meningitis (NSAIDs, TMP/SMX, amoxicillin, TNF-α inhibitors, lamotrigine, IVIG, and monoclonal antibodies) (1)[C]
- Brain/epidural abscess, inflammatory disorders (e.g., Behçet, sarcoidosis, SLE) (1)[C]

DIAGNOSTIC TESTS & INTERPRETATION
Initial Tests (lab, imaging)
- Serum labs: CBC, BMP, procalcitonin/C-reactive protein, blood cultures (3)[C]
  - CBC: normal or mildly elevated WBC
  - BMP: CSF glucose levels should be compared to plasma levels.
  - Procalcitonin/C-reactive protein: should be normal in VM (Consider BM in adults when serum PCT is elevated.)
  - Blood cultures: should be negative in VM
- Lumbar puncture (LP):
  - LP differentiates VM from BM.
    - Do not delay empiric antibiotics if there is a concern for BM. Consider use of a validated clinical decision-making tool (e.g., Bacterial Meningitis Score) in children to calculate risk of BM.
  - Contraindications/risks:
    - Signs/symptoms of increased intracranial pressure (focal neurologic findings, papilledema, altered mental status, new-onset seizure), impaired cellular immunity, local infection over potential LP site, suspected epidural abscess, use of anticoagulation or potential coagulopathy, and possibility of cardiorespiratory compromise due to patient positioning during procedure
      - Consider CT if clinical concern for increased intracranial pressure.
    - Procedural risks include cerebral herniation, post-LP headache, bleeding, infection, and pain.
  - CSF analysis:
    - Opening pressure: should be normal
    - Ensure enough CSF volume is drawn and saved so that additional workup (i.e. PCR, NAAT) can be done if preliminary CSF analysis is not diagnostic.
    - Cell count/differential:
      - 100 to 1,000 WBC/μL (can be higher in enteroviral meningitis)
      - Lymphocyte predominance (in early infection, may be PMN predominance)
      - RBCs suggest traumatic tap but may be seen in HSV meningitis/encephalitis.

○ CSF glucose: usually normal (may have mild decrease in mumps or HIV)

○ CSF protein: normal to mildly elevated

○ CSF lactate: normal (if elevated >4.2 mmol/L, highly suggestive of BM; differential diagnosis also includes TB, seizures, hemorrhage, and ischemia if elevated; lactate levels less reliable if antibiotics have been started prior to LP)

– Gram stain: should be negative for bacteria

– CSF culture:

○ Gold standard for diagnosis of BM; should be negative for bacterial pathogens in VM

– PCR/NAAT (3)[C]:

○ Improved sensitivity/specificity

○ Useful for rapid identification of multiple possible pathogens (bacteria, viruses, fungi)—sensitivity for pathogens varies by test; may allow early discontinuation of empiric therapies

– CSF IgM antibodies for arboviruses (4)[C]

Follow-Up Tests & Special Considerations

Disorders that may alter lab results:

- Diabetes: Consider current blood sugar level to correlate with CSF glucose level.
- Neurologic diseases (e.g., history of stroke or transient ischemic attack, intracranial neoplasm, demyelinating disease)

TREATMENT

GENERAL MEASURES

Management includes supportive care (e.g., pain control, IV fluids) and low threshold for empiric antibiotics for BM pending laboratory results (2)[C].

MEDICATION

First Line

- Antipyretics/analgesics (Adult doses are presented; titrate doses to pain relief.)
  – Acetaminophen (Tylenol) 500–1,000 mg PO q8h; 325 to 650 mg PR q4–6 hours (limit 3 g/24 hr)
  – Ibuprofen 400 to 800 mg PO q8h
  – Naproxen 550 mg PO BID
  – Consider short-term opioids if pain uncontrolled
- Antiemetics
  – Ondansetron (Zofran) 4 to 8 mg IV q8h
  – Promethazine (Phenergan) 12.5 to 25.0 mg PO/PR/IM/IV q4–6h (Consider maximum dose of 50 mg/24 hr to limit side effects.)
- Antiviral agents (2)[C]
  – Empiric acyclovir at 10 mg/kg IV q8h (adult dose) for patients with CSF pleocytosis, negative gram stain, and suspicion for HSV while awaiting results of definitive (e.g., HSV or VZV PCR) testing
    ○ Immunocompetent patients with HSV meningitis improve with or without antiviral therapy and can be treated with supportive care alone.
    ○ VM due to HIV will resolve with supportive care alone.

- Antibiotics (targeted to most likely pathogen)
  – Not indicated for treatment of VM
  – Empiric treatment is reasonable while ruling out BM. Initiate following blood cultures and LP if possible. Consider, especially in elderly, those pretreated with antibiotics, ill appearing, and immunocompromised patients.
    ○ If very low risk for BM, treat symptomatically and observe in the inpatient setting pending laboratory results.
- Corticosteroids (2)[C]
  – Not recommended in VM (recommended as adjunctive treatment in BM)

ISSUES FOR REFERRAL

For patients with known CSF shunts/drains, recent neurosurgery/trauma, or intrathecal pumps in the setting of possible VM or BM, an emergent neurosurgical referral is warranted (3)[C].

ADMISSION, INPATIENT, AND NURSING CONSIDERATIONS

- Initial inpatient management includes:
  – Pain management and empiric therapies (pending lab results); IV fluids (based on hydration status and clinical presentation); neurologic monitoring for changes in mental status, fever, neck stiffness, headache; contact precautions and private room until BM ruled out
- Discharge depends on clinical parameters (dehydration, emesis, pain control, functional level, social circumstances, and ability to follow up). VM in stable patients can be managed in the outpatient setting.

ONGOING CARE

FOLLOW-UP RECOMMENDATIONS

- Close follow-up to ensure resolution of all symptoms.
  – A small portion of adult patients suffer from ongoing neuropsychological morbidities (cognitive dysfunction, sleep disturbances, decreased psychomotor speed, impaired visuoconstructive functions, and impaired executive functioning) following VM, with the degree of disability dependent on the causative virus.
- Developmental surveillance after VM in children as children are more likely to have severe complications of disease.

Patient Monitoring

- Monitor for relapse or exacerbation of symptoms.
- Monitor for neurologic complications:
  – Seizures, altered mental status, new onset weakness; assess ability to have companion monitor change in mental/neurologic status if patient discharged

DIET

Push fluids; diet as tolerated

PATIENT EDUCATION

- Discuss very low probability of transmission to close contacts. Encourage hand washing.
- Recurrence of headache, myalgia, and weakness is possible over 2 to 3 weeks.

PROGNOSIS

- Recovery generally within 7 to 10 days
  – In some patients, return to work may be delayed and quality of life may take months to return to baseline, as headaches and other neurologic symptoms may intermittently persist for weeks to months.
- There is a low mortality rate from VM.
- Very young children and some adults suffer from prolonged neuropsychological disabilities as a result of VM.

COMPLICATIONS

- Common: fatigue, irritability, muscle weakness
- Rare: neuropsychological problems and developmental delay

REFERENCES

1. Shahan B, Choi EY, Nieves G. Cerebrospinal fluid analysis. *Am Fam Physician*. 2021;103(7):422–428.
2. Kohil A, Jemmieh S, Smatti MK, et al. Viral meningitis: an overview. *Arch Virol*. 2021;166(2):335–345.
3. Poplin V, Boulware DR, Bahr NC. Methods for rapid diagnosis of meningitis etiology in adults. *Biomark Med*. 2020;14(6):459–479.
4. Hudson JA, Broad J, Martin NG, et al. Outcomes beyond hospital discharge in infants and children with viral meningitis: a systematic review. *Rev Med Virol*. 2020;30(2):e2083.

CODES

ICD10

- A87.9 Viral meningitis, unspecified
- A87.1 Adenoviral meningitis
- A87.0 Enteroviral meningitis

CLINICAL PEARLS

- VM cannot be reliably distinguished from BM based on clinical findings alone.
- Hospitalize potential meningitis cases for evaluation and treatment with broad-spectrum antibiotics until BM has been ruled out.
- VM is more common than BM, especially when vaccination rates are high.
- Morbidity and mortality with VM is low

M

MENINGOCOCCAL DISEASE

Han Q. Bui, MD, MPH

BASICS

DESCRIPTION

- Meningococcemia is a blood-borne infection caused by *Neisseria meningitidis*.
- Bacteremia without meningitis: Patient is acutely ill and may have skin manifestations (rashes, petechiae, and ecchymosis) and hypotension. Bacteremia with meningitis: sudden onset of fever, nausea, vomiting, headache, decreased ability to concentrate, and myalgias
- Disease progresses rapidly (within hours).
- Skin findings and hypotension may be present.
  - A petechial rash appears as discrete lesions 1 to 2 mm in diameter; most frequently on the trunk and lower portions of the body; seen in >50% of patients on presentation
  - Purpura fulminans is a severe complication of meningococcal disease and occurs in up to 25% of cases. It is characterized by acute onset of cutaneous hemorrhage and necrosis due to vascular thrombosis and disseminated intravascular coagulopathy (DIC).

EPIDEMIOLOGY

Incidence

- The mortality rate is ~13%.
  - 11–19% of survivors suffer serious sequelae, including deafness, neurologic deficits, or limb loss.
- Disease is seasonal, peaks in December/January.
- Atypical clinical presentations include abdominal symptoms, septic arthritis, and bacteremic pneumonia.
- Peak incidence occurs in the first year of life; 35–40% of cases occur in children aged <5 years. A second peak occurs in adolescence.
- In 2021 (most recent CDC data), there were 210 cases of reported meningococcal disease (incidence rate of ~0.2 cases per 100,000 persons) (1); most common in adolescents and young adults, followed by infants <1 year

ETIOLOGY AND PATHOPHYSIOLOGY

- *N. meningitidis* is a fastidious, aerobic, gram-negative diplococcus with at least 13 serotypes.
- *N. meningitidis* has an outer coat that produces disease-causing endotoxin. Virulence factors promote invasive disease.
- Humans are the only known reservoir for *N. meningitidis*.
- Major serogroups in the United States are B, C, Y, and W-135.
  - Serogroup B is the predominant cause of meningococcemia in children aged <1 year.
  - Serogroup C is the most common cause of meningococcal disease in the United States.
  - Serogroup Y is the predominant cause of meningococcemia in the elderly (2).
- Major serogroups worldwide are A, B, C, Y, and W-135.
  - W-135 is the major cause of disease in the "meningitis belt" of sub-Saharan Africa.

Genetics

Late complement component deficiency has an autosomal recessive inheritance.

RISK FACTORS

- Age: 3 months to 1 year
- Late complement component deficiency (C5, C6, C7, C8, or C9)
- Asplenia (1)
- Living in close quarters (e.g., household contacts, nursery/daycare, dormitories, military barracks)
- Exposure to active (and/or) passive tobacco smoke (1)

GENERAL PREVENTION

- Meningococcal ACWY Vaccines (MenACWY):
  - Infants and children: routine vaccination for high-risk children aged 2 months and older
  - Adolescents: first dose typically at age 11 or 12 years, with a booster at age 16 years. Teens and young adults (16 through 23 years old) may also receive a serogroup B meningococcal vaccine.
  - At-Risk adults: Adults with certain risk factors or who are in an area with an outbreak should also be vaccinated.
- Meningococcal B vaccines (MenB):
  - Infants and children: not routinely recommended for all children but may be given to those at increased risk
  - Adolescents and young adults: may be administered to individuals aged 16 to 23 years (preferred age is 16 to 18 years) who are not at increased risk, based on shared clinical decision-making
  - At-risk individuals: recommended for individuals 10 years and older who are at increased risk
  - Special populations: Individuals with certain medical conditions, laboratory workers, or travelers to areas where meningococcal disease is common might also need vaccination.
  - Protective levels of antibody are achieved ~7 to 10 days after primary immunization (2).
  - CDC international travel advisory: vaccine required for Hajji pilgrims >2 years of age; given to travelers to sub-Saharan Africa ("meningitis belt")

DIAGNOSIS

HISTORY

Symptoms

- Sudden onset of fever, nausea, vomiting, headache, myalgias, chills, rigor, and/or sore throat (nonsuppurative)
  - Pharyngitis may be mistaken for streptococcal disease (strep throat).
  - Myalgia may be mistaken for severe "flu," which also has a peak incidence in winter.
- Changes in mental status, decreased ability to concentrate, stiff neck, convulsions
- Assess possible exposures.
- Other

PHYSICAL EXAM

- Fever, hypotension, tachycardia
- Neurologic: nuchal rigidity, focal neurologic findings, coma, seizure
  - Focal neurologic findings and seizures are more commonly seen with *Haemophilus influenzae* or *Streptococcus pneumoniae*.
- Cardiopulmonary: signs of heart failure with pulmonary edema—gallop, rales
- Dermatologic: maculopapular rash, petechiae, ecchymosis, purpura
- Onset of specific meningitis symptoms (e.g., neck stiffness, photophobia, bulging fontanelle) can occur within 12 to 15 hours.
- Late signs of meningitis (e.g., unconsciousness, delirium, or seizures) occur after ~15 hours in infants <1 year and after ~24 hours in older children.

DIFFERENTIAL DIAGNOSIS

- Sepsis; bacterial meningitis (other organisms)
- Acute bacterial endocarditis
- Rocky Mountain spotted fever
- Hemolytic uremic syndrome
- Gonococcal arthritis dermatitis syndrome
- Influenza

DIAGNOSTIC TESTS & INTERPRETATION

ALERT

- Isolation of *N. meningitidis* from a sterile site (blood or CSF) is the gold standard
- Antibiotic administration may render blood and/or CSF culture negative within 2 hours.

Initial Tests (lab, imaging)

- Definitive diagnosis is through culture (blood, CSF or other sterile site)
- CBC with differential
  - Leukocytosis (left shift; toxic granulation) or leukopenia, thrombocytopenia
- Lactic acidosis
- Procalcitonin; often elevated in bacterial meningitis (3)
- Coagulation studies
  - Prolonged prothrombin time/partial thromboplastin time
  - Low fibrinogen; elevated fibrin degradation products
- Blood culture
  - Blood culture positive for *N. meningitidis*; cultures positive in 50–60% of cases
- CSF
  - Grossly cloudy
  - Increased WBCs with polymorphonuclear predominance
  - Gram stain showing gram-negative diplococci
  - Glucose-to-blood glucose ratio <0.4; protein >45 mg/dL
  - Positive for *N. meningitidis* antigen (MAT or PCR)
  - CSF culture positive in 80–90% of cases
- Head CT prior to lumbar puncture (LP) if concern for space-occupying lesions or if focal neurologic findings

TREATMENT

MEDICATION

First Line

- Antibiotics (3)[A]
  - Begin treatment as soon as meningococcal meningitis is suspected.
  - Age guides empiric treatment.
    - Preterm to <1 month: ampicillin plus cefotaxime or ampicillin plus gentamicin
      - Cefotaxime
        - 0 to 7 days: 50 mg/kg q12h
        - 8 to 28 days: 50 mg/kg q8h
      - Ampicillin
        - >2,000 g
          - 0 to 7 days: 50 mg/kg q8h
          - 8 to 28 days: 50 mg/kg q6h
        - <2,000 g
          - 0 to 7 days: 50 mg/kg q12h
          - 8 to 28 days: 50 mg/kg q8h
    - 1 month to 50 years: cefotaxime or ceftriaxone plus vancomycin
      - If severe penicillin allergy: chloramphenicol plus trimethoprim-sulfamethoxazole (TMP-SMX) plus vancomycin
    - >50 years of age or patients with significant comorbidity, alcohol abuse, or impaired immunity: ampicillin plus ceftriaxone plus vancomycin
      - Ampicillin: 2 g IV q4h
      - Ceftriaxone: 2 g IV q12h
      - Vancomycin: 30 to 45 mg/kg/day IV divided q6h
      - If severe penicillin allergy: TMP-SMX plus vancomycin
  - Penicillin G
    - Effective if the isolate is penicillin-sensitive minimum inhibitory concentration [MIC] <0.1 μg/mL)
    - Penicillin can be used if the isolate has a penicillin MIC of <0.1 μg/mL.
    - For isolates with a penicillin MIC of 0.1 to 1 μg/mL, a 3rd-generation cephalosporin is preferred.
    - Penicillin G: 4 million units IV q4h (pediatric dose: 0.25 mU/kg/day IV divided q4–6h) or ampicillin: 2 g IV q4h (pediatric dose: 200 to 300 mg/kg/day IV divided q6h)
    - Duration of treatment: 7 days
- Dexamethasone
  - Indications
    - Known or suspected pneumococcal meningitis in selected adults
    - Children with H. influenzae type B meningitis
  - Dexamethasone is often given initially in adults and children with suspected bacterial meningitis while awaiting microbiologic study results.
  - Dexamethasone has not been shown to be of benefit in meningococcal meningitis and should be discontinued once the diagnosis is established.
  - Dosage
    - Infants and children >6 weeks old: IV 0.15 mg/kg/dose q6h for the first 2 to 4 days of antibiotic treatment
    - Start 10 to 20 minutes before or with the first dose of antibiotic.

- Chemoprophylaxis
  - Indications
    - Close contacts: those with prolonged (>8 hours) close contact (<3 feet) to the patient or those directly exposed to the patient's oral secretions between 1 week before the onset of the patient's symptoms and until 24 hours after initiation of appropriate antibiotic therapy (2)
    - No chemoprophylaxis is indicated for casual contacts, including most health care workers, unless exposed to respiratory secretions.
  - Timing
    - Ideally <24 hours after case identification; Chemoprophylaxis not indicated if >14 d from exposure.
  - Prophylactic regimens; ciprofloxacin-resistant, β-lactamase-producing N. meningitidis serogroup Y cases are on the rise in the United States (1); the CDC recommends considering antimicrobial susceptibility testing on meningococcal isolates to inform prophylaxis decisions.
    - Rifampin, ciprofloxacin, and ceftriaxone
      - Ceftriaxone
        - Recommended for pregnant women
        - Adults: 250 mg IM as a single dose; <15 years of age: 125 mg IM as a single dose
      - Rifampin (meningococcal prophylaxis)
        - Adult: 600 mg IV or PO q12h for 2 days
        - Pediatric
          - <1 month: 10 mg/kg/day in divided doses q12h for 2 days
          - Infants and children: 20 mg/kg/day in divided doses q12h for 2 days (max 600 mg/dose)
      - Ciprofloxacin
        - Adults: 500 mg PO as a single dose
- Vaccination
  - For household contacts (if the case is from a vaccine-preventable serogroup)
- Precautions
  - Adjust the dosage of medications in patients with severe renal dysfunction.
  - Additional treatment may be needed to eliminate nasopharyngeal colonization.

Second Line

- For meningitis
  - Chloramphenicol: 1 g IV q6h (pediatric dose: 75 to 100 mg/kg/day divided q6h) or ceftriaxone 2 g IV q12h (pediatric dose: 80 to 100 mg/kg/day divided q12–24h)
  - In large outbreaks, a single dose of long-acting chloramphenicol has been used. Single-dose ceftriaxone shows equal efficacy in one randomized controlled trial.
- Precautions
  - Ceftriaxone should not be used in patients with a history of anaphylactic reactions to penicillin (e.g., hypotension, laryngeal edema, wheezing, hives).
  - Chloramphenicol may cause aplastic anemia.

ISSUES FOR REFERRAL

Potential complications

- Seizure activity
- DIC; acute respiratory distress syndrome
- Renal failure; adrenal failure; multisystem organ failure

ADMISSION, INPATIENT, AND NURSING CONSIDERATIONS

- Begin antibiotics (± corticosteroids) and obtain LP immediately if meningitis is suspected.
- Droplet isolation for 24 hours after starting antibiotics
- IV fluids: Replace volume as needed; with septic shock, large volumes of crystalloid may be required.

 ONGOING CARE

PATIENT EDUCATION

Educate family and close contacts regarding the risk of contracting meningococcal infection.

PROGNOSIS

Overall mortality is 13%. Factors associated with poor prognosis include young age, hypotension, thrombocytopenia, altered mental status and leukopenia.

COMPLICATIONS

- DIC
- Acute tubular necrosis
- Neurologic: sensorineural hearing loss, cranial nerve palsy, seizures
- Obstructive hydrocephalus
- Subdural effusions
- Acute adrenal hemorrhage
- Waterhouse-Friderichsen syndrome

REFERENCES

1. Centers for Disease Control and Prevention. Meningococcal disease: technical and clinical information. https://www.cdc.gov/meningococcal/clinical-info.html. Accessed September 28, 2023.
2. Deghmane A-E, Taha S, Taha M-K. Global epidemiology and changing clinical presentations of invasive meningococcal disease: a narrative review. Infect Dis (Lond). 2021;54(1):1–7.
3. Fitzgerald D, Waterer GW. Invasive pneumococcal and meningococcal disease. Infect Dis Clin North Am. 2019;33(4):1125–1141.

 CODES

ICD10

- A39.4 Meningococcemia, unspecified
- A39.0 Meningococcal meningitis
- A39.2 Acute meningococcemia

CLINICAL PEARLS

- Invasive meningococcal disease can be rapidly fatal. Rapid identification and early treatment with antibiotics is essential to promote good clinical outcomes. Treat then test in suspected cases.
- Provide chemoprophylaxis to close contacts.
- All adolescents and children in high-risk groups should receive MenACWY vaccine. Meningitis B vaccines are recommended for high-risk children aged 10 years or older.

M

MENISCAL INJURY

Jennifer Schwartz, MD

BASICS

DESCRIPTION
- The menisci are fibrocartilaginous structures between the femoral condyles and the tibial plateaus.
- The menisci help to stabilize the knee (with the anterior cruciate ligament [ACL]) and distribute forces across the joint to provide shock absorption.
- Meniscal tears can lead to knee pain and disability and, ultimately, are a risk factor for the development of knee osteoarthritis (OA).

Pediatric Considerations
- Meniscal injuries are less common in children aged <10 years. In this population, they are often due to a discoid meniscus.
- MRI is still the study of choice but is less sensitive and specific for diagnosing meniscal tears in children aged <12 years.
- Increased BMI in pediatric patients correlates with more complex tears and lower repair success rates.

EPIDEMIOLOGY
Bimodal age distribution—young athletes (traumatic) and older patients (degenerative)

Incidence
Medial meniscus more commonly injured

Prevalence
- One of the most common musculoskeletal injuries
- Meniscal surgery is the most common type of orthopedic surgery performed in the United States.

ETIOLOGY AND PATHOPHYSIOLOGY
- Traumatic tears are acute. They generally occur due to a twisting motion of the knee with foot planted.
  - Common in younger patients (aged <40 years) without underlying knee OA
  - Manifests with sudden pain
- Degenerative tears are chronic. They generally occur with overuse and minimal trauma.
  - There is an age related increase in prevalence, and they are often comorbid with knee OA.
  - Symptoms evolve slowly.

Genetics
No specific gene locus has been identified.

RISK FACTORS
- Nonmodifiable risk factors: male, discoid meniscus, ligamentous laxity
- Traumatic tear:
  - High degree of physical activity (especially cutting sports)
  - ACL insufficiency
- Degenerative tear:
  - Increased age (>60 years)
  - Obesity
  - Work-related kneeling/squatting/climbing stairs

GENERAL PREVENTION
- Treatment and rehabilitation of previous knee injuries, particularly ACL injuries
- Strengthening and increased flexibility of quadriceps and hamstring muscles
- Weight management

COMMONLY ASSOCIATED CONDITIONS
- Traumatic tear: ACL concomitantly torn in 1/3 of cases
- Degenerative tear: OA, Baker cyst (greater association with medial meniscal tears)

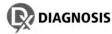DIAGNOSIS

HISTORY
- Medial or lateral knee pain and swelling (increased with knee flexion)
- Noncontact twisting mechanism of injury (if trauma present)
- ±Mechanical symptoms (i.e., locking, catching)
  - In young patients, it is often due to entrapped meniscal tissue after a trauma; in older patients, may also be due to degenerative factors or OA

PHYSICAL EXAM
- Effusion—typically >24 hours postinjury
- Joint line tenderness (medial and/or lateral)
- Decreased range of motion of knee, pain with full flexion (posterior horn tear) or extension (anterior horn tear)
- Accuracy of special tests (McMurray test, Apley grind test) varies.

DIFFERENTIAL DIAGNOSIS
- ACL or collateral ligament tear
- Pathologic plica
- Osteochondritis dissecans
- Loose body or fracture
- OA
- Patellofemoral syndrome

DIAGNOSTIC TESTS & INTERPRETATION
- Plain radiographs can detect fractures, loose bodies, or arthritic changes.
- Ultrasound may help to identify meniscal tears.
- MRI is the primary imaging test for detecting meniscal tears.

Follow-Up Tests & Special Considerations
Meniscal tears are often found incidentally on MRI and may not always be the cause of a patient's symptoms—important to correlate history, physical exam, and imaging findings.
- Asymptomatic tears are more common in middle-aged/older patients and those with OA.

Diagnostic Procedures/Other
Arthroscopy may be needed if the MRI is indeterminate.

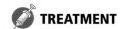TREATMENT

GENERAL MEASURES
- Nonoperative management is recommended as first-line treatment for most meniscal tears. This includes the following:
  - Rest, ice, activity modification
  - OTC medication
  - Physical therapy (PT)
  - Intra-articular corticosteroid injections
- Multiple trials have shown no increased benefit to surgery versus PT in patients aged >40 years with degenerative meniscal tears (1)[A].
- In young/active patients with meniscal tears, early surgery is not always superior to PT.

MEDICATION
First Line
- NSAIDs (i.e., ibuprofen up to 800 mg PO TID, naproxen [Naprosyn] 500 mg PO BID) or acetaminophen (Tylenol)
- Corticosteroid injection (5 cc lidocaine plus 1 cc methylprednisolone acetate [Depo-Medrol] [80 mg/mL] or equivalent)

ISSUES FOR REFERRAL
Surgical consultation for patients not improving with PT or wishing surgical repair

ADDITIONAL THERAPIES
- Weight control
- Platelet-rich plasma (PRP) injections may improve symptoms from degenerative meniscal tears.

SURGERY/OTHER PROCEDURES
- Consider surgical intervention if:
  - Concurrent injuries (i.e., ACL tear)
  - Mechanical symptoms (knee "catching" or "locking")
    - Early surgery may be most effective in alleviating subjective mechanical symptoms in patients aged <40 years (2)[B].
    - No benefit to early surgery for alleviating mechanical symptoms in older patients.
  - No improvement with conservative treatment
- Meniscal preservation surgery (i.e., meniscal repair or replacement) is preferred in older patients and may have better outcomes than meniscectomy (3)[B].
  - Will better preserve knee biomechanics and delay progression of OA
- Meniscectomy (removal of injured portion of meniscus) can lead to articular cartilage degeneration and OA.

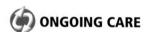 ONGOING CARE

FOLLOW-UP RECOMMENDATIONS
Return to play requires the athlete to be pain free, have full range of motion, and have full strength.

PATIENT EDUCATION
Patients should be aware of the risks and benefits of surgery compared with conservative treatment.

PROGNOSIS
Following meniscal repair, patients can generally return to activities in 3 to 6 months. Prognosis is better if tear is peripheral/lateral and <2.5 cm.

COMPLICATIONS
Meniscectomies increase the risk of developing OA.

REFERENCES
1. Rotini M, Papalia G, Setaro N, et al. Arthroscopic surgery or exercise therapy for degenerative meniscal lesions: a systematic review of systematic reviews. *Musculoskel Surg*. 2023;107(2):127–141.
2. Damsted C, Thorlund JB, Hölmich P, et al. Effect of exercise therapy versus surgery on mechanical symptoms in young patietns with a meniscal tear: a secondary analysis of the DREAM trial. *Br J Sports Med*. 2023;57(9):521–527.
3. Husen M, Kennedy NI, Till S, et al. Benefits of meniscal repair in selected patients aged 60 years and older. *Orthop J Sports Med*. 2022;10(9).

ADDITIONAL READING
- Noorduyn JCA, van de Graaf VA, Willigenburg NW, et al. Effect of physical therapy vs arthroscopic partial meniscectomy in people with degenerative meniscal tears: five-year follow-up of the ESCAPE randomized clinical trial. *JAMA Netw Open*. 2022;5(7):e2220394.
- Rohde MA, Shea KG, Dawson T, et al. Age, sex, and BMI differences related to repairable meniscal tears in pediatric and adolescent patients. *Am J Sports Med*. 2023;51(2):389–397.
- Sihvonen R, Paavola M, Malmivaara A, et al; for FIDELITY (Finnish Degenerative Meniscus Lesion Study) Investigators. Arthroscopic partial meniscectomy for a degenerative meniscus tear: a 5-year follow-up of the placebo-surgery controlled FIDELITY (Finnish Degenerative Meniscus Lesion Study) trial. *Br J Sports Med*. 2020;54(22):1332–1339.

 SEE ALSO

Algorithm: Knee Pain

 CODES

ICD10
- S83.209A Unsp tear of unsp meniscus, current injury, unsp knee, init
- S83.249A Oth tear of medial meniscus, current injury, unsp knee, init
- S83.289A Oth tear of lat mensc, current injury, unsp knee, init

CLINICAL PEARLS
- Chronic/degenerative meniscal tears are common in patients >40 years old and are associated with knee OA.
- Acute/traumatic meniscal tears are more common in young athletes.
- Conservative management is generally preferred as first-line treatment for meniscal tears. This includes PT/education with the option of later surgery.
- MRI is imaging modality of choice to identify meniscal tears.
- In patients opting for surgery, meniscal repairs have a better functional outcome and a decreased risk of OA compared with meniscectomy.

M

MENOPAUSE
Madeline Taskier, MD

BASICS

DESCRIPTION
- Natural menopause: 12 consecutive months of amenorrhea in a nonpregnant person with a uterus ≥40 years old; mean age of 51 years; resulting from loss of ovarian activity
- Perimenopause/menopausal transition (MT): the onset of irregular menses to the final menstrual cycle; begins on average 4 years before menopause; mean age of 47 years
- Postmenopause: usually >1/3 of a woman's life
- Primary ovarian insufficiency: irregularity or cessation of ovulatory cycles before age 40 years
- Surgical menopause: removal of hormone-producing ovaries leading to immediate menopause

EPIDEMIOLOGY
- The median age of menopause is 51 years in the United States.
- 5% of people with a uterus undergo menopause after age 55 years; another 5% between ages 40 and 45 years
- Occurs earlier in Hispanic patients and later in Japanese American patients as compared with Caucasians

Incidence
In the United States, 1.3 million patients reach menopause annually.

ETIOLOGY AND PATHOPHYSIOLOGY
- As women age, the number of ovarian follicles decreases. Ovarian production of estrogen varies and then decreases. Follicle-stimulating hormone (FSH) production varies and then increases.
- Insufficient estradiol production leads to the absence of the luteinizing hormone (LH) surge, resulting in anovulation. Anovulation causes lack of progesterone production.
- Failure to produce estradiol leads to thinning of endometrial lining and eventually menstruation ceases.
- Estrone (produced by adipose tissue) becomes the dominant form of estrogen during menopause.

RISK FACTORS
Oophorectomy/hysterectomy; sex chromosome abnormalities (e.g., Turner syndrome and fragile X syndrome); family history of early menopause; smoking (earlier age of onset by 2 years); chemotherapy and/or pelvic radiation; low body mass index (BMI)

GENERAL PREVENTION
Menopause is a physiologic event and cannot be prevented. It is associated with increased risk of long-term medical issues, including cardiovascular disease (CVD) and osteoporotic fractures.
- Decrease risk of CVD by increasing exercise; maintaining healthy diet and a healthy weight; avoiding tobacco use; and treating hypertension, hyperlipidemia, and diabetes mellitus.
- Decrease risk of osteoporotic fractures with weight-bearing exercise and fall prevention, avoidance of smoking and excessive alcohol intake, dietary calcium of 1,200 mg/day, and adequate vitamin D intake.

DIAGNOSIS

12 consecutive months of amenorrhea in a nonpregnant woman ≥40 years of age

HISTORY
- Cessation of menses: generally preceded by irregular cycles with heavy bleeding followed by diminished bleeding
- Vasomotor symptoms reported by 80%:
  - Sudden unpleasant feeling of heat and sweating, most commonly over face, neck, and chest, typically lasting 1 to 5 minutes; intervals unpredictable (1)
  - Associated with clamminess, anxiety, and heart palpitations
  - Generally begin 2 years before the final menstrual period, peak during 1 year after the final menstrual period, and then diminish
  - Frequency and duration vary: 87% of women who report flushes experience them daily; ~33% have >10 per day. Mean duration of symptoms lasts 4 to 10.2 years and may begin during MT and extend well past menopause.
  - Varies with ethnicity: greatest in African and Hispanic women and least in Asian women
  - More common in patients with comorbid obesity
- Genitourinary syndrome of menopause:
  - Vulvovaginal atrophy in 50%:
    ○ Vaginal/vulvar dryness, itching, dyspareunia, and possible sexual dysfunction
    ○ Alkaline vaginal pH and atrophy increases risk of vaginal infections and urinary tract infections.
- Anxiety/depression: New diagnosis of depression is 2.5 times more likely during the MT as compared to premenopause.
- Sleep disturbance: arousal from sleep, chronic sleep disruption, and chronic insomnia
- Change in intensity and severity of migraines
- Skin thinning, mild hirsutism, brittle nails

Geriatric Considerations
Vaginal bleeding in postmenopausal patients is abnormal; endometrial cancer/endometrioid adenocarcinoma (EAC) must be ruled out.

PHYSICAL EXAM
- Decrease in breast size and change in breast texture
- Genitourinary exam: atrophic vulva and vaginal mucosa; possible signs of uterine prolapse with Valsalva maneuvers

DIFFERENTIAL DIAGNOSIS
Pregnancy, thyroid diseases, pituitary adenoma, Sheehan syndrome, hypothalamic dysfunction, anorexia nervosa, Asherman syndrome, and obstruction of uterine outflow tract

DIAGNOSTIC TESTS & INTERPRETATION
Initial Tests (lab, imaging)
- Lab testing for menopause is not required; age and symptoms establish the diagnosis.
- Lab tests appropriate in age <45 years if premature/early menopause suspected or to rule out other causes of oligomenorrhea/amenorrhea:
  - Elevated serum FSH level >30 mIU/mL indicates ovarian failure.
  - Symptoms may precede lab changes.
- Infertility evaluation: may use elevated day 3 FSH, decreased antimüllerian hormone levels, and decreased antral follicle count to predict decreased ovarian reserve
- Estrogens, androgens, and oral contraceptive pills (OCPs) may alter lab results.

Follow-Up Tests & Special Considerations
- Pregnancy test
- TSH and prolactin level if pituitary disease is suspected
- Abnormal uterine bleeding, including postmenopausal bleeding, should be evaluated by TVUS and/or EMB. If endometrial stripe is <5 mm on TVUS, EAC is unlikely.
- Breast cancer screening: U.S. Preventive Services Task Force (USPSTF) recommends mammogram every 2 years from ages 50 to 74 years. Women with a strong family history of breast cancer in a first-degree relative may warrant earlier screening. The American College of Obstetricians and Gynecologists (ACOG) recommends mammogram every 1 to 2 years from ages 40 to 75 years. The American Cancer Society recommends annual mammogram for ages 45 to 54 years and then every other year for ages ≥55 years until life expectancy is <10 years.
- Osteoporosis screening: USPSTF recommends bone mineral density (BMD) screening with dual energy x-ray absorptiometry (DEXA) scan in women >65 years or <65 years if the risk for fracture is equivalent to that of a 65-year-old woman (using the FRAX tool to assess, https://www.sheffield.ac.uk/FRAX/). Risk factors include a previous history of fractures, low body weight, cigarette smoking, and family history of osteoporotic fracture.

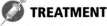

TREATMENT

GENERAL MEASURES
Behavioral modifications to manage vasomotor symptoms including lowering ambient temperature settings, wearing layered clothing, and avoiding possible triggers (heat, stress, caffeine, alcohol, tobacco, spicy foods); during vasomotor episodes, portable fans or ice packs and relaxation techniques such as deep breathing have also been shown to be helpful.

MEDICATION
First Line
Hormone therapy (HT): most effective treatment for vasomotor symptoms and has been shown to prevent bone loss and fracture (2); developing an individual risk-benefit profile is essential, factoring in age, time from menopause, severity of symptoms, and CVD risk factors (3). For patients who are <60 years old or within 10 years of menopause onset, the risk-benefit profile is more favorable for HT. Treatment goal is to minimize menopausal symptoms to improve quality of life (2).
- HT can reduce weekly hot flush frequency by ~75%.
- HT may also help with disrupted sleep and urogenital atrophy.
- Long-term use of hormone replacement therapy has more risks than benefits, including breast, ovarian, and endometrial cancer; venous thromboembolism; CVD; and gallbladder disease.

- Less worrisome side effects include breast tenderness, vaginal bleeding, bloating, headaches.
- HT should be individualized with the lowest effective dose for the shortest duration of time needed to relieve vasomotor symptoms (1). Lower doses have similar symptom reduction profiles for many patients. Results of ultra-low-dose regimens are mixed.
- Estrogen is available orally, transdermally (patch, gel, or spray), intravaginally (rings), or intramuscularly. Treatment regimens include but are not limited to:
  - Low dose: conjugated equine estrogen (CEE) 0.30 to 0.45 mg/day or micronized estradiol 17β 0.5 mg/day or transdermal estradiol 17β 0.025 mg/day
  - Max dose: CEE 0.625 mg/day or micronized estradiol 17β 1.0 mg/day or transdermal estradiol 17β 0.10 mg/day
  - Transdermal estradiol spray: 1.53 mg per spray; start at 1 spray per day and increase to 3 sprays per day. Transdermal estradiol gel should be applied on a large area of skin.
  - Intravaginal estradiol: vaginal ring, inserted every 3 months, releasing 0.05 to 0.10 mg/day
  - Injectable estrogen: estradiol cypionate 1 to 5 mg or estradiol valerate 10 to 20 mg every 4 weeks
- In patients with an intact uterus, give estrogen with progestin because unopposed estrogen carries an increased risk of EAC. Micronized progesterone 100 to 200 mg/day can be used as progestin; alternative: medroxyprogesterone acetate (MPA) 2.5 mg/day
- Combination forms are available as oral pills or transdermally. Oral pills are available with CEE, estradiol, or micronized estradiol as the estrogen source and drospirenone, MPA, norethindrone, or norgestimate as the progestin source. Combination estradiol/progestin transdermal treatments have either levonorgestrel or norethindrone as progestin source.
- Tissue-selective estrogen complex: bazedoxifene (selective estrogen receptor modulator [SERM]) + conjugated estrogens; provides endometrial protection without need for progesterone for relief of vasomotor symptoms and bone loss prevention
- MenoPro app is from The North American Menopause Society (NAMS). It has two modes: one for clinicians and one for patients to aid in shared decision-making to evaluate CVD and cancer risk.
- Precautions:
  - The Women's Health Initiative (WHI) study demonstrated that women who take CEE with MPA versus placebo had increased CHD events, invasive breast cancer, stroke, pulmonary embolism, dementia, gallbladder disease, and urinary incontinence; benefits included decreased hip fractures, diabetes, and vasomotor symptoms.
  - Breast cancer risk is not seen until 5 years of use.
  - Women on estrogen alone had no increased risk of invasive breast cancer but did increase abnormal mammograms requiring follow-up investigations.
  - HRT should not be used for cardioprotective benefit as risk outweighs benefit.

  - Higher doses of estrogen can cause hypercoagulability, breast tenderness, gallbladder disease, and hypertension.
  - Contraindications to HT: estrogen-dependent malignancies; unexplained uterine bleeding or untreated endometrial hyperplasia; history of thromboembolism, stroke, or other coagulopathy; coronary artery disease; active liver disease; untreated hypertension; current or past breast cancer; smoking
- For genitourinary syndrome of menopause:
  - Topical estrogen reverses vaginal atrophy, enhances blood flow, and reduces urinary tract infections. Continue for as long as distressing symptoms remain. Initiate treatment daily for 1 to 2 weeks and then decrease to 2 times weekly; comes as estradiol cream, tablet, or ring; no evidence of difference in efficacy between various intravaginal estrogenic preparations; apply vaginally:
    - Ospemifene: 60 mg PO daily; SERM for moderate to severe dyspareunia associated with vaginal atrophy
    - Estradiol cream 0.01% (1 g), conjugated estrogen 0.625 mg/g (0.5 g), vaginal tablet (10 μg) used twice weekly, or vaginal ring (7.5 μg daily lasting for 3 months)
    - Nonestrogen vaginal lubricant may be as effective as topical estrogen for some.

Second Line
Nonhormonal treatments may be helpful to treat vasomotor symptoms:
- Paroxetine (7.5 mg/day): approved for treatment of vasomotor symptoms; shows modest decrease in hot flushes
- Other SSRI/SRNIs: Venlafaxine (37.5 to 100.0 mg/day) or fluoxetine (20 mg/day) and citalopram (20 mg/day) reduce hot flushes compared to placebo.
- Gabapentin (300 to 900 mg/day) decreases hot flushes compared to placebo.
- Clonidine (0.05 mg BID) may be used to treat mild hot flashes, less effective than SSRI/SRNIs.
- Note that most trials of second-line therapies have been brief (i.e., a few months).

COMPLEMENTARY & ALTERNATIVE MEDICINE
- Phytoestrogens, herbs, and other supplements do not have clear benefit in relieving menopause symptoms compared to placebo. Some may interact with anticoagulants, like warfarin, so they should be used with caution.
- Hypnotherapy and mindfulness meditation may provide relief for some.
- Acupuncture has not been shown to be more effective than simulated acupuncture for relieving hot flashes.
- Yoga has not been shown to relieve hot flashes but may be helpful for some symptoms associated with menopause.
- Compounded bioidentical HT should be avoided, given concerns about safety, including possibility of overdosing or underdosing, lack of efficacy and safety studies, and lack of a label providing risks (2).
- Overall, most data involve short-term trials, so little is known about their long-term safety. But, mind-body practices such as acupuncture, hypnosis, meditation, and yoga generally have good safety records.

ONGOING CARE

FOLLOW-UP RECOMMENDATIONS
Patient Monitoring
If HRT is initiated, consider decrease or discontinuation after 3 to 5 years to minimize risks.

DIET
Calcium-rich diet and vitamin D supplementation (800 to 1,000 IU/day) to prevent osteoporosis.

PATIENT EDUCATION
- Smoking cessation, reducing alcohol intake
- Exercise >30 minutes, 3 times weekly
- Healthy nutrition to prevent CVD and maintain healthy BMI

PROGNOSIS
If untreated, vasomotor symptoms will resolve, but vaginal/vulvar atrophy will worsen.

COMPLICATIONS
- Osteoporosis: accelerated bone loss up to 3–5% per year for 5 to 7 years
- Increased risk of CVD following menopause

REFERENCES
1. ACOG Practice Bulletin No. 141: management of menopausal symptoms. *Obstet Gynecol*. 2014;123(1):202–216.
2. North American Menopause Society. The 2022 hormone therapy position statement of the North American Menopause Society. *Menopause*. 2022;29(7):767–794.
3. Cobin RH, Goodman NF; for AACE Reproductive Endocrinology Scientific Committee. American Association of Clinical Endocrinologists and American College of Endocrinology position statement on menopause–2017 update. *Endor Pract*. 2017;23(7):869–880.

 CODES

ICD10
- E28.310 Symptomatic premature menopause
- N95.1 Menopausal and female climacteric states
- Z78.0 Asymptomatic menopausal state

CLINICAL PEARLS
- Menopause is usually diagnosed by history alone.
- HT can be used short term for relief of moderate to severe vasomotor symptoms. Use the lowest effective dose for the shortest duration of time.
- In patients with an intact uterus, give estrogen with progestin because unopposed estrogen increases the risk of endometrial hyperplasia or cancer.

M

MENORRHAGIA (HEAVY MENSTRUAL BLEEDING)

Daniel R. Matta, MD • Thandi Walters, MD

 BASICS

This topic will focus on heavy menstrual bleeding (HMB) in nonpregnant reproductive-aged women.

DESCRIPTION

- HMB is a form of abnormal uterine bleeding (AUB) and is an abnormality of the volume of menstrual blood loss; this volume as defined by clinical trials is >80 mL of blood lost per cycle.
- Clinically, menstrual blood loss is not commonly measured, and HMB is more subjectively defined as "excessive menstrual blood loss that physically, emotionally, socially, and financially affects the quality of life of women." It is based on how this deviation from normal menstrual blood volume causes disruption of the patient's life.
- There is a consensus to abandon the use of the term *menorrhagia* as it is found to be confusing.

EPIDEMIOLOGY

- AUB is a common complaint with a prevalence of 20–30% and is one of the leading causes of outpatient gynecological visits. About 1 in 5 women in the United States experience HMB. The prevalence varies with age and is higher in adolescence and during the 5th decade of life.
- A 2019 study of 306 women conducted in the outpatient internal medicine department of a training and research university hospital found that a prevalence of HMB in women of reproductive age was 37.9%.
- HMB is linked to decreased quality of life and increased health care costs.

Incidence

HMB can present as an acute or chronic condition.

ETIOLOGY AND PATHOPHYSIOLOGY

- Any process that interferes with normal hemostatic, endocrine, or paracrine functions of the endometrium or interferes with myometrial contractility can cause HMB.
- The pathophysiology of HMB is outlined with reference to the International Federation of Gynecology and Obstetrics (FIGO) PALM-COEIN classification system of AUB. More research needs to be done to elaborate the many causes of this condition.
- HMB can be caused by structural issues such as the PALM acronym:
  – Polyp (AUB-P)
  – Adenomyosis (AUB-A)
  – Leiomyoma (AUB-L)
  – Malignancy/hyperplasia (AUB-M)
- Excessive estrogen stimulation likely causes polyps, which are abnormal outgrowths of hypertrophied endometrial tissue. It does not demonstrate the normal cyclical changes of normal endometrium causing irregular and intermenstrual HMB.
- Adenomyosis may cause HMB by affecting normal myometrial contraction, but the exact cause is unknown.

- Leiomyomas are common benign myometrial neoplasms thought to form as a result of chromosomal abnormalities and grow in response to estrogen and progesterone. The exact cause for HMB lacks sufficient evidence to support the many proposed theories.
- Excess estrogen can promote endometrial hyperplasia.
- It can also be caused by nonstructural causes which include COEIN acronym:
  – Coagulopathy (AUB-C)
  – Ovulatory (AUB-O)
  – Endometrial (AUB-E)
  – Iatrogenic (AUB-I)
  – Not yet classified (AUB-N)
- Ovulatory dysfunction is associated with a thick stratum functionalis caused by excessive estrogen stimulation of the endometrium. Endometrial shedding tends to be noncyclical with irregular bleeding noted.
- HMB can also be classified as ovulatory or anovulatory bleeding.

Genetics

Pediatric Considerations

Due to immaturity of the hypothalamic-pituitary-ovarian axis, adolescents are at risk of irregular and HMB. Of note, adolescents with heavy bleeding should be evaluated for possible bleeding disorders, especially von Willebrand disease and qualitative platelet dysfunction.

RISK FACTORS

Obesity

GENERAL PREVENTION

- Combined oral contraceptives may prevent HMB particularly when progesterone is dominant. Lower estrogen doses result in less menstrual bleeding.
- Progesterone-only contraceptives may reduce overall blood loss but often result in irregular bleeding.

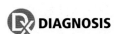 **DIAGNOSIS**

The first part of diagnosis involves a thorough history and physical exam.

HISTORY

- It is important to obtain a proper understanding of the patient's bleeding episode and to ask questions focused on PALM-COEIN etiologies to determine the patient's cause of abnormal bleeding.
- Menstrual history should try to estimate cycle length, duration, variability and quantity of blood loss. To determine the quantity of blood loss, pads changed every 2 to 3 hours represents at least 80 mL of blood loss. The presence and size of clots or the sensation of "flooding" are also surrogate indicators of excessive blood loss.

- There are screening tools which can be used to identify possible coagulopathy as a cause of heavy bleeding.
- This includes identifying HMB since menarche; two or more of family history of bleeding symptoms, frequent gum bleeding, epistaxis 1 to 2 times per month, or bruising 2 times per month; plus one of the following: bleeding associated with dental work, surgery-related bleeding, or postpartum hemorrhage
- The screen is positive if the patient answered yes to any of the above categories and warrants further testing and hematology referral.
- Anovulatory bleeding is noted to be irregular and unpredictable, and the patient lacks typical ovulatory symptoms such as midcycle pain or premenstrual symptoms.

PHYSICAL EXAM

- If the patient has acute blood loss, the exam should begin by assessing for life-threatening signs of hemodynamic instability.
- One can look for possible causes of AUB by observing obesity, assessing the thyroid gland, and examining the skin for signs of bleeding disorders such as petechiae and ecchymoses. Also, assess for signs of hyperandrogenism such as hirsutism and acne.
- Perform a speculum examination and look for other sites of bleeding by thoroughly inspecting the vulva, urethra, vagina, anus, and perineum. Note signs of trauma like lacerations. It is also prudent to note any hemorrhoids as a possible source of bleeding.
- Bimanual exam is done to feel for uterine or cervical abnormalities or enlargement. Pelvic and adnexal masses would also be palpated during this exam.

DIFFERENTIAL DIAGNOSIS

- Normal menses
- Complication of pregnancy
- Other sources of bleeding (e.g., cervical, vaginal, gastrointestinal)

DIAGNOSTIC TESTS & INTERPRETATION

Initial Tests (lab, imaging)

- Initial testing on all patients should include pregnancy test and CBC.
- If the patient is acutely bleeding heavily, type and crossmatch should be ordered.
- Other tests may include PT/INR, PTT, TSH with reflex T_4, CMPi, Iron studies, and STI panel.
- Labs to consider in select cases; for suspected coagulopathy:
  – Workup for von Willebrand disease: plasma vWF antigen, plasma vWF activity (ristocetin cofactor activity)
  – vWF: RCo activity and vWF collagen binding, factor VIII, and other factor testing (1)
  – For ovulatory dysfunction: thyroid function testing, human chorionic gonadotropin, prolactin, and follicle-stimulating hormone
- Transvaginal ultrasound; additional imaging at clinicians discretion

Follow-Up Tests & Special Considerations
- Saline infusion sonohysterography, diagnostic hysterography, and hysterosalpingography can be performed to diagnose endometrial polyps and submucosal leiomyoma (1).
- MRI can be performed to better visualize the changes of adenomyosis and determine if uterine-sparing treatment is an option in patients with leiomyoma (1). MRI can also detect leiomyosarcoma.

Diagnostic Procedures/Other
If a patient is aged >40 years or <40 years with high risk factors endometrial biopsy with or without hysteroscopy is performed for possible endometrial hyperplasia or carcinoma (2).

TREATMENT

MEDICATION

First Line
- Acute bleeding
  - Conjugated equine estrogen 25 mg IV q4–6h for 24 hours with IV antiemetic agents
  - Monophasic 35-mg estrogen-containing OCP TID for 7 days and then 1 daily
  - Medroxyprogesterone 20 mg or norethindrone 20 mg TID for 7 days
  - Tranexamic acid 10 mg/kg IV (maximum of 600 mg per dose) or 1.5 g PO q8h for 5 days
- Chronic bleeding
  - Ibuprofen 600 mg q6h or 800 mg q8h; naproxen 500 mg initially and repeat 3 to 5 hours later and then 250 to 500 mg BID; mefenamic acid 500 mg TID (with food)
  - Monophasic 30- to 35-mg estrogen-containing OCP daily with or without inert pills
  - Medroxyprogesterone 5 to 10 mg or norethindrone 5 to 10 mg daily
  - Depot medroxyprogesterone 150 mg subcutaneously q3mo; levonorgestrel 19.5- to 52.0-mg intrauterine devices (3)[A] (19.5-mg LNG IUS is a slightly smaller device); etonogestrel subdermal implant

Second Line
Danazol, GnRH agonists, aromatase inhibitors, selective estrogen receptor modulators (SERMs), and selective progesterone receptor modulators (SPRMs) are used as second-line agents in management of bleeding caused by leiomyoma and adenomyosis. Of note, SPRMs are not currently available in the United States.

ISSUES FOR REFERRAL
Refer to gynecology if a primary care physician is uncomfortable placing an intrauterine device, performing endometrial sampling, there is persistent bleeding despite treatment, or malignancy is suspected.

ADDITIONAL THERAPIES
- Iron replacement therapy PO (preferred) or IV (if unable to tolerate oral) for anemia
- MRI-guided focused ultrasound (MgFUS) had been approved by the FDA for the treatment of uterine fibroids and has been used with success in decreasing bleeding in patients with adenomyosis.

SURGERY/OTHER PROCEDURES
- Dilation and curettage can be considered in the setting of acute severe bleeding.
- Surgical procedures are directed to the specific identified pathology.
  - Endometrial and cervical polyps—polypectomy
  - Adenomyosis—hysterectomy
  - Leiomyoma—for women who do not desire fertility, laparoscopic radiofrequency ablation, uterine artery embolization, or hysterectomy can be performed; for women who desire fertility, myomectomy is preferred.
  - Malignancy—hysterectomy with or without adjuvant chemotherapy and radiotherapy
- Conservative surgery (i.e., myomectomy, endometrial ablation, or uterine artery embolization) is more effective for controlling bleeding symptoms at 1 and 2 years than oral medications or the levonorgestrel-releasing IUD, but by 5 years, there is no difference in long-term results or patient satisfaction.
- Hysterectomy is curative but with more severe adverse effects and is typically reserved for failure of medical management or presence of another indication such as malignancy.

REFERENCES

1. Marnach ML, Laughlin-Tommaso SK. Evaluation and management of abnormal uterine bleeding. *Mayo Clin Proc.* 2019;94(2):326–335.
2. Cheong Y, Cameron IT, Critchley HO. Abnormal uterine bleeding. *Br Med Bull.* 2019;131(1):119.
3. Sangkomkamhang US, Lumbiganon P, Pattanittum P. Progestogens or progestogen-releasing intra-uterine systems for uterine fibroids (other than preoperative medical therapy). *Cochrane Database Syst Rev.* 2020;11(11):CD008994.

ADDITIONAL READING

Centers for Disease Control and Prevention. Bleeding disorders in women: free materials about signs and symptoms. https://www.cdc.gov/ncbddd/blooddisorders/women/materials/better-you-know-freematerials.html. Accessed September 25, 2023.

 CODES

ICD10
- N92.0 Excessive and frequent menstruation with regular cycle
- N92.3 Ovulation bleeding
- N92.2 Excessive menstruation at puberty

CLINICAL PEARLS
- HMB is often associated with a structural uterine disorder.
- A thorough history and physical examination is a key part of determining the cause of AUB.
- The treatment of AUB should take the cause of the bleeding into consideration as well as the severity of symptoms and the patient's desire for fertility.
- The goal of initial therapy is to stop bleeding, to treat anemia, and to restore quality of life.

M

MESOTHELIOMA

William Edwin Martin, MD, MBA, MPH • Kristen EB Said, MD, MPH

 BASICS

DESCRIPTION

- Mesothelioma is a rare, insidious, and aggressive malignancy of the mesothelial or serous tissues primarily found in the pleura (80–95%), peritoneum (5–20%), and rarely, the tunica vaginalis and pericardium (1–2%).
- Inhalation of asbestos is the predominant cause of mesothelioma, most often from remote occupational exposure (≥20 years earlier).
- Histologically, there are three types of malignant mesothelioma: epithelioid type (most common and least aggressive), sarcomatoid type (most aggressive), and biphasic type.
- Mesothelioma has a rapidly fatal course (median survival 17 to 25 months for resectable pleural mesothelioma) (1).

EPIDEMIOLOGY

Incidence

- The incidence in the United States has recently begun to decline, a trend attributable to the delayed effects of the asbestos ban initiated in the 1970s.
- Globally, areas of endemic clustering persist, typically in regions with high levels of ongoing asbestos-related industry. Incidence rates are not available, however, due to lack of quality reporting data.
- Incidence increases with age, peaking in the 5th and 6th decade of life, with 70% of pleural disease occurring in males. Peritoneal involvement is slightly higher in women.
- There are 3,000 cases of mesothelioma diagnosed in the United States annually (1).

Prevalence

In the United States, 1 case per 100,000 persons without asbestos industry exposure and 2 to 3 per 100,000 persons with asbestos exposure (1).

ETIOLOGY AND PATHOPHYSIOLOGY

- The predominant cause of mesothelioma is exposure to asbestos (hydrated magnesium silicate fibrous minerals).
- The majority of asbestos fibers are either amphibole (needle-like) or serpentine (curved). All types are capable of causing mesothelioma, although amphiboles (particularly crocidolite and amosite) are more carcinogenic. Serpentine fibers, the predominant fiber type in the United States, are mostly found in ships, buildings, brake lining, and ceiling tiles (2).
- There is a long latent period, typically 20 to 50 years, between exposure and the development of mesothelioma (3).
- The pathogenesis of mesothelioma is multifactorial and not fully understood, but the predominant cause is via inhaled or ingested asbestos fibers becoming trapped in pleural or peritoneal membranes, causing irritation and inflammation. This continued tissue damage and inflammation leads to tumor formation (3).
- Tumors coalesce with a gradual progression from the parietal to visceral pleura and eventual invasion of surrounding structures (2).
- In addition to asbestos, tumors have arisen after prior radiation or exposure to talc, erionite, or mica or in patients with familial Mediterranean fever and diffuse lymphocytic leukemia.

Genetics

- A substantial percentage (>10%) of patients harbor germline mutations in cancer predisposition genes, notably BAP1. BAP1 mutations are linked to an inherited susceptibility to mesothelioma and a pattern of familial cancers. Patients may report an elevated personal or familial history of cancers, especially mesothelioma and uveal melanoma (1),(4).
- In addition to BAP1, other mutations have been associated with genetic predisposition, including MLH1, MLH3, TP53, BRAC2 (1),(4).

RISK FACTORS

- The predominant risk factor is exposure to asbestos with a dose-dependent risk.
- Occupational exposures involve mining or milling of fibers; work with textiles, cement, friction materials, or insulation; or shipbuilding.
- Nonoccupational exposures include renovation or destruction of asbestos-containing buildings, exposure to industrial sources in the community or natural geologic sources, or exposure to soiled clothing of asbestos workers.
- Radiation exposure, proximity to naturally occurring asbestos deposits, or inhalation of other fibrous silicates can contribute to malignant mesothelioma.
- In contrast to lung cancer and asbestosis, it appears to be no synergistic effect between smoking and the development of mesothelioma.

GENERAL PREVENTION

- Avoidance of asbestos exposure
- Strict adherence to protective protocols for workers in buildings where asbestos is found
- Continued aggressive remediation of asbestos-affected buildings and homes

DIAGNOSIS

Most often presenting symptoms are nonspecific; so, a thorough exposure history supported by imaging is most helpful.

HISTORY

- Symptoms are usually nonspecific and occur when disease is advanced, leading to delays in presentation.
- Pleural mesothelioma presents with gradual onset of pulmonary symptoms, such as, chest pain (chest wall invasion), breathlessness (pleural infusion), and cough. Fatigue, night sweats, anorexia, and weight loss may also be present and worsen with disease progression (3).
- Peritoneal disease presents with vague abdominal pain, increased abdominal girth, nausea, anorexia, and weight loss.
- Establishing a history of asbestos exposure is a challenge as patients may not remember potential exposure events 30 years prior. Asbestos-specific questionnaires may be helpful (2).
- Community and paraoccupational exposures must also be included. Questions pertaining to household contacts from workers, home renovations, non-industrial settings (e.g., schools), and nearby asbestos industries (e.g., mines and factories) (2),(3).

PHYSICAL EXAM

- Pulmonary findings consistent with pleural effusion, including decreased breath sounds, dullness to percussion, and asymmetric chest wall expansion
- Abdominal findings consistent with ascites, including abdominal distension, fluid wave, and tenderness are found in cases involving the peritoneum.
- Clubbing may be found in extremities.
- Neurologic findings consistent with spinal cord compression are possible.

DIFFERENTIAL DIAGNOSIS

- Pleural mesothelioma's differential diagnosis includes inflammatory reactions (empyema, pleural effusion), metastatic tumor from other sites, fibrosarcoma, malignant fibrous histiocytoma, sarcomatoid carcinoma, and synovial sarcoma.
- Peritoneal mesothelioma's differential diagnosis includes peritoneal carcinomatosis, serous peritoneal carcinoma, ovarian carcinoma in women, lymphomatosis, and tuberculous peritonitis.

DIAGNOSTIC TESTS & INTERPRETATION

Initial Tests (lab, imaging)

- Biomarkers may be elevated in mesothelioma, such as mesothelin; however, they require further study and do not have an established routine use in diagnosis or monitoring response to therapy (3).
- Chest x-ray is insensitive and nonspecific. Further imaging is often required (3).
- Pleural mesothelioma diagnosis requires tissue. Thoracentesis for cytology and closed pleural biopsy may be adequate, but often, more invasive procedures such as video-assisted thoracoscopic surgery (VATS) is needed to obtain an adequate specimen (1).

Follow-Up Tests & Special Considerations

- Seeding of biopsy sites and tracks may occur in mesothelioma. The usage of prophylactic radiotherapy has largely been discontinued in the wake of negative results from randomized controlled studies (3).
- Immunohistochemical panels help support the histopathologic diagnosis (3).

Diagnostic Procedures/Other

- Chest x-ray is insensitive and nonspecific. Common findings include unilateral pleural effusion, thickening, or calcifications. Further imaging is often required, with CT of the chest and abdomen being the initial test of choice (2),(3).
- CT, MRI, PET, or integrated PET-CT helps with clinical staging in pleural and peritoneal disease (2),(3).
- Mediastinoscopy and thoracoscopy can assist when diagnostic uncertainty remains and in the full surgical staging of pleural disease (3).
- Pleural mesothelioma diagnosis requires tissue. Thoracentesis for cytology and closed pleural biopsy may be adequate, but often, more invasive procedures such as VATS is needed to obtain an adequate specimen (4).

Test Interpretation

- Initial clinical staging is conducted through imaging. However, as evidenced by postmortem studies, clinical staging frequently underrepresents the actual extent of the disease (3).
- The tumor, node, metastasis (TNM) staging system is widely used, although alternative staging systems are adopted by some centers. The TNM system facilitates treatment selection by quantifying the progression of the disease based on the extent of pleural infiltration, the level of lymph node involvement, and the existence of metastases (3).
- The Butchart staging system, being the oldest, continues to be employed in certain regions of the world. The system seeks to define the resectability and the degree of lymph node involvement.

 TREATMENT

Treatment is generally ineffective with a median survival of 9 to 12 months. However, multidisciplinary approaches are essential to prolonging life and palliation.

GENERAL MEASURES

- A multidisciplinary team is important in management and should include thoracic surgery, oncology, pathology, pulmonary, and radiology for patient-specific planning of management.
- Pain assessment and control should follow principles of cancer pain management.

MEDICATION

First Line

- Chemotherapy remains the mainstay treatment in pleural disease; combined therapy with cisplatin + gemcitabine, pemetrexed, or raltitrexed are all associated with longer median survival than cisplatin alone (1),(3),(5).
- Addition of bevacizumab to cisplatin and pemetrexed in pleural disease showed a small survival advantage but was never filed for licensing, and doubt remains on its value (3).
- Hyperthermic intraoperative or early postoperative intraperitoneal chemotherapy can increase drug concentration in the peritoneum and decrease systemic side effects. Use cisplatin, mitomycin C, fluorouracil, doxorubicin, and/or paclitaxel (1).

Second Line

- Palliative benefit in pleural disease with mitomycin C, vinblastine, cisplatin, and pemetrexed alone or in combination with carboplatin (1)
- Radiation therapy continues to evolve as part of the multidisciplinary approach to mesothelioma and may also be considered for palliation or as an adjunct to surgery. However, survival benefits have not been demonstrated in randomized controlled studies (3),(6).

ISSUES FOR REFERRAL

- Pulmonary, oncology, and surgical follow-up after discharge as indicated
- Psychological services and support should be offered.

ADDITIONAL THERAPIES

- Nivolumab and ipilimumab combined immunotherapy have shown superiority as a front-line treatment when compared to standard chemotherapy and is the first systemic therapy approved for pleural mesothelioma since 2004 (3).
- Gene therapy, photodynamic therapy, noninvasive delivery of alternating electric fields

SURGERY/OTHER PROCEDURES

- For pleural mesothelioma, the role of surgery remains controversial due to its modest amount of data, lack of standardization, and no proven survival benefit for aggressive surgical treatments. Most patients are not offered surgery due to their degree of disease progression and functional status. Instead, most are offered palliative chemotherapy (1).
- Pleurectomy/decortication (P/D) and extrapleural pneumonectomy (EPP) does reduce tumor load, but there remains no clear effect on mortality (1).
- Surgical multimodality therapy remains a common approach for stages I to III pleural mesothelioma. The surgery for mesothelioma after radiation therapy (SMART), which has promising results, combines radiation therapy and surgery. The most common multimodal approach combines P/D or EPP and intraoperative lavage of chemotherapeutic agents (1),(6).
- For aggressive treatments, the first prospective randomized control trial, mesothelioma and radical surgery (MARS), failed to demonstrate any added survival benefit with the addition of surgery to chemotherapy. However, the trial was criticized for its design, which the ongoing MARS 2 trial aims to address (1),(3).

 ONGOING CARE

FOLLOW-UP RECOMMENDATIONS

- Smoking cessation
- Immunization for pneumococcal pneumonia and influenza

Patient Monitoring

Monitor for paraneoplastic phenomenon, including fever, thrombocytosis, malignancy-related thrombosis, hypoglycemia, and rare Coombs-positive hemolytic anemia.

PROGNOSIS

- Prognosis must be individualized and is based on gender, stage, histology, and level of completeness of cytoreduction. Stage and histology are the most important predictors in prognosis (1),(2).
- Poorly differentiated tumor grade, advanced age, and male gender are all independent predictors of poorer prognosis (1),(2).

COMPLICATIONS

Relapses and progression, infection and dysphagia

Geriatric Considerations

Age >65 years is associated with significantly increased morbidity and mortality.

REFERENCES

1. Carbone M, Adusumilli PS, Alexander HR Jr, et al. Mesothelioma: scientific clues for prevention, diagnosis, and therapy. *CA Cancer J Clin*. 2019;69(5):402–429.
2. Brims F. Epidemiology and clinical aspects of malignant pleural mesothelioma. *Cancers (Basel)*. 2021;13(16):4194.
3. Janes SM, Alrifai D, Fennell DA. Perspectives on the treatment of malignant pleural mesothelioma. *N Engl J Med*. 2021;385(13):1207–1218.
4. Panou V, Gadiraju M, Wolin A, et al. Frequency of germline mutations in cancer susceptibility genes in malignant mesothelioma. *J Clin Oncol*. 2018;36(28):2863–2871.
5. Scagliotti GV, Gaafar R, Nowak AK, et al. Nintedanib in combination with pemetrexed and cisplatin for chemotherapy-naive patients with advanced malignant pleural mesothelioma (LUME-Meso): a double-blind, randomised, placebo-controlled phase 3 trial. *Lancet Respir Med*. 2019;7(7):569–580.
6. Gomez DR, Rimner A, Simone CB, et al. The use of radiation therapy for the treatment of malignant pleural mesothelioma: expert opinion from the National Cancer Institute Thoracic Malignancy Steering Committee, International Association for the Study of Lung Cancer, and Mesothelioma Applied Research Foundation. *J Thorac Oncol*. 2019;14(7):1172–1183.

 CODES

ICD10

- C45.1 Mesothelioma of peritoneum
- C45.2 Mesothelioma of pericardium
- C45.0 Mesothelioma of pleura

CLINICAL PEARLS

- Mesothelioma remains a rare but universally fatal disease in part due to long latency.
- Multimodal treatment has decreased recurrence rates and has extended survival time.
- The main risk factor is asbestos exposure.

M

METABOLIC SYNDROME

Naomi Parrella, MD, FAAFP, Dipl. ABOM • Sylvia M. Robinson, MD

 BASICS

DESCRIPTION

- Metabolic syndrome (MetS) represents a cluster of progressive metabolic abnormalities demonstrating insulin resistance, a proinflammatory and prothrombotic state that together, correlate with an increased risk of premature morbidity including complications associated with COVID-19, type 2 diabetes mellitus (T2DM), cardiovascular disease (CVD), stroke, nonalcoholic fatty liver disease (NAFLD), certain cancers, and all-cause mortality.
- Multiple definitions for MetS exist. The most commonly accepted are from WHO 1999, National Cholesterol Education Program (NCEP) ATP3 2005, and International Diabetes Federation (IDF) 2006.

EPIDEMIOLOGY

Incidence
Parallels the incidence of obesity and T2DM.

Prevalence
Global prevalence is estimated at approximately one quarter of the world population as of 2015 and over one third of the U.S. adult population as of 2016.

ETIOLOGY AND PATHOPHYSIOLOGY

- Increase in intra-abdominal and visceral adipose tissue with abnormal fatty acid metabolism leading to hormone dysregulation including:
  - Decreased levels of adiponectin and ghrelin
  - Development of resistance to chronically elevated levels of insulin and leptin
- Systemic inflammation (increased IL-6, tumor necrosis factor-α [TNF-α], resistin, CRP), vascular endothelial dysfunction, and a prothrombotic state (increased tissue plasminogen activator inhibitor-1), elevated renin-angiotensin system activation, oxidative stress leading to HTN, atherosclerosis
- Genetic factors and obesogen exposures appear to contribute to the predisposition promoting obesity and MetS. Parental obesity at the time of conception and epigenetic changes may play a significant role in promoting MetS in offspring.

RISK FACTORS

- Birth status: small for gestational age (SGA) and large for gestational age (LGA), gestational diabetes mellitus (DM)
- Demographics: older age; ethnicity; family history of MetS, T2DM, stroke, and CVD
- Lifestyle factors: physical inactivity, high consumption of sugar/fructose/sugar-sweetened beverages and alcohol; smoking; poor sleep
- Alteration of gut microbiome; disordered sleep
- Weight-promoting medications (corticosteroids, antipsychotics, β-blockers)

GENERAL PREVENTION
Maintenance of healthy weight, regular physical activity, Limiting processed carbohydrates and sugars, limiting alcohol consumption, smoking cessation

COMMONLY ASSOCIATED CONDITIONS
PCOS, obesity, acanthosis nigricans, NAFLD, obstructive sleep apnea (OSA), depression and anxiety, cognitive impairment, Alzheimer disease, GERD, gallstones, chronic renal disease, erectile dysfunction, hyperuricemia, and gout

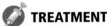 **DIAGNOSIS**

MetS: a cluster of progressive metabolic abnormalities that manifest with at least three of the following:

- Abdominal obesity or waist circumference (WC): waist-to-hip ratio >0.90 men, >0.85 women, or BMI >30 kg/m² (WHO), WC in men ≥94 cm (90 cm for South Asian/Chinese/Japanese), women ≥80 cm (IDF); men ≥102 cm, women ≥88 cm (NCEP), WC ≥90th percentile for age and sex (IDF); >90th percentile for age, gender, and ethnicity (NCEP)
- Elevated blood pressure (BP): (>130/85 mm Hg [NCEP and IDF], >140/90 mm Hg [WHO]) ≥ the 90th percentile for age, height, and sex (NCEP)
- Dislipidemia:
  - Elevated triglycerides (TG): ≥150 mg/dL or treatment NCEP TG ≥100 mg/dL; IDF criteria are the same with adults.
  - Decreased high-density lipoprotein (HDL): men <35 mg/dL, women <39 mg/dL (WHO); men <40 mg/dL, women <50 mg/dL (NCEP and IDF); <40 mg/dL (<50 mg/dL in women >aged 16 years) (IDF); <50 mg/dL (<45 mg/dL in men aged 15 to 19 years) (NCEP)
- Elevated fasting glucose ≥100 mg/dL (consistent across WHO, NCEP, and IDF); criteria are the same with adults (IDF).

PHYSICAL EXAM
WC, BP, exam findings suggestive of insulin resistance—acanthosis nigricans, hirsutism, acrochordons

DIFFERENTIAL DIAGNOSIS
Thyroid dysfunction, Cushing syndrome, and medication effect (especially psychotropic, some anticonvulsants, chronic steroid exposure, β-blockers, and thiazide diuretic medications)

DIAGNOSTIC TESTS & INTERPRETATION
Initial Tests (lab, imaging)
Fasting lipid panel or treatment of dyslipidemia; fasting glucose, hemoglobin A1c (HbA1c), or treatment for hyperglycemia; fasting insulin (optional)

Follow-Up Tests & Special Considerations
- Formal 75-mg (1.75 g/kg up to max dose of 75g*) oral glucose tolerance test or hemoglobin A1C for diagnosis of impaired glucose tolerance (IGT) or prediabetes
- Consider measurement of fasting insulin levels and/or calculation of TG-to-HDL ratio (elevated in insulin resistance) or HOMA-IR.
- Liver function tests to assess for NAFLD
- Consider evaluation for hyperuricemia, hs-CRP, and microalbuminuria.
- Consider detailed lipid analysis and APOE-4 genotype testing.
- Consider evaluation for OSA.
- *Pediatric consideration

 TREATMENT

MEDICATION
Metformin and GLP-1RA/GIP may also be effective in treating insulin resistance. If CAD or T2DM is already diagnosed, treat as per guidelines. Consider vitamin B_{12} supplementation as needed for patients using metformin.

First Line
Prevent or reduce insulin resistance, obesity, and cardiometabolic risk factors with aggressive lifestyle modifications (diet, exercise, and sleep), which are considered as first-line therapy.

- Clinically effective if ≥7% (fat mass) weight loss, which can improve and/or reverse MetS risk factors (1)[A]
- Diet: Minimize alcohol intake. Optimize timing (avoid night eating), frequency (limit snacking/grazing), and intake of proteins, fats, and carbohydrates (limit highly processed foods, added sugars, and sugar-sweetened beverages).
  - Consider Mediterranean or dietary approaches to stop hypertension (DASH) diet.
  - Consider time-restricted feeding or intermittent fasting. Time-restricted feeding may improve the individual components of MetS (2).
- Physical activity: Interrupt sedentary time; 30 to 60 minutes of moderate-intensity aerobic activities such as walking 5 to 7 days per week, with resistance training 1 to 2 days per week; shorter bursts of exercise several times a day also contribute to health benefits (3).
- For IGT and/or prediabetes, intensive lifestyle interventions including low carbohydrate diets +/− metformin +/− GLP1-RA to decrease the risk of progression to T2DM*
- Evaluate and treat cardiac risk factors including elevated TG, low HDL, uncontrolled HTN, or DM
- *Pediatric consideration: metformin has not been shown to decrease the progression of IGT to T2DM in youth

ISSUES FOR REFERRAL
- Liver function tests suggesting liver disease
- Suspected OSA
- Mental health services: mood disorders, disordered eating, traumatic experiences
- Worsening comorbid conditions may benefit from consideration for bariatric surgery.

ADDITIONAL THERAPIES
An FDA-approved device, the superabsorbent hydrogel capsules, can be used together with water for two meals per day to reduce total food intake, which can help with weight loss.

SURGERY/OTHER PROCEDURES
Bariatric surgery can treat MetS in severely obese patients who have failed trials of lifestyle modification and pharmacotherapy if BMI >40 kg/m² or BMI >35 kg/m² with obesity-related comorbidities.

COMPLEMENTARY & ALTERNATIVE MEDICINE
Insufficient evidence on the use of garlic, resveratrol, cinnamon, berberine, green tea, L-carnitine, plant sterols, or zinc supplementation for improved insulin sensitivity; there is some evidence that probiotics and synbiotics may be beneficial.

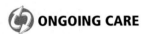 ONGOING CARE

FOLLOW-UP RECOMMENDATIONS
Patient Monitoring
Regular monitoring of weight, WC, BP, fasting TG, HDL, and glucose (or HbA1c)

DIET
See "Treatment" section.

COMPLICATIONS
Progression of CVD and T2DM; an increased risk of NAFLD, stroke, chronic kidney disease, cognitive decline, and developing certain cancers including breast cancer in women, pancreatic cancer, and colon cancer among others

REFERENCES
1. Fechner E, Smeets ETHC, Schrauwen P, et al. The effects of different degrees of carbohydrate restriction and carbohydrate replacement on cardiometabolic risk markers in humans—a systematic review and meta-analysis. *Nutrients*. 2020;12(4):991.
2. Wang X, Li Q, Liu Y, et al. Intermittent fasting versus continuous energy-restricted diet for patients with type 2 diabetes mellitus and metabolic syndrome for glycemic control: a systematic review and meta-analysis of randomized control trials. *Diab Res Clin Pract*. 2021;179:109003.
3. Liang M, Pan Y, Zhong T, et al. Effects of aerobic, resistance, and combined exercise on metabolic syndrome parameters and cardiovascular risk factors: a systematic review and network meta-analysis. *Rev Cardiovasc Med*. 2021;22(4)1523–1533.

ADDITIONAL READING
- Noubiap JJ, Nansseu JR, Lontchi-Yimagou E, et al. Geographic distribution of metabolic syndrome and its components in the general adult population: a meta-analysis of global data from 28 million individuals. *Diab Res Clin Prac*. 2022;188:109924.
- Suglia SF, Koenen KC, Boynton-Jarrett R, et al; for American Heart Association Council on Epidemiology and Prevention, Council on Cardiovascular Disease in the Young, Council on Functional Genomics and Translational Biology, Council on Cardiovascular and Stroke Nursing, Council on Quality of Care and Outcomes Research. Childhood and adolescent adversity and cardiometabolic outcomes: a scientific statement from the American Heart Association. *Circulation*. 2018;137(5):e15–e28.
- Świątkiewicz I, Woźniak A, Taub PR. Time-restricted eating and metabolic syndrome: current status and future perspectives. *Nutrients*. 2021;13(1):221.
- Watanabe M, Risi R, Masi D, et al. Current evidence to propose different food supplements for weight loss: a comprehensive review. *Nutrients*. 2020;12(9):2873.
- Zimmet P, Alberti G, Kaufman F, et al. The metabolic syndrome in children and adolescents. *Lancet*. 2007;369(9579):2059–2061.

  SEE ALSO

Diabetes Mellitus, Type 2; Hypertension, Essential; Obesity; Sleep Apnea, Obstructive; Polycystic Ovarian Syndrome (PCOS)

CODES

ICD10
E88.81 Metabolic syndrome

CLINICAL PEARLS
- Consider further evaluation for MetS when history and/or physical exam demonstrates findings consistent with sedentary lifestyle, sleep apnea, increasing WC, elevation of BP, increased TG-to-HDL ratio, evidence of insulin resistance, or abnormal screening labs or treatment for lipids or blood glucose.
- Reduction of obesity and cardiovascular risk factors is the cornerstone of management of MetS. Aggressive lifelong lifestyle modification is the first-line and most potent treatment for all patients.
- Consider alternatives for medications known to increase risk of weight gain and/or MetS such as atypical antipsychotic medications and chronic steroids.
- Advance interventions early to prevent progression and further complications. Add medications and/or refer to obesity medicine specialists or endocrinologists early if no improvement despite initial efforts.

M

METATARSALGIA

Ammar Shahid, MD • Marc McKenna, MD, CAQSM

BASICS

DESCRIPTION
- Metatarsalgia is defined as pain in the forefoot under one or more metatarsal heads.
- There are three groups:
  - Primary: due to anatomic issues between the metatarsal and other parts of the foot
  - Secondary: due to conditions that increase metatarsal loading via indirect mechanisms, such as chronic synovitis or fracture or injury to the metatarsophalangeal (MTP) joint
  - Iatrogenic usually after a prior forefoot surgery, such as with halux valgus surgery

EPIDEMIOLOGY
Incidence
The overall incidence in the general population is 5–36%; especially common in athletes engaging in high-impact sports (running, jumping, dancing), in rock climbers (12.5%), and in older active adults; most common in women aged 3 to 60 years.

Prevalence
Common

ETIOLOGY AND PATHOPHYSIOLOGY
- The 1st metatarsal head bears significant weight when walking or running. A normal metatarsal arch ensures this balance. The 1st metatarsal head normally has adequate padding to accommodate increased forces.
- Reactive tissue can build a callus around the metatarsal head, compounding the pain.
  - Excessive or repetitive stress; Forces are transmitted to the forefoot during several stages (midstance and push off) of walking and running. These forces are translated across the metatarsal heads at nearly 3 times the body weight.
  - A pronated splayfoot disturbs this balance, causing equal weight-bearing on all metatarsal heads.
  - Any foot deformity changes distribution of weight, impacting areas of the foot that do not have sufficient padding.
  - Soft tissue dysfunction: intrinsic muscle weakness, laxity in the Lisfranc ligament
  - Abnormal foot posture: forefoot varus or valgus, cavus or equinus deformities, loss of the metatarsal arch, splayfoot, pronated foot, inappropriate footwear
  - Dermatologic: warts, calluses (1)[C]
- Great toe
  - Hallux valgus (bunion), either varus or rigidus
- Lesser metatarsals
  - Freiberg infraction (i.e., aseptic necrosis of the metatarsal head usually due to trauma in adolescents who jump or sprint)
  - Hammer toe or claw toe
  - Morton syndrome (i.e., long 2nd metatarsal)

RISK FACTORS
- Obesity
- Forefoot surgery or trauma
- High heels, narrow shoes, or overly tight-fitting shoes (rock climbers typically wear small shoes)
- Competitive athletes in weight-bearing sports (e.g., ballet, basketball, running, soccer, baseball, football)
- Foot deformities or changes in range of motion (ROM) (e.g., pes planus, pes cavus, tight Achilles tendon, tarsal tunnel syndrome, hallux valgus, prominent metatarsal heads, excessive pronation, hammer toe deformity, tight toe extensors) (1)[C]

Geriatric Considerations
- Concomitant arthritis
- Metatarsalgia is common in older athletes.
- Age-related atrophy of the metatarsal fat pad may increase the risk for metatarsalgia.

Pediatric Considerations
- Muscle imbalance disorders (e.g., Duchenne muscular dystrophy) causing foot deformities in children.
- In adolescent girls, consider Freiberg infraction.
- Salter-Harris type I injuries may affect subsequent growth and healing of the epiphysis.

Pregnancy Considerations
- Forefoot pain during pregnancy usually results from change in gait, center of mass, and joint laxity.
- Wear properly fitted low-heeled shoes.

GENERAL PREVENTION
- Wear properly fitted shoes with good padding.
- Start weight-bearing exercise programs gradually.
- Adequate stretching, particularly of the calf muscles
- Weight loss, if overweight

COMMONLY ASSOCIATED CONDITIONS
- Arthritis
- Morton neuroma
- Sesamoiditis
- Plantar keratosis—callus formation

DIAGNOSIS

HISTORY
- Pain gradually develops and persists over the heads of one or more metatarsals. Pain is usually on the plantar surface and worsen during midstance gait phase.
- Pain is often chronic.
- Predisposition with pes cavus and hyperpronation
- Pain often described as walking with a pebble in the shoe; aggravated during midstance or propulsion phases of walking or running

PHYSICAL EXAM
- Point tenderness over plantar metatarsal heads
- Pain in the interdigital space or a positive metatarsal squeeze test suggests Morton neuroma.
- Plantar keratosis
- Tenderness of the metatarsal head(s) with pressure applied by the examiner's finger and thumb
- Erythema and swelling (occasionally)

DIFFERENTIAL DIAGNOSIS
- Stress fracture (most commonly 2nd metatarsal)
- Morton neuroma (i.e., interdigital neuroma)
- Tarsal tunnel syndrome
- Sesamoiditis or sesamoid fracture
- Salter-Harris type I fracture in children
- Arthritis (e.g., gouty, rheumatoid, inflammatory, osteoarthritis, septic, calcium pyrophosphate dihydrate crystal deposition disease [CPPD])
- Lisfranc injury
- Avascular necrosis of the metatarsal head
- Ganglion cyst
- Foreign body
- Vasculitis (diabetes)
- Bony tumors

DIAGNOSTIC TESTS & INTERPRETATION
Often a clinical diagnosis; testing is not always required

Initial Tests (lab, imaging)
- Weight-bearing radiographs: anteroposterior, lateral, and oblique views:
  - Occasionally, metatarsal or sesamoid axial films (to rule out sesamoid fracture) or skyline view of the metatarsal heads to assess the plantar declination of the metatarsal heads: obtained with the MTP joints in dorsiflexion (to evaluate alignment)
- Ultrasound and MRI in recalcitrant cases especially if concern for stress fracture (2)[C]
- MR arthrography of the MTP joint can delineate capsular tears, typically of the distal lateral border of the plantar plate (an often underrecognized cause of metatarsalgia).
- Only if diagnosis is in question
  - Erythrocyte sedimentation rate or C-reactive protein
  - Rheumatoid factor
  - Uric acid
  - Glucose
  - CBC with differential

Diagnostic Procedures/Other
Plantar pressure distribution analysis may help distinguish pressure distribution patterns due to malalignment.

TREATMENT

Treatment for metatarsalgia is typically conservative.
- Relieve pain
- Ice initially
- Rest: temporary alteration of weight-bearing activity; use of cane or crutch; for more physically active patients, suggest an alternative exercise or cross-training:
  – Moist heat later
  – Taping or using gel metatarsal cushion
  – Stiff-soled shoes will act as a splint.
  – Gastrocnemius stretching exercises
- Relieve the pressure beneath the area of maximal pain by redistributing the pressure load of the foot, which can be achieved through orthotics.
- Weight loss, if overweight

MEDICATION
Nonsteroidal anti-inflammatory medications for 7 to 14 days if no contraindications

ISSUES FOR REFERRAL
High-level athletes may benefit from early podiatric or orthopedic evaluation.

ADDITIONAL THERAPIES
- Physical therapy to restore normal foot biomechanics
- Low-heeled (<2 cm height) wide-toe-box shoes
- Metatarsal bars, pads, and arch supports; metatarsal bars are often more effective than pads; if hallux valgus present, may try a valgus splint
- Orthotics/rocker bar (Prescriptive orthotics have been shown to be an effective treatment.)
- Thick-soled shoes
- Shaving the callus may provide temporary relief. Callus excision is not recommended.
- Corticosteroid injection may benefit interdigital neuritis but should be used with caution because it may cause MTP instability and fat pad atrophy.
- Improve flexibility and strength of the intrinsic muscles of the foot with:
  – Exercises (e.g., towel grasps, pencil curls)
  – Physical therapy to maintain ROM and restore normal biomechanics

SURGERY/OTHER PROCEDURES
- If no improvement with conservative therapy for 3 months, refer to foot/ankle orthopedic surgeon or podiatrist.
- Surgery may help correct anatomic abnormality: bunionectomy, partial osteotomy, or foot fusion surgery (arthrodesis). Success rates vary depending on procedure.
- Direct plantar plate repair (grade II medial collateral ligament tear) combined with Weil osteotomy can restore normal alignment of the MTP joint, leading to diminished pain with improved functional scores.
- Callus removal is generally not recommended.

- Morton neurectomy and ultrasound-guided alcohol ablation of Morton neuroma are options (3)[C].
- Surgery only as a last resort if no anatomic abnormality is present.

COMPLEMENTARY & ALTERNATIVE MEDICINE
Magnetic insoles are not effective for chronic nonspecific foot pain.

ADMISSION, INPATIENT, AND NURSING CONSIDERATIONS
Patients generally admitted only for surgery

ONGOING CARE

FOLLOW-UP RECOMMENDATIONS
Patient Monitoring
If stress fracture has been ruled out and patient's condition has not improved >3 months of conservative treatment, consider surgical evaluation or corticosteroid injection (depending on the condition).

PATIENT EDUCATION
- Instruct about wearing proper shoes and gradual return to activity.
- Cross-training until symptoms subside. Goal is to restore normal foot biomechanics, relieve abnormal pressure on the plantar metatarsal heads, and relieve pain (4)[C].

PROGNOSIS
Outcome depends on the severity of the problem and whether surgery is required to correct it.

COMPLICATIONS
- Back, knee, and hip pain due to change in gait
- Transfer metatarsalgia following surgical intervention, which subsequently transfers stress to other areas.

REFERENCES
1. DiPreta JA. Metatarsalgia, lesser toe deformities, and associated disorders of the forefoot. *Med Clin North Am*. 2014;98(2):233–251.
2. Besse JL. Metatarsalgia. *Orthop Traumatol Surg Res*. 2017;103(1S):S29–S39.
3. Musson RE, Sawhney JS, Lamb L, et al. Ultrasound guided alcohol ablation of Morton's neuroma. *Foot Ankle Int*. 2012;33(3):196–201.
4. Espinosa N, Brodsky JW, Maceira E. Metatarsalgia. *J Am Acad Orthop Surg*. 2010;18(8):474–485.

ADDITIONAL READING
- Birbilis T, Theodoropoulou E, Koulalis D. Forefoot complaints—the Morton's metatarsalgia. The role of MR imaging. *Acta Medica (Hradec Kralove)*. 2007;50(3):221–222.

- Burns J, Landorf KB, Ryan MM, et al. Interventions for the prevention and treatment of pes cavus. *Cochrane Database Syst Rev*. 2007;2007(4):CD006154.
- Deshaies A, Roy P, Symeonidis PD, et al. Metatarsal bars more effective than metatarsal pads in reducing impulse on the second metatarsal head. *Foot (Edinb)*. 2011;21(4):172–175.
- Pace A, Scammell B, Dhar S. The outcome of Morton's neurectomy in the treatment of metatarsalgia. *Int Orthop*. 2010;34(4):511–515.
- Park CH, Chang MC. Forefoot disorders and conservative treatment. *Yeungnam Univ J Med*. 2019;36(2):92–98.
- Thomas JL, Blitch EL IV, Chaney DM, et al; for Clinical Practice Guideline Forefoot Disorders Panel. Diagnosis and treatment of forefoot disorders. Section 2. Central metatarsalgia. *J Foot Ankle Surg*. 2009;48(2):239–250.
- Cooke R, Manning C, Palihawadana D, et al. Metatarsalgia: anatomy, pathology and management. *Br J Hosp Med (Lond)*. 2021;82(9):1–8.

SEE ALSO

Morton Neuroma (Interdigital Neuroma)

CODES

ICD10
- M77.40 Metatarsalgia, unspecified foot
- G57.60 Lesion of plantar nerve, unspecified lower limb
- M77.42 Metatarsalgia, left foot

CLINICAL PEARLS
- Metatarsalgia refers to pain of the plantar surface of the forefoot in the region of the metatarsal heads.
- Metatarsalgia is common in athletes who participate in high-impact sports involving the lower extremities.
- Patients describe as "walking with a pebble in the shoe." Pain is worse during midstance or propulsion phases of walking or running. The most common physical finding is point tenderness over the plantar metatarsal heads.
- Typical treatment is conservative, including rest and ice, activity modification, and ensuring proper padding under the foot.
- Pregnant patients should wear properly fitted, low-heeled shoes to reduce incidence of metatarsalgia.

M

MILD COGNITIVE IMPAIRMENT

Birju B. Patel, MD, FACP

BASICS

DESCRIPTION
- Mild cognitive impairment (MCI) is defined as significant cognitive impairment in the absence of dementia, as measured by standard memory tests:
  - Concern regarding change in cognition
  - Preservation of independence in functional activities of daily living (ADLs)
  - Impairment in ≥1 cognitive domains (attention, executive dysfunction, memory, learning, visuospatial, language)
  - Other terms used in the literature relating to MCI: cognitive impairment not dementia (CIND); mild cognitive disorder; some of these conditions do not progress to dementia. *DSM-5* mentions "mild neurocognitive disorder" (mNCD), which may be a precursor to Alzheimer disease and has many of the same features as MCI.
- Older adults with MCI are 3 times more likely to progress to dementia in 2 to 5 years than age-matched cohorts (1)[A].

EPIDEMIOLOGY
Incidence
- Predominant sex: male > female
- Predominant age:
  - Higher in older persons and in those with less education
  - 12 to 15/1,000 person-years in those aged ≥65 years
  - 50 to 75/1,000 person-years in those aged ≥75 years

Prevalence
- MCI is more prevalent than dementia in the United States.
- 12–18% for those aged ≥60 years; ~25% for ages 80 to 84 years; prevalence increases with age and for those with lower educational level (2).

ETIOLOGY AND PATHOPHYSIOLOGY
- Subtypes of MCI:
  - Single-domain amnestic
  - Multiple-domain amnestic
  - Single-domain nonamnestic
  - Multiple-domain nonamnestic
- The amnestic subtypes are higher risk for progression to Alzheimer disease.
- Vascular, neurodegenerative, traumatic, metabolic, psychiatric, or a combination

Genetics
In certain subsets of MCI where the disease will progress to Alzheimer disease, one must consider apolipoprotein (APO) E4 genotype: Various pathways exist leading to amyloid accumulation and deposition thought to be associated with Alzheimer disease.

RISK FACTORS
- Diabetes; hypertension; hyperlipidemia; cerebrovascular disease
- Smoking
- Sleep apnea
- APO E4 genotype
- Low educational levels
- Depression
- Sedentary lifestyle

GENERAL PREVENTION
Optimize vascular risk factors and focus on a healthy, active lifestyle.

COMMONLY ASSOCIATED CONDITIONS
See "Risk Factors."

DIAGNOSIS

HISTORY
- Focus on cognitive deficits and impairment. MCI is meant to reflect a change in cognition and not a lifelong impaired cognition.
- Review all medications that may affect cognition with emphasis given to anticholinergic medications (patients on these may mistakenly be classified as having MCI).
- Rule out depression. The prevalence of depression in patients with MCI is higher than age-matched cohorts.
- Assess function (ADLs, instrumental ADLs) and subtle changes in daily function (e.g., in the workplace).
- Impact on interpersonal relationships and caregiver stress
- Assess vascular risk factors (hypertension, diabetes, hyperlipidemia, and cerebrovascular disease).
- Assess behavioral changes (agitation, aggression, impulsivity, disinhibition, apathy, and others).
- Olfactory dysfunction may be associated with amnestic MCI and progression to Alzheimer disease. This can be easily evaluated in patients with memory impairment (3).

PHYSICAL EXAM
- A general exam focusing on clinical clues in identifying vascular disease (e.g., bruits, abnormal BP)
- Neurologic exam to rule out reversible CNS causes of cognitive impairment or other causes of cognitive impairment
- Office measures of cognitive function, depression, and functional status

DIFFERENTIAL DIAGNOSIS
- Normal aging (age-related cognitive impairment, age-associated memory impairment)
- Delirium; dementia; depression
- "Reversible" cognitive impairment
  - Medications (anticholinergics and medications with anticholinergic properties)
  - Hypothyroidism
  - Vitamin B$_{12}$ deficiency
- Give consideration to sleep conditions, especially sleep apnea, that can contribute to cognitive deficits.

DIAGNOSTIC TESTS & INTERPRETATION
- Formal screening with standardized cognitive tests is important (e.g., Montreal Cognitive Assessment [MoCA] and Saint Louis University Mental Status [SLUMS]); MoCA may be more sensitive for detecting and following MCI.
- Neuropsychological testing is recommended for all patients with presumed MCI.

Initial Tests (lab, imaging)
- Complete blood count
- Comprehensive metabolic profile
- Thyroid-stimulating hormone
- Vitamin B$_{12}$
- Syphilis and HIV testing
- Imaging tests are helpful when there are focal neurologic deficits or rapid or atypical presentations:
  - CT scan can detect structural CNS conditions leading to cognitive impairment:
    ○ Subdural hematoma; normal pressure hydrocephalus; metastatic disease; cerebrovascular accident
  - MRI further evaluates vascular, infectious, neoplastic, and inflammatory conditions.

Follow-Up Tests & Special Considerations
- Document progression of functional impairment, cognitive decline, concurrent depression, and comorbid conditions.
- Advanced care planning while patient is competent
- Early education of caregivers on safety, maintaining structure, managing stress, support, and future planning
- Focus on driving ability and safety.
- Work-related issues should be explored and optimized as best possible.
- Neuropsychological testing should be done at 1- to 2-year intervals depending on subjective concerns and ongoing diagnosis of MCI.
- If early Alzheimer disease is being considered and antiamyloid therapies are being considered, confirmatory testing is needed (lumbar puncture for cerebrospinal fluid [CSF] biomarkers, amyloid specific scans, ApoE testing, etc.). This workup may not be readily available, and referral to specialized centers may be necessary.

Test Interpretation
- Little is known about MCI pathology due to a lack of longitudinal studies and heterogeneity of population studied.
- Alzheimer disease pathophysiology:
  - Neurofibrillary tangles in hippocampus
  - Senile plaques (amyloid deposition)
  - Neuronal degeneration
- Those with MCI have intermediate amounts of pathologic findings of Alzheimer disease with amyloid deposition and neurofibrillary tangles in the mesial temporal lobes compared with those with dementia.
- Amnestic MCI is associated with white matter hyperintensity volume on MRI, whereas nonamnestic MCI is associated with infarcts.

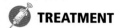

TREATMENT

GENERAL MEASURES
Atherosclerotic risk factors should be treated aggressively.

MEDICATION
The use of cholinesterase inhibitors (ChEIs) in MCI is not associated with any delay in the onset of Alzheimer disease or dementia. Moreover, the safety profile showed that the risks associated with ChEIs are significant. Therefore, ChEIs are not routinely recommended (1)[B]. Antiamyloid therapies require confirmatory diagnosis of Alzheimer disease and should not be used in MCI.

ISSUES FOR REFERRAL
Consider referral to a memory specialist (i.e., geriatrician, neurologist, geropsychiatric, neuropsychologist) to evaluate and differentiate subtypes of MCI and specific cognitive deficits.

ADDITIONAL THERAPIES
There may be benefit in terms of improvement in performance on tests for global cognitive functioning with cognitive training and physical exercise.

COMPLEMENTARY & ALTERNATIVE MEDICINE
- No evidence suggests the efficacy of vitamin E in the prevention or treatment of people with MCI.
- Long-term use of *Ginkgo biloba* extract has shown to have no benefit in the treatment of MCI and in terms of progression to dementia. In addition, *Ginkgo biloba* can be associated with increase in bleeding risk including CNS bleeds (4)[B].

ADMISSION, INPATIENT, AND NURSING CONSIDERATIONS
Delirium is more common in patients hospitalized with all forms of cognitive impairment.
- Avoid medications that may worsen or precipitate cognitive decline (e.g., anticholinergics, antihistamines, and sedatives).
- Patients may be extremely sensitive to the hospital environment:
  - Moderate level of stimulation is best.
  - Avoid sensory deprivation. Make sure that patients have access to hearing aids and eyeglasses.
  - Use frequent cueing and have caregivers or family in the room whenever possible with patient.
  - Frequently orient patients to date and time.

ONGOING CARE

FOLLOW-UP RECOMMENDATIONS
Reevaluate every 6 to 12 months to determine if symptoms are progressing.

Patient Monitoring
Appropriate cognitive and functional testing should be used to evaluate progression, along with clinical history and exam. If a medication is started, patients need to be followed more frequently to evaluate for efficacy, side effects, dose titration, and so forth. Declining executive function may be an early marker to progression of MCI to dementia, and clinicians should monitor and advise patients and families proactively to look for this. Impairments in ADL function is a good clue to progression to dementia from MCI. Attempts should be made to wean medications that can impact cognition.

DIET
Diet to minimize atherosclerotic risk factors should be emphasized.

PATIENT EDUCATION
- Long-term planning topics should be discussed including advanced directives, firearm safety, driving safety, finances, and estate planning.
- Encourage lifestyle changes:
  - Physical activity, such as walking 30 minutes daily on most days of the week, as exercise modestly improved some measures of cognition in some studies
  - Mental activity that stimulates language skills and psychomotor coordination should be encouraged. Computer activities, reading books, crafts, crossword puzzles, and games may be linked to decreased risk of development of MCI (5)[C].
- Cognitive rehabilitation strategies may be beneficial in helping with daily activities relating to memory tasks in MCI.
- Treatment of vascular risk factors (hypertension, diabetes, cerebrovascular disease, and hyperlipidemia) is important in lowering risk of progression to dementia (e.g., intensive blood pressure lowering in the Sprint Mind Study reduced incidence of MCI with target SBP of 120 mm Hg).
- There are no FDA-approved medications or dietary agents currently for MCI shown to have benefit.
- In those with sleep apnea, compliance with CPAP improves cognition.
- Good dental hygiene and regular dental evaluation must be maintained. Significant periodontal disease is associated with MCI.
- Excessive alcohol consumption, above recommended limits, worsens cognition.

PROGNOSIS
- Older adults with MCI have 3 times higher risks of progression to dementia in 2 to 5 years.
- Amnestic subtypes of MCI are most likely to progress to dementia.
- Neuropsychological testing measures, CSF biomarkers, and neuroimaging studies are being used in specialty settings to predict conversion to dementia. These are not widely available or cost effective and are not used in general use.
- Women are more likely to progress to dementia.

- Olfactory dysfunction can be higher risk for progression to dementia.
- Patients with neuropsychiatric symptoms, such as anxiety or depression, are higher risk for progression to Alzheimer disease. This may be helpful in identifying higher risk MCI patients (6)[C].

REFERENCES
1. Petersen RC, Lopez O, Armstrong MJ, et al. Practice guideline update summary: mild cognitive impairment: report of the Guideline Development, Dissemination, and Implementation Subcommittee of the American Academy of Neurology. *Neurology.* 2018;90(3):126–135.
2. Petersen RC. Mild cognitive impairment. *Continuum (Minneap Minn).* 2016;22(2):404–418.
3. Roberts RO, Christianson TJH, Kremers WK, et al. Association between olfactory dysfunction and amnestic mild cognitive impairment and Alzheimer disease dementia. *JAMA Neurol.* 2016;73(1): 93–101.
4. Vellas B, Coley N, Ousset PJ, et al; for GuidAge Study Group. Long-term use of standardised *Ginkgo biloba* extract for the prevention of Alzheimer's disease (GuidAge): a randomised placebo-controlled trial. *Lancet Neurol.* 2012;11(10):851–859.
5. Marshall GA, Rentz DM, Frey MT, et al; for Alzheimer's Disease Neuroimaging Initiative. Executive function and instrumental activities of daily living in mild cognitive impairment and Alzheimer's disease. *Alzheimers Dement.* 2011;7(3):300–308.
6. Roberto N, Portella MJ, Marquié M, et al. Neuropsychiatric profiles and conversion to dementia in mild cognitive impairment, a latent class analysis. *Sci Rep.* 2021;11(1):6448.

 CODES

ICD10
G31.84 Mild cognitive impairment, so stated

CLINICAL PEARLS
- Amnestic MCI affects primarily memory and is more likely to progress to Alzheimer dementia.
- Screen for reversible factors, particularly anticholinergic medications, depression, and sleep disorders.
- Look closely at vascular risk factors and modify them as best as possible.
- ChEIs should not be used routinely unless memory complaints are affecting quality of life in patients. Potential side effects of these medications should be thoroughly discussed with patients and their families. A baseline ECG should be done prior to initiation of ChEIs due to risk of bradycardia and syncope.
- Neuropsychological testing is recommended in individuals suspected of having MCI. Patients with MCI and with prominent subjective complaints should have follow-up testing to evaluate for progression between 1 and 2 years after the initial assessment.

M

MISCARRIAGE (EARLY PREGNANCY LOSS)

Clara M. Keegan, MD

BASICS

DESCRIPTION
- Miscarriage, also known as early pregnancy loss (EPL) or spontaneous abortion (SAb), is the failure or loss of a pregnancy before 13 weeks' gestational age (WGA).
- Related terms
  - Anembryonic gestation: gestational sac on ultrasound (US) without visible embryo after 6 WGA
  - Complete abortion: entire contents of uterus expelled
  - Ectopic pregnancy: pregnancy outside the uterus
  - Embryonic or fetal demise: cervix closed; embryo or fetus present in the uterus without cardiac activity
  - Incomplete abortion: abortion with retained products of conception, generally placental tissue
  - Induced or therapeutic abortion: evacuation of uterine contents or products of conception medically or surgically
  - Inevitable abortion: cervical dilatation or rupture of membranes in the presence of vaginal bleeding
  - Recurrent abortion: three or more consecutive pregnancy losses at <15 WGA
  - Threatened abortion: vaginal bleeding in the 1st trimester of pregnancy
  - Septic abortion: a spontaneous or therapeutic abortion complicated by pelvic infection; common complication of illegally performed induced abortions
- Synonym(s): SAb
  - Missed abortion and blighted ovum are used less frequently in favor of terms representing the sonographic diagnosis.

EPIDEMIOLOGY
Predominant age: increases with advancing age, especially >35 years; at age 40 years, the loss rate is twice that of age 20 years.

Incidence
- Threatened abortion (1st-trimester bleeding) occurs in 20–25% of clinical pregnancies.
- Between 10% and 15% of all clinically recognized pregnancies end in EPL, with 80% of these occurring within 12 weeks after last menstrual period (LMP) (1).
- When both clinical and biochemical (β-hCG detected) pregnancies are considered, about 30% of pregnancies end in EPL.
- One in four people with a uterus will have an EPL during their lifetime (1).

ETIOLOGY AND PATHOPHYSIOLOGY
Chromosomal anomalies (50% of cases), congenital anomalies, trauma, maternal factors: uterine abnormalities, infection (toxoplasma, other viruses, rubella, cytomegalovirus, herpesvirus), maternal endocrine disorders, hypercoagulable state

Genetics
Approximately 50% of 1st-trimester EPLs have significant chromosomal anomalies, with 50% of these being autosomal trisomies and the remainder being triploidy, tetraploidy, or 45X monosomies.

RISK FACTORS
Most cases of EPL occur in patients without identifiable risk factors; however, risk factors include the following: chromosomal abnormalities, advancing maternal age, uterine abnormalities, and maternal chronic disease (antiphospholipid antibodies, uncontrolled diabetes mellitus, polycystic ovarian syndrome, obesity, hypertension, thyroid disease, renal disease); other possible contributing factors include smoking, alcohol intake, cocaine use, infection, and luteal phase defect.

GENERAL PREVENTION
- Insufficient evidence supports the use of aspirin and/or other anticoagulants, bed rest, hCG, immunotherapy, uterine muscle relaxants, or vitamins for general prevention of EPL, before or after threatened abortion is diagnosed.
- By the time the hemorrhage begins, half of pregnancies complicated by threatened abortion already have no fetal cardiac activity.
- In threatened abortion, oral progestogens may reduce the risk of EPL (RR 0.73, 95% CI 0.59–0.92) and possibly increase the rate of live birth (RR 1.07, 95% CI 1–1.15).
- Antiphospholipid syndrome: The combination of unfractionated heparin and aspirin reduces risk of EPL in women with antiphospholipid antibodies and a history of recurrent abortion.

DIAGNOSIS

HISTORY
- The possibility of pregnancy should be considered in a reproductive-aged person with a uterus who presents with nonmenstrual vaginal bleeding.
- Vaginal bleeding
  - Characteristics (amount, color, consistency, associated symptoms), onset (abrupt or gradual), duration, intensity/quantity, and exacerbating/precipitating factors
  - Document LMP if known: It allows calculation of estimated gestational age.
- Abdominal pain/uterine cramping, as well as associated nausea/vomiting/syncope
- Rupture of membranes
- Passage of products of conception
- Prenatal course: toxic or infectious exposures, family or personal history of genetic abnormalities, past history of ectopic pregnancy or EPL, endocrine disease, autoimmune disorder, bleeding/clotting disorder

PHYSICAL EXAM
- Orthostatic vital signs to estimate hemodynamic stability
- Abdominal exam for tenderness, guarding, rebound, bowel sounds (Peritoneal signs are more likely with ectopic pregnancy.)
- Speculum exam for visual assessment of cervical dilation, blood, and products of conception (confirms diagnosis of EPL)
- Bimanual exam to assess for uterine size–dates discrepancy and adnexal tenderness or mass

DIFFERENTIAL DIAGNOSIS
- Ectopic pregnancy: potentially life-threatening; must be considered in any woman of childbearing age with abdominal pain and vaginal bleeding
- Physiologic bleeding in normal pregnancy (implantation bleeding)
- Subchorionic bleeding
- Cervical polyps, neoplasia, and/or inflammatory conditions
- Hydatidiform mole pregnancy
- hCG-secreting ovarian tumor

DIAGNOSTIC TESTS & INTERPRETATION
Initial Tests (lab, imaging)
- Quantitative hCG
  - Particularly useful if intrauterine pregnancy (IUP) has not been documented by US
  - Serial quantitative serum hCG measurements can assess viability of the pregnancy. Serum hCG should rise at least 53% every 48 hours through 7 weeks after LMP. An inappropriate rise, plateau, or decrease of hCG suggests abnormal IUP or possible ectopic pregnancy.
- Complete blood count (CBC) with differential
- Cultures: gonorrhea/chlamydia
- US exam to evaluate fetal viability and to rule out ectopic pregnancy
  - hCG >2,000 mIU/mL necessary to detect IUP via transvaginal US (TVUS), >5,500 mIU/mL for abdominal US
  - TVUS criteria for nonviable intrauterine gestation: 7-mm fetal pole without cardiac activity or 25-mm gestational sac without a fetal pole, IUP with no growth over 1 week, or previously seen IUP no longer visible
  - Structures and timing: with TVUS, gestational sac of 2 to 3 mm generally seen around 5 WGA; yolk sac by 5.5 WGA; fetal pole with cardiac activity by 6 WGA

Follow-Up Tests & Special Considerations
- In the case of vaginal bleeding with no documented IUP and hCG <2,000 mIU/mL, follow serum hCG levels weekly to zero.
- If levels plateau, consider ectopic pregnancy or retained products of conception. If levels are very high, consider gestational trophoblastic disease.
- If initial hCG level does not permit documentation of IUP by TVUS, follow serum hCG in 48 hours to document appropriate rise.
- Repeat US once hCG is at a level commensurate with visualization on US (see above).
- Provide the patient with ectopic precautions in interim: worsening abdominal pain, dizziness/syncope, nausea/vomiting.
- In a pregnancy of unknown location with hCG rise <53% in 48 hours, offer methotrexate for treatment of presumed ectopic pregnancy.

Diagnostic Procedures/Other
- Fetal heart tones can be auscultated with Doppler US. starting between 10 and 12 WGA in a viable pregnancy.
- In threatened abortion, fetal cardiac activity at 7 to 11 WGA is 90–96% predictive of continued pregnancy (1).

TREATMENT

GENERAL MEASURES
- Discuss contraception plan at the time of diagnosis of EPL, as ovulation can occur prior to resumption of normal menses.
- Expectant management ("watchful waiting") is 90% effective for incomplete abortion, although it may take several weeks for the process to be complete (1). This approach is only recommended in the 1st trimester and is more effective in women with symptoms of impending pregnancy loss.

MEDICATION
- Rates of complete miscarriage and of need for surgical evacuation are equivalent with expectant management and medication.
- Long-term conception rate and pregnancy outcomes are similar for women who undergo expectant management, medical treatment, or surgical evacuation.
- Infection rates are lower with medical versus surgical management.

First Line
- Misoprostol: most common agent for inducing passage of tissue in incomplete abortion or embryonic demise
  – Off-label use; has not been submitted to the FDA for consideration for use in treatment of early pregnancy failure; recognized by the World Health Organization (WHO) as a life-saving medication for this indication
  – Efficacy: Complete expulsion of products of conception in 71% by day 3 and 84% by day 8.
  – Efficacy depends on route of administration, gestational age of pregnancy, and dose.
  – Recommended dose is 800 mcg vaginally; alternate regimens include the WHO regimen of 600 mcg sublingually q3h for up to 3 doses; multidose regimens and oral dosing (including buccal and sublingual) may result in increased side effects.
  – The addition of mifepristone 200 mg, if available, given 24 hours before misoprostol increases the efficacy to 83.8% (ARR 16.7%, 95% CI 7.1–26.3%) (2)[A].
- Common adverse effects include abdominal pain/cramping, nausea, and diarrhea. Pain increases at higher doses but is manageable with oral analgesia.
- Recommended for stable patients who decline surgery but do not want to wait for spontaneous passage of products of conception.

Second Line
Patients with evidence of anemia should receive iron supplementation.

ISSUES FOR REFERRAL
Patients should be monitored for up to 1 year for the development of pathologic grief. There is an insufficient evidence to support counseling to prevent development of anxiety or depression related to grief following EPL.

ADDITIONAL THERAPIES
Rh immunoglobulin is not required for Rh-negative patients with EPL in the 1st trimester.

SURGERY/OTHER PROCEDURES
- Uterine aspiration (suction dilation and curettage [D&C] or manual uterine aspiration [MUA], also known as manual vacuum aspiration [MVA]) is the conventional treatment.
- Indications: septic abortion, heavy bleeding, hypotension, persistent IUP after medical or expectant management, patient's choice

- Risks (all rare): anesthesia (usually local), uterine perforation, intrauterine adhesions, cervical trauma, infection that may lead to infertility or increased risk of ectopic pregnancy
- When compared with expectant management, surgical intervention leads to fewer days of vaginal bleeding, with a lower risk of incomplete abortion and heavy bleeding and a similar risk of infection, but with a higher cost. It is appropriate to prioritize the patient's preference in determining management.
- Vacuum aspiration (manual or electric) is considered preferable to sharp curettage, as aspiration is less painful, takes less time, involves less blood loss, and does not require general anesthesia. The WHO supports use of suction curettage over rigid metal curettage.
- Although data from induced abortions suggest that antibiotic prophylaxis with doxycycline 200 mg in a single dose reduces the already rare risk of postprocedure infection, data are insufficient to support use of antibiotics before aspiration for EPL.

COMPLEMENTARY & ALTERNATIVE MEDICINE
A systematic review of Chinese herbal medicine alone and in conjunction with Western medicine showed benefit over Western medicine alone in achieving continued viability at 28 weeks (number needed to treat [NNT] = 4.8 pregnancies with combined therapy). However, the available studies did not meet international standards for reporting quality.

ADMISSION, INPATIENT, AND NURSING CONSIDERATIONS
- If the patient has orthostatic vital signs, initiate resuscitation with IV fluids and/or blood products, if needed.
- Hemodynamically unstable patients may require IV fluids and/or blood products to maintain BP.

ONGOING CARE

FOLLOW-UP RECOMMENDATIONS
All patients should be offered follow-up in 2 to 6 weeks to monitor for resolution of bleeding, return of menses, and symptoms related to grief, as well as to review the contraception plan.

Patient Monitoring
- If EPL occurs in setting of previously documented IUP and abortion is completed with resumption of normal menses, it is not necessary to check or follow serum hCG to 0.
- After medical management, confirm complete expulsion with US or serial serum β-hCG.
- If pregnancy is not immediately desired, offer effective contraception. Immediate insertion of an intrauterine device is both acceptable and safe.
- If pregnancy is desired, provide preconception counseling. There is no evidence that it is necessary to wait a certain number of cycles before attempting conception again.

DIET
NPO if patient will undergo D&C under general anesthesia

PATIENT EDUCATION
- Pelvic rest for 1 week after D&C or MUA; advise the patients to call if there is an excessive bleeding (soaking two pads per hour for 2 hours), fever, pelvic pain, or malaise, which could indicate retained products of conception or endometritis.
- A patient fact sheet on miscarriage is available through the American Academy of Family Physicians: https://www.aafp.org/afp/2011/0701/p85.html
- Additional patient references are available through the Reproductive Health Access Project:
  – https://www.reproductiveaccess.org/resource/what-is-a-miscarriage
  – https://www.reproductiveaccess.org/resource/miscarriage-treatment-options/

PROGNOSIS
- Prognosis is excellent once bleeding is controlled.
- Recurrent miscarriage: prognosis depends on etiology; up to 70% rate of success with subsequent pregnancy

COMPLICATIONS
- D&C or MUA: uterine perforation, bleeding, adhesions, cervical trauma, and infection that may lead to infertility or increased risk of ectopic pregnancy. Bleeding and adhesions are more common with D&C than with MUA; all complications are rare.
- Retained products of conception

REFERENCES
1. Prine LW, MacNaughton H. Office management of early pregnancy loss. *Am Fam Physician.* 2011;84(1):75–82.
2. Schreiber CA, Creinin MD, Atrio J, et al. Mifepristone pretreatment for the medical management of early pregnancy loss. *N Engl J Med.* 2018;378(23):2161–2170.

ADDITIONAL READING
American College of Obstetricians and Gynecologists. ACOG practice bulletin No. 200; early pregnancy loss. *Obstet Gynecol.* 2018;132(5):e197–e207.

SEE ALSO
- Ectopic Pregnancy
- Algorithm: Recurrent Pregnancy Loss

CODES

ICD10
- O03.9 Complete or unspecified spontaneous abortion without complication
- O03.4 Incomplete spontaneous abortion without complication
- O02.1 Missed abortion

CLINICAL PEARLS
- Any pregnant woman with abdominal pain and/or vaginal bleeding must be evaluated to rule out ectopic pregnancy, which is potentially life-threatening.
- As all options have similar long-term outcomes, patient's preference should determine whether management is expectant, medical, or procedural.

M

MITRAL REGURGITATION

Yongkasem Vorasettakarnkij, MD, MSc

BASICS

DESCRIPTION
- Disorder of mitral valve (MV) closure, either primary, secondary (functional), or mixed, resulting in a backflow of the left ventricular (LV) stroke volume into the left atrium (LA); uncompensated, this leads to LV and LA enlargement, elevated pulmonary pressures, atrial fibrillation (AF), heart failure (HF), and sudden cardiac death.
- Types of mitral regurgitation (MR):
  - Acute versus chronic
  - Primary versus secondary (functional) and mixed
    - Primary: abnormalities at any level of the MV structures (annulus, leaflets, chordae tendineae, and papillary muscles)
    - Secondary: No valvular abnormalities are found. The abnormal and dilated LV causes papillary muscle displacement, resulting in leaflet tethering with annular dilatation that prevents coaptation.
    - Mixed: mixed abnormalities of both primary and secondary types
- System(s) affected: cardiac; pulmonary

EPIDEMIOLOGY
Moderate to severe MR affects 2.5 million people in the United States (2000 data). It is the most common valvular disease and is expected to double by 2030.

Prevalence
- By severity on echocardiography:
  - Mild MR: 19% (up to 40% if trivial jets included)
  - Moderate MR: 1.9%
  - Severe MR: 0.2%
- By category: degenerative (myxomatous disease, annular calcification): 60–70%, ischemic: 20%, endocarditis: 2–5%, rheumatic: 2–5%

ETIOLOGY AND PATHOPHYSIOLOGY
- Acute MR
  - Leaflet perforation: infective endocarditis, trauma
  - Chordae tendineae rupture: trauma, spontaneous rupture, infective endocarditis, or rheumatic fever
  - Papillary muscle rupture or dysfunction: acute myocardial infarction (MI), severe myocardial ischemia, or trauma
- Chronic MR
  - Primary—degenerative (mitral annular calcification, MV prolapse [MVP]), infective endocarditis, rheumatic heart disease (RHD), inflammatory diseases (lupus, eosinophilic endocardial disease), toxin induced (anorectic drugs), congenital
  - Secondary (functional)
    - Ischemic: coronary artery disease (CAD)/MI
    - Nonischemic: cardiomyopathy from any cause, annular dilatation from chronic AF, dyssynchrony from right ventricular pacing
- Acute MR: Acute MV damage leads to sudden LA and LV volume overload. Sudden rise in LV volume load without LV remodeling results in impaired forward cardiac output and possible cardiogenic shock.
- Chronic MR: LV eccentric hypertrophy compensates for increased regurgitant volume to maintain forward cardiac output and alleviate pulmonary congestion. However, LV remodeling can result in LV dysfunction. LA compensatory dilatation for the larger regurgitant volume predisposes patients to develop AF.
- Ischemic MR: papillary muscle rupture, ischemia during acute MI, and incomplete coaptation of leaflets or restricted valve movement from chronic ischemia

RISK FACTORS
Age, hypertension, RHD, endocarditis, anorectic drugs, radiation

GENERAL PREVENTION
- Risk factor modification for CAD
- Antibiotic prophylaxis for poststreptococcal RHD
- Routine dental endocarditis prophylaxis is no longer recommended.

COMMONLY ASSOCIATED CONDITIONS
MVP with MR common in Marfan syndrome

DIAGNOSIS

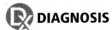

HISTORY
- Associated conditions: RHD, prior MI, connective tissue disorder
- Acute MR; sudden onset of dyspnea; orthopnea, paroxysmal nocturnal dyspnea
- Chronic MR; exertional dyspnea, fatigue; palpitation: paroxysmal/persistent AF

PHYSICAL EXAM
- Acute MR
  - Rapid and thready pulses
  - Signs of poor tissue perfusion with peripheral vasoconstriction
  - Hyperdynamic precordium without apical shift
  - S_3 and S_4 (if in sinus rhythm)
  - Systolic murmur at left sternal border and base: early, middle, or holosystolic murmur; often soft, low-pitched decrescendo murmur
  - Rales
- Chronic MR
  - Brisk upstroke of arterial pulse; leftward displaced LV apical impulse
  - Systolic thrill at the apex (suggests severe MR); soft S_1 and widely split S_2, S_3 gallop; loud P_2 (if pulmonary hypertension)
  - Holosystolic murmur at apex that radiates to axilla or to left parasternal border
  - Ankle edema, jugular venous distension, and ascites, if development of right-sided HF

DIFFERENTIAL DIAGNOSIS
- Aortic stenosis (AS): usually midsystolic but can be long; difficult to distinguish from holosystolic, at apical area, and radiating to the carotid arteries (unlike MR)
- Tricuspid regurgitation: holosystolic but at left lower sternal border, does not radiate to axilla, and may increase in intensity with inspiration (unlike MR)
- Ventricular septal defect (VSD): harsh holosystolic murmur at lower left sternal border but radiates to right sternal border (not axilla)

DIAGNOSTIC TESTS & INTERPRETATION
Initial Tests (lab, imaging)
- Chest x-ray (CXR)
  - Acute MR: pulmonary edema, normal heart size
  - Chronic MR: LA and LV enlargement
- ECG
  - Acute MR: varies depending on etiologies (e.g., acute MI)
  - Chronic MR
    - P mitrale from LA enlargement, AF
    - LV hypertrophy
    - Q waves from prior MI
- Cardiac enzymes: brain natriuretic peptide, if appropriate

- Transthoracic echocardiogram (TTE)
  - Indications for TTE
    - Baseline evaluation of LV size and function, right ventricular function, LA size, pulmonary artery pressure, and severity of MR
    - Delineation of the mechanism of MR
    - Surveillance of asymptomatic moderate to severe LV dysfunction (ejection fraction [EF] and end-systolic dimension [ESD])
    - Evaluate MV apparatus and LV size and function after a change in sign/symptom in MR patient.
    - Evaluate after MV repair or replacement.
  - Findings in acute MR
    - Evidence of etiology: flail leaflet or vegetations
    - Normal LA and LV size
  - Findings in chronic MR
    - Evidence of degenerative, rheumatic, ischemic, congenital, and other causes
    - Enlarged LA and LV

Follow-Up Tests & Special Considerations
- Intervals for follow-up TTE: See "Follow-Up Recommendations."
- Cardiovascular magnetic resonance (CMR):
  - TTE results are not satisfactory to assess LV and right ventricular volumes, function, or MR severity.
- Transesophageal echocardiogram (TEE)
  - Intraoperatively to define the anatomic basis of MR and to guide repair
  - Nondiagnostic information about severity, mechanism of MR, and/or status of LV function from noninvasive imaging
- Exercise hemodynamics with either Doppler echocardiography or cardiac catheterization.
  - Discrepancy between symptoms and the severity of MR from resting TTE in symptomatic patients with chronic primary MR
- Exercise treadmill testing
  - To establish symptom status and exercise tolerance in asymptomatic patients with chronic primary MR
- Noninvasive imaging (stress nuclear/positron emission tomography, CMR, stress echocardiography, cardiac CT angiography)
  - To establish etiology of chronic secondary MR and/or to assess myocardial viability

Diagnostic Procedures/Other
Cardiac catheterization
- Left ventriculography and hemodynamic measurement
  - Noninvasive tests are inconclusive regarding the severity of MR, LV function, and the need for surgery.
- Coronary angiography: prior to MV surgery in patients at risk for CAD

Test Interpretation
Quantification of severe MR requires an integration of the following structural parameters:
- LA size: dilated, unless acute
- LV size: dilated, unless acute
- MV morphology: flail leaflet, ruptured papillary muscle, large perforation, severe retraction, poor leaflet coaptation
- Doppler parameters: large central jet (>50% of LA), pulmonary vein systolic flow reversal
- Quantitative parameter: effective regurgitant orifice area ≥0.4 cm², regurgitation volume ≥60 mL, regurgitation fraction ≥50%

TREATMENT

MEDICATION
- Acute, severe MR
  - Medical therapy has a limited role and is aimed to stabilize hemodynamics preoperatively.
  - Vasodilators (nitroprusside, nicardipine): to improve hemodynamic compensation but is often limited by systemic hypotension (1),(2)
- Chronic MR
  - Primary
    - Asymptomatic and normal LV systolic function: no proven long-term medical therapy
    - Symptomatic or asymptomatic with LV systolic dysfunction: diuretics, β-blockers, angiotensin-converting enzyme inhibitors (ACE-I) or angiotensin receptor blockers (ARBs) or angiotensin receptor-neprilysin inhibitor (ARNI), and aldosterone antagonists as indicated in standard therapy for HF (1),(2)
  - Secondary: LV dysfunction or symptomatic (stages B to D): ACE-I or ARBs or ARNI, β-blockers, and aldosterone antagonists, as indicated in standard therapy for HF (1)

SURGERY/OTHER PROCEDURES
- Isolated MV surgery is not indicated for patients with mild to moderate MR.
- Acute, severe MR secondary to acute MI
  - Acute rupture of papillary muscle: emergency MV repair/replacement
  - Papillary muscle displacement: aggressive medical stabilization and intra-aortic balloon pump; valve surgery usually required in addition to revascularization
- Chronic severe MR
  - Severe primary MR
    - MV surgery
      - Symptomatic patients (stage D): absence of severe LV dysfunction (EF >30%); may be considered if presence of severe LV dysfunction (EF ≤30%)
      - Asymptomatic patients
        - Mild/moderate LV dysfunction (EF 30–60% and/or ESD ≥40 mm, stage C2)
        - Preserved LV function (EF ≥60% and ESD ≤40 mm): MV repair is reasonable for asymptomatic patients (stage C1) if the likelihood of a successful and durable repair without residual MR is >95% and expected mortality is <1% when performed at a heart valve center of excellence (1).
        - Progressive increase in LV size or decrease in EF on ≥3 serial imaging studies (1)
      - Nonrheumatic MR with new onset of AF or resting pulmonary hypertension (pulmonary artery systolic pressure >50 mm Hg) and the likelihood of a successful and durable repair is high (2).
      - MV repair is recommended over MV replacement in patients with MR limited to the posterior leaflet or MR involving the anterior leaflet or both leaflets when a successful and durable repair can be accomplished.

  - Transcatheter edge-to-edge repair (TEER): may be considered for severely symptomatic patients (NYHA class III/IV) despite optimal GDMT for HF, who have favorable anatomy for the repair, and a reasonable life expectancy but a prohibitive surgical risk from severe comorbidities (1),(2)
  - Severe secondary MR
    - MV surgery
      - Undergoing coronary artery bypass graft (CABG) (1),(2)
      - Undergoing aortic valve replacement
      - May be considered for severely symptomatic patients (NYHA classes III and IV) despite optimal GDMT for HF (1),(2)
      - Chordal-sparing MVR is preferred over downsized annuloplasty repair in ischemic MR patients (1).
    - Cardiac resynchronization therapy is recommended for symptomatic patients (stages B to D) who meet the indications for device therapy (1),(2).
    - TEER: is reasonable for persistent symptoms despite maximally tolerated GDMT as assessed by a multidisciplinary experienced team in the evaluation and treatment of HF and MV disease, who have LVEF 20–50%, LV end-systolic diameter ≤7.0 cm, and pulmonary artery systolic pressure ≤70 mm Hg (1)

Geriatric Considerations
Medical therapy alone for patients >75 years of age with MR is preferred, owing to increased operative mortality and decreased survival (compared with those with AS), especially with preexisting CAD or need for MV replacement. MV repair is preferable than MV replacement.

ADMISSION, INPATIENT, AND NURSING CONSIDERATIONS
Acute MR: Stabilize airway, breathing, and circulation (ABCs). Obtain urgent surgical consultation.

 ONGOING CARE

FOLLOW-UP RECOMMENDATIONS
- Chronic MR with new-onset or changing symptoms: TTE
- Chronic MR: asymptomatic patients with normal LV function
  - Mild MR with normal LV size and no pulmonary hypertension: annual clinical evaluation and TTE every 3 to 5 years or more frequently depending on course
  - Moderate MR: annual clinical evaluation and TTE every 1 to 2 years
  - Severe MR: clinical evaluation and TTE every 6 to 12 months; biomarkers and/or global longitudinal strain may be considered.
  - Consider serial CXRs and ECGs and consider stress test if exercise capacity is doubtful.

PATIENT EDUCATION
- Exercise after MV repair: Avoid sports with risk for bodily contact or trauma. Low-intensity competitive sports are allowed.
- Competitive athletes with MR: asymptomatic with normal LV size and function, normal pulmonary artery pressures, and sinus rhythm: no restrictions; mildly symptomatic and those with LV dilatation: activities with low to moderate dynamic and static cardiac demand allowed; AF and anticoagulation: no contact sports

PROGNOSIS
- Acute, severe MR: Mortality risk with surgery is 50%; mortality risk with medical therapy alone is 75% in the first 24 hours and 95% at 2 weeks.
- Chronic MR: asymptomatic severe MR with normal LVEF: 10% yearly rate of progression to symptoms and subnormal resting LVEF; symptomatic severe MR: 8-year survival rate, 33% without surgery; mortality rate, 5% yearly

Pregnancy Considerations
MR with NYHA functional classes III and IV at high risk for maternal and/or fetal risk

COMPLICATIONS
Acute pulmonary edema, CHF, AF, bleeding risk with anticoagulation, endocarditis, sudden cardiac death

REFERENCES
1. Otto CM, Nishimura RA, Bonow RO, et al. 2020 ACC/AHA guideline for the management of patients with valvular heart disease: a report of the American College of Cardiology/American Heart Association Joint Committee on Clinical Practice Guidelines. *Circulation*. 2021;143(5):e72–e227.
2. Vahanian A, Beyersdorf F, Praz F, et al; for ESC/EACTS Scientific Document Group. 2021 ESC/EACTS guidelines for the management of valvular heart disease. *Eur Heart J*. 2022;43(7):561–632.

CODES

ICD10
- I34.0 Nonrheumatic mitral (valve) insufficiency
- I05.1 Rheumatic mitral insufficiency
- Q23.3 Congenital mitral insufficiency

CLINICAL PEARLS
Follow-up for mild to moderate MR: serial exam and/or echo (mild, every 3 to 5 years; moderate, 1 to 2 years) unless LV structural changes; severe primary MR is usually managed with MV repair.

M

MITRAL STENOSIS

Parul Chaudhri, DO • Sourabh Prabhakar, MD

BASICS

DESCRIPTION
- Mitral stenosis (MS) is narrowing of the mitral valve area causing obstruction of left ventricular (LV) inflow, resulting in increased left atrial (LA) pressures and consequent elevation of pulmonary venous pressure. The most common etiology for MS is rheumatic heart disease (RHD).
- Normal valve orifice is 4 to 6 cm^2; symptoms typically seen when orifice is <2.5 cm^2
- Staging of the disease is used to guide appropriate treatment regimen.
  - Stage A: "at risk of MS"—mild valve doming with normal flow velocity and NO hemodynamic obstruction or symptoms; no symptoms or echocardiographic changes
  - Stage B: "progressive MS"—increased diastolic doming, increased flow velocity, but MVA >1.5 cm^2, diastolic pressure 1/2 time <150 ms; no symptoms; mild to moderate LA enlargement and normal pulmonary pressures at rest on echo
  - Stage C: "asymptomatic severe MS"—diastolic doming, MVA <1.5 cm^2, diastolic pressure half time >150 ms, severe LA enlargement, PASP >30 mm Hg, but NO symptoms; severe LA enlargement and elevated PA systolic pressures >50 mm Hg on echo
  - Stage D: "symptomatic severe MS"—stage C with dyspnea on exertion and decreased exercise tolerance; severe LA enlargement and elevated PA systolic pressures >50 mm Hg on echo

EPIDEMIOLOGY
Global prevalence of RHD is 40.5 million cases. There are 305,000 deaths attributed to RHD annually. Incidence of rheumatic disease in the continental United States remains low (<2 per 100,000 school-aged children).

ETIOLOGY AND PATHOPHYSIOLOGY
- Narrowing of the mitral valve orifice leads to obstruction of blood flow between LA and LV. This impairs LV filling during diastole and causes increased LA pressure.
- Increased LA pressure is transmitted passively ("back pressure") to the pulmonary circulation causing pulmonary hypertension (HTN) and pulmonary congestion over time, leading to right-sided failure.
- Chronic LA pressure overload results in atrial dilation and fibrosis, resulting in atrial fibrillation.
- Rheumatic fever: most common cause (See "Risk Factors.")
  - Pathognomonic commissural fusion, leaflet thickening, and "fish mouth appearance" seen with RHD
  - The anatomic changes of severe MS is thought to be secondary to recurrent episodes of ARF as well as a chronic autoimmune process caused by cross-reactivity between a streptococcal protein and valve tissue.
- Aging (extension of mitral annular calcification)

- Rare causes: congenital (associated with mucopolysaccharidoses); autoimmune: systemic lupus erythematosus (SLE), rheumatoid arthritis, malignant carcinoid, Whipple disease, methysergide therapy; and other acquired: LA myxoma, LA thrombus, endomyocardial fibrosis

RISK FACTORS
- ARF and RHD are the greatest risk factors. ARF occurs 2 to 3 weeks after an episode of untreated pharyngitis caused by rheumatogenic group A streptococci (GAS) organism in a genetically susceptible host.
  - 30–40% of rheumatic fever patients eventually develop MS, presenting 20 years after diagnosis of ARF.
  - Recurrent infections can accelerate the progression of the disease.
  - Low socioeconomic status (i.e., crowded conditions) favors the spread of streptococcal infection.
- Aging (increasing valvular calcification)
- Chest irradiation (increasing tissue fibrosis)
- Use of drugs: MDMA (ecstasy), ergot alkaloids

GENERAL PREVENTION
- Prompt recognition and treatment of GAS infection in at-risk populations; recognition of cardinal signs and symptoms of ARF via Jones criteria
- Transthoracic echo (TTE) screening has been shown to increase diagnosis of RHD in asymptomatic patients residing in areas of high prevalence.

COMMONLY ASSOCIATED CONDITIONS
Atrial fibrillation (30–40% of symptomatic patients), other valvular problems (aortic stenosis and insufficiency), pulmonary HTN and right heart failure, systemic embolism, infective endocarditis

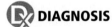

DIAGNOSIS

HISTORY
- History of ARF or RHD
- Severity depends on valve area; most early cases will be asymptomatic.
- Mean age of symptom onset in rheumatic valvular disease is in the late 30s to 40s. Latent period is 20 to 40 years after infection. Rapid progression can be seen in some high prevalence areas.
- Presenting features usually include dyspnea on exertion, decrease exercise tolerance, chest pain, palpitations, hoarseness, hemoptysis, fatigue, paroxysmal nocturnal dyspnea, orthopnea, atrial fibrillation, and embolic events.
- In advanced disease, symptoms of pulmonary HTN and right heart failure predominate: jugular venous distention, hepatomegaly, ascites, and peripheral edema.
- Not infrequently, symptoms are first noted in pregnancy: mitral facies, plethoric cheeks, and bluish patches.

PHYSICAL EXAM
- Elevated jugular venous pressure, diastolic thrill in the left lateral decubitus position; a right ventricle lift may be felt in the left parasternal area in patients with pulmonary HTN.
- Auscultation
  - Classic murmur: accentuated S$_1$, opening snap (OS), apical early decrescendo diastolic rumble with presystolic accentuation (presystolic accentuation of murmur is lost with atrial fibrillation). Murmur is low pitch and best heard at the apex in the left lateral decubitus position.
  - Murmur is accentuated with exercise and decreased with rest and Valsalva. With mobile, noncalcified valve, murmur persists throughout diastole and S$_1$, and the OS remains loud. With increasing severity of MS, murmur often is difficult to hear. Duration of murmur is reflective of severity. S$_1$ and the OS may be soft to absent. A shorter S$_2$ to OS interval indicates more severe MS (<70 ms).
- If pulmonary HTN is present: Increased P$_2$, high-pitched decrescendo diastolic murmur of pulmonic insufficiency is heard (Graham Steell murmur); may have signs of right heart failure; RV lift can also be seen.
- May also find associated aortic or tricuspid murmurs due to involvement from RHD

DIAGNOSTIC TESTS & INTERPRETATION
Initial Tests (lab, imaging)
- ECG: LA enlargement ("P mitrale"), atrial fibrillation, and right ventricular hypertrophy may be seen.
- Chest radiograph: LA enlargement, straightening of the left heart border, a "double density" on right, and elevation of the left main stem bronchus; prominent pulmonary arteries at the hilum with rapid tapering, RVH, and edema pattern with Kerley A and B lines (late presentation)
- TTE is recommended in all patients with signs of symptoms of MS. It is used to diagnose and assess for concomitant valvulopathies
- Transesophageal echocardiogram (TEE) should be performed if TTE images are nondiagnostic or if being considered for a percutaneous mitral balloon commissurotomy (PMBC) or valvuloplasty (PMBV) to exclude thrombus in LA and evaluate severity of MR.
- Exercise stress testing with Doppler echocardiography can also be considered in patients with MS who have a discrepancy in their symptoms and signs and resting echo findings.
- Cardiac catheterization and the use of Gorlin formula to assess LA and LV pressures are indicated when echo is inconclusive or if there is a discrepancy between the echo, symptoms, and severity (class I).
- CT imaging: provides MVA estimates, LA cavity size; useful prior to surgery, to evaluate for concomitant coronary artery disease (CAD)

Follow-Up Tests & Special Considerations
- If valve area >1.5 cm^2 and mean pressure gradient <5 mm Hg, clinical follow-up in 3 to 5 years is recommended.

- Otherwise, follow-up is usually symptom based. Symptomatic patients with severe MS need further evaluation for interventional/surgical treatment.
- Holter monitor placement to rule out paroxysmal atrial fibrillation

Diagnostic Procedures/Other
- Exercise testing is recommended for those with clinical discrepancy.
- Wilkins score evaluates valvular anatomy from a TTE in order to see if the patient is a candidate for surgery.

Test Interpretation
- Rheumatic fever–induced pathologic changes: leaflet thickening, leaflet calcification, commissural fusion, chordal shortening
- MV area defined: normal: 4 to 6 cm^2, progressive MS: >1.5 cm^2, asymptomatic severe MS: <1.5 cm^2, severe MS: <1.5 cm^2, very severe MS: <1.0 cm^2

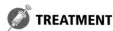 TREATMENT

GENERAL MEASURES
- Treatment is dependent on severity of stenosis and symptoms.
- Patients who have a valvular area >1.5 cm^2 and no symptoms can be managed medically.
- MS is generally progressive, and medical therapy only delays the need for definitive therapy. It entails:
  – Treatment to prevent recurrence of rheumatic fever
  – Treatments aimed at improving dyspnea and exercise tolerance
  – Controlling the ventricular rate whether in sinus rhythm or atrial fibrillation
  – Anticoagulation for prevention of thromboembolic events

MEDICATION
First Line
- Use of anticoagulation for prevention of thromboembolism
  – Class I recommendations: MS and atrial fibrillation or history of atrial fibrillation, MS and prior embolic event, or MS and LA thrombus
  – Class IIB recommendations: patients with enlarged LA and spontaneous contrast on echo
- Warfarin is the accepted modality for anticoagulation in patients with rheumatic MV disease (international normalized ratio range 2 to 3). Factor Xa inhibitors and direct thrombin inhibitors are not approved for use in atrial fibrillation with patients that have moderate-to-severe MS (1),(2).
- Heparin is used for anticoagulation with atrial fibrillation.
- Antibiotic prophylaxis against rheumatic fever and/or carditis is recommended for patients with history of rheumatic fever. Secondary prophylaxis is dependent on many factors: number of previous attacks, time since previous infection, risk for getting GAS, age of patient, and absence or presence of cardiac involvement.
- Diuretics for congestive symptoms and symptomatic heart failure
- β-Blockers or nondihydropyridine calcium channel blockers used for controlling heart rate both in sinus rhythm and atrial fibrillation to allow adequate diastolic filling and decrease LA diastolic pressure, tachycardia or exertional symptoms (class IIa)

- Ivabradine *helpful because it doesn't affect myocardial contraction*
- Consider cardioversion, especially in patients with mild MS and recent diagnosis of atrial fibrillation (<6 months).

Second Line
Consider amiodarone or digitalis if β-blockers and calcium channel blockers are not beneficial in controlling rapid ventricular rate. Consider digitalis in patients with symptomatic systolic dysfunction.

SURGERY/OTHER PROCEDURES
- Surgical techniques include balloon valvotomy, open mitral commissurotomy, or closed mitral commissurotomy and mitral valve replacement.
- Patients with severe MS and symptoms consistent with NYHA classes III and IV are candidates for surgery.
- Any patient with a valve area >1.5 cm^2, LA thrombus, moderate or severe MR, severe or bicommissural calcifications, severe aortic valve disease, moderate TR or TS, and concomitant CAD requiring bypass surgery are NOT candidates for PMBC or PMBV.
- Per the 2014 AHA/ACC valvular heart disease guidelines (which is similar to the 2017 European Society of Cardiology Guidelines) (3), PMBC or PMBV is recommended for patients with the following: symptomatic severe MS (MVA <1.5 cm^2) and favorable valve morphology; symptomatic severe MS with severe (NYHA III/IV) symptoms who have suboptimal valve anatomy and are not candidates or are high risk for surgery; asymptomatic very severe MS (MVA <1 cm^2) and favorable valve anatomy in the absence of contraindications; asymptomatic very severe MS (MVA <1 cm^2) and favorable valve anatomy in the absence of contraindications; asymptomatic severe MS and favorable valve morphology with new-onset atrial fibrillation in absence of contraindications; symptomatic patients with MVA >1.5 cm^2 if there is an evidence of hemodynamically significant MS during exercise
- Patient's age, bleeding risk, and other comorbidities prior to deciding if patient should have a prosthetic versus mechanical valve

Pregnancy Considerations
- Volume expansion during pregnancy can exacerbate heart failure symptoms. For patients with known severe MS, prepregnancy discussions should be pursued with a cardiologist.
- Warfarin (Coumadin) is considered relatively safe in the 2nd and 3rd trimesters if anticoagulation is required. However, unfractionated heparin is preferred prior to labor and delivery.

 ONGOING CARE

FOLLOW-UP RECOMMENDATIONS
- Counsel patients that MS usually is slowly progressive but can have sudden onset of atrial fibrillation, which could become rapidly fatal. Call 911 for marked worsening of symptoms.
- Echocardiographic surveillance in asymptomatic patients in any degree of MS: very severe (MVA <1 cm^2) MS: yearly, severe (MVA ≤1.5 cm^2) MS: every 1 to 2 years, mild or moderate MS (MVA >1.5 cm^2): every 3 to 5 years

- Follow-up will depend on the severity of the MS and the patient's symptoms. Asymptomatic patients will need annual history and examination. Symptomatic patients are followed closely based on clinical response to adjust therapy and plan definitive treatment.

DIET
Salt restriction for pulmonary congestion

PROGNOSIS
- Asymptomatic latent period after rheumatic fever for 10 to 30 years; 10-year survival for asymptomatic or minimally symptomatic patients is 80%. 10-year survival after onset of debilitating symptoms is only 0–15%. Mean survival with significant pulmonary HTN is <3 years.
- Commissurotomy is an effective means of reducing stenosis but is not curative. Restenosis sometimes occurs and can be early (<5 years) or late (>20 years).

COMPLICATIONS
Left and right heart failure, atrial fibrillation and systemic embolic events, pulmonary HTN, hepatic congestion, and infective endocarditis

REFERENCES
1. Otto CM, Nishimura RA, Bonow RO, et al. 2020 ACC/AHA guideline for the management of patients with valvular heart disease: executive summary: a report of the American College of Cardiology/American Heart Association Joint Committee on Clinical Practice Guidelines. *Circulation*. 2021;143(5):e35–e71.
2. January CT, Wann LS, Calkins H, et al. 2019 AHA/ACC/HRS focused update of the 2014 AHA/ACC/HRS guideline for the management of patients with atrial fibrillation: a report of the American College of Cardiology/American Heart Association Task Force on Clinical Practice Guidelines and the Heart Rhythm Society. *J Am Coll Cardiol*. 2019;74(1):104–132.
3. Nishimura RA, Otto CM, Bonow RO, et al. 2017 AHA/ACC focused update of the 2014 AHA/ACC guideline for the management of patients with valvular heart disease: a report of the American College of Cardiology/American Heart Association Task Force on Clinical Practice Guidelines. *J Am Coll Cardiol*. 2017;70(2):252–289.

CODES

ICD10
- I01.1 Acute rheumatic endocarditis
- Q23.2 Congenital mitral stenosis
- I34.2 Nonrheumatic mitral (valve) stenosis

CLINICAL PEARLS
- Asymptomatic patients may be followed clinically with yearly exams for development of symptoms with periodic echo to evaluate valve area and PA systolic pressure.
- Once symptoms of MS develop, initiate appropriate medical therapy and advise patient that surgical therapy may be needed to prolong survival. Almost all cases of MV stenosis progress in severity over time.

M

MITRAL VALVE PROLAPSE
Justin T. Ertle, MD • Timothy A. Scully, DO

BASICS

DESCRIPTION
- Mitral valve prolapse (MVP) is the billowing of one or both mitral valve leaflets into the left atrium (LA) during ventricular systole.
- MVP can be classified in different ways, including by etiology (primary or secondary; see "Etiology and Pathophysiology") or by morphology (classic MVP and nonclassic MVP; see "Test Interpretation").
- MVP is often asymptomatic and often has a benign clinical course; however, it may occasionally be associated with symptoms, such as palpitations, or complications, such as mitral regurgitation (MR) (see "Complications").
- Synonym(s): systolic click-murmur syndrome, billowing mitral cusp syndrome, myxomatous mitral valve, floppy valve syndrome, redundant cusp syndrome, Barlow syndrome.

EPIDEMIOLOGY
Prevalence
- Estimated 1–3% of the population (1),(2)
- Equally distributed by gender (1),(2)
- Typically found in adults, although not at a certain stage of adulthood (1),(2)

ETIOLOGY AND PATHOPHYSIOLOGY
- The pathophysiology of MVP typically involves myxomatous degeneration of the mitral valve leaflets, characterized by expansion of the valve spongiosa layer, structural alterations in collagen, and structurally abnormal chordae (1),(3).
- Papillary muscle or chordae disruption, dysfunction, or rupture may also cause MVP; this can occur without a process causing myxomatous degeneration or as part of the natural history of a process causing myxomatous degeneration.
- The etiology of MVP is multifactorial and includes the following (1):
  – Primary MVP: sporadic or familial
  – Secondary MVP
    ○ "Syndromic" MVP: myxomatous degeneration associated with connective tissue disorders, for example Marfan syndrome, Ehlers-Danlos syndrome, osteogenesis imperfecta, pseudoxanthoma elasticum, Loeys-Dietz syndrome
    ○ Associated with congenital heart disease: atrial septal defect, Ebstein anomaly
- Papillary/chordae disruption, dysfunction or rupture: infarction, endocarditis, rheumatic fever, trauma, hypertrophic cardiomyopathy

Genetics
- In primary MVP, both autosomal dominant and X-linked instances have been found.
  – Autosomal dominant: variable penetrance; several genetic loci so far identified (1)
    ○ *MMVP1:* chromosome 16 p11.2–p12.1
    ○ *MMVP2:* chromosome 11 p15.4
    ○ *MMVP3:* chromosome 13 q31.3–q32.1
  – X-linked: One gene has been identified: filamin A gene, Xq28 (1).
- Connective tissue disorders, which often have a genetic basis, are associated with secondary MVP (see "Etiology and Pathophysiology").

RISK FACTORS
- Medical conditions implicated in the development of MVP include both heritable and sporadic congenital abnormalities as well as other disease processes. (See "Etiology and Pathophysiology.")
- MVP is more common with leaner BMI (1).

COMMONLY ASSOCIATED CONDITIONS
- Conditions implicated in the development of MVP include both heritable and sporadic congenital abnormalities as well as other disease processes. (See "Etiology and Pathophysiology.")
- MVP is implicated in the development of other medical conditions/complications, such as MR and stroke. (See "Complications.")
- Some associated conditions that are less clearly either (i) a cause of MVP or (ii) caused by MVP include von Willebrand disease; primary hypomastia; thoracic skeletal abnormalities; and prolapse of the tricuspid, pulmonic, or aortic valves.

DIAGNOSIS

HISTORY
- Most patients with MVP are asymptomatic.
- Symptoms that occur may be related to MVP itself, to MR as a result of MVP, or to other complications of MVP such as stroke, arrhythmia, etc.
- Symptoms related to MVP include palpitations (most commonly associated symptom), atypical chest pain, fatigue, exercise intolerance, orthostasis/presyncope, and neuropsychiatric symptoms such as panic attacks.
- Symptoms related to progression of MR: fatigue, dyspnea, exercise intolerance, orthopnea, paroxysmal nocturnal dyspnea

PHYSICAL EXAM
- The principal auscultatory finding is a midsystolic click, although not heard in all cases (1).
- This may also be followed by mid- to late-systolic murmur, loudest at the apex (1).
- Dynamic auscultation may help differentiate between similar systolic sounds.
  – Maneuvers that decrease end-diastolic volume move the click and murmur toward S1: standing up, Valsalva.
    ○ Note: Valsalva maneuver may help differentiate hypertrophic obstructive cardiomyopathy (HOCM) from MVP as it increases the intensity of the murmur in HOCM, whereas it increases the duration of the murmur in MVP.
  – Maneuvers that increase end-diastolic volume move the click and murmur toward S2: squatting, leg raise.
- Exam findings may also reflect the presence of MR as a result of MVP.
  – MR holosystolic murmur best heard at the apex, with radiation to the left axilla
  – The duration of the murmur corresponds with the severity of MR. Presence of an S3 may indicate severe regurgitation.

DIFFERENTIAL DIAGNOSIS
- Ejection clicks (do not change timing with systole)
- Papillary muscle dysfunction
- MR
- Tricuspid regurgitation
- Hypertrophic cardiomyopathy

DIAGNOSTIC TESTS & INTERPRETATION
Initial Tests (lab, imaging)
- Transthoracic echocardiogram (TTE) is the diagnostic modality of choice after an appropriate physical exam; echocardiogram is required for definitive diagnosis.
  – In asymptomatic patients with physical signs of MVP, echocardiography is indicated for the diagnosis of MVP and assessment of MR, leaflet morphology, and ventricular compensation.
  – Echocardiography is not indicated to exclude MVP in asymptomatic patients with ill-defined symptoms in the absence of a constellation of clinical symptoms or physical findings suggestive of MVP, or a positive family history.
- Electrocardiogram (ECG) may be considered but is not required in the workup of MVP, without other indication.
  – Palpitations are a common symptom, which should prompt ECG.
  – ECG in MVP is typically normal; however, ECG findings in MVP can include nonspecific ST-T wave changes, T-wave inversions, prominent Q waves, and even prolonged QT.

Follow-Up Tests & Special Considerations
- Ambulatory heart rhythm monitor should be considered if patient has palpitations but is not indicated for asymptomatic MVP.
- Transesophageal echocardiography (TEE), particularly with 3D imaging, may be considered to further visualize anatomy if intervention is planned or there is limited visibility of the mitral valve on TTE.
- Angiography is rarely used for diagnostic purposes but may be recommended for hemodynamic assessment when noninvasive options are inconclusive.
- Patients with MVP and severe MR may require coronary angiography and TEE if cardiac surgical referral is planned (see "Indications for Referral").
- Cardiac MRI and/or electrophysiology studies may be indicated in patients with findings that may indicate an elevated risk of sudden cardiac death (SCD) (see "Complications") (2)[C].

Test Interpretation
MVP is defined as anterior, posterior, or bileaflet prolapse of at least 2-mm superior displacement into the LA during systole on the parasternal long-axis annular plane of the valve on echocardiogram, with or without associated leaflet thickening (1).
- Morphologic classification (1):
  – Classic MVP (a.k.a. Barlow syndrome): prolapse with >5 mm of leaflet thickening
  – Nonclassic MVP (fibroelastic deficiency): prolapse with <5 mm of leaflet thickening
- "Flail" mitral prolapse is the term for a severe form in which a segment or segments of a leaflet protrude into the LA during systole; typically, this is associated with torn chordae or ruptured papillary muscle.

TREATMENT

GENERAL MEASURES

- Reassurance is appropriate for patients with milder forms of prolapse and low symptom burden; normal lifestyle and regular exercise is encouraged.
- If MVP is associated with palpitations, fatigue, or anxiety, patients are encouraged to limit alcohol, cigarettes, and caffeine.
- MVP with orthostatic symptoms may be managed by liberalizing fluid and salt intake. Support stockings may also be beneficial.

MEDICATION

- Aspirin (75 to 325 mg daily) may be considered for MVP with "high-risk" echocardiographic features (thickening >5 mm or valve redundancy).
- Aspirin (75 to 325 mg daily) is recommended for patients with MVP and transient ischemic attacks (TIAs).
- Warfarin may be considered for patients with MVP and TIAs who continue to experience TIAs despite aspirin.
- Aspirin (75 to 325 mg daily) is considered for patients with MVP and history of stroke, without high-risk echocardiographic features (thickening >5 mm or valve redundancy), MR, atrial fibrillation, or left atrial thrombus.
- Warfarin is considered for patients with MVP and history of stroke, who do have either high-risk echocardiographic features (thickening >5 mm or valve redundancy), MR, atrial fibrillation, or atrial thrombus.
- Patients with MVP and palpitations may be treated with β-blockers.

ISSUES FOR REFERRAL

- Cardiology referral is indicated in MVP with significant symptoms, high-risk features, or concomitant cardiac diagnoses. Electrophysiologist referral would be recommended for significant arrhythmia.
- Cardiothoracic surgery referral is indicated in patients with indication for surgical repair.
- Genetic counselling is considered when a heritable condition is suspected.

SURGERY/OTHER PROCEDURES

MVP and myxomatous valve degeneration are the most common causes of chronic primary MR requiring surgery in high-income countries.

- Referral for consideration of mitral valve surgery is indicated for the following:
  - Severe primary MR with symptoms
  - Asymptomatic MR patients with LV systolic dysfunction (LVEF ≤60%, LVESD ≥40mm)
- Minimally invasive surgery and surgery for asymptomatic patients without LV systolic dysfunction is an area of ongoing research.
  - Asymptomatic patients with atrial fibrillation or pulmonary hypertension may be considered for surgical intervention.
- In general, if surgery is indicated for MR, mitral valve repair is preferred over replacement when possible, due to lower rates of operative mortality and long-term complications.

 ONGOING CARE

FOLLOW-UP RECOMMENDATIONS

- Periodic monitoring with TTE is recommended in asymptomatic patients with known valvular heart disease, at intervals depending on valve lesion, severity, ventricular size, and ventricular function.
  - Asymptomatic MVP with no significant MR can be followed every 3 to 5 years.
  - Patients who are symptomatic or have high-risk features on initial echocardiogram, including moderate to severe MR, may need serial echocardiograms and should be followed clinically at least once per year.

PATIENT EDUCATION

- Patients can be counselled that MVP is often a benign condition.
- Patients should be counselled that there is no contraindication to pregnancy based on the diagnosis of MVP alone.
- Patients should be counselled to promptly report any change in symptom status, which may require repeat echocardiography.
- Educate patients on occasional familial MVP occurrence.
- Restriction from high-intensity competitive sports is recommended if a patient has MVP with any one of the following features:
  - Moderate LV enlargement or LV dysfunction
  - Uncontrolled tachyarrhythmias
  - Prolonged QT interval
  - Unexplained syncope
  - Prior resuscitation from cardiac arrest
  - Aortic root enlargement

PROGNOSIS

- Prognosis is excellent for asymptomatic patients without complications; MVP is often benign with a normal life expectancy.
- Overall, the prognosis of MVP is closely tied to whether MR develops and how it progresses as well as occurrence of other serious complications (1).
- Ventricular arrhythmias and SCD both occur more often with MVP that in the general population but are still rare (see "Complications"). SCD occurs in the community at 0.06–0.08% per year; in MVP, this appears to be 1.75 to 2.3 times higher; per 100 patient-years, there is an estimated 0.14 SCD events in patients with MVP (2).

COMPLICATIONS

- MR—MVP and myxomatous valve degeneration is the most common cause of chronic primary MR in high-income countries.
  - Many additional complications may arise as a consequence of severe MR:
    - Heart failure
    - Pulmonary hypertension with associated RV dysfunction
    - Left atrial dilatation with associated paroxysmal supraventricular tachycardias (including atrial fibrillation)

- Arrhythmias, including premature atrial complexes, supraventricular tachycardias, ventricular ectopy, and ventricular arrhythmias in general (2)
- SCD occurs more often with MVP than in the general population; still very rare (See "Prognosis.")
  - Patients with MVP who have bileaflet prolapse, cardiac fibrosis, ST-T wave abnormalities, complex ventricular ectopy, or ventricular arrhythmias seem to specifically have elevated risk of SCD (2).
- Cerebrovascular ischemia (stroke and TIAs)
- Infective endocarditis

REFERENCES

1. Delling FN, Vasan RS. Epidemiology and pathophysiology of mitral valve prolapse: new insights into disease progression, genetics, and molecular basis. *Circulation*. 2014;129(21):2158–2170.
2. Nalliah CJ, Mahajan R, Elliott AD, et al. Mitral valve prolapse and sudden cardiac death: a systematic review and meta-analysis. *Heart*. 2019;105(2):144–151.
3. Otto CM, Nishimura RA, Bonow RO, et al. 2020 ACC/AHA guideline for the management of patients with valvular heart disease: a report of the American College of Cardiology/American Heart Association Joint Committee on Clinical Practice Guidelines. *Circulation*. 2021;143(5):e72–e227.

ADDITIONAL READING

- Guy TS, Hill AC. Mitral valve prolapse. *Annu Rev Med*. 2012;63:277–292.
- Nishimura RA, Vahanian A, Eleid MF, et al. Mitral valve disease—current management and future challenges. *Lancet*. 2016;387(10025):1324–1334.

CODES

ICD10

- I34.1 Nonrheumatic mitral (valve) prolapse
- I05.8 Other rheumatic mitral valve diseases

CLINICAL PEARLS

- MVP is the billowing of one or both mitral valve leaflets into the LA during ventricular systole.
- The principal auscultatory finding is a midsystolic click, although this is not heard in all cases; the click may also be followed by mid- to late-systolic murmur, loudest at the apex.
- Echocardiogram is required for definitive diagnosis.
- The etiology of MVP is multifactorial and can be secondary to a diverse range of other conditions such as connective tissue disorders, congenital heart disease, infarction, endocarditis, rheumatic fever, and trauma.

M

MOLLUSCUM CONTAGIOSUM

Dongsheng Jiang, MD, MSc

 BASICS

DESCRIPTION
Molluscum contagiosum is a common, benign, viral (poxvirus) skin infection, characterized by small (2 to 5 mm), waxy white or flesh-colored, dome-shaped papules often with central umbilication. Lesions contain a cheesy grayish white material. Molluscum contagiosum is highly contagious and spreads by autoinoculation, skin-to-skin contact, sexual contact, and shared clothing/towels. Molluscum contagiosum is a self-limited infection in immunocompetent patients but can be difficult to treat and disfiguring in immunocompromised patients.

EPIDEMIOLOGY
Prevalence
- 1% in the United States, occurring mainly in children aged 2 to 15 years and sexually active young adults
- 5–18% HIV population

ETIOLOGY AND PATHOPHYSIOLOGY
- DNA virus; Poxviridae family
- Four genetic virus types, clinically indistinguishable
- Virions invade and replicate in cytoplasm of epithelial cells causing abnormal cell proliferation.
- Genome encodes proteins to evade host immune system.
- Incubation period: 2 to 6 weeks
- Time to resolution: 6 to 24 months
- Not associated with malignancy
- No cross-hybridization or reactivation by other poxviruses

RISK FACTORS
- Skin-to-skin contact with infected person
- Contact sports
- Swimming
- Atopic dermatitis
- Sexual activity with infected partner
- Immunocompromised: HIV, chemotherapy, corticosteroid therapy, transplant patients, patients on biologics

GENERAL PREVENTION
- Avoid skin-to-skin contact with host (e.g., contact sports, sexual activity).
- Avoid sharing clothing and towels.

COMMONLY ASSOCIATED CONDITIONS
- Atopic dermatitis
- Immunosuppression medications: corticosteroids, biologics, chemotherapy, etc.
- HIV/AIDS

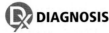 DIAGNOSIS

HISTORY
- Contact with known infected person
- Participation in contact sports
- Sexual activity

PHYSICAL EXAM
- Perform thorough skin exam including conjunctiva and anogenital area.
- Discrete, firm papules with a central umbilication
- White curd-like core under umbilicated center
- Lesions are flesh-colored, pearly, or red in color and frequently located in intertriginous areas.
- May have surrounding erythema or dermatitis
- Immunocompetent hosts: average of 11 to 20 lesions, 2 to 5 mm diameter (range: 1 to 10 mm)
- Immunocompromised hosts may have hundreds of widespread lesions or "giant" molluscum (lesions >1 cm)
- Sexually active: inner thighs, anogenital area

Pediatric Considerations
- Infants <3 months: Consider vertical transmission. If vertical transmission, lesions often located on scalp
- Children: fever, >50 lesions, limited response to therapy; consider immunodeficiency.
- Children: anogenital lesions; most likely autoinoculation if lesions present elsewhere on body. However, provider should consider possible sexual abuse.

DIFFERENTIAL DIAGNOSIS
- Verruca vulgaris
- Chickenpox
- Milia
- AIDS patients: *Cryptococcus neoformans*, penicilliosis, histoplasmosis, coccidioidomycosis
- Basal cell carcinoma
- Benign appendageal tumors: syringomas, hidrocystomas, ectopic sebaceous glands
- Condyloma acuminatum
- Dermatofibroma

- Eyelid: abscess, chalazion, foreign-body granuloma
- Folliculitis/furunculosis
- Keratoacanthoma
- Oral squamous cell carcinoma
- Trichoepithelioma
- Warty dyskeratoma
- Amelanotic melanoma
- Papular urticaria

DIAGNOSTIC TESTS & INTERPRETATION
Initial Tests (lab, imaging)
- Virus cannot be cultured.
- Culture lesion if concern is secondary infection.
- Sexual transmission: Test for other sexually transmitted infections, including HIV.
- Microscopy: scrape lesion
  - Core material has characteristic Henderson-Paterson intracytoplasmic viral inclusion bodies.
  - Crush prep with 10% potassium hydroxide will show characteristic inclusion bodies as well.
  - Alternatively, hematoxylin-eosin-stained formalin-fixed tissue shows same confirmatory features.

Diagnostic Procedures/Other
Clinical exam generally diagnostic, but dermatoscopy can be helpful.

Test Interpretation
Characteristic dermoscopic findings:
- Central pore or umbilication, white-to-yellow polylobular structure, and crown vessels

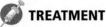 TREATMENT

GENERAL MEASURES
- In healthy patients, molluscum contagiosum is generally self-limited and resolves spontaneously; therefore, treatment is optional (1)[A].
- No single intervention is shown to be convincingly more effective than any other in treating molluscum contagiosum (1)[A].
- There are no FDA-approved treatments for molluscum contagiosum.
- Treatment decision is typically based on patient's age, location, number of lesions, comorbidities, availability, and cost.
- Three categories of treatment: destructive, immune-enhancing, and antiviral

MEDICATION

First Line

Cantharidin 0.7–0.9% solution: In office application to lesions, cover with dressing; wash off in 2 to 6 hours or sooner if blistering. Repeat treatment every 2 to 4 weeks until lesions resolve (1)[A].

- Not commercially available in the United States but may be prepared in the United States by compounding pharmacy from powder; might be available as solution from Canada
- Adverse effects: blistering, erythema, pain, pruritus develop after the office visit. Initially no discomfort, so this medication may be particularly useful in children.
- Precautions: Do not use on face or on genital mucosa.

Second Line

- Benzoyl peroxide 10% cream: Apply to each lesion twice daily for 4 weeks (1)[A].
  - Inexpensive, available over the counter
  - Adverse effects: mild dermatitis
- Imiquimod 5% cream: 3–5 times per week for 12 weeks
  - Adverse effects: mucositis, leukopenia, vitiligo (2)
- Other topicals reported: podophyllotoxin, trichloroacetic acid, salicylic acid, lactic acid, glycolic acid, and tretinoin (3)
- Cimetidine: oral; 25–40 mg/kg/day (3)
- For immunocompromised patients (including HIV) with refractory lesions, consider
  - Cidofovir: topical cream or IV

ISSUES FOR REFERRAL

Immunocompromised patients not responding to first- or second-line treatment

SURGERY/OTHER PROCEDURES

- Cryotherapy: 1 or 2 cycles of 10 to 20 seconds (3); repeat every 3 to 4 weeks as needed until lesions disappear.
  - Adverse effects: erythema, edema, pain, blistering
  - Contraindications: cryoglobulinemia, Raynaud disease
- Curettage under local or topical anesthesia (1)[A]
  - Adverse effects: pain, scarring
- Intralesional immunotherapy:
  - Candida antigen, PPD, vitamin D, MMR
  - Benefits: low to no recurrence
  - Adverse effects: erythema, edema, allergic reaction, anaphylaxis

COMPLEMENTARY & ALTERNATIVE MEDICINE

- Australian lemon myrtle oil: Apply 10% solution once daily for 21 days (1)[A].
- Potassium hydroxide 5–10% solution: Apply 1 to 2 times a day until the lesions disappeared completely (1)[A].

Pediatric Considerations

- Treatment is optional for immunocompetent children.
- Surgical interventions: second line in small children due to associated pain
- Pain control: Pretreat with topical lidocaine or EMLA before surgical treatment.
- Note: adverse effect: lidocaine or EMLA over large body surface area: methemoglobinemia and CNS toxicity. Refer to manufacturer's recommendations on dosing and use in children.

Pregnancy Considerations

Treatments safe in pregnancy: curettage, cryotherapy, incision, and expression

 ONGOING CARE

FOLLOW-UP RECOMMENDATIONS

Patient Monitoring

Depends on type of treatment

PATIENT EDUCATION

- Cover lesions to prevent spread.
- Avoid scratching to prevent autoinoculation.
- Avoid sharing towels and clothing.
- Practice safe sex or avoid sexual activity when lesions present.

PROGNOSIS

- Immunocompetent: self-limited, resolves in 3 to 12 months (range: 2 months to 4 years)
- Immunocompromised: lesions difficult to treat; may persist for years

COMPLICATIONS

- Secondary infection
- Scarring, hyper-/hypopigmentation (generally only occurs as a result of treatment, not when lesions resolve spontaneously)

REFERENCES

1. van der Wouden JC, van der Sande R, Kruithof EJ, et al. Interventions for cutaneous molluscum contagiosum. *Cochrane Database Syst Rev.* 2017;5(5):CD004767.
2. DiBiagio JR, Pyle T, Green JJ. Reviewing the use of imiquimod for molluscum contagiosum. *Dermatol Online J.* 2018;24(6):13030/qt3b4606qt.
3. Meza-Romero R, Navarrete-Dechent C, Downey C. Molluscum contagiosum: an update and review of new perspectives in etiology, diagnosis, and treatment. *Clin Cosmet Investig Dermatol.* 2019;12:373–381.

ADDITIONAL READING

- Clebak KT, Malone MA. Skin Infections. *Prim Care.* 2018;45(3):433–454.
- Nowicka D, Bagłaj-Oleszczuk M, Maj J. Infectious diseases of the skin in contact sports. *Adv Clin Exp Med.* 2020;29(12):1491–1495.

 CODES

ICD10

B08.1 Molluscum contagiosum

CLINICAL PEARLS

- Observation is preferred treatment in healthy patients as lesions will spontaneously resolve.
- Reassure parents that a child's lesions will heal naturally and generally resolve without scarring.
- No specific treatment has been identified as superior to any other, and no treatment is FDA approved.
- Consider topical corticosteroids for pruritus or associated dermatitis.

M

MORTON NEUROMA (INTERDIGITAL NEUROMA)

Lee A. Mancini, MD, CSCS*D, CSN

 BASICS

DESCRIPTION
- Painful condition of the webbed spaces of the toes
- Features perineural fibrosis of the common digital nerve as it passes between metatarsals
  - The interspace between the 3rd and 4th metatarsals is most commonly affected.
  - The interspace between the 2nd and 3rd metatarsals is the next most common site.
- Systems affected: musculoskeletal, nervous
- Synonyms: plantar digital neuritis; Morton metatarsalgia; intermetatarsal neuroma

EPIDEMIOLOGY

Prevalence
- Unknown
- Mean age: 45 to 50 years
- Predominant sex: female > male (8:1)

ETIOLOGY AND PATHOPHYSIOLOGY
- Lateral plantar nerve joins a portion of medial plantar nerve, creating a nerve with a larger diameter than those going to other digits.
- Etiology not fully understood; four main theories:
  - Chronic traction damage
  - Inflammatory environment due to intermetatarsal bursitis
  - Compression by the deep transverse intermetatarsal ligament
  - Ischemia of vasa nervorum
- Nerve lies in SC tissue, deep to the fat pad of foot, just superficial to the digital artery and vein.
- Superficial to the nerve is the strong, deep transverse metatarsal ligament that holds the metatarsal bones together.
- With each step the patient takes, the inflamed nerve becomes compressed between the ground and the deep transverse metatarsal ligament. This can generate perineural fibrotic reaction with subsequent neuroma formation.

RISK FACTORS
- High-heeled shoes
  - Transfer more weight to the forefoot.
- Shoes with tight toe boxes
  - Cause lateral compression
- Pes planus (flat feet)
  - Pulls nerve medially, increasing irritation
- Obesity

- Female gender
- Ballet dancing, particularly associated with the demi-pointe position
- Basketball, aerobics, tennis, running, and similar activities
- Hyperpronation

GENERAL PREVENTION
- Wear properly fitting shoes.
- Avoid high heels and shoes with narrow toe boxes.

Ⓡ DIAGNOSIS

HISTORY
- Most common complaint is pain localized to interspace between 3rd and 4th toes.
- Pain is less severe when not bearing weight.
- Pain, cramping, or numbness of the forefoot during weight-bearing or immediately after strenuous foot exertion
- Radiation of pain to the toes
- Pain is relieved by removing shoes and massaging the foot.
- Patients often complain of "walking on a marble."
- Burning pain in the ball of the foot radiating to the toes
- Tingling or numbness in the toes
- Aggravated by wearing tight or narrow shoes

PHYSICAL EXAM
- Intense pain when pressure applied between metatarsal heads, sometimes with a palpable nodule
- Assess midfoot motion and digital motion to determine if arthritis or synovitis.
- Palpate along metatarsal shafts to assess for metatarsalgia or stress fractures.
- Special testing (See "Diagnostic Procedures/Other.")

DIFFERENTIAL DIAGNOSIS
- Stress fracture
- Hammer toe
- Metatarsophalangeal synovitis
- Metatarsalgia
- Arthritis
- Traumatic neuroma
- Osteomyelitis
- Bursitis
- Foreign body

- Freiberg infraction (avascular necrosis of the metatarsal head, most commonly in adolescent females at the 2nd metatarsal)
- Neoplasm (malignancy, osteochondroma, neurofibroma)
- Gout

DIAGNOSTIC TESTS & INTERPRETATION

Initial Tests (lab, imaging)
- Predominantly a clinical diagnosis; imaging should be reserved for when the diagnosis is unclear.
- Imaging may be helpful if more than one web space is involved.
- Radiographs may help to rule out osseous pathology if diagnosis is in question, but plain films usually are normal in patients with a Morton neuroma.
- Ultrasound (US) has 79% specificity and 99% sensitivity for Morton neuromas but is poor at assessing the size of the lesion. Specificity declines to 50% for lesions <6 mm.
- MRI can rule out an osseous tumor and help with surgical planning; MRI has a sensitivity of 83% and a specificity of 99% for diagnosis of Morton neuroma.

Diagnostic Procedures/Other
- Five special tests have been described: thumb index finger squeeze test, Mulder sign, foot squeeze test, plantar percussion test, and toe tip sensation deficit.
  - Thumb index finger squeeze test is the most sensitive and specific (96% and 96%, respectively); positive when pain elicited by squeezing the symptomatic intermetatarsal space between the index finger and thumb
  - Mulder sign is a painful "click" produced by squeezing the metatarsal heads together while compressing the neuroma between the thumb and index finger of the other hand; sensitivity 40–84%
  - Foot squeeze test is positive when pain is induced in the symptomatic web space when the metatarsal heads are compressed by grasping the foot; sensitivity 40%
  - Plantar and dorsal percussion tests are positive when percussion of the affected web space elicits pain.
  - Toe tip sensation deficit exists when the sensation of the toe distal to the affected web space is decreased relative to the other toes.
- More than one of the above tests being positive increases the diagnostic accuracy.

Test Interpretation
Pathologic examination shows chronic fibrosis and thickening within and around the digital nerve. Arterial thickening and thrombosis of the common digital artery are sometimes present.

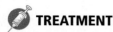 **TREATMENT**

GENERAL MEASURES
- Stepwise treatment, with typical progression from conservative measures followed by infiltrative treatment and ultimately surgical treatment
- Surgical treatments are the most successful (89%) followed by infiltrative (84%) then conservative (48%) as assessed by patient satisfaction with pain reduction at ≥6 months.
- Conservative treatments include the following:
  – Flat shoes with a roomy toe box
  – Plantar pads or metatarsal bar may help with alignment of metatarsal heads to provide relief.
  – There is no role for varus or valgus footwear padding.
  – There is no role for extracorporeal shock wave therapy (ESWT).
- NSAIDs for temporary symptom relief (1)[A]

MEDICATION
First Line
- Injectable steroids (e.g., betamethasone phosphate/acetate or methylprednisolone): number needed to treat (NNT) for significant benefit over conservative measures at 6 months = 2.3 (2)[A]
- One study demonstrated clinically significant improvement in use of US guidance versus palpation for corticosteroid injection.

Second Line
US-guided alcohol ablation therapy to sclerose the nerve is effective and has a lower complication rate than surgery.

ISSUES FOR REFERRAL
- Continued pain despite conservative treatments and injections
- Large interdigital neuromas (>5 mm diameter) or young patients who may benefit from earlier operative intervention
- One study demonstrated a cut-off value of 6.3 mm or larger Morton neuroma was associated with failure of corticosteroid injection.

SURGERY/OTHER PROCEDURES
- Surgical removal of the neuroma or shortening of the metatarsals, with or without release of the transverse metatarsal ligament, have an 89% success rate at 6 months defined by satisfaction scores.
- Small trials have been conducted using other invasive, nonsurgical techniques including injection with botulinum toxin, cryoablation, radiofrequency ablation, and platelet-rich plasma, but evidence is limited at this time.

 ONGOING CARE

FOLLOW-UP RECOMMENDATIONS
At diagnosis or if no improvement after 3 months of conservative treatment, consider corticosteroid injection.
- May repeat injection if no improvement after 2 to 4 weeks or consider referring for surgical management
- 21–51% of patients receiving a single corticosteroid injection require surgical intervention within 2 to 4 years.
- Size >5 mm and younger patients are more likely to undergo invasive treatment.

PATIENT EDUCATION
Wear properly fitting comfortable shoes.

PROGNOSIS
- 48% satisfaction rate with conservative treatment
- 85% satisfaction rate with infiltrative treatment
- 89% satisfaction rate with operative treatment

COMPLICATIONS
- Hip and knee pain can develop secondary to gait changes.
- Complications vary by treatment type.
- Failure rate is 47% with conservative treatment; 9–23% with invasive, nonsurgical treatment; and 4% with surgical treatment.
- Surgical complications vary by specific procedure and include keloid, CRPS, and stiffness. There was a global complication rate of 21% with operative treatment.

REFERENCES
1. Thomson CE, Gibson JNA, Martin D. Interventions for the treatment of Morton's neuroma. *Cochrane Database Syst Rev*. 2004;2004(3):CD003118.
2. Saygi B, Yildirim Y, Saygi EK, et al. Morton neuroma: comparative results of two conservative methods. *Foot Ankle Int*. 2005;26(7):556–559.

ADDITIONAL READING
Jain S, Mannan K. The diagnosis and management of Morton's neuroma: a literature review. *Foot Ankle Spec*. 2013;6(4):307–317.

 CODES

ICD10
- G57.60 Lesion of plantar nerve, unspecified lower limb
- G57.61 Lesion of plantar nerve, right lower limb
- G57.62 Lesion of plantar nerve, left lower limb

CLINICAL PEARLS
- Morton neuroma is usually a clinical diagnosis but can be further evaluated with US or MRI.
- Typical treatment is stepwise with conservative, then infiltrative, and then operative treatment.
- Morton neuromas with >5 mm diameter are more likely to require operative treatment.
- Younger patients are more likely to require operative treatment.
- Neurectomy is the definitive treatment. Patients should be aware of surgical complications.

MOTION SICKNESS

Kristina Gracey, MD, MPH

BASICS

DESCRIPTION
- Motion sickness is a physiologic response in affected individuals to a situation in which sensory conflict about body motion exists among visual receptors, vestibular receptors, and body proprioceptors.
- Often induced when patterns of motion differ from those previously experienced or expected
- Differs from "cybersickness" or "virtual reality sickness" (symptoms, including dizziness, that result from exposure to computer based stimuli) in the fact that some form of actual movement is generally required to diagnose motion sickness
- Systems affected: nervous, gastrointestinal
- Synonym(s): car sickness; sea sickness; air sickness; space sickness; physiologic vertigo; kinetosis

EPIDEMIOLOGY
Incidence
Predominant sex: female > male

Prevalence
Estimation is complex; syndrome occurs in ~25% due to travel by air, ~29% by sea, and ~41% by road. Estimates for vomiting are 0.5% by air, 7% by sea, and 2% by road.

ETIOLOGY AND PATHOPHYSIOLOGY
- Precise etiology unknown; thought to be due to a mismatch of vestibular and visual sensations
- Rotary, vertical, and low-frequency motions produce more symptoms than linear, horizontal, and high-frequency motions.
- Nausea and vomiting occur as a result of increased levels of dopamine and acetylcholine, which stimulate chemoreceptor trigger zone and vomiting center in CNS. Other signals which can be involved in this process include histamine, norepinephrine, and γ-aminobutyric acid (1).

Genetics
Heritability estimates range from 55% to 75%.

RISK FACTORS
- Motion (auto, plane, boat, amusement rides)
- Visual stimuli (e.g., moving horizon)
- Poor ventilation (fumes, smoke, carbon monoxide)
- Emotions (fear, anxiety)
- Zero gravity
- Pregnancy, menstruation, oral contraceptive use
- History of migraine headaches, especially vestibular migraine

GENERAL PREVENTION
See "General Measures."

Pediatric Considerations
- Rare in children <2 years of age
- Incidence peaks between 6 and 12 years of age.
- Antihistamines may cause excitation in children.

Geriatric Considerations
- Age confers some resistance to motion sickness.
- Elderly are at increased risk for anticholinergic side effects from treatment.

Pregnancy Considerations
- Pregnant patients are more likely to experience motion sickness.
- Treatment with medications is thought to be safe during morning sickness (e.g., meclizine, dimenhydrinate).
- Scopolamine, meclizine, diphenhydramine, and promethazine are generally considered safe during breastfeeding.

COMMONLY ASSOCIATED CONDITIONS
- Migraine headache
- Vestibular syndromes

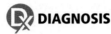

DIAGNOSIS

HISTORY
Presence of the following signs and symptoms in the context of a typical stimulus (2):
- Nausea
- Vomiting
- Stomach awareness (feeling of fullness in epigastrium)
- Diaphoresis
- Facial and perioral pallor
- Hypersalivation
- Yawning, hyperventilation
- Anxiety, panic
- Malaise/fatigue/lethargy
- Weakness
- Confusion
- Dizziness

PHYSICAL EXAM
No specific findings

DIFFERENTIAL DIAGNOSIS
- Mountain sickness
- Vestibular disease, central and peripheral
- Gastroenteritis
- Metabolic disorders
- Toxin exposure
- Concussion
- Hypoglycemia

DIAGNOSTIC TESTS & INTERPRETATION
None usually indicated

Initial Tests (lab, imaging)
Can consider pregnancy test or fingerstick glucose to rule out hypoglycemia

Follow-Up Tests & Special Considerations
Multiple online questionnaires (such as the Motion Sickness Susceptibility Questionnaire) are available to help patients recognize their susceptibility to motion sickness and what situations are most likely to cause symptom development.

TREATMENT

- Follow guidelines under "General Measures" section to prevent motion sickness (2)[C].
- Premedicate before travel with antidopaminergic, anticholinergic, or antihistamine agents (2)[A]:
  - For extended travel, consider treatment with scopolamine transdermal patch (3)[A].
- Benzodiazepines suppress vestibular nuclei but would not be considered first line due to sedation and addiction potential (4)[C].
- Serotonin receptor agonist (rizatriptan) may be effective for migraineurs with motion sickness (5)[C].

GENERAL MEASURES
- Avoid noxious types of motions; travelling in inclement weather may exacerbate symptoms.
- Improve ventilation; avoid noxious stimuli.
- Eat before travel (light, soft, bland, low-fat, and low-acid foods); avoid alcohol; avoid empty stomach.
- Increase airflow around face.
- Use semirecumbent seating or lay supine.
- Fix vision on horizon; avoid fixation on moving objects; keep eyes fixed on still, distant objects.
- Avoid reading while actively traveling.
- Frequent and graded exposure to stimulus that triggers nausea (habituation)
- Counsel patient on minimizing motion (airplanes: sit over the wing; automobiles: driver or sit in front passenger seat, facing forward; boat: sit facing toward the waves, away from rocking bow, near surface of the water; buses: sit near the front, at lowest level, facing forward; trains: sit at the lowest level, facing forward).

MEDICATION

First Line

- Scopolamine transdermal patch (Transderm Scop): Apply 2.5-cm^2 (4 mg) patch behind ear over the mastoid at least 4 hours (preferably 6 to 12 hours) before travel and replace every 3 days (3)[A].
- Promethazine (Phenergan): Take 30 to 60 minutes before travel.
  - Adults: 25 mg PO q12h; 25 to 50 mg IM if already developed severe motion sickness
  - Children and adolescents: 0.5 mg/kg PO q12h, maximum 25 mg BID; *caution:* increased risk of dystonic reaction in this age group
- Dimenhydrinate (Dramamine): Take 30 to 60 minutes before travel.
  - Adults and adolescents: 50 to 100 mg PO q4–6h, maximum 400 mg/day
  - Children 6 to 12 years of age: 25 to 50 mg PO q6–8h, maximum 150 mg/day
  - Children 2 to 5 years of age: 12.5 to 25 mg PO q6–8h, maximum 75 mg/day
- Meclizine (Travel Ease): Take 60 minutes before travel.
  - Adults and adolescents >12 years of age: 25 to 50 mg PO q24h
  - Children <12 years of age: not recommended
- Diphenhydramine (Benadryl): Take 30 minutes before travel.
  - Adults and adolescents: 25 to 50 mg PO q6–8h, maximum 300 mg/day
  - Children 6 to 12 years of age: 5 mg/kg or 12.5 to 25 mg PO q4–6h, maximum 150 mg/day
- Contraindications: patients at risk for acute angle-closure glaucoma
- Precautions:
  - Young children
  - Elderly
  - Pregnancy
  - Urinary obstruction
  - Pyloric duodenal obstruction
- Adverse reactions:
  - Drowsiness
  - Dry mouth
  - Blurred vision
  - Confusion/delirium
  - Headache
  - Urinary retention
  - Constipation
- Significant possible interactions:
  - Sedatives (antihistamines, alcohol, antidepressants)
  - Anticholinergics (belladonna alkaloids)

Second Line

- Benzodiazepines: Take 1 to 2 hours before travel.
  - Diazepam 2 to 10 mg PO q6–12h
  - Lorazepam 1 to 2 mg PO q8h
- Contraindications:
  - Severe respiratory or liver dysfunction
- Precautions:
  - Alcohol/drug abuse
  - Elderly
  - Sedation
  - Addiction is possible.

COMPLEMENTARY & ALTERNATIVE MEDICINE

- Acupressure on point PC6 (*Neiguan* on pericardium meridian) has been shown to reduce feelings of nausea and vomiting during pregnancy, after surgery, and in cancer chemotherapy. However, limited evidence of efficacy has been found for motion sickness; point PC6: 2 cm proximal of transverse crease of palmar side of wrist between tendons of the palmaris longus and the flexor carpi radialis (6)[B].
- Ginger: 1 to 1.5 g per 24 hours (250 mg PO 4 times a day); take 4 hours before travel; studies have shown ginger to be an effective treatment for nausea and vomiting (7)[B].

 ## ONGOING CARE

DIET

- Eat before travel, avoid empty stomach; eat light, soft, bland, low-fat, and low-acid foods.
- Avoid alcohol.

PROGNOSIS

- Symptoms should resolve when motion exposure ends.
- Resistance to motion sickness seems to increase with age.

COMPLICATIONS

- Hypotension
- Dehydration
- Depression
- Panic
- Syncope

REFERENCES

1. Leung AK, Hon KL. Motion sickness: an overview. *Drugs Context*. 2019;8:2019-9-4.
2. Brainard A, Gresham C. Prevention and treatment of motion sickness. *Am Fam Physician*. 2014;90(1):41–46.
3. Spinks AB, Wasiak J. Scopolamine (hyoscine) for preventing and treating motion sickness. *Cochrane Database Syst Rev*. 2011;(6):CD002851.
4. Soto E, Vega R. Neuropharmacology of vestibular system disorders. *Curr Neuropharmacol*. 2010;8(1):26–40.
5. Furman JM, Marcus DA, Balaban CD. Rizatriptan reduces vestibular-induced motion sickness in migraineurs. *J Headache Pain*. 2011;12(1):81–88.
6. Lee EJ, Frazier SK. The efficacy of acupressure for symptom management: a systematic review. *J Pain Symptom Manage*. 2011;42(4):589–603.
7. Marx W, Kiss N, Isenring L. Is ginger beneficial for nausea and vomiting? An update of the literature. *Curr Opin Support Palliat Care*. 2015;9(2):189–195.

 SEE ALSO

Algorithm: Dizziness

 CODES

ICD10
T75.3XXA Motion sickness, initial encounter

CLINICAL PEARLS

- The scopolamine transdermal patch is the first line for prevention of motion sickness. It should be applied at least 4 hours before travel, although it is most effective if placed 12 hours before departure.
- First-generation antihistamines are also effective, although sedating. They should be administered 30 to 60 minutes before departure.
- Nonsedating antihistamines, ondansetron, and ginger root are not effective in the prevention or treatment of motion sickness.
- Although acupressure wristbands have been found to be effective by systematic reviews in postoperative and chemotherapy-induced nausea and vomiting, as well as hyperemesis gravidarum, conflicting data exist for use with motion sickness.

M

MULTIPLE MYELOMA

Michael Haddadin, MD

BASICS

DESCRIPTION
- Multiple myeloma (MM) is a malignant proliferation of a single clone of plasma cells. These malignant cells produce monoclonal protein (immunoglobulin [Ig]) that can be detected in the blood and/or urine as it is filtered in the kidneys.
- MM is characterized by bony lytic lesions, hypercalcemia, increased susceptibility to infections, and renal impairment.
- Monoclonal gammopathy of undetermined significance (MGUS) is a common disorder with limited monoclonal plasma cell proliferation that can progress to smoldering MM (SMM) or symptomatic MM at rate of ~1% per year.

EPIDEMIOLOGY
- MM affects the older adults with a median age of 65 to 74 years.
- Accounts for nearly 2% of all cancers and 17% of hematologic malignancies in the United States
- African Americans about 2 to 3 times more commonly affected than Caucasians; less common in Asians

Incidence
7 cases per 100,000 in the United States annually

Prevalence
In 2018, there were ~160,000 recognized cases worldwide.

ETIOLOGY AND PATHOPHYSIOLOGY
- It is most likely caused by genetic alteration involving chromosomal abnormalities and sporadic mutations.
- Genetic damage in developing B lymphocytes occur at time of isotype switching.
- Chromosomal abnormalities involve Ig heavy chain translocations, with cyclin D1 t(11;14) the most common, and deletion of 17p13 (p53 locus).

Genetics
MM rarely occurs in familial clusters. A rare form of paratarg-7 protein might have pathogenic role.

RISK FACTORS
- Most cases have no known risks associated.
- Old age; immunosuppression; and exposure to chemicals, heavy metals, and ionizing radiation increase the risk of MM.

COMMONLY ASSOCIATED CONDITIONS
Secondary amyloidosis can be associated with MM and polyneuropathy, organomegaly, endocrinopathy, monoclonal protein, skin changes (POEMS).

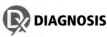

DIAGNOSIS

HISTORY
- 34% of patients are asymptomatic at the time of presentation.
- Anemia (73%) is the most common presentation of MM.

- Hypercalcemia (28%): anorexia, abdominal pain, somnolence, polydipsia, polyuria, dehydration
- Elevated creatinine (48%), acute kidney injury in MM can occur due to multiple different mechanisms.
- Bony lesions (80%): lytic lesions causing bone pain (58%) (1)[C], osteoporosis, or pathologic fracture (26–34%)
- Other symptoms: fatigue (32%), peripheral neuropathy (PN), weight loss (24%), recurrent infections, hyperviscosity syndrome, and spinal cord compression. Those are rare presentation but warrant immediate intervention.

PHYSICAL EXAM
- Dehydration, pallor, and bone tenderness
- Hyperviscosity syndrome in 7%: retinal hemorrhages, prolonged bleeding, neurologic changes
- Extramedullary plasmacytomas can present as large, purplish, subcutaneous masses.
- Skin findings of amyloidosis: waxy papules or plaques that may be evident in the eyelids, retroauricular region, neck, or inguinal and anogenital regions

DIFFERENTIAL DIAGNOSIS
- Reactive plasmacytosis
- MGUS
- SMM: no end organ damage (CRAB: hypercalcemia, renal insufficiency, anemia, bone lesions) features
- Metastatic carcinoma (kidney, breast, non–small cell lung cancer)
- Waldenström macroglobulinemia
- Reactive plasmacytosis
- AL amyloidosis
- Solitary plasmacytoma
- POEMS syndrome

DIAGNOSTIC TESTS & INTERPRETATION
Criteria for diagnosis: The diagnosis of MM requires the following:
- Bone marrow (BM) involvement with ≥10% of plasma cells or the presence of a plasmacytoma and one or more of the following myeloma-defining events:
  – Evidence of end-organ damage that can be attributed to the underlying plasma cell proliferative disorder, specifically:
    ○ Hypercalcemia: serum calcium >0.25 mmol/L (>1 mg/dL) higher than the upper limit of normal or >2.75 mmol/L (>11 mg/dL)
    ○ Renal insufficiency: creatinine clearance <40 mL/min or serum creatinine >177 μmol/L (>2 mg/dL)
    ○ Anemia: hemoglobin value of >2 g/dL below the lower limit of normal or a hemoglobin value <10 g/dL
    ○ Bone lesions: one or more osteolytic lesions on skeletal radiography, CT, or PET-CT
  – Any one or more of the following findings is considered an MM-defining event (SLiM criteria):
    ○ Clonal BM plasma cell percentage ≥60% (S)
    ○ Involved: uninvolved serum free light chain (FLC) ratio ≥100 (Li) or <0.01%
    ○ >1 focal lesion on MRI studies, or PET-CT (M)

Initial Tests (lab, imaging)
- CBC with differential to evaluate anemia and other cytopenias
- BUN, creatinine, serum electrolytes, albumin, and calcium
- Serum lactate dehydrogenase (LDH), β_2-microglobulin
- Serum protein electrophoresis (SPEP), serum immunofixation electrophoresis (SIFE): M protein level elevated
- Quantitative serum Ig levels: IgG, IgA, and IgM
- Quantitative serum FLC levels: κ and λ chains
- ESR, C-reactive protein: elevated
- Urinalysis: 24-hour urine for protein, urine protein electrophoresis (UPEP), urine immunofixation electrophoresis (UIFE); 20% positive urine protein (1)[C]:
  – Urinalysis dip is often negative for protein because this test identifies albumin, and the protein in MM is Bence Jones (BJ) monoclonal protein.
- Cross-sectional imaging (whole-body low-dose CT) is preferred over plain radiographs for the detection of bone involvement.
- Skeletal surveys are reserved for patients who are unable to undergo whole-body low-dose CT, MRI, and PET.
- BM biopsy: plasma cell percentage, histology, immunohistochemistry, flow cytometry, cytogenetics, and fluorescence in situ hybridization (FISH)

Follow-Up Tests & Special Considerations
- For patients with suspected SMM, a whole-body MRI or MRI of the spine and pelvis is recommended to evaluate for spinal cord compression.
- For patients with suspected extramedullary disease outside of the spine, a whole-body PET/CT is recommended.
- Baseline bone densitometry may be indicated.
- BM aspiration and biopsy to monitor response to treatment
- SPEP with SIFE: M-protein helps to track progression of myeloma and response to treatment.
- Serum Igs and FLCs can be used to monitor response or relapse.

Diagnostic Procedures/Other
Staging to determine disease burden, multiple staging systems are used. The most common one is the Revised International Staging System (R-ISS). Durie-Salmon staging system is rarely used nowadays.
- International Staging System (ISS)
  – Stage I: albumin ≥3.5 g/dL and β_2-microglobulin <3.5 μg/mL
  – Stage II: neither stage I nor stage III
  – Stage III: β_2-microglobulin ≥5.5 μg/mL
- Mayo Stratification of Myeloma and Risk-Adapted Therapy (mSMART)
  – Standard risk: >t(11;14), t(6;14), and hyperdiploidy
  – Intermediate risk: t(4;14), del(13q) by cytogenetics, hypodiploidy
  – High risk: t(14;16), t(14;20), del(17 p)
- R-ISS combines ISS information with chromosomal abnormalities and LDH to provide better prognostic information for MM.

TREATMENT

- Key factors to consider prior to initiation of treatment: patient's characteristics and comorbidities (i.e., cardiac and renal function), cytogenetic risk, and autologous stem cell transplant (ASCT) eligibility.
- Induction chemotherapy followed by ASCT is considered standard of care for eligible patients. In some high-risk MM patients allogeneic transplant maybe considered. Patients who are ineligible for ASCT or who do not have access are treated with an extended course of induction chemotherapy and maintenance.

GENERAL MEASURES
Maintain adequate hydration to prevent renal insufficiency. Most patients will require some form of antimicrobial prophylaxis during treatment.

MEDICATION
- Treatment for MM consists of three different phases: induction phase, consolidation (often ASCT for those who are eligible), and maintenance phase.
- Agents include chemotherapy, proteasome inhibitors (PIs), immunomodulatory agents, steroids, bispecific antibodies, monoclonal antibodies, and chimeric antigen receptor (CAR)-T cell therapy.
- Induction phase for ASCT eligible patient can be composed of a 3- or 4-drug combination, such as bortezomib/lenalidomide/dexamethasone, bortezomib/cyclophosphamide/dexamethasone, daratumumab/bortezomib/lenalidomide or thalidomide/dexamethasone or carfilzomib/lenalidomide/dexamethasone, with or without daratumumab.
- Induction chemotherapy for ASCT-ineligible patients is similar either with doublet or triplet (e.g., lenalidomide/low-dose dexamethasone or bortezomib/dexamethasone or daratumumab/lenalidomide/dexamethasone).
- Maintenance treatment: Lenalidomide is the most preferred agent for maintenance therapy after induction or transplant. Additional agents are being investigated. There are ongoing studies investigating the use of two or more agents for maintenance.

First Line
- PIs
  - Blocks ubiquitin-proteasome catalytic pathway in cells by binding to the 20S proteasome complex
  - Consider herpes simplex virus (HSV) prophylaxis with acyclovir.
  - Bortezomib: PI, IV or SC; SC has lower risk of PN; toxicity: PN, cytopenia, nausea, anorexia, leukopenia, thrombocytopenia, rash
  - Carfilzomib: IV, 2nd-generation PI; toxicity: cardiomyopathy and other cardiac adverse events, fever, diarrhea, thrombotic microangiopathy, fatigue; can have hypersensitivity reaction after infusion
  - Ixazomib—oral PI; toxicity: PN, diarrhea, thrombocytopenia, neutropenia, back pain, edema
- Cyclophosphamide
  - Nitrogen mustard–derivative alkylating agent
  - Toxicity: cytopenia, anaphylaxis, interstitial pulmonary fibrosis, hemorrhagic cystitis, impaired fertility

- Immunomodulators: thalidomide, lenalidomide, and pomalidomide
  - Antiangiogenesis inhibition, immunomodulation
  - Toxicity: birth defects (thalidomide), deep vein thrombosis (DVT), neuropathy, rash, nausea, bradycardia
- Dexamethasone: dose (40 mg/week)
- Daratumumab: IgGκ1 monoclonal antibodies against CD38; toxicity: fatigue, back pain, lymphocytopenia, neutropenia, anemia including Coomb positive hemolytic anemia, thrombocytopenia, cough, flulike symptoms, and infusion-related reaction
- Bisphosphonates
  - No effect on mortality but decrease pain, pathologic vertebral fractures, and fractures of other bones
  - Dose-adjust/monitor renal function.
  - Monitor for osteonecrosis of jaw.

Second Line
- Progression of MM is usually identified by a rise in monoclonal M protein in the serum or the urine or in the serum FLC ratio with new or worsening end-organ damage.
- Not all patients with laboratory progression need to change treatment, rather the whole clinical picture and patient's goals.
- Multiple regimens can be used as salvage therapy to treat relapsed or refractory myeloma.
- Regimen of choice depends on the previously failed lines; if relapse occurs >6 months after completing initial primary treatment, can use same regimen for retreatment
- Most patients with relapsed or refractory MM should undergo transplant if not attempted previously and/or evaluation for a clinical trial.
- MM is a disease that tends to relapse quite frequently, and require subsequent treatments.
- Regimens can include, but not limited to, daratumumab if not previously used, pomalidomide (immunomodulator), elotuzumab, venetoclax, or combination of chemotherapy.
- Several other agents have been in development for second and subsequent relapses. Options include selinexor, bispecific antibodies, and CAR-T cell therapy.
- Bispecific antibodies are monoclonal antibodies and a bispecific B-cell maturation antigen (BCMA)-directed T cell engager. These agents can be used for fourth and higher disease recurrence.
- BCMA can also be targeted through the two recently FDA-approved CAR-T cell therapy agents: idecabtagene vicleucel and ciltacabtagene autoleucel.

ISSUES FOR REFERRAL
- For spinal or other bone pathology, refer to orthopedics for support.
- Referral to a large center is recommended after three lines of treatment for trial evaluation.

ADDITIONAL THERAPIES
- Local radiation therapy for uncontrolled bone pain or plasmacytoma
- Effective pain management; avoid NSAIDs due to nephrotoxicity.
- Aspirin 81 to 325 mg is recommended for patients treated with immunomodulators for DVT prophylaxis.

- Erythropoietin for selected patients with anemia
- IVIg infusion for patients with recurrent life-threatening infections
- Patients should receive vaccines for pneumococcus, influenza, and SARS-CoV-2.
- Do not administer live-virus vaccines (1).

SURGERY/OTHER PROCEDURES
Kyphoplasty/vertebroplasty: Consider for symptomatic vertebral compressions.

ADMISSION, INPATIENT, AND NURSING CONSIDERATIONS
Indications: pain, infections, cytopenia, renal failure, bone complications, spinal cord compression
- Adequate hydration and practice caution for contrast-induced nephropathy; manage hypercalcemia.

 ## ONGOING CARE

PATIENT EDUCATION
International Myeloma Foundation: https://myeloma.org/Main.action

PROGNOSIS
- The survival depends heavily on the cytogenetic risk and stage of the disease.
- Median survival by R-ISS stage:
  - Stage I: has not been reached
  - Stage II: 83 months
  - Stage III: 43 months

COMPLICATIONS
Patients with MM are prone to many complications related to the disease and the treatment. Complications include infections, pain, fractures, hypercalcemia, hyperuricemia, spinal cord compression, hyperviscosity syndrome, amyloidosis, and dialysis.

REFERENCE
1. Palumbo A, Anderson K. Multiple myeloma. *N Engl J Med*. 2011;364(11):1046–1060.

 ## CODES

ICD10
- C90.0 Multiple myeloma
- C90.00 Multiple myeloma not having achieved remission
- C90.01 Multiple myeloma in remission

CLINICAL PEARLS
- MM is a plasma cell malignancy that causes end-organ damage.
- Look for presence of "CRAB."
- Suspect MM if high total protein-to-albumin ratio is present.
- Avoid nephrotoxins (radiographic contrast material, NSAIDs, dehydration).
- Patients with MM are immunocompromised.

M

MULTIPLE SCLEROSIS

Afsha Rais Kaisani, MD • Tasaduq Hussain Mir, MD, FAAFP • Sana W. Qureshi, DO

BASICS

Multiple sclerosis (MS) is an autoimmune disease directed against components of the neural myelin sheath causing demyelination. This leads to progressive axonal loss and CNS atrophy affecting primarily white matter but may also damage grey matter and overlying meninges.

DESCRIPTION

Subtypes of MS (1):

- Clinically isolated syndrome (CIS): Patient's initial symptoms are characteristic of CNS demyelination that may be due to MS but does not fulfill the criteria of dissemination in time; ~80% of patients with CIS will later relapse and be diagnosed with MS.
- Radiologically isolated syndrome (RIS): incidental brain or spinal cord MRI findings highly suggestive of MS in an asymptomatic patient; no evidence of clinical attacks suggestive of MS; ~30–40% of patients with RIS later meet criteria for CIS or MS.
- Relapsing-remitting MS (RRMS): most common type of disease onset; defined by relapse (attacks or exacerbations) followed by partial or complete improvement; recovery of residual deficits may ensue following each episode.
- Secondary progressive MS (SPMS): progressive worsening of neurologic function following initial RRMS; may be associated with acute exacerbations; often diagnosed retrospectively
- Primary progressive MS (PPMS): progressive decline in disease status and accumulation of disability from onset of disease without initial relapsing-remitting disease course (~10% of patients) (2)

Pregnancy Considerations

- If treatment is clinically necessary during pregnancy, preferred treatments include interferon-β and glatiramer acetate (3).
- Natalizumab may be continued with reduced infusion regimen for patients with high risk of relapse (3).
- Majority of patients experience reduced disease exacerbations during pregnancy but relapse in the postpartum period.
- All drugs licensed for MS treatment are contraindicated during breastfeeding.

EPIDEMIOLOGY

Most often affects Caucasian women during their 2nd and 3rd generations of life.

Incidence

2.1 per 100,000 person-years (1)

Prevalence

- Differs by latitude, higher rates among those living further from the equator (1)
- America: 117.49 per 100,000 people
- Worldwide: 43.95 per 100,000 people

ETIOLOGY AND PATHOPHYSIOLOGY

- Predominately an autoimmune process driven by T cells and B cells against the myelin sheath. Dysregulation and mistaken antigen identity lead CD4 T cells to cross the blood–brain barrier and recognize proteins on the surface of the myelin sheath. Cytokines, interferon-γ, and tumor necrosis factor-α are subsequently released, and activation of macrophages and B cells leads to oligodendrocyte and myelin destruction, resulting in slower saltatory nerve conduction velocities.
- Oligodendrocytes, which have survived or formed from precursor cells, are able to partially remyelinate stripped axons, producing scars which overtime can lead to irreversible axonal loss and brain atrophy.
- The majority of axons are typically lost from the lateral corticospinal (motor) tracts of the spinal cord (2).

Genetics

Over 100 genetic loci have been associated with MS, suggesting that it is ultimately an antigen-specific autoimmune process. Most commonly, these are mapped to the class II region of the HLA gene clusters. The most common is the HLA-DRB1 locus on chromosome 6, which produces major histocompatibility complexes with high-binding affinity for myelin basic proteins.

RISK FACTORS

- Age: peak incidence ages 20 to 40 years, but can present at any age (slightly earlier in women than men)
- Sex: female > male
- Race: Caucasian > Afro-Caribbean > East Asian
- Prior infections: Epstein-Barr virus; mononucleosis
- Substance: tobacco smoking
- Historically, proximity to the equator and its correlation with increased vitamin D exposure were inversely proportional to MS incidence. However, this association has been less noted and may be due to lifestyle changes leading to decreased sun exposure in these areas (2).
- Anti-TNF-α inhibitors like etanercept and infliximab have been associated with developing MS.

COMMONLY ASSOCIATED CONDITIONS

Internuclear ophthalmoplegia, optic neuritis, transverse myelitis, association with other autoimmune processes

DIAGNOSIS

A person with MS may present with a number of neurologic signs and symptoms depending on the locations of the lesion. The essential means of diagnoses is to demonstrate evidence of CNS lesions that are separated by both time and space that are not due to a separate disease process.

HISTORY

Common symptoms may include but not limited to the following: cognitive dysfunction, fatigue, dizziness, visual disturbances, facial palsy, dysphagia, muscle weakness or spasms, hyperesthesia or paresthesia, pain, bowel or bladder incontinence, urinary frequency or retention, or sexual dysfunction (2).

PHYSICAL EXAM

- Weakness, internuclear ophthalmoplegia, gait disturbance, hyperesthesia or paresthesia, cerebellar dysarthria (scanning speech), and spasticity (especially in lower extremities)
- Uhthoff phenomenon: Symptoms are worse with exposure to higher than usual temperature.
- Lhermitte phenomenon (barber chair phenomenon): Electric-like shocks extending down the spine caused by neck movement, especially flexion

DIFFERENTIAL DIAGNOSIS

- Infectious: Lyme disease, syphilis, acute disseminated encephalomyelitis, progressive multifocal leukoencephalopathy (PML), Guillain-Barré syndrome, primary cerebral angiitis, amyotrophic lateral sclerosis, Huntington disease, and HIV
- Autoimmune: systemic lupus erythematosus, antiphospholipid antibody syndrome, neurosarcoidosis, Behçet disease, vasculitis, and Bell palsy
- CNS: neuromyelitis optica, neoplasms, stroke, migraine, and normal pressure hydrocephalus
- Medications and illicit substances: Alcohol, anticholinergic drugs, cocaine, etanercept, infliximab, isoniazid, methanol
- Other: cobalamin (vitamin B_{12}) deficiency, manganese toxicity, paraneoplastic disease, hypothyroidism, psychiatric disease (anxiety disorder, conversion disorder), Charcot-Marie-Tooth disease

DIAGNOSTIC TESTS & INTERPRETATION

- Blood tests to rule out alternative diagnosis: antinuclear antibody, antineutrophil cytoplasmic antibody, anti–double-stranded DNA antibody, antiphospholipid antibody, erythrocyte sedimentation rate, immunoglobulin G, immunoglobulin M, rheumatoid factor, HIV screening, rapid plasma reagin, thyroid-stimulating hormone (TSH), vitamin B_{12} level, complete blood count (CBC), Lyme disease antibody (2)[B]
- MRI of head/spine: Periventricular and callosal lesions are relatively specific for MS; addition of gadolinium can help identify active lesions.
- Lumbar puncture: cerebrospinal fluid (CSF) with elevated or normal protein levels; oligoclonal immunoglobulin G bands are seen in approximately 90% of MS but may be absent in early disease process. Positive findings are not diagnostic for MS but may be beneficial if other diagnostic criteria are equivocal.
- McDonald criteria for diagnosing MS (4): apply primarily when clinical suspicion for MS; not used for ruling out other neurologic conditions; dependent on number of attacks and number of CNS lesions:
  – Two or more clinical attacks and two or more lesions with objective clinical evidence; MS is confirmed; may start treatment *or*
  – Two or more attacks and one lesion, with dissemination in space on MRI or an additional relapse causing new symptoms that effect another CNS region *or*
  – One attack and two lesions, with dissemination in time on MRI or another disease relapse or a positive test for oligoclonal bands in the CNC (3) *or*
  – One attack and one lesion, with dissemination in space and time
  – Formal diagnosis of PPMS can be made if symptoms gradually progress for at least 1 year and two of the following criteria are met:
    ○ At least one lesion in the brain is detected on MRI.
    ○ At least two spinal cord lesions are detected on MRI.
    ○ Oligoclonal bands in CSF

Initial Tests (lab, imaging)
MRI of the brain/spine

Follow-Up Tests & Special Considerations
Lumbar puncture, EMG

Diagnostic Procedures/Other
Evoked potentials: Assess function of visual, auditory, and somatosensory motor CNS pathways; measure CNS electric potentials evoked by neural stimulation. A marked delay, without a clinical manifestation, is suggestive of demyelinating disorder. Visual evoked potentials are delayed in 80–90% of individuals with MS (1).

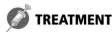 TREATMENT

GENERAL MEASURES
- Multidisciplinary team approach is paramount, including physical, occupational, and speech therapy; mental health specialist; pharmacists; urologist; neurologist; and dietitian.
- Three main categories currently exist for treatment: treatment for acute relapses, reducing MS-related activity using disease-modifying agents, and symptomatic therapy.
- Steroids: treatment for initial presentation and acute episodes of MS (1).
- Disease-modifying treatments (DMT) early in the disease process are likely to slow overall disease progression; should be managed by MS specialist (2)[C]
- Smoking cessation is encouraged due to possible decrease in disability progression (1).

MEDICATION
- Acute relapse treatment—high-dose short-term glucocorticoid therapy (2)[A]
  - Methylprednisolone 1 g PO/IV daily for 3 to 5 days; without subsequent tapering; a second course may be given.
    ○ Side effects (S/E): infection risk, adrenal insufficiency, Cushing syndrome, fluid retention, hypokalemia, GI disturbances, headache, emotional lability, delirium, osteoporosis, hyperglycemia
  - Alternative therapy for those who cannot tolerate high-dose glucocorticoids: ACTH gel 80 to 120 units IM/SC daily for 1 week followed or not followed by taper
  - Plasmapheresis
- Disease-modifying treatment: initiated to decrease clinical attacks and delay disability progression (1),(2)[B]
  - Platform injection therapies
    ○ IFN-β_{1a} (Avonex) 30 μg IM weekly or IFN-β_{1a} (Rebif) 22 or 44 μg SC 3 times per week; IFN-β_{1b} (Betaseron/Betaferon/Extavia) 250 μg SC every other day
      ■ Monitor CBC, LFTs, TSH
      ■ S/E: flulike symptoms, depression, skin site reactions, thyroid dysfunction, liver enzyme abnormalities
    ○ Glatiramer acetate (Copaxone) 20 mg SC daily
      ■ S/E: skin site reactions, postinjection reaction, lipoatrophy

- Monoclonal antibodies (monitor CBC, LFTs, TSH)
  ○ Rituximab (Rituxan) 1 g IV once every 2 weeks × 2 doses; repeat 1 g once q6–12mo. Rule out hepatitis B prior to use; S/E: hypogammaglobulinemia, infection, and PML
  ○ Natalizumab (Tysabri) 300 mg IV q4wk
    ■ S/E: dizziness, nausea, increased risk of infection, PML
    ■ Alemtuzumab (Lemtrada) 12 mg/day for 5 days; after 12 months, 12 mg/day for 3 days
      □ S/E: infusion reaction, increased risk of infection, thyroid problems, blood clots, immune thrombocytopenia
- Oral therapies—for those who prefer self-administered oral medication
  ○ Dimethyl fumarate (Tecfidera) 120 to 240 mg PO BID for 7 days and then 240 mg BID
    ■ Monitor CBC, LFTs; S/E: diarrhea, cramps, nausea, flushing
  ○ Teriflunomide (Aubagio) 7 to 14 mg PO daily
    ■ Monitor CBC, LFTs, UA; S/E: headache, diarrhea, fatigue, arthralgia, hair thinning nausea
    ■ Fingolimod (Gilenya) 0.5 mg PO daily
      □ Monitor ECG, CBC, LFTs, eye exam; S/E: 1st-degree AV block, arrhythmia, infection risk
- Symptomatic therapies (1),(2)[B]
  - Spasticity: baclofen, dantrolene, tizanidine, cannabis extract (nabiximols), botulinum toxin, benzodiazepines, physiotherapy
  - Pain: amitriptyline, pregabalin, gabapentin, cannabis extract (nabiximols), capsaicin
  - Trigeminal neuralgia: carbamazepine, oxcarbazepine, baclofen, gabapentin
  - Bladder dysfunction: imipramine, muscarinics, cannabis extract, catheterization, intravesical botulinum toxin; avoid spicy, acidic foods, caffeine, and alcohol for detrusor spasm.
  - Fatigue: amantadine, modafinil, SSRI
  - Tremors: diazepam, β-blockers
  - Depression: SSRI, SNRI, TCA
  - Movement disorder: ataxia (baclofen, dantrolene, tizanidine, deep brain stimulation); impaired walking (behavioral change therapy, physiotherapy)

ISSUES FOR REFERRAL
- Neurology: diagnosis and treatment
- Physical therapy & rehabilitation: physical therapy

ADDITIONAL THERAPIES
- Hematopoietic stem cell transplants are being tested in clinical trials and may alter treatment and prevention of MS in the future (2).
- Multiple trials are investigating remyelination and neuroprotection to prevent, reverse, or slow the progression of the disease.

 ONGOING CARE

FOLLOW-UP RECOMMENDATIONS
Patient Monitoring
Assessing the severity of neurologic impairment from MS can be done using the Kurtzke Expanded Disability Status Scale (EDSS): The EDSS quantifies severity of disability using eight functional systems (FS): pyramidal, cerebellar, brainstem, sensory, bowel and bladder, visual, and cerebral. EDSS scoring system is as follows:
- 1.0: no disability, minimal signs in 1 FS
- 2.0: minimal disability in 1 FS
- 3.0: moderate disability in 1 FS; mild disability in 3 to 4 FS but fully ambulatory
- 4.0: ambulatory without aid or rest for ~500 m
- 5.0: ambulatory without aid or rest for ~200 m
- 6.0: intermittent/constant unilateral aid (cane, crutch); must be able to walk 100 m
- 7.0: unable to walk beyond 5 m even with aid; restricted to wheelchair for ~12 hr/day, wheels self and transfers alone
- 8.0: essentially restricted to bed, chair, or wheelchair; may be out of bed most of the day; retains self-care functions, generally effective use of arms
- 9.0: helpless, bedbound; can communicate and eat
- 10: death due to MS

PROGNOSIS
Average life expectancy is 5 to 10 years less than the unaffected population (2).

COMPLICATIONS
Mortality secondary to MS relapse is unusual; death is more commonly associated with a complication of MS such as infection.

REFERENCES
1. Saguil A, Iv EAF, Jordan TS. Multiple sclerosis: a primary care perspective. *Am Fam Physician*. 2022;106(2):173–183.
2. Raffel J, Wakerley B, Nicholas R. Multiple sclerosis. *Medicine*. 2016;44(9):537–541.
3. Varytė G, Arlauskienė A, Ramašauskaitė D. Pregnancy and multiple sclerosis: an update. *Curr Opin Obstet Gynecol*. 2021;33(5):378–383.
4. Thompson AJ, Banwell BL, Barkhof F, et al. Diagnosis of multiple sclerosis: 2017 revisions of the McDonald criteria. *Lancet Neurol*. 2018;17(2):162–173.

 CODES

ICD10
G35 Multiple sclerosis

CLINICAL PEARLS
- MS is an immune-mediated inflammatory disease-causing demyelination, neuronal loss, and scarring within the CNS
- Most common cause of nontraumatic neurologic disability in young adults.
- Diagnosis is made with the McDonald criteria
- Treatment is complex and rapidly changing; MS specialist and multiprofessional therapy is necessary.

M

MUMPS
Donna Kaminski, DO, MPH, FAAFP • Brandis Belt, MD, MPH

BASICS

An acute, self-limited, generalized paramyxovirus infection, typically presenting with parotitis

DESCRIPTION
- Asymptomatic in up to 30% of the nonimmune individuals and 60% of previously vaccinated individuals.
- Painful parotitis in 95% of symptomatic mumps cases
- Epidemics in late winter and in spring
- Transmission by respiratory droplets or contact with saliva
- Incubation period is 12 to 25 days, followed by 2 to 3 days of symptomatic phase.

EPIDEMIOLOGY
- 85% of mumps cases occur prior to 15 years of age.
- Adult cases are typically more severe; predominant sex: male = female; geriatric population: Most U.S. adults are immune.
- Acute epidemic mumps: highly contagious in susceptible populations, R0 = 10
  - Most cases occur in unvaccinated children 5 to 15 years of age.
- Mumps is unusual in children <2 years of age.
- Period of maximal communicability is 24 hours before to 72 hours after onset of parotitis.

Incidence
- Worldwide, 169,799 cases of mumps were reported in 2019. In the United States, 3,474 cases of mumps were reported in 2019. In 2020, the COVID-19 pandemic year, only 616 cases were reported in the United States, followed by 154 cases in 2021, possibly due to social distancing or other COVID-19 preventative measures. In 2022, there were a total of 322 cases reported in the United States.
- Since 1967 (start of U.S. national vaccination program), case rate globally has dropped from 100/100,000 to 1.1/100,000.
- Occasional regional epidemic outbreaks occur among individuals who have been fully vaccinated, primarily in settings with intense or frequent close contact, such as universities and correctional facilities.

Prevalence
0.0064/100,000 persons in United States; 90% of adults in the United States are seropositive.

ETIOLOGY AND PATHOPHYSIOLOGY
Mumps is an RNA virus *(Rubulavirus)* of the *Paramyxovirus* genus. Mumps virus replicates in glandular epithelium of parotid gland, pancreas, and testes, and rarely kidneys, leading to interstitial edema and inflammation.
- Interstitial glandular hemorrhage may occur.
- Pressure caused by testicular edema against the tunica albuginea can lead to necrosis and loss of function.

RISK FACTORS
- Global travel: One-third of countries in Africa, South Asia, Southeast Asia, and Japan do *not* mandate mumps vaccination and continue to have pediatric epidemics (roughly every 4 years). Many areas of South and Central America do not have high mumps vaccine coverage. Travel from an area of recent epidemic should be noted.
- Crowded environments such as dormitories, barracks, or detention facilities show an increase risk of transmission. It is considered a human-only virus, but infectious viral particles have been found in bats.
- Immunity wanes rapidly after single-dose vaccination. With a 2-dose schedule, immunity drops from 95% to 86% after 9 years.

GENERAL PREVENTION
- Vaccination is effective and essential, especially for pediatric travelers (1) and should be considered 3 months post cancer chemotherapy if antibody titers are low.
  - 2 doses of live attenuated mumps vaccine or mumps, measles, rubella (MMR, or with varicella MMR-V) vaccine are recommended, first at aged 12 to 15 months and second at aged 4 to 6 years. May start early at 6 months of age if travel is planned, but this dose does not count toward their 2-dose schedule.
  - 95% effective in clinical studies; field trials show 68–95% efficacy, which may be insufficient for herd immunity to prevent spread due to high contagiousness of mumps.
  - Prevention may require 95% first-dose and >80% second-dose adherence. Vaccine failure may increase 10–27% each year after vaccination.
  - Adverse effects of Jeryl-Lynn vaccine: seizure 25/100,000; fever 8/100,000; thrombocytopenic purpura 3/100,000
  - *No relationship between MMR vaccine and autism celiac disease or multiple sclerosis; recent data show a reduced autism risk in girls after MMR vaccination (aHR 0.79, overall for both genders aHR 0.93) (2).*
- Immunoglobulin (Ig) post exposure does not prevent mumps. Postexposure vaccination does not protect from recent exposure.
- Institute respiratory droplet isolation for hospitalized patients for 5 days after onset of parotitis.
- Isolate nonimmune individuals for 26 days after last case onset (social quarantine) due to incubation period as long as 25 days.
- In an epidemic situation, a third dose of MMR is indicated to decrease the attack rate (3)[A]. The boosted immunity from a 3rd dose has been observed to last up to 3 years (4).
- The neutralizing antibodies from vaccination are still effective against variant strains of mumps virus.
- Although there are no reports of disseminated mumps from MMR vaccine in HIV patients, live vaccines (MMR) are contraindicated in immunocompromised patients (e.g., HIV patients with CD4 <200).

Pregnancy Considerations
- Live viral vaccines are typically contraindicated in pregnancy; however, vaccination of children should not be delayed if a family member is pregnant. MMR and MMR-V given to breastfeeding mothers have not shown adverse effects in their infants.
- Immunization of contacts protects against future (but not current) exposures.

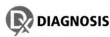

DIAGNOSIS

HISTORY
- Up to 50% of cases are mild. Parotid swelling peaks in 1 to 3 days; lasts 3 days usually, rarely up to 7 days; if complications occur, they occur after the parotitis.
- Clinical diagnosis: swelling of one or both parotid glands possibly 12 to 25 days after exposure.
  - Parotid pain lasting ≥2 days
  - Meningitis without parotitis (rare; 1–10%)
- 30% of individuals with mumps may be asymptomatic.
- Rare prodrome of fever, neck ache, myalgias, malaise, and anorexia
- Sour foods cause pain in parotid gland region.
- Moderate fever, usually not >104°F (40°C):
  - High fever often is associated with complications.

PHYSICAL EXAM
- Painful parotid swelling (95% bilateral) obscures angle of mandible and elevates earlobe.
- Often redness at opening Stensen (buccal surface opposite the upper second molar) duct without pus
- Meningeal signs (15%); rare altered consciousness or seizures from encephalitis (<1%), rare bilateral optic neuritis
- Rare maculopapular, erythematous rash
- Rare sternal swelling (pathognomonic for mumps)

DIFFERENTIAL DIAGNOSIS
- If not epidemic, consider testing for other viruses in addition to mumps such as influenza, parainfluenza parotitis, Epstein-Barr virus, coxsackievirus, adenovirus, parvovirus B19, influenza parotitis—several hundred reported in 2016.
- Suppurative parotitis: often associated with *Staphylococcus aureus* (Presence of pus within Wharton duct with parotid massage essentially excludes diagnosis of mumps.)
- Recurrent allergic parotitis; salivary calculus with intermittent swelling (usually unilateral)
- Lymphadenitis from any cause, including HIV infection; cytomegalovirus parotitis (immunocompromised)
- Mikulicz syndrome: chronic, painless parotid and lacrimal gland swelling of unknown cause that occurs in tuberculosis, sarcoidosis, lupus, leukemia, lymphosarcoma, and salivary gland tumors
- Sjögren syndrome, diabetes mellitus, uremia, malnutrition
- Drug-related parotid enlargement (iodides, guanethidine, phenothiazine)
- Mumps orchitis must be differentiated from testicular torsion and from chlamydial or bacterial orchitis.

DIAGNOSTIC TESTS & INTERPRETATION
Buccal swab and serum tests are recommended: https://www.cdc.gov/mumps/lab/specimen-collect.html
- Swab of fluid from parotid duct or other affected salivary ducts after gland massage for rRT-PCR plus viral culture—send to state lab or CDC; most sensitive at day 1 to day 3 of parotitis, especially important for vaccinated persons
- IgM titer (positive by day 5 in 100% of nonimmunized patients), rapid EIA for IgM, low sensitivity in previously immunized persons

- Rise in IgG titer samples; if not previously immunized: first, sample within 5 days of onset and second, 2 weeks later; previously vaccinated persons may not mount a 4-fold IgG increase, nor a significant IgM.
- Urine for PCR (not as sensitive as oral specimens); may not be positive until ≥4 days after symptom onset; 50 mL in sterile container; send to state lab (or recognized public health lab).
- Other potential findings: elevated serum amylase; CSF leukocytosis or leukopenia
- Testicular ultrasound may help differentiate mumps orchitis from testicular torsion.

Initial Tests (lab, imaging)
Buccal or oral swab PCR for mumps is recommended, especially in an epidemic setting as is an acute-phase serum specimen (mumps IgM, IgG, or rRT-PCR). If not epidemic, consider testing for influenza in addition to mumps virus.

Follow-Up Tests & Special Considerations
Mumps is a reportable disease. Contact local health department.

Diagnostic Procedures/Other
If meningitis symptoms present, lumbar puncture to exclude bacterial process; CSF pleocytosis, usually lymphocytic, in 65% of patients with parotitis

Test Interpretation
Periductal edema and lymphocytic infiltration of affected glands would be expected for mumps on biopsy.

TREATMENT

- No specific antiviral therapy; supportive care (3)[A]
- Immediately place mask on patients with any suspected mumps exposures who present for evaluation to decrease transmission.
- Analgesics to relieve pain
- Avoid corticosteroids for mumps orchitis because they can reduce testosterone and increase testicular atrophy.
- IVIG can reduce certain autoimmune-based sequelae such as:
  – Postinfectious encephalitis; Guillain-Barré syndrome; ITP
- Interferon-α2b improves bilateral orchitis but not testicular atrophy.

GENERAL MEASURES
- Hospitalize patients with high fever, pancreatitis, or CNS symptoms for supportive care, steroids, or interferon. Mask the patient and use respiratory droplet isolation precautions.
- Orchitis
  – Ice packs to scrotum can help to relieve pain.
  – Scrotal support with adhesive bridge while recumbent and/or athletic supporter while ambulatory

MEDICATION
First Line
- Analgesics and anti-inflammatory medications (acetaminophen, nonsteroidal anti-inflammatory drugs [NSAIDs]) may diminish pain and swelling in acute orchitis and arthritis of mumps.
- May use acetaminophen for fever and/or pain
- Precautions: Avoid aspirin for pain in children (previously associated with Reye syndrome).

Second Line
Interferon-α2b for severe orchitis

COMPLEMENTARY & ALTERNATIVE MEDICINE
Medicinal herbs or acupuncture have not shown benefit in randomized controlled trials.

ADMISSION, INPATIENT, AND NURSING CONSIDERATIONS
- Hospitalize only if CNS symptoms or severe complications occur. Use respiratory droplet precautions.
- Provide outpatient supportive care if no complications.
- Give IV fluids if severe nausea or vomiting accompanies pancreatitis.

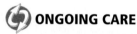

ONGOING CARE

FOLLOW-UP RECOMMENDATIONS
Mumps orchitis:
- Bed rest and local supportive clothing (e.g., two pairs of briefs) or adhesive-tape bridge
- Withhold from school until no longer contagious (5 days after onset of parotid pain).
- Any unvaccinated school contacts should be excluded for 26 days.

Patient Monitoring
Most cases will be mild. Monitor hydration status.

DIET
Liquid diet if unable to chew

PATIENT EDUCATION
Orchitis is common in older children but rarely results in sterility, even if bilateral.

PROGNOSIS
- Complete recovery is typical; immunity is lifelong.
- Transient sensorineural hearing loss in 4% of adults; some degree of permanent unilateral hearing loss in 1/1,000 children; mumps is the most common cause of pediatric hearing loss in some countries.
- Recurrence after 2 weeks may be nonepidemic nonmumps viral parotitis, but mumps RNA has been found in some recurrent parotitis swabs.

COMPLICATIONS
- Orchitis is more common (20–30%) in postpubertal boys:
  – Starts within 8 days of onset of parotitis; impaired fertility in 13%; absolute sterility is rare.
- Meningitis may present 5 to 10 days after the first symptoms. Aseptic meningitis is typically mild, but meningoencephalitis may lead to seizures, paralysis, hydrocephalus, or death (in 2% of encephalitis cases).

- Acute cerebellar ataxia has been reported after mumps infections; self-resolving in 2 to 3 weeks
- Oophoritis in 7% of postpubertal females; no decreased fertility. Mastitis has been reported in females. Pancreatitis, (usually mild), nephritis, thyroiditis, and arthralgias are rare.
- Myocarditis: usually mild but may depress ST segment; may be linked to endocardial fibroelastosis
- Deafness: 1/15,000 unilateral nerve deafness unrelated to encephalitis; may be permanent

Pediatric Considerations
- Orchitis is more common in adolescents. Young children are less likely to develop complications.
- Most complications occur in postpubertal group. Avoid aspirin use in children with viral symptoms.

Pregnancy Considerations
May increase risk of spontaneous pregnancy loss in first trimester. Perinatal mumps often has a benign course.

REFERENCES

1. Bangs AC, Gastañaduy P, Neilan AM, et al. Clinical and economic impact of measles-mumps-rubella vaccinations to prevent measles importations from US pediatric travelers returning from abroad. *J Pediatric Infect Dis Soc*. 2022;11(6):257–266.
2. Hviid A, Hansen JV, Frisch M, et al. Measles, mumps, rubella vaccination and autism. *Ann Intern Med*. 2019;171(5):388.
3. Lam E, Rosen JB, Zucker JR. Mumps: an update on outbreaks, vaccine efficacy, and genomic diversity. *Clin Microbiol Rev*. 2020;33(2):e00151–19.
4. Kaaijk P, Wijmenga-Monsuur AJ, Hulscher HIT, et al. Antibody levels at 3-years follow-up of a third dose of measles-mumps-rubella vaccine in young adults. *Vaccines (Basel)*. 2022;10(1):132.

 SEE ALSO

CDC Surveillance Manual. https://www.cdc.gov /vaccines/pubs/surv-manual/index.html

 CODES

ICD10
- B26.3 Mumps pancreatitis
- B26.2 Mumps encephalitis
- B26.81 Mumps hepatitis

CLINICAL PEARLS

- Mumps is a clinical diagnosis based on swelling of ≥1 parotid glands for ≥2 days without other obvious cause. Confirm with buccal swab PCR, viral culture, and IgM and IgG serology to identify early in epidemic setting. Work with local health authorities to ensure appropriate specimen collection and report positive results to public health authorities.
- Ultrasound helps distinguish testicular torsion from testicular pain in the setting of mumps orchitis.
- A history of vaccination with MMR does not exclude mumps, especially if vaccination more than 9 years prior
- The MMR vaccine is 68–95% effective after two immunizations. Immunity wanes over time.

M

MYALGIC ENCEPHALOMYELITIS/CHRONIC FATIGUE SYNDROME (CFS)

Allison H. Ferris, MD • Michael Mamone, MD

 BASICS

DESCRIPTION

- A chronic and complex physical illness characterized by a new or definitive onset of debilitating fatigue that persists for >6 months with moderate to severe intensity at least half of the time, which significantly reduces a person's ability to perform activities, and can't be fully explained by an underlying medical condition
- Key features include impaired memory or concentration, joint/muscle pain, nonrestorative sleep, postexertional malaise (PEM), orthostatic intolerance.
- Synonyms: myalgic encephalomyelitis (ME)/chronic fatigue syndrome (CFS), chronic Epstein-Barr virus syndrome, postviral fatigue syndrome, chronic fatigue immune dysfunction, systemic exertion intolerance disease

EPIDEMIOLOGY

- Can affect all ages; incidence peaks at 10 to 19 years and 30 to 39 years.
- Females are twice as likely to be affected.

Prevalence

- Affects all racial and ethnic groups; more prevalent in minority and low socioeconomic
- Estimated at 519 to 1,038 diagnosed per 100,000; 1.7 to 3.4 million patients may have ME/CFS.
- Up to 90% of cases may stay undiagnosed (1).

ETIOLOGY AND PATHOPHYSIOLOGY

The cause is unknown and likely multifactorial.

- Suspected initiating stressors:
  - Viral, bacterial, or parasitic infection: Epstein-Barr virus, retroviruses, Lyme disease, Q fever, human herpesvirus type 6 (HHV6), enteroviruses, Ross River virus, Borna disease virus
  - Recent vaccination; overexertion, chronic sleep deprivation; toxin exposure (e.g., organophosphate pesticides) or an atypical adverse reaction to a medication; significant physical or emotional trauma
- Hypothesized contributing factors:
  - Cellular metabolism (e.g., reduced oxidative phosphorylation and mitochondrial function in T cells); neuroendocrine system (e.g., diminished cortisol response to increased corticotropin); immune system (e.g., increased proinflammatory cytokines, C-reactive protein, and β_2-microglobulin); muscular system (e.g., reduced oxygen uptake); autonomic system (e.g., orthostatic hypotension); serotonergic system (e.g., upregulation of serotonin receptors); gastrointestinal system (e.g., increased wall permeability, altered gut microbiota, irritable bowel syndrome [IBS] comorbidity)

Genetics

- Higher concordance in monozygotic twins
- Genetic polymorphisms in several neuroimmunoendocrine-related genes may contribute to developing disease.

RISK FACTORS

- Family history of ME or CFS
- Personality characteristics (neuroticism and introversion); comorbid depression or anxiety
- Long-standing medical and/or mental health conditions in childhood; childhood inactivity or overactivity; childhood trauma (emotional, physical, or sexual abuse)
- Prolonged idiopathic chronic fatigue

COMMONLY ASSOCIATED CONDITIONS

- Fibromyalgia
- IBS
- Gynecologic conditions (pelvic pain, endometriosis) and surgeries (hysterectomy, oophorectomy)
- Anxiety disorders and/or major depressive disorders; posttraumatic stress disorder (PTSD), including physical and/or past sexual abuse; domestic violence; attention deficit hyperactivity disorder (ADHD)
- Postural orthostatic tachycardia syndrome (POTS); sleep disorders, including obstructive sleep apnea (OSA)
- Reduced left ventricular size and mass; prolapsed mitral valve; temporomandibular joint syndrome
- Multiple chemical sensitivities; migraines, myofascial pain syndrome
- Hashimoto thyroiditis, Raynaud phenomenon; interstitial cystitis, sicca syndrome, allergies

 DIAGNOSIS

HISTORY

A thorough medical history and psychosocial history is required for an accurate diagnosis. The 2015 diagnostic criteria proposed by the Institute of Medicine (IOM) require three symptoms and at least one of two additional manifestations:

- A substantial reduction or impairment in the ability to engage in preillness levels of activity (occupational, educational, social, or personal life) that:
  - Lasts for 6 months and is accompanied by fatigue that is often profound, of new onset (not lifelong), not the result of ongoing or unusual excessive exertion, and not substantially alleviated by rest
- PEM—worsening of symptoms after physical, mental, or emotional exertion that would not have caused a problem before the illness; often causes relapse lasting for days, weeks, or longer
- Nonrestorative sleep—may not feel better even after a full night of sleep despite the absence of objective sleep alterations
- And at least one of the following two additional manifestations must be present:
  - Cognitive impairment—problems with thinking, memory, executive function, and information processing; attention deficit; and impaired psychomotor functions
  - Orthostatic intolerance—worsening of symptoms on assuming and maintaining upright posture as measured by objective heart rate and blood pressure abnormalities during standing, bedside orthostatic vital signs, or head-up tilt testing

PHYSICAL EXAM

Complete physical exam (including mental status) to rule out other medical causes for symptoms. A complete mental status examination should be performed as well.

DIFFERENTIAL DIAGNOSIS

- Idiopathic chronic fatigue (i.e., fatigue of unknown cause for >6 months without meeting criteria for CFS)
- Psychiatric disorders: depression, anxiety, somatization disorder, substance abuse
- Physiologic: poor sleep hygiene, menopause, pregnancy until 3 months postpartum
- Sleep disorders: insomnia, OSA, narcolepsy
- Endocrine disorders: hypothyroidism or hyperthyroidism, primary adrenal insufficiency, hypercortisolism, diabetes mellitus, hypercalcemia)
- Chronic infections: Lyme disease, chronic hepatitis B or C, fungal disease (e.g., histoplasmosis, coccidioidomycosis), parasitic disease (e.g., amebiasis, giardiasis, helminth infestation), HIV, tuberculosis, chronic or subacute bacterial diseases (e.g., endocarditis, occult abscess), long COVID-19
- Acute infections: Epstein-Barr virus, parvovirus B19, Q Fever, West Nile virus
- Iatrogenic (e.g., medication side effects), toxic agent exposure, substance abuse
- Rheumatologic diseases: systemic lupus erythematosus, rheumatoid arthritis, polymyositis, polymyalgia rheumatica
- Chronic inflammatory diseases: sarcoidosis, granulomatosis with polyangiitis, celiac disease, inflammatory bowel disease
- Neurologic disorders: multiple sclerosis, myasthenia gravis, Parkinson disease, traumatic brain injury
- Cardiovascular diseases: cardiomyopathy, pulmonary hypertension, valvular heart disease, arrhythmias
- Other: small intestinal bacterial overgrowth, obesity, malignancy

DIAGNOSTIC TESTS & INTERPRETATION

There is no validated diagnostic test. An abnormal result does not always indicate the cause of fatigue. Renew the search if the suspected problem is treated and the patient remains fatigued.

Initial Tests (lab, imaging)

Standard laboratory tests are recommended to rule out other causes for symptoms:

- CBC; CMP; urinalysis; TSH and free T_4
- ESR or CRP; magnesium and phosphorus; vitamin B_{12}; serum folate; creatine kinase
- 25-hydroxy-cholecalciferol (vitamin D); serum iron, iron-binding capacity, ferritin

Follow-Up Tests & Special Considerations

- Additional laboratory studies, based on clinical features:
  - Antinuclear antibodies and rheumatoid factor, tuberculin skin test, salivary cortisol, HIV, RPR, Lyme serology, IgA tissue transglutaminase, urine drug screen

- Age/gender-appropriate cancer screening
- Electroencephalogram and/or magnetic resonance imaging if CNS symptoms
- Polysomnography and/or multiple sleep latency test if features of sleep disorder
- Assess for personality and psychosocial factors and maladaptive coping styles.

Diagnostic Procedures/Other
Potential biomarkers (e.g., HHV6 infection markers and antibodies against adrenergic and muscarinic receptors) are emerging.

 TREATMENT

- While large numbers of randomized clinical trials have not been performed, those that have suggest more positive results with nonpharmacologic treatments than pharmacologic treatments (2)[A]; most recommendations are based on expert opinion and standard symptom management (e.g., sleep disturbances, depression, and pain).
- Patients commonly use earplugs, earphones, sunglasses, and eye glasses to relieve sensitivity to light and sound (1).
- Focus on changes in lifestyle and insight with a goal to avoid complicating treatments (e.g., addictive medications, invasive testing) or interventions that support secondary gain. A multidisciplinary approach is recommended.
- Evidence surrounding cognitive-behavior therapy (CBT) and graded exercise therapy (GET) has been mixed, with some studies showing benefit and others not (1)[A],(2)[A]; pacing has been suggested as an individualized approach to combat PEM (2)[A].

GENERAL MEASURES
Treatment involves symptom control and guided self-management. The aim is to reduce symptoms and improve quality of life. Identify the most troublesome symptoms (typically pain and insomnia) and address those first.

- Individual CBT: not curative; may improve coping strategies and/or assist in rehabilitation (e.g., social, occupational)
- GET: Track amount of exercise patient can do without exacerbating symptoms and gradually increase intensity and duration. Strike a balance between activity and rest. GET should only be performed in the presence of a trained professional to prevent illness exacerbation.
- Pacing: to mitigate the frequency, duration, and severity of PEM; individualized plans to conserve energy and manage activities

MEDICATION
- There are no established pharmacologic treatments. Medications used are primarily for specific symptoms.
- Use lowest effective dose; increase cautiously.

- Attempt to use medications that treat more than one symptom to limit polypharmacy (1)[C].
  - Studies have been conducted with antivirals, antidepressants, immunoglobulins, steroids (hydrocortisone or fludrocortisone), modafinil, staphylococcus toxoid, methylphenidate, melatonin, gabapentin and galantamine. None show clear benefit.
  - Agomelatine, an antidepressant with agonist activity at melatonin receptors, has been promising in early studies.
- If insomnia is present, the use of nonaddicting sleep aids (hydroxyzine, trazodone, doxepin, etc.) may improve outcomes.

ISSUES FOR REFERRAL
Psychiatrist for comorbid behavioral disorders; rehabilitative medicine; sleep or pain management specialist

COMPLEMENTARY & ALTERNATIVE MEDICINE
- Acupuncture, massage, and chiropractic have been shown to benefit some patients.
- Other helpful nonpharmacologic interventions may include physical therapy, stretches, hydrotherapy, yoga, tai chi, qigong, meditation, hot or cold packs, warm baths, electrical massagers, and transcutaneous electrical nerve stimulations.
- Equivocal evidence for homeopathy and biofeedback

 ONGOING CARE

FOLLOW-UP RECOMMENDATIONS
Patient Monitoring
No consensus exists; periodic reevaluation is appropriate for support, reevaluation, and assessment for other causes of symptoms.

DIET
- No particular diet program has been shown to be effective for treatment of CFS.
- Whether weight loss improves symptoms in obese CFS patients is still unknown.

PATIENT EDUCATION
- Gradually increase exercise tolerance. Explain PEM and aerobic metabolism impairment for patients to not exceed their "energy envelope" (1). "Paced" activity management can help patients not exceed their energy limits (1).
- Avoid extended periods of rest, but ensure adequate rest between sessions. Relaxation techniques may also be helpful.
- Promote the benefits of cognitive therapies, lifestyle changes, and pharmacologic therapy. Educate patient's family on the condition and assist with applications for disability (1).
- The Solve ME/CFS Initiative: https://solvecfs.org/; Centers for Disease Control and Prevention, Myalgic Encephalomyelitis/Chronic Fatigue Syndrome: https://www.cdc.gov/me-cfs/

PROGNOSIS
- Disease severity can be classified as mild, moderate, severe, or very severe.
- A fluctuating course with relapse is common. Improvement is generally slow over months to years.
- Up to 75% of patients are unable to return to work, and 25% remain bedridden or housebound.

COMPLICATIONS
- Reduced physical activity out of fear that it may worsen symptoms
- Depression
- Polypharmacy
- Unemployment: <1/3 of patients in trials return to work even if improved symptoms. The Social Security Administration considers CFS to be a disability. Receipt of third-party disability pay (secondary gain) has been associated with treatment nonresponse.
- Chronic immune activation or associated infection may increase risk for non-Hodgkin lymphoma in elderly (aged >80 years).

REFERENCES
1. Bateman L, Bested AC, Bonilla HF, et al. Myalgic encephalomyelitis/chronic fatigue syndrome: essentials of diagnosis and management. *Mayo Clin Proc*. 2021;96(11):2861–2878.
2. Kim DY, Lee JS, Park SY, et al. Systematic review of randomized controlled trials for chronic fatigue syndrome/myalgic encephalomyelitis (CFS/ME). *J Transl Med*. 2020;18(1):7.

ADDITIONAL READING
Gravelsina S, Vilmane A, Svirskis S, et al. Biomarkers in the diagnostic algorithm of myalgic encephalomyelitis/chronic fatigue syndrome. *Front Immunol*. 2022;13:928945.

 SEE ALSO

Algorithm: Fatigue

 CODES

ICD10
R53.82 Chronic fatigue, unspecified

CLINICAL PEARLS
- Use the IOM criteria for diagnosis.
- There are many more patients with idiopathic chronic fatigue than true CFS.
- No pharmacologic agents (e.g., antidepressants, immune modulators) are consistently effective for treating CFS.
- Management focuses on reducing the burden of disease and improving quality of life by managing symptoms, assessing patient needs, and providing support.

M

MYASTHENIA GRAVIS
Melody A. Jordahl-Iafrato, MD, FAAFP • Jennifer R. Collins, PharmD

BASICS

DESCRIPTION
A disorder of neuromuscular transmission characterized by fluctuating muscle weakness:
- Ocular myasthenia gravis (MG) (15%): weakness limited to eyelids and extraocular muscles
- Generalized MG (85%): commonly affects ocular as well as a variable combination of bulbar, proximal limb, and respiratory muscles
- 50% of patients who present with ocular symptoms develop generalized MG within 2 years.
- Onset may be sudden and severe, but it is typically mild and intermittent over many years, maximum severity reached within 3 years for 85%.
- System(s) affected: neurologic, hematologic, lymphatic, immunologic, musculoskeletal

EPIDEMIOLOGY
Occurs at any age but a bimodal distribution to the age of onset:
- Female: 20 to 40 years old
- Male: 60 to 80 years old

Prevalence
In the United States, 70 to 320/1 million; increasing over the past 5 decades

Pediatric Considerations
A transient form of neonatal MG seen in 10–20% of infants born to mothers with MG; it occurs as a result of the transplacental passage of maternal antibodies that interfere with function of the neuromuscular junction; resolves in weeks to months; autoimmune juvenile MG makes up 10–15% of cases of MG in North America.

ETIOLOGY AND PATHOPHYSIOLOGY
An autoimmune disorder resulting in the reduction in the function of acetylcholine receptors (AChRs) at muscle end plates, resulting in insufficient neuromuscular transmission
- Seropositive/antiacetylcholine receptor (anti-AChR): a humoral, antibody-mediated, T-cell–dependent attack of the AChRs or receptor-associated proteins at the postsynaptic membrane of the neuromuscular junction; found in 85% of generalized MG and 50% of ocular MG; thymic abnormalities common (1)
- Muscle-specific kinase (MuSKs): 5% of generalized MG patients; typically females; is a severe form, respiratory and bulbar muscles involved; thymic abnormalities are rare (1).
- In remainder of seronegative, 12–50% with anti-LRP4, a molecule that forms a complex with MuSK, mild generalized weakness most common (1)
- Seronegative MG (SNMG): 5%; may have anti-AChR detectable by cell-based assay; clinically similar to anti-AChR; thymic hyperplasia may be present (1).
- Also documented immediately after viral infections (measles, Epstein-Barr virus [EBV], HIV, and human T-lymphotropic virus [HTLV])

Genetics
Familial predisposition is seen in 5% of cases.

RISK FACTORS
- Familial MG
- D-penicillamine (drug-induced MG)
- Other autoimmune diseases

COMMONLY ASSOCIATED CONDITIONS
- Thymic hyperplasia (60–70%)
- Thymoma (10–15%)
- Autoimmune thyroid disease (3–8%)

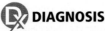

DIAGNOSIS

Myasthenia Gravis Foundation of America Clinical Classification:
- Class I: any eye muscle weakness, possible ptosis, no other evidence of muscle weakness elsewhere
- Class II: eye muscle weakness of any severity; mild weakness of other muscles:
  - Class IIa: predominantly limb or axial muscles
  - Class IIb: predominantly bulbar and/or respiratory muscles
- Class III: eye muscle weakness of any severity; moderate weakness of other muscles:
  - Class IIIa: predominantly limb or axial muscles
  - Class IIIb: predominantly bulbar and/or respiratory muscles
- Class IV: eye muscle weakness of any severity; severe weakness of other muscles:
  - Class IVa: predominantly limb or axial muscles
  - Class IVb: predominantly bulbar and/or respiratory muscles (can also include feeding tube without intubation)
- Class V: intubation needed to maintain airway

HISTORY
The hallmark of MG is fatigability.
- Fluctuating weakness, often subtle, that worsens during the day and after prolonged use of affected muscles; may improve with rest
- Early symptoms are transient with asymptomatic periods lasting days or weeks.
- With progression, asymptomatic periods shorten, and symptoms fluctuate from mild to severe.
- >50% of patients present with ocular symptoms (ptosis and/or diplopia). Eventually, 90% of patients with MG develop ocular symptoms.
- Ptosis might be unilateral, bilateral, or shifting from eye to eye.
- 15% present with bulbar symptoms.
- <5% present with proximal limb weakness alone.

ALERT
Myasthenic crisis: respiratory muscle weakness producing respiratory insufficiency and pending respiratory failure

PHYSICAL EXAM
- Ptosis may worsen with propping of opposite eyelid (curtain sign) or sustained upward gaze.
- "Myasthenic sneer," in which the midlip rises but corners of mouth do not move
- Muscle weakness is usually proximal and symmetric.
- Test for muscle fatigability by repetitive or prolonged use of individual muscles.
- Important to test and monitor respiratory function

DIFFERENTIAL DIAGNOSIS
- Thyroid ophthalmopathy
- Oculopharyngeal muscular dystrophy
- Myotonic dystrophy
- Brainstem and motor cranial nerve lesions

- Botulism
- Motor neuron disease (e.g., amyotrophic lateral sclerosis [ALS])
- Dermatomyositis/polymyositis

DIAGNOSTIC TESTS & INTERPRETATION

Initial Tests (lab, imaging)
- Anti-AChR antibody (74–85% are seropositive):
  - Generalized myasthenia: 75–85%
  - Ocular myasthenia: 50%
  - MG and thymoma: 98–100%
  - Poor correlation between antibody titer and disease severity (1)[C]
  - False-positive results in thymoma without MG, Lambert-Eaton myasthenic syndrome, small cell lung cancer, and rheumatoid arthritis treated with penicillamine
- Anti-MuSK antibody:
  - Used if MG is suspected and the patient is seronegative for AChR antibodies
  - Strong correlation between titer and disease severity (1)[C]
- LRP4 and clustered anti-AChR:
  - Used if MG is suspected and the patient is seronegative for AChR antibodies
- Thyroid and other autoimmune testing anti-striated muscle (anti-SM) antibody:
  - Present in 84% of patients with thymoma who are <40 years of age
  - Can be present without thymoma in patients >40 years of age
- Chest radiographs or CT scans may identify a thymoma.
- MRI of brain and orbits to rule out other causes of cranial nerve deficit

Diagnostic Procedures/Other
- Tensilon (edrophonium) test:
  - Rarely done as edrophonium no longer available in the United States and many other countries
  - A positive test shows improvement of strength within 30 seconds of administration.
  - Sensitivity 80–90% (2)[C]
  - Cardiac disease and bronchial asthma are relative contraindications, especially in elderly.
  - Atropine: 0.4 to 0.6 mg IV may rarely be required as antidote; must be available
- Ice pack test:
  - Ice pack applied to closed eyelid for 60 seconds and then removed; extent of ptosis immediately assessed
  - Ice will decrease the ptosis induced by MG.
  - Sensitivity 80% in patients with prominent ptosis
- Electrophysiology testing:
  - Repetitive nerve stimulation (RNS):
    - Widely available, most frequently used
    - Sensitivity generalized MG 76%; ocular MG 50% (2)[C]
  - Single-fiber electromyogram (SFEMG):
    - Assesses temporal variability between two muscle fibers within same motor unit (jitter)
    - Sensitivity 99%
    - Technically difficult to perform; limited availability, use if suspected and negative RNS (2)[C]

Test Interpretation

- Lymphofollicular hyperplasia of thymic medulla occurs in 65% of patients with MG, thymoma in 15%.
- Immunofluorescence: IgG antibodies and complement on receptor membranes in seropositive patients

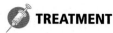 TREATMENT

GENERAL MEASURES

Three basic approaches: symptomatic, immunosuppressive, and supportive. Most should receive symptomatic treatment along with immunosuppressive and/or supportive modalities.

MEDICATION

First Line

Symptomatic treatments (anticholinesterase agents)

- Pyridostigmine bromide (Mestinon):
  - *Most commonly prescribed because available in oral tablet*
  - Starting dose of 60 mg PO TID with food
  - Maximum dose: 120 mg q3–4h
  - Long acting is available, but effect is not consistent.
  - Side effects are common, which can result in dose reduction or slower titration of dose: gastrointestinal disturbances, hypotension, syncope, urinary frequency (3).
- Neostigmine methylsulfate (Prostigmin):
  - Starting dose of 0.5 mg SC or IM q3h
  - Titrate dosage to clinical need.
  - Useful for patients who cannot absorb medications orally
  - May cause excessive salivary secretions, which may exacerbate swallowing difficulties (3)
- Patients with anti-MuSK may not respond well to these medications.

Second Line

- Immunosuppressants: Oral corticosteroids are the first choice of drugs when immunosuppression is necessary.
  - Prednisone:
    - May exacerbate symptoms short-term in up to 50% of patients
    - If inpatient and on other acute treatment, start with 60 mg/day PO.
    - If outpatient, start at lower dose (10 to 20 mg/day PO).
    - Titrate dose by 5 mg every 3 to 7 days to attain lowest effective dose (4)[B].
    - Use caution regarding long-term side effects from corticosteroids, including but not limited to weight gain, fluid retention, gastritis, ulcer formation, hyperglycemia, risk of infection, and osteoporosis.
- Azathioprine: 100 to 200 mg/day PO (4)[B]
  - *Most frequently used for long-term immunomodulation*, similar efficacy to steroids and IVIG
  - Consider screening for thiopurine S-methyltransferase (TPMT) levels prior to initiation of azathioprine.

- Benefit may not be apparent for up to 18 months after initiation of therapy.
  - Prednisolone + azathioprine may be effective when used as a corticosteroid-sparing agent.
- Mycophenolate: 1 g PO or IV BID
- Cyclosporine: dosing varies; may be given IV or PO (Use caution due to nephrotoxicity and drug interactions.)
- Acute immunomodulating treatments:
  - Plasmapheresis: bulk removal of 2 to 3 L of plasma 3 times per week, repeated until rate of improvement plateaus
    - Improves weakness and can last up to 3 months
  - Immunoglobulin: 2 g/kg IV over 2 to 5 days (4)[B]
  - *Plasmapheresis and immunoglobulin have comparable efficacy in treating moderate to severe MG.*
  - Rapid onset of effect but short duration of action
  - Used for acute worsening of MG to improve strength prior to surgery, prevent acute exacerbations induced by corticosteroids, and as a chronic intermittent treatment to provide relief in refractory MG
- Other immunosuppressant therapies, typically used in refractory cases:
  - Eculizumab
  - Efgartigimod alfa: only for use in AChR antibody positive MG
  - Ravulizumab
  - Rituximab:
    - Seronegative MuSK-antibody positive MG patients may have better response to rituximab than conventional therapies.
  - Tacrolimus
  - Cyclophosphamide

ALERT

Use caution with drugs that can precipitate weakness: aminoglycosides, fluoroquinolones, β-blockers, calcium channel blockers, neuromuscular blockers, statins, diuretics, oral contraceptives, gabapentin, phenytoin, lithium, among others.

SURGERY/OTHER PROCEDURES

Thymectomy recommended for thymic abnormalities

Pediatric Considerations

- Infants with severe weakness from transient neonatal myasthenia may be treated with oral pyridostigmine; general support is necessary until the condition clears.
- Corticosteroids limited only to severe disease

ADMISSION, INPATIENT, AND NURSING CONSIDERATIONS

- Management of pulmonary infections
- Myasthenic/cholinergic crises
- Plasmapheresis
- IV γ-globulin

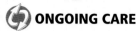 ONGOING CARE

PATIENT EDUCATION

Myasthenia Gravis Foundation of America (MGFA): https://www.myasthenia.org/

PROGNOSIS

- Overall good but highly variable
- Myasthenic crisis associated with substantial morbidity and 4% mortality
- Seronegative patients are more likely to have purely ocular disease, and those with generalized SNMG have a better outcome after treatment.

COMPLICATIONS

Acute respiratory arrest; chronic respiratory insufficiency

REFERENCES

1. Berrih-Aknin S, Frenkian-Cuvelier M, Eymard B. Diagnostic and clinical classification of autoimmune myasthenia gravis. *J Autoimmun*. 2014; 48–49:143–148.
2. Pasnoor M, Dimachkie MM, Farmakidis C, et al. Diagnosis of myasthenia gravis. *Neurol Clin*. 2018;36(2):261–274.
3. Farrugia ME, Goodfellow JA. A practical approach to managing patients with myasthenia gravis—opinions and a review of the literature. *Front Neurol*. 2020;11:604.
4. Gotterer L, Li Y. Maintenance immunosuppression in myasthenia gravis. *J Neurol Sci*. 2016;369: 294–302.

ADDITIONAL READING

Menon D, Barnett C, Bril V. Novel treatments in myasthenia gravis. *Front Neurol*. 2020;11:538.

 CODES

ICD10

- G70.01 Myasthenia gravis with (acute) exacerbation
- G70.00 Myasthenia gravis without (acute) exacerbation
- G70.0 Myasthenia gravis

CLINICAL PEARLS

- An autoimmune disease, marked by abnormal fatigability and weakness of selected muscles, which is relieved by rest
- >50% of patients present with ocular symptoms (ptosis and/or diplopia).
- Anticholinesterase medication and a thymectomy lessen symptom severity.
- Steroid therapy, plasma exchange, or immunoglobulin can be used in severely affected patients.

M

MYELODYSPLASTIC SYNDROMES (MDS)

Tara Baney, MS, CRNP • Frank J. Domino, MD

BASICS

DESCRIPTION
- Myelodysplastic syndromes (MDSs) are a heterogeneous group of clonal stem cell disorders characterized by dysplastic cells and peripheral blood cytopenias: anemia, thrombocytopenia, and/or neutropenia
- Dysplasia refers to an abnormality of development or differentiation in specific cell lines within the bone marrow. MDS has similar pathological/cellular characteristics with acute myelogenous leukemia (AML). MDS has a lower percentage of blast (<20%) in the peripheral blood and bone marrow. MDS has the ability to transform into AML and is a premalignant condition.

EPIDEMIOLOGY
Incidence
The incidence in the United States is approximately 4.9 cases per 100,000 population and increases with age (majority >80 years)

ETIOLOGY AND PATHOPHYSIOLOGY
- MDS arises from mutations in hematopoietic stem cell lines due to various genetic/chromosomal abnormalities. Mutations are due to genetic abnormalities/damage to hematopoietic cells. Bone marrow is replaced with mutated cells which crowd out the normal cells and cause cytopenias of one or more cell lines.
- 80% of cases have no know cause or exposure.
- Environmental exposures: benzenes
- Chemotherapy and/or radiation therapy have been known to cause MDS which is classified as iatrogenic/secondary MDS. MDS can occur up to 10 years after treatment.
- De novo MDS or primary MDS may occur due to somatic mutations.
- Two classification systems of MDS exist.
  - World Health Organization (WHO)
  - International Consensus Classification (ICC) includes cytogenetics/karyotype abnormalities, degree of dysplasia, and percentage of blast. Recent changes: MDS/AML 10–19% blast, MDS with multiple hit PT53 mutations, and MDS due to cytotoxic agents (1).

Genetics
- Cytogenetic anomalies are observed in >90% of MDS patients which include translocations or aneuploidy (loss or gain of a chromosome).
- Deletion of the long arm of chromosome 5 (5q) is the most common abnormal karyotype due to either treatment-related MDS with 5q deletion associated with chemotherapeutic agents versus de novo isolated 5q deletion. Patients with 5q deletion due to exposure to chemotherapeutic agents usually have other cytogenetic abnormalities and/or TP53 mutations. These tend to have a poorer prognosis. Isolated 5q deletion without other cytogenetic anomalies generally have better prognosis. Other cytogenetic anomalies commonly studied include normal karyotype, deletion 7q (-7), and trisomy 8 and -Y (1).

RISK FACTORS
- Age: increased risk in patients >60 years old
- Tobacco use
- Chronic exposure to chemicals: benzene, pesticides, insecticides, and petroleum
- Prior chemotherapy or radiation therapy
- Inherited disorders: Fanconi anemia, Shwachman-Diamond syndromes, severe congenital neutropenia, and familial platelet disorder
- Autoimmune disorders such as vasculitis, connective tissue disease, and inflammatory arthritis
- End-stage renal disease on dialysis.

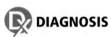

DIAGNOSIS

HISTORY
- The clinical course of MDS patients is driven by the type and degree of cytopenias.
- Recurrent infections, bleeding issues, fatigue, weight loss, and exertional dyspnea
- Fatigue is the most common symptom and tends to be out of proportion to anemia.
- Fevers, night sweats, and weight loss are not common.
- Evaluate for toxin exposure, including alcohol or previous chemotherapy.

PHYSICAL EXAM
- Generalized pallor, fatigue, petechiae, and ecchymosis as result of the anemia and thrombocytopenia.
- Hepatosplenomegaly, although rare, as consequence of extramedullary hemopoiesis is present, especially in MDS/MPN overlapping syndromes
- Lymphadenopathies are not common.

DIFFERENTIAL DIAGNOSIS
- Acute leukemia: AML or AMML
- Vitamin B$_{12}$ and folate deficiencies
- HIV
- Chronic liver disease
- Excessive alcohol use
- Infections of the bone marrow: HIV, tuberculosis, atypical mycobacterium, and Epstein-Barr virus
- Other hematopoietic disorders that do not fulfill diagnostic criteria for MDS such as idiopathic cytopenia of unknown significance, idiopathic dysplasia of unknown significance, clonal hematopoiesis of indeterminate potential (CHIP), and clonal cytopenia of unknown significance

DIAGNOSTIC TESTS & INTERPRETATION
Initial Tests (lab, imaging)
A complete blood count with peripheral smear, peripheral flow cytometry, chemistry, viral studies (HIV and hepatitis panel), erythropoietin levels, and vitamin levels (B$_{12}$ and folate) should be evaluated.

Diagnostic Procedures/Other
- *Histopathology.* A bone marrow evaluation to distinguish MDS from AML and to perform karyotype studies, fluorescent in situ hybridization (FISH), and mutational studies
  - Blast %: <20% is consistent with MDS; ≥20% is diagnostic of AML.
- *Cytogenetics.* Clonal chromosome abnormalities are observed in 30–80% of MDS patients. In the rest of the patients (20–70%), submicroscopic alterations (microdeletions, point mutations) provide diagnostic evidence.

Test Interpretation
- Hematologic findings in the blood smear include macrocytic anemia with possible basophilic stippling, hyposegmented neutrophils (pseudo Pelger-Huet), and thrombocytopenia.
- A low reticulocyte index reflects the hypoproliferative nature of the disease.

TREATMENT

GENERAL MEASURES

- Treatment is based on severity of symptoms and cytopenias, MDS classification, prognostic category, co-morbidities, and patient preferences (2).
- IPSS-M or IPSS-R scoring system should be used to guide treatment.
  - Lower-risk MDS—Treatment is based on severity of cytopenias and symptoms.
  - Asymptomatic—monitoring rather than immediate treatment
  - Symptomatic patients
- Anemia—symptoms related to anemia (e.g., dyspnea, fatigue, weakness) and hemoglobin (Hb) <10 g/dL
- Thrombocytopenia—platelets <20,000/μL or excessive bleeding or bruising with platelets <50,000/μL
- Neutropenia—recurrent and/or severe infections with absolute neutrophil count (ANC) <500 neutrophils/μL or ANC <1,000 neutrophils/μL with recurrent infections

MEDICATION

First Line

- MDS-related anemia
  - Blood transfusions and erythropoiesis-stimulating agents (ESA) (2)
    - ESA have a 30–60% response rate in LR-MDS; indications: Hb <10 g/dL and erythropoietin level <500; uncommon complications: worsening hypertension and thromboembolism
    - Need to be mindful of transfusions of packed red blood cells (PRBCs) as can cause iron overload
  - Lenalidomide; used in anemia in MDS with isolated deletion (5q); decreased need for transfusions (2)
  - Luspatercept anemia requiring 2 or more PRBCs over 8 weeks in low- to intermediate-risk MDS (2).
- MDS-related thrombocytopenia and neutropenia (2)
  - Thrombopoietin receptor agonists (romiplostim, eltrombopag) (close monitoring for leukemic transformation)
  - Neutropenia may be managed with G-CSF/antibiotics.

- Low-intensity chemotherapy
  - In LR-MDS with lack of response to supportive therapy, can use hypomethylating agents (HMA)
    - Azacitidine and decitabine (2)
- High-intensity chemotherapy with stem cell transplant (SCT)
  - Allogenic SCT only curative treatment option but reserved for high-risk disease in medically appropriate; rarely used (2)

ADDITIONAL THERAPIES

Management of iron overload. Iron chelation is often considered in patient with transfusion dependency.

ADMISSION, INPATIENT, AND NURSING CONSIDERATIONS

Complications such as bleeding, neutropenic fever, and undergoing SCT, warrant a hospital admission.

 ONGOING CARE

FOLLOW-UP RECOMMENDATIONS

Patient Monitoring

- Complete blood count to monitor cytopenias
- Repeat bone marrow examination for worsening cytopenias or evaluate response to therapy.
- Temperature and other vital signs to assess for signs of infection, bleeding and anemia
- Quality of life assessment

DIET

Alcohol consumption, meat, vegetable and fruit intake do not appear to have significant influence in the risk of developing disease.

PATIENT EDUCATION

- Regular follow-up and compliance with medications; smoking cessation
- Instruct about symptoms that should prompt the patient to seek out medical care for treatment of infection, bleeding, and/or anemia.

PROGNOSIS

Overall, the outcome of MDS patients is variable, with medial survival ranging from 6 months to >5 years depending on classification.

COMPLICATIONS

- Infection and bleeding are the leading causes of death, rather than AML conversion.
- Increased risk of cardiovascular disease either secondary to iron overload or chronic anemia
- Possibility of hepatic dysfunction from iron overload

REFERENCES

1. Arber DA, Orazi A, Hasserjian RP, et al. International Consensus Classification of Myeloid Neoplasms and Acute Leukemias: integrating morphologic, clinical, and genomic data. *Blood*. 2022;140(11):1200–1228.
2. Garcia-Manero G, Chien KS, Montalban-Bravo G. Myelodysplastic syndromes: 2021 update on diagnosis, risk stratification and management. *Am J Hematol*. 2020;95(11):1399–1420.

 CODES

ICD10

- D46.9 Myelodysplastic syndrome, unspecified
- D46.4 Refractory anemia, unspecified
- D46.B Refract cytopenia w multilin dysplasia and ring sideroblasts

CLINICAL PEARLS

- MDSs are a heterogeneous group of clonal stem cell disorders characterized by blood cytopenias and tendency for leukemic transformation.
- Different molecular and genetic mechanisms of pathogenesis translate into the same phenotypic manifestation of the disease.
- Infection and bleeding are the leading causes of death.
- Allogeneic SCT is ultimately the only curative treatment.

M

MYELOPROLIFERATIVE NEOPLASMS

Justin T. Ertle, MD

 BASICS

DESCRIPTION
- Myeloproliferative neoplasms (MPNs) are a group of clonal disorders that all originate in the pluripotent hematopoietic stem cell. This topic focuses on chronic myelogenous leukemia (CML), polycythemia vera (PV), essential thrombocythemia (ET), and primary myelofibrosis (PMF).
  - The 2016 World Health Organization (WHO) MPN classification also includes chronic neutrophilic leukemia (CNL), chronic eosinophilic leukemia-not otherwise specified (CEL-NOS), and MPN-unclassifiable, all more rare.
  - CML is characterized by uninhibited proliferation of myeloid precursor cells.
  - PV is characterized by erythrocytosis.
  - ET is characterized by thrombocytosis.
  - PMF is characterized by bone marrow fibrosis and extramedullary hematopoiesis.
    - As MPNs share common origins, they often share common features, and they can transform into one another.
- The natural history can last decades, but each MPN carries the risk of complications.

EPIDEMIOLOGY
The median age of diagnosis is >60 years.

Incidence
- CML: 1.6/100,000/year
- PV: 0.8/100,000/year
- ET: 1.0/100,000/year
- PMF: 0.5/100,000/year

ETIOLOGY AND PATHOPHYSIOLOGY
Genetic mutations activating hematopoiesis result in proliferation of cells of myeloid, erythroid, and/or megakaryocyte lineages.

Genetics
- CML is characterized by a 9:22 translocation (the Philadelphia chromosome) resulting in the oncogenic BCR-ABL1 fusion gene producing the constitutively active tyrosine kinase leading to cell proliferation, particularly of granulocytes.
- PV, ET, and PMF share "driver" mutations, most often of JAK2, MPL, and CALR genes, that activate hematopoiesis. Mutation in one of these three genes is found in >90% of BCR-ABL negative MPNs.
  - Janus kinase 2 (JAK2) mutations: JAK2 specifically regulates hematopoiesis via erythropoietin (EPO), GM-CSF, thrombopoietin, growth hormone, leptin, and IL-3 and IL-5 signaling (1). Mutations constitutively activating the JAK2 protein lead to cell proliferation and prolonged survival.
    - JAK2 V617F mutations: 95% of PV, 55% of ET, and 65% of PMF cases (1)
    - JAK2 exon 12 mutations: 4% of PV cases (1)
  - Myeloproliferative leukemia protein (MPL) gene mutations: The MPL gene encodes the thrombopoietin receptor, which regulates hematopoietic stem cells, especially megakaryocytes; mutations can cause cell overproduction.
    - MPL mutations: 3% of ET, 5% of PMF (1)
  - Calreticulin (CALR) gene mutations: specific frameshift mutations of CALR, which encodes calreticulin protein, lead to activated hematopoiesis, particularly of the megakaryocyte lineage. The mechanism may be via constitutive activation of the thrombopoietin receptor (1).
    - CALR mutations: 25% of ET, PMF cases (1)

RISK FACTORS
- Any factor that increases risk of somatic mutations, such as ionizing radiation.
- Although a large majority of MPNs are due to somatic mutations, familial cases occur (1).
- PV, ET, and PMF can transform into one another.

COMMONLY ASSOCIATED CONDITIONS
- Thrombotic events (e.g., CVA, TIA, DVT, Portal Vein Thrombosis)
- Major and minor hemorrhagic events (e.g., acquired von Willebrand disease)
- Anemia
- Bone marrow fibrosis, osteosclerosis
- Extramedullary hematopoiesis
- Blast transformation into acute leukemia

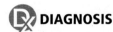 **DIAGNOSIS**

HISTORY
Constitutional symptoms are common, although a significant minority are asymptomatic.
- Any MPN may have these symptoms (1):
  - Constitutional: fatigue, weakness, night sweats, fevers, weight loss
  - Gastrointestinal: abdominal fullness, discomfort, or pain; early satiety
  - Musculoskeletal: bone pain
  - Neurologic: headaches, dizziness, trouble concentrating, transient visual disturbances
  - Psychiatric: depression, sexual dysfunction, insomnia
- Symptoms more common with certain MPNs:
  - CML: excess sweating, gout
  - PV: aquagenic pruritus, erythromelalgia, facial plethora, gout, tinnitus
  - PMF: abdominal fullness or pain, early satiety, gastrointestinal bleeding, weight loss, arthralgias, bone pain
  - ET: lightheadedness, transient visual disturbance, atypical chest pain, erythromelalgia, livedo reticularis, pregnancy loss

PHYSICAL EXAM
- Any MPN may present with pallor, splenomegaly, hepatomegaly.
- Signs more common with certain MPNs:
  - CML: gouty tophi
  - PMV: gouty tophi, increased blood pressure, conjunctival injection, facial plethora
  - ET: petechiae, livedo reticularis
  - PMF: petechiae, lymphadenopathy, marked splenomegaly

DIFFERENTIAL DIAGNOSIS
Generally, when one MPN is suspected, every MPN may be considered a possibility.
- CML: leukemoid reaction, other leukemias
- PV: secondary polycythemia, EPO receptor activating mutations
- ET: reactive thrombocytosis, myelodysplastic syndrome, thrombopoietin gene mutations
- PMF: secondary myelofibrosis, multiple myeloma, lymphoma, autoimmune disorders

DIAGNOSTIC TESTS & INTERPRETATION
Initial Tests (lab, imaging)
- Complete blood count and peripheral smear
- Renal and liver function, electrolytes)
- Lactate dehydrogenase (LDH), uric acid

Follow-Up Tests & Special Considerations
- Testing for BCR-ABL (Philadelphia chromosome)
  - Karyotype to detect the 9:22 translocation
  - Detecting the BCR-ABL gene
- Testing for JAK2, MPL, CALR gene mutants
- Bone marrow biopsy (BMBx) and aspiration
- Depending on the clinical scenario, consider the following:
  - EPO level, for detecting secondary causes of polycythemia
  - Iron studies (ferritin, transferrin, iron level)
  - von Willebrand factor, for detecting acquired von Willebrand disease, and assessing for increased bleeding risk

Diagnostic Procedures/Other
BMBx and aspiration is often used in establishing an MPN diagnosis.

Test Interpretation
- CML
  - Leukocytosis, granulocytosis (neutrophil predominant), and mature and immature forms in peripheral blood
  - The Philadelphia chromosome/BCR-ABL fusion gene establishes the diagnosis.
  - Chronic CML can progress to an accelerated phase or a blast crisis phase.
    - CML accelerated phase—there are eight hematologic/cytogenetic criteria in the WHO guidelines.
    - CML blast phase—WHO criteria
      - ≥20% blasts in PB or BM, or
      - Infiltrative proliferation of blasts at an extramedullary site
- PV—WHO criteria
  - Either all three major criteria, or the first two major criteria and the minor criterion
    - Major criteria
      - Hemoglobin >16.5 g/dL in men >16.0 g/dL in woman; or hematocrit >49%/48%; or increased red cell mass (RCM)
      - BMBx showing hypercellularity for age with trilineage growth including prominent erythroid, granulocytic, and megakaryocytic proliferation with pleomorphic, mature megakaryocytes
      - Presence of JAK2V617F or JAK2 SH2
    - Minor criterion: subnormal serum EPO level
- ET—WHO criteria
  - Either all four major criteria or the first three major criteria and the minor criterion
    - Major criteria
      - Platelet count ≥450 × 10⁹/L
      - BMBx showing proliferation mainly of the megakaryocyte lineage with increased numbers of enlarged, mature megakaryocytes with hyperlobulated nuclei; no significant increase or left shift in neutrophil granulopoiesis or erythropoiesis and very rarely minor (grade 1) increase in reticulin fibers
      - Not meeting WHO criteria for BCR-ABL1+ CML, PV, PMF, myelodysplastic syndromes, or other myeloid neoplasms
      - Presence of JAK2, CALR, or MPL mutation

○ Minor criterion: presence of a clonal marker or absence of evidence for reactive thrombocytosis
- PMF
  - PMF has been subdivided into prefibrotic/early stage and overt fibrotic stage.
  - Overt PMF—WHO criteria
    ○ Diagnosis requires all three major criteria, and at least one minor criterion
    ○ Major criteria
      ■ Presence of megakaryocytic proliferation and atypia, accompanied by either reticulin and/or collagen fibrosis grades 2 and 3
      ■ Not meeting WHO criteria for ET, PV, BCR-ABL1+ CML, MPNs, or other myeloid neoplasms
      ■ Presence of JAK2, CALR, or MPL mutation or in the absence of these mutations, presence of another clonal marker, or absence of reactive myelofibrosis
    ○ Minor criteria: presence of at least one of the following, confirmed in two consecutive determinations:
      ■ Leukoerythroblastosis
      ■ LDH above upper limit of normal
      ■ Palpable splenomegaly
      ■ Leukocytosis ≥11 × 10⁹/L
      ■ Anemia not attributed to other condition

 TREATMENT

GENERAL MEASURES
- PV:
  - Phlebotomy is the first line; goal hematocrit <45% in men and <42% in women (1)[A]
    ○ Achieving goal hematocrit decreases mortality from cardiovascular or thrombotic events 4-fold (1)
- PMF:
  - Transfusions for symptomatic anemia or thrombocytopenia
- As MPNs confer increased risk of thromboembolic events, reduce cardiovascular risk (address hypertension, hyperlipidemia, diabetes, smoking, etc.).

MEDICATION
- CML:
  - First-line medications:
    ○ Tyrosine kinase inhibitors (TKIs) are the first line for chronic phase, accelerated phase, and in the blast phase while evaluating for stem cell transplant.
    ○ The first-generation TKI (1GTKI) is imatinib; second-generation TKIs (2GTKI) include nilotinib, dasatinib, bosutinib; third-generation TKI (3GTKI) is ponatinib.
      ■ In low-risk chronic phase, 1GTKI or 2GTKI is recommended; choice influenced by patient and medication factors.
      ■ In high-risk chronic phase, 2GTKI may be preferred.
      ■ In accelerated phase, 2GTKI or 3GTKI is preferred; stem cell transplant may be considered.
      ■ In blast phase, TKIs are recommended, often in combination with induction chemotherapy, while evaluating for stem cell transplant.
  - Second-line medications
    ○ Active areas of research include adding other agents (e.g., interferon-α, ruxolitinib, venetoclax) in combination with TKIs as well as development of new TKIs.

- PV:
  - First-line medications:
    ○ All patients: aspirin (81 to 100 mg); aids in prevention of thrombotic complications and treatment of microvascular episodes such as ocular migraine, transient ischemic attacks, and erythromelalgia (1)[A]
    ○ High-risk PV patients (older age or history of thrombosis): cytoreduction with hydroxyurea or interferon-α (1)[C]
  - Second-line medications:
    ○ For low-risk patients who do not tolerate phlebotomy for cytoreduction, consider hydroxyurea.
    ○ For high-risk patients with inadequate response to cytoreductive medication, consider JAK2 inhibitor ruxolitinib (1)[C].
- ET:
  - First-line medications:
    ○ Aspirin (81 to 100 mg) is indicated in patients with prior history of thrombosis, JAK2 mutation, microvascular complications, or vasomotor symptoms (1)[C].
    ○ Cytoreduction in hydroxyurea is indicated for high-risk ET patients (thrombosis, or age >60 + JAK2 mutation), or patients with progressive thrombocytosis, acquired von Willebrand syndrome, significant bleeding, or splenomegaly (1)[C].
  - Second-line medications
    ○ When cytoreduction is indicated and an alternative to hydroxyurea is warranted, consider interferon-α or anagrelide (1)[C].
    ○ For symptoms not controlled with aspirin alone, cytoreduction with hydroxyurea can be considered.
- PMF:
  - First-line medications:
    ○ If transplant is not planned, and platelets ≥50 × 10⁹/L, consider the JAK2 inhibitor ruxolitinib (1)[A].
  - Second-line medication therapy:
    ○ Low-risk patients with bothersome symptoms may consider ruxolitinib, hydroxyurea, or interferon-α (1)[C].
    ○ Patients with disease progression on ruxolitinib may be considered for a newer JAK2 inhibitor (1)[C].
    ○ Patients with anemia who are not adequately responsive to nutrient repletion and/or transfusion (1)[C]:
      ■ EPO <500 mUmL: erythropoiesis-stimulating agents
      ■ EPO >500 mUmL: Consider danazol, prednisone, lenalidomide, thalidomide.

SURGERY/OTHER PROCEDURES
- Allogeneic stem cell transplant may be considered in CML accelerated phase and blast crisis as well as in high-risk PMF (1)[A].
- Splenectomy may be considered in severe cases, most often in PMF (1)[C].
- Palliative radiation can be considered for foci of extramedullary hematopoiesis.

 ONGOING CARE

PATIENT EDUCATION
- Avoid situations increasing risk of thrombosis.
- With splenomegaly, patients are advised to avoid activities increasing risk of rupture.

PROGNOSIS
- CML prognosis is strongly tied to disease phase (chronic, accelerated, blast) and therapy response.
  - Patients in chronic phase responding well to therapy have a near-normal lifespan.
  - Patients in blast phase have a median overall survival of 1 year.
- Though PV, ET, and PMF share driver mutations, prognosis varies considerably:
  - PV: median survival 14 years (24 years if age <60 years) (1)
  - ET: median survival 20 years (33 years if age <60 years) (1)
  - PMF: median survival 6 years (15 years if age <60 years) (1)
    ○ Driver mutation affects prognosis: CALR generally confers a better prognosis, whereas JAK2 or "triple-negative" (no JAK2, MPL, or CALR mutation) status confers worse prognoses (1).
  - Transformation from PV or ET into overt PMF confers a worse prognosis.
  - Transformation into acute leukemia confers a poor prognosis; occurs most often in PMF (20%) and less often in PV and ET (8%) (1)

REFERENCE

1. Patel AB, Vellore NA, Deininger MW. New strategies in myeloproliferative neoplasms: the evolving genetic and therapeutic landscape. *Clin Cancer Res*. 2016;22(5):1037–1047.

ADDITIONAL READING

Grinfeld J, Nangalia J, Baxter EJ, et al. Classification and personalized prognosis in myeloproliferative neoplasms. *N Engl J Med*. 2018;379(15):1416–1430.

 SEE ALSO

Leukemia, Chronic Myelogenous; Polycythemia Vera

CODES

ICD10
- D47.1 Chronic myeloproliferative disease
- C92.10 Chronic myeloid leukemia, BCR/ABL-positive, not having achieved remission
- D45 Polycythemia vera

CLINICAL PEARLS

- MPNs result from mutations that activate hematopoiesis, resulting in proliferation of cells of myeloid, erythroid, and/or megakaryocyte lineages.
- CML is characterized by granulocytosis, PV is characterized by erythrocytosis, ET is characterized by thrombocytosis, and PMF is characterized by bone marrow fibrosis and extramedullary hematopoiesis, often also with thrombocytosis.
- As MPNs share common mutational origins, multiple cell lines may be increased, they often share common symptoms (such as constitutional symptoms) and clinical features, and they can transform into one another.
- Often, the natural history lasts decades, but each MPN carries the risk of complications, such as thrombotic events, as well as transformation into acute leukemia or bone marrow fibrosis.

M

NARCOLEPSY

Waiz Wasey, MD

BASICS

DESCRIPTION

- Narcolepsy is a neurologic sleep disorder characterized by excessive daytime sleepiness (EDS) and may be associated with cataplexy (sudden loss of muscle control), hypnagogic hallucinations (vivid perceptual experiences while falling asleep), hypnopompic (vivid perceptual experiences while waking up from sleep), or sleep paralysis (temporary inability to move or speak that happens during transition from sleeping to awake state).
- Mainly two types identified by American Academy of Sleep Medicine: type 1 (60–70%) (formerly narcolepsy with cataplexy) and type 2 (formerly narcolepsy without cataplexy)
- No cure, symptomatic management

EPIDEMIOLOGY

Incidence
- Bimodal distribution; age of onset peak at 15 years and again at 35 years of age with male predominance
- African Americans are more likely to present without cataplexy and at a younger age.

Prevalence
- Narcolepsy type 1: 25 to 50/100,000 people
- Narcolepsy type 2: 20 to 34/100,000 people

ETIOLOGY AND PATHOPHYSIOLOGY

- Primarily caused by degeneration of hypothalamic neurons that produce orexin (hypocretin); postmortem studies show 85% loss of these neurons in type 1 and about 33% loss in type 2.
- Orexin is crucial to promote wakefulness; it stimulates the reticular activating system (RAS) and inhibits rapid eye movement (REM). Loss of orexin leads to disorganization of sleep-wake cycle, leading to sleepiness.
- Neurodegeneration may be caused by autoimmune process, probably stimulated by infections (such as influenza A or group A *Streptococcus*) or environmental factors (occurs commonly in late spring).
- *International Classification of Sleep Disorders*, 3rd edition (ICSD-3) classification:
  - Narcolepsy
  - Narcolepsy type 1
  - Narcolepsy type 2
  - Narcolepsy due to medical conditions
- Cataplexy is a result of hypocretin cell deficiency.

Genetics
- Usually sporadic but increased incidence in families with positive history
- 98% of patients with narcolepsy type 1 have human leukocyte antigen (HLA) DQB1*0602; 40–50% of patients with narcolepsy type 2 express this antigen. HLA-DQB1*0602 is present in 12–30% of the general population.
- Autosomal recessive inheritance pattern
- Affects 12% of Asians and 25% of whites, and 38% of African Americans are gene carriers

RISK FACTORS

Age (peaks at 15 and 35 years), usually underdiagnosed before age of 18 years; obesity, head trauma, CNS infections, psychological stress, positive Family history, recent influenza A, streptococcal infection, or H1N1 vaccine; no evidence of COVID-19 leading to narcolepsy yet (1)

COMMONLY ASSOCIATED CONDITIONS
Obstructive sleep apnea (OSA) (up to 25%), obesity, anxiety

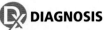

DIAGNOSIS

HISTORY

- Classic pentad of EDS, cataplexy, sleep paralysis, and hypnagogic/hypnopompic hallucinations, and disrupted/fragmented nocturnal sleep (five most common symptoms): Only 10–20% have all five.
- EDS and sleep attacks (cardinal symptom):
  - EDS is present in 100% of patients, usually the first initial symptom.
  - ICSD-3 classification for both type 1 and 2 requires EDS occurring almost daily for at least 3 months.
  - Patients may report refreshing daytime naps, with a possible return of EDS in 1 to 2 hours.
  - Sudden sleep attacks (seconds) during stimulating situations such as driving and walking
- Cataplexy (65–75% patients)
  - Mainly associated with type 1 narcolepsy, type 2 may develop in the long run
  - Sudden transient (seconds to minutes) episodes of total or partial loss of motor tone (buckling of knees, head dropping, sagging of jaw or weakness in arms, slurred speech, facial droop or grimace, etc.), triggered by strong emotions (such as laughing, anger, or fright).
  - Symptoms can be subtle as much as slurred speech to loss of muscle strength leading to collapse.
  - Consciousness and memory are not impaired.
- Sleep paralysis
  - Transient (several minutes) inability to move, speak, or open the eyes either while falling asleep or on awakening
  - During the event, breathing may be difficult because intercostal muscles are paralyzed and chest feels heavier.
  - Patients are aware of their surroundings and are able to recall the event.
  - Seen in 67% of patients who have narcolepsy with cataplexy and 49% narcolepsy without cataplexy
- Hypnagogic or hypnopompic hallucinations:
  - Vivid dreamlike experience in 30–60% patients with type 1 narcolepsy occurs during awakening (hypnopompic hallucinations) or at sleep onset (hypnagogic). Hypnopompic hallucinations are more indicative of narcolepsy than hypnagogic.
  - Hallucination is commonly visual, tactile, or auditory.
  - Characteristic hallucinations include being attacked by animals.
  - 15% of type 2 patients experience these as well.
- Other reported history
  - Nocturnal insomnia and sleep fragmentation
  - Retrograde amnesia
  - Increased periodic limb movements
  - Dream enactment behaviors
  - Weight gain seen with progression

PHYSICAL EXAM

- Unremarkable, but complete exam may help rule out other causes
- Deep tendon reflexes are either diminished or absent during an episode of cataplexy.

DIFFERENTIAL DIAGNOSIS

EDS is present in 4–28% of the general population, although most individuals are not narcoleptic:
- Sleep apnea syndromes
- Epileptic seizures and syncope
- Idiopathic hypersomnia (5–10% with EDS)
- Psychiatric (depression, bipolar II, and substance abuse/withdrawal)
- Sleep-related movement disorders (restless leg syndrome, periodic limb movements of sleep)
- Iatrogenic/secondary to medication (benzodiazepines; barbiturates; opioids; antihistamines; β-blockers; and some antipsychotics, antidepressants, and anticonvulsants)
- Poor sleep hygiene and habits leading to sleep deficit and chronic sleep deprivation
- Circadian rhythm disorders (jet lag, shift work, delayed or advanced sleep phase disorders)
- Cataplexy disorders (Niemann-Pick type C, Prader-Willi syndrome, Norrie disease)
- Hypersomnia in Parkinson disease
- Stroke (slurred speech and facial sagging seen in partial cataplexy)

Pediatric Considerations
Narcolepsy is rare before the age of 5 years. EDS is more often attributable to OSA, poor sleep hygiene, and the increased sleep requirements early in life. The recommended amount of sleep decreases with age: newborns, 16 to 18 hr/day; preschool-aged children, 11 to 12 hr/day; school-aged children and teens, 10 hr/day; adults, 7 to 8 hr/day. Children can gain excessive weight, from 20 to 40 lb (2). Symptoms of EDS, sleep paralysis, and cataplexy might last longer than compared to adult population.

DIAGNOSTIC TESTS & INTERPRETATION

- Sleep log/actigraphy: First, ensure patient is getting 6 hours of sleep at night for at least 7 to 14 days.
- Prerequisites for valid multiple sleep latency test (MSLT) → normal polysomnography (PSG) with at least 360 minutes of sleep, free of drugs that may alter REM sleep for at least 2 weeks, standardized sleep schedule for 7 days
- Primary diagnostic tool
  - An overnight PSG to rule out other causes of EDS
  - MSLT: performed the day after PSG if at least 6 hours of sleep and no sleep disorder explained by PSG
    - 4 to 5 20-minute naps at 2-hour intervals
    - Positive if rapid onset of REM (<15 minutes) in at least 2 of 5 sleeps (including baseline PSG) and shortened mean sleep latency (<8 minutes)
    - If MSLT is negative, but strong clinical suspicion, repeat the test.
    - Antidepressants and stimulants should be discontinued for at least 2 weeks prior to the test.
- Scoring tools
  - Epworth Sleepiness Scale (ESS): scored 0 to 24: >10 is suggestive of a sleep disorder rather than generalized fatigue; helpful for detecting response to medications
  - Narcolepsy Severity Scale: a 15-item scale to assess the frequency, severity, and consequences of symptoms of narcolepsy type 1

Follow-Up Tests & Special Considerations
- Lumbar puncture for orexin level; <110 pg/mL in the cerebrospinal fluid (CSF) is indicative of narcolepsy; rarely performed
- HLA typing (HLA-DQB1*06:02): particularly in children; it is supportive of diagnosis, lacks specificity; generally not recommended because 30% of healthy patient population has the gene (1)

Diagnostic Procedures/Other
- Narcolepsy type 1
  - EDS daily for ≥3 months
  - One of the following:
    - Cataplexy with positive MSLT
    - Low CSF orexin level <110 pg/mL or <1/3 of mean values in normal subjects
- Narcolepsy type 2
  - All the above (with or without cataplexy) and normal CSF orexin level

TREATMENT

GENERAL MEASURES
- Medications do not cure, but the goal is to minimize EDS and cataplectic episodes.
- Drug therapy, if used, should be supplemented by various behavioral strategies.
- Proper sleep hygiene and a regular sleep schedule
- Well-timed 20-minute naps may be helpful.
- Avoid stimulants (alcohol, heavy meals, caffeine, nicotine).
- Maneuvers such as altering thoughts, placing tension on muscles, or pressing against a firm support might rapidly terminate cataplectic episodes.
- Use safety precautions, particularly when driving. Untreated patients are at 10-fold at risk of accidents.

MEDICATION
First Line
- EDS
  - Modafinil (Provigil):
    - Works on dopaminergic, adrenergic, and histaminergic receptors of hypothalamus
    - Adult dose: 200 mg/day; start with 100 mg/day; max dose of 400 mg/day
    - Adverse effects: headache, GI upset, tachycardia, increased metabolism of oral contraceptives with less rebound hypersomnolence and does not affect blood pressure (BP); tolerance limited
    - Caution with oral contraceptive use as it decreases the efficacy
  - Armodafinil (Nuvigil):
    - Enantiomeric form of modafinil with the same half-life, but lower adverse effect profile
    - Adult Dose: 150 to 250 mg every morning
    - Headache, xerostomia, Stevens-Johnson syndrome, and toxic epidermal necrolysis
  - Pitolisant (Wakix): FDA approved for narcolepsy and cataplexy; doses up to 35.6 mg demonstrated effectiveness (2).

- Solriamfetol (Sunosi):
  - Start with 75 mg QD; increase dose based on response every 3 days to a max dose of 150 mg/day.
  - Contraindicated with concomitant or recent MAOI use
  - Abuse potential: Use caution in patients with a history of drug use.
- Clarithromycin: acts on GABA-A receptor; can be used for hypersomnia if alternative primary medication fails; dose of 500 mg BID (start with a 2-week trial period); adverse effect: GI distress
- Cataplexy:
  - Sodium oxybate (Xyrem):
    - Only medication FDA-approved for both EDS and cataplexy; now approved for ages ≥7 years
    - For moderate to severe cases and best option for improving nighttime sleep
    - Dose: 6 to 9 g/day divided BID; start with 2.25 g and increase by 1.5 g/day qwk; max dose: 9 g/day
    - May take 8 to 12 weeks for a full response
    - Is a date rape drug; abuse potential
    - May worsen sleep-disordered breathing in patients with OSA
  - Sodium oxybate, calcium, magnesium, potassium (Xywav) (3):
    - Approved by FDA for cataplexy and EDS in children aged ≥7 years
    - Once a day dosing options available
  - Sodium oxybate (Lumryz)
    - Once a day dosing
  - Tricyclic antidepressants
    - Clomipramine: dose: 25 to 75 mg/day
    - Anticholinergic side effect profile: dry mouth, sedation, urinary retention, impotence
  - Serotonin-norepinephrine reuptake inhibitors
    - Venlafaxine: dose: 75 to 300 mg/day; start at 37.5 mg, max dose of 375 mg/day. Taper dose to discontinue.
    - Fluoxetine: dose: 20 to 80 mg/day

Second Line
EDS
- Amphetamines: used if first line fail or patient unable to tolerate
  - Methylphenidate (Ritalin): dose: initial dose of 5 to 10 mg/day divided BID or TID; max dose of 60 mg/day, short-acting, most potent amphetamine available; can be used in combination with modafinil and armodafinil
  - Dextroamphetamine: dose: initial dose of 10 mg/day; can increase by 10 mg qwk to a max dose of 60 mg/day divided BID or TID
  - Adverse reactions: headaches, irritability, HTN, psychosis, anorexia, habituation, rebound hypersomnia
- Frequent nocturnal awakenings
  - Temazepam: Dose 15 to 30 mg at bedtime once helps with preventing frequent nocturnal awakenings and improving daytime sleepiness.

ISSUES FOR REFERRAL
Unresponsiveness to primary medication and severe cataplexy may benefit from neurology referral.

 ONGOING CARE

FOLLOW-UP RECOMMENDATIONS
Patient Monitoring
Monitoring using scoring tools to gauge treatment effectiveness and symptom control

PATIENT EDUCATION
- National Institute of Neurological Disorders and Stroke: https://www.ninds.nih.gov/Disorders/Patient-Caregiver-Education/Fact-Sheets/Narcolepsy-Fact-Sheet
- Narcolepsy Network: https://narcolepsynetwork.org/

PROGNOSIS
Improvements seen in 60–80% of patients; symptoms can worsen with aging. In women, symptoms can improve after menopause.

REFERENCES
1. Anderson D. Narcolepsy: a clinical review. *JAAPA*. 2021;34(6):20–25.
2. Meskill GJ, Davis CW, Zarycranski D, et al. Assessment of the clinical benefits of pitolisant on excessive daytime sleepiness and cataplexy in adults with narcolepsy. *Sleep*. 2021;44(Suppl 2):A189–A199.
3. Bogan RK, Thorpy MJ, Dauvilliers Y, et al. Efficacy and safety of calcium, magnesium, potassium, and sodium oxybates (lower-sodium oxybate [LXB]; JZP-258) in a placebo-controlled, double-blind, randomized withdrawal study in adults with narcolepsy with cataplexy. *Sleep*. 2021;44(3):zsaa206.

 CODES

ICD10
- G47.429 Narcolepsy in conditions classified elsewhere w/o cataplexy
- G47.411 Narcolepsy with cataplexy
- G47.419 Narcolepsy without cataplexy

CLINICAL PEARLS
- Narcolepsy is an incurable, REM disorder.
- The classic tetrad includes EDS, cataplexy, sleep paralysis, and hypnagogic hallucinations, only cataplexy is pathognomonic for the disorder.

NASAL POLYPS

Daniel Perez, MD • Sagar Saoji, MD

BASICS

- Painless benign inflammatory and hyperplastic lesions of sinonasal mucosa (1)
- Arise from near the ethmoid sinus but can infrequently arise from maxillary sinus mucosa
- Usually associated with chronic rhinosinusitis (CRS)

DESCRIPTION

- Appearance of edematous pedunculated mass in the nasal cavity or within the paranasal sinus
- Often causes symptoms of blockage, discharge, or loss of smell
- Most commonly bilateral; if unilateral, malignancy should be on differential.

EPIDEMIOLOGY

Incidence

- Typical age at diagnosis ranges from 40 to 60 years.
- Increases with age to a peak in the sixth decade
- Men are more commonly affected, although women are more likely to have severe disease.

Prevalence

- ~1–4% in general population (2)
- Much rarer in children: ~0.1% and associated with cystic fibrosis
- Asthma is present in up to 65% of patients.

ETIOLOGY AND PATHOPHYSIOLOGY

- Separate T helper 1–driven and T helper 2–driven pathways
- In the Western Hemisphere, nasal polyps are due to the T helper 2–driven eosinophilia, IgE causing inflammation, and elevated levels of interleukin-5, which is often associated with environmental and/or seasonal allergic triggers.

Genetics

Patients with nasal polyps are more likely than controls to report having a first-degree relative with nasal polyps (3)[B].

RISK FACTORS

- An increased prevalence of nasal polyps has been described among textile workers who have been exposed to occupational dust, particularly among those with longer-duration exposure (3)[B].
- Nasal irritants such as smoke and other common allergens

GENERAL PREVENTION

- Use of intranasal corticosteroids after polyp removal surgery has shown effectiveness against recurrence.
- Using a humidifier will help keep your nasal passages moist. This can help improve flow of mucus in your sinuses and prevent blockage or inflammation, thus preventing nasal polyps from occurring or recurring.

COMMONLY ASSOCIATED CONDITIONS

- Asthma
- Bronchiectasis
- Aspirin hypersensitivity
- Allergic rhinitis
- Chronic sinusitis
- Allergic fungal sinusitis
- Cystic fibrosis (pediatric patients)
- Primary ciliary dyskinesia (Kartagener syndrome)
- Laryngopharyngeal reflux

DIAGNOSIS

- Made on the basis of the presence of sinonasal symptoms for >3 months and the visualization of polyps in the nasal cavity, usually initially via nasal endoscopy
- CT or MRI scans of the sinuses can also be used.
- Biopsy of the mass may be done to help differentiate a benign versus malignant growth.

HISTORY

Symptoms

- Rhinorrhea
- Nasal congestion
- Postnasal drainage
- Hyposmia/anosmia
- Inability to breathe through nose
- Dull headaches
- Facial pain/pressure over the middle third of the face
- Sleep disturbance
- In some cases, there may be no symptoms.

PHYSICAL EXAM

Besides rhinorrhea, sinus tenderness to palpation, and/or visualization of polyp, there are no other definitive physical exam findings.

DIFFERENTIAL DIAGNOSIS

- CRS without nasal polyps, rhinitis, structural abnormalities of the nose, and neurologic causes of hyposmia
- Other benign or malignant tumors (e.g., fibroma, hemangioma, osteoma, chondroma, encephalocele)
- Squamous cell carcinoma
- Malignant melanoma
- Meningocele
- Nasal foreign body

DIAGNOSTIC TESTS & INTERPRETATION

Initial Tests (lab, imaging)

Anterior rhinoscopy shows pale, translucent mass

- Most commonly on lateral wall of middle meatus

Follow-Up Tests & Special Considerations

- If large posterior nasal polyps, examine tympanic membrane for eustachian tube dysfunction.
- If unilateral polyp, a biopsy should be done to exclude malignancy.
- Test for cystic fibrosis in children with polyps.
- Sinus CT scan:
  - May be helpful to corroborate history and endoscopic findings
  - Unable to differentiate polyp from other soft tissue masses
  - Reveals extent of disease and is necessary to formulate a plan for surgical intervention if indicated
- MRI:
  - May aid in diagnosis if concern for neoplasia, mycetoma, or encephalocele

Diagnostic Procedures/Other

Flexible/rigid endoscopy is required to assess the nasal cavity fully (3).

- Gold standard for diagnosis

TREATMENT

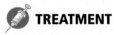

GENERAL MEASURES

- Goal is to reduce the size or eliminate nasal polyps because they can obstruct the nasal cavity and impair sense of smell, restrict breathing ability through nose, and obstruct drainage of sinuses.
- Assess symptom severity with 22-item Sinonasal Outcome Test (SNOT-22) or the Visual Analog Scale in primary care settings.

MEDICATION

First Line

Daily intranasal corticosteroid use with saline irrigation is the first-line therapy (4)[A].

- In patients who do not have significant nasal blockage by polyps, intranasal saline and intranasal glucocorticoids can be administered for 1 to 3 months.
- Intranasal corticosteroids shown to decrease nasal polyp size, lessen sinonasal symptoms, and improve quality of life
  - Budesonide 256 µg/day (one 64 µg spray in each nostril twice daily)
  - Beclomethasone dipropionate 168 to 320 µg/day (1 to 2 sprays per nostril twice daily)
  - Fluticasone propionate 400 to 744 µg/day (1 to 2 sprays per nostril twice daily)
  - Mometasone furoate 400 µg/day (2 sprays per nostril twice daily)
  - For children, mometasone furoate is preferred.

Second Line
- In patients with severe symptoms or those who cannot tolerate intranasal steroids, consider short course of oral corticosteroids (14 to 21 days) and/or doxycycline (21 days) (4)[B].
  - Prednisone 30 to 50 mg daily (taper when indicated)
  - Prednisolone 20 to 60 mg daily (taper when indicated)
  - Doxycycline 200 mg once, followed by 100 mg daily (contraindicated in pregnancy or if breast-feeding)
- There are more risks associated with use of oral steroids; can lead to serious side effects such as elevated blood sugar, cataracts, glaucoma, osteoporosis, bone fractures, and heart problems

ISSUES FOR REFERRAL
- If unilateral polyp, send for biopsy.
- Consider referral to otorhinolaryngologist for endoscopic sinus surgery if severe obstruction symptoms or conservative management ineffective.

ADDITIONAL THERAPIES
Patients with persistent symptoms and have concurrent allergic rhinitis, consider:
- Injectable steroids—steroid medication can be injected directly into the nasal polyp. It is generally as effective as oral steroids but has less associated side effects (5).
  - One major side effect that can occur, though, is short-term vision loss.
- Systemic antihistamine—does not treat nasal polyps directly but can help reduce associated symptoms.
- Leukotriene pathway antagonist
- Allergy immunotherapy
- Aspirin desensitization
- Intralesional bleomycin A5 (BLE) injection may treat eosinophilic-type nasal polyps.
- Biologics:
  - Based on two multicentered randomized double-blinded studies, adding dupilumab to daily mometasone furoate nasal spray reduced polyp size, sinus opacification, and symptom severity; it was well-tolerated and decreased systemic corticosteroid treatment and surgery (6)[B].
  - Dupilumab works by blocking interleukin-4 and interleukin-13.
  - Other biologics that have efficacy and/or relief of symptoms: omalizumab, mepolizumab (7)

SURGERY/OTHER PROCEDURES
- Most surgeries are approached endonasally.
  - The external (Caldwell-Luc) approach is used for more difficult cases but carries higher risk of complications.
- Functional endonasal sinus surgery has slightly lower revision rate than intranasal polypectomy. Both modalities provide effective symptom relief.
- Postoperative use of nasal corticosteroids delays the recurrence of nasal polyps and hence the timing of revision surgery.
- Postoperative use of steroid-releasing stents to prevent polyp recurrence by decreasing mucosal inflammation

 ## ONGOING CARE

- Recurrence up to ~40% (3)
- Use of intranasal corticosteroids after polyp removal surgery has shown effectiveness against recurrence.
- Recurrence twice as likely in those with asthma

PROGNOSIS
Persons who undergo surgery have great improvements in symptoms, but recurrence rate is high (8),(9)[B].

COMPLICATIONS
- Acute/chronic sinus infections
- Heterotrophic bone formation within the sinus cavity may occur.

REFERENCES
1. del Toro E, Portela J. Nasal polyps. In: *StatPearls* [Internet]. Treasure Island, FL: StatPearls Publishing; 2023.
2. Raciborski F, Arcimowicz M, Samoliñski B, et al. Recorded prevalence of nasal polyps increases with age. *Postepy Dermatol Alergol*. 2021;38(4):682–688.
3. Hopkins C. Chronic rhinosinusitis with nasal polyps. *N Engl J Med*. 2019;381(1):55–63.
4. Rudmik L, Soler ZM. Medical therapies for adult chronic sinusitis: a systematic review. *JAMA*. 2015;314(9):926–939.
5. Zamzam SM, Elshazly M, Salah M, et al. Comparative study between intrapolyp steroid injection and oral steroid for treatment of sinonasal polyposis in Egyptian patients. *Egyptian J Otolaryngol*. 2020;36(59).
6. Bachert C, Han JK, Desrosiers M, et al. Efficacy and safety of dupilumab in patients with severe chronic rhinosinusitis with nasal polyps (LIBERTY NP SINUS-24 and LIBERTY NP SINUS-52): results from two multicentre, randomised, double-blind, placebo-controlled, parallel-group phase 3 trials. *Lancet*. 2019;394(10209):1638–1650.
7. Han JK, Bachert C, Fokkens W, et al. Mepolizumab for chronic rhinosinusitis with nasal polyps (SYNAPSE): a randomised, double-blind, placebo-controlled, phase 3 trial. *Lancet Respir Med*. 2021;9(10):1141–1153.
8. Sharma R, Lakhani R, Rimmer J, et al. Surgical interventions for chronic rhinosinusitis with nasal polyps. *Cochrane Database Syst Rev*. 2014;(11):CD006990.
9. Rimmer J, Fokkens W, Chong LY, et al. Surgical versus medical interventions for chronic rhinosinusitis with nasal polyps. *Cochrane Database Syst Rev*. 2014;(12):CD006991.

CODES

ICD10
- J33.9 Nasal polyp, unspecified
- J33.0 Polyp of nasal cavity
- J33.8 Other polyp of sinus

CLINICAL PEARLS
- Intranasal corticosteroid use has been demonstrated to reduce polyp size and recurrence as well as to improve nasal congestion.
- Short-course oral corticosteroids may be considered in those with persistent symptoms.
- Asthma is a common concomitant diagnosis and is often previously undiagnosed.
- Aggressive medical and surgical treatment improves asthma outcomes.
- Allergy testing can be helpful.
- If unilateral nasal polyp, refer for biopsy.

NEPHROTIC SYNDROME
Hanadi Abou Dargham, MD

BASICS

DESCRIPTION
- A constellation of clinical and laboratory features defined by the presence of massive proteinuria (>3.5 g/1.73 m²/24 hr), hypoalbuminemia (<3 g/dL), severe hyperlipidemia (total cholesterol often >10 mmol/L) (380 mg/dL), and peripheral edema, with risk for thrombotic disease
- It can be due to intrinsic renal disease or secondary to congenital infections, diabetes mellitus, systemic lupus erythematosus, neoplasia, or certain drug use.
- Associated with many types of kidney disease

EPIDEMIOLOGY
- Diabetic nephropathy (1)
- Minimal change disease (MCD)
  - Most common cause of nephrotic syndrome in children aged <10 years (90%)
  - Idiopathic condition in adults associated with NSAID use or Hodgkin lymphoma
- Amyloidosis: 4–17% of idiopathic nephrotic syndrome—two renal types are primary (AL) and secondary (AA)
- Lupus nephropathy (LN): Adult women are affected about 10 times more often than men.
- Focal segmental glomerulosclerosis (FSGS)
  - 35% of nephrotic syndrome in adults; most common primary nephrotic syndrome in African Americans
  - Has both primary (idiopathic) and secondary forms (associated with HIV, morbid obesity, reflux nephropathy, previous glomerular injury)
- Membranous nephropathy
  - Most common cause of primary nephrotic syndrome in adults (40%)
  - Most often primary (idiopathic) but can be secondary associated with malignancy, hepatitis B, autoimmune diseases, thyroiditis, and certain drugs including NSAIDs, penicillamine, gold, and captopril
- Membranoproliferative glomerulonephritis (MGN)
  - May present in the setting of a systemic viral or rheumatic illness

Incidence
Approximately 3 cases per 100,000 per year in adults and 2 to 7 per 100,000 in Caucasian children <18 years of age. There is increased incidence and development of severe disease in African American and Hispanic populations.

ETIOLOGY AND PATHOPHYSIOLOGY
- Increased glomerular permeability to protein macromolecules, especially albumin
- Edema results primarily from renal salt retention, with arterial underfilling from decreased plasma oncotic pressure playing an additional role.
- The hypercoagulable state that can occur in some nephrotic states is likely due to loss of antithrombin III in urine.
- Primary renal disease (e.g., MCD, FSGS, MGN, IgA nephropathy)
- Secondary renal disease (e.g., diabetic nephropathy, amyloidosis, and paraproteinemias)

Genetics
Mutations in genes regulating podocyte proteins identified in families with inherited nephrotic syndrome.

RISK FACTORS
- Drug addiction (e.g., heroin [FSGS])
- Hepatitis B and C, HIV, CMV, parvovirus B19, toxoplasmosis, other infections
- Immunosuppression
- Nephrotoxic drugs (lithium, bisphosphonates, interferon therapy, gold, bucillamine, and penicillamine)
- Vesicoureteral reflux (FSGS)
- Cancer (usually MGN, may be MCD)
- Chronic analgesic use/abuse (NSAIDs)
- Preeclampsia
- Diabetes mellitus

GENERAL PREVENTION
Avoidance of known causative medications including NSAIDs, gold, penicillamine, and captopril; avoidance of heroin abuse; avoidance of high-risk sexual behaviors and tight glycemic control

DIAGNOSIS

HISTORY
- Inquire about signs or symptoms of systemic disease: joint complaint, rash, edema, infectious complaint, fevers, anorexia, oliguria, foamy or frothy urine, acute flank pain, and hematuria.
- Obtain a recent drug history for medications that may be causative, especially NSAIDs.
- Inquire about any prior history of venous thromboembolism as it could be the first indication of nephrotic syndrome.

PHYSICAL EXAM
- Fluid retention: abdominal distention, abdominal fluid shift, lower extremity edema, puffy eyelids, scrotal swelling, weight gain, shortness of breath; pericardial rub and decreased breath sounds with pleural effusions may develop.
- Arterial hypertension is found in 25% of the cases.
- Orthostatic hypotension
- Macroscopic hematuria is rare, but microscopic hematuria is present in 20% of the cases.

ALERT
The potential for thromboembolic disease leading to pulmonary embolism is one of the most life-threatening aspects of a patient who is actively nephrotic.

DIFFERENTIAL DIAGNOSIS
- Edema and proteinuria: See "Etiology and Pathophysiology."
- Edema alone: congestive heart failure, cirrhosis, hypothyroidism, nutritional hypoalbuminemia, protein-losing enteropathy

DIAGNOSTIC TESTS & INTERPRETATION
No guidelines are available for the investigation of nephrotic syndrome. Blood workup should be based on the clinical presentation.

Initial Tests (lab, imaging)
- Confirm proteinuria if present: by urine dipstick initially (3+ or 4+ readings) and then quantitate by 24-hour urine or spot urine protein-to-creatinine ratio.
- Urine culture
- CBC and coagulation screen
- Renal function tests
- Glucose
- Serum albumin that is often <2.5 g/dL
- Lipid panel
- Liver function tests
- Antinuclear antibody and/or antidouble-stranded DNA positivity suggest lupus.
- Complement levels (C3/C4 and total hemolytic complement): A low C3 may suggest a postinfectious or membranoproliferative process, whereas both low C3 and C4 point to lupus.
- Serum protein electrophoresis/urine immune electrophoresis to rule in a paraproteinemia
- Hepatitis B and C, HIV, and syphilis serology
- Renal US to verify the presence of two kidneys of normal shape and size
- Chest x-ray to detect presence of pleural effusion or infection
- Doppler US of the lower extremities if deep vein thrombosis (DVT) is suspected

Follow-Up Tests & Special Considerations
Consider genetic testing for the NPHS1 and NPHS2 mutations for infants and testing for NPHS2 in children who are resistant to steroid therapy.

Diagnostic Procedures/Other
Renal biopsy to determine the underlying cause of nephrotic syndrome and treatment
- Rarely done in children with first episode of nephrotic syndrome because MCD is common and empiric steroid therapy is the standard of care
- Contraindications to renal biopsy include small kidneys, renal tumor or bilateral renal cysts, active infection, severe malignant hypertension, hydronephrosis, bleeding diathesis, and uncooperative patient.

Test Interpretation
- Light microscopy
  - May see nothing (e.g., MCD)
  - Sclerosis (e.g., FSGS or diabetic nodules in diabetes)
  - Diffuse mesangial hypercellularity suggests a proliferative disease such as IgA nephropathy, LN, or postinfectious GN.
- Immunofluorescence: Mesangial IgA suggests IgA nephropathy, or Henoch-Schönlein purpura; other staining patterns are specific for other disease processes.

TREATMENT

Depends on the type of renal pathology and varies between children and adults; KDIGO issued guidelines in 2012 on the treatment for nephrotic syndrome in adults and children (2).

GENERAL MEASURES

Weight, height, and blood pressure should be monitored closely prior and during therapy along with urine output.

MEDICATION

First Line

- Edema: salt restriction and salt-wasting diuretics (loop and thiazide diuretics) (3)[A]:
  – Salt restriction to <2 to 3 g sodium per day
  – Restrict fluid intake to <1.5 L/day if hyponatremic.
  – Target weight loss of 0.5 to 1 kg/day (1 to 2 lb/day)
- Edema should be corrected slowly to avoid acute hypovolemia, electrolyte disturbances, acute renal failure, and thromboembolism as a result of hemoconcentration.
- Hyperlipidemia is often reversed with resolution of the disease.
  – Statins have been shown to improve endothelial function (3)[A] and may decrease proteinuria with the exception to rosuvastatin that can worsen proteinuria, but effect on GFR and preservation of renal function is small. The major role for statin use is in cardiovascular risk reduction.
- Proteinuria:
  – ACE inhibitors or angiotensin II receptor blockers are thought to reduce proteinuria, hyperlipidemia, thrombotic tendencies, progression of renal failure, and to control hypertension, if present (4)[A].
  – Protein restriction can slow the progression of the disease, but evidence is unclear.
- For steroid-responsive disease (MCD and FSGS), steroids dosed in consultation with a nephrologist

Second Line

- Many of the nephrotic diseases will require escalation in therapy above steroids. These include rapidly relapsing forms as well as MGN, LN, and IgA nephropathy. Bolus steroids and other immunosuppressives are required in this circumstance (cyclophosphamide, mycophenolate mofetil, chlorambucil, cyclosporine) (5)[A].
- Rituximab, anti–CD20 and abatacept, anti–B7-1, combined with steroids or other immunosuppressive agents, has demonstrated early promise in the treatment of refractory nephrotic syndrome (6)[B].
- Randomized controlled data have been insufficient to determine which patients require prophylactic anticoagulation (7)[A] and for how long. Common practice is to anticoagulate with heparin and then warfarin in patients who have persistent nephrotic-range proteinuria. This decision is made based on the patient's history of edema, hypoalbuminemia, thromboembolism, or immobility.
- Corticotropin injection is a potential treatment for steroid-resistant nephrotic syndrome; however, data is only based on retrospective and observational studies.
- Hypocalcemia from vitamin D loss should be treated with oral vitamin D.

ISSUES FOR REFERRAL

Nephrology for renal biopsy to confirm diagnosis and to assist with management

ADDITIONAL THERAPIES

Ambulation or range of motion exercises to lower risk of DVT

ADMISSION, INPATIENT, AND NURSING CONSIDERATIONS

Admission criteria/initial stabilization: respiratory distress, sepsis/severe infection, thrombosis, renal failure, hypertensive urgency/emergency, or other complications

ONGOING CARE

Adjustment in the doses of diuretics and angiotensin antagonists depends on the degree of edema and proteinuria.

FOLLOW-UP RECOMMENDATIONS

Patient Monitoring

- Frequent monitoring is required for relapse, disease progression, and for detecting signs of toxicity of medical management.
- Reevaluate for azotemia, urine protein, hypertension, edema, loss of renal function, cholesterol, and weight.
- Routine immunizations should be deferred until there are no relapses and the patient has been off immunosuppressants for at least 3 months.

DIET

Muscle wasting and malnutrition are major problems in severe nephrotic syndrome. Optimal diet includes:

- Normal protein (1 g/kg/day)
- Low fat (cholesterol)
- Reduced sodium (<2 g/day)
- Supplemental multivitamins and minerals, especially vitamin D and iron
- Supplemental dietary proteins are of no value.
- Fluid restriction if hyponatremic

PATIENT EDUCATION

https://www.niddk.nih.gov/health-information/kidney-disease/children/childhood-nephrotic-syndrome

PROGNOSIS

- Nephrotic syndrome in children (MCD) is typically self-limited and carries a good prognosis.
- Complete remission is expected if the basic disease is treatable (infection, malignancy, drug induced); otherwise, a relapsing and remitting course is possible, with progression to dialysis seen in more aggressive forms (diabetic glomerulosclerosis and FSGS).

COMPLICATIONS

- Deep vein, renal vein, or central venous thrombosis may occur.
- Pleural effusion, ascites
- Hyperlipidemia, cardiovascular disease
- Acute renal failure, progressive renal failure
- Protein malnutrition/muscle wasting

REFERENCES

1. Kodner C. Diagnosis and management of nephrotic syndrome in adults. *Am Fam Physician*. 2016;93(6):479–485.
2. Kidney Disease: Improving Global Outcomes (KDIGO) Glomerulonephritis Work Group. KDIGO Clinical practice guideline for glomerulonephritis. *Kidney Inter Suppl*. 2012;2(2):139–274.
3. Crew RJ, Radhakrishnan J, Appel G. Complications of the nephrotic syndrome and their treatment. *Clin Nephrol*. 2004;62(4):245–259.
4. Kunz R, Friedrich C, Wolbers M, et al. Meta-analysis: effect of monotherapy and combination therapy with inhibitors of the renin angiotensin system on proteinuria in renal disease. *Ann Intern Med*. 2008;148(1):30–48.
5. Hodson EM, Willis NS, Craig JC. Interventions for idiopathic steroid-resistant nephrotic syndrome in children. *Cochrane Database Syst Rev*. 2010;(11):CD003594.
6. Kamei K, Okada M, Sato M, et al. Rituximab treatment combined with methylprednisolone pulse therapy and immunosuppressants for childhood steroid-resistant nephrotic syndrome. *Pediatr Nephrol*. 2014;29(7):1181–1187.
7. Kulshrestha S, Grieff M, Navaneethan SD. Interventions for preventing thrombosis in adults and children with nephrotic syndrome (protocol). *Cochrane Database Syst Rev*. 2006;(2):CD006024.

SEE ALSO

Acute Kidney Injury; Amyloidosis; Diabetes Mellitus, Type 1; Diabetes Mellitus, Type 2; Glomerulonephritis, Acute; HIV/AIDS; Lupus Erythematosus, Discoid; Multiple Myeloma

CODES

ICD10

- N04.0 Nephrotic syndrome with minor glomerular abnormality
- N04 Nephrotic syndrome
- N04.3 Nephrotic syndrome with diffuse mesangial proliferative glomerulonephritis

CLINICAL PEARLS

- Nephrotic syndrome is a clinical syndrome of >3.5 g/day proteinuria, hypoalbuminemia, hyperlipidemia, and edema often associated with diabetes and NSAIDs use.
- Pediatric nephrotic syndrome typically carries a good prognosis and is more easily treated with steroids, although recurrences are common.
- Nondiabetic adults with nephrotic syndrome will require a renal biopsy to determine cause.
- Have a high index of suspicion for symptoms that may represent an embolic event in patients with nephrotic syndrome.

N

NEUROPATHIC PAIN
Raye Reeder, MD, MPH

 BASICS

DESCRIPTION
- The term *neuropathic pain* represents a broad spectrum of pain syndromes and encompasses a wide variety of peripheral and central disorders.
- Defined as injury of the nociceptive pathway in the central or peripheral nervous system (CNS and PNS) that results in either impairment, absence, or paradoxically augmentation of pain sensation
- Symptoms are usually burning, tingling, sharp, stabbing, shooting, and electric shock-like quality.
- Often severe and resistant to standard treatments for pain

EPIDEMIOLOGY
Incidence
There is an insufficient evidence on the general incidence rate of neuropathic pain as most studies target a single type of neuropathic pain. In a Dutch study targeted between 1996 and 2003, 9,135 new cases of neuropathic pain out of 362,693 persons contributing to the study were identified, yielding 8.2 new cases per 1,000 person-years (PY). The study approximates an annual incidence of almost 1% of the general population, affecting more women and middle-aged population.

Prevalence
Includes chronic conditions that affect up to 10% of the population, accounting for 20 to 25% of individuals with chronic pain.
- Malignancy—up to 20% have neuropathic pain from either cancer or treatment.
- Poststroke patients—up to 8%
- Spinal cord injury—60–69%, a large majority of whom present with a syringomyelia
- Herpes zoster—lifetime incidence ~25%; up to 10% develop chronic postherpetic neuralgia
- HIV—up to 50% have neuropathic pain
- Diabetes—~50% will eventually develop neuropathy; 34% will develop neuropathic pain.

ETIOLOGY AND PATHOPHYSIOLOGY
- A variety of mechanisms contribute to neuropathic pain, and many are still poorly understood.
- One proposed mechanism suggests that damaged primary afferents, including nociceptors, become highly sensitive to mechanical stimuli and may generate impulses in the absence of stimulation. This increase in sensitivity and spontaneous activation without apparent stimulation is thought to be caused by an increase in the density of sodium channels in the damaged nerve fibers, leading to increased excitability and signal transduction.

Genetics
Studies have demonstrated that $Na_v1.7$ and $Na_v1.8$, two types of voltage-gated sodium channels encoded by the *SCN9A* and *SCN10A* genes, respectively, are expressed at high levels on the peripheral nociceptive neurons in the dorsal root ganglion.

RISK FACTORS
- General risk factors include older age, female, physical inactivity, and manual occupation.
- Diabetes mellitus types 1 and 2, multiple sclerosis, Guillain-Barré syndrome, herpes zoster, trigeminal neuralgia, HIV, Lyme disease, malignancy/chemotherapy, nutrition (B_6 and B_{12} deficiencies), medications (isoniazid, ethambutol, chloroquine, paclitaxel, cisplatin, amiodarone, vincristine).

GENERAL PREVENTION
- Use of herpes zoster vaccines, which reduces both herpes zoster infections in patients >50 years of age and postherpetic neuralgia
- Use of antiviral or analgesic treatment in patients with herpes zoster infection
- Perioperative treatment of surgical patients to prevent chronic postsurgical pain; use of multimodal analgesia with gabapentin and local anesthetics to prevent acute and chronic pain after breast surgery for cancer
- Proper management of associated health conditions, such as diabetes mellitus

COMMONLY ASSOCIATED CONDITIONS
Depression and anxiety, sleep disturbances, substance abuse, impaired cognition, polypharmacy, and suicidal ideation

DIAGNOSIS

Diagnosis is based primarily on clinical history and the findings on physical examination.

HISTORY
- Onset and duration of symptoms, location, intensity (0 to 10), exacerbating factors
- Pain often described as burning, shooting, tingling, or electric shock-like
- Temporal profile: Symptoms become worse toward the end of the day.
- Sensory descriptors: numbness; weakness; reduced sensation to touch, pinprick, temperature, or vibration; decreased proprioception
- Effect on function: effect on sleep, ambulation, self-care, and sexual function
- Past medical, surgical, and psychosocial history, substance use (especially alcohol)
- Previous treatments: Neuropathic pain is generally resistant to acetaminophen or NSAIDs.
- Different screening tools in the form of questionnaires have emerged: Leeds Assessment of Neuropathic Symptoms and Signs, Douleur Neuropathique 4 questions, Neuropathic Pain Questionnaire, PainDETECT, Neuropathic Pain Symptom Inventory.

PHYSICAL EXAM
- Positive symptoms
  - Hyperalgesia (abnormally increased pain response to stimulus) evoked by sharp or blunt pressure, heat or cold
  - Allodynia (pain from nonpainful stimulus) evoked by light touch, clothing, or bed sheets
- Negative symptoms
  - Hypoesthesia (abnormally reduced sensation of a tactile stimulus) to touch or temperature
- Gross motor examination
  - Weakness, fatigue, decreased range of motion, stiffness, and muscle spasm
  - Hypotonia, tremor, dystonia, ataxia, hyporeflexia/hyperreflexia, motor neglect
- Sensory examination
  - Light touch, pinprick, vibration sense, and proprioception may be either diminished or amplified.
  - Sensory disturbance may extend beyond a discrete nerve territory.
- Skin examination
  - Alterations in temperature, color, sweating, and hair growth suggestive of sympathetic nervous system involvement, such as in complex regional pain syndrome (CRPS)
  - Residual dermatomal scars can indicate previous herpes zoster infection.
  - Acanthosis nigricans can indicate diabetes.

DIFFERENTIAL DIAGNOSIS
- Nociceptive pain due to actual tissue damage
- Somatic symptom disorder
- Conversion disorder

DIAGNOSTIC TESTS & INTERPRETATION
Neurologic testing establishes distribution but does not yet provide benefit in determining treatment (1)[C].
- Confirmatory tests include the following (in order of increasing invasiveness):
  - Sensory assessment—touch, pinprick, pressure, cold, heat, vibration, temporal summation
  - Quantitative sensory testing—uses standardized mechanical and thermal stimuli to test the afferent nociceptive and nonnociceptive systems
  - Blink reflex testing—assesses trigeminal afferent system
  - Nerve conduction study/electromyography—assesses nonnociceptive large fibre function of the peripheral nerves
  - Somatosensory-evoked potentials and laser-evoked potentials (LEP)—assess afferent fibre function
  - Skin biopsy—assesses quantification of the intraepidermal nerve fiber
  - Corneal confocal microscopy—assesses corneal innervation and small nerve fibres
- CT/MRI—facilitate specific diagnosis such as herniated disc, nerve compression by tumor

Initial Tests (lab, imaging)
None specifically for neuropathic pain but can rule in or out a possible cause: serum vitamin B_{12}, TSH, syphilis screening, fasting glucose/HbA1C, CBC, CMP, Lyme serology, HIV testing

TREATMENT

GENERAL MEASURES

- Due to multiple neuropathic pain pathways, all medications have limited efficacy, and minority of patients have significant benefit at tolerable doses.
- Physical and occupational therapy can help with functional goals.

MEDICATION

- The efficacy of systemic drug treatments is generally not dependent on the etiology of the underlying disorder.
- Combined therapy are likely more effective than increasing dose of a single medicine.
- Thought to be resistant to acetaminophen and NSAIDs but often used with some benefit in treatment of acute pain (2)[C]

First Line

- Calcium channel $\alpha2\delta$ ligands
  - Gabapentin: number needed to treat (NNT) = 7 for significant pain improvement (3)[A]
    - Dosing: up to 3,600 mg in 3 divided doses
    - Precautions: requires renal dosing
    - Common side effects: sedation, dizziness, peripheral edema, weight gain
    - Also in the form of extended release or enacarbil
  - Pregabalin: NNT = 8 (3)[A]
    - Dosing: up to 600 mg in 2 doses
    - Precautions: requires renal dosing
    - Common side effects: sedation, dizziness, peripheral edema, weight gain
- Tricyclic antidepressants: NNT = 4 (3)[A]
  - Nortriptyline, desipramine, amitriptyline clomipramine, imipramine
    - Dosing: Start 10 to 25 mg at bedtime and then increase by 10 to 25 mg every 4 to 7 days up to 150 mg/day as tolerated.
    - Precautions: cardiac disease, glaucoma, prostatic adenoma, seizure, tramadol use
    - Geriatric: falls; limit dose to <75 mg.
    - Common side effects: somnolence, weight gain, anticholinergic effects, cardiac conduction block
    - Increased suicidality warning in children, adolescents, and young adults
- Serotonin norepinephrine reuptake inhibitors (SNRIs): NNT = 6 (3)[A]
  - Duloxetine
    - Dosing: 20 mg once daily to 60 mg twice daily; effective doses 60 to 120 mg/day
    - Precautions: hepatic disorder, tramadol use, hypertension
    - Common side effect: nausea, constipation; relatively the safest medication for neuropathic pain
  - Venlafaxine
    - Dosing: 37.5 mg to 225.0 mg/day
    - Effective doses: 150 to 225 mg/day
    - Precautions: cardiac disease, tramadol use, hypertension
    - Common side effects: nausea, hypertension at higher doses

Second Line

- Lidocaine, 5% patches (3)[B]
  - As effective as pregabalin for localized neuropathic pain from diabetes or herpes
  - Dosage: 1 to 3 patches for 12 hours daily to cover the painful area
  - Common side effects: local erythema, itch, rash
- Capsaicin high-concentration patches (8%): NNT = 11 (3)[A]
  - Dosing: 1 to 4 patches to cover the painful area; 30 minutes application to feet, 60 minutes application to remainder of the body; avoid use on face; benefits for up to 3 months
  - Common side effects: pain (initial increase), erythema, itching, rare cases of hypertension, progressive neuropathy
  - No benefit from low concentration capsaicin cream

Third Line

- Botulinum toxin type A (3)[B]
  - Limited evidence based on small studies, no quality of life improvement
    - Dosage: 50 to 200 units subcutaneously to the painful area; repeat every 3 months.
    - Common side effects: pain and infection at injection site, weakness
- Cannabinoids (dronabinol and nabilone): low quality evidence
  - NNT = 20 for 50% improvement in pain
  - Number needed to harm (NNH) = 3 for adverse events
    - NNH = 25 for withdrawal due to adverse events
- Opioids (including tramadol): no proven long-term benefit; utility for neuropathic pain is questioned (4)[A].
  - Chronic opioids decrease the number and sensitivity of μ-opioid receptors, increasing hyperalgesia.

ISSUES FOR REFERRAL

Refer to pain clinic if refractory to initial treatment for trial of additional therapies.

ADDITIONAL THERAPIES

- Interventional pain management (epidural or peripheral nerve injections) will provide partial, lasting relief in 40–60% of patients (1)[B].
- Spinal cord stimulation (SCS): Pain that is continuous and unchanging responds best; best evidence for failed back surgery syndrome with leg pain (1)[B]
- Intrathecal drug delivery: reserved for refractory pain; ziconotide has demonstrated efficacy (1)[B].
- Transcutaneous electrical nerve stimulation is widely used; evidence shows slight benefit (1)[B],(3)[B].
- Cognitive behavioral and mindfulness therapies have some benefit as an adjunct to other therapies, especially in postherpetic neuropathy (1)[B],(3)[B].

SURGERY/OTHER PROCEDURES

Nerve destructive procedures haven't shown effectiveness and may cause additional insult/injury (an exception is treatment of terminal cancer) (1)[B].

- Sympathectomy dorsal root entry zone lesion (dorsal rhizotomy)
- Lateral cordotomy
- Trigeminal nerve ganglion ablation

COMPLEMENTARY & ALTERNATIVE MEDICINE

Acupuncture: limited evidence for improvement in pain

 ONGOING CARE

PROGNOSIS

Chronic course of pain symptoms often requires management with numerous medications and adjunctive therapies. Pain management requires ongoing evaluation, patient education, and reassurance. Complete pain relief is rare.

COMPLICATIONS

Long-term disability and drug addiction are possible.

REFERENCES

1. Jones RCW III, Lawson E, Backonja M. Managing neuropathic pain. *Med Clin North Am*. 2016;100(1):151–167.
2. Gilron I, Baron R, Jensen T. Neuropathic pain: principles of diagnosis and treatment. *Mayo Clin Proc*. 2015;90(4):532–545.
3. Moisset X, Bouhassira D, Avez Couturier J, et al. Pharmacological and non-pharmacological treatments for neuropathic pain: systematic review and French recommendations. *Rev Neurol (Paris)*. 2020;176(5):325–352.
4. Zhang Y, Ahmed S, Vo T, et al. Increased pain sensitivity in chronic pain subjects on opioid therapy: a cross-sectional study using quantitative sensory testing. *Pain Med*. 2015;16(5):911–922.

ADDITIONAL READING

- Colloca L, Ludman T, Bouhassira D, et al. Neuropathic pain. *Nat Rev Dis Primers*. 2017;3:17002.
- Fornasari D. Pharmacotherapy for neuropathic pain: a review. *Pain Ther*. 2017;6(Suppl 1):25–33.

 CODES

ICD10

- M79.2 Neuralgia and neuritis, unspecified
- E10.40 Type 1 diabetes mellitus with diabetic neuropathy, unsp
- E11.40 Type 2 diabetes mellitus with diabetic neuropathy, unsp

CLINICAL PEARLS

- Neuropathic pain is a common syndrome, affecting up to 10% of the population with major impacts on quality of life.
- Due to numerous mechanisms in neuropathy, potential benefit from any single treatment is limited.
- Narcotics likely have more harm than benefit; chronic use will likely increase pain.
- Functional goals and realistic pain targets are essential.

N

NEUROPATHY, PERIPHERAL

Christine S. Persaud, MD, MBA • Daniel Scura, DO

 BASICS

A disease of the peripheral nervous system (PNS) that has multiple etiologies including diabetes, neurotoxic agents, alcohol use, nutrition deficiencies, immune-mediated causes, nerve compression, nerve injury, genetic mutations, and idiopathic (1)

DESCRIPTION

- A functional or structural disorder of the PNS, affecting any combination of motor, sensory, or autonomic nerves
- Peripheral motor involvement causes muscle atrophy, weakness, cramps, and fasciculations.
- Disorders of sensory nerves produce negative phenomena (loss of sensibility, lack of balance) or heightened phenomena (tingling or pain). Large sensory fiber dysfunction impairs touch and vibration sensation, whereas small fiber sensory neuropathy (SFSN) affects pin and thermal sensation and causes neuropathic pain.
- The autonomic nervous system (ANS) dysfunction causes cardiovascular, gastrointestinal, and sudomotor symptoms.
- Peripheral neuropathy (PN) can be subdivided as mononeuropathies, multifocal neuropathies, and polyneuropathies.

EPIDEMIOLOGY

- Diabetic PN is the most common cause of neuropathy globally (2).
- Approximately 50% of Diabetics will develop PN (3).
- Chemotherapy-induced PN (CIPN) is a frequent side effect of chemotherapeutic agents with an estimated 30% of patients experiencing CIPN at 6 months after chemotherapy (1).

ETIOLOGY AND PATHOPHYSIOLOGY

- The most common cause of acquired PN is diabetes mellitus, which manifests most commonly at approximately 75% in the pattern of a distal sensory polyneuropathy (DSP).
- Other causes include:
  - Vascular: ischemia, vasculitis
  - Infectious: HIV, hepatitis C, cryoglobulinemia, Lyme disease, varicella zoster
  - Traumatic: compression, crush, stretch, or transection (e.g., due to broken or dislocated bones, slipped disks between vertebrae, arthritis)
  - Autoimmune: rheumatoid arthritis, Sjögren syndrome, lupus
  - Metabolic: renal failure, hypothyroidism, vitamin B_{12} deficiency, celiac disease, porphyria
  - Iatrogenic/toxic: chemotherapy, platinum, taxanes, metronidazole, colchicine, infliximab, lead, alcoholism
  - Neoplastic/paraneoplastic: paraproteinemia, Waldenström macroglobulinemia, multiple myeloma, amyloidosis, neurofibromatosis

Genetics
Approximately 50% of undiagnosed PN is hereditary.

RISK FACTORS
Diabetes and alcoholism

GENERAL PREVENTION
Management of underlying preventable causes of PN such as glycemic control, nutritional deficiencies, and avoiding neurotoxic agents

DIAGNOSIS

Diagnosis is made by a detailed patient history, clinical symptoms, laboratory tests and diagnostic testing of nerve conductions studies/electromyography (NCS/EMG), and possibly nerve biopsy (4).

HISTORY

- A detailed inquiry for symptoms of sensory, motor, or autonomic dysfunction:
  - Numbness, tingling, prickling, burning pain, a "tightly wrapped" sensation, and an "unsteady gait"
  - Distal weakness manifests as foot drop (tripping, foot slapping) or difficulty with grip; proximal weakness (e.g., difficulty arising from a chair) is less common.
  - Orthostatic dizziness, abnormal sweating, constipation, erectile dysfunction, or voiding difficulties
- Symptom onset:
  - Acute: Consider infection (e.g., Lyme disease), postinfectious dysimmune process (e.g., GBS), ischemia (e.g., vasculitis), toxin, or trauma.
  - Subacute: Consider metabolic, neoplastic, paraneoplastic, or dysimmune processes.
  - Chronic: Consider dysimmune process (CIDP), idiopathic, or hereditary.
- Progression: stable or indolent; slowly or rapidly progressive; monophasic or relapsing or remitting
- Anatomic pattern: focal, multifocal, diffuse
- Inquire about family history and comorbidities to help determine if condition is inherited.

PHYSICAL EXAM

- Based on exam, a functional (*sensory*: small fiber vs. large fiber vs. mixed, *sensorimotor*, *motor*, *autonomic*) and anatomic pattern of PN (*distal symmetric*, *multifocal*, or *focal*) should be established.
- Cognition is preserved in isolated PN.
- Cranial nerves may be involved with focal or multifocal PN (e.g., bifacial weakness may occur with GBS, Lyme disease, sarcoidosis, among other causes).
- Stocking/glove sensory loss is typical of distal symmetric sensory PN (e.g., diabetes).
- Isolated reduced pin or thermal sensation or allodynia suggests a pure SFSN.

- Reduced vibration and proprioception suggests large-fiber sensory neuropathy; when severe, a Romberg sign is present, and gait is wide based or ataxic.
- Distal muscle atrophy and weaknesses of toe extension and finger abduction are often present with distal symmetric axonal PN.
- In acquired demyelinating PN (e.g., GBS or CIDP), weakness is commonly both proximally and distally.
- Deep tendon reflexes may be reduced or absent, distally at the ankles in large-fiber axonal PN, or diffusely in demyelinating PN.
- High arched or flat feet or hammer toes suggest hereditary PN.

ALERT
Hyperreflexia and spasticity are upper motor neuron signs not seen with isolated PN.

DIFFERENTIAL DIAGNOSIS
- Mononeuropathy most likely due to compression, entrapment, or trauma
- Mononeuropathy multiplex (plexopathy, polyradiculopathy)

DIAGNOSTIC TESTS & INTERPRETATION
Initial Tests (lab, imaging)
- CBC, Cr, HbA1C, vitamin B_{12} with methylmalonic acid, LFTs, serum protein immunofixation electrophoresis, TSH
- NCS (the gold standard for the diagnosis of diabetic painful neuropathy [DPN]) (5) and EMG delineate axonal versus demyelinating, anatomic pattern, chronicity, and severity of PN.
- Autonomic reflex screen, testing of sweat function, quantitative sensory testing, and epidermal skin biopsy to evaluate small nerve fiber function (6)
- Specialized epidermal skin biopsy if suspected SFN and NCS/EMG is normal
- Neuroimaging generally not indicated in evaluation of PN but useful in evaluation of brachial plexopathies, radiculopathies, or where findings are attributable to the CNS

Follow-Up Tests & Special Considerations
- Based on the medical history, the PN type, and NCS/EMG findings; such as vitamin A, D, and E; zinc; copper; ESR; CRP; ANA; Hep B/C; antitissue transglutaminase
- Screen for alcohol use with distal symmetric PN.

Diagnostic Procedures/Other
Nerve biopsy (sural or superficial peroneal nerve): useful if vasculitis, amyloidosis, granulomatous disorders, or neoplastic infiltration is suspected; rarely helpful in late-onset chronic, slowly progressive distal symmetric PN

Test Interpretation

- Demyelinating PN: disproportionate slowing of conduction velocities, conduction block, increased temporal dispersion, or prolonged distal latencies on NCS; EMG findings including decreased recruitment and myokymia
- Axonal PN: reduced amplitude in sensory or motor responses, with relatively preserved conduction velocities and distal latency on NCS; EMG findings include abnormal spontaneous activity, decreased recruitment, increased duration and amplitude, and polyphasicity.
- Reduced ENFD on distal leg skin biopsies is supportive of SFN.

TREATMENT

GENERAL MEASURES

- Counsel on foot care and monitoring for signs of skin breakdown.
- Targeted treatment for underlying systemic conditions

MEDICATION

First Line

Treatment of neuropathic pain: evidence of efficacy derived from clinical trials in DPN, postherpetic neuralgia (PHN), or trigeminal neuralgia:

- Anticonvulsants: gabapentin, for PHN; pregabalin, for DPN and PHN; gabapentin (off-label), for DPN; oxcarbazepine for DPN; carbamazepine, for trigeminal neuralgia
- SNRI: duloxetine or venlafaxine for DPN
- Tricyclic antidepressants (TCA): amitriptyline or nortriptyline
- Patches: lidocaine 5%, capsaicin 8%
- Supplements: α-lipoic acid, acetyl-L-carnitine

Second Line

Mexiletine

Third Line

Tapentadol: for DPN

ISSUES FOR REFERRAL

- Neurology for rapidly progressive symptoms
- Rheumatology for vasculitic PN
- Hematology/skeletal survey for paraproteinemia
- Physical therapy for gait and balance training

ADDITIONAL THERAPIES

- Combination therapy (e.g., gabapentin with TCA, venlafaxine, or tramadol) can be more effective than monotherapy for neuropathic pain.
- Botulinum toxin subcutaneous, intradermal, or direct nerve injections can be considered for trigeminal neuralgia, DPN, or complex regional pain syndrome (CRPS) (7)[A].

- Additional immunosuppressant agents (e.g., cyclophosphamide) may be used in refractory chronic dysimmune PN.
- Immunotherapy for dysimmune PN
  - Intravenous immunoglobulin (IVIG): within the first 2 weeks of GBS to hasten recovery (8)[A]; as a first-line alternative to corticosteroids for treatment of CIDP; and for prevention of secondary axonal loss in MMN
  - Plasma exchange: first agent shown to improve functional outcome for patients with GBS (9)[A]; short-term benefit in CIDP (9)[A]
  - Corticosteroids: a first-line option in treatment of CIDP (9)[C]; oral or pulsed IV regimen can induce remission.
- Treatment of autonomic symptoms
  - Compression stockings, abdominal binder, hydration, midodrine, and fludrocortisone for orthostatic hypotension
  - Pyridostigmine for immune-mediated dysautonomia (off-label)

SURGERY/OTHER PROCEDURES

Decompressive surgery for entrapment neuropathy (e.g., carpal tunnel syndrome) syndrome

COMPLEMENTARY & ALTERNATIVE MEDICINE

Low-intensity transcutaneous electrical nerve stimulation (TENS), acupuncture, meditation, and supplements (G-agmatine, methylcobalamin, inositol) may be helpful.

ALERT

Vitamin B_6 supplementation may cause peripheral neurotoxicity and should be avoided except for a deficiency state.

ONGOING CARE

FOLLOW-UP RECOMMENDATIONS

- Exercises to improve muscle strength
- Avoid flu vaccination in the 1st year following GBS.

DIET

Assess for B_{12} deficiency, ingestion of heavy metal toxins, thiamine deficiency in those with alcohol use disorder, and high carbohydrate intake for those with diabetes.

PROGNOSIS

- Late-onset idiopathic distal symmetric axonal PNs are indolent.
- 80% of GBS have a near complete or good recovery. 80% of CIDP have moderate or good response with treatment but can be relapsing.

COMPLICATIONS

PN is related to an increase in fall risk.

REFERENCES

1. Zajączkowska R, Kocot-Kępska M, Leppert W, et al. Mechanisms of chemotherapy-induced peripheral neuropathy. *Int J Mol Sci.* 2019;20(6):1451.
2. Iqbal Z, Azmi S, Yadav R, et al. Diabetic peripheral neuropathy: epidemiology, diagnosis, and pharmacotherapy. *Clin Ther.* 2018;40(6):828–849.
3. Hicks CW, Selvin E. Epidemiology of peripheral neuropathy and lower extremity disease in diabetes. *Curr Diab Rep.* 2019;19(10):86.
4. Castelli G, Desai KM, Cantone RE. Peripheral neuropathy: evaluation and differential diagnosis. *Am Fam Physician.* 2020;102(12):732–739.
5. Selvarajah D, Kar D, Khunti K, et al. Diabetic peripheral neuropathy: advances in diagnosis and strategies for screening and early intervention. *Lancet Diabetes Endocrinol.* 2019;7(12):938–948.
6. Barrell K, Smith AG. Peripheral neuropathy. *Med Clin North Am.* 2019;103(2):383–397.
7. Park J, Park HJ. Botulinum toxin for the treatment of neuropathic pain. *Toxins (Basel).* 2017;9(9):260.
8. Hughes RAC, Swan AV, van Doorn PA. Intravenous immunoglobulin for Guillain-Barré syndrome. *Cochrane Database Syst Rev.* 2014;2014(9): CD002063.
9. Nobile-Orazio E, Gallia F. Update on the treatment of chronic inflammatory demyelinating polyradiculoneuropathy. *Curr Opin Neurol.* 2015;28(5):480–485.

CODES

ICD10

- G62.9 Polyneuropathy, unspecified
- G60.9 Hereditary and idiopathic neuropathy, unspecified
- G60.8 Other hereditary and idiopathic neuropathies

CLINICAL PEARLS

- Diagnosis is made by history and physical exam, targeted laboratory testing, NCS/EMG, skin biopsy, or ANS testing.
- Consider hereditary neuropathy if patient has an early age of PN symptom onset, family history of PN, or foot deformity.
- GBS is monophasic and progresses for up to 4 weeks; CIDP progresses beyond 8 weeks, and if untreated, usually has a progressive course.

N

NICOTINE ADDICTION

Boyd S. Malphrus, BA, MPAS • Kristen EB Said, MD, MPH • Elizabeth H. Carver, DNP, FNP-BC, CNE

BASICS

DESCRIPTION
Nicotine addiction is characterized by the compulsive use of nicotine products coupled with a lack of control over using, withdrawal symptoms, and/or continued use despite knowledge of or experiencing adverse consequences.

EPIDEMIOLOGY
Prevalence
- In 2019, an estimated 50.6 million U.S. adults (20.8% of the adult population) used tobacco; 14% of the U.S. adult population are actively smoking cigarettes, and 4.5% are using e-cigarettes (1).
- In 2016, 7.2% of women who gave birth smoked cigarettes during their pregnancy.
- In 2020, 19.6% of U.S. high school students and 4.7% of U.S. middle school students—a total of 3.6 million youth—reported current use (use in the past 30 days) of e-cigarettes (2). E-cigarettes have been the most commonly used tobacco product annually among youth since 2014 and have been associated with nicotine addiction in adulthood.
- Sociodemographic factors: Smoking rates are particularly high in non-Hispanic American Indian/Alaska Native persons; lesbian, gay, or bisexual adults; adults whose highest level of educational attainment is a GED certificate; persons who are uninsured or those with Medicaid; adults with a disability; and persons with mild, moderate, or severe generalized anxiety symptoms (1).

ETIOLOGY AND PATHOPHYSIOLOGY
- Similar to other addictive drugs, nicotine affects neural pathways that control reward and pleasure.
- Nicotine exerts its biologic effects through nicotinic acetylcholine receptors (nAChRs), which modulate neurotransmission with acetylcholine and other chemical messengers including glutamate, GABA, dopamine, serotonin, acetylcholine, and norepinephrine. In this way, it induces euphoria, assists in information processing, reduces anxiety, and mitigates fatigue.
- Upregulation of these receptors occurs over time, leading to tolerance and dependence.
- Polymorphisms in neuronal nAChR genes are associated with increased susceptibility to dependence.
- Nicotine is metabolized by cytochrome P450 2A6 (CYP2A6). Individuals who are fast metabolizers tend to smoke more cigarettes, are more likely to suffer intense withdrawal symptoms, and have a lower probability of quitting than slow metabolizers.
- Nicotine withdrawal involves the release of corticotropin-releasing factor in the amygdala, which induces the perception of anxiety and stress.

Pregnancy Considerations
- Smoking is a risk factor associated with placenta previa, abruptio placentae, decreased maternal thyroid function, preterm premature rupture of membranes, and ectopic pregnancy.
- Carbon monoxide and nicotine interfere with fetal oxygen supply, resulting in decreased birth weights and intrauterine growth restriction.
- Maternal smoking adversely affects fetal lung development, with lifelong decreases in pulmonary function and increased risk of asthma.
- Maternal smoking is associated with increased risk for sudden infant death syndrome, learning and behavioral problems, and obesity.

RISK FACTORS
- Mental illness (depression, posttraumatic stress disorder, bipolar disorder, and schizophrenia)
- Low socioeconomic status, low educational status
- Early firsthand nicotine experience, home and peer influence
- Concurrent substance abuse

GENERAL PREVENTION
- The U.S. Preventive Services Task Force (USPSTF) strongly recommends the following:
  - Screening all adults for tobacco use, providing cessation interventions for those who screen positive
  - Screening all pregnant women for tobacco use and providing pregnancy-tailored counseling to those who screen positive
- The USPSTF recommends that clinicians provide interventions, including education or brief counseling to prevent initiation of tobacco use among school-aged children and adolescents.

DIAGNOSIS

HISTORY
- Identify types, amount, and duration of nicotine products used.
- Review previous attempts to quit (methods used and duration of cessation).

PHYSICAL EXAM
- Pulmonary exam: wheezing, decreased breath sounds, prolonged expiration
- Cardiovascular exam: tachycardia, hypertension
- HEENT exam: epithelial dysplasia, squamous cell carcinoma, leukoplakia, stained teeth, hoarseness
- Skin exam: In combustible tobacco users, yellow-brown staining of the digits, "Harlequin nail" (bicolor nail seen after acute illness cause cessation of tobacco consumption, as unstained nail bed grows in), and clubbing may be seen.

DIAGNOSTIC TESTS & INTERPRETATION
- Lung cancer screening with low-dose CT is recommended annually by USPSTF for patients between 50 and 80 years old with a history of >20 pack-years of tobacco use who are currently smoking or have quit within the past 15 years (except those with life-limiting comorbidities).
- Neither spirometry nor regular chest x-rays are recommended for routine screening.

TREATMENT

Counseling
- Counseling interventions (individual, telephone, or group) improve quit rates compared to minimal support.
- More intensive interactions (i.e., motivational interviewing, close follow-up) may result in higher rates of quitting.
- Brief strategies to help the patient willing to quit tobacco—use the "5 As":
  - Ask patient if he or she uses nicotine.
  - Advise him or her to quit.
  - Assess willingness to make a quit attempt.
  - Assist those willing to make a quit attempt.
  - Arrange follow-up contact to prevent relapse.

- Users should be given a choice of methods to quit.
- Quit rates appear to be higher with abrupt quitting rather than gradual reduction prior to the quit date.

MEDICATION
- There are currently seven FDA-approved medications: nicotine replacement therapy (NRT), both long-acting (i.e., patch) and short-acting (i.e., gum, inhaler, lozenge, nasal spray) types, and non-NRT meds, bupropion SR and varenicline.
- With few exceptions, the choice of a first-line medication depends on patient's preference.
- Duration of nicotine addiction controller therapy is strongly recommended to be >12 weeks.
- Varenicline is a nicotinic acetylcholine partial agonist (pregnancy Category C). It is probably the single most effective pharmacologic intervention for smoking cessation; contraindications: known history of skin reactions or hypersensitivity; associated neuropsychiatric symptoms may include vivid dreams, sleepwalking, depression, suicidal ideation/attempts in patients with and without preexisting psychiatric conditions—close monitoring is recommended.
  - Starter pack: 0.5 mg/day for 3 days, 0.5 mg BID for 4 days, 1 mg/day starting day 7
  - Maintenance pack of 1 mg BID for 12 weeks; if successful, may continue for another 12 weeks
  - Varenicline is strongly recommended over nicotine patch or bupropion monotherapy.
  - Varenicline + NRT is more effective at 6 months than varenicline alone (NNT 6).
  - Clinicians should start varenicline in adults even if they are not ready to quit.
- Varenicline + bupropion is not more effective than either alone and confers increased side effects.
- Bupropion SR is an atypical antidepressant and norepinephrine-dopamine reuptake inhibitor (pregnancy Category C). Contraindications: history of seizure, stroke, brain injury, brain tumors, anorexia/bulimia, recent use of MAOI (within 14 days)
  - Start 1 week before target quit date due to time needed to reach steady state.
  - Use 150 mg/day for 3 days and then 150 mg BID for 7 to 12 weeks.
- Nortriptyline (off-label use) is a tricyclic antidepressant (pregnancy Category D); contraindications: narrow-angle glaucoma, heart disease (CAD, heart block, long QT)
  - Start 25 mg/day, gradually increase to 75 to 100 mg/day and continue for 12 weeks.
  - Set quit date 2 to 4 weeks after initiation.
- NRT (Gum: pregnancy Category C; all other formulations are Category D.)
  - Patch: For <10 cigarettes per day or <2 cans per pouches of smokeless tobacco, start with 14 mg/day for 6 weeks and then 7 mg/day for 2 weeks; for 10 to 29 cigarettes per day or 2 to 3 cans per pouches of tobacco, start 21 mg/day for 6 weeks, then 14 mg/day for 2 weeks, and then 7 mg/day for 2 weeks; for 30 to 39 cigarettes per day or >3 pouches per cans of tobacco, start 35 mg (21 mg/day + 14 mg/day patch) for 4 weeks and then 21 mg/day for 2 weeks, 14 mg/day for 2 weeks, 7 mg/day for 2 weeks; for >40 cigarettes per day, start 42 mg (21 mg/day patch for 2 weeks) for 4 weeks and then 21 mg/day for 2 weeks, 14 mg/day for 2 weeks, 7 mg/day for 2 weeks. Extending use of the patch beyond 8 to 10 weeks may improve abstinence rates.

– Gum: For >25 cigarettes per day, start 4 mg gum q1–2h for 6 weeks; for <25 cigarettes per day, start 2 mg gum q1–2h for 6 weeks; then double dosing interval every 3 weeks (i.e., q2–4h and then q4–8h). Chew then tuck between cheek and gingiva once nicotine flavor is released and repeat for up to 30 minutes and then discard. Avoid using with acidic foods (i.e., coffee, soda), which decrease nicotine absorption.

– Lozenges: For patients who smoke their first cigarette within 30 minutes of waking, start 4 mg lozenge PO q1–2h for 6 weeks; if first cigarette >30 minutes after waking, start 2 mg lozenge PO q1–2h for 6 weeks; then double dosing interval every 3 weeks (i.e., q2–4h and then q4–8h).

– Nasal spray: Start 1 to 2 sprays (0.5 mg per spray) each nostril q1h for 8 weeks and then taper; max of 10 sprays per hour and 80 sprays per day

– Inhaler: 6 to 16 cartridges inhaled (4 mg per cartridge) per day for 6 to 12 weeks and then taper; incorporates the behavioral and sensory aspects of smoking

• Combination NRT: All forms of NRT increase quit rate 50–70%. Combining long-acting maintenance with short-acting breakthrough NRTs is more effective than using any single method alone. If combining patch with lozenge or gum, limit to one to three 2 mg. Avoid combined NRT use for patients with serious arrhythmias, unstable angina, MI within the prior 2 weeks, or those age <18 years old.

• E-cigarette is an electronic device that delivers aerosolized liquid with or without nicotine and includes various flavorings and other chemicals. Insufficient evidence exists regarding this product's safety and efficacy. Low-quality evidence suggests that e-cigarettes can help patients cut down on the number of cigarettes smoked but not nicotine consumption. Other research demonstrates poor efficacy of abstinence with long-term follow-up. Long-term safety has not been established.

Pregnancy Considerations

• Tobacco cessation prior to 15 weeks' gestation provides the greatest benefit for both the woman and the fetus, but quitting any time is beneficial. ACOG recommends that pregnant and breastfeeding women be offered behavioral therapy and education as first-line treatment. NRT and medications should be reserved for patients in need of additional assistance given limited safety data.

• NRT is metabolized faster in pregnant women, which may lead to higher dose requirements.

• Pregnant women may perceive e-cigarettes to be safer than conventional cigarettes; however, given limited evidence regarding this NRT and concerns regarding fetal nicotine exposure, e-cigarettes are not recommended in pregnancy.

Pediatric Considerations

• Behavioral therapy (including CBT) is recommended as first-line treatment. There is an evidence that group counseling is superior to individual counseling and group messaging for tobacco cessation in youth. There are currently no FDA-approved pharmacologic treatments for youth. AAP recommends using NRT only for youth with moderate to severe substance use disorder.

• Risk of long-term addiction is much higher when smoking is initiated in adolescence than later in life, likely reflecting changes induced by nicotine in the developing brain. The biology of addiction, including withdrawal, occurs with fewer daily cigarettes in teens than in adults. Explanation of these biologic factors may help adolescents to stop or defer smoking.

• E-cigarette use in adolescents is reliably associated with subsequent smoking. An intervention to reduce smoking initiation was found to reduce the likelihood of ever smoking, suggesting there is a role for interventions to reduce smoking initiation even in adolescents who use e-cigarettes.

COMPLEMENTARY & ALTERNATIVE MEDICINE

• Acupuncture: no consistent evidence of efficacy
• Hypnotherapy: no consistent evidence of efficacy

ADMISSION, INPATIENT, AND NURSING CONSIDERATIONS

• Consider NRT for inpatients who use nicotine to decrease withdrawal symptoms (use with caution in patients with unstable angina, serious arrhythmias, or MI within the previous 2 weeks).

• Bupropion may not adequately control acute withdrawal symptoms.

 ONGOING CARE

FOLLOW-UP RECOMMENDATIONS

• Patients who have initiated therapy should follow up after 1 to 2 weeks to monitor response and side effects.

• Monitor for signs of nicotine withdrawal syndrome and start medication-assisted treatment or adjust dosage:

– Increased appetite/weight gain (4 to 5 kg over 10 weeks)

– Dysphoric, depressed mood, or anhedonia; insomnia, irritability, frustration, or anger, anxiety

– Difficulty concentrating, restlessness

• Follow-up should continue periodically in person or via telephone, especially during the first 3 months.

• Pharmacotherapy is generally recommended for 3 months duration.

PATIENT EDUCATION

• Smokefree: http://smokefree.gov
• 1-800-QUIT-NOW (1-800-784-8669)
• BecomeAnEX: https://www.becomeanex.org
• Text Messaging Support—National Texting Portal; Text "QUITNOW" to 333888.
• Smartphone App—quitSTART app

PROGNOSIS

• Roughly 50% of all smokers will die from a tobacco-related illness.

• Former smokers have a 50% reduction in risk of CAD 1 year after quitting, a 50% reduction in head and neck cancers by 2 to 5 years, and a 50% reduction in lung cancer mortality by 10 years. The risk of stroke is reduced to that of nonsmokers 2 to 5 years after quitting.

• 22% of smokers relapse within 3 months of quitting. Multiple attempts are often required.

• Individuals receiving support from significant others are more likely to quit.

COMPLICATIONS

• Chronic obstructive pulmonary disease (COPD) (emphysema and chronic bronchitis)
• Cancers (i.e., lung, oral/pharyngeal, kidney, bladder, cervical, anal, squamous cell)
• Atherosclerotic disease, peptic ulcer disease, periodontal disease
• Osteoporosis and hip fracture (in women), delayed wound healing
• Others (listed above)

REFERENCES

1. Cornelius ME, Wang TW, Jamal A, et al. Tobacco product use among adults—United States, 2019. *MMWR Morb Mortal Wkly Rep.* 2020;69(46):1736–1742.

2. Wang TW, Neff LJ, Park-Lee E, et al. E-cigarette use among middle and high school students—United States, 2020. *MMWR Morb Mortal Wkly Rep.* 2020;69(37):1310–1312.

3. U.S. Department of Health and Human Services. *E-Cigarette Use Among Youth and Young Adults: A Report of the Surgeon General.* Rockville, MD: U.S. Department of Health and Human Services, Centers for Disease Control and Prevention, National Center for Chronic Disease Prevention and Health Promotion, Office on Smoking and Health. https://www.cdc.gov/tobacco/sgr/e-cigarettes/pdfs/2016_sgr_entire_report_508.pdf. Accessed September 26, 2023.

CODES

ICD10

• F17.200 Nicotine dependence, unspecified, uncomplicated
• F17.201 Nicotine dependence, unspecified, in remission
• F17.203 Nicotine dependence unspecified, with withdrawal

CLINICAL PEARLS

• Nicotine dependence is a chronic disease and will often require repeated interventions and multiple cessation attempts.

• No single type of medication is best; thus, the choice should be based on patient's preference and risk factors for side effects.

• Although considerable progress has been made in reducing cigarette smoking among U.S. adults and youth, the tobacco product landscape continues to evolve to include a variety of tobacco products, including smoked, smokeless, and electronic products, such as e-cigarettes (3).

N

NONALCOHOLIC FATTY LIVER DISEASE (NAFLD)

Jill T. Wei Doherty, MD • Anita Wong, MD • Daniel T. Lee, MD, MA

BASICS

- A spectrum of fatty liver diseases ranging from nonalcoholic fatty liver (NAFL), to nonalcoholic steatohepatitis (NASH), to fibrosis and cirrhosis, not due to other cause of fatty infiltration of liver (such as alcohol use)
- Most common chronic liver disease in the United States and other industrialized nations; implicated in up to 90% of patients with asymptomatic, mild aminotransferase elevation not caused by alcohol, viral hepatitis, or medications

DESCRIPTION
- NAFL (1)
  - Reversible condition in which large vacuoles of triglyceride fat accumulate in hepatocytes
  - Liver biopsy: fatty deposits in cells without hepatocellular injury (no hepatocyte ballooning, no necrosis, no fibrosis)
  - ALT and AST normal or <3 to 4 ULN
  - Minimal risk of progressing to cirrhosis or liver failure
  - Synonym: steatosis
- NASH: progressive form of NAFL (1)
  - Liver biopsy: fatty deposits in cells with hepatocellular injury (ballooning, acute/chronic inflammation, ± fibrosis); may be histologically indistinguishable from alcoholic steatohepatitis
  - ALT and AST elevated, generally <3 to 4 ULN
  - 30% with NASH may progress to fibrosis over 5 years and may progress to cirrhosis, liver failure, and rarely hepatocellular cancer
- NASH cirrhosis: presence of cirrhosis with current or previous histologic evidence of steatosis or steatohepatitis

EPIDEMIOLOGY
- Most common chronic liver disease in industrialized Western countries
- Predicted to become the most frequent indication for liver transplantation by 2030 (2)
- Predominant age: 40s to 50s; can occur in children
- Predominant sex: male = female

Incidence
Estimates vary widely from 31 to 86 cases of NAFLD per 10,000 person-years to 29/100,000 person-years (1).

Prevalence
- United States estimate: 10–46%
- Present in 58–74% of obese (BMI ≥30 kg/m²); 90% of morbidly obese (BMI ≥40 kg/m²); 69–87% with type 2 DM; 50% with dyslipidemia (1)

ETIOLOGY AND PATHOPHYSIOLOGY
Primary mechanism is thought to be *insulin resistance*, leading to increased lipolysis, triglyceride synthesis, and increased hepatic uptake of fatty acids. Thus, there is international momentum to rename this condition metabolic-associated fatty liver disease (MAFLD).
- NAFL: excessive triglyceride accumulation in the liver and impaired ability to remove fatty acids
- NASH: multiple hit theory (insulin resistance, adipose tissue hormones, oxidative stress damage, genetic factors, intestinal bacteria) that causes inflammation and acts on liver parenchymal cells leading to steatohepatitis

Genetics
- Largely unknown: some familial clustering and increased heritability
- NAFL: more first-degree relatives with cirrhosis than matched controls
- NASH: 18% with affected first-degree relative (1)

RISK FACTORS
- Obesity (BMI >30 kg/m²), visceral obesity (waist circumference >102 cm for men or >88 cm for women), hypertension, high triglycerides and low high-density lipoprotein (HDL) levels, metabolic syndrome
- Type 2 diabetes mellitus (DM), cardiovascular disease, and chronic kidney disease
- Protein–calorie malnutrition; total parenteral nutrition (TPN) >6 weeks
- Severe weight loss (starvation, bariatric surgery)
- Organic solvent exposure (e.g., chlorinated hydrocarbons, toluene); vinyl chloride; hypoglycin A
- Gene for hemochromatosis/other conditions with increased iron stores
- Smoking
- Drugs: tetracycline, glucocorticoids, tamoxifen, methotrexate, amiodarone, antiretroviral agents for HIV, valproic acid, fialuridine, many chemotherapy regimens, nucleoside analogues
- History of cholecystectomy
- Increasing age associated with increased prevalence, severity, advanced fibrosis, and mortality

Pregnancy Considerations
Acute fatty liver of pregnancy: rare but serious complication in 3rd trimester—50% of cases are associated with preeclampsia

Pediatric Considerations
- Pediatric NAFLD
  - Increasing prevalence of NAFLD among children parallels rise in pediatric obesity, with prevalence of 9.6% (1)
  - Vitamin E of possible benefit
- Reye syndrome: fatty liver syndrome with encephalopathy usually following viral illness and aspirin use

GENERAL PREVENTION
- Avoid excess alcohol: ≤2 units per day (men); ≤1 unit per day (women). One unit equals 10 mL or 8 g of pure alcohol, which is around the amount of alcohol the average adult can process in an hour. 1 shot of spirits = 1 unit; 12 oz beer = ~1.7 units; glass of wine = 2 units.
- Maintain appropriate BMI.
- Prevention and optimal management of diabetes
- Avoid hepatotoxic medications.

COMMONLY ASSOCIATED CONDITIONS
Central obesity; hypertension; type 2 diabetes; insulin resistance; hyperlipidemia; preeclampsia in pregnancy; CVD and arrhythmias; hypothyroidism; hypogonadism; OSA; chronic kidney disease; growth hormone deficiency; polycystic ovary syndrome (1)

DIAGNOSIS

- Routine screening not recommended because of lack of effective drug treatment and unclear long-term benefits of screening (2)
- Consider NAFLD in patients with asymptomatic aminotransferase elevations (1)[A].
- NAFLD has no distinguishing historical/lab features to differentiate from other chronic liver disorders.
- Index of suspicion is higher with risk factors, such as metabolic syndrome or obesity
- May present as cryptogenic cirrhosis
- Noninvasive biomarkers of steatosis/fibrosis are not sufficiently reliable.
- Liver biopsy is the definitive diagnostic test but should only be considered if results will change management.

HISTORY
- Typically asymptomatic
- Possible fatigue and/or abdominal fullness
- Vague right upper quadrant pain
- History of medications, family history

PHYSICAL EXAM
Usually normal, but signs may include the following:
- Liver tenderness
- Mild to marked hepatomegaly
- Splenomegaly
- In advanced cases: cutaneous stigmata of chronic liver disease or portal hypertension (e.g., palmar erythema, spider angiomata, ascites); jaundice

DIFFERENTIAL DIAGNOSIS
- Viral hepatitis; drug- or toxin-induced hepatitis; autoimmune hepatitis
- Alcoholic liver disease
- Celiac disease
- Muscle disease, if nonhepatic cause of elevated enzymes is possible
- Hemochromatosis; Wilson disease; lipodystrophy

DIAGNOSTIC TESTS & INTERPRETATION
The diagnosis of NAFLD (2) requires:
- Demonstration of hepatic steatosis by imaging or biopsy
- No history of significant alcohol consumption
- Exclusion of other causes of hepatic steatosis
- Absence of coexisting chronic liver disease

Initial Tests (lab, imaging)
- ALT and AST may be elevated.
  - Nonalcoholic, usually AST/ALT <1
  - Nonspecific enzyme abnormalities may exist or may be normal with advanced cirrhosis (1).
  - Level of enzyme elevation does NOT correlate with degree of fibrosis (1).
- Elevated ferritin (1.5 times normal)
- Elevated alkaline phosphatase, total/direct biliburin
- Lipid abnormalities: elevated total cholesterol, elevated LDL, elevated triglycerides, decreased HDL
- If cirrhosis present: decreased serum albumin, elevated PT, thrombocytopenia
- Serum labs to exclude other causes of liver disease: celiac, α₁-antitrypsin, iron, copper, hepatitis serologies, anti-smooth muscle antibody, ANA, serum γ-globulin (1)[B]
- Ultrasound (US) is first-line imaging: fatty liver appears hyperechogenic (1)[B].

Follow-Up Tests & Special Considerations

Other modalities can help noninvasively quantify fibrosis by estimating liver stiffness, but no modality accurately distinguishes simple steatosis from steatohepatitis (1).

- Clinical decision aids: NAFLD fibrosis score, FIB-4 index, APRI score (2)
- Serum biomarkers: enhanced liver fibrosis panel, FibroTest, HepaScore
- Imaging: vibration controlled transient elastography (VCTE) or FibroScan, acoustic radiation force impulse (ARFI), magnetic resonance elastography (MRE, most reliable measurement, but expensive)

Diagnostic Procedures/Other

Liver biopsy: gold standard for diagnosis and prognosis—must have likelihood of changing management prior to biopsy (1)[B]

Test Interpretation

- NAFLD activity score (NAS): used to grade diagnosis, based on three histologic features: steatosis (0 to 3), inflammation (0 to 3), and hepatocyte ballooning (0 to 2), for score between 0 and 8. NASH is very likely with scores ≥5.
- Steatosis Activity Fibrosis: staging scale (0 to 4) based on degree of fibrosis (1)

 ## TREATMENT

Emphasis on early management of metabolic risk factors, NAFLD associated with increased cardiovascular morbidity and mortality

GENERAL MEASURES

- Weight loss for those who are overweight or obese is the only therapy that has good evidence of benefits and safety. Aim for sustained weight loss (5–10% body weight) (1).
- Diet modification: Mediterranean diet has been shown to reduce liver fat (1). Avoid or limit alcohol consumption.
- Aerobic exercise 5 times per week for a total of 150 minutes per week (1)[B]
- Tight diabetes control (1)
- Treat metabolic syndrome—hypertension, dyslipidemia, and obesity
- Vaccination for hepatitis A and B for those nonimmune
- Pneumococcal and annual influenza vaccinations
- Avoid hepatotoxic medications (1)[B].

MEDICATION

- Currently no definitively effective medication treatment to treat NAFL or NASH (1)
- Some promising agents include the following:
  – Thiazolidinediones (pioglitazone) (3)
    ○ Improves liver histology
    ○ Can be used in patients with and without type 2 DM but preferentially use only with type 2 DM
  – Vitamin E 800 IU daily (3)
    ○ Only use with biopsy-proven NASH and those without diabetes (1)[C]
    ○ Long-term safety concerns at high doses, avoid in patients at higher risk for prostate cancer or hemorrhagic stroke.

– GLP-1 receptor agonists (semaglutide, liraglutide) (3)
    ○ Histological reduction in steatosis, less progression to fibrosis, and helps with weight loss
    ○ Can be used in patients with and without type 2 DM
  – Statins (3)
    ○ Improve cardiovascular risk and decrease fatty infiltration
    ○ Benefits outweigh minimal risk of liver failure even in patients with compensated cirrhosis.
  – Sodium-glucose cotransporter-2 (SGLT-2) inhibitors (3)
    ○ Show reduction in steatosis by imaging, unclear effect on progression to fibrosis
    ○ Use in patients with type 2 DM.
- Agents that have shown +/− benefit
  – Metformin, ursodeoxycholic acid
  – Pentoxifylline, probiotics
  – Obeticholic acid and Tropifexor
  – Omega-3 fatty acids
  – Aspirin, caffeine/coffee
  – Lipogenesis inhibitors (e.g., aramchol, firsocostat)
  – Fibroblast growth factor-19 analogues (e.g., aldafermin)
  – Silymarin (milk thistle)

ISSUES FOR REFERRAL

Refer to hepatology if persistent AST/ALT elevations, advanced fibrosis (stage F3 or greater) on liver scan, or fibrosis on liver biopsy (1)[A].

SURGERY/OTHER PROCEDURES

- Bariatric surgery: may be considered in obese patients with NAFLD, NASH, or advanced fibrosis who do not achieve weight loss goals after adequate trial of lifestyle modifications.
- Liver transplant: NAFLD is second most common cause for liver transplant; however, NAFLD will recur in the transplanted liver in 80–100% of patients.

 ## ONGOING CARE

FOLLOW-UP RECOMMENDATIONS

- Annual monitoring of LFTs (1)
- Surveillance with US or CT to evaluate for disease progression every 2 to 4 years, or sooner if increasing metabolic risk factors
- Routine liver biopsy is not recommended but may be repeated 5 years after baseline biopsy if progression of fibrosis is suspected (1).
- Hepatic fibrosis staging is the strongest predictor for mortality in patients with histologically confirmed NAFLD (2).
- Screening for hepatocellular carcinoma in noncirrhotic NAFLD is yet to be determined (2).

DIET

Low in saturated and trans fat; low in simple carbohydrates; avoid excessive alcohol or abstinence preferred (protective or worsening effect of light/moderate consumption inconclusive).

PATIENT EDUCATION

Extensive counseling on sustained lifestyle changes in nutrition, exercise, and alcohol use

PROGNOSIS

Within the spectrum of NAFLD, only NASH has been shown to be progressive, potentially leading to cirrhosis, hepatocellular carcinoma, cholangiocarcinoma, and/or liver failure.

- Cirrhosis develops in up to 20% of patients. Up to 42% of patients develop hepatocellular carcinoma without showing cirrhosis.
- Transplantation is effective, but NASH often recurs after due to ongoing risk factors.

COMPLICATIONS

Progressive disease may lead to decompensated cirrhosis and portal hypertension with complications such as ascites, encephalopathy, bleeding varices, and hepatorenal or hepatopulmonary syndromes.

REFERENCES

1. Chalasani N, Younossi Z, Lavine JE, et al. The diagnosis and management of nonalcoholic fatty liver disease: practice guidance from the American Association for the Study of Liver diseases. *Hepatology*. 2018;67(1):328–357.
2. Ando Y, Jou JH. Nonalcoholic fatty liver disease and recent guideline updates. *Clin Liver Dis (Hoboken)*. 2021;17(1):23–38.
3. Rinella ME, Neuschwander-Tetri BA, Siddiqui MS, et al. AASLD practice guidance on the clinical assessment and management of nonalcoholic fatty liver disease. *Hepatology*. 2023;77(5):1797–1835.

ADDITIONAL READING

Kumar R, Priyadarshi RN, Anand U. Non-alcoholic fatty liver disease: growing burden, adverse outcomes and associations. *J Clin Transl Hepatol*. 2020;8(1):76–86.

 ## SEE ALSO

- Alcohol Use Disorder (AUD); Cirrhosis of the Liver; Diabetes Mellitus, Type 2; Metabolic Syndrome
- Algorithm: Weight Loss, Treatment

CODES

ICD10

K76.0 Fatty (change of) liver, not elsewhere classified

CLINICAL PEARLS

- NAFLD is a major cause of liver disease, and is increasing every year with increasing rates of overweight and obesity.
- Spectrum ranges from NAFL to NASH, advanced fibrosis, and cirrhosis.
- NAFLD is the most common chronic liver disease in children; there has been a parallel rise in childhood obesity and NAFLD.
- Lifestyle changes with targeted weight loss are the cornerstones of therapy for NAFLD.

N

NONFATAL DROWNING
Nergess T. Taheri, DO, MSBI

 BASICS

DESCRIPTION
Respiratory impairment resulting from submersion or immersion in liquid; a drowning event in which the process of respiratory impairment is stopped before death and the victim survives

EPIDEMIOLOGY
Incidence
- From 2011 to 2020, an average of 4,012 fatal unintentional drownings and an average of 8,061 emergency room (ER) visits due to nonfatal drowning occurred each year in the United States (1)
- Three age-related peaks: toddlers and young children (1 to 5 years old), adolescents and young adults (15 to 25 years old), and the elderly
- Nearly 80% of people who die from drowning are male (1).
- In swimming pools, black children aged 10 to 14 years drown at rates 7.6 times higher than white children, whereas in natural water, American Indian or Alaska Native children drown at rates 2.7 times higher than white children (1).

Prevalence
- Most common injury-related cause of death for children aged 1 to 4 years in the United States (2)
- Second most common injury-related cause of death for children aged 5 to 14 years in the United States after motor vehicle crashes (1)
- For every child aged <18 years who dies from drowning, seven more children are seen in the ER for nonfatal submersion injuries (1).

ALERT
Proper water supervision and safety techniques are critical in avoiding morbidity and mortality from drowning.

ETIOLOGY AND PATHOPHYSIOLOGY
Hypoxemia via aspiration and/or reflex laryngospasm causing cerebral hypoxia and multisystem organ dysfunction
- 10–20% of victims drown without aspiration, likely due to prolonged laryngospasm; bathtub and bucket drowning in children aged <1 year; swimming pool drowning in children and young adults; motor vehicle accidents (vehicle submerged in water); head trauma while swimming or diving
- Pulmonary: morbidity primarily caused by hypoxia; aspiration of 1 to 3 mL/kg of liquid causes dilution of surfactant with decreased gas transfer across alveoli, atelectasis, development of intrapulmonary right-to-left shunting; acute respiratory distress syndrome (ARDS); obstruction due to laryngospasm and bronchospasm (2)
- Cardiac: hypoxic-ischemic injury and arrhythmia (primary or secondary); renal: acute tubular necrosis from hypoxemia, shock, hemoglobinuria, myoglobinuria
- Neurologic: hypoxic-ischemic brain injury with damage especially to the hippocampus, insular cortex, and basal ganglia; cerebral edema and increased intracranial pressure
- Coagulation: hemolysis and coagulopathy

RISK FACTORS
- Inadequate physical barriers surrounding pools, alcohol ingestion, male sex, low socioeconomic status
- Use of illicit drugs, seizure disorder, inability to swim or overestimation of swimming capabilities, hyperventilation prior to underwater swimming
- Boating mishaps and trauma during water sports, particularly when not wearing a life jacket; scuba diving
- Inadequate adult supervision of children, lack of appropriate instruction on how to swim, concomitant stroke or myocardial infarction (MI), hypothermia
- Cardiac arrhythmias: familial long QT and polymorphic ventricular tachycardia (VT)

GENERAL PREVENTION
- Periodic education regarding proper supervision and drowning prevention for caretakers of young children; proper adult supervision of children, particularly around water; pool alarms, buddy system; knowledge of water safety guidelines
- Mandatory physical barriers surrounding pools; four-sided fencing; self-closing gate at least 48 inches above the ground (1)
- Avoid alcohol or recreational drugs around water; swimming instruction at an early age; cardiopulmonary resuscitation (CPR) instruction for pool owners and parents; boating safety knowledge; personal flotation device and rescue equipment (e.g., pre-server, if necessary)

Pediatric Considerations
Children should never be left alone near water. Young children can drown in very small amounts of water (bathtubs, buckets of water, and toilets).

COMMONLY ASSOCIATED CONDITIONS
- Trauma, seizure disorder, alcohol or illicit drug use
- Hypothermia, concomitant stroke or MI, cardiac arrhythmias: familial long QT and familial polymorphic VT, hyperventilation
- Pneumonia, hypotension

DIAGNOSIS

HISTORY
The Revised Utstein-style approach provides a standardized template for evaluating drowning incidents and provides guidance for the history, physical exam, and appropriate management by categorizing information into core (considered important and feasible to be reported in most systems worldwide) and supplemental data:
- Victim information core data: (i) victim identifier—unique number or code; (ii) sex; (iii) age; (iv) incident date and time of day; (v) precipitating event; (vi) Was the face submerged at any time before or at the time of rescue? (vii) preexisting illness; supplemental: (viii) race/ethnicity
- Scene information core data: (i) water temperature; (ii) Who witnessed the drowning? (iii) Was bystander (non-EMS) CPR performed? (iv) Was bystander ventilation given? (v) Did a trained first responder perform CPR or ventilation only? (vi) vital status at first trained responder assessment: Was the victim responsive? Breathing normally? Pulse palpable? (vii) initial cardiac rhythm; supplementary data: (viii) vital signs at first EMS assessment; (ix) pulmonary status at first EMS assessment; (x) type of water/liquid; (xi) body of water

- Time points and intervals from EMS core data: (i) time face was first seen to be underwater; (ii) time victim was removed from water; (iii) duration underwater (submersion duration); (iv) time of first trained responder treatment; (v) time trained responder started CPR on scene; (vi) time return of spontaneous circulation achieved; (vii) time first conscious/awake; (viii) interval from face first submerged to first treatment/CPR

PHYSICAL EXAM
- Airway status and degree of respiratory distress
- Pulse: absent, weak, or normal; vital signs, including pulse oximetry
- Pulmonary: rales, wheezing; cardiac: rate, rhythm; neurologic examination

DIFFERENTIAL DIAGNOSIS
Syncopal event, head trauma, arrhythmia, seizure, MI, stroke, alcohol or other substance overdose, nonaccidental trauma

DIAGNOSTIC TESTS & INTERPRETATION
Initial Tests (lab, imaging)
- Primary focus starts with the respiratory system, get pulse oximetry and arterial blood gas (ABG). Further testing will be unnecessary if GCS and pulse oximetry are normal (and remain so for 6 to 8 hours).
- Otherwise consider:
  - CBC with differential. ABG: hypoxia, hypercarbia, acidosis
  - Electrolytes: hypokalemia, hyponatremia, hypernatremia; blood glucose: increased levels may impair neurologic recovery after ischemic brain injury; BUN, creatinine: acute tubular necrosis
  - ECG, cardiac monitoring, and serial troponin: MI; creatine kinase (CK) and urine myoglobin: rhabdomyolysis; coagulation studies: coagulopathy
  - Toxicology screen; blood alcohol level
  - Chest x-ray (CXR) unnecessary if:
    ○ Normal initial GCS and pulse oximetry; no evidence of respiratory distress; no change after 4 to 6 hours of observation
  - CXR may show evidence of aspiration, atelectasis, pneumothorax, or ARDS in more severe cases.
  - Head CT and/or C-spine imaging for trauma

Follow-Up Tests & Special Considerations
- Observe patients with an initial GCS of 15 and pulse oximetry >95% for 4 to 6 hours in the emergency department (ED). Four factors predicted safe discharge: normal mentation, normal respiratory rate, absence of dyspnea, and hypotension (3).
- CXR findings may be minimal or absent early on.

Diagnostic Procedures/Other
Continuous cardiac monitoring and pulse oximetry; continuous core temperature monitoring if hypothermic; 12-lead ECG; central venous pressure (CVP) monitoring for critically ill with hypotension refractory to IV fluids; electroencephalogram (EEG) if seizure suspected

TREATMENT

Early resuscitation and reversal of hypoxemia/acidosis are key.

GENERAL MEASURES
- Prehospital
  - Never approach a struggling victim alone. Initiate basic life support (BLS) and advanced cardiovascular life support (ACLS) evaluation. Rescue breathing may be helpful if the victim is in the water and cannot be removed; chest compressions not as effective while in the water and may harm the rescuer and the victim
  - Remove the victim from the water and begin effective resuscitation as quickly as possible. Immediate CPR (airway, breathing, and circulation [ABC] sequence)
  - Start CPR if pulse is not definitely felt within 10 seconds, even in the hypothermic victim whose heart rate may be severely bradycardic. Routine cervical collar use and spinal precautions are not needed unless trauma is suspected; supplemental oxygen and early intubation with mechanical ventilation, if needed
  - Rapid crystalloid infusion if there is hypotension that is not corrected by oxygenation
  - Ventricular fibrillation is rare in drowning, but if an AED is available, use during the initial resuscitation phase; AED use is not contraindicated in a wet environment (3). If patient is breathing on his or her own and does not need spinal precautions, consider placing in the right lateral decubitus position to prevent aspiration of vomit or gastric contents. Evacuate patients with abnormal lung sounds, severe cough, frothy sputum, foamy material in the airway, depressed mentation, or hypotension to advanced medical care (3).
  - An asymptomatic patient with normal lung exam can be considered for release from the scene if another person can be with them for the next 4 to 6 hours for symptom monitoring (3).
- ED
  - Oxygen, as needed, to maintain saturation between 92% and 96%
  - Continuous positive airway pressure (CPAP), bilevel positive airway pressure (BiPAP), or intubation if supplemental oxygen alone is inadequate
  - If intubation is indicated, employ lung-protective ventilator settings (lower end-inspiratory airway pressures, lower tidal volumes of 6 mL/kg, higher positive end-expiratory pressures of 6 to 12 cm H_2O) to avoid barotrauma.
  - Indications for intubation
    ○ Neurologic deterioration; inability to protect the airway; inability to maintain oxygen saturation >90% or PaO_2 >60 mm Hg on high-flow supplemental oxygen; $PaCO_2$ >50 mm Hg
  - Remove wet clothing and initiate rewarming
  - Obtain core temperature to rule out hypothermia.
  - If hypothermic, rewarm with minimally invasive core techniques such as warm IV fluids, warm/humidified oxygen, and external blanketing.
  - Active core rewarming only for refractory cases

MEDICATION
First Line
- High-flow oxygen, as needed
- For bronchospasm: aerosolized bronchodilator (2)[C]: albuterol (Proventil, Ventolin), 3 mL of 0.083% solution or 0.5 mL of 0.5% solution diluted in 3 mL of saline
- Vasopressors, as needed, for hypotension refractory to IV fluid resuscitation
- Prophylactic antibiotics are not recommended.

Second Line
For pneumonia: antibiotics based on sputum or endotracheal lavage culture

ADMISSION, INPATIENT, AND NURSING CONSIDERATIONS
- Admit all symptomatic patients or patients with abnormal vital signs, mental status, oxygenation, CXR, or laboratory analysis.
- Monitor vital signs and reassess neurologic status, continuous cardiac, and pulse oximetry monitoring.
- After initial resuscitation, induce hypothermia with core temperature maintained between 32°C and 34°C for 24 hours; may be neuroprotective for patients that remain comatose or have neurologic deterioration
- Patients can be discharged from the ED after 4 to 6 hours if they have a normal mental status and respiratory function with no further deterioration (3).

 ONGOING CARE

FOLLOW-UP RECOMMENDATIONS
Appropriate follow-up with primary care provider, orthopedic, neurologic, cardiac, pulmonary, and additional specialists as indicated

Patient Monitoring
- ABG monitoring, as indicated
- A pulmonary artery catheter may be needed for hemodynamic monitoring in unstable patients (2)[C].
- Intracranial pressure monitoring in selected patients (2)[C]
- Serum electrolyte determinations

DIET
NPO until mental status normalizes

PATIENT EDUCATION
Reemphasize preventive measures on discharge from hospital and educate parents regarding supervision and preventive practices.

PROGNOSIS
- 75% of drowning victims survive; 6% will have residual neurologic deficits.
- Patients with an initial GCS ≥13 and an oxygen saturation ≥95% have a low risk of complications and an excellent chance for a full recovery.
- Patients who are comatose or receiving CPR at the time of presentation and those who have dilated and fixed pupils and no spontaneous respiratory activity have a poor prognosis.
- Neurogenic pulmonary edema may occur within 48 hours of initial presentation.

COMPLICATIONS
- Early
  - Bronchospasm, vomiting, aspiration
  - Hypoglycemia, hypothermia, seizures
  - Hypovolemia, electrolyte abnormalities
  - Arrhythmia from hypoxia or hypothermia (rarely from electrolyte imbalance)
  - Hypotension
- Late
  - ARDS, pneumonia, lung abscess, empyema
  - Anoxic encephalopathy, barotrauma, seizure
  - Renal failure, coagulopathy, sepsis

REFERENCES
1. Girasek DC, Hargarten S. Prevention of and emergency response to drowning. *N Engl J Med.* 2022;387(14):1303–1308.
2. Mott TF, Latimer KM. Prevention and treatment of drowning. *Am Fam Physician.* 2016;93(7):576–582.
3. Schmidt AC, Sempsrott JR, Hawkins SC, et al. Wilderness Medical Society clinical practice guidelines for the treatment and prevention of drowning: 2019 update. *Wilderness Environ Med.* 2019;30(4S):S70–S86.

ADDITIONAL READING
Peri F, De Nardi L, Canuto A, et al. Drowning in children and predictive parameters: a 15-year multicenter retrospective analysis. *Pediatr Emerg Care.* 2023;39(7):516–523.

CODES

ICD10
- T75.1XXA Unsp effects of drowning and nonfatal submersion, init
- T75.1XXD Unsp effects of drowning and nonfatal submersion, subs
- T75.1XXS Unsp effects of drowning and nonfatal submersion, sequel

CLINICAL PEARLS
- The most important treatment for near-drowning victims is prompt reversal of hypoxia.
- Water safety education (physical and behavioral modifications) helps prevent drowning.
- Encourage pool owners and parents with young children to become CPR certified.
- Patients remain at risk for ARDS for hours after submersion. All resuscitated patients require careful monitoring.
- Use lung-protective ventilator settings for intubated patients to prevent barotrauma.
- Patients with an initial GCS ≥13 and an oxygen saturation ≥95% have a low risk of complications and an excellent chance for a full recovery.

N

OBESITY
Justin Chu, MD • Jordan Patrick Hilgefort, MD • David Neuberger, MD

 BASICS

DESCRIPTION
- A complex, multifactorial disease characterized by excess adipose tissue to the extent that health may be impaired, typically quantified in adults by body mass index (BMI) (kg/m^2), $\geq$30 kg/m^2
- Overweight: BMI 25 to 29.9 kg/m^2
- Obesity is categorized into three classes:
  - Class 1 obesity is BMI 30 to 34.9 kg/m^2.
  - Class 2 obesity is BMI 35 to 39.9 kg/m^2.
  - Class 3 obesity (also called severe obesity) is BMI $\geq$40 kg/m^2.
- Obesity is preventable and associated with negative health outcomes. Abdominal obesity increases the risk of morbidity and mortality.
- Obesity is sometimes associated with various eating disorders.

Geriatric Considerations
Aging is associated with changes in body composition including sarcopenia, decreased bone mineral density, and accumulation of visceral fat.

EPIDEMIOLOGY
Predominant age: Incidence rises in the early 20s and peaks at middle-aged adults 40 to 59 years old.

Prevalence
42% of U.S. adults and 20% of children and adolescents (2 to 19 years old) meet BMI criteria for obesity.

Pediatric Considerations
- The United States Preventive Services Task Force (USPSTF) recommends screening for obesity in children and adolescents $\geq$6 years old and referring those with positive screens to comprehensive, intensive behavioral interventions (grade B recommendation).
- Pediatric classifications by age- and sex-specific WHO or CDC growth curves:
  - Overweight: BMI $\geq$85th to <95th percentile
  - Obesity (Class I): BMI $\geq$95th to 119th percentile
  - Severe Obesity:
    - Class II: BMI $\geq$120th to 139th percentile of the 95th percentile
    - Class III: BMI $\geq$140th percentile of the 95th percentile
- Obesity affects 1 in 6 children before they enter school.
- Obesity during adolescence is strongly associated with obesity in adulthood, largely in part to eating habits, lifestyle choices, and metabolic set points.
- Obesity in children is associated with mental health and psychological issues, low self-esteem, and impaired quality of life.

ETIOLOGY AND PATHOPHYSIOLOGY
- Multifactorial process where genetic, environmental, behavioral, and psychosocial issues lead to an imbalance between energy intake and expenditure.
- Adipocytes (fat cells) produce peptides called adiponectin and leptin. Adiponectin improves insulin sensitivity and the absence of leptin has been associated with severe obesity.
- After obesity has developed, an individual's neuronal signaling is altered to decrease satiety, and adipocyte hypertrophy leads to both local and systemic inflammation.

Genetics
- Genetic syndromes such as Prader-Willi and Bardet-Biedl are found in a minority of people with obesity.
- Multiple genes are implicated in obesity and certain genotypes may account for differences in weight loss response following dietary changes.

RISK FACTORS
- Parental obesity
- Sedentary lifestyle and lack of regular physical activity
- Poor nutrition, especially consumption of calorie-dense food, and limited access to fresh produce/foods
- Stress and mental illness

GENERAL PREVENTION
- Encourage regular physical activity with a goal of at least 150 minutes of moderate-intensity activity per week (e.g., 30 minutes of exercise, 5 days/week), and a well-balanced diet with appropriate portion sizes.
- Avoid calorie-dense and nutrient-poor foods such as sugar-sweetened beverages and processed foods.
- Early preventive counseling, especially in children and young adults

COMMONLY ASSOCIATED CONDITIONS
- Type 2 diabetes, HTN, hyperlipidemia
- Coronary artery disease, congestive heart failure
- Obstructive sleep apnea
- Osteoarthritis
- Nonalcoholic fatty liver disease
- Mood disorders: anxiety, depression
- Polycystic ovarian syndrome

 DIAGNOSIS

HISTORY
- Diet and exercise habits
- Reported readiness to change lifestyle, previous attempts at weight loss
- Life stressors, social support, and resources; screen for eating disorder and eating-disordered behaviors.

PHYSICAL EXAM
- Physical Activity Vital Sign: Assess if patient achieves a minimum goal of 150 minutes of moderate-intensity physical activity per week.
- Waist circumference:
  - May be more important than BMI to assess obesity-associated health risks, especially in the elderly (sarcopenia)
  - Recommend measuring in patients with BMI 25 to 35 kg/m^2.
  - Measure at the level of the umbilicus; elevated:
    - Male: >40 inches (102 cm)
    - Female: >35 inches (88 cm)
- Common abnormal findings: large neck habitus, acanthosis nigricans, striae

DIFFERENTIAL DIAGNOSIS
- Cushing syndrome
- Hypothyroidism
- Undiagnosed concomitant primary psychiatric disorder

DIAGNOSTIC TESTS & INTERPRETATION
- Screen for underlying physiologic causes as well as associated comorbid conditions
- Fasting blood glucose, hemoglobin A1C, lipid panel
- Thyroid function tests
- LFTs (nonalcoholic fatty liver disease)

Follow-Up Tests & Special Considerations
Fatigue may be related to underlying obstructive sleep apnea and may warrant further investigation with sleep study.

TREATMENT
GENERAL MEASURES
- Assess:
  - Motivation to lose weight and patient-specific goals of therapy, interest in medication and/or surgery
  - Nutritional intake and physical activity habits
- Goal: Achieve and sustain loss of at least $\geq$5% of body weight.
  - Weight loss is curvilinear with rapid weight loss at first and then slows until plateau.
- USPSTF recommendation: "Encourage clinicians to promote behavioral interventions as the primary focus of the effective interventions for weight loss in adults."
- Treat obesity-related comorbidities.

MEDICATION
- Guidelines suggest at least 3 to 6 months of nonpharmacologic treatment with comprehensive lifestyle intervention alone prior to starting medications.
- Insufficient evidence for children <12 years old
- Consider pharmacotherapy in patients with a history of failure to achieve clinically meaningful weight loss ($\geq$5% total body weight) and to sustain lost weight in patients who meet the following criteria:
  - BMI $\geq$30 kg/m^2
  - BMI $\geq$27 kg/m^2 + comorbidities (e.g., CAD, diabetes, sleep apnea, HTN, hyperlipidemia)
- Meta-analyses of randomized trials comparing pharmacologic therapy with placebo demonstrated that all active drug interventions are effective at reducing weight compared with placebo (1).
- USPSTF found that pharmacotherapy combined with behavioral interventions was associated with greater weight loss and maintenance over 12 to 18 months than behavioral treatment alone. Long-term use is necessary for maintenance in most people.

First Line
- There are 9 FDA-approved medications for weight loss (5 for long-term use and 4 for short-term). A combination of medications from different classes may be needed for greater weight loss.
- The most common side effects are GI related (nausea, vomiting, diarrhea, abdominal pain), unless otherwise specified.

- Long-term treatment:
  – Liraglutide (Saxenda, Victoza):
    ○ GLP-1 agonist and preferred drug for patients with diabetes and cardiovascular disease; can be prescribed for adolescents ≥12 years old
    ○ Dose: 0.6 mg SC daily for 1 week and then increase at weekly intervals to target dose of 3 mg daily
  – Semaglutide (Ozempic, Rybelsus, Wegovy):
    ○ GLP-1 agonist FDA approved for obesity, in addition to diabetes; likely the most effective medication for weight loss
    ○ Dose: 0.25 mg SC once weekly ×4 weeks and then increase dose at 4-week intervals to a target dose of 2.4 mg once weekly
  – Phentermine/topiramate (Qysmia)—likely most effective oral medication available:
    ○ Phentermine reduces appetite through increasing norepinephrine in the hypothalamus, and topiramate reduces appetite through its effect on GABA receptors. Schedule IV medication.
    ○ Dose: phentermine 3.75 mg/topiramate 23 mg once daily for 14 days and then titrate up to 15 mg/92 mg once daily
    ○ Adverse effects: misuse potential, tachycardia, mood disorders, dry mouth; and topiramate is associated with fetal toxic effects (oral clefts)
  – Orlistat (Xenical):
    ○ Inhibitor of pancreatic lipase that reduces intestinal absorption of fat and increases excretion; FDA approved for ≥12 years old
    ○ Dose: 120 mg 3 times daily with fat-containing meals
    ○ Adverse effects: GI side effects (cramps, flatus, fecal incontinence, oily spotting) often not tolerated; should be taken with vitamin supplements because of slight decrease in fat-soluble vitamins (A, D, E, and K)
  – Naltrexone/bupropion (Contrave):
    ○ Naltrexone is an opioid antagonist that blocks effects of β-endorphins to reduce food intake. Bupropion reduces food intake by acting on adrenergic and dopaminergic receptors in the hypothalamus.
    ○ Dose: naltrexone 8 mg/bupropion 90 mg once daily for the first week and up titrate to a goal of 16 mg/180 mg twice daily by week 4
    ○ Adverse effects: increased blood pressure, dry mouth, headache, insomnia
  – Superabsorbent hydrogel (Plenity)—oral hydrogel of cellulose and citric acid creates feeling of fullness; taken twice daily, 30 minutes before lunch and dinner with at least 16 oz of water; relatively inexpensive; listed as an FDA approved medical device and not a medication

Second Line
Short-term use medications (<12 weeks) are older, sympathomimetic drugs that reduce food intake by causing early satiety. Adverse effects include increase in heart rate, blood pressure, insomnia, and dry mouth.
- Phentermine: (Schedule IV medication)
  – Dose: 15.0 to 37.5 mg daily or divided twice daily
- Diethylpropion: (Schedule IV medication)
  – Dose: 25 mg 3 to 4 times daily before meals
- Benzphetamine: (Schedule III medication)
  – Dose: Start at 25 mg once daily and may titrate up to max dose of 50 mg 3 times daily
- Phendimetrazine: (Schedule III medication)
  – Dose: 17.5 to 35.0 mg 2 or 3 times daily taken 1 hour before meals

ADDITIONAL THERAPIES
- Physical activity
  – Results in additional 11.5 kg weight loss over 1 year in addition to dietary intervention alone
  – Aerobic versus resistance or high intensity versus low intensity does not seem to affect overall weight loss.
  – Dose-response relationship between duration of physical activity and weight loss, although still some inter-individual variability
  – Should be individualized to patient's goals, physical capacity, exercise history, motivation, and overall health status
- Comprehensive behavioral therapy (CBT)
  – Components: (i) prescription of a moderately reduced-calorie diet, (ii) program of increased physical activity, and (iii) behavioral strategies to facilitate adherence to diet and activity recommendations
  – Most effective in-person with high intensity (≥14 sessions in 6 months) by a trained interventionist

SURGERY/OTHER PROCEDURES
- A referral for bariatric surgery is considered when other treatments have failed, BMI ≥35 kg/m^2 + comorbidities, or BMI ≥40 kg/m^2
- Associated with significant improvement in diabetes, sleep apnea, quality of life, depression, pain, and physical function
- Surgical procedures include biliopancreatic diversion, Roux-en-Y gastric bypass, sleeve gastrectomy, laparoscopic adjustable gastric banding, vagal blocking therapy, and gastric aspiration (AspireAssist).

 ONGOING CARE

FOLLOW-UP RECOMMENDATIONS
- Continue to discuss weight and lifestyle modifications, and address both current and new goals. Long-term treatment is needed to maintain weight loss.
- A new treatment plan should be implemented if no clinical meaningful weight loss after 3 to 4 months.

DIET
- Long-term studies suggest net calorie reduction (~500 kcal/day) with a diet that a patient can adhere to is the best; goal for women: 1,200 to 1,500 kcal/day, men: 1,500 to 1,800 kcal/day; a reduction of 500 kcal/day can result in ~1 lb (0.45 kg) weight loss per week.
- Very low calorie diet (200 to 800 kcal/day) produced significantly greater short-term weight loss but had similar long-term weight loss compared to low-calorie diets; requires medical supervision
- Mediterranean: primarily plant-based foods, olive oil, nuts, legumes, whole grain, fruits, and vegetables; fish and poultry multiple times per week; meta-analysis showed decrease in bodyweight, BMI, hemoglobin A1c, fasting glucose, and cardiovascular disease risk.
- Balanced-nutrient, moderate calorie: usually 1,200 to 1,800 kcal/day; for example, DASH diet: based on MyPyramid food guide with emphasis on low saturated fat and ample fruits, vegetables, and fiber

PATIENT EDUCATION
- American Medical Society for Sports Medicine: https://www.sportsmedtoday.com/exercise-prescription-va-156.htm
- Build a healthy eating routine: https://health.gov/sites/default/files/2021-08/DGA-FactSheet-2021-03-26-compressed.pdf

PROGNOSIS
- Patients who are obese compared to those with a normal weight are at an increased risk for many serious health conditions.
- Patient motivation is associated with successful weight loss.

COMPLICATIONS
Cardiovascular disease, osteoarthritis, slipped capital femoral epiphysis (SCFE) in children, higher death rates from cancer: colon, breast, prostate, endometrial, gallbladder, liver, kidney

REFERENCE
1. Khera R, Murad MH, Chandar AK, et al. Association of pharmacological treatments for obesity with weight loss and adverse events: a systematic review and meta-analysis. *JAMA*. 2016;315(22):2424–2434.

ADDITIONAL READING
- Hampl SE, Hassink SG, Skinner AC, et al. Clinical practice guideline for the evaluation and treatment of children and adolescents with obesity. *Pediatrics*. 2023;151(2):e2022060640.
- U.S. Department of Agriculture, U.S. Department of Health and Human Services. *Dietary Guidelines for Americans, 2020–2025*. 9th Edition. Washington, DC: U.S. Department of Agriculture; 2020. https://www.dietaryguidelines.gov/sites/default/files/2021-03/Dietary_Guidelines_for_Americans-2020-2025.pdf. Accessed October 4, 2023.

 SEE ALSO

Algorithm: Weight Loss, Treatment

CODES

ICD10
- E66.9 Obesity, unspecified
- E66.3 Overweight
- R63.5 Abnormal weight gain

CLINICAL PEARLS
- A majority of American adults are overweight or obese, and the percentage is increasing.
- Modification in dietary and physical activity patterns remains the cornerstone of therapy. Consider bariatric surgery in patients with a BMI >40 kg/m^2 who have failed conservative treatment, particularly if there are associated risk factors.
- Medication may be indicated when nonpharmacologic treatment for 3 to 6 months has been ineffective, and the patient has a BMI >30 kg/m^2 or a BMI >27 kg/m^2 with associated risk factors.

OBSESSIVE-COMPULSIVE DISORDER (OCD)

Matthew J. Filippo, DO • Chelsea Karson, MD

BASICS

DESCRIPTION
- A behavioral disorder characterized by pathologic obsessions (recurrent intrusive thoughts, ideas, or images) and/or compulsions (repetitive, ritualistic behaviors or mental acts) causing significant distress
- Not to be confused with obsessive-compulsive (anankastic) personality disorder

EPIDEMIOLOGY
Incidence
- Three subtypes: child/adolescent-onset (age <18 years), adult-onset (ages 18 to 39 years) and late-onset (age ≥40 years).
- Child/adolescent-onset in 50% of cases (usually by age 18 years) (1)
- ~2% lifetime prevalence; slight female predominance when including postpartum OCD

Pediatric Considerations
Consider pediatric autoimmune neuropsychiatric disorders associated with streptococcal (PANDAS) in acute presentation of OCD and tics in children (2).

Geriatric Considerations
Consider neurologic or neurodegenerative disorders in new-onset OCD.

ETIOLOGY AND PATHOPHYSIOLOGY
- Dysregulation of serotonergic, catecholaminergic and glutamatergic pathways
- Dysfunction of cortico-striatal-thalamo-cortical (CSTC) circuit, involving the orbitofrontal cortex (OFC) and anterior cingulate cortex (ACC)
- Brain injury (physical trauma, stroke, etc.)

Genetics
- Prevalence rates of 7–15% in first-degree relatives of children/adolescents with OCD
- ~45–65% of the variance of OCD is explained by genetics

RISK FACTORS
- Family history of OCD
- Advanced paternal and maternal age
- Coexisting psychiatric disorders, most commonly anxiety disorders and schizophrenia
- Low serotonin levels (Antipsychotics with greater anti-serotoninergic mechanism, such as clozapine and olanzapine, have been associated with onset of OCD.)
- Brain insult (i.e., encephalitis, pediatric streptococcal infection, or head injury)
- History of childhood traumatic events, including social isolation and physical abuse

GENERAL PREVENTION
Early diagnosis and treatment can decrease patient's distress and impairment.

COMMONLY ASSOCIATED CONDITIONS
- Major depressive disorder
- Anxiety disorders including panic disorder/phobia/social phobia/generalized anxiety disorder
- Tourette syndrome/tic syndromes
- Substance abuse/eating disorder/body dysmorphic disorder
- Other obsessive-compulsive spectrum disorders including body-focused repetitive behaviors (trichotillomania, excoriation disorder), body dysmorphia, and hoarding disorder

DIAGNOSIS

HISTORY
- Obsessions, compulsions, or both, which cause marked distress, are time-consuming (>1 hr/day), and cause significant occupational/social impairment.
- Two criteria support the diagnosis of obsessions:
  - Presence of recurrent, persistent, intrusive and inappropriate thoughts, causing significant anxiety and distress
  - The individual makes attempts to suppress or neutralize such thoughts with some other thought or activity (i.e., by performing a compulsion).
  - The context of obsessions tends to change over time; for example, religious obsessions are common in adolescence while sexual obsessions are more common in adulthood.
- Two criteria support the diagnosis of compulsions:
  - Repetitive, rigid behaviors (e.g., handwashing) or mental acts (e.g., counting silently) performed in response to an obsession
  - Although aimed at reducing stress, the response is either not realistically connected with the obsession or is excessive.
  - In children, check for precedent streptococcal infection.
- The average time to treatment is 11 years. Individuals with OCD may have significant embarrassment over the intrusive thoughts and be reluctant to admit them. It is important to build rapport and maintain a safe space with open dialogue.

PHYSICAL EXAM
The following may be observed in affected individuals. OCD is highly comorbid with body focused repetitive behaviors including trichotillomania and excoriation disorder. These may be thought of as part of an obsessive-compulsive spectrum.
- Chapped hands caused by excessive handwashing
- Scars and/or sores from skin picking and/or biting
- Patchy hair loss caused by compulsive pulling/picking/twisting of hair
- Weight loss from food restriction due to contamination fears

DIFFERENTIAL DIAGNOSIS
- Impulse-control disorders, involving compulsive gambling, sex, or substance use
- Tic disorder and stereotypic movement disorder (tics are often preceded by premonitory sensations and not aimed at neutralizing the obsession)
- Generalized anxiety disorder, phobic disorders, separation anxiety (excessive worry/anxious rumination but without compulsion)

DIAGNOSTIC TESTS & INTERPRETATION
With obsession and/or compulsions, DSM-5 diagnostic criteria are used to confirm a diagnosis of OCD.
- Obsessions are defined as persistent "unwanted" thoughts that cause significant anxiety for the individual. Often attempts are made to ignore such thoughts or to counteract intrusive thoughts by doing some other action, which are referred to as "compulsions."
- Compulsions are further defined as unusual behaviors such as repetitive pacing or handwashing or thought processes such as praying or silently counting. These behaviors are done in an attempt to reduce the anxiety and distress caused by the abnormal obsessive thoughts.
- Many individuals understand that their OCD beliefs are unlikely to be true and have good insight into their thought processes, whereas others may believe that their OCD beliefs are real.
- Some with OCD behaviors are accompanied by a tic disorder.

Initial Tests (lab, imaging)
No testing is typically necessary. This is a clinical diagnosis based on the history with a structured interview process.

Diagnostic Procedures/Other
- Free-form interviews are the most common method for determining an OCD diagnosis.
- Yale-Brown Obsessive-Compulsive Scale (Y-BOCS) to assess severity of OCD and monitor progress

Test Interpretation
- Common obsessive themes
  - Harm (i.e., being responsible for an accident)
  - Doubt (i.e., whether doors/windows are locked or the iron is turned off)
  - Blasphemous thoughts (i.e., in a devoutly religious person)
  - Sexual obsessions (i.e., unwanted, forbidden sexual thoughts)
  - Contamination, dirt, or disease
  - Symmetry/orderliness
- Common rituals or compulsions
  - Handwashing, cleaning
  - Checking, counting, ordering, arranging
  - Hoarding
  - Repeating
- Neither obsessions nor compulsions are related to another mental disorder (i.e., thoughts of food and presence of eating disorder).
- 80–90% of patients with OCD have obsessions and compulsions.
- 10–19% of patients with OCD are pure obsessional.

TREATMENT

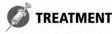

GENERAL MEASURES
- Exposure with response (ritual) prevention (ERP), a type of cognitive-behavioral therapy (CBT) composed of typically graded exposures with response prevention and cognitive therapy is recommended as first-line treatment.
- Combined use of medications and CBT is most effective.
- Electroconvulsive therapy (ECT) and deep transcranial magnetic stimulation (TMS) for severe illness.

MEDICATION

First Line

- Adequate trial of antidepressants for at least 10 to 12 weeks
- Doses may exceed typical doses for depression.
- Varying degrees of efficacy between agents; no one SSRI is superior to the other.
- SSRIs are recommended first-line agents.
  - Fluoxetine (Prozac)
    - Adults: 20 mg/day; increase by 10 to 20 mg every 4 to 6 weeks until response (20 to 80 mg/day)
    - Children (7 to 17 years of age): 10 mg/day; increase gradually every 4 to 6 weeks until response (20 to 60 mg/day).
  - Sertraline (Zoloft)
    - Adults: 50 mg/day; increase by 50 mg every 4 to 7 days until response; range: 50 to 200 mg/day; may divide if >100 mg/day
    - Children (6 to 17 years of age): 25 mg/day; increase by 25 mg every 7 days until response (50 to 200 mg/day).
  - Fluvoxamine (Luvox)
    - Adults: 50 mg QHS initially; may increase by 50 mg/day q4–7 days up to 100 to 300 mg/day
    - Doses >100 mg/day should be divided q12h.
- Precautions: Watch for suicidal behavior/worsening depression during first few months of therapy/after dosage changes with antidepressants, particularly in children, adolescents, and young adults.

Pregnancy Considerations

All SSRIs are pregnancy Category C, except paroxetine, which is Category D.

Second Line

- Try switching to another SSRI:
  - 40–70% of patients show an adequate response to a trial of SSRI, with a remission rate of 10–40%.
  - Citalopram/escitalopram do not have FDA approvals for OCD but are effective. Given dose-related QTc concerns, these are best reserved as second-line options.
  - Paroxetine is FDA approved for OCD. Given a higher side effect burden including weight gain, sedation, sexual side effects, and rebound discontinuation syndrome from missed doses, this is best reserved as a second-line option.
- If no response, switch to the tricyclic antidepressant (TCA), clomipramine (Anafranil).
  - Adults: 25 mg/day; increase gradually over 2 weeks to 100 mg/day and then to 250 mg/day (max dose) over next several weeks, as tolerated
  - Children (10 to 17 years of age): 25 mg/day; titrate as needed and tolerated up to 3 mg/kg/day or 200 mg/day (whichever is less).

- Absolute clomipramine contraindications
  - Within 6 months of a myocardial infarction (MI)
  - Hypersensitivity to clomipramine or other TCA
  - Concomitant use within 14 days of a MAOI
  - 3rd-degree atrioventricular (AV) block
- Relative clomipramine contraindications
  - Narrow-angle glaucoma
  - Prostatic hypertrophy
  - 1st- or 2nd-degree AV block, bundle branch block, and congestive heart failure
  - Pregnancy Category C
- Precautions
  - Pretreatment ECG for patients >40 years of age; potential arrhythmia
  - Watch for suicidal behavior/worsening depression during first few months of therapy or after dosage changes with antidepressants, particularly in children, adolescents, and young adults.
  - May cause drowsiness and dizziness when therapy is initiated

ISSUES FOR REFERRAL

- Referral for ERP (in vivo exposure and prevention of compulsions)
- Psychiatric evaluation if significantly interfering with patient's functioning

ADDITIONAL THERAPIES

- Antipsychotic agents alone are not effective in treating OCD. They can augment serotonergic agent(s) for treatment-resistant OCD; clozapine is known to worsen OCD symptoms.
  - Risperidone (Risperdal): initial dose: 0.5 mg/day; target dose: 0.5 to 2 mg/day for at least 8 weeks
  - Aripiprazole (Abilify): initial dose: 5 mg/day; target dose: 10 mg/day for at least 8 weeks
    - If no response, consider switching to novel glutamatergic agents such as N-acetylcysteine or memantine.
    - Serotonin-norepinephrine reuptake inhibitor (SNRI) including venlafaxine and atypical antidepressants such as mirtazapine show efficacy as well.
- Deep transcranial magnetic stimulation (dTMS) is FDA approved for OCD by directly targeting deep neuronal pathways.

SURGERY/OTHER PROCEDURES

For severe treatment resistant cases, consider neurosurgical procedure(s) including anterior cingulotomy or capsulotomy. These can be done via neurosurgery or via stereotactic radiotherapy (SRT).

ONGOING CARE

FOLLOW-UP RECOMMENDATIONS

- Y-BCOS survey to track progress
- Continue medication 1 to 2 years at full dose, the taper of 12.5–25% q1–2 mo.

Patient Monitoring

Monitor for decrease in obsessions and time spent performing compulsions.

PATIENT EDUCATION

- International OCD Foundation: https://iocdf.org/
- Obsessive Compulsive Anonymous: http://obsessivecompulsiveanonymous.org

PROGNOSIS

- Chronic waxing and waning course in most patients
- 50% have suicidal thoughts.
- Early onset is a poor predictor.
- Pharmacotherapy is recommended for 1 to 2 years after remission is achieved.
- Discontinuation of medication is associated with high relapse rate.

COMPLICATIONS

- Depression, anxiety, and panic attacks
- Avoidant behavior (Children may drop out of school; adults may become homebound.)

REFERENCES

1. Goodman WK, Grice DE, Lapidus KA, et al. Obsessive-compulsive disorder. *Psychiatr Clin North Am.* 2014;37(3):257–267.
2. American Psychiatric Association. *Practice Guideline for the Treatment of Patients with Obsessive-Compulsive Disorder.* Arlington, VA: American Psychiatric Association; 2007.

CODES

ICD10

- F42 Obsessive-compulsive disorder
- F42.2 Mixed obsessional thoughts and acts
- F42.3 Hoarding disorder

CLINICAL PEARLS

- ERP, a type of CBT composed of graded exposures with response prevention and cognitive therapy is recommended as first-line treatment.
- ERP plus an SSRI is the treatment choice for more severe OCD.
- The majority of patients with OCD respond to treatment with an SSRI and ERP.
- Improvement in symptoms is often partial, ranging from 25% to 60%.

OCULAR CHEMICAL BURNS

Jonathan Tsui, MD • Vincent Huang, MD • Clare W. Teng, MD

BASICS

DESCRIPTION

- Chemical exposure to the eye can result in rapid, devastating, and permanent damage and is one of the true emergencies in ophthalmology.
  - Alkali burns: more severe; alkaline compounds are lipophilic and penetrate rapidly into eye tissue; saponification of cell membranes leads to necrosis and may cause injury to lids, conjunctiva, cornea, sclera, iris, and lens.
  - Acid burns: less severe; associated anions from acidic compounds cause protein denaturation, creating a barrier to further acid penetration (hydrofluoric acid is an exception to this rule; see below). Injury is often limited to lids, conjunctiva, and cornea.
- System(s) affected: nervous, skin/exocrine
- Synonym(s): chemical ocular injuries

EPIDEMIOLOGY

Incidence

- Estimated 5 to 6 cases/100,000 persons per year (accounting for 11–22% of all ocular injuries)
- Median age is 32 years, but children between the ages of 1 and 2 years represent the highest-risk group.
- Male > female
- Most common in workplace and residential settings

ETIOLOGY AND PATHOPHYSIOLOGY

- Alkaline compounds (pH >7)
  - Alkali burns are twice as common as acid burns.
  - Typical sources include ammonia (most common), calcium hydroxide (lime), sodium/potassium hydroxide (lye), and ammonium hydroxide.
  - Lipophilic compounds that penetrate into deep structures dissociate into cations and hydroxide. Hydroxide causes saponification of fatty acids in cell membranes, leading to cell death. Cations cause hydration of glycosaminoglycans, leading to hydration of collagen, rapid shortening and thickening of collagen fibrils, and resultant corneal opacification and acute elevation in intraocular pressure (IOP).
  - Long-term elevation in IOP may occur from accumulation of inflammatory debris within the trabecular meshwork.
  - Penetration into deep structures may affect perfusing vessels, leading to ischemia.
- Acidic compounds (pH <7)
  - Typical sources include sulfuric acid (most common), sulfurous acid, hydrochloric acid, acetic acid, hydrofluoric acid.
  - Anion leads to protein denaturing and protective barrier formation by coagulation necrosis forming an eschar. This more superficial mechanism of injury reduces further tissue penetration but may lead to more prominent scarring.
  - Hydrofluoric acid is an exception. In its nonionized form, it behaves like an alkaline substance that can penetrate the corneal stroma and lead to extensive anterior segment lesions. When ionized, it may combine with intracellular calcium and magnesium to form insoluble complexes, leading to potassium ion movements and cell death. Once systemically absorbed, severe hypocalcemia can occur.

RISK FACTORS

- Industrial work, including in chemical labs
- Construction work (plaster, cement, whitewash)
- Use of cleaning agents (drain cleaners, ammonia)
- Automobile battery explosions (sulfuric acid)
- Any risk factor for assault

GENERAL PREVENTION

- Safety glasses/goggles to safeguard eyes
- Safe handling training for occupational exposures

COMMONLY ASSOCIATED CONDITIONS

Facial (including eyelids) cutaneous chemical or thermal burns

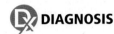 DIAGNOSIS

HISTORY

- Patient presents with pain, photophobia, blurred vision, and foreign body sensation.
- Ask about chemical involved, temperature, volume, timing and duration of exposure, velocity of impact, and involved area.
- In alkali burns, can have initial pain that later diminishes

PHYSICAL EXAM

- Alkaline compounds may present with corneal opacification secondary to glycosaminoglycan hydration; however, severe acid burns may also present with this finding.
- Acidic compound may present with a ground-glass appearance secondary to superficial scar formation.

DIFFERENTIAL DIAGNOSIS

- Thermal burns
- Ruptured globe
- Traumatic corneal abrasion or epithelial defects
- Infectious keratoconjunctivitis
- Intraocular/superficial ocular foreign body
- Ocular cicatricial pemphigoid

DIAGNOSTIC TESTS & INTERPRETATION

Initial Tests (lab, imaging)

- Examine the eye before initiating irrigation to rule out open globe (may require emergent surgical exploration if high index of suspicion for open globe that would be exacerbated by irrigation).
- Measure pH of tear film on both eyes and immediately initiate irrigation (if nonneutral) prior to additional tests.
- Imaging is not necessary unless suspicion of intraocular or orbital foreign body is present. In this case, CT should be used—MRI is contraindicated.

Follow-Up Tests & Special Considerations

- Complete ophthalmic exam include measuring visual acuity, IOP, and examining both anterior and posterior segments
- Grade the degree of injury based on corneal, conjunctival, and limbal involvement using the Roper-Hall or Dua classification schemes to guide prognosis and treatment. It is important to establish baseline at time of injury and document changes over time as the patient is followed.
- Stem cell survival is the rate limiting mechanism of recovery after corneal injury; limbal ischemia is a surrogate measure to estimate the degree of stem cell loss.

Diagnostic Procedures/Other

- Measure pH of tear film with litmus paper or electronic probe: Irrigating fluid with nonneutral pH (e.g., normal saline has pH of 4.5) may alter results; wipe away all excess topical anesthetics before measuring.
- Careful slit-lamp exam, fundus ophthalmoscopy, tonometry, and measurement of visual acuity
- Using fluorescein to evaluate the state of the corneal epithelium is essential.
- Examination of posterior segment may be challenging but should be attempted carefully using nonvasoconstrictive mydriatics to avoid potential worsening of ischemia.
- Full extent of damage from alkali burns may not be apparent until 48 to 72 hours after exposure.

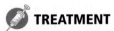 TREATMENT

Immediate copious irrigation and removal of corneal or conjunctival foreign bodies are always the initial treatment and paramount to minimizing long-term sequelae (1),(2),(3)[A]:

- Passively open patient's eyelid and have patient look in all directions while irrigating.
- Remove all chemical reservoirs from the eyes via lid eversion while flushing.
- Continue irrigation until the tear film and superior/inferior cul-de-sac is of neutral pH (7.2 ± 0.1) and stable, testing every 30 minutes (1)[A]:
  - Severe burns should be irrigated for at least 15 to 30 minutes and up to 2 to 4 hours; this irrigation should not be interrupted during transportation to hospital (1)[B].
  - Irrigation via Morgan lens (polymethylmethacrylate scleral lens) is a good way to achieve continuous irrigation over a prolonged period of time.
- Perform initial pH testing on both eyes even if the patient claims to only have unilateral ocular pain/irritation so that a contralateral injury is not overlooked.
- Use any available nontoxic fluid for irrigation on scene including bottled or tap water. In the clinic/hospital, sterile water, normal saline, normal saline with bicarbonate, balanced salt solution (BSS), or lactated Ringer solution may be used.
- A topical anesthetic can be used to provide patient comfort (e.g., proparacaine, tetracaine).
- Sweep the conjunctival fornices every 12 to 24 hours to prevent symblepharon formation and adhesions.

MEDICATION

First Line

- After initial irrigation, further treatment aims to decrease inflammation and collagen degradation and aid in collagen synthesis and recovery of corneal epithelium. Selection of medications depends on severity and associated conditions.
  - Topical prophylactic antibiotics: any broad-spectrum agent (e.g., bacitracin–polymyxin B ointment q2–4h, ciprofloxacin drops q2–4h)
    - Some experts suggest adding systemic tetracycline such as doxycycline 100 mg PO BID to encourage healing and prevent corneal ulceration (1),(2)[C].
  - Preservative-free artificial tears: carboxymethylcellulose (Refresh Plus) drops q1h for first 24 hours
    - Promotes reepithelialization, reduces recurrent erosion risk, and increases visual rehab (1),(2)[A]
  - Cycloplegics for photophobia and/or uveitis: cyclopentolate 1% TID (3)[C]
  - Topical corticosteroids for intraocular inflammation: prednisolone 1% or equivalent q1–2h for 7 to 10 days; and if severe, prednisone 20 to 60 mg PO daily for 5 to 7 days; taper rapidly if epithelium is intact, by day 10 to 14 (1)[C].
  - Vitamin C (ascorbic acid) 500 mg PO QID and topical 10% q2h ascorbate solution in artificial tears
    - Using vitamin C in conjunction with steroids reduces incidence of corneal thinning, ulceration, and perforation (1),(2)[A].
  - Acetylcysteine (Mucomyst) 10–20% topically q4h may promote wound healing (1)[B].
  - Ocular antihypertensives for IOP >30 to reduce risk of optic nerve damage: latanoprost 0.005% QHS, timolol 0.5% BID or levobunolol 0.5% BID, and/or acetazolamide 125 to 250 mg PO q6h or methazolamide 25 to 50 mg PO BID (2)[B]
  - Bandage contact lens: After initial injury, lenses with high oxygen permeability and hydrophilic properties may aid in epithelial migration/adhesion and basement membrane regeneration (3)[B].
- Precautions
  - Timolol and levobunolol: history of cardiac/pulmonary disease including bradycardia and asthma/COPD
  - Acetazolamide and methazolamide: history of nephrolithiasis or metabolic acidosis
  - Mannitol: history of heart failure, renal failure, or sickle cell
  - Scopolamine: history of urinary retention
  - Ascorbic acid: history of renal impairment
  - Tetracycline/doxycycline: Avoid systemic use in children <8 years old and pregnant patients.
  - Topical corticosteroids: Use with caution in the presence of damaged corneal epithelium because iatrogenic infection can occur. Use of corticosteroids >6 days may inhibit repair and cause corneoscleral melt (1)[B]. Daily follow-up or consultation with an ophthalmologist is recommended.

- Consider adjunctive treatments and corneal subspecialty referral in advanced cases.
  - Biologic fluids with consultation to ophthalmology: umbilical cord serum 20% q2–3h, autologous serum 20% q2–3h, platelet-rich plasma q2–3h, or amniotic membrane suspension 30–50% q1h; these contain growth factors, vitamins, cytokines, and anti-inflammatory factors to improve dry eyes and to reduce pain, persistent epithelial defects, recurrent erosion syndrome, and neurotrophic ulcers (1),(2)[B].

SURGERY/OTHER PROCEDURES

- The goals of subacute treatment are restoration of the normal ocular surface anatomy and corneal clarity and control of glaucoma.
- Surgical options include the following:
  - Débridement of necrotic tissue and inflammatory debris (1),(3)[A]
  - Conjunctival/tenon advancement (tenoplasty) to restore vascularity in severe burns
  - Tissue adhesive (e.g., cyanoacrylate) for impending or actual corneal perforation
    - Tectonic keratoplasty for acute perforation >1 mm
  - Limbal autograft transplantation for epithelial stem cell restoration
  - Amniotic membrane transplantation or umbilical cord serum drops to promote faster epithelial regeneration and improvement in visual acuity (1)[B]
  - Conjunctival or mucosal membrane transplant to restore ocular surface in severe injury
  - Corneal transplant (penetrating keratoplasty, anterior lamellar keratoplasty) for extensive scarring
  - Enucleation for blind, painful eyes

ADMISSION, INPATIENT, AND NURSING CONSIDERATIONS

Based on ophthalmologic consultation, therapy compliance assessment, and concomitant burn injuries

 # ONGOING CARE

FOLLOW-UP RECOMMENDATIONS

Patient Monitoring

- Ranges from daily to weekly visits initially depending on severity of ocular injury
- May need to be admitted if noncompliant or pediatric patient
- If on mannitol or prednisone, consider frequently checking serum electrolytes

PATIENT EDUCATION

- Need for immediate ocular irrigation with water following ocular chemical exposure
- Shield at all times during acute care
- Safety glasses for future protection

PROGNOSIS

- Depends on severity of initial injury: increased limbal involvement in clock hours and greater percentage of conjunctival involvement correlate with poorer prognosis (Dua classification system)
- For mildly injured eyes, complete recovery is common.
- For severely injured eyes, permanent loss of vision is not uncommon.

COMPLICATIONS

- Orbital compartment syndrome
- Keratoconjunctivitis sicca (dry eye)
- Corneal ulcer/perforation/scarring
- Cicatricial ectropion/entropion
- Symblepharon
- Glaucoma
- Cataract
- Phthisis bulbi
- Blindness

REFERENCES

1. Sharma N, Kaur M, Agarwal T, et al. Treatment of acute ocular chemical burns. *Surv Ophthalmol*. 2018;63(2):214–235.
2. Baradaran-Rafii A, Eslani M, Haq Z, et al. Current and upcoming therapies for ocular surface chemical injuries. *Ocul Surf*. 2017;15(1):48–64.
3. Eslani M, Baradaran-Rafii A, Movahedan A, et al. The ocular surface chemical burns. *J Ophthalmol*. 2014;2014:196827.

 SEE ALSO

Burns

CODES

ICD10

- T26.50XA Corrosion of unsp eyelid and periocular area, init encntr
- T26.60XA Corrosion of cornea and conjunctival sac, unsp eye, init
- S05.00XA Inj conjunctiva and corneal abrasion w/o fb, unsp eye, init

CLINICAL PEARLS

- Prompt irrigation of all chemical burns, with any available nontoxic fluid such as water, as soon as possible (prior to arrival in the emergency department), is essential to ensure the best outcomes.
- All patients with ocular chemical injuries should have urgent ophthalmology evaluation.
- Prognosis is guarded depending on type of chemical injury.

ONYCHOMYCOSIS

Karl T. Clebak, MD, MHA, FAAFP • Huong N. Nguyen, DO, MS

BASICS

DESCRIPTION
- Fungal infection of fingernails/toenails
- Caused mostly by dermatophytes but also yeasts and nondermatophyte molds
- Toenails are more commonly affected than fingernails.
- Synonym: tinea unguium

EPIDEMIOLOGY
Prevalence
- Worldwide prevalence is approximately 5.5%.
- More common in adults than children; prevalence increases with age; 35% of adults aged >65
- Rare before puberty
- Prevalence 15–40% in persons with human immunodeficiency virus (HIV)
- Estimated 50% of all nail disorders in the outpatient setting

ETIOLOGY AND PATHOPHYSIOLOGY
- Inoculation of nail with dermatophytes, nondermatophyte molds, or yeasts
- Dermatophytes: *Trichophyton* (*Trichophyton rubrum* most common), *Epidermophyton*, *Microsporum*
- Yeasts: *Candida albicans* (most common), *Candida parapsilosis*, *Candida tropicalis*, *Candida krusei*
- Molds: *Scopulariopsis brevicaulis*, *Hendersonula toruloidea*, *Aspergillus* sp., *Alternaria tenuis*, *Cephalosporium*, *Scytalidium hyalinum*
- Dermatophytes, notably *Trichophyton*, cause 90% of toenail and 75% of fingernail onychomycoses.
- Yeasts, especially *Candida*, may involve fingernails (not uncommonly) or toenails.

RISK FACTORS
- Older age, occlusive footwear, tinea pedis
- Cancer/diabetes/psoriasis
- Peripheral vascular disease
- Living with others with onychomycosis, communal swimming pools
- Peripheral vascular disease
- Smoking
- Immunodeficiency
- Autosomal dominant genetic predisposition

GENERAL PREVENTION
- Keeping feet cool and dry
- Avoiding occlusive footwear
- Using sandals in public locker rooms and swimming pools
- Discarding or treating of infected footwear and socks (1)

COMMONLY ASSOCIATED CONDITIONS
- Immunodeficiency (acquired immune deficiency syndrome and transplant patients) and chronic metabolic disease (e.g., diabetes)
- Tinea pedis/manuum

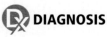

DIAGNOSIS

HISTORY
Discoloration of nail plate with thickening and onycholysis

PHYSICAL EXAM
- Dermatophytes: commonly preceded by dermatophyte infection at another site; 80% involve toenails, especially hallux; simultaneous infection of fingernails and toenails is rare. Five clinical forms occur:
  – Distal/lateral subungual onychomycosis (most common): mainly due to *T. rubrum*; spreads from distal/lateral margins to nail bed to nail plate, causing linear channels or "spikes" subungual hyperkeratosis; onycholysis; nail dystrophy; discoloration—yellow-white or brown-black, *bois vermoulu* ("worm-eaten wood"); onychomadesis
  – Proximal subungual onychomycosis (rare <1% of cases): typically caused by *T. rubrum* and *Fusarium* spp; can affect hands/feet; leukonychia—begins at proximal part of nail plate near cuticle and distally, appearing to occur from the proximal underside of the nail (or direct invasion of the nail plate from above); spreads to nail plate and lunula; seen with immunosuppressive conditions
  – Superficial onychomycosis (~10% of cases): infection of surface of nail plate; merging opaque white spots on nail plate eventually can involve entire surface of the nail; most commonly due to *Trichophyton mentagrophytes*
  – Endonyx onychomycosis involves interior of nail plate, sparing nail bed. Nail develops milky appearance with indentations and lamellar splitting. Subungual hyperkeratosis is absent.
  – Total dystrophic onychomycosis causes complete destruction of nail plate by fungus, resulting in thickened and ridged nail bed covered with keratotic debris; considered end-stage that may follow any subtype
- Candidal
  – Hands, 70% of all candida nail infections, especially for the dominant hand; middle finger is most common.
  – Pain is mild, unless secondarily infected; increases on prolonged contact with water
  – Primarily affects tissue surrounding nail
  – Begins with cuticle detachment and produces white or white-yellow nail discoloration
  – Secondary ungual changes: convex, irregular, striated nail plate with dull, rough surface
  – Onycholysis, especially on hands; distal subungual onychomycosis may occur.
  – Primary involvement of the nail plate is uncommon.
  – Periungual edema/erythema may occur (club-shaped, bulbous fingertips).
- Molds (nondermatophyte)
  – More common in those >60 years of age, more common in nails of hallux
  – Resembles distal and lateral onychomycosis

Pediatric Considerations
- Candidal infection presents more commonly as superficial onychomycosis.
- The U.S. Food and Drug Administration (FDA) has not approved any systemic antifungal agents for treatment of onychomycosis in children.

DIFFERENTIAL DIAGNOSIS
- Psoriasis (most common alternate diagnosis)
- Traumatic dystrophy
- Lichen planus
- Onychogryphosis ("ram's horn nails")
- Eczematous conditions
- Hypothyroidism
- Drugs and chemicals
- Yellow nail syndrome
- Neoplasms (0.7–3.5%) of all melanoma cases are subungual. In a brownish yellow nail, if dark pigment extends into periungual skin fold, consider subungual melanoma.
- Alopecia areata
- Chronic paronychia
- Pemphigus vulgaris

DIAGNOSTIC TESTS & INTERPRETATION
- Accurate diagnosis includes both laboratory and clinical evidence. Diagnostic accuracy ranges from 66% to 75%.
- About 50% of nail dystrophy seen on visual inspection is not fungal in origin.
- A nail plate biopsy or partial/full removal of nail with culture is needed to diagnose proximal subungual onychomycosis.

Initial Tests (lab, imaging)
- Direct microscopy with potassium hydroxide (KOH) preparation from nail sample
- Cultures: false-negative finding in 30%; results may take 3 to 6 weeks.
- In-office dermatophyte test, medium culture indicates dermatophyte growth; results in 3 to 7 days; limited studies
- Histologic examination of nail clippings/nail plate punch biopsy: proximal lesions; stain both with periodic acid–Schiff (PAS) stain
- Polymerase chain reaction (PCR) increases sensitivity of detection of dermatophytes in nail specimen; results available within 3 days; not widely available
- Fluorescence microscopy can be used as a rapid screening tool for identification of fungi in nail specimens.
- Commercial laboratories may use KOH with calcofluor white stain to improve view of fungal elements in fluorescent microscopy.
- Discontinue all topical medication for at least 1 week before obtaining a sample.

Follow-Up Tests & Special Considerations
Laboratory confirmation prior to treatment is cost-effective and should be considered to avoid misdiagnosis and unnecessary treatment.

Test Interpretation
Pathogens within the nail keratin

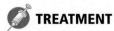

TREATMENT

GENERAL MEASURES
- Avoid factors that promote fungal growth (i.e., heat, moisture, occlusion, tight-fitting shoes).
- Treat underlying disease risk factors.
- Treat secondary infections.

MEDICATION

Pregnancy Considerations
Oral antifungals and ciclopirox are pregnancy Category B (terbinafine, ciclopirox) or C (itraconazole, fluconazole, and griseofulvin). Griseofulvin is not advised in pregnancy due to risks of teratogenicity. Ideally, postpone treatment of onychomycosis until after pregnancy.

First Line
- Oral antifungals are preferred due to higher rates of cure and shorter courses of treatment but have systemic adverse effects and many drug–drug interactions; recommended when >50% of nail is affected, multiple nails, involvement of nail matrix, or presence of dermatophytoma; recurrence following treatment is common—25–50% within 5 years.
- Terbinafine: 250 mg/day PO for 6 weeks for fingernails and 12 weeks for toenails; terbinafine offers the most effective clinical and mycological cure rates compared to other treatments (2)[A]. Continuous terbinafine treatment has similar efficacy as pulse treatment.
- Alternative therapies for terbinafine resistant infections include posaconazole, voriconazole and itraconazole.
- Itraconazole pulse: 200 mg PO BID for 1 week and then 3 weeks off; repeat for two cycles for fingernails and 3 to 4 cycles for toenails; does not need to monitor liver function tests (LFTs) with pulse dosing
- Itraconazole continuous: 200 mg/day PO for 6 weeks for fingernails and 12 weeks for toenails (less effective than itraconazole pulse for dermatophytes, more effective than terbinafine for *Candida* and molds)

Second Line
- Fluconazole pulse: 150 to 300 mg PO weekly for 6 months; not FDA-approved for onychomycosis
- Griseofulvin: 500 to 1,000 mg/day PO for up to 18 months; less effective with significant adverse events
- Posaconazole: 100, 200, or 400 mg once daily for 24 weeks; 400 mg once daily for 12 weeks; higher cost
- Topical agents: use limited to disease not involving the lunula (proximal nail plate) or when <3 nails are affected; topical therapy does not cause systemic toxicity but is much less effective than oral therapy.
- Efinaconazole 10% solution: apply directly to the affected nails once daily for 48 weeks; complete or almost-complete cure after 48 weeks in range of 15–18%
- Ciclopirox: 8% nail lacquer: Apply once daily to the affected nails for up to 48 weeks; remove lacquer with alcohol every 7 days and then file loose nail material and trim nails; application after PO treatment may reduce recurrences; systematic review >60% failure rate after 48 weeks of use (3)[A]
- Tavaborole 5% solution: indicated for onychomycosis of the toenails due to *T. rubrum* or *T. mentagrophytes*; complete or almost-complete cure 15–18% after 48 weeks; reserve topical treatment for those with less extensive disease and no proximal involvement who wish to avoid oral medication.

- Contraindications for oral antifungals
  - Hepatic disease
  - Pregnancy
  - Current/history of congestive heart failure (CHF) (itraconazole)
  - Ventricular dysfunction (itraconazole)
  - Porphyria (griseofulvin)
- Precautions/adverse effects:
  - Oral antifungals: rhinitis (itraconazole); CHF, peripheral edema, pulmonary edema (itraconazole), chronic kidney disease (avoid terbinafine for patients with creatinine clearance [CrCl] <50 mL/min; decrease fluconazole dose), photosensitivity, lupus-like symptoms, proteinuria (griseofulvin), hypersensitivity, hepatotoxicity/neutropenia
  - Oral agents: numerous significant drug–drug interactions; need to check each medication
- Ciclopirox topical: side effects: rash, nail disorders; avoid contact with skin except along nail edge; caution with broken skin or vascular compromise

ADDITIONAL THERAPIES
Laser therapy is promising although data is lacking to support routine use.

SURGERY/OTHER PROCEDURES
- Trimming, avulsion, débridement, or nail abrasion to reduce fungal load and enhance penetration of antifungal agents
  - Mechanical: File with abrasive stone or curette.
  - Chemical: Protect peripheral tissue with adhesive strips; apply ointment of 30% salicylic acid, 40% urea, or 50% potassium iodide under occlusive dressing.
  - Débridement may be combined with topical antifungal therapy.
  - Surgical avulsion if few nails are involved for pain control
- Laser treatment has shown some positive results but poor statistical power and limited efficacy or safety data.
- Limited data with using photodynamic therapy using topical photosensitizing agents and irradiation
- Keratolytic agents including urea, salicylic acid, and papain applied to the nail prior to topical agents proposed to enhance penetration

COMPLEMENTARY & ALTERNATIVE MEDICINE
Melaleuca alternifolia (tea tree oil): Cochrane Review found no evidence of benefit (3)[A]. Vicks VapoRub application to nails daily for 48 weeks has been found safe, but efficacy is uncertain.

ONGOING CARE

FOLLOW-UP RECOMMENDATIONS
Formation of a new fingernail takes 4 to 6 months, and a new toenail takes 12 to 18 months.

Patient Monitoring
- Topical agents: slow response is expected; visits every 6 to 12 weeks
- Terbinafine, griseofulvin: baseline and as needed; LFTs and CBC
- Itraconazole continuous: baseline and as needed; LFTs

PATIENT EDUCATION
Advise the patient to keep the affected area clean and dry, to avoid occlusive footwear, to wear absorbent socks, to discard old sneakers, and to avoid sharing nail implements and using on both infected and uninfected nails. Cure may not be attainable.

PROGNOSIS
- Complete clinical cure in 25–50% (higher mycologic cure rates) with oral therapy
- Recurrence is 10–50% (relapse/reinfection).
- Poor prognostic factors
  - Areas of nail involvement >50%
  - Significant proximal/lateral disease
  - Subungual hyperkeratosis >2 mm
  - White/yellow or orange/brown streaks in the nail (includes dermatophytoma)
  - Total dystrophic onychomycosis (with matrix involvement)
  - Nonresponsive organisms (e.g., *Scytalidium* mold)
  - Patients with immunosuppression
  - Diminished peripheral circulation

COMPLICATIONS
- Secondary infections with progression to soft tissue infection/osteomyelitis
- Toenail discomfort/pain that can limit physical mobility or activity
- Anxiety, negative self-image

REFERENCES
1. Lipner SR, Scher RK. Onychomycosis: treatment and prevention of recurrence. *J Am Acad Dermatol*. 2019;80(4):853–867.
2. Kreijkamp-Kaspers S, Hawke K, Guo L, et al. Oral antifungal medication for toenail onychomycosis. *Cochrane Database Syst Rev*. 2017;7(7):CD010031.
3. Crawford F, Hollis S. Topical treatments for fungal infections of the skin and nails of the foot. *Cochrane Database Syst Rev*. 2007;(3):CD001434.

CODES

ICD10
- B35.1 Tinea unguium
- B37.2 Candidiasis of skin and nail

CLINICAL PEARLS
- Psoriasis and chronic nail trauma are commonly mistaken for fungal infection.
- Diagnosis should be based on both clinical and mycologic laboratory evidence.
- Oral medication is much more effective than topical, but recurrence following treatment is common.

OPIOID USE DISORDER

Laurel Banach, MD

BASICS

DESCRIPTION

Opioids are a class of medication that are commonly used for analgesia or pain relief with the concurrent potential for central nervous system depression and/or feelings of euphoria. The diagnosis of opioid use disorder (OUD) refers to the misuse of prescription opioids or use of illicit opioids, such as heroin that may result in self-harm including death. OUD is considered a chronic illness.

EPIDEMIOLOGY

Prevalence

In 2018, an estimated 10,250,000 people reported opioid misuse (3.7% of population ≥12 years old).

- 2,028,000 of those met the *Diagnostic and Statistical Manual of Mental Disorders*, 5th edition (*DSM-5*) criteria for a diagnosis of OUD (0.7% of population ≥12 years old) (1).

RISK FACTORS

- Prior history of substance use disorder
- More severe reported pain
- Co-occurring mental disorders (2)

GENERAL PREVENTION

- Opioid prescriptions have been reduced by 29% between 2006 and 2018, which reduces access to prescription opioids.
- Harm reduction practices can prevent complications from OUD such as clean needle exchanges and safe injection sites.
- Access to intranasal naloxone can prevent opioid-related deaths.

COMMONLY ASSOCIATED CONDITIONS

- Mood disorders
- Personality disorders
- Posttraumatic stress disorder (PTSD)
- Other substance use disorders
- Sexually transmitted infections
- Hepatitis A, B, C
- HIV

DIAGNOSIS

HISTORY

A majority of the diagnostic criteria can be obtained by history alone. Diagnosis of OUD is outlined in the *DSM-5* by exhibiting at least two of the following criteria in a 12-month period:

- Opioids are taken in larger amounts or longer period than intended.
- Strong craving or desire to use opioids
- Spending larger amounts of time to obtain, use, or recover from opioid effects
- Persistent desire or efforts to cut down opioid use
- Continued opioid use despite persistent interpersonal problems related to opioid use
- Recurrent opioid use resulting in a failure to fulfill major role obligations
- Reduced important social, occupational, or recreational activities because of opioid use
- Continued opioid use despite knowledge of a physical or psychological problem caused by the substance
- Opioid use in hazardous situations
- Developing a tolerance to opioids
- Demonstrating withdrawal symptoms to opioids

PHYSICAL EXAM

- Physical exam is of use for distinguishing between a substance use disorder and dependence. Exhibiting tolerance and withdrawal alone cannot be used for diagnosis of OUD because these represent signs of dependence. These signs may be exhibited on physical exam or found through history taking.
- Tolerance is either:
  - The need for increasing doses or frequency of opioid medication to achieve similar effect
  - Decreasing effectiveness with the same dose of prescription opioid
- Withdrawal is defined as the experience of pain or undesired symptoms with the absence of the opioid. Common undesired symptoms include sweating, restlessness, body aches, pupil dilation, tremor, anxiety, and diarrhea.

DIFFERENTIAL DIAGNOSIS

- Physical dependence on an opioid
- Disorders causing psychosis
- Mood disorders
- Effects of trauma including PTSD
- Another substance use disorder
- Polysubstance use disorder

DIAGNOSTIC TESTS & INTERPRETATION

One could make the diagnosis of OUD without additional testing; however, a medical professional may choose to obtain data from a prescription drug monitoring program or by urine or saliva drug testing.

TREATMENT

GENERAL MEASURES

- Treatment mainstays include both medications for opioid use disorder (MOUD) and a variety of therapy interventions performed by trained professionals.
- Intranasal naloxone (Narcan) should be prescribed to all patients.
  - Family, friends, and bystanders can administer in the setting of an overdose with a brief training.
  - Narcan reverses the effects of opioids causing respiratory and central nervous system depression almost immediately.
  - Narcan, given to a person without experiencing an opioid overdose, has minimal side effects.

MEDICATION

First Line

- Opioid agonists act by binding the opioid receptors stronger than prescription or illicit opioids. These medications include the following:
  - Methadone: a long-acting, full opioid agonist whose half-life allows for once daily dosing; available in an oral solution or tablet, methadone for maintenance medication-assisted treatment (MAT) is only available at designated distribution sites, but can also be used as a chronic pain agent
  - Buprenorphine: a partial mu-opioid agonist; buprenorphine is available in transmucosal films or tablets as well as newer products including implants and injectable solutions; it is often paired with naloxone (Suboxone), to discourage abuse of buprenorphine
    - Injectable buprenorphine is now available and widely used as a MOUD.
- Opioid antagonists are also a potential therapy and include naltrexone, which comes in both injectable and oral forms. As full antagonists, these medications have the potential to send patients into withdrawal if they have not been off of opioids for roughly 1 week.

ISSUES FOR REFERRAL

Pregnancy Considerations

- Will face challenges with pain management and potential for neonatal abstinence syndrome (NAS) in newborns
- The American College of Obstetricians and Gynecologists recognizes that usual prenatal guidelines may need adjustment for women with co-occurring OUD and therefore may benefit from a provider with more experience caring for pregnant women with OUD.
- Newborns born to mothers with OUD, even on MAT, should be monitored by a provider trained in evaluating for NAS.

ADDITIONAL THERAPIES

Patients are also recommended engaging with psychosocial interventions. These psychosocial interventions should be individualized and patient autonomy to decline these interventions should be respected (3).

ADMISSION, INPATIENT, AND NURSING CONSIDERATIONS

Pain management is challenging with patients diagnosed with OUD or who have a history of opioid misuse and may require higher doses of opioid analgesia or alternative medications.

 ONGOING CARE

PATIENT EDUCATION

- All patients with OUD should discuss harm reduction practices to reduce chronic illnesses, including using needle exchanges or pharmacies to obtain clean needles for injecting and intranasal or oral opioid use as opposed to IV administration.
- Intranasal naloxone (Narcan) prescriptions should be sent to all patients with OUD and close acquaintances.

PROGNOSIS

Mortality is high due to death by unintentional overdose and significant medical complications.

- In the United States in 2017, 47,600 died of an opioid-related overdose (age-adjusted rate being 14.9 per 100,000 people).
  - 43,036/47,600 were considered unintentional overdoses (1).

REFERENCES

1. Centers for Disease Control and Prevention. *Annual Surveillance Report of Drug-Related Risks and Outcomes—United States, 2019.* Atlanta GA: Centers for Disease Control and Prevention, U.S.
2. Department of Health and Human Services; 2019.
3. Kaye AD, Jones MR, Kaye AM, et al. Prescription opioid abuse in chronic pain: an updated review of opioid abuse predictors and strategies to curb opioid abuse: part 1. *Pain Physician.* 2017;20(2S):S93–S109.
4. Cunningham C, Edlund MJ, Fishman M, et al. The ASAM national practice guideline for the treatment of opioid use disorder: 2020 focused update. *J Addict Med.* 2020;14(2S Suppl 1):1–91.

 CODES

ICD10
- F11.10 Opioid abuse, uncomplicated
- F11.90 Opioid use, unspecified, uncomplicated
- F11.1 Opioid abuse

CLINICAL PEARLS

- Treatment includes both MAT and therapy interventions performed by trained professionals.
- Intranasal naloxone (Narcan) should be prescribed to all patients and close acquaintances.

OPTIC NEURITIS
Navpreet K. Singh, MD

BASICS

DESCRIPTION
- Inflammation of the optic nerve (cranial nerve II)
- The most common form is acute demyelinating optic neuritis (ON), but other causes include infectious disease and systemic autoimmune disorders.
- Optic disc may be normal in appearance at onset (retrobulbar ON, 67%) or swollen (papillitis, 33%).
- Key features:
  – Abrupt visual loss (typically monocular)
  – Periorbital pain with eye movement (90%)
  – Pain in the distribution of the first division of the trigeminal nerve
  – Dyschromatopsia: color vision deficits
  – Relative afferent pupillary defect (RAPD)
- Usually unilateral in adults; bilateral disease more common in children
- Associated with multiple sclerosis (MS), presenting complaint (25% MS patients)
- In children, headaches are common.
- System(s) affected: nervous
- Synonym(s): papillitis, demyelinating optic neuropathy; retrobulbar ON

EPIDEMIOLOGY
Incidence
- 5/100,000 cases per year
- More common in whites than in other races
- Predominant age: 18 to 45 years; mean age of 30 years
- Predominant sex: female > male (3:1)

ETIOLOGY AND PATHOPHYSIOLOGY
- In both MS-associated and isolated monosymptomatic ON, the cause is presumed to be a demyelinating autoimmune reaction.
- Neuromyelitis optica (NMO) IgG autoantibody, which targets the water channel aquaporin-4
- Viral infections: measles, mumps, varicella-zoster, coxsackievirus, adenovirus, hepatitis A and B, HIV, herpes simplex virus, cytomegalovirus, SARS-CoV-2 (myelin oligodendrocyte glycoprotein [MOG] antibody-associated ON and myelitis in COVID-19) (1)
- Nonviral infections: syphilis, tuberculosis, meningococcus, cryptococcosis, cysticercosis, bacterial sinusitis, Group B Streptococcus, Bartonella, typhoid fever, Lyme disease, fungus
- Systemic inflammatory disease: sarcoidosis, systemic lupus erythematosus, vasculitis
- Local inflammatory disease: intraocular or contiguous with the orbit, sinus, or meninges
- Toxic: lead, methanol, arsenic, radiation
- Medications: ethambutol, chloroquine, isoniazid, chronic high-dose chloramphenicol, tumor necrosis factor α-antagonist, infliximab (Remicade), adalimumab (Humira), etanercept (Enbrel)

Genetics
Genetics: Some people have genetic mutations that increase their chance of ON (i.e., MS) and several immune-mediated inflammatory diseases (IMIDs).

COMMONLY ASSOCIATED CONDITIONS
- MS (common): ON is associated with an increased risk of MS.
- Other demyelinating diseases: Guillain-Barré syndrome, Devic NMO, multifocal demyelinating neuropathy, acute disseminated encephalomyelitis

DIAGNOSIS

- Clinical criteria: A: monocular, subacute loss of vision associated with orbital pain worsening on eye movements, reduced contrast and colour vision, and relative afferent pupillary deficit; B: painless with all other features of (A); C: binocular loss of vision with all features of (A) or (B)
- Paraclinical criteria: OCT: corresponding optic disc swelling acutely or an intereye difference in the mGCIPL of >4% or >4 μm or in the pRNFL of >5% or >5 μm within 3 months after onset; MRI: contrast enhancement of the symptomatic optic nerve and sheaths acutely or an intrinsic signal (looking brighter) increase within 3 months; biomarker: AQP4, MOG, or CRMP5 antibody seropositive or intrathecal CSF IgG (oligoclonal bands [OCBs])
- Application of the clinical and paraclinical criteria: definite ON: A: one paraclinical test: B: two paraclinical tests of different modality: C: two different paraclinical tests of which one is MRI; possible ON: (A), (B), or (C) if seen acutely but in absence of paraclinical tests, with fundus examination typical for ON and consistent with the natural history during follow-up; positive paraclinical test or tests, with a medical history suggestive of ON (2)

HISTORY
- *Decreased visual acuity*, deteriorating in hours to days, usually reaching lowest level after 1 week
- Usually unilateral but can also be bilateral
- Brow ache, globe tenderness, deep orbital *pain* exacerbated by *eye movement* (92%)
- Retro-orbital pain may precede visual loss.
- Desaturation of color vision (dull or faded colors), especially red tones
- Apparent dimness of light intensities
- Impairment of depth perception (80%); worse with moving objects (*Pulfrich phenomenon*)
- Transient increase in visual symptoms with increased body temperature and exercise (*Uhthoff phenomenon*)
- *Phosphenes*: fleeting colors and flashes of light (30%)
- May present with a recent flulike viral syndrome
- Detailed history and review of systems, looking for a history of demyelinating, infectious, or systemic inflammatory disease

PHYSICAL EXAM
Complete general exam, full neurologic exam, and ophthalmologic exam (with vision testing) looking for the following:
- Decreased visual acuity and color perception
- Central, cecocentral, arcuate, or altitudinal visual field deficits

- Papillitis: (1/3) swollen disc ± peripapillary flame-shape hemorrhage or often (2/3) normal disc exam
- Temporal disc pallor seen later *at 4 to 6 weeks* (3)[A]
- *RAPD*: The pupil of the affected eye dilates with a swinging light test unless disease is bilateral.

DIFFERENTIAL DIAGNOSIS
- Demyelinating disease, especially MS, the distribution and appearance of inflammatory lesions on orbital MRI have been reported to show significant differences between ON associated with AQP4-IgG-seropositive NMO spectrum disorders (NMOSD-ON), MOG-IgG encephalomyelitis (MOG-ON), and seronegative MS-ON (4).
- MOG-antibody disease (MOG-AD)
- Infectious/systemic inflammatory disease
- Acute papilledema (bilateral disc edema)
- Compression from a tumor/abscess compressing the optic nerve
- Temporal arteritis or other vasculitides
- Diabetic papillopathy

DIAGNOSTIC TESTS & INTERPRETATION
Initial Tests (lab, imaging)
- In typical presentations, erythrocyte sedimentation rate (ESR) is standard, but other labs are unnecessary. Antinuclear antibodies (ANAs), angiotensin-converting enzyme (ACE) level, fluorescent treponemal antibody absorption (FTA-ABS), and chest x-ray (CXR) have been shown to have no value in typical cases (3),(5)[A].
- In atypical presentations, including absence of pain, a very swollen optic nerve, >30 days without recovery, or retinal exudates, labs (CBC, ANA, rapid plasma reagin [RPR], SARS-CoV-2 PCR) may be indicated to rule out underlying disorders.
- MRI of brain and orbits to evaluate risk of etiology of ON from MS
- Lumbar puncture (LP): to evaluate cerebrospinal fluid (CSF) composition and oligoclonal bands (OCBs)
- CT scan of chest to rule out sarcoidosis if clinical suspicion is high

Follow-Up Tests & Special Considerations
- Optical coherence tomography (OCT) of the retinal nerve fiber layer (RNFL); a noninvasive imaging technique of the optic nerve; may serve as a diagnostic tool to quantify thickness of the nerve fiber layer objectively and thus monitor structural change (axonal loss) of the optic nerve in the course of the disease
- Antibody testing: Serum NMO antibody testing is suggested for individuals with recurrent ON, particularly if the MRI brain is negative for any abnormal T2/FLAIR lesions outside of the affected optic nerve(s).
- Visual field test (Humphrey 30-2) to evaluate for visual field loss: diffuse and central visual loss more predominant in the affected eye at baseline (3)[A]
- OCT of the optic nerve RNFL to detect and monitor axonal loss in the anterior visual pathways

- Low-contrast visual acuity (as a measure of disease progression)
- A blood test serum marker: *NMO-IgG* checks for antibodies for NMO

Diagnostic Procedures/Other
- In atypical cases, including bilateral deficits, young age, or suspicion of infectious etiology, LP with neurology consultation is indicated.
- LP for suspected MS is a physician-dependent decision. Some studies indicate that it may not add value to MRI for MS detection (3)[A], but no consensus on the subject exists.

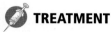 TREATMENT

Most recover spontaneously.

MEDICATION
First Line
- IV methylprednisolone has been shown to speed up the rate of visual recovery but without significant long-term benefit; consider for patients who require fast recovery (i.e., monocular patients or those whose occupation requires high-level visual acuity). For significant vision loss, parenteral corticosteroids may be considered on an individualized basis: Optic Neuritis Treatment Trial (ONTT):
  – Observation and corticosteroid treatment are both acceptable courses of action.
  – High-dose IV methylprednisolone (250 mg q6h for 3 days) followed by oral corticosteroids (1 mg/kg/day PO for 11 days, taper over 1 to 2 weeks) (5),(6)[A]
- Others use IV Solu-Medrol infusion (1 g in 250 mL D_5 1/2 normal saline infused over 1 hour daily for 3 to 5 days):
  – No evidence of long-term benefit (6)[A]
  – May decrease recovery time (6)[A]
  – May decrease risk of MS at 2 years but not 5 years (6)[A]
- Discuss the benefits and potential side effects of corticosteroids with patient (i.e., weight gain, osteoporosis, mood changes, gastrointestinal disturbances, hyperglycemia, insomnia).

ALERT
Avoid oral prednisone alone as the primary treatment because this may increase the risk for recurrent ON.

Second Line
- Disease-modifying agents, such as interferon-β1a (IFN-β1a; Avonex, Rebif) and IFN-β1b (Betaseron), are used to prevent or delay the development of MS in people with ON who have ≥2 brain lesions evident on MRI (7)[B].
- *Eculizumab (Soliris)* is FDA approved for NMOSD in patients who are anti-aquaporin-4 (AQP4) antibody positive. The most common symptoms of NMOSD are ON and transverse myelitis.
- Vitamin D_3 supplements for ON patients with low serum vitamin 25 (OH) D levels may delay the onset of a second clinical attack and the subsequent conversion to MS (8).

Pediatric Considerations
- Optic disc swelling and bilateral disease are more common in children as severe loss of visual acuity (20/200 or worse).
- Obtain serological marker for antibodies to MOG antibody (MOG-Ab) (9).
- No systematic study defining high-dose corticosteroids in children with pediatric ON (PON) has been conducted.
  – Consensus recommends: 3 to 5 days of IV methylprednisolone (4 to 30 mg/kg/day), followed by a 2- to 4-week taper of oral steroids
- Consider infectious and postinfectious causes of optic nerve impairment.

ISSUES FOR REFERRAL
Referral to a neurologist and/or ophthalmologist

ADMISSION, INPATIENT, AND NURSING CONSIDERATIONS
In acute visual loss, admit to expedite workup for initial diagnostic testing and referral to ophthalmology.

 ONGOING CARE

FOLLOW-UP RECOMMENDATIONS
Patient Monitoring
Monthly follow-up to monitor visual changes and steroid side effects

PATIENT EDUCATION
North American Neuro-Ophthalmology Society (NANOS): http://www.nanosweb.org/files/Patient%20Brochures/English/OpticNeuritis_English.pdf (available in other languages)

PROGNOSIS
- Orbital pain usually resolves within 1 week.
- Improvement of visual acuity begins over 2 to 4 weeks and steadily continues over 6 to 12 weeks. Visual acuity often returns to normal (20/40 or better) within 1 year (90–95%), even after near blindness.
- Other visual disturbances (e.g., contrast sensitivity, stereopsis) often persist after acuity returns to normal.
- Recurrence risk of 35% within 10 years: 14% affected eye, 12% contralateral, 9% bilateral; recurrence is higher in MS patients (48%).
- ON is associated with an increased risk of developing MS: 35% risk at 7 years, 58% at 15 years.
- Poor prognostic factors:
  – Absence of pain
  – Low initial visual acuity
  – Involvement of intracanalicular optic nerve
- Children with bilateral visual loss have a better prognosis than adults.

COMPLICATIONS
Permanent loss of vision

REFERENCES
1. Benito-Pascual B, Gegúndez JA, Díaz-Valle D, et al. Panuveitis and optic neuritis as a possible initial presentation of the novel coronavirus disease 2019 (COVID-19). *Ocul Immunol Inflamm.* 2020;28(6):922–925.
2. Petzold A, Fraser CL, Abegg M, et al. Diagnosis and classification of optic neuritis. *Lancet Neurol.* 2022;21(12):1120–1134.
3. Balcer LJ. Clinical practice; optic neuritis. *N Engl J Med.* 2006;354(12):1273–1280.
4. Horton L, Bennett JL. Acute management of optic neuritis: an evolving paradigm. *J Neuroophthalmol.* 2018;38(3):358–367.
5. Vedula SS, Brodney-Folse S, Gal RL, et al. Corticosteroids for treating optic neuritis. *Cochrane Database Syst Rev.* 2007;(1):CD001430.
6. Keltner JL, Johnson CA, Cello KE, et al; for Optic Neuritis Study Group. Visual field profile of optic neuritis: a final follow-up report from the optic neuritis treatment trial from baseline through 15 years. *Arch Ophthalmol.* 2010;128(3):330–337.
7. Balk LJ, Cruz-Herranz A, Albrecht P, et al. Timing of retinal neuronal and axonal loss in MS: a longitudinal OCT study. *J Neurol.* 2016;263(7):1323–1331.
8. Derakhshandi H, Etemadifar M, Feizi A, et al. Preventive effect of vitamin D3 supplementation on conversion of optic neuritis to clinically definite multiple sclerosis: a double blind, randomized, placebo-controlled pilot clinical trial. *Acta Neurol Belg.* 2013;113(3):257–63.
9. Zhou S, Jones-Lopez EC, Soneji DJ, et al. Myelin oligodendrocyte glycoprotein antibody–associated optic neuritis and myelitis in COVID-19. *J Neuroophthalmol.* 2020;40(3):398–402.

SEE ALSO

Multiple Sclerosis

 CODES

ICD10
- H46.9 Unspecified optic neuritis
- H46.00 Optic papillitis, unspecified eye
- H46.10 Retrobulbar neuritis, unspecified eye

CLINICAL PEARLS
- Key features include an abrupt visual loss (typically monocular), with periorbital pain with eye movement.
- MRI is the procedure of choice for determining relative risk and possible therapy for MS prevention.
- High-dose IV methylprednisolone followed by oral prednisone accelerated visual recovery but does not improve 1-year visual outcome, whereas treatment with oral prednisone alone did not improve the outcome and was associated with an increased rate of recurrence of ON.

OSGOOD-SCHLATTER DISEASE (TIBIAL APOPHYSITIS)

David P. Sealy, MD, CAQSM, FAAFP, FAMSSM • Jacob Ringenberg, MD, CAQSM, MUSC, AHEC

BASICS

DESCRIPTION
- Osgood-Schlatter disease (OSD) is a syndrome associated with traction apophysitis and patellar tendinosis that is most common in adolescent boys and girls.
- Patients classically present with pain and swelling of the anterior tibial tubercle.
- System(s) affected: musculoskeletal
- Synonym(s): tibial tubercle apophysis

EPIDEMIOLOGY
Incidence
The incidence in girls is rising with increased participation in organized youth sports; almost equal to boys in the United States

Prevalence
- A common apophysitis in childhood and adolescence affecting athletes more frequently than nonathletes
- Estimated point prevalence of 10% in the general population aged 12 to 15 years

ETIOLOGY AND PATHOPHYSIOLOGY
Traction apophysitis of the tibial tubercle due to repetitive strain on the secondary ossification center of the tibial tuberosity; concurrent patellar tendinosis, disruption of the proximal tibial apophysis, and avulsion microfractures at the tibial tuberosity are contributing factors.
- Jumping and pivoting sports place the highest strain on the tibial tubercle. Repetitive trauma and deceleration with an eccentric load are the most likely inciting factors.
- Likely biomechanical association with tight iliopsoas, quadriceps, and hamstring muscles; increased quadriceps strength relative to hamstring strength in adolescence contributes.

RISK FACTORS
- Affects children and adolescents most commonly from the ages of 8 to 18 years
  - Girls 8 to 13 years old
  - Boys 10 to 15 years old
- OSD is slightly more common in boys than girls but likely equally common with similar sports participation.
- Early sport specialization increases the risk of OSD by 4-fold.
- Rapid skeletal growth
- Weak core stabilizing muscles
- Increased weight/BMI/height
- Patellofemoral malalignment
- Overload training volume
- Quadriceps tightness and/or shortening

- Hamstring tightness or relative weakness in ratio to the quadriceps
- Participation in repetitive-jumping sports and sports with heavy quadriceps activity (football, volleyball, basketball, hockey, soccer, skating, gymnastics)
- Ballet (2-fold risk compared with nonathletes)

GENERAL PREVENTION
- Avoid sports with heavy quadriceps loading (especially deceleration activities and eccentric loading).
- Patients may compete if pain is minimal.
- Increase hamstring and quadriceps flexibility.
- Reduce sports specialization.
- Increase cross-training.

COMMONLY ASSOCIATED CONDITIONS
- Shortened (tight) rectus femoris found in 75% with OSD
- Hamstring tightness
- Possible association with ADD/ADHD; adolescents with ADD/ADHD are at risk for other musculoskeletal injuries.
- Sinding-Larsen-Johansson apophysitis
- Calcaneal apophysitis (Sever disease)

DIAGNOSIS

HISTORY
- Unilateral or bilateral (30%) pain of the tibial tuberosity
- Pain exacerbated by exercise; particularly jumping, landing, and squatting
- Pain upon kneeling on the affected side(s)
- Antalgic or straight-legged gait
- Heavy or increasing intensity of jumping/cutting sports

PHYSICAL EXAM
- Knee pain with squatting or crouching
- Absence of effusion or condyle tenderness
- Tibial tuberosity swelling and tenderness
- Pain increased with resisted knee extension or kneeling
- Erythema over tibial tuberosity
- Hamstring/quadriceps tightness
- Core muscle weakness
- Functional testing: Single-leg squat (SLS) and standing broad jump reproduce pain.

DIFFERENTIAL DIAGNOSIS
- Stress fracture of the proximal tibia
- Pes anserinus bursitis
- Quadriceps tendon avulsion
- Patellofemoral stress syndrome

- Chondromalacia patellae (retropatellar pain)
- Proximal tibial neoplasm
- Osteomyelitis of the proximal tibia
- Tibial plateau fracture
- Sinding-Larsen-Johansson syndrome (patellar apophysitis)—pain over inferior patellar tendon
- Patellar fracture or stress fracture
- Infrapatellar bursitis
- Patellar tendinitis—pain over inferior patellar tendon and inferior pole of patella
- Osteochondroma of the tibial tubercle
- Tibial tuberosity fracture
- Patellar tendon lipoma
- Bacterial apophysitis
- Osteosynchondroses
- Osteochondritis dissecans
- Iliotibial band syndrome
- Hoffa disease (infrapatellar fat pad syndrome)
- Saphenous neuritis

DIAGNOSTIC TESTS & INTERPRETATION
Initial Tests (lab, imaging)
- Generally a clinical diagnosis; no tests are indicated unless other diagnoses are under consideration.
- Radiographic imaging of the proximal tibia and knee may show heterotopic calcification in the patellar tendon and primarily serves to rule out other pathology:
  - X-rays are rarely diagnostic, but appearance of a separate fragment at the tibial tuberosity identifies candidates for potential surgical intervention.
  - Calcified thickening of the tibial tuberosity with irregular ossification at tendon insertion on the tibial tubercle, fragmentation of the apophysis (1)[B]

Diagnostic Procedures/Other
- Bone scan may show increased uptake in the area of the tibial tuberosity:
  - Increased uptake in apophysitis is normal in children, but with OSD, there may be more uptake on the affected side.
- Ultrasound is a useful imaging modality, showing thickening of the distal patellar tendon, occasional infrapatellar bursa effusion, irregular ossification, and neovascularity of the patellar tendon insertion (1)[B].
- MRI shows fragmentation of the tibial tubercle and hyperintense T2 signal of the apophysis and patellar tendon insertion in more advanced cases.

Test Interpretation
Biopsy is not necessary but would show osteolysis and fragmentation of the tibial tubercle.

TREATMENT

GENERAL MEASURES

- No randomized controlled studies have been published to demonstrate clear benefit of any treatment over another.
- Frequent ice applications 2 to 3 times per day for 15 to 20 minutes
- Rest and activity modification—avoid activities that increase pain and/or swelling.
- Physical therapy helps with hamstring and quadriceps strengthening and stretching.
- Open- and closed-chain eccentric quadriceps strengthening
- Avoid aggressive stretching if pain is significant to avoid risk of tibial tubercle avulsion.
- Consult orthopedic surgery for tibial tuberosity fracture or complete avulsion.
- Electrical stimulation and iontophoresis have been reported (1)[B].
- Patients with marked midfoot pronation may benefit from orthotics.
- Various bracing and straps have been used including patellar straps.
- With more severe disease, longer term removal from sports may be indicated.

MEDICATION

First Line

- Common OTC analgesics may be considered.
- NSAIDs may be beneficial for pain relief.
- Opioids are not recommended as first line.

Second Line

- More potent analgesics, such as opioids, may *only* be considered for short-term use in extreme situations.
- Corticosteroid injections are not recommended.
- Hyperosmolar dextrose injections (prolotherapy) have shown benefit in randomized controlled trials (2)[B].
- Autologous conditioned platelet rich plasma have shown benefit in case studies (3)[C].

ISSUES FOR REFERRAL

When conservative therapy is unsuccessful and symptoms persist into adulthood, consider surgical referral.

SURGERY/OTHER PROCEDURES

- Débridement of a thickened, cosmetically unsatisfactory tibial tubercle (rare) or removal of mobile heterotopic bone
- Surgical excision of a painful tibial tubercle is rarely needed (<5%) and may be successfully done with bursoscopy instead of an open procedure.

- Recent report of successful pain elimination in OSD with percutaneous screw fixation of the tibial tuberosity (1)[C]
- Reduction wedge osteotomy has been recently reported as 100% successful in a small case series.

COMPLEMENTARY & ALTERNATIVE MEDICINE

Acupuncture has been used successfully as a treatment modality.

ONGOING CARE

FOLLOW-UP RECOMMENDATIONS

- Athletes may return to play if pain is controlled.
- Presence of pain does not preclude competition.

Patient Monitoring

With worsening of symptoms only

PATIENT EDUCATION

- Avoid jumping sports or reduce activities that increase pain and swelling.
- Assure patients and their family that symptoms and physical findings will diminish with time and rest.
- Patients can safely play sports with mild pain.
- Quadriceps and hamstring stretching and strengthening are important.
- Surgical options are rarely needed, but good results can be expected.

PROGNOSIS

- Usually, this is a self-limiting condition that resolves within 2 years of full skeletal maturation. However, recent data suggest that many are affected into adulthood and must reduce sports and physical activity.
- Most patients with OSD will have residual "knots" on their tibial tubercles that never completely resolve.

COMPLICATIONS

- Rarely, a heavily fragmented and inflamed tibial ossicle will avulse and require surgery.
- Although 90% are reported to resolve, recent studies suggest that chronic pain and reduction of activity may continue into adulthood.
- Rare complications in adulthood include pseudarthrosis of the tibial tubercle, genu recurvatum, patella alta, and ossicle fragmentation possibly leading to osteoarthritis of the knee.

REFERENCES

1. Ladenhauf HN, Seitlinger G, Green DW. Osgood-Schlatter disease: a 2020 update of a common knee condition in children. *Curr Opin Pediatr*. 2020;32(1):107–112.
2. Wu Z, Tu X, Tu Z. Hyperosmolar dextrose injection for Osgood-Schlatter disease: a double-blind, randomized controlled trial. *Arch Orthop Trauma Surg*. 2022;142(9):2279–2285.
3. Danneberg DJ. Successful treatment of Osgood-Schlatter disease with autologous-conditioned plasma in two patients. *Joints*. 2017;5(3):191–194.

ADDITIONAL READING

Guldhammer C, Rathleff MS, Jensen HP, et al. Long-term prognosis and impact of Osgood-Schlatter disease 4 years after diagnosis: a retrospective study. *Orthop J Sports Med*. 2019;7(10):2325967119878136.

CODES

ICD10

- M92.50 Juvenile osteochondrosis of tibia and fibula, unsp leg
- M92.51 Juvenile osteochondrosis of tibia and fibula, right leg
- M92.52 Juvenile osteochondrosis of tibia and fibula, left leg

CLINICAL PEARLS

- Infrapatellar pain in an adolescent athlete is most commonly OSD, patellar tendinosis, or Sinding-Larsen-Johansson syndrome.
- Always consider lumbar disc disease, osteogenic sarcoma, or hip pathology in the differential diagnosis of OSD.
- OSD is generally self-limited. Athletes should modify activity based on pain. Mild pain is not a contraindication to athletic participation.
- Treatment focuses on strengthening and stretching of the hamstrings and quadriceps.
- ≥10% of adolescents with OSD will be symptomatic as adults.
- Persistent employment hampering symptoms in adults often require surgical intervention.

OSTEOARTHRITIS

Patrick Wakefield Joyner, MD, MS • Frederic Baker Mills IV, MD, MS

 BASICS

DESCRIPTION
- Progressive loss of articular cartilage with reactive changes at joint margins and in subchondral bone
- Primary osteoarthritis (OA)
  - Idiopathic: categorized by clinical features (localized, generalized, erosive)
- Secondary OA
  - Posttraumatic (e.g., ACL rupture, distal radius fracture, shoulder dislocation)
  - Childhood anatomic abnormalities (e.g., congenital hip dysplasia, slipped capital femoral epiphysis [SCFE])
  - Inheritable metabolic disorders (e.g., Wilson disease, alkaptonuria, hemochromatosis)
  - Neuropathic arthropathy (Charcot joints)
  - Endocrinopathies: acromegalic arthropathy, hyperparathyroidism, hypothyroidism
  - Paget disease
  - Noninfectious inflammatory arthritis (e.g., rheumatoid arthritis [RA], spondyloarthropathies)
  - Gout, calcium pyrophosphate deposition disease (pseudogout)
- Synonym(s): osteoarthrosis; degenerative joint disease (DJD)

EPIDEMIOLOGY
- Most common joint disease in United States
- Symptomatic OA most common in patients aged >40 years
- Leading cause of disability in patients aged >65 years
- Predominant sex: male = female
- Predominantly impacts weight-bearing joints

Incidence
- Hip (symptomatic)—88 per 100,000 per year
- Knee (symptomatic)—240 per 100,000 per year

Prevalence
- >30 million patients affected in United States
- Increases with age; radiographic evidence of OA is present in many patients >65 years old.
- 16–20% of patients >65 years old have radiographic evidence of glenohumeral OA.
- Moderate to severe hip OA in 3–6% of whites; <1% in East Indians, blacks, Chinese, and Native Americans

ETIOLOGY AND PATHOPHYSIOLOGY
Failure of chondrocytes to maintain the balance between degradation and synthesis of extracellular collagen matrix. Collagen loss results in alteration of proteoglycan matrix and increased susceptibility to degenerative change.

Genetics
- Up to 65% of OA cases may have a genetic component.
- The heritability of end-stage hip OA is up to 27%.
- >100 polymorphic DNA variants have been associated with OA; these variants account for >20% OA heritability.

RISK FACTORS
- Increasing age: >50 years
- Age as a risk factor is greatest for hip, knee, and shoulder OA.

- Obesity (weight-bearing joints); BMI >35 kg/m^2
- Trauma, infection, or inflammatory arthritis
- Female gender (knee and hand)

GENERAL PREVENTION
Weight management; regular physical activity, peri-joint muscle strengthening ("prehabbing")

COMMONLY ASSOCIATED CONDITIONS
- Obesity
- History of trauma
- Shoulder arthritis can be associated with a rotator cuff tear.

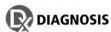 **DIAGNOSIS**

HISTORY
- Distinguish OA from other types of arthritis by:
  - Absence of systemic findings
  - Minimal articular inflammation
  - Distribution of involved joints (e.g., distal and proximal interphalangeal joints)
- OA characterized by slowly developing joint pain. Pain often described as aching or burning in nature. Anecdotally, many patients describe pain changes with alterations in weather conditions.
- Transient stiffness (especially after awakening in morning and after sitting) that tends to lessen 10 to 15 minutes after joint movement
- Most common joints in hand are as follows:
  - Distal interphalangeal > thumb carpometacarpal > PIP > MCP

PHYSICAL EXAM
- Joint bony enlargement
- Decreased range of motion of affected joints
- Mechanical symptoms (clicking, locking) may be present, especially in knees with degenerative meniscal injury.
- Meniscus tear in the setting of severe/end-stage knee OA is an OA problem and should be treated as an OA ailment in the absence of the mechanical symptoms.
- Local pain and stiffness with OA of spine; radicular pain (if compression of nerve roots)
- Changes in joint alignment (genu varum [bowlegs] and genu valgum [knock-knees])

DIFFERENTIAL DIAGNOSIS
- Crystalline arthropathies (gout; pseudogout): inflammatory arthritides (RA), spondyloarthropathies (reactive arthritis; psoriatic arthritis), septic arthritis
- Fibromyalgia; avascular necrosis; Lyme disease

DIAGNOSTIC TESTS & INTERPRETATION
Initial Tests (lab, imaging)
- Routine chemistries are not helpful in diagnosis.
- X-rays are usually normal early in disease process.
- As OA progresses, plain films show:
  - Narrowed, asymmetric joint space, osteophyte formation, subchondral bony sclerosis, subchondral cyst formation
- MRI may particularly demonstrate chondral degeneration and associated meniscal tears. 5–10% weight loss is associated with slowing of arthritic changes and decreased chondral loss on follow-up studies, subchondral bone edema.

Follow-Up Tests & Special Considerations
- Monitor treatment with NSAIDs (renal insufficiency and GI bleeding).
- In secondary OA, abnormal lab results associated with underlying disorder (e.g., hemochromatosis [abnormal iron studies])

Diagnostic Procedures/Other
Joint aspiration (not usually necessary for diagnosis)
- OA: cell count usually <500 cells/mm^3, predominantly mononuclear
- Inflammatory: cell count usually >2,000 cells/mm^3, predominantly neutrophils
- Birefringent crystals in gout (−) and pseudogout (+)

Test Interpretation
- Patchy cartilage damage and bony hypertrophy
- Histologic phases:
  - Extracellular matrix edema and cartilage microfissures, subchondral fissuring and pitting, erosion and formation of osteocartilaginous loose bodies
- Subchondral bone trabecular microfractures and sclerosis with osteophyte formation

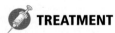 **TREATMENT**

GENERAL MEASURES
- Weight management combined with exercise/physical therapy to maintain or regain joint motion and muscle strength
  - Quadriceps strengthening for knee OA—closed not open chain exercises
  - Periscapular strengthening and range of motion for shoulder OA
  - Abductor and core strengthening as well as gait mechanics for hip OA
- Transition to non–weight-bearing exercises (i.e., elliptical, stationary bike, swimming)
- Exercise must be maintained; benefits are lost 6 months after exercise cessation.
- Bracing, joint supports, or insoles in patients with biomechanical instability:
  - Bracing is more beneficial in patients with unicompartmental disease of the knee.
- For knee OA in particular, several nonpharmacologic modalities are strongly recommended: aerobic, aquatic, and/or resistance exercise and weight loss.

MEDICATION
First Line
- Weight management
  - 1 lb of weight loss reduces pressure on lower extremities by ~4 lb.
- Manage pain and inflammation:
  - Acetaminophen up to 1,000 mg TID: effective for pain relief in OA of knee and hip
  - Topical NSAID gels, creams have short-term (<4 weeks) benefits. Topical NSAIDs are a core treatment for hand and joints with minimal soft tissue–coverage (i.e., elbow, ankle, AC joint) OA.

– If acetaminophen or topical NSAIDs are insufficient, consider an oral NSAID/COX-2 inhibitor. Use the lowest effective dose for the shortest time possible.

– May use nonacetylated salicylates (e.g., salsalate, choline magnesium salicylate) or low-dose ibuprofen ≤1,600 mg/day. Consider a once-daily NSAID, if necessary, to help maintain compliance.

ALERT
NSAIDs are associated with an increased risk of adverse cardiovascular events. The absolute risk is dependent on patient age, comorbidities, particular NSAID used, dose, and duration of use.

- All PO NSAIDs/COX-2 inhibitors have analgesic effects of a similar magnitude but vary in their potential GI and cardiorenal toxicity. Avoid NSAIDs in patients with renal disease, CHF, HTN, active peptic ulcer disease, and previous hypersensitivity to an NSAID or aspirin. Combination of NSAIDs and full-strength aspirin (325 mg) is contraindicated. In patients at high cardiovascular risk: Combination of a nonselective NSAID and low-dose aspirin (81 mg) is recommended. Oral or parenteral corticosteroids are contraindicated.
- Precautions:
  – If PO NSAID/COX-2 inhibitor use is necessary for a patient aged >65 years or a patient <65 years with increased GI bleeding risk factors, proton pump inhibitors are recommended.
  – Significant possible interactions:
    ○ NSAIDs reduce effectiveness of ACE inhibitors and diuretics. Aspirin and NSAIDs (except COX-2 inhibitors) may increase effects of anticoagulants. Salicylates reduce effectiveness of spironolactone (Aldactone) and uricosurics. Corticosteroids and some antacids increase salicylate excretion, whereas ascorbic acid and ammonium chloride reduce salicylate excretion and may cause toxicity.

Pregnancy Considerations
- ASA and NSAIDs have reported fetal risk during 1st and 3rd trimesters of pregnancy.
- Compatible with breastfeeding

Second Line
- Topical NSAIDs, CBD, and capsaicin can lower gastric and renal risks associated with oral NSAIDs.
- Bracing; medial and lateral unloader braces are effective; long leg alignment x-rays can help determine the appropriate brace.
- TENS modalities for pain may be more beneficial than hyaluronic acid (HA) injection.

Third Line
- Intra-auricular corticosteroid injections can be used for acute flares and for patients failing first- and second-line treatments. Minimize injections (≤3 per joint per year).
- Platelet-rich plasma (PRP) for patients with mild to moderate OA and patellofemoral OA

- In selected patients, PRP and Bone Marrow Aspirate Concentrate (BMAC) are equivalent in providing better and longer outcomes than HA injections alone (1).
- Biologic injections demonstrate no difference in patient outcome in knee OA when compared to saline injections, in patients with severe OA (complete loss of joint space on X-ray, bone on bone).
- Cryotherapy with physical therapy is better than physical therapy alone for knee arthritis (1).

ISSUES FOR REFERRAL
Disease that fails conservative management. Concern for a septic joint or gout. Musculoskeletal injury as a result of OA

ADDITIONAL THERAPIES
Address psychosocial factors (i.e., self-efficacy, coping skills). Screen for and appropriately treat anxiety and depression. Improve social support.

SURGERY/OTHER PROCEDURES
- Total knee arthroplasty (TKA); total hip arthroplasty (THA), total shoulder arthroplasty (TSA), reverse total shoulder arthroplasty (RTSA), and total ankle arthroplasty (TAA) all remain options for patients that fail conservative management for these respective joints. Total elbow arthroplasty (TEA) carries the highest complication and failure rate. TEA also results in lifelong weightbearing limitation of 5 lb.
- Ligament reconstruction and tendon interposition (LRTI) is an option for patients failing conservative treatment of the carpo-metacarpal joints.
- Knee arthroscopy is not routinely recommended for the treatment of OA in the absence of clear mechanical symptoms (i.e., locking, clicking, etc.).
- Patients possible too young for TKA can consider an osteotomy, or unicompartmental knee arthroplasty (UKA)

COMPLEMENTARY & ALTERNATIVE MEDICINE
- Nutritional supplements (glucosamine and chondroitin sulfate) may benefit some patients and have low toxicity. There is lack of standardized outcome assessments. Trial results using glucosamine and chondroitin have been mixed. If no response is apparent within 6 months, discontinue use.
- TENS, yoga, and acupuncture have shown benefit.

 ## ONGOING CARE

FOLLOW-UP RECOMMENDATIONS
- Follow-up at 3-month intervals for assessment of conservative management treatment and future options
- Recommend plain films of effected joint annually.

Patient Monitoring
Regularly assess range of motion and functional status. Monitor for GI blood loss and cardiac, renal, and mental status in older patients on NSAIDs or aspirin; periodic CBC, renal function tests, stool for occult blood in patients on chronic NSAID therapy

DIET
Continue to ensure patients have adequate Vitamin D intake and levels to maximize bone health.

PATIENT EDUCATION
- American College of Rheumatology: https://www.rheumatology.org/I-Am-A/Patient -Caregiver/Diseases-Conditions/Osteoarthritis
- Arthritis Foundation: http://www.arthritis.org

PROGNOSIS
- Progressive and chronic disease: early in course, pain relieved by rest; later, pain may persist at rest and at night.
- Joint effusions and enlargement may occur (especially in knees) as disease progresses.
- Osteophyte (spur) formation, especially at joint margins

COMPLICATIONS
- Leading cause of musculoskeletal pain and disability
- Decompensated CHF, GI bleeding, decreased renal function on chronic NSAID or aspirin therapy

REFERENCE
1. Belk JW, Lim JJ, Keeter C, et al. Patients with knee osteoarthritis who receive platelet-rich plasma or bone marrow aspirate concentrate injections have better outcomes than patients who receive hyaluronic acid: systematic review and meta-analysis. *Arthroscopy*. 2023;39(7):1714–1734.

CODES

ICD10
- M19.239 Secondary osteoarthritis, unspecified wrist
- M19.9 Osteoarthritis, unspecified site
- M19.212 Secondary osteoarthritis, left shoulder

CLINICAL PEARLS
- Patients with OA typically have morning stiffness lasting for <15 minutes.
- OA most commonly affects the hips, knees, and hands (proximal interphalangeal and distal interphalangeal joints).
- NSAID use is associated with increased risk of cardiovascular events.
- If used, intra-articular steroid injections should be limited to no more than 2 per joint per year.
- Biologics are (higher cost) options for early-stage knee OA.
- PRP and BMAC appear to be better options than HA alone in patients with mild to moderate OA.
- Long-term OA therapy is individualized to patient pain management and activity goals.

OSTEOMYELITIS
Andrew McBride, MD

BASICS

DESCRIPTION
- An acute or chronic bone infection with associated inflammation; can occur as a result of hematogenous seeding, contiguous spread of infection, or direct inoculation into intact bone (trauma or surgery)
- Two major classification systems:
  - Lew and Waldvogel classification: classified according to duration (acute or chronic) and source of infection (hematogenous or contiguous)
  - Cierny-Mader classification: based on the portion of bone affected, physiologic status of the host, and risk factors
- Special situations
  - Vertebral osteomyelitis
    - Results from hematogenous seeding (most common), direct inoculation, or contiguous spread; back pain is the most common initial symptom. Lumbar spine is the most commonly involved, followed by thoracic spine.
  - Prosthetic joint infections
    - X-ray and three-phase bone scan; MRI/CT is of limited use with prostheses.
  - Posttraumatic infections
    - Risk factors include type and severity of fracture as well as contamination. Tibia is the most common location.

EPIDEMIOLOGY
- More common in older adults; predominant sex: male > female
- Hematogenous osteomyelitis
  - Adults (mostly >50 years of age): vertebral
  - Children: long bones
- Contiguous osteomyelitis: related to diabetic foot infections (DFIs), decubitus ulcers, and infected total joint arthroplasties in older adults; trauma and surgery in younger adults
- *Mycobacterium tuberculosis* (MTB) is the most common cause of vertebral osteomyelitis worldwide. It is more likely to involve multiple vertebral bodies—especially of the thoracic spine—and is associated with paraspinal abscess formation.

Incidence
Generally low; normal bone is resistant to infection. The incidence of vertebral osteomyelitis has been estimated at 2.4 cases per 100,000 population, with an increasing incidence with advancing age.

Prevalence
Up to 66% of diabetics with foot ulcerations

ETIOLOGY AND PATHOPHYSIOLOGY
- Acute: suppurative infection of bone with edema and vascular compromise leading to sequestrum (segments of necrotic bone, may contain pus)
- Chronic: presence of necrotic bone or sequestrum or recurrence of previous infection
- Hematogenous osteomyelitis (typically monomicrobial)
  - *Staphylococcus aureus* (most common); coagulase-negative staphylococci and aerobic gram-negative bacteria; *Pseudomonas aeruginosa* (intravenous [IV] drug user); *Salmonella* sp. (sickle cell disease); MTB and fungal (rare; in endemic areas or in immunocompromised hosts)
- Contiguous focus osteomyelitis (polymicrobial)
  - Diabetes or vascular insufficiency
    - Coagulase-positive and coagulase-negative staphylococci; streptococci, gram-negative bacilli, anaerobes (*Peptostreptococcus* sp.)
  - Sacral decubitus ulcer
    - Pressure-related skin ulceration and necrosis
  - Puncture wound through shoe
    - *P. aeruginosa*
- Prosthetic device
  - Coagulase-negative staphylococci and *S. aureus*

RISK FACTORS
- Diabetes mellitus (particularly, diabetic foot ulcer); recent trauma/surgery; foreign body (e.g., prosthetic implant)
- Neuropathy and vascular insufficiency; immunosuppression (including dialysis); sickle cell disease; injection drug use; previous osteomyelitis; bacteremia

GENERAL PREVENTION
- Comprehensive annual foot exam for diabetic patients; screen for peripheral artery disease; optimize glycemic control in diabetes.
- Antibiotic prophylaxis for posttraumatic infection
  - Clean bone surgery
    - Administer IV antibiotics within an hour of skin incision, keep at therapeutic level throughout surgery, and continue ≤24 hours postprocedure.
  - Closed fractures
    - Cefazolin, cefuroxime, clindamycin (β-lactam allergy), or vancomycin (β-lactam allergy or MRSA infection)
  - Open fractures
    - In patients who can receive antibiotics within 3 hours of injury with prompt operative treatment, 1st-generation cephalosporins are preferred (clindamycin or vancomycin if allergic); ceftriaxone for type III fractures; add metronidazole if associated with soil or fecal matter contamination.

DIAGNOSIS

HISTORY
- Fever, chills, pain, swelling, and erythema, particularly in acute osteomyelitis. These features may be absent in chronic osteomyelitis.
- Hematogenous osteomyelitis
  - Elicit a history of conditions predisposing to bacteremia (diabetes, hemodialysis, invasive procedures, IV drug use, immunosuppression).
- Contiguous osteomyelitis and vascular insufficiency
  - Recent trauma/surgery within 1 to 2 months; presence of prosthetic device; history of diabetes/DFI
- Chronic osteomyelitis
  - History of acute osteomyelitis; draining sinus tract

PHYSICAL EXAM
- Fever, restricted range of motion, tenderness, signs of localized inflammation. Motor and sensory deficits can be seen with vertebral infection in 1/3 of patients. Exposed bone in the setting of DFI is highly suspicious.
- Classic signs and symptoms of infection may be masked in diabetics due to vascular disease and neuropathy.

DIFFERENTIAL DIAGNOSIS
Systemic infection from other source, aseptic bone infarction, localized inflammation or infection of overlying skin and soft tissues (e.g., gout), Brodie abscess (subacute osteomyelitis), neuropathic joint disease (Charcot foot), fractures/trauma, tumor

DIAGNOSTIC TESTS & INTERPRETATION
Initial Tests (lab, imaging)
Labs
- WBC is not reliable (can be normal or elevated) (1).
- A normocytic normochromic anemia may be present in chronic cases (1).
- CRP is usually elevated (nonspecific). ESR is high in most cases:
  - ESR >70 mm/hr increases likelihood >10-fold.
- Procalcitonin may also be elevated.
- For vertebral/hematogenous osteomyelitis, definitive diagnosis is made by vertebral disc aspiration or blood culture.
- Patients with positive blood cultures (with a pathogen likely to cause vertebral/hematogenous osteomyelitis) and with radiographic evidence of osteomyelitis do not need bone biopsy. Antibiotics given prior to culture may alter results.
- Immunosuppression (including diabetes), chronic inflammatory disease, and other sites of infection may alter lab results.
- Routine radiography is first-line imaging: Classic triad for osteomyelitis is demineralization, periosteal reaction, and bone destruction:
  - Bone destruction is not apparent on plain films until after 10 to 21 days of infection.
  - Bone scan is first test after plain x-ray for evaluation of prosthesis-related infection.
- Radionuclide scanning (e.g., technetium, indium, or gallium) helps if diagnosis is ambiguous or unsure of extent of disease; limited by low sensitivity/specificity
- MRI
  - Best for visualization of septic arthritis, spinal infection, and DFI
  - T1-weighted image: low signal intensity; T2-weighted image: high signal intensity; MRI: sensitivity 90% and specificity 80% for osteomyelitis in diabetic foot ulcers
  - Not as accurate for diagnosis of osteomyelitis with presence of Charcot neuroarthropathy joint disease or after recent surgery
  - MRI does not help assess the response to therapy due to persistence of bony edema.
- CT
  - Better than standard radiography to evaluate bony fragments and sequestration; inferior to MRI for soft tissue and bone marrow assessment

Follow-Up Tests & Special Considerations
- A persistently elevated CRP (4 to 6 weeks) can be associated with osteomyelitis but is nonspecific. CRP decreases faster than ESR, but a decrease in ESR after treatment is a good prognostic sign.
- Monitor patients receiving prolonged antimicrobial therapy with weekly labs.

Diagnostic Procedures/Other

- Probe-to-bone test in DFI has high pooled sensitivity and specificity for osteomyelitis of 0.87 (95% CI 0.75–0.93) and 0.83 (95% CI 0.65–0.93), respectively.
- A probe-to-bone test can be used to help diagnose osteomyelitis. A sterile blunt metal instrument deep in the wound—positive if a hard gritty sensation is felt.
- Ulcer >2-cm wide and >2-cm deep increases likelihood for osteomyelitis in DFI.
- Positive probe-to-bone test and ulcer area >2 cm^2 are physical exam findings that best support osteomyelitis in the setting of DFI.
- Bone biopsy
  - For contiguous osteomyelitis, definitive diagnosis is made by bone biopsy for culture and histology.
  - Avoid wound swabs or needle aspiration in DFI and decubitus ulcers because these do not correlate well with bone biopsy culture (1)[A].
  - Can obtain bone biopsy at same time as surgical débridement

Test Interpretation
Pathology of bone revealing inflammatory process with pyogenic bacteria and necrosis is diagnostic.

 TREATMENT

GENERAL MEASURES
Adequate nutrition, smoking cessation, glycemic control, foot care, IV drug use cessation

MEDICATION
- In clinically stable patients, delay initiation of empiric antibiotics until biopsy and/or blood cultures have been obtained.
- Direct empiric therapy toward probable organism and tailor according to culture results. Optimal antimicrobial concentration at infected site is essential (consider vascular perfusion). Adjust antibiotic dosing according to renal function.
- 4 to 6 weeks of therapy is appropriate for most cases of acute osteomyelitis. In the setting of amputation or complete removal of infected bone, a 2-week course of pathogen-directed antibiotics may be adequate (1)[C].
- Uncomplicated acute hematogenous vertebral osteomyelitis can be treated with 6 weeks of antibiotics.
- If a prosthetic joint or other orthopedic hardware cannot be removed or is completely débrided, a prolonged 6-week course of parenteral antibiotics is indicated.
- Consider longer treatment courses for chronic osteomyelitis or MRSA infection (minimum of 8 weeks).
- Empiric therapy:
  - For vertebral/hematogenous osteomyelitis, include coverage for MRSA and gram-negative organisms.
  - IV vancomycin plus 3rd- or 4th-generation IV cephalosporin +/− metronidazole for DFI/contiguous osteomyelitis

First Line
- *S. aureus* or coagulase-negative staphylococci
  - MSSA: β-lactam at high dose (nafcillin or oxacillin 2 g IV q4h) *or* cefazolin 1 to 2 g IV q8h (use 2 g for patients >80 kg)
  - MRSA: vancomycin 15 to 20 mg/kg IV q8–12h (use q8h interval if CrCl >70 mL/min) with target trough of 15 to 20 μg/mL, not to exceed 2 g/dose
- *Streptococcus* sp.
  - Ceftriaxone 2 g IV q24h or cefazolin 2 g IV q8h
- *Enterobacter* sp.
  - Ciprofloxacin 750 mg PO q12h (or 400 mg IV q12h) or cefepime 2 g IV q12h
- *P. aeruginosa*
  - Cefepime 2 g IV q8h or ciprofloxacin 750 mg PO q12h (or 400 mg IV q8h)

Second Line
- *S. aureus*
  - MSSA: ceftriaxone 2 g IV q24h
  - MRSA: linezolid 600 mg PO/IV q12h *or* daptomycin 6 mg/kg IV q24h
- *Streptococcus* sp.
  - Penicillin G 4 million U q4–6h
- *P. aeruginosa*
  - Piperacillin-tazobactam 3.375 g IV q6h

> **ALERT**
> The combination of vancomycin plus piperacillin-tazobactam can increase risk of acute renal failure (number needed to harm = 11).

ADDITIONAL THERAPIES
Recent studies have demonstrated that there may be benefit of hyperbaric oxygen therapy in the management of chronic osteomyelitis.

SURGERY/OTHER PROCEDURES
- Surgical drainage, minimizing dead space, adequate soft tissue coverage, restoration of blood supply, and removal of necrotic tissues improve cure rates. Surgery indicated with presence of neurologic symptoms or infection of spinal implant; surgical débridement to healthy bone and/or soft tissue coverage/surgical flap (1)[C].
- Evidence suggests antibiotics alone may be sufficient for DFI.
- Use of antibiotic-loaded cement or antibiotic coated polymethyl methacrylate cement beads for patients with vascular insufficiency to manage dead space and help control the infection.

ADMISSION, INPATIENT, AND NURSING CONSIDERATIONS
- Off-load pressure
- Discharge criteria: clinical and laboratory evidence of resolving infection and appropriate outpatient therapy

 ONGOING CARE

FOLLOW-UP RECOMMENDATIONS
Patient Monitoring
Antimicrobial levels, ESR, CRP, and repeat plain radiography as clinical course dictate; CRP correlates better with clinical response than ESR.

DIET
Glycemic control for diabetics; proper nutrition for malnourished patients

PATIENT EDUCATION
Diabetic glycemic control and foot care; IV drug use cessation

PROGNOSIS
- Superficial and medullary osteomyelitis treated with antimicrobial and surgical therapy have a response rate of 90–100%.
- Up to 36% recurrence rate in diabetics; increased mortality after amputation

COMPLICATIONS
- Abscess formation; bacteremia; fracture/nonunion; loosening of prosthetic implant; postoperative infection
- Sinus tract formation can be associated with neoplasms (e.g., Marjolin ulcer), especially in presence of long-standing infection.

REFERENCE
1. Schmitt SK. Osteomyelitis. *Infect Dis Clin North Am*. 2017;31(2):325–338.

 CODES

ICD10
- M86.03 Acute hematogenous osteomyelitis, radius and ulna
- M86.032 Acute hematogenous osteomyelitis, left radius and ulna
- M86.01 Acute hematogenous osteomyelitis, shoulder

CLINICAL PEARLS
- Hematogenous osteomyelitis is usually monomicrobial. Osteomyelitis due to contiguous spread or direct inoculation is usually polymicrobial.
- Pain associated with acute osteomyelitis is typically gradual in onset.
- Treatment of chronic osteomyelitis often requires both surgical débridement and ≥6 weeks of antimicrobial therapy.
- Unlike diabetic foot ulcers, a positive probe-to-bone test (or frankly exposed bone) and abnormal MRI findings are not diagnostic of osteomyelitis in stage IV sacral pressure ulcers. Definitive treatment of osteomyelitis in stage IV sacral pressure ulcers often requires surgical débridement to healthy bone.
- Follow-up MRI is not needed for patients who are clinically improving with appropriate treatment.
- In diabetic foot wounds with no signs or symptoms of soft tissue or bone infection, antibiotic therapy is unnecessary.

OSTEOPOROSIS AND OSTEOPENIA

Ramanpreet Grewal, MD

 BASICS

DESCRIPTION
A metabolic bone disease characterized by low bone mass, with deterioration of bone microarchitecture leading to compromised bone strength and increased risk of fragility fracture

EPIDEMIOLOGY
Prevalence
- 10.2 million Americans have osteoporosis (1).
- >43.3 million Americans have low bone mass (1).
- Women >50 years of age: osteoporosis 19.6% and osteopenia 51.5%
- Men >50 years of age: osteoporosis 4.4% and osteopenia 33.5%

ETIOLOGY AND PATHOPHYSIOLOGY
Imbalance between bone resorption and formation results in a net loss of bone mass and density over time, leading to weakened and porous bones.

Genetics
- Familial predisposition
- More common in Caucasians and Asians than in African Americans and Hispanics

COMMONLY ASSOCIATED CONDITIONS
- Malabsorption syndromes: gastrectomy, inflammatory bowel disease, celiac disease
- Hypoestrogenism: menopause, hypogonadism, eating disorders, etc.
- Endocrinopathies: hyperparathyroidism, hyperthyroidism, hypercortisolism, diabetes mellitus
- Hematologic disorders: sickle cell disease, multiple myeloma, thalassemia, hemochromatosis
- Many other chronic diseases including end-stage renal disease
- Medications: chemotherapy agents, antiepileptics, aromatase inhibitors (raloxifene), chronic corticosteroids (equivalent to at least 5 mg of prednisone daily for at least 3 months), medroxyprogesterone acetate, heparin, SSRIs, thyroid hormone (in supraphysiologic doses), PPIs

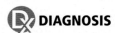 DIAGNOSIS

HISTORY
- Review modifiable (smoking, excessive alcohol intake, physical inactivity, and poor nutrition) and nonmodifiable (age, gender, race, and family history) risk factors.
- History of fragility fracture
- Online risk factor assessment tool (FRAX): https://www.shef.ac.uk/FRAX/
- Assess for commonly associated conditions.

PHYSICAL EXAM
- Thoracic kyphosis (stooped posture) and rounded shoulders also known as "Dowager hump"
- Poor balance, deconditioning (loss of strength and mobility)
- Historical height loss >4 cm (difference between current height and peak height at age 20 years)
- Prospective height loss >2 cm (difference between current height and previously documented height)

DIFFERENTIAL DIAGNOSIS
- Primary hyperparathyroidism
- Multiple myeloma/other neoplasms
- Paget's disease of bone

DIAGNOSTIC TESTS & INTERPRETATION
Initial Tests (lab, imaging)
- Dual energy x-ray absorptiometry (DEXA) of the lumbar spine/hip is considered the gold standard for measuring BMD and for diagnosing osteoporosis. BMD is expressed in terms of T-scores and Z-scores:
  - T-Score: The T-score compares an individual's BMD to that of healthy young adult of the same sex. The World Health Organization (WHO) criteria classify bone health based on T-scores:
    - T-score between +1 and −1: normal bone density
    - T-score between −1 and −2.5: osteopenia (low bone density)
    - T-score ≤ −2.5: Osteoporosis
  - Z-Score: The Z-score compares BMD to an age-matched group of individuals of the same sex. A Z-score < −2 SD may indicate secondary causes of bone loss, such as underlying medical conditions or medications.
- A minimum of 2 years is needed to reliably measure a change in BMD.
- Trabecular bone score (TBS) can stratify those with osteopenic range BMD.
- Initial laboratory tests:
  - Complete chemistry profile (including calcium, phosphorus, alkaline phosphatase)
  - Complete blood count
  - 25-hydroxyvitamin D
- Plain radiographs lack sensitivity to diagnose osteoporosis, but an abnormality (e.g., widened intervertebral spaces, rib fractures, vertebral compression fractures) should prompt evaluation.

Follow-Up Tests & Special Considerations
Consider further lab work based on initial evaluation, Z-score ≤ −2.5 or young age:
- 24-hour urine for calcium, creatinine, and free cortisol
- Serum and urine protein electrophoresis
- Follicle-stimulating hormone (FSH), luteinizing hormone (LH), prolactin
- Magnesium, 1,25-dihydroxyvitamin D
- Intact parathyroid hormone (PTH), thyroid-stimulating hormone (TSH)
- Celiac screen
- Erythrocyte sedimentation rate, rheumatoid factor
- Ferritin and carotene levels; iron and total iron binding capacity
- Serum tryptase and histamine levels, homocysteine
- Skin biopsy for connective tissue disorders
- Consider bone marrow biopsy.

 TREATMENT

- Treatment involves lifestyle modifications (weight-bearing exercise, resistance training, balanced diet, avoiding smoking and excessive alcohol), calcium and vitamin D supplements, medications, and fall prevention.
- The treatment of osteopenia aims to slow down bone loss, increase bone density, and reduce the risk of developing osteoporosis.
- Criteria for patients who benefit from treatment for their osteoporosis include the following:
  - Patient's T-score ≤ −2.5 with no risk factors
  - All postmenopausal women and men >50 years old with history of fracture of vertebrae (clinical or subclinical), hip, wrist, pelvis, or humerus
  - All postmenopausal women who have BMD values consistent with osteoporosis (T-score ≤2.5) at the lumbar spine, femoral neck, or total hip region
  - Postmenopausal women and men aged >50 years with osteopenia (i.e., T-score between −1 and −2.5) at the femoral neck or spine and a 10-year probability of hip fracture ≥3% or a 10-year probability of any major osteoporosis-related fracture ≥20% based on the United States–adapted WHO algorithm

MEDICATION
1,200 mg of calcium (total of diet and supplement) and at least 800 international units of vitamin D daily

First Line
Bisphosphonates:
- Inhibit bone resorption by osteoclasts in skeletal tissue, reducing the incidence of vertebral and nonvertebral fractures
  - Alendronate 10 mg PO daily or 70 mg PO weekly
  - Risedronate 5 mg PO daily, 35 mg PO weekly, or 150 mg PO monthly
  - Zoledronic acid 5 mg IV yearly or 5 mg IV every 18 months
- For primary prevention, zoledronate (once every 18 month) reduced both vertebral (RR 0.46, 95% CI 0.28–0.74) and nonvertebral (HR 0.66, 95% CI 0.51–0.85) fractures (2)[A].
- For secondary prevention of mild/moderate osteoporosis, oral bisphosphonates are preferred (2)[A].
- Side effects include esophagitis and gastritis.
- Osteonecrosis of the jaw is a risk, primarily seen in patients with cancer who receive high doses and those who receive IV treatment (3).
- There is a possible risk of atypical femur fractures in patients receiving bisphosphonates for >5 years (4)[A].
- Avoid oral bisphosphonates in patients with:
  - Delayed esophageal emptying
  - Inability to stand/sit upright for at least 30 to 60 minutes after taking the bisphosphonates
  - Hypocalcemia (Correct prior to initiating therapy.)
  - Severe renal impairment (creatinine clearance [CrCl] ≤30 for risedronate and ≤35 mL/min for alendronate and zoledronic acid)

Second Line

- Monoclonal antibody therapy:
  - Denosumab 60 mg SC every 6 months
    - Human monoclonal antibody receptor activator of nuclear factor κ-B ligand (RANKL) receptor, blocking, inhibiting osteoclast formation and decreasing bone resorption
    - Can be considered as an initial therapy option if higher fracture risk or not candidates for an oral bisphosphonate and is the agent of choice in patients with renal insufficiency (4)[B]
    - Side effects can include dermatologic reactions, musculoskeletal pain, hypocalcemia, and less commonly osteonecrosis of the jaw, atypical femur fracture, and serious infections.
    - Potentially, an increased risk for rebound bone turnover following discontinuation; therefore, consideration of subsequent bisphosphonate or alternative therapy is recommended.
  - Romosozumab 210 mg (split in two separate injections) once monthly
    - Monoclonal antibody that inhibits sclerostin, leading to increased bone formation
    - Romosozumab therapy (12 months) followed by alendronate for women with severe osteoporosis or at high risk for fractures (2)[B]
    - May increase risk of adverse cardiovascular events (pairing with a bisphosphonate may reduce this risk)
- Recombinant formulations of PTH—anabolic agents that stimulate bone through osteoblastic activation:
  - Preferred in severe osteoporosis patients due to their capability of reducing fracture risk more quickly
    - Teriparatide 20 mg SC daily
      - Use is limited to high risk for fractures (or previous therapy unsuccessful) as only approved for use up to 2 years in duration (4)[B]
      - Bone loss may rapidly occur after discontinuation; therefore, sequential therapy with antiresorptive agent (bisphosphonate) is recommended (2)[A].
    - Abaloparatide 80 μg SC daily
      - Similar safety profile to teriparatide

ISSUES FOR REFERRAL

- Endocrinology referral for severe disease, young age of onset, rapid bone loss, poor response to treatment
- Dental referral for oral examinations

ADDITIONAL THERAPIES

- Calcitonin: although not commonly used can help reduce bone breakdown and pain in some cases
- Hormone replacement therapy (HRT): Consider for select cases in postmenopausal women.

SURGERY/OTHER PROCEDURES

Surgical options for compression fractures:

- Vertebroplasty: Orthopedic cement is injected into the compressed vertebral body.
- Kyphoplasty: A balloon is expanded within the compressed vertebral body; cement is injected.

COMPLEMENTARY & ALTERNATIVE MEDICINE

- Acupuncture may help manage pain associated with osteoporosis.
- Yoga and tai chi can improve balance, strength, and flexibility, which may reduce the risk of falls and fractures.

 ONGOING CARE

- Regular bone density monitoring, medication management, lifestyle modifications, fall prevention strategies, nutritional support, and patient education to optimize bone health and reduce fracture risk
- The duration of medication therapy is determined based on treatment guidelines and involves shared decision-making with the patient, considering the balance between treatment benefits and potential risks.

FOLLOW-UP RECOMMENDATIONS
Patient Monitoring

- Yearly height measurement assists treatment efficacy. Patients who lose >2 cm in height should have a repeat vertebral imaging (5).
- Most recommendations suggest repeating a DEXA scan to assess BMD 2 years after starting bisphosphonate therapy.
- Perform a risk assessment after 3 to 5 years of treatment. If BMD T-score at the hip is ≥2.5 and there has not been a hip or vertebral fracture, consider stopping treatment. If BMD remains low or high risk for fractures, the patient may benefit by continuing treatment >5 years (6)[B].
- Patients on bisphosphonates for 5 years (3 years of IV of zoledronic acid) and if a stable BMD, no prior fracture, and a low risk for fracture, can be considered for a drug holiday (4)[B]
- Patients on bisphosphonates for 5 years at high fracture risk (prior fragility fracture, older age, frailty, and high fall risk) should be continued on therapy and a drug holiday can be reconsidered after 6 to 10 years (4)[B].
- Physicians prescribing bisphosphonates should advise patients of the small risk of osteonecrosis of the jaw and encourage dental examinations (6)[C].

DIET

- Calcium-rich foods: dairy products like milk, yogurt, and cheese; fortified plant milks (soy, almond, oat) for lactose intolerant or plant-based options; leafy greens such as kale, collard greens, and spinach
- Vitamin D sources: fatty fish (salmon, mackerel), egg yolks, and fortified cereals
- Limit sodium and caffeine: Excessive sodium intake can lead to calcium loss from bones. Excessive caffeine consumption can interfere with calcium absorption.
- Moderate alcohol consumption: Excessive alcohol consumption can weaken bones and increase fracture risk.

PATIENT EDUCATION

- Bone Health & Osteoporosis Foundation: https://www.bonehealthandosteoporosis.org/about-us/about-bhof/
- International Osteoporosis Foundation: https://www.osteoporosis.foundation/educational-hub/topic/calcium-calculator

PROGNOSIS

- With treatment, 80% increase bone mass and mobility and have reduced pain.
- 15% of vertebral and 20–40% of hip fractures may lead to chronic care and/or premature death.

COMPLICATIONS

- Recurrent fractures (spine, hips, wrists, ribs)
- Chronic back pain and loss of height
- Reduced mobility and muscle weakness
- Decreased quality of life and independence
- Hospitalization and surgical interventions
- Higher mortality risk, especially with hip fractures

REFERENCES

1. Sarafrazi N, Wambogo EA, Shepherd JA. Osteoporosis or low bone mass in older adults: United States, 2017–2018. *NCHS Data Brief*. 2021;(405):1–8.
2. Wen F, Du H, Ding L, et al. Clinical efficacy and safety of drug interventions for primary and secondary prevention of osteoporotic fractures in postmenopausal woman: network meta-analysis followed by factor and cluster analysis. *PLoS ONE*. 2020;15(6):e0234123.
3. Zhou J, Ma X, Wang T, et al. Comparative efficacy of bisphosphonates in short-term fracture prevention for primary osteoporosis: a systematic review with network meta-analyses. *Osteoporos Int*. 2016;27(11):3289–3300.
4. Anthamatten A, Parish A. Clinical update on osteoporosis. *J Midwifery Womens Health*. 2019;64(3):265–275.
5. Qaseem A, Forciea MA, McLean RM, et al; for Clinical Guidelines Committee of the American College of Physicians. Treatment of low bone density or osteoporosis to prevent fractures in men and women: a clinical practice guideline update from the American College of Physicians. *Ann Intern Med*. 2017;166(11):818–839.
6. McClung M, Harris ST, Miller PD, et al. Bisphosphonate therapy for osteoporosis: benefits, risks, and drug holiday. *Am J Med*. 2013;126(1):13–20.

ADDITIONAL READING

Camacho PM, Petak SM, Binkley N, et al. American Association of Clinical Endocrinologists/American College of Endocrinology clinical practice guidelines for the diagnosis and treatment of postmenopausal osteoporosis—2020 update. *Endocrine Pract*. 2020;26(Suppl 1):1–46.

 CODES

ICD10

- M85.80 Other specified disorders of bone density and structure, unspecified site
- M81.0 Age-related osteoporosis w/o current pathological fracture
- M80.00XA Age-rel osteopor w current path fracture, unsp site, init

CLINICAL PEARLS

Choosing Wisely recommendations related to osteoporosis:

- Don't do DEXA screening for osteoporosis in women aged <65 years or men aged <70 years with no risk factors.
- Don't routinely repeat DEXA scans more often than once every 2 years.
- Don't use bone-building drugs (bisphosphonates) for >5 years in low-risk patients.
- Don't use bone-building drugs (bisphosphonates) as a first-line treatment in postmenopausal women with osteopenia (mild bone density loss).
- Don't routinely use bone turnover marker testing to assess osteoporosis risk or monitor treatment.
- Don't prescribe calcitonin for osteoporosis treatment.

OTITIS EXTERNA

Christine A. Quartuccio-Carran, DO, FAAFP

BASICS

DESCRIPTION

Inflammation of the external auditory canal:

- Acute diffuse otitis externa (AOE) (<6 weeks): most common form; infectious etiology most commonly bacterial (*Pseudomonas aeruginosa* and *Staphylococcus aureus*); less commonly fungal (*Aspergillus* and *Candida*)
- Chronic otitis externa (>3 months): commonly due to inadequately treated acute otitis externa, persistent allergies, or chronic skin conditions
- Eczematous otitis externa: may accompany typical atopic eczema or other primary skin conditions
- Malignant (necrotizing) otitis externa: an infection that extends into the deeper tissues adjacent to the canal; may include osteomyelitis of the mastoid or temporal bone; a medical emergency requiring urgent referral; can be life-threatening; rare, especially in children (1)
- Synonym: swimmer's ear

EPIDEMIOLOGY

Incidence
- Annual incidence of ~1% (2)
- Higher in the summer months and in warm, wet climates
- Can affect all age groups but has a peak incidence in 7- to 12-year-olds (3)

Prevalence
Lifetime prevalence of 10% (2)

ETIOLOGY AND PATHOPHYSIOLOGY

- Factors associated with pathogenesis:
  - Skin, cerumen, and surrounding structures provide protection for the integrity of external auditory canal.
  - Cerumen, being a hydrophobic and sticky substance, provides a physical barrier against many foreign particles. Normal cerumen production also creates an environment that is slightly acidic and not favorable for most pathogens.
  - Disruption of the protective skin-cerumen barrier, followed by the subsequent inflammation, swelling, and obstruction of the canal, and impaired cerumen production, are all factors in the development of acute otitis externa.
- AOE, infectious etiology (3):
  - Bacterial infection (>90%): *P. aeruginosa* (22–62%), *Staphylococcus aureus* (11–34%); polymicrobial infection is common.
  - Fungal infection (<10%, more commonly associated with chronic otitis externa): *Aspergillus* (60–90%), *Candida* species (10–40%)
- Chronic otitis externa etiology: often occurs due to inadequately treated acute otitis externa, persistent allergies, or chronic skin conditions (2)

- Eczematous otitis externa (associated with primary skin disorder) etiology:
  - Eczema, seborrhea, psoriasis
  - Contact dermatitis
  - Purulent otitis media
  - Sensitivity to topical medications
- Malignant (necrotizing) otitis externa etiology (1):
  - Invasive bacterial infection: *Pseudomonas*, increasing incidence of methicillin-resistant *Staphylococcus aureus* (MRSA)
  - Associated with patients with diabetes or immunosuppression

RISK FACTORS

- Acute and chronic otitis externa
  - Water exposure—typically swimming in fresh water
  - Hot, humid weather; sweating
  - Trauma to the external canal—cleaning, scratching, use of instruments
  - Foreign body
  - Use of external devices—hearing aids, ear plugs
  - Anatomic abnormalities—narrow canal, exostoses
  - Dermatologic conditions—eczema, seborrhea, psoriasis
  - Cerumen buildup
  - Excessive hair in canal
  - Previous ear surgery
  - Previous local radiotherapy
- Eczematous: primary skin disorder
- Necrotizing otitis externa in adults
  - Advanced age
  - Diabetes mellitus
  - Immunosuppression (e.g., AIDS, malignancy)

GENERAL PREVENTION

- Avoid prolonged exposure to moisture.
- Use a hair dryer on a low setting to dry the canal.
- Use a head-tilt maneuver to remove excess water.
- Treat predisposing skin conditions.
- Eliminate self-inflicted trauma to canal with cotton swabs and other foreign objects.
- Treat underlying systemic conditions.
- Ear plugs when swimming.

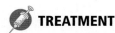**DIAGNOSIS**

HISTORY

- Associated symptoms: ear pain (70%), itching (60%), fullness (22%), +/− conductive hearing loss *32%), +/− jaw pain (1)
- Onset: rapid (within 48 hours), within the past 3 weeks
- Duration of symptoms: acute lasting <6 weeks, chronic lasting >3 months
- Assess: risk factors, predisposing conditions, history of prior ear infections or known tympanic membrane perforation, prior surgeries, local radiation therapy (1)
- Consider malignant otitis externa in older patients with a history or diabetes or an immunocompromised state that present with refractory purulent discharge and severe pain (2)

PHYSICAL EXAM

- Inspect the ear for erythema, swelling, discharge, signs of trauma, condition of the skin in and around the canal
- Pain on manipulation of the pinnae (when pulled) and/or tragus (when pushed) is a classic finding. Pain is often disproportionate to visual findings.
- Palpate mastoid area and surrounding lymph nodes.
- Otoscopy—assess for signs of otitis media (pneumatic otoscopy or tympanometry can differentiate between otitis media vs. otitis externa); determine if the tympanic membrane is intact, an important factor for treatment options as the treatment options are more limited if the tympanic membrane is perforated (1),(2),(4).
- Assess for cranial nerve (VII, IX to XII) involvement (rare).
- Granulation tissue in the external canal, particularly at the bone–cartilage junction, is a clinical finding of malignant otitis externa (1),(2).

DIFFERENTIAL DIAGNOSIS

- Otitis media +/− perforation
- Seborrheic dermatitis
- Psoriasis
- Eczema
- Contact dermatitis
- Furunculosis (infected hair follicle)
- Viral infections (varicella, measles, or herpes virus)
- Herpes zoster oticus (Ramsay-Hunt syndrome)
- Myringitis
- Otomycosis
- Cholesteatoma
- Temporomandibular joint (TMJ) syndrome
- Dental pathologies (caries, impacted molars) or other sources of referred pain
- Malignant otitis externa (osteomyelitis)
- Basal cell or squamous cell carcinoma

DIAGNOSTIC TESTS & INTERPRETATION

Initial Tests (lab, imaging)
Acute otitis externa is a clinical diagnosis based on the patient's history and physical exam findings (2).

Follow-Up Tests & Special Considerations
- Culture otorrhea if (2):
  - No improvement after initial treatment, the patient has predisposing risk factors, or there is concern for extension beyond the external canal
- Radiologic evaluation of deep tissues with high-resolution CT scan, MRI, gallium scan, and bone scan if concerns for necrotizing otitis externa (1)

TREATMENT

GENERAL MEASURES

- Clean the external canal (aural toilet)—helps to facilitate the delivery of otic drops and healing process
- Analgesics as appropriate for pain—acetaminophen, nonsteroidal anti-inflammatory drugs, or, in rare cases, a short-term opioid (4)

MEDICATION

- For diffuse, uncomplicated AOE, topical antibiotic preparations with or without topical corticosteroids are recommended for initial therapy (1).
  - Limited evidence to show that one preparation is more effective than another.
  - If there is a known or suspected perforation of the tympanic membrane, recommend a non-ototoxic topical preparation (ofloxacin or ciprofloxacin).
  - Advise patient on proper administration of topical preparations:
    - Patient lies down with affected side facing up. Topical preparation is administered into the canal (patient can gently move the pinna around to facilitate delivery). Patient is to remain in this position for 3 to 5 minutes.
- If the canal is obstructed, perform an aural toilet and/or place a wick using either compressed cellulose or ribbon gauze.
- Use systemic antibiotics only if the infection extends outside the external canal, if the patient has specific predisposing risk factors (diabetes, immunocompromised states, prior local radiotherapy, etc.), if unable to deliver topical preparation effectively, or if the patient fails initial therapeutic option (1),(2).
- Reassess diagnosis and treatment adherence within 48 to 72 hours if the patient does not respond to the initial therapeutic option (1),(2).

First Line

- Acute bacterial otitis externa, uncomplicated
  - Ciprofloxacin/dexamethasone 0.3%/0.1% suspension: children >6 months of age and adults: 4 drops instilled in affected ear twice daily for 7 days
  - Ofloxacin 0.3% solution (generic): children aged 6 months to 13 years: 5 drops instilled in affected ear once a day for 7 days; for patients aged 13 years and older: 10 drops instilled in affected ear once a day for 7 days
  - Neomycin/polymyxin B/hydrocortisone otic (Cortisporin, generic): children: 3 drops in affected ear(s) 3 to 4 times daily for 7 days; adults: 4 drops in affected ear(s) 3 to 4 times daily for 7 days. Do not continue for longer than 10 days.
  - Acetic acid 2%: children aged >3 years and adults: 3 to 5 drops every 4 to 6 hours with ear wick for 24 hours; wick may be removed after 24 hours then instill 5 drops 3 to 4 times a day for a total of 7 days. Recommend lower end of dosage range for children due to smaller capacity of the ear canal.
- Acute bacterial otitis externa, complicated—for severe or refractory cases, infection spreading beyond the ear canal, or patient with predisposing conditions (diabetes, immunocompromised states, etc.)
  - Topical and systemic treatment
  - Systemic options: Consider ciprofloxacin, amoxicillin, or amoxicillin/clavulanate.
- Chronic otitis externa
  - Treat the underlying cause; remove any offending agents.
  - Consider the use of a corticosteroid (topical vs. systemic) for inflammation.

- Fungal otitis externa
  - Clean external canal.
  - If the tympanic membrane is intact:
    - Can use acidifying agents (acetic acid topical preparations)
    - If the patient fails acidifying agents, consider topical antifungal (clotrimazole topical 1%).
- Malignant otitis externa
  - Seek emergent otolaryngology consultation and hospitalization.
  - IV antibiotics
  - Debridement

ISSUES FOR REFERRAL

Severe and/or resistant cases, concerns for malignant otitis externa (medical emergency), or those requiring surgical intervention

SURGERY/OTHER PROCEDURES

For malignant (necrotizing) otitis externa or furuncle

ADMISSION, INPATIENT, AND NURSING CONSIDERATIONS

Malignant (necrotizing) otitis media requiring parenteral antipseudomonal antibiotics, hospitalization, and emergent otolaryngology referral

 ONGOING CARE

FOLLOW-UP RECOMMENDATIONS

Patient Monitoring

For acute otitis externa, reassess diagnosis and treatment adherence within 48 to 72 hours if the patient does not respond to the initial therapeutic option (1). For chronic otitis externa, return every 2 to 3 weeks for repeated cleansing of canal.

PROGNOSIS

- With repeated cleansing and antibiotic therapy, most cases of chronic otitis externa will resolve. Occasionally, surgical intervention is required for resistant cases.
- Malignant (necrotizing otitis externa) managed inpatient with débridement and antipseudomonal antibiotics. Surgical intervention may be necessary in resistant cases or if there is cranial nerve involvement (1).

COMPLICATIONS

- Malignant (necrotizing) otitis externa may spread to infect contiguous bone causing osteomyelitis and infect other CNS structures, including causing cranial nerve palsies.
- Acute otitis externa may spread to pinna, causing chondritis.

REFERENCES

1. Rosenfeld RM, Schwartz SR, Cannon CR, et al. Clinical practice guideline: acute otitis externa. *Otolaryngol Head Neck Surg*. 2014;150(1 Suppl):S1–S24.
2. Schaefer P, Baugh RF. Acute otitis externa: an update. *Am Fam Physician*. 2012;86(11):1055–1061.
3. Wiegand S, Berner R, Schneider A, et al. Otitis externa. *Dtsch Arztebl Int*. 2019;116(13):224–234.
4. Jackson EA, Geer K. Acute otitis externa: rapid evidence review. *Am Fam Physician*. 2023;107(2):145–151.

 SEE ALSO

Algorithm: Ear Pain/Otalgia

CODES

ICD10

- H60.523 Acute chemical otitis externa, bilateral
- H60.593 Other noninfective acute otitis externa, bilateral
- B37.84 Candidal otitis externa

CLINICAL PEARLS

- For diffuse, uncomplicated AOE, topical preparations with or without topical corticosteroids are recommended for initial therapy.
- If there is a known or suspected perforation of the tympanic membrane, recommend a non-ototoxic topical preparation (ofloxacin or ciprofloxacin).
- If the canal is obstructed, perform an aural toilet and/or place a wick (use either compressed cellulose or ribbon gauze).
- Use systemic antibiotics only if the infection extends outside the external canal, if the patient has specific predisposing risk factors (diabetes, immunocompromised states, prior local radiotherapy, etc.), if unable to deliver topical preparation effectively, or if the patient fails initial therapeutic option.
- Reassess diagnosis and treatment adherence within 48 to 72 hours if the patient does not respond to the initial therapeutic option.
- Consider malignant otitis externa in older patients with a history or diabetes or an immunocompromised state that present with refractory purulent discharge and severe pain. Malignant otitis externa is a medical emergency that requires urgent referral and treatment.

OTITIS MEDIA
Sahil Mullick, MD • Mina Soliman, MD

BASICS

DESCRIPTION
- Inflammation of the middle ear; usually accompanied by fluid collection
- Acute otitis media (AOM): inflammation of the middle ear; rapid onset; cause may be infectious, either viral (AOM-v) or bacterial (AOM-b) also known as suppurative otitis media, but there is also a sterile etiology (AOM-s)
- Recurrent AOM: ≥3 episodes in 6 months or ≥4 episodes in 1 year with ≥1 in the past 6 months
- Otitis media with effusion (OME): fluid in the middle ear without signs or symptoms of infection. This is also referred to as serous, secretory, or nonsuppurative otitis media.
- Chronic suppurative otitis media (CSOM) also known as chronic otitis media: recurrent or chronic infection of the middle ear and mastoid cavity without an intact tympanic membrane; may present with or without cholesteatoma
- System(s) affected: nervous

EPIDEMIOLOGY
Incidence
- AOM
  - Predominant age: 6 to 24 months; declines >7 years; rare in adults
  - 50%–85% of children have had at least 1 episodes of AOM by age 3 years; 24% have had 3 or more episodes.
- OME
  - 90% of children have had at least one episode by age 4 years

ETIOLOGY AND PATHOPHYSIOLOGY
- AOM-b (bacterial): Usually, a preceding viral upper respiratory infection (URI) can produce eustachian tube dysfunction, leading to reduced clearance.
  - *Streptococcus pneumoniae, Haemophilus influenzae,* and *Moraxella catarrhalis* are the most frequent pathogens and account for 80% of AOM-b infections. *Streptococcus pyogenes, Mycoplasma* spp., *Chlamydia,* anaerobes, and other organisms are less frequent.
- AOM-v (viral): 15–44% of AOM infections are caused primarily by viruses (e.g., rhinovirus, respiratory syncytial virus, parainfluenza, influenza, enteroviruses, adenovirus, human metapneumovirus, and bocavirus).
- AOM-s (sterile/nonpathogens): 25–30%
- OME: middle ear inflammation and eustachian tube dysfunction; allergic causes are rarely substantiated.

Genetics
Immunologic defects and genetic disorders (e.g., Down syndrome) can predispose changes in physical anatomy (e.g., more horizontal ear canals) that increase the likelihood of developing otitis media.

RISK FACTORS
- Developing AOM prior to 1 year of age is a risk for recurrent AOM
- Bottle feeding while supine; pacifier use
- Routine daycare attendance

- Family history of AOM
- Environmental smoke exposure
- Absence of breastfeeding during the first 6 months of life
- Low socioeconomic status
- Atopy (such as eczema, asthma)
- Underlying ENT abnormalities (e.g., cleft palate)

GENERAL PREVENTION
- PCV-7, PCV-13, and influenzae vaccines (1)[B]
- Breastfeeding for ≥6 months is protective (1)[B].
- Avoiding supine bottlefeeding, passive smoke, and pacifiers >6 months may be helpful.
- Secondary prevention: Adenoidectomy and adenotonsillectomy for recurrent AOM have limited short-term efficacy and are associated with their own adverse risks.

COMMONLY ASSOCIATED CONDITIONS
URI

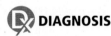

DIAGNOSIS

HISTORY
- AOM:
  - Otalgia
  - Preceding or accompanying URI symptoms
  - Decreased hearing
- AOM in adults can present with only otalgia without fever, or unilateral hearing loss.
- AOM in infants and toddlers may present with only irritability in early months of life.
- OME: usually asymptomatic and may only present with decreased hearing and, less frequently, complaints of tinnitus and ear-fullness (2)

PHYSICAL EXAM
- AOM:
  - Fever (not required for diagnosis)
  - Decreased eardrum mobility (with pneumatic otoscopy)
  - Moderate to severe bulging of tympanic membrane
  - Red, yellow, or cloudy tympanic membrane
  - Otorrhea
- OME:
  - Eardrum often dull but not bulging
  - Decreased eardrum mobility (pneumatic otoscopy)
  - Presence of air-fluid level
  - Weber test lateralizes to affected ear for an ear with effusion
  - Tympanometry if pneumatic otoscopy has no findings

DIFFERENTIAL DIAGNOSIS
- Tympanosclerosis
- Trauma
- Otitis externa
- Temporal arteritis in adults

DIAGNOSTIC TESTS & INTERPRETATION
Initial Tests (lab, imaging)
AOM is largely a clinical diagnosis requiring middle ear effusion (MEE) and signs of middle ear inflammation on exam.

Diagnostic Procedures/Other
- Otoscopy—to document the presence of middle ear fluid
- Pneumatic otoscopy—to detect middle ear fluid (can be supplemented with tympanometry and acoustic reflex measurement). Pneumatic otoscopy is contraindicated with known tympanic perforation.
- Hearing testing is recommended when hearing loss persists for ≥3 months or at any time suspecting language delay.
- Tympanocentesis for microbiologic diagnosis warranted if the child appears toxic, is immunocompromised, or has failed previous courses of antibiotic therapy; may be followed by myringotomy

Test Interpretation
Pneumatic otoscopy—tympanic mobility will be impaired if middle ear fluid is present.

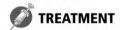

TREATMENT

GENERAL MEASURES
- Assess pain and if present, recommend treatment to decrease otalgia.
- Two-thirds of children will recover without any antibiotic treatment.
- AOM: Observation with watchful waiting for those >6 months with mild AOM. Prescribe antibiotics if no improvement or clinical worsening within 24 to 48 hours (3)[C].
- OME watchful waiting for 3 months, and if no improvement, then refer to ENT for possible surgery. Antibiotics, decongestants, antihistamines, and steroids are not recommended.

MEDICATION
First Line
- Controversy exists about the usefulness of antibiotic treatment for this often self-resolving condition. Overdiagnosis of AOM is widespread, which can lead to the injudicious use of antibiotics and contributes to antibiotic resistance (4). Studies suggest number needed to treat for an additional beneficial outcome (NNTB) is 20 when looking at relief of pain at 2 to 3 days after start of antibiotics; the number needed to harm (primarily diarrhea and vomiting) is 9.
- AAP/AAFP recommends:
  - Treatment for <6 months of age: Treat with amoxicillin if >2 weeks old.
  - >6 months: Antibacterial therapy is recommended with severe otitis media (i.e., moderate to severe otalgia, otalgia >48 hours or fever ≥39°C) (5)[B] or otorrhea or bilateral otitis media between 6 months and 2 years of age.
- Observation is an option with nonsevere otitis media at >6 months to 2 years (otalgia <48 hours, temperature <39°C). However, there is a high risk of treatment failure and antibiotics are recommended (6)[C].
- Immunocompetent children aged >2 years can be observed. Parents/guardians must understand risks/benefits of observation.

- AOM: AAP/AAFP consensus guideline recommends treating with antibiotics if:
  - Between 2 weeks and 6 months, *or*
  - If >6 months with severe otitis media (e.g., moderate to severe otalgia, otalgia >48 hours, or fevers >39°C) *or*
  - Otorrhea *or*
  - Bilateral otitis media in infants between 6 months and 23 months of age without severe signs/symptoms.
- Treat with amoxicillin, 90 mg/kg/day in 2 divided doses (maximum of 3 g/day) in those without risk of antibiotic resistance (5)[B]. Use a 10-day course for children aged <2 years; 5- to 7-day course for children aged ≥2 years (7)[C]
- If penicillin allergic:
  - Cefdinir, 14 mg/kg/day in 1 to 2 doses (maximum 600 mg/day)
  - Cefpodoxime, 10 mg/kg/day in 2 divided doses (maximum 400 mg/day) for 10 days *or*
  - Cefuroxime 30 mg/kg/day in 2 divided doses (maximum 1 g/day) for 10 days *or*
  - Ceftriaxone 50 mg/kg IM/IV per day for 1 to 3 days depending on symptomatic improvement (5)
  - Azithromycin 10 mg/kg on day 1 and 5 mg/kg days 2 to 5
- OME: no apparent benefit to medications which promote transitory resolution in 10–15%, but the effect is short-lived (8)[B].

Second Line
- Alternative antibiotics are indicated for the following:
  - Persistent symptoms after 48 to 72 hours of amoxicillin
  - AOM within 1 month of amoxicillin therapy
  - Severe earache
  - Age <6 months with high fever
  - Immunocompromised
    - Amoxicillin-clavulanate; 90 mg/kg/day of amoxicillin, with 6.4 mg/kg/day of clavulanate in 2 divided doses; recommended in children who have taken amoxicillin in the previous 30 days and those with concurrent purulent conjunctivitis or history of AOM unresponsive to amoxicillin
    - Ceftriaxone, 50 mg/kg IM or IV q24h for 2 to 3 consecutive days can be reserved for those who are too sick to take oral medications or who unsuccessfully took amoxicillin-clavulanate.
- Neither erythromycin nor trimethoprim-sulfamethoxazole should be used as a second-line agent in treatment failures.
- Recurrent AOM: Antibiotic prophylaxis for recurrent AOM (>3 distinct, well-documented episodes in 6 months) is not recommended (1)[B].

ISSUES FOR REFERRAL
- If hearing loss occurs for >2 weeks after AOM resolution, follow up with audiogram.
- If >2 episodes in a 6-month period, consider ENT referral for fiberoptic nasopharyngoscopy to rule out malignancy.
- Refer to ENT for recurrent COM for consideration of tympanostomy tubes.

ADDITIONAL THERAPIES
Pain control: acetaminophen, ibuprofen, topical procaine, or lidocaine for children >2 years but should not be used with tympanic perforation

SURGERY/OTHER PROCEDURES
- Recurrent AOM: no definitive guidelines agreed upon as indications for surgery
- Tympanostomy tubes may be effective in children <2 years with recurrent AOM.
- Adenotonsillectomy reduced the rate of AOM by 0.7 episode per child only in the 1st year after surgery and had a 15% complication rate.
- COM: Referral for surgery for tympanostomy should be individualized. It can be considered if >4 to 6 months of bilateral OME and/or >6 months of unilateral OME and/or hearing loss >25 dB or for high-risk individuals at any time.
- Tympanostomy tubes may reduce recurrence of AOM minimally, but it does not lower the risk of hearing loss (5)[B].

ADMISSION, INPATIENT, AND NURSING CONSIDERATIONS
Outpatient management except AOM in febrile infants aged <2 months or children requiring ceftriaxone who also require monitoring for 24 hours.

 ## ONGOING CARE

FOLLOW-UP RECOMMENDATIONS
Patients with otitis media who do not respond within 48 to 72 hours should be reevaluated. Consider changing the antibiotic.

Patient Monitoring
- AOM: Up to 40% may have persistent MEE at 1 month, with 10–25% at 3 months.
- OME/COM: Repeat otoscopic or tympanometric exams at 3 months, as indicated, as long as OME persists or sooner if there are red flags (see earlier discussion).

PROGNOSIS
Most cases of uncomplicated, nonsevere AOM resolve without antibiotics.

COMPLICATIONS
- AOM: tympanic membrane perforation/otorrhea, acute mastoiditis, facial nerve paralysis, otitic hydrocephalus, meningitis, labyrinthitis and hearing impairment, myringosclerosis, petrositis, brain abscess, epidural or subdural abscess, lateral or cavernous sinus thrombosis, or cholesteatoma
- COM: Speech and language disabilities may occur. Hearing loss is not caused by OME, but in children who are at risk for speech, language, or learning problems (e.g., autism spectrum, syndromes, craniofacial disorders, developmental delay, and children already with speech/language delay), it could lead to further problems because they are less tolerant of a hearing impairment.
- Recurrent AOM and COM: atrophy and scarring of eardrum, chronic perforation and otorrhea, cholesteatoma, permanent hearing loss, chronic mastoiditis, other intracranial suppurative complications

REFERENCES

1. Lieberthal AS, Carroll AE, Chonmaitree T, et al. The diagnosis and management of acute otitis media. *Pediatrics*. 2013;131(3):e964–e999.
2. Lee D-H, Yeo S-W. Clinical diagnostic accuracy of otitis media with effusion in children, and significance of myringotomy: diagnostic or therapeutic? *J Korean Med Sci*. 2004;19(5):739–743.
3. Sakulchit T, Goldman RD. Antibiotic therapy for children with acute otitis media. *Can Fam Physician*. 2017;63(9):685–687.
4. Jamal A, Alsabea A, Tarakmeh M, et al. Etiology, diagnosis, complications, and management of acute otitis media in children. *Cureus*. 2022;14(8):e28019.
5. Harmes KM, Blackwood RA, Burrows HL, et al. Otitis media: diagnosis and treatment. *Am Fam Physician*. 2013;88(7):435–440.
6. Hoberman A, Ruohola A, Shaikh N, et al. Acute otitis media in children younger than 2 years. *JAMA Pediatr*. 2013;167(12):1171–1172.
7. Hoberman A, Paradise JL, Rockette HE, et al. Shortened antimicrobial treatment for acute otitis media in young children. *N Engl J Med*. 2016;375(25):2446–2456.
8. Venekamp RP, Burton MJ, van Dongen TMA, et al. Antibiotics for otitis media with effusion in children. *Cochrane Database Syst Rev*. 2016;(6):CD009163.

 ## SEE ALSO

Algorithm: Ear Pain/Otalgia

CODES

ICD10
- H65 Nonsuppurative otitis media
- H65.0 Acute serous otitis media
- H65.00 Acute serous otitis media, unspecified ear

CLINICAL PEARLS
- Pneumatic otoscopy is the single most specific and clinically useful test for diagnosis.
- Consider a delay of antibiotics for 24 to 48 hours in uncomplicated presentations (>6 months of age) who do not have severe illness or otorrhea.
- First-line treatment is amoxicillin, 80 to 90 mg/kg/day for 10 days for children aged <2 years; consider a 5- to 7-day course in >2 years of age.
- Erythema and effusion can persist for weeks.
- Antibiotics, antihistamines, and steroids are not indicated for COM.
- OME rarely develops in adults. Persistent unilateral effusion should be investigated to rule out neoplasm, particularly if there is a cranial nerve palsy.

OTITIS MEDIA WITH EFFUSION

Hobart Lee, MD, FAAFP

BASICS

DESCRIPTION

- Also called serous otitis media, secretory otitis media, nonsuppurative otitis media, "ear fluid," or "glue ear"
- Otitis media with effusion (OME) is defined as the presence of fluid in the middle ear in the absence of acute signs or symptoms of infection.
- More commonly, a pediatric disease
- May occur spontaneously from poor eustachian tube function or as an inflammatory response after acute otitis media (AOM)

EPIDEMIOLOGY

Approximately 90% of children have OME before school age, mostly between the ages of 6 months and 4 years.

Incidence

Approximately 2.2 million new cases annually in the United States

Prevalence

Less prevalent in adults and is usually associated with an underlying disorder

ETIOLOGY AND PATHOPHYSIOLOGY

- Chronic inflammatory condition where an underlying stimulus causes an inflammatory reaction with increased mucin production creating a functional blockage of the eustachian tube and thick accumulation of mucin-rich middle ear effusion
- Young children are more prone to OME due to shorter and more horizontal eustachian tubes, which become more vertical around 7 years of age.
- Biofilms, anatomic variations, and AOM caused by viruses or bacteria have been implicated as stimuli causing OME. The common pathogens causing AOM include nontypeable *Haemophilus influenzae*, *Streptococcus pneumoniae*, and *Moraxella catarrhalis*.
- In adults, OME is often associated with paranasal sinus disease (66%), smoking-induced nasopharyngeal lymphoid hyperplasia and adult-onset adenoidal hypertrophy (19%), or head and neck tumors (4.8%).

RISK FACTORS

- Risk factors include a family history of OME, early daycare, exposure to cigarette smoke, bottle-feeding, and low socioeconomic status (1).
- Eustachian tube dysfunction may be a predisposing factor, although the evidence is unclear (2).
- Gastroesophageal reflux is associated with OME (2).

GENERAL PREVENTION

OME is generally not preventable, although lowering smoke exposure, breastfeeding, and avoiding daycare centers at an early age may decrease the risk.

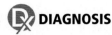**DIAGNOSIS**

HISTORY

- OME is transient and asymptomatic in many pediatric patients.
- Most common reported symptom is hearing loss (2). There may be mild discomfort present in the ear, fullness, or "popping."
- Infants may have ear rubbing, excessive irritability, sleep problems, or failure to respond appropriately to voices or sounds.
- Clinical features may include "a history of hearing difficulties, poor attention, behavioral problems, delayed speech and language development, clumsiness, and poor balance" (2).
- There may be a history of recent or recurrent episodes of AOM or a recent upper respiratory tract infection (2).

PHYSICAL EXAM

- Cloudy tympanic membrane (TM) with distinctly impaired mobility; air-fluid level or bubble may be visible in the middle ear (1),(2).
- Color may be abnormal (yellow, amber, or blue), and the TM may be retracted or concave (2).
- Distinct redness of the TM may be present in approximately 5% of OME cases (1).
- Clinical signs and symptoms of acute illness should be absent in patients with OME (1).

DIFFERENTIAL DIAGNOSIS

- AOM
- Bullous myringitis
- Tympanosclerosis (may cause decreased/absent motion of the TM)
- Sensorineural hearing loss

DIAGNOSTIC TESTS & INTERPRETATION

Initial Tests (lab, imaging)

The primary standard to make the diagnosis is pneumatic otoscopy, which demonstrates reduced/absent mobility of the TM secondary to fluid in the middle ear. Pneumatic otoscopy has 94% sensitivity and 80% specificity for diagnosing OME. Accuracy of diagnosis with an experienced examiner is between 70% and 79% (1)[C].

Follow-Up Tests & Special Considerations

- Tympanometry may also be used to support or exclude the diagnosis in infants >4 months old, especially when the presence of middle ear effusion is difficult to determine (1)[C].
- Acoustic reflectometry (64% specificity and 80% sensitivity) may be considered instead of tympanometry (3)[B].
- Audiogram may show mild conductive hearing loss (2)[C].
- Hearing tests are recommended for OME lasting >3 months (1)[C].
- Language testing is recommended for children with abnormal hearing tests (1)[C].

Diagnostic Procedures/Other

Myringotomy is the gold standard but is not practical for clinical use (2)[C].

TREATMENT

- OME improves or resolves without medical intervention in most patients within 3 months, especially if secondary to AOM (1)[C].
- Current guidelines support a 3-month period of observation with optional serial exams, tympanometry, and language assessment during that wait time (1),(2)[C].
- Adults found to have OME should be screened for an underlying disorder and treated accordingly (2)[C].

MEDICATION

- The 2016 AAOHNS guideline recommends against routine use of antibiotics in treatment of OME. A 2016 Cochrane review, however, found that children treated with oral antibiotics were more likely to have tympanogram confirmed OME resolution in 2 to 3 months (number needed to treat = 5). Adverse events included diarrhea, vomiting, skin rash, and allergic reactions (number needed to harm = 20). Importantly, there were no reported patient-oriented outcomes (e.g., cognitive development, language, quality of life, or speech). Outcomes regarding short-term hearing, reduction of AOM infections, or need for ventilation tubes are unknown (1)[C],(4)[A].
- The 2016 AAOHNS and a 2006 Cochrane review found that antihistamines and decongestants have no benefit over placebo in OME treatment with possible adverse side effects such as insomnia, hyperactivity, and drowsiness (5)[A].

- The 2016 AAOHNS guideline recommends against administering oral or intranasal corticosteroids. No long-term benefit was shown, and adverse side effects such as weight gain and behavioral changes are possible (1)[C].
- In adults, eustachian tube dysfunction secondary to allergic rhinitis or recent upper respiratory infection can be the cause of OME. It is unknown whether decongestants, antihistamines, or nasal steroids improve outcomes in adults.

ISSUES FOR REFERRAL

The following are indications for referral to a surgeon for evaluation of tympanostomy tube placement:

- Chronic bilateral OME (≥3 months) with hearing difficulty
- Chronic OME with symptoms (e.g., vestibular problems, poor school performance, behavioral issues, ear discomfort, or reduced quality of life)
- At-risk children (speech, language, or learning problems due to baseline sensory, physical, cognitive, or behavioral factors) with chronic OME or type B (flat) tympanogram

ADDITIONAL THERAPIES

Hearing aids may be an acceptable alternative to surgery (2)[C].

SURGERY/OTHER PROCEDURES

- Tympanostomy tubes are recommended as initial surgery. Risks include purulent otorrhea, myringosclerosis, retraction pockets, and persistent TM perforations (1)[C].
- Adenoidectomy with myringotomy has similar efficacy to tympanostomy tubes in children >4 years of age but with added surgical and anesthetic risks (1)[C],(6).
- Adenoidectomy should not be performed in children with persistent OME alone unless there is a distinct indication for the procedure for another problem (e.g., adenoiditis/chronic sinusitis/nasal obstruction) (1)[C].
- Adenoidectomy (and concurrent tube placement) may be considered when repeat surgery for OME is necessary (e.g., when effusion recurs after tubes have fallen out or are removed). In these cases, adenoidectomy has been shown to decrease the need for future procedures for OME (1),(2)[C].
- Tonsillectomy or myringotomy alone is not recommended for treatment (1)[C].

COMPLEMENTARY & ALTERNATIVE MEDICINE

Autoinflation, which refers to the process of opening the eustachian tube by raising intranasal pressure (e.g., by forced exhalation with closed mouth and nose), may be beneficial in improving patients' tympanogram or audiometry and quality of life scores.

 ONGOING CARE

FOLLOW-UP RECOMMENDATIONS
Patient Monitoring

- Children who are at risk for developmental difficulties should be evaluated for OME at the time of diagnosis and at 12 to 18 months (if initial diagnosis occurred <12 months). At-risk conditions include permanent hearing loss independent of OME, suspected or confirmed speech and language delay, autism spectrum disorder or other pervasive developmental disorder, Down syndrome or other craniofacial disorder, blindness or other uncorrectable visual impairment, cleft palate, and unspecified developmental delay (1)[C].
- For patients diagnosed with OME, reevaluation and repeat hearing tests should be performed every 3 to 6 months until the effusion has resolved or until the child develops an indication for surgical referral (1)[C].

PROGNOSIS

Approximately 50% of children >3 years of age have OME resolution within 3 months.

COMPLICATIONS

- The most significant complication of OME is permanent hearing loss, leading to possible language, speech, and developmental delays.
- Underventilation of the middle ear can cause a cholesteatoma (1)[C].

REFERENCES

1. Rosenfeld RM, Shin JJ, Schwartz SR, et al. Clinical practice guideline: otitis media with effusion executive summary (update). *Otolaryngol Head Neck Surg.* 2016;154(2):201–214.
2. Qureishi A, Lee Y, Belfield K, et al. Update on otitis media—prevention and treatment. *Infect Drug Resist.* 2014;7:15–24.
3. Shekelle P, Takata G, Chan LS, et al. Diagnosis, natural history, and late effects of otitis media with effusion. *Evid Rep Technol Assess (Summ).* 2002;(55):1–5.
4. Venekamp RP, Burton MJ, van Dongen TMA, et al. Antibiotics for otitis media with effusion in children. *Cochrane Database Syst Rev.* 2016;2016(6):CD009163.
5. Griffin G, Flynn CA. Antihistamines and/or decongestants for otitis media with effusion (OME) in children. *Cochrane Database Syst Rev.* 2011;2011(9):CD003423.
6. Casselbrant ML, Mandel EM, Rockette HE, et al. Adenoidectomy for otitis media with effusion in 2–3-year-old children. *Int J Pediatr Otorhinolaryngol.* 2009;73(12):1718–1724.

CODES

ICD10

- H65.90 Unspecified nonsuppurative otitis media, unspecified ear
- H65.00 Acute serous otitis media, unspecified ear
- H65.20 Chronic serous otitis media, unspecified ear

CLINICAL PEARLS

- OME is defined as the presence of a middle ear effusion in the absence of acute signs of infection.
- In children, OME most often arises following an AOM. In adults, it often occurs in association with eustachian tube dysfunction.
- The primary standard for diagnosis is pneumatic otoscopy.
- There is no benefit in antihistamines, decongestants, or corticosteroids for the treatment of OME in children.
- Management usually includes watchful waiting and surgery (when indicated); which strategy is chosen depends on many factors, including the risk/presence of any associated speech, language, or learning delays, and on the severity of any associated hearing loss.

OVARIAN CYST, RUPTURED

Kristina Gracey, MD, MPH

BASICS

- Ovarian cysts are frequent in reproductive-aged women.
- Patients with a symptomatic ruptured cyst usually complain of acute onset unilateral lower abdominal pain.
- Rupture can be caused by sexual intercourse, luteal phase, exercise, trauma, or pregnancy, or it can be idiopathic.
- Evaluation of the patient should include exclusion of other emergent causes: ectopic pregnancy, ovarian torsion, and nongynecologic sources of acute unilateral lower abdominal pain.
- Once the diagnosis of a ruptured cyst is confirmed, most patients can be managed conservatively as outpatients with adequate pain control. Surgical intervention is rarely indicated.

DESCRIPTION

Most ovarian cysts are benign physiologic follicles created by the ovary at the time of ovulation. Ovarian cysts can cause symptoms when they become enlarged and exert a mass effect on surrounding structures, or when they rupture and the cyst contents irritate the peritoneum or nearby pelvic organs.

EPIDEMIOLOGY

- The actual incidence of ovarian cysts is difficult to calculate as many ruptured cysts are asymptomatic or found incidentally.
- Ovarian cysts can be seen on transvaginal ultrasounds in nearly all premenopausal women and in up to 18% of postmenopausal women. The vast majority of these cysts are benign or functional.
- About 13% of ovarian masses in reproductive-aged women are malignant, as opposed to 45% in postmenopausal women. About 70% of ovarian malignancies are diagnosed at a late stage.
- Ruptured ovarian cysts most commonly affect the right ovary, 63%.

Incidence

About 7% of women worldwide experience a symptomatic cyst during their lifetime.

Prevalence

During pregnancy, prevalence varies from 1 to 5.3%; of those, just 0.63% are symptomatic and 1% are malignant.

ETIOLOGY AND PATHOPHYSIOLOGY

Normal ovulation occurs when a follicle matures and ruptures, releasing an oocyte, leaving a corpus luteum, which subsequently involutes. If the follicle fails to rupture and continues to grow, a follicular cyst is formed. If a corpus luteum fails to involute and continues to grow, then a corpus luteum cyst occurs. These are the most common cysts. Both types are physiologic (termed "functional") without malignant potential. Other cyst types include endometriomas (filled with menstrual blood), dermoid cysts that contains mature tissue of ectodermal, mesodermal, and/or endodermal origin, and ovarian malignancy originating from any of the structures of the ovary.

RISK FACTORS

Medications or conditions associated with increased ovulation and/or increased risk of cyst rupture.

- Ovulation induction agents (i.e., clomiphene [Clomid], aromatase inhibitors, GnRH agonists)
- Tamoxifen increases the risk of ovarian cysts in reproductive-aged women.
- Polycystic ovarian syndrome (PCOS) (common), fibrous dysplasia/McCune-Albright syndrome (rare)
- Ovarian endometriosis

GENERAL PREVENTION

Ovulation suppression with combined hormonal contraceptives is the mainstay therapy for prevention of recurrent ovarian cyst.

COMMONLY ASSOCIATED CONDITIONS

- Endometriomas located on or adjacent to the ovaries are found in 20–55% of women with endometriosis.
- PCOS

DIAGNOSIS

The characteristic symptoms of ruptured cyst may resemble ectopic pregnancy. Ectopic pregnancy should be ruled out when a ruptured cyst is suspected (1)[C].

HISTORY

- Questions that should be addressed if a ruptured ovarian cyst is suspected include:
  – Onset and characteristics of pain
  – Pain associated with timing of sexual intercourse, strenuous activity, or trauma
  – Date of last menstrual period
  – Presence or absence of vaginal bleeding
  – Nausea or vomiting
  – Shoulder or upper abdominal pain due to subphrenic extravasation
- Symptoms of hypotension/hypovolemia, including palpitations, shortness of breath, sensation of being hot or clammy, dizziness
- Additional information that will guide diagnosis should include patient age, known or previous ovarian cysts, and reproductive history.

ALERT

Patients with bleeding diathesis or undergoing anticoagulation therapy may experience significant bleeding from hemorrhagic cysts.

PHYSICAL EXAM

- Vital signs are usually normal unless significant blood loss has occurred.
- Rupture characterized by significant blood loss may be present in the form of pallor, pale mucosal membranes, and tachycardia.
- Patients will have significant tenderness to palpation or an acute abdomen if the peritoneum is irritated or inflamed.
- On some occasions, a palpable adnexal mass can be felt on bimanual exam. Care should be taken not to cause further injury with a forceful exam.

DIFFERENTIAL DIAGNOSIS

Includes all causes of acute abdominal pain, both gynecologic and nongynecologic

- Ectopic pregnancy should always be excluded with a negative pregnancy test (1)[C].
- Common gynecologic etiologies include:
  – Functional ovarian cysts
  – Ovarian torsion
  – Tubo-ovarian abscess
  – Teratomas
  – Degenerating fibroids
  – Endometrioma
  – Cystadenoma (mucinous or serous)
  – Hydrosalpinx
- Malignant gynecologic etiologies can usually be attributed to the various gynecologic cancers of the reproductive tract.
- Benign nongynecologic causes of acute lower abdominal pain include:
  – Appendicitis
  – Diverticulitis
  – Infections of the urinary tract
  – Renal colic
- Malignant nongynecologic causes of acute lower abdominal pain can be attributed to neoplastic processes of the lower GI tract.

DIAGNOSTIC TESTS & INTERPRETATION

- In all premenopausal women, pregnancy must be ruled out by a urine test.
- Complete blood count may reveal a significant drop in hematocrit if there is ongoing hemorrhage (2)[B]. Leukocytosis should raise the suspicion of an infectious process (1)[C].
- Urinalysis and STD testing should be obtained to evaluate for infectious causes, PID, or symptomatic renal stones (1)[C].
- A type and screen is indicated if surgical intervention is planned or blood products are being considered.

Initial Tests (lab, imaging)

- Ultrasonography
- Serial quantitative β-hCG if pregnancy of unknown location
- Complete blood count
- Urinalysis and STD Testing

Follow-Up Tests & Special Considerations

Computed tomography (CT) or magnetic resonance imaging (MRI) may narrow the differential diagnosis when ultrasonography is indeterminate.

- Sonographic imaging along with CT and MRI can aid in diagnosis of gynecologic emergencies (3)[C].
- CT is useful to confirm a hemoperitoneum, and MRI can assist when the diagnosis remains unclear after CT and ultrasound (3)[C].
- Ultrasound and CT imaging for diagnosis has decreased the need for diagnostic surgical intervention (2)[B].
- Additionally, ultrasound is useful in confirming normal Doppler flow to the affected ovary and adnexa (1)[C].

Diagnostic Procedures/Other

Laparoscopy may be diagnostic and therapeutic in emergent cases.

TREATMENT

GENERAL MEASURES
- For many patients, pain associated with a ruptured cyst will be transient and self-limiting.
- Cyst rupture in a stable healthy patient can be managed conservatively in 80% of cases (2)[B].
- Patient with anticoagulation can also be managed conservatively with cyst rupture using a multidisciplinary team (4)[C].

MEDICATION
Scheduled NSAIDs or oral narcotics can be prescribed depending on pain severity.

First Line
For patients with multiple episodes or a single severe occurrence, OCPs can be considered for ovulation suppression and prevention. They are not effective for treatment of ovarian cysts which are already present.

ISSUES FOR REFERRAL
- Obstetrician (OB)/GYN
  - Consider referral to an obstetrician if an adnexal mass is diagnosed during pregnancy. Such masses have a low risk of malignancy or acute complication for the pregnancy.
  - Most cysts resolve without intervention within 2 to 3 weeks; those that do not resolve in 12 weeks require referral for surgical assessment (5)[A].
  - Unstable patients with hemodynamic compromise or patients with significant hemoperitoneum should be resuscitated, and laparoscopy or a laparotomy should be considered. Surgical exploration should also be considered if there is a concern for malignancy.
- Gynecologic oncology: Referral to a gynecologic oncologist should be considered for complex adnexal masses with an elevated CA-125 and associated symptoms concerning for malignancy such as ascites, thick septation noted on ultrasound, early satiety, pleural effusion, enlarging abdominal mass, or bowel obstruction.
- General surgery: Acute lower abdominal pain that is nongynecologic and suspicious for bowel involvement should be referred to general surgery or a gastroenterologist.

ADDITIONAL THERAPIES
Guided cyst aspiration is not recommended for either diagnosis or treatment but could be considered in patients at high risk who are not good surgical candidates.

SURGERY/OTHER PROCEDURES
- Although the need for surgical intervention is rare, it is usually of an emergent nature.
- Patients with a low diastolic blood pressure and a large amount of hemoperitoneum often need surgery (2)[B].
- In most cases, laparoscopy is diagnostic and therapeutic. The decision to proceed with cystectomy or oophorectomy should be made intraoperatively after a thorough evaluation of the intra-abdominal environment has been completed.

- The advantages of a laparoscopic approach include a shorter length of stay, faster recovery, small scar, and few adhesions. Postoperative recovery time as well as patient satisfaction is significantly improved with a minimally invasive approach.
- Laparotomy should be performed in cases of critical hemodynamic instability or lack of laparoscopically trained surgeons. If there is a concern for malignancy or metastases, laparotomy may be the preferred method of surgery.

ADMISSION, INPATIENT, AND NURSING CONSIDERATIONS
Patients who require inpatient management should be managed with serial abdominal exams, analgesia, and intravenous resuscitation as indicated by their initial presentation.

 ONGOING CARE

FOLLOW-UP RECOMMENDATIONS
- Follow-up for patients managed conservatively should be scheduled in 72 hours from the initial onset of symptoms. Patients should present sooner for new or worsening symptoms.
- Patients with complete resolution of symptoms within a few days can follow up as needed. However, these patients should be counseled on risk of reoccurrence and options for prevention.
- In patients who had surgery, postop follow-up should be scheduled 2 weeks from the date of surgery.
- Patients in whom an ovarian cyst was diagnosed incidentally should follow-up based on the size of their cyst.

Pregnancy Considerations
- The management of adnexal masses during pregnancy is controversial.
- Most adnexal masses in pregnancy can be managed expectantly because the risk of malignancy is low (1)[C]. If there is a risk for ruptured endometriotic cyst, early surgical intervention can reduce the risk of cyst fluid leakage, thus preventing adhesions and preserving fertility. MRI can help further characterize a mass safely in pregnancy (1)[C]. However, the possible risk of torsion or rupture should not be considered as an indication for surgery.

PATIENT EDUCATION
Reassurance of the benign nature of most ovarian cysts is an important cornerstone of patient education.

COMPLICATIONS
- Surgical procedure complications related to any laparoscopic surgery
- Ovarian reserve reduction may occur following any ovarian surgery. Desire for future fertility should be factored into surgical decisions. Cysts with a diameter of ≥5 cm can themselves cause compromise in ovarian reserve. It is unclear if the effect is temporary or permanent.

REFERENCES
1. Biggs WS, Marks ST. Diagnosis and management of adnexal masses. *Am Fam Physician*. 2016;93(8):676–681.
2. Kim JH, Lee SM, Lee JH, et al. Successful conservative management of ruptured ovarian cysts with hemoperitoneum in healthy women. *PLoS One*. 2014;9(3):e91171.
3. Iraha Y, Okada M, Iraha R, et al. CT and MR imaging of gynecologic emergencies. *Radiographics*. 2017;37(5):1569–1586.
4. Gupta A, Gupta S, Manaktala U, et al. Conservative management of corpus luteum haemorrhage in patients on anticoagulation: a report of three cases and review of the literature. *Arch Gynecol Obstet*. 2015;291(2):427–431.
5. Seehusen DA, Earwood JS. Oral contraceptives are not an effective treatment for ovarian cysts. *Am Fam Physician*. 2014;90(9):623.

ADDITIONAL READING
American College of Obstetricians and Gynecologists, Committee on Practice Bulletins—Gynecology. Practice Bulletin No. 174: evaluation and management of adnexal masses. *Obstet Gynecol*. 2016;128(5):e210–e226.

 CODES

ICD10
- N83.20 Unspecified ovarian cysts
- N83.0 Follicular cyst of ovary
- N83.1 Corpus luteum cyst

CLINICAL PEARLS
- Functional ovarian cysts are very common in reproductive-aged women and are usually self-limiting.
- Always exclude ectopic pregnancy.
- Management of symptomatic ruptured cysts is usually accomplished with outpatient pain control and follow-up.
- Combined hormonal contraception is the mainstay of preventive treatment.

PALLIATIVE CARE

Erika Zimmons, DO, MS

 BASICS

Palliative care focuses on preventing and alleviating the suffering of patients (and their families) living at any stage of a life-limiting illness.

DESCRIPTION
- The principal goal of palliative care is to prevent and alleviate suffering—whether physical (pain, breathlessness, nausea, etc.), emotional, social, or spiritual regardless of the underlying etiology.
- Palliative care is an interdisciplinary approach to caring for patients and families.
- Palliative care aims to improve or maintain quality of life for patients and families despite serious illness.
- The palliative care team helps to identify goals of care based on patient's preferences and values.
- Palliative care is available for patients with serious, life-limiting illness, at any stage of their disease, with or without concurrent curative care. Patients and their families may access palliative care services in the hospital, rehabilitation or skilled nursing facility, and ambulatory setting.
- Hospice: In the United Sates, hospice is available for patients whose average life expectancy is ≤6 months and whose principal goal is to stay at home (including long-term care or assisted living facility), avoid hospitalizations, and forego disease-directed care with a curative intent. Unlike regular home nursing services, hospice does not require a patient to be homebound. Hospice offers backup support for patients 24 hours a day and 7 days per week. Hospice will also provide bereavement support for family and friends for 1 year after the patient's death.

COMMONLY ASSOCIATED CONDITIONS
Common symptoms/syndromes encountered in palliative care:
- Pain: chronic pain, neuropathic pain, pain from bone metastases
- GI symptoms: ascites, anorexia/cachexia, bowel obstruction, constipation and stool impaction, diarrhea, dysphagia, mucositis/stomatitis, sialorrhea, xerostomia, nausea and vomiting
  - For nausea and vomiting, consider underlying etiology and treat accordingly.
    - GI causes: constipation, bowel (full or partial) obstruction, ileus, reflux, inflammation
    - Intrathoracic causes: cardiac, effusions (cardiac, pulmonary), mediastinal causes, esophageal disease

- Autonomic dysfunction
- Centrally mediated: intracranial pressure change, inflammation, cerebellar, vestibular, medication or metabolic cause stimulating vomiting center, and/or chemoreceptor trigger zone
- Medication side effects
- General medical symptoms: delirium and fatigue
- Pulmonary symptoms: cough and breathlessness or dyspnea
- Psychological symptoms: anxiety, depression, insomnia
- Skin: decubitus ulcer, pruritus, complex wounds

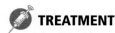 **DIAGNOSIS**

A useful tool in palliative care is the PEACE tool. This tool evaluates (1):
- **P**hysical symptoms
- **E**motive and cognitive symptoms
- **A**utonomy and related issues
- **C**ommunication: contribution to others and closure of life affairs–related issues
- **E**conomic burden and other practical issues, including transcendent and existential concerns

HISTORY
A comprehensive palliative care assessment includes the following:
- Underlying medical conditions and associated physical symptoms
- Communication with empathic inquiry and open-ended questions
  - Framework for breaking bad news—SPIKES (**S**et up interview, assess **P**erception, obtain **I**nvitation, impart **K**nowledge, address **E**motions with empathic responses, **S**trategy and summary) (2)
- Comprehensive pain assessment and review of systems (e.g., Edmonton Symptom Assessment Scale)
- Psychological symptom assessment
- Cultural, social, financial, and practical concerns
- Spiritual and existential issues
  - FICA assessment (**F**aith, **I**mportance and influence, **C**ommunity, **A**ddress—how does the patient wish these items to be addressed?) (3)

- Presence and sources of suffering
- Goals of care: posthospital care, practical needs, hopes, and fears
- Prognosis: functional status and interest in knowing prognosis

PHYSICAL EXAM
The physical examination is directed by underlying diagnosis, symptoms, and functional decline in the context of meeting the goals of the patient and family to maximize function, comfort, and support.

DIAGNOSTIC TESTS & INTERPRETATION
Initial Tests (lab, imaging)
Laboratory and radiology testing depends on the underlying diagnosis and any associated symptoms. Avoid unnecessary testing.

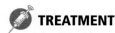 **TREATMENT**

GENERAL MEASURES
- Targeted interventions to maximize quality of life and minimize symptom burden considering patient values, goals, fears, and social setting
- Treatment should involve an interdisciplinary team to address potential and realized suffering (physical, emotional, social, and/or spiritual).

MEDICATION
- Minimize polypharmacy; discontinue medications that offer little improvement in the quality of life.
- Focus the use of medications for symptom management. Continue the use of disease-modifying medications especially if they lessen symptom burden and enhance immediate quality of life.
- In patients with cognitive impairment, consider that they may not be able to verbalize symptoms.

- Consider medications to address symptoms:
  - *Pain*
    - Use immediate-release opioids—titrate to adequate control.
    - Once pain is controlled, convert to long-acting opioids with short-acting agents made available because tolerance develops and/or patient develops breakthrough pain.
  - Bone pain: NSAIDs added to narcotics are more effective than narcotics alone.
  - Neuropathic pain: may use adjuvant treatment, such as gabapentin or other anticonvulsants

ALERT
Avoid morphine in patients with renal failure; can induce delirium, hyperalgesia, agitation, and seizures

- *Vomiting* associated with a particular opioid may be relieved by substitution with an equianalgesic dose of another opioid or a sustained-release formulation.
  - Dopamine receptor antagonists (metoclopramide, prochlorperazine) may improve nausea symptoms.
  - Droperidol: insufficient evidence on the use for the management of nausea and vomiting
- *Constipation*: Consider prophylactic stimulants (bisacodyl or senna) or osmotic laxatives. Avoid nonessential medications that may cause constipation.

ALERT
Consider laxatives with opioid treatment to avoid constipation.

- Subcutaneous methylnaltrexone may be used for inducing bowel movements without inducing withdrawal in opioid-induced constipation.
- Dyspnea: Consider oxygen. Consider benzodiazepines if there is an increased anxiety.
  - Treat the underlying cause of breathlessness. In addition, as the disease advances, low-dose opioids may be beneficial to patients. Immediate-release opioids PO/IV treat dyspnea effectively and typically at doses lower than necessary for the relief of moderate pain.

- *Delirium*: consider review of medications or other causes that may be contributing to delirium; lowest doses of antipsychotics (haloperidol, risperidone, etc.) or, in some cases, benzodiazepines (only when necessary)
  - Monitor the patient's safety and use nonpharmacologic strategies to assist orientation (clocks, calendars, environment, and redirection).
- Pruritus: no optimal therapy; general measures include moisturizing the skin and avoiding irritants.
- Anxiety: insufficient data for recommendations of specific medication
- Megestrol acetate improves appetite and slight weight gain in patients with anorexia-cachexia syndrome. However, consider possible side effects.

ISSUES FOR REFERRAL
- Referral to palliative care
  - Any patient with a serious, life-limiting illness who could use help with burdensome symptoms or suffering and/or complex goals of care discussion
  - Early referral to palliative care may improve quality of life and longevity for patients with advanced cancer.
- Referral to hospice care
  - Any patient with an average life expectancy of ≤6 months
  - Consider patients who have multiple hospitalizations and/or emergency department visits in the prior 6 months.
  - Refer to local hospice guidelines for additional disease-specific criteria.

 ONGOING CARE

PATIENT EDUCATION
- Hospice Foundation of America: https://hospicefoundation.org/
- National Institute on Aging, "What Are Palliative Care and Hospice Care?": https://www.nia.nih.gov/health/what-are-palliative-care-and-hospice-care

REFERENCES
1. ElMokhallalati Y, Bradley SH, Chapman E, et al. Identification of patients with potential palliative care needs: a systematic review of screening tools in primary care. *Palliat Med.* 2020;34(8):989–1005.
2. Baile WF, Buckman R, Lenzi R, et al. SPIKES—a six-step protocol for delivering bad news: application to the patient with cancer. *Oncologist.* 2000;5(4):302–311.
3. Borneman T, Ferrell B, Puchalski CM. Evaluation of the FICA tool for spiritual assessment. *J Pain Symptom Manage.* 2010;40(2):163–173.

ADDITIONAL READING
Marshall C, Virdun C, Phillips JL. Evidence-based models of rural palliative care: a systematic review. *Palliat Med.* 2023;37(8):1129–1143.

 CODES

ICD10
Z51.5 Encounter for palliative care

CLINICAL PEARLS
- Palliative care is a holistic approach to providing comfort to patients with life-limiting illness.
- Early referral to palliative care helps enhance the quality of life of patients living with serious illness.
- The addition of adjuvant treatments may be more effective than narcotics alone for managing pain.
- Use laxatives with opioid treatment to avoid constipation.

PANCREATITIS, ACUTE

Robert L. Frachtman, MD, FACG • Marni L. Martinez, APRN

 BASICS

DESCRIPTION

Acute inflammation of the pancreas with variable involvement of regional tissue or remote organ systems

- Symptoms relate to intrapancreatic activation of enzymes with pain, nausea and vomiting, and associated intestinal ileus.
- Complete structural and functional recovery if there is no necrosis or pancreatic ductal disruption.

EPIDEMIOLOGY

Incidence
1 to 5/10,000, with no predominant age or sex

Prevalence
- 19/10,000
- It is the most common gastrointestinal diagnosis for inpatient hospitalization.

ETIOLOGY AND PATHOPHYSIOLOGY

- Alcohol—most common in adults (ages 30 to 50 years)
- Gallstones (including microlithiasis)—most common in adults (median age of 69 years)
- Trauma/surgery—most common in adults (median age of 65 years)
- Acute discontinuation of medications for diabetes or hyperlipidemia
- Following endoscopic retrograde cholangiopancreatography (ERCP)
- Medications (most common, not an exhaustive list)
  - ACE inhibitors; angiotensin receptor blockers (ARBs); thiazide diuretics and furosemide
  - Antimetabolites (mercaptopurine and azathioprine) and checkpoint inhibitors
  - Corticosteroids; glyburide; exenatide
  - Mesalamine; sulfamethoxazole/trimethoprim, pentamidine; valproic acid; statins
- Metabolic causes
  - Hypertriglyceridemia (classically >1,000 mg/dL); even nonfasting levels as low as ~≥177 mg/dL
  - Hypercalcemia; acute renal failure
  - Diet with high glycemic load
  - Systemic lupus erythematosus/polyarteritis/other vascular disease
  - Autoimmune; type I with elevated IgG4 and type II with normal IgG4
  - Infections
    ○ Mumps, coxsackievirus, CMV, EBV, cryptosporidiosis, ascaris, clonorchis, SARS-CoV-2
- Penetrating peptic ulcer (rare)
- AIDS
- Cystic fibrosis, CFTR gene mutations, and other mutations
- Tumors (e.g., pancreatic, ampullary)
- Miscellaneous obstruction
  - Celiac disease; Crohn disease; pancreas divisum; sphincter of Oddi dysfunction; choledochocele
- Scorpion venom
- Acute fatty liver of pregnancy
- Pancreatic fat deposition
- Associated coexisting risk factors
  - Obesity; type II diabetes; smoking

- Pathophysiology—enzymatic autodigestion of the pancreas with interstitial edema and third spacing of fluid. Possible sequelae include necrosis, pseudocyst formation, pancreatic ductal disruption, pancreatic ascites, multiorgan failure (early or late), walled off necrosis (late), and injury to surrounding vascular structures such as splenic vein thrombosis and splenic artery pseudoaneurysm.
- Cellular injury alters membrane trafficking, which alters lysosomal function leading to trypsin formation and zymogen activation. A robust inflammatory response ensues resulting in increased vascular permeability, hemorrhage, edema, and necrosis.
- The severity of the first episode of acute pancreatitis, alcohol abuse, and smoking all increase the risk of acute recurrent pancreatitis, which, in turn, increases the risk of progression to chronic pancreatitis.
- Clinical features associated with an increasing severity of acute pancreatitis: age ≥60 years; obesity; long-term, heavy alcohol use

Genetics
Hereditary pancreatitis is rare; autosomal dominant

GENERAL PREVENTION
- Avoid excess alcohol consumption.
- Tobacco cessation
- Correct underlying metabolic processes (hypertriglyceridemia or hypercalcemia).
- Discontinue offending medications.
- Cholecystectomy (symptomatic cholelithiasis)
- Diet: There is an increased risk of gallstone pancreatitis with diets high in saturated fats, cholesterol, red meat, and eggs.

COMMONLY ASSOCIATED CONDITIONS
- Alcohol withdrawal, alcoholic hepatitis, diabetic ketoacidosis, and ascending cholangitis
- Morbid obesity, a proinflammatory state, increases severity and adverse outcomes (organ failure, mortality).

Rx DIAGNOSIS

Symptoms don't always correlate with objective findings.

HISTORY
- Acute onset of "boring" epigastric pain, which may radiate posteriorly
- Nausea/vomiting
- Alcohol use
- Personal or family history of gallstones
- Medication use—look for inciting medications.
- Abdominal trauma
- Recent significant rapid weight loss

PHYSICAL EXAM
- Vital signs—assess hemodynamic stability, fever, tachycardia, and hypotension.
- Abdominal findings: epigastric tenderness, loss of bowel sounds, peritoneal signs
- Other findings: jaundice, rales/percussive dullness
- Rare (with hemorrhagic pancreatitis)
  - Flank discoloration (Grey Turner sign) or umbilical discoloration (Cullen sign)

DIFFERENTIAL DIAGNOSIS
- Penetrating peptic ulcer
- Acute cholecystitis or cholangitis
- Macroamylasemia, macrolipasemia
- Mesenteric vascular occlusion and/or infarction
- Intestinal obstruction, perforated viscus
- Aortic aneurysm (dissecting or rupturing)
- Inferior wall myocardial infarction
- Lymphoma

DIAGNOSTIC TESTS & INTERPRETATION
- Interpret laboratory and radiographic findings in the context of the clinical history.
- Bedside Index for Severity in Acute Pancreatitis (BISAP) score
  - Patients receive 1 point for each element in the first 24 hours: BUN >25 mg/dL, impaired mental status, systemic inflammatory response syndrome (SIRS)—a score of 0 predicts mortality of <1%, and a score of 5 correlates with a mortality rate of 22%.
- Ranson criteria is an older model of predicting severity of pancreatitis. It includes 11 criteria, 5 of which are measured at admission, and 6 are measured in the following 48 hours. A score of ≤3 represents mild pancreatitis, and as the score increases, the mortality rises sharply.
- American College of Gastroenterology requires at least two of the three elements to make a diagnosis of acute pancreatitis: characteristic abdominal pain, specific radiographic findings, and lipase level 3 times the upper limit of normal (ULN).
- Elevated serum amylase >3 times ULN (Severity is not related to degree of elevation. Amylase is not specific to pancreatitis.)
- Elevated serum lipase >3 times ULN. Lipase is more specific to the pancreas than amylase.
- Elevated total bilirubin. If >3 mg/dL, consider common bile duct obstruction.
- A 3-fold elevation in the alanine aminotransferase (ALT) in the setting of acute pancreatitis has a 95% positive predictive value for gallstone pancreatitis. Triglyceride levels >1,000 mg/dL suggest hypertriglyceridemia as the cause.
- Glucose and calcium increased in severe disease.
- WBC elevation to 10,000 to 25,000/μL possible and not indicative of active infection
- Elevated baseline hematocrit >44 or rising hematocrit is poor prognostic sign (severe third spacing with associated hemoconcentration).

Initial Tests (lab, imaging)
- Use follow-up labs to assess renal function, hydration, sepsis, biliary obstruction, and tissue oxygenation.
- Chest x-ray (CXR) to evaluate for early acute respiratory distress syndrome (ARDS), pleural effusion, and perforation
- Ultrasound to look for gallbladder/biliary stones

- CT scan
  - Confirms the diagnosis, assesses severity, establishes a baseline, provides prognostic information, and rules out most other pathologies (excluding noncalcified cholelithiasis)
  - IV contrast is not essential for the initial CT scan; avoid contrast in volume-depleted patients.
  - The presence of gas in the peripancreatic collection is a strong evidence for infection, but its absence does not rule it out.
- Magnetic resonance cholangiopancreatography (MRCP) helps assess choledocholithiasis, pancreas divisum, dilated pancreatic duct, and ductal changes.
- Esophagogastroduodenoscopy (EGD) is useful to rule out a penetrating duodenal ulcer or an obstructing ampullary neoplasm.
- ERCP may be necessary to decompress common bile duct due to an impacted stone.
- Endoscopic ultrasonography (EUS) is useful if patients present with "idiopathic pancreatitis."
- EUS-guided fine needle aspiration if autoimmune pancreatitis is suspected

Follow-Up Tests & Special Considerations
If renal function is stable, a contrast-enhanced CT scan at day 3 to assess for necrosis; CT guidance assists aspiration and drainage of abscess—mainly recommended if a fungal or drug-resistant infection is suspected.

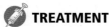 TREATMENT

GENERAL MEASURES
Many cases of acute pancreatitis require hospitalization; ICU if multiorgan dysfunction or hypotension/respiratory failure; 15–20% of cases of acute pancreatitis progress from mild to severe (including persistent organ failure).

- Fluid resuscitation
  - Significant volume deficit due to third spacing
  - Infuse bolus of 10 mL/kg, followed by 1.5 mL/kg/hour. Larger volumes may be required for patients presenting with severe pancreatitis, preferably with CVP monitoring (1)[A].
  - Target urine output should be 0.5 to 1.0 mL/kg/hr. 4 L should be the maximum total fluid on day 1.
  - Fluid resuscitation is of limited value after 24 hours, and fluid overload results in significant complications.
- Eliminate unnecessary medications, especially those implicated as causes of pancreatitis.
- Nasogastric (NG) tube for intractable emesis
- Follow renal function, volume status, calcium, and oxygenation. Organ failure is more important prognostic indicator than pancreatic necrosis.
- Begin oral alimentation after pain, tenderness, and ileus have resolved; small amounts of high-carbohydrate, low-fat, and low-protein foods; advance as tolerated; in cases of mild pancreatitis, a soft low-fat diet may be started even before enzymes elevation and pain have completely resolved (2)[A].
- Enteral nutrition at level of ligament of Treitz if oral feeding not possible within 5 to 7 days; discontinue with increases in pain, increases in amylase/lipase levels, or fluid retention.
- TPN (without lipids if triglycerides are elevated) if oral or nasoenteric feedings are not tolerated

MEDICATION
First Line
- Analgesia: no consensus; *avoid* meperidine (Demerol) due to the potential of accumulation of a toxic metabolite.
- Antibiotics
  - In the clear absence of infection, the use of prophylactic antibiotics is no longer recommended.
  - In patients with ascending cholangitis or necrotizing pancreatitis, if there is a strong suspicion of active infection, consider empiric imipenem class or β-lactam/β-lactamase inhibitor (e.g., piperacillin/tazobactam 4.5 g IV q8h) for initial treatment before cultures (especially aspirates) return.
  - Levofloxacin 500 mg QD IV if cholangitis and there is an allergy to penicillin
  - Watch for fungal superinfections when giving prophylactic antibiotics.

ISSUES FOR REFERRAL
Refer to a tertiary center if pancreatitis is severe or actively evolving and when advanced imaging or endoscopic therapy is being considered.

SURGERY/OTHER PROCEDURES
- Consider cholecystectomy before discharge in patients with cholelithiasis and nonnecrotizing pancreatitis to reduce risk of recurrence.
- Necrosectomy should be performed nonsurgically for either infected or noninfected necrosis. Walled-off necrosis should be observed for 4 weeks and treated with antibiotics if infected.
- ERCP early if evidence of acute cholangitis or at 72 hours if evidence of ongoing biliary obstruction; ERCP with pancreatic ductal stent placement if ductal disruption persists longer than 1 to 2 weeks
- Plasma exchange with insulin within 24 hours of presentation if severe necrotizing pancreatitis secondary to hypertriglyceridemia (2)

ADMISSION, INPATIENT, AND NURSING CONSIDERATIONS
Discharge criteria
- Pain controlled
- Tolerating oral diet
- Alcohol rehabilitation and tobacco cessation
- Low-grade fever and mild leukocytosis do not necessarily indicate infection and may take weeks to resolve. Infections may occur even after 10 days (33% of patients with necrotizing pancreatitis) due to secondary infection of necrotic material, requiring surgical débridement.

 ONGOING CARE

FOLLOW-UP RECOMMENDATIONS
- Follow-up imaging in several weeks if the original CT scan showed a fluid collection or necrosis or if the amylase/lipase continue to be elevated. Follow-up findings may include:
  - Pseudocyst (occurs in 10%) or abscess (sudden onset of fever): Conservative management is an option for asymptomatic pseudocysts up to 6 cm in diameter.
  - Splenic vein thrombosis in 16–18% with necrotizing pancreatitis
  - Pseudoaneurysm (splenic, gastroduodenal, intrapancreatic) hemorrhage can be life threatening.

- Mild exocrine and endocrine dysfunction is usually subclinical. Patients with necrotizing pancreatitis, steatorrhea, or ductal obstruction, however, should receive enzyme supplementation.
- After the first episode of acute pancreatitis, the risk of lifetime diabetes doubles, the risk of developing acute recurrent pancreatitis is ~17%, and the risk for developing chronic pancreatitis is ~8%.

DIET
Advance diet as tolerated; reduce fat, alcohol, and added sugars.

PROGNOSIS
85–90% of cases of acute pancreatitis resolve spontaneously; 3–5% mortality (17% in necrotizing pancreatitis)

REFERENCES
1. Gardner TB. Fluid resuscitation in acute pancreatitis—going over the waterfall. *N Engl J Med*. 2022;387(11):1038–1039.
2. Gulati A, Papachristou GI. Update on the management of acute pancreatitis and its complications. *New Gastroenterol*. 2017;2017:12–17.

ADDITIONAL READING
Hey-Hadavi J, Velisetty P, Mhatre S. Trends and recent developments in pharmacotherapy of acute pancreatitis. *Postgrad Med*. 2022:1–11.

CODES
ICD10
- K85.9 Acute pancreatitis, unspecified
- K85.8 Other acute pancreatitis
- K85.2 Alcohol induced acute pancreatitis

CLINICAL PEARLS
- Gallstones and alcohol misuse are the leading causes of pancreatitis.
- The BISAP score is easier to apply than Ranson criteria and just as accurate for predicting mortality.
- Review all medications and discontinue any that may cause (or contribute to) pancreatitis.
- Start oral feeding as soon as possible in the absence of severe pain, vomiting, or ileus.
- Mild pancreatitis can progress to severe pancreatitis over the initial 48 hours, often due to inadequate fluid replacement.
- Refer to tertiary center if acute pancreatitis is severe or evolving/worsening.

PANIC DISORDER

Jay Winner, MD, FAAFP

 BASICS

DESCRIPTION
- A classic panic attack is characterized by rapid onset of a brief period of sympathetic nervous system hyperarousal accompanied by intense fear.
- In panic disorder, multiple panic attacks occur (including at least two without a recognizable trigger). Patients experience at least 1 month of worried anticipation of additional attacks and/or maladaptive (e.g., avoidance) behaviors.

EPIDEMIOLOGY
Incidence
Median age of onset is 24 years. Prevalence significantly decreases after age 60 years; predominant sex: female > male (2:1)

Prevalence
Lifetime prevalence: 4.7%

ETIOLOGY AND PATHOPHYSIOLOGY
Patients resist the initial surge of adrenaline which exacerbates the symptoms—in essence, they get anxious about being anxious.

Genetics
There is a higher incidence of panic disorder among family members.

RISK FACTORS
- Life stressors of any kind can precipitate attacks, including history of sexual or physical abuse.
- Substance abuse, smoking, bipolar disorder, major depression, obsessive-compulsive disorder (OCD), and simple phobia

GENERAL PREVENTION
- Healthy lifestyle, including healthy diet, regular exercise, and stress-reduction techniques (such as mindfulness), are useful.
- The USPSTF now recommends screening children and teens for anxiety in ages 8 to 18. In September 2022, the USPTF made a draft recommendation to screen adults aged ≤64 years.

COMMONLY ASSOCIATED CONDITIONS
- Other psychiatric diagnoses: PTSD, social phobia, simple phobia, major depression, bipolar disorder, substance abuse, OCD, separation anxiety disorder
- More common in patients with asthma, migraine headaches, hypertension, mitral valve prolapse, reflux esophagitis, interstitial cystitis, irritable bowel syndrome, fibromyalgia, nicotine dependence
- Panic disorder increases the risk of suicide attempts and ideation.

DIAGNOSIS

- Panic attack: an abrupt surge of intense fear, reaching a peak within minutes in which ≥4 of the following symptoms develop abruptly: (i) palpitations, pounding heart, or accelerated heart rate; (ii) sweating; (iii) trembling or shaking; (iv) sensation of shortness of breath or smothering; (v) a choking sensation; (vi) chest pain or discomfort; (vii) nausea or abdominal distress; (viii) feeling dizzy, unsteady, light-headed, or faint; (ix) derealization (feelings of unreality) or depersonalization (feeling detached from oneself); (x) fear of losing control or going crazy; (xi) fear of dying; (xii) paresthesias; and (xiii) chills or hot flashes (1)[C]
- Panic disorder: recurrent panic attacks, at least two without known trigger, not better accounted for by another psychiatric condition (e.g., PTSD, OCD, separation anxiety disorder, social anxiety disorder, or specific phobia) *and* not induced by drugs of abuse, medical conditions, or prescribed drugs *and* with >1 month of at least one of the following: (i) worry about additional attacks or worry about the implications of the attack (e.g., losing control, having a heart attack, "going crazy") and (ii) a significant maladaptive change in behavior related to the attacks (1)[C]

HISTORY
- Obtain a good history through tactful, nonjudgmental questioning. Information should be elicited about physical and emotional symptoms, current life stress, separations, recent deaths, patient's concerns and fears, and interpersonal problems.
- A thorough medication and substance abuse history is important.
- Review *DSM*-5 diagnostic criteria. Ask for avoidance patterns that have developed since the onset of panic attacks.

PHYSICAL EXAM
- During an attack, there can be tachycardia, hyperventilation, and diaphoresis.
- Thyroid exam for fullness or nodules; look for exophthalmos or lid lag.
- Cardiac exam for murmur or arrhythmias
- Lung exam to rule out asthma (limited airflow, wheezing)

DIFFERENTIAL DIAGNOSIS
- Medication use may mimic panic disorder and create anxiety: Paradoxically, antidepressants used to treat panic may, initially, worsen panic; antidepressants in bipolar patients can cause anxiety/mania/panic; short-acting benzodiazepines (alprazolam), β-blockers (propranolol), and short-acting opioids can cause interdose rebound anxiety; benzodiazepine treatment causes panic when patients take too much and run out of these medicines early; bupropion, levodopa, amphetamines, steroids, albuterol, sympathomimetics, fluoroquinolones, and interferon can cause panic; rare medication side effect syndromes such as serotonin syndrome or malignant hyperthermia
- Substance withdrawal or abuse

- Medical conditions: cardiovascular, pulmonary, endocrine (hypothyroidism/hyperthyroidism, premenstrual dysphoric disorder, menopause, pregnancy, hypoglycemia [in diabetes], carcinoid syndrome, pheochromocytoma, Cushing syndrome, hyperaldosteronism, hyperparathyroidism), neurologic (transient ischemic attacks [TIAs], preictal and postictal states), and others. Note: It is unusual to have a first panic attack after the age of 40 years, making it more important to consider other medical conditions for those patients.
- Psychiatric conditions that have overlapping symptomatology include mood, anxiety, and personality disorders such as major depression, bipolar disorder, PTSD, borderline personality disorder, social phobia, OCD, and generalized anxiety disorder. In PTSD, there is always a recollection or visual image that precedes the panic attack. In social phobia, fear of scrutiny precedes the panic attack. In bipolar disorder, major depression, borderline personality disorder, and particularly substance abuse, the patient often complains first of panic symptoms and anxiety and minimizes other potentially relevant symptoms and behaviors.

DIAGNOSTIC TESTS & INTERPRETATION
No specific lab tests are indicated except to rule out conditions in the differential diagnosis.
- If chest discomfort, do appropriate workup; electrocardiogram (ECG) and pulse oximetry; consider Holter monitoring, stress testing, and/or chest CT in select patients.
- Fingerstick blood sugar test in acute setting in a diabetic patient
- Thyroid-stimulating hormone (TSH), complete metabolic panel, CBC
- If nocturnal panic attacks, consider sleep study to evaluate for possible sleep apnea.
- Other testing as indicated, for instance, if typical signs and symptoms of rare conditions like pheochromocytoma or carcinoid

Diagnostic Procedures/Other
- If a medical cause of anxiety is strongly suspected, do the workup appropriate for that condition.
- Panic Disorder Severity Scale (PDSS) can be used for monitoring changes in severity of symptoms and response to treatment. Also, the PHQ-PD can be used if screening is desired.

 TREATMENT

Combined antidepressant therapy and psychotherapy is superior to either alone during initial treatment for panic disorder (2)[A]. Most effective therapy includes cognitive-behavioral therapy (CBT), mindfulness-based therapy, and exposure therapy. Psychotherapy provides long-lasting treatment, often without subsequent need for medications.

GENERAL MEASURES

Patient education is a vital part of treatment. A useful mnemonic is HR BET (think of Babe Ruth as the person you would have betted on to get a home run or your "HR BET").

- Harmless: Explain to patients why they are having their symptoms. For instance, hyperventilation may change the acid–base balance of the blood causing dizziness, extremity tingling, and odd out-of-body sensations.
- Resistance: Explain how resistance can prolong the panic and make it worse. People get anxious about being anxious.
- Breathing: Teach mindful diaphragmatic breathing (paying attention to the sensation of one breath at a time, with the abdomen expanding with each inhalation).
- Energy: Discuss that adrenaline can be felt as anxiety or excitement. Instead of calling it a panic attack, reframe it as an energy burst and see if patients can feel the energy flowing through their veins.
- Thoughts: Develop the skill of noticing thoughts without believing them all. People can also be taught to dispute irrational thoughts and beliefs (e.g., disputing "I'm dying now," with "I've had many of these attacks before; they have been thoroughly evaluated by my doctor, and they are not harmful; if I don't resist them and just do my diaphragmatic breathing, they resolve more quickly.").

MEDICATION

- Medication management is indicated if psychotherapy is not successful and/or if symptoms are severe and may be combined with psychotherapy.
- Selective serotonin reuptake inhibitor (SSRI), serotonin-norepinephrine reuptake inhibitor (SNRI), tricyclic antidepressant (TCA), monoamine oxidase inhibitor (MAOI), and benzodiazepines have shown efficacy in treating panic disorder.
- It is recommended that medications should be maintained for at least 1 year after symptom control to reduce risk of relapse.

First Line

- SSRIs and SNRIs are first line given efficacy, relatively benign side effect profile, and lack of abuse potential.
- Start a low-dose SSRI or SNRI, for example, fluoxetine 5 to 10 mg, paroxetine 10 mg, sertraline 25 mg, citalopram 10 mg, escitalopram 5 mg, or venlafaxine extended release (ER) 37.5 mg once daily in the morning. (If sedation occurs, this can be changed to nightly dosing.). Titrate up slowly every 1 to 2 weeks to therapeutic doses. If indicated, further dose increases usually happen no more frequently than monthly. Side effects include irritability, diarrhea, and sexual dysfunction, with less frequent side effects such as hyponatremia, GI bleeding, manic episodes (if patient is bipolar), elevated LFTs, QT prolongation (more often with citalopram), and serotonin syndrome. Warn people who are starting escitalopram that nausea is very frequent but usually resolves after 1 week of treatment. Suicidality can be seen in young patients. When stopping SSRI, taper over several weeks or months because of risk of discontinuation syndrome. This is more important for medications with a shorter half-life like paroxetine and venlafaxine compared with medications such as fluoxetine.
- Among SNRIs, venlafaxine ER, if not effective after a month of 75 mg/day, can be slowly titrated up to a maximum dose of 225 mg/day with risk of hypertension at higher doses. Other side effects are similar to SSRIs. SNRIs such as desvenlafaxine or duloxetine can also be tried.

Second Line

- Mirtazapine can be used starting at 15 mg QHS and potentially increasing to 30 mg QHS. Side effects of sedation and weight gain may limit use, but for people suffering from weight loss and insomnia, this medication could be helpful.
- TCAs, particularly imipramine, may be an option but are seldom used (because of difficulty in dosing, more side effects, and greater risk associated with overdose compared with SSRIs). Screen for cardiac conduction system in patients >40 years of age with an ECG.
- MAOIs like phenelzine and tranylcypromine are also efficacious compared to placebo. Avoid with serotonergic agents given risk for serotonin syndrome. There are also dietary restrictions and multiple other drug interactions that limit use of these medications.
- Benzodiazepines should be either avoided or used only for crisis and short-term relief of severe symptoms. Alprazolam (start 0.25 mg TID PRN) and clonazepam (start at 0.5 mg BID PRN) are FDA-approved for panic disorder. Clonazepam has a longer half-life, less interdose anxiety, and lower abuse potential than alprazolam. Benzodiazepines are associated with sedation, dependence, increased falls, increased car accidents, and increased mortality. Prescribing benzodiazepines to patients on opiates increases risk of overdose.

ISSUES FOR REFERRAL

- Refer to a counselor who treats anxiety with CBT, mindfulness-based therapy, and/or exposure therapy.
- Consider psychiatrist referral for comorbid bipolar disorder, borderline personality disorder, schizophrenia, suicidality, alcohol, substance abuse, or for patients unresponsive to initial treatment.

ADDITIONAL THERAPIES

- Aerobic exercise, yoga, or tai chi may reduce symptoms.
- Mindfulness meditation can be learned with stress reduction classes such as Mindfulness-Based Stress Reduction (MBSR), apps such as Ten Percent Happier, Headspace, and UCLA Mindful; free meditations also at StressRemedy.com/audio; one study showed that an 8-week MBSR class was as effective as escitalopram in treating anxiety disorders.

COMPLEMENTARY & ALTERNATIVE MEDICINE

There is limited data supporting the use of supplements for the treatment of anxiety disorders. Kava kava should be avoided because of the risks of liver failure. A 2018 meta-analysis did show potential reduction in anxiety from omega-3 fatty acids 2 g daily with EPA <60% (would start at 1 g daily) (3)[C].

ADMISSION, INPATIENT, AND NURSING CONSIDERATIONS

If a panic disorder patient has concrete suicidal ideation, a psychiatric admission is indicated.

 ONGOING CARE

FOLLOW-UP RECOMMENDATIONS

Full therapeutic effect of antidepressants often does not occur until 4 to 6 weeks. Monitor (usually within 1 to 2 weeks) for suicidal ideation when starting antidepressants in patients aged ≤24 years.

DIET

A primarily whole-food, plant-based diet and limiting caffeine may be helpful.

PATIENT EDUCATION

- Video on "Dealing with Panic and Anxiety" at StressRemedy.com/videos
- National Institute of Mental Health: http://www.nimh.nih.gov/health/publications/panic-disorder-when-fear-overwhelms/index.shtml

PROGNOSIS

Remission occurs in 64.5% of patients with a mean time to remission of about 5.7 months. Recurrence does occur in 21.4% in those who achieved remission. Predictors of remission are female gender, absence of ongoing stressors, and a low initial frequency of attacks.

COMPLICATIONS

- Iatrogenic benzodiazepine dependence
- Iatrogenic mania in bipolar patients treated for panic with unopposed antidepressants

REFERENCES

1. American Psychiatric Association. *Diagnostic and Statistical Manual of Mental Disorders*. 5th ed. Arlington, VA: American Psychiatric Association; 2013.
2. Furukawa TA, Watanabe N, Churchill R. Combined psychotherapy plus antidepressants for panic disorder with or without agoraphobia. *Cochrane Database Syst Rev*. 2007;2007(1):CD004364.
3. Su KP, Tseng PT, Lin PY, et al. Association of use of omega-3 polyunsaturated fatty acids with changes in severity of anxiety symptoms: a systematic review and meta-analysis. *JAMA Netw Open*. 2018;1(5):e182327.

ADDITIONAL READING

DeGeorge KC, Grover M, Streeter GS. Generalized anxiety disorder and panic disorder in adults. *Am Fam Physician*. 2022;106(2):157–164.

 SEE ALSO

Algorithm: Anxiety

CODES

ICD10

F41.0 Panic disorder [episodic paroxysmal anxiety]

CLINICAL PEARLS

First-line pharmacological treatment is usually an SSRI or SNRI; patient education is also important and counseling, particularly CBT, is often helpful. Consider assessing suicidality because patients with panic disorder are at increased risk for suicide, particularly if depressed.

PARKINSON DISEASE

Svitlana Zhukivska, MD

BASICS

DESCRIPTION
- An adult-onset, progressive, neurodegenerative disorder caused by loss of dopaminergic neurons in the substantia nigra and other dopaminergic regions of the brain
- Cardinal symptoms include resting tremor, rigidity, bradykinesia, and postural instability.

EPIDEMIOLOGY
Prevalence
- Second most common neurodegenerative disease after Alzheimer disease
- Average age of onset: ~60 years; slightly more common in men than women
- 1 to 2/1,000 persons; 0.3% of general population and 1 to 2% of those ≥60 years of age and up to 4% of those ≥80 years of age; affects >1 million people in the United States and >6 million worldwide

ETIOLOGY AND PATHOPHYSIOLOGY
Dopamine depletion in the substantia nigra and the nigrostriatal pathways results in the classic motor signs of PD such as tremor, bradykinesia, and rigidity.
- Loss of neurons accompanied by presence of Lewy bodies (hyaline inclusion bodies) and Lewy neuritis

Genetics
Mutations in multiple autosomal dominant and autosomal recessive genes are linked to PD/parkinsonian syndrome particularly when the age at symptom onset is <50 years.

RISK FACTORS
Age and family history of PD or tremor; lifelong pesticide use (rotenone, carbamate) is associated with risk of developing PD; repeated head trauma and living in rural areas, drinking well water; high dietary iron intake, low vitamin D level, and low bone density/osteoporosis in women (1)

GENERAL PREVENTION
Caffeine consumption, cigarette smoking, and physical activity have been linked to decreased risk of development of PD include weight training, running, dancing, yoga, and traditional Chinese martial arts (2).

COMMONLY ASSOCIATED CONDITIONS
Cognitive abnormalities, autonomic dysfunction (e.g., constipation, urinary urgency), sleep disturbances, mental status changes (depression, psychosis, hallucinations, dementia), orthostatic hypotension, and pain

DIAGNOSIS

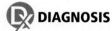

- Diagnosis is based on clinical features (rest tremor, rigidity, bradykinesia, postural instability) and response to dopaminergic therapy.
- PD is a clinical diagnosis, and the gold standards for diagnosis are history and neuropathologic exam.
- Generally, bradykinesia plus either tremor or rigidity must be present.
- Idiopathic rapid eye movement sleep behavior disorder is a possible prodrome for PD.

HISTORY
Symptoms often subtle or attributed to aging
- Decreased emotion displayed in facial features
- General motor slowing and stiffness (One or both arms do not swing with walk.)
- Resting tremor (often initially one hand)
- Speech soft/mumbling
- Falls/difficulty with balance; seen with disease progression
- Psychiatric symptoms including depression, anxiety, hallucinations, and dementia
- Urinary symptoms including increased frequency and urgency; constipation

PHYSICAL EXAM
- Tremor
  - Resting tremor (4 to 6 Hz) that is often asymmetric; disappears with voluntary movement; frequently emerges in a hand while walking and may present as pill rolling; frequently also present in jaw, chin, lips, tongue
- Bradykinesia—generalized slowness of movements
- Rigidity: cogwheel (catching and releasing) or lead pipe (continuously rigid); tested by passively manipulating the limbs
- Postural instability—decreased ability to prevent falling

DIFFERENTIAL DIAGNOSIS
- Essential tremor: bradykinesia is not present; often symmetric and occurs mostly during action or when holding hands outstretched, nonresponsive to levodopa
- Depression can cause psychomotor slowing that may appear similar to bradykinesia in PD.
- Dementia with Lewy bodies: characterized clinically by visual hallucinations, fluctuating cognition, and parkinsonism; dementia occurs concomitantly with or before the development of parkinsonism.
- Multiple system atrophy: presets with parkinsonism and varying degrees of dysautonomia, cerebellar involvement, and pyramidal signs; poor response to levodopa
- Progressive supranuclear palsy: impairment in vertical eye movements (particularly down gaze), hyperextension of neck, and early falling; pseudobulbar palsy
- Associated neurodegenerative disorders: late stages of Alzheimer disease, Huntington disease, frontotemporal dementia, spinocerebellar ataxias
- Secondary parkinsonism (drug induced: reversible; may take weeks/months after offending medication is stopped; often bilateral symptoms): neuroleptics (most common); antiemetics (e.g., prochlorperazine and promethazine), metoclopramide; SSRIs; calcium channel blockers; amiodarone; lithium/valproic acid; amphotericin B; estrogens.

DIAGNOSTIC TESTS & INTERPRETATION
Initial Tests (lab, imaging)
- Diagnosis is mainly clinical, and there are no confirmatory physiologic or blood tests.
- Reduction in α-synuclein and DJ-1 protein can act as a qualitative feature in PD diagnosis.
- MRI of brain is nondiagnostic but can be used to rule out structural abnormalities.

Follow-Up Tests & Special Considerations
Single-photon emission computerized tomography (SPECT) might be helpful to differentiate PD from secondary parkinsonism.

Diagnostic Procedures/Other
PET and MR Spectroscopy are not recommended.

Test Interpretation
Diagnosis is clinical, and no tests are recommended to confirm diagnosis of PD.

TREATMENT

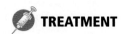

GENERAL MEASURES
Multidisciplinary rehabilitation with standard physical and occupational therapy components to improve functional outcomes

MEDICATION
- PD treatment goal: Improve motor and nonmotor symptoms. Start treatment when symptoms impair functioning or quality of life.
- Agents are chosen based on patient's age and symptoms present.
- "Off" periods describe the development of symptoms (often dyskinesias) while patient is on PD medication. This especially occurs among elderly patients taking levodopa medications.

First Line
- First-line agents in early PD: levodopa, dopamine agonists, monoamine oxidase B (MAO-B) inhibitors (3)[A],(4)[A]
  - Levodopa combined with carbidopa is still the most effective treatment for symptoms of PD, particularly bradykinesia. Levodopa by itself requires frequent dosing because of peripheral conversion.
  - Levodopa versus dopamine agonist is controversial:
    ○ Most patients eventually will develop involuntary motor fluctuations or dyskinesias with levodopa.
    ○ Older patients are often less able to tolerate the adverse events of dopamine agonists.
    ○ All patients eventually will require levodopa.
  - For patients who experience dyskinesias while on levodopa, they can consider MAO-B inhibitors (rasagiline) or catechol O-methyltransferase (COMT) inhibitors (entacapone) as adjuvants.
- Carbidopa + levodopa (Carbidopa inhibits peripheral conversion of levodopa.)
  - Immediate release (Sinemet)
  - Orally disintegrating (Parcopa)
- Carbidopa + levodopa + entacapone (Stalevo)
  - Addition of entacapone as a single agent should be initiated prior to use of this combination:
    ○ Once daily dose of carbidopa/levodopa has been identified, may convert to Stalevo
  - Side effects are the same, plus diarrhea and brownish orange urine.

- Dopamine-receptor agonists (nonergot): use when mild symptoms; preference for once-daily medication and in younger patients; side effects: nausea, vomiting, hypotension, sedation, vivid dreaming, compulsive behavior, confusion, light-headedness, and hallucinations:
  – Pramipexole (Mirapex)
  – Ropinirole (Requip)
  – Rotigotine (transdermal patch)
- Selective MAO-B inhibitors: side effects: insomnia, jitteriness, hallucinations; mostly found with selegiline; rasagiline similar adverse events as placebo in clinical trials; rasagiline is metabolized via *CYP1A2*; caution with other medications using this enzyme system (e.g., ciprofloxacin):
  – Selegiline (Eldepryl)
  – Rasagiline (Azilect)

Second Line
- Second-line agents in early PD: β-adrenergic antagonists (postural tremor), amantadine, anticholinergics (young patients with tremor); lack of good evidence for symptom control
- Dopamine agonists (ergot): increased adverse event profile makes these agents nonpreferred to nonergot dopamine agonists; bromocriptine (Parlodel)
- Treatment of levodopa-induced motor complications
  – End of dose wearing off (i.e., decreased responsiveness to PD medication resulting in return of PD symptoms)
  – Entacapone (with each levodopa dose) or rasagiline preferred
  – Dyskinesias: typically occur at peak dopamine level
  – Amantadine may be considered; however, efficacy is questionable.
  – The FDA has approved istradefylline (Nourianz) as the first adenosine A2A receptor antagonist to be approved in the United States an oral agent for use as an adjunct to carbidopa/levodopa in adults with PD who experience "off" episodes.
- Anticholinergic agents: avoided due to lack of efficacy (only useful for tremor) and increased adverse event profile: trihexyphenidyl; benztropine (Cogentin)
- *N*-methyl-D-aspartic acid antagonist: exact mechanism unknown, efficacy is questionable; may be useful for dyskinesias; side effects: confusion, dizziness, dry mouth, livedo reticularis, and hallucinations:
  – Amantadine (Symmetrel)
- COMT inhibitors: entacapone preferred due to hepatotoxicity associated with tolcapone; adverse events include nausea and orthostatic hypotension: entacapone (Comtan); tolcapone (Tasmar).
  – Requires LFT monitoring
- Apomorphine (Apokyn): nonergot-derived dopamine agonist given SC for "off" episodes in advanced disease; adverse events: nausea, vomiting, dizziness, hallucinations, orthostatic hypotension, somnolence
  – Only for "off" episodes with levodopa therapy

ISSUES FOR REFERRAL
Neurology for suspected PD

ADDITIONAL THERAPIES
- Emotional and psychological support of patient and family; refer patients to community resources to promote social engagement.
- Physical therapy and endurance exercise to improve balance, muscle strength, and walking speed
- Speech therapy: may be helpful in improving speech volume and maintaining voice quality
- Treatment of nonmotor symptoms:
  – Psychosis
    ○ In 2016, the FDA approved pimavanserin (Nuplazid) as the first drug specifically designed to treat PD psychosis
    ○ Quetiapine (Seroquel) had been widely used for people with PDP before pimavanserin.
    ○ Insomnia: rotigotine: FDA-approved in transdermal form to treat insomnia in PD
    ○ Orthostatic hypotension: in addition to increasing salt and fluid intake, can also use FDA-approved droxidopa
      ■ Can also consider midodrine, fludrocortisone, use of compression stockings
    ○ Dementia: rivastigmine can be considered for cognitive impairment (i.e., mild to moderate dementia in PD)
    ○ Depression in PD: can consider pramipexole, nortriptyline, desipramine, venlafaxine, and CBT

SURGERY/OTHER PROCEDURES
- Deep brain stimulation (DBS) is an effective therapeutic option for patients with motor complications refractory to the best medical treatment who are healthy, have no significant comorbidities, are responsive to levodopa, and do not have depression or dementia.
- Patients, who are not candidates for DBS, might benefit from MRI-guided focused ultrasound lesioning (unilateral pallidotomy) for relief from disabling motor symptoms.

COMPLEMENTARY & ALTERNATIVE MEDICINE
Music therapy may help to improve quality of life and motor symptoms in PD patients.

ADMISSION, INPATIENT, AND NURSING CONSIDERATIONS
- Fall risk precaution when admitted
- Note that small variation in medication dosage can impact PD symptoms. Make sure patient has home PD medications and takes them at the correct time.
- Avoid dopamine-blocking agents such as antipsychotics and antiemetics (prochlorperazine, metoclopramide).

ONGOING CARE

FOLLOW-UP RECOMMENDATIONS
- Avoid drug holidays if patient is having "off" time on levodopa.
- Consider switching to dopamine agonist (nonergot preferred), MAO-B inhibitors, or COMT inhibitors if patient develops dyskinesias on levodopa/carbidopa therapy.
- Severe motor symptoms; at this point, patient should not be allowed to drive for himself or herself. This should be noted and reported to licensing agency.

Patient Monitoring
If on dopamine agonists—monitor for development of impulse control behaviors.

DIET
- For dysphagia, consider soft food, swallowing evaluation, and increased time for meals.
- Avoid large, high-fat meals that slow digestion and interfere with medication absorption.

PATIENT EDUCATION
- Parkinson's Foundation: https://www.parkinson.org/
- For caregivers: https://www.caregiver.org/resource/parkinsons-disease-caregiving/

PROGNOSIS
- PD is a chronic progressive disease; prognosis varies based on patient-specific symptoms.
- Increased mortality in PD; on average, survival rate is reduced by 5% every year of follow-up.

REFERENCES
1. Park KY, Jung JH, Hwang HS, et al. Bone mineral density and the risk of Parkinson's disease in postmenopausal women. *Mov Disord*. 2023;38(9):1606–1614.
2. Fan B, Jabeen R, Bo B, et al. What and how can physical activity prevention function on Parkinson's disease? *Oxid Med Cell Longev*. 2020;2020:4293071.
3. Halli-Tierney AD, Luker J, Carroll DG. Parkinson Disease. *Am Fam Physician*. 2020;102(11): 679–691.
4. Drugs for Parkinson's disease. *Med Lett Drugs Ther*. 2021;63(1618):25–32.

ADDITIONAL READING
Miyasaki JM, Martin W, Suchowersky O, et al. Practice parameter: initiation of treatment for Parkinson's disease: an evidence-based review: report of the Quality Standards Subcommittee of the American Academy of Neurology. *Neurology*. 2002;58(1):11–17.

CODES

ICD10
- G21.11 Neuroleptic induced parkinsonism
- G21.8 Other secondary parkinsonism
- G21.4 Vascular parkinsonism

CLINICAL PEARLS
- The classic description for PD is shaky (pill-rolling tremor at rest), stiff (cogwheel rigidity), slow (bradykinesia), and stumbling (shuffling gait).
- No cure—the goals are to delay disease progression and to relieve symptoms.
- Emphasize the importance of exercise and movement to help preserve function.
- Pharmacotherapeutic regimens need to be individualized based on age/specific symptoms.

PARONYCHIA

Nancy V. Nguyen, DO

 BASICS

DESCRIPTION
- Superficial inflammation of the lateral and posterior nail folds surrounding the fingernail or toenail. Develops after breakdown of barrier between nail plate and the adjacent nail fold
- Acute: characterized by pain, erythema, and swelling (1) lasting <6 weeks; usually a bacterial infection appearing after nail biting, trauma, manicures, ingrown nails, and hangnail manipulation. It also occurs as an adverse effect from several drugs. It can progress to abscess formation.
- Chronic: characterized by swelling, tenderness, cuticle elevation, and nail dystrophy and separation lasting at least 6 weeks, or recurrent episodes of acute eponychial inflammation and drainage
- Chemotherapy-associated paronychia (CAP) starts 4 to 8 weeks after chemotherapy initiation (2).
- May be considered work-related among bartenders, restaurant servers, dishwashers, nurses, and others who often wash their hands
- Usually involves one finger but drug-induced paronychia may involve multiple fingers
- Relevant anatomy: nail bed, nail plate, and perionychium
- Synonym(s): eponychia, perionychia, retronychia

Pediatric Considerations
Less common in pediatric age groups; commonly caused by trauma to periungual skin, such as thumb/finger-sucking or other injuries (*Staphylococcus aureus* and group A *Streptococcus* may be present). Paronychia is also a frequent adverse effect of BRAF and MEK inhibitor anticancer drugs.

EPIDEMIOLOGY
Incidence
- One of the most common hand infections in the United States
- Predominant age: all ages
- Predominant sex: female > male

ETIOLOGY AND PATHOPHYSIOLOGY
- Acute: mixed aerobic and anaerobic bacterial flora in 50% of cases. *Staphylococcus aureus* most common and *Streptococcus pyogenes*; less frequently, *Pseudomonas aeruginosa* and other gram-negative bacteria (with chronic paronychia)
- Chronic: eczematous reaction with secondary *Candida albicans* (~95%)
- Pediatric age groups: mixed anaerobic (*Fusobacterium, Peptostreptococcus*) and aerobic infections (*Eikenella corrodens, S. aureus,* streptococci) from oral flora
- A paronychial infection commonly starts in the lateral nail fold.
- Acute paronychia of the fingers is often due to trauma; acute paronychia of the toes is often due to ingrown nails (3).
- Recurrent inflammation, persistent edema, and fibrosis of nail folds cause nail folds to round up and retract, exposing nail grooves to irritants, allergens, and pathogens.

- Inflammation compromises ability of proximal nail fold to regenerate cuticle leading to decreased vascular supply. This can cause decrease efficacy of topical medications.
- Early in the course, cellulitis alone may be present.
- An abscess can form if the infection does not resolve quickly.

RISK FACTORS
- Acute: direct or indirect trauma to cuticle or nail fold, manicured/sculptured nails, nail biting, thumb sucking, manipulating a hangnail, ingrown toenail
- Chronic: frequent immersion of hands in water with excoriation of the lateral nail fold (e.g., chefs, bartenders, housekeepers, swimmers, dishwashers, nurses)
- Predisposing conditions such as diabetes mellitus (DM) and immunosuppression
- Medications such as EGFR inhibitors, systemic retinoids, chemotherapy, and antiretroviral agents

GENERAL PREVENTION
- Acute: Avoid trauma such as nail biting or manipulating a hangnail. Prevent ingrown toenails.
- Chronic: Avoid exposure to allergens and contact irritants; keep fingers/hands dry; wear rubber gloves with a cotton liner. Prevent excoriation of the skin.
- Keep nails short; avoid manicures.
- Apply moisturizer after washing hands.

COMMONLY ASSOCIATED CONDITIONS
DM, eczema or atopic dermatitis, immunosuppression

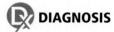 **DIAGNOSIS**

HISTORY
- Localized pain or tenderness, swelling, and erythema of posterior or lateral nail folds
  - Acute: fairly rapid onset (2 to 5 days after trauma)
  - Chronic: at least 6 weeks' duration
- Previous trauma (i.e., bitten nails, ingrown nails, manicured nails)
- Contact with herpes infections
- Contact with allergens or irritants (frequent water immersion, latex)
- Immunosuppressive therapy

PHYSICAL EXAM
- Acute: red, warm, tender, tense posterior or lateral nail fold ± abscess
- Chronic:
  - Initially appears as swollen, tender, boggy nail fold ± abscess
  - Later appears as retraction of nail fold and absence of adjacent healthy cuticle, thickening of nail plate with prominent transverse ridges known as Beau lines and discoloration; multiple digits typically involved
- Occasional elevation of nail bed or separation of nail fold from nail plate
- Fluctuance, purulence at the nail margin, or purulent drainage
- An untreated infection of the toe may lead to the formation of granulation tissue around the nail fold (3).

- Secondary changes of nail platelike discoloration
- Suspect *Pseudomonas* if with green changes in nail (chloronychia).

DIFFERENTIAL DIAGNOSIS
- Felon (abscess of fingertip pulp; urgent diagnosis required)
- Cellulitis
- Eczema
- Herpetic whitlow (similar in appearance, very painful, often associated with vesicles)
- Allergic contact dermatitis (latex, acrylic)
- Psoriasis (especially acute flare)
- Proximal/lateral onychomycosis (nail folds not predominantly involved)
- Retronychia
- Pemphigus vulgaris
- Acute osteomyelitis of the distal phalanx
- Reiter disease
- Pustular psoriasis
- Dermatomyositis
- Malignancy: squamous cell carcinoma of the nail, malignant melanoma, metastatic disease

DIAGNOSTIC TESTS & INTERPRETATION
None required unless condition is severe; resistant to treatment or if recurrence or methicillin-resistant *S. aureus* (MRSA) is suspected, then
- Gram stain
- Culture and sensitivity
- Potassium hydroxide wet mount plus fungal culture especially in chronic paronychia
- Drugs that may alter lab results: use of over-the-counter antimicrobials or antifungals

Initial Tests (lab, imaging)
Consider ultrasonography if uncertain about presence of an abscess.

Diagnostic Procedures/Other
- Incision and drainage recommended for suppurative cases or cases not responding to conservative management or empiric antibiotics
- Tzanck testing or viral culture in suspected viral cases
- Biopsy in cases not responding to conservative management or when malignancy suspected

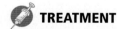 **TREATMENT**

GENERAL MEASURES
- Acute inflammation without abscess: warm water soaks or antiseptic soaks, and topical antibiotics (2). Consider oral antibiotics for more severe cases that do not respond to topical treatment alone.
- Abscesses should be drained.
- Antibiotics may not be necessary for successful I&D of uncomplicated infections.
- Chronic: Keep fingers dry; apply moisturizing lotion after hand washing; avoid exposure to irritants; improved diabetic control
- Pediatric cases should be treated with systemic antibiotics.

MEDICATION

First Line

- Acute paronychia (mild cases, no abscess formation):
  - Warm water soaks or antiseptic soaks (chlorhexidine, povidone-iodine) multiple times a day for 10 to 15 minutes each time, and topical antibiotics with *S. aureus* coverage (triple antibiotic ointment, mupirocin, bacitracin)
  - Antibiotic cream applied TID–QID after warm soak for 5 to 10 days
  - If eczematous: high-potency topical steroid applied BID (e.g., betamethasone 0.05% cream) for 7 to 14 days
- Acute paronychia (no abscess formation, not responding to topical treatment). Treat for 5 to 7 days.
  - Dicloxacillin 250 mg QID
  - Cephalexin 500 mg TID–QID
- Acute paronychia (exposure to oral flora, no abscess formation). Treat for 7 days. Cover for Eikenella.
  - Amoxicillin-clavulanate: 875 mg/125 mg BID; pediatric, 45 mg/kg q12h (for <40 kg) *or*
  - One of the following for Eikenella coverage:
    ○ Doxycycline 100 mg BID
    ○ Trimethoprim/sulfamethoxazole BID
    ○ Penicillin VK 500 mg QID
    ○ Ciprofloxacin 500 to 750 mg BID (Reserve fluoroquinolones for severe infection due to risks from this class of antibiotic.)
  - *PLUS* one of the following for anaerobic coverage:
    ○ Clindamycin 450 mg TID (pediatric, 10 mg/kg q8h)
    ○ Metronidazole 500 mg TID
- Acute paronychia (with risk factors for MRSA including but not limited to: recent hospitalization, recent surgery, ESRD on hemodialysis, HIV/AIDS, IVDU, resident of long term care facility). Treat for 7 days.
  - Trimethoprim/sulfamethoxazole 160 mg/800 mg BID
  - Doxycycline 100 mg BID
  - Clindamycin 300 to 450 mg TID–QID
- Acute paronychia with abscess formation:
  - Incision and drainage
    ○ Consider digital block anesthesia. Then, insert nail elevator, #11 scalpel blade, or hypodermic needle along nail plate at junction of the affected nail fold and nail to facilitate drainage. If no drainage occurs, use a needle or scalpel to open skin directly above abscess.
  - If ingrown nail involved or abscess extends to nail bed, consider partial nail removal.
  - Consider oral antibiotics for extension of cellulitis. Otherwise, usually no antibiotics indicated after I&D

Pediatric Considerations

- Without abscess formation: use systemic antibiotics as first-line treatment. Empiric treatment with beta-lactamase-resistant antibiotics (e.g., dicloxacillin, cloxacillin).
- With abscess formation: incision and drainage
- Chronic paronychia: Stop source of irritation, control inflammation, and restore natural protective barrier.
  - Topical high-potency steroids: betamethasone 0.05%; applied BID for 7 to 14 days
  - Topical antifungal: clotrimazole or nystatin; applied topically TID for up to 30 days
  - Topical calcineurin inhibitor: Tacrolimus 0.1% ointment BID for up to 21 days has been shown to be more effective than betamethasone but is more expensive.

- For paronychia caused by EGFR inhibitors, treat with topical antibiotics and potent topical corticosteroids without discontinuing the EGFR inhibitor for mild cases. For more severe cases, discontinue EGFR inhibitor temporarily.
- For paronychia caused by oncology pharmacotherapy, treat with corticosteroid ointment and phenol chemical matricectomy. Prompt treatment enables patients to continue anticancer drug treatment without impairing their quality of life.

Second Line

- Systemic antifungals (rarely needed, use if topical fails)
  - Itraconazole 200 mg for 90 days (may have longer action because it is incorporated into nail plate); pulse therapy may be useful (i.e., 200 mg BID for 7 days, repeated monthly for 2 months).
  - Terbinafine 250 mg/day for 6 weeks (fingernails) or 12 weeks (toenails)
  - Fluconazole 100 mg daily for 7 to 14 days
  - Ciclopirox 0.77% topical suspension BID for 2 to 4 weeks along with strict irritant avoidance
- Antipseudomonal drugs (e.g., ceftazidime, aminoglycosides) when pseudomonas is suspected

ISSUES FOR REFERRAL

- Acute: Severe infection may spread to underlying tendons, requiring evaluation and treatment by a hand surgeon as it often involves débridement, washout, or amputation, based on the severity of the infection.
- Chronic: In treatment failure, consider biopsy and/or, in cases of chronic paronychia, referral for possible partial excision of the nail fold or eponychial marsupialization with or without complete nail removal or Swiss roll technique.
- Failure to respond to therapy or chronic redness, tenderness and swelling of nail folds without abscess can be concerning for malignancy. Consider biopsy (3).

ADDITIONAL THERAPIES

Topical betaxolol 0.25% eye drops once daily on paronychia and pyogenic granuloma-like lesions covered with bandage

SURGERY/OTHER PROCEDURES

- Incision and drainage of abscess, if present. A subungual abscess or ingrown nail requires partial or complete removal of nail with phenolization of germinal matrix.
- Swiss roll technique for chronic and severe acute paronychia with runaround abscess involving both nail folds
- Recalcitrant cases may also need nail removal.

COMPLEMENTARY & ALTERNATIVE MEDICINE

Nail braces as a noninvasive alternative to nail extraction for patients with severe paronychia induced by EGFR inhibitors

 ONGOING CARE

FOLLOW-UP RECOMMENDATIONS

- Acute: Postdrainage care consists of warm soaks or antiseptic soaks. Follow up in 24 to 48 hours after I&D to monitor for worsening infection.
- Chronic: Avoid frequent immersion, triggers, allergens, nail biting, or finger sucking.

DIET

Maintain good glucose control.

PATIENT EDUCATION

- Avoid trimming cuticles; avoid nail trauma; and stress importance of good diabetic control and diabetic education.
- Avoid contact irritants; use rubber gloves with cotton liners to avoid exposure to excess moisture.
- Use moisturizing lotion after washing hands; do not bite nails/suck on fingers.

PROGNOSIS

- With adequate treatment and prevention, healing can be expected in 1 to 2 weeks.
- Chronic paronychia may respond slowly to treatment, taking weeks to months.
- If no response in chronic lesions, rarely benign or malignant neoplasm may be present and referral to dermatology should be considered.

COMPLICATIONS

- Acute: subungual abscess
- Chronic: nail thickening, discoloration of nail, and nail loss

REFERENCES

1. Leggit JC. Acute and chronic paronychia. *Am Fam Physician*. 2017;96(1):44–51.
2. Relhan V, Bansal A. Acute and chronic paronychia revisited: a narrative review. *J Cutan Aesthet Surg*. 2022;15(1):1–16.
3. Lomax A, Thornton J, Singh D. Toenail paronychia. *Foot Ankle Surg*. 2016;22(4):219–223.

 SEE ALSO

Onychomycosis, Retronychia

CODES

ICD10

- L03.019 Cellulitis of unspecified finger
- L03.039 Cellulitis of unspecified toe
- L03.011 Cellulitis of right finger

CLINICAL PEARLS

- Consider incision and drainage when appropriate.
- For chronic paronychia, topical steroid is the first-line treatment. Consider other differentials in non-responders (e.g., rare causes: Raynaud, metastatic cancer, psoriasis, drug toxicity).
- Consider presence of more than one nail disease at the same time (e.g., paronychia and onychomycosis).

PAROTITIS, ACUTE AND CHRONIC
Tamara L. Gayle, MD, MEd

BASICS

DESCRIPTION
- Parotitis is caused by inflammation of the parotid gland due to infection, systemic illnesses, mechanical obstruction, or medications.
- The parotid gland is the largest salivary gland, located lateral and anterior to the masseter muscle, and extends posteriorly over the sternocleidomastoid muscle behind the angle of the mandible. It produces serous secretions, which lack bacteriostatic properties, making it more susceptible to infection than other salivary glands.
- The parotid duct, also called the Stensen duct, pierces the buccinator muscle and enters the buccal mucosa opposite to the maxillary second molar.
- The branches of the facial nerve bisect the gland into lobes.

EPIDEMIOLOGY
- Viral parotitis is the most common cause of parotitis in children; incidence has decreased since the advent of the mumps vaccine.
- Incidence of viral parotitis has increased overall due to SARS-CoV-2 infections.
- Acute bacterial parotitis is less common but occurs more frequently in elderly patients, neonates, and postoperative patients.
- Juvenile recurrent parotitis (JRP): second most common inflammatory cause of parotitis in children in the United States; first episode usually occurs between ages 3 and 6 years.
- Chronic parotitis primarily affects adults; typically presents between ages 40 and 60 years
- Chronic bilateral parotid enlargement is a common manifestation of HIV infection.

ETIOLOGY AND PATHOPHYSIOLOGY
- Acute viral parotitis begins as a systemic infection that localizes to the parotid gland, resulting in inflammation and swelling.
  - Mumps, or paramyxovirus, has a predilection for the parotid gland and classically has been linked to parotitis 16 to 18 days after infection. Mumps is a nationally reportable disease.
  - Other viral pathogens: parainfluenza, enterovirus, echovirus, influenza A, coxsackievirus, Epstein-Barr virus (EBV), human herpesvirus 6 (HHV-6)
  - Parotiditis more common in pediatric patients with SARS-CoV-2 infection in the setting of multisystem inflammatory system
- Acute bacterial parotitis results from stasis of salivary flow that allows retrograde introduction of bacterial pathogens into the gland, resulting in localized infection.
  - Staphylococcus aureus is the most common, followed by Streptococcus pneumoniae and anaerobes. Less common are Streptococcus viridans, Escherichia coli, and Haemophilus influenzae.
  - Klebsiella, Enterobacter, and Pseudomonas can be seen in chronically ill or hospitalized patients.
  - Consider Bartonella henselae with cat exposure.
  - May be a manifestation of late-onset group B Streptococcus (rare)
  - Mycobacterium tuberculosis has been seen in immunocompromised patients.

- Fungal
  - Candida has been isolated in chronically ill or hospitalized patients.
  - Actinomyces in patients with a history of trauma or dental caries
- Acute, recurrent parotitis
  - Mechanical: Repeated sialolith formation leads to ductal wall damage, fibrosis, and stricture formation.
  - Pneumoparotitis occurs when air is trapped in the parotid gland ducts; seen in wind instrument players, glassblowers, scuba divers, and rarely with dental cleaning
- "Anesthesia mumps": may be due to transient mechanical compression of the Stensen duct by airway devices, loss of muscle tone around the Stensen orifice after neuromuscular relaxants, increased salivary secretion, and increased flexion or rotation of the head during general anesthesia
- Chronic parotitis in patients with HIV can be due to presence of benign lymphoepithelial cysts, follicular hyperplasia of parotid lymph nodes, or diffuse infiltrative lymphocytosis syndrome, causing infiltration of the parotid gland by CD8 cells. Parotitis may be secondary to immune reconstitution after initiation of antiretroviral therapy.
- There are case reports of acute parotitis as a symptom of Kawasaki disease.

RISK FACTORS
- Immunosuppression, HIV, chemotherapy, radiation, malnutrition, alcoholism
- Acute viral parotitis: lack of mumps, measles, and rubella (MMR) vaccination
- Acute bacterial parotitis: dehydration, debilitation, poor oral hygiene, Sjögren syndrome, cystic fibrosis, bulimia/anorexia, sialolithiasis (stones), ductal stenosis, trauma
- Neonatal parotitis: prematurity, dehydration, low birth weight, ductal obstruction, oral trauma, structural abnormalities
- JRP: dental malocclusion, congenital duct malformation, immunologic anomalies, disrupted enzyme activity
- Drug-induced parotitis: anticholinergics, ACE inhibitors (captopril), antihistamines, tricyclic antidepressants, antipsychotics (phenylbutazone, thioridazine, clozapine), iodine (contrast media), and L-asparaginase
- Chronic parotitis: ductal stenosis, HIV, tuberculosis, sarcoidosis, uremia, diabetes, gout, and atopy

GENERAL PREVENTION
- Complete MMR vaccine series; childhood vaccination does not guarantee prevention, possibly due to waning immunity.
- Those without documented mumps immunity should receive 2 doses of the MMR vaccine, 28 days apart.
- Pregnant women should not receive the mumps vaccine. Pregnancy should be avoided for 4 weeks after vaccination.
- Maintain adequate hydration, good dental hygiene, smoking cessation, abstinence from alcohol, and avoidance of chronic purging.

COMMONLY ASSOCIATED CONDITIONS
Mumps, HIV, Sjögren syndrome, sarcoidosis, sialolithiasis

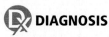

DIAGNOSIS

HISTORY
- Acute parotitis presents with sudden-onset pain and swelling of the cheek.
  - Viral parotitis is usually bilateral and accompanied by malaise, anorexia, headaches, myalgias, arthralgias, and fever.
  - Bacterial parotitis is associated with fever.
- JRP is usually unilateral, with pain and swelling resolving within 2 weeks.
- Other symptoms: trismus, pain exacerbated by chewing or worsened by foods that stimulate production of saliva, dry mouth with abnormal taste, difficulty with drinking/eating, anorexia, or dehydration
- Sialolithiasis is characterized by recurrent acute swelling and pain, exacerbated by eating. It may be associated with swelling around the Stensen duct.
- Chronic parotitis presents with recurrent or chronic nontender swelling of one or both parotid glands.

PHYSICAL EXAM
- Swelling or enlargement of the parotid gland(s); it may obscure the angle of the mandible or cause the ear to protrude upward and outward.
- Palpate with one hand starting at the attachment of the earlobe and proceed anteriorly and inferiorly along the mandibular ramus while the other hand simultaneously palpates the Stensen duct inside the oral cavity.
  - Bilateral tenderness suggests viral etiology, whereas unilateral tenderness, erythema, and warmth suggest a bacterial etiology.
  - Chronic parotitis is typically nontender.
- Trismus, halitosis, and dental decay may be noted.
- Drainage from the Stensen duct suggests bacterial parotitis or superinfection.
- In JRP, the Stensen duct is often enlarged, dilated, erythematous, and swollen.
- Facial nerve palsy can be seen in severe cases.

DIFFERENTIAL DIAGNOSIS
Lymphoma, neoplasm, lymphangitis, cervical adenitis, otitis externa, odontogenic infections, Ludwig angina, and cellulitis

DIAGNOSTIC TESTS & INTERPRETATION
- History and exam are sufficient for diagnosis.
- Perform aerobic culture of purulent drainage from Stensen duct or aerobic and anaerobic culture from fine-needle aspiration of gland or abscess.
  - Anaerobic culture from the Stensen duct will likely contain oropharyngeal contamination, thus perform anaerobic cultures only through fine-needle aspiration.
- Acute bacterial parotitis can be associated with leukocytosis and elevated amylase.

- For suspected mumps, the CDC recommends collecting a buccal swab for mumps RT-PCR if ≤3 days of symptom onset. If >3 days since onset of symptoms, obtain both buccal swab and a serum specimen for IgM.
  - Mumps RT-PCR is best obtained from a buccal swab performed after massaging the parotid gland for 30 seconds. In areas of high vaccination rates, IgM may be falsely negative necessitating correlation with clinical symptoms.
  - If initial IgM and RT-PCR obtained ≤3 days of symptom onset are negative and there is a strong clinical suspicion for mumps, consider repeating serum testing as IgM response may not be detectable for 5 days after symptom onset.
- Send CMV titers in immunocompromised patients.
- For chronic, recurrent, or nontender parotitis, obtain HIV testing, PPD, SS-A/SS-B antibodies, rheumatoid factor, and antinuclear antibodies to evaluate for underlying etiology.

Initial Tests (lab, imaging)
- Imaging may be used to assess for abscess, masses, ductal stenosis, or sialolithiasis.
- Ultrasound is the first-line diagnostic modality for detecting sialadenitis and has high sensitivity for identifying abscess and ductal lithiasis (1)[B]. CT or MRI may also be used.

Follow-Up Tests & Special Considerations
Consider sialography in chronic parotitis to assess the anatomy and functional integrity of the gland (diagnostic and therapeutic) (1)[C].

Diagnostic Procedures/Other
- Consider biopsy or fine-needle aspiration if there is a suspicion for tuberculosis, Sjögren syndrome, or sarcoidosis.
- Noncaseating granulomas may be seen in sarcoidosis. Caseating granulomas may be seen in tuberculosis and *B. henselae* infections.

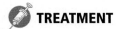 **TREATMENT**

GENERAL MEASURES
- Usually a self-limited course; treat with supportive care: rest, hydration, analgesia, and antipyretics.
  - Stimulate saliva production by eating hard candies.
  - Local heat application and gentle massage
  - Chronic parotitis: Encourage good dental hygiene and treat the underlying etiology.
- Patients with mumps should be isolated with standard and droplet precautions for 5 days after onset of parotid swelling.
- During a mumps outbreak, the CDC recommends administration of MMR vaccine even in fully vaccinated individuals, as a 3rd vaccine dose can decrease risk, especially in those whose second MMR was given >13 years ago (2)[A].

MEDICATION
- Viral parotitis: no evidence for the use of immunoglobulin for postexposure prophylaxis or treatment; may initiate antibiotics if patient is toxic appearing

- Acute bacterial parotitis
  - Outpatient: amoxicillin/clavulanate or ciprofloxacin and clindamycin
  - Chronically ill or hospitalized: ampicillin/sulbactam or cefuroxime and metronidazole; if MRSA is probable, consider vancomycin or linezolid.
- Sjögren syndrome recurrent parotitis: Pilocarpine and cevimeline can stimulate saliva production and inhibit ascending infection and provide symptomatic relief. Alternatively, botulism toxin injection may be a consideration in these patients because it limits production of saliva and sialectasis (3)[B].

ISSUES FOR REFERRAL
- For sialolithiasis, ductal stenosis, chronic obstruction due to Sjögren syndrome, or >1 recurrence per year, consult otolaryngologist for possible sialendoscopy, duct ligation, ductoplasty, or parotidectomy (4)[B].
- Refer to otolaryngology if parotid mass is seen, malignancy is suspected, or no improvement with antibiotics.

SURGERY/OTHER PROCEDURES
- Consider fine-needle aspiration for bacterial parotitis with abscess, or clinical deterioration with increasing pain, erythema, and swelling not responding to medication.
- Consider superficial parotidectomy for severe recurrent parotitis in patients with underlying predisposing etiology.
- JRP: sialography; sialendoscopy with steroid irrigation is effective and safe for the treatment; performing US is recommended first to differentiate JRP from ductal stones (4)[A].
- Sclerotherapy with methyl violet or tetracycline is effective in the treatment of cysts in HIV parotitis and is also considered definitive treatment for chronic parotitis (5)[C].

ADMISSION, INPATIENT, AND NURSING CONSIDERATIONS
Admit those with comorbidities, systemic involvement, inability to tolerate PO, or neonates.

 ONGOING CARE

FOLLOW-UP RECOMMENDATIONS
Antibiotic therapy for bacterial parotitis combined with adequate hydration should result in improvement within 48 hours; if not, patient should be reevaluated.

DIET
Ensure adequate fluid intake and promote salivary flow with hard or sour candy.

PROGNOSIS
- Viral infection in immunocompetent individuals often resolves with excellent prognosis.
- Parotid cysts in patients with HIV are usually benign lymphoepithelial lesions with infrequent malignant transformation.
- There is an increased incidence of malignant lymphoma or lymphoepithelial carcinoma in patients with Sjögren syndrome.

COMPLICATIONS
- Complications of mumps may include orchitis, oophoritis, mastitis, aseptic meningitis, encephalitis, pancreatitis, myocarditis, sensorineural hearing loss, and nephritis.
- Untreated bacterial parotitis can lead to abscess formation and facial paralysis.
- Neoplasm can result from chronic autoimmune parotitis.
- Facial nerve paralysis can result from chronic inflammatory parotitis.

REFERENCES
1. Nation J, Panuganti B, Manteghi A, et al. Pediatric sialendoscopy for recurrent salivary gland swelling: workup, findings, and outcomes. *Ann Otol Rhinol Laryngol*. 2019;128(4):338–344.
2. Cardemil CV, Dahl RM, James L, et al. Effectiveness of a third dose of MMR vaccine for mumps outbreak control. *N Engl J Med*. 2017;377(10): 947–956.
3. O'Neil LM, Palme CE, Riffat F, et al. Botulinum toxin for the management of Sjögren syndrome-associated recurrent parotitis. *J Oral Maxillofac Surg*. 2016;74(12):2428–2430.
4. Wood J, Toll EC, Hall F, et al. Juvenile recurrent parotitis: review and proposed management algorithm. *Int J Pediatr Otorhinolaryngol*. 2021;142:110617.
5. Berg EE, Moore CE. Office-based sclerotherapy for benign parotid lymphoepithelial cysts in the HIV-positive patient. *Laryngoscope*. 2009;119(5):868–870.

ADDITIONAL READING
Hernandez S, Busso C, Walvekar RR. Parotitis and sialendoscopy of the parotid gland. *Otolaryngol Clin North Am*. 2016;49(2):381–393.

CODES

ICD10
- K11.20 Sialoadenitis, unspecified
- K11.21 Acute sialoadenitis
- K11.23 Chronic sialoadenitis

CLINICAL PEARLS
- History and physical exam are sufficient for diagnosis (parotid swelling, tenderness, with or without purulent drainage from the Stensen duct).
- *S. aureus, S. pneumoniae,* and anaerobes are the most common organisms isolated in acute bacterial parotitis.
- In recurrent or chronic cases, consider other underlying etiologies, such as HIV.
- Usually self-limited with supportive care (local heat and gentle massage of gland, adequate hydration, analgesia, and antipyretics)
- Encouraging good oral hygiene and hydration in chronically ill, debilitated, and hospitalized patients can reduce risk of occurrence.

PARVOVIRUS B19 INFECTION
Christina Conrad, DO • Priya Prasher, MBBS

 BASICS

DESCRIPTION
- Human parvovirus B19 is the cause of erythema infectiosum (fifth disease, morbus quintus).
- Individuals with increased red blood cell (RBC) turnover (sickle-cell anemia, spherocytosis, thalassemia) are more susceptible to transient aplastic crisis (TAC). In immunocompromised individuals, pure red cell aplasia may lead to transfusion-dependent anemia. In immunocompetent individuals, arthritis and arthralgias are common complications of parvovirus B19 infection.
- Systems affected: hematologic/lymphatic/immunologic, musculoskeletal, skin/exocrine, central nervous system, cardiac, renal, hepatobiliary

Pregnancy Considerations
Documented acute infection during pregnancy should prompt referral to maternal-fetal medicine specialist. There is a 30% chance of fetal transmission with acute maternal infection—this may be higher during epidemic outbreaks. 30–40% of pregnant women do not have antibodies to parvovirus B19 and thus are considered susceptible to infection (1).

EPIDEMIOLOGY
- Common in childhood; may be asymptomatic
- Erythema infectiosum has an extremely low mortality rate.
- Peak age for erythema infectiosum is 4 to 12 years.
- Males and females are equally affected.
- Women are more likely to develop postinfectious arthritis.
- No known racial predilection
- In temperate climates, infections often occur from late winter to early summer.
- Local outbreaks may occur every 2 to 5 years.
- Parvovirus B19 DNA has been isolated from human remains over 6,900 years old.

Prevalence
Based on serologic studies, infection with parvovirus B19 is extremely common throughout the world. By age 5 years, 2–15% of individuals in the United States and Western Europe are IgG positive. This steadily increases to 70–85% seropositivity by >40 years of age.

ETIOLOGY AND PATHOPHYSIOLOGY
- First described in 1974, parvovirus B19 is a small (20 to 25 nm) nonenveloped, single-stranded DNA virus in the *Erythrovirus* genus of the *Parvoviridae* family
- Parvovirus B19 spreads primarily through respiratory droplets.
- Children 4 to 10 years of age are most often affected.
- The incubation period is typically 4 to 14 days.
- Prodromal symptoms are usually mild and include low-grade fever, headache, malaise, and myalgia. The characteristic rash usually presents in several stages. The first stage is the characteristic "slapped cheek." During the second stage, the rash spreads to the trunk and extremities in a diffuse, macular, erythematous pattern sparing the palms and soles. Central clearing leads to a commonly seen lacy/reticulated appearance. Within 3 weeks, the rash typically resolves.

- Rash and joint symptoms usually occur 2 to 3 weeks after initial infection. These are thought to be due to immune complex formation and are associated with viral clearance (and decreased risk of transmission).
- Patients infected with parvovirus B19 are most contagious 5 to 10 days after exposure, well before the rash typically manifests.
- Cytotoxic infection of erythroid progenitor cells decreases RBC production, which can lead to TAC in patients with increased RBC turnover.

Genetics
Erythrocyte P antigen–negative individuals (approximately 1 in 200,000 people) are resistant to infection.

RISK FACTORS
- School-related epidemic and nonimmune household contacts have a secondary attack rate of 20–50%.
- Highest secondary attack rates are for daycare providers and school personnel in contact with affected children.
- Conditions with increased RBC turnover (spherocytosis, sickle-cell anemia, thalassemia) increase the risk of TAC.
- Immunodeficiency (congenital, due to HIV or malignancy) increases risk of pure red cell aplasia and chronic anemia.
- As many as 40% of pregnant women are not immune; 1.5% seroconversion rate per year

GENERAL PREVENTION
- Respiratory spread; hand washing, cough/sneeze hygiene, and barrier precautions
- Droplet precautions are recommended around patients with TAC and in immunocompromised patients.
- Difficult to eliminate exposure because the period of maximal contagion occurs prior to the onset of the typical rash
- No significant risk of infection based on occupational exposure if proper isolation precautions are followed; exclusion from the workplace is neither necessary nor recommended.
- No preventive vaccine is currently available.

COMMONLY ASSOCIATED CONDITIONS
- Nondegenerative arthritis
  - In children, joint symptoms are uncommon and typically involve the knees and ankles (symmetric or asymmetric joint involvement).
  - In adults, joint symptoms are much more common, usually symmetric, involving the hands, with less frequent involvement of larger joints. Women are affected with joint symptoms more often than men.
  - Joint symptoms generally resolve within 3 weeks but may persist for months or years. Longer duration symptoms are more common in women. Routine radiography is not necessary.
- TAC
  - Involves patients with increased RBC turnover (sickle-cell disease, spherocytosis, thalassemia) or decreased RBC production (iron deficiency anemia)
  - Presents with fatigue, weakness, lethargy, and pallor (symptoms of anemia); may have dyspnea/shortness of breath

- Aplastic event may be life-threatening but is typically self-limited. Reticulocytes typically reappear in 7 to 10 days with full recovery in 2 to 3 weeks.
  - In children with sickle cell hemoglobinopathies and hereditary spherocytosis, fever is the most common symptom (73%); rash is uncommon in these patients.
- Chronic anemia
  - Seen in immunocompromised individuals (HIV, cancer, transplant) with poor antibody response
  - Usually no clinical manifestations (fever, rash, or joint symptoms)
  - Patients may be transfusion-dependent.
- Fetal/neonatal infection (1)
  - Risk of transplacental spread of virus is ~30% in infected mothers.
  - Up to 50% of infected pregnant women may be asymptomatic, but vertical transmission can still occur.
  - Check IgM and IgG levels in pregnant women with symptoms consistent with parvovirus B19 infection.
  - Test pregnant women with known exposure to individuals with acute parvovirus B19.
    - If IgG positive and IgM negative, consider immune, and no further intervention is needed.
    - If IgM and IgG negative, repeat serologic testing in several weeks to look for seroconversion.
    - If IgM positive, test further to determine if acute infection is present (false-positive result).
  - Overall fetal death may occur in 5–10% of fetal infections and can occur with or without fetal hydrops.
  - Fetal bone marrow is primarily impacted. RBC survival is shortened resulting in anemia and (potentially) high-output cardiac failure. Other complications can result from fetal hypoalbuminemia, myocarditis, hepatitis, and placentitis.
  - The risk of fetal loss is highest in 1st trimester (19%).
  - Intrauterine fetal RBC transfusion can decrease fetal loss rate if fetal hydrops is present.
  - Infants who have undergone intrauterine transfusions are at risk for delays in psychomotor development.
- Parvovirus has also been associated with a gloves and socks syndrome (2).
  - Typically in younger adults, there is symmetric painful erythema and edema of feet and hands.
  - Gradually progresses to petechiae/purpura/vesicles/bullae and then skin sloughing
  - May have no other symptoms but can have fevers or arthralgias
  - Generally resolves in 1 to 3 weeks without scarring

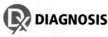 **DIAGNOSIS**

HISTORY
- May have a prodrome of fever, coryza, pharyngitis, headache, rhinorrhea, nausea
- Rash and arthralgias develop after these symptoms.
- Arthralgias may last for weeks or longer.

PHYSICAL EXAM

- Typical "slapped cheek" appearance that spares the nasolabial folds
- A secondary lacy, reticular rash on the trunk, buttocks, and limbs often follows 1 to 4 days later, may last 1 to 6 weeks. This secondary rash may be pruritic and recurrent, exacerbated by bathing, exercise, sun exposure, heat, or emotional stress.
- B19 may manifest as painful pruritic papules and purpura on the hands and feet (glove and sock distribution).

DIFFERENTIAL DIAGNOSIS

- Rubella, measles, enteroviral disease
- Systemic lupus erythematosus, drug reaction, rheumatoid arthritis

DIAGNOSTIC TESTS & INTERPRETATION

Initial Tests (lab, imaging)

- No need for routine lab studies in typical cases. Diagnosis is clinical, and the illness is mild and self-limiting.
- IgG and IgM serology in immunocompetent patients
- B19-specific DNA polymerase chain reaction (PCR) testing for fetal infection (via cord blood or amniotic fluid) as well as for patients with chronic infection or those who are immunocompromised
- For patients with TAC, anemia and reticulocytopenia are present. IgM antibodies are noted by day 3, and IgG antibodies are detectable at time of clinical recovery. PCR shows high levels of viremia.
- Pregnant women exposed to B19 require serologic testing to assess fetal risk.

Follow-Up Tests & Special Considerations

Fetal/neonatal infection (3)[C]

- To exclude congenital B19 in infants with negative B19 IgM, follow IgG serology over the 1st year of life.
- Serial fetal ultrasound to assess for hydrops in cases of documented acute maternal infection in the 1st trimester
- Weekly peak systolic velocity measurements of the middle cerebral artery by Doppler US is recommended to evaluate for heart failure, fetal anemia, and the potential need for intrauterine transfusion (>1.5 MoM).

 ## TREATMENT

GENERAL MEASURES

- No therapy is usually needed.
- Cessation of immunosuppressive therapy allows some patients to clear chronic infections.
- B19-associated anemia in HIV-positive patients may resolve with antiretroviral therapy and immune reconstitution.

MEDICATION

First Line

- Anti-inflammatory agents for arthritic symptoms
- Antipyretics for fever

Second Line

- May require RBC transfusions for TAC
- Intravenous immunoglobulin (IVIG) for B19-related refractory anemia or PRAC, especially in immunodeficient states
- Consider reduction of immunosuppressive therapy while on IVIG therapy.
- Intrauterine RBC transfusions reduce mortality in cases of fetal hydrops.

ISSUES FOR REFERRAL

- Acute infection during pregnancy should prompt referral to a maternal–fetal medicine specialist.
- Patients with chronic or abnormal B19 infections may benefit from consultation with immunology or infectious disease specialists.

ADMISSION, INPATIENT, AND NURSING CONSIDERATIONS

- Outpatient management is typical for erythema infectiosum.
- Inpatient management for aplastic crisis, which may require RBC transfusions
- In the inpatient setting, droplet isolation is appropriate for acute infections, TAC, and chronic infections in the immunocompromised.

 ## ONGOING CARE

FOLLOW-UP RECOMMENDATIONS

Patient Monitoring

Periodic blood counts for anemic patients until they have reticulocyte recovery

PATIENT EDUCATION

- Parvovirus B19: https://www.cdc.gov/parvovirusB19/fifth-disease.html
- Parvovirus B19 and pregnancy: https://www.cdc.gov/parvovirusB19/pregnancy.html
- Healthy Children.org: Parvovirus: https://www.healthychildren.org/English/health-issues/conditions/skin/Pages/fifth-disease-parvovirus-b19.aspx
- Children with typical rash are no longer infectious and may attend childcare or school.

PROGNOSIS

- Usually self-limited
- Joint symptoms usually subside within 3 weeks but may last months to years.
- ~20% of infections result in delayed virus elimination and viremia persisting for several months to years.
- Full recovery from aplastic crisis in 2 to 3 weeks

COMPLICATIONS

Conditions associated with B19 but where causality is unconfirmed

- Hepatitis—may predispose to acute fulminant hepatic failure
- Neurologic manifestations
- Myocarditis, pericarditis
- Membranoproliferative glomerulonephritis, focal segmental glomerulosclerosis, nephrotic syndrome
- Henoch-Schönlein purpura, idiopathic thrombocytopenic purpura, vasculitis, lymphocytic histiocytosis/hemophagocytic syndrome

REFERENCES

1. Ornoy A, Ergaz Z. Parvovirus B19 infection during pregnancy and risks to the fetus. *Birth Defects Res*. 2017;109(5):311–323.
2. Leung AKC, Lam JM, Barankin B, et al. Erythema infectiosum: a narrative review. *Curr Pediatr Rev*. Published online ahead of print April 28, 2023.
3. De Jong EP, Lindenburg IT, van Klink JM, et al. Intrauterine transfusion for parvovirus B19 infection: long-term neurodevelopmental outcome. *Am J Obstet Gynecol*. 2012;206(3):204.e1–204.e5.

ADDITIONAL READING

Moosazadeh M, Alimohammadi M, Mousavi T. Seroprevalence and geographical distribution of parvovirus B19 antibodies in pregnant women: a-meta analysis. *J Immunoassay Immunochem*. 2023;44(2):103–116.

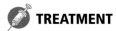 ## CODES

ICD10

- B34.3 Parvovirus infection, unspecified
- B08.3 Erythema infectiosum [fifth disease]

CLINICAL PEARLS

- Parvovirus B19 infection is usually a benign, self-limited illness with no long-term effects.
- Patients are no longer infectious by the time the "slapped cheek" rash of erythema infectiosum appears.
- Patients with increased RBC turnover (sickle cell disease, thalassemia, spherocytosis) are at risk for TAC.
- Immunocompromised patients are at risk for chronic anemia, which may be transfusion-dependent.
- Documentation of acute infection in pregnant women merits maternal–fetal consultation.

PATELLOFEMORAL PAIN SYNDROME (PFPS)

David L. Lee, MD

BASICS

DESCRIPTION
- Pain in or around the patella that is aggravated with increased patellar loading (e.g., prolonged sitting, squatting, kneeling, or ascending/descending stairs); not attributable to other causes
- Synonyms: anterior knee or retropatellar pain syndrome, chondromalacia patellae, runner's knee
- System(s) affected: musculoskeletal

EPIDEMIOLOGY
Prevalence
- Incidence between 2007 and 2011 in the United States was ~6%.
  - 55% of patients were female.
  - More cases were identified in the southern portion of the United States, compared to other regions of the country (1).
- In a military population, prevalence of 12% in males and 15% in females (2).

ETIOLOGY AND PATHOPHYSIOLOGY
Increased patellofemoral joint loading, which is often multifactorial (3):
- Patellar malalignment or maltracking (3)
- Abnormal anatomy (e.g., patella alta, trochlear dysplasia) (3)
- Quadriceps asymmetry, weakness and/or tightness (3)
- Hamstring tightness (3)
- Laxity of the patellofemoral joint or a tight lateral retinaculum (3)
- Increased hip joint internal rotation (3)
- Altered tibiofemoral joint mechanics (3)

RISK FACTORS
- Activities such as running, squatting, and climbing up and down stairs
- Sudden increase in activities
- Female gender
- Dynamic valgus
- Patellar instability
- Quadriceps weakness
- Foot abnormalities (e.g., pes pronatus, rearfoot eversion) (1)
- In adolescents: increased hip adduction strength, although this may represent increased activity level
- Factors of uncertain significance: age, height, weight, body mass index, body fat, Q angle, and hip weakness

GENERAL PREVENTION
Strengthening and stretching exercises, particularly hip abductors and terminal extension of the quadriceps

COMMONLY ASSOCIATED CONDITIONS
- Overuse injury
- Knee ligament injury/surgery
- Patellar tendinopathy
- Prolonged synovitis
- Iliotibial band friction syndrome

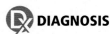 DIAGNOSIS

HISTORY
- An accurate history to differentiate between pain and instability (pain quality, location, swelling, giving way, locking, grinding, inciting events, overuse, changes in activity/training, and history of trauma)
- Most common symptom: diffuse anterior knee pain exacerbated during or after physical activity
- Pain with squatting, descending or ascending stairs, ambulating over uneven surfaces, or running (2)

PHYSICAL EXAM
- Evaluate knee range of motion (ROM) and for effusion.
- Palpation: pain on palpation of the patellar edges (medial or lateral)
- Compression/patellar grind test: With patient supine, place one hand superior to the patella and push the patella inferiorly. Ask the patient to contract the quadriceps; pain on contraction is consistent with PFPS; grinding may indicate chondromalacia of the patellofemoral joint.
- Single leg squat: 80% of patients with PFPS will demonstrate pain with this maneuver (2)[A]. Also helpful in assessing for dynamic valgus
- Patellar apprehension test: With the patient supine with the knee flexed to 30 degrees, medial pressure is applied to the patella (to displace it laterally); pain or apprehension with passive patellar displacement is a positive test. Not sensitive for PFPS (7–32%), but specific (86–92%)

- Passive patellar tilt test: With the patient supine with the knee extended, the patella is grasped, and the examiner lifts the lateral edge of the patella from the lateral femoral condyle, assessing for a tight lateral retinacular restraint. Not sensitive for PFPS (42%), but specific (92%)
- Gait and posture may indicate any imbalances (e.g., femoral internal rotation, hip height, scoliosis, quadriceps atrophy) that may contribute to PFPS.
- Footwear evaluation may detect pes pronatus or rearfoot eversion which could contribute to PFPS (1).

DIFFERENTIAL DIAGNOSIS
- Prepatellar bursitis
- Patellar and quadriceps tendinopathy
- Chondromalacia patellae
- Patellofemoral arthrosis
- Patellar subluxation and dislocation
- Knee ligamentous and meniscal pathology
- Iliotibial band syndrome
- Plica syndrome
- Osteochondral defect
- Osteochondritis dissecans
- Sinding-Larsen-Johansson syndrome
- Osgood-Schlatter disease
- Knee infection
- Neuroma or nerve entrapment
- Benign or malignant tumors
- Referred pain from hip or spine

DIAGNOSTIC TESTS & INTERPRETATION
- None indicated. In general, imaging is not necessary for the diagnosis of PFPS. If imaging is indicated because of severity, atypical symptoms, or persistence of symptoms despite treatment, plain films with four views of the knee are recommended to view patellar tilt and to rule out other etiologies of anterior knee pain:
  - Lateral
  - Merchant or sunrise
  - Standing anteroposterior
  - Posteroanterior tunnel views
- CT can be used to grade patellar malalignment.
- Radiographic findings may not correlate with symptoms.

Follow-Up Tests & Special Considerations

Radiographic images may be normal until late stages, when the posterior patellar surface becomes irregular and cartilage erosion is radiographically detectable.

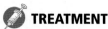 **TREATMENT**

GENERAL MEASURES

- Conservative therapy of physical therapy, rehabilitation, and NSAIDs is the gold standard (4)[A].
- Initial goal of therapy is to increase strength, flexibility, and ROM to enable practice of correct motion.
- Supervised therapy should focus on hip abductors and external rotators, knee extensors, and core muscles (4)[A].
- Stretching of the muscles surrounding the hip and knee, particularly proprioceptive neuromuscular facilitation stretches (4)[A]

MEDICATION

- Acetaminophen or NSAIDs for pain management
- The evidence for oral glucosamine and chondroitin sulfate and hyaluronic acid injections is lacking and is not routinely recommended for treatment of patellofemoral pain.

ISSUES FOR REFERRAL

- Referral for surgery after all conservative measures fail. Surgery is rarely needed.
- Recalcitrant cases can be associated with psychosocial issues including depression, catastrophization, and central sensitization. Multimodal care including referral to a mental health care professional may be necessary.

ADDITIONAL THERAPIES

- Combination therapy in addition to an exercise program with other modalities such as patellar taping or manual therapy may be beneficial (5)[A].
- Ankle and foot orthoses may offer some relief in the short term, but there is lack of strong evidence to support its use, particularly in the long term (4)[B],(5).

SURGERY/OTHER PROCEDURES

- Exercise therapy is first line.
- For patients with a tight lateral retinaculum and lateral patellar tilt: operative realignment of the patella
- For patients with a defect in the cartilage of the patellofemoral joint: cartilage resurfacing/restoration

 ONGOING CARE

PATIENT EDUCATION

- Patient education materials including home exercise programs may be provided but this should not be considered a replacement for formal physical therapy.
- Educate patient on importance of participation and compliance in a specialized exercise program with a physical therapist.
- Provide a list of physical therapy locations for the patient.

PROGNOSIS

- PFPS may not be self-limiting and can become chronic (6).
- Patellofemoral pain for longer than 12 months duration is associated with long-term pain (6).
- Long-term PFPS has not clearly been linked to structural patellofemoral joint OA (6).

REFERENCES

1. Gaitonde DY, Ericksen A, Robbins RC. Patellofemoral pain syndrome. *Am Fam Physician*. 2019;99(2):88–94.
2. Crossley KM, Stefanik JJ, Selfe J, et al. 2016 Patellofemoral pain consensus statement from the 4th International Patellofemoral Pain Research Retreat, Manchester. Part 1: terminology, definitions, clinical examination, natural history, patellofemoral osteoarthritis and patient-reported outcome measures. *Br J Sports Med*. 2016;50(14):839–843.
3. Powers CM, Witvrouw E, Davis IS, et al. Evidence-based framework for a pathomechanical model of patellofemoral pain: 2017 patellofemoral pain consensus statement from the 4th International Patellofemoral Pain Research Retreat, Manchester, UK: part 3. *Br J Sports Med*. 2017;51(24):1713–1723.
4. van der Heijden RA, Lankhorst NE, van Linschoten R, et al. Exercise for treating patellofemoral pain syndrome. *Cochrane Database Syst Rev*. 2015;(1):CD010387.
5. Collins NJ, Barton CJ, van Middelkoop M, et al. 2018 Consensus statement on exercise therapy and physical interventions (orthoses, taping and manual therapy) to treat patellofemoral pain: recommendations from the 5th International Patellofemoral Pain Research Retreat, Gold Coast, Australia, 2017. *Br J Sports Med*. 2018;52(18):1170–1178.
6. Lankhorst NE, van Middelkoop M, Crossley KM, et al. Factors that predict a poor outcome 5–8 years after the diagnosis of patellofemoral pain: a multicentre observational analysis. *Br J Sports Med*. 2016;50(14):881–886.

ADDITIONAL READING

- Bolgla LA, Boling MC, Mace KL, et al. National Athletic Trainers' Association position statement: management of individuals with patellofemoral pain. *J Athl Train*. 2018;53(9):820–836.
- Saltychev M, Dutton RA, Laimi K, et al. Effectiveness of conservative treatment for patellofemoral pain syndrome: a systematic review and meta-analysis. *J Rehabil Med*. 2018;50(5):393–401.
- Willy RW, Hoglund LT, Barton CJ, et al. Patellofemoral pain. *J Orthop Sports Phys Ther*. 2019;49(9):CPG1–CPG95.

 SEE ALSO

Algorithm: Knee Pain

 CODES

ICD10

- M25.569 Pain in unspecified knee
- M25.561 Pain in right knee
- M25.562 Pain in left knee

CLINICAL PEARLS

- PFPS is the most common cause of anterior knee pain in active adults.
- The clinical diagnosis is made by an accurate history and physical exam.
- Well-designed exercises geared at core, hip, and lower extremity flexibility and strength are the most effective evidence-based treatments.

PEDICULOSIS (LICE)

Sangili Chandran, MD • Damini Patel, DO • Hiba A. Khan, DO

BASICS

DESCRIPTION
- A contagious parasitic infection caused by ectoparasitic blood-feeding insects (lice)
- Two species of lice infest humans:
  - *Pediculus humanus* has two subspecies: the head louse (var. *capitis*) and the body louse (var. *corporis*). Both species are 1 to 3 mm long, flat, and wingless and have three pairs of legs that attach closely behind the head.
  - *Pthirus pubis* (pubic or crab louse): resembles a sea crab and has widespread claws on the 2nd and 3rd legs

EPIDEMIOLOGY
Incidence
- In the United States: 6 to 12 million new cases per year
- Head lice are most common in children 3 to 11 years of age; more common in girls than boys. Pubic lice are more common in adults.

Prevalence
Head lice: 1–3% in industrialized countries

ETIOLOGY AND PATHOPHYSIOLOGY
- Characteristics of lice:
  - Adult louse is dark grayish and moves quickly by crawling (does not jump or fly). It has claws that allow it to cling to individual strands of hair. Eggs (nits) camouflage with the individuals' hair color and are cemented to the base of the hair shaft (within 4 mm of the scalp). Nits (empty egg casings) appear white (opalescent) and remain cemented to the hair shaft.
  - Lice feed solely on human blood by piercing the skin, injecting saliva (anticoagulant properties to allow for blood meal), and then ingesting blood.
  - Itching is a delayed hypersensitivity reaction to the saliva of the feeding louse, which may take 4 to 6 weeks to develop after the first exposure. Subsequent exposures may take 1 to 2 days for symptoms to develop (1).
- Transmission: direct human-to-human contact
  - Head lice: direct head-to-head contact or contact with infected fomite (less likely)
  - Body lice: contact with contaminated clothing or bedding
  - Pubic lice: typically transmitted sexually (fomite transmission much less likely)

RISK FACTORS
- General: overcrowding and close personal contact
- Head lice
  - School-aged children, gender (girls; longer hair); sharing combs, hats (including helmets), clothing, and bed linens
- Body lice: poor hygiene, homelessness
- Pubic lice: promiscuity (very high transmission rate)

GENERAL PREVENTION
- Environmental measures: Wash, dry-clean, or vacuum items that may have contacted infected individuals.
- Screen and treat affected household contacts.
- Head lice: Follow-up by school nurses may help to prevent recurrence and spread. Pubic lice: Limit the number of sexual partners (condoms do not prevent transmission nor does shaving pubic hair). Body lice: proper body hygiene

COMMONLY ASSOCIATED CONDITIONS
Up to 30% of patients with pubic lice have at least one concomitant STI.

DIAGNOSIS

HISTORY
- Pruritus is common, often worse at night.
- Often associated with "outbreak" in school settings
- Investigate contacts of infected individuals.

PHYSICAL EXAM
- Diagnosis is confirmed by visualization of live lice.
- *P. humanus capitis* (head lice)
  - Found most often on the back of the head and neck and behind the ears (warmer areas)
  - Eyelashes may be involved.
  - Eggs, found cemented on the base of a hair shaft, are difficult to remove.
  - Pruritus may be accompanied by local erythema and small papules.
  - May see excoriations around hairline
  - Scratching can cause inflammation and secondary bacterial infection.
  - Pyoderma and lymphadenopathy may occur in severe infestation.
- *P. humanus corporis* (body lice)
  - Poor general hygiene
  - Adult lice and nits in the seams of clothing
  - Intense pruritus involving area covered by clothing (trunk, axillae, and groin)
  - Uninfected bites present as erythematous macules, papules, and wheals. Pyoderma and excoriation may be seen.
  - Transmit *Bartonella quintana* (trench fever) and *Borrelia recurrentis* (louse-borne relapsing fever) and *Rickettsia prowazekii* (epidemic typhus)
- *P. pubis* (pubic lice)
  - Pubic hair is the most common site, but lice may spread to hair around anus, abdomen, axillae, chest, beard, eyebrows, and eyelashes.
  - Eggs are present at the base of hair shafts. Anogenital pruritus; blue macules may be seen in surrounding skin.
  - Delay in treatment may lead to development of groin infection and regional adenopathy.

DIFFERENTIAL DIAGNOSIS
- Scabies and other mite species that can cause cutaneous reactions in humans
- Dandruff and other hair debris sometimes look like head lice eggs and nits but are less adherent.

DIAGNOSTIC TESTS & INTERPRETATION
- Diagnosis is based on visualization of live louse.
- Head lice: Comb hair thoroughly with a fine-toothed louse comb (0.2 to 0.3 mm between teeth) to identify live lice (2)[C]. Wet the hair to limit static electricity, which repels lice. Simple visual inspection has same sensitivity as wet combing but is only ~25% as effective as dry combing with a metal comb (3).
- Body lice: Examine the seams of clothing to locate lice and eggs.
- Lice and eggs are more easily visualized with a microscope.
- In contrast to dandruff, eggs and nits cannot be removed easily from a hair shaft.

Follow-Up Tests & Special Considerations
- Empty nits remain on hair shafts for months after eradication of the live infestation. Wood lamp exam: Live nits fluoresce white, and empty nits fluoresce gray.
- Pubic lice: Evaluate for concurrent STIs.

TREATMENT

GENERAL MEASURES
- Head lice: Clean items that have been in contact with the head of the infected individual within 48 hours.
- Wash all beddings, towels, clothes, headgears, combs, brushes, and hair accessories in hot water (>60°C).
- Vacuum furniture and carpets. Seal any personal articles that cannot be washed in hot water, dry-cleaned, or vacuumed in a plastic bag and store for at least 2 weeks. Examine and treat household members and close contacts concurrently.
- Insecticide sprays are not necessary. Pubic lice: Avoid sexual activity until all partners are successfully treated.
- Nit and egg removal:
  - Remove eggs within 1 cm of the scalp to prevent reinfestation. After treatment with shampoo or lotion, eggs and nits remain in the scalp or pubic hair until mechanically removed. Hair conditioner facilitates nit removal. Eggs and nits best removed with a fine nit comb

MEDICATION
Permethrin (over the counter [OTC]), synergized pyrethrin (OTC), spinosad (Rx), benzyl alcohol (Rx), malathion (Rx), and topical ivermectin (Rx) are all effective for head lice (2)[A],(3)[C]. Permethrin, synergized pyrethrin, and malathion are effective for pubic lice (3)[C]:
- Permethrin is generally preferred because it may have residual activity for up to 3 weeks. However, use of newer shampoos and conditioners may reduce the residual effect (2)[C].
- Malathion and spinosad are considered second line for head lice but may not require a second application due to ovicidal activity (2)[B],(3)[C].
- Ivermectin 0.5% lotion and benzyl alcohol 5% lotion are also effective for head lice (2),(3)[C].

First Line
- Head and pubic lice:
  - Pyrethrum insecticides: Permethrin 1% (Nix Crème Rinse) or pyrethrins 0.33% with piperonyl butoxide 4% (synergized pyrethrin, Rid, Pronto) are first line unless there is proven resistance in the community.
    - Apply for 10 minutes and then wash. Reapply synergized pyrethrin in 7 to 10 days (day 9 is optimal); also be necessary with permethrin, if live lice are observed
    - Side effects: application-site erythema, ocular erythema, and application-site irritation
- Body lice: best treated with synergized pyrethrin lotion applied once and left on for several hours
- Eyelash infestation: Apply petroleum jelly BID for 10 days.

- Precautions:
  - Pyrethrin: Avoid in patients with ragweed allergy (may cause respiratory symptoms).
  - Pediculicides should never be used to treat eyelash infections.

Second Line
- Head lice and pubic lice
  - Malathion 0.5% lotion (Ovide)
    - Apply for 8 to 12 hours and then wash off.
      - Flammable and has a bad odor. Despite ovicidal activity, a second application may be necessary after 7 to 10 days (day 9 is optimal) if live lice are observed.
  - Abametapir 0.74%, lotion
    - Apply once in age group ≥6 months. Mechanism of action: inhibits metalloproteinases in adult lice and eggs; side effects: erythema, rash, and skin burning sensation
  - Lindane 1% shampoo, no longer recommended
    - Apply for 4 minutes and then wash (do not repeat).
    - Side effects: neurotoxicity (seizures, muscle spasms), aplastic anemia
    - Contraindications: uncontrolled seizure disorder, premature infants
    - Precautions: Do not use on excoriated skin, in immunocompromised patients, conditions that increase seizure risk, or with medications that decrease seizure threshold.
    - Possible interactions: concomitant use with medications that lower the seizure threshold
- Head lice
  - Spinosad 0.9% lotion (Natroba)
    - Apply to dry hair and scalp for 10 minutes and then rinse with warm water. Repeat in 7 days if live lice are observed.
    - Side effects: application-site erythema, ocular erythema, and application-site irritation
  - Benzyl alcohol 5% lotion (Ulesfia)
    - Apply to dry hair using enough amount to saturate scalp and hair (amount depends on hair length), rinse after 10 minutes; repeat in 1 week.
    - Side effects: pruritus, erythema, pyoderma, ocular irritation, application-site irritation
  - Ivermectin 0.5% lotion (Sklice)
    - Apply to dry hair by using enough to saturate the scalp and hair (max. 4 oz) and then rinse after 10 minutes.
    - Side effects: burning sensation at application site, dandruff, dry skin, eye irritation
- Mechanical removal of lice and nits by wetting hair and then systematically combing with a fine-toothed comb every 3 to 4 days for 2 weeks to remove all lice as they hatch

ALERT
Lindane: FDA black box warning of severe neurologic toxicity (use only when first-line agents have failed). The National Pediculosis Association strongly advises against using lindane at all.

Pediatric Considerations
- Ivermectin lotion 0.5% and abametapir lotion 0.74% recently approved by FDA for children aged ≥6 months. Benzyl alcohol is also approved for children >6 months.
- Avoid synergized pyrethrin and permethrin in infants <2 months of age. Avoid topical ivermectin, and spinosad in children <6 months of age and avoid malathion in children <2 years of age.
- Lindane: not recommended

Pregnancy Considerations
Permethrin, synergized pyrethrin, malathion, spinosad, and benzyl alcohol are pregnancy Category B. Lindane and topical ivermectin are pregnancy Category C.

ADDITIONAL THERAPIES
- For "difficult to treat" cases of head lice, oral ivermectin 400 μg/kg (not approved by the FDA for lice), given twice at a 7-day interval, is superior to topical 0.5% malathion lotion (4)[B].
- Ivermectin: 200 μg/kg PO repeated after 10 days or 300 μg/kg PO repeated after 7 days; should not be used in children <15 kg; pregnancy Category C; not approved by the FDA for lice
- Dual therapy with permethrin 1% and oral trimethoprim/sulfamethoxazole (TMP/SMX) only for cases of multiple treatment failures or suspected cases of lice-related resistance to therapy (TMP/SMX is not approved by the FDA for lice.)
- Permethrin 5% cream (Rx) is not FDA approved for lice and is unlikely to be effective for lice that are resistant to 1% cream rinse (2)[B].

COMPLEMENTARY & ALTERNATIVE MEDICINE
- Cetaphil lotion: dry-on, suffocation-based pediculicide (not approved by the FDA for lice)
  - Apply thoroughly to hair, comb, and then dry with hair dryer; shampoo after 8 hours. Repeat once a week until cured, up to a maximum of three applications.
- Dimethicone 4% lotion: Apply to hair for 8 hours; repeat in 1 week (not approved by the FDA for lice).
- No home remedies (e.g., vinegar, isopropyl alcohol, olive oil, ylang ylang oil, mayonnaise, melted butter, and petroleum jelly) are proven effective.
- Herbal shampoos and pomades have not been evaluated in clinical trials. Lavender oil and tea tree oil have been implicated in triggering prepubertal gynecomastia in boys and should not be used to treat lice.
- Electronic louse combs have not proven effective and are not approved by the FDA.
- Repellents: A placebo-controlled clinical trial demonstrated that rosemary, citronella, and piperonal essential oils were clinically effective as repellents when applied topically to the head of children.

 ## ONGOING CARE

FOLLOW-UP RECOMMENDATIONS
Children may return to school after completing topical treatment, even if nits remain in place. No-nit policies are unnecessary.

Patient Monitoring
Drug resistance should be suspected if no dead lice are observed 8 to 12 hours after treatment.

PATIENT EDUCATION
- National Pediculosis Association: https://www.headlice.org/
- CDC: https://www.cdc.gov/parasites/lice/index.html
- National Guideline Clearinghouse: https://www.guideline.gov/content.aspx?id=46429&search=lice

PROGNOSIS
- With appropriate treatment, >90% cure rate
- Recurrence is common, mainly from reinfection or treatment nonadherence. Resistance to synthetic pyrethroids is increasing.

COMPLICATIONS
- Poor sleep due to pruritus. Persistent itching may be caused by too frequent use of the pediculicide.
- Missed school; social stigma
- Secondary bacterial infections; body lice can transmit typhus and trench fever.

REFERENCES
1. Gunning K, Kiraly B, Pippitt K. Lice and scabies: treatment update. *Am Fam Physician*. 2019;99(10):635–642.
2. Devore CD, Schutze GE; for Council on School Health and Committee on Infectious Diseases, American Academy of Pediatrics. Head lice. *Pediatrics*. 2015;135(5):e1355–e1365.
3. Coates SJ, Thomas C, Chosidow O, et al. Ectoparasites: pediculosis and tungiasis. *J Am Acad Dermatol*. 2020;82(3):551–569.
4. Feldmeier H. Treatment of pediculosis capitis: a critical appraisal of the current literature. *Am J Clin Dermatol*. 2014;15(5):401–412.

 SEE ALSO

Arthropod Bites and Stings; Scabies

CODES

ICD10
- B85.0 Pediculosis due to Pediculus humanus capitis
- B85.1 Pediculosis due to Pediculus humanus corporis
- B85.3 Phthiriasis

CLINICAL PEARLS
- School-based no-nit policies are not necessary because empty nits may remain on hair shafts for months after successful eradication.
- Improper product application is a common cause of treatment failure.
- Prevalence of resistant infestations is increasing; if no dead lice are observed 8 to 12 hours after treatment, suspect resistance and use an alternative agent.
- Routine retreatment on day 9 is recommended for nonovicidal products (permethrin and synergized pyrethrin).
- With all treatment options, reinspect hair after 7 to 9 days, and if live lice are detected, repeat treatment on day 9.

PELVIC INFLAMMATORY DISEASE

Chirag N. Shah, MD • Daniel Scott Morrison, MD • Malhar Desai, DO, MS, BA

 BASICS

DESCRIPTION
- Pelvic inflammatory disease (PID) is an infection of the upper female genital tract, including the uterus, fallopian tubes, ovaries, and adjacent pelvic structures. PID is most commonly an ascending polymicrobial infection acquired through retrograde movement of microorganisms from the lower genital tract (1)[C].
- PID is clinically concerning due to its consequences for future fertility.
- Mild to moderate PID is characterized by the absence of a tubo-ovarian abscess (TOA). Severe disease is defined as severe systemic symptoms OR the presence of a TOA (2)[C].
- Diagnosis may be challenging due to nonstandardized definitions and guidelines, lack of a single definitive diagnostic test, and variation in signs and symptoms. Many patients with PID have subtle or nonspecific symptoms (2)[C].

EPIDEMIOLOGY
Most commonly affects sexually active patients aged <30 years

Incidence
More than one million patients are diagnosed with PID annually (1)[C].

Prevalence
Estimated prevalence of lifetime PID is 4.4% in sexually active cisgender women aged 18 to 44 years. Approximately 2.5 million women of reproductive age in the United States have had a PID diagnosis.
- Lifetime prevalence has decreased steadily since 1995.
- Without history of prior STI, lifetime prevalence is higher in black versus white women (6% vs. 2.7%). Among patients with a prior STI, lifetime prevalence was similar across race (10% vs. 10.3%). This disparity suggests black patients might be more likely to have had an undiagnosed STI, subsequently developing PID.

ETIOLOGY AND PATHOPHYSIOLOGY
Multiple organisms cause PID, and polymicrobial infections are common.
- *Chlamydia trachomatis* and *Neisseria gonorrhoeae*, previously thought to be the most commonly implicated pathogens in PID, are now identified in only 22–50% of cases (2)[C]. Genital tract mycoplasmas (particularly *Mycoplasma genitalium*) have similar incidence rates as *C. trachomatis* in recent studies of patients with PID, although their role in the pathophysiology of PID is unclear.
- Common flora and causes of bacterial vaginosis including aerobic and anaerobic (*Bacteroides fragilis*) species and vaginal microbes (e.g., *Prevotella*, peptostreptococci, *Gardnerella vaginalis*, *Escherichia coli*, *Haemophilus influenzae*) are increasingly implicated (2)[C].
- Possible mechanisms for ascent from the lower genital tract include (i) travel from cervix to endometrium to salpinx to peritoneal cavity; (ii) lymphatic spread via infection of the parametrium (from an IUD); and (iii) hematogenous route, although this is rare.

RISK FACTORS
- Sexually active and age <25 years
- New sexual partner or sexual partner with symptoms or a known diagnosis of STI
- Two or more sexual partners within the last year
- Inconsistent condom use
- Gynecologic procedures that break the cervical barrier such as endometrial biopsy, curettage, hysterosalpingography, hysteroscopy, in vitro fertilization, and insertion of IUD in the last 3 weeks (3)[C]
- Other factors associated with PID:
  - Previous history of PID; 20–25% will have a recurrence.
  - Cervical ectopy
  - History of *C. trachomatis*; 10–40% will develop PID.
  - History of gonococcal cervicitis; 10–20% will develop PID.

GENERAL PREVENTION
- Educational programs about safe sex practices such as barrier contraceptives, especially condoms.
- The U.S. Preventive Services Task Force recommends annual screening for chlamydia in all sexually active women aged <25 years and in those aged ≥25 years at increased risk (new sex partner/multiple sex partners). Moderate-quality evidence suggests that chlamydia screening reduces cases of PID (3)[C].
- Routine STI screening in pregnancy
- Early medical care with the occurrence of genital lesions or abnormal discharge

COMMONLY ASSOCIATED CONDITIONS
- In a patient with an IUD and a pelvic abscess, suspect *Actinomyces* infection requiring penicillin treatment.
- Rupture of an adnexal abscess is rare but is life-threatening. Early surgical exploration is mandatory (2)[C].
- Chlamydial or gonococcal perihepatitis, called Fitz-Hugh-Curtis (FHC) syndrome, may occur with PID. FHC syndrome is characterized by severe pleuritic right upper quadrant pain and complicates 4–6% of PID cases (2)[C].

℞ DIAGNOSIS
- Clinical diagnosis, with the positive predictive value of clinical diagnosis approaching 65–90% compared with laparoscopy (3)[C]
- The CDC recommends empiric treatment for PID in females at risk with pelvic/lower abdominal pain of unknown etiology and one or more of the following: cervical motion tenderness, uterine tenderness, and adnexal tenderness.
- Additional criteria enhance specificity: fever >101°F, new/abnormal cervical mucopurulent discharge or cervical friability, presence of abundant WBCs on wet prep, elevated C-reactive protein (CRP), elevated ESR, and laboratory documentation of genitourinary infection with *N. gonorrhoeae* or *C. trachomatis* (3)[C].
- Tubal thickening on ultrasound or MRI is a highly specific finding (>90%) (2)[C].

HISTORY
- Lower abdominal/pelvic pain: dull, aching or crampy, bilateral, constant; exacerbated by motion, exercise, or coitus
- New/abnormal vaginal discharge (~75% of cases)
- Fever, chills, cramping, dyspareunia
- Low back pain
- Urinary discomfort
- Unanticipated vaginal bleeding, often postcoital, is reported in about 40% of cases.
- Recent hysterosalpingogram (HSG) or other procedure breaking the uterine barrier
- IUD insertion within the past 21 days

PHYSICAL EXAM
Fever; lower abdominal pain; cervical motion, uterine, or adnexal tenderness; evidence of cervicitis with/without vaginal discharge

DIFFERENTIAL DIAGNOSIS
Appendicitis, constipation, gastroenteritis, ectopic pregnancy, ovarian tumor/torsion, hemorrhagic/ruptured ovarian cyst, endometriosis/dysmenorrhea, functional pelvic pain, inflammatory bowel disease, diverticulitis, UTI/pyelonephritis, nephrolithiasis

DIAGNOSTIC TESTS & INTERPRETATION
Initial Tests (lab, imaging)
- Pregnancy test to rule out ectopic pregnancy and complications of an intrauterine pregnancy
- Chlamydia and gonorrhea testing (urine or cervical swab nucleic acid amplification test [NAAT] and/or ligase chain reaction); a negative result does not exclude PID.
- Urinalysis
- Saline microscopy of vaginal fluid (for WBC, bacterial vaginosis, and trichomoniasis)
- HIV test and syphilis screening test
- Transvaginal ultrasound may show thickened, fluid-filled tubes (hydrosalpinges) ± free fluid, or TOA.

Pediatric Considerations
Consider sexual abuse in children presenting with symptoms of PID.

Follow-Up Tests & Special Considerations
Follow-up ultrasound as an outpatient for resolution of adnexal abscess

Diagnostic Procedures/Other
- Laparoscopy only in the following situations: ill patient with competing diagnosis (e.g., appendicitis); ill patient who has failed outpatient treatment; any patient not improving after 72 hours of inpatient treatment
- Endometrial biopsy (indicated only if laparoscopy shows no evidence of salpingitis): reveals endometritis

Test Interpretation
Since NAAT test results may not be immediately available, empiric treatment is recommended if suspicion for PID is high.

TREATMENT

- Patient education: Avoid intercourse until patient and partner(s) have been adequately treated. Counsel patients and partners on possible long-term implications.
- Outpatient treatment is recommended, if clinically appropriate.
- Criteria for hospitalization and parenteral treatment are described below.

GENERAL MEASURES
- IUD removal is NOT required for PID unless no clinical improvement occurs within 48 to 72 hours of initiating treatment (3)[C].
- Treatment should cover principal pathogens (CT, NG, and polymicrobial infections with anaerobic coverage), regardless of the test results.

MEDICATION
First Line
Outpatient treatment regimen: long-acting cephalosporin, macrolide or tetracycline, and metronidazole.

- Ceftriaxone 500 mg IM single dose *plus* doxycycline 100 mg PO BID for 14 days plus metronidazole 500 mg BID for 14 days; patients weighing >150 kg need 1 g of ceftriaxone.
- As of 2021, CDC recommends that oral metronidazole be added to standard outpatient regimen (3)[C].
- Due to the rise of fluoroquinolone resistance, CDC does not recommend fluoroquinolones as 1st or 2nd-line treatment of gonococcal infections including PID.

Second Line
- Because of emerging resistance, a culture for sensitivity testing and a test of cure 2 weeks after completion of treatment is advisable (2)[C].
- Outpatient treatment regimen
  - Cefoxitin 2 g IM single dose and probenecid 1 g PO single dose, or cefotaxime (1 g IM) or ceftizoxime (1 g IM) *plus* doxycycline 100 mg PO BID for 14 days *plus* metronidazole 500 mg PO BID for 14 days
- In persons with documented severe allergic reactions to penicillin:
  - Skin testing is important to confirm or refute penicillin allergy.
  - Cross-reactivity between penicillin and third-generation cephalosporins is low (<1%) (3).
  - Levofloxacin 500 mg PO BID for 14 days can be substituted for cephalosporins (2)[C].
- Special consideration
  - Refer sex partners from the last 60 days for treatment. Even if last sexual intercourse was >60 days, the most recent sex partner should be treated. Expedited partner therapy should be administered where available (3)[C].
  - HIV-infected patients with acute PID should be treated similarly to non–HIV-infected patients (2)[C], although they are at higher risk for TOA, especially if they have a low CD4 count (<200/mm³).

SURGERY/OTHER PROCEDURES
Reserved for failures of medical treatment and for suspected ruptured adnexal abscess with resulting acute surgical abdomen.

ADMISSION, INPATIENT, AND NURSING CONSIDERATIONS
- Criteria for hospitalization if any of the following (3)[C]:
  - Surgical emergencies (e.g., appendicitis) cannot be excluded.
  - Pregnancy
  - TOA
  - Severe illness, nausea or vomiting, unable to follow or tolerate outpatient regimen, or fever >101°F
  - Failure to respond clinically within 72 hours of oral antibiotics
- For inpatient treatment of PID, the CDC recommends the following treatment regimens (3)[C]:
  - Parenteral regimen A
    - Ceftriaxone 1 g IV every 24 hours plus doxycycline 100 mg PO or IV every 12 hours plus metronidazole 500 mg PO or IV every 12 hours
    - Alternatively, cefotetan 2 g IV every 12 hours or cefoxitin 2 g IV every 6 hours plus doxycycline 100 mg PO or IV every 12 hours; this regimen does not require additional anaerobic coverage with metronidazole.
    - Parenteral therapy for 24 to 48 hours after clinical improvement; oral doxycycline should be preferred when possible due to similar bioavailability to IV. Continue doxycycline and metronidazole for a total of 14 days.
  - Parenteral regimen B
    - Clindamycin 900 mg IV every 8 hours plus gentamicin loading dose IV or IM (2 mg/kg of body weight) followed by a maintenance dose (1.5 mg/kg) every 8 hours or single daily dosing at 3 to 5 mg/kg can be substituted.
    - Parenteral therapy may be discontinued 24 hours after clinical improvement, and oral therapy with doxycycline as aforementioned or clindamycin 450 mg PO QID for a total of 14 days should be continued.
  - Parenteral regimen C: ampicillin/sulbactam 3 g IV every 6 hours plus doxycycline 100 mg PO or IV every 12 hours
- PID is rare in pregnant patients but requires hospitalization, infectious disease consultation, and parenteral antibiotics due to high risk for maternal morbidity, perinatal mortality, and preterm delivery (2)[C],(3)[C].

 ## ONGOING CARE

FOLLOW-UP RECOMMENDATIONS
Patient Monitoring
- Follow up 72 hours after initiation of treatment, particularly for patients with moderate or severe clinical presentation (3)[C].
- Observe for worsening symptoms (fever, abdominal pain, and cervical motion tenderness).
- Retest for gonorrhea and chlamydia in 3 months after treatment (3)[C].
- Follow adnexal abscess size and position with serial ultrasounds.

PATIENT EDUCATION
- Abstinence from any type of sexual contact until treatment of patient/partner is complete
- Consistent and correct condom use should be encouraged.

- Hepatitis B and human papillomavirus (HPV) vaccines should be given to patients who meet criteria.
- Advise comprehensive STI screening (3)[C].
- Offer HIV preexposure prophylaxis (PrEP) to patients presenting with new STI or PID.
- IUD insertion presents a low risk of PID in the setting of prior/current STI diagnosis.

PROGNOSIS
- PID has a high morbidity; about 18% of affected patients become infertile, 29% develop chronic pelvic pain, and 0.6% have an ectopic pregnancy.
- Good prognosis if the patient receives early effective therapy and further infection is avoided.
- Poor prognosis with delayed treatment
- Nongonococcal, nonchlamydial PID is associated with severe PID and a worse prognosis for future fertility.

COMPLICATIONS
- TOA occurs in 7–16% of patients before presentation; 1/3 of patients hospitalized with PID
- Recurrent infection occurs in 20–25% of patients.
- Risk of ectopic pregnancy is increased 7- to 10-fold among patients with a history of PID.
- Tubal infertility in 8%, 19.5%, and 40% of patients after 1, 2, and 3 episodes of PID, respectively.
- Chronic pelvic pain in 20–30% of cases is related to adhesions, chronic salpingitis, or recurrent infection.
- Hydrosalpinx: After PID resolves, fallopian tube fills with sterile fluid and becomes blocked; associated with pain and infertility

REFERENCES
1. Yusuf H, Trent M. Management of pelvic inflammatory disease in clinical practice. *Ther Clin Risk Manag*. 2023;19:183–192.
2. Taira T, Broussard N, Bugg C. Pelvic inflammatory disease: diagnosis and treatment in the emergency department. *Emerg Med Pract*. 2022;24(12):1–24.
3. Workowski KA, Bachmann LH, Chan PA, et al. Sexually transmitted infections treatment guidelines, 2021. *MMWR Recomm Rep*. 2021;70(4):1–187.

CODES

ICD10
- N70.0 Acute salpingitis and oophoritis
- N70 Salpingitis and oophoritis
- N71.0 Acute inflammatory disease of uterus

CLINICAL PEARLS
- PID often starts with gonorrhea or chlamydia infection, but it can be polymicrobial.
- Treat based on clinical suspicion (pelvic pain, cervical motion, or adnexal or uterine tenderness) without waiting for confirmatory testing.
- PID is a common cause of infertility.
- Complications include hydrosalpinx, adhesions, pelvic pain, and a 10-fold increased risk of ectopic pregnancy.

PEPTIC ULCER DISEASE

Afsha Rais Kaisani, MD • Tasaduq Hussain Mir, MD, FAAFP • Bremmy L. Alsbrooks, DO, MPH

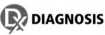

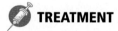

BASICS

Peptic ulcer disease (PUD) is characterized by defects in the stomach and/or duodenal mucosa, leading to inflammation and erosion of the underlying tissue by gastric acid and pepsin.

DESCRIPTION
- Esophageal ulcers: located in the distal esophagus; usually secondary to gastroesophageal reflux disease (GERD); also seen with gastrinoma
- Duodenal ulcer: the most common form of PUD; usually located in the anterior wall of proximal duodenum (duodenal bulb)
- Gastric ulcer: less common than duodenal ulcer in absence of NSAID use; often located along lesser curvature of the antrum
- Multiple ulcers/ulcers distal to the second portion of duodenum and/or jejunum raise possibility of gastrinoma (Zollinger-Ellison syndrome [ZES]).
- Ectopic gastric mucosal ulceration: caused by residual columnar epithelium of the embryonic esophagus; often seen in the upper esophagus; can be seen with Meckel diverticulum (1)

EPIDEMIOLOGY
The global prevalence of PUD has dramatically decreased in the past decade due to improved sanitary conditions, effective treatment of *Helicobacter pylori* infection, and careful NSAID use (1).

Incidence
- PUD can affect any age group.
- Duodenal ulcers typically appear between age 30 and 50 years and are more common in men.
- Gastric ulcers tend to occur after age 60 years and affect women more than men.
- Duodenal/gastric ulcer incidence increases with age in both sexes.
- Peptic ulcer: 500,000 new cases per year
- Recurrence: 4 million per year
- Global incidence rate 0.1–0.19%; overall decrease from improved sanitary conditions, effective treatment and careful NSAIDs use.
- Lifetime risk globally: 5–10%

Prevalence
PUD affects 4 million people worldwide annually and has an estimated lifetime prevalence of 5–10% in the general population. Prevalence increases to 10–20% in *H. pylori*–positive patients.

ETIOLOGY AND PATHOPHYSIOLOGY
Genetics
Increased incidence in families due to familial clustering of *H. pylori* infection and inherited genetic factors reflecting response to the bacteria

RISK FACTORS
- Most common cause: *H. pylori* (gram-negative bacteria) infection
- Second most common cause: NSAIDs use (including aspirin and COX-2 inhibitors)
- Other medications: corticosteroids (high dose; prolonged therapy), bisphosphonates, potassium chloride, clopidogrel, sirolimus chemotherapeutic agents

- Hypersecretion syndromes: gastrinoma (ZES), systemic mastocytosis, cystic fibrosis, hyperparathyroidism, carcinoid syndrome, antral G-cell hyperplasia
- Others factors: tobacco use, alcohol use, stress (e.g., acute illness, ventilator support, extensive burns, head injury), radiation therapy, obesity

GENERAL PREVENTION
- Educate patients about harmful agents like NSAIDs, aspirin, alcohol, tobacco, caffeine.
- NSAID ulcers: discontinue use of NSAIDs, use acetaminophen instead when appropriate, or add proton pump inhibitor [PPI] in patients with previous NSAID-related ulcer.
  - If NSAIDs necessary, use the lowest possible dose with a PPI or misoprostol.
  - To reduce ulcer risk, consider testing for and eradicating *H. pylori*.
- Maintenance therapy with PPIs or H$_2$ blockers is indicated for history of ulcer complications, recurrences, refractory ulcers, or persistent *H. pylori* infection.
- Consider maintenance PPI treatment in patients with *H. pylori*–negative, non–NSAID-induced ulcers.
- Strong association between obesity and PUD; counsel patients on weight loss.

COMMONLY ASSOCIATED CONDITIONS
Gastrinoma (ZES); multiple endocrine neoplasia type 1; carcinoid syndrome

DIAGNOSIS

HISTORY
- 70% of peptic ulcers are asymptomatic.
- Common symptoms: midepigastric pain; gnawing or burning, nonradiating, recurring pain that is often episodic
  - Duodenal ulcer: often have nocturnal pain; relieved by food or antacids.
  - Gastric ulcer: aggravated by food, relieved by antacids
- Nonspecific dyspeptic symptoms: indigestion, nausea, vomiting, loss of appetite, heartburn, and epigastric fullness
- Red flag or alarming symptoms: onset of symptoms after age 55 years, progressive dysphagia, overt GI bleeding, iron deficiency anemia, persistent/recurrent vomiting, severe abdominal pain, unintentional weight loss, anorexia, and/or family history of gastric malignancy
- NSAID-induced ulcers are often silent; initial presentation likely perforation or bleeding

PHYSICAL EXAM
Check vital signs for hemodynamic stability; conjunctival pallor (anemia); epigastric tenderness (absent in ~30% of older patients); heme-positive stool from occult blood loss

DIFFERENTIAL DIAGNOSIS
- Functional dyspepsia, gastritis, GERD, biliary colic, gastroenteritis, pancreatitis, cholecystitis, Crohn disease, GI malignancy
- Possibly life-threatening conditions: myocardial infarction, mesenteric ischemia, mesenteric vasculitis

DIAGNOSTIC TESTS & INTERPRETATION
Initial Tests (lab, imaging)
- Depending on the differential, can obtain CBC, liver function tests, amylase, and lipase
- *H. pylori* test: urea breath test, stool antigen test; false-negative results may occur if patient was recently treated with antibiotics, bismuth, or PPIs, or in patients with active bleeding.
  - Stop antibiotics and bismuth for at least 4 weeks and PPIs for at least 2 weeks prior to testing.
- Urea breath test: identifies active infection; used for screening and posttreatment testing; high positive predicted (PPV) and negative predicted value (NPV) (sensitivity 93%; specificity 92%)
- Stool antigen: identifies active infection; used for screening and posttreatment testing; sensitivity 87%; specificity 70%; patients may not want to collect full stool sample.
- Serology: inexpensive; used in untreated patients, not used to document successful eradication; sensitivity 88%; specificity 69%

Follow-Up Tests & Special Considerations
If multiple/refractory ulcers, consider fasting serum gastrin to rule out ZES.

Diagnostic Procedures/Other
- Esophagogastroduodenoscopy (EGD): sensitivity >90%; specificity >95%; most accurate test for diagnosing PUD and active *H. pylori* infection. Patients of age >50 years with dyspepsia symptoms and any patient with alarm symptoms should have an EGD. EGD is costly and invasive (1)[B].
- Can obtain barium swallow if EGD contraindicated or not possible

TREATMENT

MEDICATION
First Line
- Acid suppression
  - PPIs: higher efficacy; most duodenal ulcers heal within 4 weeks.
    - Oral: omeprazole 20 mg/day; lansoprazole 30 mg/day; rabeprazole 20 mg/day; esomeprazole 40 mg/day; pantoprazole 40 mg/day; dexlansoprazole 30 mg/day
    - Length of treatment: 4 to 8 weeks
    - Precautions (2)
      - May decrease bone density—obtain interval bone densitometry with long-term use
      - Associated with development of community-acquired pneumonia
      - Associated with increased risk of *Clostridium difficile* infection
      - May cause hypomagnesemia.
      - Despite concerns, PPIs do not appear to decrease the efficacy of clopidogrel.
  - H$_2$ blockers
    - Oral: ranitidine or nizatidine 150 mg twice daily (BID) or 300 mg bedtime; cimetidine 400 mg BID or 800 mg bedtime; famotidine 20 mg BID or 40 mg bedtime; decrease dose by 50% if CrCl <50 mL/min.
    - Length of treatment: 4 to 8 weeks
    - Safer long-term option that PPI

- NSAID-induced or aspirin-induced ulcers
  - PPIs, H_2 blockers, sucralfate, or misoprostol can be given for NSAID-induced ulcers, but PPIs are most effective of all these options (3).
  - Discontinue NSAID or switch to lower dose.
  - Treat with PPIs for 6 to 8 weeks, may use as maintenance for patients with recurrent, complicated, or idiopathic ulcers; or in patients who require long-term aspirin or NSAID use.
- *H. pylori*–induced ulcers: Use one of the following 14-day regimens:
  - Clarithromycin triple therapy: PPI standard or double dose BID, clarithromycin 500 mg BID, amoxicillin 1 g BID *or* metronidazole 500 mg TID
  - Concomitant therapy: PPI standard or double dose BID, clarithromycin 500 mg BID, amoxicillin 1 g BID, nitroimidazole 500 mg BID
  - Bismuth subsalicylate 300 mg QID, metronidazole 500 mg TID, tetracycline 500 mg QID, levofloxacin 500 mg daily, rifabutin 300 mg daily
  - Bismuth-based quadruple therapy: standard dose PPI + bismuth + tetracycline + metronidazole (3)
  - Clarithromycin-based quadruple therapy: standard dose PPI + clarithromycin + amoxicillin + metronidazole
  - Clarithromycin-based triple therapy: double dose PPI + clarithromycin + amoxicillin (if allergic to penicillin, replace amoxicillin with metronidazole)

Second Line

- *H. pylori* eradication: use one of the following regimens (for 14 days) if the first-line regimen fails:
  - Levofloxacin triple therapy: PPI standard or double dose BID, amoxicillin 1 g BID, levofloxacin 500 mg daily
  - Levofloxacin sequential therapy: PPI standard or double dose BID *plus* amoxicillin 1 g BID for 5 to 7 days, followed by PPI standard or double dose BID *plus* amoxicillin 1 g BID plus levofloxacin 500 mg QD plus nitroimidazole* 500 mg BID for additional 5 to 7 days
  - Levofloxacin quadruple therapy: PPI double dose QD, levofloxacin 250 mg daily, nitazoxanide 500 mg BID, doxycycline 100 mg daily
  - Sequential therapy: PPI standard dose BID *plus* amoxicillin 1 g BID for 5 to 7 days followed by PPI standard dose BID *plus* clarithromycin 500 mg BID *plus* nitroimidazole 500 mg BID for additional 5 to 7 days
  - Hybrid therapy: PPI standard dose BID *plus* amoxicillin 1 g BID for 7 days followed by PPI standard dose BID *plus* amoxicillin 1 g BID plus Clarithromycin 500 mg BID plus nitroimidazole* 500 mg BID for additional 7 days
  - Alternative ulcer-healing drugs: sucralfate and antacids
- Significant possible interactions:
  - Cimetidine inhibits cytochrome P450 isozymes (avoid with theophylline, warfarin, phenytoin, and lidocaine).
  - Omeprazole may prolong elimination of diazepam, warfarin, and phenytoin.
  - Sucralfate reduces absorption of tetracycline, norfloxacin, ciprofloxacin, and theophylline; it leads to subtherapeutic levels.

Pregnancy Considerations

- PPIs are *not* associated with increased risk of major birth defects, spontaneous abortions, or preterm delivery.
- Breastfeeding: Both ranitidine and esomeprazole are secreted in breast milk at considerably lower doses than used for treatment in infants with reflux disease. Use in breastfeeding women is generally safe.

ISSUES FOR REFERRAL

Refer for endoscopy if red flag signs are present: onset of symptoms after age 55 years, progressive dysphagia, overt GI bleeding, iron deficiency anemia, persistent/recurrent vomiting, severe abdominal pain, unintentional weight loss, anorexia, and/or family history of gastric malignancy.

SURGERY/OTHER PROCEDURES

- Endoscopy: indicated for patients aged >55 years with new onset dyspeptic symptoms, in treatment failure, and those with red flag symptoms
- During endoscopy:
  - Biopsy stomach for *H. pylori* testing
  - Biopsy ulcer margin to exclude malignancy
  - Interventions to stop active bleeding or prevent rebleeding: injection with epinephrine, heater probe treatment, or placement of endoscopic clips (2)
- Nonemergent surgery indications: ulcers refractory to treatment; patients at high risk for complications (e.g., transplant recipients, on chronic steroids/NSAIDs); bleeding not responding to endoscopic therapy
- Surgical options:
  - Duodenal ulcers: truncal vagotomy and drainage (pyloroplasty/gastrojejunostomy), selective vagotomy (preserving the hepatic and/or celiac branches of the vagus) and drainage, or highly selective vagotomy (1)
  - Gastric ulcers: partial gastrectomy, Billroth I or II
- Emerging options: Vonoprazan is a novel acid blocker that is noninferior to PPIs.

ADMISSION, INPATIENT, AND NURSING CONSIDERATIONS

- Discontinue ulcerogenic agents (e.g., NSAIDs).
- Bleeding peptic ulcers
  - If patient is hemodynamically stable, administer a PPI to reduce transfusion requirements, the need for surgery, and length of hospital stay.
  - Oral PPIs have shown to be equivalent to IV PPIs after endoscopic treatment.
- Emergent surgery is the treatment for ulcer perforation (laparoscopy/open patching) (1).

 ONGOING CARE

FOLLOW-UP RECOMMENDATIONS

Patient Monitoring

- *H. pylori* eradication is expected in >90% (with double antibiotic regimen); confirm eradication 4 weeks after completing therapy with urea breath test or fecal antigen test.
- Acute duodenal ulcer: Monitor clinically.
- Acute gastric ulcer: Confirm healing via endoscopy in 6 to 8 weeks; if ulcer not healed, obtain biopsy to rule out gastric cancer (3).

PATIENT EDUCATION

Important to discuss lifestyle modifications: smoking cessation, decreased alcohol and caffeine consumption, weight loss, limited NSAID use

PROGNOSIS

- NSAID or aspirin-induced ulcer: Healing occurs >85% of the time with full PPI course and discontinuing offending medication (3).
- Once *H. pylori* is successfully eradicated, there is a low risk of recurrence. If recurrence does occur, consider other causes such as NSAID or tobacco use.
- Recurrence of PUD is common (up to >60%).

COMPLICATIONS

- Hemorrhage (up to 25% of patients), perforation (<5%), gastric outlet obstruction (up to 5% of duodenal or pyloric channel ulcers; male predilection), refractory PUD (5–10% after eradication of *H. pylori* or completion of 12 weeks of PPI)
- Risk of gastric adenocarcinoma is increased in *H. pylori*–infected patients.

REFERENCES

1. Lanas A, Chan FKL. Peptic ulcer disease. *Lancet*. 2017;390(10094):613–624.
2. Neumann I, Letelier LM, Rada G, et al. Comparison of different regimens of proton pump inhibitors for acute peptic ulcer bleeding. *Cochrane Database Syst Rev*. 2013;(6):CD007999.
3. Narayanan M, Reddy KM, Marsicano E. Peptic ulcer disease and *Helicobacter pylori* infection. *Mo Med*. 2018;115(3):219–224.

CODES

ICD10

- K27.9 Peptic ulc, site unsp, unsp as ac or chr, w/o hemor or perf
- K26.9 Duodenal ulcer, unspecified as acute or chronic, without hemorrhage or perforation
- K25.9 Gastric ulcer, unspecified as acute or chronic, without hemorrhage or perforation

CLINICAL PEARLS

- PPIs: higher efficacy than H_2 blockers for healing duodenal ulcers
- Eradicate *H. pylori* to assist healing and reduce the risk of recurrence.
- EGD indications: patients with suspected peptic ulcers, red flag symptoms, treatment failure

PERICARDITIS
Munima Nasir, MD • Kyle Burke, DO

BASICS

DESCRIPTION
Inflammation of the pericardium, with or without associated pericardial effusion; myopericarditis or perimyocarditis refers to cases that have myocardial involvement in addition to involvement of the pericardium.

EPIDEMIOLOGY
Incidence
- Incidence is approximately 27.7 cases per 100,000 per year (1).
- After the first episode of acute pericarditis, about 30% of patients will experience recurrence within next 18 months.

ETIOLOGY AND PATHOPHYSIOLOGY
- Inflammation of the pericardial sac can be *acute*, incessant, *chronic*, or recurrent (2).
- Can lead to production of serous/purulent fluid/dense fibrinous material, which may or may not lead to hemodynamic compromise
- Idiopathic: 85–90% of cases; likely related to viral infection, which may trigger immune-related process
- Infectious
  - Viral (80–85% of cases): coxsackievirus, echovirus, adenovirus, Epstein-Barr virus, cytomegalovirus, hepatitis viruses, influenza virus, HIV, measles, mumps, varicella, SARS-CoV-2 (1.5% of cases), parvovirus B19
  - Bacterial: *Mycobacterium tuberculosis* (common in endemic countries); fungal (more common in immunocompromised populations): *Blastomyces dermatitidis, Candida* sp., *Histoplasma capsulatum*; parasites: *Echinococcus*
- Noninfectious causes (15–20% of cases)
  - Acute MI (2 to 4 days after MI), Dressler syndrome (weeks to months after MI); aortic dissection; renal failure, uremia, dialysis-associated: malignancy (e.g., breast cancer, lung cancer, Hodgkin disease, leukemia, lymphoma); radiation therapy; trauma; after cardiac procedures (e.g., catheterization, pacemaker placement, ablation, pericardiotomy)
  - Autoimmune disorders: connective tissue disorders, systemic lupus erythematosus (SLE), rheumatoid arthritis, scleroderma, hypothyroidism, inflammatory bowel disease, Wegener granulomatosis, spondyloarthropathies, sarcoidosis, IgG4-related disease
  - Suspected vaccination associations: smallpox, influenza, SARS-CoV-2 mRNA vaccine (incidence of ~4.8 per 1 million)
- Medication-induced: dantrolene, doxorubicin, hydralazine, isoniazid, mesalamine, methysergide, penicillin, phenytoin, procainamide, rifampin

Genetics
Familial Mediterranean fever, tumor necrosis factor receptor-associated periodic syndrome (TRAPS) both particularly related to recurrent pericarditis (3)

RISK FACTORS
Thoracic surgery, chronic kidney disease, pneumonia, autoimmune diseases, lung or breast cancer especially if treated with radiation therapy

DIAGNOSIS

- Acute pericarditis (at least two of four criteria)
  - New/increasing pericardial effusion (60–80% of cases) seen on imaging
  - ECG changes with widespread (nonregional) ST-segment elevations (up to 60% of cases)
  - Pericardial friction rub (<33% of cases)
  - Typical (pleuritic) chest pain
- Incessant pericarditis: symptoms above persist for >4 to 6 weeks but <3 months; recurrent pericarditis: return of symptoms after a 4- to 6-week symptom-free interval; chronic pericarditis: symptoms >3 months
- Myopericarditis: definite pericarditis *plus*
  - Symptoms (dyspnea, chest pain, or palpitations) and ECG changes not previously documented (ST/T wave abnormalities, supraventricular/ventricular tachycardia) or focal/diffuse depressed left ventricular (LV) function documented on imaging study
  - Absence of evidence of other cause
  - One of the following: elevated cardiac enzymes (creatine kinase [CK]-MB, troponin I or T) or new focal/diffuse depressed LV function or abnormal imaging consistent with myocarditis (MRI with gadolinium, gallium-67 scanning, antimyosin antibody scanning)

HISTORY
Prodrome of fever, malaise, myalgias, recent viral upper respiratory infection; acute, sharp/stabbing chest pain, pathognomonic if pain radiates to trapezius; duration typically hours to days; pleuritic pain; pain reduced by leaning forward, worsened by lying supine; shortness of breath

PHYSICAL EXAM
Pericardial friction rub: coarse, high-pitched sound best heard during end expiration at left lower sternal border with patient leaning forward; highly specific for diagnosis (but not sensitive); may be transient and mono-, bi-, or triphasic; new S_3 may suggest myopericarditis

DIFFERENTIAL DIAGNOSIS
Myocardial ischemia/acute coronary syndrome, pulmonary embolism, aortic dissection, gastroesophageal reflux disease, pneumonia

DIAGNOSTIC TESTS & INTERPRETATION
Initial Tests (lab, imaging)
- CBC: typically shows leukocytosis
- Inflammatory markers: elevated erythrocyte sedimentation rate (ESR), C-reactive protein (CRP), and lactate dehydrogenase (LDH)
- Cardiac biomarkers: typically elevated CK, troponins; elevated troponins associated with younger age, male sex, pericardial effusion at presentation, and ST segment elevation on ECG; adverse outcomes are not predicted by elevated troponin.
- ECG: Findings include widespread upward concave ST-segment elevation (in all or most leads, a diffuse, nonregional process) and PR-segment depression that may evolve through four stages. ECG may be normal/show nonspecific abnormalities; may demonstrate low voltage and electrical alternans with large effusions and tamponade

- Transthoracic echocardiogram is recommended to evaluate for the presence of pericardial effusion, tamponade, or myocardial disease.
- Chest x-ray (CXR) is performed to rule out pulmonary/mediastinal pathology. Enlarged cardiac silhouette suggests large pericardial effusion (at least 300 mL).
- CT and MRI allow visualization of pericardium to assess for complications; can assist in planning of pericardiectomy if necessary
- Additional testing (if clinically appropriate based on history or atypical presentation or course) may include thyroid stimulating hormone (TSH), tuberculin skin test, sputum cultures, rheumatoid factor, antinuclear antibody, and HIV serology.

Diagnostic Procedures/Other
Pericardiocentesis indicated for cardiac tamponade; for suspected purulent, tuberculous, or neoplastic pericarditis; and for effusions >20 mm on echocardiography

Test Interpretation
- Microscopic examination may reveal hyperemia, leukocyte accumulation, or fibrin deposition.
- Purulent fluid with neutrophilic predominance if bacterial etiology; lymphocytic predominance in viral, tuberculous, and neoplastic pericarditis
- Do not use Light criteria (set of three criteria to determine if pleural fluid is exudative) for evaluation of pericardial fluid (3)[C].

TREATMENT

GENERAL MEASURES
Specific therapy directed toward underlying disorder for patients with identified cause; restrictions of physical activity are an important part of treatment for recurrences.

MEDICATION
First Line
- NSAIDs are considered the mainstay of therapy for acute pericarditis:
  - Ibuprofen 600 mg TID for 7 to 10 days (2 to 4 weeks for recurrence) then taper (1)[C]
  - Aspirin 1,000 mg TID for 7 to 10 days (2 to 4 weeks for recurrence) then taper; preferable for patients with recent MI because other NSAIDs impair scar formation in animal studies (1)[C]
  - Indomethacin 50 mg TID for 7 to 10 days (2 to 4 weeks for recurrence) then taper; should avoid in elderly and those with coronary artery disease (1)[C]
  - GI protection should be provided (proton pump inhibitor) (1)[C].
  - Tapering should be done only if the patient is asymptomatic and CRP/ESR are normal. Repeat CRP/ESR every 1 to 2 weeks (1)[C].
  - Monitoring: NSAIDs: CBC and CRP at baseline and weekly until CRP normalizes
  - Contraindications: hypersensitivity to aspirin or NSAIDs, active peptic ulcer/GI bleeding
  - Precautions: Use with caution in patients with asthma, 3rd-trimester pregnancy, coagulopathy, elderly, and renal/hepatic dysfunction.

- Colchicine:
  – Use in combination with NSAIDs to decrease incidence of recurrence, treatment failure, and for faster symptomatic response; not recommended for monotherapy (2)[A]
  – 0.5 to 0.6 mg BID for up to 3 months (up to 6 months for recurrence); taper is not required. Adjust for weight, renal, and hepatic function (1)[C],(3)[C].
  – This is the only agent proven to prevent recurrences in RCTs. Adjunctive therapy can reduce rate of recurrence by 50% (2)[A].
  – Monitoring: Consider CBC, transaminases, CK, and creatinine at baseline and after 1 month at a minimum; follow CRP weekly until normalizes (1)[C]
  – Adverse reactions: diarrhea, abdominal pain, nausea
- Pregnancy: <20 weeks' gestation: Aspirin is the first choice, but NSAIDs and prednisone are also allowed; >20 weeks' gestation: Prednisone is allowed with avoidance of NSAIDs, aspirin, and colchicine (3)[C].

Second Line
- Corticosteroid treatment is indicated in connective tissue disease, tuberculous pericarditis, contraindications to NSAIDs or colchicine, or severe recurrent symptoms unresponsive to NSAIDs or colchicine. Steroids should be avoided in uncomplicated acute pericarditis or if infectious etiology is suspected. *Corticosteroid use alone has been found to be an independent risk factor for recurrence.*
- Use low dose (0.2 to 0.5 mg/kg/day) until resolution of symptoms and normalization of CRP and then perform slow tapering (1)[C].
- Consider adequate prophylaxis treatment with calcium/vitamin D, and conditionally use bisphosphonates in men or postmenopausal women for osteoporosis prevention (1)[C].
- If recurrence while tapering, try to not increase dose or restart corticosteroids
- Intrapericardial administration of steroids may be effective and limits systemic side effects.
- Anakinra (interleukin-1 [IL-1] antagonist)— for recurrent pericarditis
  – 2 mg/kg (up to 100 mg) subcutaneously daily for 2 to 6 months; adjust for renal function.
  – Decreased incidence of recurrence in one small RCT (2)[A]
  – Adverse reactions—injection site reactions, elevated liver enzymes, herpes zoster reactivation
- Rilonacept (IL-1 antagonist)—for recurrent pericarditis
  – 320 mg subcutaneous injection once followed by 160 mg dose weekly for 12 weeks
  – Decreased recurrence rate compared to placebo (3)[C]
  – Adverse effects—injection site reactions, increased risk for upper respiratory tract infections

ISSUES FOR REFERRAL
Hospitalization is recommended for any patient with major medical comorbidities, refractory cases, uremic/dialysis related cases, suspected or threatened tamponade, poor prognostic factors, or presentation that suggests an underlying systemic inflammatory disease (1)[C].

SURGERY/OTHER PROCEDURES
- Pericardiocentesis is indicated in cases of cardiac tamponade, high likelihood of tuberculous/purulent/neoplastic pericarditis, and moderate-to-large symptomatic effusions refractory to medical therapy.
- Pericardial biopsy may be considered for diagnosis in those with persistent worsening pericarditis without a definite diagnosis.
- Pericardial window may be performed in cases of recurrent cardiac tamponade with large pericardial effusion despite medical therapy.
- Pericardiectomy is the standard of care for chronic constrictive pericarditis with persistent symptoms, such as NYHA class III or IV. Mortality is high at 6–12% so is reserved only after careful evaluation by experienced surgeons at hospitals with specific interest in pericardial diseases.

ADMISSION, INPATIENT, AND NURSING CONSIDERATIONS
- Inpatient therapy is recommended for pericarditis associated with clinical predictors of poor prognosis:
  – Fever >38°C, subacute onset, large pericardial effusion, cardiac tamponade, lack of response to NSAID/aspirin therapy after at least 1 week, immunosuppressed state, trauma, oral anticoagulation therapy, myopericarditis
- IV fluids considered for hypotension or in the setting of pericardial tamponade

 ONGOING CARE

FOLLOW-UP RECOMMENDATIONS
- 1 week to check response to treatment, CBC, CRP
- Those with clinical predictors of poor prognosis may require closer follow-up based on lab data and echocardiographic findings.

Patient Monitoring
Myopericarditis
- Use lower doses of anti-inflammatory drugs to control symptoms for 1 to 2 weeks while minimizing deleterious effects.
- Exercise restrictions for 4 to 6 weeks or until symptoms resolved and biomarkers normalized; for athletes, exercise restriction should be a minimum of 3 months after symptom onset.
- Echocardiographic monitoring at 1, 6, and 12 months (especially in those with LV dysfunction)

PROGNOSIS
Overall good prognosis but depends on underlying etiology; disease usually benign and self-limiting; purulent and tuberculosis pericarditis with high mortality

COMPLICATIONS
- Recurrent pericarditis: occurs in 15–30% of patients, with most instances resulting from idiopathic, viral, or autoimmune pericarditis; inadequate treatment of the initial attack; and, less commonly, neoplastic etiologies; recurrence usually within 1st week following initial episode but may occur months to years later
- Cardiac tamponade: rare complication with increased incidence in neoplastic, purulent, and tuberculous pericarditis
- Effusive-constrictive pericarditis: reported in 24% of patients undergoing surgery for constrictive pericarditis and in 8% of patients undergoing pericardiocentesis and cardiac catheterization for cardiac tamponade; failure of right atrial pressure to fall by 50% or to a level <10 mm Hg after pericardiocentesis is diagnostic
- Constrictive pericarditis: rare complication in which rigid pericardium produces abnormal diastolic filling with elevated filling pressures; pericardiectomy remains definitive therapy; found to be associated with incessant pericarditis; mortality for those without diagnosis reaches up to 90%.
- Atrial fibrillation/flutter

REFERENCES
1. Lazarou E, Tsioufis P, Vlachopoulos C, et al. Acute pericarditis: update. *Curr Cardiol Rep.* 2022;24(8):905–913.
2. Melendo-Viu M, Marchán-Lopez Á, Guarch CJ, et al. A systematic review and meta-analysis of randomized controlled trials evaluating pharmacologic therapies for acute and recurrent pericarditis. *Trends Cardiovasc Med.* 2023;33(5):319–326.
3. Bizzi E, Picchi C, Mastrangelo G, et al. Recent advances in pericarditis. *Eur J Intern Med.* 2022;95:24–31.

CODES

ICD10
- I31.9 Disease of pericardium, unspecified
- I30.9 Acute pericarditis, unspecified
- I30.1 Infective pericarditis

CLINICAL PEARLS
Therapy aimed at symptomatic relief and NSAIDs with colchicine are first-line treatment. Colchicine has been shown to decrease risk of recurrence by 50%.

PERIODIC LIMB MOVEMENT DISORDER (PLMD)

Denise Sharon, MD, PhD, FAASM • Rochelle Zak, MD

 BASICS

DESCRIPTION

Sleep-related movement disorder characterized by periodic limb movements of sleep (PLMS) with significant sleep disturbance and/or daytime functional impairment:

- PLMS demonstrated during polysomnography
- PLMS are repetitive contractions of tibialis anterior muscles occurring mainly in non–rapid eye movement (NREM) sleep.
- Movements consist of unilateral or bilateral, simultaneous or not, rhythmical extension of the big toe and ankle dorsiflexion.
- Sometimes, knee and hip flexion are noted.
- Arm movements or more generalized movements occur less commonly.
- Movements might be associated with cortical arousals from sleep unbeknownst to the patient (PLMs with arousals—PLMA).
- A clinical history of significant sleep disturbance and/or functional impairment is necessary for diagnosis.
- Complaints include insomnia, nonrestorative sleep, daytime fatigue, and somnolence.
- Bed partner may complain of patient's movements.
- Other sleep disorders such as obstructive sleep apnea (OSA), narcolepsy, and restless legs syndrome (RLS) do not explain the PLMS.
- No associated restlessness or dysesthesia while awake
  - If there is an associated sensory perception or restlessness, the diagnosis is not PLMD but possibly RLS.
- System(s) affected: musculoskeletal, nervous
- Synonym(s) referring to the PLMS: nocturnal myoclonus; sleep myoclonus

EPIDEMIOLOGY

Incidence
- PLMD is rare, affecting children and adults (1).
- PLMS occurs in >15% of insomnia patients.
- PLMS are frequent in narcolepsy, RBD, OSA, and during initiation of CPAP.

Prevalence
- PLMS increases with age: 45% of patients aged >65 years exhibit PLMS >5/hr but not PLMD.
- PLMD is much less common: <5% of adults but also underdiagnosed (1)
- 85% of RLS patients have PLMS (2).

ETIOLOGY AND PATHOPHYSIOLOGY
- Understudied; most data reports on PLMS as it pertains to RLS:
  - CNS dopamine dysregulation supported by increased incidence of PLMS in untreated Parkinson disease (PD) and decreased incidence of PLMS in schizophrenia
- Triggering and exacerbating factors:
  - Peripheral neuropathy
  - Arthritis
  - Renal failure
  - Spinal cord injury
  - Pregnancy

- Medication side effects:
  - Most antidepressants (except bupropion or desipramine) and lithium
  - Some antipsychotic and antidementia medications
  - Antiemetics (antidopaminergic)
  - Sedating antihistamines

Genetics
BTBD9 on chromosome 6p associated with PLMS in patients with or without RLS but not in RLS patients without PLMS

RISK FACTORS
- Family history of RLS
- Iron deficiency and associated conditions
- History of prematurity

GENERAL PREVENTION
- Promoting adequate sleep
- Avoid PLMS triggers such as iron deficiency, frequently observed in children (3).

COMMONLY ASSOCIATED CONDITIONS
- Narcolepsy
- End-stage renal disease; cardiovascular disease; stroke
- Gastric surgery
- Pregnancy
- Arthritis
- Lumbar spine disease; spinal cord injury
- Peripheral neuropathy
- Insomnia, insufficient sleep, parasomnias
- ADHD, anxiety, oppositional behaviors

Pediatric Considerations
- PLMD may precede overt RLS by years (3).
- Association with RLS is more common.
- Association and differential diagnosis with restless sleep disorder, ADHD, oppositional behaviors, mood disorders, growing pains (3)

Pregnancy Considerations
- May be secondary to iron, folate deficiency
- Most severe in the 3rd trimester
- Usually resolves after delivery

Geriatric Considerations
- May cause or exacerbate circadian disruption and "sundowning"
- PLMS may increase risk of atrial fibrillation in elderly.

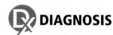 **DIAGNOSIS**

HISTORY
Sleep disturbance:
- Insomnia: difficulty maintaining sleep
- Nonrestorative sleep
- Daytime fatigue, tiredness, somnolence
- Oppositional behaviors
- Memory impairment
- Depression
- ADHD, particularly in children (3)

PHYSICAL EXAM
No specific findings

DIFFERENTIAL DIAGNOSIS
- PLMS occurring with RLS, RBD, and narcolepsy are secondary to the sleep disorder, not PLMD.
- PLMS occurring with OSA may be associated with respiratory events and is not PLMD.
- Sleep starts: nonperiodic, generalized, only at wake–sleep transition, <0.2-inch duration
- Sleep-related leg cramps: isolated, painful, muscle knots
- Fragmentary myoclonus: 75 to 150 ms of electromyographic (EMG) activity, minimal movement, no periodicity
- Nocturnal seizures: epileptiform EEG, motor pattern incongruent with PLMs
- Fasciculations, tremor: no sleep association
- Sleep-related rhythmic movement disorder: voluntary movement during wake–sleep transition; higher frequency than PLMs
- Restless sleep disorder—large body movements, no periodicity

DIAGNOSTIC TESTS & INTERPRETATION
Polysomnography (PSG) demonstrating PLMS:
- Tibialis ant EMG activation lasting 0.5 to 10.0 inches
- EMG amplitude increase >8 μV from baseline
- Movements occur in a sequence of ≥4 at intervals of 5 to 90 seconds.
- Associated with heart rate variability from autonomic-level arousals
- Most PLMs episodes occur in the first hours of NREM sleep.
- Night-to-night PLMS variability is common.

Initial Tests (lab, imaging)
Serum iron stores including ferritin, transferrin, iron-binding capacity, serum iron

Follow-Up Tests & Special Considerations
Repeat iron stores, at least ferritin if suspected change, or nonresponsive to treatment

Diagnostic Procedures/Other
EMG, nerve conduction studies for peripheral neuropathy/radiculopathy if indicated

Test Interpretation
On PSG: PLMSI >5/hr children, and >15/hr adults

 TREATMENT

Treatment paradigm similar to that for RLS, except that all medications are off-label for PLMD (2),(4),(5)[B]

GENERAL MEASURES
- Assess for and correct iron insufficiency.
- Adequate nightly sleep
- Regular exercise, low impact in the evening
- Weighted blanket, warm the legs (long socks, leg warmers, electric blanket, etc.)
- Hot/leg baths, warm soaks before bedtime
- Avoid caffeine and alcohol.

MEDICATION

- Use minimum effective dose.
- Goals of medication:
  - Improve subjective sleep quality.
  - Control PLMS and their effect on sleep.
- Consider risks, side effects, and interactions in different populations (e.g., benzodiazepines in elderly).
- Treatment should decrease daytime somnolence.

First Line

- Voltage-gated calcium channel $\alpha 2\delta$ subunit ligands: useful for associated neuropathy; decrease PLMS and improve sleep architecture; caution with renal impairment (2)[C],(4)
  - Gabapentin enacarbil (Horizant): 600 mg early evening
  - Gabapentin (Neurontin) 300 to 600 mg HS
  - Pregabalin (Lyrica): 75 to 300 mg HS
- Dopamine agonists reduce PLMS and increase sleep efficiency; start low and titrate slow (2),(4),(5)[C]; caveat: no data on long-term effects of DA on PLMD
  - Pramipexole (Mirapex): 0.125 to 0.500 mg; titrate by 0.125 mg; take 2 hours HS
  - Ropinirole (Requip): 0.25 to 4.00 mg; titrate by 0.25 mg; take 1/2 to 1 hour HS; preferred in renal impairment
  - Transdermal rotigotine (Neupro): 1 to 3 mg/24 hr patch; initiate with 1 mg/24 hr; titrate up by 1 mg slowly to effectiveness.
- Avoid dopamine agonists in psychotic patients, especially if taking dopamine antagonists.
- Dopamine agonists may exert a stimulant effect, further disturbing sleep.

Second Line

Benzodiazepines and agonists (2)[C],(4); most commonly used because of their effect on sleep; caution in the elderly

- Clonazepam (Klonopin): 0.5 to 2.0 mg QHS
- Zaleplon, zolpidem, temazepam, triazolam, alprazolam, diazepam

ISSUES FOR REFERRAL

To sleep medicine clinic, neurology and movement disorders clinic:

- High-dose medications
- Worsening of Sx while on medications
- Intractable iron deficiency
- Uncontrolled symptoms in adults and special populations

Pediatric Considerations

- First-line treatment: nonpharmacologic (3)[C]
- Assess/correct iron deficiency (6)[B].
- Consider low-dose clonidine 0.1 to 0.3 mg HS; caution: orthostatic hypotension (3)[C]

Pregnancy Considerations

- Initial approach: iron supplementation, nonpharmacologic therapies (5)
- In 2nd and 3rd trimesters, can use clonazepam 0.25 to 1.00 mg QHS
- CarbiDOPA/levoDOPA 25/100 to 50/200 ER
- Refractory PLMD—may use oxycodone in 2nd and 3rd trimesters: Discontinue 2 weeks prior delivery.

Geriatric Considerations

In weak or frail patients, avoid medications that may cause dizziness or unsteadiness.

ADDITIONAL THERAPIES

- If iron deficient, iron supplementation:
  - 325 mg ferrous sulfate with 200 mg vitamin C between meals QD
  - Repletion may require months of treatment.
- Clonidine 0.05 to 0.30 mg/day

SURGERY/OTHER PROCEDURES

Correction of orthopedic, neuropathic, or peripheral vascular problems

COMPLEMENTARY & ALTERNATIVE MEDICINE

Vitamin/mineral supplements, including calcium, magnesium, vitamin D, vitamin B_{12}, and folate, maybe helpful

 ONGOING CARE

FOLLOW-UP RECOMMENDATIONS

Patient Monitoring

- At monthly intervals until stable
- Assess symptom severity, medication side effects, and augmentation.
- Annual and PRN follow-up thereafter
- Repeat iron blood work if previously low.

DIET

Avoid caffeine, alcohol, more so late in the day.

PATIENT EDUCATION

- National Sleep Foundation: https://www.thensf.org
- American Academy of Sleep Medicine: https://www.sleepeducation.org/

PROGNOSIS

- Primary PLMD: lifelong, no current cure
- Secondary PLMD: may subside with resolution of cause(s) such as low iron stores
- Current therapies usually control symptoms.
- PLMD often precedes the emergence of RLS.

COMPLICATIONS

- Tolerance to meds requiring increased dose
- Augmentation (increased PLMs and sleep disturbance, emergence of RLS) from dopamine agonists:
  - Higher doses increase risk.
  - Iron deficiency increases augmentation risk.
  - Add alternative medication and then gradually discontinue dopaminergic agent.
- Iatrogenic PLMD (from antidepressants, etc.)

REFERENCES

1. Hornyak M, Feige B, Riemann D, et al. Periodic leg movements in sleep and periodic limb movement disorder: prevalence, clinical significance and treatment. *Sleep Med Rev.* 2006;10(3):169–177.
2. Fulda S. The role of periodic limb movements during sleep in restless legs syndrome: a selective update. *Sleep Med Clin.* 2015;10(3):241–248.
3. Sharon D, Walters AS, Simakajjornboon N. RLS and PLMD in children in sleep disorders in children. *J Child Sci.* In press.
4. Aurora RN, Kristo DA, Bista SR, et al; for American Academy of Sleep Medicine. The treatment of restless legs syndrome and periodic limb movement disorder in adults—an update for 2012: practice parameters with an evidence-based systematic review and meta-analyses: an American Academy of Sleep Medicine clinical practice guideline. *Sleep.* 2012;35(8):1039–1062.
5. Garcia-Borreguero D, Silber MH, Winkelman JW, et al. Guidelines for the first-line treatment of restless legs syndrome/Willis-Ekbom disease, prevention and treatment of dopaminergic augmentation: a combined task force of the IRLSSG, EURLSSG, and the RLS-foundation. *Sleep Med.* 2016;21:1–11.
6. Gingras JL, Gaultney JF, Picchietti DL. Pediatric periodic limb movement disorder: sleep symptom and polysomnographic correlates compared to obstructive sleep apnea. *J Clin Sleep Med.* 2011;7(6):603A–609A.

ADDITIONAL READING

American Academy of Sleep Medicine. Periodic limb movement disorder. In: *International Classification of Sleep Disorders*. 3rd ed. Darien, IL: American Academy of Sleep Medicine; 2014:292–299.

 SEE ALSO

Restless Legs Syndrome

 CODES

ICD10

G47.61 Periodic limb movement disorder

CLINICAL PEARLS

- Many patients with PLMs may not require treatment; when sleep disturbance associated with PLMs causes insomnia and/or daytime consequences, PLMD should be treated.
- Assuring adequate iron stores, with a ferritin >75 is advised.
- Many antidepressants and some antihistamines cause or exacerbate PLMs.

PERIPHERAL ARTERIAL DISEASE
Pooja Gandhi, DO • Tyler D. Sharpe, MD • Jennifer Koch, MD

 BASICS

DESCRIPTION
Peripheral arterial disease (PAD) represents an athero-sclerotic occlusive disease of the peripheral arteries, most commonly in the lower extremities. Following coronary artery disease and cerebrovascular disease, PAD is the third leading source of atherosclerotic vascular morbidity. PAD manifests as intermittent claudication (IC) or atypical leg pain and is commonly diagnosed with a resting ankle-brachial index (ABI) of <0.90 (1).

EPIDEMIOLOGY
- Age: ≥65 years, 50 to 64 years with atherosclerosis risk factors (e.g., diabetes mellitus [DM], hyperlipe-demia [HLD], hypertension [HTN], history of smok-ing) or family history of PAD, or <50 years, with DM and one additional atherosclerosis risk factor
- Individuals with known atherosclerotic disease in another vascular bed (e.g., coronary, carotid, subcla-vian, renal, mesenteric artery stenosis, or AAA)

Incidence
Incidence increases with age and the presence of cardiovascular risk factors.

Prevalence
- Data from the National Health and Nutrition Examination Survey (1999–2004) show that 5.9% of the U.S. population ≥40 years has a low ABI (<0.9) indicating the presence of PAD. In 2021, the American College of Cardiology estimated 238 million people are living with PAD worldwide.
- However, the true prevalence of PAD is difficult to establish because more than half of persons are asymptomatic.

ETIOLOGY AND PATHOPHYSIOLOGY
- In PAD, arterial occlusion is most commonly a result of underlying chronic atherosclerotic disease.
- The association between PAD and cardiovascular morbidity and mortality has been well established, with a lower ABI being an independent predictor.
- Other etiologies for PAD include phlebitis, trauma, or autoimmune/vasculitic diseases.
- Arterial narrowing results in insufficient oxygen delivery to the muscle during periods of increased demand (i.e., exercise), causing claudication and limiting exercise. Reperfusion at rest following ischemia can result in subsequent physiologic changes, including inflammation, oxidant stress, endothelial dysfunction, and mitochondrial injury.

Genetics
Several of the risk factors for PAD (as noted below) are heritable, and genome-wide association studies to isolate PAD-specific single nucleotide polymorphisms are being explored (2).

RISK FACTORS
- Older age, atherosclerotic disease of any vascular bed, current or history of smoking, DM, HTN, HLD, chronic kidney disease (CKD)
- Heritable conditions: chylomicronemia, hypercholes-terolemia, hyperhomocysteinemia, and pseudoxan-thoma elasticum

GENERAL PREVENTION
- Regular aerobic exercise program, smoking cessa-tion, blood pressure (BP) and diabetes control
- Statin therapy is indicated in patients with clinical PAD for secondary prevention of atherosclerotic cardiovascular disease.

COMMONLY ASSOCIATED CONDITIONS
In addition to the aforementioned risk factors, PAD is associated with other forms of atherosclerotic disease including myocardial infarction (MI), transient ischemic attack (TIA), and cerebrovascular accident (CVA).

 DIAGNOSIS

HISTORY
- 20–40% of patients will be asymptomatic (3).
- 10–35% of patients present with classic IC (painful, aching, cramping, uncomfortable, or tired feeling in legs during walking, relieved by rest) (3).
- Reduced exercise or mobility to avoid pain
- 1–2% of patients will develop critical limb ischemia. This may present subacutely as nonhealing wounds/ulcerations, or as acute limb ischemia due to acute thrombosis/embolism, which is a medical emergency.
- Skin discoloration
- Erectile dysfunction (in conjunction with IC and absent or diminished femoral pulses constitutes Leriche syndrome, caused by severe atherosclerosis of the distal abdominal aorta, iliac arteries and femoral and popliteal arteries)
- Mesenteric ischemia caused by severe atherosclero-sis of abdominal vessels

PHYSICAL EXAM
- Pallor with leg elevation, dependent rubor
- Pale atrophic skin with hair thinning or loss (seen with chronic PAD)
- Brittle or hypertrophic nails
- Moderate to severe PAD can cause reduced/absent extremity pulses. Distal extremities may feel cool.
- Severe PAD may present non-healing ulcers and wounds on distal toes or heels. May present as gangrene.
- Acute limb ischemia may present with pulselessness, pallor, paraesthesias, and skin discoloration.

DIFFERENTIAL DIAGNOSIS
- Arterial aneurysm or dissection
- Deep vein thrombosis (DVT)
- Thromboangiitis obliterans (Buerger disease) or other vasculopathies
- Arterial embolism
- Peripheral neuropathy
- Spinal stenosis or nerve root compression (pseudoclaudication)
- Popliteal entrapment syndrome

DIAGNOSTIC TESTS & INTERPRETATION
Screening
- Current AHA/ACC guidelines recommend resting ABI testing for symptomatic patients and also state that it could be reasonable to test asymptomatic patients with increased risk of PAD (patients with known atherosclerotic disease or risk factors of atherosclerosis including DM, HTN, HLD, smoking and age ≥65 years). USPSTF recommends against routine screening for asymptomatic adults due to insufficient evidence (I).

Initial Tests (lab, imaging)
- Risk factor identification with fasting lipid profile and basic metabolic profile
- Exercise treadmill ABI is useful in patients who are symptomatic but have normal resting ABI.

Follow-Up Tests & Special Considerations
Imaging is reserved for patients who have lifestyle-limiting symptoms (IC) despite appropriate guideline-directed management and therapy.
- Duplex ultrasound, magnetic resonance angiography (MRA), and computed tomography angiography (CTA) are recommended in symptomatic patients who are being considered for revascularization.
- Invasive angiography is recommended in patients with critical limb ischemia and is reasonable in those with symptomatic PAD who are candidates for revascularization.

Diagnostic Procedures/Other
- Doppler ABI: ratio of systolic BP taken with Doppler flowmeter at the ankle (dorsalis pedis or posterior tibial artery) divided by the systolic BP at the brachial artery
- Toe-brachial index (TBI) is recommended when ABI is ≥1.40, suggesting a noncompressible vessel.

Test Interpretation
- ABI <0.9 abnormal, diagnostic for PAD and <0.4 is severe PAD/critical limb ischemia
- ABI 0.91 to 0.99 borderline, correlated clinically, and consider additional testing
- 1 to 1.4 normal, >1.4 concern for incompressible arteries, association with DM

 TREATMENT

GENERAL MEASURES
- The treatment of PAD is multifactorial and includes a supervised exercise program, guideline-based medical therapy, and risk factor modification. Recommendations below are based primarily on AHA/ACC Guideline (1)[C].
- Assess functional status via the Fontaine or Rutherford classification systems. Anatomic classification of complexity is determined by the Trans-Atlantic Inter-Society Consensus (TASC). This classification may be used to guide management.

- Cardiovascular risk factor modification, especially in the setting of smoking cessation
  - High-intensity statin (lipid-lowering therapy) is recommended for all patients with PAD and has been shown to reduce all-cause mortality. Goal LDL <100.
  - Goal BP <140/90 mm Hg
  - ACE-inhibitors or ARBs can be effective to reduce the risk of cardiovascular ischemic events in patients with PAD (moderate strength recommendation from AHA/ACC).
  - Counseling on smoking cessation and offering pharmacologic agents (varenicline, bupropion, nicotine replacement therapy) and behavioral counselling
- Supervised exercise training, which takes place in a hospital or outpatient facility, is the initial treatment modality recommended in patients with IC. Patients are instructed to walk for a minimum of 30 to 45 minutes (with rest when symptomatic) 3 times per week for a minimum of 12 weeks. A structured community or home-based exercise program can be beneficial and is recommended when a supervised program is not possible.

MEDICATION

First Line

- Antiplatelet monotherapy is recommended in symptomatic PAD without bleeding risk contraindications (4)[A]. Aspirin (75 to 325 mg) or clopidogrel (75 mg) are acceptable first-line antiplatelet agents.
  - It is reasonable to prescribe antiplatelet monotherapy in asymptomatic patients who have an ABI diagnostic of PAD.
  - In asymptomatic patients with borderline ABIs (0.91 to 0.99), the utility of antiplatelet therapy is not well established.
- Dual antiplatelet therapy (DAPT; aspirin and clopidogrel) should be prescribed only following endovascular intervention; the data for efficacy is not well established, and bleeding risk is increased.
- Data is emerging for the combination of aspirin and low-dose 2.5 mg rivaroxaban in those with symptomatic PAD and high risk for cardiovascular comorbidities/limb complications. This must be balanced against the bleeding risk.
- Statins are recommended by AHA/ACC and AAFP guidelines for all individuals with symptomatic and asymptomatic PAD to LDL goal of at least less than 100 mg/dL, individualized depending on comorbid conditions (1),(3).
- Cilostazol (100 mg orally twice daily) has been shown to improve walking distance and should be considered in all patients with claudication that impacts daily living.
- The above medications can be prescribed concurrently with the initiation of an exercise program.

Second Line

- Pentoxifylline (400 mg 3 times daily) was previously considered first line for symptomatic relief of claudication; however, evidence is of poor quality and benefit is uncertain (Cochrane, other reviews).
- Vorapaxar (a protease-activated receptor antagonist) acts against thrombin receptors to reduce cardiovascular and PAD-associated complications. New information is emerging on which patient population this is best for and is not routinely prescribed.

SURGERY/OTHER PROCEDURES

Percutaneous and surgical interventions should be considered in patients who had an inadequate response to less-invasive modalities (i.e., exercise and pharmacotherapy), have significant disability from their claudication, and have a favorable risk-benefit ratio.

- Percutaneous intervention involves accessing the artery with a wire or catheter and balloon angioplasty with possible stent placement to widen the stenosed arterial lumen. Balloons and stents may be drug-eluting.
- Preferred for patients with aortoiliac disease and reasonable for femoropopliteal disease
- Current data are insufficient regarding infrapopliteal lesions, but ongoing studies are comparing efficacy between endovascular and surgical intervention.
- Surgical intervention involves using a bypass graft to revascularize the artery distal to the stenosis.

COMPLEMENTARY & ALTERNATIVE MEDICINE

- Chelation therapy and B-complex vitamins are not recommended in patients with PAD.
- Additional studies on *Ginkgo biloba*, L-arginine, propionyl-L-carnitine, omega-3 fatty acids, and vitamin E have been studied, and in general, their efficacy is uncertain.

 ONGOING CARE

FOLLOW-UP RECOMMENDATIONS

- At follow-up, patients should undergo thorough history and physical examinations. They should be asked about their progress with risk-factor modification (i.e., smoking, glucose control, HTN), exercise endurance and program compliance, and effectiveness of pharmacotherapy.
- After endovascular or surgical intervention, patients should receive regular assessment of symptoms via resting and exercise ABIs.

DIET

- A heart-healthy diet is recommended in all patients with PAD or risk factors.
- Balanced diets consisting of vegetables, fruit, nuts, protein, and healthy fats (such as the Mediterranean diet) are likely best.

PROGNOSIS

- Limb ischemia and IC: 15–20% will have worsening claudication, 5–10% will require endovascular or surgical intervention, and 2–5% will undergo amputation (most commonly smokers and diabetics).
- At 5 years, 20% of patients with PAD will experience a nonfatal cardiovascular event, and 15–20% will die, most commonly of cardiovascular disease.

REFERENCES

1. Gerhard-Herman MD, Gornik HL, Barrett C, et al. 2016 AHA/ACC guideline on the management of patients with lower extremity peripheral artery disease: executive summary: a report of the American College of Cardiology/American Heart Association Task Force on Clinical Practice Guidelines. *Circulation*. 2017;135(12):e686–e725.
2. Virani SS, Alonso A, Aparicio HJ, et al. Heart disease and stroke statistics—2021 update: a report From the American Heart Association. *Circulation*. 2021;143(8):e254–e743.
3. Firnhaber JM, Powell CS. Lower extremity peripheral artery disease: diagnosis and treatment [published correction appears in *Am Fam Physician*. 2019;15;100(2):74]. *Am Fam Physician*. 2019;99(6):362–369.
4. Wong PF, Chong LY, Mikhailidis DP, et al. Antiplatelet agents for intermittent claudication. *Cochrane Database Syst Rev*. 2011;(11):CD001272.

CODES

ICD10

- I73.9 Peripheral vascular disease, unspecified
- I70.209 Unsp athscl native arteries of extremities, unsp extremity
- I70.219 Athscl native arteries of extrm w intrmt claud, unsp extrm

CLINICAL PEARLS

- USPSTF (2018): Insufficient evidence to suggest routine screening for PAD with ABI.
- Patients who fail noninvasive therapy with a supervised exercise program and pharmacotherapy should be referred to vascular surgery. Patients with CLI (pain at rest, gangrene, ulceration) should be referred.
- Antiplatelet therapy (aspirin or clopidogrel) and cilostazol for symptomatic relief are at the cornerstone of pharmacotherapy. Additionally, management of HLD and BP control are indicated in all patients. ACE-inhibitors or ARBs should be considered due to associated reduction in cardiovascular ischemic events.

PERITONITIS, ACUTE

Marie L. Borum, MD, EdD, MPH • Junseo Bernard Lee, MD

 BASICS

DESCRIPTION
- Definition: inflammation of the peritoneum
- Classification:
  – Aseptic: chemical irritation or systemic inflammation of peritoneum
  – Bacterial: infection of peritoneal fluid
- Bacterial peritonitis types:
  – Primary/spontaneous bacterial peritonitis (SBP): infection of ascitic fluid in the absence of an intra-abdominal source
  – Secondary bacterial peritonitis: infection of ascitic fluid from a detectable intra-abdominal source
    ○ Secondary bacterial peritonitis can be further classified as either perforation peritonitis or nonperforation peritonitis.
  – Tertiary bacterial peritonitis: >48 hours of infection despite source control
  – Peritoneal dialysis–associated (PD) peritonitis

EPIDEMIOLOGY
Incidence
Annual incidence of SBP is around one-third in hospitalized patients with cirrhosis (1).

Prevalence
- In asymptomatic patients with cirrhosis and ascites, the prevalence of SBP is low in the outpatient setting.
- In patients with cirrhosis and ascites, 5% of peritonitis is secondary.
- Secondary peritonitis is the most common cause of sepsis in surgical ICU patients.

ETIOLOGY AND PATHOPHYSIOLOGY
- Mechanism
  – SBP:
    ○ Bacterial translocation via lymphatic spread through mesenteric lymph nodes
    ○ Often develops in the setting of large-volume ascites in patients with advanced cirrhosis
    ○ Cirrhotic patients have:
      ■ Alterations to gut microbiota with higher prevalence of pathogenic organisms
      ■ Small intestinal bacterial overgrowth (SIBO) and increased intestinal mucosal permeability to bacteria
      ■ Decreased cellular and humoral immunity limiting peritoneal bacterial clearance
  – Secondary:
    ○ Translocation of bacteria from inflamed or perforated intraperitoneal (IP) organs or introduction of bacterial through instrumentation
  – Tertiary: evolves from secondary peritonitis
  – PD peritonitis:
    ○ Contamination with pathogenic skin flora during exchanges or exit-site infection
- Microbiology
  – Most cases of SBP are monomicrobial.
    ○ Most common gram-negative pathogens are *Escherichia coli* and *Klebsiella* species.
    ○ Most common gram-positive pathogens are *Streptococcus* and *Staphylococcus* species.

– Secondary: perforation of a viscus, small bowel strangulation, necrotizing pancreatitis. Organism depends on cause of peritonitis; gram-positive organisms more common with upper GI pathology whereas gram-negative organisms more common with lower GI pathology. Common species include *E. coli*, *Klebsiella*, *Proteus*, *Streptococcus*, *Enterococcus*, *Bacteroides*, and *Clostridium* (1).
  – PD peritonitis is most commonly due to *Staphylococcus epidermidis* and *Staphylococcus aureus* (2).

RISK FACTORS
- SBP: advanced cirrhosis with ascites, malnutrition, variceal hemorrhage, acid-suppressive therapy, and prior SBP (1)
  – Acid suppression (most commonly with PPIs) promotes gut bacterial growth and translocation.
  – 70% of SBP cases are in patients with Child-Pugh class C cirrhosis.
  – Low ascites protein (<1 g/dL) increases risk.
- Secondary:
  – *Helicobacter pylori* or NSAID-induced ulcers, vascular disease causing bowel ischemia, alcohol-related pancreatitis, trauma, or IBD causing bowel perforation
- PD peritonitis:
  – Nonsterile technique
  – Recent instrumentation

GENERAL PREVENTION
- SBP prophylaxis decreases mortality in patients at high risk (e.g., ascitic fluid protein concentration <1 g/dL, esophageal varices, or history of previous SBP).
  – Primary prophylaxis: antibiotics including norfloxacin, ciprofloxacin, trimethoprim-sulfamethoxazole
  – Patients with cirrhotic ascites who have low ascitic fluid protein (<1.5 g/dL), renal impairment (creatinine ≥1.2 mg/dL, BUN ≥25 mg/dL, serum sodium [Na] ≤130 mEq/L) or liver failure (Child-Pugh score ≥9 and serum bilirubin ≥3 mg/dL) should receive SBP prophylaxis (1).
- Limit use of PPI therapy.
- PD peritonitis:
  – Adherence to sterile technique
  – Antibiotic prophylaxis prior to selected procedures

COMMONLY ASSOCIATED CONDITIONS
SBP almost always occurs in the setting of decompensated cirrhosis (3).

 DIAGNOSIS

HISTORY
- SBP: history of cirrhosis and/or ascites, fever, chills, mental status changes, abdominal pain (diffuse, continuous; may be subtle due to presence of ascites), nausea/vomiting, diarrhea, GI bleeding
- Secondary: may be clinically indistinguishable from SBP unless history of perforation, abscess, other intra-abdominal pathology, or recent surgical intervention is present
- Tertiary: persistent signs and symptoms despite initial treatment or history of recurrent peritonitis
- PD peritonitis: presumptive diagnosis in PD patients with cloudy effluent (2)

ALERT
Up to one-third of patients are asymptomatic (3).

PHYSICAL EXAM
- Tachycardia, tachypnea, altered mental status (can be subtle), hypotension, hyperthermia, or hypothermia
- Abdominal pain and distention, ascites, abdominal wall guarding, rebound tenderness, hypoactive/absent bowel sounds, diarrhea, ileus
  – There is no rigidity because ascites separates parietal layer of peritoneum from visceral layer.

DIFFERENTIAL DIAGNOSIS
- Liver disease: hepatitis, decompensated cirrhosis
- Luminal disease: abscess formation, ileus, volvulus, intussusception, mesenteric adenitis, pancreatitis, cholecystitis, malignancy, peritoneal carcinomatosis, IBD
- Extraluminal disease: ruptured ectopic pregnancy, tubo-ovarian abscess, PID, UTI, pyelonephritis
- Systemic disease: tuberculosis, pneumonia, MI, porphyria, SLE

DIAGNOSTIC TESTS & INTERPRETATION

ALERT
Early diagnosis and immediate evaluation reduces mortality.

Initial Tests (lab, imaging)
- CBC: leukocytosis, anemia
  – Thrombocytopenia <100,000/mL predicts SBP (4)[B]
- BMP: metabolic acidosis, azotemia
- LFTs, coagulation panel often abnormal at baseline in patients with cirrhosis
- CRP >60 mg/L + cirrhotic ascites is highly specific for SBP (96.5%) (4)[B].
- Secondary:
  – Abdominal x-rays or CT may show free air or source of infection (abscess, perforation, etc.).

Follow-Up Tests & Special Considerations
- Obtain ascites, blood, and urine cultures before antibiotics are given.
- If culture is monomicrobial but PMN <250, colonization generally resolves if patient asymptomatic but generally progresses to SBP if patient symptomatic (1).
- If culture is polymicrobial but PMN <250, cause is likely traumatic paracentesis (1).
- If culture negative but PMN >250, still likely to be SBP and requires broad-spectrum antibiotics (1)
- Alcoholic hepatitis and SBP can occur concurrently.

Diagnostic Procedures/Other
- Most important is diagnostic paracentesis with ascites fluid analysis: culture, Gram stain, cell count with differential, albumin; for secondary peritonitis, include LDH, total protein, glucose, alkaline phosphatase (ALP), and CEA.
- SBP:
  – PMN >250 cells/mm³ (3)
  – Serum-ascites albumin gradient <1.1 g/dL rules out portal hypertension, making SBP unlikely.
- Secondary peritonitis: PMN >250 cells/mm³ on ascitic fluid analysis with polymicrobial culture and/or two of the following (Runyon criteria): ascitic fluid total protein >1 g/dL, glucose <50 mg/dL, and LDH > upper limit of normal for serum
  – Effluent amylase level may suggest intra-abdominal pathology (2).

- PD peritonitis:
  - Two of: positive effluent culture, consistent clinical features, and peritoneal fluid WBC >100 mm³ with PMN >50% (2)

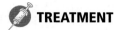 **TREATMENT**

GENERAL MEASURES
- Control ascites with salt restriction, spironolactone ±, furosemide, albumin infusion after large-volume paracentesis, and/or lactulose for encephalopathy.
- Discontinue β-blockers in SBP in patients who are hypotensive and/or have acute kidney injury (AKI).
- Avoid nephrotoxic medications.

MEDICATION
- SBP
  - First line: If low prevalence of multidrug-resistant organisms (MDRO): 3rd-generation cephalosporins, preferably IV cefotaxime
  - In absence of previous quinolone use/prophylaxis, vomiting, shock, hepatic encephalopathy, or serum creatinine >3 mg/dL: can substitute oral fluoroquinolones (must be renally dosed) for cefotaxime (1)
  - Consider broader coverage if high prevalence of MDRO and/or for critically ill patients (1)
- SBP with renal or hepatic impairment (serum creatinine >1 mg/dL, BUN >30 mg/dL, or total bilirubin >5 mg/dL): Add albumin 1.5 g/kg within 6 hours and 1 g/kg on day 3 to prevent progression of AKI (3).
- If hypotension (MAP <65 mm Hg) or AKI, clinicians should hold nonselective β-blockers.
- Reassess patient after 2 days of antibiotic therapy with repeat paracentesis.
  - If <25% decrease in PMN from baseline, indicates lack of response. Consider broadening antibiotic coverage and evaluate for secondary bacterial peritonitis.
- Secondary:
  - Empiric broad-spectrum antibiotic coverage for polymicrobial infection; IV cefotaxime or other 3rd- to 4th-generation cephalosporin plus metronidazole.
- Tertiary:
  - If no unrepaired perforations or leaks, continue with medical management: broad-spectrum antibiotics (guided by susceptibilities), early enteral nutrition to prevent atrophy
  - Consider adding antifungal coverage.
  - Consider removing catheter if recurrent or persistent PD-associated infection (2).
- PD peritonitis:
  - IP route for antibiotics preferred over IV route unless patient is septic.
  - Gram-positive coverage: vancomycin or a 1st-generation cephalosporin (e.g., cefazolin)
  - Gram-negative coverage: 3rd-generation cephalosporin (e.g., ceftazidime, cefepime), an aminoglycoside, or a carbapenem
  - Most patients usually improve within 48 hours of initiation of antibiotic therapy.
    - Clinical improvement, less cloudy efferent, and/or lower cell count in peritoneal fluid all demonstrate infection is resolving.
  - PD does not have to be discontinued (2).
  - Remove catheter if:
    - Fungal or mycobacterial peritonitis
    - Culture-negative peritonitis with persistent symptoms and elevated WBC in peritoneal fluid
    - PD effluent is not clear after a 5-day course of antibiotics (refractory peritonitis).

- Peritonitis recurrence within 4 weeks of completion of antibiotic course
- Laparotomy required
- If catheter removed, can be replaced after 2 weeks if symptoms have resolved (2)

SURGERY/OTHER PROCEDURES
- SBP:
  - Medical management only (high mortality if patient with SBP receives exploratory laparotomy)
- Secondary:
  - Emergent surgical management, including source control with open laparotomy to repair any perforated viscus and eradicate infected material
- Tertiary:
  - If there are no unrepaired perforations or leaks, additional surgery for severe abdominal infection correlates with deterioration and mortality.

ADMISSION, INPATIENT, AND NURSING CONSIDERATIONS
- Acute peritonitis typically warrants hospitalization.
- In patients with cardiogenic or septic shock, use invasive monitoring with goal-directed fluid therapy.
- Patients who present with peritonitis can be severely hypovolemic and volume resuscitation is critical.
- Patients with cirrhosis are often on β-blockers. During an episode of SBP, β-blockers can increase mortality, hepatorenal syndrome, and hospital stay.

 ONGOING CARE

FOLLOW-UP RECOMMENDATIONS
Patient Monitoring
Normalization of vital signs with resolution of leukocytosis is a sign of improvement.
- PMN decrease >25% is expected if repeat paracentesis is performed after 48 hours.

DIET
- NPO, total parental nutrition (TPN) as necessary, especially in secondary peritonitis
- Resume enteral feeding after return of bowel function.
- Sodium restriction can reduce future development of ascites.

PROGNOSIS
- SBP:
  - Mortality is low with prompt diagnosis and treatment.
  - Prognosis improves if antibiotics are started early and prior to onset of shock or renal failure.
  - Renal insufficiency is the strongest negative prognostic indicator (5).
- Secondary:
  - In-hospital mortality is generally higher with secondary peritonitis than those with SBP.
  - Prognosis is worse in perforation peritonitis (vs. nonperforation peritonitis) and mortality of perforation approaches 100% if not treated surgically.
- PD peritonitis
  - 2–6% mortality (highest in fungal, gram-negative, and S. aureus infections) (2)
  - 5–20% transition to hemodialysis

COMPLICATIONS
- Renal and hepatic failure, encephalopathy, coagulopathy, secondary infection, iatrogenic infection, abscess, fistula formation, abdominal compartment syndrome
- Sepsis/septic shock, cardiovascular collapse, adrenal insufficiency, respiratory failure, ARDS

- Complications related to diagnostic paracentesis (e.g., bleeding, infection)

REFERENCES
1. Dever JB, Sheikh MY. Review article: spontaneous bacterial peritonitis—bacteriology, diagnosis, treatment, risk factors and prevention. *Aliment Pharmacol Ther*. 2015;41(11):1116–1131.
2. Li PK, Chow KM, Cho Y, et al. ISPD peritonitis guideline recommendations: 2022 update on prevention and treatment. *Perit Dial Int*. 2022;42(2):110–153.
3. Biggins SW, Angeli P, Garcia-Tsao G, et al. Diagnosis, evaluation, and management of ascites, spontaneous bacterial peritonitis and hepatorenal syndrome: 2021 practice guidance by the American Association for the Study of Liver Diseases. *Hepatology*. 2021;74(2):1014–1048.
4. MacIntosh T. Emergency management of spontaneous bacterial peritonitis—a clinical review. *Cureus*. 2018;10(3):e2253.
5. Tandon P, Garcia-Tsao G. Renal dysfunction is the most important independent predictor of mortality in cirrhotic patients with spontaneous bacterial peritonitis. *Clin Gastroenterol Hepatol*. 2011;9(3):260–265.

ADDITIONAL READING
- Aithal GP, Palaniyappan N, China L, et al. Guidelines on the management of ascites in cirrhosis. *Gut*. 2021;70(1):9–29.
- Mattos AA, Wiltgen D, Jotz RF, et al. Spontaneous bacterial peritonitis and extraperitoneal infections in patients with cirrhosis. *Ann Hepatol*. 2020;19(5):451–457.

 SEE ALSO

Appendicitis, Acute; Cirrhosis of the Liver; Diverticular Disease; Peptic Ulcer Disease

 CODES

ICD10
- K65.0 Generalized (acute) peritonitis
- K65.2 Spontaneous bacterial peritonitis
- K65.8 Other peritonitis

CLINICAL PEARLS
- Maintain a high index of suspicion for SBP in cirrhotic patients with ascites (up to one-third of cases may be asymptomatic) and start empiric antibiotic therapy early.
- SBP is usually monomicrobial. Paracentesis is the gold standard for diagnosis.
- *E. coli* is the most common bacterial isolate from cases of SBP. Third-generation cephalosporins are first-line treatment.
- Ascitic fluid analysis stratifies patients at risk for secondary peritonitis who require additional imaging.
- Renal function is an important prognostic indicator for SBP.

PERTUSSIS

Susan McDiarmid, EdD, MS, PA-C • Michelle E. Duffelmeyer, MD

BASICS

- Highly contagious respiratory illness among close contacts
- Synonyms: whooping cough, "the cough of 100 days"

DESCRIPTION
- Host: humans
- Most common reservoir: adults
- Ages: all
- Distribution: worldwide
- Pattern: endemic or epidemic with outbreaks every 3 to 5 years
- Seasonality: peaks late summer–autumn; can occur year-round
- Transmission: person to person via aerosolized droplets
- Effective vaccine: available
- Immunity: neither 100% nor lifelong immunity with either infection or vaccine
- System(s) affected: respiratory
- Classic clinical manifestations include paroxysmal cough, inspiratory whoop, and posttussive emesis.

EPIDEMIOLOGY
- Caused by *Bordetella pertussis*
- Typical incubation period: 7 to 10 days

Incidence
- United States (2012 most recent peak year): 48,277 cases reported
- Worldwide: 24.1 million cases and about 160,700 deaths per year

ETIOLOGY AND PATHOPHYSIOLOGY
- Toxin mediated
- Infectious process with predilection for ciliated respiratory epithelium
- Common organisms:
  - *B. pertussis*
  - *Bordetella parapertussis*

Genetics
No known genetic predisposition

RISK FACTORS
- Exposure to a confirmed case
- Non- or underimmunized infants and children
- Premature birth
- Chronic lung disease
- Immunodeficiency (e.g., AIDS)
- Obesity and pre-existing asthma
- Age <6 months (accounts for ~90% pediatric pertussis hospitalizations) (1)

GENERAL PREVENTION
- Public health measures
  - Surveillance
  - Outbreak management
  - Care of exposed individuals
- Prevention programs
- Immunizations
  - Primary childhood immunization series against pertussis followed by boosters
  - Maternal immunization during each pregnancy
  - Adults, including health care providers in close contact with infants <1 year of age, should be immunized.

Pediatric Considerations
Strategies to reduce neonatal pertussis:
- Tdap with each pregnancy, ideally between 27 and 36 weeks' gestation
- Cocooning
- Tdap recommended for all persons in close contact with infants <1 year of age

Geriatric Considerations
Older adults are at increased risk for pertussis complications due to (2):
- Age-related changes in immunity
- Comorbid medical conditions

COMMONLY ASSOCIATED CONDITIONS
- Apnea in infants
- Secondary bacterial pneumonia
- Sinusitis
- Seizures
- Encephalopathy
- Urinary incontinence
- Death

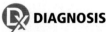 DIAGNOSIS

HISTORY
- Exposure to pertussis
- Insidious onset
- Classic clinical manifestations include paroxysmal cough, inspiratory whoop, and posttussive emesis.
- Incubation period of 7 to 10 days (range: 5 to 21 days)

PHYSICAL EXAM
- Classic pertussis has three phases, which occur over 6 to 10 weeks:
  - Catarrhal phase: rhinorrhea, mild cough, and low-grade fever
  - Paroxysmal phase: Cough occurs in bursts, with increased frequency and intensity, often followed by an inspiratory whoop and/or posttussive vomiting.
  - Convalescent phase: Coughing paroxysms decrease in frequency and intensity.
- Classic presentation is more common in adults and unvaccinated children.

DIFFERENTIAL DIAGNOSIS
Sporadic, prolonged cough can also be caused by:
- *B. parapertussis*
- *Mycoplasma pneumoniae*
- *Chlamydia trachomatis*
- *Chlamydia pneumoniae*
- *Bordetella bronchiseptica*
- *Bordetella holmesii*
- Respiratory syncytial virus
- Adenovirus

DIAGNOSTIC TESTS & INTERPRETATION
Initial Tests (lab, imaging)
- Nasopharyngeal culture (gold standard): best results within 2 weeks of cough onset
- False results can occur in:
  - Previously immunized individuals
  - After initiation of appropriate antibiotic
  - After 2 weeks from cough onset
  - With incorrect collection or handling
- Polymerase chain reaction (PCR) assays: rapid turnaround time; good within first 3 weeks
- Serology:
  - Commercially available assay
  - Not FDA-approved for diagnosis

Follow-Up Tests & Special Considerations
- Evaluation and follow-up for associated conditions and complications
- Chest radiograph (two views) to evaluate for the presence of pneumonia
- EEG/neuroimaging may be considered in infant with seizure or apparent life-threatening events (ALTEs).
- Infants <1 month of age who are treated with macrolides should be monitored for the possible development of hypertrophic pyloric stenosis.

TREATMENT

GENERAL MEASURES
- Hospitalization with continuous cardiopulmonary monitoring is recommended for neonates with pertussis.
- Supplemental oxygen and/or mechanical ventilatory support may be needed.

MEDICATION

- Start empiric antibiotic therapy once diagnostic testing is performed in cases with strong clinical suspicion or in those at high risk for complications.
- Antibiotic therapy after cough is established may help to limit spread but is not expected to change clinical symptoms.
- Preferred antibiotics:
  - For patients >6 months:
    ○ Azithromycin, clarithromycin, or erythromycin
  - For infants <1 month of age, azithromycin is preferred but with caution

First Line
Azithromycin is the first line for treatment and for postexposure prophylaxis (5-day course).

ALERT
- Infantile hypertrophic pyloric stenosis has been associated with the use of macrolides in infants <1 month of age.
- Consultation and monitoring are recommended.

ALERT
- *Fatal cardiac dysrhythmias* have been reported with azithromycin.
- Caution is recommended in individuals with prolonged QT and proarrhythmic conditions.

Second Line
Trimethoprim/sulfamethoxazole (TMX/SMX) (for persons >2 months of age) if:
- Macrolide intolerance
- Macrolide resistance

ALERT
- TMP/SMX is *contraindicated* in infants <2 months of age.
- Clarithromycin is not recommended in infants <1 month of age.

ISSUES FOR REFERRAL
Evaluation and treatment of infants <6 months of age, especially those born prematurely, who are unimmunized, and those who require hospitalization

ADDITIONAL THERAPIES
Symptomatic treatment of the cough in pertussis (e.g., corticosteroids, β_2-adrenergic agonists) has not shown consistent benefit (3).

ADMISSION, INPATIENT, AND NURSING CONSIDERATIONS

- In infants, considerations for hospitalization include respiratory distress, evidence of pneumonia, inability to feed, cyanosis, apnea, seizures, and age <4 months.
- Small, frequent meals may be necessary to ensure adequate nutrition.
- IV fluids indicated for dehydration and when oral fluids are either contraindicated or poorly tolerated
- In addition to standard precautions, hospitalized patients should be isolated with respiratory precautions for 5 days after the initiation of effective antibiotic treatment and for 3 weeks after the onset of paroxysms in older patients if antibiotics are not used.
- Gentle suctioning of nasal secretions
- Avoid stimuli that trigger paroxysms.
- Respiratory monitoring, including pulse oximetry
- Educate each family about the importance of immunization.
- Discuss chemoprophylaxis with each family.

 ONGOING CARE

FOLLOW-UP RECOMMENDATIONS
- Monitor infants who received EES or azithromycin for hypotrophic pyloric stenosis.
- Neurologic and/or pulmonary follow-up as necessary

Patient Monitoring
ICU care may be necessary for severely ill or compromised patients.

DIET
IV fluids/nutrition may be required to treat dehydration or to supplement poor oral intake.

PATIENT EDUCATION
- American Academy of Pediatrics: https://www.aap.org/
- Centers for Disease Control and Prevention: https://www.cdc.gov/pertussis/materials/index.html

PROGNOSIS
- Complete recovery in most cases
- Most severe morbidity and highest mortality in infants <6 months of age
- Worldwide overall mortality estimated at 160,799 deaths/year

COMPLICATIONS
- Highest and most severe in infants; may include apnea, cyanosis, and sudden death
- In children: may include conjunctival hemorrhage, inguinal hernia, pneumonia, and seizures
- More frequent in adults than adolescents: may include sinusitis, otitis media, pneumonia, weight loss, fainting, rib fracture, urinary incontinence, seizures, and encephalopathy

REFERENCES

1. Lopez MA, Cruz AT, Kowalkowski MA, et al. Trends in hospitalizations and resource utilization for pediatric pertussis. *Hosp Pediatr*. 2014;4(5):269–275.
2. Burke M, Rowe T. Vaccinations in older adults. *Clin Geriatr Med*. 2018;34(1):131–143.
3. Polinori I, Esposito S. Clinical findings and management of pertussis. *Adv Exp Med Biol*. 2019;1183:151–160.

ADDITIONAL READING

American Academy of Pediatrics. Pertussis (whooping cough). In: Kimberlin DW, Barnett ED, Lynfield R, Sawyer MH, eds. *Red Book: 2021–2024 Report of the Committee on Infectious Diseases*. 32nd ed. Itasca, IL: American Academy of Pediatrics; 2021:578–589.

 CODES

ICD10
- A37.10 Whooping cough due to Bordetella parapertussis without pneumonia
- A37 Whooping cough
- A37.91 Whooping cough, unspecified species with pneumonia

CLINICAL PEARLS

- Classic clinical manifestations include paroxysmal cough, inspiratory whoop, and posttussive emesis.
- Hospitalizations for pertussis is highest in infants <4 months of age.
  - Maternal Tdap is effective in protecting young infants against pertussis, especially during the first 2 months of life.
- Neither immunization nor active infection confers lifelong immunity.

PHARYNGITIS

Munima Nasir, MD • Alyssa Anderson, MD

BASICS

DESCRIPTION
- Synonym(s): sore throat; tonsillitis; "strep throat"
- Acute or chronic inflammation of the pharyngeal mucosa and underlying structures of the throat
- Group A *Streptococcus* (GAS) pharyngitis is notable for preventable suppurative (e.g., retropharyngeal or peritonsillar abscess) and nonsuppurative (e.g., rheumatic sequelae) complications.

EPIDEMIOLOGY
- ~15 million cases are diagnosed yearly.
- Accounts for 1–2% of all outpatient visits and 6% of all pediatric visits to primary care physicians
- Most commonly viral (40–60% of cases)
- GAS is the most common bacterial cause of acute pharyngitis, accounting for 15–30% of pediatric cases (with peak incidence in 5- to 11-year-olds) and 5–15% of adult cases. The incubation period ranges from 24 to 72 hours.
- Less common causes of pharyngitis includes *Fusobacterium necrophorum*, nongroup A (group C or G) *Streptococcus*, and, if sexually active, *Neisseria gonorrhoeae*
- Rheumatic fever is a serious sequelae but is rare in the United States (<1 case per 100,000). Early antibiotic use has diminished occurrence.
- 3,000 to 4,000 patients with group A β-hemolytic streptococcal infection must be treated to prevent one case of acute rheumatic fever.

Pediatric Considerations
The highest incidence of rheumatic fever is in children aged 5 to 18 years as a rare sequela of streptococcal pharyngitis.

ETIOLOGY AND PATHOPHYSIOLOGY
- Acute, viral (associated with lower grade fever)
  - Rhinovirus; adenovirus (associated with conjunctivitis); parainfluenza virus; coxsackievirus (hand-foot-and-mouth disease); coronavirus; echovirus
  - Herpes simplex virus (vesicular lesions); Epstein-Barr virus (EBV; mononucleosis); cytomegalovirus (CMV)
  - HIV
- Acute, bacterial (associated with higher fevers)
  - Group A β-hemolytic streptococcus
  - *N. gonorrhoeae*; *Corynebacterium diphtheriae* (diphtheria); *Haemophilus influenzae*
  - *Moraxella catarrhalis*; *Chlamydia pneumonia*
  - *F. necrophorum* (20% young adult cases); group C or G *Streptococcus*
  - *Arcanobacterium haemolyticum*; *Mycoplasma pneumoniae*; *Francisella tularensis* (tularemia)
- Acute, noninfectious
  - Various caustic, mechanical, or trauma-related (including endotracheal intubation)
- Chronic, more likely noninfectious
  - Chemical irritation (GERD)
  - Smoking
  - Neoplasms
  - Vasculitis
  - Radiation changes

Genetics
Patients with a family history of rheumatic fever have a higher risk of rheumatic sequelae following an untreated group A β-hemolytic streptococcal infection.

RISK FACTORS
- Epidemics of group A β-hemolytic streptococcal disease
- Cold and flu season (late fall through early spring)
- Age (rheumatic fever possible, especially in children/adolescents aged 5 to 15 years)
- Close contact with infected individuals (home, daycare, military barracks)
- Immunosuppression
- Smoking/secondhand smoke exposure
- Acid reflux
- Oral sex
- Diabetes mellitus
- Recent illness (secondary postviral bacterial infection)
- Chronic colonization of bacteria in tonsils/adenoids

GENERAL PREVENTION
- Avoid close contact with infectious patients.
- Wash hands frequently.
- Avoid firsthand or secondhand smoke.
- Manage preventable causes (e.g., GERD).

DIAGNOSIS

HISTORY
- Sore throat
- Difficulty swallowing (dysphagia) or pain on swallowing (odynophagia)
- Cough (uncommon in GAS pharyngitis)
- Hoarseness; "hot potato" voice
- Fever
- Anorexia
- Chills
- Malaise; fatigue
- Headache
- Dysuria and arthralgias (suggest gonococcal etiology)
- Sick contacts with similar symptoms or confirmed diagnosis

PHYSICAL EXAM
- Enlarged tonsils with or without exudate
- Pharyngeal erythema; palatal petechiae
- Unilateral tonsillar swelling or uvular deviation (concern for peritonsillar abscess)
- Trismus; stridor; drooling (concern for peritonsillar or retropharyngeal abscess)
- Cervical adenopathy (anterior suggestive of GAS, posterior most commonly associated with infectious mononucleosis)
- Fever (higher in bacterial infections)
- Pharyngeal ulcers (CMV, HIV, Crohn disease, other autoimmune vasculitides)
- Scarlet fever rash: punctate erythematous macules with reddened flexor creases and circumoral pallor suggests streptococcal pharyngitis
- Tonsillar/soft palate petechiae with hepatosplenomegaly suggest infectious mononucleosis (EBV/CMV).
- Gray oral pseudomembrane suggests diphtheria and occasionally infectious mononucleosis (EBV/CMV).
- Characteristic erythematous-based clear vesicles suggest HSV or coxsackie A virus infection (herpangina).
- Conjunctivitis suggests adenovirus.

DIFFERENTIAL DIAGNOSIS
- Viral infection, including acute HIV, EBV, CMV infections
- Streptococcal infection
- Allergic rhinitis/postnasal drip
- GERD
- Malignancy (lymphoma or squamous cell carcinoma)
- Irritants/chemicals (detergent/caustic ingestion)
- Atypical bacterial (e.g., gonococcal, chlamydial, syphilis, pertussis, diphtheria)
- Oral candidiasis (patients typically complain mostly of dysphagia)
- Thyroiditis (can be painful or painless, possibly associated with hyperthyroid syndrome)
- Epiglottitis (associated with stridor, drooling, and progressive respiratory distress)

DIAGNOSTIC TESTS & INTERPRETATION
- Prediction rules determine the need for further testing (see below).
- Additional testing generally not needed if viral-like clinical features (e.g., cough, rhinorrhea, hoarseness, oral ulcers, diarrhea, conjunctivitis, rash) (1)[A]
- Avoid testing for GAS pharyngitis in children aged <3 years as acute rheumatic flare is rare, unless there is a close sick contact who is GAS-positive (1)[B].
- Modified Centor clinical prediction rule for group A streptococcal infection:
  - +1 point: tonsillar exudates
  - +1 point: tender anterior chain cervical adenopathy
  - +1 point: absence of cough
  - +1 point: fever by history
  - +1 point: age <15 years
  - 0 point: age 15 to 45 years
  - −1 point: age >45 years
- Scoring:
  - If 4 points, positive predictive value of ~80%; treat empirically.
  - If 2 to 3 points, positive predictive value of ~50%, rapid strep antigen; treat if GAS-positive.
  - If 0 or 1 point, positive predictive value <20%; do not test; treat symptomatically with follow-up as needed.

Initial Tests (lab, imaging)
- Testing, if performed, is usually for GAS. Options include the following:
  - Rapid antigen streptococcus test (RAST); quick adjunct to throat culture with 96% specificity and 86% sensitivity (although sensitivity varies by modality kit) (2)[A]
  - Blood agar throat culture from swab; gold standard—90–95% sensitivity (2)[A]
    - Backup throat cultures are not needed for adults with negative RAST. They are recommended for children with negative RAST due to the higher likelihood of complications but can be omitted if a highly sensitive immunoassay or molecular test was used.
  - Antistreptolysin O titer test is not recommended for routine diagnosis.
- Special tests if history suggests a different diagnosis
  - NAAT for *N. gonorrhoeae*
  - Viral cultures for HSV
  - Monospot for EBV
  - IgM serology for CMV
  - HIV viral load

Follow-Up Tests & Special Considerations

Recurrent GAS infection may indicate β-lactamase production by host and may require antibiotic with anti-beta-lactamase activity.

Test Interpretation

Bacitracin disk sensitivity of hemolytic colonies suggests group A β-hemolytic streptococcus.

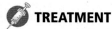 TREATMENT

Treatment is largely for symptomatic relief, unless bacterial infection is confirmed or highly suspected.

GENERAL MEASURES

Conservative therapy is recommended for most cases (unless bacterial etiology is suspected):

- Salt water gargles
- Acetaminophen 10 to 15 mg/kg/dose q4h PRN pain or fever (pediatric); in adults, do not exceed >3 g/day.
- Nonsteroidal anti-inflammatory drugs (NSAIDs) for pain or fever (more effective than acetaminophen for GAS pharyngitis)
- Anesthetic lozenges
- Cool-mist humidifier
- Hydration (PO or IV if PO is not tolerated)
- Viscous lidocaine (2%) 5 to 10 mL PO q4h swish/spit (severe pain)

Pediatric Treatment Considerations

- Opioids are not recommended due to black box warnings.
- Lower threshold to start antibiotics due to higher risk of rheumatic fever.
- Avoid aspirin for symptom relief in pediatric patients due to risk of Reye syndrome.

MEDICATION

- Antibiotics (particularly penicillin) are used primarily to prevent complications.
  - 60–70% primary care visits by children with pharyngitis result in antibiotic prescriptions (3). Empiric therapy results in antibiotic overuse.
  - Treatment duration is generally 10 days (1)[A].
  - Antibiotics do not reduce the risk of poststreptococcal glomerulonephritis.
  - Antibiotics shorten the duration of symptoms by approximately 16 hours.
  - Antibiotics may prevent pharyngitis/fever by day 3 (NNT 4 if GAS-positive, 6.5 if GAS-negative, 14.4 if untested).
- Ulcers related to autoimmune diseases usually require systemic or intralesional injectable steroids.
- HIV-related ulcers are due to decreasing counts of CD4 and respond when patients' CD4 titers increase.
- Corticosteroids, when used concomitantly with antibiotics, may provide a small reduction in the duration of symptoms (24 hours). Routine use is not currently recommended (1)[B],(2)[B].

First Line

Recommended first-line therapies (1)[A]:

- Penicillin V: children (<27 kg): 250 mg PO TID (BID dosing sufficient if good compliance); adolescents and adults (>27 kg): 250 mg PO QID or 500 mg PO BID
- Penicillin G benzathine: children <60 lb (<27 kg): 600,000 units intramuscularly 1 dose; children ≥60 lb (≥27 kg) and adults: 1.2 million units intramuscularly 1 dose
- Amoxicillin: 50 mg/kg PO once daily (max of 1,000 mg per dose) or 25 mg/kg PO BID (max of 500 mg per dose)

ALERT
Use with caution if diagnosis is unclear because using amoxicillin with EBV infection may induce rash.

Second Line

- If type IV hypersensitivity but no history of anaphylactic penicillin allergy:
  - Cephalexin 20 mg/kg PO BID or (children) 25 to 50 mg/kg/day divided BID or (adults) 1,000 mg PO QID (max of 4 g/day)
  - Cefadroxil 30 mg/kg PO once daily (max of 1 g/day)
- If history of anaphylactic penicillin allergy (type I hypersensitivity):
  - Azithromycin 12 mg/kg PO once daily for 5 days (max of 500 mg per dose)
  - Clarithromycin 7.5 mg/kg PO BID (max of 250 mg per dose) or (adults) 250 to 500 mg PO BID
  - Clindamycin 7 mg/kg PO TID (max of 300 mg per dose) or (children) 10 to 30 mg/kg/day PO divided TID–QID or (adults) 150 to 450 mg PO TID–QID
- Penicillin is most commonly used to prevent rheumatic sequelae; cephalosporins have a lower rate of antimicrobial failure for streptococcal pharyngitis.
- Newer macrolides are effective against streptococcal pharyngitis; they are also more expensive and unproven at preventing rheumatic complications.
- Macrolide-resistant strains of GAS are currently <10% in the United States but more prevalent worldwide.
- For children with lab confirmed recurrence of GAS pharyngitis, you can treat with the same agent or an alternative agent such as a cephalosporin, amoxicillin-clavulanic acid, or a macrolide.
- Repeatedly positive GAS tests may represent a chronic carrier status of GAS. Antibiotics to eradicate GAS carriage are not routinely recommended as risk of complications and transmission to others is low.

ISSUES FOR REFERRAL

- Document each GAS-confirmed episode to support the need for future tonsillectomy and adenoidectomy.
- Tonsillectomy is recommended for patients who have had seven or more throat infections (viral or bacterial) in 1 year, five or more infections per year for the past 2 years, or three or more infections per year for the past 3 years. Tonsillectomy is also recommended in patients who are difficult to treat medically, including those who are allergic to multiple antibiotics or with history of peritonsillar abscess.

 ONGOING CARE

FOLLOW-UP RECOMMENDATIONS

- Complete the full course of antibiotic therapy, regardless of symptom response.
- Patients are generally noninfectious after 24 hours of antibiotics.
- Follow-up culture for GAS is not recommended (1)[A].

DIET

As tolerated; encourage the consumption of fluids.

PROGNOSIS

- Streptococcal pharyngitis runs a 5- to 7-day course with peak fever at 2 to 3 days.
- Symptoms will resolve spontaneously without treatment, but rheumatic complications are still possible.

COMPLICATIONS

- Rheumatic fever (e.g., carditis, valve disease, arthritis)
- Poststreptococcal glomerulonephritis
- Peritonsillar abscess (a.k.a. quinsy tonsillitis): considered a clinical diagnosis and does not warrant ultrasound/computed tomography; will generally require percutaneous/transoral drainage; surgery may also involve a quinsy (acute) tonsillectomy. Most sources recommend resolution of the acute infection before surgery.
- Acute airway compromise (rare) can typically be bypassed with nasal trumpets. Consult anesthesiologist/otolaryngologist.
- Repeated episodes of GAS pharyngitis may represent recurrent viral infections in a chronic pharyngeal GAS carrier (1)[B]. IDSA recommends against repeated diagnostic efforts/antibiotic therapy in a known chronic pharyngeal GAS carrier, as they are seldom contagious or at risk for serious complications.

REFERENCES

1. Shulman ST, Bisno AL, Clegg HW, et al. Clinical practice guideline for the diagnosis and management of group A streptococcal pharyngitis: 2012 update by the Infectious Diseases Society of America. *Clin Infect Dis*. 2012;55(10):1279–1282.
2. Sauve L, Forrester AM, Top KA. Group A streptococcal pharyngitis: a practical guide to diagnosis and treatment. *Paediatr Child Health*. 2021;26(5):319–320.
3. Robinson JL. Paediatrics: how to manage pharyngitis in an era of increasing antimicrobial resistance. *Drugs Context*. 2021;10:2020-11-6.

ADDITIONAL READING

Supper I, Gratadour J, François M, et al. A critical appraisal of acute sore throat guidelines using the AGREE II instrument: a scoping review. *Fam Pract*. 2023;cmad060.

 SEE ALSO

- Herpes Simplex; Infectious Mononucleosis, Epstein-Barr Virus Infections; Rheumatic Fever
- Algorithm: Pharyngitis

CODES

ICD10

- J31.1 Chronic nasopharyngitis
- A54.5 Gonococcal pharyngitis
- B08.5 Enteroviral vesicular pharyngitis

CLINICAL PEARLS

- Most cases of pharyngitis are viral and do not require antibiotics.
- The risk associated with undiagnosed and untreated group A streptococcal infection is for rheumatic sequelae—a rare complication.
- The use of the Modified Centor Score helps to guide testing and treatment.
- Penicillin is the preferred first-line therapy for group A streptococcal infection.

PILONIDAL DISEASE
Tam T. Nguyen, MD

 BASICS

DESCRIPTION
- Pilonidal disease results from an abscess, or sinus tract, in the upper part of the natal (gluteal) cleft.
- Synonym(s): jeep disease

EPIDEMIOLOGY
Incidence
- 16 to 26/100,000 per year
- Predominant sex: male > female (3 to 4:1)
- Predominant age: 2nd to 3rd decade, rare in age >45 years
- Ethnic consideration: whites > blacks > Asians

Prevalence
Surgical procedures show male:female ratio of 4:1, yet incidence data are 10:1.

ETIOLOGY AND PATHOPHYSIOLOGY
Pilonidal means "nest of hair"; hair in the natal cleft allows hair to be drawn into the deeper tissues via negative pressure caused by movement of the buttocks (50%); follicular occlusion from stretching and blocking of pores with debris (50%) creating a pilonidal cyst
- Inflammation of SC gluteal tissues with secondary infection and sinus tract formation
- Polymicrobial, likely from enteric pathogens given proximity to anorectal contamination

Genetics
- Congenital dimple in the natal cleft/spina bifida occulta
- Follicular-occluding tetrad: acne conglobata, dissecting cellulitis, hidradenitis suppurativa, pilonidal

RISK FACTORS
- Sedentary/prolonged sitting
- Excessive body hair
- Obesity/increased sacrococcygeal fold thickness
- Congenital natal dimple
- Trauma to coccyx

GENERAL PREVENTION
- Weight loss
- Trim hair in/around gluteal cleft weekly.
- Hygiene
- Ingrown hair prevention/follicle unblocking

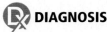 **DIAGNOSIS**

HISTORY
Three distinct clinical presentations
- Asymptomatic: painless cyst or sinus at the top of the gluteal cleft; fever is rare.
- Acute abscess: severe pain, swelling, and/or discharge from the top of the gluteal cleft that may or may not have drained spontaneously
- Chronic abscess: persistent drainage from a sinus tract at the top of the gluteal cleft

PHYSICAL EXAM
- Common: inflamed cystic mass at the top of the gluteal cleft with limited surrounding erythema ± drainage or a sinus tract
- Inflamed sinus accompanied with one or more pits with or without hair debris
- Less common: significant cellulitis of the surrounding tissues near the gluteal cleft

DIFFERENTIAL DIAGNOSIS
- Furunculosis or folliculitis
- Hidradenitis suppurativa
- Anal fistula
- Perirectal abscess
- Crohn disease

DIAGNOSTIC TESTS & INTERPRETATION
Generally, no tests are needed since it can be diagnosed clinically.

Initial Tests (lab, imaging)
- Consider CBC and wound culture but generally not necessary for less severe infections.
- Ultrasound or MRI might be considered to differentiate between perirectal abscess and pilonidal disease.

Follow-Up Tests & Special Considerations
None

Diagnostic Procedures/Other
Wound culture if infection is suspected

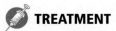 **TREATMENT**

GENERAL MEASURES
- Shave hair area; remove hair from crypts weekly.
- Asymptomatic disease does not need surgical treatment.

MEDICATION
- Antibiotics are not indicated unless there is a significant cellulitis (1).
- If antibiotics are needed, a culture to direct therapy might be useful.
- Cefazolin plus metronidazole or amoxicillin-clavulanate are often used empirically if cellulitis is suspected.

ISSUES FOR REFERRAL
- Patients who cannot comply with frequent dressing changes required after incision and drainage (I&D)
- Patients who have recurrence after I&D
- Patients who have complex disease with multiple sinus tracts

ADDITIONAL THERAPIES

- I&D with only enough packing to allow the cyst to drain; overpacking is not indicated.
- Antibiotics only if significant cellulitis and abscess; temporizing, not curative
- Negative pressure wound therapy
- Laser epilation of hair in the gluteal fold (2)[B]
- Phenol infusion treatment can be used, especially for recurring disease.

SURGERY/OTHER PROCEDURES

- Several surgical techniques have proposed with limited data on superiority of one over another.
- Six levels of care based on severity or recurrence of disease; recent innovations in technique are aimed at expediting healing and minimizing recurrence.
  - I&D, remove hair, curette granulation tissue (3)[A]
  - Excision of midline "pits" allows drainage of lateral sinus tracts (pit picking).
  - Pilonidal cystotomy: Insert probe into sinus tract, excise overlying skin, and close wound (4)[B].
  - Marsupialization: Excise overlying skin and roof of cyst, and suture skin edges to cyst floor (3),(5)[B].
  - Excision: use of flap closure; no clear benefit for open healing over surgical closure
  - Off-midline surgical excision (cleft lift or modified Karydakis procedure): A systematic review showed a clear benefit in favor of off-midline rather than midline wound closure. When closure of pilonidal sinuses is the desired surgical option, off-midline closure should be the standard management (3)[A].
  - Endoscopic pilonidal sinus treatment (EPSiT): minimally invasive procedure (6)
- Endoscopic treatment such as EPSiT (endoscopic pilonidal sinus surgery)
- Fibrin glue in conjunction with some type of minimally excision

ADMISSION, INPATIENT, AND NURSING CONSIDERATIONS

- Severe cellulitis
- Large area excision

 ONGOING CARE

FOLLOW-UP RECOMMENDATIONS

- Frequent dressing changes are required after I&D.
- Follow-up wound checks to assess for recurrence

Patient Monitoring

Monitor for fever; more extensive cellulitis

PATIENT EDUCATION

- Wash area briskly with washcloth daily.
- Shave the area weekly.
- Remove any embedded hair from the crypt.
- Avoid prolonged sitting.

PROGNOSIS

- Simple I&D has a 55% failure rate; median time to healing is 5 weeks.
- More extensive surgical excisions involve hospital stays and longer time to heal.

COMPLICATIONS

Malignant degeneration is a rare complication of untreated chronic pilonidal disease.

REFERENCES

1. Mavros MN, Mitsikostas PK, Alexiou VG, et al. Antimicrobials as an adjunct to pilonidal disease surgery: a systematic review of the literature. *Eur J Clin Microbiol Infect Dis*. 2013;32(7):851–858.
2. Loganathan A, Arsalani Zadeh R, Hartley J. Pilonidal disease: time to reevaluate a common pain in the rear! *Dis Colon Rectum*. 2012;55(4):491–493.
3. Humphries AE, Duncan JE. Evaluation and management of pilonidal disease. *Surg Clin North Am*. 2010;90(1):113–124.
4. da Silva JH. Pilonidal cyst: cause and treatment. *Dis Colon Rectum*. 2000;43(8):1146–1156.
5. Aydede H, Erhan Y, Sakarya A, et al. Comparison of three methods in surgical treatment of pilonidal disease. *ANZ J Surg*. 2001;71(6):362–364.
6. Meinero P, Stazi A, Carbone A, et al. Endoscopic pilonidal sinus treatment: a prospective multicentre trial. *Colorectal Dis*. 2016;18(5):O164–O170.

 CODES

ICD10

- L05.91 Pilonidal cyst without abscess
- L05.92 Pilonidal sinus without abscess
- L05.01 Pilonidal cyst with abscess

CLINICAL PEARLS

- Avoid prolonged sitting.
- Lose weight.
- Trim hair in gluteal cleft weekly.
- Refer recurring infections for more definitive surgical management.

PINWORMS

Jonathan Edward MacClements, MD, FAAFP

BASICS

DESCRIPTION
- Intestinal infection with *Enterobius vermicularis*
  - Characterized by perineal and perianal itching
  - Usually worse at night
- System(s) affected: gastrointestinal; skin/exocrine
- Synonym(s): enterobiasis

EPIDEMIOLOGY
Predominant age: 5 to 14 years

Prevalence
- Most common helminthic infection in the United States
  - 20 to 42 million people harbor the parasite.
- ~30% of children are infected worldwide.

Pediatric Considerations
More common in children, who are more likely to become reinfected

ETIOLOGY AND PATHOPHYSIOLOGY
- Small white worms (2 to 13 mm) inhabit the cecum, appendix, and adjacent portions of the ascending colon following ingestion; associated with multiple case reports of appendicitis
- Female worms migrate to the perineal areas at night to deposit eggs; this causes local irritation and itching.
- Scratching leads to autoingestion of the eggs and continuation of pinworm's life cycle within the host. Eggs incubate 1 to 2 months in the host small intestine. When mature, female pinworms migrate to the colon where they lay eggs around the anus at night, and the lifecycle continues.
- Infestation by the intestinal nematode *E. vermicularis* (1)

RISK FACTORS
- Institutionalization (prevalence >50%)
- Crowded living conditions
- Poor hygiene
- Warm climate
- Handling of infected children's clothing or bedding

GENERAL PREVENTION
- Hand hygiene, especially after bowel movements
- Clip and maintain short fingernails.
- Wash anus and genitals at least once a day, preferably during shower.
- Avoid scratching anus and putting fingers near nose (pinworm eggs can also be inhaled) or mouth.

COMMONLY ASSOCIATED CONDITIONS
- Pruritus ani
- Appendicitis

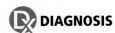

DIAGNOSIS

HISTORY
Many patients are asymptomatic. Common symptoms include the following:
- Perianal or perineal itching
- Vulvovaginitis
- Dysuria
- Abdominal pain (rare)
- Insomnia (typically due to pruritus)

PHYSICAL EXAM
Perineal and perianal exam; particularly in early morning to look for evidence of migrating worms

DIFFERENTIAL DIAGNOSIS
- Idiopathic pruritus ani
- Atopic dermatitis, contact dermatitis
- Psoriasis; lichen planus
- Human papillomavirus (HPV)
- Herpes simplex virus (HSV)
- Fungal infections; erythrasma
- Scabies
- Vaginitis; hemorrhoids
- Chron disease; ulcerative colitis

DIAGNOSTIC TESTS & INTERPRETATION
- Adhesive tape test
  - Place cellophane tape on the perianal skin in the early morning before bathing and affix to a microscope slide to look for pinworm eggs.
  - 90% sensitivity if performed on three consecutive mornings
  - Alternatively, use anal swabs or a pinworm paddle coated with adhesive material.
  - Scrapings from under fingernails of affected individuals can reveal pinworm eggs.
- Digital rectal exam with saline slide preparation of stool on gloved finger
- Stool samples are not helpful.
- *Routine stool examination for ova and parasites is positive in only 10–15% of infected patients.*

Initial Tests (lab, imaging)
Serologic tests are currently not available for diagnosing pinworm infections.

Test Interpretation
Identification of ova on low-power microscopy or direct visualization of the female worm (10-mm long); ova are asymmetric, flat on one side, and measure $56 \times 27 \ \mu m$.

TREATMENT

MEDICATION

First Line

- Treatment options include the following:
  - Albendazole (Albenza): 400 mg PO as a single dose in adults and children >20 kg; may repeat in 2 weeks; 200 mg PO as a single dose repeated in 2 weeks in children ≤20 kg (1)[A]
  - Mebendazole (Emverm, Vermox): chewable 100-mg tablet as a single dose in adults and children >2 years of age; may repeat in 2 to 3 weeks; use with caution in children <2 years of age (1)[A].
  - Pyrantel pamoate (Pin-X, Reese Pinworm Medicine): oral liquid or tablet 11 mg/kg as a single dose in adults and children >2 years of age; maximum dose 1 g. Use with caution in children <2 years of age (1)[A].
- Repeat treatment after 2 weeks is often recommended due to the high frequency of reinfection. Refractory cases may (rarely) require retreatment every 2 weeks for 4 to 6 cycles.
- All symptomatic family members should be treated.

Pregnancy Considerations

Avoid drug therapy in pregnancy as all three drugs are FDA Pregnancy Category C. Treat after delivery but may consider treating in 3rd trimester if infection is compromising the pregnancy. Breastfeeding is allowed during mebendazole therapy (1)[A].

ONGOING CARE

FOLLOW-UP RECOMMENDATIONS

Unnecessary unless symptoms recur after initial therapy

PATIENT EDUCATION

- Take medicine with food.
- Practice good hygiene: handwashing and perianal hygiene; particularly after bowel movements

- Encourage frequent and careful handwashing.
- Clip fingernails.
- Wash clothing and bedding after diagnosis to prevent reinfection. Do not shake linen and clothing before laundering because this may spread the eggs.
- Do not share washcloths.
- Do not allow children to cobathe during treatment and for 2 weeks after treatment; showering is preferred.

PROGNOSIS

- Asymptomatic carriers are common.
- Drug therapy is 90% curative.
- Reinfection is common, especially among children.

COMPLICATIONS

- Perianal scratching may lead to bacterial superinfection.
- Females: vulvovaginitis, urethritis, endometritis, and salpingitis (2)
- UTIs
- Appendicitis
- Rarely: ectopic disease with granulomas of the pelvis, genitourinary tract, and appendix; colonic intussusception (3)

REFERENCES

1. The Medical Letter. *Enterobius vermicularis* (pinworm) infection. In: Drugs for Parasitic Infection. *Treat Guidel Med Lett*. 2013;11(143):e7.
2. Kang W-H, Jee S-C. *Enterobius vermicularis* (pinworm) infection. *N Engl J Med*. 2019;381:e1.
3. Sousa J, Hawkins R, Shenoy A, et al. Enterobius vermicularis-associated appendicitis: a 22-year case series and comprehensive review of the literature. *J Pediatr Surg*. 2022;57(8):1494–1498.

ADDITIONAL READING

Centers for Disease Control and Prevention. Parasites—enterobiasis (also known as pinworm infection). https://www.cdc.gov/parasites/pinworm/health_professionals/index.html. Updated August 28, 2019. Accessed June 26, 2023.

 SEE ALSO

Pruritus Ani

 CODES

ICD10

B80 Enterobiasis

CLINICAL PEARLS

- Nocturnal or early morning perianal itch with restless sleep or insomnia (particularly in children) is the hallmark of symptomatic pinworm infection.
- Treatment includes of mebendazole, albendazole, or pyrantel pamoate.
- Treat close contacts.
- Retreatment after 2 weeks is generally recommended.

PITUITARY ADENOMA

Anup Sabharwal, MD, MBA, FACE, FASPC, FNLA

 BASICS

DESCRIPTION
Typically benign, slow-growing tumors that arise from cells in the pituitary gland
- Presenting symptoms include neurologic deficits, visual changes including diplopia, and headaches.
- Subtypes (hormonal): prolactinoma (PRL) 25–40%, nonfunctioning pituitary adenomas 30%, somatotroph adenoma (growth hormone [GH]) 15–20%, corticotroph adenoma (adrenocorticotropic hormone [ACTH]) 5–10%, thyrotroph adenoma (thyroid-stimulating hormone [TSH]) <1%, gonadotropinoma (luteinizing hormone/follicle-stimulating hormone [LH/FSH]), mixed (1)[A]
- Defined as microadenoma <10 mm and macroadenoma ≥10 mm
- May secrete hormones and/or cause mass effects or visual changes

EPIDEMIOLOGY
Incidence
- Autopsy studies have found microadenomas in 3–27% and macroadenomas in <0.5% of people without any pituitary disorders.
- Clinically apparent pituitary tumors are seen in 18/100,000 persons.

ETIOLOGY AND PATHOPHYSIOLOGY
- Monoclonal adenohypophysial cell growth
- Hormonal effects of functional microadenomas often prompt diagnosis before mass effect.
- PRL increased by functional PRLs or inhibited dopaminergic suppression by stalk effect

Genetics
Familial isolated pituitary adenomas: ~15% have mutations in the aryl hydrocarbon receptor–interacting protein gene (*AIP*); present at a younger age and are larger in size (2)

RISK FACTORS
Multiple endocrine neoplasias

COMMONLY ASSOCIATED CONDITIONS
- McCune-Albright syndrome
- Multiple endocrine neoplasia type 1 (MEN1)

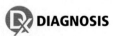 **DIAGNOSIS**

HISTORY
- Common
  - Hyperprolactinemia: infertility, amenorrhea, galactorrhea, gynecomastia, impotence
  - Headache (sellar expansion)
  - Visual disturbances: bitemporal hemianopsia
- Less common
  - Hypersomatotropinemia: acromegaly (coarse facial features, hand/foot swelling, carpal tunnel syndrome, hyperhidrosis, left ventricular hypertrophy)
  - Hyposomatotropinemia: failure to thrive (FTT) (children), asymptomatic (adults)

- Intracranial pressure (ICP) elevation: headache, nausea, seizures
- Hypercorticotropinemia: Cushing disease (supraclavicular/dorsocervical fat pad thickening, moon face, hirsutism, acne, plethora, abdominal striae, centripetal obesity with thin limbs, easy bruising and bleeding, hyperglycemia)
- Rare
  - Apoplexy: headache, sudden collapse
  - Secondary hyperthyroidism: palpitations, diaphoresis, heat intolerance, diarrhea
  - Secondary adrenal insufficiency: weakness, irritability, anorexia, nausea/vomiting
- Hypothalamic compression: temperature, thirst/appetite disorders

PHYSICAL EXAM
- Common
  - Visual disturbances: bitemporal hemianopsia
  - Hyperprolactinemia: hypogonadism, galactorrhea, gynecomastia
  - Hypersomatotropinemia: acromegaly (coarse features, hand/foot swelling, diaphoresis)
  - Hyposomatotropinemia: FTT (children)
- Less common
  - ICP elevation: papilledema, dementia
  - Cushing disease: centripetal obesity, supraclavicular fat pad thickening, moon face, hirsutism, acne
- Rare
  - Apoplexy: hypotension, hypoglycemia, tachycardia, oliguria
  - Secondary hyperthyroidism: tachycardia, tachypnea, diaphoresis, warm/moist skin, tremor
  - Adrenal crisis: orthostatic hypotension
- Hypothalamic compression: temperature dysregulation, obesity, increased urination

DIFFERENTIAL DIAGNOSIS
Pituitary hyperplasia (e.g., pregnancy, primary hypothyroidism, menopause), Rathke cleft cyst, granulomatous disease (e.g., tuberculosis), lymphocytic hypophysitis, metastatic tumor, germinoma, craniopharyngioma

DIAGNOSTIC TESTS & INTERPRETATION
- Somatotrophic (GH secreting: 40 to 130/million)
  - Acromegaly/hypersomatotropinemia: serum IGF-1 elevated; oral glucose tolerance test with GH given at 0, 30, and 60 minutes (normally suppresses GH to <1 g/L)
  - Hyposomatotropinemia: low GH-releasing hormone response
  - Macimorelin is a noninvasive oral test to evaluate for adult GH deficiency (3)[A].
- Corticotropic
  - Cushing disease/hypercorticotropinemia
  - 24-hour urinary-free cortisol >50 μg
  - Overnight low-dose dexamethasone suppression test (DMST): normal free plasma cortisol (FPC) >1.8 μg/dL at 8 AM (after 1 mg given at 11 PM on night prior)

- ACTH level assay (if DMST results abnormal): <20 pg/mL = adrenal tumor; ≥20 pg/mL = ectopic/pituitary source
- Hypocorticotropinemia/secondary glucocorticoid deficiency: high-dose corticotropin stimulation test: FPC <10 g/dL at baseline, with an increase of <25% 1 hour after 250 μg; metyrapone test: 11-deoxycortisol <150 ng/L after 2 g given (Prepare to give steroids because test may worsen insufficiency.)
- Gonadotrophic/hypogonadotropism: gonadotropin-releasing hormone stimulation of LH/FSH blunted in pituitary hypergonadism but increased in primary hypogonadism
- Lactotrophic (PRL secreting): hyperprolactinemia: serum PRL >20 ng/mL
- Thyrotrophic (TSH secreting): hyper-/hypothyroidism: TSH and free T_4 both increased for pituitary hyperthyroidism and both decreased for pituitary hypothyroidism

Initial Tests (lab, imaging)
- A typical panel for asymptomatic tumors: PRL, GH, IGF-1, ACTH, 24-hour urinary-free cortisol or overnight DMST, β-HCG, FSH, LH, TSH, free T_4
- MRI preferred (>90% sensitivity and specificity) after biochemically confirmed
- Octreotide scintigraphy is useful in identifying tumors with somatostatin receptors (4)[B].

 TREATMENT

Medical therapy is primary therapy for PRLs and adjunct for other tumors.

MEDICATION
First Line
- Hyperprolactinemia: Dopamine agonists increase dopaminergic suppression of PRL.
  - Cabergoline (Dostinex): D_2 receptor–specific
    ○ Initial dose: 0.25 mg PO once or twice weekly
    ○ Maintenance dose: Increase q4wk by 0.25 mg 2 times per week per PRL (max 2 mg/week).
    ○ Contraindications: hypersensitivity (ergots), uncontrolled hypertension (HTN), pregnancy
    ○ Precautions: caution with liver impairment
    ○ Interactions: may be inhibited by tricyclic antidepressants, phenothiazines, opiates
    ○ Adverse reactions: orthostatic hypotension, vertigo, dyspepsia, hot flashes
  - Bromocriptine (Parlodel): D_2 receptor–specific
    ○ Initial dose: 1.25 to 2.50 mg PO daily (give with food)
    ○ Maintenance dose: Increase by 2.5 mg/day q2–7d (max 15 mg/day).
    ○ Contraindications: hypersensitivity (ergots), uncontrolled HTN, pregnancy; preferred over cabergoline if required
    ○ Precautions: caution with liver impairment
    ○ Interactions: may be inhibited by tricyclic antidepressants, phenothiazines, opiates
    ○ Adverse reactions: orthostatic hypotension, seizures, hallucinations, stroke, myocardial infarction

- Somatotropinoma
  - Long-acting analogues of somatostatin (Sandostatin LAR and lanreotide Autogel)
    - Sandostatin LAR: 20 mg q28d (4)[A]; lanreotide Autogel 90 mg q28d; titrate per package insert.
    - Contraindication: hypersensitivity
    - Precautions: caution with biliary, thyroid, cardiac, liver, or kidney disease
    - Interactions: Pimozide increases risk of QT prolongation; variable effects with β-blockers, diuretics, oral glycemic agents
    - Adverse reactions: ascending cholangitis, arrhythmias, congestive heart failure, glycemic instability
    - More effective as adjuvant than as primary treatment for somatotropinomas
    - Consider use of somatostatin analogue or pegvisomant in patients with severe residual disease (4)[A].
    - Consider use of cabergoline in patients with mild residual disease (5)[B].
  - Pegvisomant (Somavert): GH receptor antagonist
    - Initial dose: 40 mg SC × 1 and then 10 mg daily and titrate by 5 mg every 4 to 6 weeks based on IGF-1 levels (max 30 mg/day maintenance dose)
    - Contraindication: hypersensitivity
    - Precautions: caution if GH-secreting tumors, diabetes mellitus, impaired liver function
    - Interactions: NSAIDs, opiates, insulins, oral glycemic agents
    - Adverse reactions: hepatitis, tumor growth, GH secretion
- Corticotropinemia: peripheral inhibitors
  - Mitotane (Lysodren)
    - Initial dose: 2 to 6 g/day divided PO TID (max 19 g/day)
    - Maintenance dose: 2 to 16 g TID
    - Contraindication: hypersensitivity
    - Precautions: caution with liver dysfunction and brain damage
    - Interactions: contraindicated with rotavirus vaccine; caution with other vaccines
    - Adverse reactions: HTN, orthostatic hypotension, hemorrhagic cystitis, rash
  - Ketoconazole
    - Dosing: 200 mg PO TID (max 1,200 mg/day)
    - Contraindications: hypersensitivity, achlorhydria, fungal meningitis, impaired liver function
    - Precautions: caution with liver dysfunction
    - Interactions: contraindicated with dronedarone, methadone, statins, pimozide, sirolimus; caution with other antifungals
    - Adverse reactions: adrenal insufficiency, thrombocytopenia, hepatic failure, hepatotoxicity, anaphylaxis, leukopenia, hemolytic anemia
  - Pasireotide (Signifor)
    - Dosing: initially, 0.6 to 0.9 mg twice daily and then 0.3 to 0.9 mg twice daily
    - Contraindication: none
    - Precautions: hypocortisolism, hyperglycemia, bradycardia or QT prolongation, liver test elevations, cholelithiasis, and other pituitary hormone deficiencies

- Mifepristone (Korlym)
  - Dosing: Administer PO once daily with a meal. The recommended starting dose is 300 mg once daily; not to exceed 600 mg daily in renal impairment
  - Contraindication: pregnancy, use of simvastatin or lovastatin and CYP3A substrates with narrow therapeutic range, concurrent long-term corticosteroid use, women with history of unexplained vaginal bleeding, women with endometrial hyperplasia with atypia or endometrial carcinoma
  - Precautions: adrenal insufficiency, hypokalemia, vaginal bleeding and endometrial changes, QT interval prolongation, use of strong CYP3A inhibitors
  - Interactions: potential interactions with drugs metabolized by CYP3A, CYP2C8/9, CYP2B6, and hormonal contraceptives. Nursing mothers should discontinue drug or discontinue nursing.
- Gonadotropinemia
  - Bromocriptine: See above
- Thyrotropinemia
  - Somatostatin analogues: See above

Second Line
- Corticotropinemia: peripheral inhibitors
  - Metyrapone
    - Dose: 250 mg PO QID
    - Contraindication: porphyria
    - Precautions: caution in liver/thyroid disease
    - Interactions: Dilantin increases metabolism.
    - Adverse reactions: nausea, hypotension
- Gonadotropinemia
  - Octreotide: See above

ISSUES FOR REFERRAL
Neurosurgery consultation for symptomatic tumors (except for PRL)

ADDITIONAL THERAPIES
- Fractionated radiotherapy: often effective as adjunctive when surgery is inadequate (5)[B]
- Stereotactic radiosurgery: alternative to surgery in high-risk patients or as adjunct (5)[B]

SURGERY/OTHER PROCEDURES
Most are now done endoscopically via translabial/transsphenoidal approach (6)[A].

 ONGOING CARE

FOLLOW-UP RECOMMENDATIONS
Patient Monitoring
- Follow-up MRIs at 6 and 12 months after surgery
- Involved hormone(s) are followed postoperatively, especially after radiation because hypopituitarism may develop 10 to 15 years after treatment.

PROGNOSIS
Depends on type, size, symptoms, therapy

COMPLICATIONS
- Postoperative diabetes insipidus and/or hypogonadism (usually transient/common)
- Pituitary apoplexy (acute/uncommon): acute hemorrhagic pituitary infarction; adrenal crisis with severe headache; surgical decompression required to prevent shock, coma, and death
- Nelson syndrome (subacute/uncommon): rapid adenoma growth postadrenalectomy
- Pituitary hormone insufficiency (chronic/uncommon): often years after treatment
- Optic nerve neuropathy and brain necrosis after >60 Gy radiotherapy (chronic/rare)

REFERENCES
1. Dworakowska D, Grossman AB. The pathophysiology of pituitary adenomas. *Best Pract Res Clin Endocrinol Metab.* 2009;23(5):525–541.
2. Georgitsi M, Raitila A, Karhu A, et al. Molecular diagnosis of pituitary adenoma predisposition caused by aryl hydrocarbon receptor-interacting protein gene mutations. *Proc Natl Acad Sci U S A.* 2007;104(10):4101–4105.
3. Agrawal V, Garcia JM. The macimorelin-stimulated growth hormone test for adult growth hormone deficiency diagnosis. *Expert Rev Mol Diagn.* 2014;14(6):647–654.
4. Tichomirowa MA, Daly AF, Beckers A. Treatment of pituitary tumors: somatostatin. *Endocrine.* 2005;28(1):93–100.
5. Mondok A, Szeifert GT, Mayer A, et al. Treatment of pituitary tumors: radiation. *Endocrine.* 2005;28(1):77–85.
6. Buchfelder M. Treatment of pituitary tumors: surgery. *Endocrine.* 2005;28(1):67–75.

 SEE ALSO

Cushing Disease and Cushing Syndrome; Galactorrhea

 CODES

ICD10
D35.2 Benign neoplasm of pituitary gland

CLINICAL PEARLS
- An incidentaloma is an asymptomatic microadenoma found on imaging. General labs include PRL, GH, IGF-1, ACTH, 24-hour urinary-free cortisol/overnight DMST, β-subunit FSH, LH, TSH, and free T_4. Obtain follow-up MRIs at 6 and 12 months if normal, but consult endocrinology if not.
- Initial treatment selected for symptomatic pituitary adenoma includes a dopamine agonist for PRLs and surgical resection for all others.
- Pituitary apoplexy is a rapid hemorrhagic pituitary infarction due to compression of the blood supply. It is fatal within hours unless surgically decompressed.

PLANTAR FASCIITIS

Krystyna Guinevere Golden, MD • Nolan P. Feola, MD • Meghan Plunkett, MD

BASICS

DESCRIPTION
- Degenerative change of plantar fascia at origin on medial tuberosity of calcaneus
- Classically presents as pain on plantar surface of the foot, usually at calcaneal insertion of plantar fascia with weight-bearing, especially in morning or on initiation of walking after prolonged rest
- Synonym(s): plantar fasciopathy, plantar heel pain syndrome, plantar fasciosis, and painful heel syndrome

EPIDEMIOLOGY
Incidence
Estimated 1 million patient visits yearly in the United States
Prevalence
- Most common cause of plantar heel pain
- Lifetime: 10–15% of population; peak incidence between ages 40 and 60 years; earlier in runners

ETIOLOGY AND PATHOPHYSIOLOGY
- Plantar fascia is composed of fibrous and dense connective tissue.
  - Three bands: medial, lateral, and central
  - Supports longitudinal plantar arch, assists intrinsic foot musculature, may assist in energy storage
- Repetitive microtrauma and collagen degeneration of plantar fascia
- Chronic degenerative change (-osis/-opathy rather than -itis) of plantar fascia generally at insertion on medial tuberosity of calcaneus

RISK FACTORS
- Intrinsic
  - Age (40 to 60 years)
  - Female, pregnancy
  - Obesity (BMI >30 kg/m^2)
  - Pes planus (flat feet), pes cavus (high arch), overpronation, leg length discrepancy
  - Hamstring, calf, and Achilles tightness
  - Calf and intrinsic foot muscle weakness
  - Decreased ankle range of motion with dorsiflexion (equinus or tight heel cord; <15 degrees of dorsiflexion)
  - Systemic connective tissue disorders
- Extrinsic
  - Dancers, runners, court sport athletes (e.g, tennis, volleyball)
  - Occupations with prolonged standing, especially on hard surfaces (nurses, letter carriers, warehouse/factory workers)
  - Overuse and rapid increase in activities involving repetitive loading

GENERAL PREVENTION
- Maintain normal body weight.
- Avoid training errors (increasing intensity, distance, duration, and frequency of high-impact activities too rapidly); avoid overtraining.
- Proper footwear (appropriate cushion/arch support)
- Runners should replace footwear every 250 to 500 miles.

COMMONLY ASSOCIATED CONDITIONS
- Heel spurs commonly seen but are not a marker of severity nor pathognomonic and surgical removal of unclear benefit
- Posterior tibial neuropathy

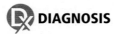

DIAGNOSIS

HISTORY
- Pain on plantar surface of foot, usually at fascial insertion at calcaneus (medial calcaneal tubercle), but can have pain anywhere along length of plantar fascia
- Pain is typically worse with first few steps in the morning or after prolonged rest or standing (post-static dyskinesia).
- Pain typically improves after first few steps only to recur toward the end of the day or after prolonged ambulation.
- Pain commonly unilateral but can be bilateral in 1/3 of cases
- Pain can be dull and constant in chronic cases.
- Limp with excessive toe walking
- Numbness and burning of medial hindfoot are more suggestive of posterior tibial nerve compression.

PHYSICAL EXAM
- Point tenderness on medial tuberosity of calcaneus at insertion of plantar fascia
- Pain along plantar fascia with dorsiflexion of foot
- Windlass test: Extend MTP while allowing passive flexion of IP joint of hallux—pain indicates a positive test; high specificity, low sensitivity; sensitivity improves (13.5 → 31.8%) if performed while standing.
- Dorsiflexion-eversion test: pain with dorsiflexion plus eversion of the subtalar joint
- Decreased passive range of motion with dorsiflexion
- Loss of heel fat pad suggests heel fat pad syndrome.
- Point tenderness on posterosuperior aspect of heel suggests Achilles tendinopathy.

DIFFERENTIAL DIAGNOSIS
- Calcaneal stress fracture
- Heel fat pad syndrome (painful or atrophic heel pad)
- Longitudinal arch strain
- Nerve entrapment (posterior tibial nerve—tarsal tunnel syndrome, medial calcaneal branch of posterior tibial nerve, abductor digiti quinti)
- Achilles tendinopathy
- Calcaneal contusion
- Plantar calcaneal bursitis
- Tendonitis of posterior tibialis
- Plantar fascia tear
- S1 radiculopathy
- Adolescents: calcaneal apophysitis (Sever disease)

DIAGNOSTIC TESTS & INTERPRETATION
- Usually not necessary; typically a clinical diagnosis
- Consider applying a navicular sling; improvement confirms pronation induced plantar fasciitis.
- Consider imaging only to rule out other causes or persistent heel pain after 4 to 6 months of conservative therapy.
- Radiographs: two views of foot to evaluate for fracture, tumor, cyst, periostitis, bony erosions; weight-bearing films preferred; calcaneal spurs common but not diagnostic
- Ultrasound: hypoechoic at insertion, thickened plantar fascia (≥4 mm); may additionally see partial thickness tears
- MRI can evaluate for other soft tissue etiologies.
- CT or technetium-99m bone scan can rule out calcaneal stress fracture and evaluate for infection.
- Nerve conduction studies can rule out nerve entrapment.
- Inflammatory markers: can consider if bilateral heel pain or young patients

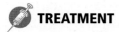

TREATMENT

GENERAL MEASURES
- Weight reduction if BMI >25 kg/m^2
- Intrinsic foot muscle strengthening to stabilize the arch
- Strengthen calf and intrinsic foot muscles using the towel drag/pickup exercise and barefoot single leg balance.
- Relative rest/activity modification with avoidance of high-impact causative activities
- Stretching: Plantar fascia stretches are more effective than Achilles tendon/gastrocnemius-soleus stretches; non–weight-bearing stretches are preferable.

- Plantar fascia mobilization done in office and taught to patients
  - Foot to inversion; compress tender point while moving foot to eversion; repeat along plantar fascia.
- Ice (frozen water bottle roll) and massage (golf or tennis ball roll) of tibialis anterior
- Supportive footwear with stable midfoot or orthoses may be helpful.
  - For relief of acute pain (2 to 3 weeks), continued use may contribute to continued intrinsic muscle weakness.
  - Options include heel cup, soft heel pad, navicular pad, medial heel wedge, Thomas heel, and night splint (1).
  - Custom orthoses show no benefit over prefabricated orthoses and are more costly.
  - Improved effectiveness of night splints when used in association with orthotics
- Surgical treatment of "heel spurs" is not indicated.

MEDICATION
First Line
- NSAIDs scheduled for 2 to 3 weeks: naproxen 500 mg PO BID or ibuprofen 600 to 800 mg PO TID PRN for pain
- Acetaminophen 1,000 mg PO TID PRN for pain

ISSUES FOR REFERRAL
- Physical therapy for patient instruction on proper stretching and strengthening techniques, manipulative treatments (joint and soft tissue mobilization), and massage; for chronic cases, consider analysis of gait and biomechanical factors.
- Podiatry: Consider if conservative measures fail after 3 to 6 months.
- Surgery: Consider if conservative measures fail after 6 to 12 months.

ADDITIONAL THERAPIES
- Corticosteroid injections (provides short-term pain relief)
  - Risk for plantar fascia rupture and calcaneal fat pad atrophy with resultant permanent heel pain
- Platelet-rich plasma (PRP) injections
  - May lead to greater improvement in pain and functional outcomes compared to CSI
- Extracorporeal shock wave therapy (ESWT)
  - Is an effective alternative to CSI in relieving pain and improving function
  - High-energy flux density ESWT for high sessions is more effective than low-energy flux density ESWT for low sessions

- Dextrose prolotherapy
  - Inferior in short-term pain relief when compared to corticosteroid injection but may be more effective long term and associated with lower risk of complication
- Radiofrequency thermal lesioning (RTL) (2)
  - CSI and RTL yielded better therapeutic outcomes compared to ESWT.
- Low-dye and calcaneal taping
- Short walking cast

SURGERY/OTHER PROCEDURES
- Necessary in <10% of patients; more likely beneficial in severely obese
- Recommended if conservative treatment fails after 6 to 12 months and pain is unrelenting.
- Open/endoscopic plantar fasciotomy (less risk and complications with endoscopic technique but requires specialized equipment and skills; not widely used)

COMPLEMENTARY & ALTERNATIVE MEDICINE
Acupuncture may reduce pain in short term but insufficient evidence for the long-term treatment of plantar fasciitis

 ONGOING CARE

FOLLOW-UP RECOMMENDATIONS
- Ensure patient adherence to proper stretching technique.
- Following 3 to 6 months of unsuccessful conservative treatment, consider additional therapies or referrals.

PATIENT EDUCATION
- Weight reduction if BMI >25 kg/m^2
- Home plantar fascia mobilization exercises
- Strengthen foot muscles: place a towel on the floor, pull toward yourself with ball of foot and toes without lifting the heel; progressive one-leg standing
- Proper footwear (adequate cushion and arch support)
- Stretch plantar fascia: Pull toes into dorsiflexion prior to walking after prolonged sitting or sleep.
- Ice the foot using a frozen water bottle: Roll foot over bottle for 10 minutes in the morning and after work.
- Decrease repetitive stress.

PROGNOSIS
Self-limited (resolves within 12 months) in up to 80–90% of patients

COMPLICATIONS
- Rupture of plantar fascia (more common with repeated corticosteroid injections)
- Chronic pain, gait abnormality

REFERENCES
1. Choo YJ, Park CH, Chang MC. Rearfoot disorders and conservative treatment: a narrative review. *Ann Palliat Med*. 2020;9(5):3546–3552.
2. Erden T, Toker B, Cengiz O, et al. Outcome of corticosteroid injections, extracorporeal shock wave therapy, and radiofrequency thermal lesioning for chronic plantar fasciitis. *Foot Ankle Int*. 2021;42(1):69–75.

ADDITIONAL READING
Li Z, Yu A, Qi B, et al. Corticosteroid versus placebo injection for plantar fasciitis: a meta-analysis of randomized controlled trials. *Exp Ther Med*. 2015;9(6):2263–2268.

 SEE ALSO

Algorithm: Heel Pain

CODES

ICD10
M72.2 Plantar fascial fibromatosis

CLINICAL PEARLS
- Plantar fasciitis occurs due to degeneration of plantar fascia at origin (medial calcaneal tuberosity).
- Plantar medial heel pain with weight-bearing (most noticeable with initial steps in the morning or after period of inactivity) is hallmark presentation.
- Generally, self-limited (within 12 months)
- Strengthen intrinsic foot muscles, modify activity, stretch plantar fascia, ice (water bottle roll), and massage (golf ball roll).
- Weight loss for BMI ≥25 kg/m^2
- Trial of over-the-counter orthoses

PLEURAL EFFUSION

Erik Colegrove, MD

 BASICS

Abnormal accumulation of fluid in the pleural space

DESCRIPTION
Types: transudate (low protein/low specific gravity) and exudate (high protein and cellular debris); transudate: commonly caused by congestive heart failure (CHF): 40%; exudates: pneumonia 25%, malignancy 15%, and pulmonary embolism (PE) 10%

EPIDEMIOLOGY
Incidence
Estimated 1.5 million cases per year in the United States; CHF: 500,000; pneumonia: 300,000; malignancy: 150,000; PE: 150,000; cirrhosis: 150,000; tuberculosis (TB): 2,500; pancreatitis: 20,000; collagen vascular disease: 6,000

Prevalence
Estimated 320 cases per 100,000 people in industrialized countries; in hospitalized patients with AIDS, prevalence is 7–27%; no gender predilection: ~2/3 of malignant pleural effusions occur in women.

ETIOLOGY AND PATHOPHYSIOLOGY
- Imbalance between pleural fluid formation and pleural fluid absorption due to and imbalance between oncotic and hydrostatic pressures between the vascular and pleural space
  - Favors pleural effusion: hydrostatic pressure in vessel greater than pleural space, oncotic pressure vessel less than pleural space, elevated capillary permeability from baseline
  - Favors fluid retention in the vessel: hydrostatic pressure in vessel less than pleural space, oncotic pressure vessel greater than pleural space, decreased capillary permeability from baseline
- Transudates: pleural fluid migration that results from imbalances in hydrostatic/oncotic forces, increase in capillary permeability, lymphatic obstruction/impaired drainage, translocation of fluid from another compartment (e.g., peritoneal or retroperitoneal)
- Transudates: CHF: 40% of transudative effusions; 80% bilateral; constrictive pericarditis, atelectasis; superior vena cava syndrome.; cirrhosis (hepatic hydrothorax), nephrotic syndrome, hypoalbuminemia; myxedema; urinothorax, central line misplacement; peritoneal dialysis; Dressler syndrome (postmyocardial infarction syndrome); yellow nail syndrome: yellow nails, lymphedema, and pleural effusion; SARS-CoV-2
- Exudates: lung parenchyma infection: bacterial (parapneumonic, tuberculous pleurisy), fungal, viral, parasitic (amebiasis, *Echinococcus granulosus*); cancer: lung cancer, metastases (breast, lymphoma, ovaries), mesothelioma; PE: 25% of PEs are transudate; collagen vascular disease: rheumatoid arthritis, systemic lupus erythematosus (SLE), Wegener granulomatosis, sarcoidosis, Churg-Strauss syndrome, Sjogren syndrome, granulomatosis with polyangitis; GI: pancreatitis, esophageal rupture, abdominal abscess, after liver transplant; chylothorax: thoracic

duct tear, malignancy; hemothorax: trauma, PE, malignancy, coagulopathy, aortic aneurysm; others: after coronary artery bypass graft, uremia, asbestos exposure, radiation, drugs; drugs: nitrofurantoin, bromocriptine, amiodarone, procarbazine, hydralazine, procainamide, quinidine, methotrexate, methysergide, interleukin-2, mitomycin, practolol, minoxidil, bleomycin, cyclophosphamide, procarbazine, imatinib, all-trans retinoic acid, gemcitabine, dantrolene, valproic acid, sulfasalazine, minocycline, acebutolol, phenytoin, practolol, minoxidil, methysergide, L-tryptophan, dasatinib, docetaxel, filgrastim, ergot alkaloids
  - Meigs syndrome; yellow nail syndrome; ovarian stimulation syndrome; lymphangiomatosis; acute respiratory distress syndrome (ARDS); chylothorax: thoracic duct tear, malignancy, associated with lymphoma
  - Pleural effusions of extravascular origin (PEEVO)
  - Transudative PEEVO: hepatic hydrothorax, peritoneal dialysis, urinothorax, extravascular migration of central venous catheter, duropleural fistula, ventriculoperitoneal and ventriculopleural shunts, glycinothorax
  - Exudative PEEVO: esophageal or gastric perforation, misplaced enteral feeding tube, pancreaticopleural fistula and pancreatic pseudocyst, bilothorax

RISK FACTORS
Occupational exposures/drugs; PE, TB, bacterial pneumonias; opportunistic infections (in HIV patients when CD4 count is <150 cells/μL)

COMMONLY ASSOCIATED CONDITIONS
Hypoproteinemia, heart failure, cirrhosis, kidney disease

 DIAGNOSIS

Presumptive diagnosis in 50% of cases; small pleural effusions; radiographic area <2 intercostal spaces (<300 mL) are asymptomatic

HISTORY
Dyspnea, fever, malaise, and weight loss; chest pain, cough, hemoptysis, and dull pain

PHYSICAL EXAM
- Pleural effusion >300 mL: tachypnea, asymmetric expansion of the thoracic cage; decrease/absent tactile fremitus; dullness to percussion; decreased/inaudible breath sounds, egophony, pleural friction rub
- Ascites suggest hepatic hydrothorax, ovarian cancer, and Meigs syndrome. If associated with unilateral swelling in lower extremity, consider DVT with PE. Lymphadenopathy may suggest malignancy.

DIFFERENTIAL DIAGNOSIS
Pseudochylothorax: accumulation of cholesterol or lecithin-globulin complexes in pleural space

DIAGNOSTIC TESTS & INTERPRETATION
Initial Tests (lab, imaging)
- Thoracocentesis: Use of thoracic ultrasound lowers rate of pneumothorax (4% vs. 9.5%); ultrasonography (US): detects as little as 5 to 50 mL of pleural fluid; identifies loculated effusions; site for thoracentesis, pleural biopsy, or pleural drainage; chest CT scan with contrast for patients with undiagnosed pleural effusion; CT pulmonary angiography if PE is suspected; CT scan of the chest with contrast is recommended if the pleural fluid has complex ultrasonographic features such as septations and loculations.
- Pleural fluid: appearance, pH, WBC differential, total protein, lactate dehydrogenase (LDH), glucose, Gram stain and culture, and acid-fast bacilli staining; consider polymerase chain reaction (PCR) for *Mycobacterium tuberculosis* and *Streptococcus pneumoniae*. If comorbidities implying risk, consider amylase, triglycerides, cholesterol, LE cells, cytology, antinuclear antibodies (ANAs), adenosine deaminase, tumor markers, rheumatoid factor, cytology, creatinine
  - PH ≤7.2, high risk of infection, insert intercostal drain
  - PH >7.2 <7.4, intermediate risk of infection, measure LDH, consider drain if LDH >900 IU/L
  - PH ≥7.4, low risk of pleural infection, ICD (drain) not needed
- Light criteria, transudate versus exudate (98% sensitivity; 80% specificity); fluid is considered an exudate if any of the following: ratio of pleural fluid-to-serum protein levels >0.5; ratio of pleural fluid-to-serum LDH levels >0.6; pleural fluid LDH level >2/3 the upper limit for serum LDH level; 99.5% sensitive for detecting exudative effusion; Light criteria may misdiagnose as high as 20% of transudates as exudative, thus clinical correlation remains important.
- Other exudate criteria: serum-effusion albumin gradient ≤1.2 (sensitivity 87%; specificity 92%); cholesterol effusion >45 mg/dL and LDH effusion >200 mg/dL (sensitivity 90%; specificity 98%); empyema: pus, putrid odor; culture; a putrid odor suggests an anaerobic empyema: LDH levels >1,000 IU/L (normal serum = 200 IU/L); glucose, <60 mg/dL; low pH; malignancy: cytology, red, bloody; glucose, normal to low, depending on the tumor burden; RBCs, >100,000/mm³
- Lupus pleuritis: LE cells present; pleural fluid-to-serum ANAs ratio >1; glucose <60 mg/dL; pleural fluid-to-serum glucose ratio <0.5; fungal: positive KOH, culture; peritoneal dialysis: protein, <1 g/dL; glucose, 300 to 400 mg/dL; urinothorax: creatinine: pleural/blood >0.5; high LDH pleural fluid, with low protein levels
- Hemothorax: hematocrit: pleural/blood >0.5; benign asbestos effusion: unilateral, exudative; have elevated eosinophil count

- TB pleuritis: lymphocytes >80% predominance effusion; elevated levels of adenosine deaminase (ADA) >50 U/L and interferon-γ >140 pg/mL; positive acid-fast bacillus (AFB) stain, culture; total protein >4 g/dL; nuclear acid amplification (NAA), LDH levels elevated in about 75% of patients (often >500 units/L)
  - High prevalence populations: use ADA +/− IFN gamma
- Low prevalence populations use ADA (i.e., lower risk of a false positive).
- Chylothorax: milky; triglycerides >110 mg/dL; lipoprotein electrophoresis (chylomicrons); pseudo-chylothorax: cholesterol level >200 mg/dL or presence of cholesterol crystals; amebic liver abscess: anchovy paste effusion; Waldenström macroglobulinemia and multiple myeloma: protein >7 g/dL
- Esophageal rupture: high salivary amylase; pleural fluid acidosis, pH <6; amylase rich: acute pancreatitis, chronic pancreatic pleural effusion, malignancy, esophageal rupture; rheumatoid pleurisy: glucose <60 mg/dL; pleural fluid/serum glucose <0.5
- Lymphocytosis: tuberculous pleurisy, lymphoma, sarcoidosis, chronic rheumatoid pleurisy, yellow nail syndrome, or chylothorax (80–95% of the nucleated cells); carcinomatosis in half of cases (50–70% are lymphocytes.)
- Neutrophils >50% suggest parapneumonic effusion, empyema, PE, abdominal disease, malignant pleural effusion, and acute TB pleurisy. COVID-19 5.88% of pleural effusion
- Eosinophilia (>10% of total nucleated cells): pneumothorax, hemothorax, malignancy, drugs, pulmonary infarction, parasitic infection (lung fluke, amoebiasis, and echinococcus/ruptured hydatid cyst), fungal (coccidioidomycosis, cryptococcosis, histoplasmosis), benign asbestos pleural effusion
- Low glucose (<60 mg/dL): TB, malignancy, rheumatoid pleurisy, parapneumonic, empyema, hemothorax, paragonimiasis, Churg-Strauss syndrome. RBC count >100,000/mm³: trauma, malignancy, PE, injury after cardiac surgery, asbestos pleurisy, pancreatitis, TB
- Pleural fluid LDH >1,000 IU/L: suggests empyema, malignant effusion, rheumatoid effusion, or pleural paragonimiasis; pH >7.3: rheumatoid pleurisy, empyema, malignant effusion, TB, esophageal rupture, or lupus nephritis pH <7.2 necessitates fluid drainage in patient with parapneumonic effusion.
- Mesothelial cells in exudates: TB is unlikely if there are >5% of mesothelial cells. ADA >35 units/L suggest TB pleurisy, empyema, complicated parapneumonic effusion, and malignancy. ADA >250 units/L consider empyema or lymphoma over TB. *S. pneumoniae* accounts for 50% of cases of parapneumonic effusions in AIDS patients, followed by *Staphylococcus aureus, Haemophilus influenzae, Mycoplasma pneumoniae, Legionella, Nocardia,* and *Bordetella bronchiseptica*; exudate with low count of nucleated cells. *Pneumocystis jiroveci* is an uncommon cause in HIV. Usually, it is a small effusion, unilateral or bilateral, and serous to bloody in appearance. Demonstration of the trophozoite or cyst

is mandatory; cancer-related HIV pleural effusion: Kaposi sarcoma, Castleman disease, and primary effusion lymphoma; Kaposi sarcoma: mononuclear predominance, exudate, pH >7.4; LDH, 111 to 330 IU/L; glucose >60 mg/dL
- Comparison of specific imaging modalities
- Chest x-ray (CXR): posteroanterior–anteroposterior views: upright x-rays show a concave meniscus in the costophrenic angle that suggests >250 mL of pleural fluid; homogeneous opacity, with visibility of pulmonary vessels through diffuse haziness and absence of air bronchogram; 75 mL of fluid will obliterate the posterior costophrenic sulcus. Lateral x-rays show blunting of the posterior costophrenic angle and the posterior gutter; decubitus x-rays to exclude a loculated effusion and underlying pulmonary lesion or pulmonary thickening; supine x-rays show costophrenic blunting, haziness, obliteration of the diaphragmatic silhouette, decreased visibility of the lower lobe vasculature, and widened minor fissure.
- Chest US: uses artifacts in the lung fields to determine underlying level of free-flowing fluid, consolidation; increasing levels of consolidation results in more echogenic (whiter) tissue.
- Chest CT: better location of loculations and pleural thickening compared to x-ray, resulting in the "split pleural sign" enhancement of visceral and parietal layers at the margin of the effusion
- Chest MRI: Distinguish between transudates and exudates and evaluate for extent of tissue extension.

Diagnostic Procedures/Other
Diagnostic thoracentesis indicated for the following: clinically significant pleural effusion (>10-mm thick on US or lateral decubitus x-ray with no known cause)

 ## TREATMENT

MEDICATION

First Line
CHF: diuretics (75% clearing in 48 hours); parapneumonic effusion: antibiotics; rheumatologic conditions/inflammation: steroids and NSAID

Second Line
Intrapleural treatments for fibrinopurulent stage
- Fibrinolytic/enzymatic therapy
- Streptokinse (250,000 IU per day)
- Patients with pleural infection: no benefit on mortality, rate of surgery, length of hospital stay
- Urokinase (100,000 to 200,000 IU per day)
  - More expensive than tPA/DNAase but lower hemothorax rate
- tPA (5 to 10 mg BID, 10 mg QD)
- DNAase
- Saline washes
- Intrapleural irrigation with saline in the pleural space, then manual aspiration until clear, reduces intrapleural enzyme administration and shortens chest tube removal time (1).

ISSUES FOR REFERRAL
Uncertain etiology; malignant effusion; high-risk diagnostic thoracentesis; decortication

ADDITIONAL THERAPIES
Pleurodesis for symptomatic patients whose pleural effusion reaccumulates too quickly for repeat therapeutic thoracentesis

SURGERY/OTHER PROCEDURES
- Percutaneous pleural biopsy if a cause is not clear after thoracentesis
- Contraindications for thoracentesis: anticoagulation, bleeding diathesis, thrombocytopenia <20,000/mm³, mechanical ventilation
- Bronchoscopy: when malignancy is suspected (pulmonary infiltrate or mass on CXR or CT scan, hemoptysis, massive pleural effusion, or shift of the mediastinum toward the side of effusion)
- Video-assisted thoracoscopic surgery may reduce length of hospital stay and have better overall surgical outcomes compared to thoracostomy.

 ## ONGOING CARE

COMPLICATIONS
Pleural effusion: constrictive fibrosis, pleurocutaneous fistula; 40% of pneumonia patients will developed up to 40% parapneumonic effusion, and close to 10% will progress to empyema. Mortality approaches 20% and up to 30% in patients with comorbidities; thoracentesis: pneumothorax (5–10%); hemothorax (~1%); empyema; spleen/liver laceration; reexpansion pulmonary edema (REPE) (if >1.5 L is removed); complications related to large-volume thoracentesis include REPE and pneumothorax ex vacuo.

REFERENCE
1. Sorino C, Mondoni M, Lococo F, et al. Optimizing the management of complicated pleural effusion: from intrapleural agents to surgery. *Respir Med*. 2022;191:106706.

 ## CODES

ICD10
- J86.9 Pyothorax without fistula
- J86.0 Pyothorax with fistula
- J91.0 Malignant pleural effusion

CLINICAL PEARLS
Rare causes of pleural exudates include constrictive pericarditis, urinothorax, and Meigs syndrome. Most common pleural exudates include malignancy, parapneumonic effusions, TB, and empyema.

PNEUMONIA, BACTERIAL

Jocelyn C. Young, DO, MSc • Lukas D. Kost, MD

BASICS

Bacterial pneumonia is an acute infection of the pulmonary parenchyma by a bacterial organism.

DESCRIPTION
Bacterial pneumonia can be classified as the following:
- Community acquired pneumonia (CAP) is classified by severity:
  - CAP in an outpatient setting
  - Nonsevere CAP in an inpatient setting
  - CAP in an intensive care unit (ICU) or severe CAP is based on illness severity criteria and is defined as the presence of one major criterion or at least three minor criteria.
    - Major criteria: septic shock requiring vasopressors, respiratory failure requiring mechanical ventilation
    - Minor criteria: respiratory rate (RR) $\geq$30 breaths/min, PaO$_2$/FiO$_2$ ratio $\leq$250, multilobar infiltrates, confusion, BUN $\geq$20, WBC $\leq$4, platelets <100,000, hypothermia, and hypotension requiring aggressive fluid resuscitation
- Nosocomial pneumonia: acquired in health care settings
  - Hospital-acquired pneumonia (HAP): occurs $\geq$48 hours after admission and did not appear to be incubating at the time of admission
  - Ventilator-associated pneumonia (VAP): develops $\geq$48 hours after endotracheal intubation

EPIDEMIOLOGY
- In the United States, the annual incidence of CAP is 24.8 cases per 10,000 adults with higher rates as age increases. Pneumonia is the eighth leading cause of death and is the first among infectious causes of death.
- Worldwide, pneumonia kills more children than any other infectious disease, claiming the lives of >700,000 children aged <5 years every year. Respiratory viruses are the most commonly detected causes of pneumonia.

Incidence
- CAP: 5 to 6 cases per 1,000 persons with increased incidence occurring in the winter months
- HAP: 5 to 20 cases per 1,000 admissions; incidence increases 6- to 20-fold in ventilated patients.

ETIOLOGY AND PATHOPHYSIOLOGY
- Adults, outpatient CAP
  - Typical (85%): *Streptococcus pneumoniae, Haemophilus influenzae, Staphylococcus aureus,* group A *Streptococcus, Moraxella catarrhalis*
  - Atypical (15%): *Legionella* sp., *Mycoplasma pneumoniae, Chlamydophila pneumoniae*
- Adults, inpatient nonsevere or severe CAP, HAP, VAP
  - Aerobic gram-negative bacilli: *Pseudomonas aeruginosa, Escherichia coli, Klebsiella pneumoniae,* and *Acinetobacter* sp.
  - Gram-positive cocci: *Streptococcus* sp. and *S. aureus* (including MRSA)
- Pediatric
  - Birth to 3 weeks: *E. coli,* group B streptococci, *Listeria monocytogenes*
  - <3 months: *Chlamydia trachomatis, S. pneumoniae, H. influenzae*
  - 3 months to 18 years: typical: *S. pneumoniae;* atypical: *C. pneumoniae, M. pneumoniae*

RISK FACTORS
- Immunosuppression:
  - Chronic steroid use (>20 mg/day or >2 mg/kg/day of prednisone for >14 days)
  - HIV/immunoglobulin deficiencies/solid organ transplant/TNF-α inhibitor therapy
- Chronic health conditions: asthma, COPD, type 2 diabetes mellitus (DM), chronic renal failure, CHF, liver disease, tobacco use
- Age >65 years, antibiotic therapy in the past 6 months/resistance to antibiotics
- Hospitalization for $\geq$2 days during past 90 days
- Poor functional status

GENERAL PREVENTION
Vaccination recommendations:
- All children 2 to 59 months of age should be vaccinated with pneumococcal conjugate (PCV13); given at 2, 4, 6, and 12 to 15 months of age
- Pneumococcal vaccination is recommended for all adults aged $\geq$65 years. For those who have never received vaccine before, give 1 dose of PCV20. For those with previous vaccination in adulthood, additional vaccinations are recommended per the Centers for Disease Control and Prevention (CDC)
- Adults aged 19 to 64 years with chronic diseases, defined by the CDC, should receive 1 dose of PCV20. For those who have only received PPSV23, give PCV20 1 year after their most recent PPSV23.
- Annual influenza vaccine

DIAGNOSIS

HISTORY
- Fever, chills, rigors, malaise, fatigue, dyspnea, cough (with/without sputum), pleuritic chest pain, myalgias, GI symptoms
- Pediatric patients: lethargy, hypotonia, poor feeding, dry mucus membranes, vomiting

> **ALERT**
> - High fever (>104°F [40°C]), male sex, multilobar involvement, and GI and neurologic abnormalities have been associated with CAP caused by *Legionella*.
> - History of advanced neurodegenerative disease or dementia who develop sudden high fever and cough should raise suspicion for aspiration pneumonia.

Geriatric Considerations
Older adults with pneumonia present with weakness, mental status change, agitation, or history of falls.

PHYSICAL EXAM
- Vitals: fever >100.4°F (38°C), tachypnea, tachycardia, hypoxemia
  - Severe cases may also present with hypothermia, bradycardia, or hypotension.
- Pulmonary exam: decreased breath sounds unilaterally with rales, rhonchi, egophony, increased fremitus, bronchial breath sounds, dullness to percussion, asymmetric breath sounds, abdominal tenderness
- Pediatric exam findings: grunting, retractions

DIFFERENTIAL DIAGNOSIS
Viral pneumonia, bronchitis, asthma or COPD exacerbation, pulmonary edema, lung cancer, pulmonary tuberculosis, pneumonitis, rheumatologic etiologies (i.e., sarcoidosis)

DIAGNOSTIC TESTS & INTERPRETATION
Initial Tests (lab, imaging)
- Outpatient setting:
  - No routine laboratory testing or imaging in outpatients is indicated.
  - Clinical diagnosis with fever, tachypnea, and physical exam findings
- Inpatient and noncritical care setting:
  - CBC, CRP, chest x-ray
  - Procalcitonin is no longer recommended.
  - Urine *Legionella* antigen testing if there is travel to an endemic area or exposure to an outbreak
- Inpatient and critical care setting or severe CAP:
  - CBC, CRP, chest x-ray
  - Blood culture and sputum culture are recommended for severe CAP, history of MRSA or *P. aeruginosa* infections, active MRSA/*P. aeruginosa* infections, or hospitalized and treated with parental antibiotics within the previous 90 days.
  - For intubated patients, endotracheal aspirates have a higher yield of microbiological organisms compared to sputum culture.
  - Urine pneumococcal and *Legionella* antigen testing should be performed.
  - Procalcitonin is no longer recommended.
  - If MRSA is suspected, nasal testing for rapid MRSA is preferred, and if negative, coverage for MRSA is not indicated.
  - Evidence of necrotizing/cavitary pneumonia should raise suspicion for MRSA pneumonia.

Follow-Up Tests & Special Considerations
- Viral testing including influenzae as up to 80% of children aged <2 years old will have a viral cause.
- Obtain blood cultures only if no improvement on antibiotics or with severe CAP.
- Follow-up imaging is not indicated for patients with CAP symptoms improved in 5 to 7 days.

Diagnostic Procedures/Other
For HAP and VAP: By bronchoscopic or nonbronchoscopic means, obtain a lower respiratory tract sample for culture prior to initiation/change of therapy.

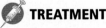

TREATMENT

GENERAL MEASURES

> **ALERT**
> Use a risk calculator to determine the need for hospitalization and efficacy of treatment:

- Pneumonia Severity Index (PSI) Calculator: https://www.thecalculator.co/health/Pneumonia -Severity-Index-(PSI)-Calculator-977.html
- CURB-65 Score for Pneumonia Severity: https://www.mdcalc.com/curb-65-score -pneumonia-severity

MEDICATION

First Line

- Adults (1)
  - CAP, outpatient empiric treatment: no risk factors for MRSA or *P. aeruginosa* and no comorbidities
    - Doxycycline 100 mg BID
    - Azithromycin 500 mg on day 1 and then 250 mg/day, if local resistance <25%
  - CAP, outpatient empiric treatment: with comorbidities but without risk factors for MRSA or *P. aeruginosa*
    - Combination therapy:
      - Doxycycline 100 mg BID *plus*
      - Amoxicillin/clavulanate 875 mg/125 mg BID, cefpodoxime 200 mg BID, or cefuroxime 500 mg BID
    - Monotherapy with a respiratory fluoroquinolone
  - Minimum duration of therapy is 5 days.
- CAP, inpatient: nonsevere pneumonia without risk factors for MRSA or *P. aeruginosa*
  - IV antibiotics initially, transition to PO with improvement
  - Minimum duration of therapy is 5 days.
  - Combination of:
    - β-Lactam (ampicillin/sulbactam 1.5 to 3.00 g IV q6h or cefotaxime 1 to 2 g IV q8h or ceftaroline, 600 mg IV q12h or ceftriaxone, 1 to 2 g IV daily) *plus*
    - Macrolide (azithromycin 500 mg PO/IV daily or clarithromycin 500 mg PO q12h) *or*
  - Monotherapy with a respiratory fluoroquinolone (levofloxacin 750 mg/day or moxifloxacin 400 mg/day)
  - If contraindications to macrolides and fluoroquinolones, use doxycycline 100 mg BID with β-lactam.
- CAP, inpatient: severe pneumonia without risk factors for MRSA or *P. aeruginosa*
  - β-Lactam *plus* macrolide
  - β-Lactam *plus* respiratory fluoroquinolone
- CAP, inpatient: severe pneumonia with locally validated risk factors for MRSA or *P. aeruginosa*
  - Add appropriate coverage as follows:
  - For MRSA risk factors: linezolid or vancomycin
  - For *P. aeruginosa* risk factors: aztreonam or cefepime or meropenem or piperacillin/tazobactam or ceftazidime
- Corticosteroids are indicated only in cases with refractory shock.
- Routine administration of anaerobic coverage for suspected aspiration pneumonia is not recommended except in patients who have empyema or lung abscess concerns.
- When there is clinical and radiographic evidence of CAP in patients who tested positive for influenza, antibacterial and anti-influenza treatments are recommended.
- HAP, inpatient (2)
  - Patients without MRSA risk factors and not at high risk of mortality, choose one of the following:
    - Piperacillin-tazobactam 4.5 mg IV q6h or cefepime 2 g IV q8h or levofloxacin 750 mg IV q24h or imipenem 500 mg IV q6h or meropenem 1 g IV q8h
  - Patients with MRSA risk factors: add either vancomycin 15 mg/kg IV q8–12h based on trough or linezolid 600 mg IV q12h

- VAP, inpatient (2)
  - Empirically cover *S. aureus*, *P. aeruginosa*, and other gram-negative bacilli.
  - Cover MRSA if at risk for antimicrobial resistance or if prevalence of MRSA is not known.
  - Include double pseudomonas coverage from two different classes if at risk for antimicrobial resistance or in an ICU where susceptibility rates are not known.
- Pediatric, outpatient (≥3 months)
  - Antibiotic treatment in preschool-aged children is not routinely required because viral pathogens are more common.
  - 5 days of antibiotic therapy is recommended and 7 days duration for those aged <6 months.
  - Presumed typical bacterial pneumonia
    - Amoxicillin 90 mg/kg/day PO BID (max of 4 g/day) or amoxicillin-clavulanate 90 mg/kg/day PO BID (max of 4 g/day)
    - For patients with penicillin allergy, clindamycin 13 mg/kg per dose PO TID
    - For children who are not up to date with vaccination and have penicillin allergy, levofloxacin if aged <5 years, 10 mg/kg per dose IV/PO BID (max of 375 mg per dose); for children aged >5 years, 10 mg/kg per dose IV/PO daily (max of 750 mg per dose)
  - Presumed atypical bacterial pneumonia
    - Doxycycline 1 to 2 mg/kg per dose PO BID if >7 years old
    - Azithromycin 10 mg/kg PO on day 1 (max of 500 mg) and then 5 mg/kg/day (max of 250 mg) on days 2 to 5
    - Clarithromycin 15 mg/kg/day PO BID (max of 1 g/day) or erythromycin 40 mg/kg/day PO daily
- Pediatric, inpatient (≥3 months)
  - Uncomplicated CAP
    - First-line empirical treatment is ampicillin 50 mg/kg per dose IV q6h.
    - For low- or medium-risk penicillin allergy/not fully immunized, ceftriaxone 50 to 100 mg/kg/day IV q12–24h (max of 2,000 mg)
    - For high-risk allergy, levofloxacin, 10 mg/kg per dose
  - Complicated CAP
    - First-line empirical treatment is ceftriaxone 100 mg/kg once followed by 50 mg/kg per dose IV q12h.
    - Add vancomycin or clindamycin if suspecting community-acquired MRSA.
    - Due to inferior in vitro activity of oral cephalosporins, transition from empiric ceftriaxone should be to amoxicillin-clavulanate.
    - For high-risk allergy, substitute levofloxacin, 10 mg/kg per dose and vancomycin
    - Presumed atypical bacterial pneumonia
      - Azithromycin 10 mg/kg IV daily on days 1 and 2 (max of 500 mg) and then 5 mg/kg/day PO (max of 250 mg) on days 3 to 5
      - Alternatives: clarithromycin, erythromycin, doxycycline (if >8 years old), levofloxacin (if reached growth maturity)

ADMISSION, INPATIENT, AND NURSING CONSIDERATIONS

- Analgesia and antipyretics, chest physiotherapy, IV fluids (and conversely, diuretics) if indicated
- Pulse oximetry and oxygen supplementation
- Positioning minimize aspiration risk

Pediatric Considerations

- Approximately 15% of all deaths worldwide in children <5 years of age can be traced back to CAP.
- Tachypnea along with high temperature lasting >3 days with cyanosis and respiratory distress are highly indicative of pneumonia.
- Inpatient treatment is recommended for infants aged ≤3 to 6 months or for those with presence of respiratory distress.
- Discharge criteria: clinical stability for 12 to 24 hours including temperature ≤100°F (37.8°C); HR ≤100 beats/min; RR ≤24 breaths/min; O₂ sat ≥90% on room air; maintain oral intake; normal mental status

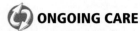 ONGOING CARE

PATIENT EDUCATION

Smoking cessation, vaccinations

COMPLICATIONS

Necrotizing pneumonia, respiratory failure, empyema, abscesses, cavitation, bronchopleural fistula, sepsis

REFERENCES

1. Metlay JP, Waterer GW, Long AC, et al. Diagnosis and treatment of adults with community-acquired pneumonia. An official clinical practice guideline of the American Thoracic Society and Infectious Diseases Society of America. *Am J Respir Crit Care Med.* 2019;200(7):e45–e67.
2. Kalil AC, Metersky ML, Klompas M, et al. Management of adults with hospital-acquired and ventilator-associated pneumonia: 2016 clinical practice guidelines by the Infectious Diseases Society of America and the American Thoracic Society. *Clin Infect Dis.* 2016;63(5):e61–e111.

CODES

ICD10

- J15.9 Unspecified bacterial pneumonia
- J15.4 Pneumonia due to other streptococci
- J14 Pneumonia due to Hemophilus influenzae

CLINICAL PEARLS

Severity of illness score is helpful in determining the need for hospitalization but does not replace clinical judgment.

PNEUMONIA, MYCOPLASMA

Kenneth A. Ballou, MD

BASICS

DESCRIPTION
- Bronchopulmonary infection caused by one of several *Mycoplasma* spp.; *Mycoplasma pneumoniae* being the most common pathogen of the class
- Smallest, free-living organism; fastidious and slow-growing; first isolated in cattle in 1898
- Most frequently affects children/young adults but can also occur in the elderly; often causes epidemics in close communities (i.e., skilled nursing facilities, dormitories, military barracks)
- Infection may be asymptomatic, most often confined to the upper respiratory tract; however, may progress to pneumonia (5–10%) (1)
- Course is usually acute with an incubation period of 1 to 4 weeks.
- Synonym(s): primary atypical pneumonia (PAP); Eaton agent pneumonia; cold agglutinin–positive pneumonia; walking pneumonia

Pediatric Considerations
- Increased incidence of asthma exacerbation in older children
- Infants 3 to 6 months old with suspected bacterial pneumonia should be hospitalized.

EPIDEMIOLOGY
Incidence
- ~1 million cases/year in United States; annual infection rate of 1% in United States
- 20% of CAP requiring hospitalizations annually
- Most frequently in autumn/winter seasons

Prevalence
- Predominant sex: male = female
- Predominant age group affected: 5 to 20 years
  - May occur at any age
  - Rare in children <5 years of age
- Responsible for up to 15–20% of all cases of CAP yearly
  - Most common cause of pneumonia in school children and young adults who do not have a chronic underlying condition

ETIOLOGY AND PATHOPHYSIOLOGY
- *M. pneumoniae* is a short-rod mucosal pathogen, which lacks a cell wall and thus not visible on Gram stain.
- Can grow under both aerobic and anaerobic conditions
- Highly contagious, transmitted by aerosol droplets
- Pathogenicity linked to its filamentous tips, which adhere selectively to respiratory epithelial cell membrane proteins with production of H_2O_2 and superoxide radicals, damaging cilia
- Decreased ciliary movement produces prolonged paroxysmal, hacking cough.
- Incubation period is 2 to 3 weeks.

ALERT
- *M. pneumoniae* infection may worsen asthma symptoms as well as cause wheezing in children without asthma.
- *M. pneumoniae* infection may worsen chronic obstructive pulmonary disease (COPD) or other chronic pulmonary condition symptoms in adults.

RISK FACTORS
- Immunocompromised state (e.g., HIV, transplant recipients, chemotherapy)
- Smoking
- Close communal living (e.g., military barracks, prisons, hospitals, dormitories, schools, household contacts, skilled nursing facilities)

COMMONLY ASSOCIATED CONDITIONS
- Asthma exacerbations as a result of proinflammatory cytokine release
- COPD

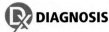DIAGNOSIS

HISTORY
- Infection may be asymptomatic.
- Gradual onset of headache, malaise, low-grade fevers, chills
- Symptoms of upper respiratory infection, including incessant, nonproductive cough, worsening cough (which may become mildly productive late in the disease) and pleurisy; rhinorrhea, pharyngitis, and otalgia; sinusitis may subsequently occur (2).
- Pneumonia may occur with associated pleural effusion.
- The presence of pleuritic chest pain warrants a higher suspicion of *M. pneumoniae*.
- Extrapulmonary findings may develop in 5–10% of patients, including arthralgias, skin rashes, cervical adenopathy, hemolysis, congestive heart failure (CHF), and cardiac conduction abnormalities.
- Neurologic symptoms develop more commonly in children and may include encephalitis, aseptic meningitis, cranial nerve palsies, cerebellar ataxia, ascending paralysis, and coma.
- Persistent cough is common during convalescence; other sequelae are rare.

PHYSICAL EXAM
- Hacking/pertussis-like cough may be present along with fever and lassitude.
- Normal lung findings with early infection, but rhonchi, rales, and/or wheezes may develop several days later.
- Mild pharyngeal injection without exudates
- Minimal/no cervical adenopathy
- Some patients may develop an audible pleural friction rub.
- Various exanthems, including erythema multiforme and Stevens-Johnson syndrome

DIFFERENTIAL DIAGNOSIS
- Viral/bacterial/fungal pneumonia
- Tuberculosis
- Other atypical pneumonias, including *Chlamydia pneumoniae, Chlamydophila psittaci, Coxiella burnetii* (Q fever), *Francisella tularensis* (tularemia), *Pneumocystis jiroveci, Legionella pneumophila,* and other community-acquired pneumonias
- Must differentiate from COVID-19–related pulmonary infection; COVID-19 testing recommended

DIAGNOSTIC TESTS & INTERPRETATION
- *M. pneumoniae* is typically a clinical diagnosis and treated empirically; however, when specific pathogen testing is indicated, polymerase chain reaction (PCR) is the test of choice.
- No clinical or radiographic findings can differentiate between *M. pneumoniae* and other atypical pneumonia pathogens (*Chlamydia/Legionella*).

Initial Tests (lab, imaging)
- WBC count may be normal or elevated.
- Hemolytic anemia is rare.
- Elevated erythrocyte sedimentation rate (ESR) may be present but is nonspecific.
- Procalcitonin (PCT) levels is not recommended.
- When indicated, PCR for *M. pneumoniae* DNA in nasopharyngeal and throat swabs as well as bronchoalveolar lavage respiratory secretions, CSF, and tissue samples may be the most sensitive and specific.
- Radiography of the chest shows reticulonodular pattern with patchy areas of lower lobe consolidation. Small pleural effusion may be present in 10–15% cases.

Follow-Up Tests & Special Considerations
- Sputum Gram stains are not helpful because *M. pneumoniae* lacks a cell wall and cannot be stained.
- *M. pneumoniae* is difficult to culture and requires 7 to 21 days to grow; does not provide information to guide treatment.
- Complement fixation serologic assay shows 4-fold rise in IgM antibody titer at 2 to 4 weeks after symptom onset; this is an older technique.
- Positive cold agglutinins (titer of ≥1:128 or rising 4-fold) in 50% of infections but can take 1 to 2 weeks to develop; not sensitive/specific; not routinely recommended
- CT of chest may show a combination of patchy tree-in-bud opacities with segmental ground glass opacities.

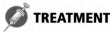TREATMENT

GENERAL MEASURES
- Supportive care indicated, especially for very ill patients who may require inpatient treatment
- Treatment is initially empiric and must be comprehensive to cover all likely pathogens in the context of the clinical setting.
- Calculation of pneumonia severity score (CAP score: http://www.mdcalc.com/psi-port-score-pneumonia-severity-index-adult-cap) may be helpful in determining inpatient versus outpatient treatment.

ALERT
There is insufficient evidence regarding the efficacy of antibiotics in pediatric patients <24 months of age infected with *M. pneumoniae*. However, some studies show benefit to treating with a macrolide and amoxicillin to cover *M. pneumoniae* in addition to other likely agents causing CAP.

Pregnancy Considerations
- Azithromycin: pregnancy Category B (preferred treatment)
- Clarithromycin, levofloxacin, and moxifloxacin: pregnancy Category C

MEDICATION
First Line
- Doxycycline (drug of choice for CAP)
  - Children <8 years of age: not recommended
  - Children >8 years of age (≤45 kg): 2 to 4 mg/kg/day up to 200 mg/day PO divided BID for 10 to 14 days
  - Children >8 years of age (≥45 kg): Refer to adult dosing.
  - Adults: 100 mg PO BID ×14 days
  - Useful in macrolide-resistant strains of *M. pneumoniae*
- Clarithromycin
  - Children <6 months of age: not established
  - Patients >6 months of age: 15 mg/kg/day PO divided q12h for 10 to 14 days
  - Adults: 500 mg PO BID for 14 to 21 days
- Azithromycin
  - <3 months of age: not established (2)
  - >3 months of age: day 1, 10 mg/kg PO × 1 (not to exceed 500 mg); days 2 to 5: 5 mg/kg PO daily (not to exceed 250 mg/day)
  - Adults: 500 mg PO on the first day, followed by 250 mg PO daily × 4 days
- Erythromycin
  - Children: 20 to 50 mg/kg/day (base) PO divided q6–8h for 10 to 14 days
  - Adults: 500 mg (base) PO q6h × 14 to 21 days

Second Line
- Levofloxacin
  - Children <18 years of age: not recommended
  - Adults: 750 mg PO/IV daily × 5 days
- Moxifloxacin
  - Children <18 years of age: not recommended
  - Adults: 400 mg PO/IV daily for 7 to 14 days
- Gemifloxacin
  - Children <18 years of age: not recommended
  - Adults: 320 mg PO daily for 5 to 7 days
- Levofloxacin and moxifloxacin show good activity against *M. pneumoniae*. Consider use with comorbid conditions and other pneumonia pathogens; also useful if macrolide resistance is suspected

ADDITIONAL THERAPIES
- Albuterol inhaler: 2 puffs q4–6h as needed for wheezing
- Dexamethasone may downregulate cytokine release, particularly if symptoms outside the respiratory tract are present.
- Supplemental oxygen as needed; up to 10.9% of hospitalized patients may require mechanical ventilation.
- Plasmapheresis in cases of severe hemolytic anemia

ADMISSION, INPATIENT, AND NURSING CONSIDERATIONS
- CAP score risk class IV/V
- Advanced age with comorbidities
- Complicating neoplastic disease
- Significant cerebrovascular, cardiac, renal, liver, or GI symptoms
- Altered mental status
- Inability to maintain oxygen saturation
- Tachycardia/tachypnea
- Hypotension
- Neurologic symptoms
- Signs of Stevens-Johnson syndrome
- Significant hemolysis (autoimmune hemolytic anemia, cold agglutinin disease)
- Change from IV to PO antibiotic may be made when:
  - Respiratory distress and hypoxia have resolved.
  - Patients are tolerating oral hydration.
  - No significant complications are present.
  - Utilization of PCT may aid in this decision.
- Generally, no need for 24-hour observation on PO antibiotics prior to discharge.

 ## ONGOING CARE

FOLLOW-UP RECOMMENDATIONS
- Clearing of condition on CXR should be documented in patients >50 years of age.
- In smokers, document a clear CXR in 6 to 8 weeks.
- Worsening symptoms/development of rash or meningeal/neurologic signs should prompt immediate presentation to medical attention.
- Antibiotic prophylaxis for exposed contacts is not routinely recommended.
- For household contacts who may be predisposed to severe mycoplasmal infection, macrolide or doxycycline prophylaxis should be used.

DIET
Ensure adequate hydration.

PATIENT EDUCATION
- Smoking cessation
- Contact and droplet precautions
- Adequate handwashing techniques

PROGNOSIS
- Symptoms usually resolve in 2 weeks.
- Some constitutional symptoms may persist for several weeks.
- With correct therapy, even most severe cases can expect complete recovery.

COMPLICATIONS
- All complications are rare, except reactive airway disease, hemolytic anemia, and erythema multiforme.
- Reactive airway disease may persist indefinitely and can cause acute chest syndrome in patients with sickle cell anemia.
- Meningoencephalitis, aseptic meningitis
- Peripheral neuropathy
- Transverse myelitis/acute transverse myelitis
- Cerebellar ataxia
- Acute disseminated encephalomyelitis
- Guillain-Barré syndrome
- Encephalitis (especially in children)
- Polyneuritis/polyarthritis
- Stevens-Johnson syndrome
- Pericarditis/myocarditis
- Respiratory distress syndrome
- Cerebral ataxia
- Thromboembolic phenomena
- Pleural effusion
- Nephritis
- Occasional deaths occur primarily among the elderly and persons with sickle cell disease.

REFERENCES
1. Jiang Z, Li S, Zhu C, et al. *Mycoplasma pneumoniae* infections: pathogenesis and vaccine development. *Pathogens.* 2021;10(2):119.
2. Miyashita N. Atypical pneumonia: pathophysiology, diagnosis, and treatment. *Respir Investig.* 2022;60(1):56–67.

ADDITIONAL READING
Garin N, Marti C, Skali Lami A, et al. Atypical pathogens in adult community-acquired pneumonia and implications for emperic antibiotic treatment: a narrative review. *Microorganisms.* 2022;10(12):2326.

 ## CODES

ICD10
J15.7 Pneumonia due to Mycoplasma pneumoniae

CLINICAL PEARLS
- Mycoplasma (*M. pneumoniae*) is one of the most common atypical respiratory pathogens seen in community-acquired pneumonia.
- Atypical pneumonia is usually a clinical diagnosis.
- Atypical pneumonia with *M. pneumoniae* usually responds to empiric treatment (doxycycline).
- Outbreaks of *M. pneumoniae* can be seen in close communities (i.e., dormitories).

PNEUMONIA, PNEUMOCYSTIS JIROVECI

Thomas J. Hansen, MD

BASICS

DESCRIPTION
- *Pneumocystis jiroveci* causes pneumonia primarily in immunocompromised patients.
- The fungus that causes this pneumonia in humans was previously called *Pneumocystis carinii*.
- The name was formally changed to *P. jiroveci* in 2001, following the discovery that the fungus that infects humans is unique and distinctive from the fungus that infects animals.
- *P. jiroveci* is extremely resistant to traditional antifungal agents, including both amphotericin and azole agents.
- To prevent confusion, the term PCP, which used to represent *P. carinii* pneumonia, now represents *Pneumocystis* pneumonia.

ALERT
No combination of symptoms, signs, blood chemistries, or radiographic findings is diagnostic of *P. jiroveci* pneumonia (1).

EPIDEMIOLOGY
- *P. jiroveci* has a worldwide distribution, and most children have been exposed to the fungus by 2 to 4 years (2).
- The reservoir and mode of transmission for *P. jiroveci* is still unclear.
  - Human studies favor an airborne transmission model, with person-to-person spread being the most likely mode of infection acquisition (1).

Incidence
- Infants with HIV infection have a peak incidence of PCP between 2 and 6 months (2).
- HIV-infected infants have a high mortality rate, with a median survival of only 1 month.

Prevalence
- The prevalence of *P. jiroveci* colonization among healthy adults is 0–20%.
- Recent studies have demonstrated the transient nature of *P. jiroveci* colonization in asymptomatic, immunocompetent patients (1).
- 50% of patients with PCP are coinfected with ≥2 strains of *P. jiroveci* (2).
- There is evidence that distinct strains are responsible for each episode in patients who develop multiple episodes of PCP (2).

ETIOLOGY AND PATHOPHYSIOLOGY
Mode of transmission is unknown; likely respiratory from infected host

RISK FACTORS
Individuals at risk (1)
- Patients with HIV infection, especially if not receiving prophylactic treatment for PCP
- Patients who are receiving high doses of glucocorticoids
- Patients who have an altered immune system not due to HIV

- Patients who are receiving chronic immunosuppressive medications
- Patients who have hematologic or solid malignancies resulting in malignancy-related immune depression

GENERAL PREVENTION
- Indications for prophylaxis
  - HIV-infected adults (2)
    - Should start when CD4 count is <200 cells/μL or if the patient develops oropharyngeal candidiasis
  - HIV-infected children (2)
    - Prophylaxis should be provided for children aged ≥6 years based on adult guidelines.
    - For children aged 1 to 5 years, start when CD4 count is <500 cells/μL.
    - For infants 4 to 6 weeks to 12 months old, prophylaxis for first year of life.
  - Non–HIV-infected adults receiving immunosuppressive medications or with underlying immune system deficits should receive PCP prophylaxis, but currently, there are no specific guidelines on when to start this.
- Medication
  - Trimethoprim-sulfamethoxazole (TMP-SMX)
    - Adults: 1 double-strength tablet daily (preferred regimen) or 1 double-strength tablet 3 times per week
    - Children 4 weeks old and older: TMP 5 to 10 mg/kg/day; and sulfamethoxazole, 25 to 50 mg/kg per day, orally. The total daily dose should not exceed 320 mg TMP and 16,000 mg SMX. Acceptable dosing intervals and schedules: in divided doses twice daily, 3 days per week on consecutive or alternate days; in divided doses twice daily, 2 days per week on consecutive or alternate days; total dose once daily, given 7 days per week.
  - Atovaquone suspension
    - Adults: 1,500 mg PO once daily with food
    - Children: not to exceed 1,500 mg/day
      - 1 to 3 months: 30 mg/kg/day PO once daily
      - 4 to 24 months: 45 mg/kg/day PO once daily
      - >24 months: 30 mg/kg/day PO once daily
      - Adolescents aged ≥13 years: Refer to adult dosing.
  - Dapsone
    - Adults only: 50 mg twice daily or 100 mg once daily
    - Children 1 month or older: 2 mg/kg (maximum 100 mg), orally, once a day or 4 mg/kg (maximum 200 mg), orally every week.
  - Pentamidine
    - Adults only: 300 mg aerosolized every 4 weeks
- Discontinuation of prophylaxis
  - Discontinue if combined antiretroviral therapy has been administered for 6 months or more and the CD4+ T-lymphocyte cell count is >200 cells/μL or greater and have been sustained for >3 consecutive months in patients aged ≥6 years.
  - In children aged 1 to 5 years, discontinue if combined antiretroviral therapy has been administered for 6 months or more and the CD4+ T-lymphocyte cell count is 500 cells/μL or greater and have been sustained for >3 consecutive months.

COMMONLY ASSOCIATED CONDITIONS
- HIV Infection
- Chronic obstructive pulmonary disease (COPD)
- Interstitial lung disease
- Connective tissue diseases treated with corticosteroids
- Cancer and organ transplant patients on immunosuppressive medication

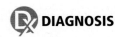

DIAGNOSIS

HISTORY
- HIV-infected patients
  - Subacute onset over several weeks
    - Progressively worsening dyspnea
    - Tachypnea
    - Cough: nonproductive or productive of clear sputum
    - Low-grade fever, chills
    - Weakness, fatigue, malaise
- Non–HIV-infected immunocompromised patients
  - More acute onset with fulminant respiratory failure
    - Abrupt tachypnea, dyspnea
    - Fever
    - Dry cough

PHYSICAL EXAM
- Fever
- Tachypnea
- Tachycardia
- Lung exam is normal or near normal.

DIFFERENTIAL DIAGNOSIS
- Tuberculosis
- Bacterial pneumonia
- Fungal pneumonia
- Viral pneumonia

DIAGNOSTIC TESTS & INTERPRETATION
P. jiroveci cannot be cultured. Therefore, a diagnosis relies on detection of the organism by colorimetric or immunofluorescent stains or by polymerase chain reaction (PCR) (2)[C].
- ABG: reveals hypoxemia and increased alveolar–arterial gradient that varies with severity of disease
- LDH: Serum lactate dehydrogenase is frequently increased (nonspecific; likely due to underlying lung inflammation and injury).
- CD4 cell count is generally <200 cells/μL in HIV-infected patients with PCP.
- S-adenosylmethionine levels are significantly lower in a patient with PCP. The levels increase with successful treatment.
- Comprehensive metabolic profile

- Chest x-ray (CXR) (1)[C]
  - Bilateral, symmetric, fine, reticular interstitial infiltrates involving perihilar areas; becomes more homogeneous and diffuse as severity of infection progresses
  - Less common patterns include upper lobe involvement in patients receiving aerosolized pentamidine, solitary or multiple nodular opacities, lobar infiltrates, pneumatoceles, and pneumothoraces.
  - May be normal in up to 30% of patients with PCP
- High-resolution CT is more sensitive than CXR.

Diagnostic Procedures/Other

- Fiberoptic bronchoscopy with bronchoalveolar lavage (BAL) is the preferred diagnostic procedure to obtain samples for direct fluorescent antibody staining.
  - Sensitivities range from 89% to >98%.
- *Pneumocystis* trophic forms or cysts obtained from induced sputum, BAL fluid, or lung tissue, which can be visualized using conventional stains
- PCR can detect *Pneumocystis* from respiratory sources, but the potential remains for false positives (1)[C].

TREATMENT

The recommended duration of therapy differs in patients who are with/without AIDS:

- In patients with PCP who do not have AIDS, the typical duration of therapy is 14 days.
- Treatment of PCP in patients who have AIDS was increased to 21 days due to the risk for relapse after only 14 days of treatment (1)[C].

MEDICATION

First Line

- TMP-SMX (1)[C]
- Adult dosing
  - TMP-SMX: 15 to 20 mg/kg/day, PO or IV, divided into three or four divided doses
- Pediatric dosing (>2 months) (1)[C]
  - TMP: 15 to 20 mg/kg/day in divided doses q6–8h
- Reduce doses of TMP-SMX in patients with renal failure.
- Patients should receive 21 days of therapy.
- Treatment response to *Pneumocystis* therapy often requires at least 7 to 10 days before clinical improvement is documented.
- Pregnancy risk factor: category C (1)[C]
- Precautions
  - History of sulfa allergy
  - There is an emergence of drug-resistant PCP, especially against TMP-SMX.

Second Line

- Pentamidine (for moderate to severe cases)
  - Adults and children: 4 mg/kg IV once daily
- Dapsone + trimethoprim (adults only)
  - Dapsone 100 mg PO once daily, *plus*
  - Trimethoprim 5 mg/kg PO TID
    - Check the glucose-6-phosphate dehydrogenase level before beginning dapsone because hemolysis may result.
- Clindamycin + primaquine (adults only)
  - Clindamycin 900 mg IV q8h or 600 mg IV q6h or 600 mg PO TID or 450 mg PO QID, *plus*
  - Primaquine 30 mg PO once daily
- Atovaquone
  - Adults: 750 mg PO BID (>13 years of age)
  - Children: 40 mg/kg/day PO divided BID (max 1,500 mg)
- Note: Pentamidine has greater toxicity than TMP-SMX: hypotension, hypoglycemia, pancreatitis (1)[C].

ADDITIONAL THERAPIES

Adjunctive corticosteroid (prednisone or methylprednisolone) (1)[C]

- Adjunctive corticosteroids are shown to provide benefits in patients who have HIV and symptoms of moderate to severe PCP.
- Corticosteroids provide the greatest benefit to HIV patients who have hypoxemia manifested as a partial pressure of arterial oxygen <70 mm Hg or an alveolar–arterial gradient >35 mm Hg on room air.
- Adults and children >13 years of age: prednisone, 40 mg PO BID on days 1 to 5; 40 mg daily on days 6 to 11; 20 mg daily on days 12 to 21

ADMISSION, INPATIENT, AND NURSING CONSIDERATIONS

- No set criteria for hospital admission
- Five predictors of mortality in HIV-associated *Pneumocystis* pneumonia
  - Increased age of the patient
  - Recent IV drug use
  - Total bilirubin >0.6 mg/dL
  - Serum albumin <3 g/dL
  - Alveolar–arterial oxygen gradient ≥50 mm Hg

ONGOING CARE

FOLLOW-UP RECOMMENDATIONS

In patients with HIV/AIDS: Patients with previous episodes of PCP should receive lifelong secondary prophylaxis unless they respond well to highly active antiretroviral therapy (HAART) and have a CD4 count >200 cells/μL for at least 3 months.

Patient Monitoring

Serum lactate dehydrogenase levels, pulmonary function test results, and ABG measurements generally normalize with treatment.

DIET

No special diet needed

PATIENT EDUCATION

- Centers for Disease Control and Prevention: https://www.cdc.gov/dpdx/pneumocystis/index.html
- FamilyDoctor.org: http://familydoctor.org/familydoctor/en/diseases-conditions/hiv-and-aids/complications/pneumocystis-pneumonia-pcp-and-hiv.html

REFERENCES

1. Krajicek BJ, Thomas CF Jr, Limper AH. Pneumocystis pneumonia: current concepts in pathogenesis, diagnosis, and treatment. *Clin Chest Med*. 2009;30(2):265–278.
2. Kovacs JA, Masur H. Evolving health effects of Pneumocystis: one hundred years of progress in diagnosis and treatment. *JAMA*. 2009;301(24):2578–2585.

ADDITIONAL READING

Green H, Paul M, Vidal L, et al. Prophylaxis for Pneumocystis pneumonia (PCP) in non-HIV immunocompromised patients. *Cochrane Database Syst Rev*. 2007;(3):CD005590.

 SEE ALSO

HIV/AIDS

CODES

ICD10

B59 Pneumocystosis

CLINICAL PEARLS

- Colonization with *P. jiroveci* is common in the pediatric population.
- PCP only occurs in immunocompromised patients.
- Patients with HIV are at risk once their CD4 count is <200 cells/μL. At that time, TMP-SMX should be initiated as prophylaxis. Prophylaxis may end after HAART has been initiated and the CD4 count is >200 cells/μL for 3 months.
- Patients who are immunocompromised are also at risk. Currently, no clear clinical guidelines are available as to when to initiate or end prophylaxis.
- The first-line treatment is TMP-SMX. The typical duration of therapy is 14 days in non–HIV-infected patients and 21 days in HIV-infected patients.

POLYARTERITIS NODOSA

Ratnesh Chopra, MD • Yevgeniy Popov, DO, MPH

 BASICS

DESCRIPTION

- Polyarteritis nodosa (PAN) is an antineutrophil cytoplasmic antibody (ANCA)-negative necrotizing arteritis of medium-sized muscular arteries and (occasionally) small arteries. Arterioles, capillaries, and venules are spared (1).
- Involved systems include gastrointestinal (GI) tract, peripheral nervous system (sensory and motor), CNS, genitourinary, skin, and cardiovascular. Glomerulonephritis and pulmonary capillaritis are rare (1),(2).
- Features depend on location of vasculitis: for example, mesenteric ischemia–related symptoms, new onset or worsening hypertension (HTN), mononeuritis multiplex, purpuric or nodular skin lesions, or livedo reticularis (2).
- Renal disease in PAN usually manifests as HTN and mild proteinuria with/without azotemia (2).
- PAN formerly encompassed several distinct entities (classic PAN, microscopic PAN, and cutaneous PAN). With ANCA testing, microscopic PAN appears pathophysiologically unrelated to the other two.
  - Idiopathic generalized PAN (classic PAN) is clinically variable, ranging from single organ involvement to polyvisceral failure (1).
  - HBV-associated PAN patients are positive for active hepatitis B infection and can present in similar fashion to idiopathic generalized PAN (1).
  - Microscopic PAN has ANCAs directed against myeloperoxidase (MPO) and involvement of small arterioles (microscopic polyangiitis [MPA]). This is now classified as ANCA-associated vasculitis.
  - Cutaneous (or limited) PAN is generally limited to the deep dermal and subcutaneous (SC) levels of the skin with characteristic histopathologic features of PAN. There are few systemic manifestations, although myalgias and peripheral motor neuropathy (mononeuritis multiplex) or sensory neuropathy may be present (2).

EPIDEMIOLOGY

Incidence
Incidence of 0 to 1.6 cases per million; predominant age: peaks in 5th to 6th decade; incidence rises with age. Mean age at diagnosis is 50 years; male predominance

Prevalence
Rare: up to 31 cases per 1 million adults (1)

ETIOLOGY AND PATHOPHYSIOLOGY

- Segmental, transmural, necrotizing inflammation of medium and small muscular arteries, with intimal proliferation, thrombosis, and ischemia of the end-organ/tissue supplied by the affected vessels; aneurysm formation at vessel bifurcations (2)
- Hepatitis B–related PAN results in direct vessel injury due to viral replication or deposition of immune complexes, with complement activation and subsequent inflammatory response (2).
- Most cases are idiopathic; 20% are related to hepatitis B or C infection.
- In patients with PAN and hepatitis B, HBsAg has been recovered from involved vessel walls.

Genetics
Mutations of adenosine deaminase 2 (ADA 2) have been identified in families with PAN (1).

RISK FACTORS
Hepatitis B > hepatitis C infection (cutaneous PAN)

COMMONLY ASSOCIATED CONDITIONS
- Hepatitis B (strong association with classic PAN); hepatitis C (less strongly linked to cutaneous PAN)
- Hairy cell leukemia; rare following hepatitis B vaccination
- Minocycline (symptoms resolve on stopping drug, reoccur if rechallenged); case-based associations with CMV infection, amphetamines, and interferon

 DIAGNOSIS

- There are no formal diagnostic criteria for PAN (2).
- Suspect PAN with:
  - Acute, sometimes fulminant multisystem disease with a relatively short prodrome (i.e., weeks to months); vasculitic skin rash with sensorimotor symptoms/findings; recent-onset HTN with systemic symptoms; unexplained sensory and/or motor neuropathy with systemic symptoms; hepatitis B infection with multisystem disease

HISTORY
Symptoms reflect specific organ involvement (2).
- Constitutional symptoms (fever, weight loss, malaise)
- Organ-specific symptoms
  - Focal muscular weakness/extremity numbness; myalgia and arthralgia
  - Rash (nodules, purpura, livedo)
  - Recurrent postprandial pain, intestinal angina, nausea, vomiting, and bleeding
  - Altered mental status, headaches, mononeuritis multiplex
  - Testicular/epididymal pain, neurogenic bladder (rare)

PHYSICAL EXAM
Findings/course reflect specific organ involvement (2).
- Peripheral nervous system: peripheral neuropathy, mononeuritis multiplex
- Renal: HTN
- Skin: purpura, urticaria, polymorphic rashes, SC nodules (uncommon but characteristic), livedo reticularis; deep skin ulcers, especially in lower extremities; Raynaud phenomenon (rare); single digit gangrene (rare)
- GI: acute abdomen; rebound, guarding, tenderness
- CNS: seizures, altered mental status, papillitis
- Lung: signs of pleural effusion—dullness to percussion; decreased breath sounds
- Cardiac: signs of congestive heart failure and/or myocardial infarction—S_3 gallop; pericarditis (Friction rub is rare).
- Genitourinary: testicular/epididymal tenderness (can mimic testicular torsion)
- Musculoskeletal: arthritis (usually large joint in lower extremities)

DIFFERENTIAL DIAGNOSIS
- Other forms of vasculitis (ANCA-associated, such as granulomatosis with polyangiitis [GPA—formerly Wegener granulomatosis], Churg-Strauss syndrome, and MPA; Henoch-Schönlein purpura, drug-induced vasculitis, cryoglobulinemia, Goodpasture syndrome)
- Buerger disease; systemic lupus erythematosus (SLE); embolic disease (atrial myxoma, cholesterol emboli); thrombotic disease (antiphospholipid antibody syndrome); dissecting aneurysm; Ehlers-Danlos syndrome; multiple sclerosis, systemic amyloidosis; infection (subacute endocarditis, HIV infection, trichinosis, rickettsial diseases)
- Fibromuscular dysplasia; ergotamine use; segmental arterial mediolysis

DIAGNOSTIC TESTS & INTERPRETATION
- No specific laboratory abnormalities; confirm diagnosis with biopsy if possible.
- Angiography (conventional, CT angiography, or MR angiography) may reveal microaneurysms and/or beading of bifurcating blood vessels.
- Avoid contrast in renal disease.
- Nonspecific laboratory abnormalities:
  - Elevated ESR and CRP; mild proteinuria, elevated creatinine
  - Hepatitis B surface antigen positive in 10–50%; hepatitis C antibody/hepatitis C virus RNA
  - ANCA, anti-proteinase 3 (PR3), and anti-MPO are negative. Positive ANCA argues against PAN. Rheumatoid factor may be positive.
  - Anemia of chronic disease (2)

Initial Tests (lab, imaging)
Look for evidence of systemic disease and rule out other causes (2)
- CBC (thrombocytosis), ESR, and CRP (elevated)
- Chemistries: elevated creatinine/BUN
- Hepatitis B serology: often positive; hepatitis C is less commonly positive.
- LFTs: abnormal if associated hepatitis B, C, or involvement of hepatobiliary tract
- Urinalysis: proteinuria/hematuria, generally no cellular casts or active urinary sediment
- ANA, cryoglobulins
- ANCA, anti-MPO, and anti-PR3
- Complement levels (C3, C4)
- Angiographic demonstration of aneurysmal changes/beading of small and medium-sized arteries

Diagnostic Procedures/Other
- Electromyography and nerve conduction studies in patients with suspected mononeuritis multiplex; if abnormal, consider sural nerve biopsy.
- Arterial/tissue biopsy (least invasive approach preferable)
- Skin biopsy from edges of ulcers; include deep dermis and SC fat to assess small muscular artery involvement (excisional *not* punch biopsy) (2).

Test Interpretation

- Necrotizing inflammation with fibrinoid necrosis of small- and medium-sized muscular arteries; segmental, often at bifurcations and branchings; venules are not involved in classic PAN.
- Capillaritis/other lung parenchymal involvement by vasculitis *strongly suggests* another process (microscopic PAN, GPA, Churg-Strauss syndrome, or antiglomerular basement membrane disease).
- Acute lesions with infiltration of polymorphonuclear cells through vessel walls into perivascular area; necrosis, thrombosis, and infarction of involved tissue
- Aneurysmal dilatations, including aortic dissection
- Peripheral nerves: 50–70% (vasa nervorum with necrotizing vasculitis)
- Testicular vessels involved in symptomatic males
- *The key differences from other necrotizing vasculitides are lack of granuloma formation and sparing of veins and pulmonary arteries (2).*

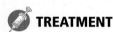 **TREATMENT**

GENERAL MEASURES
Treat HTN aggressively to prevent complications (stroke, myocardial infarction, heart failure).

MEDICATION

First Line
- Severe (life-threatening) disease: corticosteroids (CS) (high-dose oral prednisone [1 mg/kg/day] or intravenous [IV] methylprednisolone [0.5 to 1.0 g/day] for 3 days, then transition to prednisone 1 mg/kg/day, and taper according to response) (1)[A].
  - Only 50% of patients achieve and maintain remission with CS. Other patients require additional immunosuppressive therapy, and CS monotherapy is not recommended (1).
  - IV cyclophosphamide (0.6 g/m² every 2 weeks for 3 doses and then monthly for 4 to 12 months) in combination with CS: improves survival and spares use of chronic steroids in moderate/severe PAN (1)[A].
    - Cyclophosphamide has risk of infertility and malignancy.
  - Plasma exchange for severe refractory disease, such as progressive renal disease or catastrophic disease; the benefit of plasma exchange is unknown (1)[A].
- Less severe disease: CS alone ± other immunosuppressive agents (azathioprine 2 mg/kg/day, methotrexate 20 to 25 mg/week, mycophenolate mofetil 2,000 to 3,000 mg daily); hydroxychloroquine (5 mg/kg/day) use has been reported.
- Cutaneous PAN: Nonsteroidal anti-inflammatory drugs, dapsone, and colchicine are used.
- HBV-associated PAN: antiviral agents, short-term CS, plasma exchange
- Tocilizumab has been reported in treatment refractory, hepatitis B–negative PAN.
- Tumor necrosis inhibitors should be used in patients with clinical manifestations of deficiency of the enzyme Adenosine Deaminase 2 (DADA2) (1).

Second Line
- There is no well-defined second-line therapy in PAN.
- Infliximab (3 to 5 mg/kg IV at 0, 2, and 6 weeks, and every 4 to 8 weeks thereafter) and rituximab (1,000 mg IV on days 0 and 14 and then every 6 months *or* 375 mg/m² IV weekly for 4 weeks) anecdotally reported to be of benefit in refractory PAN.

ADDITIONAL THERAPIES
- For patients receiving IV cyclophosphamide, mercaptoethanesulfonate reduces bladder exposure to carcinogenic metabolites.
- Prophylactically treat patients on cyclophosphamide for *Pneumocystis jiroveci (carinii)* pneumonia with trimethoprim-sulfamethoxazole (use dapsone 100 mg/day or atovaquone 1,500 mg/day in intolerant/allergic patients).

COMPLEMENTARY & ALTERNATIVE MEDICINE
Physical therapy is recommended for patients with muscular or nerve disease (1).

ADMISSION, INPATIENT, AND NURSING CONSIDERATIONS
Depends on extent and involvement of specific organs

 ONGOING CARE

FOLLOW-UP RECOMMENDATIONS
- For patients with severe abdominal disease who become asymptomatic, follow-up vascular imaging is recommended (1).
- For patients with peripheral motor neuropathy symptoms, serial neurologic exams over periodic EMGs are recommended (1).

Patient Monitoring
- CBC, urinalysis, renal, and hepatic function tests; acute-phase reactants (e.g., ESR, CRP) may help monitor disease activity.
- The Five Factor Score (FFS) can predict mortality and guide treatment strategies. Factors used in the evaluation of patients with PAN include age, renal insufficiency, cardiac involvement, and GI manifestations. The fifth factor, ENT manifestations, is only applied to patients with ANCA-associated vasculitis.
- Be alert for side effects of immunosuppressant medications; delayed appearance of neoplasms, especially bladder malignancy in patients treated with cyclophosphamide (check annual U/A, urinary cytology with urologic evaluation if microscopic hematuria); steroid-induced osteoporosis

DIET
- Low-salt diet (HTN); Mediterranean diet for cardiovascular health
- Calcium and vitamin D–rich diets for patients on CS therapy

PATIENT EDUCATION
ACR Web site: https://www.rheumatology.org

PROGNOSIS
- Expected outcome of untreated PAN is poor. Patients presenting with proteinuria, renal insufficiency, GI tract involvement, cardiomyopathy, CNS involvement, or aged >65 years have a worse prognosis.
- Steroid and cytotoxic treatment increases 5-year survival rate to 75–80% (2).
- Survival is greater for hepatitis B–related PAN as a result of the introduction of antiviral treatments.

COMPLICATIONS
- End-organ damage from ischemia
- Complications from immunosuppressive agents

REFERENCES
1. Chung SA, Gorelik M, Langford CA, et al. 2021 American College of Rheumatology/Vasculitis Foundation guideline for the management of polyarteritis nodosa. *Arthritis Rheumatol.* 2021;73(8):1384–1393.
2. Pagnoux C, Seror R, Henegar C, et al; for French Vasculitis Study Group. Clinical features and outcomes in 348 patients with polyarteritis nodosa: a systematic retrospective study of patients diagnosed between 1963 and 2005 and entered into the French Vasculitis Study Group database. *Arthritis Rheum.* 2010;62(2):616–626.

 SEE ALSO

Hepatitis B; Hepatitis C

 CODES

ICD10
- M30.0 Polyarteritis nodosa
- M30.1 Polyarteritis with lung involvement [Churg-Strauss]
- M30.8 Other conditions related to polyarteritis nodosa

CLINICAL PEARLS

- PAN is a necrotizing vasculitis of small- to medium-sized muscular arteries with lack of granuloma formation that spares veins and pulmonary arteries.
- Clinical features of PAN depend on target organ involvement
- Skin biopsies at ulcer edges (include deep dermis and SC fat) improve diagnostic yield.
- Check hepatitis B and C serologies.
- ANCA is negative in classic PAN.
- At diagnosis, the revised FFS can determine prognosis and guide therapy.
- Treatment involves use of immunosuppressive drugs; the choice depends on the extent and severity of disease.

POLYCYSTIC KIDNEY DISEASE

Anila Khaliq, MD

 BASICS

DESCRIPTION
- A group of monogenic disorders that results in renal cyst development
- Autosomal dominant polycystic kidney disease (ADPKD) and autosomal recessive polycystic kidney disease (ARPKD)
- ADPKD is one of the most common human genetic disorders.

EPIDEMIOLOGY
- ADPKD is generally late onset with end-stage kidney disease (ESKD) developing in older adults.
- ARPKD is usually present in infants.

Prevalence
As ESKD, ADPKD: 8.7/1 million in the United States; 7/1 million in Europe

ETIOLOGY AND PATHOPHYSIOLOGY
- ADPKD results from *PKD1* and *PKD2* mutations, which encode for polycystin 1 (PC1) and polycystin 2 (PC2). The disrupted polycystin function results in fluid-filled cysts that progressively increase in size, leading to gross enlargement of the kidney, and distortion of the renal architecture.
- ARPKD secondary to *PKHD1* mutations

Genetics
- ADPKD: autosomal dominant inheritance
  - *PKD1* on chromosome 16p13.3 (85% of patients) encodes PC1.
  - *PKD2* on chromosome 4q21 (15% of patients) encodes PC2.
- ARPKD: autosomal recessive inheritance
  - Gene *PKHD1* on chromosome 6p21.1–p12 encodes fibrocystin.

RISK FACTORS
Family history

GENERAL PREVENTION
Genetic counseling

COMMONLY ASSOCIATED CONDITIONS
- ADPKD
  - Cysts in other organs
    - Polycystic liver disease in 58% of young age group to 94% of 45-year-olds
    - Pancreatic (5%); seminal (40%); arachnoid (8%)
  - Vascular manifestations
    - Intracerebral aneurysms in 6% of patients without family history and in 16% with family history
    - Aortic root dilation, dissections
  - Cardiac manifestations:
    - Mitral valve prolapse (25%); left Ventricular Hypertrophy
  - Diverticular disease
- ARPKD: liver involvement: affected in inverse proportion to renal disease; congenital hepatic fibrosis with portal HTN

DIAGNOSIS

HISTORY
- ADPKD
  - Positive family history (15% are de novo mutations.)
  - Flank pain: 60%
  - Hematuria
  - UTI
  - HTN: 50% aged 20 to 34 years; 100% with ESKD
  - Renal failure
  - Presymptomatic screening of ADPKD is not currently recommended for at-risk children (1).
- ARPKD
  - 30% of affected neonates die:
    - Enlarged echogenic kidneys and oligohydramnios are diagnosed in utero.
    - Later in childhood: HTN
  - Adolescents and adults present with complications of portal HTN: esophageal varices
  - Hypersplenism

PHYSICAL EXAM
- HTN
- Flank masses

DIFFERENTIAL DIAGNOSIS
- ADPKD and ARPKD
- Tuberous sclerosis: prevalence 1/6,000
- Von Hippel-Lindau syndrome: prevalence 1/36,000
- Nephronophthisis: accounts for 10–20% of cases of renal failure in children; medullary cystic kidney disease
- Renal cystic dysplasias: multicystic dysplastic kidneys: grossly deformed kidneys; most common type of bilateral cystic diseases in newborns (prevalence: 1/4,000)
- Simple cysts: most common cystic abnormality
  - Localized or unilateral renal cystic disease
  - Medullary sponge kidney
  - Acquired renal cystic disease
- Renal cystic neoplasms: benign multilocular cyst (cystic nephroma)

DIAGNOSTIC TESTS & INTERPRETATION
Electrolytes, BUN/creatinine, urinalysis plus urinary citrate

Initial Tests (lab, imaging)
- ADPKD
  - Renal dysfunction
    - Impaired renal concentration (2), hypocitraturia aciduria
    - Hyperfiltration
    - Elevated creatinine
  - Urinalysis: hematuria and mild proteinuria
- ARPKD
  - Electrolyte abnormalities and renal insufficiency
  - Anemia, thrombocytopenia, leukopenia

- ADPKD
  - US: It is the easiest diagnostic method; however, it is suboptimal for disease exclusion at age <40 years (1)[C].
    - Renal enlargement is universal.
    - In at-risk patients: By age 30 years, two renal cysts (bilateral or unilateral) are 100% diagnostic. In children, it sometimes appears similar to ARPKD; may be diagnosed in utero
    - Presence of hepatic cysts in young adults is pathognomonic for ADPKD.
    - In the absence of family history, bilateral renal enlargement and cysts make the diagnosis.
    - In subjects between ages 16 and 40 years and without an established family history, the presence of >10 cysts is considered diagnostic.
  - CT scan/MRI ideally should be part of the initial evaluation (1)[C].
    - Kidney volume assessed by CT or MRI is a main predictor of progression.
    - Helpful in identifying cysts in other organs
    - In subjects aged <40 years, fewer than five cysts by MRI excludes the diagnosis (1)[B].
    - In at-risk subjects aged <40 years, 10 ≥ cysts by MRI is considered sufficient for diagnosis with a sensitivity and specificity of 100%
- ARPKD
  - US: Kidneys are enlarged, homogeneously hyperechogenic (cortex and medulla).
  - CT scan is more sensitive if diagnosis is in doubt.
  - Presence of hepatic fibrosis helps the diagnosis.

Follow-Up Tests & Special Considerations
- Diagnosis and prevention of secondary problems because of renal and liver abnormalities
- Beyond age 2 years, renal size decreases in ARPKD but continues to grow in ADPKD at an average rate of 5.27% per year. Total kidney volume identifies patients with progressive disease (1).
- Consensus recommendations advise HTN screening in children with a family history of ADPKD from the age of 5 years onward with an interval of 3 years in cases where the child is normotensive.

Diagnostic Procedures/Other
- Genetic testing is available for *PKD1* and *PKD2* in ADPKD when imaging results are equivocal and for potential living related donors (3)[C].
- For *PKHD1* in ARPKD, a prenatal diagnosis is feasible in about 72% of patients.

Test Interpretation
- ADPKD
  - Kidneys are diffusely cystic and, although enlarged, retain their general shape.
  - Cysts range from a few millimeters to several centimeters and are distributed evenly throughout the cortex and medulla.

- They arise in all segments of the nephron, although they arise initially from the collecting ducts.
  - One kidney may be larger than the other.
  - In patients without established family history, the detection of more than ten cysts per kidney by ultrasonography is usually considered diagnostic.
- ARPKD
  - Disease is a spectrum, ranging from severe renal disease with mild liver damage to mild renal disease with severe liver damage.
  - Renal enlargement is due to fusiform dilatation of the collecting ducts in the cortex and medulla in the newborn period.
  - Liver lesion is diffuse but limited to fibrotic portal areas.
  - Diagnosis is likely based on clinical imaging in severe neonatal or infantile cases on the basis of enlarged echogenic kidneys, a negative family history, and lack of additional features.
  - Molecular diagnostic analysis is the gold standard for diagnosing this disorder.
  - Kidneys decrease in size over time as the amount of fibrosis increases.

 ## TREATMENT

GENERAL MEASURES
- HTN: moderate sodium restriction, weight control, and regular exercise
- Aggressive blood pressure control (<110/75 mm Hg) in subjects <50 years of age with preserved eGFR and no cardiovascular comorbidities is associated with a reduction in kidney volume over time and improved markers of left ventricular mass index and urinary albumin excretion.
- Medications: ACE inhibitors; angiotensin receptor blockers (ARBs)
- Pain: narcotics and other analgesics; bed rest; limit NSAIDs (they worsen renal function).
- Urolithiasis: treated with alkalinization of urine and hydration therapy; surgery as needed
- UTIs/infections of cysts: lipid-soluble antibiotics more effective (e.g., trimethoprim-sulfamethoxazole and chloramphenicol); fluoroquinolones are also useful
- Dialysis for ESKD patients
- Hematuria: Reduce physical activity.

MEDICATION
- Treatments that directly target cytogenic mechanisms such as decreasing cAMP levels in cystic tissues are now available. Tolvaptan slowed the rate of kidney growth and estimated GFR decline in patients with early ADPKD.
- Monitoring hepatic safety should be considered when prescribing tolvaptan
- HTN: should be very well controlled to prevent complications. ACE inhibitors are preferred if no contraindications are present.
- The use of antihypertensive medications has been found to decrease mortality (4)[B].
- Hyperlipidemia: statins preferred

ISSUES FOR REFERRAL
- Nephrologist primary management
- Urologic consultation for management of symptomatic/infected cysts
- Genetic counseling is critical.

SURGERY/OTHER PROCEDURES
- Indications for surgical intervention
  - Uncontrollable HTN
  - Severe back and loin pain, abdominal fullness
  - Renal deterioration due to enlarging cysts
  - Hematuria/hemorrhage or recurrent UTI
- Open and laparoscopic cyst unroofing: may decrease pain and narcotics requirements; has not been proven to prevent renal failure or to prolong current renal function
- Percutaneous cyst aspiration ± injection of sclerosing agent; not usually performed secondary to recurrent fluid accumulation
- Renal transplant for ESKD

ADMISSION, INPATIENT, AND NURSING CONSIDERATIONS
Severe pain, gross hematuria with clots

 ## ONGOING CARE

FOLLOW-UP RECOMMENDATIONS
None in early stages of the disease; avoid vigorous activity if disease advances. Recurrent gross hematuria is secondary to trauma, associated with faster decline of renal function.

Patient Monitoring
- Monitor BP and renal function. Encourage hydration. Treat UTI and stone disease aggressively.
- Avoid nephrotoxic drugs.
- Creatinine and BP monitoring at least twice a year; more often as needed
- Screening for intracranial aneurysms (5)
- No matter the severity of the disease, GFR remains within normal limits for decades, reducing its practicality as a marker for prognosis and progression of the disease state.

DIET
- Low-protein diet may retard renal insufficiency.
- Limit caffeine because this might increase cyst growth.
- High water intake to decrease ADH >3 L/day (6)[C]
- Limiting salt intake to ≤5 g per day

PROGNOSIS
- Renal failure in 2% by age 40 years; 23% by age 50 years; 48% by age 73 years
- ADPKD accounts for 10–15% of dialysis patients.
- No increased incidence of renal cell cancer
- Prognosis is variable and progression to ESRD is not predestined. Certain patients with PKD2 genotype or atypical PCKD may never progress to ESRD

COMPLICATIONS
- Cyst rupture, infection, or hemorrhage
- Progression to renal failure
- Renal calculi
- Cholangitis

REFERENCES
1. Chapman AB, Devuyst O, Eckardt KU, et al. Autosomal-dominant polycystic kidney disease (ADPKD): executive summary from a Kidney Disease: Improving Global Outcomes (KDIGO) controversies conference. *Kidney Int*. 2015;88(1):17–27.
2. Zittema D, Boertien WE, van Beek AP, et al. Vasopressin, copeptin, and renal concentrating capacity in patients with autosomal dominant polycystic kidney disease without renal impairment. *Clin J Am Soc Nephrol*. 2012;7(6):906–913.
3. Harris PC, Rossetti S. Molecular diagnostics for autosomal dominant polycystic kidney disease. *Nat Rev Nephrol*. 2010;6(4):197–206.
4. Patch C, Charlton J, Roderick PJ, et al. Use of antihypertensive medications and mortality of patients with autosomal dominant polycystic kidney disease: a population-based study. *Am J Kidney Dis*. 2011;57(6):856–862.
5. Rozenfeld MN, Ansari SA, Shaibani A, et al. Should patients with autosomal dominant polycystic kidney disease be screened for cerebral aneurysms? *AJNR Am J Neuroradiol*. 2014;35(1):3–9.
6. Mahnensmith RL. Novel treatments of autosomal dominant polycystic kidney disease. *Clin J Am Soc Nephrol*. 2014;9(5):831–836.

 ### SEE ALSO

Chronic Kidney Disease

 ### CODES

ICD10
- Q61.3 Polycystic kidney, unspecified
- Q61.2 Polycystic kidney, adult type
- Q61.1 Polycystic kidney, infantile type

CLINICAL PEARLS
- Most PKD patients eventually develop ESKD. No specific treatment has been proven to prevent ESKD, but hydration and control of BP are reasonable goals.
- Patients may benefit from a nephrology consultation after the initial diagnosis to counsel regarding disease progression prevention. Then, they can be followed by primary care if the disease was an incidental finding or no significant kidney dysfunction is present.

POLYCYSTIC OVARIAN SYNDROME (PCOS)

Loreal Dolar, DO • Jennifer A. Meeks, DO

 BASICS

DESCRIPTION

- Polycystic ovarian syndrome (PCOS) is a common endocrine disorder with heterogeneous manifestations that affects 6–10% of the U.S. population. It is characterized by hyperandrogenism, insulin resistance, and anovulation, typically presenting as amenorrhea or oligomenorrhea.
- Diagnostic clinical characteristics include menstrual dysfunction, infertility, hirsutism, acne, obesity, and metabolic syndrome. The ovaries are often polycystic on imaging but are not required for diagnosis.
- The etiology of PCOS is unknown, but presentation and course can be modified by lifestyle factors.
- System(s) affected: reproductive, endocrine/metabolic, skin/exocrine
- Synonym(s): Stein-Leventhal syndrome; polycystic ovary disease

ALERT
- Obesity may amplify PCOS, but it is not diagnostic. 20% of women with PCOS are not obese.
- Predisposes to and is associated with obesity, hypertension, diabetes, metabolic syndrome, hyperlipidemia, infertility, insulin-resistance syndrome, endometrial hyperplasia, and uterine cancer

EPIDEMIOLOGY

Incidence
Incidence and prevalence are still highly debated due to a wide spectrum of diagnostic features; the National Institutes of Health (NIH) criteria require chronic anovulation and hyperandrogenism.

Prevalence
The prevalence based on NIH criteria is 7% of reproductive age women.

ETIOLOGY AND PATHOPHYSIOLOGY

- Recent evidence points to a primary role for insulin resistance with hyperinsulinemia.
- Increased GnRH pulsations in the hypothalamus lead to increased production of LH with limited production of FSH.
- Hyperandrogenism: Ovaries are the main source of excess androgens (75% of circulating testosterone originates in the ovary). Polycystic ovaries have thickened thecal layers and overexpressed LH receptors, which cause excess androgen secretion.
- Ovarian follicles: Abnormal androgen signaling may account for abnormal folliculogenesis causing polycystic ovaries.
- Obesity results in compensatory hyperinsulinemia: Women with PCOS have insulin resistance similar to that in type 2 diabetes. Elevated levels of insulin decrease sex hormone–binding globulin (SHBG), increasing bioavailability of testosterone. Insulin may also act directly on adrenal glands, ovaries, and hypothalamus to enhance androgen production.
- Insulin resistance causes elevated insulin levels and the frequently associated metabolic syndrome or frank diabetes mellitus.

Genetics
Likely a combination of polygenic and environmental factors. Implicated genes include *DENND1A* and *THADA*.

RISK FACTORS
See "Commonly Associated Conditions"; cause and effect are difficult to extricate in this disorder.

GENERAL PREVENTION
None known; focus on early diagnosis and treatment to prevent long-term complications.

COMMONLY ASSOCIATED CONDITIONS
Infertility, obesity, obstructive sleep apnea, hypertension, diabetes mellitus, endometrial hyperplasia/carcinoma, fatty liver disease, mood disturbances and depression, hirsutism

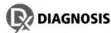 **DIAGNOSIS**

HISTORY
A comprehensive history, including a family history of diabetes and premature onset of cardiovascular disease, is important in the differential diagnosis. Focus on the onset and duration of the various signs of androgen excess, menstrual history, and concomitant medications, including the use of exogenous androgens. Unpredictable, heavy, or absent menstrual cycles

PHYSICAL EXAM
- Vital signs: elevated body mass index (BMI), hypertension
- General appearance: central obesity, hirsutism, acne
- Skin: male hair pattern, balding, acne, seborrhea, acanthosis nigricans
- Pelvic: ovarian enlargement, clitoromegaly

ALERT
Look specifically for signs of virilization, such as hair pattern, deepened voice, and clitoromegaly because they indicate significant testosterone levels beyond that of PCOS.

DIFFERENTIAL DIAGNOSIS
- Cushing syndrome, androgen-secreting ovarian or adrenal tumor
- HAIR-AN syndrome
- Thyroid disease, acromegaly, Prolactin-producing pituitary adenoma
- Adult-onset adrenal hyperplasia, partial congenital adrenal hyperplasia (21-hydroxylase deficiency)
- 11β-Hydroxylase deficiency or 17β-Hydroxysteroid dehydrogenase deficiency
- Drug-induced hirsutism, oligo-ovulation (e.g., danazol, steroids, valproic acid)
- Idiopathic hirsutism

DIAGNOSTIC TESTS & INTERPRETATION
- Most commonly used diagnostic criteria is the Rotterdam criteria (need any 2 of 3): Oligomenorrhea or amenorrhea, clinical and/or biochemical signs of hyperandrogenism, transvaginal ultrasonographic evidence of polycystic ovaries
- The value of measurement of circulating androgens to document PCOS is uncertain but should include calculating free testosterone concentration using mass spectrometry of total testosterone and measurement of SHBG.

- Must exclude other etiologies including Cushing disease, congenital adrenal hyperplasia, and androgen-secreting tumors
- Ultrasonographic polycystic ovaries are not necessary for the diagnosis of PCOS.
- More recent criteria also focus on similar criteria while acknowledging that there may be forms of PCOS without overt evidence of hyperandrogenism.

Initial Tests (lab, imaging)
- Screening workup should rule out pregnancy, thyroid disease, hyperprolactinemia, congenital adrenal hyperplasia, and premature ovarian failure. Serum testing includes human chorionic gonadotropin (hCG), TSH, prolactin, 17-OH progesterone, and FSH.
- Hirsute women should have a free testosterone determination (total testosterone minus SHBG) and a DHEA-S.
- Workup to rule out hypothalamic amenorrhea (LH and FSH), androgen-secreting tumors (FSH, estradiol, testosterone, DHEA-S), Cushing syndrome (24-hour urinary free cortisol), and acromegaly (IGF-1) should be considered based on clinical characteristics (1).
- Typical findings in PCOS include testosterone increased but <200 ng/dL (6.94 nmol/L), mild elevation in DHEA-S but <800 μg/dL (20.8 μmol/L), mild increase in 17-OH progesterone level, increased estrogen level, and decreased SHBG.
- Anovulation can be determined by a midluteal phase progesterone level (>3 ng/mL if the woman has ovulated).
- LH/FSH level ≥2.5 to 3 in ~50% of women with PCOS, but such testing is not generally necessary.
- Drugs that may alter lab results: oral contraceptive pills (OCPs), steroids, antidepressants
- Transvaginal ultrasound findings: one or both ovaries with ≥12 follicles measuring 2 to 9 mm or increased ovarian volume to 10 cm³

Follow-Up Tests & Special Considerations
- Consider fasting serum glucose, insulin level, and plasminogen activator inhibitor-1 determinations to establish presence of insulin resistance and glucose intolerance, especially if diagnosis is in doubt.
- Endometrial biopsy to rule out hyperplasia and/or carcinoma, if indicated
- If the syndrome is diagnosed, determination of fasting glucose and fasting lipid levels should be performed and formal glucose tolerance test is considered.

ALERT
Prolonged or heavy bleeding should prompt an endometrial biopsy for evaluation of endometrial hyperplasia and possible cancer.

Test Interpretation
- Ovary is usually enlarged with a smooth white glistening capsule.
- Ovarian cortex is lined with follicles in all stages of development but most atretic.
- Thecal cell proliferation with an increase in the stromal compartment

TREATMENT

GENERAL MEASURES

Lifestyle changes including appropriate nutrition and exercise to decrease body weight by as little as 5% can restore ovulation and increase insulin sensitivity (1)[A]. Treatment plans should be individualized based on patient needs and desires.

MEDICATION

- The goal of treatment in PCOS depends on symptoms and patient's goals for fertility.
- Treatment can be divided into four main categories: (i) restore menses, (ii) decrease insulin resistance, (iii) ameliorate androgen excess, and (iv) assist in fertility.

First Line

- Restore menses when pregnancy not desired:
  - OCPs and progestins provide improvement in menstrual irregularity and provide endometrial protection.
  - Low-dose OCPs (30 to 35 μg); newer formulations containing progestins with lower androgenicity (e.g., norethindrone, desogestrel, norgestimate, drospirenone) may be particularly beneficial, but all OCPs increase SHBG and decrease excess androgens. Discuss benefits and balance against slightly increased thrombotic potential of third- and fourth-generation progestins as compared with older progestins.
  - Levonorgestrel IUD offers endometrial protection and pregnancy prevention but will not counteract hyperandrogenism (2).
  - If unable to tolerate OCPs, then intermittent medroxyprogesterone (Provera) 10 mg PO, or micronized progesterone (Crinone and Prometrium) 200 mg PO, for 10 to 14 days can be given every 1 to 3 months (2)[C]. These offer endometrial protection. However, these will not counteract hyperandrogenism or protect against pregnancy.
- Decrease insulin resistance:
  - Metformin may help to correct metabolic abnormalities in women who are insulin resistant. Initial dose is 500 mg daily for 1 week, increasing by 500 mg/week to a total of 1,500 to 2,000 mg/day divided BID; take with food.
    - Overall, data support the usefulness of metformin on both cardiometabolic risk, weight loss, and reproduction assistance in women with PCOS.
    - Thiazolidinediones may increase likelihood of ovulation and treat insulin resistance but do not increase live birth rate.
- If pregnancy is desired:
  - Letrozole (an aromatase inhibitor) has increased ovulation rates, clinical pregnancy rates, and live birth rates compared to clomiphene (Clomid). Live birth rate with letrozole is 27.5%. Dosing starts on day 3, 4, or 5 with 2.5 mg daily for 5 days; can increase to 5 mg daily with max dose 7.5 mg daily for 5 days
  - Counsel patients that letrozole is not approved by the FDA for ovulation induction.

- Metformin: 500 to 2,000 mg PO divided BID has been shown to improve hyperandrogenism and restore ovulation. Some providers will choose to continue metformin throughout the 1st trimester or the entire pregnancy if there is a history of spontaneous abortion or glucose intolerance. It does improve ovulation rates and insulin resistance but does not improve live birth rates alone or in combination with clomiphene when used for ovulation induction.
- Metformin reduces the incidence of gestational diabetes.
- All ovulation induction drugs increase the risk of multiple births and obstetric complications, such as preterm birth and hypertensive disorders.

Second Line

- Acne:
  - OCPs with low-androgenicity progestins for example, norethindrone, desogestrel, norgestimate, drospirenone
  - Spironolactone: 50 to 200 mg daily in 1 to 2 divided doses for acne and hirsutism not addressed by OCP therapy. This medication is unsafe in pregnancy, and potassium levels must be followed when used.
- Hirsutism:
  - Eflornithine hydrochloride 13.9% cream BID
  - Finasteride 2.5 to 5 mg daily; must be on very reliable contraception as this medication is teratogenic

ISSUES FOR REFERRAL

To reproductive endocrinologist for all women who cannot achieve pregnancy with clomiphene (Clomid) or letrozole

ADDITIONAL THERAPIES

If excess hair is uncomfortable, mechanical means of hair removal, including laser, electrolysis, waxing, and depilatory, may improve cosmesis.

SURGERY/OTHER PROCEDURES

Ovarian wedge resection and laparoscopic laser drilling are considered second line therapies but can be considered controversial and are rarely used today.

 ONGOING CARE

FOLLOW-UP RECOMMENDATIONS

6-month intervals to evaluate response to therapy and to monitor weight and medication side effects

Patient Monitoring

- Counsel patient about the risk of endometrial and breast carcinoma, insulin resistance, and diabetes as well as obesity and its role in infertility.
- See patient frequently throughout the menstrual cycle, depending on which drug combination is used to induce ovulation.
- All patients with PCOS who have not received medication or IUD for endometrial protection and have been amenorrheic for 1 year should undergo endometrial biopsy.

DIET

In overweight patients, weight loss is the most successful therapy because it improves cardiovascular risk, insulin sensitivity, menstrual patterns, and infertility: counsel on lifestyle dietary changes; consider referral to nutritionist and weight center. No specific diet plan is proven to be better than another.

PATIENT EDUCATION

- Provide patient with information about PCOS, such as from http://www.acog.org/.
- Review the importance of exercise and weight loss, if applicable. Modest weight loss of 5–10% of initial body weight has been demonstrated to improve many of the features of PCOS.

PROGNOSIS

- Fertility prognosis is good but may need assisted reproductive technologies.
- Proper follow-up and screening can prevent endometrial carcinoma.
- Early detection of diabetes may decrease morbidity and mortality associated with cardiovascular risk factor.

COMPLICATIONS

- Predisposes to endometrial hyperplasia and as high as 9% lifetime risk of endometrial cancer
- Women with PCOS appear to be at increased risk of complications of pregnancy including gestational diabetes and hypertensive disorders.

REFERENCES

1. Tang T, Lord JM, Norman RJ, et al. Insulin-sensitising drugs (metformin, rosiglitazone, pioglitazone, D-chiro-inositol) for women with polycystic ovary syndrome, oligo amenorrhoea and subfertility. *Cochrane Database Syst Rev*. 2012;(5):CD003053.
2. McCartney CR, Marshall JC. Clinical practice. Polycystic ovary syndrome. *N Engl J Med*. 2016; 375(1):54–64.

 SEE ALSO

Algorithm: Amenorrhea, Secondary

 CODES

ICD10

- E28.2 Polycystic ovarian syndrome
- L68.0 Hirsutism

CLINICAL PEARLS

- PCOS is diagnosed based on 2 of 3 of (i) oligoovulation, (ii) signs of hyperandrogenism, and (iii) polycystic ovaries. Polycystic ovaries are not required for the diagnosis of PCOS.
- Treat chronic anovulation to reduce risk of endometrial hyperplasia.

POLYCYTHEMIA VERA

Alexander Sasha Rackman, MD • Lislie Lisete Gonzalez Veitia, MD

BASICS

DESCRIPTION
- Polycythemia vera (PV) is a myeloproliferative clonal stem cell disorder marked by increased production of red blood cells (erythrocytosis) with excessive erythroid, myeloid, and megakaryocytic elements in the bone marrow.
- Morbidity and mortality are primarily related to complications from blood hyperviscosity leading to thrombosis development as well as malignant transformation. Untreated patients may survive 6 to 18 months. Adequate treatment may extend life to >10 years.
- Myelofibrosis (MF) can develop in the bone marrow, leading to progressive hepatosplenomegaly.
- Synonyms: primary polycythemia; maladie de Vaquez disease; primary PV; PV rubra; polycythemia, splenomegalic; Vaquez-Osler disease

EPIDEMIOLOGY
Incidence
- Predominant age: 50 to 75 years; however, can occur in early adulthood and childhood
- Predominant sex: male > female (slightly)
- Incidence in the United States in 2012: 2.8/100,000 population of men and 1.3/100,000 population of women; highest for men 70 to 79 years at 23.5/100,000 persons per year

Prevalence
In the United States in 2010, estimates ranged from 45 to 57 cases per 100,000 patients.

ETIOLOGY AND PATHOPHYSIOLOGY
JAK2 V617F mutation associated with clonal proliferative disorder

Genetics
JAK2 V617F (tyrosine kinase) mutation: >97% of patients with PV have an activating mutation; this is helpful in differentiating from secondary erythrocytosis. Homozygote carriers will have higher incidence of symptoms such as pruritus but will not have higher incidence of disease than heterozygotes.

RISK FACTORS
- PV may be slightly more prevalent among Jews of Eastern European descent than other Europeans or Asians.
- Familial history is rare.

COMMONLY ASSOCIATED CONDITIONS
- Budd-Chiari syndrome
- Ischemic digits
- Mesenteric artery thrombosis
- Myocardial infarction
- Cerebrovascular accident or transient ischemic attack
- Venous thromboembolism and pulmonary embolism

DIAGNOSIS

HISTORY
- Patients may be asymptomatic or present with nonspecific complaints, including fatigue, malaise, weight loss, sweating, and subjective weakness.
- Erythromelalgia (burning pain of feet/hands, occasionally with erythema, pallor, cyanosis, or paresthesias)
- Pruritus, especially after bathing (aquagenic pruritus)
- Arterial and venous occlusive events
- Headaches
- Blurred vision or blind spots
- Tinnitus, vertigo, dizziness
- Spontaneous bruising/bleeding
- Peptic ulcer disease (due to alterations in gastric mucosal blood flow)
- Early satiety due to enlarged spleen
- Bone pain (ribs and sternum)
- Gout
- Insomnia
- Depressed mood

PHYSICAL EXAM
- Hypertension (46%)
- Splenomegaly (75%), palpable spleen (36%)
- Hepatomegaly (30%)
- Facial plethora (ruddy cyanosis)
- Bone tenderness (especially ribs and sternum)
- Skin excoriations from significant pruritus
- Gouty tophi or arthritis
- Injection of the conjunctival small vessels and/or engorgement of the veins of the optic fundus

DIFFERENTIAL DIAGNOSIS
- Essential thrombocytopenia
- Secondary erythrocytosis:
  - Sleep apnea
  - Emphysema
  - Cigarette smoking
  - Renal artery stenosis
  - Carbon monoxide poisoning
  - Drugs: diuretics, testosterone replacement, erythropoietin (EPO)
- Hemoglobinopathy
- Ectopic EPO production
- Spurious polycythemia

DIAGNOSTIC TESTS & INTERPRETATION
- CBC; if suspicion is high, then obtain EPO level and gene testing for *JAK2 V617F*.
- If the only indication of PV is elevated hemoglobin (Hgb)/hematocrit (Hct), a CBC should be repeated. Further testing is unnecessary if the Hgb/Hct return to normal.

Initial Tests (lab, imaging)
- 2016 World Health Organization diagnostic criteria requires all three major criteria or the first 2 major criteria and the minor criterion* (1).
  - Major criteria:
    - Hgb >16.5 g/dL (men); Hgb >16 g/dL (women) or Hct >49% (men); Hct >48% (women) or increased cell mass (>25% above mean normal predictive value)
    - Bone marrow biopsy showing hypercellularity for age with trilineage growth (panmyelosis) including prominent erythroid, granulocytic, and megakaryocytic proliferation with pleomorphic, mature megakaryocytes (difference in sizes)
    - Presence of *JAK2 V617F* or similar mutation such as *JAK2* exon 12 mutation
  - Minor criteria:
    - Serum EPO level below normal *criterion number 2 (bone marrow biopsy) may not be required in cases with substantive absolute erythrocytosis: Hgb >18.5 g/dL in men (Hct, 55.5%) or >16.5 g/dL in women (Hct, 49.5%) if major criterion 3 and minor criterion are present. However, initial MF (present in up to 20% of points) can only be detected by performing a bone marrow biopsy; this finding may predict a more rapid progression to overt myelofibrosis (post-PV MF).
- Other lab findings that are common but not specific
  - Hyperuricemia
  - Hypercholesterolemia
  - Elevated serum vitamin B_{12} levels
  - Prolonged PT, aPTT due to low plasma volume
  - Thrombocytosis (>400,000 platelets/mm^3)
  - Leukocytosis (>12,000/mm^3)
  - Leukocyte alkaline phosphatase (100,000 U in the absence of fever or infection)
- CT or US to assess for splenomegaly, although not necessary for diagnosis
- Arterial oxygen saturation (<92% SaO_2) and carboxyhemoglobin (COHb)
- Bone marrow biopsy is not necessary. There is no staging system for this disease.

Diagnostic Procedures/Other
- Bone marrow aspiration if performed shows hypercellularity of erythroid, granulocytic and megakaryocytic lines, or myelofibrosis.
- Cytogenetic testing (*JAK2 V617F*)

Test Interpretation
- If *JAK2 V617F* mutation testing is negative and the EPO level is normal or high, then PV is excluded; investigate causes of secondary erythrocytosis.
- *JAK2 V617F* mutation in exon 14 is a distinguishing feature versus secondary polycythemia but not specific to PV as it can also be present in essential thrombocytopenia and primary myelofibrosis.
- Other causes of erythrocytosis such as ectopic EPO production from a renal tumor, hypoxia from chronic lung, or cyanotic heart disease can be excluded with low or undetectable serum EPO level and normal oxygen saturation.

TREATMENT
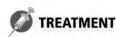

GENERAL MEASURES
- Risk factors: Patients aged >60 years with history of thrombosis are high risk. Those who are <60 years of age with no history of thrombosis but with elevated platelets (>150,000) are intermediate risk. Those who are <60 years of age, with normal platelets, and no history of thrombosis are low risk.
- Phlebotomy and low-dose aspirin is first-line therapy for all patients.

- Although not curative, modern therapy for PV can relieve symptoms and prolong survival.
- If secondary PV, address etiology: aggressive treatment of obstructive sleep apnea, COPD (especially smoking cessation), renal disease; consider lowering dose in testosterone replacement.
- Phlebotomy reduces the blood hyperviscosity, improves platelet function, restores systemic pressures, and decreases risk of thrombosis.
- Phlebotomy:
  - Reduce Hct to <45%; will significantly lower rate of cardiovascular death and major thrombosis (2)[A]
  - Performed initially as often as every 2 to 3 days until normal Hct reached; phlebotomies of 250 to 500 mL (1 unit—500 mL—phlebotomy should reduce Hct by 3 percentage points). Reduce to 250 to 350 mL in elderly patients or patients with cerebrovascular disease.
  - Frail patients should have volume replaced with saline solution to avoid postural hypotension.
  - High risk for thrombosis or presence of elevated platelet count is indication for cytoreductive therapy.
  - Complications of phlebotomy: chronic iron deficiency (symptomatology: pica, angular stomatitis, and glossitis), possible muscle weakness, and dysphagia that is the result of esophageal webs (very rare)
- Other therapies:
  - Maintain hydration.
  - Pruritus therapy: H_1 and H_2 blockers, SSRIs, oatmeal baths, interferon α-2b
  - Uric acid reduction therapy

MEDICATION

First Line
- Primary therapies:
  - Low-dose aspirin 81 mg PO has been associated with a statistically nonsignificant reduction in the risk of fatal thrombotic events without increasing bleeding complications when used in conjunction with phlebotomy (3)[A]. Aspirin should not be used in those with acquired von Willebrand disease or those with other contraindications.
  - Hydroxyurea is recommended for patients at high risk for thrombosis (age >60 years or history of thrombotic event) and with splenomegaly and hepatomegaly. Common starting dose 500 to 1,500 mg PO daily, titrating to control Hct and platelet count. Be aware that hydroxyurea can lead to skin ulcer, myelosuppression, and higher risk of leukemic transformation (4)[A].
  - Ruxolitinib is approved for refractory PV or for patients who are intolerant to hydroxyurea.
  - Radioactive phosphorus (^{32}P) may control Hgb level and platelet count by destroying overactive marrow cells. May take up to 3 months before affecting cells. Consider for patients intolerant or nonadherent to hydroxyurea or short expected survival due to mutagenic potential.
  - Pegylated interferon α-2a is effective in controlling erythrocytosis, although dosing is generally limited secondary to intolerable side effects; usually recommended for younger patients (<40 years old) and those who might become pregnant (4)
  - Refer to hematologist/oncologist for further dosing and instructions.

- Symptomatic/adjunctive:
  - Allopurinol 300 mg/day PO for uric acid reduction
  - Cyproheptadine 4 to 16 mg PO daily as needed for pruritus
  - H_2 receptor blockers or antacids for GI hyperacidity; cimetidine is also used for pruritus.
  - Low-dose aspirin also used for pruritus/erythromelalgia
  - SSRIs (paroxetine or fluoxetine) have shown some efficacy in controlling pruritus.
  - Ultraviolet light therapy may help with pruritus.

Second Line
Myelosuppression: chlorambucil or busulfan; busulfan at 2 to 4 mg daily may be effective option for elderly patients with advanced PV refractory or intolerant to other agents such as hydroxyurea and interferon, but significant rate of transformation was observed.

ISSUES FOR REFERRAL
Referral to a hematologist to assist in diagnosis and management.

COMPLEMENTARY & ALTERNATIVE MEDICINE
Osteopathic manipulative medicine to promote circulation

ADMISSION, INPATIENT, AND NURSING CONSIDERATIONS
DVT prophylaxis should be given.

 ONGOING CARE

FOLLOW-UP RECOMMENDATIONS
Monitor for secondary malignancies such as myeloproliferative neoplasms.

Patient Monitoring
Monitor Hct often and phlebotomize as needed to maintain target goal.

DIET
- Avoid high-sodium diet; can cause fluid retention
- Avoid iron supplement; a permissive chronic state of iron deficiency can help decrease blood production.

PATIENT EDUCATION
- Perform leg and ankle exercises to prevent clots.
- Continuous education regarding possible complications and seeking treatment early for any change or increase in symptoms

PROGNOSIS
- PV cannot be cured but can be controlled with treatment.
- Survival is >15 years with treatment.
- Patients are at risk for developing postpolycythemic myelofibrosis (PPMF) and an increased risk of malignant transformation.

COMPLICATIONS
- Splenomegaly or hepatomegaly
- Budd-Chiari syndrome
- Vascular thrombosis (major cause of death) (20%)
- Transformation to acute leukemia (5%)
- Transformation to myelofibrosis (10%)

- Hemorrhage
- Peptic ulcer
- Uric acid stones
- Secondary gout
- Increased risk for complications and mortality from surgical procedures; assess risk/benefits and ensure optimal control of disorder before any elective surgery.

REFERENCES
1. Arber DA, Orazi A, Hasserjian R, et al. The 2016 revision to the World Health Organization classification of myeloid neoplasms and acute leukemia. *Blood.* 2016;127(20):2391–2405.
2. Marchioli R, Finazzi G, Specchia G, et al; for CYTO-PV Collaborative Group. Cardiovascular events and intensity of treatment in polycythemia vera. *N Engl J Med.* 2013;368(1):22–33.
3. Squizzato A, Romualdi E, Passamonti F, et al. Antiplatelet drugs for polycythaemia vera and essential thrombocythaemia. *Cochrane Database Syst Rev.* 2013;(4):CD006503.
4. Mascarenhas J, Mughal TI, Verstovsek S. Biology and clinical management of myeloproliferative neoplasms and development of the JAK inhibitor ruxolitinib. *Curr Med Chem.* 2012;19(26):4399–4413.

ADDITIONAL READING
Kim T-Y, Kwag D, Lee JH, et al. Clinical features, gene alterations, and outcomes in prefibrotic and overt primary and secondary myelofibrotic patients. *Cancers (Basel).* 2022;14(18):4485.

 SEE ALSO

Myeloproliferative Neoplasms

 CODES

ICD10
D45 Polycythemia vera

CLINICAL PEARLS
- Erythrocytosis: Hgb >16.5 g/dL in men, >16 g/dL in women
- *JAK2* mutations are an important component of myeloproliferative disorders.
- *Bone marrow biopsy can help in diagnosis showing hypercellularity and trilineage growth.*
- Common complications include thrombosis, malignant transformation, and MF.
- All patients should take low-dose aspirin unless there is major bleeding or GI intolerance.
- Phlebotomy is first-line treatment, and consultation with an experienced hematologist is recommended.

POLYMYALGIA RHEUMATICA
Juliana Chang, MD

BASICS

DESCRIPTION
- An inflammatory clinical syndrome characterized by pain and morning stiffness of the shoulder, hip girdles, and neck; primarily impacts patients aged >50 years; associated with morning stiffness and elevated markers of inflammation
- Can be associated with giant cell arteritis (GCA)
- System(s) affected: musculoskeletal; hematologic/lymphatic/immunologic
- Synonym(s): senile rheumatic disease; polymyalgia rheumatica (PMR) syndrome; pseudo-polyarthrite rhizomélique

Geriatric Considerations
Incidence increases with age (age >50 years).

Pediatric Considerations
Rare in patients <50 years of age (1)

EPIDEMIOLOGY
Incidence
- Incidence increases after age 50 years. Incidence of PMR and GCA in the United States is 50 and 18 per 100,000 people, respectively.
- Predominant sex: female > male (2 to 3:1)
- Most common in Caucasians, especially those of Northern European ancestry and in Scandinavian countries
- Peak incidence occurs between ages 70 and 80 years.

Prevalence
Prevalence in those >50 years old: 700/100,000

ETIOLOGY AND PATHOPHYSIOLOGY
- Unknown; symptoms relate to enhanced immune system and periarticular inflammatory activity.
- Pathogenesis
  - Polygenic; involves multiple environmental and genetic factors
  - Significant association between histologic evidence of GCA and parvovirus B19 DNA in temporal artery specimen

Genetics
Associated with human leukocyte antigen determinants (HLA-DRB1*04 and DRB1*01 alleles)

RISK FACTORS
- Aged >50 years
- Presence of GCA

COMMONLY ASSOCIATED CONDITIONS
Concurrent GCA (temporal arteritis) in ~15–30% of patients; more commonly in females than males

DIAGNOSIS

HISTORY
- Suspect PMR in elderly patients with new onset of proximal limb pain and stiffness (neck, shoulder, hip). Patients may use the term "stiffness" and "pain" interchangeably (2). Shoulder pain is most typically present.
- Symptoms often have a rapid onset.
- Difficulty rising from chair or combing hair (proximal muscle involvement) or putting on clothes like shirt or coat
- Nighttime pain
- Can be unilateral; however, soon it becomes symmetrical
- Severe morning stiffness
- Nonspecific systemic symptoms in ~25% (fatigue, weight loss, low-grade fever, depression, anorexia)
- Carpal tunnel syndrome can be seen in 10–15% of patients.
- Duration is usually >2 weeks.

PHYSICAL EXAM
- Decreased range of motion (ROM) of shoulders, neck, and hips
- Muscle strength is usually normal—may be limited by pain and/or stiffness.
- Muscle tenderness
- Disuse atrophy
- Synovitis of the small joints and tenosynovitis; feet and ankles are never affected.
- Coexisting carpal tunnel syndrome

DIFFERENTIAL DIAGNOSIS
- Rheumatoid arthritis (RA)
- Palindromic rheumatism
- Late-onset seronegative spondyloarthropathies (e.g., psoriatic arthritis, ankylosing spondylitis)
- Systemic lupus erythematosus; Sjögren syndrome; fibromyalgia
- Polymyositis-dermatomyositis (Check creatine phosphokinase and aldolase.)
- Thyroid disease; hyperparathyroidism, hypoparathyroidism
- Hypovitaminosis D
- Osteoarthritis
- Rotator cuff syndrome; adhesive capsulitis
- RS3PE syndrome (remitting seronegative symmetrical synovitis with pitting edema)
- Occult infection or malignancy (e.g., lymphoma, leukemia, myeloma, solid tumor)
- Myopathy (e.g., steroid, alcohol, electrolyte depletion)
- Depression; fibromyalgia

DIAGNOSTIC TESTS & INTERPRETATION
ACR/EULAR classification criteria (3):
- Patients aged ≥50 years with bilateral shoulder aching and abnormal C-reactive protein concentrations or ESR, plus at least 4 points (without ultrasonography) or 5 points or more (with ultrasonography) from:
  - Morning stiffness for >45 minutes (2 points)
  - Hip pain or restricted ROM (1 point)
  - Absence of rheumatoid factor (RF) or anti–citrullinated protein antibodies (ACPAs) (2 points)
  - Absence of other joint involvement (1 point)
  - If ultrasonography is available, at least one shoulder with subdeltoid bursitis, biceps tenosynovitis, or glenohumeral synovitis (either posterior or axillary); and at least one hip with synovitis or trochanteric bursitis (1 point)
  - If ultrasonography is available, both shoulders with subdeltoid bursitis, biceps tenosynovitis, or glenohumeral synovitis (1 point)
- Temporal artery biopsy if symptoms of GCA is present
- ESR (Westergren) elevation >40 mm/hr
  - ESR generally elevated, sometimes >100 mm/hr
  - ESR normal (<40 mm/hr) in 7–22% of patients
- Elevated C-reactive protein
- Normochromic/normocytic anemia
- Anti–cyclic citrullinated peptide (anti-CCP) antibodies are usually negative (in contrast to elderly-onset RA).
- RF: negative (5–10% of patients aged >60 years have positive RF without RA.)
- Mild elevations in liver function tests, especially alkaline phosphatase
- Antibodies to ferritin peptide may be a useful diagnostic marker.
- Prednisone may alter lab results.
- Other disorders may cause elevation of ESR (e.g., infection, neoplasm, renal failure).
- Normal EMG
- Normal muscle histology
- CK is always normal.

Initial Tests (lab, imaging)
- ESR (usually >40 mm/hr); C-reactive protein; CBC (normocytic anemia)
- MRI is not necessary for diagnosis but may show periarticular inflammation, tenosynovitis, and bursitis.
- US may show bursitis, tendinitis, and synovitis.
- MRI, PET, and temporal artery US may help in diagnosis of PMR.
- ACR/EULAR classification criteria help confirm the clinical diagnosis.
- ¹⁸F-fluorodeoxyglucose PET scan prior to therapy improves diagnostic accuracy.

- A scoring algorithm was devised consisting of the following: morning stiffness >45 minutes (2 points), hip pain/limited ROM (1 point), absence of RF and ACPA (2 points), and absence of peripheral joint pain (1 point).
- A score of >4 has 68% sensitivity and 78% specificity for PMR.

Diagnostic Procedures/Other
Temporal artery biopsy in patients with symptoms suggestive of GCA; treat empirically pending results.

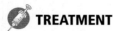

TREATMENT

GENERAL MEASURES
- Address risk of steroid-induced osteoporosis.
  - Obtain dual energy x-ray absorptiometry, and check 25-OH vitamin D levels if necessary.
  - Consider antiresorptive therapies (bisphosphonates) for treatment of corticosteroid-induced osteoporosis.
- Encourage adequate calcium (1,500 mg/day) and vitamin D (800 to 1,000 U/day) supplementation.
- Physical therapy for ROM exercises, if needed

MEDICATION
First Line
- Prednisone: 10 to 20 mg/day PO initially; expect a dramatic (diagnostic) response within days. 15 mg/day is effective in almost all patients.
  - May increase to 20 mg/day if no immediate response
  - If no response to 10 to 20 mg/day within a week, reconsider diagnosis.
- Divided-dose steroids (BID or TID) may be useful initially (especially if symptoms recur in the afternoon).
- Consider using delayed-release prednisone taken at bedtime, which may help treat morning stiffness compared to immediate-release prednisone.
- Begin slow taper by 2.5 mg decrements every 2 to 4 weeks to a dose of 7.5 to 10.0 mg/day. Below this dose, taper by 1 mg/month to prevent relapse.
- Increase prednisone for symptom relapse (common).
- Corticosteroid treatment often lasts for several years.
- May stop after 6 to 12 months if symptom free and ESR is normal
- Contraindications
  - Use steroids with caution in patients with chronic heart failure, diabetes mellitus (or other immunocompromised state), and systemic fungal or bacterial infection.
  - Treat any concurrent infections.
- Precautions
  - Long-term steroid use (>2 years) is associated with sodium and water retention, exacerbation of chronic heart failure, hypokalemia, increased susceptibility to infection, osteoporosis, fractures, hypertension, cataracts, glaucoma, avascular necrosis, depression, and weight gain.

- Patients may develop temporal arteritis while on low-dose corticosteroid treatment for PMR. This requires an increase in prednisone dosing (up to 40 to 60 mg).
  - Alternate-day steroids are not effective.

Second Line
- Routine use of adjunctive therapy is not recommended.
- NSAIDs usually are not adequate for pain relief.
- Methotrexate modestly reduces relapse rate and lowers the cumulative dose of steroid therapy but has not been formally studied in PMR.
- Tocilizumab (IL-6 inhibitor) has been reported in case reports and small studies.
- There is a conflicting evidence for anti-tumor necrosis factor (anti-TNF) agents (infliximab, etanercept).
- Rituxan (rituximab) may have a role in treatment based on a small proof of concept trial (4).
- Corticosteroid injections (primarily for the shoulder) may help reduce the pain and the duration of morning stiffness, allowing for increased levels of activity.

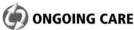

ONGOING CARE

FOLLOW-UP RECOMMENDATIONS
Patient Monitoring
- Monthly evaluations initially and during medication taper; every 3 months otherwise
- Follow ESR as steroids are tapered; ESR and C-reactive protein should decline as symptoms improve.
- Follow up immediately for symptoms of GCA (e.g., headache, visual loss, diplopia).
- Monitor the side effects of corticosteroid therapy (osteoporosis, hypertension, and hyperglycemia).
- If patient is asymptomatic, do not treat elevated ESR (do not increase steroid dose to normalize ESR).

DIET
- Regular diet
- Adequate calcium and vitamin D intake

PATIENT EDUCATION
- Review adverse effects of corticosteroids.
- Discuss the symptoms of GCA (headache, visual loss, diplopia) and present immediately if any occur.
- Follow up if symptoms recur during steroid taper.
- Do not abruptly stop steroids.
- Ensure adequate calcium and vitamin D intake.
- Patient resources:
  - Arthritis Foundation: https://www.arthritis.org/
  - American College of Rheumatology: https://www.rheumatology.org/I-Am-A/Patient-Caregiver/Diseases-Conditions/Polymyalgia-Rheumatica

PROGNOSIS
- Most patients require at least 2 years of corticosteroid treatment.
- Exacerbation or relapse is common if steroids are tapered too quickly.

- Prognosis is very good with proper treatment.
- Relapse is common (in 25–50% of patients).
- Higher age at diagnosis, female sex, high baseline ESR, increased levels of soluble IL-6 receptor, and high initial steroid dose have been associated with a prolonged disease course and more disease flares.

COMPLICATIONS
- Complications related to chronic steroid use
- Exacerbation of disease with taper of steroids; development of GCA (may occur when PMR is being treated adequately)

REFERENCES

1. El Chami S, Springer JM. Update on the treatment of giant cell arteritis and polymyalgia rheumatica. *Med Clin North Am*. 2021;105(2):311–324.
2. Lally L, Spiera R. Management of difficult polymyalgia rheumatica and giant cell arteritis: updates for clinical practice. *Best Pract Res Clin Rheumatol*. 2018;32(6):803–812.
3. Dasgupta B, Cimmino MA, Maradit-Kremers H, et al. 2012 Provisional classification criteria for polymyalgia rheumatica: a European League Against Rheumatism/American College of Rheumatology collaborative initiative. *Ann Rheum Dis*. 2012;71(4):484–492.
4. Espígol-Frigolé G, Dejaco C, Mackie SL, et al. Polymyalgia rheumatica. *Lancet*. 2023;402(10411):1459–1472.

ADDITIONAL READING

Figus FA, Skoczyńska M, McConnell R, et al. Imaging in polymyalgia rheumatica: which technique to use? *Clin Exp Rheumatol*. 2021;39(4):883–888.

 SEE ALSO

Arteritis, Temporal; Arthritis, Rheumatoid (RA); Depression; Fibromyalgia; Osteoarthritis; Polymyositis/ Dermatomyositis

 CODES

ICD10
- M35.3 Polymyalgia rheumatica
- M31.5 Giant cell arteritis with polymyalgia rheumatica

CLINICAL PEARLS
- Consider PMR in patients aged >50 years who present with hip, neck, and/or shoulder pain and stiffness.
- A normal ESR does not exclude PMR.
- Corticosteroids are the treatment of choice. If there is no dramatic and rapid response, reconsider the diagnosis.
- Adjust steroids according to symptoms, not ESR.

POLYMYOSITIS/DERMATOMYOSITIS

Christopher M. Wise, MD • Nehal R. Shah, MD

BASICS

DESCRIPTION
- Systemic connective tissue disease characterized by inflammatory and degenerative changes in proximal muscles, sometimes accompanied by characteristic skin rash
  - If skin manifestations (Gottron sign [symmetric, scaly, violaceous, erythematous eruption over the extensor surfaces of the metacarpophalangeal and interphalangeal joints of the fingers]; heliotrope [reddish violaceous eruption on the upper eyelids]) are present, it is designated as dermatomyositis.
  - Different types of myositis include the following (1):
    ○ Idiopathic polymyositis
    ○ Idiopathic dermatomyositis
    ○ Polymyositis/dermatomyositis as an overlap (usually with lupus or systemic sclerosis or as part of mixed connective tissue disease)
    ○ Myositis associated with malignancy
    ○ Necrotizing autoimmune myositis (often statin associated)
    ○ Inclusion body myositis (IBM), a variant with atypical patterns of weakness and biopsy findings
- System(s) affected: cardiovascular, musculoskeletal, pulmonary, skin/exocrine
- Synonym(s): myositis; inflammatory myopathy; antisynthetase syndrome (subset with certain antibodies)

EPIDEMIOLOGY
Incidence
- Estimated at 1.2 to 19 per million population per year
- Predominant age: 5 to 15 years, 40 to 60 years, peak incidence in mid-40s
- Predominant sex: female > male (2:1)

Prevalence
2.4 to 33.8 patients per 100,000 population

Geriatric Considerations
Elderly patients with myositis or dermatomyositis are at increased risk of neoplasm.

Pediatric Considerations
Childhood dermatomyositis is likely a separate entity associated with cutaneous vasculitis and muscle calcifications.

ETIOLOGY AND PATHOPHYSIOLOGY
- Inflammatory process, mediated by T cells and cytokine release, leading to damage to muscle cells (predominantly skeletal muscles)
- In patients with IBM, degenerative mechanisms may be important.
- Unknown; potential viral, genetic factors

Genetics
Mild association with human leukocyte antigen (HLA)-DR3, HLA-DRw52

RISK FACTORS
Family history of autoimmune disease (e.g., systemic lupus erythematosus (SLE), myositis) or vasculitis

COMMONLY ASSOCIATED CONDITIONS
- Malignancy more common in dermatomyositis subtype, older patients
- Progressive systemic sclerosis
- Vasculitis
- SLE
- Mixed connective tissue disease

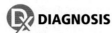

DIAGNOSIS

HISTORY
- Symmetric proximal muscle weakness causing difficulty when
  - Arising from sitting or lying positions
  - Climbing stairs
  - Raising arms
- Joint pain/swelling
- Dysphagia
- Dyspnea
- Rash on face, eyelids, hands, arms

PHYSICAL EXAM
Proximal muscle weakness
- Shoulder muscles
- Hip girdle muscles (trouble standing from seated or squatting position, weak hip flexors in supine position)
- Muscle swelling, stiffness, induration
- Distal muscle weakness is seen only in patients with IBM.
- Rash over face (eyelids, nasolabial folds), upper chest, dorsal hands (especially knuckle pads), fingers ("mechanic's hands")
- Periorbital edema
- Calcinosis cutis (childhood cases)
- Mesenteric arterial insufficiency/infarction (childhood cases)
- Cardiac impairment; arrhythmia, heart failure

DIFFERENTIAL DIAGNOSIS
- Vasculitis
- Progressive systemic sclerosis
- SLE
- Rheumatoid arthritis
- Muscular dystrophy
- Lambert-Eaton syndrome
- Sarcoidosis
- Amyotrophic lateral sclerosis
- Endocrine disorders
  - Thyroid disease
  - Cushing syndrome
- Infectious myositis (viral, bacterial, parasitic)
- Drug-induced myopathies:
  - Cholesterol-lowering agents (statins)
  - Colchicine
  - Corticosteroids
  - Ethanol
  - Chloroquine
  - Zidovudine
- Electrolyte disorders (magnesium, calcium, potassium)
- Heritable metabolic myopathies
- Sleep apnea syndrome

DIAGNOSTIC TESTS & INTERPRETATION
- Diagnosis of muscle component (myositis) usually relies on four findings:
  - Weakness
  - Creatine kinase (CK) and/or aldolase elevation
  - Abnormal electromyogram (EMG) results
  - Findings on muscle biopsy
- Presence of compatible skin rash of dermatomyositis
- There is an emerging role for myositis-specific antibody (MSA) profiles. MSAs can be used to guide the appropriate workup for malignancy and interstitial lung disease (ILD) (2).

Initial Tests (lab, imaging)
- Increased CK, aldolase
- Increased serum aspartate aminotransferase (AST)
- Increased lactate dehydrogenase (LDH)
- Myoglobinuria
- Increased ESR
- Positive rheumatoid factor (<50% of patients)
- Positive antinuclear antibody (ANA) (>50% of patients)
- Leukocytosis (<50% of patients)
- Anemia (<50% of patients)
- Hyperglobulinemia (<50% of patients)
- Anti-3-hydroxy-3-methylglutaryl-coenzyme A reductase (HMGCR) and anti-SRP antibodies seen in patient with necrotizing autoimmune myositis
- Antisynthetase antibodies (anti–Jo-1 and non–Jo-1 synthetases) present in antisynthetase syndrome
  - Associated with an increased incidence of ILD
- Anti–MDA-5 antibody seen in overlap myositis with atypical rashes and severe ILD
- Anti–U1-RNP, anti-PM/Scl, and anti-Ku antibodies seen in overlap myositis
- Chest radiograph as part of initial evaluation to assess for associated pulmonary involvement or malignancy

Follow-Up Tests & Special Considerations
- Changes in muscle enzymes (CK or aldolase) correlate with improvement and worsening.
- MRI to assess muscle edema and inflammation may be used in some patients to determine best biopsy site or response to therapy.

Diagnostic Procedures/Other
- EMG: muscle irritability, low-amplitude potentials, polyphasic action potentials, fibrillations
- Muscle biopsy (deltoid or quadriceps femoris)

Test Interpretation
- Microscopic findings:
  - Muscle fiber degeneration
  - Phagocytosis of muscle debris
  - Perifascicular muscle fiber atrophy
  - Inflammatory cell infiltrates in adult form
  - Via electron microscopy: inclusion bodies (IBM only)
  - Sarcoplasmic basophilia
- Muscle fiber increased in size
- Vasculopathy (childhood polymyositis/dermatomyositis)

TREATMENT

GENERAL MEASURES
Approach to treatment has varied by specialty involved (dermatology, rheumatology, neurology). Treatment approach should be informed by lesion type, degree of muscle involvement, presence of systemic symptoms, presence of MSAs, and patient's age (2)[C],(3).

MEDICATION
First Line
- Prednisone
  - 0.5–1 mg/kg/day PO in divided doses
  - IV pulse dose methylprednisone 1,000 mg daily for 3 to 5 days in acute and severe cases
  - Consolidate doses and reduce prednisone slowly when enzyme levels are normal.
  - Probably need to continue 5 to 10 mg/day for maintenance in most patients
- Immunosuppressive maintenance therapy in parallel to steroids—recommended in most patients:
  - Azathioprine 1 to 2 mg/kg PO (arthritis dose) once daily or BID, or
  - Methotrexate 10 to 25 mg PO weekly, or
  - Mycophenolate mofetil 2 to 3 mg daily
- Rash of dermatomyositis may require topical steroids or oral hydroxychloroquine.
- Patients with IBM have very poor response to steroids and other first- and second-line drugs in general.

Second Line
- Other immunosuppressant drugs (e.g., cyclophosphamide, chlorambucil, cyclosporine, tacrolimus) can be added to steroids in refractory cases. Adrenocorticotropic (ACTH) gel may have a role in refractory cases.
- Combination methotrexate and azathioprine also may be useful in refractory cases.
- IVIG and rituximab have been reported to be helpful in a small series of patients with refractory disease. Rituximab (Rituxan) may be more effective in patients with autoantibodies positive myositis (especially anti–Jo-1 and anti–Mi-2). IVIG can be a reasonable alternative in patients whom steroids or other immunosuppressive drugs are contraindicated such as infection and neoplasm.
- Cyclophosphamide is usually reserved for severe cases with lung or heart involvement.
- Contraindications: Methotrexate is contraindicated with previous liver disease, alcohol use, pregnancy, and underlying renal disease (use with extreme caution in patients with serum creatinine >1.5 mg/dL in general).
- Precautions
  - Prednisone: Adverse effects associated with long-term steroid use include adrenal suppression, sodium and water retention, hypokalemia, osteoporosis, cataracts, and increased susceptibility to infection.
  - Azathioprine: Adverse effects include bone marrow suppression, increased liver function tests, and increased risk of infection.
  - Methotrexate: Adverse effects include stomatitis, bone marrow suppression, pneumonitis, and risk of liver fibrosis and cirrhosis with prolonged use.

ISSUES FOR REFERRAL
- Diagnostic uncertainty, usually related to elevated muscle enzymes without typical symptoms of findings of muscle weakness
- Poor response to initial steroid therapy
- Excessive steroid requirement (unable to taper prednisone to <20 mg/day after 4 to 6 months)

SURGERY/OTHER PROCEDURES
None indicated, other than initial biopsy

COMPLEMENTARY & ALTERNATIVE MEDICINE
Benefits and harms of physical therapy are not well established, especially in active muscle disease (4)[A], although there is some suggestion of benefit in quiescent disease (5)[A]. Research is of low quality in this area.

ADMISSION, INPATIENT, AND NURSING CONSIDERATIONS
- Inability to stand, ambulate, respiratory difficulty, fever, or other signs of infection
- Inpatient evaluation seldom needed

ONGOING CARE

FOLLOW-UP RECOMMENDATIONS
Patient Monitoring
- Follow muscle enzymes along with muscle strength and functional capacity.
- Monitor for steroid-induced complications (e.g., hypokalemia, hypertension, and hyperglycemia).
- Bone densitometry and consideration of calcium, vitamin D, and bisphosphonate therapy
- If azathioprine, methotrexate, or other immunosuppressant is used, appropriate laboratory monitoring should be done periodically (e.g., hematology, liver enzymes, and creatinine).
- Attempt to decrease and/or discontinue steroid dose as patient responds to therapy.
- Maintain immunosuppression until patient's muscle strength stabilizes for prolonged period depending on individual patient parameters, risks of medication, and risk of relapse; time period undefined (months, years)

DIET
Moderation of caloric and sodium intake to avoid weight gain from corticosteroid therapy

PATIENT EDUCATION
Curtail excess physical activity in early phases when muscle enzymes are markedly elevated. Emphasize range of motion exercises. Gradually introduce muscle strengthening when muscle enzymes are normal or improved and stable.

PROGNOSIS
- Residual weakness: 30%, persistent active disease: 20%
- 5-year survival is 65–75%, but mortality is 3- to 5-fold higher than general population. Most of the increase in mortality occurs in the 1st year after diagnosis. Survival is worse for women and African Americans and those with dermatomyositis, IBM, or cancer.
- Most patients improve with therapy.
- Patient with ILD have poor prognosis.
- Patients with IBM respond poorly to most therapies.
- 20–50% have full recovery.

COMPLICATIONS
Pneumonia, infection, myocardial infarction, carcinoma (especially breast, lung), severe dysphagia, respiratory impairment due to muscle weakness, ILD, aspiration pneumonitis, steroid myopathy, steroid-induced diabetes, hypertension, hypokalemia, osteoporosis

REFERENCES
1. Senécal JL, Raynauld JP, Troyanov Y. Editorial: a new classification of adult autoimmune myositis. *Arthritis Rheumatol*. 2017;69(5):878–884.
2. Waldman R, DeWane ME, Lu J. Dermatomyositis: diagnosis and treatment. *J Am Acad Dermatol*. 2020;82(2):283–296.
3. Lundberg IE. Expert perspective: management of refractory inflammatory myopathy. *Arthritis Rheumatol*. 2021;73(8):1394–1407.
4. Voet NB, van der Kooi EL, van Engelen BG, et al. Strength training and aerobic exercise training for muscle disease. *Cochrane Database Syst Rev*. 2019;12(12):CD003907.
5. Van Thillo A, Vulsteke JB, Van Assche D, et al. Physical therapy in adult inflammatory myopathy patients: a systematic review. *Clin Rheumatol*. 2019;38(8):2039–2051.

ADDITIONAL READING
Mammen AL. Statin-associated autoimmune myopathy. *N Engl J Med*. 2016;374(7):664–669.

CODES

ICD10
- M33.20 Polymyositis, organ involvement unspecified
- M33.90 Dermatopolymyositis, unspecified, organ involvement unspecified
- M33.92 Dermatopolymyositis, unspecified with myopathy

CLINICAL PEARLS
- Corticosteroids alone may be sufficient in patients who have rapid improvement in weakness and muscle enzymes. However, most patients require azathioprine, methotrexate, or other immunosuppressive medications.
- Elevated muscle enzymes (e.g., CK and aldolase) are seen frequently as transient phenomena in patients with febrile illness and injuries; may return to normal on repeat
- In patients with persistently elevated muscle enzymes and symptoms and findings of muscle weakness, EMG followed by muscle biopsy should be the initial studies considered.
- Suspect IBM in older patients with very slow onset and progression of symptoms, poor response to steroids and immunosuppressive therapy, and atypical patterns (asymmetric, sometimes distal) of muscle weakness.

POPLITEAL (BAKER) CYST

Shane L. Larson, MD • Christopher Morrow, PA-C

BASICS

DESCRIPTION
- A fluid-filled synovial sac arising in the popliteal fossa as a distention of (typically) the gastrocnemial-semimembranous bursa; not a true cyst
- Can be unilateral or bilateral
- Most frequent cystic mass around the knee
- Primary cysts are a distention of the bursa (arise independently without an intra-articular disorder).
- Secondary cysts occur if there is a communication between the bursa and knee joint, allowing articular fluid to fill the cyst.
- Associated with synovial inflammation

EPIDEMIOLOGY
Incidence
- Bimodal distribution
  - Children ages 4 to 7 years
  - Adults increasing with age
- Primary cysts usually seen in children <15 years
- Secondary cysts seen in adults

Prevalence
- Variable adult prevalence of 19–47% in symptomatic knees and 2–5% in asymptomatic knees
- In children: 6.3% in symptomatic knees; 2.4% in asymptomatic knees

ETIOLOGY AND PATHOPHYSIOLOGY
Associated intra-articular pathology includes
- Meniscal tears, mostly of the posterior horn
- Anterior cruciate ligament (ACL) insufficiency
- Degenerative articular cartilage lesions
- Rheumatoid arthritis (20%)
- Osteoarthritis (50%)
- Osteochondritis
- Gout (14%)
- Other potential factors
  - Infectious arthritis
  - Polyarthritis
  - Villonodular synovitis
  - Lymphoma
  - Sarcoidosis
  - Connective tissue diseases

- Extension or herniation of synovial membrane of the knee joint capsule or connection of normal bursa with the joint capsule
- May result from increased intra-articular pressure
- Commonly seen with knee effusions
- Direct trauma to the bursa is likely the primary cause in children because of no communication between the bursa and the joint.
- A valve-like mechanism allowing one-way passage of fluid from the joint to the bursal connection has been described.

RISK FACTORS
- Osteoarthritis of knee (most common)
- Rheumatoid arthritis
- Meniscal degeneration or tear
- Advancing age
- Ligamentous trauma
- Ligamentous insufficiency

COMMONLY ASSOCIATED CONDITIONS
Any condition causing knee joint effusion

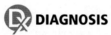

DIAGNOSIS

HISTORY
- Painless mass arising in the popliteal fossa
- Most cysts are asymptomatic.
- Dull ache if cyst is large enough to impede joint motion—typically a restriction of flexion
- Painful if cyst ruptures
- Large cysts may cause entrapment neuropathy of the tibial nerve.
- Vascular compression, most commonly of the popliteal vein, may produce claudication or thrombophlebitis.
- Activity alters the cyst size.

PHYSICAL EXAM
- Examine in full extension and 90 degrees of flexion.
- Foucher sign: Mass increases with extension and disappears with flexion.
- Most commonly found in medial aspect of popliteal fossa lateral to the head of the gastrocnemius and medial to the neurovascular bundle

- Cyst is easiest to palpate when knee is slightly flexed and may occasionally be fluctuant or tender.
- Transillumination helps distinguish cyst from solid mass.
- Ruptured cysts are typically painful with associated swelling and bruising over the ipsilateral calf and ankle at the medial malleolus (crescent sign).
- Ruptured cysts also are associated with pseudothrombophlebitis, and rarely, compartment syndrome (1).

DIFFERENTIAL DIAGNOSIS
- Deep venous thrombosis
- Infection/abscess
- Ganglion cyst
- Hematoma
- Thrombophlebitis
- Lipoma, liposarcoma
- Fibroma, fibrosarcoma
- Vascular tumor
- Popliteal vein varices
- Xanthoma
- Aneurysm (rare)
- Muscular herniation (rare, related to trauma)

DIAGNOSTIC TESTS & INTERPRETATION
Initial Tests (lab, imaging)
- CBC, ESR (if septic arthritis suspected)
- Ensure not a popliteal aneurysm prior to aspiration. Send aspirate for cell count and culture to determine if fluid is infectious, inflammatory, or mechanical.
- Ultrasound confirms presence and size; Doppler can differentiate Baker cysts from popliteal vessel aneurysms, DVT, or soft tissue tumors (2).
- MRI helps assess derangements of internal joint structures and to identify cyst leakage.

Follow-Up Tests & Special Considerations
- Consider observation over invasive testing in children.
- Radiographs may show soft tissue density posteriorly.
- Arthrography may demonstrate communication with joint capsule or rupture.
- CT arthrography is superior for visualizing cystic details and can help distinguish lipomas, aneurysms, and malignancies from cysts.

TREATMENT

GENERAL MEASURES
- No treatment if asymptomatic
- Treat any associated underlying conditions.
- Compressive wrap or sleeve for comfort

MEDICATION
If etiology is identified from cellular fluid examination, treat the underlying condition.

First Line
Analgesics and NSAIDs for symptomatic relief

ADDITIONAL THERAPIES
- Physical therapy improves knee ROM and strength, particularly with coexisting pathology.
- Temporary relief with needle aspiration; recurrence common
- Improvement in joint ROM, knee pain, swelling, accompanied reduction in bursa size after aspiration, and intra-articular/intracystic corticosteroid injection (3)[B]
- A combination of physical therapy and corticosteroid injection with or without aspiration leads to best improvements in pain, function, and reduction in cyst size (4)[A].
- Sclerotherapy injections of ethanol or dextrose/sodium morrhuate shown to have good results in small studies (5)[B].

SURGERY/OTHER PROCEDURES
- Consider excision when symptoms persist despite treatment or no etiology is found.
- Surgery usually not required in children
- Recurrence after standard surgery is common and is highest if chondral lesions are present.
- Arthroscopic surgery is highly successful if a valvular mechanism is identified and intra-articular pathology is treated (6)[B].
- Excision via arthroscopy or open procedure often requires concomitant treatment of underlying pathology.

 ## ONGOING CARE

PROGNOSIS
- Variable; many cysts remain asymptomatic.
- Some cysts resolve with treatment of underlying etiology (e.g., gout, rheumatoid arthritis).
- In children, most cysts resolve without treatment.

COMPLICATIONS
- Compartment syndrome in ruptured cyst
- Thrombophlebitis from compression of the popliteal vein
- Infection of popliteal cyst
- Hemorrhage into cyst if on anticoagulants

REFERENCES

1. Chatzopoulos D, Moralidis E, Markou P, et al. Baker's cysts in knees with chronic osteoarthritic pain: a clinical, ultrasonographic, radiographic and scintigraphic evaluation. *Rheumatol Int.* 2008;29(2):141–146.
2. Sanchez JE, Conkling N, Labropoulos N. Compression syndromes of the popliteal neurovascular bundle due to Baker cyst. *J Vasc Surg.* 2011;54(6):1821–1829.
3. Acebes JC, Sánchez-Pernaute O, Díaz-Oca A, et al. Ultrasonographic assessment of Baker's cysts after intra-articular corticosteroid injection in knee osteoarthritis. *J Clin Ultrasound.* 2006;34(3):113–117.
4. Di Sante L, Paoloni M, Dimaggio M, et al. Ultrasound-guided aspiration and corticosteroid injection compared to horizontal therapy for treatment of knee osteoarthritis complicated with Baker's cyst: a randomized, controlled trial. *Eur J Phys Rehabil Med.* 2012;48(4):561–567.
5. Centeno CJ, Schultz J, Freeman M. Sclerotherapy of Baker's cyst with imaging confirmation of resolution. *Pain Physician.* 2008;11(2):257–261.
6. Lie CW, Ng TP. Arthroscopic treatment of popliteal cyst. *Hong Kong Med J.* 2011;17(3):180–183.

ADDITIONAL READING

- Akagi R, Saisu T, Segawa Y, et al. Natural history of popliteal cysts in the pediatric population. *J Pediatr Orthop.* 2013;33(3):262–268.
- Akgul O, Guldeste Z, Ozgocmen S. The reliability of the clinical examination for detecting Baker's cyst in asymptomatic fossa. *Int J Rheum Dis.* 2014;17(2):204–209.
- Han JH, Bae JH, Nha KW, et al. Arthroscopic treatment of popliteal cysts with and without cystectomy: a systematic review and meta-analysis. *Knee Surg Relat Res.* 2019;31(2):103–112.
- Su C, Kuang S-D, Zhao X, et al. Clinical outcome of arthroscopic internal drainage of popliteal cysts with or without cyst wall resection. *BMC Musculoskelet Disord.* 2020;21(1):440.
- Van Nest DS, Tjoumakaris FP, Smith BJ, et al. Popliteal cysts: a systematic review of nonoperative and operative treatment. *JBJS Rev.* 2020;8(3):e0139.

 ## SEE ALSO

Algorithm: Knee Pain

CODES

ICD10
- M71.20 Synovial cyst of popliteal space [Baker], unspecified knee
- M71.21 Synovial cyst of popliteal space [Baker], right knee
- M71.22 Synovial cyst of popliteal space [Baker], left knee

CLINICAL PEARLS

- Baker cyst: a fluid-filled synovial sac arising in the popliteal fossa as a distention of (typically) the gastrocnemial-semimembranous bursa; not a true cyst; often secondary to meniscal tear, osteoarthritis, etc.
- Conservative treatment of Baker cysts is preferred in children, as most will spontaneously resolve.
- In adults, treatment of underlying cause may resolve Baker cysts.
- Pain, bruising, and swelling over the medial malleolus (crescent sign) suggest cyst rupture.

PORTAL HYPERTENSION

Walter M. Kim, MD, PhD

BASICS

DESCRIPTION
- Increased portal venous pressure >5 mm Hg that occurs in association with splanchnic vasodilatation, portosystemic collateral formation, and hyperdynamic circulation
- Most commonly secondary to elevated hepatic venous pressure gradient (HVPG; the gradient between portal and central venous pressures)
- Course is progressive, with risk of acute variceal bleeding, ascites, hepatic encephalopathy, portopulmonary syndrome, and hepatorenal syndrome.

EPIDEMIOLOGY
Prevalence
- Prevalence: <200,000 persons in the United States
- Predominant sex: male > female adults

ETIOLOGY AND PATHOPHYSIOLOGY
- Develops as a consequence of resistance to blood flow in the portal venous system
- Causes generally classified as follows:
  - Prehepatic (portal vein thrombosis or obstruction)
  - Intrahepatic (most commonly cirrhosis or schistosomiasis)
  - Posthepatic (hepatic vein thrombosis, Budd-Chiari syndrome, right-sided heart failure)
- 90% of intrahepatic cases are due to cirrhosis secondary to the following:
  - Virus (hepatitis B, hepatitis C, hepatitis D)
  - Alcoholism
  - Nonalcoholic fatty liver disease
  - Schistosomiasis
  - Wilson disease
  - Hemochromatosis
  - Primary biliary cholangitis (PBC)
  - Sarcoidosis
- Increased HVPG results in venous collateral formation in the distal esophagus, proximal stomach, rectum, and umbilicus.
- Progression of portal hypertension results in splanchnic vasodilation and angiogenesis.
- Gastroesophageal variceal formation is found in 40% of patients with portal hypertension.

RISK FACTORS
Pediatric Considerations
Portal vein thrombosis is the most common extrahepatic cause; intrahepatic causes are more likely to be biliary atresia, viral hepatitis, and metabolic liver disease.

COMMONLY ASSOCIATED CONDITIONS
- Alcoholism
- Cirrhosis
- Nonalcoholic fatty liver disease
- Schistosomiasis
- Extrahepatic portal vein thrombosis

DIAGNOSIS

HISTORY
- Ascites; symptoms of heart failure including chest pain, shortness of breath, and/or edema
- Hematemesis
- Melena
- Oliguria
- Jaundice
- Weakness/fatigue
- History of chronic liver disease
- Alcoholic hepatitis
- Alcohol abuse

PHYSICAL EXAM
- Exam findings may be general or related to specific complications.
- General
  - Pallor
  - Icterus
  - Digital clubbing
  - Palmar erythema
  - Splenomegaly
  - Caput medusa
  - Spider angioma
  - Abdominal bruit
  - Hemorrhoids
  - Gynecomastia
  - Testicular atrophy
- Gastroesophageal varices
  - Hypotension
  - Tachycardia
- Ascites
  - Distended abdomen
  - Fluid wave
  - Shifting dullness with percussion
- Hepatic encephalopathy
  - Confusion/coma
  - Asterixis
  - Hyperreflexia

DIFFERENTIAL DIAGNOSIS
- Gastroesophageal varices with hemorrhage
  - Portal hypertensive gastropathy
  - Hemorrhagic gastritis
  - Peptic ulcer disease
  - Mallory-Weiss tear
- Ascites
  - Spontaneous bacterial peritonitis (SBP)
  - Pancreatic ascites
  - Peritoneal carcinomatosis
  - Tuberculous peritonitis
  - Hepatic malignancy
  - Fluid overload from heart failure
  - Nephrotic syndrome
- Hepatic encephalopathy
  - Delirium tremens
  - Intracranial hemorrhage
  - Sedative abuse
  - Uremia
- Hepatorenal syndrome
  - Drug nephrotoxicity
  - Renal tubular necrosis

DIAGNOSTIC TESTS & INTERPRETATION
Initial Tests (lab, imaging)
Direct calculation of HVPG (approximation of the gradient in pressure between portal vein and inferior vena cava) is the gold standard in diagnosing portal hypertension:
- HVPG = wedged hepatic venous pressure (WHVP) − free hepatic venous pressure (FHVP)
- WHVP is estimated by occlusion of the hepatic vein by a balloon catheter and measurement of the proximal static column of blood.
- FHVP is estimated by direct measurement of the patent hepatic vein, intra-abdominal inferior vena cava, or right atrium.
- Esophageal varices generally develop when HVPG >10 mm Hg in compensated cirrhosis and HVPG >16 mm Hg in decompensated cirrhosis.
- Nonspecific changes associated with underlying disease:
  - Hypersplenism: anemia (also may be due to malnutrition or bleeding), leukopenia, thrombocytopenia
  - Hepatic dysfunction
    - Hypoalbuminemia
    - Hyperbilirubinemia
    - Elevated alkaline phosphatase
    - Elevated liver enzymes (AST, ALT)
    - Abnormal clotting (prothrombin time, international normalized ratio, partial thromboplastin time)
  - GI bleeding
    - Iron deficiency anemia
    - Elevated serum ammonia
    - Fecal occult blood
    - Thrombocytopenia
  - Hepatorenal syndrome
    - Elevated serum creatinine (Cr), blood urea nitrogen (BUN)
    - Urine sodium <5 mEq/L (<5 mmol/L)
  - US and CT scan/MRI may detect cirrhosis, splenomegaly, ascites, and varices.
  - US/duplex Doppler
    - Can determine presence and direction of flow in portal and hepatic veins
    - Useful in diagnosing portal vein thrombosis, shunt thrombosis, or the presence of ascites
  - CT scan/MRI: angiographic measurement of hepatic venous wedge pressure via jugular or femoral vein
    - Correlates with portal pressure
    - Risk of variceal bleeding is increased if HVPG >12 mm Hg.
  - Transient elastography is a noninvasive method to determine hepatic fibrosis/cirrhosis and to predict portal hypertension.

Follow-Up Tests & Special Considerations
- If portal hypertension is diagnosed in a patient with no risk factors, the patient should first be evaluated for cirrhosis.
- HVPG response to nonselective β-blockers is associated with a significant reduction in risk of variceal bleeding and decompensation.

Diagnostic Procedures/Other

- Diagnostic paracentesis and calculation of the serum-ascites albumin gradient (SAAG) can differentiate portal hypertensive (SAAG >1.1 g/dL) from nonportal hypertensive (SAAG <1.1 g/dL) causes of ascites.
- Upper endoscopy should be performed in patients with cirrhosis for variceal screening and can diagnose the presence of esophageal and gastric varices and portal hypertensive gastropathy.

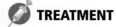 **TREATMENT**

GENERAL MEASURES

- Avoid sedatives that may precipitate encephalopathy.
- Limit sodium intake because cirrhotic patients avidly retain sodium (<2 g sodium per day).

MEDICATION

First Line

- Prophylaxis against variceal bleeding:
  - Nonselective β-blockade
    - Nadolol: 20 to 40 mg PO once-daily dosing
    - Propranolol: Start with 20 to 40 mg PO BID to TID.
  - May consider carvedilol: 6.25 mg PO once-daily dosing as an alternative β-blocker
  - Doses may be titrated up as tolerated to maximum recommended doses; goal resting heart rate of 55 to 60 beats/min
- Therapy for acute variceal hemorrhage:
  - Octreotide: 50 μg IV bolus followed by 50 μg/hr continuous infusion; pediatric dose: 1 μg/kg bolus followed by 1 μg/kg/hr is used traditionally; treat for up to 5 days.
  - Vasopressin: Start with 0.2 to 0.4 U/min IV; increase to maximum dose 0.8 U/min as needed; pediatric dose: 0.002 to 0.005 U/kg/min; do not exceed 0.01 U/kg/min. After bleeding stops, continue at same dose for 12 hours and then taper off over 24 to 48 hours.
- For prevention of recurrence and for overall reduction in mortality:
  - Nadolol: 40 to 80 mg/day PO reduces portal venous blood inflow by blocking the adrenergic dilatation of the mesenteric arterioles.
  - Propranolol: 10 to 60 mg/day PO BID–QID; pediatric dose: 0.5 to 1.0 mg/kg/day PO divided q6–8h
  - Tetrandrine, a calcium channel blocker, also has been found to reduce the rate of rebleeding with fewer side effects.
- Initial treatment for ascites (along with salt and fluid restriction):
  - Furosemide: 20 to 40 mg/day PO; pediatric dose: 1 to 2 mg/kg/dose PO
  - Spironolactone: 50 to 100 mg/day PO; pediatric dose: 1 to 3 mg/kg/day PO

Second Line

- Terlipressin (2 mg IV q4h; titrate down to 1 mg IV q4h once hemorrhage is controlled; may be used for up to 48 hours) is a more selective splanchnic vasoconstrictor and may be associated with fewer complications. It is currently used when standard therapy with somatostatin or octreotide fails.
- Addition of nitrates, such as nitroglycerin or isosorbide mononitrate, reduces portal pressures and bleeding rates and has been shown to reduce mortality. Because the risk–benefit ratio is not clear, nitrates are not considered first-line treatment.

SURGERY/OTHER PROCEDURES

- Treatments available for specific complications of portal hypertension (in addition to or if refractory to medications):
  - Gastroesophageal varices without hemorrhage
    - Endoscopic variceal ligation (EVL) is the preferred therapy for prevention of bleeding of large (grade II or III) varices and requires serial interventions every 2 to 8 weeks until the varices are eradicated.
  - Gastroesophageal varices with hemorrhage
    - EVL or sclerosis (the first-line treatment in many cases for acute hemorrhage) within 12 hours of presentation (1)[A]
    - Balloon tamponade (not used commonly when endoscopic treatment is available)
    - Transjugular intrahepatic portosystemic shunt (TIPS)
    - Portacaval shunting
  - Ascites refractory to medical management
    - Large-volume paracentesis
    - Peritoneovenous shunt
    - TIPS (relatively contraindicated in patients with acute or recurrent hepatic encephalopathy)
- Liver transplantation should be considered for patients with advanced disease.

ADMISSION, INPATIENT, AND NURSING CONSIDERATIONS

- Acute bleeding from the intestinal tract, either vomiting or per rectum
- Acute confusional state/mental status changes
- If acute variceal bleeding:
  - Type and cross patient's blood.
  - Initial resuscitation with isotonic fluid until packed RBCs are available
  - Correct coagulopathy with vitamin K and fresh frozen plasma (FFP).
  - Upper endoscopy as soon as the patient is stabilized (for diagnosis and treatment)
  - Avoid sedatives that may precipitate encephalopathy.
  - Limit sodium administration because cirrhotic patients avidly retain sodium.
  - Restrict protein only if encephalopathic.

ALERT

If the patient is an active alcohol drinker, assess for alcoholic hepatitis and watch for signs and symptoms of withdrawal. Follow inpatient protocols for alcohol withdrawal management.

- Use isotonic fluid for hydration.
- Discharge criteria
  - For GI bleeding:
    - No active bleeding in 24 hours
    - Stable hemoglobin and hematocrit
    - Hemodynamically stable (especially heart rate)
  - For encephalopathy: Improvement in or resolution of mental status changes to baseline.

 ONGOING CARE

DIET

- In cirrhosis, patients retain sodium, so restrict sodium intake to <2 g daily.
- Alcohol abstinence

PROGNOSIS

- Hepatic reserve defined by Child-Pugh classification: rating based on encephalopathy, ascites, bilirubin, albumin, prothrombin
- Variceal bleeding
  - 1/3 of patients with known varices will bleed eventually.
  - 50% rebleed, usually within 2 years, unless portal pressure is reduced by surgical or TIPS procedure.
  - 15–20% mortality rate
- Ascites and encephalopathy often recur.
- Prognosis of patients with ascites is poor: 50% 1-year survival without liver transplant (compared with 90% for patients with cirrhosis and no ascites).

COMPLICATIONS

- Acute gastroesophageal variceal bleed
- Ascites
- Hepatic encephalopathy
- Hepatic hydrothorax
- Hepatorenal syndrome
- Portal hypertensive gastropathy
- Portopulmonary hypertension
- Splenomegaly
- SBP

REFERENCE

1. de Franchis R; for Baveno VI Faculty. Expanding consensus in portal hypertension: report of the Baveno VI Consensus Workshop: stratifying risk and individualizing care for portal hypertension. *J Hepatol*. 2015;63(3):743–752.

 CODES

ICD10

K76.6 Portal hypertension

CLINICAL PEARLS

- Portal hypertension can be diagnosed based on physical examination in the setting of known risk factors, specifically cirrhosis.
- Endoscopic treatment is successful for acute variceal hemorrhage 85% of the time.
- Prognosis of patients with ascites is poor: 50% 1-year survival without liver transplant (compared with 90% for patients with cirrhosis and no ascites).

POSTCONCUSSION SYNDROME (MILD TRAUMATIC BRAIN INJURY)

Vicki R. Nelson, MD, PhD

 BASICS

DESCRIPTION

- Postconcussion syndrome (PCS) is a constellation of symptoms involving physical, cognitive, and/or behavioral symptoms persisting after a concussion (synonymous with mild traumatic brain injury [mTBI]) that may continue for weeks to years.
- It is difficult to define when concussive symptoms transition to postconcussive syndrome. A recent consensus suggests persistent symptoms lasting >10 to 14 days in adults and 4 weeks in children (1).
- PCS may present with any symptoms of concussion including:
  - Cognitive
    o Poor attention
    o Poor memory
    o Diminished academic/intellectual performance
    o Slowed response time
  - Physical
    o Headache
    o Nausea
    o Visual changes
    o Light or noise sensitivity
    o Dizziness and balance problems
    o Fatigue and sleep disturbance
  - Behavioral
    o Depression
    o Anxiety
    o Irritability/emotional lability
    o Apathy
    o Increased sensitivity to alcohol
- Diagnosis is based on history and clinical symptoms.

EPIDEMIOLOGY

Incidence
The reported frequency of patients with concussion who develop PCS varies widely between 5% and 80%.
- Largely due to difficulty differentiating postconcussion *symptoms* from PCS
- 80–90% of individuals with concussion recover from postconcussion *symptoms* within 7 to 10 days, longer in children/adolescents. A diagnosis of PCS is made in patients with persistent concussive symptoms.

Prevalence
Predominant sex: Females are slightly more likely to experience prolonged symptoms following a concussive injury.

ETIOLOGY AND PATHOPHYSIOLOGY
- Controversial; exact mechanism(s) unknown
- Because the pathophysiology of PCS is not well understood and because of symptom overlap with other psychiatric conditions, PCS remains difficult to diagnose and to manage.
  - Only some individuals with mTBI develop PCS; it is unclear what causes postconcussion symptoms to persist, leading to PCS.

- Behavioral factors are commonly associated with (and may play a role in) the development of PCS. It can be challenging to differentiate some preexisting behavioral disorders from PCS. Neuropsychiatry evaluation can be helpful.
- Patients who reported high symptom burden following mTBI are at increased risk of PCS (2).

RISK FACTORS
- Strongest predictor of prolonged recovery and development of PCS is severity of initial concussion symptoms (1).
- Initial symptoms including retrograde amnesia, difficulty concentrating, disorientation, insomnia, loss of balance, sensitivity to noise, or visual disturbance (3)
- Preexisting psychiatric disorders including depression, anxiety, personality disorder, and posttraumatic stress disorder (PTSD)
- Preexisting expectation of poor outcomes following mTBI
- Nonsport concussion/mTBI
- Unclear if previous history of concussion(s) is a risk factor for PCS
- Low socioeconomic status
- Loss of consciousness is NOT predictive of PCS.

GENERAL PREVENTION
- Early clinical evaluation and treatment can help reduce time of recovery. Identified concussion symptom constellations should be addressed and treated early.
- Education of players, coaches, parents, and athletic trainers about concussion, PCS, and appropriate safety rules
- Head injury precautions are advised. Evidence is lacking that these decrease incidence of mTBI/PCS.
- Screening and intervention for preexisting comorbidities such as anxiety, depression, attention disorders, migraines, or insomnia early in concussion treatment may reduce the likelihood of transitioning from concussion to PCS.

COMMONLY ASSOCIATED CONDITIONS
- PTSD
- Anxiety
- Depression
- Fibromyalgia
- Personality disorders (namely, compulsive, histrionic, and narcissistic)
- ADHD

DIAGNOSIS

HISTORY
- Detailed history of recent impact and closed head injury, including:
  - Mechanism
  - Timing of injury related to symptoms
  - Previous head injuries, including concussion, and timing of those injuries
  - Previous medical, psychiatric, or social history
  - Thorough characterization of associated symptoms, intensity, and duration
- Report of neurologic, cognitive, or behavioral symptoms by patient/family

PHYSICAL EXAM
Complete neurologic exam, including the following:
- Glasgow Coma Scale (GCS)
- Many screening and diagnostic tools are available (e.g., Sport Concussion Assessment Tool [SCAT], NFL Sideline Concussion Assessment Tool) and may be used for diagnosis of concussion (1).
- Vestibular/ocular assessment
  - for example, Vestibular Ocular Motor Screening (VOMS)
- Anxiety/depression screening
  - for example, Patient Health Questionnaire-9 (PHQ-9) for depression
  - for example, Generalized Anxiety Disorder-7 (GAD-7) for anxiety
- Computerized neuropsychiatric (CNP) testing may be useful for determining treatment course and effectiveness.

DIFFERENTIAL DIAGNOSIS
- Concussion/mTBI
- PTSD
- Anxiety/depression
- Personality disorders
- Migraine headaches
- Chronic fatigue syndrome, fibromyalgia
- Evolving intracranial hemorrhage
- Exposure to toxins, including prescription and recreational drugs
- Endocrine/metabolic abnormality

DIAGNOSTIC TESTS & INTERPRETATION
Initial Tests (lab, imaging)
- Consider infection, intoxication, and endocrine or metabolic abnormality in appropriate clinical setting.
- Brain imaging both on initial evaluation of mTBI and PCS is not routinely indicated.
- Imaging to evaluate for bleeding is appropriate with comorbidities or anticoagulation therapy at the time of injury.
- Imaging indicated if cervical spine injury is suspected at the time of initial injury

Follow-Up Tests & Special Considerations
- Several CNP tests are available to help guide treatment, academic accommodations, and return-to-play decisions.
- Formal neuropsychiatric evaluations are superior to CNP testing when available. None of these tests should be used in isolation for decision-making, especially if a patient is still symptomatic (1).
- Common neuropsychological testing programs
  - Immediate Post-Concussion Assessment and Cognitive Testing (ImPACT)
  - CNS Vital Signs
  - Axon Sports Computerized Cognitive Assessment Tool (CCAT)
  - Automated Neuropsychological Assessment Metrics (ANAM)

TREATMENT

GENERAL MEASURES

- Return to full activity should progress according to existing evidence-based recommendations for return to activity (work, school, sport) after concussion (1).
- When possible, controlling cognitive stress or stimuli-rich environments by providing school accommodations can be beneficial in the setting of prolonged cognitive deficits or symptom exacerbation in the learning environment (1).
- Restrict individuals with PCS from sport activity until symptoms have resolved and patients have been weaned from any medications that might mask PCS symptoms. Noncontact, aerobic activity that does not exacerbate symptoms can be beneficial to recovery (1).
- Physical therapy for coexisting cervical and vestibular injuries is beneficial.
- Cognitive-behavioral therapy helps with persistent mood disturbances, anxiety symptoms, or PTSD (2).
- Limited evidence that pharmacotherapy is beneficial

MEDICATION

First Line

- Headache/neck pain
  - Nonopioid pain control (e.g., NSAIDs) preferred
    - With the use of opioid medications, sedation obscures cognitive evaluation.
    - Possible association between the use of opiates and increased risk of anxiety/depression in PCS patients
    - Consider occipital nerve block.
  - Propranolol or amitriptyline alone or in combination for headache prophylaxis
- Emotional dysregulation (irritability, sadness, anxiety, depression)
  - Anxiety/depression screening starting in the 1st week post-mTBI
    - SSRIs (e.g., sertraline 25 mg daily titrated to effective dose with maximum of 200 mg/day) for persistent depressive symptoms
  - Consider referral to behavioral health specialist(s).
- Sleep dysregulation
  - Sleep hygiene
  - Melatonin (up to 3 mg in older children and 5 mg in adolescents and adults)
  - Trazodone (25 to 50 mg at night)
  - Amitriptyline, especially where dual benefit from headache prevention may be achieved
- Cognitive disorders (poor concentration, fogginess, drowsiness)
  - Neuropsychological evaluation
  - Consider preexisting conditions such as learning difficulties or attention disorders.
  - Neurostimulants, such as amantadine (100 mg BID), methylphenidate, atomoxetine; preexisting attention disorders may benefit from temporary modification of existing treatments.

ISSUES FOR REFERRAL

- Neuropsychiatric therapy including comprehensive cognitive evaluation for potential TBI rehabilitation
- Cognitive-behavioral therapy for anxiety and depression symptoms
- Occupational therapy for vocational rehabilitation
- Physical therapy for vestibular/ocular rehabilitation, neck pain
- Neurology referral if primary care interventions for seizures, headache, vertigo, or cognition are unsuccessful
- Substance abuse counseling, if needed

COMPLEMENTARY & ALTERNATIVE MEDICINE

- Massage therapy, osteopathic manipulative treatment, acupuncture for headache and neck pain
- Potential benefits shown with hyperbaric oxygen therapy in military veterans with concurrent PCS and PTSD

ONGOING CARE

FOLLOW-UP RECOMMENDATIONS

Schedule regular follow-up to evaluate for persistent symptoms, efficacy of and/or need for neuropsychiatric evaluation, and the efficacy of and/or need for pharmacologic therapy.

Patient Monitoring

- Consider serial neuropsychological testing.
- Follow return-to-play guidelines for resuming physical activity and sport (1).

PATIENT EDUCATION

- Centers for Disease Control and Prevention: https://www.cdc.gov/headsup/
- Brain Injury Association of America: https://www.biausa.org/; (800) 444-6443

PROGNOSIS

- Prognosis generally is good. Most patients improve within 3 months.
- Adolescents may recover more slowly than adults.

COMPLICATIONS

- Repeat head injury or return to sport before resolution of PCS can worsen/prolong symptoms.
- Case studies of second-impact syndrome, a rare but potentially fatal condition owing to a second head injury soon after the first, have been reported.

REFERENCES

1. Patricios JS, Schneider KJ, Dvorak J, et al. Consensus statement on concussion in sport: the 6th International Conference on Concussion in Sport—Amsterdam, October 2022. *Br J Sports Med*. 2023;57(11):695–711.
2. Déry J, Ouellet B, de Guise É, et al. Prognostic factors for persistent symptoms in adults with mild traumatic brain injury: an overview of systematic reviews. *Syst Rev*. 2023;12(1):127.
3. Kerr ZY, Zuckerman SL, Wasserman EB, et al. Factors associated with post-concussion syndrome in high school student-athletes. *J Sci Med Sport*. 2018;21(5):447–452.

ADDITIONAL READING

- Miutz LN, Burma JS, Lapointe AP, et al. Physical activity following sport-related concussion in adolescents: a systematic review. *J Appl Physiol (1985)*. 2022;132(5):1250–1266.
- Neelakantan M, Ryali B, Cabral MD, et al. Academic performance following sport-related concussions in children and adolescents: a scoping review. *Int J Environ Res Public Health*. 2020;17(20):7602.

 SEE ALSO

Concussion (Mild Traumatic Brain Injury)

CODES

ICD10

- F07.81 Postconcussional syndrome
- S06.9X0A Unsp intracranial injury w/o loss of consciousness, init
- S06.9X9A Unsp intracranial injury w LOC of unsp duration, init

CLINICAL PEARLS

- Imaging is rarely useful for PCS.
- Coordinate multidisciplinary treatment plans for patients with persistent symptoms.
- A full return to sport/physical activity should not occur until the individual is fully asymptomatic. Graduated return to daily activities, driving, work, and academics should be advanced as symptoms permit and may require accommodations.

POSTTRAUMATIC STRESS DISORDER (PTSD)

Siddhi Bhivandkar, MD

 BASICS

A psychiatric disorder that may occur in people who have experienced or witnessed a traumatic event or who have been threatened with death, sexual violence, or serious injury

DESCRIPTION

- The disorder can appear at any age. In children >6 years of age, young adults, and adults, it presents with four trauma-associated symptom groups:
  - Intrusion symptoms such as flashbacks, nightmares, distressing recollections
  - Avoidance of anything related to the traumatic event and/or numbing of general responsiveness
  - Increased arousal and reactivity
  - Negative alterations in mood and cognition
- Symptoms of PTSD usually develop within 3 months after a trauma.
- Onset of symptoms can be delayed 6 months to years after trauma exposure.
- For diagnosis of PTSD, symptoms should be present for more than 1 month.

EPIDEMIOLOGY

- Probability of PTSD was assessed in about 29 types of traumatic experiences, divided into groups: sexual relationship violence, interpersonal violence, exposure to organized violence, participation in organized violence, and other life-threatening traumatic experiences.
- Unexpected death of loved one, rape, and other sexual assault were associated with the highest rate of PTSD.
- 16% of children and adolescents exposed to trauma develop PTSD.

Incidence
~7.7 million American adults aged ≥18 years (3.5% of this age group) are diagnosed with PTSD each year.

Prevalence
The lifetime prevalence of PTSD was 6.8%.

ETIOLOGY AND PATHOPHYSIOLOGY

- Biologic dimensions: hypersensitivity of catecholamine pathways and overactivity of the central opioid pathways is seen; the amygdala and hippocampus dysfunction, with possible atrophy from overexposure to catecholamines, serotonergic dysregulation, glutamatergic dysregulation, and increased thyroid activity
- Learning theory: Life-threatening fear is classically conditioned by event exposure; any internal or external cue reminiscent of the event produces an intense "fight-or-flight" fear response.
- Cognitive theories: These models suggest that severe trauma becomes represented in complex memory structures. The activation of these memories triggers intense thoughts and emotions that cause discomfort and dysfunction.
- Psychodynamic theory: Traumatic memories overwhelm defense mechanisms. Repeated recall of the traumatic event with associated fear is an effort to understand the event in a less threatening way.

RISK FACTORS

- Preexisting factors:
  - Female sex
  - Younger age
  - Psychiatric history
  - Low socioeconomic status
- Peritrauma factors:
  - Severity of the trauma
  - Peritrauma emotionality
  - Perception of threat to life
  - Perpetration of the trauma
- Posttrauma environment:
  - Perceived injury severity
  - Medical complications
  - Perceived social support
  - Persistent dissociation from traumatic event
- Subsequent exposure to trauma-related stimuli

GENERAL PREVENTION

Trauma-focused cognitive-behavioral therapy (CBT) and modified prolonged exposure delivered within weeks of a potentially traumatic event for people showing signs of distress have the most evidence in the prevention of PTSD.

COMMONLY ASSOCIATED CONDITIONS

- Major depressive disorder
- Alcohol/substance abuse
- Panic disorder/agoraphobia/social phobia/obsessive-compulsive disorder
- Smoking (especially with assaultive trauma)
- Major neurocognitive disorders, dementia, or amnesia/traumatic brain injury

Pediatric Considerations
Oppositional defiant disorder and separation anxiety are common comorbid conditions.

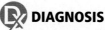 **DIAGNOSIS**

Diagnosis is based on *DSM-5* criteria (1):

- Criterion A: exposure to trauma (≥1 of the following):
  - Direct experience of a traumatic event
  - In-person witnessing of a traumatic event
  - Learning of a traumatic event involving a close friend or family member
  - Repeated exposure to details of a traumatic event
- Criterion B: intrusive symptoms associated with the traumatic event (≥1 of the following):
  - Recurrent, involuntary, and intrusive distressing memories of the event
  - Recurrent distressing dreams related to the event
  - Dissociative reactions that simulate a recurrence of the event
  - Intense or prolonged distress to stimuli that resemble an aspect of the event
- Criterion C: avoidance of stimuli associated with the trauma (≥1 of the following):
  - Avoidance of memories, thoughts, or feelings about the event
  - Avoidance of external reminders that trigger memories, thoughts, or feelings about the event

- Criterion D: negative cognitive and mood changes associated with the trauma (≥2 of the following):
  - Inability to remember aspects of event
  - Persistent and exaggerated negative opinion of self, others, or the world
  - Distorted beliefs about the cause or consequences of the event
  - Negative emotional state
  - Diminished interest in significant activities
  - Feeling detached from others
  - Inability to experience positive emotions
- Criterion E: hyperarousal (≥2 of the following):
  - Difficulty sleeping/falling asleep
  - Decreased concentration
  - Hypervigilance
  - Outbursts of anger/irritable mood
  - Exaggerated startle response
  - Self-destructive behavior
- Criterion F: Duration of the relevant criteria symptoms should be >1 month.
- Criterion G: clinically significant distress/impairment in functioning
- Criterion H: relevant criteria not attributed to substance effects or other medical conditions

Pediatric Considerations
- Reactions can include a fear of being separated from a parent or regressive behavior.
- Older children may show extreme withdrawal, disruptive behavior, and/or an inability to pay attention. Regressive behaviors, nightmares, sleep problems, irrational fears, irritability, refusal to attend school, outbursts of anger, fighting, somatic complaints with no medical basis, and decline in schoolwork performance.
- Parental posttraumatic stress has been shown to be a robust predictor of pediatric PTSD (2)[A].

HISTORY
Symptoms of intrusion, avoidance, alternations of mood and cognition, and hyperarousal must have lasted >1 month.

PHYSICAL EXAM
- Patients may present with physical injuries from the traumatic event.
- Mental status examination:
  - Thoughts and perceptions (e.g., hallucinations, delusions, suicidal ideation, phobias)
  - General appearance: disheveled, poor hygiene
  - Behavior: agitation; startle reaction extreme
  - Psychological numbness
  - Orientation may be affected.
  - Memory: forgetfulness, especially concerning the details of the traumatic event
  - Poor concentration
  - Poor impulse control
  - Altered speech rate and flow
  - Mood and affect may be changed: depression, anxiety, guilt, and/or fear.

Pediatric Considerations
Elevated heart rate immediately following trauma is associated with development of PTSD (2)[A].

DIFFERENTIAL DIAGNOSIS
- Generalized anxiety disorder/adjustment disorder
- Obsessive-compulsive disorder
- Schizophrenia
- Major depressive disorder/mood disorder with psychotic features
- Substance abuse
- Personality/dissociative/conversion disorders
- Factitious disorder or malingering

DIAGNOSTIC TESTS & INTERPRETATION
- Diagnosis is based on *DSM-5* criteria (1).
- Primary Care PTSD Screen for *DSM-5* (PC-PTSD-5) (3)
- Trauma Screening Questionnaire (TSQ)

 TREATMENT

The combination of psychotherapy and pharmacotherapy, initiated soon after the trauma, results in better prognosis.

MEDICATION
Both paroxetine and sertraline are FDA-approved drugs for the treatment of PTSD, but other SSRIs are also effective.

First Line
- Depression, panic attacks, startle response, and sleep disruption may improve with SSRIs (4)[A]:
  - Sertraline: 50 to 200 mg every day (FDA-approved)
  - Paroxetine: starting dose: 10 mg every day; maybe increased in 10-mg increments at intervals ≥1 week (FDA-approved)
  - Fluoxetine: 20 mg every day/BID not to exceed 80 mg/day (demonstrates some efficacy for all three symptom clusters)
- Sleep disruption: sleep disruption due to hyperarousal is ubiquitous in PTSD; standard sedatives, such as trazodone 50 to 300 mg at bedtime, mirtazapine 7.5 to 30.0 mg QHS, or amitriptyline 25 to 100 mg QHS
- Nightmares/nighttime hyperarousal: prazosin 2 to 15 mg QHS (5)[A], clonidine 0.1 to 0.2 mg QHS, amitriptyline 25 to 100 mg QHS

Second Line
Refractory/residual symptoms: Consider augmentation with:
- Depression: mirtazapine 15 to 45 mg/day; consider switch to a serotonin-norepinephrine reuptake inhibitor (SNRI), such as venlafaxine XR 37.5 to 300.0 mg/day, duloxetine 60 to 120 mg/day, or desvenlafaxine 50 to 100 mg/day. Nefazodone 300 to 600 mg/day in divided doses can be very effective but requires quarterly LFTs.
- Reexperiencing/intrusive thoughts: 1st-/2nd-generation antipsychotic medications: aripiprazole 5 to 15 mg/day, risperidone 0.5 to 2.0 mg/day, olanzapine 2.5 to 10.0 mg/day, quetiapine 50 to 400 mg/day (6)[A]. 2nd-generation Rx less prone to extrapyramidal symptoms (EPS): cognitive dulling

- Hyperarousal: clonidine, start 0.05 mg BID/TID; slowly titrate to as much as 0.45 mg/day divided doses; guanfacine 1 to 3 mg/day in divided doses (long-acting forms of both clonidine and guanfacine now available). Also consider 2nd-generation antipsychotics quetiapine, risperidone, and olanzapine as above; divided doses are often more helpful.
- Impulsivity/explosiveness: anticonvulsants: valproic acid 500 to 2,000 mg/day, carbamazepine 200 to 600 mg/day, topiramate 50 to 200 mg/day
- Anxiety: Benzodiazepines (especially short-acting) should be avoided given the risk of substance abuse and questionable benefit in PTSD (7)[A]. Consider hydroxyzine 25 to 50 mg TID/QID PRN or risperidone 0.25 to 0.50 mg TID PRN.

ADDITIONAL THERAPIES
- Exposure therapies have shown the highest effectiveness for treatment of PTSD (8)[A]:
  - Behavioral and CBT: Early CBT, including virtual exposure, has been shown to speed recovery. CBT is considered the standard of care for PTSD by the U.S. Department of Defense.
  - Eye movement desensitization and reprocessing (EMDR) has been shown to benefit patients with PTSD.
- Telemedicine-based collaborative care (nurse, case manager, pharmacy, psychology, psychiatry)

Pediatric Considerations
Little evidence to support use of pharmacologic interventions for pediatric PTSD

 ONGOING CARE

- The initial stabilization phase can be prolonged.
- Ongoing exposure to trauma can undermine the improvement.
- Patients with a history of childhood sexual abuse (complex PTSD) are often challenging to treat; they have significant difficulties with affect regulation and trust.
- It can take years for patients of complex PTSD to build trust and develop a relationship with the therapist.

PATIENT EDUCATION
National Center for PTSD: https://www.ptsd.va.gov

PROGNOSIS
- In 50% of cases, the symptoms spontaneously remit after 3 months; however, symptoms may persist and cause long-term impairment in life functioning.
- Factors associated with a good prognosis include:
  - Rapid engagement of treatment
  - Early and ongoing social support
  - Avoidance of retraumatization
  - Absence of other psychiatric disorders/substance abuse

COMPLICATIONS
- Increased risk for panic disorder, agoraphobia, obsessive-compulsive disorder, social phobia, specific phobia, major depressive disorder, somatization disorder; impulsive behavior, suicide, and homicide
- Victims of sexual assault are at especially high risk for developing mental health problems and committing suicide.

REFERENCES

1. American Psychiatric Association. *Diagnostic and Statistical Manual of Mental Disorders*. 5th ed. Arlington, VA: American Psychiatric Association; 2013.
2. Brosbe MS, Hoefling K, Faust J. Predicting posttraumatic stress following pediatric injury: a systematic review. *J Pediatr Psychol*. 2011;36(6):718–729.
3. Prins A, Ouimette P, Kimerling R, et al. The primary care PTSD screen (PC-PTSD): development and operating characteristics. *Primary Care Psychiatry*. 2003;9(1):9–14.
4. Stein DJ, Ipser JC, Seedat S. Pharmacotherapy for post traumatic stress disorder (PTSD). *Cochrane Database Syst Rev*. 2006;(1):CD002795.
5. Writer BW, Meyer EG, Schillerstrom JE. Prazosin for military combat-related PTSD nightmares: a critical review. *J Neuropsychiatry Clin Neurosci*. 2014;26(1):24–33.
6. Han C, Pae C-U, Wang S-M, et al. The potential role of atypical antipsychotics for the treatment of posttraumatic stress disorder. *J Psychiatr Res*. 2014;56:72–81.
7. Jeffreys M, Capehart B, Friedman MJ. Pharmacotherapy for posttraumatic stress disorder: review with clinical applications. *J Rehabil Res Dev*. 2012;49(5):703–715.
8. Kornør H, Winje D, Ekeberg Ø, et al. Early trauma-focused cognitive-behavioural therapy to prevent chronic post-traumatic stress disorder and related symptoms: a systematic review and meta-analysis. *BMC Psychiatry*. 2008;8:81.

 CODES

ICD10
- F43.10 Post-traumatic stress disorder, unspecified
- F43.11 Post-traumatic stress disorder, acute
- F43.12 Post-traumatic stress disorder, chronic

CLINICAL PEARLS

Treatment is often best accomplished with a combination of psychotherapy and pharmacotherapy.

PREECLAMPSIA AND ECLAMPSIA (TOXEMIA OF PREGNANCY)

Ann M. Aring, MD, FAAFP

BASICS

DESCRIPTION
- Preeclampsia: A disorder of pregnancy occurring after 20 weeks' gestation characterized by new-onset hypertension (HTN), new-onset proteinuria, ± impaired organ function
- Eclampsia: new-onset grand mal seizure activity with no history of underlying neurologic disease
- Most postpartum cases of preeclampsia and eclampsia occur within 48 hours of delivery but can occur up to 6 weeks postpartum.

EPIDEMIOLOGY
Incidence
Preeclampsia occurs in 5–8% of all pregnancies.

Prevalence
- Predominant age
  - Most in younger women, primiparous women
  - Older (aged >40 years) patients with pre-eclampsia have 4 times the incidence of seizures compared with patients in their 20s.
- 40% of eclamptic seizures occur before delivery; 16% occur >48 hours after delivery.
- Eclampsia is a main cause of perinatal mortality and morbidity (2–8% of all pregnancies).

ETIOLOGY AND PATHOPHYSIOLOGY
- Cause of preeclampsia is becoming clearer.
  - Genetic predisposition and abnormal placental implantation
  - Angiogenic factors
  - Vascular endothelial damage and oxidative stress
- Systemic disorders in eclampsia include the following:
  - Cardiovascular: generalized vasospasm
  - Hematologic: decreased plasma volume, increased blood viscosity, hemoconcentration, coagulopathy
  - Renal: decreased glomerular filtration rate
  - Hepatic: periportal necrosis, hepatocellular damage, subcapsular hematoma
  - CNS: cerebral vasospasm and ischemia, cerebral edema, cerebral hemorrhage

Genetics
2 to 4 times increased risk in pregnant women with family history of preeclampsia

RISK FACTORS
- Nulliparity
- Age >40 years
- Family history of preeclampsia
- Maternal medical problems: diabetes, chronic HTN, chronic renal disease, obesity, systemic lupus erythematosus
- Multiple gestation
- Prior pregnancy with preeclampsia
- In vitro fertilization

GENERAL PREVENTION
- Adequate prenatal care
- Good control of preexisting HTN
- Low-dose aspirin (ASA) (60 to 80 mg): ASA started early after 12 weeks' gestational age (GA) may lower the risk of developing preeclampsia and the rate of preterm delivery and neonatal death in moderate- to high-risk patients (1)[C] (see "Risk Factors" as mentioned earlier).
- Low-dose calcium supplementation has been shown to reduce the risk and severity of preeclampsia in calcium-deficient populations.

COMMONLY ASSOCIATED CONDITIONS
Abruptio placentae, placental insufficiency, fetal growth restriction, preterm delivery, fetal demise maternal seizures (eclampsia), maternal pulmonary edema, maternal liver/kidney failure, or maternal death

DIAGNOSIS

- Preeclampsia diagnosis:
  - New-onset elevated blood pressure (BP): systolic BP (SBP) ≥140 mm Hg or diastolic BP (DBP) ≥90 mm Hg (on two occasions at least 4 hours apart) after 20 weeks' gestation *and new onset of one or more of the following:*
    - Proteinuria
      - Proteinuria >300 mg/24 hr
      - Spot protein: creatinine ≥0.3
      - Urine dipstick ≥2+ if quantitative measurement is not available
    - Or, without proteinuria and new onset of at least one of these features:
      - Platelets <100,000/μL
      - Liver transaminase levels >2 times normal +/− right upper quadrant (RUQ) pain
      - Creatinine >1.1 mg/dL or doubling of serum creatinine levels
      - Pulmonary edema
      - Headache or visual symptoms
  - Preeclampsia with severe features occurs with new-onset BP ≥160/110 mm Hg after 20 weeks of gestation and new onset of one or more of the following:
    - Platelets <100,000/μL
    - Severe persistent right upper quadrant (RUQ)/epigastric pain, or both
    - Creatinine >1.1 mg/dL or doubling of serum creatinine levels
    - Visual symptoms
    - New-onset severe headache
    - Pulmonary edema
- Eclampsia diagnosis:
  - New-onset tonic-clonic, focal, or multifocal seizures
  - No history of neurologic disease

HISTORY
- May be asymptomatic. In some cases, rapid excessive weight gain (>5 lb/week; >2.3 kg/week); more severe cases are associated with epigastric/RUQ pain, headache, altered mental status, and visual disturbance. Note: Headache, visual symptoms, and epigastric or RUQ pain often precede seizure.
- Seizures may occur once/repeatedly.

PHYSICAL EXAM
BP criteria:
- Preeclampsia *without* severe features: elevated BP ≥140/90 mm Hg
- Preeclampsia *with* severe features: Elevated BP: SBP ≥160 mm Hg or DBP 110 mm Hg
- Normal BP, even in response to treatment; does not rule out potential for seizures

DIFFERENTIAL DIAGNOSIS
- Chronic HTN: HTN before pregnancy; high BP before the 20th week
- Chronic HTN with superimposed preeclampsia

- Gestational HTN: Increased BP first discovered after 20 weeks, often close to term, with no proteinuria and without evidence of organ dysfunction. BP becomes normal by 12 weeks postpartum, or it is reclassified as chronic HTN.
- Seizures in pregnancy: epilepsy, cerebral tumors, meningitis/encephalitis, and ruptured cerebral aneurysm. Until other causes are proven, all pregnant women with seizures should be considered to have eclampsia.

DIAGNOSTIC TESTS & INTERPRETATION
Initial Tests (lab, imaging)
- Urinalysis for protein should be done at each prenatal visit, especially for patients at higher risk.
- Complete blood count (CBC) with platelets, serum creatinine, serum transaminase levels, lactate dehydrogenase (LDH), and uric acid
- 24-hour urine or spot protein/creatinine ratio if urine protein dips 1+ on more than one occasion, or if preeclampsia is being considered
- Coagulation studies (PT/PTT/fibrinogen) are not routine. Order if bleeding, severe liver dysfunction, thrombocytopenia, or placental abruption.
- Daily fetal movement monitoring by mother ("kick counts")
- US imaging is used to monitor growth and cord blood flow; perform, as indicated, based on clinical stability and laboratory findings.
- Nonstress test (NST) at diagnosis and then twice weekly until delivery
- Biophysical profile (BPP) if NST is nonreactive
- US imaging for growth progress every 3 weeks, and amniotic fluid volume at least once weekly.
- With seizures, CT scan and MRI should be considered if focal findings persist or uncharacteristic signs/symptoms are present.

Follow-Up Tests & Special Considerations
Disseminated intravascular coagulation, thrombocytopenia, liver dysfunction, and renal failure can complicate preeclampsia associated with HELLP (hemolysis, elevated liver enzymes, low platelet) syndrome.

Test Interpretation
CNS: cerebral edema, hyperemia, focal anemia, thrombosis, and hemorrhage. Cerebral lesions account for 40% of eclamptic deaths.

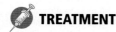 TREATMENT

GENERAL MEASURES
- Health care providers must balance timing of delivery with maternal and fetal risks.
- Delivery recommended for preeclampsia of any severity at ≥37 weeks' gestation.
- Preeclampsia without severe features:
  - Consider outpatient care.
  - Maternal: daily BP monitoring; daily weights; weekly labs (CBC, creatinine, liver function test [LFT])
  - Fetal:
    - Patient-measured: daily "kick counts"
    - NST/BPP/US (see "Initial Tests [lab, imaging]" section above)
    - Induction of labor at 37 0/7 weeks' gestation (1)[C]
    - Steroids for gestation <37 weeks

- Preeclampsia with severe features:
  - Inpatient care
  - Maternal:
    - Daily labs (CBC, serum creatinine, LFTs)
    - Use magnesium sulfate (MgSO$_4$) IV as seizure prophylaxis and continue 24 hours after delivery.
    - Antihypertensive therapy titrated to keep SBP <160 mm Hg and DBP <110 mm Hg (some recommend <150/100 mm Hg postpartum)
  - Fetal:
    - Continuous heart monitoring
    - Daily US with BPP
    - Check amniotic fluid levels and fetal growth.
  - Definitive management (delivery) depends on GA (1)[C].
  - At 23 to 34 weeks:
    - Antihypertensives
    - Evaluate maternal–fetal condition.
    - Use steroids such as betamethasone 12 mg IM daily × 2 doses or dexamethasone 6 mg every 12 hours × 4 doses to accelerate fetal lung maturity
    - Plan delivery at 34 weeks with MgSO$_4$ prophylaxis.
    - If HELLP syndrome (full or partial), severe oligohydramnios, significant renal dysfunction, persistent symptoms, fetal growth restriction, onset of labor, or premature rupture of membranes (PROM), proceed to delivery.
  - At ≥34 weeks: Delivery is recommended. Start MgSO$_4$ IV. Do not delay delivery to give steroids in the late preterm period.

ALERT
- A severe BP reading ≥160/110 mm Hg requires pharmacologic treatment within 30 to 60 minutes of confirming the diagnosis.
- Regardless of GA, emergent delivery is recommended if there are signs of maternal hypertensive crisis, abruptio placentae, uterine rupture, or fetal distress. Delivery is the definitive treatment.
- Seizures: control of convulsions, correction of hypoxia and acidosis, lowering of BP, steps to delivery baby as soon as convulsions are controlled

MEDICATION
First Line
- Seizure prophylaxis for women with severe preeclampsia but normal renal function: MgSO$_4$ loading dose 4 to 6 g IV in 200 mL normal saline over 20 to 30 minutes; maintenance dose 1 to 2 g/hr IV continuous infusion
- BP control:
  - Antihypertensives are not advised for mildly elevated BP without severe features.
  - Start antihypertensive treatment for severe HTN ≥160/110 mm Hg within 30 minutes of meeting diagnostic criteria.
    - Labetalol (IV): 20 mg over 2 minutes followed at 20 to 30 minutes intervals with doses of 20 to 80 mg titrated to keep BP <160/110 mm Hg; max of 300 mg/24 hr (contraindicated in asthma, heart disease, congestive heart failure)

- Hydralazine (IV): 5 to 10 mg over 2 minutes, followed at 20 minutes intervals with 5 to 10 mg IV boluses; titrated to keep BP <160/110 mm Hg; max of 25 mg/24 hr
- Nifedipine immediate release 10 mg oral followed by 20 mg in 20 minutes if needed for severe range (1)[C]. Sustained release (PO) (used in the postpartum): 30 to 120 mg/day (caution with combination of nifedipine and MgSO$_4$ resulting in hypotension and neuromuscular blockade)
- Eclampsia/seizures:
  - MgSO$_4$ for seizures
    - 4 to 6 g IV over 15 to 20 minutes followed by 1 to 2 g/hr infusion
    - Further boluses of magnesium may be given for recurrent convulsions with the amount given based on the neurologic examination and patellar reflexes.
    - Contraindications: myasthenia gravis, renal failure, pulmonary edema
  - Levels of 6 to 8 mEq/mL are considered therapeutic, but monitor clinical status of:
    - Patellar reflexes are present.
    - Respirations are not depressed.
    - Urine output is ≥25 mL/hr.
  - May be given safely, even in the presence of renal insufficiency
- Fluid therapy
  - Ringer lactated solution with 5% dextrose at 60 to 120 mL/hr, with careful attention to fluid volume status
- Calcium gluconate or chloride (1 g, administered slowly IV) may reverse magnesium-induced respiratory depression.

Second Line
For refractory seizures unresponsive to MgSO$_4$, consider using:
- Diazepam 2 mg/min until resolution or 20 mg given or
- Lorazepam 1 to 2 mg/min up to total of 10 mg or
- Phenytoin 15 to 20 mg/kg at a maximum rate of 50 mg/min or
- Phenobarbital 20 mg/kg infused at 50 mg/min; may repeat with additional 5 to 10 mg/kg after 15 minutes

ONGOING CARE

FOLLOW-UP RECOMMENDATIONS
Women with a history of preeclampsia should report this to physicians caring for them in later life. It is an important cardiovascular disease risk factor.

DIET
Do not recommend salt restriction because the patient often experiences intravascular hypovolemia.

PATIENT EDUCATION
American College of Obstetricians and Gynecologists: http://www.acog.org/

PROGNOSIS
- For nulliparous women with preeclampsia before 30 weeks of gestation, the recurrence rate for the disorder may be as high as 40% in future pregnancies.
- 25% of eclamptic women will have HTN during subsequent pregnancies.
- Preeclamptic, multiparous women may be at higher risk for subsequent essential HTN; they also have higher mortality during subsequent pregnancies than do primiparous women.

COMPLICATIONS
- Most women do not have long-term sequelae from eclampsia, although many may have transient neurologic deficits.
- Maternal and/or fetal death

REFERENCE
1. American College of Obstetricians and Gynecologists. ACOG Committee Opinion No. 767: Emergent therapy for acute-onset, severe hypertension during pregnancy and the postpartum period. *Obstet Gynecol*. 2019;133(2):e174–e180.

ADDITIONAL READING
- Abalos E, Duley L, Steyn DW. Antihypertensive drug therapy for mild to moderate hypertension during pregnancy. *Cochrane Database Syst Rev*. 2014;(2):CD002252.
- Duley L, Meher S, Jones L. Drugs for treatment of very high blood pressure during pregnancy. *Cochrane Database Syst Rev*. 2013;(7):CD011449.

CODES

ICD10
- O14.90 Unspecified pre-eclampsia, unspecified trimester
- O15.00 Eclampsia in pregnancy, unspecified trimester
- O14.00 Mild to moderate pre-eclampsia, unspecified trimester

CLINICAL PEARLS
- Management of preeclampsia depends on both the severity of the condition and the GA of the fetus.
- MgSO$_4$ is the drug of choice for preeclampsia with severe features.
- Start daily low-dose ASA in the late 1st trimester in high-risk patients to prevent preeclampsia.
- Continue to monitor maternal BP postpartum. The patient is still at risk for developing preeclampsia.

PREMENSTRUAL SYNDROME (PMS) AND PREMENSTRUAL DYSPHORIC DISORDER (PMDD)

Ulunma Natalie Umesi, MD, MBA • Ambreka Benons, MD • Frantz Aubry, MD

 BASICS

DESCRIPTION
- Premenstrual syndrome (PMS), a complex of physical and emotional symptoms sufficiently severe to interfere with everyday life, occurs cyclically during the luteal phase of menses.
- Premenstrual dysphoric disorder (PMDD) is a severe form of PMS characterized by severe recurrent depressive and anxiety symptoms, with premenstrual (luteal phase) onset, that remits a few days after the start of menses as defined in the *Diagnostic and Statistical Manual of Mental Disorders*, 5th edition (*DSM-5*).
- System(s) affected: endocrine/metabolic, nervous, reproductive

EPIDEMIOLOGY
Prevalence
- Many women have some physical and psychological symptoms before menses that can encompass a spectrum from mild molimina to severe and disabling symptoms.
- The prevalence of PMS is reported anywhere between 20% and 30% of menstruating women. 1.2% to 6.4% of women have PMDD based on *DSM-5* criteria (1) with upward of 18% of menstruating women meeting partial *DSM* criteria (2).

ETIOLOGY AND PATHOPHYSIOLOGY
Although not yet fully understood, there are two main views on the pathophysiology (1):
- Changing levels of the progesterone metabolite allopregnanolone interacts with serotonin and γ-aminobutyric acid (GABA) receptors, provoking downstream effects of decreased GABA-mediated inhibition and decreased serotonin levels.
- Decreased function of the serotonin system (in particular the serotonin transporter) serves as the primary abnormality and thus when modulated by sex hormones leads to decreased serotonin levels in patients with PMS/PMDD.

Genetics
- The role of genetic predisposition is controversial; however, twin studies do suggest a genetic component.
- Involvement of gene coding for the serotonergic *5HT1A* receptor and allelic variants of the estrogen receptor-α gene (*ESR1*) is suggested.

RISK FACTORS
- Age: usually presents in the late 20s to mid-30s
- History of mood disorder (major depression, bipolar disorder), anxiety disorder, personality disorder, or substance abuse
- Family history
- Low parity
- Cigarette smoking and other nicotine-containing products
- Psychosocial stressors/history of trauma
- High BMI (>27.5)

COMMONLY ASSOCIATED CONDITIONS
There is a high prevalence of comorbid mood disorders and/or anxiety disorders in patients with PMS/PMDD.

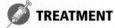 **DIAGNOSIS**

HISTORY
- Criteria for the diagnosis of PMS has been established by the International Society for Premenstrual Disorders (ISPMD) and include the following:
  – Physical or emotional symptoms
  – Symptoms are present during the luteal phase and abate as menstruation begins
  – A symptom-free week
  – Symptoms are associated with significant impairment during the luteal phase.
- Criteria for the diagnosis of PMDD was established by the American Psychiatric Association in 2013 and included in the *DSM-5*.
- Symptoms occur 1 week before menses, improve in the first few days after menses begin, and are minimal/absent in the week following menses (over most menstrual cycles during the past year).
- ≥5 of the following (1 must be among the first 4):
  – Marked depressed mood, feelings of hopelessness, or self-deprecating thoughts
  – Marked anxiety, tension, and/or feelings of being keyed up or on edge
  – Marked affective lability (mood swings)
  – Marked irritability or anger or increased interpersonal conflicts
  – Decreased interest in usual activities and social withdrawal
  – Lethargy, easy fatigability, or lack of energy
  – Appetite change, overeating, food cravings
  – Hypersomnia or insomnia
  – Feeling out of control or overwhelmed
  – Subjective difficulty concentrating
  – Physical symptoms, such as abdominal bloating, breast tenderness, headaches, weight gain, and joint/muscle pain
- Emotional symptoms must be sufficiently severe to interfere with work, school, usual social activities, or relationships with others.
- Symptoms may be superimposed on an underlying psychiatric disorder but may not be an exacerbation of another condition, such as panic disorder/major depression.
- Criteria should be confirmed by prospective patient record of symptoms for a minimum of two consecutive menstrual cycles (without confirmation, "provisional" should be noted with diagnosis).
- Symptoms should not be attributable to drug abuse, medications, or other medical conditions.
- Diagnosis can be established through the use of a validated tool such as the Daily Record of Severity of Problems (available online at https://psychscenehub.com/wp-content/uploads/2020/10/Daily-Record-of-Severity-of-Problems-PMDD.pdf) or similar inventory.

PHYSICAL EXAM
No specific physical exam is required; may consider thyroid and pelvic exams if indicated by additional patient symptoms

DIFFERENTIAL DIAGNOSIS
- Premenstrual exacerbation of underlying psychiatric disorder
- Psychiatric disorders (especially bipolar disorder, major depression, anxiety)
- Thyroid disorders
- Perimenopause
- Premenstrual migraine
- Chronic fatigue syndrome
- Irritable bowel syndrome (painful symptoms)
- Seizures
- Anemia
- Endometriosis (painful symptoms)
- Drug/alcohol abuse

DIAGNOSTIC TESTS & INTERPRETATION
- The repetitive nature of symptoms precludes the need for labs if a classic history is present.
- Consider
  – Hemoglobin to rule out anemia
  – Serum thyroid-stimulating hormone (TSH) to rule out hypothyroidism
- Imaging with pelvic ultrasound to diagnose causes of pelvic pain and dysmenorrhea may be needed.

TREATMENT

GENERAL MEASURES
Exercise increases β-endorphins in the brain, but the role of physical activity in the treatment of premenstrual disorders remains unclear (3).

MEDICATION
First Line
- SSRIs are recommended as the first-line therapy in the treatment of physical, functional, and behavioral symptoms of PMS and PMDD compared to placebo (4)[A]:
  – Both intermittent luteal phase dosing and continuous full-cycle dosing are effective with no clear evidence of a difference between modes of administration (4)[A].
  – All SSRIs tested appeared effective (4)[A].
  – SSRIs are effective at low doses but may require titration of the dose for the desired response in certain patients. Higher doses have increased effect but are accompanied by increased side effects (4)[A].
- Fluoxetine (Prozac, Sarafem) 20 mg/day every day or 20 mg/day only during the luteal phase, or 90 mg once a week for 2 weeks in the luteal phase
- Sertraline (Zoloft) 50 to 150 mg/day every day or 50 to 150 mg/day only during the luteal phase
- Citalopram (Celexa) 10 to 30 mg/day every day or 10 to 30 mg/day only during the luteal phase
- Adverse effects (number needed to harm [NNH] with moderate-dose SSRI): nausea (NNH = 7), asthenia (NNH = 9), somnolence (NNH = 13), fatigue (NNH = 14), decreased libido (NNH = 14), and sweating (NNH = 14) (4)[A]
- Contraindications: patients taking monoamine oxidase inhibitors (MAOIs)
- Precautions
  – Increased risk of suicidal thinking and behavior in children and adolescents with depressive disorders; uncertain if this risk applies to those taking SSRIs for PMDD
  – Bipolar disorder

- Seizure disorder
- QTc prolongation (with citalopram)
- Hepatic dysfunction
- Renal dysfunction

Second Line
Alternative therapies should be considered if no response to SSRIs:

- Spironolactone (Aldactone) 50 to 100 mg/day for 7 to 10 days during the luteal phase; helpful for fluid retention.
  - Adverse reactions: lethargy, headache, irregular menses, hyperkalemia
  - Regular monitoring of electrolytes is recommended due to the risk of hyperkalemia.
- Oral contraceptive pills (OCPs)
  - OCPs can cause adverse effects similar to PMDD symptoms.
  - Extended-cycle use of OCPs (e.g., 12 weeks on and 1 week off) or a shorter placebo interval (e.g., 24 active pills with 4 placebo days [24/4] compared with 21/7 preparations) may be beneficial.
  - OCPs containing the progestin drospirenone (structurally similar to spironolactone) may improve physical symptoms and mood changes associated with PMDD. Caution: Side effects (5)[A] and the risk of venous thromboembolism may be modestly higher than with other OCPs.
  - Continuous administration of levonorgestrel/ethinyl estradiol may improve patient symptoms in PMDD.
  - Suggested OCP formulations:
    - Ethinyl estradiol 0.02 to 0.03 mg/drospirenone 3 mg (Gianvi/Loryna/Nikki/Ocella/Syeda/Vestura/Yasmin/Yaz Zarah): 1 tablet/day
    - Ethinyl estradiol 0.02 to 0.03 mg/drospirenone 3 mg/levomefolate 0.451 mg (Beyaz/Safyral): 1 tablet/day
    - Levonorgestrel 90 μg/ethinyl estradiol 20 μg (Amethyst/Lybrel): 1 tablet/day
- Anxiolytics
  - Alprazolam (Xanax) 0.25 mg TID–QID only during luteal phase; taper at the onset of menses (other benzodiazepines not studied for PMDD); caution: addictive potential
  - Buspirone (BuSpar) 10 to 30 mg/day divided BID–TID in the luteal phase
- Ovulation inhibitors
  - Gonadotropin-releasing hormone (GnRH) agonists: leuprolide (Lupron) depot 3.75 mg/month IM; precautions: menopause-like side effects (e.g., osteoporosis, hot flashes, headaches, muscle aches, vaginal dryness, irritability) limit treatment to 6 months; may be the first step if considering bilateral oophorectomy for severe, refractory PMDD
  - Danazol (Danocrine) 300 to 400 mg BID; adverse reactions: androgenic and antiestrogenic effects (e.g., amenorrhea, weight gain, acne, fluid retention, hirsutism, hot flashes, vaginal dryness, emotional lability)
  - Estrogen, transdermal preferred, 100 to 200 μg:
    - Precautions: increased risk of blood clots, stroke, heart attack, and breast cancer
    - Requires concomitant progesterone add-back therapy to protect against uterine hyperplasia and endometrial cancer
- Progesterone: insufficient evidence to support use

ISSUES FOR REFERRAL
Short-term follow-up (within 1 to 3 months) can assess if the patient has an adequate response to treatment. If not, referral to a psychiatrist may be indicated for further evaluation.

ADDITIONAL THERAPIES
Cognitive-behavioral therapy (CBT) is theoretically helpful for PMS/PMDD given its application for symptom reduction in other mood disorders, but direct evidence is lacking.

SURGERY/OTHER PROCEDURES
Bilateral oophorectomy, usually with concomitant hysterectomy, is an option for rare, refractory cases with severe, disabling symptoms.

COMPLEMENTARY & ALTERNATIVE MEDICINE
Acupuncture demonstrated superiority to progestins, anxiolytics, and sham acupuncture with no evidence of harm (6)[A].

- Some data support the use of the following:
  - Calcium: 600 mg BID
  - Vitamin B$_6$: 50 to 100 mg/day
  - Chasteberry (*Vitex agnus-castus*): 4 mg/day of extract containing 6% of agnuside (or 20 to 40 mg/day of fruit extract)
  - Omega-3 fatty acids 2 g/day
- Data insufficient regarding the following:
  - Magnesium: 200 to 400 mg/day
  - Vitamin D: 2,000 IU/day
  - Vitamin E: 400 IU/day
  - Manganese: 1.8 mg/day
  - St. John's wort: 900 mg/day
  - Soy: 68 mg/day isoflavones
  - Ginkgo: 160 to 320 mg/day
  - Saffron: 30 mg/day
- Evidence supporting efficacy and/or safety of herbal products is lacking; the following products/interventions have not been found useful for PMS/PMDD, although not all studies are of high quality and able to eliminate the possibility of benefit completely:
  - Evening primrose oil
  - Black currant oil
  - Black cohosh
  - Wild yam root
  - Dong quai
  - Kava kava
  - Light-based therapy

 ## ONGOING CARE

FOLLOW-UP RECOMMENDATIONS
Patient Monitoring
Increased risk of suicidal thinking and behavior in children and adolescents with depressive disorders on initiation of SSRIs; uncertain if this risk applies to those taking SSRIs for PMDD

DIET
- Reduce consumption of salt, sugar, caffeine, dairy products, and alcohol (anecdotal reports).
- Eat small, frequent portions of food high in complex carbohydrates (limited data).

PATIENT EDUCATION
- Counsel patients to eat a balanced diet rich in calcium, vitamin D, and omega-3 fatty acids and low in saturated fat and caffeine.
- Counsel patients to quit tobacco and other nicotine use (more research is needed on the benefit of smoking cessation in PMS and PMDD).
- Counsel women that they are not "crazy." PMDD is a real disorder with a physiologic basis.
- Although incompletely understood, successful treatment is often possible.

PROGNOSIS
- Many patients can have their symptoms adequately controlled. PMS disappears at menopause.
- PMS can continue after hysterectomy if ovaries are left in place.

REFERENCES

1. Yonkers KA, Simoni MK. Premenstrual disorders. *Am J Obstet Gynecol*. 2018;218(1):68–74.
2. Carlini SV, Deligiannidis KM. Evidence-based treatment of premenstrual dysphoric disorder: a concise review. *J Clin Psychiatry*. 2020;81(2):19ac13071.
3. Lanza di Scalea T, Pearlstein T. Premenstrual dysphoric disorder. *Med Clin North Am*. 2019;103(4):613–628.
4. Marjoribanks J, Brown J, O'Brien PMS, et al. Selective serotonin reuptake inhibitors for premenstrual syndrome. *Cochrane Database Syst Rev*. 2013;2013(6):CD001396.
5. Ma S, Song SJ. Oral contraceptives containing drospirenone for premenstrual syndrome. *Cochrane Database Syst Rev*. 2023;6(6):CD006586.
6. Kim SY, Park HJ, Lee H, et al. Acupuncture for premenstrual syndrome: a systematic review and meta-analysis of randomized controlled trials. *BJOG*. 2011;118(8):899–915.

CODES

ICD10
N94.3 Premenstrual tension syndrome

CLINICAL PEARLS
- Have the patient keep a daily log of her symptoms and menses. Symptoms beginning in the week before menses and abating before the end of menses, occurring over at least 2 months, and sufficiently severe to interfere with daily functioning are diagnostic of PMS.
- Treatment only during the luteal phase is likely as effective as continuous-cycle treatment with SSRIs but has fewer adverse effects.

PRENATAL CARE AND TESTING

Henry Del Rosario, MD

BASICS

The goal of prenatal care is to ensure the well-being of mother and baby using the best available evidence and a patient-centered approach. General concepts include estimating the gestational age (GA) accurately; identifying risk for complications; encouraging and empowering the patient for motherhood, newborn care, and breastfeeding; and intervening when fetal abnormalities are present to prevent morbidity and mortality.

GENERAL PREVENTION

In the United States, the typical prenatal visit schedule consists of monthly visits for weeks 4 to 28 of pregnancy, visits twice monthly from 28 to 36 weeks, weekly after week 36 (until delivery, typically at weeks 38 to 41).

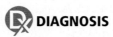 DIAGNOSIS

HISTORY

Collect the following histories in the initial prenatal visit and continually update throughout the pregnancy (1),(2):

- Medical history, with an emphasis on the following but not limited to prediabetes/DM, obesity/overweight, thyroid disorders, pregestational hypertension (HTN) or history of hypertensive disease in pregnancy (e.g., chronic HTN, gestational HTN, pre-eclampsia with or without severe features, HELLP syndrome), maternal age at delivery, previous DVT/PE, known uterine anomaly, autoimmune disease (e.g., systemic lupus erythematosus, rheumatoid arthritis, Sjögren), strong family history of diseases in pregnancy or congenital/inheritable conditions
- Obstetrical history, including but not limited to:
  - History of preterm delivery or PTL
  - History of hypertensive disease in pregnancy
  - History of gestational diabetes (GDM) or early onset GDM
  - Other medical conditions raising maternal risk: HIV/AIDS or other STIs in the past, sickle cell disease, intrahepatic cholestasis of pregnancy
  - Personal history of delivering a newborn with birth defects/trisomies or congenital/inheritable condition
- Psychosocial history, including but not limited to:
  - Depression screening (use EPDS or PHQ-9), intimate partner violence (ACOG guidelines: Screen *all* pregnant patients at the first prenatal visit, 1x/trimester, and at postpartum checkup.)
  - Tobacco, alcohol, and drug use
  - Lifestyle, nutrition, toxin exposures, travel to areas with endemic diseases, stressors/supports; potential barriers to care (preferred language, housing, transportation, child care issues, economic constraints, work schedule)

PHYSICAL EXAM

- A full physical exam on intake (1),(2)
- At each subsequent prenatal visit, the following should be recorded (1),(2):
  - Weight gain recommendations (2009 IOM)
    - BMI <18.5 kg/m^2 (underweight): 28 to 40 lb (12.5 to 18 kg)
    - BMI 18.5 to 24.9 kg/m^2 (normal weight): 25 to 35 lb (11.5 to 16 kg)
    - BMI 25 to 29.9 kg/m^2 (overweight): 15 to 25 lb (7 to 11.5 kg)
    - BMI ≥30 kg/m^2 (obese): 11 to 20 lb (5 to 9 kg)
  - BP (mm Hg): Assess for mild (≥140 to <160/≥90 to <110) or severe range (≥160/≥110) BP if not normal
  - Fundal height: Start after weeks 20 to 24.
  - Fetal heart rate: usually audible by 8 to 12 weeks' GA with a Doppler device
  - Pelvic/cervical exam if indicated
  - Fetal position by Leopold maneuver at weeks 32 to 36; confirm by ultrasound (US) if available.

DIAGNOSTIC TESTS & INTERPRETATION

- First prenatal visit (1):
  - Lab tests
    - Hematocrit or hemoglobin, blood type, Rhesus type, and antibody screen
    - Hemoglobin electrophoresis: Screen for sickle cell disease, SCT, or thalassemia.
    - Urine culture
    - Ab titers for Rubella and Varicella
    - STI screen: RPR/VDRL, GC/C, hepatitis B, HIV
    - Not recommended: routine screening for bacterial vaginosis, toxoplasmosis, CMV, and parvovirus; thyroid and vitamin D deficiency
  - Carrier screening (including, but not limited to):
    - Cystic fibrosis screening: Counseling is needed first, and screening should be offered when one partner is of Caucasian, European, or Ashkenazi Jewish descent.
    - Spinal muscular atrophy
    - Hemoglobinopathies (i.e., risk for sickle cell disease, thalassemia)
  - Screening for fetal aneuploidy:
    - Counseling should be provided before any shared decision-making on testing.
    - All women should be offered screening or diagnostic testing, regardless of maternal age.
    - US nuchal translucency (NT): measures thickness at the back of the neck of the fetus
    - Blood screens: human chorionic gonadotropin (hCG), pregnancy-associated plasma protein A (PAPP-A), quadruple test: α-fetoprotein (AFP), unconjugated estriol (UE3), hCG, dimeric inhibin-A (DIA)
    - Cell-free DNA testing: should not be used as a substitute for diagnostic testing due to potential for false-positive or false-negative results; all women with positive screening test should have a diagnostic procedure before any irreversible action is taken.
    - 1st-trimester "combined test" between 11 and 13 weeks' GA using both NT and hCG/PAPP-A blood testing is an effective protocol; may be performed either as a single combined stand-alone test (US NT 1 blood [HCG and PAPP-A]) or as part of a sequential "step-by-step" 1st- and 2nd-trimester screening process (See the following discussion.)

- Women who undergo 1st-trimester screening should be offered 2nd-trimester assessment for open fetal defects and US screening for other fetal structural defects.
- 2nd-trimester screening: Obtain quadruple test ideally at weeks 15 to 18 but can be done as late as week 22.
- If risk is found, all pregnant women should be offered invasive prenatal diagnostic testing regardless of maternal age or other risk factors (3); diagnostic tests for genetic disorders:
  - CVS: 1st trimester: usually done weeks 10 to 12; small sample of the placenta; chorionic tissue sample obtained either transcervical (TC) or transabdominal (TA)
  - Amniocentesis: usually done weeks 15 to 18; small sample of amniotic fluid from the amniotic sac surrounding the developing fetus is obtained by a US-guided TA approach.
  - The rate of procedure-related pregnancy loss that is attributable to a prenatal diagnostic procedure is 0.1–0.3% when performed by experienced health care providers (3).
  - Chromosomal microarray analysis: can detect a pathogenic copy number variant in about 1.7% of patients with normal US and normal karyotype; make available to any patient choosing to undergo invasive diagnostic testing; primary test for patients undergoing diagnostic testing for indication of a fetal structural abnormality detected by US examination (3)
- Cervical cancer screening:
  - A Pap smear or approved high-risk HPV screen should be obtained when indicated by standard Pap screening guidelines, regardless of gestation, to start at age 21 years.
  - Squamous intraepithelial lesions can progress during pregnancy but often regress postpartum.
  - LSIL/CIN1 in pregnancy: Colposcopy is preferred, but it is acceptable to defer colposcopy to 6 weeks postpartum.
  - CIN 2 or CIN 3 in pregnancy: In the absence of invasive disease or advanced pregnancy, additional colposcopic and cytologic examinations are acceptable; repeat biopsy is recommended only if appearance of lesion worsens or if cytology suggests invasive cancer; it is acceptable to defer reevaluation until 6 weeks postpartum.
  - Endocervical sampling is contraindicated in pregnancy.
- Subsequent prenatal visits (1),(2):
  - Urinalysis for glucose and protein: limited evidence for benefit or harm; the baseline during initial intake may be useful for high-risk patients (e.g., chronic HTN).
- 24- to 28-week prenatal visits (1),(2):
  - Obtain diabetes screen.
  - Repeat hematocrit or hemoglobin, and repeat antibody screen in Rh-negative mother prior to receiving prophylactic Rh immunoglobulin. Repeat syphilis testing in the 3rd trimester around 28 weeks in all cases (2018 CDC, ACOG and AAP guidelines due to rising cases of congenital syphilis). Retest for HIV at 28 weeks in high-risk cases. Retest for syphilis and HIV at delivery in high-risk cases.

– GDM screening (2)
  ○ The ADA and ACOG define increased risk of diabetes in pregnancy who need earlier screening based on BMI ≥25 kg/m² (≥23 kg/m² in Asian Americans) plus one or more of the following:
    ▪ Previous pregnancy history of GDM, fetal macrosomia (≥4,000 g BW prior delivery), or stillbirth
    ▪ HTN (140/90 mm Hg or being treated for HTN)
    ▪ HDL cholesterol ≤35 mg/dL (0.90 mmol/L)
    ▪ Fasting triglyceride ≥250 mg/dL (2.82 mmol/L)
    ▪ Hemoglobin A1C ≥5.7%, impaired glucose tolerance or impaired fasting glucose
    ▪ PCOS, acanthosis nigricans, nonalcoholic steatohepatitis, morbid obesity prepregnancy BMI ≥40 kg/m², and other conditions associated with insulin resistance
    ▪ Current or past history of cardiovascular disease
    ▪ Family history of diabetes—first-degree relative (parent or sibling)
    ▪ High-risk ethnicity or communities
  ○ Early onset diagnosis is made via 2-step testing (see below) ideally between weeks 12 to 16 of pregnancy for at risk cases.
  ○ For typical low-risk cases, employ 2-step testing starting week 24 to 28: Screen using a 1-hour glucola test and, if needed and appropriate (see below*), a 3-hour diagnostic test.
  ○ The risk of developing type 2 diabetes with the personal history of GDM is up to 50% in the next 20 years after delivery. Therefore, a fasting 75-g 2-hour oral glucose tolerance test (OGTT), because it is only 1 step, may be helpful in diagnosing postpartum diabetes or glucose intolerance. It is unclear if the 75-g 2-hour GTT is comparable to the 2-step approach in diagnosing GDM*.
  ○ Assess for readiness for change in diet +/− exercise. Provide counseling, nutrition, and other support on diagnosis of GDM. Continue to support during the postpartum period and beyond.
  ○ Diagnosing GDM (ACOG and AAFP guidelines):
    ▪ Setting cutoff for "elevated 1-hour GCT": Setting the cutoff at 130 or 135 may be prudent for a practice with higher local prevalence of GDM. Setting the cutoff at 140 may be prudent for a practice with low local prevalence of GDM.
    ▪ Routine screening for GDM (~week 24 to 28): 50 g PO nonfasting glucose load with blood glucose testing 1 hour later; if elevated, then proceed to 3-hour testing for diagnosis.
      □ *Each practice or institution may have internal guidelines for 1-hour results if ≥180 to 185 and proceed with fasting BG monitoring instead of proceeding with 3-hour GTT.
    ▪ Diagnostic test: 3-hour GTT is achieved, on a separate day from 1-hour GCT, by 100 g PO glucose load after fasting for ≥8 hours with blood drawn: fasting, 1, 2, and 3 hours after ingestion of glucose. A positive diagnosis of GDM requires that ≥2 positive thresholds by either of the criteria listed below.
      □ NDDG standard: ≥105 (fasting), ≥190 (1-hour), ≥165 (2-hour), ≥145 (3-hour)
      □ Carpenter and Coustan standard: ≥95 (fasting), ≥180 (1-hour), ≥155 (2-hour), ≥140 (3-hour)

    ▪ ACOG states, due to known adverse events, one elevated value from the 3-hour GTT may be sufficient to demonstrate evidence of glucose intolerance.
    ▪ 1-step approach (75-g OGTT) on all women will increase the diagnosis of GDM, but sufficient prospective studies demonstrating improved outcomes are still lacking and need further research. ACOG does acknowledge that some centers may opt for "1 step" if warranted based on their population.
- 35 to 37 week prenatal visits (1):
  – Group B *Streptococcus* (GBS) culture: Screen all low-risk cases at 35 to 37 weeks' GA to identify women colonized with GBS. For cases requiring induction at 37 weeks or earlier, screen as soon as possible.
  – High-risk patients: High-risk patients should be screened again for gonorrhea, chlamydia, syphilis, and HIV.
- Postterm pregnancy:
  – The rate of stillbirth increases with GA by 1/3,000 per week at 41 weeks, 3/3,000 per week at 42 weeks, and 6/3,000 per week at 43 weeks. In one meta-analysis, routine induction of labor at 41 weeks' GA reduced rates of perinatal death without increased rates of cesarean delivery.
  – For prenatal care >41 to 42 weeks, fetal well-being should be assessed with nonstress testing and US assessment of amniotic fluid volume.

TREATMENT

ISSUES FOR REFERRAL
Abnormal screening labs or imaging may prompt referral to maternal–fetal medicine specialist or other medical specialists as indicated.

ONGOING CARE

PATIENT EDUCATION
- Immunizations during pregnancy per CDC:
  – Tdap during each pregnancy (should be given between 27 and 36 weeks' GA); hepatitis B and influenza; likely safe include meningococcal, rabies; contraindicated or safety not established: live vaccines including BCG, MMR, and varicella
  – Vaccination against COVID-19 is recommended in pregnancy. COVID-19 increases the risk for patient and fetus.
- Recommendations for use of dietary supplements in pregnancy (1),(2)
  – Folic acid 0.4 mg/day beginning at least 1 month prior to attempting conception and continuing throughout pregnancy; 1 to 4 mg for women at higher risk of having child with neural tube defect beginning 1 to 3 months before conception, continued through first 12 weeks of gestation, and then reduced to 0.4 mg/day
  – Calcium: 1,000 to 1,300 mg/day; supplement may be beneficial for women with high risk for gestational HTN or communities with low dietary calcium intake.

  – Caffeine: Limit to <200 mg/day; more research needed
  – Iron: Screen for anemia (hemoglobin/hematocrit) and order extra iron supplementation if necessary.
  – Vitamin A: Pregnant women in industrialized countries should limit to <5,000 IU/day.
  – Vitamin D: 200 to 1,200 IU (dose in standard prenatal vitamin) is recommended until more evidence is available to support different dose.
- Other important counseling topics during pregnancy (2):
  – Airline travel: generally safe until up to week 35; >2 hours without ambulation increases the risk of thrombosis.
  – Exercise: Healthy women with uncomplicated pregnancies should continue to exercise.
  – Seat belts/airbags: Wear lap and shoulder seatbelts; working airbags (ACOG and AAFP)
  – Sexual activity: Intercourse while pregnant is not associated with adverse outcomes. Avoiding sex may be necessary in cases of low-lying placenta, placenta previa, or vasa previa.
  – Alcohol, cigarettes, and illicit drugs are injurious to fetal and maternal health.
  – Pregnancy-safe medications (teratogenicity)
  – Avoid large fish such as shark, tuna, swordfish, and mackerel (high levels of mercury).
  – Preconception counseling offers the opportunity to discuss individualized risks.

REFERENCES

1. Zolotor AJ, Carlough MC. Update on prenatal care. *Am Fam Physician*. 2014;89(3):199–208.
2. Kilpatrick SJ, Papile L, Macones GA, et al, eds. *Guidelines for Perinatal Care*. 8th ed. Elk Grove Village, IL: American Academy of Pediatrics, 2017.
3. American College of Obstetricians and Gynecologists' Committee on Practice Bulletins—Obstetrics, Committee on Genetics, Society for Maternal-Fetal Medicine. Practice Bulletin No. 162: prenatal diagnostic testing for genetic disorders. *Obstet Gynecol*. 2016;127(5):e108–e122.

CODES

ICD10
- Z34.90 Encntr for suprvsn of normal pregnancy, unsp, unsp trimester
- Z36 Encounter for antenatal screening of mother
- Z34.00 Encntr for suprvsn of normal first pregnancy, unsp trimester

CLINICAL PEARLS

Given the complexity of screening and counseling, checklists and team-based care help ensure consistent application of recommended interventions.

Andrew Grimes, MD

BASICS

DESCRIPTION

- Preoperative medical evaluation should determine the presence of established or unrecognized disease or other factors that may increase the risk of perioperative morbidity and mortality in patients undergoing surgery.
- Specific assessment goals include the following:
  - Conducting a thorough medical history and physical exam to assess the need for further testing and/or consultation
  - Recommending strategies to reduce risk and optimize patient condition prior to surgery
  - Encouraging patients to optimize their health for possible improvement of both perioperative and long-term outcomes
- Synonym(s): preoperative diagnostic workup; preoperative preparation; preoperative general health assessment

EPIDEMIOLOGY

Overall patient morbidity and mortality related to surgery may be decreasing. One large study of inpatients found major adverse cardiovascular and cerebrovascular events (MACCE) has gone from 3.1% of hospitalizations in 2004 to 2.6% in 2013. Perioperative acute myocardial infarction (MI) and death decreased but the rate of ischemic stroke increased (1). Preoperative patient evaluation and subsequent optimization of perioperative care can reduce both postoperative morbidity and mortality.

RISK FACTORS

- Functional capacity (2): Exercise tolerance is one of the most important determinants of cardiac risk:
  - Self-reported exercise tolerance may be an extremely useful predictive tool when assessing risk. Patients unable to meet a 4–metabolic equivalents (METs) demand (see "Diagnosis" section) during daily activities have increased perioperative cardiac and long-term risks. A study compared physicians' subjective assessment of functional capacity to objective measures of functional capacity. It found that the subjective assessment tended to misclassify high-risk patients as low risk. Structured questionnaires such as the Duke Activity Status Index had much better prognostic accuracy to assess functional status (3).
  - Patients who report good exercise tolerance require minimal, if any, additional testing.
- Levels of surgical risk
  - An increased risk for major adverse cardiac events (MACE) is associated with procedures that are intrathoracic, intra-abdominal, or vascular procedures that are suprainguinal in nature.
- Clinical risk factors: history of ischemic heart disease, the presence of compensated heart failure or a history of prior congestive heart failure (CHF), cerebrovascular disease, diabetes mellitus (DM), and renal insufficiency; these risk factors plus surgical risk can dictate the need for further cardiac testing.
- Age: Patients >70 years of age are at higher risk for perioperative complications and mortality and have a longer length of stay in the hospital postoperatively (likely attributed to increasing medical comorbidities with increasing age). Age alone should not be a deciding factor in the decision to proceed or not to proceed with surgery.

DIAGNOSIS

HISTORY

- Evaluate pertinent medical records and interview the patient. Many institutions provide standard patient questionnaires that screen for preoperative risk factors:
  - History of present illness and treatments
  - Past medical and surgical history
  - Patient and family anesthetic history and associated complications
  - Current medications (including over-the-counter [OTC] medications, vitamins, supplements, and herbals) as well as reasons for use
  - Allergies (including specific reactions)
  - Social history: tobacco, alcohol, drug use, and cessation
- Systems (both history and current status)
  - Cardiovascular: Inquire about exercise capacity.
    - 1 MET: can take care of self, eat, dress, and use toilet; walk around house indoors; walk a block or two on level ground at 2 to 3 mph
    - 4 METs: can climb two flights of stairs or walk uphill, walk on level ground at 4 mph, run a short distance, do heavy work around house, participate in moderate recreational activities
    - 10 METs: can participate in strenuous sports such as swimming, singles tennis, football, basketball, or skiing
  - Note presence of CHF, cardiomyopathy, ischemic heart disease (stable vs. unstable), valvular disease, hypertension (HTN), arrhythmias, murmurs, pericarditis, history of pacemaker or implantable cardioverter defibrillator (ICD):
    - Rhythm management devices (pacemakers and automatic ICDs [AICDs]) affect the perioperative course. Most importantly, the following information needs to be available for proper management: name of cardiologist who manages the device, type of device, manufacturer, last interrogation, and any problems that have occurred recently. Based on this information and the location and type of surgery, a perioperative plan of management will be made.
    - Stents: Patients with coronary stents are maintained on dual antiplatelet therapy (DAPT) for a prescribed period of time. This is typically done with a thienopyridine, such as clopidogrel, in combination with aspirin. The perioperative period is associated with a prothrombotic state. Premature discontinuation of DAPT markedly increases the risk of acute stent thrombosis, MI, and death. Elective surgery should be delayed and DAPT continued for a minimum of 30 days after bare metal stent placement. Duration of DAPT following drug-eluting stent (DES) placement depends on the type of stent and risk of thrombosis. DAPT has been advised for 6 to 12 months following DES, but shorter durations may be possible for newer stents. Several caveats to these recommendations exist. Any perioperative disruption in the patient's DAPT regimen needs to be discussed with the patient's cardiologist and surgeon. The risk of perioperative bleeding must be weighed against the risks of discontinuation of DAPT prior to surgery.

- Pulmonary: Patient risk factors for postoperative pulmonary complications are age, smoking status, poorly controlled asthma, COPD, CHF, pulmonary HTN, nutritional status, and dependent functional status. Active disease processes should be addressed:
  - Sleep apnea: Patients with obstructive sleep apnea (OSA) are at increased risk for perioperative adverse events. Screening tools (such as the STOP-Bang questionnaire) can help risk stratify patients. Additional evaluation should be considered if a patient has associated significant systemic disease, hypoventilation syndrome, severe pulmonary HTN, or resting hypoxemia (4).
  - Often, patients with an existing diagnosis of OSA who use positive airway pressure (PAP) at night are asked to bring their PAP machine to the hospital or surgery center when they are admitted for surgery. For patients with suspected but previously undiagnosed OSA, PAP therapy should be considered on a case-by-case basis.
  - Some studies suggest that even short periods (3 weeks) of treatment with PAP can improve some indices of ventilation and therefore may reduce postoperative morbidity.
- GI: hepatic disease, gastric ulcer, inflammatory bowel disease, hernias (especially hiatal), significant weight loss, nausea, vomiting, history of postoperative nausea, and vomiting: Any symptoms consistent with gastroesophageal reflux disease (GERD) should be optimally treated.
- Hematologic: anemia, serious bleeding, clotting problems, blood transfusions, hereditary disorders
- Renal: kidney failure, dialysis, infections, stones, changes in bladder function
- Endocrine: nocturia, parathyroid, pituitary, adrenal disease, thyroid disease
  - Diabetes: Multiple lines of evidence show that hyperglycemia in the perioperative period is associated with increased perioperative complications. Although recommendations vary, most experts recommend keeping perioperative blood glucose levels <180 mg/dL.
- Neurologic/psychiatric: seizures, stroke, paralysis, tremor, migraine headaches, nerve injury, multiple sclerosis, extremity numbness, psychiatric disorders (e.g., anxiety, depression)
- Musculoskeletal: arthritis, lower back pain
- Frailty is increasingly recognized as a perioperative risk factor. Research is being done on various screening tools and interventions that can decrease perioperative mortality and morbidity in the frail population.
- Reproductive: possibility of pregnancy in women of childbearing potential
- Mouth/upper airway: dentures, crowns, partials, bridges, teeth (loose, chipped, cracked, capped)

PHYSICAL EXAM

- Assess vital signs, including arterial BP bilaterally.
- Check carotid pulses; auscultate for bruits.
- Examine lungs by auscultating all lung fields and listening for rales, rhonchi, wheezes, or other sounds indicating disease.
- Examine cardiovascular system by auscultating heart and noting any irregular rhythms or murmurs; precordial palpation
- If a regional anesthesia technique is being contemplated, perform a relevant, focused neurologic exam.

DIAGNOSTIC TESTS & INTERPRETATION
Initial Tests (lab, imaging)
- Laboratory testing should never be "routine" prior to surgery. Tests should be obtained only when indicated by specific conditions or risk factors. "Routine" testing results in unnecessary delays and disruptions to planned surgery. Specific tests should be requested if the evaluator suspects findings from the clinical evaluation that may influence perioperative patient management.
- Labs performed within the past 4 months prior to evaluation are reliable, unless the patient has had an interim change in clinical presentation or is taking medications that require monitoring of plasma level or effect.
- CBC
  - Hemoglobin: if a patient has symptoms of anemia or is undergoing a procedure with major blood loss; extremes of age; liver or kidney disease
  - WBC count: if symptoms suggest infection or myeloproliferative disorder or the patient is at risk for chemotherapy-induced leukopenia
  - Platelet count: if history of bleeding, myeloproliferative disorder, liver or renal disease, or the patient is at risk for chemotherapy-induced thrombocytopenia
- Serum chemistries (electrolytes, glucose, renal and liver function tests) should be obtained for extremes of age; in known renal insufficiency, CHF, liver dysfunction, or endocrine abnormalities; or the patient is on medications that alter electrolyte levels, such as diuretics. Cr is indicated for patients taking nephrotoxic medications.
- PT/PTT: if history of a bleeding disorder, chronic liver disease, or malnutrition, or those with recent or chronic antibiotic or anticoagulant use
- Urinalysis: Routine urinalysis is not recommended preoperatively.
- Pregnancy test: controversial; should be *considered* for all female patients of childbearing age
- CXR is not generally indicated unless there is a history of significant heart or lung disease or there is a recent change of symptoms.

Diagnostic Procedures/Other
- ECG
  - Preoperative resting 12-lead ECG is reasonable for patients with known coronary disease, known peripheral vascular disease, significant arrhythmia, or known significant structural heart disease.
  - ECGs are not indicated for asymptomatic patients undergoing low-risk procedures.
- ECHO
  - Routine preoperative ECHO evaluation of LV function is not recommended. Per American College of Cardiology (ACC)/American Heart Association (AHA) guidelines, it is reasonable for patients who have dyspnea of unknown origin or CHF with worsening symptoms. Additionally, it is recommended for patients with moderate to severe valve disease who had a significant change in clinical status or have not had an ECHO evaluation in more than a year.

- AHA guidelines recommend using the Revised Cardiac Risk Index or the ACS NSQIP online risk calculator to make an estimate of risk of MACE in the perioperative period. If the risk of MACE is low (<1%), then proceed with surgery. If the risk is >1%, the functional capacity needs to be considered. For patients with a functional capacity of >4 METs, then proceed with surgery. If the functional capacity is <4 METs or unknown, consider pharmacologic stress testing if it will change management.
- PFTs: Definitive data regarding the efficacy of preoperative testing are lacking except for thoracic surgery.

TREATMENT

MEDICATION
- Reducing cardiac risk
  - Elective surgery should be delayed or cancelled if the patient has any of the following: unstable coronary syndromes (unstable or severe angina), recent MI (<30 days), decompensated heart failure, significant arrhythmias, or severe valvular disease.
  - Timing of elective noncardiac surgery after ischemic stroke or MI can have a significant effect on perioperative morbidity and mortality. The AHA/ACC guidelines recommend waiting at least 60 days after a MI if the patient did not require a coronary intervention. The guidelines also recommend waiting at least 6 months and preferably 9 months after a stroke to have elective nonurgent surgery.
  - Perioperative β-blockade has been shown to reduce mortality and the incidence of perioperative MIs in high-risk patients. Studies conflict, however, in which patients need to be treated, the dosage and timing of treatment, and for what surgeries. *Patients chronically on* β-blockers should have the medication continued in the perioperative period. When β-blockers are discontinued in the perioperative period, 30-day mortality increases. It is not recommended to start β-blockers on the day of surgery in β-blocker–naïve patients.
- Reducing pulmonary risk
  - Recommend cigarette cessation for at least 8 weeks prior to elective surgery.
  - Patients with asthma should not be wheezing and should have a peak flow of at least 80% of their predicted or personal-best value.
  - Treatment of COPD and asthma should focus on maximally reducing airflow obstruction and is identical to treatment of nonsurgical patients.

REFERENCES

1. Smilowitz NR, Gupta N, Ramakrishna H, et al. Perioperative major adverse cardiovascular and cerebrovascular events associated with noncardiac surgery. *JAMA Cardiol*. 2017;2(2):181–187.
2. Fleisher LA, Fleischmann KE, Auerbach AD, et al. 2014 ACC/AHA guideline on perioperative cardiovascular evaluation and management of patients undergoing noncardiac surgery: executive summary: a report of the American College of Cardiology/American Heart Association Task Force on practice guidelines. Developed in collaboration with the American College of Surgeons, American Society of Anesthesiologists, American Society of Echocardiography, American Society of Nuclear Cardiology, Heart Rhythm Society, Society for Cardiovascular Angiography and Interventions, Society of Cardiovascular Anesthesiologists, and Society of Vascular Medicine endorsed by the Society of Hospital Medicine. *J Nucl Cardiol*. 2015;22(1):162–215.
3. Wijeysundera DN, Pearse RM, Shulman MA, et al. Assessment of functional capacity before major noncardiac surgery: an international, prospective cohort study. *Lancet*. 2018;391(10140):2631–2640.
4. Chan MTV, Wang CY, Seet E, et al. Association of unrecognized obstructive sleep apnea with postoperative cardiovascular events in patients undergoing major noncardiac surgery. *JAMA*. 2019;321(18):1788–1798.

 SEE ALSO

Algorithm: Preoperative Evaluation of Noncardiac Surgical Patient

CODES

ICD10
- Z01.818 Encounter for other preprocedural examination
- Z01.811 Encounter for preprocedural respiratory examination
- Z01.812 Encounter for preprocedural laboratory examination

CLINICAL PEARLS

- The preoperative evaluation should include medical record evaluation, patient interview, and physical exam.
- Functional capacity, the level of surgical risk, and clinical risk factors determine if further cardiac testing is needed.
- No preoperative tests are or should be routine.
- Active cardiac conditions should lead to delay or cancellation of nonemergent surgery.

PRESBYCUSIS

Darnel Viray Dabu, MD, MPH, FAAFP • Sabari Nair, DO

 BASICS

DESCRIPTION

- Age-related hearing loss (HL); it often presents as difficulty communicating in noisy conditions.
- Represents a lifetime of insults to the auditory system from toxic noise exposure and natural decline resulting in gradual, progressive, bilateral HL.
- Usually presents as high-frequency HL with tinnitus (ringing)
- Impacts the "clarity" of sounds (i.e., ability to detect, identify, and localize sounds) making it difficult to hear in noisy conditions and reduced ability to understand speech.
- Central and peripheral causes:
  - Central presbycusis: age-related change in the auditory portions of the central nervous system, negatively impacting auditory perception, speech-communication performance, or both
  - Peripheral presbycusis: age-related, bilateral sensorineural HL (SNHL) typically symmetric
- No cure for presbycusis exists to date; management consists of mitigating risk factors and auditory amplification.
- Hearing aids (HAs) are the mainstay of treatment and are now sold over the counter for mild-to-moderate HL.
- Can lead to adverse effects on physical, cognitive, emotional, behavioral, and social function in the elderly (e.g., depression, social isolation) and is a contributor to all-cause dementia (1)

EPIDEMIOLOGY

Prevalence
- Increases with age—age 60 to 69 years: 27%; age 70 to 79 years: 55%; age >80 years: 81%
- Predominant sex: male > female

ETIOLOGY AND PATHOPHYSIOLOGY
- The external ear transmits sound energy to the tympanic membrane. The middle ear ossicles amplify and conduct the sound waves into the inner ear (cochlea) via the oval window. The organ of Corti, located in the cochlea, contains hair cells that detect these vibrations and depolarize, producing electrical signals that travel through the auditory nerve to the brain. These hair cells are susceptible to damage from a variety of insults and cannot be regenerated leading to cell death and permanent HL.
- Presbycusis is caused by the accumulated effects of noise exposure, systemic disease, oxidative damage, ototoxic drugs, and genetic susceptibility.

Genetics
Presbycusis has a clear familial aggregation:
- Genetic polymorphisms in genes encoding detoxification enzymes have been linked to age-related HL including GSTM1, GSTT1, and NAT2*6A (2).
- Other genes linked to age-related HL include GRM7, GRHL2, DFNA5, MYO6, and KCNQ4 (2)
- Mitochondrial DNA mutations/deletions have also been implicated in age-related HL (3).

RISK FACTORS
- Advancing age
- Noise exposure (military, industrial, leisure etc.)
- Ototoxic substances (organic solvents, heavy metals, carbon monoxide)
- Drugs (aminoglycosides, cisplatin [dose dependent], salicylates, NSAIDs, diuretics, antimalarials)
- Cigarette smoking
- Alcohol abuse
- Lower socioeconomic status
- Family history of presbycusis
- Head trauma (temporal bone fractures)
- Cardiovascular disease (hypertension, atherosclerosis, hyperlipidemia)
- Diabetes mellitus
- Autoimmune disease (auto cochleitis/labyrinthitis)
- Metabolic bone disease
- Endocrine medical conditions: levels of aldosterone
- Otologic conditions (e.g., Ménière disease or otosclerosis)

GENERAL PREVENTION
- Avoid hazardous noise exposure.
- Use hearing protection (earmuffs, earplugs).
- Screening
  - Based on a 2021 review, according to the USPSTF, there is an insufficient evidence to assess the relative benefits and harms of HL screening in adults aged ≥50 years.
  - Hearing Handicap Inventory for the Elderly Screening (4)
  - RCT published in 2010 on screening for HL, HA use was significantly higher in three screened groups (4.1% in those using a questionnaire, 6.3% using handheld audiometry, and 7.4% using both modalities) versus unscreened control participants (3.3%) at 1-year follow-up (5)[B].

COMMONLY ASSOCIATED CONDITIONS
- Accelerated multidomain cognitive decline, cognitive impairment, and dementia (6)[A]
- A variety of cognitive, behavioral, and psychosocial disorders (7)

DIAGNOSIS

HISTORY
- Reduced hearing sensitivity and speech understanding in noisy/public environments
- Impaired localization of sound sources
- Increased difficulty understanding conversations, especially with women, due to higher frequency of spoken voice
- Presents bilaterally and symmetrically
- If unilateral HL, alternative diagnosis should be pursued.
- Cardiac risk factors
- Exposure to ototoxic medications
- Family history of age-related HL

- Additional history if HL is suspected or detected:
  - Time course of HL
  - Symptoms of tinnitus, otalgia, otorrhea, or vertigo
  - History of noise exposure, ear trauma, or head trauma
  - Presence of any neurologic deficit
- Reports from patient/family/caregiver
  - Confusion in social situations
  - Excessive volume of television/radio/computer
  - Social withdrawal
  - Anxiety in group settings

PHYSICAL EXAM
- Whispered voice test
- Otoscopic examination to rule out other etiologies like infection, tumors, cerumen impaction, or tympanic membrane perforation
- Pneumatic otoscopy to evaluate for simple middle ear effusion as cause of conductive HL
- Rinne and Weber tests are helpful for determining conductive versus SNHL but not recommended for general screening.

DIFFERENTIAL DIAGNOSIS
- Complete canal occlusion (cerumen, foreign body)
- Large external or middle ear tumors
- Chronic otitis media or effusion
- Cholesteatoma
- Otosclerosis
- Osteogenesis imperfecta
- Perilymph fistula (trauma/iatrogenic)
- Ménière disease
- Acoustic neuroma (usually unilateral)
- Vascular anomaly
- Acute noise-induced traumatic loss (explosion)
- Autoimmune HL

DIAGNOSTIC TESTS & INTERPRETATION
- Central: synthetic sentence identification test with ipsilateral competing message and the dichotic sentence identification test (4)[C]
- Peripheral: handheld audiometry; insert probe in ear (sealing canal) and have patient indicate if tones can be heard.
  - Positive likelihood ratio (LR) range, 3.1 to 5.8; negative LR range, 0.03 to 0.4
- Screening audiometry
  - Symmetric high-frequency HL in descending slope pattern
  - SNHL frequencies >2 KHz initially
  - Essential to determine global clinical hearing status and if etiology is conductive HL versus SNHL or pseudohypacusis (conversion)

Initial Tests (lab, imaging)
Imaging studies are not indicated for the diagnosis of presbycusis.

Follow-Up Tests & Special Considerations
Asymmetric HL should have evaluation via MRI for acoustic neuroma.

TREATMENT

- Treatment consists of HAs, cochlear implants (CIs), active middle ear implants (AMEIs), electrical acoustic stimulation, hearing assistive technologies, and aural rehabilitation.
- Analog HA: picks up sound waves through a microphone; converts them into electrical signals; amplifies and sends them through the ear canal to the tympanic membrane
- Digital HA: programmable; may reduce acoustic feedback, reduce background noise, detect and automatically accommodate different listening environments, control multiple microphones
  - HAs have an average decibel gain of 16.3 dB.
  - Associated with hypersensitivity to loud sounds ("loudness recruitment")
- Hearing-assistive technologies (HATs) (4)
  - Can be used alone or in combination with HAs (for difficult listening conditions)
  - Addresses face-to-face communication, broadcast or other electronic media (radio, TV), telephone conversation, sensitivity to alerting signals and environment stimuli (doorbell, baby's cry, alarm clock, etc.)
  - Includes personal FM systems, infrared systems, induction loop systems, hardwired systems, telephone amplifier, telecoil, telecommunication device for the deaf (TDD), situation-specific devices (e.g., television), alerting devices
- Aural rehabilitation (also known as audiologic orientation or auditory training)
  - Adjunct to HA or HATs
  - Involves education regarding proper use of amplification devices, coaching on how to manage the auditory environment, training in speech perception and communication, and counseling for coping strategies to deal with the difficulties of HAs or HATs

ISSUES FOR REFERRAL
- Sudden SNHL is atypical and an otologic emergency warranting urgent otolaryngologic evaluation/audiometry.
- Refer to audiologist for formal evaluation and optimal fitting of HAs and/or HATs

ADDITIONAL THERAPIES
- Gene therapy: Ongoing research targets include investigation of various transcription factors, cell cycle modulators, and cyclin-dependent kinase inhibitors associated with formation and regeneration of hair cells and maintenance of supporting cells.
- Pharmacotherapy: Ongoing research includes cellular signaling pathways and molecules as the most investigated targets for pharmacotherapy. Wnt and Notch signaling cascades are implicated in proliferation of supporting cells and associated with limited hair cell growth.
- Stem cell therapy: Mesenchymal stem cells have also shown success in regenerating cochlear spiral ganglion neurons. Endogenous stem cells show the most promising results (4).

SURGERY/OTHER PROCEDURES
- CIs
  - Bypasses the ear canal, middle ear, and hair cells in the cochlea to provide electric stimulation directly to the auditory nerve
  - Indications include hearing no better than identifying ≤50% of keywords in test sentences in the best aided condition in the worst ear and 60% in the better ear.
  - Incoming sounds are received through the microphone in the audio processor component (resembles a small HA), which converts them into electrical impulses and sends them to the magnetic coil (located on the skin). The impulses transmit these across intact skin via radio waves to the implanted component (directly subjacent to the coil). The pulses travel to the electrodes in the cochlea and stimulate the cochlea at high rates.
  - Receiving a unilateral CI is most common; some may receive bilateral CIs (either sequentially or in the same surgery). Others may wear a CI in one ear and an HA in the contralateral ear (bimodal fit).
  - Younger age at CI placement derives the greatest benefit.
- AMEIs
  - Suitable for elderly adults who cannot wear conventional HAs for medical or personal (cosmetic) reasons and whose HL is not severe enough for a CI
  - Different models available and may include components that are implantable under the skin
- Electric acoustic stimulation: use of CI and HA together in one ear
  - Addresses the specific needs of patients presenting with good low-frequency hearing (a mild-to-moderate sensorineural HL in frequencies up to 1,000 Hz) but poorer hearing in the high frequencies (sloping to 60 dB or worse HL >1,000 Hz)
    - Contraindications: progressive HL, autoimmune disease; HL related to meningitis, otosclerosis, or ossification; malformation of the cochlea; a gap in air conduction and bone conduction thresholds of >15 dB; external ear contraindications, active infection, or unwillingness to use amplification device (4)

 ONGOING CARE

FOLLOW-UP RECOMMENDATIONS
Patient Monitoring
- Check for proper fit of HA and assess and address any patient concerns to improve compliance as 25–40% of adults will either stop wearing them or use them only occasionally.
- Annual audiograms

PATIENT EDUCATION
- Should be face-to-face; spoken clearly and unhurriedly, without competing background noise (e.g., radio, TV); and include a confirmation that the message is received
- Formal speech reading classes may be beneficial.

REFERENCES

1. Deal JA, Sharrett AR, Albert MS, et al. Hearing impairment and cognitive decline: a pilot study conducted within the atherosclerosis risk in communities neurocognitive study. *Am J Epidemiol*. 2015;181(9):680–690.
2. Wang J, Puel JL. Presbycusis: an update on cochlear mechanisms and therapies. *J Clin Med*. 2020;9(1):218.
3. Yamasoba T, Someya S, Yamada C, et al. Role of mitochondrial dysfunction and mitochondrial DNA mutations in age-related hearing loss. *Hear Res*. 2007;226(1–2):185–193.
4. Vaisbuch Y, Santa Maria PL. Age-related hearing loss: innovations in hearing augmentation. *Otolaryngol Clin North Am*. 2018;51(4):705–723.
5. Yueh B, Collins MP, Souza PE, et al. Long-term effectiveness of screening for hearing loss: the screening for auditory impairment—which hearing assessment test (SAI-WHAT) randomized trial. *J Am Geriatr Soc*. 2010;58(3):427–434.
6. Loughrey DG, Kelly ME, Kelley GA, et al. Association of age-related hearing loss with cognitive function, cognitive impairment, and dementia: a systematic review and meta-analysis. *JAMA Otolaryngol Head Neck Surg*. 2018;144(2):115–126.
7. Fishman J, Fisher EW. Impact of coronavirus disease 2019 on otolaryngological practice, effect of presbylarynx and presbycusis in the elderly, and suicidal ideation in patients with tinnitus. *J Lar Otol*. 2021;135(12):1035–1036.

CODES

ICD10
- H91.10 Presbycusis, unspecified ear
- H91.13 Presbycusis, bilateral
- H91.11 Presbycusis, right ear

CLINICAL PEARLS
- Presbycusis is an age-related HL, showing increased prevalence with age. It is often bilateral and initially begins as high-frequency HL. It presents as difficulty communicating in noisy conditions.
- HL is significantly associated with social isolation, depression, and progressive cognitive impairment leading to dementia.
- Early audiology referral for individuals with suspected HL may improve treatment efficacy.
- The use of auditory assistive devices such as HAs, CIs, and AMEIs are associated with improvement in cognitive function, social isolation, and depression.

P

PRESSURE ULCER

Ramanpreet Grewal, MD

BASICS

DESCRIPTION
- Breakdown in a localized area of skin or underlying tissue, primarily caused by prolonged pressure and/or shear
- Usually over a bony prominence where the skin is in proximity with the underlying bone (e.g., sacrum, calcaneus, ischium)
- Classified in stages according to the National Pressure Injury Advisory Panel (NPIAP):
  - Stage I: nonblanchable erythema—intact skin with nonblanchable redness; darkly pigmented skin may not have visible blanching.
  - Stage II: partial-thickness skin loss—shallow open ulcer with a viable red-pink, moist wound bed, without slough; or intact or open/ruptured serum-filled blister
  - Stage III: full-thickness skin loss—subcutaneous fat may be visible, but bone, tendon, or muscle is not exposed; slough, if present, does not obscure depth of tissue loss.
  - Stage IV: full-thickness tissue loss—exposed bone, tendon, or joint; slough or eschar may be present but does not completely obscure wound base.
  - Unstageable: depth unknown—base of the ulcer is covered by slough and/or eschar in the wound bed.
  - Suspected deep tissue injury: depth unknown—purple or maroon area of intact skin or blood-filled blister. Pain and temperature change precede skin color changes.
- Synonyms: bedsores, decubitus ulcers, pressure sores, pressure injuries, pressure wounds, pressure points, pressure damage, pressure-related skin injuries, skin breakdown, ischemic ulcers

EPIDEMIOLOGY
Incidence
Ranges widely depending on setting and population: 0–53.4% (1)

Prevalence
Ranges widely depending on setting and population: 0–72.5% (1)

ETIOLOGY AND PATHOPHYSIOLOGY
Complex process of risk factors interacting with external forces (pressure and/or shear, friction, and moisture)

RISK FACTORS
- Mobility impairment
- Malnutrition
- Reduced skin perfusion
- Sensory impairment
- Medical devices

GENERAL PREVENTION
- Structured risk assessment
- Skin and tissue assessment
- Preventive skin care
- Nutrition screening
- Repositioning
- Early mobilization
- Support surfaces
- Microclimate control
- Prophylactic dressings
- Electrical stimulation of the muscles

COMMONLY ASSOCIATED CONDITIONS
- Advanced age
- Immobility
- Trauma
- Hip fractures
- Diabetes
- Cerebrovascular and cardiovascular disease
- Incontinence

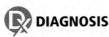

DIAGNOSIS

HISTORY
- Risk factors
- Nutritional assessment
- Pain assessment
- Date of ulcer diagnosis
- Treatment course

PHYSICAL EXAM
- Full skin examination on initial contact and repeatedly throughout visits
- Assess location, stage, size (length, width, depth), identify the presence of sinus tracts, undermining, tunneling, exudate, necrosis, odor, and signs of healing (e.g., granulation tissue) (1).
- Identify factors that may affect healing (impaired perfusion, sensation, presence of infection).

DIFFERENTIAL DIAGNOSIS
- Venous ulcers
- Arterial ulcers
- Diabetic foot ulcer
- Cellulitis and erysipelas
- Incontinence associated dermatitis
- Skin tears
- Intertrigo
- Neuropathic ulcers
- Cutaneous squamous cell carcinomas
- Hypertensive ulcers
- Pyoderma gangrenosum, cancers, vasculitides, and other dermatologic conditions

DIAGNOSTIC TESTS & INTERPRETATION
Initial Tests (lab, imaging)
- Laboratory tests:
  - Complete blood count (CBC) and consider C-reactive protein (CRP) to check for infection/inflammation or anemia
  - Albumin and prealbumin to assess nutritional status
  - Electrolytes to assess overall metabolic status
  - Blood urea nitrogen (BUN) and creatinine to assess kidney function
  - Hemoglobin A1c (HbA1c) to assess long-term blood sugar control
  - Wound culture: Do not culture surface drainage. If culture is necessary, do deep tissue culture/bone biopsy.
- Imaging studies:
  - X-rays, MRI, or ultrasound may be used to assess the depth of the ulcer and determine if there is underlying bone involvement.
  - Ankle-brachial index and Doppler ultrasound (for lower extremity wounds)

Follow-Up Tests & Special Considerations
- Nutrition management: Ensure adequate nutrition, especially in at-risk patients.
- Pressure redistribution: Use support surfaces to reduce pressure on vulnerable areas.
- Diabetes management: Monitor and manage blood sugar in diabetic patients.
- Mobility and positioning: Encourage regular position changes to prevent ulcers.
- Patient education: Educate patients and caregivers on wound care and prevention.
- Addressing underlying causes: Manage medical conditions contributing to ulcers.
- Physical therapy: Involve physical therapists to improve mobility and healing.
- Pain management: Address pain to improve patient comfort.
- Patient compliance: Encourage adherence to the treatment plan and follow-up appointments.

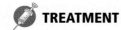

TREATMENT

GENERAL MEASURES
- Comprehensive initial assessment of the patient
- Pressure reduction/redistribution (2)[A]
- Nutritional support (e.g., protein-containing supplements) (3)[B]
- Wound assessment and treatment
  - Wound bed preparation (tissue management, infection and inflammation control, moisture balance, epithelial edge advancement) (1)
  - Wound cleansing (1)[C]
  - Debridement (1)[C]
- Address immobility.
- Manage incontinence.
- Address pain.
- Assess goals of care and advance directives.

MEDICATION
First Line
- Wound dressings as appropriate for the category of ulcer (transparent film, hydrocolloid, hydrogel, alginate, foam, silver-impregnated, honey-impregnated, cadexomer iodine, gauze, silicone, collagen matrix, composite) (1)[C].
- Individual studies comparing dressings are generally of low quality. Systematic reviews comparing dressings have been unable to find superiority of one dressing over another (4)[A].
- Enzymatic débriding agents

Second Line
- Activated charcoal
- Topical antiseptics (hydrogen peroxide, Dakin solution, povidone-iodine)

ISSUES FOR REFERRAL
- Consider referral to a wound care specialist (if available) for complex or nonhealing wounds.
- Consider vascular surgery for improvement of blood flow to wound via vascular bypass if appropriate.
- Consider a surgical consultation for possible urgent drainage and/or débridement if advancing cellulitis; suspected source of sepsis; undermining, tunneling, sinus tracts, and/or extensive necrotic tissue that cannot otherwise be removed by nonsurgical debridement methods; or for stage III or IV that are not closing with conservative management (1)[C].
- Consider plastic surgery for skin graft/flap if appropriate.
- Consider dermatology referral if suspected pyoderma gangrenosum, cancer, vasculitis, or other dermatologic conditions.

ADDITIONAL THERAPIES
- Direct contact electrical stimulation for recalcitrant stage II and any category/stage III and IV (1)[C]
- Electromagnetic field for recalcitrant category/stage II and any stage III and IV (1)[C]
- Pulsed radio frequency energy for recalcitrant stage II and any stage III and IV (1)[C]

SURGERY/OTHER PROCEDURES
- Débridement: removal of dead or infected tissue from the ulcer
- Flap surgery: transplanting healthy tissue from nearby areas to cover the ulcer
- Skin grafting: using healthy skin from another part of the body to cover the ulcer
- Negative pressure wound therapy (NPWT): applying vacuum to the wound to promote healing
- Muscle flap rotation: rotating a muscle with its blood supply to cover the wound
- Implants and bioengineered tissues: Using surgical implants or bioengineered tissues to aid healing

COMPLEMENTARY & ALTERNATIVE MEDICINE
- Low-frequency ultrasound for débridement of necrotic soft tissue (not eschar) (1)[C]
- High-frequency ultrasound as adjunct for infected pressure ulcers (1)[C]
- NPWT as an early adjuvant treatment for deep, stage III and IV (1)[C]
- Consider course of hydrotherapy with pulsed lavage with suction for wound cleansing and débridement (1)[C].
- Phototherapy: short-term UVC light if traditional therapies fail (1)[C]; laser not recommended; infrared is not recommended (1)[C].

- Hyperbaric and topical oxygen therapy not recommended for routine use (1)[C]
- Hydrotherapy with whirlpool should not be considered for routine use (1)[C].
- Vibration therapy not recommended (1)[C]
- Consider sterile maggot débridement therapy.

ADMISSION, INPATIENT, AND NURSING CONSIDERATIONS
- Admission criteria/initial stabilization: refractory cellulitis, osteomyelitis, systemic infection, advanced nutritional decline, suspected patient mistreatment, inability to care for self
- Dressing changes 1 to 3 times daily based on wound assessment and plan of care
- Assess risk factors according to scales.
- Assess for changing or new wounds.
- Discharge criteria: clinical improvement in wound and systemic illness; when applicable, safe and appropriate location for discharge

ONGOING CARE

FOLLOW-UP RECOMMENDATIONS
- Wound assessment: Regularly assess the pressure ulcer for progress and changes.
- Wound measurement: Periodically measure the ulcer's dimensions to track healing and treatment effectiveness.

Patient Monitoring
- Home health nursing
- Change plan of care if no improvement in 2 to 3 weeks.

DIET
- Approximately 1.0 to 1.5 kg/day of protein
- Strict glycemic control
- Include micronutrients in diet or as supplements (vitamin C and zinc).

PATIENT EDUCATION
- Check skin regularly.
- Signs and symptoms of infection
- Report new or increased pain.
- Prevention of new wound where old wound healed
- Skin care, moisture prevention
- Smoking cessation

PROGNOSIS
Variable, depending on the following:
- Removal of pressure
- Nutrition
- Wound care

COMPLICATIONS
- Infection
- Amputation
- Increased mortality

REFERENCES
1. Haesler E, ed. *Prevention and Treatment of Pressure Ulcers: Clinical Practice Guideline*. Osborne Park, Western Australia: Cambridge Media; 2014.
2. Bergstrom N, Horn SD, Rapp MP, et al. Turning for Ulcer Reduction: a multisite randomized clinical trial in nursing homes. *J Am Geriatr Soc*. 2013;61(10):1705–1713.
3. Smith ME, Totten A, Hickam DH, et al. Pressure ulcer treatment strategies: a systematic comparative effectiveness review. *Ann Intern Med*. 2013;159(1):39–50.
4. Westby MJ, Dumville JC, Soares MO, et al. Dressings and topical agents for treating pressure ulcers. *Cochrane Database Syst Rev*. 2017;6(6):CD011947.

ADDITIONAL READING
- Pieper B, ed. *Pressure Ulcers: Prevalence, Incidence, and Implications for the Future*. Washington, DC: NPUAP; 2012.
- Qaseem A, Humphrey LL, Forciea MA, et al; for Clinical Guidelines Committee of the American College of Physicians. Treatment of pressure ulcers: a clinical practice guideline from the American College of Physicians. *Ann Intern Med*. 2015;162(5):370–379.
- Reddy M, Gill SS, Rochon PA. Preventing pressure ulcers: a systematic review. *JAMA*. 2006;296(8):974–984.
- Stansby G, Avital L, Jones K, et al. Prevention and management of pressure ulcers in primary and secondary care: summary of NICE guidance. *BMJ*. 2014;348:g2592.

CODES

ICD10
- L89.95 Pressure ulcer of unspecified site, unstageable
- L89.91 Pressure ulcer of unspecified site, stage 1
- L89.92 Pressure ulcer of unspecified site, stage 2

CLINICAL PEARLS
- Create assessment and prevention protocols for all patients.
- Identify risk factors, reduce/redistribute pressure, maximize nutrition, regular skin checks, and assess and treat wounds appropriately.
- All care needs to be done in a time-sensitive, patient-centered fashion.

PRETERM LABOR

Bindusri Paruchuri, MD

 BASICS

Preterm birth is defined as birth between 20 0/7 and 36 6/7 weeks' gestation.

DESCRIPTION

Regular contractions occurring between 20 0/7 and 36 6/7 weeks' gestation with either a change in effacement and cervical dilation or cervical dilation of ≥2 cm on presentation

EPIDEMIOLOGY

Preterm birth is the leading cause of perinatal morbidity and mortality in the United States.

Incidence

- 10–15% of pregnancies experienced at least one episode of preterm labor.
- Causes of preterm births in the United States: spontaneous preterm labor makes up 40–45% of preterm births, preterm premature rupture of membranes makes up 30–35% of preterm births, medically indicated delivery due to maternal or neonatal etiology associated with 30–35% of preterm births, and multiple gestation

Prevalence

- Non-Hispanic blacks are 50% more likely to have a preterm birth than Hispanic or white patients.
- 10% of all births in the United States in 2019 were preterm: 50% of preterm deliveries are due to spontaneous preterm labor, 25% following preterm prelabor rupture of membranes, and 25% due to maternal or fetal medical indications due to complications (1).

ETIOLOGY AND PATHOPHYSIOLOGY

- Premature formation and activation of myometrial gap junctions
- Abnormal placental implantation/placental abruption/placental ischemic disease (preeclampsia and fetal growth restriction)
- Systemic inflammation/infections (e.g., UTI, autoimmune conditions)/immunopathology (e.g., antiphospholipid antibodies)
- Local inflammation/infections (e.g., intraamniotic infections, group B *Streptococcus* [GBS]—colonization with infectious organism noted in 25–40% of all preterm births
- Uterine abnormalities/overdistension (multiple gestation, polyhydramnios)/cervical insufficiency/premature dilation
- Preterm premature rupture of membranes
- Trauma
- Fetal abnormalities
- Hypertensive disorders of pregnancy

Genetics

Familial predisposition; numerous gene candidates mediating various pathways have been identified, but causality and gene–environment interactions are not well-defined.

RISK FACTORS

- Prior preterm delivery (most significant risk factor): >3-fold if previous preterm birth
- Demographic factors, including social and economic disadvantages and black race with concern for chronic stress from structural racism
- Short interpregnancy interval (<18 months)
- Prepregnancy weight <45 kg (<100 lb), body mass index <18.5

- Substance abuse (e.g., cocaine, tobacco)
- Unintended pregnancy
- Cervical insufficiency/short cervical length of <25 mm
- Abdominal surgery/trauma during pregnancy; history of dilation and curettage
- Uterine structural abnormalities, such as large fibroids or müllerian abnormalities
- Serious maternal infections/diseases; bacterial vaginosis and genital tract infections; bacteriuria
- Multiple gestation; intrauterine growth restriction; polyhydramnios
- Placenta previa; vaginal bleeding; premature placental separation (abruption)

GENERAL PREVENTION

- Patient education at each visit in 2nd and 3rd trimesters for those at risk and periodically in the last two trimesters for the general population
- For women with a singleton pregnancy and no history of spontaneous preterm births, visualization of the cervix on routine fetal anatomical scan between 18 0/7 and 22 6/7 weeks' gestation should be performed. If found to be shortened, a transvaginal ultrasound should be done for further evaluation (1)[C]. This recommendation is the same for multiple gestation and women with a history of medically induced preterm birth. Twin pregnancies are more likely to have a shortened cervix during the 2nd trimester, and women with a history of medically induced preterm birth are more likely to have a subsequent preterm birth (1).
- For women with history of spontaneous preterm birth and singleton pregnancy, a screening transvaginal ultrasound to evaluate cervix length should be done at 16 0/7 weeks' gestation and repeated every 1 to 4 weeks (protocols vary) until 24 0/7 weeks (1).
- Primary prevention involves counseling on: interval contraception to optimize pregnancy spacing and smoking cessation; if previous preterm birth, evaluate if etiology is likely to recur and target intervention to specific condition. Women with history of spontaneous preterm birth and singleton pregnancy should be offered vaginal or intramuscular progesterone to prevent preterm birth with a shared decision model (1).
- Secondary prevention:
  - For patients with a cervix of <25 mm in length with or without a history of previous spontaneous preterm delivery and singleton pregnancy, it has been recommended to give vaginal progesterone if not already on progesterone. Most protocols give 200 mg/day at diagnosis at 18 0/7 to 25 6/7 weeks' gestation to continue until 36 to 37 weeks (1). An FDA advisory committee voted in late 2022 to withdraw approval of 17-hydroxy progesterone and its generic equivalents based on results from postmarket confirmatory trial data in the PROLONG study, released in October 2019, showing lack of efficacy. Data is insufficient to recommend vaginal progesterone for multiple gestation (1).
  - Women with a singleton pregnancy and history of spontaneous preterm birth with shortened cervix should be considered for a cerclage (1). Cerclage can be considered for any patient who is noted to have cervical insufficiency on physical exam (1).
- Tocolysis

 DIAGNOSIS

- Diagnosis is generally based on a combination of significant cervical changes (such as dilation, effacement) with regular contractions. However, there is no single test that will reliably diagnose or predict true preterm labor.
- ACOG defines preterm labor as regular contractions noted with change in cervical dilation, effacement, or both, or regular contractions and cervical dilation of at least 2 cm at presentation.

HISTORY

- Address risk factors
- Regular uterine contractions or cramping; dull, low backache or pain; intermittent lower abdominal pain; increased low pelvic pressure
- Change in vaginal discharge; vaginal bleeding
- Amniotic fluid leakage

PHYSICAL EXAM

- Sterile speculum exam for membrane rupture evaluation, cultures, and cervical inspection
- Bimanual cervical exam if intact membranes

ALERT
Avoid bimanual examination when possible if rupture of the membranes is suspected.

DIFFERENTIAL DIAGNOSIS

- Braxton-Hicks contractions/false labor
- Round ligament pain
- Lumbosacral muscular back pain
- UTI or vaginal infections
- Adnexal torsion
- Appendicitis
- Nephrolithiasis

DIAGNOSTIC TESTS & INTERPRETATION

Initial Tests (lab, imaging)

- There are no specific tests that completely or accurately predict preterm birth, although they help with risk stratification.
- In symptomatic women from 22 to 34 weeks' gestation with intact membranes and no intercourse or bleeding in the past 24 hours, obtain a fetal fibronectin (fFN) swab from the posterior vaginal fornix.
  - If results are positive (≥50 ng/mL), patient is at a modest increased risk of preterm birth (positive predictive value [PPV] 13–30% for delivery within 2 weeks). However, if results are negative, >97% of patients will not deliver in 14 days, so can consider avoiding complicated or high-risk interventions.
  - fFN and shortened cervix alone has low predictive value, so other data should be used as well in acute management of patient (2).
- Urinalysis and urine culture; cultures for gonorrhea, chlamydia, and wet prep
- Vaginal introitus and rectal culture for GBS if indicated
- pH and fern test of vaginal fluid to evaluate for rupture of membranes
- CBC with differential and Kleihauer-Betke test if abruption suspected

- US to identify number of fetuses and fetal position, confirm gestational age, estimate fetal weight, quantify amniotic fluid, and look for conditions that contraindicate tocolysis
- Transvaginal US to evaluate cervix length, funneling, and dynamic changes after obtaining fFN (if clinical assessment of the cervix is uncertain or if the cervix is closed on digital exam); ACOG and Society for Maternal-Fetal Medicine (SMFM) recommend transvaginal cervical length screening in patients with history of previous spontaneous preterm birth.

Diagnostic Procedures/Other
Monitor contractions with external tocodynamometer.

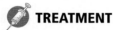

TREATMENT

GENERAL MEASURES
Treat underlying risk factors. Hospitalization is necessary if the patient needs IV tocolysis.

MEDICATION
Tocolysis may allow time for interventions such as transfer to tertiary care facility and administration of corticosteroids but may not prolong pregnancy significantly (2).

First Line
- Corticosteroids (2):
  - Corticosteroids decrease neonatal respiratory distress, intraventricular hemorrhage, necrotizing enterocolitis, and overall perinatal mortality.
  - Give if the mother is at 24 to 34 weeks' gestation and is at risk for delivery in the next 7 days (2); can consider if mother is at 23 0/7 to 23 6/7 weeks' gestation and at risk for delivery in the next 7 days
  - Rescue course considered if <34 weeks' gestation, at risk of delivery in the next 7 days, and previous course of corticosteroids was administered 14 days prior (2)
  - Betamethasone 12 mg IM × 2 doses 24 hours apart or dexamethasone 6 mg IM q12h for 4 doses (2)
  - Steroids may reduce the risk of respiratory morbidities in singleton infants born to nondiabetic mothers in the late preterm period (34 0/7 to 36 6/7 weeks' gestation). If delivery is likely during this time period, administration of steroids may be considered as above. Tocolysis is not recommended.
- Tocolysis: reserved for women who benefit from a 48-hour delay to receive corticosteroids as there is no evidence showing tocolysis causes improvement in neonatal outcomes up to 34 weeks' gestation (2)
  - Nifedipine is a calcium channel blocker (CCB) that can be used for tocolysis: 20 mg PO loading dose and then 10 to 20 mg q4–6h for 48 hours (do not use sublingual route); check BP often and avoid hypotension; concurrent use with magnesium sulfate is discouraged due to the theoretical risk of neuromuscular blockade (3); contraindications: hypotension, preload dependent cardiac abnormalities such as aortic insufficiency (2)

- Indomethacin is a nonsteroidal anti-inflammatory drug (NSAID) used for tocolysis: 50 to 100 mg PO initial dose and then 25 to 50 mg q6–8h; best to use in combination with magnesium if it is being used for neuroprotection (2),(3); consider for use up to 32 weeks (2); contraindications: platelet dysfunction, bleeding disorder, gastrointestinal ulcerative disease, and asthma (if hypersensitive to aspirin) (2)
- Terbutaline is a β-adrenergic receptor agonist given for tocolysis; given via SC administration; if contractions persist or pulse >120 beats/min, change to another tocolytic agent (3). Due to reports of serious cardiovascular events and maternal deaths, PO or long-term SC administration of terbutaline should not be given (3); contraindications: tachycardia-sensitive maternal cardiac disease and poorly controlled diabetes mellitus (2)
- Contraindications to tocolysis: severe preeclampsia, eclampsia, hemorrhage with hemodynamic instability, preterm premature rupture of membranes, chorioamnionitis, advanced labor, intrauterine growth restriction, fetal distress, or lethal fetal abnormalities
- Magnesium sulfate: recommended for imminent delivery prior to 32 weeks for neuroprotection as it reduces the risk and severity of cerebral palsy
- Antibiotics for GBS prophylaxis if culture is indicated

Second Line
- Magnesium sulfate by IV infusion has not been shown to be superior to placebo in prolonging pregnancy >48 hours. The side effects are generally greater than those with CCBs or NSAIDs. Therefore, this agent should be used cautiously; contraindication: myasthenia gravis
- Antibiotics should not be used as tocolysis or to improve neonatal outcomes for preterm labor with intact membranes and may be associated with harm.

ISSUES FOR REFERRAL
- If delivery is inevitable but not immediate, consider transport to a tertiary care center or hospital equipped with a neonatal ICU.
- Consider consultation with maternal–fetal medicine specialist.

ADDITIONAL THERAPIES
- Data to prove efficacy of pelvic rest (e.g., no douching or intercourse) is lacking. Bed rest and hydration have not been shown to be effective in the prevention of preterm delivery and are not recommended (2).
- If there is preterm premature rupture of membranes, latency antibiotics are indicated.

SURGERY/OTHER PROCEDURES
Consider cerclage with history of recurrent 2nd trimester losses and diagnosis of cervical insufficiency, ultrasound finding of shortened cervix (<25 mm) and history of preterm birth, and rescue cerclage can be done emergently when cervical insufficiency is noted in patient with threatened preterm labor.

ADMISSION, INPATIENT, AND NURSING CONSIDERATIONS
Suspected/threatened preterm labor management: IV access with IV hydration, continuous fetal and contraction monitoring, assessing cervical dilatation and effacement, and monitoring for fluid overload

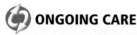

ONGOING CARE

FOLLOW-UP RECOMMENDATIONS
Patient Monitoring
- Weekly office visits with contraction monitoring, cervical checks, or cervical US if at high risk for recurrence
- Routine use of maintenance tocolysis is ineffective in preventing recurrent preterm labor or preterm birth.

PATIENT EDUCATION
Call physician or proceed to hospital whenever regular contractions last >1 hour, bleeding, increased vaginal discharge or fluid, decreased fetal movement.

PROGNOSIS
- If membranes are ruptured and no infection is confirmed, delivery often occurs within 3 to 7 days.
- If membranes are intact, 20–50% deliver preterm.

COMPLICATIONS
Labor resistant to tocolysis, pulmonary edema, intraamniotic infection

REFERENCES
1. American College of Obstetricians and Gynecologists. Prediction and prevention of spontaneous preterm birth: ACOG Practice Bulletin, Number 234. Obstet Gynecol. 2021;138(2): e65–e90.
2. American College of Obstetricians and Gynecologists. Practice Bulletin No. 171 summary: management of preterm labor. Obstet Gynecol. 2016;128(4):931–933.
3. Rundell K, Panchal B. Preterm labor: prevention and management. Am Fam Physician. 2017;95(6): 366–372.

 CODES

ICD10
- O60.03 Preterm labor without delivery, third trimester
- O60.0 Preterm labor without delivery
- O60.02 Preterm labor without delivery, second trimester

CLINICAL PEARLS
- Treatment of preterm labor/tocolysis may delay delivery to facilitate short-term interventions such as administration of corticosteroids, which improve neonatal outcomes.
- Magnesium sulfate is recommended for neuroprotection for imminent deliveries prior to 32 weeks.

PRIAPISM

Dongsheng Jiang, MD, MSc • Joseph P. Wiedemer, MD, FAAFP

 BASICS

DESCRIPTION

- Penile (or less common clitoral) erection lasting for >4 hours and unrelated to sexual stimulation or arousal
- Classification:
  - Ischemic (low-flow, veno-occlusive): accounts for 95% of priapism cases. It is associated with ischaemia of the corpora cavernosa.
  - Nonischemic (high-flow, arterial): less common and often painless and does not require urgent treatment
  - Recurrent ischemic ("stuttering") priapism: episodic, short-lived, and may not require intervention
- Malignant priapism: rare, resulting most commonly from penile metastases related to primary bladder, prostatic, rectosigmoid, and renal tumors
- System(s) affected: reproductive and vascular
- Functional impairment: neurophysiologic, sexual, psychosocial

Pediatric Considerations
In children, the most common etiology is sickle cell disease (SCD) (63% of cases). Less common etiologies, occurring more typically in the adolescent years, are leukemia, idiopathic, penile trauma (e.g., post circumcision), or illicit drugs (up to 35% of cases).

EPIDEMIOLOGY
Incidence
- About 5.3 per 100,000 men per year
- Age: There has been an age shift since 2008 toward men in their 40s. The incidence doubles in men aged >40 years (2.9 vs. 1.5/100,000 person-years).
- Race: 61.1% African American (correlated with incidence of SCD), 30% Caucasian, 6.3% Hispanic

ETIOLOGY AND PATHOPHYSIOLOGY
- Anatomy and physiology:
  - The penis consists of three longitudinally oriented corpora: two dorsolaterally paired corpora cavernosa that are responsible for penile erection and a single ventral corpus spongiosum that surrounds the glans penis and extends distally to form the glans penis.
  - In general, the penile artery supplies the penis. It divides into three branches: dorsal artery, bulbar artery (supplies the corpus spongiosum), and cavernosal artery (the main blood supply to the erectile tissue).

- In ischemic priapism, decreased venous outflow results in increased intracavernosal pressure. This leads to erection, decreased arterial inflow, blood stasis, local hypoxia, and acidosis (a compartment syndrome). Penile tissue necrosis and fibrosis may occur if priapism persists >24 hours. Pathophysiology mechanisms thought to contribute to impaired smooth muscle relaxation and decreased venous outflow include dysregulation of the NO/cGMP, RhoA/Rho kinase, and opiorphin signaling pathways as well as excessive adenosine signaling (1).
- In nonischemic priapism, increased arterial flow without decreased venous outflow results in a sustained, nonpainful, partially rigid erection.
- Causes:
  - Ischemic priapism:
    - Idiopathic: about 50% cases
    - Hematologic dyscrasias: SCD, thalassemia, leukemia, multiple myeloma, fat emboli during hyperalimentation, hemodialysis, glucose-6-phosphate dehydrogenase (G6PD) deficiency, factor V Leiden mutation
    - Infections (toxin mediated): urinary tract infections, scorpion sting, spider bite, rabies, malaria
    - Metabolic disorders: nephrolithiasis, amyloidosis, Fabry disease, gout
    - Neurogenic disorders: syphilis, spinal cord injury, cauda equina syndrome, autonomic neuropathy, lumbar disc herniation, spinal stenosis, cerebrovascular accident, brain tumor, spinal anesthesia
    - Neoplasms: penis, urethra, bladder, prostate, kidney and rectum
    - Medications:
      - Vasoactive erectile agents (i.e., papaverine, phentolamine, prostaglandin E1/alprostadil)
      - α-Adrenergic receptor antagonists (i.e., prazosin, terazosin, doxazosin, tamsulosin)
      - Antidepressants and antipsychotics (i.e., trazodone, bupropion, fluoxetine, sertraline, lithium, clozapine, risperidone, olanzapine, chlorpromazine, thioridazine, phenothiazines)
      - Antihypertensives (i.e., hydralazine, guanethidine, propranolol)
      - Hormones (i.e., gonadotropin-releasing hormone, testosterone)
      - Anxiolytics (hydroxyzine)
      - Anticoagulants (heparin, warfarin)
      - Recreational drugs (i.e., alcohol, marijuana, cocaine)
  - Nonischemic priapism (2):
    - Almost universally associated with penile or perineal trauma resulting in a fistula between the cavernous artery and the corpus cavernosum
    - Acute spinal cord injury
    - Treatment of ischemic priapism

RISK FACTORS
- SCD has a lifetime risk of ischemic priapism 29–42%.
- Dehydration correlated with SCD or trait
- Prior history of priapismic episodes

GENERAL PREVENTION
- Avoid dehydration (SCD cases).
- Avoid excessive sexual stimulation.
- Avoid or limit causative drugs.
- Avoid trauma to the genital area

COMMONLY ASSOCIATED CONDITIONS
- SCD (42.9%) or sickle cell trait (2.5%)
- Drug abuse (7.9%)
- G6PD deficiency
- Leukemia
- Neoplasm

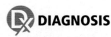 **DIAGNOSIS**

HISTORY
- Prior priapism episodes or prolonged erections after waking and degree of pain
- Duration of erection
- Perineal or penile trauma (blunt force or needle injury)
- Urination difficult during erection
- History of any hematologic abnormalities (e.g., SCD or trait)
- Cardiovascular disease
- Medications
- Recreational drug use

PHYSICAL EXAM
- In general, physical examination should include the following:
  - A complete penile, scrotal, and perineal exam to identify the presence of trauma, gangrene (rare), or prosthesis
  - An abdominal and lymph noted exam to rule out underlying conditions
- Common findings:
  - Ischemic (or stuttering): Penis is fully erect, painful, or tender; corpora cavernosa are rigid; and corpora spongiosum and glans are flaccid.
  - Nonischemic: Penis is partially erect (not tender or painful), and the corpora cavernosa are semirigid and nontender, with the glans and corpora spongiosum flaccid.

DIAGNOSTIC TESTS & INTERPRETATION
- CBC with reticulocyte count
- Sickling hemoglobin (Hgb) solubility test and Hgb electrophoresis
- Coagulation profile
- Urinalysis/urine toxicology

- Corporal blood gas (CBG): Nonischemic blood gas analysis is identical to normal arterial blood, whereas the following is concerning for ischemic priapism: pH <7.25, pO_2 <30 mm Hg, and pCO_2 >60 mm Hg.
- A color Doppler ultrasound:
  – Ischemic—low arterial flow
  – Nonischemic—high arterial flow
- Penile arteriography can be used to identify the presence and arterial cavernous fistula or pseudoaneurysms (nonischemic).
- Penile MRI can be used for cases >48- to 72-hour duration to evaluate for corporal smooth muscle necrosis and candidacy for immediate penile prosthesis implantation.

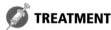 TREATMENT

- Based on the type:
  – Ischemic priapism: requires immediate treatment and urology consultation
    ○ Initial conservative management with encouraging ejaculation, vigorous physical exercise, cold bath, icing
    ○ Cold enemas are *not* recommended especially if those measures lead to delay in starting more evidence based treatment (2).
    ○ Cavernosal aspiration with a large-bore needle
    ○ Cavernosal injection of phenylephrine 200 μg repeated to a maximum of 1,500 μg (with BP monitoring)
    ○ If this fails, shunt procedures are considered.
  – Nonischemic priapism: not an emergency
    ○ Observation, icing, site specific compression; causative fistula may close spontaneously.
    ○ If persists, may consider selective arteriography and embolization (2)
  – Stuttering priapism
    ○ The initial goal is to prevent recurrence. But, if the episode is prolonged, there is a risk of conversion to ischemic priapism.
    ○ Initial conservative treatment including ejaculation, physical exercise, icing, and/or cold shower.
    ○ Manage acute episodes as ischemic cases—aspiration then intracavernous injections of:
      ▪ Phenylephrine: 200 μg every 3 to 5 minutes to a maximum of 1 mg within 1 hour
      ▪ Etilefrine: 2.5 mg diluted in 1 to 2 mL saline
      ▪ Adrenaline: 2 mL of 1/100,000 solution given up to 5 times in a 20-minute period
      ▪ Methylene blue: 50 to 100 mg
- In all cases, particularly SCD cases, treat the underlying condition (e.g., SCD does not delay intracavernous treatment).
- Although blood transfusion is an option, particularly in SCD cases, other interventions should be explored and exhausted first.

GENERAL MEASURES
- Treat any underlying cause or disease process.
- In SCD cases: IV hydration; supplemental oxygen; partial exchange or repeated transfusions to reduce percentage of sickle cells to <50%

MEDICATION
- Analgesics (e.g., opioids) for pain, if needed
- May try oral pseudoephedrine or terbutaline while waiting for intracavernous injection

Second Line
- Ischemic priapism:
  – Etilefrine (intracavernous) is the second most used sympathomimetic.
  – Methylene blue (intracavernous) can be used for pharmacologically induced priapism (cGMP inhibitor).
  – Epinephrine (intracavernous) has a higher success rate than phenylephrine but greater cardiovascular side effects.
- Stuttering priapism:
  – Prevention of recurrence with daily oral medications:
    ○ Adrenergic agonists: pseudoephedrine and etilefrine
    ○ Androgen suppression: antiandrogens, 5α-reductase inhibitors (finasteride), and ketoconazole
    ○ PDE5 inhibitors: sildenafil
    ○ Smooth muscle regulation: digoxin or terbutaline
    ○ Others: gabapentin, baclofen, hydroxyurea

ISSUES FOR REFERRAL
A urologist should be consulted in all cases of suspected priapism.

SURGERY/OTHER PROCEDURES
- For ischemic priapism, surgical options after medical therapy include the following:
  – Distal cavernoglandular shunts
    ○ Percutaneous: Ebbehoj, Winter, or T shunt
    ○ Open: Al-Ghorab or Burnett
  – Proximal cavernoglandular shunts
    ○ Open: Quackles or Sacher
  – Venous shunts
    ○ Grayhack (saphenous vein shunt)
    ○ Barry (deep dorsal vein shunt)
  – Immediate penile prothesis placement: Relative indications include failure of intracavernous therapies or corporal smooth muscle necrosis or MRI/biopsy; early surgery avoids cavernosus fibrosis, which offers the opportunity to maintain penile size, and prevent penile curvature due to cavernosal fibrosis.
- For nonischemic priapism, surgical options include the following:
  – Selective embolization with autologous blood clot, absorbable (gel foam or sponge) or nonabsorbable materials (coils or acrylic glue), or surgical ligation as a last resort

 ONGOING CARE

PROGNOSIS
- Even with excellent treatment for a prolonged priapism, complete detumescence may require several weeks secondary to edema.
- Impotence due to irreversible corporal fibrosis is likely in ischemic priapism and is up to 90% if the priapism lasts >24 hours.

COMPLICATIONS
- Patient can have mental illnesses such as suicidality, depression, and anxiety. When treating those condition, drugs such as fluoxetine, citalopram, and trazodone should be avoided due to potential in precipitating priapism (3).
- Erectile dysfunction

REFERENCES

1. Anele UA, Morrison BF, Burnett AL. Molecular pathophysiology of priapism: emerging targets. *Curr Drug Targets*. 2015;16(5):474–483.
2. Ericson C, Baird B, Broderick GA. Management of priapism: 2021 update. *Urol Clin North Am*. 2021;48(4):565–576.
3. Idris IM, Burnett AL, DeBaun MR. Epidemiology and treatment of priapism in sickle cell disease. *Hematology Am Soc Hematol Educ Program*. 2022;2022(1):450–458.

 SEE ALSO

Anemia, Sickle Cell; Erectile Dysfunction

 CODES

ICD10
- N48.30 Priapism, unspecified
- N48.39 Other priapism
- N48.31 Priapism due to trauma

CLINICAL PEARLS
- If priapism lasts >24 hours, it likely results in permanent sexual impairment.
- Priapism can occur in children, particularly in SCD. Treatment should address both the underlying disease as well as developmental needs.
- In evaluating priapism, the clinician must distinguish ischemic from nonischemic priapism by history and physical exam as well as cavernosal blood gas and possibly ultrasound or MRI, if indicated.
- Ischemic priapism is an emergent condition that requires immediate urologic evaluation and treatment.

PROSTATE CANCER

Dylan Buller, MD • Joseph R. Wagner, MD

 BASICS

DESCRIPTION

- The prostate is a male reproductive gland that contributes seminal fluid to the ejaculate.
- Prostate gland is approximately the size of a walnut, 20 to 25 g in an adult male; enlarges after age 50 years
- Three distinct zones delineate the functional anatomy of the prostate: peripheral zone (largest, neighbors rectal wall, palpable on digital rectal exam [DRE], most common location for prostate cancer), central zone (contains the ejaculatory ducts), and transition zone (located centrally, adjacent to the urethra).
- Prostatic epithelial cells produce prostate-specific antigen (PSA), which is used as a tumor marker and in screening.

EPIDEMIOLOGY

Incidence

An estimated 288,300 men in the United States will be newly diagnosed with carcinoma of the prostate (CaP) in 2023, representing 15% of all new cancer diagnoses.

Prevalence

- An estimated 34,700 men in the United States will die of CaP in 2023, representing 5.7% of all cancer deaths.
- Median age at diagnosis is 67 years; probability of CaP 10.9% (1 in 9) ≥70 years
- Autopsy studies find foci of latent CaP in 50% of men in their 8th decade of life.

ETIOLOGY AND PATHOPHYSIOLOGY

- Adenocarcinoma: >95%; nonadenocarcinoma: <5% (most common transitional cell carcinoma)
- Location of CaP: 70% peripheral zone, 20% transitional zone, 5–10% central zone

RISK FACTORS

Age >50 years, African American race, positive family history

GENERAL PREVENTION

Finasteride use associated with moderate risk reduction in CaP but associated with an increased risk of high-grade disease

ALERT

Screening for prostate cancer is controversial:
- U.S. Preventive Services Task Force (USPSTF): "For men aged 55 to 69 years, the decision to undergo periodic PSA-based screening for prostate cancer should be an individual one and should include discussion of the potential benefits and harms of screening with their clinician. Screening offers a small potential benefit of reducing the chance of death from prostate cancer in some men. However, many men will experience potential harms of screening" (1)[A]. USPSTF recommends against PSA screening for men ≥70 years old (1).
- The American Urological Association (AUA) panel recommends for men aged 55 to 69 years shared decision-making between physician and patient regarding PSA screening.

- PSA screening is not recommended in men aged <40 years or any man with <10 years of estimated life expectancy.
- When providing informed consent, data shows if you screen 1,000 men between ages 55 and 69 years:
  – 240 will have a positive result; only ~100 will truly have CaP; of the 100 with cancer, 80 will agree to treatment.
  – Treatment will result in one less person dying, but 50 will develop erectile dysfunction (ED); 15 permanent incontinence

 DIAGNOSIS

HISTORY

Symptoms of bladder outlet obstruction and other voiding symptoms

PHYSICAL EXAM

DRE to assess for prostatic masses, firmness, or asymmetry

DIFFERENTIAL DIAGNOSIS

Benign prostatic hyperplasia, prostatitis, prostatic intraepithelial neoplasia (PIN), prostate stones, atypical small acinar proliferation (ASAP)

DIAGNOSTIC TESTS & INTERPRETATION

Initial Tests (lab, imaging)

- In general, total PSA ≥4 ng/mL is concerning for CaP (sensitivity of 21% and specificity of 91%).
  – Rectal manipulation will not significantly elevate PSA.
  – 5-α-Reductase inhibitors decrease PSA by ~50%.
  – Consider MRI to guide biopsy.
- Other PSA metrics used to aid in CaP diagnosis:
  – Total PSA velocity: ≥0.75 ng/mL/year or >20% baseline for higher values increases CaP risk.
  – Free PSA and age-/race-adjusted PSA are helpful in evaluating risk. With PSA 4 to 10 ng/mL, a low percent free PSA is associated with higher risk of CaP.
  – PSAD ≥0.15 associated with higher prevalence of CaP
- Prostate biopsy
  – Decision to biopsy involves PSA, DRE, MRI, and consideration of comorbidities and life expectancy
  – Standard biopsy: systematic random cores from peripheral zone base, mid-gland, and apex, 8 to 12 cores
  – Prebiopsy MRI used to identify suspicious prostate lesions
    ○ The Gleason grade ranks specimens from 1 (most differentiated) to 5 (least differentiated).
    ○ Primary and secondary patterns are identified and reported, and the sum is the Gleason score (e.g., 3 + 4 = 7).
    ○ Most prostate cancer are scored 6 to 10, with 10 having the worst prognosis.
    ○ Grade group 1 = Gleason 6; grade group 2 = Gleason 3 + 4 = 7; grade group 3 = Gleason 4 + 3 = 7; grade group 4 = Gleason 8; grade group 5 = Gleason 9 and 10

- Staging
  – TNM (tumor, node, and metastasis) staging is used to generate a clinical and pathologic stage, which directs treatment. Clinical staging is as follows:
    ○ T1: cancer found incidentally on TURP or found on biopsy for elevated PSA
    ○ T2: cancer found on DRE but confined to the prostate
    ○ T3: cancer found to be extended locally outside of the prostate and/or the seminal vesicle
    ○ T4: cancer invading adjacent organs
    ○ N1: denotes local lymph node spread
    ○ M1: distant metastasis

Follow-Up Tests & Special Considerations

- PSMA-PET has increased sensitivity and specificity over conventional imaging.
- Germline and/or somatic testing can be undertaken based on factors related to personal/family history or pathologic features.

TREATMENT

- Use Prostate Predict Calculator to help patient consider treatment options: https://prostate.predict.nhs.uk/.
- Treatment options include the following:
  – Watchful waiting: monitoring with expectation to provide palliation with symptoms
  – Active surveillance: close monitoring of PSA, DRE, and repeat biopsy at regular intervals
    ○ ProtecT trial (2016) found that watchful waiting had equal cancer-specific and all-cause mortality compared to surgery or radiotherapy. In the treatment arms, there was less disease progression (including metastatic disease) but resulted in significantly more morbidity (urinary and bowel dysfunction, ED).
  – Radical prostatectomy: ± pelvic lymph node dissection (PLND)
  – Radiation therapy: external beam (EBRT)
  – Brachytherapy: radioactive implants placed in prostate; option for early clinical stage localized to the prostate
  – Antiandrogen therapy
    ○ Bilateral orchiectomy (surgical castration)
    ○ Gonadotropin-releasing hormone (GnRH) agonist, antagonist, or antiandrogen (medical castration)
    ○ Abiraterone: 17α-hydroxylase inhibitor (CYP17A adrenal androgen production)
    ○ Bicalutamide/nilutamide/flutamide/ enzalutamide/apalutamide: androgen receptor antagonists
  – Chemotherapy: includes multiple chemotherapeutic agents used to treat castrate-resistant prostate cancer (CRPC)
  – Risk factors
    ○ Treatment options based on risk: very low-, low-, favorable intermediate-, unfavorable intermediate-, high-, and very high-risk categories; this is based on risk of recurrence after definitive treatment
    ○ Must meet all three criteria to be low risk; any one criterion moves patient to a higher risk group: risk category clinical stage/serum PSA (ng/mL)/grade group: low T1–T2a/<10/1; intermediate T2b–T2c/10–20/2–3; high T3a/>20/4–5

- Very low- and very-high risk categories, as well as differentiating favorable versus unfavorable intermediate risk, are based on additional clinical/pathologic criteria.
- Updated risk stratification algorithms include additional groups of very low risk, favorable and unfavorable intermediate risk, and very high risk.
- Localized CaP
  - Very low and low risk:
    - □ Mainstay of therapy is active surveillance.
    - □ Radical prostatectomy and radiation therapy may be offered.
  - Intermediate risk:
    - □ Mainstay of therapy is radical prostatectomy or radiation therapy.
    - □ Radical prostatectomy has shown a possible survival benefit in intermediate prostate cancer.
    - □ Active surveillance may be offered to patients in the favorable intermediate risk group.
  - High and very high risk:
    - □ Mainstay of therapy is radical prostatectomy or radiation therapy.
    - □ Adjuvant radiation may be considered based on adverse pathologic findings after prostatectomy.
  - Patients with unfavorable intermediate disease or worse are recommended to undergo additional staging evaluation with soft tissue and bone imaging.

ALERT
Life expectancy determination and risks and benefits of surveillance and treatment options is critical.

- Locally advanced CaP:
  - Mainstay of therapy is androgen deprivation therapy (ADT) and radiation; surgery and adjuvant radiation are also used.
  - Adding abiraterone + prednisone in patients commencing long-term ADT for high-risk (T3–T4, Gleason 8 to 10, PSA >40), locally advanced prostate cancer has been shown to significantly increase overall survival.
- Metastatic CaP:
  - Mainstay of therapy is RT and ADT.
  - Early chemotherapy (docetaxel) with ADT may be considered for high-volume disease; ADT with abiraterone + prednisone for lower volume disease
  - ADT specifics:
    - GnRH agonists include leuprolide, goserelin, histrelin, or triptorelin.
    - GnRH antagonists include degarelix: an alternative to GnRH agonists; suppresses testosterone production and avoids flare phenomenon observed with GnRH agonists
    - Side effects of ADT: osteoporosis, gynecomastia, ED, decreased libido, obesity, lipid alterations, diabetes, and cardiovascular disease
    - Flare phenomenon (disease flare: hot flashes, fatigue) can occur owing to transient increase in testosterone levels on initiation of GnRH agonist therapy.
    - If spinal cord metastases are present, the concern for cord compression with a testosterone flare can be avoided by starting antiandrogen therapy prior to initiation of a GnRH agonist.
    - Combined androgen blockade with GnRH agonist and antiandrogen (e.g., bicalutamide, nilutamide, or flutamide) may be used to prevent flare.

- CRPC: CRPC is defined as progression of disease following ADT. Treatment includes the following:
  - Treatment (prior docetaxel, prior novel hormone therapy):
    - 177Lu-PSMA-617 for patients with metastases seen on PSMA-PET imaging
    - Cabazitaxel, docetaxel rechallenge (preferred if visceral metastases)
    - Cabazitaxel/carboplatin, mitoxantrone, olaparib, pembrolizumab, radium-223, rucaparib in specific patient populations
    - Abiraterone, enzalutamide, or other secondary hormone therapies are also recommended.
  - Treatment (prior docetaxel, no prior novel hormone therapy):
    - Abiraterone, cabazitaxel, or enzalutamide is preferred.
    - Mitoxantrone, cabazitaxel/carboplatin, radium-223, sipuleucel-T in specific patient populations
    - Other secondary hormone therapies are also recommended.
  - Treatment (no prior docetaxel, prior novel hormone therapy):
    - Docetaxel preferred
    - Sipuleucel-T, cabazitaxel/carboplatin, olaparib, rucaparib, radium-223 in specific patient populations
    - Abiraterone, abiraterone + dexamethasone, enzalutamide, or other secondary hormone therapies are also recommended.
  - Treatment (no prior docetaxel, no prior novel hormone therapy):
    - Docetaxel: chemotherapeutic that inhibits microtubules
    - Enzalutamide: androgen receptor inhibitor
    - Abiraterone: inhibitor of CYP17A (adrenal androgen production), used with prednisone
    - Radium-223 (radiopharmaceutical) for patients with symptomatic bony metastases
    - Sipuleucel-T: immunotherapy
    - Other secondary hormone therapies are also recommended.
  - Metastatic: Tumor and germline testing are recommended.
  - Nonmetastatic
    - Continue ADT; add antiandrogen (apalutamide, darolutamide, or enzalutamide).
- Bone health: Men with prostate cancer, especially on ADT, are at elevated risk of pathologic fractures; consider bone density.
  - Denosumab (RANK-ligand inhibitor—prevents osteoclast activation) and zoledronic acid (bisphosphonate) can be offered for prevention.
- Targeted therapies (i.e., poly[ADP-ribose] polymerase [PARP] inhibitors) are generally used in CRCP.
  - Immunotherapy (i.e., sipuleucel-T or pembrolizumab)—therapies meant to boost the body's immune system to attack prostate cancer, generally used in advanced/metastatic disease
  - Cryotherapy (use of very cold temperatures to freeze and kill prostate cancer cells as well as prostate tissue)

 ## ONGOING CARE

FOLLOW-UP RECOMMENDATIONS
- Prostatectomy: PSA and DRE; some combination of CT/MRI/PET/bone scan is obtained at recurrence. If the PSA recurrence is due to local disease, salvage radiation +/− ADT is considered. For metastatic disease, androgen deprivation is considered.
- XRT: PSA and DRE are recommended at regular intervals. Biochemical recurrence is defined as PSA increase ≥2 ng/mL above nadir; some combination of CT/MRI/PET/bone scan is usually obtained. If the PSA recurrence is thought to be from local disease, salvage prostatectomy, cryosurgery, brachytherapy, or high-intensity focused ultrasound (HIFU) is considered. For metastatic disease, androgen deprivation is considered.

PROGNOSIS
- Localized disease is frequently curable; advanced disease has a favorable prognosis if lesions are hormone sensitive.
- 5-year CaP survival by stage: local 100%, regional 100%, distant 30.2%
- Recurrence risk increased if: extraprostatic extension, seminal vesicle invasion, positive surgical margins

COMPLICATIONS
- Prostatectomy: Urinary incontinence and ED are the most common long-term issues.
- Radiation therapy: urinary incontinence, ED, radiation cystitis, and radiation proctitis
- Treatment options for ED: PDE5 inhibitors, intracavernosal injections, intraurethral suppositories, vacuum pump, penile prosthesis
- Treatment options for incontinence: oral medications, urethral sling, artificial sphincter

REFERENCE

1. Grossman DC, Curry SJ, Owens DK, et al; for US Preventive Services Task Force. Screening for prostate cancer: US Preventive Services Task Force recommendation statement. *JAMA*. 2018;319(18):1901–1913.

 ## CODES

ICD10
- C61 Malignant neoplasm of prostate
- Z80.42 Family history of malignant neoplasm of prostate
- D07.5 Carcinoma in situ of prostate

CLINICAL PEARLS
- The use of PSA for CaP screening is controversial; shared decision-making is recommended.
- Care must be taken when interpreting PSA levels in patients taking 5-α-reductase inhibitors.
- Decision to treat localized CaP is based on risk group and patient factors. Survival outcomes are excellent for patients with localized CaP, but treatment can carry significant morbidity impacting quality of life.

PROSTATIC HYPERPLASIA, BENIGN (BPH)

Michael T. Partin, MD • Sahel Uddin, DO

BASICS

- Benign prostatic hyperplasia (BPH) is due to proliferation of both smooth muscle and epithelial cell lines of the periurethral prostate which causes increased prostate volume and may lead to compression of the urethra and obstructive symptoms.
- BPH presents clinically with storage and/or voiding symptoms known collectively as lower urinary tract symptoms (LUTS). These include difficulty initiating a urinary stream, frequency, urgency, nocturia, and/or dysuria.
- Symptoms do not directly correlate to prostate volume. It is estimated that only half of all men with histologic evidence of BPH experience moderate to severe LUTS.
- Progression may result in upper and lower urinary tract infections and may progress to direct bladder outlet obstruction and acute renal failure (ARF).

EPIDEMIOLOGY
Age related with nearly universal development in men

Incidence
Incidence increases with age with an estimated prevalence varying from 70% to 90% by the age of 80 years (estimated at 8–20% by the age of 40 years).

ETIOLOGY AND PATHOPHYSIOLOGY
- Unknown etiology
- Develops in prostatic periurethral or transition zone
- Hyperplastic nodules of stromal and epithelial components increase glandular components.

RISK FACTORS
- Increasing age
- Higher free prostate-specific antigen (PSA) levels, heart disease, and use of β-blockers
- Low androgen levels from cirrhosis/chronic alcoholism reduce the risk of BPH.
- Obesity and sedentary lifestyle can worsen LUTS.
- No evidence of increased or decreased risk with smoking, alcohol, or any dietary factors

GENERAL PREVENTION
Symptoms can be managed through weight loss, regulation of fluid intake (especially in the evening), decreased intake of caffeine, and increased physical activity.

COMMONLY ASSOCIATED CONDITIONS
- LUTS can be divided into two groups:
  - Filling/storage symptoms: frequency, nocturia, urgency, and urge incontinence
  - Voiding symptoms: difficulty initiating urinary stream, incomplete voiding, or weak stream
- Sexual dysfunction, including erectile dysfunction and ejaculatory disorders
- LUTS can also be secondary to cardiovascular, respiratory, or renal disease (1).

DIAGNOSIS

HISTORY
- Screen for other causes such as infection, procedural history, or neurogenic causes.
- Evaluate symptom severity with the American Urological Association Society Symptom Index (AUA-SI) or the International Prostate Symptom Score (IPSS).
- Evaluate for comorbid conditions such as diabetes, congestive heart failure (CHF), or Parkinson disease.
- Review medication list and family history of BPH/prostate cancer.
- Screen for gross hematuria.
- Nocturia >2 times per night warrants a frequency/volume chart for 2 to 3 days to detect urinary patterns.

PHYSICAL EXAM
- Digital rectal exam (DRE): symmetrically enlarged prostate (*Size does not always correlate with symptoms.*)
- Signs of renal failure due to obstructive uropathy (edema, pallor, pruritus, ecchymosis, nutritional deficiencies)

DIFFERENTIAL DIAGNOSIS
- Obstructive
  - Prostate cancer
  - Urethral stricture or valves
  - Bladder neck contracture (usually secondary to prostate surgery)
  - Inability of bladder neck or external sphincter to relax appropriately during voiding
- Neurogenic
  - Spinal cord injury or stroke
  - Parkinsonism
  - Multiple sclerosis
- Medical
  - Poorly controlled diabetes mellitus
  - CHF
- Pharmacologic
  - Diuretics (increased urine production)
  - Decongestants (increased sphincter tone)
  - Opioids (impaired autonomic function)
  - Tricyclic antidepressants (anticholinergic)
- Other
  - Bladder carcinoma
  - Overactive bladder
  - Nocturnal polyuria
  - Bladder calculi
  - UTI and prostatitis
  - Urethritis/sexually transmitted infections
  - Obstructive sleep apnea (OSA) (nocturia)
  - Caffeine

DIAGNOSTIC TESTS & INTERPRETATION
Initial Tests (lab, imaging)
- Urinalysis (UA) in all patients presenting with LUTS to evaluate other etiologies such as bladder/kidney stones, cancer, UTI, or urethral strictures.
- PSA (especially for men with a life expectancy of ≥10 years who would be surgical candidates if prostate cancer was identified)
- PSA levels correlate with prostate volume which can help guide treatment choice.
- With bladder cancer risk factors (smoking history or hematuria), obtain urine cytology, CT urogram, and/or cystoscopy.
- If nocturia is the main concern, consider using a frequency volume chart for urine output.
- Uroflow: volume voided per unit time (Peak flow <10 mL/sec is abnormal.)
- Postvoid residual (PVR): either with catheterization or bladder ultrasound (>100 mL = incomplete emptying)
- Sleep study if OSA or primary nocturnal polyuria is suspected

Follow-Up Tests & Special Considerations
- No additional testing is recommended in uncomplicated LUTS.
- Further testing if symptoms do not respond to medical management or if initial evaluation suggests underlying disease
- Transrectal ultrasound or cross-sectional imaging (MRI/CT): assessment of prostate gland size; not necessary in the routine evaluation
- Abdominal ultrasound: can demonstrate increased PVR or hydronephrosis; not necessary in the routine evaluation

Diagnostic Procedures/Other
- Pressure-flow studies (urine flow vs. voiding pressures) to determine etiology of symptoms
  - Obstructive pattern shows high voiding pressures with low-flow rate.
- Cystoscopy
  - Demonstrates presence, configuration, cause (stricture, stone), and site of obstructive tissue
  - Not recommended in routine evaluation unless other factors, such as hematuria, are present

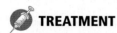 TREATMENT

GENERAL MEASURES
- The treatment ranges from watchful waiting to lifestyle modifications, medications, or surgical management.
- Mild symptoms (score of <7) or moderate symptoms (scores 8 to 15) on IPSS that are nonbothersome require no treatment with repeat evaluation performed annually.
- For moderate to severe symptoms, attempt lifestyle interventions including regulation of fluid intake, avoidance of alcohol and caffeine, exercise, diet, and eliminating/reducing contributing medications.

MEDICATION

- α-Adrenergic antagonists:
  - First-line option for moderate/severe and bothersome LUTS (2)
  - Affects contraction of smooth muscle in the prostatic urethra and bladder neck
  - Clinical improvement typically takes 2 to 4 weeks.
  - May affect blood pressure and lead to orthostatic hypotension
  - AUA recommends alfuzosin (Uroxatral), doxazosin (Cardura), and tamsulosin (Flomax) because they are thought to be more selective and have less effect on blood pressure. Prazosin (Minipress) and phenoxybenzamine (Dibenzyline) have insufficient evidence and are not recommended.
    - Tamsulosin (Flomax): 0.4 to 0.8 mg/day PO
    - Alfuzosin (Uroxatral): 10 mg/day PO
    - Terazosin (Hytrin): Start at 1 mg PO daily at bedtime, max of 20 mg/day.
    - Doxazosin (Cardura): 1 to 8 mg/day PO
  - Terazosin and doxazosin are nonuroselective and require dose titration to avoid vascular-related events.
  - **Contraindications:**
    - Use caution in patients who are also using phosphodiesterase type 5 inhibitors for erectile dysfunction.
    - Do not use in men pursuing cataract surgery until they are postoperative due to the risk for perioperative floppy iris syndrome.
    - Do not use concomitantly with other α-adrenergic antagonists.
- **5-α-Reductase inhibitors**
  - Blocks conversion of testosterone to dihydrotestosterone to gradually reduce prostatic volume
  - Greatest clinical benefit when prostate volume exceeds 30 mL and thus recommended to avoid use without evidence of enlarged prostate
  - Generally requires 6 months to show clinical benefits
    - Finasteride (Proscar): 5 mg/day PO
    - Dutasteride (Avodart): 0.5 mg/day PO
  - Shows reduced risk of acute urinary retention and less need for surgical intervention
  - Used in patients with refractory hematuria after other causes have been ruled out
  - Side effects include decreased libido, depressive symptoms, and erectile dysfunction; low risk of prostate cancer (3)[C]

ALERT
A PSA value in a patient taking a **5-α-reductase inhibitors will be artificially reduced by up to 50%.** Test before and after initiating treatment.

- Combination therapy of α-blocker plus 5-α-reductase inhibitor is superior to monotherapy with an α-blocker only in men with evidence of enlarged prostates.
- Anticholinergic agents are appropriate for moderate to severe predominant storage LUTS without an elevated PVR. Options include solifenacin (VESIcare), tolterodine (Detrol LA), or oxybutynin (Ditropan XL); should be avoided in patients with PVR >250 mL
- β3 adrenergic agonists combined with an α-blocker is a treatment option for patients with moderate to severe storage LUTS (3)[C].
- Phosphodiesterase-5 inhibitors lead to mild improvement of LUTS; can use tadalafil (Cialis): 5 mg/day PO but avoid use in combination with α-blockers or in those with CrCl <30 mL/min irrespective of comorbid erectile dysfunction (3)[B]

Geriatric Considerations
Use caution with anticholinergics, antihistamines, sympathomimetics, tricyclic antidepressants, and opioids.

ISSUES FOR REFERRAL
- Moderate or severe LUTS that do not respond to medical management
- BPH-related complications such as recurrent UTIs or hematuria, renal insufficiency, and urinary retention
- Abnormal PSA or prostate exam
- Any history of urethral trauma or stricture, or neurologic disease of the bladder/urinary system

SURGERY/OTHER PROCEDURES
- Indications for surgery
  - Recurrent urinary retention due to prostatic obstruction refractory to medical therapy
  - Intractable symptoms secondary to prostatic obstruction with AUA score of >8
  - Obstructive uropathy (renal insufficiency)
  - Recurrent or persistent UTIs due to prostatic obstruction
  - Recurrent gross hematuria due to enlarged prostate
  - Bladder calculi
- Surgical procedures: TURP remains the gold standard surgical procedure; however, for selected patient populations, there are other options available.
- Common complications of TURP:
  - Bleeding, retrograde ejaculation, urinary incontinence
  - TURP syndrome: hyponatremia secondary to absorption of hypotonic irrigation fluid
- Other options include transurethral vaporization of the prostate (TUVP), transurethral microwave thermotherapy (TUMT), transurethral incision of the prostate (TUIP), photoselective vaporization of the prostate (PVP), prostatic urethral lift (PUL), water vapor thermal therapy (WVTT), laser enucleation, and robotic waterjet treatment (RWT).
- Holmium laser enucleation (HoLEP), thulium laser enucleation of the prostate (ThuLEP), and PVP are options for patients on anticoagulation (4).
- PUL and WVTT can be offered as a treatment option for patients who prefer conservation of erectile and ejaculatory function (4)[C].
- Transurethral needle ablation and prostate artery embolization are not supported by current data (4)[C].

COMPLEMENTARY & ALTERNATIVE MEDICINE
- There are no recommended complementary or alternative treatments for BPH (2).
- Saw palmetto (Serenoa repens) has been thoroughly studied in a Cochrane review and did not improve LUTS.

 ONGOING CARE

FOLLOW-UP RECOMMENDATIONS
Patient Monitoring
- DRE and PSA yearly in patients who choose watchful waiting; PSA should not be checked while the patient is in retention, recently catheterized, or within a week of any prostate related surgery.
- Consider monitoring PVR, if elevated.

DIET
Large boluses of oral/IV fluids, alcohol, or caffeine may exacerbate LUTS.

PATIENT EDUCATION
National Institute of Diabetes and Digestive and Kidney Diseases Clearinghouses & Health Information Center: https://www.niddk.nih.gov/health-information/community-health-outreach/information-clearinghouses

PROGNOSIS
- Symptoms improve or stabilize in 70–80% of patients.
- 25% of men with LUTS will have persistent storage symptoms after prostatectomy.
- Of men with BPH, 11–33% have occult prostate cancer.

COMPLICATIONS
- Urinary retention (acute or chronic)
- Bladder stones, prostatitis, hematuria

REFERENCES

1. McVary KT, Roehrborn CG, Avins AL, et al. Update on AUA guideline on the management of benign prostatic hyperplasia. J Urol. 2011;185(5): 1793–1803.
2. Pearson R, Williams PM. Common questions about the diagnosis and management of benign prostatic hyperplasia. Am Fam Physician. 2014;90(11): 769–774.
3. Lerner LB, McVary KT, Barry MJ, et al. Management of lower urinary tract symptoms attributed to benign prostatic hyperplasia: AUA GUIDELINE PART I—initial work-up and medical management. J Urol. 2021;206(4):806–817.
4. Lerner LB, McVary KT, Barry MJ, et al. Management of lower urinary tract symptoms attributed to benign prostatic hyperplasia: AUA GUIDELINE PART II—surgical evaluation and treatment. J Urol. 2021;206(4):818–826.

CODES

ICD10
- N40.0 Enlarged prostate without lower urinary tract symptoms
- N40.1 Enlarged prostate with lower urinary tract symptoms

CLINICAL PEARLS
- Although medical therapy has changed the management of BPH, it has only delayed the need for TURP by 10 to 15 years, not eliminated it.
- Urinary retention, obstructive uropathy, recurrent UTIs, elevated PSA, bladder calculi, hematuria, and failure of medical therapy are indications for surgical management of BPH.

PROSTATITIS
Ross C. Stanton, MD, JD, MPH • Julie A. Creech, DO

 BASICS

DESCRIPTION
- Painful or inflammatory condition affecting the prostate gland with or without bacterial etiology, often characterized by urogenital pain, voiding symptoms, and/or sexual dysfunction
- National Institutes of Health's (NIH) classifications:
  - *Class I: acute bacterial prostatitis*: symptomatic with fever, perineal pain, dysuria, and obstructive symptoms; polymorphonuclear leukocytes (PMNL) and bacteria in urine
  - *Class II: chronic bacterial prostatitis*: symptomatic chronic or recurrent bacterial infection with pain and voiding disturbances; PMNL and bacteria in expressed prostatic secretions (EPS), or urine after prostate massage, or in semen
  - *Class III: chronic prostatitis/chronic pelvic pain syndrome* (CP/CPPS)
    - Inflammatory (subtype IIIA): chronic symptoms with PMNL in EPS/urine after prostate massage or in semen
    - Noninflammatory (subtype IIIB): chronic symptoms without presence of PMNL in EPS/urine after prostate massage or in semen
  - *Class IV: asymptomatic inflammatory prostatitis*: incidental finding during prostate biopsy; presence of PMNL and/or bacteria in EPS/urine after prostatic massage or in semen
- System(s) affected: genitourinary, renal, reproductive

EPIDEMIOLOGY
Incidence
- 2 million cases annually in the United States, with bimodal distribution: 20 to 40 and >60 years old
- CD is more common after 50 years.
- Bacterial prostatitis is more frequent in HIV.

Prevalence
- Affects approximately 16%, up to 10% of those are acute bacterial prostatitis
- Accounts for 8% of visits to urologists and 1% of visits to primary care physicians

ETIOLOGY AND PATHOPHYSIOLOGY
- Acute bacterial prostatitis (NIH class I)
  - Most likely from ascending urethral infection with intraprostatic reflux of infected urine into prostatic ducts, often associated with cystitis
  - Can occur after instrumentation of prostate
  - Usually, gram-negative bacteria (*Escherichia coli* [most common]; *Proteus, Klebsiella, Serratia,* and *Enterobacter* species; *Pseudomonas aeruginosa*); Rarely, gram-positive (*Staphylococcus aureus, Streptococcus,* and *Enterococcus* spp.)
  - Staphylococcal prostatitis warrants evaluation for hematogenous spread (endovascular).
  - Atypical bacteria include *Chlamydia trachomatis, Trichomonas vaginalis, Ureaplasma urealyticum, Mycobacterium tuberculosis* and fungal etiologies in immunocompromised hosts.
  - Consider *Neisseria gonorrhoeae* or *C. trachomatis* in sexually active men aged <35 years.
- Chronic bacterial prostatitis (NIH class II)
  - Similar pathogens as NIH class I
  - Often recurrent episodes of same organism
  - Progression from acute to CP is poorly understood.

- CP/CPPS (NIH class III): most common
  - Unclear etiology
  - Inciting agent may cause inflammation or neurologic damage around the prostate and leads to pelvic floor neuromuscular and/or neuropathic pain.
  - No correlation between histologic inflammation of prostate and presence or absence of symptoms
  - Patients with chronic inflammation on histology have shorter time to symptomatic progression.

RISK FACTORS
- Urinary tract infections (including STIs)
- HIV infection
- Prostatic calculi
- Urethral stricture
- Urinary catheterization: indwelling and intermittent
- Genitourinary instrumentation: prostate biopsy (especially with prior quinolone intake), transurethral resection of the prostate (TURP), cystoscopy
- Urinary retention
- Benign prostatic hyperplasia
- Unprotected sexual intercourse
- Prostate cancer

GENERAL PREVENTION
- Antibiotic prophylaxis for genitourinary instrumentation and prostatic biopsy
- Increased physical activity associated with reduced risk for CP/CPPS

COMMONLY ASSOCIATED CONDITIONS
- Benign prostatic hyperplasia, cystitis, urethritis
- Sexual dysfunction (erectile dysfunction, premature ejaculation)

 DIAGNOSIS

HISTORY
- Acute prostatitis (NIH class I):
  - Acutely ill with fever, chills, malaise
  - Low back pain, myalgias
  - Nausea, vomiting
  - Frequency, urgency, dysuria, nocturia
  - Prostatodynia, pelvic pain, perineal pain
  - Cloudy urine
  - Obstructive voiding symptoms: poor stream, hesitancy, retention, urge incontinence
  - Recent prostate instrumentation
- CP (NIH classes II and III) (symptoms vary from patient to patient and may include the following):
  - More insidious presentation than class I
  - Symptoms for 3 of 6 previous months
  - High caffeine and alcohol intake
  - Low-grade fever (class II only)
  - Prostatodynia, perineal pain
  - Dysuria, frequency, urgency
  - Lower abdominal pain
  - Low back, testicular, and/or penile pain
  - Hematospermia
  - Sexual dysfunction/painful ejaculation

PHYSICAL EXAM
- Vital signs (Unstable vitals suggest sepsis.)
- Back exam (CVA tenderness)
- Abdominal exam (bladder distension)

- Prostate exam
  - NIH class I (acute bacterial prostatitis): Prostate is very tender, warm, firm, and edematous.
  - NIH class II (chronic bacterial prostatitis): Prostate is often normal, but it is occasionally enlarged, tender, edematous, and nodular.
  - NIH class III (CP/CPPS): often normal prostate

ALERT
Avoid vigorous massage of the prostate in acute bacterial prostatitis; may induce iatrogenic bacteremia

DIFFERENTIAL DIAGNOSIS
- Lower urinary tract infection
- Pyelonephritis
- Cystitis (bacterial, interstitial) and urethritis
- Epididymitis
- Proctitis
- Prostatic abscess
- Acute/chronic urinary retention
- Benign prostatic hyperplasia or malignancy (prostate, bladder)
- Obstructive calculi
- Prostate cancer

DIAGNOSTIC TESTS & INTERPRETATION
Initial Tests (lab, imaging)
- Suspected acute prostatitis (NIH class I)
  - Urinalysis, urine culture and sensitivity
  - Complete blood count with differential, blood culture if immunocompromised or concerns for sepsis
  - Prostate-specific antigen (PSA) is not recommended unless specific indications.
  - Imaging is optional and used as indicated to rule out complications; for example, transrectal ultrasound (TRUS) or CT scan of abdomen to rule out abscess, pelvic ultrasound (US)/bladder scan if symptoms of urinary retention; initial imaging of prostate is not recommended.
  - STI testing (higher risk in men <35 years or men >35 years with high risk sexual behavior)
- Suspected chronic bacterial prostatitis (NIH class II)
  - Microbiologic localization cultures of lower urinary tract 4- or 2-glass test (pre- and post-massage urine culture)
  - Semen cultures are not recommended.
  - TRUS is not recommended.
  - Urodynamics studies are optional and could help to document obstruction/bladder problems.
- Suspected CP/CPPS (NIH class III)
  - Diagnosis of exclusion (especially to rule out urinary tract infection/STI with history/physical exam and appropriate laboratory investigation if indicated)
  - Administration of NIH Chronic Prostatitis Symptom Index (NIH-CPSI): Nine-question symptom survey (http://www.prostatitis.org/symptomindex.html) is useful for symptom evaluation (not diagnosis) at diagnosis and with ongoing treatment.
  - 4- or 2-glass test pre- and postmassage test with urine microscopy considered optional (prostatic massage rarely and anecdotally associated with sepsis; proceed with caution)
  - Urodynamic studies are optional and could be helpful to investigate obstructive symptoms.
  - Semen cultures are not recommended.

- Cystoscopy may be indicated for select patients (i.e., with hematuria or obstructive symptoms refractory to treatment).
- TRUS is not recommended.
- Serum PSA levels are not recommended unless specific indications (e.g., abnormal DRE, age >45 years, family history of prostate cancer or risk factors)
- Psychological assessment
- If the following additional symptoms are present, consider the following additional work-up:
  ○ Hematuria: urine cytology, cystoscopy, CT urography with or without contrast
  ○ Urethral symptoms (dysuria, discharge, penile pain): urethral swab
  ○ Concomitant abdominal pain: CT scan
  ○ Testicular pain: scrotal US
  ○ Lumbar radiculopathy: MRI of spine

Follow-Up Tests & Special Considerations
If not improving: US, CT scan, TRUS, MRI, or urology referral

Diagnostic Procedures/Other
- Urodynamic testing if obstructive symptoms present
- Cystoscopy

TREATMENT

GENERAL MEASURES
- NSAIDs for analgesia
- α_1-Blockers for lower urinary tract symptoms (obstructive/voiding symptoms)
- Antipyretics/stool softeners/hydration
- Sitz baths to relieve pain and spasm
- Urinary drainage for urine retention

MEDICATION
First Line
- Acute bacterial NIH class I (outpatient)
  - Fluoroquinolones are preferred first-line agents (1)[B].
    ○ Ciprofloxacin 500 mg PO q12h or levofloxacin 500 to 750 mg PO once daily
    ○ Trimethoprim-sulfamethoxazole 160/800 mg PO q12h (Consider local *E. Coli* resistance rates.)
  - Duration of therapy is 2 to 4 weeks (some support for 4 to 6 weeks).
  - If at risk for STI: ceftriaxone 250 mg IM for 1 dose (or cefixime 400 mg PO 1 dose) plus doxycycline 100 mg PO q12h for 10 days
  - α_1-Blockers for symptomatic relief of lower urinary tract symptoms and NSAIDs for analgesia
- Acute bacterial NIH class I (inpatient)
  - Urinary drainage (indwelling, intermittent, or suprapubic catheterization)
  - Obtain both blood and urine cultures.
  - Initial broad-spectrum IV antibiotic therapy in acutely ill patients:
    ○ Not severely ill (2)[B]:
      ▪ Ceftriaxone 1 to 2 g IV q24h + levofloxacin 500 to 750 mg IV q24h *or*
      ▪ Piperacillin and tazobactam (Zosyn) 3.375g IV q6h

  ○ Severely ill (2)[B]:
    ▪ Piperacillin and tazobactam (Zosyn) q6h + aminoglycoside *or*
    ▪ Cefotaxime 2g q4h + aminoglycoside *or*
    ▪ Ceftazidime 2g q8h + aminoglycoside
  - De-escalate to oral regimen pending blood/urine culture results and with clinical improvement for additional 2 to 4 weeks of therapy.
- Chronic bacterial NIH class II
  - Ciprofloxacin 500 mg PO q12h or levofloxacin 500 to 750 mg PO daily for 4 to 6 weeks or trimethoprim-sulfamethoxazole (160/800 mg PO q12h for 8 to 12 weeks).
  - If gram-positive bacteria (*Enterococcus faecalis*) and failed ciprofloxacin or levofloxacin consider moxifloxacin 400 mg PO once daily or linezolid 600 mg PO q12h.
  - Refractory cases: can consider intermittent antimicrobial treatment of acute symptomatic episodes (cystitis), low-dose antimicrobial suppression, radical TURP, or open prostatectomy if all options failed
  - α-Blockers combined with antimicrobial therapy reduce the high recurrence rate and optimal for patients with obstructive symptoms.
- CP/CPPS NIH class III
  - Unclear source of disease, limited evidence on effective treatment
  - Treatment choice is patient-centered, focusing on symptom relief in four domains: pain, lower urinary tract symptoms, psychological stress, and sexual dysfunction.
  - Empiric trial of eliminating caffeine and alcohol
  - α-Blockers (tamsulosin 0.4 mg PO daily) can be beneficial, especially in men with lower urinary tract symptoms; however, studies do not show statistically significant differences.
  - Fluoroquinolones (ciprofloxacin 500 mg PO BID) may help for symptoms in patients, but studies do not show that it is statistically significant.
  - NSAIDs can help with symptoms.

ISSUES FOR REFERRAL
Urology referral if antibiotic treatment fails, symptoms persist (especially obstructive voiding symptoms), hematuria, or elevated PSA; or for surgical drainage, if an abscess persists after ≥1 week of therapy

ADDITIONAL THERAPIES
- Cognitive-behavioral therapy (CBT) for psychosocial stressors or sexual dysfunction
- Pudendal nerve block or neurolysis if due to pudendal nerve entrapment

SURGERY/OTHER PROCEDURES
Surgical resection may be considered for refractory cases of recurrent bacterial prostatitis or to drain an abscess.

ADMISSION, INPATIENT, AND NURSING CONSIDERATIONS
- Sepsis
- PO intolerance
- Urinary retention
- Proven or suspected abscess
- Risk factors for resistance (recent prostatic instrumentation or recent fluoroquinolone use)
- Immunocompromised

ONGOING CARE

FOLLOW-UP RECOMMENDATIONS
Negative urine culture at 7 days predictive of cure after completion of treatment course

PROGNOSIS
- Fever and dysuria usually resolve in 2 to 6 days.
- Acute infection usually improves in 3 to 4 weeks.
- Course of CP is often prolonged; 55–97% cure rate depending on population and drug used
- 20% have reinfection or persistent infection.
- 10% with acute bacterial prostatitis may progress to CP.

COMPLICATIONS
- Prostatic abscess (common in patients with HIV)
- Pyelonephritis
- Urinary retention
- Epididymitis
- Infertility
- Chronic bacterial prostatitis (following acute prostatitis)
- Metastatic infection (spinal, sacroiliac)
- Erectile dysfunction

REFERENCES
1. Marquez-Algaba E, Pigrau C, Bosch-Nicolau P, et al. Risk factors for relapse in acute bacterial prostatitis: the impact of antibiotic regimens. *Microbiol Spectr*. 2021;9(2):e0053421.
2. Coker TJ, Dierfeldt DM. Acute bacterial prostatitis: diagnosis and management. *Am Fam Physician*. 2016;93(2):114–120.

 SEE ALSO

- Prostate Cancer; Prostatic Hyperplasia, Benign (BPH); Urinary Tract Infection (UTI) in Males
- Algorithm: Hematuria

 CODES

ICD10
- N41.8 Other inflammatory diseases of prostate
- N41 Inflammatory diseases of prostate
- N41.4 Granulomatous prostatitis

CLINICAL PEARLS
- Prostatic massage is contraindicated in acute prostatitis.
- Fluoroquinolones are recommended first-line antibiotic for bacterial prostatitis.
- 14 to 30 days of antibiotic therapy is required for acute prostatitis; longer for chronic prostatitis

PROTEIN C DEFICIENCY
Kyle J. Fletke, MD

 BASICS

Protein C deficiency (PCD) is a rare heritable disorder or acquired risk factor resulting in a prothrombotic state. Symptoms range from an asymptomatic presentation to recurrent venous thromboembolism (VTE), life-threatening neonatal purpura fulminans, or severe disseminated intravascular coagulation (DIC).

DESCRIPTION
- Protein C is a vitamin K–dependent anticoagulant protein synthesized in an inactive form by the liver.
- Activated protein C (APC) inhibits generation of thrombin by inactivating factors Va and VIIIa, using protein S as a cofactor.
- Deficiency in protein C activity therefore leads to a prothrombotic state.
- System(s) affected: cardiovascular, pulmonary, integumentary, hematologic, and immunologic

EPIDEMIOLOGY
Incidence
The estimated incidence is between 1 in 200 and 1 in 500 (1). Clinically substantial PCD is estimated to be 1 in 20,000. Severe PCD is rare, predicted in 1 in 4 million infants.

Prevalence
- 0.3% of the general population
- 3–5% of persons with VTE
- Mean age of first thrombosis is 45 years.
- There is no known gender predominance.

ETIOLOGY AND PATHOPHYSIOLOGY
- PCD can be inherited or acquired.
- Genetic mutations can lead to two types of PCD; however, the distinction between the two is clinically irrelevant.
  - Type I (most common) results in the reduction of protein C levels.
  - Type II results in a decreased functionality, despite having normal levels of protein C.
- Acquired PCD is more common and can occur in many disease states such as:
  - Liver disease
  - DIC
  - Severe infections (especially meningococcemia)
  - Autoantibody inhibitors directed toward protein C
  - Cancer and chemotherapy (i.e., L-asparaginase, 5-FU, methotrexate, and cyclophosphamide)
  - Initial use of vitamin K antagonists (warfarin)
  - Vitamin K deficiency (secondary to malnutrition or malabsorption of fat-soluble vitamins)
- Heterozygous PCD and mild deficiency can cause a wide range of symptom severity from asymptomatic to recurrent thromboses.
  - There is an increased risk of DVT, PE, and sequelae such as ischemic arterial stroke and pregnancy-associated thrombosis.

Genetics
- Autosomal dominant inheritance pattern with incomplete penetrance
- At least 270 genetic mutations have been described in the protein C (PROC) gene that can lead to a functional deficiency.

- Heterozygous patients often have mild or asymptomatic disease.
- Homozygous patients, or those with another coexisting genetic thrombophilia, often have more severe disease.
- Additionally, mutations in other genes (GCKR, EDEM2, BAZ1B, etc.) are associated with variability in the levels of protein C expression in the general population, although their clinical significance is currently unknown.
- Patients with PCD who start warfarin without concomitant heparin are at increased risk of developing warfarin-induced skin necrosis (WISN). This is thought to be due to the shorter half-life of protein C (5 to 8 hours) compared to other vitamin K–dependent clotting factors. However, not all patients who develop WISN have PCD.

ALERT
The prevention of warfarin necrosis has been achieved by avoiding loading doses of warfarin and the use of heparin bridging. Screening all patients for inherited or acquired forms of PCD prior to initiating warfarin is neither cost-effective nor prognostic because many patients with documented deficiency do not progress to WISN.

RISK FACTORS
Acquired conditions such as heart failure, severe liver disease, DIC, vitamin K antagonists

GENERAL PREVENTION
Because PCD is usually a congenital disease, there are no preventive measures.

COMMONLY ASSOCIATED CONDITIONS
- VTE at any site, often spontaneous
- Arterial thrombosis is rare, and a causative relationship has not been clearly demonstrated.
- Homozygosity can be associated with catastrophic thrombotic complications at birth (e.g., purpura fulminans).
- Recurrent pregnancy losses

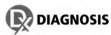 **DIAGNOSIS**

HISTORY
- Recurrent VTE
- VTE at <40 years of age
- Thrombosis in unusual locations (e.g., mesentery, sagittal sinus, portal vein)
- Thrombosis at a young age (<50 years)
- Family history of thrombosis, spontaneous abortion, or WISN

PHYSICAL EXAM
Normal unless patient is presenting with active thrombosis and/or has physical stigmata of illness associated with PCD

DIFFERENTIAL DIAGNOSIS
- Factor V Leiden
- Protein S deficiency
- Antithrombin deficiency
- Dysfibrinogenemia

- Dysplasminogenemia
- Hyperhomocysteinemia
- Prothrombin G20210A mutation
- Elevated factor VIII, IX, or XI levels
- Antiphospholipid antibody syndrome
- DIC
- Heparin-induced thrombocytopenia (HIT)

DIAGNOSTIC TESTS & INTERPRETATION
PCD can be diagnosed using clotting assays, ELISA, and chromogenic tests to assess protein C levels. PROC gene mutational analysis is also available.

Initial Tests (lab, imaging)
- CBC with peripheral smear, INR, aPTT, hepatic and renal function tests, appropriate imaging
- Testing for heritable causes of thrombophilia in unselected patients presenting with a first-time VTE (provoked or unprovoked) is not indicated (2).
- Consider screening for antiphospholipid syndrome rather than other thrombophilia (PCD) for women with recurrent early pregnancy loss (three loses prior to 10 weeks' gestation) (3)[B].

Follow-Up Tests & Special Considerations
- Testing for heritable or acquired thrombophilia is suggested in the following circumstances:
  - First episode of VTE and patient age <40 years
  - Recurrent VTE regardless of the presence of risk factors
  - Patients with VTE at unusual sites
- Testing for PCD should be considered in patients with history of WISN.
- Testing for protein C and S deficiencies should be done urgently in neonates and children suspected to have purpura fulminans (2).
- Testing for hereditary thrombophilia should only be considered in asymptomatic first-degree relatives of those with proven hereditary thrombophilia if they are female, of childbearing age, and have no history of prior pregnancy complications (3)[C].
- When ordering additional testing for hereditary or acquired thrombophilia, the following conditions should be considered:
  - Antiphospholipid antibody syndrome
  - Antithrombin III deficiency
  - Factor V Leiden
  - PCD
  - Protein S deficiency
  - Prothrombin G20210A mutation

Diagnostic Procedures/Other
Testing for PCD is done using two separate lab tests:
- An immunoassay for a quantitative assessment of protein C levels
- A functional activity assay using a snake venom protease to activate protein C

Test Interpretation
- Drugs that may alter lab results:
  - Oral contraceptives can raise protein C levels.
  - Warfarin reduces protein C levels and should be discontinued 2 to 3 weeks before reliable testing.
- Liver disease reduces protein C levels.

ALERT
Acute thrombosis can lower protein C levels. Repeat confirmatory test of low protein C level at a separate time is advisable. If a normal level of protein C is obtained at presentation, then deficiency can be excluded.

 TREATMENT

GENERAL MEASURES
- Individuals with PCD should be educated regarding signs and symptoms of VTE.
- Women with any of the following history should avoid estradiol-containing contraceptives and hormone replacement therapy during menopause:
  - Diagnoses of PCD
  - First-degree relative with PCD
  - First-degree relative with VTE at age <50 years
- Women may use progestin-only hormonal contraception options.
- Routine anticoagulation for asymptomatic patients with PCD is not recommended (3)[C].
- Anticoagulation is recommended for at least 3 months in patients with inherited thrombophilia following their first VTE (2). Shared decision-making should be used to discuss duration of therapy >3 months.
- Treat VTE as an outpatient when possible if clinically stable (3)[B].
- Severe congenital PCD may be treated with protein C concentrates.

Pregnancy Considerations
- The VTE risk per pregnancy in patients with no prior history of VTE is 0.1–1.7%. The VTE risk per pregnancy in patients with prior VTE is 4–17%.
- Heparin-based products should be used during pregnancy when therapeutic or prophylactic treatment of VTE is needed.
- For pregnant women with known PCD but no personal history of VTE or additional thrombotic risk factors (i.e., family history of VTE in first-degree relative <50 years of age, obesity, prolonged immobility), antepartum and postpartum clinical monitoring is recommended over prophylactic therapy.
- For pregnant women with known PCD, no personal history of VTE but with an additional thrombotic risk factor, antepartum surveillance is recommended with postpartum prophylactic therapy for 6 weeks of either prophylactic or intermediate dose. Individuals with a high risk of thrombosis may be treated with protein C concentrate at the time of surgery or delivery.
- For pregnant women with known PCD and previous VTE, it is recommended to treat antepartum and postpartum patients with either prophylactic or intermediate-dose LMWH/UFH.

MEDICATION
First Line
- LMWH (3)[A]: initially started with warfarin for a minimum of 5 days and two consecutive INRs between 2 and 3 to bridge; additionally, LMWH may be started 5 to 10 days prior to starting dabigatran or edoxaban.
  - Enoxaparin (Lovenox) 1 mg/kg SC BID or 1.5 mg/kg/day SC
  - Tinzaparin (Innohep): 175 anti-Xa IU/kg/day SC
  - Dalteparin (Fragmin) 200 U/kg/day
- Novel oral anticoagulants (NOACs):
  - Rivaroxaban (Xarelto) 15 mg PO BID with food for 21 days and then 20 mg PO QD with food
  - Apixaban (Eliquis) 10 mg PO BID for 7 days and then 5 mg PO BID
  - Dabigatran (Pradaxa) 150 mg PO BID (after 5 to 10 days of parenteral anticoagulation)
  - Edoxaban (Savaysa) 60 mg PO QD (after 5 to 10 days of parenteral anticoagulation)
- Oral vitamin K antagonist:
  - Warfarin (Coumadin) titrated to an INR of 2.0 to 3.0 (3)[A]
- Factor Xa inhibitors:
  - Fondaparinux (Arixtra) <50 kg: 5 mg/day SC; 50 to 100 kg: 7.5 mg/day SC; >100 kg: 10 mg/day SC; contraindicated if CrCl <30 mL/min
- Contraindications
  - Active bleeding
  - Risk of bleeding is a relative contraindication to long-term anticoagulation.
- Precautions
  - Observe patient for signs of embolization, further thrombosis, or bleeding.
  - Monitor kidney function, drug–drug interactions, and CBC (including platelets to monitor for HIT).

Second Line
- Heparin 80 U/kg IV bolus followed by 18 U/kg/hr; adjust dose depending on PPT.
- In patients requiring large daily doses of heparin, measure an anti-Xa level for dose guidance.
- Alternatively, and for outpatients, unfractionated heparin can be given at 333 U/kg and then 250 U/kg SC, without monitoring (3)[C].
- May be treatable with replacement protein C concentrate; neonatal purpura fulminans can be controlled with protein C replacement from fresh frozen plasma (FFP).

SURGERY/OTHER PROCEDURES
- Anticoagulation may be held for surgical interventions.
- In patients with acute proximal DVT of the lower extremity *and* an absolute contraindication to anticoagulation, inferior vena cava (IVC) filters are recommended; otherwise, the use of an IVC filter in addition to anticoagulants is not recommended (3)[B].

ADMISSION, INPATIENT, AND NURSING CONSIDERATIONS
- Life-threatening VTE
- Significant bleeding while on anticoagulant therapy

 ONGOING CARE

FOLLOW-UP RECOMMENDATIONS
Patient Monitoring
- Warfarin requires periodic monitoring of the INR to maintain a range of 2.0 to 3.0 (monthly, after initial stabilization).
- LMWH is the treatment of choice in pregnancy. Periodic monitoring with anti-Xa levels is recommended in these patients.

DIET
Unrestricted (except if on warfarin—avoid varying diet with foods that have significant amounts of vitamin K)

PATIENT EDUCATION
- Patients should be educated about signs and symptoms of VTE as well as the use of oral anticoagulant therapy if taking such.
- Avoid NSAIDs while on warfarin.
- Avoid estrogen containing OCPs because of increased risk of thrombosis.

PROGNOSIS
When compared with normal individuals, persons with PCD have normal life spans.

COMPLICATIONS
Primary or recurrent VTE

REFERENCES
1. Tait RC, Walker ID, Reitsma PH, et al. Prevalence of protein C deficiency in the healthy population. *Thromb Haemost.* 1995;73(1):87–93.
2. Baglin T, Gray E, Greaves M, et al; for British Committee for Standards in Haematology. Clinical guidelines for testing for heritable thrombophilia. *Br J Haematol.* 2010;149(2):209–220.
3. Guyatt GH, Akl EA, Crowther M, et al; for American College of Chest Physicians Antithrombotic Therapy and Prevention of Thrombosis Panel. Executive summary: antithrombotic therapy and prevention of thrombosis, 9th ed: American College of Chest Physicians evidence-based clinical practice guidelines. *Chest.* 2012;141(Suppl 2):7S–47S.

 CODES

ICD10
D68.59 Other primary thrombophilia

CLINICAL PEARLS
- Screening of asymptomatic family members is not justified with the possible exception of females of childbearing age with no previous history of pregnancy complications.
- Asymptomatic patients with PCD do not need prophylactic anticoagulation because the risk of thrombosis is low.
- Patients with PCD presenting with first-time VTE should be anticoagulated for at least 3 months. Other risk factors and shared decision-making should be used to determine if anticoagulation should be used for a longer duration.
- Recurrent VTE is an indication for indefinite anticoagulation.

PROTEIN S DEFICIENCY

Opeoluwa Olukorede, MD

 BASICS

DESCRIPTION
- Protein S is a vitamin K–dependent glycoprotein, produced mainly in the liver that acts as a cofactor for protein C. It is also produced by megakaryocytes and endothelial cells.
- Protein C becomes activated when thrombin binds to the endothelial receptor, thrombomodulin.
- Activated protein C, with protein S (a cofactor), inactivates clotting factors Va and VIIIa enhancing fibrinolysis.
- Protein S is also able to directly inhibit factors Va, VIIa, and Xa independently of activated protein C.
- Protein S deficiency is a congenital thrombophilia, which increases the risk of thromboembolism.
- It primarily affects the venous system.
- System(s) affected: cardiovascular, hematologic/immunologic, pulmonary

EPIDEMIOLOGY
Incidence
- Mean age of first thrombosis: 2nd decade
- Predominant sex: male = female

Prevalence
- ~0.2% of general population
- Found in ~1% of persons with venous thrombosis embolism (VTE)

ETIOLOGY AND PATHOPHYSIOLOGY
- It is an autosomal dominant disease.
- Only the free form of protein S (30–40%) acts as a cofactor for activated protein C. Protein S reversibly binds to the C4b protein, which leads to conditions in which free protein S is low, but total protein S is normal. These individuals are prone to thrombosis.
- Conditions with reduced protein S: pregnancy, disseminated intravascular coagulation (DIC), liver disease, nephrotic syndrome, HIV, acute thrombosis, and acute varicella-zoster virus infection
- Drugs: oral contraceptives, warfarin, and L-asparaginase chemotherapy

Genetics
- Due to mutations in the PROS1 gene on chromosome 3; most individuals are heterozygous.
- Heterozygotes have an odds ratio (OR) of VTE of 1.6 to 11.5.
- Homozygosity or compound heterozygosity, if untreated, is usually incompatible with adult life.
- Homozygotes can have a fulminant thrombotic event in infancy, termed *neonatal purpura fulminans*.

RISK FACTORS
- Oral contraceptives, pregnancy, and the use of hormone replacement therapy (HRT) increase the risk of VTE in patients with protein S deficiency.
- Patients with protein S deficiency and other prothrombotic states have further increased rate of thrombosis.
- Arterial thrombosis is more frequent in patients with protein S deficiency who smoke.
- Patients heterozygous for protein S deficiency who are initiated on warfarin without concomitant heparin can develop warfarin-induced skin necrosis because the half-life of other vitamin K–dependent clotting factors (e.g., prothrombin, factor IX, and factor X) is much longer than the anticoagulant protein S (4 to 8 hours), leading to a transient hypercoagulable state when protein S becomes depleted. These patients develop extremely low levels of protein S and develop necrosis of the skin over central areas of the body such as the breast, abdomen, buttocks, and genitalia.

Pregnancy Considerations
Increased thrombotic risk and pregnancy losses

GENERAL PREVENTION
There are no preventive measures.

COMMONLY ASSOCIATED CONDITIONS
- Deep and superficial VTE, often unprovoked
- Up to 50% of homozygotes will have thrombosis.
- Homozygosity is associated with catastrophic thrombotic complications at birth: *neonatal purpura fulminans*.
- Sites of thrombosis can be unusual, including the mesentery, cerebral veins, and axillary veins.
- Arterial thrombosis is rare but reported in several case reports.
- Skin necrosis in patients treated with warfarin
- Recurrent pregnancy losses

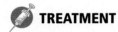 **DIAGNOSIS**

HISTORY
Inherited thrombophilias should be suspected in:
- Unprovoked VTE at age <50 years
- VTE with a strong family history of VTE or known familial protein S deficiency
- VTE in unusual sites as mesenteric or cerebral vein
- Recurrent VTE

PHYSICAL EXAM
Normal

DIFFERENTIAL DIAGNOSIS
Other inherited thrombophilias:
- Factor V Leiden (most common; usually in Caucasians)
- Protein C deficiency (in Caucasians)

- Antithrombin deficiency
- Dysfibrinogenemia
- Dysplasminogenemia
- Homocystinemia
- Prothrombin G20210A mutation
- Elevated factor VIII levels
- Acquired VTE risk factors: surgery, immobility, cancer, myeloproliferative neoplasms, trauma, antiphospholipid syndrome, paroxysmal nocturnal hemoglobinuria, pregnancy, HRT, postpartum, DIC

DIAGNOSTIC TESTS & INTERPRETATION
Initial Tests (lab, imaging)
- For evaluation of new clot in a patient at risk: CBC with peripheral smear, PT/INR, aPTT, thrombin time, lupus anticoagulant, antiphospholipid antibodies, anticardiolipin antibody, anti-β_2-glycoprotein I antibody, activated protein C resistance, protein S antigen and resistance, antithrombin III assay, fibrinogen, factor V Leiden, prothrombin G20210A
- Immunoassay for quantitative assessment of total and free protein S levels
- Protein S activity assay (mainly after obtaining activated protein C resistance)
- Disorders that may alter lab results: acute thrombosis, vitamin K antagonists (VKA), any acute illness response, liver disease, and pregnancy-reduced protein S levels; direct oral anticoagulants affect protein S activity assay.
- Heparin and low-weight heparin do not alter lab results.
- Total protein S levels are markedly decreased in newborns and young infants; use age-adjusted norms.

 TREATMENT

GENERAL MEASURES
- Routine anticoagulation for asymptomatic patients with protein S deficiency is not recommended.
- Antithrombotic therapy recommendations for patients with protein S deficiency can be guided by antithrombotic therapy for VTE disease guidelines.
- Patients with unprovoked VTE and who have a low or moderate bleeding risk are suggested to receive extended anticoagulant therapy (no scheduled stop date) >3 months of therapy (1), and those who have a high bleeding risk are recommended to receive 3 months of anticoagulant therapy (1),(2)[B].
- Patients with a second unprovoked VTE and who have a low-to-moderate bleeding risk are recommended to receive extended anticoagulant therapy >3 months (1),(2)[B]; those who have high bleeding risk are suggested to receive 3 months of anticoagulant therapy (1).

- Patients with VTE and no history of cancer are suggested to receive dabigatran, rivaroxaban, apixaban, or edoxaban over VKA therapy as long-term (first 3 months) anticoagulant therapy; VKA therapy over low-molecular-weight heparin (LMWH) (1)
- Patients with VTE and active cancer are suggested to receive LMWH, rivaroxaban, or edoxaban for long-term anticoagulation (3). It is recommended that these patients receive extended anticoagulant therapy (1).
- Treatment of thrombosis with LMWH is recommended over unfractionated heparin, unless the patient has severe renal failure.
- Treat as outpatient, if possible.
- Prophylaxis should be considered in risk situations such as surgery, immobility, or postpartum, especially in patients with family history.
- The role of family screening for protein S deficiency is unclear because most patients with this mutation do not have thrombosis. Screening should be considered for women considering oral contraceptives or pregnancy and who have a family history of protein S deficiency (4)[B].

MEDICATION
- LMWH
  - Enoxaparin (Lovenox) 1 mg/kg SC BID
    ○ Alternatively, 1.5 mg/kg/day SC
  - Tinzaparin (Innohep) 175 anti-Xa U/kg/day SC
  - Dalteparin (Fragmin) 200 U/kg/day SC divided QD–BID
- Factor Xa inhibitor
  - Fondaparinux (Arixtra) <50 kg: 5 mg/day SC; 50 to 100 kg: 7.5 mg/day SC; >100 kg: 10 mg/day SC; contraindicated if CrCl <30 mL/min
- Dual oral anticoagulants (DOACs):
  - Dabigatran 150 mg PO BID (after 5 to 10 days of parenteral anticoagulation)
  - Rivaroxaban 15 mg PO BID for 21 days and then 20 mg PO QD
  - Apixaban 10 mg PO BID for 7 days and then 5 mg PO BID
  - Edoxaban: person weighs ≤60 kg: 30 mg PO QD; >60 kg: 60 mg PO QD (after 5 to 10 days of parenteral anticoagulation)
- Oral anticoagulant: warfarin (Coumadin): 2 to 5 mg PO QD then adjusted to an INR of 2 to 3; LMWH initially for a minimum of 5 days and two consecutive INRs between 2 and 3, at which time it can be stopped; contraindications
  - Active bleeding precludes anticoagulation; risk of bleeding is a relative contraindication to long-term anticoagulation.
  - Warfarin is contraindicated in patients with a prior history of warfarin-induced skin necrosis.
- Precautions
  - Observe patient for signs of embolization, further thrombosis, or bleeding.
  - Avoid IM injections.

- Periodically, check stool and urine for occult blood; monitor CBC, including platelets.
  - Heparin: thrombocytopenia and/or paradoxical thrombosis with thrombocytopenia
  - Warfarin: necrotic skin lesions (typically breasts, thighs, and buttocks)
  - LMWH: Adjust dose in renal insufficiency.
- Significant possible interactions
  - Agents that intensify the response to oral anticoagulants: ethanol, allopurinol, amiodarone, anabolic steroids, androgens, many antimicrobials, cimetidine, chloral hydrate, disulfiram, NSAIDs, sulfinpyrazone, tamoxifen, levothyroxine, vitamin E, ranitidine, salicylates, and acetaminophen
  - Agents that diminish the response to oral anticoagulants: aminoglutethimide, antacids, barbiturates, carbamazepine, cholestyramine, diuretics, griseofulvin, rifampin, and oral contraceptives

ISSUES FOR REFERRAL
- Patients with suspected protein S deficiency should be seen by a hematologist.
- Screening and prophylactic treatment of asymptomatic family members is not justified (5).

SURGERY/OTHER PROCEDURES
- Anticoagulation must be held for surgical interventions.
- For most patients with DVT, recommendations are against routine use of vena cava filter in addition to anticoagulation. IVC filter is only recommended in case of contraindication to anticoagulation (1)[A].

COMPLEMENTARY & ALTERNATIVE MEDICINE
Diet modifications if taking VKA

ADMISSION, INPATIENT, AND NURSING CONSIDERATIONS
- Life-threatening VTE
- Significant bleeding while on anticoagulant therapy
- Look for signs of bleeding while on anticoagulation therapy.

ONGOING CARE

FOLLOW-UP RECOMMENDATIONS
Patient Monitoring
- Warfarin requires periodic (monthly after initial stabilization) monitoring of the INR.
- Periodic measurement of INR to maintain a range of 2 to 3
- LMWH is the treatment of choice in pregnancy. Periodic monitoring with anti-Xa levels is recommended in some cases, such as overweight and borderline renal failure.

DIET
Unrestricted, unless taking VKA

PATIENT EDUCATION
- Patients should be educated about the use of oral anticoagulant therapy if taking such.
- Patients undergoing warfarin therapy should avoid drinking alcohol on a daily basis.
- Avoid NSAIDs while on warfarin.

PROGNOSIS
- Persons with protein S deficiency have normal lifespan.
- By the age of 45 years, 50% of the people heterozygous for protein S deficiency will have VT; half will be spontaneous.

COMPLICATIONS
Recurrent thrombosis (requires indefinite anticoagulation)

REFERENCES
1. Kearon C, Akl EA, Ornelas J, et al. Antithrombotic therapy for VTE disease: CHEST Guideline and Expert Panel Report. *Chest*. 2016;149(2):315–352.
2. Moll S. Thrombophilias—practical implications and testing caveats. *J Thromb Thrombolysis*. 2006;21(1):7–15.
3. Key NS, Khorana AA, Kuderer NM, et al. Venous thromboembolism prophylaxis and treatment in patients with cancer: ASCO clinical practice guideline update. *J Clin Oncol*. 2020;38(5):496–520.
4. Langlois NJ, Wells PS. Risk of venous thromboembolism in relatives of symptomatic probands with thrombophilia: a systematic review. *Thromb Haemost*. 2003;90(1):17–26.
5. Hornsby LB, Armstrong EM, Bellone JM, et al. Thrombophilia screening. *J Pharm Pract*. 2014;27(3):253–259.

ADDITIONAL READING
Ameku K, Higa M. Rivaroxaban treatment for warfarin-refractory thrombosis in a patient with hereditary protein S deficiency. *Case Rep Hematol*. 2018;2018:5217301.

CODES

ICD10
D68.59 Other primary thrombophilia

CLINICAL PEARLS
- Asymptomatic patients with protein S deficiency do not require prophylactic anticoagulation because the risk of thrombosis is low; asymptomatic patients do not require anticoagulation.
- Patients with protein S deficiency and DVT should be anticoagulated for at least 6 months, especially if first episode.

PROTEINURIA
Samantha Carroll, MD • Christian Soeharsono, MD

BASICS

DESCRIPTION
- Proteinuria: urinary protein excretion of >150 mg/day
- Nephrotic-range proteinuria: Urinary protein excretion of ≥3.5 g/day; also called heavy proteinuria

Pediatric Considerations
- Proteinuria: Normal is daily excretion of up to 100 mg/m² (body surface area) for children. For neonates, daily excretion may be up to 300 mg/m² due to decreased reabsorption of filtered proteins.
- Nephrotic-range proteinuria: daily excretion of >1,000 mg/m² (body surface area)

Pregnancy Considerations
- Proteinuria in pregnancy >20 weeks' gestation is a hallmark of preeclampsia/eclampsia and demands further workup.
- Proteinuria in pregnancy before 20 weeks' gestation is suggestive of underlying renal disease.

EPIDEMIOLOGY
Prevalence
The prevalence of proteinuria varies based on the definition used; maybe as high as 10% in school-aged children

ETIOLOGY AND PATHOPHYSIOLOGY
Normal protein filtration up to 150 mg/day, of which approximately 20 mg is albumin
- Glomerular proteinuria: increased glomerular capillary wall permeability due to both the increased size of glomerular basement membrane pores and loss of negatively charged barrier from glycosaminoglycans
  - Primary glomerulonephropathy
    ○ Minimal-change disease
    ○ Idiopathic/primary membranous glomerulonephritis
    ○ Focal segmental glomerulosclerosis/ glomerulonephritis
    ○ Membranoproliferative glomerulonephritis
    ○ IgA nephropathy (Berger disease)
  - Secondary glomerulonephropathy
    ○ Chronic disease (diabetes, hypertension, chronic kidney disease)
    ○ Autoimmune/collagen vascular disorders (e.g., lupus nephritis, Henoch-Schönlein purpura, Goodpasture syndrome)
    ○ Genetic disorders (Alport syndrome, Fabry disease)
    ○ Amyloidosis, sarcoidosis
    ○ Preeclampsia
    ○ Infection (HIV, CMV, hepatitis B and C, post-streptococcal, endocarditis, syphilis, malaria)
    ○ Malignancy (GI, lung, lymphoma)
    ○ Renal transplant rejection
    ○ Structural (reflux nephropathy, polycystic kidney disease)
    ○ Drug-induced (NSAIDs, penicillamine, lithium, heavy metals, gold, heroin)
    ○ Sickle cell disease

- Tubulointerstitial proteinuria: Tubulointerstitial disease prevents proximal tubular reabsorption of smaller proteins (β_2-microglobulin, immunoglobulin [Ig] light chains, retinol-binding protein, amino acids).
  - Medications (NSAIDs, aminoglycosides, penicillins, cephalosporins, quinolones, sulfonamides, amphotericin B, cisplatin, radiocontrast media)
  - Toxins (lead, copper, mercury)
  - Uric acid nephropathy
  - Interstitial nephritis
  - Fanconi syndrome
  - Acute tubular necrosis
- Overflow proteinuria: Plasma concentration of low-molecular-weight proteins exceed capacity of the tubules to reabsorb filtered protein.
  - Multiple myeloma (light chains; also tubulotoxic)
  - Hemoglobinuria
  - Myoglobinuria (in rhabdomyolysis)
  - Lysozyme (in acute monocytic leukemia)
- Benign proteinuria
  - Functional (fever, exercise, cold exposure, stress, dehydration, seizures, CHF)
  - Idiopathic transient
  - Orthostasis (postural)—usually found in older children and adolescents

GENERAL PREVENTION
Control of weight, BP, and blood glucose reduces the risk of chronic disease that leads to proteinuria.

COMMONLY ASSOCIATED CONDITIONS
Nephrotic syndrome, glomerulonephritis, chronic kidney disease

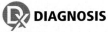

DIAGNOSIS

HISTORY
- Fever
- Frothy/foamy urine
- Change in urine output
- Blood- or cola-colored urine
- Recent weight change
- History of UTIs
- Dysuria, flank pain
- Swelling
- Rule out systemic illness: diabetes, heart failure, autoimmune, recent streptococcal infection.
- If pregnant: swelling of hands or face, headaches, blurry vision, abdominal pain

PHYSICAL EXAM
- Vitals (temperature, BP)
- Weight
- Peripheral edema
- Periorbital/facial edema
- Abdominal or CVA tenderness
- Ascites
- Palpation of kidneys
- Check lungs and heart for signs of CHF.

DIFFERENTIAL DIAGNOSIS
Includes all causes listed under "Etiology and Pathophysiology"

DIAGNOSTIC TESTS & INTERPRETATION
All patients with CKD risk factors should be screened via serum creatine determination for GFR estimation and analysis of random urine sample for proteinuria.

Initial Tests (lab, imaging)
- Urinalysis (UA) quantitatively estimates proteinuria:
  - Only sensitive to albumin; will not detect low-molecular proteins of overflow/tubular etiologies
  - False-positive: if urine pH >7, highly concentrated (specific gravity [SG] >1.015), gross hematuria, mucus, semen, leukocytes, iodinated contrast agents, penicillin analogues, sulfonamide metabolites
  - False-negative: if urine is dilute (SG 1.005), albumin excretion <20 to 30 mg/dL, urinary protein is low-molecular weight
  - Sensitivity, 32–46%; specificity, 97–100%
  - Negative urine dipstick with positive sulfosalicylic acid test may indicate Bence-Jones protein.
- Protein results interpretation on dipstick UA
  - 1+ = 30 mg/dL
  - 2+ = 100 mg/dL
  - 3+ = 300 mg/dL
  - 4+ = 1000 mg/dL
- If UA shows trace to 2+ protein, rule out transient proteinuria with repeat UA at another visit:
  - More common than persistent proteinuria
  - Reassure the patient that transient proteinuria is benign and requires no further workup.
- If initial UA shows 3+ to 4+ protein or repeat UA is positive, measure creatinine clearance and quantify proteinuria with first morning spot urine to calculate urine protein-to-creatinine (P/C) ratio, which is preferred over 24-hour urine test due to inconsistent collection and inconvenience to patients (1),(2),(3)[A]. 24-hour urine test remains the gold standard.
  - Numerical P/C ratios correlate with total protein excreted in grams per day (i.e., ratio of 0.2 correlates with 0.2 g during a 24-hour collection).
  - Consider orthostatic proteinuria if P/C ratio <0.3 after recumbent position and P/C ratio >0.3 after prolonged standing activity.

Follow-Up Tests & Special Considerations
If urine P/C ratio >0.3, consider further evaluation, which can include the following:
- CBC, ferritin, ESR, serum iron
- Electrolytes, LFTs
- Lipid profile (ideally, fasting)
- Prothrombin time/international normalized ratio to assess for concurrent coagulopathy
- Antiphospholipase A2 receptor antibody: positive in ~70% of primary membranous nephropathy
- Antinuclear antibodies: elevated in lupus
- Antistreptolysin O titer: elevated after streptococcal infection
- Complement C3/C4: low in most glomerulonephritis
- HIV, syphilis, and hepatitis serologies: all associated with glomerular proteinuria
- Serum and urine protein electrophoresis: abnormal in multiple myeloma

- Patients with persistent proteinuria not explained by orthostatic changes should undergo renal ultrasound to rule out structural abnormalities (e.g., reflux nephropathy, polycystic kidney).
- Patients with nephrotic-range proteinuria are at increased risk for hypercholesterolemia and thromboembolic events (~25% of adult patients) with the highest risk in membranous nephropathy. Optimal duration of prophylactic anticoagulation is unknown but may extend for the duration of the nephrotic state (4).
- Proteinuric pregnant patients >20 weeks' gestation should be examined for other signs/symptoms of preeclampsia (e.g., hypertension, thrombocytopenia, elevated liver transaminases).

 TREATMENT

- Treat any identified underlying etiology
- BP goal for both diabetic and nondiabetic is ≤140/90 mm Hg (5)[C].
- Proteinuria goal is <0.5 g/day (6)[A].
- BP goal of 130/80 mm Hg for patients with normal urinary albumin concentration.
- BP goal of 125/75 mm Hg for patients with ≥1 g/24 hr proteinuria.

GENERAL MEASURES
- Limit protein intake to 0.8 g/kg/day in adults with DM or without DM and glomerular filtration rate (GFR) <30 mL/min/1.73 m². Soy protein may be renoprotective. Monitor protein intake with 24-hour urine urea excretion (6)[A].
- Limit sodium chloride intake to <2 g/day to optimize antiproteinuric medications (5)[B].
- Effect on BP is further protective (6)[A].
- Limit fluid intake for urine output goal of <2 L/day. Larger urine volumes are associated with increased proteinuria and later GFR decline (6)[B],(7).
- Smoking cessation: Smoking is associated with increased proteinuria and faster kidney disease progression (6)[B].
- Encourage supine posture (up to 50% reduction vs. upright) (6)[B].
- Discourage severe exertion (6)[B].
- Encourage weight loss (6)[B].

MEDICATION
First Line
Loop diuretics, ACE inhibitors (ACEi), or Angiotensin II receptor blockers (ARBs) use is a conservative management approach with nephrotic syndrome.
- ACEi: first-line therapy; if persistent proteinuria >0.5 g/day, use maximally tolerated doses; use even if normotensive (6),(8)[A].
- ARBs: proven antiproteinuric and renoprotective; ARBs are first choice if ACEi are not tolerated (6)[A].
  – Combination ACEi and ARB should not be used. Although shown to reduce proteinuria, combination does not reduce poor CV outcomes and does increase risk of adverse drug reactions (7),(9)[A].
  – May continue therapy with ACEi or ARB up to 30% increase in serum creatinine (8)
- Loop diuretics: first-line therapy if edema is present; may be used as additional therapy for BP control and proteinuria reduction

Second Line
- β-Blockers: antiproteinuric and cardioprotective (6)[A]
- Non-dihydropyridine calcium channel blockers (non-DHCCBs): antiproteinuric, may be renoprotective (6)[B]
- Aldosterone antagonists: antiproteinuric independent of BP control (6)[B]
- NSAIDs: antiproteinuric but also nephrotoxic; generally should be avoided (6)

ISSUES FOR REFERRAL
Consider nephrology referral for possible renal biopsy if impaired creatinine clearance, nephrotic-range proteinuria, or unclear etiology

ADDITIONAL THERAPIES
Corticosteroids: There is no proven benefit in mortality or the need for renal replacement in adults with nephrotic syndrome, although steroids are recommended in some patients who do not respond to conservative treatment. Classically, children with nephrotic syndrome respond better than adults, especially those with minimal-change disease (7)[A].

COMPLEMENTARY & ALTERNATIVE MEDICINE
- Regular exercise and smoking cessation
- Antioxidant therapy: may be antiproteinuric in diabetic nephropathy (6)[C]
- Avoid excessive caffeine consumption: antiproteinuric in diabetic rat models (6)[C].
- Avoid iron overload (6)[C].

 ONGOING CARE

FOLLOW-UP RECOMMENDATIONS
Patient Monitoring
All patients with persistent proteinuria should be followed with serial BP checks, UA, and renal function tests.

DIET
- Restrict dietary sodium to <2 g/day.
- Restrict caloric intake to achieve normal BMI with target 35 kcal/kg/day.
- Restrict dietary fat to <30% of total calories.

PROGNOSIS
- Transient and orthostatic proteinuria are benign conditions.
- Clinical significance of persistent proteinuria varies greatly and depends on underlying etiology.
- Degree of proteinuria is associated with disease progression in chronic kidney disease.
- Independent of GFR, higher levels of proteinuria likely convey an increased risk of mortality, myocardial infarction, and progression to kidney failure.

COMPLICATIONS
- Progression to chronic renal failure
- Hypercholesterolemia
- Hypercoagulable state
- Increased risk for infection for patient with nephrotic syndrome

REFERENCES
1. Mazaheri M, Assadi F. Simplified algorithm for evaluation of proteinuria in clinical practice: how should a clinician approach? *Int J Prev Med*. 2019;10:35.
2. Hull RP, Goldsmith DJA. Nephrotic syndrome in adults. *BMJ*. 2008;336(7654):1185–1189.
3. National Kidney Foundation. K/DOQI clinical practice guidelines for chronic kidney disease: evaluation, classification and stratification: guideline 5. Assessment of proteinuria. https://www.kidney.org/sites/default/files/docs/ckd_evaluation_classification_stratification.pdf. Accessed October 24, 2023.
4. Kerlin BA, Ayoob R, Smoyer WE. Epidemiology and pathophysiology of nephrotic syndrome-associated thromboembolic disease. *Clin J Am Soc Nephrol*. 2012;7(3):513–520.
5. James PA, Oparil S, Carter BL, et al. 2014 Evidence-based guideline for the management of high blood pressure in adults: report from the panel members appointed to the Eighth Joint National Committee (JNC 8). *JAMA*. 2014;311(5):507–520.
6. Wilmer WA, Rovin BH, Hebert CJ, et al. Management of glomerular proteinuria: a commentary. *J Am Soc Nephrol*. 2003;14(12):3217–3232.
7. Kodner C. Diagnosis and management of nephrotic syndrome in adults. *Am Fam Physician*. 2016;93(6):479–485.
8. Rovin BH, Adler SG, Barratt J, et al. KDIGO 2021 clinical practice guideline for the management of glomerular diseases. *Kidney Int*. 2021;100(4S): S1–S276.
9. Fried LF, Emanuele N, Zhang JH, et al; for VA NEPHRON-D Investigators. Combined angiotensin inhibition for the treatment of diabetic nephropathy. *N Engl J Med*. 2013;369(20):1892–1903.

 CODES

ICD10
- R80.9 Proteinuria, unspecified
- R80.2 Orthostatic proteinuria, unspecified
- R80.1 Persistent proteinuria, unspecified

CLINICAL PEARLS
- Transient and orthostatic proteinuria are benign conditions that do not convey a poor prognosis.
- Proteinuria >2 g/day likely represents glomerular malfunction and warrants a nephrology consultation.
- Clinical course varies greatly but, in general, the degree of proteinuria correlates with kidney disease progression.
- First-line therapy for persistent proteinuric patients is a high-dose ACE inhibitor.

PROTHROMBIN 20210 (MUTATION)

Touqir Zahra, MD, FACP • Raksha Sharma, MD

 BASICS

DESCRIPTION
- The G20210A is a gain of function mutation where adenine is substituted for a guanine at the 20210 noncoding position of the prothrombin (a.k.a. factor II) gene.
- Prothrombin 20210 mutation is the second most common venous thrombophilia after the factor V Leiden mutation.
- The mechanism of increasing the risk of thrombosis is incompletely understood but has been attributed to increased prothrombin or factor II levels in circulation by increased prothrombin protein translation without changing the levels of prothrombin mRNA transcription.
- Autosomal dominant condition, where heterozygotes have a 30% higher prothrombin level and a 3- to 4-fold increased risk of venous thromboembolism (VTE)
- System(s) affected: cardiovascular, hematologic/lymphatic/immunologic, nervous, pulmonary, reproductive, and hepatic
- Synonym(s): prothrombin G20210A mutation; prothrombin G20210A gene polymorphism; prothrombin gene mutation; and factor II A^{20210} mutation

EPIDEMIOLOGY
- Mean age of first thrombosis is in the 2nd decade of life.
- Inheritance is similar between both genders (autosomal).

Incidence
In patients with the prothrombin 20210 mutation, the cumulative incidence of VTE complications after 10 years was 61.3% (1).

Prevalence
- Found largely in Caucasian population with a prevalence ranging between 1% and 6%, but overall, it is about 2%.
- In patients presenting with a VTE, prothrombin 20210 mutation has a prevalence that ranges from 4.6% to 18% with increased prevalence attributed to highly thrombophilic families.

ETIOLOGY AND PATHOPHYSIOLOGY
- Noncoding substitution of adenine for guanine at the 20210 position at the terminal nucleotide of the 3' resulting in a gain of function of prothrombin gene, leading to increased levels of prothrombin (factor II), by increased translation of prothrombin mRNA but not transcription
- The base change location is in the 3' terminal nucleotide of the untranslated region associated with the mRNA sequence for polyadenylation. The gain of function is possible due to increased rate of processing, alteration of the site of cleavage, or increased mRNA stability.

- In the coagulation cascade, prothrombin (factor II) is the precursor of thrombin, which cleaves fibrinogen to fibrin. Elevated prothrombin activity leads to elevated thrombin levels and subsequent clot formation.
- The majority of thrombus formation occurs in the venous circulation: deep venous thrombosis (DVT)/PE, mesenteric, and cerebral. Recent studies have shown that prothrombin 20210 mutation did not correlate with Budd-Chiari syndrome or a portal or hepatic vein thrombosis.
- G20210A mutation is not known to be a risk factor for some arterial thrombotic events (myocardial infarction or acute ischemic stroke); however, studies have shown an increased prevalence of the mutation in patients with critical limb ischemia.

Genetics
- Caused by the G20210A mutation of the *F2* gene (prothrombin gene) located in the short (p) arm of chromosome 11 that causes a gain of function
- Heterozygotes have a 30% increased levels of prothrombin levels, with a 3- to 4-fold increase of VTE events. Homozygotes are at an even greater risk.
- There are three other prothrombin mutations not related to the G20210A area:
  - Yukuhashi: missense mutation G1787T, arginine for leucine at amino acid 596, leading to prolonged procoagulant activity
  - C20209T: adjacent to G20210A mutation, primarily found in African individuals; newer studies have suggested a possible relationship between this mutation and recurrent pregnancy loss, although it is not fully understood.
  - A19911G: located in the intron of the prothrombin gene; may affect the G20210A mutation by increasing the odds ratio of the venous thromboembolic event. Mechanism is still unknown.

RISK FACTORS
- Being a hereditary condition, the presence of such mutation in the parents poses risk of transmission to offspring.
- Regarding the risk of developing VTE:
  - Patients with both the prothrombin 20210 mutation and factor V Leiden mutation increases the odds ratio of VTE by 20-fold.
  - Virchow triad of thrombogenesis consists of stasis, endothelial injury, and thrombophilia. Any condition that promotes stasis and endothelial injury will consequently increase the risk of VTE, for example, oral contraceptive, pregnancy, malignancy, orthopedic surgery, congestive heart failure, cerebrovascular accident in the past 3 months, air travel, obesity, and smoking.

Pregnancy Considerations
- Increased thrombotic risk in patients with prothrombin 20210 mutation during pregnancy and in the postpartum state is attributed to relative stasis.
- Anticoagulation should begin in the 1st trimester because the risk of VTE increases early in pregnancy and should be discontinued at onset of labor or before scheduled induction/cesarean delivery. Postpartum risk of VTE is usually greater, and anticoagulation can resume 4 to 6 hours after a vaginal delivery or 6 to 12 hours after surgery. Warfarin may begin immediately due to slow onset of action.
- C20209T mutation may have some relation with recurrent pregnancy loss; however, it is not well studied.

GENERAL PREVENTION
Asymptomatic individuals with the mutation do not require any prophylactic anticoagulation. Exceptions are generally made for pregnant women with very high-risk thrombophilic mutations (usually factor V Leiden) with a strong family history. After the first VTE, lifelong prophylaxis may be warranted if some features are present: unprovoked or in a nontraditional area like hepatic, portal, mesenteric, or cerebral.

COMMONLY ASSOCIATED CONDITIONS
- VTE
- Factor V Leiden

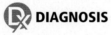 **DIAGNOSIS**

HISTORY
- Previous VTE
- Family history of VTE
- Family history of prothrombin 20210 mutation

PHYSICAL EXAM
- Unilateral swollen, erythematous, and tender calf is significant for a possible DVT.
- Positive Homans sign, sensitivity of 10–54%, specificity of 39–89% for DVT
- Tachycardia is the most common sign of a pulmonary embolism; however, patients may have chest pain and hypotension depending on the severity of the pulmonary embolus.
- A tender abdomen may be indicative of mesenteric veins thrombosis; however, other causes of an acute abdomen should be worked up as appropriate.

DIFFERENTIAL DIAGNOSIS
- Factor V Leiden mutation
- Protein C deficiency
- Protein S deficiency
- Antithrombin deficiency
- Other causes of activated protein C resistance (e.g., antiphospholipid antibodies)
- Dysfibrinogenemia
- Dysplasminogenemia
- Homocystinemia
- Elevated factor VIII levels

DIAGNOSTIC TESTS & INTERPRETATION

Screening for prothrombin G20210A mutation in asymptomatic individuals is not recommended, except for those with very strong family history. Testing can take place in patients with thrombosis at a very early age, recurrent unprovoked VTE, or those with thrombosis in unusual locations.

Initial Tests (lab, imaging)

- This mutation can be diagnosed using PCR with electrophoresis or immunoassays.
- Imaging should be obtained as appropriate for the suspected site of thrombosis: ultrasound with Doppler, computed tomography scan with contrast to evaluate venous phase, and V/Q scan.
- Testing for an inherited thrombophilic condition is reliable during an acute embolic event or with anticoagulation use.

Follow-Up Tests & Special Considerations

Although prothrombin levels are elevated, this is not a sensitive test to make the diagnosis.

Diagnostic Procedures/Other

MR angiography (MRA), venography, or arteriography to detect thrombosis

Test Interpretation

Imaging is likely to show presence of arterial or venous thrombus.

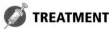 ## TREATMENT

GENERAL MEASURES

Management of patients with a first-time VTE with or without an acquired thrombophilic condition remains overall very similar.

MEDICATION

Is directed to treat those patients with VTE (prophylactic doses may vary). We recommend the reader to check the most updated doses, dose adjustments, and contraindications for the medications listed below. The doses listed apply to most adults.

First Line

In adult patients without cancer, the following oral anticoagulants are preferred over warfarin and low-molecular-weight heparin (LMWH): dabigatran, rivaroxaban, apixaban, or edoxaban is preferred over warfarin.

- Apixaban (Eliquis): Initial dose is 10 mg BID for 7 days, followed by 5 mg BID.
- Dabigatran (Pradaxa): requires initial parenteral anticoagulation for 5 to 10 days, followed by 150 mg BID
- Edoxaban (Savaysa): requires initial parenteral anticoagulation for 5 to 10 days, followed by 60 mg daily
- Rivaroxaban (Xarelto): Initial dose is 15 mg BID with food for 21 days, followed by a daily dose of 20 mg with food.

Second Line

For patients without cancer that cannot be treated with DOAC, warfarin is preferred over LMWH.

- Warfarin (Coumadin): Initial dose may range from 2 to 10 mg PO daily and then adjusted to an INR of 2 to 3.
- Enoxaparin (Lovenox): 1 mg/kg SC injection every 12 hours

ISSUES FOR REFERRAL

- Recurrent thrombosis on anticoagulation
- Difficulty anticoagulating
- Genetic counseling

SURGERY/OTHER PROCEDURES

- Anticoagulation must be held for surgical interventions.
- For most patients with DVT, recommendations are against routine use of vena cava filter in addition to anticoagulation, except in case with contraindication to anticoagulation.
- Thrombectomy may be necessary in some cases.

ADMISSION, INPATIENT, AND NURSING CONSIDERATIONS

- Admission criteria/initial stabilization: complicated thrombosis, such as pulmonary embolus; required heparin drip
- Patient can be safely discharged if patient is stable on anticoagulation.

 ## ONGOING CARE

- Compression stockings for prevention
- DVT prophylaxis as appropriate if patient admitted to hospital

FOLLOW-UP RECOMMENDATIONS

Patient Monitoring

- Warfarin use requires periodic (weekly and then monthly after initial stabilization) INR measurements, with a goal of 2 to 3.
- Heterozygosity for the prothrombin 20210 mutation increases the risk for recurrent VTE only slightly; thus, its presence does not alter the length of anticoagulation treatment decision.

DIET

- No restrictions; unless taking warfarin
- Food rich in vitamin K may interfere with warfarin anticoagulation.
- Grapefruit and St. John's wort interfere with the cytochrome P450 and can alter the levels and clearance of anticoagulant therapy.

PATIENT EDUCATION

Patients should be educated about:

- Use of oral anticoagulant therapy
- Signs and symptoms of acute blood loss
- Avoidance of NSAIDs while on warfarin

PROGNOSIS

When compared with normal individuals, persons with prothrombin 20210 have normal lifespans.

COMPLICATIONS

- Recurrent thrombosis on anticoagulation
- Bleeding on anticoagulation
- Complications are usually location dependent and can lead to death, possibly from a massive pulmonary embolism.
- Venous stasis ulcers

REFERENCE

1. Simioni P, Prandoni P, Lensing AW, et al. Risk for subsequent venous thromboembolic complications in carriers of the prothrombin or the factor V gene mutation with a first episode of deep-vein thrombosis. *Blood*. 2000;96(10):3329–3333.

ADDITIONAL READING

- Kearon C, Akl EA. Duration of anticoagulant therapy for deep vein thrombosis and pulmonary embolism. *Blood*. 2014;123(12):1794–1801.
- Moll S. Thrombophilias—practical implications and testing caveats. *J Thromb Thrombolysis*. 2006;21(1):7–15.
- Wells PS, Forgie MA, Rodger MA. Treatment of venous thromboembolism. *JAMA*. 2014;311(7):717–728.

 ## SEE ALSO

Antithrombin Deficiency; Deep Vein Thrombophlebitis; Factor V Leiden; Protein C Deficiency; Protein S Deficiency

CODES

ICD10

D68.52 Prothrombin gene mutation

CLINICAL PEARLS

- Prothrombin 20210 mutation is the second most common inherited risk factor for VTE after factor V Leiden mutation.
- Asymptomatic patients with prothrombin 20210 mutation do not need anticoagulation or screening.
- Management of VTE is no different with or without the prothrombin G20210A mutation. However, indefinite anticoagulation may be considered in people with an unprovoked VTE or thrombus in a nontraditional area (mesenteric or cerebral).

PRURITUS ANI

Marie L. Borum, MD, EdD, MPH • Justin Paul Canakis, DO • Jacob Thomas Newman, DO

 BASICS

DESCRIPTION
- Intense anal/perianal itching and/or burning
- Usually acute (defined as <6 weeks of symptoms)
- Classified as primary (idiopathic) or secondary (25–75% of cases) to anorectal pathology

EPIDEMIOLOGY
Incidence
- 1–5% of the general population
- Predominant age: 30 to 50 years; although seen in all age groups
- Predominant sex: male > female (4:1)

Prevalence
Difficult to estimate because many patients do not report symptoms; affects 1–5% of the population

ETIOLOGY AND PATHOPHYSIOLOGY
- Multiple etiologies categorized by inflammatory, infectious, systemic, neoplastic, anorectal disorders, neuropathic, neurogenic, and psychogenic causes (1),(2)
- Most cases are idiopathic (25–90%), which are likely due to trauma from wiping or scratching and perianal fecal contamination.
  - Soilage can be due to an abnormality of rectoanal inhibitory reflex and a lower threshold or transient internal anal sphincter relaxation.
- Depending on underlying etiology, itch pathway may be histamine mediated or nonhistamine mediated (1).
- Pruritus ani is typically intensely perceived by the patient due to dense innervation.
- Etiologies of secondary pruritus ani:
  - Inflammatory dermatologic diseases:
    ○ Allergic contact dermatitis (soaps, perfumes, or dyes in toilet paper, topical anesthetics, oral antibiotics)
    ○ Atopic dermatitis ± lichen simplex chronicus (Patients may also have asthma and/or eczema.)
    ○ Psoriasis (Lesions tend to be poorly demarcated, pale, and nonscaling.)
    ○ Seborrheic dermatitis
    ○ Scleroderma
    ○ Lichen planus (may be seen in patients with ulcerative colitis and myasthenia gravis)
    ○ Hidradenitis suppurativa
    ○ Radiation dermatitis (2)
  - Colorectal/anorectal diseases: rectal prolapse, hemorrhoids, fissures or fistulas, proctitis, chronic diarrhea/constipation, polyps
  - Infectious etiologies may be sexually transmitted: bacteria (gonorrhea, chlamydia, syphilis), viruses (herpes simplex virus [HSV], condyloma acuminata from human papillomavirus [HPV], molluscum), parasites (pinworms, lice, scabies, or bed bugs), fungi (*Candida* or dermatophytes like tinea); other bacteria (*Staphylococcus aureus*, β-hemolytic *Streptococcus*, *Corynebacterium minutissimum* [erythrasma]) (2)

- Malignancies: melanoma, basal cell/squamous cell carcinoma, colorectal cancer, leukemia, lymphoma, or (uncommon) the presenting symptom of Bowen or Paget disease
- Mechanical factors: vigorous cleaning and scrubbing, tight-fitting clothes, synthetic undergarments
- Systemic diseases (often presents as generalized pruritus): diabetes mellitus (most common), cholestasis, chronic liver disease, renal failure, hyperthyroidism, anemia, HIV, vitamin or iron deficiencies, lumbosacral radiculopathy (particularly in the elderly)
- Chemical irritants: local anesthetics, chemotherapy, diarrhea (often from antibiotic use)
- Dietary elements (citrus, milk products, coffee, tea, cola, chocolate, beer, wine, tomatoes, nuts)
- Psychogenic factors: anxiety–itch–anxiety cycle

RISK FACTORS
- Obesity
- Excess perianal hair growth and/or perspiration
- Underlying anorectal pathology
- Atopic disease
- Underlying anxiety disorder
- Caffeine intake has been correlated with symptoms.

GENERAL PREVENTION
- Good perianal hygiene; avoid overzealous cleaning.
- Avoid mechanical irritation of skin (vigorous cleaning or rubbing with dry toilet paper or baby wipes, harsh soaps or perfumed products, excessive scratching with fingernails, or tight/synthetic undergarments).
- Minimize moisture in perianal area (absorbent cotton in anal cleft may help keep area dry).
- Avoid laxative use (loose stool is an irritant).

COMMONLY ASSOCIATED CONDITIONS
- Psoriasis is seen in 5–55% of patients with pruritus ani.
- Coexisting anorectal disease, such as hemorrhoids, can be seen in up to 52% of patients with pruritus ani.

DIAGNOSIS

HISTORY
- Patients present with complaints of anal and/or perianal itching, burning, or excoriation.
- Inquire about:
  - Timing (when it started, when it is worse)
  - Perianal hygiene (frequency of cleansing and products used)
  - Change in bowel habits
  - Bleeding (spotting of toilet paper, melena, hematochezia)
  - Recent antibiotic use
  - Skin disorders (psoriasis, eczema)
  - Rectal or vaginal discharge, menstrual cycle
  - Dietary history: Focus on the "C's": caffeine, coffee, cola, chocolate, citrus, calcium (dairy) (2).

- Medical history (hepatitis, iron deficiency anemia, and diabetes in particular)
- Family history of colorectal cancer
- Anal receptive intercourse
- Change in toiletry products
- Household members (particularly children) with itching (possible pinworms)
- Pets
- Clothing preference (tight, synthetic) (3)

PHYSICAL EXAM
- Perianal visual inspection for erythema, hemorrhoids, anal fissures, maceration, lichenification, warts, polyps, excoriations, neoplasia, stool seepage
- Classification based on gross appearance
  - Stage 1: erythema, inflamed appearance
  - Stage 2: lichenification
  - Stage 3: lichenification, coarse skin, potential fissures or ulcerations (3)
- Digital rectal exam to evaluate for masses, internal sphincter tone, pain
- Valsalva to evaluate for prolapse
- Anoscopy to evaluate for hemorrhoids, fissures, other internal lesions

DIFFERENTIAL DIAGNOSIS
"ITCHeS" acronym (4)
- **I**nfection: *Candida*, parasites (scabies, pinworms), HPV, HSV, bacterial (gram-positive bacteria, gonorrhea, chlamydia, syphilis)
- **T**opical irritants: soaps/detergents, garments, deodorants, perfumes, stool leakage
- **C**utaneous/**C**ancer/**C**olorectal: eczema, psoriasis, lichen planus, lichen sclerosus, seborrhea, skin cancer, extramammary Paget disease, Bowen disease, fistula, fissure, prolapse, hemorrhoids, colorectal cancer
- **H**ypersensitivity: foods, medications (colchicine, quinidine, mineral oil)
- e**S**ystemic: diabetes, iron deficiency anemia, uremia, cholestasis, hematologic malignancy

DIAGNOSTIC TESTS & INTERPRETATION
Initial Tests (lab, imaging)
Use history and exam to suggest a specific etiology, and guide testing:
- Pinworm tape test; stool for ova and parasites
- CBC, comprehensive metabolic panel, A1c, thyroid studies to identify underlying systemic disease
- Wood lamp examination will show coral-red fluorescence in erythrasma (2).
- Skin scraping with potassium hydroxide (KOH) prep for dermatophytes or candidiasis (as etiology or as superinfection) and mineral oil prep for scabies
- Perianal skin culture (bacterial superinfection)
- Hemoccult testing of stool

Pediatric Considerations
Pinworms are common in children. Consider perianal Crohn disease.

Follow-Up Tests & Special Considerations

Anal DNA polymerase chain reaction (PCR) probe for gonorrhea and chlamydia; may perform anal speculum exam and test for anal HPV if receptive anal intercourse; HIV testing in patients with HIV risk factors

Diagnostic Procedures/Other

- Biopsy suspicious lesions (e.g., lichenification, ulcerated epithelium, refractory cases) to exclude neoplasia; evaluate etiology.
- Consider colonoscopy if history, exam, or testing suggests colorectal pathology (family history of colorectal disease, especially if age >40 years, weight loss, rectal bleeding, change in bowel habits).

Geriatric Considerations

- Stool incontinence may be a predisposing factor.
- Consider systemic disease.
- Higher likelihood of colorectal pathology

 TREATMENT

GENERAL MEASURES

- Proper anal/perianal hygiene; avoid vigorous rubbing while cleansing after bowel movement. Use cotton swabs moistened with warm water instead of tissue paper. Avoid chemical and mechanical irritants and wear proper undergarments.
- High-fiber diet and/or bowel regimen to maintain regular bowel movements
- Avoid tight-fitting clothing. Use cotton undergarments.
- Avoiding moisture; absorbent cotton, talcum powder, or cornstarch if there is an excess moisture; can use hair dryer on cool setting to dry anal area (3)[C]
- Cotton gloves at night to control nocturnal scratching

MEDICATION

First Line

- Treat underlying infections: fungal or dermatophyte infection with topical imidazoles, bacterial infection with topical antibacterials.
- Treat underlying anorectal anatomic pathology: banding of prolapsing internal hemorrhoids, treat fistulas, or fissures.
- Break itch–scratch cycle with low-potency steroid cream such as hydrocortisone 1% ointment applied sparingly up to 4 times daily (3)[C]. Discontinue when itching subsides. Avoid use >2 weeks due to risk of skin atrophy.
- If no response with low-potency steroid, consider high-potency steroid cream.
- Antihistamines, particularly sedating antihistamines, may be useful in reducing nighttime itching until local measures take effect. Avoid in elderly patients due to anticholinergic properties.
- Tricyclic antidepressants may reduce nighttime scratching. SSRIs or gabapentin may be used in resistant cases (1)[C].
- Zinc oxide can be used after steroid course for barrier protection (2); petroleum jelly is another barrier. Avoid mineral oil as it can worsen pruritus.
- Albendazole for pinworm

Second Line

- Low-dose topical capsaicin cream in combination with steroid cream if refractory symptoms (3)[C]
- 0.03% tacrolimus ointment can be considered in cases not responsive to high potency steroids (3)[C].
- Intradermal methylene blue injections, sometimes known as anal tattooing, may be used to destroy nerve endings and create permanent anesthesia in cases not responsive to medical management (3)[C].
- Biologics, such as the IL-4 inhibitor dupilumab, show promise for recalcitrant cases, although there is limited data currently.

ISSUES FOR REFERRAL

- Intractable pruritus: Consider referral to gastroenterology (for colonoscopy) or dermatology (for additional treatment, possibly injections, or biopsies). Refractory or persistent symptoms should signal the possibility of underlying neoplasia because pruritus ani of long duration is associated with a greater likelihood of colorectal pathology.
- Refer for colonoscopy if at risk for colon cancer.

SURGERY/OTHER PROCEDURES

As above, especially if concern for malignancy is identified

 ONGOING CARE

FOLLOW-UP RECOMMENDATIONS

- See patient every 2 weeks if not improving.
- Ensure proper hygiene and avoidance of irritants.
- Work up for systemic disease, and check for persistent lichenification. If refractory pruritus or lichenification does not resolve, consider underlying malignancy.

DIET

- Eliminate foods and beverages known or suspected to exacerbate symptoms: coffee, tea, chocolate, beer, cola, vitamin C tablets in excessive doses, citrus fruits, tomatoes, or spices.
- Eliminate foods or drugs contributing to loose bowel movements or dermatitis.
- Add fiber supplementation to bulk stools and prevent fecal leakage in patients who have fecal incontinence or partially formed stools.

PATIENT EDUCATION

- Review proper anal hygiene:
  – Resist overuse of soap and rubbing.
  – Avoid products with irritating perfumes and dyes.
  – Avoid use of ointments and mineral oil.
  – Wear loose, light cotton clothing.
  – If moisture is a problem, use cotton, unmedicated talcum powder, or cornstarch to keep the area dry.
  – Cleanse perianal area after bowel movements with water-moistened cotton.
  – Dry the area after bathing by patting with a soft towel or by using a hair dryer on cool setting (3)[C].
- Avoid medications that cause diarrhea or constipation.
- Avoid caffeine, cola, chocolate, citrus, tomatoes, tea, alcohol, nuts, and milk products (2).
- Use barrier protection if engaging in anal intercourse.
- If unable to completely empty rectum with defecation, use small plain-water enema (infant bulb syringe) after each bowel movement to prevent soiling and irritation.
- If persists, consider underlying medical disease.

PROGNOSIS

- Conservative treatment successful in ~90% of cases
- Idiopathic pruritus ani is often chronic—waxes and wanes.

COMPLICATIONS

- Bacterial superinfection at site of excoriations and potential abscess formation or penetrating infection via self-inoculation with colonic pathogens
- Lichenification
- Significant effect on quality of life

REFERENCES

1. Jakubauskas M, Dulskas A. Evaluation, management and future perspectives of anal pruritus: a narrative review. *Eur J Med Res*. 2023;28(1):57.
2. Sacks OA, Beresneva O. Causes and management of pruritus ani. *Dis Colon Rectum*. 2023;66(1):10–13.
3. Ortega AE, Delgadillo X. Idiopathic pruritus ani and acute perianal dermatitis. *Clin Colon Rectal Surg*. 2019;32(5):327–332.
4. Andrade A, Kuah CY, Martin-Lopez JE, et al. Interventions for chronic pruritus of unknown origin. *Cochrane Database Syst Rev*. 2020;1(1):CD013128.

ADDITIONAL READING

- Davies D, Bailey J. Diagnosis and management of anorectal disorders in the primary care setting. *Prim Care*. 2017;44(4):709–720.
- Felemovicius I, Ganz RA, Saremi M, et al. SOOTHER TRIAL: observational study of an over-the-counter ointment to heal anal itch. *Front Med (Lausanne)*. 2022;9:890883.

 SEE ALSO

Pinworms; Pruritus Vulvae

 CODES

ICD10
L29.0 Pruritus ani

CLINICAL PEARLS

- Pruritus ani is characterized by anal/perianal itching and/or burning. It is a skin irritation with itch–scratch–itch cycle.
- Conservative treatment with perianal hygiene and reassurance is successful in 90% of patients.
- Consider trial of dietary elimination of "C's"—citrus, vitamin C supplements, calcium products, caffeine, coffee, cola, chocolate.
- Rule out infection (viral, bacterial, parasitic) in immunosuppressed patients.
- Consider underlying malignancy if refractory.

PRURITUS VULVAE

Sareena Singh, MD, FACOG

BASICS

DESCRIPTION
- Pruritus vulvae is a symptom or can be a primary diagnosis.
- If a primary diagnosis, other etiologies must be excluded
- Pruritus vulvae as a primary diagnosis may also be more appropriately documented as vulvodynia (see "Vulvodynia" topic) or burning vulva syndrome.

EPIDEMIOLOGY
Symptoms may occur at any age during a woman's lifetime.
- Young girls most commonly have infectious or hygiene etiology.
- The primary diagnosis is more common in post-menopausal women.

Incidence
The exact incidence is unknown, although most women complain of vulvar pruritus at some point in their lifetime.

ETIOLOGY AND PATHOPHYSIOLOGY
Vulvar tissue is more permeable than exposed skin due to differences in structure, occlusion, hydration, and susceptibility to friction. It is particularly vulnerable to irritants such as (1)
- Perfumes
- Soaps
- Vaginal hygiene products
- Topical medications
- Dyes
- Body fluids

RISK FACTORS
- High-risk sexual behavior
- Immunosuppression
- Obesity

GENERAL PREVENTION
- Avoid irritants.
- Tight-fitting clothing should be avoided.
- Only cotton underwear should be worn.

COMMONLY ASSOCIATED CONDITIONS
- Infectious etiology
  - Vaginal or vulvar candida
  - *Gardnerella vaginalis*
  - *Trichomonas*
  - Human papillomavirus
  - Herpes simplex virus
- Vulvar vestibulitis
- Lichen sclerosus
- Lichen planus
- Lichen simplex chronicus (squamous cell hyperplasia)
- Malignant or premalignant conditions
- Psoriasis
- Fecal or urinary incontinence
- Dermatophytosis
- Parasites: scabies, *Pthirus pubis*
- Extramammary Paget
- Dietary: methylxanthines (e.g., coffee, cola), tomatoes, peanuts
- Autoimmune progesterone dermatitis: perimenstrual eruptions
- Irritant or allergic contact dermatitis
- Atopic dermatitis

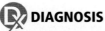

DIAGNOSIS

Pruritus vulvae is a diagnosis of exclusion. Delay in diagnosis is common due to patient hesitancy to seek treatment or provider delay in biopsy. Delayed diagnosis can have profound negative effect on women's sexual comfort and quality of life (2).

HISTORY
- Persistent itching
- Persistent burning sensation over the vulva or perineum
- Change in vaginal discharge
- Postcoital bleeding
- Dyspareunia

PHYSICAL EXAM
- Visual inspection of the vulva, vagina, perineum, and anus
  - Superior surfaces of the labia majora—extending from mons to the anal orifice—are most involved.
  - Vulvar skin is leathery or lichenified in appearance.
  - Papillomatosis may be a sign of chronic inflammation.
- Cotton swab–applied pressure to area of pain and to vestibular glands
- Musculoskeletal evaluation to confirm not contributing if persistent vulvar pain

DIAGNOSTIC TESTS & INTERPRETATION
- Sodium chloride: *Gardnerella* or *Trichomonas*
- 10% potassium hydroxide: *Candida*
- Viral culture or polymerase chain reaction: herpes simplex virus
- Directed biopsy recommended (3)[B]: human papillomavirus, lichen, malignancy, chronic inflammation
- Colposcopy with acetic acid or Lugol solution of vagina and vulva

Follow-Up Tests & Special Considerations

- A patch test may be performed by a dermatologist to assist in identifying a causative agent if contact dermatitis is suspected or if topical products are suspected as source of dermatitis (4)[A].
- Exam-directed tissue biopsies are essential in the postmenopausal population to rule out malignancy.

Diagnostic Procedures/Other

Biopsies should be collected from any ulceration, discoloration, raised areas, macerated areas, and the area of most intense pruritus.

Test Interpretation

- Only in the absence of pathologic findings can the primary diagnosis of pruritus vulvae be made.
- Biopsies of visible lesions most commonly show lichen simplex chronicus (25%), lichen sclerosus (20%), or chronic inflammation (15%) (3).

 TREATMENT

Identify the underlying cause or disease to target treatment.

- Stop all potential irritants.
- Eliminate bacterial and fungal infection.
- Cool the affected area: Use cool gel packs (not ice packs, which may cause further injury).
- Sitz baths and bland emollients to soothe fissured or eroded skin

MEDICATION

First Line

- Topical steroids (1),(5)
  - Triamcinolone 0.1% applied daily for 2 to 4 weeks and then twice weekly
  - Hydrocortisone 1–2.5% cream applied 2 to 4 times daily
  - Avoid long-term use due to risk of atrophy.
- 1st-generation antihistamines
  - Hydroxyzine: Initiate with 10 mg before bedtime (slowly increase up to 100 mg).
  - Doxepin: Initiate with 10 mg before bedtime.
  - 2nd-generation antihistamines are of little benefit.

Second Line

- SSRI such as citalopram 20 to 40 mg for resistant cases
- Calcineurin inhibitors such as 1% pimecrolimus (5)[A]

ISSUES FOR REFERRAL

- Persistent symptoms should prompt additional investigation and referral to a gynecologist or gynecologic oncologist.
- Gynecologic oncology referral for proven or suspected malignancy
- Dermatology referral for patch testing to evaluate for contact dermatitis

ADDITIONAL THERAPIES

- Sacral neuromodulation device
- Laser therapy
- GnRH analogues
- Naltrexone

 ONGOING CARE

- Frequent evaluation, repeat cultures, and biopsies are necessary for cases resistant to treatment.
- Refractory cases may require referral to gynecologist or gynecologic oncology for further management.

DIET

Dietary alterations include avoidance of the following:

- Coffee and other caffeine-containing beverages
- Tomatoes
- Peanuts

PATIENT EDUCATION

- American College of Obstetricians and Gynecologists: https://www.acog.org
- National Vulvodynia Association: https://www.nva.org

PROGNOSIS

Conservative measures and short-term topical steroids control most patients' symptoms.

COMPLICATIONS

Malignancy

REFERENCES

1. Stockdale CK, Boardman L. Diagnosis and treatment of vulvar dermatoses. *Obstet Gynecol*. 2018;131(2):371–386.
2. Kellogg Spadt S, Kusturiss E. Vulvar dermatoses: a primer for the sexual medicine clinician. *Sex Med Rev*. 2015;3(3):126–136.
3. Ozalp SS, Telli E, Yalcin OT, et al. Vulval pruritus: the experience of gynaecologists revealed by biopsy. *J Obstet Gynaecol*. 2015;35(1):53–56.

4. Corazza M, Virgili A, Toni G, et al. Level of use and safety of botanical products for itching vulvar dermatoses. Are patch tests useful? *Contact Dermatitis*. 2016;74(5):289–294.
5. Chi CC, Kirtschig G, Baldo M, et al. Systematic review and meta-analysis of randomized controlled trials on topical interventions for genital lichen sclerosus. *J Am Acad Dermatol*. 2012;67(2):305–312.

ADDITIONAL READING

- Böttcher B, Wildt L. Treatment of refractory vulvovaginal pruritus with naltrexone, a specific opiate antagonist. *Eur J Obstet Gynecol Reprod Biol*. 2014;174:115–116.
- Hill AJ, Paraiso MFR. Resolution of chronic vulvar pruritus with replacement of a neuromodulation device. *J Minim Invasive Gynecol*. 2015;22(5):889–891.
- Pichardo-Geisinger R. Atopic and contact dermatitis of the vulva. *Obstet Gynecol Clin North Am*. 2017;44(3):371–378.
- Savas JA, Pichardo RO. Female genital itch. *Dermatol Clin*. 2018;36(3):225–243.

 CODES

ICD10

- L29.2 Pruritus vulvae
- N94.819 Vulvodynia, unspecified

CLINICAL PEARLS

- Pruritus vulvae is a common complaint.
- Pruritus vulvae is a diagnosis of exclusion once other causes of itching have been ruled out.
- Exam-directed biopsies from any ulceration, discoloration, raised areas, macerated areas, and the area of most intense pruritus are essential to rule out malignancy.
- Initial treatment is conservative.

PSEUDOFOLLICULITIS BARBAE

Maurice Duggins, MD, FAAFP

 BASICS

DESCRIPTION
- Foreign body inflammatory reaction from an ingrown hair resulting in the appearance of papules and pustules. This is found mainly in the bearded area (barbae) but may occur in other hairy locations such as the scalp, axilla, or pubic areas where shaving is done (1).
- A mechanical problem: extrafollicular and transfollicular hair penetration
- System(s) affected: skin/exocrine
- Synonym(s): chronic sycosis barbae; pili incarnati; folliculitis barbae traumatica; razor bumps; shaving bumps; tinea barbae

EPIDEMIOLOGY
- Predominant age: postpubertal, middle age (14 to 25 years)
- Predominant sex: male > female (can be seen in females of all races who wax/shave)

Incidence
- Adult male African Americans: unknown
- Adult male whites: unknown

Prevalence
- Widespread in Fitzpatrick skin types IV to VI (darker complexions) who shave
- 45–83% of African American soldiers who shave (1)

ETIOLOGY AND PATHOPHYSIOLOGY
- Transfollicular escape of the low-cut hair shaft as it tries to exit the skin is accompanied by inflammation and often an intraepidermal abscess.
- As the hair enters the dermis, more severe inflammation occurs, with downgrowth of the epidermis in an attempt to sheath the hair.
- A foreign body reaction forms at the tip of the invading hair, followed by abscess formation.
- Shaving too close
- Plucking/tweezing or wax depilation of hair may cause abnormal hair growth in injured follicles.

Genetics
- People with curly hair have an asymmetric accumulation of acidic keratin hHa8 on hair shaft.
- Single-nucleotide polymorphism (disruption Ala12Thr substitution) affects keratin of hair follicle.

RISK FACTORS
- Curly hair
- Shaving too close or shaving with multiple razor strokes

- Plucking/tweezing hairs
- South Mediterranean/American, Middle Eastern, Asian, or African descent (skin types IV to VI)

GENERAL PREVENTION
- Prior to shaving, rinse face with warm water to hydrate and soften hairs.
- Use adjustable hair clippers that leave very low hair length above skin.
- Shave with either a manual adjustable razor at coarsest setting (avoids close shaves), a single-edge blade razor (e.g., Bump Fighter), a foil-guarded razor (e.g., PFB razor), or electric triple "O-head" razor.
- Empty razor of hair frequently.
- Shave in the direction of hair growth. Do not over-stretch skin when shaving.
- Use a generous amount of the correct shaving cream/gel (e.g., Ef-Kay shaving gel, Edge shaving gel, Aveeno therapeutic shave gel, Easy Shave medicated shaving cream).
- Daily shaving reduces papules/pruritus.
- Regular use of depilatories

COMMONLY ASSOCIATED CONDITIONS
- Keloidal folliculitis
- Pseudofolliculitis nuchae

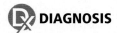 **DIAGNOSIS**

HISTORY
Pain on shaving; pruritus of shaved areas, irritated "razor bumps"

PHYSICAL EXAM
- Tender, exudative, erythematous follicular papules or pustules in beard area (less commonly in scalp, axilla, and pubic areas); range from 2 to 4 mm
- Hyperpigmented "razor or shave bumps"
- Alopecia
- Lusterless, brittle hair

DIFFERENTIAL DIAGNOSIS
- Bacterial folliculitis
- Impetigo
- Acne vulgaris
- Tinea barbae
- Sarcoidal papules

DIAGNOSTIC TESTS & INTERPRETATION
Initial Tests (lab, imaging)
- Clinical diagnosis
- Culture of pustules: usually sterile; may show coagulase-negative *Staphylococcus epidermidis* (normal skin flora)
- Additional hormonal testing may be indicated in females with hirsutism and/or polycystic ovary syndrome: dehydroepiandrosterone sulfate, luteinizing hormone (LH)/follicle-stimulating hormone (FSH), and free and total testosterone (2)[C].

Test Interpretation
Follicular papules and pustules

 TREATMENT

- Mild cases
  - Stop shaving or avoid close shaving for 30 days while keeping beard groomed and clean (1),(3).
  - Consider 5% benzoyl peroxide after shaving and application of 1% hydrocortisone cream at bedtime (or LactiCare-HC lotion after shaving).
  - Tretinoin 0.025% cream; apply daily (1)[C].
- Moderate cases
  - Chemical depilatories (barium sulfide; Magic shaving powder); first test on forearm for 48 hours (for irritation) (1),(2)[B]
  - Consider eflornithine HCl cream (Vaniqa) to reduce hair growth and stiffness in combination with other therapies (1),(4)[B].
- Severe cases
  - Laser therapy: Longer wavelength laser (e.g., neodymium [Nd]:YAG) is safer for dark skin (5)[B].
  - Avoid shaving altogether; grow beard (1),(2)[C].

GENERAL MEASURES
Acute treatment
- Dislodge embedded hair with sterile needle/tweezers.
- Discontinue shaving until red papules have resolved (minimum 3 to 4 weeks; longer if moderate or severe); can trim to length >0.5 cm during this time
- Massage beard area with washcloth, coarse sponge, or a soft brush several times daily.
- Hydrocortisone 1–2.5% cream to relieve inflammation
- Selenium sulfide if seborrhea is present and to help reduce pruritus
- Systemic antibiotics if secondary infection is present

Pregnancy Considerations
Do not use tretinoin (Retin-A), tetracycline, or benzoyl peroxide.

MEDICATION
First Line
- Topical or systemic antibiotic for secondary infection
  - Application of clindamycin (Cleocin T) solution BID or topical erythromycin
  - Low-dose erythromycin or tetracycline 250 to 500 mg PO BID for more severe inflammation
  - Benzoyl peroxide 5%–clindamycin 1% gel BID: Administer until papule/pustule resolves.
- Mild cases: tretinoin 0.025% cream at bedtime; combination of the above therapies
- Moderate disease/chemical depilatories
  - Disrupt cross-linking of disulfide bonds of hair to produce blunt (less sharp) hair tip.
  - Apply no more frequently than every third day: 2% barium sulfide (Magic shaving cream) or calcium thioglycolate (Surgex); calcium hydroxide (Nair)
- Contraindications
  - Clindamycin: hypersensitivity history; history of regional enteritis or ulcerative colitis; history of antibiotic-associated colitis
  - Erythromycin, tetracycline, tretinoin: history of hypersensitivity
- Precautions
  - Clindamycin: colitis, eye burning and irritation, skin dryness; pregnancy Category B
  - Erythromycin: Use cautiously in patients with impaired hepatic function; GI side effects, especially abdominal cramping; pregnancy Category B (erythromycin base formulation)
  - Chemical depilatories: Use cautiously; frequent use and prolonged application may lead to irritant contact dermatitis and chemical burns.
  - Tetracycline: Avoid in pregnancy.
  - Tretinoin: Avoid in pregnancy; severe skin irritation
  - Benzoyl peroxide: skin irritation and dryness, allergic contact dermatitis
  - Hydrocortisone cream: local skin irritation, skin atrophy with prolonged use, lightening of skin color
- Significant possible interactions
  - Erythromycin: increases theophylline and carbamazepine levels; decreases clearance of warfarin
  - Tetracycline: depresses plasma prothrombin activity

Second Line
Chemical peels with either glycolic acid or salicylic acid

ISSUES FOR REFERRAL
- Worsening or poor response to the above therapies after 4 to 6 weeks should prompt dermatology consultation.
- Occupational demands may also prompt earlier referral to dermatology for more aggressive therapy.

SURGERY/OTHER PROCEDURES
Laser treatment with long-pulsed Nd:YAG is helpful for severe cases.

 ## ONGOING CARE

FOLLOW-UP RECOMMENDATIONS
Patient Monitoring
- As needed
- Educate patient on curative and preventive treatment.

DIET
- No restrictions
- No dietary studies available

PATIENT EDUCATION
https://skinofcolorsociety.org/patient-dermatology-education/1408-2/

PROGNOSIS
- Good, with preventive methods
- Prognosis is poor in the presence of progressive scarring and foreign body granuloma formation.

COMPLICATIONS
- Scarring (occasionally keloidal)
- Foreign body granuloma formation
- Disfiguring postinflammatory hyperpigmentation (use sunscreens; can treat with hydroquinone 4% cream, Retin-A, clinical peels)
- Impetiginization of inflamed skin
- Epidermal (erythema, crusting, burns with scarring) and pigmentary changes with laser

REFERENCES
1. Bridgeman-Shah S. The medical and surgical therapy of pseudofolliculitis barbae. *Dermatol Ther*. 2004;17(2):158–163.
2. Quarles FN, Brody H, Johnson BA, et al. Pseudofolliculitis barbae. *Dermatol Ther*. 2007;20(3):133–136.
3. Nussbaum D, Friedman A. Pseudofolliculitis barbae: a review of current treatment options. *J Drugs Dermatol*. 2019;18(3):246–250.
4. Xia Y, Cho S, Howard RS, et al. Topical eflornithine hydrochloride improves the effectiveness of standard laser hair removal for treating pseudofolliculitis barbae: a randomized, double-blinded, placebo-controlled trial. *J Am Acad Dermatol*. 2012;67(4):694–699.
5. Weaver SM III, Sagaral EC. Treatment of pseudofolliculitis barbae using the long-pulse Nd:YAG laser on skin types V and VI. *Dermatol Surg*. 2003;29(12):1187–1191.

ADDITIONAL READING
- Daniel A, Gustafson CJ, Zupkosky PJ, et al. Shave frequency and regimen variation effects on the management of pseudofolliculitis barbae. *J Drugs Dermatol*. 2013;12(4):410–418.
- Kindred C, Oresajo CO, Yatskayer M, et al. Comparative evaluation of men's depilatory composition versus razor in black men. *Cutis*. 2011;88(2):98–103.
- Kundu RV, Patterson S. Dermatologic conditions in skin of color: part II. Disorders occurring predominantly in skin of color. *Am Fam Physician*. 2013;87(12):859–865.
- Taylor SC, Barbosa V, Burgess C, et al. Hair and scalp disorders in adult and pediatric patients with skin of color. *Cutis*. 2017;100(1):31–35.

 ## SEE ALSO

Folliculitis; Impetigo

 ## CODES

ICD10
- L73.1 Pseudofolliculitis barbae
- B35.0 Tinea barbae and tinea capitis
- L73.8 Other specified follicular disorders

CLINICAL PEARLS
- Electrolysis is not recommended as a treatment. It is expensive, painful, and often unsuccessful.
- Combination of laser therapy with eflornithine is more effective than laser alone.
- The unpleasant smell of sulfur could be a problem with some depilatory products.
- Have patient test for skin sensitivity with a small (coin sized) amount of the depilatory on the bearded area or forearm.

PSEUDOGOUT (CALCIUM PYROPHOSPHATE DIHYDRATE)

Juliana Chang, MD

BASICS

DESCRIPTION
- Autoinflammatory disease triggered by calcium pyrophosphate dihydrate (CPPD) crystal deposition within joints
- One of many diseases associated with pathologic deposition of crystal; mineralization and ossification
  - CPPD crystal deposition = chondrocalcinosis (calcification of hyaline or fibrocartilage), pseudogout, and pyrophosphate arthropathy
  - Monosodium urate crystal deposition = gout
  - Hydroxyapatite deposition = ankylosing spondylitis, osteoarthritis, and vascular calcification
- Suspect pseudogout with arthritis and a pattern of joint involvement inconsistent with degenerative joint disease (e.g., metacarpophalangeal joints, wrists).
- Clinical presentation is broad:
  - Asymptomatic CPPD (incidentally identified on radiograph with or without additional findings of osteoarthritis)
  - Acute CPPD arthritis (acute onset, self-limiting, synovitis)
    ○ Knee is affected in >50% of all acute attacks versus MTP in gout.
    ○ Can be brought on my trauma, medical illness, or surgery (after parathyroidectomy) (1)
  - Chronic CPPD crystal inflammatory arthritis (2)[C]
  - Osteoarthritis with CPPD
- Chronic CPPD crystal deposition may cause a progressive degenerative arthritis in numerous joints; usually large joints; primarily in elderly patients
- Symptom onset is usually insidious.
- Definitive diagnosis requires the identification of CPPD crystals in synovial fluid.
- System(s) affected: endocrine/metabolic; musculoskeletal
- Synonyms: pseudogout; CPPD; pyrophosphate arthropathy; chondrocalcinosis

EPIDEMIOLOGY
Prevalence
- Thought to affect 4–7% of adults in Europe and United States; 80% of patients >60 years
- No gender predominance; men more likely to present acutely; women more likely to present atypically
- Chondrocalcinosis present in 1:10 adults aged 60 to 75 years, 1:3 age >80 years; only a small percentage develop arthropathy.

ETIOLOGY AND PATHOPHYSIOLOGY
- Arthropathy results from an acute autoinflammatory reaction to CPPD crystals in the synovial cavity.
- CPPD crystal deposition occurs in three stages:
  - Overproduction of anionic pyrophosphate (PPi) in articular cartilage
  - PPi binds calcium to form CCPD crystals, eliciting an inflammatory response. Neutrophils engulf CPPD crystals, inducing extracellular trap formation.
  - Increased CPPD crystal deposition causes inflammation and damage (3)[C].

Genetics
Most cases are sporadic; rare familial pattern with autosomal dominant inheritance (<1% of patients); mutation in *ANKH* gene increases risk for calcium crystal formation.

RISK FACTORS
Advanced age; joint trauma

GENERAL PREVENTION
Colchicine 0.6 mg BID may be used prophylactically to reduce frequency of episodes in recurrent CPPD.

COMMONLY ASSOCIATED CONDITIONS
- Gout
- Hyperparathyroidism
- Amyloidosis
- Hemochromatosis; ochronosis
- Hypothyroidism
- Wilson disease
- Hypomagnesemia
- Familial hypocalciuric hypercalcemia
- X-linked hypophosphatemic rickets
- Acromegaly

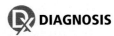

DIAGNOSIS

HISTORY
- Presentation often mimics gout ("pseudogout").
- Acute CPPD: pain and swelling of ≥1 joints; knee involved 50% of the time; ankle, wrist, toe, and shoulder are also common.
- Proximal joint involvement (mimicking polymyalgia rheumatica), often with tibiofemoral and ankle arthritis and tendinous calcifications
- Multiple symmetric joint involvement (mimicking RA) in <5% of cases
- May develop after intra-articular injection of hyaluronic acid (Hyalgan, Synvisc)
- Chronic CPPD: progressive degenerative arthritis with superimposed acute inflammatory attacks

PHYSICAL EXAM
- Inflammation (erythema, warmth, tender to touch), joint effusion, decreased range of motion (ROM)
- 50% associated with fever

DIFFERENTIAL DIAGNOSIS
- Illnesses that may cause acute inflammatory arthritis in a single or multiple joint(s): gout, septic arthritis, trauma
- Other acute inflammatory arthritides: Reiter syndrome, lyme disease, acute RA

DIAGNOSTIC TESTS & INTERPRETATION
Initial Tests (lab, imaging)
Synovial fluid analysis shows an inflammatory effusion:
- Cell count 2,000 to 100,000 WBCs/mL
- Neutrophil predominance (80–90%)
- >50,000 WBC count increases likelihood of septic arthritis; >100,000 WBCs/mL
- Polarized microscopy shows small number of positively birefringent crystals; high false-negative rate
- Consider the following to exclude underlying disease:
  - Serum calcium, phosphorus, and magnesium
  - Serum alkaline phosphatase
  - Serum parathormone (i-PTH)
  - Serum iron, total iron-binding capacity, and serum ferritin
  - Serum thyroid-stimulating hormone (TSH) level
- Plain radiograph:
  - Radiographic findings in pseudogout are neither sensitive nor specific.
  - Punctate and linear calcifications in fibrocartilage, particularly of knees, hips, symphysis pubis, and wrists
  - Chronic CPPD: subchondral cysts and loose bodies in joints not typically affected by degenerative joint disease
- Ultrasound: joint effusion, synovial thickening, and hyperechoic deposits
  - May be more useful than plain radiography for the diagnosis of pseudogout in peripheral joints, with a positive predictive value of 92% and negative predictive value of 93% (4)[C]
- MRI: chondrocalcinosis evident as hypointense lesions, particularly of knee menisci

Diagnostic Procedures/Other

> **ALERT**
> Synovial fluid analysis with demonstration of CPPD crystals is required for diagnosis; aspiration may help relieve symptoms and speed resolution.

Test Interpretation
CPPD crystal deposition in articular cartilage, synovium, ligaments, and tendons

TREATMENT

GENERAL MEASURES
Target symptom relief (reduce inflammation):
- Rest and elevate affected joint(s).
- Apply ice/cool compresses to affected joints.
- Non–weight-bearing on affected joint while painful; use crutches or a walker.

MEDICATION

First Line

- Acute attacks: ice packs, rest, and joint aspiration with or without steroid injection
- Chronic CPPD: prophylactic management with oral NSAIDs and/or colchicine (4)[C]
- Oral NSAIDs
  - Ibuprofen 600 to 800 mg PO TID–QID with food; maximum of 3.2 g/day
  - Naproxen 500 mg PO BID with food
  - Other NSAIDs are effective, although indomethacin has higher complication rates (relative risk [RR] = 2.2) compared with ibuprofen (RR = 1.2).
- Contraindications:
  - History of hypersensitivity to NSAIDs or aspirin
  - Active peptic ulcer disease or history of recurrent upper GI lesions
  - Avoid in renal insufficiency.
  - Serious GI bleeding can occur without warning; patient should be instructed on signs/symptoms. Administer proton pump inhibitor (PPI) or misoprostol 200 μg PO QID in patients at risk for NSAID-induced gastric ulcers.
  - Caution in cardiovascular disease, particularly heart failure or difficult to control hypertension
  - Avoid in concomitant aspirin and anticoagulant use.
- Oral colchicine: 0.5 mg up to 3 to 4 times daily, with or without 1 mg initial dose; 1.2 mg at the first sign of flare, followed in 1 hour
- Intra-articular steroid injection: prednisolone sodium phosphate 4 to 20 mg or triamcinolone diacetate 2 to 40 mg with local anesthetic
- Supportive measures for symptomatic relief (application of ice or cool packs) and immobilization

Second Line

- Oral prednisone: 30 to 50 mg/day for 7 to 10 days
- IM triamcinolone acetonide 40 mg; if necessary, may repeat in 1 to 4 days
- Consider referring patients with large space-occupying tophaceous lesions for surgical removal.
- Alternative therapies for chronic CPPD
  - ACTH, anakinra (anti–IL-1), hydroxychloroquine, infliximab, probenecid, magnesium, and ethylenediaminetetraacetic acid (EDTA) have all been suggested. Large scale studies are needed to evaluate effectiveness (5)[C].

ALERT

Recent randomized trial showed no significant effect of methotrexate in chronic-recurrent CPPD (6)[B].

ISSUES FOR REFERRAL

Consider consultation with orthopedist or rheumatologist if septic joint or patient is not responding.

ADDITIONAL THERAPIES

Physical therapy

- Isometric exercises to maintain muscle strength during the acute stage
- Begin joint ROM exercises as inflammation and pain subside.
- Resume weight bearing when pain subsides.

SURGERY/OTHER PROCEDURES

Perform arthrocentesis and joint fluid analysis.

ADMISSION, INPATIENT, AND NURSING CONSIDERATIONS

Consider admission for septic arthritis if:

- Synovial fluid WBC count >50,000/mL
- Treat with appropriate antibiotics pending culture results.

 ONGOING CARE

FOLLOW-UP RECOMMENDATIONS

Patient Monitoring

Reevaluate response to therapy 48 to 72 hours after beginning treatment; reexamine in 1 week then as needed.

DIET

No known relationship to diet

PATIENT EDUCATION

- Rest the affected joint.
- Symptoms usually resolve in 7 to 10 days.

PROGNOSIS

- Acute attack usually resolves in 10 days; prognosis for resolution of acute attack is excellent.
- Patients may experience progressive joint damage and functional limitation with recurrent attacks.

COMPLICATIONS

- Recurrent acute attacks
- Osteoarthritis

Geriatric Considerations

Elderly patients treated with NSAIDs require careful monitoring and are at higher risk for GI bleeding and acute renal insufficiency; no loading dose for colchicine due to high rates of renal insufficiency in elderly patients

REFERENCES

1. Bilezikian JP, Connor TB, Aptekar R, et al. Pseudogout after parathyroidectomy. *Lancet*. 1973;1(7801):445–446.
2. Zhang W, Doherty M, Bardin T, et al. European League Against Rheumatism recommendations for calcium pyrophosphate deposition. Part I: terminology and diagnosis. *Ann Rheum Dis*. 2011;70(4):563–570.
3. Rosenthal AK, Ryan LM. Nonpharmacologic and pharmacologic management of CPP crystal arthritis and BCP arthropathy and periarticular syndromes. *Rheum Dis Clin North Am*. 2014;40(2):343–356.
4. Zhang W, Doherty M, Pascual E, et al. EULAR recommendations for calcium pyrophosphate deposition. Part II: management. *Ann Rheum Dis*. 2011;70(4):571–575.
5. Pascart T, Richette P, Flipo RM. Treatment of non-gout joint deposition diseases: an update. *Arthritis*. 2014;2014:375202.
6. Finckh A, Mc Carthy GM, Madigan A, et al. Methotrexate in chronic-recurrent calcium pyrophosphate deposition disease: no significant effect in a randomized crossover trial. *Arthritis Res Ther*. 2014;16(5):458.

ADDITIONAL READING

- Bruges-Armas J, Bettencourt BF, Couto AR, et al. Effectiveness and safety of infliximab in two cases of severe chondrocalcinosis: nine years of follow-up. *Case Rep Rheumatol*. 2014;2014:536856.
- Daoussis D, Antonopoulos I, Andonopoulos AP. ACTH as a treatment for acute crystal-induced arthritis: update on clinical evidence and mechanisms of action. *Semin Arthritis Rheum*. 2014;43(5):648–653.
- Demertzis JL, Rubin DA. MR imaging assessment of inflammatory, crystalline-induced, and infectious arthritides. *Magn Reson Imaging Clin N Am*. 2011;19(2):339–363.
- Macmullan P, McCarthy G. Treatment and management of pseudogout: insights for the clinician. *Ther Adv Musculoskelet Dis*. 2012;4(2):121–131.
- Sattui SE, Singh JA, Gaffo AL. Comorbidities in patients with crystal diseases and hyperuricemia. *Rheum Dis Clin North Am*. 2014;40(2):251–278.

CODES

ICD10

- M11.20 Other chondrocalcinosis, unspecified site
- M11.269 Other chondrocalcinosis, unspecified knee
- M11.29 Other chondrocalcinosis, multiple sites

CLINICAL PEARLS

- Suspect CPPD in arthritis cases that do not follow a pattern typical of degenerative joint disease.
- Perform arthrocentesis to confirm diagnosis.
- If septic arthritis is suspected, treat empirically with antibiotics while awaiting culture.
- NSAIDs are preferred pharmacologic treatment for acute flare.
- Oral steroids are useful if NSAIDs are contraindicated.
- Intra-articular steroids can be used *if* septic arthritis has been excluded.

PSORIASIS

Karl T. Clebak, MD, MHA, FAAFP • Roland W. Newman II, DO

BASICS

DESCRIPTION
- A chronic, inflammatory disorder commonly characterized by cutaneous erythematous plaques with silvery scale, and varying phenotypes and severity
- Clinical phenotypes:
  - Plaque (vulgaris): most common variant (~80% of cases); well-demarcated, red plaques with silvery scale; symmetrically distributed commonly on the scalp, extensor surfaces, and trunk.
  - Guttate: <2% of psoriasis patients, usually in patients <30 years of age; presents abruptly with 1- to 10-mm droplet-shaped erythematous papules with fine scale over trunk and extremities; often preceded by group A β-hemolytic streptococcal infection 2 to 3 weeks prior. Most cases resolve spontaneously.
  - Inverse: affects intertriginous areas and flexural surfaces; pink-to-red plaques with minimal scale; absence of satellite pustules distinguishes it from candidiasis.
  - Erythrodermic: generalized erythema and scaling, affecting 90% of body surface area (BSA) or more; associated with desquamation; hair loss; nail dystrophy; and systemic symptoms such as fever, chills, malaise, lymphadenopathy, and/or high-output cardiac failure.
  - Pustular: sterile pustules; several forms including generalized pustular psoriasis, localized pustular psoriasis, and impetigo herpetiformis (in pregnancy); generalized type can result in life-threatening bacterial superinfections.
  - Nail disease: pitting, oil spots, and onycholysis; nails involved in 50% with psoriasis at diagnosis with lifetime incidence of 80–90% with cutaneous psoriasis; increased association with psoriatic arthritis.

EPIDEMIOLOGY
Incidence
Predominant age: two peaks of incidence between the ages of 20 to 30 years and 50 to 60 years

Prevalence
- 3.2% prevalence in the United States
- In the United States, the most commonly affected demographic group is non-Hispanic Caucasian.

ETIOLOGY AND PATHOPHYSIOLOGY
Psoriasis is a complex immune-mediated disorder with interactions between dendritic cells, T lymphocytes, neutrophils, and keratinocytes that results from a polygenic predisposition in the setting of environmental triggers; associated with relapsing flares related to systemic, psychological, infectious, and environmental factors

Genetics
- Genetic predisposition (polygenic)
- 40% have psoriasis in a first-degree relative.
- Multiple susceptibility loci contain genes involved in immune system regulation.
- HLA-C*06 is most strongly correlated with early onset psoriasis.

RISK FACTORS
- Family history
- Obesity
- Local trauma; local irritation (Koebner phenomenon)
- HIV
- Streptococcal infection
- Stress (may contribute to exacerbation)
- Medications (lithium, antimalarials, β-blockers, interferon, TNF-α inhibitors, withdrawal of steroids)
- Smoking
- Alcohol abuse
- Dysbiosis of gut microbiota

GENERAL PREVENTION
Control cardiovascular risk factors. Avoid triggers including trauma, sunburns, smoking, and exposure to certain medications, alcohol, and stress. Avoid excess dietary saturated fats, simple sugars, and red meats.

COMMONLY ASSOCIATED CONDITIONS
- Psoriatic arthritis
- Seborrheic dermatitis
- Obesity, metabolic syndrome, diabetes, chronic kidney disease
- Cardiovascular disease, atherosclerotic disease
- Nonalcoholic fatty liver disease (NAFLD)
- Other autoimmune conditions: Crohn disease, ulcerative colitis, ankylosing spondylitis
- Psychiatric/psychological conditions: depression, anxiety, suicidal ideation, poor self-esteem, emotional burden/anxiety, alcohol abuse, sexual dysfunction
- Myopathy

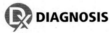

DIAGNOSIS

HISTORY
- May include sudden onset of clearly demarcated, erythematous plaques with overlying silvery scales or exacerbation of chronic plaques, especially on extensor surfaces and scalp; typically, no or mild pruritus. Triggers may include recent streptococcal infection or trauma.
- Family history of similar condition

PHYSICAL EXAM
- Well-demarcated salmon pink-to-red erythematous papules and plaques with silvery scale
- Distribution favors scalp, auricular conchal bowls and postauricular area, extensor surface of extremities, especially knees and elbows, umbilicus, lower back, intergluteal cleft, and nails.
- Nail findings: pitting, oil spots, onycholysis
- Auspitz sign: pinpoint bleeding with removal of scale
- Koebner phenomenon: new psoriatic lesions arising at sites of skin injury/trauma
- Woronoff ring is a pale blanching ring that may be seen around a psoriatic lesion.
- Sebopsoriasis: Psoriasis can overlap with seborrheic dermatitis as greasy scales on the scalp, eyebrows, nasolabial folds, postauricular, and presternal areas.

DIFFERENTIAL DIAGNOSIS
- Plaque: seborrheic dermatitis (may coexist), nummular eczema, atopic dermatitis, contact dermatitis, lichen simplex chronicus (may coexist), tinea, pityriasis rubra pilaris, dermatomyositis, squamous cell carcinoma in situ, reactive arthritis, pityriasis rosea, lichen planus, lichen sclerosis et atrophicus
- Guttate: secondary syphilis, pityriasis rosea, pityriasis lichenoides chronica, small plaque parapsoriasis
- Inverse: cutaneous candidiasis, tinea, seborrheic dermatitis, contact dermatitis
- Pustular: subcorneal pustulosis, acute generalized exanthematous pustulosis, folliculitis
- Erythrodermic: cutaneous T-cell lymphoma, drug-induced erythroderma, pityriasis rubra pilaris

DIAGNOSTIC TESTS & INTERPRETATION
Initial Tests (lab, imaging)
- Clinical diagnosis based on history and physical exam.
- Labs generally not needed, although KOH to rule out tinea helpful, especially in inverse psoriasis.
- Biopsy is rarely needed unless diagnosis is unclear.
- Consider x-rays if complaints of joint pain to evaluate for psoriatic arthritis.

Diagnostic Procedures/Other
- Psoriasis Area and Severity Index (PASI) evaluates overall severity and BSA involvement.
- Dermatology Life Quality Index (DLQI)

Test Interpretation
Biopsy findings: thickening of the stratum corneum (hyperkeratosis) with retention of nuclei (parakeratosis); elongation, thickening, and clubbing of rete ridges; dilated tortuous capillary loops in the dermal papillae; perivascular lymphocytic infiltrate, Munro microabscesses: neutrophils in stratum corneum

TREATMENT

GENERAL MEASURES
Adequate topical hydration (emollients); avoidance of triggers; weight loss

MEDICATION
Choice of management is based on severity of psoriasis and presence of inflammatory arthritis.

First Line
- Assess for concurrent psoriatic arthritis; if present, start with therapies with dual approval for psoriasis and psoriatic arthritis, even if skin manifestations are mild due to risk of joint destruction secondary to psoriatic arthritis (1)[C].
- Mild-to-moderate disease
  - Emollients: petrolatum/ointments to maintain skin hydration and minimize pruritus and risk of koebnerization
  - Topical corticosteroids
    - Anti-inflammatory, antiproliferative, immunosuppressive, and vasoconstrictive effects
    - Local side effects: skin atrophy, hypopigmentation, striae, acne, folliculitis, and purpura. Systemic side effects: Risk is higher, with higher potency formulations used over a large surface for a prolonged period; pregnancy Category C

- Applications are typically twice daily until lesions flatten/resolve and then taper to PRN use for maintenance.
- Scalp: high potency in solution/foam vehicle; shampoos and sprays also available
- Face, intertriginous areas, infants: low-potency corticosteroids: 1% hydrocortisone
- Adult initial therapy: medium-potency corticosteroids daily: 0.1% mometasone or triamcinolone; high-potency corticosteroids: 0.05% betamethasone or fluocinonide daily; superpotent corticosteroids: clobetasol, halobetasol; caution with use over 2 to 4 weeks; avoid occlusive dressings; reserved for recalcitrant plaques
- Vitamin D analogues: calcipotriene 0.005% cream daily to BID; may be used in combination with a superpotent corticosteroid; should not be used with products that can alter pH (e.g., topical lactic acid) local side effects: burning, pruritus, edema, peeling, dryness, and erythema; pregnancy Category C
- Topical retinoids: tazarotene 0.05% or 0.1% (Tazorac) daily; may be combined with corticosteroids; side effects: local irritation, photosensitivity; pregnancy Category X
- Topical calcineurin inhibitors: Tacrolimus 0.1% or pimecrolimus 1% may be used as steroid-sparing agents, especially in facial and intertriginous areas.
- Comparison of topical therapies: Vitamin D analogues have slower onset of action than topical corticosteroids but longer disease-free periods for body plaques; for scalp, potent and superpotent steroids are more effective (2)[A].
- Combination of superpotent steroids and vitamin D analogues has better efficacy than either as monotherapy.
- Severe disease: may need combination therapy
  - Light therapy: UVB (broad/narrowband [BB, NB]) or PUVA: Treatment protocols are skin type dependent. PUVA with GI SE, photosensitivity, and increased risk of nonmelanoma skin cancers; can be used as adjunct therapy
  - Oral systemic therapies
    - Methotrexate: start with 5-mg test dose, then increase to 7.5 to 15 mg/week IV, PO, IM, or SC, and then increase 2.5 mg every 2 to 3 weeks, up to 25 mg; contraindicated in pregnancy and use caution in women of childbearing age; supplement with folic acid 1 mg/day baseline chest x-ray, monitor LFTs, renal function, CBC, testing for latent tuberculosis (TB); consider liver biopsy when cumulative dose reaches 3.5 to 4 g; avoid alcohol and medications that interfere with folic acid metabolism including trimethoprim—sulfamethoxazole (Bactrim), NSAIDs, sulfamethoxazole, or hepatotoxic agents (e.g., retinoids).
    - Cyclosporine: Start 2.5 mg/kg/day; if insufficient response after 4 weeks, increase by 0.5 mg/kg/day; additional dosage increases every 2 weeks (max dose: 5 mg/kg/day); pregnancy Category C; side effects: renal toxicity and hypertension, limit use to 6 months to 1 year; monitor renal function and electrolytes with Mg^{2+}, CBC, lipids, and blood pressure.

- Acitretin (Soriatane): Start at 10 to 25 mg/day; effective for pustular psoriasis and as a maintenance therapy after stabilization with other agents; pregnancy Category X: pregnancy test before starting; two forms of contraception 1 month before, during, and for at least 3 years after treatment; avoid alcohol; side effects: alopecia, xerosis, cheilitis, hepatotoxicity, hyperlipidemia, cataracts; monitor LFTs, renal function, lipid profile, CBC, regular eye exams.
- Phosphodiesterase-4 enzyme inhibitor: Apremilast (Otezla): 10 mg PO, titrate up by 10 mg/day on days 2 to 5 to maintenance dose of 30 mg BID starting on day 6. Routine lab monitoring not required; very expensive. Most common SE are GI symptoms, depression; pregnancy Category C
- Biologics—Achieve remission for patients with moderate to severe disease; very expensive and long-term outcomes, and safety data not available (3)[A]
  - General guidelines: Screen for latent TB at baseline and yearly, hepatitis panel at baseline, avoid live vaccines; monitor CBC with differential, signs/symptoms of infections, heart failure, malignancy, drug-induced lupus, demyelinating disorder. All should be considered effective first-line treatments; pregnancy Category B
    - TNF-α inhibitors: also approved for treatment of psoriatic arthritis. Options include etanercept (Enbrel), adalimumab (Humira), infliximab (Remicade), and certolizumab pegol (Cimzia).
    - IL-12/IL-23 antagonist: ustekinumab (Stelara); also approved for treatment of psoriatic arthritis
    - IL-17 antagonists: secukinumab (Cosentyx), brodalumab (Siliq), ixekizumab (Taltz); also approved for the treatment of psoriatic arthritis. Avoid in patients with inflammatory bowel disease.

Second Line
- Immunosuppressives: azathioprine, hydroxyurea, 6-thioguanine, fumaric acid esters
- Topicals: salicylic acid, anthralin, coal tar

ISSUES FOR REFERRAL
Refer patients with psoriasis >20% of BSA, psoriatic arthritis, pustular psoriasis, severe extremity involvement, or disease not responding to topical therapy.

SURGERY/OTHER PROCEDURES
Psoriasis and psoriatic medications can affect wound healing postoperatively.

COMPLEMENTARY & ALTERNATIVE MEDICINE
Balneotherapy, climatotherapy, and stress management interventions

ADMISSION, INPATIENT, AND NURSING CONSIDERATIONS
Rule out sepsis; restoration of barrier function of skin with cleaning and bandaging; intensive topical corticosteroid therapy, initiate systemic therapy; management of electrolytes

 ONGOING CARE

FOLLOW-UP RECOMMENDATIONS
Measure BSA involvement to determine if therapy is working; change therapy or add agent if no improvement is seen.

DIET
- Heart healthy diet and exercise to limit cardiovascular risk factors
- Evidence for efficacy is inconsistent. Diet may be adjunctive to medical treatment. Limit saturated fats, simple sugars, and red meats. Encourage fatty fish.

PATIENT EDUCATION
National Psoriasis Foundation: https://www.psoriasis.org; (800) 723-9166

PROGNOSIS
Guttate form may be self-limited and remit after months; chronic plaque type is lifelong, with intermittent spontaneous remissions and exacerbations; erythrodermic and generalized pustular forms may be severe and persistent.

COMPLICATIONS
- Psoriatic arthritis, generalized pustular psoriasis, erythrodermic psoriasis.
- Cardiovascular disease

REFERENCES
1. Armstrong AW, Read C. Pathophysiology, clinical presentation, and treatment of psoriasis: a review. *JAMA*. 2020;323(19):1945–1960.
2. Mason AR, Mason J, Cork M, et al. Topical treatments for chronic plaque psoriasis. *Cochrane Database Syst Rev*. 2013;(3):CD005028.
3. Sbidian E, Chaimani A, Guelimi R, et al. Systemic pharmacological treatments for chronic plaque psoriasis: a network meta-analysis. *Cochrane Database Syst Rev*. 2023;7(7):CD011535.

ADDITIONAL READING
Clebak KT, Helm L, Helm MF, et al. The many variants of psoriasis. *J Fam Pract*. 2020;69(4):192–200.

 SEE ALSO

Arthritis, Psoriatic

 CODES

ICD10
- L40.2 Acrodermatitis continua
- L40.5 Arthropathic psoriasis
- L40.59 Other psoriatic arthropathy

CLINICAL PEARLS
Lifelong condition with remissions and exacerbations; set realistic expectations with patient. Disease burden is not limited to skin. Control cardiovascular risk factors.

PSYCHOSIS
Matthew J. Filippo, DO

BASICS

DESCRIPTION
A disorder where thoughts and emotions are disrupted; seen in schizophrenia, mood disorders, substance use, medical problems, delirium, and dementia;
- Positive symptoms: hallucinations and delusions (fixed false beliefs not typical of cultural background)
- Negative symptoms: anhedonia, poverty of speech, lack of motivation, social withdrawal, affective blunting
- Cognition: poor working memory, information processing, inattention, disorganized speech and/or behavior

EPIDEMIOLOGY
Prevalence
- Schizophrenia: peak onset: males: 18 to 25 years old; females: 25 to 35 years old
- 1% of the U.S. population; similar percentage worldwide
- Seen in ~50% of bipolar cases and 20% of unipolar depression cases

ETIOLOGY AND PATHOPHYSIOLOGY
- Many causes including psychiatric, medical, and/or substance use
- Positive symptoms: excessive dopaminergic activity in the mesolimbic pathway
- Negative symptoms: diminished dopaminergic activity in mesocortical pathway

Genetics
Schizophrenia: 50% concordance in monozygotic twins; many genes involved

RISK FACTORS
Substance use (particularly stimulants and THC), family history of psychosis, lower socioeconomic status

GENERAL PREVENTION
Community interventions for early detection and treatment of prodromal symptoms.

COMMONLY ASSOCIATED CONDITIONS
- Associated with metabolic syndrome, autonomic dysfunction, sudden cardiac death, and breast and lung cancer
- Substance use, including nicotine dependence

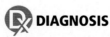

DIAGNOSIS

Rule out delirium: Unlike delirium, psychosis should not have fluctuating mentation.

HISTORY
- Delusions: persecutory, bizarre, somatic, referential, or grandiose
- Hallucinations: auditory, visual, tactile, gustatory, or olfactory

- Bipolar, unipolar depression, and dementia are associated with psychosis.
- Screen for drugs of abuse and history of epileptiform activity or TBI.
- Suicidality: higher risk with comorbid depression/mania, previous attempts, drug use, agitation/akathisia, poor adherence to medications

PHYSICAL EXAM
- Mental status exam: disorganized speech, behavior, and/or thought process; thought blocking; response latency; blunted affect; social withdrawal; lack of initiative; poverty of thought/speech; hallucinations
- Pay attention to focal neurologic signs, parkinsonism, tardive dyskinesia, and akathisia.
- May present with catatonia: lack of movement or extreme excitement, posturing, mutism, grimacing, waxy flexibility

DIFFERENTIAL DIAGNOSIS
- Schizophrenia: positive symptoms and negative symptoms, prodrome of social withdrawal, cognitive impairment
- Mood disorder with psychotic features: occur in mania and depression; mood congruent; psychosis remits as mood improves.
- Substance-induced: alcohol and benzodiazepine withdrawal, intoxication with cocaine, bath salts, PCP, THC, amphetamines, hallucinogens, and alcohol; may persist beyond acute intoxication
- Posttraumatic stress disorder: psychosis associated with traumatic recollections; often visual hallucinations
- Psychosis due to general medical condition
- Medication-induced psychosis: steroids especially >40 mg prednisone equivalent, L-dopa, anticholinergics, antidepressants in bipolar patients, interferon, digoxin, stimulants

DIAGNOSTIC TESTS & INTERPRETATION
Labs: CBC, CMP, thyroid-stimulating hormone (TSH), lipid panel, ECG, pregnancy test, urine drug screen. Consider rapid plasma reagin (RPR), HIV, ANA, ESR, vitamin B_{12}, vitamin D, urinalysis

Initial Tests (lab, imaging)
- Imaging: not necessary for diagnosis. Consider CT or MRI if focal neurological signs, first break or new onset in elderly or adolescents; sudden onset of symptoms, especially with comorbid fever or headache.
- Consider ECG to assess QTc interval.

Follow-Up Tests & Special Considerations
- Consider Wilson disease, porphyria, metachromatic leukodystrophy, and inflammatory conditions.
- Consider lumbar puncture if unable to distinguish from delirium and/or rapid-onset psychosis.
- Consider electroencephalogram (EEG) for seizures and psychosis associated with ictal events.
- Consider anti-NMDA receptor antibodies in suspected autoimmune encephalitis.

TREATMENT

GENERAL MEASURES
Ensure safety of person and environment and rule out medical causes particularly delirium.

MEDICATION
- Antipsychotics are the mainstay of treatment (1),(2)[B].
- For mania with psychotic features, a mood stabilizer may be used with an antipsychotic.
- For depression with psychotic features, antidepressant and antipsychotic combination improves response more than either alone. In delirium, must treat underlying cause; may not require antipsychotic therapy
- Side effects
  - Acute dystonia: benztropine 1 to 3 mg IM/IV then 0.5 to 2 mg BID–TID or diphenhydramine 50 to 100 mg IM/IV BID–TID max 400 mg/day
  - Parkinsonism: Lower antipsychotic dose; switch to atypical (particularly, quetiapine or clozapine) and/or add benztropine 0.5 to 2.0 mg PO BID–TID
  - Akathisia (intense restlessness): lower antipsychotic dose; treat with β-blocker or benzodiazepine; may switch to antipsychotic with lower akathisia risk such as quetiapine or clozapine
  - Tardive dyskinesia: seen in ~1/3 of those treated long term with typicals, ~1/8 with atypicals. Switch to clozapine or quetiapine. Otherwise, minimize dose. Symptomatic treatment has been tried with low-dose benzodiazepines, botulinum toxin, and VMAT-2 inhibitors such as valbenazine and deutetrabenazine.
  - Neuroleptic malignant syndrome: potentially fatal; rigidity, tremor, fever, autonomic instability, mental status changes; discontinue neuroleptic; ICU; volume resuscitation; cooling blankets; no anticholinergics/antihistamines; consider dantrolene, amantadine, bromocriptine, and electroconvulsive therapy (ECT).
  - Metabolic syndrome, sudden cardiac death (risk higher IM/IV droperidol, IV haloperidol), stroke, heart failure, PNA (elderly), pulmonary embolus. Can minimize metabolic risk by using anorexigenics and behavioral counselling.

First Line
- Atypical antipsychotics lower risk of extrapyramidal symptoms and dyskinesias (clozapine, quetiapine);
- Greater risk of weight gain, diabetes, and hyperlipidemia especially with olanzapine and clozapine
- Acute psychotic agitation:
  - Olanzapine 5 to 10 mg IM NTE 30 mg/day; do not administer with IM/IV benzodiazepine
  - Ziprasidone 10 mg IM q2h or 20 mg q4h, NTE 40 mg/day
  - Haloperidol 2 to 5 mg +/– lorazepam 2 mg IM, can be given with 1 mg IM benztropine, NTE 20 mg haloperidol and 8 mg lorazepam per day;

– Droperidol, 2.5 to 5.0 mg IV or IM; high risk of QT prolongation
– Dexmedetomidine (sublingual) 120 to 180 μg q2h, NTE 360 μg/day
– Risperidone (ODT), 1 to 2 mg PO
– Loxapine: inhaled powder, 10 mg via oral inhaler; single dose in 24-hour period; can cause bronchospasm, especially in patients with preexisting lung disease
• Psychosis in schizophrenia
– Risperidone: Start 1 to 2 mg QD; target dose of 2 to 8 mg/day reached over 1 to 2 weeks; >6 mg rarely more effective and higher risk of parkinsonism; higher risk of prolactinemia/parkinsonism due to D_2 blockade
– Ziprasidone: Start 20 to 40 mg PO BID with at least 500 calories. Target dose 100 to 160 mg/day in divided doses over 2 weeks; prolongs QTc; less likely to cause weight gain than other atypicals; higher risk of akathisia/parkinsonism
– Aripiprazole: Start 10 to 15 mg QD, may increase to 30 mg/day over 1 to 2 weeks; less weight gain but high rates of akathisia; lowers QTc
– Lurasidone: Start 20 to 40 mg QD with at least 350 calories, increase up to 160 mg qhs over 2 to 4 weeks; less weight gain but high rates of akathisia/parkinsonism

Second Line
• Olanzapine: Start 5 to 10 mg qhs; target dose 5 to 20 mg/day within 2 days; more likely weight gain, hyperlipidemia, and hyperglycemia than other atypicals except clozapine; sedating; drug metabolism increased 50% by tobacco use
• Quetiapine: Start 25 mg BID, increase 25 to 50 mg q8–12h days 2 and 3, up to 3–400 mg by day 4; can then increase 50 to 100 mg/day, NTE 800 mg/day divided BID–TID; less risk of parkinsonism but more weight gain; sedation, restless legs syndrome; gradual titration better tolerated; prolongs QTc
• Paliperidone: Start 3 to 6 mg QD; target dose 6 to 12 mg QD; titrate over 1 to 2 weeks; higher risk of prolactinemia/parkinsonism than others; minimal hepatic metabolism, ideal for hepatic impairment
• Asenapine: Start 5 mg QHS or BID sublingually, increase to 10 mg BID if needed over 1 to 2 weeks; less weight gain than some, high rates of akathisia/parkinsonism; sedation, orthostatic hypotension; transdermal patch available, start on 3.8 mg/24 hours, may increase to 5.7 or 7.6/24 hours if needed after 1 week.
• Iloperidone: Start 1 mg BID, may increase by 2 mg daily, but slower can be better due to significant orthostasis (max 12 mg BID); little akathisia/parkinsonism, less weight gain but long titration, orthostasis, sedation; prolongs QTc
• Brexpiprazole: Start 1 mg QD for first 4 days, 2 mg QD days 5 to 7, can increase dose up to 4 mg/day based on response; lower rates of akathisia than aripiprazole but higher rates than others; less weight gain than others

• Cariprazine: Start at 1.5 mg QD, can be increased to 3 mg QD on day 2, dosed up to 6 mg QD based on response; in 6-week study, fasting glucose, cholesterol, triglycerides and weight were similar to placebo.
• Lumateperone: 42 mg daily; no titration required; mild average weight loss; moderate sedation and dry mouth
• First-generation antipsychotics such as haloperidol which can be started at 0.5 to 2.0 mg q8–12hr; target dose of 10 mg QD or less divided doses; high rates of tardive dyskinesia; decreased rates of metabolic syndrome
• Olanzapine/samidorphan: Start at 5 mg/10 mg QD. Increase olanzapine at weekly intervals of 5 mg pending response, up to 20 mg/10 mg QD. Less weight gain risk attributed to samidorphan—a novel opioid-system modulator, similar to naltrexone.

Geriatric Considerations
Antipsychotics increase risk of death in the elderly with dementia. Pimavanserin is approved for Parkinson disease psychosis.

ADDITIONAL THERAPIES
Psychotherapy, vocational, art, and group are effective adjuvants to antipsychotics (2)[B].

COMPLEMENTARY & ALTERNATIVE MEDICINE
• Vitamin treatments if there is a deficiency (common with folic acid, vitamins B_6 and B_{12}, D), omega 3 supplements, glycine
• THC can precipitate psychosis.

ADMISSION, INPATIENT, AND NURSING CONSIDERATIONS
Admission if at risk for harm to self or others; extreme functional impairment; new-onset psychosis

 ONGOING CARE

Medication management, psychotherapy

FOLLOW-UP RECOMMENDATIONS
Close follow-up for inpatient discharge (high risk for suicide); use therapy, exercise, smoking cessation, AIMS testing.

Patient Monitoring
• For patients treated with antipsychotics screen initially for metabolic syndrome (lipid panel, glucose, HgbA1c, CBC, CMP, LFTs, weight, waist circumference) and AIMS testing. Continue monitoring with long-term use.
• EPS: Evaluate once a week until dose is stable for 2 weeks. Once stabilized, assess EPS and TD at least q6–12 months.

DIET
Avoid alcohol and sugar-sweetened beverages.

PATIENT EDUCATION
National Alliance on Mental Illness: https://www.nami.org/

PROGNOSIS
• Schizophrenia: fluctuating course; 70% first-episode psychosis patients improve in 3 to 4 months, 20–40% attempt suicide; 7% die of suicide.
• Medications are a mainstay of treatment but are only one component; others include psychosocial interventions, cognitive behavioral therapy, self-help-based interventions, and motivational enhancement techniques.

COMPLICATIONS
• Metabolic disturbances secondary to antipsychotic medications, sedentary lifestyle, and smoking
• Life expectancy reduced over a decade compared to general population (largely mediated by heart disease)

REFERENCES
1. American Psychiatric Association. Clinical practice guidelines. https://www.psychiatry.org/psychiatrists/practice/clinical-practice-guidelines. Accessed October 24, 2023.
2. National Institute for Health and Care Excellence. Psychosis and schizophrenia in adults: prevention and management. http://www.nice.org.uk/guidance/cg178. Accessed July 17, 2023.

 SEE ALSO

Delirium; Schizophrenia

CODES

ICD10
• F29 Unsp psychosis not due to a substance or known physiol cond
• F20.9 Schizophrenia, unspecified
• F39 Unspecified mood [affective] disorder

CLINICAL PEARLS
• Antipsychotics are the mainstay of treatment; decrease all-cause mortality and increase quality of life
• Aripiprazole shortens QTc.
• Clozapine and long-acting injectables may increase adherence.

PULMONARY ARTERIAL HYPERTENSION

Nasheena Jiwa, MD

BASICS

DESCRIPTION
Pulmonary arterial hypertension (PAH) is characterized by abnormalities in the small pulmonary arteries (precapillary pulmonary hypertension [PH]) that produce increased pulmonary arterial pressure (PAP) and vascular resistance, eventually resulting in right-sided heart failure.

- Previously, PH was classified as primary PH (without cause, now idiopathic PAH [IPAH]) or secondary PH (with cause or associated condition); now, it is clear that some types of secondary PH closely match primary PH (IPAH) in their histology, natural history, and response to treatment. Therefore, WHO classifies PH into five groups based on mechanism, with PAH as group 1 in this classification.
- PAH is diagnosed by right-heart catheterization and defined by a mean PAP $\geq$20 mm Hg at rest and a pulmonary vascular resistance (PVR) of $\geq$3 Wood units when other groups of PH are ruled out; pulmonary capillary wedge pressure $\leq$15 mm Hg (excludes PH owing to left heart disease; i.e., group 2 PH) without:
  – Mild or absent chronic lung disease or other causes of hypoxemia (excludes PH owing to lung disease or hypoxemia; i.e., group 3 PH)
  – Venous thromboembolic disease (excludes chronic thromboembolic PH [CTEPH]; i.e., group 4 PH)
  – Systemic disorder (like sarcoidosis), hematologic disorders (like myeloproliferative disease), and metabolic disorders (like glycogen storage disease) (excludes group 5 PH)
- PAH is divided into following main categories:
  – Idiopathic: sporadic, with no family history or risk factors
  – Heritable: IPAH with mutations or familial cases with or without mutations
  – Drug or toxin induced: mostly associated with anorectics (e.g., fenfluramine), rapeseed oil, L-tryptophan, dasatinib (Bcr-Abl tyrosine kinase inhibitor), and illicit drugs such as methamphetamine, cocaine
  – Associated: connective tissue diseases (e.g., systemic lupus erythematosus, rheumatoid arthritis, scleroderma), HIV infection, portal hypertension, congenital heart disease, schistosomiasis (chronic hemolytic anemia added to group 5 PH—unclear/multifactorial mechanisms)
  – Pulmonary veno-occlusive disease (PVOD) and/or pulmonary capillary hemangiomatosis (PCH) and persistent PH of the newborn (PPHN) are classified as separate categories due to more differences than similarities with PAH.
    ○ PVOD and/or PCH: rare cause of PH characterized by extensive diffuse occlusion of the pulmonary veins (unlike PAH which involves the small muscular pulmonary arterioles)

EPIDEMIOLOGY
- Age: can occur at any age; mean age 37 years
- Sex (IPAH): female > male (female:male ratio ranges from 1.7 to 4.8:1)

Incidence
- Overall PAH: 5 to 52 cases per million
- IPAH: low, ~2 to 6 per million
- Drug-induced PAH: 1/25,000 with >3 months of anorectic use
- HIV associated: 0.5/100
- Portal hypertension associated: 1 to 6/100
- Scleroderma associated: 6–60%

Prevalence
PAH: ~15 to 50 cases per million; IPAH: ~6 cases per million

ETIOLOGY AND PATHOPHYSIOLOGY
- Pulmonary: inflammation, vasoconstriction, endothelial dysfunction, and intimal proliferation causing remodeling of pulmonary arteries produced by increased cell proliferation and reduced rates of apoptosis lead to obstruction
- Cardiovascular: Right ventricular hypertrophy (RVH), eventually leading to right-sided heart failure and right ventricular (RV) ischemia due to reduced right coronary artery flow causes RV remodeling associated with PAH.
- IPAH: by definition, unknown. True IPAH is mostly sporadic or sometimes familial in nature.
- Pulmonary arteriolar hyperactivity and vasoconstriction, occult thromboembolism, or autoimmune (high frequency of antinuclear antibodies)

Genetics
75% of heritable PAH (HPAH) cases and 25% of IPAH cases have mutations in *BMPR2* (autosomal dominant).

RISK FACTORS
Female sex, previous illicit anorectic drug use, recent pulmonary embolism, first-degree relatives of patient with familial PAH

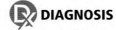

DIAGNOSIS

HISTORY
Dyspnea, weakness, syncope, dizziness, chest pain, palpitations, lower extremity edema

PHYSICAL EXAM
- Pulmonary component of S_2 (at apex in >90% of patients)
- Early systolic click of pulmonary valve
- Pansystolic murmur of tricuspid regurgitation
- Diastolic murmur of pulmonic insufficiency (Graham Steell murmur)
- Edema as jugular vein distention, ascites, hepatomegaly, or peripheral edema

DIFFERENTIAL DIAGNOSIS
Other causes of dyspnea:
- Pulmonary parenchymal disease such as chronic obstructive pulmonary disease, interstitial lung disease, or restrictive lung disease
- Pulmonary vascular disease such as pulmonary thromboembolism
- Cardiac disease such as cardiomyopathy

DIAGNOSTIC TESTS & INTERPRETATION
- Echocardiography (ECG): RVH and right axis deviation, or RV strain (increased P wave amplitude, incomplete right bundle branch block pattern, an R-to-S ratio >1 in lead V_1)
- Pulmonary function testing: reduced diffusion capacity
- Arterial blood gas: arterial hypoxemia, hypocapnia
- Ventilation/perfusion (V/Q) scan: Look for proximal pulmonary artery emboli and CTEPH; rule out group 4 PH.
- Exercise test: reduced maximal O_2 consumption, high-minute ventilation, low anaerobic threshold, increased PO_2 alveolar–arterial gradient; correlation to severity of disease with 6-minute walk distance (6MWD) test
- Antinuclear antibody test: positive (up to 40% of patients)
- LFTs: Evaluate for portopulmonary hypertension as a complication of chronic liver disease.
- HIV test, thyroid function tests, sickle cell disease screening
- Elevated brain natriuretic peptide (BNP) and N-terminal-proBNP may be useful for early detection of PAH in young, otherwise healthy patients with mild symptoms. It can also be used to assess disease severity and prognosis.
- Chest radiograph
  – Prominent central pulmonary arteries with peripheral hypovascularity of pulmonary arterial branches
  – RV enlargement is a late finding.
- Echo Doppler: should be performed with suspicion of PAH; echo suggests, but does not diagnose, PAH; most commonly used screening tool
  – Important to rule out underlying cardiac disease such as atrial septal defect with secondary PH or mitral stenosis
  – Right atrial and RV enlargement; tricuspid regurgitation
  – Estimates mean PAP and assesses cardiac structure and function, excludes congenital anomalies
- In patients at risk for HPAH, screen for gene mutations *BMPR2*.
- Polysomnography: for suspected symptoms of obstructive sleep apnea

Diagnostic Procedures/Other
- Pulmonary angiography
  – Should be done if V/Q scan suggests CTEPH
  – Use caution; can lead to hemodynamic collapse; use low-osmolar agents, subselective angiograms
- Right-sided cardiac catheterization (gold standard for diagnosis of PAH)
- Essential to confirm diagnosis and determine severity and prognosis by measuring PAPs and hemodynamics: Rule out underlying cardiac disease (e.g., left-sided heart disease) and assess response to vasodilator therapy.
- 6MWD: classifies severity of PAH and estimates prognosis

TREATMENT

- Treat underlying diseases/conditions that may cause PAH to relieve symptoms and improve quality of life and survival.
- Reasonable goals of therapy include:
  - Modified NYHA functional class (FC) I or II
  - ECG/CMR of normal/near-normal RV size and function
  - Hemodynamic parameters showing normalization of the RV function (right arterial pressure [RAP] <8 mm Hg and cardiac index [CI] >2.5 to 3 L/min/m^2)
  - 6MWD of >380 to 440 m
  - Cardiopulmonary exercise testing, including peak oxygen consumption of >15 mL/min/kg and EqCO$_2$ <45 L/min
  - Normal BNP levels (1)[C]

GENERAL MEASURES

- Supervised exercise training; avoid strenuous physical activity; psychosocial support (2)[C].
- Avoid pregnancy (2)[C].
- Influenza and pneumococcal immunization (2)[C]
- Oxygen—maintain arterial blood O$_2$ pressure >60 mm Hg (2)[C]

MEDICATION

- Acute vasodilator test during heart catheterization for all patients who are potential candidates for long-term oral calcium channel blocker (CCB) therapy (2)[C]
  - Screens for pulmonary vasoreactivity/responsiveness using inhaled nitrous oxide; epoprostenol (IV) or adenosine (IV): Positive response may be a prognostic indicator.
  - Contraindicated in right-sided heart failure or hemodynamic instability
- Chronic vasodilator therapy
  - If IPAH with positive response to acute vasodilator test (a fall in mean PAP of ≥10 mm Hg and to a value <40 mm Hg, with unchanged/increased cardiac output), use CCBs.
    - Adequate response confirmed after 3 to 4 months of treatment
    - ~13% will initially respond. Long-term clinical response to CCB therapy is small (~7%) (2)[C].
    - CCBs include nifedipine (long-acting), diltiazem, and amlodipine.
    - Avoid verapamil due to its significant negative inotropic effect.
  - CCBs are contraindicated in patients with a cardiac index of <2 L/min/m^2 or a right atrial pressure >15 mm Hg if PAH with negative response to acute vasodilator test or worsening on therapy; specific vasodilator choice based on risk stratification (2)[C]
    - Nonresponders to acute vasoreactivity who are in WHO-FC II should be treated with an oral compound (2)[B].
    - Nonresponders who remain or progress to WHO-FC III should be considered for treatment with any approved PAH drugs (2)[B].
    - Continuous IV epoprostenol is recommended as first-line therapy for WHO-FC IV PAH due to survival benefit (NNT = 5) (2)[A].

- In case of inadequate clinical response, sequential combination therapy should be considered. Therapy includes ERA plus a phosphodiesterase type 5 (PDE5) inhibitor or a prostanoid plus ERA or a prostanoid plus a PDE5 inhibitor (2)[A].
  - WHO-FC II PAH-approved drugs: ambrisentan, bosentan, macitentan, riociguat, sildenafil, tadalafil (2)[B]
  - WHO-FC III PAH-approved drugs: ambrisentan, bosentan, epoprostenol (IV), macitentan, riociguat, sildenafil, tadalafil, treprostinil (SC, inhaled) (2)[B]
  - WHO-FC IV PAH-approved drugs: epoprostenol (IV) (2)[A]
  - Drug classes:
    - Prostacyclins: improve exercise capacity, cardiopulmonary hemodynamics: epoprostenol (IV), treprostinil (IV, SC, or inhaled), iloprost, beraprost
    - Prostacyclin IP: receptor agonist—selexipag
    - Endothelin receptor antagonists: improve exercise capacity; reducing mortality has been noted: bosentan (PO), ambrisentan (PO), macitentan. Pregnancy Category X; monitor LFTs monthly.
    - PDE5 inhibitor: suggested improvement in exercise capacity, cardiopulmonary hemodynamics, and symptoms (2)[C]: sildenafil (PO), tadalafil (PO), vardenafil
    - Guanylate cyclase stimulant: stimulators of the nitric oxide receptor, improves exercise capacity: riociguat (PO)
- Anticoagulation
  - Improved survival originally suggested in patients with IPAH only. Newer studies show some evidence for favorable effects of anticoagulation on survival in IPAH, HPAH, or PAH associated with anorexigens (2)[C].
  - Warfarin with international normalized ratio of 1.5 to 2.5 shows survival advantage in patients in multiple observational studies.
    - Contraindications: Avoid in patients with syncope or significant hemoptysis; consider drug interactions.
- Diuretics indicated in patients with RV volume overload (e.g., peripheral edema or ascites) (2)[B]
- Digoxin has little long-term data in PAH: used in RV failure and/or atrial dysrhythmias, increases cardiac output, and preserves RV contractility

ISSUES FOR REFERRAL

Refer to a pulmonologist and/or a cardiologist for further evaluation/treatment if PAH is suspected.

SURGERY/OTHER PROCEDURES

- Balloon atrial septostomy for severe PAH with right-sided heart failure despite optimized medical therapy to relieve symptoms prior to lung transplant or as a treatment on its own
- Heart–lung or lung transplantation

ADMISSION, INPATIENT, AND NURSING CONSIDERATIONS

Medical therapy is primarily palliative.

 ONGOING CARE

FOLLOW-UP RECOMMENDATIONS

Exercise: walking or low-level aerobic activity, as tolerated, once stable; respiratory training

DIET

Fluid and salt restrictions, especially with RV failure

PATIENT EDUCATION

Discuss prognosis, lifestyle changes, and all therapeutic options (including transplant).

PROGNOSIS

- Median survival is 2 to 3 years from diagnosis; 5-year survival rate is 34% (NIH registry); newer data show 5-year survival ~70% with new treatment.
- Mode of death: right-sided heart failure (most common), pneumonia, sudden death, cardiac death
- Poor prognostic factors
  - Rapid symptom progression
  - Clinical evidence of RV failure
  - WHO functional PAH class IV (or NYHA functional class III or IV)
  - 6MWD <300 m
  - Peak VO$_2$ during cardiopulmonary exercise testing <10.4 mL/kg/min
  - ECG with pericardial effusion, significant RV enlargement/dysfunction, right atrial enlargement
  - Mean right atrial pressure >20 mm Hg
  - Cardiac index <2 L/min/m^2
  - Elevated mean PAP
  - Significantly elevated BNP and NT-proBNP; other markers also show promise in predicting survival: RDW, GDF-15, interleukin-6, creatinine.
  - Scleroderma spectrum of diseases

COMPLICATIONS

- Thromboembolism, heart failure, pleural effusion, and sudden death
- Pregnancy should be avoided due to high maternal mortality (30–50%) and fetal wastage.

REFERENCES

1. McLaughlin VV, Gaine SP, Howard LS, et al. Treatment goals of pulmonary hypertension. *J Am Coll Cardiol.* 2013;62(Suppl 25):D73–D81.
2. Galiè N, Corris PA, Frost A, et al. Updated treatment algorithm of pulmonary arterial hypertension. *J Am Coll Cardiol.* 2013;62(Suppl 25):D60–D72.

 CODES

ICD10

- I27.0 Primary pulmonary hypertension
- I27.2 Other secondary pulmonary hypertension

CLINICAL PEARLS

- PAH involves abnormalities in the small pulmonary arteries (precapillary PH) which increase PAP and vascular resistance leading to right heart failure. Diagnosis is made by right heart catheterization.
- For positive vasodilator test, CCBs are the first-line agents to manage IPAH.

PULMONARY EMBOLISM
Jasmine S. Beria, DO, MPH

BASICS

Pulmonary embolism (PE) is an acute cardiovascular disorder that causes pulmonary vascular bed obstruction, resulting in acute right ventricular failure.

DESCRIPTION
- PE is the most serious presentation of venous thromboembolism (VTE).
- Classified based on severity:
  - Low-risk PE: acute and absence of clinical markers of adverse prognosis
  - Submassive PE: no systemic hypotension, but there is either myocardial necrosis (elevated troponin) or right ventricle (RV) dysfunction (RV dilation or systolic dysfunction on echocardiography [echo], RV/LV ratio >1 on computed tomography [CT], elevation of B-type natriuretic peptide [BNP] or N-terminal pro-BNP, or consistent electrocardiogram [ECG] changes)
  - Massive PE: hemodynamic instability with sustained hypotension; pulselessness; or persistent bradycardia, cardiogenic shock, acute manifesting RV failure

EPIDEMIOLOGY
Third leading cause of vascular death (after MI and stroke); case fatality rates vary (1–60%); ~11% at 2 weeks

Incidence
- Approximately 30 to 80/100,000, with higher incidence in African Americans and lower in Asians; >100,000 cases annually in the United States
- Incidence increases with age, most occurring at 60 to 70 years of age.
- 250,000 hospitalizations per year in the United States, 10–60% in hospitalized patients (highest risk for orthopedic and cancer patients; 1:1,000 pregnancies)

Prevalence
Within hospitalized patients: 17.3% prevalence of PE in hospitalized adults who were admitted for first episode of syncope (between 2012 and 2014) (1)

ETIOLOGY AND PATHOPHYSIOLOGY
- Venous stasis, endothelial damage, and changes in coagulation properties generate thrombus formation
- Thrombus causes increased pulmonary vascular resistance, impaired gas exchange, and decreased pulmonary compliance. RV failure due to pressure overload is usually the primary cause of death.
- The most common source (85%) of PE is proximal lower extremity deep vein thrombosis (DVT).

Genetics
- Factor V Leiden: most common thrombophilia; >5.5% in Caucasian, 2.2% in Hispanics, 1.2% in African American, 0.5% in Asian; associated with 20% of VTE
- Prothrombin G20210A: 3% of Caucasians; rare in African American, Asian, and Native American; 6% in patients with VTE
- Rarely, deficiencies in protein C, S, and antithrombin

RISK FACTORS
- Older age, obesity, prolonged immobilization, surgery (total hip and knee arthroplasty, hip fracture cancer), major trauma, joint replacement, spinal cord injury, active cancer, hormonal replacement therapy, pregnancy/puerperium, previous thrombosis, antiphospholipid syndrome, genetics
- Oral contraceptive is the most frequent risk factor in women.

GENERAL PREVENTION
- Low VTE risk: early ambulation after surgery, compression stockings, and intermittent pneumatic compression
- The use of thromboprophylaxis in COVID-19 infection is not commonly done but may be considered in those at high risk (prior VTE, recent surgery, limb immobilization, recent trauma, etc.).
- Hip or knee arthroplasty (high VTE risk): ≥10 days prophylaxis with low-molecular-weight heparin (LMWH), fondaparinux, apixaban, dabigatran, rivaroxaban, or low-dose unfractionated heparin (UFH)
- Spinal cord injury, hip fracture surgery, and trauma surgery (high VTE risk): 28 to 35 days with LMWH, fondaparinux, UFH, or vitamin K antagonists (VKA)
- Long-distance travel (>8 hours): hydration, walking, avoidance of constrictive clothing and frequent calf exercises, compression stockings below knee
- Patients with factor V Leiden and prothrombin *G20210A* with no previous thrombosis do not need prophylaxis.

COMMONLY ASSOCIATED CONDITIONS
COVID-19 infection, cancer, sepsis, illnesses leading to hospitalizations, surgery

Dx DIAGNOSIS

Establish a pretest probability based on clinical criteria.
- Wells score (each predictor is +1; PE unlikely if 0 to 1, PE likely if >2)
- Geneva score (Each predictor is +1 except for heart rate >95 beats/min, which is +2; PE unlikely if 0 to 2 and PE likely if >3)
- If unlikely score: D-dimer fibrin degradation product; levels are adjusted for age or adjusted to the YEARS algorithm for ruling out PE or the Wells score
- PE rule-out criteria (PERC rule): Physicians can use this to rule out a need for imaging for PE where the clinical gestalt is low risk. All of these points should be negative to rule out a PE (age, HR >100, O₂ Sat <95% on RA, unilateral leg swelling hemoptysis, recent surgery or trauma, prior PE or DVT, oral hormone therapy).

HISTORY
- Determine if the presentation is provoked or idiopathic. Approximately 30% of cases develop without identifiable risk factor.
- Bleeding risk (previous anticoagulation, history of bleeding, recent interventions/surgeries, liver disease, kidney disease)
- Sudden onset dyspnea (>85%), chest pain (>50%), cough (20%), syncope (14%), hemoptysis (7%)

PHYSICAL EXAM
- Dyspnea, syncope, hemoptysis, tachycardia, tachypnea, accentuated S₂; pleuritic chest pain, pleural friction rub, rales
- Signs of DVT: leg swelling, tenderness, visible collateral veins
- Signs of RV failure: jugular vein distention, S₃ or S₄, systolic murmur at left sternal edge, hepatomegaly

DIFFERENTIAL DIAGNOSIS
- Pulmonary: pneumonia, bronchitis, pneumothorax, pneumonitis, chronic obstructive pulmonary disease exacerbation, pulmonary edema
- Cardiac/vascular: myocardial infarction, pericarditis, congestive heart failure, aortic dissection
- Musculoskeletal: rib fracture(s), chest wall pain

DIAGNOSTIC TESTS & INTERPRETATION
- D-dimer ELISA: In patients with low pretest probability, it can rule out PE if it is negative (high NPV). It is not diagnostic if positive (low positive predictive value [PPV]), and it is not helpful if pretest probability is intermediate or high.
- CBC, creatinine, aPTT and PT, ABG: In young patients with idiopathic, recurrent, or significant family history of VTE, consider hypercoagulable test.
- Do not test for protein C, S, factor VIII, or antithrombin in the acute setting.
- Patients with intermediate or high pretest probability *or* low probability with elevated D-dimer need further diagnostic testing.
- Chest x-ray (CXR): Westermark sign (lack of vessels in an area distal to the embolus), Hampton hump (wedge-shaped opacity with base in pleura), Fleischner sign (enlarged pulmonary arteries), pleural effusion, hemidiaphragm elevation
- ECG: right heart strain, S1Q3T3
- CT pulmonary angiography: sensitivity 96–100%, specificity 86–89%; NPV 99.8%; if normal, it excludes PE if low or intermediate clinical probability.
- Ventilation/perfusion scintigraphy (V/Q scan): Use if CT angiography is not available or contraindicated. A high-probability V/Q scan makes the diagnosis of PE; normal V/Q scan excludes PE.
- Pulmonary angiography: gold standard invasive and technically difficult: 2% morbidity and <0.01 mortality risk
- Echo: assesses RV function and thrombus in transit
- Magnetic resonance (MR) angiography: lower sensitivity and specificity than CT angiography
- Compression venous ultrasound (CUS): noninvasive; sensitivity >90%, specificity ~95%; it confirms the diagnosis of PE in patients with clinical suspicion.
- CT venography: can be done at the same time as CT angiography; increases diagnostic yield

ALERT
If preclinical probability is intermediate or high and patient has a low bleeding risk, start treatment while waiting for results.

Diagnostic Procedures/Other
Pulmonary angiography—definitive test

Test Interpretation

- D-dimer (performed if Wells criteria for PE is ≤4): Normal: PE is ruled out; high: Move on to imaging (spiral CTA).
- Spiral CTA (performed if Wells is >4 or D-dimer is high): diagnostic/positive: Treat for PE; nondiagnostic/contraindicated: Perform V/Q scan and CUS.
- V/Q scan, CUS: negative: TEE or MR or pulmonary angiography; positive: Treat for PE.

TREATMENT

- Patients with acute PE should be treated for at least 3 to 6 months.
- Treatment is based on risk stratification (2).
  - Low-risk PE → Use anticoagulation or inferior vena cava (IVC) filter. Assessment for outpatient treatment guided by PE severity index (PESI) score or the Hestia score
  - Intermediate-risk PE → anticoagulation (LMWH is recommended.)
  - High-risk PE → Anticoagulation + definite INR consult for thrombolysis/embolectomy catheter/ surgery

GENERAL MEASURES
Goal to maintain SaO$_2$ at >92%

MEDICATION

First Line
- Rivaroxaban (first line): 15 mg BID for 3 weeks and then 20 mg once daily to complete treatment; compared to warfarin, it has less major bleeding side effects while having same efficacy; ok to use in heparin-induced thrombocytopenia (HIT)
- Apixaban (first line): 10 mg BID for 7 days, then 5 mg once daily; less major bleeding episodes; ok to use in HIT
- Warfarin (second line) on day 1, if possible; 5 mg/ day for 3 days in hospitalized or older patients and at a dose of 10 mg in <60 years of aged patients; adjust dose to maintain an INR of 2 to 3; needs to overlap with UFH, LMWH, or fondaparinux: 5 to 7 days, until 2 consecutive days of therapeutic INR
- LMWH (third line): preferred due to lower risk of major bleeding and HIT
  - Enoxaparin (Lovenox) 1 mg/kg/dose SC q12h or 1.5 mg/kg/dose SC qday
  - Dalteparin (Fragmin) 200 U/kg SC q24h
  - Fondaparinux (Arixtra) 5 mg (body weight <50 kg), 7.5 mg (body weight 50 to 100 kg), or 10 mg (body weight >100 kg) SC q24h
- UFH: IV bolus of 80 U/kg or 5,000 U followed by continuous infusion (initially 18 U/kg/hr or 1,300 U/hr) with dose adjustments to maintain aPTT that corresponds to anti-Xa levels of 0.3 to 0.7
- LMWH or DOAC are preferred over warfarin in patients with cancer.

Pregnancy Considerations
- Warfarin: teratogenic; safe while breastfeeding
- LMWH: Dalteparin, enoxaparin, and fondaparinux are Category B; heparin is Category C: Use if the benefit outweighs risks.
- UFH: requires aPTT monitoring; can cause osteoporosis if used for prolonged period
- Rivaroxaban is Category C.
- Edoxaban and apixaban: Category B; increase risk of hemorrhage
- Dabigatran: Category C; only if benefit > risk

Second Line
High-risk PE: thrombolytics if shock, end-organ hypoperfusion, hypotension or cardiac arrest and low bleeding risk, intracranial hemorrhage risk: 0.7–6.4%:
- IV systemic thrombolysis with weight-based dose of tenecteplase, alteplase at a dose of 0.6 mg per kilogram of body weight or alteplase at a dose of 100 mg administered over 1 to 2 hours.
- Absolute contraindications: intracranial hemorrhage, intracranial cerebrovascular or malignancy, ischemic stroke <3 months, possible aortic dissection, bleeding diathesis, active bleeding, recent neurosurgery, or major trauma

SURGERY/OTHER PROCEDURES
- IVC filter placement if absolute contraindication for anticoagulation or recurrent PE despite adequate anticoagulation treatment
- Emergency embolectomy can be considered in patients with massive PE with contraindications for thrombolysis.
- Consider US-assisted catheter-directed thrombolysis with intermediate risk of death or submassive PE.

ADMISSION, INPATIENT, AND NURSING CONSIDERATIONS
In selected, low-risk acute PE population (PESI score class I or II), patients could be managed safely and effectively in the outpatient setting with close follow-up.

ONGOING CARE

Duration of anticoagulation
- Provoked PE (trigger no longer present): 3 months
- Unprovoked PE: >3 months; consider long-term or prolonged secondary prophylaxis if bleeding risk is low. HERDOO2 Score provides guidance to determine duration of therapy in women with first unprovoked VTE. Low risk (0 to 1 criteria) can safely stop treatment after 6 months.

- Cancer-related PE: LMWH first 3 to 6 months; consider secondary prophylaxis as long as the patient has active cancer.
- Recurrent unprovoked PE: long-term anticoagulation

FOLLOW-UP RECOMMENDATIONS
If concomitant DVT, consider 30 to 40 mm Hg knee-high compression stockings

Patient Monitoring
- INR should be checked regularly; target is 2 to 3.
- aPTT needs to be monitored in SC UFH.
- Anti-Xa can be checked in special circumstances if treated with LMWH, including pregnancy, younger patients, and renal disease.

PROGNOSIS
- Mortality: submassive 6–14%; massive PE 15–60%
- PESI score predicts 30-day mortality.
- Any one of the following defines high risk: age >80 years, cancer, chronic cardiopulmonary disease, heart rate 110 beats/min, systolic blood pressure <100 mm Hg, and O$_2$ saturation <90%.

COMPLICATIONS
Post-PE syndrome: permanent pulmonary vasculature changes, chronic dyspnea, reduced exercise capacity

REFERENCES

1. Lee LH, Gallus A, Jindal R, et al. Incidence of venous cerebroembolism in Asian populations: a systematic review. *Thromb Haemost*. 2017;117(12): 2243–2260.
2. Kahn SR, de Wit K. Pulmonary embolism. *N Engl J Med*. 2022;387(1):45–57.

CODES

ICD10
- I26.02 Saddle embolus of pulmonary artery with acute cor pulmonale
- I26.92 Saddle embolus of pulmonary artery without acute cor pulmonale
- I26.01 Septic pulmonary embolism with acute cor pulmonale

CLINICAL PEARLS
- In low pretest probability patients, a negative D-dimer can rule out PE (high NPV).
- In moderate to high pretest probability, obtain CT pulmonary angiography.

PULMONARY FIBROSIS

Avignat S. Patel, MD

 BASICS

DESCRIPTION

- Pulmonary fibrosis (PF) is an interstitial lung disease (ILD), a family of >200 different lung diseases, characterized by inflammation, cellular proliferation, and fibrosis within lung interstitium and bronchial walls. If no cause identified, ILD is called idiopathic interstitial pneumonia.
- The most common idiopathic interstitial pneumonia is idiopathic PF (IPF).
- IPF is defined as a form of progressive fibrotic ILD associated with the histologic and/or radiologic appearance of usual interstitial pneumonia (UIP) when other causes have been excluded.

EPIDEMIOLOGY

- Most common ILD prevalent worldwide (25–30% of all ILD)
- Most common in men >60 years of age

Incidence

Higher in North America and Europe (3 to 9 cases per 100,000 person-years) than in South America and East Asia (fewer than 4 cases per 100,000 person-years)

Prevalence

In the United States, the prevalence has been reported to range from 10 to 60 cases per 100,000 person-years.

ETIOLOGY AND PATHOPHYSIOLOGY

- A favored model for the pathogenesis of IPF is that recurrent, alveolar epithelial damage with accelerated cell senescence leads to abnormal cellular repair and deposition of interstitial fibrosis by myofibroblasts.
- Causes of nonidiopathic PF include occupational and environmental exposures, drugs, and connective tissue diseases.

Genetics

- The role of host genetic factors and their interactions with environmental factors is unknown.
- Mutations in genes involved in maintenance of telomere length are associated with increased risk of IPF.
- An SNP in the MUC5B promoter leads to gene overexpression and is associated with increased risk of IPF. However, the mechanism linking MUC5B and IPF is not clear.

RISK FACTORS

- Family history of IPF
- Smoking—most significant association
- GERD, OSA
- Occupational and environmental exposures: wood (pine), metal dusts (lead, brass, steel), farming, birds, hairdressing, stone cutting, exposure to livestock, vegetable and animal dust, air pollution, mold

GENERAL PREVENTION

Avoidance of above risk factors

COMMONLY ASSOCIATED CONDITIONS

- Pulmonary hypertension: 30–80% of patients with IPF
- GERD
- Nonidiopathic PF may be related to connective tissue diseases (RA and systemic sclerosis).

DIAGNOSIS

HISTORY

- Gradual onset
- Exertional breathlessness and nonproductive cough
- Constitutional symptoms (weight loss, fever, fatigue, myalgias, arthralgias) are uncommon.
- History of exposure (See "Risk Factors" section.)

PHYSICAL EXAM

- Lung auscultation: bibasilar fine, late inspiratory crackles: "Velcro" crackles
- Clubbing in late stages, cyanosis (rare)
- Findings of pulmonary hypertension and right ventricular (RV) failure (elevated JVP, RV parasternal heave, loud P_2, LE edema)
- Signs of connective tissue disorders (skin/nail fold changes, arthritis)

DIFFERENTIAL DIAGNOSIS

- Other ILDs such as chronic hypersensitivity pneumonitis, nonspecific interstitial pneumonia, occupational lung disease, connective tissue disease-associated ILD (CTD-ILD), cryptogenic organizing pneumonia, post-COVID-19 ILD
- See below for histologic differential diagnosis of UIP.

DIAGNOSTIC TESTS & INTERPRETATION

Initial Tests (lab, imaging)

- Blood tests: Most labs are normal.
- Chest radiograph:
  - Reduced lung volumes and reticular opacities mostly at lung bases
  - Coarse reticular pattern and honeycombed cysts in advanced stages
- Pleural abnormalities (such as pleural plaques and effusions) are uncommon.

Follow-Up Tests & Special Considerations

- Chest CT scan:
  - Once diagnosis of IPF is suspected, obtain high-resolution CT (HRCT) of chest, including inspiratory and expiratory images with thin <1.25 mm slices and prone images if subtle subpleural basal changes present.
  - In diagnosing IPF, HRCT is categorized into one of four patterns: UIP, probable UIP, indeterminate for UIP, and alternative diagnosis (1)[C].
  - UIP pattern requires bilateral, primary peripheral, basilar reticulation AND honeycombing with or without traction bronchiectasis. UIP pattern on HRCT is diagnostic of IPF without need for surgical lung biopsy.
  - Probable UIP pattern has changes described previously with traction bronchiectasis but without honeycombing.
  - Atypical features on HRCT include upper- or mid-lung predominance, predominant consolidation, ground-glass opacities, and diffuse nodules or cysts; these increase the likelihood of an ILD other than IPF.
- Serologic testing for connective tissue diseases to exclude nonidiopathic causes: ANA; RF; anti-CCP antibodies; anti–Scl-70, anti-Ro, anti-La, anti–U1-RNP, and anti–Jo-1 antibodies; and antisynthetase antibodies
- Echocardiogram to assess cardiac function, RV function, and pulmonary hypertension

Diagnostic Procedures/Other

- Pulmonary function test (PFT):
  - PFTs in all patients undergoing evaluation and treatment of IPF/ILD
  - Findings include:
    - Decreased diffusion capacity for carbon monoxide (DLCO)
    - Decreased lung volumes (TLC, RV, FRC)
    - Decreased spirometric values: FVC and FEV_1 due to reduced lung volumes with preserved FEV_1/FVC ratio.
- ABG may show hypoxemia and respiratory alkalosis.
- 6-minute walk distance (6MWD): reduced distance and exertional hypoxemia
- Bronchoscopy:
  - Bronchoalveolar lavage (BAL):
    - Can be helpful in excluding other diagnoses like infection, malignancy, etc.
    - ATS/ERS does not recommend routine use of BAL for diagnosis of IPF.
  - Bronchoscopic transbronchial biopsy:
    - Not recommended for diagnosis of IPF as sensitivity and specificity is poor
    - May help exclude other ILDs
    - A genomic classifier run on transbronchial biopsy specimens can assist in diagnosing patients whose CT is not definite for UIP.
  - Transbronchial lung cryobiopsy is a potential alternative to thoracoscopic biopsy (1)[B].
- Surgical lung biopsy:
  - Gold standard for diagnosis of ILD
  - When the combination of clinical and imaging data is not diagnostic, a thoracoscopic lung biopsy can be considered.
  - Biopsy samples should be taken from multiple lobes, avoiding the most severely affected areas as they will show nondiagnostic fibrosis.
  - Procedure should not be performed in high-risk patients, including:
    - High oxygen requirements (>2 L/min)
    - Significant pulmonary hypertension
    - Rapid disease progression
    - Severely reduced FVC or DLCO

Test Interpretation

- Histopathology
  - Gross pathology distinctive nodular pleural surface
  - Histopathologic pattern in IPF is UIP.
    - UIP pattern requires dense fibrosis with architectural distortion, subpleural, and basal distribution, spatial and temporal heterogeneity, fibroblastic foci, and honeycomb changes plus absence of features suggestive of alternate diagnosis.
    - Differential diagnosis of UIP histologic pattern includes IPF, CTD-ILD, chronic hypersensitivity pneumonitis, asbestosis, chronic radiation pneumonitis, Hermansky-Pudlak syndrome, and neurofibromatosis.

- Diagnostic strategies:
  - As per ATS/ERS statement of IPF in 2018, diagnosis of IPF requires (2)[C]:
    - Exclusion of other known causes of ILD and either of the following:
      - UIP pattern on HRCT
      - Specific combinations of HRCT patterns and histopathology patterns
  - UIP pattern on HRCT would be diagnostic with all histology patterns except alternate diagnosis findings.
  - UIP pattern on histology would be diagnostic with all HRCT patterns except alternate diagnosis findings.
  - Per ATS/ERS, for patients suspected of having IPF, a multidisciplinary discussion (pulmonologists, radiologists, pathologists, rheumatologists) is recommended for diagnostic decision-making.

TREATMENT

GENERAL MEASURES
- Smoking cessation
- Vaccinations: pneumococcus, influenza, SARS-CoV-2
- Pulmonary rehabilitation
- Referral to a transplant center
- Supplemental oxygen: Clinical practice guidelines strongly recommend supplemental oxygen if SpO_2 <88%.

MEDICATION
Two medications, nintedanib and pirfenidone, have been shown to be safe, effective, and are recommended in the treatment of IPF.

- In placebo-controlled, randomized trials, each drug slowed the rate of FVC decline by approximately 50% over the course of 1 year.
- Both have shown some efficacy in reducing severe respiratory events such as acute exacerbations and hospitalization.
- Pooled data and meta-analyses also suggest reduced mortality.
- The cost of each medication is estimated to exceed $100,000 annually.

First Line
- Nintedanib:
  - Mechanism of action: tyrosine kinase inhibitor that targets growth factor pathways including VEGF, FGF, and PDGF receptors
  - Most common side effect is diarrhea (>2/3 of patients). It is also associated with a small risk of bleeding and should be used cautiously, if at all, in patients on therapeutic anticoagulation.
  - Liver function should be monitored as liver toxicity has been reported.
  - Also approved for progressive fibrotic ILDs other than IPF and systemic sclerosis-ILD
- Pirfenidone:
  - Mechanism of action: anti-inflammatory and antifibrotic effects, including inhibition of collagen synthesis, down regulation of TGF-β and TNF-α, and reduction in fibroblast proliferation
  - Common side effects: anorexia, nausea, vomiting, photosensitive rash, abnormal liver function
- Cannot recommend one agent over the other because there have been no head-to-head comparisons, and the efficacy is similar

Second Line
- No second-line agents available.
- Treatment guidelines for IPF by ATS/ERS include:
  - Strong recommendations against use of:
    - Anticoagulation (warfarin)
    - Combination prednisone + azathioprine + N-acetyl cysteine (NAC)
    - Selective endothelin receptor antagonist (ambrisentan)
    - Imatinib, a tyrosine kinase inhibitor with one target
  - Conditional recommendations against:
    - Dual endothelin receptor antagonists (macitentan, bosentan)
    - Phosphodiesterase-5 inhibitor (sildenafil)
    - NAC monotherapy

ISSUES FOR REFERRAL
- Referral to pulmonologist for diagnosis and management
- Thoracic surgeon referral is indicated if patient cannot be diagnosed by ATS clinical and radiographic criteria.
- Referral to lung transplant center is indicated early for patients showing progressive worsening of the disease.

ADDITIONAL THERAPIES
Several investigational therapies are being studied in randomized controlled trials.

SURGERY/OTHER PROCEDURES
Lung transplant:
- Can prolong survival and improve quality of life for highly selected candidates
- Only a minority of patients with IPF receive lung transplants.
- Only 66% of lung transplant recipients survive for >3 years after transplant and only 53% survive for >5 years.
- Common complications include primary graft dysfunction, acute and chronic allograft rejection, opportunistic infections, and cancer.

COMPLEMENTARY & ALTERNATIVE MEDICINE
No proven benefit of any complementary and alternative medications

ADMISSION, INPATIENT, AND NURSING CONSIDERATIONS
- Patient with acute exacerbation of IPF should be admitted to the hospital for management.
- Need for mechanical ventilation portends a poor prognosis and should be avoided if possible.
- Palliative care consult is appropriate for all patients diagnosed with IPF.

ONGOING CARE

FOLLOW-UP RECOMMENDATIONS
- Pulmonary clinic and, if possible, at an ILD clinic
- Monitoring with serial HRCT (at least yearly), PFT (at least every 6 months)
- If on antifibrotic medications, monitor LFTs.

PROGNOSIS
IPF carries a poor prognosis with a median survival of 3.8 years among adults ≥65 years of age in the United States.

COMPLICATIONS
- Acute exacerbation of IPF
  - 10–20% per patient per year
  - It is characterized by worsening hypoxemia, new bilateral ground-glass opacities, consolidation, or both on HRCT imaging that are not fully explained by volume overload or infection.
  - Triggers: infection, aspiration, drug toxicity, or idiopathic
  - Treatment: Available guidelines make weak recommendations for the use of glucocorticoids (no definitive benefit based on available data) and do not recommend the use of mechanical ventilation. Consider palliative care referral.
- Increased risk for VTE, lung cancer, and pulmonary hypertension
  - Management of pulmonary hypertension should be in consultation with a pulmonary hypertension specialist. A recent study of inhaled treprostinil in ILD, including IPF, demonstrated a clinical benefit and can be considered.

REFERENCES
1. Raghu G, Remy-Jardin M, Richeldi L, et al; for American Thoracic Society, European Respiratory Society, Japanese Respiratory Society, Latin American Thoracic Society. Idiopathic pulmonary fibrosis (an update) and progressive pulmonary fibrosis in adults: an official ATS/ERS/JRS/ALAT clinical practice guideline. *Am J Respir Crit Care Med*. 2022;205(9):e18–e47.
2. Raghu G, Remy-Jardin M, Myers JL, et al; for American Thoracic Society, European Respiratory Society, Japanese Respiratory Society, Latin American Thoracic Society. Diagnosis of idiopathic pulmonary fibrosis. An official ATS/ERS/JRS/ALAT clinical practice guideline. *Am J Respir Crit Care Med*. 2018;198(5):e44–e68.

CODES

ICD10
- J84.10 Pulmonary fibrosis, unspecified
- J84.112 Idiopathic pulmonary fibrosis

CLINICAL PEARLS
- IPF is the most common idiopathic ILD and frequently misdiagnosed or has delayed diagnosis.
- HRCT scan is the cornerstone for diagnosis.
- Two anti-fibrotic drugs are the only approved therapy for IPF.
- Oxygen supplementation, pulmonary rehab, anti-reflux treatment, vaccinations against pneumococcus, influenza, and SARS-CoV2 should be considered in all patients.
- Referral to pulmonary clinic, ILD clinic, and lung transplant center should be considered early.

PYELONEPHRITIS

Dana G. Carroll, PharmD, BCPS, CDCES, BCGP • Randi Cheree Melton, DO • Jacquelynn P. Luker, MD

 BASICS

DESCRIPTION
- A syndrome caused by infection of the renal parenchyma and/or renal pelvis, often producing localized flank/back pain combined with systemic symptoms, such as fever, chills, nausea and vomiting; there is a wide spectrum of illness ranging from mild symptoms to septic shock.
- Chronic pyelonephritis is the result of progressive inflammation of the renal interstitium and tubules, due to recurrent infection, vesicoureteral reflux, or both.
- Pyelonephritis is considered uncomplicated if the infection is caused by a typical pathogen in an immunocompetent patient with normal urinary tract anatomy and renal function.

Geriatric Considerations
May present as altered mental status; absence of fever is common in older adults. Older patients with diabetes and pyelonephritis are at higher risk of bacteremia, prolonged hospitalization, and mortality. The high prevalence of asymptomatic bacteriuria (ABU) in older adults makes the use of urine dipstick less reliable for diagnosing UTI in this population. Culture and sensitivity data are more useful in guiding antimicrobial therapy for pyelonephritis in older adults and should therefore be obtained.

Pregnancy Considerations
Pyelonephritis affects 1–2% of all pregnancies and is the most common medical complication requiring hospitalization during pregnancy. Pregnant patients with untreated ABU have a 20–30% risk of developing acute pyelonephritis. Patients with pyelonephritis are at increased risk of developing acute respiratory distress syndrome (ARDS) and spontaneous preterm labor. Pregnant women with acute pyelonephritis should be strongly considered for hospitalization and treated initially with a 2nd- or 3rd-generation intravenous cephalosporin.

Pediatric Considerations
UTI is present in ~5% of patients aged 2 months to 2 years with fever and no apparent source on history and physical exam. A urine specimen, preferably by catheterization or suprapubic aspiration, should be obtained and sent for urinalysis prior to antibiotics being initiated. Treatment (PO or IV; inpatient or outpatient) should be based on the clinical situation and patient toxicity.

EPIDEMIOLOGY
Incidence
Community-acquired acute pyelonephritis: 3 to 4 cases per 10,000 males; 15 to 17 cases per 10,000 females; 28 cases per 10,000 women aged 18 to 49 years

Prevalence
Adult cases: 250,000/year, with 200,000 hospitalizations

ETIOLOGY AND PATHOPHYSIOLOGY
- *Escherichia coli* (>80%); other gram-negative pathogens: *Proteus*, *Klebsiella*, *Serratia*, *Clostridium*, *Pseudomonas*, and *Enterobacter* spp.; *Enterococcus* spp.
- *Staphylococcus*: *Staphylococcus epidermidis*, *Staphylococcus saprophyticus* (number 2 cause in young women), and *Staphylococcus aureus*; *Candida* spp.

RISK FACTORS
- Underlying urinary tract abnormalities; indwelling catheter/recent urinary tract instrumentation; nephrolithiasis; immunocompromised, including diabetes; elderly, institutionalized patients (particularly women); prostatic enlargement; stress incontinence
- Childhood UTI; acute pyelonephritis within the prior year; recent sexual intercourse; spermicide use; new sex partner within the prior year; pregnancy; hospital-acquired infection; symptoms >7 days at time of presentation

COMMONLY ASSOCIATED CONDITIONS
Indwelling catheters, renal calculi; benign prostatic hyperplasia

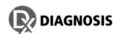 **DIAGNOSIS**

HISTORY
- In adults: fever; flank pain; nausea ± vomiting; malaise, anorexia, myalgia; dysuria, urinary frequency, urgency; suprapubic discomfort; mental status changes (older adults)
- In infants and children: fever, irritability, poor feeding; GI symptoms

PHYSICAL EXAM
- In adults
  - Presentation ranges from no physical findings to septic shock; fever: ≥38°C (100.4°F)
  - Costovertebral angle tenderness
  - Mental status changes are common in older adults. Depending on presentation, consider a pelvic exam in women to exclude pelvic inflammatory disease.
- In infants and children: lethargy, fever, poor skin perfusion; inadequate weight gain/weight loss; jaundice; pallor; gray skin color

DIFFERENTIAL DIAGNOSIS
- Obstructive uropathy; acute bacterial pneumonia (lower lobe); cholecystitis, acute pancreatitis, appendicitis
- Perforated viscus; aortic dissection; pelvic inflammatory disease; ectopic pregnancy; kidney stone; diverticulitis

DIAGNOSTIC TESTS & INTERPRETATION
Initial Tests (lab, imaging)
- Urinalysis: pyuria (>5 WBC/HPF) ± leukocyte casts, hematuria, nitrites (sensitivity 35–85%; specificity 92–100%), and mild proteinuria; urine leukocyte esterase positive (sensitivity 74–96%; specificity 94–98%); urine Gram stain; urine culture (>100,000 colony forming units/mL or >100 colony forming units/mL + symptoms) and sensitivities
- Complete blood count, blood urea nitrogen, creatinine, glomerular filtration rate (GFR), and pregnancy test (if indicated)
- C-reactive protein levels correlate with prolonged hospitalization and recurrence; serum albumin <3.3 g/dL also associated with increased risk for hospital admission
- Imaging is not necessary in routine cases.
- Pediatrics: Guidelines recommend renal/bladder US (not voiding cystourethrogram) after first febrile UTI between ages 2 and 24 months.

Follow-Up Tests & Special Considerations
- Catheterization/suprapubic aspirate to obtain samples from non–toilet-trained children; blood culture(s): if hospitalized, diagnosis uncertain, suspected hematogenous source or immunosuppression; recent antibiotic use may alter lab results.
- If patient's condition does not improve within 72 hours, if obstruction/anatomic abnormality is suspected, in patients with immunosuppression or multiple comorbidities, and/or if certain lab abnormalities are present (urine pH >7, GFR <40, 50% decline in renal function), consider CT scan of abdomen and pelvis ± contrast. Contrast-enhanced computed tomography (CECT) is typically the image of choice for children and adults with acute pyelonephritis. US of kidneys, ureter, or bladder is not as sensitive as CT but is cheaper and more readily available; cystoscopy with ureteral catheterization

Test Interpretation
- Acute: abscess formation with neutrophil response
- Chronic: fibrosis with reduction in renal tissue

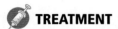 **TREATMENT**

- ≤7 days of treatment is equivalent to longer regimens in adults (including those with bacteremia) without urogenital abnormalities (1)[A].
- IV antibiotics for inpatients who are toxic appearing or unable to tolerate oral antibiotics

GENERAL MEASURES
- Broad-spectrum antibiotics initially based on severity of illness, health status, and risk factors for resistant pathogens; tailor to culture and sensitivity results.
  - Risk factors for a multidrug-resistant (MDR) pathogens/infections if present within last 3 months: history of urinary MDR pathogen; inpatient stay at a health care facility (hospital, nursing home, etc.); use of fluoroquinolone, trimethoprim-sulfamethoxazole (TMP-SMX), or broad-spectrum β-lactam; travel to geographic regions with significant incidence of MDR pathogens (e.g., Asia, Middle East, Africa); obstructive uropathy (2)[A]
- Consider urinary analgesics (e.g., phenazopyridine 200 mg q8h) for dysuria.

MEDICATION
- For empiric oral therapy, a fluoroquinolone is recommended. Should fluoroquinolone resistance exceed 10% ceftriaxone 1 g IV daily for 10 days or if the patient has nausea/vomiting, a single initial IV dose of a long-acting antibiotic such as ceftriaxone 1 g IV daily is recommended until oral agents can be used.
- For parenteral therapy, fluoroquinolone, an aminoglycoside with or without ampicillin, an extended-spectrum cephalosporin with or without a β-lactamase inhibitor, an extended-spectrum penicillin with or without an aminoglycoside, or a carbapenem are recommended.

- Contraindications: Known drug allergy; fluoroquinolones are not recommended in children, adolescents, and pregnant women unless other alternatives are not available. Nitrofurantoin does not achieve reliable tissue levels to treat pyelonephritis.
- Precautions
  - Adjust antibiotic dosages in patients with renal insufficiency. Monitor aminoglycoside levels and renal function.
  - If *Enterococcus* is suspected based on Gram stain, ampicillin ± gentamicin or piperacillin-tazobactam are good empiric choices; unless patient is penicillin allergic, then use vancomycin. If outpatient, add amoxicillin to fluoroquinolone, pending culture results and sensitivity. Do not use a 3rd-generation cephalosporin for suspected/proven enterococcal infections.
  - >20% *E. coli* strains are resistant to ampicillin and TMP-SMX in community-acquired infections.
  - Extended-spectrum β-lactamase (ESBL)-producing strains should be treated with a carbapenem ± β-lactamase inhibitor or ceftolozane-tazobactam or plazomicin.

First Line
- Adults
  - Oral (initial outpatient treatment)
    ○ Ciprofloxacin: 500 mg q12h for 5 to 7 days; ciprofloxacin XR: 1,000 mg/day for 5 to 7 days
    ○ Levofloxacin: 750 mg/day for 5 to 7 days
    ○ TMP-SMX (160/800 mg): 1 tablet q12h for 10 to 14 days provided uropathogen known to be susceptible ± ceftriaxone 1 g initial IM/IV dose
  - IV (initial inpatient treatment for patients with no risk factors for MDR organisms)
    ○ Ciprofloxacin: 400 mg q12h; levofloxacin: 750 mg/day
    ○ Cefotaxime: 1 g q8–12h up to 2 g q4h; ceftriaxone: 1 to 2 g/day; cefepime: 1 to 2 g q12h
    ○ Gentamicin: 5 to 7 mg/kg body weight daily
    ○ Piperacillin-tazobactam: 3.375 g q6–8h
    ○ Ampicillin: 2 g q6h ± gentamicin for *Enterococcus*
  - IV (initial inpatient treatment for patients with at least one risk factor for MDR organisms)
    ○ Antipseudomonal carbapenem: meropenem: 1 g q8h; imipenem: 500 mg q6h; doripenem: 500 mg q8h
    ○ Add vancomycin for methicillin-resistant *S. aureus* (MRSA) or daptomycin or linezolid for vancomycin-resistant *Enterococcus* (VRE).
  - Severe illness: IV therapy until afebrile for 24 to 48 hours and tolerating PO intake; switch to oral agents to complete up to a 2-week course.
- Pediatric
  - Oral: cefdinir: 14 mg/kg/day for 10 to 14 days; ceftibuten 9 mg/kg/day for 10 to 14 days; cefixime 8 mg/kg/day for 10 to 14 days
  - IV (General indication for IV therapy is age <2 months or clinical concern in other ages.)
    ○ Ceftriaxone: 75 mg/kg/day (IM use acceptable in outpatient setting); cefotaxime: 150 mg/kg/day divided in 3 to 4 doses; ampicillin: 100 mg/kg/day divided in 4 doses + gentamicin 7.5 mg/kg/day divided in 3 doses

Second Line
Adults
- Oral
  - Use oral β-lactams with caution; if used, longer courses of therapy (10 to 14 days) are recommended.
  - Cefpodoxime: 200 mg q12h
  - Amoxicillin-clavulanate: 875/125 mg q12h or 500/125 mg q8h
- IV
  - Ticarcillin-clavulanate: 3.1 g q4–6h
  - Targeted therapy for MDR organisms
    ○ Ceftazidime-avibactam: 2.5 g q8h; Ceftolozane-tazobactam: 1.5 g q8h; Meropenem-vaborbactam: 4 g q8h

Pediatric Considerations
- Treat children <2 years of age and children with febrile or recurrent UTI for 10 to 14 days.
- Initial empiric antibiotic choice should cover *E. coli*. Add ampicillin if *Enterococcus* is suspected.
  - Oral antibiotics (ceftibuten, cefixime, and amoxicillin/clavulanic acid) may be used alone, *or*
  - IV antibiotics (single daily dosing if an aminoglycoside is chosen) for 2 to 4 days, followed by oral antibiotics for a total of 10 to 14 days
- Complete outpatient antibiotic course.

Pregnancy Considerations
- Acute pyelonephritis should be aggressively treated. Hospital admission should be considered, and parenteral therapy may be required.
- May consider low-dose suppressive antibiotics (nitrofurantoin or cephalexin) for the remainder of pregnancy following treatment of pyelonephritis (3)[A]

ISSUES FOR REFERRAL
Acute pyelonephritis unresponsive to therapy; chronic pyelonephritis, abnormal urogenital anatomy

SURGERY/OTHER PROCEDURES
Perinephric abscess may require surgical drainage.

ADMISSION, INPATIENT, AND NURSING CONSIDERATIONS
- Inpatient therapy for severe illness, risk factors for complicated pyelonephritis, pregnancy, or extremes of age
- Consider transitioning from IV to oral therapies after the patient is afebrile for 24 hours; outpatient therapy if mild to moderate illness, uncomplicated course, and tolerating oral intake; IV fluids for dehydration; blood cultures for patients admitted with pyelonephritis; discharge on oral agent after the patient is afebrile for 24 to 48 hours to complete up to 2 weeks of therapy.

ONGOING CARE

FOLLOW-UP RECOMMENDATIONS
Adults and children: Patients treated in the outpatient setting should have follow-up at 48 to 72 hours to evaluate for improvement and consideration of further evaluations and/or broadening coverage if not improving. Repeat urine culture only needed for complicated cases.

Patient Monitoring
If no response within 48 to 72 hours (5% of patients): Reevaluate and review cultures, CT scan, or US to review anatomy; adjust therapy as needed; urologic or infectious disease consult; the two most common causes of failure to respond are a resistant organism and nephrolithiasis.

DIET
Encourage fluid intake.

PROGNOSIS
95% of treated patients respond within 48 hours.

COMPLICATIONS
Renal abscess; perinephric abscess; metastatic infection: skeletal system, endocardium, eye, meningitis with subsequent seizures; septic shock and death; acute/chronic renal failure

REFERENCES
1. Eliakim-Raz N, Yahav D, Paul M, et al. Duration of antibiotic treatment for acute pyelonephritis and septic urinary tract infection—7 days or less versus longer treatment: systematic review and meta-analysis of randomized controlled trials. *J Antimicrob Chemother*. 2013;68(10): 2183–2191.
2. Talan DA, Takhar SS, Krshnadasan A, et al; for EMERGENcy ID Net Study Group. Fluoroquinolone-resistant and extended-spectrum β-lactamase producing *Eschericia coli* infections in patients with pyelonephritis, United States. *Emerg Infect Dis*. 2016;22(9):1594–1603.
3. Schneeberger C, Geerlings SE, Middleton P, et al. Interventions for preventing recurring urinary tract infections during pregnancy. *Cochrane Database Syst Rev*. 2015;2015(7):CD009279.

CODES

ICD10
- N12 Tubulo-interstitial nephritis, not spcf as acute or chronic
- N10 Acute tubulo-interstitial nephritis
- N11.9 Chronic tubulo-interstitial nephritis, unspecified

CLINICAL PEARLS
- Urine culture is helpful for targeting antibiotic therapy and should be obtained when possible.
- The most common causes of poor response to treatment are antibiotic resistance and coexisting nephrolithiasis.
- Fluoroquinolones are generally the initial antibiotic of choice for pyelonephritis. Oral β-lactams are less effective. Parenteral β-lactams may be used in cases of complicated UTIs.

PYLORIC STENOSIS

Shani H. Cunningham, DO, MEd, FAAP • Katelyn Hernandez, DO

BASICS

DESCRIPTION
Acquired narrowing of the pyloric canal due to progressive hypertrophy of pyloric muscle leading to obstruction

EPIDEMIOLOGY
- Presentation is most common between 2 and 8 weeks of age, with a median presentation of 6 weeks
- The most common condition requiring surgical intervention in the 1st year of life

Incidence
- Highest incidence found in first-born males
- Overall 1.56 per 1,000 live births
- Higher in Caucasian and Hispanic children

ETIOLOGY AND PATHOPHYSIOLOGY
- Impaired physiologic relaxation of the pyloric muscle leads to hypertrophy.
- Gastric outflow is obstructed, leading to gastric distension and forceful projectile postprandial vomiting.

RISK FACTORS
- Maternal smoking during pregnancy
- C-section delivery
- Prematurity
- Formula feeding which may cause higher serum levels associated with pylorospasm
- Postnatal macrolide antibiotics, especially if administered in the first 2 weeks of life
- Multiple gestations:
  - 200-fold increased risk if monozygotic twin affected
  - 20-fold increased risk if dizygotic twin affected

GENERAL PREVENTION
Breast milk contains increased vasoactive intestinal peptides which are agents of smooth muscle relaxation.

COMMONLY ASSOCIATED CONDITIONS
Hiatal and inguinal hernias

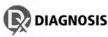

DIAGNOSIS

HISTORY
- Nonbilious projectile vomiting immediately after feeding with increasing in frequency and severity
- Hunger and irritability due to inadequate nutrition
- Weight loss
- Median duration of symptoms is 10 days.

PHYSICAL EXAM
- Firm "olive-like" mass palpable in the right upper quadrant
- Visible peristalsis after feeding
- Late signs include dry mucous membranes, poor skin turgor, tachycardia, and irritability.
- Rarely, jaundice when starvation leads to an elevated indirect hyperbilirubinemia.

DIFFERENTIAL DIAGNOSIS
- Inappropriate feeding
- GERD
- Gastritis
- Adrenal crisis
- Antral or gastric web

DIAGNOSTIC TESTS & INTERPRETATION
Initial Tests (lab, imaging)
- Labs:
  - Hypokalemic, hypochloremic, metabolic alkalosis
- Pyloric ultrasound is the study of choice:
  - Pathologic limits are 3-mm pyloric muscle thickness, 15-mm pyloric length, 11-mm pyloric diameter, and 12-mL pyloric volume with muscle thickness being the key factor. Although these measurements remain diagnostic, they may exclude younger (<3 weeks old), smaller infants who can be clinically diagnosed (1)[B].
- Upper GI series: rarely indicated
  - Strong gastric contractions; pyloric canal outlined by string of contrast material (string sign) and parallel lines of barium in the narrow channel separated by mucosa (double-tract sign or railroad track sign)

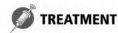

TREATMENT

GENERAL MEASURES
- Pyloric stenosis is a medical emergency but not a surgical emergency.
- Ensure proper nutrition and hydration; treat alkalosis or electrolyte deranges preoperatively if present.
- Definitive treatment is surgical pyloromyotomy.

ADDITIONAL THERAPIES

Medical treatment with oral or IV atropine is an alternative to surgical treatment (2)[A].

- Oral atropine: initial dose of 0.05 mg/kg/day and increased to max of 0.1 mg/kg/day
- IV atropine: initial dose of 0.1 mg/kg/day and increased by 0.01 mg/kg/day until vomiting ceases then change to oral atropine at twice the effective IV dose
- Recommended for use in patients when anesthesia or surgery is not possible
- Takes 5 to 15 months for pyloric muscle to normalize on medical therapy, although vomiting will usually cease within 7 days
- Associated with lower success rates and longer stays as compared to surgery

SURGERY/OTHER PROCEDURES

- Pyloromyotomy (Ramstedt procedure) is curative.
  - The entire length of hypertrophied muscle is divided, with preservation of the underlying mucosa.
- Laparoscopic approach results in less postoperative pain, shorter hospital stays, shorter postoperative recovery, lower complication rates, improved cosmesis, and can be performed with no increase in operative time or complications (2),(3)[A],(4)[B].

ADMISSION, INPATIENT, AND NURSING CONSIDERATIONS

- Fluid resuscitation:
  - Initially, ≥1 20 mL/kg boluses is needed.
  - For optimal resuscitation in infants, use D5 1/2 NS with 20 mEq of KCl
  - Usually then placed on 1.5 to 2 times maintenance fluids
- Correct electrolyte abnormalities prior to anesthesia due to metabolic alkalosis reducing inspiratory drive and potentially causing postoperative apnea.

ONGOING CARE

FOLLOW-UP RECOMMENDATIONS

Discharge following surgery when tolerating 2 to 3 full feeds (5)[C].

Patient Monitoring

- Postoperative monitoring including monitoring for pain, emesis, apnea
- If significant emesis present after 1 to 2 weeks, then upper GI studies needed to rule out incomplete pyloromyotomy or duodenal leak (5)[C]

DIET

- Ad-lib feedings are recommended after pyloromyotomy as they decrease length of stay.
- Timing of first feed is not significant, but early feeding is associated with increased potential for emesis without impacting length of stay (6)[A].

PATIENT EDUCATION

Counsel caregivers on postoperative emesis, signs and symptoms of infection, and assessment of hydration status

PROGNOSIS

Surgery is curative.

COMPLICATIONS

- Dehydration
- Failure to thrive
- Jaundice
- Chronic abdominal pain and pain-associated functional GI disorders following surgery
- Incomplete pyloromyotomy
- Mucosal perforation

REFERENCES

1. Said M, Shaul DB, Fujimoto M, et al. Ultrasound measurements in hypertrophic pyloric stenosis: don't let the numbers fool you. *Perm J.* 2012;16(3):25–27.
2. Wu SF, Lin HY, Huang FK, et al. Efficacy of medical treatment for infantile hypertrophic pyloric stenosis: a meta-analysis. *Pediatr Neonatol.* 2016;57(6):515–521.
3. Oomen MWN, Hoekstra LT, Bakx R, et al. Open versus laparoscopic pyloromyotomy for hypertrophic pyloric stenosis: a systematic review and meta-analysis focusing on major complications. *Surg Endosc.* 2012;26(8):2104–2110.
4. Mahida JB, Asti L, Deans KJ, et al. Laparoscopic pyloromyotomy decreases postoperative length of stay in children with hypertrophic pyloric stenosis. *J Pediatr Surg.* 2016;51(9):1436–1439.
5. Peters B, Oomen MWN, Bakx R, et al. Advances in infantile hypertrophic pyloric stenosis. *Expert Rev Gastroenterol Hepatol.* 2014;8(5):533–541.
6. Sullivan KJ, Chan E, Vincent J, et al; for the Canadian Association of Paediatric Surgeons Evidence-Based Resource. Feeding post-pyloromyotomy: a meta-analysis. *Pediatrics.* 2016;137(1).

CODES

ICD10

Q40.0 Congenital hypertrophic pyloric stenosis

CLINICAL PEARLS

- Pyloric stenosis is the most common condition requiring surgical intervention in the 1st year of life.
- The condition classically presents between 1 and 5 months of life, with projectile vomiting after feeds and a firm, mobile mass in the right upper quadrant.
- Abdominal US is the study of choice.
- Surgery (laparoscopic Ramstedt pyloromyotomy is the preferred method) is curative, but conservative medical management with atropine can be safe and effective as well.

RAPE CRISIS SYNDROME

Ulunma Natalie Umesi, MD, MBA • Frantz Aubry, MD • Ambreka Benons, MD

 BASICS

- Known also as rape trauma syndrome
- Refers to trauma following sexual assault
- May be experienced by all sexual and gender identities

DESCRIPTION

- Definitions (vary by jurisdiction on local, state, and national levels):
  - Rape (a legal term), sexual assault (a medical term), or sexual violence (a general term): any form of sexual activity that occurs without consent between a victim and perpetrator(s)/suspect(s)
  - Rape/sexual assault/sexual violence: may be associated with the use of force and/or threats, alcohol, and/or illicit and/or prescription drugs
  - Rape crisis syndrome is a historical term that has previously been used to define what is now known as the following, differentiated by time lapsed since the inciting event:
  - Acute stress reaction (ASR)—up to 3 days following event (no longer recognized in *DSM*)
  - Acute stress disorder (ASD)—3 days to 1 month following event (*DSM-5*)
  - Posttraumatic stress disorder (PTSD)—>1 month following event (*DSM-5*)
- Psychological responses to sexual violence range from transient to chronic and debilitating.

EPIDEMIOLOGY

- In the United States, 33% of women and 25% of men have reported experiencing sexual violence during their lifetime.
- The following populations are especially vulnerable:
  - Adolescents and young children
  - Persons with disabilities
  - Elderly adults
  - Those with a low socioeconomic status and/or that are homeless
  - Sex workers and persons being trafficked
  - People living in institutions/areas of conflict/ training environments
- 33% of female victims first experienced sexual violence before age of 18 years; 13% first experienced it before age of 10 years
- 25% of male victims first experienced sexual violence before age of 18 years; 25% first experienced it before age of 10 years
- Only 16–38% of victims report to law enforcement, and only 17–43% of victims obtain a medical evaluation.

RISK FACTORS

- History of sexual violence, psychological aggression, physical violence, trafficking, and/or stalking
- Early initiation of sexual activity
- Engagement in high-risk sexual behavior
- Exposure to familial and/or environmental violence
- Consumption of alcohol/use of illicit drugs
- Belief in traditional gender roles

GENERAL PREVENTION

- Primary prevention: Promoting gender equality, teaching skills to prevent sexual violence, empowering and supporting females, and creating protective environments decrease the occurrence of sexual violence perpetration.

- Secondary prevention:
  - HARK screening tool, which includes questions that assess if a patient has felt humiliated (H) and/or afraid (A), and been raped (R) and/or kicked (K) within the past year, is 81% sensitive and 95% specific for intimate partner violence as well as clinically useful (1).

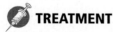 **DIAGNOSIS**

History and/or objective physical exam findings concerning for sexual violence

HISTORY

- Medical and forensic histories and exams should ideally be performed by providers with specialized training in providing medical and forensic care (e.g., Sexual Assault Nurse Examiners [SANEs]) who should be willing to testify in court on behalf of the patient, if indicated.
- States usually require the completion of specific forms for documenting the history of a victim and/or suspect/perpetrator of sexual violence.
- Use a trauma-informed approach to patient care in order to help prevent retraumatization by incorporating the "four Rs" (1): (i) realizing the widespread impact of trauma; (ii) recognizing signs and symptoms of trauma; (iii) responding by integrating knowledge about trauma into practices, procedures, and policies; and (iv) resisting retraumatization (2)
- Avoid questioning that may imply that a patient is at fault and/or be interpreted as investigative.
- Inquire about patient safety.
- Record answers in the patient's own words, and request clarification on unclear terminology.
- Describe all types of physical trauma and sexual contact and whether it was actual/attempted and with/without use of force.
- Inquire about any alcohol and/or illicit drug use before and/or after the episode of sexual violence.
- Document the time of occurrence of activities that could potentially alter biologic specimens (e.g., taking a bath or shower, using a douche or mouthwash, brushing teeth, eating/drinking, and/or changing clothes).
- Obtain a thorough gynecologic history, including the LMP, last consenting sexual contact, last use of contraception, and prior surgeries.
- Inquire about a recent history of strangulation.
  - If positive, advise obtaining angiographic neck imaging (e.g., a CT angiogram [CTA]) to assess for a potential carotid artery dissection, embolus, hematoma, and/or edema around the larynx and/or trachea.

PHYSICAL EXAM

- Request for exams to be performed by SANEs, if available.
- Document all atypical physical findings and/or signs concerning for sexual and/or physical trauma.
- Document the patient's mental status and emotional state during the exam.
- In patients with a recent history of strangulation, examine the patient's scalp, eyes, eyelids, ears, face, oropharynx, neck, and chest; and assess for any neurologic, respiratory, voice, and throat-related changes.

- Obtain the patient's consent prior to each step of the examination, as it is both mandatory and empowering to patients.
- Pending the patient's preferences, may obtain confidential medical photographs (i.e., on a secure digital camera that is reserved solely for use on this unique patient population) prior to swabbing and physically examining the patient
- May use a UV light (Wood lamp) and orange-tinted forensic goggles to detect biologic specimens on clothing and/or skin prior to swabbing and physically examining the patient

ALERT

- A medical and forensic SAFE Kit (previously referred to as a "rape kit") contains sterile cotton swabs that can be used to collect biologic specimens from the oropharyngeal cavity, anogenital regions, and other bodily sites as clinically indicated.
- Perform a complete oropharyngeal, genital, and rectal exam and assess for physical signs concerning for physical and sexual trauma, blood and/or other biologic fluids, and/or foreign objects.
  - Use a nonlubricated, water-moistened speculum for patients with a vagina.
  - Perform testing and/or collect biologic specimens as indicated based on the patient's history and physical exam.

DIAGNOSTIC TESTS & INTERPRETATION

- Pregnancy test
- Drug and/or alcohol testing as indicated
- Testing for sexually transmitted infections (STIs) is medically indicated but not required prior to prescribing treatment.

Follow-Up Tests & Special Considerations

- Screen for safety following treatment, including suicidality.
- Counsel regarding pregnancy or transmission of STI following sexual assault.

TREATMENT

GENERAL MEASURES

- Employ enhanced sensitivity and privacy measures as well as a trauma-informed care approach.
- All cases of sexual violence must be reported immediately to the appropriate law enforcement agency.
- With a victim's permission, enlist the help of personnel from local support agencies (e.g., sexual violence/"rape crisis" support centers) and in-house social services (e.g., SANEs, victim advocates, sexual assault response and care coordinators, sexual assault care providers, behavioral health specialists, and chaplains).
- Sensitivity of treatment may be best executed with the use of a designated Sexual Assault Response Team (SART).
  - National Sexual Violence Resource Center offers both free and certificate courses (3).
- Discuss risks of STI exposure and test/treat as indicated.
- Evaluate for psychological sequelae, and refer for a further evaluation and treatment by behavioral health specialists.

MEDICATION

First Line

- Empirically and prophylactically, treat STIs (especially gonorrhea, chlamydia, trichomoniasis, bacterial vaginosis, hepatitis B, and human papillomavirus [HPV]), as well as considering treatment for human immunodeficiency virus (HIV) and syphilis, depending on a patient's level of risk (4). Cultures are not required before treatment.
- Gonorrhea: (adult dosing) (i) weight <150 kg: ceftriaxone 500 mg IM single dose, (ii) weight ≥150 kg: ceftriaxone 1 g IM single dose; (pediatric dosing) (i) weight ≤45 kg: ceftriaxone 25 to 50 mg/kg IV or IM single dose (not to exceed 250 mg), (ii) weight >45 kg: refer to adult dosing.
- Chlamydia: (adult dosing) azithromycin 1 g PO single dose, or doxycycline 100 mg PO BID for 7 days, or levofloxacin 500 mg PO daily for 7 days; (pediatric dosing) (i) age ≥8 years: azithromycin 1 g PO single dose, or doxycycline 100 mg PO BID for 7 days, (ii) age <8 years with weight ≥45 kg: azithromycin 1 g PO single dose, (iii) age <8 years with weight <45 kg: erythromycin base or ethylsuccinate 50 mg/kg/day PO divided into 4 doses daily for 14 days
- Trichomoniasis: (adult and pediatric dosing) (i) men: metronidazole or tinidazole 2 g PO single dose, (ii) women: metronidazole 500 mg BID for 7 days, or tinidazole 2 g PO single dose
- Bacterial vaginosis: (adult and pediatric dosing) metronidazole 500 mg PO BID for 7 days, or metronidazole gel 0.75% 5 g (one full applicator) intravaginally daily for 5 days, or clindamycin cream 2% 5 g (one full applicator) intravaginally nightly for 7 days
- HIV: postexposure prophylaxis (nPEP) for victims with a high-risk of HIV exposure (e.g., the suspect/perpetrator's HIV status is positive and/or history is positive for IV drug use)
  - nPEP options: (5)
    - Tenofovir disoproxil fumarate (Viread) 300 mg PO daily with emtricitabine (Truvada) 200 mg PO daily for 28 days plus
    - Raltegravir (Isentress) 400 mg PO BID or dolutegravir (Tivicay) 50 mg PO daily for 28 days
    - Pregnant: Dolutegravir should be cautiously prescribed, especially during the first 28 days, given the potential risk of congenital neural tube defects; recommend consulting an infectious disease (ID) provider.
    - Nonpregnant women: nPEP should be cautiously prescribed in nonpregnant women of childbearing age who are effectively using birth control.
    - Children (aged ≤12 years): Consult an ID provider.
  - Treatment is most effective if started within 4 hours of an episode of sexual assault and can reduce HIV transmission by ~80%; it is unlikely to be beneficial, if started after 72 hours.
- Hepatitis B: hepatitis B immunoglobulin 0.06 mL/kg IM single dose and initiate a 3 dose-total hepatitis B virus immunization series
  - No treatment if the victim has received a complete hepatitis B vaccine series and has documented levels of immunity.
- HPV: HPV vaccination is recommended for all victims between 9 and 26 years of age and may be considered after shared clinical decision-making in victims between 27 and 45 years of age. Administer 1st dose at initial exam.
- Syphilis: Patients with a high-risk of contracting syphilis may be treated with benzathine penicillin G 2.4 million units IM single dose.

Pregnancy Considerations

Discuss termination-related options listed in order of increasing effectiveness (6).

- Levonorgestrel 0.75 mg PO q12h × 2 doses (Plan B) or 1.5 mg PO single dose (Plan B One-Step); effective up to 72 hours
- Ulipristal acetate (Ella) 30 mg PO single dose; lacks a hormonal component; effective up to 120 hours; preferred for use in overweight and obese
- Copper IUD (Paragard) 313.4 mg IU single device; lacks a hormonal component; effective up to 120 hours

ADMISSION, INPATIENT, AND NURSING CONSIDERATIONS

Patients expressing suicidal or homicidal ideation meet criteria for inpatient psychiatric admission

 ONGOING CARE

FOLLOW-UP RECOMMENDATIONS

Patient Monitoring

Follow-up medical care:

- 1 to 2 weeks: counseling, pregnancy and gonorrhea and chlamydia retesting, and vaginitis assessment
- 6, 12, and 24 weeks: syphilis and HIV retesting
- 4 to 8 weeks: HPV anogenital wart assessment

DIET

Higher prevalence in disordered eating following sexual assault in female victims of younger age

PATIENT EDUCATION

Provide community resources for support.

COMPLICATIONS

- PTSD
- MDD

REFERENCES

1. Nelson HD, Bougatsos C, Blazina I. *Screening Women for Intimate Partner Violence and Elderly and Vulnerable Adults for Abuse: Systematic Review to Update the 2004 U.S. Preventive Services Task Force Recommendation*. Rockville, MD: Agency for Healthcare Research and Quality; 2012. Evidence synthesis no. 92. AHRQ publication no. 12-05167-EF-1.
2. Ravi A, Little V. Providing trauma-informed care. *Am Fam Physician*. 2017;95(10):655–657.
3. National Sexual Violence Resource Center (NSVRC). National Sexual Violence Resource Center Web site. https://www.nsvrc.org/. Accessed December 5, 2023.
4. Meehan PJ, Rosenstein NE, Gillen M, et al. Responding to detection of aerosolized Bacillus anthracis by autonomous detection systems in the workplace. *MMWR Recomm Rep*. 2004;53(RR-7):1–12.
5. Centers for Disease Control and Prevention, U.S. Department of Health and Human Services. *Updated Guidelines for Antiretroviral Postexposure Prophylaxis After Sexual, Injection Drug Use, or Other Nonoccupational Exposure to HIV—United States, 2016*. Atlanta, GA: U.S. Department of Health and Human Services; 2016.
6. Cheng L, Che Y, Gülmezoglu AM. Interventions for emergency contraception. *Cochrane Database Syst Rev*. 2012;(8):CD001324.

 CODES

ICD10

- T74.21XA Adult sexual abuse, confirmed, initial encounter
- T74.22XA Child sexual abuse, confirmed, initial encounter
- Z04.41 Encounter for exam and obs following alleged adult rape

CLINICAL PEARLS

- Employ enhanced sensitivity and privacy measures, as well as a trauma-informed care approach, when providing care.
- All cases of sexual violence must be reported immediately to the appropriate law enforcement agency.

RAYNAUD PHENOMENON

Kelsey E. Phelps, MD

BASICS

DESCRIPTION
- Idiopathic intermittent episodes of vasoconstriction of digital arteries, precapillary arterioles, and cutaneous arteriovenous shunts in response to cold, emotional stress, or blunt trauma
  - A triphasic color change of the fingers (occasionally the toes, rarely nipples) is the principal physical manifestation.
    - The initial color is *white* from extreme pallor, then *blue* from cyanosis, and finally with warming/vasodilatation, the skin appears *red*.
    - Thumbs are rarely involved.
  - Swelling, throbbing, and paresthesias are associated symptoms.
  - Primary
    - 80% of patients have primary disease.
    - Episodes are bilateral and nonprogressive.
    - Diagnosis confirmed if after 2 years of symptoms, no underlying connective tissue disease develops
  - Secondary
    - Progressive and asymmetric
    - Vascular spasm is more frequent and more severe over time. Ulceration is rare; gangrene does not develop; 13% progress to digital fat pad atrophy and ischemic fingertip changes.
    - Typically associated with an underlying connective tissue disorder
- System(s) affected: hematologic, lymphatic, immunologic, musculoskeletal, dermatologic, exocrine

Pregnancy Considerations
- Raynaud phenomenon can appear as breast pain in lactating women.
- Positive breast milk bacterial culture distinguishes mastitis from Raynaud phenomenon.

Geriatric Considerations
Initial appearance of Raynaud phenomenon after age 40 years suggests underlying connective tissue disease.

Pediatric Considerations
Associated with systemic lupus erythematosus (SLE) and scleroderma

EPIDEMIOLOGY
Incidence
- Primary
  - Predominant age: 14 years; ~1/4 begin >40 years
  - Predominant sex: female > male (4:1)
- Secondary
  - Predominant age: >40 years
  - Predominant sex: no gender predilection

Prevalence
- Primary: 3–12% of men; 6–20% of women (based on clinical history)
- Secondary: ~1% of population

ETIOLOGY AND PATHOPHYSIOLOGY
Unknown. Dysregulation of vascular control mechanisms leads to imbalance between vasodilation and vasoconstriction. There is a reduced endothelin-dependent vasodilation activity and an increased vasoconstriction in peripheral vessels by overproduction of endothelin-1. 5-HT$_2$ serotonin receptors may be involved in secondary Raynaud phenomenon. Platelet and blood viscosity abnormalities in secondary disease contribute to ischemic pathology.

Genetics
Some studies suggest dominant inheritance pattern. ~1/4 of patients with primary condition also have a first-degree relative with Raynaud phenomenon.

RISK FACTORS
- Existing autoimmune or connective tissue disorder
- End-stage renal disease with hemodialysis may increase risk if a steal phenomenon develops in association with the arteriovenous shunt.
- Primary and secondary disease associated with elevated homocysteine levels
- Smoking is not associated with increased risk of Raynaud phenomenon but may worsen symptoms.

GENERAL PREVENTION
- Avoid cold exposure.
- Tobacco cessation
- No relationship has been established between Raynaud phenomenon and vibratory tool use.
- Stress and anxiety can trigger attacks.

COMMONLY ASSOCIATED CONDITIONS
Secondary Raynaud
- Scleroderma; SLE; polymyositis
- Sjögren syndrome; occlusive vascular disease
- Cryoglobulinemia

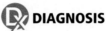

DIAGNOSIS

HISTORY
- Primary
  - Symmetric attacks involving fingers
  - Family history of connective tissue disorder
  - Absence of tissue necrosis, ulceration, or gangrene
  - If after ≥2 years of symptoms, no abnormal clinical or laboratory signs have developed, secondary disease is unlikely.
- Secondary
  - Onset typically after 40 years of age
  - Asymmetric episodes more intense and painful
  - Arthritis, myalgias, fever, dry eyes and/or mouth, rash, or cardiopulmonary symptoms
  - History of medication and/or recreational drug use
  - Exposure to toxic agents
  - Repetitive trauma

PHYSICAL EXAM
Pallor (whiteness) of fingertips with cold exposure, then cyanosis (blue), and then redness and pain with warming
- Ischemic attacks evidenced by demarcated or cyanotic skin limited to digits; usually starts on one digit and spreads symmetrically to remaining fingers of both hands. The thumb is typically spared.
- Rarely involves other tissues (e.g., tongue) (1),(2)
- Beau lines: transverse linear depressions in nail plate on most or all fingernails that occurs after exposure to cold or any insult that disrupts normal nail growth
- Livedo reticularis: mottling of the skin of the arms and legs; benign and reverses with warming
- Primary
  - Normal physical exam
  - Nail bed capillaries have normal appearance: Place 1 drop of type B immersion oil on skin at base of fingernail and view capillaries with handheld ophthalmoscope at 10 to 40 diopters.

- Secondary
  - Skin changes, arthritis, and abnormal lung findings suggest connective tissue disease.
  - Ischemic skin lesions: ulceration of finger pads (autoamputation in severe, prolonged cases)
  - Nail bed capillary distortion including giant loops, avascular areas, and increased tortuosity
  - Abnormal Allen test (Have patient open and close hand several times and then tightly into a fist. Sequentially occlude the ulnar and radial arteries while the patient opens hand to reveal the return of color as a measure of circulation.)

DIFFERENTIAL DIAGNOSIS
- Thromboangiitis obliterans (Buerger disease): primarily affects men; smoking related
- Rheumatoid arthritis (RA)
- Progressive systemic sclerosis (scleroderma): Raynaud phenomenon precedes other symptoms.
- SLE
- Carpal tunnel syndrome; thoracic outlet syndrome
- Hypothyroidism
- CREST syndrome (calcinosis cutis, Raynaud phenomenon, esophageal dysmotility, sclerodactyly, and telangiectasias)
- Cryoglobulinemia; Waldenström macroglobulinemia
- Acrocyanosis
- Polycythemia
- Occupational (e.g., especially from vibrating tools, masonry work, exposure to polyvinyl chloride)
- Drug induced (e.g., clonidine, ergotamine, methysergide, amphetamines, bromocriptine, bleomycin, vinblastine, cisplatin, cyclosporine)

DIAGNOSTIC TESTS & INTERPRETATION
Provocative test (e.g., ice water immersion) unnecessary
- Primary
  - Antinuclear antibody: negative
  - ESR: normal
- Secondary
  - Tests for secondary causes (e.g., CBC, ESR)
  - Positive autoantibody has low positive predictive value for connective tissue disease (30%).
  - Antibodies to specific autoantigens (e.g., scleroderma with anticentromere or antitopoisomerase antibodies)
  - Nailfold videocapillaroscopy is gold standard (200 times magnification).

Follow-Up Tests & Special Considerations
Periodic assessments for a connective tissue disorder

Diagnostic Procedures/Other
Diagnosis is determined by history and physical exam.

TREATMENT

Assess using a Raynaud Condition Score.

GENERAL MEASURES
- Dress warmly, wear gloves, avoid cold temperatures.
- During attacks, rotate the arms in a windmill pattern or place the hands under warm water or in a warm body fold to alleviate symptoms.
- Tobacco cessation

- Avoid β-blockers, amphetamines, ergot alkaloids, OTC medications containing pseudoephedrine, and sumatriptan.
- Temperature-related biofeedback may help patients increase hand temperature. 1-year follow-up is no better than control.
- Finger guards to protect ulcerated fingertips
- Recognition and avoidance of stressful situations

MEDICATION

First Line

- Calcium channel blockers (CCBs); nifedipine is the best studied and most frequently used. 30 to 180 mg/day (sustained-release form); seasonal (winter) use is effective with up to 75% of patients experiencing improvement.
- Compatible with breastfeeding
- Contraindications: allergy to drug, pregnancy, CHF
- Precautions: may cause headache, dizziness, light-headedness, edema, or hypotension
- Significant possible interactions
  – Increases serum level of digoxin

Second Line

- Amlodipine (5 to 10 mg/day) and nicardipine are effective and may have fewer adverse effects.
- No data exist to support switching CCB if initial drug is ineffective.
- Small studies support benefit from losartan and fluoxetine.
- Phosphodiesterase type 5 inhibitors (sildenafil, vardenafil) may reduce symptoms without increasing blood flow.
- Parenteral iloprost, a prostacyclin, in low doses (0.5 ng/kg/min over 6 hours), has improved ulcerations with severe Raynaud phenomenon when CCBs failed. Oral prostacyclin has not proven useful.
- Nitroglycerin patches may be helpful, but use is limited by the incidence of severe headache. Nitroglycerin gel has shown promise as a topical therapy.
- Topical sildenafil cream may also improve digital arterial blood flow in patients with secondary Raynaud phenomenon (3).
- Prazosin (1 to 2 mg TID) is the only well-studied α1-adrenergic receptor blocker with modest effect; adverse effects may outweigh any benefit.
- ACE inhibitors are no longer recommended.

ISSUES FOR REFERRAL

If an underlying disease is suspected, consider rheumatology consultation for evaluation and treatment.

ADDITIONAL THERAPIES

- Botulinum toxin has shown promising evidence in the treatment of primary Raynaud phenomenon as well as systemic sclerosis-associated Raynaud phenomenon, including treatment of ischemic ulcers (4).
- Aspirin

- Digital or wrist block with lidocaine or bupivacaine (without epinephrine) for pain control
- Short-term anticoagulation with heparin if persistent critical ischemia, evidence of large-artery occlusive disease, or both

SURGERY/OTHER PROCEDURES

Surgical intervention is rare in Raynaud phenomenon. Effect of cervical sympathectomy is transient; symptoms return in 1 to 2 years. Digital fat grafting is a novel modality that has shown improved symptomatology.

COMPLEMENTARY & ALTERNATIVE MEDICINE

- *Ginkgo biloba* with unclear benefit
- Fish oil supplements may increase digital systolic pressure and time to onset of symptoms after exposure to cold; not proven in controlled trials
- Vitamin D supplementation led to improvement in self-reported symptoms in vitamin D–deficient patients with Raynaud phenomenon (5)[B].
- Evening primrose oil reduced severity of attacks in one study.
- Oral arginine is no better than placebo.
- Acupuncture and acupressure found to be helpful in symptom reduction, but studies have been small and evidence is not statistically significant (6).
- Traditional Chinese medicine (TCM) may have a positive effect on primary Raynaud phenomenon, but evidence is inconclusive due to weak methodology (7).
- Biofeedback is not likely helpful.

 ## ONGOING CARE

FOLLOW-UP RECOMMENDATIONS

Avoid exposure to cold; reassess for secondary causes.

Patient Monitoring

Manage fingertip ulcers and rapidly treat infection.

DIET

No special diet

PATIENT EDUCATION

- Tobacco cessation
- Avoid triggers (e.g., trauma, vibration, cold).
- Dress warmly; wear gloves.
- Warm hands when experiencing vasospasm.

PROGNOSIS

- Attacks may last from several minutes to a few hours.
- 2/3 of attacks resolve spontaneously.
- ~13% of Raynaud phenomenon patients develop a secondary disorder, typically connective tissue diseases.

COMPLICATIONS

- Primary: very rare
- Secondary: gangrene, autoamputation of fingertips

REFERENCES

1. Wigley FM, Flavahan NA. Raynaud's phenomenon. *N Engl J Med*. 2016;375(6):556–565.
2. Devgire V, Hughes M. Raynaud's phenomenon. *Br J Hosp Med (Lond)*. 2019;80(11):658–664.
3. Wortsman X, Del Barrio-Díaz P, Meza-Romero R, et al. Nifedipine cream versus sildenafil cream for patients with secondary Raynaud phenomenon: a randomized, double-blind, controlled pilot study. *J Am Acad Dermatol*. 2018;78(1):189–190.
4. Ennis D, Ahmad Z, Anderson MA, et al. Botulinum toxin in the management of primary and secondary Raynaud's phenomenon. *Best Pract Res Clin Rheumatol*. 2021;35(3):101684.
5. Hélou J, Moutran R, Maatouk I, et al. Raynaud's phenomenon and vitamin D. *Rheumatol Int*. 2013;33(3):751–755.
6. Gladue H, Berrocal V, Harris R, et al. A randomized controlled trial of acupressure for the treatment of Raynaud's phenomenon: the difficulty of conducting a trial in Raynaud's phenomenon. *J Scleroderma Relat Disord*. 2016;1(2):226–233.
7. Zhang J, Hu J, He X, et al. Effectiveness of Chinese herbal medicine for primary Raynaud's phenomenon: a systematic review and meta-analysis of randomized controlled trials. *J Tradit Chin Med*. 2020;40(4):509–517.

ADDITIONAL READING

Herrick AL. Evidence-based management of Raynaud's phenomenon. *Ther Adv Musculoskelet Dis*. 2017;9(12):317–329.

 ## SEE ALSO

Algorithm: Raynaud Phenomenon

CODES

ICD10

- I73.00 Raynaud's syndrome without gangrene
- I73.01 Raynaud's syndrome with gangrene

CLINICAL PEARLS

- Raynaud phenomenon is a clinical diagnosis.
- Provocative testing is not recommended.
- Initial presentation of Raynaud phenomenon after age 40 years suggests underlying (secondary) disease.
- Cold avoidance and stress reduction are foundational in treating Raynaud phenomenon.
- Digital ulcers are not normal and always merit a workup for secondary disease.
- Acute digital ischemia is a medical emergency.

REACTIVE ARTHRITIS (REITER SYNDROME)

Laura Marsh, MD, CAQSM

 BASICS

Reiter syndrome is a seronegative, multisystem, inflammatory disorder classically involving joints, the eye, the lower genitourinary (GU) tract, and the skin. It is an inflammatory arthritis that is triggered by an infection, usually in the gastrointestinal or GU tract. Lower limb joint, axial joint (e.g., spine, sacroiliac joints), and dermatologic manifestations are common (1)[C].

DESCRIPTION

The classic triad includes arthritis, conjunctivitis/iritis, and either urethritis or cervicitis ("can't see," "can't pee," "can't bend my knee"). The diagnosis is primarily clinical, and there are no formal diagnostic criteria.

- The epidemiology is similar to other reactive arthritides, typically characterized by sterile joint inflammation associated with infections originating at nonarticular sites. Active *Chlamydia* spp. have been detected in the joint fluid of some affected patients, although this is not the norm. A fourth feature (dermatologic involvement) may include buccal ulceration, balanitis, or a psoriasiform skin eruption. (Having only two features does not rule out the diagnosis.)
- Two forms of Reiter syndrome:
  - Sexually transmitted: Symptoms emerge 7 to 14 days after exposure to *Chlamydia trachomatis* and other sexually acquired pathogens.
  - Postenteric infection (including traveler's diarrhea)
- In individuals with new or frequent sexual partners, the triggering infection is likely sexually transmitted (rather than enteric). The infection has often been cleared by the time rheumatic symptoms appear, and genital chlamydia is often asymptomatic.
- In individuals with a history of recent enteric illness, the triggering event is more likely to be a bacterial enteric infection rather than sexual transmission.
- System(s) affected: musculoskeletal, renal/urologic, dermatologic/exocrine
- Synonym(s): idiopathic blennorrheal arthritis; arthritis urethritica; urethro-oculo-synovial syndrome; Fiessinger-Leroy-Reiter disease; reactive arthritis

Pediatric Considerations
Juvenile rheumatoid arthritis (RA) has many of the same clinical features as Reiter syndrome.

Pregnancy Considerations
No special considerations; usual drug precautions

EPIDEMIOLOGY
- Predominant age: 20 to 40 years
- Predominant sex: male > female

Incidence
- 0.2–1% incidence after bacterial dysentery outbreaks
- Complicates 1–2% of nongonococcal urethritis cases

Prevalence
~3–5 cases per 100,000 individuals per year

ETIOLOGY AND PATHOPHYSIOLOGY
- The pathophysiology of all the seronegative reactive arthritis syndromes and the immunologic role of infectious diseases as precipitants for clinical illness are incompletely understood.
- Proinflammatory cytokines lead to synovitis. Toll-like receptors (TLRs) have been implicated in the recognition of gram-negative lipopolysaccharide as part of the disease cascade.
- The role of HLA-B27 is incompletely understood, but there is an increased risk of developing reactive arthritis if patients are HLA-B27–positive. In these patients, the disease is more likely to be severe and longer lasting.
- Avoiding precipitant infections and early management of multiorgan inflammation is important.
- *C. trachomatis* is the most common sexually transmitted infection associated with Reiter syndrome.
- Dysentery-associated Reiter syndrome follows infection with *Shigella, Salmonella, Yersinia*, and *Campylobacter* spp. Enteric-associated Reiter syndrome is more common in women, children, and the elderly than the postvenereal form.

Genetics
HLA-B27 tissue antigen is present in 60–80% of patients, suggesting a genetic predisposition.

RISK FACTORS
- New or high-risk sexual contacts 1 to 4 weeks before the onset of clinical presentation; the primary infection may be subclinical and undiagnosed.
- Food poisoning or bacterial dysentery due to travel or incorrectly prepped/stored food

GENERAL PREVENTION
- Avoidance of infectious precipitants is the most important general precaution (and potentially the most difficult to achieve).
- Safe sexual practices; proper food and water hygiene

COMMONLY ASSOCIATED CONDITIONS
- Enteric disease
  - Shigellosis; Salmonellosis; Campylobacteriosis
  - Enteric infection with *Yersinia* spp.
- Urogenital infection
  - *Chlamydia* urethritis/cervicitis (2)
  - *Mycoplasma* or *Ureaplasma* spp.
- HIV/AIDS

DIAGNOSIS
- Clinical presentation with joint, eye, and GU inflammation ("classic triad") and negative serologic testing for rheumatoid factor.
- Classic symptoms are not always present.
- HLA-B27 testing is not required for diagnosis.

HISTORY
The presence of the clinical syndrome plus
- Diarrhea, dysentery, urethritis, or genital discharge and appropriate exposure history
- Exposure risks, including travel or migration history and potential infectious exposure
- Arthritis associated with urethritis for >1 month (84% sensitive; 98% specific for diagnosis)
- Urethritis occurs 1 to 15 days after sexual exposure.
- Reiter syndrome onset within 10 to 30 days of either enteric infection or STI
- Mean duration of symptoms is 19 weeks.

PHYSICAL EXAM
- Musculoskeletal
  - Asymmetric arthritis (especially knees, ankles, and metatarsophalangeal joints)
  - Enthesopathy (inflammation at tendinous insertion into bone, such as plantar fasciitis, digital periostitis, polydactylitis and Achilles tendinitis)
  - Spondyloarthropathy (spine and sacroiliac joint involvement)
- Urogenital tract
  - Urethritis; prostatitis; cystitis (rare)
  - Balanitis
  - Cervicitis: usually asymptomatic
- Eye
  - Conjunctivitis of one or both eyes
  - Occasionally, scleritis, keratitis, and corneal ulceration
  - Rarely, uveitis and iritis
- Skin
  - Mucocutaneous lesions (small, painless superficial ulcers on oral mucosa, tongue, or glans penis)
  - Keratoderma blennorrhagica (hyperkeratotic skin lesions of palms and soles and around nails—can be mistaken for psoriasis)
- Cardiovascular: occasionally, pericarditis, murmur, conduction defects, and aortic incompetence
- Nervous system: rarely, peripheral neuropathy, cranial neuropathy, meningoencephalitis, and neuropsychiatric changes
- Constitutional
  - Fever, malaise, anorexia, and weight loss
  - Patient can appear seriously ill (e.g., fever, rigors, tachycardia, and exquisitely tender joints).

DIFFERENTIAL DIAGNOSIS
- Seropositive arthritides: RA and others
- Ankylosing spondylitis
- Arthritis associated with inflammatory bowel disease
- Psoriatic arthritis
- Juvenile RA
- Bacterial arthritis, including gonococcal
- Rheumatic fever

DIAGNOSTIC TESTS & INTERPRETATION

- Blood
  - Negative rheumatoid factor
  - Leukocyte count: 10,000 to 20,000 cells/mm³
  - Neutrophil predominance
  - Elevated ESR and/or CRP
  - Moderate normochromic, normocytic anemia
  - Hypergammaglobulinemia
- Synovial fluid
  - Leukocyte count: 1,000 to 8,000 cells/mm³
  - Bacterial culture negative
  - Crystals negative
- Supportive tests
  - Cultures, antigens, or PCR positive for *C. trachomatis* or stool test positive for *Salmonella*, *Shigella*, *Yersinia*, or *Campylobacter* spp.
  - HIV serology positive (acute retroviral syndrome)
  - HLA-B27 histocompatibility antigen is positive in 60–80% of cases in non–HIV-related Reiter syndrome; HLA testing is not required or recommended for diagnosis.
  - Rheumatoid factor is negative.
  - Screening for STI if indicated
  - Screening for enteric infections is rarely useful and generally not indicated.
- X-ray
  - Periosteal proliferation, thickening
  - Articular bony spurs; erosions at articular margins
  - Joint space narrowing
  - Soft tissue swelling
  - Syndesmophytes (spine); sacroiliitis

Test Interpretation

- Villous formation within joints; hyperemia, and inflammation
- Prostatitis and seminal vesiculitis
- Skin biopsy similar to psoriasis

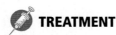 TREATMENT

GENERAL MEASURES

Treatment is determined by symptoms.

- Conjunctivitis does not require specific treatment.
- Iritis requires treatment.
- Mucocutaneous lesions do not require treatment.
- Physical therapy (PT) aids recovery.
- Arthritis may become prominent and disabling during the acute phase.

MEDICATION

First Line

- Symptomatic management:
  - NSAIDs, including indomethacin, naproxen, and others
    - Contraindications
      - GI bleeding
      - Peptic ulcer, gastritis, or ulcerative colitis
      - Renal insufficiency

- Intra-articular or systemic corticosteroids for refractory arthritis and enteritis
- Specific treatment of isolated microorganism:
  - *C. trachomatis*: doxycycline 100 mg PO BID for 7 to 14 days (*Note*: All STIs should be treated whether associated with Reiter syndrome or not.)
  - *Salmonella*, *Shigella*, *Yersinia*, and *Campylobacter* infections: ciprofloxacin 500 mg PO BID for 5 to 10 days (*Note*: Emerging antimicrobial resistance will limit the utility of ciprofloxacin. Antibiotic treatment does not reduce GI symptoms or duration of infection or prevent carrier state [Salmonella only]).
  - Antibiotic treatment following onset of syndrome does not appear to benefit inflammatory joint, eye, or urinary tract symptoms, but it may be needed for the triggering infection.
- GI upset: antacids
- Iritis: intraocular steroids
- Keratitis: topical steroids

Second Line

- Sulfasalazine is promising but not FDA-approved.
- Methotrexate or azathioprine in severe cases (experimental, not approved or known to be effective); immunosuppressive therapy is relatively contraindicated in HIV-related Reiter syndrome.
- Specialty consultation is recommended, particularly if considering immunomodulatory agents such as sulfasalazine, methotrexate, or azathioprine or for treatment with anti-TNF medications (etanercept and infliximab), which have shown benefit in isolated case reports.
- No published evidence supports the beneficial effect of antibiotics on the long-term outcome in patients with Reiter syndrome.

ISSUES FOR REFERRAL

Joint and eye complications; complex cases—consider consultation with rheumatology; ophthalmology

ADMISSION, INPATIENT, AND NURSING CONSIDERATIONS

- Based on severity of disease and associated complications
- Inpatient care may be needed during acute phase.

 ONGOING CARE

FOLLOW-UP RECOMMENDATIONS

Activity modification until joint inflammation subsides.

Patient Monitoring

Monitor clinical response to anti-inflammatory medications. Observe for complications, particularly with sulfasalazine and immunosuppressive drugs.

PATIENT EDUCATION

- Educate on risk factors for exposure and recurrence.
- Home PT program
- National Institute of Arthritis and Musculoskeletal and Skin Diseases: https://www.niams.nih.gov/

PROGNOSIS

Acute reactive arthritis typically lasts from 3 to 5 months. Approximately 25% of patients develop chronic reactive arthritis (longer than 6 months). Patients may develop secondary arthritis in the peripheral joints. Prognosis is poor in cases involving the heel, eye, or heart.

COMPLICATIONS

- Chronic or recurrent disease in 5–50% of patients
- Ankylosing spondylitis develops in 30–50% of patients who test positive for HLA-B27 antigen.
- Urethral strictures
- Cataracts and blindness
- Aortic root necrosis

REFERENCES

1. Schmitt SK. Reactive arthritis. *Infect Dis Clin North Am.* 2017;31(2):265–277.
2. Jubber A, Moorthy A. Reactive Arthritis: a clinical review. *J R Coll Physicians Edinb.* 2021;51(3):288–297.

 SEE ALSO

Ankylosing Spondylitis; Arthritis, Psoriatic; Behçet Syndrome

CODES

ICD10

- M02.30 Reiter's disease, unspecified site
- M02.39 Reiter's disease, multiple sites

CLINICAL PEARLS

- Diagnosis of reactive arthritis is based on the clinical presentation of the classic triad of joint, eye, and GU inflammation and negative serologic testing for rheumatoid factor (signs and symptoms may not all be present at the same time).
- Screen for STI (including HIV) if sexually acquired. Enteric studies are rarely clinically indicated.
- Refer patients with a chronic or recurrent course and those who have clinical complications.
- Treatment focuses on symptom relief and treating any underlying infection.

RENALTUBULAR ACIDOSIS

Mark B. Stephens, MD, MS, FAAFP • Lewjain Sakr, MD

BASICS

DESCRIPTION
- Renal tubular acidosis (RTA) is a group of disorders characterized by an inability of the kidney to resorb bicarbonate (HCO_3)/secrete hydrogen ions, resulting in normal anion gap metabolic acidosis. Renal function must be normal or near normal.
- Several types have been identified:
  - Type I (distal) RTA: inability of the distal tubule to acidify the urine due to impaired hydrogen ion secretion, increased back leak of secreted hydrogen ions, or impaired sodium reabsorption; urine pH >5.5
  - Type II (proximal) RTA: defect of the proximal tubule in HCO_3 reabsorption; proximal tubular HCO_3 reabsorption is absent; plasma HCO_3 concentration stabilizes at 12 to 18 mEq/L due to compensatory distal HCO_3 reabsorption; urine pH <5.5
  - Type III RTA: extremely rare autosomal recessive syndrome with associated osteopetrosis, cerebral calcification, and intellectual disability.
  - Type IV RTA (hypoaldosteronism): due to aldosterone resistance/deficiency that results in hyperkalemia; urine pH is usually <5.5.

EPIDEMIOLOGY
Incidence
Predominant sex: male > female (with regard to type II RTA with isolated defect in HCO_3 reabsorption)

ETIOLOGY AND PATHOPHYSIOLOGY
- Type I RTA—caused by conditions and medications that impair adequate urine acidification at the distal tubule:
  - Autoimmune diseases: Sjögren syndrome, rheumatoid arthritis (RA), systemic lupus erythematosus (SLE), thyroiditis
  - Medications: amphotericin B, lithium, ifosfamide, foscarnet, triamterene, trimethoprim, pentamidine; obstructive uropathy (hyperkalemic); genetic inheritance (see below); other familial disorders: Ehlers-Danlos syndrome, glycogenosis type III, Fabry disease, Wilson disease; hematologic diseases: sickle cell disease (hyperkalemic), hereditary elliptocytosis; toxins: toluene, glue
  - Incomplete distal RTA—a form in which patients are unable to appropriately acidify their urine, however are able to excrete sufficient acid to maintain normal serum HCO_3 and pH (1). Cause and pathophysiology is poorly understood.
  - Voltage-dependent RTA—a form of distal RTA in which the impairment in urine acidification is due to poor delivery of Na^+ to the distal tube, leading to disruption of favorable transepithelial voltage gradient, and retention of K^+ and H^+. This form will lead to hyperkalemia, as opposed to hypokalemia in classic distal RTA (2).
    ○ Amiloride causes voltage-dependent RTA rather than classic distal RTA (2).

- Type II RTA—caused by conditions and medications that impair adequate HCO_3 reabsorption in the proximal convoluted tubule:
  - Genetic inheritance (see below); primary Fanconi syndrome
  - Systemic diseases causing Fanconi syndrome: multiple myeloma and other dysproteinemic states, amyloidosis, paroxysmal nocturnal hemoglobinuria, tubulointerstitial nephritis
  - Medications
    ○ Carbonic anhydrase inhibitors: acetazolamide, methazolamide and dichlorphenamide; chemotherapy agents: ifosfamide, oxaliplatin, cisplatin; antiretroviral medications: tenofovir, didanosine; anticonvulsant medications: topiramate, valproic acid; antibiotics: sulfanilamide, outdated tetracycline, aminoglycosides; other miscellaneous medications: deferasirox, apremilast, heavy metals
  - Familial (cystinosis, tyrosinemia, hereditary fructose intolerance, galactosemia, glycogen storage disease type I, Wilson disease, Lowe syndrome, inherited carbonic anhydrase deficiency)
  - Defects in calcium metabolism (hyperparathyroidism)
- Type IV RTA
  - Medications: NSAIDs, ACE inhibitors, ARBs, heparin/low-molecular-weight (LMW) heparin (hyperkalemia in 5–10% of patients), ketoconazole, tacrolimus, cyclosporine, spironolactone, eplerenone
  - Diabetic nephropathy; tubulointerstitial nephropathies; primary adrenal insufficiency; markedly decreased distal Na^+ delivery; pseudohypoaldosteronism (PHA) (end-organ resistance to aldosterone)

Genetics
- Type I RTA: hereditary forms due to mutations affecting intercalated cells in collecting tubules; loss of function mutations of a chloride-bicarbonate exchanger (AE1) found in the kidney and red blood cells is inherited in autosomal dominant and recessive manners and may be associated with hemolytic anemia, spherocytosis, or ovalocytosis.
- Type II RTA: Autosomal dominant form is extremely rare. Autosomal recessive form is associated with mutation in a basolateral electrogenic sodium-bicarbonate cotransporter (NBCe1) and can be seen with severe growth retardation, ophthalmologic abnormalities, and intellectual disability.
- Type IV RTA: Some cases are familial, such as PHA type I (autosomal dominant).

GENERAL PREVENTION
Careful use/avoidance of causative agents

COMMONLY ASSOCIATED CONDITIONS
- Type I RTA in children: hypercalciuria leading to rickets, nephrocalcinosis
- Type I RTA in adults: autoimmune diseases (Sjögren syndrome, RA, SLE), obstructive uropathy, hypercalciuria

- Type II RTA: Fanconi syndrome (generalized proximal tubular dysfunction resulting in glycosuria, aminoaciduria, hyperuricosuria, phosphaturia, bicarbonaturia)
- Type II RTA in adults: multiple myeloma, carbonic anhydrase inhibitors, aminoglycosides
- Type IV RTA: diabetic nephropathy, solid-organ transplant (due to calcineurin inhibitors)

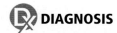

DIAGNOSIS

HISTORY
- Often asymptomatic (particularly type IV); in children: failure to thrive, rickets
- Anorexia, nausea/vomiting, constipation; weakness or polyuria (due to hypokalemia or hypercalciuria)
- Polydipsia; osteomalacia in adults

DIFFERENTIAL DIAGNOSIS
- Plasma anion gap should be normal. If not, evaluate for causes of anion-gap metabolic acidosis: ketoacidosis, ingestions (ASA, methanol, ethylene glycol, propylene glycol), lactic acidosis, D-lactic acidosis, uremia, pyroglutamic acid.
- Extrarenal HCO_3 losses
  - Chronic diarrhea; small bowel, pancreatic, or biliary fistulas; urinary diversion (e.g., ureterosigmoidostomy, ileal conduit)
- Acidosis of chronic renal failure (develops when GFR ≤20 to 30 mL/min)
- Excessive administration of acid load via chloride salts, including dilutional acidosis via normal saline ($NaCl$, HCl, NH_4Cl, lysine HCl, $CaCl_2$, $MgCl_2$)

DIAGNOSTIC TESTS & INTERPRETATION
Initial Tests (lab, imaging)
- Serum chemistries and electrolytes
  - Hyperchloremic metabolic acidosis with a normal anion gap (anion gap = $Na^+ - [Cl^- + HCO_3]$)
  - Plasma potassium:
    ○ Low: in type I RTA (due to impaired distal H^+ secretion/increased H^+ back leak) and type II RTA
    ○ High: in type IV RTA and type I (if due to voltage-dependent RTA)
  - BUN and Cr should be normal/near baseline to rule out renal failure as a cause of acidosis.
  - Electrolyte abnormalities of Fanconi syndrome (hypophosphatemia, hyponatremia, hypoglycemia, hypoproteinemia) may be seen in type II RTA (2).
- Urine studies (2)
  - Urine pH >5.5 in the presence of hyperchloremic metabolic acidosis is strongly suggestive of type I RTA and type II RTA if serum HCO_3^- is above resorptive threshold of distal tubules (12 to 18 mEq/L). Urine pH is typically <5.5 in type IV RTA.

– Urine calcium is typically high in type I RTA (2). Increased fractional excretion of phosphate, uric acid, glucose, amino acids, low molecular weight proteins, and presence of urinary retinol-binding protein 4 (not readily available in most places) are sensitive for type II RTA.

– Urine anion gap (UAG; $U_{Na} + U_K − U_{Cl}$) is inversely related to urine NH_4^+ excretion (NH_4^+ cannot be directly measured in urine). Positive UAG in acidemic patient indicates impaired urine acid excretion and is a sign of types I and IV RTA.

  ○ Accurate UAG requires U_{Na} >25 mEq/L. UAG will also be positive in renal failure, in which acid excretion is impaired. There is a limited utility of UAG in type II RTA, as patients may not have maximal ammonium excretion during acidosis, and UAG may not be appropriately negative.

Pediatric Considerations
Audiogram to evaluate hearing loss or MRI/CT to evaluate presence of enlarged vestibular aqueducts in type I RTA (1)

Pregnancy Considerations
Studies have identified severe acid–base disturbances in pregnant women with inherited type I RTA, who presented with severe hypokalemia and metabolic acidosis.

Diagnostic Procedures/Other
• Helpful to measure urine pH on fresh sample with pH meter for increased accuracy instead of dipstick; pour film of oil over urine to avoid loss of CO_2 if pH cannot be measured quickly.
• HCO_3 loading test is the gold standard for diagnosis for type II RTA. Fractional excretion of HCO_3 >15% during 1 mEq/kg/h HCO_3 infusion is diagnostic of type II RTA. <5% excludes type II RTA (2).

 TREATMENT

MEDICATION
First Line
• Provide oral alkali to raise serum HCO_3 to normal. Start at a low dose and increase until HCO_3 is normal. Give as sodium bicarbonate (HCO_3) (7.7 mEq $NaHCO_3$/650 mg tab), sodium citrate (oral solution, 1 mEq HCO_3 equivalent/mL), sodium/potassium citrate (oral solution), or potassium citrate (tablet, powder, or oral solution: 2 mEq K/mL, 2 mEq HCO_3/mL), depending on need for potassium.
• Type I RTA: typical doses of 1 to 2 mEq/kg/day (in adults), 3 to 4 mEq/kg/day (in children) HCO_3 equivalent divided 3 to 4 times per day (require much higher doses if HCO_3 wasting is present); may require K^+ supplementation
• Type II RTA: typical doses of 10 to 15 mEq/kg/day HCO_3 equivalent, divided 4 to 6 times per day; very difficult to restore plasma HCO_3 to normal, as renal HCO_3 losses increase once plasma HCO_3 is corrected above resorptive threshold; exogenous HCO_3 increases K^+ losses, requiring supplemental K^+; often need supplemental PO_4 and vitamin D due to proximal PO_4 losses

• Type IV RTA: Avoid inciting medications and treat the underlying cause of hypoaldosteronism; restrict dietary K^+. May augment K^+ excretion with loop diuretic, thiazide diuretic, or polystyrene sulfonate (Kayexalate); correcting hyperkalemia increases activity of the urea cycle, augmenting renal ammoniagenesis and adding substrate for renal acid excretion; if necessary, 1 to 5 mEq/kg/day alkali divided 2 to 3 times per day; if mineralocorticoid deficiency, fludrocortisone: 0.1 to 0.3 mg/day
• Precautions
  – Sodium-containing compounds will increase urinary calcium excretion, potentially increasing the risk of nephrolithiasis. Mineralocorticoids and sodium-based alkali may lead to hypertension and/or edema. Aluminum-containing medications (antacids, sucralfate) should be avoided if solutions containing citric acid are prescribed because citric acid increases aluminum absorption. $NaHCO_3$ may cause flatulence because CO_2 is formed, whereas citrate is metabolized to HCO_3 in the liver, avoiding gas production.

Second Line
• Thiazide diuretics may be used as adjunctive therapy in type II RTA (after maximal alkali replacement) to induce mild hypovolemia, which increases proximal $Na^+/HCO_3^−$ reabsorption and reduces amount of alkali replacement needed but are likely to further increase urinary K^+ losses. They can also be considered in type I RTA to reduce calcium excretion; however, they carry the same risk of hypokalemia (1).
• Indomethacin can also be considered to reduce severity of polyuria and hypokalemia in type I RTA (1).
• Recent case reports and case studies have described the safety and efficacy of low-dose fludrocortisone in normalizing recurrent hyperkalemia in type IV RTA in the context of diabetes, amyloidosis, and patients undergoing renal transplant or newly entering dialysis.

SURGERY/OTHER PROCEDURES
If distal, RTA is due to obstructive uropathy

ADMISSION, INPATIENT, AND NURSING CONSIDERATIONS
Admit if severe acidosis patient unreliable, emesis persistent, or infant with severe failure to thrive

 ONGOING CARE

FOLLOW-UP RECOMMENDATIONS
Patient Monitoring
Electrolytes 1 to 2 weeks following initiation of therapy, monthly until serum HCO_3 corrected to desired range, and then as clinically indicated; poor compliance is common due to 3 to 6 times per day alkali dosing schedule.

DIET
Varies based on serum K^+ level and volume status

PATIENT EDUCATION
National Kidney Foundation: https://www.kidney.org/

PROGNOSIS
Depends on associated disease:
• Type I RTA: The amount of alkali supplementation decreases with age due to increased release of H^+ from bone during skeletal growth. Primary disease is permanent and will require lifelong alkali replacement.
• Type II RTA: Long-term compliance to therapy is poor due to large amounts of supplementation required. Prognosis depends on cause; sporadic cases can improve over time and therapy stopped.
• Type IV RTA: Treatment and prognosis depends on underlying cause.

COMPLICATIONS
Nephrocalcinosis, nephrolithiasis (type I); hypercalciuria (type I); hypokalemia (type I, type II if given HCO_3); hyperkalemia (type IV, some causes of type I); osteomalacia (type II due to phosphate wasting), osteopenia (due to buffering of acid in bone)

REFERENCES
1. Mohebbi N, Wagner CA. Pathophysiology, diagnosis and treatment of inherited distal renal tubular acidosis. *J Nephrol.* 2018;31(4):511–522.
2. Yaxley J, Pirrone C. Review of the diagnostic evaluation of renal tubular acidosis. *Ochsner J.* 2016;16(4):525–530.

 CODES

ICD10
N25.89 Oth disorders resulting from impaired renal tubular function

CLINICAL PEARLS
• Consider RTA in cases of normal anion gap metabolic acidosis with normal renal function.
• Type I RTA: urine pH >5.5 in setting of acidemia; positive UAG; acidemia can be severe.
• Type II RTA: urine pH <5.5 unless HCO_3 raised above reabsorptive threshold (12 to 18 mEq/L)
• Type IV RTA: most common subtype; hyperkalemia; urine pH <5.5; acidemia usually mild.
• Treatment includes avoidance of inciting causes, provision of oral alkali (HCO_3 or citrate), and measures to supplement (type II, many type I) or restrict (type IV) potassium.

RESPIRATORY DISTRESS SYNDROME, ACUTE (ARDS)

Caleb J. Mentzer, DO • Tyler Johnson, DO • Rachel C. Murphy, DO

 BASICS

DESCRIPTION

- Acute respiratory distress syndrome (ARDS) is defined as the onset of acute hypoxemia within 7 days of a known clinical insult, or new or worsening respiratory symptoms with bilateral opacities (patchy, diffuse, or homogenous) consistent with pulmonary edema on imaging. It is a diagnosis of exclusion.
- Severity of ARDS is defined by the severity of hypoxia present, measured with a ratio of partial pressure of arterial oxygen (PaO_2) to fraction of inspired oxygen (FiO_2) at a positive end-expiratory pressure (PEEP) or continuous positive airway pressure (CPAP) of at least 5 cm H_2O.
  - Mild—200 mm Hg $< PaO_2/FiO_2 \leq 300$ mm Hg
  - Moderate—100 mm Hg $< PaO_2/FiO_2 \leq 200$ mm Hg
  - Severe—$PaO_2/FiO_2 \leq 100$ mm Hg
- Synonym(s): acute lung injury; increased-permeability pulmonary edema; noncardiac pulmonary edema
- Systems affected: pulmonary, cardiovascular

EPIDEMIOLOGY

Incidence

- The incidence of ARDS in the United States is estimated to range from 64.2 to 78.9 cases/100,000 person-years.
- An estimated 10–15% of all ICU patients and approximately 23% of ventilator dependent patients meet the criteria for the diagnosis of ARDS.
- 25% of ARDS cases are classified as mild at the time of diagnosis, whereas 75% are classified as moderate to severe. Females sex is a risk factor for ARDS.

ETIOLOGY AND PATHOPHYSIOLOGY

- ARDS is a response to direct or indirect alveolar injury leading to diffuse alveolar damage.
  - Direct
    - Pneumonia (bacterial, viral, fungal, or opportunistic)
    - Aspiration of gastric contents
    - Near drowning
    - Pulmonary contusion
    - Inhalation injury
  - Indirect
    - Sepsis (nonpulmonary)
    - Shock
    - Transfusion of blood products
    - Major burn injury
    - Nonthoracic trauma
    - Drug overdose
    - Cardiopulmonary bypass
    - Reperfusion edema after lung transplant or embolectomy
- Progression of the diffuse alveolar damage in ARDS is divided into three phases.
  - Exudative phase—The initial highly inflammatory phase when alveolar macrophages are activated due to lung injury, leading to complement activation, release of proinflammatory mediators, and activation of neutrophils. This causes epithelial–endothelial barrier disruption, leading to intra-alveolar and extra-alveolar flooding with fluid. This is followed by hyaline membrane formation leading to alveolar collapse.
  - Proliferative phase—The second phase characterized by fibroblasts, myofibroblasts, and alveolar epithelial cell (ACE) II mediated repair. Formation of new matrix, differentiation into ACE I, and formation of cellular junctions begins which leads to expression of aquaporin and ion channels, aiding in the reabsorption of fluid.
  - Fibrotic phase—The final phase, not experience by every patient, is characterized by prolonged mechanical ventilation and associated with increased mortality.

Genetics

No single gene has been identified for clinical use.

RISK FACTORS

- Patients who are at low risk may be identified by a lung injury prevention score; however, this score is less accurate in high-risk patients.
- There are several risk factors that predispose patients to developing ARDS. These include advanced age, female sex, smoking, alcohol use, aortic or cardiovascular surgeries, and traumatic brain injury.
- Increased levels of markers of systemic inflammation have been associated with adverse outcomes.

GENERAL PREVENTION

To date, there has been no effective strategy proven to prevent developing ARDS; however, measures can be taken to mitigate risk factors. Early lung protective ventilation and sepsis management have both been shown to improve clinical outcomes in ARDS.

COMMONLY ASSOCIATED CONDITIONS

- Pneumonia, sepsis, and aspiration of gastric contents cause 85% of ARDS cases.
- Other causes can include:
  - Trauma
  - Burns
  - Cardiothoracic surgery
  - Pancreatitis
  - Inhalational injuries and near drownings
  - Transfusion-related acute lung injury (TRALI)
  - Shock
  - Medication toxicity

DIAGNOSIS

HISTORY

Precipitating event (see "Etiology and Pathophysiology") followed by abrupt onset of respiratory distress and hypoxemia.

PHYSICAL EXAM

- Tachypnea and tachycardia during the first 12 to 24 hours
- Increased oxygen requirements
- Decreased breath sounds with or without rales

DIFFERENTIAL DIAGNOSIS

- Bilateral pneumonia (including COVID-19)
- Congestive heart failure
- Interstitial and airway diseases
- Hypersensitivity pneumonitis
- Endobronchial tuberculosis
- Diffuse alveolar hemorrhage
- Veno-occlusive disease
- Mitral stenosis: intravascular volume overload
- Drug-induced lung disease especially vascular leak syndrome with immunotherapy

DIAGNOSTIC TESTS & INTERPRETATION

Initial Tests (lab, imaging)

- Initial labs should include a CBC, CMP, and ABG with evidence of hypoxemia.
- ECG: can show sinus tachycardia; nonspecific ST–T wave changes
- Chest x-ray (CXR): bilateral opacities; air bronchograms can be common.
- Chest CT scan: diffuse interstitial opacities.

Follow-Up Tests & Special Considerations

- Blood cultures, Sputum cultures, COVID-19 PCR.
- Consider transthoracic echocardiography (TTE) in patients when the diagnosis of cardiac failure cannot be excluded.
- Consider bronchoscopy when the cause of ARDS cannot be clearly identified.

Diagnostic Procedures/Other

- Old approach: Invasive monitoring of pulmonary artery wedge pressure (PAWP) has fallen out of favor after clinical trials have shown no increased benefit and an increase in catheter-related complications.
- New approach: Measuring esophageal pressure with a manometer to estimate pleural pressure allows for adjustment of PEEP to achieve a positive end-expiratory transpulmonary pressure gradient, an approach that is increasingly used in clinical care and especially useful in the morbidly obese (1)[C].

Test Interpretation

- With introduction of the Berlin criteria, a diagnosis of ARDS can be made with a calculated PaO_2/FiO_2 of ≤ 300 mm Hg along with radiologic evidence of new bilateral infiltrates. If an ABG is not available, the oxygen saturation can be used as a surrogate for the PaO_2.
- Severity of ARDS is based on the Berlin criteria:
  - Mild—200 mm Hg $< PaO_2/FiO_2 \leq 300$ mm Hg
  - Moderate—100 mm Hg $< PaO_2/FiO_2 \leq 200$ mm Hg
  - Severe—$PaO_2/FiO_2 \leq 100$ mm Hg

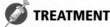 **TREATMENT**

GENERAL MEASURES

- Identify and treat the cause of ARDS.
- Lung protective ventilation and conservative fluid therapy
- Using tidal volumes of 6 mL/kg of predicted body weight with a plateau pressure goal of ≤ 30 cm H_2O has shown a decrease in mortality in comparison to higher volumes.
- Tidal volumes can be reduced to 4 mL/kg if plateau pressures exceed 30 cm H_2O (1)[A].
- Respiratory rate can be set to maintain adequate minute ventilation. Permissive hypercapnia is allowed as long as pH >7.30. Recent data supports lower respiratory rates (1)[C].

- No clear guideline for PEEP has been established. No clinical trial has shown consistent benefit of high PEEP. There is a possible benefit of reduced mortality in patients with moderate to severe ARDS with high PEEP (1)[C].
- In patients with early moderate to severe ARDS (PaO$_2$/FiO$_2$ <150 mm Hg), use of neuromuscular blockade with sedation compared with placebo resulted in a mortality benefit. Proposed mechanisms include prevention of breath stacking and limiting patient-ventilator dyssynchrony along with increased efficacy of lung protective ventilation.
- Prone positioning has shown a decrease in mortality and has led to early extubation in patients with moderate to severe ARDS (PaO$_2$/FiO$_2$ <150 mm Hg and PEEP >5 cm H$_2$O) who have been intubated for <36 hours. Patients are placed in a prone position for 16 consecutive hours a day for up to 28 days or until a PaO$_2$/FiO$_2$ ratio is ≥150 mm Hg. While in the supine position, patients need a PEEP of ≤10 cm H$_2$O and an FiO$_2$ of ≤0.6 for >4 hours. The benefit of prone positioning is reduction in deleterious effects of positive pressure ventilation on nondependent and less injured airspaces.
- Extracorporeal membrane oxygenation (ECMO) is reserved for severe ARDS after standard supportive measures have failed. One randomized controlled trial suggested improved mortality in select individuals with ARDS referred to an ECMO center (1)[C].
- In patients with very severe ARDS (PaO$_2$/FiO$_2$ <80 mm Hg), the use of early ECMO versus conventional mechanical ventilation that included ECMO as a rescue therapy had no difference in 60-day mortality (2)[A].

MEDICATION

No single medication or combination of medications prevents or improves clinical outcomes in ARDS. Treatment is aimed at addressing the underlying cause and is mostly supportive.

ADDITIONAL THERAPIES

- For fluid management, central venous pressure (CVP) can be used to estimate fluid status. Liberal fluid management strategy targeting CVP of 10 to 14 cm H$_2$O was compared to conservative fluid management strategy targeting CVP of 4 cm H$_2$O. The conservative approach led to increased ventilator-free days and a decreased stay in the ICU with no change in mortality.
- High-frequency oscillation ventilation showed increased mortality in a clinical trial, although a meta-analysis suggested some benefit when patients with PaO$_2$/FiO$_2$ <60 mm Hg (1)[C].
- Airway pressure release ventilation may improve oxygenation, but studies have shown no mortality benefit (1)[C].
- Noninvasive ventilation in patients with severe hypoxemia may increase the risk of ventilation-induced lung injury in ARDS (1)[C].
- Corticosteroids may improve airway pressures and oxygenation, but there is not a consensus on mortality benefit in ARDS. There is potential harm when started after 14 days in the disease course (1)[C].
- Inhaled nitric oxide, surfactant, statins, nonsteroidal anti-inflammatory agents, antioxidants, albuterol, and neutrophil elastase inhibitor have not shown any benefit in clinical trials (1)[C].
- Clinical trials for additional therapies such as dexamethasone, vitamin D, aspirin, mesenchymal stem cells, and others are underway.

Pregnancy Considerations

Supportive care while identifying the underlying cause of ARDS continues to be important in the management of pregnant women with ARDS. However, fetal well-being, possible need for delivery, and physiologic changes associated with pregnancy must be considered. All pregnant patient should be followed by an obstetrician.

ADMISSION, INPATIENT, AND NURSING CONSIDERATIONS

All patients with ARDS should be managed in an ICU setting.

- Use lung protective ventilation while providing adequate PEEP.
- Consider prone positioning and paralysis if PaO$_2$/FiO$_2$ <120 to 150 mm Hg.
- If failing initial supportive measures, consider early referral to an ECMO center.
- If perfusion is inadequate after restoration of intravascular volume (e.g., septic shock), vasopressor therapy is indicated.
- Early physical therapy
- Nursing care may include any or all of the following:
  – Skin, eye, and mouth care
  – Deep vein thrombosis (DVT) prophylaxis
  – Stress ulcer prophylaxis
  – Suctioning of endotracheal tube
  – Adequate care while changing position of patient from supine to prone and vice versa
  – Ensure adequate level of sedation and/or paralysis while on mechanical ventilation.
  – Tracheostomy care
- Discharge criteria
  – Resolution or improvement of underlying cause, improving respiratory status, and return to baseline oxygen status

 ## ONGOING CARE

FOLLOW-UP RECOMMENDATIONS
Patient Monitoring

- Driving pressure and static lung compliance are important measures of lung mechanics.
- Daily labs are needed until the patient is no longer critical.
- Daily CXRs are not needed but should be ordered when evaluating for endotracheal tube placement, the presence of progressing infiltrates, catheter placement, worsening hypoxia, or complications of mechanical ventilation (e.g., air leaks).

DIET

Trophic and full-calorie enteral nutrition have shown no difference in mortality, whereas early parenteral nutrition might be harmful (1)[C].

PATIENT EDUCATION

https://www.thoracic.org/patients/patient-resources/resources/acute-respiratory-distress-syndrome.pdf

PROGNOSIS

- Mortality rate is up to 45% with a significant increase across the severity categories.
- Mortality is 34.9% in mild ARDS, 40.3% in moderate, and 46.1% in severe ARDS.

COMPLICATIONS

- Short-term complications include:
  – Barotrauma
  – Nosocomial infection
  – Delirium
  – Catheter-related infection
  – DVT
  – Gastrointestinal bleeding due to stress ulcer
  – Poor nutrition
  – Multiple organ dysfunction syndrome
  – Death
- Long-term complications are related to the age and comorbidities of the patient.
  – Pulmonary dysfunction
  – Reduced health-related quality of life
  – Persistent reticular pattern/ground glass opacities on radiographic imaging
  – Neuropsychological disability, such as depression and PTSD

REFERENCES

1. Thompson BT, Chambers RC, Liu KD. Acute respiratory distress syndrome. *N Engl J Med*. 2017;377(6):562–572.
2. Combes A, Hajage D, Capellier G, et al; for EOLIA Trial Group, REVA, ECMONet. Extracorporeal membrane oxygenation for severe acute respiratory distress syndrome. *N Engl J Med*. 2018;378(21):1965–1975.

ADDITIONAL READING

Matthay MA, McAuley DF, Ware LB. Clinical trials in acute respiratory distress syndrome: challenges and opportunities. *Lancet Respir Med*. 2017;5(6):524–534.

 ## SEE ALSO

http://www.ardsnet.org/

CODES

ICD10
J80 Acute respiratory distress syndrome

CLINICAL PEARLS

- ARDS is the acute onset of hypoxemia secondary to alveolar injury with a PaO$_2$/FiO$_2$ ≤300 mm Hg and bilateral infiltrates on CXR.
- Treatment includes identifying and treating the underlying cause.
- Lung protective mechanical ventilation can improve morbidity and mortality.
- Prone positioning and paralytics can be considered in PaO$_2$/FiO$_2$ <150 mm Hg.

RESPIRATORY DISTRESS SYNDROME, NEONATAL

Elizabeth T. Nguyen, MD • Lena Dung Doan, DO • Nikhil Jaiswal, MD

 BASICS

DESCRIPTION
- Neonatal respiratory distress syndrome (NRDS) is a disorder primarily of prematurity manifested by respiratory distress. However, it can occur in early term neonates as well.
- System(s) affected: respiratory
- Synonym(s): hyaline membrane disease; surfactant deficiency

ALERT
A disorder of the neonatal period

EPIDEMIOLOGY
Incidence
- >90% incidence in infants born ≤28 weeks' gestation
- 1% all newborns, 10% of preterm infants
- Inversely proportional to gestational age
- Gender: male predominance
- Eighth leading cause of infant death in the United States in 2021: 11.3 infant deaths per 100,000 live births (1)

ETIOLOGY AND PATHOPHYSIOLOGY
- Impaired surfactant synthesis and secretion
  - Usually secondary to deficient surfactant (dipalmitoyl lecithin) production in immature lungs
  - Leads to low lung compliance, low lung volume, and increased lung resistance
- High oxygen exposure and barotrauma during treatment can cause further damage to alveolar epithelium.

Genetics
No known genetic pattern

RISK FACTORS
- Premature birth
- Low birth weight
- Infants of diabetic mothers
- Infants of hypertensive mothers
- Perinatal asphyxia
- History of RDS in a sibling
- Cesarean delivery or operative vaginal delivery
- Assisted reproductive technology
- Lack of prenatal care

GENERAL PREVENTION
- Prevention of premature birth:
  - Education
  - Regular prenatal care
  - Management of maternal medical conditions
- Promote healthy behaviors during pregnancy focusing on:
  - Diet
  - Exercise
  - Avoidance of exposure to tobacco smoke, alcohol, and illegal drugs
- Antenatal corticosteroids:
  - For babies born between 24 weeks' and 31 6/7 weeks, gestational age, antenatal corticosteroid use when administered 2 to 7 days prior decreased the risk of NRDS, surfactant use, and death.
  - For women at risk for preterm delivery within 24 0/7 and 33 6/7, weeks' gestation, including those with ruptured membranes and multiple gestations

COMMONLY ASSOCIATED CONDITIONS
- Patent ductus arteriosus (PDA)
- Bronchopulmonary dysplasia (BPD)
- Pneumothorax
- Recurrent wheezing, asthma, respiratory infections, and PFT abnormalities

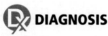 **DIAGNOSIS**

HISTORY
- Preterm neonates with worsening respiratory distress beginning at or shortly after birth and progressing over first few hours of life
- Early interventions can modify classic course.

PHYSICAL EXAM
- Tachypnea
- Tachycardia
- Expiratory grunting
- Low oxygen saturation
- Nasal flaring
- Subcostal and intercostal retractions
- Cyanosis
- Decreased breath sounds
- Pallor
- Diminished pulses
- Peripheral edema
- Decreased urine output

DIFFERENTIAL DIAGNOSIS
- Bacterial pneumonia
- Transient tachypnea of newborn
- Interstitial lung disease
- Persistent pulmonary hypertension
- Cyanotic congenital heart disease
- Meconium aspiration syndrome

DIAGNOSTIC TESTS & INTERPRETATION
Initial Tests (lab, imaging)
- Arterial blood gases (ABGs)
  - Evaluate for evidence of acid-base abnormalities (respiratory acidosis, metabolic acidosis), hypoxemia, and hypercarbia.
- Chest x-ray (CXR):
  - Microatelectasis
  - Diffuse reticulogranular pattern (ground-glass appearance)
  - Air bronchograms
  - Low lung volumes

Follow-Up Tests & Special Considerations
- Complete blood count with differential
- Blood culture
- Blood glucose

Diagnostic Procedures/Other
- Echocardiogram: Consider if murmur is present to evaluate for PDA and contribution to lung disease due to L → R shunting.
- Lung pathology (autopsy findings)
  - Macroscopically: uniformly ruddy, airless appearance of lungs
  - Microscopically: diffuse atelectasis and hyaline membranes (eosinophilic and fibrinous membrane lining air spaces)

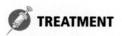 **TREATMENT**

GENERAL MEASURES
- Delivery Room
  - Delayed cord clamping if possible to allow time for placental transfusion and improvement in hemodynamic transition
  - Optimal thermoregulation of delivery room
- Respiratory support
  - If no respiratory failure: early initiation of continuous positive airway pressure (CPAP)
  - If respiratory failure: Intubate, ventilate as needed, and administer pulmonary surfactant.
- Respiratory monitoring options
  - Noninvasive
    ○ Transcutaneous monitor or end tidal CO_2 monitor
    ○ Pulse oximetry: target >90% to <94% O_2 saturation
  - Invasive
    ○ Umbilical artery catheter placement
      ■ Direct sampling of ABGs

- Empiric antibiotic therapy with ampicillin and gentamicin pending evaluation of blood cultures
- Supportive care:
  - Thermoneutral environment
  - Maintain adequate perfusion.
  - Optimize fluid and electrolyte balance (avoid overhydration).
  - Routine use of diuretics is not indicated.
  - Provide for nutritional needs.

MEDICATION
- Pulmonary surfactant
  - Poractant alfa (Curosurf)—porcine lung minced extract
  - Calfactant (Infasurf)—bovine lung lavage extract
  - Beractant (Survanta)—bovine lung minced extract
  - Each surfactant has specific protocols for delivery; consult local standards.
    - Trials show similar efficacy among surfactants; possible survival advantage of poractant alfa at a higher dose
    - Possible benefit of surfactant with added budesonide to reduce BPD but further studies needed
  - Administer within the first 30 to 60 minutes of life; should be balanced with less invasive forms of respiratory support
  - Strong evidence for use with gestational age <30 weeks, especially if requiring intubation for stabilization
  - LISA is the preferred method of surfactant administration for spontaneously breathing babies on CPAP.
  - Side effects
    - Bradycardia
    - Hypotension
    - Airway obstruction/endotracheal tube blockage with administration
    - Rapid changes in tidal volume (due to increased compliance) can cause a pneumothorax and small risk of pulmonary hemorrhage.
    - Transient adverse effects indicate that surfactant administration should be temporarily stopped until neonate is stable and dosing can be continued.
  - Contraindications: presence of congenital anomalies incompatible with life beyond neonatal period; infant with laboratory evidence of lung maturity
- Caffeine: Early therapy may improve respiratory effort and improve neurodevelopmental outcomes in low-birth-weight infants requiring mechanical ventilation.

- Inhaled nitrous oxide (INO) limited to those with documented pulmonary hypertension with severe respiratory distress; should stop if no response
- No current data to support routine diuretic use

ISSUES FOR REFERRAL
Comorbid conditions associated with prematurity
- PDA (cardiology consult)
- Necrotizing enterocolitis (NEC) (gastroenterology)
- Retinopathy of prematurity (ROP) (ophthalmology)

ADDITIONAL THERAPIES
Treat associated problems of prematurity.

ADMISSION, INPATIENT, AND NURSING CONSIDERATIONS
- All neonates with respiratory distress require immediate evaluation, monitoring, and treatment in the delivery room with transfer to a NICU.
- Supportive care
  - Thermoneutral environment
  - Respiratory monitoring
  - Establish relationship with family to provide education and emotional support.
- Discharge criteria
  - Should have stable vital signs and pulse oximetry before discharge
  - Medical home and support services should be in place.

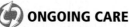 ONGOING CARE

FOLLOW-UP RECOMMENDATIONS
Following discharge, infants should be followed closely by their physicians to monitor growth and respiratory symptomatology.

PATIENT EDUCATION
- Educate parents regarding the risks in subsequent pregnancies.
- Advise parents regarding potential issues with chronic lung disease.

PROGNOSIS
- Progressive worsening of clinical picture during first 2 days of life (2)
- Prognosis and outcome are highly dependent on gestational age; significant neurodevelopmental delays in almost half infants ≤25 weeks' gestation

COMPLICATIONS
- Complications specific to NRDS
  - Pneumothorax
  - Chronic lung disease, BPD
  - Pulmonary interstitial edema (PIE)
- Additional complications may occur related to therapeutic interventions and comorbid conditions.

REFERENCES
1. Xu J, Murphy SL, Kochanek KD, et al. Mortality in the United States, 2021. *NCHS Data Brief*. 2022;(456):1–8.
2. Sweet DG, Carnielli VP, Greisen G, et al. European consensus guidelines on the management of respiratory distress syndrome: 2022 update. *Neonatology*. 2023;120(1):3–23.

ADDITIONAL READING
- Lemyre B, Laughon M, Bose C, et al. Early nasal intermittent positive pressure ventilation (NIPPV) versus early nasal continuous positive airway pressure (NCPAP) for preterm infants. *Cochrane Database Syst Rev*. 2016;12(12):CD005384.
- Roberts D, Brown J, Medley N, et al. Antenatal corticosteroids for accelerating fetal lung maturation for women at risk of preterm birth. *Cochrane Database Syst Rev*. 2017;3(3):CD004454.

 CODES

ICD10
P22.0 Respiratory distress syndrome of newborn

CLINICAL PEARLS
- NRDS is a disorder primarily of prematurity manifested by respiratory distress.
- Early treatment with CPAP or pulmonary surfactant can modify clinical course.
- Prognosis and outcome are highly dependent on gestational age.

R

RESPIRATORY SYNCYTIAL VIRUS (RSV) INFECTION

Sahil Mullick, MD • Sudeshna Dutta, MD

BASICS

Respiratory syncytial virus (RSV) is a medium-sized, membrane-bound RNA virus that causes acute respiratory tract illness in patients of all ages.

DESCRIPTION
- In adults, RSV typically causes upper respiratory tract infection (URTI) but can progress to pneumonia or worsening of asthma and/or chronic obstructive pulmonary disease (COPD).
- In infants and children, RSV commonly presents as lower respiratory tract infection (LRTI) that manifests as bronchiolitis and rarely pneumonia, respiratory failure, and death.

Pediatric Considerations
90–95% of children are infected by 24 months; leading cause of pediatric bronchiolitis (50–90%); premature infants and infants aged <6 months are at increased risk.

EPIDEMIOLOGY
- Seasonality: Outbreaks of RSV disease occur each winter (October to late January).
- Morbidity and mortality: RSV infection leads to >100,000 annual hospitalizations. In the United States, 2.1 million outpatient visits for RSV in children aged <5 years.

Incidence
- Worldwide, RSV is responsible for approximately 33 million LRTI per year and up to 199,000 childhood deaths.
- Annually, RSV causes an estimated 33.1 million acute LRTI worldwide and 3.2 million hospitalizations in children aged <5 years.
- RSV cases are particularly increasing in the wake of the COVID-19 pandemic.

Prevalence
Difficult to conclude accurately

ETIOLOGY AND PATHOPHYSIOLOGY
- RSV is a single-stranded, negative-sense RNA virus belonging to the *Paramyxoviridae* family.
- Two subtypes, A and B, are simultaneously present in most outbreaks with A subtypes causing more severe disease.
- RSV is spread via direct contact or droplet aerosols. Incubation period ranges from 2 to 8 days, mean 4 to 6.
- Natural RSV infections result in incomplete immunity; recurrent infections are common.
  - RSV causes a neutrophil-intensive inflammation of the airway. RSV develops in the cytoplasm of infected cells and matures by budding from the plasma membrane. RSV is a major cause of asthma exacerbation and COPD.

Genetics
- Severe RSV infections may be associated with polymorphisms in cytokine-related genes, including *CCR5*, *IL4*, *IL8*, *IL10*, and *IL13*.
- RSV replicates in apical ciliated bronchial epithelial cells. The airway epithelium produces chemokines, which recruit neutrophils.

RISK FACTORS
Significant association with RSV-associated acute LRTI
- Infants born before the 35 weeks' gestation; low birth weight, male gender; underlying cardiopulmonary disease; HIV; Down syndrome
- Any age group with persistent asthma; children aged <5 years with socioeconomic vulnerability; immunodeficiency; siblings with asymptomatic RSV infection; secondhand smoke; history of atopy, no breastfeeding; adult patients with COPD or functional disability
- Other risk factors: daycare center attendance; exposure to indoor and environmental air pollutants; multiple births, malnutrition, higher altitude

GENERAL PREVENTION
- Hand hygiene is the most important step to prevent the spread of RSV (1)[B].
  - Use alcohol-based rubs for hand decontamination when caring for children with bronchiolitis. When alcohol-based rubs are not available, wash the hands with soap and water (1)[B].
- Avoid passive smoke exposure (1)[B].
- Isolate patients with proven or suspected RSV.
- Palivizumab is a humanized monoclonal antibody for the prevention of severe RSV in high-risk children (2)[A]: preterm infants born ≤28 weeks, 6 days of gestation, or who are <12 months at start of RSV season; infants with bronchopulmonary dysplasia who are <1 year or <23 months of age and requiring treatment; infants ≤12 months of age who are being medically treated for acyanotic heart disease or have moderate to severe pulmonary hypertension
- Nirsevimab is a long acting monoclonal antibody recently approved by FDA. A single injection of nirsevimab administered before the RSV season protected healthy late-preterm and term infants from medically attended RSV-associated LRTI. Target populations for immunization include older infants and young children (e.g., those born prematurely or with cardiopulmonary disease or immunodeficiency).
- Nirsevimab offers a large advantage over current therapy with palivizumab, which has an involved treatment regimen of 5 monthly doses.
- Probiotics protect against RSV infection in neonatal mice through a microbiota-AM axis, suggesting that the probiotics may be a promising candidate to prevent and treat RSV infection, and deserve more research and development in the future.
- Prophylactic use is indicated for infants and children <24 months of age with:
  - Chronic lung disease (CLD) of prematurity
  - Hemodynamically significant congenital heart disease
    - Congenital abnormalities of the airway or neuromuscular disease
- AAP guidelines (2)[A]: preterm infants born <29 weeks' gestational age (WGA) and <1 year of age at the RSV season start date; infants in the 1st year of life with CLD of prematurity; infants with HS-CHD <1 year of age at the season start date

- Dosage: maximum of 5 monthly doses beginning in November or December at 15 mg/kg per dose IM
- Breastfeeding can significantly reduce hospitalizations due to respiratory infections.

COMMONLY ASSOCIATED CONDITIONS
In hospitalized infants:
- Pulmonary infiltrates/atelectasis (42.8%); otitis media (25.3%); hyperinflation (20.8%); respiratory failure (14%)
- Hyperkalemia (10.1%, defined as K+ >6); apnea (8.8%); bacterial pneumonia (7.6%)

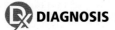 DIAGNOSIS

HISTORY
- History of prematurity, secondhand tobacco smoke exposure, daycare, number and age of siblings
- Immunization history
- Family history of respiratory disease
- Children: nasal congestion, cough, and coryza; low-grade fever, wheezing; nasal flaring, chest wall retraction
- Adults: young adults present with URI symptoms; mild fever, cough in 90%, wheeze in 40%

PHYSICAL EXAM
- Vital signs: fever, signs of increased work of breathing (tachypnea, grunting, flaring, retracting), apnea, pulse rate; pulse oximetry
- Dry mucous membranes; skin turgor (dehydration); serous otitis or acute otitis
- Upper respiratory findings: rhinorrhea, nasal congestion, cough, sneezing, and sometimes fever and myalgia
- Lower respiratory tract involvement with various permutations of the classic findings of bronchiolitis: rhonchus breath sounds, tachypnea; accessory muscle use, wheezes and crackles; prolonged expiration

Pediatric Considerations
- Young infants with bronchiolitis may develop apnea.
- Hospital admission based on apnea, hypoxia, respiratory failure, reduced oral intake, and hydration status

DIFFERENTIAL DIAGNOSIS
- Mild illness/URTI: other respiratory viral infections: parainfluenza virus, metapneumovirus, influenza virus, rhinovirus, coronavirus, human bocavirus, and adenovirus; coinfection with other viruses (e.g., adenovirus, influenza), mycoplasma, or bacteria, including Bordetella pertussis, should be considered; allergic rhinitis, sinusitis; asthma exacerbation, croup
- Severe illness/LRTI: bronchiolitis, asthma; pneumonia, foreign body aspiration

DIAGNOSTIC TESTS & INTERPRETATION

Initial Tests (lab, imaging)

- The diagnosis of RSV is clinical and does not require confirmatory testing or imaging. However, it is recommended in hospitalized patients being treated prophylactically with palivizumab.
  - If obtained, WBC count normal or elevated; virologic tests for RSV rarely change management decisions or outcomes.
- Septic workups are not necessary, unless the child is toxic in appearance.
- When obtained, typical CXR findings include hyperinflation and peribronchiolar thickening; atelectasis, interstitial infiltrates; segmental or lobar consolidation

Follow-Up Tests & Special Considerations

Real-time PCR have superior sensitivity and specificity compared with antigen detection assays and tissue culture.

Diagnostic Procedures/Other

Evidence of inadequate feeding or fluid intake, history of apnea, lethargy, or moderate to severe respiratory distress (nasal flaring, tachypnea, grunting, retractions or cyanosis), and/or an $SpO_2 \leq 92\%$ in room air (cutoffs for acceptable SpO_2 vary per country), warrant hospitalization, ideally in a secondary care level hospital

Test Interpretation

Antigen test for RSV: Sensitivity ranges from 72% to 94% and specificity of 95–100%, in children up to 32 months of age, but sensitivity is 0–25% in older children and adults.

 ## TREATMENT

GENERAL MEASURES

- Treatment for patients with RSV is supportive.
- Nasal suction and lubrication; antipyretics for fever; treat dehydration (oral or intravenous/nasogastric)—particularly in infants; oxygen for hypoxia, with an SpO_2 of 92% as the cutoff for supplementation

MEDICATION

First Line

Oxygen as needed, control of fever and pain with acetaminophen and ibuprofen; encourage fluid intake to prevent dehydration.

Second Line

- Do not administer albuterol (or salbutamol) to infants and children with a diagnosis of bronchiolitis (1)[B].
- Do not administer epinephrine to infants and children with diagnosis of bronchiolitis (1)[B].
- Do not administer systemic corticosteroids to infants with a diagnosis of bronchiolitis (1)[A].
- Do not administer nebulized hypertonic saline to infants with bronchiolitis in the emergency department (1)[B].
- May choose not to administer supplemental oxygen if the oxyhemoglobin saturation exceeds 90% in infants and children with a diagnosis of bronchiolitis (1)[C].
- Do not use chest physiotherapy for infants and children with a diagnosis of bronchiolitis (1)[B].

- Do not administer antibacterial medications to infants and children with bronchiolitis, unless there is a concomitant bacterial infection or a strong suspicion of one (1)[B].
- Clinicians should administer nasogastric or intravenous fluids for infants with a diagnosis of bronchiolitis who cannot maintain hydration orally (1)[A].
- Routine use of ribavirin is discouraged but can be considered on case-by-case basis.
- Ribavirin should be considered for treatment of RSV and LRTI in hematologic subjects. Oral formulation appears to be an easier, safe, and cost-effective alternative to aerosolized ribavirin.
- Suctioning is often used to reduce secretions in nasopharynx. However, studies have shown that it prolongs the duration of hospitalization particularly in infant aged 2 to 12 months.

ADDITIONAL THERAPIES

Bulb suctioning of the nares

Pediatric Considerations

Over-the-counter (OTC) cough and cold medications should not be used in children aged <6 years. If a hospitalized infant cannot receive oral feedings, use a nasogastric tube to restore adequate feeding and hydration.

COMPLEMENTARY & ALTERNATIVE MEDICINE

No complementary, alternative, or integrative therapies are of proven benefit.

ADMISSION, INPATIENT, AND NURSING CONSIDERATIONS

- The main goal is to achieve an adequate fluid balance and normal oxygen saturation levels. Patients with worsening despite oxygen supplementation may benefit from CPAP.
- Mechanical ventilation is required in about 5% of infants hospitalized with RSV.
- Nursing considerations/education:
  - Educate the family on hand washing.
  - Cleaning of environmental surfaces; universal precautions
- No set criteria for discharge; patients should be recovering and demonstrate: stable respiratory status with no oxygen requirement; ability to maintain oral intake and hydration status; adequate follow-up and patient education

 ## ONGOING CARE

- Ad26.RSV.preF demonstrated protection from RSV infection through immunization in a human challenge model and therefore could potentially protect against natural RSV infection and disease.
- RSVpreF vaccine was effective against symptomatic RSV infection and viral shedding. No evident safety concerns were identified. Recently, FDA has approved bivalent RSVpreF vaccine in individuals 60 years and older. CDC recommends that adults aged ≥60 years should receive a single dose of RSV vaccine. Maternal RSVpreF vaccine is in clinical trials.
- RSV vaccination be given during pregnancy (Pfizer's bivalent RSVpreF vaccine) recommended for use during pregnancy (maternal RSV vaccine). It is given during RSV season to people who are 32 through 36 weeks pregnant)

FOLLOW-UP RECOMMENDATIONS

Patient Monitoring

- Adequate fluid intake
- Maintaining oxygen saturation

PATIENT EDUCATION

- Bronchiolitis and Your Child: https://familydoctor.org/condition/bronchiolitis/
- Parent education—emphasize the use of alcohol-based hand gels/wash and/or to wash hands with soap and water. Clean surfaces with gloves and avoid daycare/kindergarten during recovery.

PROGNOSIS

Most patients recover fully within 7 to 10 days. Reinfection is common.

COMPLICATIONS

- The overall mortality for RSV is <1% with <400 deaths attributed to RSV each year.
- Infants hospitalized for RSV may be at increased risk for recurrent wheezing, allergic sensitization, and reduced pulmonary function, particularly during the 1st decade of life.
- Studies have shown early RSV infection is linked with development of childhood asthma (3).

REFERENCES

1. Ralston SL, Lieberthal AS, Meissner HC, et al. Clinical practice guideline: the diagnosis, management, and prevention of bronchiolitis [published correction appears in *Pediatrics*. 2015;136(4):782]. *Pediatrics*. 2014;134(5):e1474–e1502.
2. Binns E, Koenraads M, Hristeva L, et al. Influenza and respiratory syncytial virus during the COVID-19 pandemic: time for a new paradigm? *Pediatr Pulmonol*. 2022;57(1):38–42.
3. Harris E. RSV infection during infancy tied to asthma later. *JAMA*. 2023;329(20):1731.

ADDITIONAL READING

- Centers for Disease Control and Prevention. For healthcare providers. https://www.cdc.gov/rsv/clinical/index.html. Accessed October 7, 2023.
- Munro APS, Martinón-Torres F, Drysdale SB, et al. The disease burden of respiratory syncytial virus in infants. *Curr Opin Infect Dis*. 2023;36(5):379–384.

CODES

ICD10

- B97.4 Respiratory syncytial virus causing diseases classd elswhr
- J06.9 Acute upper respiratory infection, unspecified
- J21.0 Acute bronchiolitis due to respiratory syncytial virus

CLINICAL PEARLS

- RSV causes 50–90% of pediatric bronchiolitis.
- Hand sanitation (alcohol-based rubs are preferred) is the key to RSV prevention.
- The diagnosis of RSV is typically clinical. Routine laboratory or radiology studies are not necessary.
- Treatment of RSV is usually supportive.
- Palivizumab should be used to prevent RSV in high-risk patients.
- Consider RSV vaccination for individuals aged ≥60 years.

RESTLESS LEGS SYNDROME

Denise Sharon, MD, PhD, FAASM • Rochelle Zak, MD

BASICS

DESCRIPTION

- Sensorimotor disorder consisting of a strong, nearly irresistible urge to move the limbs; legs are usually affected initially but may involve arms or other body parts.
- The symptoms (Sx) begin or worsen during rest or inactivity and are relieved by movement or at least as long as the activity continues. If not current, previous relief by movement
- Occur preferentially in the evening/night; if not currently, previously reported circadian aspect
- Involuntary leg jerks reported during wake/sleep
- Early onset phenotype: 40–92% familial, stable, slow progression of Sx
- Late onset phenotype: more aggravating factors; rapid progression is common.
- Synonym(s): Willis-Ekbom disease

EPIDEMIOLOGY

Incidence

- 0.8–2.2% annually
- Onset at any age
- Parous females have twice the prevalence of males.
- Temperature (cold weather, other environmental factors may increase incidence/trigger Sx)

Pregnancy Considerations

- 10–30% prevalence; triggers/exacerbates RLS
- Predictors: past history (Hx), family Hx, iron deficiency (ID), Hgb ≤11 g/dL (1)[C]
- Peaks in 3rd trimester
- Most are relieved by 1-month postpartum.

ETIOLOGY AND PATHOPHYSIOLOGY

- Brain ID (BID), from either low serum iron or impaired transport of iron into the brain, leading to CNS dopamine (DA) dysregulation:
  - Higher than normal DA levels in the morning leading to DA D_2 receptors downregulation
  - Lower than normal DA at night
  - Increased glutamate and decreased adenosine leading to hyperarousal and insomnia
- Sensorimotor pathways abnormalities and increased motor excitability
- Triggered by prolonged immobility, such as hospitalizations
- Medication induced:
  - Most antidepressants (except bupropion)
  - DA-blocking antiemetics (e.g., metoclopramide, prochlorperazine)
  - Phenothiazine antipsychotics (risperidone, clozapine, olanzapine, quetiapine, etc.); possible exception: aripiprazole (partial D_2 agonist)
  - PPIs, H_2 blockers (increase risk)
  - Theophylline and other xanthines
  - Sedating α-histamines

Genetics

- Susceptibility loci: 2p14, 2q, 6p21.2, 9p, 12q, 14q, 15q23, and 20p
- Genes: MEIS1, BTBD9, PTPRD, TOX3, MAP2K5/LBXCOR1

RISK FACTORS

- ID; vitamin D deficiency
- Family Hx
- Chronic renal failure

GENERAL PREVENTION

- Regular physical activity/exercise during the day, low-impact activity at night such as stretches and walks
- Adequate sleep quality and quantity; delay wake time if possible.
- Avoid caffeine, alcohol, and nicotine mainly in the evening.
- Avoid use of meds that may trigger RLS (2)[C].

COMMONLY ASSOCIATED CONDITIONS

- Insomnia, sleep walking, delayed sleep phase
- ID, renal disease/uremia/dialysis, gastric surgery, IBS
- Parkinson disease, multiple sclerosis, peripheral neuropathy, Machado-Joseph disease, migraine
- Anxiety, depression, ADHD
- Cardiovascular disease, coronary artery disease, and stroke
- Venous insufficiency/peripheral vascular disease
- Pulmonary hypertension, lung transplantation, chronic obstructive pulmonary disease (COPD)
- Orthopedic problems, arthritis, fibromyalgia

DIAGNOSIS

Clinical, based on Hx, "difficult to describe"; all criteria must be met for RLS diagnosis (3)[C]:

- An urge to move the legs, usually accompanied by or thought to be caused by uncomfortable and unpleasant sensations in the legs; the urge must:
  - Begin or worsen during periods of rest or inactivity such as lying down or sitting
  - Be partially or totally relieved by movement such as walking or stretching at least as long as the activity continues. Relief by movement may not be noticeable but must have been previously reported.
  - Occur exclusively or predominantly in the evening or night rather than during the day; circadian aspect may not be noticeable but must have been previously reported.
- The above features are not solely accounted for by "mimics" or another sleep, medical, or behavioral condition. (Mimics include leg cramps, positional discomfort, habitual foot tapping, arthralgias/arthritis, myalgias, leg edema, peripheral neuropathy, and radiculopathy; even though some may coexist.)
- The Sx of RLS cause concern/distress; sleep disturbance; or impairment in mental, physical, social, occupational, educational, behavioral, or other areas of functioning.

HISTORY

- Signs/Sx (see also "Description") (4)[A]
  - Painful in ~35% of patients
  - Example descriptions: antsy, burning, achy, itching, "can't get comfortable"
  - Urge to move may be the only "discomfort."
  - Some patients must get up and walk.
  - PLMS in ~80% of patients
  - Insomnia, fatigue, anxiety, depression
- Severity range: from rare, minor problem to daily, mild to moderate, to severe impact on quality of life

Pediatric Consideration

Additional supportive findings (3)[A],(4):

- Insomnia or sleep disturbance
- RLS in immediate biologic relative
- PLMS

PHYSICAL EXAM

Usually normal

DIFFERENTIAL DIAGNOSIS

- Vascular compression: Single position change eliminates discomfort without requiring repetitive movements.
- Claudication: Movement doesn't relieve pain.
- Motor neuron disease: fasciculation/tremor, no discomfort or circadian pattern
- Peripheral neuropathy: prominent daytime component unresponsive to DA agonists (DAs)
- Dermatitis/pruritus: movement only to scratch; no circadian pattern
- Sleep-related leg cramps: muscle knot
- PLMD, RSD: no wake time urge to move
- Growing pains: no urge to move or relief by movement

DIAGNOSTIC TESTS & INTERPRETATION

Assessment of serum iron stores: ferritin, transferrin saturation, iron-binding capacity, serum iron (see "General Measures") (5)[C]

Diagnostic Procedures/Other

- Sleep study (PSG) helpful but not required
  - Frequent, PLM during wake, prior to sleep and
  - Frequent PLMS on PSG support diagnosis
- Suggested immobilization test (SIT) or multiple SIT (m-SIT)
  - Conducted before or without nocturnal PSG
  - Patient attempts to sit still in bed for 1 hour (SIT) or four 1-hour periods, every 2 hours (m-SIT) while completing every 10 min a visual analogue scale (VAS) or m-SIT disturbance scale.
  - SIT of >40 movements per hour suggests RLS.

TREATMENT

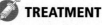

GENERAL MEASURES

- If iron insufficient, supplement (2)[C]:
  - 325 mg $FeSO_4$ + 100 mg vitamin C QHS
  - Repletion requires months till serum ferritin >75 ng/mL and TSAT >16%.
  - IV iron: LMWD 1,000 mg and ferumoxytol 1,020 mg
- Daily exercise; avoid activities that exacerbate RLS.
- Avoid exacerbating factors; maintain regular sleep.
- Treat obstructive sleep apnea (OSA) if present.
- Hot baths, warm soaks, leg massage (6)[C]
- In bed: long socks, electric blanket, weighted blanket
- Intense mental activity (games, puzzles, etc.)

MEDICATION

- Consider not initiating medications in mild to moderate cases until general measures have failed. Use minimum dose necessary to control Sx, including sleep disturbance.
- Assess Sx severity every encounter using a scale (e.g., sIRLS, IRLS, JHRLSS).
- Opt for longer acting/extended-release options (2),(5),(6)[C].
- Refractory RLS may require combination therapy Tx.

First Line

$\alpha2\delta$ Ligands—less risk for augmentation and more effective in DA-naive patients (2),(5),(6)[C]:

- Gabapentin enacarbil (Horizant): 300 to 1,200 mg QD ~5:00 PM FDA APPR (2),(5)[C]
- Pregabalin (Lyrica): 50 to 450 mg/day (off-label)
- Gabapentin (Neurontin): 100 to 2,400 mg/day (off-label)

Second Line

- Off-label: opiates (2),(5),(6)[C]
  - Buprenorphine/naloxone 2.0/0.5 mg, 1.25 to 2.00 strips QD
  - Methadone 2.5 to 20.0 mg; oxycodone (IR or ER) 5 to 30 mg
- DAs (FDA approved)—increased risk for augmentation (Rx-induced worsening of Sx, Sx occur earlier and spread to other body parts); at every encounter, assess for augmentation and impulse-control disorders (ICD) (2),(5),(6)[C].
  - Pramipexole: ER 0.375 mg tablet; IR (Mirapex): 0.125 to 0.500 mg 1 to 2 hours before Sx; titrate by 0.125 mg q 4 days.
  - Ropinirole: XL 2 mg; IR (Requip) 0.25 to 4.00 mg 0.5 to 1.0 hour before Sx; titrate by 0.25 mg q 4 days.
  - Transdermal rotigotine (Neupro): 1 to 3 mg/24 hr patch; start at 1 mg/d; titrate by 1 mg/week.
- Short-acting DAs for occasional Sx
  - Carbidopa/levodopa (Sinemet or Sinemet CR): 10/100 to 25/250; PRN up to twice per week
- Avoid DAs in psychotic patients, particularly if taking dopamine antagonists.
- Avoid exceeding DA-recommended dose.
- Benzodiazepines and agonists if insomnia/anxiety
  - Clonazepam (Klonopin): 0.5 to 3.0 mg/day
  - Temazepam, triazolam, alprazolam, zaleplon, zolpidem, and diazepam

Pregnancy Considerations

- Nonpharmacologic therapies, assess/correct ID, vitamin D, folate
- If severe and failed above, 2/3 trimesters, consider low-dose clonazepam, clonidine, carbidopa/levodopa, or opioids (1)[B].

Pediatric Considerations

- First-line treatment: nonpharmacologic therapies, healthy sleep habits, assess/correct ID
- Consider low-dose, age-adjusted gabapentin, clonidine, or melatonin for sleep.

Geriatric Considerations

- Avoid medications causing dizziness/unsteadiness.
- Many medications trigger/worsen RLS in the elderly.

ISSUES FOR REFERRAL

Severe, intractable Sx

ADDITIONAL THERAPIES

- Noninvasive peroneal nerve stimulator
- Vitamin/suppl: Mg, vitamin D, folate

SURGERY/OTHER PROCEDURES

For orthopedic, neuropathic, or lower extremities vein disease (laser ablation, sclerotherapy)

COMPLEMENTARY & ALTERNATIVE MEDICINE

Compression stockings, pneumatic compression devices for the legs

ADMISSION, INPATIENT, AND NURSING CONSIDERATIONS

Prolonged hospitalization can trigger/worsen RLS.

 ONGOING CARE

FOLLOW-UP RECOMMENDATIONS

Patient Monitoring

- At 1- to 4-week intervals until stable and then annually
- If taking iron, reassess iron stores, at least ferritin.
- If the status changes, assess for augmentation, ICD, associated conditions, and medications.

DIET

Avoid caffeine and alcohol, mainly in the evening.

PATIENT EDUCATION

- RLS Foundation: https://www.rls.org
- National Sleep Foundation: https://www.sleepfoundation.org/
- American Academy of Sleep Medicine: https://sleepeducation.org/

PROGNOSIS

- Early onset: lifelong condition with no current cure
- Late onset/secondary: may subside with resolution of precipitating factors, otherwise chronic, progressive
- Current therapies usually control Sx.

COMPLICATIONS

- Augmentation of Sx following DA therapy to be assessed at every visit (5)[C]:
  - 4-hour time advance of Sx or 2 to 4 hours advance of Sx together with shorter latency at rest; Sx spread to other body parts or have greater intensity.
  - Higher doses increase risk, and increasing the dose makes Sx worse.
  - Greater risk with meds with shorter half-lives
  - ID increases risk.
  - Down-titrate and discontinue DAs for at least 10 days, may add alternative medication then or to continue treatment
- The potential for ICD/Sx needs to be assessed at every visit in patients receiving DA (5)[C].
- Iatrogenic RLS (following blood loss or donation)

REFERENCES

1. Picchietti DL, Hensley JG, Bainbridge JL, et al; for International Restless Legs Syndrome Study Group. Consensus clinical practice guidelines for the diagnosis and treatment of restless legs syndrome/Willis-Ekbom disease during pregnancy and lactation. *Sleep Med Rev.* 2015;22:64–77.
2. Garcia-Borreguero D, Silber MH, Winkelman JW, et al. Guidelines for the first-line treatment of restless legs syndrome/Willis-Ekbom disease, prevention and treatment of dopaminergic augmentation: a combined task force of the IRLSSG, EURLSSG, and the RLS-foundation. *Sleep Med.* 2016;21:1–11.
3. American Academy of Sleep Medicine. Restless legs syndrome. In: *International Classification of Sleep Disorders.* 3rd ed. Darien, IL: American Academy of Sleep Medicine; 2014:281–291.
4. Allen RP, Picchietti DL, Garcia-Borreguero D, et al; for International Restless Legs Syndrome Study Group. Restless legs syndrome/Willis-Ekbom disease diagnostic criteria: updated International Restless Legs Syndrome Study Group (IRLSSG) consensus criteria—history, rationale, description, and significance. *Sleep Med.* 2014;15(8):860–873.
5. Trotti LM, Goldstein CA, Harrod CG, et al. Quality measures for the care of adult patients with restless legs syndrome. *J Clin Sleep Med.* 2015;11(3):293–310.
6. Sharon D. Nonpharmacologic management of restless legs syndrome (Willis-Ekbom disease): myths or science. *Sleep Med Clin.* 2015;10(3):263–278.

ADDITIONAL READING

Silber MH, Buchfuhrer MJ, Earley CJ, et al; for Scientific and Medical Advisory Board of the Restless Legs Syndrome Foundation. The management of restless legs syndrome: an updated algorithm. *Mayo Clin Proc.* 2021;96(7):1921–1937.

 SEE ALSO

- Periodic Limb Movement Disorder (PLMD)
- International Restless Legs Syndrome Study Group: https://irlssg.org/

 CODES

ICD10

G25.81 Restless legs syndrome

CLINICAL PEARLS

- Iron supplement is an often well-tolerated, easily available treatment for RLS.
- $\alpha2\delta$ (gabapentinoids) should be considered as initial therapy.
- To avoid augmentation, titrate DAs only up to the minimum dose necessary to control Sx.
- Antidepressants, antipsychotics, antiemetics, and sedating antihistamines can trigger or worsen RLS.
- Severity and change in Sx can be monitored using a severity scale such as sIRLS, IRLS, or JHRLSS.
- Insomnia is often a Sx of RLS.

RETINAL DETACHMENT
Tony Cha Her, MD

 BASICS

DESCRIPTION
- Separation of the sensory retina from the underlying retinal pigment epithelium
- Rhegmatogenous retinal detachment (RRD): most common type; occurs when the fluid vitreous gains access to the subretinal space through a break in the retina (Greek *rhegma*, "rent")
- Exudative or serous detachment: occurs in the absence of a retinal break, usually in association with inflammation or a tumor
- Traction detachment: Vitreoretinal adhesions mechanically pull the retina from the retinal pigment epithelium. The most common cause is proliferative diabetic retinopathy.
- System(s) affected: nervous

EPIDEMIOLOGY
Incidence
- Incidence increases with age.
- Predominant sex: male > female (3:2)
- Per year: 1/10,000 in patients who have not had cataract surgery
- 1–3% develop a retinal detachment (RD) after cataract surgery.

ETIOLOGY AND PATHOPHYSIOLOGY
- Traction from a posterior vitreous detachment (PVD) causes most retinal tears. With aging, vitreous gel liquefies, leading to separation of the vitreous from the retina. Vitreoschisis (lamellar separation of the posterior vitreous cortex) commonly precedes a complete PVD. The vitreous gel remains attached at the vitreous base, in the retinal periphery, resulting in vitreous traction that produces tears in the retinal periphery. There is an ~15% chance of developing a retinal tear from a PVD.
- PVD associated with vitreous hemorrhage has a high incidence of retinal tears.
- Exudative detachment
  - Tumors
  - Inflammatory diseases
  - Miscellaneous (central serous retinopathy, uveal effusion syndrome, malignant hypertension, drugs—ipilimumab, topiramate)
- Traction detachment
  - Proliferative diabetic retinopathy
  - Cicatricial retinopathy of prematurity
  - Proliferative sickle-cell retinopathy
  - Proliferative vitreoretinopathy (PVR)
  - Pars planitis
- Penetrating trauma

Genetics
There is an increased risk of RRD if a sibling has been affected by this condition. The risk increases with higher levels of myopia in the family history.

RISK FACTORS
- Myopia (>5 diopters)
- Aphakia or pseudophakia
  - In patients undergoing small-incision coaxial phacoemulsification with high myopia (axial length ≥26 mm), the incidence of RD is 2.7%.
- PVD

- RD in fellow eye
- Lattice degeneration: a vitreoretinal abnormality found in 6–10% of the general population
- Glaucoma: 4–7% of patients with RD have chronic open-angle glaucoma.
- The risk of RD after intravitreal injection for age-related macular degeneration or retinal vein occlusion is low with a rate of approximately 1 in 7,500 injections (1)[B].

GENERAL PREVENTION
Pediatric Considerations
Usually associated with underlying vitreoretinal disorders and/or retinopathy of prematurity

COMMONLY ASSOCIATED CONDITIONS
- Lattice degeneration
- High myopia
- Glaucoma

Pregnancy Considerations
Preeclampsia/eclampsia may be associated with exudative RD. No intervention is indicated, provided that hypertension is controlled. Prognosis is usually good.

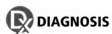 **DIAGNOSIS**

HISTORY
- Sudden flashes of light (photopsia)
- Shower of floaters
- Visual field loss: "curtain coming across vision"
- Central vision will be preserved if the macula is not detached.
- Poor visual acuity (20/200 or worse), with loss of central vision when macula is detached

PHYSICAL EXAM
- Elevation of the neurosensory retina from the underlying retinal pigment epithelium
- Elevation of retina associated with ≥1 retinal tears in RRD or elevation of the retina without tears in exudative detachment
- In 3–10% of patients with presumed RRD, no definite retinal break is found.
- Tenting of the retina without retinal tears in traction detachment
- Pigmented cells within the vitreous ("tobacco dust")

DIFFERENTIAL DIAGNOSIS
Retinoschisis (splitting of the retina)

DIAGNOSTIC TESTS & INTERPRETATION
Visual field testing: differentiates RRD from retinoschisis

Initial Tests (lab, imaging)
- Ultrasound (US) can demonstrate a detached retina and may be helpful when the retina cannot be visualized directly (e.g., with cataracts or vitreous hemorrhage).
- Fluorescein dye leakage can be seen in exudative RD; caused by central serous retinopathy and other inflammatory conditions
- Optical coherence tomography (OCT) to detect PVD and RD

 TREATMENT

GENERAL MEASURES
- Not all retinal tears or breaks need to be treated:
  - Flap or horseshoe tears in symptomatic patients (e.g., patients with flashes or floaters) are treated frequently.
  - Operculated holes in symptomatic patients are treated sometimes.
  - Asymptomatic atrophic round holes are rarely treated.
- Lattice degeneration with or without holes within the lattice in an asymptomatic patient with prior RD in the fellow eye may be treated prophylactically.
- Flap retinal tears in asymptomatic patients frequently are treated prophylactically.
- Exudative detachments are usually managed by treating underlying disorder.
- Traction detachments are usually managed by observation. If the fovea is involved, a vitrectomy is needed.

MEDICATION
First Line
The following may be used at the time of surgery to facilitate repair of the RRD:
- Intraocular gases (air, perfluoropropane, sulfur hexafluoride)
- Perfluorocarbon liquids
- Silicone oil (SO)
- Contraindications to intraocular gas: patients with poorly controlled glaucoma
- Precautions with intraocular gas: Expanding intraocular gas bubble increases intraocular pressure; therefore, avoid higher altitudes.
- Significant possible interactions with intraocular gas: Nitrous oxide used in general anesthesia can expand an intraocular gas bubble.

Second Line
Steroids can treat some causes of exudative RD. Steroids may cause worsening of central serous retinopathy.

SURGERY/OTHER PROCEDURES
- Timing of repairs
  - Macula attached: within 24 hours if possible; if the detachment is peripheral and does not have features suggestive of rapid progression (e.g., large and/or superior tears), repair can be performed within a few days.
    - Preoperative posturing consisting of bed rest and positioning is frequently prescribed to patients with macula-on RD. Preoperative posturing can reduce the progression of macula-on RDs.
- Macula recently detached: within 10 days of development of a macula-off RD (2)[B]
  - Old macular detachment: elective repair within 2 weeks
- If a retinal break has led to the development of an RD, surgery is needed. Surgical options (and combinations) include the following:
  - Demarcation laser treatment
  - Pneumatic retinopexy (PR) is when air or gas is injected intraocularly in the office: Head positioning is required postoperatively.

– Scleral buckle (SB)
– Pars plana vitrectomy (PPV)
– Perfluorocarbon liquids, especially for giant tears (circumferential tears ≥90 degrees)
– SO for complex repairs
• RRD may have >1 break. If any retinal break is not closed at the time of surgery, the surgery will fail.
• In patients ≥50 years of age, there is a higher incidence of inferior retinal breaks and inferior RDs in pseudophakic eyes compared to phakic eyes (3)[A].
• Additional surgery may be required if the retina redetaches secondary to a new retinal break or because of PVR.
• If a vitreous hemorrhage is present, presumably from a retinal tear and the fundus cannot be well visualized, consideration can be given for early vitrectomy.
– Patients who underwent PPV within the 1st week of presentation had a significantly lower risk of having a macula-off RD.
– Both phakic and pseudophakic patients had a similar chance of developing an RD. Phakic patients who underwent PPV had a higher chance of requiring subsequent cataract surgery.
• There is a trend toward primary vitrectomy in the management of RRD. Eyes undergoing PPV for primary RRD repair may not need the addition of an SB.
• In patients with RRD who are at high risk for PVR (RD in two or more quadrants, retinal tears >1 clock hour, preoperative PVR, or vitreous hemorrhage), PPV + SB were associated with higher rates of anatomical success compared to PPV alone.
• The single-procedure anatomic success rate of PPV, retinectomy, and SO tamponade without SB for PVR-related recurrent RRD is comparable to similar surgery incorporating an SB (4)[C].

⚡ ONGOING CARE

FOLLOW-UP RECOMMENDATIONS

Postoperatively, if intraocular gas has been used, the patient may need specific head positioning and should not travel to high altitudes to avoid expanding the intraocular gas bubble.

Patient Monitoring

• Alert ophthalmologist if there is new onset of floaters or flashes, increase in floaters or flashes, sudden shower of floaters, curtain or shadow in the peripheral visual field, or reduced vision.
• Patients with acute symptomatic PVD should be reexamined by the ophthalmologist in 3 to 4 weeks. Delayed retinal breaks and RRDs can occur for several months after an acute PVD, so the patient should be monitored and be given the warning signs of an RRD (5)[B].
• If acute symptomatic PVD is associated with gross vitreous hemorrhage that interferes with complete visualization of the retinal periphery by indirect ophthalmoscopy, the patient should be reexamined at shorter intervals with indirect ophthalmoscopy until the entire retinal periphery can be observed. Early PPV can be considered.
• If the examiner is not certain whether the retina is detached in the presence of opaque medium, US should be performed.

PROGNOSIS

• RRD
– 90% of RDs can be reattached successfully after ≥1 surgical procedures. Postoperative visual acuity depends primarily on the status of the macula preoperatively. Also important is the length of time between the detachment and the repair (75% of eyes with macular detachments of <1 week will obtain a final visual acuity of 20/70 or better).
– 87% of eyes with an RD not involving the macula attain a visual acuity of 20/50 or better postoperatively. 37% of eyes with a detached macula preoperatively attain 20/50 or better vision postoperatively.
– In 10–15% of successfully repaired RDs not involving the macula preoperatively, visual acuity does not return to the preoperative level. This decrease is secondary to complications such as macular edema and macular pucker.
– Failed primary PR selects for RDs that are inherently more difficult to reattach.
• Risk factors associated with primary RRD repair failure include choroidal detachment, significant hypotony, grade C-1 PVR or worse, four detached quadrants, and large or giant retinal breaks. Additional risk factors associated with primary RRD repair failure include increased number of breaks and inferior location of retinal breaks.
• 18% of patients undergoing primary RRD repair by either laser barricade, PR, PPV, or SB required a secondary procedure within 90 days. PR was associated with the highest rate of reoperation of 29%. Most secondary repairs were performed by PPV (6)[A].
• Tractional RD
– When not involving the fovea, the patient usually can be observed because it is uncommon for these to extend into the fovea.
• Exudative RD
– Management is usually nonsurgical.
– The presence of shifting fluid is highly suggestive of an exudative RD. Fixed retinal folds, which are indicative of PVR, are seen rarely in exudative RD. If the underlying condition is treated, the prognosis generally is good.

COMPLICATIONS

• PVR is the most common cause of failed RD repair; 10–15% of retinas that reattach initially after retinal surgery will redetach subsequently, usually within 6 weeks, as a result of cellular proliferation and contraction on the retinal surface.
• Partial or total loss of vision due to macular detachment and/or PVR
• Moderate-to-severe forms of PVR usually are treated with PPV and fluid–gas exchange. If a segmental SB was placed at the initial procedure, it may need to be revised.
• Primary retinectomy can be used in cases of PVR without an SB.
• SBs may erode the overlying conjunctiva and lead to an infection.
• Optic neuropathy after PPV for macula-sparing primary RRD.

REFERENCES

1. Storey PP, Pancholy M, Wibbelsman TD, et al. Rhegmatogenous retinal detachment after intravitreal injection of anti-vascular endothelial growth factor. *Ophthalmology*. 2019;126(10):1424–1431.
2. Hassan TS, Sarrafizadeh R, Ruby AJ, et al. The effect of duration of macular detachment on results after the scleral buckle repair of primary, macula-off retinal detachments. *Ophthalmology*. 2002;109(1):146–152.
3. Ferrara M, Mehta A, Qureshi H, et al; for BEAVRS Retinal Detachment Outcomes Group. Phenotype and outcomes of phakic versus pseudophakic primary rhegmatogenous retinal detachments: cataract or cataract surgery related? *Am J Ophthalmol*. 2021;222:318–327.
4. Deaner JD, Aderman CM, Bonafede L, et al. PPV, retinectomy, and silicone oil without scleral buckle for recurrent RRD from proliferative vitreoretinopathy. *Ophthalmic Surg Lasers Imaging Retina*. 2019;50(11):e278–e287.
5. Uhr JH, Obeid A, Wibbelsman TD, et al. Delayed retinal breaks and detachments after acute posterior vitreous detachment. *Ophthalmology*. 2020;127(4):516–522.
6. Reeves MGR, Afshar AR, Pershing S. Need for retinal detachment reoperation based on primary repair method among commercially insured patients, 2003–2016. *Am J Ophthalmol*. 2021;229:71–81.

 SEE ALSO

Retinopathy, Diabetic

 CODES

ICD10

• H33.059 Total retinal detachment, unspecified eye
• H33.20 Serous retinal detachment, unspecified eye
• H33.0 Retinal detachment with retinal break

CLINICAL PEARLS

• If a patient complains of the new onset of floaters or flashes of light, the patient should undergo a dilated eye exam to rule out a retinal tear or RD.
• There is an increased risk of RD after cataract surgery.

RETINOPATHY, DIABETIC

Richard W. Allinson, MD • Hunter Grey, OD

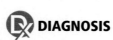 **BASICS**

DESCRIPTION
- Most patients with diabetes mellitus (DM) will develop diabetic retinopathy (DR). It is the leading cause of new cases of legal blindness among residents in the United States between the ages of 20 and 64 years.
- DR can be divided into three stages:
  - Nonproliferative diabetic retinopathy (NPDR) (background)
  - Severe NPDR (preproliferative)
  - Proliferative diabetic retinopathy [PDR]

Pregnancy Considerations
Pregnancy can exacerbate condition.

EPIDEMIOLOGY
Incidence
- Peak incidence of type 1, juvenile-onset DM is between the ages of 12 and 15 years.
- Peak incidence of type 2, adult-onset DM is between the ages of 50 and 70 years.

Prevalence
- Worldwide, DR affects 1 out of 3 persons with DM.
- 2/3 of type 1 DM (T1DM) patients who have had DM for at least 35 years will develop PDR, and 1/3 will develop diabetic macular edema (DME). Proportions are reversed for type 2 DM (T2DM).

ETIOLOGY AND PATHOPHYSIOLOGY
- Related to development of diabetic microaneurysms and microvascular abnormalities
- Vascular endothelial growth factor (VEGF) is elevated in patients with hypoxic retina. Intraocular levels of VEGF are elevated in patients with retinal or iris NV. Retinal hypoxia also contributes to DME, and VEGF is a major contributor to DME.

RISK FACTORS
- Renal disease
- Systemic hypertension (HTN)
- Smoking
- Elevated lipid levels

GENERAL PREVENTION
- Monitor and control of blood glucose.
- Schedule yearly ophthalmologic eye exams.

COMMONLY ASSOCIATED CONDITIONS
- Glaucoma; cataracts
- Retinal detachment; vitreous hemorrhage (VH)
- Disc edema (diabetic papillopathy)

 DIAGNOSIS

PHYSICAL EXAM
- Eye exam: measurement of visual acuity (VA) and documentation of the status of the iris, lens, vitreous, and fundus
- NPDR (background)
  - Microaneurysms
  - Intraretinal hemorrhage
  - Lipid deposits

- Severe NPDR (preproliferative)
  - Nerve fiber layer infarctions ("cotton wool spots")
  - Venous beading
  - Venous dilatation
  - Intraretinal microvascular abnormalities (IRMA)
  - Extensive retinal hemorrhage
  - The Early Treatment Diabetic Retinopathy Study (ETDRS) developed the 4:2:1 rule for severe NPDR. Severe NPDR was defined as having any one of the following features:
    - Severe intraretinal hemorrhages and microaneurysms in four quadrants
    - Venous beading in two or more quadrants
    - IRMAs in one or more quadrants
- PDR
  - New blood vessel proliferation: NV can be found on the retinal surface, optic nerve, and iris.
  - Visual loss caused by VH, traction retinal detachment; contraction of fibrovascular tissue on a vitreous scaffold can lead to VH and traction retinal detachment.

DIFFERENTIAL DIAGNOSIS
Other causes of retinopathy (e.g., radiation, retinal venous obstruction, HTN)

DIAGNOSTIC TESTS & INTERPRETATION
Diagnostic Procedures/Other
- Fluorescein angiography demonstrates retinal nonperfusion, retinal leakage, and PDR.
- Optical coherence tomography (OCT) can be used to help detect DME by measuring retinal thickness. Swept-source optical coherence tomography angiography (SS-OCTA) can detect diabetic NV. OCT angiography (OCTA) can visualize the retinal vasculature.

 TREATMENT

GENERAL MEASURES
- The Diabetes Control and Complications Trial (DCCT) recommended that for most patients with T1DM with insulin-dependent DM, blood glucose levels should be as close to the nondiabetic range as is safe to reduce the risk and rate of progression of DR.
- The United Kingdom Prospective Diabetes Study (UKPDS) demonstrated patients with T2DM had slower progression of DR with intensive blood glucose control. It also showed that intensive control of blood pressure slowed progression of DR.
- Microvascular complications, including PDR, are increased when blood sugar levels are ≥200 mg/dL.
- Cataract surgery can cause retinopathy to worsen and increase the risk for development of DME.

- HTN has a detrimental effect on DR and must be controlled.
- Severe obstructive sleep apnea (OSA) is a risk factor for DME in patients with T2DM. Refractory DME is more frequent in patients with severe OSA. Continuous positive airway pressure (CPAP) may help prevent refractory DME in patients with OSA (1)[B].

MEDICATION
- Treatment of HTN with the angiotensin receptor blocker candesartan has been shown to result in regression of DR in some patients.
- Statin therapy in patients with T2DM is associated with a decreased risk of DR. T2DM patients on lipid-lowering medications are less likely to develop NPDR, PDR, or DME.

SURGERY/OTHER PROCEDURES
- Preventive treatment of moderate to severe NPDR without centered-involved diabetic macular edema (CI-DME) with intravitreal aflibercept injection (IAI) reduced the development of PDR or vision-reducing CI-DME. After 2 years of follow-up, preventive treatment with IAI did not confer VA benefit compared with observation plus IAI only after development of PDR or vision-reducing CI-DME (2)[A].
- Treatment for DME
  - Intravitreal anti-VEGF is first-line treatment for DME:
    - Ranibizumab, an antibody fragment that binds VEGF, can be used to treat DME when injected intravitreally. Ranibizumab 0.3 mg (0.05 mL) injected intravitreally monthly resulted in improved vision and reduced central foveal thickness.
      - Anti-VEGF treatment by intravitreal injection (IVI) results in superior clinical outcomes compared to laser photocoagulation for DME.
      - Intravitreal ranibizumab injections (IRIs) are beneficial for patients with DME and concurrent macular nonperfusion.
      - IRI for DME may also improve DR severity and reduce the risk of DR progression.
      - Treat and extend dosing for IRI decreased the number of injections while giving similar visual and anatomic outcomes compared with monthly dosing at 1 year.
      - As-needed treatment after a loading dose of 3 monthly injections has been shown to result in comparable results to more frequent treatments.
      - Topical povidone-iodine prophylaxis is important to help prevent endophthalmitis from IVIs from anti-VEGF treatment.
    - Bevacizumab, a full-length antibody that binds VEGF, can be used to treat DME when injected intravitreally. Intravitreal bevacizumab injection (IBI) is an off-label use.

○ Aflibercept, a decoy receptor for VEGF that inhibits all isoforms of VEGF-A and placental growth factor. Aflibercept 2 mg (0.05 mL) injected intravitreally every 4 weeks for the first 5 injections followed by 2 mg (0.05 mL) intravitreally once every 8 weeks; it is indicated for patients with DME and for DR in patients without DME.
  ■ IAI has demonstrated significant superiority in functional and anatomic end points over macular laser photocoagulation.
  ■ At worse levels of initial VA (20/50 or worse) in patients with DME, IAI was more effective in improving vision than ranibizumab or bevacizumab with 1-year follow-up. When the initial vision loss was mild (20/32 to 20/40) in patients with DME, there was no significant difference between aflibercept, ranibizumab, and bevacizumab.
    □ Aflibercept had superior 2-year VA outcomes compared with bevacizumab. The superiority of aflibercept over ranibizumab, noted at 1 year, was no longer seen at 2 years of follow-up.
  ■ Among eyes with CI-DME and good VA (20/25 or better), there was no significant difference in vision loss whether eyes were initially managed with observation plus IAI only if VA decreased, or with initial focal laser treatment plus IAI only if VA decreased, or prompt IAI. Observation without treatment unless VA worsens may be a reasonable plan of action for CI-DME (3)[A].
  ■ As-needed IAI has been shown to maintain vision and reduce treatment frequency.
○ Brolucizumab, a humanized single-chain antibody fragment that inhibits all isoforms of VEGF-A. It is injected intravitreally, at a dose of 6 mg every 6 weeks for the first 5 doses, followed by 1 injection every 8 to 12 weeks. There are reports of retinal vasculitis and/or retinal vascular occlusion after IVI of brolucizumab.
○ Faricimab inhibits both angiopoietin-2 and VEGF-A. It is injected intravitreally, at a dose of 6 mg monthly for the first 4 doses. Treatment is extended or reduced based on outcomes, with a range of 1 to 4 months between doses (4)[A].
– Focal laser treatment
– Vitrectomy may benefit some with diffuse macular edema. This may apply especially to eyes with vitreomacular traction found on OCT and with persistent DME.
– Intravitreal triamcinolone may be used for DM-related macular edema that fails laser treatment; no long-term benefit of intravitreal triamcinolone relative to focal/grid photocoagulation in patients with DME. When anti-VEGF treatment is inappropriate or ineffective for DME, intravitreal corticosteroid treatment and/or macular focal/grid laser photocoagulation may be used.
– Intraocular steroid implants for DME; either a dexamethasone implant or a fluocinolone acetonide implant; complications of these implants include cataract and glaucoma.

• Treatment for PDR:
  – Thermal laser photocoagulation in a panretinal pattern is a common form of treatment for PDR. The goal of panretinal photocoagulation (PRP) is regression or involution of NV. PRP destroys ischemic retina and decreases the neovascular stimulus.
    ○ The Diabetic Retinopathy Study demonstrated that when PRP was used to treat PDR or severe NPDR, eyes treated with PRP had a reduction of ≥50% in the rates of severe vision loss compared with untreated control eyes. In certain subgroups, the incidence of severe visual loss in untreated eyes was as high as 36.9% at 2 years.
    ○ Patients with DME and high-risk proliferative disease can have simultaneous focal and PRP without adversely affecting the visual outcome.
  – Both IRI and IAI are alternative therapies to PRP for PDR. They can be used in conjunction with PRP to treat PDR.
  – Initial IAI or pars plana vitrectomy (PPV) with PRP can be used to treat PDR-related VH (5)[A].
  – IVI of anti-VEGF therapy for PDR does not increase the risk for TRD.
  – PPV recommended for patients with severe PDR, traction retinal detachment involving the macula, and nonclearing VH:
    ○ The Diabetic Retinopathy Vitrectomy Study (DRVS) demonstrated the benefits of early PPV (1 to 6 months after onset of VH) in T1DM and for eyes with very severe PDR.
    ○ Immediate PPV with endolaser may be considered for PDR-associated VH (<30 days).
    ○ Preoperative IBI can be used as an adjuvant to vitrectomy for complications of PDR. This is an off-label use.

 ONGOING CARE

FOLLOW-UP RECOMMENDATIONS
Patient Monitoring
Scheduled ophthalmologic eye exams
• Yearly follow-up if no retinopathy
• Every 6 months with background DR
• At least every 3 to 4 months with pre-PDR
• Every 2 to 3 months with active PDR
• Patients with DME should be followed every 4 to 6 weeks.

DIET
In middle-aged and older individuals with T2DM, intake of at least 500 mg/day of dietary long-chain omega-3 polyunsaturated fatty acids, achievable with 2 weekly servings of oily fish, is associated with a decreased risk of DR.

PATIENT EDUCATION
• Advise regular ophthalmic exams.
• Stress importance of glucose control.

PROGNOSIS
If the condition is diagnosed and treated early in development, outlook is good. If treatment is delayed, blindness may result.

COMPLICATIONS
• Repeated IVI of anti-VEGF therapy may increase the risk of sustained intraocular pressure elevation and the possible need for ocular hypotensive treatment.
• Blindness

REFERENCES
1. Chiang JF, Sun MH, Chen KJ, et al. Association between obstructive sleep apnea and diabetic macular edema in patients with type 2 diabetes. *Am J Ophthalmol*. 2021;226:217–225.
2. Maturi RK, Glassman AR, Josic K, et al. Effect of intravitreous anti-vascular endothelial growth factor vs sham treatment for prevention of vision-threatening complications of diabetic retinopathy: the Protocol W randomized clinical trial. *JAMA Ophthalmol*. 2021;139(7):701–712.
3. Glassman AR, Baker CW, Beaulieu WT, et al. Assessment of the DRCR Retina Network approach to management with initial observation for eyes with center-involved diabetic macular edema and good visual acuity: a secondary analysis of a randomized clinical trial. *JAMA Ophthalmol*. 2020;138(4):341–349.
4. Wykoff CC, Abreu F, Adamis AP, et al. Efficacy, durability, and safety of intravitreal faricimab with extended dosing up to every 16 weeks in patients with diabetic macular oedema (YOSEMITE and RHINE); two randomised, double-masked, phase 3 trials. *Lancet*. 2022;399(10326):741–755.
5. Glassman AR, Beaulieu WT, Maguire MG, et al. Visual acuity, vitreous hemorrhage, and other ocular outcomes after vitrectomy vs aflibercept for vitreous hemorrhage due to diabetic retinopathy: a secondary analysis of a randomized clinical trial. *JAMA Ophthalmol*. 2021;139(7):725–733.

 CODES

ICD10
• E11.319 Type 2 diabetes mellitus with unspecified diabetic retinopathy without macular edema
• E10.319 Type 1 diabetes mellitus with unspecified diabetic retinopathy without macular edema
• E10.329 Type 1 diab w mild nonprlf diabetic rtnop w/o macular edema

CLINICAL PEARLS
• Schedule yearly ophthalmologic eye exams.
• Options for the treatment of DME include focal laser treatment, intravitreal triamcinolone, intravitreal ranibizumab, intravitreal bevacizumab (off-label), intravitreal aflibercept, intraocular steroid implants, and vitrectomy.

RHABDOMYOLYSIS

Chirag N. Shah, MD • Artika Saharan, MD • Daniel Scott Morrison, MD

BASICS

DESCRIPTION
- Breakdown of muscle and release of intracellular contents into the bloodstream
- Most commonly caused by traumatic muscle injury
- Typically presents with muscle pain, weakness, and reddish brown (tea-colored) urine
- Up to 50% of patients are asymptomatic.

EPIDEMIOLOGY
Most common among
- Males; <10 years old; >60 years old; BMI >40 kg/m^3

Incidence
- 25,000 reported cases annually in the United States
- Although muscle-related side effects of statins are the most common reason for discontinuation of statins, rhabdomyolysis is only seen in 0.5% of patients.

ETIOLOGY AND PATHOPHYSIOLOGY
- Direct muscle trauma (most common cause)
  - Crush injuries; fractures; extended periods of muscle pressure (during surgery, unconscious from alcohol ingestion, coma); burns, electrocution, lightning strike
- Muscle exertion
  - New strenuous and/or prolonged physical exercise (marathon runners, athletes, contact sports); seizures; delirium tremens; malignant hyperthermia; neuroleptic malignant syndrome (NMS)
- Drugs and toxins
  - Alcohol; cocaine (most common recreational drug), methamphetamine, phencyclidine, heroin, bath salts (1)[B], and synthetic marijuana has been associated with severe rhabdomyolysis; antipsychotics (due to NMS, malignant hyperthermia, and dystonia); zidovudine; antimalarials; HMG-CoA reductase inhibitors (statins)— develops about 2 to 3 weeks after initiating therapy (risk <0.01%, elevated with higher doses and in combination with fibrates); colchicine; corticosteroids; carbon monoxide; snake envenomation; scorpion bites
- Muscle ischemia
  - Thrombosis, embolism, sickle cell disease; compartment syndrome; tourniquets
- Infections
  - Viral: influenza A and B, coxsackievirus, HIV, varicella
  - Bacterial: *Streptococcus* or *Staphylococcus* sepsis, gas gangrene, necrotizing fasciitis, *Salmonella*, *Legionella*
  - Malaria
- Hypothermia; hyperthermia
- Autoimmune disorders
  - Polymyositis, dermatomyositis
- Metabolic and endocrinologic:
  - Hypothyroidism or thyrotoxicosis; electrolyte imbalances (e.g., hyponatremia, hypernatremia, hypokalemia, hypocalcemia, hypophosphatemia); diabetic ketoacidosis; hyperosmolar state

Genetics
Hereditary causes of rhabdomyolysis are rare but should be suspected in children; patients with recurrent attacks; or patients who have attacks after minimal exertion, mild illness, or starvation.
- Genetic disorders
  - Muscular dystrophies; disorders of lipid metabolism (e.g., carnitine palmitoyltransferase deficiency)
  - Disorders of carbohydrate metabolism (i.e., phosphofructokinase deficiency, phosphoglycerate mutase, myophosphorylase deficiency, a.k.a. McArdle disease/deficiency); glycogen storage diseases (e.g., phosphorylase B kinase deficiency) and others (e.g., lactate dehydrogenase A deficiency, phosphofructokinase deficiency)
  - Mitochondrial disorders; sickle cell trait

GENERAL PREVENTION
- Avoid excessive exertion; ensure adequate hydration.
- Avoid precipitating drugs, metabolic and electrolyte abnormalities.

DIAGNOSIS

HISTORY
- Crush injuries
  - Direct trauma and/or prolonged compression/immobility
    - Motor vehicle accidents (MVA) and entrapment in collapsed buildings; the elderly are more susceptible to crush injury due to immobility and falls.
- Overexertion and/or use of drug/toxin (e.g., cocaine, amphetamine, statins), particularly in warm environments; agitation while patients are in restraints; prolonged periods of lying on a hard surface (e.g., intoxicated or obtunded individuals)
- Common symptoms
  - Malaise, muscle aches, weakness, cramps, or fatigue; nausea, vomiting, diarrhea, fever
- Urinary symptoms—brown or "tea colored" urine; decreased urine output in severe cases
- Encephalopathy and confusion in severe cases

PHYSICAL EXAM
- Vital sign abnormalities
  - Low-grade temperature; tachycardia in severe cases
- Obvious crush injury; discoloration or blisters seen in cases of prolonged pressure necrosis; neurovascular compromise in severe cases with compartment syndrome
- May have muscle tenderness usually in the proximal muscles such as thighs, calves, and lower back with weakness and/or swelling on exam; the muscle exam may also be completely normal.
- Tea-colored urine is indicative of myoglobinuria.

DIFFERENTIAL DIAGNOSIS
- Traumatic injuries
- Other diseases with dark urine:
  - Kidney stones; nephritic syndromes; hemoglobinuria; porphyria
- Inflammatory myopathies; infection (bacterial or viral); phosphorylase, phosphofructokinase, carnitine palmityl transferase, phosphoglycerate mutase deficiency; Guillain-Barré syndrome; myocardial infarction

DIAGNOSTIC TESTS & INTERPRETATION

Initial Tests (lab, imaging)
- 12-lead ECG (hyperkalemia/peaked T-waves, may induce fatal arrhythmias)
- Creatine kinase (total CK) is the diagnostic test of choice: elevated >5 times the upper limit of normal or >1,000 U/L to diagnose rhabdomyolysis
  - CK levels >5,000 U/L are causally related to acute renal failure (ARF) (1)[A] and should prompt aggressive fluid resuscitation.
  - CK levels rise within 12 hours, peak within 24 to 72 hours, and return to normal in 3 to 5 days.
    - As a result, CK is a more sensitive marker than myoglobin, although myoglobin is responsible for renal damage (1)[C].
    - Serum myoglobin levels peak within a few hours and return to normal after ~24 hours. Normal myoglobin levels do not rule out rhabdomyolysis (due to rapid clearance).
- Urinalysis: Dipstick test positive for blood without erythrocytes (RBCs) in sediment suggests injury from either hemoglobin or myoglobin.
  - Absence of myoglobinuria does not rule out rhabdomyolysis as the myoglobin can be cleared within 1 to 6 hours (2)[A].
  - Urine pH usually acidic; often positive for protein
- Other lab/electrolyte abnormalities:
  - Hyperkalemia: elevations of serum potassium from muscle injury can be compounded by ARF.
  - Calcium:
    - Initial hypocalcemia: Calcium enters the injured muscle cells and precipitates as calcium phosphate, leading to calcification of ischemic muscle cells.
      - Only correct initial hypocalcemia if patient is symptomatic or has ECG changes; resolves during the renal recovery phase
    - Hypercalcemia during renal recovery phase: unique to rhabdomyolysis-induced ARF for 20–30% of patients (1)[A]; as renal function improves, there is a mobilization of the precipitated calcium.
  - Extreme hyperuricemia may or may not be present and can cause acute uric acid nephropathy.
  - Elevations in BUN and creatinine suggest ARF.
  - Transaminitis: reversible hepatic dysfunction
    - Elevations in alanine aminotransferase (ALT), aspartate aminotransferase (AST), and lactic dehydrogenase are likely due to muscle injury rather than hepatic injury.

– Hyperphosphatemia
– Increased PT/PTT, fibrin degradation products, and D-dimer with decreases in platelets and fibrinogen indicate disseminated intravascular coagulation (DIC).

Follow-Up Tests & Special Considerations
McMahon Scoring Tool can predict mortality and patients who will require renal replacement therapy (RRT). Delayed renal failure/electrolyte abnormalities despite normal initial levels; ongoing muscle injury is manifested by rising creatine phosphokinase (CPK). Renal imaging shows findings similar to other mechanisms of ARF.

Diagnostic Procedures/Other
- Muscle compartment pressures if compartment syndrome is suspected
- Ultrasound imaging can show muscle thickening, ground glass opacity, traits of edema, and anechoic areas.
- If the patient requires intubation, rocuronium is the paralytic of choice as patients can have severe hyperkalemia from rhabdomyolysis.

Test Interpretation
Muscle necrosis; myoglobin-related renal injury may resemble acute tubular necrosis from other causes.

TREATMENT

GENERAL MEASURES
- Address underlying cause (e.g., medications cessation, temperature control, trauma, infection).
- Aggressive hydration with large volumes of IV fluids is often necessary.
  – In severe muscle trauma (crush injuries), up to 12 L of fluid may be sequestered in the muscles.
- Monitor CK levels, renal function, and electrolytes.
  – Follow potassium levels due to the potential for arrhythmias. Treat hyperphosphatemia and hypocalcemia cautiously as treatment may worsen calcium precipitation in the muscle tissue.
- Treat DIC or hepatic dysfunction appropriately.
  – Both should be transient and resolve over a few days.
- Recognize and treat compartment syndrome promptly.

MEDICATION
First Line
Aggressive fluid resuscitation is the most important intervention: normal saline (NS) and 5% glucose solution
- Target urine output of 200 to 300 mL/hr; alternating NS and 5% glucose is recommended to prevent volume overload. Infusion rate should be 500 mL/hr.

Second Line
- Alkalinization of the urine may decrease myoglobin-induced nephrotoxicity in the tubules (sodium bicarbonate to increase urine pH >6.5).
  – Use is controversial. Side effects include worsening hypocalcemia. Sodium bicarbonate helps patients with very high CK levels, acidosis, or coexisting hyperkalemia.
  – 150 mEq (3 ampules) $NaHCO_3$ in 1 L of D5W and infuse at 200 mL/hr

- IV mannitol as a bolus if urine output remains low, 1 to 2 g/kg, not to exceed 200 g in 24 hours with a cumulative dose of 800 g; it is used to prevent ARF only if diuresis is not adequate (<200 mL/hr) despite fluid therapy.
  – An osmotic agent, filtered but not reabsorbed by the tubules; this may remove necrotic cell debris and prevent the rise in compartment pressures. Use of mannitol is controversial.
  – Consider adding furosemide to force diuresis if necessary (40 to 120 mg/day). Do not diurese in anuric renal failure; caution also in the elderly and patients with heart disease
- Hyperkalemia can result from massive release of intracellular potassium stores or ARF. Severe hyperkalemia may be life-threatening; treatment when ECG changes are present (tall, thin T waves; PR prolongation; QRS widening; P wave flattening)
  – Calcium gluconate: to stabilize the cardiac membrane; IV 1 to 2 ampules (0.5 mL 10% calcium gluconate = 4 mg elemental calcium; give 4 mg/kg/hr for 4 hours.)
  – If acidosis is present: 1 to 2 ampules (2 to 3 mL/kg) sodium bicarbonate IV; sodium bicarbonate can worsen hypocalcemia. If tolerated: Oral sodium polystyrene sulfonate (Kayexalate) as much as 20 g (1 g/kg) can be given via enema. Insulin and albuterol transiently drive potassium into the cells. Administration of glucose can prevent the hypoglycemic effects of insulin. Precautions: continuous monitoring of potassium levels to prevent overcorrecting with potential hypokalemia and arrhythmias
  – Indications for dialysis include resistant and symptomatic hyperkalemia (ECG), oliguria (<0.5 mL/kg over 12-hour period), anuria, volume overload, or persistent acidosis (pH <7.1).

ISSUES FOR REFERRAL
Usually managed as an inpatient; diagnosis of compartment syndrome merits surgical consultation for consideration of fasciotomy. Renal dialysis may be indicated in ARF.

ADDITIONAL THERAPIES
During the oliguric phase, symptomatic hypocalcemia (rare) may benefit from IV calcium gluconate.

SURGERY/OTHER PROCEDURES
For muscle entrapment/compartment syndrome

ADMISSION, INPATIENT, AND NURSING CONSIDERATIONS
- Patients with significant elevations of CK or any signs of renal injury should be admitted for IV hydration and clinical monitoring; volume expansion with NS to increase urine output to at least 150 mL/hr
- CK usually peaks 24 to 36 hours after muscle injury; so, monitoring should confirm that the CK is trending down. Renal function should be stable/improving. Electrolytes should be normal.
- Patients with mild CK elevation, normal renal function, clear etiology, and adequate follow-up may be discharged after observation phase and hydration if CK is trending down.

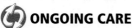

ONGOING CARE

FOLLOW-UP RECOMMENDATIONS
Follow up within a few days to recheck CK, electrolytes, and renal function.

Patient Monitoring
Contingent on disease: essential for metabolic myopathies; myotoxic drugs should be discontinued/monitored closely.

DIET
With renal failure, restrict protein intake to lower BUN level. Limit potassium intake. With anuria, it is essential to restrict volume intake.

PROGNOSIS
Contingent on primary cause of rhabdomyolysis and on recovery from ARF without complications

COMPLICATIONS
- Death, especially from hyperkalemia/renal failure
- With prompt initiation of fluids for IV rehydration, dialysis, and supportive care, the prognosis is very good.

REFERENCES
1. Long B, Koyfman A, Gottlieb M. An evidence-based narrative review of the emergency department evaluation and management of rhabdomyolysis. *Am J Emerg Med*. 2019;37(3):518–523.
2. Stahl K, Rastelli E, Schoser B. A systematic review on the definition of rhabdomyolysis. *J Neurol*. 2020;267(4):877–882.

ADDITIONAL READING
- Cabral BMI, Edding SN, Portocarrero JP, et al. Rhabdomyolysis. *Dis Mon*. 2020;66(8):101015.
- Knafl EG, Hughes JA, Dimeski G, et al. Rhabdomyolysis: patterns, circumstances, and outcomes of patients presenting to the emergency department. *Ochsner J*. 2018;18(3):215–221.

 SEE ALSO

Algorithm: Acute Kidney Injury (Acute Renal Failure)

 CODES

ICD10
- M62.82 Rhabdomyolysis
- T79.6 Traumatic ischemia of muscle
- T79.6xxS Traumatic ischemia of muscle, sequela

CLINICAL PEARLS
- Elevation of CK is the diagnostic hallmark of rhabdomyolysis.
- The cornerstone of treatment of rhabdomyolysis is aggressive fluid administration.
- Initial serum creatinine predicts mortality.
- Electrolyte abnormalities, acute kidney injury, hepatic injury, compartment syndrome, and (rarely) DIC are the most worrisome complications of rhabdomyolysis.

RHABDOMYOSARCOMA

Bryan G. Beutel, MD

 BASICS

DESCRIPTION
- Rhabdomyosarcoma (RMS) is a malignant soft tissue tumor presumed to originate from a mesenchymal cell line shared with striated skeletal muscle.
- Occurs mainly as primary malignancy but can also be a component of heterogeneous neoplasms
  - WHO classification of soft tissue tumors describes four main RMS subtypes:
    - Embryonal RMS (ERMS): 60% of RMS cases
      - Early onset and the most common subtype in children
      - Commonly presents in the head, neck, and genitourinary areas
      - Subdivided into:
        - Classic
        - Botryoid (6% overall embryonal): seen in infants, although can happen in <4-year-old patients
        - Spindle cell: 3% of cases and affects young children
        - Both botryoid and spindle cell variants have better prognosis than the classic variant
    - Alveolar RMS (ARMS): 20% of pediatric cases
      - Aggressive subtype
      - More common in the trunk, perineum/perianal area, and extremities
    - Spindle/Sclerosing: approximately 10% of cases
      - Mostly found in the paratesticular region
    - Anaplastic (children)/pleomorphic (adults): <10% of cases
      - Typically seen in patients aged 30 to 50 years (rarely in pediatric population)
      - Associated with Li-Fraumeni symptoms
      - Demonstrates hyperchromatic enlarged nuclei
  - Pathologic and molecular studies have now delineated up to five or six distinct subfamilies of RMS.
  - Common primary sites:
    - Head and neck (25%) presentation (common in young children, usually embryonal type)
    - Genitourinary (31%, mostly embryonal type)
    - Musculoskeletal (13%, most common in extremities primary sites in adolescents and adults, alveolar subtype)

EPIDEMIOLOGY
- RMS is the most common soft tissue sarcoma in pediatric population.
- Common metastatic sites: bone marrow, lung, lymph nodes

Incidence
- 4.5 cases of RMS per 1 million children per year
- Accounts for 50% of all soft tissue sarcomas in children and adolescents
  - 50% of pediatric cases occur before the age of 10 years (often before age 6 years).

Prevalence
- Represents 3% of all pediatric tumors and 1% of all adult tumors
- Slight predilection for males (1.3:1 male-to-female ratio)
- More common in the African-American population

ETIOLOGY AND PATHOPHYSIOLOGY
- Originates from rhabdomyoblast cell
- Tumor is often >5 cm in size with poorly circumscribed border, white coloration, and infiltrative features.

Genetics
Genetic characteristics vary according to the RMS subtype:
- Alveolar:
  - Linked to recurrent Forkhead box O1 (FOXO1) fusions (identified in 90% of cases)
  - t(1;13)(p36;q14), causing formation of the fusion oncogenes *PAX7-FOXO1*
  - t(2;13)(q35;q14), causing formation of the fusion oncogenes *PAX3-FOXO1*
- Embryonal:
  - Multiple complex genetic aberrations, including *MYOD1* mutations
  - Loss or uniparental disomy of 11p15.5 +2, +8, +11, +12, +13, +20 affecting genes *IGF-2*, *H19*, *CDKN1C*, and/or *HOTS*
- Spindle cell/sclerosing:
  - 8q13 rearrangements involving *SRF-NCOA2* and *TEAD1-NCOA2*

RISK FACTORS
Largely unknown; however, appears to be increased risk of RMS in setting of:
- Rapid growth in utero
- Radiation exposure in utero
- Lower socioeconomic status
- Recreational drug use during pregnancy

COMMONLY ASSOCIATED CONDITIONS
- Beckwith-Wiedemann syndrome (11p15 mutations)
- Costello syndrome (germline *HRAS* mutations)
- Li-Fraumeni syndrome (germline *TP53*; known as *p53* mutations)
- Neurofibromatosis type I (*NF1* mutations)
- Noonan syndrome (*PTPN11* mutations)

DIAGNOSIS

Thorough history and physical examination necessary but typically requires molecular genetic, immunohistochemical (ICH), and/or structural techniques to confirm diagnosis of RMS

HISTORY
Initial presenting symptoms variable based on location of mass, age of patient, etc.
- Manifests as a progressive, palpable mass
- When in the head/neck region, patients may report diplopia, recurrent sinusitis, or persistent nasal discharge.
- RMS of genitourinary tissue may present as urinary obstruction, hematuria, polyuria, or potentially vaginal bleeding in females.
- Other symptoms may be noted due to the mass effect of the primary/metastatic lesions.
- Personal or family history of genetic syndromes (e.g., Li-Fraumeni syndrome, Noonan syndrome)

PHYSICAL EXAM
- Painless, enlarging mass when in head/neck region but may be painful when present in the extremities (with overlying erythema of skin)
- Polypoid mass protruding from the vagina (suggests botryoid subtype)
- Exophthalmos and chemosis (seen with orbital involvement)
- Abdominal pain and mass effect symptoms include seizures, visual field defects, nerve palsy, headaches, etc.

DIFFERENTIAL DIAGNOSIS
- Osteosarcoma
- Ewing sarcoma
- Liposarcoma
- Lipoma
- Wilms tumor
- Lymphoproliferative disorder
- Lymphadenopathy
- Neurofibromatosis type I

DIAGNOSTIC TESTS & INTERPRETATION
Initial Tests (lab, imaging)
- Laboratory studies: Complete blood count, serum chemistries, liver function test, and coagulation profile should be obtained for clinical optimization prior to initiating treatment.
- Imaging studies should include the following:
  - MRI with/without contrast (or CT) of the primary tumor (to define anatomy)
  - CT chest and abdomen/pelvis
  - Bone scan
- Additional staging workup:
  - Lymph node biopsy
  - Bone marrow aspirate and biopsy

Follow-Up Tests & Special Considerations
Biopsy of the suspected RMS tumor is necessary for diagnosis.

Diagnostic Procedures/Other
- For pathologic diagnosis:
  - Core needle biopsy, incisional biopsy, or excisional biopsy (based on size of the mass)
  - RMS tumors typically demonstrate eccentric eosinophilic cytoplasm with abundant thick/thin filaments.

Table 1. TNM Staging System for RMS

Stage	Site(s)	T	Tumor Diameter	N	M
1	Orbit; head and neck (excluding parameningeal), genitourinary—nonbladder and nonprostate, biliary tract	T1 or T2	a or b	Any N	M0
2	Bladder or prostate, extremity, cranial parameningeal, other	T1 or T2	a	N0 or NX	M0
3a	Bladder or prostate, extremity, cranial parameningeal, other	T1 or T2	a	N1	M0
3b	Bladder or prostate, extremity, cranial parameningeal, other	T1 or T2	b	Any N	M0
4	All sites (metastatic)	T1 or T2	a or b	N0 or N1	M1

T1, confined to organ of origin; T2, extends outside the organ of origin; a, ≤5 cm in diameter; b, >5 cm in diameter; M0, no distant metastasis; N0, regional nodes not clinically involved; NX, clinical status of regional nodes unknown; N1, regional nodes clinically involved by neoplasm; M1, distant metastasis.

- Histologic classification:
  - Alveolar: rhabdomyoblasts grossly mimicking pulmonary alveoli arranged in interseptal nests within a network of intersecting fibrous septae
  - Embryonal: typically displays a myxoid matrix
    - Classic: rhabdomyoblasts configured in sheets, large nest, eosinophilic cytoplasm
    - Botryoid: "grape-like" appearance with notable clustering in subepithelium forming the cambium layer
    - Spindle cell: rhabdomyoblasts with spindle-like appearance
  - Anaplastic/pleomorphic: rhabdomyoblast with large hyperchromatic nuclei and multipolar mitotic morphologies
- ICH markers:
  - Positive for desmin, sarcomeric actin, myogenin, myoglobin
  - Usually negative for CD99, CK, S100, NKX2.2, NSE
- Molecular testing for PAX/FOXO1 fusion (tested by PCR and fluorescence in situ hybridization) (1)[A]
- Genetic profiling likely to become gold standard for diagnosis and prognosis
- Staging is based on the site, size, regional nodal involvement, and degree of spread (Table 1).

 ## TREATMENT

- Spans surgical resection, radiation, and chemotherapy
- Treatment should be performed by interdisciplinary team that includes oncologist, surgeon, and radiologist

GENERAL MEASURES

The development of multimodal therapy protocols has led to improved outcomes

SURGERY/OTHER PROCEDURES

- Surgery:
  - Local resection of tumor along with metastases and nodal resection (2)[C]
  - Lymph node sampling is intended to identify unknown metastasis and guide decision for postoperative radiation.

- Radiation therapy: recommended to enhance local control, except in patients with embryonal type
  - Emergent therapy only considered in patients with compression symptoms
  - Ionizing radiation shown to decrease recurrence rates, especially in higher stage classifications
- Chemotherapy:
  - Selected based on prognosis/risk stratification (i.e., low, intermediate, or high)
    - "VAC" regimen consists of vincristine, actinomycin D (dactinomycin), and cyclophosphamide
    - "IVA" regimen includes ifosfamide, vincristine, and actinomycin D.
  - Most common adverse reactions are the following:
    - Vincristine: peripheral neuropathy
    - Dactinomycin: myelosuppression and hepatotoxicity
    - Cyclophosphamide: hemorrhagic cystitis (mesna is used for prophylaxis), transitional cell carcinoma, myelosuppression with leukopenia, and infertility
- In addition, ifosfamide, topotecan, doxorubicin, etoposide, and irinotecan may be used in alternative regimens.
- Administration protocol depends on risk stratification but, generally, ranges from 12 to 24 months given in separate cycles (up to 15 cycles).

 ## ONGOING CARE

FOLLOW-UP RECOMMENDATIONS

- Physical examination and imaging surveillance for the first 5 years (CT/MRI/x-ray) to assess for recurrence, metastatic disease, or development of secondary malignancies
  - Imaging should be done every 3 months for the 1st year, every 4 months for the following 2 years, and finally every 6 months for the subsequent 2 years.
- After first 5 years, no more imaging surveillance is typically required.

DIET

There are no specific dietary limitations.

PATIENT EDUCATION

National Cancer Institute: https://www.cancer.gov/types/soft-tissue-sarcoma/patient/rhabdomyosarcoma-treatment-pdq

PROGNOSIS

- RMS (overall) 5-year survival: 61% (children) and 27% (adults)
- Metastatic RMS overall survival <25%
- RMS of extremities and parameningeal RMS have worse prognosis.

COMPLICATIONS

- Recurrence
- Secondary neoplasm
- Growth abnormalities

R

REFERENCES

1. Gallagher KPD, van Heerden W, Said-Al-Naief N, et al. Molecular profile of head and neck rhabdomyosarcomas: a systematic review and meta-analysis. *Oral Surg Oral Med Oral Pathol Oral Radiol*. 2022;134(3):354–366.
2. Skapek SX, Ferrari A, Gupta AA, et al. Rhabdomyosarcoma. *Nat Rev Dis Primers*. 2019;5(1):1.

ADDITIONAL READING

Leiner J, Le Loarer F. The current landscape of rhabdomyosarcomas: an update. *Virchows Arch*. 2020;476(1):97–108.

 ## CODES

ICD10

- C49.9 Malignant neoplasm of connective and soft tissue, unsp
- C49.0 Malignant neoplasm of connective and soft tissue of head, face and neck
- C49.5 Malignant neoplasm of connective and soft tissue of pelvis

CLINICAL PEARLS

- RMS is more common in children but can develop in adults, the latter having higher mortality.
- Genetic disorders and congenital syndromes increase risk of RMS.
- If a localized tumor is identified with concurrent lymph node involvement, implement more aggressive therapy.
- The most common site of metastasis is the lung, followed by bone marrow/bone and peritoneum.

RHEUMATIC FEVER

Robert J. Casey, MD

 BASICS

DESCRIPTION

- Acute rheumatic fever (ARF) is an autoimmune, inflammatory response to infection with group A *Streptococcus* (GAS) that affects multiple organ systems.
- Untreated acute disease can lead to chronic rheumatic heart disease (RHD).
- Recurrence is common without adequate antibiotic treatment.

Pediatric Considerations

Most cases occur in children aged 5 to 15 years; rare in children aged <5 years

EPIDEMIOLOGY

- ARF and RHD are largely restricted to low-income countries and marginalized sections of wealthy countries.
- Male = female; females more likely to develop chorea and RHD.
- Endemic regions include South Pacific, indigenous populations of Australia and New Zealand, Africa, and Asia (1).

Incidence

- Worldwide, incidence has been declining for 25 years. The large majority of new cases are in developing countries (1).
- Mean worldwide incidence ranges from 8 to 51/100,000 school-aged children; in endemic regions, prevalence can be >1,000 cases per 100,000 people (1).
- Incidence of ARF in the United States is currently <3.4 to 2/100,000 school-aged children (1).

Prevalence

- In developing areas, RHD affects >33 million people and is the leading cause of cardiovascular death during the first 5 decades of life.
- Prevalence has been rising due to improved medical care and longer survival.

ETIOLOGY AND PATHOPHYSIOLOGY

- ARF most commonly occurs 2 to 3 weeks after GAS pharyngitis infection, but GAS impetigo may also be a proceeding infection.
- Although pathogenicity is not completely understood, expert consensus implicates genetic and molecular mimicry leading to an inflammatory cascade as key to disease development.
- Immune cross reactive response contributes to joint involvement due to accumulation of immune complexes.

Genetics

- Susceptibility is associated with certain indigenous populations.
- ARF is heritable, polygenic, and displays variable and incomplete penetrance.

RISK FACTORS

Poverty, household crowding, genetic susceptibility, ethnic predisposition, and social disadvantage are the strongest risk factors.

GENERAL PREVENTION

- Primary prevention: Appropriate treatment of streptococcal infection prevents ARF in most cases.
- Secondary prevention: long-term antibiotic prophylaxis (up to 5 to 10 years) to prevent recurrence (1)

 DIAGNOSIS

- 2015 revised Jones criteria and lab evidence of preceding GAS infection are used for diagnosis.
- Initial ARF: 2 major *or* 1 major + 2 minor
- Recurrent ARF: 2 major *or* 1 major + 2 minor *or* 3 minor
- Sydenham chorea is independently sufficient to diagnosis ARF, even without lab evidence of preceding infection.

Low-Risk Population	Moderate- and High-Risk Population
Major criteria:	Major criteria:
• Carditis: clinical or subclinical (echocardiogram)	• Carditis: clinical or subclinical (echocardiogram)
• Polyarthritis ONLY	• Polyarthritis OR monoarthritis
• Chorea	• Chorea
• Erythema marginatum	• Erythema marginatum
• Subcutaneous nodules	• Subcutaneous nodules
Minor criteria:	Minor criteria:
• Polyarthralgia	• Monoarthralgia
• Fever ≥38.5°C	• Fever ≥38°C
• ESR ≥60 mm/hr	• ESR ≥30 mm/hr
• CRP ≥3 mg/dL	• CRP ≥3 mg/dL
• ↑PR interval	• ↑PR interval

- The revised criteria distinguish between low-risk and moderate- to high-risk patient populations. Patients can be considered low risk if they are from and among a low-incidence group.
- Subclinical carditis can be diagnosed with echocardiographic evidence of mitral or aortic valve regurgitation and can be supported by chest x-ray demonstrating cardiomegaly or left atrial enlargement.

HISTORY

- ARF typically presents 2 to 3 weeks following GAS pharyngitis or impetigo.
- Polyarthritis (knees, ankles, elbows, wrists) (35–66%) is self-limited and often the first symptom; each resolves in days, thus seems to "migrate." Rapid improvement occurs with aspirin or NSAIDs, which may mask initial symptoms. Moderate- and high-risk patients may only have monoarthritis.
- Fever
- Erythema marginatum rash
- Pancarditis or valvulitis (50–70%) can be subclinical (asymptomatic without auscultatory findings) or clinically apparent.
- Sydenham chorea (late manifestation [1 to 6 months after infection] in 10–30%): purposeless, involuntary, nonstereotypical movements, most commonly involving the face and hands
  - More common in 5- to 15-year-olds, females
  - Improves or ceases during sleep
  - Can have associated muscular weakness, may manifest as deteriorating handwriting
  - Psychiatric symptoms may have onset prior to chorea, with emotional lability and obsessive-compulsive symptoms.
  - Self-resolves over several months and can relapse

PHYSICAL EXAM

- Neuro: Sydenham chorea: Involuntary movements may be general or unilateral and involve the face. "Milkmaid grip" is intermittent hypotonia on test of grip strength.
- Cardiac: pericardial friction rub, holosystolic murmur of mitral/aortic regurgitation, rarely diastolic; rarely evidence of heart failure
- Skin
  - Subcutaneous nodules (<10%): firm, painless protuberances on extensor surfaces involving knees, elbows, wrists, occiput, and spinous process of thoracic and lumbar vertebrae; more common in severe ARF, persists several weeks
  - Erythema marginatum (5–13%): evanescent, pink rash with pale centers and rounded/serpiginous margins found on trunk and proximal extremities; rare to be found on face; typically nonpruritic; blanches with pressure and can be induced with heat

DIFFERENTIAL DIAGNOSIS

- Systemic lupus erythematosus
- Poststreptococcal reactive arthritis
- Juvenile rheumatoid arthritis
- Infectious arthritis
- Myocarditis (viral or idiopathic)
- Innocent cardiac murmur
- Cardiomyopathy
- Tourette syndrome
- Kawasaki syndrome
- Pediatric autoimmune neuropsychiatric disorders associated with streptococcal infections (PANDAS)
- Lyme disease
- Henoch-Schönlein purpura
- Wilson disease
- Substance abuse
- Tic disorder
- Encephalitis
- Huntington chorea
- Drug reaction

DIAGNOSTIC TESTS & INTERPRETATION

Initial Tests (lab, imaging)

- Serologic evidence of GAS infection is needed whenever possible, and diagnosis is in question when it cannot be obtained (chorea and chronic indolent rheumatic carditis being the exception due to delayed onset).
  - Rapid streptococcal antigen test with high pretest probability
  - Positive GAS throat culture
  - Elevated or rising antistreptococcal antibody titer (ASO or ADB); ASO peaks 3 to 5 weeks postinfection, ADB 6 to 8 weeks. A rise in titer is better than a single titer result.
- ESR and CRP are acute-phase reactants; almost always increased in ARF
- CBC with differential: leukocytosis, normocytic anemia
- ECG: PR prolongation, AV block, signs of pericarditis
- Joint aspiration and synovial fluid evaluation is indicated if significant effusion or septic arthritis is suspected.
- Echocardiogram: chamber size and function, pericardial effusion, and valve disease
- All cases of confirmed *or* suspected ARF should have an echocardiogram within 12 weeks due to 18% prevalence of subclinical carditis.

Follow-Up Tests & Special Considerations

- CRP is useful to monitor the acute disease process and can initially be trended twice weekly, followed by every 1 to 2 weeks until normalized.
- Due to morbidity associate with untreated cardiac disease, all confirmed cases of ARF should have serial echocardiograms, even if the initial screen was negative for carditis (1)[C].
- All household contacts should be screened with GAS throat cultures. Positive results should be treated with antibiotics, even if asymptomatic.

Test Interpretation

Prior treatment with aspirin or steroids may lead to falsely negative lab results.

 TREATMENT

GENERAL MEASURES

- Antibiotic
- Anti-inflammatory agent (aspirin or naproxen)
- Manage other manifestations as indicated (e.g., chorea, dysrhythmia, carditis, or heart failure).

MEDICATION

First Line

- Eradication: GAS infection treatment should begin within 9 days of illness to prevent ARF. If ARF diagnosis is confirmed, begin secondary prophylaxis.
- If no penicillin allergy:
  - Penicillin VK 250 mg PO BID for 10 days, benzathine penicillin G IM for 1 day, or amoxicillin 50 mg/kg PO for 10 days (preferred in children)
- If penicillin allergy:
  - 1st-generation cephalosporin PO for 10 days, azithromycin 12 mg/kg PO for 5 days, clindamycin 7 mg/kg/dose PO for 10 days, or clarithromycin 7.5 mg/kg/dose PO for 10 days
- Arthritis: Naproxen 10 to 20 mg/kg/day divided BID is now recommended over aspirin, given superior side-effect profile and less risk of Reye syndrome.
- Carditis: If heart failure, 3rd-degree AV block, or other severe manifestations, appropriate traditional management should be initiated as indicated.
- NSAIDs, glucocorticoids, and IVIG are not recommended for carditis, although glucocorticoids can be considered in severe carditis with acute cardiac failure.
- Chorea: generally self-limited, not requiring treatment. Valproic acid or carbamazepine may be used for severe cases. IVIG and glucocorticoids are restricted to failure of initial management. Antipsychotics are not routinely used due to extrapyramidal side effects.

Second Line

- Penicillin allergy and severity should be confirmed prior to starting a second line agent.
- If severe penicillin allergy is present, erythromycin is preferred by the New Zealand Guidelines Group but not by the Infectious Diseases Society of America.

ISSUES FOR REFERRAL

- A cardiologist should be involved in management of ARF.
- Pediatric neurologist or movement specialist can help guide therapy with severe chorea.

SURGERY/OTHER PROCEDURES

Valve stenosis is a late sequela resulting from fibrosis and calcification; mainstay of therapy is surgical correction (1).

ADMISSION, INPATIENT, AND NURSING CONSIDERATIONS

- Initial hospitalization may be helpful for diagnosis and to ensure stability.
- Heart failure requires prompt hospitalization.
- IV fluids
  - Only if signs of dehydration or hypotension; use caution in heart failure.
- Nursing
  - Activity as tolerated

 ONGOING CARE

FOLLOW-UP RECOMMENDATIONS

- Secondary prophylaxis: antibiotic therapy from time of diagnosis until at least age 21 years, or 5 years after diagnosis (whichever comes later)
- In patients with ARF with carditis, antibiotic therapy from time of diagnosis until at least age 21 years, or 10 years after diagnosis (whichever comes later)
- Indefinite prophylactic antibiotics can be indicated if valvular disease is present, as recurrence of disease can worsen severity of carditis.
  - First-line prophylaxis is long-acting benzathine penicillin G monthly IM injections.
  - Penicillin V PO 250 mg BID is an alternative.
  - If penicillin allergy, sulfadiazine 0.5 to 1 g daily
  - If penicillin and sulfa drug allergy, azithromycin
  - Patients on penicillin prophylaxis who develop GAS pharyngitis while on penicillin should be treated with clindamycin.
- If ARF is possible, but uncertain, treat with 1 year of secondary antibiotic prophylaxis until repeat echocardiogram (1)[C].
- Routine antibiotic prophylaxis for dental procedures is no longer recommended for patients with RHD.

Patient Monitoring

Weekly monitoring after the initial diagnosis; every 6 months thereafter, based on clinical stability.

Pediatric Considerations

Use aspirin with caution in children given the risk of Reye syndrome.

Pregnancy Considerations

May exacerbate valve disease, particularly mitral stenosis in RHD. Refer pregnant patients to a cardiologist.

DIET

No dietary restrictions; low-sodium if heart failure present

PATIENT EDUCATION

American Heart Association: https://www.heart.org

PROGNOSIS

Long-term sequelae are generally limited to the heart and depend on the severity of carditis during an acute attack. Recurrence is most common in the first year after diagnosis (1).

COMPLICATIONS

- Recurrence of ARF due to GAS reinfection
- RHD can occur 10 to 20 years after ARF, with mitral more common than aortic regurgitation, can lead to mitral stenosis. Heart failure is the worst complication.
- Jaccoud arthropathy is chronic and involves painless deformities of hands/feet.
- Patients with a history of ARF have a higher incidence of infective endocarditis in the future.

REFERENCE

1. Kumar RK, Antunes MJ, Beaton A, et al; for the American Heart Association Council on Lifelong Congenital Heart Disease and Heart Health in the Young; Council on Cardiovascular and Stroke Nursing; and Council on Clinical Cardiology. Contemporary diagnosis and management of rheumatic heart disease: implications for closing the gap: a scientific statement from the American Heart Association. *Circulation*. 2020;142(20):e337–e357.

 CODES

ICD10

- I00 Rheumatic fever without heart involvement
- I01.9 Acute rheumatic heart disease, unspecified
- I01.0 Acute rheumatic pericarditis

CLINICAL PEARLS

- ARF is an autoimmune, inflammatory disease that follows a GAS pharyngeal infection and affects multiple organ systems, most notably, the heart.
- Modified Jones criteria now delineates between low-risk and moderate-/high-risk patients. Diagnosis requires two major or one major plus two minor manifestations in the context of a preceding documented GAS infection.
- Early echocardiogram evaluation for subclinical carditis can expedite initial diagnosis and improve clinical outcomes.
- Treatment involves acute antibiotic eradication, ideally within 9 days of illness, followed immediately by long-term antibiotic prophylaxis to prevent chronic RHD. Supportive care includes NSAIDs such as naproxen or aspirin.

RHINITIS, ALLERGIC

Madhavi Singh, MD

 BASICS

Allergic rhinitis is the collection of symptoms involving mucous membranes of nose, eyes, ears, and throat after an exposure to allergens such as pollen, dust, or dander.

DESCRIPTION

- IgE-mediated inflammation of the nasal mucosa following exposure to an extrinsic protein; an immediate symptomatic response is characterized by sneezing, congestion, and rhinorrhea followed by a persistent late phase dominated by congestion and mucosal hyperreactivity.
- Allergic rhinitis can be classified into seasonal or perennial and can be intermittent or persistent.
- Seasonal responses are usually due to outdoor allergens such as tree pollen, flowering shrubs in spring, grasses and flowering plants in summer, and ragweed and mold in fall.
- Perennial responses, or year-round symptoms, are usually associated with indoor allergens like dust mites, mold, and animal dander.
- Occupational allergic rhinitis is caused by allergens at the workplace and can be sporadic or year-round.
- Nonallergic rhinitis (e.g., vasomotor, rhinitis of pregnancy, and rhinitis medicamentosa [RM]) can occur.

Pediatric Considerations
Chronic nasal obstruction can result in facial deformities, dental malocclusions, and sleep disorders.

Pregnancy Considerations
Physiologic changes during pregnancy may aggravate all types of rhinitis, frequently in the 2nd trimester.

EPIDEMIOLOGY

- Onset usually in first 2 decades, rarely before 6 months of age, with tendency declining with advancing age
- The mean age of onset is 8 to 11 years, and about 80% of cases have established allergic rhinitis by age 20 years.

Prevalence
- ~10–25% of the U.S. adult population and 9–42% of the U.S. pediatric population are affected.
- 44–87% of patients with allergic rhinitis have mixed allergic and nonallergic rhinitis, which is more common than either pure form (1).

ETIOLOGY AND PATHOPHYSIOLOGY

- Aeroallergen-driven mucosal inflammation due to resident and infiltrating inflammatory cells as well as vasoactive and proinflammatory mediators (e.g., cytokines)
- Inhalant allergens:
  – Perennial: house dust mites, indoor molds, animal dander, cockroach/insect detritus
  – Seasonal: tree, grass, and weed pollens; outdoor molds
  – Occupational: latex, plant products (e.g., baking flour), sensitizing chemicals, and certain animals for people working in farms and vet clinics

RISK FACTORS

- Family history of atopy, with a greater risk if both parents have atopy
- Higher socioeconomic status
- Tobacco smoke can exacerbate symptoms and increase risk of developing asthma.
- Unclear evidence regarding risk due to early, repeated exposure to offending allergen and early introduction of solid food
- Pets in house and houses infested with cockroaches can cause perennial allergic rhinitis.
- Male sex
- Exposure to pollutants increase the risk of Ige-mediated allergic disease

GENERAL PREVENTION

- Primary prevention of atopic disease has not been proven effective by maternal diet or maternal allergen avoidance.
- Exclusive breastfeeding to 6 months of age lowers risk of some atopic disorders.
- Symptomatic control by environmental avoidance is the "first-line treatment."
- No evidence to support use of acaricides with mite-proof mattress and pillow covers, carpet and drape removal, removal of plants in the home, and pet control
- Air conditioning and limited outside exposure during allergy season (1)[B]
- HEPA air cleaners and vacuum bags of unclear efficacy
- Close doors and windows during allergy season.
- Use a dehumidifier to reduce indoor humidity.

COMMONLY ASSOCIATED CONDITIONS
Other IgE-mediated conditions: asthma, atopic dermatitis, allergic conjunctivitis, food allergy

DIAGNOSIS

Diagnosis is made primarily by history and physical exam.

HISTORY

- History of atopic dermatitis and/or food allergies
- History of nasal congestion; rhinorrhea; pruritus of nose, eyes, ears, and/or palate; sneezing; itching; and watering eyes
- Family history of allergic diseases
- History of environmental and occupational exposure and various nasal stimuli can help differentiate between allergic and vasomotor rhinitis.

PHYSICAL EXAM
Many findings are suggestive of but not specific for allergic rhinitis:

- Dark circles under eyes, "allergic shiners" (infraorbital venous congestion)
- Transverse nasal crease from rubbing nose upward; typically seen in children
- Rhinorrhea, usually with clear discharge
- Pale, boggy, blue-gray nasal mucosa
- Postnasal mucus discharge
- Oropharyngeal lymphoid tissue hypertrophy

DIFFERENTIAL DIAGNOSIS

- Infectious rhinitis: usually viral, commonly with secondary bacterial infection
  – Usually associated with sinusitis and is known as rhinosinusitis
  – Viral rhinitis averages six episodes per year from ages 2 to 6 years.
  – IgA deficiency with recurrent sinusitis
- RM:
  – Rebound effect associated with continued use of certain medications; topical decongestant drops and sprays are the most common.
  – Other medications that may indue RM include ACE inhibitors, reserpine, β-blockers, oral contraceptive pills (OCPs), guanethidine, methyldopa, aspirin, and NSAIDs.
- Vasomotor (idiopathic) rhinitis caused by numerous nasal stimuli such as warm or cold air, scents and odors, light or particulate matter
  – Hormonal: pregnancy, thyroid, OCPs
  – Nonallergic rhinitis with eosinophilia syndrome (NARES)
  – Gustatory: watery rhinorrhea in response to alcohol or food
  – "Skier's nose": watery rhinorrhea in response to cold air
- Conditions associated with rhinitis:
  – Nasal polyps, tumor
  – Septal/anatomic obstruction
    ○ Adenoidal hypertrophy, particularly in children
    ○ Septal abnormality or deflected nasal septum (DNS) in adults

DIAGNOSTIC TESTS & INTERPRETATION
- Lab tests rarely needed
- Skin testing is done to identify the allergen for immunotherapy.

Initial Tests (lab, imaging)
- Testing is rarely indicated.
- If diagnosis implies other causes, consider the following:
  – CBC with differential may show elevated eosinophils.
  – Increased total serum IgE level
  – Nasal probe smear may show elevated eosinophils.
- Medications that may alter lab results:
  – Corticosteroids may decrease eosinophilia.
  – Antihistamines suppress reactivity to skin tests; stop antihistamines 7 days before testing.

Diagnostic Procedures/Other
- Consider testing in only those cases where allergic symptoms do not respond to 1st- and 2nd-line treatments and/or considering immunotherapy.
- Specific allergen sensitivity with allergen skin testing or radioallergosorbent test (RAST); clinical correlation based on history is essential in interpreting results.
- Diagnostic allergen prick tests are used to select agent to determine appropriate environmental control measures as well as to direct immunotherapy:
  – Prick or puncture: superficial injury to epidermis with application of test antigen
  – Intradermal

- RAST: more expensive and less sensitive than skin testing; typically used in patients to whom skin testing is not practical or a severe reaction is possible
- Rhinoscopy: useful to visualize intranasal and posterior pharyngeal structures, including adenoids, polyps, and larynx
- CT scan of sinuses is not routinely done but can be used to check for complete opacity, fluid level, and mucosal thickening.

Test Interpretation
- Nasal washing/scraping: eosinophils predominate but may see basophils, mast cells
- Nasal mucosa: submucosal edema but without destruction; eosinophilic infiltration; congested mucous glands and goblet cells

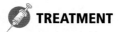 TREATMENT

There are three mainstays of treatment of allergic rhinitis:
- Allergen avoidance
- Medication
- Allergy immunotherapy

GENERAL MEASURES
Limit exposure to offending allergen.

MEDICATION
First Line
- Mild symptoms: 2nd-generation nonsedating antihistamines are the first-line therapy for mild to moderate allergic rhinitis (1).
  – Adverse effects: mild sedation, mild anticholinergic effects
  – Generic (cetirizine, fexofenadine, loratadine, levocetirizine)
- Intranasal antihistamine spray and intranasal steroid spray can also be used.
- Moderate to severe symptoms: Intranasal corticosteroids are first-line therapy for moderate to severe allergic rhinitis (1):
  – Beclomethasone dipropionate, budesonide, flunisolide, fluticasone propionate, mometasone furoate, and triamcinolone acetonide
  – Most effective drug class for symptoms of allergic rhinitis
  – Use nasal sprays after showering and direct the spray away from septum to improve deposition on mucosal surface.
  – May be used as needed; however, more effective with daily use (1)
  – Adverse effects: nosebleed, nasal septal perforation, and systemic corticosteroid effects
- Ciclesonide is a new-generation corticosteroid with previously demonstrated efficacy in the treatment of asthma when delivered through a metered-dose inhaler. Ciclesonide is also currently in clinical development as an intranasal formulation for use in the treatment of allergic rhinitis.
- Systemic steroids should be considered only in urgent cases and only for short-term use.
- Patients with comorbid moderate-to-severe asthma treated with omalizumab and dupilumab show improvement in symptoms.

Second Line
- Nasal antihistamines effective but may be systemically absorbed and may cause sedation: azelastine, olopatadine
- Intranasal anticholinergics such as ipratropium nasal spray: 2 sprays per nostril BID–TID
- Intranasal anticholinergics can increase efficacy in combination with steroid use.
- Leukotriene antagonists such as montelukast 10 mg/day PO
  – Should generally be used as an adjunct, not monotherapy
  – May be first line in those with concomitant asthma
- Mast-cell stabilizers such as cromolyn nasal spray: 1 spray per nostril TID–QID
  – May take 2 to 4 weeks of therapy for optimal efficacy
  – May be ineffective in patients with nonallergic rhinitis and nasal polyps
- 3rd-generation antihistamines, such as the following:
  – Brompheniramine: 12 to 24 mg PO BID
  – Chlorpheniramine: 4 mg PO q4–6h PRN
  – Clemastine: 1 to 2 mg PO BID PRN
  – Diphenhydramine: 25 to 50 mg PO q4–6h PRN:
    ○ May precipitate urinary retention in men with prostatism and/or hypertrophy
    ○ Adverse effects: sedation, prolonged QT interval, performance impairment, and anticholinergic effect
  – Decongestants
    ○ Phenylephrine: 10 mg PO q4h PRN
    ○ Pseudoephedrine: 60 mg PO q4–6h PRN
    ○ Oxymetazoline nasal spray (Afrin): 2 to 3 sprays per nostril q10–12h PRN (max of 3 days); intranasal agents should not be used for >3 days due to rebound rhinitis. Discourage use in patients with hypertension (HTN) or cardiac arrhythmia.
- Nasal saline sprays or irrigation used as needed, daily or twice a day for increased symptoms

ISSUES FOR REFERRAL
Refer to allergist for consideration of immunotherapy.

ADDITIONAL THERAPIES
- Nasal saline use has evidence of efficacy as sole agent or as adjunctive treatment (1).
- Other treatment strategies
  – When initiating intranasal steroids, consider starting with a "burst," using 2 sprays in each nostril daily for 2 weeks and then decreasing to 1 spray in each nostril daily thereafter.
  – To mitigate long-term side effects of intranasal steroids, consider a "5 days on, 2 days off" strategy, with the days off being the days of lowest exposure to allergens.
  – Allergen immunotherapy (desensitization)
    ○ Reserved when symptoms are uncontrollable with medical therapy or have a comorbidity (e.g., asthma)
    ○ Specific allergen extract is injected SC in increasing doses to induce patient tolerance.

 ONGOING CARE

DIET
Some patients with severe sensitivity to seasonal pollens may have oral allergy syndrome, which is associated with itching in the mouth with the ingestion of fresh fruits that may cross-react with the allergens.

PATIENT EDUCATION
- Asthma and Allergy Foundation of America: https://www.aafa.org/
- Other helpful information available at ACAAI: http://www.acaai.org/ and AAAAI: http://www.aaaai.org/home.aspx

PROGNOSIS
- Acceptable control of symptoms is the goal.
- Treatment is helpful to reduce the risk of comorbidities, such as sinusitis and asthma.

COMPLICATIONS
- Secondary infection such as otitis media or sinusitis
- Epistaxis
- Nasopharyngeal lymphoid hyperplasia
- Airway hyperreactivity with allergen exposure
- Asthma
- Facial changes, especially in children who are mouth breathers
- Sleep disturbance

REFERENCE
1. Wallace DV, Dykewicz MS, Bernstein DI, et al; for Joint Task Force on Practice Parameters for Allergy and Immunology. The diagnosis and management of rhinitis: an updated practice parameter. *J Allergy Clin Immunol*. 2008;122(Suppl 2):S1–S84.

 SEE ALSO

Conjunctivitis, Acute

 CODES

ICD10
- J30.89 Other allergic rhinitis
- J30.81 Allergic rhinitis due to animal (cat) (dog) hair and dander
- J30.2 Other seasonal allergic rhinitis

CLINICAL PEARLS
- Nasal saline irrigation (flushing 6 to 8 oz) may be very helpful in clearing upper airway of secretions and may precede the use of nasal corticosteroids.
- 2nd-generation antihistamines and intranasal corticosteroids are first-line therapies for allergic rhinitis.

ROCKY MOUNTAIN SPOTTED FEVER

Lisa C. Martinez, MD • Michael Mamone, MD

BASICS

Tick-borne rickettsial diseases include spotted fever rickettsiosis (SFR), ehrlichiosis, and anaplasmosis. In the United States, Rocky Mountain spotted fever (RMSF) is the SFR associated with the most severe and fatal outcomes (1)[A].

DESCRIPTION

- RMSF is a tick-borne illness caused by the bacterium *Rickettsia rickettsii* (2)[C].
- Symptoms include fever, headache, and a petechial or maculopapular rash that typically begins at wrists and ankles, spreading toward palms, soles, and the trunk.
- System(s) affected: cardiovascular, musculoskeletal, skin, CNS, renal, hepatic, and pulmonary

EPIDEMIOLOGY

In the United States, ticks are both vectors and main reservoirs. Important species in the United States include the American dog tick, *Dermacentor variabilis* (the most common vector) found in eastern, central, and pacific coastal areas; the Rocky Mountain wood tick, *Dermacentor andersoni*, found in the western United States; and the brown dog tick, *Rhipicephalus sanguineus*, distributed throughout all states. Although it can be seen throughout the United States, RMSF is the most common in the southeastern and south-central United States (1)[A].

Incidence

- In the United States, the annual incidence of SFR increased from 1.7 cases per million persons in 2000 to 13.2 in 2016. Cases have been reported in all states except Hawaii and Alaska. RMSF is also seen in Canada, Mexico, and throughout Central and South America (3)[B].
- Arkansas, Missouri, North Carolina, Tennessee, and Virginia account for >50% of SFR cases. There has also been increasing prevalence in Arizona, likely due to the brown dog tick (1).
- Cases occur year round. Most cases are reported from May through August during the peak of outdoor activity.
- Highest incidence occurs in those aged >40 years. Highest number of reported deaths is in children aged <10 years.

Prevalence

In the United States, 5,207 cases were reported in 2019, although the highest peak was in 2017 with 5,248.

ETIOLOGY AND PATHOPHYSIOLOGY

- An adult tick releases *R. rickettsii*, from its salivary glands after 6 to 10 hours of feeding.
- Pathogens infect vascular endothelial cells, causing small and medium vessel injury throughout the body leading to disseminated inflammation. Subsequent vascular permeability can cause pulmonary edema, cerebral edema, and hyponatremia. Local consumption of platelets and the small vessel injury results in the characteristic petechial rash.

- Subsequent end-organ injury may also result in meningoencephalitis, acute renal failure, acute respiratory distress syndrome, shock, arrhythmia, and seizure (1).
- It is unknown whether *R. rickettsii* crosses the placenta and causes in utero infection.
- RMSF can rarely be caused by direct inoculation of tick blood or fluid into open wounds or conjunctivae or through inhalation of contaminated aerosols.

RISK FACTORS

- Known tick bite, engorged tick, or presence of tick for >20 hours.
- Tick crushed during removal
- Accumulated outdoor exposure or residence in wooded areas; contact with outdoor pets, particularly dogs, or wild animals

GENERAL PREVENTION

- Limit tick exposure; highest tick exposure is in tall grasses, open areas of low bushy vegetation, or wooded areas.
- Wear light-colored clothing, long sleeves, pants, socks, and closed-toed shoes. Use 20–30% DEET-containing insect repellents.
- Permethrin spray on clothing
- Regular tick checks, prompt and proper tick removal; do not use bare hands to remove ticks.
- Wash hands and site of bite with soap and water after tick removal to avoid potential mucosal inoculation.
- Protect pets through ectoparasite control (1)[A].

DIAGNOSIS

- Maintain high incidence of suspicion for Rickettsial infections when patients present with "influenza-like" symptoms during summer months regardless of a known history of tick exposure (2)[C].
- Delay of empirical therapy increases risk of long-term sequelae and mortality.

HISTORY

Consider RMSF in acute febrile illness and rash, particularly with a history of potential tick exposure within previous 14 days, outdoor activities or travels to an endemic area, during late spring or summer months. *The tick bite goes unnoticed 30–50% of the time, and the lack of a clear history of a tick bite should not exclude the diagnosis.*

- Typically presents like a viral illness in the first 1 to 4 days with sudden onset of fever, severe frontal headache, malaise, myalgia, anorexia, nausea, vomiting, abdominal pain and photophobia (1)
- Rash typically appears 2 to 4 days after onset of fever; starts as a small blanching, pink macules on wrist and ankles before spreading to the trunk where rash may become maculopapular in appearance
- Involvement of palms and soles usually present by 5th to 6th day, along with generalized petechial rash; a sign of advanced disease. Rash generally spares the face. The rash is not pruritic.

- Although children more frequently (>90%) have a rash, the classic triad of fever, rash, and tick bite occurs in <60% of children with RMSF. 10% of patients never develop a rash, and the decision to treat should not be based solely on presence of rash (1)[A].
- Other symptoms include conjunctival injection, mental status impairments, restlessness, arthralgia, peripheral or periorbital edema, calf pain, and hearing loss (1)[A].

PHYSICAL EXAM

- Fever is typically >102°F.
- The rash typically starts as an erythematous, macular, or maculopapular exanthema (1 to 5 mm in diameter); 50% become petechial or purpuric; rash can be difficult to visualize on dark skin.
  - In severe cases, the rash can involve the entire body (including mucous membranes) and may progress to necrotic or gangrenous lesions, appearing similar to meningococcemia.
- AMS, focal neurologic deficits, lymphadenopathy, hepatosplenomegaly, and edema of dorsum of hands or feet can occur.

DIFFERENTIAL DIAGNOSIS

- Viral exanthema (e.g., hand-foot-and-mouth disease, measles, rubella, roseola)
- Viral gastroenteritis, appendicitis, mononucleosis, upper respiratory infection
- TTP/ITP, toxic shock syndrome
- Meningoencephalitis, meningococcemia
- Other tick-borne infections: typhus, ehrlichiosis, Lyme disease, babesiosis, boutonneuse fever, leptospirosis
- Drug reaction or serum sickness
- Kawasaki disease, idiopathic vasculitides, infective endocarditis

DIAGNOSTIC TESTS & INTERPRETATION

Most cases of RMSF are diagnosed based on IgM and IgG serologic response to *R. rickettsiae,* in conjunction with a high degree of clinical suspicion. Do not delay therapy awaiting results, as confirmation can take weeks (2)[C],(3)[A].

Initial Tests (lab, imaging)

- Specific laboratory diagnosis
  - Indirect fluorescent antibody (IFA) testing is the gold standard; requires one sample in the 1st week and a repeat in 2 to 4 weeks later to see a 4-fold change in antibody titers (3)
  - Sensitivity of IFA in the first 10 to 12 days of illness is low. 2 weeks after onset of illness, the sensitivity is 94% but cannot distinguish between *R. rickettsii* and other spotted fever-group rickettsii (3)[A],(4)[C].
  - Due to seroprevalence, it is impossible to differentiate a single elevated IgG titer associated with acute illness from previous infections (3)[B].
  - Polymerase chair reaction (PCR) of blood samples or skin biopsy can also be used for definitive diagnosis (2).

- Nonspecific laboratory tests:
  - WBC count: variable, frequently normal
  - Thrombocytopenia (<150,000 cells/μL) in 60% of children
  - Hyponatremia <135 mEq/dL
  - Elevated hepatic transaminases
  - Anemia, increase in blood urea nitrogen/creatinine, PT/PTT, hyperbilirubinemia, and hypoalbuminemia may also be present.
  - CSF may have lymphocytic pleocytosis, elevated protein, and normal glucose (1)[A].
- Imaging procedures are rarely helpful.

Diagnostic Procedures/Other
Skin biopsy can offer definitive diagnosis; a 3-mm punch biopsy to perform a rapid direct fluorescent antibody (DFA) test (sensitivity 70%, specificity 100%); however, the results are often delayed and should not preclude initiation of treatment.

Test Interpretation
- Test acute and convalescent phase sera in tandem.
- Early treatment may limit antibody formation.
- Seropositivity increases with age in endemic states. In such situations, positive spotted fever–group *Rickettsia* serologies do not necessarily signify an acute infection (this is why the 4-fold change is necessary for definitive diagnosis).

 TREATMENT

MEDICATION

First Line
Doxycycline is the treatment of choice in both adults and children (1)[A],(2)[C].

- Untreated rickettsial infections have a high rate of morbidity and mortality (20–30% without prompt antibiotic treatment). Antibiotics should not be delayed while awaiting confirmatory testing (1)[A]. Other antibiotics are considerably less effective (2)[C].
- Dosing:
  - Adults and children who are >100 lb (>45 kg): doxycycline 100 mg PO or IV q12h until 3 days after the fever subsides and there is a clinical improvement (1)[A]
  - Children who are <100 lb (<45 kg), including those <8 years old: doxycycline 2.2 mg/kg PO or IV q 12h until 3 days after fever subsides and there is a clinical improvement (1)[A]
- Typical course of treatment is 5 to 7 days, at a minimum, possibly longer if severe or complicated disease (1)[A].
- RMSF resistance to doxycycline has not been documented.
- Adverse effects may include the following:
  - Dyspepsia; take medication with food and water. Avoid dairy, iron, or antacids, as they may inhibit drug absorption.
  - Photosensitivity may occur. Minimize sun exposure and use sunscreen.
  - No risk of dental staining in children <8 years old (1)[A],(2)[C]
- Severe allergy is a contraindication to doxycycline; rapid desensitization may be considered for life-threatening disease in severe illness.

Second Line
In patients with allergies to tetracyclines/doxycycline, a thorough history to determine extent of allergy should be obtained because doxycycline is the best treatment. In setting of anaphylaxis or other contraindication to tetracyclines, chloramphenicol 50 to 75 mg/kg IV divided into 4 doses daily for 7 days is the second-line therapy. Chloramphenicol is the alternative to treat RMSF; associated with adverse hematologic effects (e.g., aplastic anemia) and increased case mortality (1)[A]

Pregnancy Considerations
- Doxycycline is appropriate for this life-threatening infection in pregnancy if suspicion is high. No current data have found evidence of teratogenicity, although studies are limited. There are some data on fatty liver of pregnancy with high dose doxycycline, but these doses exceeded what is used for RMSF (1)[A].
- Short-term doxycycline is compatible with breastfeeding (1)[A].
- Chloramphenicol may be considered but should be avoided in the 3rd trimester due to risk for gray baby syndrome.

ISSUES FOR REFERRAL
- Consider infectious disease consult along with immunology/allergist if patient is severely allergic to doxycycline.
- Report cases of RMSF to public health authorities.

ADDITIONAL THERAPIES
Patients with neurologic injury may require prolonged physical and cognitive therapy.

ADMISSION, INPATIENT, AND NURSING CONSIDERATIONS
- Admission criteria/initial stabilization
  - CNS dysfunction
  - Nausea/vomiting preventing oral antibiotic therapy
  - Immunocompromised patients
  - Specific acute organ failure
  - Failure of oral pain management
  - ICU for patients with shock
  - Severe allergy to tetracycline/doxycycline
- Discharge criteria
  - Resolution of fever
  - Ability to take oral therapy and nutrition

 ONGOING CARE

FOLLOW-UP RECOMMENDATIONS
- Patients with mild disease may be treated as outpatients if close follow-up is available.
- Hospitalize patients with moderate to severe disease.
- Infection does not confer lifelong immunity.

Patient Monitoring
- Follow patients treated as outpatients every 2 to 3 days until symptoms resolve.
- Follow-up CBC, electrolytes, LFTs if clinically indicated.

DIET
Consider nutritional supplementation if intake is poor.

PATIENT EDUCATION
General prevention and caution regarding tick avoidance during outside activities in endemic areas

PROGNOSIS
- Prognosis is closely related to timely administration of appropriate antibiotics.
- Delay in treatment may increase mortality by 3-fold if delayed to 5th day of illness (1)[A].
- When treated promptly, prognosis is excellent with resolution of symptoms and no sequelae.
- Children aged <10 years and elderly aged >70 years are at higher risk of morbidity and/or mortality.
- Patients with G6PD deficiency are at high risk for fulminant RMSF, in which death can occur ≤5 days.

COMPLICATIONS
- Encephalopathy, most commonly transient impaired level of consciousness or meningismus
- Seizures, focal neurologic deficit
- Renal injury leading to acute renal failure
- Hepatitis, congestive heart failure (CHF), respiratory failure
- Proximal muscle weakness, changes in personality, paresthesias, deafness, secondary thromboses, and tissue necrosis may also be seen.

REFERENCES

1. Biggs HM, Behravesh CB, Bradley KK, et al. Diagnosis and management of tickborne rickettsial diseases: Rocky Mountain spotted fever and other spotted fever group rickettsioses, ehrlichioses, and anaplasmosis—United States. *MMWR Recomm Rep.* 2016;65(2):1–44.
2. Pace EJ, O'Reilly M. Tickborne diseases: diagnosis and management. *Am Fam Physician.* 2020;101(9):530–540.
3. Binder AM, Nichols Heitman K, Drexler NA. Diagnostic methods used to classify confirmed and probable cases of spotted fever rickettsioses—United States, 2010–2015. *MMWR Morb Mortal Wkly Rep.* 2019;68(10):243–246.
4. Blanton LS. The rickettsioses: a practical update. *Infect Dis Clin North Am.* 2019;33(1):213–229.

CODES

ICD10
A77.0 Spotted fever due to Rickettsia rickettsii

CLINICAL PEARLS

- Diagnosis of RMSF requires a high index of clinical suspicion.
- Tick bites are often unnoticed, and some patients may never develop a rash.
- Begin treatment immediately without waiting for confirmatory testing in suspected cases. Doxycycline is drug of choice for RMSF in both adults and children. The only absolute contraindication is severe allergy to the drug.
- There is no evidence to support prophylaxis against RMSF in patients with known tick bite.

ROSEOLA
Jeffrey D. Quinlan, MD, FAAFP

 BASICS

Omnipresent infection occurring in infancy and childhood; majority of cases are caused by human herpesvirus 6 (HHV-6); may be associated with other diseases including encephalitis

DESCRIPTION
- Acute infection of infants or very young children (1)
- Causes a high fever followed by a skin eruption as the fever resolves (1)
- Transmission via contact with salivary secretions or respiratory droplet (1)
- Incubation period of 9 to 10 days (1)
- System(s) affected: skin/exocrine, metabolic, gastrointestinal, respiratory, neurologic
- Synonym(s): roseola infantum, exanthem subitum; pseudorubella; sixth disease; 3-day fever (1)

Pediatric Considerations
A disease of infants and very young children (2)

EPIDEMIOLOGY
- Predominant age
  - HHV-6
    - Infants and very young children (<2 years old)
    - Peak age infection 6 to 9 months, rarely congenital or perinatal infection (1)
    - 95% of children have been infected with HHV-6 by 2 years of life.
  - HHV-7
    - Later childhood
    - Mean age of infection is 26 months.
    - >90% population with HHV-7 by 10 years (1)
- Predominant sex: male = female (1)
- No seasonal variance

Incidence
Common—accounts for 20% ED visits for febrile illness among children aged 6 to 8 months

Prevalence
- Peak prevalence is between 9 and 21 months.
- Nearly 100% population carrying HHV-6 by 3 years (1)
- Approximately 20% patients with primary HHV-6 have roseola.

ETIOLOGY AND PATHOPHYSIOLOGY
- HHV-6 and HHV-7 (2)
- Majority of cases (60–74%) due to HHV-6
  - HHV-6B > HHV-6A (2)
  - HHV-6A seen in children in Africa
  - HHV-6 binds to CD46 receptors on all nucleated cells (2).
- Primary infection typically through respiratory droplets or saliva
- Congenital infection/vertical transmission occurs in 1% of cases (1).
  - Transplacental transmission
  - Chromosomal integration (clinical significance unknown)
- Lifelong latent or persistent asymptomatic infection occurs after primary infection (1).
  - 80–90% of population intermittently sheds HHV-6/HHV-7 in saliva (2).
  - Patients are viremic from 2 days prior to fever until defervescence and onset of rash.
  - HHV-6 latency is also implicated in CSF.

Genetics
HHV-6 is integrated into the chromosomes of 0.2–3.0% of the population. This leads to vertical transmission of the virus. Clinical significance of this is unknown (1).

RISK FACTORS
- Female gender
- Having older siblings
- At-risk adults: immunocompromised
  - Renal, liver, other solid organ, and bone marrow transplant (BMT)
  - HHV-6 reactivation can occur in 1st week posttransplant. HHV-6 viremia occurs in 30–45% of BMT within the first several weeks after transplantation.
    - Usually asymptomatic
    - Up to 82% of HHV-6 reactivation/reinfection in solid organ transplant
- Nonrisk factors
  - Child care attendance
  - Method of delivery
  - Breastfeeding (HHV does not appear to pass through breast milk.)
  - Maternal age
  - Season

DIAGNOSIS

HISTORY
- 3 to 5 days abrupt fever 102.2–104.0°F (39–40°C) not associated with a rash (1)
- The child may be fussy during this prodrome (1).
- Sudden drop of fever associated with appearance of rash (1)
  - Rash on trunk then spreads centrifugally mainly to neck, possibly also to peripheral extremities, and face
- Diarrhea
- Mild upper respiratory symptoms
- Rhinorrhea
- Febrile seizure occurs in 13% of cases (1).

PHYSICAL EXAM
- Rash (exanthem subitum) (1)
  - Rose-pink macules and/or papules that blanch
  - First appears on the trunk then peripherally
  - May occur up to 3 days after fever resolves (1)
  - Fades within 2 days
  - Occurs in approximately 20% of patients in the United States (1)
- Mild inflammation of tympanic membrane, pharynx, and/or conjunctiva (1)
- Ulcers on soft palate and uvula (Nagayama spots) (1)
- Cervical lymphadenopathy (1)
- Periorbital edema (2)

DIFFERENTIAL DIAGNOSIS
- Enterovirus infection
- Adenovirus infection (1)
- Epstein-Barr virus
- Fifth disease—parvovirus B19
- Rubella (1)
- Scarlet fever (1)
- Drug eruption (1)
- Measles (1)

DIAGNOSTIC TESTS & INTERPRETATION
- Primarily a clinical diagnosis not requiring laboratory or radiologic testing (1)[C]
- Tests often cannot differentiate latent or active disease (1)[C].
- Specific diagnosis only necessary in severe cases, unclear diagnosis where more serious disease needs to be ruled out, or if considering antiviral therapy (1)[C]

Initial Tests (lab, imaging)

- If necessary, HHV-6 and HHV-7 by PCR (1)
  - Serum, whole blood, CSF, or saliva
  - Becoming more widely available
  - Not required in nonimmunocompromised individuals
- HHV-6 IgM immunofluorescence (1)
- Diagnostic for acute infection
  - Spike seen in 1st week of illness
- HHV-6 IgG immunofluorescence (1)
  - Check at diagnosis and then 2 weeks later.
  - Use with IgM to show primary infection.
  - Negative initial test and rise on follow-up suggest primary infection.
- Viral culture
  - Rarely done
  - No clinical use (very time-consuming)
- Other laboratory findings (1)
  - Decreased total leukocytes, lymphocytes, and neutrophils
  - Elevated transaminases
  - Thrombocytopenia

Diagnostic Procedures/Other

- Urine culture: to rule out UTI as source of fever (2)
- Chest x-ray (CXR): if a child has respiratory symptoms

TREATMENT

No treatment necessary, resolves without sequelae (1)[C]

GENERAL MEASURES

- Symptomatic relief including antipyretics (1)[C]
- Hydration (1)[C]

MEDICATION

First Line

- No specific first-line treatment in immunocompetent hosts beyond supportive measures (2)[C]
  - Antivirals are not recommended in immunocompetent.
- No approved antiviral treatment in immunocompromised (2)[C]
- Second-line IV ganciclovir, cidofovir, foscarnet tested in vitro studies in stem cell transplant patients
  - HHV-6B susceptible: ganciclovir and foscarnet
  - HHV-6A and HHV-7 are more resistant to ganciclovir.
- Antivirals suggested in individual cases of encephalitis (associated with reactivation of HHV-6)
- In bone marrow and stem cell transplant recipients receiving immunosuppression, ganciclovir prophylaxis is effective in preventing reactivation of HHV-6.

ONGOING CARE

FOLLOW-UP RECOMMENDATIONS

Patient Monitoring

- During febrile prodrome, monitor for dehydration.
- None after typical rash appears and fever resolves
- Mean duration of illness is 6 days.
- If febrile seizures occur, they will cease after fever subsides and will not likely recur.
- Symptomatic reactivation in immunocompromised (1)

DIET

Encourage fluids.

PATIENT EDUCATION

- Parental reassurance that this is usually a benign, self-limited disease (1)
- There is no specific, recommended period of exclusion from out-of-home care for affected children.
- Patient is viremic a few days prior to fever until time of defervescence and rash onset.

PROGNOSIS

- Course: acute, complete recovery without sequelae (1)
- Reactivation in immunocompromised patients is common.

COMPLICATIONS

- Febrile seizures
  - 13% patients with roseola (1)
  - Accounts for 1/3 of primary seizures in children <2 years old (1)
- Medication hypersensitivity syndromes (drug reaction with eosinophilia and systemic symptoms) (2)
- Reactivation can occur in transplant patients, HIV-1 infected individuals, and other immunocompromised individuals.
- Meningoencephalitis occurs in immunocompetent and in immunosuppressed patients; poor association with multiple sclerosis
- Pityriasis rosea (1)
- Possible association with progressive multifocal leukoencephalopathy

REFERENCES

1. Stone RC, Micali GA, Schwartz RA. Roseola infantum and its causal human herpesviruses. *Int J Dermatol*. 2014;53(4):397–403.
2. Wolz MM, Sciallis GF, Pittelkow MR. Human herpesviruses 6, 7, and 8 from a dermatologic perspective. *Mayo Clin Proc*. 2012;87(10):1004–1014.

ADDITIONAL READING

- Ablashi DV, Devin CL, Yoshikawa T, et al. Review part 3: human herpesvirus-6 in multiple non-neurological diseases. *J Med Virol*. 2010;82(11): 1903–1910.
- Caselli E, Di Luca D. Molecular biology and clinical associations of roseoloviruses human herpesvirus 6 and human herpesvirus 7. *New Microbiol*. 2007;30(3):173–187.
- Fölster-Holst R, Kreth HW. Viral exanthems in childhood—infectious (direct) exanthems. Part 1: classic exanthems. *J Dtsch Dermatol Ges*. 2009;7(4): 309–316.

 CODES

ICD10

- B08.20 Exanthema subitum [sixth disease], unspecified
- B08.21 Exanthema subitum [sixth disease] due to human herpesvirus 6
- B08.22 Exanthema subitum [sixth disease] due to human herpesvirus 7

CLINICAL PEARLS

- Roseola infection should be suspected if an infant or young child presents with a high temperature without other clinical findings.
- As the fever abates, a macular rash will be seen on the trunk, with eventual spread to the face and extremities in 20% of patients.
- Roseola is a clinical diagnosis, and laboratory testing is not necessary for most children with classic presentation.
- For atypical presentations, complications, and immunocompromised hosts, several laboratory tools are available, including serologic testing for antibody, viral PCR testing, and viral culture.
- Infection is typically self-limiting and without sequelae.
- Usually, only symptomatic treatment is needed.
- Consider prophylaxis in patients undergoing bone marrow or stem cell transplant and receiving immunosuppressive therapy.

ROTATOR CUFF IMPINGEMENT SYNDROME

Faren H. Williams, MD, MS • Minjin Fromm, MD

 BASICS

DESCRIPTION

- Compression of rotator cuff tendons and subacromial bursa between the humeral head and the structures comprising the coracoacromial arch and proximal humerus
- Most common cause of atraumatic shoulder pain in patients >25 years of age
- Primary symptom is pain that is most severe when the arm is abducted between 60 and 120 degrees (the "painful arc").
- Classically divided into three stages:
  - Stage I: acute inflammation, edema, or hemorrhage of the underlying tendons due to overuse (typically in those aged <25 years)
  - Stage II: progressive tendinosis that leads to partial rotator cuff tear along with underlying thickening or fibrosis of surrounding structures (commonly, ages 25 to 40 years)
  - Stage III: full-thickness tear (typically in patients aged >40 years)

EPIDEMIOLOGY

Incidence

- Shoulder pain accounts for 1% of all primary care visits.
- Peak incidence of 25/1,000 patients per year occurs in patients aged 42 to 46 years.
- Impingement responsible for 18–74% of shoulder pain diagnoses

Prevalence

Prevalence of shoulder pain in general population ranges from ~7% to 30%.

RISK FACTORS

- Repetitive overhead motions (throwing, swimming)
- Glenohumeral joint instability or muscle imbalance
- Acromioclavicular arthritis or osteophytes
- Thickened coracoacromial ligament
- Shoulder trauma
- Increasing age
- Smoking

GENERAL PREVENTION

- Proper throwing and lifting techniques
- Proper strengthening to balance rotator cuff and scapula stabilizer muscles

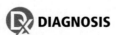 **DIAGNOSIS**

HISTORY

- Gradual increase in shoulder pain with overhead activities (Sudden onset of sharp pain suggests a tear.)
- Night pain is common, exacerbated by lying on the affected shoulder or sleeping with the affected arm above the head.
- Anterolateral shoulder pain with overhead activities
- May progress to weakness and decreased range of motion if shoulder is not used through full range of motion

PHYSICAL EXAM

- Examine patient for atrophy/asymmetry. Observe how the patient takes off his or her shirt during exam.
- Neer impingement test: Examiner stabilizes the scapula and moves the affected upper extremity through a flexion arc. Positive is pain with flexion of the shoulder. Sensitivity: 78%; specificity: 58% (1)[A]
- Hawkins-Kennedy impingement test: Examiner places the arm in 90 degrees of forward flexion and then gently internally rotates the arm. End point for internal rotation is when the patient feels pain or when the rotation of the scapula is felt or observed by the examiner. Test is positive when patient experiences pain during the maneuver. Sensitivity: 74%; specificity: 57% (1)[A]
- Empty can test (supraspinatus): Examiner asks the patient to elevate and internally rotate the arm with thumbs pointing downward in the scapular plane. Elbow should be fully extended. Examiner applies downward pressure on upper surface of the arm. Test is positive when patient complains of pain with resistance. Sensitivity: 69%; specificity: 62% (1)[A]
- Lift-off test (subscapularis): Patient internally rotates the shoulder, placing the back of the hand on ipsilateral buttock, and then lifts hand off buttock against resistance. A tear in the subscapularis muscle produces weakness of this action. Sensitivity: 42%; specificity: 97% (1)[A]
- Drop-arm test: Patient fully elevates arm and then slowly reverses the motion. If the arm is dropped suddenly or the patient has extreme pain, the test is positive for a possible rotator cuff tear. Sensitivity: 21%; specificity: 92% (1)[A]
- Resisted external rotation: weakness suggestive of infraspinatus and/or teres minor tendon involvement
- Apprehension-relocation test for anterior glenohumeral joint instability: Have the patient supine or sitting; abduct the arm to 90 degrees and flex the patient's elbow to 90 degrees; examiner slowly rotates the humerus (pushes hand posteriorly while the patient resists and then anteriorly while the patient resists). If the patient becomes anxious or has apprehension from this maneuver, test is positive implying instability and risk for dislocation. If pain is present, rather than instability, consider labral tear and/or impingement syndrome.
- Examine cervical spine to rule out cervical pathology as source of shoulder pain.
- Neurovascular exam of the upper extremity

DIFFERENTIAL DIAGNOSIS

- Labral injury
- Acromioclavicular arthritis (more common in older patients; positive cross-arm test—pain when affected arm is fully adducted across the chest in the horizontal plane)
- Adhesive capsulitis (rotator cuff tendonitis leads to decreased use and atrophy of rotator cuff muscles, followed by contracture; linked to diabetes and potentially prior trauma)
- Anterior shoulder instability (prior trauma; more common in patients <25 years old)
- Multidirectional instability
- Biceps tendonitis or rupture (Perform Speed and Yergason tests and look for visible or palpable defect of biceps—"Popeye sign.")
- Calcific tendonitis
- Cervical radiculopathy (spinal or foraminal stenosis, can test with Spurling maneuver)
- Glenohumeral arthritis (Evaluate with plain films.)
- Suprascapular nerve entrapment (Look for focal muscle atrophy of supra- or infraspinatus.)
- Traumatic rotator cuff tear

DIAGNOSTIC TESTS & INTERPRETATION

Initial Tests (lab, imaging)

- Plain-film radiographs of the shoulder (three views): anteroposterior, axillary, scapular Y views
- Plain films may reveal:
  - Osteoarthritis of the acromioclavicular and glenohumeral joints
  - Superior migration of the humeral head (indicative of a large rotator cuff tear)
  - Cystic change of the humeral head and sclerosis of the inferior acromion (indicative of chronic rotator cuff disease)
  - Calcific tendonitis
- MRI is used to definitively assess rotator cuff tendinopathy, partial tears, and complete tears.
- MR arthrogram is preferred for labral pathology.
- Ultrasound is sensitive and specific for rotator cuff tears but is highly operator dependent.
- CT scan is preferred for bony pathology or for those unable to undergo MRI.

Diagnostic Procedures/Other

- Lidocaine injection test
  - Inject lidocaine into the subacromial space:
    - Repeat impingement tests; if pain is completely relieved and range of motion is improved, likely impingement syndrome (rather than cuff tear)
  - Allows for more accurate strength testing on physical examination:
    - If strength is intact, rule out rotator cuff tear.
    - If range of motion does not improve in any plane, more likely adhesive capsulitis

- Some pain relief and improved range of motion occur after lidocaine injection with
  - Glenoid labral tear
  - Capsular strain
  - Glenohumeral osteoarthritis
  - Glenohumeral instability
- A lack of any pain relief suggests other sources (i.e., cervical radiculopathy) or inappropriate placement of injection.

Test Interpretation
May have tendinosis, tendonitis, or muscle/tendon tear

 TREATMENT

Pain control in combination with aggressive rehabilitation improves and fully resolves rotator cuff tendonitis in most patients.

GENERAL MEASURES
- Rest initially and then mandatory supervised physical therapy for 6 to 8 weeks
- Ice or heat for symptom relief
- Activity modification, with avoidance of aggravating activities, particularly overhead motions
- Range of motion exercises
- Rotator cuff and adjacent muscle strengthening to enhance stability and prevent further injuries

MEDICATION
First Line
NSAIDs or other analgesic, often for 6 to 12 weeks

ISSUES FOR REFERRAL
Failure of conservative treatment, persistent pain, weakness, full thickness, or complete tear of rotator cuff

ADDITIONAL THERAPIES
- Supervised- or home-exercise regimens provide significant pain reduction and improve function (2)[A].
- Physical therapy is effective for short-term and long-term recovery of function (3)[A]:
  - Initial goal is to restore range of motion.
  - After pain resolves, gradually strengthen rotator cuff muscles in internal rotation, external rotation, and abduction.

SURGERY/OTHER PROCEDURES
- Steroid injections may have a significant benefit on pain and function in the short term but do not appear to have a significant long-term effect (4)[A].
- No evidence that surgery is superior to conservative management or that one surgical technique is superior to another for impingement syndrome

- Platelet-rich therapies for musculoskeletal soft tissue injuries are increasingly common.
  - No apparent effect of platelet-rich plasma injection during arthroscopic rotator cuff repair on overall retear rates or shoulder-specific outcomes
- Extracorporeal shock wave therapy is currently under study as an emerging treatment for calcific tendonitis.

COMPLEMENTARY & ALTERNATIVE MEDICINE
Acupuncture is potentially beneficial for reducing pain and improving function, particularly when used with physical therapy (5)[A].

 ONGOING CARE

PATIENT EDUCATION
- Physical rehabilitation is necessary, both in conservative course of treatment (i.e., NSAIDs, physical therapy, home exercises) and in surgical intervention.
- An aggressive trial of rehabilitation should be encouraged prior to extensive testing or surgical intervention. Providing pain relief prior to beginning a program of physical therapy improves adherence and outcomes.
- Symptoms often recur if not fully addressed.

PROGNOSIS
- Variable, depends on underlying pathology
- Most patients improve with conservative management. Recovery can be slow.
- Patients with more severe symptoms—those with symptoms for >1 year—are less likely to respond well with conservative therapies.

COMPLICATIONS
- Progression of injury
- Tendon retraction in complete rotator cuff tear

REFERENCES
1. Alqunaee M, Galvin R, Fahey T. Diagnostic accuracy of clinical tests for subacromial impingement syndrome: a systematic review and meta-analysis. *Arch Phys Med Rehabil*. 2012;93(2):229–236.
2. Kuhn JE. Exercise in the treatment of rotator cuff impingement: a systematic review and a synthesized evidence-based rehabilitation protocol. *J Shoulder Elbow Surg*. 2009;18(1):138–160.
3. Green S, Buchbinder R, Hetrick S. Physiotherapy interventions for shoulder pain. *Cochrane Database Syst Rev*. 2003;2003(2):CD004258.
4. Gaujoux-Viala C, Dougados M, Gossec L. Efficacy and safety of steroid injections for shoulder and elbow tendonitis: a meta-analysis of randomised controlled trials. *Ann Rheum Dis*. 2009;68(12):1843–1849.
5. Vas J, Ortega C, Olmo V, et al. Single-point acupuncture and physiotherapy for the treatment of painful shoulder: a multicentre randomized controlled trial. *Rheumatology (Oxford)*. 2008;47(6):887–893.

R

CODES

ICD10
- M75.40 Impingement syndrome of unspecified shoulder
- M75.110 Incmpl rotatr-cuff tear/ruptr of unsp shoulder, not trauma
- M75.120 Complete rotatr-cuff tear/ruptr of unsp shoulder, not trauma

CLINICAL PEARLS
- Consider impingement syndrome in patients who engage in activities with repetitive overhead motions (e.g., swimming, throwing) who present with shoulder pain.
- Atraumatic shoulder pain in middle age often represents rotator cuff tendonitis.
- The supraspinatus tendon is most commonly affected in impingement syndrome.
- Neer and Hawkins tests specifically check for shoulder impingement.
- The empty can maneuver tests for weakness of supraspinatus muscle.
- The drop-arm test is specific for rotator cuff tear.
- Physical therapy over 6 to 12 weeks promotes return to function.
- Most patients with shoulder impingement respond well to conservative management.

SALIVARY GLAND CALCULI/SIALADENITIS

Sahil Mullick, MD • Antoine Sioufi, MD

BASICS

DESCRIPTION
- Inflammation of one or more salivary glands
- Infectious, obstructive, or autoimmune
- "Sialolithiasis" is characterized by a painful swelling of the affected gland when eating due to an obstructing stones within the salivary glands or ducts.
- "Sialadenitis" is inflammation of the salivary gland classified as acute or chronic sialadenitis.
  - Acute can be caused by a primary infection (viral/bacterial) or secondary infection.
  - Chronic sialadenitis is due to repeated episodes of inflammation resulting in progressive loss of salivary gland function.
- Parotid gland and submandibular glands are commonly affected by sialadenitis. However, parotid gland is affected mostly by acute suppurative sialadenitis. The submandibular gland is more commonly affected (80–90% of cases) by stones than the parotid gland due to higher mucinous content of saliva, longer course of Wharton duct, and slow salivary flow against gravity.

EPIDEMIOLOGY
Incidence
- Peak incidence is 30 to 60 years; rarely in children
- Most common in debilitated and dehydrated patients
- 70% of the stones are single; 30% bilateral

ETIOLOGY AND PATHOPHYSIOLOGY
- Stagnation of salivary flow and elevated calcium concentrations are thought to be important.
- Decreased salivary outflow from anticholinergics, dehydration, or radiation
- Salivary calculi are composed of calcium phosphate and hydroxyapatite with smaller amounts of magnesium, potassium, and ammonium.
- Predisposing factors include inflammation of the salivary gland or duct, salivary stasis, retrograde bacterial contamination from the oral cavity, increased alkalinity of saliva, and physical trauma to salivary duct or gland.
- Gout is associated with salivary stone development. In gout, sialoliths are composed of uric acid.
- Bacterial sialadenitis tends to be unifocal caused by *Staphylococcus aureus*, *Streptococcus viridans*, *Streptococcus pyogenes*, *Haemophilus influenzae*, *Escherichia coli*, *Pseudomonas aeruginosa*, and group B streptococci (neonates and children).
- Viral sialadenitis tends to be multifocal caused by mumps, cytomegalovirus, Epstein-Barr virus, HIV, and enteroviruses.
- Other common causes include radioiodine use, positive pressure ventilation use with anesthesia, Sjögren syndrome, and sarcoidosis (1).

Pediatric Considerations
Common causes of sialadenitis in children are mumps and idiopathic juvenile recurrent parotitis.

RISK FACTORS
- Hypovolemia
- Diuretic use
- Anticholinergic use
- Trauma
- Gout
- History of nephrolithiasis
- Poor oral hygiene, malnutrition, smoking, dehydration
- Head/neck radiation

GENERAL PREVENTION
- Maintain proper oral care and hygiene.
- Avoid anticholinergics and other causes of xerostomia.

COMMONLY ASSOCIATED CONDITIONS
- Radiation or drug-induced xerostomia
- Sjögren syndrome, Mikulicz syndrome
- Hypercalcemia

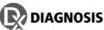

DIAGNOSIS

Diagnosis is most often clinical based on physical exam and characteristic history, which is often described as sudden onset swelling and pain in the affected gland. Pain is often worse with eating. Most (75–80%) salivary gland stones occur in the submandibular glands, 6–20% occur in the parotid gland, and 1–2% occur in the sublingual or minor salivary glands. Submandibular stones are more often located in the duct. Parotid stones tend to be smaller than mandibular stones, are more often multiple, and are located within the gland itself (1).

HISTORY
- Review history for
  - Alcoholism, bulimia, malnutrition; radiation therapy, past malignancy; TB or HIV exposure
- Acute onset of pain and swelling over the affected salivary gland, especially postprandial or following the anticipation of eating
- Dental pain, discharge, foul breath (halitosis) hypersalivation, and pain with chewing
- Xerostomia
- 33% of the patients with submandibular sialolithiasis present with painless swelling and 10% with pain but not swelling.
- Worsening pain, erythema, and/or fever may indicate secondary infection.
- Pus drainage through the gland duct into the mouth

PHYSICAL EXAM
- Visual inspection of the glands and ducts; for submandibular gland, a stone may be felt within the Wharton duct or seen near the frenulum of the tongue. For parotid glands, a stone may be felt within Stensen duct or seen at the orifice.
- Bimanual exam of oral cavity palpating all salivary glands, floor of mouth, tongue, and neck to assess symmetry, tenderness, induration, edema, presence of stones, lymphadenopathy, and the number of glands involved. A functioning gland is usually spongy and elastic.
- Examine duct openings for purulent discharge and presence of saliva. Purulent discharge at the orifice raises concern for acute bacterial sialadenitis.
- Gently palpate the gland to express normal, thin, absent, or reduced amounts of saliva; assess for bubbling appearance or purulent drainage.
- Examine eyes for interstitial keratitis.
- Evaluation of facial nerve (CN VII) function, which is at risk for compromise if parotid gland is involved

Pediatric Considerations
Stones in children are often within the distal duct. Ultrasound with sialendoscopy is diagnostic and therapeutic.

DIFFERENTIAL DIAGNOSIS
- Bacterial parotitis
- Idiopathic juvenile recurrent parotitis; cystic fibrosis
- Mumps; tularemia
- Collagen vascular disease
- Metal poisoning
- Salivary gland tumors; lymphoma

DIAGNOSTIC TESTS & INTERPRETATION
Sialolithiasis is a clinical diagnosis based on a characteristic history and physical examination. There is typically sudden onset of swelling and pain in the affected gland associated with eating or anticipation of eating. A stone may be seen at the opening of the affected salivary duct or palpated along the course of the duct. Imaging is helpful when physical exam is equivocal or if there is a concern for tumor formation.

Initial Tests (lab, imaging)
- Consider CBC.
- Culture and sensitivity of any expressed pus
- Ultrasound is able to detect up to 90% of stones 2 mm or larger (2)[C].
- CT scan with IV contrast is more sensitive but has radiation exposure (3)[C].
- MR sialography for patients with an inconclusive ultrasound and persistent symptoms without the use of intraductal contrast
- Sonopalpation (concurrent ultrasound with transoral palpation) proved to have a sensitivity and specificity of 96.6% and 90%, respectively, in finding a calculus (3)[B].

Follow-Up Tests & Special Considerations

- If autoimmune process is suspected, order rheumatoid factor (RF) and antinuclear antibodies (ANAs) (4)[C].
- Salivary gland biopsy

Diagnostic Procedures/Other

- Sialography to evaluate sialolithiasis and other obstructive lesions
- Sialendoscopy to find and remove sialoliths; in one study, sialendoscopy confirmed 221 (79%) parotid and 812 (93%) submandibular stones (5)[A].
- One study revealed that sonography, cone beam CT, and sialendoscopy all had excellent specificity and positive predictive value in diagnosing stones (3)[B].
- When sialendoscopy fails, a novel ultrasound-guided needle localization approach has been proposed.
- Technetium-99m-pertechnetate scintigraphy showed decreased gland excretion and decreased uptake in patients with sialolithiasis.

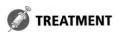 TREATMENT

GENERAL MEASURES

- Maintain hydration.
- Apply warm compresses.
- Massage the gland and milk the duct.
- Sialagogues (agents that promote salivary flow) like tart, lemon juice, and hard candies (lemon drops) may be helpful. Use throughout the day as tolerated.
- Maintain good oral hygiene.
- Chlorhexidine 0.12% mouth rinses 3 times a day will help to reduce the bacterial burden in oral cavity and will promote oral hygiene.
- Discontinue medications with anticholinergic effects that reduce salivary flow.

MEDICATION

- Pain management with NSAIDs
- Antibiotics for suspected secondary infection (fever, purulent discharge)

First Line

- Antistaphylococcal antibiotics such as dicloxacillin 500 mg or cephalexin 500 mg QID for 7 to 10 days
- If no improvement within 5 to 7 days, a culture of the duct discharge should be obtained and the antibiotic coverage broadened by substituting amoxicillin/clavulanate or clindamycin.
- Penicillin-allergic: Use clindamycin 300 mg PO q8h.
- Gram negative: 3rd-generation cephalosporin or fluoroquinolone
- Anaerobic: metronidazole or clindamycin

Second Line

- 1st-generation cephalosporin (cephalexin or cefazolin) or clindamycin is also indicated for empiric coverage.
- If MRSA, then vancomycin

ISSUES FOR REFERRAL

- Dental referral if poor dentition/dental abscess
- ENT referral if failure to improve with conservative management, recurrent symptoms (6)

ADDITIONAL THERAPIES

In the case of chronic sialadenitis with strictures, consider sialostent placement.

SURGERY/OTHER PROCEDURES

- Submandibular stones found in the anterior floor of the mouth can be excised intraorally (sialodochoplasty), whereas those in the hilum require gland excision. Parotid stones usually require parotidectomy (4)[A].
- Good results in patient symptom relief, quality of life, and safety have been reported in sialadenitis and sialolithiasis using sialendoscopy (4),(5). Complications include strictures, ranulas, and lingual nerve injury. However, sialendoscopy is contraindicated in acute sialadenitis.
- A combined approach using limited intraoral incision with sialendoscopy has shown an 86% success rate.
- Incision and drainage of parotid abscess is indicated after failing 3 to 5 days of medical management (7).
- Sialoliths larger than 4 mm and stenoses can be successfully treated by radiologically or fluoroscopically controlled or sialendoscopically based methods in ~80% of cases. Extracorporeal shock wave lithotripsy (ESWL) is successful in up to 50% of cases.
- Transoral duct slitting for extraparenchymal submandibular stones; 90% success rate

COMPLEMENTARY & ALTERNATIVE MEDICINE

Consider lemon drops or other sialogogues to promote salivation. In one study, postoperative use of sialogogues nearly halved rates of sialadenitis (4)[C].

ADMISSION, INPATIENT, AND NURSING CONSIDERATIONS

- Parotid abscess
- Inability to tolerate PO intake

 ONGOING CARE

FOLLOW-UP RECOMMENDATIONS

Avoid prescribing medications that cause xerostomia.

Patient Monitoring

Monitor patients with chronic sialadenitis because decreased salivary gland function due to fibrosis and loss of acini can lead to acute exacerbations.

DIET

- Avoid sialogogues during acute attacks.
- Maintain adequate hydration.

PATIENT EDUCATION

Maintaining excellent oral hygiene/hydration

PROGNOSIS

- Acute symptoms are usually resolving in about a week with appropriate treatment. Complete resolution is expected after conservative outpatient treatment.
- Patients with autoimmune etiology may have prolonged course due to systemic involvement.
- In patients who undergo transoral surgical stone removal, recurrence has been reported in 18%.

COMPLICATIONS

- Local spreading of infection, causing cellulitis or Ludwig angina
- Facial nerve impingement, hypoglossal and lingual nerve injuries
- Dental decay: Hypofunction of salivary gland causes decrease protection from acid erosion, promoting dental decay.

REFERENCES

1. Kao WK, Chole RA, Ogden MA. Evidence of a microbial etiology for sialoliths. *Laryngoscope*. 2020;130(1):69–74.
2. Goncalves M, Mantsopoulos K, Schapher M, et al. Ultrasound supplemented by sialendoscopy: diagnostic value in sialolithiasis. *Otolaryngol Head Neck Surg*. 2018;159(3):449–455.
3. Schwarz D, Kabbasch C, Scheer M, et al. Comparative analysis of sialendoscopy, sonography, and CBCT in the detection of sialolithiasis. *Laryngoscope*. 2015;125(5):1098–1101.
4. Wilson KF, Meier JD, Ward PD. Salivary gland disorders. *Am Fam Physician*. 2014;89(11):882–888.
5. Atienza G, López-Cedrún JL. Management of obstructive salivary disorders by sialendoscopy: a systematic review. *Br J Oral Maxillofac Surg*. 2015;53(6):507–519.
6. Wallace E, Tauzin M, Hagan J, et al. Management of giant sialoliths: review of the literature and preliminary experience with interventional sialendoscopy. *Laryngoscope*. 2010;120(10):1974–1978.
7. Capaccio P, Torretta S, Pignataro L, et al. Salivary lithotripsy in the era of sialendoscopy. *Acta Otorhinolaryngol Ital*. 2017;37(2):113–121.

CODES

ICD10

- K11.5 Sialolithiasis
- K11.20 Sialoadenitis, unspecified
- K11.21 Acute sialoadenitis

CLINICAL PEARLS

- Mainstay of treatment is hydration, good oral hygiene, sialogogues, and possible surgical excision.
- Nonpharmacologic agents that promote salivary flow like tart and hard candies such as lemon drops may be helpful and should be used throughout the day.

SALMONELLA INFECTION

Marie L. Borum, MD, EdD, MPH • Cyrus Adams-Mardi, MD, MS

BASICS

DESCRIPTION
- Infection caused by any serotype of the bacterial genus *Salmonella*, a gram-negative facultatively anaerobic bacillus
- Nontyphoidal *Salmonella* typically causes gastroenteritis via foodborne infection and sporadic outbreaks; less commonly causes infection outside the gastrointestinal (GI) tract
- Clinical syndromes
  - Enteric fever (see "Typhoid Fever")
  - Nontyphoidal gastroenteritis
    ○ Chronic carrier state (>1 year)
  - Nontyphoidal invasive disease
    ○ Bacteremia
      ▪ Endovascular complications; localized infection outside GI tract (i.e., osteomyelitis, abscess)

Geriatric Considerations
Patients >65 years old have increased risk of invasive disease with bacteremia and endovascular complications due to comorbidities (atherosclerotic endovascular lesions, prostheses, etc.) that increase risk of bacterial seeding.

Pediatric Considerations
Neonates (<3 months) are more susceptible to invasive disease and complications.

EPIDEMIOLOGY
Incidence
- Global incidence of nontyphoidal *Salmonella enteritidis* was estimated to be ~94 million per year (mostly foodborne).
  - Wide variation by region from 40 to 3,980 estimated cases per 100,000
- Global incidence of invasive nontyphoidal *Salmonella* infection was estimated to be 535,000 cases in 2017.
- Most commonly identified foodborne bacterial illness in the United States and a common cause of traveler's diarrhea
  - Estimated 1.4 million cases per year in the United States, with annual incidence of 15 illnesses per 100,000
  - Estimated 25,000 hospitalizations and 420 deaths per year (1)[A]
- Second most common bacteria isolated from stool cultures in diarrheal illness (following *Campylobacter*) in the United States; highest incidence of bacteremia in children <5 years old; hospitalization rates higher in patients >50 years old; peak frequency: July to November

ETIOLOGY AND PATHOPHYSIOLOGY
- *Salmonella enterica*
  - Most pathogenic species in humans; 2,500 different serotypes
- Etiology
  - ~95% of cases are foodborne.
- Pathophysiology
  - Typical infectious dose in immunocompetent patients is ingestion of 1 million bacteria but can be lower in patients taking antibiotics or in the setting of gastric acid reduction. Bacteria ingested invade the distal ileal and proximal colonic mucosa to produce an inflammatory and cytotoxic response. Bacteria can enter the mesenteric lymphatic system and then the systemic circulation to cause disseminated/invasive disease.

RISK FACTORS
Recent travel to underdeveloped nations; consumption of undercooked meat, egg, or unpasteurized dairy products; nonanimal products have also been implicated in outbreaks. Contact with live reptiles or poultry; contact with human carrier (*Salmonella* fecal shedding); impaired gastric acidity: H_2 receptor blockers, antacids, proton pump inhibitors (PPIs), gastrectomy, achlorhydria, pernicious anemia, infants; recent antibiotic use; reticuloendothelial blockade: sickle cell disease, malaria, bartonellosis; immunosuppression: HIV, diabetes, corticosteroid or other immunosuppressant use, chemotherapy; impaired phagocytic function: chronic granulomatous disease, hemoglobinopathies, malaria

GENERAL PREVENTION
Proper hygiene in production, transport, and storage of food (e.g., refrigeration during food storage and thoroughly cooking food prior to consumption); control of animal reservoirs: Avoid contact with high-risk animals, feces, and polluted waters; hand hygiene; CDC tracks outbreaks (https://www.cdc.gov/salmonella/index.html)

COMMONLY ASSOCIATED CONDITIONS
Gastroenteritis; bacteremia: immunocompromised or patients with underlying disease (e.g., cholelithiasis, prostheses); osteomyelitis: higher incidence in sickle cell disease; abscesses: higher incidence with malignant tumors; reactive arthritis

DIAGNOSIS

HISTORY
- *Salmonella* infections are typically asymptomatic or may result in mild, self-limited gastroenteritis.
- Exposure history: travel; contact with infected human, reptile, or poultry; improper food preparation; local outbreaks; host factors: age, immune status, other risk factors; symptoms typically begin 8 to 72 hours after ingestion and resolve within 4 to 10 days.
- Acute uncomplicated illness
  - Sudden onset of diarrhea
    ○ Not typically grossly bloody, but can be bloody especially among pediatric patients
  - Vomiting is infrequent. Abdominal cramping; headache; myalgias; fever.

PHYSICAL EXAM
- Fever
- Evidence of hypovolemia; abdominal tenderness; heme-positive stool in some patients; hepatosplenomegaly in some patients

DIFFERENTIAL DIAGNOSIS
Viral gastroenteritis; bacterial enteritis due to other organisms; pseudomembranous colitis; inflammatory bowel disease

DIAGNOSTIC TESTS & INTERPRETATION
Initial Tests (lab, imaging)
- Gastroenteritis
  - Stool culture for *Salmonella*, *Escherichia coli*, *Shigella*, and *Campylobacter* (2)[C] (Optimal specimen is a diarrheal stool sample.)
  - Indications for stool culture include the following:
    ○ Severe diarrhea (≥6 loose stools daily) (2)[C]
    ○ Diarrhea >1 week in duration
    ○ Fever (2)[C]
    ○ Diarrhea containing blood or mucous (2)[C]
    ○ Multiple cases suggesting an outbreak (2)[C]
  - Fecal leukocytes: positive
  - Blood cultures are warranted in:
    ○ Infants <3 months; people of any age with signs of septicemia or other systemic manifestations of infection; cases where enteric fever is suspected; immunocompromised patients
- Bacteremia
  - Blood cultures if febrile (2)[C]
  - Stool cultures: may also be positive (2)[C]
  - Culture CSF if patient is <3 months of age with positive blood culture.
- Endovascular infection
  - Consider angiography in bacteremic patients >50 years of age if aortic or vascular source is suspected.
- Local infections
  - Wound culture; consider CT or MRI for soft tissue or bone infections (2)[C].
- Chronic carrier state
  - Stool culture positive for >1 year (2)[C]
  - Urine culture may be positive in chronic carriers.

Follow-Up Tests & Special Considerations
- Look for other causes in diarrhea lasting >14 days. Asymptomatic excretion of *Salmonella* may occur for weeks after infection; follow-up fecal cultures are routinely not indicated for patients with uncomplicated gastroenteritis (2).
- Follow-up blood cultures suggested for patients with bacteremia (2)[C]

Test Interpretation
Intestinal biopsies (if taken) may show mucosal ulceration, hemorrhage, and necrosis seen on along with reticuloendothelial hypertrophy/hyperplasia.

TREATMENT

- Treatment is supportive for nonsevere nontyphoidal *Salmonella* gastroenteritis in immunocompetent patients between 12 months and 50 years of age. The illness is typically self-limited. There is no proven benefit for treatment of mild disease. Treatment can suppress the host immunologic response. Higher rates of relapse have also been reported and there is a potential to extend asymptomatic carriage (2)[C].
- Consider antibiotics in immunocompetent hosts with severe diarrhea, high fever, or those requiring hospitalization (2)[C].

- Patients at increased risk of bacteremia benefit from antibiotics:
  - Infants <3 months of age (2)[C]
  - Patients >50 years old (risk particularly increases after age 65 years) (2)[C]
  - HIV-infected patients; cancer patients, especially those with hematologic, gastrointestinal, or genitourinary malignancies
  - Patients with hemoglobinopathies, atherosclerotic lesions, and prosthetic valves, grafts, or joints or any immunosuppressed state (2)[C]
- Chronic carriage of nontyphoidal *Salmonella*
  - 4 to 6 weeks of antimicrobial therapy; prophylactic therapy in immunocompromised patients

GENERAL MEASURES

- Hydration and electrolyte replacement; hand washing and barrier precautions for inpatients
- Avoid antimotility drugs in patients with fever or dysentery. Antimotility drugs may increase contact time of the enteropathogen in the gut mucosa (2)[C].

MEDICATION

First Line

- Gastroenteritis, uncomplicated: No specific medications are necessary; supportive care
- Gastroenteritis, complicated (due to illness severity or host risk factors such as immunocompromised)
  - Adults (Treat for 14 days if immunocompromised.)
    - Levofloxacin: 500 mg/day PO for 1 to 3 days *or* ciprofloxacin: 750 mg/day PO for 1 day or 500 mg/day PO for 3 days *or* ofloxacin: 400 mg/day PO for 1 to 3 days *or*
    - Azithromycin: 500 mg/day PO for 3 days or 1 g followed by 500 mg daily for 3 days
      - Preferred agent for febrile diarrhea or dysentery
  - Children
    - Ceftriaxone: 100 mg/kg/day IV or IM in 2 equally divided doses for 7 to 10 days *or*
    - Azithromycin: 20 mg/kg PO for first dose and then 10 mg/kg/day for subsequent doses daily for 7 days
  - HIV patients
    - Increased duration (range of 2 to 6 weeks) of antimicrobial therapy and/or zidovudine may decrease relapse.
- Bacteremia: Due to resistance trends, treat life-threatening infections in adults with a fluoroquinolone *or* a 3rd-generation cephalosporin until susceptibilities are determined.
  - Adults
    - Ciprofloxacin (or other fluoroquinolone): 400 mg IV BID for 10 to 14 days *plus* ceftriaxone: 1 to 2 g/day IV for 10 to 14 days *or* cefotaxime: 2 g IV q8h for 10 to 14 days
  - Children
    - Amoxicillin: 30 mg/kg/dose TID for 10 to 14 day; trimethoprim-sulfamethoxazole: 8 to 12 mg/kg/day of trimethoprim component in 2 divided doses for 10 to 14 days *or* ceftriaxone: 50 mg/kg/day (max of 1 g) BID for 10 to 14 days

- Localized infection (e.g., septic arthritis, osteomyelitis, cholangitis, and pneumonia); surgical drainage or débridement in addition to a minimum of 3 weeks of antimicrobial therapy
  - In sustained bacteremia, prolonged local infection, or immunocompromised patients, give antibiotics PO for 4 to 6 weeks.
- Chronic carrier state (shedding >1 year duration)
  - Amoxicillin: 1 g PO TID for 12 weeks *or* trimethoprim-sulfamethoxazole 160 mg/800 mg PO BID for 12 weeks *or*
  - Ciprofloxacin: 500 mg PO BID for 4 weeks *or* levofloxacin 500 mg/day for 4 weeks *or* norfloxacin 400 mg PO BID for 4 weeks if gallstones are present

ALERT

- Strains resistant to ampicillin, chloramphenicol, and trimethoprim-sulfamethoxazole have been reported.
- Fluoroquinolone resistance is increasing, perhaps due to increasing use in livestock.
- Pet reptiles were identified as having a 48% carrier-rate, 72% of which were multidrug-resistant organisms.

Second Line

- Aztreonam is an alternative agent that may be useful in patients with multiple allergies or if the organism demonstrates an unusual resistance pattern.
- Fluoroquinolones are now routinely given to children for 5 to 7 days in areas of the world where multidrug-resistant *Salmonella typhi* is common.

SURGERY/OTHER PROCEDURES

- Surgical excision and drainage for infected tissue sites, followed by a minimum of 3 weeks of antibiotic therapy
- If biliary tract disease is present, a preoperative 10- to 14-day course of parenteral antibiotics is recommended prior to cholecystectomy.

ONGOING CARE

FOLLOW-UP RECOMMENDATIONS

Patient Monitoring

- Asymptomatic shedding of *Salmonella* may occur for weeks after infection. Follow-up fecal cultures are generally not indicated for patients with uncomplicated gastroenteritis. Requirements may differ during a *Salmonella* outbreak.
- Criteria may vary by state and local regulations. Some public health departments require negative stool cultures for health workers and food handlers prior to returning to work. Shedding may last from 4 to 8 weeks.
- Serotyping of isolates can be performed at public health laboratories. Genomic techniques are available to identify and monitor outbreaks.

DIET

Easily digestible foods

PATIENT EDUCATION

Meticulous hand hygiene; caution handling raw meat, poultry, and eggs; fruits and vegetables should be thoroughly washed prior to consumption. Thoroughly cooking meats eliminates *Salmonella*; caution when handling animals with high fecal carriage rates.

PROGNOSIS

Most cases of *Salmonella* gastroenteritis are self-limited and have an excellent prognosis. Increased mortality is seen in the young (<3 months), elderly (>65 years), and immunocompromised. Increased mortality is seen with bacteremia and other invasive infections. Mortality is increased in multidrug-resistant strains.

COMPLICATIONS

Toxic megacolon, hypovolemic shock, metastatic abscess formation, endocarditis, infectious endarteritis, meningitis, septic arthritis, reactive arthritis, osteomyelitis, pneumonia, appendicitis, cholecystitis

REFERENCES

1. Centers for Disease Control and Prevention. Salmonella. https://www.cdc.gov/salmonella/index.html. Accessed September 28, 2022.
2. Shane AL, Mody RK, Crump JA, et al. 2017 Infectious Diseases Society of America clinical practice guidelines for the diagnosis and management of infectious diarrhea. *Clin Infect Dis*. 2017;65(12):e45–e80.

SEE ALSO

Gastroenteritis; Typhoid Fever

CODES

ICD10

- A02.25 Salmonella pyelonephritis
- A01.02 Typhoid fever with heart involvement
- A01.3 Paratyphoid fever C

CLINICAL PEARLS

- Nontyphoidal *Salmonella* infection is typically a foodborne infection associated with a self-limited gastroenteritis.
- Clinical syndromes include gastroenteritis, bacteremia, endovascular infection, localized infection outside the GI tract, and a chronic carrier state.
- Those at greatest risk of complications from *Salmonella* infection include the young, the elderly, and the immunocompromised patients.
- Uncomplicated gastroenteritis in healthy patients can be treated with supportive care.
- Antibiotics should be used in infants, the elderly, immunocompromised patients, and for invasive infections such as bacteremia outside the GI tract.

SARCOIDOSIS
Donnah Mathews, MD, FACP

BASICS

DESCRIPTION
- Sarcoidosis is a noninfectious, multisystem, granulomatous disease of unknown cause.
  - Frequently presents with bilateral hilar adenopathy, pulmonary infiltrates, ocular or skin lesions
  - In ~50% of cases, it is diagnosed in asymptomatic patients with abnormal chest x-rays (CXRs).
- System(s) affected: primarily pulmonary but also cardiovascular, gastrointestinal, hematologic, endocrine, renal, neurologic, dermatologic, ophthalmologic, musculoskeletal
- Synonym(s): Löfgren syndrome (erythema nodosum [EN], hilar adenopathy, fever, arthralgias); Heerfordt syndrome (uveitis, parotid enlargement, facial palsy, fever); lupus pernio; Besnier-Boeck disease; Boeck sarcoid; Scheuermann disease (1)

EPIDEMIOLOGY
Incidence
Estimated 6/100 person-years

Prevalence
- Estimated 10 to 20 cases per 100,000 persons, although recent evidence suggests it could be more prevalent
- 11/100,000 annual incidence rate for women (1)
- Usually occurs in younger persons, with the peak age of incidence for women aged 50 to 69 years and for men aged 40 to 59 years; rare in children

ETIOLOGY AND PATHOPHYSIOLOGY
Despite extensive research, etiology is unknown; thought to be due to exaggerated cell-mediated immune response to unknown antigen(s)

Genetics
- Reports of familial clustering, with genetic linkage to a section within MHC on short arm of chromosome 6
- Although worldwide in distribution, increased prevalence in Scandinavians, Japanese, Black Americans, and women
- In Northern Europe, 5 to 40 cases per 100,000 persons; in Black Americans, 35 cases per 100,000 persons; in Caucasian Americans, 11 cases per 100,000 persons

RISK FACTORS
Exact etiology and pathogenesis remain unknown.

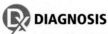

DIAGNOSIS

Diagnosis is based on three criteria: clinical presentation, nonnecrotizing granulomatous inflammation in tissue samples (although not always required), and exclusion of other diagnoses.

HISTORY
- Patients may be asymptomatic.
- Patients may have nonspecific complaints, such as the following:
  - Nonproductive cough or shortness of breath
  - Fever or night sweats
  - Weight loss
  - General fatigue
  - Eye pain
  - Chest pain/palpitations/arrhythmias
  - Skin lesions
  - Polyarthritis
  - Encephalopathy, seizures, hydrocephalus (rare)
  - Patients >70 years old are more likely to have systemic symptoms.

PHYSICAL EXAM
- Many patients have a normal physical exam.
- Lungs may reveal wheezing/fine interstitial crackles.
- ~30% of patients have extrapulmonary manifestations, including the following:
  - Uveitis, retinitis, or other eye findings: conjunctival nodules, lacrimal gland enlargement, cataracts, glaucoma, papilledema
  - Cranial nerve palsies, especially 7th nerve
  - Salivary gland swelling or lymphadenopathy
  - Arrhythmias
  - Hepatosplenomegaly
  - Polyarthritis
  - Rashes
    - Maculopapular of nares, eyelids, forehead, base of neck at hairline, and previous trauma sites
    - Waxy nodular of face, trunk, and extensor surfaces of extremities
    - Plaques (lupus pernio) of nose, cheeks, chin, and ears
    - EN (component of Löfgren syndrome)

DIFFERENTIAL DIAGNOSIS
- Infectious granulomatous disease, such as tuberculosis, nontuberculous mycobacteria, and fungal infections
  - Bacterial pneumonia, such as *Brucella*, *Tropheryma whipplei*, *Francisella tularensis*, *Bartonella henselae*, *Coxiella burnetii*
  - Viral, such as herpes zoster
  - Parasitic, such as *Toxoplasma gondii*, schistosomiasis, leishmaniasis
- Lymphoma
- Autoimmune such as vasculitides, Langerhans cell histocytosis, inflammatory bowel disease
- Hypersensitivity pneumonitis

DIAGNOSTIC TESTS & INTERPRETATION
No definitive test for diagnosis, but diagnosis is suggested by the following:
- Clinical and radiographic manifestations
- Exclusion of other diagnoses
- Histopathologic detection of noncaseating granulomas (not always required)

Initial Tests (lab, imaging)
- Screening for extrapulmonary disease:
  - CBC, HIV
  - Creatinine (renal sarcoidosis)
  - Alkaline phosphatase (hepatic sarcoidosis) +/− transaminase testing
  - Calcium
  - 25- and 1,25-OH vitamin D levels to determine if replacement needed
- Baseline eye exam
- Baseline ECG
- Serum ACE elevated in >75% of patients but is not diagnostic or exclusionary and testing not recommended
- CXR or CT scan may reveal granulomas/hilar adenopathy. CXRs are staged using Scadding classification.
  - Stage 0 = normal
  - Stage 1 = bilateral hilar adenopathy alone
  - Stage 2 = bilateral hilar adenopathy + parenchymal infiltrates (primarily upper lobes)
  - Stage 3 = parenchymal infiltrates with shrinking hilar adenopathy
  - Stage 4 = parenchymal infiltrates with volume loss, bronchiectasis, calcification, or cyst formation
- High-resolution chest CT scan may reveal peribronchial disease.
- Positron emission tomography (PET) scan can indicate areas of disease activity in lungs, lymph nodes, and other areas of the body but does not differentiate between malignancy and sarcoidosis.
- For patients with extracardiac disease, cardiac MRI is recommended over cardiac PET scan. If cardiac MRI is not available, dedicated PET scan may be used.
- For patients with suspected pulmonary hypertension, transthoracic echocardiogram is suggested and may lead to right heart catheterization if indicated.

Follow-Up Tests & Special Considerations
Patients with asymptomatic bilateral hilar lymphadenopathy
- If high clinical suspicion for sarcoidosis (i.e., Lofgren syndrome, lupus pernio, Heerfordt syndrome), biopsy not needed
- If tissue sampling determined to be necessary, endobronchial ultrasound (EBUS)-guided lymph node sampling preferred over mediastinoscopy

Diagnostic Procedures/Other
- Pulmonary function tests (PFTs) may reveal restrictive pattern with decreased carbon monoxide diffusing capacity (DLCO).
- Ophthalmologic examination may reveal uveitis, retinal vasculitis, or conjunctivitis.
- ECG
- Tuberculin skin test
- Biopsy of lesions should reveal noncaseating granulomas.
- If lungs are affected, bronchoscopy with biopsy of central and peripheral airways is helpful. EBUS—guided transbronchial needle aspiration may have a better diagnostic yield.

Test Interpretation

Noncaseating epithelioid granulomas without evidence of fungal/mycobacterial infection

 TREATMENT

- Many patients undergo spontaneous remission.
- No treatment may be necessary in asymptomatic individuals, but treatment may be required for cardiac, CNS, renal, or ocular involvement.
- No treatment is indicated for asymptomatic patients with stages I to III radiographic changes with normal/mildly abnormal lung function, although close follow-up recommended.
- Treatment of pulmonary manifestations is done on the basis of impairment.
  - Worsening pulmonary symptoms and deteriorating lung function and/or worsening radiographic findings

MEDICATION

Systemic therapy is indicated for hypercalcemia or cardiac, neurologic, or eye disease.

First Line

- No FDA-approved treatment for sarcoidosis
- Systemic corticosteroids in the symptomatic individual or with worsening lung function or radiographic findings
  - Optimal dose of glucocorticoids is not known; prior to initiating glucocorticoids, must exclude tuberculosis
  - Usually prednisone, 0.3 to 0.6 mg/kg ideal body weight (20 to 40 mg/day) for 4 to 6 weeks
  - If stable, taper by 5 mg/week to 10 to 20 mg/day over the next 6 weeks.
  - If no relapse, 10 to 20 mg/day for 8 to 12 months; relapse is common.
  - Higher doses (80 to 100 mg/day) may be warranted in patients with acute respiratory failure and cardiac, neurologic, or ocular disease.
- In patients with skin disease, topical steroids may be effective.
- Inhaled steroids (budesonide 800 to 1,600 μg BID) may be of some clinical benefit in early disease with mild pulmonary symptoms.
  - Contraindications and significant possible interactions: Refer to the manufacturer's profile of each drug (2).

Second Line

- All alternative agents to glucocorticoids carry substantial risk for toxicity, including myelosuppression, hepatotoxicity, and opportunistic infection. Prior to using these medications, assess for adherence to steroid therapy, comorbid disease, or other complicating factors contributing to steroid failure. Referral to specialist is recommended.
- Alternative immunosuppressants:
  - Methotrexate: initially 7.5 mg/week, increasing gradually to 10 to 15 mg/week; cannot be used with underlying liver disease
  - Other immunosuppressants include azathioprine, leflunomide, or mycophenolate.
  - If tolerated, continue low dose prednisone (<20 mg/day)
  - Use of immunosuppressants requires regular monitoring of CBC and LFTs.
- Antimalarial agents have been trialed without clear benefit, such as chloroquine or hydroxychloroquine.
- Tumor necrosis factor antagonists, such as infliximab, have been useful in refractory cases.

ISSUES FOR REFERRAL

May be followed by a pulmonologist, with referrals to other specialists as dictated by involvement of other organ systems; if requiring a second-line therapy

SURGERY/OTHER PROCEDURES

Lung transplantation in severe, refractory cases; long-term outcomes are unknown.

 ONGOING CARE

FOLLOW-UP RECOMMENDATIONS

Patient Monitoring

- Approximately 23% of patients with sarcoidosis will develop a new disease manifestation within 3 years of baseline evaluation.
- Monitor serum calcium, creatinine, and alkaline phosphatase annually.
- Patients on prednisone for symptoms should be seen every 1 to 2 months while on therapy.
- Patients not requiring therapy should be seen every 3 months for at least the first 2 years after diagnosis, obtaining a history and physical exam, laboratory testing tailored to sites of disease activity, PFTs, and ambulatory pulse oximetry.
- If on hydroxychloroquine, obtain ophthalmologic exam every 6 to 12 months
- Other testing per individual patient's symptoms, including HRCT, echocardiogram, Holter monitoring, urinalysis (UA), thyroid-stimulating hormone (TSH), bone density, MRI of brain, ophthalmologic exam

PATIENT EDUCATION

- American Lung Association: https://www.lung.org/lung-health-diseases/lung-disease-lookup/sarcoidosis
- MedlinePlus: https://medlineplus.gov/sarcoidosis.html

PROGNOSIS

- 50% of patients will have spontaneous resolution within 2 years.
- 25% of patients will have significant fibrosis but no further worsening of the disease after 2 years.
- 25% of patients (higher in some populations, including Black Americans) will have chronic disease.
- Patients on corticosteroids for >6 months have a greater chance of having chronic disease.
- Overall death rate: <5%; however, subset analysis suggests that Black American women have a higher mortality.

COMPLICATIONS

- Patients may develop significant respiratory involvement, including cor pulmonale. Pulmonary hemorrhage from infection with aspergillosis in the damaged lung is possible.
- Other organs, especially the heart (congestive heart failure, arrhythmias), eyes (rarely blindness), and CNS, can be involved with serious consequences.

REFERENCES

1. Dumas O, Abramovitz L, Wiley AS, et al. Epidemiology of sarcoidosis in a prospective cohort study of U.S. women. *Ann Am Thorac Soc.* 2016;13(1):67–71.
2. Melani AS, Bigliazzi C, Cimmino FA, et al. A comprehensive review of sarcoidosis treatment for pulmonologists. *Pulm Ther.* 2021;7(2):325–344.

 CODES

ICD10

- D86.89 Sarcoidosis of other sites
- D86.81 Sarcoid meningitis
- D86.2 Sarcoidosis of lung with sarcoidosis of lymph nodes

CLINICAL PEARLS

- Sarcoidosis is a noninfectious, multisystem, granulomatous disease of unknown cause, typically affecting young and middle-aged adults.
- Diagnosis is based on clinical findings, exclusion of other disorders, and pathologic detection of noncaseating granulomas.

SCABIES

Roland W. Newman II, DO • Matthew J. Kor, MD

BASICS

DESCRIPTION

- A contagious parasitic infection of the skin caused by the mite *Sarcoptes scabiei*, var. *hominis*
- Typically, a clinical diagnosis based on history and physical exam
- System(s) affected: skin/exocrine

EPIDEMIOLOGY

Incidence

- Predominant age: children, sexually active young adults, and the elderly
- Male children from lower income quartiles were more likely to visit the ED in a retrospective analysis of nationally representative National Emergency Department Sample for 2013 to 2015, whereas older male patients, insured by Medicare, from the highest income quartile in the Midwest/West were most likely to be admitted to the hospital.

Prevalence

Prevalence varies substantially worldwide but is more common in resource-poor settings.

- More prevalent in areas of overcrowding and in developing countries, particularly tropical climates
- Added to World Health Organization's list of neglected tropical diseases in 2017

ETIOLOGY AND PATHOPHYSIOLOGY

- *S. scabiei*, var. *hominis*
  - An obligate human parasite
  - Primarily transmitted by prolonged human-to-human direct skin contact
  - Infrequently transmitted via fomites (e.g., bedding, clothing, or furnishings)
- Female mite lays eggs in burrows in the stratum corneum and epidermis.
- Itching is caused by a delayed type IV hypersensitivity reaction to the mite saliva, eggs, or excrement.

RISK FACTORS

- Prolonged skin-to-skin contact (e.g., sexual, overcrowding, nosocomial infection)
- Poor nutritional status, poverty, and homelessness
- Hot, tropical climates
- Seasonal variation: Incidence may be higher in the winter than in the summer (due to overcrowding).
- Immunocompromised patients (drug-induced), those with leukemia, lymphoma, or those with congenital immune deficiencies, including those with HIV/AIDS, are at increased risk of developing severe (crusted/Norwegian) scabies (1).

GENERAL PREVENTION

Prevent outbreaks by prompt treatment and cleansing of fomites (see "General Measures").

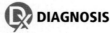**DIAGNOSIS**

HISTORY

- Generalized itching is often severe and worse at night.
- Identify potential contact with infected individuals.
- Initial/primary infection is usually asymptomatic for the first 3 to 4 weeks (until sensitivity occurs).
- Subsequent reinfection typically develops symptoms after only 1 to 3 days.

PHYSICAL EXAM

- Lesions (inflammatory, erythematous, pruritic papules) most commonly located in the finger webs, flexor surfaces of the wrists, elbows, axillae, buttocks, genitalia, feet, and ankles; often spares the head/neck in adults
- Burrows (thin, curvy lines in the upper epidermis that measure 1 to 10 mm in length)—a pathognomonic sign of scabies most common in hands and wrists
- Secondary erosions and excoriations from scratching
- Pustules (if secondarily infected)
- Pruritic papular or nodular lesions in covered areas (buttocks, groin, axillae) resulting from an exaggerated scratching due to hypersensitivity reaction (1)
- Crusted scabies (or Norwegian scabies) is a psoriasiform dermatosis occurring with hyperinfestation with thousands/millions of mites (more common in immunosuppressed patients).

Geriatric Considerations

The elderly often itch more severely despite fewer cutaneous lesions and are at risk for extensive infestations, perhaps related to a decline in cell-mediated immunity. There may be back involvement in those who are bedridden.

Pediatric Considerations

Infants and very young children often present with vesicles, papules, and pustules and have more widespread involvement, including the hands, palms, feet, soles, body folds, and head (rare for adults).

DIFFERENTIAL DIAGNOSIS

- Atopic dermatitis
- Contact dermatitis
- Dermatitis herpetiformis
- Eczema
- Folliculitis/impetigo
- Insect bites
- Papular urticaria
- Pediculosis corporis
- Psoriasis (crusted scabies)
- Pyoderma
- Seborrheic dermatitis
- Syphilis
- Tinea corporis

DIAGNOSTIC TESTS & INTERPRETATION

- Based on 2018 IACS (International Alliance Control for Scabies) Criteria for the Diagnosis of Scabies:
  - Confirmed scabies diagnosis: based on microscopic identification of mites, eggs, or fecal pellets (scybala) *or* visualization of mite with dermoscopy
  - Clinical scabies diagnosis: detection of burrows, *or* typical lesions on male genitalia, *or* typical lesions in a typical distribution with two history features of itch and known infectious contact
  - Suspected scabies diagnosis: typical lesions in a typical distribution with one history feature of itch or known infectious contact, *or* atypical lesions or atypical distribution with two history features of itch and known infectious contact
- A failure to find mites does not rule out scabies.

Initial Tests (lab, imaging)

CBC is rarely needed but may show eosinophilia.

Diagnostic Procedures/Other

- Examination of skin with dermoscopy
  - Simplest and fastest method to identify the pathogen (1)
  - Look for typical burrows in finger webs, on flexor aspect of the wrists, and on the penis.
  - Look for a dark point at the end of the burrow (the mite, also known as "delta wing sign").
- Skin scraping
  - Place a drop of mineral oil over a nonexcoriated lesion or burrow.
  - Scrape the lesion with a surgical blade (no. 15).
  - Examine scrapings under a microscope for mites, eggs, egg casings, or feces.
  - Scraping under fingernails may be positive.
  - When mite is not found with scraping, biopsy may reveal mite, eggs, or feces (2).
- Potassium hydroxide (KOH) wet mount NOT recommended because it can dissolve mite pellets
- Burrow ink test
  - If burrows are not obvious, apply gentian violet or India ink to an area of rash. Wash off the ink with alcohol. A burrow should remain stained and become more evident. Then apply mineral oil, scrape, and observe microscopically, as noted previously.

Test Interpretation

Skin biopsy of a nodule (although performed rarely) will reveal portions of the mite in the corneal layer.

TREATMENT

GENERAL MEASURES

- Treat all intimate contacts (including close household and family members).
- Treat items in contact with skin. Wash all clothing, bed linens, and towels in hot (60°C) water and dry in hot dryer. Personal items that cannot be washed should be sealed in a plastic bag for at least 7 days.
- Itching and dermatitis can persist for up to 4 weeks despite appropriate treatment and can be treated with oral antihistamines and/or topical/oral corticosteroids. It is important to educate patients that this is likely not a sign of treatment failure. However, persistent symptoms greater than 4 weeks posttreatment may need further workup for an alternative diagnosis, failure of initial treatment, or irritation secondary to treatment (2).

MEDICATION

First Line

- Permethrin 5% cream (Elimite) is generally accepted as first-line therapy (3)[A].
  - After bathing or showering, apply cream from the neck to the soles of the feet, paying particular attention to areas that are most involved and then wash off after 8 to 14 hours.
  - It is recommended to repeat treatment 1 to 2 weeks later.
  - The adult dose is usually 30 g per treatment.
  - Side effects include itching, stinging, erythema, and burning (minimal absorption).

- Ivermectin (Stromectol) (3)[A]
  - Not FDA-approved for scabies
  - 200 μg/kg PO as a single dose, which may be repeated in 2 weeks, is an option according to the CDC. Failure of a second dose of ivermectin has been shown to be a predictor of unsuccessful treatment (4)
  - Take with food to improve bioavailability and enhance penetration into the epidermis.
  - May need higher doses or may need to use in combination with topical scabicide for HIV-positive patients
  - Side effects may include headache and nausea (5).
- Both permethrin and ivermectin are associated with high clearance rates in the treatment of scabies without highly significant differences between the two (5).
- Choice between either permethrin or ivermectin can be based on availability, practicality, and associated cost depending on the individual situation (5).
- Crusted scabies often require more frequent application of permethrin (q2–3d for 1 to 2 weeks) in combination with repeated doses of PO ivermectin on days 1, 2, 8, 9, and 15. Severe cases may need further dosing of ivermectin on days 22 and 29.

Pediatric Considerations

- Permethrin may be used on infants >2 months of age. In children <5 years of age, the cream should be applied to the head and neck as well as to the entire body.
- PO ivermectin should be avoided in children aged <5 years and in those weighing <15 kg.

Second Line

- Crotamiton (Eurax) 10% cream may be used on infants >3 months of age.
  - Apply from the neck down for 24 hours, rinse off, reapply for an additional 24 to 48 hours, and then thoroughly wash off.
  - Nodular scabies: Apply to nodules for 24 hours, rinse off, reapply for an additional 24 hours, and then thoroughly wash off.
- Precipitated sulfur 2–10% in petrolatum
  - Not FDA-approved for scabies
  - Apply to the entire body from the neck down for 24 hours, rinse by bathing and then repeat for 2 more days (3 days total). It is malodorous and messy but is thought to be safer than lindane, especially in infants <6 months of age and safer than permethrin in infants <2 months of age.
- Lindane (γ-benzene hexachloride, Kwell) 1% lotion
  - Apply a thin layer to all skin surfaces from the neck down and wash off 6 to 8 hours later.
  - Two applications 1 week apart are recommended but may increase the risk of toxicity.
  - 2 oz is usually adequate for an adult.
  - Side effects: neurotoxicity (seizures, muscle spasms), aplastic anemia
  - Contraindications: uncontrolled seizure disorder, premature infants
  - Precautions: Do not use on excoriated skin, on immunocompromised patients, in conditions that may increase risk of seizures, or with medications that decrease seizure threshold.

- Possible interactions: concomitant use with medications that lower the seizure threshold
- Some instances of lindane-resistant scabies have been reported. These cases do respond to permethrin.

ALERT

Lindane: FDA black box warning of severe neurologic toxicity; use only when all other agents have failed.

Pediatric Considerations

- The FDA recommends caution when using lindane in patients who weigh <50 kg. It is not recommended for infants and is contraindicated in premature infants.
- Infants <2 months should be treated with crotamiton or sulfur preparation.

Pregnancy Considerations

- Permethrin is pregnancy Category B, and lindane, ivermectin, and crotamiton are Category C.
- Permethrin is considered compatible with lactation, but if permethrin is used while breastfeeding, the infant should be bottle-fed until the cream has been thoroughly washed off.

ISSUES FOR REFERRAL

Consider referral to dermatology if unable to confirm diagnosis and/or resistant to repeated treatments.

ADDITIONAL THERAPIES

- Crusted scabies may require use of keratolytics to improve penetration of permethrin.
- Nodular scabies may require intralesional steroids for complete resolution, if they persist for several weeks after treatment.
- Benzyl benzoate lotion (not available in the United States but used widely in developing countries)
  - Not FDA-approved for scabies
  - Dose for adults is 25–28%; dilute to 12.5% for children and 6.25% for infants.
  - After bathing, apply lotion from the neck to soles of feet for 24 hours.
- Topical ivermectin 1% lotion (investigational, moderate level of certainty); not FDA-approved for scabies; apply to affected sites and wash off 8 hours later (3)[A].

COMPLEMENTARY & ALTERNATIVE MEDICINE

Tea tree oil (TTO) derived from the plant Melaleuca alternifolia is a safe, effective, and generally well tolerated alternative option as a treatment for scabies. 5% TTO has proven efficacy as a scabicidal agent in vitro. Topical application of TTO is generally associated with a low incidence of adverse effects (irritant or localized reactions to the oil). Most irritant skin reactions can be avoided by use of TTO concentrations of less than 20%.

 ONGOING CARE

FOLLOW-UP RECOMMENDATIONS

Patient Monitoring

Recheck patient at weekly intervals only if rash or itching persists. Scrape new lesions and retreat if mites or products are found.

PATIENT EDUCATION

Patients should be instructed on proper application and cautioned not to overuse the medication when applying it to the skin. A patient fact sheet is available from the CDC: https://www.cdc.gov/parasites/scabies/fact_sheet.html

PROGNOSIS

Lesions begin to regress in 1 to 2 days, but eczema and itching may persist for up to 4 weeks after treatment.

COMPLICATIONS

- Nodules (nodular scabies) may persist for weeks to months after treatment.
- Postscabetic pruritus; poor sleep due to pruritus
- Pyoderma; secondary bacterial infection (more common in developing countries); impetigo due to group A Streptococci and *Staphylococcus aureus* may lead to sepsis, poststreptococcal glomerulonephritis, and rheumatic heart disease.
- Social stigma

REFERENCES

1. Sunderkötter C, Wohlrab J, Hamm H. Scabies: epidemiology, diagnosis, and treatment. *Dtsch Arztebl Int.* 2021;118(41):695–704.
2. Gunning K, Kiraly B, Pippit K. Lice and scabies: treatment update. *Am Fam Physician.* 2019;99(10):635–642.
3. Rosumeck S, Nast A, Dressler C. Ivermectin and permethrin for treating scabies. *Cochrane Database Syst Rev.* 2018;4(4):CD012994.
4. Aussy A, Houivet E, Hébert V, et al. Risk factors for treatment failure in scabies: a cohort study. *Br J Dermatol.* 2019;180(4):888–893.
5. Rosumeck S, Nast A, Dressler C. Evaluation of ivermectin vs permethrin for treating scabies—summary of a Cochrane review. *JAMA Dermatol.* 2019;155(6):730–732.

 SEE ALSO

Arthropod Bites and Stings; Pediculosis (Lice)

CODES

ICD10
B86 Scabies

CLINICAL PEARLS

- Prior to diagnosis, the use of a topical steroid to treat pruritic symptoms may mask symptoms and is termed *scabies incognito*.
- Eczema and itching may persist for up to 4 weeks after treatment, causing many patients to falsely believe that they have failed treatment or are being reinfected.
- In patients with actual reinfection, it is possible that the patient has not applied the medication properly or, more likely, the index patient has not been identified and treated.

SCARLET FEVER

Christina Scartozzi, DO

BASICS

DESCRIPTION

- A disease (typically in childhood) characterized by fever, pharyngitis, and rash caused by group A β-hemolytic *Streptococcus pyogenes* (GAS) that produces erythrogenic toxin
- Incubation period: 1 to 7 days
- Duration of illness: 4 to 10 days
- Rash (erythematous, blanchable 1 to 2 mm papules; "sand paper") usually appears within 24 to 48 hours after symptom onset.
- Rash first appears in the groin, trunk, and axillae accompanied by strawberry tongue and circumoral pallor and then rapidly spreads outward all over the body, sparing palms and soles.
- Rash clears at the end of the 1st week and is followed by several weeks of desquamation.
- Rash is not dangerous but is a marker for GAS infection with suppurative and nonsuppurative complications.
- System(s) affected: head, eyes, ears, nose, throat, skin/exocrine
- Synonym(s): scarlatina

EPIDEMIOLOGY

Incidence

- In developed countries, 15% of school-aged children and 4–10% of adults have an episode of GAS pharyngitis each year.
- Scarlet fever is rare in infancy because of maternal antitoxin antibodies.
- Predominant age: 6 to 12 years
- Peak age: 4 to 8 years
- Predominant sex: male = female
- Rare in the United States in persons aged >12 years because of high rates (>80%) of life-long protective antibodies to erythrogenic toxins

Prevalence

- 15–30% of cases of pharyngitis in children are due to GAS; 5–15% in adults
- <10% of children with streptococcal pharyngitis develop scarlet fever.

ETIOLOGY AND PATHOPHYSIOLOGY

- Erythrogenic toxin production is necessary for scarlet fever to develop clinically.
- Three toxin types: A, B, C
- Toxins damage capillaries (producing rash) and act as superantigens, stimulating cytokine release.
- Antibodies to toxins prevent development of rash but do not protect against underlying infection.
- Primary site of streptococcal infection is usually within the tonsils, but scarlet fever may also occur with infection of skin, surgical wounds, or uterus (puerperal scarlet fever).

RISK FACTORS

- Winter/early spring seasonal increase
- More common in school-aged children
- Contact with infected individual(s)
- Crowded living conditions (e.g., lower socioeconomic status, barracks, child care, schools)

GENERAL PREVENTION

- Spread by contact with airborne respiratory droplets, saliva, and nasal secretions
- Foodborne outbreaks have been reported but are rare.
- Asymptomatic contacts do not require cultures/prophylaxis.

- Symptomatic contacts of a child with documented GAS infection who have recent or current clinical evidence of a GAS infection should undergo appropriate laboratory tests and should be treated if test results are positive.
- Children should not return to school/daycare until they are afebrile and have received 24 hours of antibiotic therapy.

COMMONLY ASSOCIATED CONDITIONS

- Pharyngitis
- Impetigo
- Rheumatic fever
- Glomerulonephritis

℞ DIAGNOSIS

HISTORY

Prodrome 1 to 2 days

- Sore throat
- Headache
- Myalgias
- Malaise
- Fever (>38°C [100.4°F])
- Vomiting
- Abdominal pain (may mimic acute abdomen)
- Rash—scarlatiniform erythematous punctate eruption
- Cough, conjunctivitis, hoarseness, diarrhea, coryza, oral ulceration, and rhinorrhea are more commonly associated with viral infections.

PHYSICAL EXAM

- Oral exam
  - Beefy red tonsils and pharynx with/without exudate
  - Petechiae on palate
  - White coating on tongue: White strawberry tongue appears on days 1 to 2. This sheds by days 4 to 5, leaving a red strawberry tongue, which is shiny and erythematous with prominent papillae.
- Exanthem (appears within 1 to 5 days)
  - Scarlet, nonconfluent, 1 to 2 mm papules with generalized erythema; blanches when pressed
  - Orange-red punctate skin eruption with sandpaper-like texture, "sunburn with goose pimples"
  - Coarse "sandpaper" rash, initially appearing in groin, upper trunk, and axillae, and then spreading outward to extremities; prominent in skin folds, flexural surfaces (e.g., axillae, groin, buttocks), with sparing of palms and soles
  - Flushed face with circumoral pallor, red lips
  - Pastia lines: transverse red streaks in skin folds of abdomen, antecubital space, and axillae
  - Desquamation begins on face after 7 to 10 days and proceeds over trunk to hands and feet; may persist for 6 weeks
  - In severe cases, small vesicular lesions (miliary sudamina) may appear on abdomen, hands, and feet.

DIFFERENTIAL DIAGNOSIS

- Viral exanthem: measles; rubella; roseola; erythema infectiosum (fifth disease)
- Infectious mononucleosis
- *Mycoplasma* pneumonia
- Secondary syphilis
- Toxic shock syndrome
- Staphylococcal scalded-skin syndrome
- Kawasaki disease

- Acute systemic lupus erythematosus
- Juvenile arthritis
- Drug hypersensitivity
- Severe sunburn

DIAGNOSTIC TESTS & INTERPRETATION

- The signs and symptoms of streptococcal and nonstreptococcal pharyngitis overlap too broadly for diagnosis to be made with precision on clinical grounds alone. Even patients with all clinical features are confirmed to have streptococcal pharyngitis only about 35–50% of the time, particularly in children.
- Use results from rapid antigen detection testing (RADT) or polymerase chain reaction (PCR)-based rapid testing.
- Modified Centor clinical decision rule
  - Absence of cough — 1 point
  - Swollen, tender anterior cervical nodes — 1 point
  - Temperature 38°C (100.4°F) — 1 point
  - Tonsillar exudate or swelling — 1 point
  - Age:
    - 3 to 14 years — 1 point
    - 15 to 44 years — 0 point
    - ≥45 years — −1 point
- Cumulative score:
  - 0: risk of GAS pharyngitis 1–2.5%—no further testing or antibiotics indicated
  - 1: risk of GAS pharyngitis 5–10%—no further testing or antibiotics indicated—option to perform throat culture or RADT—treat if positive.
  - 2: risk of GAS pharyngitis 11–17%—perform throat culture or RADT—treat if positive.
  - 3: risk of GAS pharyngitis 28–35%—perform throat culture or RADT—treat if positive.
  - 4+: risk of GAS pharyngitis 51–53%—consider empiric treatment with antibiotics.
- Testing for GAS pharyngitis is *not recommended* for patients with symptoms suggesting a viral etiology (e.g., cough, coryza, diarrhea, conjunctivitis, rhinorrhea, hoarseness, oral ulcers).

Initial Tests (lab, imaging)

- RADT: diagnostic if positive, sensitivity approaches that of culture, 95% specific; in children, negative RADT should be confirmed by throat culture (not necessary in adults). Positive RADT does not require confirmatory culture.
- PCR: diagnostic if positive, 100% sensitive, 94.1% specific, 84.1% positive predictive value, 100% negative predictive value; positive PCR does not require confirmatory culture.
- Throat culture is the gold standard to confirm streptococcal infection (99% specific, 90–97% sensitive; 5–10% of healthy individuals are carriers).
- Serologic tests (antistreptolysin O titer and streptozyme tests, antihyaluronidase): confirm recent GAS infection; not helpful or recommended for diagnosis of acute disease
- Gram stain: gram-positive cocci in chains
- CBC may show elevated WBC count (12,000 to 16,000/mm³); eosinophilia later (second week)
- Follow-up (posttreatment) throat cultures or RADT/PCR is not routinely recommended.
- Diagnostic testing and empiric treatment of asymptomatic household contacts of patients with acute streptococcal pharyngitis is not routinely recommended (1)[B].

Follow-Up Tests & Special Considerations
- Recent antibiotic therapy may impact culture results.
- Within 5 days of symptoms, antibiotics can delay/abolish antistreptolysin O response.

Test Interpretation
Skin lesions reveal characteristic inflammatory reaction, specifically hyperemia, edema, and polymorphonuclear cell infiltration.

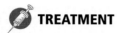

TREATMENT

GENERAL MEASURES
Supportive care; analgesic/antipyretic such as acetaminophen or NSAID for moderate to severe symptoms or to control fever; symptomatic treatment can include medicated throat lozenges and topical anesthetics.

MEDICATION
First Line
The primary reason for treating GAS is to decrease the risk of acute rheumatic fever. Early treatment decreases duration of symptoms by 1 to 2 days and decreases the period of contagiousness. Penicillin is the drug of choice for GAS pharyngitis given its proven efficacy, safety, narrow spectrum, and low cost.
- Penicillin (PO; penicillin V and others) for 10 days
  - 250 mg PO BID or TID for <27 kg (60 lb); 250 mg QID or 500 mg BID for >27 kg (60 lb) adolescents and adults (2)[A],(3)
  - If compliance is questionable, use penicillin G benzathine: single IM dose 600,000 U for <27 kg (60 lb); 1.2 mU for those >27 kg
- Amoxicillin (PO) 50 mg/kg (max dose of 1,000 mg) once daily or 25 mg/kg (max dose of 500 mg) twice daily for 10 days (Use only for definitive GAS because it can induce rash with some viral infections.)
  - Contraindications: penicillin allergy
  - Amoxicillin has similar efficacy to penicillin and is more palatable for children.
- Precautions: Avoid in patients with penicillin allergy (anaphylaxis).

Second Line
For patients allergic to penicillin
- Type IV hypersensitivity to penicillin:
  - Oral cephalosporins: Many are effective, but 1st-generation cephalosporins are less expensive:
    ○ Cephalexin 20 mg/kg dose twice daily for 10 days; max of 500 mg q12h
    ○ Cefadroxil 30 mg/kg once daily; max of 1,000 mg for 10 days
- Type I hypersensitivity to penicillin:
  - Azithromycin (Zithromax, Z pack): 12 mg/kg/day (max of 500 mg) for 5 days (2)[A]
  - Clarithromycin (Biaxin): children aged >6 months: 7.5 mg/kg BID for 10 days; adults: 250 mg BID for 10 days
  - Clindamycin 7 mg/kg (max of 300 mg per dose) TID for 10 days (2)[B]
- Tetracyclines and sulfonamides should not be used.

ALERT
Avoid aspirin in children due to risk of Reye syndrome.

ISSUES FOR REFERRAL
Peritonsillar abscess/retropharyngeal abscess; shock symptoms: hypotension, disseminated intravascular coagulation (DIC), cardiac, liver, renal dysfunction

SURGERY/OTHER PROCEDURES
- Tonsillectomy is recommended with recurrent bouts of pharyngitis (six or more positive strep cultures in 1 year).
- Although children still may get streptococcal pharyngitis ("strep throat") after a tonsillectomy, the procedure reduces the frequency and severity of infections.

 ## ONGOING CARE

FOLLOW-UP RECOMMENDATIONS
Follow-up throat culture not needed unless symptomatic

Patient Monitoring
GAS is uniformly susceptible to penicillin; treatment failures are typically due to the following:
- Poor adherence to recommended antibiotic therapy
- β-Lactamase oral flora hydrolyzing penicillin
- GAS carrier state and concurrent viral rash (requires no treatment)
- Repeat exposure to carriers in family: Streptococci persist on unrinsed toothbrushes and orthodontic appliances for up to 15 days.
- Retreat recurrent GAS pharyngitis with the same agent, an alternative oral agent, or IM penicillin G.

DIET
No special diet

PATIENT EDUCATION
- Delay in treatment awaiting culture results does not increase the risk of rheumatic fever.
- Complete the entire course of antibiotics.
- Children should not return to school/daycare until they have received >24 hours of antibiotic therapy.
- Can spread person to person; personal hygiene is important (wash hands, don't share utensils).
- "Recurring strep throat: When is tonsillectomy useful?" (https://www.mayoclinic.org/diseasesconditions/strep-throat/expert-answers/recurringstrep-throat/faq-20058360)

PROGNOSIS
- Treatment shortens symptoms by 12 to 24 hours.
- Recurrent attacks are possible (different erythrogenic toxins).

COMPLICATIONS
- Suppurative
  - Sinusitis
  - Otitis media/mastoiditis
  - Cervical lymphadenitis
  - Peritonsillar abscess/retropharyngeal abscess
  - Pneumonia
  - Bacteremia with metastatic infectious foci: meningitis, brain abscess, osteomyelitis, septic arthritis, endocarditis, intracranial venous sinus thrombosis, necrotizing fasciitis
- Nonsuppurative
  - Rheumatic fever: Therapy prevents rheumatic fever when started as long as 10 days after onset of acute GAS infection.
  - Glomerulonephritis: due to nephritogenic strain of *Streptococcus*; prevention even after adequate treatment of GAS is less certain.
  - Streptococcal toxic shock syndrome: fever; hypotension; DIC; and cardiac, liver, and/or kidney dysfunction due to other toxin-mediated sequelae
  - Poststreptococcal reactive arthritis—a reactive arthritis following a pharyngeal streptococcal infection with a symptom free interval and subsequent aseptic inflammation of one or more joints typically without cardiac involvement

- Cellulitis
- Weeks to months later, may develop transverse grooves in nail plates and hair loss (telogen effluvium)
- Pediatric autoimmune neuropsychiatric disorder associated with GAS (PANDAS); a subset of children has been recognized whose symptoms of obsessive-compulsive disorder (OCD) or tic disorders are exacerbated by GAS infection.

REFERENCES
1. Shulman ST, Bisno AL, Clegg HW, et al. Clinical practice guideline for the diagnosis and management of group A streptococcal pharyngitis: 2012 update by the Infectious Diseases Society of America. *Clin Infect Dis*. 2012;55(10):1279–1282.
2. Gerber MA, Baltimore RS, Eaton CB, et al. Prevention of rheumatic fever and diagnosis and treatment of acute streptococcal pharyngitis: a scientific statement from the American Heart Association Rheumatic Fever, Endocarditis, and Kawasaki Disease Committee of the Council on Cardiovascular Disease in the Young, the Interdisciplinary Council on Functional Genomics and Translational Biology, and the Interdisciplinary Council on Quality of Care and Outcomes Research: endorsed by the American Academy of Pediatrics. *Circulation*. 2009;119(11):1541–1551.
3. van Driel ML, De Sutter AI, Thorning S, et al. Different antibiotic treatments for group A streptococcal pharyngitis. *Cochrane Database of Syst Rev*. 2021;3(3):CD004406.

ADDITIONAL READING
Mohapatra RK, Kutikuppala LVS, Mishra S, et al. Rising global incidence of invasive group A streptococcus infection and scarlet fever in the COVID-19 era—our knowledge thus far. *Int J Surg*. 2023;109(3):639–640.

 ## SEE ALSO
- Pharyngitis
- Algorithm: Pharyngitis

CODES

ICD10
- A38.9 Scarlet fever, uncomplicated
- J02.0 Streptococcal pharyngitis
- A38.0 Scarlet fever with otitis media

CLINICAL PEARLS
- Consider scarlet fever in the differential diagnosis of children with fever and an exanthematous rash.
- Key clinical findings include strawberry tongue, circumoral pallor, and a coarse sandpaper rash.
- Desquamation (7 to 10 days after symptom onset) may last for several weeks following scarlet fever.
- Diagnose GAS pharyngitis using a validated clinical decision rule (modified Centor score) and selective use of RADT.
- Penicillin remains the drug of choice; however, amoxicillin is as effective as penicillin and is more palatable for children.

S

SCHIZOPHRENIA

Cerrone A. Cohen, MD

BASICS

A severe and persistent mental illness characterized by delusions, hallucinations, disorganization of thought and behavior, cognitive dysfunction, and impairment in reality testing

DESCRIPTION
- Major psychiatric disorder with a variable course, typically involving prodromal, active, and residual psychotic symptoms with disturbances in thought, speech, affect, behavior, and perception
- *DSM-5* eliminated subcategories of schizophrenia (paranoid, disorganized, catatonic, etc.).
- System(s) affected: central nervous system (CNS)

EPIDEMIOLOGY
Prevalence
- 0.3–0.7% of the population >18 years old
- Age of onset: typically <30 years, earlier in males (late teens to mid-20s) than females (early 20s to early 30s)

ETIOLOGY AND PATHOPHYSIOLOGY
- A complex interaction between genetic and environmental factors
- Overstimulation of mesolimbic dopamine D_2 receptors, deficient prefrontal dopamine, and aberrant prefrontal glutamate (NMDA) activity result in perceptual disturbances, disordered thought process, and cognitive impairments.

Genetics
If first-degree biologic relative has schizophrenia, risk is 8–10%.

RISK FACTORS
- Antenatal risk factors include prenatal infection or malnutrition, obstetric complications leading to hypoxia, winter births, postnatal infections requiring hospitalization, urban birth, and advanced paternal age.
- Risk factors across the lifespan include adolescent cannabis use, childhood trauma, urban residence, autoimmune disorders, severe and repeated stress, lower socioeconomic status, minority status, being a first- or second-generation immigrant, and inadequate social support.

GENERAL PREVENTION
Educate all patients on the risks around cannabis use, especially those in a potential prodromal period or those with a family history of psychosis.

COMMONLY ASSOCIATED CONDITIONS
- Nicotine dependence (>50%) and substance use disorders
- Metabolic syndrome, diabetes mellitus, and obesity

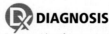DIAGNOSIS

Focus on identifying an insidious social and functional decline over a ≥6-month period (differentiates schizophrenia from brief psychotic and schizophreniform disorders).

HISTORY
At least two of the following core symptoms must be present for ≥1 month and at least one of these symptoms must be delusions, hallucinations, or disorganized speech (1):
- Delusions (fixed, false beliefs)
- Hallucinations (Auditory are more common than visual disturbances.)
- Disorganized speech (derailed or incoherent speech)
- Grossly disorganized/catatonic behavior (hyper- or hypoactive movements that are often repetitive)
- Negative symptoms (diminished emotional expression, poverty of speech and thought, amotivation, lack of social interest)

PHYSICAL EXAM
No physical findings characterize the illness; however, chronic treatment with neuroleptic agents may result in extrapyramidal symptoms, including dystonia (sustained muscle contractions), akathisia (restlessness), parkinsonism (tremor, shuffling gait), or tardive dyskinesia (repetitive, involuntary movements, not limited to but, often involving the face and mouth).

DIFFERENTIAL DIAGNOSIS
- Substance-induced psychosis
  - 25% of patients with substance-induced psychosis will transition to schizophrenia. Highest transition rates are associated with cannabis use (2)[A].
- Personality disorders: paranoid, schizotypal, schizoid, borderline personality disorders
- Mood disorders: bipolar disorder, major depressive disorders with psychotic features or catatonia
- Posttraumatic stress disorder
- Autism spectrum disorder or neurodevelopmental disorders

DIAGNOSTIC TESTS & INTERPRETATION
Imaging (MRI), EEG, LP, and laboratory tests may be indicated to rule out other causes and may be used as clinical presentation warrants.

Initial Tests (lab, imaging)
- The following labs are often used to rule out a medical etiology of psychotic symptoms (3):
  - Thyroid-stimulating hormone (TSH), complete blood count (CBC), blood chemistries
  - Vitamin levels (thiamine, vitamin D, methylmalonic acid/vitamin B_{12}, folate)
  - Drug/alcohol screen of blood and urine, urinalysis
  - Syphilis screen, HIV
  - Heavy metal blood test: lead, mercury
  - Ceruloplasmin, urine porphobilinogen as indicated
  - Erythrocyte sedimentation rate, antinuclear antibody
  - Hepatitis B and C
- The following labs are used to assess for comorbidities and baseline values prior to antipsychotic initiation:
  - Electrocardiogram (ECG) for baseline QTc
  - CBC, blood chemistries, TSH, hemoglobin A1C,
  - Lipid panel
  - Pregnancy test, if indicated

Follow-Up Tests & Special Considerations
Clinical and laboratory tests for routine monitoring, at least yearly, if using antipsychotic medications:
- Weight, waist circumference, and blood pressure
- CBC, hemoglobin A1C, lipid panel
- Pregnancy test and prolactin level, if indicated
- ECG, monitoring for QTc prolongation
- Clinical assessment of extrapyramidal symptoms using a standardized test such as the Abnormal Involuntary Movement Scale (AIMS)

Diagnostic Procedures/Other
Neuropsychological testing: not a routine part of assessment but can help assess cognitive level to predict functioning and need for assistance

Test Interpretation
Ventriculomegaly is frequently seen on MRI with whole brain gray matter loss and white matter loss in medial temporal lobe structures preferentially.

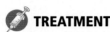TREATMENT

GENERAL MEASURES
- Pharmacologic treatments are the mainstay of the treatment.
- If accessible, psychosocial intervention and rehabilitative therapies can help with successful community functioning.

MEDICATION
First Line
- Two classes of antipsychotic medications: typical and atypical; first-line treatment is with an atypical antipsychotic given lower potential for extrapyramidal side effects.
  - Atypical (2nd generation)
    - Risperidone, olanzapine, ziprasidone, aripiprazole, quetiapine, paliperidone, iloperidone, asenapine, lurasidone, clozapine, brexpiprazole, cariprazine, pimavanserin (Parkinson disease–related psychosis)
  - Typical (1st generation)
    - Haloperidol, chlorpromazine, fluphenazine, trifluoperazine, perphenazine, thioridazine, thiothixene, loxapine
- Medication choice is based on clinical and subjective responses and side-effect profile (4).
  - Sensitivity to extrapyramidal adverse effects: atypical
  - For least risk of tardive dyskinesia: quetiapine, clozapine
  - For least risk of metabolic syndrome: aripiprazole, ziprasidone, lurasidone, perphenazine, brexpiprazole
  - For least risk of QTc prolongation: aripiprazole
    - Avoid use of thioridazine and ziprasidone in patients with a prolonged QT interval.
- For poor compliance/high risk of relapse: Injectable form of long-acting antipsychotic may be used.
  - Haloperidol, fluphenazine, risperidone, olanzapine, aripiprazole, and paliperidone

- Usual maintenance daily range (Initiation is commonly at a lower dose.)
  - Chlorpromazine: 200 to 800 mg/day divided BID/TID/QID
  - Aripiprazole: 10 to 30 mg/day
  - Asenapine: 5 to 10 mg BID (sublingual), once daily patch (FDA approved in October 2019)
  - Fluphenazine: 5 to 20 mg/day
  - Haloperidol: 5 to 20 mg/day
  - Lurasidone: 40 to 80 mg/day (with meal)
  - Olanzapine: 10 to 30 mg/day
  - Paliperidone: 3 to 12 mg/day
  - Perphenazine: 24 mg/day divided BID/TID
  - Quetiapine: 200 to 400 mg BID
  - Risperidone: 2 to 8 mg/day
  - Ziprasidone: 20 to 80 mg BID (with meal)
  - Cariprazine: 1.5 to 6.0 mg/day
  - Brexpiprazole: 2 to 4 mg/day
  - Pimavanserin (for Parkinson disease–related psychosis): 34 mg/day
  - Clozapine: 200 mg BID
    - Typical dosage range is 300 to 600 mg/day split into BID dosing.
    - The gold-standard treatment for refractory schizophrenia
    - Effective in treatment of suicidal patients
    - Serious risk of agranulocytosis mandates registration with National Clozapine Registry and weekly to monthly monitoring of CBC with differential.
    - Significant risk of seizure at higher doses
    - SE can include myocarditis, DVT, sialorrhea, tachycardia, orthostasis, severe constipation, and weight gain.

ALERT
All antipsychotics are associated with weight gain and carry the risk of tardive dyskinesia.

- Managing adverse effects of antipsychotics
  - Dystonic reaction (especially of head and neck): diphenhydramine 25 to 50 mg IM or benztropine 1 to 2 mg IM
  - Akathisia (restlessness): propranolol 20 to 30 mg BID or lorazepam 0.5 to 1.0 mg BID
  - Parkinsonism: trihexyphenidyl 2 mg BID (up to 15 mg daily) or benztropine 0.5 BID (1 to 4 mg/day); amantadine 100 mg daily (up to 300 mg daily)
  - Tardive dyskinesia: consider switching to clozapine; otherwise, deutetrabenazine (6 to 24 mg BID), valbenazine (80 mg daily), or tetrabenazine (25 to 50 mg TID)
  - Neuroleptic malignant syndrome: hyperthermia, autonomic dysfunction, and extrapyramidal symptoms; requires hospitalization and supportive management (IVF and cessation of offending neuroleptic)
  - Weight gain/metabolic syndrome: Metformin up to 2,000 mg daily may attenuate weight gain (5).
  - Geriatric considerations: All antipsychotics carry a black box warning for increased mortality risk in elderly patients with dementia.
- Adjunctive treatments
  - Benzodiazepines
    - May be effective adjuncts to antipsychotics during acute phase of illness, especially when anxiety is prominent
    - First line for the treatment of catatonia

- Withdrawal reactions with psychosis or seizures; risk for dependence and cognitive impairment
- Best when used only in the short term; high cumulative exposure to benzodiazepines may be associated with a significantly increased risk of death in patients with schizophrenia.
  - Mood stabilizers
    - Valproic acid may be effective adjunct for those with agitated/violent behavior (4).
    - Lithium may be effective adjunct for patients with prominent affective symptoms or suicidal ideation (4).
  - Antidepressants:
    - Useful if comorbid depression and/or anxiety are present
    - Associated with a lower risk of psychiatric hospitalization when added to antipsychotic monotherapy compared to adding a second antipsychotic (6)[B]

ISSUES FOR REFERRAL
- Consider referral in cases of suicidality, coexistence of a substance use disorder, difficulty in engagement, or poor self-care.
- Family members often benefit from referral to family advocacy organizations such as National Alliance on Mental Illness (NAMI).

ADDITIONAL THERAPIES
- Psychoeducation and psychotherapy for patient and family: These include specific treatments to reduce the impact of psychotic symptoms, enhance social functioning, and reduce risk of symptom exacerbation. Cognitive-behavioral therapy has been shown to be effective for specific symptoms of schizophrenia (4).
- Vocational support programs
- Negative symptoms typically respond better to these nonpharmacologic interventions than they do to medications.

SURGERY/OTHER PROCEDURES
Electroconvulsive therapy (ECT) should be considered for patients presenting with catatonic features, severe depression, or aggression and suicidality.

ADMISSION, INPATIENT, AND NURSING CONSIDERATIONS
The decision to admit is based on the risk of self-harm or harm to others and the inability to care for self.

ONGOING CARE

FOLLOW-UP RECOMMENDATIONS
Monitoring is based on evaluation of symptoms (including safety and psychotic symptoms), looking for the emergence of comorbidities, medication side effects, and prevention of complications.

PATIENT EDUCATION
NAMI: https://www.NAMI.org

PROGNOSIS
- Typical course is one of remissions and exacerbations.
- About 20% attempt and 5–6% die of suicide.
- Decreased lifespan related to medical comorbidities

COMPLICATIONS
- Medication side effects (tardive dyskinesia, orthostatic hypotension, QTc prolongation, metabolic syndrome)
- Comorbid substance use disorders

REFERENCES
1. American Psychiatric Association. Schizophrenia spectrum and other psychotic disorders. In: *Diagnostic and Statistical Manual of Mental Disorders. 5th ed.* Washington, DC: American Psychiatric Association; 2022.
2. Murrie B, Lappin J, Large M, et al. Transition of substance-induced, brief, and atypical psychoses to schizophrenia: a systematic review and meta-analysis. *Schizophr Bull.* 2020;46(3):505–516.
3. Skikic M, Arriola JA. First episode psychosis medical workup: evidence-informed recommendations and introduction to a clinically guided approach. *Child Adolesc Psychiatr Clin N Am.* 2020;29(1):15–28.
4. Hasan A, Falkai P, Wobrock T, et al; for WFSBP Task Force on Treatment Guidelines for Schizophrenia. World Federation of Societies of Biological Psychiatry (WFSBP) guidelines for biological treatment of schizophrenia—a short version for primary care. *Int J Psychiatry Clin Pract.* 2017;21(2):82–90.
5. Agarwal SM, Stogios N, Ahsan ZA, et al. Pharmacologic interventions for prevention of weight gain in people with schizophrenia. *Cochrane Database Syst Rev.* 2022;10(10):CD013337.
6. Stroup TS, Gerhard T, Crystal S, et al. Comparative effectiveness of adjunctive psychotropic medications in patients with schizophrenia. *JAMA Psychiatry.* 2019;76(5):508–515.

 SEE ALSO

Algorithm: Delirium

CODES

ICD10
- F20.3 Undifferentiated schizophrenia
- F20.5 Residual schizophrenia
- F20.2 Catatonic schizophrenia

CLINICAL PEARLS
- Schizophrenia is a severe and persistent mental illness that impacts cognition and functioning and requires a multidisciplinary team approach to assist with coping, treatment, and to promote recovery.
- Schizophrenia is characterized by positive symptoms, including hallucinations and delusions, and negative symptoms, including flattened affect, anhedonia, amotivation, and social withdrawal.
- Comprehensive care should include treatment of the whole person, not just their mental health. Tobacco use, diabetes, dyslipidemia, and obesity occur at higher rates in individuals with schizophrenia and are associated with reduced life expectancy.

SCLERITIS
Nioti R. Karim, MD

BASICS

DESCRIPTION
- Scleritis is a painful, inflammatory process of the sclera, part of the eye's outer coat.
  - Categorized into anterior or posterior and diffuse, nodular, or necrotizing
  - Commonly associated with systemic disorders
  - Potentially vision threatening
- In contrast, episcleritis is a self-limited inflammation of the superficial episclera with only mild discomfort.
- System(s) affected: ocular

EPIDEMIOLOGY
- Mean age is 54 years (ranges from 12 to 96 years).
- Predominant sex: female > male (1.6:1)

Incidence
Estimated to be 6 cases per 100,000 people in the general population

Prevalence
- Anterior scleritis, about 94% of cases (1)
  - Diffuse anterior scleritis, about 75% (most common)
- Remaining 6% have posterior scleritis.

ETIOLOGY AND PATHOPHYSIOLOGY
- Frequently associated with a systemic illness (1)[B]
  - Most commonly associated with rheumatoid arthritis
  - In about 38% of cases, scleritis is the presenting manifestation of an underlying systemic disorder.
  - Necrotizing scleritis has the highest association with systemic disease.
- Other etiologies
  - Proposed pathogenesis is dependent on type of scleritis. In necrotizing scleritis, the predominant mechanism is likely due to the activity of matrix metalloproteinases.
  - Drug-induced scleritis has been reported in patients on bisphosphonate therapy.
  - Surgically induced necrotizing scleritis is exceedingly rare and occurs after multiple surgeries.
  - Infectious scleritis occurs most commonly after surgical trauma, and *Pseudomonas aeruginosa* in poorly controlled diabetic patients is the most common causative organism (2)[B].

RISK FACTORS
Individuals with autoimmune disorders are most at risk.

COMMONLY ASSOCIATED CONDITIONS
- Rheumatoid arthritis (most common)
- Sjögren syndrome
- Granulomatosis with polyangiitis
- HLA-B27–associated ankylosing spondylitis
- Systemic lupus erythematosus
- Behçet disease
- Juvenile idiopathic arthritis
- Cogan disease
- Relapsing polychondritis
- Polyarteritis nodosa
- Sarcoidosis
- Inflammatory bowel disease
- Herpes zoster, herpes simplex
- HIV, syphilis, Lyme disease, tuberculosis

DIAGNOSIS

HISTORY
- Redness and inflammation of the sclera
  - Can be bilateral in about 40% of cases (1)
- Photophobia and tearing
- Pain ranging from mild discomfort to extreme localized tenderness
  - May be described as constant, deep, boring, or pulsating
  - Pain may be referred to the eyebrow, temple, or jaw.
  - Pain may awaken patient from sleep in early hours of morning.
  - Severe pain is most commonly associated with necrotizing scleritis (1)[B].

PHYSICAL EXAM
- Examine sclera in all directions of gaze by gross inspection.
  - A bluish hue may suggest thinning of sclera.
  - Inspect for degree of injection and extent of thinning.
- Check visual acuity.
  - Decrease in visual acuity of two or more Snellen lines occurs in about 16% of patients (1)[B].
- Slit-lamp exam
  - Episcleritis: conjunctival and superficial vascular plexuses displaced anteriorly; blanches with phenylephrine
  - Scleritis: Deep episcleral plexus is the maximum site of vascular congestion, displaced anteriorly due to edema of underlying sclera; characteristic blue or violet color, absent in patients with episcleritis

- Dilated fundus exam to rule out posterior involvement
- A complete physical exam, particularly of the skin, joints, heart, and lungs, should be done to evaluate for associated conditions.

DIFFERENTIAL DIAGNOSIS
- Conjunctivitis
- Episcleritis
- Iritis (anterior uveitis)
- Posterior uveitis
- Blepharitis
- Ocular rosacea

DIAGNOSTIC TESTS & INTERPRETATION
- Routine tests to exclude systemic disease: CBC, serum chemistry, urinalysis, ESR, and/or C-reactive protein, blood, and urine cultures
- Specific tests for underlying systemic illness: Rheumatoid factor, anticyclic citrullinated peptide antibodies, ACE level, HLA-B27, antineutrophil cytoplasmic antibodies, PPD or QuantiFERON-TB level, fluorescent treponemal antibody absorption (FTA-ABS), rapid plasma regain (RPR), Lyme titers, and antinuclear antibody may aid in the diagnosis.
- Further imaging studies, such as a chest x-ray, sacroiliac joint films, colonoscopy, may be useful if a specific systemic illness is suspected.
- B-scan US to detect posterior scleritis; look at thickness of sclera and for T-sign (fluid in Tenon space at interface between the optic nerve and sclera).
- MRI/CT scan may provide additional diagnostic benefit and detect orbital disease (3)[C].
- Different subtypes of scleritis are associated with varying presentations and distinct findings:
  - Diffuse anterior scleritis: widespread inflammation
  - Nodular anterior scleritis: immovable, inflamed nodule
  - Necrotizing anterior scleritis: "with inflammation": Sclera becomes transparent; scleromalacia perforans without inflammation: painless and often associated with rheumatoid arthritis
  - Posterior scleritis: associated with retinal and choroidal complications; adjacent swelling of orbital tissues may occur.

Diagnostic Procedures/Other
Biopsy is not routinely required, unless diagnosis remains uncertain after above investigations. Culture if suspect infectious etiology.

TREATMENT

GENERAL MEASURES
If scleral thinning, glasses/eye shield should be worn to prevent perforation; should be managed by an appropriate eye care professional

MEDICATION
- First-line therapies for noninfectious scleritis (4)[C]
  - Oral NSAID therapy, choice based on availability, example is ibuprofen 600 to 800 mg PO TID–QID or indomethacin 50 mg PO TID provided no contraindications exists; about 37% successful (5)[B]
  - Systemic steroids (initial if necrotizing scleritis and preferentially IV if vision threatening, otherwise use if failure of NSAIDs), prednisone 40 to 60 mg PO QD or 1 mg/kg/day, taper over 4 to 6 weeks; use caution if suspect infectious etiology.
  - Antimetabolites including methotrexate, azathioprine, mycophenolate mofetil, cyclophosphamide, and cyclosporine may be used as steroid-sparing agents. They are generally recommended if steroids cannot be tapered below 10 mg PO QD (5)[C].
- Second-line therapies (5)[C],(6)[A],(7)[C]
  - Immunomodulatory agents such as infliximab, rituximab, and adalimumab can be used if patient has failed or is not a candidate for antimetabolites or calcineurin inhibitors. These agents are preferred over etanercept due to higher treatment success and its potential paradoxic effect on ocular inflammation.
- Adjunct therapy considerations
  - Topical steroids: prednisolone acetate 1% or difluprednate 0.05% under ophthalmologist care
  - Subconjunctival triamcinolone acetonide injection only for nonnecrotizing, 40 mg/mL, 97% improvement after one injection; increased risk of ocular HTN, cataract, and globe perforation
- Necrotizing anterior scleritis and posterior scleritis
  - May require immunosuppressive therapy in addition to systemic steroids
  - Treat aggressively due to possible complications if left untreated; may need patch grafting to maintain globe integrity
- Infectious
  - Antibiotic therapy resolves about 18% of cases, whereas the remaining often requires surgical intervention such as débridement (2)[B].

ISSUES FOR REFERRAL
- All patients with scleritis should be managed by an ophthalmologist familiar with this condition.
- Rheumatology referral for coexistent systemic disease is helpful for long-term success.

ADDITIONAL THERAPIES
Immunosuppressants used for autoimmune and collagen vascular disorders may be of help in active scleritis.

SURGERY/OTHER PROCEDURES
- In rare cases, scleral biopsy may be indicated to confirm infection or other etiology.
- Ocular perforation requires scleral grafting.

 ONGOING CARE

FOLLOW-UP RECOMMENDATIONS
Avoid contact lenses—wear only if there is corneal involvement, which is rare.

Patient Monitoring
- Patient in the active stage of inflammation should be followed very closely by an ophthalmologist to assess the effectiveness of therapy.
- Medication use mandates close surveillance for adverse effects.

PATIENT EDUCATION
The Ocular Immunology and Uveitis Foundation. Scleritis. https://www.uveitis.org/patient_articles/scleritis/

PROGNOSIS
Scleritis is indolent, chronic, and often progressive.
- Diffuse anterior scleritis (best prognosis)
- Necrotizing anterior scleritis (worst prognosis)
- Recurrent bouts of inflammation may occur.
- Scleromalacia perforans has the highest risk of perforation of the globe.

COMPLICATIONS
- Decrease in vision, anterior uveitis, ocular HTN, and peripheral keratitis
- Cataract and glaucoma can result from disease or treatment with steroids.
- Ocular perforation can occur in severe stages.

REFERENCES
1. Sainz de la Maza M, Molina N, Gonzalez-Gonzalez LA, et al. Clinical characteristics of a large cohort of patients with scleritis and episcleritis. *Ophthalmology*. 2012;119(1):43–50.
2. Hodson KL, Galor A, Karp CL, et al. Epidemiology and visual outcomes in patients with infectious scleritis. *Cornea*. 2013;32(4):466–472.
3. Diogo MC, Jager MJ, Ferreira TA. CT and MR imaging in the diagnosis of scleritis. *AJNR Am J Neuroradiol*. 2016;37(12):2334–2339.
4. Beardsley RM, Suhler EB, Rosenbaum JT, et al. Pharmacotherapy of scleritis: current paradigms and future directions. *Expert Opin Pharmacother*. 2013;14(4):411–424.
5. Sainz de la Maza M, Molina N, Gonzalez-Gonzalez LA, et al. Scleritis therapy. *Ophthalmology*. 2012;119(1):51–58.
6. Levy-Clarke G, Jabs DA, Read RW, et al. Expert panel recommendations for the use of anti-tumor necrosis factor biologic agents in patients with ocular inflammatory disorders. *Ophthalmology*. 2014;121(3):785.e3–796.e3.
7. Cao JH, Oray M, Cocho L, et al. Rituximab in the treatment of refractory noninfectious scleritis. *Am J Ophthalmol*. 2016;164:22–28.

 CODES

ICD10
- H15.009 Unspecified scleritis, unspecified eye
- H15.019 Anterior scleritis, unspecified eye
- H15.039 Posterior scleritis, unspecified eye

CLINICAL PEARLS
- Episcleritis is a self-limited inflammation of the eye with mild discomfort.
- Scleritis is a painful, severe, and potentially vision-threatening condition.
- Although both conditions can be associated with underlying inflammatory diseases, 35% of scleritis cases are associated with a systemic disease such as rheumatoid arthritis. Necrotizing scleritis has the highest association.

SCLERODERMA

Jeremy Golding, MD, FAAFP • Ann M. Lynch, PharmD, RPh, AE-C

BASICS

DESCRIPTION
- Scleroderma (systemic sclerosis [SSc]) is a chronic disease of unknown cause involving connective tissue, characterized by diffuse fibrosis of skin and visceral organs and vascular abnormalities.
- Most manifestations have vascular features (e.g., Raynaud phenomenon), but frank vasculitis is rarely seen.
- Can range from a mild disease, affecting the skin, to a systemic disease that can cause death in a few months
- The disease is categorized into two major clinical variants (1).
  - Diffuse: distal and proximal extremity and truncal skin thickening
  - Limited
    ○ Restricted to the fingers, hands, and face
    ○ CREST syndrome (calcinosis, Raynaud phenomenon, esophageal dysmotility, sclerodactyly, telangiectasia)
- System(s) affected: include, but not limited to skin, renal, cardiovascular, pulmonary, musculoskeletal, gastrointestinal (GI)

Geriatric Considerations
Uncommon >75 years of age

Pediatric Considerations
Rare in this age group

Pregnancy Considerations
- Safe and healthy pregnancies are common and possible despite higher frequency of premature births.
- High-risk management must be standard care to avoid complications, specifically renal crisis.
- Diffuse scleroderma causes greater risk for developing serious cardiopulmonary and renal problems. Pregnancy should be delayed until disease stabilizes.

EPIDEMIOLOGY
Incidence
- In the United States: 1 to 5/100,000 per year
- Predominant age
  - Young adult (16 to 40 years old); middle-aged (40 to 75 years old); peak onset 30 to 50 years old
  - Symptoms usually appear in the 3rd to 5th decades of life.
- Predominant sex: female > male (4:1)

Prevalence
In the United States: 1 to 25/100,000

ETIOLOGY AND PATHOPHYSIOLOGY
Pathophysiology involves both a vascular component and a fibrotic component. Both occur simultaneously. The inciting event is unknown, but there is an increase in certain cytokines after endothelial cell activation that are profibrotic (TGF-β and PDGF).
- Unknown
- Possible alterations in immune response
- Possibly some association with exposure to quartz mining, quarrying, vinyl chloride, hydrocarbons, toxin exposure
- Treatment with bleomycin has caused a scleroderma-like syndrome, as has exposure to rapeseed oil.

Genetics
Familial clustering is rare but has been seen.

RISK FACTORS
Unknown

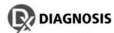

DIAGNOSIS

HISTORY
- Raynaud phenomenon is generally the presenting complaint (differentiated from Raynaud disease, generally affecting younger individuals and without digital ulcers).
- Skin thickening, "puffy hands," pruritus, and gastroesophageal reflux disease (GERD) are often noted early in the disease process.

PHYSICAL EXAM
- Skin
  - Digital ulcerations
  - Digital pitting
  - Tightness, swelling, thickening of digits
  - Hyperpigmentation/hypopigmentation
  - Narrowed oral aperture
  - SC calcinosis
- Peripheral vascular system
  - Telangiectasia
- Joints, tendons, and bones
  - Flexion contractures
  - Friction rub on tendon movement
  - Hand swelling
  - Joint stiffness
  - Polyarthralgia
  - Sclerodactyly
- Muscle
  - Proximal muscle weakness
- GI tract
  - Dysphagia
  - Esophageal reflux due to dysmotility (most common systemic sign in diffuse disease)
  - Malabsorptive diarrhea
  - Nausea and vomiting
  - Weight loss
  - Xerostomia
- Kidney
  - Hypertension
  - May develop scleroderma renal crisis: acute renal failure (ARF)
- Pulmonary
  - Dry crackles at lung bases
  - Dyspnea
- Nervous system
  - Peripheral neuropathy
  - Trigeminal neuropathy
- Cardiac (progressive disease)
  - Conduction abnormalities
  - Cardiomyopathy
  - Pericarditis
  - Secondary cor pulmonale

DIFFERENTIAL DIAGNOSIS
- Mixed connective tissue disease/overlap syndromes
- Scleredema
- Nephrogenic systemic fibrosis

- Toxic oil syndrome (Madrid, 1981, affecting 20,000 people)
- Eosinophilia–myalgia syndrome
- Diffuse fasciitis with eosinophilia
- Scleredema of Buschke

DIAGNOSTIC TESTS & INTERPRETATION
Initial Tests (lab, imaging)
- Nail fold capillary microscopy—drop out is the most significant finding.
- CBC
- Creatinine
- Urinalysis (albuminuria, microscopic hematuria)
- Antinuclear antibodies (ANA): positive in >90% of patients
- Anti-Scl-70 (anti-topoisomerase [ATA]) antibody is highly specific for systemic disease and confers a higher risk of interstitial lung disease (ILD).
- Anticentromere antibody is usually associated with CREST variant.
- Chest radiograph
  - Diffuse reticular pattern
  - Bilateral basilar pulmonary fibrosis
- Hand radiograph
  - Soft tissue atrophy and acroosteolysis
  - Can see overlap syndromes such as rheumatoid arthritis
  - SC calcinosis

Follow-Up Tests & Special Considerations
- Pulmonary function tests (PFTs)
  - Decreased maximum breathing capacity
  - Increased residual volume
  - Diffusion defect
- Antibodies to U3-RNP—higher risk for scleroderma-associated pulmonary hypertension
- Anti–PM-Scl antibodies (for myositis)
- Anti-RNA polymerase III—higher risk for diffuse cutaneous involvement and renal crisis
- ECG (low voltage): possible nonspecific abnormalities, arrhythmia, and conduction defects
- Echocardiography: pulmonary hypertension or cardiomyopathy
- Nail fold capillary loop abnormalities
- Upper GI
  - Distal esophageal dilatation
  - Atonic esophagus
  - Esophageal dysmotility
  - Duodenal diverticula
- Barium enema
  - Colonic diverticula
  - Megacolon
- High-resolution CT scan for detecting alveolitis, which has a ground-glass appearance or fibrosis predominant in bilateral lower lobes

Diagnostic Procedures/Other
- Skin biopsy
  - Compact collagen fibers in the reticular dermis and hyalinization and fibrosis of arterioles
  - Thinning of epidermis, with loss of rete pegs, and atrophy of dermal appendages
  - Accumulation of mononuclear cells is also seen.
- Right-sided heart catheterization: Pulmonary hypertension is an ominous prognostic feature.

Test Interpretation
- Skin
  - Edema, fibrosis, or atrophy (late stage)
  - Lymphocytic infiltrate around sweat glands
  - Loss of capillaries
  - Endothelial proliferation
  - Hair follicle atrophy
- Synovium
  - Pannus formation
  - Fibrin deposits in tendons
- Kidney
  - Small kidneys
  - Intimal proliferation in interlobular arteries
- Heart
  - Endocardial thickening
  - Myocardial interstitial fibrosis
  - Ischemic band necrosis
  - Enlarged heart
  - Cardiac hypertrophy
  - Pulmonary hypertension
- Lung
  - Interstitial pneumonitis
  - Cyst formation
  - Interstitial fibrosis
  - Bronchiectasis
- Esophagus
  - Esophageal atrophy
  - Fibrosis

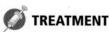 TREATMENT

GENERAL MEASURES
- The treatment is symptomatic and supportive.
- Esophageal dilation may be used for strictures.
- Avoid cold; dress appropriately in layers for the weather; be wary of air conditioning.
- Avoid smoking (crucial).
- Avoid fingersticks (e.g., blood tests).
- Elevate the head of the bed during sleep to help relieve GI symptoms.
- Use softening lotions, ointments, and bath oils to help prevent dryness and cracking of skin.
- Dialysis may be necessary in renal crisis.

MEDICATION
First Line
- ACE inhibitors (ACEIs): for preservation of renal blood flow and for treatment of hypertensive renal crisis
- Dihydropyridine calcium channel blockers (e.g., nifedipine, amlodipine) for Raynaud phenomenon
- Corticosteroids: for disabling myositis, pulmonary alveolitis, or mixed connective tissue disease (not recommended in high doses due to increased incidence of renal failure)
- NSAIDs: for joint or tendon symptoms; caution with long-term concurrent use with ACEIs (potential renal complications)
- Antibiotics: for secondary infections in bowel and active skin infections
- Antacids, proton pump inhibitors: for gastric reflux
- Metoclopramide: for intestinal dysfunction
- Hydrophilic skin ointments: for skin therapy

- Topical clindamycin, erythromycin, or silver sulfadiazine, and PDE5 inhibitors for prevention of recurrent infectious cutaneous ulcers
- Consider immunosuppressives for treatment of life-threatening or potentially crippling scleroderma or interstitial pneumonitis such as cyclophosphamide for ILD.
- Nitrates, dihydropyridine calcium channel blockers, PDE5 antagonists, and fluoxetine for Raynaud phenomenon (2)[C]
- Avoidance of caffeine, nicotine, and sympathomimetics may ease Raynaud symptoms.
- PDE5 antagonists (e.g., sildenafil), prostanoids, and endothelin-1 antagonists are changing the management of pulmonary hypertension.
- Alveolitis: immunosuppressants and alkylating agents (e.g., cyclophosphamide)

ADDITIONAL THERAPIES
- Anti–TNF-α therapy: Preliminary suggestion is that this may reduce joint symptoms and disability in inflammatory arthritis, but small sample sizes and observational biases lend to the need for further well-designed, adequately powered, longitudinal clinical trials.
- Physical therapy to maintain function and promote strength
- Heat therapy to relieve joint stiffness

SURGERY/OTHER PROCEDURES
- Some success with gastroplasty for correction of GERD
- Limited role for sympathectomy for Raynaud phenomenon
- Lung transplantation for pulmonary hypertension and ILD
- Hematopoietic stem cell transplantation for selected patients with rapidly progressive SSc (2)

 ONGOING CARE

FOLLOW-UP RECOMMENDATIONS
Patient Monitoring
- Monitor every 3 to 6 months for end organ and skin involvement and medications. Provide encouragement.
- Echocardiology and PFTs yearly

DIET
- Drink plenty of fluids with meals.
- Adjust eating habits if GI symptoms are present.

PATIENT EDUCATION
- Stay as active as possible, but avoid fatigue.
- Printed patient information available from the Scleroderma Federation, 1725 York Avenue, No. 29F, New York, NY 10128; (212) 427–7040; https://scleroderma.org/
- Advise the patient to report any abnormal bruising or nonhealing abrasions.
- Assist the patient about smoking cessation, if needed.

PROGNOSIS
- Possible improvement but incurable
- Prognosis is poor if cardiac, pulmonary, or renal manifestations present early.

COMPLICATIONS
- Renal failure
- Respiratory failure
- Flexion contractures
- Disability
- Esophageal dysmotility
- Reflux esophagitis
- Arrhythmia
- Megacolon
- Pneumatosis intestinalis
- Obstructive bowel
- Cardiomyopathy
- Pulmonary hypertension
- Possible association with lung and other cancers
- Death

REFERENCES
1. van den Hoogen F, Khanna D, Fransen J, et al. 2013 Classification criteria for systemic sclerosis: an American College of Rheumatology/European League against Rheumatism collaborative initiative. *Arthritis Rheum*. 2013;65(11):2737–2747.
2. Kowal-Bielecka O, Fransen J, Avouac J, et al; for EUSTAR Coauthors. Update of EULAR recommendations for the treatment of systemic sclerosis. *Ann Rheum Dis*. 2017;76(8):1327–1339.

ADDITIONAL READING
- Fernández-Codina A, Walker KM, Pope JE; for Scleroderma Algorithm Group. Treatment algorithms for systemic sclerosis according to experts. *Arthritis Rheumatol*. 2018;70(11):1820–1828.
- Foeldvari I, Culpo R, Sperotto F, et al. Consensus-based recommendations for the management of juvenile systemic sclerosis. *Rheumatology (Oxford)*. 2021;60(4):1651–1658.

 SEE ALSO

Morphea

 CODES

ICD10
- M34.2 Systemic sclerosis induced by drug and chemical
- M34.9 Systemic sclerosis, unspecified
- M34.0 Progressive systemic sclerosis

CLINICAL PEARLS
- Raynaud phenomenon is frequently the initial complaint.
- Skin thickening, "puffy hands," and GERD are often noted early in disease.
- Patients must be followed proactively for development of pulmonary hypertension or ILD.

S

SEASONAL AFFECTIVE DISORDER

Matthew J. Filippo, DO • Janki Thakkar, MD

 BASICS

DESCRIPTION

- Seasonal affective disorder (SAD) describes mood episodes that occur as a part of major depressive or bipolar disorder in a seasonal pattern. Patients may more commonly experience depressive or less commonly hypomanic to manic episodes.
- Depressive episodes typically occur during winter months (fall-winter onset), with full remission in the spring and summer. Less commonly, patients may experience a spring-summer onset with remission in the fall-winter months.
- Ranges from a milder form (winter blues) to a seriously disabling illness

EPIDEMIOLOGY

Incidence

- Affects up to 500,000 Americans every winter
- Up to 30% of patients visiting a primary care physician (PCP) during winter may report winter depressive symptoms.
- Predominant age: occurs at any age; peaks in 20s and 30s
- Predominant sex: female > male (3:1)

ETIOLOGY AND PATHOPHYSIOLOGY

- Photoperiod and phase shift hypothesis note that during the winter months, the period of natural daylight is shorter. When there is less sunlight, the pineal gland increases melatonin secretion, which can lead to a phase shift in circadian rhythm. This process has been linked to symptoms of depression. Light therapy in the morning or evening can suppress melatonin secretion to correct the phase shift and improve symptoms of depression. Reduced sunlight may also decrease vitamin D levels, which may contribute to symptoms of depression.
- Serotonin dysregulation hypothesis is a suspected dysregulation of serotonin, particularly increased clearance from the synaptic cleft and reduced secretion, contributes to SAD pathophysiology. Central acting serotonergic agents such as SSRIs appear to reverse SAD symptoms.

Genetics

- Twin studies suggest a genetic component.
- Studies also indicate an association with melanopsin gene (OPN4) and GPR50 melatonin receptor variants.

RISK FACTORS

- Most common during months of January and February
- Working in a building without windows or other environments without significant sunlight exposure

GENERAL PREVENTION

- Consider use of light therapy at the start of winter (if prior episodes begin in October), increase time outside during daylight hours, or move to a more southern location.
- Bupropion (Wellbutrin) is the only FDA-approved antidepressant for the prevention of SAD.
- Although studies show mixed results, low-dose evening melatonin may help prevent symptoms of depression from occurring.

COMMONLY ASSOCIATED CONDITIONS

Comorbid psychiatric disorders such as alcohol use disorder, ADHD, and binge eating

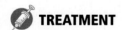 **DIAGNOSIS**

Under *DSM-5*, SAD is denoted by adding the "with seasonal pattern" specifier to a diagnosis of major depressive disorder, bipolar I disorder, or bipolar II disorder.

- Remission of symptoms during nonseasonal months (usually spring and summer)
- Symptoms have occurred for the past 2 years.
- Seasonal episodes substantially outnumber any nonseasonal depressive episodes in the patient's lifetime.
- Carefully document the presence or absence of prior manic episodes.
- Screen for the existence of any suicidal ideation and safety risk factors.

HISTORY

- Symptoms of depression meeting the criteria for major depressive disorder are the following:
  - Sleep disturbance: either too much or too little
  - Lack of interest in life and absence of pleasure from hobbies/activities
  - Guilt: feelings of guilt or worthlessness
  - Energy: fatigue or constantly feeling tired
  - Concentration: difficulty with concentration and memory
  - Appetite: changes in appetite and weight
  - Psychomotor retardation: Patients feel slowed down with decreased activity.
  - Suicidal thoughts: Patients report thoughts of suicide.

- In SAD episodes with fall-winter onset, hypersomnia, hyperphagia (craving for carbohydrates and sweets), and weight gain usually predominate. Despite sleeping more, patients report daytime sleepiness and fatigue. Cravings may lead to binge eating and weight gains >20 lb.
- In SAD episodes with spring-summer onset, depression symptoms of insomnia and loss of appetite are more common.
- Obtain collateral history if patient is unable to provide insight into the seasonal component.

PHYSICAL EXAM

Use exam to exclude other organic causes for symptoms. Neurologic deficits, signs of endocrine dysfunction, or stigmata of substance abuse should prompt further testing.

DIFFERENTIAL DIAGNOSIS

- Organic causes of low energy and fatigue, such as hypothyroidism, anemia, autoimmune disorders, and mononucleosis (or other viral syndromes), need to be considered
- Substance use disorders

DIAGNOSTIC TESTS & INTERPRETATION

- Thyroid-stimulating hormone, CBC, electrolytes, glucose, and
- 25-OH vitamin D level
- Pregnancy test for women of childbearing potential
- Urine toxicology screen if substance use is a concern
- Imaging is not useful unless focal neurologic finding or looking to exclude an organic cause.

Follow-Up Tests & Special Considerations

Polysomnography generally shows that REM sleep is increased in patients with SAD compared to controls.

TREATMENT

MEDICATION

There is a lack of evidence to determine whether light therapy or medication should be the first-line agent. Both are strongly supported by the literature and may have equal efficacy. The combination of medication and light therapy has been shown to be more efficacious than monotherapy. Adherence to both remains a critical issue. The ultimate choice depends on the acuity of the patient and the comfort level of the prescribing clinician with each treatment modality (1).

First Line

- SSRIs can be effective as first-line treatments for SAD. It may be reasonable to decrease a patient's dose during nonseasonal months when patients do not experience symptoms of depression (2)[C].
- SSRIs such as sertraline (Zoloft), paroxetine (Paxil), fluoxetine (Prozac), citalopram (Celexa), and escitalopram (Lexapro) can be used at typical antidepressant doses.
- Bupropion (Wellbutrin) is the only antidepressant currently approved by the FDA for the prevention of SAD.
- There is evidence that suggests low-dose melatonin given in the early evening (not at nighttime) paired with early morning light therapy helps shift one's circadian rhythm and reduces SAD symptoms.
- There is no definitive evidence showing low-dose melatonin as an effective preventative treatment for SAD.

Second Line

Short-acting β-blockers in the early morning given before sunrise suppress melatonin release and can be helpful in reducing SAD symptoms in treatment-resistant cases.

ISSUES FOR REFERRAL

- Patients with ocular disease should be referred for an ophthalmologic exam before phototherapy and for serial monitoring.
- Patients who fail to respond or who develop manic symptoms or suicidal ideation once treatment is initiated should be considered for psychiatric referral.

ADDITIONAL THERAPIES

- Phototherapy, using special light sources, has been shown to be effective in 60–90% of patients and can be considered a first-line treatment, often providing relief with a few sessions.
- Variables that can regulate effect of bright light therapy are the following:
  - Light intensity: At least 2,500 lux is suggested (domestic lights emit, on average, 200 to 500 lux). There is stronger evidence using 7,000 to 10,000 lux.
  - Treatment duration is dependent on the intensity of light source, with daily sessions of 30 minutes to a few hours. Treatment should continue into the season of remission until symptoms improve.
  - Time of treatment: Most patients respond better by using the light therapy early in the morning.
  - Color of light source: Emerging data suggest that shorter sessions of lower intensity light-emitting diodes enriched in the blue spectrum have equal efficacy to the traditional white-light treatment.
- A light box (with an ultraviolet filter) is placed on table several feet away, and the light is allowed to shine onto the patient's retinas (sunglasses should be avoided).

- Most common side effects are eye strain and headache. Insomnia can result if the light box is used too late in the evening. Light boxes can rarely precipitate mania in some patients but can still be used in patients with bipolar disorder.
- Dawn simulation machines gradually increase illumination while the patient sleeps, simulating sunrise while using a significantly less intense light source. These devices have been shown in studies to improve SAD symptoms similar to bright light therapy and are more effective than placebo.

COMPLEMENTARY & ALTERNATIVE MEDICINE

- Work to reduce stress levels through meditation, progressive relaxation exercises, and/or lifestyle modification.
- Currently, there is a lack of consistent research to satisfactorily demonstrate that vitamin D supplementation improves SAD symptoms. Typically, maintenance doses are between 400 and 800 IU/day.

ADMISSION, INPATIENT, AND NURSING CONSIDERATIONS

Consider for suicidal ideation or the loss of ability to function secondary to depression or mania.

ONGOING CARE

FOLLOW-UP RECOMMENDATIONS

Regular monitoring for response to treatment; rarely, patients may become manic when treated with SSRIs or light therapy.

Patient Monitoring

Monitor weekly when initiating light or pharmacotherapy to monitor treatment results, side effects, and any increased suicidal thoughts if using SSRIs.

DIET

Patients with SAD may find themselves craving carbohydrates and feeling energized with increased carbohydrate intake.

PATIENT EDUCATION

- Increase time outdoors during daylight.
- Rearrange home or work environment to get more direct sunlight through windows.

PROGNOSIS

Symptoms, if untreated, generally remit within 5 months with exposure to spring light, only to return in subsequent winters. If treated, patients usually respond within 3 to 6 weeks.

COMPLICATIONS

Development of suicidal ideation and mania are two outcomes the clinician needs to monitor.

REFERENCES

1. Lam RW, Levitt AJ, Levitan RD, et al. The Can-SAD study: a randomized controlled trial of the effectiveness of light therapy and fluoxetine in patients with winter seasonal affective disorder. *Am J Psychiatry*. 2006;163(5):805–812.
2. Nussbaumer-Streit B, Thaler K, Chapman A, et al. Second-generation antidepressants for treatment of seasonal affective disorder. *Cochrane Database Syst Rev*. 2021;3(3):CD008591.

SEE ALSO

- Bipolar I Disorder; Bipolar II Disorder; Depression
- Algorithm: Depressive Episode, Major

CODES

ICD10

- F33.9 Major depressive disorder, recurrent, unspecified
- F33.0 Major depressive disorder, recurrent, mild
- F33.1 Major depressive disorder, recurrent, moderate

CLINICAL PEARLS

- SAD is a subtype of unipolar and bipolar depression, with seasonal pattern. Once the patient has a diagnosed mood disorder, ask whether the symptoms vary in a seasonal pattern to qualify for the diagnosis of SAD. Generally, these patients will report sleeping too much, eating too much (especially carbs and sweets), and gaining weight during winter months.
- Ensure that symptoms are not due to an organic process or better explained by substance use.
- Guidelines suggest using SSRIs first if the patient is more acute or has contraindications to light therapy.
- Light therapy boxes are available from numerous online suppliers but are not extensively regulated; practitioners should take care to ensure that patients are using devices from reputable suppliers. Dawn simulation therapy can be used as an alternative if bright light therapy is less tolerable.
- If using SSRIs, recent studies indicate some patients may experience increased suicidal thoughts after starting therapy; these patients need to be monitored closely as outpatients every 1 to 2 weeks.

S

SEIZURE DISORDER, ABSENCE

John F. Emerson, MD

BASICS

DESCRIPTION

A type of generalized nonmotor seizure characterized by a brief lapse of awareness; classified by the International League Against Epilepsy (ILAE) (1):

- Typical has an abrupt onset and offset of behavioral arrest, loss of awareness, and blank staring, sometimes with eyelid movements, eye-opening, or oral automatisms (e.g., lip smacking).
  – Typically occurs at 3 Hz, lasts 5 to 30 seconds, with immediate return to normal consciousness with no aura or postictal phase
- Atypical has a less abrupt onset and offset and often associated with loss of muscle tone or subtle myoclonic jerks.
  – Typically occurs at <2.5 Hz, lasts 10 to 45 seconds, with often incomplete impairment of consciousness with continued purposeful activity, albeit done more slowly
  – Brief postictal confusion can sometimes occur.
- Myoclonic has an abrupt onset and offset of staring and loss of awareness with continuous rhythmic jerks of shoulders, arms, legs, head, or perioral muscles.
  – Typically occurs at 2.5 to 4.5 Hz, lasts 10 to 60 seconds, with impairment of consciousness varying from complete loss of awareness to retained awareness
- Eyelid myoclonia has an abrupt onset and offset of repetitive, rhythmic jerks of the eyelids with simultaneous upward deviation of the eyeballs and extension of the head.
  – Typically occurs at 4 to 6 Hz, lasts <6 seconds, with incomplete impairment of consciousness and often with awareness mostly retained

EPIDEMIOLOGY

- Predominant age of onset: between 4 and 10 years, with peak onset between 5 and 7 years
- Predominant gender: female > male (2:1) with male predominance in myoclonic absence seizure

Incidence

- 6 to 8/100,000 person-years in children up to 15 years of age
- Prevalence: 5 to 50/10,000

ETIOLOGY AND PATHOPHYSIOLOGY

- Mainly genetic with complex, multifactorial inheritance; however, may be secondary to a variety of congenital or acquired brain disorders such as hypoxia–ischemia, trauma, CNS infection, cortical malformations, or inborn errors of metabolism
- Absences are triggered in the cortico-thalamo-cortical system when γ-aminobutyric acid (GABA)-mediated activity induces prolonged hyperpolarization and activates T-type ("low threshold") calcium channels, resulting in sustained-burst firing of these neurons, causing absence seizures.

Genetics

- 75% concordance occurs in monozygotic twins; 84% share EEG features (2).
- 15–44% of patients with childhood absence epilepsy (CAE) have a family history of epilepsy.
- Mutations of GABA-A/B receptors—involved in spike wave discharges
- Mutations in calcium channels (CACNA1 A, CACNA1 H, CACNA1 I, CACNG3)—thalamocortical dysrhythmia
- Mutations of SLC21A, which encodes GLUT1—associated with a worse prognosis

RISK FACTORS

- Lack of medication compliance
- Lack of sleep
- Alcohol use
- Medications that lower seizure threshold
- Hyperventilation

COMMONLY ASSOCIATED CONDITIONS

Difficulties in visual attention and visuospatial skills, verbal learning and memory, fine motor skills, executive functions, reduced language abilities, ADHD, anxiety, depression, social isolation, and low esteem

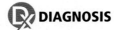DIAGNOSIS

HISTORY

- Detailed description of episode, including activity at onset, any automatisms, duration of episode, frequency of episodes, aura or postictal state, age of onset, and birth and developmental history
- Teachers report that child seems to daydream or zone out frequently and, during episodes, becomes unresponsive and unaware with a blank stare.
- Pallor is frequently reported.
- Child will forget portions of conversations.
- Child with normal IQ underperforms in school.

ALERT
Seizures are often so brief that untrained observers are not aware of the occurrence.

PHYSICAL EXAM

- Unless a child has another genetic or acquired abnormality, a neurologic exam usually is normal. Abnormal physical exam indicates the need for further diagnostic workup (e.g., MRI, metabolic, genetic testing).
- Seizures may be induced by hyperventilation:
  – Have the child blow on a pinwheel or similar exercise for 3 to 5 minutes to provoke seizure.
  – Alternatively, ask the patient to perform hyperventilation with eyes closed and count. Patient will open eyes at onset of seizure and stop counting.

ALERT
Absence seizures are not associated with sensitivity to light or other photic stimuli (e.g., strobe lights).

DIFFERENTIAL DIAGNOSIS

- Juvenile absence epilepsy (JAE)
- Juvenile myoclonic epilepsy (JME)
- Focal seizures with or without awareness
- Psychogenic nonepileptic seizures
- ADHD
- Confusional states and acute memory disorders
- Migraine variants
- Panic/anxiety attacks
- Breath-holding spells
- Nonepileptic staring spells
- Febrile seizures
- Status epilepticus

DIAGNOSTIC TESTS & INTERPRETATION

Initial Tests (lab, imaging)

- Video-EEG monitoring, including sleep and awake with hyperventilation resulting in spike-wave complexes from <2.5 to 6 Hz, depending on type of absence seizure, is standard for diagnosis (3)[B].
- Imaging is not routinely indicated in children with typical absence and normal neurologic exam and cognition. If imaging is performed, MRI is preferable to CT scan due to higher sensitivity for anatomic abnormalities (3)[B].
- Presently, no laboratory values can definitively prove or rule out the diagnosis of an absence seizure. However, labs such as electrolytes, creatinine, liver and renal function tests, TSH, CBC, and toxicology screen can rule out endocrine, metabolic, toxic, or infectious etiologies (4)[C].

Follow-Up Tests & Special Considerations

- Drug levels are useful in evaluating symptoms of toxicity or for breakthrough seizures.
- Follow blood chemistry, hepatic function, blood counts, etc., specific to drug regimen.

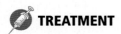TREATMENT

GENERAL MEASURES

ALERT
Patients should refrain from activities that would put them at risk if a seizure occurred (e.g., climbing heights, swimming unsupervised, cycling on busy roads, driving, operating heavy machinery, cooking with stoves unsupervised). Providers should be familiar with state laws concerning driving with epilepsy.

MEDICATION

ALERT
- Certain common anticonvulsants may exacerbate absence including carbamazepine, oxcarbazepine, phenytoin, phenobarbital, tiagabine, vigabatrin, pregabalin, and gabapentin.
- 30% of children are pharmacoresistant (2).

First Line
- Ethosuximide blocks T-type calcium channels:
  - High efficacy (5)[A], fastest onset of efficacy (6)[B], and fewer adverse attentional effects compared to valproic acid (5)[A]; however, it is only effective against absence seizures.
  - Side effects: vomiting, diarrhea, abdominal discomfort, hiccups, headache, sedation
  - Adverse effects: aplastic anemia, skin reactions, and renal/hepatic impairment; monitor CBC and CMP (7)[C].
- Valproic acid (alternative first line)
  - Attention deficits persist more frequently with valproic acid monotherapy compared to ethosuximide or lamotrigine.
  - Adverse effects: teratogenicity, behavior/cognitive abnormalities, hepatotoxicity, pancreatitis; monitor CMP, amylase, and lipase (7)[C]; reduced bone mineral density and increased risk of osteoporosis and fractures
  - Side effects: tremor, drowsiness, dizziness, weight gain, alopecia, sedation, vomiting
  - Very effective but has highest rate of adverse events leading to treatment discontinuation, including negative attentional effects and weight gain (5)[A]; it is considered broad spectrum due to effective against absence and comorbid seizure types such as myoclonic, tonic-clonic, and partial.

Second Line
Lamotrigine affects sodium channels:
- Controls seizures but may be less efficacious than ethosuximide or valproic acid (5)[A]
- Side effects: rash, diplopia, headache, insomnia, dizziness, nausea, vomiting, diarrhea
- Adverse effects: rare Stevens-Johnson rash, more often when coadministered with valproic acid

ISSUES FOR REFERRAL
Failure to gain seizure control for at least 1 year with two AEDs (whether as monotherapy or in combination) should prompt referral to neurologist for confirmation of the diagnosis for seizure and/or syndrome classification and, if appropriate, for consideration of epilepsy surgery (6)[B].

Pediatric Considerations
- Prescribe vitamin D supplementation (usual dose of 400 to 1,000 IU/day) in children taking valproic acid due to AE of reduced bone mineral density (8)[A].
- Fatal hepatotoxicity with valproic acid risk is greatest in <2 years old (7)[C].

Pregnancy Considerations
- Anticonvulsants, especially valproic acid, are associated with an increase in fetal malformations. Use of valproic acid in women of childbearing age, who are not using adequate birth control, is contraindicated.
- Pregnant women with epilepsy can enroll in The North American Antiepileptic Drug Pregnancy Registry: https://www.aedpregnancyregistry.org.

SURGERY/OTHER PROCEDURES
- Epilepsy surgery including ablation and resection for medically refractive absence epilepsy
- Vagal nerve stimulator (VNS) may be considered as an option for medically refractory absence epilepsy.

COMPLEMENTARY & ALTERNATIVE MEDICINE
A ketogenic diet can reduce seizure frequency by 50% in children with drug-resistant epilepsy (9).

ADMISSION, INPATIENT, AND NURSING CONSIDERATIONS
Status epilepticus requires inpatient care.

ONGOING CARE

PATIENT EDUCATION
- Caregivers should be informed that tonic-clonic seizures are rare in absence seizures but should be taught how to manage a generalized tonic-clonic seizure.
- Caregivers who question the need to treat these seizures should be informed that although brief, these can interfere with learning and daily activities and can increase the risk of accidents.
- Sarah Jayne Has Staring Moments: a fictional children's book for child absence seizure epilepsy by Kate Lambert

PROGNOSIS
- Prognosis for CAE is excellent with 56–84% remission rate.
- Remission is less common in JAE, JME, and those who progress to generalized tonic-clonic seizures or myoclonic seizures.
- Patients whose shortest pretreatment EEG seizures are >20 seconds in duration are more likely to achieve seizure freedom, regardless of treatment.
- Typical absence seizures generally cease spontaneously by age 12 years or sooner.

COMPLICATIONS
- Reported frequencies of typical absence status epilepticus range from 5.8% to 9.4%.
- <10% develop generalized tonic-clonic seizures.

REFERENCES

1. Fisher RS, Cross JH, D'Souza C, et al. Instruction manual for the ILAE 2017 operational classification of seizure types. *Epilepsia*. 2017;58(4):531–542.
2. Matricardi S, Verrotti A, Chiarelli F, et al. Current advances in childhood absence epilepsy. *Pediatr Neurol*. 2014;50(3):205–212.
3. Uysal-Soyer O, Yalnizoğlu D, Turanli G. The classification and differential diagnosis of absence seizures with short-term video-EEG monitoring during childhood. *Turk J Pediatr*. 2012;54(1):7–14.
4. Nass RD, Sassen R, Elger CE, et al. The role of postictal laboratory blood analyses in the diagnosis and prognosis of seizures. *Seizure*. 2017;47:51–65.
5. Glauser TA, Cnaan A, Shinnar S, et al; for Childhood Absence Epilepsy Study Team. Ethosuximide, valproic acid, and lamotrigine in childhood absence epilepsy: initial monotherapy outcomes at 12 months. *Epilepsia*. 2013;54(1):141–155.
6. Mohanraj R, Brodie MJ. Early predictors of outcome in newly diagnosed epilepsy. *Seizure*. 2013;22(5):333–344.
7. Posner E. Absence seizures in children. *Am Fam Physician*. 2015;91(2):114–115.
8. Crepeau AZ, Moseley BD, Wirrell EC. Specific safety and tolerability considerations in the use of anticonvulsant medications in children. *Drug Healthc Patient Saf*. 2012;4:39–54.
9. Martin-McGill KJ, Bresnahan R, Levy RG, et al. Ketogenic diets for drug-resistant epilepsy. *Cochrane Database Syst Rev*. 2020;6(6):CD001903.

 CODES

ICD10
- G40.409 Other generalized epilepsy and epileptic syndromes, not intractable, without status epilepticus
- G40.419 Oth generalized epilepsy, intractable, w/o stat epi
- G40.401 Oth generalized epilepsy, not intractable, w stat epi

CLINICAL PEARLS
- Children with CAE can exhibit cognitive, behavioral, and psychosocial comorbidities. For these children, attentional deficits are the most important marker of cognitive dysfunction and often associated with reduced academic performance, anxiety, depression, and behavioral disorders.
- If parents are unable to determine the cause of a staring spell, try suggesting that parents mention something exciting or unexpected like "ice cream" during a spell to get the child's attention rather than calling his or her name.
- Ethosuximide and valproic acid are first-line agents in treatment of absence seizures.
- If failure to gain seizure control for at least 1 year with two AEDs, consider referral to neurologist for confirmation of seizure disorder and/or additional/alternative therapies including ketogenic diet, VNS, and surgery.
- Maintain a seizure diary to help identify type and cause of seizures (https://diary.epilepsy.com/login).
- Review seizure precautions and create a seizure response plan: https://www.epilepsy.com/sites/core/files/atoms/files/GENERAL%20Seizure%20Action%20Plan%202020-April7_FILLABLE.pdf.

S

SEIZURE DISORDER, FOCAL

Zaiba Jetpuri, DO, MBA, FAAFP • Hamid Kadiwala, MD

BASICS

DESCRIPTION
- Seizures occur when abnormal synchronous neuronal discharges in the brain cause transient cortical dysfunction.
- Focal or localization-related seizures have previously been referred to as partial seizures and originate from a discrete focus limited to one cerebral hemisphere.
- Focal seizures are further divided into aware versus unaware and motor versus nonmotor.
- Presence of impaired awareness is defined as the inability to respond normally to exogenous stimuli due to altered awareness and/or responsiveness:
  - Focal seizures with impairment of awareness (formerly "complex partial seizures")
  - Focal seizures without impairment of awareness (formerly "simple partial seizures")

EPIDEMIOLOGY
Prevalence
Focal seizures occur in 20/100,000 persons in the United States.

ETIOLOGY AND PATHOPHYSIOLOGY
- Focal seizures begin when a localized seizure focus produces an abnormal, synchronized depolarization within a neuronal network limited to one cerebral hemisphere; it may stay discretely localized or be widely distributed throughout that hemisphere.
- The area of cortex involved in the seizure determines the symptoms; for example, an epileptogenic focus in motor cortex produces contralateral motor symptoms.
- Most common etiologies vary by life stage:
  - Early childhood: developmental/congenital malformation, trauma
  - Young adults: developmental, infection, trauma
  - Adults 40 to 60 years of age: cerebrovascular insult, infection, trauma
  - Adults >60 years of age: cerebrovascular insult, trauma, neoplasm

Genetics
Benign rolandic epilepsy, has an autosomal dominant inheritance pattern

RISK FACTORS
- History of traumatic brain injury (TBI)
- Thiamine-deficient formula

COMMONLY ASSOCIATED CONDITIONS
Depression

DIAGNOSIS

Duration: seconds to minutes, unless status epilepticus develops; status epilepticus may present as focal/generalized convulsions/altered mental status without convulsions.

- Focal seizures without impairment of awareness (simple partial seizures)
  - Motor onset: Seizure activity in motor strip causes contraction (tonic) or rhythmic jerking (clonic) movements that may involve one entire side of body or may be more localized (i.e., hands, feet, or face).
    - Jacksonian march: As discharge spreads through motor cortex, tonic–clonic activity spreads in predictable fashion (i.e., beginning in hand and progressing up arm and to the face).
  - Nonmotor onset:
    - Todd paralysis: after motor seizure, residual, temporary weakness in the affected area
    - Parietal lobe: sensory loss/paresthesias, dizziness
    - Temporal lobe: déjà vu, rising sensation in epigastrium, auditory hallucinations/forced memories, unpleasant smell/taste
    - Occipital: visual hallucinations
- Focal seizures with impairment of awareness (complex partial seizures):
  - May have aura; indicates the onset of the seizure
  - Amnesia for the event, postictal confusion
  - Most often, focus is temporal/frontal.
  - Motor manifestations may include dystonic posturing/automatisms (i.e., simple, repetitive movements of face and hands such as lip smacking, picking, or more complex actions such as purposeless walking).
  - Frontal lobe seizure is characterized by brief, bilateral complex movements, vocalizations, often with onset during sleep.

HISTORY
- A detailed description of the seizure should be obtained from an observer.
- Review medication list for drugs that lower seizure threshold (e.g., tramadol, bupropion, theophylline).
- Obtain history of drugs of abuse (e.g., cocaine) that may lower seizure threshold.
- Review history of prior TBI.

PHYSICAL EXAM
Include neurologic exam, with attention to lateralizing signs suggestive of structural lesion.

DIFFERENTIAL DIAGNOSIS
- Syncope/postanoxic myoclonus
- Hypoglycemia
- Psychogenic nonepileptic seizure
- For hemiparesis following event: TIA, hemiplegic migraine

DIAGNOSTIC TESTS & INTERPRETATION
- CBC; complete metabolic panel; urinalysis; urine drug screen; levels of antiepileptic drugs; chest x-ray
- Elevated prolactin, if measured within 10 to 20 minutes of suspected seizure, or elevated creatine phosphokinase; if measured within 6 to 24 hours, may help to differentiate generalized/focal seizure from psychogenic nonepileptic seizure (1)[B]
- Emergency evaluation of new seizure: CT scan to screen for hemorrhage and stroke
- CSF exam if infection is suspected
- EEG should be considered in patients with first time unprovoked seizure (2)[B].
- Yield of EEG is increased by being obtained in the first 24 hours following seizure and by sleep deprivation.
- If difficulty with diagnosis, continuous video–EEG monitoring may be appropriate.
- In patients without recent neuroimaging, consider CT or MRI (2)[B].

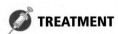 TREATMENT

GENERAL MEASURES
Maintain a seizure diary, noting potential triggers, such as stress, sleep deprivation, drug use, discontinuation of alcohol/benzodiazepines, menses.

MEDICATION
- Current guidelines do not recommend for or against starting an AED after a single unprovoked seizure. Patients should be counseled that AEDs will reduce risk of repeat seizure over 2 years but have no effect on long-term remission (3)[C].
- Initiating an AED after a single unprovoked seizure lowers the probability of recurrence within 5 years but does not have an effect on remission or mortality. Additionally, there is increased risk of adverse effects with immediate treatment (4).
- AEDs act on voltage-gated ion channels, affect neuronal inhibition via enhancement of γ-aminobutyric acid (GABA, an inhibitory neurotransmitter), or decrease neuronal excitation. End result is to decrease the abnormal synchronized firing and to prevent seizure propagation.
- 50% of those with newly diagnosed focal seizures respond to, and tolerate, first AED trial. Up to 50% of those who fail the first AED trial will also fail a second AED trial (5)[B].
- Choose AED based on seizure type, side effect profile, and patient characteristics. Increase dose until seizure control is obtained/side effects become unacceptable.
- Attempt monotherapy, but many patients will require adjunctive agents. Multiple effective add-on agents are available, but there is no clear evidence for one AED over another.
- AEDs may prevent seizures after a TBI in the short term, although they provide no efficacy in long-term prevention (6)[B].
- Several AEDs induce/inhibit cytochrome P450 enzymes (watch for drug interactions).

First Line

- Carbamazepine: affects sodium channels
  - Side effects include GI distress, hyponatremia, diplopia, dizziness, rare pancytopenia/marrow suppression, and exfoliative rash.
  - Patients of Asian ancestry should be screened for HLA-B*1502 prior to initiation to reduce risk of Stevens-Johnson or toxic epidermal necrolysis.
- Oxcarbazepine: affects sodium channels; side effects include dizziness, diplopia, hyponatremia, and headache.
- Lamotrigine: affects sodium channels
  - Side effects include insomnia, dizziness, and ataxia.
  - Risk of Stevens-Johnson reaction (potentially fatal exfoliative rash), especially when given with valproate, requires slow titration.
- Levetiracetam: multiple mechanisms; side effects include sedation, ataxia, and irritability.

Second Line

- Phenytoin: affects sodium channels; side effects include ataxia, dizziness, diplopia, tremor, GI upset, gingival hyperplasia, and fever.
- Phenobarbital: multiple mechanisms; side effects include sedation and withdrawal seizures.
- Valproate: multiple mechanisms; side effects include GI upset, weight gain, alopecia, and tremor; less common, thrombocytopenia, hepatitis, pancreatitis
- Topiramate: multiple mechanisms; side effects include anorexia, cognitive slowing, sedation, nephrolithiasis, and anhidrosis.
- Gabapentin: multiple mechanisms; side effects include sedation, dizziness, and ataxia.
- Pregabalin: affects calcium channels; side effects include sedation, dizziness, and weight gain.
- Zonisamide: affects sodium channels
  - Side effects include sedation, anorexia, nausea, dizziness, ataxia, anhidrosis, and nephrolithiasis.
  - Cross-reaction with sulfa allergy

Pregnancy Considerations

- Folate should be prescribed for all women of childbearing age who are taking AEDs. AED therapy during the 1st trimester is associated with doubled risk for major fetal malformations (6% vs. 3%).
- Phenytoin in pregnancy may result in fetal hydantoin syndrome.
- Valproate is associated with neural tube defects and should be avoided in pregnancy when possible.
- Fetal insult from seizures following withdrawal of therapy also may be severe. Risk-to-benefit balance should be evaluated with high-risk pregnancy and neurology consultations. Most patients remain on anticonvulsants.
- AED levels should be monitored at least every trimester.

ISSUES FOR REFERRAL

Epilepsy specialist for refractory seizures

ADDITIONAL THERAPIES

- Vagal nerve stimulator provides periodic stimulation to vagus nerve. High-frequency stimulation in adults provides greater reduction in seizure frequency than low-frequency stimulation but also has greater rates of side effects (7)[B].
- Deep brain stimulation may decrease seizure frequency in medically refractive epilepsy.
- Repetitive magnetic transcranial stimulation may reduce seizures with refractory focal seizures.

SURGERY/OTHER PROCEDURES

- For refractory focal seizures with identifiable focus
- Preoperative testing, such as Wada test, should be done to decrease likelihood of inducing aphasia and memory loss.
- 34–74% will be seizure free after temporal lobe surgery. Prognosis varies for surgical resection of extratemporal foci.
- Goal of surgical intervention is to reduce reliance on medications; most patients remain on anticonvulsants postoperatively.

ADMISSION, INPATIENT, AND NURSING CONSIDERATIONS

Admit for unremitting seizure (status epilepticus).

 ONGOING CARE

FOLLOW-UP RECOMMENDATIONS

- Most states have restrictions on driving for those with seizure disorders.
- Depending on seizure manifestation, may also recommend against activities such as swimming, climbing to heights, or operating heavy machinery

Patient Monitoring

AED levels if concern over toxicity, noncompliance, or for breakthrough seizures

DIET

Ketogenic or low-glycemic index diet may improve seizure control in some patients.

PATIENT EDUCATION

Avoid potential triggers such as alcohol or drug use and sleep deprivation.

PROGNOSIS

- Risk of seizure recurrence: ~30% after first seizure; of these, 50% will occur in the first 6 months, 90% in the first 2 years.
- Depends on seizure type; rolandic epilepsy has a good prognosis; temporal lobe epilepsy is more likely to be persistent.
- ~25–30% of all seizures are refractory to current medications.
- AEDs initiated after an initial seizure have been shown to decrease the risk of seizure over the first 5 years but are not demonstrated to reduce long-term risk of recurrence or mortality.
- The risk of developing seizure after mild TBI remains high for a long period (>10 years).

COMPLICATIONS

- Risk of accidental injury
- Depression, anxiety, memory impairment

REFERENCES

1. Brigo F, Igwe SC, Erro R, et al. Postictal serum creatine kinase for the differential diagnosis of epileptic seizures and psychogenic non-epileptic seizures: a systematic review. *J Neurol*. 2015;262(2):251–257.
2. Krumholz A, Wiebe S, Gronseth G, et al. Practice parameter: evaluating an apparent unprovoked first seizure in adults (an evidence-based review): report of the Quality Standards Subcommittee of the American Academy of Neurology and the American Epilepsy Society. *Neurology*. 2007;69(21):1996–2007.
3. Krumholz A, Wiebe S, Gronseth GS, et al. Evidence-based guideline: management of an unprovoked first seizure in adults: report of the Guideline Development Subcommittee of the American Academy of Neurology and the American Epilepsy Society. *Neurology*. 2015;84(16):1705–1713.
4. Leone MA, Giussani G, Nevitt SJ, et al. Immediate antiepileptic drug treatment, versus placebo, deferred, or no treatment for first unprovoked seizure. *Cochrane Database Syst Rev*. 2021;5(5):CD007144.
5. Bonnett LJ, Tudur Smith C, Donegan S, et al. Treatment outcome after failure of a first antiepileptic drug. *Neurology*. 2014;83(6):552–560.
6. Thompson K, Pohlmann-Eden B, Campbell LA, et al. Pharmacological treatments for preventing epilepsy following traumatic head injury. *Cochrane Database Syst Rev*. 2015;(8):CD009900.
7. Panebianco M, Rigby A, Marson AG. Vagus nerve stimulation for focal seizures. *Cochrane Database Syst Rev*. 2022;7(7):CD002896.

ADDITIONAL READING

Gavvala JR, Schuele SU. New-onset seizure in adults and adolescents: a review. *JAMA*. 2016;316(24):2657–2668.

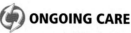 CODES

ICD10

- G40.109 Local-rel symptc epi w simp prt seiz,not ntrct, w/o stat epi
- G40.209 Local-rel symptc epi w cmplx prt seiz,not ntrct,w/o stat epi
- G40.119 Local-rel symptc epi w simple part seiz, ntrct, w/o stat epi

CLINICAL PEARLS

- Focal seizures originate from a discrete focus limited to one hemisphere in the cerebral cortex and are further divided into aware versus unaware and motor versus nonmotor, depending on patient presentation.
- It is controversial whether AED treatment is indicated after a first seizure. Treatment should be strongly considered when a clear structural cause is identified/risk of injury from seizure is high (e.g., osteoporosis, anticoagulation).
- An EEG and neuroimaging (CT or MRI) should be considered in evaluating a first unprovoked seizure.
- Postictal elevation in prolactin and CPK levels can help distinguish physiologic from psychogenic nonepileptic seizures.

S

SEIZURE DISORDERS
Sahil Mullick, MD • Mohamad Khalil, MD

 BASICS

DESCRIPTION
- Seizure: sudden and transient symptoms (altered level of consciousness, motor manifestations) due to abnormal neuronal electrical activity in the brain
- Epilepsy: two or more unprovoked seizures apart in a >24-hour period or one unprovoked seizure with a risk of further seizures that is similar to the risk after two unprovoked seizures (at least 60%)
- Status epilepticus: an epileptic seizure that lasts >5 minutes or multiple seizures without returning to normal between them; classifications: generalized, simple and complex partial, absence, nonconvulsive; based on three key features:
  - Seizure origin: focal (previously partial), focal to bilateral, generalized
  - Awareness: aware, focal impaired, or generalized
  - Clinical features: motor, nonmotor (absence, behavior, cognitive, autonomic)
- System(s) affected: nervous
- Synonym(s): convulsion, attacks, spells

EPIDEMIOLOGY
Incidence
200,000 new cases of epilepsy are diagnosed in the United States annually with 45,000 new cases in children <15 years of age.

Prevalence
In 2015, 1.2% of the total U.S. population had active epilepsy.

ETIOLOGY AND PATHOPHYSIOLOGY
- Synchronous and excessive firing of neurons, resulting in an imbalance of regulatory mechanisms in favor of excitatory activity
- Acute symptomatic seizures: triggered by an acute insult to the brain, medical illness, metabolic disturbance, substance/medication ingestion, or withdrawal (such seizures do not necessarily define the presence of epilepsy)
  - Stroke, subdural hematoma, subarachnoid bleed, traumatic brain injury, hypoxic-ischemic injury, acute infection
  - Metabolic and endocrine disorders, drug intoxication/poisoning/overdose
  - Medications: opioids, anticancer drugs, various antibiotics, hypoglycemic agents, immunosuppressants, psychotropic medications, and decongestants
- Vascular malformations
- Familial/genetic seizure syndromes
- Benign neonatal seizures, benign familial neonatal epilepsy, EME, Ohtahara syndrome
- Infancy (age <2 years): febrile seizures, metabolic causes (e.g., hypoglycemia, vitamin B_6 deficiency)
- Childhood (age 2 to 10 years): absence or febrile seizure
- Adolescent (age 10 to 18 years): AV malformation
- Late adulthood (age >60 years); stroke, metabolic disturbances (hypoglycemia, uremia, hepatic failure, electrolyte abnormality), and drugs

Genetics
Family history increases risk by 3-fold.

RISK FACTORS
History of congenital brain malformations, CNS infections, head trauma, stroke, tumors

GENERAL PREVENTION
Prevent head injuries. Avoid sleep deprivation, excessive alcohol intake, and dehydration.

COMMONLY ASSOCIATED CONDITIONS
Genetic syndromes (Angelman, tuberous sclerosis, Sturge-Weber), infections, tumors, drug abuse, alcohol and drug withdrawal, trauma, metabolic disorders, and hormonal changes related to menstrual cycle

 DIAGNOSIS

Conventional classification of seizures
- Generalized seizures
  - Tonic–clonic: tonic phase: sudden loss of consciousness; clonic phase: sustained contraction followed by rhythmic contractions of all four extremities; postictal phase: headache, confusion, fatigue; clinically hypertensive, tachycardic, and otherwise hypersympathetic
  - Absence: impaired awareness and responsiveness
  - Atonic: abrupt loss of muscle tone
  - Myoclonic: repetitive muscle contractions
- Focal seizures with retained awareness (previously called simple partial seizures): Symptoms vary depending entirely on the part of the cortex involved; they can present with auras and a postictal phase
- Focal seizures with impaired awareness (previously called complex partial seizures): most common type of seizure in adults with epilepsy; can stare into space, motionless, or engage in automatisms and then postictal phase
- Both focal seizures may propagate diffusely to cause bilateral tonic–clonic seizures.
- Nonconvulsive status epilepticus: most commonly seen in ICU patients; no tonic–clonic activity seen so diagnose with bedside EEG
- Status epilepticus: repetitive generalized seizures without recovery between seizures; considered a neurologic emergency
- PNES: nonrhythmic pattern of movement, eye closure during the event, anterior tongue biting, history of psychiatric disorders; patients can also have coexisting epilepsy.
- Febrile seizures
  - Usually ≤6 years; fever without evidence of any other defined cause of seizures

HISTORY
- Eyewitness descriptions of the event; patient impressions of what occurred before, during, and after the event
- Screen for etiologies, including provoking/ameliorating factors for the event, such as sleep deprivation.
- Ask about bowel/bladder incontinence (urinary incontinence has low specificity and sensitivity), tongue biting, other injury, automatisms, or prior seizure activity.
- Ictal behaviors are useful for localization.
- Evaluate for medication or substance use.

PHYSICAL EXAM
Thorough neurologic exam
- Lateral tongue biting is suggestive of generalized seizure, whereas the tip of the tongue is more suggestive of a nonepileptic event.
- Tongue biting lacks sensitivity but has high specificity to differentiate from PNES and syncope.

DIFFERENTIAL DIAGNOSIS
- Syncope, orthostatic hypotension, convulsive syncope
- Transient ischemic attack, stroke
- Complicated migraine
- Sleep disorders: cataplexy, narcolepsy
- Psychiatric disorders: conversion, malingering, panic

DIAGNOSTIC TESTS & INTERPRETATION
A negative EEG does not rule out a seizure disorder. Interictal EEG sensitivity may be as low as 20%; multiple EEGs (at least three) may increase sensitivity to 80% (1)[C].
- Sleep deprivation may be helpful prior to EEG, and hyperventilation and photic stimulation during recording may increase sensitivity.
- Video EEG monitoring is used to differentiate PNES from true cortical events.
- EEG is necessary for the diagnosis of nonconvulsive status epilepticus.

Initial Tests (lab, imaging)
- Glucose, sodium, potassium, calcium, phosphorus, magnesium, BUN, ammonia; drug and toxin screens
- AED levels (if a patient is taking antiepileptic medication)
- CBC, UA, ECG, lumbar puncture if needed: Rule out infection.
- Serum prolactin has limited use; may be useful in differentiating generalized tonic–clonic and focal seizure from PNES
- Imaging is recommended for new-onset seizures. MRI is preferred to CT.
  - CT scan of the brain: indicated routinely as an initial evaluation, especially in the ER
  - Brain MRI: superior in evaluation of the temporal lobes, strokes, and other structural abnormalities

Diagnostic Procedures/Other
A lumbar puncture for spinal fluid analysis may be necessary to rule out meningitis.

 TREATMENT

- Older adults are more sensitive to side effects from AEDs; use lower initial dosing (2).
- After an initial unprovoked seizure, 21–45% will have a recurrence within 2 years (3).
- Starting antiepileptic medications is likely to reduce recurrences of seizures but does not alter long-term outcomes or improve quality of life (3).
- Patients with a single unprovoked seizure and associated risk factors that increase recurrence risk up to 60% (abnormal EEG, neurologic exam, or neuroimaging) can potentially benefit from starting therapy.

GENERAL MEASURES
- Most seizures remit spontaneously within 2 minutes.
- Treat metabolic and infectious etiologies.
- Main goals: Control seizures, avoid side effects, and restore quality of life.

MEDICATION
- AED: Select based on the type of seizure, potential adverse effects/drug interactions, and comorbid medical conditions.
- Treatment should begin with a single agent and the dose titrated until seizures are controlled or side effects become problematic. Consider switching to a different agent versus adding a second agent.
- Patients treated with loading doses of AED in status epilepticus can be started on a maintenance dose of a different AED.

First Line
Treatment options include the following:
- Levetiracetam (Keppra): 1,000 to 4,000 mg/day in 2 doses
- Carbamazepine (Tegretol): 100 to 200 mg/day, 2 to 4 doses; therapeutic range of 4 to 12 mg/L
- Lamotrigine (Lamictal): 25 mg/day, titrated by 50 mg/day every 1 to 2 weeks to 225 to 375 mg/day in 2 doses for immediate release or 300 to 400 mg/day for extended release
- Oxcarbazepine (Trileptal): 900 to 2,400 mg/day in 2 to 3 doses
- Lacosamide (Vimpat): 200 to 400 mg/day in 2 doses
- Ethosuximide (Zarontin): 20 to 40 mg/kg/day in 1 to 3 doses, therapeutic concentration of 40 to 100 μg/mL
- Generalized status epilepticus:
  - Lorazepam 4 mg IV, repeat once in 5 to 10 minutes if seizure continues (4); midazolam/diazepam 10 mg IV, repeat once in 5 to 10 minutes if seizure continues
  - Fosphenytoin 20 mg phenytoin equivalents/kg load
  - Valproic acid 15 to 45 mg/kg administered at ≤6 mg/kg/min
  - Levetiracetam 60 mg/kg up to a max of 4.5 g infused over 10 minutes
  - Lacosamide 10 mg/kg (max dose of 200 mg) loading dose, then 12 hours later start 100 mg BID

Second Line
- Phenytoin (Dilantin): 300 to 400 mg/day in 1 to 3 doses; therapeutic range of 10 to 20 mg/L
- Valproic acid (Depakene): 750 to 3,000 mg/day in 1 to 3 doses to begin at 15 mg/kg/day; therapeutic range of 50 to 125 μg/mL
- Topiramate (Topamax): 50 mg/day; adjust weekly to effect; 400 mg/day in 2 doses, max of 1,600 mg/day
- Gabapentin (Neurontin):1,800 to 3,600 mg in 3 doses for adjunct therapy
- Pregabalin (Lyrica): 150 to 300 mg/day in 2 to 3 doses
- Zonisamide (Zonegran): 100 to 600 mg/day in 1 to 2 doses
- Perampanel (Fycompa): 4 to 12 mg/day
- Clonazepam (Klonopin): 1.5 to 8.0 mg in 2 to 3 doses (max of 20 mg/day)
- Clobazam (Onfi): 20 to 40 mg in 1 to 2 doses
- Rufinamide (Banzel): 3,200 mg in 2 doses
- Brivaracetam (Briviact) (an analog of levetiracetam): 50 to 200 mg/day in 2 doses
- Caution about increased risk of suicide but risk of untreated seizures is far greater
- Patients are susceptible to sudden unexpected death in epilepsy (SUDEP), possibly due to cardiac arrhythmia.

Pregnancy Considerations
- Pregnancy: Avoid valproate if possible. Monitor AED levels every trimester for dose adjustment, continue folic acid supplementation, and screen for congenital abnormalities.
- Levetiracetam, topiramate, and lamotrigine are alternatives for women of childbearing potential (5).

ISSUES FOR REFERRAL
- Psychological therapies may be used in conjunction with AED therapy. Cognitive-behavioral therapy, relaxation, biofeedback, and yoga may help as adjunctive therapy.
- Neurology referral for first-time seizure patients, unless clearly provoked and initial studies unremarkable

SURGERY/OTHER PROCEDURES
If traditional therapy fails: lobectomy, resection, laser ablation, and vagus nerve stimulation

COMPLEMENTARY & ALTERNATIVE MEDICINE
Complementary supplements may induce drug interactions with prescribed AEDs.

ADMISSION, INPATIENT, AND NURSING CONSIDERATIONS
- Admit for status epilepticus, prolonged postictal state, or serious seizure-related injury.
- Admissions to epilepsy monitoring units for video EEG monitoring may benefit patients with events that pose a diagnostic challenge or patients with intractable seizures already on two AED.

ONGOING CARE

FOLLOW-UP RECOMMENDATIONS
Maintain adequate drug therapy; ensure compliance and/or access to medication. Drug therapy withdrawal and tapering of doses may be done after a seizure-free 2-year period. Expect a 33% relapse rate in the following 3 years.

Patient Monitoring
- Monitor drug levels and seizure frequency.
- CBC and lab values (e.g., calcium, vitamin D) as indicated; BMD
- Monitor for side effects and adverse reactions.
- All patients taking any AED should be monitored closely for notable changes in behavior that could indicate the emergence/worsening of suicidal thoughts/behavior/depression.

DIET
Ketogenic diet may be beneficial in children in conjunction with AED therapy and refractory seizures. Low-sugar and high-fat diet alter the excitability of the brain, causing a decrease in the seizure threshold.

PATIENT EDUCATION
- Seizure precautions: Be aware of common triggers or precipitating factors to avoid.
- Unsupervised activities can be dangerous with a sudden loss of consciousness.
- Emphasize the danger of driving unless seizure free for a certain period. Laws vary by state: https://www.epilepsy.org.

PROGNOSIS
- Depending on the type of seizure disorder: ~70% will become seizure free with treatment. The number of seizures within 6 months after the first presentation is a prognostic factor for remission.
- ~90% with an unprovoked seizure attain a 1- to 2-year remission within 4 or 5 years of the initial event.
- Life expectancy is shortened in persons with epilepsy.
- Case fatality rate for status epilepticus: 20%

COMPLICATIONS
SUDEP

REFERENCES
1. Fisher RS, Acevedo C, Arzimanoglou A, et al. ILAE official report: a practical clinical definition of epilepsy. *Epilepsia*. 2014;55(4):475–482.
2. Lee SK. Epilepsy in the elderly: treatment and consideration of comorbid diseases. *J Epilepsy Res*. 2019;9(1):27–35.
3. Rizvi S, Ladino LD, Hernandez-Ronquillo L, et al. Epidemiology of early stages of epilepsy: risk of seizure recurrence after a first seizure. *Seizure*. 2017;49:46–53.
4. Sathe AG, Tillman H, Coles LD, et al. Underdosing of benzodiazepines in patients with status epilepticus enrolled in established status epilepticus treatment trial. *Acad Emerg Med*. 2019;26(8):940–943.
5. Perucca E, Tomson T. The pharmacological treatment of epilepsy in adults. *Lancet Neurol*. 2011;10(5):446–456.

SEE ALSO

Seizures, Febrile; Status Epilepticus

CODES

ICD10
- G40.B1 Juvenile myoclonic epilepsy, intractable
- G40.804 Other epilepsy, intractable, without status epilepticus
- G40.A0 Absence epileptic syndrome, not intractable

CLINICAL PEARLS
- Treatment depends on the type of seizure, underlying risk factors, and risk of recurrence.
- Semiology of event is very important for diagnosis of seizures versus PNES (these patients can have concomitant epileptic seizures).
- Patients in status epilepticus who receive a loading dose of one AED do not require to be continued on the same medication.
- New-onset seizures can raise suspicion of a presentation or complication of COVID-19 infection or other causative factors.

SEIZURES, FEBRILE

Christina Conrad, DO • Priya Prasher, MBBS

 BASICS

DESCRIPTION

Febrile seizures (FS) occur in children aged 6 months to 6 years with fever ≥100.4°F (38°C) in the absence of an underlying neurologic abnormality, metabolic condition, or intracranial infection. There are three distinct categories (1),(2),(3),(4):

- Simple febrile seizure (SFS) (70–75%; must meet all criteria):
  - Generalized clonic or tonic–clonic seizure activity without focal features
  - Duration <15 minutes
  - Does not recur within 24 hours
  - Resolves spontaneously
  - No history of previous afebrile seizure, seizure disorder, or other neurologic problem
- Complex febrile seizure (CFS) (20–25%; only one criterion must be met):
  - Partial seizure, focal activity
  - Duration >15 minutes but <30 minutes
  - Recurrence within 24 hours
  - Postictal focal neurologic abnormalities (e.g., Todd paralysis)
- Febrile status epilepticus (FSE) (5%):
  - Lasts >30 minutes

EPIDEMIOLOGY

Incidence

- About 500,000 FS in the United States annually
- Occurs in 3–5% of children aged 6 months to 6 years of age; peak incidence is 18 months of age with 90% of children having their first FS before age 3 years. Only 6% of FS occur before age 6 months (4).
- Seasonal pattern that mirrors peaks of febrile respiratory (November to January) and gastrointestinal infections (June to August)

ETIOLOGY AND PATHOPHYSIOLOGY

The pathophysiology of FS remains unclear, but current research suggests the following mechanisms that lower seizure threshold:

- Age-dependent vulnerability of developing nervous system (3)
- Increased neuronal activity (i.e., seizures) secondary to temperature-sensitive ion channels and secretion of cytokines from inflammatory processes such as fever-promoting pyrogen interleukin-1β
- Hyperthermia-induced hyperventilation and alkalosis, which provokes neuronal excitability

Genetics

- FS are more common in children with first-degree relatives who have had FS. Monozygotic twins have a higher concordance rate than dizygotic twins (in whom the rate is similar to other siblings) (2).
- Certain genes that have been identified as risk factors for family epilepsy syndromes may also increase the risk of FS (2).

RISK FACTORS

- Most common risk factors for developing first FS (2),(5):
  - Height of fever, more so than rate of rise
  - Viral infection (80% of FS caused by virus)—human herpesvirus 6 (HHV-6), influenza A, adenovirus, and parainfluenza are commonly associated viruses.
  - Recently immunized, particularly with MMR and DTwP
  - Family history of FS.
    - As many as 25–40% of cases have a positive family history of FS. Risk increases with number of affected first-degree (OR = 4.5%) and second-degree relatives (OR = 3.6%); greater concordance rate in monozygotic than dizygotic twins (2)
- Other general risk factors for FS: nicotine exposure in utero, NICU stay for >28 days, developmental delay, or daycare attendance
- Risk is slightly increased for males (3).
- Recent vaccination
  - Certain vaccines (e.g., MMR, DTwP, PCV13), method of preparation, vaccine coadministration, and associated age of administration have shown to increase risk of FS (4).
  - No evidence of increased risk with isolated influenza vaccination.
- Perhaps increased risk with iron deficiency anemia and low zinc levels (2)

GENERAL PREVENTION

- Choose vaccines with lower risk of developing FS, and ask if the child has ever had a history of FS after vaccine administration (4),(5).
  - Increased risk of FS if vaccine administrations are delayed
  - Separate MMR and varicella vaccine and administer between 12 and 15 months of age.
  - Administer DTaP (acellular) rather than DTwP (whole cell) vaccine.

COMMONLY ASSOCIATED CONDITIONS

- Viral infections are the cause of fever in nearly 80% of FS cases, particularly HHV-6, influenza, parainfluenza, adenovirus, and respiratory syncytial virus (RSV) (4).
- Bacterial infections: otitis media, pharyngitis, urinary tract infection (UTI), pneumonia, and gastroenteritis (specifically with *Shigella*)
- Vaccinations (4)
  - MMRV vaccination had 2-fold increase in risk of FS compared to separation of MMR and varicella vaccine.
  - DTwP vaccine had roughly 15% greater chance of causing FS compared to DTaP (1 per 2,835 vaccines and 1 per 19,496 vaccines, respectively).
  - There is a small increased risk for FS when activated influenza vaccine (flu shot) is given at the same time as either the PCV13 (pneumococcal) or the DTaP vaccine.
    - Also, small increased risk with PCV13 given alone
    - No increased risk if influenza vaccine or DTaP vaccine is given alone

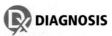 **DIAGNOSIS**

HISTORY

- Symptoms of underlying infection or neurologic deficits
- Onset, duration, type, and number of seizure
  - A SFS is generalized and associated with tonic–clonic movements of the limb and rolling back of the eyes. It may last a few seconds to 15 minutes, although generally <5 minutes, and does not recur within 24 hours.
- Presence of postictal state (such as weakness or paralysis).
  - Postictal drowsiness should resolve within 5 to 10 minutes. Encephalopathy beyond this range raises suspicion of CNS or systemic infection.
- Any interventions made to stop seizure
- Past medical history:
  - Immunization status, recent vaccines
  - Preexisting conditions: developmental delay, cerebral palsy, metabolic disorders, injury
  - Recent antibiotic course
- Family history: FS, afebrile seizures, epilepsy, metabolic disorders, and other neurologic conditions
- Factors concerning for child abuse or trauma

PHYSICAL EXAM

- Monitoring vital signs and close observation of neurologic status/change are essential in all children (2).
  - Unstable vital signs or toxic appearance warrants further evaluation.
  - Look for tachypnea, hypoxemia, lesions in oropharynx, or viral exanthem.
    - Observe for presence of closed eyes and a deep breath to indicate cessation of seizure. Children with persistently open and deviated eyes may still be seizing in absence of convulsive motor activities.
    - Average duration of FSE is 67 minutes.
  - Assess mental status and signs of meningitis—obtunded or comatose mental state, nuchal rigidity, prolonged focal seizure or petechial rash, and multiple seizures.
  - Duration of seizures >30 minutes, presence of postictal drowsiness, and neurologic deficits were predictive factors for meningitis.
- A thorough physical exam should not be deferred until postictal state has resolved. Although exam may be limited, prompt evaluation may reveal focal neurologic deficits or Todd paresis (3)[A].
- Assess for nonaccidental trauma with skin inspection, palpation for occult trauma, and retinal exam.

DIFFERENTIAL DIAGNOSIS

- Seizures due to other etiology: meningitis, encephalitis, primary epilepsy, intracranial mass, trauma, electrolyte abnormality, hypoglycemia, metabolic disorder.
- Seizure mimics: rigors, crying, breath-holding spell, choking episode, tic disorder, parasomnia, dystonic reaction, shaking chills (shivering)

DIAGNOSTIC TESTS & INTERPRETATION
Initial Tests (lab, imaging)
- Routine laboratory tests not routinely recommended if the child is well appearing (5)
  - Blood workup if other symptoms, such as vomiting, diarrhea, and poor fluid intake that points toward another etiology for seizure
  - Urinalysis only if indicated by current UTI rates in children with SFS are comparable to febrile children without seizure
- Lumbar puncture (LP) not necessary in well-appearing children who quickly return to baseline
  - Following situations may warrant LP:
    o Meningeal signs and symptoms (5); infant 6 to 12 months of age without known *Haemophilus influenzae* type b (Hib) or *Streptococcus pneumoniae* immunization (5)
    o Child was treated with antibiotics as it can mask the signs and symptoms of meningitis (5).
- Neuroimaging is not routinely recommended to identify the cause of an FS (3)[A],(5).
  - Studies demonstrate limited use of emergent imaging in most patients with FS; no advantage of MRI versus CT for management of FS in ED
  - Warranted if strong indication of acute/subacute bleeding or structural lesion
  - Nonurgent, outpatient MRI brain is recommended for patients with focal CFS especially with postictal neurologic deficits
    o No evidence to support routine use of neuroimaging in absence of interictal or postictal focality
- Check for anemia if iron deficiency is suspected.

Follow-Up Tests & Special Considerations
If there is a need to perform both EEG and MRI for a child presenting with FS, do EEG first. MRI in children will most often require complete sedation, which may alter the results of an EEG.

 ## TREATMENT

Most FS are self-limited; however, if health care professionals are able to witness the FS, acute abortive treatment should be no different than any other seizure treatment. FSE rarely stops spontaneously and often requires more than one medication to control. Early intervention with AEDs is important for duration of FSE and outcome (3)[A].

GENERAL MEASURES
During an acute seizure management, continue to monitor patient's ABCs (2):
- Airway: Position the patient laterally, suction secretions, and place a nasopharyngeal airway.
- Breathing: Administer oxygen for cyanosis; consider bag-mask ventilation or intubation for inadequate ventilation.
- Circulation: Establish IV access for any medication and fluid bolus.

MEDICATION
First Line
- Treat seizures of ≥5 minutes duration with anticonvulsants. If seizures continue 5 minutes after administration of medication, can repeat dose (3):
  - Out of hospital (e.g., home or paramedics on route): rectal diazepam 0.5 mg/kg, buccal midazolam (0.2 to 0.4 mg/kg), or nasal midazolam (0.2 mg/kg).
  - In hospital: IV or IM lorazepam 0.05 to 0.1 mg/kg or IV diazepam 0.1 to 0.2 mg/kg; "out of hospital" options can also be used if IV option is not available.
- If seizures are prolonged or recurrent, administer IV fosphenytoin (20 mg PE/kg); if seizures persist after 10 minutes of loading dose, can give additional dose (5 to 10 mg phenytoin equivalent/kg) (3)
  - There is some evidence that fosphenytoin should be avoided due to risk of worsening seizures in patients with SCN1A mutations (3).
- Antipyretics should be used to reduce fever as it often helps with overall comfort level of patients (2).
  - In one study, rectal acetaminophen (10 mg/kg, q6h for 24 hours) showed potential to prevent FS recurrence during same fever episode (2).
  - Prophylactic antipyretics before vaccination is not recommended as it is not effective and could decrease immune response to certain vaccines.

Second Line
IV phenobarbital (15 to 20 mg/kg), valproic acid (20 to 40 mg/kg), or levetiracetam (20 to 60 mg/kg)

ISSUES FOR REFERRAL
Neurology consultation if persistent neurologic deficits, recurrent FS, or abnormal exam on evaluation (3)

ADMISSION, INPATIENT, AND NURSING CONSIDERATIONS
Abnormal or concerning findings on history or physical exam or prolonged/delayed recovery

 ## ONGOING CARE

FOLLOW-UP RECOMMENDATIONS
Anticonvulsant prophylaxis during subsequent febrile episodes is not recommended as adverse effects of anticonvulsants outweigh benefits (1)[A],(5).

PATIENT EDUCATION
Guidance for parents should focus on reassurance, emphasizing the benign nature of FS, overall excellent prognosis of the disease, and basic guidelines on interventions if FS were to reoccur (2).
- FS often do not cause brain damage, have a low risk for sequelae, and do not have a negative impact on intellect, behavior, or risk of death (6).
- The benefits of vaccinations greatly outweigh the side effects. The vaccine-induced FS risk is more affected by personal and family history rather than the sole act of receiving the vaccination (4).

PROGNOSIS
Favorable for children with normal neurodevelopmental status (6).
- A second FS occurs in about 1/3 of the patients; a third FS in 15% of patients.
- Risk factors for recurrent FS (1)[A],(2),(3):
  - Age of onset: younger the age, higher the risk
  - Relatively low temp (<104°F) at time of first FS
  - Shorter interval (<1 hour) between onset of fever and seizure
  - First-degree relative with history of FS or epilepsy
  - First FS has CFS features, particularly focal or prolonged CFS (continued topic of debate)
- Risk of FS developing into epilepsy (1),(2):
  - Age >3 years at time of first FS
  - Developmental delay or abnormal neurologic exam prior to onset of first FS
  - CFS
  - Family history of epilepsy
  - Fever duration of 1 hour before seizure onset
- An unprovoked, afebrile seizure (epilepsy) after FS is estimated to be 1% for SFS and 4–6% for CFS.

REFERENCES
1. Steering Committee on Quality Improvement and Management, Subcommittee on Febrile Seizures American Academy of Pediatrics. Febrile seizures: clinical practice guideline for the long-term management of the child with simple febrile seizures. *Pediatrics*. 2008;121(6):1281–1286.
2. Smith DK, Sadler KP, Benedum M. Febrile seizures: risks, evaluation, and prognosis. *Am Fam Physician*. 2019;99(7):445–450.
3. Whelan H, Harmelink M, Chou E, et al. Complex febrile seizures—a systematic review. *Dis Mon*. 2017;63(1):5–23.
4. Deng L, Gidding H, Macartney K, et al. Postvaccination febrile seizure severity and outcome. *Pediatrics*. 2019;143(5):e20182120.
5. Subcommittee on Febrile Seizures, American Academy of Pediatrics. Neurodiagnostic evaluation of the child with a simple febrile seizure. *Pediatrics*. 2011;127(2):389–394.
6. Mewasingh LD, Chin RFM, Scott RC. Current understanding of febrile seizures and their long-term outcomes. *Dev Med Child Neurol*. 2020;62(11):1245–1249.

 ## CODES

ICD10
- R56.00 Simple febrile convulsions
- R56.01 Complex febrile convulsions
- G40.901 Epilepsy, unsp, not intractable, with status epilepticus

CLINICAL PEARLS
- FS are generally benign and without sequelae if the underlying causes are ruled out.
- Labs, LP, neuroimaging, and EEG not routinely recommended in an acute setting in the absence of suspicion for underlying pathology.
- Prophylaxis with anticonvulsants or antipyretics during subsequent febrile episodes is not recommended.

SEROTONIN SYNDROME

Michael T. Partin, MD • Karl T. Clebak, MD, MHA, FAAFP • Munima Nasir, MD

BASICS

DESCRIPTION

- A potentially life-threatening drug-induced syndrome that results from synaptic increase in serotonin (5-hydroxytryptamine [5-HT]) concentrations and stimulation of peripheral and CNS serotonergic receptors
- Classic triad of symptoms that include mental status changes, neuromuscular hyperactivity, and autonomic instability
- Onset is usually within 24 hours with the majority occurring within 6 hours of exposure to, or change in, dosing of a serotonergic agent; rarely, reported weeks after discontinuation of serotonergic agents
- It is a concentration-dependent toxicity that can develop in any individual who has ingested drug combinations that synergistically increase synaptic 5-HT.
- Serotonin toxicity occurs in three main settings: (i) therapeutic drug use, which often results in mild to moderate symptoms; (ii) intentional overdose of a single serotonergic agent, which typically leads to moderate symptoms; and (iii) as the result of a drug interaction between numerous serotonergic agents (most commonly, selective serotonin reuptake inhibitors [SSRIs], serotonin noradrenergic reuptake inhibitors [SNRIs], and monoamine oxidase inhibitors [MAOIs]), most often associated with severe serotonin toxicity.

Geriatric Considerations
Increased risk through polypharmacy given frequent use of serotonergic analgesics, antibiotics, and antidepressants

Pediatric Considerations
- Similar manifestations and management in children and adults
- Consider toxic ingestion of serotonergic agents prescribed to caregivers of pediatric patients.
- Symptoms in neonates may include tremors, increased muscle tone, jitteriness, shivering, feeding/digestive disturbances, irritability, agitation, sleep disturbances, increased reflexes, excessive crying, and respiratory disturbances.

Pregnancy Considerations
Serotonin levels are increased from baseline during an uncomplicated pregnancy with preeclamptic patients demonstrating a 10-fold increase in serotonin levels.

EPIDEMIOLOGY
Seen in approximately 14–16% of SSRI overdose patients

Incidence
In a 2008 study, SSRIs were responsible for adverse events in 18.8% of cases, with 55.7% due to intentional causes, 39.5% unintentional, and remainder of causes unknown. 46.6% had symptoms requiring hospitalization, and significant toxic effects occurred in 90 patients with two resultant deaths (1).

ETIOLOGY AND PATHOPHYSIOLOGY
- Increased synaptic 5-HT or agonist concentration as a result of one or more of the following mechanisms: (i) decreased 5-HT breakdown (e.g., MAOI), (ii) decreased 5-HT reuptake (e.g., SSRI), (iii) increased 5-HT agonists (e.g., tryptophan), (iv) increased 5-HT release (e.g., amphetamines), and (v) CYP2D6 and CYP3A4 inhibitors (e.g., erythromycin)

- Risk is mediated in a dose-related manner to the action of 5-HT/5-HT agonists on 5-HT$_{1A}$ and/or 5-HT$_{2A}$ receptors.
- A number of drugs are associated with serotonin syndrome, which usually involves combination with an SSRI. These include SSRIs (e.g., citalopram, escitalopram, fluoxetine, fluvoxamine, paroxetine, sertraline); MAOIs; SNRIs (duloxetine, venlafaxine, desvenlafaxine); tricyclic antidepressants (e.g., amitriptyline, clomipramine); other antidepressants (nefazodone, trazodone, mirtazapine); anxiolytic (buspirone); lithium; triptans; anticonvulsants (divalproex [Depakote]); analgesics (fentanyl, meperidine, pentazocine, tramadol); antibiotics/antivirals (linezolid, tedizolid [weak MAOI], ritonavir); over-the-counter (OTC) cough medications (dextromethorphan); some antipsychotics (risperidone, olanzapine); antiemetics (ondansetron, granisetron); other medications, such as metoclopramide, cyclobenzaprine, L-dopa; dietary supplements (tryptophan); herbal supplements (St. John wort, nutmeg); methylene blue; and drugs of abuse (e.g., methylenedioxymethamphetamine [MDMA], cocaine, D-lysergic acid diethylamide [LSD], amphetamine) (2)[A]

RISK FACTORS
- Recent dose adjustments or overdose of drugs associated with serotonin syndrome
- The greatest number of adverse events are associated with SSRIs in combination with other substances, and the combination of SSRIs and MAOIs carries the greatest risk of developing serotonin toxicity.

GENERAL PREVENTION
- Consider drug–drug interactions when a multidrug regimen is required and avoid if possible.
- Caution patients about taking SSRIs with OTC medications (e.g., dextromethorphan) or herbal supplements (e.g., St. John wort) prior to consulting a physician.
- Avoid serotonergic agents for nonpsychiatric disorders (e.g., tramadol for pain relief).

DIAGNOSIS

- Serotonin syndrome is a clinical diagnosis.
- *Hunter Toxicity Criteria Decision Rules* (3) aid in the diagnosis of clinically significant serotonin toxicity (sensitivity, 84%; specificity, 97%). A patient who took a serotonergic agent must have one of the following:
  - Spontaneous clonus
  - Inducible clonus with agitation or diaphoresis
  - Ocular clonus with agitation or diaphoresis
  - Hypertonia and hyperthermia (temperature >38°C) with inducible clonus or ocular clonus (3)[A]
  - Tremor and hyperreflexia

HISTORY
- Obtain a thorough drug history including OTC remedies, dietary and herbal supplements, and illicit drugs. Ask about dose, formulation, and recent changes.
- Review comorbidities (e.g., depression, chronic pain).
- Address possibility of drug overdose and obtain collateral information if intentional overdose is suspected.
- Elicit description of symptoms, including onset and progression.

PHYSICAL EXAM
Initially, patients can develop a peripheral tremor, confusion, and ataxia; systemic signs follow (e.g., agitation, diaphoresis, hyperreflexia, shivering). Severe signs include fever, jerking, and diarrhea.
- Neuromuscular abnormalities:
  - Mild: hyperreflexia, myoclonus, and tremor all greater in lower extremities; bilateral Babinski sign
  - Moderate: opsoclonus, spontaneous, or inducible clonus (involuntary muscle contractions, most commonly tested by rapid dorsiflexion of foot)
  - Severe: rigidity, respiratory failure, tonic–clonic seizure
- Autonomic dysfunction:
  - Mild: diaphoresis, mydriasis, tachycardia
  - Moderate: hyperactive bowel sounds, diarrhea, nausea, vomiting, hyperthermia (<40°C)
  - Severe: hyperthermia (≥40°C), labile blood pressure (BP)
- Mental status changes:
  - Mild: anxiety, akathisia (restlessness), insomnia
  - Moderate: agitation
  - Severe: coma, delirium, confusion (4)[B]
- Severe cases have led to altered level of consciousness, rhabdomyolysis, metabolic acidosis, disseminated intravascular coagulation (DIC), and acute respiratory distress syndrome (ARDS) (3)[A].

DIFFERENTIAL DIAGNOSIS
- Neuroleptic malignant syndrome (NMS): lead pipe rigidity and extrapyramidal features without clonus or hyperreflexia
- Anticholinergic fever (e.g., benztropine, diphenhydramine, oxybutynin, nifedipine, famotidine, atropine, scopolamine; plant poisoning from belladonna/"deadly nightshade"): urinary retention, decreased bowel sounds, normal reflexes
- Malignant hyperthermia: generally following administration of anesthetics or depolarizing muscle relaxants
- CNS infection (e.g., meningitis, encephalitis) and heat stroke
- Sympathomimetic toxicity (e.g., cocaine, methamphetamine, PCP)
- Hyperthyroidism (thyroid storm)
- Tetanus and rabies

DIAGNOSTIC TESTS & INTERPRETATION
- Serum serotonin levels do not correlate with clinical findings.
- Nonspecific lab findings may include:
  - Elevated WBC, creatine phosphokinase, hepatic transaminases
  - Decreased serum bicarbonate
- Consider urine toxicology screening for illicit drugs.

TREATMENT

Supportive care is the mainstay of therapy: administrating oxygen and aggressive IV fluids, continuous cardiac monitoring, monitoring urine output, and stabilizing vital signs.
- Benzodiazepines may be effective for the management of agitation.
- Administration of serotonin antagonists: Cyproheptadine may be useful if supportive measures and sedation (benzodiazepines) are unable to control agitation and correct vital signs. This agent does not reduce the duration of serotonin syndrome.

- Mild cases (afebrile, tachycardia, shivering, diaphoresis, mydriasis, hyperreflexia, intermittent tremor, or myoclonus)
  - Discontinue precipitating agent(s).
  - Supportive care and sedation
  - Observe for 12 to 24 hours.
- Moderate cases (temperature >38°C, autonomic instability, hyperactive bowel sounds, diarrhea, diaphoresis, ocular clonus, hyperreflexia, tremor, mild agitation, or hypervigilance)
  - Interventions as listed earlier for mild cases
  - Aggressive treatment of autonomic instability
  - Treatment with cyproheptadine should be initiated if agitation and vital sign abnormalities are unimproved with benzodiazepines and supportive care.
  - Hypotension from MAOI interactions should be treated with low doses of direct-acting sympathomimetics (e.g., norepinephrine, phenylephrine, epinephrine); indirect serotonin agonists, such as dopamine, should be avoided.
  - Severe hypertension and tachycardia should be treated with short-acting agents, such as nitroprusside or esmolol.
- Severe cases (temperature >41.1°C, autonomic instability, delirium, muscular rigidity, and hypertonicity)
  - Discontinue precipitating agent(s).
  - Immediate sedation and endotracheal intubation as indicated
  - Paralysis as clinically indicated (maintained with nondepolarizing continuous paralytic agents such as vecuronium, cisatracurium, rocuronium)
  - Succinylcholine should not be used in cases of rhabdomyolysis to avoid exacerbation of hyperkalemia (5)[A].
  - Antipyretic medications are not effective (4)[A]; the increased body temperature is due to muscle activity, not an alteration in the hypothalamic set point.
  - Avoid physical restraints because it can worsen hyperthermia and lactic acidosis in agitated patients (5)[A].

MEDICATION
- Benzodiazepines may be used to manage agitation in serotonin syndrome and also may correct mild increases in BP and heart rate. Use with caution in patients with delirium, given the known paradoxical effect of exacerbating delirium.

- Cyproheptadine (Periactin):
  - Adult: initial dose of 12 mg PO (can also be crushed and given via nasogastric [NG] tube) followed by 2 mg q2h until clinical response is observed; 12 to 32 mg of drug may be required in a 24-hour period.
  - Pediatric:
    ○ Age <2 years: 0.06 mg/kg q6h
    ○ Ages 2 to 6 years: 2 mg q6h
    ○ Ages 7 to 14 years: 4 mg q6h
- Use of antipsychotics with 5-HT$_{2A}$ antagonist activity, such as olanzapine and chlorpromazine, is not recommended (4)[B].

ISSUES FOR REFERRAL
- Psychiatry: for assistance with medication management and follow-up care (inpatient psychiatric care vs. outpatient psychiatric follow-up)
- Toxicology/clinical pharmacology service
- Poison control center

ADMISSION, INPATIENT, AND NURSING CONSIDERATIONS
- ICU admission is often indicated in severe cases.
- Discharge when mental status has returned to baseline, with stable vital and neurologic (e.g., clonus) signs. Ensure close follow-up.

ONGOING CARE

FOLLOW-UP RECOMMENDATIONS
- In mild cases, address risks and benefits of restarting offending agents. Serotonergic medications need to be titrated slowly, and patients must have close outpatient follow-up.
- In severe cases, the offending agent should likely not be resumed unless precipitant for serotonin syndrome is found (e.g., combination with another serotonin agonist); the patient can be carefully monitored, or there is a clear benefit versus risk of restarting the medication.

PROGNOSIS
Most cases resolve within 24 hours of discontinuation of serotonergic agents; this can be longer depending on the drug's half-life:
- MAOIs can result in toxicity for several days.
- SSRIs can result in toxicity for up to several weeks after discontinuation.

COMPLICATIONS
Adverse outcomes, including death, are usually the consequence of poorly treated hyperthermia and may include acute renal failure, ARDS, arrhythmia, coma, DIC, seizure, metabolic acidosis, multiorgan failure, myoglobinuria, respiratory arrest, and rhabdomyolysis.

REFERENCES
1. Bronstein AC, Spyker DA, Cantilena LR Jr, et al. 2008 Annual report of the American Association of Poison Control Centers' National Poison Data System (NPDS): 26th annual report. *Clin Toxicol (Phila)*. 2009;47(10):911–1084.
2. Moss MJ, Hendrickson RG; for Toxicology Investigators Consortium (ToxIC). Serotonin toxicity: associated agents and clinical characteristics. *J Clin Psychopharmacol*. 2019;39(6):628–633.
3. Dunkley EJC, Isbister GK, Sibbritt D, et al. The Hunter Serotonin Toxicity Criteria: simple and accurate diagnostic decision rules for serotonin toxicity. *QJM*. 2003;96(9):635–642.
4. Buckley NA, Dawson AH, Isbister GK. Serotonin syndrome. *BMJ*. 2014;348:g1626.
5. Heitmiller DR. Serotonin syndrome: a concise review of a toxic state. *R I Med J (2013)*. 2014;97(6):33–35.

ADDITIONAL READING
Mas Serrano M, Pérez-Sánchez JR, Portela Sánchez S, et al. Serotonin syndrome in two COVID-19 patients treated with lopinavir/ritonavir. *J Neurol Sci*. 2020;415:116944.

 ## CODES

ICD10
G25.79 Other drug induced movement disorders

CLINICAL PEARLS

Consider serotonin syndrome in patients with recent use of a serotonergic agent (particularly if multiple proserotonergic agents are involved) presenting with unexplained tachycardia, hypertension, hyperthermia, clonus, hyperreflexia, and change in mental status.

SEXUAL DYSFUNCTION IN WOMEN

Rachel Kristina Moyer, MD • Emily A. Yocom, DO • Shelby Takeshita, MD

BASICS

- Female sexual dysfunction (FSD) is a common multidisciplinary concern faced by ~43% of women in the United States.
- The evaluation should include exploration across biomedical, sexual, and psychosocial etiologies.

DESCRIPTION

- According to the *DSM-5*, FSD is defined as sexual concerns arising from desire, arousal, orgasm, or sexual pain (1).
  - For diagnosis, symptoms must be present for >6 months, be present >75% of the time, and cause distress.
- The focus of this discussion will be on individuals assigned female at birth, with the understanding that sexual dysfunction can occur across all genders with similar and unique challenges as those described below.
- FSD may arise from a variety of conditions discussed in depth below.

EPIDEMIOLOGY

According to ACOG, 43% of women disclose sexual function concerns, and about 12% of women feel that it causes personal distress.

Incidence

- Sexual dysfunction can occur at any age, but rates vary by age.
- FSD can be lifelong, acquired, generalized, or situational depending on the underlying cause.
- 74% incidence in women with gynecologic cancers
- 83% of women experience problems in first 3 months after childbirth (1).

Prevalence

- Sexual dysfunction prevalence varies by age, with the highest prevalence in women aged 45 to 65 years (15%)
- Prevalence in women aged 18 to 44 years is 10%, whereas prevalence in women aged 65 to 85 years is 9% (2).

ETIOLOGY AND PATHOPHYSIOLOGY

The female sexual response follows a circular model requiring motivation, arousal (physical and subjective), willingness, and neural inputs (2). Thus, pathophysiology of sexual dysfunction is complex and multifactorial, with underlying cause varying between patients. These may include the following:

- Changes in sex hormones: Sex hormones are important in creating a neurochemical sexual response in the central nervous system as well as at the urogenital level, leading to changes in lubrication, clitoral engorgement, neurovasculature to the pelvis, and pelvic floor function.
- Central nervous system: Neuroendocrine circuits impact the emotional and behavioral aspects of sexual function including arousal, orgasm, and desire (3).
- Comorbid illness: Comorbidities such as diabetes, cardiovascular disease, malignancy, or neurologic disease can impact the above processes and alter an individual's view of themselves.

- Psychological: mood disorders, stress, alcohol/substance use
- Individual factors: sleep, relationship concerns, body image, trauma, societal attitudes toward sexuality

Genetics

Sexual dysfunction in women is a multifactorial issue, often including a combination of biologic and psychosocial causes.

RISK FACTORS

- Menopause: changing body image, genitourinary syndrome of menopause
- Lack of knowledge about sexual stimulation and response
- Psychological: mood disorders, personality disorders, or psychopathies
- Chronic medical problems: cardiovascular disease; endocrine, dermatologic, and neurologic disorders; malignancy
- Gynecologic issues: childbirth, pelvic floor or bladder dysfunction, endometriosis, uterine fibroids, chronic vulvovaginal candidiasis/vaginal infections, female genital mutilation, breastfeeding
- Relationship factors: safety, intimate partner violence, discrepancies in partners' expectations, cultural attitudes toward sexuality, sexual trauma
- Medications or substance abuse

GENERAL PREVENTION

Ways to help evaluate for, support, and assist in prevention are to:

- Practice trauma informed care in clinic.
- Perform sexual dysfunction screening in annual wellness visits.
- Assess patient safety at every visit (2)[C].

COMMONLY ASSOCIATED CONDITIONS

History of sexual trauma, marital/relationship discord, psychiatric disorders, malignancy, menopause, pregnancy/childbirth, abnormal uterine bleeding, pelvic pain, incontinence, pelvic organ prolapse

DIAGNOSIS

- Take a thorough sexual history and perform trauma-informed genitourinary exam based on areas of concern from history.
- Diagnosis will require assessment of the above multifactorial etiologies for FSD to determine cause/management.
- Screening tools: Female Sexual Function Index, Female Sexual Distress Scale

HISTORY

- Thorough sexual history including questions on safety, pain, sexuality, sexual partners, lubrication, arousal, libido, and orgasm
- Obtain current medical, obstetric, and psychiatric history.
- Evaluate current medication list.
- Discuss current life stressors and social circumstances.

PHYSICAL EXAM

- Follow trauma-informed principles during physical exam, allowing patient to guide speed and content of exam.
- Examine vulva visually for rashes/lesions, and evaluate for pain with cotton swab on vestibule.
- Perform speculum exam to evaluate for lesions, prolapse, or cervical abnormalities.
- Perform bimanual exam, with focus on tense or painful pelvic floor muscles, cervical motion tenderness, or pelvic masses.
- During exam, pay attention to vascular and neurologic findings.

DIFFERENTIAL DIAGNOSIS

- Pelvic floor and uterine disorders: fibroids, endometriosis, sexually transmitted infection (STI), cancer, pregnancy, urinary incontinence, vaginismus, female orgasmic disorder, genito-pelvic pain disorder
- Vulvar disorders: genitourinary syndrome of menopause, lichen sclerosis, genital mutilation
- Hormonal concerns: menopause, pregnancy, breastfeeding
- Psychosocial concerns: stressors, mental health disorders, prior abuse, body image, societal stereotypes
- Cardiovascular history: hypertension, heart failure, vascular disease
- Neurologic disorders: stroke, multiple sclerosis, spinal cord injury
- Gastrointestinal disorders: irritable bowel disease, liver failure
- Endocrine disorders: diabetes, adrenal insufficiency, thyroid disease
- Iatrogenic: selective serotonin reuptake inhibitors (SSRIs), chemotherapy, surgical menopause, steroids

DIAGNOSTIC TESTS & INTERPRETATION

Labs and imaging can assist in identifying causes for FSD.

Initial Tests (lab, imaging)

- Laboratory testing is typically not necessary in initial evaluation unless undiagnosed medical etiology is suspected (2)[C]
- Labs to consider based on unique patient history: FSH, estradiol, free androgen index and sex hormone binding globulin, thyroid function, prolactin, ferritin, lipid panel, HbA1c, STI screening (2)
- Can consider pelvic or abdominal imaging if concern for structural issue

Follow-Up Tests & Special Considerations

As there is no standard workup for FSD, testing must be individualized to the symptoms described.

Test Interpretation

Tests should be interpreted in the clinical context of the individual patient and their symptoms.

TREATMENT

Treatment should be multifactorial in nature and tailored to the patient. It is important to address underlying medical/psychiatric conditions, and use a mixture of the medical and lifestyle therapies discussed below.

GENERAL MEASURES
- Identify if patient has underlying medical conditions influencing sexual function or if they are taking medications such as SSRIs which may impact function.
- Provide education on vulvovaginal care and on use of lubricants that are similar to vaginal pH and osmolarity (2)[C].
- Educate patient on relationship safety and communication.
- Lifestyle education surrounding sleep, nutrition, decreased alcohol/substance use, and smoking cessation

MEDICATION
- Hormonal medications:
  - Low dose vaginal estrogen: assists in postmenopausal dryness and pain by improving lubrication and vaginal pH
    ○ Preferred hormonal treatment for FSD due to genitourinary syndrome of menopause (2)[C]
  - Transdermal testosterone: can assist with libido, and short-term use can be considered for postmenopausal women with sexual interest or arousal disorders; stop if the patient has no response after 3 to 6 months of trial (2)[C]; insufficient evidence for use in premenopausal women
- Tibolone: synthetic steroid uses for menopausal symptoms; however, can have increased risk of stroke
- Ospemifene: selective estrogen receptor modulator (SERM) approved for postmenopausal dryness and pain; can be considered in individuals who are not responsive to vaginal estrogen (2)[C].
- Estrogen or SERM therapy is not recommended for treatment of FSD that is not due to hypoestrogenic state (2)[C].
- Vascular and muscular medications:
  - Tizanide: muscle relaxant being researched for high-tone pelvic floor
  - PDE5 inhibitors (sildenafil): possible vasodilatory effect, although there is a poor evidence for efficacy in women and this is currently not recommended outside clinical trials (2)[C]
- Central nervous system medications:
  - Bupropion: adjunct for SSRI-induced sexual dysfunction
  - Flibanserin: Serotonin agonist is approved for hypoactive desire disorder in premenopausal women without depression (2)[C]. Patients should be counseled that they cannot drink alcohol while on this therapy.

First Line
- First-line therapy should include lifestyle counseling and nonpharmacologic interventions.
- For postmenopausal dysfunction, vaginal estrogen is included in first-line therapies unless contraindicated.

Second Line
Second line therapy will vary based on the underlying cause of FSD

ISSUES FOR REFERRAL
Referrals are warranted for underlying muscular, structural, social, or psychological basis of pain.

ADDITIONAL THERAPIES
Nonpharmacologic therapies play a large role in managing FSD, including:
- Pelvic floor physical therapy: helps patients with self-awareness, strength, control, and confidence while decreasing vaginismus and improving libido (2)[C]
- Vaginal dilators: helpful with vaginismus or vaginal stenosis; initiating treatment with a small dilator under supervision of a specialist or in combination with other therapies is the most beneficial.
- Psychotherapy: cognitive behavioral therapy, psychosexual counseling, couples therapy, mindfulness-based therapy (2)[C]

SURGERY/OTHER PROCEDURES
Surgical interventions such as laser therapy and trigger point injections are under investigation and are currently not recommended outside clinical trials (2)[C].

COMPLEMENTARY & ALTERNATIVE MEDICINE
- Self-stimulation devices
- Yoga
- Relaxation techniques or mindfulness-based practices
- Hypnotherapy

ADMISSION, INPATIENT, AND NURSING CONSIDERATIONS
Indications depend on individual's underlying cause of dysfunction.

ONGOING CARE

Multiple visits may be necessary due to issues identified which require further exploration and to help destigmatize discussion of sexual function (2)[C]

FOLLOW-UP RECOMMENDATIONS
As needed for continued lifestyle and medication-based interventions

Patient Monitoring
Follow up with patients as needed for symptom level and for underlying comorbid conditions

DIET
Encourage patient to consume healthy diet and maintain ideal body weight.

PATIENT EDUCATION
- American Association of Sexuality Educators, Counselors, and Therapists: https://www.aasect.org/
- HealthyWomen: https://www.healthywomen.org/
- Meet Rosy: https://meetrosy.com/; online platform and app for sexual wellness
- International Society for the Study of Women's Sexual Health: https://www.isswsh.org/

PROGNOSIS
Prognosis depends on the underlying cause for FSD. Certain therapies such as pelvic floor PT have been proven to improve function in 39% of women after 6 months of therapy.

COMPLICATIONS
If untreated, FSD can lead to decreased quality of life, relationship conflict, and mood-based symptoms.

REFERENCES
1. Kershaw V, Jha S. Female sexual dysfunction. *Obstet Gynecol*. 2022;24(1):12–23.
2. American College of Obstetricians and Gynecologists. Female sexual dysfunction: ACOG Practice Bulletin Summary, Number 213. *Obstet Gynecol*. 2019;134(1):203–205.
3. Nappi RE, Tiranini L, Martini E, et al. Medical treatment of female sexual dysfunction. *Urol Clin North Am*. 2022;49(2):299–307.

CODES

ICD10
- R37 Sexual dysfunction, unspecified
- F52.0 Hypoactive sexual desire disorder
- N94.1 Dyspareunia

CLINICAL PEARLS
- FSD is a common, complex, multifactorial problem.
- The causes of FSD can be identified with thorough history and physical exam.
- Symptoms of sexual dysfunction peak in women aged 45 to 64 years.
- Combination of behavioral, physical, and medical therapy leads to greater treatment success.

S

SHOULDER PAIN

Lee A. Mancini, MD, CSCS*D, CSN • Nicholas R. Martin, MD • Michael J. Maddaleni, MD

BASICS

DESCRIPTION
- Shoulder pain commonly affects patients of all ages.
- Causes include acute trauma, overuse during sports, infection, and activities of everyday living.
- Age plays an important role in determining the etiology of shoulder pain.
- Onset and characteristics of pain, mechanism of injury, and limitation in activity or sport narrow the differential diagnosis.

EPIDEMIOLOGY
- Shoulder pain accounts for 16% of all musculoskeletal (MSK) complaints.
- The lifetime prevalence of shoulder pain is ~70%.
- Predominant etiology varies with age:
  - <30 years old: shoulder instability, overuse injuries
  - 30 to 60 years old: rotator cuff (RTC) disorder, impingement syndrome, partial tears
  - >60 years old: full-thickness tear, glenohumeral OA

Incidence
The incidence of shoulder pain is 7 to 25 cases per 1,000 patients, with a peak incidence in the 4th to 6th decades of life.

ETIOLOGY AND PATHOPHYSIOLOGY
Pathology varies with cause:
- Trauma—fracture, dislocation, ligament/tendon tear, acromioclavicular (AC) separation
- Overuse—RTC pathology, biceps tenosynovitis, bursitis, muscle strain, apophyseal injuries, labral injuries
- RTC disorders most commonly result from repetitive overhead activity, leading to RTC impingement with a three-stage progression:
  - Stage I: tendinopathy
  - Stage II: partial RTC tear
  - Stage III: full-thickness RTC tear
- Subacromial bursitis can occur with RTC disorders but is rarely an isolated diagnosis.
- Age related: In pediatric athletes, instability and physeal injuries are more common. With increasing age, the incidence of AC and glenohumeral joint OA, adhesive capsulitis, and RTC tear rises.
- Rheumatologic: rheumatoid arthritis, polymyalgia rheumatica, fibromyalgia
- Infectious: septic arthritis
- Referred pain: neck, gallbladder, diaphragm

RISK FACTORS
- Repetitive overhead activity
- Overhead and upper extremity weight-bearing sports (baseball, softball, swimming, tennis, volleyball)
- Weight lifting: AC joint disorders
- Rapid increases in training frequency or load (often associated with improper technique)
- Muscle weakness or imbalance
- Trauma or fall onto the shoulder
- Diabetes, thyroid disorders and other autoimmune diseases, female gender, and ages 40 to 60 years are the risk factors for adhesive capsulitis.

GENERAL PREVENTION
- Maintain strength and range of motion (ROM).
- Avoid repetitive overhead activities such as pitch counts in younger baseball athletes.
- Proper technique (pitching, weight lifting)

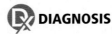

DIAGNOSIS

HISTORY
- Pain characteristics location:
  - Superior: AC pathology, trapezius strain
  - Lateral: RTC pathology, deltoid pathology
  - Anterior: proximal biceps tendinosis, labrum pathology
  - Diffuse pain: RTC pathology, adhesive capsulitis, glenohumeral OA
- Descriptors:
  - Night pain, worse lying on affected side: RTC pathology, adhesive capsulitis, glenohumeral OA
  - Stiff shoulder, limited ROM: adhesive capsulitis, glenohumeral OA
- Aggravating movements:
  - Cross-body adduction, "scarf test": AC pathology
  - Abduction/external rotation (reaching behind): instability, RTC pathology, glenohumeral OA
  - Overhead activity: RTC pathology, AC pathology, labrum pathology, glenohumeral OA
  - Turning neck, pain past elbow: cervical pathology
- Mechanism of injury
  - Forceful abduction and external rotation: traumatic shoulder instability/dislocation
  - Fall directly onto lateral shoulder: AC joint sprain or separation, clavicular fracture
  - Repetitive overhead activity: RTC pathology
  - Fall on outstretched hand (FOOSH): shoulder separation; forearm/wrist fracture
- Age
  - Shoulder instability (subluxation, dislocation, multidirectional instability) is the most common cause of shoulder pain in young athletes (<30 years old).
  - RTC disorders are the most common cause of shoulder pain in patients >30 years old. Severity of RTC disorder increases with age.
  - Older patients (>60 years old) commonly have OA.
  - Trauma in a young person aged <40 years is more commonly associated with dislocation/subluxation. In patients aged >40 years, trauma is more commonly associated with RTC tear.

PHYSICAL EXAM
- Three main joints combine to create the shoulder: glenohumeral, AC, sternoclavicular.
- Four RTC muscles/tendons (SITS): supraspinatus (abduction), infraspinatus (external rotation), teres minor (external rotation, adduction), and subscapularis (adduction, internal rotation)
- Observe face and shoulder movements as patient disrobes, moves arm, and shakes hand.
- Inspect for malalignment, muscle atrophy, asymmetry, erythema, ecchymosis, and swelling. Scapular winging suggests long thoracic nerve or muscular (trapezius, serratus anterior) dysfunction. Prominent scapular spine with scalloped infraspinatus fossa suggests infraspinatus atrophy.

- Palpate SC joint, AC joint, acromion, biceps tendon for tenderness, warmth, or bony step-offs.
- Evaluate active *and* passive ROM and flexibility.
- Decreased active *and* passive ROM is more common with adhesive capsulitis. Normal abduction is to 180 degrees.
- Pain from 60 to 180 degrees suggests subacromial impingement; 120 to 180 degrees suggests AC joint pathology (1).
- Mildly decreased active and/or passive ROM may also indicate glenohumeral OA.
- Decreased active ROM with full passive ROM: RTC pathology
- Evaluate for muscle strength, including grip, biceps, triceps, and deltoid.
- Test RTC strength: supraspinatus (empty can test), infraspinatus/teres minor (resisted external rotation, external lag test), subscapularis (lift-off test, belly press, resisted internal rotation).
- Pain with RTC strength testing indicates RTC pathology. Weakness could suggest tear.
- Special diagnostic tests
  - Neer RTC impingement test: Examiner stabilizes the scapula and internally rotates the patient's arm and flexes the shoulder through the full ROM or until the patient reports pain.
  - Hawkins RTC impingement test: Examiner internally rotates the shoulder with the elbow, and shoulder is flexed to 90 degrees to the end of ROM or until the patient reports pain.
  - Drop-arm test for RTC tear: positive if patient is unable to smoothly control the lowering of their arm or to hold the arm in 90 degrees of abduction
  - Cross-arm adduction (Scarf Test) is painful in AC joint arthritis or sprain.
  - Speed test for biceps tendinopathy: With arm 30 degrees of flexion and palm supinated, patient attempts to flex the elbow against resistance. Pain over biceps is positive.
  - Yergason test for biceps tendinopathy: With the elbow stabilized to the patient's side and flexed to 90 degrees, place the patient's forearm in pronation and resist against supination.
  - Apprehension, relocation test for anterior glenohumeral joint instability: Examiner supports the elbow of the patient and with the other hand holding the wrist, slowly externally rotates the humerus with the shoulder at 90 degrees abduction, patient apprehension with maneuver.
  - Sulcus sign for inferior glenohumeral joint instability: Examiner pulls down with the hand grasping the subject's elbow, positive if significant inferior movement of the arm, relative to shoulder.
  - O'Brien, clunk test for labral pathology: Move arm at 90 degrees of flexion, 10 degrees of adduction, and thumb pointed down (arm in internal rotation); examiner resists flexion distally. Maintain the same position and have the patient turn thumb up. Pain with thumb down and no pain with thumb up is positive.
  - Spurling test for cervical pathology: rotation of head toward side of symptoms along with neck extension with applied downward force to reproduce radicular symptoms

DIFFERENTIAL DIAGNOSIS

- Fracture (clavicle, humerus, scapula), contusion
- RTC disorder: impingement, tear, calcific tendonitis
- Subacromial bursitis
- Scapulothoracic dyskinesis
- AC joint pathology (AC separation/OA, osteolysis)
- Biceps tenosynovitis or tear
- Acromial apophysitis or os acromiale
- Glenohumeral joint OA
- Glenohumeral joint instability (acute dislocation or chronic multidirectional instability)
- Adhesive capsulitis
- Labral tear or associated bony pathology
- Muscle strain (trapezius, deltoid, biceps)
- Cervical radiculopathy
- Other: autoimmune, rheumatologic, referred pain, septic joint (biliary/splenic, cardiac, pneumonia/lung mass)

DIAGNOSTIC TESTS & INTERPRETATION

Initial Tests (lab, imaging)

- A history of significant trauma, prolonged symptoms, or red flags (older age, fever, rest pain) suggests a need for imaging.
- Adults with nontraumatic shoulder pain of <4 weeks duration may not require initial imaging.
- Plain radiographs anteroposterior, scapular Y, axillary views
- EMG study of the upper extremity may help differentiate referred cervical pain and brachial plexopathy from a primary shoulder disorder.
- Obtain ECG if any suspicion for cardiac etiology.
- Serologic tests if autoimmune etiology is suspected

Follow-Up Tests & Special Considerations

- CT or MRI can rule out an occult fracture.
- MRI is gold standard for noninvasive soft tissue imaging, including RTC, biceps tendon.
- MR arthrogram may be necessary to assess for labral tears.
- Ultrasound (US) can assess for RTC tears, biceps tendinopathy, and AC joint pathology.
- US is operator dependent but in the hands of a good technician can be equivalent to MRI in detecting full-thickness tears (sensitivity 92%, specificity 94%) and partial-thickness tears (sensitivity 67%, specificity 94%) (1).

Diagnostic Procedures/Other

Consider diagnostic arthroscopy after failing conservative management if structural injury is suspected.

Test Interpretation

- Tendinosis rather than tendonitis is common with stage I impingement.
- Capsular scarring is the hallmark of adhesive capsulitis.
- RTC enthesophytes visualized with calcific tendonitis
- Tear enlargement and pain development in asymptomatic tears are more common with involvement of the dominant shoulder.

 TREATMENT

- Treatment is based on underlying diagnosis.
- In general, conservative therapy includes activity modification, analgesics, and/or anti-inflammatory medicines in association with appropriate rehabilitative programs.
- Physical therapy almost always required for full resolution

MEDICATION

First Line

- Analgesics and anti-inflammatory medications for symptomatic relief include NSAIDs, such as ibuprofen, naproxen, and meloxicam. Acetaminophen may also be used especially if the patient has a history of a GI bleed.
- Corticosteroid injections (subacromial, glenohumeral, AC, subscapular bursa) can be used to acutely relieve pain due to RTC pathology, adhesive capsulitis, OA, or scapulothoracic dyskinesis.
- Steroid injections can improve ability to engage in rehabilitative activities.
- US guidance improves accuracy of anatomic placement of corticosteroid injections; long-term outcomes have thus far been shown to be similar between US-guided versus nonguided injections (2).

ISSUES FOR REFERRAL

- If etiology remains unclear, patient is not responsive to conservative care, for complicated or displaced fractures.
- Full-thickness RTC tears >1 cm (acute or chronic) in patients <65 years old or any tear with significant changes in functional status require surgical referral. These tears have a high rate of progression, fatty infiltration, or retraction with nonoperative care.

ADDITIONAL THERAPIES

- Physical therapy can benefit persistent RTC disorders, adhesive capsulitis, and shoulder instability.
- Manual therapy and exercises may improve pain and increase function in RTC disease.
- Manual manipulative therapy (MMT) by chiropractors, osteopathic physicians, or physical therapists improves pain with adhesive capsulitis, RTC, and soft tissue disorders. In adhesive capsulitis, MMT is generally less effective than glucocorticoid injections at 6-week mark, but both have similar long-term outcomes. Acupuncture may improve short-term pain and function in RTC impingement.

SURGERY/OTHER PROCEDURES

- Surgery is recommended for shoulder pain caused by acute displaced fractures, large RTC tears (criteria as above). It may also be recommended for multiple shoulder dislocation in patients <20 years of age.
- Surgery can be considered for shoulder pain unresponsive to conservative measures >3 to 6 months. Surgery is not more effective than active nonsurgical treatment in impingement syndrome.
- Platelet-rich therapies need more conclusive evidence before routine use in treatment of MSK soft tissue injuries.

COMPLEMENTARY & ALTERNATIVE MEDICINE

Acupuncture may help with acute shoulder pain. There is no conclusive evidence for the effectiveness of acupuncture.

 ONGOING CARE

FOLLOW-UP RECOMMENDATIONS

Limit overhead activity to reduce impingement symptoms.

PATIENT EDUCATION

Refer to specific diagnosis for shoulder pain.

PROGNOSIS

Shoulder pain generally has a favorable outcome with conservative care, but recovery can be slow, with 40–50% of patients complaining of persistent pain or recurrence at 12 months.

REFERENCES

1. Greenberg DL. Evaluation and treatment of shoulder pain. *Med Clin North Am*. 2014;98(3):487–504.
2. Daniels EW, Cole D, Jacobs B, et al. Existing evidence on ultrasound-guided injections in sports medicine. *Orthop J Sports Med*. 2018;6(2):2325967118756576.

ADDITIONAL READING

Littlewood C, Ashton J, Chance-Larsen K, et al. Exercise for rotator cuff tendinopathy: a systematic review. *Physiotherapy*. 2012;98(2):101–109.

 CODES

ICD10

M25.519 Pain in unspecified shoulder

CLINICAL PEARLS

- RTC disorders (tendinopathy, tears) are the most common cause of shoulder pain in individuals >30 years of age.
- Shoulder instability (acute dislocation/subluxation or chronic instability) is the most common source of shoulder pain in individuals <30 years of age.
- Patients with diabetes are at increased risk for adhesive capsulitis.
- Most patients do well with a structured program of pain control and rehabilitation.

S

SINUSITIS

Chirag N. Shah, MD • Grant Wei, MD, FACEP • Daniel Idahosa, MD, BS

BASICS

DESCRIPTION
- Acute sinusitis is a symptomatic inflammation of ≥1 paranasal sinuses of <4 weeks duration resulting from impaired drainage and retained secretions accompanied by obstruction, facial pain/pressure/fullness, or both. Because rhinitis and sinusitis usually coexist, "rhinosinusitis" is the preferred term.
- Disease is subacute when symptomatic for 4 to 12 weeks, recurrent acute when ≥4 annual episodes without persistent symptoms in between, and chronic when symptomatic for >12 weeks.
- Uncomplicated rhinosinusitis has no extension of inflammation beyond paranasal sinuses and nasal cavity.

EPIDEMIOLOGY
- Affects 1 in 8 adults (>30 million people in the United States yearly diagnosed with rhinosinusitis)
- Acute bacterial rhinosinusitis remains the fifth leading reason for prescribing antibiotics.
- Viral cause in 90–98% of cases with 0.5–2% having a bacterial superinfection

Incidence
Incidence is highest in early fall through early spring (related to the incidence of viral upper respiratory infection [URI]). Adults have 2 to 3 viral URIs per year; 90% of colds are accompanied by viral rhinosinusitis. It is the fifth most common diagnosis during family physician visits.

ETIOLOGY AND PATHOPHYSIOLOGY
- Important features
  - Inflammation and edema of the sinus mucosa lead to obstruction of the sinus ostia causing impaired mucociliary clearance and stagnation of secretions that become hospitable to bacterial growth.
- Neutrophil influx and release of cytokines damage mucosal surfaces.
- Viral: majority of cases (rhinovirus; influenza A and B; parainfluenza; respiratory syncytial, adeno-, corona-, and enteroviruses)
- Bacterial (complicates 0.5–2% of viral cases)
  - More likely if symptoms worsen within 5 to 6 days after initial improvement
  - No improvement within 10 days of symptom onset
  - >3 to 4 days of fever >102°F and facial pain and purulent nasal discharge
  - *Streptococcus pneumoniae, Haemophilus influenzae*, and *Moraxella catarrhalis* are the most common bacterial pathogens.
  - Overdiagnosis may lead to overuse of and increasing resistance to antibiotics.
  - Methicillin-resistant *Staphylococcus aureus* present in 0–15.9% of patients
- Fungal: seen in immunocompromised hosts (uncontrolled diabetes, neutropenia, use of corticosteroids) or as a nosocomial infection; most common etiology is aspergillus.

RISK FACTORS
- Viral URI
- Allergic rhinitis
- Asthma
- Cigarette smoking
- Dental infections and procedures
- Anatomic variations
  - Tonsillar and adenoid hypertrophy
  - Turbinate hypertrophy, nasal polyps
  - Cleft palate
  - Septal deviations
- Immunodeficiency (e.g., HIV)
- Cystic fibrosis (CF)
- Prolonged supine positioning (i.e., ICU patients)

GENERAL PREVENTION
Hand washing, vaccinations, avoiding symptomatic individuals, avoid smoking, and exposure to second-hand smoke.

DIAGNOSIS

- History and physical exam suggest and establish diagnosis but rarely helpful in distinguishing bacterial from viral causes.
- Use a constellation of symptoms rather than a particular sign or symptom in diagnosis.

HISTORY
- Symptoms somewhat predictive of bacterial sinusitis (1)[C]
  - Worsening of symptoms for >5 to 6 days after initial improvement
  - Persistent symptoms for ≥10 days
  - Persistent purulent nasal discharge
  - Unilateral upper tooth or facial pain
  - Unilateral maxillary sinus tenderness
  - Fever
- Associated symptoms
  - Headache
  - Nasal congestion
  - Retro-orbital pain
  - Otalgia
  - Hyposmia
  - Halitosis
  - Chronic cough
- Symptoms requiring urgent attention
  - Visual disturbances, especially diplopia
  - Periorbital swelling or erythema
  - Altered mental status

PHYSICAL EXAM
- Fever
- Edema and erythema of nasal mucosa
- Purulent discharge
- Tenderness to palpation over sinus(es)
- Pain localized to sinuses bending forward
- Transillumination of the sinuses may confirm fluid in sinuses (helpful if asymmetric; not helpful if symmetric exam).

Pediatric Considerations
- Sinuses are not fully developed until 20 years of age; maxillary and ethmoid sinuses at birth; frontal sinuses last to develop
- Children are at risk for developing sinusitis because they have an average of 6 to 8 colds per year.

DIFFERENTIAL DIAGNOSIS
- Dental disease
- CF
- Wegener granulomatosis
- HIV infection
- Neoplasm
- Nasal foreign body
- Allergic rhinitis
- Headache: tension, cluster, or migraine

DIAGNOSTIC TESTS & INTERPRETATION
Diagnostic tests are not routinely recommended; no diagnostic test adequately differentiates viral and bacterial rhinosinusitis (2)[C].
- None indicated in routine evaluation
- Routine use of sinus radiography is discouraged because of the following:
  - ≥3 clinical findings have similar diagnostic accuracy as imaging.
  - Imaging does not distinguish viral from bacterial etiology.
- Limited coronal CT scan in recurrent infection or failure of medical therapy (CT paranasal sinuses if a CNS or orbital involvement is suspected)
- Culture and biopsy are indicated for chronic bacterial sinusitis and fungal sinusitis.

Test Interpretation
- Inflammation, edema, thickened mucosa
- Polyps

TREATMENT

Most cases resolve with supportive care (treating pain and nasal symptoms). Antibiotics should be reserved for symptoms that persist for >10 days, onset with severe symptoms (high fever, purulent nasal discharge, facial pain) for at least 3 to 4 consecutive days, or worsening signs/symptoms that were initially improving (1)[C],(2)[C].

GENERAL MEASURES
- Hydration
- Steam inhalation 20 to 30 minutes TID
- Saline irrigation (Neti pot) or nasal drops
- Sleep with the head of the bed elevated.
- Avoid caffeine, alcohol, and exposure to cigarette smoke or fumes.
- Acute viral sinusitis is self-limited; antibiotics only when findings suggest bacterial infection
- Analgesics, NSAIDs

MEDICATION
First Line
- Decongestants
  - Pseudoephedrine HCl
  - Phenylephrine nasal spray (limited use)
  - Oxymetazoline nasal spray (e.g., Afrin) (not to be used for >3 days)
- Analgesics
  - Acetaminophen
  - NSAIDs
- Intranasal steroids (3)[C]
  - Budesonide (Rhinocort)
  - Mometasone furoate (Nasonex)
  - Fluticasone (Flonase)

- Antibiotics
  - Antibiotics can shorten time to cure but only in 5 to 11 people per 100 (4)[A]; most improve without antibiotics.
  - Reserve antibiotic use for patients with moderate to severe disease.
  - Antibiotics have not been shown to prevent recurrences or complications.
  - Chronic rhinosinusitis requires a 3-month course of antibiotics to achieve minimal symptom improvement.
  - Choice should be based on understanding of antibiotic resistance in the community.
  - Infectious Disease Society of America (IDSA) recommends the following (1)[C]:
    - Start antibiotics as soon as a clinical diagnosis of acute bacterial sinusitis is made.
    - Use amoxicillin-clavulanate rather than amoxicillin alone.
    - Amoxicillin-clavulanate 875/125 mg q12h; 2 g PO BID in regions with high rates of resistant *S. pneumoniae*
    - Doxycycline: 100 mg PO BID; an alternative to amoxicillin-clavulanate for initial therapy (adults only)
    - Trimethoprim-sulfamethoxazole (TMP/SMX) and 3rd-generation cephalosporins not recommended due to high rate of resistance
    - Treat adults for 5 to 7 days if uncomplicated bacterial rhinosinusitis (IDSA low- to moderate-quality evidence). Treat children 10 to 14 days if uncomplicated bacterial rhinosinusitis (IDSA low- to moderate-quality evidence).
  - American Academy of Pediatrics recommends the following (5):
    - Amoxicillin: 45 to 90 mg/kg/day in 2 divided doses if uncomplicated acute bacterial sinusitis in children
    - Amoxicillin-clavulanate: 80 to 90 mg/6.4 mg/kg/day in 2 divided doses for children with severe illness, recent antibiotics, or attending daycare
    - Levofloxacin: 10 to 20 mg/kg/day, max of 750 mg/day for severe PCN allergy
    - Clindamycin (30 to 40 mg/kg/day) + cefixime (8 mg/kg/day in 2 divided doses) or cefpodoxime (10 mg/kg/day in 2 divided doses) for non-type 1 PCN allergy (1)[C]
    - Ceftriaxone: 50 mg/kg IM single dose if not able to tolerate oral meds
- Because allergies may be a predisposing factor, some patients may benefit from the use of the following agents:
  - Oral antihistamines
    - Loratadine (Claritin), fexofenadine (Allegra), cetirizine (Zyrtec), desloratadine (Clarinex), or levocetirizine (Xyzal)
    - Chlorpheniramine (Chlor-Trimeton)
    - Diphenhydramine (Benadryl)
  - Leukotriene inhibitors (montelukast sodium [Singulair], zafirlukast [Accolate]), especially in patients with asthma

Second Line
- Levofloxacin (Levaquin): 750 mg/day for 5 days or moxifloxacin 400 mg/day for 5 to 7 days (adults only) (1)[C]

- No response to first-line therapy >72 hours
  - Broaden antibiotic coverage or switch to a different class; evaluate for resistant pathogens or other causes.
- *Note:* Bacteriologic failure rates of up to 20–25% are possible with use of azithromycin and clarithromycin.
- If lack of response to 3 weeks of antibiotics, consider CT scan of sinuses and ENT referral.

ISSUES FOR REFERRAL
Complications such as periorbital edema, cranial nerve palsies, vision changes, and meningeal signs or failure of treatment

ALERT
- Meta-analyses have demonstrated no benefit of newer antibiotics over amoxicillin or doxycycline.
- Higher antibiotic doses and antibiotic therapy taken longer than a standard 5-day course do not curtail symptom degree or duration.
- Antibiotic recommendations vary with different guidelines. Patients seen by specialists are different from those in a primary care setting. Patients usually do not have complicated sinusitis in a primary care setting.
  - American Academy of Otolaryngology—Head and Neck Surgery Foundation recommends the following (2)[C]:
    - Consider watchful waiting without antibiotics in patients with uncomplicated mild illness (mild pain and temperature <101°F) with assurance of follow-up within 7 days.
- PCV-13 pneumococcal vaccine can be helpful in reducing chronic sinusitis in children.
- Use of intranasal steroids with small but significant improvement in symptoms when used alone or with antibiotics
- The use of systemic steroids is not indicated.
- Precautions
  - Decongestants can exacerbate hypertension.
  - Intranasal decongestants limited to 3 days to avoid rebound nasal congestion

Pregnancy Considerations
- Nasal irrigation with saline, pseudoephedrine, most antihistamines, and some nasal steroids are safe during pregnancy and lactation.
- Antibiotics safe in pregnancy and lactation: amoxicillin, amoxicillin-clavulanate, cephalosporins
- Antibiotic contraindicated: doxycycline, fluoroquinolones
- Antibiotic safe in lactation but not pregnancy: levofloxacin

ADDITIONAL THERAPIES
Topical ipratropium to decrease secretions and expectorants such as guaifenesin to thin mucous secretions

SURGERY/OTHER PROCEDURES
- If medical therapy fails, consider sinus irrigation.
- Functional endoscopic sinus surgery is the preferred treatment for medically recalcitrant cases.
- Absolute surgical indications include massive nasal polyposis, subperiosteal or orbital abscess, frontal soft tissue spread of infection, mucocele or mucopyocele, invasive or allergic fungal sinusitis, suspected obstructing tumor, or CSF rhinorrhea.

ADMISSION, INPATIENT, AND NURSING CONSIDERATIONS
Hospitalization for complications (e.g., meningitis, orbital cellulitis or abscess, brain abscess)

ONGOING CARE

FOLLOW-UP RECOMMENDATIONS
Return if no improvement after 72 hours or no resolution of symptoms after 10 days of antibiotics.

PROGNOSIS
Alleviation of symptoms within 72 hours with complete resolution within 10 to 14 days

COMPLICATIONS
Serious complications (meningitis, orbital cellulitis, brain abscess, cavernous sinus thrombosis, osteomyelitis, subdural empyema) are rare.

REFERENCES
1. Chow AW, Benninger MS, Brook I, et al; for Infectious Diseases Society of America. IDSA clinical practice guideline for acute bacterial rhinosinusitis in children and adults. *Clin Infect Dis*. 2012;54(8):e72–e112.
2. Rosenfeld RM, Piccirillo JF, Chandrasekhar SS, et al. Clinical practice guideline (update): adult sinusitis. *Otolaryngol Head Neck Surg*. 2015;152(Suppl 2): S1–S39.
3. Hayward G, Heneghan C, Perera R, et al. Intranasal corticosteroids in management of acute sinusitis: a systematic review and meta-analysis. *Ann Fam Med*. 2012;10(3):241–249.
4. Lemiengre MB, van Driel ML, Merenstein D, et al. Antibiotics for acute rhinosinusitis in adults. *Cochrane Database Syst Rev*. 2018;9(9):CD006089.
5. Wald ER, Applegate KE, Bordley C, et al; for American Academy of Pediatrics. Clinical practice guideline for the diagnosis and management of acute bacterial sinusitis in children aged 1 to 18 years. *Pediatrics*. 2013;132(1):e262–e280.

CODES

ICD10
- J01.41 Acute recurrent pansinusitis
- J01.0 Acute maxillary sinusitis
- J01.80 Other acute sinusitis

CLINICAL PEARLS

- Most cases resolve with supportive care (treating pain, nasal symptoms).
- Reserve antibiotics for symptoms >10 days, or if 3 to 4 consecutive days of severe symptoms (high fever, purulent nasal discharge, facial pain).
- Multiple meta-analyses have demonstrated *no* benefit of newer antibiotics over amoxicillin or doxycycline.
- Significant patient symptom relief with nasal saline spray or drops or irrigation (Neti pot).

SJÖGREN SYNDROME

Julie A. Creech, DO • Alexander Vavra, DO

BASICS

- First described by Swedish ophthalmologist Henrik Sjögren; chronic autoimmune disorder characterized by inflammation from lymphocytic infiltration of exocrine organs (especially lacrimal and salivary glands) resulting in decreased gland function; typically presents with sicca symptoms such as dry eyes (xerophthalmia), dry mouth (xerostomia), and parotid enlargement
- Extraglandular manifestations: arthralgia, myalgia, Raynaud phenomenon, pulmonary disease, GI disease, leukopenia, anemia, lymphadenopathy, vasculitis, renal tubular acidosis, lymphoma, CNS involvement with longitudinal transverse myelitis (>4 vertebral segments), and optic neuritis associated with anti–aquaporin-4 antibodies, PNS involvement with small fiber neuropathy
- Primary Sjögren: not associated with other diseases; *HLA-DRB1*0301* and *HLA-DRB1*1501* are the most common.
- Secondary Sjögren: occurs in conjunction with other autoimmune rheumatic disorders, such as rheumatoid arthritis (most common); associated with HLA-DR4, systemic lupus erythematous (SLE), or systemic sclerosis

EPIDEMIOLOGY

Incidence
Annual incidence: ~4/100,000

- No racial or geographic predilection; predominant sex: female > male (9:1); predominant age at onset: 4th to 5th decades of life

Prevalence
Sjögren syndrome (SS) affects 1 to 4 million people in the United States.

ETIOLOGY AND PATHOPHYSIOLOGY

- Etiology is unknown; theorized to be a viral trigger (Epstein-Barr virus [EBV], HCV, HTLV-1) in genetically predisposed people
- Pathophysiology involves multifactorial systemic autoimmune process characterized by infiltration of glandular tissue predominately by CD4 T lymphocytes.
  - Theorized that glandular epithelial cells present antigen to the T cells inducing cytokine production, ultimately leading to B-cell dysregulation and resulting in autoantibody production, chronic inflammation, and increased incidence of B-cell malignancies.

Genetics
A familial tendency suggests a genetic predisposition.

RISK FACTORS
There are no known modifiable risk factors.

GENERAL PREVENTION
No known prevention; complications can be prevented by early diagnosis and treatment. Oral health providers play a key role in early detection and management of salivary dysfunction.

COMMONLY ASSOCIATED CONDITIONS
Secondary SS associated with rheumatoid arthritis, scleroderma, SLE, polymyositis, HIV, hepatitis C, MCTD, PBC, hypergammaglobulinemic purpura, necrotizing vasculitis, autoimmune thyroiditis, chronic active hepatitis, mixed cryoglobulinemia

Pregnancy Considerations
Pregnant SS patients with high anti-SSA Abs have increased risk of delivering a fetus with congenital heart block. Currently, there are no established evidence-based protocols for screening, prophylaxis, or treatment.

DIAGNOSIS

- 2016 ACR/EULAR classification criteria (1)[A]:
  - Based on five objective tests/items
  - Inclusion criteria is applicable if the patient is positive for one ocular/oral dryness symptom (based on the AECG questions) or at least one positive domain from the EULAR SS disease activity index questionnaire and a total score of ≥4 from the following:
    ○ Positive serum anti-SSA/Ro antibody—3 points; focal lymphocytic sialadenitis with a focus score ≥1 foci/4 mm² from labial salivary gland biopsy—3 points; abnormal ocular staining score of ≥5 or van Bijsterveld score of ≥4—1 point; Schirmer test result of ≤5 mm/5 min—1 point; an unstimulated salivary flow rate of ≤0.1 mL/min—1 point
- Ocular signs and symptoms
  - Troublesome dry eyes daily for ≥3 months; recurrent sandy/gritty ocular sensation; use of tear substitute ≥3 times per day
- Oral signs and symptoms
  - Daily symptoms of dry mouth for ≥3 months; recurrent feeling of swollen salivary glands; need to drink liquid to help swallow dry foods
- Exclusion criteria: prior diagnosis would exclude SS diagnosis:
  - History of head and neck radiation; active hepatitis C infection (positive PCR); AIDS; sarcoidosis/amylodosis; graft versus host disease
- Other manifestations: chronic arthritis, type 1 RTA, tubular interstitial nephritis, rheumatoid arthritis, vasculitis, vaginal dryness, pleuritis, pancreatitis

HISTORY

- Decreased tear production; burning, scratchy sensation in eyes; difficulty speaking or swallowing, dental caries, xerotrachea; enlarged or intermittent swelling of parotid glands (bilateral)
- Dyspareunia; vaginal dryness
- From consensus criteria and EULAR questionnaire:
  - Have you had daily, persistent, troublesome dry eyes for >3 months?
  - Do you have a recurrent sensation of sand or gravel in the eyes?
  - Do you use tear substitutes >3 times a day?
  - Have you had a daily feeling of dry mouth for >3 months?
  - Do you frequently drink liquids to aid in swallowing dry food?

PHYSICAL EXAM

- Eye exam: dry eyes (keratoconjunctivitis sicca), decreased tear pool in the lower conjunctiva, dilated conjunctival vessels, mucinous threads, and filamentary keratosis (slit-lamp examination)
- Oral exam: dry mouth (xerostomia); decreased sublingual salivary pool (tongue may stick to the tongue depressor); frequent oral caries (sometimes in unusual locations such as the incisor surface and along the gum line [cervical portion of the teeth]); dark red tongue from prolonged xerostomia
- Ear, nose, and throat exam: parotid enlargement, submandibular enlargement
- Skin exam: nonpalpable or palpable vasculitic purpura (typically 2 to 3 mm in diameter and on the lower extremities)

DIFFERENTIAL DIAGNOSIS

- Causes of ocular dryness: hypovitaminosis A, decreased tear production unrelated to autoimmune process (i.e., age related), chronic blepharitis or conjunctivitis, impaired blinking (i.e., due to Parkinson disease or Bell palsy), infiltration of lacrimal glands (i.e., amyloidosis, lymphoma, sarcoidosis), low estrogen levels
- Causes of oral dryness: medications (anticholinergics, antihistamines, antidepressants), dehydration, anxiety, sialadenitis due to chronic obstruction, chronic viral infections (e.g., hepatitis C or HIV), radiation of head/neck
- Causes of salivary gland swelling: unilateral: obstruction, chronic sialadenitis, bacterial infection, neoplasm; bilateral (asymmetric): IgG4-related disease, HIV; bilateral (symmetric): hepatic cirrhosis, DM, anorexia/bulimia, acromegaly, alcoholism, hypolipoproteinemia, chronic pancreatitis, acute or chronic viral infection (i.e., mumps, EBV), coxsackievirus, echovirus, granulomatous diseases (i.e., tuberculosis, sarcoidosis)

DIAGNOSTIC TESTS & INTERPRETATION

- Schirmer test (<5-mm wetness after 5 minutes); Rose Bengal test (slit lamp) to obtain ocular surface staining and tear break-up time (TBUT); minor salivary gland biopsy (gold standard); autoantibodies: +antinuclear antibodies (ANAs) (95%), +RF (75%)
- In primary SS: +anti-Ro (anti-SSA, 56%) and +anti-La (anti-SSB, 30%)

Initial Tests (lab, imaging)
Preliminary lab workup

- Basic labs: CBC with differential, chemistry panel, erythrocyte sedimentation rate (ESR), C-reactive protein (CRP), urinalysis
- Special labs: ANA, rheumatoid factor (RF), anti-Ro/SSA, anti-La/SSB
- Anti-SSA and anti-SSB antibodies present in 33–74% and 23–52% of SS patients, respectively.
- Imaging may include:
  - Imaging for xerostomia: salivary gland scintigraphy (insensitive but highly specific); parotid gland sialography (should not be used in acute parotitis); MRI (correlates well with salivary gland biopsy)
  - Salivary gland US (SGUS), highly specific for salivary gland involvement in SS

Diagnostic Procedures/Other

Salivary gland biopsy: used to confirm suspected diagnosis of SS or to exclude other causes of xerostomia and bilateral glandular enlargement; parotid biopsy if malignancy is suspected; lymph node biopsy to rule out pseudolymphoma or lymphoma if suspected

Test Interpretation

- Salivary gland histology shows focal collections of lymphocytes; immunocytology shows CD4+ T-cell lymphocyte predominance.
- SGUS parameters include:
  - Parenchymal nonhomogeneity—the most useful diagnostic marker
  - US inflammatory findings include hypoechoic and hyperechoic bands; real-time sonoelastography (RTS) to quantify tissue rigidity and assess glandular damage

 ## TREATMENT

- Goals of treatment: symptom palliation, improved quality of life, monitor and treat systemic manifestations
- Prior to treatment of oral dryness, assess baseline salivary gland function. Avoid medications that may worsen oral dryness (i.e., anticholinergics, antidepressants). Promote good oral hygiene and routine dental care. Address fatigue and pain.

MEDICATION

- Therapy for dry mouth:
  - Nonpharmacologic: gustatory stimulants (sugar-free candies, lozenges, xylitol), mechanical stimulants (xylitol containing sugar-free gum), fluoride-containing mouth wash/gel/spray or artificial saliva preparations such as Salivart, Saliment, Xero-Lube, Mouth Kote.
  - Pharmacologic: cevimeline (Evoxac) or pilocarpine (Salagen) work via stimulation of salivary flow
  - Not recommended: immunosuppressive therapies, hydroxychloroquine (HCQ), oral glucocorticoids, or rituximab
- Therapy for dry eyes:
  - Nonpharmacologic: artificial tears with hydroxy-ethylcellulose or dextran are more viscous and can last longer; (opt for preservative free), topical gel/ointment (assist in controlling nighttime symptoms take prior to going to bed)
  - If unresponsive to nonpharmacologic, consider ophthalmology evaluation to guide use of pharmacologic options such as topical NSAIDs/corticosteroids and topical Cyclosporin A (CyA). The evidence of serum teardrop benefits is inconsistent.
- Therapy for MSK-related pain
  - Inflammatory MSK pain: HCQ is first line.
  - In acute MSK pain: short course of acetaminophen or NSAIDs for <7 to 10 days
- Tumor necrosis factor inhibitors are strongly discouraged in sicca treatment and in most other primary Sjögren's clinical contexts.

First Line

- Xerostomia: sugar-free lozenges, especially malic acid, artificial saliva; pilocarpine 5 mg PO starting at QD with titration to QID or cevimeline 30 mg PO TID
- Keratoconjunctivitis sicca: artificial tears and ocular lubricants for symptomatic relief

Second Line

- Xerostomia: Interferon-α lozenges may enhance salivary gland flow.
- Keratoconjunctivitis sicca: topical glucocorticoids or topical NSAIDs (Use with caution—avoid long-term use—consider ophthalmic supervision.)
- Inflammatory MSK pain: If unresponsive to HCQ, consider methotrexate (MTX) alone or MTX and HCQ. If unresponsive, consider short term (<1 month) of corticosteroids or cyclosporine.
- For life-threatening extraglandular manifestations, cyclophosphamide (PO or IV), mycophenolate mofetil, and azathioprine are often used.

ISSUES FOR REFERRAL

Rheumatology to help manage systemic manifestations or resistant symptoms; oral health: At a minimum, patients should undergo annual dental examination with twice yearly dental cleanings; ophthalmology for grading of severity and management of xerophthalmia

ADDITIONAL THERAPIES

- Gynecologic conditions:
  - Vaginal dryness: moisturizers (e.g., Replens, Vagisil) and lubricants (e.g., Sylk, Silken Secret); if unresponsive to above measures, vaginal estrogen creams/rings/tablets are options.
  - Be vigilant for and treat vaginal yeast infections.
- Keratoconjunctivitis sicca:
  - Conserve tears with side shields or ski/swim goggles, humidifiers, and warm moist compresses.
- Fatigue:
  - Dehydroepiandrosterone (DHEA) does not offer improvement in fatigue and well-being above placebo.
  - Counsel on exercise and role of reducing fatigue.

SURGERY/OTHER PROCEDURES

Punctal plug/occlusion: If keratoconjunctivitis is refractory to artificial tears, consider punctal plug.

COMPLEMENTARY & ALTERNATIVE MEDICINE

Some studies show that acupuncture benefits saliva production and symptoms of xerostomia.

ADMISSION, INPATIENT, AND NURSING CONSIDERATIONS

More likely from extraglandular manifestations such as cardiopulmonary disease, renal involvement, and CNS manifestations (e.g., optic neuritis, transverse myelitis, vasculitis, or ischemic stroke)

 ## ONGOING CARE

FOLLOW-UP RECOMMENDATIONS

Frequency of follow-up depends on severity.

Patient Monitoring

Monitor for complications, systemic manifestations, and relief of symptoms. Medicolegal pitfalls: Monitor for parotid tumor or lymphoma.

DIET

No specific diet identified to contribute to formation of SS. It is recommended to reduce sugar intake and avoid nonwater drinks between meals and 1 hour prior to bedtime.

PATIENT EDUCATION

In most cases, nonpharmacologic measures are adequate: humidifiers, adequate water intake, chewing gum, artificial tears, smoking cessation.

PROGNOSIS

Hypocomplementemia is an independent risk factor for premature death. Extraglandular involvement is associated with decreased quality of life and increased mortality. Primary SS is associated with increased risks of malignancy, non-Hodgkin lymphoma, and thyroid cancer.

COMPLICATIONS

Complications include dental caries, gum disease, dysphagia, salivary gland calculi, keratitis, conjunctivitis, and scarring of the ocular surface.

REFERENCE

1. Shiboski CH, Shiboski SC, Seror R, et al; for International Sjögren's Syndrome Criteria Working Group. 2016 American College of Rheumatology/European League Against Rheumatism classification criteria for primary Sjögren's syndrome: a consensus and data-driven methodology involving three international patient cohorts. *Arthritis Rheumatol.* 2017;69(1):35–45.

 ## CODES

ICD10

- M35.01 Sjögren syndrome with keratoconjunctivitis
- M35.03 Sjögren syndrome with myopathy
- M35.00 Sjögren syndrome, unspecified

CLINICAL PEARLS

- Many symptoms of SS can be treated with nonpharmacologic interventions such as artificial tears and sugar-free candy/lozenges.
- Coordinate care management with rheumatology, ophthalmology, and oral health.
- Consider SS in patients with unexplained lung disease and +ANA.
- Patients with primary SS may have an increased risk of lymphoma and incidence of celiac disease.

°S

SLEEP APNEA, OBSTRUCTIVE

Thomas J. Hansen, MD

BASICS

DESCRIPTION
- Obstructive sleep apnea (OSA) is defined as repetitive episodes of cessation of airflow (apnea) through the nose and mouth during sleep due to obstruction at the level of the pharynx.
  - Repetitive apneas produce sleep disruption, leading to excessive daytime sleepiness (EDS).
  - Associated with oxygen desaturation and nocturnal hypoxemia
- System(s) affected: cardiovascular; nervous; pulmonary
- Synonym(s): sleep apnea syndrome; nocturnal upper airway occlusion

EPIDEMIOLOGY
Prevalence
- The estimated prevalence rated of moderate to severe sleep-disordered breathing has substantially increased over the last 2 decades. The current prevalence is 10% among 30- to 49-year-old men and 17% among 50- to 70-year-old men. In women, the prevalence is 3% among 30- to 49-year-old women and 9% among 50- to 70-year-old women.
- Highest in obese/hypertensive patients

ETIOLOGY AND PATHOPHYSIOLOGY
OSA occurs when the naso- or oropharynx collapses passively during inspiration. Anatomic and neuromuscular factors contribute to pharyngeal collapse, which leads to hypoxic arousal.
- Anatomic abnormalities, such as increased soft tissue in the palate, tonsillar hypertrophy, macroglossia, and craniofacial abnormalities, predispose the airway to collapse by decreasing the area of the upper airway or increasing the pressure surrounding the airway.
- During sleep, decreased muscle tone in the naso- or oropharynx contributes to airway obstruction and collapse.
- Upper airway narrowing may be due to the following:
  - Obesity, redundant tissue in the soft palate
  - Enlarged tonsils/uvula or a low soft palate; large/posteriorly located tongue
  - Craniofacial abnormalities or neuromuscular disorders
  - Alcohol/sedative use before bedtime

RISK FACTORS
- Obesity (strongest risk factor)
- Age >40 years
- Alcohol/sedative intake before bedtime
- Smoking
- Nasal obstruction (due to polyps, rhinitis, or deviated septum)
- Anatomic narrowing of nasopharynx
- Hypothyroidism
- Neurologic syndromes (e.g., muscular dystrophy, cerebral palsy)

GENERAL PREVENTION
Weight control and avoidance of alcohol and sedatives at night can help.

COMMONLY ASSOCIATED CONDITIONS
- Hypertension
- Obesity
- Daytime sleepiness
- Metabolic syndrome
Rare:
- Cardiac arrhythmias
- Cardiovascular disease
- Congestive heart failure
- Pulmonary hypertension
- Nasal obstructive problems

DIAGNOSIS

HISTORY
- Elicit a complete history of daytime and nighttime symptoms. Symptoms can be insidious and may have been present for years.
- Daytime symptoms
  - EDS or fatigue (cardinal symptom)
    - Mild symptoms are those that occur during quiet activities (e.g., reading, watching television).
    - More severe symptoms are those that occur during dynamic activities (e.g., work, driving).
  - Tired on morning awakening "nonrestorative sleep"
  - Sore/dry throat
  - Poor concentration, memory problems, irritability, mood changes, behavior problems (in children)
  - Morning headaches
  - Decreased libido
  - Depression
- Nighttime symptoms
  - Loud snoring (present in 60% of people with OSA)
  - Snort/gasp that arouses patient from sleep but not usually to full consciousness
  - Disrupted sleep
  - Witnessed apneic episodes at night

PHYSICAL EXAM
- OSA is commonly associated with obesity.
- Focused head and neck exam
  - Short neck with large circumference
  - Oropharynx
    - Narrowing of the lateral airway wall
    - Tonsillar hypertrophy; macroglossia
    - Micrognathia/retrognathia
    - Soft palate edema; high, arched hard palate
    - Long/thick uvula
  - Nasopharynx
    - Deviated nasal septum; poor nasal airflow

DIFFERENTIAL DIAGNOSIS
- Other causes of EDS such as the following:
  - Narcolepsy
  - Idiopathic daytime hypersomnolence
  - Inadequate sleep time
  - Depressive episodes with EDS
  - Periodic limb movements disorder
- Respiratory disorders with nocturnal awakenings such as the following:
  - Asthma
  - Chronic obstructive pulmonary disease
  - Congestive heart failure
- Central sleep apnea (Respiratory effort is absent as compared to OSA where effort is present.)
- Sleep-related choking/laryngospasm
- Gastroesophageal reflux
- Sleep-associated seizures (temporal lobe epilepsy)

DIAGNOSTIC TESTS & INTERPRETATION
Initial Tests (lab, imaging)
When clinically indicated
- Thyroid-stimulating hormone; CBC to evaluate anemia and polycythemia, which can indicate nocturnal hypoxemia; fasting glucose in patients with obesity
- Rare: arterial blood gases to evaluate daytime hypercapnia

Diagnostic Procedures/Other
- The gold standard for OSA is a full-night, in-laboratory polysomnography (PSG), a nighttime sleep study (1)[B].
  - Demonstrates severity of hypoxemia, sleep disruption, and cardiac arrhythmias associated with OSA and elevated end-tidal CO_2
  - Shows repetitive episodes of cessation/marked reduction in airflow despite continued respiratory efforts
  - Apneic episodes must last at least 10 seconds and occur 10 to 15 times per hour and cause decreased oxygen saturation to be considered clinically significant.
  - Complete PSG is expensive, and health insurance may not cover the cost.
- Multiple sleep latency testing is a diagnostic tool used to measure the time it takes from the start of a daytime nap period to the first signs of sleep (sleep latency). It provides an objective measurement of daytime sleepiness.
- The apnea-hypopnea index (AHI) is defined as the total number of apneas and hypopneas divided by the total sleep time in hours.
  - Mild OSA: AHI = 5 to 15
  - Moderate OSA: AHI = 15 to 30
  - Severe OSA: AHI >30
- Split-night PSG (as compared to a full-night PSG) occurs when patients are diagnosed with OSA within the first part of the night, and then positive pressure device titration is initiated during the second half of the night.
- Drugs that may alter the test results include benzodiazepines and other sedatives that can amplify the severity of apnea seen during the sleep study.
- Early data suggest that home-based diagnosis using portable monitoring devices may be an alternative to laboratory-based PSG if the test is of sufficient duration.

TREATMENT

- Lifestyle modification: weight loss; exercise; and avoidance of alcohol, smoking, and sedatives, especially before bedtime
- Weight loss decreases the severity of symptoms in patients with obesity. Lifestyle modifications should be seen as adjunctive rather than curative therapy (2)[A], and a lack of improvement of symptoms with lifestyle modification should not preclude patients from receiving other therapy such as continuous positive airway pressure (CPAP).
- Position changes—if OSA is present only when supine, keep the patient off his or her back when sleeping (e.g., tennis ball worn on back of nightshirt or using a sleep position trainer).
- Positive airway pressure—the most effective therapy for mild, moderate, or severe OSA is CPAP (3)[A]. Treatment with CPAP uses a mask interface and a flow generator to prevent airway collapse, thus helping to prevent apnea, hypoxia, and sleep disturbance.
- Several types of mask interfaces, including nasal masks, oral masks, and nasal pillows, exist for CPAP therapy. Short-term data suggest that nasal pillows are the preferred interface in almost all patients. In patients with compliance difficulty, a different choice of interface may be appropriate.
- Hypoglossal nerve stimulation is an option for patients who fail or are intolerant of CPAP therapy. Indications include a diagnosis of moderate-to-severe OSA with an AHI between 15 and 65 events per hour, a body mass index <35 kg/m^2, and absence of complete concentric collapse at the level of velopharynx or soft palate on drug-induced sleep endoscopy.
- Oral appliances to treat OSA are available and often subjectively preferred by patients (mandibular advancement devices vs. tongue retaining devices). Although oral appliances have been shown to improve symptoms compared with inactive controls, they are not as effective for reduction of respiratory disturbances as CPAP over short-term data. Treatment with oral appliances may be considered in patients who fail to comply with or decline CPAP therapy.

MEDICATION
Medications are yet to be proven effective in treating OSA.

ISSUES FOR REFERRAL
If sleep apnea is suspected, patient should be referred for a sleep study evaluation.

 ONGOING CARE

Lifelong compliance with weight loss or CPAP is necessary.

DIET
Overweight patients should be encouraged to lose weight.

PATIENT EDUCATION
- Weight loss and avoidance of alcohol and sedatives
- Significantly sleepy patients should not drive a motor vehicle/operate dangerous equipment.

PROGNOSIS
- Lifelong compliance with weight loss or CPAP is necessary for effective treatment of OSA, but long-term adherence is poor.
- Morbidity usually due to motor vehicle accidents or secondary to cardiac complications, including arrhythmias, cardiac ischemia, and hypertension; data are insufficient on whether treatment changes outcomes.

COMPLICATIONS
Untreated OSA may increase the risk for development of hypertension, stroke, myocardial infarction, diabetes, cardiovascular disease, and work-related and driving accidents, but it is unclear that treatment reduces or prevents any of these problems.

Pediatric Considerations
- The most common cause is tonsillar hypertrophy. Additional causes are obesity and craniofacial abnormalities along with neuromuscular diseases such as cerebral palsy and spinal muscular atrophy.
- Signs and symptoms
  - Nighttime: loud snoring, restlessness, and sweating
  - Daytime: hyperactivity and decreased school performance

- Diagnosis is with PSG. Abnormal AHI is different in children: >1 per hour is abnormal.
- Surgery is the first-line treatment in cases due to adenotonsillar hypertrophy. For cases due to obesity/craniofacial abnormalities, patients can use CPAP treatment.

Geriatric Considerations
The presence of sleep apnea in the geriatric population may be associated with earlier onset of mild cognitive impairment as well as Alzheimer disease at an earlier age.

REFERENCES

1. Kapur VK, Auckley DH, Chowdhuri S, et al. Clinical practice guideline for diagnostic testing for adult obstructive sleep apnea: an American Academy of Sleep Medicine clinical practice guideline. *J Clin Sleep Med*. 2017;13(3):479–504.
2. Anandam A, Akinnusi M, Kufel T, et al. Effects of dietary weight loss on obstructive sleep apnea: a meta-analysis. *Sleep Breath*. 2013;17(1):227–234.
3. Giles TL, Lasserson TJ, Smith BJ, et al. Continuous positive airways pressure for obstructive sleep apnoea in adults. *Cochrane Database Syst Rev*. 2006;(1):CD001106.

CODES

ICD10
- G47.33 Obstructive sleep apnea (adult) (pediatric)
- G47.30 Sleep apnea, unspecified

CLINICAL PEARLS

- OSA is characterized by repetitive episodes of apnea often terminating in a snort/gasp.
- Laboratory PSG is the key to diagnosis.
- CPAP is the most effective form of treatment for both mild-to-moderate and moderate-to-severe OSA.
- Central sleep apnea may mimic OSA.

SLEEP DISORDER, SHIFT WORK

Jennifer W. Caceres, MD

BASICS

DESCRIPTION

Shift work disorder (SWD), classified as a circadian rhythm sleep-wake disorder, is characterized by symptoms of insomnia and/or excessive sleepiness when required to work during usual sleep times. SWD is caused by a misalignment between the internal circadian rhythm and the required sleep-wake schedule defined by nontraditional work shifts including night shifts, afternoon or evening shifts, early morning shifts, irregular shifts, and rotating shifts (1).

EPIDEMIOLOGY

Prevalence
- In the United States, ~20% of employed adults are shift workers, particularly in service-related occupations such as health care, protective services, transportation, and food services (1).
- 1 in 3 shift workers is affected by insomnia or some form of sleep disturbance. ~90% of shift workers note daytime sleepiness or fatigue. SWD has an estimated prevalence of approximately 2–5% in the general population of the United States (1).
- Prevalence of SWD rises with age, particularly for adults age >50 years.

ETIOLOGY AND PATHOPHYSIOLOGY
In shift workers, there is a misalignment between one's endogenous circadian rhythm of sleep and wakefulness and a sleep-wake schedule based on nontraditional shift work. Dyssynchrony results in excessive sleepiness during the work shift and/or insomnia during desired sleep time (1),(2).

Genetics
One possibly genetically linked trait is a person's preference for the morning versus evening. This is partially linked to the polymorphism of the clock gene PERIOD3 (PER3) involved in sleep-wake regulation (1).

RISK FACTORS
- Age >50 years (1)
- Strong competing social and domestic needs

GENERAL PREVENTION
- Reduce or eliminate shift work. Try to rotate shifts forward if shifts must be rotated. Use bright light during shifts.
- Improve sleep hygiene. Schedule regular sleep including naps (<1 hour) just before a shift or, if possible, during a shift.

COMMONLY ASSOCIATED CONDITIONS
- SWD has been associated with functional consequences including impaired immediate free recall, decreased processing speed, and selective attention impairments.
- SWD has been associated with higher risk of vehicular accidents, job-related injuries.
- SWD has been associated with poor physical health (including increased incidence of gastrointestinal [GI] disorders, cardiovascular disease [CVD], diabetes, and possible increase risk of cancers) as well as poor mental health (including increased incidence of substance use disorders and mood disorders).

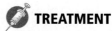**DIAGNOSIS**

- This is a clinical diagnosis. Criteria for circadian rhythm disorder per *Diagnostic and Statistical Manual of Mental Disorders*, 5th edition (*DSM-5*) include all three of the following:
  - A persistent or recurrent pattern of sleep disruption that is primarily due to an alteration of the circadian system or to a misalignment between the endogenous circadian rhythm and sleep-wake schedule required by an individual's physical environment or social or professional schedule.
  - The sleep disruption leads to excessive sleepiness or insomnia, or both.
  - The sleep disturbance causes clinically significant distress or impairment in social, occupational, and other important areas of functioning.
- Additional specification per *DSM-5* for SWD includes:
  - Insomnia during the major sleep period and/or excessive sleepiness (including inadvertent sleep) during the major awake period associated with a shift work schedule (i.e., requiring unconventional work hours).
  - The disorder is classified as to whether it is episodic (symptoms at least 1 month but <3 months), persistent (symptoms at least 3 months or longer) or recurrent (two or more episodes occurring within 1 year).

HISTORY
- A careful history is critical. Assess work history, detailed sleep history, level of sleepiness, safety risk, and performance impairments during work shifts.
- Note the following in particular (2)[C]:
  - Sleep/wake habits, sleep environment; degree of alertness or sleepiness; light exposure before, during, and after the shift; job-related factors: occupation, work schedule, years of shift work, length of shift, number of consecutive shifts, and commute after shift; sedating or stimulating medications or substance use; impact on social and domestic responsibilities (including drowsy driving)

- Evaluate for symptoms of other sleep disorders, which often coexist and can exacerbate SWD such as the following (2):
  - Loud snoring and pauses in breathing during sleep (obstructive sleep apnea [OSA]); sudden sleep attacks and leg symptoms (restless legs syndrome [RLS]); falling asleep at inappropriate times, drop attacks, and daytime fatigue (narcolepsy)

PHYSICAL EXAM
Evaluate for findings suggestive of mood disorders, GI disease, diabetes, CVD, cancer signs of OSA such as obesity, and large neck (2)[C].

DIFFERENTIAL DIAGNOSIS
- Other primary sleep disorders: insomnia, sleep-related breathing disorders, central disorders of hypersomnolence, parasomnias, sleep-related movement disorders (2)
- Other circadian rhythm sleep disorders such as delayed sleep phase type or irregular sleep-wake type. Distinguishing among these can be challenging.

DIAGNOSTIC TESTS & INTERPRETATION
No diagnostic testing is required for the diagnosis. If concern for another sleep disorder, consider polysomnography or multiple sleep latency testing (testing for narcolepsy). Given possible increased risk, consider screen for potential medical comorbidities as discussed above including mood disorders and metabolic disorders among shift workers (1),(2).

Diagnostic Procedures/Other
- Sleep diaries can help identify sleep-wake disturbances related to shift work and should be recorded for 2 weeks.
- Standardized measures of sleepiness can be obtained using several tools including the Insomnia Severity Index (ISI) and Epworth Sleepiness Scale (ESS).

Test Interpretation
Sleep diaries often reveal:
- Increased sleep latency; decreased total sleep time; frequent awakenings
- Most people revert to nocturnal sleeping on their days off. Every work week, they must "start over" to shift circadian rhythms to align with work schedules.

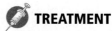**TREATMENT**

- The only standard recommendation by the American Academy of Sleep Medicine (AASM) is planned (prescribed) sleep schedules.
- Other commonly used strategies include promoting wakefulness while at work with bright light exposure, caffeine or rarely other stimulants, and/or promoting sleep with sleep hygiene optimization, melatonin, and hypnotics.

GENERAL MEASURES

- Sleep hygiene: an important first step in approaching the treatment of sleep disorders. This includes minimizing exposure to bright light before and during scheduled sleep periods (maintain a dark sleeping space, wear dark sunglasses following work shift, wear an eye mask to sleep), maintaining a quiet sleep environment (wear ear plugs to sleep, disconnect phone/doorbell, use a white noise generator), maintaining cool sleeping quarters to help retrain core body temperature to align with modified sleep-wake cycle, and avoiding use of stimulants during second half of work shift.
- Sleep time: protected time for sleep prior to and following work shifts with strategic naps where possible. Shift workers, particularly night shift workers, should be aware of postnap sleep inertia and avoid driving when drowsy (1).
- Anchor sleep: Schedule sleep periods so that at least 1 to 2 hours of designated sleep time overlap on work days and nonwork days. Anchor sleep can help increase sleep duration as well as allow workers to maintain time for socialization and recreation.
- Work/social/domestic factors: Treat psychosocial stress, depression; encourage healthy eating habits; limit substance use; increase exercise to at least 30 minutes, 5 times per week (not within 2 to 4 hours of bedtime). Seek family member and social support for protected sleep time (1).
- Work-related interventions: If possible, reduce number of consecutive shifts (<4) or reduce shift duration (<12 hours), allow adequate time between shifts (>11 hours), move heavy workload outside circadian nadir (04:00 PM to 07:00 PM).
- Light exposure: Timed bright light exposure can delay the physiologic nadir of alertness and thus, promote alertness during the night/early shift and possibly reduce circadian misalignment. Light avoidance during the day may also help with circadian adaption and improve sleep (1),(2).

MEDICATION

- Sleep-promoting medications:
  - Melatonin may help shift circadian rhythms and can increase the quality and duration of sleep as well as increase alertness during the work shift. AASM recommends 3 mg of melatonin for daytime sleep for shift workers (1); clinical effectiveness of melatonin is unclear.
  - Ramelteon (Rozerem), a melatonin receptor agonist, is FDA approved to treat insomnia, and may also provide benefit in SWD.
  - Doxepin (tricyclic antidepressant) given at low doses may improve sleep without residual daytime impairment. Trazodone is a non–first-line agent for treatment of insomnia; it may also provide some benefit in SWD.
  - Intermediate-acting hypnotics such as zolpidem (Ambien) or eszopiclone (Lunesta) can cause post-sleep sedation. Long-term use is discouraged due to potential dependence. Additionally, side effects such as anxiety or irritability may affect sleep (1).

- Wakefulness-promoting medications:
  - Modafinil (Provigil) and armodafinil (Nuvigil) are FDA approved for excessive sleepiness in patients with SWD and can reduce daytime sleepiness and improve cognitive performance. Notably, modafinil has been tied to rare instances of Stevens-Johnson syndrome (2).
  - Prophylactic caffeine use immediately prior to and during work shift. Limiting caffeine to the first half of the night shift is recommended to limit disruption of daytime sleep (2).

First Line
Circadian shift/sleep promoting: melatonin 3 mg PO or sublingual, 30 minutes before daytime sleep period. Take only when the patient is home and able to go to bed.

Second Line
- Wakefulness promoting:
  - Modafinil initially 200 mg PO 1 hour prior to work shift; armodafinil 150 mg PO 1 hour prior to work shift; long-acting (12 to 16 hours, depending on food intake) use judiciously in SWD to impede the patient's ability to sleep after the shift
- Sleep promoting:
  - Nonbenzodiazepine hypnotics:
    - Zolpidem 5 to 10 mg or eszopiclone 1 to 3 mg immediately prior to bed; suvorexant 10 to 20 mg PO 30 minutes prior to bed
  - Antidepressants
    - Doxepin (3 to 6 mg) and trazodone (25 to 150 mg), 1 to 2 hours prior to bed
  - Benzodiazepines: Estazolam, flurazepam, quazepam, temazepam, and triazolam are FDA approved for the treatment of insomnia. Due to high risk of tolerance/withdrawal, use cautiously for short-term treatment of insomnia.
  - In general, hypnotics may improve daytime sleep but does not appear to improve sleep maintenance or nighttime alertness. They may also cause residual sedation during work hours. This may worsen SWD symptoms.

ISSUES FOR REFERRAL
Refer to a sleep specialist for suspicion of other primary sleep disorders or dependence on hypnotics, alcohol, or stimulants.

ADDITIONAL THERAPIES
- Bright light therapy: Blue wavelengths are more effective and higher intensities (>2,000 lux) are recommended (1),(2).
- Cognitive-behavioral therapy for insomnia (CBT-I): It has been shown to have positive effects on sleep latency and total sleep time in small studies, but has not been evaluated in large, high-powered randomized control trials as of yet (2).
- Notably, there have been no high-powered, long-term studies to evaluate what effect these therapies have on comorbidities associated with SWD.

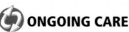

ONGOING CARE

PATIENT EDUCATION
Discuss sleep hygiene and optimizing the sleep environment. Shift workers who sleep in the daytime should ensure a cool, dark, quiet sleep environment. Reserve bedroom for sleeping and intimacy only. Remove televisions, cell phones, tablets, and laptop computers from the bedroom. When going to sleep, turn clock away from bed and discourage prolonged reading in bed. Blackout shades help achieve the proper darkness. Symptoms are associated with shift work and should resolve if shift work is eliminated, this may not be feasible for patients. Fatigue risk management programs to educate shift workers, especially night shift workers, about sleep and the hazards associated with sleep deficiency.

REFERENCES
1. Wickwire EM, Geiger-Brown J, Scharf SM, et al. Shift work and shift work sleep disorder: clinical and organizational perspectives. *Chest*. 2017;151(5):1156–1172.
2. Cheng P, Drake C. Shift work disorder. *Neurol Clin*. 2019;37(3):563–577.

ADDITIONAL READING
HelpGuide. Weekly sleep diary. https://www.helpguide.org/wp-content/uploads/2018/12/sleep-diary.pdf. Accessed November 6, 2022.

CODES

ICD10
G47.26 Circadian rhythm sleep disorder, shift work type

CLINICAL PEARLS
- SWD has been associated with increased risk for metabolic disorders and mood disorders.
- The first diagnostic step in SWD is to obtain a comprehensive sleep history and work history. Sleep diaries are helpful tools to assess sleep-wake patterns.
- Shift workers are at greater risk for accidents during night and early morning shifts.

S

SMELL AND TASTE DISORDERS
Beth K. Mazyck, MD • Daniel B. Kurtz, PhD, BS

 BASICS

DESCRIPTION
- Physiologically, the senses of smell and taste aid in normal digestion by triggering GI secretions.
- Loss of smell occurs more frequently than loss of taste, and patients frequently confuse the concepts of flavor loss (as a result of smell impairment) with taste loss (an impaired ability to sense sweet, sour, salty, or bitter).
- Smell depends on the functioning of CN I (olfactory nerve) and CN V (trigeminal nerve).
- Taste depends on the functioning of CNs VII, IX, and X. Because of these multiple pathways, total loss of taste (ageusia) is rare.
- Systems affected: nervous, upper respiratory

EPIDEMIOLOGY
Incidence
There are ~200,000 patient visits a year for smell and taste disturbances.

Prevalence
- Predominant sex: male > female. Men begin to lose their ability to smell earlier in life than women.
- Predominant age:
  – Age >80 years: 80% have major olfactory impairment; nearly 50% are anosmic.
  – Ages 65 to 80 years: 60% have major olfactory impairment; nearly 25% are anosmic.
  – Age <65 years: 1–2% have smell impairment.
- Prior to the COVID-19 pandemic, an estimated >2 million affected in the United States.
- Commonly occurs with SARS-CoV-2, the virus responsible for COVID-19

ETIOLOGY AND PATHOPHYSIOLOGY
- Smell and/or taste disturbances:
  – COVID-19: common in mildly symptomatic patients (~65%) but even more common in patients needing hospitalization (85%) (1),(2),(3). Unexplained chemosensory loss is a good predictor of COVID-19 (4),(5)[B].
  – Nutritional factors (e.g., malnutrition, vitamin deficiencies, liver disease, pernicious anemia)
  – Endocrine disorders (e.g., thyroid disease, diabetes mellitus, renal disease)
  – Migraine headache (e.g., gustatory aura, olfactory aura)
  – Sjögren syndrome
  – Toxic exposures
  – Neurodegenerative diseases (e.g., multiple sclerosis, Alzheimer disease, cerebrovascular accident, Parkinson disease)
  – Infections
- Smell-specific disturbance:
  – Nasal and sinus disease (e.g., allergies, rhinitis, rhinorrhea, URI)
  – Cigarette smoking
  – Cocaine abuse (intranasal)
  – Hemodialysis
  – Neoplasm (e.g., brain tumor, nasal polyps, intranasal tumor)
  – Systemic lupus erythematosus (SLE)
  – Bell palsy

- Taste-specific loss:
  – Oral appliances, procedures
  – Intraoral abscess, gingivitis
  – Damage to CNs VI, IX, or X
  – Stroke (especially frontal lobe)
- Selected medications:
  – Antibiotics: amikacin, ampicillin, azithromycin, ciprofloxacin, clarithromycin, doxycycline, griseofulvin, metronidazole, ofloxacin, tetracycline, terbinafine, β-lactamase inhibitors
  – Anticonvulsants: carbamazepine, phenytoin
  – Antidepressants: amitriptyline, doxepin, imipramine, nortriptyline
  – Antihistamines and decongestants: zinc-based cold remedies (Zicam)
  – Antihypertensives and cardiac medications: acetazolamide, amiloride, captopril, diltiazem, hydrochlorothiazide, nifedipine, propranolol, spironolactone
  – Anti-inflammatory agents: auranofin, gold, penicillamine
  – Antimanic drugs: lithium
  – Antineoplastics: cisplatin, doxorubicin, methotrexate, vincristine
  – Antiparkinsonian agents: levodopa, carbidopa
  – Antiseptic: chlorhexidine
  – Antithyroid agents: methimazole, propylthiouracil
  – Lipid-lowering agents: statins

Genetics
Unknown

RISK FACTORS
- Poor nutritional status
- Smoking

GENERAL PREVENTION
- Well-balanced diet
- Maintain good oral and nasal health.
- Avoid tobacco products, chemical exposures.

Geriatric Considerations
Anosmia also may be an early sign of degenerative disorders and has been shown to predict increased 5-year mortality (6)[B].

Pediatric Considerations
- In developing countries with poor nutrition (particularly zinc depletion), smell and taste disorders may occur.
- Delayed puberty in association with anosmia (± midline craniofacial abnormalities, deafness, or renal abnormalities) suggests the possibility of Kallmann syndrome (hypogonadotropic hypogonadism).

Pregnancy Considerations
Many women report increased sensitivity to odors during pregnancy as well as an increased dislike for bitterness and a preference for salty substances.

COMMONLY ASSOCIATED CONDITIONS
URI, allergic rhinitis, dental abscesses

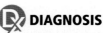 **DIAGNOSIS**

Smell and taste disturbances are symptoms; it is essential to look for possible underlying causes.

HISTORY
- Symptoms of URI, environmental allergies
- Fever, cough, sore throat suggestive of COVID-19 infection
- Oral pain, other dental problems
- Cognitive/memory difficulties
- Current medications
- Nutritional status, ovolactovegetarian
- Weight loss or gain
- Frequent infections (impaired immunity)
- Worsening of underlying medical illness
- Increased use of salt and/or sugar to increase taste of food
- Neurodegenerative disease

PHYSICAL EXAM
Thorough HEENT exam

DIFFERENTIAL DIAGNOSIS
- Epilepsy (gustatory or olfactory aura)
- Memory impairment
- Psychiatric conditions

DIAGNOSTIC TESTS & INTERPRETATION
Initial Tests (lab, imaging)
Consider (Not all patients require all tests.)
- SARS-CoV-2
- CBC, chemistry panel
- Vitamin B_{12} level
- Thyroid-stimulating hormone (TSH)
- Serum IgE
- CT scanning is the most useful and cost-effective technique for assessing sinonasal disorders and is superior to an MRI in evaluating bony structures and airway patency. Coronal CT scans are particularly valuable in assessing paranasal anatomy (7)[B].

Follow-Up Tests & Special Considerations
Diagnosis of smell and taste disturbances is usually possible through history; however, the following tests can be used to confirm:
- Olfactory tests
  – Smell identification test: evaluates the ability to identify 40 microencapsulated scratch-and-sniff odorants (8)[B]
  – Brief smell identification test (9)[B]
  – Taste tests (more difficult because no convenient standardized tests are presently available): Solutions containing sucrose (sweet), sodium chloride (salty), quinine (bitter), and citric acid (sour) are helpful.
  – An MRI is useful in defining soft tissue disease; therefore, a coronal MRI is the technique of choice to image the olfactory bulbs, tracts, and cortical parenchyma; possible placement of an accessory coil (TMJ) over the nose to assist in imaging

TREATMENT

GENERAL MEASURES
- Appropriate treatment for underlying cause
- Quit smoking.
- Treatment of underlying nasal congestion with nasal decongestants and/or nasal/oral steroids (10)[B]
- Surgical correction of nasal blockage/nasal polyps
- Drug-related smell or taste loss can be reversed with cessation of the offending medication, but it may take many months.
- Proper nutritional and dietary assessment (7)[C]
- Formal dental evaluation

MEDICATION
- Treat underlying causes as appropriate. Idiopathic cases will often resolve spontaneously.
- Consider trial of corticosteroids topically (e.g., fluticasone nasal spray daily to BID) and/or systemically (e.g., oral prednisone 60 mg daily for 5 to 7 days) (10)[B].
- Zinc and vitamins (A, B complex) when deficiency is suspected

ISSUES FOR REFERRAL
Consider referral to an otolaryngologist or neurologist for persistent cases.

 ONGOING CARE

DIET
- Weight gain/loss is possible because the patient may reject food or may switch to calorie-rich foods that are still palatable.
- Ensure a nutritionally balanced diet with appropriate levels of nutrients, vitamins, and essential minerals.

PATIENT EDUCATION
- Caution patients not to overindulge as compensation for the bland taste of food. For example, patients with diabetes may need help in avoiding excessive sugar intake as an inappropriate way of improving food taste.
- Patients with chemosensory impairments should use measuring devices when cooking and should not cook by taste.
- Optimizing food texture, aroma, temperature, and color may improve the overall food experience when taste is limited.
- Patients with permanent smell dysfunction must develop adaptive strategies for dealing with hygiene, appetite, safety, and health.

- Natural gas and smoke detectors are essential; check for proper function frequently.
- Check food expiration dates frequently; discard old food.

PROGNOSIS
- COVID-19 infection–associated smell loss:
  - Recovery of smell by 30, 60, 90, or 120 days was reported by 74%, 86%, 90%, and 96%, respectively (11). A small number will experience long-term loss, although recovery can still occur beyond 6 months.
- A small number of those who lost smell due to COVID-19 experience phantosmia or parosmia (phantom smells, or previously pleasant smells become foul).
- In general, the olfactory system regenerates poorly after a head injury. Most patients who recover smell function following head trauma do so within 12 weeks of injury.
- Patients who quit smoking typically recover improved olfactory function and flavor sensation.
- Many taste disorders (dysgeusias) resolve spontaneously within a few years of onset.
- Phantosmias that are flow dependent may respond to surgical ablation of olfactory mucosa.
- Conditions such as radiation-induced xerostomia and Bell palsy generally improve over time.

COMPLICATIONS
- Permanent loss of ability to smell/taste
- Psychiatric issues with dysgeusias and phantosmia

REFERENCES
1. Spinato G, Fabbris C, Polesel J, et al. Alterations in smell or taste in mildly symptomatic outpatients with SARS-CoV-2 infection. *JAMA*. 2020;323(20):2089–2090.
2. Menni C, Valdes AM, Freidin MB, et al. Real-time tracking of self-reported symptoms to predict potential COVID-19. *Nat Med*. 2020;26(7): 1037–1040.
3. Vaira LA, Hopkins C, Petrocelli M, et al. Smell and taste recovery in coronavirus disease 2019 patients: a 60-day objective and prospective study. *J Laryngol Otol*. 2020;134(8):703–709.
4. Parma V, Ohla K, Veldhuizen MG, et al. More than smell—COVID-19 is associated with severe impairment of smell, taste, and chemesthesis. *Chem Senses*. 2020;45(7):609–622.
5. Gerkin RC, Ohla K, Veldhuizen MG, et al. The best COVID-19 predictor is recent smell loss: a cross-sectional study. *medRxiv*. 2020;2020.07.22.20157263.
6. Pinto JM, Wroblewski KE, Kern DW, et al. Olfactory dysfunction predicts 5-year mortality in older adults. *PLoS One*. 2014;9(10):e107541.
7. Malaty J, Malaty IAC. Smell and taste disorders in primary care. *Am Fam Physician*. 2013;88(12):852–859.
8. Doty RL, Shaman P, Dann M. Development of the University of Pennsylvania Smell Identification Test: a standardized microencapsulated test of olfactory function. *Physiol Behav*. 1984;32(3):489–502.
9. Jackman AH, Doty RL. Utility of a three-item smell identification test in detecting olfactory dysfunction. *Laryngoscope*. 2005;115(12):2209–2212.
10. Seiden AM, Duncan HJ. The diagnosis of a conductive olfactory loss. *Laryngoscope*. 2001;111(1):9–14.
11. Tan BKJ, Han R, Zhao JJ, et al. Prognosis and persistence of smell and taste dysfunction in patients with COVID-19: Meta-analysis with parametric cure modelling of recovery curves. *BMJ*. 2022;378:e069503.

 CODES

ICD10
- R43.9 Unspecified disturbances of smell and taste
- R43.1 Parosmia
- R43.2 Parageusia

CLINICAL PEARLS
- Smell loss is often the first and only symptom of mild cases of COVID-19.
- Smell disorders are often mistaken as decreased taste by patients.
- Most temporary smell loss is due to nasal passage obstruction.
- Actual taste disorders are often related to dental problems or medication side effects.
- Gradual smell loss is very common in the elderly; extensive workup in this population may not be indicated if no associated signs/symptoms are present but may be predictive of 5- to 13-year mortality.
- Sudden unexplained smell loss may be a predictor of COVID-19.

SOMATIC SYMPTOM (SOMATIZATION) DISORDER

William G. Elder, PhD

 BASICS

DESCRIPTION

- Somatic symptom disorders (SSD) are a pattern of one or more somatic symptoms recurring or persisting for >6 months that are distressing or result in significant disruption of daily life.
- Designation of a symptom as somatic means that it appears to be physical problem or complaint yet is medically unexplained.
- Conceptualization and diagnostic criteria for somatic symptom presentations were significantly modified with the advent of *Diagnostic and Statistical Manual, 5th edition (DSM-5)*. SSD is similar in many aspects to the former somatization disorder, which required presentation with multiple physical complaints; no longer based on symptoms counts; current diagnosis is based on the way the patient presents and perceives his or her symptoms.
- SSD now includes most presentations that would formerly be considered hypochondriasis. Hypochondriasis has been replaced by illness anxiety disorder, which is diagnosed when the patient presents with significant preoccupation with having a serious illness in the absence of illness-related somatic complaints.
- Somatization increases disability independent of comorbidity, and individuals with SSD have health-related functioning that is 2 standard deviations below the mean.
- Symptoms may be specific (e.g., localized pain) or relatively nonspecific (e.g., fatigue).
- Symptoms sometimes may represent normal bodily sensations or discomfort that does not signify serious disease.
- Suffering is authentic. Symptoms are not intentionally produced or feigned.
- SSDs are sometimes referred to as "functional disorders" to denote their nonphysical basis and with the assumption that the illness behavior is a function of the environment.

EPIDEMIOLOGY

Incidence
- Usually, first symptoms appear in adolescence.
- Predominant sex: female > male (10:1)
- Type and frequency of somatic complaints may differ among cultures, so symptom reviews should be adjusted based on culture; more frequent in cultures without Western/empirical explanatory models

Prevalence
- Expected 2% among women and <0.2% among men
- Somatization is seen in up to 29% of patients presenting to primary care offices.
- Somatic concerns may increase, but other features of the presentation decrease such that prevalence declines after age 65 years.

ETIOLOGY AND PATHOPHYSIOLOGY
Patients with SSD demonstrate different patterns of heart rate variability. Although this cannot be used to clinically differentiate, it does point to the differences in psychophysiology of SSD. Also, not to be used clinically, patients with SSD display differences in brain functional connectivity, with the possibility that deficits in attention distort perception of external stimuli, affecting regulation of externally responsive body functioning (1)[C]. Reduced density in the form of decreased cell counts and radiologic signaling have also been detected in brain areas related to somatic sensation and emotional experience.

Genetics
Consanguinity studies and single nucleotide polymorphism genotyping indicate that both genetic and environmental factors contribute to the risk of SSD.

RISK FACTORS
- Child abuse, particularly sexual abuse, has been shown to be a risk factor for somatization.
- Symptoms begin or worsen after losses (e.g., job, close relative, or friend).
- Greater intensity of symptoms often occurs with stress.

COMMONLY ASSOCIATED CONDITIONS
Comorbid with other psychiatric conditions is yet to be determined but is likely to be 20–50% with anxiety, depression, or personality disorders.

DIAGNOSIS

- Determining that a somatic symptom is medically unexplained is unreliable, and it is inappropriate to diagnose a mental disorder solely because a medical diagnosis is not demonstrated. Rely on symptoms and presentation rather than ruling out medical causes in making the SSD diagnosis.
- Up to 10% of patients meeting criteria for SSD will be false positives for these diagnoses (2)[B].
- Illness anxiety and somatic distress are independent but often co-occur.

HISTORY
- One or more somatic complaints, with sometimes a grossly positive review of symptoms
- SSD involves patient's unrealistic thoughts, feelings, or behaviors associated with symptoms or associated health concerns manifested by at least one of the following:
  – Disproportionate and persistent thoughts about the seriousness of the symptoms
  – Persistent high level of anxiety about health or symptoms
  – Excessive time or energy devoted to symptoms or health concerns

- Diagnoses no longer rely on symptom counts, but common symptoms include:
  – Pain symptoms related to different sites such as head, abdomen, back, joints, extremities, chest, or rectum, or related to body functions such as menstruation, sexual intercourse, or urination
  – Gastrointestinal symptoms such as nausea, bloating, vomiting (not during pregnancy), diarrhea, intolerance of several foods
  – Sexual symptoms such as indifference to sex, difficulties with erection or ejaculation, irregular menses, excessive menstrual bleeding, or vomiting throughout all 9 months of pregnancy
  – Pseudoneurologic symptoms such as impaired balance or coordination, weak or paralyzed muscles, lump in throat or trouble swallowing, loss of voice, retention of urine, hallucinations, numbness (to touch or pain), double vision, blindness, deafness, seizures, amnesia or other dissociative symptoms, loss of consciousness (other than with fainting); none of these is limited to pain.
- Patients with SSD frequently use alternative treatments, which should be explored for their effects on health and physical functioning.

PHYSICAL EXAM
Physical exam remarkable for absence of objective findings to explain the many subjective complaints

DIFFERENTIAL DIAGNOSIS
- Other psychiatric illnesses must be ruled out:
  – Depressive disorders
  – Anxiety disorders
  – Schizophrenia
  – Other somatic disorders: illness anxiety disorder, conversion disorder
  – Factitious disorder
  – Body dysmorphic disorder
- Malingering
- General medical conditions, with vague, multiple, confusing symptoms, must be ruled out.
  – Systemic lupus erythematosus
  – Hyperparathyroidism
  – Hyper- or hypothyroidism
  – Lyme disease
  – Porphyria

DIAGNOSTIC TESTS & INTERPRETATION
Several screening tools are available that help to identify symptoms as somatic:
- Patient Health Questionnaire (PHQ)-15 (screens and monitors symptoms)
- Minnesota Multiphasic Personality Inventory (MMPI) (identifies somatization)

Initial Tests (lab, imaging)
- Laboratory test results do not support the subjective complaints.
- Imaging studies do not support the subjective complaints.

Test Interpretation
None are identified.

TREATMENT

GENERAL MEASURES
- The goal of treatment is to help the person learn to control the symptoms.
- Do not tell patients that the problems are in their head and that their symptoms are imaginary. Enhanced or structured care can be as effective as psychological interventions in adults.
- The involvement of a single provider is important because a history of seeking medical attention and "doctor shopping" is common.
- Patients usually receive the most benefit from primary care providers who accept the limitations of treatment, listen to their patient's concerns, and provide reassurance.
- A supportive relationship with a sympathetic health care provider is the most important aspect of treatment:
  – Regular scheduled appointments should be maintained to review symptoms and the person's coping mechanisms (at least 15 minutes once a month).
  – Acknowledge and explain test results.
- Antidepressant or antianxiety medication and referral to a support group or mental health provider can help patients who are willing to participate in their treatment.

MEDICATION
Antidepressants (e.g., SSRIs) help to treat comorbid depression and anxiety. Fluoxetine has been shown to have efficacy with illness anxiety disorder (formerly hypochondriasis), although >50% of those patients did not respond to the medication.

ISSUES FOR REFERRAL
- Discourage referrals to specialists for further investigation of somatic complaints.
- Referrals to support groups or to a mental health provider may be helpful.

ADDITIONAL THERAPIES
- Treatments have not been evaluated for this recently reformulated disorder. However, there are numerous studies with positive outcomes for child and adult patients with various forms of somatization or medically unexplained symptoms.
- Treatment typically includes long-term therapy, which has been shown to decrease the severity of symptoms.

- Individual or group cognitive-behavioral therapy addressing health anxiety, health beliefs, and health behaviors has been shown to be the most efficacious treatment for SSD. Cognitive processes modified in therapy include patient tendencies to ruminate and catastrophize.
- For children, SSD can result in missing school. School avoidance (malingering) and school anxiety should be your first considerations. Psychological interventions reduce symptom numbers and severity, disability, and school absence.
- Consideration should be given to providing integrated multidisciplinary care. For example, for patients with a functional gastrointestinal disorder, inclusion of dietitians, gut-focused hypnotherapists, psychiatrists, and behavioral (biofeedback) physiotherapists has been shown to improve symptoms, specific functional disorders, psychological state, quality of life, and cost of care for the treatment of functional gastrointestinal disorders.

 ONGOING CARE

FOLLOW-UP RECOMMENDATIONS
Patients should have regularly scheduled follow-up with a primary care doctor, psychiatrist, and/or therapist.

PATIENT EDUCATION
Encourage interventions that decrease stressful elements of the patient's life:
- Psychoeducational advice
- Increase in exercise
- Pleasurable private time

PROGNOSIS
- Chronic course, fluctuating in severity
- Full remission is rare.
- Individuals with this disorder do not experience any significant difference in mortality rate or significant physical illness.
- Patients with this diagnosis do experience substantially greater functional disability and role impairment than nonsomatizing patients.

COMPLICATIONS
- May result from invasive testing and from multiple evaluations that are performed while looking for the cause of the symptoms
- A dependency on pain relievers or sedatives may develop.

REFERENCES

1. Kim SM, Hong JS, Min KJ, et al. Brain functional connectivity in patients with somatic symptom disorder. *Psychosom Med*. 2019;81(3):313–318.
2. Henningsen P. Management of somatic symptom disorder. *Dialogues Clin Neurosci*. 2018;20(1): 23–31.

ADDITIONAL READING

Elder WG. Personality disorders. In: South-Paul JE, Matheny SC, Lewis EL, eds. *Current Diagnosis & Treatment: Family Medicine*. 5th ed. New York, NY: McGraw-Hill Education, 2020.

 CODES

ICD10
- F45.9 Somatoform disorder, unspecified
- F45.20 Hypochondriacal disorder, unspecified
- F45.22 Body dysmorphic disorder

CLINICAL PEARLS
- Diagnosis is based on a pattern of symptoms rather than an absence of medical explanation.
- A clue is accumulation of several diagnoses with >13 letters (e.g., chronic fatigue syndrome, fibromyalgia syndrome, reflex sympathetic dystrophy, temporomandibular joint syndrome, carpal tunnel syndrome, mitral valve prolapse).
- Inability of more than three physicians to make a meaningful diagnosis suggests somatization.
- Acknowledge the patient's pain, suffering, and disability.
- Do not tell patients that the symptoms are "all in their head."
- Emphasize that this is not a rare disorder.
- Discuss the limitations of treatment while providing reassurance that there are interventions that will lessen suffering and reduce symptoms.

S

SPINAL STENOSIS

Stephen W. Line, DO, CAQ-SM • Victoria Allon Nutting, DO, MS • Laura Marsh, MD, CAQSM

BASICS

DESCRIPTION
- A condition characterized by narrowing of either the central spinal canal, lateral recess, and/or neural foramen
- Symptoms may include pain, numbness, tingling, and muscle weakness.

EPIDEMIOLOGY
Prevalence
The prevalence of acquired spinal stenosis increases with age.
- Approximately 11–38% of adults will have some degree of lumbar stenosis on imaging (aged 19 to 93 years; mean age 62 years) (1).
- Lumbar spinal stenosis affects more than 200,000 people in the United States and is one of the most common reasons for spinal surgery in patients >65 years old (2).

ETIOLOGY AND PATHOPHYSIOLOGY
- Spinal stenosis can result from congenital or acquired causes (1).
  - Congenital spinal stenosis:
    o Developmentally short pedicles, achondroplasia, spinal dysraphism, spina bifida, and spondyloepiphyseal dysplasias.
  - Acquired spinal stenosis:
    o Spondylosis, spondylolisthesis (degenerative or due to pars interarticular fracture), trauma, postoperative changes, inflammatory arthropathy (e.g., ankylosing spondylitis, rheumatoid arthritis), and space-occupying lesions (tumors, cysts)
- The most common cause of acquired spinal stenosis is degenerative spondylosis.
  - May involve the lumbar, cervical, thoracic spine (in order of prevalence)
    o Within the lumbar spine, the L4–L5 and L5–S1 levels are the most frequently involved.
  - Degenerative changes leading to spinal cord and nerve root compression include disc degeneration, facet arthropathy, osteophyte formation, and ligamentum flavum hypertrophy (3).
    o Disc dehydration leads to loss of height with bulging of the disc annulus and ligamentum flavum into the spinal canal.
    o Increased facet loading causes reactive sclerosis and osteophyte formation which compresses neural structures.
  - Not all patients with radiographic spinal stenosis are symptomatic, and the degree of radiographic stenosis does not always correlate with the patients symptoms.
  - Symptomatic spinal stenosis is likely caused by mechanical compression and ischemia of spinal nerve roots. Increased intrathecal pressure may also lead to development of symptoms (3).

RISK FACTORS
Spinal trauma, spinal surgery, spine inflammatory arthropathy, vitamin B_{12} deficiency, osteoporosis, renal osteodystrophy, Cushing disease, acromegaly, and Paget disease

COMMONLY ASSOCIATED CONDITIONS
- Cervical or lumbosacral radiculopathy
- Degenerative spondylolisthesis
- Pars interarticular fracture
- Scoliosis
- Cauda equina syndrome

DIAGNOSIS

The diagnosis of spinal stenosis can be made clinically based on typical features and symptoms but is more commonly diagnosed radiographically. Anatomical narrowing can be seen in the absence of clinical symptoms.

HISTORY
- Insidious onset and slow progression are typical; discomfort with standing, paresthesias, and weakness (often bilateral) (3)
- Symptoms *worsen with extension* (prolonged standing, walking downhill or downstairs).
- Symptoms *improve with flexion* (sitting, leaning forward while walking, walking uphill or upstairs, lying in a flexed position, pushing a shopping cart, biking).
- Neurogenic claudication (i.e., pain, tightness, numbness, aching, and cramping of lower extremities) may mimic vascular claudication (2).
- The Zurich Claudication Questionnaire (ZCQ) is a self-administered measure to evaluate symptom severity, physical function, and satisfaction after treatment (2).

PHYSICAL EXAM
Neurologic exam may be normal. Key exam areas include the following:
- Inspection of spinal alignment:
  - Positive finding: loss of lordosis or scoliosis
- Palpation of the spinal region:
  - Positive finding: midline tenderness or paraspinal muscle tenderness
  - Most patients will not exhibit significant pain to palpation.
- Assessment of active or passive range of motion:
  - Positive finding: limitation in flexion, extension, sidebending, or rotation
  - Pain with extension of lumbar spine is typical.
- Muscle strength testing:
  - L4–L5 nerve root impingement may lead to weakness in hip abduction and great toe flexion.
  - S1 nerve root impingement may lead to hip extension weakness.
- Neurovascular evaluation:
  - Sensory changes (C5–T1 or L3–S1) may be detectable on light touch.
  - Deep tendon reflexes may be decreased.
  - About 50% of patients with LSS will have decreased Achilles reflex testing.
- Specialty testing:
  - Straight leg raise and Trendelenburg may be positive in nerve root impingement.
  - Positive Romberg test in the setting of low back pain (3)
  - FABER, FADIR, Ober, and log roll testing can help to rule out hip pathology
- Gait assessment:
  - A forward flexed gait, wide-based gate, or antalgic gait pattern is common.

DIFFERENTIAL DIAGNOSIS
- Vascular claudication
- Disc herniation or bulge
- Degenerative joint disease of the upper extremity (shoulder, elbow, or wrist)
- Degenerative joint disease of the lower extremity (hip, knee, or ankle)
- Peripheral neuropathy
- Cervical myelopathy

DIAGNOSTIC TESTS & INTERPRETATION
Generally, diagnosis is clinical. Diagnostic imaging is used to stage severity and formulate treatment plan.

Initial Tests (lab, imaging)
- CBC, ESR, C-reactive protein (if considering infection or malignancy)
- Plain radiographs (AP, lateral, oblique views)
  - Assists in excluding other causes of new back pain (e.g., malignant lytic lesions, vertebral compression fractures, degenerative spondylolisthesis, and scoliosis).
- MRI without contrast is the modality of choice (2),(3).

Follow-Up Tests & Special Considerations
- New back pain lasting >2 weeks or back pain accompanied by neurologic findings in patients >50 years generally warrants further evaluation, including evaluation for potential metastatic disease.
- CT myelography is an alternative to MRI but is invasive and has higher risk of complications.

Diagnostic Procedures/Other
- Electromyelography and nerve conduction studies are not required for diagnosis but may assist in ruling out other diagnosis such as peripheral neuropathy or cervical myelopathy.
- Ankle brachial index (ABI) testing can help diagnose or rule out peripheral arterial disease.

Test Interpretation
- Common radiograph findings include decreased disc height, facet hypertrophy, osteophyte formation, and spinal canal and/or foraminal narrowing.
- MRI will detail the extent and location of central canal stenosis, neuroforaminal stenosis, lateral recess stenosis, disc herniation/bulge, and other features of degenerative disc and spine disease.
- Radiologic abnormalities in general do not correlate with the clinical severity.

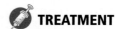

TREATMENT

- In general, nonoperative interventions are first line in the absence of progressive or debilitating neurologic symptoms:
  - Multimodal rehabilitation interventions, such as physical therapy, home exercise program, weight management (1)
  - Targeted injections (e.g., epidural steroid injections, facet joint injections) and radiofrequency ablation procedures (e.g., medial branch ablations) can help reduce symptoms (2),(3).
  - Expert consensus does not recommend the use of long-term NSAIDs, opioids, and adjunctive analgesics such as acetaminophen, methylcobalamin, and calcitonin in patients with LSS and neurogenic claudication (1).

- When conservative measures fail, neurosurgical or orthopedic spine consultation is warranted to prevent further neuropathy or myelopathy.
  - Patients should understand that the benefits of surgery may diminish over time.

MEDICATION

When pharmacotherapy is used, it is important to consider duration of treatment and the etiology of the symptoms as treatment of acute and low back pain can have varying recommendations.

First Line

- Nonsteroidal anti-inflammatory drugs (NSAIDs)
  - NSAIDs have been shown to provide modest relief in acute low back pain.
  - Consider potential for GI side effects, fluid retention, and renal failure. Use with caution in elderly.
  - COX-2 selective NSAIDs are associated with increased risk of serious cardiovascular events.
  - Typical treatment duration is 2 to 4 weeks and dose should be reduced once tolerated. Use with chronic low back pain is not recommended (1).
- Acetaminophen
  - Historically, acetaminophen has been considered a first-line medication for acute and chronic low back pain but recent evidence has shown mixed efficacy. Consider risk for hepatotoxicity (1).

Second Line

- Nonbenzodiazepine muscle relaxants
  - Have been shown to provide short-term effect symptomatic relief in acute low back pain
  - Provide mild analgesia in muscle spasm and modest skeletal muscle relaxation.
  - Side effect of sedation and dizziness is common.
    - Use with caution in geriatric population and those operating heavy machinery.
    - Consider dosing at bedtime to reduce sedation side effect.
- Management of chronic pain
  - Several medications may play a role in chronic pain management after assessment of risk profile. The following medications may be a reasonable option in select patients when contraindications exist to other pharmacotherapy options.
    - Gabapentin
    - Pregabalin
    - Duloxetine
    - Opiates (Tramadol often selected as first choice in this class)
      - Side effects of opioids include constipation, confusion, urinary retention, drowsiness, nausea, vomiting, and the potential for dependence and abuse. Use with caution in elderly.
  - Oral steroids, benzodiazepines, and antidepressants have inconsistent evidence for chronic pain and are typically not recommended as second-line agents.

ISSUES FOR REFERRAL

Nonsurgical patients with unremitting pain would benefit from pain management consultation. Consultation with neurosurgery or orthopedic spine specialist should be considered in patients with ongoing pain, progressive myelopathy, or worsening radicular symptoms that are refractory to conservative treatment.

ADDITIONAL THERAPIES

- Physical activity, core exercises, and gentle back mobility exercises are encouraged to prevent deconditioning.
- Modified exercise regimen (e.g., aquatic therapy, recumbent biking, walking, yoga, or Pilates)
- Lumbar spine bracing is controversial due to lack of evidence and due to concern for paraspinal muscle weakening with prolonged use.

SURGERY/OTHER PROCEDURES

- Surgery may be required for pain relief to increase mobility and improve quality of life.
- Surgical decompression is definitive for patients who are symptomatic after nonoperative treatment.
- Cognitive impairment, multiple comorbidities, and osteoporosis may increase the risk of perioperative complications.
- Surgical options include minimally invasive lumbar decompression (MILD), decompression with interspinous process spacers (IPS), and decompressive laminectomy (with or without fusion) (2),(3).

COMPLEMENTARY & ALTERNATIVE MEDICINE

Osteopathic manipulation, chiropractic techniques, acupuncture, massage, heat therapy, and cryotherapy can be considered.

- Severe spinal stenosis is a contraindication to high-velocity manipulation techniques.
- More clinical research is needed on these complementary modalities.

ADMISSION, INPATIENT, AND NURSING CONSIDERATIONS

- Admission criteria/initial stabilization: acute or progressive neurologic deficit.
- Discharge criteria: improved pain or after neurologic deficit has been addressed.

 ONGOING CARE

FOLLOW-UP RECOMMENDATIONS

- Follow-up is based on stability or progression of symptoms.
- No specific limitations to activity; patients may be as active as tolerated.

DIET

Optimize nutrition for weight management as obesity can significantly contribute to progression of symptoms (3).

PATIENT EDUCATION

Educate on common symptoms, treatments, and diagnostic options. Maintaining and active lifestyle should be encouraged. Discuss monitoring for red flags of low back pain, including bowel/bladder dysfunction, saddle anesthesia, progressive extremity numbness, or weakness.

PROGNOSIS

- Spinal stenosis can usually be managed conservatively, but the pain can lead to limitation in ADLs and progressive disability.
- Surgery usually improves pain and symptoms in patients who fail nonoperative treatment.
- Surgical outcomes are similar in terms of pain relief and functional improvement for patients of all ages.

COMPLICATIONS

- Severe spinal stenosis can lead to bowel and/or bladder dysfunction and disabling weakness.
- Surgical complications include infection, neurologic injury, chronic pain, and disability.

REFERENCES

1. Bussierès A, Cancelliere C, Ammendolia C, et al. Non-surgical interventions for lumbar spinal stenosis leading to neurogenic claudication: a clinical practice guideline. *J Pain*. 2021;22(9):1015–1039.
2. Diwan S, Sayed D, Deer TR, et al. An algorithmic approach to treating lumbar spinal stenosis: an evidence-based approach. *Pain Med*. 2019;20(Suppl 2):S23–S31.
3. Deer TR, Sayed D, Michels J, et al. A Review of Lumbar Spinal Stenosis with Intermittent Neurogenic Claudication: Disease and Diagnosis. *Pain Med*. 2019;20(Suppl 2):S32–S44.

ADDITIONAL READING

Comer C, Ammendolia C, Battié MC, et al. Consensus on a standardised treatment pathway algorithm for lumbar spinal stenosis: an international Delphi study. *BMC Musculoskelet Disord*. 2022;23(1):550.

 SEE ALSO

Algorithm: Low Back Pain, Acute

CODES

ICD10

- M48.00 Spinal stenosis, site unspecified
- M48.06 Spinal stenosis, lumbar region
- M48.04 Spinal stenosis, thoracic region

CLINICAL PEARLS

- Spinal stenosis most commonly affects the lumbar spine.
- Typical symptoms present as neurogenic claudication (pain, tightness, numbness, and subjective weakness of lower extremities). Flexion of the spine generally relieves symptoms associated with spinal stenosis, whereas extension of the spine tends to worsen symptoms.
- MRI is the diagnostic modality of choice.
- All patients with spinal stenosis should pursue lifestyle modifications.
- Additional conservative measures include physical therapy, home exercise programs, oral medications, and targeted epidural steroid injections. Consider surgical referral for decompression when spinal stenosis fails conservative management.

SPRAIN, ANKLE

Shane L. Larson, MD • Briana Lindberg, MD, CAQSM • Brock A. Benedict, DO

BASICS

DESCRIPTION

The most common cause of ankle injury comprising a significant proportion of injuries in the athletic and general populations:

- There are three types of ankle sprains: lateral, medial, and syndesmotic ("high ankle sprain"):
  - Lateral ankle sprains (LAS) are the most common. The anterior talofibular ligament (ATFL) is the most likely to be injured, followed by the calcaneofibular ligament (CFL) and then posterior talofibular ligament (PTFL) (1).
  - Medial ankle sprains (MAS) are the second most common and result from an injury to the deltoid ligament.
  - Syndesmotic injuries are the least common ankle sprains. These injuries result from injury to the syndesmosis between the distal tibia and distal fibula bones, consisting of the anterior, posterior, and transverse tibiofibular ligaments; the interosseous ligament; and interosseous membrane.
- Ankle sprains are classified according to the degree of ligamentous disruption:
  - Grade I: mild stretching of a ligament with possible microscopic tears
  - Grade II: incomplete tear of a ligament
  - Grade III: complete ligament tear

Geriatric Considerations
Increased risk of fracture in patients with preexisting bone weakness (osteoporosis/osteopenia)

Pediatric Considerations
- Increased risk of physeal injuries instead of ligament sprain because ligaments have greater tensile strength than physes
- Inversion ankle injuries in children may have a concomitant fibular physeal injury (Salter-Harris type I or higher fracture).
- Consider tarsal coalition with recurrent ankle sprains.

EPIDEMIOLOGY

Incidence
- Ankle sprains are very common in the general population and are some of the most commonly reported sport-related injuries. Nearly half of all ankle sprains occur during sports participation (1).
- The highest incidence of LAS occur in indoor/court sports (basketball, volleyball, tennis), followed by field sports such as football and soccer (1),(2).
- High ankle sprains are reported most frequently in men's football, wrestling, and soccer (1).

Prevalence
- 11–17% of high school and collegiate sports-related injuries in the United States (2)
- Although common in the general population, ankles sprains occur more frequently with athletic participation.

ETIOLOGY AND PATHOPHYSIOLOGY
- LAS result from an inversion force with the ankle in plantar flexion.
- MAS are due to forced eversion while the foot is in dorsiflexion.
- Syndesmotic sprains result from eversion stress/extreme dorsiflexion along with internal rotation of tibia.

RISK FACTORS
- Intrinsic risk factors
  - Limited ankle dorsiflexion range of motion
  - Reduced ankle proprioception
  - Decreased postural core strength/balance
  - Female gender
  - Low body mass index (BMI)
  - Poor strength, cardiorespiratory endurance, and/or coordination
  - Anatomical abnormalities of the knee, ankle, and/or foot
- Extrinsic risk factors
  - Type of sport played:
    ○ LAS: basketball, indoor volleyball, field sports and climbing
    ○ MAS: collegiate men's/women's soccer, men's football, women's gymnastics
    ○ Syndesmotic injury: football, wrestling, ice hockey
  - Higher heel height on footwear
- Prior history of ankle sprain may contribute to chronic ankle instability and increased risk for repeated ankle sprain (2).

GENERAL PREVENTION
- Address modifiable risk factors and improve overall physical conditioning:
  - Training in agility and flexibility
  - Single-leg balancing
  - Proprioceptive training
- Taping and/or bracing may help reduce the risk of both primary injury in selected sports (i.e., volleyball, basketball, football) or reinjury (1),(2). Taping and bracing do not reduce sprain severity.

COMMONLY ASSOCIATED CONDITIONS
- Contusions
- Fractures
  - Fibular head fracture/dislocation (Maisonneuve)
  - Fracture of the base of the 5th metatarsal
  - Distal fibula physeal fracture (includes Salter-Harris fractures in pediatric patients; most common type of pediatric ankle fracture)

DIAGNOSIS

HISTORY
- Elicit specific mechanism of injury (inversion vs. eversion).
- Popping/snapping sensation during the injury
- Previous history of ankle injuries
- Ability to ambulate immediately after the injury
- Rapid onset of pain, swelling, or ecchymosis
- Location of pain (lateral/medial)
- Difficulty bearing weight
- Past medical history of systemic disorders

PHYSICAL EXAM
- Timing: Initial assessment for laxity may be difficult due to pain, swelling, and muscle spasm. Repeating the exam ~5 days after injury often improves sensitivity.
- Compare to uninjured ankle for swelling, ecchymosis, weakness, and laxity.
- Assess the ability to bear weight, gait, and inspect for evidence of swelling, bruising, deformity, or other visible injuries.

- Palpate ATFL, CFL, PTFL, and deltoid ligament for tenderness.
- Palpate lateral and medial malleolus, base of 5th metatarsal, navicular, and entire fibula (concern for fibular head fracture with syndesmotic injury).
- Assess active and passive ankle range of motion with dorsiflexion, plantarflexion, inversion, and eversion.
- Determine strength in all ranges of motion.
- Evaluate neurovascular status.
- Special tests:
  - Anterior drawer test to check for ATFL laxity
  - Talar tilt test to check laxity in CFL (with inversion) or deltoid ligament (eversion)
  - Squeeze test: compress tibia and fibula midcalf to check for syndesmotic injury; sensitivity, 30%; specificity, 93.5%
  - Dorsiflexion/external rotation test: positive test is pain at syndesmosis with rotation; sensitivity, 20%; specificity, 85%
- Grade the injury.
  - Grade I sprain: mild swelling and pain; no laxity; able to bear weight/ambulate without pain
  - Grade II sprain: moderate swelling and pain; mild laxity with firm end point is noted; weight-bearing/ambulation is painful.
  - Grade III sprain: severe swelling, pain, and bruising; laxity with no end point; significant instability and loss of function/motion; unable to bear weight/ambulate

DIFFERENTIAL DIAGNOSIS
- Tendinopathy/tendon tear
- Fracture and/or dislocation of the ankle/foot
- Hindfoot/midfoot injuries
- Nerve injury
- Contusion

DIAGNOSTIC TESTS & INTERPRETATION
Initial Tests (lab, imaging)
- Ottawa ankle rules (sensitivity, 86–99%; specificity, 25–46%) may help determine need for radiographs to rule out ankle fractures (patient must be aged 18 to 55 years; certain patients, e.g., diabetics with diminished sensation, may still need radiographs):
  - Pain in malleolar zone
  - Inability to bear weight (walk ≥4 steps) immediately and in the exam room
  - Bony tenderness at distal 6 cm of the posterior edge of the lateral and/or medial malleolus
  - Bony tenderness with palpation of navicular
  - Tenderness on palpation at the base of 5th metatarsal
  - Although Ottawa ankle rules are highly sensitive, they should not overrule clinical judgment.
- If radiographs are indicated, obtain anteroposterior, lateral, and mortise views of the ankle.
  - Small avulsion fractures are associated with grade III sprains.
  - Stress views may assist in establishing the diagnosis of syndesmotic or deltoid ligament injuries (1).
- Ultrasound (US) is comparable to MRI in identifying major ligamentous injury, although it is operator-dependent. US also allows for dynamic assessment for stability and/or functional deficits (1).

- Consider CT if radiographs are negative but suspicion for occult fracture is high.
- MRI is the gold standard for soft tissue imaging but is expensive and rarely necessary.

Follow-Up Tests & Special Considerations
If the patient's condition does not improve in 6 to 8 weeks, consider CT, MRI, or US. Failure to resolve could indicate an injury such as a missed fracture, osteochondral defect, or syndesmotic injury.

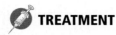 TREATMENT

GENERAL MEASURES
- Most grades I, II, and III lateral ankle sprains can be managed conservatively.
- Relative rest, ice, compression, and elevation (RICE) is a reasonable intervention in the acute phase (1)[A]. However, there is no evidence that RICE alone, cryotherapy alone, or compression alone impacts pain, swelling, or function for LAS but may improve pain, swelling, and function when used along with exercise (2)[A].
- Functional bracing (i.e., lace-up bracing) combined with exercise improves has better functional outcomes over immobilization (2)[A]. For significant pain/swelling, a short period of immobilization (<10 days) may improve pain and function prior to mobilization. For medial and syndesmosis sprains, a period of immobilization and protected weight-bearing for up to 2 weeks may prevent secondary injury (1)[B].
- Manual therapies (i.e., talocrural glides, talocrural distraction) following acute injury can improve ankle dorsiflexion, pain, and function (1)[A].
- Neuromuscular/proprioceptive training implemented within the first week following injury improves pain, swelling, return to activity, and it reduces the rate of reinjury when compared to RICE therapy (1)[A].

MEDICATION
- NSAIDs may be used judiciously in the acute phase to help with pain and swelling; however, there are some concerns that NSAID use may impair the normal inflammatory process necessary for healing (1),(2)[A].
  – Topical forms (e.g., 1% diclofenac gel) may be used to minimize gastrointestinal, renal, and cardiac side effects. PRN NSAID dosing has similar outcomes to scheduled dosing with improved safety profile.
  – Example: naproxen 500 mg BID PRN
- Acetaminophen 650 mg q4–6h (max outpatient therapy dose: 3,250 mg/day) is a reasonable alternative to NSAIDs to assist with reducing the pain in the first two weeks. Acetaminophen may be combined with NSAIDs without the risk of adverse drug interaction.

- Opioids (<5 days) if severe pain (rarely needed)
- Platelet-rich plasma (PRP) injections into the ATFL following LAS may improve short-term pain and function over bracing alone but are nonsuperior in the longer term. There is a limited evidence that PRP injection for syndesmosis injuries may lead to faster return to play over standard rehabilitation protocols (1)[A].

ISSUES FOR REFERRAL
- Malleolar/talar dome fracture
- Syndesmotic sprain
- Dislocation/subluxation
- Tendon rupture
- Ongoing instability
- Uncertain diagnosis

ADDITIONAL THERAPIES
Physical therapy:
- After the acute phase of the injury, early initiation of physical therapy can increase range of motion, strength, and flexibility, and it can improve proprioceptive balance (wobble board/ankle disk).
- Functional rehabilitation through physical therapy may prevent chronic instability and speeds healing.
- Athletes should undergo sport-specific rehabilitation before returning to play.

SURGERY/OTHER PROCEDURES
- Surgery is typically reserved for treatment of complicated recurrent sprains and certain syndesmotic sprains.
- Patients with chronic ankle instability who fail functional rehabilitation or with poor tissue quality may need anatomic repair/reconstructive surgery.

 ONGOING CARE

FOLLOW-UP RECOMMENDATIONS
- After an ankle sprain, consider ankle-stabilizing orthoses (air-stirrup braces, lace-up supports, athletic taping, etc.) for athletes participating in high-risk sports to prevent future ankle sprains.
- Moderate and severe sprains require ankle orthoses for ≥6 months during sports participation.
- Gradual return to play for athletes with a grade I lateral ankle sprain can generally be accomplished in 1 to 2 weeks; grade II sprain return to play time is 2 to 3 weeks; grade III sprain is approximately 4 weeks.
- Syndesmotic sprains take longer (~8 to 9 weeks) to heal than lateral ankle sprains.

Patient Monitoring
If athletes continue to have symptoms when they return to play or if a patient has pain for 6 to 8 weeks after injury, repeat examination and imaging.

PATIENT EDUCATION
- Crutch training
- Provide training on proper use of elastic bandages, brace, and/or orthoses.
- Demonstrate mobilization exercises (alphabet trace and towel grab).

PROGNOSIS
- Earlier physical therapy and mobilization with bracing allow for faster return to daily living and/or sports.
- Higher grade sprains, older patient age, and initial non–weight-bearing status have poorer prognosis and longer recovery.
- Ligamentous strength does not return for months after the injury.

COMPLICATIONS
- Joint instability
- Intermittent swelling/pain if not properly treated
- 5–33% continue to have pain 1 year postinjury.
- Accumulation of cartilage damage, leading to degenerative changes

REFERENCES
1. Chen ET, Borg-Stein J, McInnis KC. Ankle sprains: evaluation, rehabilitation, and prevention. *Curr Sports Med Rep*. 2019;18(6):217–223.
2. Vuurberg G, Hoorntje A, Wink LM, et al. Diagnosis, treatment and prevention of ankle sprains: update of an evidence-based clinical guideline. *Br J Sports Med*. 2018;52(15):956.

ADDITIONAL READING
- Caldemeyer LE, Brown SM, Mulcahey MK. Neuromuscular training for the prevention of ankle sprains in female athletes: a systematic review. *Phys Sportsmed*. 2020;48(4):363–369.
- D'Hooghe P, Cruz F, Alkhelaifi K. Return to play after a lateral ligament ankle sprain. *Curr Rev Musculoskelet Med*. 2020;13(3):281–288.
- Ortega-Avila AB, Cervera-Garvi P, Marchena-Rodriguez A, et al. Conservative treatment for acute ankle sprain: a systematic review. *J Clin Med*. 2020;9(10):3128.

CODES

ICD10
- S96.919A Strain of unsp msl/tnd at ank/ft level, unsp foot, init
- S93.499A Sprain of other ligament of unspecified ankle, init encntr
- S93.419A Sprain of calcaneofibular ligament of unsp ankle, init

CLINICAL PEARLS
- Children are at an increased risk of physeal injuries because ligaments are stronger than physes.
- Conditioning, including proprioceptive training, before participating in sports and throughout the season helps to prevent ankle sprains.
- Functional rehabilitation, rather than total immobilization, is recommended for quicker return to sport and work.
- Patients who do not adequately rehabilitate an ankle sprain are at increased risk for recurrence and chronic ankle instability.
- If patient's condition is not improving in 6 to 8 weeks, consider advanced imaging with CT, MRI, or US.

SPRAINS AND STRAINS

Lee A. Mancini, MD, CSCS*D, CSN • Alec L. Tributino, DO • Grant Pierre, MD, CAQSM

 BASICS

DESCRIPTION
- *Sprains* are complete or partial ligamentous injuries either within the body of the ligament or at the site of attachment to bone.
  - Classified as grade 1, 2, or 3 (AMA Ligament Injury Classification)
    - Grade 1: stretch injury without ligamentous laxity
    - Grade 2: partial tear with increased ligamentous laxity but firm end point on exam
    - Grade 3: complete tear with increased ligamentous laxity and no firm end point on exam
  - Usually secondary to trauma (e.g., falls, twisting injuries, motor vehicle accidents)
  - Physical exam is the key to accurate diagnosis.
- *Strains* are partial or complete disruptions of the muscle, muscle–tendon junction, or tendon.
  - Classified as
    - First degree: minimal damage to muscle, tendon, or musculotendinous unit
    - Second degree: partial tear to the muscle, tendon, or musculotendinous unit
    - Third degree: complete disruption of the muscle, tendon, or musculotendinous unit
  - Often associated with overuse injuries

Geriatric Considerations
More likely to see associated bony injuries due to decreased joint flexibility and increased prevalence of osteoporosis and osteopenia

Pediatric Considerations
- Sprains and strains account for 24% of pediatric injuries.
- 3 million pediatric sports injuries occur annually.
- Consider physeal/apophyseal injuries in the skeletally immature patient.

EPIDEMIOLOGY
Incidence
~80% of all U.S. athletes experience a sprain or strain at some point.

Prevalence
- Ankle sprains are among the most common injuries in primary care, accounting for ~30% of sports medicine clinic visits. Most ankle sprains are due to inversion injuries (lateral sprains) involving the anterior talofibular ligament; account for 650,000 annual ER visits in the United States
- Predominant age
  - Sprains: any age in physically active patient
  - Strains: usually 15 to 40 years of age
- Predominant sex: male > female for most; female > male for sprain of anterior cruciate ligament (ACL)

ETIOLOGY AND PATHOPHYSIOLOGY
- Trauma, falls, motor vehicle accidents
- Excessive exercise; poor conditioning
- Improper footwear
- Inadequate warm-up and stretching before activity
- Prior sprain or strain

RISK FACTORS
- Prior history of sprain or strain is the greatest risk factor for future sprain/strain.
- Change in or improper footwear, protective gear, or environment (e.g., surface)
- Sudden increase in training schedule or volume
- Tobacco use, medication adverse effects

GENERAL PREVENTION
- Appropriate warm-up and cool-down exercises
- Use proper equipment and footwear.
- Balance training programs improve proprioception and reduce the risk of ankle sprains.
- Semirigid orthoses may prevent ankle sprains during high-risk sports, especially in athletes with history of sprain.
- Proprioception and strength training decrease injury risk; stretching does not

COMMONLY ASSOCIATED CONDITIONS
- Effusions, ecchymosis, hemarthrosis
- Stress, avulsion, and/or other fractures
- Syndesmotic injuries
- Contusions
- Dislocations/subluxations

 DIAGNOSIS

HISTORY
- Obtain a thorough description of mechanism of injury including activity, trauma, baseline conditioning, and prior musculoskeletal injuries.
- May describe feeling or hearing pop or snap

PHYSICAL EXAM
- Inspect for swelling, asymmetry, ecchymosis, and gait disturbance.
- Evaluate for neurovascular compromise.
- Palpate for tenderness.
- Evaluate for decreased range of motion (ROM) of joint and joint instability/laxity.
- Evaluate for strength.
- Sprains
  - Grade 1: tenderness without laxity; minimal pain, swelling; little ecchymosis; can bear weight
  - Grade 2: tenderness with increased laxity on exam but firm end point; more pain, swelling; often ecchymosis; some difficulty bearing weight
  - Grade 3: tenderness with increased laxity on exam and no firm end point; severe pain, swelling; obvious ecchymosis; difficulty bearing weight

DIFFERENTIAL DIAGNOSIS
- Tendonitis
- Bursitis
- Contusion
- Hematoma
- Fracture
- Osteochondral lesion
- Rheumatologic process

DIAGNOSTIC TESTS & INTERPRETATION
- Ankle
  - Anterior drawer test assesses integrity of anterior talofibular ligament.
  - Talar tilt test assesses integrity of calcaneofibular ligament.
  - Squeeze test assesses for syndesmotic injury.
  - Palpate lateral and medial malleoli.
- Knee
  - Lachman and anterior drawer tests assess integrity of ACL. Posterior drawer and sag tests assess integrity of posterior cruciate ligament.
  - Valgus/varus stress tests assess integrity of medial and lateral collateral ligaments, respectively.
- Shoulder
  - Load and shift test; sulcus sign; and the apprehension, relocation, surprise test assess for instability of the glenohumeral joint.
- Radiographs help rule out bony injury; stress views may be necessary. Obtain bilateral radiographs in children to rule out growth plate injuries.
- Use Ottawa Foot and Ankle Rules (ages 18 to 55 years) to determine if radiographs are necessary.
- Ottawa Ankle Rules: x-ray required if pain in the malleolar zone *and*
  - Bone tenderness in posterior aspect distal 6 cm of tibia or fibula *or*
  - Unable to bear weight immediately or in emergency department
- Ottawa Foot Rules: x-ray required if midfoot zone pain is present *and*
  - Bone tenderness at base of 5th metatarsal *or*
  - Bone tenderness at navicular *or*
  - Inability to bear weight immediately or in emergency department

Follow-Up Tests & Special Considerations
- Can consider repeat x-rays in 1 to 2 weeks if symptoms not improved to rule out occult fracture
- CT scan can be considered if occult fracture is suspected.
- MRI is the gold standard for imaging soft tissue structures, including muscle, ligaments, and intra-articular structures. If tibiofibular syndesmotic disruption is suspected, MRI is highly accurate for diagnosis. Contrast is usually not necessary for diagnosis of most ligamentous and labral injuries.
- Ultrasound evaluation of a variety of muscles, tendons, and ligaments by a skilled operator allows for dynamic evaluation of potential sprain/strain that can add to traditional diagnostic imaging.

Diagnostic Procedures/Other
Surgery may be required for some partial and complete sprains depending on location, mechanism, and chronicity.

TREATMENT

GENERAL MEASURES

- Acute: *p*rotection, relative *r*est (activity modification), *i*ce, *c*ompression, *e*levation, *m*edications, *m*odalities (PRICEMM) therapy
- Ankle sprains: should consist of functional support, possibly augmented by nonsteroidal anti-inflammatory drugs in the early phases after injury
- Grades 1 and 2 ankle sprain: functional treatment with brace, orthosis, taping, elastic bandage wrap
  - Ankle braces (lace-up, stirrup-type, air cast) are a more effective functional treatment than elastic bandages or taping (1)[A].
- Grade 3 ankle sprain: Short period of immobilization may be needed. Consider short walking boot and/or crutches.
- Refer for early physical therapy.
- For high-level athletes with more extensive damage (e.g., biceps or pectoralis disruption), consider surgical referral.

MEDICATION

First Line

- Acetaminophen: not to exceed 3 g/day
- NSAIDs
  - Ibuprofen: 200 to 800 mg TID
  - Naproxen: 250 to 500 mg BID
  - Diclofenac: 50 to 75 mg BID
- Acetaminophen and NSAIDs have similar efficacy in reducing pain after soft tissue injuries with less GI side effects; NSAIDs are better than narcotics.
- Topical diclofenac, ibuprofen, and ketoprofen are effective for pain related to strains and sprains, especially in gel form or patch (2)[A].

Second Line

- Platelet-rich plasma injections may aid recovery in treatment of muscle strains, but more studies are needed.
- Opioids should rarely be considered acutely for severe pain, but discretion is advised.

ISSUES FOR REFERRAL

- ACL sprain in athletes/physically active
- Salter-Harris physeal fractures
- Joint instability especially if chronic
- Tendon disruption (i.e., Achilles, biceps, ACL)
- Lack of improvement with conservative measures

ADDITIONAL THERAPIES

- Physical therapy is a useful adjunct after a sprain, particularly if early mobilization is crucial.
  - Proprioception retraining
  - Core strengthening
  - Eccentric exercises
  - Thera-Band exercises
- After hamstring strain, frequent daily stretching and progressive agility and trunk stabilization exercises may speed recovery and reduce risk of reinjury (3)[A]. Rehab protocols emphasizing eccentric/lengthening exercises are more effective than conventional exercises (4)[B].

SURGERY/OTHER PROCEDURES

- Casting and surgery are reserved for select partial and complete sprains. Need for surgery depends on the neurovascular supply to the injured area as well as the ability to attain full ROM and stability of the affected joint. The need for surgery also depends on activity level and patient preference.
- For primary management of acute lateral ankle sprains, there is no difference between surgical versus conservative therapy. Risks are increased with surgical intervention.
- Chronic ankle instability affects 10–20% of people who sustain an acute sprain. If conservative management fails and laxity is present, surgery is considered (5)[A].
- Percutaneous needle tenotomy versus surgical tenotomy are available as options for chronic tendinosis (chronic, recurrent strains).

 ONGOING CARE

FOLLOW-UP RECOMMENDATIONS

If the affected joint has full strength and ROM, the patient can advance activity as tolerated using pain as a guide for return to activity.

Patient Monitoring

After initial treatment, consider early rehabilitation. Limit swelling and work on increasing ROM.

DIET

Weight loss if overweight

PATIENT EDUCATION

- Injury prevention through proprioceptive training and physical therapy
- ROM and strengthening exercises to restore functional capacity

PROGNOSIS

Favorable with appropriate treatment and rest. Duration of recovery depends on the severity and location of injury.

COMPLICATIONS

- Chronic joint instability
- Arthritis
- Muscle contracture
- Chronic tendinopathy

REFERENCES

1. Petersen W, Rembitzki IV, Koppenburg AG, et al. Treatment of acute ankle ligament injuries: a systematic review. *Arch Orthop Trauma Surg*. 2013;133(8):1129–1141.
2. Derry S, Moore RA, Gaskell H, et al. Topical NSAIDs for acute musculoskeletal pain in adults. *Cochrane Database Syst Rev*. 2015;2015(6):CD007402.
3. Pas HIMFL, Reurink G, Tol JL, et al. Efficacy of rehabilitation (lengthening) exercises, platelet-rich plasma injections, and other conservative interventions in acute hamstring injuries: an updated systematic review and meta-analysis. *Br J Sports Med*. 2015;49(18):1197–1205.
4. Askling CM, Tengvar M, Tarassova O, et al. Acute hamstring injuries in Swedish elite sprinters and jumpers: a prospective randomised controlled clinical trial comparing two rehabilitation protocols. *Br J Sports Med*. 2014;48(7):532–539.
5. McCriskin BJ, Cameron KL, Orr JD, et al. Management and prevention of acute and chronic lateral ankle instability in athletic patient populations. *World J Orthop*. 2015;6(2):161–171.

ADDITIONAL READING

- Hamilton BH, Best TM. Platelet-enriched plasma and muscle strain injuries: challenges imposed by the burden of proof. *Clin J Sport Med*. 2011;21(1):31–36.
- Kim TH, Lee MS, Kim KH, et al. Acupuncture for treating acute ankle sprains in adults. *Cochrane Database Syst Rev*. 2014;(6):CD009065.
- Monk AP, Davies LJ, Hopewell S, et al. Surgical versus conservative interventions for treating anterior cruciate ligament injuries. *Cochrane Database Syst Rev*. 2016;4(4):CD011166.
- Seah R, Mani-Babu S. Managing ankle sprains in primary care: what is best practice? A systematic review of the last 10 years of evidence. *Br Med Bull*. 2011;97:105–135.

 SEE ALSO

Tendinopathy

 CODES

ICD10

- S93.6 Sprain of foot
- S93.4 Sprain of ankle
- S93.5 Sprain of toe

CLINICAL PEARLS

For acute injury, remember PRICEMM:

- Protection of the joint
- Relative rest (activity modification)
- Apply ice.
- Apply compression.
- Elevate joint.
- Medications/ice for pain
- Other modalities as needed
- Wean out of brace as tolerated to limit atrophy of stabilizing muscles.

S

SQUAMOUS CELL CARCINOMA, CUTANEOUS

Sujitha Yadlapati, MD

BASICS

DESCRIPTION

Cutaneous squamous cell cancer is the second most common nonmelanoma skin cancer after basal cell carcinoma.

EPIDEMIOLOGY

Nonmelanoma skin cancer is the most common malignancy worldwide. Historically, squamous cell carcinoma (SCC) has been thought to account for 20% of nonmelanoma skin cancers, thus being the second most common malignancy after basal cell carcinoma. However, recent data indicate that the ratio of basal cell carcinoma to SCC is 1 in the U.S. Medicare population. An accurate incidence of cutaneous SCC is not known because this is not required to be reported to national cancer registries.

Incidence
- The average age for incidence is around 60 years, more common in men.
- Incidence increases the closer the person gets to the equator or higher altitude.

ETIOLOGY AND PATHOPHYSIOLOGY

Genetics
Some hereditary disorders have genes that are associated with cutaneous squamous cell cancer. They include:
- Xeroderma pigmentosum
- Oculocutaneous albinism
- Epidermodysplasia verruciformis
- Genes mutated include TP53, CDKN2A, NOTCH1, Ras, TP53 (most common gene involved in cutaneous SCC).

RISK FACTORS
- SCCs arise in:
  – Sun-damaged skin of elderly white individuals of European ancestry
  – Gender (more common in men)
  – Increasing age (average age of onset is the mid-60s)
  – Preexisting lesions of actinic keratosis (AK)
  – UV exposure
  – Preexisting conditions
  – Immunosuppression
    ○ Solid organ transplantation
    ○ HIV/AIDS, non-Hodgkin lymphoma, and chronic lymphocytic leukemia have increasing rates of developing cutaneous squamous cell cancer.
- Chronic skin conditions
  – Burn scars, hidradenitis suppurativa, chronic osteomyelitis, discoid lupus erythematosus, lichen planus, lichen sclerosis et atrophicus
- Inherited genetic conditions
  – Albinism, epidermolysis bullosa, xeroderma pigmentosum
- Ionizing radiation exposure
- Arsenic exposure

- Ulcers
- Bowen disease (SCC in situ)
- Erythroplasia of Queyrat (SCC in situ of the penis)
- HPV infection (6, 11, 16, 18)
- Treatment with BRAF inhibitors (vemurafenib and dabrafenib)

GENERAL PREVENTION
- Protect skin from sun exposure.
- Wear sunscreen, hats, and UV-protective clothing.
- Vitamin B_3 (nicotinamide) can repair DNA by preventing UV-induced adenosine triphosphate depletion.

COMMONLY ASSOCIATED CONDITIONS
AK is the precursor of cutaneous squamous cell cancer, Bowen disease, and erythroplasia of Querat.

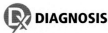**DIAGNOSIS**

- Histopathology remains the gold standard for the diagnosis of SCC. A punch or shave biopsy can be used to obtain a sample (1).
- Dermoscopy is a noninvasive technique that can help improve diagnostic accuracy (1).

PHYSICAL EXAM
- Lesions occur mainly in chronically exposed areas:
  – Face (especially lips, ear, nose, cheek, and eyelid)
- Lesions occur chiefly in chronically sun-exposed areas:
  – Face and backs of the forearms and hands
  – Bald areas of the scalp and top of ears in men
  – The sun-exposed "V" of the neck as well as the posterior neck below the occipital hairline
  – In elderly females, lesions tend to occur on the legs and other sun-exposed locations.
  – In African Americans, equal frequency in sun-exposed and unexposed areas
- Clinical appearance
  – Generally slow-growing, firm, hyperkeratotic papules, nodules, or plaques
  – Most SCCs are asymptomatic, although bleeding, pain, and tenderness may be noted.
  – Lesions may have a smooth, verrucous, or papillomatous surface.
  – Varying degrees of ulceration, erosion, crust, or scale
  – Color is often red to brown, tan, or pearly (indistinguishable from basal cell carcinoma).
- Clinical variants of SCC
  – Bowen disease (SCC in situ): a solitary lesion that resembles a scaly psoriatic plaque
  – Invasive SCC: often a raised, firm papule, nodule, or plaque. Lesions may be smooth, verrucous, or papillomatous, with varying degrees of ulceration, erosion, crust, or scale.

  – Cutaneous horn: SCC with an overlying cutaneous horn. A cutaneous horn represents a thick, hard, fingernail-like keratinization produced by the SCC. Bowen disease may also have a cutaneous horn on its surface.
  – Erythroplasia of Queyrat refers to Bowen disease of the glans penis, which manifests as one or more velvety red plaques.
  – Subungual SCC appears as hyperkeratotic lesions under the nail plate or surrounding periungual skin, often mimicking warts.
  – Marjolin ulcer: an SCC evolving from a new area of ulceration or elevation at the site of a scar or ulcer
  – HPV-associated SCC: virally induced; present as new or enlarging warty growth on the penis, vulva, perianal area, or periungual region
  – Verrucous carcinoma: a subtype of SCC that is extremely well differentiated, can be locally destructive, but rarely metastasizes. Lesions are "cauliflower-like" verrucous nodules or plaques.
  – Basaloid SCC: less common than typical SCC; seen more often in men aged 40 to 70 years

DIFFERENTIAL DIAGNOSIS
- AK
- Basal cell carcinoma

DIAGNOSTIC TESTS & INTERPRETATION
- Biopsy of the lesion will demonstrate characteristic histologic findings. Shave biopsy, punch biopsy, or excisional biopsy can be used (1).
- Histopathologic findings are as follows (1):
  – Pleomorphic, hyperchromatic squamous cells with nuclear pleomorphism (1)
  – Aggregates of glassy, eosinophilic keratinocytes (1)
  – Full-thickness atypia of the epidermis (1)
  – Keratinocyte mitoses (1)
  – Squamous pearls (1)
  – Inflammatory infiltrate of lymphocytes and plasma cells may be seen (1).
- Factors associated with local recurrence and metastases (2)
  – Tumor diameter >2 cm, associated with disease-specific death (2)
  – Perineural involvement of nerves more than 0.1 mm is associated with an increased risk of nodal metastases and increased mortality (2).
  – Poorly differentiated tumor (2)
  – Previously treated or recurrent SCC (2)
  – SCC arising in a scar (2)
  – Immunosuppression (1)
- Current staging systems
  – The American Joint Committee on Cancer's (AJCC) staging system published on October 2016, introduced the 8th edition.
  – Brigham and Women's Hospital tumor staging system
    ○ Proposed in 2013, offers an alternative T classification but does not include N or M staging criteria

o Strengths of this staging: better for prognostication when compared to AJCC-7. Most poor outcomes occur at staging T2b or higher (2).

o The weakness of this staging is that it is based on two large institutional studies only and has not been compared against AJCC-8 in a large population-based cohort (2).

Follow-Up Tests & Special Considerations

- For high-risk cutaneous squamous cell cancer:
  – Complete skin exam and lymph node exam required every 2 to 6 months
  – Every 6 to 12 months for the next 3 years
  – Annually after 5 years
- For high-risk cutaneous squamous cell cancer with regional disease: These are the follow-up recommendations:
  – Complete skin exam and lymph node exam every 1 to 3 months.
  – Every 2 to 4 months for the next year
  – Every 4 to 6 months until the 5th year
  – Every 6 to 12 months for the patient's lifetime

 TREATMENT

Selecting the most appropriate treatment options should involve consideration of the following:
- Tumor location and characteristics
- High-risk areas
- Recurrence rate
- Patient expectations
- Patient's functional status and life expectancy

MEDICATION

First Line

- First-line treatment for cutaneous SCC is complete surgical excision with histopathologic control of excision margins.
- Surgical excision provides these benefits:
  – Shorter healing time
  – Cure rate as high as 95%
- Mohs micrographic surgery (MMS) is the treatment for high-risk tumors instead of surgical excision.
  – MMS is the gold standard for treatment of high-risk SCC.
  – SCC with a low risk of metastasis can be treated with wide local excision, electrodesiccation, curettage, or cryosurgery.
  – Cryotherapy is used to treat small squamous cell cancers.
  – Cryotherapy or radiation can be used to treat patients who have bleeding disorders or contraindications to surgery.
  – MMS offers the highest cure for patients who have recurrent or high-risk primary squamous cell cancer.

Second Line

Advances in the management of cutaneous SCC
- Monoclonal antibodies (cetuximab, panitumumab)
- Tyrosine kinase inhibitors (erlotinib)

- Chemotherapy—used in locally advanced or metastatic skin squamous cell cancer
- Chemotherapeutic drugs used are methotrexate, bleomycin, doxorubicin, and cisplatin.
- Oral retinoids decrease the incidence of actinic keratosis and cutaneous squamous cell cancer.

SURGERY/OTHER PROCEDURES

- For high-risk cutaneous squamous cell cancer patients, who have tumors in inoperable locations and are poor candidates for surgery, they have the option of radiation therapy.
- Radiation therapy side effects include:
  – Malaise
  – Nausea
  – Radiation-induced erythema
  – Telangiectasia
  – Hypopigmentation
  – Epidermal atrophy
  – Soft tissue necrosis
  – Radiation-induced malignancy

ADMISSION, INPATIENT, AND NURSING CONSIDERATIONS

Examine sentinel lymph nodes for early detection of metastasis. This can decrease disease-related morbidity and mortality.

 ONGOING CARE

PROGNOSIS

- Patients with high-risk cutaneous squamous cell cancer have an increased risk of recurrence, lymph node, or distant metastases.
- From the lesions at risk, 7–80% will locally recur or metastasize within the first two years and 95% within the first five years of initial diagnosis.
- 30–50% of high-risk cutaneous squamous cell cancer patients will develop second skin cancer within five years.
- Cutaneous squamous cell cancer has an increased risk of metastasis if these characteristics below are present:
  – Tumor recurrence
  – Diameter ≥2 cm
  – Thickness >2 mm
  – Poorly differentiated histology
  – Invasion of subcutaneous tissue or structures such as perineural, vascular, or lymphatic
  – If the tumor is located on
    o Eye
    o Vermilion lip
    o "Mask areas" of the face
    o Hands
    o Feet
    o Genitalia
- MMS provides cure rate of 97% for primary cutaneous squamous cell cancer and 94% for recurrent cutaneous squamous cell cancer.
- MMS is very beneficial for treating high-risk cutaneous squamous cell cancers and preventing local recurrence.

- Staging is essential for treating high-risk cutaneous SCC.
- High-risk factors include:
  – Diameter ≥0.1 mm
  – Poorly differentiated histology
  – Tumor invasion beyond fat
  – Perineural invasion ≥0.1 mm
- After recurrence, the prognosis is inferior. There is a risk of distant metastasis and metastasis to regional lymph nodes.
- After resection of cancer, recurrent cancers have twice the risk of recurrence.
- For patients with metastatic disease, the long-term prognosis is poor.
  – For patients having distant metastasis, 10-year survival rates are <10%.
  – For patients having regional lymph node involvement, 10-year survival rates are <20%.
- Distant metastasis occurs in 15% of cases and involves these sites:
  – Brain
  – Lungs
  – Liver
  – Skin
  – Bone

COMPLICATIONS

- Local recurrence
- Metastasis

REFERENCES

1. Combalia A, Carrera C. Squamous cell carcinoma: an update on diagnosis and treatment. *Dermatol Pract Concept.* 2020;10(3):e2020066.
2. Que SKT, Zwald FO, Schmults CD. Cutaneous squamous cell carcinoma: incidence, risk factors, diagnosis, and staging. *J Am Acad Dermatol.* 2018;78(2):237–247.

 CODES

ICD10

- C44.92 Squamous cell carcinoma of skin, unspecified
- C44.320 Squamous cell carcinoma of skin of unspecified parts of face
- C44.42 Squamous cell carcinoma of skin of scalp and neck

CLINICAL PEARLS

- Cutaneous SCC associated with UV light exposure and immunosuppression
- The head and neck are the most common regions for invasive cutaneous SCC.
- MMS provides cure rates of 97% for primary cutaneous SCC.

STRESS FRACTURE

Dongsheng Jiang, MD, MSc • Joanna Jiang, MD

BASICS

DESCRIPTION
- Stress fractures are overuse injuries caused by cumulative microdamage from repetitive bone loading.
- Stress fractures occur in different situations:
  - Fatigue fracture: abnormal repetitive stress applied to normal bone (e.g., young college athletes or new military recruits with increased physical activity demands and inadequate conditioning); common sites include tibia, fibula, metatarsals, femoral neck, and navicular.
  - Insufficiency fracture: normal stress applied to structurally abnormal bone (e.g., femoral neck fracture in osteopenic bone, metabolic bone disease); common sites include spine, sacrum, femoral neck, and medial femoral condyle.
  - Combination fracture: abnormal stress applied to abnormal bone (e.g., female long-distance runners with premature osteoporosis from athletic triad)
- Weight-bearing bones of the lower extremity are most commonly affected at the following sites:
  - Tibia/fibula (most common)
  - Metatarsals (second most)
  - Navicular
  - Femoral neck
  - Pars interarticularis
- High-risk stress fractures occur in zones of tension or areas with poor blood supply and are more likely to result in fracture displacement and/or nonunion. High-risk sites include the following:
  - Femoral neck
  - Anterior tibial diaphysis
  - Sesamoids
  - Pars interarticularis of lumbar spine (L4, L5)
  - 5th metatarsal at metaphyseal–diaphyseal junction
  - Proximal 2nd metatarsal
  - Medial malleolus
  - Tarsal navicular
  - Patella
  - Talar neck
- Synonym(s): march fracture; fatigue fracture

EPIDEMIOLOGY
Incidence
- Greatest incidence in 15- to 27-year-olds
- Females > males
- Accounts for up to 20% of visits to sports medicine and orthopedic clinics

Prevalence
- Lifetime athletic stress fracture is 10% (1).
- Affects up to 6.9% of male and 21.0% of female military members

ETIOLOGY AND PATHOPHYSIOLOGY
- Bone is dynamic and constantly remodeling in response to applied physiologic stress.
- Repetitive loading or overuse causes microfractures that fail to heal due to imbalance between bone resorption and bone formation.
- If microdamage accumulates in excess of reparation, bony fatigue leads to stress fracture.

RISK FACTORS
- Intrinsic
  - Females are at 2.3 times higher risk than males.
  - Female athlete triad
  - Small tibial width
  - Later menarche, amenorrhea, or irregular menses
  - History of stress fracture
  - History of osteoporosis, osteomalacia, rheumatoid arthritis, prolonged corticosteroid therapy
  - BMI <19 kg/m²
  - Skeletal malalignment: pes cavus/planus, leg length discrepancies, excessive forefoot varus, tarsal coalitions, prominent posterior calcaneal process, tight heel cords
  - Biomechanical factors such as increased vertical loading rate (e.g., heel-to-toe running instead of forefoot striking)
- Extrinsic
  - High-risk exercises—track and field, cross country
  - Training regimen—running >20 miles/week or training >5 hr/day
  - Nutritional—inadequate caloric intake or history of eating disorder
  - Chronic low vitamin D
  - Rapid increase in mileage, running pace, or training volume
  - Inappropriate footwear
  - Hard training/running surface
  - Inadequate recovery or rest and training with fatigued muscle
  - Lifestyle: high alcohol intake or smoking
  - Meds: glucocorticoids, anticonvulsants, antidepressants, depot-medroxyprogesterone acetate (DMPA), methotrexate, antiretrovirals, chronic cannabis use, >5 years of bisphosphonate use

GENERAL PREVENTION
- Prevention is the key especially in adolescent athletes (1).
- Graduated increments in training load intensity: no >10% per week
- Optimize energy balance.
- Diversify sports participation (minimizing sports specialization).
- Reduce intensity and duration of activity if new-onset pain.
- Proper footwear (Athletes should have a gait analysis prior to training.)
- Increasing dynamic physical activity (jumping; plyometric training) increases bone density and resistance to mechanical stress.
- Decrease vertical loading rate either by switching to forefoot strike running or (if continuing with heel-to-toe strike) by using a heel pad insert.
- Vitamin D supplementation (800 IU/day) in combination with calcium (2,000 mg/day)

COMMONLY ASSOCIATED CONDITIONS
- Osteoporosis/osteopenia
- Female athlete triad
- Metabolic bone disorders

DIAGNOSIS

HISTORY
- Insidious onset of vague bony pain over a period of weeks; pain is typically worse with physical activity.
- Initially relieved by rest and then pain persists with rest or slight activity
- If untreated, pain progresses and may occur earlier during training sessions. With time and repetitive loading, the pain also becomes more localized.
- History of recent change in training intensity, alteration in training terrain, and/or footwear
- Assess dietary practices: energy availability, disordered eating, weight fluctuations, and calcium and vitamin D intake.
- In female athletes, assess menstrual history: menarche, oligomenorrhea, or amenorrhea.

PHYSICAL EXAM
- Height, weight, BMI, and any stigmata of disordered eating (cold extremities, hypercarotenemia, lanugo hair, calluses on back of fingers, poor oral hygiene, parotid gland hypertrophy, or orthostatic hypotension)
- Antalgic gait (limp; limiting weight on affected leg)
- Point or percussion tenderness over injury site: A vibrating tuning fork over the fracture site may intensify pain.
- Swelling may be present.
- Specific tests:
  - Hop test for tibial stress fracture: With a stress fracture, the patient cannot hop on one leg 10 times; if able to perform test, consider shin splints (medial tibial stress syndrome).
  - Fulcrum test for femoral stress fracture: With patient seated, provoke pain by applying downward force on the distal femur while the other hand is under the midthigh on femoral shaft (if clinical suspicion is high, defer or use only with extreme caution to avoid completing a femoral neck stress fracture).
  - Single-leg hyperextension (Stork) test for pars interarticularis fracture of lumbar spine: Stand on one leg and extend lumbar spine; positive if painful on symptomatic side
- Anatomic malalignment may be present (leg length discrepancy, scoliosis, pes planus/cavus).

DIFFERENTIAL DIAGNOSIS
- Shin splints (medial tibial stress syndrome—pain resolves with rest; stress fracture pain does not)
- Infection (osteomyelitis)
- Soft tissue injury (sprain, tendonitis, and periostitis)
- Exertional compartment syndrome
- Bony fracture, pathologic fracture, insufficiency fracture
- Neoplasm (osteoid osteoma)
- Nerve entrapment syndromes
- Intermittent claudication

DIAGNOSTIC TESTS & INTERPRETATION
Initial Tests (lab, imaging)
- Laboratory tests are not required unless clinically indicated for suspected disease (e.g., female athlete triad, hyperparathyroidism, vitamin D deficiency).
- May consider CBC, CMP, TSH, 25-hydroxyvitamin D(25[OH]D), FSH, LH plus 24-hour urine calcium and PTH

- Plain films (x-ray):
  - First line in suspected stress fracture
  - Findings typically seen 2 to 8 weeks after pain onset
  - High false negative rate during early stages (1 to 2 weeks)
  - May see periosteal callus, "gray cortex sign" (region of decreased cortical intensity), osteopenia, endosteal reaction, or ill-defined cortical margin
  - Severe cases may show discrete fracture.

Follow-Up Tests & Special Considerations
- MRI:
  - Gold standard for imaging stress fractures
  - Early signs (edema of bone and surrounding soft tissue) can be identified as early as 1 to 2 days after the onset of symptoms.
  - Sensitivity is up to 88%; specificity up to 100%, accuracy 90% (1)
- Bone scan:
  - Sensitive but has potential for false positives
  - Can show signs of stress fracture as early as 3 to 5 days after onset of symptoms
  - Useful for suspected rib or spine stress fractures
  - Should not be used to assess healing
- CT scan:
  - Less sensitive than MRI or bone scan for early stress fractures but has an important role in evaluating longitudinal fracture lines and occult fractures of foot, tibia, carpal scaphoid, and pars interarticularis
  - Can distinguish conditions (osteoid osteoma, malignancy, and osteomyelitis) that mimic stress fracture on bone scan; useful when fractures are chronic and are associated with low bone turnover
  - Bony detail provided by CT scan allows differentiation of complete versus incomplete fracture, especially if MRI is equivocal
- US: not routinely used but beneficial for superficial stress fracture
- Classification by radiographic findings (CT, MRI, bone scan, or x-ray)
  - Grade I: asymptomatic stress reaction; no pain, periosteal edema only, no fracture line
  - Grade II: symptomatic stress reaction; pain on exam, bone marrow edema, no fracture line seen on imaging
  - Grade III: nondisplaced fracture; pain on exam, nondisplaced fracture line seen on imaging
  - Grade IV: displaced fracture; pain on exam, displaced fracture >2 mm seen on imaging
  - Grade V: nonunion; pain on exam, nonunion characteristics on imaging, long-standing symptoms

 ## TREATMENT

- Low-risk stress fractures are generally treated nonoperatively with a 2-phase protocol (2):
  - Cessation of sport activity for 6 to 8 weeks
  - After a period of pain-free rest of 10 to 14 days, gradually return to activity over the subsequent weeks, including continued physical therapy.
    - Protection, rest, ice, compression, and elevation (PRICE) for acute pain and edema
    - Activity modification: Decrease activity to the level of pain-free functioning.

- Start alternative lower load exercises, such as hydrotherapy or swimming, antigravity treadmill cycling, and elliptical workouts, to maintain fitness.
    - Consider temporarily immobilizing patients who have pain at rest or with gentle range of motion.
    - If patients have pain with ambulation, use crutches with periodic walking trial to monitor readiness for nonaided (pain free) ambulation.
    - Pneumatic leg brace is effective in decreasing the return-to-play time for tibial shaft stress fracture.
    - Adequate recovery time is important to ensure proper healing of all stress fractures. The patient should be pain free before starting rehabilitation.
- High-risk fractures: typically require immediate immobilization and a period of non–weight-bearing; may require early surgical intervention to avoid nonunion and facilitate earlier return to sport
- Criteria for allowing an athlete to return:
  - A low-grade stress fracture at a high-risk location must heal fully prior to returning to full activity.
  - Complete resolution of symptoms with activities of daily living
  - 10 to 14 days after the patient is pain free
  - Radiographic evidence of healing
  - No tenderness to palpation at the injury site
  - Optimization of the athlete's nutritional, biomechanical, hormonal, and psychological status

MEDICATION
First Line
- Calcium (up to 2 g/day through diet sources)
- Vitamin D (800 to 4,000 IU/day) to maintain 25(OH)D levels between 32 ng/mL and 50 ng/mL (2)[C]
- Acetaminophen is useful for pain.
- NSAIDs are beneficial for pain and inflammation but may adversely affect fracture healing.

Second Line
- Bisphosphonates such as IV pamidronate or ibandronate may be useful (2)[C].
- Parathyroid hormone analog teriparatide is effective (2)[C].
- Oral contraceptives do not restore bone density in athletes (1).

ISSUES FOR REFERRAL
- Multidisciplinary team approach should always be considered to include parents, coaches, athletic trainers, PT, school nurse, nutritionist, rehab, team physician, PCP, gynecology, endocrinology, and orthopedics.
- Orthopedic consultation for high-risk fractures, failure to improve with standard treatment, evidence of nonunion within 3 to 4 weeks, or inability to tolerate rehabilitation

ADDITIONAL THERAPIES
- Electrical stimulation may be an adjunct for delayed union and nonunion.
- Extracorporeal shock wave therapy (ESWT) and pulsed US require additional study.
- Physical therapy

 ## ONGOING CARE

FOLLOW-UP RECOMMENDATIONS
Once the patient is pain free, low-impact training can be started and be advanced gently as tolerated.

Patient Monitoring
Imaging every 4 to 6 weeks to assess healing

DIET
- Adequate caloric intake
- Adequate calcium and vitamin D

PATIENT EDUCATION
Correct training errors with gait retraining.

COMPLICATIONS
- Delayed union
- Nonunion

REFERENCES
1. Beck B, Drysdale L. Risk factors, diagnosis and management of bone stress injuries in adolescent athletes: a narrative review. *Sports (Basel).* 2021;9(4):52.
2. da Rocha Lemos Costa TM, Borba VZC, Correa RGP, et al. Stress fractures. *Arch Endocrinol Metab.* 2022;66(5):765–773.

 ### SEE ALSO

Algorithm: Foot Pain

CODES

ICD10
- M84.38XA Stress fracture, other site, initial encounter for fracture
- M84.369A Stress fracture, unsp tibia and fibula, init for fx
- M84.376A Stress fracture, unspecified foot, init encntr for fracture

CLINICAL PEARLS
- The diagnosis of stress fractures requires a high index of suspicion. X-rays are often negative initially.
- Identify and treat female athletic triad or underlying metabolic conditions.
- To help prevent stress fractures, gradually increase training volume and avoid sudden increases in high-impact activity or running mileage. Ensure adequate nutrition intake including calcium, vitamin D.
- High-risk fractures require immediate immobilization and non–weight-bearing.
- Ensure gradual return to training with proper rehabilitation protocol for all stress fractures. Treat any underlying metabolic causes and mitigate risk factors.

STROKE, ACUTE (CEREBROVASCULAR ACCIDENT [CVA])

Mark B. Stephens, MD, MS, FAAFP

BASICS

DESCRIPTION
The sudden onset of a focal neurologic deficit(s) resulting from either ischemia/infarction or hemorrhage within the brain
- Two broad categories: ischemic (thrombotic or embolic) (87%) and hemorrhagic (13%)
- Hemorrhage: intracerebral or subarachnoid

Pediatric Considerations
Incidence: 2 to 13/100,000; frequent risk factors: arteriopathies (53%), cardiac disorders (31%), and infection (24%) (1)

EPIDEMIOLOGY
Incidence
Annual incidence in the United States is ~795,000.

Prevalence
Prevalence in the United States: 550/100,000. Predominant age: Risk increases >45 years of age. Highest during the 7th and 8th decades. Predominant sex: male > female at younger age but higher incidence in women with age ≥75 years.

ETIOLOGY AND PATHOPHYSIOLOGY
- 87% of strokes are ischemic; three main subtypes: thrombosis, embolism, and systemic hypoperfusion.
- 13% of strokes are hemorrhagic; most commonly due to hypertension (HTN)

Genetics
Stroke is a polygenic multifactorial disease.

RISK FACTORS
- Uncontrollable: age, gender, race, family history/genetics, prior stroke or TIA
- Controllable/modifiable/treatable
  - Metabolic: diabetes, dyslipidemia; lifestyle: smoking, alcohol, cocaine/amphetamine use, physical inactivity; cardiovascular: HTN, atrial fibrillation, valvular heart disease, endocarditis, recent MI, severe carotid artery stenosis, hypercoagulable states, patent foramen ovale (2)

GENERAL PREVENTION
Smoking cessation, regular exercise, avoid prolonged physical inactivity, weight control to maintain BMI <30 kg/m² and maximize glucose control, low-salt diet, moderate alcohol use; control BP; manage hyperlipidemia; antiplatelet therapy (e.g., aspirin) in high-risk persons; treat anticoagulation therapy for nonvalvular atrial fibrillation.

COMMONLY ASSOCIATED CONDITIONS
Coronary artery disease is the major cause of death in the first 5 years after a stroke.

DIAGNOSIS

HISTORY
- Determining time course is critical: Assess onset of symptoms. History from witnesses may be helpful.
- Acute onset of focal arm/leg weakness, facial weakness, difficulty with speech or swallowing, vertigo, visual disturbances, diminished consciousness

- Assess risk factors.
- Vomiting and severe headache favor hemorrhagic stroke (2).

PHYSICAL EXAM
- Assess airway, breathing, and circulation (ABC).
- Vital signs—pulse (character and rate) and BP
- Cardiovascular exam: bruits, pulses (regularity); murmurs; gallops; peripheral stigmata
- Pulmonary exam: signs of fluid overload or bronchospasm
- Neurological exam:
  - Anterior cerebral artery: motor/sensory deficit: (leg > face/arm), gait apraxia; abulia (inability to act willfully)
  - Middle cerebral artery:
    ○ Dominant: aphasia (inability to speak); motor/sensory deficit (face > arm > leg > foot); homonymous hemianopia
    ○ Nondominant: neglect, motor/sensory deficit (face/arm > leg > foot), homonymous hemianopia
  - Posterior cerebral artery: homonymous hemianopia; visual hallucinations; visual palsies; motor/sensory deficits; alexia (inability to read—"word blindness") without agraphia (inability to write)
  - Posterior (vertebrobasilar) circulation: diplopia, vertigo, gait and limb ataxia, facial paresis, Horner syndrome, dysphagia, dysarthria, alternating sensory loss
- The three most predictive findings for stroke on physical examination are (i) facial paresis, (ii) arm weakness or drift, and (iii) abnormal speech.
- National Institutes of Health Stroke Scale (NIHSS): stroke.nih.gov/documents/NIH_Stroke_Scale_508C.pdf

DIFFERENTIAL DIAGNOSIS
- Migraine (complicated); postictal state (Todd paralysis); systemic infection, including meningitis or encephalitis (infection may uncover or enhance previous deficits); toxic or metabolic disturbance (hypoglycemia, acute renal failure, liver failure, drug intoxication); brain tumor, primary or metastases; head trauma, encephalopathy, septic emboli (2)
- Other types of intracranial hemorrhage (epidural, subdural, subarachnoid)

DIAGNOSTIC TESTS & INTERPRETATION
Used to narrow differential and identify etiology of stroke

Initial Tests (lab, imaging)
- Serum glucose (*required* to exclude hypo/hyperglycemia prior to IV alteplase); electrocardiogram (ECG); CBC; electrolyte panel; baseline troponin; coagulation studies: PT, PTT, INR
- Emergent noncontrast head CT, within 20 minutes of arrival to the emergency department
- Subsequent multimodal CT (perfusion CT, CTA, unenhanced CT) or MRI improves diagnosis of acute ischemic stroke (AIS).

Follow-Up Tests & Special Considerations
Consider liver tests, toxicology screen, blood alcohol, ABG, lumbar puncture if suspected subarachnoid hemorrhage (SAH); EEG if suspect seizures, blood type, and cross
- Diffusion-weighted (DW) MRI is more sensitive than CT for AIS. MRI is better than CT for posterior fossa lesions.
- Prior to IV tissue plasminogen activator (tPA), a noncontrast head CT (rule out ICH) and glucose are the only required tests unless contraindications exist. MRI is not required. Multimodal imaging studies should not delay IV tPA.
- For patients who meet criteria for thrombectomy, multimodal CT and MRI to rule out large vessel occlusion is recommended. Selected patients may be treated up to 16 to 24 hours after onset of symptoms.

Diagnostic Procedures/Other
Echocardiogram (transthoracic and/or transesophageal) if there is suspicion of cardioembolic source. In cryptogenic stroke patients, perform prolonged ECG monitoring with a 30-day event monitor.

Test Interpretation
Early CT findings of ischemia: hyperdense MCA sign (increased attenuation of proximal portion of the MCA; associated with MCA thrombosis), loss of gray-white matter differentiation, sulcal effacement

TREATMENT
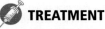

- Monitor BP closely in the first 24 hours.
  - Withhold antihypertensives unless systolic BP >220 mm Hg or diastolic BP >120 mm Hg. Goal is to lower BP ~15% in the first 24 hours if treatment. If thrombolytic therapy is planned, BP must be <185/110 mm Hg prior to administration of thrombolytics.
  - In acute spontaneous intracranial hemorrhagic stroke, goal BP is 160/90 mm Hg or MAP of 110 mm Hg
  - If there is suspicion of elevated ICP, reduce BP to a target cerebral perfusion pressure of between 61 and 80 mm Hg.
  - Start/restart antihypertensive medications 24 hours after stroke onset for patients with BP >140/90 mm Hg who are neurologically stable.
- Supplemental oxygen to maintain SaO₂ >94%
- Thrombolysis within 3 hours of onset and over the age of 18 years; severe stroke; mild but disabling stroke

- Thrombolysis if 3 to 4.5 hours from onset, between age 18 and 80 years and no history of *both* diabetes and prior stroke; NIHSS score less than 25; not taking oral anticoagulants and no imaging evidence of ischemic injury involving more than 1/3 of the middle cerebral artery territory.
  – History of ICH/symptoms suggestive of ICH; head trauma, MI or prior stroke within 3 months; GI malignancy or bleed within 21 days; major surgery within 14 days; arterial puncture at noncompressible site within 7 days; elevated BP (systolic >185 mm Hg and diastolic >110 mm Hg); active bleeding or evidence of acute trauma; taking anticoagulant and INR ≥1.7; low-molecular-weight heparin received during previous 24 hours; platelet count <100,000 mm³; blood glucose concentration <50 mg/dL; seizure with postictal neurologic impairment; multilobar infarction on CT (hypodensity >1/3 cerebral hemisphere); patient/family members unable to provide input and understand potential risks/benefits of treatment
- Extended AHA/ASA exclusion criteria for thrombolysis within 4.5 hours include the following:
  – Age >80 years; all patients taking oral anticoagulants; NIHSS >25; history of stroke and diabetes

MEDICATION

First Line

- Thrombolysis, IV administration of tPA (alteplase): Infuse 0.9 mg/kg, maximum dose 90 mg over 60 minutes with 10% of dose given as bolus over 1 minute. There is no benefit for patients with mild, nondisabling stroke symptoms (NIHSS scores 0 to 5). IV alteplase is preferred.
  – Door-to-needle time of <60 minutes. Admit to ICU or stroke unit, with neurologic exams every 15 minutes during infusion, every 30 minutes for the next 6 hours, and then hourly until 24 hours after treatment.
  – Discontinue infusion and obtain emergent CT scan if severe headache, angioedema, acute HTN, or nausea and vomiting develop.
  – Measure BP every 15 minutes for first 2 hours, every 30 minutes for next 6 hours, and then every hour until 24 hours after treatment. Maintain BP <185/105 mm Hg; follow-up CT before starting anticoagulants or antiplatelet agents
  – Obtain follow-up CT or MR at 24 hours after IV alteplase before starting anticoagulant or antiplatelet agents.
- Antiplatelet: aspirin 160 to 300 mg/day within 24 to 48 hours after AIS
- BP management options include the following:
  – Labetalol 10 to 20 mg IV over 1 to 2 minutes, may be repeated once
  – Nicardipine infusion 5 mg/hr, titrate 2.5 mg/hr at 5 to 15 minutes intervals to maximum of 15 mg/hr; reduce to 3 mg/hr when target BP is reached.

Second Line

Carotid endarterectomy (CEA) is indicated for >70% ipsilateral stenosis; may be indicated for 50–69% stenosis in carefully selected patients, depending on risk factors, and the skill and experience of the surgeon

ISSUES FOR REFERRAL

Follow-up with neurologist 1 week after discharge

ADDITIONAL THERAPIES

If no contraindications, consider a trial of fluoxetine to improve motor outcomes; deep vein thrombosis (DVT) prophylaxis; corticosteroids are *not* recommended for cerebral brain edema. Continue statin medication following acute stroke. Refer to PT, OT, and speech therapy as necessary.

SURGERY/OTHER PROCEDURES

- Ventricular drain for patients with acute hydrocephalus secondary to stroke
- Decompressive surgery is recommended for major cerebellar infarction.
- Endovascular thrombectomy (EVT) is an effective treatment for AIS patients up to 16 to 24 hours after the event.

COMPLEMENTARY & ALTERNATIVE MEDICINE

Acupuncture within 30 days of stroke onset may improve neurologic functioning.

ADMISSION, INPATIENT, AND NURSING CONSIDERATIONS

- Observe closely with frequent neurologic exams in first 24 hours for neurologic decline, particularly due to cerebral edema.
- Elevate head of bed to at least 30 degrees if elevated ICP is suspected. Patients with ischemic stroke may benefit from a horizontal bed position during the acute phase. Monitor cardiac rhythm for at least 24 hours to identify arrhythmias. Airway support and ventilatory assistance may be necessary due to diminished consciousness or bulbar involvement; reserve supplemental oxygen for hypoxic patients. Consider elective intubation for patients with malignant edema. Maintain oxygen saturation >94%. Correct hypovolemia with normal saline. Keep patients NPO until a formal swallow evaluation has been performed; to reduce risk of aspiration pneumonia, elevate head of bed to 30 degrees.
- Maintain IV hydration with normal saline until swallowing status is assessed. Hypoglycemia (especially <60 mg/dL) can cause neurologic dysfunction; correct initially. Hyperglycemia within first 24 hours of stroke is associated with poor outcomes: insulin recommended to maintain glucose levels 140 to 180 mg/dL. In patients with ICH secondary to anticoagulant use, correct an elevated INR with IV vitamin K and fresh frozen plasma or prothrombin concentrate complex.
- DVT prophylaxis; early PT and discharge planning for rehabilitation and placement; fall precautions; frequent repositioning to prevent skin breakdown
- Discharge criteria: medically stable, adequate nutritional support, neurologic status stable
- COVID-19 has been linked with hypercoagulability, with elevated D-dimer and fibrinogen levels that may explain a rise in stroke, although patients with severe disease are often older with other comorbidities that increase their risk as well.
- Admissions for mild and severe strokes have decreased since the COVID-19 pandemic, likely multifactorial, may be related to improved hygiene preventing against other infections linked to stroke or patient reluctance to visit the ED due to fear of exposure to SARS-CoV-2 virus.

 ## ONGOING CARE

FOLLOW-UP RECOMMENDATIONS

- Secondary prevention of stroke with aggressive management of risk factors; platelet inhibition using aspirin, clopidogrel, or aspirin plus extended-release dipyridamole (Aggrenox) based on physician and patient preference
- Stroke-like symptoms within 2 weeks of the initial event have a high chance of being recurrent stroke and should be followed up within 24 hours.

Patient Monitoring

Follow-up every 3 months for 1st year and then annually

DIET

Patients with impaired swallowing should receive nasogastric or percutaneous endoscopic gastrostomy feedings to maintain nutrition and hydration.

PATIENT EDUCATION

American Stroke Association (800-STROKES or http://www.stroke.org)

PROGNOSIS

Variable depends on subtype and severity of stroke; NIHSS may be used for prognosis.

COMPLICATIONS

- Acute: brain herniation, hemorrhagic transformation, MI, CHF, dysphagia, aspiration pneumonia, UTI, DVT, pulmonary embolism, malnutrition, pressure sores
- Chronic: falls, depression, dementia, orthopedic complications, contractures, OSA

REFERENCES

1. Powers WJ, Rabinstein AA, Ackerson T, et al. Guidelines for the early management of patients with acute ischemic stroke: 2019 update to the 2018 guidelines for the early management of acute ischemic stroke: a guideline for healthcare professionals from the American Heart Association/American Stroke Association. *Stroke*. 2019;50(12):e344–e418.
2. Kakkar P, Kakkar T, Patankar T, et al. Current approaches and advances in the imaging of stroke. *Dis Model Mech*. 2021;14(12):dmm048785.

 ## CODES

ICD10

- I63.9 Cerebral infarction, unspecified
- I61.9 Nontraumatic intracerebral hemorrhage, unspecified
- I63.50 Cereb infrc due to unsp occls or stenos of unsp cereb artery

CLINICAL PEARLS

- Unless stroke is hemorrhagic or patient is undergoing thrombolysis, do not lower BP acutely. This helps to maintain perfusion of penumbra region.
- IV thrombolysis (alteplase) is indicated within 4.5 hours of symptom onset for the majority of ischemic stroke patients. The earlier the treatment, the greater the patient benefit.
- Brain imaging (typically noncontrast CT) should be performed as quickly as possible for patients who are candidates for thrombolysis.

S

SUBCONJUNCTIVAL HEMORRHAGE

Nisarg Joshi, MD, BS

BASICS

DESCRIPTION

- Subconjunctival hemorrhage (SCH) is bleeding from small blood vessels underneath the conjunctiva, the thin clear skin covering the sclera (white outer layer) of the eye.
- SCH is diagnosed clinically:
  - Well-demarcated areas of extravasated blood can be seen just under the surface of the conjunctiva of the eye.
  - Lesions can be flat, elevated, or bullous.
- Typically, SCH self-resolves in a few days to weeks depending on the severity.

EPIDEMIOLOGY

Common; 3% rate of diagnosis in ophthalmology clinics (1)

Incidence

Incidence increases
- With increasing age
- In contact lenses wearers (5% of cases) (2)
- With systemic diseases such as diabetes, hypertension (HTN), and coagulation disorders
- With trauma
- During summer months, possibly due to trauma (1)

ETIOLOGY AND PATHOPHYSIOLOGY

- SCH results from damage to conjunctival and episcleral vessels from direct or indirect injury.
- Antithrombogenic and anticoagulated states (blood dyscrasias, thrombocytopenia, anemia, antiplatelet use, anticoagulant use) increase the risk and severity of SCH.
- Causes include the following:
  - Idiopathic
  - Direct trauma from
    - Blunt or penetrating injury to the eye
      - If there is a large SCH from a trauma, the patient may have underlying globe rupture and should be evaluated for this.
    - Contact lenses placement or removal; improper contact lenses wear

- Rubbing eyes
  - Commonly when sleeping, which leads to patient waking up with eye redness
  - In patient on anticoagulation, even mild eye rubbing can induce SCH.
  - Foreign body in eye
  - Ocular surgery, injection, or other procedure
  - Related to ocular surface infection (i.e., viral conjunctivitis) or ocular surface lesion
  - Valsalva maneuvers causing sudden severe venous congestion such as coughing, sneezing, vomiting, straining, severe asthma or COPD exacerbation, weight lifting, or childbirth/labor
  - Damaged vessels from atherosclerotic disease or diabetes (which is a cause of recurrent SCH without trauma)
- In patients aged >60 years, HTN is the most common etiology.
- In patients aged <40 years, trauma, Valsalva maneuver, and contact lenses use are the most common etiologies.
- In patients aged >40 years, conjunctivochalasis (redundant conjunctival folds) and presence of pinguecula are strongly associated (2).

RISK FACTORS

- Trauma
- Age
- Contact lenses wearer
- Systemic diseases (HTN, diabetes)
- Bleeding disorders (1)
- Recent ocular procedure (cataract, laser-assisted in situ keratomileusis [LASIK])

GENERAL PREVENTION

- Avoid rubbing the eyes.
- Proper cleaning and maintenance of contact lenses
- Protective eyewear during sports and hobbies
- Optimizing control of systemic diseases such as HTN, diabetes, atherosclerotic disease, and thrombocytopenia.
- Control of PT/INR in patients on warfarin therapy (3)

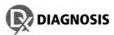

DIAGNOSIS

HISTORY

- Usually, the patient notices redness in the mirror or another person mentions it to the patient.
- Generally, patients do not have ocular symptoms like pain, light sensitivity, or decrease in vision.
- Patients may complain of mild irritation or foreign body sensation.
- Obtain history of trauma, recent ocular surgery, eye rubbing, contact lens use, eye infections, heavy Valsalva maneuvers (coughing, straining to have a bowel movement, lifting heavy objects, etc.) (1). SCH can occur 12 to 24 hours after orbital fracture (4).
- Evaluate medical history of systemic disease like diabetes mellitus, HTN, and coagulopathy.
- Ask about medications that may increase risk: aspirin, clopidogrel, other antiplatelets, and anticoagulants.
- Obtain history of other systemic symptomatology.

PHYSICAL EXAM

- Visual acuity, intraocular pressure, and pupils should be unaffected (3).
- Slit lamp exam shows bright red well-demarcated spots or patches. They are more often inferior due to gravity (2).
- Lesions can be flat, elevated, or bullous.
- The color of the conjunctiva changes over time. When the blood newly accumulates, the color is bright red. Older blood has a darker red color. The conjunctiva may have a yellow hue from blood-breakdown products as the hemorrhage dissipates.
- Fluorescein can be applied to assess for conjunctival and cornea abrasions/lacerations. Under cobalt blue light, there should be no stain uptake with a simple SCH.
- If the conjunctiva was lacerated, drops of blood can extrude from the conjunctiva onto the eyelid and periorbital skin.
- If a foreign body was involved, it could be hidden by the SCH.

- If there is a concern for penetrating or perforating ocular trauma, a shield should be placed over the eye, and the patient should be evaluated emergently by an ophthalmologist and/or trauma team.
- Measure blood pressure (BP) to evaluate for uncontrolled HTN (1).

Geriatric Considerations
In older adults, the area of SCH will be more widespread across the sclera (2). Elastic and connective tissues are more fragile with age, and underlying conditions such as HTN and diabetes may contribute.

DIFFERENTIAL DIAGNOSIS
- Viral, bacterial, allergic, or chemical conjunctivitis (enterovirus and coxsackievirus most common) (4)[B]
- Foreign body in/on the conjunctiva
- Penetrating or perforating trauma
- Recent ocular surgery/injection
- Contact lenses–induced
- Child abuse (particularly if bilateral in an infant or toddler) (4)
- Occasionally found in newborns following vaginal delivery

DIAGNOSTIC TESTS & INTERPRETATION
- Typically, no testing is indicated; SCH is a clinical diagnosis. If a foreign body is suspected, perform a fluorescein exam.
- Fluorescein exam of a patient with a SCH should show no uptake of fluorescein (3)[C].
- If an orbital fracture is suspected, an orbital/maxillofacial CT may be obtained (5)[C].

Follow-Up Tests & Special Considerations
If history and physical exam suggest a bleeding disorder (3)[C]
- CBC
- PT/INR

ALERT
- If a penetrating injury is suspected, may obtain a CT scan of the orbits
- Do not perform MRI because the foreign object may be metallic (5)[C].

 ## TREATMENT
- Reassurance is important.
- SCH self-resolves with time.
- Artificial tears can be used four times a day as needed for eye irritation (3)[C].

GENERAL MEASURES
- Control BP.
- Control blood glucose.
- Control INR.
- Wear protective eyewear.

ISSUES FOR REFERRAL
- If there is a history of any significant trauma, even blunt trauma, seek emergent ophthalmology consultation.
- If the patient complains of any decreased visual acuity or visual disturbances (i.e., new floaters), refer to an ophthalmologist as soon as possible.
- If there is no resolution of SCH within 2 weeks or if SCH are recurrent, patient may need referral to an ophthalmologist.

 ## ONGOING CARE

FOLLOW-UP RECOMMENDATIONS
- Follow up only if the SCH does not self-resolve.
- If SCH recurs, then work up patient for systemic associations such as bleeding disorders (3)[C] or diabetes.

PATIENT EDUCATION
- Reassurance of the self-limited nature of the problem and typical time frame for resolution
- Education to return to clinic if the area does not heal or recurs
- Correct cleaning and maintenance of contact lenses
- Eye lubricants for ocular irritation

PROGNOSIS
Excellent

COMPLICATIONS
Rare

REFERENCES
1. Mimura T, Usui T, Yamagami S, et al. Recent causes of subconjunctival hemorrhage. *Ophthalmologica*. 2010;224(3):133–137.
2. Mimura T, Yamagami S, Mori M, et al. Contact lens–induced subconjunctival hemorrhage. *Am J Ophthalmol*. 2010;150(5):656.e1–665.e1.
3. Cronau H, Kankanala RR, Mauger T. Diagnosis and management of red eye in primary care. *Am Fam Physician*. 2010;81(2):137–144.
4. Tarlan B, Kiratli H. Subconjunctival hemorrhage: risk factors and potential indicators. *Clin Ophthalmol*. 2013;7:1163–1170.
5. Wirbelauer C. Management of the red eye for the primary care physician. *Am J Med*. 2006;119(4):302–306.

CODES

ICD10
- H11.30 Conjunctival hemorrhage, unspecified eye
- H11.31 Conjunctival hemorrhage, right eye
- H11.32 Conjunctival hemorrhage, left eye

CLINICAL PEARLS
- SCH is a clinical diagnosis. The condition is typically asymptomatic and most will self-resolve within 2 weeks.
- Risk factors include trauma, Valsalva maneuver, HTN, and diabetes.
- Indications for immediate referral to an ophthalmologist include eye pain, changes in vision, lack of pupil reactivity, and/or suspected penetrating eye injury.
- Reassurance and comfort measures (i.e., ocular lubrication) are mainstays of treatment.

S

SUBSTANCE USE DISORDERS
S. Lindsey Clarke, MD, FAAFP • Benjamin J. Velky, MD

BASICS

DESCRIPTION
Any pattern of substance use causing significant physical, mental, or social dysfunction
- Substances of abuse include:
  – Alcohol
  – Cannabis (marijuana, hashish, cannabis oil, extracts); also sold as highly concentrated extracts for use in vaporizers
  – "Club drugs" (MDMA [ecstasy, Molly], PMMA [Superman], flunitrazepam, γ-hydroxybutyrate [GHB])
  – Dissociative drugs (ketamine, phencyclidine [PCP], tenocyclidine [TCP])
  – Hallucinogens (lysergic acid diethylamide [LSD], salvia, ayahuasca, N,N-dimethyltryptamine [DMT])
  – Inhalants (glue, paint thinners, nitrous oxide)
  – Opioids (carfentanil and other synthetic analogs of fentanyl, heroin, kratom, desomorphine [Krokodil], U-47700 [Pink])
  – Prescription medications
    ○ CNS depressants (barbiturates, benzodiazepines, hypnotics)
    ○ Dextromethorphan ("Robo tripping")
    ○ Opioids and morphine derivatives (fentanyl, hydrocodone, oxycodone, others)
    ○ Stimulants (amphetamines, methylphenidate)
  – Stimulants (cocaine, amphetamines, methamphetamines, khat)
  – Synthetic cannabinoids (Spice, K2, fake weed); often much more potent than marijuana; may be smoked or vaporized
  – Synthetic cathinones (bath salts, alpha-PVP [Flakka])
  – Tobacco

EPIDEMIOLOGY
Prevalence
- 61.2 million Americans (21.9%) reported illicit drug use in the past year in 2021.
- 14.1% of 12- to 17-year-olds; 38% of 18- to 25-year-olds
- 1 in 3 (35.4%) young adults used marijuana in the past year.

ALERT
- Opioid overdose is the leading cause of death for persons 26 to 38 years of age in the United States. More than 82% of these are due to synthetic opioids. There have been increasing cases of overdose and death related to synthetic opioids mixed with xylazine, which does not respond to naloxone administration.
- Many states require naloxone to be prescribed or offered when issuing a prescription of opioids to patients at increased risk of overdose, such as those receiving ≥50 morphine milligram equivalents per day of an opioid, those taking both opioids and benzodiazepines, and those with a history of substance abuse.

ETIOLOGY AND PATHOPHYSIOLOGY
Genetics
Substances of abuse affect dopamine and other neurotransmitter receptors. Variant alleles may account for differences in susceptibility to misuse of different substances.

RISK FACTORS
- Academic problems, school dropout
- Criminal involvement
- Depression, anxiety
- Family dysfunction or trauma
- Family history
- Peer or family use or approval
- Unemployment, low socioeconomic status

GENERAL PREVENTION
- Prescribe nonnarcotic therapies to treat pain and when necessary, use limited amounts to treat acute severe pain.
- Avoid prescribing narcotics for chronic conditions.
- Early identification and aggressive early intervention improve outcomes.
- Universal school-based interventions are modestly effective for prevention.

DIAGNOSIS
Substance use disorder (*DSM-5-TR* criteria): ≥2 of the following in the past year; severity graded by number of criteria present:
- Using more than intended
- Failed attempts to quit
- Increased time spent obtaining, using, or recovering from the substance
- Craving
- Failed obligations at work, school, or home
- Continued use despite social or interpersonal problems
- Interference with important activities
- Use in hazardous situations
- Continued use despite health problems
- Tolerance
- Withdrawal

HISTORY
- Anxiety, depression, psychosis
- Frequent visits to emergency department
- History of blackouts, insomnia, mood swings, chronic pain, repetitive trauma
- History of infections (e.g., endocarditis, hepatitis B or C, HIV, TB, STI, recurrent pneumonia)
- Incarceration
- Social or behavioral problems, including chaotic relationships and/or employment difficulties

PHYSICAL EXAM
- Abnormal vital signs
- Abnormally dilated or constricted pupils
- Cardiac dysrhythmias, pathologic murmurs
- Cutaneous needle marks
- Malnutrition
- Mental status changes

DIFFERENTIAL DIAGNOSIS
- Metabolic delirium: hypoxia, hypoglycemia, infection, thiamine deficiency, hypothyroidism, thyrotoxicosis, medication toxicity
- Mood, anxiety, and personality disorders

DIAGNOSTIC TESTS & INTERPRETATION
USPSTF recommends screening adults aged ≥18 years for unhealthy drug use when appropriate diagnosis and treatment services can be provided. USPSTF found insufficient evidence for or against such screening in adolescents.
- Substance Use Brief Screen and single-question screening tools (e.g., "How many times in the past year have you used an illegal drug or used a prescription medication for nonmedical reasons?") are sensitive (71–100%) and specific (61–96%) for identifying problem use in hospital and primary care settings (1)[A].
- CRAFFT questionnaire (sensitivity 94% with ≥2 "yes" answers):
  – C: Have you ever ridden in a CAR driven by someone (including yourself) who was "high" or who had been using alcohol or drugs?
  – R: Do you ever use alcohol or drugs to RELAX, feel better about yourself, or fit in?
  – A: Do you ever use alcohol or drugs while you are by yourself, or ALONE?
  – F: Do you ever FORGET things you did while using alcohol or drugs?
  – F: Do your FAMILY or FRIENDS ever tell you that you should cut down on your drinking or drug use?
  – T: Have you ever gotten into TROUBLE while you were using alcohol or drugs?
- American Academy of Pediatrics recommends the following screening tools for teens:
  – Screening to Brief Intervention (S2BI)
  – Brief Screener for Tobacco, Alcohol, and Other Drugs (BSTAD)

Pregnancy Considerations
- Substance abuse may cause fetal abnormalities, morbidity, and fetal or maternal death.
- Screen for substance use at the first prenatal visit with a brief intervention, and refer for treatment to improve maternal and neonatal outcomes

Initial Tests (lab, imaging)
- Blood alcohol concentration
- Urine drug screen
- Standard screening immunoassays may miss synthetic cannabinoids and opioids.
- Approximate detection limits
  – Alcohol: 6 to 10 hours
  – Amphetamines and variants: 2 to 3 days
  – Barbiturates: 2 to 10 days
  – Benzodiazepines: 1 to 6 weeks
  – Cocaine: 2 to 3 days
  – Heroin: 1 to 1.5 days
  – LSD, psilocybin: 8 hours
  – Marijuana: 1 to 7 days; up to 1 month with chronic/heavy use
  – Methadone: 1 day to 1 week
  – Opioids: 1 to 3 days
  – PCP: 7 to 14 days
  – Anabolic steroids: oral, 3 weeks; injectable, 3 months; nandrolone, 9 months
- Liver transaminases
- HIV, hepatitis B and C

Follow-Up Tests & Special Considerations
- Blood cultures, echocardiogram for endocarditis
- Head CT scan for seizure, delirium, trauma
- Right upper quadrant abdominal ultrasound for cirrhosis

TREATMENT

Determine substances abused early (may influence disposition).

GENERAL MEASURES
- Treatment should combine pharmacotherapy and cognitive behavioral therapy or another evidence-based modality when applicable (2)[A].
- Nonjudgmental, medically oriented attitude
- Motivational interviewing and brief interventions can promote change.
- Community reinforcement
- Interventional counseling
- Self-help groups to aid recovery (Alcoholics Anonymous, other 12-step programs)
- Support groups for family (Al-Anon/Alateen)

MEDICATION
- Benzodiazepine or barbiturate withdrawal
  - Gradual taper preferable to abrupt discontinuation
  - Substitution of long-acting benzodiazepine (e.g., clonazepam) or phenobarbital
- Opioid dependence
  - Buprenorphine: 8 to 24 mg SL daily, 100 to 300 mg SC monthly or as 6-month subdermal implant; may precipitate a more severe withdrawal if initiated too soon (3)[A]
  - Buprenorphine/naloxone: 2/0.5 mg to 16/4 mg SL daily; available as SL tabs and films and buccal films; combination limits abuse potential compared with buprenorphine alone.
  - Methadone: 10 to 40 mg/day PO; use restricted to inpatient settings and licensed clinics (3)[A]
  - Naltrexone: 50 mg PO daily, 100 mg PO every 2 days, 150 mg PO every 3 days, or 380 mg IM every 4 weeks; must be opioid-free for 7 to 10 days prior to treatment to avoid precipitating withdrawal
  - Naloxone: For opioid overdose, 0.4 to 2 mg IV/IM/SC, repeat every 2 to 3 minutes as needed; intranasal 4 to 8 mg, repeat every 2 to 3 minutes as needed. Refer to state mandates for coprescribing with opioid medications.
- Opioid withdrawal
  - Clonidine: 0.1 to 0.2 mg PO BID or TID for autonomic hyperactivity (3)[A]
  - Tramadol ER: 100 to 300 mg PO daily and then taper (off label) (3)[B]
- Adjuncts to therapy
  - Use all medications in conjunction with psychosocial behavioral interventions.
  - Antiemetics, nonaddictive analgesics for opioid withdrawal
  - Antidepressants, mood stabilizers, nonhabituating anxiolytics, and hypnotics for symptoms that persist after detoxification
- Contraindications
  - Buprenorphine in breastfeeding, hepatic impairment
  - Methadone in hepatic impairment
  - Naltrexone in pregnancy, breastfeeding, hepatic impairment
- Precaution: Clonidine can cause hypotension.

- Significant possible interactions
  - Buprenorphine and opioids, CNS depressants, or HIV protease inhibitors
  - Methadone and opioids, CNS depressants, or strong inhibitors of CYP3A4 (clarithromycin, ketoconazole, HIV protease inhibitors)
  - Naltrexone and opioid medications (may induce or exacerbate withdrawal)

ISSUES FOR REFERRAL
- Consider addiction specialist, especially for opioid and polysubstance abuse.
- Medication-assisted treatment for opioid dependence (e.g., methadone)
- Psychiatrist for comorbid psychiatric disorders
- Social services

ADMISSION, INPATIENT, AND NURSING CONSIDERATIONS
- Indications for inpatient detoxification
  - History of severe withdrawal (e.g., seizures)
  - Mental status changes; hallucinations or psychotic features
  - Threat of harm to self or others
  - Obstacles to close monitoring/follow-up
  - Comorbid medical illness
  - Pregnancy
- Look for signs of infection (e.g., bacterial endocarditis).
- Monitor for signs of drug use in the hospital.
- Discharge criteria
  - Detoxification is complete and a rehabilitation plan is in place.

 ONGOING CARE

FOLLOW-UP RECOMMENDATIONS
Initially frequent visits to monitor for medical stability and adherence and then progressive follow-up intervals

Patient Monitoring
Verify patient's adherence with the substance abuse treatment program.

PATIENT EDUCATION
- Substance Abuse and Mental Health Services Administration: https://www.samhsa.gov
- Alcoholics Anonymous: https://www.aa.org
- Narcotics Anonymous: https://www.na.org

PROGNOSIS
- Behavioral therapy and pharmacotherapy are most successful when used in combination.
- Patients in treatment for longer periods have higher success rates.

COMPLICATIONS
- Bacterial endocarditis
- Cirrhosis, hepatic malignancy, hepatitis, HIV, tuberculosis, syphilis
- Depression, psychosis
- Harm to self and others: accidents, violence
- Malnutrition
- Overdoses resulting in seizures, arrhythmias, cardiac and respiratory arrest, coma, death

- Sexual assault (alcohol, flunitrazepam, GHB)
- Social problems, including arrest, marital discord, and violence

REFERENCES
1. Han BH, Sherman SE, Link AR, et al. Comparison of the Substance Use Brief Screen (SUBS) to the AUDIT-C and ASSIST for detecting unhealthy alcohol and drug use in a population of hospitalized smokers. *J Subst Abuse Treat.* 2017;79:67–74.
2. Ray LA, Meredith LR, Kiluk BD, et al. Combined pharmacotherapy and cognitive behavioral therapy for adults with alcohol or substance use disorders: a systematic review and meta-analysis. *JAMA Netw Open.* 2020;3(6):e208279.
3. Srivastava AB, Mariani JJ, Levin FR. New directions in the treatment of opioid withdrawal. *Lancet.* 2020;395(10241):1938–1948.

ADDITIONAL READING
- Centers for Disease Control and Prevention. E-cigarette, or vaping, products visual dictionary. https://www.cdc.gov/tobacco/basic_information /e-cigarettes/pdfs/ecigarette-or-vaping-products -visual-dictionary-508.pdf. Accessed September 29, 2022.
- National Institute on Drug Abuse. Commonly used drugs charts. https://nida.nih.gov/research-topics /commonly-used-drugs-charts. Accessed September 29, 2022.

 SEE ALSO

Alcohol Use Disorder (AUD); Alcohol Withdrawal; Tobacco Use and Smoking Cessation

 CODES

ICD10
- F18.951 Inhalant use, unspecified with inhalant-induced psychotic disorder with hallucinations
- F11.120 Opioid abuse with intoxication, uncomplicated
- F17.201 Nicotine dependence, unspecified, in remission

CLINICAL PEARLS
- Substance use disorders are prevalent, serious, and often unrecognized in clinical practice. Comorbid psychiatric disorders are common.
- Substance abuse is distinguished by family, social, occupational, legal, or physical dysfunction that is caused by persistent use of the substance.
- Dependence is characterized by tolerance, withdrawal, compulsive use, and repeated overindulgence.
- Treatment should combine pharmacotherapy and cognitive behavioral therapy or another evidence-based modality when applicable.
- Consider referring patients with opioid dependence to an addiction specialist or to a certified outpatient treatment program.

SUICIDE

Irene Coletsos, MD • Harold J. Bursztajn, MD

BASICS

DESCRIPTION
Suicide and attempted suicide are significant causes of morbidity and mortality.

EPIDEMIOLOGY
- Women *attempt* suicide 1.5 times more often than men. Men *complete* suicide 3 times more often than women.
- In the United States; predominant age: 10 to 14 years; age 25 to 34 years (2nd leading cause of death), 11th leading cause of death overall, per 2021 Centers for Disease Control and Prevention (CDC) (latest available data as of September 2023).
- In the United States, more people died because of suicide in 2022 (>49,000) per CDC's initial review of 2022 data (the most recent available). CDC's analysis of finalized data from 2021 showed a sharp rate increase among specific populations: American Indian/Alaska Native: 42.6 per 100,000, 17% increase from 2020 to 2021; and during that same timeframe, rates increased for young adults aged 10 to 24 years. The CDC, through its Youth Risk Behavior Survey and researchers connected with the Trevor Project, which advocates for gender nonconforming youths, noted trends of increasing suicidal thoughts and behaviors (attempts) had increased—and that young adults who are gender nonconforming were 2 to 3 more times likely to have had a suicide attempt over the past year than young adults who are male and identify as gender conforming.
- Worldwide, suicide is the 4th leading cause of death among youths (ages 15 to 29 years), 15th leading cause of death per World Health Organization reports from 2020.

RISK FACTORS
- Be alert to a combination of increased emotional disturbance and access to the potential tools to cause death.
- 80% who complete suicide had a previous attempt.
- 90% who complete suicide meet *Diagnostic and Statistical Manual, 5th edition* criteria for major depression, bipolar, anorexia, panic, and personality disorders. Schizophrenia or acute onset of psychosis are also risk factors due to command hallucinations and hopelessness that can accompany these states. Delusional disorders—specifically persecutory and somatic delusions—are associated with increased depression accompanying those symptoms (1).
- Substance use and withdrawal
- Family history of suicide
- Physical illness, including head injury (associated with 20% increased risk of death by suicide)

- For teenagers: not feeling "connected" to their peers or family; being bullied; gender identity issues; poor grades
- Among veterans: childhood abuse; major depression; multiple psychiatric hospitalizations are the best predictors of suicide risk (2).
- Access to lethal means: firearms, poisons; including prescription and nonprescription drugs; pesticides

GENERAL PREVENTION
- Educate patients about 24/7 resources.
- Screen for risk: Use screening instruments *but* providers need to keep in mind risks particular to each patient, and might not be captured in some screening tools (see "Risk Factors"); and providers own biases in assessing risk. Screening instruments include the Patient Health Questionnaire-2 (PHQ-2), the PHQ-9, the Columbia Suicide Severity Rating Scale, Beck Scale for Suicide Ideation, Linehan Reasons for Living Inventory, and Motto Risk Estimator for Suicide.
- Treat underlying mental and medical illnesses and substance abuse. Continuity of care has been identified as a key protective factor. It is among the strategies in the "Perfect Depression Care" initiative out of a Detroit area HMO, and was associated with a 77% decrease in suicide rate.
- Screen for possession of means of harm, including prescribed/unprescribed drugs, poisons, and firearms
- Create a safety plan for patients at risk patients and their families, including how to access 24/7 emergency care.
- Public education about how to help others access emergency psychiatric care; suicidal people may initially confide in those they trust outside health care.
- For emergencies and imminent risk of harm, call 911.
- For additional resources, for needs ranging from quick support to educational:
  - For the military: Military Health System: Real Warriors Campaign: https://www.realwarriors.net; suggested treatments include cognitive restructuring techniques (that their experience with adversity can be a source of strength) and help with problem-solving (so the service member does not feel like a "burden"), therapeutic martial arts training, focus on vets helping others: "Power of 1" initiative (any "one" helpful contact could save a life).
  - For anyone in need within the United States: https://988lifeline.org/; text: Enter 988 to get a prompt allowing for communication via phone/text message/chat.
  - For teens, their families and their educators: CDC: https://www.cdc.gov/healthyyouth; StopBullying.gov: http://www.stopbullying.gov; https://988lifeline.org/help-yourself/youth/; text: https://988lifeline.org/chat/

- For members of "minority" populations (ethnic or gender) who are concerned that their cultures/life experiences might not be understood by the medical establishment, resources with counselors with specific knowledge/training include the following: https://988lifeline.org/help-yourself/black-mental-health/; https://988lifeline.org/help-yourself/native-americans/.
- For health care providers: multiple links available via links above; additional resources at the national Suicide Prevention Resource Center: https://sprc.org/

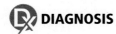

DIAGNOSIS

HISTORY
- Depressed patients should be asked about suicidal ideation and a potential plan:
  - "Have you ever felt that life isn't worth living? Do you ever wish you could go to sleep and not wake up? Are you having thoughts about killing yourself?"
- Use psychodynamic formulation: mental-state exam (including judgment, if the patient is able to make decisions, or affected by prescribed or nonprescribed drugs/drug withdrawal), history. If the patient is experiencing a loss, or is under stress, and does not have access to a previously sustaining resource (e.g., a significant other, a pet, sports ability, a job), that patient is under increased risk for suicide.
- Prior attempts: precipitants, lethality, intent to die, precautions taken to avoid being rescued, reaction to survival (A patient who is upset that the suicide was not completed is at increased risk for a subsequent attempt.)
- History of psychiatric symptoms, substance abuse
- Also note strengths, such as reasons to live, hopes for future, social supports; a patient without these strengths is at increased risk.
- Gather collateral history (from friends, family, physicians). Break confidentiality if patient is at imminent risk.

PHYSICAL EXAM
- Medical conditions: chronic illnesses (which can increase risk for hopelessness) or acute illnesses, such as delirium, intoxication, withdrawal, medication side effects, all which can impair judgment
- Psychosis
- In adults: (See "Risk Factors.")
- In teens: may not appear to be depressed; therefore, screen for chronic risk factors:
  - Adverse childhood experiences (ACEs)
  - Identification as a gender minority (LGBTQIA: Lesbian, Gay, Bisexual, Transgender, Queer/Questioning, Intersex, Asexual)

– Identification as an ethnic minority: American Indian/Alaska Native; black
– Screen for acute risk factors: substance abuse, social isolation and bullying (commonly through electronic media), poor grades.

DIFFERENTIAL DIAGNOSIS

Suicidal threats and gestures need to be immediately triaged to assess patient safety, although in some cases, the threat could be an attempt to manipulate others, such as in the case of personality disorders.

DIAGNOSTIC TESTS & INTERPRETATION
Diagnostic Procedures/Other

- PHQ-9: https://www.med.umich.edu/1info/FHP /practiceguides/depress/score.pdf
- Columbia Suicide Severity Rating Scale (C-SSRS) (clinical instructions): https://cssrs.columbia .edu/wp-content/uploads/C-SSRS_Pediatric -SLC_11.14.16.pdf
- Suicide Trigger Scale version 3 (STS-3), which measures a patient's "ruminative flooding" (self-critical, repetitive thoughts) and "frantic hopelessness" (feeling suicide is the only choice): https://www.ncbi .nlm.nih.gov/pmc/articles/PMC3443232/

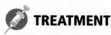 **TREATMENT**

GENERAL MEASURES

- Patients expressing active suicidal thoughts or who made an attempt require immediate evaluation for risk factors and a formal psychiatric consultation.
- Cognitive therapy decreased reattempt rate in prior suicide attempters by half (3),(4).
- Psychotherapy with suicidal patients is a challenge even for experienced clinicians. The countertransference, a clinician's feelings toward a patient, can evolve into wanting to be rid of the patient. If the patient detects this, the risk of suicide increases. Clinicians should be on the lookout for countertransference and get counseling if needed.
- Among military personnel: ACE campaign: Ask about suicidal thoughts; Care for the person, including removing access to lethal weapons; "Escort" the soldier/vet to help: an emergency room, a 911 call; call to a support hotline such as 1-800-273-TALK (8255); text: 838255

MEDICATION

- Psychopharmacology "is not a substitute for getting to know the patient."
- Patients are at increased risk of suicide at the outset of antidepressant treatment and when it is discontinued. Consider tapering/switching medicines rather than sudden discontinuation. Monitor carefully.
- Anxiety, agitation, and delusions increasing in intensity should be treated aggressively.
- In the inpatient/emergency room setting, agitated or combative patients may require sedation with IV or IM benzodiazepines and/or antipsychotics.

Pediatric Considerations
FDA posted black box warning for antidepressant use in the pediatric population after increased suicidality was noted. Weigh risks versus benefits of starting an antidepressant and closely monitor.

ISSUES FOR REFERRAL
Consider a psychiatric consultation. All decisions regarding treatment must be carefully documented and communicated to all involved health care providers.

ADMISSION, INPATIENT, AND NURSING CONSIDERATIONS

- Inpatient hospitalization if patient is suicidal with a plan, or otherwise at high risk; involuntary if at immediate risk
- Immediately after a suicide attempt, treat the medical problems resulting from the self-harm before initiating psychiatric care.
- Order lab work (e.g., solvent screen, blood and urine toxicology screen, aspirin and acetaminophen levels). Patients may not disclose ingestions.
- Risk for self-harm continues while inpatient: on arrival, patients should be searched for potentially dangerous items; be on one-to-one observation; offered medication to ease symptoms; use restraints only if necessary for patient safety.
- The period after transfer (involuntary to voluntary hospitalization; postdischarge) are times of high risk.
- Discharge when no longer considered a danger to self/others. Look for signs that the patient is truly at reduced risk, such as improved appetite, sleep, engagement with staff and group therapy.

 ONGOING CARE

FOLLOW-UP RECOMMENDATIONS
Patient Monitoring

- Increase monitoring at the beginning of treatment, when changing medications, and after hospital discharge.
- Educate family and other close contact to the warning signs of suicidality.
- Make sure that the patient is willing to accept recommended follow-up.
- Curtail access to firearms.
- Limit the number of pills to impulsive patients, but it might not prevent further attempts.

PATIENT EDUCATION
Patients who feel they are in acute danger of hurting themselves should consider one or several of these options:

- Call 911 or go directly to an emergency room.
- Contact treating therapist immediately.
- Call the National Suicide Prevention Hotline at (800) 273-TALK (8255).
- Service members and their families: call 1-800-796-9699 or 1-800-273-TALK (8255); text: 838255

PROGNOSIS
The key to a favorable prognosis is early recognition of risks, early treatment of disorders that had led to distress.

COMPLICATIONS
According to the American Association of Suicidology (AAS), the significant others of suicide victims may not seek help due to guilt or shame. It recommends counseling, including focus on the survivors' relationships. They may often seek out life partners to replace those they lost—interfering with mourning.

REFERENCES

1. González-Rodríguez A, Molina-Andreu O, Odriozola VN, et al. Suicidal ideation and suicidal behaviour in delusional disorder: a clinical overview. *Psychiatry J*. 2014;2014:834901.
2. Koola MM, Ahmed AO, Sebastian J, et al. Childhood physical and sexual abuse predicts suicide risk in a large cohort of veterans. *Prim Care Companion CNS Disord*. 2018;20(4):18m02317.
3. Brown GK, Ten Have T, Henriques GR, et al. Cognitive therapy for the prevention of suicide attempts: a randomized controlled trial. *JAMA*. 2005;294(5):563–570.
4. Ghahramanlou-Holloway M, Neely LL, Tucker J. A cognitive-behavioral strategy for preventing suicide. *Curr Psychiatr*. 2014;13(8):18–28.

 CODES

ICD10

- R45.851 Suicidal ideations
- T14.91 Suicide attempt
- Z91.5 Personal history of self-harm

CLINICAL PEARLS

- Key preventative measure is to listen to patients and take steps to keep them safe. This could include immediate hospitalization.
- Family and contacts of people who have attempted or committed suicide suffer from reactions ranging from rage to despair. Encourage counseling.
- Resources for clinicians: AAS: https://www.suicidology.org; www.suicideassessment.com
- Resources as noted in "General Prevention" section.

SUPERFICIAL THROMBOPHLEBITIS

Milap Dubal, MD, MPH

 BASICS

DESCRIPTION

- Superficial thrombophlebitis refers to a thrombosis-related inflammatory process of superficial veins.
- Most common in the lower extremities with 60–80% of total cases involving the greater saphenous vein but can occur in any location
- Classically, it was considered a benign and self-limiting process, but recent evidence associates it with increased risk of thromboembolic complications including progression to venous thromboembolism (VTE), subsequent VTE, or recurrent superficial thrombophlebitis.
- Traumatic thrombophlebitis types:
  – Injury
  – IV catheter related
  – Intentional/iatrogenic (i.e., sclerotherapy)
- Aseptic thrombophlebitis types:
  – Primary hypercoagulable states: disorders with measurable defects in the proteins of the coagulation and/or fibrinolytic systems
  – Secondary hypercoagulable states: clinical conditions with a risk of thrombosis (venous stasis, pregnancy, malignancy)
- Septic (suppurative) thrombophlebitis types:
  – Iatrogenic, long-term IV catheter use
  – Infectious, mainly syphilis and psittacosis
- Mondor disease—rare presentation of groin, penis, or anterior chest/breast veins
- System(s) affected: cardiovascular
- Synonym(s): phlebitis; phlebothrombosis, superficial vein thrombosis (SVT)

Geriatric Considerations
Septic thrombophlebitis is more common; prognosis is poorer.

Pediatric Considerations
Subperiosteal abscesses of adjacent long bone may complicate the disorder.

Pregnancy Considerations
- Associated with increased risk of aseptic superficial thrombophlebitis, especially during postpartum
- As NSAIDs are contraindicated during pregnancy, alternative therapeutic approaches are advised.

EPIDEMIOLOGY
- Mean age is 60 years old.
- 50–70% in women
- More common in those with varicose veins
- Epidemiology by thrombophlebitis types:
  – Traumatic/IV related has no predominant age/sex.
  – Suppurative and more common in extremes of ages (neonates, elderly)
  – Aseptic primary hypercoagulable state
    ○ Childhood to young adult
  – Aseptic secondary hypercoagulable state
    ○ Mondor disease: women, ages 21 to 55 years
    ○ Thromboangiitis obliterans onset: ages 20 to 50 years

Incidence
- Overall incidence is not well established. Current estimates put the incidence around 1.31 per 1,000 person-years, with increasing age associated with higher rates.
- Current incidence of catheter-associated septic thrombophlebitis is 0.5 per 1,000 days of peripherally inserted catheters.

- In pregnancy, incidence varies by trimester and postpartum. Per 1,000 person-years, incidence rates were 0.1, 0.2, 0.5, and 1.6 during the 1st, 2nd, and 3rd trimesters, and postpartum, respectively.
- Aseptic primary hypercoagulable state: Antithrombin III and heparin cofactor II deficiency incidence is 50/100,000 persons.
- Superficial migratory thrombophlebitis in 27% of patients with thromboangiitis obliterans

Prevalence
- Superficial thrombophlebitis is common with prevalence estimated between 3% and 11% of the general population.
- 1/3 of patients in a medical ICU develop thrombophlebitis that eventually progresses to the deep veins.

ETIOLOGY AND PATHOPHYSIOLOGY
- The process for thrombosis and phlebitis in superficial thrombophlebitis is variable but follows similar processes underlying thrombus formation in other vessels. These include venous stasis, vascular wall injury, microthrombi with subsequent platelet aggregation, and hypercoagulable states.
- Varicose veins play a primary role in etiology of lower extremity thrombophlebitis.
- Mondor disease pathophysiology not completely understood but thought to be related to local trauma/direct injury
- Less commonly due to infection (i.e., septic)
  – *Staphylococcus aureus, Pseudomonas, Klebsiella, Peptostreptococcus* sp.
  – *Candida* sp.
- Aseptic primary hypercoagulable state due to inherited disorders of hypercoagulability
- Aseptic secondary hypercoagulable states
  – Malignancy (Trousseau syndrome: recurrent migratory thrombophlebitis): most commonly seen in metastatic mucin or adenocarcinomas of the GI tract (pancreas, stomach, colon, and gallbladder), lung, prostate, and ovary
  – Pregnancy
  – Estrogen-based oral contraceptives
  – Behçet or Buerger disease

Genetics
Not applicable other than hypercoagulable states

RISK FACTORS
- Varicose veins
- Immobilization
- Obesity
- Advanced age
- Postoperative states
- Pregnancy or postpartum
- Hypercoagulable status
- Estrogen-based oral contraceptives
- History of previous superficial thromboembolism or venous thromboembolic event
- Trauma (IV placement/IV drug use, burns, surgery)
- Tobacco use (thromboangiitis obliterans)

GENERAL PREVENTION
- Avoid catheterization when possible, especially in the lower extremity.
- Insert catheters under aseptic conditions, secure cannulas, and replace every 3 days.

- Early mobilization and use usual deep vein thrombosis (DVT) prophylaxis in high-risk patients (i.e., ICU, immobilized)
- Minimize risk factors as able.

COMMONLY ASSOCIATED CONDITIONS
- Increasing evidence of association between superficial thrombophlebitis and VTE
- Estimated lifetime risk of VTE is 4 to 6 times higher in those with history of superficial thrombophlebitis.
- Frequently seen with concurrent DVT (6–53%)
- Symptomatic pulmonary embolism can also be seen concurrently (0–10%).
- Both DVT/PE can occur up to 3 months after onset of superficial thrombophlebitis.

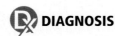 **DIAGNOSIS**

HISTORY
Patients classically complain of a section of firm, warm, and painful skin in a cord-like segment. This segment overlies the affected superficial vein. Patients may have risk factors as mentioned earlier.

PHYSICAL EXAM
- Swelling, tenderness, redness along the course of a vein or veins
- Examination often reveals a firm and tender palpable cord along the course of the vein with overlying cutaneous erythema.
- Fever in 70% of patients in septic phlebitis
- Sign of systemic sepsis in 84% of suppurative cases

DIFFERENTIAL DIAGNOSIS
- Cellulitis
- DVT
- Erythema nodosum
- Cutaneous polyarteritis nodosa
- Lymphangitis
- Contact dermatitis
- Other inflammatory vasculitides

DIAGNOSTIC TESTS & INTERPRETATION

Initial Tests (lab, imaging)
- H&P are usually adequate for diagnosis of superficial thrombophlebitis. If there is any uncertainty, venous ultrasonography can be completed.
- However, physical exam alone underestimates the extent of disease burden due to the association with DVT. Consequently, there is an increasing recommendation for a comprehensive duplex ultrasound to evaluate for the presence of DVT.

Follow-Up Tests & Special Considerations
- Patients with recurrent superficial thrombophlebitis or found with concurrent unprovoked VTE may benefit from additional testing for thrombophilia.
- If suspicious for sepsis
  – Blood cultures (bacteremia in 80–90%)
  – Consider culture of the IV fluids being infused.
  – CBC demonstrates leukocytosis.
- In migratory thrombophlebitis, have a high index of suspicion for malignancy.
- Consider repeat venous ultrasound to assess effectiveness of therapy.
  – If thrombosis is extending, more aggressive therapy required

Diagnostic Procedures/Other
Typically, additional labs and imaging are not needed.

TREATMENT

GENERAL MEASURES

- Patients with concomitant VTE should be treated per VTE standard of care.
- Suppurative thrombophlebitis treatment depends on source of infection, with typical treatment requiring source control (i.e., catheter removal), broad-spectrum antibiotics, and consultation for urgent surgical venous excision.
- Treatment of aseptic low-risk superficial thrombophlebitis is generally conservative, including NSAIDs and compression (1)[C].
  - Conservative management, antibiotics not useful
  - For varicosities, compression stockings; maintain activities.
  - Catheter/trauma associated
    ○ Immediately remove IV and culture tip.
    ○ Elevate with application of warm compresses.
    ○ If slow to resolve, consider LMWH.
- Large, severe, or septic thrombophlebitis
  - Inpatient care or bed rest with elevation and local warm compress
  - When the patient is ambulating, then start compression stockings or Ace bandages.

MEDICATION

First Line

- High-risk superficial thrombophlebitis
  - High risk defined as superficial phlebitis above the knee, age >65 years, male sex, previous VTE, cancer, autoimmune disease or SVT of non-varicose veins (2)[B]
  - Treat for 45 days with rivaroxaban 10 mg PO once daily or fondaparinux 2.5 mg SubQ once daily (3)[A]
- Otherwise, best medication(s) and duration of treatment are not well-defined, as 2018 Cochrane review found that most trials comparing NSAIDs, compression, elevation, other anticoagulation, and surgical interventions were small and of poor quality (3)[A].
- Localized, mild thrombophlebitis (usually self-limited)
  - NSAIDs and ASA for inflammation/pain to reduce symptoms and local progression
  - The use of compression stockings can also provide symptomatic relief.

Second Line

- Septic/suppurative
  - May present or be complicated by sepsis
  - Requires IV antibiotics (broad spectrum initially) and anticoagulation
- For low-risk SVT, anticoagulation with fondaparinux or rivaroxaban treatment can prevent extension of superficial venous thrombosis in addition to VTE prevention.
  - Consider if thrombus is large and close to the junction with deep veins or involves the long saphenous vein.
    ○ To prevent VTE, 4 weeks of LMWH, such as enoxaparin
    ○ 45 days of fondaparinux was found to reduce DVT and VTE by 85% (relative risk reduction) in one large study (4)[B].
- Superficial thrombophlebitis related to inherited or acquired hypercoagulable states is addressed by treating the related disease.

ISSUES FOR REFERRAL

- Severely inflamed or very large superficial thrombophlebitis should be evaluated for excision.
- Septic superficial thrombophlebitis should be urgently referred in the inpatient setting.
- Refer to vascular surgeon when patients require anticoagulation but have contraindications.

SURGERY/OTHER PROCEDURES

- Septic
  - Surgical consultation for excision of the involved vein segment and involved tributaries
  - Drain contiguous abscesses.
  - Remove all associated cannula and culture tips.
- Aseptic: Manage underlying conditions.
  - Evaluate for saphenous vein ligation to prevent deep vein extension after acute phase resolved.
  - Consider referral for varicosity excision.

ADMISSION, INPATIENT, AND NURSING CONSIDERATIONS

- Septic: inpatient
- Aseptic: outpatient

 ONGOING CARE

FOLLOW-UP RECOMMENDATIONS

Patient Monitoring

- Septic: routine WBC count and differential; target treatment based on culture result
- Aseptic
  - Some experts recommend follow up D-dimer to ensure decreasing thrombotic burden.
- Local, mild thrombophlebitis typically resolves with conservative therapy and does not require specific monitoring unless there is a failure to resolve.

DIET

No restrictions

PATIENT EDUCATION

- Review local care, elevation, and use of compression hose for acute treatment and prevention of recurrence.
- Counsel on risk of recurrence or progression.
- Counsel on signs of progression or failure of therapy.
- Counsel on need for follow-up or referral when additional workup may be required (concern for thrombophilia, migratory thrombophlebitis).

PROGNOSIS

- Septic/suppurative
  - High mortality (50%) if untreated
  - Depends on treatment delay, need for surgery, source of infection
- Aseptic
  - Usually benign course; recovery in 2 to 3 weeks
  - Depends on development of DVT and early detection of complications
  - Aseptic thrombophlebitis can be isolated, recurrent, or migratory.
  - Recurrence is likely if related to varicosity or if severely affected vein is not removed or if related to a persistent hypercoagulable state

COMPLICATIONS

- Septic: systemic sepsis, bacteremia (84%), septic pulmonary embolism (44%), metastatic abscess formation, pneumonia (44%), subperiosteal abscess of adjacent long bones in children
- Aseptic: DVT (6–53%), VTE (up to 10%), thromboembolic phenomena

REFERENCES

1. Nasr H, Scriven JM. Superficial thrombophlebitis (superficial venous thrombosis). *BMJ.* 2015;350:h2039.
2. Beyer-Westendorf J, Schellong SM, Gerlach H, et al. Prevention of thromboembolic complications in patients with superficial-vein thrombosis given rivaroxaban or fondaparinux: the open-label, randomised, non-inferiority SURPRISE phase 3b trial. *Lancet Haematol.* 2017;4(3):e105–e113.
3. Di Nisio M, Wichers IM, Middeldorp S. Treatment for superficial thrombophlebitis of the leg. *Cochrane Database Syst Rev.* 2018;2(2):CD004982.
4. Decousus H, Prandoni P, Mismetti P, et al; CALISTO Study Group. Fondaparinux for the treatment of superficial-vein thrombosis in the legs. *N Engl J Med.* 2010;363(13):1222–1232.

ADDITIONAL READING

Di Nisio M, Middeldorp S. Treatment of lower extremity superficial thrombophlebitis. *JAMA.* 2014;311(7): 729–730.

 SEE ALSO

Deep Vein Thrombophlebitis

CODES

ICD10

- I80.9 Phlebitis and thrombophlebitis of unspecified site
- I80.00 Phlbts and thombophlb of superfic vessels of unsp low extrm
- I80.8 Phlebitis and thrombophlebitis of other sites

CLINICAL PEARLS

- Mild superficial thrombophlebitis is typically self-limiting and responds well to conservative care.
- High-risk superficial thrombophlebitis should be treated with anticoagulation due to risk of extension. Lower extremity disease involving large veins or proximal saphenous vein likely benefits from anticoagulation to prevent DVT.
- Septic thrombophlebitis requires admission for antibiotics and anticoagulation. If severe, consider surgical consultation for venous excision.

SYNCOPE

Santiago O. Valdes, MD, FAAP • Alexander J. Kiener, MD

 BASICS

DESCRIPTION
- Transient loss of consciousness characterized by unresponsiveness and loss of postural tone with spontaneous recovery; usually brief and caused by cerebral hypoperfusion
- System(s) affected: cardiovascular, nervous

EPIDEMIOLOGY

Prevalence
- Approximately 20–35% of adults report ≥1 episode during their lifetime; 15% of children <18 years of age
- The prevalence in institutionalized elderly (>75 years of age) is 23%.

ETIOLOGY AND PATHOPHYSIOLOGY
Systemic hypotension secondary to decreased cardiac output and/or systemic vasodilation leads to a drop in cerebral perfusion and resultant loss of consciousness.

- Cardiac obstructions to outflow (e.g., pulmonary embolus [PE], hypertrophic cardiomyopathy, aortic stenosis)
- Cardiac arrhythmias
- Noncardiac
  - Reflex-mediated vasovagal (neurally mediated syncope [NMS]): inappropriate vasodilation leading to neurally mediated systemic hypotension and decreased cerebral blood flow; situational (micturition, defecation, cough, pain, emotions, hair combing)—most common cause in adult cases
  - Orthostatic hypotension (OHT): volume depletion, pregnancy, anemia, medications
  - Drug/alcohol induced
  - Primary autonomic failure: pure autonomic failure, Parkinson
  - Secondary autonomic failure: diabetes, amyloidosis
  - Carotid sinus hypersensitivity
- The vast majority of pediatric cases represent benign alterations in vasomotor tone.

RISK FACTORS
- Heart disease (acquired or structural)
- Dehydration
- Medications (e.g., antihypertensives, antiarrhythmics, diuretics)
- Presence of a primary autonomic degenerative disorder

 DIAGNOSIS

HISTORY
- Careful history, physical exam, and an ECG are more important than other investigations in determining the diagnosis (1).
- Make sure that the patient or witness (if present) is not referring to vertigo (i.e., sense of rotary motion, spinning, and whirling), seizure, or causes of fall without loss of consciousness. Onset of syncope is usually rapid, and recovery is spontaneous, rapid, and complete. Duration of syncopal episodes are typically brief (<60 seconds).
- Circumstances: Prolonged standing, urination, coughing, defecation, postprandial, and intense emotions are more likely to be associated with NMS. Consider carotid sinus hypersensitivity with abrupt neck movements. Consider cardiac cause with exertional syncope.
- Number of previous episodes (benign causes of syncope tend to be associated with a single episode)
- Presence of prodromal symptoms: Consider NMS.
  - Elderly patients are less likely to experience a prodrome.
- Palpitations, chest pain or dyspnea: Consider cardiac.
- Position (supine: arrhythmia; erect: NMS; supine → erect: OHT)
- Prolonged syncope: Consider psychiatric or neurologic.
- Delayed recovery: Consider neurologic (postictal).
- Ask for family history of long QT syndrome, catecholaminergic polymorphic ventricular tachycardia (VT), Brugada syndrome, implantable cardioverter-defibrillator (ICD), hypertrophic cardiomyopathy, or unexplained sudden cardiac death in young family members (<50 years).
- High-risk findings: new-onset chest discomfort, breathlessness, abdominal pain, headache, syncope during exertion or when supine, or sudden palpitations immediately followed by syncope.
- Even after careful evaluation, including diagnostic procedures and special tests, the cause will be found in only 50–60% of patients.

PHYSICAL EXAM
Check for orthostasis:
- Measure the BP and the pulse after the patient is supine for 5 minutes and then have the patient stand and repeat BP and pulse immediately, after standing 1 and 3 minutes.
  - A drop in systolic BP of ≥20 mm Hg or diastolic BP of ≥10 mm Hg is consistent with OHT. Induction of prodromal symptoms with postural changes even without vital sign changes is indicative of orthostatic intolerance.
  - Check for cardiac murmur or focal neurologic abnormality.
  - High-risk findings: unexplained systolic BP <90 mm Hg, suggestion of GI bleed on rectal exam, persistent bradycardia (<40 beats/min) in absence of physical training, or undiagnosed systolic murmur

DIFFERENTIAL DIAGNOSIS
- Drop attacks
- Vertigo
- Seizure disorder; stroke/transient ischemic attacks (TIAs)
- Psychiatric (conversion, somatization): lack hemodynamic and/or autonomic changes

DIAGNOSTIC TESTS & INTERPRETATION
Identify life-threatening conditions or those associated with significant risk of injury (2)[C].

- Evaluation of Guidelines in Syncope Study (EGSYS) Score may be used in adults, as other algorithms to suspect cardiac syncope (3)[C].

Initial Tests (lab, imaging)
- ECG: Consider cardiac cause if there are ischemic changes, bifascicular block, AV block, sinus bradycardia <40 beats/min or sinus pause >3 seconds, prolonged QTc, preexcitation, and alternating BBB.
- Other testing should be guided by history and physical:
  - CBC, electrolytes, BUN, creatinine
  - Glucose (rarely helpful if asymptomatic or presenting hours later)
  - BNP
  - Cardiac enzymes (only if history suggestive of MI or myocarditis)
  - D-dimer (for pulmonary embolism workup)
  - Urine pregnancy and urine drug screen
  - Initial cardiac or neuroimaging only if indicated
  - Lung scan or helical CT scan of chest if concern for PE

Follow-Up Tests & Special Considerations
- If history and physical suggest ischemic, valvular, or congenital heart disease (1),(2)[B]
  - Exercise stress test (if syncope with exertion) (1),(2)[C]
  - Echocardiogram (1),(2)[B]
- ECG monitoring, for example, Holter, external loop recorder, implantable loop recorder
- Head imaging, carotid US, and EEG are not recommended in routine evaluation of syncope but may be useful if history and physical is concerning for neurologic issues (1)[C].
- Tilt-table testing (1),(2)[B]
  - Provocative test for vasovagal syncope
  - High false-positive rate
  - Often, results are not reproducible.
- Psychiatric evaluation (2)[C]: indicated when syncope is thought to be psychogenic

TREATMENT

- Initial therapy consists of maintaining good hydration status and normal salt intake. Educate patients of the premonitory signs of syncope (1).
- Majority of pediatric patients improve with nonpharmacologic measures.

GENERAL MEASURES

- NMS: reassurance, education, behavior modification
- Elderly patients without previously recognized heart disease should be admitted if cardiac etiology of syncope is suspected.
- Patients without heart disease, especially young patients (age <60 years), can be worked up safely as outpatients.
- Prescribe antiarrhythmics for documented arrhythmias occurring simultaneously with syncope or symptoms of presyncope. Asymptomatic arrhythmias do not necessarily require treatment.
- The EGSYS Score may be used to help distinguish a cardiac from noncardiac syncope in adults. These include palpitations, syncope during effort or supine position, neurovegetative prodromes, and specific precipitating events. An abnormal ECG is also taken into consideration for this score (3)[C].

MEDICATION

First Line

- Geared toward specific underlying cardiac or neurologic abnormalities
- In cases of recurrent NMS and OHT (1)[B]
  - Mineralocorticoids (fludrocortisone)
  - α-Adrenergic agonists (midodrine)
  - Norepinephrine precursor (droxidopa)

Second Line

- SSRIs (1)[C] (paroxetine, sertraline, fluoxetine)
- Vagolytics (disopyramide)
- Acetylcholinesterase inhibitor (pyridostigmine)

ISSUES FOR REFERRAL

When cardiac or neurologic etiologies are suspected, obtain appropriate consultation, as indicated.

ADDITIONAL THERAPIES

For vasovagal/neurocardiogenic/NMS

- Counterpressure maneuvers and exercise improve vasovagal symptoms and recurrence (1).
- Head-up tilt sleeping (2)[C]
- Abdominal binders and/or support stockings (1),(2)[C]
- Increased fluid and salt intake to maintain intravascular volume in cases of recurrent NMS

SURGERY/OTHER PROCEDURES

- ICD placement for patients with cardiac conditions with high risk of sudden death and/or recurrent syncope on medications (e.g., long QT syndrome, Brugada syndrome, catecholaminergic polymorphic VT, hypertrophic cardiomyopathy) (1),(2)[B]
- Many recommend pacemaker implantation in patients with the following:
  - 2nd- (Mobitz type II) and 3rd-degree heart block
  - High risk of developing 3rd-degree heart block (bifascicular block, HV interval >100 ms by electrophysiology study)
  - Pacing-induced infranodal block
  - Sinus node recovery time ≥3 seconds

ADMISSION, INPATIENT, AND NURSING CONSIDERATIONS

A number of validated risk predictor tools have been published (i.e., ROSE rule) and may be useful in the determination of need for hospital admission. In the presence of one or more serious medical condition, inpatient evaluation should strongly be considered.

 ONGOING CARE

FOLLOW-UP RECOMMENDATIONS

Patient Monitoring

- Frequent follow-up visits for patients with cardiac causes of syncope, especially if on antiarrhythmics
- Patients with an unknown cause of syncope rarely (5%) are diagnosed during the follow-up.
- Home video recording with smartphone technology is recommended for recurrent episodes.

DIET

No specific diet unless the patient has heart disease or NMS (See "Additional Therapies" section.)

PATIENT EDUCATION

- Reassurance that most cardiac causes can be treated and that those with noncardiac causes do well, even if the cause is never discovered.
- Teaching of preventative and counter measures including avoidance of prolonged standing, awareness of position changes (particularly after lying or sitting), abdominal and/or leg pumping movements/contractions while standing or crossing legs upon standing
- Carefully consider whether the patient should drive while syncope is being evaluated. Physicians should be aware of pertinent local legislation.

PROGNOSIS

- The majority of patients (80%) have no recurrence of syncope.
- The identification of a cardiac etiology of syncope and/or the presence of other chronic medical conditions may alter prognosis.

COMPLICATIONS

Secondary traumatic injury from falling

REFERENCES

1. Shen WK, Sheldon RS, Benditt DG, et al. 2017 ACC/AHA/HRS guideline for the evaluation and management of patients with syncope: a report of the American College of Cardiology/American Heart Association Task Force on Clinical Practice Guidelines and the Heart Rhythm Society. *Circulation*. 2017;136(5):e60–e122.
2. Brignole M, Moya A, de Lange FJ, et al; for ESC Scientific Document Group. 2018 ESC guidelines for the diagnosis and management of syncope. *Eur Heart J*. 2018;39(21):1883–1948.
3. Albassam OT, Redelmeier RJ, Shadowitz S, et al. Did this patient have cardiac syncope?: the rational clinical examination systematic review. *JAMA*. 2019;321(24):2448–2457.

 SEE ALSO

- Aortic Valvular Stenosis; Atrial Septal Defect; Carotid Sinus Hypersensitivity; Patent Ductus Arteriosus; Pulmonary Arterial Hypertension; Pulmonary Embolism; Seizure Disorders; Stokes-Adams Attacks
- Algorithms: Syncope; Transient Ischemic Attack and Transient Neurologic Defects

 CODES

ICD10

R55 Syncope and collapse

CLINICAL PEARLS

- Careful history and physical exam are the keys to a diagnosis.
- Use the ECG/event-recorder to evaluate for arrhythmias.
- Reflex-mediated vasovagal (NMS/neurocardiogenic) is the most common cause in children and adults.
- True neurologic causes of syncope are rare.

S

SYNCOPE, REFLEX (VASOVAGAL SYNCOPE)

Melinda Kwan, DO, MPH • Norton Winer, MD

BASICS

A reversible loss of consciousness and postural tone secondary to systemic hypotension and cerebral hypoperfusion due to vasodilation and/or bradycardia (rarely, tachycardia) with spontaneous recovery and no neurologic sequelae; the term *syncope* excludes seizures, coma, shock, or other states of altered consciousness.

DESCRIPTION
• Derived from the Greek *syncopa*, "to cut short"
• Sudden, transient loss of consciousness characterized by unresponsiveness, falling, and spontaneous recovery
• Common cause of syncope in all age groups, especially in patients with no evidence of neurologic or cardiac disease
• Five main types of syncope: vasovagal or neurocardiogenic syncope, situational syncope, orthostatic hypotension, carotid sinus hypersensitivity, and glossopharyngeal/trigeminal neuralgia syncope (uncommon) (1)

EPIDEMIOLOGY
• Mortality: cardiac-related syncope 20–30% and 5% in idiopathic syncope
• Age: any age

Incidence
• Ranges from 7% in children aged <18 years and 15% in adults aged >70 years
• 36–62% of all syncopal episodes
• 30% recurrence rate

Prevalence
22% in the general population

ETIOLOGY AND PATHOPHYSIOLOGY
Cause: an abnormal response of the normal mechanisms that maintain BP in an upright posture; vasovagal syncope typically occurs when an individual is an upright position for a comparatively long duration (up to ≥10 minutes), compared with orthostatic hypotension which generally develops in a short period (such as a quick positional change).
• In normal individuals, upright posture results in venous pooling and transient decrease in BP.
• Neurally induced syncope may result from a cardio-inhibitory response, a vasodepressor response, or a combination of the two.
• Increased cardiovagal tone leads to bradycardia or asystole, and decreased peripheral sympathetic activity leads to venodilation and hypotension (2).
• Vasovagal syncope usually has a precipitating event, often related to fright, pain, panic, exercise, noxious stimuli, or heat exposure (2).
• Carotid sinus syncope is precipitated by position change, turning head, or wearing a tight collar (possible neck tumors or surgical scarring).
• Situational syncope is related to micturition, defecation, postexercise, coughing, or swallowing.
• Glossopharyngeal syncope is related to throat or facial pain.

Genetics
Vasovagal syncope is associated with certain genetic markers, particularly involving serotonin and dopamine signaling (3).

RISK FACTORS
• Low-resting BP
• Age: older age
• Prolonged supine position with resulting deconditioning of autonomic control

GENERAL PREVENTION
Avoid precipitating events or situations. Optimize diabetes control, use of elastic stockings, and adequate hydration.

COMMONLY ASSOCIATED CONDITIONS
• Cardiopulmonary disorders: CHF, MI, arrhythmias, hypertrophic obstructive cardiomyopathy, HTN, pulmonary embolism (PE)
• Neurologic disorders: autonomic dysfunction, Shy-Drager syndrome, Parkinson disease, multiple system atrophy, transient ischemic attack, vertebrobasilar insufficiency, peripheral neuropathy
• Psychiatric disorders:
  – Generalized anxiety disorder
  – Panic disorder
  – Major depression
  – Alcohol dependence

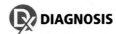

DIAGNOSIS

HISTORY
• History of syncope during or immediately after exertion is concerning for cardiac syncope.
• Neurally mediated syncope is preceded by blurred vision, palpitations, nausea, warmth, diaphoresis, or light-headedness, or there may be history of nausea, warmth, diaphoresis, or fatigue *after* syncope.
• Vasovagal syncope
  – Three phases: prodrome, loss of consciousness, and postsyncope
  – Precipitating event or stimulus is usually identified, such as panic, fright, pain, or exercise.
  – May be postexertional in athletes (diagnosis of exclusion)
  – Position: *can be preceded by prolonged standing but can occur from any position; generally resolves when the patient becomes supine*
    ○ Preceding events: as discussed above
    ○ Prodrome: as listed above for neurally mediated syncope
  – Duration: generally brief (seconds to minutes)
  – Recovery: may be prolonged with persistent nausea, pallor, and diaphoresis but without neurologic change or confusion
• Carotid sinus syncope is precipitated by position change, after turning head, or wearing a tight collar.
• Situational syncope is related to micturition, defecation, or coughing.

• Glossopharyngeal syncope (less common) is related to throat or facial pain.
  – Precipitating events or situations may include panic, pain, exercise, micturition, defecation, coughing, or swallowing.
• Pregnant women can have reflex syncope when moving from supine to lateral decubitus or upright positions.

PHYSICAL EXAM
• Vital signs, including orthostatics and bilateral BP
• Cardiac exam: volume status, murmurs, rhythm, carotid bruits
• Neurologic exam: signs of focal deficit
• Assess for occult blood loss.
• Perform Dix-Hallpike maneuver if benign paroxysmal vertigo is suspected.

DIFFERENTIAL DIAGNOSIS
• Seizure
• Arrhythmia
• Hypoglycemia
• Cardiac syncope
• Cerebrovascular syncope
• Orthostatic hypotension
• Drop attacks
• Psychiatric illness

DIAGNOSTIC TESTS & INTERPRETATION
Guided by history and physical, includes basic tests to rule out three primary causes of syncope: hypoglycemia, arrhythmia, and anemia

Initial Tests (lab, imaging)
• Blood glucose (hypoglycemia)
• ECG should be ordered for all patients. Abnormal ECG findings are common in patients with cardiac syncope (arrhythmia).
• CBC (rule out anemia)
• Head CT, MRI/MRA, carotid ultrasound only if history or physical exam suggests a neurologic cause
  – Radiology studies are not indicated for insignificant trauma in the presence of a normal neurologic exam.

Follow-Up Tests & Special Considerations
• 24-hour Holter monitoring only if a high probability of cardiac cause and/or abnormal ECG findings is present
• A low hemoglobin without obvious cause of bleed warrants stool guaiac, head CT (rule out subarachnoid hemorrhage), abdominal CT (rule out retroperitoneal bleed)
• Negative imaging prompts workup for alternative causes.
• Stroke, bleed, or carotid stenosis require appropriate disease-oriented management.
• EEG only if history or physical exam suggests seizure
• Implantable loop recorder

Diagnostic Procedures/Other
- Head-up tilt table testing:
  - Contraindicated in patients with known cardiac or neurovascular disease or in pregnancy
  - Indicated for recurrent syncope or single episode accompanied by injury or risk to others (e.g., pilots, surgeons)
  - Uses positional changes to reproduce symptoms
  - Positive test diagnostic for vasovagal syncope
- Carotid sinus massage, only in a monitored setting (i.e., BP and HR monitoring, IV access):
  - Contraindicated in patients with carotid disease (Careful auscultation prior to massage is essential.)
  - Pressure at the angle of the jaw for 5 seconds with simultaneous ECG monitoring
  - Positive tests (causing syncope or cardiac pause >3 seconds) are diagnostic of carotid sinus syncope.
- Psychiatric evaluation: to rule out anxiety, depression, and alcohol abuse

 TREATMENT

Therapy is primarily for recurrent syncope. Situational syncope does not warrant specific treatment.

GENERAL MEASURES
Identify and avoid precipitating events or situations.

MEDICATION
First Line
Nonpharmacologic treatment
- Patient counseling
  - Development of coping skills
  - Increased salt and fluid intake
- Moderate exercise training
  - Isometric muscle contractions
    - Leg crossing and buttocks clenching
    - Intense gripping of the hands and tensing of the arms
    - These maneuvers increase cardiac output and arterial BP (4).
- Tilt-table training
  - Progressively prolonged periods of enforced upright posture

Second Line
- α-Agonists are mainly used for orthostatic hypotension.
  - Midodrine is commonly used, particularly in younger, healthy patients with a high "syncope burden" (5). It increases peripheral vascular resistance and venous return. Side effects include HTN, paresthesia, urinary retention, "goose bumps," hyperactivity, dizziness, tremor, and nervousness.
- SSRIs: Paroxetine and fluoxetine are useful in treating neurocardiogenic/vasovagal syncope.
  - Serotonin affects BP and HR via the central nervous system. Serotonin decreases a sympathetic withdrawal response to rapid increases in serotonin levels.
  - Side effects include weight gain, nausea, anxiety, sexual dysfunction, and insomnia.

- Mineralocorticoids: Fludrocortisone has been found helpful mainly in orthostatic hypotension.
  - Helpful in renal sodium absorption and increasing the vasoconstrictive peripheral vascular response
  - Adverse reactions include fluid retention, HTN, CHF, peripheral edema, and hypokalemia.
- β-Blockers: metoprolol, atenolol, or pindolol mainly for postural orthostatic tachycardia syndrome (POTS)
  - Block peripheral vasodilators and ventricular mechanoreceptor stimulation
  - Stabilization of HR and BP
  - Side effects: hypotension and bradycardia (with worsening of syncope), fatigue, depression, and sexual dysfunction
  - Contraindicated in asthma

ISSUES FOR REFERRAL
Neurology or cardiology, as needed

ADDITIONAL THERAPIES
Use of support/pressure stockings

SURGERY/OTHER PROCEDURES
Pacemaker placement may be of use in patients with frequent neurocardiogenic/vasovagal syncope that is refractory to other therapies.
- Prevents prolonged bradycardia or asystole during syncopal episodes
- Long-term effect
- Invasive placement procedure

COMPLEMENTARY & ALTERNATIVE MEDICINE
Treatments for underlying heart disease or precipitating factors (e.g., anxiety); none are proven therapies.
- Nutrition and supplements: omega-3 fatty acids, multivitamin, CoQ10, acetyl-L-carnitine, α-lipoic acid, and L-arginine
- Herbs: green tea (*Camellia sinensis*), bilberry (*Vaccinium myrtillus*), ginkgo (*Ginkgo biloba*)
- Homeopathy: carbo vegetabilis, opium, sepia
- Acupuncture: It may precipitate fainting.

ADMISSION, INPATIENT, AND NURSING CONSIDERATIONS
Hospital admission or intense evaluation for:
- Severe coronary artery disease or structural heart disease (severe CHF, low ejection fraction or previous myocardial infarction, aortic stenosis)
- Arrhythmic syncope:
  - ECG may show bifascicular block, sinus bradycardia <40 without SA block or β-blockers, Brugada syndrome, abnormal QT interval, etc.
- Severe anemia or electrolyte abnormalities
- Family history of sudden death
- Isotonic crystalloids, as needed
- Vital sign monitoring
- Discharge when hemodynamically stable and workup satisfactory

 ONGOING CARE

DIET
- Increased salt intake may help if not otherwise contraindicated (2)[C].
- Maintain fluid intake.

PATIENT EDUCATION
- Identify and avoid precipitating events or situations.
- Avoid dehydration, alcohol consumption, warm environments, tight clothing, and long periods of standing motionless.
- Recognize presyncopal symptoms.
- Use behaviors, such as lying down, to avoid syncope.

PROGNOSIS
May be recurrent but not life-threatening

COMPLICATIONS
May result in injury from falls

REFERENCES
1. Zou R, Wang S, Lin P, et al. The clinical characteristics of situational syncope in children and adults undergoing head-up tilt testing. *Am J Emerg Med*. 2020;38(7):1419–1423.
2. Rocha BML, Gomes RV, Cunha GJL, et al. Diagnostic and therapeutic approach to cardioinhibitory reflex syncope: a complex and controversial issue. *Rev Port Cardiol (Engl Ed)*. 2019;38(9):661–673.
3. Sheldon RS, Gerull B. Genetic markers of vasovagal syncope. *Auton Neurosci*. 2021;235:102871.
4. Kenny RA, McNicholas T. The management of vasovagal syncope. *QJM*. 2016;109(12):767–773.
5. Sheldon R, Faris P, Tang A, et al; for POST 4 Investigators. Midodrine for the prevention of vasovagal syncope: a randomized clinical trial. *Ann Intern Med*. 2021;174(10):1349–1356.

ADDITIONAL READING
Romano S, Branz L, Fondrieschi L, et al. Does a therapy for reflex vasovagal syncope really exist? *High Blood Press Cardiovasc Prev*. 2019;26(4):273–281.

 SEE ALSO

Algorithms: Syncope; Transient Ischemic Attack and Transient Neurologic Defects

 CODES

ICD10
R55 Syncope and collapse

CLINICAL PEARLS
- A careful history of the events preceding the syncopal episode helps guide evaluation and management.
- Rule out cardiac or neurogenic syncope.
- Prodrome is common with reflex syncope.
- Recovery may be prolonged, with persistent symptoms, but there is no residual neurologic deficit or confusion.
- Patients should avoid precipitating situations or events.

SYNDROME OF INAPPROPRIATE ANTIDIURETIC HORMONE SECRETION (SIADH)

Elise Joyce Barney, DO

 BASICS

The syndrome of inappropriate secretion of antidiuretic hormone (SIADH) is a disorder with impaired water excretion (concentrated urine), caused by abnormal production of antidiuretic hormone (ADH) despite low serum osmolality.

DESCRIPTION

- Decreased urinary electrolyte-free water excretion leads to dilutional hyponatremia (total body sodium [Na] levels may be normal or near-normal, but the patient's total body water is increased).
- Often secondary to medications but may be associated with an underlying pulmonary disorder or central nervous system (CNS) disease
- Common cause of hyponatremia in hospitalized patients
- Synonym(s): SIADH; syndrome of inappropriate antidiuresis

EPIDEMIOLOGY

Incidence

- Often found in the hospital setting, especially perioperative patients in response to stress, intravenous fluids, and drugs; the incidence can be as high as 35%.
- Predominant age: elderly
- Predominate sex: females > males

ETIOLOGY AND PATHOPHYSIOLOGY

- Drugs:
  - Antidepressants (e.g., SSRIs, tricyclics, monoamine oxidase inhibitors [MAOIs])
  - Antineoplastic drugs (e.g., vincristine, vinblastine, cisplatin, cyclophosphamide)
  - Antipsychotic agents (e.g., risperidone, quetiapine, phenothiazines, haloperidol)
  - Analgesics (e.g., duloxetine, pregabalin, tramadol, NSAIDs)
  - Anticonvulsants (e.g., carbamazepine, oxcarbazepine, valproic acid, phenytoin)
  - Others (e.g., vasopressin, DDAVP, oxytocin, ciprofloxacin, α-interferon, ecstasy)
- Malignancies (ectopic ADH production):
  - Bronchogenic or small cell carcinoma of the lung
  - Lymphoma
  - Mesothelioma
  - Pancreatic adenocarcinoma
  - Thymoma
- Pulmonary conditions:
  - Asthma/COPD
  - Atelectasis/pneumothorax
  - Cystic fibrosis
  - Positive pressure mechanical ventilation
  - Pneumonia (viral, bacterial)
  - Pulmonary tuberculosis (TB)
  - Sarcoidosis
- Neurologic causes:
  - Brain tumor
  - CNS injury (i.e., subarachnoid hemorrhage, trauma, stroke, surgery)
  - CNS lupus
  - Encephalitis, meningitis
  - Epilepsy
  - Guillain-Barré syndrome
  - Multiple sclerosis

- Acute intermittent porphyria
- Delirium tremens
- HIV infection/AIDS
- Rocky Mountain spotted fever

Genetics

- 10% of patients have an X-linked mutation of vasopressin V2 receptor (V2R).
- Polymorphisms in TRPV4 gene

RISK FACTORS

- Advanced age
- Postoperative status
- Institutionalization
- Use of predisposing drugs

GENERAL PREVENTION

Avoid high-risk medications, if drug induced.

COMMONLY ASSOCIATED CONDITIONS

See "Etiology and Pathophysiology."

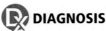 **DIAGNOSIS**

- Bartter and Schwartz criteria for SIADH:
  - Decreased osmolality (<275 mOsm/kg) with inappropriately concentrated urine (>100 mOsm/kg) and euvolemia
- Signs and symptoms depend on the acuity and severity of hyponatremia and the degree of cerebral edema.

HISTORY

Symptoms:

- Fatigue, lethargy
- Anorexia, nausea, vomiting
- Increased thirst
- Headaches
- Dizziness, changes in vision
- Unsteady gait, falls
- Myalgias/weakness
- Confusion
- Seizures, coma

PHYSICAL EXAM

- Euvolemic state
- Mild hyponatremia (serum Na 125 to 135 mEq/L)
  - Slow cognition and reaction times
  - Hyporeflexia
  - Ataxia
- Moderate to severe hyponatremia (serum Na <125 mEq/L)
  - Altered mental status, coma
  - Lethargy
  - Seizures
  - Psychosis

DIFFERENTIAL DIAGNOSIS

- Intravascular volume depletion and thiazide-diuretic induced
- Appropriate ADH secretion secondary to decreased effective arterial blood volume (e.g., congestive heart failure [CHF], nephrotic syndrome, liver cirrhosis)
- Low solute intake hyponatremia ("tea and toast" diet; beer potomania)

- Psychogenic polydipsia (water intake >10 L/day—self-correction when intake is stopped)
- Endocrinopathies (adrenal insufficiency, hypothyroidism)
- Translocational hyponatremia: caused by hyperglycemia, mannitol, sucrose, glycine
- Pseudohyponatremia (lab artifact caused by hyperlipidemia, paraproteinemias, administration of IVIG)
- Postoperative complications (nonosmotic release of ADH, stimulated by pain, nausea, vomiting, hypotension)
- Cerebral salt-wasting syndrome (hyponatremia, extracellular fluid depletion, CNS insult)

DIAGNOSTIC TESTS & INTERPRETATION

- Serum Na level: low
- Serum urea level: normal to low
- Serum osmolality: low
- Urine osmolality: high; urine osmolality >100 mOsm/kg H_2O (1)
- Urine Na concentration: high; urine Na >30 mEq/L (1)
- Fractional excretion of Na >0.5% (1)
- Serum ADH level: high (not clinically useful)
- Not usually required for diagnosis but to assist in the diagnosis and assess for other causes:
  - Serum uric acid, glucose, creatinine
  - Thyroid function
  - Morning cortisol

Initial Tests (lab, imaging)

- Serum osmolality
- Urine electrolytes (urine Na and urine potassium) and urine osmolality

Follow-Up Tests & Special Considerations

- Consider chest x-ray as part of SIADH workup to evaluate for pulmonary disease.
- Patients with nausea, vomiting, headache, vision changes, and confusion should have a head CT scan to look for signs of trauma or space-occupying lesions.

 TREATMENT

Depends on clinical picture and acute versus chronic

GENERAL MEASURES

- Treat underlying cause; remove the offending agent.
- Fluid restriction (usually <1,000 mL/day) is recommended.
- Avoid isotonic saline because this can worsen the hyponatremia.
- Correct hypokalemia.
- Mild asymptomatic hyponatremia (serum Na >125 mEq/L [>125 mmOl/L]): Restrict fluid and treat the underlying cause.
- Moderate hyponatremia (serum Na 120 to 125 mEq/L):
  - Restrict free water intake; increase oral solute intake.
  - Calculate urine/plasma electrolyte ratio ([urine Na + K] / [serum Na + serum K]) to determine efficacy of fluid restriction; ineffective if ratio >1 (2) and may need pharmacologic therapy

- Severe or with neurologic manifestations
  - Hypertonic saline (3% Na chloride [NaCl] IV bolus)
  - Can increase serum Na more rapidly with hypertonic saline by 4 to 6 mEq/L over 4 to 6 hours in the initial treatment period but not to exceed 8 mEq/L total in 24 hours (1),(3)[C]
- Chronic (≥48 hours duration)
  - Goal correction is 6 to 8 mEq/L per 24-hour period.
- Acute (<48 hours duration)
  - Can initially correct rapidly but the 24-hour goal is the same as in chronic hyponatremia (3)[C]

MEDICATION
- If severe or neurologic symptoms: IV 3% NaCl to increase serum Na cautiously (4)[B]:
  - If serum Na <120 mEq/L or severe neurologic symptoms, consider bolus of hypertonic saline to increase serum Na by 4 to 6 mEq/L over the first 4 to 6 hours.
- NaCl oral tablets
- Oral urea is an option but limited due to bitter taste.
- Loop diuretics: furosemide + potassium replacement
- V2R antagonist (the vaptans: tolvaptan, conivaptan) (4)[B]
  - Good efficacy and safety profiles in the treatment of moderate hyponatremia due to SIADH
  - Liberal fluid intake is encouraged.
  - Must be initiated in the hospital setting
  - Conivaptan only available IV and limited to 4 days maximum
  - Avoid tolvaptan in patients with liver disease.
- Demeclocycline (limited use)
  - Blocks ADH at renal tubule; produces nephrogenic diabetes insipidus
  - Dosage for long-term management: 300 to 600 mg PO BID
  - Onset of action within 1 week; therefore, not best for acute management
  - Adverse effects of GI intolerance and nephrotoxicity limit its use.
  - Paucity of evidence for efficacy
- Contraindications: Avoid tolvaptan in patients with cirrhosis due to possible liver injury. Avoid conivaptan in patients with Cr clearance <30 mL/minute.
- Precautions: Overly rapid correction (>10 mEq/L/day) can increase the risk for osmotic demyelination syndrome (ODS):
  - Permanent CNS damage in pons leading to quadriplegia and pseudobulbar palsy
  - Increased risk in women, alcoholics, malnutrition, hypoxia, chronic hyponatremia of <110 mEq/L, and hypokalemia

ALERT
Increase Na levels slowly, not >8 mEq/L/24 hr to prevent ODS (1)[C].

ISSUES FOR REFERRAL
Nephrology consultation is recommended for severe hyponatremia.

ADMISSION, INPATIENT, AND NURSING CONSIDERATIONS
Neurologic exam with vital signs if symptomatic or moderate/severe hyponatremia.

 ONGOING CARE

FOLLOW-UP RECOMMENDATIONS
Patient Monitoring
- Careful continuous clinical and laboratory monitoring of hyponatremic state during the acute phase:
  - Hourly urine output
  - Urine Na, urine potassium, urine osmolality
  - Goal Na increase is <8 mEq/L/24 hr until Na reaches 130 mEq/L (1),(3)[C].
  - If moderate/severe, check serial serum chemistry every 4 to 8 hours to ensure an appropriate rate of correction.
- Chronic management: Treat underlying cause; continue fluid restriction and NaCl tablets as needed; referral to nephrologist

DIET
Increase protein/solute intake and decrease water/fluid intake.

PATIENT EDUCATION
Diet and fluid restrictions

PROGNOSIS
- Higher risk of ICU admission and increased risk of 30-day hospital readmission in hyponatremic patients (5)
- If symptomatic (seizure, coma): high mortality due to cerebral edema if serum Na <120 mEq/L

COMPLICATIONS
- Falls and hip fractures
- Cerebral edema (see "Prognosis")
- Osmotic demyelination with overcorrection (see "Treatment" precautions): central pontine and extrapontine irreversible myelinolysis (3)
- Chronic hyponatremia is associated with osteoporosis (5)[C].

REFERENCES
1. Decaux G, Musch W. Clinical laboratory evaluation of the syndrome of inappropriate secretion of antidiuretic hormone. *Clin J Am Soc Nephrol*. 2008;3(4):1175–1184.
2. Furst H, Hallows KR, Post J, et al. The urine/plasma electrolyte ratio: a predictive guide to water restriction. *Am J Med Sci*. 2000;319(4):240–244.
3. Adrogué HJ, Madias NE. The challenge of hyponatremia. *J Am Soc Nephrol*. 2012;23(7):1140–1148.
4. Esposito P, Piotti G, Bianzina S, et al. The syndrome of inappropriate antidiuresis: pathophysiology, clinical management and new therapeutic options. *Nephron Clin Pract*. 2011;119(1):c62–c73.
5. Usala RL, Fernandez SJ, Mete M, et al. Hyponatremia is associated with increased osteoporosis and bone fractures in a large US health system population. *J Clin Endocrinol Metab*. 2015;100(8):3021–3031.

 SEE ALSO

Hyponatremia

 CODES

ICD10
E22.2 Syndrome of inappropriate secretion of antidiuretic hormone

CLINICAL PEARLS
- Treatment of the underlying cause is the key. Review all medications for potential culprits.
- ODS is a cerebral demyelination syndrome that causes quadriplegia, pseudobulbar palsy, seizures, coma, and death. It is caused by an overly rapid rate of Na correction. Increase Na levels slowly, not >8 mEq/L/24 hr, to prevent ODS.
- Safe correction of hyponatremia is important. Online calculators are available: https://www.mdcalc.com/calc/480/sodium-correction-rate-hyponatremia-hypernatremia.

S

SYPHILIS

Melissa E. Badowski, PharmD, MPH • Mahesh C. Patel, MD

BASICS

DESCRIPTION
- A chronic, systemic infectious disease caused by the spirochete *Treponema pallidum*
- Transmitted sexually by direct contact with an active lesion; also transmitted vertically (maternal–fetal) and via blood transfusions
- Untreated disease includes four overlapping stages.
  - Primary: single (usually) painless chancre at point of entry; appears in 10 to 90 days; chancre heals without treatment in 3 to 6 weeks.
  - Secondary: appears 2 to 8 weeks after primary chancre; nonpruritic rash on palms or soles of feet, mucous membrane lesions, headache, fever, lymphadenopathy, and alopecia
  - Latent: seroreactive without evidence of disease
    - Early latent: acquired within the last year
    - Late latent: exposure >12 months prior to diagnosis
  - Tertiary (late): Serology may be negative (fluorescent treponemal antibody absorption [FTA-ABS] test typically positive).
    - Gumma, cardiovascular, and late neurosyphilis; may be fatal
  - Neurosyphilis: *any* type of CNS involvement; can occur at *any* stage
    - Psychosis, delirium, dementia

Pediatric Considerations
In noncongenital cases, consider child abuse.

Pregnancy Considerations
- Screen all patients who are pregnant with venereal disease research laboratory (VDRL) test or rapid plasma reagin (RPR) test early in pregnancy, (i.e., first prenatal visit); if high risk, repeat at 28 weeks and at delivery (1)[A].
- Use the same nontreponemal test for initial screening and for follow-up (1)[A].

EPIDEMIOLOGY
Incidence
- Syphilis rates decreased through 2000 and have since increased (primarily in men who have sex with men [MSM]) (2).
  - All stages: 53 per 100,000
- Congenital: 78/100,000 live births (2)

Prevalence
- Predominant sex for primary and secondary syphilis: male (78%) > female (22%) (2)
- Highest prevalence in MSM (2)

ETIOLOGY AND PATHOPHYSIOLOGY
T. pallidum enters through intact mucous membranes or breaks in skin. The organism quickly enters the lymphatics to cause systemic disease; highly infectious; exposure to as few as 60 spirochetes is associated with ~50% chance of infection.

RISK FACTORS
MSM, multiple sexual partners, exposure to infected body fluids, injection drug use, transplacental transmission, adult individuals in custody, high-risk sexual behavior, people living with HIV (PLWH)

GENERAL PREVENTION
Education regarding safe sex; condoms reduce but do not eliminate transmission (1)[A].

COMMONLY ASSOCIATED CONDITIONS
HIV infection, hepatitis B, and other sexually transmitted infections (STIs)

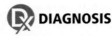

DIAGNOSIS

HISTORY
- As a "great imitator," a high index of suspicion is often required for accurate diagnosis.
- Previous sexual contact with partner with known infection or high-risk sexual behavior
- Genital lesions (chancre—primary syphilis)
- Rash, alopecia, malaise, headache, anorexia, nausea, fatigue (secondary syphilis)
- Mental status changes (tertiary syphilis)

PHYSICAL EXAM
Signs/symptoms depend on stage
- Primary: single (occasionally multiple), usually painless ulcer (chancre) in groin or at other point of entry; regional adenopathy
- Chancres begin as solitary firm, raised painless papules that erode and ulcerate. Spontaneous healing occurs in 4 to 8 weeks regardless of treatment.
- Secondary
  - Rash: skin/mucous membranes
    - Rough, red-brown macules, usually on palms and soles
    - May appear with chancre or after it has healed
    - Condylomata lata
    - Alopecia
  - Nonspecific symptoms: fever, adenopathy, malaise, headache, hair loss
- Tertiary (late) syphilis
  - Focal neurologic findings (hearing loss, vision loss; meningeal findings; loss of pain, temperature; proprioception)
  - Gummas (skin, mucous membranes, other organ systems)

DIFFERENTIAL DIAGNOSIS
- Primary: chancroid, lymphogranuloma venereum, granuloma inguinale, condylomata acuminata, herpes simplex, Behçet syndrome, trauma, carcinoma, mycotic infection, lichen planus, psoriasis, fungal infection
- Secondary: pityriasis rosea, drug eruption, psoriasis, lichen planus, viral exanthema, Stevens-Johnson syndrome
- Positive serology, asymptomatic: previously treated syphilis/other spirochetal disease (yaws, pinta)

DIAGNOSTIC TESTS & INTERPRETATION
Initial Tests (lab, imaging)
- Dark-field microscopy demonstrating *T. pallidum* spirochetes in lesion exudate/tissue biopsy is gold standard but difficult and not very sensitive (1)[A].
- Nontreponemal tests (VDRL/RPR) (2)[A]
  - Primary screening test: positive within 7 days of exposure

- Nonspecific false-positive results are common; must confirm diagnosis with treponemal tests
- Positive test should be quantified and titers followed regularly after treatment.
  - Titers usually correlate with disease activity; 4-fold change is clinically significant. Titers decrease with time/treatment; following adequate treatment for primary/secondary disease, a 4-fold decline is typical in 6 to 12 months. Absence of a 4-fold decline suggests potential treatment failure.
  - With appropriate treatment, titers should become negative (see serofast reaction).
  - Titers of patients treated in latent stages decline more gradually.
- Prozone phenomenon: negative results from high titers of antibody; test with diluted serum.
- Serofast reaction: persistently positive results years after treatment; new infection diagnosed by 4-fold rise in titer
- Conditions that may alter treponemal testing (All stages of syphilis can have a false-negative RPR result, especially in primary syphilis.)
  - Pregnancy, autoimmune disease, mononucleosis, malaria, leprosy, viral pneumonia, cardiolipin antigens, injection drug use, acute febrile illness, HIV infection; elderly can have false-positive results.
- TP-PA (*T. pallidum* particle agglutination) increasingly used for primary testing as high sensitivity overcomes challenges of nontreponemal tests
- Treponemal tests (*confirmatory test after positive nontreponemal screening test*): for example, FTA-ABS, TP-PA (*T. pallidum particle agglutination*), others (1)[A]:
  - Confirmatory test; usually positive for life after treatment; titers of no benefit; 15–25% of patients treated during primary stage revert to serologic nonreactivity after 2 to 3 years.
- Lumbar puncture (LP) indicated for (1)[A]:
  - Neurologic, ocular, or auditory manifestations; some advise LP in all secondary and early latent cases—even without neurologic symptoms. Patients with late latent/latent disease of unknown duration if nonpenicillin therapy planned; treatment failures; evidence of active tertiary syphilis (e.g., aortitis, gumma, iritis); children to rule out neurosyphilis; VDRL, not RPR, used on CSF; may be negative in neurosyphilis; highly specific but insensitive; send CSF for protein, glucose, and cell count. Monitor resolution with cell count at 6 months along with serologies (see "Patient Monitoring").
  - Negative FTA-ABS or microhemagglutination (MHA)-TP on CSF excludes neurosyphilis (highly sensitive). Positive FTA-ABS or MHA-TP on CSF is not diagnostic because of high false-positive rate. Traumatic tap, tuberculosis (TB), pyogenic/aseptic meningitis can all result in false-positive VDRL.

TREATMENT

GENERAL MEASURES

- Advise patients to notify partner(s) and to avoid intercourse until treatment is complete (1)[A].
- Test for HIV infection.
- Management of sexual contacts (3)[A]
  - Presumptively treat partners exposed within 90 days of diagnosis. Presumptively treat partners exposed >90 days before diagnosis if serologic results are not available immediately and follow-up is uncertain. Presumptively treat those exposed to a patient diagnosed with syphilis of unknown duration who has high treponemal titers (>1:32).
  - Long-term sex partners of patients with latent infection should be evaluated clinically (including serologies) and treated accordingly.

MEDICATION

ALERT
Use Bicillin L-A instead of Bicillin C-R (combination benzathine–procaine penicillin).

First Line
Parenteral penicillin G is the drug of choice. The formulation is determined by the disease stage and clinical presentation.

- Primary, secondary, and early latent <1 year (3)[A]
  - Penicillin G benzathine 2.4 million U IM × 1 dose
  - Penicillin-allergic patients: doxycycline 100 mg PO BID for 2 weeks or ceftriaxone 1 to 2 g IM or IV daily for 10 to 14 days
    ○ Azithromycin 2 g PO for 1 dose (early syphilis only; should not be used in HIV, MSM, or pregnancy); resistance and treatment failures have been noted in several U.S. regions.
- Late latent/latent of unknown duration and tertiary without evidence of neurosyphilis (3)[A]
  - Penicillin G benzathine 2.4 million U IM weekly × 3 doses
  - Penicillin-allergic patients: Attempt desensitization and treatment with penicillin or doxycycline 100 mg PO BID for 28 days; adherence may be an issue.
- Ocular or neurosyphilis (3)[A]
  - Aqueous crystalline penicillin G 3 to 4 million U IV q4h as a continuous infusion for 10 to 14 days
  - Alternative: penicillin G procaine 2.4 million U IM daily in conjunction with probenecid 500 mg PO QID for 10 to 14 days (if compliance can be ensured)
  - Penicillin-allergic patients: Attempt desensitization and treat with penicillin; ceftriaxone 2 g/day IM or IV for 10 to 14 days
  - If late latent, latent of unknown duration, or tertiary in addition to neurosyphilis, consider treating as late latent after completion of neurosyphilis treatment regimen.
- Congenital (3)[A]
  - Aqueous crystalline penicillin G 50,000 U/kg/dose IV q12h for the first 7 days of life and q8h thereafter for a total of 10 days, or penicillin G procaine 50,000 U/kg/dose IM daily for 10 days

  - If negative CSF serologies, normal physical exam, and maternal titer, then give 50,000 U/kg penicillin G benzathine IM in single dose; if >1 day of drug is missed, restart course.
  - Children (after newborn period): aqueous crystalline penicillin G 50,000 U/kg/dose IV q4–6h for 10 days; late latent, 50,000 U/kg IM as 3 doses at 1-week intervals; for contacts without symptoms: Treat as primary disease after serologies are obtained.
  - Do not give benzathine or procaine penicillins IV.
- Children (after newborn period) (3)[A]: aqueous crystalline penicillin G 50,000 U/kg/dose IV q4–6h for 10 days; late latent, 50,000 U/kg IM as 3 doses at 1-week intervals
- Pregnancy (3)[A]
  - Treatment is same as for nonpregnant patients. Some recommend second dose of penicillin G benzathine 2.4 million U IM 1 week after initial dose in 3rd trimester or with primary, secondary, or early latent syphilis.
  - Penicillin sensitivity: no proven alternatives to penicillin available for treatment during pregnancy; penicillin-allergic patients: Desensitize and treat with penicillin.
- Treat contacts without symptoms as primary disease after obtaining serologies.
- History of penicillin allergy:
  - Confirmed IgE-mediated reaction: desensitization; questionable history of IgE-mediated hypersensitivity: penicillin skin testing if major and minor penicillin determinants available
- Precautions (3)[A]
  - PLWH and patients who are pregnant may show poor response to recommended IM doses. Use IV therapy for all treatment failures in these patients.

 ONGOING CARE

FOLLOW-UP RECOMMENDATIONS
- Clinical and serologic evaluation 6 to 12 months after treatment; if >1 year duration, check at 24 months (3)[A].
- In PLWH, clinical and serologic evaluation at 3, 6, 9, 12, and 24 months after therapy (3)[A]

Patient Monitoring
- Use VDRL or RPR test to monitor therapy: 4-fold rise (two dilutions) in titer indicates new infection, whereas failure to decrease 4-fold (two dilutions) in 6 to 12 months may indicate treatment failure (although definitive criteria for cure not established); always use same test (preferably same lab) (3)[A].
- Retreatment for persistent clinical signs or recurrence, 4-fold rise in titers, or failure of initially high titer to decrease 4-fold by 6 to 12 months
- Neurosyphilis: Repeat LP every 6 months to check for normalization of CSF cell count (± CSF-VDRL and protein evaluation) (3)[A].

PATIENT EDUCATION
No intimate contacts until 4-fold titer drop

PROGNOSIS
- Excellent in all cases except patients with late syphilis complications and with HIV infection
- Syphilis in PLWH
  - Treatment same as for HIV-negative patients; more often false-negative treponemal and nontreponemal tests or unusually high titers; response to therapy less predictable; early syphilis: increased risk of neurosyphilis and higher rates of treatment failure; late neurosyphilis: harder to treat; can occur up to ≥20 years after infection

COMPLICATIONS
- Membranous glomerulonephritis; paroxysmal cold hemoglobinemia; meningitis and tabes dorsalis; cardiovascular aneurysms; valvular damage; irreversible organ damage
- Jarisch-Herxheimer reaction
  - Fever, chills, headache, myalgias, new rash; common when starting treatment (of primary/secondary disease; less common with tertiary) owing to treponemal lysis; should not be confused with drug reaction; managed with analgesics and antipyretics

REFERENCES
1. Ghanem KG, Ram S, Rice PA. The modern epidemic of syphilis. *N Engl J Med.* 2020;382(9):845–854.
2. Centers for Disease Control and Prevention. *Sexually Transmitted Disease Surveillance 2021.* Atlanta, GA: U.S. Department of Health and Human Services; 2023.
3. Workowski KA, Bachmann LH, Chan PA, et al. Sexually transmitted infections treatment guidelines, 2021. *MMWR Recomm Rep.* 2021;70(4): 1–187.

 SEE ALSO

Chlamydia Infection (Sexually Transmitted); Gonococcal Infections

CODES

ICD10
- A52.71 Late syphilitic oculopathy
- A51.0 Primary genital syphilis
- A52.74 Syphilis of liver and other viscera

CLINICAL PEARLS
- Screen all PLWH and all individuals with high-risk sexual behaviors for syphilis.
- Penicillin is the treatment of choice for syphilis.
- Syphilis rates are rising—prevalence is highest among MSM.

TARSAL TUNNEL SYNDROME

Terrence Tsui, DO

BASICS

DESCRIPTION
Tarsal tunnel syndrome is an entrapment neuropathy of the posterior tibial nerve as it passes through the tarsal tunnel (a fibro-osseous tunnel). The tarsal tunnel is located in the medial ankle posterior and inferior to the medial malleolus and deep to the flexor retinaculum (laciniate ligament).

EPIDEMIOLOGY
- Women are slightly more affected than men (56%).
- All postpubescent ages are affected.

ETIOLOGY AND PATHOPHYSIOLOGY
- Contents within the tarsal tunnel from the anterior to the posterior side include the following: the posterior tibial tendon, the flexor digitorum longus tendon, the posterior tibial artery and veins, the posterior tibial nerve, and the flexor hallucis tendon.
- The posterior tibial nerve passes through the tarsal tunnel, which is formed by three osseus structures—sustentaculum tali, medial calcaneus, and medial malleolus—covered by the laciniate ligament.
- Chronic compression of the posterior tibial nerve within the tarsal tunnel can destroy the endoneurial microvasculature, leading to edema and (eventually) fibrosis and demyelination, which results in symptoms (1),(2).
- Increased pressure in the tarsal tunnel is caused by a variety of mechanical and biochemical mechanisms. The specific cause for compression is identifiable in only 60–80% of cases (1).
- Three general categories: trauma, space-occupying lesions, deformity (1)
  - Trauma including displaced fractures, deltoid ligament sprains, or tenosynovitis
  - Varicosities
  - Hindfoot varus or valgus
  - Fibrosis of the perineurium
- Other causes:
  - Osseous prominences; osteophytes
  - Ganglia; lipoma; neurilemmoma
  - Inflammatory synovitis
  - Pigmented villonodular synovitis
  - Tarsal coalition
  - Accessory musculature
- In patients with systemic disease (e.g., diabetes), the "double crush" syndrome refers to the development of a second compression along the same nerve at a site of anatomic narrowing in patients with previous proximal nerve damage (3).

RISK FACTORS
- Tarsal tunnel syndrome is associated with certain occupations and activities involving repetitive and prolonged weight-bearing on the foot and ankle (walking, running, dancing).
- Other possible risk factors include (4):
  - Varicosities
  - Heel varus or valgus
  - Bifurcation of the posterior tibial nerve into medial and lateral plantar nerves proximal to the tarsal tunnel

COMMONLY ASSOCIATED CONDITIONS
Diabetes, systemic inflammatory arthritis, connective tissue disorders, obesity

DIAGNOSIS

Tarsal tunnel syndrome is largely a clinical diagnosis, characterized by pain and paresthesias in a predictable distribution along the medial aspect of the ankle and plantar surface of the foot (1).

HISTORY
- May have history of trauma to the foot prior to the onset of symptoms
- Pain, burning, and numbness/tingling behind medial malleolus radiating to the longitudinal arch and plantar aspect of foot including the heel (1)
- Pain usually worsens during standing or weight-bearing activities.
- Pain radiates proximally up the medial leg (Valleix phenomenon) in 33% of patients with severe compression.
- Some patients have substantial night pain (may be related to venostasis).
- Symptoms improve with rest, wearing loose footwear, and elevation.
- In advanced nerve compression, motor involvement may cause weakness, atrophy, and digital contractures of the intrinsic foot muscles (4).

ALERT
Other systemic neuropathies (diabetes, alcoholism, HIV, drug reactions) present with similar symptoms.

PHYSICAL EXAM
- Inspect: foot alignment
  - Examine for excessive foot pronation during standing or walking.
  - Examine for hindfoot varus or valgus deformity while standing.
- Palpate the tarsal tunnel and the course of the tibial nerve for tenderness and swelling.
- Tinel sign: Percussion over the tibial nerve may reproduce paresthesias that radiate distally.
- Valleix sign: Percussion over the tibial nerve may produce paresthesias that radiate proximally.
- Compression test: Applying pressure to the tarsal tunnel for 60 seconds may reproduce symptoms.
- Provocative testing: reproduction of symptoms with stretching of the nerve with exaggerated dorsiflexion and eversion of the foot/ankle or compression of the nerve with plantar flexion and inversion of the foot/ankle
- Sensory examination
  - The medial calcaneal nerve usually is spared, but numbness and altered sensation may be present in the distribution of the medial or lateral plantar nerves.
  - Vibratory sensation and two-point discrimination are decreased early in the disease process.

- Motor examination
  - Intrinsic foot muscle weakness (difficult to assess)
  - Weakness of toe plantar flexion may be present (rare).
  - Toe contractures in flexion and atrophy of the abductor hallucis or abductor digiti minimi may be seen late in the disease process.

DIFFERENTIAL DIAGNOSIS
- Peripheral neuropathies (diabetes, alcoholism, HIV, or drug related)
- Inflammatory arthritis (rheumatoid arthritis)
- Morton neuroma
- Metatarsalgia
- Subtalar joint arthritis
- Tibialis posterior tendinopathy
- Plantar fasciitis
- Plantar callosities
- Peripheral vascular disease
- Lumbar radiculopathy
- Proximal injury or compression of the tibial branch of the sciatic nerve

DIAGNOSTIC TESTS & INTERPRETATION
Initial Tests (lab, imaging)
Routine lab tests help rule out other conditions that may mimic tarsal tunnel syndrome, including diabetic neuropathy, rheumatoid arthritis, thyroid dysfunction, or other systemic illnesses (5).

- Routine weight-bearing radiographs, followed by CT (if necessary) to assess for fracture or structural abnormality
- Consider evaluation of lumbar spine x-ray if double crush (injury to lumbar nerve results in compensatory injury to posterior tibial nerve) is suspected (5).
- MRI: helps assess the tarsal tunnel for soft tissue masses or other sources of nerve compression before surgery (1)
- Ultrasound (US): gaining importance and with several advantages over MRI; dynamic testing in positions where the nerve may be stretched or compressed; can assess for space-occupying lesions (ganglia, varicose veins, lipomas, etc.) and tenosynovitis (1)

Pregnancy Considerations
- Tarsal tunnel syndrome can occur during pregnancy, typically secondary to local compression caused by fluid retention and volume changes (1).
- Care is supportive. Most cases resolve after pregnancy.

Pediatric Considerations
MRI is recommended for evaluating pediatric tarsal tunnel syndrome to exclude a neoplastic mass.

Diagnostic Procedures/Other
Electrodiagnostic studies

- Electromyography (EMG) of the intrinsic muscles of the foot can confirm the diagnosis of tarsal tunnel syndrome. A normal EMG does not exclude the diagnosis (false-negative rate is ~10%) (1).
- Nerve conduction studies (NCS) may reveal slowed conduction of the tibial nerve.
- EMG/NCS may expose a more proximal nerve compression such as a lumbar radiculopathy.

TREATMENT

Conservative management is initially recommended, except for acute onset tarsal tunnel syndrome or in the setting of a known space-occupying lesion.

MEDICATION

First Line
- Analgesics and anti-inflammatory medications
- Local corticosteroid injection into the tarsal tunnel
- Medications that alter neurogenic pain (tricyclic antidepressants, antiepileptic drugs, nerve blockers)

ADDITIONAL THERAPIES
- Physical therapy to strengthen the intrinsic and extrinsic muscles of the foot, nerve mobilization exercises, and to restore the medial longitudinal arch of the foot
- Avoiding exacerbating activities during the period of rehabilitation in physical therapy
- Immobilization with a night splint or cam walker boot
- Taping and bracing
- Orthotics or shoe modification
- Other modalities (stretching, US, massage, icing)
- Weight loss for obese patients

SURGERY/OTHER PROCEDURES
- Surgery is indicated (1),(2).
  - If nonoperative measures fail following a 6-month trial
  - In the setting of acute tarsal tunnel syndrome
  - If there are signs of motor involvement/weakness or muscle atrophy
  - If a space-occupying lesion is identified
- The surgical outcome is dependent on technique and postoperative management. 50–95% of cases have good to excellent outcomes.
- At the time of surgery, assess focal swelling, scarring, or nerve abnormalities and look for a pathologic source of compression.
- Postoperative management includes:
  - Non–weight-bearing splint until incision heals (2 to 3 weeks), followed by progressively increased weight-bearing and range of motion exercises
  - Rest, ice, compression, elevation to limit swelling

ONGOING CARE

PATIENT EDUCATION
- Discuss conservative and surgical options based on individual patient circumstance and preference.
- A decision about surgical intervention should be made with a clear understanding of risks, benefits, and potential adverse outcomes.

PROGNOSIS
Surgery is most helpful for:
- Patients with a positive Tinel sign (3)[B]
- Young patients
- Short period between occurrence of symptoms and surgery <1 year
- Localized space-occupying lesion (1)
- No motor neuron involvement

COMPLICATIONS
- The main adverse outcome is an unsuccessful surgical intervention characterized by lack of improvement or recurrence of symptoms (1).
- Causes for a failed tarsal tunnel release include:
  - Incorrect diagnosis
  - Incomplete release
  - Adhesive neuritis (external scar formation)
  - Intraneural damage (systemic disease, direct nerve injury)
  - Failure to treat all sources of nerve compression in a double crush phenomenon
- Electrodiagnostic studies are rarely helpful in determining the cause of a failed tarsal tunnel release.
- Results with surgical revision are poorer than those for the primary surgical release.

REFERENCES

1. Ahmad M, Tsang K, Mackenney PJ, et al. Tarsal tunnel syndrome: a literature review. *Foot Ankle Surg.* 2012;18(3):149–152.
2. Dellon AL. The four medial ankle tunnels: a critical review of perceptions of tarsal tunnel syndrome and neuropathy. *Neurosurg Clin N Am.* 2008;19(4):629–648, vii.
3. Dellon AL, Muse VL, Scott ND, et al. A positive Tinel sign as predictor of pain relief or sensory recovery after decompression of chronic tibial nerve compression in patients with diabetic neuropathy. *J Reconstr Microsurg.* 2012;28(4):235–240.
4. Franson J, Baravarian B. Tarsal tunnel syndrome: a compression neuropathy involving four distinct tunnels. *Clin Podiatr Med Surg.* 2006;23(3):597–609.
5. Fantino O. Role of ultrasound in posteromedial tarsal tunnel syndrome: 81 cases. *J Ultrasound.* 2014;17(2):99–112.

ADDITIONAL READING

- Abouelela AAKH, Zohiery AK. The triple compression stress test for diagnosis of tarsal tunnel syndrome. *Foot (Edinb).* 2012;22(3):146–149.
- Allen JM, Greer BJ, Sorge DG, et al. MR imaging of neuropathies of the leg, ankle, and foot. *Magn Reson Imaging Clin N Am.* 2008;16(1):117–131, vii.

- Gondring WH, Tarun PK, Trepman E. Touch pressure and sensory density after tarsal tunnel release in diabetic neuropathy. *Foot Ankle Surg.* 2012;18(4):241–246.
- Gould JS. Recurrent tarsal tunnel syndrome. *Foot Ankle Clin.* 2014;19(3):451–467.
- Imai K, Ikoma K, Imai R, et al. Tarsal tunnel syndrome in hemodialysis patients: a case series. *Foot Ankle Int.* 2013;34(3):439–444.
- Lui TH. Endoscopic resection of the tarsal tunnel ganglion. *Arthrosc Tech.* 2016;5(5):e1173–e1177.
- Patel AT, Gaines K, Malamut R, et al; for American Association of Neuromuscular and Electrodiagnostic Medicine. Usefulness of electrodiagnostic techniques in the evaluation of suspected tarsal tunnel syndrome: an evidence-based review. *Muscle Nerve.* 2005;32(2):236–240.
- Reichert P, Zimmer K, Wnukiewicz W, et al. Results of surgical treatment of tarsal tunnel syndrome. *Foot Ankle Surg.* 2015;21(1):26–29.
- Sung KS, Park SJ. Short-term operative outcome of tarsal tunnel syndrome due to benign space-occupying lesions. *Foot Ankle Int.* 2009;30(8):741–745.
- Yang Y, Du ML, Fu YS, et al. Fine dissection of the tarsal tunnel in 60 cases. *Sci Rep.* 2017;7:46351.

SEE ALSO

Algorithm: Foot Pain

CODES

ICD10
- G57.50 Tarsal tunnel syndrome, unspecified lower limb
- G57.51 Tarsal tunnel syndrome, right lower limb
- G57.52 Tarsal tunnel syndrome, left lower limb

CLINICAL PEARLS

- Tarsal tunnel syndrome typically presents with pain and numbness/tingling/burning/paresthesias of the medial ankle and plantar foot.
- Tinel sign is the most sensitive and specific physical examination test for diagnosing tarsal tunnel.
- Tarsal tunnel syndrome is a clinical diagnosis which can be supported with imaging and electrodiagnostic studies.
- Conservative management is recommended, except for patients with an acute onset tarsal tunnel syndrome or known space-occupying lesion.

T

TELOGEN EFFLUVIUM

Sahil Mullick, MD • Sreelakshmi Surendran Pillai, MD

BASICS

Acute, self-limited diffuse hair loss or hair thinning

DESCRIPTION

Telogen effluvium (TE) is a transient condition in which there is a premature conversion of a significant proportion of anagen (growth phase) hairs into telogen (resting phase) hairs resulting in subsequent increased shedding of these resting hair follicles when the follicles re-enter anagen, and the clinical appearance of moderate to severe hair thinning. Normally, each hair follicle cycles independently of others through anagen, catagen (end-of-growth transformation), and telogen, with the large majority of hair follicles in anagen at any given time.

- Five proposed types of TE:
  - Immediate anagen release: a highly common form, lasting 3 to 4 weeks, in which follicles meant to remain in anagen phase enter telogen prematurely due to a signal, including high fever, drug induced, or stress
  - Delayed anagen release: large group of hair follicles that have remained in the anagen phase for an extended period all together enter the telogen phase, resulting in hair loss; common in postpartum
  - Short anagen: a speculative type in which at least 50% of the hair follicles have an idiopathic shortening of the anagen phase; results in a doubling of the follicles in the telogen phase
  - Immediate telogen release: Normal resting club hairs remain within the hair follicle until an unknown signal causes their release, initiating the anagen stage to begin. In this type, the resting club hairs are prematurely released, ending the telogen phase abruptly and causing diffuse shedding.
  - Delayed telogen release: The presence of increased visible light, whether it be a seasonal or environmental change, is thought to end a prolonged telogen phase and initiate the anagen phase; results in diffuse shedding of hair follicles

EPIDEMIOLOGY

Most of the cases of TE are subclinical; therefore, true incidence is not clearly known. No racial predilection of the disease has been recognized, and it affects both males and females with a higher incidence rate in females. However, it should be taken into account that women take hair shedding problem more seriously than men and are likely overrepresented in seeking medical treatment. The association of TE with age is unclear; however, elderly women are known to be more susceptible to acute TE following fever, trauma, hemorrhage, or psychological stress. Studies have reported the incidence of TE in children to be around 2.7%.

Incidence

Second most common cause of alopecia

Prevalence

Unknown

ETIOLOGY AND PATHOPHYSIOLOGY

- The hair cycle consists of two predominant phases: the anagen (growth phase) and the telogen (resting phase), which last ~3 years and 3 months, respectively. In a normal scalp, ~10–15% of hairs are in the telogen phase. Due to the presence of some types of external/internal stress, there may be an increase in the percentage of telogen hairs. As new anagen hairs emerge, these telogen hair follicles are forced out. The preceding event usually occurs 2 to 3 months prior to the appearance of hair loss.
- It is hypothesized that substance P plays a key role in the pathogenesis of TE through various mechanisms. Studies have been conducted on human hair follicles in vitro and mice hair follicles in vivo, which support this theory.
- The role of substance P includes the following:
  - Upregulation of substance P receptor, NK1, at the gene and protein level, leading to premature catagen development and hair growth inhibition
  - Upregulation of nerve growth factor (NGF) and subsequently its hair apoptosis–producing receptor, p75NTR
  - Downregulation of hair growth–promoting receptor, TrkA
  - Upregulation of major histocompatibility class (MHC) I and β_2-microglobulin resulting in loss of hair follicle immune-privilege
  - Increase in tumor necrosis factor-α release by mast cells resulting in hair keratinocyte apoptosis
- Decreased cortisol levels in chronic stress states may also enhance the effects of substance P.

RISK FACTORS

- Infection
- Trauma
- Major surgery
- Thyroid disorder
- Febrile illness
- Malignancy
- Allergic contact dermatitis
- Iron deficiency anemia
- Excess vitamin A
- Protein-calorie restriction
- End-stage liver or renal disease
- Hormonal changes (including pregnancy, delivery, and estrogen-containing medications)
- Chronic stress
- Drug induced (β-blockers, anticonvulsants, antidepressants, anticoagulants, retinoids, ACE-inhibitors, etc.)
- Immunizations

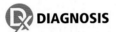

DIAGNOSIS

HISTORY

- Commonly, an inciting event 2 to 6 months previous to noted hair loss
- Fear of becoming bald
- Patients often present with evidence of hair loss with collections of hair or photographs

PHYSICAL EXAM

- Decreased density of hair on the scalp, most commonly involving the crown and temples
- In rare cases of chronic TE, there is a hair loss at the eyebrows and pubic region.
- May have diffuse shedding of hair when fingers are run through the scalp
- Shed hairs are telogen hairs, which have a small bulb of unpigmented or pigmented keratin on the root end (so-called "club" hairs).
- May affect nail growth, resulting in the appearance of Beau lines, which are transverse grooves on the nails of the hands and feet

DIFFERENTIAL DIAGNOSIS

- Hypothyroidism
- Hyperthyroidism
- Alopecia areata (diffuse pattern)
- Androgenetic alopecia
- Drug-induced alopecia
- Systemic lupus erythematosus
- Secondary syphilis
- Trichotillomania

DIAGNOSTIC TESTS & INTERPRETATION

Most often, TE is a clinical diagnosis based on typical history and exclusion of other scalp pathology and medical conditions. Blood work may be collected primarily to rule out other possible causes of hair loss. Nutritional deficiencies in iron and zinc have been associated with TE.

Initial Tests (lab, imaging)

If indicated:

- CBC, ferritin
- TSH
- Creatinine
- Consider iron profile and zinc.
- Consider hepatic enzymes.
- Consider RPR/VDRL.

Diagnostic Procedures/Other

- Hair pull test: unreliable; performed by gently pulling 25 to 30 hairs from various sites on a patient's scalp; each pull should elicit <5 normal club hairs; increased quantity may indicate possibility of TE.
- Hair clip test: performed by cutting 25 to 30 hairs from the patient's scalp and examining them under a microscope; a negative test (not indicative of TE) will demonstrate <10% of hair shafts of small diameter. A positive test will demonstrate >10% of hair shafts of small diameter.
- Trichogram: ~50 hairs are plucked using a hemostat from the patient's scalp, and the number of telogen and anagen hairs present are counted. In TE, there will be >10% of hairs in the telogen phase.
- Scalp biopsy: rarely needed; it is recommended that several 4-mm punch biopsies be obtained, all horizontally embedded to determine an accurate anagen-to-telogen ratio. Histologically, catagen-to-telogen hairs have numerous apoptotic cells in the outer sheath epithelium. >12–15% of hair follicles in telogen phase is consistent with TE.

 TREATMENT

TE is a benign, self-limited process. Identify and correct the underlying cause. The patient should be reassured that hair growth will resume in 3 to 6 months, with full growth to return in 12 to 18 months (1). No treatment is required; however, when a nutritional deficiency is identified, there may be some benefit in taking a specific supplement.

MEDICATION

- Minoxidil stimulates hair regrowth via arteriolar smooth muscle vasodilation; not effective in TE
- Oral zinc therapy: new medication that may have benefits for patients with TE through various mechanisms all essential to hair growth, including the following (2)[C]:
  - Cofactor for enzymes needed in nucleic acid and protein synthesis and cell division
  - Inhibition of the catagen phase by blocking certain enzymes involved in hair apoptosis
  - Involved in hair growth regulation via hedgehog signaling

COMPLEMENTARY & ALTERNATIVE MEDICINE

- Combination oral vitamin therapy: A formulation of zinc; biotin; iron; vitamins A, C, E, and B complex; folic acid; magnesium; and amino acids of keratin and collagen was associated with statistically significant improvement compared to a formulation of calcium pantothenate, cystine, thiamine nitrate, medicinal yeast, keratin, and aminobenzoic acid in the following measures after 180 days of use: hair loss, hair volume, scalp hair density, hair shine, and hair strength (3)[C].
- An extract from millet mixed with polar lipids has been found to enhance the cell proliferation in the hair bulb, reduce hair density in the telogen phase, improve scalp dryness, and improve hair brightness.

 ONGOING CARE

DIET

If a measurable deficiency has been found, it should be corrected. A balanced diet and stable body weight are important. Although the use of polyphenolic compounds such as those in green tea has been reported to improve hair loss in mice, no such controlled studies are available for humans.

REFERENCES

1. Malkud S. Telogen effluvium: a review. *J Clin Diagn Res*. 2015;9(9):WE01–WE03.
2. Karashima T, Tsuruta D, Hamada T, et al. Oral zinc therapy for zinc deficiency-related telogen effluvium. *Dermatol Ther*. 2012;25(2):210–213.
3. Sant'Anna Addor FA, Donato LC, Melo CSA. Comparative evaluation between two nutritional supplements in the improvement of telogen effluvium. *Clin Cosmet Investig Dermatol*. 2018;11:431–436.

ADDITIONAL READING

Mounsey AL, Reed SW. Diagnosing and treating hair loss. *Am Fam Physician*. 2009;80(4):356–362.

 CODES

ICD10
L65.0 Telogen effluvium

CLINICAL PEARLS

- TE is a self-limited form of nonscarring alopecia, most often acute.
- TE is due to a premature conversion of a significant proportion of anagen (growth phase) hairs into telogen (resting phase) hairs, resulting in increased shedding of these resting hair follicles and the clinical appearance of moderate to severe hair thinning and loss when growth resumes.
- There are many potential causes of TE, both emotional and physiologic. Often, it is hard to determine the etiology, but eliminating the stressor is the key to resolving TE and stimulating new hair growth.
- No treatment is needed. Patient should be reassured that complete hair regrowth will occur in 12 to 18 months.

T

TEMPOROMANDIBULAR JOINT DISORDER (TMD)

Akanksha Samal, DO

BASICS

DESCRIPTION
- Syndrome characterized by
  - Pain and tenderness involving the muscles of mastication and surrounding tissues
  - Sound, pain, stiffness, or grating in the temporomandibular joint (TMJ) with movement
  - Limitation of mandibular movement with possible locking or dislocation
  - Recent research suggests that TMD is a complex disorder with multiple causes consistent with a biopsychosocial model of illness.
- System(s) affected: musculoskeletal
- Synonym(s): TMJ syndrome; TMJ dysfunction; myofascial pain–dysfunction syndrome; bruxism; orofacial pain

EPIDEMIOLOGY
Incidence
- Annual first-onset incidence is 3.9%.
- Peak incidence in ages 30 to 50 years

Prevalence
- 6–12% in both adults and older children
- 2:1 female:male
- Up to 1/2 the population may have 1+ symptom of TMD, but most are not limited by symptoms, and <1:4 seek medical or dental treatment.

ETIOLOGY AND PATHOPHYSIOLOGY
- Multifactorial pathophysiology: anatomic, behavioral, emotional, and cognitive
- The American Academy of Orofacial Pain categorizes TMD according to three anatomic origins of pain. The change in name from TMJ to TMD emphasizes that many do not suffer from true articular pain.
- Muscle disorders involving the muscles of mastication
  - Occlusomuscular dysfunction (bruxism)
  - Masticatory muscle spasm
  - Myositis
  - Myofibrosis
  - Poorly fitting oral devices (dentures, splints, etc.)
  - Contracture
  - Neoplasia
- Articular disorders of the joint
  - Congenital disorders
  - Inflammatory disorders: synovitis, arthritides, capsulitis, ankyloses
  - Avascular necrosis (rare)
  - TMJ disk derangement, osteoarthritis
  - Hyper- or hypomobile TMJ
  - TMJ trauma: condylar fractures, dislocation
- Cranial bone disorder including the mandible
  - Congenital and developmental disorders
  - Acquired disorders (fracture, neoplasm)
- Current consensus is that TMD is not only a local condition, so much as a family of complex disorders that can lead to chronic pain, and often overlap with other chronic pain conditions that reflect CNS sensitization.
- OPPERA study (Orofacial Pain: Prospective Evaluation and Risk Assessment) is assessing the heterogeneity in these disorders.

Genetics
Research is ongoing in gene polymorphisms associated with TMD and other pain disorders. The catechol O-methyltransferase (COMT) gene is thought to be associated with changes in pain responsiveness.

RISK FACTORS
- Trauma to the face, jaw, and neck, including cervical whiplash injuries and hyperextension of jaw
- Rheumatologic and degenerative conditions involving the TMJ
- Psychosocial stress and poor adaptive capabilities
- Repetitive microtrauma from dental malocclusion, including inappropriate dental treatment
- Inconsistent association with bruxism and jaw/teeth clenching
- Hormonal contraceptive use

GENERAL PREVENTION
- Elimination of tension-causing oral habits
- Reduction in overall muscle tension

COMMONLY ASSOCIATED CONDITIONS
Craniomandibular disorders, somatization disorder, somatoform pain disorder, other chronic pain syndromes, fibromyalgia, juvenile idiopathic arthritis, tension headache, irritable bowel syndrome, sleep disturbance, tobacco use

DIAGNOSIS

TMD is a clinical diagnosis, and localized pain is the unifying feature.

HISTORY
- Facial and/or TMJ pain
- Locking/catching of jaw; decreased range of motion
- Noises: clicking, grinding, popping of TMJ
- Headache, earache, neck pain

PHYSICAL EXAM
- Muscle tenderness and restricted pain-free jaw opening
- Check facial symmetry, muscle hypertrophy, and intraoral exam including tooth wear.
- Palpation of muscles of mastication may reproduce pain.
- There may be tenderness over the TMJ.
- Test jaw range of motion (opening, closing, lateral, protrusive) and masticatory muscle strength.
  - Maximal (pain free) jaw opening with interincisal distance <40 mm is suggestive of joint rather than muscle pathology if accompanied by other signs and symptoms (normal 35 to 55 mm).
  - Deviation to the affected side is common.
- Clicking or crepitus of jaw with opening

DIFFERENTIAL DIAGNOSIS
- Condylar fracture/dislocation
- Trigeminal neuralgia
- Dental or periodontal conditions
- Neoplasm of the jaw, orofacial muscles, or salivary glands

- Acute, nondental infection: parotitis, sialadenitis, otitis, mastoiditis
- Jaw claudication: giant cell arteritis
- Migraine or tension-type headache
- Ramsay Hunt syndrome (zoster auricular syndrome)

DIAGNOSTIC TESTS & INTERPRETATION
Blood work only useful to rule out other conditions (CBC, CMP, ESR, CRP); not needed for diagnosis

Initial Tests (lab, imaging)
- TMD is a clinical diagnosis based primarily on history and physical exam.
- Poor correlation between pain severity and pathologic changes is seen in joint or muscle tissues. Consider the following for traumatic, infectious, severe, or treatment-resistant cases, with MR or CT more useful as part of surgical workup:
  - Panoramic dental radiographs.
  - CT scan allows fine detail of bony structures, preferred for trauma.
  - US: Effusion and findings correlate with MRI and subjective pain.
  - MRI: noninvasive study for disc position; more sensitive than US; can help determine need for surgical management

Diagnostic Procedures/Other
- Local anesthetic nerve block can differentiate orofacial pain of articular versus muscular origin.
- Arthroscopy can be diagnostic for cartilage and bony pathology.

Test Interpretation
Positive findings include:
- Condylar head displacement
- Anterior disc displacement
- Posterior capsulitis
- Loosening of disc and capsular attachments
- Chondroid metaplasia of disc leading to disc perforation and degeneration

TREATMENT

Signs and symptoms will abate without any interventions in most patients. 50% report improvement at 1 year and 85% by 3 years. With conservative therapy, symptoms resolve in 75% of cases within 3 months. Only 5–10% will require surgical intervention.

- Patient education and setting expectations are important because there is no "cure" for TMD, yet most patients will improve with limited interventions.
- Psychosocial interventions, including cognitive-behavioral therapy with or without biofeedback (1)[A]
- Behavior modification to eliminate tension-relieving oral habits including heavy chewing of food and nonfood items as well as potential strain from playing musical instruments that stress or strain the jaw (wind, brass, or string) (1)[A]
- Therapeutic exercises, especially if displacement is present, including formal physical therapy

- Occlusal adjustment cannot be recommended for the management or prevention of TMD because there is an absence of evidence from RCTs that occlusal adjustment treats or prevents TMD (2).
- Insufficient evidence exists either for or against the use of stabilization splint therapy for the treatment of TMD.
- The American Dental Association recommends a "less is often best" stepwise approach and offers the following stepwise progression for therapy:
  – Eating softer foods
  – Avoiding chewing gum and nail biting
  – Modifying pain with heat or ice
  – Relaxation techniques including meditation and biofeedback
  – Exercises to strengthen jaw muscles
  – Medications
  – Night guards and orthotics

MEDICATION

First Line
- NSAIDs:
  – Naproxen: 500 mg BID stronger evidence than for other NSAIDs
  – Ibuprofen, if osteoarthritis is suspected
  – Topical diclofenac if oral medication is contraindicated
- Gabapentin: Titrate up to 1,800 mg/day divided.
- Acetaminophen

Second Line
- Cyclobenzaprine 10 mg nightly more effective than placebo for pain reduction (3)[B]
- Tricyclic antidepressants: nortriptyline or amitriptyline
- Acupuncture and dry needling can reduce pain (2).
- Opiates should be reserved for perioperative or severe or recalcitrant cases (4)[B].
- DMARDs may benefit inflammatory arthropathies such as rheumatoid or psoriatic arthritis.
- Ineffective medications (4)[B]
  – The following medications when compared with placebo in RCTs were shown to be ineffective in improving pain and should not be used for the treatment of TMD:
    ○ Benzodiazepines
    ○ Topical capsaicin
    ○ Celecoxib

ADDITIONAL THERAPIES
Joint and muscle injections
- A systematic review of arthrocentesis with injection of hyaluronic acid and platelet rich plasma showed no clinical improvement (5).
- Steroids given >3 times annually may accelerate degenerative changes.
- Injections into inferior space or double spaces have better effect than superior space injections alone.

- A systematic review evaluating botulinum toxin type A (Botox) injections revealed mixed results (2).
- For advanced structural abnormalities, referral for discectomy, arthroplasty, or joint replacement can be considered; however, strong evidence is lacking for lavage or surgical treatments over conservative management (2).

COMPLEMENTARY & ALTERNATIVE MEDICINE
- Glucosamine may be effective if pain is secondary to osteoarthritis of the TMJ (4)[B].
- Multiple electronic diagnostic and treatment modalities are currently marketed to patients; however, the scientific literature does not support the use of electronic diagnostic and treatment devices for TMD at this time.

 ONGOING CARE

FOLLOW-UP RECOMMENDATIONS
- Relax jaw by disengaging teeth.
- Avoid wide, uncontrolled opening, such as yawning.
- Trial of soft diet
- Stress management and behavior modification counseling may be helpful.
- Be aware of any teeth-clenching or grinding habits.

Patient Monitoring
- Ongoing assessment of clinical response to conservative therapies (NSAIDs, behavior modification, occlusal splints) is necessary.
- Surgical procedure (arthroplasty, joint replacement) to correct disc displacement or replace a damaged disc may be indicated only if the patient has not responded to conservative treatment.

DIET
Soft diet to reduce chewing

PROGNOSIS
- With conservative therapy, symptoms resolve in 75% of cases within 3 months.
- Patients benefit most from a comprehensive treatment approach including the following (3):
  – Restoration of normal muscle function
  – Pain control
  – Stress management
  – Behavior modification

COMPLICATIONS
- Secondary degenerative joint disease
- Chronic TMJ dislocation
- Loss of joint range of motion
- Depression and chronic pain syndromes
- Secondary headache disorder

REFERENCES

1. Aggarwal VR, Lovell K, Peters S, et al. Psychosocial interventions for the management of chronic orofacial pain. *Cochrane Database Syst Rev*. 2011;(11):CD008456.
2. Gil-Martínez A, Paris-Alemany A, López-de-Uralde-Villanueva I, et al. Management of pain in patients with temporomandibular disorder (TMD): challenges and solutions. *J Pain Res*. 2018;11:571–587.
3. Gauer RL, Semidey MJ. Diagnosis and treatment of temporomandibular disorders. *Am Fam Physician*. 2015;91(6):378–386.
4. Mujakperuo HR, Watson M, Morrison R, et al. Pharmacological interventions for pain in patients with temporomandibular disorders. *Cochrane Database Syst Rev*. 2010;(10):CD004715.
5. Derwich M, Mitus-Kenig M, Pawlowska E. Mechanisms of action and efficacy of hyaluronic acid, corticosteroids and platelet-rich plasma in the treatment of temporomandibular joint osteoarthritis—a systematic review. *Int J Mol Sci*. 2021;22(14):7405.

 SEE ALSO

Headache, Tension

CODES

ICD10
- M26.60 Temporomandibular joint disorder, unspecified
- M26.62 Arthralgia of temporomandibular joint
- M26.63 Articular disc disorder of temporomandibular joint

CLINICAL PEARLS
- TMD refers to a number of potential underlying joint and muscle conditions involving the jaw. Characteristics of all conditions are pain and functional limitation.
- TMD is a clinical diagnosis; imaging and labs are often of limited utility.
- Cognitive-behavioral therapy reduces pain, depression, and limitation of function.
- Exercises may improve function and pain.
- Evidence is lacking to support occlusion correction or splinting.
- Naproxen, gabapentin, topical methyl salicylate, glucosamine, amitriptyline, acupuncture, and botulinum toxin injections have some evidence of efficacy.

TESTICULAR TORSION

Adedamola Ayo Omole, MD • William Pearce, MD

BASICS

DESCRIPTION
- Twisting of testis and spermatic cord, resulting in acute ischemia and loss of testis if unrecognized:
  - Intravaginal torsion: occurs within tunica vaginalis, only involves testis and spermatic cord. Most commonly seen in practice.
  - Extravaginal torsion: involves twisting of testis, cord, and processus vaginalis as a unit; typically seen in neonates
- System(s) affected: reproductive

Geriatric Considerations
Rare in this age group

Pediatric Considerations
Peak incidence at age 14 years

EPIDEMIOLOGY
Incidence
- ~1/4,000 males before age 25 years
- Predominant age:
  - Occurs from newborn period to 7th decade
  - 65% of cases occur in 2nd decade, with peak at age 14 years; rare beyond the age of 30 years
  - Second peak in neonates (in utero torsion usually occurs around week 32 of gestation)

ETIOLOGY AND PATHOPHYSIOLOGY
- Initial incomplete twisting of spermatic cord causes venous obstruction and edema of testis, leading to congestion and then to ischemia.
- Complete twisting of the spermatic cord causes arterial occlusion, in addition to the above, leading to rapid ischemia.
- Congenital bell clapper deformity, which is bilateral in at least 2/5th of cases: A high mesorchium (the posterolateral attachment of the testis to the tunica vaginalis) allows more room for the testis to twist within the tunica vaginalis and is associated intravaginal testicular torsion.
- No clear anatomic defect is associated with extravaginal testicular torsion:
  - In neonates, the tunica vaginalis is not yet well attached to scrotal wall, allowing torsion of entire testis including tunica vaginalis.
- Usually spontaneous and idiopathic
- 20% of patients have a history of trauma.
- 1/3 have had prior episodic testicular pain.
- Contraction of cremaster muscle or dartos may play a role and is stimulated by trauma, exercise, cold, and sexual stimulation.
- Increased incidence may be due to increasing weight and size of testis during pubertal development.

- Possible alterations in testosterone levels during nocturnal sex response cycle; possible elevated testosterone levels in neonates
- Testis must have inadequate, incomplete, or absent fixation within scrotum.
- Torsion may occur in either clockwise or counter-clockwise direction.

Genetics
- Unknown
- Familial testicular torsion, although previously rarely reported, may involve as many as 10% of patients.

RISK FACTORS
- May be more common in colder months
- Paraplegia
- Previous contralateral testicular torsion

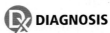

DIAGNOSIS

Testicular torsion is a clinical diagnosis. A good history and physicals are the most important and helpful tools in evaluating and managing testicular torsion. If H&P are highly suggestive of testicular torsion, imaging studies may be skipped and immediate urologic consult should be done, as time is of the utmost essence (1).

HISTORY
- Acute onset of unrelenting pain, often during period of inactivity
- Onset of pain usually sudden but may start gradually with subsequent increase in severity
- Nausea and vomiting are common:
  - Presence may increase the likelihood of testicular torsion versus other differential diagnoses.
- Prior history of multiple episodes of testicular pain with spontaneous resolution in an episodic crescendo pattern may indicate intermittent testicular torsion.

PHYSICAL EXAM
- Scrotum is enlarged, red, edematous, and painful unilaterally.
- Testicle is swollen and exquisitely tender.
- "Bell clapper" deformity: an asymmetrically high-riding testis oriented transversely instead of longitudinally occurring due to shortening spermatic cord from the torsion
- Testis may be high in scrotum with a transverse lie; this is called Brunzel sign.
- Prehn sign: when elevation of the testis does not decrease pain in the affected testicle
- Absent cremasteric reflex. Elicit cremasteric reflex by lightly stroking the inner thigh of the suspected side.

DIFFERENTIAL DIAGNOSIS
- Torsion appendix testis (this may account for 35–67% of acute scrotal pain cases in children)
- Epididymitis (8–18% of acute scrotal pain cases)
- Orchitis
- Incarcerated or strangulated inguinal hernia
- Acute hydrocele
- Traumatic hematoma
- Testicle rupture
- Idiopathic scrotal edema
- Acute varicocele
- Epididymal hypertension (venous congestion of testicle or prostate due to sexual arousal that does not end in orgasm)
- Testis tumor
- Henoch-Schönlein purpura
- Scrotal abscess
- Leukemic infiltrate

DIAGNOSTIC TESTS & INTERPRETATION
- Doppler US may confirm testicular swelling but is diagnostic by demonstrating a lack of blood flow to the testicle; PPV of 89.4%. A normal testicular US does not rule out testicular torsion.
- In boys with intermittent, recurrent testicular torsion, both Doppler US and radionuclide scintigraphy findings will be normal.

Initial Tests (lab, imaging)
Urinalysis to rule out any infection such as epididymitis, orchitis, UTI

Diagnostic Procedures/Other
- Doppler US flow detection demonstrates absent or reduced blood flow with torsion and increased flow with inflammatory process (reliable only in first 12 hours).
- Radionuclide testicular scintigraphy with technetium-99m pertechnetate demonstrates absent/decreased vascularity in torsion and increased vascularity with inflammatory processes (including torsion of appendix testes).

Test Interpretation
- Venous thrombosis
- Tissue edema and necrosis
- Arterial thrombosis
- Decreased Doppler flow also seen in hydrocele, abscess, hematoma, or scrotal hernia
- Sensitivity of radionuclide testicular scintigraphy is decreased relative to ultrasonography because hyperemia in the torsed testicle can mimic flow.

TREATMENT

- Manual reduction/detorsion: best performed by an experienced physician, especially if a surgeon is not available; may be successful, facilitated by lidocaine 1% (plain) injection at level of external ring:
  - Performed by rotating the affected testicle in a medial-to-lateral direction, described as the "open book"; 1/3 of torsion, however, is medial-to-lateral on presentation.
  - If successful will usually provide immediate relief; may need to rotate anywhere from 180 to 360 degrees, resulting in possible partial untwisting (2)
  - Difficult to determine success of manual reduction, especially after giving local anesthesia
  - Manual reduction might require sedation, and the entire process may delay definitive treatment.
  - Even if successful, must always be followed by surgical exploration, urgently but not emergently
- Surgical exploration via scrotal approach with detorsion, evaluation of testicular viability, orchidopexy of viable testicle, orchiectomy of nonviable testicle
- In boys with a history of intermittent episodes of testicular pain, scrotal exploration is warranted with testicular fixation if abnormal testicular attachments are confirmed.

GENERAL MEASURES
Early exam is crucial because necrosis of the testicle can occur after 6 to 8 hours.

MEDICATION
Studies are ongoing on medications used to prevent reperfusion injury and increase blood flow.

ISSUES FOR REFERRAL
All patients diagnosed with testicular torsion should receive urgent/emergent referral to urology

SURGERY/OTHER PROCEDURES
Operative testicular fixation of the torsed testicle after detorsion and confirmation of viability:

- At least 3- or 4-point fixation with nonabsorbable sutures between the tunica albuginea and the tunica vaginalis
- Excision of window of tunica albuginea with suture to dartos fascia
- Any testis that is not clearly viable should be removed.
- Testes of questionable viability that are preserved and pexed invariably atrophy.
- Bilateral testicular fixation is recommended by many surgeons.
- Contralateral testicle frequently has similar abnormal fixation and should be explored.

COMPLEMENTARY & ALTERNATIVE MEDICINE
No complementary or alternative medicine recommended. Patients should be educated on the acuity of illness, and the need for immediate intervention.

ADMISSION, INPATIENT, AND NURSING CONSIDERATIONS
Patients can usually be discharged from recovery.

 ONGOING CARE

FOLLOW-UP RECOMMENDATIONS
Patient Monitoring
- Postoperative visit at 1 to 2 weeks
- Yearly visits until puberty may be needed to evaluate for atrophy.
- Counsel high-risk patients during primary care visits on Emergency Room return precautions.

DIET
Regular diet

PATIENT EDUCATION
Possibility of testicular atrophy in salvaged testis with depressed sperm counts. Importantly, fertility rates in patients with one testicle remain excellent.

PROGNOSIS
- Testicular salvage:
  - Salvage is related directly to duration of torsion (85–97% if within 6 hours, 20% after 12 hours <10% if >24 hours).
  - The degree of torsion is related to testicular salvage:
    - The median degree of torsion is <360 in patients who are explored and orchidopexy performed.
- 80–94% may have depressed spermatogenesis related to duration of ischemic injury (possibly related to autoimmune-mediated injury).
- Up to 45% of patients undergoing orchidopexy for testicular torsion will develop atrophy of testicle.
- Preoperative manual detorsion is associated with improved surgical salvage in patients with testicular torsion.

COMPLICATIONS
- Possible testicular atrophy
- Abnormal spermatogenesis
- Infertility:
  - Fertility rates with one testicle remain excellent.
  - Nearly 36% of patients who experience torsion have sperm counts <20 million/mL.

REFERENCES
1. Sharp VJ, Kieran K, Arlen AM. Testicular torsion: diagnosis, evaluation, and management. *Am Fam Physician*. 2013;88(12):835–840.
2. Bowlin PR, Gatti JM, Murphy JP. Pediatric testicular torsion. *Surg Clin North Am*. 2017;97(1):161–172.

ADDITIONAL READING
Jacobsen FM, Rudlang TM, Fode M, et al. The impact of testicular torsion on testicular function. *World J Mens Health*. 2020;38(3):298–307.

 CODES

ICD10
- N44.03 Torsion of appendix testis
- N44.0 Torsion of testis
- N44.02 Intravaginal torsion of spermatic cord

CLINICAL PEARLS
- The diagnosis of testicular torsion is usually made by physical exam. Patients with suspected torsion should be taken to the OR without delay. If the diagnosis is in question, a testicular Doppler US may be done to evaluate blood flow.
- Although testicular necrosis may be present within 6 to 8 hours of torsion, this is highly variable.
- Preoperative manual detorsion is warranted and is associated with improved surgical salvage in patients with testicular torsion.
- Infertility can be a problem even if the testicle is viable. Autoimmune anti-sperm antibodies may be produced, and they may affect subsequent fertility.

T

TESTOSTERONE DEFICIENCY

Stanton C. Honig, MD • Dylan Buller, MD

BASICS

DESCRIPTION
- Testosterone (T) is the principal circulating androgen in males. Testosterone deficiency (TD) is characterized by low levels of T in addition to signs and symptoms.
- No universally accepted threshold of T concentration to distinguish eugonadal from hypogonadal men, but the U.S. Food and Drug Administration (FDA) definition is T <300 ng/dL
- T levels correlate with overall health and may be associated with sexual dysfunction.
- Synonym(s): hypogonadism, hypoandrogenism, androgen deficiency, low T

EPIDEMIOLOGY
Incidence
Overall incidence increases with age. T levels decline by 1% per year after the age of 40 years.

Prevalence
- Estimates of TD vary; typically 20% of men >60 years, 30% >70 years, and 50% >80 years of age
- Symptomatic TD in the United States in ages 40 to 69 years is 6–12.3%.
- 2.4 million men in United States ages 40 to 69 years

ETIOLOGY AND PATHOPHYSIOLOGY
Hypothalamus produces GnRH, which stimulates pituitary to produce follicle-stimulating hormone (FSH) and luteinizing hormone (LH). LH stimulates Leydig cells to produce T. Leydig cells are responsible for 90% of the body's T.
- Primary hypogonadism: Testes produce insufficient amount of T; FSH/LH levels are elevated.
- Secondary hypogonadism: low T from inadequate production of LH
- Congenital syndromes: cryptorchidism, Klinefelter, hypogonadotropic hypogonadism (Kallmann)
- Acquired: cancer, trauma, orchiectomy, steroids
- Infectious: mumps orchitis, HIV, tuberculosis
- Systemic: Cushing syndrome, hemochromatosis, autoimmune, severe illness (e.g., renal and liver disease), metabolic syndrome, obesity, obstructive sleep apnea
- Medications and drugs: LHRH agonists, corticosteroids, ethanol, marijuana, opioids, SSRIs
- Elevated prolactin: prolactinoma, dopamine antagonists (neuroleptics and metoclopramide)

Genetics
- Klinefelter syndrome: XXY karyotype
- Kallmann syndrome: abnormal GnRH secretion due to abnormal hypothalamic development

RISK FACTORS
- Obesity, diabetes, COPD, depression, thyroid disorders, malnutrition, alcohol, stress
- Chronic infections, inflammatory states, narcotic use

- Undescended testicles, varicocele
- Trauma, cancer, testicular radiation, chemotherapy, disorders of the pituitary and/or hypothalamus

GENERAL PREVENTION
General health maintenance and treatment of obesity

COMMONLY ASSOCIATED CONDITIONS
- Infertility, erectile dysfunction, low libido
- Osteopenia/osteoporosis
- Diabetes, insulin resistance, metabolic syndrome, adiposity
- Depressed mood, poor concentration, irritability

DIAGNOSIS

HISTORY
- Congenital and developmental abnormalities
- Infertility, loss of libido, erectile dysfunction
- Depression, fatigue, difficulty with concentration
- Decreased muscle strength, energy level
- Increase in body fat, development of diabetes
- Bone fractures from relatively minor trauma
- Testicular trauma, infection, radio- or chemotherapy
- Decrease in testicle size or consistency
- Headaches or vision changes
- Medications, narcotic use

PHYSICAL EXAM
- Infancy: ambiguous genitalia
- Puberty
  - Impaired growth of penis, testicles
  - Lack of secondary male characteristics
  - Gynecomastia, eunuchoid habitus
- Adulthood
  - Decreased muscular development, visceral fat distribution
  - Presence of gynecomastia
  - Small and/or soft testicles
  - Digital rectal exam and International Prostate Symptom Score (IPSS)

DIFFERENTIAL DIAGNOSIS
- Delayed puberty
- Obesity, depression, chronic illness, hypothyroidism
- Normal aging
- Prior anabolic steroid abuse

DIAGNOSTIC TESTS & INTERPRETATION
- T levels vary widely and are subject to diurnal, seasonal, and age-related variations.
- Measurement should be obtained between 6 and 10 A.M. Confirmation with a second measurement may be necessary. Free T with total T may be preferred in some cases. Measurements should not be obtained during acute illness. T circulates in blood primarily bound to SHBG or albumin. Only 2–3% of total T is found free. Free and albumin-bound T is considered bioavailable. Laboratory findings must be interpreted in the appropriate clinical setting.

Initial Tests (lab, imaging)
Morning T level is the initial test. If initial morning T is low and is confirmed on repeat test, further evaluation is appropriate.
- Evaluation should include LH and FSH to differentiate between primary versus secondary hypogonadism.
- Consider estradiol and prolactin, especially if LH is low or if with breast symptoms and gynecomastia.
- If primary hypogonadism of unknown origin and physical exam reveals severe testis atrophy, consider obtaining karyotype (Klinefelter syndrome 1:500 to 1,000 risk).
- If secondary hypogonadism, consider prolactin, iron saturation, pituitary function testing, and/or MRI.

Follow-Up Tests & Special Considerations
- Prior to initiating therapy:
  - Hemoglobin and hematocrit (to determine risk of polycythemia)
  - Prostate-specific antigen (PSA) in men >40 years of age (to exclude prostate cancer diagnosis)
  - Estradiol in men with breast symptoms or gynecomastia
- Dual energy x-ray absorptiometry (DEXA) in men with severe TD or fracture from minimal trauma
- Pituitary MRI: if there is elevation of prolactin more than twice the upper limit of normal or LH/FSH below normal range

TREATMENT

Testosterone therapy (TT) recommended for symptomatic men (e.g., low libido and/or erectile dysfunction, low energy level, constitutional symptoms) with low T levels ≤300 ng/dL obtained in the morning; not recommended for older men with low T levels in absence of signs or symptom (1)[C]
- Recent data suggest T replacement can significantly increase hemoglobin levels in men with low T and unexplained anemia.
- Recent data suggest men with low bone mineral density and low T can increase bone density and bone strength with T replacement.
- In older men with low T and age-associated memory impairment, T replacement was not seen as beneficial.

GENERAL MEASURES
- Future fertility: Impact of exogenous T should be discussed because it relates to fertility.
- Prostate cancer: Safety of TT is uncertain and a contraindication (2)[B].
  - 2018 American Urological Association (AUA) guidelines: Patients with TD and history of prostate cancer should be informed that there is inadequate evidence to quantify the risk–benefit ratio of TT (1)[B].

- 2018 endocrine guidelines: Patients with organ-confined prostate cancer who have undergone radical prostatectomy and disease free for ≥2 years with undetectable PSA may be considered for TT on an individualized basis.
- TT should be avoided in men with PSA >4 or PSA >3 and increased risk of prostate cancer (African Americans, men with first-degree relative with prostate cancer).
- TT should not be used in men with metastatic prostate cancer, breast cancer, hematocrit >54%, untreated obstructive sleep apnea, uncontrolled congestive heart failure (CHF), severe lower urinary tract symptoms with an IPSS >19 (1).
- TT is not recommended for mood or strength improvement in otherwise healthy men or asymptomatic men with low T (1).
- Cardiovascular disease (CVD) risk:
  - TD is also a risk factor for CVD (1).
  - Even in men with CVD or a high risk of developing CVD, TT was not found to cause an increased risk of cardiac events (3).
- Consider short-term TT as an adjunctive in men with HIV and low T to promote weight maintenance and gains in lean body mass and strength.

MEDICATION

ALERT
Avoid contact with females or children.

- Oral therapy with methyltestosterone is not recommended due to association with significant hepatotoxicity.
  - Oral testosterone undecanoate (Jatenzo) was FDA approved in March 2019.
- FDA cautions that TT is approved for men with confirmed low T by blood work with signs and symptoms, not solely due to aging.
- TT should NOT be started for a period of 3 to 6 months in patients with acute cardiovascular event.
- Topical gels/solutions: most common
  - Mimics normal daily circadian rhythm
  - Good absorption, 15–20% are nonresponders
- Testosterone pellets (Testopel)
  - Minor office procedure
  - Long-acting formulation, 3 to 4 months
  - 1–2% risk of infection or pellet extrusion
- Transdermal patch (Androderm)
  - Achieves less robust levels
  - High incidence of skin irritation
- Testosterone enanthate (Xyosted) SC weekly injection
  - Boxed warning for increased blood pressure
- Testosterone cypionate (IM every 1 to 3 weeks)
  - Starting dose: 100 mg/week or 200 mg/2 weeks
- Testosterone undecanoate (IM every 8 to 12 weeks)
  - Small risk of oil embolism, needs observation in office for 30 minutes postinjection

- Buccal application (Striant) BID dosing
  - Adheres to gum line, irritation in 16.3%
- Nasal gel (Natesto) TID dosing
  - Nasal irritation
  - May be protective of fertility
- Oral testosterone undecanoate (Jatenzo) BID dosing
  - FDA warning for blood pressure elevation
  - Titration required to determine appropriate dose
  - 2-year data demonstrates good efficacy, with safety profile similar to other T formulations

ISSUES FOR REFERRAL
PSA elevation, abnormal prostate exam, worsening BPH (IPSS >19), and refractory to replacement therapy should be referred to urology.

 ## ONGOING CARE

FOLLOW-UP RECOMMENDATIONS
Patient Monitoring
- 3 to 6 months after treatment initiation and then every 6 to 12 months
- Adjust dosing to achieve a total T in the middle tertile of the normal reference range.
- Measure hematocrit at baseline, at 3 to 6 months, and then annually.
- Stop treatment 3 to 6 months after starting in patients who experience normalization of T but fail to achieve symptom improvement.
- Bone mineral density after 1 to 2 years of therapy in men with osteoporosis
- Prostate exam every 6 to 12 months

DIET
Lifestyle changes and weight loss may raise T levels without the need for T replacement.

PATIENT EDUCATION
- TD can be chronic and may need lifelong therapy.
- T replacement comes with many risks, and it is very important to regularly monitor outcomes.
- Women and children must not be allowed to come in contact with TT gel products.

PROGNOSIS
There is evolving evidence that TT may improve metabolic functions such as glycosylated hemoglobin, blood sugar, total cholesterol, and visceral fat in diabetics; bone mineral density; and also unexplained anemia.

COMPLICATIONS
Complications of T replacement
- Decreased testicular volume, azoospermia in 40% of patients on TT, infertility
- Fluctuations in mood or libido
- Gynecomastia and growth of breast cancer
- Acne and oily skin

- Erythrocytosis (increased hematocrit)
- Exacerbation of sleep apnea
- Hepatotoxicity with prolonged oral use
- Possible prostate enlargement with or without worsening symptoms of BPH

REFERENCES

1. Mulhall JP, Trost LW, Brannigan RE, et al. Evaluation and management of testosterone deficiency: AUA guideline. *J Urol*. 2018;200(2):423–432.
2. Debruyne FMJ, Behre HM, Roehrborn CG, et al; for RHYME Investigators. Testosterone treatment is not associated with increased risk of prostate cancer or worsening of lower urinary tract symptoms: prostate health outcomes in the Registry of Hypogonadism in Men. *BJU Int*. 2017;119(2):216–224.
3. Lincoff AM, Bhasin S, Flevaris P, et al; TRAVERSE Study Investigators. Cardiovascular safety of testosterone-replacement therapy. *N Engl J Med*. 2023;389(2):107–117.

 ## CODES

ICD10
- E29.1 Testicular hypofunction
- E89.5 Postprocedural testicular hypofunction

CLINICAL PEARLS

- TD is common, and prevalence increases with age.
- Men with sexual dysfunction, obesity, unexplained anemia, bone density loss, chronic steroid or narcotic use, and metabolic diseases should be tested for TD.
- Initial test of choice is a morning total and free T; if low, repeat measurements.
- TT in the appropriately selected population can increase lean mass, reduce fat mass, increase bone mineral density, improve libido, improve unexplained anemia, and improve erections. However, it has not been shown to improve cognition or memory impairment in the elderly.
- Lifestyle changes such as diet and exercise may restore T levels.

T

THALASSEMIA
Garland E. Anderson II, MD

 BASICS

DESCRIPTION
- A group of inherited hematologic disorders that affect the synthesis of adult hemoglobin tetramer (HbA) (1)
- α-Thalassemia is due to a deficient synthesis of α-globin chain, whereas β-thalassemia is due to a deficient synthesis of β-globin chain:
  - The synthesis of the unaffected globin chain proceeds normally.
  - This unbalanced globin chain production causes unstable hemoglobin tetramers, which leads to hypochromic, microcytic red blood cells (RBCs), and hemolytic anemia.
- α-Thalassemia is more common in persons of Mediterranean, African, and Southeast Asian descent, whereas β-thalassemia is more common in patients of African and Southeast Asian descent.
- Types
  - Thalassemia (minor) trait (α or β): absent or mild anemia with microcytosis and hypochromia
  - α-Thalassemia major with hemoglobin Bart usually results in fatal hydrops fetalis (fluid in $\geq$2 fetal compartments secondary to anemia and fetal heart failure).
  - α-Thalassemia intermedia with hemoglobin H (hemoglobin H disease): results in moderate hemolytic anemia and splenomegaly
  - β-Thalassemia major: results in severe anemia, growth retardation, hepatosplenomegaly, bone marrow expansion, and bone deformities; transfusion therapy is necessary to sustain life.
  - β-Thalassemia intermedia: milder disease; transfusion therapy may not be needed or may be needed later in life.
- Other variants include hemoglobin E/β-thalassemia in Southeast Asians, which often mimics the severity of α-thalassemia major; δ-thalassemia; hemoglobin H Constant Spring
- System(s) affected: hematologic/lymphatic/immunologic; cardiac; hepatic
- Synonym(s): Mediterranean anemia; hereditary leptocytosis; Cooley anemia

Pediatric Considerations
- β-Thalassemia major causes symptoms during early childhood, usually starting at 6 months of age, and requires periodic transfusions to sustain life.
- Newborn's cord blood or heel stick should be screened for hemoglobinopathies with hemoglobin electrophoresis or comparably accurate test, although this primarily detects sickle cell disease.

Pregnancy Considerations
- Preconception genetic counseling is advised for couples at risk for having a child with thalassemia and for parents or other relatives of a child with thalassemia.
- Once pregnant, a chorionic villus sample at 10 to 11 weeks' gestation or an amniocentesis at 15 weeks' gestation can be done to detect point mutations or deletions with polymerase chain reaction (PCR) technology.

EPIDEMIOLOGY
Incidence
- Occurs in ~4.4/10,000 live births
- Predominant age: Symptoms start to appear 6 months after birth with β-thalassemia major.
- Predominant sex: male = female

Prevalence
- Worldwide, ~200,000 people are alive with β-thalassemia major and <1,000 patients are in the United States.
- In the worldwide population, an estimated 1.5% are β-thalassemia carriers and 5% α-thalassemia carriers (2).

ETIOLOGY AND PATHOPHYSIOLOGY
Unknown; it is unclear how the imbalance of β-globulin in α-thalassemia and α-globin in β-thalassemia results in ineffective RBC genesis and hemolysis.

Genetics
- Inherited in an autosomal recessive pattern
- α-Thalassemia results from a deletion of $\geq$1 of the 4 genes, 2 on each chromosome 16, responsible for α-globin synthesis. 1-gene deletion is a silent carrier state, 2-gene deletion is the trait, 3-gene deletion results in hemoglobin H, and 4-gene deletion results in hemoglobin Bart, causing fatal hydrops fetalis.
- Nondeletional forms do occur rarely. Hemoglobin H Constant Spring is the most common nondeletional form.
- β-Thalassemia is caused by any of >200-point mutations and, very rarely, deletions on chromosome 11; 20 alleles account for >80% of the mutations.
- Significantly disparate phenotype with the same genotype occurs because β-globin chain production can range from near-normal to absent.

RISK FACTORS
Family history of thalassemia

GENERAL PREVENTION
- Prenatal information: genetic counseling regarding partner selection and information on the availability of diagnostic tests during the pregnancy
- Complication prevention
  - For offspring of adult thalassemia patients, an evaluation for thalassemia by 1 year of age
  - Severe forms
    - Avoid exposure to sick contacts.
    - Keep immunizations up to date.
  - Promptly treat bacterial infections. (After splenectomy, patients should maintain a supply of an appropriate antibiotic to take at the onset of symptoms of a bacterial infection.)
  - Dental checkups every 6 months
  - Avoid activities that could increase the risk of bone fractures.

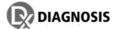 **DIAGNOSIS**

HISTORY
- Poor growth
- Excessive fatigue
- Cholelithiasis

- Pathologic fractures
- Shortness of breath

PHYSICAL EXAM
- Pallor
- Splenomegaly
- Jaundice
- Maxillary hyperplasia/frontal bossing due to massive bone marrow expansion
- Dental malocclusion

DIFFERENTIAL DIAGNOSIS
- Iron deficiency anemia
- Other microcytic anemias: lead toxicity, sideroblastic
- Other hemolytic anemias
- Other hemoglobinopathies

DIAGNOSTIC TESTS & INTERPRETATION
Special tests
- Bone marrow aspiration to evaluate for causes of microcytic anemia is rarely needed.
- Multiple indices have been evaluated to discriminate β-thalassemia trait from iron deficiency anemia, yet none is sensitive enough to exclude β-thalassemia.
- Hemoglobin: usual range 10 to 12 g/dL with thalassemia trait and 3 to 8 g/dL with β-thalassemia major before transfusions
- Hematocrit
  - 28–40% in thalassemia trait
  - May fall to <10% in β-thalassemia major
- Peripheral blood
  - Microcytosis (MCV <70 fl)
  - Hypochromia (MCH <20 pg)
  - High percentage of target cells
  - Reticulocyte count is elevated.
- Red cell distribution width (RDW)
  - A normal RDW with a microcytic hypochromic anemia is almost always thalassemia trait.
  - The RDW can be elevated in ~50% of thalassemia trait patients. This is in contrast to iron deficiency anemia, where the RDW is almost always elevated (90%).
- Hemoglobin electrophoresis
  - In α-thalassemia trait, no recognizable electrophoretic pattern occurs in adults.
  - However, in the neonatal period, 3–10% of trait patients will have hemoglobin H or hemoglobin Bart at birth, which would confirm α-thalassemia.
  - If HbA$_2$ is below normal (<2.5%) with a normal HbF level, the diagnosis is α-thalassemia intermedia (HbH disease).
  - In the neonatal period with β-thalassemia trait, the electrophoresis is normal. However, in adults, elevated HbA$_2$ levels (>4%) may be present but are usually normal.
  - β-Thalassemia major or intermedia has elevated HbA$_2$, elevated HbF, and reduced or absent HbA.
- DNA analysis
  - α-Thalassemia can definitively be diagnosed with genetic testing of hemoglobin A1 and A2 (for deletions and point mutations), but this is not routinely done due to the high cost.
  - High-performance liquid chromatography
  - Cost-effective primary screening tool for children and adolescents
  - Equivocal results should be confirmed with DNA analysis.

Pediatric Considerations

For children, calculate Mentzer index (mean corpuscular volume/RBC count).

- <13: suggests thalassemia
- >13: suggests iron deficiency anemia
- Liver iron concentrations can be assessed with MRI (FerriScan).

TREATMENT

- Outpatient for mild cases
- Inpatient for transfusion therapy

GENERAL MEASURES

- Mild cases (trait or minor) require no therapy.
- Thalassemia intermedia: No therapy is necessary unless hemoglobin falls to a level that causes symptoms; then, transfusion therapy is needed. Decision is based on patient's quality of life.
- Iron supplements should not be given unless iron deficiency occurs and is confirmed with low ferritin. Supplements increase the risk of iron overload (1)[C].
- Thalassemia major
  - A regular transfusion schedule to increase post-transfusion hemoglobin to 13 to 14 g/L and maintain a mean hemoglobin level of at least 9.3 g/dL (1.4 mmol/L) (1)[B]
  - Patients require >8 transfusion events per year. An event may be multiple transfused units.
  - Iron overload
    - Patients receiving transfusion therapy increase total body iron 4 times the normal amount.
    - Therapy is iron chelation. (See "Medication.")

MEDICATION

Thalassemia intermedia and major: folic acid supplements (1 mg/day)

First Line

β-Thalassemia major

- Iron chelation with deferoxamine (Desferal)
  - Usually continuous SC or IV infusion
  - Acute toxicity: initial—1,000 mg IV, may be followed by 500 mg every 4 hours for 2 doses; subsequent doses of 500 mg every 4 to 12 hours based on response (max of 6,000 mg/day)
  - Chronic: 20 to 40 mg/kg over 8 to 12 hours daily
  - Usually started by 5 to 8 years of age
  - Treatment lasts 3 to 5 years to reach serum ferritin <1,000 ng/mL.
- Deferasirox (Exjade): 20 to 30 mg/kg/day PO acceptable alternative; approved for transfusion and non–transfusion-dependent patients with hepatic iron concentrations ≥5 mg/g of dry weight and serum ferritin >300 μg/L; renal and hepatic monitoring is recommended.

Second Line

Chelation with deferiprone (Ferriprox) 25 mg/kg TID PO initially is an acceptable alternative for patients who have not responded to deferoxamine; may provide more cardioprotection. A drawback is weekly CBC because ~1% of patients develop agranulocytosis.

ADDITIONAL THERAPIES

β-Thalassemia intermedia

- Hydroxyurea may improve hemoglobin 1 to 2 g/dL.
- Psychological support seems appropriate for this chronic disease. However, no conclusions can be made regarding specific psychological therapies.

SURGERY/OTHER PROCEDURES

- Splenectomy
  - May be needed if hypersplenism causes an increase in the transfusion requirements (>180 to 200 mL/kg/year)
  - Defer surgery until patient is at least 4 years of age (due to increased infection risk).
  - Administer pneumococcal polyvalent-23 vaccine 1 month before splenectomy. Children should complete their pneumococcal conjugate vaccine series before surgery.
  - Daily penicillin prophylaxis, 250 mg BID, after splenectomy for 2 years for all patients and for children until age 16 years
- Bone marrow transplantation with HLA-identical related donor stem cells in children before developing hepatitis or iron overload has high likelihood of remission but may impair fertility.
- Mitapivat
  - Small molecule that activates RBC pyruvate kinase
  - Can increase hemoglobin levels for both α- and β-thalassemia patients

 ONGOING CARE

FOLLOW-UP RECOMMENDATIONS

- Thalassemia trait requires no restrictions.
- β-Thalassemia major
  - Avoid strenuous activities (e.g., football, soccer).
  - Acceptable activity levels will be determined on an individual basis depending on the severity of the disorder.

Patient Monitoring

- Thalassemia-trait patients require no special follow-up.
- For β-thalassemia major, lifelong monitoring is necessary because the therapy and disease progression have numerous potential complications.

DIET

- Thalassemia trait requires no restrictions.
- β-Thalassemia major
  - Limit intake of iron-rich foods (e.g., red meats such as liver and some cereals).

PATIENT EDUCATION

Printed patient information available from Cooley's Anemia Foundation: https://www.thalassemia.org or http://www.cooleysanemia.org

PROGNOSIS

- Thalassemia-trait patients live a normal lifespan.
- β-Thalassemia major patients live an average of 17 years and usually die by age 30 years.
- Iron overload causes most of the morbidity and mortality:
  - Cardiac events are the primary cause of death.
  - Myocardial iron deposition is best assessed with MRI T2.
  - Effective iron chelation improves longevity.

COMPLICATIONS

- Chronic hemolysis
- Susceptibility to infections after splenectomy
- Infections from blood transfusion
- Jaundice
- Leg ulcers
- Cholelithiasis
- Osteoporosis and low-trauma fractures
- Impaired growth rate
- Delayed or absent puberty
- Hypogonadism
- Hepatic siderosis
- Splenomegaly
- Cardiac disease from iron overload
- Thromboembolic phenomenon
- Aplastic and megaloblastic crises
- Increased risk of hematologic and abdominal cancer
- Increased risk of dementia

REFERENCES

1. Muncie HL Jr, Campbell J. Alpha and beta thalassemia. *Am Fam Physician*. 2009;80(4):339–344.
2. Peters M, Heijboer H, Smiers F, et al. Diagnosis and management of thalassaemia. *BMJ*. 2012;344:e228.

 CODES

ICD10

- D56.5 Hemoglobin E-beta thalassemia
- D56.3 Thalassemia minor
- D56.0 Alpha thalassemia

CLINICAL PEARLS

- Thalassemia (group of inherited hematologic disorders that affect the synthesis of adult hemoglobin tetramer) is a genetic condition; hemoglobin will not improve over time.
- α-Thalassemia is due to a deficient synthesis of the α-globin chain, whereas β-thalassemia is due to a deficient synthesis of the β-globin chain.
- Hemoglobin electrophoresis is needed for genetic counseling but not to make the diagnosis of thalassemia minor when evaluating a patient with mild hypochromic, microcytic anemia, and normal serum ferritin.
- Anemia from thalassemia minor is not due to inadequate iron availability or iron storage. Therefore, iron supplements will not improve the anemia and could be harmful due to GI distress and iron overload. If coexisting iron deficiency is proven, then iron therapy is appropriate.

THORACIC OUTLET SYNDROME

Ashley Koontz Sturts, DO • Morgan Lee Chambers, MD, MEd • Huong N. Nguyen, DO, MS

 BASICS

DESCRIPTION

- This syndrome consists of a constellation of symptoms that affect the head, neck, shoulders, and upper extremities caused by compression of the neurovascular structures (brachial plexus and subclavian vessels) at the thoracic outlet.
- Three forms of thoracic outlet syndrome (TOS) have been described:
  - Neurogenic (nTOS)
  - Venous (vTOS)
  - Arterial (aTOS)
- Synonym(s): scalenus anticus syndrome; cervical rib syndrome; costoclavicular syndrome; first rib syndrome

EPIDEMIOLOGY

- There are no universal diagnostic criteria to accurately determine epidemiology.
- nTOS
  - Approximately 90–95% of all TOS cases (1)
  - Predominant in 20- to 50-year-old females
- vTOS
  - Approximately 5–10% of all TOS cases (1)
  - Predominant in 20- to 35-year-old physically active males
- aTOS
  - Approximately 1% of all TOS cases (1)
  - No gender preference

ETIOLOGY AND PATHOPHYSIOLOGY

- TOS primarily impacts three anatomic spaces within the thoracic outlet (1):
  - Scalene triangle
    - Bordered by the anterior scalene, middle scalene, and first rib
    - Contains trunks of the brachial plexus and subclavian artery
  - Costoclavicular space
    - Bordered by the clavicle, first rib, and upper portion of the scapula
    - Contains divisions of the brachial plexus, subclavian artery, and subclavian vein
  - Subcoracoid space
    - Bordered by the pectoralis muscle, 2nd to 4th ribs and coracoid process
    - Contains cords of the brachial plexus
- Proposed etiologies include (1):
  - Congenital: cervical rib, first rib
  - Traumatic: motor vehicle accidents
  - Functional: overuse activity of the upper extremity, particularly shoulder abduction/extension

RISK FACTORS

- Trauma to the shoulder girdle
- Presence of a cervical rib (1% of population)
- Exostosis of clavicle or 1st rib
- Postural abnormalities (e.g., drooping of shoulders, scoliosis)
- Occupational exposure via repetitive activity (e.g., computer users, musicians, overhead athletes, repetitive upper body work)

GENERAL PREVENTION

Consider workplace evaluation for proper occupational ergonomics, including proper posture.

COMMONLY ASSOCIATED CONDITIONS

- Paget–von Schrötter syndrome: effort thrombosis of subclavian vein
- Gilliatt-Sumner hand: neurogenic atrophy of abductor pollicis brevis
- Pancoast tumor

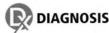 **DIAGNOSIS**

HISTORY

- nTOS
  - High index of suspicion if there is a history of neck trauma or repetitive overhead activity
  - Upper extremity pain and paresthesias are considered common presenting symptoms (1).
  - Additional symptoms:
    - Occipital and orbital headache
    - Muscle atrophy of the upper extremity
    - Raynaud phenomenon secondary to sympathic nerve irritation (1)
- vTOS
  - High index of suspicion if symptoms worsen with shoulder abduction particularly in overhead lifting athletes
  - Common symptoms: unilateral arm claudication, cyanosis, swelling, pain, venous enlargement
- aTOS
  - 85% of cases estimated to be related to cervical rib
  - Highest morbidity of all types due to risk for limb ischemia
  - Common symptoms: unilateral arm weakness, pallor, paresthesia, pain, weak or absent pulse, blood pressure asymmetry
- Sport can be an initial presentation of symptom provocation, particularly for pediatric patients (2).

PHYSICAL EXAM

- Initial considerations
  - Posture
  - Cervical alignment
  - Scapular stability
  - Inspection and palpation of thoracic outlet anatomy
  - Upper extremity and cranial nerve neurologic examination
- Specialized testing
  - Adson maneuver (aTOS)
    - Head rotation to the affected side with cervical extension and then deep inhalation
    - Positive if paresthesias occur or if radial pulse is not palpable during maneuver
  - Morley test (vTOS)
    - Positive with reproduction of an aching sensation and typical localized paresthesia
    - Manual compression of brachial plexus for 30 seconds in the supraclavicular area of the scalene triangle
  - Hyperabduction test (aTOS)
    - Elevation of arm above the head
    - Positive if diminished of radial pulse
  - Military maneuver (i.e., costoclavicular bracing)
    - Patient elevates chin and pushes shoulders posteriorly in an extreme "at-attention" position
    - Positive test reproduces symptoms.
  - 1-minute Roos test
    - Shoulders and arms are braced in a 90-degree abducted and externally rotated position; patient is required to clench and relax fists repetitively for 1 minute.
    - Positive test reproduces symptoms

DIFFERENTIAL DIAGNOSIS

- Cervical disc or carpal tunnel syndrome
- Orthopedic shoulder problems (shoulder strain, rotator cuff injury, tendonitis)
- Cervical spondylitis
- Ulnar nerve compression at elbow and hand
- Multiple sclerosis
- Spinal cord tumor/disease
- Angina pectoris
- Migraine
- Complex regional pain syndromes
- C3 to C5 and C8 radiculopathies
- Pancoast Tumor

DIAGNOSTIC TESTS & INTERPRETATION

Initial Tests (lab, imaging)

- History and physical are the strongest clinical indicators for TOS. However, additional imaging helps to confirm subtype to guide proper treatment.
- Chest x-ray is often an appropriate initial imaging modality for all subtypes (3).
- EMG may be a beneficial initial test to narrow differential between neurogenic and vascular types.
- Laboratory testing is typically not considered in the initial workup.

Follow-Up Tests & Special Considerations

- American College of Radiology recommends a variety of imaging modalities:
  - nTOS: chest MRI, can consider use of contrast although not required if contraindicated for a patient
  - aTOS: chest CTA, chest MRA, duplex US over the subclavian vessels
  - vTOS: chest CT with contrast; catheter venography of the upper extremity; duplex US of the subclavian vessels (3)
- MRI and CT assist with definitive subtype diagnosis after initial workup (4)[C]

TREATMENT

GENERAL MEASURES

- Conservative management usually involves approaches to reduce and redistribute pressure and traction on the thoracic outlet.
- Physical therapy is first-line treatment along with activity modification, rest, and NSAIDs if no vascular alarm symptoms exist (5)[B].
- Adjunctive therapies including taping, adhesive elastic bandages, moist heat, TENS, or US may be used but should not substitute active exercise and correction of posture and muscle imbalance (5)[B].

MEDICATION

No firm evidence exists for any specific pharmacologic approach to the three types of TOS.

- Anti-inflammatory (ibuprofen)
  - Adult dose: 400 to 800 mg PO q8h; not to exceed 3,200 mg/day
  - Pediatric dose:
    - <12 years: 10 mg/kg/dose q6–8h
  - Contraindications: documented hypersensitivity, active PUD, renal or hepatic impairment, recent use of anticoagulants, hemorrhagic conditions
- Neuropathic pain: Tricyclic antidepressants, carbamazepine, gabapentin, phenytoin, pregabalin; muscle relaxants such as baclofen, metaxalone, or tizanidine may be helpful.
- Severe pain: Consider procedural alternatives as listed below.

ISSUES FOR REFERRAL

- If vascular type TOS is suspected, immediate referral to vascular surgery should be made due to risk for limb ischemia.
- Sports medicine or PM&R providers can be considered for diagnostic and therapeutic injections.
- Vascular surgery (aTOS and vTOS), orthopedic surgery (nTOS) or neurosurgery (nTOS) can be considered for surgical evaluation.

SURGERY/OTHER PROCEDURES

- Botulinum toxin—type A injection therapy
  - Benefit from decreased muscular tension and pain
  - 64–69% of patients have relief for up to 3 months although with a risk for prolonged duration of symptoms (6). Alternative injection therapies show the best efficacy when combined with physical therapy modalities (6).
    - Trigger point
    - Corticosteroid
    - Local anesthetic
- Surgical options can provide greater relief to symptoms than conservative management alone (7).
- Complete 1st rib resection and anterior scalenectomy are common combined surgical interventions to provide pressure relief to the thoracic outlet structures in all subtypes.
- Thrombolytic may be necessary for acute vTOS with consideration of venoplasty thereafter.

ADMISSION, INPATIENT, AND NURSING CONSIDERATIONS

Conservative, outpatient treatment is reasonable first-line therapy except in cases of thromboembolic phenomena and acute ischemia, symptoms of chronic vascular occlusion, stenosis, arterial dilatation, or progressive neurologic deficit (8)[B].

 ONGOING CARE

FOLLOW-UP RECOMMENDATIONS

Patient Monitoring
Office follow-up visits every 3 to 4 weeks

PATIENT EDUCATION
Physical therapy, postural exercises, ergonomic workstation

PROGNOSIS
Durable long-term functional outcomes can be achieved predicated on a highly selective approach to the surgical management of patients with TOS. A majority of operated patients will not require adjunctive procedures or chronic narcotic use (9)[C].

COMPLICATIONS
- Postoperative shoulder, arm, hand pain, and paresthesias: 10%
- Patients who will have symptomatic recurrences at 1 month to 7 years postoperatively (usually within 3 months): 1.5–2%
- Patients who will have brachial plexus injury, probably due to intraoperative traction: 0.5–1%
- Reoperation is indicated for symptomatic recurrence with long posterior remnant of 1st rib (posterior approach) or with disrupted fibrous adhesions (transaxillary approach).
- Venous obstruction or arterial emboli; usually responds to thrombolytics

REFERENCES

1. Cavanna AC, Giovanis A, Daley A, et al. Thoracic outlet syndrome: a review for the primary care provider. *J Osteopath Med*. 2022;122(11):587–599.
2. Garraud T, Pomares G, Daley P, et al. Thoracic outlet syndrome in sport: a systematic review. *Front Physiol*. 2022;13:838014.
3. Zurkiya O, Ganguli S, Kalva SP, et al; for Expert Panels on Vascular Imaging, Thoracic Imaging, and Neurological Imaging. ACR Appropriateness Criteria® thoracic outlet syndrome. *J Am Coll Radiol*. 2020;17(5S):S323–S334.
4. Povlsen S, Povlsen B. Diagnosing thoracic outlet syndrome: current approaches and future directions. *Diagnostics (Basel)*. 2018;8(1):21.
5. Vanti C, Natalini L, Romeo A, et al. Conservative treatment of thoracic outlet syndrome. A review of the literature. *Eura Medicophys*. 2007;43(1):55–70.
6. Li N, Dierks G, Vervaeke HE, et al. Thoracic outlet syndrome: a narrative review. *J Clin Med*. 2021;10(5):962.
7. Balderman J, Abuirqeba AA, Eichaker L, et al. Physical therapy management, surgical treatment, and patient-reported outcomes measures in a prospective observational cohort of patients with neurogenic thoracic outlet syndrome. *J Vasc Surg*. 2019;70(3):832–841.
8. Christo PJ, Christo DK, Carinci AJ, et al. Single CT-guided chemodenervation of the anterior scalene muscle with botulinum toxin for neurogenic thoracic outlet syndrome. *Pain Med*. 2010;11(4):504–511.
9. Scali S, Stone D, Bjerke A, et al. Long-term functional results for the surgical management of neurogenic thoracic outlet syndrome. *Vasc Endovascular Surg*. 2010;44(7):550–555.

ADDITIONAL READING

- Dengler NF, Ferraresi S, Rochkind S, et al. Thoracic outlet syndrome part I: systematic review of the literature and consensus on anatomy, diagnosis, and classification of thoracic outlet syndrome by the European Association of Neurosurgical Societies' section of peripheral nerve surgery. *Neurosurgery*. 2022;90(6):653–667.
- Hock G, Johnson A, Barber P, et al. Current clinical concepts: rehabilitation of thoracic outlet syndrome [published online ahead of print November 17, 2022]. *J Athl Train*. doi: 10.4085/1062-6050-138-22.

 CODES

ICD10
G54.0 Brachial plexus disorders

CLINICAL PEARLS

- This syndrome is caused by compression of the neurovascular structures (brachial plexus and subclavian vessels) at the thoracic outlet, specifically in the area superior to the 1st rib and posterior to the clavicle.
- Three subtypes exist: neurogenic, arterial, and venous.
- Physical therapy, activity modification, rest, and NSAIDs are the first-line treatment if no alarm symptoms exist.
- If vascular type TOS (venous or arterial) is suspected, immediate referral to vascular surgery should be made due to risk for limb ischemia.

T

THROMBOPHILIA AND HYPERCOAGULABLE STATES

Touqir Zahra, MD, FACP • Raksha Sharma, MD

BASICS

DESCRIPTION

- An inherited or acquired disorder of the coagulation system predisposing an individual to thromboembolism (the formation of a venous, or less commonly, an arterial blood clot)
- Venous thrombosis typically manifests as deep venous thrombosis (DVT) of the lower extremity in the legs or pelvis and pulmonary embolism (PE).
- System(s) affected: cardiovascular, nervous, pulmonary, reproductive, hematologic
- Synonym(s): hypercoagulable disorder; prothrombotic state

EPIDEMIOLOGY

- VTE incidence is higher in ages 16 to 44 years; then, higher in men when >45 years of age
- VTE incidence is higher in African American populations.
- Inherited thrombophilias
  - An inherited thrombophilic defect or risk can be detected in up to 50% of patients with VTE.
  - Factor V Leiden (FVL) is the most common inherited thrombophilia (1/2 of all currently characterizable inherited thrombophilia cases involve the FVL mutation), and it is present in its heterozygous form in up to ~20% of patients with a first VTE.
  - Heterozygous prothrombin G20210A mutation, the second most common inherited thrombophilia, is present in up to ~8% of patients with VTE.
- Acquired thrombophilias:
  - Pregnancy: ~1 to 2/1,000 pregnancies affected by VTE
  - Cancer: ~20% of all VTEs occur in setting of active cancer; ~6% of unprovoked VTEs have undiagnosed cancer.
  - Antiphospholipid antibodies are found in ~50% of patients with systemic lupus erythematosus (SLE) and up to 5% of the general population.
  - See "Risk Factors."

Incidence

First-time thromboembolism
- ~100/100,000/year among the general population
- <1/100,000/year in those aged <15 years; ~1,000/100,000/year in those aged ≥85 years

Prevalence

- 40–80% of lower extremity orthopedic procedures can result in DVT if prophylaxis is not used.
- VTE accounts for ~1.2 to 4.7 deaths per 100,000 pregnancies.

ETIOLOGY AND PATHOPHYSIOLOGY

- Virchow triad as a cause of VTE includes venous stasis, vascular endothelial injury, and abnormalities in circulating blood constituents.
- An imbalance between the hemostatic and fibrinolytic pathways leads to thrombus formation.
- VTE is considered to be the result of inherited tendencies with other acquired risks.
- Upper extremity DVT: >60% are associated with venous catheters. Malignancy is an additional significant risk.

Genetics

- The most common genetic thrombophilias (FVL, prothrombin G20210A mutation, proteins C and S defects, and antithrombin III deficiency) are inherited in an autosomal dominant pattern.
- Homozygous mutations have a higher risk of VTE.
- FVL/activated protein C (aPC) resistance:
  - Heterozygous FVL: 3–8% prevalence in Caucasians; 1.2% in African Americans
  - Heterozygous FVL carries 3- to 5-fold increase risk in first-time VTE; mild increase risk of recurrence
  - Homozygous FVL carries 18-fold increase risk in first-time VTE compared to patients without FVL mutation.
  - Other acquired risks are synergistic.
- Prothrombin gene mutation G20210A:
  - Prevalence 6% among Caucasians, 2% of general U.S. population, 0.5% of African Americans
  - Heterozygous carriers have 3-fold increased risk in first-time VTE.
- Antithrombin deficiency: <0.2% among the general population; acquired deficiency in disseminated intravascular coagulation (DIC), sepsis, liver disease, nephrotic syndrome; relative risk (RR) of 8.1 for thrombosis
- Protein C and S deficiencies: 0.5% and 1% incidences, respectively, among the general population; homozygotes and heterozygotes are hypercoagulable; vitamin K–dependent, produced in the liver; protein C inactivates Va and VIIIa. Protein C may become an acquired deficiency in liver disease, sepsis, DIC, acute respiratory distress syndrome, and after surgery; RR of 7.3 for thrombosis; protein S is a cofactor for protein C, and it may become an acquired deficiency with oral contraceptive pill (OCP) use, pregnancy, liver disease, sepsis, DIC, HIV, and nephrosis; RR of 8.5 for thrombosis

RISK FACTORS

Acquired risk factors
- Previous thromboembolism
- First-degree relative with VTE (2- to 4-fold increased risk; regardless of relative's test results)
- Immobilization or prolonged travel (e.g., flight time >8 hours)
- Trauma
- Surgery, especially orthopedic
- Malignancies (especially pancreatic, ovarian, brain, and lymphoma)
- Pregnancy (5- to 10-fold increased RR compared to nonpregnant women)
- Postpartum state (15- to 35-fold increased risk)
- Acute medical illness: pneumonia, particularly involving SARS-CoV, MERS-CoV, SARS-CoV-2
- Exogenous female hormones/oral contraceptives
- Androgen-deprivation therapy
- Obesity
- Nephrotic syndrome, hypoalbuminemia
- APS and lupus anticoagulant
- Myeloproliferative disorders (polycythemia vera, essential thrombocythemia)
- Hyperviscosity syndromes (sickle cell, paraproteinemias)
- Hyperhomocysteinemia secondary to vitamin deficiencies (B_6, B_{12}, folic acid) also due to "Whippets"
- Tamoxifen, thalidomide, lenalidomide, bevacizumab, L-asparaginase, erythropoiesis-stimulating agents, pomalidomide, tranexamic acid
- Dehydration

- Inflammatory bowel disease
- Presence of central venous catheter
- Heart failure, congenital heart disease
- Severe liver disease
- Established genetic factors: FVL; prothrombin G20210A mutation; protein C deficiency; protein S deficiency; antithrombin III deficiency
- Rare genetic factors: dysfibrinogenemia; methylene tetrahydrofolate reductase mutation
- Indeterminate factors: elevated factor VIII
- Age: >65 years

GENERAL PREVENTION

- Consider medication prophylaxis in any hospitalized patient with VTE risk factors.
- Consider mechanical prophylaxis in patients at increased risk for VTE in whom anticoagulation may be contraindicated.
- Consider prophylaxis with low-molecular-weight heparin (LMWH) plus aspirin in pregnant patients with APS.
- Consider prophylaxis using direct oral anticoagulants (DOACs) in patients with solid tumors who have additional risk factors for VTE.
- Prophylaxis with unfractionated heparin (UFH) or LMWH should be considered in patients with genetic or acquired risks of thrombosis and an anticipated additional risk, such as the immobilization associated with surgery.
- Use caution with procoagulant medicines (e.g., OCPs) in asymptomatic individuals who have a known hereditary predisposition.

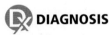

DIAGNOSIS

HISTORY

Consider prothrombotic assessment for the following:
- Recurrent VTE events
- Thrombosis at an age <50 years, particularly in the absence of provoking factors such as recent surgery, immobilization, use of combination oral contraceptives, etc.
- Strong family history of VTE suggesting multiple individuals affected with VTE; first-degree family members affected at a young age
- Purpura fulminans in children or neonates
- Skin necrosis associated with vitamin K antagonists
- Recurrent pregnancy loss

PHYSICAL EXAM

- DVT: swelling, pain, warmth, and redness, usually of one extremity
- PE: dyspnea, chest pain, hemoptysis, hypoxia, tachycardia

DIAGNOSTIC TESTS & INTERPRETATION

- Testing should be delayed until after the initial 3 months of anticoagulation.
- Rationale for screening
  - Help predict VTE recurrence risk and guide duration of therapy or future risk management
  - Help guide management of asymptomatic family members, especially in female patients seeking contraceptive counsel or who are planning pregnancy

- Appropriate tests for unprovoked VTE, recurrent VTE, VTE at age 50 years, family history of VTE, unusual sites of VTE or VTE secondary to pregnancy, OCPs or HRT:
  - FVL (aPC), protein C and S, ATIII, G20210A assays if idiopathic VTE, younger patient and/or family history of VTE
  - Antiphospholipid antibody assays if idiopathic VTE or associated autoimmune disease or no family history of VTE
- Appropriate tests for arterial thrombosis, especially if younger patient or no atherosclerosis
  - Antiphospholipid antibody assays
  - Consider FVL, G2021A, protein C and S, ATIII.
  - Consider screening for vasculitides such as antineutrophil cytoplasmic antibody (ANCA)-associated vasculitis.
  - Do not test for FVL, G2021A, protein C and S, ATIII if known atherosclerosis

Initial Tests (lab, imaging)
- CBC
- aPC profile: ≤2 implies FVL mutation; 95–100% are FVL positive; false-positive finding in pregnancy or with use of OCPs, confirm with FVL mutation testing or consider FVL mutation testing up front: aPC resistance may be unreliable while taking LMWH or UFH.
- Prothrombin G20210A genetic assay
- ATIII functional assay: will be low with acute thrombosis and on heparin therapy; may be falsely high on dabigatran, apixaban, edoxaban, and rivaroxaban
- Protein C functional assay: may be low with acute thrombosis; will be lower on warfarin, dabigatran, apixaban, edoxaban, and rivaroxaban
- Protein S antigen and functional assay and free S: may be low with acute thrombosis; will be lower on warfarin, dabigatran, apixaban, edoxaban, and rivaroxaban
- Antiphospholipid antibodies: phospholipid-dependent tests and anticardiolipin antibodies, lupus anticoagulant: may be unreliable on heparin and DOACs; risk false-positive test
- Consider evaluation for subclinical malignancy in an unprovoked thrombosis in those >40 years of age or at greater risk.
- Consider HIT antibody immunoassay or functional assay if clinical suspicion

Follow-Up Tests & Special Considerations
Special situations

- Antiphospholipid syndrome
  - Antiphospholipid syndrome can present as both arterial and venous thrombosis.
  - Other clinical manifestations can include pregnancy complications such as fetal demise, premature birth due to eclampsia or severe preeclampsia, and recurrent unexplained spontaneous abortions. Testing for lupus anticoagulant assay, anticardiolipin antibody, and anti-β-2-glycoprotein 1 antibody is recommended to meet the diagnostic criteria.
- Malignancy
  - There is an increased risk of VTE in cancer, specially with mucin-producing adenocarcinoma.
  - Thrombophilia testing is not suggested in patients with active cancer and VTE.

- Thrombosis at unusual sites
  - In patients with splanchnic veins (hepatic, portal, splenic, mesenteric) and cerebral vein thrombosis at a younger age, thrombophilia testing is recommended.
  - Consider evaluation for liver cirrhosis or extrinsic compression from a tumor in patients with portal vein thrombosis.
  - Paroxysmal nocturnal hemoglobinuria and myeloproliferative neoplasms should be considered in patients with unexplained splanchnic vein thrombosis.
- Combination oral contraceptives use: Smoking and obesity in women taking combined oral contraceptives are associated with increased risk of VTE (1).

Pediatric Considerations
- Warfarin is teratogenic and should be avoided in pregnancy.
- LMWH or UFH are preferred for all prophylactic and treatment options.
- There is lack of safety data on DOACs in pregnancy.

 TREATMENT

- Assess VTE risk:
  - Low-risk inherited thrombophilias: heterozygous FVL, heterozygous prothrombin 20210 mutation
  - High-risk inherited thrombophilias: protein C deficiency, protein S deficiency, antithrombin deficiency
- Duration of treatment
  - Heterozygosity for FVL or prothrombin 20210 mutation, as isolated risk factors, should not affect decision.
  - Consider extended thromboprophylaxis post-discharge with major prothrombotic risk factors such as history of VTE or major surgery as long as bleeding risk is not high.

MEDICATION
First Line
- DOACs: apixaban, dabigatran, edoxaban, and rivaroxaban are now recommended over vitamin K antagonists for initial and long-term oral anticoagulation.
  - Use is supported for low-risk inherited thrombophilia (i.e., FVL or prothrombin 20210 mutation).
  - Few data available to support use in rare thrombophilias such as ATIII, protein C or protein S deficiencies
  - May consider DOACs for patients with active cancer, but data are lacking to recommend over LMWH
- Parenteral anticoagulation: LMWH has largely replaced UFH as first-line therapy for VTE: Enoxaparin is preferred in patients with active cancer for a minimum of 6 months (can dose at 1.5 mg/kg SC daily), after which time the patient can be reevaluated to continue treatment.
- Vitamin K antagonist: Warfarin requires careful and frequent monitoring because of many drug–drug and drug–diet (e.g., vitamin K) interactions.
- Pregnancy: low-dose aspirin and/or LMWH or UFH; warfarin is contraindicated.
- APS: Warfarin and LMWH remain as first-line agents for anticoagulation.

Second Line
Usually indicated when contraindication to heparin or LMWH, such as heparin-associated thrombosis and thrombocytopenia
- Factor Xa inhibitors (fondaparinux)
- Direct thrombin inhibitors (argatroban)

SURGERY/OTHER PROCEDURES
Inferior vena cava filter
- Reduces short-term risk of PE in those with contraindications to anticoagulation
- May increase long-term risk of recurrent DVT

 ONGOING CARE

FOLLOW-UP RECOMMENDATIONS
Patient Monitoring
Monitor warfarin with INR goal of 2 to 3.

DIET
- Vitamin K–stable diet if patient is taking warfarin
- Rivaroxaban should be taken with a large meal to aid absorption.

PATIENT EDUCATION
Medical alert bracelets; avoid contact sports; seek evaluation for any trauma.

PROGNOSIS
- Anticoagulation should be continued for 3 months with consideration for longer in those with unprovoked VTE.
- Patients with a provoked VTE (i.e., surgery, hospitalization) not receiving chronic anticoagulation have risks of recurrence of 7% (year 1), 16% (year 5), and 23% (year 10).
- Patients with an unprovoked VTE not receiving chronic anticoagulation have risks of recurrence of 15% (year 1), 41% (year 5), and 53% (year 10).
- Currently, there are no data from randomized, controlled trials or controlled clinical trials about the benefits of thrombophilia testing to decrease the risk of recurrent VTE.

REFERENCE

1. Middeldorp S, Nieuwlaat R, Kreuziger LB, et al. American Society of Hematology 2023 guidelines for management of venous thromboembolism: thrombophilia testing. *Blood Adv*. 2023;7(22):7101–7138.

CODES

ICD10
- D68.59 Other primary thrombophilia
- D68.51 Activated protein C resistance
- D68.2 Hereditary deficiency of other clotting factors

CLINICAL PEARLS

- FVL (resistance to aPC) most common inherited thrombophilia.
- For patients <45 with VTE, suggest testing for inherited thrombotic disorders.
- Rule out malignancy, especially in those >50 years of age.

T

THROMBOTIC THROMBOCYTOPENIC PURPURA

Chirag N. Shah, MD • Grant Wei, MD, FACEP • Jay Patel, DO

BASICS

DESCRIPTION
- An acute syndrome of microangiopathic hemolytic anemia (MAHA) and consumptive thrombocytopenia with deposition of hyaline thrombi in terminal arterioles and capillaries leads to ischemic multiorgan damage.
- Thrombotic thrombocytopenic purpura (TTP) is characterized by MAHA (schistocytes on peripheral smear) and thrombocytopenia (generally <30,000), with or without the following signs and symptoms:
  - Neurologic symptoms, renal dysfunction, fever
  - Most patients do not show the historic pentad of MAHA, thrombocytopenia, renal dysfunction, neurologic abnormalities, and fever because treatment is initiated before the pentad can develop.

EPIDEMIOLOGY
Incidence
- First episode mostly in adulthood (~90%) with a median age of 41 years and 10% in childhood to adolescence (1)[C]
- Predominant sex: female > male (2:1); higher relapse in females (1)[C]
- Incidence ratio of blacks to whites is 7:1.
- Other features with increased risk: high body mass index and pregnancy
- Annual incidence of ~3 new cases per million people

Prevalence
Annual prevalence of ~10 cases per million people

ETIOLOGY AND PATHOPHYSIOLOGY
- In TTP, the aggregating agent responsible for platelet thrombi is unusually large von Willebrand factor (UL vWF) multimers, which are far larger than those found in normal plasma.
- A metalloprotease, ADAMTS13, which normally enzymatically cleaves UL vWF multimers to prevent clumping within vessels, is deficient, defective, or absent, allowing UL vWF to react with platelets. This leads to endothelial cell damage and disseminated thrombi characteristic of TTP.
- Arterioles often affected: brain, kidney, pancreas, heart, adrenal glands; lungs and liver are relatively spared.
- In familial TTP, patients have an inherited deficiency of ADAMTS13.
- In acquired idiopathic TTP, autoantibodies are directed against the metalloprotease ADAMTS13 (1)[C].
- Endothelial injury, either directly from a drug/toxin or indirectly via platelet/neutrophil activation, has been proposed as a cause of secondary TTP especially in those without ADAMTS13 deficiency.

Genetics
- TTP is most often an acquired disorder. A congenital form of inherited TTP (Upshaw-Schulman syndrome) is due to a mutation at the ADAMTS13 gene locus on chromosome 9q34. This has an autosomal-recessive pattern of inheritance.
- USS typically presents in infancy and is rarely diagnosed after 10 years of age. It does not have the female predominance seen in idiopathic TTP, more often has notable renal impairment, and there is some heterogeneity among siblings.

RISK FACTORS
- Pregnancy, oral contraceptives, AIDS and early HIV infection, bacterial infection/sepsis, acute pancreatitis
- Autoimmune disease: antiphospholipid antibody syndrome, systemic lupus erythematosus, scleroderma
- Cancer, hematopoietic stem cell transplantation, and solid organ transplant
- Drugs of abuse: MDMA, cocaine, oxymorphone ER
- Drug toxicity
  - Antimicrobials: trimethoprim, ciprofloxacin, famciclovir
  - Chemotherapy: mitomycin C and gemcitabine, pentostatin and vincristine, bleomycin and cisplatin, oxaliplatin, bevacizumab and sunitinib, adalimumab, bortezomib, carfilzomib, and ixazomib
  - Calcineurin inhibitors: tacrolimus and cyclosporine
  - Immune mediated: quinine and quinidine, ticlopidine and clopidogrel

COMMONLY ASSOCIATED CONDITIONS
- TTP/hemolytic uremic syndrome (HUS)/atypical HUS have similar presentations with MAHA and thrombocytopenia and multiorgan involvement.
- TTP generally presents with minimal renal involvement and may have neurologic abnormalities, whereas the opposite is more characteristic of HUS/atypical HUS. Creatinine of >2 to 3 is not suggestive of TTP.
- However, patients with HUS and TTP may have both prominent renal and neurologic manifestations, often making the diagnosis unclear—hence the historical hybrid name "TTP-HUS."
- ADAMTS13 levels are diminished (generally <10%) in adults with familial or acquired idiopathic TTP but are normal in children diagnosed with HUS.

DIAGNOSIS

- Screening ADAMTS13 activity level
  - <10% defines severe deficiency and makes TTP more likely. Levels of 10–20% suggest possible TTP especially if drawn after plasma exchange (PEX) has been initiated. >20% makes TTP less likely.
  - Due to the high mortality associated with TTP, do not wait for the results of ADAMTS13 determination to initiate therapy.
- Most common symptoms are nonspecific: nausea, vomiting, weakness, abdominal pain, fatigue, and fever.
- Related to thrombocytopenia: easy bruising, purpura, petechiae, epistaxis, menorrhagia, bleeding gums, GI bleeding, intracranial hemorrhage—visual symptoms are due to retinal hemorrhages
- Related to hemolytic anemia (MAHA): jaundice, fatigue; end-organ ischemia
  - Neurologic: occurs in ~60% of the patients (1)[C]; headache, altered mental status, seizures, or stroke
  - Cardiac: arrhythmia, myocardial infarction, heart failure
  - Renal: hematuria, proteinuria, oliguria, or anuria

- A scoring system (PLASMIC) was devised to predict ADAMTS13 activity <10% in adults with unexplained thrombocytopenia and MAHA. It is used to support the diagnosis of TTP while the ADAMTS13 lab test is pending; 1 point each for:
  - Platelet count <30,000/μL
  - Hemolysis (reticulocyte count >2.5%, undetectable haptoglobin, or indirect bilirubin >2 mg/dL)
  - No active cancer
  - No solid organ or stem cell transplant history
  - MCV <90 fL
  - INR <1.5
  - Creatinine <2 mg/dL
  - Score of 6 to 7 predictive of ADAMTS13 activity of <10%; score of 0 to 4 predictive of ADAMTS13 activity was >10%.

HISTORY
- Generally, acute onset of symptoms but subacute in about 1/4 of patients
- In about 50% of cases, a trigger/risk factor of some kind is identified.

PHYSICAL EXAM
- Fever
- Mental status/neurologic: confusion, coma, stupor, weakness
- HEENT: retinal hemorrhage, scleral icterus, epistaxis
- Abdomen/GI: nonspecific tenderness
- Skin: jaundice, petechiae, purpura, ecchymoses

DIFFERENTIAL DIAGNOSIS
- HUS and atypical HUS
- Antiphospholipid antibody syndrome: prolonged partial thromboplastin time (PTT) and presence of lupus anticoagulant
- Systemic lupus erythematosus
- Malignant hypertension: diastolic blood pressure >130 mm Hg, papilledema, retinal hemorrhages
- Pregnancy-associated preeclampsia/eclampsia or hemolysis, elevated liver enzymes, and low platelets (HELLP) syndrome
- Disseminated intravascular coagulation
- Idiopathic thrombocytopenic purpura (ITP): no hemolysis, normal LDH, and bilirubin, presence of antiplatelet antibodies
- Malignancy-associated microangiopathy
- Evan syndrome (autoimmune hemolytic anemia and thrombocytopenia): positive direct Coombs test
- Sclerodermal kidney

DIAGNOSTIC TESTS & INTERPRETATION
Initial Tests (lab, imaging)
- CBC
  - Hemoglobin (decreased): Average is 8 to 10 g/dL; platelets decreased in the 10 to 30,000/μL range
- High reticulocyte count (>120 × 10⁹/L)
- Undetectable haptoglobin (hemolysis)
- Peripheral smear
  - Schistocytes (prominent, >1% of RBCs)
  - Helmet cells, RBC fragments, nucleated RBCs, polychromasia (reticulocytosis)
- Coagulation studies
  - Normal in most; mild elevation in 15%; fibrinogen is normal.
- Coombs test: negative direct Coombs test
- Electrolytes, BUN/creatinine: mild elevation of BUN and creatinine (creatinine <3 mg/dL)

- Liver function studies: increased indirect bilirubin (hemolysis)
- LDH: 5 to 10 times normal
- Urinalysis
  - Proteinuria, microscopic hematuria; positive dipstick for large blood but minimal RBCs on microscopic exam
- ECG changes (10%): sinus tachycardia, heart block
- Stool for Shiga toxin
- Increased troponin in 60% of cases (>0.1 μg/L)
- HIV, hepatitis A, B, and C testing: Exclude underlying viral precipitant.
- Pregnancy test (women with inherited TTP often have their first episode during their pregnancy)
- Head CT/MRI scan: in patients with mental status changes to rule out possible intracranial pathology

 TREATMENT

ALERT

- Prompt treatment of presumptive or confirmed TTP is necessary due to the high mortality (90%).
- Complete response to treatment is defined by a platelet count >150 × 10⁹/L for 2 consecutive days, together with normal or normalizing LDH and clinical recovery (1)[C].
- In the absence of another apparent cause, the dyad of MAHA and thrombocytopenia is sufficient to begin treatment for TTP while the workup proceeds (1)[C].
  - PEX transfusion is the cornerstone of the treatment of TTP and should begin immediately.
  - The most effective therapy for TTP is PEX with fresh frozen plasma (FFP) (2)[A].
  - PEX replaces deficient or defective metalloprotease (ADAMTS13) and removes UL vWF and antimetalloprotease antibodies.
  - Optimal PEX duration is variable. Continue for 2 days after platelet count is ≥150,000 and then consider tapering.
  - FFP: temporary until PEX can be initiated; reserve for those with active bleeding.

MEDICATION

First Line

- Glucocorticoids have adjunctive benefit in some patients. The International Society on Thrombosis and Haemostasis guidelines recommend its use for all patients, due to the potential life-saving benefits compared to the adverse effects of short-term steroids (3)[C]. Steroids may work by suppressing the autoantibodies inhibiting ADAMTS13 activity.
  - May be used in patients with severe ADAMTS13 deficiency, in the setting of exacerbation when PEX is stopped or in relapse after remission; little benefit of steroids when used as monotherapy
  - Doses: prednisone 1 kg/day and taper once in remission or methylprednisolone 1 g/day IV for 3 days
- Rituximab, an anti-CD20 antibody that deletes B cells, may reduce relapse when given in conjunction with PEX and steroids; dose: 375 mg/m² IV once weekly for 4 weeks

Second Line

The following medications are used in refractory cases:

- Caplacizumab: a monoclonal antibody that inhibits vWF-glycoprotein 1b interaction; in patients with TTP, caplacizumab has been shown to reduce the time it takes for platelets to normalize, the length of the PEX, and the length of the hospital stay while not significantly raising the risk of adverse events.
- Intravenous immunoglobulin (IVIG)
- Splenectomy in the acute phase

ISSUES FOR REFERRAL

- Hematology or blood bank for PEX
- Nephrology for dialysis; cardiology for heart block or ischemia; neurosurgery for hemorrhage

ADDITIONAL THERAPIES

Recombinant ADAMTS13 is under investigation to be used as an alternative therapeutic agent.

SURGERY/OTHER PROCEDURES

Splenectomy is reserved for severe, refractory cases (1)[C].

ADMISSION, INPATIENT, AND NURSING CONSIDERATIONS

- ABCs, oxygen, IV access, telemetry
- Volume resuscitation if hypotensive/actively bleeding; packed RBCs can be transfused safely.
- Platelet transfusion may be used for the treatment of hemorrhage.
- Discharge on normalization and stabilization of neurologic symptoms, LDH, platelets, and renal function

 ONGOING CARE

FOLLOW-UP RECOMMENDATIONS

After PEX is discontinued, blood counts and ADAMTS13 activity should be monitored for months to evaluate for relapse.

PATIENT EDUCATION

- Self-monitor for signs of relapse (e.g., fever, headache, bruising) and prolonged periods of fatigue following the acute phase
- National Heart, Lung, and Blood Institute: https://www.nhlbi.nih.gov/health/thrombotic-thrombocytopenic-purpura

PROGNOSIS

- Most recover fully from idiopathic TTP when treated promptly:
  - 30-day mortality is 10% in those who receive PEX.
  - 70% respond within 14 days; 90% respond within 28 days; 80% survival in idiopathic TTP treated with PEX (1)
- Prior to widespread PEX treatment, TTP carried up to a 90% mortality rate.
- Initial LDH and platelet counts are not predictive of response to treatment.
- Final platelet count and LDH or the length or intensity of treatment do not predict relapse.
- Low levels of ADAMTS13 activity during remission are associated with higher risk of relapse (1)[C].
- Patients with severe ADAMTS13 deficiency had a risk of relapse which is estimated to be 41% at 7.5 years, with the greatest risk being in the 1st year.
- In patients with autoimmune TTP, there is a 40% relapse rate.

COMPLICATIONS

- Mild cognitive impairments in attention, concentration, and memory following ≥1 episode of TTP
- Complications of PEX: central line infections and hemorrhage, citrate toxicity, hypersensitivity reactions to frequent plasma exposure, electrolyte abnormalities

REFERENCES

1. Joly BS, Coppo P, Veyradier A. Thrombotic thrombocytopenic purpura. *Blood*. 2017;129(21):2836–2846.
2. Michael M, Elliott EJ, Ridley GF, et al. Interventions for haemolytic uraemic syndrome and thrombotic thrombocytopenic purpura. *Cochrane Database Syst Rev*. 2009;2009(1):CD003595.
3. Zheng XL, Vesely SK, Cataland SR, et al. ISTH guidelines for treatment of thrombotic thrombocytopenic purpura. *J Thromb Haemost*. 2020;18(10):2496–2502.

ADDITIONAL READING

Chen B, Li X, Xiao D, et al. Comparison of the efficacy and safety of caplacizumab versus placebo in thrombotic thrombocytopenic purpura: a meta-analysis and systematic review based on randomized controlled trials. *Ann Transl Med*. 2022;10(12):657.

 CODES

ICD10

- M31.1 Thrombotic microangiopathy
- D69.42 Congenital and hereditary thrombocytopenia purpura
- D69.3 Immune thrombocytopenic purpura

CLINICAL PEARLS

- The diagnosis of TTP is made clinically; symptoms are nonspecific: nausea; vomiting; weakness; abdominal pain; fatigue; fever; and easy bruising, purpura, or petechiae.
- The pentad of fever, neurologic symptoms, renal dysfunction, MAHA, and thrombocytopenia is not present in most patients.
- The dyad of MAHA (schistocytes on peripheral smear) and severe thrombocytopenia (<30,000) is sufficient to initiate treatment with PEX.
- Do not wait for the results of ADAMTS13 determination to initiate therapy.

T

THYROID MALIGNANT NEOPLASIA

Dana M. Vlachos, DO • Batoul Zalkout, DO • Shabia Mohammed, DO

 BASICS

DESCRIPTION

Thyroid malignant neoplasia is an uncontrolled proliferation of cells within the thyroid gland. There are several types:

- Papillary thyroid carcinoma (PTC)
  - Differentiated tumor with papillary cells with finger-like projections
  - Most common variety, 75–80% of thyroid cancers
  - Peak incidence in the 3rd or 4th decade of life
  - Associated with radiation exposure
  - Metastasizes by lymphatic route (15–30% have palpable lymphadenopathy at time of diagnosis.)
  - Many subtypes: conventional, follicular variant, oxyphilic, cribriform-morular, and more aggressive forms such as tall cell or diffuse sclerosing
- Follicular carcinoma
  - Differentiated tumor with spherical follicular cells
  - Second most common variety, 10–20% of thyroid tumors
  - Peak incidence in 5th decade of life
  - Metastasizes by the hematogenous route
  - Can be divided into invasive and minimally invasive forms based on morphology
- Hürthle cell carcinoma (variant of follicular with poorer prognosis)
  - Often considered subtype of FTC with overall poorer prognosis
  - Also known as oncocytic or oxyphilic carcinoma
  - 2–3% of thyroid malignancies
  - Usually in patients >60 years old
- Medullary thyroid carcinoma (MTC)
  - Neuroendocrine tumor arising from parafollicular C cells
  - 3–4% of all thyroid carcinoma
  - 25–35% are associated with multiple endocrine neoplasia (MEN) syndromes.
  - MTC associated with MEN2B occurs in childhood, those with MEN2A occur in young adults, and those with familial non-MEN medullary thyroid cancer (FMTC) occur in middle age.
  - Calcitonin is a serologic marker.
  - *RET* proto-oncogene mutation is used for screening; family members who carry the *RET* gene should consider early prophylactic thyroidectomy.
- Anaplastic carcinoma
  - Undifferentiated tumor arising de novo or from dedifferentiation of preexisting differentiated thyroid carcinoma
  - 1–3% of thyroid tumors
  - Most aggressive form of thyroid neoplasia
  - Almost uniformly fatal (median survival 2 to 6 months)
  - More common in elderly patients
- Poorly differentiated thyroid carcinoma (PDTC)
  - Intermediate between differentiated (follicular and papillary carcinomas) and undifferentiated (anaplastic) carcinomas
  - Aggressive tumor similar to anaplastic carcinoma but may have better treatment response
- Other: lymphoma, sarcoma, or metastatic (renal, breast, or lung)

Geriatric Considerations
Risk of malignancy (ROM) increases, and prognosis is worse >60 years old.

Pediatric Considerations
- Thyroid nodules are more frequently malignant (22–25% in children vs. 5–10% in adults).
- <2% of thyroid malignancies occur in children and adolescents.
- Increased tumor size (>4 cm), extrathyroidal extension, and multifocal disease are independent factors associated with nodal metastases in pediatric differentiated thyroid cancer and require further evaluation with FNA for suspicious nodes to consider neck dissection (1)[C].

EPIDEMIOLOGY
- Incidence: 14.5/100,000 per year in the United States
- Deaths: 0.5/100,000 per year in the United States
- In 2018, estimated 53,990 new cases and 2,060 deaths from thyroid cancer in the United States
- Predominant age: usually >40 years old
- Predominant sex: female > male (3:1) prevalence
- Lifetime risk of developing thyroid cancer is 1.2%.

ETIOLOGY AND PATHOPHYSIOLOGY
- No established etiologic factors of pathogenesis; most cases arise spontaneously.
- Radiation exposure likely has a role in the development of thyroid malignancies.

Genetics
Gene mutations that activate the MAPK pathway (e.g., *BRAF*) and PI3K-AKT pathway (e.g., PTEN) have been implicated.

RISK FACTORS
- Family history (first-degree relative)
- Radiation exposure: papillary carcinoma
- Iodine deficiency: follicular carcinoma
- MEN2: medullary carcinoma; autosomal dominant inheritance; *RET* proto-oncogene
- Previous history of subtotal thyroidectomy for malignancy: anaplastic carcinoma

GENERAL PREVENTION
- Physical exam in high-risk group
- Calcitonin stimulation screening in high-risk MEN patients
- Screening for *RET* proto-oncogene in groups at risk for MTC

COMMONLY ASSOCIATED CONDITIONS
- Papillary carcinoma: Hashimoto thyroiditis
- Medullary carcinoma: pheochromocytoma, hyperparathyroidism, ganglioneuroma of the GI tract, neuroma of mucosal membranes

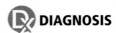 DIAGNOSIS

HISTORY
- Change in voice (dysphonia)
- Difficulty swallowing (dysphagia)
- Difficulty breathing (dyspnea)
- Stridor (in aggressive cancer)
- Growing neck mass
- Positive family history
- History of radiation exposure (environmental or radiation therapy for childhood cancer)

PHYSICAL EXAM
- Thyroid nodule/mass
- Fixation of nodule to surrounding tissues suggests malignancy.
- Cervical lymphadenopathy

DIFFERENTIAL DIAGNOSIS
- Multinodular goiter
- Thyroid adenoma
- Thyroglossal duct or dermoid cyst
- Thyroiditis
- Thyroid cyst
- Ectopic thyroid

DIAGNOSTIC TESTS & INTERPRETATION
Initial Tests (lab, imaging)
- Ultrasound (US): Nodule characteristics suggestive of malignancy include hypoechoic pattern, microcalcifications, irregular margins, and shape taller than wide (2)[A].
- Thyroid-stimulating hormone (TSH): usually normal in the setting of malignancy but recommended for all nodule workup

Follow-Up Tests & Special Considerations
- CT and MRI neck: useful to evaluate large substernal masses, extent of invasion for fixed bulky tumors, if suspicion of MTC with neck disease or calcitonin >400 pg/mL, and to evaluate for recurrent disease
- Calcitonin levels: Measure in patients with FNA results or with personal or family history of MEN2 syndrome suggestive of MTC (consider IV pentagastrin stimulation test to increase sensitivity).
- Thyroid scan: 12–15% of cold nodules are malignant; rate is higher in patients <40 years of age and those with microcalcifications on US. ^{18}F-FDG positron-emission tomographic scan can help if the cytology is indeterminant; also helpful with recurrent disease when patient has a negative ^{131}I scan and an elevated thyroglobulin (TG) level (3)[B]
- TG: not recommended in initial evaluation but used as postoperative tumor marker for recurrence

Diagnostic Procedures/Other
- Fine-needle aspiration biopsy (FNAB)
- Flexible fiberoptic laryngoscopy: if vocal cord paralysis is suspected and in high-risk disease

Test Interpretation

- FNAB: The 2017 Bethesda System for Reporting Thyroid Cytopathology classification of cytology
  - Nondiagnostic or unsatisfactory
  - Benign: 0–3% ROM
  - Atypia of undetermined significance (AUS) or follicular lesion of undetermined significance (FLUS): 10–30% ROM
  - Follicular neoplasm or suspicious for a follicular neoplasm: 25–40% ROM
  - Suspicious for malignancy: 50–75% ROM
  - Malignant: 97–99% ROM
- Papillary: psammoma bodies, anaplastic epithelial papillae
- Follicular: anaplastic epithelial cords with follicles
- Hürthle cell: large eosinophilic cells with granular cytoplasm
- Medullary: large amounts of amyloid stroma
- Anaplastic: small cell and giant cell undifferentiated tumors

 TREATMENT

GENERAL MEASURES

- Most cases of thyroid cancer are managed surgically and medically with a good prognosis (2)[A].
- Palliative support has a role in case of advanced thyroid malignancy (4)[C].
- Papillary and follicular: ^{131}I thyroid remnant ablation

MEDICATION

Postoperatively, will require thyroid hormone replacement after total thyroidectomy

- Thyroxine suppression therapy may reduce recurrence with goal to keep TSH <0.1 mU/L for high-risk patients, 0.1 to 0.5 mU/L for intermediate-risk patients, and 0.5 to 2.0 mU/L for low-risk patients (2)[A].
- Medications used for thyroid hormone replacement:
  - Levothyroxine (T$_4$, Synthroid)
  - Liothyronine (T$_3$, Cytomel)

ADDITIONAL THERAPIES

- External beam radiation or chemotherapy may be considered for radioactive iodine insensitive tumors, inoperable recurrence, and for palliative care.
- ^{131}I is used in high-risk patients with papillary and follicular tumors. The role is to ablate remnant thyroid tissue to improve specificity of future TG assays to monitor for recurrence.

SURGERY/OTHER PROCEDURES

- Papillary: total thyroidectomy with elective neck dissection for suspicious lymph nodes in central or lateral neck compartments or for large tumors (>4 cm in size); lobectomy with isthmectomy can be considered if lesion <1 cm in low-risk patient (controversial).
- Follicular and Hürthle cell: similar management as papillary carcinoma
- Medullary: total thyroidectomy with central node dissection; unilateral or bilateral modified radical neck dissection if lateral nodes are suspicious
- Anaplastic: palliative care; no adequate treatment available and surgery is controversial; consider tracheostomy (to protect airway) and clinical trials using chemotherapy/radiation.

 ONGOING CARE

FOLLOW-UP RECOMMENDATIONS
Patient Monitoring

- 10–30% of initially disease-free patients will develop recurrence and/or metastases. 80% recur in neck and 20% with distant metastases (lung).
- TSH, TG, and anti-TG antibodies at 6 months, 12 months, and then yearly after that for surveillance
- Periodic US to monitor for recurrence is recommended in intermediate- to high-risk patients and may also consider TSH-stimulated radioiodine whole body imaging in high-risk patients.
- Medullary: Calcitonin level should be done yearly with pentagastrin stimulation.
- The thyroid scan and TG level should be done with the patient in the hypothyroid state induced by 6-week withdrawal of levothyroxine or 2- to 3-week withdrawal of liothyronine.

DIET
Low-iodine diet recommended in patients undergoing radioactive iodine therapy following surgery for thyroid cancer

PATIENT EDUCATION

- National Cancer Institute: https://www.cancer.gov/types/thyroid/patient/thyroid-treatment-pdq
- American Thyroid Association: https://www.thyroid.org/thyroid-information/

PROGNOSIS

- 5-year survival of thyroid cancer is 98.1%.
- Adverse factors: age >45 years, primary tumor >4 cm, extrathyroid extension, distant metastases
- Low risk: no extrathyroidal invasion, all macroscopic tumor resected, no local or distant metastases, no vascular invasion, and no aggressive tumor histology
- Intermediate risk: microscopic extrathyroidal invasion, cervical lymph node metastases on ^{131}I update outside of thyroid bed on first whole body after remnant ablation
- High risk: macroscopic extrathyroidal tumor invasion, incomplete tumor resection, distant metastases
- Papillary carcinoma: 10-year overall survival is 93%; 30-year cancer-related death rate of 6%
- Follicular carcinoma: 10-year overall survival is 85%; histologically, microinvasive tumors parallel papillary tumor results, whereas grossly invasive tumors do far worse; 30-year cancer-related death rate of 15%
- Hürthle cell carcinoma: 93% 5-year survival rate and 83% survival rate overall; grossly invasive tumor survival <25%
- Medullary carcinoma: negative nodes, 90% 5-year survival rate and 85% 10-year survival rate; with positive nodes, 65% 5-year survival rate and 40% 10-year survival rate; prognosis worse for MEN2B compared to MEN2A; overall, 10-year survival is 75%.
- Anaplastic carcinoma: survival unexpected; long-term survivors should have original pathology reexamined.

COMPLICATIONS

- Hoarseness either from tumor invasion or iatrogenic injury to recurrent laryngeal nerve
- Hypocalcemia/hypoparathyroidism from devascularization of parathyroid glands during surgery (usually transient)

REFERENCES

1. Francis GL, Waguespack SG, Bauer AJ, et al; for American Thyroid Association Guidelines Task Force. Management guidelines for children with thyroid nodules and differentiated thyroid cancer. *Thyroid*. 2015;25(7):716–759.
2. Haugen BR, Alexander EK, Bible KC, et al. 2015 American Thyroid Association management guidelines for adult patients with thyroid nodules and differentiated thyroid cancer: the American Thyroid Association Guidelines Task Force on thyroid nodules and differentiated thyroid cancer. *Thyroid*. 2016;26(1):1–133.
3. de Koster EJ, de Geus-Oei LF, Dekkers OM, et al. Diagnostic utility of molecular and imaging biomarkers in cytological indeterminate thyroid nodules. *Endocr Rev*. 2018;39(2):154–191.
4. Goyal A, Gupta R, Mehmood S, et al. Palliative and end of life care issues of carcinoma thyroid patient. *Indian J Palliat Care*. 2012;18(2):134–137.

 SEE ALSO

Multiple Endocrine Neoplasia (MEN) Syndromes

 CODES

ICD10
C73 Malignant neoplasm of thyroid gland

CLINICAL PEARLS

- Standard workup for a patient suspected of having a thyroid cancer is a physical exam, TSH level, neck US, and FNA.
- TG levels can be elevated in several thyroid disorders. Its usefulness comes once the diagnosis of cancer has been made. It serves as a better marker for recurrent disease.
- FNA results will be benign, malignant, indeterminate, or nondiagnostic. It is very helpful in guiding the initial surgical approach.

T

THYROIDITIS

Munima Nasir, MD • Ian P. Downin, MD, MHA

 BASICS

DESCRIPTION

Painful or painless inflammatory dysfunction of the thyroid gland

- Painful thyroiditis:
  - Subacute granulomatous thyroiditis (nonsuppurative thyroiditis, de Quervain thyroiditis, giant cell thyroiditis): self-limited; viral URI prodrome, symptoms and signs of thyroid dysfunction (variable)
  - Infectious/suppurative thyroiditis is most commonly associated with *Streptococcus pyogenes*, *Staphylococcus aureus*, and *Streptococcus pneumoniae* but can be due to fungal, mycobacterial, or parasitic infections of the thyroid.
- Radiation-induced thyroiditis: from radioactive iodine therapy (1%) or external irradiation
- Painless thyroiditis
  - Hashimoto (autoimmune) thyroiditis (chronic lymphocytic thyroiditis): most common etiology of chronic hypothyroidism; 90% of patients with high-serum antithyroid peroxidase (TPO) antibodies
  - Postpartum thyroiditis (PPT): thyrotoxicosis followed by hypothyroidism in the 1st year postpartum or after spontaneous/induced abortion in women who were without clinically evident thyroid disease before pregnancy
  - Painless (silent) thyroiditis (subacute lymphocytic thyroiditis): mild hyperthyroidism, small painless goiter, and no Graves ophthalmopathy/pretibial myxedema
  - Riedel (fibrous) thyroiditis: rare inflammatory process involving the thyroid and surrounding cervical tissues; associated with various forms of systemic fibrosis; presents as a firm mass in the thyroid commonly associated with compressive symptoms (dyspnea, dysphagia, hoarseness, and aphonia) caused by local infiltration of the advancing fibrotic process with hypocalcemia and hypothyroidism
  - Drug-induced thyroiditis: interferon-α, interleukin-2, amiodarone, kinase inhibitors, or lithium

EPIDEMIOLOGY

- Subacute granulomatous thyroiditis: most common cause of thyroid pain; peaks during summer; incidence: 3/100,000/year; female > male (4:1); peak age: 40 to 50 years
- Hashimoto thyroiditis (HT): peak onset 30 to 50 years; can occur in children; female > male (7:1)
- PPT: occurs within 12 months of pregnancy in 1–18% of pregnancies
- Painless (silent) thyroiditis: accounts for 1–5% of cases; female > male (4:1) with peak age 30 to 40 years; common in areas of iodine sufficiency
- Riedel thyroiditis: female > male (4:1); highest prevalence age: 30 to 60 years; rare with estimated incidence of 1.06 cases per 100,000 patients

ETIOLOGY AND PATHOPHYSIOLOGY

- Subacute granulomatous thyroiditis: probably viral; can be associated with COVID-19 infection; the mechanism of thyroid injury can be due to direct destruction of thyroid tissue, as well as indirect immune-mediated responses and medicines used to treat COVID-19 (1).
- Hashimoto disease: Antithyroid antibodies may be produced in response to an environmental antigen and cross-react with thyroid proteins (molecular mimicry). Precipitating factors include infection, stress, sex steroids, pregnancy, iodine intake, and radiation exposure.
- PPT: autoimmunity-induced discharge of preformed hormone from the thyroid
- Painless (silent) thyroiditis: autoimmune
- Riedel (fibrous) thyroiditis: rare inflammatory process involving the thyroid and surrounding cervical tissues; associated with various forms of systemic fibrosis

Genetics

Autoimmune thyroiditis is associated with the CT60 polymorphism of cytotoxic T-cell lymphocyte–associated antigen 4; also associated with HLA-DR4, HLA-DR5, and HLA-DR6 in whites

RISK FACTORS

- Subacute granulomatous thyroiditis: recent viral respiratory infection, such as COVID-19 infection, or HLA-B35
- Hashimoto disease: family/personal history of thyroid/autoimmune disease, high iodine intake, cigarette smoking, selenium deficiency

GENERAL PREVENTION

Insufficient evidence to justify the use of vitamin D or selenium supplementation

DIAGNOSIS

HISTORY

- Hypothyroid symptoms (e.g., constipation, heavy menstrual bleeding, fatigue, weakness, dry skin, hair loss, cold intolerance)
- Hyperthyroid symptoms (e.g., irritability, heat intolerance, increased sweating, palpitations, loose stools, disturbed sleep, and lid retraction)
- Subacute granulomatous thyroiditis: sudden/gradual onset, with preceding upper respiratory infection/viral illness (fever, fatigue, malaise, anorexia, and myalgia are common); pain may be limited to thyroid region or radiated to upper neck, jaw, throat, or ears. Patients with COVID-19 infection may be more likely to have a painless presentation (1). Post–COVID-19 fatigue may be associated with hypothyroid phase of subacute thyroiditis (2).
- Classic triphasic course (thyrotoxic, hypothyroid, recovery) but variable in the following: subacute, silent, and PPT

PHYSICAL EXAM

- Hashimoto disease: 90% have a symmetric, diffusely enlarged, painless thyroid gland, with a firm, pebbly texture; 10% have atrophy.
- PPT: painless, small, nontender, firm goiter (2 to 6 months after delivery)
- Riedel thyroiditis: rock-hard, wood-like, fixed, painless goiter, often accompanied by symptoms of esophageal/tracheal compression (stridor, dyspnea, a suffocating feeling, dysphagia, and hoarseness); should be considered when restrictive and infiltrative symptoms are out of proportion of the size of the mass on exam
- Signs of hypothyroid: delayed relaxation phase of deep tendon reflexes, nonpitting edema, dry skin, alopecia, bradycardia
- Signs of hyperthyroid: moist palms, hyperreflexia, tachycardia/atrial fibrillation

DIFFERENTIAL DIAGNOSIS

Simple goiter; iodine-deficient/lithium-induced goiter; Graves disease (GD); lymphoma; oropharynx and trachea infections; thyroid cancer; amiodarone; contrast dye; amyloid

DIAGNOSTIC TESTS & INTERPRETATION

- Subacute granulomatous (de Quervain) thyroiditis
  - In the thyrotoxic phase, decreased TSH; elevated T4, ESR, CRP, WBC count; mild anemia
  - 25% of patients have low concentrations of antithyroid antibodies.
  - ESR normalizes during hypothyroid phase.
  - Consider US to rule out thyroid cancer.
- Suppurative (acute) thyroiditis (thyroid abscess)
  - Generally, patients are euthyroid; occasionally presents with destructive thyrotoxicosis
  - US or CT is usually diagnostic. Fine-needle aspiration can confirm diagnosis (3)[C]
- HT
  - Anti-TPO antibodies present in 95% of cases.
  - Antithyroglobulin antibodies present in 60–80%.
  - Ultrasonography may demonstrate decreased echogenicity and hypoechoic nodules with an echogenic rim (4)[C].
- PPT
  - Thyroid antibodies (TPOAb, TgAb) present
    - If Ab positive in the 1st trimester, higher risk of developing PPT
    - Higher Ab titers, higher risk of PPT
  - Must distinguish from thyrotoxicosis caused by GD (which has a positive TSH receptor antibody, high radioiodine uptake, and specific physical findings (e.g., goiter, ophthalmopathy)
  - After the thyrotoxic phase, obtain a TSH level in 4 to 8 weeks (or if the patient develops new symptoms) to screen for the hypothyroid phase.
  - If patient has a history of PPT, screen for permanent hypothyroidism with an annual TSH level (5)[C].

- Painless (silent) thyroiditis
  - 5–20% of patients undergo a thyrotoxic phase that lasts 3 to 4 months.
  - Thyroid function normalizes within 12 months.
  - ~50% of patients have anti-TPO antibodies.
  - Absence of TSH receptor antibodies distinguishes from Graves disease (3)[C].
- Reidel thyroiditis
  - Thyroglobulin and TPO antibody titers are elevated (likely due to simultaneous Hashimoto disease).
  - 72% of individuals have elevated CRP, and 97% have elevated ESR.
  - Parathyroid involvement can cause hypocalcemia.
  - Histology confirms diagnosis and reveals a fibroinflammatory process.
- Drug-induced thyroiditis
  - Thyroid function test results vary and depend on the offending medication. Thyrotoxicosis is common; lithium associated with hypothyroidism (3)[C]

Initial Tests (lab, imaging)
TSH, free T_4, T_3; antithyroid antibodies

Follow-Up Tests & Special Considerations
- US: shows variable heterogeneous texture, hypoechogenic in subacute, painless (silent), and PPT
- Thyroid RAIU scan: decreased in all forms of thyroiditis but not helpful in establishing diagnosis of Hashimoto disease; high RAIU in hashitoxicosis, GD
- Random urine iodine measurement may be helpful to distinguish from other causes of low RAIU.
  - Urine iodine <500 µg/L (subacute granulomatous thyroiditis)
  - Urine iodine >1,000 µg/L (in patients with exposure to excess exogenous iodine/radiocontrast material)

Diagnostic Procedures/Other
- Hashimoto with a dominant nodule should have FNA to rule out thyroid carcinoma.
- Open biopsy is necessary for a definitive diagnosis of Reidel thyroiditis.

Test Interpretation
- Subacute granulomatous thyroiditis: giant cells, mononuclear cell (granulomatous) infiltrate
- Hashimoto disease: lymphocytic infiltration with formation of Askanazy (Hürthle) cells, oxyphilic changes in follicular cells, fibrosis, thyroid atrophy
- PPT: lymphocytic infiltration, occasional germinal centers, disruption and collapse of thyroid follicles
- Painless (silent) thyroiditis: lymphocytic infiltration, but without fibrosis, Askanazy cells, and extensive lymphoid follicle formation

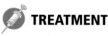

TREATMENT

GENERAL MEASURES
- If thyrotoxic and symptomatic: propylthiouracil and propranolol, except not used in PPT or painless thyroiditis
- An elevated TSH level in a woman who is pregnant or attempting to become pregnant is an indication for thyroid replacement.

MEDICATION
- Subacute granulomatous thyroiditis
  - β-Blockers and NSAIDs may be used to treat mild symptomatic cases.
  - Prednisone 40 mg/day × 1 to 2 weeks, followed by 2 to 4 week taper in severe cases
  - Levothyroxine may be used in the hypothyroid phase. Discontinue after 3 to 6 months with normalization of thyroid function (3)[C].
  - It is unclear if subacute thyroiditis is associated with COVID-19 vaccination, although evidence is low. Current limited data suggest COVID-19 vaccination should not be restricted in patients with thyroid symptoms (2)[C].
- Suppurative (acute) thyroiditis (thyroid abscess)
  - Systemic antibiotics
  - Abscess drainage or removal
  - Excision or occlusion of the pyriform sinus (3)[C]
- HT
  - Levothyroxine 1.6 to 1.8 µg/kg
- PPT
  - Treatment is guided by stage.
  - Metoprolol and propranolol for lactating women in the thyrotoxic state; antithyroid medications are not recommended.
  - If lactating or trying to conceive, treat symptomatic hypothyroidism.
  - Levothyroxine may be tapered starting at 12 months postpartum. Monitor TSH every 6 to 8 weeks. Avoid tapering if a woman is trying to conceive or is pregnant (5)[C].
- Painless (silent) thyroiditis
  - If symptomatic during hyperthyroid state, treat with β-blocker.
  - Antithyroid medications are unnecessary.
  - For severe cases, corticosteroids may reduce the severity and length of the hyperthyroid state (3)[C].
- Reidel thyroiditis (no management consensus)
  - Medical therapy is first line in absence of obstructive symptoms. Neither meds are validated by RCTs due to rarity of the condition. Glucocorticoids are first line, and tamoxifen is second line.
  - Treat hypothyroidism with levothyroxine and hypoparathyroidism with calcium and calcitriol.
  - Debulking surgery if obstruction present
- Drug-induced thyroiditis
  - Discontinue offending drug.

ONGOING CARE

FOLLOW-UP RECOMMENDATIONS

Patient Monitoring
- Subacute granulomatous thyroiditis: Repeat thyroid function tests every 3 to 6 weeks until euthyroid and then every 6 to 12 months.
- Hashimoto disease: Repeat thyroid function tests every 3 to 12 months.
- PPT: Check TSH annually.
- Reidel thyroiditis: Consider CT if extrathyroidal disease is suspected.
- Check thyroid function before and after 3 months of starting amiodarone, and then monitor every 3 to 6 months.

Pregnancy Considerations
^{131}I is contraindicated in breastfeeding women.

PROGNOSIS
- Subacute granulomatous thyroiditis: Most patients are euthyroid at 12 months. 5–15% have persistent hypothyroidism.
- Hashimoto disease: persistent goiter; eventual thyroid failure
- PPT: Thyroid function normalizes in 12 months. 10–20% of patients have persistent hypothyroidism.
- Painless (silent) thyroiditis: 5–20% of patients undergo a thyrotoxic phase that lasts 3 to 4 months.
- Reidel Thyroiditis: 90% have improvement or resolution of symptoms within 12 months. It is unclear at this time what factors contribute to poor prognosis due to the rarity of the condition.

REFERENCES
1. Meftah E, Rahmati R, Zari Meidani F, et al. Subacute thyroiditis following COVID-19: a systematic review. *Front Endocrinol (Lausanne)*. 2023;14:1126637.
2. Popescu M, Ghemigian A, Vasile CM, et al. The new entity of subacute thyroiditis amid the COVID-19 pandemic: from infection to vaccine. *Diagnostics (Basel)*. 2022;12(4):960.
3. Ross DS, Burch HB, Cooper DS, et al. 2016 American Thyroid Association guidelines for diagnosis and management of hyperthyroidism and other causes of thyrotoxicosis. *Thyroid*. 2016;26(10):1343–1421.
4. Massimo R, Angeletti D, Fiore M, et al. Hashimoto's thyroiditis: an update on pathogenic mechanisms, diagnostic protocols, therapeutic strategies, and potential malignant transformation. *Autoimmun Rev*. 2020;19(10):102649.
5. Alexander EK, Pearce EN, Brent GA, et al. 2017 Guidelines of the American Thyroid Association for the diagnosis and management of thyroid disease during pregnancy and the postpartum. *Thyroid*. 2017;27(3):315–389.

CODES

ICD10
- E06.5 Other chronic thyroiditis
- E06.0 Acute thyroiditis
- E06 Thyroiditis

CLINICAL PEARLS

HT is the most common etiology of chronic hypothyroidism.

TINEA (CAPITIS, CORPORIS, CRURIS)

Daniel Scott Morrison, MD • Laith Abushanab, MD • Chirag N. Shah, MD

 BASICS

DESCRIPTION

- Superficial fungal infections of the skin/scalp; various forms of dermatophytosis; the names relate to the particular area affected (1).
  - Tinea cruris: infection of crural fold and gluteal cleft
  - Tinea corporis: infection involving the face, trunk, and/or extremities; often presents with ring-shaped lesions, hence the misnomer *ringworm*
  - Tinea capitis: infection of the scalp and hair; affected areas of the scalp can show characteristic black dots resulting from broken hairs.
- Dermatophytes have the ability to subsist on protein, namely keratin.
- They cause disease in keratin-rich structures such as skin, nails, and hair.
- Infections result from contact with infected persons/animals.
  - Zoophilic infections are acquired from animals.
  - Anthropophilic infections are acquired from personal contact (e.g., wrestling) or fomites.
  - Geophile infections are acquired from the soil.
- System(s) affected: skin, exocrine
- Synonym(s): jock itch; ringworm

EPIDEMIOLOGY

Incidence
- Tinea cruris
  - Predominant age: any age; rare in children
  - Predominant sex: male > female
- Tinea corporis
  - Predominant age: postpubertal children and young adults
  - Predominant sex: male = female
- Tinea capitis
  - Predominant age: 3 to 9 years; almost always occurs in young children
  - Predominant sex: male = female

Prevalence
Common worldwide with dramatic increase over the past 2 decades due to more frequent international travel, socioeconomic problems, and contact with animals, specifically pets

Pediatric Considerations
- Tinea cruris is rare prior to puberty.
- Tinea capitis is common in young children.

Geriatric Considerations
Tinea cruris is more common in the geriatric population due to an increase in risk factors.

Pregnancy Considerations
Tinea cruris and capitis are rare in pregnancy.

ETIOLOGY AND PATHOPHYSIOLOGY
Superficial fungal infection of skin/scalp
- Tinea cruris: Source of infection is usually the patient's own tinea pedis, with agent being transferred from the foot to the groin via the underwear when dressing; most common causative dermatophyte is *Trichophyton rubrum*; rare cases are caused by *Epidermophyton floccosum* and *Trichophyton mentagrophytes*.

- Tinea corporis: most commonly caused by *Trichophyton rubrum*; other notable causes include *Trichophyton tonsurans*, *Microsporum canis*, *T. interdigitale*, *Microsporum gypseum*, *Trichophyton violaceum*, and *Microsporum audouinii*. It can also be caused by *E. floccosum*.
- Tinea capitis: *T. tonsurans* found in 90% and *Microsporum* sp. in 10% of patients. There may be a geographic predilection for certain organisms.

Genetics
Evidence suggests a genetic susceptibility in certain individuals.

RISK FACTORS
- Warm climates; summer months and/or copious sweating; wearing wet clothing/multiple layers (tinea cruris)
- Daycare centers/schools/confined quarters (tinea corporis and capitis)
- Depression of cell-mediated immune response (e.g., individuals with atopy or AIDS)
- Obesity (tinea cruris and corporis)
- Direct contact with an active lesion on a human, an animal, or rarely, from soil; working with animals (tinea corporis)

GENERAL PREVENTION
- Avoidance of risk factors, such as contact with suspicious lesions
- Fluconazole or itraconazole may be useful in wrestlers to prevent outbreaks during competitive season.

COMMONLY ASSOCIATED CONDITIONS
Tinea pedis, tinea barbae, tinea manus

 DIAGNOSIS

HISTORY
- Lesions range from asymptomatic to pruritic.
- In tinea cruris, acute inflammation may result from wearing occlusive clothing; chronic scratching may result in an eczematous appearance.
- Previous application of topical steroids, especially in tinea cruris and corporis, may alter the overall appearance causing a more extensive eruption with irregular borders and erythematous papules. This modified form is called *tinea incognito*.

PHYSICAL EXAM
- Tinea cruris: well-marginated, erythematous, half-moon–shaped plaques in crural folds that spread to medial thighs; advancing border is well-defined, often with fine scaling and sometimes vesicular eruptions. Lesions are usually bilateral and do not include scrotum/penis (unlike with *Candida* infections) but may migrate to perineum, perianal area, and gluteal cleft and onto the buttocks in chronic/progressive cases. The area may be hyperpigmented on resolution.
- Tinea corporis: scaling, round or oval pruritic plaques characterized by a sharply defined annular pattern with peripheral activity and central clearing (ring-shaped lesions) involving the face, trunk, and/or extremities; papules and occasionally pustules/vesicles present at border and, less commonly, in center

- Tinea capitis: commonly begins with round patches of scale involving scalp (alopecia less common). In its later stages, the infection frequently takes on patterns of chronic scaling with either little/marked inflammation or alopecia. Less often, patients will present with multiple patches of alopecia and the characteristic black-dot appearance of broken hairs. Extreme inflammation results in kerion formation (exudative, pustular nodulation).

DIFFERENTIAL DIAGNOSIS
- Tinea cruris
  - Intertrigo: inflammatory process of moist-opposed skin folds, often including infection with bacteria, yeast, and fungi; painful longitudinal fissures may occur in skin folds.
  - Erythrasma: diffuse brown, scaly, noninflammatory plaque with irregular borders, often involving groin; caused by bacterial infection with *Corynebacterium minutissimum*; fluoresces coral red with Wood lamp
  - Seborrheic dermatitis of groin
  - Psoriasis of groin ("inverse psoriasis")
  - Candidiasis of groin (typically involves the scrotum)
  - Acanthosis nigricans
- Tinea capitis
  - Psoriasis
  - Seborrheic dermatitis
  - Pyoderma
  - Alopecia areata and trichotillomania
  - Aplasia cutis congenital
- Tinea corporis
  - Pityriasis rosea
  - Eczema (nummular)
  - Contact dermatitis
  - Syphilis
  - Psoriasis
  - Seborrheic dermatitis
  - Subacute systemic lupus erythematosus (SLE)
  - Erythema annulare centrifugum
  - Erythema multiforme; erythema migrans
  - Impetigo circinatum
  - Granuloma annulare

DIAGNOSTIC TESTS & INTERPRETATION
Initial Tests (lab, imaging)
- Wood lamp exam reveals no fluorescence in most cases (*Trichophyton* sp.); 10% of infections, those caused by *T. rubrum*, will fluoresce with a green light.
- Potassium hydroxide (KOH) preparation of skin scrapings from dermatophyte leading border shows characteristic translucent, branching, rod-shaped hyphae.

Follow-Up Tests & Special Considerations
- Reevaluate to assess response, especially in resistant/extensive cases.
- Fungal culture using Sabouraud dextrose agar/dermatophyte test medium

Test Interpretation
- Skin scrapings show fungal hyphae in epidermis; best yield from scrapings from active border
- Arthrospores found in hair shafts; spores and/or hyphae seen on KOH exam

TREATMENT

GENERAL MEASURES

- Careful hand washing and personal hygiene; laundering of towels/clothing of affected individual; no sharing of towels/clothes/headgear/pillows
- Avoid predisposing conditions such as hot baths and tight-fitting clothing (boxer shorts are better than briefs).
- Avoid contact sports (e.g., wrestling) temporarily while starting treatment.
- Evaluate other family members, close contacts, or household pets (especially kittens and puppies).
- Use of prophylactic antifungal shampoo by all household members for 2 to 4 weeks in cases of tinea capitis
- Itching can be alleviated by OTC preparations such as Sarna or Prax.
- Topical steroid preparations should be avoided, unless absolutely needed to control itching and only after definitive diagnosis and initiation of antifungal treatment.
- Nystatin should be avoided in tinea infections but is indicated for cutaneous candidal infections.
- Keep area as dry as possible (talcum/powders may be beneficial).

MEDICATION

First Line

- Tinea cruris/corporis (2)[A],(3)[A]
  - Topical terbinafine 1% (Lamisil): OTC inexpensive and effective compound; can be applied once or BID for 1 to 3 weeks
  - Topical econazole 1% (Spectazole), ketoconazole (Nizoral): usually applied BID for 2 to 3 weeks
  - Topical butenafine 1% (Mentax): applied once daily for 2 weeks; also very effective. To prevent relapse, use for 1 week after resolution.
- Tinea capitis (4)[A]; PO terbinafine for 4 weeks, PO griseofulvin for 8 weeks, and PO itraconazole are about equally effective in children, although terbinafine might have a slight advantage in *Trichophtyon*, whereas griseofulvin may be preferable with *Microsporum* sp.
  - PO griseofulvin for *Trichophyton* and *Microsporum* sp.; microsized preparation available; dosage of 10 to 20 mg/kg/day (max 1,000 mg); taken BID or as a single dose daily for 6 to 12 weeks
  - PO terbinafine can be used for *Trichophyton* sp. at 62.5 mg/day in patients weighing 10 to 20 kg; 125 mg/day if weighing 20 to 40 kg; 250 mg/day if weighing >40 kg; use for 4 to 6 weeks. There is little evidence for use in children <4 years of age.
  - PO itraconazole can be used for *Microsporum* sp. and matches griseofulvin efficacy while being better tolerated; dosage of 3 to 5 mg/kg/day (maximum 400 mg daily), but most studies have used 100 mg/day for 6 weeks in children >2 years of age

Second Line

Tinea cruris/corporis (5)[A]

- Oral antifungal agents are effective but not indicated in uncomplicated tinea cruris/corporis cases. They can be used for resistant and extensive infections or if the patient is immunocompromised. If topical therapy fails, consider possible oral therapy.
- The following oral regimens have been reported in medical literature as being effective but currently are not specifically approved by FDA for tinea cruris:
  - PO terbinafine (Lamisil): 250 mg/day for 1 to 2 weeks
  - PO itraconazole (Sporanox): children 3 to 5 mg/kg/day with maximum dose of 200 mg/day; adults 100 mg BID once and repeated 1 week later
  - PO fluconazole (Diflucan): children 6 mg/kg once weekly with maximum dose of 200 mg weekly; adults 200 mg once per week for 4 weeks
- Topical terbinafine 1% solution has been studied recently and appears effective as a once daily application for 1 week.
- Oral antifungals have many interactions including warfarin, OCPs, and alcohol; advise checking for drug interactions prior to use; contraindicated in pregnancy. Monitor for liver toxicity when using oral antifungals.

ISSUES FOR REFERRAL

Refer if disease is nonresponsive/resistant, especially in immunocompromised host.

ADDITIONAL THERAPIES

Treatment of secondary bacterial infections

 ## ONGOING CARE

FOLLOW-UP RECOMMENDATIONS

Reevaluate response to treatment.

Patient Monitoring

Liver function testing prior to therapy and at regular intervals during course of therapy for patients requiring oral terbinafine, fluconazole, itraconazole, and griseofulvin

PATIENT EDUCATION

Explain the causative agents, predisposing factors, and prevention measures.

PROGNOSIS

- Excellent prognosis for cure with therapy in tinea cruris and corporis
- In tinea capitis, lesions will heal spontaneously in 6 months without treatment, but scarring is more likely.

COMPLICATIONS

- Secondary bacterial infection
- Generalized, invasive dermatophyte infection
- Secondary eruptions called dermatophytid reactions (which occur in association with primary/inflammatory skin disorders) may occur at distant sites.

REFERENCES

1. Ameen M. Epidemiology of superficial fungal infections. *Clin Dermatol*. 2010;28(2):197–201.
2. van Zuuren EJ, Fedorowicz Z, El-Gohary M. Evidence-based topical treatments for tinea cruris and tinea corporis: a summary of a Cochrane systematic review. *Br J Dermatol*. 2015;172(3): 616–641.
3. El-Gohary M, van Zuuren EJ, Fedorowicz Z, et al. Topical antifungal treatments for tinea cruris and tinea corporis. *Cochrane Database Syst Rev*. 2014;(8):CD009992.
4. Gupta AK, Mays RR, Versteeg SG, et al. Tinea capitis in children: a systematic review of management. *J Eur Acad Dermatol Venereol*. 2018;32(12): 2264–2274.
5. Leung AK, Lam JM, Leong KF, et al. Tinea corporis: an updated review. *Drugs Context*. 2020;9:2020-5-6.

ADDITIONAL READING

- Bell-Syer SEM, Khan SM, Torgerson DJ. Oral treatments for fungal infections of the skin of the foot. *Cochrane Database Syst Rev*. 2012;10(10):CD003584.
- Chen X, Jiang X, Yang M, et al. Systemic antifungal therapy for tinea capitis in children. *Cochrane Database Syst Rev*. 2016;2016(5):CD004685.

 ## CODES

ICD10

- B35.0 Tinea barbae and tinea capitis
- B35.4 Tinea corporis
- B35.6 Tinea cruris

CLINICAL PEARLS

- Tinea corporis is characterized by scaly plaque, with peripheral activity and central clearing.
- Tinea cruris is characterized by erythematous plaque in crural folds usually sparing the scrotum. Treatment of concomitant tinea pedis is advised.
- Tinea capitis is a fungal infection of the scalp affecting hair growth. Topical therapy is ineffective for this infection.

T

TINEA PEDIS

William Andrew Pleasant, MD • Chirag N. Shah, MD • Daniel Scott Morrison, MD

 BASICS

DESCRIPTION
- Superficial fungal infection of the skin of the feet caused by dermatophytes
- Most common dermatophyte infection encountered in clinical practice; contagious
- Often accompanied by tinea manuum, tinea unguium, and tinea cruris
- Clinical forms: interdigital (most common), hyperkeratotic (moccasin type), vesiculobullous (inflammatory), and rarely ulcerative
- System(s) affected: skin/exocrine
- Synonym(s): athlete's foot, foot ringworm

EPIDEMIOLOGY
- Predominant age: 20 to 50 years, although can occur at any age
- Predominant gender: males infected about 4 times as frequently as females

Prevalence
- 4–10% of the population
- >70% of population will experience during a lifetime.

Pediatric Considerations
Rare in younger children; common in adolescents

Geriatric Considerations
Elderly are more susceptible to outbreaks because of immunocompromised and impaired perfusion of distal extremities.

ETIOLOGY AND PATHOPHYSIOLOGY
Superficial infection caused by dermatophytes that release enzymes called keratinases to invade and thrive only in nonviable keratinized tissue
- *Trichophyton interdigitale* (acute)
- *Trichophyton rubrum* (chronic): most common
- *Trichophyton tonsurans*
- *Epidermophyton floccosum*

Genetics
No known genetic pattern

RISK FACTORS
- Hot, humid weather
- Sweating
- Occlusive/tight-fitting footwear
- Immunosuppression
- Prolonged application of topical steroids

GENERAL PREVENTION
- Good personal hygiene
- Wearing rubber or wooden sandals in community showers, bathing places, locker rooms
- Careful drying between toes after showering or bathing; blow-drying feet with hair dryer may be more effective than drying with towel
- Changing socks and shoes frequently
- Applying drying or dusting powder
- Applying topical antiperspirants

COMMONLY ASSOCIATED CONDITIONS
- Hyperhidrosis
- Onychomycosis
- Tinea manuum/unguium/cruris/corporis

 DIAGNOSIS

HISTORY
- Itchy, scaly rash on foot, usually between toes; may progress to fissuring/maceration in toe web spaces
- May be associated with onychomycosis and other tinea infections
- May be complicated by secondary bacterial infections

PHYSICAL EXAM
- Acute form: self-limited, intermittent, recurrent; scaling, thickening, and fissuring of sole and heel; silvery white scaling or fissuring of toe webs; or pruritic vesicular/bullous lesions between toes or on soles
- Chronic form: most common; slowly progressive, pruritic erythematous erosion/scales between toes, in digital interspaces; extension onto soles, sides/dorsum of feet (moccasin distribution); if untreated, may persist indefinitely
- Other features: strong odor, hyperkeratosis, maceration, ulceration
- Tinea pedis may occur unilaterally or bilaterally.
- Secondary presumably immune-mediated eruptions called dermatophytid reactions may occur at distant sites.

DIFFERENTIAL DIAGNOSIS
- Interdigital type: erythrasma, impetigo, pitted keratolysis, candidal intertrigo
- Moccasin type: psoriasis vulgaris, chronic contact dermatitis, eczematous dermatitis, pitted keratolysis
- Inflammatory/bullous type: impetigo, allergic contact dermatitis, dyshidrotic eczema (negative potassium hydroxide [KOH] examination of scrapings), bullous disease

DIAGNOSTIC TESTS & INTERPRETATION
Wood's lamp exam will not fluoresce unless complicated by another fungus, which is uncommon: *Malassezia furfur* (yellow to white), *Corynebacterium* (red), or *Microsporum* (blue-green)

Initial Tests (lab, imaging)
Testing is not needed in typical presentation
- Microscopic exam using KOH applied to scrapings of the affected area
- Culture (Sabouraud medium)

Follow-Up Tests & Special Considerations
Real time PCR increasingly being used; helpful in cases of recurrence as it identifies species

Test Interpretation
- KOH preparation: confirmed with detection of segmented hyphae
- Culture: dermatophyte

 TREATMENT

Treatment is generally with topical antifungal medications for up to 4 weeks and is more effective than placebo (1)[A].
- Acute treatment
  - Aluminum acetate soak (Burow solution; Domeboro, 1 pack to 1 quart warm water) to decrease itching and acute eczematous reaction
  - Antifungal cream of choice BID after soaks (allylamines slightly more effective than azoles)
- Chronic treatment:
  - Antifungal creams BID, continuing for 3 days after the rash is resolved: terbinafine 1%, clotrimazole 1%, econazole 1%, ketoconazole 2%, tolnaftate 1%, etc. (2)[A]
  - May try systemic antifungal therapy (see below); consider if concomitant onychomycosis or after failed topical treatment

GENERAL MEASURES
- Soak with aluminum chloride 30% or aluminum acetate for 20 minutes BID.
- Perform careful removal of dead/thickened skin after soaking or bathing.
- Treat shoes with antifungal powders.
- Avoid occlusive footwear.
- Chronic, extensive disease, or nail involvement requires oral antifungal medication for systemic therapy.

MEDICATION
Oral therapy indicated for extensive infections, disease refractory to topical treatment and in immunocompromised patients.

First Line
- Systemic antifungals (3)[A]:
  - Itraconazole: 200 mg PO BID for 7 days (cure rate >90%)
  - Terbinafine: 250 mg PO daily for 14 days (more efficacious than itraconazole)
- If concomitant onychomycosis:
  - Itraconazole: 200 mg PO BID for 1st week of the month for 3 months (Liver function testing is recommended.)
  - Terbinafine: 250 mg PO daily for 12 weeks, or pulse dosing: 500 mg PO daily for 1st week of the month for 3 months (not recommended if creatinine clearance <50 mL/min)

- Pediatric dosing options: weight based with treatment duration similar to adults
  - Griseofulvin: 10 to 15 mg/kg/day or divided
  - Terbinafine:
    - 10 to 20 kg: 62.5 mg/day
    - 20 to 40 kg: 125 mg/day
    - >40 kg: 250 mg/day
  - Itraconazole: 3 to 5 mg/kg/day
  - Fluconazole: 6 mg/kg/week
- Contraindications: itraconazole, pregnancy Category C
- Precautions: All systemic antifungal drugs may have potential hepatotoxicity.
- Dose reduction is required for patients with moderate to severe chronic kidney disease.
- Significant possible interactions: Itraconazole requires gastric acid for absorption; effectiveness is reduced with antacids, H_2 blockers, proton pump inhibitors, etc. Take with acidic beverage, such as soda if on antacids.
- Side effects: Itraconazole and terbinafine may lead to gastrointestinal distress including diarrhea; itraconazole may also lead to peripheral edema especially if used in conjunction with calcium channel blockers.

Second Line
- Systemic antifungals: griseofulvin V (griseofulvin microsize) 250 to 500 mg daily for 21 days
- Contraindications (griseofulvin):
  - Patients with porphyria, hepatocellular failure
  - Patients with history of hypersensitivity to griseofulvin
- Precautions (griseofulvin):
  - Should be used only in severe cases
  - Periodic monitoring of organ system functioning, including renal, hepatic, and hematopoietic
  - Possible photosensitivity reactions
  - Systemic lupus erythematosus, lupus-like syndromes, or exacerbation of existing systemic lupus erythematosus has been reported.
- Significant possible interactions (griseofulvin):
  - Decreases activity of warfarin-type anticoagulants
  - Barbiturates usually depress griseofulvin activity
  - May potentiate effect of alcohol, producing tachycardia and flush

ISSUES FOR REFERRAL
Consider dermatology referral if extensive or resistant disease, especially in immunocompromised host.

ADDITIONAL THERAPIES
- Treatment of secondary bacterial infections
- Treatment of eczematoid changes

COMPLEMENTARY & ALTERNATIVE MEDICINE
- Baking soda soak (1/2 cup in 1 quart warm water) has been shown to provide antifungal activity (4).
- White vinegar soak (1:1 white vinegar to warm water) may be used to aid in gram-negative bacterial coinfection.

 ONGOING CARE

FOLLOW-UP RECOMMENDATIONS
Avoid sweat buildup along feet.

Patient Monitoring
Evaluate for response, recognizing that infections may be chronic/recurrent.

DIET
No restrictions

PATIENT EDUCATION
See "General Prevention."

PROGNOSIS
- Often may obtain control but not completely cure
- Infections tend to be chronic with exacerbations (e.g., in hot, humid weather).
- Personal hygiene and preventive measures, such as open-toed sandals, careful drying, and frequent sock changes are essential.

COMPLICATIONS
- Secondary bacterial infections (common portal of entry for streptococcal infections, producing lymphangitis/cellulitis of lower extremity)
- Eczematoid changes/dermatophytid reactions

REFERENCES

1. Thomas B, Falk J, Allan GM. Topical management of tinea pedis. *Can Fam Physician*. 2021;67(1):30.
2. Ward H, Parkes N, Smith C, et al. Consensus for the treatment of tinea pedis: a systematic review of randomised controlled trials. *J Fungi (Basel)*. 2022;8(4):351.
3. Bell-Syer SEM, Khan SM, Torgerson DJ. Oral treatments for fungal infections of the skin of the foot. *Cochrane Database Syst Rev*. 2012;10(10):CD003584.
4. Letscher-Bru V, Obszynski CM, Samsoen M, et al. Antifungal activity of sodium bicarbonate against fungal agents causing superficial infections. *Mycopathologia*. 2013;175(1–2):153–158.

ADDITIONAL READING

- Crawford F, Hollis S. Topical treatments for fungal infections of the skin and nails of the foot. *Cochrane Database Syst Rev*. 2007;2007(3):CD001434.
- Hawkins DM, Smidt AC. Superficial fungal infections in children. *Pediatr Clin North Am*. 2014;61(2): 443–455.
- Liu X, Tan J, Yang H, et al. Characterization of skin microbiome in tinea pedis. *Indian J Microbiol*. 2019;59(4):422–427.
- Rotta I, Sanchez A, Gonçalves PR, et al. Efficacy and safety of topical antifungals in the treatment of dermatomycosis: a systematic review. *Br J Dermatol*. 2012;166(5):927–933.
- Sahoo AK, Mahajan R. Management of tinea corporis, tinea cruris, and tinea pedis: a comprehensive review. *Indian Dermatol Online J*. 2016;7(2):77–86.

 SEE ALSO

Dermatitis, Contact; Dyshidrosis

 CODES

ICD10
B35.3 Tinea pedis

CLINICAL PEARLS
- Tinea pedis is often recurrent or chronic in nature.
- Careful drying between toes after showering or bathing helps prevent recurrences; blow-drying feet with hair dryer may be more effective than drying with towel.
- Socks should be changed frequently; put on socks before underwear to prevent infection from spreading to groin (tinea cruris).
- Treatment with topical antifungal medications for up to 4 weeks is usually sufficient.
- Dusting and desiccating powders (containing antifungal agents) may help prevent recurrences.

T

TINEA VERSICOLOR

Samantha Cotler, DO, MBA

 BASICS

DESCRIPTION
- Superficial fungal infection that interferes with normal skin pigmentation resulting in macules or patches that are hypopigmented, tan, brown or salmon-colored. Tinea versicolor is usually well-demarcated, finely scaling, occurring primarily on the trunk and proximal upper extremities. Tinea versicolor is not a dermatophyte infection. It is caused by lipophilic (fat/oil-loving) *Malassezia* yeast organisms that normally inhabit the skin.
- System(s) affected: skin/exocrine
- Synonym(s): pityriasis versicolor

EPIDEMIOLOGY
Incidence
- Common, occurs worldwide, especially in tropical climates
- Predominant age: adolescents and young adults
- Predominant sex: male = female

Pediatric Considerations
Skin eruptions usually occur after puberty, when sebaceous glands are more active. However, tinea versicolor can also be seen in children, especially in tropical climates; facial lesions are more common in children.

Geriatric Considerations
Not common in the geriatric population

Prevalence
Prevalence can reach up to 50%, especially in warm climates.

ETIOLOGY AND PATHOPHYSIOLOGY
The inhibition of pigment synthesis in epidermal melanocytes leads to hypopigmented skin patches. In the hyperpigmented type, melanosomes increase in size resulting in brown or darker patches of skin of varying shades.
- Tinea versicolor is caused by saprophytic yeast: *Pityrosporum orbiculare* (also known as *Plasmodium ovale*, *Malassezia furfur*, or *Malassezia ovalis*), which is a known colonizer of all humans.
- Development of clinical disease is associated with transformation of *Malassezia* from yeast cells to pathogenic mycelial form. Several endogenous (host) and exogenous/external factors may play a role in the transformation to active disease.
- Tinea versicolor is not linked to poor hygiene.
- Tinea versicolor is generally not contagious.

Genetics
Genetic predisposition may exist.

RISK FACTORS
- Hot, humid weather
- Use of topical skin oils
- Hyperhidrosis
- HIV infection/immunosuppression
- High cortisol levels (Cushing syndrome/disease, prolonged steroid administration)
- Pregnancy
- Malnutrition
- Oral contraceptives

GENERAL PREVENTION
- Prophylaxis can be used in warm summer months and prior to tanning season in people with frequent recurrences.
- Avoiding skin oils may help.
- Tinea versicolor is not contagious.

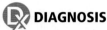 DIAGNOSIS

HISTORY
- Asymptomatic scaling macules typically affect the trunk and shoulders.
- Mild pruritus may occur.
- Skin eruptions are more prominent in summer months.
- Sun tanning accentuates lesions because affected areas usually do not tan.
- Periodic recurrences are common, especially in warm, summer months and in tropical regions.

PHYSICAL EXAM
- *Versicolor* refers to the variety and changing shades of colors. Color variations can exist between individuals and also between lesions.
- Sun exposure usually makes hypopigmented, light-colored patches more noticeable.
- In covered areas, lesions are often brown or salmon-colored.
- Usual distribution involves sebum-rich areas the chest, shoulders and back, and sometimes the face and intertriginous areas. In children, the face is more likely to be involved.
- Appearance: Tinea versicolor usually presents as small individual macules that frequently coalesce to form patches.
- Fine scales are present over the lesions and become more visible with scraping.

DIFFERENTIAL DIAGNOSIS
Other skin diseases with discolored macules and plaques or patches include the following:
- Pityriasis alba/rosea ("Christmas tree-like" distribution visible in pityriasis rosea)
- Vitiligo (presents without scaling)
- Seborrheic dermatitis (more erythematous; thicker scales)
- Nummular eczema
- Secondary syphilis
- Erythrasma
- Mycosis fungoides

DIAGNOSTIC TESTS & INTERPRETATION
Visualization of affected skin under Wood's light often appears fluorescent yellow to yellow-green.

Initial Tests (lab, imaging)
- Direct microscopy of scales with 10% potassium hydroxide (KOH) preparation shows hyphae and spores ("spaghetti and meatballs" pattern).
- Routine lab tests are usually not necessary.
- Fungal culture is not useful.

Test Interpretation
- Short, stubby, or Y-shaped hyphae
- Small, round spores in clusters on hyphae

 TREATMENT

GENERAL MEASURES
- Apply prescribed topical medications to the affected skin.
- Pigmentation/discoloration may take months to improve.
- In people with recurrences, repeat treatment each spring prior to sun exposure may be beneficial; consider monthly prophylaxis during the summer months.
- Patients who fail topical treatment can be treated with an oral/systemic medication.

MEDICATION
Topical antifungal therapy is the treatment of choice in limited disease and is safe and usually effective. Evidence is generally of poor quality, but data suggest that longer durations of treatment and higher concentrations of active agents produce greater cure rates (1)[A].

First Line

- Ketoconazole 2% shampoo applied to damp skin for 1 to 3 days and left on for 5 minutes (Ketoconazole is contraindicated in pregnancy.) *or*
- Ketoconazole 2% (Nizoral) cream applied twice daily for 2 to 4 weeks (Ketoconazole is contraindicated in pregnancy.) *or*
- Selenium sulfide shampoo 2.5% (Selsun):
  - Applied daily for 1 week to the affected areas and allowed to dry and remain on skin for 10 minutes prior to showering or
  - Allowed to remain on body once a week for 4 weeks for 12 to 24 hours prior to rinsing off or
- Clotrimazole 1% topical (Lotrimin) twice daily for 2 to 4 weeks *or*
- Miconazole 2% (Micatin, Monistat) twice daily for 2 to 4 weeks *or*
- Topical ciclopirox olamine 1% cream twice daily for 2 weeks *or*
- Terbinafine (Lamisil) 1% solution twice daily for 1 week *or*
- Terbinafine (Lamisil DermGel) once daily for 1 week
- Newer preparations include 2.25% selenium sulfide foam and ketoconazole 2% gel.
- Cure rates of topical anti-yeast preparations typically 70–80%; healing continues after active treatment. Even pigmentation may take months to return.

Second Line

- Can be used for extensive and recalcitrant disease (nonresponders)
- Oral fluconazole 300 mg once weekly for 2 weeks (2)[A]
- Itraconazole 200 mg/day PO for 1 week (7 days); cure rate >90% (2)[A]
- Oral ketoconazole is no longer recommended by the FDA due to risks of hepatotoxicity, adrenal insufficiency, and drug–drug interactions.
- Oral terbinafine or griseofulvin is not effective.

ISSUES FOR REFERRAL

- If resistant to treatment
- If extensive disease occurs in immunocompromised host

SURGERY/OTHER PROCEDURES

Photodynamic therapy and narrow-band ultraviolet B (NB-UVB) light have both been shown to be effective alternative treatments in tinea versicolor (3).

 ## ONGOING CARE

- Ketoconazole 2% or selenium sulfide 2.5% shampoo can be used weekly for maintenance or monthly for prophylaxis.
- Itraconazole 400 mg once monthly (in 2 divided dosages) during the warmer months of the year can also reduce recurrences.

FOLLOW-UP RECOMMENDATIONS

Inform patients that pigment changes/variations may remain for several months after treatment.

Patient Monitoring

- Prophylactic medication can be used in warm summer months and prior to tanning season in people with frequent recurrences.
- Failure to respond should prompt reassessment or dermatology referral.
- Resistance to treatment, frequent recurrences, or widespread disease may point to immunodeficiency.

DIET

There is no proven diet to treat and prevent recurrence of tinea versicolor.

PATIENT EDUCATION

For patient education materials on this topic, contact American Academy of Dermatology: https://www.aad.org/

PROGNOSIS

- Lesions may last for months to years.
- Lesions may recur periodically because *Malassezia* yeast organisms are known human colonizers and natural inhabitants of the skin.
- Pigment changes/variations may take months to resolve.

REFERENCES

1. Hald M, Arendrup MC, Svejgaard EL, et al. Evidence-based Danish guidelines for the treatment of *Malassezia*-related skin diseases. *Acta Derm Venereol*. 2015;95(1):12–19.
2. Gupta AK, Lane D, Paquet M. Systematic review of systemic treatments for tinea versicolor and evidence-based dosing regimen recommendations. *J Cutan Med Surg*. 2014;18(2):79–90.
3. Arce M, Gutiérrez-Mendoza D. Pityriasis versicolor: treatment update. *Curr Fungal Infect Rep*. 2018;12(2):195–200.

ADDITIONAL READING

- Bhogal CS, Singal A, Baruah MC. Comparative efficacy of ketoconazole and fluconazole in the treatment of pityriasis versicolor: a one year follow-up study. *J Dermatol*. 2001;28(10):535–539.
- Faergemann J, Todd G, Pather S, et al. A double-blind, randomized, placebo-controlled, dose-finding study of oral pramiconazole in the treatment of pityriasis versicolor. *J Am Acad Dermatol*. 2009;61(6):971–976.
- Gupta AK, Lyons DCA. Pityriasis versicolor: an update on pharmacological treatment options. *Expert Opin Pharmacother*. 2014;15(12):1707–1713.
- Hawkins DM, Smidt AC. Superficial fungal infections in children. *Pediatr Clin North Am*. 2014;61(2): 443–455.
- Köse O, Bülent Taştan H, Riza Gür A, et al. Comparison of a single 400 mg dose versus a 7-day 200 mg daily dose of itraconazole in the treatment of tinea versicolor. *J Dermatolog Treat*. 2002;13(2):77–79.

 ## CODES

ICD10

B36.0 Pityriasis versicolor

CLINICAL PEARLS

- Tinea versicolor, also called pityriasis versicolor, is characterized by noncontagious, finely scaling macules of varying colors.
- Recurrence is common in summer months.
- Lesions tend to become more apparent after tanning because they typically do not tan; hypopigmented patches become more visible.
- Inform patients that discoloration/pigment variations may remain for several months after treatment.

T

TINNITUS

Donna I. Meltzer, MD

BASICS

DESCRIPTION

- Tinnitus is a perceived sensation of sound in the absence of an external acoustic stimulus; often described as a ringing, hissing, buzzing, clicking, or whooshing
- Derived from the Latin word *tinnire*, meaning "to ring"
- May be heard in one or both ears or centrally within the head
- Two types: subjective (most common) and objective tinnitus
  - Subjective tinnitus: perceived only by the patient; can be continuous, intermittent, or pulsatile
  - Objective tinnitus: audible to the examiner; rare
- Primary tinnitus: idiopathic with or without sensorineural hearing loss (SNHL) (1)
- Secondary tinnitus: associated with a specific cause (other than SNHL)

EPIDEMIOLOGY

Incidence

- Incidence is increasing in association with excessive noise exposure.
- Higher rates of tinnitus in smokers, hypertensives, diabetics, and obese patients

Prevalence

- Tinnitus reported by 35 to 50 million adults in the United States; although underreported, 12 million seek medical care.
- Affects 10–15% of adults (2)
- Prevalence increases with age and peaks in 6th decade of life; estimated 8% prevalence reported post–COVID-19 infection
- Prevalence of 13–53% in general pediatric population
- Ethnic: whites > blacks and Hispanics
- Gender: males > females

ETIOLOGY AND PATHOPHYSIOLOGY

- Precise pathophysiology is unknown; numerous theories have been proposed. Ototoxic agents or noise exposure damage hair cells so that there is abnormal neural activity in the auditory cortex. Inflammation may play a role.
- Causes of secondary tinnitus (2):
  - Otologic: cholesteatoma, cerumen impaction, foreign body, middle ear effusion, otosclerosis, Ménière disease, vestibular schwannoma, patulous Eustachian tube
  - Medications: anti-inflammatory agents (aspirin, NSAIDs); antimalarial agents, antimicrobial drugs (aminoglycosides, macrolides); antineoplastic agents, loop diuretics, miscellaneous drugs (antiarrhythmics, antiulcer, anticonvulsants, antihypertensives); anesthetics

- Somatic: temporomandibular joint (TMJ) dysfunction, head or neck injury
- Neurologic: multiple sclerosis, spontaneous intracranial hypertension, vestibular migraine, type I Chiari malformation, palatal myoclonus, idiopathic stapedial muscle spasm
- Infectious: viral (impact of COVID-19 on tinnitus is unknown), bacterial, fungal
- Metabolic: diabetes mellitus, dyslipidemia, vitamin B_{12} deficiency
- Vascular: aortic or carotid stenosis, venous hum, arteriovenous fistula or malformation, vascular tumors, high cardiac output state (anemia)

Genetics

Limited evidence to support a genetic component

RISK FACTORS

- Hearing loss (but can have tinnitus with normal hearing)
- High-level noise exposure
- Advanced age
- Use of ototoxic medications (Some are irreversible.)
- Otologic disease (otosclerosis, Ménière disease, cerumen impaction)
- Depression and anxiety are associated with increased odds of tinnitus.

GENERAL PREVENTION

- Avoid loud noise exposure and wear appropriate ear protection to prevent hearing loss.
- Monitor ototoxic medications and avoid prescribing more than one ototoxic agent concurrently.

COMMONLY ASSOCIATED CONDITIONS

- SNHL caused by presbycusis (age-associated hearing loss) or prolonged loud noise exposure
- Conductive hearing loss due to cerumen, otosclerosis, cholesteatoma
- Psychological disorders: depression, anxiety, insomnia, suicidal ideation
- Despair, frustration, interference with concentration and social interactions, work hindrance

DIAGNOSIS

HISTORY

- Onset gradual (presbycusis) or abrupt (following loud noise exposure)
- Duration: acute versus chronic (>6 months)
- Timing: can be continuous (hearing loss) or intermittent (Ménière disease)
- Pattern: nonpulsatile > pulsatile (often vascular cause)
- Location: bilateral > unilateral (vestibular schwannoma, cerumen, Ménière disease)

- Pitch: high pitch (with SNHL) > low pitch (Ménière disease)
- Associated symptoms: hearing loss, headache, noise intolerance, vertigo, TMJ dysfunction, neck pain
- Exacerbating factors: loud noise; jaw, head, or neck movements
- Alleviating factors: hearing aid, position change, medications
- Medication use (prescription, OTC, supplements)
- Hearing and past noise exposure (occupational, military, recreational)
- Psychosocial history (depression, sleep habits)
- Impact of tinnitus: bothersome or nonbothersome; Tinnitus Handicap Inventory, Tinnitus Functional Index

PHYSICAL EXAM

- HEENT, neck, neurologic, and vascular examinations to help with etiology or guide next steps
- Ear: cerumen impaction, effusion, cholesteatoma
- Check hearing; air and bone conduction testing with 512- or 1,024-Hz tuning fork (Weber and Rinne tests)
- Eye: funduscopic exam for papilledema (intracranial hypertension) or visual field change (mass)
- TMJ: Palpate for tenderness and crepitus with movement.
- Cranial nerve, Romberg test (equilibrium), finger to nose, gait; assess for nystagmus.
- Auscultate for bruits or murmurs; compress jugular vein (suspect venous etiology if maneuver reduces tinnitus)

DIFFERENTIAL DIAGNOSIS

- Pulsatile tinnitus: carotid stenosis, aortic valve disease, AV malformation, high cardiac output state (anemia, hyperthyroidism), paraganglioma (glomus tumor)
- Nonpulsatile tinnitus: auditory hallucinations

DIAGNOSTIC TESTS & INTERPRETATION

- Tinnitus is a symptom; no objective test to confirm diagnosis
- Complete audiologic examination
  - Pure tone audiometry (air and bone conduction)
  - Tympanometry
  - Weber test, Rinne test
- Carotid Doppler ultrasonography (neck bruit)

Initial Tests (lab, imaging)

- Little evidence to support lab testing other than targeted lab studies based on history and physical exam; use clinical judgment and consider the following:
  - CBC, BUN/creatinine, fasting glucose, lipid panel
- Guidelines advise against imaging studies unless there is a unilateral and pulsatile tinnitus, focal neurologic abnormality, or asymmetric hearing loss (1)[C].

- The American College of Radiology (ACR) recently updated the evidence-based recommendations for patients presenting with tinnitus; history, physical, and associated symptoms guide initial imaging (3)[C]:
  - Pulsatile tinnitus (unilateral or bilateral) with normal otoscopy: initial imaging includes MRA of head with IV contrast, MRI of head and internal auditory canal (IAC) without and with contrast, or CTA of head alone or head and neck with IV contrast; carotid artery duplex scan is no longer recommended.
  - Pulsatile tinnitus (unilateral or bilateral) with suspected retrotympanic lesion on otoscopy: CT of temporal bone without IV contrast; might consider CTA of head and neck with IV contrast
  - Unilateral nonpulsatile tinnitus if no hearing loss and no neurologic deficit: MRI of head and IAC without and with IV contrast; might consider MRI study without contrast
  - Bilateral nonpulsatile tinnitus: imaging not indicated if no hearing loss, neurologic deficit, or trauma

Follow-Up Tests & Special Considerations
Consider TSH, HIV test, RPR, autoimmune panel, Lyme test, vitamin B_{12} level, and serum 25-hydroxyvitamin D test; low quality evidence for some of these studies (2)

Diagnostic Procedures/Other
Electronystagmography (vestibular testing for Ménière disease)

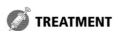 ## TREATMENT

GENERAL MEASURES
- Individualize treatment based on the severity of tinnitus and impact on function.
- Cognitive behavioral therapy (CBT), education, relaxation therapy
- Reassure patient.
- Manage treatable pathology.
- Hearing aids (corrects hearing and might mask tinnitus) can be tried if there is hearing loss and bothersome tinnitus (1)[C].
- Protect hearing against future loud noise.
- Masking sound devices or generators on discontinuation might have decreased tinnitus (residual inhibition).
- Discontinue ototoxic medications (some medications have reversible ototoxic effects).

MEDICATION
No pharmacologic agent has been shown to consistently alleviate tinnitus.

First Line
- Antidepressants (SSRIs or TCAs): probably help with psychological distress; insufficient evidence that antidepressant drug therapy improves tinnitus (2)
- Anxiolytics (benzodiazepines) do not provide consistent benefit and risk side effect of dependency (2).

Second Line
Anticonvulsants: potentially suppress central auditory hyperactivity but not recommended (1)[C]

ISSUES FOR REFERRAL
- Audiologist for comprehensive hearing evaluation and management
- Otolaryngologist, neurologist, or neurosurgeon depending on pathology
- Dental referral for TMJ treatment and dental orthotics (splint, night guard)
- Therapists for CBT, biofeedback, education, and relaxation techniques

ADDITIONAL THERAPIES
- CBT employs relaxation exercises, coping strategies, and deconditioning techniques to reduce arousal levels and reverse negative thoughts about tinnitus; might reduce negative impact of tinnitus on quality of life; recommended as beneficial based on randomized controlled trials (1)[C]
- Sound therapy (masking): Patients wear low-level noise generators to mask the tinnitus noise; optional therapy (1)[C]
- Tinnitus retraining therapy (TRT) combines counseling, education, and acoustic therapy (soft music, sound machine) to minimize bothersome nature of tinnitus. TRT might reduce tinnitus but probably no benefit over standard counseling with enriched sound.
- Internet-based technology or smartphone apps to mask tinnitus may hold promise but high-quality studies are lacking.
- Transcranial magnetic stimulation (TMS): a noninvasive method to stimulate neurons in the brain by rapidly changing magnetic fields; not recommended as randomized trials were inconclusive (1)[C]
- Botulism toxin (for palatal myoclonus)
- Intratympanic steroid injections are not recommended (1)[C].

SURGERY/OTHER PROCEDURES
- Cochlear implants (for severe SNHL) might improve severity of tinnitus.
- Ablation of cochlear nerve (destroys hearing)
- Otosclerosis: stapedectomy surgery with implantation of ossicular prosthesis
- Severe Ménière disease not alleviated by medications: installation of endolymphatic shunt, labyrinthectomy, or vestibular neurectomy
- Auditory neoplasms: surgical resection/radiation
- Pulsatile tinnitus due to atherosclerotic carotid artery disease: carotid endarterectomy

COMPLEMENTARY & ALTERNATIVE MEDICINE
Acupuncture, *Ginkgo biloba*, melatonin, zinc, or antioxidants might alleviate tinnitus in some patients; however, many conflicting studies report no benefit with these methods.

 ## ONGOING CARE

FOLLOW-UP RECOMMENDATIONS
- Audiologist: for hearing evaluation and therapy
- Counseling: as needed for psychological distress
- Family physician: as needed for support and guidance

PATIENT EDUCATION
- American Tinnitus Association: https://www.ata.org/
- National Institute on Deafness and Other Communication Disorders: https://www.nidcd.nih.gov/health/tinnitus

PROGNOSIS
- Tinnitus persisted in 80% of older patients and increased in severity in 50%.
- Focus on managing tinnitus and reducing severity, not curing.

REFERENCES

1. Tunkel DE, Bauer CA, Sun GH, et al. Clinical practice guideline: tinnitus executive summary. *Otolaryngol Head Neck Surg*. 2014;151(4):533–541.
2. Dalrymple SN, Lewis SH, Philman S. Tinnitus: diagnosis and management. *Am Fam Physician*. 2021;103(11):663–671.
3. Jain V, Policeni B, Julilano AF, et al; for American College of Radiology. ACR appropriateness criteria. Tinnitus. https://acsearch.acr.org/docs/3094199/Narrative/. Accessed June 2, 2023.

ADDITIONAL READING

Grundfast KM, Jamil TL. Evaluation and management of tinnitus: are there opportunities for improvement? *Otolaryngol Head Neck Surg*. 2023;168(1):45–58.

 ## CODES

ICD10
- H93.19 Tinnitus, unspecified ear
- H93.11 Tinnitus, right ear
- H93.12 Tinnitus, left ear

CLINICAL PEARLS

- People have different levels of tolerance to tinnitus. It may affect sleep, concentration, and emotional state. Many patients with chronic tinnitus have depression.
- To keep tinnitus from worsening, avoid loud noises and minimize stress.
- Optimal management may involve multiple strategies.

TOBACCO USE AND SMOKING CESSATION

Naureen Bashir Rafiq, MD, FAAFP

BASICS

Use of tobacco in any form

DESCRIPTION

- Nicotine sources: cigars, pipes, water pipes, hookahs, cigarettes, electronic cigarettes (e-cigarettes), and smokeless tobacco such as dip, snuff, and chewing tobacco
- Electronic nicotine delivery system (ENDS) use is on the rise.
- E-cigarettes are called e-cigs, vapes, e-hookahs, and vape pens.

EPIDEMIOLOGY

Smoking causes more deaths each year than alcohol use, motor vehicle accidents, illegal drug use, and firearm-related injuries combined.

Incidence

- >2 million new smokers annually in the United States
- More than half of new smokers are <18 years of age (6% initiation rate for teens).
- More than half of individuals who have ever smoked cigarettes have successfully quit.

Prevalence

- Age: highest among those aged 45 to 64 years (16%); gender: male > female (15% vs. 12%)
- Cigarette smoking among adults has declined significantly since the 1960s. Cigarette smoking is responsible for >480,000 deaths per year in the United States, including >41,000 deaths from secondhand smoke exposure. This is about 1 in 5 deaths annually or 1,300 deaths every day.
- Each day, about 2,000 people aged <18 years smoke their first cigarette. Each day, about 1,600 youth try their first cigarette.
- In 2018, 21% of high school students reported current use of e-cigarettes.
- In 2020, ~31 million U.S. adults were current cigarette smokers; this represents 14% of men and 11% of women. In 2019, 14% of all adults (34.1 million people) currently smoked cigarettes: 15.3% in men, 12.7% of women.
- 5% of middle school students report current e-cigarette use.

ETIOLOGY AND PATHOPHYSIOLOGY

- Addiction due to nicotine's rapid stimulation of the brain's dopamine system (teenage brain especially susceptible)
- Atherosclerotic risk due to adrenergic stimulation, endothelial damage, carbon monoxide, and adverse effects on lipids
- Direct airway damage from cigarette tar; carcinogens in all tobacco products
- E-cigarettes produce an aerosol by heating liquid nicotine, flavoring, and chemicals. Potential adverse effects of e-cigarettes are related to exposure to nicotine as well as to other vapor components produced by the devices.
- If e-cigarette, or vaping product, use is suspected as a possible etiology of a patient's lung injury, obtain detailed history regarding:
  - Substance(s) used: nicotine, cannabinoids (e.g., marijuana, THC, THC concentrates, CBD, CBD oil, synthetic cannabinoids [e.g., K2 or spice], hash oil, Dank vapes), flavors, or other substances
  - Substance source(s): commercially available liquids, homemade liquids

- Device(s) used: manufacturer; brand name; product name; model
- Vitamin E acetate is strongly linked to the EVALI outbreaks.
- Most product use-associated lung injury (EVALI) associated with products containing THC

RISK FACTORS

- Presence of a smoker in the household
- Easy access to cigarettes
- Comorbid stress and psychiatric disorders
- Low self-esteem/self-worth
- Poor academic performance
- Boys: high levels of aggression and rebelliousness; girls: preoccupation with weight and body image

GENERAL PREVENTION

- Most first-time tobacco use occurs before high school graduation; restrict minors' access to tobacco by limiting tobacco advertisements and encouraging tobacco-free sports initiatives.
- Smoking bans in public areas and workplaces
- Media campaigns
- Health warnings on tobacco products
- Peer education program
- Motivational Interviewing

COMMONLY ASSOCIATED CONDITIONS

- Coronary artery disease, cerebrovascular disease; peripheral vascular disease; abdominal aortic aneurysm (AAA)
- Chronic obstructive pulmonary disease (COPD); cancer of the lip, oral cavity, pharynx, larynx, lung, esophagus, stomach, pancreas, kidney, urinary bladder, cervix, and blood; pneumonia, osteoporosis; periodontitis; alcohol use; depression and anxiety, reduced fertility
- E-cigarette use has been associated with several cases of idiopathic acute eosinophilic pneumonia.

Pregnancy Considerations

Smoking during pregnancy can increase the risk of miscarriage, congenital anomalies, stillbirth, fetal growth restriction, preterm birth, and placental abruption. Patients are encouraged to quit smoking completely as the evidence on pharmacotherapy interventions for tobacco smoking cessation in pregnancy is insufficient.

Pediatric Considerations

Secondhand smoke increases the risk for sudden infant death syndrome, acute upper and lower respiratory tract infections, exacerbations of asthma, and otitis media. Nicotine passes through breast milk and decreases the production of milk by suppressing the prolactin levels.

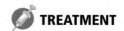**DIAGNOSIS**

HISTORY

- Ask about (and document) tobacco use and secondhand smoke exposure at every encounter.
- Type and quantity of tobacco used: "Heavy smoking" is ≥20 cigarettes per day or ≥20 pack-years.
  - Pack-years = packs/day × years
  - Assess for awareness of health risks and interest in quitting.
- Identify triggers for smoking: stress, habit, pleasure.
- Prior attempts to quit: method, duration of success, reason for relapse

PHYSICAL EXAM

- General: tobacco odor, staining of nails, hair
- Skin: premature wrinkling, especially the face
- Mouth: nicotine-stained teeth; inspect for mucosal changes, hypertrophy, fungating lesions
- Lungs: crackles, wheezing, increased or decreased volume, chronic cough
- Vessels: carotid or abdominal bruits, abdominal aortic enlargement or aneurysm, weak peripheral pulses, stigmata of peripheral vascular disease

DIAGNOSTIC TESTS & INTERPRETATION

- The U.S. Preventive Services Task Force (USPSTF) recommends that clinicians ask all adults about tobacco use, advise them to stop using tobacco, and assist with behavioral interventions and FDA-approved pharmacotherapy for cessation to nonpregnant adults who use tobacco.
- The USPSTF recommends one-time screening abdominal ultrasound (US) for AAA in men ≥65 years of age who ever smoked (number needed to screen to prevent one AAA = 500).
- USPSTF recommends yearly screening for lung cancer with low-dose CT for individuals aged 55 to 80 years with a 30 pack-years history of smoking, current smokers, or those who have quit within the past 15 years.

Initial Tests (lab, imaging)

Nicotine can be measured in the blood and urine by checking cotinine levels.

Diagnostic Procedures/Other

Pulmonary function tests (PFTs) for smokers with chronic pulmonary symptoms, such as wheezing, cough, or dyspnea

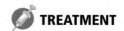**TREATMENT**

> **ALERT**
> Report cases of lung injury of unclear etiology and a history of e-cigarette or vaping product use within the past 90 days to state or local health department.

GENERAL MEASURES

- Behavioral counseling (5 A's):
  - Ask about tobacco use at every office visit.
  - Advise all smokers to quit.
  - Assess the patient's willingness to quit.
  - Assist the patient in his or her attempt to quit and provide quit line number (1-800-QUIT-NOW).
  - Arrange follow-up and support.
- 50% of adult smokers try to quit every year. Fewer than 1 in 10 succeed. <50% of adult smokers receive professional advice to quit. Even very brief advice promotes successful attempts at quitting.
- Patients ready to quit smoking should set a quit date within the next 2 weeks; no difference in success rates between patients who taper prior to their quit date and those who stop abruptly
- Behavioral interventions and use of FDA-approved pharmacotherapy for tobacco smoking cessation are effective in helping people to quit.
- Current evidence is insufficient to recommend the use of e-cigarettes for tobacco cessation in adults.

MEDICATION

Varenicline and nicotine gum therapy may each reduce relapse in patients who had stopped smoking.

First Line

- Varenicline (Chantix): 0.5 mg/day PO for 3 days, then 0.5 mg BID for 4 days, and then 1 mg BID for 11 weeks:
  - Start 1 to 4 weeks prior to smoking cessation and continue for 12 to 24 weeks.
  - Superior versus placebo and bupropion; number needed to treat = 6 and 15, respectively
  - May be combined with nicotine replacement therapy (NRT) for those with cravings
  - Side effects: nausea, insomnia, headache, depression, suicidal ideation; safety not established in adolescents or patients with psychiatric or cardiovascular disease; pregnancy Category C
- Bupropion SR (Zyban): 150 mg PO for 3 days and then 150 mg BID (1)[A]:
  - Start 1 week prior to smoking cessation and continue for 7 to 12 weeks.
  - Twice as effective as placebo
  - Drug of choice for patients with depression or schizophrenia; additional benefit of weight loss
  - May be combined with varenicline and NRT in men who smoke >1 PPD
  - Side effects: tachycardia, headache, nausea, insomnia, dry mouth; contraindicated in patients who have seizure disorders or anorexia/bulimia; pregnancy Category C
- NRT (e.g., patch, gum, lozenge, inhaler, nasal spray) (2)[A]:
  - Improves quit rates by 50–70% versus placebo
  - Available over the counter
  - Patch (NicoDerm CQ 21, 14, and 7 mg):
    ○ 1 patch q24h; start with 21 mg if smoking ≥10 cigarettes per day; otherwise, start with 14 mg.
    ○ 6 weeks on initial dose and then taper
    ○ 2 weeks each on subsequent doses
    ○ No proven benefit beyond 8 weeks
  - ENDS
    ○ Contain less nicotine than cigarette
    ○ Controversial if less "dangerous" than tobacco
    ○ Conflicting data on whether teen use increases or decreases risk to cigarette progression
    ○ Insufficient evidence to recommend as adjunct for tobacco cessation
  - Gum (Nicorette, 2 and 4 mg):
    ○ Use 4 mg if smoking ≥25 cigarettes per day.
    ○ Chew 1 piece q1–2h for 6 weeks, then 1 piece q2–4h for 3 weeks, and then 1 piece q4–8h for 3 weeks.
    ○ May use in combination with bupropion; monitor for hypertension.
    ○ Side effects: headache, pharyngitis, cough, rhinitis, dyspepsia; all mainly with inhaler and spray forms
    ○ Pregnancy Category D
  - NRT is reasonable in hospitalized smokers because NRT products immediately treat nicotine withdrawal symptoms, whereas varenicline and bupropion take time to reach steady state.

Second Line

- Nortriptyline: 25 to 75 mg/day PO or in divided doses:
  - Start 10 to 14 days prior to smoking cessation and continue for at least 12 weeks.
  - Efficacy similar to bupropion but side effects are more common; pregnancy Category D
  - The antidepressants bupropion and nortriptyline aid long-term smoking cessation.
- Clonidine: 0.1 mg PO BID or 0.1 mg/day transdermal patch weekly:
  - Side effects: hypotension, bradycardia, depression, fatigue; pregnancy Category C

ADDITIONAL THERAPIES

- Pharmacotherapy and behavior support increase success compared with minimal intervention or usual care.
- Naltrexone can be used in addition to other pharmacotherapy as it shows decreased nicotine use and craving without significant weight gain (3).

COMPLEMENTARY & ALTERNATIVE MEDICINE

- Acupuncture and hypnotherapy may help smoking cessation in short term
- Avoid situations and activities that are associated with smoking.

ADMISSION, INPATIENT, AND NURSING CONSIDERATIONS

Intense counseling interventions in hospitalized patients combined with follow-up for >1 month after discharge showed significant improvement in smoking cessation rates at ≥6 months postdischarge.

 ## ONGOING CARE

35–40% of patients relapse between years 1 and 5 after quitting. 2/3 of smokers who relapse report wanting to quit again within 30 days.

FOLLOW-UP RECOMMENDATIONS

Follow up 3 to 7 days after scheduled quit date and at least monthly for 3 months thereafter. Refraining from tobacco products for the first 2 weeks is critical to long-term abstinence. Inpatient counseling plus four postdischarge telephone calls effective for relapse prevention in hospitalized smokers

Patient Monitoring

- Short-term withdrawal symptoms include dysphoria, depressed mood, irritability, anxiety, insomnia, increased appetite, and poor concentration.
- Nicotine withdrawal syndrome: dysphoric or depressed mood, insomnia, irritability, frustration, or anger; anxiety, difficulty concentrating, restlessness, and increased appetite or weight gain; within 2 to 5 years after quitting, risk for stroke approximate to that of a nonsmoker
- Risk for cancer of the mouth, throat, esophagus, and bladder drops by half within 5 years of quitting. 10 years after quitting, the risk of dying from lung cancer drops by 50%.

DIET

Healthy eating for limiting weight gain

PATIENT EDUCATION

1-800-QUIT-NOW: https://www.cdc.gov/tobacco/

PROGNOSIS

- Smoking increases the risk for coronary heart disease (2- to 4-fold), stroke (2- to 4-fold), and lung cancer (25-fold). Smokers are more likely to die from COPD than nonsmokers (12-fold increased risk). Tobacco cessation reduces the risk of coronary heart disease sharply in the first 2 years after quitting (more slowly after that).
- Tobacco cessation slows the progression of COPD and reduces the loss of lung function over time. Tobacco cessation also reduces the risk of acute myeloid leukemia and cancers of the lung, cervix, colon, rectum, bladder, esophagus, kidney, liver, mouth, and throat. The risk of developing diabetes is 30–40% higher for active smokers than nonsmokers.
- People who quit smoking after a heart attack or cardiac surgery reduce their risk of death by 1/3. Relapse rates initially >60% but decrease to 2–4% after 2 years of abstinence. The incidence of myocardial infarction (MI) is increased by 6-fold in women and 3-fold in men who smoke at least 20 cigarettes per day, when compared with nonsmokers.
- Tobacco cessation reduces the risk of premature death and can add as much as 10 years of life expectancy.

COMPLICATIONS

- Disability and premature death due to heart attack, stroke, cancer, COPD
- Causation proven cancers associated with smoking: colorectal, head and neck, esophagus, kidney, liver, lower urinary tract, renal pelvis, ureter, bladder, lung, mesothelioma, nasal cavity, paranasal sinuses, pancreas, penis, stomach, uterine, and cervix; evidence equivocal: breast, skin
- Smoking doubles the risk of coronary artery disease and stroke.

REFERENCES

1. Howes S, Hartmann-Boyce J, Livingstone-Banks J, et al. Antidepressants for smoking cessation. *Cochrane Database Syst Rev.* 2020;4(4):CD000031.
2. Lindson N, Chepkin SC, Ye W, et al. Different doses, durations and modes of delivery of nicotine replacement therapy for smoking cessation. *Cochrane Database Syst Rev.* 2019;4(4):CD013308.
3. Green R, Bujarski S, Lim AC, et al. Naltrexone and alcohol effects on craving for cigarettes in heavy drinking smokers. *Exp Clin Psychopharmacol.* 2019;27(3):257–264.

 ## CODES

ICD10

- F17.210 Nicotine dependence, cigarettes, uncomplicated
- F17.213 Nicotine dependence, cigarettes, with withdrawal
- F17.211 Nicotine dependence, cigarettes, in remission

CLINICAL PEARLS

- Most adult cigarette smokers want to quit.
- Nicotine replacement improves cessation rates.
- Establish a quit date and provide resources to promote success (1-800-QUIT-NOW).

TOURETTE SYNDROME
Akanksha Samal, DO

BASICS

DESCRIPTION
Tourette syndrome (TS) is a childhood-onset neurobehavioral disorder characterized by the presence of multiple motor and at least one phonic tic.

- Tics are sudden, brief, repetitive, stereotyped motor movements (motor tics) or sounds (phonic tics) produced by moving air through the nose, mouth, or throat.
- Patients can suppress their tics, but this often causes inner tension that eventually results in more forceful tics.
- System(s) affected: nervous

EPIDEMIOLOGY
Incidence
- Average age of onset: 7 years with greatest tic severity between 10 and 12 years (1)
- Male > female (3:1); heterogeneous disorder, but non-Hispanic whites (2:1) compared with Hispanics and/or blacks

Prevalence
0.77% overall in children (1.06% in boys, 0.25% in girls)

ETIOLOGY AND PATHOPHYSIOLOGY
Abnormalities of dopamine neurotransmission and receptor hypersensitivity, most likely in the ventral striatum, play a primary role in the pathophysiology; may involve dysfunction of basal ganglia–thalamocortical circuits, likely involving decreased inhibitory output from the basal ganglia, which results in an imbalance of inhibition and excitation in the motor cortex

- Thought to result from a complex interaction between social, environmental, and multiple genetic abnormalities
- Controversial pediatric autoimmune neuropsychiatric disorder associated with streptococcal infection (PANDAS); TS/OCD cases linked to immunologic response to previous group A β-hemolytic *Streptococcus* (GABHS)

Genetics
- Predisposition: frequent familial history of tic disorders and OCD
- Recent studies suggest polygenic inheritance with evidence for a locus on chromosome 17q; sequence variants in *SLITRK1* gene on chromosome 13q also are associated with TS.

RISK FACTORS
- Risk of TS among relatives: 9.8–15%
- Low birth weight, maternal stress, nausea/vomiting in 1st trimester, maternal smoking (2)

COMMONLY ASSOCIATED CONDITIONS
- OCD (28–67%), ADHD (50–60%), conduct disorder, learning disabilities (23%)
- Depression/anxiety including phobias, panic attacks, and stuttering; increased risk of contemplating suicide (1)
- Impairments of visual perception, sleep disorders, restless leg syndrome, and migraine headaches
- Cardiometabolic disorders, especially obesity, circulatory system diseases, type 2 diabetes (50%) (3)

DIAGNOSIS

HISTORY
Diagnosis of TS is based on history and clinical presentation (i.e., observation of tics with/without presence of coexisting disorders). Identify comorbid conditions.

PHYSICAL EXAM
- Typically, the physical exam is normal.
- Motor and vocal tics are the clinical hallmarks.
  - Tics fluctuate in type, frequency, and anatomic distribution over time.
  - Multiple motor tics include facial grimacing, blinking, head/neck jerking, tongue protruding, sniffing, touching, and burping.
  - Vocal tics include grunts, snorts, throat clearing, barking, yelling, hiccupping, sucking, and coughing.
  - Tics are exacerbated by anticipation, emotional upset, anxiety, or fatigue.
  - Tics subside when patient is concentrating/absorbed in activities but may persist during sleep.
- *Diagnostic and Statistical Manual of Mental Disorders*, 5th edition (*DSM-5*) criteria:
  - Both multiple motor and one or more vocal tics have been present at some time, although not necessarily concurrently.
  - Tics may wax and wane in frequency but have persisted for >1 year since onset.
  - Onset before age 18 years
  - Not attributable to the physiologic effects of a substance (e.g., cocaine) or another medical condition (e.g., Huntington disease, postviral encephalitis)

DIFFERENTIAL DIAGNOSIS
- Chorea/Huntington disease
- Myoclonus
- Seizure
- Ischemic or hemorrhagic stroke
- Essential tremor
- Posttraumatic/head injury
- Headache
- Dementia
- Wilson disease
- Sydenham chorea
- Multiple sclerosis
- Postviral encephalitis
- Toxin exposure (e.g., carbon monoxide, cocaine)
- Drug effects (e.g., dopamine agonists, fluoroquinolones)

DIAGNOSTIC TESTS & INTERPRETATION
Initial Tests (lab, imaging)
- No definitive lab tests diagnose TS; based on clinical features
- Measure thyroid-stimulating hormone (TSH) due to association of tics with hyperthyroidism.
- EEG shows nonspecific abnormalities; useful only to differentiate tics from epilepsy

Test Interpretation
Smaller caudate volumes and increased striatal dopaminergic terminals

TREATMENT

GENERAL MEASURES
- The goal of treatment should be to improve social functioning, self-esteem, and quality of life. Patients should play an active role in treatment decisions and be educated that tics are not voluntary or psychiatric.
- Watchful waiting is an acceptable approach to treatment in patients without functional impairments (1)[A].
- Valid, reliable, responsive tic severity scales for treatment assessment (4): Yale Global Tic Severity Scale (most extensively used and validated (1)); Shapiro Tourette Syndrome Severity Scale; Tourette's Disorder Scale
- Educate patient, family, teachers, and friends to identify and address psychosocial stressors and environmental triggers.
- No cure for tics: Treatment is purely symptomatic, and multimodal treatment usually is indicated.
- TS clusters with several comorbid conditions; each disorder must be evaluated for associated functional impairment because patients often are more disabled by their psychiatric conditions than by the tics; choice of initial treatment depends largely on worst symptoms (tics, obsessions, or impulsivity).
- Comprehensive Behavioral Intervention for Tics (CBIT) should be offered as an initial treatment before medications (1)[B].
  - Includes habit reversal training, relaxation training, and function intervention
  - Reduced tic severity with CBIT compared to psychoeducation and supportive therapy
- When pharmacotherapy is employed, monotherapy is preferred to polytherapy. Additionally, physicians should routinely reevaluate the necessity of pharmacotherapy (1)[A].

MEDICATION
First Line
- Recommendations should be individualized based on shared decision making after considering benefits and harms along with treating comorbid conditions (1).
- Most of the data points to antipsychotics being most effective, but use is limited by side effects and other medications (i.e., α_2-agonists) are generally used first (5).
- Antipsychotics (5)
  - Haloperidol, risperidone, aripiprazole, and tiapride are probably more likely than placebo to reduce tic severity (1).
  - Pimozide and ziprasidone are possibly more likely than placebo to reduce tic severity (1).
  - Prescribe the lowest effective dose to decrease the risk of side effects (1)[A].

- Atypical (risk of weight gain an other metabolic disturbances, EPS)
  - Risperidone: Initiate 0.25 mg BID; titrate up to 4 mg/day.
  - Olanzapine: Initiate 2.5 to 5.0 mg/day; titrate up to 20 mg/day.
  - Quetiapine: Initiate 12.5 to 25.0 mg/day; titrate to 300 to 400 mg/day.
  - Ziprasidone: Initiate 5 to 10 mg/day; titrate up to 10 to 40 mg/day.
    - Must be given under ECG monitoring (1)[A]
  - Aripiprazole: Initiate 2 mg/day; titrate up to 10 to 20 mg/day.
- Typical (high risk for EPS)
  - Haloperidol: Initiate 0.5 mg/day; titrate up to 2 to 10 mg QHS.
    - FDA approved for treating tics but considered last option of typical antipsychotics due to lower efficacy and increased side effects
  - Pimozide: Initiate 0.05 mg/kg/dose; titrate up to 0.2 mg/kg/day QHS with a maximum of 10 mg/day.
    - FDA approved for treating tics; good for long-term control of tics, not exacerbations
    - Risk of cardiac toxicity (prolonged QTc) so give under ECG monitoring
  - Fluphenazine: Initiate 0.5 to 1.0 mg/day; titrate up to 3 mg/day in kids and 10 mg/day in adults.
- α_2-Adrenergic receptor agonists (6)[B]
  - Historically first line due to favorable side effects but suboptimal efficacy in limited clinical trials
  - Good choice in patients with comorbid ADHD due to efficacy in treating both conditions (1)
  - Side effects: bradycardia, sedation, and hypotension; monitor heart rate and blood pressure (1)[A]
  - Clonidine 0.1 to 0.3 mg/day given BID–TID; maximum dose of 0.5 mg/day
  - Guanfacine 1 to 3 mg/day given daily or BID
    - Less sedating and longer duration of action compared with clonidine
    - Monitor QTc interval in patients with a history of cardiac conditions, patients taking QT-prolonging drugs, or patients with family history of long QT syndrome (1)[A].
- Alternative treatments
  - Topiramate: 25 to 200 mg/day (6)[A]
  - Tetrabenazine
  - Baclofen: initiate 10 mg/day; titrate up to 10 to 80 mg/day (5).
  - Preliminary data for deutetrabenazine and valbenazine (vesicular monoamine transporter-2 [VMAT2] inhibitors) and ecopipam (novel D1 receptor antagonist) (5)
- Comorbid ADHD:
  - Stimulants: methylphenidate: 2.5 to 30.0 mg/day; dextroamphetamine: 5 to 30 mg/day
  - α_2-Adrenergic agonists: guanfacine, clonidine
  - Other medications: atomoxetine, desipramine

- Comorbid OCD (7)[B]:
  - SSRIs: fluoxetine: 10 to 80 mg/day, fluvoxamine: 50 to 300 mg/day, or sertraline: 50 to 200 mg/day
    - First-line treatment of OCD; can be used in TS as well
    - Side effects: nausea, insomnia, sexual dysfunction, headache, agitation, suicidality
    - SSRIs are not as effective in treating OCD symptoms in children with tics compared to those without tics; however, cognitive behavioral therapy was effective in both populations making this intervention first line for OCD in patients with tic disorders (1).
  - Tricyclic antidepressants: clomipramine: 25 to 200 mg/day
    - Can be used in patients refractory to SSRIs or to augment SSRIs in partial responders
    - Side effects: weight gain, dry mouth, lowered seizure threshold, and constipation; ECG changes, including QT prolongation and tachycardia

ADDITIONAL THERAPIES
- Botulinum toxin injections for localized simple motor ticks and disabling vocal tics (1)
- Habit-reversal training for tic suppression treatment: works equally for motor and vocal tics

SURGERY/OTHER PROCEDURES
Thalamic ablation and deep brain stimulation have been used experimentally and can be considered for severe, self-injurious tics (1)[C]. Patients must have failed multiple classes of medications and behavioral therapy (1)[A].

COMPLEMENTARY & ALTERNATIVE MEDICINE
- Reassurance and environmental modification
- Identification and treatment of triggers
- CBIT, hypnotherapy, biofeedback, acupuncture
- Cannabinoids: insufficient evidence to recommend; small trials show small positive effects (8).
- Physical exercise (9)

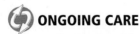 ONGOING CARE

FOLLOW-UP RECOMMENDATIONS
Patient Monitoring
Observe for associated psychiatric disorders and inquire about suicidal thoughts (1).

PATIENT EDUCATION
- Reassurance that many patients with tics do not need medication, simply education and/or therapy
- National Tourette Syndrome Association: https://www.tsa-usa.org

PROGNOSIS
- Symptoms will fluctuate throughout illness.
- Tic severity typically stabilizes by age 25 years.
- 60–75% of young adults show some improvement in symptoms; 10–40% of patients will exhibit full remission.

REFERENCES
1. Pringsheim T, Okun MS, Müller-Vahl K, et al. Practice guideline recommendations summary: treatment of tics in people with Tourette syndrome and chronic tic disorders. *Neurology*. 2019;92(19):896–906.
2. Ayubi E, Mansori K, Doosti-Irani A. Effect of maternal smoking during pregnancy on Tourette syndrome and chronic tic disorders among offspring: a systematic review and meta-analysis. *Obstet Gynecol Sci*. 2021;64(1):1–12.
3. Brander G, Isomura K, Chang Z, et al. Association of Tourette syndrome and chronic tic disorder with metabolic and cardiovascular disorders. *JAMA Neurol*. 2019;76(4):454–461.
4. Martino D, Pringsheim TM, Cavanna AE, et al; Members of the MDS Committee on Rating Scales Development. Systematic review of severity scales and screening instruments for tics: critique and recommendations. *Mov Disord*. 2017;32(3):467–473.
5. Quezada J, Coffman KA. Current approaches and new developments in the pharmacological management of Tourette syndrome. *CNS Drugs*. 2018;32(1):33–45.
6. Huys D, Hardenacke K, Poppe P, et al. Update on the role of antipsychotics in the treatment of Tourette syndrome. *Neuropsychiatr Dis Treat*. 2012;8:95–104.
7. Pringsheim T, Steeves T. Pharmacological treatment for attention deficit hyperactivity disorder (ADHD) in children with comorbid tic disorders. *Cochrane Database Syst Rev*. 2011;(4):CD007990.
8. Curtis A, Clarke CE, Rickards HE. Cannabinoids for Tourette's syndrome. *Cochrane Database Syst Rev*. 2009;2009(4):CD006565.
9. Reilly C, Grant M, Bennett S, et al. Review: physical exercise in Tourette syndrome—a systematic review. *Child Adolesc Ment Health*. 2019;24(1):3–11.

T

 CODES

ICD10
F95.2 Tourette's disorder

CLINICAL PEARLS
- TS is diagnosed by history and witnessing tics; have parent video patient's tics if not present on exam.
- Many patients require no treatment; patient should play an active role in treatment decisions.
- Nearly 50% of children with tics also have ADHD. Stimulants may be used as first-line treatment for ADHD (tics are not a contraindication, as previously believed).

TOXOPLASMOSIS
Jonathan Edward MacClements, MD, FAAFP

BASICS

- *Toxoplasma gondii* is an obligate intracellular protozoan parasite.
- Most common latent protozoan infection
- Clinically significant disease typically manifests only in pregnancy or in an immunocompromised patient.

DESCRIPTION
- Acute self-limited infection in immunocompetent individuals
- Acute symptomatic or reactivated latent infection in immunocompromised patients
- Congenital toxoplasmosis (acute primary infection during pregnancy)
- Ocular toxoplasmosis

Pediatric Considerations
- The earlier a fetal infection occurs, the more severe the resulting disease.
- Risk of perinatal death is 5% if infected in 1st trimester.

Pregnancy Considerations
- Pregnant immunocompromised and HIV-infected women should undergo serologic testing.
- Counsel pregnant women regarding risks of toxoplasmosis.
- Serologic testing during pregnancy is controversial.

EPIDEMIOLOGY

Incidence
- Prevalence of congenital toxoplasmosis in the United States: 10 to 100/100,000 live births
- Predominant sex: male > female

Prevalence
- Present in every country with prevalence differing worldwide. Seropositivity rates range from <10% to >90% (1)[A] with overall seroprevalence declining (2).
- In the United States, 11% of individuals aged 6 to 49 years are seropositive.
- Age-adjusted prevalence in the United States is 10%.
- Seroprevalence among women in the United States is 9%.
- Increasing prevalence of IgG seropositivity with age as a result of cumulative seropositivity
- Toxoplasmosis is considered a neglected parasitic infections in the United States and has been targeted by CDC for public health action.

ETIOLOGY AND PATHOPHYSIOLOGY
- *T. gondii* has two life cycles. The sexual portion of the life cycle is exclusive to felines. The asexual cycle occurs in humans. Cats become infected by eating contaminated meat (birds, mice). Oocysts form within the tract of the cat and are shed in the stool.
- Transmission to humans
  - Ingestion of raw or undercooked meat, food, or water containing tissue cysts or oocytes that is usually from soil contaminated with feline feces
  - Transplacental passage from infected mother to fetus; risk of transmission is 30% on average.
  - Blood product transfusion or solid-organ transplantation
  - Ingested *T. gondii* oocysts enter host's gastrointestinal tract where bradyzoites/tachyzoites are released, penetrate contiguous cells, replicate, and are transported to susceptible tissues causing clinical disease.

Genetics
Human leukocyte antigen (HLA) DQ3 is a genetic marker for susceptibility in HIV/AIDS patients.

RISK FACTORS
- Immunocompromised states, including HIV infection with CD4 cell count <100/μL
- Primary infection during pregnancy; risk of fetal transmission increases with gestational age at seroconversion. Transmission in the 1st trimester is associated with more severe consequences.
- Chronically infected immunocompromised pregnant women are at increased risk for transmitting congenital toxoplasmosis.

GENERAL PREVENTION
- Avoid eating undercooked meat: Cook to 152°F (66°C) or freeze for 24 hours at ≤ −12°C.
- Avoid drinking unfiltered water.
- Wash produce thoroughly.
- Wear gloves and wash hands after gardening and handling soil.
- Wear gloves and wash hands after handling raw meat or cat litter.
- Avoid shellfish (*Toxoplasma* cysts).

COMMONLY ASSOCIATED CONDITIONS
- Chorioretinitis; self-limiting, febrile lymphadenopathy; mononucleosis-like illness
- Potential association with schizophrenia

DIAGNOSIS

HISTORY
- Congenital toxoplasmosis
  - Clinical presentation varies widely; 80% of patients are asymptomatic at birth.
  - Classic triad (*uncommon*): chorioretinitis, hydrocephalus, cerebral calcifications
  - Manifestations may include prematurity, intrauterine growth retardation (IUGR).
  - Jaundice, rash with a mononucleosis-like illness
  - Mental retardation, seizures, visual defects, spasticity, sensorineural hearing loss
- Ocular toxoplasmosis
  - Chorioretinitis: focal necrotizing retinitis
  - Yellowish-white elevated cotton patch
  - Congenital disease usually bilateral; acquired is more often unilateral.
  - Symptoms include blurred vision, scotoma, pain, and photophobia.
- Acute toxoplasmosis (immunocompetent host)
  - ~90% of patients are asymptomatic.
  - Most common manifestation is bilateral, symmetric, nontender cervical lymphadenopathy.
  - Constitutional symptoms such as fever, chills, and sweats are usually mild.
  - Headaches, myalgias, pharyngitis, hepatosplenomegaly, and diffuse nonpruritic maculopapular rash may occur.
  - Pregnant women are often asymptomatic.
  - CNS: encephalitis
  - Headache; focal neurologic deficits and seizures
  - Fever usually present
  - Extracerebral toxoplasmosis: pneumonitis, chorioretinitis; rarely, GI system, liver, musculoskeletal system, heart, bone marrow, bladder, and orchitis

PHYSICAL EXAM
- In adults: fever, lymphadenopathy, nonpruritic maculopapular rash (spares palms and soles); hepatosplenomegaly; visual changes; funduscopic changes
- In newborns: hydrocephalus, neurologic abnormalities, hepatosplenomegaly, chorioretinitis, microcephaly, mental retardation

DIFFERENTIAL DIAGNOSIS
Syphilis, lymphoma, progressive multifocal leukoencephalopathy, cryptococcal meningitis, congenital TORCH infections, HIV; *Listeria* infection, tuberculosis (TB), tularemia; CMV infection; leukemia; erythroblastosis fetalis

DIAGNOSTIC TESTS & INTERPRETATION
- CBC: atypical lymphocytosis, anemia, thrombocytopenia
- Serology interpretation
  - IgM antibodies appear in the 1st week if acute infection.
  - Initial test demonstrates positive IgM and negative IgG, with both tests being positive 2 weeks later.
  - If follow-up IgG is negative 2 to 4 weeks later and IgM is positive, this is likely a false positive.
  - Negative IgG rules out prior infection (IgG persists for life).
- Types of serologic tests
  - ELISA: most commonly used
  - Sabin-Feldman dye test: Gold standard against which all other serologic assays are compared.
  - IFA test: more available in commercial labs
  - ISAGA: widely available commercially; more sensitive and specific than IFA for detecting IgM
  - Avidity testing: confirmatory test to establish if positive IgM/IgG reflects recent or chronic infection
- PCR: *T. gondii* DNA amplification in blood or amniotic fluid; used for diagnosis of fetal infection
- Culture (rarely necessary): Organism can be isolated either by cell culture or by mouse inoculation.

Initial Tests (lab, imaging)
- Diagnosis of primary infection is typically based on history and confirmed by serology.
- Serum *Toxoplasma*-specific IgG and IgM are first step.
- According to IgM result, determine IgG avidity.
- Diagnosis of maternal infection and congenital toxoplasmosis
  - Test pregnant women who have mononucleosis-like illness but negative heterophile test for toxoplasmosis.
  - Diagnose maternal infection based on two blood samples at least 2 weeks to show seroconversion.
  - High avidity of IgG during 1st trimester argues against maternal primary infection.
  - Real-time PCR analysis of amniotic fluid predicts fetal infection and guides treatment.
  - Fetal ultrasound is useful for prognosis.
  - Routine screening for toxoplasmosis is not recommended in pregnancy.
- Neonatal diagnosis of congenital toxoplasmosis
  - Serology requires repeat testing for IgM and IgA.
  - Sample cord or peripheral blood within 2 weeks
  - Ophthalmologic, auditory, and neurologic examinations; lumbar puncture and head CT
- Diagnosis of toxoplasmic encephalitis
  - Serology for IgG
  - Imaging: MRI is more sensitive than CT scan to identify characteristic ring-enhancing lesions.
- SPECT and PET scans can help distinguish toxoplasmosis from CNS lymphoma.

Diagnostic Procedures/Other
- Lymph node biopsy
- Brain biopsy in CNS disease
- Amniocentesis with PCR (risk of false negatives and false positives)
- Placental isolation of *Toxoplasma* is diagnostic.

Test Interpretation
- Confirmatory, meningocerebritis ± abscesses with necrosis, Giemsa
- Lymph node histology shows triad of:
  – Reactive follicular hyperplasia
  – Irregular clusters of epithelioid histiocytes blurring margins of germinal centers
  – Distension of sinuses with monocytoid cells
- Sensitivity of triad 63%, specificity 91%

 TREATMENT

GENERAL MEASURES
Immunocompetent patients usually require no treatment.

MEDICATION
Recommended treatment drugs for toxoplasmosis target the tachyzoite stage of the parasite and do not eradicate encysted parasites in the tissues

First Line

> **ALERT**
> *Important*: All pyrimethamine-containing regimens should include leucovorin (folinic acid 10 to 25 mg/day PO) during and 1 week after completion of pyrimethamine to prevent drug-induced hematologic toxicity (3)[A].

- Treatment in immunocompromised hosts
  – Initial regimen of choice is pyrimethamine 200 mg loading dose PO, followed by 50 mg/day plus sulfadiazine 4 to 6 g/day PO in 4 divided doses; for those intolerant or allergic to sulfadiazine, clindamycin 600 to 1,200 mg IV or 450 mg PO QID can be used instead.
  – Alternative regimens for patients intolerant to sulfadiazine and clindamycin include the following:
    ○ Pyrimethamine: 200 mg loading dose PO, followed by 50 mg/day plus azithromycin 900 to 1,200 mg PO once daily
    ○ Pyrimethamine: 200 mg loading dose PO and then 50 mg/day plus atovaquone 1,500 mg PO BID
    ○ Sulfadiazine: 1,000 to 1,500 mg QID plus atovaquone 1,500 mg BID
    ○ Trimethoprim-sulfamethoxazole: 10/50 mg/kg/day PO or IV divided BID (for 30 days) may be a cost-effective alternative.
  – Duration of therapy: typically 6 weeks, lower doses for secondary prophylaxis (3)[A]
  – Use adjunctive steroids in patients with signs of increased intracranial pressure.
  – Anticonvulsants, if there is a history of seizures
- Prophylaxis in immunocompromised patients
  – Primary prophylaxis: indicated for patients with HIV infection and CD4 count <100 cells/μL who are *T. gondii* IgG–positive
    ○ Trimethoprim-sulfamethoxazole-DS: 1 tablet PO daily. Alternative for sulfa allergy is dapsone 50 mg/day PO *plus* pyrimethamine 50 mg PO weekly *plus* leucovorin 25 mg PO weekly *or* atovaquone 1,500 mg PO daily.

– Secondary prophylaxis: Following 6 weeks of therapy, administer lower doses of drugs:
  ○ Sulfadiazine 2 to 4 g/day in 2 to 4 divided doses *plus* pyrimethamine 25 to 50 mg/day is the first choice.
  ○ Alternative regimens include clindamycin 600 mg PO q8h *plus* pyrimethamine 25 to 50 mg/day PO *or* atovaquone 750 mg PO BID to QID ± pyrimethamine 25 mg PO daily.
- Pregnant women
  – Although typically offered, it is unsure if antenatal treatment reduces congenital transmission.
  – <18 weeks' gestation: spiramycin 1 g PO q8h without food until delivery if amniotic fluid PCR is negative; does not treat infection in the fetus
  – >18 weeks' gestation: Pyrimethamine and sulfadiazine should be considered only if fetal infection is documented by positive amniotic fluid PCR (pyrimethamine is teratogenic):
    ○ Pyrimethamine: 50 mg PO q12h for 2 days, then 50 mg/day plus sulfadiazine 75 mg/kg PO × 1 dose, and then 50 mg/kg q12h (max 4 g/day)
- Treat infected newborns regardless of clinical manifestations:
  – Pyrimethamine 2 mg/kg/day (max 50 mg) for 2 days, then 1 mg/kg/day (max 25 mg) for 2 to 6 month, and then 1 mg/kg (max 25 mg) on Monday, Wednesday, and Friday; sulfadiazine 100 mg/kg/day divided BID; and leucovorin 10 mg 3 times per week during pyrimethamine and 1 week after discontinuation
- Immunocompetent nonpregnant patients generally do not require treatment unless symptoms are severe or prolonged; one of two regimens can be used:
  – Pyrimethamine: 100-mg loading dose PO, followed by 25 to 50 mg/day *plus* sulfadiazine 2 to 4 g/day in 4 divided doses
  – Pyrimethamine: 100-mg loading dose PO, followed by 25 to 50 mg/day *plus* clindamycin 300 mg PO QID

Second Line
- Clindamycin: 900 to 1,200 mg TID IV used for ocular and CNS toxoplasmosis alone and in combination with pyrimethamine; as effective as the sulfadiazine-pyrimethamine with fewer adverse effects
- Corticosteroids (prednisone 1 to 2 mg/kg/day) are added for macular chorioretinitis or CNS infection.
- Alternatives: atovaquone (Mepron), azithromycin (Zithromax), clarithromycin (Biaxin), or dapsone *plus* pyrimethamine and leucovorin
- Trimethoprim-sulfamethoxazole appears to be equivalent to pyrimethamine-sulfadiazine in AIDS patients with CNS disease.

ADDITIONAL THERAPIES
For prevention of recurrent episode of chorioretinitis, trimethoprim-sulfamethoxazole-DS q12h for 45 days

 ONGOING CARE

FOLLOW-UP RECOMMENDATIONS
Patient Monitoring
Precautions
- Monitor for bone marrow, renal, or liver toxicity.
- Good hydration: Sulfadiazine is poorly soluble and may crystallize in the urine.

- Watch for antibiotic-associated diarrhea.
- Sulfonamides may alter phenytoin and warfarin levels or interfere with oral hypoglycemic agents.

PATIENT EDUCATION
- https://www.aafp.org/pubs/afp/issues/2003/0515/p2145.html
- https://familydoctor.org/condition/toxoplasmosis/

PROGNOSIS
- Immunodeficient patients often relapse if treatment or suppression therapy is stopped.
- Treatment may prevent the development of untoward sequelae in infants with congenital toxoplasmosis.

REFERENCES
1. Dubey JP. Outbreaks of clinical toxoplasmosis in humans: five decades of personal experience, perspectives and lessons learned. *Parasit Vectors*. 2021;14(1):263.
2. Jones JL, Kruszon-Moran D, Elder S, et al. *Toxoplasma gondii* infection in the United States, 2011–2014. *Am J Trop Med Hyg*. 2018;98(2):551–557.
3. Dunay IR, Gajurel K, Dhakal R, et al. Treatment of toxoplasmosis: historical perspective, animal models, and current clinical practice. *Clin Microbiol Rev*. 2018;31(4):e00057-17.

ADDITIONAL READING
- Maldonado YA, Read JS; and AAP Committee on Infectious Diseases. Diagnosis, Treatment, and Prevention of Congenital Toxoplasmosis in the United States. *Pediatrics*. 2017;139(2):e20163860.
- Parasites—toxoplasmosis (toxoplasma infection). https://www.cdc.gov/parasites/toxoplasmosis/health_professionals/index.html. Accessed June 26, 2023.

 CODES

ICD10
- B58.9 Toxoplasmosis, unspecified
- P37.1 Congenital toxoplasmosis
- B58.2 Toxoplasma meningoencephalitis

CLINICAL PEARLS
- Toxoplasmosis is typically asymptomatic in immunocompetent patients.
- Primary prevention is important, particularly for pregnant women and immunodeficient patients.
- The most common manifestation of acute toxoplasmosis in immunocompetent host is bilateral, symmetric, nontender cervical lymphadenopathy.
- Universal screening for congenital toxoplasmosis is not currently recommended.
- Serologic testing should be performed at a reference laboratory. CDC recommends the reference laboratory at Palo Alto Medical Foundation Toxoplasma Serology Laboratory (https://www.sutterhealth.org/pamf/services/lab-pathology/toxoplasma-serology-laboratory).

T

TRACHEITIS, BACTERIAL

Stephanie Mayle Scott, DO • Justin Atwood, MD

 BASICS

DESCRIPTION
- Acute, life-threatening upper airway obstruction due to infraglottic bacterial infection following a primary viral infection (typically parainfluenza or influenza)
- Historically high mortality rates of up to 20% in children; more recent experience suggests changing epidemiology resulting in a more atypical presentation and variable course (1) but which can still result in severe, acute, upper airway obstruction.
- Affects two major groups of patients in the pediatric age range:
  – Those with a native intact airway
  – Those with an artificial airway
- Often preceded by viral infection, such as influenza, parainfluenza, or respiratory syncytial virus
- *Staphylococcus aureus* is the most common bacteria identified (1).
- Diagnostic hallmarks on endoscopy: ulceration, pseudomembranes in the trachea with thick mucopurulent exudates and mucosal sloughing (1)
- System(s) affected: pulmonary
- Synonym(s): laryngotracheobronchitis; bacterial croup; pseudomembranous croup

EPIDEMIOLOGY
Incidence
- Incidence: 4 to 8 per 1 million children
- Peak incidence in children: fall and winter
- Mean age: 5 years (2)
- Infections in adolescents and adults have been reported.

Prevalence
Methicillin-resistant *Staphylococcus aureus* (MRSA) may contribute to changing epidemiology and virulence.

ETIOLOGY AND PATHOPHYSIOLOGY
- Methicillin-sensitive *S. aureus* (MSSA) accounted for 50% cases in Casazza series (2019) (1).
- Mixed respiratory
- *Streptococcus pneumoniae*
- In children with artificial airway, most common organisms are *S. aureus, Haemophilus influenzae, S. pneumoniae, Pseudomonas aeruginosa*, and other gram-negative organisms.
- Viral-induced injury to the respiratory epithelium in conjunction with localized immune impairment can predispose individuals to bacterial superinfection.

Genetics
No known genetic predisposition

RISK FACTORS
- Periods of increased seasonal activity of respiratory viruses
- Reports following tonsillectomy, adenoidectomy, with chronic tracheal aspiration, and with evidence of other concurrent infections, including sinusitis, otitis, pneumonia, or pharyngitis

GENERAL PREVENTION
- Standard precautions, with scrupulous attention to handwashing
- Vaccination against viruses that may predispose to bacterial tracheitis

COMMONLY ASSOCIATED CONDITIONS
- Consider anatomic abnormalities and foreign bodies as well as recent pharyngeal or laryngeal surgery.
- Predisposing: Down syndrome, immunodeficiency, subglottic hemangioma, tracheoesophageal fistula repair, tracheobronchomalacia
- More common in children with tracheostomy
- Viral coinfection may occur.

Dx **DIAGNOSIS**

- Careful history and physical exam are the best methods to help distinguish bacterial tracheitis from croup and other rare causes of upper airway obstruction.
- The diagnosis of bacterial tracheitis is confirmed by flexible laryngoscopy, operative bronchoscopy, and/or autopsy. Findings include mucopurulent exudates, ulcerations, and pseudomembranes within the subglottis and/or trachea (1).

HISTORY
- Presentation can be variable from mild to severe with high fever and systemic toxicity (1).
- Classic presentation:
  – Prodromal upper respiratory tract symptoms
  – Gradual progression of mild upper airway symptoms over 1 hour to 6 days to acute, febrile phase of rapid respiratory decompensation
  – Drooling usually absent
  – No response to aerosolized epinephrine and/or systemic corticosteroids
- Individuals with artificial airways may have a more indolent case and are also more likely to experience recurrence.

PHYSICAL EXAM
- Acute onset
- High fever
- Inspiratory stridor
- Respiratory distress
- Toxic appearance
- Voice and cry usually normal
- Drooling uncommon
- Atypical presentations can also occur and some may present with URI symptoms.
- Children with artificial airways can have more indolent onset (1).

DIFFERENTIAL DIAGNOSIS
- Severe croup (viral)
- Spasmodic croup
- Diphtheria in unimmunized individuals
- Retropharyngeal abscess
- Epiglottitis
- Bronchiolitis
- Bacterial pneumonia
- Foreign body aspiration
- Angioneurotic edema

DIAGNOSTIC TESTS & INTERPRETATION
- Tracheal endoscopy (rigid bronchoscopy in children with intact airway or tracheoscopy in those with artificial airway) provides a definitive diagnosis.
- Diffuse inflammation of larynx, trachea, and bronchi
- Mucopurulent exudate; microabscesses may be present.
- Semiadherent membranes (containing numerous neutrophils and cellular debris) may be identified within the trachea.

Initial Tests (lab, imaging)
Obtain gram stain and aerobic, anaerobic, and viral cultures of tracheal secretions during the tracheal endoscopy. Bacterial cultures of tracheal secretions are required for culture isolates and sensitivities.
- Tracheal biopsy is rarely indicated but may be considered in immunodeficient child or child with ulcerative colitis.
- Routine laboratory studies are not required to make the diagnosis and are rarely helpful.
- Rapid antigen or polymerase chain reaction (PCR) based testing for respiratory viruses may be helpful.
- CBC results may vary.
  – WBC count may show marked leukocytosis or may be normal.
  – Increased band cell count
- Chest radiographs are neither definitive nor diagnostic of bacterial tracheitis but may be helpful in identifying associated pneumonia.
- Anteroposterior (AP) and lateral neck x-rays show subglottic and tracheal narrowing (i.e., steeple sign on AP film).

Follow-Up Tests & Special Considerations
- In patients with pneumonia, follow-up chest films may be required.
- Repeat bronchoscopies may be needed to remove pseudomembranes.
- Children with or at risk for acute airway obstruction should be carefully monitored in a setting and with personnel capable of securing a pediatric airway.

Diagnostic Procedures/Other
Bronchoscopy

Test Interpretation
Findings include mucopurulent exudates, ulcerations, and pseudomembranes within the subglottis and/or trachea (1).

TREATMENT

- Consider bacterial tracheitis as a potentially life-threatening airway emergency.
- Children with suspected or actual bacterial tracheitis should be cared for in a pediatric ICU (2)[C].
- Assess and monitor respiratory status; supplemental oxygen may be necessary.
- Airway protection and support, as necessary (at least 50% require intubation; some studies report up to 100% [80% require intubation; 94% admitted to PICU])
- Ventilatory support may be required.

GENERAL MEASURES
- Consider bacterial tracheitis as a potentially life-threatening airway emergency.
- Support care and monitoring in PICU care often required.
- Supplemental oxygen, endotracheal intubation, and/or mechanical ventilation may be required.

MEDICATION
- Empiric therapy should cover the most common pathogens until sensitivities are available: antistaphylococcal agent (vancomycin or clindamycin) and a 3rd-generation cephalosporin (e.g., ceftriaxone or cefotaxime).
- In the case of technology-dependent children with tracheostomy, make initial antibiotic choices based on previous tracheal culture.
- Narrow regimen when pathogens and sensitivities are available.
- Systemic or inhaled corticosteroids or racemic epinephrine have no proven efficacy in relieving airway obstruction in bacterial tracheitis.
- Contraindications: Refer to the manufacturer's literature for each drug.
- Precautions: Refer to the manufacturer's literature for each drug.
- Significant possible interactions: Refer to the manufacturer's literature for each medication.
- Complications:
  - Acute respiratory distress syndrome (1)
  - Pneumonia
  - Pneumothorax
  - Toxic shock syndrome (1)
  - Septic shock (1)
  - Disseminated intravascular coagulation (1)
  - Tracheal stenosis, especially with prolonged intubation
  - Cardiopulmonary arrest

ISSUES FOR REFERRAL
- All children with suspected or actual bacterial tracheitis should be cared for in a pediatric ICU.
- Critical care teams may include ID, ENT, and pulmonary consultants in addition to the pediatric intensivist.

SURGERY/OTHER PROCEDURES
- Therapeutic bronchoscopy may be needed to facilitate the removal of inspissated secretions and accumulated debris (2).
- Tracheostomy is usually not necessary.

COMPLEMENTARY & ALTERNATIVE MEDICINE
No evidence to support use

ADMISSION, INPATIENT, AND NURSING CONSIDERATIONS
- Diagnostic endoscopic evaluation of the upper airway
- Airway stabilization and support
- Pediatric intensive care admission

Pediatric Considerations
- Suctioning and pulmonary toilet
- Hydration
- Antibiotics as described above
- Nursing
  - Provide a calm, quiet environment for child once endoscopy and cultures are done.
  - Airway monitoring
  - Frequent suctioning
  - Monitor fluid balance.
  - Establish and maintain open lines of communication with child and parent.

 ONGOING CARE

FOLLOW-UP RECOMMENDATIONS
Patient Monitoring
Children with artificial airway will require ongoing follow-up.

DIET
Varies with clinical situations

PATIENT EDUCATION
Keep immunizations up to date.

PROGNOSIS
- Intubation generally 3 to 11 days
- Usually requires 3 to 7 days of hospitalization
- With effective early recognition and management, complete recovery can be expected.
- Cardiopulmonary arrest and death have occurred.
- Higher recurrence rates in children with artificial airways

COMPLICATIONS
Tracheal stenosis

REFERENCES

1. Casazza G, Graham ME, Nelson D, et al. Pediatric bacterial tracheitis—a variable entity: case series with literature review. *Otolaryngol Head Neck Surg*. 2019;160(3):546–549.
2. Blot M, Bonniaud-Blot P, Favrolt N, et al. Update on childhood and adult infectious tracheitis. *Med Mal Infect*. 2017;47(7):443–452.

ADDITIONAL READING

Russell CJ, Shiroishi MS, Siantz E, et al. The use of inhaled antibiotic therapy in the treatment of ventilator-associated pneumonia and tracheobronchitis: a systematic review. *BMC Pulm Med*. 2016;16:40.

 CODES

ICD10
- J04.10 Acute tracheitis without obstruction
- J04.11 Acute tracheitis with obstruction
- J05.0 Acute obstructive laryngitis [croup]

CLINICAL PEARLS
- Bacterial tracheitis is an acute, potentially life-threatening, infraglottic bacterial infection which generally follows a primary viral infection.
- Bacterial tracheitis should be suspected in croup-like cases who fail to respond to oral or inhaled corticosteroids and racemic epinephrine.
- Bronchoscopy (or tracheoscopy in the child with an artificial airway) provides a definitive diagnosis.
- Initial treatment priorities include broad-spectrum antibiotic coverage, aggressive airway protection, and supportive care.

T

TRANSGENDER HEALTH

George W. Matar, MD • Michelle Caster, MD

BASICS

DESCRIPTION

- Lesbian, gay, bisexual, and transgender individuals continue to be medically underserved and subject to unique health care disparities, including higher rates of mental and physical comorbidities and a greater need for health care services. Better education of physicians and other providers is imperative to improve the health of the transgender population. Such education begins with teaching acceptance of all human beings into health care and ensuring a welcoming and safe office environment for transgender individuals to speak openly with knowledgeable and culturally competent clinicians.
  - As of 2015, estimates indicate 0.7% of youth (age 13 to 17 years), or some 150,000 people, and 0.6% of U.S. adults, or some 1.4 million people, identify themselves as transgender, a 2-fold increase since 2011 (1).
- Gender identity, the sense of one's self as male or female, and especially gender presentation, the outward expression of gender, may or may not reflect the self-identification of a transgender and gender nonbinary (TGNB) patient. Transgender status says nothing about an individual's sexual orientation. Transgender people may be sexually oriented toward men, women, other transgender people, or any combination of the above. TGNB patients are further defined by those who have undergone surgical procedures and/or medical treatment to better align gender identity, by those who plan such procedures in the future, and by others who do not.
- Ask transgender patients how they would describe themselves and to honor terminology acceptable to each patient, specifically preferred name, preferred pronoun, preferred gender identity, and sex assigned at birth; those attributes then entered in the electronic medical record (2).
- Transgender people have a unique set of mental and physical needs (3),(4).
  - Stigma and discrimination are barriers to health care.
  - 24% of transgender persons report unequal treatment in health care environments, 19% report refusal of care altogether, 33% do not seek preventive services, and 23% delay needed care (4).
  - 91% of transgender patients want counseling and/or hormones even though only 65% ever get any of these (2).
- Many U.S. insurance companies require a diagnosis of gender dysphoria (defined as distress and unease experienced if gender identity and designated gender are not completely congruent) for reimbursement of medical and surgical interventions (5). Despite the fact that being transgender is not a behavioral health condition, codes for a transgender diagnosis are in the mental health section in the *International Classification of Diseases, 10th revision (ICD-10)*.

DIAGNOSIS

- Specific health concerns
  - Transition-related medical care, or gender-affirming therapy, including hormone therapy and surgical treatment, or gender-affirming surgery (GAS), helps patients align primary and secondary sexual characteristics with gender identity (3).
  - The World Professional Association for Transgender Health (WPATH) has published standards of care (SOCs) that include hormone therapy and GAS (3),(4),(6).
    - Hormone therapy and surgery not only treat symptoms of gender dysphoria but also help transgender patients improve quality of life, self-esteem, and anxiety (4).
    - Hormone therapy does increase risk of thromboembolic disease (venous thromboembolism [VTE]), erythrocytosis, hypertriglyceridemia, elevated liver enzymes, development of gallstones, cardiovascular (CV) disease, metabolic disease, and decreased fertility (3),(4).
    - Treatment is associated with high patient satisfaction, low prevalence of regrets, and relief of dysphoria.
- Specific diseases
  - HIV/AIDS: Among those respondents to the Transgender Discrimination Survey, 1.4% were living with HIV, which is 5 times higher than those of the general population in the United States. Worldwide, the prevalence may be 50 times higher than the background rate (1),(3).
- Psychosocial considerations
  - Transgender people are at risk of intimate partner violence and of mental health issues, including depression, anxiety, and risk of suicide.
    - 40% of transgender people have attempted suicide compared to 1.6% of the U.S. general population (3).
    - Transgender people are at greater risk of housing and workforce discrimination and are more likely to be unemployed, homeless, be victims of truancy and bullying, and lacking in social support owing to federal and state laws that inadequately protect transgender people from discrimination (3),(4).
  - Psychosocial assessment is recommended at baseline and at least annually (4).
  - Mental health and substance abuse screenings are also indicated (4).

ALERT

- Transgender patients are at increased risk of suicidal ideation, suicide attempts, and suicide (3),(4).
- Transgender patients are often reluctant to disclose gender identity or expression, owing to the risk of stigma or discrimination.
- Improving access to care
  - Barriers to health care and the need for respectful, supportive, and inclusive clinic environments by following transgender-friendly concepts
  - Financial barriers
    - According to the 2015 U.S. Transgender Survey, 29% of respondents were currently living in poverty, compared with 14% of the general U.S. population. More than half (55%) of transgender participants who completed the survey had been denied coverage for transition-related surgery, and 25% were denied coverage for hormone therapy.

HISTORY

- When assessing transgender patients for gender-affirming care, evaluate the magnitude, duration, and stability of any gender dysphoria or incongruence (3),(4).
- Evaluation of the support and safety of patients' social environment is accomplished with multidisciplinary care (3),(4).

PHYSICAL EXAM

Transgender patients may experience discomfort during the physical examination because of ongoing dysphoria or negative past experiences (4). Examinations should be based on the patient's current anatomy and specific needs for the visit and should be explained, chaperoned, and stopped as indicated by the patient's comfort level.

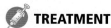

TREATMENT

GENERAL MEASURES

- Care of transgender people, including hormone therapy, is well within the scope of primary care providers.
- Education of health care providers, for physicians, and those beginning in medical school is crucial in providing optimal care to transgender patients (1).

MEDICATION

First Line

- Gender-affirming hormone therapy (Specific information on gender-affirming hormone therapy can be found in the Endocrine Society's clinical practice guidelines.) (7)
- Indications for hormone therapy (6)
  - Criteria for GAS per the WPATH include persistent, well-documented gender dysphoria; capacity to make a fully informed decision and to consent for treatment; legal age of majority in the given country; and if significant medical or mental health concerns are present, they must be well controlled.
- Hormonal therapy for transgender adolescents (7)
  - Suppress pubertal development using reversible puberty blockers, such as gonadotropin-releasing hormone (GnRH) analogues, when adolescents first exhibit pubertal physical changes (Tanner stage 2).
  - Gender-affirming hormones at about age 16 years or with adolescents presenting for gender-affirming hormone therapy after initiation of puberty
  - Initiate treatment after persistent gender dysphoria has been confirmed by a multidisciplinary team of medical and mental health providers and when the patient has the mental capacity to provide informed consent, generally by age 16 years.

- Hormonal therapy for transgender adults
  - The two major goals of hormonal therapy are to reduce endogenous sex hormone levels, and thus reduce the secondary sex characteristics of the individual's designated gender, and to replace endogenous sex hormone levels consistent with the individual's gender identity by using the principles of hormone replacement treatment of hypogonadal patients.
  - Feminizing therapy
    ○ Treatment with physiologic doses of estrogen alone is insufficient to suppress testosterone levels into the normal range for females. Androgen blockers, such as spironolactone, are often used in addition to estradiol to achieve feminizing effects.
    ○ Results in redistribution of body fat, decrease in muscle mass and strength, softening of skin/decreased oiliness, decreased sexual desire, decreased spontaneous erections, male sexual dysfunction, breast growth, decreased testicular volume, decreased sperm production, and possible scalp hair
  - Masculinizing therapy
    ○ Regimens similar to the general principle of hormone replacement treatment with testosterone in male hypogonadism; results in skin oiliness/acne, facial/body hair growth, scalp hair loss, increased muscle mass/strength, fat redistribution, cessation of menses, clitoral enlargement, vaginal atrophy, deepening of voice

SURGERY/OTHER PROCEDURES

- There are multiple surgical procedures available for gender affirmation depending on an individual's goals. Per WPATH, surgeons are recommended to work with a multidisciplinary team of medical and mental health professionals to ensure that patients are eligible (6).
  - Eligible patients meeting criteria require a single opinion for the initiation of this treatment from a professional who has the appropriate competencies (6).
  - At least 6 months of continuous hormone therapy are recommended for some procedures (e.g., genital surgery) but not for others (e.g., chest masculinization) (6).
- The rate of GAS is increasing, with some 25% of transgender patients having undergone some form of GAS (2).
- GAS has a positive impact on individual health in that it improves mental health, results in a higher quality of life, and results in a higher socioeconomic status; also increases cultural awareness and decreases social stigma (5)

 ONGOING CARE

FOLLOW-UP RECOMMENDATIONS
Patient Monitoring
- Transmasculine individuals (3),(6)
  - Breast cancer screening with annual chest wall exam is recommended for those with breast tissue with careful review of operative reports.
  - Cervical cancer screening for those who have a cervix according to age-related guidelines

- Transfeminine individuals (3)
  - Prostate cancer screening should follow the recommendations for cisgender men.
  - Breast cancer screening should begin after 50 years of age and after a minimum of 5 years of feminizing hormone use, with a health care professional–patient discussion about the potential harms of over screening.
- Routine laboratory testing and physical exam should be completed per hormone use as indicated by the Endocrine Society's clinical practice guidelines (7).
- Screening for HIV and STIs based on patient's behaviors and present anatomy; pre- and postexposure HIV prophylaxis should be considered for patients who meet criteria.
- Consider anal cancer screening with anal Pap smear for those people who have anal sex. If performed, abnormal results must be followed with high-resolution anoscopy, which is not available in all settings.
- Evaluation of CV risk factors
- Bone mineral density tests, as indicated
- Age-appropriate and behavior-specific immunizations (e.g., human papillomavirus)
- Screening for intimate partner violence
- Fertility, pregnancy, contraception, and abortion (3)
  - Fertility and parenting desires should be discussed early in the process of transition, before the initiation of hormone therapy or gender affirmation surgery; patients should be informed of out-of-pocket costs, which vary by state and insurance coverage.
  - Transmasculine individuals
    ○ Pregnancy may be achieved after cessation of testosterone, but return of fertility is not well studied and is of unknown reversibility (6).
    ○ Contraception can be underused in this population because of concerns of adverse effects or access to care.
  - Transfeminine individuals
    ○ If retaining gonads, may need to use assisted reproductive technologies to achieve pregnancy and others may have return of fertility within months of ceasing hormone therapy; it is best practice to encourage sperm banking.
  - Contraception
    ○ Gender-affirming hormone therapy is not an effective contraception. Transmasculine individuals should be consulted that lack of menses does not mean they are unable to conceive. In addition, testosterone use is not a specific contraindication in using any form of contraception. All patients should be counseled on barrier use for prevention of STIs.

PATIENT EDUCATION
- Hormone therapy and potential health risks
- Counseling for GAS
- Legal issues
  - Under the Affordable Care Act (ACA), denial of treatment of being transgender as a "preexisting condition" is banned.
  - Since 2014, Centers for Medicare & Medicaid Services (CMS) has been providing transition-related coverage (8).
  - The U.S. Department of Veterans Affairs (VA), although acknowledging the need to care for transgender veterans, denies coverage of gender-confirming surgery on the basis of a VA regulation that excludes gender alterations from the medical benefits package.

REFERENCES

1. Korpaisarn S, Safer JD. Gaps in transgender medical education among healthcare providers: a major barrier to care for transgender persons. *Rev Endocr Metab Disord*. 2018;19(3):271–275.
2. Nolan IT, Kuhner CJ, Dy GW. Demographic and temporal trends in transgender identities and gender confirming surgery. *Transl Androl Urol*. 2019;8(3):184–190.
3. American College of Obstetricians and Gynecologists' Committee on Gynecologic Practice and Committee on Health Care for Underserved Women. Health care for transgender and gender diverse individuals: ACOG Committee Opinion, Number 823. *Obstet Gynecol*. 2021;137(3):e75–e88.
4. Klein DA, Paradise SL, Goodwin ET. Caring for transgender and gender-diverse persons: what clinicians should know. *Am Fam Physician*. 2018;98(11):645–653.
5. Safer JD, Tangpricha V. Care of transgender persons. *N Engl J Med*. 2019;381(25):2451–2460.
6. Coleman E, Radix AE, Bouman WP, et al. Standards of care for the health of transgender and gender diverse people, version 8. *Int J Transgend Health*. 2022;23(Suppl 1):S1–S259.
7. Hembree WC, Cohen-Kettenis PT, Gooren L, et al. Endocrine treatment of gender-dysphoric/gender-incongruent persons: an Endocrine Society clinical practice guideline. *J Clin Endocrinol Metab*. 2017;102(11):3869–3903.
8. Williams EA, Patete CL, Thaller SR. Gender affirmation surgery from a public health perspective: advances, challenges, and areas of opportunity. *J Craniofac Surg*. 2019;30(5):1349–1351.

ADDITIONAL READING

Healthy People 2030: https://health.gov/healthypeople/objectives-and-data/browse-objectives/lgbt

CODES

ICD10
- F64.1 Gender identity disorder in adolescence and adulthood
- Z11.4 Encounter for screening for human immunodeficiency virus
- Z72.52 High risk homosexual behavior

CLINICAL PEARLS

- Health care providers must be sensitive to the unique needs of transgender patients; must be open to the care of such patients; and should, as with all patients, display an ethical, principled, and timely approach to care.
- Do use inclusive language in the care of transgender patients, assessing the individuals' preferences, and respect differences among transgender patients.

T

TRANSIENT ISCHEMIC ATTACK (TIA)

Haris Vakil, MD

 BASICS

DESCRIPTION
- A transient episode of neurologic dysfunction due to focal brain, retinal, or spinal cord ischemia without acute infarction
- 7.5–17.4% of patients with transient ischemic attack (TIA) experience a stroke within 3 months (1).
- Synonym(s): ministroke

EPIDEMIOLOGY
Prevalence
- Prevalence of TIA in general population: ~2%
- Risk increases >60 years of age; highest in 7th and 8th decades of life
- Predominant sex: male > female
- Predominant race/ethnicity: African Americans > Hispanics > Caucasians

ETIOLOGY AND PATHOPHYSIOLOGY
Temporary reduction/cessation of cerebral blood flow adversely affecting neuronal function
- Carotid/vertebral atherosclerotic disease (artery-to-artery thromboembolism, low-flow ischemia)
- Lacunar infarcts: small, deep vessel disease associated with hypertension (HTN) and diabetes mellitus (DM)
- Embolism secondary to the following:
  – Valvular (mitral valve) pathology
  – Mural hypokinesias/akinesias with thrombosis (acute anterior MI/congestive cardiomyopathies)
  – Cardiac arrhythmia (atrial fibrillation accounts for 5–20% incidence)
- Hypercoagulable states (antiphospholipid antibodies, increased estrogen [e.g., oral contraceptives], pregnancy and parturition)
- Arteritis (vasculitis)
- Sympathomimetic drugs (e.g., cocaine)
- Other causes: spontaneous and posttraumatic (e.g., chiropractic manipulation) arterial dissection
- Fibromuscular dysplasia

Genetics
Inheritance is polygenic, with tendency to clustering of risk factors within families.

RISK FACTORS
- Older age (i.e., >60 years old)
- HTN, cardiac diseases (atrial fibrillation, MI, valvular disease)
- Atherosclerotic disease (carotid/vertebral stenosis)
- Obesity, DM, hyperlipidemia
- Cigarette smoking
- Thrombophilias

GENERAL PREVENTION
- Control of medical risk factors: *DM, HTN, hyperlipidemia*
- Anticoagulation when high risk of cardioembolism (e.g., atrial fibrillation, mechanical valves)
- Blood pressure (BP) control, with antiplatelet therapy for preventing recurrence if previous TIA (2)

Geriatric Considerations
- Older patients have a higher mortality rate—highest in 7th and 8th decades of life.
- Atrial fibrillation is a frequent cause among the elderly.

Pediatric Considerations
- Congenital heart disease is a common cause among pediatric patients.
- Genetic: Marfan syndrome, moyamoya, or sickle cell disease

Pregnancy Considerations
- Preeclampsia, eclampsia, and HELLP syndrome
- Thrombotic thrombocytopenic purpura (TTP) and hemolytic uremic syndrome
- Postpartum angiopathy
- Cerebral venous thrombosis
- Hypercoagulable states related to pregnancy

COMMONLY ASSOCIATED CONDITIONS
- Atrial fibrillation, uncontrolled HTN
- Carotid stenosis
- Some disease processes mimic TIA presentation (seizures, migraines, metabolic disturbances, syncope, multiple sclerosis); difference: gradual onset with nonspecific symptoms (headache, memory loss) versus acute onset with specific neurologic deficits (TIA)

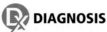 **DIAGNOSIS**

HISTORY
- Emphasis on symptom onset, progression, and recovery
- Carotid circulation (hemispheric): monocular visual loss, hemiplegia, hemianesthesia, neglect, aphasia, visual field defects (amaurosis fugax); less often, headaches, seizures, amnesia, confusion
- Vertebrobasilar (brain stem/cerebellar): bilateral visual obscuration, diplopia, vertigo, ataxia, facial paresis, Horner syndrome, dysphagia, dysarthria; also headache, nausea, and vomiting
- Past medical history, baseline functional status
- ABCD2 with imaging or ABCD3-I score: helps predict CVA risk after TIA (3)[B]
  – Score of 0 to 1: 0%; 2 to 3: 1.3%; 4 to 5: 4.1%; 6 to 7: 8.1%
    o **A**ge >65 years: 1 point
    o **B**P 140/90 mm Hg: 1 point
    o **C**linical presentation
      ▪ Unilateral weakness: 2 points
      ▪ Speech impaired without weakness: 1 point
    o **D**uration: 1 to 2 points based on time
    o **D**iabetes: 1 point
    o **Dual TIA** (within 7 days preceding): 2 points
    o **I**maging (new lesion or carotid stenosis): 2 points

PHYSICAL EXAM
- Vital signs, oxygen saturation
- Thorough neurologic and cardiac exams
- Ocular exam for examination of emboli

DIFFERENTIAL DIAGNOSIS
- Migraine (hemiplegic)
- Focal seizure (Todd paralysis)
- Bell palsy
- Neoplasm of brain, subarachnoid hemorrhage
- Intoxication
- Glucose or other electrolyte abnormalities
- Central nervous system infection
- Multiple sclerosis

DIAGNOSTIC TESTS & INTERPRETATION
Initial Tests (lab, imaging)
- Neuroimaging within 24 hours of symptom onset
- MRI, including diffusion-weighted imaging, is the preferred brain diagnostic modality to rule out stroke; if not available, then noncontrast head computed tomography (CT) (1)
- Noninvasive imaging of the cervicocephalic vessels should be performed routinely in suspected TIA by carotid US/TCD, MRA, or CTA depending on availability and expertise and characteristics of the patient (4)[B].
- Routine blood tests (CBC, chemistry, PT/PTT, UPT, coagulation screen, fasting lipid panel, ECG) are reasonable in evaluation of patient with TIA (4)[B]

Follow-Up Tests & Special Considerations
- Transesophageal echocardiogram (TEE) to identify patent foramen ovale (PFO), aortic arch atherosclerosis, and valvular disease (4)[B]
- Prolonged cardiac monitoring if unclear etiology after initial brain imaging and ECG (4)[B]
- EEG: if seizure is suspected

Diagnostic Procedures/Other
- CT is typically the first neuroimaging test. Preferred variant is noncontrast, but probability of detecting acute tissue changes after ischemic symptoms resolve within 24 hours is 4% (1).
- Diffusion-weighted MRI can identify brain ischemia within minutes of onset and is highly sensitive (88% sensitivity within 24 hours) and specific (95% specificity) for acute infarction and will guide management (1).

Test Interpretation
Clinical suspicion increases if carotid bruits are heard or emboli are noticed in the eyes.

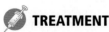 **TREATMENT**

GENERAL MEASURES
- Patients with high-risk TIAs require rapid referral and a 24-hour admission for observation and work-up.
- Outpatient investigations may be considered based on patient's stroke risk, arrangement of follow-up, and social circumstances.
- Antiplatelet therapy to prevent recurrence or future CVA
- Treatment/control of underlying associated conditions

MEDICATION

For patients with TIA, the use of antiplatelet agents rather than oral anticoagulation is recommended to reduce risk of recurrent stroke and other cardiovascular events, with the exception of cardioembolic etiologies (4)[A].

First Line

- Enteric-coated aspirin: 160 to 325 mg/day for noncardioembolic TIA and anticoagulation for cardioembolic etiology
- Antiplatelet therapy:
  - Aspirin 81 to 325 mg/day (5)[A]
    - Contraindications: active peptic ulcer disease and hypersensitivity to aspirin or NSAIDs
    - Precautions: may aggravate preexisting PUD; or worsen symptoms of asthma
  - ER dipyridamole–aspirin (Aggrenox): 25/200 mg BID (5)[B]
    - Combined therapy with dipyridamole and aspirin not proven to have greater efficacy (4)
  - Clopidogrel 75 mg/day (5)[B]
    - Can be used in patients who are allergic to aspirin (5)[B]
    - Precautions: TTP can occur and increases risk of bleeding when combined with aspirin.
    - May be very slightly more effective than aspirin alone (5)[B]
- Combined aspirin and clopidogrel therapy has shown to reduce the incidence of subsequent stroke for high-risk TIA patients by 21% without increased risk of bleeding when used for a duration of ≤1 month immediately following TIA or CVA (2)[A].
- Anticoagulation therapy
  - Direct thrombin inhibitor:
    - Dabigatran (Pradaxa)
    - Idarucizumab (Praxbind) reversal agent
  - Factor Xa inhibitors:
    - Apixaban (Eliquis)
    - Rivaroxaban (Xarelto)
    - Edoxaban (Savaysa)
  - Warfarin (INR-adjusted dose) (5)[A]

Second Line

- Aspirin 325 mg/day or aspirin 81 mg/day plus clopidogrel 75 mg/day (5)[A]:
  - Reserved for patients who cannot take anticoagulation for reasons other than bleeding risk
- Ticlopidine (Ticlid): 250 mg PO BID:
  - For patients unable to tolerate other agents
  - Contraindications: hypersensitivity, presence of hematopoietic/hemostatic disorders, conditions associated with bleeding, severe liver dysfunction
  - Precautions: neutropenia (0.8% severe), which is reversible with cessation of the drug; monitor blood counts every 2 weeks for the first 3 months. TTP can occur.

ISSUES FOR REFERRAL

Interventional radiology or vascular surgery if carotid endarterectomy appropriate

ADDITIONAL THERAPIES

- High-dose statin (4)
- BP should be reduced after 24 hours. Thiazides, ACE inhibitors, and ARBs have shown to be of benefit. β-Blockers have not shown benefit in reducing TIA recurrence or stroke.
- Patients with DM or pre-DM should be advised to maintain glycemic control.

SURGERY/OTHER PROCEDURES

Consider carotid endarterectomy if carotid artery stenosis ≥70%, recommended within 2 weeks if there are no contraindications to early revascularization.

ADMISSION, INPATIENT, AND NURSING CONSIDERATIONS

Symptoms <72 hours and the following:

- ABCD2-I score of >3
- ABCD2-I score of 0 to 3 and uncertainty that diagnostic workup can be completed within 2 days as outpatient; alternatively: if urgent imaging not available through ED or urgent neurology follow-up not available, admit ABCD2-I score ≥3 with evidence of focal ischemia

 ## ONGOING CARE

FOLLOW-UP RECOMMENDATIONS

Patient Monitoring

- Follow-up with neurologic support every 3 months for 1st year and then annually
- Strict control of BP and other CVD risk factors

DIET

- DASH diet or as appropriate for medical problems
- Any level of physical activity is beneficial, but at least 30 minutes of moderate-intensity physical activity daily is preferred (150 minutes/week).

PATIENT EDUCATION

- Keep a BP log; avoid tobacco; limit alcohol; keep a healthy weight.
- Call 911 with the following warning signs:
  - Weakness, tingling, or loss of feeling in one side of the body
  - Sudden double vision or loss of vision in one eye
  - Sudden severe headaches
  - Trouble speaking
  - Trouble understanding others

PROGNOSIS

High mortality risk associated with TIA, up to 25% of patients will die within 1 year of TIA

COMPLICATIONS

Stroke and functional impairment

REFERENCES

1. Kleindorfer DO, Towfighi A, Chaturvedi S, et al. 2021 Guideline for the prevention of stroke in patients with stroke and transient ischemic attack: a guideline from the American Heart Association/American Stroke Association. *Stroke.* 2021;52(7):e364–e467.
2. Pan Y, Elm JJ, Li H, et al. Outcomes associated with clopidogrel-aspirin use in minor stroke or transient ischemic attack: a pooled analysis of clopidogrel in high-risk patients with acute non-disabling cerebrovascular events (CHANCE) and platelet-oriented inhibition in new TIA and minor ischemic stroke (POINT) trials. *JAMA Neurol.* 2019;76(12):1466–1473.
3. Zhao M, Wang S, Zhang D, et al. Comparison of stroke prediction accuracy of ABCD2 and ABCD3-I in patients with transient ischemic attack: a meta-analysis. *J Stroke Cerebrovasc Dis.* 2017;26(10):2387–2395.
4. Coutts SB. Diagnosis and management of transient ischemic attack. *Continuum (Minneap Minn).* 2017;23(1):82–92.
5. Lansberg MG, O'Donnell MJ, Khatri P, et al. Antithrombotic and thrombolytic therapy for ischemic stroke: antithrombotic therapy and prevention of thrombosis, 9th ed: American College of Chest Physicians evidence-based clinical practice guidelines. *Chest.* 2012;141(Suppl 2):e601S–e636S.

 ## SEE ALSO

Algorithms: Stroke; Transient Ischemic Attack and Transient Neurologic Defects

CODES

ICD10

- G45.9 Transient cerebral ischemic attack, unspecified
- G45.1 Carotid artery syndrome (hemispheric)
- G45.0 Vertebro-basilar artery syndrome

CLINICAL PEARLS

- Use the ABCD2-I or ABCD3-I scoring systems to help with risk stratification.
- Encourage smoking cessation, exercise, weight loss, limited ETOH intake, and control of HTN, hyperlipidemia, and DM.
- Antiplatelet therapy (e.g., aspirin, clopidogrel, or aspirin-clopidogrel) should be initiated.
- Anticoagulation therapy (e.g., warfarin, apixaban) should be initiated in patients with atrial fibrillation or cardioembolic risk factors.

T

TRANSIENT STRESS CARDIOMYOPATHY

Adedapo Iluyomade, MD, MBA • Ana De Diego, MD

 BASICS

DESCRIPTION

- Transient stress cardiomyopathy (TSC) is a unique cause of reversible left ventricle (LV) dysfunction with a presentation indistinguishable from the acute coronary syndromes (ACS), particularly ST-segment elevation myocardial infarction (STEMI) (1).
- Typically, the patient is a postmenopausal woman who presents with acute chest pain, dyspnea, or syncope and an identifiable "trigger" (i.e., an acute emotional or physiologic stressor).
- First reported by authors from Japan as "takotsubo" (the Japanese word for octopus trap, due to the characteristic shape of the LV at the end of systole) cardiomyopathy
- Presenting clinical features include:
  - Chest pain/pressure, dyspnea, and/or syncope
  - ECG changes, including ST-segment elevations or diffuse T-wave inversions
  - Mild elevation in cardiac biomarkers (creatine kinase [CK], troponin)
  - Transient wall motion abnormalities that may involve the base, midportion, and/or lateral walls of the LV
  - The apex of the right ventricle (RV) may be affected in up to 25% of cases (1).
- Clinical features may vary on a case-by-case basis, and formal diagnostic criteria have not been established.
- Authors from the Mayo Clinic have proposed that three of the four following criteria establish the diagnosis (1):
  - Transient akinesis or dyskinesis of the LV apical and midventricular segments with regional wall motion abnormalities extending beyond a single epicardial vascular distribution
  - Absence of obstructive coronary artery disease (CAD) or angiographic evidence of acute plaque rupture
  - New ECG abnormalities, either ST-segment elevation or T-wave inversion
  - Absence of recent significant head trauma, intracranial bleeding, pheochromocytoma, obstructive epicardial CAD, myocarditis, hypertrophic cardiomyopathy
- Synonym(s): takotsubo cardiomyopathy; apical ballooning syndrome; stress cardiomyopathy; broken heart syndrome; ampulla cardiomyopathy

EPIDEMIOLOGY

Incidence

- TSC accounts for an estimated 1–3% of all and 5–6% of female patients presenting with suspected STEMI.
- In a recent prospective evaluation of patients admitted to the ICU, as many as 28% had apical ballooning, often in association with sepsis.
- Predominant sex: 82–100% of cases occur in women.
- Predominant age: The mean age of patients is 62 to 75 years.

Prevalence

2.2% of patients presenting to a referral hospital with STEMIs were found to have TSC.

ETIOLOGY AND PATHOPHYSIOLOGY

- The precise pathophysiologic mechanisms of TSC are not well understood.
- There is a considerable evidence that sympathetic stimulation is central to its pathogenesis. A clear emotional or physiologic triggering event precipitates the syndrome in most cases, and TSC has been associated with conditions of catecholamine excess (e.g., pheochromocytoma, central nervous system disorders) and activated specific cerebral regions (1).
- Occurs primarily in subjects with increased susceptibility of the coronary microcirculation and of cardiac myocytes to stress hormones leading to temporary left ventricular dysfunction with secondary myocardial inflammation (1)
- A perturbation in the brain–heart axis, originating in the insular cortex, may be the inciting event (2).
- Subsequent overwhelming activation of the sympathetic nervous system initiates a cascade of events, including the following:
  - Catecholamine-induced LV dysfunction: "biased agonism" of epinephrine for β_2-adrenergic receptors, located predominantly at the cardiac apex
  - Endothelial dysfunction and vasospasm
  - Cellular metabolic injury: myocardial norepinephrine release, calcium overload, contraction band necrosis

Genetics

No genetic associations have been described to date.

RISK FACTORS

- Female sex
- Postmenopausal state
- Emotional stress (i.e., argument, death of family member), more common in women
- Physiologic stress (i.e., acute medical illness), more common in men
- Chronic neurologic or psychiatric disease (2)

COMMONLY ASSOCIATED CONDITIONS

Death from TSC is rare, and most cases resolve rapidly within 2 to 3 days. Reported complications include:

- Left-sided heart failure, pulmonary edema
- Cardiogenic shock and hemodynamic compromise
- Dynamic LV outflow tract gradient complicated by hypotension
- Mitral regurgitation
- Ventricular arrhythmias
- LV thrombus formation
- LV free wall rupture
- Death (rare, 0–8%)

 DIAGNOSIS

Because TSC is often indistinguishable from an ACS, it should be treated initially as such: Activate emergency medical services or report to emergency department; provide oxygen if needed, IV access, and ECG monitoring; and obtain urgent cardiology consultation.

HISTORY

- In 2/3 of patients, there is an exposure to a "trigger event."
  - Emotional stress: argument, death of family member, divorce, public speaking, etc.
  - Physiologic stress: acute medical condition such as head trauma, asthma attack, seizure, etc.
- In 1/3 of patients, there is no identifiable trigger (2).
- Studies suggest preference for time of day, day of the week, and months/season of the year; summer and winter most commonly reported
- Acute onset of dyspnea or chest pain
- Palpitations
- Syncope

PHYSICAL EXAM

Exam may be unremarkable or may include any of the following: tachypnea, tachycardia, hypotension, jugular venous distension, bibasilar rales, S_3 gallop, systolic ejection murmur due to dynamic LV outflow tract gradient, holosystolic murmur of mitral regurgitation.

DIFFERENTIAL DIAGNOSIS

Acute STEMI, pulmonary embolism, myopericarditis, pheochromocytoma, hypertrophic cardiomyopathy, subarachnoid hemorrhage or stroke

DIAGNOSTIC TESTS & INTERPRETATION

The InterTAK Diagnostic Score comprises seven parameters (female sex, emotional trigger, physical trigger, absence of ST-segment depression [except in lead aVR], psychiatric disorders, neurologic disorders, and QT prolongation) ranked by their diagnostic importance with a maximum attainable score of 100 points (1)[C].

- In patients with non–ST-segment elevation, the InterTAK Diagnostic Score can be considered. Patients with a low probability (InterTAK score ≤70 points) should undergo coronary angiography with left ventriculography, whereas in patients with a high score (score ≥70), transthoracic echocardiography should be considered (1)[C].

Initial Tests (lab, imaging)

- ECG should be done urgently and may show the following:
  - Diffuse ST-segment elevations
  - Diffuse and often dramatic T-wave inversions
  - QTc interval prolongation
  - Q waves
- Laboratory tests typically reveal a mild elevation in cardiac biomarkers such as
  - CK (rarely >500 U/mL)
  - Troponin I, Troponin T, or high-sensitivity cardiac troponin
  - B-type natriuretic peptide (BNP)
  - Markers of high filling pressures (e.g., BNP) tend to be higher than markers of necrosis (e.g., CK, troponin).
  - TSC can be distinguished from AMI with 95% specificity using a BNP/TnT ratio ≥1,272 (sensitivity 52%).
- Chest radiograph: cardiomegaly, pulmonary edema

- Echocardiogram
  - Reduced LV systolic function
  - Abnormal diastolic function, including evidence of increased filling pressures
  - Regional wall motion abnormalities in one of the following patterns:
    - Classic or "takotsubo-type" ballooning of the apex with a hypercontractile base
    - "Reverse takotsubo": apical hypercontractility with basal akinesis
    - "Midventricular" akinesis with apical and basal hypercontractility
    - Focal or localized akinesis of an isolated segment
  - Dynamic intracavitary LV gradient
  - Mitral regurgitation
  - Variable involvement of the RV

Follow-Up Tests & Special Considerations
Cardiac MRI

- Reduced LV function
- Wall motion abnormalities as described for transthoracic echocardiography
- Absence of delayed hyperenhancement with gadolinium
- Allows for differentiation between reversible and irreversible changes

Diagnostic Procedures/Other
- The diagnosis of TSC is often challenging because its clinical phenotype may closely resemble STEMI regarding electrocardiographic abnormalities and biomarkers. Although a widely established noninvasive tool allowing a rapid and reliable diagnosis of TSC is currently lacking, coronary angiography with left ventriculography is considered the "gold standard" diagnostic tool to exclude or confirm TSC.
- Coronary angiography reveals nonocclusive CAD; endothelial dysfunction as measured by fractional flow reserve or TIMI frame counts; and rarely, epicardial coronary spasm.
- Left-sided heart catheterization: increased LV end-diastolic pressure to a similar degree as AMI
- Ventriculography: wall motion abnormalities as described for transthoracic echocardiography
- Right-sided heart catheterization:
  - Increased pulmonary capillary wedge pressure
  - Secondary pulmonary hypertension
  - Increased right ventricular filling pressures
  - Reduced cardiac output or cardiogenic shock (cardiac index <2 L/min/m^2 and mean arterial pressure [MAP] <60 mm Hg)

Test Interpretation
Characteristic pathologic findings of involved myocardium have not been described.

 TREATMENT

- Guidelines regarding TSC management are lacking because no prospective randomized clinical trials have been performed in this patient population. Therapeutic strategies are therefore based on clinical experience and expert consensus (3)[C].
- Activation of emergency medical services and advanced cardiac life support therapies as needed
- Oxygen, IV access, ECG monitoring

MEDICATION
After diagnostic cardiac catheterization, empirical treatment goals are as follows:

- Management of hypotension: differentiation between cardiogenic shock and dynamic LV cavity gradient
- Management of increased filling pressures and congestive states
- Attenuation of sympathetic drive

First Line
- Although β-blockers are of theoretical benefit, their use has not been associated with improved outcomes in observational cohorts (2).
- Due to the potential risk of pause-dependent torsades de pointes, β-blockers should be used cautiously, especially in patients with bradycardia and QTc >500 ms (3).
- If there is evidence of left ventricular systolic dysfunction or pulmonary edema, consider the following:
  - Furosemide: 20 to 40 mg IV/PO BID as needed to reduce LV filling pressures and dyspnea
  - The use of angiotensin-converting enzyme inhibitors or angiotensin receptor blockers was associated with improved survival at 1-year follow-up even after propensity matching (2),(3): Lisinopril 10 to 40 mg/day PO or equivalent or valsartan 80 to 160 mg PO BID has been associated with improved outcomes in observational cohorts (2)[B].

Second Line
Short-term anticoagulation should be considered in patients with severely reduced LV function to prevent LV thrombus formation; unfractionated heparin 80 U/kg IV bolus followed by 18 U/kg/hr IV or enoxaparin sodium (Lovenox) 1 mg/kg SC BID

ISSUES FOR REFERRAL
All patients with TSC generally should be comanaged with cardiology while inpatient and referred to cardiology as an outpatient.

ADDITIONAL THERAPIES
- Urgent cardiology consultation and consideration of cardiac catheterization
- Hypotension may require the following:
  - Vasopressors (e.g., dopamine or norepinephrine bitartrate [Levophed]) if there is no LV outflow tract gradient
  - Phenylephrine and IV fluids to increase afterload in the presence of an LV outflow tract gradient
  - Cardiogenic shock that is not due to an LV outflow tract gradient may require placement of an intra-aortic balloon pump.

COMPLEMENTARY & ALTERNATIVE MEDICINE
Psychiatric evaluation and treatment: Despite psychiatric disorders being recognized as a clear substrate and trigger for TSC, studies show that only 32% of patients are treated during their incident hospitalization.

ADMISSION, INPATIENT, AND NURSING CONSIDERATIONS
- Admission criteria/initial stabilization: 12-lead ECG, chest radiograph, laboratory testing, echocardiography. Patients with TSC usually are admitted for observation because the differential diagnosis includes ACS.

- Normal saline infusion to support BP, if necessary, and no evidence of heart failure
- Discharge criteria is generally considered after exclusion of ACS and resolution of congestive state, hypotension, and major impairment of systolic function.

 ONGOING CARE

FOLLOW-UP RECOMMENDATIONS
- Impairments in systolic function typically resolve in 2 to 3 days but may last as long as 1 month.
- Patients should follow up with cardiology and serial echocardiography to document improved LV function.

PROGNOSIS
- Although TSC has generally been considered a benign disease, contemporary observations show that rates of cardiogenic shock and death are comparable to ACS patients treated according to current guidelines (3).
- Recurrence is rare; it also has been reported in 0–8% of patients.

REFERENCES
1. Ghadri JR, Wittstein IS, Prasad A, et al. International expert consensus document on takotsubo syndrome (part I): clinical characteristics, diagnostic criteria, and pathophysiology. *Eur Heart J*. 2018;39(22):2032–2046.
2. Templin C, Ghadri JR, Diekmann J, et al. Clinical features and outcomes of takotsubo (stress) cardiomyopathy. *N Engl J Med*. 2015;373(10):929–938.
3. Ghadri JR, Wittstein IS, Prasad A, et al. International expert consensus document on takotsubo syndrome (part II): diagnostic workup, outcome, and management. *Eur Heart J*. 2018;39(22): 2047–2062.

 SEE ALSO

Algorithm: Chest Pain/Acute Coronary Syndrome

 CODES

ICD10
I51.81 Takotsubo syndrome

CLINICAL PEARLS
- TSC is poorly recognized and often regarded as a benign condition. However, it may be associated with severe clinical complications including death, and its prevalence is likely underestimated.
- TSC is a cause of reversible LV dysfunction with a clinical presentation indistinguishable from the ACS, particularly STEMI.
- Echocardiography may strongly suggest the diagnosis.
- Treatment is supportive and should include diuretics and ACE inhibitors in patients with CHF.

T

TRICHOMONIASIS

Michael J. Arnold, MD

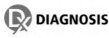 BASICS

DESCRIPTION
- Sexually transmitted urogenital infection caused by a pear-shaped, parasitic protozoan
- Causes vaginitis/urethritis in women, nongonococcal urethritis in men
- Association with infertility in epidemiologic studies
- In pregnancy, increases risk of preterm labor, preterm premature rupture of membranes, small for gestational age infant, and possibly stillbirth
- Synonym(s): trich; trichomonal urethritis

EPIDEMIOLOGY
Incidence
- The most common curable sexually transmitted infection (STI); in 2008, >275 million new cases worldwide, over half of curable STIs
- Estimated 1.1 million new cases annually in United States
  - 10–25% of vaginal infections
  - In males, up to 17% of nongonococcal urethritis; French study shows decreasing prevalence in men since 2007.
- Predominant age: middle-aged adults
  - Rare until onset of sexual activity
  - Common in postmenopausal women; age is not protective, and long-term carriage is common.

Pediatric Considerations
- Rare in prepubertal children; diagnosis should raise concern of sexual abuse.
- Neonatal infections occur most often in the lungs, also vaginal (1)

Prevalence
- 2.1% in U.S. women aged 14 to 59 years
- 0.5% of U.S. men aged 14 to 59 years
- Racial disparity demonstrated
  - 9.6% of black women versus 0.8% of other women
  - 3.4% of black men versus 0.03% of other men

ETIOLOGY AND PATHOPHYSIOLOGY
- *Trichomonas vaginalis*: pear-shaped, flagellated, parasitic protozoan
- Grows best at 35–37°C in anaerobic conditions with pH 5.5 to 6.0

- Divides by binary fission, does not have a cyst form so does not survive externally
- STI, but nonsexual transmission possible because it can survive several hours in moist environment

Genetics
No known genetic considerations

RISK FACTORS
- Multiple sexual partners
- Unprotected intercourse
- Lower socioeconomic status
- Other STIs
- Untreated partner with previous infection
- Use of douching or feminine powders
- Hormonal contraception use does NOT increase risk.

GENERAL PREVENTION
- Use of male or female condoms
- Limiting sexual partners
- Male circumcision may be protective.

COMMONLY ASSOCIATED CONDITIONS
- Other STIs, including HIV, increases risk of STI (1)
- Bacterial vaginosis (1)

DIAGNOSIS

HISTORY
- Women—up to 85% may be asymptomatic (1).
  - Yellow-green, malodorous vaginal discharge
  - Vulvovaginal pruritus
  - Dysuria
  - Symptoms often worsen during menses.
- Men—77% are asymptomatic (1).
  - Dysuria
  - Urethral discharge, often scant
  - Pruritus or burning after intercourse

PHYSICAL EXAM
- Women
  - Vaginal erythema
  - Yellow-green, frothy, malodorous vaginal discharge
  - Cervical petechiae ("strawberry cervix"; seen in <5% of patients on pelvic exam, more with colposcopy) (1)
  - Pelvic exams do not improve STI diagnosis.
- Men: penile discharge, spontaneous and with expression

DIFFERENTIAL DIAGNOSIS
- Women (other vaginitides)
  - Bacterial vaginosis
  - Vaginal candidiasis
  - Chlamydial infection
  - Gonorrheal infection
- Men (other urethritis)
  - Chlamydial infection
  - Gonorrheal infection

DIAGNOSTIC TESTS & INTERPRETATION
Initial Tests (lab, imaging)
- Wet mounts of vaginal or urethral discharge: direct visualization of motile trichomonads; most common because inexpensive and available
  - Sensitivity: as low as 26%; declines rapidly within 1 hour from collection
  - Specificity: 99.8%
- Culture: sensitivity >95%, specificity >99%; takes 4 to 7 days for growth
- Nucleic acid amplification test (NAAT)
  - Gold standard for diagnosis
  - Sensitivity and specificity 95–99%
  - Vaginal, endocervical, or urine specimens
  - British analysis shows that combined NAAT for *Trichomonas*, gonorrhea, *Chlamydia*, and *Mycoplasma genitalium* is the most cost-effective.
- Antigen detection
  - ELISA and direct fluorescent antibody tests: sensitivity of 80–90%
  - Limited clinical availability

Follow-Up Tests & Special Considerations
Detection on cervical Papanicolaou smear
- Treat because highly specific (97–99%)
- Not effective for *Trichomonas* screening—sensitivity as low as 60%

Diagnostic Procedures/Other
In males, urethral meatal swab increases *Trichomonas* detection rate by 4 times over urine.

TREATMENT
- Symptomatic individuals require treatment.
- Sexual partners should be treated presumptively.
- Patients should abstain from sexual intercourse during treatment and until they are asymptomatic.

GENERAL MEASURES

The nitroimidazole class is the only proven effective antimicrobial treatment. If metronidazole resistance is suspected, use tinidazole.

MEDICATION

It is essential to treat partners to prevent reinfection.

First Line

- Metronidazole: 500 mg PO BID for 7 days (1)
  - FDA pregnancy risk Category B
  - Cure rate: 84–98%
  - Single 2-g dose no longer recommended (1)
    - 7-day course increases cure rate with number needed to treat (NNT) of 13 compared to single 2-g dose (2)
    - Single dose has double the rate of repeat infection (1).
  - Increasing resistance—study of PID treatment showed that metronidazole did not improve *T. vaginalis* rate compared to control.
- Tinidazole: 2 g PO, 1 dose (1)
  - FDA pregnancy risk Category C
  - Abstain from breastfeeding during treatment and for 3 days after the dose.
  - More expensive
  - Reaches higher levels in genitourinary tract
  - Cure rate: 92–100%

Second Line

- Secnidazole, 2 g PO, 1 dose (1)
  - Longer half-life than metronidazole and tinidazole, approved for treatment of both *T. vaginalis* and bacterial vaginosis with single dose
  - Approval is based on study of 147 women with 92% cure rate at 6 to 12 days after single 2-g dose.
- Can dose with metronidazole or tinidazole 2 g daily for 7 days if infection persists (3)
- Consider IV dosing of metronidazole based on case report demonstrating cure after multiple failed oral regimens (3).
- Recommendations for metronidazole resistance include tinidazole with intravaginal paromomycin, intravaginal boric acid, and intravaginal metronidazole with miconazole.

Pregnancy Considerations

Metronidazole is effective for trichomoniasis infection during pregnancy but may increase risk of preterm delivery and low-birth-weight babies.

- Studies showed risk in patients receiving 4 times the standard dosing.
- Trichomoniasis is also associated with prematurity.

ISSUES FOR REFERRAL

- Multidrug-resistant organism
- Patient allergy to metronidazole: Desensitization to metronidazole is recommended.

ADDITIONAL THERAPIES

- Limited clinical trials assessing effectiveness of alternative therapies
- Intravaginal metronidazole gel is only effective if adding miconazole (3).

COMPLEMENTARY & ALTERNATIVE MEDICINE

See "Additional Therapies."

 ONGOING CARE

FOLLOW-UP RECOMMENDATIONS

- If symptoms persist after initial treatment, repeat testing.
- Repeat infections occur in up to 37% of cases, treat with metronidazole at same or higher dosage (1)
- Retest *T. vaginalis* recommended between 3 weeks and 3 months of treatment (1)
- HIV-positive patients should be screened for trichomoniasis at time of HIV diagnosis and at least annually (1).
- Patients with multiple partners should be screened annually (1).

DIET

Abstain from alcohol during treatment and for 24 hours following last dose of metronidazole or 48 to 72 hours following last dose of tinidazole due to disulfiram-like reaction.

PATIENT EDUCATION

Educate about the sexually transmitted aspect.

- Advise patient to notify sexual partner to be treated.
- Discuss STI prevention—condom use can prevent recurrence.
- Abstain from intercourse while undergoing treatment; use condoms if abstention is not feasible.
- Avoid alcohol during treatment with metronidazole or tinidazole.

PROGNOSIS

- Excellent
- Usually eliminated after one course of antibiotics although resistance is increasing

COMPLICATIONS

Pregnancy Considerations

Linked to low birth weight, preterm premature rupture of membranes, and preterm birth; associations with infertility, but not proven

REFERENCES

1. Kissinger PJ, Gaydos CA, Seña AC, et al. Diagnosis and management of *Trichomonas vaginalis*: summary of evidence reviewed for the 2021 Centers for Disease Control and Prevention sexually transmitted infections treatment guidelines. *Clin Infect Dis*. 2022;74(Suppl 2):S152–S161.
2. Muzny CA, Mena LA, Lillis RA, et al. A comparison of single-dose versus multidose metronidazole by select clinical factors for the treatment of *Trichomonas vaginalis* in women. *Sex Transm Dis*. 2022;49(3):231–236.
3. Alessio C, Nyirjesy P. Management of resistant trichomoniasis. *Curr Infect Dis Rep*. 2019;21(9):31.

ADDITIONAL READING

- Akter T, Festin M, Dawson A. Hormonal contraceptive use and the risk of sexually transmitted infections: a systematic review and meta-analysis. *Sci Rep*. 2022;12(1):20325.
- Daugherty M, Glynn K, Byler T. Prevalence of *Trichomonas vaginalis* infection among US males, 2013–2016. *Clin Infect Dis*. 2019;68(3):460–465.
- Hawkins I, Carne C, Sonnex C, et al. Successful treatment of refractory *Trichomonas vaginalis* infection using intravenous metronidazole. *Int J STD AIDS*. 2015;26(9):676–678.
- Helms DJ, Mosure DJ, Secor WE, et al. Management of *Trichomonas vaginalis* in women with suspected metronidazole hypersensitivity. *Am J Obstet Gynecol*. 2008;198(4):370.e1–377.e1.
- Kirkcaldy RD, Augostini P, Asbel LE, et al. *Trichomonas vaginalis* antimicrobial drug resistance in 6 US cities, STD Surveillance Network, 2009–2010. *Emerg Infect Dis*. 2012;18(6):939–943.

CODES

ICD10

- A59.02 Trichomonal prostatitis
- A59 Trichomoniasis
- A59.0 Urogenital trichomoniasis

CLINICAL PEARLS

- Both partners need to be treated for trichomoniasis.
- Retest patients between 3 weeks and 3 months of treatment.
- Avoid alcohol during treatment.
- Treatment in pregnancy does not reduce risk of adverse pregnancy outcomes.
- Annual screening is recommended for HIV-positive patients and patients with multiple partners.
- Not a nationally notifiable condition

T

TRIGEMINAL NEURALGIA
Daniel R. Matta, MD • William B. Bradley, MD

BASICS

DESCRIPTION
- Trigeminal neuralgia (TN) is a painful disorder of the sensory nucleus of the 5th cranial (trigeminal) nerve that commonly produces episodic, paroxysmal, severe, lancinating facial pain lasting seconds to minutes
- Often precipitated by stimulation of well-defined, ipsilateral trigger zones: usually perioral, perinasal, and occasionally intraoral (e.g., by talking, washing your face, shaving, or exposure to cold air)
- Subtypes:
  - Classical: secondary to neurovascular compression
  - Idiopathic: when the criterion for TN is met, but neither classic nor secondary TN can be diagnosed based on MRI and electrophysiological testing.
  - Secondary: diagnosed based on fulfillment of criteria for TN but attributed to a separate causative comorbid condition. The three subtypes of secondary TN are TN attributed to multiple sclerosis (MS), space-occupying lesions (such as cerebellopontine angle tumors, meningioma, neuroma, etc.), or attributed to other causes
- System(s) affected: nervous
- Synonym(s): tic douloureux; Fothergill neuralgia; trifacial neuralgia; prosopalgia

EPIDEMIOLOGY
Incidence
- 4 to 29/100,000 per year
- Incidence increases with age, mean onset of 55 years
- Female-to-male ratio 3:2

Pregnancy Considerations
Teratogenicity of medication therapy limits their use during 1st and 2nd trimesters

ETIOLOGY AND PATHOPHYSIOLOGY
- Compression of the trigeminal nerve root by an anomalous artery or vein
- Compression by tumors such as meningioma, acoustic neuroma, or arteriovenous malformation
- Demyelination from compression, or other secondary cause such as MS, leads to an ectopic impulse generation with erratic responses such as hyperexcitability of damaged nerves and transmission of action potentials along adjacent, undamaged, and unstimulated sensory fibers.
- Dysregulation of voltage gated sodium channels

RISK FACTORS
MS associated with a 20-fold increased risk of developing TN

COMMONLY ASSOCIATED CONDITIONS
- Sjögren syndrome; rheumatoid arthritis
- Acute polyneuropathy
- MS
- Charcot-Marie-Tooth neuropathy

DIAGNOSIS

HISTORY
Paroxysms of pain in the distribution of the trigeminal nerve, which include the ophthalmologic (V1), maxillary (V2), and mandibular (V3) branches. Patients typically experience unilateral pain in the V2 and V3 dermatomes, although pain can be bilateral. Attacks are stereotyped in the individual often triggered by stimuli such as light touch, chewing, talking, brushing teeth, cold air, smiling, or grimacing. Autonomic symptoms such as lacrimation, conjunctival injection, or rhinorrhea can be associated with TN. Pain can be continuous and mild between attacks. MS-associated secondary TN differs significantly in regard to classic TN. In general, it often presents at a younger age and more commonly, occurs bilaterally.

PHYSICAL EXAM
Exam findings are typically benign due to the paroxysmal nature of the disorder. Light touch to affected trigger zone(s) may elicit pain attacks.

DIFFERENTIAL DIAGNOSIS
Other forms of neuralgia usually have sensory loss. Presence of sensory loss nearly excludes the diagnosis of trigeminal neuralgia.
- Neoplasia in cerebellopontine angle
- Vascular malformation of brainstem
- Demyelinating lesion (MS)
- Migraine, cluster headache
- Giant cell arteritis
- Postherpetic neuralgia
- SUNHA (short-lasting unilateral neuralgiform headache attacks)

DIAGNOSTIC TESTS & INTERPRETATION
International Classification of Headache Disorders 3rd edition (ICHD-3) diagnostic criteria for trigeminal neuralgia:
- A. Recurrent paroxysms of unilateral facial pain in the distribution(s) of one of more divisions of the trigeminal nerve, with no radiation beyond, and fulfilling criteria B and C
- B. Pain has all of the following characteristics:
  - Lasting from a fraction of a second to 2 minutes
  - Severe intensity
  - Electric shocklike shooting, stabbing, or sharp in quality
- C. Precipitated by innocuous stimuli within the affected trigeminal distribution
- D. Not better accounted for by another ICHD-3 diagnosis
  - Additional criteria for classical: demonstration on MRI or surgical findings of neurovascular compression with nerve root changes (not simply contact)
  - Subclassifications of TN with concomitant continuous pain: presence of background pain between episodes in the same distribution; typically burning, throbbing, or aching
  - Secondary TN is caused by a demonstrable structural lesion other than vascular compression or demyelinating disease such as MS.

Initial Tests (lab, imaging)
Imaging is indicated without an obvious cause to rule out secondary causes.
- MRI, with and without contrast with trigeminal sequences, offers more detailed imaging and is preferred over CT.

Follow-Up Tests & Special Considerations
Dependent on treatment.
- Labs (e.g., electrolytes, liver and kidney function) and EKG prior to initiating medications.
- Screen for HLA-B*1502 allele in patients of Han Chinese descent before initiating carbamazepine/oxcarbazepine.

Diagnostic Procedures/Other
If MR is contraindicated, a CT scan of the head, CT cerebral angiogram and trigeminal-evoked potentials, and/or neurophysiological recordings of trigeminal reflexes should be obtained.

Test Interpretation
Diagnosis of classical TN requires imaging or surgical confirmation of morphological changes to the trigeminal nerve indicating neurovascular compression such as dislocation, distortion, atrophy, or compression of the nerve at its origin from the pons.

TREATMENT

GENERAL MEASURES
- Avoid stimulation (e.g., air, heat, cold) of trigger zones, including lips, cheeks, and gums.
- Medication treatment is first line.
- Invasive procedures are reserved for patients who fail to respond to chronic drug treatment.

MEDICATION
First Line
- Carbamazepine (Tegretol): Start 100 to 200 mg BID and increase gradually (100 mg every other day up to 1,600 mg) to avoid adverse reactions until pain relieved or side effects occur:
  - First-line therapy along with oxcarbazepine; offers meaningful and initial pain control in almost 90% of patients (1)[B]; limited by side effects that lead to withdrawal in up to 40% of patients (1).
  - Number needed to treat (NNT) for any pain relief is 1.9 and 2.6 for significant pain relief, whereas the number needed to harm is 3.4 for minor reactions and 24 for serious events (2)[A].
  - Common side effects: sedation, GI upset, hyponatremia, rash, dizziness, visual disturbance
  - Contraindications: AV block, serious blood dyscrasias
  - Precautions: Decreased dose in impaired liver function, careful when using in combination with anticholinergics in elderly and those with dementia, monitor for Steven-Johnson syndrome and toxic epidermal necrolysis, avoid use in patients with the HLA-B*1502 allele

- Oxcarbazepine (Trileptal): Start 150 to 300 mg BID; effective dose usually 375 mg BID; max dose 1,800 mg/day:
  - Efficacy, side effects, and precautions similar to carbamazepine
  - Faster, with less drowsiness and fewer drug interactions than carbamazepine
  - Often causes hyponatremia
  - Common side effects: sedation, GI upset, and hyponatremia

Second Line
- Phenytoin (Dilantin): can be used in refractory cases or as rescue therapy (off label); 250 to 1,000 mg IV at a rate no faster than 50 mg/min.
- Baclofen (Lioresal): 40 to 80 mg/day; start 5 mg TID and titrate up (as an adjunct to phenytoin or carbamazepine); maintenance dose 50 to 60 mg/day, use limited by side effects: drowsiness, weakness, nausea, vomiting
- Gabapentin (Neurontin): Start 300 mg daily; can increase dose up to 300 to 600 mg TID–QID; can be used as monotherapy or in combination with other medications
- Lamotrigine: Titrate up to 200 mg BID over weeks; use limited by medication interactions and side effects: aseptic meningitis, blood dyscrasias, hypersensitivity reactions, suicidal ideation
- Botulinum toxin injection may be beneficial.
- Pimozide: dopamine receptor agonist; can be used in refractory cases, limited by side effects: sedation, arrhythmias, anticholinergic effects, extrapyramidal symptoms, parkinsonism

ISSUES FOR REFERRAL
Initial treatment failure or positive findings on imaging studies; evaluation at pain clinic prior to surgical referral

ADDITIONAL THERAPIES
Stereotactic radiosurgery, such as Gamma Knife radiosurgery, has been shown to be effective after drug failure. Due to its noninvasive nature, it is preferred when there is no evidence of neurovascular contact, or when there are significant comorbidities limiting surgical or percutaneous procedures (1)
- 24–71% of patients achieved continued pain relief 1 to 2 years after the procedure (3)
- Most common side effect: sensory disturbance (facial numbness)

SURGERY/OTHER PROCEDURES
- Microvascular decompression of CN V at its entrance to (or exit from) brainstem
  - 68–88% of patients have pain relief 1 to 2 years after microvascular decompression, and 61–80% have pain relief at 4 to 5 years (3)[C].
  - Most common side effect: transient facial numbness and diplopia, headache, nausea, vomiting
  - Pain relief after procedure strongly correlates with the type of TN pain: Paroxysmal results in better outcomes than concomitant continuous (aching pain between paroxysms).

- Peripheral nerve ablation (multiple methods):
  - Higher rates of failure and facial numbness than decompression surgery
  - Radiofrequency thermocoagulation
  - Neurectomy; partial sensory rhizotomy
- 4% tetracaine dissolved in 0.5% bupivacaine nerve block; also, ropivacaine or lidocaine can provide temporary relief.
- Alcohol block or glycerol injection into trigeminal cistern: unpredictable side effects (dysesthesia and anesthesia dolorosa) and temporary relief
- Peripheral block or section of CN V proximal to gasserian ganglion
- Balloon compression of gasserian ganglion
- Evidence supporting destructive procedures for benign pain conditions remains limited.

COMPLEMENTARY & ALTERNATIVE MEDICINE
Acupuncture: evidence of analgesic effect in both idiopathic TN and associated secondary myofascial pain

ADMISSION, INPATIENT, AND NURSING CONSIDERATIONS
Severe acute exacerbations, with high attack frequency leading to dehydration or anorexia due to trigger avoidance.

 ## ONGOING CARE

FOLLOW-UP RECOMMENDATIONS
- Follow up, every 3 to 6 months in initial few years, to monitor symptoms and treatment efficacy.
- Patients with TN, especially those whose symptoms are proving refractory to pharmacotherapy, are best managed in multidisciplinary team setting with a neurologist specializing in headache disorders, pain specialist, neurosurgeon, nurses and psychologists.

Patient Monitoring
- Medication serum levels if indicated
- CBC and CMP
- If carbamazepine is prescribed: CBC and platelets at baseline, then weekly for a month, then monthly for 4 months, and then every 6 to 12 months if dose is stable (Regimens for monitoring vary.)
- Reduce drugs after 4 to 6 weeks to determine whether condition is in remission; resume at previous dose if pain recurs. Withdraw drugs slowly after several months, again to check for remission or if lower dose of drugs can be tolerated.

PATIENT EDUCATION
- The Facial Pain Association: https://www.facepain.org/
- Living with Facial Pain: https://www.livingwithfacialpain.org

PROGNOSIS
- 50–60% eventually fail pharmacologic treatment.
- Of those, relapse is seen in ~50% of stereotactic radiosurgeries and ~27% of surgical microvascular decompressions.
- The natural history of TN has been considered progressive; however, recent studies have suggested that patients managed in specialists centers using a multidisciplinary approach may experience disease stabilization and improvement.

COMPLICATIONS
- Mental and physical sluggishness; dizziness with carbamazepine
- Paresthesias and corneal reflex loss with stereotactic radiosurgery
- Surgical mortality and morbidity associated with microvascular decompression

REFERENCES
1. Lambru G, Zakrzewska J, Matharu M. Trigeminal neuralgia: a practical guide. *Pract Neurol*. 2021;21(5):392–402.
2. Allam AK, Sharma H, Larkin MB, et al. Trigeminal neuralgia: diagnosis and treatment. *Neurol Clin*. 2023;41(1):107–121.
3. Cruccu G, Di Stefano G, Truini A. Trigeminal neuralgia. *N Engl J Med*. 2020;383(8):754–762.

 ## CODES

ICD10
- B02.22 Postherpetic trigeminal neuralgia
- G50.0 Trigeminal neuralgia

CLINICAL PEARLS
- Patients with TN typically have a normal physical exam.
- Imaging, ideally MRI, should be obtained to rule out secondary causes in newly presenting patients with clinical suspicion of TN.
- The long-term efficacy of pharmacotherapy for TN is 40–50%.
- First-line treatment: carbamazepine or oxcarbazepine
- If pharmacotherapy fails, stereotactic radiosurgery or surgical microvascular decompression often is successful.

TRIGGER FINGER (DIGITAL STENOSING TENOSYNOVITIS)

Leigh A. Romero, MD, CAQSM • Marvin Valencia, DO

 BASICS

DESCRIPTION
Trigger finger, also known as stenosing flexor tenosynovitis, is disruption of smooth tendon gliding in the fingers/thumb that causes clicking, locking, catching, and pain with flexion and extension.

EPIDEMIOLOGY
Incidence
- Adult population: 2–3% of adults
  - Typically presents in the 5th and 6th decades of life
  - Female > male (6:1)
- Rare in children
  - Associated with mucopolysaccharidoses (MPS)
  - Female = male
- 10% of diabetic population
- Thumb is predominant digit

Prevalence
Lifetime prevalence in the general population is 2.6%.

Pediatric Considerations
- Successful treatment using nonoperative methods such as casting and splinting
- Surgical methods provided satisfactory resolution with those who failed conservative measures and are also used as initial therapy as well.

ETIOLOGY AND PATHOPHYSIOLOGY
- The result of fibrocartilaginous metaplasia of the tendon and/or pulley from prolonged inflammation causing narrowing around the pulley
- This can occur at any of the five pulleys along the flexor tendon—A1 pulley is the most common.
- If flexor tendon becomes nodular, the triggering phenomenon is worse because the nodule has difficulty passing under the A1 pulley.
- Because intrinsic flexor muscles are stronger than extensors, the finger can get stuck in the flexed position.
- No clear association with repetitive movements

RISK FACTORS
- Diabetes mellitus
- Rheumatoid arthritis
- Hypothyroidism
- Mucopolysaccharide disorders
- Amyloidosis

GENERAL PREVENTION
- Most cases are idiopathic.
- No clear association with occupational-related or repetitive activities

COMMONLY ASSOCIATED CONDITIONS
- Orthopedic conditions:
  - Rheumatoid arthritis
  - Calcific tendinitis
  - Septic tenosynovitis
  - Carpal tunnel syndrome
  - Congenital trigger thumb
- Medical conditions:
  - Diabetes
  - Amyloidosis
  - Hypothyroidism
  - Sarcoidosis
  - Gout
  - Pseudogout

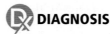 **DIAGNOSIS**

HISTORY
- Clicking, catching, snapping, or locking of a digit during flexion—usually painless initially and then progresses to painful episodes
- The finger may become locked in the flexed position requiring passive manipulation of the finger into extension in more severe cases.
- Functional limitations tend to include difficulty with grasping and holding objects, manipulating coins, or buttoning (1).
- Green classification for severity of trigger finger symptoms:
  - Grade 1: palm pain, tenderness at A1 pulley
  - Grade 2: catching of digit
  - Grade 3: locking of digit, passively correctable
  - Grade 4: fixed, locked digit

PHYSICAL EXAM
- May visualize locking/catching or "triggering" of the affected digit, specifically while flexing the digit; can be painful or painless
- If active triggering is not present, place a finger on the proximal interphalangeal (PIP) joint as the finger is actively flexed and extended, noting the presence of loss of smooth motion or a clicking sensation.
- Palpable and tender nodule may be present at the affected pulley.
- Fixed flexion of the affected joint in more severe cases

DIFFERENTIAL DIAGNOSIS
- Dupuytren contracture
- Ganglion of tendon sheath
- Osteoarthritis
- Diabetic cheiroarthropathy
- Metacarpophalangeal (MCP) joint sprain

DIAGNOSTIC TESTS & INTERPRETATION
Initial Tests (lab, imaging)
- No labs or imaging necessary
- Ultrasound and MRI may be potentially useful to rule out other conditions.

Diagnostic Procedures/Other
Ultrasound can be used for diagnostic and therapeutic purposes.

Test Interpretation
MRI/ultrasound
- Thickening of the affected pulley and alteration in echotexture of the flexor tendons that pass through the digital tunnel; possible synovial sheath effusion around the tendon

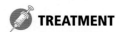 **TREATMENT**

GENERAL MEASURES
- Goals of treatment are to alleviate pain and to allow smoother movement of the digit.
- Start with conservative interventions such as oral NSAIDs, activity modification, and splinting followed by corticosteroid injection.
- Activity modification can be helpful in early disease (2).
- Splinting may be more effective in preventing recurrence than initial treatment choice.
- Splinting the MCP joint at 10 to 15 degrees of flexion for 6 weeks with the distal joints free to move
  - Splinting is more effective for fingers than thumbs (70% vs. 50%).
  - Splinting is less effective with severe symptoms, symptoms >6 months, or if multiple digits are involved.
- Most recommend attempting steroid injection prior to surgery (2).
- Injection of long-acting corticosteroid may provide symptom relief. Subsequent injections are less likely to help.
- Surgery is often successful for patients who are unresponsive to splinting/corticosteroid injections or who suffered recurrence (2).

MEDICATION
First Line
- Oral NSAIDs may reduce pain and discomfort but have not been shown to alter underlying disease.
- NSAIDs do not reduce symptoms of snapping/locking/catching.
- Steroid injection of the tendon sheath/surrounding subcutaneous tissue has 57–90% success rate.

- Triamcinolone appears more effective than dexamethasone (2).
- Injection in surrounding tissues is as efficacious as injecting into the tendon sheath (2).
- Injection into the palmar surface at the mid-proximal phalanx is associated with less pain than injection of tendon sheath at MCP joint.
- Corticosteroid injection has higher success rate than splinting; however, a systematic review quotes the efficacy of orthotic use as 47–93% effective (1).

Second Line
- Injection with diclofenac may be an alternative to corticosteroid for patients with diabetes mellitus if increase in blood sugar is a concern (2).
- Corticosteroids are more effective than diclofenac during the first 3 weeks postinjection. Efficacy is similar to other modalities by 3 months postinjection (2).

ISSUES FOR REFERRAL
Refer to a hand surgeon if symptoms are refractory to conservative measures with oral NSAIDs, physical therapy, and splinting or corticosteroid injections.

ADDITIONAL THERAPIES
- Splinting—dependent on what provides the patient the most relief; lower success rates in patients with severe or chronic symptoms
  - Can take 6 to 10 weeks
  - Can splint at distal interphalangeal (DIP) joint—resolution of 50% of symptoms (3)
  - Can splint at MCP joint with 15 degrees of flexion—resolution of 92.9% of symptoms
  - Can night splint: better compliance versus continuous splinting—resolution in 55% of grades 1 and 2 trigger finger
- Exercises—can be useful particularly after surgical release
  - Digit blocking—blocking MCP joint while allowing PIP joint to bend; can perform at DIP joint
  - Tendon gliding
  - Active range of motion
- Heat/ice, ultrasound, electric stimulation, massage, stretching, and joint motion

SURGERY/OTHER PROCEDURES
- Suggested after failure to reduce symptoms despite conservative therapy and multiple injections
- No apparent differences in success or rates of complications between surgical approaches (3),(4)
- Surgery has lower rate of recurrence than corticosteroid injection but has disadvantage of being more painful initially (5).

- Methods
  - Percutaneous release of A1 pulley
    - Can be performed using ultrasound guidance
    - Success rate >90%
    - Shorter recovery time
  - Open surgical débridement and release of the A1 pulley
    - Gold standard
    - Success rate >90%
    - Better visualization of the pulley
    - Less risk of damage to other structures

COMPLEMENTARY & ALTERNATIVE MEDICINE
Extracorporeal shock wave therapy (ESWT)
- Believed to suppress ongoing inflammation reducing thickening of the flexor tendon and its sheath

ADMISSION, INPATIENT, AND NURSING CONSIDERATIONS
Day surgery for trigger finger release

 ONGOING CARE

FOLLOW-UP RECOMMENDATIONS
- Follow-up is needed only if symptoms persist or if complications develop after surgery.
- Splinting of the affected digit to minimize flexion/extension of the MCP joint helps symptom resolution.

Patient Monitoring
Pain level, postprocedure or postoperative guidelines, and adherence to treatment regiment

PROGNOSIS
Prognosis is excellent with conservative treatment or surgical intervention. Recurrence following corticosteroid injection is more likely for patients with type 1 diabetes mellitus, younger patients, involvement of multiple digits, and history of other upper extremity tendinopathies (2).

COMPLICATIONS
- Diabetic patients may have increased blood sugar levels for up to 5 days following steroid injection.
- Other minor steroid injection complications include skin depigmentation and fat necrosis; tendon attrition or rupture is rare.
- Complications from surgery include infection, bleeding, digital nerve injury, persistent pain, and loss of range of motion of the affected finger. The rate of major complications is low (3%). The rate of minor complications (including loss of range of motion) is higher (up to 28%).
- Another surgical complication, injury to the A2 pulley, may result in bowstringing (bulging of the flexor tendon in the palm with flexion) and pain.

REFERENCES
1. Lundsford D, Valdes K, Hengy S. Conservative management of trigger finger: a systematic review. *J Hand Therapy*. 2019;(32):212–221.
2. Giugale JM, Fowler JR. Trigger finger: adult and pediatric treatment strategies. *Orthop Clin North Am*. 2015;46(4):561–569.
3. Makkouk AH, Oetgen ME, Swigart CR, et al. Trigger finger: etiology, evaluation, and treatment. *Curr Rev Musculoskelet Med*. 2008;1(2):92–96.
4. Wang J, Zhao JG, Liang CC. Percutaneous release, open surgery, or corticosteroid injection, which is the best treatment method for trigger digits? *Clin Orthop Relat Res*. 2013;471(6):1879–1886.
5. Fiorini HJ, Tamaoki MJ, Lenza M, et al. Surgery for trigger finger. *Cochrane Database Syst Rev*. 2018;(2):CD009860.

ADDITIONAL READING
Amirfeyz R, McNinch R, Watts A, et al. Evidence-based management of adult trigger digits. *J Hand Surg Eur Vol*. 2017;42(5):473–480.

CODES

ICD10
- M65.30 Trigger finger, unspecified finger
- M65.319 Trigger thumb, unspecified thumb
- M65.329 Trigger finger, unspecified index finger

CLINICAL PEARLS
- Trigger finger is the inhibition of smooth tendon gliding due to narrowing around the flexor pulley that causes pain, clicking, catching, and locking.
- Diagnosis is based on clinical presentation (history and physical exam).
- Initial conservative therapy consists of NSAIDs, splinting, physical therapy, or corticosteroid injection.
- Long-acting corticosteroid injections are effective for treatment of trigger finger but have higher recurrence rate than surgery.
- Open and percutaneous surgical release have high success rates for patients not responsive to splinting or injections.

T

TROCHANTERIC BURSITIS (GREATER TROCHANTERIC PAIN SYNDROME)

Daniel L. Warden, MD • Nicholas Moore, MD, FAAFP, CAQSM • Kyle M. Samyn, DO, MS

 BASICS

Trochanteric bursitis is often used as a general term to describe lateral hip pain and tenderness over the greater trochanter. There may be inflammation at one of a number of bursa at the lateral hip, but more commonly, the pain is due to hip abductor tendon injury and external snapping hip. More recently, there has been a shift to describe this condition as greater trochanteric pain syndrome (GTPS) (1).

DESCRIPTION
- Bursae are fluid-filled sacs found primarily at tendon attachment sites with bony protuberances:
  - Multiple bursae are in the area of the greater trochanter of the femur.
  - These bursae are associated with the tendons of the gluteus muscles, iliotibial band (ITB), and tensor fasciae latae.
  - The subgluteus maximus bursa is implicated most commonly in lateral hip pain (1).
- Other structures of the lateral hip include the following:
  - ITB, tensor fasciae latae, gluteus maximus tendon, gluteus medius tendon, gluteus minimus tendon, quadratus femoris muscle, vastus lateralis tendon, piriformis tendon
- *Bursitis* refers to bursal inflammation.
- *Tendinopathy* refers to any abnormality of a tendon, inflammatory or degenerative.
- *Enthesopathy* refers to abnormalities of the zones of attachment of ligaments and tendons to bones.

EPIDEMIOLOGY
Incidence
- 1.8/1,000 persons/year
- Peak incidence in 4th to 6th decades

Prevalence
- Predominant sex: female > male
- More common in running and contact athletes
  - Football, rugby, soccer

ETIOLOGY AND PATHOPHYSIOLOGY
- Acute: Abnormal gait or poor muscle flexibility and strength imbalances lead to bursal friction and secondary inflammation.
  - Tendon overuse and inflammation
  - Direct trauma from contact or frequently lying with body weight on hip can cause an inflammatory response.
- Chronic
  - Fibrosis and thickening of bursal sac due to chronic inflammatory process
  - Tendinopathy due to chronic overuse and degeneration: gluteus medius and minimus most commonly involved (1)

Genetics
No known genetic factors

RISK FACTORS
Multiple factors have been implicated (1):
- Female gender
- Obesity
- Tight hip musculature (including ITB)
- Direct trauma
- Total hip arthroplasty
- Abnormal gait or pelvic architecture
  - Leg length discrepancy
  - Sacroiliac (SI) joint dysfunction
  - Knee or hip osteoarthritis
  - Abnormal foot mechanics (e.g., pes planus, overpronation)
  - Neuromuscular disorder: Trendelenburg gait

GENERAL PREVENTION
- Maintain ITB, hip, and lower back flexibility and strength.
- Avoid direct trauma (use of appropriate padding in contact sports).
- Avoid prolonged running on banked or crowned surfaces.
- Wear appropriate shoes.
- Appropriate bedding and sleeping surface
- Maintain appropriate body weight loss.

COMMONLY ASSOCIATED CONDITIONS
- Biomechanical factors (1)
  - Tight ITBs, leg length discrepancy, SI joint dysfunction, pes planus
  - Width of greater trochanters greater than width of iliac wings
- Other associated pathology (1):
  - Low back pain
  - Knee and hip osteoarthritis
  - Obesity

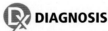 **DIAGNOSIS**

HISTORY
General history (1)
- Pain localized to the lateral hip or buttock
- Pain may radiate to groin or lateral thigh (pseudoradiculopathy).
- Pain exacerbated by:
  - Prolonged walking or standing
  - Rising after prolonged sitting
  - Sitting with legs crossed
  - Lying on affected side

- Other historical features:
  - Direct trauma to affected hip
  - Chronic low back pain
  - Chronic leg/knee/ankle/hip pain
  - Recent increase in running distance or intensity
  - Change in running surfaces

PHYSICAL EXAM
- Palpate for point tenderness with direct palpation over the lateral hip is characteristic of GTPS (1)[B].
- Other exam features have lower sensitivity (1)[B]:
  - Pain with extremes of passive rotation, abduction, or adduction
  - Pain with resisted hip abduction and external or internal rotation
  - Trendelenburg sign
- Other tests to rule out associated conditions:
  - Patrick-FABERE (flexion, abduction, external rotation, extension) test for SI joint dysfunction
  - Ober test for ITB pathology
  - Flexion and extension of hip for osteoarthritis
  - Leg length measurement
  - Foot inspection for pes planus or overpronation
  - Lower extremity neurologic assessment for lumbar radiculopathy or neuromuscular disorders
  - Hip lag sign

DIFFERENTIAL DIAGNOSIS
- ITB syndrome
- Piriformis syndrome
- Osteoarthritis or avascular necrosis of the hip
- Lumbosacral osteoarthritis/disc disease with nerve root compression
- Fracture or contusion of the hip or pelvis—particularly in setting of trauma
- Stress reaction/fracture of femoral neck—particularly in female runners
- Septic bursitis/arthritis

DIAGNOSTIC TESTS & INTERPRETATION
No routine lab testing is recommended.

Initial Tests (lab, imaging)
- Diagnosis can be made by history and exam (2).
- If imaging is ordered:
  - US can aid in diagnosis and guide aspiration and/or injection.
  - Anteroposterior and frog-leg views of affected hip to rule out specific bony pathology (OA, stress fracture, etc.)
  - Consider lumbar spine radiographs if back pain is thought to be a contributing factor.
  - MRI is image of choice in recalcitrant pain or to formally exclude stress fracture.

Follow-Up Tests & Special Considerations
- If there is a concern for a septic bursitis, then aspiration or incision and drainage may be necessary.
- Advanced imaging rarely necessary; detection of abnormalities on MRI is a poor predictor of GTPS.

 TREATMENT

GENERAL MEASURES
- Physical therapy to address underlying dysfunction and weakness
- Correct pelvic/hip instability.
- Correct lower limb biomechanics.
- Low-impact conditioning and aquatic therapy
- Gait training
- Weight loss (if applicable)
- Minimize aggravating activities such as prolonged walking or standing.
- Avoid lying on affected side.
- Runners
  - May need to decrease distance and/or intensity of runs during treatment. Some need to stop running. Amount of time is case specific but may range from 2 to 4 weeks.
  - Avoid banked tracks or roads with excessive tilt.

MEDICATION
First Line
- NSAIDs (1)[B]: Treat for 2 to 4 weeks.
  - Naproxen: 500 mg PO BID
  - Ibuprofen: 800 mg PO TID
- Corticosteroid injection is effective for pain relief (3)[C] and can be considered first-line therapy for selected cases:
  - Dexamethasone: 4 mg/mL or
  - Kenalog: 40 mg/mL; use 1 to 2 mL.
  - Consider adding a local anesthetic (short- and/or long-acting) for more immediate pain relief.
  - Can be repeated with similar effect if original treatment showed a strong response
  - Goal is pain relief.
  - Corticosteroid injections may not be effective for certain cases (4). A noninflammatory cause, such as a chronic tendinopathy or referred pain, should be considered and further explored in these cases.

ISSUES FOR REFERRAL
- Septic bursitis
- Recalcitrant bursitis
- Positive sag test concerning for gluteal tendon tear

ADDITIONAL THERAPIES
- Ice
- Low-energy shock wave therapy has been shown to be superior to other nonoperative modalities.
- Focus on achieving flexibility of hip musculature, particularly the ITB.
- Address contributing factors:
  - Low back flexibility
  - If leg length discrepancy, consider heel lift.
  - If pes planus or overpronation, consider arch supports or custom orthotics.

SURGERY/OTHER PROCEDURES
- Surgery rare but effective in refractory cases
- If surgery is indicated, potential options include:
  - Arthroscopic bursectomy
  - ITB release
  - Gluteus medius tendon repair
- Tenotomy

COMPLEMENTARY & ALTERNATIVE MEDICINE
- Acupuncture
- Prolotherapy
- Growth factor injection techniques
- Platelet-rich plasma injection

 ONGOING CARE

FOLLOW-UP RECOMMENDATIONS
4 weeks posttreatment, sooner if significant worsening

PATIENT EDUCATION
- Maintain hip musculature flexibility, including ITB.
- Correct issues that may cause abnormal gait:
  - Low back pain
  - Knee pain
  - Leg length discrepancy (heel lift)
  - Foot mechanics (orthotics)
- Gradual return to physical activity

PROGNOSIS
Depends on chronicity and recurrence, with more acute cases having an excellent prognosis

COMPLICATIONS
Bursal thickening and fibrosis

REFERENCES
1. Williams BS, Cohen SP. Greater trochanteric pain syndrome: a review of anatomy, diagnosis and treatment. *Anesth Analg.* 2009;108(5):1662–1670.
2. Chowdhury R, Naaseri S, Lee J, et al. Imaging and management of greater trochanteric pain syndrome. *Postgrad Med J.* 2014;90(1068):576–581.
3. Stephens MB, Beutler AI, O'Connor FG. Musculoskeletal injections: a review of the evidence. *Am Fam Physician.* 2008;78(8):971–976.
4. Nissen MJ, Brulhart L, Faundez A, et al. Glucocorticoid injections for greater trochanteric pain syndrome: a randomised double-blind placebo-controlled (GLUTEAL) trial. *Clin Rheumatol.* 2019;38(3):647–655.

ADDITIONAL READING
- Barratt PA, Brookes N, Newson A. Conservative treatments for greater trochanteric pain syndrome: a systematic review. *Br J Sports Med.* 2017;51(2):97–104.
- Pretell J, Ortega J, García-Rayo R, et al. Distal fascia lata lengthening: an alternative surgical technique for recalcitrant trochanteric bursitis. *Int Orthop.* 2009;33(5):1223–1227.

 CODES

ICD10
- M70.60 Trochanteric bursitis, unspecified hip
- M70.62 Trochanteric bursitis, left hip
- M70.61 Trochanteric bursitis, right hip

CLINICAL PEARLS
- Patients with GTPS often present with an inability to lie on the affected side.
- Femoral neck stress fractures are a do-not-miss diagnosis, particularly in young female runners.
- Corticosteroid injection helps as an initial therapy, particularly for pain relief to allow for aggressive physical therapy.
- Physical therapy is treatment mainstay for correcting biomechanical imbalances and restoring proper function.

T

TUBERCULOSIS

Joanna Drowos, DO, MPH, MBA

BASICS

DESCRIPTION

- Active tuberculosis (TB) infection caused by *Mycobacterium tuberculosis*
  - Primary infection or reactivation of latent infection. Risk increases with immunosuppression: highest risk first 2 years after infection. Reactivation risk increases with comorbid disease (e.g., HIV, diabetes).
  - Well-described forms: pulmonary (85%), miliary (disseminated), meningeal, abdominal, lymphadenitis (scrofula)
- Usually acquired by inhalation of airborne bacilli from an individual with active TB. Bacilli multiply in alveoli and spread via macrophages, lymphatics, and blood. Outcomes include eradication (tissue hypersensitivity stops infection; primary TB; latent TB (LTBI).

EPIDEMIOLOGY

Incidence

- Worldwide (2021): an estimated 10.6 million people equivalent to 134/100,000
- 7% of cases involve people living with HIV. Most cases in Southeast Asia and Africa.
- United States (2022): 8,300 (2.5/100,000); 71% of U.S. cases were in persons born outside of the United States. Following a 10-year decline, TB case rates rose slightly in 2022.

Prevalence

- Worldwide (2020): World Health Organization estimates 9.9 million new cases of TB in 2020.
- Mortality
  - Worldwide (2021): 1.6 million deaths due to TB; 13th leading cause of death worldwide

ETIOLOGY AND PATHOPHYSIOLOGY

- *M. tuberculosis, Mycobacterium bovis,* or *Mycobacterium africanum* are causative organisms.
- Spread by aerosol droplets and reach alveolar space. Alveolar macrophages ingest and migrate.
- Cell-mediated response by activated T lymphocytes and macrophages forms a granuloma ("tubercle") that limits bacterial replication. If bacterial replication continues, the tubercle grows with spread to regional lymph nodes. An expanding tubercle within the lung parenchyma combined with regional lymph node enlargement is called a Ranke complex.
- As the infection is contained, destruction of the macrophages produces early "solid necrosis." In 2 to 3 weeks, "caseous necrosis" develops and LTBI ensues. In the immunocompetent, granuloma undergoes "fibrosis" and calcification. In the immunocompromised, primary progressive TB develops. Cavitary lesions may form.

RISK FACTORS

- For latent infection: homeless, correctional facilities, close contact with infected person, living in areas with high incidence of active TB, health care workers; medically underserved, low income, substance abuse
- For development of disease once infected: renal failure; lymphoma; silicosis; diabetes; cancer of head, neck, or lung; children aged <5 years old; malnutrition; systemic corticosteroids; HIV; immunosuppressive drugs; IV drug abuse, alcohol abuse, cigarette smokers; <2 years since infection with *M. tuberculosis*; <90% of ideal body weight

GENERAL PREVENTION

- Screen for and treat LTBI. Report active TB to health department; test and treat all close contacts. Without treatment, LTBI will progress to active TB disease in 5–10% of affected people.
- Bacillus Calmette-Guérin (BCG) vaccine: used primarily in endemic countries; BCG is not recommended in United States for high-risk children with negative PPD and ongoing exposure.

COMMONLY ASSOCIATED CONDITIONS

Immunosuppression; HIV coinfection; malignancy

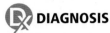

DIAGNOSIS

HISTORY

Signs and symptoms

- General: fever, night sweats, unintentional weight loss, malaise, painless lymph node swelling, arthralgias
- Pulmonary TB: unexplained cough >2 to 3 weeks, hemoptysis, pleuritic chest pain
- Abdominal TB: acutely as surgical abdomen; chronic abdominal TB varies (vague abdominal symptoms, abdominal mass, "doughy" abdomen).

PHYSICAL EXAM

- Can be normal; specific findings depend on organs involved: hepatosplenomegaly, adenopathy, rales; poor weight gain in children
- Late findings: renal, bone, or CNS disease

DIFFERENTIAL DIAGNOSIS

- Pulmonary TB: pneumonia, malignancy, actinomycosis, coccidiomycosis, sarcoidosis, tularemia, etc.
- Extrapulmonary TB: other mycobacterial infections, syphilis, cat-scratch disease, leishmaniasis, erythema nodosum, rheumatologic disease, erythema induratum

DIAGNOSTIC TESTS & INTERPRETATION

- For individuals >5 years old, interferon γ-release assay (IGRA) is generally preferred over tuberculin skin test (TST). For children <5 years old, TST is preferred over IGRA (1)[B]. IGRA favored in BCG-vaccinated children ≥2 years old.
- Don't test individuals at low risk for TB infection. In situations where required (schools, employers, etc.), IGRA is preferred. If initial test is positive in low-risk patients, a 2nd test is recommended which can be either an IGRA or TST. The patient is considered positive for TB infection only if both tests are positive (1)[C].
- TST (e.g., PPD): Measure induration at 48 to 72 hours:
  - PPD positive if induration
    - >5 mm *plus* HIV infection, recent TB contact, immunosuppressed, or positive x-ray
    - >10 mm *plus* age <5 years, moved to the United States from high prevalence country in the last 5 years, IV drug users, or other risk factors
    - >15 mm *plus* age >4 years with no risk factors
  - Two-step test, 1 to 3 weeks apart: no recent PPD, age >55 years, nursing home resident, prison inmate, or health care workers

- Context of PPD results:
  - False positive: BCG (unreliable, would still consider as positive and should not affect decision to treat)
  - False negative: HIV, steroids, gastrectomy, alcoholism, renal failure, sarcoidosis, recent viral vaccination, malnutrition, hematologic or lymphoreticular disorder, very recent exposure
  - If positive once, no need to repeat
- Interferon-γ release assays (IGRAs) measure interferon release after stimulation in vitro by *M. tuberculosis* antigens; may be falsely negative in severely immunosuppressed patients (AIDS, chemotherapy)
- TST and IGRA cannot discern LTBI from active TB.
- Annual LTBI screening of health care workers without elevated risk is no longer recommended once baseline testing complete, unless they are caring for patients at increased risk of TB.

Initial Tests (lab, imaging)

Active TB

- Three sputum samples for acid-fast bacilli (AFB) stain and mycobacterial culture by aerosol induction, gastric aspirate (children), or bronchoalveolar lavage (1)[B]
- Positive AFB: Treat immediately; culture and sensitivity guide treatment.
- Nucleic acid amplification test (NAAT): Use as an adjunct to culture and AFB smear (1)[C]. Positive result supports presumptive diagnosis of TB while culture pending. Negative NAAT does not rule out TB.
- Chest radiograph: primary TB: Infiltrate with or without atelectasis, effusion, or adenopathy.
- CT chest: good sensitivity, tree-in-bud (centrilobular nodules with branching linear opacities)

Follow-Up Tests & Special Considerations

- Baseline CBC, creatinine, liver function tests, visual acuity, and red-green color discrimination (regimens involving ethambutol [EMB])
- HIV: If positive, get baseline CD4 count, viral load and genotype. Check hepatitis B and C if injection drug users, Africa or Asia born, HIV infected or otherwise high risk.
- Extrapulmonary: urine, CSF, bone marrow, and liver biopsy for culture as indicated; interferon-γ (IFN-γ) and adenosine deaminase levels
- Nonspecific findings: anemia, thrombocytosis, SIADH, hypergammaglobulinemia, monocytosis, sterile pyuria

Diagnostic Procedures/Other

- Culture: takes several weeks for definitive results
- Xpert MTB/RIF (rapid molecular test): currently the only FDA-approved molecular assay for pulmonary TB diagnosis and detection of rifampicin resistance in areas with high prevalence of MDR TB

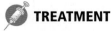

TREATMENT

GENERAL MEASURES

If clinical suspicion, treat immediately. Prescribing physician is responsible for treatment completion. Respiratory and droplet precautions, airborne isolation; not infectious if favorable clinical response after 2 to 3 weeks of therapy and each of three repeat AFB smears are negative

MEDICATION

Use ideal body weight for dosing; directly observed therapy generally preferred

First Line

- LTBI—See "Tuberculosis, Latent (LTBI)."
- Active TB infection
  - Regimen 1 (preferred regimen for patients with newly diagnosed pulmonary TB)
    - Initial phase:
      - Isoniazid (INH), rifampin (RIF), pyrazinamide (PZA), and EMB for 8 weeks (2)[B] *or*
      - INH/RIF/PZA/EMB 5 days/week for 8 weeks under DOT (2)[C]
    - Continuation phase:
      - INH/RIF daily for 18 weeks; or, if DOT, INH/RIF 5 days/week for 18 weeks (2)[B]
  - Regimen 2 (4 months in length; noninferior to standard therapy; for 12 and over with body weight >40 kg, pulmonary TB without resistance and no contraindications)
    - Initial phase:
      - INH, rifapentine (RPT), moxifloxacin (MOX), pyrazinamide (PZA)
        - INH/RPT/MOX/PZA daily for 8 weeks
    - Continuation phase:
      - INH/RPT/MOX daily for 9 weeks
  - Regimen 3 (preferred when more frequent DOT in continuation phase is difficult to achieve)
    - Initial phase:
      - INH/RIF/PZA/EMB daily for 8 weeks *or*
      - INH/RIF/PZA/EMB 5 days/week for 8 weeks
    - Continuation phase:
      - INH/RIF 3 times per week for 18 weeks (2)[C]
  - Regimen 4 (caution if HIV infected or with cavitary disease; missed doses can lead to treatment failure, relapse, and acquired drug resistance)
    - Initial phase: INH/RIF/PZA/EMB 3 times per week for 8 weeks
    - Continuation phase: INH/RIF 3 times per week for 18 weeks (2)[C]
  - Regimen 5 (do not use if HIV positive, smear positive, or cavitary disease; missed doses make therapy equivalent to once weekly therapy which is inferior)
    - Initial phase: INH/RIF/PZA/EMB daily for 14 doses and then twice a week for 12 doses
    - Continuation phase: INH/RIF twice a week for 18 weeks (2)[C]

Pregnancy Considerations

- Treatment for TB is initiated whenever the probability of maternal disease is moderate to high.
- Treat TB in pregnancy with INH/RIF/EMB/PZA; add pyridoxine 25 to 50 mg/day.
- Breastfeeding: OK while taking TB drugs; supplement with pyridoxine 25 to 50 mg/day.

Pediatric Considerations

- Children may attend school if they are taking the appropriate medications.
- Children more commonly have severe disease and faster rate of progression to disease.
- Pediatric TB treatment should be directly observed using four drugs.

ALERT

- If patient does not receive PZA for all of the first 2 months, extend treatment to 9 months.
- Continue EMB until organism susceptibility to INH plus RIF is determined.
- Initiation of ART therapy in HIV-positive patients infected with TB carries an increased risk of immune reconstitution inflammatory syndrome (IRIS) with pulmonary TB (2)[A].

Second Line

Fluoroquinolones and injectable aminoglycosides; use when MDR is suspected or patient intolerance; pretomanid approved for use in XDR-TB

ISSUES FOR REFERRAL

ALERT

Notify public health authorities for all cases of active TB. Consult infectious disease specialist for drug-resistant TB and HIV-positive patients on ART. Case management referral is recommended.

ADDITIONAL THERAPIES

- Pyridoxine: 50 mg for persons at risk for INH neuropathy; 100 mg daily to patients with pre-existing neuropathy.
- Steroids: recommended for TB meningitis; not recommended for TB pericarditis

SURGERY/OTHER PROCEDURES

For extrapulmonary complications (spinal cord compression, bowel obstruction, constrictive pericarditis)

ADMISSION, INPATIENT, AND NURSING CONSIDERATIONS

- Negative pressure isolation room with personal respirators and droplet precaution
- Three consecutive negative sputum AFB smears are necessary for release from isolation.

 ## ONGOING CARE

FOLLOW-UP RECOMMENDATIONS

Patient Monitoring

- Monthly sputum for AFB smear and culture until two consecutive cultures are negative; must confirm prior to starting continuation phase; monthly visits to monitor medication adherence and adverse effects; CXR after 2 months of treatment
- Liver enzymes monthly for chronic liver disease, alcohol use, pregnant or postpartum patients; drug-induced liver injury is most common side effect of treatment. Temporarily halt medications for enzyme increase ≥5 × ULN if asymptomatic or ≥3 × ULN if symptomatic.
- Visual acuity and red-green color monthly if on EMB >2 months or doses >20 mg/kg/day
- If culture positive after 2 months of therapy, reassess drug sensitivity, initiate DOT, coordinate care with public health authorities, and consider infectious disease consultation.

PATIENT EDUCATION

- Emphasize medication adherence. Screen and treat close contacts.
- Alert patient that health authorities must be notified.

PROGNOSIS

Few complications and full resolution of infection if medications are taken for full course as prescribed

COMPLICATIONS

- Cavitary lesions can become secondarily infected.
- Risk for drug resistance increases with HIV positive, treatment nonadherence, or residence in area with high incidence of resistance.

REFERENCES

1. Lewinsohn DM, Leonard MK, LoBue PA, et al. Official American Thoracic Society/Infectious Diseases Society of America/Centers for Disease Control and Prevention Clinical Practice Guidelines: diagnosis of tuberculosis in adults and children. *Clin Infect Dis*. 2017;64(2):111–115.
2. Nahid P, Dorman SE, Alipanah N, et al. Official American Thoracic Society/Centers for Disease Control and Prevention/Infectious Diseases Society of America Clinical Practice Guidelines: treatment of drug-susceptible tuberculosis. *Clin Infect Dis*. 2016;63(7):e147–e195.

 ## SEE ALSO

- WHO TB program: https://www.who.int/teams/global-tuberculosis-programme/overview
- Tuberculosis, CNS; Tuberculosis, Latent (LTBI); Tuberculosis, Miliary

 ## CODES

ICD10

- A15.9 Respiratory tuberculosis unspecified
- A15.0 Tuberculosis of lung
- A19.9 Miliary tuberculosis, unspecified

CLINICAL PEARLS

- TB is fully curable when treated appropriately.
- Children and elderly patients exhibit fewer classic clinical features of TB.
- TST and IGRA cannot discern active TB from LTBI.
- Notify public health authorities for all cases of active TB. Consult infectious disease for drug-resistant TB and HIV-positive patients on ART.

T

TUBERCULOSIS, LATENT (LTBI)

Laurel Banach, MD • Rebecca Thal, NP-C, AAHIVS

BASICS

DESCRIPTION
- Latent tuberculosis infection (LTBI) is an asymptomatic, noninfectious condition following exposure to an active case of tuberculosis (TB). LTBI is usually detected by a screening skin/blood test.
- Active TB occurs in 5–10% of infected individuals who have not received preventive therapy. Chance of active TB increases with immunosuppression and is highest for all individuals within 2 years of infection; 85% of the cases are pulmonary, which can be spread person-to-person via aerosol route.
- >80% of active TB cases in the United States result from untreated LTBI.
- LTBI treatment is a key component of the TB elimination strategy for the United States.

ALERT
- Nitrosamine particles have been isolated in rifampin (RIF) and rifapentine products in 2020 and through 2022. These nitrosamine particles are potential or probable carcinogens, and due to the life-threatening nature of TB, the FDA has approved ongoing production of these antimicrobials with close monitoring (1).
- The current pace of decline in TB incidence will not eliminate TB in the United States in the 21st century. Extra effort is needed to identify patients with LTBI (2).

EPIDEMIOLOGY
- Epidemiology is difficult to assess because LTBI is not a reportable infection in many states.
- In the United States, high-risk groups include immigrants from countries with a high TB rate (countries other than Canada, Australia, New Zealand, or a country in western or northern Europe); persons with a history of drug use or experiencing homelessness; HIV-infected or immunocompromised individuals; and persons living or working in high-risk congregate settings such as nursing homes, carceral facilities, and health care facilities (2).
- Newly exposed (particularly children) are also at high risk.
- On average, 5–10% of those infected with LTBI will go on to develop active TB in their lives, typically within 5 years (1).
- In 2022, there were 8,300 TB cases reported in the United States.
- The highest TB incidence for U.S.-born persons occurred among people of non-Hispanic white race/ethnicity, and the most likely medical diagnostic risk factor was a diagnosis of diabetes.

Incidence
There are no estimates for annual incidence of LTBI in the United States.

Prevalence
- Globally, ~2 billion people are estimated to be infected with TB. Globally, ~10 million people were diagnosed with active TB in 2020, of which ~1.1 million were children.
- The CDC estimates 13 million people with LTBI (3).

ETIOLOGY AND PATHOPHYSIOLOGY
Mycobacterium tuberculosis, Mycobacterium bovis, and *Mycobacterium africanum*

RISK FACTORS
Immigrants from TB-endemic countries, which include most countries of Africa, Asia, and Eastern Europe; close contact with infected individual; living or working in a congregate setting (e.g., prison, nursing home); use of illicit drugs; lower socioeconomic status or experiencing homelessness; health care workers; laboratory personnel working with mycobacteria

GENERAL PREVENTION
- Screen for LTBI and treat individuals with positive tests.
- If a person has fibrotic lung changes on imaging and no evidence of TB treatment, these patients should be screened for LTBI, regardless of their other risk factors.
- Special population: Organ donors should be screened. If donor is deceased, IGRA testing is still possible.

COMMONLY ASSOCIATED CONDITIONS
- HIV infection (see "Initial Tests [lab, imaging]")
- Immunosuppression
- IV drug use and substance use disorders

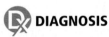
DIAGNOSIS

HISTORY
- Assess risk; history of immigration from a high-risk area including those with temporary visas for school or work (note: TB screening for this type of visa is not required, unlike regulations for those seeking permanent residence in the United States), history of IV drug use and/or drug treatment, HIV, recent incarceration or experience of homelessness, immunosuppression; known exposure to TB case; caring for an individual with TB
  - If household contact has LTBI, test all household contacts.
- Assess for active TB cough for more than of >2 to 3 weeks, fevers, night sweats, weight loss, and hemoptysis.

PHYSICAL EXAM
- No active signs of infection on exam in patients with LTBI
- Assess for active TB by performing vital signs, weight, pulmonary, and lymph node exams.

DIFFERENTIAL DIAGNOSIS
- Fungal infections; atypical mycobacteria or *Nocardia*
- Immunosuppression from conditions such as HIV

DIAGNOSTIC TESTS & INTERPRETATION
Initial Tests (lab, imaging)
- Test for TB infection with tuberculin skin (PPD) or interferon-γ release assay (IGRA) (2). IGRA is preferred for people with history of BCG vaccine and/or those who would have difficulty returning for second test (to read tuberculin skin test [TST])
- Chest x-ray to rule out active TB

- Only if concern for active disease, perform acid fast bacilli sputum smear and culture (2).
- Screen at-risk patients for HIV (2).
- Baseline lab testing prior to treatment is not required but is recommended for patients at risk for liver disease including heavy alcohol use as hepatotoxicity is the primary side effect of treatment or for patients who are HIV infected.

Follow-Up Tests & Special Considerations
- Repeat liver transaminases are recommended during LTBI treatment if symptoms develop concerning for hepatotoxicity.
- Discontinue treatment if ALT elevation is >5 × the upper limit of normal or >3 × the upper limit of normal with signs/symptoms consistent with hepatic damage.
- Without known exposure or evidence of TB transmission, health care workers in the United States do not need to serial TB screening at any interval after a baseline test.

Test Interpretation
- TST: PPD: 5 U (0.1 mL) intermediate-strength intradermal volar forearm; measure induration at 48 to 72 hours:
  - Positive if induration is (2):
    - >5 mm and patient has HIV infection (or suspected), is immunosuppressed, had recent close TB contact, or has clinical evidence of active or old disease on CXR
    - >10 mm and patient is aged <4 years or has other risk factors noted earlier
    - >15 mm and patient is aged >4 years and has no risk factors
  - Negative if induration is <5 mm on initial test and, if indicated, on second test
  - Use the two-step test (administer a second intradermal test 1 to 3 weeks after initial test; measure and interpret as usual) if patient has had no recent PPD and is aged >55 years or is a nursing home resident, prison inmate, or health care worker.
  - Preferred for children aged <2 years
- The IGRA QuantiFERON-TB and QuantiFERON-TB GOLD; T-SPOT measures the release of interferon by sensitized lymphocytes when exposed to antigens of *M. tuberculosis*.
  - It is unaffected by prior BCG vaccination; requires only one visit for the lab draw; improves sensitivity and specificity but is costly
- Special considerations
  - Measles vaccine: may suppress tuberculin activity; simultaneous PPD and measles vaccine recommended; if not simultaneous, defer PPD for 4 to 6 weeks after measles vaccine.
  - The history of BCG vaccination should not alter the management of a positive PPD test, but consider IGRA test in persons who have received the BCG vaccination.
  - Situations that may give a false-negative skin test: recent viral infection, new (<10 weeks) infection, severe malnutrition, HIV, anergy, age <6 months, active TB, steroid use.

TREATMENT

GENERAL MEASURES
- Must first exclude active TB by history, physical exam, and lung imaging; chest x-ray must be obtained within 2 months prior to starting LTBI treatment.
- Treatment for LTBI is critical for the control and elimination of TB disease. LTBI treatment decreases the risk of active TB and of potential spread to others. Treat all persons with LTBI.
- Directly observed therapy (DOT) is recommended if patient adherence is not assured. Video DOT is an effective alternative.
- Treat LTBI during pregnancy if patient has recent infection or is HIV positive (use isoniazid [INH] with pyridoxine, and monitor liver enzymes); otherwise, postpone treatment until after delivery.
- Consult public health or infectious disease specialist for suspected INH resistance in HIV patients and for complicated medication interactions, especially in the circumstance of nitrosamine products in RIF and rifapentine.

MEDICATION
The CDC and National Tuberculosis Controllers Association (NTCA) recently convened in 2020 to complete a systemic review and update the treatment recommendations.

First Line
- Rifamycin-based antimicrobials (rifamycins) have many drug interactions (via CYP3A4 pathway), and a drug-interaction tool should be used before prescribing.
  - Rifamycins can reduce the effectiveness of hormonal contraception; persons using hormonal contraception should consider the copper IUD and switch to or add a barrier method for the full duration of latent TB treatment.
  - Rifamycins can interact with warfarin—patients require increased monitoring.
  - Monitor for hypersensitivity reaction, hepatotoxicity.
  - Monitor for hypotensive or flulike reaction to weekly INH/rifapentine and discontinue if this occurs.
  - Rifamycins cause temporary red-orange discoloration of body fluids (urine, sweat, tears, saliva); this reverses on discontinuation of medication.
- INH should be closely monitored for hepatotoxicity, especially in patients with a history of alcohol use disorder, HBV, HCV, fatty liver, NASH, or other signs of liver dysfunction or injury.
  - Peripheral neuritis and hypersensitivity are possible. Consider concurrent pyridoxine (vitamin B_6) 25 to 50 mg/day.
- Regimens:
  - RIF alone
    - 4 months duration, RIF given daily
    - RIF: max daily dose of 600 mg; adults 10 mg/kg and children 15 to 20 mg/kg
  - INH + RIF daily
    - 3 months duration
    - INH: max daily dose of 900 mg; adults 15 mg/kg and children (ages 2 to 11 years) 25 mg/kg
    - RIF dosing (see above)

- Once-weekly INH + rifapentine (3HP)
  - 3 months duration, weekly administration with DOT
  - INH dosing (see above)
  - Rifapentine dosing
    - 10 to 14 kg, 300 mg
    - 14.1 to 25.0 kg, 450 mg
    - 25.1 to 32.0 kg, 600 mg
    - 32.1 to 49.9 kg, 750 mg
    - >50 kg, 900 mg (max daily dose)

Second Line
Alternative options include INH daily for 6 or 9 months.
- Reduced adherence when compared to shorter-course regimens
- Longer duration could increase risk for hepatotoxicity.
- These two durations have not been directly compared.

ISSUES FOR REFERRAL
Consult public health or infectious disease specialist for suspected INH resistance in HIV patients. Consult public health or infectious disease specialist for complicated medication interactions, especially in the circumstance of nitrosamine products in RIF and rifapentine. Consult infectious disease specialists for concerns for multidrug resistant cases.

ADDITIONAL THERAPIES
Pediatric Considerations
- Follow public health recommendations for assessing and treating newborns.
- If mother has disease and is possibly contagious, evaluate infant for congenital TB and test for HIV as well; separating newborn from mother is an individualized risk-benefit discussion.
- Treat or refer for treatment if you suspect congenital TB.

ADMISSION, INPATIENT, AND NURSING CONSIDERATIONS
Geriatric Considerations
Before entering a long-term care setting, patients should have two-step PPD using facility protocols. INH side effects are more pronounced. No isolation required.

ONGOING CARE

FOLLOW-UP RECOMMENDATIONS
Patient Monitoring
- During treatment course for LTBI, monthly visits to assess adherence and monitor for signs and symptoms of active TP or signs of adverse treatment effects (hepatitis, hypersensitivity, neuropathy); consider partnering with local public health offices for DOT monitoring if appropriate.
- Check liver enzymes if patient is symptomatic, HIV positive, has chronic liver disease, uses alcohol, or is pregnant or postpartum. Modify drugs as needed.
- In a patient who has elected to defer LTBI treatment, there is no indication to repeat chest x-ray unless symptoms develop or the patient elects to initiate treatment.

DIET
Regular; in patients treated with INH, consider pyridoxine 10 to 50 mg/day.

PROGNOSIS
Generally, there are few complications, and treatment is effective if medications are taken as prescribed. If LTBI treatment is erroneously offered to a patient with active TB, it can result in monotherapy of active disease. Nonadherence during LTBI treatment does not lead to drug resistance but does result in untreated LTBI. Retreatment is not necessary.

COMPLICATIONS
Active TB

REFERENCES
1. World Health Organization. Latent tuberculosis infection: updated and consolidated guidelines for programmatic management. https://apps.who.int/iris/handle/10665/260233. Accessed November 21, 2023.
2. Sterling TR, Njie G, Zenner D, et al. Guidelines for the treatment of latent tuberculosis infection: recommendations from the National Tuberculosis Controllers Association and CDC, 2020. *MMWR Recomm Rep*. 2020;69(1):1–11.
3. Centers for Disease Control and Prevention. Latent TB infection and TB disease. https://www.cdc.gov/tb/topic/basics/tbinfectiondisease.htm. Accessed October 30, 2023.

ADDITIONAL READING
Centers for Disease Control and Prevention. Latent tuberculosis infection: a guide for primary health care providers. https://www.cdc.gov/tb/publications/ltbi/default.htm. Accessed November 21, 2023.

SEE ALSO
Tuberculosis; Tuberculosis, Miliary

CODES

ICD10
R76.11 Nonspecific reaction to skin test w/o active tuberculosis

CLINICAL PEARLS
- Treatment of LTBI is crucial to the control and elimination of TB disease in the United States.
- Screen persons from TB-endemic countries, and treat those who are positive. Screen household contacts of patients who are LTBI positive. Screen individuals who are exposed to active cases of TB.
- The IGRA blood test is unaffected by prior BCG vaccination.

ULCER, APHTHOUS

Velyn Wu, MD, MACM

BASICS

Aphthous ulcers are the most common ulcerative disease of the oral mucosa.

DESCRIPTION

- Self-limited, painful ulcerations of the nonkera-tinized oral mucosa, which are often recurrent
  - Affects chewing, eating, and speaking
- Synonyms: canker sores; aphthae; aphthous stomatitis
  - Comes from *aphthi* meaning "to set on fire" or "to inflame" in Greek; first used by Hippocrates to categorize oral disease
- Classification based on severity
  - Simple aphthosis
    - Common, episodic, infrequent (<7 episodes annually)
    - Prompt healing (resolution in 1 to 2 weeks), few ulcers
    - Minimal pain, little disability, limited to oral cavity
    - Self-limiting, responds well to local treatments
  - Complex aphthous ulcers
    - Uncommon, episodic or continuous, slow healing
    - Few to many ulcers, frequent or continuous ulceration
    - Short or nonexistent disease-free intervals
    - Marked pain, major disability
    - Often need systemic treatments
    - May have genital aphthae
- Classification based on ulcer morphology
  - Minor aphthous ulcers (Mikulicz aphthae)
    - Age of onset 5 to 19 years
    - Usually <10 mm in diameter
    - Number of ulcers: 1 to 5
    - Self-limited, healing within 4 to 14 days
    - Distribution: lips, cheeks, tongue, floor of mouth
    - Rarely affects the roof of the mouth
    - Nonscarring
    - Affects males and females equally
  - Major aphthous ulcers (Sutton disease), 10% of all aphthae
    - Age of onset 10 to 19 years
    - Usually >10 mm in diameter
    - Number of ulcers: 1 to 10
    - Distribution: lips, soft palate, pharynx
    - May take weeks to months to heal
    - Generally more painful than minor aphthous ulcers
    - May cause scarring and be accompanied by fever and malaise
    - Affects males and females equally
  - Herpetiform ulcers, 5% of all aphthae
    - Age of onset 20 to 29 years
    - Usually 1 to 2 mm in diameter, form larger lesions when coalesced
    - No association with herpes simplex virus
    - Occur in small clusters numbering 10s to 100s, lasting 1 to 4 weeks
    - Generally more painful than minor aphthous ulcers
    - Scarring unusual
    - May also affect the palate, gingiva, and pharynx
    - Affects more females than males

EPIDEMIOLOGY

- Recurrent aphthous stomatitis (RAS) is the most common ulcerative disease of the oral mucosa and accounts for 25% of recurrent ulcers in adults and 40% in children.
- More common in patients <40 years of age, Caucasians, nonsmokers, and those of higher socioeconomic status

Incidence

5–60% depending on ethnic and socioeconomic groups

Prevalence

Lifetime prevalence of 5–85%

ETIOLOGY AND PATHOPHYSIOLOGY

Associated with stress-induced rise in salivary cortisol, multiple HLA antigens, cell-mediated immunity and inflammation

Genetics

Associations with specific HLA subtypes

RISK FACTORS

- Local trauma: sharp teeth, dental treatments, or mucosal injury secondary to toothbrushing
- Sodium lauryl sulfate–containing toothpaste
- Increased stress and anxiety
- Nutritional deficiencies: iron, zinc, vitamin B complex, and folate
- Immunodeficiency: HIV
- Recent cessation of tobacco use
- Medications (numerous)
- Endocrine alterations (i.e., menstrual cycle)
- *Helicobacter pylori* infection
- Underlying medical disorders (e.g., celiac disease, inflammatory bowel disease [IBD], Behçet syndrome)

GENERAL PREVENTION

- Avoid sodium lauryl sulfate–containing toothpaste
- Vitamin supplementation: vitamins B_{12}, D, zinc

DIAGNOSIS

HISTORY

- Patients typically complain of oral ulcerations, which are painful and exacerbated by movement of the mouth. Exacerbation may also be reported with certain foods (hot, spicy, acidic, or carbonated foods or drinks).
- May experience prodrome of burning or pruritic sensation of the oral mucosa 2 to 48 hours prior to appearance of ulcers, progressing to pain which peaks before ulceration
- Aphthae typically begin between the ages of 5 and 29 years and are recurrent.
- Ask about ulcerative lesions of other anatomic areas, family history, prior history of aphthous ulcers, and new medications prior to onset of ulcers. Ask about the risk factors and take a comprehensive review of systems in order to prioritize the differential.

PHYSICAL EXAM

- Round or ovoid ulcerations generally <10 mm in size; covered with a grayish-white pseudomembrane surrounded by an erythematous halo
- Ulcers are typically found in the buccal or lip mucosa, ventral tongue, soft palate, or oral vestibule; rarely on the roof of the mouth or lips
- Evaluate for signs of secondary infection: elevated temperature, lymphadenopathy, increased surrounding edema, or pus drainage.

DIFFERENTIAL DIAGNOSIS

- Oral trauma (biting, dentures)
- Infection
  - Herpesvirus (HSV stomatitis): vesicular lesions on keratinized tissue (dorsal tongue, vermillion border); generally not present on mucosa, often with prodromal symptoms (fever, headache, malaise, etc.)
  - HIV: Ulcerations have lengthened healing time and tend to be more painful; may be seen in acute seroconversion syndrome or in advanced disease (low CD4 count)
  - Hand-foot-and-mouth disease: small vesicles within the oral cavity, along with lesions on the hands and feet
  - COVID-19
  - Association with *H. pylori* remains controversial.
- Mucocutaneous syndromes (lichen planus, pemphigus); especially if chronic or nonhealing
- Medication induced
  - Fixed drug eruptions
  - Linear IgA bullous dermatosis: tense vesicles or bullae appearing 1 to 15 days after initiation of medication, most commonly caused by vancomycin
- Malignancy: nonhealing lesions, leukoplakia, or ipsilateral cervical lymphadenopathy
- Systemic disease should be considered, causing aphthous-like ulcerations, in adults with their first episode (late onset) or lesions elsewhere (atypical presentation).
  - Behçet syndrome: autoimmune systemic vasculitis usually involving mucous membranes
    - In 80% of Behçet syndrome, ulcers are the presenting sign.
    - Genital and oral ulceration, more likely major than minor aphthae
    - Signs and symptoms can include uveitis, arthritis, skin lesions, or central nervous system deficits.
  - Reiter syndrome: reactive arthritis, preceded by infection, usually of the genital tract, predominantly found in men
    - Uveitis; urethritis; HLA-B27–associated arthritis
  - Sweet syndrome
  - IBD: Crohn disease, ulcerative colitis
  - PFAPA syndrome: periodic fevers, aphthous ulcers, pharyngitis, adenitis, abdominal pain, and joint pain
  - Systemic lupus erythematosus (SLE): autoimmune vascular collagen disease
  - Gluten-sensitive enteropathy (celiac disease)
  - Herpangina and hand-foot-and-mouth disease

DIAGNOSTIC TESTS & INTERPRETATION

Lab work maybe useful for evaluation for other etiologies of aphthae.

Initial Tests (lab, imaging)

Consider complete blood count, zinc, folic acid, iron, ferritin, and B vitamins to evaluate for systemic causes in severe or recurrent cases (1)[C].

Follow-Up Tests & Special Considerations

- Biopsy and viral testing for nonhealing ulcers or atypical presentations
- Rheumatologic serology if underlying systemic disease is suspected
- Gastroenterology evaluation if gastroenterologic disease is suspected

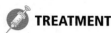 **TREATMENT**

GENERAL MEASURES

Management is symptomatic. The goals are to reduce inflammation, relieve pain, promote healing, and decrease frequency of recurrence.

MEDICATION

In general, treatment is supportive. Topicals can be helpful and effective for minor aphthae, but systemic treatment may be needed for major aphthae.

First Line

- Topical corticosteroids (to improve healing time and symptoms) (1)[C],(2)[C],(3)[C]
  - Adverse effects: may increase risk of oral candidiasis (more likely with higher potency formulations)
  - Topical steroid preparations
    - Triamcinolone acetonide 0.1% dental paste
      - Apply sparingly to ulcers 2 to 4 times daily for up to 2 weeks or until ulcer resolution.
    - Fluocinonide 0.05% gel or ointment
      - Apply sparingly to ulcer 4 times daily for up to 2 weeks or until ulcer resolution.
- Topical anesthetics (to reduce symptoms only) (1)[B],(3)[A]
  - Preparations
    - Lidocaine 5% ointment or 10% spray
      - Apply 4 times daily or prior to eating as needed for pain for up to 2 weeks or until ulcer resolution.
    - Hyaluronic acid 2.5% gel
      - Apply 2 times per day for 2 weeks until ulcer resolution.
    - Benzocaine topical (OTC)
  - Adverse effects: may cause initial stinging; benzocaine rarely causes methemoglobinemia, especially in children aged <2 years.
- Antimicrobial/antiseptic mouth rinses (improve healing time, decrease pain, and may prevent recurrence) (1)[A],(3)[A]
  - Preparations
    - Chlorhexidine aqueous mouthwash 0.12% or 0.2%
      - Use 3 times daily while lesions persist.
      - May cause superficial tooth staining

- Doxycycline
  - 100 mg in 10 mL of water
  - Use rinses for 2 to 3 minutes 4 times per day for 3 days.
  - May consider rinses of hydrogen peroxide with menthol
- Topical immunomodulators (improves healing time, reduces symptoms, and prevents recurrence when used in prodromal phase) (1)[B],(3)[A]
  - Adverse effects: may cause stinging sensation
  - Preparation
    - Amlexanox 5% oral paste
      - Apply to ulcers 4 times daily for up to 2 weeks or until ulcer resolution.
      - Not available in the United States

Second Line

Oral medications (may extend time between recurrence) (1)[B],(3)[A]

- Systemic corticosteroids—rescue therapy in acute, severe, recurrent outbreaks
  - Prednisone 0.75 mg/kg/day, tapered by 0.25 mg/kg/day every 2 weeks
- Montelukast 10 mg daily can have similar efficacy to steroids.
- Colchicine, pentoxifylline, thalidomide, and dapsone have been used with variable success but should be used with caution due to side effects.
- Levamisole—immune modulator, typically well tolerated, pregnancy Category C
- Antibiotics—penicillin G potassium, 50 mg 4 times daily for 4 days

ISSUES FOR REFERRAL

Otolaryngology or dental referral if lesions have not resolved as expected

ADDITIONAL THERAPIES

- Vitamin B_{12} 1,000 μ sublingual daily may be effective in decreasing the duration of outbreaks, number of ulcers, and level of pain (1)[B].
- Vitamin C 2,000 mg/day may also be an effective adjunctive therapy given its anti-inflammatory properties (3)[A].
- H. pylori eradication has been associated with lower number of aphthous lesions (3)[A].

SURGERY/OTHER PROCEDURES

Low-level laser therapy at wavelength of 658 nm can improve pain and promote healing (1)[A],(3)[A].

 ONGOING CARE

FOLLOW-UP RECOMMENDATIONS

Evaluation for infection, mucocutaneous or systemic disease, or malignancy should be pursued for nonhealing lesions or lesions with lymphadenopathy or unusual presentation.

Patient Monitoring

Aphthous ulcers are often recurrent, so patients should be monitored for recurrence.

DIET

Deficiencies of iron, vitamin B_{12}, and folic acid are significantly associated with recurrent aphthous ulcers.

PATIENT EDUCATION

- Avoid
  - Acidic food or drink
  - Abrasive, hard foods
  - Sodium laurel sulfate–containing toothpaste
- Behavior modification to reduce dental trauma with toothbrush or bruxism
- Maintain proper nutrition.

PROGNOSIS

Varies from single or infrequent recurrences of few, mild, self-resolving lesions to chronic, large, or deep painful lesions; symptoms improve with age.

COMPLICATIONS

- Aphthous ulcers can provide a site for infection and can leave scars.
- Disability from ulcers can affect mental health

REFERENCES

1. Lau CB, Smith GP. Recurrent aphthous stomatitis: A comprehensive review and recommendations on therapeutic options. *Dermatol Ther*. 2022;35(6):e15500.
2. Benahmed AG, Noor S, Menzel A, et al. Oral aphthous: pathophysiology, clinical aspects and medical treatment. *Arch Razi Inst*. 2021;76(5):1155–1163.
3. Edgar NR, Saleh D, Miller RA. Recurrent aphthous stomatitis: a review. *J Clin Aesthet Dermatol*. 2017;10(3):26–36.

ADDITIONAL READING

Wang Z, Cao H, Xiong J, et al. Recent advances in the aetiology of recurrent aphthous stomatitis (RAS). *Postgrad Med J*. 2022;98(1155):57–66.

 CODES

ICD10

K12.0 Recurrent oral aphthae

CLINICAL PEARLS

- Aphthous ulcers are the most common chronic disease of the oral cavity.
- Most cases are mild, self-limited episodes.
- Appropriate treatment should be aimed at symptom control and promotion of healing.
- Nonhealing ulcers, extraoral involvement, and sudden onset in adulthood require additional workup.

ULCERATIVE COLITIS

Etny Raul Candelario, MD, MS • Maureen Alvarado, DO

 BASICS

DESCRIPTION

- Ulcerative colitis (UC), one of the two inflammatory bowel disease, is a chronic disease characterized by diffuse mucosal inflammatory changes limited to the colon.
- Most cases involve the rectum or terminal colon and may extend proximally in a continuous fashion involving part or the entire large intestine (pan-ulcerative colitis) (1).
- Frequently manifested by recurrent episodes of bloody and mucoid diarrhea often associated with abdominal pain, rectal urgency, stool incontinence, fever, and weight loss
- Clinical course includes exacerbations and spontaneous or treatment-induced remissions.
- Colonic involvement is universal and may be accompanied by other systemic manifestations including large joint arthritis, ocular inflammation, skin lesions, biliary disease, liver disease, thromboembolic disease, and pulmonary complications.

EPIDEMIOLOGY

Prevalence
Because UC is commonly diagnosed in young people and has relatively low mortality, prevalence may continue to rise:
- North America: 249/100,000 persons
- Europe: 505/100,000 persons

ETIOLOGY AND PATHOPHYSIOLOGY

- Idiopathic inflammatory disorder; hypothesized to result from autoimmune dysfunction in response to colonic microbiome, genetic predisposition, and distinct risk factors
- Almost universally associated with inflammation of the terminal colon. >95% of patients have rectal involvement, 50% have disease limited to the rectum and sigmoid, and 20% have pancolitis. The absence of rectal involvement has been noted in <5% of adult patients and in up to 1/3 of pediatric patients.

Genetics
- Genetic factors contribute to IBD susceptibility.
- Several genetic syndromes have been associated with IBD (Turner syndrome, Hermansky-Pudlak syndrome, and glycogen storage disease type 1b).

RISK FACTORS

- Incidence rates were highest among persons 20 to 40 years old.
- Incidence rates of IBD are higher in white and Jewish people.
- Increasing incidence of UC in developing nations suggest that UC may be influenced by environmental factors.
- Having multiple family members with UC (2)
- Theorized risk factors include disruption of the colonic microbiome by enteric infection, dietary factors (Western diet in particular), antibiotic use, lack of breastfeeding in infant, obesity, and NSAID use.

GENERAL PREVENTION

Smoking may lower the risk of UC.

Pregnancy Considerations
- Patient should be advised to conceive during remission if planning a pregnancy.
  - Given the higher risk of thromboembolism in patients with UC, an estrogen-free contraceptive is preferred (2).

- Variable disease course in pregnancy seems to mirror disease state at conception; 3 to 6 months of remission before conceiving decreases the risks of an exacerbation during pregnancy (2).
- There is increased risk of preterm delivery and small for gestational age in women with active disease.
- Incidence rate of offspring from a UC mother of having UC is 3.7 (absolute rate of 1.6%).
- Ideally, pregnant women should be monitored by both gastroenterologist and maternal–fetal medicine specialist (2).

Pediatric Considerations
- Breastfeeding may protect against pediatric IBD.
- Pancolonic involvement is more likely at onset with shorter time from diagnosis to colectomy (median 11 years) than adults.

COMMONLY ASSOCIATED CONDITIONS

- Arthritis: large joint, sacroiliitis, ankylosing spondylitis (common)
- Aphthous ulcers (common)
- Erythema nodosum (common)
- Osteoporosis (common)
- Fatty liver (common)
- Episcleritis and uveitis (rare)
- Autoimmune liver disease (rare)
- Liver cirrhosis (rare)
- Primary sclerosing cholangitis (rare)
- Bile duct carcinoma (rare)
- Thromboembolic disease (rare)
- Pyoderma gangrenosum (rare)
- Colon cancer (rare)
- Anemia (rare)
- Pulmonary diseases (very rare)

DIAGNOSIS

HISTORY

- Symptoms may include:
  - Small frequent bloody or mucoid diarrhea associated with tenesmus, rectal urgency, fecal incontinence and abdominal pain; onset is gradual and progressive over weeks.
  - Weight loss, anorexia, fatigue, and anemia
  - Extraintestinal manifestation including joint, skin, ocular, oral, hepatobiliary-related symptoms
- Assess for potential precipitating factors:
  - Recent smoking cessation
  - NSAID use
  - Enteric infection like Clostridium difficile infection (may be a differential or superimposed with UC) (1)
- Assess for a family history of IBD.
- Predominant age of onset: 15 to 30 years; smaller peak in ages 50 to 80 years
- About 50% of all patient diagnosed with UC have a relapse or exacerbation in any year.

PHYSICAL EXAM

- Exam may often be normal.
- Weight loss
- Signs of fluid depletion (tachycardia, low blood pressure)
- Signs of anemia (pallor)
- Abdominal tenderness or tenderness
- Presence of blood on rectal exam
- Severe disease: fever, hypotension, tachycardia, pallor, loss of subcutaneous fat, muscle atrophy, peripheral edema, clubbing

DIFFERENTIAL DIAGNOSIS

- Crohn disease
- Infectious colitis: bacterial, parasitic, or viral (cytomegalovirus [CMV])
- Ischemic colitis
- Pseudomembranous colitis (C. difficile infection)
- Irritable bowel syndrome
- Diverticular colitis
- Diversion colitis in patients with prior bowel surgery
- Medication-induced colitis
- Radiation colitis
- Graft versus host disease
- Celiac disease

DIAGNOSTIC TESTS & INTERPRETATION

Initial Tests (lab, imaging)
- CBC: leukocytosis and anemia
- BMP: abnormal urea and electrolytes, especially hypokalemia
- LFTs: can be abnormal; low albumin indicates severe disease.
- ESR or CRP may be elevated, especially in more severe disease.
- Vitamin B_{12} and folate levels
- Fecal calprotectin (FC): elevated; (levels >782 μg/g differentiate acute severe colitis from mild to moderate UC). FC may also used to differentiate IBD from irritable bowel syndrome (1).
- Stool studies to rule out infectious cause: C. difficile (CDI in newly diagnosed or relapsing IBD ranges from 5% to 47%), stool cultures, Shiga toxin, ova and parasite microscopy, Giardia antigen (1)
- STI testing to rule out proctitis, particularly in men who have sexual with men
- Abdominal x-ray to exclude dangerous colonic dilation and assess disease severity

Follow-Up Tests & Special Considerations
FC can be used to monitor disease severity in relapsing UC in response to treatment (1).

Diagnostic Procedures/Other
Diagnosis of UC requires examination with lower gastrointestinal endoscopy with biopsies:
- Complete colonoscopy with at least two biopsies from each of five sites along the entire colon (unaffected and affected areas) (1)
- Complete colonoscopy in severe UC may be contraindicated due to risk of perforation or precipitation of toxic megacolon. In this case, a sigmoidoscopy with biopsy may be more appropriate (1).

Test Interpretation
- Endoscopic findings: mucosal engorgement with vascular markings, mucosal erythema, friability, erosions, and granularity. In severe UC, deep ulcerations and active bleeding may be found. Affected areas will most likely include the rectum and extend proximally and continuously (1).
- Histologic findings: mucosal separation, distortion, and atrophy of the crypts; chronic inflammatory cells in lamina propria; lymphocytes and plasma cells in crypt bases
- Rectal biopsy: Villous mucosal architecture and Paneth cells metaplasia support UC.

- Mild ileal inflammation ("backwash ileitis") may be present in UC.
- Characterize extent of disease according to Montreal classification: proctitis (within 18 cm of anal verge), left-sided colitis (sigmoid to splenic flexure), or extensive colitis (extension proximally from to the splenic flexure).

 TREATMENT

- Disease severity (see Table 1) and extent (i.e., proctitis, left-sided colitis vs. extensive colitis) dictate induction and maintenance treatment (1).
- Goals are to restore normal bowel function, reverse inflammatory changes, and to maintain a steroid-free remission without extraintestinal manifestations (1).

MEDICATION

First Line

- Induction of remission in mildly active UC:
  - Proctitis
    - Rectal 5-ASA 1 g/day (1)[A] or oral 5-ASA (1)[B]
    - If 5-ASA fails, add budesonide MMX 9 mg/day (1)[B].
    - If 5-ASA fails, use oral systemic corticosteroid (1)[C].
  - Left-sided colitis
    - Rectal 5-ASA 1 g/day (1)[A] and oral 5-ASA (1)[B]
    - If 5-ASA fails, use budesonide MMX 9 mg/day (1)[B].
    - If 5-ASA fails, use oral systemic corticosteroid (1)[C].
  - Extensive
    - Oral 5-ASA 2 g/day (1)[B]
    - If 5-ASA fails, use budesonide MMX 9 mg/day (1)[B].
    - If 5-ASA fails, use oral systemic corticosteroid (1)[C].
  - Reassess within 6 weeks to determine response to induction therapy.
- Maintenance of remission in patient with previously mild active UC:
  - Proctitis
    - Rectal 5-ASA 1 g/day (1)[B]
  - Left-side colitis
    - Oral 5-ASA (1)[B]
  - Extensive
    - Oral 5-ASA (1)[B]
- Induction of remission in moderate to severe active UC:
  - Moderate
    - Budesonide MMX (1)[B]
  - Moderate to severe

- Anti-TNF therapy (adalimumab, golimumab, infliximab) (1)[A]
  - If infliximab is used, use in addition with thiopurine (1)[B].
  - Vedolizumab (1)[B]
  - Tofacitinib 10 mg BID for 8 weeks (1)[B]
  - Oral systemic corticosteroid (1)[B]
  - If anti-TNF therapy fails, use vedolizumab or tofacitinib (1)[B].
- Maintenance of remission in patient with previously moderate to severe active UC:
  - Corticosteroid induction, use thiopurine (1)[C].
  - Anti-TNF induction, continue anti-TNF (1)[B].
  - Vedolizumab induction, continue vedolizumab (1)[B].
  - Tofacitinib induction, continue tofacitinib (1)[B].
- Maintenance of remission in patient with previously acute ulcerative colitis (ASUC):
  - Infliximab induction, continue infliximab (1)[B]
  - Cyclosporine induction, thiopurine (1)[C] or vedolizumab (1)[C]

Pediatric Considerations

- Pediatric growth and development can be affected due to malabsorption.
- Avoid live vaccines (rotavirus) in the first 6 months of life of infant born to mother with UC with exposure to biologic therapy (except certolizumab) (2).

Pregnancy Considerations

- Stop methotrexate at least 3 months prior to conceiving. It is contraindicated in pregnancy.
- In general, aminosalicylate, biologic, and immunomodulator therapies may be continued during pregnancy and lactation.

SURGERY/OTHER PROCEDURES

- Surgery is indicated for those who refractory or intolerant to medical therapy (high-dose steroids).
- Total colectomy with ileostomy is curative.

ADMISSION, INPATIENT, AND NURSING CONSIDERATIONS

Initiate IV corticosteroids and rule out infectious etiologies (*C. difficile*, CMV, *Shigella*/amoeba).

 ONGOING CARE

FOLLOW-UP RECOMMENDATIONS

Patient Monitoring

- UC patient should be screened for anxiety and depression (1).
- Assess for colorectal carcinoma (CRC) or dysplasia with surveillance colonoscopy

DIET

NPO during acute exacerbations

PATIENT EDUCATION

Crohn and Colitis Foundation of America (CCFA): http://www.ccfa.org/

PROGNOSIS

- Poor prognostic factors as measured by the likelihood of colectomy (1):
  - <40 years old at prognosis
  - Extensive UC
  - Severe endoscopic disease
  - Previous hospitalization for colitis
  - Elevated CRP
  - Low serum albumin
- Variable: Mortality for initial attack is ~5%; 75–85% experience relapse; up to 20% require colectomy.
- Colon cancer risk is the single most important factor affecting long-term prognosis.
- Left-sided colitis and ulcerative proctitis have favorable prognoses with probable normal lifespan.

COMPLICATIONS

- Perforation: Treat toxic megacolon with prompt surgery. Limit colonoscopies in severe disease.
- Obstruction
- Anemia
- Fulminant colitis
- Toxic megacolon
- Liver disease
- Stricture formation
- Osteoporosis
- Colorectal cancer

REFERENCES

1. Rubin DT, Ananthakrishnan AN, Siegel CA, et al. ACG clinical guideline: ulcerative colitis in adults. *Am J Gastroenterol*. 2019;114(3):384–413.
2. Mahadevan U, Robinson C, Bernasko N, et al. Inflammatory bowel disease in pregnancy clinical care pathway: a report from the American Gastroenterological Association IBD Parenthood Project Working Group. *Gastroenterology*. 2019;156(5):1508–1524.

 SEE ALSO

Algorithm: Hematemesis (Bleeding, Upper Gastrointestinal)

 CODES

ICD10

- K51.90 Ulcerative colitis, unspecified, without complications
- K51.919 Ulcerative colitis, unspecified with unspecified complications
- K51.80 Other ulcerative colitis without complications

CLINICAL PEARLS

- Diffuse, uninterrupted colonic mucosal inflammation
- The hallmark symptom is bloody diarrhea.
- Common medical treatments include 5-ASA, steroids, and anti–TNF-α therapy.
- Refractory disease or severe complications may require surgical intervention.
- Annual or biannual surveillance colonoscopy after 8 to 10 years of colitis due to increased risk of colorectal cancer (1)

Table 1. Activity index of UC (1)

Symptom/Labs	Remission	Mild	Moderate-Severe	Fulminant
Stools (no./d)	Formed stools	<4	>6	>10
Blood in stools	None	Intermittent	Frequent	Continuous
Urgency	None	Mild/occasional	Often	Continuous
Hemoglobin	Normal	Normal	<75% of normal	Transfusion required
ESR	<30	<30	>30	>30
CRP (mg/L)	Normal	Elevated	Elevated	Elevated
FC (μg/g)	<150–200	>150–200	>150–200	>150–200
Endoscopy (Mayo subscore)	0–1	1	2–3	3
UCEIS	0–1	2–4	5–8	7–8

Adapted from Rubin DT, Ananthakrishnan AN, Siegel CA, et al. ACG clinical guideline: ulcerative colitis in adults. *Am J Gastroenterol*. 2019;114(3):384–413.

U

Chirag N. Shah, MD • William Andrew Pleasant, MD • Ashley Asensio, DO

BASICS

DESCRIPTION
- Inflammation of the urethra
- Common manifestation of sexually transmitted infection (STI)
- Frequently associated with dysuria, pruritus, and/or urethral discharge; classified as gonococcal (caused by *Neisseria gonorrhoeae*) and nongonococcal (caused by other bacteria, or less common autoimmune disorders [Reiter syndrome], trauma, or chemical irritation)

EPIDEMIOLOGY

Incidence
- In 2021, there were 1,644,416 reported cases of chlamydia, the most commonly reported bacterial STI, which is a 4.1% increase from 2020.
- Young people aged 14 to 25 years comprise 2/3 of newly diagnosed chlamydial infections.
- About 1 in 20 young women between 14 and 24 years of age have chlamydia.
- In 2021, there were 710,151 reported cases of gonorrhea, the second most commonly reported bacterial STI; rates of gonorrhea have increased by 118% since 2009.
- For both chlamydia and gonorrhea, rates have increased among men and women, among most age groups, as well as among most racial/ethnic groups.
- In 2021, there were a total of 176,713 reported cases of syphilis.
- The number of primary and secondary syphilis cases—the most infectious stages of syphilis—increased 28.6% to 53,767 cases from 2020 to 2021.

ETIOLOGY AND PATHOPHYSIOLOGY
- Most common cause is infection via sexual transmission of *N. gonorrhoeae*, a gram-negative diplococcus.
- *N. gonorrhoeae* is a gram-negative diplococcus that interacts with nonciliated epithelial cells → cellular invasion → inflammation, neutrophil production, and bacterial cell phagocytosis.
- Sexually transmitted *Chlamydia trachomatis* infection is the most common cause of nongonococcal urethritis.
- Other established pathogens:
  - *Mycoplasma genitalium*
  - *Trichomonas vaginalis*
  - *Ureaplasma urealyticum*
  - Herpes simplex virus (rare)
  - Adenovirus (rare)
- Noninfectious causes (less common):
  - Chemical irritants (i.e., soaps, shampoos, douches, spermicides)
  - Foreign bodies
  - Urethral instrumentation

RISK FACTORS
- Age 15 to 24 years
- New sex partner
- One or more sex partner(s)
- History of coexisting STI
- Sex partner with concurrent partner(s)
- Inconsistent condom use outside a mutually monogamous relationship
- Exchanging sex for money or drugs
- Member of population with increased prevalence of infection, including incarcerated populations, military recruits, and economically disadvantaged populations

GENERAL PREVENTION
- Use of male condoms, female condoms, or cervical diaphragms
- Abstinence or reduction in the number of sex partners
- Behavioral counseling

COMMONLY ASSOCIATED CONDITIONS

> **ALERT**
> Annual chlamydia and gonorrhea screening is recommended for all sexually active women aged 24 years or younger as well as women aged 25 years and older with risk factors (B recommendation). There is insufficient evidence to recommend screening in men (1)[A].

DIAGNOSIS

- Chief complaint
  - Urethral discharge (mucopurulent suggestive of *N. gonorrhoeae*)
  - Dysuria
  - Erythema of the urethral meatus
  - Symptom onset 2 to 8 days following exposure
- History
  - Sexual history, including condom use, number of partners, sexual behaviors
  - Previous STIs
  - Substance use
  - Recent travel
  - Symptoms indicative of complications or additional sites of infection (i.e., men: testicular pain and swelling, anal itching, rectal pain or bleeding; women: lower abdominal pain, dyspareunia, irregular vaginal bleeding)
- Male genitourinary (GU) exam (possible findings)
  - Urethral discharge
  - Meatal erythema
  - Testicular tenderness
  - Palpate scrotum to check for epididymitis or orchitis.
  - Assess for ulcers.
  - Assess for inguinal lymphadenopathy.
- Female GU exam (possible findings)
  - Vaginal discharge
  - Endocervical discharge, hyperemia, and/or friability

Pediatric Considerations
Pediatric infections with gonorrhea and chlamydia after the neonatal period strongly suggest sexual contact. If indicated, investigations should be initiated promptly (2)[C].

DIFFERENTIAL DIAGNOSIS
- Other GU tract diseases:
  - Cystitis/urinary tract infection
  - Epididymitis
  - Prostatitis
  - Pelvic inflammatory disease (PID)
  - Pyelonephritis
- Vaginal atrophy, especially in postmenopausal women
- Stevens-Johnson syndrome
- Reiter syndrome: uveitis, urethritis, arthritis
- Wegener granulomatosis
- Urethral syndrome (pain without infection or purulence), longstanding or intermittent symptoms

DIAGNOSTIC TESTS & INTERPRETATION

> **ALERT**
> Health care providers are required to report all gonorrhea and chlamydia infections in accordance with local and state requirements.

Initial Tests (lab, imaging)
- Gonorrhea
  - Nucleic acid amplification test (NAAT)
  - Sensitivity: 90–100%
  - Specificity: 97–100%
  - Preferred specimen collection in first void (men) and vaginal swab (women)
  - Tissue culture was the traditional gold standard but typically only used now in cases of suspected chlamydial pneumonia or chlamydial opthalmia (2)[C].
- Chlamydia
  - NAAT
  - Sensitivity: 85–95%
  - Specificity: 93–99%
  - Preferred specimen collection is the same as for gonorrhea.
  - Tissue culture was the traditional gold standard but is currently NOT recommended.
- Gram stain diagnosis criteria:
  - Urethral secretions with ≥2 WBC per oil immersion
  - Mucopurulent or purulent discharge
  - First void urine sediment with ≥10 WBC per high-power field
  - Symptom onset 2 to 8 days following exposure
- Methylene blue/gentian violet [MB/GV]
  - Alternative to gram staining
  - Does not require heat fixation
  - Sensitivity: 97.3% (same as gram stain)
- If concern for *Trichomonas*: NAAT (urine, urethral, vaginal, or endocervical swab), wet mount, or culture
- There is no FDA-approved diagnostic test available for *M. genitalium*, an emerging pathogen with a greater prevalence than gonorrhea in many populations.

> **ALERT**
> Due to the similarity in clinical symptoms and high rates of coinfection, cotesting for gonorrhea and chlamydia infection is recommended. In addition, given that risk factors for gonorrhea and chlamydia indicate risks for other STIs, screening for HIV, syphillis (RPR), hepatitis B, and hepatitis C may also be indicated.

Follow-Up Tests & Special Considerations

- Test of cure (TOC) for chlamydia and gonorrhea is recommended in pregnant women or when treatment noncompliance is suspected.
- Repeat testing in 3 months is recommended due to rates of reinfection.
- HIV infection: Persons with HIV infection should receive the same treatment as patients without HIV infection.

Diagnostic Procedures/Other

Cystourethroscopy for cases with suspected foreign body, intraurethral warts, or urethral stricture

Test Interpretation

Urethral strictures (untreated gonorrhea), intraurethral lesions (venereal warts, congenital anomalies), PID, or tubo-ovarian abscesses are possible.

 ## TREATMENT

- Most cases can be treated in the outpatient setting.
- Single-dose regimens with direct observation preferred
- If either gonorrhea or chlamydia is suspected, treatment of BOTH gonorrhea and chlamydia is usually indicated.

MEDICATION

CDC recommendations
- Chlamydia
  - Preferred regimen:
    ○ Doxycycline 100 mg PO BID for 7 days
  - Alternative regimens:
    ○ Azithromycin 1 g PO single dose
      ■ Increasing resistance; no longer first line in the general population
      ■ Still the preferred regimen during pregnancy
    ○ Levofloxacin 500 mg PO QD for 7 days
    ○ Amoxicillin 500 mg PO TID for 7 days
  - Alternative regimen during pregnancy
- Gonorrhea
  - Preferred regimen:
    ○ Ceftriaxone 500 mg IM single dose (if weight <150 kg) OR 1 g IM (if weight >150 kg) single dose
  - Alternative regimens:
    ○ Gentamicin 240 mg IM single dose *plus* azithromycin 2 g PO single dose
    ○ Cefixime 800 mg PO single dose
- *Trichomonas*
  - Metronidazole 2 g PO single dose for men
  - Metronidazole 500 mg PO BID for 7 days for women
- Recurrent and persistent urethritis
  - If doxycycline was initially used, consider repeating doxycycline, or trial of moxifloxacin 400 mg PO QD for 7 days *or* azithromycin 1 g PO single dose, with TOC
- General considerations
  - Contraindications: sensitivity to any of the indicated medications
  - Precautions: Patients taking tetracyclines may have increased photosensitivity.
  - Significant possible interactions:
    ○ Tetracyclines should not be taken with milk products or antacids.
    ○ Oral contraceptives may be rendered less effective by oral antibiotics. Patients and partners should use a backup method of birth control for the remainder of the cycle.

Pregnancy Considerations

- Chlamydia:
  - Screen all pregnant patients.
  - All pregnant women at increased risk should be screened for chlamydia at their prenatal visit and again in the 3rd trimester.
  - TOC 3 weeks after therapy to check for chlamydial eradication and retest in 3 months
  - Azithromycin 1 g PO single dose
  - Alternative regimens:
    ○ Amoxicillin 500 mg PO TID for 7 days
- Gonorrhea:
  - Screen all pregnant patients.
  - All pregnant women at increased risk should be screened for chlamydia at their prenatal visit and again in the 3rd trimester.
  - TOC 3 weeks after therapy to check for gonococcal eradication and retest in 3 months
  - Tetracyclines and fluoroquinolones are contraindicated.
  - Ceftriaxone 500 mg IM single dose
  - If cephalosporin allergy is present, infectious disease consult is recommended.

 ## ONGOING CARE

FOLLOW-UP RECOMMENDATIONS

- Sexual activity should be avoided for 7 days following administration of single-dose therapy or until completion of multiday regimen.
- All sexual partners who came in contact with the patient within 60 days should be referred for evaluation, testing, and presumptive treatment.
- Expedited partner therapy (EPT)—the practice of treating the diagnosed patient's sex partner(s) for chlamydia or gonorrhea by providing medications to the partner(s) without clinical evaluation is an acceptable alternative.

Patient Monitoring

- Instruct patients to return if symptoms persist or recur after completing treatment.
- Screen for reinfection in all patients at 3 months.

PATIENT EDUCATION

- Behavioral counseling interventions are recommended. Evidence of benefit increases with intensity of intervention.
- Successful approaches include basic information about STIs and transmission, assess risk for transmission, include training skills (i.e., condom use, communication about safe sex, problem solving, goal setting).

PROGNOSIS

If the diagnosis is firmly established, appropriate medications are prescribed, and the patient is compliant with treatment, relief of symptoms occurs within days, and the problem should resolve without sequela.

COMPLICATIONS

- Stricture formation
- Epididymitis
- Prostatitis
- PID in women
- Disseminated gonococcal infection
- Gonococcal meningitis
- Gonococcal endocarditis
- Perinatal transmission (chlamydial conjunctivitis, chlamydial pneumonia, ophthalmia neonatorum)
- Reiter syndrome
- Chronic cervical chlamydial infection has been proposed to increase the risk of cervical cancer.

REFERENCES

1. US Preventive Services Task Force. Screening for chlamydia and gonorrhea: US Preventive Services Task Force recommendation statement. *JAMA*. 2021;326(10):949–956.
2. Workowski KA, Bachmann LH, Chan PA, et al. Sexually transmitted infections treatment guidelines, 2021. *MMWR Recomm Rep*. 2021;70(4):1–187.

 ## SEE ALSO

- Chlamydia Infection (Sexually Transmitted); Epididymitis; Gonococcal Infections; Pelvic Inflammatory Disease; Prostatitis; Urinary Tract Infection (UTI) in Females; Urinary Tract Infection (UTI) in Males; Vulvovaginitis, Estrogen Deficient; Vulvovaginitis, Prepubescent
- Algorithms: Dysuria; Genital Ulcers; Urethral Discharge

 ## CODES

ICD10

- N34.2 Other urethritis
- A56.01 Chlamydial cystitis and urethritis
- A54.01 Gonococcal cystitis and urethritis, unspecified

CLINICAL PEARLS

- Urethritis is inflammation of the urethra, frequently associated with dysuria, pruritus, and/or urethral discharge.
- NAAT preferred method of diagnosis for men and women
- If either gonorrhea or chlamydia is suspected, treatment of BOTH gonorrhea and chlamydia is usually indicated.
- In cases of gonorrhea or chlamydia infection, in-person follow-up or EPT recommended for all partners of patients within the last 60 days
- Given that risk factors for gonorrhea and chlamydia indicate risk for other STIs, screening for HIV, syphilis (RPR), hepatitis B, and hepatitis C may also be indicated.
- Repeat testing for gonorrhea and chlamydia in 3 months is recommended due to rates of reinfection.
- Treatment in persons with HIV infection is the same as in patients without HIV infection.

U

URINARY TRACT INFECTION (UTI) IN FEMALES

Akhil Das, MD, FACS • James F. Jiang, MD

 BASICS

DESCRIPTION

- Urinary tract infection (UTI) is the presence of pathogenic microorganisms within the urinary tract and associated symptoms (dysuria, urinary urgency/frequency, hematuria, new or worsening incontinence).
- Uncomplicated UTI: infection in patients with an unobstructed and anatomically normal urinary tract, with no predisposing risk factors, and whose symptoms are confined to the lower urinary tract
- Complicated UTI: infection of the urinary tract in the presence of an anatomic or functional abnormality, immunocompromised host, or presence of a multi-drug resistant organism (See "Risk Factors.")
- Recurrent UTI: symptomatic UTI that occurs following complete treatment and resolution of documented infection; two or more culture-proven infections in 6 months or three or more in 12 months; affects 20–40% of women with prior cystitis episodes (1)
- Asymptomatic bacteriuria: presence of bacteria in urine without reports of associated symptoms
- Synonym(s): cystitis

EPIDEMIOLOGY

UTI among women is an extremely common occurrence.

Incidence
- Accounts for 10.5 million office visits and 2 to 3 million emergency room visits; contributes to >100,000 hospital admissions each year with a cost of >$2.6 billion annually
- Primarily affects young adults and older adults; predominantly female > male

Prevalence
- Up to 60% of females have at least one UTI in their lifetime, and 11% report having at least one per year.
- 1/4 of women with uncomplicated UTI experience a second UTI within 6 months and half at some time during their lifetime.

ETIOLOGY AND PATHOPHYSIOLOGY
- Ascension of bacteria into the bladder via the urethra is the most common etiology.
- Pathogenic organisms possess adherence factors (pili or fimbriae) and toxins that allow initiation and propagation of genitourinary infections.
- Most UTIs are caused by bacteria originating from bowel flora:
  - *Escherichia coli* is the causative organism in 80–85% of cases of uncomplicated cystitis.
  - *Staphylococcus saprophyticus* accounts for 10–15% of infections.
  - *Klebsiella pneumoniae* and *Proteus mirabilis* each account for approximately 4%.

Genetics
Women with human leukocyte antigen 3 (HLA-3) and nonsecretor Lewis antigen have an increased bacterial adherence, which may lead to an increased risk in UTI.

RISK FACTORS
- Biologic:
  - Urinary stasis/obstruction: pelvic organ prolapse, bladder diverticula, neurogenic bladder, voiding dysfunction, urethral stricture, anatomic anomalies of the lower urinary tract
  - Urinary calculi
  - Immunosuppression: diabetes, HIV, steroid use, malignancy, malnutrition
- Behavioral practices that promote colonization: sexual intercourse, spermicide, estrogen depletion, antimicrobial use, poor hygiene

GENERAL PREVENTION
- Mitigate urinary obstruction or stasis.
- Adequate hydration
- Women with frequent or intercourse-related UTI should empty bladder immediately before and following intercourse.
- Avoid feminine hygiene sprays, diaphragms, spermicidal agents, and douches.
- Wipe urethra from front to back.
- Vaginal estrogen in postmenopausal women may aid in preventing recurrent UTI.

COMMONLY ASSOCIATED CONDITIONS
See "Risk Factors."

Geriatric Considerations
- Elderly patients are more likely to have underlying urinary tract abnormality or voiding dysfunction.
  - Poor perineal hygiene, urinary or fecal incontinence, and pelvic organ prolapse are common risk factors.
  - Decreased estrogen levels increase vaginal pH and alter microbial flora, leading to increased colonization.
- May present with atypical symptoms such as altered mental status or urinary incontinence
- Treatment of asymptomatic bacteriuria does not improve outcomes and should be avoided due to associated morbidity.

Pediatric Considerations
Bowel bladder dysfunction or congenital urinary tract abnormalities such as vesicoureteral reflux (VUR) or duplicated collecting system are risk factors.

 DIAGNOSIS

HISTORY
- Dysuria, urgency, frequency, sensation of incomplete bladder emptying, hematuria, suprapubic pain, malodorous urine, altered mental status, nocturia, sudden onset or worsening of urinary incontinence, dyspareunia
- Number of UTIs, recent sexual activity, or new sexual partner(s)

PHYSICAL EXAM
- Suprapubic tenderness
- Urethral and/or vaginal tenderness; evaluate for diverticulum or other urethral masses.
- Fever or costovertebral angle tenderness indicates upper tract infection.

DIFFERENTIAL DIAGNOSIS
Vaginal infection, STDs causing urethritis or pyuria, neoplasm, calculi, interstitial cystitis

DIAGNOSTIC TESTS & INTERPRETATION

Initial Tests (lab, imaging)
- Clean catch midstream voided urine may be contaminated with either vaginal or perineal organisms. Suspect contamination when growth of normal vaginal flora (lactobacillus) or mixed cultures with more than one organism arise.
- Urinalysis (microscopic)
  - Pyuria (>10 neutrophils/high-power field [HPF])
  - Bacteriuria (any amount on unspun urine or five bacteria/HPF on centrifuged urine)
  - Hematuria (≥3 RBCs/HPF)
  - Squamous cells indicate poor collection/quality (>15 to 20 squamous cells/HPF is suggestive of contamination).
- Dipstick urinalysis
  - Leukocyte esterase (indicates presence of 5 to 15 WBC/HPF; 75–96% sensitivity, 94–98% specificity, when >100,000 colony-forming units [CFU])
  - Nitrite tests are specific, but not sensitive, if nitrite-reducing organisms (e.g., *E. coli, Klebsiella, Proteus*) are causative.
- Urine culture: not indicated in the setting of an uncomplicated UTI; necessary for patients with either unclear diagnosis, recurrent UTI, or complicated UTI

Follow-Up Tests & Special Considerations
- Empiric antibiotics may be given without urine culture for uncomplicated UTI. Guidelines recommend urine culture for recurrent or complicated UTI.
- Imaging may be indicated for UTIs in infants, immunocompromised patients, febrile infections, signs of urinary obstruction, or recurrent UTI.
- CT or MR urogram provides detailed anatomic information but should generally only be considered in patients with recurrent UTIs or have known risk factors for anatomic abnormalities.

Pediatric Considerations
A renal bladder ultrasound or voiding cystourethrogram can evaluate pelvocaliectasis or ureteral dilatation or VUR.

Diagnostic Procedures/Other
- If the urine specimen is suspected to be contaminated, a catheterized specimen may be necessary.
- Suprapubic bladder aspiration or urethral catheterization can be used to obtain specimens from infants, although these methods are more invasive.
- Cystourethroscopy can be used to evaluate patients with recurrent UTIs, history of nephrolithiasis, previous anti-incontinence surgery, or hematuria in the absence of an active infection.

Test Interpretation
See "Initial Tests (lab, imaging)."

TREATMENT

GENERAL MEASURES
- Asymptomatic bacteriuria in a nonpregnant woman should not be treated with antibiotics (2).
- Maintain adequate hydration with at least 2 L of water daily.
- Many women with uncomplicated UTI have resolution without treatment and rarely progress to serious infections.

MEDICATION
First Line
Phenazopyridine 100 to 200 mg TID is a urinary topical analgesic and should only be used for rapid symptom relief, not definitive treatment. Urinalysis interpretation on this medication may be inaccurate by identifying the urine as nitrite positive. In addition, this medication obscures interpretation of leukocyte esterase on the urinalysis. However, urine culture results are not impacted by this medication. NSAIDs may also offer some relief of UTI symptoms.

- Uncomplicated UTI:
  – Trimethoprim/sulfamethoxazole (TMP/SMX; Bactrim): 160/800 mg PO BID for 3 days, best where resistance of *E. coli* strains <20%; rash may be higher than with other antibiotics; preferred as first line
  – Nitrofurantoin (Macrobid): 100 mg PO BID for 5 days should be used in patients with allergy to TMP/SMX and in areas where *E. coli* resistance to TMP/SMX >20%. Macrobid does not penetrate renal parenchyma and thus is ineffective in treating upper UTI. It should also be avoided if there is suspicion of early pyelonephritis or if the creatinine clearance is <30 mL/min. Its safety and efficacy have been evaluated for older women with mild renal impairment in observational studies.
  – Fosfomycin (Monurol): 3 g PO single dose; some studies have evaluated a higher dose (3 g once every 2 to 3 days for 3 doses) for infections resistant to treatment, but there is not enough evidence that this has greater efficacy than single-dose therapy (expensive).
- Lower UTI in pregnancy:
  – Nitrofurantoin: 100 mg PO BID for 7 days; discontinue at 35 weeks for risk of neonatal hemolytic anemia.
  – Cephalexin (Keflex): 500 mg PO BID for 7 days
  – TMP/SMX is avoided in pregnancy (especially in 1st and 3rd trimesters) due to risk of kernicterus.
  – Fluoroquinolones are not safe during pregnancy and are avoided in the treatment of children.
- Postcoital UTI: Single-dose TMP/SMX or cephalexin may reduce frequency of UTI in sexually active women.
- Complicated UTI: Extend course to 7 to 10 days; may begin with fluoroquinolone, TMP/SMX, or cephalosporin (Avoid using nitrofurantoin for complicated UTI due to lack of tissue penetration.)

Second Line
- Uncomplicated UTI
  – β-Lactams (amoxicillin/clavulanate, cefdinir, cefpodoxime) for 3 to 7 days
  – Fluoroquinolones should not be used in uncomplicated UTI due to risk of potentially irreversible adverse reactions, which may occur even with single doses (see FDA black box warnings regarding hypoglycemia, tendon rupture risk, neuropathy).
- Recurrent UTIs
  – Recurrent UTI treatment aims at the shortest antibiotic course with symptom resolution. Urine culture is required for these patients. Consider 3 to 6 months of daily suppressive antibiotic therapy, followed by observation for reinfection after discontinuing prophylaxis. Continuous antimicrobial prophylaxis involves daily low-dose TMP/SMX 80/400 mg or nitrofurantoin 50 to 100 mg.
  – Other options are patient-initiated treatment for early UTI symptoms (minimizes office visits, antibiotic use), postcoital prophylaxis, and intermittent-dosed prophylaxis (e.g., Monday-Wednesday-Friday).

Pediatric Considerations
Long-term antibiotics appear to reduce the risk of recurrent symptomatic UTI in susceptible children, but the benefit must be considered together with the increased risk of microbial resistance.

ISSUES FOR REFERRAL
Patients with recurrent or complicated UTIs should be referred to a urologist.

Pediatric Considerations
UTI in children, especially <1 year of age, should prompt referral to a pediatric urologist.

SURGERY/OTHER PROCEDURES
- Sepsis from urinary tract obstruction requires prompt drainage often in the setting of upper tract obstruction/dilation requiring ureteral stent or percutaneous nephrostomy tube.
- Children with febrile UTIs and VUR may be appropriate for antireflux surgery such as ureteral reimplantation.

COMPLEMENTARY & ALTERNATIVE MEDICINE
- *Vaccinium macrocarpon* (cranberry, not cranberry juice cocktail) may help to prevent and treat UTIs by inhibiting bacterial adherence to the bladder epithelium. Probiotic use for UTI prophylaxis or methenamine (Hiprex) can be used for recurrent UTIs.
- Vaginal estrogen can prevent recurrent UTIs in peri- and postmenopausal women.

ADMISSION, INPATIENT, AND NURSING CONSIDERATIONS
Inpatient evaluation is reserved for patients with complicated UTIs. Majority of uncomplicated UTIs are managed in an outpatient setting.

 ONGOING CARE

FOLLOW-UP RECOMMENDATIONS
First UTI: Reproductive-age and middle-age, nonpregnant females require no follow-up if UTI is clinically cured after 3-day therapy (2)[C]. Obtain urine culture if symptoms persist after 2 to 3 days of treatment.

Pregnancy Considerations
- During pregnancy, UTI always requires culture and usually requires a 7- to 14-day treatment.
- Following the treatment of acute infection, pregnant women warrant surveillance of urine cultures every trimester. They may receive prophylactic antibiotics for the remainder of pregnancy.

Patient Monitoring
- Repeat culture in asymptomatic patients after completing therapy for a UTI to document bacterial clearance is unnecessary and may promote overtreatment of asymptomatic bacteriuria (ASB).
- Obtain repeat urine cultures in patients with persistent symptoms after treatment. An empiric course of alternate antibiotics can be started but preferably after a urine sample is obtained.

DIET
Reduce/prevent glycosuria.

PATIENT EDUCATION
Urology Care Foundation: https://www.urologyhealth.org/

PROGNOSIS
Symptoms resolve within 2 to 3 days of antibiotic treatment in almost all patients.

COMPLICATIONS
Pyelonephritis or sepsis, renal abscess, urinary outlet obstruction

Pregnancy Considerations
Pregnant females, infants, and young children with cystitis are at higher risk of pyelonephritis.

REFERENCES
1. Gupta K, Trautner BW. Diagnosis and management of recurrent urinary tract infections in non-pregnant women. *BMJ*. 2013;346:f3140.
2. Anger J, Lee U, Ackerman AL, et al. Recurrent uncomplicated urinary tract infections in women: AUA/CUA/SUFU guideline. *J Urol*. 2019;202(2):282–289.

 SEE ALSO

Algorithm: Dysuria

CODES

ICD10
- N39.0 Urinary tract infection, site not specified
- N30.90 Cystitis, unspecified without hematuria
- N30.91 Cystitis, unspecified with hematuria

CLINICAL PEARLS
- Urine culture is generally not indicated for women with uncomplicated UTI.
- Uncomplicated UTIs should be treated for 3 days (TMP/SMX) or 5 days (nitrofurantoin). Pregnant women with bacteriuria should be treated due to risk of poor outcomes with incompletely or untreated UTI.
- Nonpregnant women with ASB should not be treated.

U

987

URINARY TRACT INFECTION (UTI) IN MALES

Suzanne Florczyk, PharmD • Laura Ross, MD

BASICS

DESCRIPTION
- Cystitis is an infection of the lower urinary tract usually resulting from a single gram-negative enteric bacteria (see also Prostatitis, Pyelonephritis, and Urethritis).
- System(s) affected: renal/urologic
- Synonym(s): urinary tract infection (UTI); cystitis
- In otherwise healthy males aged 15 to 50 years, UTI is uncommon and considered uncomplicated.
- In male newborns, infants, and elderly men, UTI is considered complicated, with associated functional/structural mechanisms.

EPIDEMIOLOGY
Incidence
- Predominant age: increases with age
- Uncommon in men <50 years of age; 6 to 8 infections per 10,000 men aged 21 to 50 years (1)

Prevalence
Lifetime prevalence approximately 14%

ETIOLOGY AND PATHOPHYSIOLOGY
- *Escherichia coli* (majority of infections)
- *Klebsiella* spp.
- *Enterobacter*
- *Enterococcus*
- *Proteus*
- *Citrobacter*
- *Providencia*
- *Streptococcus faecalis* and *Staphylococcus* sp.
- *Pseudomonas* and *Morganella* (more common in elderly and catheterized patients)
- Pathogenesis—bacterial entry into urinary tract via ascension or bladder instrumentation

Genetics
Not applicable

RISK FACTORS
- Age
- Obesity
- History of prior UTI
- Outlet obstruction
  - Benign prostatic hypertrophy (BPH)—incidence of 33% of men with UTIs (2)
  - Urethral stricture
  - Calculi
- Fecal incontinence
- Urinary incontinence
- Recent urologic surgery
- Urinary tract instrumentation/catheterization
- Infection of the prostate/kidney
- Immunocompromised
- Diabetes
- Bladder diverticula
- Neurogenic bladder
- Cognitive impairment
- Institutionalization
- Uncircumcised
- Anal intercourse
- Intercourse with an infected female partner (1)

GENERAL PREVENTION
- Prompt treatment of predisposing factors
- Use a catheter only when necessary; if needed, use aseptic technique and closed system and remove as soon as possible.
- Cranberry products are not recommended for preventing UTI.

COMMONLY ASSOCIATED CONDITIONS
- Acute bacterial pyelonephritis
- Chronic bacterial pyelonephritis
- Urethritis
- Prostatitis
- Prostatic hypertrophy
- Prostate cancer

Geriatric Considerations
Bacteriuria is more common among the elderly, usually is transient, and may be related to functional status. Of men >65 years of age, 5–10% have asymptomatic bacteriuria (ASB). If ASB is noted, no treatment is needed (1).

Pediatric Considerations
Can be associated with obstruction to normal flow of urine, such as vesicoureteral reflux. Unique diagnostic criteria and evaluation recommendations exist.

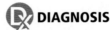**DIAGNOSIS**

HISTORY
- Urinary frequency
- Urinary urgency
- Dysuria
- Hesitancy
- Slow urinary stream
- Dribbling of urine
- Nocturia
- Suprapubic discomfort or perineal pain
- Constipation
- Low back pain
- Hematuria
- Systemic symptoms (chills, fever) or flank pain, nausea, vomiting present with concomitant pyelonephritis or prostatitis

PHYSICAL EXAM
- Suprapubic tenderness
- Costovertebral angle (CVA) tenderness and/or fever may be present with concomitant pyelonephritis/prostatitis/epididymitis.
- Perform genital examination.
- Consider digital rectal exam, including palpation of the prostate gland, to rule out bacterial prostatitis.

DIFFERENTIAL DIAGNOSIS
- Anatomic/functional pathology of the urinary tract
- Urethritis/STIs
- Infections in other sites of the genitourinary tract (e.g., epididymis, prostatitis). >90% of men with febrile UTI have concomitant prostate infection (1)[A].

DIAGNOSTIC TESTS & INTERPRETATION
- Urine dipstick/manual microscopy of clean catch midstream void showing the following:
  - Pyuria (>10 WBCs)
  - Bacteriuria
  - Leukocyte esterase is more sensitive, and nitrite is more specific in detecting UTI.
  - Positive leukocyte esterase (in males: sensitivity, 78%; specificity, 59%; positive predictive value [PPV], 71%; negative predictive value [NPV], 67%)
  - Positive nitrite (in males: sensitivity, 47%; specificity, 98%; PPV, 96%; NPV, 59%)

ALERT
All patients presenting with dysuria should be tested for STIs, as gonorrhea, chlamydia, and syphilis are epidemic in the United States.

- Automated microscopy/flow cytometry that measures cell counts and bacterial counts can be used to improve screening characteristics (sensitivity, 92%; specificity, 55%; PPV, 47%; NPV, 97%). The high NPV of these screening tests allows for more judicious use of urine culture.
- Urine culture: >100,000 colony-forming units (CFU; >10^5 CFU) of bacteria per milliliter of urine confirm diagnosis.
- Lower counts, such as >10^3 CFU, also may be indicative of infection, especially in the presence of pyuria.
- Diagnosis in infants and children <24 months old made on the basis of both pyuria and 50,000 CFU on culture
- Renal and bladder ultrasound recommended in infants and young children after first confirmed UTI

Follow-Up Tests & Special Considerations
- Consider assessing for risk factors for STIs because chlamydial/gonococcal urethritis can mimic a UTI. If risk factors are present, use urine nucleic acid amplification tests to identify gonococcal and *Chlamydia* infections and treat as necessary.
- Further urologic evaluation is warranted to rule out other disorders in men with recurrent UTI, febrile UTI, or pyelonephritis. This may include the following:
  - Ultrasound
  - Cystoscopy
  - Urodynamics
  - IV pyelography
- Value of a urologic evaluation in a single uncomplicated UTI has not been determined.
- Antibiotics prior to culture or phenazopyridine prior to urine dipstick can alter results.
- Blood cultures are not routine; perform if concern for sepsis or bacteremia.

Test Interpretation
Depends on site of infection

TREATMENT

- Catheter management: In general, avoid unnecessary catheterization.
- Minimize the use of indwelling catheters. Those who require extended catheterization should be managed by intermittent catheterization, if possible. There is no benefit of using prophylactic antibiotics to reduce the risk of catheter-associated UTIs.
- Exchange the Foley for acute infections when initiating antibiotics.

GENERAL MEASURES
- Hydration
- Analgesia, if required
- Aggressive treatment to prevent constipation with both soluble (psyllium) and insoluble (wheat germ) fiber
- Patient with indwelling catheters
  - If asymptomatic bacterial colonization, no need to treat (Sterilization of urine is not possible, and resistant organisms may take up residence.)
  - If symptomatic of acute infection, institute treatment.

MEDICATION
First Line
- Acute, uncomplicated cystitis
  - Treat empirically; strongly consider if nitrite positive, using local resistance patterns or based on culture and sensitivity results for 5–7 days.
  - For empirical therapy, a fluoroquinolone or trimethoprim-sulfamethoxazole DS usually used to treat the most likely pathogens. Fosfomycin, nitrofurantoin, and beta-lactams do not achieve reliable tissue concentration in the prostate.
- Complicated, febrile, or recurrent infection
  - Prescribe a minimum of 2 weeks antibiotics based on antimicrobial sensitivities with repeat urine check after the treatment. In men with febrile UTI or pyelonephritis, prostatic involvement also must be considered. Total duration of antimicrobial therapy generally ranges from 10 to 14 days. Five- to 7-day regiments of fluoroquinolones are comparable to longer durations. Treatment of concomitant prostatitis requires antimicrobials with good prostatic tissue and fluid penetration (fluoroquinolones).

Second Line
According to culture and sensitivity results and patient's history

ISSUES FOR REFERRAL
Further urologic evaluation and referral are warranted to rule out other disorders in male infants and men with recurrent UTI, febrile UTI, or pyelonephritis.

ADDITIONAL THERAPIES
- Probiotics
- Polyethylene glycol 3350 for constipation
- Phenazopyridine—limit use to 48 hours when used concomitantly with an antibacterial agent.

ADMISSION, INPATIENT, AND NURSING CONSIDERATIONS
- Inability to tolerate oral medications
- Acute renal failure
- Suspected sepsis

 ONGOING CARE

FOLLOW-UP RECOMMENDATIONS
Patient Monitoring
Any patients who have worsening symptoms following initiation of antimicrobials, persistent symptoms after 48 to 72 hours of appropriate therapy, or recurrent symptoms within a few weeks of treatment should have additional evaluation.

DIET
Encourage adequate fluid intake.

PATIENT EDUCATION
National Kidney Foundation: https://www.kidney.org

PROGNOSIS
Clearing of infections with appropriate antibiotic treatment

COMPLICATIONS
- Pyelonephritis
- Ascending infection
- Recurrent infection
- Prostatitis

REFERENCES
1. Wagenlehner FME, Weidner W, Pilatz A, et al. Urinary tract infections and bacterial prostatitis in men. *Curr Opin Infect Dis*. 2014;27(1):97–101.
2. Drekonja DM, Rector TS, Cutting A, et al. Urinary tract infection in male veterans: treatment patterns and outcomes. *JAMA Intern Med*. 2013;173(1):62–68.

ADDITIONAL READING
- Coupat C, Pradier C, Degand N, et al. Selective reporting of antibiotic susceptibility data improves the appropriateness of intended antibiotic prescriptions in urinary tract infections: a case-vignette randomised study. *Eur J Clin Microbiol Infect Dis*. 2013;32(5):627–636.
- Foxman B. Urinary tract infection syndromes: occurrence, recurrence, bacteriology, risk factors, and disease burden. *Infect Dis Clin North Am*. 2014;28(1):1–13.

 SEE ALSO

- Prostate Cancer; Prostatic Hyperplasia, Benign (BPH); Prostatitis; Pyelonephritis; Urethritis
- Algorithms: Dysuria; Urethral Discharge

 CODES

ICD10
- N39.0 Urinary tract infection, site not specified
- N30.90 Cystitis, unspecified without hematuria
- N30.91 Cystitis, unspecified with hematuria

CLINICAL PEARLS
- Cystitis is an infection of the lower urinary tract, usually resulting from a single gram-negative enteric bacteria.
- Risk factors/causes: age, obesity, history of UTI, BPH/outlet obstruction, incontinence, urinary tract instrumentation or catheterization, infection of the prostate/kidney, immunocompromised or diabetes, cognitive impairment, institutionalization, neurogenic bladder, uncircumcised, anal intercourse, intercourse with infected female partner
- Evaluation: urinalysis, urine culture, STI testing (e.g., gonorrhea, *Chlamydia* by culture/DNA probe)
- Treat empirically with fluoroquinolones or trimethoprim-sulfamethoxazole DS for 5 to 7 days.

U

UROLITHIASIS
Roland W. Newman II, DO

BASICS

DESCRIPTION
- Stone formation within the urinary tract: Urinary crystals bind to form a nidus, which grows to form a calculus (stone).
- Range of symptoms: asymptomatic to obstructive; febrile morbidity if result of infection

EPIDEMIOLOGY
- Vesical calculosis (bladder stones) due to malnutrition during early life is frequent in the Middle East and in Asian countries.
- Incidence in industrialized countries seems to be increasing, probably due to improved diagnostics and increasingly rich diets.
- Increased incidence in patients with surgically induced absorption issues (IBD, gastric bypass)

Incidence
- In industrialized countries: 100 to 200/100,000 per year
- Predominant age: Mean age is 40 to 60 years.
- Predominant sex: male > female (~3:1)

Prevalence
- 10–15% in the United States
- Lifetime risk of >14% in men, >6% in women
  - Incidence is increasing in female, pediatric, and adolescent populations.

ETIOLOGY AND PATHOPHYSIOLOGY
- Supersaturation and dehydration lead to high salt content in urine which congregates.
- Stasis of urine
  - Renal malformation (e.g., horseshoe kidney, ureteropelvic junction obstruction)
  - Incomplete bladder emptying (e.g., neurogenic bladder, prostate enlargement, multiple sclerosis)
- Crystals may form in pure solutions (homogeneous) or on existing surfaces, such as other crystals or cellular debris (heterogeneous).
- Balance of promoters and inhibitors: organic (Tamm-Horsfall protein, glycosaminoglycan, uropontin, nephrocalcin) and inorganic (citrate, pyrophosphate)
- Calcium oxalate and/or phosphate stones (80%)
  - Hypercalciuria
    ○ Absorptive hypercalciuria: increased jejunal calcium absorption
    ○ Renal leak: increased calcium excretion from renal proximal tubule
    ○ Resorptive hypercalciuria: mild hyperparathyroidism
  - Hypercalcemia
    ○ Hyperparathyroidism
    ○ Sarcoidosis
    ○ Malignancy
    ○ Immobilization
    ○ Paget disease

- Hyperoxaluria
  - Enteric hyperoxaluria
    ○ Intestinal malabsorptive state associated with irritable bowel syndrome, celiac sprue, or intestinal resection
    ○ Bile salt malabsorption leads to formation of calcium soaps.
  - Primary hyperoxaluria: autosomal recessive, types I and II
  - Dietary hyperoxaluria: overindulgence in oxalate-rich food
- Hyperuricosuria
  - Seen in 10% of calcium stone formers
  - Caused by increased dietary purine intake, systemic acidosis, myeloproliferative diseases, gout, chemotherapy, Lesch-Nyhan syndrome
  - Thiazides, probenecid
- Hypocitraturia
  - Caused by acidosis: renal tubular acidosis, malabsorption, thiazides, enalapril, excessive dietary protein
- Uric acid stones (10–15%): hyperuricemia causes as discussed earlier
- Struvite stones (5–10%): infected urine with urease-producing organisms (most commonly *Proteus* sp.)
- Cystine stones (<1%): autosomal recessive disorder of renal tubular reabsorption of cystine
- Bladder stones: seen with chronic bladder catheterization and some medications (indinavir)
- In children: usually due to malnutrition

Genetics
- Up to 20% of patients have a family history. However, spouses of those who form stones have higher calcium excretion rates than controls, suggesting strong dietary–environmental factors.
- Autosomal dominant: idiopathic hypercalciuria
- Autosomal recessive
  - Cystinuria, Lesch-Nyhan syndrome, hyperoxaluria types I and II
  - Ehlers-Danlos syndrome, Marfan syndrome, Wilson disease, familial renal tubular acidosis

RISK FACTORS
- White > Asian > African American
- Male
- Family history (increases risk by up to 2.5 times)
- Diet rich in protein, refined carbohydrates, and sodium; carbonated drinks; low calcium diet; low fluid intake
- Occupations associated with a sedentary lifestyle or with a hot, dry workplace
- Incidence rates peak during summer secondary to dehydration, hot climates.
- Obesity
- Surgically/medically induced malabsorption (Crohn disease, gastric bypass, celiac, primary hyperparathyroidism)
- Horseshoe kidney (incidence of 21–60%)
- Medications that can increase risk of forming calcium and uric acid stones
- Recent literature suggesting possible association between microbiome (gut and urinary) and urolithiasis

GENERAL PREVENTION
- Hydration (1)
- Decrease salt and meat intake.
- Avoid oxalate-rich foods.

Pediatric Considerations
- Increasing in prevalence due to obesity, diabetes, and hypertension
- Additional risk factor considerations include renal disease or immaturity, preterm birth, and low birth weight.
- Ultrasound should be considered in children before CT imaging to reduce radiation exposure.
- Consider additional work-up to evaluate for metabolic abnormality or hereditary etiology.
- Children with uncomplicated ureteral stones of ≤10 mm can be offered observation with or without medical expulsion therapy (MET) using α-blockers.

Pregnancy Considerations
- Pregnant women have the same incidence of renal colic as do nonpregnant women.
- Most symptomatic stones occur during the 2nd and 3rd trimesters, heralded by symptoms of flank pain/hematuria.
- Most common differential diagnosis is physiologic hydronephrosis of pregnancy. Use ultrasound to avoid irradiation. Noncontrast-enhanced CT scan also is diagnostic.
- 30% require intervention, such as stent placement.
- Pregnant women who have ureteral stones with symptoms that are generally well controlled should be offered observation as first-line therapy.

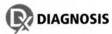

DIAGNOSIS

HISTORY
- Pain
  - Renal colic: acute onset of severe groin and/or flank pain
  - Distal stones may present with referred pain in labia, penile meatus, or testis.
- Microscopic/gross hematuria occurs in 95% of patients.
- Nausea, vomiting, tachycardia, diaphoresis, low-grade fever
- Frequency and dysuria occur with stones at the vesicoureteric junction (VUJ).

PHYSICAL EXAM
Tender costovertebral angle with palpation/percussion and/or iliac fossa

DIFFERENTIAL DIAGNOSIS
- Appendicitis
- Ruptured aortic aneurysm
- Musculoskeletal strain
- Pyelonephritis (upper UTI)
- Pyonephrosis (obstructed upper UTI; emergency)
- Perinephric abscess
- Pelvic or ovarian pathology: ectopic pregnancy, cyst, torsion
- Salpingitis
- Myocardial infarction
- Additional GI pathology: biliary colic, diverticulitis, obstruction, incarcerated hernia

DIAGNOSTIC TESTS & INTERPRETATION
- Urinalysis for RBCs, leukocytes, nitrates, pH (acidic urine <5.5 is associated with uric acid stones; alkaline >7 with struvite stones), send for culture and sensitivity
- Blood: urea, creatinine, electrolytes, calcium, and urate; consider CBC.
- Parathyroid hormone only if calcium is elevated
- Stone analysis if/when stone passed

Initial Tests (lab, imaging)
- Noncontrast-enhanced helical CT scan of the abdomen and pelvis has replaced IV pyelogram.
  - Stone is found most commonly at levels of ureteric luminal narrowing: pelviureteric junction, pelvic brim, and VUJ.
  - Acute obstruction: Proximal ureter and renal pelvis are dilated to the level of obstruction, and perinephric stranding is possible on imaging.
- Renal ultrasound may be as effective with lower radiation at diagnosis as well as identifying obstruction.
- X-ray of kidneys, ureter, and bladder to determine if stone is radiopaque or lucent
  - Calcium oxalate/phosphate stones are radiopaque.
  - Uric acid stones are radiolucent.
  - Staghorn calculi (that fill the shape of the renal calyces) are usually struvite and opaque.
  - Cystine stones are faintly opaque (ground-glass appearance).
- Ultrasound has low sensitivity and specificity but is often the first choice for pregnant women and children.

 ## TREATMENT

GENERAL MEASURES
- 75% of patients are successfully treated conservatively and pass the stone spontaneously.
- Most stones <5 mm will pass spontaneously with conservative treatment.
- Stones between 5 to 10 mm may pass with medical expulsive therapy.
- Stones >10 mm generally require surgical intervention.
- 30–50% of patients will have recurrent stones within 5 to 10 years.

MEDICATION
- Medical expulsive therapy: α_1-Antagonists (e.g., tamsulosin) may improve likelihood of spontaneous stone passage.
- Passage of larger stones (i.e., 5 to 10 mm) increased with tamsulosin
- Category C in pregnancy
- Initiation of medical expulsive therapy should factor comorbidities and medication side effects into consideration (e.g., hypotension, heart palpitations).
- Adequate pain control can be achieved with NSAIDs (anti-inflammatory effect decreases smooth muscle stimulation and spasms).

ISSUES FOR REFERRAL
- Urgent referral of patients with UTI, sepsis, acute renal failure, anuria
- Early referral of pregnant patients, children, adults aged >60 years, large stones (>8 mm), bilateral obstruction, solitary kidney, chronic renal failure, transplanted kidney

ADDITIONAL THERAPIES
- Uric acid stone dissolution therapy
  - Alkalinize urine with potassium citrate; keep pH >6.5.
  - Allopurinol 100 to 300 mg/day PO (for those who continue to form stones despite alkalinization of urine)
- Cystine stone dissolution/prevention
  - Alkalinize urine with potassium citrate; keep pH >6.5.
  - Chelating agents: captopril, α-mercaptopropionylglycine, D-penicillamine
- Consider altering medications that increase the risk of stone formation: probenecid, loop diuretics, salicylic acid, salbutamol, indinavir, triamterene, and acetazolamide.
- Vitamin D supplementation does NOT induce stone formation; calcium supplementation ≤1,200 mg/day (or as antacid) with vitamin D supplementation does not increase the risk of stone formation and may lower risk.
- Treat hypercalciuria with thiazides on an acute basis only.
- Treat hypocitraturia with potassium citrate and high-citrate juices (e.g., orange, lemon).
- Treat enteric hyperoxaluria with oral calcium/magnesium, cholestyramine, and potassium citrate.

SURGERY/OTHER PROCEDURES
- Immediate relief of obstruction is required for patients with the following conditions:
  - Sepsis, renal failure (obstructed solitary kidney, bilateral obstruction), uncontrolled pain, despite adequate analgesia
- Emergency surgery for obstruction
  - Placement of a retrograde stent (i.e., endoscopic surgery, usually requires an anesthetic)
  - Radiologic placement of a percutaneous nephrostomy tube
- Elective surgery for stone treatment
  - Extracorporeal shock wave lithotripsy
  - Ureteroscopy with basket extraction/lithotripsy (laser/pneumatic)
  - Percutaneous nephrolithotomy
    - First choice for stones >2 cm
- Open surgery is uncommon.

ADMISSION, INPATIENT, AND NURSING CONSIDERATIONS
Analgesia
- Combination of NSAIDs (ketorolac 30 to 60 mg) and oral opiate
- Parenteral opioid if vomiting or if preceding fails to control pain (morphine 5 to 10 mg IV or IM q4h)
- Antiemetic if required or prophylactically with parenteral narcotics

 ## ONGOING CARE

FOLLOW-UP RECOMMENDATIONS
- Patients being treated conservatively should be followed until imaging is clear or stone is visibly passed.
  - Strain urine and send stone for composition.
  - Tamsulosin and nifedipine in selected patients to speed passage
  - If pain management is suboptimal or if stone does not progress or pass within 4 to 6 weeks, patient should be referred to a urologist.

- Patients with recurrent stone formation should have metabolic workup: 24-hour urine for volume, pH, creatinine, calcium, cystine, phosphate, oxalate, uric acid, and magnesium.
  - PTH if serum calcium is found elevated
  - Ultrasonography to evaluate for renal anomaly if indicated

DIET
ALERT
- Increased fluid intake for life cannot be overemphasized for decreasing recurrence. Encourage intake of 2 to 3 L/day; advise patient to have clear urine rather than yellow.
- Decrease or eliminate carbonated drinks.
- Patients who form calcium stones should minimize high-oxalate foods such as green leafy vegetables, rhubarb, peanuts, chocolates, and beer.
- Decrease protein and salt intake.
- Lowering calcium intake is inadvisable and may even increase urine calcium excretion.
- Increase phytate-rich foods (natural dietary bran, legumes and beans, whole cereal)
- Avoid excessive vitamin C.

PATIENT EDUCATION
- Multiple dietary factors play a role in stone formation: hydration; carbohydrate, protein, calcium, sodium chloride, and oxalate intake.
- Reducing dietary intake of calcium oxalate is effective in correcting risk factors for stone formation (2).

PROGNOSIS
- Spontaneous stone passage depends on stone location (proximal vs. distal) and stone size (<5 mm, 90% pass; >8 mm, 10% pass).
- Stone recurrence: 50% of patients at 10 years

REFERENCES
1. Bao Y, Tu X, Wei Q. Water for preventing urinary stones. Cochrane Database Syst Rev. 2020;2(2):CD004292.
2. Siener R. Nutrition and kidney stone disease. Nutrients. 2021;13(6):1917.

 ## SEE ALSO

Algorithms: Dysuria; Renal Calculi; Urethral Discharge

CODES

ICD10
- N20.9 Urinary calculus, unspecified
- N20.0 Calculus of kidney
- N20.1 Calculus of ureter

CLINICAL PEARLS
- Medical expulsive therapy may improve likelihood of spontaneous stone passage.
- Increased fluid intake for life; 2 to 3 L/day intake
- Patients with calcium stones should minimize high-oxalate foods (e.g., green leafy vegetables, rhubarb, peanuts, chocolates, beer).
- Decrease protein and salt intake.
- Lowering calcium intake is inadvisable and may even increase urine calcium excretion.

U

URICARIA
Todd A. Wical, DO

 BASICS

DESCRIPTION

- A cutaneous lesion or lesions involving edema of the epidermis and/or dermis presenting with rapid onset and pruritus, returning to normal skin appearance within 24 hours
- Pathophysiology is primarily mast cell degranulation and subsequent histamine release.
- Angioedema may occur with urticaria, which is characterized by sudden pronounced erythematous nonpitting edema of the lower dermis and subcutis; may take up to 72 hours to remit
- Pruritus and burning are more commonly associated with urticaria; pain more often with angioedema
- Lesions can occur on any part of the body.
- Urticaria can be classified as acute or chronic.
  - Acute: if lesions recur within <6 weeks
  - Chronic: recurring lesions that persist for >6 weeks
- Three main causal categories of urticarial lesions
  - Immunoglobulin E (IgE) mediated
  - Non-IgE immunologically mediated
  - Nonimmunologically mediated
- Underlying etiology may be difficult to pinpoint, although in some cases possible.
- For those with chronic urticaria, 40% have concurrent angioedema
- Etiology of urticaria is either spontaneous or induced.
- System(s) affected: integumentary
- Synonym(s): hives; wheals

EPIDEMIOLOGY

Incidence
- Equally distributed across all ages: female > male (2:1 in chronic urticaria)
- In 20% of patients, chronic urticaria lasts >10 years.

Prevalence
- 5–25% of the population
- Of people with urticaria, 40% have no angioedema, 40% have urticaria and angioedema, and 20% have angioedema with no urticaria.
- Up to 3% of the population has chronic idiopathic urticaria.

ETIOLOGY AND PATHOPHYSIOLOGY
- Mast cell degranulation with release of inflammatory reactants, which leads to vascular leakage, inflammatory cell extravasation, and dermal (angioedema) and/or epidermal (wheals/hives) edema
- Histamine, cytokines, leukotrienes, and proteases are main active substances released.
- If release of histamine and other mediators occurs in the dermis, urticaria lesions result. If release occurs deep in the dermis, then angioedema develops.
- Acute spontaneous urticaria (ASU)
  - Bacterial infections: strep throat, sinusitis, otitis, urinary tract
  - Viral infections: rhinovirus, rotavirus, hepatitis B, mononucleosis, herpes

- Foods: peanuts, tree nuts, seafood, milk, soy, fish, wheat, and eggs; tend to be IgE-mediated; pseudoallergenic foods such as strawberries, tomatoes, preservatives, and coloring agents contain histamine.
  - Drugs: IgE-mediated (e.g., penicillin and other antibiotics), direct mast cell stimulation (e.g., aspirin, NSAIDs, opiates)
  - Inhalant, contact, ingestion, or occupational exposure (e.g., latex, cosmetics)
  - Parasitic infection; insect bite/sting
  - Transfusion reaction
- Chronic spontaneous urticaria (CSU)
  - Chronic subclinical allergic rhinitis, eczema, and other atopic disorders
  - Chronic indolent infections: *Helicobacter pylori*, fungal, parasitic (*Anisakis simplex*, strongyloidiasis), and chronic viral infections (hepatitis)
  - Collagen vascular disease (cutaneous vasculitis, serum sickness, lupus)
  - Thyroid autoimmunity, especially Hashimoto
  - Hormonal: pregnancy and progesterone
  - Autoimmune antibodies to the IgE receptor α chain on mast cells and to the IgE antibody
  - Chronic medications (e.g., NSAIDs, hormones, ACE inhibitors). NSAID sensitivity demonstrated almost in half of adults with chronic urticaria and presents with a worsening of symptoms 4 hours after ingestion.
  - Malignancy
  - Physical stimuli (cold, heat, vibration, pressure) in physical urticaria
- Chronic inducible urticaria (CIU)
  - Dermatographism: "skin writing" or the appearance of linear wheals at the site of any type of irritation. This is the most common physical induced urticaria.
  - Cold urticaria: Wheals occur within minutes of rewarming after cold exposure; 95% idiopathic but can be due to infections (mononucleosis, HIV), neoplasia, or autoimmune diseases.
  - Delayed pressure urticaria: Urticaria occurs 0.5 to 12 hours after pressure to skin (e.g., from elastic or shoes), may be pruritic and/or painful, and may not subside for several days.
  - Solar urticaria: from sunlight exposure, usually UV; onset in minutes; subsides within 2 hours
  - Heat urticaria: from direct contact with warm objects or air; rare
  - Vibratory urticaria/angioedema: very rare; secondary to vibrations (e.g., motorcycle)
  - Cholinergic urticaria: due to brief increase of core body temperature from exercise, baths, or emotional stress. This is the second most common induced urticaria.
  - Adrenergic urticaria: caused by stress; extremely rare; vasoconstricted, blanched skin around pink wheals as opposed to cholinergic's erythematous surrounding
  - Contact urticaria: wheals at sites where chemical substances contact the skin, may be either IgE-dependent (e.g., latex) or IgE-independent (e.g., stinging nettle)
  - Aquagenic and solar urticaria: small wheals after contact with water of any temperature or UV light, respectively; rare

Genetics
No consistent pattern known: Chronic urticaria has increased frequency of HLA-DR4 and HLA-D8Q MHC II alleles.

GENERAL PREVENTION
Avoidance of known triggers is the mainstay of prevention.

COMMONLY ASSOCIATED CONDITIONS
- Angioedema (common)
- Anaphylaxis (somewhat common)

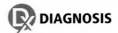 **DIAGNOSIS**

HISTORY
Rapid onset; individual lesions resolve in <24 hours, pruritus

ALERT
Important to rule out underlying anaphylaxis in those patients presenting with acute onset of urticaria (1)[C],(2)[C]

PHYSICAL EXAM
- Single/multiple raised, polymorphic indurated plaques with central pallor and edema with an erythematous flare
- Evaluate for underlying conditions including thyroid abnormalities (nodules), bacterial, viral, or fungal infection (e.g., fever).

DIFFERENTIAL DIAGNOSIS
- Anaphylaxis (may present with urticaria)
- Morbilliform or fixed drug eruptions
- Erythema multiforme
- Systemic lupus erythematosus (SLE), vasculitis, and polyarteritis
- Angioedema without urticaria
- Urticaria pigmentosa/systemic mastocytosis
- Bullous pemphigoid (urticarial stage)
- Arthropod bite
- Atopic/contact dermatitis
- Viral exanthem

DIAGNOSTIC TESTS & INTERPRETATION
- Diagnosis is usually clinical (1),(2).
- In general, only if the history or physical are suggestive of a specific underlying disease should targeted laboratory studies be utilized.

Initial Tests (lab, imaging)
- Acute: generally not indicated
- Chronic: directed by clinical suspicion of underlying cause
  - Allergy skin tests and radioallergosorbent test (RAST) for inhaled allergens, insects, drugs, or foods
  - Infection: Consider pharyngeal culture, LFTs, mononucleosis test, urinalysis in appropriate setting

Follow-Up Tests & Special Considerations

Chronic urticaria (CIU/CSU): Extensive lab testing is not indicated and has not proven to improve outcome nor is it cost-effective. Limit lab testing according to clinical history and indication. Skin or IgE testing should be limited to specific history of provoking allergen (3)[C].

- CBC, ESR, and CRP are recommended by most guidelines.
- Thyroid function tests, LFTs, and urinalysis are recommended by several guidelines.
- Consider allergy skin tests and RAST for inhaled allergens, insects, drugs, or foods; total IgE level
- Autoimmune: ESR, ANA, RF, complement (e.g., CH50, C3, C4), cryoglobulins in urticarial vasculitis
- Tests for *H. pylori* (e.g., antibodies) in dyspeptic patients. Consider stool for ova and parasites in at-risk individuals.
- Autologous serum skin testing: injection of serum under skin to test for presence of IgE receptor–activating antibodies
- Consider malignancy workup, including serum protein electrophoresis and immunofixation in the proper setting.

Diagnostic Procedures/Other

- Food and drug reactions: elimination of (or challenges with) suspected agents
- Physical and special forms of urticaria challenge tests:
  - Dermatographism: stroke skin lightly with rounded object and observe for surrounding urticaria
  - Cold urticaria: ice cube test—place ice cube on skin for 5 minutes; observe for 10 to 15 minutes.
  - Cholinergic: exercise to the point of sweating/partial immersion in 42°C bath for 10 minutes
  - Solar: exposure to different wavelengths of light
  - Delayed pressure: Apply 5-lb sandbag to back for 20 minutes; observe 6 hours later.
  - Aquagenic: Apply water at various temperatures.
  - Vibratory: Apply vibration 4 to 5 minutes with a lab mixing device; observe.
- Skin biopsy with lesions lasting >24 hours or if concern for underlying vasculitis (1)[C],(2)[C]

TREATMENT

GENERAL MEASURES

The mainstay of therapy for urticaria is the avoidance of identified triggers.

MEDICATION

First Line

2nd-generation antihistamine (H$_1$) blockers are the first-line treatment of any urticaria in which avoidance of stimulus is impossible or not feasible (1)[C],(2)[C]:

- Fexofenadine (Allegra): 180 mg/day
- Loratadine (Claritin): 10 mg/day, increasing to 30 mg/day if needed; only medication studied for safe use in pregnancy

- Desloratadine (Clarinex): 5 mg/day (4)[B]
- Cetirizine (Zyrtec): 10 mg/day, increasing to 30 mg per day if needed
- Levocetirizine (Xyzal): 5 mg/day; requires weight-based dosing in children (4)[B]
- Rupatadine: novel H$_1$ antagonist with antiplatelet-activating factor activity

Second Line

Doubling the typical 2nd-generation H$_1$ blocker dosages should be attempted before adding 1st-generation H$_1$ or H$_2$ blockers (1),(2)[C],(4)[B].

- H$_2$-specific antihistamines (beneficial as adjuvants): cimetidine, ranitidine, nizatidine, famotidine
- 1st-generation antihistamines (H$_1$; for patients with sleep disturbed by itching):
  - Older children and adults: hydroxyzine or diphenhydramine 25 to 50 mg q6h
  - Children <6 years of age: diphenhydramine 12.5 mg q6–8h (5 mg/kg/day) or hydroxyzine (10 mg/5 mL) 2 mg/kg/day divided q6–8h

Geriatric Considerations

1st-generation H$_1$ blockers may cause excessive drowsiness as well as dry mouth and eyes.

ISSUES FOR REFERRAL

Referral to an allergist, immunologist, or dermatologist for recalcitrant cases, especially if lesions consistently remain present for >24 hours

ADMISSION, INPATIENT, AND NURSING CONSIDERATIONS

Educating patient on use of EpiPen as pathophysiology is similar to anaphylaxis; if the airway is threatened, immediate consultation to evaluate for laryngeal edema and need for definitive airway management

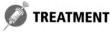 ONGOING CARE

FOLLOW-UP RECOMMENDATIONS

After initial diagnosis, follow-up is recommended within 6 weeks as nearly 1/3 of acute patient go on to have persistent urticaria.

Patient Monitoring

- Use the urticaria activity score (UAS7) for assessing CSU.
- Recently was developed urticaria control test (UCT)
  - The tool to assess disease control in patients with chronic urticaria (spontaneous and inducible) (5)[A]

PROGNOSIS

- Resolution of acute symptoms: 70% <72 hours
- Chronic urticaria: 35% symptom-free in a year; another 30% will see symptom reduction.

REFERENCES

1. Zuberbier T, Aberer W, Asero R, et al. The EAACI/GA^{2}LEN/EDF/WAO guideline for the definition, classification, diagnosis and management of urticaria. *Allergy*. 2018;73(7):1393–1414.
2. Bernstein JA, Lang DM, Khan DA, et al. The diagnosis and management of acute and chronic urticaria: 2014 update. *J Allergy Clin Immunol*. 2014;133(5):1270–1277.
3. Choosing Wisely. American Academy of Allergy, Asthma & Immunology. Don't routinely do diagnostic testing in patients with chronic urticaria. http://www.choosingwisely.org/clinician-lists/american-academy-allergy-asthma-immunology-chronic-urticaria/. Accessed July 15, 2021.
4. Staevska M, Popov TA, Kralimarkova T, et al. The effectiveness of levocetirizine and desloratadine in up to 4 times conventional doses in difficult-to-treat urticaria. *J Allergy Clin Immunol*. 2010;125(3):676–682.
5. Weller K, Groffik A, Church MK, et al. Development and validation of the urticaria control test: a patient-reported outcome instrument for assessing urticaria control. *J Allergy Clin Immunol*. 2014;133(5):1365–1372.

ADDITIONAL READING

- Dressler C, Werner RN, Eisert L, et al. Chronic inducible urticaria: a systematic review of treatment options. *J Allergy Clin Immunol*. 2018;141(5):1726–1734. doi:10.1016/j.jaci.2018.01.031.
- Poonawalla T, Kelly B. Urticaria: a review. *Am J Clin Dermatol*. 2009;10(1):9–21.
- Powell R, Leech S, Till S, et al. BSACI guideline for the management of chronic urticaria and angioedema. *Clin Exp Allergy*. 2015;45(3):547–565.
- Zuberbier T, Balke M, Worm M, et al. Epidemiology of urticaria: a representative cross-sectional survey. *Clin Exp Dermatol*. 2010;35(8):869–873.

 CODES

ICD10

- L50.9 Urticaria, unspecified
- L50.1 Idiopathic urticaria
- L50.8 Other urticaria

CLINICAL PEARLS

- Urticaria occurs rapidly, and individual lesions resolve within 24 hours, although multiple crops of lesions can occur in stages.
- Mainstay of therapy is to avoid identified triggers.
- Antihistamines are the best studied and most efficacious therapy but may require higher-than-normal doses for efficacy.
- If individual lesions last >24 hours, patient should be evaluated for urticarial vasculitis and other more serious diagnoses.

U

UTERINE AND PELVIC ORGAN PROLAPSE
Deepali Maheshwari, DO, MPH • Lauren Simms, MD

 BASICS

DESCRIPTION
- Symptomatic descent of one or more of the following (1),(2):
  – The anterior vaginal wall (bladder or cystocele)
  – The posterior vaginal wall (rectum or rectocele)
  – The uterus and cervix
  – The vaginal apex (vault or cuff scar after hysterectomy)
- Prolapse above or to the level of the hymen are generally not symptomatic.
- Associated symptoms
  – Feeling of pelvic pressure or heaviness
  – Vaginal bulge
  – Bowel or bladder symptoms
- Cost associated with treatment is >$1 billion annually (~200,000 surgeries per year).

EPIDEMIOLOGY
Incidence
- The incidence of pelvic organ prolapse (POP) ranges from 1.5 to 1.8 per 1,000 woman-years and peaks in women aged 60 to 69 years.
- In the United States, there are approximately 300,000 surgeries for POP each year, and a woman's lifetime risk of undergoing surgery for pelvic floor prolapse ranges from 6% to 18%.

Prevalence
- When POP is defined by the patient's symptoms alone, the prevalence is 2.9–8%. When defined by exam findings, the prevalence is 41.1%.
- POP is common but not always symptomatic. It does not always progress. It is estimated that 50% of women will develop prolapse, but only 10–20% of those will seek care for their condition.

ETIOLOGY AND PATHOPHYSIOLOGY
- Pelvic organs are supported by attachments between pelvic floor muscles, connective tissue, and the bony pelvis. Defects in this support can lead to prolapse in one or multiple compartments (3).
- Symptomatic women typically have defects in more than one compartment as well as damage to the levator ani muscle complex (a critical component of uterovaginal support) and its attachments to the pelvis (3).
- Gradual process that often begins long before symptoms develop

RISK FACTORS
- Vaginal childbirth: Each additional vaginal birth increases risk (1).
- Increasing age
- Family history
- Race: White and Hispanic women may be at higher risk than black or Asian women (2).

- Obesity BMI >30 kg/m²
- Chronic straining (constipation, chronic cough from pulmonary disease, repeated heavy lifting)
- History of hysterectomy

GENERAL PREVENTION
There is some evidence that pelvic floor muscle training ("Kegel exercises") may decrease the risk of symptomatic POP (3)[B]. Weight loss and proper management of conditions that cause increase in intra-abdominal pressure such as constipation may help prevent prolapse (3)[C].

COMMONLY ASSOCIATED CONDITIONS
- Constipation
- Fecal incontinence
- Urinary incontinence or retention
- Other urinary symptoms
  – Urgency
  – Frequency

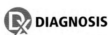 **DIAGNOSIS**

Less than half of women discuss symptoms with PCP. Only 10–12% seek medical attention. Barriers include embarrassment, social stigma, ability to cope, belief that POP is part of the aging process, belief that treatment options are limited, and fear of surgery.

HISTORY
- Common symptoms include the following:
  – Feeling a bulge in vagina
  – Something "falling out" of vagina
  – Pelvic pressure with activity or prolonged standing
  – Difficulty with voiding or defecation
  – Splinting the bulge to evacuate
  – Urinary or fecal urgency
  – Urinary frequency
  – Urinary or fecal incontinence
  – Constipation
- Document the presence, duration, and severity of coexisting urinary or bowel symptom.
- Assess impact on sexual function and quality of life.
- Assess past medical and surgical history:
  – Gravidity and parity/obstetric history
  – Chronic constipation
  – Pulmonary disease
  – Prior pelvic procedures

PHYSICAL EXAM
- Abdominal examination to document any distention or masses
- Complete pelvic and rectal examination. Patient can be evaluated in supine position. If prolapse is not well demonstrated, have the patient cough or strain in an upright (standing) position to assess maximum descent.

- The standard to measure prolapse is the validated Pelvic Organ Prolapse Quantification (POP-Q) scale.
  – Describes prolapse of each compartment in relationship to the vaginal hymen
  – Patient is supine with the head of the bed at 45 degrees, performing Valsalva.
    ○ Stage 1: prolapse in which the distal point is superior or equal to 1 cm above hymen
    ○ Stage 2: prolapse in which the distal point is between 1 cm above and 1 cm below hymen
    ○ Stage 3: prolapse in which the distal point is superior or equal to 1 cm below the hymen, but some vaginal mucosa is not everted
    ○ Stage 4: complete vaginal vault eversion ("procidentia"); entire vaginal mucosa everted
- A split speculum should be used to observe apical, anterior, and posterior compartments successively.

DIFFERENTIAL DIAGNOSIS
- Rectal prolapse
- Hemorrhoids
- Bartholin cyst
- Vaginal cyst
- Urethral diverticulum
- Cervical elongation

DIAGNOSTIC TESTS & INTERPRETATION
Initial Tests (lab, imaging)
- Urinalysis if symptomatic POP to evaluate for urinary tract infection (2)
- Postvoid residual to evaluate bladder emptying (2)

Follow-Up Tests & Special Considerations
- Consider urodynamic testing if results would alter treatment plan (e.g., if evaluating concurrent urinary retention or voiding dysfunction or if evaluating for occult stress urinary incontinence).
- Selective use of upper urinary tract imaging if observation is planned or if there is evidence of obstruction (e.g., abnormal postvoid residual) (2)
- If fecal incontinence or significant change in bowel habits, selective use of lower GI tract imaging or endoscopy (2)
- Consider defecography if severity of symptoms is out of proportion with the extent of prolapse.

 TREATMENT

GENERAL MEASURES
- Treatment is generally guided by degree of bother for the patient. It is important to document the patient's desire, goals, and expectations.
- Treatment should consider type and severity of symptoms, patient's age, other comorbid conditions, prior surgical history, sexual function, infertility, and risk of recurrence.

- Treatment for asymptomatic patients:
  - Stage 1 or 2: clinical observation
  - Stage 3 or 4: regular follow-up and evaluation (every 3 to 6 months)
- Expectant management is an acceptable option for patients without evidence of urinary or bowel obstruction.
- Treatment is indicated when there is urinary/bowel obstruction or hydronephrosis regardless of the degree of prolapse.
- A vaginal pessary should be considered in all women presenting with symptomatic prolapse.
  - There are >13 types of pessaries.
  - The most commonly used pessaries are the ring pessary and the Gellhorn pessary.
  - Most women can be successfully fitted with a pessary.
  - Satisfaction rate for patients using pessaries is very high (3).
  - Minor complications such as vaginal discharge and odor can often be treated with vaginal estrogen.
  - Vaginal erosion is rare and can be treated by removal of pessary and optional vaginal estrogen supplementation.
  - Complications such as erosions, abrasions, ulcerations, vaginal bleeding, and fistulas may be seen with neglected pessaries.

MEDICATION
- There are no data to support the use of vaginal estrogen or other medications for the prevention or treatment of POP.
- Constipation should be managed with an appropriate bowel regimen that includes daily fiber supplementation.

ISSUES FOR REFERRAL
Referral is indicated when pessary or surgery is necessary or desired by the patient.

ADDITIONAL THERAPIES
Pelvic floor muscle training: may reduce the symptoms of POP but does not affect the degree of prolapse (3)

SURGERY/OTHER PROCEDURES
- Reconstructive procedures are performed with the goal of restoration of vaginal anatomy and resolution of symptoms.
- There are a variety of surgeries for repair of the anterior, apical, and posterior compartments. Surgical approaches include vaginal, abdominal, and laparoscopic (straight stick and robot assisted).
- Reconstructive surgery using native tissue is associated with an increased rate of failure (one in three lifetime risks of repeat surgery). Procedures using surgical mesh and graft material have higher success rates.

- Surgical repair should focus on repairing all affected compartments in a single procedure.
- Coexisting stress incontinence should be addressed at the same time as the prolapse repair.
- For apical repairs:
  - Sacral colpopexy uses surgical mesh and has higher success rates and overall durability. It can be performed abdominally, laparoscopically, or robotically. The risk of recurrent prolapse is considered lower with sacral colpopexy than vaginal approaches; there may be an elevated risk of complications.
  - Concomitant hysterectomy is generally performed with prolapse repair. The risk of mesh extrusions appears to be decreased by retaining the cervix.
  - Uterine preservation via hysteropexy is also an option and may be offered by some surgeons. The risks and benefits of uterine preservation in prolapse repair remain unclear.

 ONGOING CARE

FOLLOW-UP RECOMMENDATIONS
Patient Monitoring
- Patients who choose a pessary for management should be seen regularly. There is no standard of care established for follow-up but commonly:
  - Within 7 to 14 days of initial fitting and then at 3- to 12-month intervals depending on patient's independence with the pessary, proficiency with placement and removal of pessary, and cognitive and motor abilities
  - Pessary should be removed regularly and cleaned with soap and water.
- Patients who undergo prolapse surgery should be evaluated postoperatively, and follow-up intervals vary by provider.

PATIENT EDUCATION
- Patients should have POP explained to them with diagrams and descriptions of their anatomy.
- It is important to emphasize that surgery is geared toward improving quality of life.
- Patients should be educated about potential pessary complications.
- Patients should be informed about possible symptoms of POP if they are still asymptomatic.
- Using insoluble fibers may help patients with bowel complaints such as constipation.

COMPLICATIONS
- Recurrence rates after surgery are variable and quoted between 3.4% and 29.2%.
- There is a risk of dyspareunia and pelvic pain after any surgical repair. Those repairs using mesh may also be complicated by mesh erosion.

- Potential complications of pessary use include vaginal erosion and fistula in patients that are lost to follow-up.
- Severe prolapse can lead to urinary retention and defecatory dysfunction that may go unrecognized in the elderly.

REFERENCES

1. Raju R, Linder BJ. Evaluation and management of pelvic organ prolapse. *Mayo Clin Proc*. 2021;96(12):3122–3129.
2. Dumoulin C, Hunter KF, Moore K, et al. Conservative management for female urinary incontinence and pelvic organ prolapse review 2013: summary of the 5th International Consultation on Incontinence. *Neurourol Urodyn*. 2016;35(1):15–20.
3. Hagen S, Stark D. Conservative prevention and management of pelvic organ prolapse in women. *Cochrane Database Syst Rev*. 2011;(12):CD003882.

ADDITIONAL READING

- Baessler K, Christmann-Schmid C, Maher C, et al. Surgery for women with pelvic organ prolapse with or without stress urinary incontinence. *Cochrane Database Syst Rev*. 2018;8(8):CD013108.
- Larouche M, Belzile E, Geoffrion R. Surgical management of symptomatic apical pelvic organ prolapse: a systematic review and meta-analysis. *Obstet Gynecol*. 2021;137(6):1061–1073.

CODES

ICD10
- N81.9 Female genital prolapse, unspecified
- N81.10 Cystocele, unspecified
- N99.3 Prolapse of vaginal vault after hysterectomy

CLINICAL PEARLS
- Many women do not discuss POP with their doctor—ask routinely.
- Vaginal pessary is a nonsurgical treatment option in any patients with symptomatic prolapse.
- Treatment should be guided by degree of bother and impact on patient's quality of life.

U

UTERINE MYOMAS

Sareena Singh, MD, FACOG • Kimberly Resnick, MD

BASICS

DESCRIPTION
- Uterine leiomyomas are well-circumscribed, pseudoencapsulated, benign monoclonal tumors composed mainly of smooth muscle with varying amounts of fibrous connective tissue (1).
- Three major subtypes
  - Subserous: common; external; may become pedunculated
  - Intramural: common; within myometrium; may cause marked uterine enlargement
  - Submucous: ~5% of all cases; internal, evoking abnormal uterine bleeding and infection; occasionally protruding from cervix
- Rare locations: broad, round, and uterosacral ligaments
- System affected: reproductive
- Synonym(s): fibroids; myoma; fibromyoma; myofibroma; fibroleiomyoma

EPIDEMIOLOGY
Incidence
- Cumulative incidence up to 80%
  - 60% in African American women by age 35 years; 80% by age 50 years
  - 40% in Caucasian women by age 35 years; 70% by age 50 years (1),(2)
- Incidence increases with each decade during reproductive years.
- Rarely seen in premenarchal females
- Predominant sex: females only

ETIOLOGY AND PATHOPHYSIOLOGY
- Enlargement of benign smooth muscle tumors that may lead to symptoms affecting the reproductive, GI, or genitourinary system
- Complex multifactorial process involving transition from normal myocyte to abnormal cells and then to visibly evident tumor (monoclonal expansion)
  - Hormones (1): Increases in estrogen and progesterone are correlated with myoma formation (i.e., rarely seen before menarche). Estrogen receptors in myomas bind more estradiol than normal myometrium.
  - Growth factors (1)
    - Increased smooth muscle proliferation (transforming growth factor β [TGF-β], basic fibroblast growth factor [bFGF])
    - Increase DNA synthesis (epidermal growth factor [EGF], platelet-derived growth factor [PDGF], activin, myostatin)
    - Stimulate synthesis of extracellular matrix (TGF-β)
    - Promote mitogenesis (TGF-β, EGF, insulin-like growth factor [IGF], prolactin)
    - Promote angiogenesis (bFGF, vascular endothelial growth factor [VEGF])
  - Vasoconstrictive hypoxia (1): proposed, but not confirmed, mechanism of myometrial injury during menstruation

Genetics
- A variety of somatic chromosomal rearrangements have been described in 40% of uterine myomas. Mutations in the gene encoding mediator complex subunit 12 (MED12) on the X chromosome were found in 70% of myomas in one study (3).
- Higher levels of aromatase and therefore estrogen have been found in myomas in African American women (3).

RISK FACTORS
- African American heritage: 2.9 times greater risk than Caucasian women; occur at a younger age, are more numerous, larger, and more symptomatic (1),(2)
- Early menarche (<10 years)
- Oral contraceptive use before 16 years old (2)
- Nulliparous
- Hypertension
- Familial predisposition: 2.5 times more likely in women with a first-degree relative with myomas (1)
- Obesity: Risk increases by 21% with each 10 kg of weight gain (1).
- Alcohol
- Risk decreased by parity, progesterone-only contraceptives, diet (fruits, veggies, low fat dairy) (2).

COMMONLY ASSOCIATED CONDITIONS
Endometrial and breast cancer also associated with high, unopposed estrogen stimulation

DIAGNOSIS

HISTORY
- Usually asymptomatic; 30% present with abnormal symptoms—usually enlarged uterus or heavy bleeding (2).
- Symptoms include the following:
  - Abnormal uterine bleeding: usually heavy/prolonged menses
  - Pain: infrequent; usually associated with torsion of pedunculated myoma, degeneration, or cervical dilation by submucous myoma near cervical os
  - Pressure on bladder: suprapubic discomfort, urinary frequency/obstruction
  - Pressure on rectosigmoid: may cause low back pain, constipation
  - Infertility: rare, estimated 1–2.5%; usually from submucous myoma distorting the uterine cavity or interference with implantation

ALERT
Rapid growth, particularly in perimenopausal/postmenopausal patients; may indicate sarcoma; extremely rare, 0.1–0.3% of cases

PHYSICAL EXAM
- Usually incidental finding on abdominal and pelvic exam
- Firm, smooth nodules/masses arising from uterus
- Masses are mobile without tenderness.

DIFFERENTIAL DIAGNOSIS
Intrauterine pregnancy, cancer, including ovarian, uterine, or leiomyosarcoma; cecal/sigmoid tumor, appendiceal abscess, diverticulitis, pelvic kidney, urachal cyst

DIAGNOSTIC TESTS & INTERPRETATION
Initial Tests (lab, imaging)
- Pregnancy test
- Hemoglobin
- Pelvic ultrasound: standard confirmatory test; shows characteristic hypoechoic appearance (2)
- Saline infusion hysterosonography: helps to distinguish submucosal myomas

- Hysterosalpingogram: evaluates the contour of the endometrial cavity
- CT scan or MRI: provides info on degeneration and special relationships (2); may help to differentiate complex cases or used when uterine artery embolization is planned

Follow-Up Tests & Special Considerations
Consider cancer antigen 125 (CA-125): may be slightly elevated in some cases of uterine myoma but generally more useful in differentiating myomas from various gynecologic adenocarcinomas
- IV pyelogram: if suspect ureteral distortion
- Barium enema

Diagnostic Procedures/Other
- Fractional dilation and curettage: aids in ruling out cervical/uterine carcinomas when clinically suspicious
- Hysteroscopy: helps to diagnose submucosal/intracavitary myomas
- Laparoscopy: useful in complex cases and to rule out other pelvic diseases/disorders

Test Interpretation
- Myomas are usually multiple and vary in size and location; have been reported up to 100 lb
- Gross pathology: firm tumors with characteristic whorl-like trabeculated appearance; a thin pseudocapsular layer is present.
- Microscopic: bundles of smooth muscle mixed with varying amounts of connective tissue elements running in different directions
- Cellular variant has a preponderance of muscle cells. Mitoses are rare.
- May undergo various types of degeneration
  - Hyaline degeneration: very common
  - Calcification: late result of circulatory impairment to myomas
  - Infection and suppuration: most common with submucosal myomas
  - Necrosis: most common with pedunculated myomas secondary to torsion

TREATMENT

- Treatment must be individualized and based on symptoms, fertility desires, and time until menopause.
- Medical therapy may be of benefit.
- Patients with minimal symptoms may be treated with iron preparations and analgesics.
- Conservative management of asymptomatic myomas
  - Pelvic exams and ultrasounds at ≥3-month intervals if size remains stable
  - Substantial regression usually occurs after menopause.
- Surgical options should be considered if symptomatic or worrisome myomas are unresponsive to conservative/medical management.

GENERAL MEASURES

Patients not desiring pharmacologic therapy or surgery may consider the following:

- Uterine artery embolization: averages 50% shrinkage of myomas (4)[A]; painful and may cause ovarian failure (1–2%), amenorrhea, postembolization syndrome, or other complications; shorter hospital stay and quicker recovery but no difference in satisfaction compared with hysterectomy (2); high reintervention rate (15–32% by 2 years) compared to hysterectomy/ myomectomy (7% by 2 years) (4)[A]
- MR-guided focused ultrasound (MRgFUS): noninvasive, ultrasound transducer passes through abdominal wall and causes coagulative necrosis of fibroid; up to 98% reduction in myoma volume and symptoms. Not appropriate for some types of myomas. Efficacy may be comparable with other hysterectomy-sparing procedures. Fertility has been shown to be preserved (2) although risks and outcomes data are limited (2).

MEDICATION

- Progestins may reduce overall uterine size.
  - Norethindrone 10 mg/day
  - Medroxyprogesterone 200 mg IM monthly
  - Levonorgestrel intrauterine device
- Combination oral contraceptives: may help prevent development of new fibroids and control bleeding
- Gonadotropin-releasing hormone agonists
  - Nafarelin (nasal spray), goserelin acetate, and leuprolide
  - Induces abrupt artificial menopause; may reduce myoma symptoms dramatically; induces atrophy of myomas by up to 40% in 2 to 3 months
  - May be valuable as preoperative adjunct to myomectomy/hysterectomy by allowing recovery of anemia, donation of autologous blood, and possibly converting abdominal to vaginal hysterectomy (2)[B]
  - Not recommended for use >6 months because of osteoporosis risk
  - Following discontinuation, myomas return within 60 days to pretherapy size.
- Antiprogesterones
  - Mifepristone
    - Shown to have similar reduction in myoma size as gonadotropin-releasing hormone agonists
    - Decreases heavy bleeding and increases quality of life (5)[A]
  - Selective progesterone receptor modulator (SPRM): ulipristal acetate: may be as effective as gonadotropin-releasing hormones with fewer side effects (2)[B]

ISSUES FOR REFERRAL

- Medical therapy may be initiated by a primary care physician/gynecologist after adequate pelvic examination.
- Surgical considerations may be pursued with gynecologic consultation.
- Uterine embolization may be discussed with an interventional radiologist.

SURGERY/OTHER PROCEDURES

- Surgical management is indicated in the following situations:
  - Excessive uterine size or excessive rate of growth (except during pregnancy)
  - Submucosal myomas when associated with hypermenorrhea

- Pedunculated myomas that are painful or undergo torsion, necrosis, and hemorrhage
- If a myoma causes symptoms from pressure on bladder/rectum
- If differentiation from ovarian mass is not possible
- If associated pelvic disease is present (endometriosis, pelvic inflammatory disease)
- If infertility/habitual abortion is likely due to the anatomic location of the myoma
- Surgical procedures
  - Preliminary pelvic examination, Pap smear, and endometrial biopsy should be performed to rule out malignant/premalignant conditions.
  - Hysterectomy: may be performed vaginally, laparoscopically, robotically, or by laparotomy
    - Effective in relieving symptoms and improving quality of life (2)[B]
    - Similar fertility and live birth rates between laparoscopic and abdominal myomectomy
    - FDA discourages the use of laparoscopic power morcellation during hysterectomy or myomectomy for uterine fibroids given the risk of spreading an occult malignancy and all patients should be counseled preoperatively of risk (2).
  - Abdominal, laparoscopic, robotic, or hysteroscopic myomectomy may be performed in younger women who want to maintain fertility.
  - Hysteroscopic/laparoscopic cautery/laser myoma resection can be performed in selected patients.
  - Endometrial ablation: for small submucosal myomas

ADMISSION, INPATIENT, AND NURSING CONSIDERATIONS

- Usually outpatient
- Inpatient for some surgical procedures

 ONGOING CARE

FOLLOW-UP RECOMMENDATIONS

Patient Monitoring

- Pelvic examination and ultrasound: every 2 to 3 months for newly diagnosed symptomatic/excessively large myomas
- Hemoglobin and hematocrit: if uterine bleeding is excessive
- Once uterine size and symptoms stabilize, monitor every 6 to 12 months, although no high-quality evidence exists (2).

DIET

No restrictions

PATIENT EDUCATION

- Society of Interventional Radiology: https://www.sirweb.org/patient-center/conditions-and-treatments/uterine-fibroids/
- U.S. Department of Health and Human Services: https://www.womenshealth.gov/a-z-topics/uterine-fibroids
- American Congress of Obstetricians and Gynecologists: http://www.acog.org

PROGNOSIS

- Resection of submucosal fibroids has been associated with increased fertility.
- At least 10% of myomas recur after myomectomy; however, only 25% require further treatment (2)[B].

COMPLICATIONS

- May mask other gynecologic malignancies (e.g., uterine sarcoma, ovarian cancer)
- Degenerating fibroids may cause pain and bleeding.
- May rarely prolapse through the cervix

Pregnancy Considerations

- Rapid growth of fibroids is common.
- Pregnant women may need additional fetal testing if placenta is located over or near fibroid.
- Complications during pregnancy: abortion, premature labor, 2nd-trimester rapid growth leading to degeneration/pain, 3rd-trimester fetal malpresentation, and dystocia during labor and delivery
- Cesarean section is recommended if the endometrial cavity was entered during myomectomy due to increased risk of uterine rupture.

Geriatric Considerations

Postmenopausal patients with newly diagnosed uterine myoma/enlarging uterine myomas have a high suspicion of uterine sarcoma/other gynecologic malignancy.

REFERENCES

1. Parker WH. Etiology, symptomatology, and diagnosis of uterine myomas. *Fertil Steril*. 2007; 87(4):725–736.
2. Stewart EA. Clinical practice. Uterine fibroids. *N Engl J Med*. 2015;372(17):1646–1655.
3. Bulun SE. Uterine fibroids. *N Engl J Med*. 2013;369(14):1344–1355.
4. Gupta JK, Sinha A, Lumsden MA, et al. Uterine artery embolization for symptomatic uterine fibroids. *Cochrane Database Syst Rev*. 2014;(12):CD005073.
5. Tristan M, Orozco LJ, Steed A, et al. Mifepristone for uterine fibroids. *Cochrane Database Syst Rev*. 2012;(8):CD007687.

CODES

ICD10

- D25.9 Leiomyoma of uterus, unspecified
- D25.2 Subserosal leiomyoma of uterus
- D25.1 Intramural leiomyoma of uterus

CLINICAL PEARLS

- Uterine myomas are benign smooth muscle tumors composed mainly of fibrous connective tissue.
- Usually incidental finding on pelvic exam or ultrasound but may cause pelvic pain and pressure, abnormal uterine bleeding, and/or infertility
- Management ranges from conservative to medical to surgical.

U

UVEITIS

Mikayla L. Spangler, PharmD • Laura K. Klug, PharmD • Matthew A. Halfar, MD

 BASICS

DESCRIPTION

- A nonspecific term used to describe any intraocular inflammatory disorder
- The uvea is the middle layer of the eye between the sclera and retina. The anterior part of the uvea includes the iris and ciliary body. The posterior part of the uvea is the choroid.
  - Anterior uveitis: refers to ocular inflammation limited to the iris (iritis) alone or iris and ciliary body (iridocyclitis)
  - Intermediate uveitis: refers to inflammation of the structures just posterior to the lens (pars planitis or peripheral uveitis)
  - Posterior uveitis: refers to inflammation of the choroid (choroiditis), retina (retinitis), or vitreous near the optic nerve and macula
  - Panuveitis: refers to inflammation of all of the above areas of the uvea
- System(s) affected: nervous
- Synonym(s): iritis; iridocyclitis; choroiditis; retinochoroiditis; chorioretinitis; anterior uveitis; posterior uveitis; pars planitis; panuveitis; synonyms are anatomic descriptions of the focus of the uveal inflammation

Pediatric Considerations
- Infection should be the primary consideration.
- Allergies and psychological factors (depression, stress) may serve as triggers.
- Trauma is also a common cause in this population.

EPIDEMIOLOGY
Predominant sex: male = female, except for human leukocyte antigen B27 (HLA-B27) anterior uveitis: male > female, autoimmune etiology: female > male

Incidence
Overall incidence is 17 to 52 cases/100,000 per year in the developed countries.

Prevalence
- Overall prevalence is 38 to 714 cases/100,000 population.
- Anterior uveitis is the most common (80% of cases) with iritis being 4 times more prevalent than posterior uveitis.

ETIOLOGY AND PATHOPHYSIOLOGY
- Infectious: may result from viral, bacterial, parasitic, or fungal etiologies
- Suspected immune mediated: possible autoimmune or immune complex–mediated mechanism postulated in association with systemic (especially rheumatologic) disorders
  - Autoimmune uveitis (AIU) patients should be referred to an ophthalmologist for local treatment.
- Isolated eye disease
- Undifferentiated (~25%)

- Some medications may cause uveitis. The most causative medications include rifabutin, bisphosphonates, sulfonamides, metipranolol, brimonidine, prostaglandin analogs, immune checkpoint inhibitors, TNF-α inhibitors, protein kinase inhibitors (BRAF and MEK), anti–vascular endothelial growth factor (VEGF) agents, bacillus Calmette-Guérin (BCG) vaccination, and systemic and intraocular cidofovir.
- Masquerade syndromes: diseases such as malignancies that may be mistaken for primary inflammation of the eye

Genetics
- Iritis: 50–70% are HLA-B27 positive.
- Predisposing gene for posterior uveitis associated with Behçet disease may include HLA-B51.

RISK FACTORS
No specific risk factors

COMMONLY ASSOCIATED CONDITIONS
- Viral infections: herpes simplex, herpes zoster, HIV, cytomegalovirus, congenital Zika virus
- Bacterial infections: brucellosis, leprosy, leptospirosis, Lyme disease, propionibacterium infection, syphilis, tuberculosis (TB), Whipple disease
- Parasitic infections: acanthamebiasis, cysticercosis, onchocerciasis, toxocariasis, toxoplasmosis
- Fungal infections: aspergillosis, blastomycosis, candidiasis, coccidioidomycosis, cryptococcosis, histoplasmosis, sporotrichosis
- Suspected immune mediated: ankylosing spondylitis, Behçet disease, Crohn disease, drug or hypersensitivity reaction, interstitial nephritis, juvenile rheumatoid arthritis, Kawasaki disease, multiple sclerosis, psoriatic arthritis, Reiter syndrome, relapsing polychondritis, sarcoidosis, Sjögren syndrome, systemic lupus erythematosus, ulcerative colitis, vasculitis, vitiligo, Vogt-Koyanagi (Harada) syndrome
- Isolated eye disease: acute multifocal placoid pigmentary epitheliopathy, acute retinal necrosis, birdshot chorioretinopathy, Fuchs heterochromic cyclitis, glaucomatocyclitic crisis, lens-induced uveitis, multifocal choroiditis, pars planitis, serpiginous choroiditis, sympathetic ophthalmia, trauma
- Masquerade syndromes: leukemia, lymphoma, retinitis pigmentosa, retinoblastoma

DIAGNOSIS

HISTORY
- Decreased visual acuity
- Pain, photophobia, blurring of vision (1)[C]
  - Usually acute
- Anterior uveitis
  - Generally acute in onset
  - Deep eye pain
  - Photophobia (consensual)
- Intermediate and posterior uveitis
  - Unresolving floaters
  - Generally insidious in onset
  - More commonly bilateral

PHYSICAL EXAM
Slit-lamp exam and indirect ophthalmoscopy are necessary for precise diagnosis (1)[C].

- Anterior uveitis
  - Conjunctival vessel dilation
  - Perilimbal (circumcorneal) dilation of episcleral and scleral vessels (ciliary flush)
  - Small pupillary size of affected eye
  - Hypopyon or hyphema (WBCs or RBCs pooled in the anterior chamber)
  - Frequently unilateral (95% of HLA-B27–associated cases); if first occurrence and otherwise asymptomatic, no further diagnostic testing is needed (1)[C].
  - Bilateral involvement and systemic symptoms (fever, fatigue, abdominal pain) may be associated with interstitial nephritis (1)[C].
  - Systemic disease is most likely to be associated with anterior uveitis (in one study, 53% of patients were found to have systemic disease) (1)[C].
- Intermediate and posterior uveitis
  - More commonly bilateral
  - Posterior inflammation will generally cause minimal pain or redness unless associated with an iritis.

DIFFERENTIAL DIAGNOSIS
- Acute angle-closure glaucoma
- Conjunctivitis; episcleritis; keratitis; scleritis

DIAGNOSTIC TESTS & INTERPRETATION
No specific test for the diagnosis of uveitis; tests for etiologic factors or associated conditions should be based on history and physical exam (1)[C].

Initial Tests (lab, imaging)
- CBC, BUN, creatinine (interstitial nephritis) (1)[C]
- HLA-B27 typing (ankylosing spondylitis, Reiter syndrome) (1)[C],(2)
- Antinuclear antibody, ESR (systemic lupus erythematosus, Sjögren syndrome) (1)[C],(2)
- Venereal disease research laboratory (VDRL) test, fluorescent titer antibody (syphilis) (1)[C],(2)
- Fluorescent treponemal antibody absorption (FTA-ABS) or microhemagglutination assay for antibodies to *Treponema pallidum* (MHA-TP) (1)[C]
- Purified protein derivative (PPD) tuberculin skin test (TB) (1)[C]
- Lyme serology (Lyme disease) (1)[C],(2)
- Chest x-ray (sarcoidosis, histoplasmosis, TB, lymphoma) (1)[C],(2)
- Sacroiliac radiograph (ankylosing spondylitis) (1)[C]

Diagnostic Procedures/Other
Slit-lamp exam (1)[C],(2)

Test Interpretation

- Keratic precipitates
- Inflammatory cells in anterior chamber or vitreous
- Synechiae (fibrous tissue scarring between iris and lens)
- Macular edema
- Perivasculitis of retinal vessels

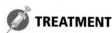 TREATMENT

GENERAL MEASURES

- Urgent ophthalmologic consultation
- Medical therapy is best initiated following full ophthalmologic evaluation.
- Treatment of underlying cause, if identified
- Anti-inflammatory therapy

MEDICATION

First Line

- The treatment depends on the etiology, location, and severity of the inflammation.
- Prednisolone acetate 1% ophthalmic suspension: 1 to 2 drops to the affected eye 2 to 4 times per day, during first 24 to 48 hours, dosing frequency may be increased or dexamethasone 0.1% ophthalmic suspension: 1 to 2 drops to the affected eye 4 to 6 times per day, may use hourly in severe disease; other corticosteroid options include prednisolone sodium phosphate 1% solution, dexamethasone sodium phosphate 0.1% solution, loteprednol etabonate 0.5% (Lotemax) suspension, and difluprednate (Durezol) 0.05% emulsion (1),(2)[C].
  - Taper prior to discontinuation
  - Contraindications
    - Hypersensitivity to the medication or component of the preparation
    - Topical corticosteroid therapy is contraindicated in uveitis secondary to infectious etiologies, unless used in conjunction with appropriate anti-infectious agents.
  - Precautions
    - Topical corticosteroids may increase intraocular pressure, increase susceptibility to infections, impair corneal or scleral wound healing, or cause corneal epithelial toxicity or crystalline keratopathy. Prolonged use may cause cataract formation and exacerbate existing herpetic keratitis, which may masquerade as iritis.
    - Significant possible interactions
- Cycloplegic agents may be used to dilate the eye and relieve pain. Agents include atropine 1% 1 to 2 drops up to QID or homatropine hydrobromide (Isopto) 5% 1 to 2 drops q3–4h (1)[C].
  - Contraindications
    - Patients known to have or be predisposed to glaucoma
  - Precautions
    - Use extreme caution in infants, young children, and elderly because of increased susceptibility to systemic effects.

Second Line

- Systemic corticosteroids are useful for maintenance therapy for patients with noninfectious posterior uveitis or for severe ocular inflammation. These should always be used with other immunosuppressive medications for steroid-sparing effects; prednisone ≤7.5 mg daily (2)[B]
- Intravitreal corticosteroid deposits may also be used for long-term maintenance; fluocinolone acetonide (Retisert [590 μg released over 30 months] and Yutiq [180 μg released over 36 months]), dexamethasone (Ozurdex) 0.7 mg released slowly >3 to 6 months (2),(3)[C]
  - Retisert has caused nearly all patients to develop cataracts and significant increases in intraocular pressure in just >75% of patients, whereas Ozurdex resulted in less occurrence of an increase in intraocular pressure and cataract development (2),(3)[C].
- Intravitreal triamcinolone acetonide injections can be given (2)[C].
- Immunosuppressive agents including antimetabolites (methotrexate, azathioprine, and mycophenolate mofetil), T-cell inhibitors (cyclosporine and tacrolimus), and alkylating agents (cyclophosphamide, chlorambucil) may be employed in cases of resistant or intolerant to initial treatment or used for their corticosteroid-sparing effect. Close monitoring is required (3),(4)[C].
- Advancing research suggests benefit of the biologic agents in refractory uveitis. Adalimumab is the only biologic agent with FDA approval for this indication. Other biologic agents, including infliximab, golimumab, certolizumab pegol, abatacept, and tocilizumab, have also been studied (2),(3),(4)[C].
  - Benefits of biologic therapy include glucocorticoid sparing effects, but limitations may include high cost and adverse effect potential.
- Systemic and ophthalmic preparations of NSAIDs may provide some symptom relief (1)[C].

ISSUES FOR REFERRAL

Caution when using empiric treatment; referral to an ophthalmologist is recommended in most cases.

SURGERY/OTHER PROCEDURES

Various surgical procedures may be used to manage complications associated with uveitis but do not reverse the underlying cause (4).

 ONGOING CARE

FOLLOW-UP RECOMMENDATIONS

Patient Monitoring

- Complete history and physical to evaluate for associated systemic disease
- Ophthalmologic follow-up as recommended by consultant

PATIENT EDUCATION

- Instruct on proper method for instilling eye drops.
- Wear dark glasses if photophobia is a problem.

PROGNOSIS

- Depends on the presence of causal diseases or associated conditions
- Uveitis resulting from infections (systemic or local) tends to resolve with eradication of the underlying infection.
- Uveitis associated with seronegative arthropathies tends to be acute (lasting <3 months) and frequently recurrent.

COMPLICATIONS

- Cycloplegia: paralysis of the ciliary muscle of the eye, resulting in a loss of accommodation
- Loss of vision as a result of the following:
  - Keratic precipitate deposition on the corneal or lens surfaces
  - Increased intraocular pressure, acute angle-closure glaucoma
  - Formation of synechiae
  - Cataract formation
  - Vasculitis with vascular occlusion, retinal infarction
  - Macular edema
  - Optic nerve damage

REFERENCES

1. Harthan JS, Opitz DL, Fromstein SR, et al. Diagnosis and treatment of anterior uveitis: optometric management. *Clin Optom (Auckl)*. 2016;8:23–35.
2. Burkholder BM, Jabs DA. Uveitis for the non-ophthalmologist. *BMJ*. 2021;372:m4979.
3. Pleyer U, Neri P, Deuter C. New pharmacotherapy options for noninfectious posterior uveitis. *Int Ophthalmol*. 2021;41(6):2265–2281.
4. Dick AD, Rosenbaum JT, Al-Dhibi HA, et al; for Fundamentals of Care for Uveitis International Consensus Group. Guidance on noncorticosteroid systemic immunomodulatory therapy in noninfectious uveitis: Fundamentals of Care for UveitiS (FOCUS) initiative. *Ophthalmology*. 2018;125(5):757–773.

ADDITIONAL READING

- Abdalla Elsayed MEA, Kozak I. Pharmacologically induced uveitis. *Surv Ophthalmol*. 2021;66(5): 781–801.
- Majumder PD, Biswas J. Pediatric uveitis: an update. *Oman J Ophthalmol*. 2013;6(3):140–150.

 SEE ALSO

Conjunctivitis, Acute; Glaucoma, Primary Closed-Angle; Scleritis

CODES

ICD10

- H20.9 Unspecified iridocyclitis
- H30.90 Unspecified chorioretinal inflammation, unspecified eye
- H20.019 Primary iridocyclitis, unspecified eye

CLINICAL PEARLS

- Symptoms vary depending on depth of involvement and associated conditions but should be suspected when eye pain is associated with visual changes.
- Severe or unresponsive uveitis may require therapy, including periocular injection of corticosteroids, sustained-release corticosteroid implants, systemic corticosteroids, cytotoxic agents, immunosuppressive agents, immunomodulatory agents, or tumor necrosis factor inhibitors.

VAGINAL ADENOSIS

Sareena Singh, MD, FACOG • Kimberly Resnick, MD

BASICS

DESCRIPTION
- The normal vagina is lined with squamous epithelium. Adenosis is characterized by the presence of columnar epithelium or glandular tissue in the wall of the vagina.
- Around week 15 of embryologic development, the müllerian system, which forms the upper 2/3 of the vagina, fuses with the invaginating cloaca or urogenital sinus to form the lower 1/3 of the vagina. Squamous metaplasia from the cloacal region then produces squamous epithelium within the vagina (1).
- *Adenosis* occurs when this squamous epithelium fails to epithelialize the vagina completely.
- Three main types of adenosis epithelium:
  - Endocervical
  - Endometrial
  - Tubal
- System(s) affected: reproductive

Geriatric Considerations
- Adenosis is a disorder of the young female. By menopause, the vagina and cervix should be completely epithelialized.
- In a postmenopausal patient, the presence of glandular epithelium is an indication for excision and evaluation, given the risk of well-differentiated adenocarcinoma.

Pregnancy Considerations
Pregnancy produces a wide eversion of the transformation zone of the cervix. This can become so widely everted that it will extend onto the vaginal fornices, leading to the impression of adenosis. This will resolve after pregnancy.

EPIDEMIOLOGY
Incidence
- Although the cumulative incidence of vaginal adenosis is unknown, the incidence of cloacal malformations is 1/20,000 to 1/25,000 live births.
- Although spontaneous vaginal adenosis appears to be fairly common (10% of adult women), it is mostly an insignificant coincidental finding. Widespread symptomatic involvement is rare (2).

Prevalence
- In the United States, adenosis is common in young women, affecting 10–20%. As maturation progresses with puberty, epithelialization occurs.
- Predominant age
  - Age <1 month: 15%
  - Prepubertal: typically absent
  - Age 13 to 25 years: 13%
  - Age >25 years: decreasing prevalence, uncommon beyond age 30 years (2)

ETIOLOGY AND PATHOPHYSIOLOGY
- In most young females, the etiology is incomplete squamous metaplasia or epithelialization. This occurs as a natural phenomenon and resolves with age.
- Described as congenital or acquired:
  - Congenital: proliferation of the remnant müllerian epithelium in the vagina due to exposure to diethylstilbestrol (DES) in utero ("DES daughters"). DES is a synthetic, nonsteroidal estrogen used to prevent miscarriage or premature deliveries from 1938 to 1971 (3). An estimated 5 million women were prescribed DES during this period (4).
  - Transformation-related protein 63 (TRP63/p63) marks the cell fate of müllerian duct epithelium to become squamous epithelium in the cervix and vagina. DES disrupts the TRP63 expression and induces adenosis lesions (4). It has also been suggested that DES induces vaginal adenosis by inhibiting the BMP4/Activin A-regulated vaginal cell fate through a downregulation of RUNX1 (5).
  - Acquired: trauma and inflammation causing spontaneous de novo changes or changes in an acquired lesion in the vaginal epithelium
  - Additional reports documented adenosis subsequent to sulfonamide-induced Stevens–Johnson syndrome and after treatment of vaginal condylomas with 5-fluorouracil (6).

RISK FACTORS
Adenosis of the vagina/cervix may arise in up to 90% of DES daughters and has a 40-fold increased risk of developing into clear cell adenocarcinoma (3).

GENERAL PREVENTION
None: Last DES exposure was in the 1970s.

COMMONLY ASSOCIATED CONDITIONS
DES exposure
- Adenosis from DES exposure should lead to an evaluation of other DES-related abnormalities.
- Müllerian tract anomalies associated with DES exposure include cervical hood, cervical ridge, shortened cervix, incompetent cervix, and T-shaped uterine cavity.
- Patients with known DES exposure should have their reproductive tract evaluated prior to conception.
- Most patients with adenosis have not been DES-exposed and do not require evaluation of the reproductive system.
- The FDA issued a drug bulletin in 1971 advising physicians to stop prescribing DES to pregnant women because of its link to vaginal clear cell adenocarcinoma in DES daughters (3).

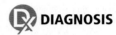

DIAGNOSIS

HISTORY
- Maternal DES exposure
- Complaints of
  - Profuse mucoid vaginal discharge from the glandular epithelium
  - Pruritus
  - Pain/soreness of the vaginal introitus
  - Postcoital bleeding
  - Dyspareunia

PHYSICAL EXAM
On pelvic exam, adenosis appearance is varied: patchy or diffuse red stippling, granularity or nodularity, single or multiple cysts, erosions, ulcers, or warty protuberances that may even extend to the vulva.

DIFFERENTIAL DIAGNOSIS
- Erosive lichen planus
- Fixed drug eruption
- Erythema multiforme
- Bullous skin disease
- Adenocarcinoma

DIAGNOSTIC TESTS & INTERPRETATION
Initial Tests (lab, imaging)
Four-quadrant Pap smear should be used liberally to isolate quadrants of the vagina that may contain abnormalities. No imaging is indicated, unless diagnosed with underlying malignancy.

Follow-Up Tests & Special Considerations

Pap smear can be followed by colposcopy and biopsy.

Diagnostic Procedures/Other

- Colposcopy should be used to outline areas of adenosis to ensure that no malignancy is present.
- A thorough evaluation for adenocarcinoma of the vagina arising in adenosis should be done.
- A biopsy may be necessary to ensure that the process represents only benign adenosis.

Test Interpretation

- Biopsy will show benign glandular epithelium.
- Biopsies may show areas of ongoing squamous metaplasia.

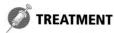 TREATMENT

GENERAL MEASURES

- Unless malignancy is present, treatment is conservative.
- In most young females with this condition, it will resolve with expectant management.
- Treatment is warranted in women with severe subjective symptoms that impair the quality of life.
- First-line treatment: If indicated in patients with focal lesions and no history of DES exposure, simple excision is an effective treatment (6).

ISSUES FOR REFERRAL

Malignancy found on biopsy warrants referral to gynecologic oncology specialist.

SURGERY/OTHER PROCEDURES

- Aggressive therapy, such as laser or surgical excision, is necessary if premalignant or malignant changes arise (5).
- Symptomatic treatment has been performed with carbon dioxide laser coagulation, unipolar coagulation, or vaginal resection.

ADMISSION, INPATIENT, AND NURSING CONSIDERATIONS

Outpatient management

 ONGOING CARE

FOLLOW-UP RECOMMENDATIONS

Patient Monitoring

If the initial colposcopy is normal, a yearly four-quadrant Pap smear of the vagina and of the cervix should be performed.

DIET

No special diet is recommended.

PATIENT EDUCATION

- No limitations
- It is not necessary to avoid intercourse or placing objects in the vagina.
- The patient should be educated to keep normal guideline-recommended pelvic and Pap smear appointments. In most situations, this is benign, and expectant management is all that is necessary.
- http://www.acog.org/

PROGNOSIS

- Most patients will have squamous metaplasia and epithelialization with complete resolution of the adenosis.
- The rare patient, 1/1,000 to 1/10,000, may develop adenocarcinoma in the adenosis and will require definitive therapy as for vaginal cancer.
  - Cumulative incidence of progression of adenosis to adenocarcinoma is 1.5/1,000 for DES daughters (3).

COMPLICATIONS

- Infertility with DES association
- Adverse pregnancy outcome with DES association
- Adenocarcinoma of vagina
- Clear cell adenocarcinoma with DES association

REFERENCES

1. Reich O, Fritsch H. The developmental origin of cervical and vaginal epithelium and their clinical consequences: a systematic review. *J Low Genit Tract Dis*. 2014;18(4):358–360.
2. Kranl C, Zelger B, Kofler H, et al. Vulval and vaginal adenosis. *Br J Dermatol*. 1998;139(1):128–131.
3. National Toxicology Program, Department of Health and Human Services. Diethylstilbestrol. In: *Report on Carcinogens*. 12th ed. Research Triangle Park, NC: National Toxicology Program, U.S. Department of Health and Human Services; 2011:159–161.
4. Laronda MM, Unno K, Butler LM, et al. The development of cervical and vaginal adenosis as a result of diethylstilbestrol exposure in utero. *Differentiation*. 2012;84(3):252–260.
5. Laronda M, Unno K, Ishi K, et al. Diethylstilbestrol induces vaginal adenosis by disrupting SMAD/RUNX1-mediated cell fate decision in the Müllerian duct epithelium. *Dev Biol*. 2013;381(1):5–16.
6. Martin AA, Atkins KA, Lonergan CL, et al. Vaginal adenosis as a dermatologic complaint. *J Am Acad Dermatol*. 2013;69(2):e92–e93.

ADDITIONAL READING

Bamigboye AA, Morris J. Oestrogen supplementation, mainly diethylstilbestrol, for preventing miscarriages and other adverse pregnancy outcomes. *Cochrane Database Syst Rev*. 2003;(3):CD004353.

 SEE ALSO

Vaginal Malignancy

 CODES

ICD10

- Q52.4 Other congenital malformations of vagina
- N89.8 Other specified noninflammatory disorders of vagina
- T38.5X5A Adverse effect of other estrogens and progestogens, initial encounter

CLINICAL PEARLS

- Adenosis is characterized by the presence of columnar epithelium or glandular tissue in the wall of the vagina.
- Adenosis is common among the daughters of women exposed to DES.
- Rarely, adenosis can be associated with an underlying vaginal malignancy.

V

VAGINAL BLEEDING DURING PREGNANCY

Morgan J. Parker, DO • Elizabeth J. Trout, MD, MLS

 BASICS

DESCRIPTION
- Vaginal bleeding during pregnancy has many causes and ranges in severity from benign with normal pregnancy outcome to life-threatening for both infant and mother.
- Etiology can be from the vagina, cervix, uterus, fetus, or placenta. The differential diagnosis is guided by the gestational age of the fetus.

EPIDEMIOLOGY
Prevalence
- In early pregnancy: 7–25% of patients
- In late pregnancy: 0.3–2% of patients

ETIOLOGY AND PATHOPHYSIOLOGY
- Many times, the cause is unknown.
- Anytime in pregnancy:
  - Cervicitis (infectious or noninfectious)
  - Vaginitis (infectious or noninfectious)
  - Vaginal or cervical trauma (including postcoital)
  - Cervical lesion (including polyps or warts) or neoplasia
  - Hyperemia of cervix (increased blood flow from pregnancy)
- Early pregnancy:
  - For up to 50% of early pregnancy bleeding, no cause is ever found.
  - Ectopic pregnancy: leading cause of 1st-trimester maternal death in the United States—must be excluded in every pregnant patient with bleeding. Risk factors: previous ectopic, trauma to fallopian tubes (tubal surgery, infection, tumor), congenital anomaly of tubes, in utero diethylstilbestrol (DES) exposure, current use of IUD, history of infertility, tobacco use
  - Spontaneous abortion: risk factors: advanced maternal age (AMA), alcohol use, tobacco use, anesthetic gas, heavy caffeine use, cocaine use, chronic maternal diseases (poorly controlled diabetes mellitus [DM], celiac disease, autoimmune diseases such as antiphospholipid syndrome), short interconception time (3 to 6 months), current use of IUD, maternal infection (e.g., herpes simplex virus [HSV], gonorrhea, chlamydia, toxoplasmosis, listeriosis, HIV, syphilis, malaria), medications (e.g., retinoids, methotrexate, NSAIDs), multiple previous therapeutic abortions, previous spontaneous abortion, toxins (arsenic, lead, polyurethane), uterine abnormalities (congenital, adhesions, fibroids); bleeding may be a cause and/or a consequence of early pregnancy loss.
  - Loss of one fetus from a multiple gestation ("vanishing twin")
  - Implantation bleeding: benign, about 6 days after fertilization
  - Uterine fibroids
  - Subchorionic bleeding (or hematoma): in late 1st trimester
  - Low-lying placenta
  - Gestational trophoblastic disease: hydatidiform mole (most common), choriocarcinoma, or placental-site trophoblastic tumors

- Late pregnancy:
  - Bloody show of labor (loss of mucus plug)
  - Placenta previa: painless bleeding; occurs in 0.4% deliveries in the United States. Risk factors: previous history of placenta previa, previous uterine surgery (cesarean section, D&C), chronic hypertension, multiparity, multiple gestation, tobacco use, AMA
  - Placental abruption: (typically) painful bleeding; occurs in 1–2% deliveries in the United States. Risk factors: previous placental abruption, 1st-trimester bleeding, hypertension, preeclampsia, multiple gestation, tobacco, cocaine or methamphetamine use, unexplained elevated maternal α-fetoprotein, poly- or oligohydramnios, AMA, trauma to abdomen, premature rupture of membranes, thrombophilia, short umbilical cord, male fetus, chorioamnionitis, nutritional deficiency
  - Vasa previa: minimal bleeding with fetal distress; rare (1:2,500 deliveries). Risk factors: in vitro fertilization, multiple gestations, placental abnormalities (low-lying position, bilobate, succenturiate lobe, velamentous insertion of umbilical cord)
  - Placenta accreta, increta, percreta: risk factors: uterine scar (e.g., from cesarean section, endometrial ablation, or D&C), current placenta previa, AMA, tobacco use, multiparity, uterine anomalies, uterine fibroids, hypertension
  - Uterine rupture: typically presents with vaginal bleeding, abnormal fetal heart rate, and disordered or hypertonic uterine contractions with or without pain. Risk factors: previous cesarean section (most common), trauma, use of oxytocin or prostaglandins, multiparity, external cephalic version, placental abruption, shoulder dystocia, placenta percreta, müllerian duct anomalies, history of pelvic radiation

RISK FACTORS
See specific etiologies in earlier discussion.

GENERAL PREVENTION
- Address modifiable risk factors such as domestic violence and tobacco and drug use.
- If placenta or vasa previa, nothing per vagina

 DIAGNOSIS

HISTORY
- Anytime in pregnancy: quality of pregnancy dating, context (e.g., following bowel movement, during voiding, after intercourse, drug use, or trauma including domestic violence), amount of bleeding, obstetrical history, personal or family history of inherited bleeding disorders
- Early pregnancy: severe nausea/vomiting (can be associated with molar pregnancy); amount of bleeding, pelvic pain, or suprapubic cramping (e.g., spontaneous abortion, ectopic) complications in previous pregnancies (e.g., spontaneous abortion, abruption, 1st-trimester vaginal bleeding)
- Late pregnancy: contractions (labor), abdominal pain especially between contractions (abruption, uterine rupture), presence or absence of fetal movement, rupture of membranes
- See "Etiology and Pathophysiology" for additional pertinent history.

PHYSICAL EXAM
- Vital signs: When present, signs of hemodynamic instability are first tachycardia and tachypnea and then hypotension and thready pulse.
- Abdomen: uterine tenderness, fundal height (increasing fundal height may be associated with placental abruption)
- Speculum: Visualize cervix and identify source of bleeding (from cervical os or from within vagina).
- Cervix: Assess for dilation; required to assess for labor but should not be performed until placenta previa ruled out via ultrasound
- Fetal monitoring: Doppler heart tones in early pregnancy; external fetal monitoring for gestational age >26 weeks

DIFFERENTIAL DIAGNOSIS
- Hematuria (UTI, kidney stones)
- Rectal bleeding

DIAGNOSTIC TESTS & INTERPRETATION
Initial Tests (lab, imaging)
- CBC
- Blood type and screen if more than minimal bleeding; if significant hemorrhage, type and crossmatch
- Quantitative β-human chorionic gonadotropin (β-hCG):
  - Prior to 12 weeks, levels can be followed serially every 2 days with following trends:
    ○ Doubles or at least 66% rise in 48 hours in normal pregnancy
    ○ Falls in spontaneous abortion
    ○ Rises gradually (<50% in 48 hours) or plateaus in ectopic pregnancy
    ○ Extremely high in molar pregnancy
- Transvaginal ultrasound should be used to confirm an intrauterine pregnancy (IUP) when the quantitative β-hCG >2,000 (1)[A].
- Other lab tests based on clinical scenario:
  - Wet mount, gonorrhea/chlamydia/trichomoniasis, Pap smear
  - Progesterone level occasionally used to determine viability in threatened abortion (<5 indicates not viable, >25 indicates viability, 5 to 25 is equivocal)
  - Prothrombin time with international normalized ratio (INR), partial thromboplastin time, fibrinogen, and fibrin split products: if suspect coagulopathy or abruption
  - Kleihauer-Betke: assesses for fetal–maternal hemorrhage; low sensitivity and specificity for abruption; helpful for dosing RhoGAM
- Transvaginal ultrasound is the preferred imaging modality.
  - Early pregnancy:
    ○ Gestational sac seen at 5 to 6 weeks; fetal heartbeat observed by 8 to 9 weeks
    ○ Diagnostic of ectopic with nearly 100% sensitivity when β-hCG level is 1,500 to 2,000 mIU/mL; if no IUP is present and ultrasound does not confirm ectopic pregnancy, serial quantitative β-hCG values should be followed (2)[C].
  - Late pregnancy:
    ○ Proceed to rule out placenta previa with ultrasound, labor with serial cervical exams, and abruption with external fetal monitoring.

TREATMENT

MEDICATION

First Line

- Treat underlying cause of bleeding, if identified.
- If mother is Rh-negative, give RhoGAM to prevent autoimmunization. In late pregnancy, dose according to the amount of estimated fetal–maternal hemorrhage.
- If cause of bleeding is preterm labor, consider betamethasone for fetal lung maturity if <36 weeks' gestation. Tocolytics may be used to prolong pregnancy to allow for course of steroids.
- If threatened abortion: Consider progesterone (relative risk 0.53) (3)[A]; shown to improve live birth outcomes in subgroups of pregnant patients in 1st trimester, namely women with history of three or more spontaneous abortions
- If mother has an inherited bleeding disorder or if bleeding is severe, consider recombinant or donor blood products.

SURGERY/OTHER PROCEDURES

- Cesarean section may be indicated for recurrent or uncontrolled bleeding with placenta previa or vasa previa.
- If ectopic is diagnosed, immediate surgical treatment may be needed. Some early ectopic pregnancies can be treated medically if certain criteria are met (2)[C].
- Surgical uterine evacuation is necessary for molar pregnancy due to malignant potential (4)[C].
- Incomplete or inevitable spontaneous abortion: Management is patient centered and should include psychological support. In the absence of infection, patient may elect expectant, medical, or surgical management. If expectant management, typically wait 2 weeks for patient to complete abortion; most complete by 9 days. If at 2 weeks, abortion is not completed or medical management has failed, surgical intervention (D&C or aspiration) is generally indicated (5)[A]; may send tissue to pathology to confirm

ADMISSION, INPATIENT, AND NURSING CONSIDERATIONS

- In early pregnancy: based on quantity of bleeding, need for surgical treatment for ectopic pregnancy, or presence of infection in case of spontaneous abortion
- In late pregnancy, consider admission if there is significant bleeding and/or presence of maternal or fetal compromise.
- In late pregnancy, consider admission with trauma, if ≥2 contractions per 10 minutes.

- In late pregnancy, may discharge when bleeding has stopped; labor, previa, and abruption have been ruled out; and fetal heart tracing is normal
- After trauma in late pregnancy, may discharge home if normal fetal heart tracing for ≥4 hours with <2 contractions per 10 minutes

 ONGOING CARE

FOLLOW-UP RECOMMENDATIONS

Patient Monitoring

- Patient should be instructed to report any increase in the amount or frequency of bleeding and to seek immediate care if experiencing fever, dizziness, abdominal pain, or sudden increased bleeding. Patient should save any tissue passed vaginally for examination.
- Frequency of outpatient follow-up as indicated based on etiology of bleeding

PATIENT EDUCATION

- American Academy of Family Physicians (AAFP): https://www.familydoctor.org
- American College of Obstetricians and Gynecologists (ACOG): https://www.acog.org/

PROGNOSIS

- Prognosis depends on the etiology of vaginal bleeding, severity of bleeding, and rapidity of diagnosis.
- Maternal mortality is 31.9 deaths per 100,000 ectopic pregnancies.
- 1/2 of patients with early pregnancy bleeding miscarry; if fetal heart activity (ultrasound) present in 1st-trimester bleeding, <10% chance of pregnancy loss
- Heavy bleeding in early pregnancy, particularly when accompanied by pain, is associated with higher risk of spontaneous abortion. Spotting and light episodes are not, especially if lasting only 1 to 2 days. There may be a decreased risk of pregnancy loss if the patient experiences nausea/vomiting.
- Subchorionic bleeding has about 2- to 3-fold increased risk of spontaneous abortion. Smaller hemorrhage and presence of viable fetal heart rate confer lower risk of loss; most resolve spontaneously.
- Women with early pregnancy bleeding have an increased risk of preterm delivery, premature rupture of membranes, manual removal of placenta, placental abruption, elective cesarean delivery, and term labor induction later in the same pregnancy. These women also have an increased risk of adverse pregnancy outcomes, including hyperbilirubinemia, congenital anomalies, NICU admission, and reduced neonatal birth weight. Finally, there is an increased risk in subsequent pregnancies of recurrence of early pregnancy bleeding.
- Bed rest has not been shown to affect the outcome of bleeding in early pregnancy but may be indicated for bleeding in late pregnancy with placenta or vasa previa or with maternal hypertension.

REFERENCES

1. Crochet JR, Bastian LA, Chireau MV. Does this woman have an ectopic pregnancy? the rational clinical examination systematic review. *JAMA*. 2013;309(16):1722–1729.
2. Deutchman M, Tubay AT, Turok D. First trimester bleeding. *Am Fam Physician*. 2009;79(11):985–994.
3. Wahabi HA, Fayed AA, Esmaeil SA, et al. Progestogen for treating threatened miscarriage. *Cochrane Database Syst Rev*. 2011;(12):CD005943.
4. Snell BJ. Assessment and management of bleeding in the first trimester of pregnancy. *J Midwifery Womens Health*. 2009;54(6):483–491.
5. Nanda K, Lopez LM, Grimes DA, et al. Expectant care versus surgical treatment for miscarriage. *Cochrane Database Syst Rev*. 2012;2012(3):CD003518.

ADDITIONAL READING

- Al-Ma'ani W, Solomayer EF, Hammadeh M. Expectant versus surgical management of first-trimester miscarriage: a randomised controlled study. *Arch Gynecol Obstet*. 2014;289(5):1011–1015.
- Chi C, Kadir RA. Inherited bleeding disorders in pregnancy. *Best Pract Res Clin Obstet Gynaecol*. 2012;26(1):103–117.
- Prine LW, MacNaughton H. Office management of early pregnancy loss. *Am Fam Physician*. 2011;84(1):75–82.

 SEE ALSO

Abnormal Pap and Cervical Dysplasia; Abruptio Placentae; Cervical Malignancy; Cervical Polyps; Cervicitis, Ectropion, and True Erosion; Chlamydia Infection (Sexually Transmitted); Ectopic Pregnancy; Miscarriage (Early Pregnancy Loss); Placenta Previa; Preterm Labor; Trichomoniasis; Vaginal Malignancy

V

CODES

ICD10

- O20.9 Hemorrhage in early pregnancy, unspecified
- O46.90 Antepartum hemorrhage, unspecified, unspecified trimester
- O20.0 Threatened abortion

CLINICAL PEARLS

- Obtain blood type and screen all women presenting with vaginal bleeding in pregnancy after 8 to 9 weeks' gestation and administer RhoGAM to all Rh-negative patients.
- For up to 50% of early pregnancy bleeding, no cause is ever found.
- Always consider ectopic pregnancy in 1st-trimester bleeding.
- Do not perform digital exam in late pregnancy bleeding until placenta has been located on ultrasound.

VAGINAL MALIGNANCY

Sareena Singh, MD, FACOG

 BASICS

DESCRIPTION

- Carcinomas of the vagina are uncommon: 2–3% of gynecologic malignancies; 2,300 new cases annually.
- Vaginal intraepithelial neoplasia (VAIN), defined by squamous cell atypia, is classified by the depth of epithelial involvement:
  - VAIN 1: 1/3 thickness
  - VAIN 2: 2/3 thickness
  - VAIN 3: >2/3 thickness
  - Carcinoma in situ (CIS): designating full-thickness neoplastic changes without invasion through the basement membrane
- Invasive malignancies: Vaginal malignancies include squamous cell carcinoma (85–90%), adenocarcinoma (5–10%), sarcoma (2–3%), and melanoma (2–3%). Clear cell carcinoma is a subtype of adenocarcinoma. Invasive squamous cell carcinoma has the potential for metastasis to the lungs and liver.
- To be classified as a vaginal malignancy, only the vagina can be involved. If the cervix or vulva is involved, then the tumor is classified as a primary cancer arising from the cervix or the vulva. Additionally, if the patient has had a diagnosis of invasive cervical or vulvar cancer in the preceding 5 years, it can not be classified as a primary vaginal malignancy.
- Most vaginal malignancies are metastatic tumors from other primary sites (e.g., cervix, vulva, endometrium, breast, ovary).
- Most common sites of primary vaginal cancer metastases: lung, liver, bone

Pregnancy Considerations
This malignancy is not typically associated with pregnancy.

EPIDEMIOLOGY

Incidence
Predominant age
- CIS: mid-40 to 60 years
- Invasive squamous cell malignancy: mid-60 to 70 years
- Adenocarcinoma: any age; 50 years is the mean age. Peak incidence is between 17 and 21 years of age.
- Clear cell adenocarcinoma occurs most often in females aged <30 years with a history of exposure to diethylstilbestrol (DES) in utero.
- Mixed müllerian sarcomas and leiomyosarcomas in the adult population: mean age is 60 years

Pediatric Considerations
Vaginal tumors are extremely rare. Rhabdomyosarcoma (botryoid and embryonal subtype) is the most common malignant neoplasm of the vagina. Less common entities are germ cell tumor and clear cell adenocarcinoma.

Prevalence
In the United States, it is one of the rarest of all gynecologic malignancies (3%).

ETIOLOGY AND PATHOPHYSIOLOGY

- Women with a history of cervical malignancy have a higher probability of developing squamous cell malignancy in the vagina, even after hysterectomy.
- Human papillomavirus (HPV) is found in 80–93% of patients with vaginal CIS and 50–65% of the patients with invasive vaginal carcinoma.
- HPV-16 is the most common, found in 66% of CIS and 55% of invasive vaginal cancers.
- Smokers have a higher incidence.
- Clear cell adenocarcinoma of the vagina in young women has been associated with DES exposure. The incidence, however, is exceedingly rare, estimated at 1/1,000 to 1/10,000 exposed females.
- Metastatic lesions can involve the vagina, spreading from the other gynecologic organs.
- Although rare, renal cell carcinoma, lung adenocarcinoma, GI cancer, pancreatic adenocarcinoma, ovarian germ cell cancer, trophoblastic neoplasm, and breast cancer can all metastasize to the vagina.

Genetics
No known genetic pattern

RISK FACTORS
- Similar risk factors as cervical cancer
- Age
- African American
- Smoking
- Multiple sex partners, early age of first sexual intercourse
- History of squamous cell cancer of the cervix or vulva
- HPV infection
- Vaginal adenosis
- Vaginal irritation
- DES exposure in utero
- Immunocompromised, HIV
- Prior pelvic radiation

COMMONLY ASSOCIATED CONDITIONS
Due to the field effect, patients with vaginal cancer are more likely to develop malignancy in the cervix or vulva and should be followed closely.

 DIAGNOSIS

HISTORY
- Abnormal bleeding is the most common symptom.
- Postcoital bleeding can result from direct trauma to the tumor.
- Vaginal discharge
- Dyspareunia
- Urinary symptoms, including hematuria and increased frequency
- Constipation
- Pain along with symptoms and signs of hydroureter are late findings when the tumor has spread into the paravaginal tissues and extends to the pelvic sidewall.

Pediatric Considerations
In children, sarcomas can present either as a mass protruding from the vagina or as an abnormal genital bleeding.

PHYSICAL EXAM
Pelvic examination
- The vagina, uterus, adnexa (fallopian tubes and ovaries), bladder, and rectum should be evaluated for unusual changes.
- Vaginal malignancies are found most commonly on the posterior wall in the upper 1/3 of the vagina.

DIFFERENTIAL DIAGNOSIS
- Premalignant changes: VAIN 1, 2, and 3 and CIS
- Adequate biopsies ensure that invasive lesions are not overlooked. Invasive lesions penetrate the basement membrane and cannot be treated conservatively.
- Other malignancies, such as endometrial, cervix, bladder, or colon cancer, can invade directly into the vagina or metastasize to the vagina.
- In the childbearing years, trophoblastic disease should be considered.
  - The vagina is a common site of metastases; however, biopsy should typically be avoided because the implants are very vascular and may hemorrhage if sampled.
  - The clinical presentation is typically obvious so histopathologic confirmation before treatment is not required.

DIAGNOSTIC TESTS & INTERPRETATION

Initial Tests (lab, imaging)
- Pap smear may incidentally detect asymptomatic lesions.
- Biopsy suspicious lesions
- Chest x-ray (CXR): to evaluate for metastatic disease
- CT scan and/or MRI: to evaluate the liver and retroperitoneum, especially the lymph nodes in the pelvic and periaortic area
- PET scan detects primary and secondary metastatic lesions more often than CT scan.

> **ALERT**
> PET scan correlation with CT scan lesions strongly suggests malignancy.

Follow-Up Tests & Special Considerations
- Lymphoscintigraphy (sentinel lymph node mapping) as part of the pretreatment evaluation can result in a change in the radiation fields and improve comprehensive treatment planning in women with vaginal cancer.
- HPV vaccination: Implementation of prophylactic HPV vaccination could prevent ~2/3 of the intraepithelial lesions in the lower genital tract but is yet to be proven.

Diagnostic Procedures/Other
- Colposcopy with directed biopsies for small lesions
- Wide excision under anesthesia of superficial disease may be necessary to ensure that invasive cancer is not present.
- Cystoscopy to rule out bladder invasion
- Proctosigmoidoscopy to rule out rectal invasion

Test Interpretation
Tumors are staged clinically:
- Stage 0: VAIN and CIS
- Stage I: carcinoma limited to the vaginal wall (26%)
- Stage II: involves the subvaginal tissues but has not extended to the pelvic wall (37%)
- Stage III: extends to the pelvic wall (24%)
- Stage IV: extends beyond the true pelvis (13%)
  - IVa: Tumor invades bladder and/or rectal mucosa and/or direct extension beyond the true pelvis.
  - IVb: spread to distant organs

TREATMENT

GENERAL MEASURES
Treatment methods for VAIN and CIS include the following:
- Wide local excision
- Partial or total vaginectomy
- Intravaginal chemotherapy with 5% fluorouracil cream
- Laser therapy
- Intracavitary radiation therapy

MEDICATION
- Imiquimod
  - In a review of the effectiveness of 5% imiquimod cream in the treatment of VAIN (1), the following results were reported:
    - ○ 26–100% of patients had complete regression.
    - ○ 0–60% of patients had partial regression.
    - ○ 0–37% of patients experienced recurrence.
- Contraindications
  - The diagnosis must be established with certainty prior to treatment.
  - If there is any doubt that a process beyond in situ disease exists, vaginectomy must be performed. These patients are often elderly, and aggressive therapy is limited by the patient's performance status and ability to tolerate radical surgery, chemotherapy, or radiation.

ISSUES FOR REFERRAL
Patients should be treated and followed by a gynecologic oncologist and/or a radiation oncologist.

ADDITIONAL THERAPIES
- Treatment with radiotherapy depends on the stage of disease (2)[A]. This treatment option should be discussed with physicians experienced with this malignancy.
- It is common to use radiotherapy and sensitizing chemotherapy (chemoradiation) for better cancer control.
- Early-stage primary squamous cell carcinoma treated with radiation alone has shown good results.
- Stage III vaginal cancer may benefit from combined radiation and hyperthermia.

- Patients with advanced squamous cell carcinoma or adenocarcinoma receive concurrent irradiation and cisplatin-based chemotherapy.
- Neoadjuvant chemotherapy followed by radical surgery may benefit selected patients.
- In most tumor types, metastatic disease from the vagina to other sites is only minimally responsive to chemotherapy.
- With one exception, no chemotherapeutic agents have shown a survival advantage. The exception is childhood sarcomas, which have been treated with combinations of the following: vincristine, dactinomycin (actinomycin-D), cyclophosphamide (Cytoxan), cisplatin, etoposide (VP-16)

SURGERY/OTHER PROCEDURES
- Whenever there is a doubt as to the presence or absence of invasive disease, vaginectomy must be performed.
- Invasive lesions usually are treated by radiation therapy, but stage I lesions can be treated with radical hysterectomy or radical vaginectomy with pelvic lymph node dissection (2)[A].
- If the lesion involves the lower vagina, inguinal node dissection also must be done because cancer involving the lower vagina can metastasize to the groin region (inguinal–femoral nodes).
- Premenopausal women who desire to retain ovarian function are better candidates for radical surgery for early-stage disease, with vaginal reconstruction possible afterward.
- Patients who have not completed their family can occasionally be treated with limited resection and localized radiation to the area (3).
- Sarcomas are treated by radiation therapy followed by pelvic exenteration if persistent disease is present.

Pediatric Considerations
The treatment of vaginal tumors today mainly consists of neoadjuvant chemotherapy followed by local control with surgery or radiotherapy.

Geriatric Considerations
Older patients, many with a long history of smoking, are at a higher risk for malignancies requiring surgical treatments.

ONGOING CARE

FOLLOW-UP RECOMMENDATIONS
- Patients are usually ambulatory and able to resume full activity by 6 weeks after surgery.
- Most patients are fully active while receiving chemotherapy and radiation therapy.

Patient Monitoring
- Pelvic examination and Pap smear every 3 months for 2 years, then every 6 months for the next 3 years, and then yearly thereafter
- Annual CXR

PATIENT EDUCATION
- American College of Obstetricians and Gynecologists: http://www.acog.org
- American Cancer Society: https://www.cancer.org/
- MedlinePlus: http://www.nlm.nih.gov/medlineplus/vaginalcancer.html

PROGNOSIS
Stage and 5-year survival (4)
- I: 77.6%
- II: 52.2%
- III: 42.5%
- IVA: 20.5%
- IVB: 12.9%
- Stage is the most important determinant of survival.
- Tumor size >2 cm, correlated with worse survival outcome

COMPLICATIONS
- Those typically associated with major abdominal surgery or radiation therapy
- Common complications of treatment include rectovaginal or vesicovaginal fistulas, rectal/vaginal strictures, radiation cystitis, and/or proctitis.
- Most recurrences occur within the first 2 years after initial diagnosis.

REFERENCES
1. Iavazzo C, Pitsouni E, Athanasiou S, et al. Imiquimod for treatment of vulvar and vaginal intraepithelial neoplasia. *Int J Gynaecol Obstet*. 2008;101(1):3–10.
2. Guerri S, Perrone AM, Buwenge M, et al. Definitive radiotherapy in invasive vaginal carcinoma: a systematic review. *Oncologist*. 2019;24(1):132–141.
3. Gadducci A, Fabrini MG, Lanfredini N, et al. Squamous cell carcinoma of the vagina: natural history, treatment modalities and prognostic factors. *Crit Rev Oncol Hematol*. 2015;93(3):211–224.
4. Adams TS, Cuello MA. Cancer of the vagina. *Int J Gynaecol Obstet*. 2018;143(Suppl 2):14–21.

ADDITIONAL READING
Wolfson AH, Reis IM, Portelance L, et al. Prognostic impact of clinical tumor size on overall survival for subclassifying stages I and II vaginal cancer: a SEER analysis. *Gynecol Oncol*. 2016;141(2):255–259.

CODES

ICD10
- C52 Malignant neoplasm of vagina
- D07.2 Carcinoma in situ of vagina
- N89.3 Dysplasia of vagina, unspecified

CLINICAL PEARLS
- Vaginal cancer is rare; 85–90% of vaginal cancers are squamous cell.
- Vaginal malignancies are found most commonly on the posterior wall in the upper 1/3 of the vagina.
- Most vaginal malignancies are metastatic (from cervix, vulva, endometrium, breast, or ovary).

V

VAGINITIS AND VAGINOSIS
Brett Johnson, MD • Katherine E. Bouchard, DO

BASICS

DESCRIPTION
- "Vaginosis" and "vaginitis" are broad terms indicating any disease process of the vagina caused by or leading to infection, inflammation, or changes in the normal vaginal flora. The difference between vaginitis and vaginosis is the presence (vaginitis) or absence (vaginosis) of inflammation.
- The most common causes of vaginitis and vaginosis are bacterial vaginosis (BV), vulvovaginal candidiasis (VVC), and trichomoniasis. Noninfectious causes (<10%) can include atrophic, irritant, allergic, and inflammatory vaginitis.
- Diagnosis of vaginitis relies on a thorough history, physical exam, and clinical assessment.
- Normal physiologic vaginal discharge is clear to white, not malodorous, and not associated with pain or pruritus, and the quantity varies during the menstrual cycle.

EPIDEMIOLOGY
- Vaginal symptoms are common in the general population and are one of the most frequent reasons women present to their medical care providers, accounting for approximately 10 million office visits each year (1).
- BV is the most common cause of vaginal discharge in reproductive-aged women (2).
- VVC is the second most common cause of vaginitis in reproductive-aged women (2).

Incidence
An estimated 7.4 million cases of BV occur yearly in the United States (1).

Prevalence
- Prevalence rates of BV are of 15% in pregnant women, 20–25% young females at student health clinics, and up to 30–40% among women seen at sexually transmitted infection (STI) clinics (1).
- Nonwhite women have higher rates of BV (African American 51%, Mexican Americans 32%) than white women (23%).
- 29–40% of all females report at least one episode of VVC.
- VVC is uncommon in prepubescent girls and postmenopausal women and is often overdiagnosed in these populations.
- Vaginal trichomoniasis is a common STI with 3 to 5 million cases diagnosed in the United States yearly (2).
- African American women are 10 times more commonly affected by vaginal trichomoniasis when compared to white and Hispanic women (2).
- Desquamative inflammatory vaginitis (DIV) is found in 2–20% of pregnant and nonpregnant women (1).

ETIOLOGY AND PATHOPHYSIOLOGY
- BV is caused by a change in the normal vaginal flora (2). Lactobacilli responsible for maintaining the acidic vaginal pH are overcome by facultative anaerobic organisms and lack of hydrogen peroxide producing lactobacilli (2).
  - Increase in the pH and a malodorous, clear, white, or gray discharge and a fishy odor
  - Organisms generally implicated in BV infections: *Gardnerella vaginalis, Prevotella* species, *Porphyromonas* species, *Bacteroides* species, *Peptostreptococcus* species, *Mycoplasma hominis, Ureaplasma urealyticum, Mobiluncus* species, *Fusobacterium* species, *Atopobium vaginae*
  - Not directly caused by sexual transmission
- VVC is caused by *Candida* species, particularly *Candida albicans* (80–92%) and *Candida glabrata* (<10%).
  - *Candida* can be identified in the lower genital tract in healthy women, and it is thought to gain access via rectal and perianal colonization and migration.
  - Symptoms occur when candidal organisms overwhelm the normal vaginal flora and invade the superficial vaginal epithelial cells.
  - Complicated VVC should be considered in pregnant patients and patients with diabetes or immunocompromising conditions. Those who experience four or more episodes of VVC in a year or who have only budding yeast on wet mount may also be considered to have complicated VVC.
- Trichomoniasis is caused by an infection via *Trichomonas vaginalis*. The organism infects the squamous epithelium of the vagina as well as the urethra and paraurethral glands; primarily transmitted during intercourse
- DIV—a chronic, purulent vaginitis with an uncertain etiology or pathogenesis; inflammation is the cardinal feature. The vagina is colonized with facultative bacteria, not the obligate anaerobic bacteria that colonize the vagina in BV (1).
- Atrophic vaginitis—genitourinary symptoms resulting from a lack of estrogen
- Irritant/allergic vaginitis—vaginal symptoms can result from mechanical, chemical, or allergic irritation.

RISK FACTORS
- BV
  - Sexual activity; although not considered an STI
  - Women who have sex with women, smoking, vaginal douching, low socioeconomic status, the presence of STIs such as HSV-2, the use of an IUD
  - Male circumcision decreases risk.
- VVC—diabetes, recent use of antibiotics, immunosuppression, higher estrogen levels, estrogen-containing contraceptives
- Trichomoniasis—inconsistent use of barrier contraception, multiple sexual partners, limited education and low socioeconomic status, illicit drug use, smoking, coexistent STIs, douching, incarceration (2)
- Other risk factors associated with vaginitis and vaginosis: decreased estrogen; smoking; use of vaginal douches, creams, gels, or lubricants; tight-fitting clothing; poor hygienic practice; changes in diet; condoms, sex toys, tampons

GENERAL PREVENTION
- Vulvar hygiene with warm water and unscented cleanser; advise patients not to douche. Wear cotton underwear.
- Except in cases of trichomoniasis, treatment of sexual partners is not recommended but may be considered in recurrent cases.

COMMONLY ASSOCIATED CONDITIONS
- STIs (gonorrhea, chlamydia, HSV, or HIV)
- Vaginal intraepithelial neoplasia and cancer can present with symptoms of vaginitis.

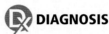

DIAGNOSIS

HISTORY
- General principles:
  - It is important to distinguish vulvar versus vaginal symptoms.
  - Onset, timing, severity, duration, and character of the vaginal symptoms are important to discern.
  - Symptomatic patients complain of itching, burning, irritation, dyspareunia, and abnormal discharge.
  - Other topics to discuss: age, menstrual status and relation to cycle, discharge characteristics (color, consistency, amount, odor), recurrence of symptoms, sexual history (including risk factors for STIs, number of partners, gender identification, specific sexual practices), vulvovaginal hygiene practices (shaving, douching), self-treatment (OTC medications), and other underlying medical conditions (DM, HIV, IBD) (2)
- BV—thin, homogenous discharge with characteristic "fishy" odor; pain and pruritus are uncommon.
- VVC—symptomatic women report itching, burning, irritation, dyspareunia, dysuria, and a white thick discharge; odor is uncommon.
- Trichomoniasis: A majority of patients will have minimal or no genitourinary symptoms (70–85%). Symptomatic patients will complain of abnormal discharge, itching, burning, or postcoital bleeding (2).
- DIV: purulent vaginal discharge with burning, dyspareunia, and/or introital pain; homogenous yellowish discharge with no fishy smell (1); symptoms may last for a long period of time and fluctuate (1).

PHYSICAL EXAM
- Physical exam should begin with a thorough evaluation of the vulva and the skin surrounding the anus (2).
- BV—thin, watery discharge that can range from clear to gray or tan colored; an amine or "fishy" smell may be present. Vaginal epithelium should appear normal and noninflamed; does not affect vulva
- VVC—erythema and swelling of the vulva and vaginal mucosa. Severely affected patients may have vulvar excoriations and fissures. Typically, cottage cheese-like, discharge can vary from watery to homogenously thick; lack of odor
- Trichomoniasis—yellow or green frothy discharge with foul odor; discharge can appear purulent. Vulvar or vaginal erythema can be visualized. Rarely, punctate hemorrhages can be seen on the cervix ("strawberry cervix").
- DIV—purulent discharge and vaginal inflammation; submucosal cervico-vaginal petechiae; no fishy smell

DIFFERENTIAL DIAGNOSIS

Physiologic discharge; leukorrhea of pregnancy; STIs; foreign body; contact dermatitis; cervicitis; urinary tract infection; atrophic vaginitis; dermatoses: lichen sclerosus, lichen planus, seborrheic dermatitis, psoriasis; genitourinary syndrome of menopause (2)

DIAGNOSTIC TESTS & INTERPRETATION

Initial Tests (lab, imaging)

- BV
  - Symptomatic patients complain of an abnormal vaginal discharge and a fishy odor.
  - Clinical diagnosis is established with Amsel criteria; positive diagnosis can be made if meeting 3 out of 4:
    ○ Thin, homogenous discharge that smoothly coats vaginal wall
    ○ Vaginal pH >4.5
    ○ A positive amine or "Whiff" test with use of KOH solution added to discharge
    ○ >20% of the epithelial cells identified as "clue cells"; most reliable indicator
- VVC
  - Visualization of blastospores or pseudohyphae on saline or 10% KOH microscopy
  - Positive culture in a symptomatic patient (2)
- Trichomoniasis
  - Visualization of motile trichomonads on saline microscopy
  - Nucleic acid amplification test (NAAT) is preferred as microscopy has limited sensitivity (50–60%) (2).
  - Several POC tests, including patient performed, are available with increased sensitivity compared to microscopy but are expensive.
- DIV
  - Wet mount with increase in inflammatory cells and parabasal (immature) squamous epithelial cells, pH >4.5
  - Wet mount is the preferred diagnostic method.

Follow-Up Tests & Special Considerations

BV/VVC/trichomoniasis—new testing modalities such as oligonucleotide probes and NAATs may be used in some settings for patient comfort, but outcomes are not clearly improved compared to more standard diagnostic methods and treatment, and the tests are expensive.

 TREATMENT

GENERAL MEASURES

- Avoid douching and tight-fitting clothing.
- Regular use of condoms may help to prevent BV (2).
- Asymptomatic, pregnant women generally do not require treatment for BV.
- Consider avoiding use of tampons during intravaginal treatment to ensure adequate dispersion of medication.

MEDICATION

Medication recommendations are based on CDC treatment guidelines and American College of Obstetricians and Gynecologists (ACOG) Practice Bulletin (2)[C].

First Line

- BV
  - Metronidazole 500 mg orally BID for 7 days, 0.75% gel 1 full applicator (5 g) vaginally daily for 5 days, or clindamycin 2% cream vaginally daily for 5 to 7 days
  - Recurrent infection may require repeated treatment (e.g., 1 week monthly for 6 months). Advise patients to avoid alcohol during treatment with oral metronidazole and for 24 hours following.
- VVC
  - Uncomplicated infections can be treated with a one-time dose of fluconazole 150-mg tab. Topical/vaginal suppository antifungal regimens include butoconazole, clotrimazole, miconazole, terconazole, or nystatin creams. Treatment can range from 3 to 7 days; recurrent infection: fluconazole 150 mg 3 times in 1st week and then weekly for up to 6 months
  - Avoid oral azoles in pregnant women.
  - Advise patients that topical medications may weaken rubber or latex condoms.
- Trichomoniasis
  - Metronidazole 500 mg orally BID for 7 days
  - Partner should be treated as well and counseled to abstain from sex until both patients have completed treatment and are asymptomatic.
  - Test of cure is not necessary, although retesting 3 months after initial treatment is acceptable.
  - Advise to avoid alcohol during treatment with oral metronidazole and for 24 hours following.
- DIV
  - Address estrogen deficiency.
  - Clindamycin 2% cream intravaginally at bedtime for 1 to 3 weeks
  - May need additional maintenance therapy

Second Line

- BV—secnidazole 2 g orally once or tinidazole/clindamycin orally ranging from 2 to 5 days; avoid alcohol during treatment with and 72 hours after tinidazole.
- VVC
  - Recurrent infections benefit from speciation to help determine treatment course.
  - Nonalbican candidiasis may require longer duration of treatment with topical or oral azoles or boric acid (vaginal suppository 600 mg daily for 7 days for acute VVC, 2 weeks for recurrent VVC).
- Trichomoniasis—one-time, 2-g oral dose of either tinidazole or metronidazole
- DIV—topical glucocorticoid such as hydrocortisone cream 300 to 500 mg intravaginally nightly for 3 weeks or clobetasol intravaginally nightly for 1 week

 ONGOING CARE

FOLLOW-UP RECOMMENDATIONS

- Delay sexual relations until symptoms are clear or discomfort resolves. The use of condoms may reduce the recurrence of BV.
- Consider suppressive therapy for recurrent infection. Monthly treatment may help reduce colonization of bacteria associated with BV (3)[C].

Patient Monitoring

No specific follow-up needed; if symptoms persist or recur within 2 months, repeat pelvic exam and culture.

PATIENT EDUCATION

ACOG: https://www.acog.org

PROGNOSIS

VVC: 80–90% of uncomplicated cases cured with appropriate treatment; 30–50% of recurrent infections return after discontinuation of maintenance therapy; high spontaneous remission rate of untreated symptoms as well

COMPLICATIONS

- BV has been associated with an increased risk of HIV and other STIs.
- BV has been associated with increased risk of preterm birth, chorioamnionitis, postpartum and postabortal endometritis, and pelvic inflammatory disease.
- VVC may occur following treatment of BV.

REFERENCES

1. Paavonen J, Brunham RC. Bacterial vaginosis and dequamative inflammatory vaginitis. *N Engl J Med*. 2018;379:2246–2254.
2. American College of Obstetricians and Gynecologists. Vaginitis in nonpregnant patients: ACOG Practice Bulletin, Number 215. *Obstet Gynecol*. 2020;135(1):e1–e17.
3. Balkus JE, Srinivasan S, Anzala O, et al. Impact of periodic presumptive treatment for bacterial vaginosis on the vaginal microbiome among women participating in the preventing vaginal infections trial. *J Infect Dis*. 2017;215(5):723–731.

 SEE ALSO

Algorithm: Vaginal Discharge

 CODES

ICD10

- N76.0 Acute vaginitis
- B37.3 Candidiasis of vulva and vagina
- N95.2 Postmenopausal atrophic vaginitis

CLINICAL PEARLS

- Most women experience relief of symptoms with appropriate therapy chosen.
- Vaginal pH is underused as a diagnostic tool for evaluation of vaginitis.

V

VARICOSE VEINS

Bliss Puthenpurayil, MD • Amrutha Pavle, MD

 BASICS

Varicose veins (VV), or varicosities, are dilated subcutaneous veins of at least 3 mm in diameter, measured with patient in upright position. They are part of a spectrum of chronic venous disorders ranging from telangiectasias to chronic venous insufficiency. Ovarian vein failure can also cause pelvic VV and subsequently pelvic congestion syndrome.

DESCRIPTION
- Lower extremities venous drainage is accomplished via a network of superficial veins > small perforator veins > deep veins; diseases in any of these systems may result in VV.
- VV usually form in the greater and lesser saphenous veins and sometimes their branches.

Geriatric Considerations
- Surgeries have low morbidity and mortality in patients aged >60 years, with significant self-reported improvement despite more advanced disease on presentation.
- High-risk geriatric patients should avoid hybrid procedures and general anesthesia when possible.

Pregnancy Considerations
External compression is the first-line treatment in pregnant female.

EPIDEMIOLOGY
Treatment of VV late complications such as chronic venous ulcerations results in an estimated 3 billion per year to treat in the United States.

Prevalence
- Approximately 23% of U.S. adult have VV.
- VV affect an estimate of 22 million women and 11 million men between 40 and 80 years old; of which, 2 million will develop symptom.

ETIOLOGY AND PATHOPHYSIOLOGY
Exact pathophysiology is debated, but it involves venous hypertension, valves dysfunction, structural changes in the vessel wall, inflammation, alteration of shear wall stress, and genetic disposition.

- Venous hypertension is caused by reflux from valvular incompetence, outflow obstruction, calf muscle failure, or increased intra-abdominal pressure from pregnancy, obesity, chronic constipation, tumor, or other proximal obstruction.
- Valve dysfunction may be due to deformation, tearing, thinning or adhesion of the valve leaflets, the vein wall stiffening with failure of the leaflet to fit together, trauma, deep thrombophlebitis, and congenital valvular incompetence.
- Structural changes in the vein wall (disruption of smooth muscle cells and elastic fibers, etc.) leads to vessels weakening and dilation.
- Turbulent flow, reflux, and increases in shear stress promote inflammatory and prothrombotic changes that further contribute to the loss of wall and leaflet integrity.
- Deep venous insufficiency can lead to secondary VV via enlarging collaterals.

Genetics
VV is highly polygenic; a cohort study of >500,000 individuals has generated a list of genetic associations that include 30 new loci, with the strongest associations occurring in intron region CASZ1 (implicated in blood pressure) and 16q24 (contains genes that encode a vascular mechanosensory channel).

RISK FACTORS
- Inherited: tall height (>180 cm), congenital syndromes
- Acquired: age, deep vein thrombosis (DVT), pregnancy, decreased leg impedance
- Lifestyle: prolonged standing and/or sitting, tobacco use, obesity
- Hormonal: female gender (high estrogen state)
- Socioeconomic: lower education level

GENERAL PREVENTION
- Maintain a healthy body mass index.
- Avoid sitting or standing for prolonged periods of time.
- Wear compression stockings.

COMMONLY ASSOCIATED CONDITIONS
- Stasis dermatitis
- Lipodermatosclerosis
- Venous ulceration (usually near medial malleolus/gaiter area)

 DIAGNOSIS

HISTORY
- Symptoms range from asymptomatic, minor annoyance/cosmetic concern to debilitating complaints.
- Localized symptoms: pain/tingling, burning, itching
- Generalized symptoms: leg cramp, fatigue, swelling, and heaviness
- Symptoms often worse at the end of the day and after prolonged standing.
- Women are more prone to symptoms due to hormonal influences; symptom is usually worse during menses.

PHYSICAL EXAM
- Inspection
  – Performed while the patient is standing; VV in proximal femoral ring and distal legs may not be visible when the patient is supine.
  – Telangiectasias (spider veins) are small, dilated blood vessels (arteriole, venule, or capillary).
  – VV features:
    ○ Dilated, tortuous superficial veins, ≥3 mm in diameter
    ○ Dark purple/blue in color, raised above the surface of the skin
    ○ Often twisted, bulging, and can look like cords
    ○ Most commonly found on the posterior/medial lower extremity
  – Skin changes may include erythema, eczema, hemosiderosis, atrophie blanche, lipodermatosclerosis, and ulcers (most often above the medial malleus).
  – Edema of the affected limb may be present.

- Atrophy blanche, fan-shaped VV in ankle (corona phlebectatica), and lipodermatosclerosis are signs of advanced venous disease.
- Vulva, perineal, or groin VV may be a sign of pelvic vein incompetence or obstruction due to abdominal, pelvic, or renal mass.
- Palpation
  – Palpate saphenofemoral junction (SFJ)—~4 cm inferolateral to pubic tubercle—for any saphena varix.
- Beside tests, including tap and cough test, have limited value.
  – Tap test: Examiner places one finger on the SFJ and uses another hand to tap along the VV. A thrill will be felt on the SFJ if the examiner taps on a defective vein. A healthy valve will block the transmission of the thrill.
  – Cough test: Examiner palpates the SFJ for thrill when the patient cough.
- Duplex ultrasound has largely replaced the tourniquet tests.
  – Trendelenburg test locates the defective valves. Patient starts by laying spine and elevating the leg. Once the patient's venous blood is drained, the examiner ties a tourniquet on the leg and the patient stands up. If the VV remains flat, the defect is above the tourniquet level. If the VV fills back up, the problem is below the tourniquet level. The examiner repeats the test till the site of the defect is found.
  – Perthes test access the deep system. Patient starts by laying supine. The examiner ties a tourniquet around the patient's upper thigh. Patient will walk for 5 minutes. Persistent VV indicates deep vein pathology. VV disappears with competent deep venous system.

DIFFERENTIAL DIAGNOSIS
- For lower extremity pain: arthritis, peripheral neuritis, DVT, superficial thrombophlebitis, ischemia
- For lower extremity ulcers: arterial/venous insufficiency, neuropathic, infection, trauma, vasculitis, drugs (e.g., warfarin skin necrosis, heparin-induced thrombocytopenia), inflammatory disorders (e.g., pyoderma gangrenosum, panniculitis)

DIAGNOSTIC TESTS & INTERPRETATION
Initial Tests (lab, imaging)
Venous duplex ultrasonography is recommended for severe disease requiring intervention. It can determine saphenous junction competency, the junction diameter, the extent of the reflux, and the location and size of the affected vein. It can also assess for DVT and thrombophlebitis (1).

Follow-Up Tests & Special Considerations
- Lab tests are only needed to rule out other differentials.
- Magnetic resonance imaging, venography, and plethysmography are only used if venous ultrasound is inconclusive or for more complex surgical situations.

Test Interpretation

- The CEAP (clinical, etiologic, anatomical, patho-physiologic) classification is the gold standard of classification of chronic venous disorders.
- Uncomplicated:
  - C0: no visible or palpable signs of venous disease
  - C1: telangiectasias or reticular veins
- Local symptoms and complication:
  - C2: VV; CV2r recurrent VV
  - C3: edema
- Complex varicose disease:
  - C4a: pigmentation or eczema; C4b Lipodermatosclerosis or atrophie blanch, C4c Corona phlebectatica
  - C5: healed venous ulcer
  - C6: active venous ulcer; C6r recurrent active venous ulcer

TREATMENT

- VV is not curable because chronic venous insufficiency causes irreversible damages to the veins and valves.
- Indications for treatment include pain, aching, heaviness, fatigue, burning, edema, stasis dermatitis, recurrent superficial phlebitis, or ulceration.
- Management options (most treatment involves multiple modalities and repetition): lifestyle modifications, compression therapy, local ablative therapies, surgery, and endovenous ablative therapies
- Lifestyle modification
  - Elevation of feet to at least heart level for 30 minutes 4 times daily
  - Avoid prolonged standing and sitting.
  - Weight loss, exercise such as walking and foot flexion exercises to improve calf muscle pump function
- Compression stockings while awake; nonadherence rate up to 60% due to difficulty with applying the stocking; mostly recommended if interventional treatment is ineffective, presence of active or healed venous ulcer, and as first line in pregnant women; trial of compression therapy may be required before approval of interventional treatments by insurance.

MEDICATION

- Low-dose diuretics have minimal effect.
- Topical steroid is helpful with stasis dermatitis.
- Oral and topical therapies called phlebotonics may reduce symptoms of chronic venous insufficiency. Vasculera is the only prescription formulation available in the United States.
- Horse chestnut seed extract may reduce pain, edema, and itching, although long-term studies of the safety and effectiveness of phlebotonics are lacking (1)[C].

ISSUES FOR REFERRAL

National Institute for Health and Care Excellence (NICE) recommends referral of patients with:
- Symptomatic primary (or recurrent) VV
- Skin changes
- Superficial venous thrombosis
- Active and healed leg ulcers

ADDITIONAL THERAPIES

- Activity modification
  - If standing is necessary, shift weight from side to side.
  - Never sit with legs hanging down.
- Physical therapy

SURGERY/OTHER PROCEDURES

- Sclerotherapy, surgery, and endovenous ablation: indicated if noninvasive measures fail or if the patient has cosmetic concerns, recurrent hemorrhage, and superficial thrombophlebitis; contraindicated in pregnancy, acute venous thromboembolism, peripheral artery disease (ankle brachial index <0.9); sclerotherapy is likely safe and at least somewhat effective for cosmesis and symptoms (2)[A].
- Local ablative therapy: for telangiectasias and reticular vein
  - Rely on chemical (sclerotherapy) or heat-based (thermoregulation, cutaneous laser) endothelial injury resulting in fibrosis of the veins
  - Liquid or foam sclerotherapy
    - Results in cosmetic improvement in 70% of patients and a patient satisfaction rate >70%
    - Best result when compression stocking are worn 7 to 10 days after the procedure
    - Complications include allergic reactions to the sclerosants, hyperpigmentation, superficial thread-like capillaries causing a bluish discoloration (matting), cellulitis, and rarely ulceration or thromboembolism.
    - Ultrasound-guided sclerotherapy is useful in treating perforator vein reflux.
  - Limited efficacy studies with thermal or cutaneous laser but helpful in patients who prefer needleless procedure
  - Surgery: for large branch, residual postablation VV and saphenous VV
    - CHIVA/stab phlebectomy:
      - French acronym for Conservatrice Hémodynamique de l'Insuffisance Veineuse en Ambulatoire (ambulatory conservative hemo-dynamic treatment venous insufficiency)—a procedure aim to alleviate signs and symptoms without destroying the vein
      - The surgeon maps the affected veins with ultrasound, makes a few small incisions, and ties off the veins.
      - Only requires local anesthesia and leaves minimal scar; reduces VV recurrence and produces fewer side effects than vein stripping
    - Surgical Stripping
      - Less used with the development of less invasive procedures
      - Recurrence is up to 50% of the patients by 5 years
      - Complications include extensive ecchymosis, scarring, hematoma, lymphocele, infection, nerve damage, and DVT; endovenous ablation—indicated for saphenous VV
- Radiofrequency ablation (RFA) uses thermal energy (85–120°C) to seal the incompetent vein via heat damage; endovenous laser ablation (EVLA) uses laser and fiber-optic catheter to generate thermal energy (up to 800°C).
  - 3 years estimated pooled success rates of 84% for RFA, 94% for EVLA compared to 78% in surgical stripping
  - Recommended by NICE as first-line treatment of truncal vein incompetence
  - RFA has a much lower subsequence incidence of thromboembolism and peripheral artery disease compared to other treatment.
- Mechanochemical endovenous ablation (MOCA) is a hybrid system composed of a rotating tip with simultaneous injection of liquid sclerosant.

COMPLEMENTARY & ALTERNATIVE MEDICINE

Phlebotonics including horse chestnut seed extract may ease symptoms, but long-term studies for safety and efficacy is lacking.

ADMISSION, INPATIENT, AND NURSING CONSIDERATIONS

- Compression stockings or sequential compression
- Encourage ambulation, VTE prevention

 # ONGOING CARE

DIET
Weight-loss diet if obesity is a problem

PATIENT EDUCATION

- Avoid long periods of standing and crossing legs.
- Exercise (walking, running) regularly to improve leg strength and circulation.
- Maintain a healthy weight.
- Wear elastic support stockings.
- Avoid clothing that constricts legs.

PROGNOSIS

- Will progress to advanced chronic venous diseases without treatment or correction to underlying cause
- Associated with a 7-fold increased risk of DVT

COMPLICATIONS

- Chronic edema
- Petechial hemorrhages
- Venous stasis dermatitis, pigmentation, lipodermatosclerosis
- Venous ulcers +/− superimposed infection
- Recurrence after surgical treatment

REFERENCES

1. Raetz J, Wilson M, Collins K. Varicose veins: diagnosis and treatment. *Am Fam Physician*. 2019;99(11):682–688.
2. de Ávila Oliveira R, Riera R, Vasconcelos V, et al. Injection sclerotherapy for varicose veins. *Cochrane Database Syst Rev*. 2021;12(12):CD001732.

ADDITIONAL READING

Alsaigh T, Fukaya E. Varicose veins and chronic venous disease. *Cardiol Clin*. 2021;39(4):567–581.

 # CODES

ICD10

- I83.90 Asymptomatic varicose veins of unspecified lower extremity
- I83.009 Varicose veins of unsp lower extremity w ulcer of unsp site
- I83.10 Varicose veins of unsp lower extremity with inflammation

CLINICAL PEARLS

RFA and EVLA have been demonstrated to be superior to open surgical techniques for VV treatment with similar improvement in quality of life.

V

VASCULITIS
Irene J. Tan, MD, FACR

BASICS

DESCRIPTION
An inflammatory disorder of blood vessels
- Clinical features result from the destruction of blood vessel walls with subsequent thrombosis, ischemia, bleeding, and/or aneurysm formation.
- Vasculitis is a heterogeneous group of diseases classified by the size, type, and location of involved blood vessels.
  - Small-vessel vasculitis
    - Microscopic polyangiitis (MPA)
    - Granulomatosis with polyangiitis (GPA; formerly Wegener granulomatosis)
    - Eosinophilic GPA (EGPA; formerly Churg-Strauss syndrome)
    - Antiglomerular basement membrane (anti-GBM) disease
    - Cryoglobulinemic vasculitis
    - IgA vasculitis (formerly Henoch-Schönlein purpura [HSP])
    - Hypocomplementemic urticarial vasculitis
  - Medium-vessel vasculitis
    - Polyarteritis nodosa (PAN)
    - Kawasaki disease (KD)
  - Large-vessel vasculitis
    - Takayasu arteritis (TAK)
    - Giant cell arteritis (GCA)
- Vasculitis occurs as a primary disorder or secondary to infection, a drug reaction, malignancy, or connective tissue disease.
  - Variable vessel vasculitis
    - Behçet disease
    - Cogan syndrome
  - Single-organ vasculitis
    - Cutaneous leukocytoclastic angiitis
    - Cutaneous arteritis
    - Primary CNS vasculitis
  - Vasculitis associated with systemic disease
    - Lupus vasculitis
    - Rheumatoid vasculitis
    - Sarcoid vasculitis
  - Vasculitis associated with other etiology
    - Hepatitis C–associated cryoglobulinemic vasculitis
    - Hepatitis B–associated vasculitis
    - Syphilis-associated aortitis
    - Drug-induced immune complex vasculitis
    - Drug-induced antineutrophil cytoplasmic antibodies (ANCA)-associated vasculitis
    - Cancer-associated vasculitis
- Protean features often delay definitive diagnosis.

EPIDEMIOLOGY
Highly variable, depending on the particular syndrome
- Hypersensitivity vasculitis is most commonly encountered in clinical practice.
- KD, IgA vasculitis, and dermatomyositis are more common in children.
- TAK is most prevalent in young Asian women. GPA, MPA, and EGPA are more common in middle-aged males.
- GCA occurs exclusively in those >50 years of age and is rare in the African-American population.

Incidence
Annual incidence in adults (unless otherwise specified)
- IgA vasculitis: 200 to 700/1 million in children <17 years of age
- GCA: 100 to 170/1 million in Caucasians aged >50 years
- KD: depends on race/age; ~200/1 million
- PAN: 2 to 33/1 million
- GPA: 4 to 15/1 million
- MPA: 1 to 24/1 million
- EGPA: 1 to 3/1 million
- TAK: 2/1 million
- Primary CNS vasculitis: 2/1 million in adults
- Hypersensitivity vasculitis: depends on drug exposure
- Viral-/retroviral-associated vasculitis: unknown; >90% of cases of cryoglobulinemic vasculitis are associated with hepatitis C.
- Connective tissue disorder–associated vasculitis: variable

ETIOLOGY AND PATHOPHYSIOLOGY
- Three major immunopathogenic mechanisms
  - Immune-complex formation: systemic lupus erythematosus (SLE), IgA vasculitis (HSP), and cryoglobulinemic vasculitis
  - ANCA autoantibodies: GPA, MPA, and EGPA
  - Pathogenic T-lymphocyte response: GCA and TAK
- Pathophysiology best understood where known drug triggers have been identified (e.g., antibiotics, sulfonamides, and hydralazine)

Genetics
- Mutation in CECR1 encoding adenosine deaminase 2 is associated with PAN.
- Behçet syndrome is associated with HLA-B*51.
- IgA vasculitis is associated with HLA-DQA1*01:01, HLA-DQB1*05:01, and HLA-DRB1*01:01.

RISK FACTORS
A combination of genetic susceptibility and environmental exposure likely triggers onset.

GENERAL PREVENTION
Early identification is the key to prevent irreversible organ damage in severe forms of systemic vasculitis.

COMMONLY ASSOCIATED CONDITIONS
Hepatitis C (cryoglobulinemic vasculitis), hepatitis B (PAN), cytomegalovirus (CMV), Epstein-Barr virus (EBV), HIV (viral-/retroviral-associated vasculitis), SLE, rheumatoid arthritis (RA), Sjögren syndrome, mixed connective tissue disease (MCTD), dermatomyositis, ankylosing spondylitis, Behçet disease, relapsing polychondritis (CTD-associated vasculitis), respiratory tract methicillin-resistant *Staphylococcus aureus* (MRSA) in GPA, levamisole-adulterated cocaine; medications: propylthiouracil, methimazole, hydralazine, minocycline; SARS-CoV-2 infection

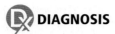

DIAGNOSIS

HISTORY
- Consider age, gender, and ethnicity.
- Comprehensive medication history
- Family history of vasculitis
- Constitutional symptoms: fever, weight loss, malaise, fatigue, diminished appetite, sweats
- CNS/PNS: mononeuritis multiplex, polyneuropathy, headaches, visual loss, tinnitus, stroke, seizure, encephalopathy
- Heart/lung: myocardial infarction, cardiomyopathy, pericarditis, cough, chest pain, hemoptysis, dyspnea
- Renal: hematuria, hypertension
- GI: abdominal pain, hematochezia, perforation
- Musculoskeletal: arthralgia, myalgia
- Miscellaneous: unexplained ischemic or hemorrhagic events, chronic sinusitis, and recurrent epistaxis
- Note the organs affected, and estimate the size of blood vessels involved.
- Demographics, clinical features, and the predominant vessel size/organ involvement help identify specific type of vasculitis.
- Vasculitis is a presenting condition in SARS-CoV-2/COVID-19 infection.

PHYSICAL EXAM
- Vital signs: blood pressure (hypertension) and pulse (regularity and rate)
- Skin: palpable purpura, livedo reticularis, nodules, ulcers, gangrene, nail bed capillary changes
- Neurologic: cranial nerve exam, sensorimotor exam
- Ocular exam: visual fields, scleritis, episcleritis
- Cardiopulmonary exam: rubs, murmurs, arrhythmias
- Abdominal exam: tenderness, organomegaly

DIFFERENTIAL DIAGNOSIS
- Fibromuscular dysplasia
- Embolic disease (atheroma, cholesterol emboli, atrial myxoma, mycotic aneurysm with embolization)
- Drug-induced vasospasm (cocaine, amphetamines, ergots)
- Thrombotic thrombocytopenic disorders (disseminated intravascular coagulation [DIC], thrombotic thrombocytopenic purpura [TTP], antiphospholipid syndrome, heparin- or warfarin-induced thrombosis), thromboangiitis obliterans
- Systemic infection (infective endocarditis, fungal infections, disseminated gonococcal infection, Lyme disease, syphilis, Rocky Mountain spotted fever [RMSF], bacteremia, ehrlichiosis, babesiosis)
- Malignancy (lymphomatoid granulomatosis, angioimmunoblastic T-cell lymphoma, intravascular lymphoma)
- Miscellaneous (Goodpasture syndrome, sarcoidosis, amyloidosis, Whipple disease, congenital coarctation of aorta)

DIAGNOSTIC TESTS & INTERPRETATION

ALERT
Renal involvement is often clinically silent. Routine serum creatinine and urinalysis with microscopy are needed to identify underlying glomerulonephritis.

- Initial tests exclude alternate diagnoses and guide therapy.
- Routine tests
  - CBC, serum creatinine, liver enzymes, urinalysis with microscopy, random urine for protein and creatinine
  - Specific serology when appropriate
    ○ Antinuclear antibodies (ANA); C3, C4
    ○ Rheumatoid factor (RF); cryoglobulin
    ○ Rapid plasma reagin/venereal disease reaction level (RPR/VDRL)
    ○ RMSF titers; Lyme titers
    ○ ANCA, antiproteinase 3 (anti-PR3) and antimyeloperoxidase (anti-MPO) antibodies
    ○ Hepatitis screen for B and C; HIV test
    ○ Anti-GBM titer; SARS-CoV-2 RT-PCR and antigen test
    ○ Serum and urine protein electrophoresis
- Miscellaneous
  - ESR, C-reactive protein; drug screen; creatine kinase (CK); blood culture; ECG
- CXR, CT scan, MRI, and arteriography may be required to delineate extent of organs involved.

Diagnostic Procedures/Other
- Electromyography with nerve conduction can document neuropathy and target nerve for biopsy.
- Biopsy of affected site confirms diagnosis (e.g., temporal artery, sural nerve, renal biopsy).
- If biopsy is not practical, angiography may be diagnostic for large- and medium-vessel vasculitides.
- Bronchoscopy may be required to differentiate pulmonary infection from potentially life-threatening hemorrhagic vasculitis in patients with hemoptysis.

Test Interpretation
Blood vessel biopsy shows immune cell infiltration into vessel wall layers with varying degrees of necrosis and granuloma formation in some, depending on the type.

 TREATMENT

GENERAL MEASURES
- Discontinue offending drug (hypersensitivity vasculitis).
- Simple observation for mild cases of pediatric IgA vasculitis
- ANCA-associated vasculitis has two-phase treatment: initial induction followed by maintenance (steady tapering of corticosteroids with immunosuppressants or immunomodulators).

MEDICATION

First Line
- Corticosteroids are usually the initial anti-inflammatory of choice.
- Patients with large vessel vasculitis are often treated with an initial (induction) course of 1 mg/kg of prednisone for ~4 weeks followed by a gradual taper.

Second Line
Cytotoxic medications, immunomodulatory, or biologic agents (e.g., cyclophosphamide (1)[B], methotrexate, azathioprine, leflunomide, mycophenolate mofetil (1)[B], and rituximab) are often required in combination with corticosteroids for rapidly progressive vasculitis with significant organ involvement or inadequate response to corticosteroids. Rituximab and avacopan are FDA-approved treatments for ANCA-associated vasculitis. Tocilizumab is the first FDA-approved treatment for GCA. Mepolizumab is the first FDA-approved treatment for EGPA. Intravenous immunoglobulins (IVIg) is FDA-approved treatment for KD in combination with aspirin. Apremilast is FDA-approved for oral ulcers in Behçet disease.

ISSUES FOR REFERRAL
- Rheumatology for comanagement with biologic agents
- Nephrology referral for persistent hematuria or proteinuria, rising creatinine, or a positive ANCA titer
- Pulmonary referral for persistent pulmonary infiltrate unresponsive to antibiotic therapy or if gross hemoptysis

ADDITIONAL THERAPIES
Plasma exchange does not improve mortality or progression to ESRD in severe ANCA-associated vasculitis.

SURGERY/OTHER PROCEDURES
Rarely, corrective surgery is required to repair tissue damage as a result of aggressive vasculitis.

ADMISSION, INPATIENT, AND NURSING CONSIDERATIONS
- Hemoptysis, acute renal failure, intestinal ischemia, any organ-threatening symptoms or signs, and/or need for biopsy
- Initial therapy is guided by the organ system involved.
  - If pulmonary hemorrhage is present, life-saving measures may include mechanical ventilation and immunosuppression.
  - If acute renal failure is present, attend to electrolyte and fluid balance and immunosuppression.
  - If signs of intestinal ischemia are present, make NPO and consider immunosuppression and parenteral nutrition.
- Discharge criteria: stabilization or resolution of potential life-threatening symptoms

 ONGOING CARE

FOLLOW-UP RECOMMENDATIONS
If significant coronary artery disease is involved in KD, moderate activity restriction may be of benefit.

Patient Monitoring
Frequent clinical follow-up supported by patient self-monitoring to identify disease relapse

DIET
Alter diets for patients with renal involvement or hyperglycemia/dyslipidemia.

PROGNOSIS
Prognosis is good for patients with limited organ involvement. Relapsing courses, renal, intestinal, or extensive lung involvement have a poorer prognosis.

COMPLICATIONS
Early morbidity/mortality is due to active vasculitic disease; delayed morbidity/mortality may also be secondary to complications of chronic therapy with cytotoxic medications or subsequent tissue scarring.

REFERENCE
1. Sunderkötter CH, Zelger B, Chen KR, et al. Nomenclature of cutaneous vasculitis: dermatologic addendum to the 2012 revised International Chapel Hill Consensus Conference nomenclature of vasculitides. *Arthritis Rheumatol*. 2018;70(2):171–184.

ADDITIONAL READING
- Iba T, Connors JM, Levy JH. The coagulopathy, endotheliopathy, and vasculitis of COVID-19. *Inflamm Res*. 2020;69(12):1181–1189.
- Walsh M, Merkel PA, Peh CA, et al; for PEXIVAS Investigators. Plasma exchange and glucocorticoids in severe ANCA-associated vasculitis. *N Engl J Med*. 2020;382(7):622–631.

CODES

ICD10
- M31.7 Microscopic polyangiitis
- M31.30 Wegener's granulomatosis without renal involvement
- M31.9 Necrotizing vasculopathy, unspecified

CLINICAL PEARLS
- Suspect vasculitis in patients with a petechial rash, palpable purpura, glomerulonephritis, pulmonary-renal syndrome, intestinal ischemia, or mononeuritis multiplex.
- Exclude silent renal involvement by routinely obtaining serum creatinine, urinalysis with microscopy, and random urine and creatinine.
- Vasculitis has "skip" lesions, which may complicate diagnostic biopsy.
- In patients with vasculitis, look for an underlying inciting process such as medication, infection, thrombosis, or malignancy.

V

VENOUS INSUFFICIENCY ULCERS

Daud Lodin, MD, MPH

BASICS

- Venous insufficiency is a condition that occurs when the venous wall and/or valves in the leg veins are not working effectively, making it difficult for blood to return to the heart and causing stasis.
- Signs of chronic venous insufficiency include edema, bulging veins, hyperpigmentation, dermatitis, woody fibrosis, lipodermatosclerosis, and ulcers.
- Venous stasis ulcers are the most serious consequence of chronic venous insufficiency.
- Venous stasis ulcers affect up to 3% of adults in developed countries at some point during their lives.
- The annual estimated treatment cost of chronic venous ulcers is 2.5 to 3.5 billion dollars per year.

DESCRIPTION
- Irregular and shallow skin defect with surrounding hyperpigmentation and well-defined borders
- Most frequently located in the lower leg or ankle over the bony prominences
- Present for >30 days and fails to heal spontaneously
- May only have mild pain unless infected

EPIDEMIOLOGY
80% of leg ulcers are caused by venous disease versus 10–25% arterial disease.

Incidence
- The overall incidence of venous ulcers is 18/100,000 persons; more common in women than men (20.4 vs. 14.6/100,000); incidence increases with age in both men and women.
- >20,000 patients are newly diagnosed with venous ulcers in the United States yearly.

Prevalence
- Venous ulcers are seen in ~1% of the adult population and up to 4% in adults ≥80 years old in industrialized countries.
- 70% of ulcers recur within 5 years of closure.

ETIOLOGY AND PATHOPHYSIOLOGY
- In a diseased venous system, venous pressure in the deep system fails to fall with ambulation, causing venous hypertension.
- Venous hypertension comes from the following:
  - Venous obstruction
  - Incompetent venous valves in the deep or superficial system
  - Inadequate muscle contraction (e.g., arthritis, myopathies, neuropathies)
- Venous pressure transmitted to capillaries leads to venous hypertensive microangiopathy and extravasation of RBCs and proteins (especially fibrinogen).
- Increased RBC aggregation leads to reduced oxygen transport, slowed arteriolar circulation, and ischemia at the skin level, contributing to ulcers.
- Leukocytes aggregate to the hypoxic areas and increase local inflammation.
- Prolonged chronic inflammation and bacterial infection promote the persistence of ulcers.

Genetics
- Autosomal dominant trait with variable penetrance with no specific gene or gene set identified
- Forkhead box protein C2 identified as possible marker in patients with varicose veins

RISK FACTORS
- History of leg injury, age >55 years, high BMI
- Congestive heart failure (CHF)
- History of deep venous thrombosis (DVT)
- Failure of the calf muscle pump (e.g., ankle fusion, inactivity)
- Previous varicose vein surgery or ulcers
- Smoking, prolonged standing, pregnancy

GENERAL PREVENTION
- After DVT: compression hose for at least 2 years (≥20 to 30 mm Hg compression)
- For recurrent ulceration: compression, treat underlying problem, exercise.
- Avoid triple antibiotic ointment, including anything containing neomycin sulfate.

DIAGNOSIS

HISTORY
- Recent trauma
- Prevalent features: cramping, pruritus, prickling, and throbbing sensation
- Pain that may improve with leg elevation
- Duration of wound and over-the-counter (OTC) treatments already attempted
- History of DVTs (especially factor V Leiden mutation; strongly associated with ulceration)
- History of leg edema that improves overnight (Edema that does not improve overnight is more likely lymphedema.)

PHYSICAL EXAM
- Look for evidence of venous insufficiency:
  - Pitting edema
  - Hemosiderin staining (red and brown diffuse pigment changes)
  - Stasis dermatitis
  - Atrophie blanche, ivory-colored stellate scars
  - Lipodermatosclerosis ("bottleneck" narrowing in the lower leg from fibrosis and scarring)
- Look for evidence of significant lymphedema (i.e., dorsal foot or toe edema, edema that does not resolve overnight or with elevation). This may require referral for comprehensive lymph therapy.
- Examine for palpable pulses.
- Examine wound for the following:
  - Length, width, and depth to monitor wound healing rate
  - Presence of necrotic tissue
  - Presence of biofilms or infection: fever, chills, purulent material in the wound, increased amount of odorous exudate, and/or spreading cellulitis

- Get initial and interim girth measurements (ankle and midcalf) to monitor edema.
- Important to rule out poor arterial circulation because compression dressings cannot be used in patients with ankle-brachial index (ABI) <0.8

DIFFERENTIAL DIAGNOSIS
- Arterial insufficiency ulcer
- Neuropathic ulcer
- Lymphedema
- Cellulitis (unilateral, febrile, patient feels ill, area warm, erythema without hyperpigmentation)
- Malignancy
- Sickle cell ulcer
- Vasculitic ulcer
- Rare: cryoglobulinemia, leishmaniasis, cutaneous tuberculosis, calciphylaxis
- Pyoderma gangrenosum
- Collagen vascular disease

DIAGNOSTIC TESTS & INTERPRETATION
No uniform staging system for venous insufficiency ulcers although Clinical-Etiology-Anatomy-Pathophysiology (CEAP) classification commonly used to help direct therapy

Initial Tests (lab, imaging)
Fasting glucose, consider Factor V Leiden (associated with venous ulcers), and ABIs are recommended (1)[C].

Follow-Up Tests & Special Considerations
Biopsy of leg ulcers that fail to heal or have atypical features

Diagnostic Procedures/Other
- Biopsy of leg ulcers that fail to heal or have atypical features
- Venography

Test Interpretation
- ABI <0.8 or >1.3 will need referral to vascular surgeon for revascularization as full compression stocking therapy may be detrimental at these levels until arterial disease is treated.
- Venography is used to identify thrombus or valvular insufficiency, which is seen with reflux time >0.5 seconds.

TREATMENT

- Treatment options: conservative management, mechanical treatment, medications, and surgical options
- Goals: Reduce edema, improve ulcer healing, and prevent recurrence.

GENERAL MEASURES
- Compression therapy is the standard of care for venous ulcers and chronic venous insufficiency and should be started as early as possible (2)[C].
- Leg elevation above the level of the heart 30 minutes, 3 to 4 times a day.

- Dressings are used under compression bandages to promote faster healing and prevent adherence of the bandage to the ulcer.
- To prevent maceration of surrounding skin, use a barrier ointment/cream.
- Compression therapy methods: inelastic, elastic, and intermittent pneumatic compression
  - Outcome: reduces edema, improves venous reflux, enhances healing, and reduces pain
  - Barriers: pain, drainage, application difficulty, and physical limitations (obesity and contact dermatitis)
  - Contraindications: clinically significant arterial disease (ABI <0.8) and uncompensated heart failure
  - Inelastic compression therapy: provides pressure during ambulation and muscle contraction but no resting pressure; most common: Unna boot (zinc oxide moist bandage that hardens after application)
  - Elastic compression therapy: sustains compression during rest and activity; compression stockings: Pressure should be at least 20 to 30 mm Hg and preferably 30 to 40 mm Hg. They should be removed at night and should be replaced every 6 months. Elastic bandages (i.e., Profore) are alternatives to compression stockings.
  - Intermittent pneumatic compression: generally reserved for bedridden patients because it is expensive and requires immobilization
  - Compression stockings reduce the risk of venous insufficiency ulcer reoccurrence.

MEDICATION
- Micronized purified flavonoid fraction, pentoxifylline, and sulfoxide all have been proven to aid in healing venous limb ulcers and are recommended as effective adjuvant therapies to compression therapy (2).
- Evidence is inconsistent regarding the benefits of aspirin (1).
- Oral antibiotic therapy is indicated if infection is suspected (1)[C].

ALERT
Routine use of antibiotics for all venous ulcers is not recommended.

First Line
Compression therapy, medical management, lifestyle changes and local wound care

Second Line
- Surgical therapy generally reserved for patients who have failed conservative management for 4 to 6 weeks
- Sclerotherapy, endovenous ablation, open vascular surgery, and radiofrequency ablation are generally reserved for after failed conservative measures.
- Recent studies have shown that endovenous ablation done early resulted in faster healing and improved time free of ulcer compared to those who waited until after ulcer healing or chronicity of >6 months.
- Other therapies for venous ulcers include negative pressure wound therapy to prepare wound followed by skin graft. Platelet rich plasma is an alternate therapy to surgery that is a promising therapy for ulcer healing (2).

ISSUES FOR REFERRAL
- With prominent toe or foot edema, consider lymphedema. Refer to a certified lymphedema therapist (CLT).
- Refer to a wound clinic for complex, large, or poorly healing ulcers (>3 months or >10 cm).
- Refer to a vascular specialist for recurrent ulcers and/or ABI <0.8.
- Use home health nurses to help with immobile patients needing frequent wrapping/dressing changes.

ADDITIONAL THERAPIES
- Exercise (e.g., activation of calf muscle pump with ankle flexion and extension)
- Infection control if likelihood is high (elevated WBC, unilateral, sudden onset, patient ill, etc.)
  - Débridement of necrotic tissue
  - Treat cellulitis (usually gram-positive bacteria) with bactericidal systemic antibiotics. Suspect local infection when there is pain or no improvement in the wound after 2 weeks of compression.
  - Treatment of critical colonization with topical antimicrobials, such as cadexomer iodine (Silver dressings and honey are widely used, but definitive data are lacking.) (2)
- Hyperbaric oxygen therapy may be effective as adjuvant to venous intervention in treatment of chronic resistant venous limb ulcers (3).

SURGERY/OTHER PROCEDURES
- Current evidence does not support the superiority of surgical interventions (open or endovascular) versus compression alone for ulcer healing and recurrence.
- If necrotic tissue, consider sharp, enzymatic, mechanical, larval, or autolytic débridement (1)[A].
- Skin grafting generally is not effective if there is a persistent edema and the underlying venous disease is not addressed.
- Autologous split-thickness skin grafting is the first choice to treat large venous limb ulcers (2).

 ONGOING CARE

FOLLOW-UP RECOMMENDATIONS
When ulcers are nearly healed and edema is controlled, switch from compression bandages to compression hose. (Consider referral for compression hose fitting early because insurance may not reimburse for the hose unless an ulcer is present.)

Patient Monitoring
Monitor the ulcer for healing by measuring its size; expect at least a 10% reduction every 2 weeks.

DIET
Low-sodium diet and weight loss for patients with a high BMI

PATIENT EDUCATION
Patient education on the underlying mechanism and appropriate wound care

PROGNOSIS
- Venous insufficiency is a lifelong medical problem.
- Poor prognostic factors
  - Ulcer duration >3 months
  - Ulcer >10 cm
  - Presence of arterial disease in the lower limbs
  - Advanced age
  - Elevated BMI

COMPLICATIONS
Venous insufficiency ulcers significantly reduce health-related quality of life, increase higher health-related expenditures, and increase work absenteeism (1)[B].

REFERENCES
1. Bonkemeyer Millan S, Gan R, Townsend PE. Venous ulcers: diagnosis and treatment. *Am Fam Physician*. 2019;100(5):298–305.
2. Ren SY, Liu YS, Zhu GJ, et al. Strategies and challenges in the treatment of chronic venous leg ulcers. *World J Clin Cases*. 2020;8(21):5070–5085.
3. Elsharnoby AM, El-Barbary AH, Eldeeb AE, et al. Resistant chronic venous leg ulcers: effect of adjuvant systemic hyperbaric oxygen therapy versus venous intervention alone [published online ahead of print May 16, 2022]. *Int J Low Extrem Wounds*. 2022.

CODES

ICD10
- I87.2 Venous insufficiency (chronic) (peripheral)
- I83.009 Varicose veins of unsp lower extremity w ulcer of unsp site
- I89.0 Lymphedema, not elsewhere classified

CLINICAL PEARLS
- The diagnosis of venous ulcers is clinical; however, exams such as ABI and color duplex ultrasonography may be helpful if the diagnosis is unclear.
- Compression therapy is the standard of care for venous ulcers and chronic venous insufficiency but may be contraindicated if ABI <0.8.
- Treat critical colonization with topical antimicrobials (avoid neomycin).
- Refer patients with recurrent or venous ulcers failing to heal after 4 to 6 weeks of moist wound care and compression to a wound specialist.
- Early referral to vascular surgeon for severe venous ulcer disease including wounds, bleeding varicosities, elevated CEAP score, and those with concomitant arterial disease

V

VENTRICULAR SEPTAL DEFECT

Jeremy Golding, MD, FAAFP • Luay Sarsam, MD

 BASICS

DESCRIPTION

- Congenital (usually) or acquired defect in the inter-ventricular septum that allows communication of blood between the left and the right ventricles
- Second most common congenital heart malformation reported in infants and children. It can also occur as a late complication of acute myocardial infarction (MI).
- Severity of the defect is correlated with its size, with large defects being the most severe.
- Blood flow across the defect typically is left to right, depending on defect size and pulmonary vascular resistance (PVR).
- Prolonged left-to-right shunting of blood can lead to pulmonary hypertension (HTN). This may eventually lead to a reversal of flow across the defect and cyanosis (Eisenmenger complex).

Geriatric Considerations
Almost entirely associated with late complication of MI

Pediatric Considerations
Congenital defect

ALERT
- Pregnancy may exacerbate symptoms and signs of a ventricular septal defect (VSD).
- Can be tolerated during pregnancy if VSD is small
- May be associated with an increased risk of pre-eclampsia in women with an unrepaired VSD

EPIDEMIOLOGY

Incidence
- Congenital defect: no gender predilection, occurs in ~2/1,000 live births and accounts for 30% of all congenital cardiac malformations
- Post-MI: Some studies suggest that gender may play a role.

Prevalence
In the United States:
- Occurs in ~50% of all children with congenital heart disease
- Low prevalence in adults (~0.3 per 1,000) due to spontaneous closure
- Post-MI complication in ~0.2–3% of cases

ETIOLOGY AND PATHOPHYSIOLOGY
- Congenital
- In adults, late complication of MI
- Some reports of iatrogenic causes

Genetics
Multifactorial etiology; autosomal dominant and recessive transmissions have been reported.

RISK FACTORS
- Congenital VSD:
  - Risk of sibling being affected: 4.2%
  - Risk of offspring being affected: 4%
  - Prematurity
- Post-MI VSD:
  - Advanced age
  - Arterial HTN
  - First MI
  - Most frequent within 1st week after MI
  - Most commonly after anterior wall acute MI

GENERAL PREVENTION
Avoid prenatal exposure to known risk factors (ibuprofen cyclooxygenase [COX] inhibitors, marijuana, organic solvents, febrile illness). For adults, avoid risk factors for MI and obtain evaluation before pregnancy.

COMMONLY ASSOCIATED CONDITIONS
- Congenital:
  - Tetralogy of Fallot
  - Aortic valvular deformities, especially aortic insufficiency and bicuspid aortic valve
  - Down syndrome (trisomy 21), endocardial cushion defect
  - Transposition of great arteries
  - Coarctation of aorta
  - Tricuspid atresia
  - Truncus arteriosus
  - Patent ductus arteriosus
  - Atrial septal defect
  - Pulmonic stenosis
  - Subaortic stenosis
- Adult: coronary artery disease

 DIAGNOSIS

HISTORY
- Presentation depends on degree of shunting across the defect; may be completely asymptomatic with small defects
- Respiratory distress, tachypnea, tachycardia
- Diaphoresis with feeds, poor weight gain in infants

PHYSICAL EXAM
- Small defect:
  - Harsh holosystolic murmur loudest at left lower sternal border
  - Detected after PVR drops at 4 to 8 weeks of life
- Moderate defect:
  - Harsh holosystolic murmur at left lower sternal border associated with a thrill
  - Forceful apical impulse with lateral displacement
  - Increased intensity of P_2
  - Diastolic rumble at apex due to increased flow across the mitral valve
- Large defect:
  - Holosystolic murmur heard throughout the precordium with diastolic rumble at apex with precordial bulge and hyperactivity, although large defects may have little or no murmur initially
  - If congestive heart failure (CHF) exists: tachycardia, tachypnea, and hepatomegaly
  - If pulmonary HTN exists: cyanosis with exertion
  - If severe, irreversible pulmonary HTN (Eisenmenger complex) exists: cyanosis, clubbing, syncope, arrhythmias, and polycythemia

DIFFERENTIAL DIAGNOSIS
- Patent ductus arteriosus, atrial septal defect
- Children: tetralogy of Fallot
- Adults: mitral regurgitation

DIAGNOSTIC TESTS & INTERPRETATION

Initial Tests (lab, imaging)
- A 12-lead ECG may show left ventricular hypertrophy and left atrial enlargement initially. As pulmonary HTN develops, right ventricular hypertrophy and right atrial enlargement may be seen.
- A chest x-ray (CXR) may demonstrate increased pulmonary vascularity and/or cardiomegaly.
- A 2D echocardiogram using color Doppler and bubble study for visualization of location, size of defect, and shunt direction
- Color flow Doppler for direction and velocity of VSD jet; may be used to estimate right ventricular pressure
- Ventriculography in conjunction with above imaging modalities can aid in characterization of VSD but is invasive

Follow-Up Tests & Special Considerations
- Weight and hematocrit check
- Serial echocardiograms
- Cardiac catheterization performed occasionally for perioperative planning or to assess need for closure of defect

Diagnostic Procedures/Other
- Cardiac catheterization (left and right sides of heart) can confirm the diagnosis, document number of defects, quantify ratio of pulmonary blood flow to systemic blood flow (Qp/Qs), and determine PVR.
- Demonstration of an oxygen saturation step up from the right atrium to the distal pulmonary artery

Test Interpretation
- Congenital VSD (four major anatomic types)
  - Membranous (70%)
  - Muscular (20%)
  - Atrioventricular canal type (5%)
  - Supracristal (5%; higher in Asians)
- Post-MI VSD predominantly involves muscular septum.
- Right bundle branch block is common after surgical repair

TREATMENT
- Small VSD tends to close spontaneously during childhood and has low risk for complications.
- Larger VSD tends to persist into adulthood and has more risk for complications.
- Start diuretic therapy if signs of fluid overload.
- Minimize IV fluids.
- Consider ACE inhibitor and/or digoxin.
- Nasogastric feeds for neonates
- Correct anemia via iron supplementation or a possible RBC transfusion.

GENERAL MEASURES
- Appropriate health care maintenance
- Outpatient, until surgical repair is indicated
- Inpatient management in setting of acute MI
- Inpatient for treatment of severe CHF

MEDICATION

First Line

- Per the 2007 American Heart Association guidelines, endocarditis antibiotic prophylaxis is not recommended for most VSDs. It is recommended for VSDs associated with complex cyanotic heart disease, during the first 6 months after surgical repair, or for residual VSDs located near the patch following surgery.
- Pediatric: Medications aim to control pulmonary edema, decrease work of breathing, and allow for growth:
  - Furosemide 1 to 2 mg/kg PO/IV once to twice a day
  - Spironolactone 1 to 2 mg/kg/day divided BID
  - Captopril
    - Infants: oral: 0.3 to 2.5 mg/kg/day divided every 8 to 12 hours; max 2 mg/kg/day
    - Children and adolescents: oral: 0.3 to 6.0 mg/kg/day divided every 8 to 12 hours; maximum daily dose: 150 mg/day
  - Digoxin: infants <2 years of age, 10 μg/kg/day PO divided BID; children, 2 to 10 years of age, 5 to 10 μg/kg/day PO divided BID; children >10 years of age, 2 to 5 μg/kg/day PO divided BID
- Adults: Digoxin and diuretics may be beneficial in some circumstances.
- Side effects:
  - Drugs that increase systemic vascular resistance may increase left-to-right shunting and cause signs and symptoms of pulmonary overcirculation.
  - HTN

Second Line

- Surgical closure is indicated if the pulmonic-to-systemic flow is >2:1 or with poorly controlled pulmonary overcirculation despite maximal medical and dietary interventions.
- If an infant with a VSD has persistent pulmonary HTN or failure to grow, surgical repair is recommended prior to 6 months of age even if patient is otherwise asymptomatic.
- For post-MI VSDs, afterload reduction, inotropic support, intra-aortic balloon pump, and left ventricular assist device may be used to stabilize the patient prior to surgery. Surgical repair includes septal débridement and patch placement.

ISSUES FOR REFERRAL

Close follow-up of a congenital VSD is necessary until primary intracardiac repair is performed to ensure that significant pulmonary HTN does not develop.

ADDITIONAL THERAPIES

- Infant caloric requirements up to 150 kcal/kg/day or more for adequate weight gain
- Treatment of iron deficiency anemia to increase oxygen-carrying capacity

SURGERY/OTHER PROCEDURES

- Surgical correction with either a VSD patch or repair is commonly used. Postsurgical outcomes for isolated VSD are excellent. Complications are rare and include reoperation for residual VSD, extended hospital stay, arrhythmias, valve injury, depressed ventricular function, and heart block (1).
- Percutaneous transcatheter device closure has become a safe and effective option for some children with small to moderate VSDs. Complications include valvular regurgitation, residual defects, and heart block. There is a greater risk of conduction abnormality with this technique compared to surgical closure. Recent studies have shown steroids may decrease this risk (2)[C].
- Perventricular device closure (hybrid technique) of some subtypes of isolated VSDs without cardiopulmonary bypass is feasible under transesophageal echocardiographic (TEE) guidance. Complications are similar to percutaneous closure (3)

ADMISSION, INPATIENT, AND NURSING CONSIDERATIONS

- Failure to thrive
- Pulmonary overcirculation/CHF
- Stabilize airway.
- Reduce temperature stress.
- Frequent vital sign monitoring; daily weight and calorie counts
- Discharge criteria: CHF stabilization, weight gain, or successful repair

 ONGOING CARE

FOLLOW-UP RECOMMENDATIONS

- Small VSDs without evidence of CHF or pulmonary HTN generally can be followed every 1 to 5 years after the neonatal period.
- Moderate to large VSDs require more frequent follow-up.
- Potential complications of VSDs include right ventricular outflow obstruction and aortic valve prolapse.

Patient Monitoring

- Physical growth and development monitoring
- Influenza vaccine for children >6 months of age
- RSV prophylaxis with nirsevimab for children <24 months of age with hemodynamically significant lesions entering both 1st and 2nd RSV season. Children with small VSDs do not need RSV prophylaxis beyond that recommended for healthy infants.

DIET

- Low sodium in heart failure
- High calorie in failure to thrive

PATIENT EDUCATION

- No activity restriction in absence of pulmonary HTN
- Parents need support and instructions for prevention of complications until the child is ready for surgery.

PROGNOSIS

- Congenital:
  - Course is variable depending on the size of the VSD.
  - Small VSD: Many will close spontaneously by age 3 years. Muscular defects are more likely to close spontaneously.
  - Large VSD: CHF or failure to thrive in infancy necessitating surgical repair
  - 20-year cumulative survival rate after surgery for isolated VSD is 87%; 40 years is 78%.
  - Progressive pulmonary vascular disease and pulmonary HTN are the most feared complications of VSD caused by left-to-right shunting and may eventually lead to reversal of the shunt (Eisenmenger complex). Death usually occurs in the 4th decade of life if untreated.
- Post-MI:
  - With medical management alone, 80–90% mortality in the first 2 weeks
  - Prognosis worse with inferior MI compared with anterior MI

COMPLICATIONS

- CHF
- Aortic insufficiency
- Sudden death
- Hemoptysis
- Cerebral abscess
- Paradoxical emboli
- Cardiogenic shock
- Heart block rarely may accompany surgical closure.
- Pulmonary HTN, particularly Eisenmenger complex

REFERENCES

1. Scully BB, Morales DLS, Zafar F, et al. Current expectations for surgical repair of isolated ventricular septal defects. *Ann Thorac Surg.* 2010;89(2):544–549.
2. Yang L, Tai B-C, Khin LW, et al. A systematic review on the efficacy and safety of transcatheter device closure of ventricular septal defects (VSD). *J Interv Cardiol.* 2014;27(3):260–272.
3. Yin S, Zhu D, Lin K, et al. Perventricular device closure of congenital ventricular septal defects. *J Card Surg.* 2014;29(3):390–400.

ADDITIONAL READING

Penny DJ, Vick GW III. Ventricular septal defect. *Lancet.* 2011;377(9771):1103–1112.

 SEE ALSO

Acute Coronary Syndromes: NSTE-ACS (Unstable Angina and NSTEMI); Down Syndrome; Tetralogy of Fallot

CODES

ICD10

- Q21.0 Ventricular septal defect
- I23.2 Ventricular septal defect as current comp following AMI
- Q21.3 Tetralogy of Fallot

CLINICAL PEARLS

- A loud 2/6 to 3/6 low-pitched harsh holosystolic murmur at the left lower sternal border is typical.
- A diastolic rumble at the apex indicates moderate to large VSD or ratio of pulmonary to systemic blood flow (Qp/Qs) >2:1, which likely will require surgical or percutaneous closure.
- Disappearance of the murmur could be secondary to spontaneous closure of the defect or the development of pulmonary HTN.

V

VERTIGO
James J. Arnold, DO, FACOFP

BASICS

DESCRIPTION
- Vertigo is a sensation of perceived motion with no motion is happening; differs from dizziness, which is a disturbance of orientation without movement (1)
- A symptom, not a disease process; causes can be peripheral or central (1)
- Often described as a sensation of movement (room spinning) when no movement is actually occurring (1)
- One of the four types of dizziness (vertigo, presyncope, lightheadedness, disequilibrium) (1),(2)
- System(s) affected: nervous, cardiovascular, psychiatry
- Synonym(s): dizziness

EPIDEMIOLOGY
Incidence
- Vertigo/dizziness accounts for >4 million ED visits a year in the United States, of which only 15% has a serious underlying condition (2),(3).
- Women are three times more likely to experience vertiginous migraine (2).

Geriatric Considerations
- Higher index of suspicion for cardiovascular disease, arrhythmias, and orthostatic hypotension
- Benign paroxysmal positional vertigo (BPPV) is more common in ages 50 to 70 years.
- Medications are implicated 1/4 of the time (1),(2).

ETIOLOGY AND PATHOPHYSIOLOGY
- Dysfunction of the rotational velocity sensors of the inner ear results in asymmetric central processing; combination of sensory disturbance of motion and malfunction of the central vestibular apparatus (1)
- Peripheral causes: acute vestibular neuritis, BPPV caused by otoliths in the posterior canal 85–95% and lateral canal 5–15%, Ménière disease, otosclerosis, acute labyrinthitis, cholesteatoma, perilymphatic fistula, superior canal dehiscence syndrome, motion sickness; BPPV, vestibular neuritis, and Ménière disease account for the majority of peripheral causes (1).
- Central causes: cerebellar tumor, stroke, migraine, vestibular ischemia (1)
- Numerous drug causes (1),(2)

Genetics
Unknown

RISK FACTORS
- History of migraines
- History of CVD/risk factors for CVD
- Use of ototoxic medications
- Trauma/barotrauma
- Perilymphatic fistula
- Heavy weight-bearing
- Psychosocial stress/depression
- Exposure to toxins

GENERAL PREVENTION
If due to motion sickness, consider pretreatment with anticholinergics, such as scopolamine.

DIAGNOSIS

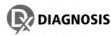

HISTORY
- Review current medications, specifically any recent additions or change in dosage as medication are a common cause of vertigo (1).
- Do not rely on symptom quality—often unreliable. Focus on timing and triggers.
  - TiTrATE is a clinically useful evaluation tool: **Ti**ming, **Tr**iggers, **A**nd a **T**argeted **E**valuation (3).
  - **Ti**ming: episodic or continuous; episodic may last seconds to a few days; continuous lasts days to weeks (3)
    - If continuous, assess for trauma or toxins (including prescribed and recreational).
    - To further evaluate continuous, spontaneous vertigo, perform HINTS exam (see "Physical Exam").
    - If episodic, assess for triggers.
  - **Tr**iggers: present or absent (3)
    - If triggers, perform Dix-Hallpike maneuver (see "Physical Exam").
    - Do not confuse *worsening* of symptoms with motion to be the same as triggering. Many central vertigos are worse with movement.
    - If no triggers, assess for hearing loss, migraines, or psych symptoms. Cardiovascular causes may also fall into this category.
  - **A**nd a **T**argeted **E**valuation: See "Physical Exam" for more details (3).
- Specific history items that suggest a diagnosis:
  - Unilateral hearing loss suggests Ménière disease. Further assess to determine if sensorineural versus conductive because the latter suggests otosclerosis.
  - Symptoms triggered by sudden change in head position suggest BPPV.
  - Symptoms triggered when going from sitting to standing suggests orthostatic hypotension.
  - History of migraines suggests vestibular migraine. Differentiate from nonmigrainous headaches, which can also be present with CNS tumors.
  - Depressed mood/anxiety with episodic vertigo that has since become continuous suggests psychiatric causes.
  - History of unilateral sensory or motor symptoms indicates a central cause such as TIA or CVA until proven otherwise.
  - Onset after decompression (diving, flying) suggests decompression sickness or barotrauma and warrants emergency evaluation (1),(2),(3).

PHYSICAL EXAM
- Cardiovascular: orthostatic blood pressure assessment on patients with episodic symptoms (1)
- HEENT: may identify barotrauma, otosclerosis, cholesteatoma; also check Rinne and Weber tests if hearing loss (1)
- Neurologic: Assess for nystagmus in all patients (1),(2),(3).
  - Vertical nystagmus is almost always of central origin.
  - Nystagmus of peripheral origin may be horizontal or rotational.
- Dix-Hallpike maneuver: for episodic, triggered vertigo: Rapidly move the patient from a seated to supine position with the head turned 45 degrees to the right and held just over (below) the edge of the exam table. Observe for nystagmus and patient report of vertigo. Nystagmus/vertigo may not appear immediately. Wait until symptoms resolve and then return the patient to the sitting position. Repeat on the left (1),(2).
  - The presence of extinguishing horizontal nystagmus (transient, upbeat) is a positive test for BPPV. If induced nystagmus does not subside however, consider central causes and perform HINTS (1),(3).
  - Vertical nystagmus always indicates a central cause even if triggered by Dix-Hallpike maneuver.
  - If Dix-Hallpike is negative, check for lateral canal BPPV with a log roll test.
  - If duration and trigger of symptoms are not consistent with BPPV, do not perform Dix-Hallpike maneuver to avoid overlooking a central cause.
  - A negative Dix-Hallpike maneuver does not rule out BPPV if symptoms are consistent and suspicion for other cause is unlikely (1),(2).
- HINTS exam: Perform for continuous, spontaneous vertigo with spontaneous nystagmus (3).
  - Horizontal **H**ead **I**mpulse: Rapidly and repeatedly bring patient's head to midline from 20 degrees. Patients with vestibular neuritis will show rapid saccades to refocus on a target. With normal peripheral nervous function, eyes stay on target, raising concern for central causes.
  - Direction changing **N**ystagmus: Having already assessed for presence and direction of nystagmus, now check for changing direction. Nystagmus that changes direction with eye motion indicates a central lesion.
  - Test of **S**kew: Vertical eye movement during cover-uncover test indicates a central lesion. A normal test has no movement.
  - A combination of these findings is 96.8% sensitive and 98.5% specific for CVA/other central cause (HINTS positive).
  - If a patient meets criteria for HINTS exam, do not perform Dix-Hallpike maneuver.
- Perform a full neuro exam if diagnosis is not already clear, paying attention to sensation, gait, and Romberg testing (1),(2).

DIFFERENTIAL DIAGNOSIS

Causes (1),(2):

- BPPV (episodic, triggered, positive Dix-Hallpike maneuver)
- Orthostatic hypotension (episodic, triggered, positive orthostatic blood pressure drop)
- Ménière disease (episodic, spontaneous, associated with unilateral sensorineural hearing loss)
- Vestibular migraine (episodic, associated with migraine HA)
- CVD (continuous, spontaneous; HINTS exam shows normal horizontal head impulse, direction-changing nystagmus, or vertical skew on cover-uncover)
- Posterior fossa tumor (continuous, spontaneous)
- Psychiatric (associated psych symptoms)
- Medication/toxin (continuous, medication/substance history, evaluation otherwise negative)
- Other CVD such as arrhythmia (episodic, often no triggers or triggered by exertion)
- Hypoglycemia (episodic, associated medications or comorbidities)
- Degenerative neurologic disease (often progressive by history, associated neurologic findings)
- Peripheral neuropathy

DIAGNOSTIC TESTS & INTERPRETATION

Initial Tests (lab, imaging)

- Labs not routinely necessary unless abnormal neuro exam, and identify a cause in <1% of patients (1),(2)
- Obtain STAT MRI if a central cause is suspected to rule out stroke. CT cannot reliably see the posterior fossa and will not show changes in the early stages of an infarct. Vertigo may be the only symptom of acute stroke (1)[C].
- Ear, nose, and throat (ENT) specialist/audiologist referral if Ménière disease is suspected for electronystagmography (1),(2)[C]
- If acoustic neuroma is suspected, either CT or MRI to evaluate internal auditory canal (1),(2)[C]

Diagnostic Procedures/Other

Audiometry if acoustic neuroma or Ménière disease is suspected (1),(2)[C]

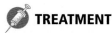 TREATMENT

GENERAL MEASURES

Treatments depend on cause (1),(2).

- If medication is likely the cause: Stop medication and reassess.
- BPPV: Epley maneuver and modified Epley maneuver (Epley maneuver—YouTube) (1),(2)[B]
- Vestibular neuritis and labyrinthitis (See separate topic.)
  - Vestibular-suppressant medications
  - Vestibular rehabilitation exercises
  - No evidence to support improvement of symptoms with corticosteroid use
- Ménière disease (see separate topic):
  - Low-salt diet (<1 to 2 g/day)
  - Diuretics such as hydrochlorothiazide
- Perilymphatic fistula, canal dehiscence—consult ENT.

- Vascular ischemia: prevention of future events through blood pressure reduction, lipid lowering, smoking cessation, antiplatelet therapy, and anticoagulation, if necessary; MRI or CT if suspected
- Vertiginous migraines: dietary and lifestyle modifications, vestibular rehab, prophylactic and abortive medications
- Psychological: SSRIs are better than benzodiazepines for anxiety-related vertigo. Use slow titration to avoid worsening symptoms.

MEDICATION

Avoid use of medication in mild cases. Use for a few days only because longer use may impair adaptation/compensation by the brain; medications not recommended for BPPV (1),(2)[C]

- Meclizine: 12.5 to 50.0 mg PO q4–8h
- Dimenhydrate: 50 mg PO q6h
  - Precautions: prostatic hyperplasia, glaucoma
- Prochlorperazine: 5 to 10 mg PO or IM q6–8h; 25 mg rectally q12h; 5 to 10 mg by slow IV over 2 minutes
  - Contraindications: blood dyscrasias, age <2 years, hypotension
  - Precautions: acutely ill children, glaucoma, breast cancer history, impaired cardiac function, prostatic hyperplasia
- Metoclopramide: 5 to 10 mg PO q6h, 5 to 10 mg slow IV q6h
  - Contraindications: concomitant use of drugs with extrapyramidal effects, seizure disorders
  - Precautions: history of depression, Parkinson disease, hypertension
- Psychiatric causes
  - SSRIs preferred for frequent vertigo related to depression/anxiety
  - Lorazepam (Ativan) 0.5 to 2.0 mg PO, IM, or IV q4–8h for short-term relief of more severe anxiety-related vertigo
  - Diazepam (Valium) 2 to 10 mg PO or IV q4–8h for short-term relief of more severe symptoms

Geriatric Considerations

Use vestibular-suppressant medications with caution due to increased risk of falls and urinary retention.

Pregnancy Considerations

Meclizine and dimenhydrinate are pregnancy Category B.

ISSUES FOR REFERRAL

Consider referral to otolaryngologist, ENT specialist, vestibular rehabilitation therapist, or neurologist if patient requires further care.

ADDITIONAL THERAPIES

- Epley maneuver/modified Epley maneuver for BPPV to displace calcium deposits in the semicircular canals
  - Effective for short-term symptomatic improvement and for converting patient from positive to negative Dix-Hallpike maneuver; some studies suggest long-term relief.
- Lateral canal BPPV may respond to barbecue roll maneuver.
- Vestibular rehabilitation exercises: ball toss, lying-to-standing, target-change, thumb-tracking, tightrope, walking turns

---

 ONGOING CARE

FOLLOW-UP RECOMMENDATIONS

Balance exercises should be adhered to for symptom reduction and return to normal activities of daily living (ADLs).

Patient Monitoring

After 1 to 2 weeks, assess for the following:

- Recurrence or new symptoms
- Medication-related adverse effects

DIET

- Restricted salt intake for Ménière disease
- Dietary modifications for vertiginous migraine

PATIENT EDUCATION

Avoid triggers such as caffeine/alcohol (vertiginous migraine).

PROGNOSIS

Depends on diagnosis and response to treatment

COMPLICATIONS

- Anxiety, depression
- Disability, injuries from falls

REFERENCES

1. Rogers TS, Noel MA, Garcia B. Dizziness: evaluation and management. *Am Fam Physician.* 2023;107(5):514–523.
2. Muncie HL, Sirmans SM, James E. Dizziness: approach to evaluation and management. *Am Fam Physician.* 2017;95(3):154–162.
3. Newman-Toker DE, Edlow JA. TiTrATE: a novel, evidence-based approach to diagnosing acute dizziness and vertigo. *Neurol Clin.* 2015;33(3): 577–599, viii.

 SEE ALSO

- Ménière Disease; Motion Sickness; Vertigo, Benign Paroxysmal Positional (BPPV)
- Algorithm: Dizziness

 CODES

ICD10

- R42 Dizziness and giddiness
- H81.10 Benign paroxysmal vertigo, unspecified ear
- H81.49 Vertigo of central origin, unspecified ear

CLINICAL PEARLS

- Ensure no medications are cause of symptoms.
- TiTrATE your assessment.
- Acute, spontaneous, continuous vertigo with a normal horizontal head impulse, direction-changing nystagmus, and skew deviation (HINTS positive) is highly sensitive and specific for CVA.
- Episodic, triggered vertigo with positive Dix-Hallpike test is consistent with BPPV.
- If patient warrants a HINTS exam, do not perform Dix-Hallpike maneuver because central cause can also produce a positive Dix-Hallpike.
- The Epley maneuver is recommended for the treatment of BPPV.
- Medications are not recommended for BPPV.

VERTIGO, BENIGN PAROXYSMAL POSITIONAL (BPPV)

Chirag N. Shah, MD • Daniel Scott Morrison, MD • Michael DiGaetano, MD

 BASICS

DESCRIPTION

- Benign paroxysmal positional vertigo (BPPV) is a mechanical disorder of the inner ear characterized by a brief period of vertigo experienced when the position of the patient's head is changed relative to gravity.
- Vertigo results from the mismatch of the perception of movement by the visual, vestibular, and proprioceptive symptoms when none exist.
- The brief period of vertigo is caused by abnormal stimulation of ≥1 of the 3 semicircular canals of the inner ear, with the posterior canal most commonly affected.
- BPPV is the single most common cause of vertigo.

EPIDEMIOLOGY

- Age of onset is typically between the 5th and 7th decades of life.
- Incidence increases with each decade of life.
- Prevalent sex: female > male
- BPPV affects the quality of life of elderly patients and is associated with reduced activities of daily living scores, falls, and depression.

Incidence
1-year incidence 0.6%

Prevalence
Lifetime prevalence 2.4%

ETIOLOGY AND PATHOPHYSIOLOGY

- In BPPV, calcite particles (otoconia) that normally weigh the sensory membrane of the maculae become dislodged and settle into the semicircular canal, changing the dynamics of the canal. Reorientation of the canal relative to gravity causes the otoconia to move to the lowest part of the canal, causing displacement of the endolymph, deflection of the cupula, and activation of the primary afferent. This results in the generation of nystagmus and the associated sensation of vertigo.
- BPPV may be idiopathic, posttraumatic, or associated with viral neurolabyrinthitis.

RISK FACTORS
Female gender, vitamin D deficiency, osteoporosis, migraine, head trauma, and high total cholesterol level (1)[A]

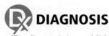 DIAGNOSIS

- The diagnosis is established based on history and findings on positional testing, clarified by Dix and Hallpike in 1952.
- Positional tests place the plane of the canal being tested into the plane parallel with gravity.
- Systematic approach to prevent misdiagnosis or failure to recognize a stroke, notably posterior stroke

HISTORY

- Most common form of triggered episodic vestibular syndrome
- Brief in duration with head motion intolerance
- Patients present with a usual chief complaint of dizziness, light-headedness, and/or feeling "off balance."
- Brief episodes of vertigo (sensation that the room is spinning) are associated with
  - Rolling over in bed
  - Getting out of bed
  - Looking up (referred to as "top-shelf syndrome")
  - Bending forward
  - Quick head movements
- Frequently, patients complain of nausea and, if severe enough, vomiting.

PHYSICAL EXAM

- The Dix-Hallpike test (DHT) is used to diagnose BPPV. The test provokes the characteristic nystagmus associated with the symptoms of vertigo, with an estimated sensitivity of 79% (95% CI 65–94) and specificity of 75% (95% CI 33–100).
  - To perform the DHT, rapidly move the patient from seated to supine position with the head turned 45 degrees to the right and held extended just over the edge of the exam table. This position is maintained for 45 to 60 seconds. Observe for nystagmus and patient report of vertigo. Nystagmus/vertigo may not appear immediately. Wait until symptoms resolve and then return the patient to the sitting position. Repeat on the left.
- The direction of the fast phase of the nystagmus, along with any latency period before onset and duration of the nystagmus, before it ceases is recorded.
- BPPV is consistent with a latency period of <30 seconds between lowering the head and the subsequent onset of nystagmus; the eye movements peak then slowly resolve within 40 seconds. The direction of the nystagmus reverses when the patient's head is brought back upright and to the neutral position. Repeated testing results in diminished vertiginous symptoms and nystagmus fatigue.
- The following characteristics help to distinguish a peripheral etiology for the patient with vertigo versus a central cause:
  - Triggered nystagmus (vs. spontaneous or gaze)
  - Onset is sudden (vs. sudden or slow).
  - Severity of intense spinning (vs. less intense)
  - Pattern is paroxysmal (vs. constant).
  - Symptoms are aggravated by movement (vs. variable).
  - Nausea or diaphoresis is frequent (vs. variable).
  - Nystagmus has rotatory-vertical, horizontal eye movements (vs. vertical).
  - Symptoms fatigue (vs. ongoing)
  - Hearing loss or tinnitus may occur (vs. not typically an associated symptom).
  - An abnormal TM may be seen (vs. this is not an associated finding).
  - CNS symptoms are not associated (vs. CNS findings usually present).

- Red flags in vertigo
  - Neurologic deficit, ipsilateral hearing loss, gait abnormality, direction-changing nystagmus (nystagmus that changes its direction with different body and head positions)
- Head Impulse Nystagmus Test of Skew (HINTS) + no hearing loss
  - Head impulse test of vestibulo-ocular reflex function
    ○ Normally, eye movement will correct with rapid head movement so that the center of the vision remains on a target. This reflex fails in peripheral causes of vertigo.
    ○ Have the patient fix their eyes on your nose, and move their head in the horizontal plane to the left and then to the right.
    ○ When the head is turned toward the normal side, the vestibulo-ocular reflex remains intact and the eyes are fixated on the examiner's nose.
    ○ When the head is turned toward the affected side, the vestibulo-ocular reflex fails and the eyes make a corrective saccade to refixate on the examiner's nose.
    ○ It is reassuring if the reflex is *abnormal* (due to dysfunction of the peripheral nerve).
  - Unidirectional gaze-evoked nystagmus
  - Test for skew deviation "vertical dysconjugate gaze."
    ○ Skew deviation is a fairly specific predictor of a central lesion in patients with acute vestibular syndrome.
    ○ The presence of skew may help identify stroke when a positive head impulse test falsely suggests a peripheral lesion.
    ○ Have the patient look at your nose with their eyes and start by covering one eye and then rapidly move to cover the other eye; do this rapidly back and forth.
    ○ When each eye is uncovered, quickly look to see if the eye has movement or refixation. Horizontal is normal; vertical is not.
  - In the setting of dizziness and vertigo, HINTS substantially outperforms ABCD2 for stroke diagnosis and outperforms MRI obtained within the first 2 days after symptom onset (2)[B].
  - The use of HINTS is limited in evaluation in the ED to specifically rule out a stroke in those presenting with acute vestibular syndromes.

DIFFERENTIAL DIAGNOSIS

- Orthostatic hypotension and other disorders that cause low BP; symptoms usually occur when the patient stands up.
- Damage to the brainstem or cerebellum can cause positional vertigo but is accompanied by other neurologic signs and usually has a different pattern of nystagmus.
- Low spinal fluid pressure may cause positional symptoms that are better when the patient lies down.
- Migraine-associated vertigo
- Traumatic brain injury
- Brain tumors, hemorrhage, or infarction
- Vestibular neuronitis

DIAGNOSTIC TESTS & INTERPRETATION

Systematic approach: Triage, TiTrATE, then treatment

- TiTrATE approach: Timing, Triggers, and Targeted examinations
  - Timing classifies the disease processes into episodic versus continuous.
  - Triggers further seek to find underlying causes by looking at exam findings (e.g., DHT).
  - Targeted examination and ancillary tests are based on findings.
- Combination of all this information allows the clinician to further evaluate with CT or MRI.

TREATMENT

- The Canalith Repositioning Procedure (CRP) or Epley maneuver is effective in the treatment of posterior canal BPPV. Using a particle repositioning maneuver, the clinician moves the patient through a series of positions. Most studies evaluating the effectiveness of CRP have been performed in specialist clinics. However, in a randomized controlled trial out of primary care offices, a single CRP administered by a general practitioner demonstrated significant improvement in symptoms compared to a sham maneuver.
- The clinician moves the patient through a series of four provoking positions:
  - Placement of the right posterior canal (involved canal) in the right head-hanging position of the DHT
  - The head is then rotated a total of 90 degrees toward the left (uninvolved side) into 45 degrees of left head rotation.
  - Maintaining 45 degrees of left head rotation, the patient is rolled onto the left side (uninvolved side) with the head slightly elevated from the supporting surface.
  - The patient then sits up and flexes the neck 36 degrees. Each position is maintained for a minimum of 45 seconds or as long as the nystagmus lasts.
- CRP is the best maneuver for posterior BPPV and should be offered to all age groups.
- Semont maneuver is also another maneuver, less superior when performed alone.
- Lempert roll maneuver
- Contraindications are cervical spine disease, carotid vascular disease, and retinal detachment. If the CRP is ineffective, self-administered CRP is performed at home. The patient performs the CRP on the bed with the head extended over the edge of a pillow. Better outcomes are achieved with a combination of CRP with self-administered CRP.
- CRP and Semont maneuver are ineffective for horizontal BPPV; variations of the Lempert maneuver, barbecue roll, or Gufoni maneuver are widely used treatment methods for horizontal BPPV.
- Postmaneuver activity restrictions were previously advocated, but in controlled trials, they did not differ in clinical outcomes.

MEDICATION

- Vestibular suppressant medications are not recommended for the treatment of BPPV, other than for the short-term management of vegetative symptoms (3)[A].
- Antiemetics such as ondansetron may be considered for prophylaxis for patients who have had severe nausea or vomiting with the DHT.
- Vestibular suppressants such as benzodiazepines and antihistamine anticholinergics such as meclizine should be avoided because they may suppress nystagmus during the DHT and treatment.

ISSUES FOR REFERRAL

Consider a referral to a specialist if BPPV is unresponsive to treatment or if the patient is diagnosed with atypical BPPV involving the anterior or lateral canal. Consider referring to a physical therapist, a neurologist, or otolaryngologist.

ADDITIONAL THERAPIES

- Vestibular rehabilitation therapy (VRT) has been shown to have some efficacy in reducing symptom burden on quality of life in patients with BPPV. This therapy modality consists of exercises that focus on strengthening vestibular compensation to changes in positioning.
- Hypertension, diabetes mellitus, hyperlipidemia, osteoporosis, and vitamin D deficiency have been identified as potential risk factors for recurrence of BPPV. It is possible that the management of these comorbidities may help prevent recurrence of symptoms.
- Surgical intervention is rarely indicated, except for refractory BPPV, and includes posterior canal occlusion and singular neurectomy.

ONGOING CARE

FOLLOW-UP RECOMMENDATIONS

The patient should follow up within a week after treatment to ensure resolution.

PATIENT EDUCATION

A number of illustrative YouTube videos are available for education and self-administered CRP maneuvers.

PROGNOSIS

80% cure rate with CRP maneuvers, with a 30% recurrence rate at 1 year, and 44% redevelop BPPV within 2 years

COMPLICATIONS

During the maneuvers, a canal conversion may occur. The debris from the canal being treated may reflux into another canal.

REFERENCES

1. Chen J, Zhao W, Yue X, et al. Risk factors for the occurrence of benign paroxysmal positional vertigo: a systematic review and meta-analysis. *Front Neurol*. 2020;11:506.
2. Newman-Toker DE, Kerber KA, Hsieh YH, et al. HINTS outperforms ABCD2 to screen for stroke in acute continuous vertigo and dizziness. *Acad Emerg Med*. 2013;20(10):986–996.
3. Sharif S, Khoujah D, Greer A, et al. Vestibular suppressants for benign paroxysmal positional vertigo: a systematic review and meta-analysis of randomized controlled trials. *Acad Emerg Med*. 2023;30(5):541–551.

ADDITIONAL READING

- Ballvé JL, Carrillo-Muñoz R, Rando-Matos Y, et al. Effectiveness of the Epley manoeuvre in posterior canal benign paroxysmal positional vertigo: a randomised clinical trial in primary care. *Br J Gen Pract*. 2019;69(678):e52–e60.
- Bhattacharyya N, Gubbels SP, Schwartz SR, et al. Clinical practice guideline: benign paroxysmal positional vertigo (update). *Otolaryngol Head Neck Surg*. 2017;156(Suppl 3):S1–S47.
- Epley JM. The canalith repositioning procedure: for treatment of benign paroxysmal positional vertigo. *Otolaryngol Head Neck Surg*. 1992;107(3):399–404.
- Kattah JC, Talkad AV, Wang DZ, et al. HINTS to diagnose stroke in the acute vestibular syndrome: three-step bedside oculomotor examination more sensitive than early MRI diffusion-weighted imaging. *Stroke*. 2009;40(11):3504–3510.
- Shah VP, Silva LOJE, Farah W, et al. Diagnostic accuracy of the physical examination in emergency department patients with acute vertigo or dizziness: a systematic review and meta-analysis for GRACE-3. *Acad Emerg Med*. 2023;30(5):552–578.
- Shaphe MA, Alshehri MM, Alajam RA, et al. Effectiveness of Epley—Canalith repositioning procedure versus vestibular rehabilitation therapy in diabetic patients with posterior benign paroxysmal positional vertigo: a randomized trial. *Life (Basel)*. 2023;13(5):1169.

CODES

ICD10

- H81.10 Benign paroxysmal vertigo, unspecified ear
- H81.12 Benign paroxysmal vertigo, left ear
- H81.11 Benign paroxysmal vertigo, right ear

CLINICAL PEARLS

- The diagnosis of BPPV is based on history and findings on positional testing.
- The typical presentation is a report of transient episodes of vertigo (sensation that the room is spinning) associated with a change in position of the head relative to gravity.
- BPPV may be treated effectively with particle-repositioning maneuvers in the office and at home.
- Vestibular suppressant medications and antiemetics are not recommended for the treatment of BPPV, other than for the short-term management of symptoms.
- Patients should always be ambulated in order to verify normal gait prior to discharge.

V

VINCENT STOMATITIS

Daniel V. Girzadas Jr., MD • Nicolas Semenchuk, MD, MS

 BASICS

A distinct form of periodontal disease due to inflammatory infection of the gingiva, characterized by pain, ulcerations, and necrotizing damage to interdental papillae

DESCRIPTION

- Caused by an imbalance of oral flora, resulting in a predominance of anaerobic bacteria that invade the gingival mucosa and form a gray pseudomembranous exudate
- Clinical presentation includes oral pain, fetid breath, gingival ulcerations, necrosis, and bleeding
- Differentiated from other periodontal diseases by rapid onset, pain, ulcerated gingival mucosa, and "punched out" crater-like lesions of interdental papillae (1)
- The most common bacteria include *Fusobacterium* spp., *Prevotella intermedia*, and spirochetes. Concomitant infection with Epstein-Barr virus, herpes simplex virus, and type 1 human cytomegalovirus is common.
- Synonym(s): Vincent angina; Vincent disease; trench mouth; fusospirochetal gingivitis; acute necrotizing ulcerative gingivitis (ANUG); necrotizing ulcerative gingivitis (NUG)
- Necrotizing gingivitis, necrotizing periodontitis, and necrotizing stomatitis are classified together under the umbrella term "necrotizing periodontal disease (NPD)." Necrotizing gingivitis is confined to the gingiva without a loss of peridontal attachment or alveolar bone support.

EPIDEMIOLOGY

Incidence

- Predominant age: 18 to 30 years in developed countries, malnourished children ages 3 to 14 years
- Affects both genders with similar frequency
- Historically, incidence increased in military personnel due to poor battlefield conditions and psychological stress (1)

Prevalence

- The true prevalence is unknown but likely <1% overall (1).
- Worldwide prevalence has declined since World War II (1).
- A rare disease in developed countries; however, in recent data, prevalence rate was 6.7% in Chilean students between ages 12 and 21 years and approaching 25% in children in sub-Saharan African countries (2),(3).

ETIOLOGY AND PATHOPHYSIOLOGY

- Impaired host immunologic response due to immunocompromised state or malnutrition
- Disruption of normal oral flora with a predominance of invasive anaerobic bacteria (*Treponema* spp., *Selenomonas* spp., *Fusobacterium* spp., and *Prevotella intermedia*) (2)

- Endogenous bacteria produce metabolites such as collagenase, endotoxins, and fibrinolysin that destroy tissue, leading to loss of integrity and necrosis of the gingival mucosa and interdental papillae (4)
- Stress increases adrenocortical hormones and reduces gingival microcirculation and salivary flow, which alters leukocyte and lymphocyte function. Stress may also result in behavioral changes that lead to poor oral hygiene and malnutrition (2).
- Increased bacterial attachment with active herpesvirus infection

RISK FACTORS

- Malnutrition
- Immunosuppression (diabetes, alcohol use, HIV, cancer, chemotherapy, steroid use)
- Low socioeconomic status
- Tobacco use
- Poor oral hygiene, infrequent or absent dental care
- Orthodontics
- Herpesvirus infection
- Psychological stress

GENERAL PREVENTION

- Appropriate nutrition
- Proper oral hygiene
- Regular dental care
- Prompt recognition and institution of therapy
- Management of medical problems such as cancer and HIV infection
- Smoking cessation
- Stress management

COMMONLY ASSOCIATED CONDITIONS

- Most commonly seen in malnourished patients, patients undergoing cancer treatment, or those from underdeveloped countries
- Bacteremia
- Tooth loss
- Chronic gingivitis
- Noma (cancrum oris), a gangrenous infection of the oral mucosa
- Aspiration pneumonia

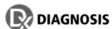 **DIAGNOSIS**

HISTORY

- Presentation typically includes the triad of rapid onset of gingival pain, bleeding, and ulcerations/necrosis of interdental papillae (4).
- Fetid odor of breath, metallic taste in the mouth
- Systemic symptoms: regional lymphadenopathy, fever, malaise

- Presence of risk factors including tobacco use, poor oral hygiene, malnourishment, and immunocompromise
- Active herpesvirus infection or HIV

PHYSICAL EXAM

- Fever
- Fetid odor of the breath
- Ulceration of gingival mucosa
- Inflamed, erythematous gingiva
- Necrosis of interdental papillae
- Gingival bleeding
- Formation of gray, pseudomembranous exudate
- Cervical and submandibular lymphadenopathy

DIFFERENTIAL DIAGNOSIS

- Herpes simplex virus
- Recurrent aphthous stomatitis
- Medication side effects
- Oral malignancy
- Diphtheria
- Lymphoma/leukemia
- Primary syphilis
- Ascorbic acid deficiency
- Behçet disease or granulomatosis with polyangiitis
- Oral histoplasmosis

DIAGNOSTIC TESTS & INTERPRETATION

Initial Tests (lab, imaging)

Diagnosis is primarily based on clinical presentation, but if systemic illness or invasive spread to deeper tissue or bone is suspected, the following studies should be considered:

- Aerobic and anaerobic cultures of inflamed or débrided tissue
- Group A strep rapid antigen detection assay or throat culture
- Blood cultures if systemic involvement
- Dental radiographs
- CT imaging of the face and neck if there is a concern that the infection has spread to deeper tissue

Diagnostic Procedures/Other

Although biopsy could be performed for histopathology, the diagnosis is largely clinical in nature. Microbiology testing often does not add relevant diagnostic information given that many of these bacterial pathogens are typical of healthy gingiva and other nonspecific cases of gingivitis and periodontitis (1).

 TREATMENT

The goals of care include sequential steps of alleviating the acute phase, managing the preexisting conditions, and treating disease sequelae (2).

GENERAL MEASURES

- The initial phase of treatment aims to control the acute phase of the disease through a multimodal treatment approach with superficial débridement, oral hygiene, antimicrobial mouthwash, and consideration for oral antibiotics in those with poor response to débridement or those with symptoms of systemic involvement (fever, malaise, vomiting).
  - Débridement can be accomplished by a cotton-topped swab soaked with hydrogen peroxide for gentle local débridement, rinse with hydrogen peroxide or chlorhexidine, ultrasonic débridement with a dental specialist, or surgical débridement under local anesthesia.
- Once the acute disease is controlled, the patient will require ongoing outpatient dental cleanings, specifically scaling and root planing.
- Elimination of tobacco, improved nutritional status, and improved immunologic status will increase the rate of healing and reduce the risk of future gingival disease.

MEDICATION

Most cases are treatable on an outpatient basis. Severe disease with systemic effects and/or neck involvement requires inpatient treatment. Other than chlorhexidine, there is no role for topical antibiotics given that they cannot effectively penetrate the periodontal tissue (2).

First Line

- Chlorhexidine gluconate 0.12% 15 mL 30 seconds rinse/spit twice daily (1)[C]
- The following antibiotics can be considered for patients with signs and symptoms of systemic infection:
  - Penicillin V potassium 250 to 500 mg PO q6h PO for 5 to 7 days for adults and children >12 years of age or
  - Metronidazole 250 to 500 mg PO or IV q8h for 7 to 10 days (1)[C],(2)[C],(4)[C]; pediatric dosing: 30 to 50 mg/kg/day divided q8h (3)[A] or
  - Amoxicillin 250 to 500 mg PO q8h PO for 7 days (4)[C]; pediatric dosing: 25 to 45 mg/kg/day divided q12h or
  - Amoxicillin-clavulanate 875 mg PO q12h for 7 to 10 days; pediatric dosing: 25 to 45 mg/kg/day divided q12h amoxicillin or
  - Clindamycin 450 mg PO or 600 mg IV q8h for 7 to 10 days; pediatric dosing: 8 to 25 mg/kg/day divided q6–8h
  - Some historical data suggest combination therapy of metronidazole with either amoxicillin or penicillin V potassium.
  - Ampicillin/sulbactam offers effective coverage for immunocompromised patients requiring hospitalization.

Second Line

- Tetracycline 250 to 500 mg QID PO for 10 days (do not use for children <8 years of age); pediatric dosing: 25 to 50 mg/kg/day divided q6h or
- Erythromycin 250 to 500 mg q6–12h PO for 10 days; pediatric dosing: 30 to 50 mg/kg/day divided q6–8h

Pediatric Considerations

- Chlorhexidine and alcohol mouth rinses are generally avoided due to the risk of ingestion, but chlorhexidine may be prescribed in gel form for topical application.
- Alternatively, can consider 3% hydrogen peroxide diluted by half with water as a safer mouthwash in children to help remove the pseudomembranous coating and decrease bleeding (3)
- In addition to amoxicillin or amoxicillin-clavulanate, metronidazole may be considered as first-line oral therapy (refer to dosing above) (3)[A].

ISSUES FOR REFERRAL

Severe disease requires débridement by a consultant dentist, oral surgeon, or ENT specialist.

ADDITIONAL THERAPIES

- Warm saline rinses q2h
- Sodium bicarbonate toothpaste, brush q2h
- Viscous lidocaine 2% 1 tbsp rinse/spit q6–8h
- NSAID medications q4–12h
- Opioid analgesics q4–6h (severe pain)
- Treatment of underlying immunodeficiency (if present)

SURGERY/OTHER PROCEDURES

- Débridement of inflamed/necrotic gingival tissue
- Dental extraction
- Gingival restoration
- Adjuvant therapies
  - Low-level laser therapy (LLLT) has been shown in one case series to decrease pain and accelerate healing.
  - Photochemotherapy has been shown to reduce bleeding ulcers and bacterial counts compared to conventional therapy alone.

COMPLEMENTARY & ALTERNATIVE MEDICINE

3% hydrogen peroxide and warm sterile saline in a 1:1 ratio q2–3h as an oral rinse (1)[C]

ADMISSION, INPATIENT, AND NURSING CONSIDERATIONS

- Severe disease, failure of oral antibiotics, or ongoing comorbidities
- Parenteral antibiotics, analgesia requirement, or inability to tolerate PO

ONGOING CARE

FOLLOW-UP RECOMMENDATIONS

- Close dental follow-up
- Specialty follow-up (if underlying immunodeficiency)

DIET

- Soft diet until healed
- Balanced nutritional diet with multivitamin supplementation

PATIENT EDUCATION

- Oral hygiene with emphasis on twice daily brushing, flossing, and routine dental care
- Proper nutrition
- Tobacco cessation

PROGNOSIS

- Lack of treatment can lead to rapid tissue destruction, necrotizing ulcerative periodontitis, and cancrum oris, an often fatal gangrenous orofacial infection
- The maintenance of adequate oral hygiene is needed to prevent recurrence.

COMPLICATIONS

- Malnutrition/dehydration
- Gingival/tooth loss
- Deep infection of neck

REFERENCES

1. Dufty J, Gkranias N, Donos N. Necrotising ulcerative gingivitis: a literature review. *Oral Health Prev Dent*. 2017;15(4):321–327.
2. Malek R, Gharibi A, Khlil N, et al. Necrotizing ulcerative gingivitis. *Contemp Clin Dent*. 2017;8(3):496–500.
3. Marty M, Palmieri J, Noirrit-Esclassan E, et al. Necrotizing periodontal diseases in children: a literature review and adjustment of treatment. *J Trop Pediatr*. 2016;62(4):331–337.
4. Atout RN, Todescan S. Managing patients with necrotizing ulcerative gingivitis. *J Can Dent Assoc*. 2013;79:d46.

CODES

ICD10

A69.1 Other Vincent's infections

CLINICAL PEARLS

- Diagnosis is largely clinical based on symptoms of oral pain, fetid breath, gingival ulcerations, interdental papillary necrosis, and grayish exudate on the gingival surface.
- Immunosuppression, malnourishment, smoking, and poor oral hygiene are key risk factors for NUG.
- Most patients experience rapid improvement following appropriate treatment with gentle débridement, chlorhexidine rinses, improved oral hygiene, and oral antibiotics.
- Smoking cessation and treatment of malnutrition or underlying illness are additional important treatment considerations.
- Severe disease requires extensive débridement of necrotic gingival tissue and close follow-up with a periodontal specialist or oral surgeon to limit recurrence and prevent rapid destruction of the periodontium.

V

VITAMIN B$_{12}$ DEFICIENCY

Sahil Mullick, MD • Aya Allam, MD

BASICS

- Vitamin B$_{12}$ deficiency is related to inadequate intake or absorption of cobalamin.
- Cobalamin is critical for central nervous system myelination, red blood cell production, immune cell cytogenesis, and DNA synthesis (1).
- Deficiency can cause megaloblastic anemia, bone marrow dysfunction, cytopenia including lymphopenia, and diverse and potentially irreversible neuropsychiatric changes.
- Neuropsychiatric disorders are due to demyelination of cervical, thoracic dorsal, and lateral spinal cords; white matter; and cranial and peripheral nerves.
- Elevated MMA and homocysteine levels MMA are more sensitive and specific and persist for several days even after treatment.

DESCRIPTION

Normal vitamin B$_{12}$ absorption and diet recommendations

- Vitamin B$_{12}$ is a water-soluble vitamin present in animal-source foods and foods fortified with vitamin B$_{12}$.
- Dietary vitamin B$_{12}$ (cobalamin) bound to food is cleaved by acids in stomach and bound to haptocorrin that are secreted in saliva (commonly known as R-factor).
- Pancreatic proteases cleave vitamin B$_{12}$ from haptocorrin.
- In duodenum, vitamin B$_{12}$ uptake depends on binding to intrinsic factor (IF) secreted by gastric parietal cells.
- Vitamin B$_{12}$-IF complex is absorbed by terminal ileum into portal circulation.
- Small amount of ingested vitamin B$_{12}$ (<1 percent) can be absorbed by passive diffusion and is the basis for use of high dose oral vitamin B$_{12}$ in pernicious anemia (PA).
- Total body stores of vitamin B$_{12}$ are in 2 to 5 mg range. Most of it are stored in liver.
- Vitamin B$_{12}$ excreted in bile is effectively reabsorbed through enterohepatic circulation.
- Typical Western diet: 5 to 30 mg/day; however, only 1 to 5 mg/day is effectively absorbed.
- Recommend 2.4 mg/day for adults and 2.6 mg/day during pregnancy and 2.8 mg/day during lactation (most prenatal vitamins contain vitamin B$_{12}$).

EPIDEMIOLOGY

Prevalence

- National Health and Nutrition Examination Survey documented 6.9% and 15% prevalence of B$_{12}$ deficiency in U.S. adults aged 51 to 70 and >70 years, respectively (2).
- Morbidity increases vitamin B$_{12}$ deficiency occurrence, ranging from 4% to 5% in community-living elderly to about 30–40% in institutionalized subjects with multiple comorbidities.
- Prevalence in those <60 years old is 6% versus 20% in those >60 years.
- Increasing recognition in breastfed-only infants with vitamin B$_{12}$–deficient mothers
- Among patients with clinical macrocytosis (defined as a mean corpuscular volume [MCV] >100), 18–20% were due to vitamin B$_{12}$ deficiency (3).

- Vitamin B$_{12}$ deficiency due to PA is more common in people of Northern European ancestry and lower in people of African descent.

ETIOLOGY AND PATHOPHYSIOLOGY

- Decreased oral intake
  - Vegetarians and vegans: Vitamin B$_{12}$ is found in animal-source foods.
- Decreased IF
  - PA: can be associated with autoantibodies directed against gastric parietal cells and/or IF; 15–30% of all cases; most frequent cause of severe disease; neurologic disorders are common presenting complaints.
  - Chronic atrophic gastritis: autoimmune attack on gastric parietal cells causing autoimmune gastritis and leading to decreased IF production
  - Gastrectomy: removal of entire or part of stomach
- Decreased absorption
  - Crohn disease: Terminal ileal inflammation decreases body's ability to absorb vitamin B$_{12}$.
  - Chronic alcoholism: decreases body's ability to absorb vitamin B$_{12}$
  - Gluten hypersensitivity (celiac disease) intestinal villi atrophy and subsequent malabsorption
  - Ileal resection
  - Pancreatic insufficiency: Pancreatic proteases are required to cleave the vitamin B$_{12}$–haptocorrin bond to allow vitamin B$_{12}$ to bind to IF.
  - *Helicobacter pylori* infection: impairs release of vitamin B$_{12}$ from bound proteins
- Medications:
  - Proton pump inhibitors (PPIs), H$_2$ antagonists, and antacids decrease gastric acidity, inhibiting vitamin B$_{12}$ release from dietary protein; metformin
  - Metformin usage can cause calcium-dependent membrane inhibition, interfering with vitamin B$_{12}$–IF absorption
- Hereditary (rare): transcobalamin II deficiency

Genetics

Imerslund-Gräsbeck disease (juvenile megaloblastic anemia) caused by mutations in the amnionless (AMN) or cubilin (CUBN) genes with autosomal recessive pattern of inheritance; inadequate ileal uptake of vitamin B$_{12}$-IF complex and decreased vitamin B$_{12}$ renal protein reabsorption.

COMMONLY ASSOCIATED CONDITIONS

- Gastric abnormalities: PA, gastritis, gastrectomy/bariatric surgery
- Small bowel disease: malabsorption syndrome, ileal resection, IBD, celiac disease
- Pancreatic insufficiency
- Diet: breastfed infant in vitamin B$_{12}$ deficient mother, strict vegan diet
- Medications: neomycin, metformin, PPI, histamine 2 receptor antagonists, nitrous oxide (N$_2$O) abuse

DIAGNOSIS

- Asymptomatic; incidental finding of anemia or elevated MCV.
- Neuropsychiatric
  - Frequent: sensory polyneuritis, paresthesias, positive Babinski sign, weakness, gait unsteadiness,

loss of proprioception (impaired vibratory sensation, positive Romberg, ataxia, hyperreflexia)
  - Classic but uncommon: subacute combined degeneration of spinal cord associated with PA; areflexia, ataxia, proprioception and vibration loss, bowel and bladder incontinence, orthostatic hypotension, decreased memory, mania, delirium, psychosis, depression
- Digestive
  - Classic: Hunter glossitis, jaundice, and high lactate dehydrogenase and bilirubin
  - Possible: abdominal pain, dyspepsia, nausea, vomiting, diarrhea
  - Rare: mucocutaneous ulcers
- Other
  - Frequent: fatigue with exertion, skin pallor, palpitations, edema, jaundice

HISTORY

- Underlying disease associated with vitamin B$_{12}$ deficiency
- Fatigue, anorexia, depression
- Falls (due to diminished proprioception), loss of sensation in "stocking-glove" distribution
- Glossitis/loss of sense of taste

PHYSICAL EXAM

- Lymphadenopathy, hepatosplenomegaly, enlarged tongue (glossitis)
- Neurologic exam: impaired vibratory sense, altered proprioception possible ataxia, diminished sensations in light touch, and/or weakness

DIFFERENTIAL DIAGNOSIS

Folate deficiency, copper deficiency, hypothyroidism, syphilis, multiple sclerosis, HIV myelopathy

DIAGNOSTIC TESTS & INTERPRETATION

- Measurement of vitamin B$_{12}$, complete blood count (MCV)
- Measurement of vitamin B$_{12}$ may be low or low normal depending on cutoff value.
  - 95–97% sensitive levels <200 pg/mL
  - May need additional tests such as MMA and homocysteine if vitamin B$_{12}$ level is low normal (<350 pg/mL)
- MCV is often increased, although it is not necessarily present if the condition is associated with other kinds of anemia.
- Measurement of MMA
  - More sensitive and specific than homocysteine
  - Levels increased in renal failure and volume depletion
- Measurement of homocysteine
  - Levels increased in folate deficiency, renal failure, homocystinuria; vitamin B$_6$ deficiency and hypothyroidism
- MMA and homocysteine levels only reliable in an untreated patient because levels fall with supplementation
- Other tests: folate and other markers of anemia (iron studies)
- Holotranscobalamin (holo-TC) accounts for approximately 10% of the circulating vitamin B$_{12}$ and is the earliest marker showing vitamin B$_{12}$ depletion. It is also known as active vitamin B$_{12}$, the only form of vitamin B$_{12}$ that is taken up and used by the cells in the body.

- Low levels of vitamin B$_{12}$ are seen in folate deficiency, HIV, and multiple myeloma.
- Elevated levels of vitamin B$_{12}$ are seen in renal disease, occult malignancy, and alcoholic liver disease.
- Macrocytosis may be due to folate deficiency, reticulocytosis, medications, bone marrow dysplasia, and hypothyroidism or be masked by concomitant microcytic anemia.
- In asymptomatic individuals, vitamin B$_{12}$ deficiency is associated with reductions in the binding protein haptocorrin. However, this condition may be difficult to discriminate from true vitamin B$_{12}$ deficiency in the presence of symptoms.
- Check antibody to IF; positive test is confirmatory for PA, but sensitivity is only 50–70%.
- Antibodies to parietal cells, present in 90% of patients with PA, are less specific and can occur in simple atrophic gastritis and in autoimmune thyroid disease.
- For patients with negative anti-IF result and high suspicion for PA, check serum gastrin level (elevated in PA).

Pregnancy and Newborn Considerations
- Pregnant women with low vitamin B$_{12}$ have higher risk of having children with neural tube defects, developmental delay, failure to thrive, hypotonia, ataxia, and anemia.
- Exclusively breastfed infants of mothers who are vitamin B$_{12}$ deficient are at risk of developing vitamin B$_{12}$ deficiency. Infants might not show signs or symptoms until 4 to 6 months of age, which may include developmental regression, feeding difficulties, lethargy, or hypotonia.
- Children born to mothers with normal to high folate levels and low serum vitamin B$_{12}$ values have higher truncal adiposity and insulin resistance which may influence long-term risk of development of type 2 diabetes and cardiovascular disease.
- Low vitamin B$_{12}$ has a negative influence on children's development and cognitive functioning, may cause growth and motor retardation.
- Untreated severe vitamin B$_{12}$ deficiency during pregnancy can lead to severe anemia, peripheral neuropathy, cognitive decline, and a variety of neuropsychiatric manifestations.
- May also manifest with microangiopathic hemolytic anemia and thrombocytopenia, mimicking other thrombotic microangiopathy disorders such as atypical hemolytic uremic syndrome, HELLP syndrome, and thrombotic thrombocytopenic purpura

Initial Tests (lab, imaging)
Vitamin B$_{12}$, MMA, and homocysteine levels

Diagnostic Procedures/Other
Bone marrow exam is usually unnecessary.

Test Interpretation
- If vitamin B$_{12}$ level is:
  - >400 pg/mL, no deficiency

  - Between 150 to 399 pg/mL, obtain MMA level and homocysteine level.
  - <150 pg/mL, deficiency is present
- If MMA and homocysteine level testing is warranted
  - If MMA levels and homocysteine levels are high, vitamin B$_{12}$ deficiency is confirmed.
  - If MMA levels are normal but homocysteine levels are high, folate deficiency is confirmed.
  - If both are normal, vitamin B$_{12}$ deficiency is unlikely.

TREATMENT

All individuals with documented vitamin B$_{12}$ deficiency should be treated, unless there's a strong reason not to such as patient refusal or palliative care setting.

GENERAL MEASURES
- Repleting deficiency can be done over weeks, must be done urgently in symptomatic patients, unless there is a strong reason not to do so (e.g., palliative care setting or patient refusal).
- If asymptomatic, repletion can be instituted over a period of weeks
- Urgent replacement with:
  - Symptomatic anemia or neurologic or neuropsychiatric findings, due to risk of adverse events and irreversibility of neurologic deficits
  - Pregnancy, as the developing fetus may be affected
  - Neonates and infants, whose development may be impacted

MEDICATION
- Parenteral cyanocobalamin replacement recommended in patients with severe neurologic symptoms or severe anemia: IM cyanocobalamin
  - 1,000 μg injected every other day for 1 to 2 weeks, then
  - 1,000 μg every week for 1 month, then
  - 1,000 μg once a month for life
- Can also use high-dose, daily oral cyanocobalamin at doses of 1,000 to 2,000 μg

ONGOING CARE

FOLLOW-UP RECOMMENDATIONS
Patient Monitoring
- Hematologic
  - Reticulocytosis in 1 week
  - Hemoglobin will usually return to normal in 6 to 8 weeks.
  - Monitor potassium in profoundly anemic patients.

- Neurologic: improvement within 6 weeks to 3 months of treatment; however, maximum improvement noticed at 6 to 12 months; some symptoms may be irreversible.

DIET
Meat, animal protein, foods fortified with vitamin B$_{12}$ unless contraindicated

PROGNOSIS
- Deficiency typically resolves by 4 to 8 weeks.
- It takes longer to resolve and might not completely resolve in severe or longstanding illness. If expected response is not achieved, then additional testing should be indicated.

COMPLICATIONS
- Vision problems
- Memory loss
- Pins and needles (paraesthesia)
- Loss of physical coordination (ataxia)
- Peripheral neuropathy, particularly in the legs

REFERENCES

1. Layden AJ, Täse K, Finkelstein JL. Neglected tropical diseases and vitamin B$_{12}$: a review of the current evidence. *Trans R Soc Trop Med Hyg*. 2018;112(10):423–435.
2. Vincenti A, Bertuzzo L, Limitone A, et al. Perspective: practical approach to preventing subclinical B$_{12}$ deficiency in elderly population. *Nutrients*. 2021;13(6):1913.
3. Devi A, Rush E, Harper M, et al. Vitamin B$_{12}$ status of various ethnic groups living in New Zealand: an analysis of the Adult Nutrition Survey 2008/2009. *Nutrients*. 2018;10(2):181.

 CODES

ICD10
- D51 Vitamin B$_{12}$ deficiency anemia
- D51.3 Other dietary vitamin B$_{12}$ deficiency anemia
- D51.8 Other vitamin B$_{12}$ deficiency anemias

CLINICAL PEARLS
- Vitamin B$_{12}$ deficiency can coexist with other anemia; thus, MCV can be normal, decreased, or increased.
- Common presenting symptoms include fatigue, depression, falls, glossitis/loss of taste, stocking/glove neuropathy.
- For PA, cyanocobalamin must be lifelong.

V

VITAMIN D DEFICIENCY

Ramanpreet Grewal, MD

BASICS

This topic covers the commonly acquired vitamin D deficiency and not type II vitamin D–resistant rickets/type I pseudovitamin D–resistant rickets (both rare autosomal recessive disorders).

DESCRIPTION
- Vitamin D is a hormone and a fat-soluble vitamin.
- Vitamin D undergoes a series of metabolic processes to become calcitriol, which is the biologically active form.
- The skin synthesizes vitamin D_3 (cholecalciferol) by exposure to sunlight (ultraviolet B), and vitamin D_2 (Ergocalciferol) can be obtained from certain foods or supplements.
- D_2 and D_3 are hydroxylated in the liver to 25 vitamin D (calcidiol), the major circulating form.
- Calcidiol is further hydroxylated in the kidney to the active metabolite 1,25 vitamin D (calcitriol).
- Hypocalcemia stimulates parathyroid hormone (PTH) secretion, which prompts increased conversion of 25 vitamin D to 1,25 vitamin D.
- 1,25 vitamin D decreases renal calcium and phosphorus excretion, increases intestinal calcium and phosphorus absorption, and increases osteoclast activity. The net result is an increase in serum calcium.

EPIDEMIOLOGY
The overall prevalence rate of vitamin D deficiency has been reported to be around 40%.
- Geographical variation: more common in regions with limited sunlight; higher prevalence in northern latitudes
- Seasonal variability: lower vitamin D levels in winter; higher levels in summer with more sun exposure
- Age and life stage: Infants, children, and adolescents are at risk. Older adults can have reduced skin synthesis.
- Skin pigmentation: Darker skin may lead to reduced vitamin D production. Rates are the highest in blacks (82%), followed by Hispanics (69%).
- Cultural practices and clothing: Covered skin for religious or cultural reasons can increase risk.
- Obesity and health conditions: Obesity may reduce vitamin D bioavailability. Some health conditions and medications can affect vitamin D metabolism.
- Dietary intake: Limited access to vitamin D-rich foods increases risk. Fortified foods can help address deficiencies.
- Public health interventions: Some countries implement supplementation and fortification policies. Targeted interventions for at-risk populations are in place.

Pediatric Considerations
NHANES data suggest 70% of children do not have sufficient 25-OH vitamin D serum levels (9% deficient and 61% insufficient); deficiency has been associated with an increase in BP and decrease in high-density lipoprotein (HDL) cholesterol.

ETIOLOGY AND PATHOPHYSIOLOGY
- Inadequate sun exposure: Lack of sufficient sunlight exposure is one of the primary causes of vitamin D deficiency. The skin produces vitamin D when exposed to ultraviolet B rays from the sun.
- Dietary insufficiency: A strict vegetarian diet or a diet low in vitamin D-rich foods that include fatty fish (e.g., salmon, mackerel), egg yolks, and cod liver oil can contribute to deficiency.
- Malabsorption disorders: Certain medical conditions that affect the gastrointestinal (GI) tract, such as celiac disease, Crohn disease, and inflammatory bowel disease (IBD), can impair the absorption of vitamin D from the diet. Conditions like liver disease can also affect the conversion of vitamin D into its active form.
- Obesity: Vitamin D is a fat-soluble vitamin, and excess body fat can sequester vitamin D, making it less bioavailable to the body.
- Medications: Certain medications, such as anticonvulsants, glucocorticoids, and weight-loss drugs, can interfere with vitamin D metabolism and absorption, leading to deficiency.
- Chronic kidney disease: The kidneys play a crucial role in converting vitamin D into its active form. Individuals with chronic kidney disease may have impaired vitamin D activation, leading to deficiency.
- Pregnancy and lactation: Pregnancy and breastfeeding increase the body's demand for vitamin D, and women who do not receive adequate sun exposure or dietary sources may become deficient.
- Inflammatory conditions: Chronic inflammatory conditions, such as rheumatoid arthritis, can lead to increased breakdown of vitamin D and reduced effectiveness.
- Excessive alcohol consumption: Chronic excessive alcohol intake can impair the liver's ability to convert vitamin D into its active form.

Genetics
Vitamin D–dependent rickets type 1 occurs due to inactivating mutation of the 1α-hydroxylase gene; as a result, calcidiol is not hydroxylated to calcitriol.

GENERAL PREVENTION
- Adequate exposure to sunlight and dietary sources of vitamin D (plants, fish); many foods are fortified with vitamins D_2 and D_3.
- The recommended intake of vitamin D can vary depending on factors like age, gender, and life stage. In general, the recommended dietary allowance (RDA) for vitamin D in the United States is as follows:
  - Infants (ages 0 to 12 months): 400 to 1,000 IU (10 to 25 μg) per day
  - Children and adolescents (ages 1 to 18 years): 600 to 1,000 IU (15 to 25 μg) per day
  - Adults (ages 19 to 70 years): 600 to 800 IU (15 to 20 μg) per day
  - Older adults (ages $\geq$71 years): 800 to 1,000 IU (20 to 25 μg) per day
  - Pregnant and lactating women: 600 to 800 IU (15 to 20 μg) per day

Pediatric Considerations

ALERT
- The American Academy of Pediatrics (AAP) recommends all breastfed babies receive 400 IU/day of vitamin D beginning "within the first few days of life."
- 2016 Global Consensus Recommendations suggest all infants, regardless of feeding method, begin vitamin D 400 IU within a few days of birth.

- Midgestational vitamin D deficiency doubled the risk of autism spectrum disorder in European cohort.
- The AAP states percentage of U.S. infants who meet the AAP's guidelines for vitamin D intake has not increased; only 27% of infants overall and <40% of infants in nearly all demographic subgroups met intake recommendations.

Pregnancy Considerations
Insufficient data to recommend routine screening of all pregnancies; only "at risk" should be screened; it is safe to take 1,000 to 2,000 IU/day during pregnancy.

COMMONLY ASSOCIATED CONDITIONS
- Osteomalacia, osteoporosis
- Premenstrual syndrome
- Rickets
- Celiac disease; gastric bypass
- Chronic renal disease
- Bacterial vaginosis in pregnant women
- Hypertension
- Cohort study found that vitamin D deficiency is correlated with increased risk of all-cause mortality.

ALERT
Vitamin D deficiency is associated with risk of myocardial infarction (MI) and all-cause mortality.

DIAGNOSIS
- Nonspecific musculoskeletal complaints
- Weak antigravity muscles
- Fracture with minimal trauma

HISTORY
- Senior citizens at risk of falling
- Renal disease
- GI (malabsorption) disorders; liver dysfunction
- Immigration from tropical to colder climates
- Dark-skinned/veiled individuals
- Housebound patients
- Women at perimenopause

PHYSICAL EXAM
- Vague neurologic signs: numbness, proximal myopathy, paresthesias, muscle cramps, laryngospasm
- Chvostek sign: contraction of the facial muscles by tapping along the facial nerve
- Trousseau phenomenon: carpal spasms and paresthesia produced by pressure on nerves and vessels of the upper arm, by inflation of a BP cuff
- Tetany, seizures
- Bowed legs

DIFFERENTIAL DIAGNOSIS

- Malabsorptive disease (e.g., IBD, gastric bypass, celiac disease)
- Malnutrition

DIAGNOSTIC TESTS & INTERPRETATION

Initial Tests (lab, imaging)

- Only test those at increased risk of deficiency (those lacking dietary exposure, sun exposure, etc.) or if suspected due to risk factors (malabsorption, meds, symptoms, etc.)
- 25-OH vitamin D (most sensitive measure of vitamin D status)
- Vitamin D deficiency
  - IOM: <20 ng/mL
  - Endocrine Society, National Osteoporosis Foundation (NOF), International Osteoporosis Foundation (IOF), American Geriatrics Society (AGS) suggest a minimum level of 30 ng/mL.
- PTH elevation: not routinely obtained unless severe deficiency
- Low-normal/low calcium and phosphorous
- Elevated alkaline phosphatase (in later disease)
- Plain radiographs: If atypical fracture, radiographs may show osteomalacia (pseudofractures/looser zones) in pelvis, femur, and fibula.
- Osteoporosis screen
  - Women aged ≥65 years with no risk factors
  - Women aged ≥60 years at risk: body weight <70 kg (best predictor)
  - Less evidence: smoking, low body mass index, family history, decreased activity, alcohol, or caffeine use
  - African American women have higher bone density than Caucasians.

 TREATMENT

- Treatment goals remain unclear, but current "normal" 25-OH vitamin D levels are based on the suppression of PTH.
- Obesity: Treatment of VDD in obesity, especially to those who are obese and depressed, improves depressive symptoms and may improve weight loss.

ALERT

All-cause mortality: A Cochrane Systematic Review found that vitamin D supplementation lowers all-cause mortality (1)[A]. Recent long-term data shows treatment to 25 vitamin D levels >30 ng/mL lowered both MI and all-cause mortality risk.

Geriatric Considerations

In senior citizens, serum 25-OH vitamin D of 20 ng/mL resulted in improved physical performance scores; recent data suggest supplementation may not improve fracture risk and remains unclear about a true benefit.

MEDICATION

- Vitamin D sufficient (25-OH vitamin D ≥20 ng/mL)
  - Vitamin D 800 to 2,000 IU/day D_2/D_3
  - D_3 (animal derived) may be slightly more effective than D_2 (plant derived).
  - Calcium supplementation: unclear benefit and may increase some CHD risk in patients; no supplementation currently required (see below)
- Vitamin D deficiency (25-OH vitamin D <20 ng/mL)
  - D_2 50,000 IU/week for 8 to 12 weeks, followed by 1,000 to 2,000 IU/day of vitamin D_3
- Calcium: Meta-analysis data support dietary intake of calcium rather than calcium supplementation.
  - Dietary intake of ~700 mg/day leads to best outcomes; higher doses did NOT decrease risk of osteoporotic fractures.
  - Dietary calcium may be more beneficial than calcium supplementation. Supplementary calcium is associated with an increased risk of MI, especially in women, but this data remain controversial.
  - Supplementation of both vitamin D and calcium may increase risk of renal stone formation.

ISSUES FOR REFERRAL

Endocrinology if no response to treatment

ADDITIONAL THERAPIES

Aggressive calcium in ICU patients with ionized calcium <3.2 mg/dL or if symptomatic (tetany, seizures, QT prolongation, bradycardia, or hypotension or ventilated patient with decreased diaphragmatic function)

ADMISSION, INPATIENT, AND NURSING CONSIDERATIONS

- Symptoms of severe hypocalcemia
- Malabsorption syndromes

 ONGOING CARE

FOLLOW-UP RECOMMENDATIONS

Follow-up of abnormal 25-OH vitamin D not required

DIET

- Cod liver oil is the most potent source of vitamin D and has ~1,300 IU vitamin D/tablet/tbsp.
- Fatty fish (tuna, salmon)
- Fortified milk (100 IU/8 oz), cereal, and foods

PROGNOSIS

ALERT

- Cancer:
  - Systematic review of 63 observational studies found adequate 25-OH vitamin D levels correlate with lower rates of colon, breast, and prostate cancer.
  - Observational data show inverse relationship between serum 25-OH vitamin D levels and breast cancer.
  - Serum level >30 ng/mL lowered the risk of bladder cancer.
  - Vitamin D supplementation lowers cancer mortality and all-cause mortality (2).

- Cardiovascular disease: A serum 25 vitamin D level >30 ng/mL may lower MI risk and CV mortality.
- Asthma:
  - A Cochrane Systematic Review found that vitamin D supplement reduced the risk of severe asthma attacks requiring hospital admission or emergency department from 6% to ~3% and that vitamin D supplementation reduced the rate of asthma attacks needing treatment with steroids.
- Upper respiratory infections (URI): Vitamin D supplementation lowers the risk of URI.
- Fractures: Vitamin D_3 supplementation in general population of midlife and older adults did not result in a significantly lower risk of fractures versus placebo who were not selected for vitamin D deficiency, low bone mass, or osteoporosis (3)
- Other outcomes: Adequate vitamin D levels may lower pain scores in osteoarthritis of the knee, decrease PMS symptoms, lower risk of metabolic syndrome in women, lower dementia risk, and improve depression symptoms.

REFERENCES

1. Bjelakovic G, Gluud LL, Nikolova D, et al. Vitamin D supplementation for prevention of mortality in adults. *Cochrane Database Syst Rev.* 2011;(7):CD007470.
2. Zhang Y, Fang F, Tang J, et al. Association between vitamin D supplementation and mortality: systematic review and meta-analysis. *BMJ.* 2019;366:l4673.
3. LeBoff MS, Chou SH, Ratliff KA, et al. Supplemental vitamin D and incident fractures in midlife and older adults. *N Engl J Med.* 2022;387(4):299–309.

 CODES

ICD10

- E55 Vitamin D deficiency
- E55.0 Rickets, active
- E55.9 Vitamin D deficiency, unspecified

CLINICAL PEARLS

- Common risk factors for vitamin D deficiency include inadequate sun exposure or dietary intake, black or Hispanic ethnicity, and obesity.
- 25-OH vitamin D (most sensitive measure of vitamin D status) is the most sensitive laboratory test for diagnosis.
- Vitamin D deficiency is defined by serum levels <20 ng/mL.
- Up to 2,000 IU/day of supplemental vitamin D is safe in healthy adults without risk of toxicity.
- The AAP recommends all breastfed babies receive 400 IU/day of vitamin D beginning within a few days of birth.

V

VITAMIN DEFICIENCY

Tricia Bautista, MD • Jyothi R. Patri, MD, MHA, FAAFP, HMDC

BASICS

DESCRIPTION

- Vitamins are essential micronutrients required for normal metabolism, growth, and development.
- Vitamin supplementation in food products, adequate food security, and availability of supplements make vitamin deficiencies less common in developed countries. Certain populations are at increased risk.
- Toxicity is rare for water-soluble vitamins. It is possible for fat-soluble vitamins (A, D, E, K).

EPIDEMIOLOGY

Incidence

- Higher incidence seen in geriatric patients, pregnant women, exclusively breastfed infants, individuals with highly restricted diets or certain chronic disease states
- True incidence is unknown because most vitamin deficiencies are asymptomatic.

Prevalence

- Varies by age groups, comorbid conditions, geography, and setting (i.e., urban, rural)
- The prevalence of vitamin B_{12} deficiency is ~6% in patients <60 years old and increases to ~20% after the age of 60 years (1).
- Vitamin D deficiency prevalence is increased in individuals with darker skin pigmentation, obesity, low dietary intake of vitamin D, or low sunlight exposure. This deficiency is seen in ~5% of the general population, with non-Hispanic Blacks having the highest prevalence.

ETIOLOGY AND PATHOPHYSIOLOGY

- Deficiency usually develops from one of five mechanisms: reduced intake, diminished absorption, increased use, increased demand, increased demand or increased excretion
- Chronic disease states: HIV, malabsorption (i.e., celiac sprue, short bowel syndrome), chronic liver and kidney disease, alcoholism, malignancies, pernicious anemia, inborn errors of metabolism
- Bariatric surgeries: gastric bypass, gastrectomy, small or large bowel resection
- Certain drugs predispose to vitamin deficiencies: prednisone, phenytoin, isoniazid, protease inhibitors, methotrexate, phenobarbital, alcohol, nitrous oxide, H_2 receptor antagonists, metformin, colchicine, cholestyramine, 5-fluorouracil, 6-mercaptopurine, azathioprine, chloramphenicol, proton pump inhibitors, chronically used antibiotics, penicillamine, hydralazine
- Malnutrition, imbalanced nutrition, obesity, fad diets, extreme vegetarianism, total parenteral nutrition, bulimia/anorexia, other eating disorders, parasitic infection

Genetics

- Cystic fibrosis
- Hartnup disease, A-β-lipoproteinemia
- Rare genetic predisposition
  - Autoimmune disease (i.e., pernicious anemia)
  - Congenital enzyme deficiencies (i.e., biotinidase or holocarboxylase synthetase deficiency)
  - Transcobalamin II deficiency
  - Ataxia with vitamin E deficiency (AVED)

RISK FACTORS

Poverty, malnutrition, chronic excessive alcohol intake, chronic disease states, advanced age, dietary restrictions, bariatric surgery, certain medications, and exclusively breastfed infants

GENERAL PREVENTION

- Ingesting large and varied amounts of vitamin supplements increases risk of toxicity and drug–drug interactions and is not recommended.
- Antioxidant supplements have not been shown to impact cancer incidence; *increased* mortality risk seen in some studies
- Avoid restrictive diets.
- USPSTF recommends against low-dose supplementation with vitamin D (<400 IU) and calcium (<1,000 mg) to reduce fracture risk in community-dwelling postmenopausal women.
- USPSTF concludes current evidence is insufficient to assess benefits and harms of daily supplementation with doses >400 IU of vitamin D and >1000 mg of calcium for primary prevention of fractures in:
  - Community-dwelling, postmenopausal women
  - Men and premenopausal women
  - Note: The above recommendations are not applicable if there is a history of osteoporotic fractures, increased risk for falls or diagnosis of osteoporosis, or vitamin D deficiency.
- USPSTF recommends all women planning or capable of pregnancy take a daily supplement containing 0.4 to 0.8 mg of folic acid (2)[A].
- USPSTF recommends against using β-carotene or vitamin E supplements for the prevention of cardiovascular disease or cancer.
- Adults without regular, effective sun exposure year round should consume 600 to 800 IU/day of vitamin D_3. Elderly confined indoors and other high-risk groups may require higher doses (800 to 1,000 IU/day).
- All infants should receive 400 IU/day of vitamin D soon after birth if exclusively or partially breastfed.

COMMONLY ASSOCIATED CONDITIONS

Anemia, neuropathies, dermatitis, visual disturbances

DIAGNOSIS

HISTORY

- Review dietary intake and supplement use.
- Decreased visual acuity, night blindness
- Poor wound healing, easy bruising
- Skin changes, new rash
- Neuropathy
- Abnormal food cravings (pica)
- Osteomalacia, history of pathologic fracture
- Birth of a child with spina bifida
- Previous GI or bariatric surgery (1)
- Recurrent or persistent vomiting or diarrhea
- Prior or current medical conditions
  - Tuberculosis (TB), HIV infection, hepatitis, cancer
  - Hypermetabolic state: thyrotoxicosis, 2nd- or 3rd-degree burns, extensive or chronic wound, any systemic infection
- Chronic disease requiring steroids, disease-modifying antirheumatic drugs (DMARDs), or immunosuppressants

- Malabsorptive or chronic GI disorder: celiac disease, sprue, Crohn disease, ulcerative colitis, GERD
- Parenteral or enteral nutrition via tube feeding
- Pregnancy
- Amenorrhea or infertility issues
- Medications, supplements
- Food allergies or intolerances, fad or restrictive diet

PHYSICAL EXAM

- Neurologic exam: gait, memory/cognitive impairment, reflexes, sensory or motor impairment, peripheral neuropathy (1)
- Oropharyngeal exam: glossitis, bleeding gums, hyperemic pharynx, stomatitis, cheilitis (1)
- Skin exam: maculosquamous dermatitis, photosensitive pigmented dermatitis, ecchymosis, petechiae
- Visual assessment

DIFFERENTIAL DIAGNOSIS

Multiple conditions mimic signs and symptoms of vitamin deficiencies.

- Diabetes mellitus, thyroid disorders, hyperparathyroidism, heart failure, Alzheimer disease, multiple sclerosis, substance abuse, toxic ingestions, hematologic disorders/malignancies

DIAGNOSTIC TESTS & INTERPRETATION

Initial Tests (lab, imaging)

- No routine screening indicated
- Test if symptomatic, history indicates high risk, or clinical characteristics are present:
  - 25-OH vitamin D
    - Sufficient levels are >20 ng/mL (20 to 50 ng/mL is a level that is safe and sufficient for skeletal health).
    - Vitamin D insufficiency is 12 to 20 ng/mL.
    - Vitamin D deficiency is <12 ng/mL (increased risk of rickets and osteomalacia) (3).
  - Prothrombin time (PT)/partial thromboplastin time (PTT)
  - Vitamin B_{12} and folate levels (1)
  - Serum homocysteine and methylmalonic acid (if high suspicion of vitamin B_{12} deficiency with normal B_{12} level)
  - Retinol serum level, retinol-binding protein
- Cyanocobalamin, thiamine, vitamin A
- Ancillary tests:
  - BUN, calcium, phosphorus, magnesium
  - Albumin, liver function tests
  - CBC
  - Parathyroid hormone
- Bone densitometry for:
  - Women ≥65 years old without previous fractures or risk factors
  - Women <65 years old whose 10-year fracture risk is equal to a 65-year-old white woman without additional risk factors
- Disease states from vitamin deficiency
  - Vitamin A (retinol): night blindness, complete blindness, xerophthalmia
  - Vitamin B_1 (thiamine)
    - Wernicke encephalopathy: acute syndrome with memory disturbance, truncal ataxia, nystagmus, ophthalmoplegia
    - Korsakoff syndrome: anterograde and retrograde amnesia, confabulation

○ Dry beriberi: symmetric motor and sensory peripheral neuropathy, paresthesias, loss of reflexes

○ Wet beriberi: neuropathy with cardiovascular symptoms of peripheral vasodilation, high-output failure, dyspnea, and tachycardia

○ Infantile beriberi: loud piercing cry, cyanosis, tachycardia, cardiomegaly, dyspnea, vomiting, seizures

– Vitamin B_2 (riboflavin): glossitis, stomatitis, cheilitis, hyperemia of the pharyngeal mucosal membranes, normocytic-normochromic anemia

– Vitamin B_3 (niacin): pellagra = photosensitive pigmented dermatitis, dementia, and diarrhea

– Vitamin B_5 (pantothenic acid): paresthesias and dysesthesias ("burning feet syndrome"), anemia

– Vitamin B_6 (pyridoxine): dermatitis, cheilosis, atrophic glossitis, stomatitis, neuropathy

– Vitamin B_9 (folate): megaloblastic anemia, rarely manifest neurologic symptoms

– Vitamin B_{12} (cobalamin): pernicious anemia, leukopenia, pancytopenia, shuffling broad-based gait, atrophic glossitis, loss of vibration and position sense, cognitive impairment, areflexia, olfactory impairment, peripheral neuropathy, hyperpigmentation, jaundice, vitiligo

– Vitamin C (ascorbic acid): scurvy = ecchymoses, bleeding gums and petechiae; hyperkeratosis, arthralgias, impaired wound healing

– Vitamin D (calciferol): rickets, osteomalacia

– Vitamin E: neuromuscular disorders and hemolysis

– Vitamin K: easy bruising, mucosal bleeding, melena, hematuria

– Biotin: changes in mental status, dysesthesias, nausea, maculosquamous dermatitis of the extremities

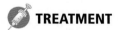 TREATMENT

MEDICATION

- Ask patients about supplement use; encourage patients to bring vitamin and supplement bottles for review.
- Assess for potential adverse drug effects/reactions. Patients with alcohol use disorders should receive thiamine, folic acid, and MVI.
- Give patients with suspected thiamine deficiency 100 mg thiamine prior to IV fluids containing glucose to prevent precipitating Korsakoff psychosis.
- Treat vitamin D deficiency with weekly 50,000 IU of oral ergocalciferol for 6 to 8 weeks. Recommended daily supplementation for children, adolescents, and adults up to age 70 years is 600 IU/day. Those aged >71 years is 800 IU/day.
- If there is concomitant B_{12} and folate deficiency, start vitamin B_{12} first to avoid precipitating subacute combined degeneration of the spinal cord (1).

- Consider obtaining prealbumin/albumin levels and a dietary consult for malnourished patients.
- Bariatric surgery patients will need lifelong vitamin supplementation; there are no consensus practice guidelines for supplement dosing regimens.

Geriatric Considerations

- Vitamin B_{12} deficiency exists in ~20% of patients aged >60 years. Treat symptomatic or severe deficiency with an IM injection of cyanocobalamin 1,000 μg/day 3 times a week for 2 weeks. For neurologic symptoms, give same dose every other day for 3 weeks or until symptom resolution. To prevent recurrence or treat mild deficiency, take daily oral vitamin B_{12} 1,000 μg or monthly IM vitamin B_{12} 1,000 μg every month. High-dose (1,000 to 2,000 μg/day) oral treatment is as effective as monthly IM injections, but use caution with malabsorption or compliance issues (1)[C].
- Vitamin D deficiency target level of >30 ng/mL minimizes risk of falls and fractures in the elderly.

Pediatric Considerations

- Vitamin K deficiency increases bleeding risk.
  – More common in neonates because they lack intestinal flora that produces vitamin K during the 1st week of life
  – Condition peaks 2 to 10 days after birth: bleeding from the umbilical stump and/or circumcision site, generalized bruising, and GI hemorrhage.
  – Infrequent in developed countries due to routine injection of newborns with vitamin K (1 mg)
- Vitamin D deficiency increases risk of rickets.
  – Vitamin D supplementation (400 IU/day) is recommended for all infants starting in the first few days of life.
  – 600 IU/day of vitamin D is recommended for children aged >12 months and adults either through diet or supplementation.
  – Morbidly obese and minority children are at increased risk for vitamin D deficiency.
- In children aged >6 months in developing countries, vitamin A supplementation has been shown to decrease mortality.

Pregnancy Considerations

All pregnant women and women of childbearing age considering pregnancy are strongly encouraged to take a multivitamin containing at least 0.4 mg folic acid daily to prevent neural tube defects (2)[A].

 ONGOING CARE

DIET

Vitamins are best used by the body from food intake. Supplements should be used where it is not feasible to ingest the recommended amount of a particular vitamin.

PATIENT EDUCATION

- Drug–drug interactions may occur between vitamins and medications. Patients should report all supplements and medications to their health care provider.
- Risk of vitamin toxicity is most common with fat-soluble vitamins (A, D, E, K).

PROGNOSIS

Most vitamin deficiencies are fully reversible if treated without undue delay.

COMPLICATIONS

- Vitamin toxicities, liver failure (vitamins A, D, E, K), desquamation of skin (vitamin A), neuropathy (vitamin B_6)
- Kidney stones (vitamin C, vitamin D), hypercoagulability (vitamin K), pseudohyperparathyroidism (vitamin D)
- Masking of pernicious anemia (folic acid)

REFERENCES

1. Langan RC, Goodbred AJ. Vitamin B12 deficiency: recognition and management. *Am Fam Physician*. 2017;96(6):384–389.
2. Bibbins-Domingo K, Grossman DC, Curry SJ, et al; for U.S. Preventive Services Task Force. Folic acid supplementation for the prevention of neural tube defects: US Preventive Services Task Force recommendation statement. *JAMA*. 2017;317(2):183–189.
3. Giustina A, Adler RA, Binkley N, et al. Controversies in vitamin D: summary statement from an international conference. *J Clin Endocrinol Metab*. 2019;104(2):234–240.

 CODES

ICD10

- E56.9 Vitamin deficiency, unspecified
- E56.0 Deficiency of vitamin E
- E55.9 Vitamin D deficiency, unspecified

CLINICAL PEARLS

- In healthy adults, multivitamins have no value if dietary intake is adequate.
- Vitamin D supplementation (400 IU/day) is recommended for all infants.
- No routine screening for Vitamin D deficiency is indicated.

V

VITILIGO

Amanda M. DiSabato, DO • Emily Ann Gorman, DO

 BASICS

DESCRIPTION
- An acquired depigmentation of the skin, which correlates with a loss of epidermal melanocytes. There are two major clinical variants, each with subtypes.
- Nonsegmental vitiligo: depigmented macules of varying size
  - Acrofacial: on distal extremities and face
  - Generalized: progressive, with flares, commonly associated with autoimmunity. Common locations are acral, periorificial, and in sites sensitive to pressure/friction (Koebner phenomenon).
  - Mixed: coexistence of nonsegmental and segmental
  - Mucosal (multifocal): only mucosal surfaces
  - Rare variants:
    - Ponctué: discrete, confetti-like macules
    - Inflammatory: peripheral erythematous rim
    - Trichrome: Tan zone is present between normal and depigmented skin.
    - Quadrichrome: as above but with marginal/perifollicular hyperpigmentation
    - Blue: Dermal melanophages give blue hue in areas affected by prior postinflammatory hyperpigmentation.
  - Universal: involves >80% of the body surface area (BSA). Most likely to have family history; comorbidities are common and associated with poorest quality-of-life (QOL).
- Segmental vitiligo: Lesions occur within a dermatome (often trigeminal) or may follow Blaschko lines. Lesions usually stop abruptly at the midline; typically occurs earlier than nonsegmental vitiligo, is rapidly progressive, and involves melanocytes of hair follicles.
  - Bisegmental: bilaterally distributed
  - Plurisegmental: multiple segments
  - Unisegmental: single segment
- Undetermined/unclassified:
  - Focal: few lesions, random distribution; may be able to later classify as one of the forms above after 1 to 2 years
  - Mucosal (focal type): only mucosal surfaces

EPIDEMIOLOGY
- 50% begin before age 20 years; females in 1st decade; males in 5th decade; onset earlier with positive family history; can appear as early as 6th weeks of life
- Predominance: male = female; however, females are more likely to seek treatment.
- No race or socioeconomic predilection

Prevalence
~1% in the United States and Europe (1); 0.1–8% in the world; highest in Gujarat, India at 8.8% (1)

ETIOLOGY AND PATHOPHYSIOLOGY
Most likely, a spectrum of disorders with a common phenotype and multiple mechanisms contribute to the pathology (convergence theory).
- Autoimmune: humoral autoantibodies and skin-homing T cells
- Neural: local or systemic dysregulation leading to excess neurotransmitters

- Viral: direct melanocyte toxicity, cytomegalovirus (CMV), hepatitis C, and Epstein-Barr virus (EBV) found in lesion biopsies
- Oxidative stress from elevated H_2O_2 and NO and decreased catalase and erythrocyte glutathione

Genetics
- Polygenic/multifactorial inheritance
- 20% of patients report affected relative; monozygotic twins have only 23% concordance.
- HLA haplotypes, small nucleotide polymorphisms, and specific genes are all possible contributors.

RISK FACTORS
- Family history of vitiligo/autoimmune disorders
- Personal history of associated conditions

COMMONLY ASSOCIATED CONDITIONS
- Most common
  - Endocrine: thyroid disease (hypo-/hyperthyroidism), hypoparathyroidism, Addison disease, insulin-dependent diabetes
  - Dermatologic: psoriasis, atopic dermatitis, alopecia areata, chronic urticaria, halo nevi, ichthyosis
  - Pernicious anemia
  - Hypoacusis, rheumatoid arthritis
  - Ocular abnormalities in up to 40%
  - High antinuclear antibodies in up to 40%
  - Elevated thyroperoxidase antibodies in 50%
- Less common
  - Systemic lupus erythematosus
  - Inflammatory bowel disease
  - Melanoma and other skin cancers
  - Syndromes: Alezzandrini; mitochondrial encephalomyopathy, lactic acidosis, and stroke-like episodes (MELAS); Schmidt; and autoimmune polyendocrinopathy-candidiasis-ectodermal dystrophy (APECED)
- Age >50 years at onset should prompt investigation for associated conditions.

Pediatric Considerations
Associated with Hashimoto thyroiditis in a significant portion of children; screening at onset and possibly annually may be beneficial.

 DIAGNOSIS

HISTORY
- Inquire about recent history of sunburns, pregnancy, skin trauma, or emotional stress.
- Discuss family history of premature graying, vitiligo, and autoimmune disorders.
- Complete a review of systems for relative associated conditions.
- Ascertain psychological impact on QOL, Dermatology Life Quality Index (DLQI).

PHYSICAL EXAM
- Complete a full-body skin exam with Wood lamp to accentuate lesions and distinguish depigmentation from hypopigmentation.
- Lesions are well-demarcated, uniform, white macules and patches.
- Look for evidence of repigmentation (most commonly around hair follicles).

DIFFERENTIAL DIAGNOSIS
- Infectious: tinea versicolor, leprosy, leishmaniasis, onchocerciasis, treponematoses
- Postinflammatory hypopigmentation: psoriasis, atopic dermatitis, pityriasis alba, systemic lupus erythematosus, scleroderma
- Inherited hypomelanoses: piebaldism, tuberous sclerosis, Waardenburg syndrome, hypomelanosis of Ito, Vogt-Koyanagi-Harada disease
- Malformations: nevus anemicus, nevus depigmentosus
- Paraneoplastic: mycosis fungoides, melanoma-associated leukoderma
- Occupational and chemical induced
  - Occupational: phenolic/catechol derivatives and arsenic-containing compounds
  - Chemical: numerous, including cosmetics, cleansers, insecticides, and even medications (imatinib, topical corticosteroids [TCS])
- Melasma: Normal skin may be confused as vitiligo in the setting of surrounding hyperpigmentation.
- Halo nevi
- Lichen sclerosus et atrophicus
- Idiopathic guttate hypomelanosis
- Progressive-acquired macular hypomelanosis

DIAGNOSTIC TESTS & INTERPRETATION
Initial Tests (lab, imaging)
- Obtain TSH, CBC, ANA.
- Consider antithyroid peroxidase, antithyroglobulin antibodies, hemoglobin, vitamin B_{12}.

Follow-Up Tests & Special Considerations
- Monitor for disease progression/flares.
- Monitor for symptoms of related conditions.

Diagnostic Procedures/Other
- Skin biopsy is rarely needed. Highest yield is with comparison of lesional/perilesional.
- Consider ophthalmologic and audiologic evaluations.

Test Interpretation
Few or no epidermal melanocytes. At margins, melanocytes may be larger, vacuolated, and dendritic. Early lesions show inflammation and later, degeneration, including adnexa and nerves.

TREATMENT

The variant of vitiligo may affect response.
- If untreated, progression is the natural course for those with mucosal involvement, family history, koebnerization, and nonsegmental variants.
- Lesions that respond best are on the face, of recent onset, in darker skin type, and in younger patients.

GENERAL MEASURES
- Sunscreen to decrease sunburn and prevent accentuation of uninvolved skin
- Corrective camouflage as cover-up (Cover FX, Dermablend)

MEDICATION

- Individualize therapy depending on age, extent, distribution, and rate of progression.
- Many therapies are considered "off-label" and not FDA-approved for vitiligo, although they are often considered first-line therapy.
- Corticosteroids: Midpotency TCS (mometasone furoate, fluticasone propionate) applied daily as monotherapy is first line. Do not use on face/axilla/groin. Pediatric: for children >12 years of age. Side effects include atrophy, telangiectasia, hypertrichosis, acneiform eruptions, and striae; regular steroid holidays are recommended (1).
  - Combination of light therapy and TCS is the most effective treatment overall.
  - Addition of tretinoin 0.025–0.05% BID can decrease potential skin atrophy.
  - Systemic corticosteroids can be helpful, but dosage and safety parameters have not been fully evaluated for long-term treatment (2)[A].
- Topical calcineurin inhibitors: slightly inferior to TCS as monotherapy but better side-effect profile (3)[A]; can be used as adjunctive to light therapy; carries a controversial black box warning for a theoretical risk of lymphoma or skin cancer. Local reactions include burning sensation, pruritus, erythema, and rare transient hyperpigmentation (2).
  - Tacrolimus 0.03% or 0.1% ointment BID; pediatric: 0.03% ointment BID for children >2 years of age
  - Pimecrolimus 1% cream BID; pediatric: for children >2 years of age
- Topical vitamin D_3 analogs: less effective than TCS alone but in combination with TCS or phototherapy can shorten time until, and improve stability of, repigmentation (2),(3)[B]
  - Calcipotriene ointment 1 to 2 times per day
  - Available as a combination formulation, betamethasone dipropionate 0.064%/calcipotriene 0.005% ointment daily, max dose of 100 g/week for 4 weeks, not for >30% BSA, and not for face/axilla/groin
- Oral vitamin D_3: reported to induce repigmentation; oral vitamin D_3 35,000 IU once daily plus low-calcium diet for 6 months
- Phototherapy: Narrow band UVB (NBUVB) is superior to UVA and indicated for lesions involving >15–20% BSA (3)[A].
  - Psoralen plus UVA (PUVA) may increase the incidence of skin cancers. Pediatric: Oral PUVA is contraindicated.
  - Khellin plus UVA may be less carcinogenic but is associated with liver toxicity.
- Laser therapy: Excimer laser (308 nm) is superior to other light therapy. Helium–neon laser works for segmental vitiligo (3)[A].
- Antioxidants: may have protective role in preventing melanocyte degradation from reactive oxygen species. Options include vitamin C, vitamin E, Vitix, *Polypodium leucotomos* extracts, and *Ginkgo biloba* (3)[A].

First Line

- Avoidance of triggering factors plus TCS alone or in combination with NBUVB
- Topical calcineurin inhibitors (preferred for face, neck, axilla, and groin)
- PUVA in adults
- Camouflage and psychotherapy to all patients at any stage

Second Line

- Recommended: photochemotherapy with psoralens or vitamin D analogues
- Topical vitamin D analogues
- Targeted phototherapy
- 308-nm laser in combination with topical steroids, topical calcineurin inhibitors, or vitamin D analogues
- Oral corticosteroids (pulse therapy)
- Surgery for stable 2- to 3-cm lesions, refractory to other treatments (3)[B]

ISSUES FOR REFERRAL

- Dermatologist: facial/widespread vitiligo
- Ophthalmologist: ocular symptoms
- Endocrinologist: associated conditions
- Psychologist: for severe distress
- Medical geneticist: associated conditions

ADDITIONAL THERAPIES

- Depigmentation therapy with monobenzone, hydroquinone, or Q-switched ruby laser
- Pseudocatalase with addition of NBUVB (1)[B]
- Prostaglandin E for short-duration disease and localization to face and scalp
- Cosmetic tattooing for localized stable vitiligo

SURGERY/OTHER PROCEDURES

- Transport melanocytes from other areas of the skin. Methods include punch, blister, or split-thickness skin grafting, or transplantation of autologous melanocytes (4)[A].
- Dermabrasion and curettage alone or with 5-fluorouracil may induce follicular melanocyte reservoirs (3)[A].
- Patients who koebnerize or form keloids may be worse, and permanent scarring is a risk.

COMPLEMENTARY & ALTERNATIVE MEDICINE

- *Ginkgo biloba* 60 mg PO daily may improve extension and spreading (2)[B].
- *P. leucotomos* may help with repigmentation with NBUVB and aid in reducing phototoxic reactions (3)[B].

 ONGOING CARE

FOLLOW-UP RECOMMENDATIONS

- Monitor for symptoms of related conditions.
- With topical steroids, follow at regular intervals to avoid steroid atrophy, telangiectasia, and striae distensae.

DIET

No restrictions

PATIENT EDUCATION

- Disease course, progression, and cosmesis
- Trauma/friction and Koebner phenomenon

PROGNOSIS

- Spontaneous repigmentation is uncommon.
- Generalized vitiligo is often progressive with flares. Focal vitiligo often has rapid onset and then stabilizes.

COMPLICATIONS

- Adverse effects of each treatment modality
- Psychiatric morbidity: depression, adjustment disorder, low self-esteem, sexual dysfunction, and embarrassment in relationships (1)
- Different cultures may have different perceptions/social stigmas about vitiligo.

REFERENCES

1. Ezzedine K, Eleftheriadou V, Whitton M, et al. Vitiligo. *Lancet*. 2015;386(9988):74–84.
2. Bacigalupi RM, Postolova A, Davis RS. Evidence-based, non-surgical treatments for vitiligo: a review. *Am J Clin Dermatol*. 2012;13(4):217–237.
3. Whitton ME, Pinart M, Batchelor J, et al. Interventions for vitiligo. *Cochrane Database Syst Rev*. 2015;(2):CD003263.
4. Ju HJ, Bae JM, Lee RW, et al. Surgical interventions for patients with vitiligo: a systematic review and meta-analysis. *JAMA Dermatol*. 2021;157(3):307–316.

ADDITIONAL READING

- Bergqvist C, Ezzedine K. Vitiligo: a review. *Dermatology*. 2020;236(6):571–592.
- Kussainova A, Kassym L, Akhmetova A, et al. Vitiligo and anxiety: a systematic review and meta-analysis. *PLoS One*. 2020;15(11):e0241445.
- Salloum A, Bazzi N, Maalouf D, et al. Microneedling in vitiligo: a systematic review. *Dermatol Ther*. 2020;33(6):e14297.

CODES

ICD10

- L80 Vitiligo
- H02.739 Vitiligo of unspecified eye, unspecified eyelid and periocular area
- H02.735 Vitiligo of left lower eyelid and periocular area

CLINICAL PEARLS

- Vitiligo can be a psychologically devastating skin disease.
- Screen for associated diseases, particularly if onset occurs later in life.
- Treatment should be individualized based on BSA, skin type, and patient goals.
- Consult dermatology for extensive disease, facial involvement, and when advanced treatments are considered.

VON WILLEBRAND DISEASE

Ashten Duncan, MD, MPH, CPH • William McCormick Bowen, MD • Nora Elizabeth Kratz, MD

 BASICS

DESCRIPTION

- von Willebrand disease (vWD) is a lifelong bleeding disorder resulting from either a quantitative or qualitative (e.g., structural or functional) defect in von Willebrand factor (vWF).
- vWF is a large glycoprotein that plays an essential role in primary hemostasis, which facilitates the adherence of platelets to the injured blood vessel. It also serves as a carrier for factor VIII (FVIII) circulating in the blood.
- The most common clinical consequences mucocutaneous bleeding, bleeding during childbirth, dental procedures, easy bruising, and menorrhagia.
- vWD is most commonly diagnosed as an autosomal-dominant condition but can also be autosomal recessive. In rare cases, this condition can also be acquired (AvWD).
- vWD can be broken down into three different types:
  - Type 1: mildest type—associated with a mild-to-moderate quantitative vWF deficiency
  - Type 2: qualitative defect in vWF (e.g., issues with the protein folding, binding, polypeptide chain structure)
  - Type 3: most severe type—associated with a complete deficiency in vWF

EPIDEMIOLOGY

Prevalence

- vWD is the most common inherited bleeding disorder.
- Prevalence of the inherited forms of vWD is about 109 to 2,200 per 100,000 of the general population with men and women acquiring the disorder at equal frequency.
- Women are diagnosed more often due to the increased bleeding that is seen during menstrual periods, during pregnancy, and after childbirth.
- Exact prevalence of the AvWD is unknown but is estimated to be up to 0.1% of the general population (1).

ETIOLOGY AND PATHOPHYSIOLOGY

- vWF is a large, multimeric glycoprotein that is released from endothelial cells and stored within the α-granules of platelets.
- vWF binds to subendothelial collagen at sites of vascular injury and facilitates platelet adhesion to these sites via its interaction with the platelet GP1b receptor. This process forms a platelet plug, allowing for the initial arrest of bleeding (i.e., primary hemostasis). The formation of a fibrin clot follows the creation of a platelet plug, which requires normal amounts of and function of coagulation factors (i.e., secondary hemostasis).
- vWF acts as a carrier for FVIII in the circulation, protecting it from degradation. A deficiency in vWF may result in decreased FVIII levels.
- When vWF is deficient or dysfunctional, primary hemostasis is compromised, resulting in the clinical symptoms described above.

- There are three distinct types of inherited vWD. Within this classification scheme, type 2 vWD has several subtypes, described below. Whereas types 1 and 3 are associated with quantitative deficiencies in vWF (decreased in type 1, absent in type 3), type 2 vWD results from functional defects in the glycoprotein.
  - Type 1, the most common and mildest form, represents 70–80% of cases.
  - Type 2, caused by qualitative defects in vWF, accounts for 10–15% of cases. The various subtypes are described below:
    ○ Type 2A results from the absence of high- and intermediate-molecular-weight vWF multimers.
    ○ Type 2B occurs due to a gain-of-function mutation in vWF, which increases its affinity for the platelet GP1b receptor. Complexes of platelets and vWF form as a result and are subsequently removed from circulation. Removal of these aggregates results in loss of the high-molecular-weight vWF multimers as well as thrombocytopenia.
    ○ Type 2M results from a defect in the platelet-binding domain of vWF; however, in contrast to types 2A and 2B, the entire vWF multimer remains intact.
    ○ Type 2N results from a mutation in the FVIII binding domain of vWF, resulting in low FVIII levels with an intact multimer.
  - Type 3 represents 1–5% of cases, the least common and most severe form.
    ○ Most severe form with markedly decreased to undetectable levels of vWF and FVIII
  - Platelet-type vWD (PLT-vWD), also known as pseudo-vWD, results from a hyperaffinity mutation in the platelet GP1b receptor gene, causing increased binding to vWF. Consequently, many platelet-vWF complexes form, which are then cleared from circulation. Similar to vWD type 2B, these patients demonstrate loss of high-molecular-weight vWF multimers in addition to thrombocytopenia.
  - AvWD may be due to cardiovascular, hematologic, or autoimmune conditions as well as tumors and medications. The pathophysiology of AvWD is related to underlying quantitative and/or qualitative changes in vWF and may result from shear-induced cleaving of vWF in cardiovascular conditions, increased adsorption of vWF by certain tumor cells or activated platelets, or presence of anti-vWF autoantibodies in hematologic disorders.

Genetics

- The 178-kb gene for vWF is located on the short arm of chromosome 12.
- Most cases of type 1 vWD follow an autosomal-dominant inheritance pattern, with variable expressivity. Rarer occurrences of type 1 are inherited in an autosomal-recessive manner.
- Types 2A, 2B, and 2M are inherited in an autosomal-dominant manner, whereas 2N is inherited in an autosomal-recessive manner.
- Type 3 follows an autosomal-recessive inheritance pattern.

RISK FACTORS

- Inherited vWD: personal and/or family history of bleeding disorders.
- AvWD: Risk factors include lymphoproliferative disorders, myeloproliferative disorders, autoimmune disorders, states of high vascular flow (e.g., aortic stenosis, presence of LVAD or ventricular septal defect).

COMMONLY ASSOCIATED CONDITIONS

Individuals with type O blood have accelerated clearance of vWF leading to vWF levels that are 25–30% lower than other those with blood type A, B, or AB. Therefore, type 1 disease is diagnosed more frequently in individuals with type O blood.

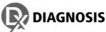 **DIAGNOSIS**

- For patients with low probability of vWD: Use a validated bleeding assessment tool (BAT) as first-line screening prior to ordering laboratory studies (https://www1.wfh.org/docs/en/Resources/Assessment_Tools_ISTHBAT.pdf).
- For patients with moderate to high probability of vWD (e.g., family history of bleeding disorders, personal history of unusual bleeding diathesis, abnormal initial laboratory tests): In addition to screening with a BAT, also order the following:
  - vWF antigen (vWF:Ag), platelet-dependent vWF activity (e.g., VWF:GPIbM), and FVIII:C lab studies
  - vWF is an acute-phase reactant that increases in response to a variety of stimuli (e.g., bleeding, trauma, pregnancy). vWD diagnostic testing should be performed when patients are at a baseline state of health.

HISTORY

- A positive family history of a bleeding disorder is the most common and suggestive finding.
- vWD should be in the differential diagnosis for heavy menstrual bleeding at any age.

PHYSICAL EXAM

Common locations of bleeding include oral mucosa, gingiva, endometrium, and gastrointestinal mucosa.

DIFFERENTIAL DIAGNOSIS

Congenital thrombocytopenia, qualitative platelet defects, coagulation factor deficiencies, hemophilia, dysfibrinogenemias, fibrinolytic disorders, liver disease, uremia, connective tissue disorders, coagulation factor inhibitors

DIAGNOSTIC TESTS & INTERPRETATION

- Initial evaluation of a suspected bleeding abnormality
  - Complete blood count (CBC)
  - Prothrombin time (PT/INR)
  - Partial thromboplastin time (PTT)
  - Fibrinogen level
  - Peripheral blood smear
- Initial evaluation of suspected inherited vWD
  - vWF:Ag: determines total amount of vWF present
  - vWF activity (vWF:RCo): functional assay tests vWF function by assessing its ability to agglutinate platelets in the presence of the antibiotic ristocetin
  - FVIII: C level
- Note: Multimeric analysis is not recommended in the initial evaluation of vWD.

Follow-Up Tests & Special Considerations

vWF is an acute-phase reactant, so elevations may be seen in proinflammatory conditions, liver disease, pregnancy (which may correct mild deficits), or with estrogen use. vWF levels also increase with age; however, it is unclear if this decreases bleeding risk.

Condition	Description	vWF:RCo (IU/dL)	vWF:Ag (IU/dL)	FVIII	vWF:RCo/ VWF:Ag
Type 1	Partial quantitative vWF deficiency (75% of symptomatic vWD patients)	<30*	<30*	↓ or Normal	>0.5–0.7
Type 2A	↓ vWF-dependent platelet adhesion with selective deficiency of high-molecular-weight multimers	<30*	<30–200*†	↓ or Normal	<0.5–0.7
Type 2B	↑ Affinity for platelet GPIb	<30*	<30–200*†	↓ or Normal	Usually <0.5–0.7
Type 2M	↓ vWF-dependent platelet adhesion without selective deficiency of high-molecular-weight multimers	<30*	<30–200*†	↓ or Normal	<0.5–0.7
Type 2N	Markedly decreased binding affinity for FVIII	30–200	30–200	↓↓	>0.5–0.7
Type 3	Virtually complete deficiency of vWF (Severe, rare)	<3	<3	↓↓↓ (<10 IU/dL)	Not applicable
"Low vWF"**		30–50	30–50	Normal	>0.5–0.7
Normal		50–200	50–200	Normal	>0.5–0.7

↓ refers to a decrease in the test result compared to the laboratory reference range. ↑ refers to an increase in the test result compared to the laboratory reference range.

*<30 IU/dL is designated as the level for a definitive diagnosis of vWD; some patients with type 1 or 2 vWD have levels of vWF:RCo and/or vWF:Ag of 30–50 IU/dL.

†The vWF:Ag in the majority of individuals with type 2A, 2B, or 2M vWD is <50 IU/dL.

**This does not preclude the diagnosis of vWD in patients with vWF:RCo of 30–50 IU/dL if there is supporting clinical and/or family evidence for vWD. This also does not preclude the use of agents to increase vWF levels in those who have vWF:RCo of 30–50 IU/dL and who may be at risk for bleeding.

 TREATMENT

GENERAL MEASURES

- Minor bleeding episodes generally do not require therapeutic intervention. Individuals receive treatment prior to undergoing surgeries, dental procedures, and following injury.
- In mild disease, trauma-related and spontaneous bleeding events may be managed with desmopressin acetate (DDAVP)
- Chronic menorrhagia can be managed with hormonal contraception (i.e., oral contraceptive pills [OCPs], progestin-containing intrauterine device [IUD]), endometrial ablation (for women no longer desiring future pregnancy), DDAVP, or antifibrinolytic agents.

MEDICATION

First Line

- Desmopressin (i.e., DDAVP)
  - Enhances release of vWF from endothelial cells
  - Effective for type 1 vWD; not indicated in type 2B or type 3
  - Trial of DDAVP should initially be measured in nonbleeding state to determine response.
- Factor-replacement therapy (i.e., vWF and/or FVIII concentrates)
  - Most effective treatment for patients with types 2 and 3 vWD
  - In cases of PT-vWD, administration of exogenous platelets is the treatment of choice
  - Dose of vWF concentrate may be adjusted for FVIII levels and ristocetin cofactor activity.
  - FVIII levels should be monitored to avoid supranormal levels and possible venous thromboembolism (VTE).

- Contraindicated if patient develops alloantibodies to vWF
- In patients with severe bleeding phenotype, prophylactic treatment is used.
- Antifibrinolytics (i.e., aminocaproic acid and tranexamic acid)
  - Contraindicated in patients with hematuria due to risk of retention of large blood clots in the renal collecting system
  - Given as adjunct to DDAVP
- Recombinant FVIIa (NovoSeven)
  - Used for patients who develop alloantibodies to vWF
  - Used effectively in the treatment of patients with type 3 vWD

Second Line

- OCPs and progestin-containing IUDs can raise vWF and FVIII levels in the blood and also have a role in the treatment of chronic menorrhagia.
- Platelets may be given as an adjunct to factor concentrates if hemostasis has not been achieved during an active bleeding event.
- Intravenous immunoglobulin has been useful in some patients with AvWD associated with monoclonal gammopathy.

ADMISSION, INPATIENT, AND NURSING CONSIDERATIONS

- If the patient is being admitted to observation for condition(s) with low thrombotic risk, mechanical VTE prophylaxis (i.e., sequential compression devices) or regular ambulation on the unit is preferred.
- If the patient is being admitted for a long hospitalization requiring immobilization and/or for a condition with high thrombotic risk, VTE chemoprophylaxis (e.g., low-molecular-weight heparin) can be considered if the patient has largely preserved qualitative and quantitative vWF levels with close monitoring for bleeding.

 ONGOING CARE

FOLLOW-UP RECOMMENDATIONS
Patients should be seen by a hematologist prior to invasive procedures to reduce risk of excessive bleeding.

Patient Monitoring

- Repeat laboratory studies only for patients with moderate to severe vWD if frequency of their bleeding events changes.
- Aspirin and other NSAIDs should be avoided to prevent bleeding events.

DIET
No dietary restrictions are recommended.

PATIENT EDUCATION

- National Bleeding Disorders Foundation: https://www.hemophilia.org/NHFWeb/MainPgs/MainNHF.aspx?menuid=182&contentid=47&rptname=bleeding
- Centers for Disease Control and Prevention: https://www.cdc.gov/ncbddd/vwd/facts.html

PROGNOSIS

- Most patients with vWD have normal life expectancy. Shortened life expectancy is often a direct result of massive hemorrhage from a major injury (e.g., high-velocity motor vehicle collision, extremity crush injuries).
- In the United States, about 15% of individuals with vWD will experience one or more major bleeding events within a 4-year period. Of these events, almost 90% will be gastrointestinal bleeds with many resulting in hospitalizations.

COMPLICATIONS
Multiple transfusions may result in alloantibodies against vWF.

REFERENCE

1. Du P, Bergamasco A, Moride Y, et al. Von Willebrand disease epidemiology, burden of illness and management: a systematic review. *J Blood Med*. 2023;14:189–208.

 SEE ALSO

Algorithms: Bleeding Gums; Ecchymosis

 CODES

ICD10
D68.0 Von Willebrand's disease

CLINICAL PEARLS

- vWD is the most common inherited bleeding disorder in American adults
- Treatment should be administered for recurrent bleeding episodes in all types of vWD, but prophylaxis is not required for minor bleeding events.
- First-line therapies for vWD include DDAVP, factor-replacement therapy, antifibrinolytics, and recombinant FVIIa.

VULVAR MALIGNANCY

Sareena Singh, MD, FACOG • Kimberly Resnick, MD • Lauren A. Hutka, DO

 BASICS

DESCRIPTION

- Premalignant lesions of the vulva are collectively known as vulvar intraepithelial neoplasia (VIN).
- Exposure to human papillomavirus (HPV) has been linked to >70% of VIN.
- Invasive squamous cell carcinoma is the most common malignancy involving the vulva (90% of patients).
- Melanoma is the second most common type of vulvar malignancy (8%), and sarcoma is the third.
- Other invasive cell types include basal cell carcinoma, Paget disease, adenocarcinoma arising from Bartholin gland or apocrine sweat glands, adenoid cystic carcinoma, small cell carcinoma, verrucous carcinoma, and sarcomas.
- Sarcomas are usually leiomyosarcoma and probably arise at the insertion of the round ligament in the labium major; however, sarcoma can arise from any structure of the vulva, including blood vessels, skeletal muscle, and fat.
- Rarely, breast carcinoma has been reported in the vulva and is thought to arise from ectopic breast tissue.
- System(s) affected: reproductive

Geriatric Considerations

- The surgery is usually well tolerated.
- Patients who are not surgical candidates can be treated with combination chemotherapy and/or radiation.
- In the very elderly, palliative vulvectomy provides relief of symptoms for ulcerating symptomatic advanced disease.

EPIDEMIOLOGY

Incidence

- Estimated 6,020 new cases and 1,150 deaths in 2017
- Mean age at diagnosis is 65 years; in situ disease: mean age is 40 years; invasive malignancy: mean age is 60 years.

ETIOLOGY AND PATHOPHYSIOLOGY

- Patients with cervical cancer are more likely to develop vulvar cancer later in life, secondary to "field effect" phenomenon with a carcinogen involving the lower genital tract.
- HPV has been associated with squamous cell abnormalities of the cervix, vagina, and vulva; 55% of vulvar cancers are attributable to oncogenic HPV, predominantly HPV 16 and 33; vaginal intraepithelial neoplasia (VAIN) and anal intraepithelial neoplasia (AIN) are attributable to HPV.
- Squamous cell carcinoma
  - There are two etiologic pathways for developing vulvar squamous cell carcinoma: lichen sclerosus and HPV.
  - The International Society for the Study of Vulvovaginal Disease (ISSVD) proposed a revised terminology in 2015: low-grade squamous intraepithelial lesion (LSIL), which includes flat condyloma and HPV effect; high-grade squamous intraepithelial lesion (HSIL); and VIN differentiated type (dVIN). The ISSVD previously used a three-level system grading VIN as 1, 2, 3, which has been abandoned.

- Differentiated type occurs in older age groups, is associated with lichen sclerosus and chronic venereal diseases, and is not related to HPV. It carries a higher risk of progression to malignancy.
- The warty basaloid type, also known as bowenoid type, is related to HPV infection and occurs in younger women. Melanoma, second most common histology, often identified in postmenopausal women; often pigmented but can be amelanotic, arising de novo, often found on clitoris or labia minora. Prognosis is poor, 5-year survival <50%.
- Smoking is associated with squamous cell disease of the vulva, possibly from direct irritation of the vulva by the transfer of tars and nicotine on the patient's hands or from systemic absorption of carcinogen.

Genetics

No known genetic pattern

RISK FACTORS

- VIN or cervical intraepithelial neoplasia (CIN)
- Smoking
- Lichen sclerosus (vulvar dystrophy)
- HPV infection, condylomata, or sexually transmitted diseases (STD) in the past
- Low economic status
- Autoimmune processes
- Immunodeficiency syndromes or immunosuppression
- Northern European ancestry
- Risk factors for recurrence: age >50 years, positive excision margins, concurrent VAIN

GENERAL PREVENTION

- HPV vaccination has the potential to decrease vulvar cancer by 60%.
- Abstinence from smoking/smoking cessation counseling

COMMONLY ASSOCIATED CONDITIONS

- Patients with invasive vulvar cancer are often elderly and have associated medical conditions.
- High rate of other gynecologic malignancies

 DIAGNOSIS

HISTORY

Complaints of pruritus or raised lesion in the vaginal area, vaginal bleeding, discharge

PHYSICAL EXAM

- In situ disease: a small raised area associated with pruritus, single vulvar plaque, ulcer, or mass on labia majora, perineum, clitoris; most commonly found on labia majora
- Vulvar bleeding, dysuria, enlarged lymph nodes less common symptomatology
- Invasive malignancy: an ulcerated, nonhealing area; as lesions become large, bleeding occurs with associated pain and foul-smelling discharge; enlarged inguinal lymph nodes indicative of advanced disease

DIFFERENTIAL DIAGNOSIS

- Infectious processes can present as ulcerative lesions and include syphilis, lymphogranuloma venereum, and granuloma inguinale.
- Disorder of Bartholin gland, seborrheic keratosis, hidradenomas, lichen sclerosus, epidermal inclusion cysts

- Crohn disease can present as an ulcerative area on the vulva.
- Rarely, lesions can metastasize to the vulva.

DIAGNOSTIC TESTS & INTERPRETATION

Initial Tests (lab, imaging)

- Hypercalcemia can occur when metastatic disease is present.
- Squamous cell antigen can be elevated with invasive disease.

Follow-Up Tests & Special Considerations

- Upon examination, any suspicious lesions should be biopsied.
- Diagnosis based on histologic findings following vulvar biopsy
- The vulva can be washed with 3% acetic acid to highlight areas and visualized with a colposcope, which allows for visualization of acetowhite lesions and vascular lesions.
- For patients with new onset of pruritus, the area of pruritus should be biopsied.
- Liberal biopsies must be used to diagnose in situ disease prior to invasion and to diagnose early invasive disease.
- The patient should not be treated for presumed benign conditions of the vulva without full exam and biopsy, including Pap smear and colposcopy of cervix, vagina, and vulva.
- When symptoms persist, reexamine and rebiopsy.
- Treatment of benign condyloma of the vulva has not been shown to decrease the eventual incidence of in situ or invasive disease of the vulva.
- CT scan to evaluate pelvic and periaortic lymph node status if tumor >2 cm or if suspicion of metastatic disease

Diagnostic Procedures/Other

Office vulvar biopsy is done to establish the diagnosis.

Test Interpretation

A surgical staging system is used for vulvar cancer (International Federation of Gynecology and Obstetrics Classification).

- Stage I: tumor confined to the vulva
  - Stage IA: lesions ≤2 cm in size, confined to the vulva or perineum and with stromal invasion ≤1 mm, no node metastasis
  - Stage IB: lesions >2 cm in size or with stromal invasion >1 mm, confined to the vulva or perineum, with negative nodes
- Stage II: tumor of any size with extension to adjacent perineal structures (lower 1/3 urethra, lower 1/3 vagina, anus) with negative nodes
- Stage III: tumor of any size with or without extension to adjacent perineal structures (lower 1/3 urethra, lower 1/3 vagina, anus) with positive inguinofemoral lymph nodes
- Stage IIIA
  - With 1 lymph node metastasis (≥5 mm), or
  - 1 to 2 lymph node metastases (<5 mm)
- Stage IIIB
  - With ≥2 lymph node metastases (≥5 mm), or
  - ≥3 lymph node metastases (<5 mm)
- Stage IIIC: with positive nodes with extracapsular spread

- Stage IV: Tumor invades other regional (upper 2/3 urethra, upper 2/3 vagina) or distant structures.
- Stage IVA: Tumor invades any of the following:
  – Upper urethral and/or vaginal mucosa, bladder mucosa, rectal mucosa, or fixed to pelvic bone
  – Fixed or ulcerated inguinofemoral lymph nodes
- Stage IVB: any distant metastasis, including pelvic lymph nodes

 TREATMENT

GENERAL MEASURES
- Wide excision can be performed for carcinoma in situ, and any suspicious lesion should be excised for definitive diagnosis.
- Cystoscopy and sigmoidoscopy should be performed if there is a question of invasion into the urethra, bladder, or rectum.

MEDICATION
- Neoadjuvant therapy is being investigated with bleomycin-cisplatin and paclitaxel-based regimens showing high-response rates and tolerable side effects.
- As an adjuvant therapy, fluorouracil (Efudex) cream for in situ disease can produce occasional results but is not well tolerated because of irritation of the vulva.
- Chemoradiotherapy with cisplatin and 5-fluorouracil (5-FU) has been successful in advanced or recurrent disease, although local morbidity is increased.
- Contraindications: elderly patients: If chemotherapeutic agents are used, pay close attention to the patient's performance status and ability to tolerate aggressive chemotherapy.

ADDITIONAL THERAPIES
- Preoperative radiation therapy can be used in those with advanced vulvar cancer.
- Adjuvant radiation should be considered with tumor size >4 cm, evidence of lymphovascular invasion, positive surgical margins, or lymph node involvement.
- Preoperative chemoradiation allows for a less radical surgical procedure in patients who are not surgical candidates.
- Postoperative radiation decreases recurrence frequency and may improve survival.
- Radiation is contraindicated with verrucous carcinoma because it induces anaplastic transformation and increases metastases.

SURGERY/OTHER PROCEDURES
- In situ disease can be treated with wide excision or laser vaporization of the affected area. Laser vaporization is preferable in the younger patient, whereas wide excision is preferable in the elderly patient, in whom the risk of invasive disease.
- If tumor extension within <1 cm from structures that will not be removed, preoperative radiation to prevent inadequate surgical margins prior to excision 1-cm tumor-free margin is required because smaller margin would increase risk of recurrence.

- Inguinofemoral lymphadenectomy: removal of superficial inguinal and deep femoral lymph nodes
- Targeted dissection of grossly involved nodes, termed "nodal debulking," is being investigated due to high rates of complication after full inguinofemoral lymphadenectomy.
- Stage IA: radical local excision without lymph node dissection
- Stage IB: radical local excision with either sentinel lymph node biopsy (SLNB) or ipsilateral inguinofemoral lymph node dissection because the risk of metastases is >8%
- Stage II: modified radical vulvectomy and/or chemoradiation and groin node dissection
- Stages III and IV: neoadjuvant chemoradiation and less radical surgery
- Pelvic exenteration after radiation provides effective therapy for advanced or recurrent malignancies involving the bladder or rectum.
- More limited surgery has been undertaken for early invasive lesions, especially in young patients, to preserve the clitoris and sexual function.
- SLNB also has been advocated for early invasive lesion (stage IB or higher). It has shown to accurately diagnose groin metastases in women with early vulvar cancer and unknown groin node status. This will limit the surgical morbidity associated with inguinofemoral lymphadenectomy in those with early stage disease.
- Radical vulvectomy with bilateral groin node dissection through separate incisions provides better cosmetic results than en bloc technique.
- Unilateral lymphadenectomy should be considered when lesion <2 cm, lateral lesion >2 cm from vulvar midline, or no palpable groin nodes.

ADMISSION, INPATIENT, AND NURSING CONSIDERATIONS
- Concurrent chemotherapy with radiation is considered standard of care.
- In advanced malignancy involving the urethra and rectum, concomitant cisplatin/5-FU chemotherapy with radiation produces a significant decrease in size of the primary tumor, usually obviating the need for pelvic exenteration.

 ONGOING CARE

FOLLOW-UP RECOMMENDATIONS
Patient Monitoring
- Early stage, treated with surgery alone: clinical exam of the groin nodes and vulvar area every 6 months for 2 years and then annually
- Following chemoradiation, assessment for further treatment within 6 to 12 weeks of therapy completion

- Advance stage, clinical exam of the groin nodes and vulvar area every 3 months for 2 years, then every 6 months for 3 years, and then annually
- Cervical and/or vaginal cytology annually
- Majority of relapses occur within 1st year.

PATIENT EDUCATION
American College of Obstetricians and Gynecologists: https://www.acog.org/

PROGNOSIS
The 5-year survival is based on stage:
- Stage I: 78.5%
- Stage II: 58.8%
- Stage III: 43.2%
- Stage IV: 13.0%
- Inguinal and/or femoral node involvement is the most important determinant of survival.

COMPLICATIONS
- The major complications are wound breakdown, lymphedema, urinary stress incontinence, and psychosexual consequences.
- In the immediate postoperative period, ~50% of patients experience breakdown of the wound. This requires aggressive wound care by visiting nurses as often as twice a day. The wounds usually granulate and heal over a period of 6 to 10 weeks.
- ~15–20% of patients experience some form of mild to moderate lymphedema after the groin node dissection. These patients should be instructed in the use of leg elevation and support hose. <1% of patients experience severe, debilitating lymphedema.

ADDITIONAL READING
Hinten F, Molijn A, Eckhardt L, et al. Vulvar cancer: two pathways with different localization and prognosis. *Gynecol Oncol*. 2018;149(2):310–317.

CODES

ICD10
- C51.9 Malignant neoplasm of vulva, unspecified
- D07.1 Carcinoma in situ of vulva
- C51.0 Malignant neoplasm of labium majus

CLINICAL PEARLS
- 55% of vulvar cancers are attributable to oncogenic HPV. VAIN and AIN are attributable to HPV. Therefore, HPV vaccination has the potential to decrease vulvar cancer by 1/3.
- Biopsy all suspicious or nonhealing vulvar lesions.

V

VULVODYNIA

Andrea B. Dotson, MD, MSPH

BASICS

DESCRIPTION
- Vulvar pain ≥3 months duration, without visible findings, lab abnormalities, or an identifiable neurologic disorder
- Provoked vulvodynia is often described as the sensation that something is blocking the vagina or the vagina is too small for penetration
- Unprovoked vulvodynia is described as constant burning or stinging in the absence of any sexual activity.

EPIDEMIOLOGY
- Can occur at any age but most women diagnosed between age 20 and 40 years (1)
- Nearly half of women opt not to seek treatment (2).
- Women with and without vulvodynia have similar rates of marital satisfaction, but women with vulvodynia have poorer sexual satisfaction.

Incidence
- Annual rate of new onset vulvodynia is 1.8%.
- Lifetime incidence approaches 15%, suggesting nearly 14 million U.S. women will experience vulvar discomfort at some point in their lives (3).
- Provoked vulvodynia is the most common cause of sexual pain in women <30 years old.

Prevalence
- Between 8.3% and 16% (2)
- Latina women are 80% more likely to present with vulvar pain compared with white and black women.

ETIOLOGY AND PATHOPHYSIOLOGY
- Multifactorial with unknown exact cause
- Neuropathically mediation:
  - Neurogenic inflammation sensitizes afferent nerves and transmits impulses to the CNS, whereas reinforcing signals sustain pain loop.
  - Vulvar biopsy specimens show increased neuronal proliferation and branching.
- Pelvic floor pathology:
  - Hypertonic pelvic floor at the superficial muscle layer, weaker vaginal muscle contraction, and decreased relaxation after contraction (3).
- Other contributing factors:
  - Recurrent vulvovaginal candidiasis or other infections
  - Immune-mediated chronic neuroinflammatory process within vulvar tissues
  - Chemical exposure (trichloroacetic acid) or physical trauma
  - Reduced estrogen receptor expression/changes in estrogen concentration

  - CNS etiology, similar to other regional pain syndromes
  - Trauma: episiotomy, forceps delivery, abuse, pelvic floor injury

RISK FACTORS
- Recurrent vulvovaginal infections, specifically candidiasis (2)
- Hormonal factors: Pain onset or increased severity may be associated with perimenopause/menopause.
- Pelvic floor dysfunction
- Interstitial cystitis/painful bladder syndrome
- Childhood physical or sexual abuse (3)
- Depression and anxiety (2)
- Other neuropathic and chronic pain disorders, including regional pain syndrome

GENERAL PREVENTION
- Wear 100% cotton underwear in the daytime and no underwear to sleep.
- Avoid douching and other vulvar irritants such as perfumes, dyes, and detergents.
- Avoid abrasive activities and tight, synthetic clothing.
- Avoid panty liners.
- Clean the vulva with water only and pat area dry after bathing.
- Avoid use of hair dryers in the vulvar area.

COMMONLY ASSOCIATED CONDITIONS
Chronic pain syndromes, chronic cystitis, irritable bowel syndrome, fibromyalgia, migraines, depression, anxiety, endometriosis, low back pain, pelvic floor dysfunction (2)

DIAGNOSIS

- Vulvodynia is a clinical diagnosis; there is no definitive test for diagnosis.
- Pain should be characterized using a standard measure such as the McGill Pain Questionnaire.
- Use physical exam to rule out other causes of vulvovaginal pain. Negative fungal culture, along with relevant history and positive cotton swab test, confirms diagnosis.

HISTORY
Adequate sexual, social, and pain history should be taken to assess degree of symptoms. Visual pain scales and pain diaries may be helpful (4)[B]:
- Pain may be described as generalized and unprovoked or feeling that the vagina is blocked or too small during penetrative intercourse.
- Quality of pain is burning or stinging (2).

- Screen for bowel or bladder dysfunction.
- History of trauma or abuse
- History of infections, including herpes, candidiasis, other STIs
- Assess for precipitants of vulvar pain: tight garments, bicycle riding, tampon use, prolonged sitting, perfumed or deodorant soaps, and douching (2).
- Assess for complaints of dyspareunia: vaginismus (involuntary vaginal muscle spasm), adequate lubrication, anorgasmia, partner problems, and abuse.

PHYSICAL EXAM
- Ask patient to show where pain is localized or most painful.
- Examine for lesions suggestive of lichen planus or lichen sclerosus.
- Vaginal exam:
  - Vulva may be erythematous, especially at the vestibule; discomfort with separation of the labia minora
  - Spontaneous or elicited pain at the lower 1/2 of anterior vaginal wall suggests bladder etiology.
- Bulbocavernosus and anal wink reflexes to assess for peripheral neuropathy

DIFFERENTIAL DIAGNOSIS
- Infections: candidiasis, herpes, human papillomavirus (HPV), bacterial vaginosis, trichomoniasis, dermatophytes
- Inflammation: lichen planus, immunobullous disorder, allergic vulvitis, lichen sclerosus, atrophic vaginitis
- Neoplasia: Paget disease, vulvar or vaginal intraepithelial neoplasia, squamous cell carcinoma
- Neurologic/muscular: herpes neuralgia, spinal nerve compression, vaginismus

DIAGNOSTIC TESTS & INTERPRETATION
- Tampon test: reproduces pain in real-life settings
- Test for concurrent infections
- Biopsy skin lesions

Initial Tests (lab, imaging)
- Vaginal pH, wet mount, and yeast culture are recommended to rule out vaginitis.
- Gonorrhea and chlamydia with risk factors present
- No need for advanced testing or other imaging unless symptoms dictate

TREATMENT

GENERAL MEASURES

- Multidisciplinary treatment has best outcomes.
- Combination of medical treatments and psychotherapy, physical therapy, and complementary treatments alleviate symptoms more than medication alone.
- Cognitive-behavioral therapy (CBT) superior to supportive therapy (4)[C]

MEDICATION

- Oral therapies
  - Tricyclic antidepressants (TCAs): first-line treatment for unprovoked vulvodynia (4)[B]; fatigue, constipation, sweating, palpitations, and weight gain are the most common side effects.
    - Amitriptyline, nortriptyline: start at 10 mg daily; dose titrated to pain control; average effective dose is 60 mg/day. In one study, a 47% complete response rate was recorded (5)[B].
  - Anticonvulsant therapies:
    - Gabapentin: 300 mg QHS and increase by 300 mg every 3 days; maximum recommended dose is 3,600 mg/day divided into 3 doses.
    - Topiramate and lamotrigine have been recommended if other therapies are not effective.
  - Selective serotonin reuptake inhibitor/serotonin norepinephrine reuptake inhibitors: not commonly used but there is some benefit for generalized vulvodynia (6); consider use in patients who cannot tolerate TCAs.
  - Opioids/nonsteroidal anti-inflammatory drugs: not recommended
- Topical therapies
  - Preferred with provoked vulvodynia (6)
  - Lidocaine 5% ointment: for provoked vestibulodynia
    - Apply 15 to 20 minutes before intercourse. Penile numbness and possible toxicity with ingestion can occur.
    - Overnight (average of 8 hours) QHS for 6 to 8 weeks; resulted in nonpainful intercourse for 76% of women (3)[C]
  - Cromolyn 4% cream: decreases mast cell degranulation in vulvar tissue; recommended application TID (2)[C]
  - Capsaicin 0.025%: decreases discomfort and increases frequency of intercourse with 20-minute daily application (3)[B]
  - Topical amitriptyline 2% combined with baclofen 2% is helpful in patients with comorbid vaginismus.
  - Topical corticosteroids and testosterone creams have not been shown to alleviate symptoms of vulvodynia.
  - Topical estrogen
- Botulinum toxin A injectable may be helpful.

ISSUES FOR REFERRAL

A team approach is recommended for most effective management. Referral to psychosexual medicine, psychology, partner therapy, and pain management teams should be strongly considered (4)[B].

ADDITIONAL THERAPIES

- CBT: associated with a 30% decrease in vulvar discomfort with sexual intercourse (7)[B]
- Biofeedback/pelvic floor physical therapy: treats both generalized and localized vulvar pain; treatment duration of 12- to 16-weeks is recommended.
- Vaginal dilators

SURGERY/OTHER PROCEDURES

- Vestibulectomy surgery may be considered for patients with localized/provoked symptoms who have failed to respond to other measures; not recommended for generalized vulvodynia (4)[B]
- 60–80% of women who undergo surgery report a significant reduction in pain symptoms; however, when surveyed, patients prefer behavioral therapies than surgical intervention.
- Vestibulectomy is less successful in patients with vaginismus (6).
- Surgical approaches
  - Local excision: precise localization of painful areas; tissue closed in elliptical fashion
  - Total vestibulectomy: Tissue is removed from Skene ducts to perineum. The vagina is then brought down to cover defect.
  - Perineoplasty: vestibulectomy plus removal of perineal tissue; incision usually terminated above the anal orifice; reserved for severe cases (2)[B]

COMPLEMENTARY & ALTERNATIVE MEDICINE

Acupuncture significantly reduces pain for some women (4)[C].

ONGOING CARE

PATIENT EDUCATION

- Reassure patients that vulvodynia is not transmissible and does not predispose to cancer (4)[C].
- The goal of treatment is symptom control, not cure. Remission can be achieved but can relapse.
- Encourage treatment with home remedies, including ice packs, sitz baths with baking soda, olive oil, and barrier cream to preserve moisture after bathing.

PROGNOSIS

- Traditionally viewed as a chronic pain disorder, but new evidence suggests remission is possible.
- 1 in 10 vulvodynia patients reported remission regardless of treatment.

REFERENCES

1. Sadownik LA. Etiology, diagnosis, and clinical management of vulvodynia. *Int J Womens Health*. 2014;6:437–449.
2. Shah M, Hoffstetter S. Vulvodynia. *Obstet Gynecol Clin North Am*. 2014;41(3):453–464.
3. Boardman LA, Stockdale CK. Sexual pain. *Clin Obstet Gynecol*. 2009;52(4):682–690.
4. Nunns D, Mandal D, Byrne M, et al; for British Society for the Study of Vulval Disease Guideline Group. Guidelines for the management of vulvodynia. *Br J Dermatol*. 2010;162(6):1180–1185.
5. Stockdale CK, Lawson HW. 2013 Vulvodynia guideline update. *J Low Genit Tract Dis*. 2014;18(2):93–100.
6. Stenson AL. Vulvodynia: diagnosis and management. *Obstet Gynecol Clin North Am*. 2017;44(3):493–508.
7. De Andres J, Sanchis-Lopez N, Asensio-Samper JM, et al. Vulvodynia—an evidence-based literature review and proposed treatment algorithm. *Pain Pract*. 2016;16(2):204–236.

CODES

ICD10

- N94.819 Vulvodynia, unspecified
- N94.818 Other vulvodynia
- N94.810 Vulvar vestibulitis

V

CLINICAL PEARLS

- Vulvodynia is a clinical diagnosis; it should be suspected in any woman with chronic pain at the introitus and vulva.
- A decrease in pain may take weeks to months and may not be complete.
- No single treatment is proven in all women; improvement over time is common even without treatment.

VULVOVAGINITIS, ESTROGEN DEFICIENT
Mark T. Nadeau, MD, MBA • Kristen R. Canady, MD, PhD

BASICS

DESCRIPTION
- Estrogen-deficient vulvovaginitis is a hypoestrogenic state with external genital, urologic, and sexual sequelae.
- Estrogen deficiency affects all tissues in the female body; however, the genital tissues are especially hormone responsive and are most affected.
- Decreased estrogen leads to decreased blood flow to vaginal tissues and thinning of vaginal tissues, dryness, and atrophy. Patients with estrogen-deficient vulvovaginitis may present with urinary incontinence, vaginal burning and itching, dyspareunia, increased urinary frequency, recurrent UTIs, or various other symptoms.
- This condition is also referred to as genitourinary syndrome of menopause when associated with the postmenopausal state, although this condition may occur in women of all ages.
- System(s) affected: reproductive

EPIDEMIOLOGY
Incidence
Predominant age: postmenopausal females. The average age of menopause in the United States is 51.3 years but ranges from 45 to 55 years old.

Prevalence
- Approximately 40–54% of postmenopausal women are affected.
- Approximately 15% of premenopausal women are also affected.
- This condition is likely underdiagnosed because patients may be reluctant to report symptoms because of embarrassment or the misconception that symptoms should be accepted as a natural part of aging (1).

ETIOLOGY AND PATHOPHYSIOLOGY
- Estrogen is vasoactive, increasing blood flow to target tissues, lubrication, and elasticity. The duration of estrogen deficiency is a major factor in the development and severity of genitourinary syndrome of menopause.
- Decreased estrogen levels in the vagina and vulva result in decreased blood flow and decreased lubrication and elasticity of vaginal and vulvar tissues as well as thinning of these tissues.
- Decreased cellular maturation results in decreased glycogen stores, which affects the normal vaginal flora and consequently the pH.
- The resulting increased pH impairs the viability of the normal flora, permitting the proliferation of fecal and other flora, resulting in UTIs and vaginal infections (1)[C].
- Estrogen deficiency is caused by the following:
  – Menopause (surgical or natural)
  – Premature ovarian failure (chemotherapy, radiation, autoimmune, anorexia, genetic)
  – Postpartum estrogen deficiency in lactating women
  – Medications that alter hormonal concentration, such as gonadotropin-releasing hormone agonists or antagonists, tamoxifen, danazol, medroxyprogesterone, and aromatase inhibitors
  – Elevated prolactin from hypothalamic–pituitary disorders with subsequent reduction in estrogen secretion

- Abstinence from sexual activity appears to exacerbate atrophic changes, whereas regular sexual activity can help to preserve the vaginal epithelium, presumably by increasing blood flow and tissue elasticity.

Genetics
No known pattern

RISK FACTORS
- Estrogen-deficient states, including lactation
- Smoking
- Alcohol abuse
- Sexual abstinence or decreased frequency of coital activity
- Lack of exercise
- Absence of vaginal childbirth
- Chemotherapy
- Radiation therapy

COMMONLY ASSOCIATED CONDITIONS
- Urge and stress urinary incontinence
- Pelvic organ prolapse
- Frequent UTIs
- Bacterial or fungal vulvovaginitis
- Vaginal stenosis
- Loss of libido
- Dyspareunia

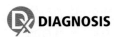

DIAGNOSIS

HISTORY
- All female patients should be asked about symptoms because many women are embarrassed to discuss these issues with their health care providers (1).
  – Vaginal dryness
  – Dyspareunia
  – Pruritus
  – Burning
  – Pressure
  – Tenderness
  – Vaginal discharge (leukorrhea or yellow/malodorous)
  – Urinary symptoms: dysuria, hematuria, frequency, infections, stress, and urge urinary incontinence
- Ask about exposure to radiation therapy and medications.
- Ask about self-treatment and products used.
- Determine exposure to irritants (e.g., soaps, feminine sprays, lotions, lubricants, constant pad use).

PHYSICAL EXAM
Evidence for the diagnosis includes the following:
- Loss of pubic hair
- Decreased elasticity
- Prominence of urethral meatus
- Decreased secretions/lubrication
- Decreased vulvar and vaginal fullness
- Fusion or resorption of labia minora
- Vulvar erythema or ecchymosis
- Decreased vulvar subcuticular fat and moisture
- Pale-appearing, shiny, smooth vaginal and urethral epithelium
- Vaginal shortening, intolerance to speculum exams
- Loss of vaginal rugation
- Pelvic organ prolapse

- Urethral atrophy
- Atrophy of Bartholin glands
- Cervical atrophy and stenosis of os

DIFFERENTIAL DIAGNOSIS
- Malignancy
- Sexual trauma
- Infection secondary to foreign bodies (e.g., piercings)
- Dermatologic conditions of vulva and vagina:
  – Dermatitis
  – Lichen sclerosis
  – Lichen planus
- Bacterial or fungal vulvovaginitis

DIAGNOSTIC TESTS & INTERPRETATION
Because vulvovaginitis is a clinical diagnosis, labs are not always necessary, but if a dermatologic or oncologic condition is suspected, biopsy is recommended (2)[C].

Initial Tests (lab, imaging)
Lab tests are generally unnecessary to make the diagnosis. However, the following labs and imaging may be obtained as corroborative of clinical impression:
- Follicle-stimulating hormone (FSH) and estrogen levels. FSH rises and estrogen drops with menopause.
- Evaluate for infections via wet preparation and vaginal pH (usually >5).
- Urinalysis if suspected concomitant UTI
- Cytology for maturation index: Higher proportion of parabasal cells and lower proportion of intermediate and superficial cells indicate decreased maturation index.
- Transvaginal ultrasound: Endometrial stripe <5 mm indicates loss of estrogen stimulation.

Follow-Up Tests & Special Considerations
Drugs that may alter lab results:
- Estrogen therapy will alter the maturation index but may improve symptoms.
- Digoxin has estrogen-like properties.
- Tamoxifen may produce menopausal-type symptoms but also may act on genital tissues as a weak estrogen agonist.
- Progestins, danazol, and gonadotropin-releasing hormone agonists may produce a reversible pseudo-menopausal state.

TREATMENT

GENERAL MEASURES
- Wear loose-fitting, undyed cotton underwear.
- Avoid prolonged pad use, especially scented pads.
- Avoid feminine deodorant sprays and douching.
- Symptomatic relief, if needed (e.g., cool baths or compresses)
- Increase coital activity.
- Smoking cessation

MEDICATION

- Nonhormonal vaginal moisturizers and lubricants are generally regarded as first-line therapy for mildly symptomatic estrogen-deficient vulvovaginitis (1)[C], although one recent study has shown that neither nonhormonal vaginal moisturizers nor lubricants and vaginal estrogen provided greater benefit than placebo gel or tablet (3)[B]. Importantly, nonhormonal vaginal moisturizers will not reverse most atrophic vaginal changes.
  - Estrogen therapy is preferred for moderate to severe symptoms: Local hormonal therapy (vaginal estrogen) is the first-line hormonal treatment and can reverse atrophic changes and alleviate symptoms (1)[C].
    - Vaginal cream: Insert via applicator 2 to 4 g daily for 1 to 2 weeks, then 1 to 2 g daily for 1 to 2 weeks and then 1 g 1 to 3 times a week.
    - Vaginal estradiol 10-μg tablet: Insert via preloaded applicator each night for 14 days and then twice weekly.
    - Estradiol-containing vaginal ring 2 mg: Insert into vagina and replace every 3 months.
    - Adverse side effects are uncommon, but patients may complain of vaginal irritation, vaginal bleeding, or breast tenderness.
  - Systemic hormonal therapy is typically reserved for patients wanting treatment for vasomotor symptoms associated with estrogen deficiency in addition to atrophic vulvovaginitis.
  - Transdermal preparations may be safer from a cardiovascular standpoint than oral preparations. Systemic estrogen therapy should be used in the lowest possible dose for the shortest duration of time (4)[C].
  - Long-term therapy may be necessary due to the chronic nature of estrogen-deficient vulvovaginitis (5)[A].
  - Contraindications:
    - Breast or estrogen-dependent cancers
    - Undiagnosed vaginal bleeding
    - Thromboembolic disorders
    - Endometrial hyperplasia or cancer
    - Hypertension
    - Hyperlipidemia
    - Liver disease
    - History of stroke
    - Coronary heart disease
    - Smoking in ages >35 years
    - Migraines with neurologic symptoms
    - Acute cholecystitis/cholangitis
    - Pregnancy
- Nonestrogen therapy:
  - Ospemifene (Osphena) 60-mg tablet daily; recommended for women with estrogen-deficient vulvovaginitis not responsive to nonpharmacologic therapies and who cannot or prefer not to use a vaginal estrogen (1)[C],(6)[B]
    - Contraindications:
      - Breast or estrogen-dependent carcinoma
      - Undiagnosed vaginal bleeding
      - Thromboembolic disorders
      - Thrombophlebitis
      - Hepatic impairment
- Precautions: Any abnormal vaginal bleeding must be evaluated. Monitor for DVT and stroke.

ISSUES FOR REFERRAL

- Refer to urogynecologist for evaluation if symptomatic due to pelvic organ prolapse and/or refractory stress and urge urinary incontinence.
- Recurrent UTIs should be further evaluated and may require a referral to urogynecology and/or urology.

ADDITIONAL THERAPIES

- Laser therapy with fractional CO_2 has demonstrated promise in initial studies. Benefits thought to be due to modeling of vaginal tissue; however, randomized controlled trials with long-term follow-up are still needed (1)[C]. This method is not FDA approved. Adverse effects can include vaginal burns, dyspareunia, and recurring/chronic pain.
- Lasofoxifene (Fablyn, Oporia) and oxytocin vaginal gel (Vagitocin) are under development but not yet approved (1)[C].

ADMISSION, INPATIENT, AND NURSING CONSIDERATIONS

Management of this condition occurs primarily in the outpatient setting.

 ONGOING CARE

FOLLOW-UP RECOMMENDATIONS

Follow up as needed to determine response to treatment and for adjustment of treatment regimen.

Patient Monitoring

Instruct the patient that symptoms should improve within 30 to 60 days. If they do not, reevaluate and reexamine for other causes.

DIET

Increased consumption of cranberry juice or extract to prevent recurrent UTIs has been recommended but is not well supported by evidence.

PATIENT EDUCATION

- American College of Obstetricians and Gynecologists (ACOG), 409 12th St., SW, Washington, DC 20024-2188; 800-762-ACOG: http://www.acog.org/
- Lactating postpartum women with high levels of prolactin are in a hypoestrogenic state. These women should be instructed to use lubrication for symptoms of dyspareunia and reassured that the symptoms will resolve when they are no longer breastfeeding.

PROGNOSIS

The prognosis is good. Most symptoms will be alleviated with vaginal estrogen replacement therapy.

COMPLICATIONS

- Recurrent UTIs may occur in women with vaginal atrophy.
- Vaginal atrophy predisposes patients to vaginal infections.

REFERENCES

1. Gandhi J, Chen A, Dagur G, et al. Genitourinary syndrome of menopause: an overview of clinical manifestations, pathophysiology, etiology, evaluation, and management. *Am J Obstet Gynecol*. 2016;215(6):704–711.
2. Johnston SL, Farrell SA, Bouchard C, et al; for SOGC Joint Committee-Clinical Practice Gynaecology and Urogynaecology. The detection and management of vaginal atrophy. *J Obstet Gynaecol Can*. 2004;26(5):503–515.
3. Mitchell CM, Reed SD, Diem S, et al. Efficacy of vaginal estradiol or vaginal moisturizer vs placebo for treating postmenopausal vulvovaginal symptoms: a randomized clinical trial. *JAMA Intern Med*. 2018;178(5):681–690.
4. Ibe C, Simon JA. Vulvovaginal atrophy: current and future therapies (CME). *J Sex Med*. 2010;7(3):1042–1050.
5. Suckling J, Lethaby A, Kennedy R. Local oestrogen for vaginal atrophy in postmenopausal women. *Cochrane Database Syst Rev*. 2006;(4):CD001500.
6. Constantine G, Graham S, Portman DJ, et al. Female sexual function improved with ospemifene in postmenopausal women with vulvar and vaginal atrophy: results of a randomized, placebo-controlled trial. *Climacteric*. 2015;18(2):226–232.

ADDITIONAL READING

- Pitsouni E, Grigoriadis T, Falagas ME, et al. Laser therapy for the genitourinary syndrome of menopause. A systematic review and meta-analysis. *Maturitas*. 2017;103:78–88.
- Ruan X, Mueck AO. Impact of smoking on estrogenic efficacy. *Climacteric*. 2015;18(1):38–46.

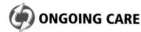 CODES

ICD10

- N95.2 Postmenopausal atrophic vaginitis
- E28.39 Other primary ovarian failure

CLINICAL PEARLS

- Estrogen-deficient vulvovaginitis affects virtually all postmenopausal women to some degree as well as some premenopausal women.
- This disorder is associated with genital, urologic, and sexual symptoms including vaginal itching, vaginal dryness, urinary incontinence, increased urinary frequency, recurrent UTIs, and dyspareunia.
- Estrogen-deficient vulvovaginitis is a clinical diagnosis; lab tests are generally unnecessary.
- Vaginal moisturizers and lubricants are first-line therapy for mild symptoms, and vaginal estrogen preparations, rather than systemic preparations, are the preferred hormonal therapy for women with moderate to severe symptoms of estrogen-deficient vulvovaginitis.

V

VULVOVAGINITIS, PREPUBESCENT
Simon B. Griesbach, MD • Haley Bodette, MD

 BASICS

DESCRIPTION
- Vulvitis is inflammation of the external genitalia.
- Vaginitis is inflammation involving the vaginal mucosa and can be characterized with or without odor or bleeding.
- In premenarchal girls, vulvitis is usually primary with secondary extension into the vagina.
- Vulvovaginitis can be classified as either nonspecific (not likely infectious but rather hygienic/behavioral cause) or specific (likely infectious cause).
- Systems affected: reproductive, integumentary
- Clinical features: vaginal/vulvar itching, soreness, dysuria, redness, discharge, odor, and pain

EPIDEMIOLOGY
Incidence
Unknown

Prevalence
Most common gynecologic problem in prepubertal girls

ETIOLOGY AND PATHOPHYSIOLOGY
- In the prepubertal child, levels of estrogen are low, leading to thin, immature, and fragile vaginal epithelium.
- Anatomically, underdeveloped labia minora, absence of pubic hair, minimal adiposity of the labia majora, and close proximity of the introitus to the anus make contamination more likely (1).
- The prepubertal child also has an alkaline vaginal pH due to a relative deficiency of lactobacilli (which is lactic acid forming) as compared to adolescent and adult females (1).
- Infectious organisms causing vulvovaginitis are typically respiratory, enteric, or rarely sexually transmitted.
- Most cases (~75%) of pediatric vulvovaginitis are classified as nonspecific vulvovaginitis and do not have an infectious etiology.
- Nonspecific vulvovaginitis causes include:
  – Poor perineal hygiene (wiping back to front) (2)
  – Chemical irritants (bubble baths, scented soaps, wipes, laundry detergents)
  – Tight-fitting clothing or underwear made of synthetic materials
- Specific vulvovaginitis causes include:
  – Bacterial:
    ○ The most common respiratory pathogen is *Streptococcus pyogenes*. Vulvitis may occur in the absence of respiratory symptoms.
    ○ *Escherichia coli* is the most common fecal pathogen.
    ○ *Shigella* vaginitis is associated with mucopurulent bloody discharge and is not always accompanied by a history of diarrhea.

ALERT
Presence of *Neisseria gonorrhoeae* or *Chlamydia trachomatis* strongly suggests sexual transmission and should prompt consideration of sexual abuse.

- *Enterobius vermicularis* (pinworms)
  – Most common symptom is nocturnal perineal itching.
  – Should be considered in children with vaginal itching and irritation
  – Very common in young children and certain populations
- Considerations for recurrent/chronic vulvovaginitis:
  – Anatomic abnormalities could include double vagina with fistula, ectopic ureter, and urethral prolapse.
  – Systemic inflammatory diseases
  – Other conditions, such as Crohn disease, lichen sclerosus, vitiligo, psoriasis, and atopic dermatitis are possible.
  – Foreign body
    ○ Presents with foul-smelling, bloody, or brown discharge from the vagina
    ○ Should be considered in patients with recurrent vulvovaginitis after other causes are ruled out
    ○ Most common objects: toilet paper, small toys, hair clips
    ○ If there is a gray watery discharge, consider possibility of battery as foreign body (1).

RISK FACTORS
- Inadequate hand washing or perineal cleansing after urination and defecation (2)
- Wearing of tight-fitting or wet clothing
- Obesity
- Immunosuppression
  – Diabetes
  – Recent antibiotic use
- Anatomic abnormalities

GENERAL PREVENTION
- Good perineal hygiene (including wiping from front to back)
- Urination with legs spread apart and labia separated
- Avoidance of tight-fitting clothing and nonabsorbent underwear
- Avoidance of irritants such as harsh/perfumed soaps and bubble baths

COMMONLY ASSOCIATED CONDITIONS
- Urinary tract infections are common in children with vulvovaginitis.
- Constipation predisposes to vulvovaginitis and vice versa.

DIAGNOSIS

HISTORY
- In taking the history from pediatric patient, develop good rapport with the patient and family as both the history and physical exam are sensitive to discuss.
- Symptoms may include:
  – Vaginal discharge
  – Vaginal or anal itching, burning or discomfort
  – Vulvar redness
  – Dysuria or perineal pain during urination
  – Prepubertal vaginal bleeding
  – Enuresis or encopresis
- Obtain careful history addressing any recent respiratory or enteric infections in the patient or close contacts.

- Ask questions to determine character of any vaginal discharge, if present.
- Determine exposure to irritants that may predispose to vulvovaginitis.
- Question when symptoms most often occur/worsen.
- Inquire about patient's toileting habits:
  – Wiping technique
  – Position of legs while urinating
  – If rushing to the bathroom and inadequate voiding
  – If not voiding/stooling while away at school

PHYSICAL EXAM
- Inform patients and family that exam may be embarrassing and uncomfortable but not painful.
- Explain physical exam thoroughly to the patient and her caregivers prior to beginning, giving opportunities to ask questions.
- If exam provokes significant anxiety, consider deferring exam or, for urgent/emergent concerns, performing exam under anesthesia.
- Examine pediatric patients in two positions for best visualization:
  – Supine in frog-leg position: provides view of external anatomy; Valsalva brings distal vagina into view.
  – Prone in knee-chest position: taking deep breath separates vaginal walls and provides view of internal vagina and cervix; foreign body can be seen in this position.
- Look for excoriation, erythema, swelling of the introitus, discharge, foreign body, and lichenification of external skin, and evaluate degree of estrogenized tissue.
- Perform rectovaginal exam if there is a vaginal bleeding, abdominal pain, or in cases concerning for tumor or foreign body.
- Perform culture collection if necessary.

DIFFERENTIAL DIAGNOSIS
- Lichen sclerosus
- Contact dermatitis
- Eczema
- Psoriasis

DIAGNOSTIC TESTS & INTERPRETATION
Diagnosis is often clinical with testing only necessary in patients with history or exam concerning for an infectious cause.

Initial Tests (lab, imaging)
- Definitive diagnosis of bacterial vulvovaginitis requires a culture of vulvar and vaginal secretions.
  – Collect this specimen with a moistened small-diameter collection swab.
- Perform PCR for STI or herpesvirus if suspected.
- Potassium hydroxide and saline smears of vaginal discharge, if present, can aid in diagnoses of fungal or certain bacterial causes. They have limited sensitivity and specificity.
- Urinalysis and urine culture can be considered; evaluate for concurrent urinary infection.
- Tape test can be considered to evaluate for pinworm; some treat based on history and exam alone due to low sensitivity of testing.

Diagnostic Procedures/Other

- Exploration of the vagina for a foreign body may be necessary in cases of persistent, recurrent symptoms.
- If an anatomic abnormality is suspected, imaging may be necessary to confirm.
- If available, consider referral to a pediatric or adult gynecologist provider with specific training/experience to determine next steps.

Test Interpretation
Culture often reveals organisms identical to those cultured in asymptomatic individuals.

 # TREATMENT

- Treatment is appropriate in the outpatient health care setting, except where systemic illness requires hospital care.
- No specific infectious cause is identified in 75% of patients. In this case, treating clinicians should recommend general hygiene/behavioral changes as first-line treatment, with recommendations tailored to patient's history.
- A known concomitant respiratory illness or visualized purulent vaginal discharge suggests infection. Obtain a culture and use antibiotic directed against the species with the highest colony count.

GENERAL MEASURES
- Avoid irritants, including scented soaps, wipes, and bubble baths.
- Soak the vulva/perineum in a small amount of clear, warm water for 15 minutes 1 to 4 times per day.
- Recommend the patient to avoid wearing underwear to bed or to instead wear loose-fitting boxer-shorts bottoms with loose pajamas.

MEDICATION
- Nonantibiotic options
  - To break the itching–scratching–infection cycle, consider clobetasol priopionate 0.05% as initial treatment and hydrocortisone cream 1% to follow for short-term maintenance.
  - For estrogen deficiency with labial adhesion/agglutination or urethral prolapse: estrogen cream 0.625 mg to fused area nightly for 2 weeks
  - Emollients or barrier creams (unscented) may offer symptomatic relief.
- Antibiotic options
  - Antibiotic use should be restricted to cases of bacterial infection only and based on culture and sensitivity analysis when available. Most durations will be 5 to 10 days (1).
  - Common bacterial organisms include *S. pyogenes*, *Streptococcus pneumoniae*, *Haemophilus influenzae*, *Staphylococcus aureus*, *Shigella* spp., and *E. coli*.
    ○ *C. trachomatis*:
      ▪ ≤45 kg: erythromycin base, 50 mg/kg/day QID for 14 days
      ▪ ≥45 kg and <8 years old: azithromycin, 1 g PO single dose
      ▪ ≥45 kg and ≥8 years old: azithromycin, 1 g PO single dose or doxycycline 100 mg BID for 7 days

    ○ *N. gonorrhoeae*:
      ▪ ≤45 kg: ceftriaxone, 25 to 50 mg/kg up to 250 mg IM or IV once
      ▪ >45 kg: ceftriaxone, 500 mg IM or IV once
      ▪ Consider treatment for chlamydia if not excluded.
    ○ *Trichomonas vaginalis*:
      ▪ Metronidazole, 500 mg PO divided TID for 7 days
    ○ *Candida* spp:
      ▪ Topical nystatin, miconazole, clotrimazole, or terconazole
    ○ Pinworms:
      ▪ Mebendazole, 100 mg PO once, repeated in 2 weeks

ISSUES FOR REFERRAL
- Suspected sexual abuse
- Suspected anatomic abnormality (except minor labial agglutination)
- Persistent, severe, or recurrent infections
- Inability to tolerate physical exam with serious cause suspected

COMPLEMENTARY & ALTERNATIVE MEDICINE
Consider the need for further psychological support for both parent (most often mother) and child:

- Parents play a large role in trial and error process of hygiene changes for their child which adds stress. Normalize this is not something the parent did wrong.
- Often, this can feel a "taboo" subject. Offer psychological support if there have been lifestyle changes that have affected socialization of the child (e.g., scared to go to sleep overs without parental support overnight).
- Delays in diagnosis may result in traumatic experiences and cause sequelae such as vaginismus.

 # ONGOING CARE

FOLLOW-UP RECOMMENDATIONS
Patient Monitoring
Monitor for fever, pruritus, and vaginal discharge.

DIET
- Healthy balanced diet, high in fiber to prevent constipation
- Adequate fluid intake

PATIENT EDUCATION
Hygiene
- Urinate with legs apart, sitting forward to decrease likelihood urine will collect in the vagina.
  - Consider facing "backward" on toilet seat to facilitate this.
- Wipe front to back after elimination and avoid reuse of toilet paper.

- Avoid bubble baths and other irritating products, including all scented products.
- Clean daily with mild soap and water and dry gently with soft towel or cool hair dryer.
- Defer hair shampooing to the end of bath time; consider washing hair while standing up.
- Apply unscented ointments or barrier creams for skin protection.
- Avoid tight clothing, underwear made of synthetic materials, sitting in wet swimsuits, or wearing full body sleeper pajamas.

COMPLICATIONS
- If an STI is identified and not treated effectively, the patient is at risk for pelvic inflammatory disease (PID).
- Untreated vulvovaginitis can cause labial adhesions.
- Vaginismus

REFERENCES
1. Romano ME. Prepubertal vulvovaginitis. *Clin Obstet Gynecol*. 2020;63(3):479–485.
2. Cemek F, Odabaş D, Şenel Ü, et al. Personal hygiene and vulvovaginitis in prepubertal children. *J Pediatr Adolesc Gynecol*. 2016;29(3):223–227.

CODES

ICD10
- N76.0 Acute vaginitis
- N77.1 Vaginitis, vulvitis and vulvovaginitis in dis classd elswhr

CLINICAL PEARLS
- Vulvovaginitis is the most common gynecologic problem in prepubescent girls.
- The hypoestrogenic state and prepubescent anatomy may increase susceptibility to vulvar and vaginal infection.
- Treatment is typically supportive (avoid scratching, warm soaks) but may require antibiotics if a bacterial infection is suspected.
- Isolating an infection with known sexual transmission should prompt further investigation.
- Recurrent or persistent vulvovaginitis, especially with foul-smelling discharge, should prompt a skilled exam of the vagina for a retained foreign body (most common is toilet paper).
- Good perineal hygiene will limit this condition.

V

WARTS

Karl T. Clebak, MD, MHA, FAAFP • Rensa Chen, DO

BASICS

- Warts (verrucae) are benign growths that are confined to the epidermis. All warts are caused by the human papillomavirus (HPV). Warts can appear on any area of the skin or mucous membranes. Common warts are predominantly seen in children and young adults.
- Clinically, warts are described as follows:
  – Common warts (verrucae vulgaris)
  – Plantar warts (verrucae plantaris)
  – Flat warts (verrucae plana)
  – Genital warts (condyloma acuminatum)
  – Epidermodysplasia verruciformis is a rare, lifelong hereditary disorder characterized by chronic infection with HPV.

DESCRIPTION

- Common warts are most often found at sites subject to frequent trauma, such as the hands and feet. Because warts often vary widely in shape, size, and appearance, the various descriptive names for them generally reflect their clinical appearance, location, or both.
- For example: Filiform (fingerlike) warts are thread-like, planar warts are flat, and plantar warts are located on the plantar surfaces (soles) of the feet.
- Genital warts, or condyloma acuminata, may be large and cauliflower-like, or they may consist of small papules.
- Warts on mucous membranes (mucosal papillomas), such as those in the mouth or vagina, tend to be white in color due to moisture retention.

EPIDEMIOLOGY

Incidence
- Predominant age: young adults and children
- No sex predominance: female = male

Prevalence
- ~7–10% of the U.S. population
- ~10% of all school children and young adults experience common warts.
- Common warts appear 2 times as frequently in whites compared with blacks or Asians.

ETIOLOGY AND PATHOPHYSIOLOGY

- HPV is a double-stranded, circular, nonenveloped, supercoiled DNA virus that infects epidermal keratinocytes, stimulating cell proliferation.
- Various strains of DNA HPV: To date, >200 different subtypes have been identified.
- The virus is passed primarily through skin-to-skin contact or from the recently shed virus kept intact in a moist, warm environment.

RISK FACTORS

- HIV/AIDS and other immunosuppressive diseases (e.g., lymphomas)
- Immunosuppressive drugs that decrease cell-mediated immunity (e.g., prednisone, cyclosporine, chemotherapeutic agents)
- Pregnancy
- Handling raw meat, fish, or other types of animal matter in one's occupation (e.g., butchers)
- Previous wart infection
- Use of communal shower room

- Close contact recreational activities
- Close contact with affected person
- Trauma

GENERAL PREVENTION

- Avoid sharing shoes, socks, towels, and tools (nail file, razors).
- Maintain personal hygiene; keep feet clean and dry.
- Wear breathable footwear.
- Wear footwear in communal shower room.
- Avoid scratching or manipulating warts.

COMMONLY ASSOCIATED CONDITIONS

Warts, hypogammaglobulinemia, infections, myelokathexis (WHIM) syndrome; warts, immunodeficiency, lymphedema, dysplasia (WILD) syndrome; hyper-IgE recurrent infection syndrome

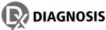

DIAGNOSIS

Most often made on clinical appearance

HISTORY

History of a growing skin lesion; usually asymptomatic; however, warts on soles of feet or around nails may cause discomfort.

PHYSICAL EXAM

- Distribution of warts is generally asymmetric, and lesions are often clustered or may appear in a linear configuration due to scratching (autoinoculation).
- Common wart: rough-surfaced, hyperkeratotic, papillomatous, raised, skin-colored to tan papules, 5 to 10 mm in diameter; several may coalesce into a larger cluster (mosaic wart); most frequently seen on hands, knees, and elbows; usually asymptomatic but may cause cosmetic disfigurement or tenderness
- Filiform warts: These are long, slender, delicate, fingerlike growths, usually seen on the face around the lips, eyelids, or nares.
- Plantar warts often have a rough surface and appear on the plantar surface of the feet in children and young adults.
  – Can be tender and painful; extensive involvement on the sole of the foot may impair ambulation, particularly when present on a weight-bearing surface.
  – Most often seen on the metatarsal area, heels, and toes in an asymmetric distribution (pressure points)
  – Pathognomonic "black dots" (thrombosed dermal capillaries); punctate bleeding becomes more evident after paring with a no. 15 blade.
  – Both common and plantar warts generally demonstrate the following clinical findings:
    ○ A loss of normal skin markings (dermatoglyphics) such as finger, foot, and hand prints
    ○ Lesions may be solitary or multiple, or they may appear in clusters (mosaic warts).
- Flat warts: slightly elevated, smooth, numerous, flat-topped, skin-colored or tan papules, small (1 to 3 mm) in diameter
  – Commonly found on the face, arms, dorsa of hands, knees, and shins (women)
  – Sometimes exhibit a linear configuration caused by autoinoculation
  – In men, shaving spreads flat warts.
  – In women, they often occur on the shins where leg shaving spreads lesions.

- Epidermodysplasia verruciformis (rare): Widespread flat, reddish brown pigmented papules and plaques that present in childhood with lifelong persistence on the trunk, hands, upper and lower extremities, and face are characteristics.
- Focal epithelial hyperplasia (rare): multiple painless, 1- to 5-mm whitish painless, soft, sessile papules or plaques on the oral mucosa, gingiva, tongue, or lips

DIFFERENTIAL DIAGNOSIS

- Molluscum contagiosum, seborrheic keratosis, epidermal nevus, acrochordon (skin tag), solar keratosis, cutaneous horn, acquired digital fibrokeratoma, squamous cell carcinoma (SCC), keratoacanthoma, lichen planus, lichen nitidus, talon noir (black heel)
- Corns/calluses
  – Corns (clavi) are sometimes difficult to distinguish from plantar warts. Like calluses, corns are thickened areas of the skin and most commonly develop at sites subjected to repeated friction and pressure, such as the tops and the tips of toes and along the sides of the feet.

ALERT

- A melanoma on the plantar surface of the foot can mimic a plantar wart.
- Verrucous carcinoma, a slow-growing, locally invasive, well-differentiated SCC, also may be easily mistaken for a common or plantar wart.

DIAGNOSTIC TESTS & INTERPRETATION

Initial Tests (lab, imaging)
Diagnosis

- HPV cannot be cultured, and lab testing is rarely necessary.
- Definitive HPV diagnosis can be achieved by the following:
  – Electron microscopy
  – Viral DNA identification employing Southern blot hybridization is used to identify the specific HPV type present in tissue.
  – Polymerase chain reaction may be used to amplify viral DNA for testing.

Follow-Up Tests & Special Considerations
Skin biopsy if suspicious for malignancy or if the diagnosis is unclear

Test Interpretation
In the granular layer, HPV-infected cells may have coarse keratohyalin granules and vacuoles surrounding wrinkled-appearing nuclei. These koilocytic (vacuolated) cells are pathognomonic for warts.

TREATMENT

The abundance of therapeutic modalities described next is a reflection that none is uniformly or clearly effective in trials. Placebo treatment response rate is significant, and quality of evidence in general is poor. Although first-line treatments with salicylic acid and cryotherapy have low cure rates, other treatments such as cantharidin-podophyllin-salicylic acid (CPA) formulation, immunotherapy, and intralesional bleomycin have higher cure rates with need for further high-quality research (1)[A].

GENERAL MEASURES
- There is no ideal treatment.
- In children and immunocompetent adults, most warts regress spontaneously.
- In many adults and immunocompromised patients, warts are often difficult to eradicate.
- Painful, aggressive therapy should be avoided unless there is a need to eliminate the wart(s).
- For surgical procedures, especially in anxious children, pretreat with anesthetic cream such as EMLA (emulsion of lidocaine and prilocaine).

MEDICATION
First Line
- Self-administered topical therapy
  - Keratolytic (peeling) agents: The affected area(s) should be hydrated first by soaking in warm water for 5 minutes before application. Apply daily for 12 weeks. Most over-the-counter agents contain salicylic acid 17–50% and/or lactic acid: agents such as Duofilm, Occlusal-HP, Trans-Ver-Sal, and Mediplast. Salicylic acid had a mean cure of 13.6% (1)[A]. Avoid use on face due to hyper- and hypopigmentation.
- Office based:
  - Cryotherapy is effective and can be used as second-line treatment with mean cure rate of 45.6% (1)[A].
  - Cantharidin 0.7%, an extract of the blister beetle that causes epidermal necrosis and blistering but may be difficult to obtain as a solution in the United States; it may be compounded in compounding pharmacies.
  - Plantar warts had high rates of clearance with combination of cantharidin 1%, salicylic acid 20–30%, and podophyllin resin 5% in flexible collodion even after single treatment. Warts were thoroughly débrided, applied a thin topical coat, occluded for several hours, and then washed off with reported mean cure rate of 97.8% (1)[A].
  - Generally well tolerated and effective
  - Potential adverse effects: pain, blistering, scarring, hyper-/hypopigmentation

Second Line
- Home based:
  - Imiquimod 5% (Aldara) cream, a local inducer of interferon, is applied at home by the patient. It is approved for external genital and perianal warts and is used off-label and may be applied to warts under duct tape occlusion. It is applied at bedtime and washed off after 6 to 10 hours; applied to flat warts without occlusion. Use 5 times a week up to 16 weeks.
  - Topical retinoids (e.g., tretinoin 0.025–0.1% cream or gel) for flat warts
- Office based:
  - Immunotherapy: induction of delayed-type hypersensitivity with the following:
    - Diphenylcyclopropenone (DPCP) or diphencyprone (DCP): cure rate 44–88%; mutagenic effects in vitro
    - Dinitrochlorobenzene (DNCB): cure rate 66–95%. Its mutagenicity limits its use.
    - Squaric acid dibutylester (SADBE): cure rate 58–86%; there is possible mutagenicity; side effects: erythema, edema, itching, burning
    - Efficacy compared to other treatment modalities requires further research. Contact immunotherapy requires sensitization before rechallenge.
  - Intralesional injections using mumps, *Candida* antigen; bleomycin, interferon, and MTB antigen are used occasionally.
  - Oral therapy
    - Oral high-dose cimetidine: possibly works better in children (40 mg/kg/day; max 1,600 mg)
    - Acitretin or isotretinoin (oral retinoids)
  - Other treatments (All have been used with varying results.)
    - Dichloroacetic acid, trichloroacetic acid, podophyllin, formic acid, aminolevulinic acid in combination with blue light, 5-fluorouracil, silver nitrate, formaldehyde, levamisole, topical cidofovir or IV cidofovir for recalcitrant warts in the setting of HIV, and glutaraldehyde
  - The quadrivalent HPV vaccine has cleared recalcitrant, chronic oral, and cutaneous warts.

ISSUES FOR REFERRAL
Consider referral to dermatology for immunocompromised patients who do not respond to initial treatments.

SURGERY/OTHER PROCEDURES
- Cryotherapy with liquid nitrogen (LN₂) may be applied with a cotton swab or with a cryotherapy gun (Cryogun). Aggressive cryotherapy may be more effective than salicylic acid (2)[A], but it is associated with increased adverse effects (blistering and scarring).
- Light electrocautery with or without curettage
- Photodynamic therapy: Topical 5-aminolevulinic acid is applied to warts followed by photoactivation; better cosmetic outcome for recalcitrant facial flat warts
- CO₂ laser ablation: expensive; clearance rate 50–200%; adverse effects: postprocedure pain, delayed wound healing, scarring, pigment changes (3)
- Pulse-dye laser: expensive; clearance rate 32–92%; adverse effects: mild pain, dyspigmentation, mild scarring; safe for children and adults (3)
- For filiform warts: Dip hemostat into LN₂ for 10 seconds and then gently grasp the wart for 10 seconds and repeat. Wart sheds in 7 to 10 days.

COMPLEMENTARY & ALTERNATIVE MEDICINE
- Duct tape: Cover wart with waterproof tape (e.g., duct tape). Leave the tape on for 6 days and then soak, pare with emery board, and leave uncovered overnight; then reapply tape cyclically for eight cycles; unclear efficacy as single agent
- Hyperthermia: safe and inexpensive approach; immerse affected area into 45°C water bath for 30 minutes 3 times per week.
- Oral daily zinc therapy at a maximum dose of 600 mg/day increased clearance rates compared to placebo.

Pregnancy Considerations
The use of some topical chemical approaches may be contraindicated during pregnancy or in women who are likely to become pregnant during the treatment period.

ONGOING CARE

FOLLOW-UP RECOMMENDATIONS
Patient Monitoring
1/3 of the warts of epidermodysplasia may become malignant.

PATIENT EDUCATION
- The HPV types causing common, plantar, or flat warts are usually different from HPV causing genital warts.
- Vaccine is available to protect against those causing genital warts.

PROGNOSIS
- More often than not (especially in children), warts tend to "cure" themselves over time.
- In many adults and immunocompromised patients, warts often prove difficult to eradicate.

COMPLICATIONS
- Autoinoculation (pseudo-Koebner reaction)
- Scar formation
- Chronic pain after plantar wart removal or scar formation
- Nail deformity after injury to nail matrix

REFERENCES
1. García-Oreja S, Álvaro-Afonso FJ, García-Álvarez Y, et al. Topical treatment for plantar warts: a systematic review. *Dermatol Ther*. 2021;34(1):e14621.
2. Kwok CS, Holland R, Gibbs S. Efficacy of topical treatments for cutaneous warts: a meta-analysis and pooled analysis of randomized controlled trials. *Br J Dermatol*. 2011;165(2):233–246.
3. Leerunyakul K, Thammarucha S, Suchonwanit P, et al. A comprehensive review of treatment options for recalcitrant nongenital cutaneous warts. *J Dermatalog Treat*. 2022;33(1):23–40.

 CODES

ICD10
- A63.0 Anogenital (venereal) warts
- B07 Viral warts
- B07.9 Viral wart, unspecified

CLINICAL PEARLS
- No single therapy for warts is uniformly effective or superior; thus, treatment involves a certain amount of trial and error.
- Because most warts in children tend to regress spontaneously within 2 years, benign neglect is often a prudent option.
- Conservative, nonscarring, least painful, and least expensive treatments are preferred.

W

ZOLLINGER-ELLISON SYNDROME

Mark B. Stephens, MD, MS, FAAFP • Justin T. Ertle, MD

 BASICS

DESCRIPTION

- Zollinger-Ellison syndrome (ZES) triad
  - Markedly elevated gastric acid secretion
  - Peptic ulcer disease
  - A gastrinoma or non-β islet cell tumor of the pancreas or duodenal wall that produces gastrin (hypergastrinemia)
    ○ Gastrinomas (at the time of diagnosis) may be single or multiple (1/2 to 2/3), large or small, benign or malignant (2/3), sporadic (70–75%) or associated with *multiple endocrine neoplasia type 1* (MEN1) (25–30%).
- System(s) affected: endocrine/metabolic, gastrointestinal
- Synonym(s): Z-E syndrome; pancreatic ulcerogenic tumor syndrome; multiple endocrine neoplasia, partial; ulcerogenic islet cell tumor

EPIDEMIOLOGY

Incidence
- 1 to 3 per million per year in the United States
- Predominant age: middle age (30 to 65 years). Mean age of onset is 43 years; presents a decade earlier in patients with ZES/MEN1
- Predominant sex: male > female (1.3:1)

Pediatric Considerations
Aggressive cases have been reported in teenagers.

Pregnancy Considerations
Rare, pregnancy alters medication choices and surgical timing.

ETIOLOGY AND PATHOPHYSIOLOGY

- Gastrinoma is found the head of the pancreas (20–30%) and the first or second portion of the duodenum (70–80%); if in the pancreas, the lesion is more likely to metastasize to the liver.
- Hypergastrinemia results in gastric mucosal hypertrophy and increased acid production. Increased acid production causes mucosal ulceration. Diarrhea (60%) and malabsorption are also common in ZES.
- Increasing number found in stomach wall, up to 8%; may be due to increased surveillance and/or increased PPI use masking symptoms
- Also may be found rarely in the mesentery, peritoneum, spleen, skin, or mediastinum (possibly metastasis with primary not identified)

Genetics
- ~25–30% of cases occur in association with the autosomal dominant MEN1 syndrome—tumors of pancreas, pituitary, and parathyroid.
- Can occur sporadically as well

RISK FACTORS
- MEN1
- Family history of ulcer disease

GENERAL PREVENTION
Screen first-degree relatives of patients with MEN1.

COMMONLY ASSOCIATED CONDITIONS
- MEN1
- Insulinoma
- Carcinoid tumors

DIAGNOSIS

HISTORY
Average of 5 years of symptoms (including recurrent ulcers) before diagnosis is made
- Abdominal pain is the most common symptom (80%).
- Diarrhea (postprandial and fasting) (70%)
- Heartburn (60%)
- Nausea (30%)
- Reflux esophagitis
- Vomiting that is unresponsive to standard therapy
- Weight loss

PHYSICAL EXAM
- Hepatomegaly with metastasis
- Conjunctival pallor if anemic
- Jaundice (tumor compressing common bile duct)
- Epigastric tenderness
- Dental erosions
- Heme + stools on rectal exam
- Complications of severe peptic ulcer disease, including hemorrhage, perforation, and obstruction
- Signs of MEN1 are hypercalcemia, hyperparathyroidism, and Cushing syndrome.

Geriatric Considerations
Consider the diagnosis in a patient with persistent or recurring peptic ulcer disease; it is a less aggressive disease if it appears after 65 years.

DIFFERENTIAL DIAGNOSIS
- Elevated serum gastrin with hypochlorhydria/achlorhydria
  - Atrophic gastritis
  - Drug-induced (associated with proton pump inhibitors [PPIs])
  - Gastric cancer
  - Pernicious anemia
  - Postvagotomy
- Elevated serum gastrin with normal or increased gastric acid
  - Antral G-cell hyperfunction
  - Chronic renal failure
  - *Helicobacter pylori* infection
  - Gastric outlet obstruction
  - Retained gastric antrum
- Consider gastrinoma in all patients with:
  - Recurrent or refractory ulcer disease
  - Gastric hypertrophy and ulcers
  - Duodenal and jejunal ulcers
  - Ulcers and diarrhea
  - Ulcers and kidney stones
  - Hypercalcemia and ulcers
  - Pituitary disease
  - Family history of ulcer disease or endocrine tumors suggestive of MEN1

DIAGNOSTIC TESTS & INTERPRETATION
- Secretin stimulation test is preferred: gastrin level >120 pg/mL (>120 ng/L); may be difficult to find lab that can do this
- Some gastrin assays undermeasure serum gastrin; if have strong index of suspicion but gastrin levels low, may need to repeat with a different lab
- Gastric secretory studies: basal acid output
- Elevated fasting serum gastrin: >1,000 pg/mL with ulcers diagnostic; >200 pg/mL with ulcers is suggestive.
- Elevated basal gastric acid output: >15 mEq/hr (>15 mmol/hr)
- A serum gastrin level >1,000 pg/mL, with gastric pH <2, is diagnostic.
- Check serum calcium, phosphorus, cortisol, and prolactin to rule out MEN1.
- Drugs may alter lab results:
  - Histamine (H_2) blockers and PPIs may increase gastric pH and serum gastrin.
  - Hold PPIs 7 days and H_2 blockers 2 days prior to drawing gastrin level.
- Endoscopic US: finds 24–38% of primary tumors in pancreas, much less effective in duodenum
- Endoscopic findings include esophagitis, duodenal ulceration with multiple ulcers, and prominent gastric and duodenal folds.
- Used to localize tumor for possible resection
- Much more likely to find tumors >3 cm (95%) than <1 cm (<15%)
- Abdominal CT scan: most useful for pancreatic tumors and metastasis >3 cm
- Abdominal US, MRI, and angiography are not typically useful except in large tumors.
- Somatostatin receptor scintigraphy (SRS): more sensitive than radiologic studies, still only finds 30% of small tumors
- Newest modality is ^{68}Gallium-labeled somatostatin PET/CT scanning which is showing excellent sensitivity and specificity
- Portal venous sampling and selective venous sampling for gastrin can localize the area of tumor and metastasis (80–90% sensitivity) for surgical intervention.
- Brain imaging (MRI) and serum calcium are useful if MEN1 is suspected.
- Because pancreatic tumors are most likely to be large and to metastasize to the liver (worse prognosis), SRS and an abdominal CT scan are suggested to look for resectable tumors. Resection improves prognosis.

Initial Tests (lab, imaging)
- Diagnosis is based on elevated fasting plasma gastrin levels and gastric pH <2 in the absence of PPI or H2 blockers.
- Radiologic studies help locate and identify tumors for resection.

Follow-Up Tests & Special Considerations

Annual radiologic studies to look for recurrent or growing tumors and liver metastasis that may require reoperation

Diagnostic Procedures/Other

Endoscopy may reveal tumors in the duodenal or stomach wall; multiple ulcers, including jejunal ulcers; and prominent gastric and duodenal folds.

Test Interpretation

- 90% of gastrinomas are found in the gastric triangle (bordered by the bile duct, the junction of second and third portions of the duodenum, and the junction of the head and body of pancreas).
- ~30% of gastrinomas are in the head of the pancreas (more likely >3 cm, metastasis to liver).
- ~70% of gastrinomas are in the wall of the first or second portion of duodenum (more likely small and solitary).
- 2/3 of gastrinomas are malignant.
- 50% of gastrinomas stain positive for adrenocorticotropic hormone (ACTH), vasoactive intestinal polypeptide, insulin, or neurotensin
- 1/3 of patients have metastasis on presentation: regional nodes > liver > bone, > peritoneum, spleen, skin, and mediastinum.
- Biopsy shows hyperplasia of antral gastrin-producing cells; histology appears similar to carcinoid.

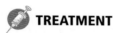 TREATMENT

GENERAL MEASURES

- Goals are to control acid hypersecretion and resect the tumor.
- Advanced imaging initially to evaluate for resection
- Surgical removal when primary tumor can be identified and as adjunct to control symptoms. Surgical resection of primary may enable stopping acid secretion and need for medical treatment.
- Medical treatment for symptom control when primary tumor is not found or metastasis on initial diagnosis

MEDICATION

- PPIs are the first-line treatment; add H_2 blockers if PPI not tolerated or insufficient.
- Medications heal 80–85% of ulcers, most of which recur. Lifelong medication use should be anticipated.
- 4- to 8-fold higher H_2 dose often necessary. May need up to double dose of PPI
  - Start at a lower dose and titrate to symptoms (or maximum recommended dosage).
- If hyperparathyroidism is present (MEN1), correct hypercalcemia.

First Line

- PPIs
  - Omeprazole 60 to 120 mg/day
  - Lansoprazole 60 to 180 mg/day (doses >120 mg need to be divided BID)
  - Rabeprazole 60 to 100 mg/day up to 60 mg BID
  - Pantoprazole 40 to 240 mg/day PO; 80 to 120 mg q12h IV
- H_2 blockers
  - Cimetidine 300 mg q6h up to 2.4 g/day
  - Ranitidine 150 mg q12h up to 6 g/day
  - Famotidine 20 mg q6h; up to 640 mg/day
- Contraindications
  - Known hypersensitivity to the drug
  - H_2 blockers: antiandrogen effects, drug interactions due to cytochrome P450 inhibition
  - PPIs: none
- Precautions
  - Adjust doses for geriatric patients and patients with renal insufficiency.
  - Gynecomastia has been reported with high-dose cimetidine (>2.4 g/day).
  - PPIs may induce a profound and long-lasting effect on gastric acid secretion, thereby affecting the bioavailability of drugs depending on low gastric pH (e.g., ketoconazole, ampicillin, iron).
- Significant possible interactions: Consider drug–drug interactions and consult prescribing materials accordingly.

Second Line

- Octreotide may slow growth of liver metastases, or (occasionally) promote regression. Octreotide LAR can be given every 28 days.
- Chemotherapy regimens using streptozocin, 5-fluorouracil, and doxorubicin shows limited response.
- Interferon shows a limited response but may be useful in combination with octreotide.

SURGERY/OTHER PROCEDURES

- Laparotomy to search for resectable tumors unless patient has liver metastasis on presentation or MEN1; surgery improves outcomes.
- Definitive therapy: removal of identifiable gastrinomas (95% of tumors are found at the time of surgery; 5-year cure is 40% when all are removed.) Second surgeries are worth considering if there is radiologic evidence of new or growing tumors and resection may prolong life span.
- Total gastrectomy is rarely indicated.
- In MEN1, parathyroidectomy, by lowering calcium, may also decrease acid production and decrease antisecretory drug use. Gastrinomas in MEN1 are generally small, benign, and multiple, and surgery is not usually curative in this situation.

ADMISSION, INPATIENT, AND NURSING CONSIDERATIONS

- Titrate medication to symptom control.
- Appropriate surveillance postoperatively to look for metastasis

 ONGOING CARE

FOLLOW-UP RECOMMENDATIONS

Patient Monitoring

- Longitudinal follow-up to evaluate for metastases. Reoperation may be considered.
- Titrate medical therapy to control symptoms.
- Advise patients of potential danger of stopping antisecretory treatment. Rare cases have been reported of severe adverse outcomes within 2 days of stopping PPIs. Gastric acid analysis can help guide medical therapy to maintain basal gastric acid output at <10 mEq/hr (<2 mEq/hr if patient has complications such as perforation or esophagitis).

DIET

Restrict foods that aggravate symptoms.

PATIENT EDUCATION

Inform patients as to the nature of disease and prognosis.

PROGNOSIS

- Overall survival rate: 5 to 10 years: 69–94%
- The prognosis improves with complete surgical removal of the tumor.
- If liver metastasis is present on initial surgery, 5-year survival is 30–40%; 10-year survival is 25%.
- Mortality is directly related to liver metastasis, tumor size and presence of pancreatic tumors.

COMPLICATIONS

- Complications of peptic ulcer disease (bleeding, perforation, obstruction)
- 2/3 of gastrinomas are malignant with metastasis.
- Paraneoplastic phenomena (e.g., production of ACTH with resulting Cushing syndrome) is possible.
- Decrease in vitamin B_{12} levels is possible with long-term PPI use.

 CODES

ICD10

E16.4 Increased secretion of gastrin

CLINICAL PEARLS

- Consider ZES if peptic ulcers recur or if unusually high doses of PPI are needed to control symptoms.
- Abdominal pain and diarrhea should be totally controllable with adequate medical treatment.
- ~25–30% of cases of ZES occur in association with MEN1.
- Once ZES is diagnosed, search for gastrinomas in the head of the pancreas and the first or second portion of the duodenum.
- PPIs heal ZES ulcers. Patients should anticipate lifelong therapy.

Z

INDEX

NOTE: Page numbers preceded by A- indicate Algorithms.